SAUNDERS MANUAL of SMALL ANIMAL PRACTICE

STEPHEN J. BIRCHARD, D.V.M., M.S., DIPLOMATE, A.C.V.S.
Associate Professor of Small Animal Surgery
Department of Veterinary Clinical Sciences
The Ohio State University
Columbus, Ohio

ROBERT G. SHERDING, D.V.M., DIPLOMATE, A.C.V.I.M.
Professor of Small Animal Internal Medicine
Chair, Department of Veterinary Clinical Sciences
The Ohio State University
Columbus, Ohio

SAUNDERS MANUAL of SMALL ANIMAL PRACTICE

2nd Edition

W.B. SAUNDERS COMPANY
A Harcourt Health Sciences Company
Philadelphia London New York St. Louis Sydney Tokyo

W.B. SAUNDERS COMPANY
A Harcourt Health Sciences Company

The Curtis Center
Independence Square West
Philadelphia, Pennsylvania 19106

Library of Congress Cataloging-in-Publication Data

Saunders manual of small animal practice / [edited by] Stephen J. Birchard, Robert G. Sherding.—2nd ed.

p.   cm.

ISBN 0–7216–7078–4

1. Pet medicine—Handbooks, manuals, etc.   2. Dogs—Diseases—Handbooks, manuals, etc.   3. Cats—Diseases—Handbooks, manuals, etc.   I. Birchard, Stephen J.   II. Sherding, Robert G.

SF981.S34 1999

636.089—dc21   98–26528

Aquisitions Editor: Ray Kersey
Developmental Editor: Melissa Dudlick
Supervisory Copy Editor: Carol DiBerardino
Illustration Coordinator: Robert Quinn

SAUNDERS MANUAL OF SMALL ANIMAL PRACTICE, 2nd Edition   0–7216–7078–4

Printed in the United States of America

Last digit is the print number: 9   8   7   6   5   4   3   2   1

We dedicate this book to our families.

To my wife Susan Crisp, my son Justin, and my daughter Mary Elizabeth.
(SJB)

In thanks for the support of my wife Sherrie, and my son Cameron.
(RGS)

Contributors

Nancy L. Anderson, D.V.M., Diplomate A.B.V.P.C. (Avian)
Graduate Research Associate, Department of Evolution, Ecology, and Organismal Biology, The Ohio State University, Columbus, Ohio
Pet Rodents; Basic Husbandry and Medicine of Pet Reptiles

Richard K. Anderson, D.V.M., Diplomate A.C.V.D.
Clinical Associate Professor, Department of Clinical Sciences, Tufts University School of Veterinary Medicine, North Grafton, Massachusetts; Staff Dermatologist, Angell Memorial Animal Hospital, Boston, Massachusetts
Scabies, Notoedric Mange, and Cheyletiellosis

Dennis N. Aron, D.V.M., Diplomate A.C.V.S.
Professor, Small Animal Surgery, Department of Small Animal Medicine, College of Veterinary Medicine, University of Georgia, Athens, Georgia
Luxation, Subluxation, and Shearing Injuries of the Tarsal Joint

Joseph W. Bartges, B.S., D.V.M., Ph.D., Diplomate A.C.V.I.M., D.A.C.V.N.
Associate Professor of Medicine and Nutrition, Department of Small Animal Clinical Sciences, College of Veterinary Medicine, The University of Tennessee; Internist and Nutritionist, Veterinary Teaching Hospital, The University of Tennessee, Knoxville, Tennessee
Diseases of the Urinary Bladder

Shane W. Bateman, D.V.M., D.V.Sc. Diplomate A.C.V.E.C.C.
Assistant Professor—Clinical, Department of Veterinary Clinical Sciences, The Ohio State University; Director, Critical Care Service, Veterinary Teaching Hospital, The Ohio State University, Columbus, Ohio
Fluid Therapy for Dogs and Cats

Karin Muth Beale, D.V.M., Diplomate A.C.V.D.
Staff Dermatologist—Gulf Coast Veterinary Specialists, Houston, Texas; Dermatology Consultant, ANTECH Diagnostics, Irvine, California
Dermatophytosis

Jamie R. Bellah, D.V.M., Diplomate A.C.V.S.
Staff Surgeon, Affiliated Veterinary Specialists, Orange Park, Florida
Surgery of Intertriginous Dermatoses

Larry Berkwitt, D.V.M., Diplomate A.C.V.I.M.
Director of Medicine, Veterinary Referral and Emergency Center, Norwalk, Connecticut
Diagnostic Methods in Respiratory Disease

David S. Biller, D.V.M., Diplomate A.C.V.R.
Professor of Radiology, Department of Clinical Sciences, College of Veterinary Medicine, Kansas State University, Manhattan, Kansas
Radiographic and Ultrasonographic Techniques

Stephen J. Birchard, D.V.M., M.S., Diplomate A.C.V.S.
Associate Professor of Small Animal Surgery, Department of Veterinary Clinical Sciences, The Ohio State University, Columbus, Ohio
Diseases of the Thyroid Gland; Selected Skin Graft and Reconstructive Techniques; Pleural Effusion; Principles of Thoracic Surgery; Surgery of the Liver and Biliary Tract; Diseases and Surgery of the Exocrine Pancreas; Peritonitis

Dale E. Bjorling, D.V.M., M.S., Diplomate A.C.V.S.
Professor and Chair, Department of Surgical Sciences, School of Veterinary Medicine, University of Wisconsin, Madison, Wisconsin
Thoracic Trauma; Surgery of the Kidney and Ureter; Surgery of the Urethra

John D. Bonagura, D.V.M., M.S. Diplomate A.C.V.I.M. (Internal Medicine, Cardiology)
Gilbreath-McLorn Professor of Veterinary Cardiology, Department of Veterinary Medicine and Surgery, University of Missouri, Columbia, Missouri
Cardiovascular Radiography; Drugs for Treatment of Cardiovascular Diseases; Heart Failure; Valvular Heart Disease; Cardiomyopathy; Vascular Diseases; Congenital Heart Disease; Respiratory Infections

Harry W. Boothe, D.V.M., M.S., Diplomate A.C.V.S.
Professor of Surgery, Department of Veterinary Small Animal Medicine and Surgery, College of Veterinary Medicine, Soft Tissue Surgeon, Texas Veterinary Medical Teaching Hospital, Texas A&M University, College Station, Texas
Surgery of the Prostate Gland; Surgery of the Testes and Scrotum; Surgery of the Penis and Prepuce; Surgery for Otitis Media and Otitis Interna

Randy J. Boudrieau, D.V.M., Diplomate A.C.V.S.
Professor of Surgery, Department of Clinical Sciences, Tufts University School of Veterinary Medicine, North Grafton, Massachusetts
Delayed Unions, Nonunions, and Malunions

Bernard M. Bouvy, D.V.M., Ph.D., DrMedVet, MSc, Diplomate ECVS, Diplomate ACVS
Co-Head of Surgery, Clinique Vétérinare Frégis, Arcueil (Paris) France
Neoplasia of Thoracic and Pelvic Limbs

Ronald M. Bright, D.V.M., M.S., Diplomate A.C.V.S.
Affiliate Professor, Department of Clinical Sciences, College of Veterinary Medicine, Colorado State University; Staff Surgeon, Surgical Referral Services, Ft. Collins, Colorado; Staff Surgeon, Veterinary Specialties Consultation Services, Inc, Knoxville, Tennessee
Surgery of the Esophagus; Diseases of the Stomach; Surgery of the Stomach; Surgery of the Intestines; Anorectal Surgery

Marjory Brooks, D.V.M.,
Associate Director, Comparative Coagulation Section, Diagnostic Laboratory, College Veterinary Medicine, Cornell University, Ithaca, New York
Coagulation Diseases

Susan A. Brown, D.V.M.
Partner/Staff Veterinarian, Midwest Bird and Exotic Animal Hospital, West Chester, Illinois
Ferrets

Steven C. Budsberg, D.V.M., M.S., Diplomate A.C.V.S.
Professor of Surgery, Department of Small Animal Medicine, University of Georgia, Athens, Georgia
Orthopedic Disorders of the Distal Extremities

C.A. Tony Buffington, D.V.M., Ph. D., Diplomate A.C.V.N.
Professor, Department of Veterinary Clinical Sciences, The Ohio State Unversity, Columbus, Ohio
Critical Care Techniques

Clay A. Calvert, D.V.M., Diplomate A.C.V.I.M.
Professor, Department of Small Animal Medicine and Surgery, College of Veterinary Medicine, University of Georgia, Athens, Georgia
Heartworm Disease

Marcia Carothers, D.V.M., Diplomate A.C.V.I.M. (Internal Medicine)
Staff Veterinarian, Akron Veterinary Referral and Emergency Center, Akron, Ohio
Diseases of the Parathyroid Gland and Calcium Metabolism; Respiratory Neoplasia

Dennis Chew, D.V.M., Diplomate A.C.V.I.M.
Professor, Department of Veterinary Clinical Sciences, College of Veterinary Medicine, The Ohio State University, Columbus, Ohio
Fluid Therapy for Dogs and Cats; Diseases of the Parathyroid Gland and Calcium Metabolism

C. Guillermo Couto, D.V.M., Diplomate A.C.V.I.M.
Professor, Department of Veterinary Clinical Sciences, The Ohio State University, Columbus, Ohio
Rickettsial Diseases; Tumors of the Skin and Subcutaneous Tissues

M. Susan Crisp, D.V.M., Diplomate A.C.V.I.M. (Internal Medicine)
Midwest Veterinary Specialty, Columbus, Ohio
Critical Care Techniques

Steven E. Crow, D.V.M., Diplomate A.C.V.I.M. (Internal Medicine: Oncology)
Staff Oncologist and Internist, Sacramento Animal Medical Group, Inc., Carmichael, California
Pericardial Diseases and Cardiac Neoplasia

Charles E. DeCamp, D.V.M., M.S., Diplomate A.C.V.S.
Professor, Michigan State University, East Lansing, Michigan
Open Fractures

R. Tass Dueland, D.V.M., M.S., Diplomate A.C.V.S.
Professor, Orthopedic Surgery, Affiliate Professor, Division of Orthopedic Surgery, Medical School, University of Wisconsin–Madison, Madison, Wisconsin
Orthopedic Disorders of the Stifle

Joan Dziezyc, D.V.M., Diplomate A.C.V.O.
Associate Professor, Department of Small Animal Medicine and Surgery, College of Veterinary Medicine; Staff Ophthalmologist, Veterinary Medical Teaching Hospital, Texas A&M University, College Station, Texas
Diseases of the Retina, Choroid, and Optic Nerve

Erick L. Egger, D.V.M., Diplomate A.C.V.S.
Affiliate Faculty, Colorado State University; Veterinary Orthopedic Consultant, Surgical Referral Services, Ft. Collins, Colorado
Fractures of the Tibia and Fibula

William R. Fenner, D.V.M., Diplomate A.C.I.M. (Neurology)
Associate Professor, College of Veterinary Medicine, The Ohio State University, Columbus, Ohio
Diagnostic Approach to Neurologic Disease

Roger B. Fingland, D.V.M., M.S., Diplomate A.C.V.S.
Professor of Surgery, Director, Veterinary Medical Teaching Hospital, College of Veterinary Medicine, Kansas State University, Manhattan, Kansas
Obstructive Upper Airway Disorders; Surgery of the Urinary Bladder; Surgery of the Ovaries and Uterus; Surgery of the Vagina and Vulva

S. Dru Forrester, D.V.M., M.S., Diplomate A.C.V.I.M. (Internal Medicine)
Associate Professor, Department of Small Animal Clinical Sciences; Small Animal Internist, Veterinary Teaching Hospital, Director of Student Affairs, Virginia-Maryland Regional College of Veterinary Medicine, Virginia Polytechnic Institute and State University, Blacksburg, Virginia
Diseases of the Kidney and Ureter

Margi Gilmour, D.V.M., Diplomate A.C.V.O.
Cascade Veterinary Specialists, Issaquah, Washington
Diseases of the Lens

Stephen D. Gilson, D.V.M., Diplomate A.C.V.S.
Sōnorā Veterinary Specialists, Scottsdale, Arizona
Principles of Oncology

Mary B. Glaze, D.V.M., M.S., Diplomate A.C.V.O.
Professor of Veterinary Ophthalmology, Louisiana State University, Veterinary Clinical Sciences; Veterinary Ophthalmologist, Veterinary Teaching Hospital and Clinic, Louisiana State University, Baton Rouge, Louisiana
Diseases of the Orbit

Justin M. Goggin, D.V.M.
Radiologist, Veterinary Referral Center, Little Falls, New Jersey
Radiographic and Ultrasonographic Techniques

Joanne C. Graham, D.V.M., M.S., Diplomate A.C.V.I.M. (Oncology)
Assistant Professor and Staff Oncologist, Iowa State University, Ames, Iowa
Soft Tissue Sarcomas and Mast Cell Tumors

Deborah S. Greco, D.V.M., Ph.D., Diplomate A.C.V.I.M.
Associate Professor, Department of Clinical Sciences, College of Veterinary Medicine and Biological Sciences, Colorado State University, Fort Collins, Colorado
Diabetes Mellitus

Craig E. Griffin, D.V.M., Diplomate A.C.V.D
Partner, Clinician, Animal Dermatology Clinic, San Diego, California and Garden Grove, California
Flea Allergy Dermatitis

Amy M. Grooters, D.V.M., Diplomate A.C.V.I.M.
Assistant Professor and Chief, Companion Animal Medicine, Veterinary Clinical Sciences, School of Veterinary Medicine, Louisiana State University, Baton Rouge, Louisiana

Diseases of the Ovaries and the Uterus; Diseases of the Vagina and Vulva

Tom Van Gundy, B.S., D.V.M., M.S., Diplomate A.C.V.S.
Staff Surgeon, Animal Surgical Practice of Portland, Portland, Oregon
Diseases of the Parathyroid Gland and Calcium Metabolism

Robert L. Hamlin, D.V.M., Ph.D., Diplomate A.C.V.I.M. (Cardiology)
Professor of Veterinary Biosciences and Professor of Biomedical Engineering, The Ohio State University, Columbus, Ohio
Auscultation and Physical Diagnosis

Callum W. Hay, D.V.M., Diplomate A.C.V.S.
Surgeon, Florida Veterinary Associates, Tampa, Florida
Osteoarthritis; Immune-Mediated Arthritis

Cheryl S. Hedlund, D.V.M., M.S., Diplomate A.C.V.S.
Professor and Chief, Companion Animal Surgery and Anesthesia, Veterinary Clinical Sciences, School of Veterinary Medicine, Louisiana State University, Baton Rouge, Louisiana
Surgery of the Nasal Cavity and Sinuses

Karen Helton-Rhodes, D.V.M., Diplomate A.C.V.D.
Dermatology Consultations, Animal Emergency and Referral Center, West Caldwell, New Jersey
Immune-Mediated Dermatoses

Elizabeth V. Hillyer, D.V.M.
Writer and Editor, PIA Ltd., Levittown, Pennsylvania
Avian Dermatology; Ferrets

Paul E. Howard, D.V.M., M.S., Diplomate A.C.V.S.
Vermont Veterinary Surgical Center, Burlington, Vermont
Fractures and Dislocations of the Mandible; Fractures of the Maxilla; Neoplasia of the Maxilla and Mandible

John A. Hubbell, D.V.M., M.S., Diplomate A.C.V.A.
Professor of Veterinary Clinical Sciences, Associate Dean for Academic Affairs, The College of Veterinary Medicine, The Ohio State University, Columbus, Ohio
Practical Methods of Anesthesia

Karen Dyer Inzana, D.V.M., Ph.D., Diplomate A.C.V.I.M. (Neurology)
Associate Professor, Virginia-Maryland Regional College of Veterinary Medicine, Virginia Polytechnic Institiute and State University, Blacksburg, Virginia
Peripheral Nerve Disorders

Joshua Jackson, D.V.M.
Veterinarian, Veterinary Specialty Hosptial, Rancho, Sante Fe, California
Osteochondrosis

Kenneth A. Johnson, M.V.Sc., Ph.D, F.A.C.V.Sc., M.R.C.V.S., Diplomate A.C.V.S., E.C.V.S.
Professor of Companion Animal Studies, University of Bristol, Department of Clinical Veterinary Science, Langford, Bristol, England
Fractures of the Pelvis; Osteomyelitis

Lynelle R. Johnson, D.V.M., M.S., Diplomate A.C.V.I.M.
Research Assistant Professor, Department of Veterinary Biomedical Sciences, University of Missouri, Columbia, Missouri
Bronchopulmonary Disease

Susan E. Johnson, D.V.M., M.S., Diplomate A.C.V.I.M.
Associate Professor, Department of Veterinary Clinical Sciences, College of Veterinary Medicine; The Ohio State University, Columbus, Ohio
Diseases of the Esophagus and Disorders of Swallowing; Diseases of the Stomach; Diseases of the Intestines; Diseases of the Liver and Bilary Tract; Diseases and Surgery of the Exocrine Pancreas

Denise Jones, B.S., D.V.M.
Practitioner, Findlay Animal Clinic, Findlay, Ohio
History and Physical Examination

Renee L. Kaswan, D.V.M., M.S., Diplomate A.C.V.O.
Professor, College of Veterinary Medicine, University of Georgia, Athens, Georgia; Ophthalmologist, Georgia Veterinary Specialists, Atlanta, Georgia
Diseases of the Lacrimal Apparatus

Nancy D. Kay, D.V.M., Diplomate A.C.V.I.M.
Owner, Internal Medicine, Support Services, Sebastopol, California; Animal Care Center, Rehnert Park, California
Diseases of the Prostate Gland

Thomas J. Kern, D.V.M., Diplomate A.C.V.O.
Associate Professor of Ophthalmology, Department of Clinical Sciences, College of Veterinary Medicine, Cornell University, Ithaca, New York
Diseases of the Cornea and Sclera

Peter R. Kintzer, D.V.M., Diplomate A.C.V.I.M.
Clinical Assistant Professor, School of Veterinary Medicine, Tufts University, North Grafton, Massachusetts; Staff Internist, Boston Road Animal Hospital, Springfield, Massachusetts
Diseases of the Adrenal Gland

Susan E. Kirschner, D.V.A., Diplomate A.C.V.O.
The Animal Eye Doctor, Oregon Veterinary Referral Center, Portland, Oregon
Diseases of the Eyelid

David Knapp, D.V.M., Diplomate A.C.V.S.
Staff Surgeon, The Angell Memorial Animal Hospital Boston, Massachusetts
Management of the Open Wound

Donald R. Krawiec, D.V.M., M.S., Ph.D., Diplomate A.C.V.I.M.
Internist, North County Specialty Animal Hospital, Hospital Director, North County Emergency Animal Clinic/Specialty Animal Hospital; San Marcos, California
Diseases of the Urethra

Gail A. Kunkle, D.V.M., Diplomate A.C.V.D.
Professor, Department Small Animal Clinical Sciences, College of Veterinary Medicine, University of Florida, Gainesville, Florida
Necrotizing Skin Diseases

Kenneth W. Kwochka, D.V.M.
Associate Professor of Dermatology, Department of Veterinary Clinical Sciences; Dermatology Service Chief, College of Veterinary Medicine, The Ohio State University, Columbus, Ohio
Keratinization Defects

Mary Anna Labato, D.V.M., Diplomate A.C.V.I.M.
Foster Hospital for Small Animals, Clinical Associate Professor, Department of Clinical Sciences, Tufts University School of Veterinary Medicine, North Grafton, Massachusetts
Disorders of Micturition

Linda B. Lehmkuhl, D.V.M., M.S., Diplomate A.C.V.I.M. (Cardiology)
Assistant Professor, The Ohio State University; Clinical Cardiologist, Veterinary Teaching Hospital, Columbus, Ohio
Cardiomyopathy

Timothy M. Lenehan, D.V.M., Diplomate A.C.V.S.
Staff Surgeon, Veterinary Surgical Specialists, San Diego, California
Osteochondrosis

Patricia J. Luttgen, D.V.M., M.S., Diplomate, A.C.V.I.M. (Neurology)
Staff Neurologist, Neurological Center for Animals, Denver, Colorado
Disorders of the Spinal Cord

Paul A. Manley, D.V.M., M.S., Diplomate A.C.V.S.
Associate Professor, Department of Surgical Sciences, School of Veterinary Medicine, University of Wisconsin, Madison, Wisconsin
Lyme Borrelioses; Fractures of the Pelvis; Amputation of the Digit; Pediatric Fractures; Osteoarthritis; Immune-Mediated Arthritis

Philip A. March, D.V.M., M.S., Diplomate A.C.V.I.M. (Neurology)
Assistant Professor, Department of Veterinary Clinical Sciences, The Ohio State University, Columbus, Ohio
Diseases of the Brain

Sandra Manfra Marretta, D.V.M., Diplomate A.C.V.S., A.V.D.C.
Associate Professor, Small Animal Surgery and Dentistry, College of Veterinary Medicine, University of Illinois, Urbana, Illinois
Dentistry and Diseases of the Oropharynx

Kurt J. Matushek, D.V.M., M.S., Diplomate A.C.V.S.
Associate Editor, American Veterinary Medical Association, Schaumburg, Illinois
Fractures and Dislocations of the Carpus

John McCall, B.S., M.S., Ph.D.
Professor of Parasitology, Department of Medical Microbiology and Parasitology, College of Veterinary Medicine, University of Georgia, Athens, Georgia
Heartworm Disease

Scott McDonald, D.V.M.
Staff Veterinarian, Midwest Bird Exotic Animal Hospital, Westchester, Illinois
Disorders of the Avian Digestive System

Margaret C. McEntee D.V.M., Diplomate A.C.V.I.M. (Medical Oncology) A.C.V.R. (Radiation Oncology)
Assistant Clinical Professor, University of California, Davis, School of Veterinary Medicine, Davis, California
Diseases of the Spleen

Matthew W. Miller, D.V.M., M.S., Diplomate A.C.V.I.M. (Cardiology)
Associate Professor of Cardiology, Department of Small Animal Medicine and Cardiology Service Chief, College of Veterinary Medicine, Texas A&M University, College Station, Texas; Adjunct Assistant Professor of Pediatric Cardiology, Department of Pediatrics, Baylor College of Medicine, Houston, Texas
Congenital Heart Disease

Michael S. Miller, M.S., V.M.D., Diplomate A.B.V.P.
Director, Cardiology-Ultrasound Referral Service, Thornton, Pennsylvania
Electrocardiography; Disorders of Cardiac Rhythm

Nicholas J. Millichamp, B.S.C., B. Vet. Med., Ph.D., DVOpthal., Diplomate A.C.V.O., M.R.C.S.
Associate Professor of Small Animal Medicine and Surgery, College of Veterinary Medicine; Staff Opthalmologist, Veterinary Teaching Hospital, Texas A&M University, College Station, Texas
Diseases of the Retina, Choroid, and Optic Nerve

Cecil P. Moore, D.V.M., M.S., Diplomate A.C.V.O.
Professor of Veterinary Ophthalmology; Interim Department Chairman and Director of Veterinary Medical Teaching Hospital, Department of Veterinary Medicine and Surgery, College of Veterinary Medicine, University of Missouri, Columbia, Missouri
Diseases of the Conjunctiva

Peter Muir, B.V.Sc. M. Vet. Clin. Stud., Ph.D. M.A.C.V.Sc., M.R.C.V.S., Diplomate A.C.V.S. and Diplomate E.C.V.S.
Lecturer in Orthopaedics, The Royal Veterinary College, Department of Small Animal Medicine and Surgery, North Mymms, Hertfordshire, United Kingdom
Fractures of the Pelvis

William Muir, III, D.V.M., M.Sc., Ph.D., Diplomate A.C.V.A. and A.C.V.E.C.C.
Professor, Department of Veterinary Clinical Science, The Ohio State University, Columbus, Ohio
Drugs for Treatment of Cardiovascular Diseases; Cardiopulmonary Cerebral Resuscitation

Holly S. Mullen, D.V.M., Diplomate A.C.V.S.
Chief of Surgery, California Veterinary Surgical Practice, San Diego, California
Diseases of the Adrenal Gland

Alan C. Mundell, D.V.M., Diplomate A.C.V.D.
Owner, Animal Dermatology Service, Seattle, Washington
Mycobacteriosis; Demodicosis

Wendy Myer, D.V.M., M.S.
Associate Professor Emeritus, The Ohio State University, Columbus, Ohio
Cardiovascular Radiography; Diagnostic Imaging in Respiratory Disease

Richard W. Nelson, D.V.M.
Professor, Internal Medicine, Department of Medicine and Epidemiology, School of Veterinary Medicine, University of California, Davis, Davis, California
Pancreatic Beta Cell Neoplasia

Rhett Nichols, D.V.M., Diplomate A.C.V.I.M.
Internal Medicine Consultant, Antech Diagnostics, Farmingdale, New York
Diseases of the Hypothalamus and Pituitary

James O. Noxon, D.V.M.
Professor, Department of Veterinary Clinical Sciences, College of Veterinary Medicine, Iowa State University, Ames, Iowa; Adjunct Professor, Department of Companion Animals, Atlantic Veterinary College, University of Prince Edward Island, Charlottetown, PEI, Canada
Otitis Externa

Richard R. Nye, B.S., D.V.M.
University of Illinois College of Veterinary Medicine, Champaign, Illinois; Owner and Partner, Midwest Bird and Exotic Animal Hospital, Westchester, Illinois
Avian Respiratory System

Gregory K. Ogilvie, D.V.M., Diplomate A.C.V.I.M. (Oncology)
Professor, Comparative Oncology Unit, Veterinary Teaching Hospital, Colorado State University, Department of Clinical Sciences, College of Veterinary Medical and Biomedical Sciences, Ft. Collins, Colorado
Lymphoid Neoplasia

Barbara L. Oglesbee, D.V.M., Diplomate A.B.V.P. (Avian)
Associate Professor—Clinical, College of Veterinary Medicine, The Ohio State University, Columbus, Ohio
Avian Techniques; Avian Infectious Diseases; Avian Digestive System Disorders

Deborah A. O'Keefe, D.V.M., M.S., Diplomate A.C.V.I.M (Internal Medicine, Oncology)
Oncologist, Michigan Veterinary Specialists, Southfield, Michigan
Soft Tissue Sarcomas and Mast Cell Tumors

Marvin L. Olmstead, D.V.M., M.S., Diplomate A.C.V.S.
Professor of Small Animal Orthopedics, Department of Veterinary Clinical Sciences, The Ohio State University, Columbus, Ohio
Disorders of the Coxofemoral Joint

Philip A. Padriud, D.V.M.
Associate Professor of Medicine, Committee on Immunology; Chief of Academic Programs, Comparative Medicine and Pathology, University of Chicago, Department of Medicine, Chicago, Illinois
Bronchopulmonary Disease

Rodney L. Page, D.V.M., M.S., Diplomate A.C.V.I.M. (Internal Medicine, Oncology)
Professor (Oncology), North Carolina State University, Raleigh, North Carolina
Diseases of the Spleen; Principles of Oncology

David L. Panciera, D.V.M., M.S., Diplomate A.C.V.I.M.
Associate Professor, Department of Small Animal Clinical Sciences, Virginia-Maryland Regional College of Veterinary Medicine, Virginia Polytechnic Institute and State University, Blacksburg, Virginia
Diseases of the Thyroid Gland

Robert B. Parker, D.V.M., Diplomate A.C.V.S.
Chairman, Department of Surgery, The Animal Medical Center, New York, New York
Fracture of the Humerus

Steven W. Petersen, D.V.M., Diplomate A.C.V.S.
Staff Surgeon, Director of Interns, Alameda East Veterinary Hospital, Denver, Colorado
Surgery of the Skeletal Muscle and Tendons

Janet L. Peterson, D.V.M., Diplomate A.C.V.I.M. (Oncology)
Staff Veterinarian, Mission MedVet, Mission, Kansas
Tumors of the Skin and Subcutaneous Tissues

Mark E. Peterson, D.V.M., Diplomate A.C.V.I.M.
Head of Endocrinology, Department of Medicine, The Animal Center, New York, New York
Diseases of the Thyroid Gland; Diseases of the Adrenal Gland; Diseases of the Hypthalamus and Pituitary

Michael Podell, M.S., D.V.M., Diplomate A.C.V.I.M. (Neurology)
Associate Professor and Director, Comparative Neurology Service, Department of Veterinary Clinical Sciences, College of Veterinary Medicine, The Ohio State University, Columbus, Ohio
Seizures

James C. Prueter, D.V.M., Diplomate A.C.V.I.M.
Hospital Director, The Veterinary Referral Clinic, Cleveland, Ohio
Diagnostic Methods in Respiratory Disease

Katherine E. Quesenberry, D.V.M.
Service Head, Avian and Exotic Pet Service, The Animal Medical Center, New York, New York
Disorders of the Avian Nervous System; Rabbits

John F. Randolph, D.V.M., Diplomate A.C.V.I.M.
Associate Professor of Medicine, College of Veterinary Medicine; Small Animal Internist, Companion Animal Hospital, Cornell University, Ithaca, New York
Diseases of the Hypothalamus and Pituitary

Rose E. Raskin, D.V.M., Ph.D., Diplomate A.C.V.P.
Associate Professor, Clinical Pathology, Department of Physiological Sciences; Service Chief, Clinical Pathology, Veterinary Medical Teaching Hospital, University of Florida, Gainesville, Florida
Erythrocytes, Leukocytes, and Platelets

Clarence A. Rawlings, D.V.M., M.S., Ph.D., Diplomate A.C.V.S.
Professor and Department Head, Department of Small Animal Medicine and Surgery, University of Georgia, College of Veterinary Medicine, Athens, Georgia
Heartworm Disease

John R. Reed, M.S., D.V.M., Diplomate A.C.V.I.M. (Cardiology)
Staff Cardiologist, Sacramento Animal Medical Group-NPC, Carmichael, California
Pericardial Diseases and Cardiac Neoplasia

Wayne S. Rosenkrantz, B.S., D.V.M., Diplomate A.C.V.D.
Owner, Animal Dermatology Clinics of Southern California, Garden Grove and San Diego, California
Miliary Dermatitis and Eosinophilic Granuloma Complex

Edmund J. Rosser, Jr., D.V.M., Diplomate A.C.V.D.
Professor of Dermatology, Department of Small Animal Clinical Sciences, Michigan State University, College of Veterinary Medicine, East Lansing, Michigan
Pyoderma

Walter J. Rosskopf, Jr., D.V.M., Diplomate A.B.V.P. (Avian)
Co-owner and Practicing Veterinarian, Avian and Exotic Animal Hospital of Los Angeles County, Hawthorne, California
Avian Obstetric Medicine

James K. Roush, D.V.M., M.S., Diplomate A.C.V.S.
Associate Professor and Section Head, Small Animal Surgery, Department of Clinical Services, College of Veterinary Medicine, Kansas State University, Manhattan, Kansas
Miscellaneous Diseases of the Bone

John E. Rush, D.V.M., M.S., Diplomate A.C.V.I.M. (Cardiology), A.C.V.E.C.C.
Associate Professor and Associate Chair, Department of Clinical Sciences, Section Head, Emergency and Critical Care Medicine, Tufts University School of Veterinary Medicine, North Grafton; Medical Director, Veterinary Emergency Treatment Services of Walpole, Walpole, Massachusetts
Heart Failure

S. Kathleen Salisbury, D.V.M., M.S., Diplomate A.C.V.S.
Professor, Small Animal Surgery, Department of Veterinary Clinical Sciences, School of Veterinary Medicine, Purdue University, West Lafayette, Indiana
Pancreatic Beta Cell Neoplasia

Randall H. Scagliotti, D.V.M., M.S., Diplomate A.C.V.O.
Associate Clinical Professor, Department of Surgical and Radiological Sciences, School of Veterinary Medicine, University of California—Davis, Davis, California; Staff Ophthalmologist—Sacramento Animal Medical Group, Carmichael, California
Neuro-ophthalmology

Vicki J. Scheidt, D.V.M., Diplomate A.C.V.D.
Hanover Veterinary Clinic, Hanover, New Hampshire
Feline Symmetric Alopecia

Eric R. Schertel, D.V.M., Ph.D., Diplomate A.C.V.S.
MedVet Associates Inc., Columbus, Ohio
Surgical Correction of Patent Ductus Arteriosus; Shock; Principles of Thoracic Surgery

Mary P. Schick, B.S., D.V.M.
Owner of Atlanta Animal Allergy and Dermatology, Atlanta, Georgia
Skin Biopsy; Diseases of the Pinna

Robert O. Schick, D.V.M., Diplomate A.C.V.D.
Owner, Animal Allergy, Skin and Ear Specialists, West Palm Beach, Florida
Skin Biopsy; Diseases of the Pinna

Lynn P. Schmeitzel, D.V.M., Diplomate A.C.V.D.
Associate Professor of Dermatology, Department of Small Animal Clinical Sciences, College of Veterinary Medicine, University of Tennessee, Knoxville, Tennessee
Growth Hormone–Responsive Alopecia and Sex Hormone–Associated Dermatoses

Linda G. Shell, D.V.M., Diplomate A.C.V.I.M. (Neurology)
Professor Neurology, Department of Small Animal Clinical Sciences, Virginia-Maryland Regional College of Veterinary Medicine, Virginia Polytechnic Institute and State University, Blacksburg, Virginia
Otitis Media and Otitis Interna; Peripheral Nerve Disorders

G. Diane Shelton D.V.M., Ph.D., Diplomate A.C.V.I.M.
Associate Adjunct Professor, Department of Pathology, School of Medicine, University of California, San Diego, La Jolla, California
Disorders of the Muscle and Neuromuscular Junction

Robert G. Sherding D.V.M., Diplomate A.C.V.I.M.
Professor of Small Animal Internal Medicine, Chair, Department of Veterinary Clinical Sciences, The Ohio State University, Columbus, Ohio
Feline Leukemia Virus; Feline Immunodeficiency Virus; Feline Infectious Peritonitis; Feline Infectious Respiratory Disease; Canine Infectious Tracheobronchitis (Kennel Cough Complex); Canine Distemper; Intestinal Viruses; Rabies and Pseudorabies; Miscellaneous Viral Diseases; Leotospirosis, Brucellosis, and Other Bacterial Infectious Diseases; Systemic Mycoses; Toxoplasmosis, Neosporosis, and Other Multisystemic Protozoal Infections; Respiratory Infections; Pleural Effusion; Diseases of the Esophagus and Disorders of Swallowing; Diseases of the Stomach; Diseases of the Intestines; Diseases of the Liver and Biliary Tract; Diseases and Surgery of the Exocrine Pancreas; Anorectal Diseases

Peter Shires, B.V.Sc., M.S., Diplomate A.C.V.S.
Professor of Small Animal Surgery, Director of Veterinary Educational Technologies, Virginia-Maryland Regional College of Veterinary Medicine, Virginia Polytechnic Institute and State University, Blacksburg, Virginia
Fractures of the Femur

David Sisson, D.V.M., Diplomate A.C.V.I.M. (Cardiology)
Associate Professor of Cardiology, Director, Cardiology Service, University of Illinois, College of Veterinary Medicine, Urbana, Illinois
Valvular Heart Disease

Daniel D. Smeak, D.V.M., Diplomate A.C.V.S.
Professor, Small Animal General Surgery; Head Small Animal Surgery, College of Veterinary Medicine, The Ohio State University, Columbus, Ohio
Surgery of the External Ear Canal and Pinna; Selected Skin Graft and Reconstructive Techniques

Francis W.K. Smith, Jr., D.V.M., Diplomate A.C.V.I.M. (Internal Medicine and Cardiology)
Clinical Assistant Professor, Department of Medicine, Tufts University, School of Veterinary Medicine, North Grafton, Massachusetts; Chief of Medicine, Cardiopet, Floral Park, New Jersey
Electrocardiography; Disorders of Cardiac Rhythm

Mark M. Smith, V.M.D., Diplomate A.C.V.S., A.V.D.C.
Associate Professor, Department of Small Animal Clinical Sciences, Virginia-Maryland Regional College of Veterinary Medicine, Virginia Polytechnic Institute and State University, Blacksburg, Virginia
Fractures of the Skull; Neoplasia of the Axial Skeleton

Susan F. Soderberg, D.V.M., Diplomate A.C.V.I.M.
East Detroit Animal Hospital, Eastpointe, Michigan
Diseases of the Testes and Scrotum; Diseases of the Penis and Prepuce; Infertility and Disorders of Breeding

Rebecca L. Stepien, D.V.M., M.S., Diplomate A.C.V.I.M. (Cardiology)
Clinical Assistant Professor, University of Wisconsin, School of Veterinary Medicine, Clinical Cardiologist, University of Wisconsin Veterinary Medical Teaching Hospital, Madison, Wisconsin
Vascular Diseases

Elizabeth Arnold Stone, D.V.M., Diplomate A.C.V.S.
Professor and Head, Department of Clinical Sciences, College of Veterinary Medicine, North Carolina State University, Raleigh, North Carolina
Mammary Gland Neoplasia

Steven F. Swaim, D.V.M., M.S.
Professor of Small Animal Surgery, College of Veterinary Medicine, Auburn University, Auburn, Alabama
Management of the Traumatic Wound by Primary Closure

Robert A. Taylor, B.S., D.V.M., M.S., Diplomate A.C.V.S.
Clinical Affiliate, Veterinary Teaching Hospital, Colorado State University, Fort Collins, Colorado; Chief Surgeon, Alameda East Veterinary Hospital, Denver, Colorado
Scapulohumeral Luxation

James P. Thompson, D.V.M., Ph.D., Diplomate A.C.V.I.M. (Internal Medicine Oncology)
Associate Professor, Small Animal Medicine, University of Florida, Gainesville, Florida
Systemic Immune-Mediated Diseases

Larry Patrick Tilley, D.V.M., Diplomate, A.C.V.I.M. (Internal Medicine)
Director, Veterinary Specialty Referral Center, President, Vet Med-Dr. Tilley and Associates, Santa Fe, New Mexico
Electrocardiography; Disorders of Cardiac Rhythm

James Tomlinson, D.V.M., M.V.Sc., Diplomate A.C.V.S.
Associate Professor of Surgery, University of Missouri, Columbia, Missouri
Fractures and Growth Deformities of the Radius and Ulna, Luxation of the Elbow

Thomas M.Turner, D.V.M., Diplomate A.C.V.S.
Assistant Professor, Department of Orthopedics, Rush-Presbyterian-St. Luke's Medical Center, Chicago, Illinois; Staff Surgeon, VCA Berwyn Animal Hospital, Berwyn, Illinois
Fractures of the Shoulder

David M. Vail, D.V.M., M.S., Diplomate A.C.V.I.M. (Oncology)
Associate Professor of Oncology; Member, Comprehensive Cancer Center, University of Wisconsin-Madison, Madison, Wisconsin
Lymphoid Neoplasia

Raymund F. Wack, D.V.M., Diplomate A.C.Z.M.
Director of Animal Health, Columbus Zoo, Powell, Ohio
Basic Husbandry and Medicine of Pet Reptiles

Stanley D. Wagner, D.V.M., M.S.
Associate Professor, Iowa State University, Ames, Iowa
Fractures and Dislocation of the Spine

Ken Warthen, D.V.M.
Featherquest Farms, Pembroke, Virginia
Disorders of the Avian Digestive System

Patricia D. White, D.V.M., M.S., Diplomate A.C.V.D.
Owner, Clinical Dermatologist, Atlanta Veterinary Skin and Allergy Clinic, P.C., Atlanta, Georgia
Atopy

Stephen D. White, D.V.M., Diplomate A.C.V.D.
Professor, College of Veterinary Medicine and Biomedical Sciences, Colorado State University, Ft. Collins, Colorado
Food Hypersensitivity

David A. Wilkie, D.V.M., M.S., Diplomate A.C.V.O.
Associate Professor and Head, Comparative Ophthalmology, Department of Veterinary Clinical Sciences, Ohio State University, Columbus, Ohio
Ophthalmic Equipment and Techniques; Diseases of the Lens; Uvea; Glaucoma

Richard W. Woerpel, M.S., D.V.M.
Co-owner and Practicing Veterinarian, Avian And Exotic Animal Hospital of Los Angles County, Hawthorne, California
Avian Obstetric Medicine

Preface

In the first edition of the *Saunders Manual of Small Animal Practice,* we attempted to condense an enormous amount of clinical information into a concise, practical, user-friendly text. The book had to be one volume and written in a way that allowed busy practitioners and students to glean essential information quickly and efficiently. We did this by using a semioutline format rather than standard paragraphs, by including many consistent titles and subtitles to allow rapid location of subject areas, by liberally using tables and simple illustrations, highlighting Key Points, and writing in a style that uses the active rather than passive voice. Based on the hundreds of verbal or written comments we have received since publication of the first edition, we believe that we have succeeded in our goal. We would be remiss if we did not thank all the students, residents, and practitioners who provided their thoughtful and useful feedback on the first edition. We hope the second edition continues to fulfill the objective of helping readers quickly find useful information and solve clinical problems.

Because of the success of the first edition, we have not made major changes in the format or subject areas in the second edition. The information is still predominantly organized by systems, with a section on general principles of patient management added in the beginning of the book. Although the book emphasizes disorders of dogs and cats, a large section on avian and exotic pets is included. The outline format for medicine and surgery chapters remains as it was in the first edition. However, several things have been done to make the second edition more current, and even more user friendly. First, all chapters have been completely revised and updated. In the editorial process, we tried to polish the concise writing style and consistency of format. We included even more titles and subtitles to break up the text and make for more interesting reading. Chapter cross-referencing was done even more extensively than in the first edition. Also, many new illustrations have been added to complement the existing ones that depict commonly performed techniques. Last, drugs and dosages that are cited in the chapters have now been placed in a table at the end of the book. We hope that this table will serve to make drug information even more accessible and convenient.

As we mentioned in the preface to the first edition, the chapter authors and section editors make up the core of this book, and we are very grateful to them for their excellent work. Not only did they provide current and useful information but they were very tolerant of our editorial idiosyncrasies. We also wish to thank the students, residents, and faculty of The Ohio State University College of Veterinary Medicine for their continuous support and wise advice as we prepared this new edition. A project like this would frankly be impossible without the skilled and experienced editorial staff at W.B. Saunders, particularly editors Melissa Dudlick and Ray Kersey. We also wish to thank the copy editors for their detailed review of text, our very talented medical illustrator Felecia Paras, and our student assistant Chrystal Gilmore.

We view the *Saunders Manual of Small Animal Practice* as a work in progress. We welcome comments, criticisms, and suggestions to help make future editions a worthwhile part of the veterinary clinician's library.

STEPHEN J. BIRCHARD, DVM, MS
ROBERT G. SHERDING, DVM

Contents

Section 4

Endocrine and Metabolic Disorders   235

Mark E. Peterson

Section 5

Skin and Ear Diseases   305

Richard Anderson

Section 8

Disorders of the Urogenital System   913
Daniel Smeak

Section 9

Skeletal System   1060
Paul A. Manley

Section 10

Nervous System   1233
Michael Podell

Section 11

Ophthalmology   1311
David A. Wilkie

Section 12

Diseases of Avian and Exotic Pets   1396
Barbara L. Oglesbee

NOTICE

Companion animal practice is an ever-changing field. Standard safety precautions must be followed, but as new research and clinical experience grow, changes in treatment and drug therapy become necessary or appropriate. The authors and editors of this work have carefully checked the generic and trade drug names and verified drug dosages to assure that dosage information is precise and in accord with standards accepted at the time of publication. Readers are advised, however, to check the product information currently provided by the manufacturer of each drug to be administered to be certain that changes have not been made in the recommended dose or in the contraindications for administration. This is of particular importance in regard to new or infrequently used drugs. Recommended dosages for animals are sometimes based on adjustments in the dosage that would be suitable for humans. Some of the drugs mentioned here have been given experimentally by the authors. Others have been used in dosages greater than those recommended by the manufacturer. In these kinds of cases, the authors have reported on their own considerable experience. It is the responsibility of those administering a drug, relying on their professional skill and experience, to determine the dosages, the best treatment for the patient, and whether the benefits of giving a drug justify the attendant risk. The editors cannot be responsible for misuse or misapplication of the material in this work.

THE PUBLISHER

1 Patient Management

Stephen J. Birchard

1 History and Physical Examination

Denise Jones

Veterinarians are faced with many diagnostic challenges on a daily basis. By far the most important diagnostic tool that veterinarians possess is their ability to obtain a complete history and thorough physical examination. This information, when accurately interpreted, lays the foundation for a logical diagnostic and therapeutic plan. A systematic and thorough history and physical examination prevents unnecessary diagnostic testing and resultant needless cost to the owner.

GENERAL HISTORY

- Obtain both objective and subjective information when collecting the history. Objective data consist of the signalment, environment, diet, and medical history. For a patient's first visit, determine the length of ownership and the place of origin.
- Subjective data include a description of the primary complaint and a historical overview of the patient's general health. The owner often may not realize how a seemingly unimportant observation may be related to the primary problem. Tailor specific questions to the individual case.

Signalment

- The signalment consists of the patient's age, species, breed, and gender. Note whether the patient is intact or neutered.
- Verify that previously recorded data are correct and up-to-date. For example, the patient may have been neutered since its last visit or the physical examination may indicate that the recorded age is questionable.

Environment

- Gather environmental information as a routine part of the patient's history. In many circumstances, where the pet is kept becomes a vital clue in diagnosis.
- Determine whether the pet is free roaming or confined to a yard or house. If the patient is confined to a yard, ask the owner if the yard is fenced, if the pet is chained, and if an escape has been possible in the recent past. The free-roaming or recently escaped pet may have had access to toxins or have been subject to trauma, which is unlikely for an indoor pet. For example, in a dyspneic patient, diaphragmatic hernia ranks higher on the differential diagnosis list for a free-roaming pet than for a strictly indoor pet.
- Determine the geographic origin of the pet and any record of recent travels. This becomes paramount if the patient has been exposed to diseases endemic to certain regions but not prevalent in the current environment, such as systemic mycoses and rickettsial diseases.
- Determine the pet's water source and the access to any toxins or ingestible foreign bodies. Source of water may be important if the pet has access to toilet-bowl water treated with cleansers or deodorants or if the pet has limited access to water. This information is unimportant if the presenting complaint does not suggest toxicity or foreign body ingestion.

Dietary History

- Always include dietary information in the routine database. Question the owner about the patient's appetite and evidence of any weight gain or loss. Also note whether the owner watches the pet eat.

- Determine the following pertinent facts in the dietary history:
  - Type of diet (e.g., dry, moist, semimoist, or table food)
  - Brand name of food
  - Type of snacks
  - Method of feeding (i.e., free-choice or individual meals)
  - Amount.

Preventive Health Care Status

- Evaluate the patient's preventive health care status. Review the patient's prior medical record.
- Record all previous vaccinations received and the dates of each. Avoid simply asking if the patient is current on vaccinations because many clients are unfamiliar with vaccination recommendations. Inform the client of what vaccinations are available as well as the indications and booster intervals for each (see Chaps. 6, 8 to 13, 16, and 17).
- For the feline patient, discuss the subject of feline leukemia virus (FeLV), including the dates and results of previous testing. Exposure to FeLV-positive patients may also be relevant.
- For the canine patient, record heartworm test dates and results. If the patient is receiving heartworm preventive therapy, note the type, frequency, and dose (see Chap. 68).

Prior Medical History: Previous Illnesses and Surgeries

- Often the patient's prior or ongoing health problems play a role in its presenting ailment; therefore, review the information previously recorded in the medical record and discuss previous problems managed by another veterinarian.
- Record the dates of the previous illness or surgery, followed by a brief description of the problem, how it was managed, and the response to treatment.
- Discern the relevance of these problems prior to obtaining all the details; otherwise, the history may become unnecessarily lengthy and confusing.

Primary Complaint

- Use the history to identify and localize the primary problem. Much of this information is subjective, based mostly on the owner's interpretation of the pet's clinical symptoms and behavior. Be aware that some owners are extremely observant of their pet and others are not. The astute clinician collects all data and subjectively analyzes this information in respect to the owner's perceptivity.
- Encourage the owner to describe the patient's problem from its onset so that a chronologic picture is obtained.
- Avoid leading questions that might result in a deceptive history. For example, ask if there has been any change in frequency of defecation. Do not ask if the patient is defecating more frequently than normal.
- Certain data are essential to the clinician's diagnostic

and therapeutic approach. This information aids in ranking the differential diagnoses in order of preference.

- Determine the last period of normalcy. This influences how rapidly or aggressively the problem is to be approached.
- Determine the onset (acute versus chronic) of the problem. For example, intestinal intussusception is a likely differential for a puppy presenting with an acute episode of frequent vomiting. A gastric foreign body is more likely in a similar patient with chronic intermittent vomiting.
- Determine treatments and response. For example, a dog presenting with pruritus unresponsive to previous treatment with corticosteroids is a more likely candidate for food allergy dermatitis than for atopy. Determine what medication was given, the dosage, the duration of treatment, and the level of response observed.
- Determine the duration and progression of the clinical signs. For example, a patient presenting with a history of seizures is managed more aggressively when the seizures are increasing in frequency and length than when they have been the same for months or years.
- Determine the intervening signs that may also provide a clue to the most likely differential diagnosis. For example, a cat with chronic diarrhea and intermittent episodes of fever is considered a more likely candidate for infectious disease than for dietary intolerance.
- Further define and localize the problem, if possible, depending on its nature. For example, characterize diarrhea as originating in the small or large bowel before proceeding to a diagnostic or therapeutic plan. Questions regarding frequency, appearance (color and consistency), and presence or absence of straining help to localize this problem. Specific questions oriented by body systems follow in the next section.

HISTORY ORIENTED BY BODY SYSTEMS

For a complete history, include a system-by-system review of the patient's general health. This can be accomplished by the experienced clinician as the physical examination is performed. The novice may prefer to obtain the entire history before proceeding with the physical examination. Develop a consistent and systematic method. One method is to begin with questions concerning the patient's head and proceed caudally, as demonstrated in the following text. It is left to the clinician's discretion as to how in-depth the client is questioned on systems that do not appear to affect the primary complaint. Apply the general principles described in the previous section in the approach to all body systems (e.g., onset and duration).

Eyes

- Ask if any ocular discharge has been noted. If so, describe the discharge (serous, mucoid, mucopurulent) and determine if it has been unilateral or bilateral.

- Determine if ocular pain or discomfort is present as indicated by blepharospasm, face rubbing or pawing, or photophobia.
- Ask about ocular redness, swelling, and asymmetry.
- Ask if the owner has noticed a color change in the pet's eye. This change can occur with anterior uveitis and iriditis, in which hyphema may be present or the iridial color may be altered. A localized color change in the iris may occur with an iris cyst or melanoma.
- Determine if visual loss has been noticed.

See also Section 11.

Head, Neck, Ears, Nose, and Oral Cavity

- Record any history of swelling and asymmetry of the head and neck region.
- Inquire about head shaking, ear scratching, and otic discharge or odor that may indicate the possibility of otitis or a foreign body in the ear. Determine if hearing loss has been noted.
- Ask if any nasal discharge has been present. Note the character of any such discharge (serous, mucoid, mucopurulent, hemorrhagic) as well as whether it has been unilateral or bilateral. Record any history of sneezing, nose rubbing, nasal asymmetry, and stridor.
- Request information relating to the oral cavity, such as odor, difficulty eating or swallowing, abnormal swellings involving the gingiva or tongue, and changes in gingival pigmentation. Ask if there has been any change in the patient's bark or meow.

Cardiopulmonary System

- Ask if cough, exercise intolerance, weakness, or fainting have been observed. These may indicate cardiopulmonary disease.

▼ *Key Point* Differentiate syncope from seizures based on the owner's description of the event.

- Characterize coughing as productive or nonproductive, moist or dry, harsh or honking. Some owners may confuse a productive cough with vomiting; therefore, ask if abdominal heaving occurs prior to the production of fluid or foam, or if coughing and gagging are more typical. Yellow-stained fluid indicates vomitus containing bile. The circumstances surrounding the cough are often relevant. For example, cough associated with tracheal collapse is often elicited with excitement or pulling on the patient's collar. Coughing secondary to congestive heart failure may be exacerbated with the pet in a sternal position.
- Determine if dyspnea has been observed. If the owner describes difficult breathing, discern whether it is panting or true dyspnea.

See also Chapter 59.

Skin

An accurate and a detailed history is essential for successful management of dermatologic problems. Some clinicians prefer the owner to fill out a standardized dermatologic history form prior to specific questioning. Include the following questions on such a form, or directly ask the owner.

- Any observation of hair loss? Did hair loss involve the undercoat or maincoat?
- Is there evidence of pruritus (scratching, biting, licking)?
  - If so, how severe? Have the owner grade the degree of pruritus on a scale of 1 to 10, with 10 being the most severe. This helps subsequent evaluation of treatment response.
  - Continuous or seasonal? If seasonal, when?
  - Has the owner noticed fleas? What flea products have been used? Has the pet been on monthly preventive treatment? If so, which product?
  - What type of bedding does the pet use?
  - Any exposure to feathers?
  - What type of carpet is in the house (wool, synthetic, cotton)?
  - What is the diet? Are treats given?
  - Any indoor plants?
  - Is the pruritus worse indoors or outdoors?
  - Is there any exposure to tobacco smoke?
  - Has the pet ever had any drug reactions? (describe)
- Describe odors, pigment changes, or texture changes of the skin or haircoat.
- Any dandruff? If so, what areas are involved?
- How often is the patient groomed (clipped, brushed, combed)?
- How often is the patient bathed? When was the last bath and what was used?
- Other pets in the household? Are they affected?
- Do any members of the household have skin problems?
- Do any of the pet's close relatives have skin problems?
- Any previous treatment? When was the pet last treated? What was the name of the drug, the dose, the route of administration, and the frequency of treatment? What level of response was noted?

See also Section 5.

Digestive System

Most problems related to the digestive system are clinically manifested as regurgitation, vomiting, diarrhea, constipation, weight loss, or their combination. Determine which clinical sign is actually being exhibited because the owner may incorrectly interpret what is observed. For example, an owner often assumes that the patient is constipated if it is observed straining to defecate, when diarrhea may be the actual cause. Include the following specific information in approaching a digestive system problem.

- Review dietary history, as previously described. Specifically ask about treats or access to garbage.
- Record environmental history, as previously described.
  - Any exposure to toxins, drugs, or plants?

- Any toys or other objects that the pet may have ingested?
- Note vaccination status.
- Has any vomiting been observed (onset, progression)?
  - Has the owner actually observed the pet vomiting?
  - How frequently is the pet vomiting?
  - What is the relationship of vomiting to eating, if any?
  - What is produced when the pet vomits? Describe the vomitus—digested or undigested food, fluid, foam, and color.
  - Is any retching or abdominal component observed?
- Is any diarrhea observed (onset, progression)?
  - Has the owner witnessed the patient defecating?
  - How frequently does the animal defecate?
  - Is the stool persistently loose?
  - What is the owner's description of the stool in regard to color and consistency (formed but soft, cow patty–like, watery)?
  - Is there any blood or mucus present?
  - What volume of stool is produced?
  - Does the animal strain while defecating?
  - Does the animal consume its own stool?
- Does the owner believe that the patient is constipated?
  - How long since the last observed bowel movement?
  - Consistency of last stool?
  - Does the owner witness all eliminations (leash walks, access to yard, or free roaming)?

See also Section 7.

Urinary System

Often, the owner complaint may be that the pet is urinating excessively. The following questions help to distinguish whether excessive urination is due to polyuria or to pollakiuria.

- Has there been any change in the quantity of water that the pet consumes?
- Are there other pets in the household that have access to the same water source?
- Has there been any change in frequency of urination?
- Is the pet urinating inside the house?
  - Are these urinations observed? (The owner should verify that this is the pet having the accidents versus another pet in the household.)
  - Do they occur while the animal is awake or asleep?
  - Does the patient seem to be consciously aware of the act?
  - Does the animal dribble urine without seeming to be aware?
- What quantity of urine is produced?
- Does the animal appear to strain while urinating?
- Has the owner noticed any blood in the urine? If so, is it before, after, or during urination?

See also Section 8.

Genital System

The reproductive status of the patient was previously noted with the patient's signalment. If the patient is intact, consider the following questions:

- If female, when was the patient's last heat cycle?
- Was the animal intentionally bred or is there any possibility of an incidental breeding? Was the breeding successful? Difficulty whelping?
- Have the heat cycles been at regular intervals?
- Any vulvar discharge noted (describe amount, consistency, color, odor)?
- If male, has the patient been used for breeding? If so, when?
- Any litters sired?
- Any preputial or penile discharge noted (describe amount, consistency, color, odor)?
- For both the male and female dog, has the patient been tested for brucellosis? When? Was the mate previously tested?

See also Section 8.

Musculoskeletal System

- History relating to the musculoskeletal system focuses on lameness. When lameness has been observed, discern if the patient has been bearing weight on the affected leg. Determine if lameness has been previously observed in the other limbs. Determine if there are any other signs of illness in addition to the lameness.
- Ascertain any possibility of trauma preceding the lameness. In some cases, the owner may have witnessed the traumatic incident. In others, the patient may have been unsupervised during the time in question. If the animal was free roaming and unobserved, determine for how long and the probability of exposure to automobiles or other sources of trauma.
- Determine if the owner has observed loss of muscle mass, asymmetry of the limbs, or swollen joints.
- Ask if the patient has demonstrated any difficulty on rising, climbing stairs, or descending stairs. Determine if these signs improve or worsen with exercise.
- In regions endemic for Lyme disease, ask if any ticks have been observed on the pet. Check vaccination status regarding Lyme disease. In nonendemic areas obtain a travel history.

See also Section 9.

Nervous System

Many questions related to the nervous system may have been previously asked while taking the history of the other body systems. Diseases of the central nervous system (CNS) may be reflected by abnormalities in other systems (e.g., blindness and hearing loss). With a presenting complaint of rear limb "weakness," the clinician does not know if the primary problem is related to the musculoskeletal system or to the nervous system until the history and physical examination are completed. Consider the following points in regard to the nervous system:

- Ask if any behavioral changes, such as aggression and dementia, have been observed.
- Record any history of seizures, including their duration and the time interval between them. Obtain a description of the seizure.
- Determine if any abnormalities in posture or ambulation have been observed, such as the pet's tendency to fall to one side, to circle to one side, to knuckle over, or to drag its toes.

See also Section 10.

Swelling or Masses

Ask if any abnormal swellings have been observed that have not been previously mentioned. Note the location, how long the mass or swelling has been present, and any change in appearance, character, or size.

PHYSICAL EXAMINATION

General Observation of Patient

- To begin the physical examination, watch the patient as it enters the room.
- Continue the visual evaluation of the patient while the history is collected. Observe the general body condition and abnormalities in behavior, attitude, posture, ambulation, and respiratory pattern. During this time, the patient may be placed on the examination table or allowed to roam the examination room.

Vital Signs

Initially, record the vital signs and current body weight on every patient.

- Body temperature
  - Obtain the rectal temperature early in the course of the examination to help avoid an elevation of temperature that may result from anxiety or excitement. In emergency situations, attend to hypothermia or hyperthermia early in the course of the examination.
  - Note any blood or melena on the thermometer.
- Pulse and heart rate
  - Record the pulse rate and evaluate the pulse quality.
  - Determine if arrhythmias and pulse deficits are present.
- Capillary refill
  - Lift up the upper lip, press on the mucous membranes, and determine how long it takes for the membranes to resume normal pink color (normal is ≤2 seconds).
- Respiratory rate
  - Evaluate the respiratory pattern as the rate is taken.
  - If moderate or severe dyspnea is present, observe caution in continuing with the remainder of the examination. The additional stress of restraint and examination may result in life-threatening respiratory compromise. Administer oxygen therapy followed by a rapid oral examination and thoracic auscultation to help determine the source of the dyspnea and appropriate emergency therapy. After stabilizing respiratory function, continue with the remainder of the physical examination.
- Hydration
  - Note if the eyes appear sunken or if the third eyelids are protruding bilaterally.
  - Note if the mucous membranes are dry or tacky.
  - Evaluate skin turgor by gently lifting the skin over the dorsal thorax. Geriatric or cachectic patients may appear to be dehydrated based on their skin turgor alone because of the loss of the skin's natural elasticity.

Body Systems Approach

The physical examination should follow the same logical pattern as the history. A consistent approach is taken so that no part of the examination is overlooked. For example, analyze one body system at a time, starting with the patient's head, and proceed caudally.

Head

- Examine the head carefully for evidence of asymmetry or localized swellings. Palpation is necessary to assess the nature of any swelling or mass (firm or fluctuant, mobile or attached).
- Evaluate the posture of the head and neck. Ventroflexion may be observed in cats with hypokalemia, chronic organophosphate toxicity, thiamine deficiency, and polymyopathies. Reluctance to lift the head may be noticed in a dog with cervical intervertebral disc protrusion. Gently manipulate the head dorsally, ventrally, and to either side to look for evidence of pain or resistance.

Eyes

- Determine if abnormalities are present unilaterally or bilaterally. If only one eye is affected, examine the normal eye first.
- Note evidence of pain such as blepharospasm, photophobia, and pawing or rubbing the eye(s).
- Observe size and symmetry of the eyes. Congenital microphthalmia or acquired phthisis bulbi results in a smaller than normal eye, whereas chronic glaucoma results in a larger than normal eye.
- Examine the position of the eyes for evidence of enophthalmos, exophthalmos, or strabismus. Enophthalmos may be secondary to microphthalmia, loss of the orbital fat pad (e.g., cachexia), Horner syndrome, dehydration, or acute ocular pain (e.g., anterior uveitis). Exophthalmos may be due to space-occupying lesions of the orbit (neoplasia, abscess, cellulitis), buphthalmos (glaucoma), myositis, or breed predisposition.
- Note ocular discharge and characterize it as serous, mucoid, or mucopurulent.
- Note swelling or masses involving the eyelids as well as distichiasis, entropion, or ectropion.
- Evaluate the conjunctiva for hyperemia, chemosis, pallor, or jaundice of the underlying sclera. The su-

perior conjunctiva is more reliable for evaluating hyperemia than the inferior conjunctiva, which may normally appear reddened. Note any abnormal pigmentation or masses involving the sclera or conjunctiva.

- Protrusion of the third eyelid may be a reflection of enophthalmos or Haw syndrome in cats. Note any masses associated with the nictitans or prolapse of the gland of the nictitans. Apply gentle pressure to the superior globe to aid in exposing the nictitans. Apply topical anesthesia and grasp the third eyelid gently with forceps, so that the posterior surface of the third eyelid can be examined for foreign bodies or follicular hyperplasia.
- Examine the cornea for cloudiness, pigmentation, vascularization, or obvious defects.
- Evaluate the anterior chamber for aqueous flare, hypopyon, hyphema, or abnormal masses. If a slit lamp is not available, use a magnifying lens and a penlight to produce a narrow beam of light so that subtle aqueous flare can be detected when the anterior chamber is viewed from the lateral aspect.
- Evaluate pupil size and symmetry and direct and consensual pupillary light reflexes. A darkened room aids in this examination. Persistent pupillary membranes may also be identified.
- Evaluate the iris for pigmentary changes, hyperemia, roughening, swelling, or synechia. Any of these changes can be seen with anterior uveitis. Tumors or cysts may occasionally occur on the iris.
- Evaluate the lens via direct or indirect ophthalmoscopy for lenticular sclerosis, cataract, or displacement.
- For a complete fundic examination, dilate the pupil with a short-acting mydriatic. Evaluate the fundus for vascularity, areas of hemorrhage, pigmentary changes, chorioretinal dysplasia or hypoplasia, and retinal detachment. Evaluate the optic disc for color, size, vascularity, fissures or colobomas, and abnormal masses. Practice and experience are the keys to retinal examinations.
- Evaluate vision by dropping a cotton ball in front of the patient or by rolling a cotton ball across the table or floor. Evaluate the menace response. Remember that young puppies and kittens normally do not respond appropriately to menace.

See also Section 11.

Oral Cavity

- Perform a thorough oral examination if the patient's demeanor allows (Fig. 1–1). If this examination is indicated but the patient is uncooperative or aggressive, sedation (see Chaps. 2 and 84) may be necessary.
- Always carefully evaluate the mucous membranes for color, moisture, and capillary refill time in order to assess the hydration status. Hyperemia, congestion, cyanosis, jaundice, pallor, or petechiae can provide vital diagnostic clues.
- Note gingival masses, ulcerations, inflammation, or pigmentary changes.

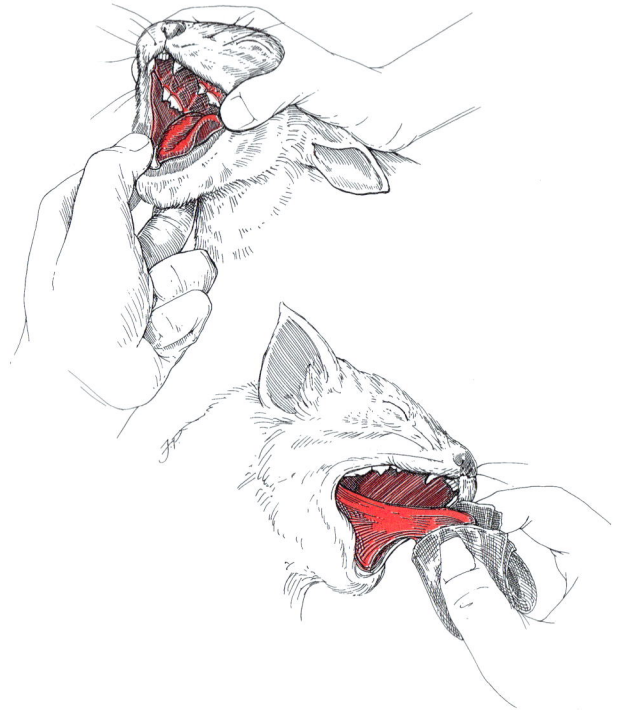

Figure 1–1.   Oral examination of the feline mouth and tongue.

- Examine the teeth for calculus or exudate at the gingival margin. Digital pressure applied to the gingiva may aid in expressing exudate when a tooth root abscess is suspected.
- Examine the tongue for evidence of trauma or masses when unexplained oral hemorrhage has been observed. In the feline patient that presents for vomiting, examine the sublingual area for evidence of a linear foreign body, using one of the following two methods:
  - Open the patient's mouth and, with the middle finger of the hand depressing the mandible, apply pressure between the mandibular rami from the ventral aspect. In this manner, the tongue is elevated so that the sublingual surface can be seen (see Fig. 1–1, *top*).
  - Occasionally, string can be overlooked with this first method. The sublingual tissue can overlap a thin string that has been drawn taut so that it is not seen. In this case, the second method is to grasp the tongue with a gauze sponge and pull the tongue out and laterally, so that it can be seen more completely (see Fig. 1–1, *bottom*).
- Examine the hard palate in the neonate for clefts. Evaluate the soft palate (if possible) for elongation or masses.
- Examine the pharyngeal region for asymmetry, masses, or foreign bodies or for evidence of inflammation or trauma. Examine the tonsils for enlargement. Depress the caudal aspect of the tongue to see the caudal pharynx.
- In the cat, if pharyngeal polyps are a differential diagnosis, examine the soft palate for evidence of

bulging. For a more complete exam, sedate the patient to look under the soft palate.

See also Chapter 84.

Nose

- Examine the nose for asymmetry or swelling. If a mass or swelling is present, palpate it carefully to determine whether it is firm or fluctuant.
- Note evidence of nasal discharge. Examine the nares closely to determine if the discharge is unilateral or bilateral and to characterize it as serous, mucoid, mucopurulent, or hemorrhagic. It may be beneficial to gently swab the external nares to detect a subtle discharge.
- If either nasal swelling or discharge is present, evaluate the patency of each nostril by wiping the examination table with an alcohol swab and positioning the patient's nose close to the table to observe condensation of the patient's breath on the surface. Alternately, place a wisp of cotton in front of each nostril to observe movement from air flow.

See also Chapter 76.

Ears

- Inspect both the external and inner surfaces of the pinna for skin lesions, hair loss, erythema, or swelling.
- Examine the external ear canals for erythema, discharge, and odor prior to an otoscopic examination. Palpate the ear canal cartilages for masses, pain, or other abnormalities.
- An otoscopic exam is invaluable in assessing an ear-related problem.
  - Otoscopic technique requires practice to be successful. Sedation of the pet may be required.
  - Lift the pinna and gently place the otoscopic cone in the vertical canal from a dorsal approach and direct it ventrally (Fig. 1–2). As the otoscope is guided deeper into the vertical canal, pull the pinna and otoscope horizontally to bring the horizontal ear canal and tympanic membrane into view.
  - Examine both the horizontal and vertical canals for masses, foreign bodies, discharges, and parasites (ear mites and ticks). Assess the tympanic membrane for rupture or evidence of otitis media (erythema or protrusion).

See also Chapters 54 to 56.

Neck

- Palpate the paratracheal area from the larynx to the thoracic inlet.
  - In middle-aged to older cats, this palpation is especially important because of the high incidence of hyperthyroidism caused by thyroid adenomas. The normal thyroid is not palpable.
  - Stand behind the cat with it standing or sitting, extend the neck, and point the nose upward. Place your thumb and forefinger on each side of the tra-

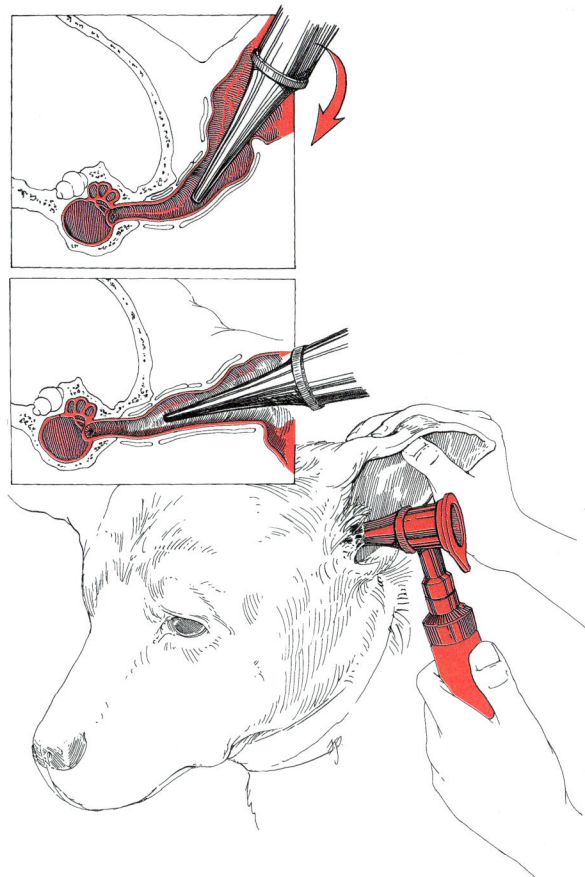

Figure 1–2. Otoscopic examination.

chea. Starting at the larynx, slide them down the length of the trachea using gentle pressure. The typical thyroid nodule will "pop" as your thumb and forefinger slip over the caudal pole (Fig. 1–3A).
  - Alternatively, palpate each side individually. Turn the patient's head slightly to one side and place your forefinger between the trachea and the adjacent muscles on the opposite side (Fig. 1–3B). Once again start at the larynx and slide your finger down to the thoracic inlet. Turn the patient's head to the opposite side and repeat the procedure on the second side. Repeated palpation may be necessary to detect subtle nodules.
  - In dogs, palpation may detect a thyroid tumor.
- Palpate the trachea for collapse, soft cartilage, or flattening.
- Attempt to elicit a cough by gently encircling the trachea with one hand and applying pressure on the tracheal muscle dorsally. If a cough is produced by this method, it suggests tracheal collapse or tracheobronchitis. Conduct this part of the examination after the thorax has been auscultated because it may induce paroxysms of coughing.
- Evaluate the jugular veins for distention or a jugular pulse extending more than one third the way up the neck. It may be necessary to moisten this area with alcohol or to clip the hair to detect these abnormalities.

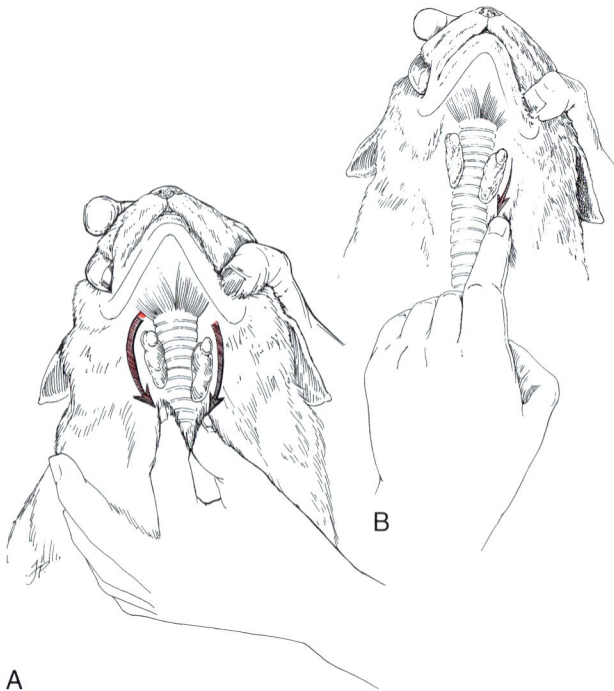

Figure 1–3. *A,* Paratracheal palpation of the thyroid. *B,* Alternatively, palpate each side of the thyroid gland individually.

Lymph Nodes and Subcutaneous Masses

- Palpate all external lymph nodes (Fig. 1–4). Generalized lymphadenopathy usually indicates a systemic disease (systemic fungal infections, immune-mediated diseases, neoplasia), whereas local lymph node enlargement usually indicates a regional infection (abscess).
  - The mandibular lymph nodes are located at the angle of the mandible, slightly cranial and ventral to the parotid and submaxillary salivary glands.

The nodes are generally smooth and ovoid in contrast to the irregular texture of the salivary glands. Practice distinguishing these lymph nodes from salivary glands.

- The superficial cervical or prescapular lymph nodes can usually be palpated just in front of the cranial border of the scapula. Grasp them by palpating beneath the scapular border. They may be more difficult to palpate in the obese or heavily muscled patient.
- The axillary lymph nodes are not always palpable because of their disc-like shape and surrounding musculature.
- The superficial inguinal lymph nodes are located at the junction of the abdominal wall and the medial thigh and may be difficult to palpate in the obese patient.
- The popliteal lymph nodes are usually palpable caudal to the stifle joint. The surrounding subcutaneous fat may make these nodes seem larger than their actual size, especially in cats.
- Palpate the trunk and extremities for abnormal masses or swelling. When a mass is found, note the location, size, and consistency. Determine which tissues are involved (dermal-epidermal, subcutaneous, underlying tissue). Note whether the mass is freely movable or attached to the underlying muscle, fascia, or bone.

Skin

- Inspect the general appearance of the haircoat for luster and fullness and areas of hair loss. Note symmetric alopecia as seen with endocrinopathy. Inspect areas of alopecia for broken hairs as seen with pruritic or psychogenic conditions. Check for erythema.
- When approaching a pet with a dermatologic problem, examine all areas of the body. Location of skin lesions often aids in the diagnosis. For example, lo-

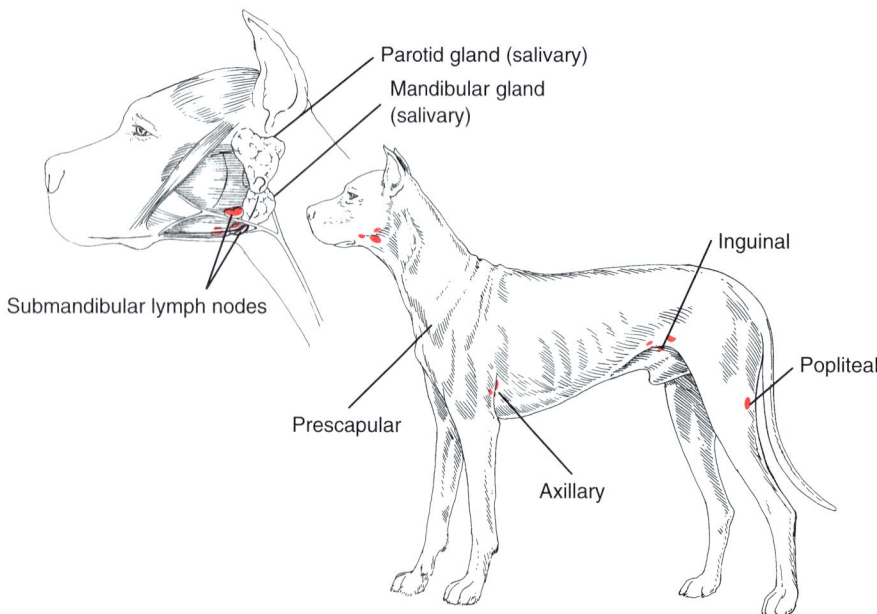

Parotid gland (salivary)
Mandibular gland (salivary)
Submandibular lymph nodes
Prescapular
Axillary
Inguinal
Popliteal

Figure 1–4. Commonly palpated lymph nodes.

calized demodicosis causes patches of alopecia involving the head and forelegs. Sarcoptic mange typically causes scaling and partial alopecia of the pinnae, elbows, and hocks. Do not overlook the interdigital areas and the foot pads. Examine mucocutaneous junctions (lips, anus, vulva, prepuce) for evidence of an immune-mediated disease.

- Identify all skin lesions and categorize them as primary or secondary. Primary lesions include papules, pustules, nodules, wheals, macules, and vesicles. Common secondary lesions are scales, crusts, ulcers, excoriations, lichenifications, hyperpigmentations, and hyperkeratoses.
- Note evidence of external parasites. If fleas are not seen, search the patient for flea dirt, especially in the tail head region. A flea comb is often helpful in discovering small amounts of flea dirt. Repetitive combing may be necessary to find small amounts of flea dirt in the flea allergy dermatitis patient. Do this while talking to the owner regarding flea control.

See also Section 5.

Thorax

- As previously described, evaluate the respiratory rate, rhythm, and effort.
- Palpate the thorax for evidence of fractured ribs, congenital malformations (pectus excavatum), subcutaneous emphysema, and masses. Palpate the areas between the fourth and sixth intercostal spaces on either side of the thorax for the point of maximum intensity (PMI) of the heart beat and for cardiac thrills.
- Perform auscultation in a quiet room with a calm patient. Have the patient standing during the examination, so that the heart is in its normal position. Evaluate the heart independently from the lungs.
  - Disregard artifactual sounds. These include rumbles due to shivering and crackles from the stethoscope rubbing against the hair. Close the patient's mouth for short periods of time to reduce upper respiratory noise.
  - Auscultate the heart initially over the PMI and identify the first and second heart sounds. Characterize the cardiac rhythm. Sinus arrhythmias are typified by increases in cardiac rate during inspiration and decreases during expiration. Evaluate the femoral pulses for quality and deficits while auscultating the heart. Note split heart sounds, murmurs, and clicks. Auscultate all cardiac valve areas, because some murmurs are localized, such as the mitral, aortic, and pulmonic on the left hemithorax and the tricuspid on the right (see also Chapter 59).
  - Note muffled heart sounds that may be due to obesity, pleural effusion, pericardial effusion, thoracic mass, or diaphragmatic hernia.
  - Pulmonary auscultation requires practice and persistence. Normal bronchovesicular sounds may be increased, decreased, or normal. They may be intensified in the nervous or tachypneic patient. These sounds are heard equally on both sides of the chest. Abnormally quiet or dull areas are sug-

gestive of pleural effusion, pneumothorax, thoracic mass, and pulmonary consolidation. Crackles are abnormal discontinuous sounds resulting from popping open of small airways or air moving through airway secretions. Wheezes are abnormal continuous, musical sounds resulting from passage of air through narrowed or partially obstructed airways.

- Percussion is a technique for evaluating the resonance (pitch and tone) of sound produced by a series of quick taps of uniform force at various points on the chest wall using a finger or a percussion hammer. Increased resonance (tympany) is indicative of pneumothorax, and decreased resonance (dull sounding) suggests pleural effusion, diaphragmatic hernia, large pulmonary mass, or area of consolidation.

See also Chapter 59.

Abdomen

- Examine the external appearance of the abdomen for distention or asymmetry. If distention appears, perform percussion to determine if it is a result of peritoneal effusion, air (gastric dilatation or volvulus), obesity, or a mass.
- Palpate the abdomen systematically proceeding in a cranial-to-caudal direction with the animal standing. (Fig. 1–5). For small animals, use a one-handed technique. With larger patients, two hands are needed, one on each side of the abdomen. Gentle but steady pressure yields the best results.
- Palpate the cranial abdomen for evidence of gastric distention (see also Chap. 87). The normal stomach is rarely palpable. Tympany indicates gastric dilatation or volvulus, and diagnosis and treatment are pursued aggressively. Overeating may result in a doughy or fluid-filled stomach in the left middle region of the cranial abdomen.
- The liver may be difficult to palpate in the normal patient (see also Chap. 91). The caudal edges are barely palpable, smooth, and well defined. Hepatomegaly results in a liver that extends past the costal arch. The edges may be rounded rather than sharp. Palpation with the animal in lateral recumbency or standing on the hind legs may be helpful.
- The spleen is located in the mid-abdomen and may not always be palpable (see also Chap. 23). If splenomegaly is present, it is usually palpable. Determine if the spleen is irregular or if a palpable mass is present.
- Other organs in the mid-abdomen include the mesenteric lymph nodes and intestines. The mesenteric lymph nodes are not usually palpable unless markedly enlarged, as with lymphoma.
- Palpate the thickness of the bowel wall and the presence of gas, fluid, foreign bodies, or masses (see also Chap. 89). Plication and clumping of the intestines may be palpated in cats with a linear (string) intestinal foreign body.
- The kidneys can be palpated in the feline patient in the dorsal region of the abdomen. The right kidney

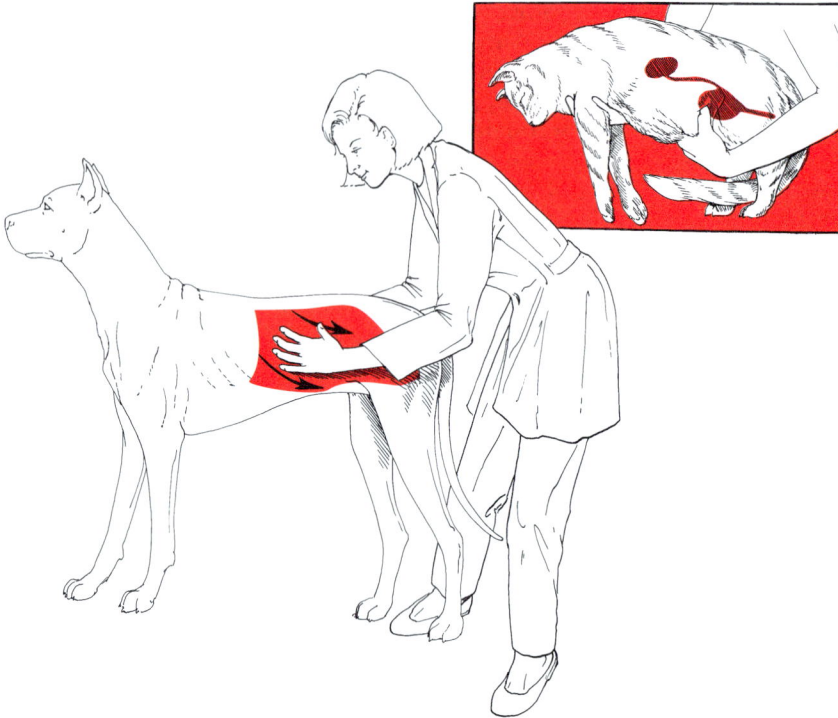

Figure 1–5. Perform abdominal palpation with two hands or with one hand (inset).

tends to be farther cranial than the left and may actually be obscured by the last ribs. Elevate the cat's thorax with one hand, while palpating with the other. This maneuver allows the kidneys to fall into a palpable position (Fig. 1–6). Palpate both kidneys and compare them for size, shape, firmness, and surface irregularities. The left kidney is especially movable. Do not mistake it for a mid-abdominal mass. The kidneys are not as readily palpable in the dog. Sometimes, the caudal poles or lateral aspect can be identified. Kidney palpation is also discussed in Chapter 97.

- Palpate the colon in the dorsal-caudal abdomen, and note the presence of feces. To determine if the palpable structure is feces or a mass, apply gentle pressure to test for deformability of the stool. Evaluate quantity and consistency of the feces to aid in the diagnosis of constipation.
- The urinary bladder can usually be palpated in the ventral caudal abdomen (see also Chap. 99). The patient does not usually resist palpation of the normal bladder. Assess size, turgidity, and thickness of the bladder wall. The normal urinary bladder is thin-walled. Careful palpation may reveal cystic calculi.
- The normal uterus usually cannot be palpated (see also Chap. 110). If it is markedly enlarged, because of pyometra or late pregnancy, the uterus is found in the mid-to-ventral abdomen, often extending from the pelvic inlet to the diaphragm. The uterus often is tubular in shape with pyometra or late pregnancy. In mid-gestation, the individual fetuses may be palpated.
- The prostate in intact male dogs can occasionally be palpated in the caudal abdomen ventral to the colon and caudal to the urinary bladder (see also Chap.

104). If found in this location, evaluate the prostate for size, shape, and surface irregularities.

External Genitalia

- In the female patient, palpate the mammary glands carefully for masses. If the history indicates a possibility of pseudopregnancy, gently express the nipples for signs of discharge or milk. In the nursing bitch or queen, examine the mammary glands for abnormal swelling, firmness, or heat, as seen with abscessed glands.
- In the female patient, examine the vulva for conformational abnormalities, swelling, or discharge. Determine the color, consistency, and odor of the dis-

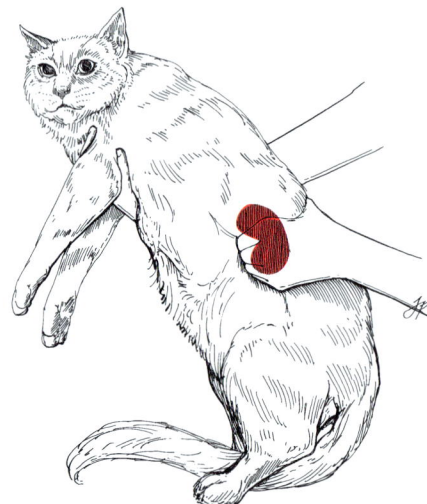

Figure 1–6. Renal palpation in the cat.

charge. Examine the vulvar mucous membranes for evidence of jaundice, cyanosis, petechiae, or ulceration. In dystocia, a vaginal examination is indicated.

- In the male canine, examine the prepuce and penis. Retract the preputial sheath caudal to the bulb so that the entire penis can be examined for any signs of trauma or masses. Inspect the penis for jaundice, cyanosis, petechiae, ulceration, or masses. Examine the tip of the feline penis for evidence of obstruction (discoloration or the presence of plug material), if so indicated by the history.
- In the male intact patient, palpate both testicles for symmetry, firmness, and irregularity. If both testicles are not present in the scrotum, examine the inguinal region for the presence of a retained testicle and palpate the abdomen for masses.

See also Section 8.

Rectal Examination

- Perform a rectal examination in all mature intact male dogs to evaluate the prostate. The normal prostate is bilobed (characterized by the presence of the median raphe), symmetric, smooth, and nonpainful. If the prostate is enlarged, it may extend slightly over the brim of the pelvis or fall into the abdomen, as previously described for the palpation of the caudal abdomen.
- In female dogs, abnormal masses associated with the uterus or urethra may sometimes be detected on rectal palpation.
- During a rectal examination, palpate the sublumbar lymph nodes in the dorsal aspect of the pelvic canal. Enlargement is usually suggestive of metastatic neoplasia.
- Note the symmetry of the pelvis for palpable fractures during the rectal examination. This is always indicated in a trauma victim. Evaluate abnormal masses in the pelvic canal for size, position, and consistency.
- During the rectal examination, observe the perineal and perianal regions for herniations or abnormal masses.
- Evaluate the anal sacs for evidence of distention or masses.
- Examine any fecal material obtained for consistency, color, and presence of blood or mucus.

Musculoskeletal System

- Initially evaluate the musculoskeletal system by observing for lameness with the patient in motion. Observe the patient's posture with special attention to head carriage, arching of the back, or stilted gait.
- A complete musculoskeletal examination is not necessary unless evidence of lameness or pain are noted in the history or on initial observation of the patient.
- If lameness is present, examine the affected limb systematically to attempt to localize the area involved. First, examine the foot for evidence of traumatized or abnormal toenails or nail beds. Evaluate each interdigital area for erythema, swelling, or draining tracts, which may be indicative of a foreign body. Palpate each toe individually and note swelling or pain.
- Palpation proceeds proximally. Evaluate each long bone for pain, swelling, abnormal masses, or palpable fractures.
- Evaluate each joint for evidence of effusion, soft tissue swelling, crepitation, or pain with flexion and extension.
- In examining the stifle, note the position of the patella in extension and flexion. If the patella is in its normal location, attempt to luxate it medially and laterally. Extension of the stifle usually aids in mobilizing the patella. Palpate the stifle for evidence of a cranial drawer sign (see Chap. 129).
- Evaluate each coxofemoral joint for a positive Ortolani sign, if the patient's breed is at risk for hip dysplasia (see Chap. 127 for more details).
- Palpate the vertebral column for signs of a pain response. Pressure applied to either side of the dorsal spinal process of each vertebra may be necessary to elicit pain (see Chap. 119, 147).

Nervous System

- As with the musculoskeletal system, a complete neurologic examination is not necessary unless specifically indicated by the history or the general physical examination. The details of the neurologic examination are discussed in Chapter 144. A brief overview of the basic procedures for localization of lesions is provided here.
- Observe mental status and behavior as previously described.
- Evaluate the gait and posture while the patient is walking and standing. Pay particular attention to strength, symmetry, and coordination.
- Always perform a complete cranial nerve examination when evaluating neurologic problems (see Chaps. 144 and 145).
- Evaluate and compare postural reactions in all limbs, including proprioception, "wheelbarrowing," hopping, extensor postural thrust, and placing reaction.
- Evaluate and compare spinal reflexes with the calm patient in lateral recumbency. Important segmental reflexes include the triceps, biceps, patellar, and cranial tibial reflexes, as well as the flexor (withdrawal) reflexes of the thoracic and pelvic limbs. Evaluate the panniculus reflex by needle stimulation of the thoracic or lumbar skin (see Chap. 144).

SUPPLEMENTAL READINGS

Bistner SI, Shaw D: Examination of the eye. Vet Clin North Am Small Anim Pract 11:595, 1981.

Crow SE, Walshaw SO: Restraint of dogs and cats. In Crow SE, Walshaw SO, eds.: Manual of Clinical Procedures in the Dog and Cat. Philadelphia: JB Lippincott, 1987, pp 3–14.

McCurnin DM, Poffenbarger EM: Small Animal Physical Diagnosis and Clinical Procedures. Philadelphia: WB Saunders, 1991.

Schaer M: The medical history, physical examination, and physical restraint. In Sherding RG, ed.: The Cat: Diseases and Clinical Management, 2nd Ed. New York: Churchill Livingstone, 1994, pp 7–23.

Practical Methods of Anesthesia

John A. E. Hubbell

Anesthesia is an integral part of the practice of companion animal medicine. In addition to surgical applications, some form of anesthesia may be required for a wide variety of procedures, such as radiography, endoscopy, cerebrospinal fluid collection, and bone marrow aspiration.

▼ **Key Point** The keys to successful anesthesia include (1) an understanding of what is "normal" in the various species; (2) a working knowledge of the pharmacology of anesthetic drugs; and (3) a systematic evaluation and reevaluation of the patient's status (monitoring) during the period of anesthesia.

The understanding of what is "normal" comes with experience. Several excellent texts describe the pharmacology of anesthetic drugs (see Supplemental Readings at the end of this chapter). Monitoring is a matter of establishing a routine and maintaining the discipline to adhere to the routine. This chapter suggests some basic anesthetic techniques and protocols that can be used in small animal practice.

GENERAL PRINCIPLES

Preoperative Assessment (Table 2–1)

- A history of vomiting or a recent meal is an indication for postponing surgery or using techniques that produce rapid induction allowing rapid endotracheal intubation which minimizes the potential for aspiration of gastric contents.
  - On an elective basis, withhold food 6–8 hours before the administration of anesthetic drugs.
  - Do not withhold water.
  - Potential problems that are discovered from the history include exercise intolerance or cough, as an indicator of cardiorespiratory dysfunction; polyuria or polydipsia, as an indicator of endocrine or renal dysfunction; or any other recent change in the animal's physical status.
- Perform a physical examination with emphasis on the cardiovascular and respiratory systems (Table 2–2 provides normal values).
  - Evaluate traumatized patients more extensively because of the potential for blood loss, cardiac arrhythmias (ventricular tachycardia), and thoracic trauma (pneumothorax).

- Evaluate abnormalities discovered after auscultation, percussion, palpation, and examination of mucous membranes with ancillary tests, such as thoracic radiography and electrocardiography.
  - The pertinent abnormalities associated with each metabolic disease are discussed with the disease syndrome.
- Weigh the animal. Estimate the lean body weight if the animal is obese to more accurately calculate correct anesthetic drug doses.
- Determine packed cell volume and total plasma protein to establish a baseline for reference if hemorrhage occurs. Check renal function with blood urea nitrogen (BUN) or creatinine concentrations in older (>7 years) animals. Increases in BUN or creatinine values may dictate a more careful perianesthetic fluid management to prevent further renal dysfunction (see Table 2–2).

Intravenous Catheterization

Place an intravenous (IV) catheter before induction of anesthesia to provide a convenient pathway for the administration of drugs, to allow for fluid or blood administration if required, and to ensure access to the vascular space if an emergency occurs.

Endotracheal Intubation

A patent airway is essential to any anesthetic protocol.

- Place a cuffed endotracheal tube in the trachea soon after induction of anesthesia.
- Alternatively, use drugs that maintain the swallowing reflex (ketamine, tiletamine/zolazepam).
- Clean, thoroughly rinse, and dry endotracheal tubes between uses. Sterilization of endotracheal tubes between uses is not necessary on a routine basis. Use chemical sterilization if a known pathogen is present. Glutaraldehyde is a safe disinfectant if the tubes are thoroughly rinsed following sterilization.
- See Table 2–3 for the range of sizes of endotracheal tubes for dogs and cats.

PRODUCING A TRACTABLE ANIMAL

Many procedures, such as radiography and cystocentesis, do not require complete anesthesia. In these instances, the combination of appropriate sedation and

Table 2–1. PREANESTHETIC CHECKLIST

History and Physical Examination

Age
Body weight
Temperature
Auscultation
Respiratory rate
Pulse rate, rhythm, and strength
Hydration, mucous membrane color, and capillary refill time
Mentation
Current medication history
Cardiopulmonary, renal, and nervous system disease history

Laboratory Data

Packed cell volume
Total plasma protein
Blood urea nitrogen, creatinine, or serum dipstick analysis (Azostick) if >7 yr
Other tests optional dependent on primary disease

Drugs

Appropriate anesthetic drugs
Sufficient oxygen supply
Emergency drugs
    Atropine or glycopyrrolate
    Lidocaine
    Epinephrine
    Sodium bicarbonate
    Intravenous fluids
    Dopamine
    Doxapram

Equipment

Syringes, needles, and catheters
Leak-tested anesthetic machine
Cuffed endotracheal tubes
Optional monitoring equipment
    Electrocardiogram
    Blood pressure monitor (pulse detector)
    Stethoscope
    Pulse oximeter

physical restraint can facilitate the completion of the procedure with minimal stress to the patient and minimal drug-induced cardiopulmonary depression. The choice of drugs is based on species, the patient's temperament, physical status, the veterinarian's familiarity with the drug, and the intended purpose. The agents that follow are employed as components of many anesthetic protocols.

The dosages of drugs alone and in combination are listed in Table 2–4 (dogs) and Table 2–5 (cats).

Tranquilizers

Acepromazine

- A potent phenothiazine tranquilizer that produces sedation in the dog. It also has antiemetic and antiarrhythmic properties.
- Not an analgesic itself, but it may potentiate other drugs that are analgesics.
- Produces hypotension through alpha-adrenergic blockade, particularly in large doses.
- Potentiates hypothermia.
- Epinephrine reversal (i.e., hypotension after epinephrine administration) can occur.
- Calms excitable dogs. Aggressive dogs or cats may not become tractable. Combine with opioids or cyclohexamines to produce the desired effect (see Tables 2–4 and 2–5).
- Avoid in animals with epilepsy, shock, bleeding disorders (inhibition of platelet function), or liver disease.
- Reduce the dose or choose another agent in stressed or older animals because effects may be exaggerated. Cats are calmed but usually still resist restraint.

Table 2–2. NORMAL VALUES

	Dogs		Cats	
	Awake	Anesthetized (If Different)	Awake	Anesthetized (If Different)
Temperature (°F)	99.5–102.5		100–102.5	
Heart rate (beats/min)	70–180	60–180	145–200	100–200
Respiratory rate (breaths/minute)	20–40	8–20	20–40	10–30
Capillary refill time (seconds)	<1.5		<1.5	
Packed cell volume (%)	35–54		27–46	
Total plasma protein (g/100 ml)	5.7–7.3		6.3–8.3	
Total leukocytes (6,000–17,000/μl)	6–18		6–20	
Albumin (g/100 ml)	2.1–3.6		2.3–3.6	
Sodium (mEq/L)	140–155		149–162	
Potassium (mEq/L)	3.8–5.3		3.6–5.4	
Chloride (mEq/L)	105–121		105–135	
Calcium (mg/100 ml)	8.8–11.3		8.3–11.3	
Creatinine (mg/100 ml)	0.3–1.3		0.8–1.8	
Blood urea nitrogen (mg/100 ml)	8–25		15–35	
Arterial pH	7.30–7.43		7.27–7.40	
Arterial pCO_2 (mm Hg)	30–49		35–49	
Arterial pO_2 (mm Hg)	91–97	90–500 (>50% inspired O_2)	91–97	100–500 (>50% inspired O_2)
Arterial HCO_3 (mEq/L)	18–22		18–25	
Arterial base excess (mEq/L)	−3–+3		−6–+1.5	
CO_2 combining power (mEq/L)	15–25		16–30	

Table 2–3. APPROXIMATE ENDOTRACHEAL TUBE SIZES

	Weight (kg)	Cuffed Tube Diameter (mm)
Dogs	3–7	3.0–5.0
	7–15	5.0–7.5
	15–30	7.5–9.5
	>30	9.5–12.0
Cats		2.5–4.0

Xylazine

- An alpha₂-adrenergic agonist that produces sedation with muscle relaxation and analgesia.
- Produces an obtunded state from which the patient is difficult to arouse.
- Produces analgesia for minor procedures. Is not usually sufficient for surgery.
- Produces profound cardiopulmonary depression, including bradycardia, first- and second-degree atrio-

Table 2–4. ANESTHETIC DRUGS AND DOSAGES IN DOGS

Drug	Intravenous Dosage (mg/kg)	Intramuscular or Subcutaneous Dosage (mg/kg)
Anticholinergics		
Atropine	0.02–0.04	0.02–0.04
Glycopyrrolate	0.005–0.01	0.005–0.01
Tranquilizer/Sedatives		
Acepromazine	0.05–0.2	0.1–0.3
Xylazine	0.3–0.8	0.5–1.5
Medetomidine	0.007–0.02	0.01–0.04
Diazepam	0.1–0.25	0.1–0.25
Midazolam	0.05–0.2	0.1–0.2
Analgesics		
Morphine	NR*	0.2–0.5
Oxymorphone	0.05–0.1	0.1–0.3
Fentanyl	0.002–0.005	0.004–0.008
Meperidine	0.4–2.0	1.0–4.0
Butorphanol	0.1–0.2	0.1–0.4
Nalbuphine	0.5–2.0	0.5–2.0
Buprenorphine	0.005	0.005
Anesthetics		
Tiletamine/ zolazepam (Telazol)	0.5–4.0	4–10
Thiopental	6–10	NR
Etomidate	1–4	NR
Propofol	2–6	NR
Combinations		
Acepromazine/ oxymorphone	0.05–0.1/0.01–0.02	0.1–0.2/0.1–0.2
Acepromazine/ butorphanol	0.05–0.1/0.1–0.2	0.1–0.2/0.1–0.2
Acepromazine/ ketamine	0.05–0.1/2–5	0.1–0.2/5–10
Xylazine/ketamine	0.1–0.8/1–5	0.3–1.5/5–10
Diazepam/ketamine (50:50)	1 ml/10 kg	NR

*NR, not recommended.

Table 2–5. ANESTHETIC DRUGS AND DOSAGES IN CATS

Drug	Intravenous Dosage (mg/kg)	Intramuscular or Subcutaneous Dosage (mg/kg)
Anticholinergics		
Atropine	0.02–0.04	0.02–0.04
Glycopyrrolate	0.005–0.01	0.005–0.01
Tranquilizer/Sedatives		
Acepromazine	0.05–0.2	0.1–0.3
Xylazine	0.4–1.0	0.8–1.8
Medetomidine	0.01–0.03	0.03–0.08
Diazepam	0.1–0.25	0.1–0.25
Midazolam	0.05–0.2	0.1–0.2
*Analgesics**		
Oxymorphone	0.01–0.04	0.05–0.1
Butorphanol	0.05–0.2	0.1–0.3
Nalbuphine	0.5–1.5	0.5–1.5
Buprenorphine	0.005	0.005
Anesthetics		
Ketamine	4–10	10–20
Tiletamine/ zolazepam (Telazol)	0.5–4.0	4–12
Thiopental	6–10	NR†
Etomidate	1.0–4.0	NR
Propofol	2–6	NR
Combinations		
Acepromazine/ oxymorphone	0.05–0.07/0.01–0.04	0.1–0.2/0.05–0.2
Acepromazine/ butorphanol	0.05–0.07/0.07–0.15	0.1–0.2/0.1–0.2
Acepromazine/ ketamine	0.05–0.1/4–8	0.1–0.2/7–15
Xylazine/ketamine	0.1–0.8/4–8	0.3–1.5/7–15
Diazepam/ketamine (50:50)	1 ml/10 kg	NR

*Higher doses can be associated with nervousness and excitement.
†NR, not recommended.

ventricular blockade, catecholamine sensitization, and decreased respiratory rate.
- Combine with an anticholinergic (atropine or glycopyrrolate).
- Do not use in patients with preexisting cardiac, liver, or kidney disease, or with shock.
- Reverse effects with yohimbine, tolazoline, or atipamezole (see Table 2–8 for dosages).
- Vomiting occurs in approximately 25% of dogs and 50% of cats.
- See Tables 2–4 and 2–5 for dosages.

Medetomidine

- An alpha₂-adrenergic agonist that produces sedation with muscle relaxation and analgesia.
- Similar to but approximately 100 times more potent than xylazine with a longer duration of action.
- Produces analgesia for minor procedures. Combine with ketamine or opioids to enhance analgesia.
- Produces dose dependent cardiopulmonary depression including bradycardia, decreased arterial blood pressure, and slowing of respiratory rate.

- Combine with an anticholinergic (atropine or gly-copyrrolate).
- Do not use in patients with preexisting cardiac or kidney disease or with shock.
- Reverse with yohimbine, tolazoline, or atipamezole.
- Vomiting, diuresis, and muscle jerking may occur.
- See Tables 2–4, 2–5, and 2–8 for dosages.

Diazepam and Midazolam

- Benzodiazepine derivatives that produce mild sedation in dogs and cats. Neither is effective in calming an excited patient when used alone. Both are anticonvulsants.
- Use to enhance tractability in depressed patients or in combination with other agents (primarily opioids).
- Administer diazepam intramuscularly (IM) or slowly IV with caution. The drug is solubilized in a propylene glycol base that can produce bradycardia and hypotension.
- Administer water-soluble midazolam via IV, subcutaneous (SC), or IM route.
- Use in patients with cardiorespiratory compromise or other metabolic disease. Both agents produce minimal cardiopulmonary side effects and provide muscle relaxation.
- Use both drugs as premedicants to parenteral or inhalation anesthesia.
- Occasionally, paradoxical responses occur, including disorientation and aggression.
- Diazepam can be given as an appetite stimulant in cats.
- See Tables 2–4 and 2–5 for dosages and suggested combinations.

Analgesic Drugs

Nonsteroidal Anti-Inflammatory Drugs (NSAIDs)

- Use NSAIDs for chronic pain associated with inflammation. They reduce pain by inhibiting prostaglandin formation.
- Potentiate the action of other analgesics.
- Use carprofen orally to provide analgesia, antipyresis, and as an anti-inflammatory. Oral dosage is 2 mg/kg q12h. Available as an injectable in other countries.
- NSAIDs can cause gastrointestinal injury and renal damage. Carprofen is the safest NSAID currently available.

Opioids

- Use in dogs and cats to augment the effects of sedatives and tranquilizers and to provide analgesia.
- Minimal or no sedation produced when administered alone, except for morphine and meperidine. Use in combination with tranquilizers or sedatives.
- Use lower dosages in cats compared with dogs (Tables 2–4 and 2–5), because higher dosages have the potential to cause excitement and disorientation.
- Morphine, oxymorphone, fentanyl, and meperidine are opioid agonist drugs frequently used in small animal practice. Regulations require rigorous record keeping and security.

Fentanyl

- Fentanyl can be administered transdermally using a patch developed for human use. Time from patch application until full effect is 2–6 hours in cats and 12–24 hours in dogs.
- The skin must be clipped (or shaved) to facilitate absorption, but absorption varies considerably. Duration of action may be as long as 5 days. Prevent ingestion by the animal or humans.

Other Opioids

- Butorphanol, nalbuphine, and buprenorphine are opioid agonist/antagonist or partial agonist drugs. This classification means that these compounds produce analgesia but have less addictive potential.
- Vagal tone is increased (bradycardia), and respiration is depressed.
- Sensations of touch or vision are not diminished. Sensitivity to sound may be increased.
- May cause vomiting and defecation.
- Reverse agonists and agonist/antagonists with naloxone. Partial reversal of the respiratory and central nervous system (CNS) depressant effects of agonists can be accomplished with agonist/antagonists (e.g., butorphanol), which reverse the deleterious effects of the agonists while providing the animal with some analgesia.

Dissociative Anesthetics
Ketamine and Tiletamine/Zolazepam

- Ketamine and tiletamine/zolazepam (Telazol, Ft. Dodge) produce a unique form of sedation/anesthesia that has been called dissociative anesthesia.
- These maintain swallowing and ocular reflexes, increase muscle tone, and produce amnesia, superficial analgesia, and catatonia.
- They stimulate the cardiovascular system resulting in increased heart rate and arterial blood pressure.
- They produce an apneustic (breath-holding) respiratory pattern. The intensity is dose related.
- Use low dosages of ketamine (up to 6 mg/kg IM) in the cat to produce an obtunded state with malleable rigidity of the limbs, dilated pupils, and hypersalivation. Use higher dosages (14–20 mg/kg IM) to intensify the effect so that surgery can be performed.
- Use Telazol to produce a state similar to that of ketamine with the addition of muscle relaxation. The drug is approved for IM use in both the dog and the cat. At low dosages (2–4 mg/kg IM) it provides helpful restraint in both the dog and cat. Higher doses can produce a state resembling general anesthesia but is associated with prolonged recovery that can be stormy, particularly in the dog.
- Use ketamine in combination with other agents (acepromazine, diazepam, xylazine) in both the dog and the cat. Do not give ketamine alone in the dog, because of resultant muscle rigidity and seizure activity. See Tables 2–4 and 2–5 for dosages.

Table 2–6. SUGGESTED ANESTHETIC PROTOCOLS FOR DOGS

Patient (Agent)	Dosage	Comments
Healthy (Elective Procedure)		
Acepromazine	0.02 mg/kg SQ or IM	Total dose not to exceed 4 mg
Thiopental	6–10 mg/kg IV	Give 6 mg/kg initially, increase in 2 mg/kg increments
Halothane* (or)	0.5–3.5%, inhaled	Adjust to anesthetic depth
Methoxyflurane*	0.3–3%, inhaled	Adjust to anesthetic depth
Aged Patient		
Intravenous fluids		
Diazepam/ketamine (or)	1 ml/10 kg (50:50) IV	Short duration of action
Propofol	2–4 mg/kg IV	
Halothane* (or)	0.5–3.5%, inhaled	
Methoxyflurane* (or)	0.3–3%, inhaled	
Isoflurane*	0.5–3.5%, inhaled	
Patient in Pain		
Intravenous fluids		
Acepromazine	0.01–0.02 mg/kg IM	Can be mixed with oxymorphone
Oxymorphone	0.05–0.02 mg/kg IM	Watch for bradycardia
Thiopental	4–8 mg/kg IV	Dose is reduced after premedicant. Start with 4 mg/kg
Halothane* (or)	0.5–3.5%, inhaled	
Methoxyflurane* (or)	0.3–3%, inhaled	
Isoflurane*	0.5–3.5%, inhaled	
Critical Patient		
Intravenous fluids		
Diazepam and	0.02 mg/kg IV	Give slowly
Propofol (or)	2–4 mg/kg IV	Give to effect
Diazepam/ketamine (50:50)	1 ml/10 kg IV	
Halothane* (or)	0.5–3.5%, inhaled	
Isoflurane*	0.5–3.5%, inhaled	

*Concentration required is dependent on fresh gas flow rate. The lower the flow rate, the higher the concentration required.

INJECTABLE DRUGS FOR SHORT-TERM ANESTHESIA

A variety of injectable drugs and drug combinations can be used for short-term anesthesia or restraint in dogs (Table 2–6) and cats (Table 2–7). Many of these combinations employ the drugs previously described. Earlier or coadministration of sedatives or tranquilizers with drugs that produce anesthesia allows a reduction in the dose of the anesthetic drug. Anesthetic drugs tend to produce more depression of cardiopulmonary function than do sedatives or tranquilizers, thus the patient benefits from the decreased dose. Thiobarbiturates are the primary addition to the list of drugs already discussed. Newer drugs, such as etomidate and propofol, offer potential advantages, such as fewer cardiopulmonary effects and lack of cumulative effects, but are expensive. Although endotracheal intubation is not required for the delivery of injectable anesthetic drugs, patients can benefit from intubation for protection of the airway and for oxygen supplementation.

Thiobarbiturates (Thiopental)

- Sedative/hypnotic agents that produce short-term IV anesthesia.
- Barbiturates produce CNS depression that ranges from drowsiness to coma.
- Not good analgesics at subhypnotic doses. When doses are increased to produce unconsciousness, anesthesia is produced.
- Cause respiratory depression and some arterial blood pressure depression.
- Sensitize the heart to catecholamine-induced arrhythmias. Ventricular bigeminy is noted but resolves without treatment.
- Duration of effect primarily determined by redistribution away from the brain into muscle and lean body tissues. Level and duration of anesthesia produced by a given dose is dependent on what other drugs have been administered, the rate administered, and the level of awareness of the animal at the time administered.
- Use with caution in patients with preexisting cardiovascular disease, hypotension, or shock.
- Administer to effect, beginning with dosages in the range of 4–6 mg/kg, increasing in 2 mg/kg increments. Onset of action is within 30 seconds.
- Do not mix with other drugs because of extreme alkalinity. Can cause sloughing of tissues if administered perivascularly.
- Use for induction to inhalation anesthesia. Compatible with all of the agents previously described. Reduce the dose by approximately half if sedatives/tranquilizers are given prior to administration.
- Duration of action is prolonged by hypoproteinemia and acidosis. Administer IV fluids to shorten dura-

Table 2–7. SUGGESTED ANESTHETIC PROTOCOLS FOR CATS

Patient (Agent)	Dosage	Comments
Healthy (Elective Procedure)		
Acepromazine (with)	0.01–0.02 mg/kg SC, IM	Mix acepromazine with ketamine
Ketamine (and)	4–8 mg/kg IM	
Thiopental (or)	5–10 mg/kg IV	Give to effect
Tiletamine/zolazepam (with)	3–5 mg/kg IM	Tiletamine/zolazepam may be sufficient for intubation
Thiopental	3–7 mg/kg IV	
Halothane* (or)	0.5–3.5%, inhaled	
Methoxyflurane*	0.3–3.5%, inhaled	
Aged or Renally Compromised Patient		
Intravenous fluids	0.05 mg/kg IM	
Midazolam (with)	0.1–0.2 mg/kg IM	Drugs can be mixed
Oxymorphone		
Ketamine (or)	1–2 mg/kg IV	
Thiopental (or)	3–7 mg/kg IV	
Propofol	2–4 mg/kg	Give slowly to effect
Halothane* (or)	0.5–3.5%, inhaled	
Isoflurane*	0.5–3.5%, inhaled	
Critical Patient		
Intravenous fluids		
Diazepam/ketamine (50:50)	0.5 ml/5 kg IV	Administer slowly
Halothane* (or)	0.5–3.0%, inhaled	
Isoflurane*	0.5–3.5%, inhaled	

*Use a nonrebreathing anesthetic system (Bain or Ayres T-piece).

tion by promoting diuresis and $NaHCO_3$ (2 mEq/kg) to shorten it by alkalinizing the urine.

Ketamine Mixtures

Use ketamine in combination with sedatives and tranquilizers to provide short-term injectable anesthesia.

Ketamine/Diazepam

- Administer ketamine with diazepam in a 50:50 volume/volume mixture at a dosage of 1 ml/10 kg IV. Give for brief periods (5–10 minutes) of restraint. Provides enough analgesia for minor surgical procedures. Readminister as needed to effect.
- Works well in depressed or geriatric patients. May not be effective in young, excited, or aggressive animals. Produces moderate muscle relaxation, cardiopulmonary support, and increased salivation. Ocular and swallowing reflexes are maintained, but orotracheal intubation can be accomplished.

Ketamine/Acepromazine

- Use ketamine with acepromazine to produce a quieter recovery than that with ketamine/diazepam but with less muscle relaxation. Usually produces enough anesthesia for minor surgery but visceral analgesia is not prominent.

Ketamine/Xylazine

- Use ketamine with xylazine to produce muscle relaxation, sedation, and analgesia that are improved over other combinations.
- Bradycardia and depression of cardiac contractility and respiration occur. Coadminister an anticholinergic. Use in young animals with good cardiopulmonary reserve. Avoid in animals with preexisting cardiovascular disease, particularly those with cardiac conduction abnormalities.

Tiletamine/Zolazepam

- Use IV or IM to produce anesthesia.
- Produces muscle relaxation and support of hemodynamics, but also produces respiratory depression.
- Maintains oropharyngeal reflexes. Recovery is prolonged with increasing doses. Recovery is usually uneventful in the cat but may be stormy in the dog.
- Administer low doses of acepromazine to quiet the difficult recovery.

Propofol

- A phenolic compound that produces hypnosis similar to thiopental.
- Depresses hemodynamics comparable to thiobarbiturates, but does not sensitize the myocardium to epinephrine-induced arrhythmias.
- Depresses respiration. Administer slowly IV over a 30–60 second period to minimize the potential for apnea.
- Use with analgesics for painful procedures. Anesthesia can be maintained using propofol as a continuous IV infusion (0.4–0.8 mg/kg/min).
- Noncumulative, so that recovery following multiple doses or an infusion occurs within the same time frame as that following a single dose.
- Available in 20-ml ampules (10 mg propofol/ml). Relatively insoluble. Formulated in a mixture of soybean oil, egg phosphatide, and glycerol without a preservative. Supports microbial growth if contaminated. Discard unused drug.
- Useful for induction of anesthesia in sight hounds and patients requiring cesarean section. Useful in compromised patients because of the lack of residual effects.

Etomidate

- A nonbarbiturate hypnotic that can be used for short-term IV anesthesia.
- Produces a hypnotic state with little cardiovascular effect.
- Etomidate is expensive. Limit to patients with significant cardiovascular and respiratory disease.
- Recovery can be stormy, with vomiting and muscle tremors. Premedicate the animal with sedatives or tranquilizers to minimize these effects.

Anticholinergics

- Used to reduce salivation, block vagal inhibition of the heart, and quiet the digestive tract if indicated.

- Not innocuous. Respiratory dead space is increased (bronchodilation). Ventricular arrhythmias are more likely to occur.
- Use if bradycardia occurs or is likely to occur.
- Not routinely indicated in anesthesia. Myocardial oxygen consumption is increased owing to tachycardia. Secretions become more viscous.
- Glycopyrrolate is more potent and has a longer duration of action than atropine. Does not cross the placental or blood-brain barrier.
- Give IM, SC, or IV when expediency is important. Atropine dose is 0.02–0.04 mg/kg. Glycopyrrolate dose is 0.01 mg/kg.

ANESTHESIA FOR MAJOR PROCEDURES

Anesthesia for major procedures, requiring optimal hypnosis, analgesia, and muscle relaxation for relatively long periods, usually incorporates the inhalant anesthetics. Although inhalant drugs can be given as the sole source of anesthesia, injectable drugs are usually given to facilitate induction and endotracheal intubation. The injectable drugs and drug combinations previously described, with the possible exception of xylazine/ketamine combinations, can be used to induce anesthesia. Xylazine/ketamine combinations produce significant cardiopulmonary depression that can be extreme when inhalant anesthetic drugs are added.

Inhalant Anesthetics

- Inhalant anesthetics have several advantages including the coadministration of oxygen, the ease with which anesthesia depth is changed, and the fact that recovery is not dependent on metabolism. The agents are primarily eliminated by exhalation. Administer via breathing circuits, with circle anesthetic systems being the most common.

Equipment

Circle Anesthetic Systems

- A carbon dioxide absorber removes carbon dioxide from the exhaled gas.
- Exhaled gas is rebreathed, making the system an economic one.
- Use 4–7 ml/kg/min as the minimum fresh gas flow rate for oxygen. This rate matches the animal's metabolic need for oxygen. Increase the fresh gas flow rate for oxygen to 10–20 ml/kg/minute if nitrous oxide is given. Add the nitrous oxide flow to the oxygen flow rate. The pop-off valve in the circle system needs to be open to vent the excess gas at this flow rate.

Nonrebreathing Anesthetic Systems (Bain and Ayres T-Piece) (Intertech, Ft Myers, Florida) (Surgivet, Waukesha, Wisconsin)

- Use for patients less than 3–5 kg, because less resistance to respiration is produced.
- Use a fresh gas flow of 1.5 times the minute ventilation (approximately 150 ml/kg/min). Fresh gas flow rates are higher because the fresh gas removes carbon dioxide from the system.

Scavenging Equipment

▼ *Key Point* Use of inhalation anesthetics mandates the removal of expired and waste gases from the operating room environment.

- Exhaust waste gases via suction systems or vent them to the outside via a hole in an exterior wall.
- Directing gases to the floor is insufficient.
- Use activated charcoal canisters as alternatives to absorb halogenated compounds. This is not effective for nitrous oxide.

Methoxyflurane

- Once the most commonly used inhalant agent in small animal practice.
- Most potent of the inhalation agents and least volatile.
- Induction and recovery can be prolonged owing to high blood solubility.
- Best muscle relaxant of the commonly used inhalation agents.
- Produces dose-dependent respiratory and cardiovascular depression.
- Administered using in-the-circle or out-of-the-circle vaporizers.
- Maximum attainable concentration at room temperature is approximately 3%.
- Use for long procedures in which muscle relaxation is important (orthopedics).
- Highly metabolized but the clinical relevance of this quality is questionable.
- Administer at concentrations of 3% for induction followed by maintenance at 0.3–1.5%.
- No longer used in humans because it is associated with postanesthetic renal failure. However, this has not been a problem in normal animals. Avoid, if possible, in animals with renal disease or those receiving nephrotoxic drugs.

Halothane

- A halogenated hydrocarbon that produces anesthesia when administered at concentrations of 0.5–3%, depending on the fresh gas flow rate.
- Induction and recovery are more rapid than with methoxyflurane. Can be used for mask or chamber induction of anesthesia.
- Use precision out-of-the-circle vaporizers. Can be administered using wickless in-the-circle vaporizers.
- Maximum attainable concentration at room temperature is approximately 30%.
- Produces dose-dependent cardiopulmonary depression with moderate degrees of muscle relaxation. Adequate ventilation is usually maintained. Potentiates ventricular arrhythmias in susceptible patients. Cardiac contractility and cardiac output are depressed.
- Termination of clinical effects is primarily due to redistribution and exhalation of the gas, which is metabolized by the liver.

- Incriminated in a syndrome characterized by hepatic failure in humans. Not proven to occur in animals.

Isoflurane

- Halogenated ether that produces anesthesia when inhaled in concentrations of 1.0–3.0%.
- Produces very rapid induction and recovery; relatively insoluble in blood.
- Vapor pressure similar to that of halothane.
- Use in precision out-of-the-circle vaporizers. Can be employed in wickless in-the-circle vaporizers.
- Better maintenance of cardiac output but produces respiratory depression similar to that for halothane. Arterial blood pressure is usually more depressed than that with halothane. Ventricular arrhythmias are not enhanced.
- Use in patients with metabolic disease, in geriatric patients, and in patients prone to cardiac arrhythmias. Expensive but provides significant advantages.
- Is minimally metabolized (<1%).

Nitrous Oxide

- A nonirritant gas that produces some analgesia when inhaled in concentrations of 50–70%.
- Cannot produce anesthesia when administered alone. Can reduce the required concentration of the other, more potent, gases (halothane, isoflurane) by approximately one-third when coadministered.
- Coadministration speeds the uptake of the second gas and thus speeds the induction to anesthesia.
- Recovery can be complicated by diffusion hypoxia. Oxygen should be supplemented for 3–5 minutes after cessation of nitrous oxide administration.
- Total fresh gas flow rate must be increased if nitrous oxide is given.
- Not employed widely in veterinary practice because of its limited potency and potential problems with hypoxia.

▼ *Key Point* Do not use nitrous oxide in patients with pneumothorax, gastric torsion, or intestinal obstruction because it will diffuse into closed gas spaces and enlarge them.

MONITORING THE ANESTHETIZED PATIENT

Monitoring is the cornerstone of safe anesthetic practice. Because irreversible CNS changes can occur within 4–5 minutes of cardiac arrest, a convenient monitoring interval of 5 minutes seems appropriate. The skills needed in basic monitoring of anesthetized patients parallel those needed in performing a physical examination.

Anesthetic Record

- Prompts the anesthetist to evaluate the patient at regular intervals. Serves as a legal document.
- Contains the following information, at minimum:
  - Summary of preoperative physical examination
  - Purpose of anesthesia

- Drugs administered including dose, route, and time
- Regular recording of heart or pulse rate and respiratory rate

Heart Rate

- Measured by auscultation using an esophageal (Malinckrodt) or precordial stethoscope.
- Palpate a peripheral pulse to determine heart rate and provide additional subjective information concerning the strength of cardiac contraction. Feel the pulse on the ventral side of the tongue (lingual pulse). Alternatively, use the femoral pulse if the animal's head is covered.
- Administer anticholinergics (atropine or glycopyrrolate) if the heart rate falls to less than 60 beats/min in dogs and 90 beats/min in cats.
- Evaluate the patient for hypotension or anesthetic plane that is too light if the heart rate is >150 in dogs or >180 in cats.
- Evaluate patients with irregular heart beats or heart beats of variable intensity with an electrocardiogram for abnormal cardiac rhythms.

Respiratory Rate

- Measure respiratory rate by watching the movements of the thoracic wall or the rebreathing bag of the anesthetic machine.
  - Most anesthetics are respiratory depressants.
  - Increases in rate or depth of respirations or panting usually indicate a plane of anesthesia that is too light.
  - Check the anesthetic depth in patients with irregular respirations; this can be a sign of excessive medullary depression. An apneustic pattern is expected after ketamine or tiletamine administration.

Capillary Refill Time and Mucous Membrane Color

- Gives further information on homeostasis.
- Capillary refill time should be <1.5–2 seconds.
- May be altered by the anesthetic agent chosen.

Other Monitoring Parameters

- Assess jaw tone to determine the degree of muscle relaxation present. This is an index of anesthetic depth.
  - Gently push the jaws apart and note the resistance to movement.
  - Halothane produces less muscle relaxation in an equivalent degree of anesthesia compared with other agents.
  - Dissociative agents do not produce muscle relaxation.
- Pinch a toe and look for a withdrawal response to check the depth of anesthesia prior to incision.

Monitoring Equipment

A wide variety of instruments are available to aid in monitoring patients.

Stethoscope

- Use esophageal stethoscopes (Mallinckrodt) to hear heart and respiratory sounds. Amplified stethoscopes are also available.

Electrocardiogram

- Use ECG to measure heart rate and to determine if cardiac arrhythmias are present.
- ECGs do not always ensure that the heart is beating or producing effective cardiac output.

Blood Pressure Monitors

- Use Doppler flow probes (Parks Electronics, Aloha, Oregon) to detect peripheral pulses. Place the probe over a peripheral artery. An audible signal is created, as pulses of blood pass under the probe and the sound waves emitted by the Doppler are altered. Place an occlusive cuff proximal to the Doppler probe to obtain an estimate of systolic arterial blood pressure. This monitor is reliable as a pulse detector but unreliable as an estimator of blood pressure.
- Oscillometric units (Dinamap; Criticon, Tampa Bay, Florida) can record heart rate and estimate systolic, mean, and diastolic blood pressures. The units inflate an occlusive cuff and slowly release pressure. Characteristic pressure fluctuations during deflation are used to estimate blood pressure. These monitors are expensive and tend to lose accuracy as blood pressure falls.
- Dorsal pedal artery can be catheterized with an over-the-needle catheter to directly measure arterial blood pressures. Connect an aneroid manometer to the catheter as a simple way to determine the mean arterial blood pressure. Use a pressure transducer to make more definitive measurements.

Pulse Oximetry

- Detects pulses and uses reflectance or absorbance of light to estimate hemoglobin saturation.
- Most units also display pulse rate.
- Values should be in excess of 90%.
- Probes are usually placed on the tongue.
- Reposition the probe periodically as needed to maintain signal.

Blood Gas Analysis

- More definitive monitoring of respiratory and metabolic integrity is accomplished by measuring arterial pH and blood gas values.

See Chapter 5 for the treatment of acid-base disorders.

RECOVERY AND POSTOPERATIVE COMPLICATIONS

Watch the patient after anesthesia until it can remain in sternal recumbency without being assisted.

Table 2–8. ANTAGONISTS USED TO REVERSE ANESTHESIA

Benzodiazepine (Diazepam, Midazolam, Lorazepam) Antagonists
Flumazenil   0.01–0.02 mg/kg IV

Alpha$_2$-Adrenergic (Xylazine, Medetomidine) Antagonists
Yohimbine   0.1–0.4 mg/kg IV
Tolazoline   0.5–2.0 mg/kg IV
Atipamezole   0.2–0.4 mg/kg IV

Narcotic Analgesic (Opioid) Antagonist
Naloxone   0.003–0.01 mg/kg IV IM

- If reversible drugs have been given, the administration of antagonists speeds recovery (Table 2–8). Do not administer an antagonist indiscriminately.
- Doxapram (1–5 mg/kg) is a nonspecific stimulant of respiration and the CNS. Doxapram can be given to effect arousal in an emergency, but it can also produce undesirable excitement.
- Animals recovering from isoflurane anesthesia may go through a period of emergence delirium. This period apparently results from a rapid return to consciousness with disorientation. The animal may or may not be in pain. Many animals respond to a reassuring voice and petting. Provide analgesia and/or sedation for animals that do not respond to these actions.
- Check the animal's temperature. Most animals lose body heat during anesthesia.
  - Some animals do not return to consciousness until body temperature is restored to 95°–97°F (35°–36.1°C).
  - Warm animals by placing them on recirculating, warm-water heating pads or by providing radiant heat from a lamp.
  - Take care to not burn the patient, particularly when heating lamps are used.
  - Oxygen utilization increases dramatically with shivering. Monitor the patient, and provide oxygen if necessary.
- Leave the endotracheal tube in place until the animal regains the oropharyngeal reflexes (i.e., begins to swallow). Give oxygen if necessary.
- Remove IV catheters, if no longer necessary, after the patient is rewarmed and conscious. Postoperative hypotension can occur, particularly if the patient does not rapidly return to consciousness.
- Monitor the patient periodically until it can stand unassisted.

SUPPLEMENTAL READINGS

Muir WW, Hubbell JAE, Skarda R: Handbook of Veterinary Anesthesia, 2nd Ed. St. Louis: CV Mosby, 1995.
Sawyer, DC: The Practice of Small Animal Anesthesia. Philadelphia: WB Saunders, 1982.
Short CE: Principles and Practice of Veterinary Anesthesia. Baltimore: Williams & Wilkins, 1987.
Thurmon JC, Tranquilli WJ, Benson GJ: Lumb and Jones' Veterinary Anesthesia, 3rd Ed. Baltimore: Williams & Wilkins, 1996.

3 Critical Care Techniques

M. Susan Crisp / C.A. Tony Buffington

This chapter describes commonly used techniques in emergency and critical care medicine. See appropriate chapters for information on the diseases that require critical care.

INTRAVENOUS CATHETERIZATION BY CUTDOWN

Indication

For intravenous (IV) administration of drugs and/or fluids in animals that cannot be catheterized percutaneously.

▼**Key Point** In an animal with cardiopulmonary arrest, rapidly proceed with cutdown procedure after one to two unsuccessful attempts at percutaneous placement.

Objective

To establish vascular access for the administration of fluids and drugs.

Equipment

- Minor surgical pack
  - Scalpel blade (#10) and handle
  - Mosquito forceps
  - Mayo scissors
- Intravenous catheter
  - Jelco (Pittman-Moore) or Angiocath (Becton, Dickinson & Co.) over-the-needle catheter (18–22 gauge)
- Silk or chromic catgut 3–0 or 4–0 suture

Technique

In an emergency situation, when time is critical (e.g., cardiac arrest; see Chap. 73), modify the sterile procedure described next by doing the following: use the jugular or cephalic vein; dispense with aseptic preparation—simply clip the area and swab with alcohol; secure the catheter with tape and leave the incision open; place a sterile intravenous catheter in another vein and remove the nonsterile catheter after successful cardiopulmonary resuscitation (CPR).

1. Use the jugular, cephalic, or lateral saphenous vein for catheterization.

2. Prepare the catheterization site for an aseptic procedure, including field drapes, cap, mask, and gloves.
3. Make a 2- to 4-cm skin incision parallel and slightly lateral to the vein to be catheterized.
4. Locate the vein and dissect it from surrounding tissues with mosquito forceps (Fig. 3–1A).
5. Place two stay sutures around the vein. Pass a double strand of suture underneath the vein and cut the looped end to result in two equal strands around the vein (Fig. 3–1B).
6. Insert the over-the-needle catheter into the vein while stabilizing the vessel with the stay sutures.
7. Tie the stay sutures around the catheterized vein (Fig. 3–1C). Tie one suture just below the catheter hub; tie the other suture more proximally. Connect the catheter to a syringe or fluid-administration set.
8. Close the skin incision in a routine fashion.
9. Place an antiseptic ointment and a sterile bandage over the catheterization site.
10. Change the catheter after 3 days to help prevent thrombophlebitis and infection.

CENTRAL VENOUS PRESSURE MEASUREMENT

Indications

- For determination of increased venous pressure associated with right-sided heart dysfunction or pericardial disease.
- For monitoring of fluid therapy in animals in hypovolemic shock (see Chap. 72).
- For monitoring of poor-risk surgical patients during anesthesia and surgery.

Objectives

- Central venous pressure (CVP) in dogs and cats is normally 0 to 5 cm H_2O. The rate of fluid administration can be adjusted to maintain the normal CVP.
- The trend of the CVP changes is more valuable than the absolute measurements. Adjust the treatment (IV fluid administration) based on the changes in the CVP values.

Equipment

- Jugular catheter (I-Cath, Delmed, Inc.; 18.5 or 22 gauge; 8- or 12-inch length)

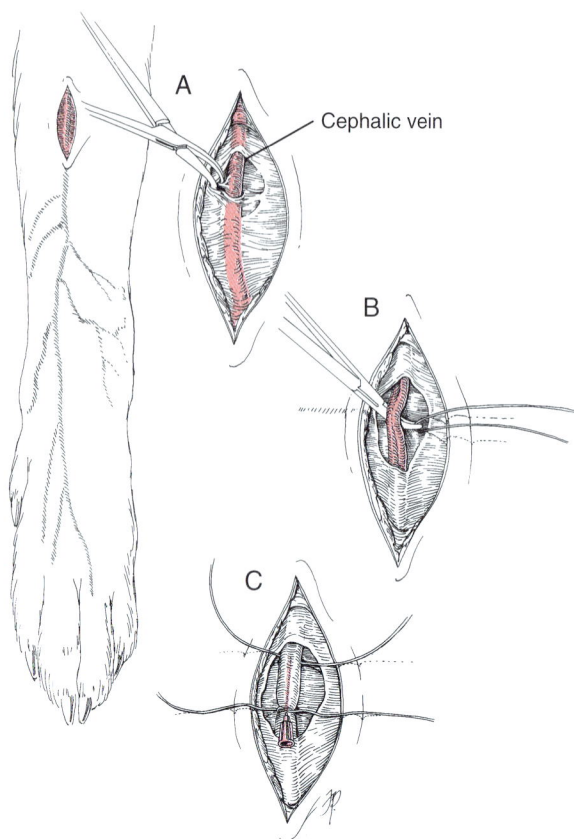

Figure 3–1. Intravenous catheterization by cutdown. *A*, Dissection of cephalic vein; *B*, threading for two stay sutures; *C*, catheter placement relative to stay sutures.

- Water manometer (Central Venous Pressure Monitor, American Pharmaseal Co.)
- Three-way stopcock
- Intravenous extension set
- Sterile isotonic fluid

Technique

1. Aseptically prepare the right or left jugular vein area for catheterization.
2. Place the IV catheter. The tip of the catheter is advanced to about the second intercostal space—just proximal to the right atrium. Secure the catheter to the neck and cover with a sterile, padded bandage.
3. Place an extension set on the catheter and connect to a stopcock. Connect the manometer to the stopcock and connect the fluid bag to the stopcock using a fluid administration set (Fig. 3–2). Do not allow air bubbles into the system.
4. Place the manometer so that the 0 level is approximately at the level of the right atrium (sternal recumbency—level of thoracic inlet; lateral recumbency—level of sternum).
5. Flush the IV line to remove any obstructions. Turn the stopcock so that it is closed to the patient and open from the IV fluid bag to the manometer. Fill the manometer to greater than 15 cm H_2O (Fig. 3–3A).

6. Turn the stopcock so that it is closed to the IV fluid administration set and open from the manometer to the patient (Fig. 3–3B).
7. Allow the fluid level in the manometer to equilibrate with the right atrium; read the resultant value from the meniscus of the column of fluid.
8. Adjust the stopcock to open the fluid line between the fluid bag and the IV catheter (closed to the manometer) (Fig. 3–3C) to allow fluid to flow to the patient.

TEMPORARY TRACHEOSTOMY

Indications

- For upper airway obstruction (e.g., acute laryngeal edema, brachycephalic syndrome, laryngeal paralysis, and pharyngeal or laryngeal foreign body or neoplasia).
- For facilitation of artificial respiration in animals exhibiting hypoventilation.
- For insurance of a patent airway either before or after major surgery of the upper airways.

Objectives

- To establish a patent airway.
- To maintain patency of the airway by frequent cleaning or replacement of the tracheostomy tube.

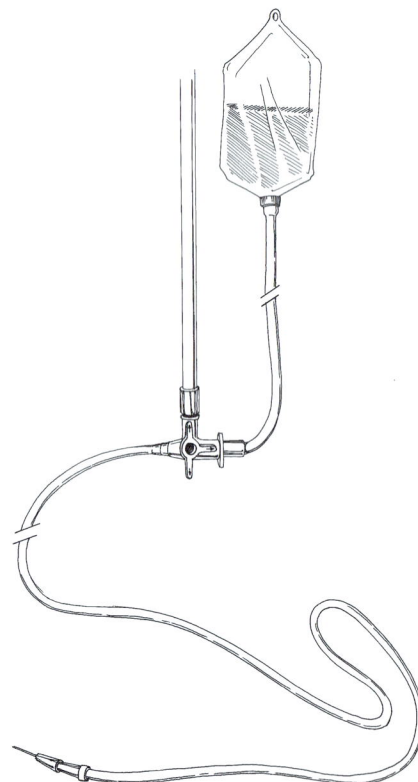

Figure 3–2. Manometer, stopcock, and catheter for central venous pressure measurement.

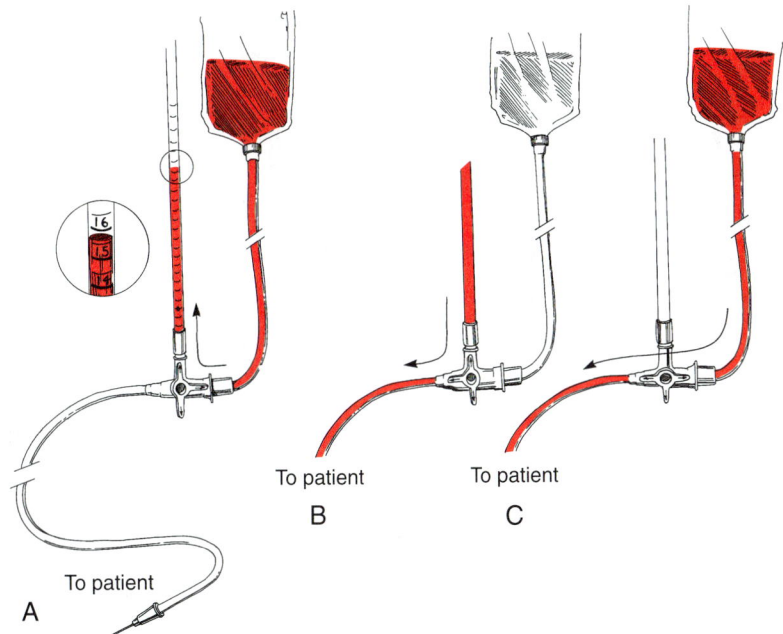

Figure 3–3. Central venous pressure measurement. See text for details.

Equipment

- Minor surgical pack (see IV cutdown procedure)
- Shiley (Shiley, Inc.) or Portex (Portex, Inc.) tracheostomy tubes (Fig. 3–4)
- Suture
  - 3–0 or 4–0 polypropylene or nylon (Prolene or Ethilon; Ethicon)
  - 3–0 absorbable (Vicryl; polydioxanone suture [PDS]; Ethicon)
- Umbilical tape

Technique

1. Place the animal in dorsal recumbency with the head extended and a rolled towel or sandbag under the neck.
2. Prepare the ventral cervical area for aseptic

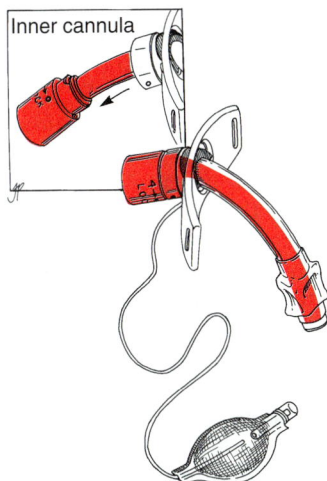

Figure 3–4. Shiley tracheostomy tube showing replaceable inner cannula.

surgery. If this is an emergency situation, simply clip the hair and swab with alcohol.
3. Make a 6- to 8-cm skin incision in the ventral cervical midline from the caudal aspect of the larynx caudally.
4. Expose the sternohyoid and sternothyroid muscles.

▼ *Key Point* Divide the muscles precisely on the midline to prevent excessive hemorrhage and poor exposure.

5. Make a transverse incision in the annular ligament between the third and fourth tracheal rings or caudal to the obstruction. Incise one half to two thirds of the circumference of the trachea. Avoid trauma to the recurrent laryngeal nerves. Place nonabsorbable stay sutures on the third and fourth tracheal rings to allow separation of the rings. Leave long tags on the stay sutures (Fig. 3–5A).
6. Place the tracheostomy tube through the incision and pass caudally. Do not use too large a tube because improper fit can produce pressure necrosis of the dorsal and/or ventral tracheal mucosa (Fig. 3–5B).
7. Secure the tracheostomy tube, passing umbilical tape around the animal's neck. Close the muscle layer with 3–0 Vicryl or PDS in a simple continuous pattern. Close the subcutaneous layer in the same fashion as for the muscle; close the skin up to the level of the tube in a routine fashion.
8. Do not bandage the tracheostomy tube because this interferes with the replacement of the tube when it becomes obstructed with mucus.

Postoperative Care and Complications

- Check the tube for patency every 1 to 2 hours or more frequently, if necessary.

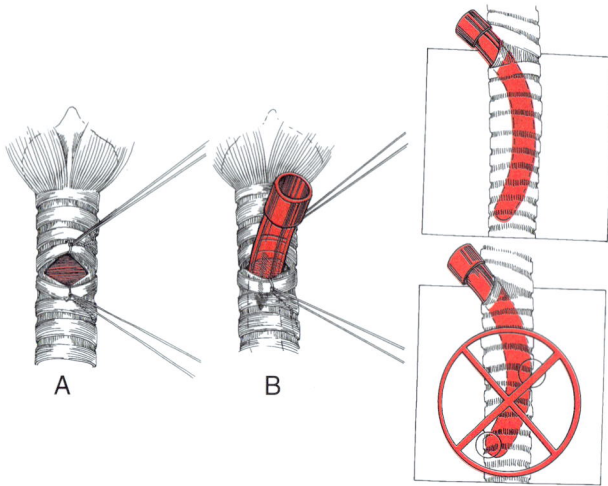

Figure 3–5. Placement of tracheostomy tube. *A,* Stay sutures retract tracheal rings; *B,* tube should slip easily through the incision. Note that a tube that is too large can cause pressure necrosis of the tracheal mucosa.

- Clean the tube every 2 hours or more frequently, if necessary. When a double-lumen tube (Shiley) is used, remove the inner cannula, clean off mucus with hydrogen peroxide, and rinse with distilled water or sterile saline. Disinfect the cannula by soaking in chlorhexidine (Nolvasan) solution for 5 minutes. Rinse again with sterile saline and replace inside the outer cannula.
- If a single-lumen tracheostomy tube is in place, change the tube at least every 2 hours. One tube is kept in cold sterilization (Nolvasan); the other tube is kept in the patient. At the time of tube change, prepare the replacement tube by rinsing with sterile saline to *completely* remove all disinfectant. Remove the soiled tracheostomy tube from the patient. By using the tracheal ring stay sutures, open the tracheal stoma and insert the clean tube. Clean the soiled tube with hydrogen peroxide, rinse with distilled water, and place it in cold sterilization until the next tube change.
- Do not apply active suction to the tracheostomy tube unless necessary. Suctioning shortly after eating can induce vomiting.
- Acetylcysteine (a mucolytic agent) is contraindicated because it is irritating to the tracheal mucosa.
- Keep the animal well hydrated to decrease the viscosity of secretions. Humidify inspired air, if possible.
- Monitor the animal for subcutaneous emphysema by palpating the head, neck, and body. Monitor the ventral neck area for evidence of irritation due to serum discharge. Apply petrolatum (Vaseline) to the area, if necessary.
- After removal, temporarily cover the tracheal stoma to ensure that the animal will be able to ventilate adequately without the tube. Allow the incision to heal as an open wound. Lightly bandage the wound, if necessary, to prevent self-trauma.

OXYGEN THERAPY VIA NASAL CATHETER

Indications

- For severe, acute respiratory or cardiovascular failure (dysfunction) causing hypoxia and hypoxemia.
- For ventilation-perfusion mismatches (e.g., pneumonia, pneumothorax, and airway obstruction).
- For supportive care for animals in shock.
- For any disease causing hypoxemia (PaO_2 < 70 mm Hg) with normal packed cell volume (PCV); or PaO_2 < 80 mm Hg with PCV < 20%.
- Hypoventilation is *not* an indication for nasal oxygen. Animals with poor ventilation require tracheal intubation and positive pressure ventilation.

Objectives

- To elevate arterial oxygen by increasing the inspired concentration of oxygen.
- To provide a nasal catheter that is effective yet comfortable for the patient.

Equipment

- Nasal catheter: 5- to 8-Fr. infant feeding tube (Davol) or 5- to 8-Fr. red rubber feeding tube and urethral catheter (Sovereign)
- Monofilament 2-0 or 3-0 nylon suture
- Adhesive tape
- Lidocaine (2%) or proparacaine (Alcaine, Alcon) 0.5%
- Sterile lubricant (K-Y jelly)
- Elizabethan collar (optional)

Technique

1. With the animal's nose pointing upward, instill 1 ml of lidocaine (dogs) or 5 drops of proparacaine (cats) into one nostril. Repeat after 1 minute.
2. Measure the tube from the external nares to carnassial tooth.
3. Lubricate the catheter tip with sterile lubricant (K-Y jelly).
4. Insert the catheter into the ventral nasal meatus to the level of the carnassial tooth. Direct the tube caudomedially ventral to the alar fold. As the nasal planum is pressed upward (Fig. 3–6*A*), direct the tube ventrally and caudally to allow entry into the ventral nasal meatus.
5. Apply tape to the catheter, in butterfly fashion, and suture to the skin immediately adjacent to the alar fold (Fig. 3–6*B*).
6. Position the tube between the animal's eyes and secure it to the top of the head in a similar fashion (see Fig. 3–6*B*).
7. Connect extension tubing to the nasal catheter. Humidify the oxygen through a bubble humidifier (Chemetron Medical Products) attached to an oxygen wall outlet or, if oxygen is not available through a wall outlet, construct a humidifier. Attach an IV administration set to the extension set (on the nasal catheter). Place the opposite end in

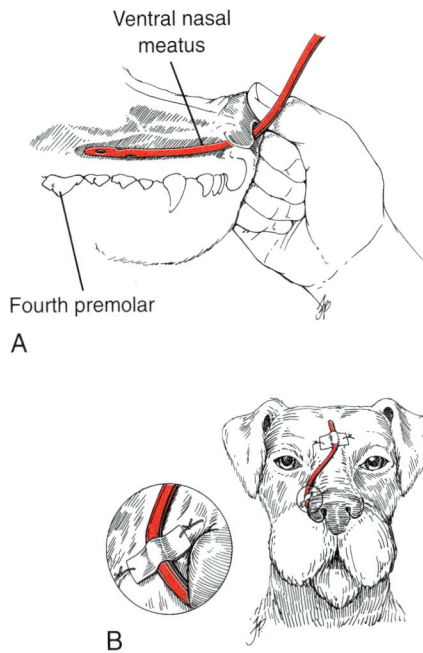

Figure 3–6. *A*, Placement of nasal catheter; *B*, method of securing the nasal catheter.

a fluid administration bottle that is half filled with sterile saline or water. Attach an oxygen line to the vent hole in the lid of the bottle, and bubble oxygen through the liquid.

8. Administer oxygen at a flow rate of 50 to 100 ml/min/kg to maintain tracheal concentrations of greater than or equal to 40%.

Postoperative Care and Complications

- Prevent dislodgement of the tube by placing an Elizabethan collar, if necessary.
- Nasal hemorrhage may occur if the catheter is placed improperly.
- Gagging may occur if the catheter is placed too far caudally.
- Gastric distension can occur if the flow rate is too high or if the catheter is placed too far caudally.

THORACOCENTESIS

Indications

- For pneumothorax, if causing a clinical problem
- For hydrothorax

Objectives

- To evacuate fluid or air from the pleural space
- To avoid iatrogenic pneumothorax or trauma to the lungs, heart, and intercostal blood vessels

Equipment

- Sterile butterfly needle (19–22 gauge) for small or thin animals; over-the-needle catheter (20–22 gauge) for large or obese animals

- Intravenous extension set
- Three-way stopcock
- Syringe

Technique

1. The animal is either standing or in sternal recumbency.
2. Clip and aseptically prepare the appropriate site on the thoracic wall.
3. Generally, perform the thoracocentesis between the seventh and ninth intercostal spaces. Based on radiographic evaluation, it sometimes may be necessary to enter the thorax at a different space.
4. To avoid the intercostal vessels and nerve, which lie along the caudal border of each rib, place the needle just cranial to the rib.
5. To evacuate pleural air, perform the thoracocentesis in the dorsal half of the thorax; to evacuate pleural fluid, perform the thoracocentesis in the ventral half of the thorax.
6. Connect the tubing of the butterfly needle to the stopcock or connect the catheter to the extension set and place the stopcock at the end of the extension set. Turn off the stopcock toward the patient.
7. Carefully place the needle into the pleural space. A slight "pop" usually can be felt when the pleura is entered. When the needle is into the thorax, angle the needle so that the point is facing slightly cranially or caudally and not aiming directly at the lung. A friction rub will be felt with each inspiration if the needle is touching the lung.
8. Connect a syringe to the stopcock. Open the stopcock from the patient to the syringe. Apply gentle negative pressure (3 to 5 ml) to evacuate the thorax.
9. If no air or fluid is obtained, redirect the needle or tap one or two alternative areas.

CHEST TUBE PLACEMENT

Indications

- For persistent pneumothorax or hydrothorax requiring repeated thoracocentesis
- For more complete evacuation of the thorax than that possible with thoracocentesis
- For tension pneumothorax
- For postoperative thoracotomy (see Chap. 83)
- For administration of intrathoracic medications

Objectives

- To aseptically place an indwelling thoracic drain tube without causing iatrogenic trauma to thoracic viscera
- To minimize iatrogenic pneumothorax
- To place the tube such that it effectively drains the pleural fluid or air

Equipment

- Chest tubes
  - Argyle trocar catheter (Sherwood)

- Red rubber feeding tube and urethral catheter (Sovereign)
- Minor surgical pack plus Kelly or Carmalt hemostatic forceps
- Three-way stopcock and Pharmaseal plastic tubing connector (Baxter)
- Monofilament nylon 2-0 or 3-0 suture
- Bandage material
- Antiseptic ointment

Technique

1. Provide local or general anesthesia depending on the patient's status and compliance. If local anesthesia (2% lidocaine) is used, infiltrate the area of the skin incision and the chest wall at the point of tube entry including the parietal pleura.
2. Place the animal in lateral or sternal recumbency.
3. Clip and aseptically prepare the lateral thoracic wall from the 5th to the 12th ribs.
4. Select an appropriately sized chest tube, i.e., approximately the diameter of a main stem bronchus.
5. Measure and mark the chest tube from the skin incision (10th intercostal space) to the point of the ipsilateral elbow.
6. Cut additional holes in the chest tube and be certain that the last hole is within the thoracic cavity.
7. Make a stab incision in the skin over the 10th in-

tercostal space in the dorsal third of the thorax and insert the tube through the incision into the subcutis (Fig. 3–7A).
8. Advance the tube subcutaneously in a cranioventral direction and enter the thoracic cavity at the seventh or eighth intercostal space, at the level of the junction between the dorsal third and middle third of the thorax (Fig. 3–7B).
9. Avoid the caudal border of the rib to prevent the possibility of trauma to the intercostal vessels and nerve.
10. To enter the thoracic cavity, grasp the trocar chest tube firmly in one hand so that the hand acts as a guard to prevent the trocar from penetrating too deeply into the chest cavity. Hold the chest tube perpendicular to the thoracic wall and firmly "smack" the tube through the thoracic wall with the other hand (Fig. 3–7C).
11. Once the tube is through the thoracic wall, place the tube parallel to the chest wall. While holding the trocar, advance the chest tube into the thoracic cavity to the premeasured point. Direct the tube ventrally to evacuate fluid and dorsally to evacuate air (Fig. 3–7D).
12. Quickly remove the trocar and clamp the tube to limit the development of pneumothorax.
13. Place one or two cerclage sutures around the tube in the subcutaneous tunnel.
14. Place a pursestring suture around the tube at the skin incision site.

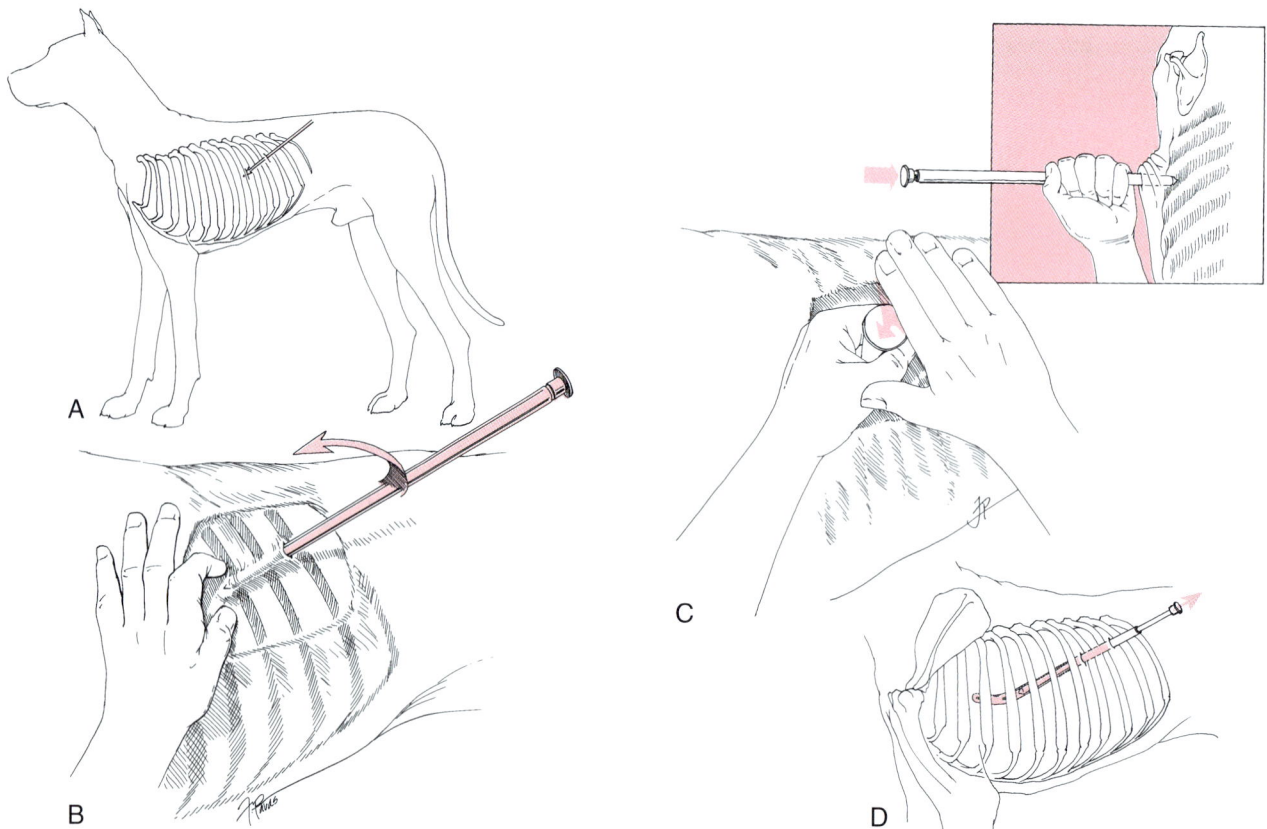

Figure 3–7. Chest tube placement. *A,* General view of direction and angle of chest tube placement; *B,* subcutaneous advancement of the tube to the entrance into thoracic wall; *C,* entering thoracic cavity; *D,* removing trocar once tube is in place.

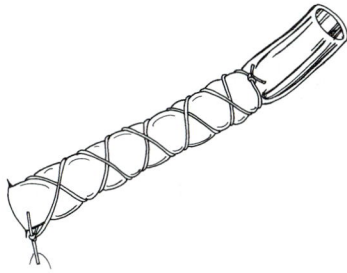

Figure 3–8.   Chinese finger trap suture.

15. Secure the tube with a Chinese finger trap suture. Place an anchoring suture through the skin adjacent to the tube's exit. Tie a square knot and leave long suture tags. Place a surgeon's throw over the top of the tube and pull snugly enough to slightly indent the tube. Cross the suture material underneath the tube, and place another surgeon's throw over the top of the tube as before. Continue this pattern 5 to 10 times and end with a square knot on top of the tube (Fig. 3–8).

16. Place a Pharmaseal plastic tubing connector into the flared end of the chest tube. Cut the flared end from a red rubber feeding tube, and place it over the other end of the tubing connector. Attach a stopcock to the narrow end of the cut red rubber feeding tube. Place ligatures around all connections from the chest tube to the stopcock (Fig. 3–9).

17. Place antiseptic ointment and a 4 × 4-gauze over the tube exit site.

18. Wrap the thoracic wall with Kling and Vet-Wrap and place the bandage material around one or both front legs to prevent bandage slippage. Apply a small amount of Elasticon at the cranial edge of the bandage for adherence to the haircoat.

19. Apply gentle suction (3–5 ml pressure) or attach the chest tube apparatus to a continuous suction unit (Pleur-Evac, Deknatel, Pfizer Inc.).

20. If a trocar catheter is unavailable, a red rubber feeding tube can be used for thoracic drainage. The tip of the catheter is grasped in the tip of Kelly or Carmalt forceps and advanced through the subcutaneous tissue as previously described. The technique for placement into the thoracic cavity is the same as that for the trocar catheter.

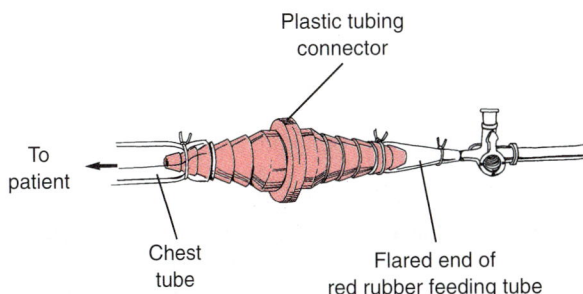

Figure 3–9.   Pharmaseal plastic tubing connector and attachment to chest tube.

Once the thoracic wall is penetrated, spread the tips of the forceps to allow passage of the tube into the thoracic cavity. The remainder of the technique is the same as that for the trocar catheter.

Postoperative Care and Complications

▼ *Key Point* Animals with indwelling chest tubes require constant supervision. Damage to the tube can cause life-threatening tension pneumothorax.

- Use an Elizabethan collar on the animal, if necessary, to prevent damage to the tube.
- Change the bandage every other day or more often if necessary. Check the position of the tube during bandage changes. Radiograph the thorax, if necessary, to check tube position in the pleural space.
- The chest tube itself can create pleural effusion. Pleural effusion ≤ 1 to 2 ml/kg/24 hours can be attributed to the presence of the chest tube. When the effusion has decreased to this volume, remove the chest tube.
  - Remove the sutures and pull the chest tube from the thorax smoothly and quickly. The tip of the tube can be cultured, if necessary.
  - Apply antiseptic ointment and a light bandage to the skin incision.

ABDOMINOCENTESIS

Indications

- For determination of organ damage associated with abdominal trauma
- For evaluation of any disease causing the development of peritoneal fluid

Objectives

- To aseptically obtain fluid from the abdominal cavity for analysis and/or culture
- To avoid causing trauma to any of the abdominal viscera

Equipment

- Butterfly needle (19–22 gauge) or needle and IV extension set
- 12-cc syringe

Technique

1. The animal can be standing or in lateral recumbency.
2. Aseptically prepare a small area (approximately 6 cm^2) in each of the four abdominal quadrants.
3. Slowly insert the needle into the abdominal cavity until it is felt to enter the peritoneal cavity.
4. Let the fluid drain by gravity flow or connect the syringe to the butterfly needle and gently aspirate. Do not drain all the fluid out of the abdomen if it is ascitic.

5. Place fluid in ethylenediaminetetra-acetic acid (EDTA) and clot tubes for analysis. Save some fluid for Gram staining and bacterial culture.

DIAGNOSTIC PERITONEAL LAVAGE

Indications

- For early detection of organ damage in an animal with an acute abdomen, when abdominocentesis results are negative.

Objectives

- To obtain fluid or debris from the abdomen
- To avoid causing trauma to the abdominal viscera

Equipment

- Local anesthetic (2% lidocaine)
- Scalpel blade (#15) and handle
- Peritoneal dialysis catheter (Travenol Laboratories)
- Intravenous extension set
- 500 ml of sterile saline
- 12-cc syringe

Technique

1. Place the animal in dorsal recumbency.
2. Empty the urinary bladder.
3. Aseptically prepare the abdomen (a 6-cm² area caudal to the umbilicus).
4. Infiltrate the subcutaneous tissue, rectus fascia, and peritoneum with 2% lidocaine.
5. Make a stab incision with the scalpel 1 to 2 cm caudal to the umbilicus—through the skin, subcutaneous tissue, and fascia down to the level of the linea alba.
6. Aim the catheter in a dorsocaudal direction. With one hand, grasp the catheter and stylet to guard against penetrating too deeply into the abdomen (see Fig. 3–7C on chest tube placement). Use a controlled push to advance the catheter and stylet through the linea alba. Once the peritoneal cavity has been entered, hold the stylet and advance the catheter off the stylet to the dorsal lumbar region. Be sure all fenestrations are within the abdominal cavity. If a celiotomy scar is present, enter the abdomen off the midline. The abdominal organs may have adhesions with the scar.
7. Infuse 20 ml/kg of sterile saline into the peritoneal cavity through the catheter.
8. Plug the catheter and gently roll the dog or cat from side to side.
9. Aspirate the fluid from the abdomen through the catheter and save a sample for analysis.
10. Fluid analysis.
    - PCV > 2% or RBC count ≥ 200,000 mm³ indicates significant hemorrhage—PCV > 1% but <2% is equivocal, and PCV < 1% is insignificant.
    - The normal neutrophil count is <500/mm³. The neutrophil count after uncomplicated abdominal surgery can be 750 to 1500/mm³ but may be higher if peripheral leukocytosis exists. Leukocyte response requires 2 to 4 hours for intraperitoneal accumulation after irritation or sepsis.
    - Biochemical tests can be performed to check for the presence of urea, creatinine, bilirubin, amylase, or lipase. The Azostick (for urea) and Ictotest (for bilirubin) (Ames Laboratories) can be employed as rapid tests.
    - Examine the fluid microscopically for the presence of bacteria or vegetable material.
    - Submit an aliquot of the lavage fluid for bacterial culture and sensitivity testing.
11. If the results are equivocal, the catheter can be sutured in place. Lavage and aspiration can be repeated several hours later.
12. After the catheter is removed, close the incision routinely.

▼*Key Point* This procedure is contraindicated in patients with ileus or a gravid uterus.

NUTRITIONAL MANAGEMENT OF THE CRITICAL CARE PATIENT

Animals require water, energy, proteins, minerals, and vitamins for normal body metabolism. If these are not ingested by the animal, they must be provided by the animal's own body tissue. Nutritional support via enteral or parenteral feeding can prevent this "autodigestion" and its subsequent complications, which include impaired immunity, muscular weakness, decreased wound strength, decreased resistance to infection, and death.

Indications for Nutritional Support: Patient Selection

History

- Recent weight loss
- Decreased food intake
- Increased nutrient needs—recent trauma or surgery, burns, fever
- Increased losses—vomiting, diarrhea, burns
- Homemade diet that may be nutritionally incomplete or imbalanced.

Physical Examination

- Underweight
  - Loss of subcutaneous fat
  - Muscle wasting
  - Hair that is easily plucked.
- Overweight
  - Edema
  - "Overcoat syndrome," which is a disproportionate loss of lean body tissue that leaves an overcoat of fat, giving the impression of a better body condition than what actually exists.
- Inability to eat

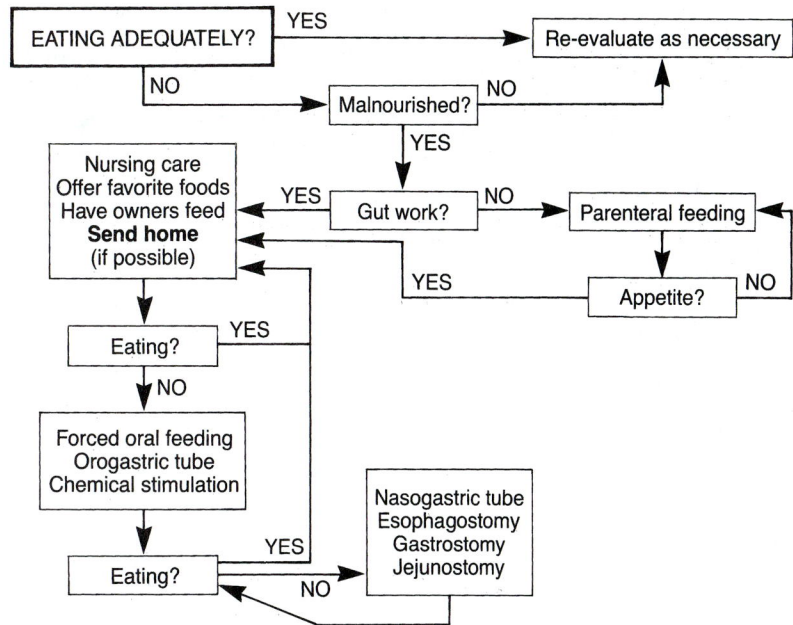

Figure 3–10. Route selection for nutritional support.

Absence of Indication for Starvation

- There are no indications for starvation.

Route Selection

See Figure 3–10.

What to Feed: Categories of Enteral Diets

See Table 3–1 for sources of dietary products and nutritional devices. Polymeric or intact macronutrients (protein, fat, carbohydrate, caloric density ~1 kcal/ml) for patients with normal or near-normal gastrointestinal function.

- High fat (>50% of kcal; caloric density ~1.5 kcal/ml) for high-energy needs, volume restriction, or diarrhea caused by high-carbohydrate (>50% kcal) products.
- Fiber-containing diets for improved consistency of feces compared with those resulting from high-carbohydrate diets.

Defined-formula diets or diets specifically modified for patients with impaired organ function.

- *Impaired gastrointestinal function, including >2 weeks' anorexia.* Diet contains peptides, medium-chain triglycerides, and glucose polymers versus intact macronutrient sources. Usually causes diarrhea if given for more than than 2 to 3 days.
- *Impaired liver function.* Diet with reduced protein (<18% of kcal). High branched-chain and aromatic amino acid content formulas are available, but their efficacy is questionable.
- *Impaired kidney function.* A diet of reduced protein (<18% of kcal). Formulas supplemented with alpha-ketoacids of some essential amino acids are available, but their efficacy is disputed.
- Stress diets are of high branched-chain amino acid

content and high (>1 kcal/ml) caloric density. Efficacy is disputed.

Nutrient Modifications for Specific Disease Problems

Energy

- Total calories (<1 kcal/ml)
  - Restricted—obesity, uncontrollable hyperglycemia (rare)
  - Increased (>1 kcal/ml)—disease-induced increases in requirements from severe trauma, burns, sepsis, hyperthyroidism, malignancy
- Carbohydrate
  - Increased (>50% of kcal)—prolonged anorexia (>2 weeks), fat maldigestion, malabsorption
  - Decreased (<30% of kcal)—diarrhea, glucose intolerance
- Fat
  - Increased (>50% of kcal)—diarrhea due to high-carbohydrate feedings, increased energy needs
  - Decreased (<30% of kcal)—same as increased carbohydrate
  - *Triglycerides.* Long chain—adequate pancreatic and intestinal function. Medium chain—severely impaired pancreatic or intestinal function, chylothorax, or lymphangiectasia

Protein

- Restricted (<18% of kcal)—impaired liver or kidney function
- Increased (>22% of kcal)—losses via intestinal tract, draining wounds, trauma
- Form
  - Intact—adequate pancreatic and intestinal function
  - Hydrolyzed—intact protein not tolerated

Table 3–1. MANUFACTURERS OF NUTRITIONAL DEVICES AND DIETARY PRODUCTS

Kendall Healthcare Products (A)
15 Hampshire St.
Mansfield, MA 02048
508-261-8000

Corpak Company (A, B)
100 Chaddick Dr.
Wheeling, IL 60090
837-537-4601

B-Braun Medical (A)
2525 McGaw Ave.
P.O. Box 19791
Irvine, CA 92623-9791
800-227-2862

Upjohn Pharmaceuticals (B)
7000 Portage Rd.
Kalamazoo, MI
800-253-8600

Cook Critical care (A, C)
P.O. Box 48
Bloomington, IN 47402
812-339-2235

Wyeth Ayerst Laboratories (B)
Central Customer Service
31 Morehall Rd
Frazer, PA 19355
800-666-7248

Procter & Gamble Pharmaceuticals (B)
P.O. Box 191
Norwich, NY 13815-0231
607-335-2111

Novartis Nutrition (B, D, E, F)
5320 W. 23rd St.
Minneapolis, MN 55440
612-925-2100

Abbott Laboratories (B)
1401 Sheridan Road
North Chicago, IL 60064-4000
888-299-7416

*A, tubes; B, feeding products; C, guidewires; D, carbohydrate modules; E, fat modules; F, protein modules.

- Specific amino acids for cats
  - Arginine—recommend 2.5 mg/kcal/day. Human formulas are supplemented with 1 mg/kcal/day.
  - Taurine—not necessary for short-term feeding. Add 0.1 mg/kcal/day for long-term feeding.

Electrolytes

Electrolytes (sodium, potassium, chlorine) ~40 mEq/L have been adequate. Adjust amounts based on laboratory determinations.

Minerals and Vitamins

Minerals and vitamins—use National Research Council (NRC) recommendations in the absence of specific information to the contrary

Osmolality

- Normal serum albumin of <650 mOsm/kg
- Hypoalbuminemia of 250 to 650 mOsm/kg, depending on severity. The lower the serum albumin level, the lower the diet osmolality.

Feeding Rates for Enteral Diets

The calculations for feeding liquid diets follow. If the tube size is ≥14 Fr., blenderized commercial canned pet food may be fed.

▼ *Key Point* Proceed with feeding only as patient tolerance allows.

Bolus Feeding—Determine BEE and Number of Feedings Per Day (Figure 3–11)

Day 1
First feeding—water at ½ BEE* ÷ number of feedings
Subsequent feedings—diet at ½ BEE ÷ number of feedings
Day 2
BEE ÷ number of feedings
Day 3
Advance to GEE† as tolerance permits

Continuous—Determine BEE and Hourly Feeding Rate

Day 1
First feeding—water at ~2 ml per pound to assess tolerance. If no vomiting occurs in 2 hours, proceed to continuous feeding of the chosen diet at ½ BEE.
Day 2
BEE/24
Day 3
Advance to GEE as tolerance permits

For formulas containing 1.5 kcal/ml, divide energy needs by 1.5 to get volume to feed. Use this value to replace energy needs in the previously listed calculations.
Sample Calculation. A moderately stressed 30-lb dog's energy needs are estimated at 500 (basal) × 1.5 = 750 kcal/day. (Round off calculations to the nearest 5.)

For four-times daily feeding, the schedule is as follows:

Day 1

Feeding				
	1	Water	(0.5 × 500) ÷ 4 =	65 ml
	2	Diet	same as feeding 1	65 ml
	3	Diet	same as feeding 1	65 ml
	4	Diet	500 ÷ 4	125 ml
		Total		320 ml
				(255 kcal)

*BEE (basal energy estimate), found in Figure 3–11.
†GEE (goal energy estimate) = BEE × stress estimate (see Fig. 3–11).

How much to feed (kcal/day)
A. To meet basal needs-see graph:

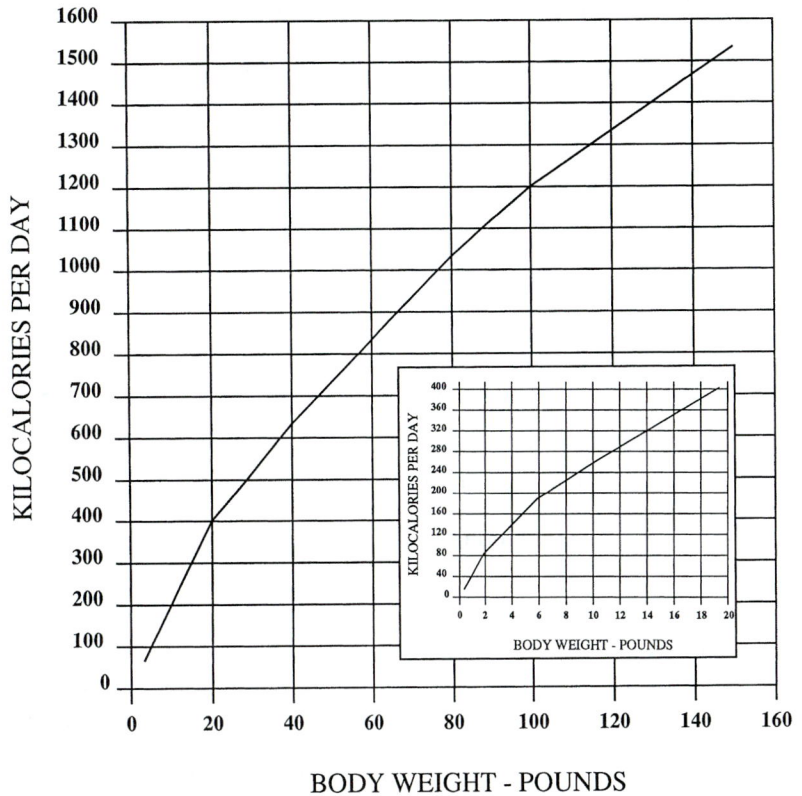

Figure 3–11. Graph for calculating caloric requirements to fill basal energy needs and to meet increased needs of stress. (BEE, basal energy estimate.)

BODY WEIGHT - POUNDS

B. **To meet increased needs of stress**
1. Mild stress-25% increase above BEE
2. Moderate stress-50% increase above BEE
3. Severe stress-100% increase above BEE

Day 2

Feeding	1	$500 \div 4$	125 ml
	2	$\dfrac{500 + \dfrac{750 - 500}{2}}{4}$	160 ml
	3	Same as feeding 2	160 ml
	4	$750 \div 4$	190 ml
	Total		635 ml (635 kcal)

Day 3

All feedings		$750 \div 4$	190 ml
	Total		760 ml (760 kcal)

For continuous feeding, the schedule is as follows:

Day 1

12 hours	Water	$(0.5 \times 500) \div 24 =$	10 ml/hr = 120 ml
12 hours	Diet	As above	10 ml/hr = 120 ml
	Total		240 ml (120 kcal)

Day 2

12 hours	Diet	$500 \div 24$	20 ml/hr = 240 ml
12 hours	Diet	$\dfrac{500 + \dfrac{750 - 500}{2}}{24}$	25 ml/hr = 300 ml
	Total		540 ml (540 kcal)

Day 3

	Diet	$750 \div 24$	30 ml/hr = 720 ml (720 kcal)

FEEDING DEVICES

Nasogastric Tube

Indications

See general indications for nutritional support. See Figure 3–10.

Objectives

- To successfully pass a nasogastric tube from the external nares to the stomach.
- To provide an adequate nutritional intake via the nasogastric tube.

Equipment

- Nasogastric tubes
  - Polyvinylchloride—inexpensive but may harden after prolonged (>2 weeks) contact with canine stomach contents.
  - Polyurethane, silicone—expensive but do not harden in the stomach; preferred for long-term placement.
  - Weighted tubes are not necessary to maintain placement and are more difficult to pass.
  - Tubes must be radiopaque to facilitate radiographic confirmation of placement.
  - Sizes are 3.5 Fr. × 15″—puppies, kittens; 5 Fr. × 36″ or 6 Fr × 22″—cats and dogs (≤20 lb); 8 Fr. × 42″ or 8 Fr × 43″—large cats and dogs (>20 lb).
- Guide wire
  - Generally necessary for placement of tubes in dogs. (Some tubes are available with stylet [Corpak].)
  - For 5 Fr. × 36″, use 0.025″ × 100 cm angiography guide wire.
  - For 8 Fr. × 42″, use 0.035″ × 120 cm angiography guide wire.
- 2% lidocaine or 0.5% proparacaine
- Lubricant (K-Y jelly)
- Monofilament nylon 2–0 or 3–0 suture
- Adhesive tape
- Elizabethan collar

Technique

1. Lubricate the angiography guide wire with mineral oil to use as stylet.
2. Before passing the tube, measure the distance from the external nares to the last rib (level of the stomach) and mark the tube.
3. Ensure patency of the nostrils.
4. Apply lubricant to the catheter tip.
5. With the animal's nose pointed upward, instill 1 ml of lidocaine (dogs) or 5 drops of proparacaine (cats) into one nostril.
6. Hold the animal's head in a normal, neutral position to avoid tracheal intubation.
7. Insert the catheter into the ventral nasal meatus. Direct the tube caudomedially, ventral to the alar fold. As the nasal planum is pushed upward, direct the tube ventrally and caudally to allow entry into the ventral nasal meatus (see Fig. 3–6).
8. Once the tube is believed to be in the stomach, a small bolus of water (3–6 ml) is injected into the tube. The animal is observed for coughing. Tube position can be confirmed by radiography.
9. Apply tape to the catheter in butterfly fashion and suture to the skin immediately adjacent to the alar fold (see Fig. 3–6B). Bring the tubing between the animal's eyes, and suture with butterfly tape to the

top of the animal's head (see Fig. 3–6). An Elizabethan collar or bucket may be needed to protect the tube from removal.

Postoperative Care and Complications

Feeding Instructions

- Check the position of continuous feeding tubes at least daily; check the position of bolus tubes before each feeding.
- Measure body weight daily. It should remain stable.
- Other laboratory determinations should be ordered as necessary.
- Bolus feeding instructions for *each feeding*
  - Inject a small bolus of air through the tube and auscultate over the cranial abdomen for sounds indicating that the tube is placed properly.
  - Inject water through the tube to produce coughing if the tube is placed improperly.
  - Aspirate the tube. If more than half of the previous feeding returns, do not feed and reassess at the next scheduled feeding.
  - When satisfied that the animal can be fed, place it in sternal or right lateral recumbency. The solution should be warmed and fed slowly.

▼ **Key Point** If the animal vomits, stop feeding.

- After feeding, flush the tube with 1 to 2 ml of warm water. Cap the tube so that a column of water is left to prevent food from drying and occluding the tube.
- Observe the animal for discomfort, colic, or diarrhea for a few minutes.
- Record all feedings (Fig. 3–12).

Complications of enteral feeding are listed in Table 3–2.

Esophagostomy Tube

Indications

- See general indications for nutritional support.
- See Figure 3–10 in previous section.
- To bypass the nasal passages or oral cavity because of trauma, tumors, or other conditions.

Objectives

- To pass and maintain an indwelling tube from the proximal esophagus to the distal esophagus.
- To provide adequate nutritional intake via the esophagostomy tube.

Equipment

- Minor surgical pack
- Long-handled right-angle forceps
- 10- to 18-Fr. red rubber feeding tube and urethral catheter (Sovereign)
- Monofilament 2–0 or 3–0 nylon suture
- Bandage material or stockinette

Technique

1. Anesthetize the patient and place in right lateral recumbency.

FOOD INTAKE RECORD

INSTRUCTIONS:
1. Weigh the food and container using the gram scale that is located on the counter in the ICU. Record this weight in the "offered" column.
2. When uneaten food is removed from cage, weigh as above (the food and container!). Record this weight in the "removed" column.
3. Subtract amount that was removed from amount that was offered. Record this weight in the "eaten" column.
4. Write down what was fed (and if it was canned, dry, liquid, etc.) in the last column.

DATE/TIME	INITIALS	AMOUNT OF FOOD (grams)			What was fed?
		offered	removed	eaten	
	example:	100	25	75	Chicken baby food

Figure 3–12. Example of a food intake record chart as used by the Nutritional Support Service of The Ohio State University Veterinary Hospital.

2. Clip and aseptically prepare the left cervical region.
3. Measure and mark the rubber feeding tube from the cervical entry site to the eighth rib.
4. Place the right-angle forceps through the mouth and into the esophagus so that the forceps tip can be palpated through the skin in the mid-cervical region.
5. Make a small incision over the instrument tip.

▼ *Key Point* When making the incision, be careful to avoid the jugular vein.

6. Push the tip of the forceps through the incision, grasp the distal end of the feeding tube in the forceps, and pull the tube out through the mouth.
7. Turn the tube around and direct it down the esophagus, stopping at the level of the premeasured mark.
8. Secure to the skin using a Chinese finger trap suture (see #15 under chest tube placement technique).
9. Place a light bandage around the neck to help protect the tube, and place a plug in the end of the tube. A hypodermic needle cap may be used.

Postoperative Care and Complications

- Keep the incision site clean.
- See section on nasogastric tube in this section for instructions and complications of enteral feeding.
- Complications of esophagostomy tube include inci-

Table 3–2. COMPLICATIONS OF ENTERAL FEEDING AND THEIR MANAGEMENT

Clogged tube	Flush with water; use pancreatic enzyme slurry, tube unclogging devices, replace tube if necessary.
Aspiration of stomach contents	Stop feeding.
Vomiting and bloating	Reduce flow rate; give metoclopramide (0.2–0.4 mg/kg PO or SC q8h; or 1–2 mg/kg/24h constant rate IV infusion); stop feeding.
Diarrhea	Reduce flow rate; add fat or fiber, dilute solution, add antidiarrheal drug.
Hyperglycemia and glucosuria	Reduce flow rate; administer insulin.
Sneezing after placing NG tube	Instill 1–2 drops local anesthetic into nostril q4–6h

sional inflammation, abscess (rare), and vomiting of
the tube followed by aspiration pneumonia.

Percutaneous Endoscopic Gastrostomy (PEG) Tube

Indications

- See Indications for Nutritional Support for route.
- See Figure 3–10.
- To provide nutrition in patients in which the nasal
  passages, oral cavity, or esophagus is bypassed.

Objectives

- To allow access to the stomach for nutritional support.
- To provide a leakage-free chronic indwelling gastric
  catheter.

Equipment

- Endoscope
- Grasping forceps
- Bard urologic catheter (18–24-Fr. Pezzer mushroom-tip model)
- Indwelling catheter (14 gauge), needle (16 gauge) (Sovereign)
- Three-way stopcock
- Suture (Vetafil) 2–0 (3 ft.)
- #11 blades (2)
- 20 gauge × 1-inch needle
- 1¼-inch rubber tubing
- 1-inch tape
- Cast padding (3-inch)
- Kling (3-inch)
- Vet Wrap (4-inch)
- Stockinette (cut to fit for "sweater")

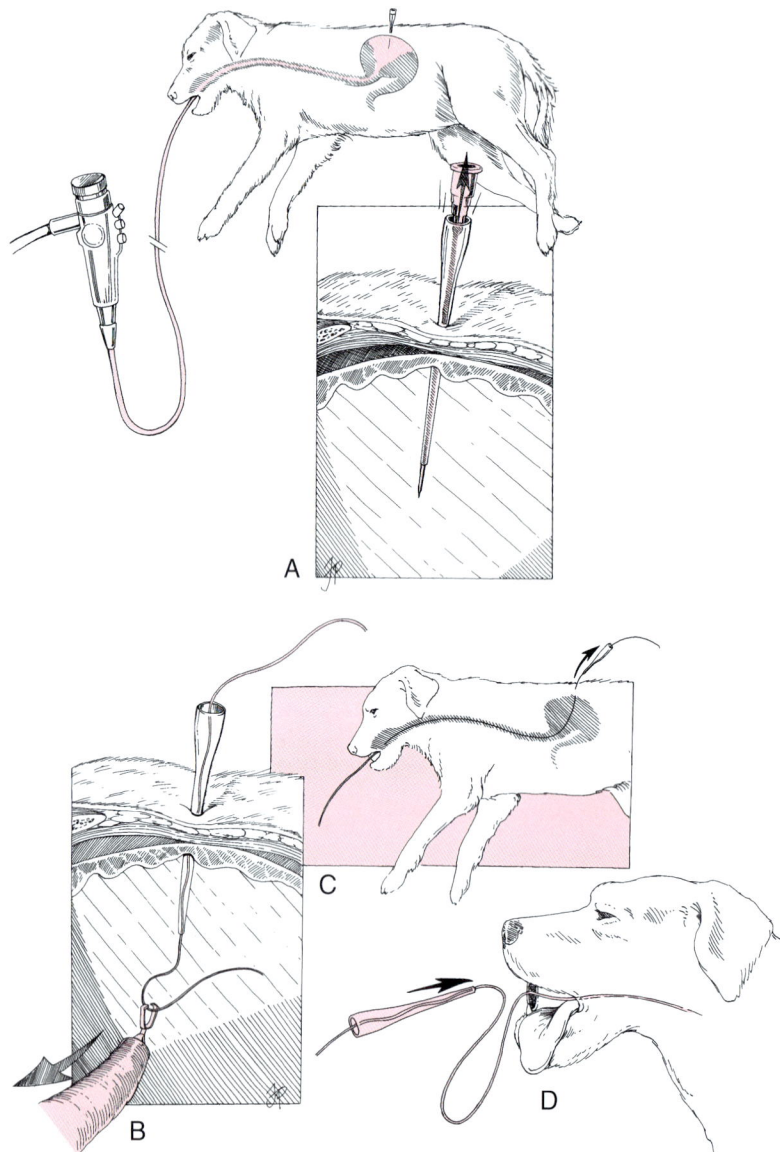

Figure 3–13. Placement of percutaneous endoscopic gastrostomy (PEG) tube. *A,* Over-the-needle catheter is placed through the skin and into the air-distended stomach; *B,* suture threaded through the catheter is grasped by endoscopic forceps and pulled out through the mouth *(C); D,* over-the-needle catheter is threaded onto the suture, which is tied to the gastrostomy tube.

- Scissors
- Hemostats
- Nolvasan

Technique

1. To prepare materials
   - Soak a 1¼-inch piece of tubing in Nolvasan solution for at least 10 minutes before procedure.
   - Using a #11 blade, cut an approximate 1-cm slice (stab) through the center of this tubing piece.
   - Remove the flared end (opposite the mushroom end), and cut this end at a 60° angle.
2. Place anesthetized animal in right lateral recumbency, and clip and prepare a 12-cm² area caudal to the costal arch.
3. Insert an endoscope and distend the stomach with air.
4. Locate the skin incision site over the gastric fundus on the left side caudal to the last rib by pressing with a finger and using the endoscope for visual guidance. Be sure that the penetration site is far enough away from the pylorus.
5. Insert an over-the-needle IV catheter through the body wall into the distended stomach while viewing through the endoscope. Withdraw the needle, leaving the cannula in place in the stomach (Fig. 3–13A).
6. Thread Vetafil suture material through the cannula into the stomach.
7. Using grasping forceps via the channel of the endoscope, grasp the Vetafil suture and withdraw the entire endoscope, along with the luminal end of the suture, out through the mouth (Fig. 3–13B). Continue holding the percutaneous end of the suture so that it remains in place through the body wall.
8. Withdraw the cannula from the animal's body wall while leaving the suture in place (Fig. 3–13C). Slide the cannula, narrow end first, over the suture coming out of the mouth (Fig. 3–13D).
9. Tie the end of the suture coming out of the mouth to the proximal end (end opposite the mushroom tip) of the gastrostomy tube and pull the tube up into the end of the cannula to fit together snugly (Fig. 3–13E).
10. Lubricate the cannula and the gastrostomy tube.
11. Pull the percutaneous end of the suture until the cannula and the gastrostomy tube are pulled all the way out through the body wall and the mushroom end is up against the inside wall (mucosal surface) of the stomach (Fig. 3–13F).
12. Check the position with the endoscope.
13. To anchor the PEG tube in place, slide the piece of 1¼-inch rubber tubing as a cross-piece over the outside of the tube for a snug fit (not too tight) against the body wall (Fig. 3–13G).
14. Butterfly a 1-inch piece of tape around the PEG tube above the cross-piece of rubber tubing to secure it in place.
15. Plug the end of the PEG tube with a catheter adapter (Becton-Dickinson) and Surflo lock-type injection plug (Terumo Medical). Apply antibiotic ointment to the skin at the tube exit site.

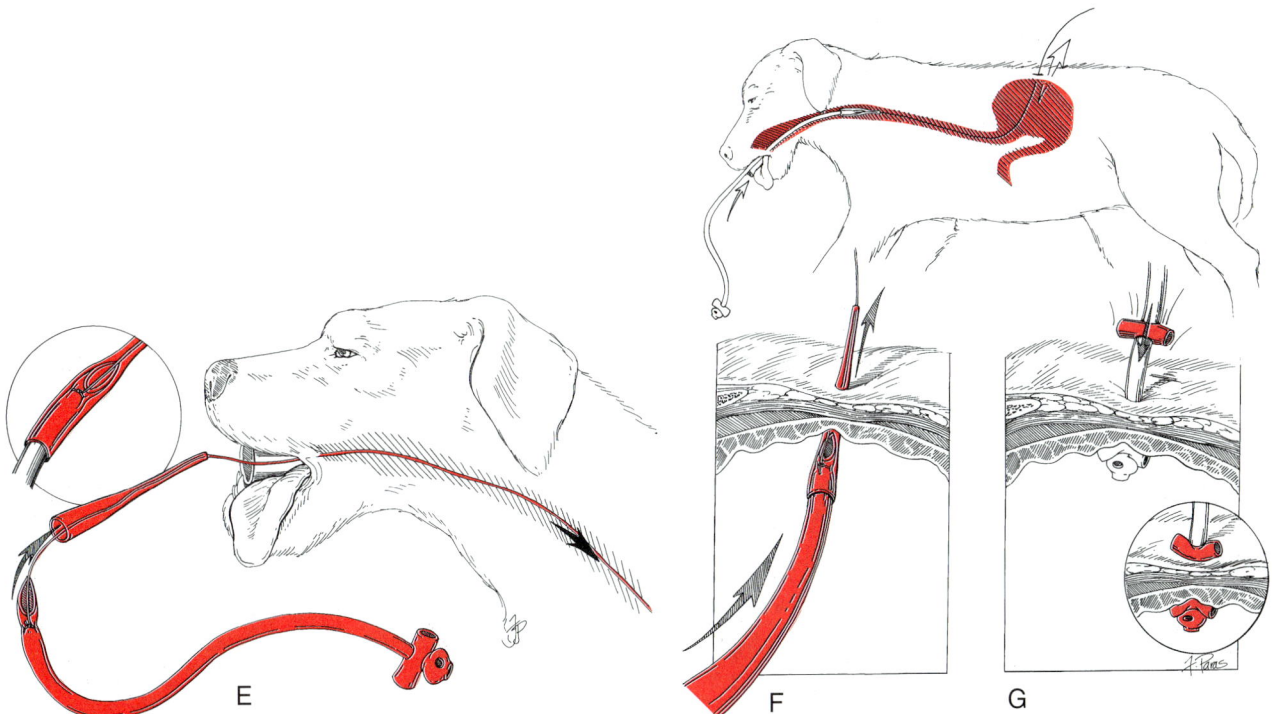

Figure 3–13.   *Continued (E)* and subsequently pulled into the stomach and out the gastric and body wall. The flange at the end of the gastrostomy tube should press snugly against the gastric mucosa. See text for *F* and *G*.

16. Put the stockinette sweater on the animal.

Postoperative Care and Complications

- See Nasogastric Tube in this chapter for feeding instructions and complications of enteral feeding.
- Allow 12 to 24 hours before beginning feeding.
- Once a PEG tube is placed, it should not be removed for at least 7–10 days to ensure a good adhesion between the serosa and abdominal wall. To remove the tube, one method is to place moderate traction on the tube and cut the tube as close to the skin as possible. Force the tip of the tube completely into the stomach using a cotton-tipped applicator. The tip eventually migrates down the intestinal tract and passes in the feces. In cats and small dogs, consider the endoscopic removal of the tip to prevent intestinal obstruction.
- Another method of removal uses a blunt stylet inserted into the tube and forced up against the mushroom tip to stretch the mushroom so that the entire tube with intact mushroom can be extracted percutaneously through the stoma.
- Complications of PEG tubes include mutilation of the tube by the animal; leakage of liquid diet intraperitoneally or subcutaneously (very rare using described technique); and obstruction of the pylorus, subsequent to the migration of the tip of the tube (also very rare).

Nonendoscopic Percutaneous Gastrostomy Tube

Gastrostomy tubes can also be placed without endoscopic visualization using the Eld gastrostomy tube applicator (Jorgensen Laboratories, Loveland, CO). This device allows placement of suture, replacing steps #3 through #7 in the PEG technique. The remainder of the technique and equipment used is the same as described for the PEG tube.

SUPPLEMENTAL READINGS

Abood SK, Buffington CA: Improved nasogastric intubation technique for administration of nutritional support in dogs. J Am Vet Med Assoc 199:577, 1991.

Crane SW: Diagnostic peritoneal lavage. *In* Kirk RW, ed.: *Current Veterinary Therapy IX*. Philadelphia: W.B. Saunders, 1986, p 3.

Grandage J: The oral cavity and pharynx. *In* Slatter DH, ed.: *Textbook of Small Animal Surgery*. Philadelphia: W.B. Saunders, 1985, p 639.

Nelson AW: Lower respiratory system. *In* Slatter DH, ed.: *Textbook of Small Animal Surgery*. Philadelphia: W.B. Saunders, 1985, p 1007.

4 Radiographic and Ultrasonographic Techniques

David S. Biller / Justin M. Goggin

The purpose of the radiograph is to provide a lasting record of maximum information. The sequence of the major operations involved in transforming the altered morphology and tissue density within a diseased animal into a two-dimensional, black-and-white radiograph and then reaching a diagnosis is complex and includes the following steps: (1) making a properly exposed and positioned radiograph; (2) recording the x-ray picture with the assistance of accessory equipment; (3) reviewing radiographs in proper conditions and in a systematic and detailed manner; (4) recognizing lesions—therefore [requiring] a knowledge of normal radiographic anatomy and its variation by age, species, and breed and the ability to recognize and understand artifacts; and (5) evaluating radiographic abnormalities with respect to clinical and laboratory findings.

Dr. Peter Suter

X-RAY MACHINE

Milliampere-Second and Kilovolt Peak

- The *mA (milliampere)* × *seconds (time)* = *mAs* (milliampere-second), which affects the degree of blackness (density) of the radiograph with no effect on contrast. A direct relationship exists between mA and radiographic density. Time and mA both influence the number of x-rays produced but have no effect on the penetrating ability of the beam. To quickly check the adequacy of the mAs on a film, hold the film up to room light and place a white sheet of paper about 1 inch behind the film. Place a finger between the film and paper. If the finger can be readily seen through the film in the black area (most exposed), increase the mAs.
- The *kVp (kilovolt peak)* is the only machine factor that influences radiographic contrast and has some control over the amount of radiographic density (blackness). The contrast can be expressed as being low, which means that there are many shades of gray (long scale) between the extremes of black and white. The term *high contrast* means that there are few shades of gray (short scale). Lowering the kVp increases the contrast, and raising the kVp reduces the contrast.

- To adjust technique to alter film contrast while maintaining the same radiographic density, consider the following:
  - The mAs and kVp have to be in balance.
  - As mAs increases, kVp must decrease.
  - As kVp increases, mAs must decrease.
  - Doubling radiographic density requires doubling the mAs or increasing kVp by 10% in the 40–100 kVp range or 15% in the ≥100 kVp range.

Recommendations

- The *300-mA machine* may have adjustable mA stations of 25, 50, 100, 200, and 300 and two (1 and 2 mm or smaller) focal spots.
- An ideal kVp range is 40–120 and is adjustable in 1 or 2 kVp per step.
- A *timing device* is necessary to control the duration of an x-ray exposure. Modern x-ray machines have electronic timers with ranges that can control motion in the patient and prevent blurring. With a timed exposure of $\frac{1}{120}$ second, all significant motion is stopped.
- The *line voltage compensator* is automatic or manual.
- The *tube stand* moves along the full length of the table and has an adjustable height from 0–60 inches (152 cm). The tube is able to rotate 90° around the vertical axis and 180° around the horizontal axis.
- The *table* is 5–6 feet in length with a top that has floating motion in four directions.
- The *collimator* at the region of interest decreases scatter radiation and human and patient exposure, while increasing film quality. Always leave a clear margin of collimation on every film. The collimator is lighted and has a centering mark. A high-quality, dial-adjustable, multileaf lead shutter collimator is highly recommended.
- The *filters* have the primary function of reducing patient radiation dose by removing scatter radiation and increasing (mean beam energy) quality. Most x-ray equipment has inherent filtration equal to 1.5–2.0 mm aluminum. Increased film quality can be obtained by adding an additional 2.0-mm aluminum filtration. Total filtration must be at least 2.5-mm aluminum.
- The *grids* consist of a flat plate with a series of lead foil strips separated by transparent spacers. They are

made in various sizes and improve the diagnostic quality of radiographs by absorbing the greater part of the scatter radiation. Position grids between the patient and cassette, usually under the table. Use only for body parts thicker than 10 cm. The reciprocating grid (Potter-Bucky diaphragm) includes a mechanism that moves the grid during exposure, in order to eliminate grid lines from the radiograph. This grid is optional equipment but recommended for the best-quality radiographs.

- Grids can be classified in three ways: the lead content (g/cm^2), the number of lines per inch, and the ratio of lead strip height to the space between the lead strips. Generally, high-ratio grids absorb scatter better but are more expensive. More lines per inch give better quality, because the lead strips are narrower and therefore lines become less prominent; however, they cost more. The most common grid is an 8:1 with 103 lines per inch.
- A grid is not used with machines of less than 100 mA because the lead in the grid absorbs a portion of the primary beam, requiring a higher exposure (increased mAs) to produce diagnostic radiographs. Machines of 100–300 mA use a grid with a ratio of 8:1 or 10:1.
- The higher the grid ratio the more critical is the x-ray tube alignment. Always stay within the focal

zone of the grid. This is usually written on the grid and is 36–42 inches (90–105 cm) in most instances.
- The *exposure switches* include the two-position exposure switch on the console and two-position exposure foot switch, with a cord of sufficient length.
- The *high-frequency x-ray machines* have a few advantages over single-phase x-ray machines. A 150-mA high-frequency generator can produce a quantity of x-rays equal to that of a 300-mA, single-phase x-ray machine. Many of the units use 110 volts. They are reliable, with less downtime than single-phase machines. Their cost, at present, is greater than that of single-phase machines but most likely will decrease in the future.
- For a listing of x-ray machine manufacturers see Table 4–1.

ACCESSORY RADIOGRAPHIC EQUIPMENT

Intensifying Screens

The screen is a suspension of phosphor crystals in a binder. The phosphor in the screen converts x-ray photons into visible light, to which the film is more sensitive. A latent image is created by exposure of the film to this light. This technique reduces x-ray exposure to the patient by at least 10 times and the time of x-ray exposure, thus decreasing the chance of blurring.

- Screen speed is dependent on the thickness of the phosphor layer, size of phosphor crystals, and efficiency of phosphor crystals at absorbing x-rays and converting them to light.
- Screen classification varies, as each company has a slightly different system for labeling screen speed. Resolution ability of the screen is inversely related to speed. Increased speed gives decreased resolution. Have a technique chart available for each screen speed. Par speed is the starting point for comparison of screens. High speed has a speed two times that of par speed. Ultra (super) speed is four times par speed. High detail speed is half that of par speed.
- Types of screens
  - Calcium tungstate screens reduce the amount of radiation necessary to expose film by 10 times, compared to film exposed without a screen. They are also less expensive than rare earth screens. Calcium tungstate emits a broad spectrum of light in the ultraviolet and blue range.
  - Rare earth screens are more expensive than calcium tungstate screens. The light emitted is in the ultraviolet, green, or blue range. The major advantage of rare earth over calcium tungstate screens is that rare earth screens are fast, because of a more efficient production of light. Therefore, they decrease the production of scatter, the exposure time, the radiation dosage, the chance of motion and subsequent blurring, and the wear and tear on the x-ray tube.
- System speed is the speed of film and screen in combination. It is not an additive system. A very low system speed results when screens and films with differ-

Table 4–1. X-RAY MACHINE MANUFACTURERS

Bennett X-Ray Technologies
54 Railroad Ave.
Copiague, NY 11726
516-691-6100

Continental X-ray
2000 S. 25th Ave.
Broadview, IL 60153
708-345-3050

Control-X Medical
West Pointe Business Park
2289 W. Brooke Dr.
Columbus, OH 43228
614-777-0476

Fischer Imaging
12300 North Grant St.
Denver, CO 80241
303-452-6800

MinXray Inc.
3611 Commercial Ave.
Northbrook, IL 60062-1822
847-564-0323

Summit Industries
2901 W. Lawrence Ave.
Chicago, IL 60625
800-729-9729

Universal
11550 W. King St.
Franklin Park, IL 60131
847-288-7000

X-ray Marketing Associates
1205 Lakeview Ct.
Romeoville, IL 60446
800-325-8880

ent color spectrum sensitivities are put together. Ask the film dealer what speed system you have with your particular screens and film. The higher the system speed number, the more sensitive it is and the less radiation necessary to make an exposure. System speeds can vary from 50–3200 and higher. The higher the system speed number, the less radiation to the patient and to personnel within the room; however, the lower the system speed number, the better the resolution qualities. When you know the system speed, changing the technique chart is simpler. If the system speed doubles, change the mAs on the technique chart by half. If the system speed decreases by 50%, double the mAs on the technique chart.

- Exposure time
  - Always use the shortest exposure times possible to eliminate blurring.
  - For thoracic radiographs, exposure times of $\frac{1}{60}$ of a second or shorter stop the effects of respiratory and heart motion.
  - For abdominal radiographs, employ exposure times of $\frac{1}{40}$ second or shorter in order to eliminate gastrointestinal motion.
  - For extremity radiographs, exposure times of $\frac{1}{20}$ second or shorter eliminate the effects of patient motion.
- Rare earth screens have a system speed that allows the shortest exposure times possible to eliminate motion problems and to lower radiation exposure to patient and personnel. Generally, when using a 300-mA machine, a 400–800 speed system with an 8:1, 103 lines per inch grid gives good-quality radiographs, including for large breed dogs. In a feline practice, a slower system, such as a 100–250 speed system, provides excellent quality. As the crystal size gets larger, the system gets faster but resolution is reduced.
- Clean screens with the product recommended by the manufacturer on a regular schedule (monthly) and whenever debris is noted on the radiographs.

Film

Radiographic film provides a permanent record containing the maximum amount of diagnostic information.

- Film is made of a light-sensitive emulsion, composed of gelatin and silver halide with other ingredients attached to a plastic (polyester) base. The silver halides are sensitive to light and change when exposed to light to produce a latent image. The process of developing changes silver ions into black silver, thus producing the radiographic image. Fixer removes all the unexposed silver from the film. The emulsion may be attached to one or both sides of the base. X-ray film may be most sensitive to direct x-ray exposure (nonscreen film), or to blue, green, or ultraviolet light.
- Films vary in their contrast. Some films appear more black and white after exposure and development. Use the film that is recommended by your screen manufacturer to match the spectrum of light produced by your screens. Choose a film that results in the contrast range that is most pleasing to you. Use a film that gives you a system speed that results in quality radiographs. Make sure to match film, screens, and processing chemicals.
- Film must be sensitive to the type of light emitted by the screens in use. Film speed determines the amount of light required to produce an image on the radiograph. Fast film has large crystals (silver halide), requires less exposure, and produces a grainy image. Slow film has small crystals, requires greater exposure, and produces a less grainy or sharper-defined image.
- Screen film is manufactured with crystals that are sensitive to fluorescent light. Nonscreen film is a direct exposure type film and is manufactured to be sensitive to x-rays. Nonscreen film requires 10 to 25 times more radiation than screen film.
- Film is available in both metric and nonmetric measurements. The most common sizes used in small animal practice are 8 × 10 inches, 10 × 12 inches, and 14 × 17 inches.
- X-ray film is sensitive not only to light and x-ray photons but also to humidity, chemicals, and physical stress. Film is stored on end to reduce pressure on the face of the film. High humidity causes film fogging, and low humidity causes film static; therefore, between 30% and 40% humidity is appropriate for film storage. Storage temperature should not exceed 50°–70°F (10°–21.1°C). Store the film away from developing chemicals and ionizing radiation. Do not put pressure on the film when loading or unloading film.
- Film and screen companies are provided in Table 4–2.

Cassettes

Cassettes are used primarily to contain and protect film. Two basic types are available: rigid cassettes that contain both the film and screen and cardboard cassettes that hold nonscreen film.

Table 4–2. FILM AND SCREEN COMPANIES

Agfa Gavert Corp. 2803 Butterfield Rd. Suite 200 Oak Brook, IL 60521 708-593-8787	Konica Medical Corporation 411 Newark Pompton Turnpike Wayne, NJ 07470 201-633-1500
Eastman Kodak Company Health Sciences Division Rochester, NY 14650 800-926-1519	Picker International Inc. 595 Miner Rd. Highland Heights, OH 44143 216-473-3000
Fuji Medical Systems 90 Viaduct Rd. Stamford, CT 06907 800-431-1850	Sterling Diagnostic Imaging Inc. P.O. Box 19048 Greenville, SC 29602-9048 Greenville, SC 800-252-9099
	3M Medical Imaging System 3M Center Building 223-2S St. Paul, MN 55144-1000 612-733-1110

Table 4–3. RADIOGRAPHIC ACCESSORY COMPANIES

Bar-ray Products, Inc. 237 Twenty-fifth St. Brooklyn, NY 11232 718-965-7000	Picker International Inc. 595 Miner Rd. Highland Heights, OH 44143 216-473-3000
Burkhart Roentgen, Inc. 3 River Rd. South Cornwall Bridge, CT 06754 800-872-9729	Radiation Concepts Inc. 4131 S.W. 47th Ave. Suite 1406 Davie, FL 33314 954-587-9222
Cone Instruments 5201 Naimen Parkway Solon, OH 44139 800-321-6964	S. & S. X-ray Products Inc. 1101 Linwood St. Brooklyn, NY 11208 800-221-6634
Fischer Industries, Inc. P.O. Box 570 2630 Kaneville Ct. Geneva, IL 60134 800-356-5911	Shielding International Inc. 182 Earl St. P.O. Box 578 Madras, OR 97741-0069 800-292-2247
Hale X-ray Company Inc. 222-224 E. 14th St. Cincinnati, OH 45210 513-241-4357	3M Animal Care Products 3M Center, Building 275-3E-03 St. Paul, MN 55144-1000 612-733-1110
Medical I.D. Systems Inc. 3954 44th St. Grand Rapids, MI 49512 616-698-0535	Wolf X-ray Corp. 420 Hempstead Turnpike West Hempstead, NY 11552 516-485-7000

- Rigid cassettes protect both screens and film from physical damage and film from exposure to light. The cassette provides snug contact between the film and screens. The front of the cassette is usually a rigid plastic, aluminum, or other substance that absorbs relatively few x-ray photons. Usually, a small rectangle in the corner of the cassette acts to shield the film from x-rays to allow an unexposed area for film identification. The back of the cassette is lined with lead to absorb backscatter radiation. The back of the cassette is also equipped with latches to provide a lightproof seal.
- Cassette for a nonscreen film only protects the film from light exposure. It is usually made from cardboard.
- Cassettes are numbered. When defects are noted on a radiograph, they can be traced to the correct cassette. Dropping a cassette causes warping and results in poor film-screen contact and a distorted radiographic image.

Miscellaneous Accessories

- Use the screen cleaner that is recommended by your screen manufacturer.
- Use safety devices (lead aprons, lead gloves, glasses, and lead thyroid shield) when personnel are required in the x-ray room for patient positioning.
- Film markers consist of right and left lead film markers; Mitchell markers (for horizontal radiographs); and time markers (for upper gastrointestinal and intravenous urography radiographs).

- A device capable of measuring body part thickness and determining kVp for exposure is needed.
- Positioning devices include sponge wedges; sandbags; Plexiglas trough; rope; tape; and agents for chemical restraint to avoid human exposure associated with hand-holding whenever possible.
- Film filing envelopes are needed.
- Contrast media (see Contrast Studies section and Table 4–6).
- Monitoring devices (film badges) for employees and room monitoring, film viewer (at least one double bank), and hot light (high-intensity light) are needed.
- Radiographic accessory companies are listed in Table 4–3.

CHECKING X-RAY MACHINE ACCURACY

mA Station Check

- Use an aluminum step wedge to check mA station (setting) accuracy. Use the step wedge to determine if your mA stations are linear. It cannot determine if all your mA stations are off by the same amount. A step wedge (see Table 4–3 for sources) gives a general idea about the mA stations. A step wedge is inexpensive ($100) and easy to use. Place the step wedge on a loaded cassette; make many separate exposures of the step wedge, changing mA but always having the same mAs and kVp. If you cannot keep the same mAs throughout all the mA stations, do as many as possible at one mAs setting then go back and check the rest at another mAs.

Example

25 mA	$\frac{1}{10}$ sec	2.5 mAs	70 kVp
50 mA	$\frac{1}{20}$ sec	2.5 mAs	70 kVp
100 mA	$\frac{1}{40}$ sec	2.5 mAs	70 kVp
300 mA	$\frac{1}{120}$ sec	2.5 mAs	70 kVp
100 mA	$\frac{1}{60}$ sec	1.7 mAs	70 kVp
200 mA	$\frac{1}{120}$ sec	1.7 mAs	70 kVp

Compare the densities of all exposures. They should be the same for all mA stations taken at the same mAs. An exposure that varies from the average shows that there is a problem with that mA station. This test does not tell you if all the mA stations are accurate, but it does tell you if a particular station has a problem.
- A digital electronic mA checking device is the most accurate way to compare your mA stations.

kVp Check

- The only accurate way to check kVp is the Wisconsin test cassette ($1300; see Table 4–3 for sources). The Wisconsin test cassette has many kVp settings listed on the front of the cassette. Under each of these settings is a certain amount of material to attenuate the beam. After exposure and processing, this film provides information to determine if the kVp settings are accurate.
- Another less accurate way to obtain a general check of kVp accuracy is to vary mAs and kVp. Go through

all the kVp settings employing density changing factors to keep the densities the same throughout all these exposures.

Example

100 mAs at 50 kVp	3.1 mAs at 81 kVp
50 mAs at 55 kVp	1.5 mAs at 90 kVp
25 mAs at 61 kVp	0.8 mAs at 99 kVp
12.5 mAs at 67 kVp	0.4 mAs at 108 kVp
6.2 mAs at 74 kVp	0.2 mAs at 124 kVp

If your mA stations and kVp settings are working correctly, these exposures have the same density but the contrast range of each is different. Remember to employ density changing factors when necessary.

Exposure Timer Check (Single-Phase Machine)

Use a spinning top test tool. It can be purchased from the same company as the machine (see Table 4–1) or from an accessory company (see Table 4–3). This tool is inexpensive ($50) and easy to use. It is a flat metal spinning top with a hole in one side. The top is set on a loaded cassette and spun. Take an exposure at $\frac{1}{120}$ second. Move the top over to another corner of the film, spin again, and expose at $\frac{1}{60}$ second. This maneuver is repeated at $\frac{1}{40}$ and $\frac{1}{30}$ second. At $\frac{1}{120}$ second, only one dot should be seen; at $\frac{1}{60}$, two dots; at $\frac{1}{40}$, three dots; and at $\frac{1}{30}$, four dots. If more or less dots are on the film than expected, the timer is not accurate.

Line Voltage

Line voltage is the amount of current coming into the machine. This amount of current may vary, depending on electrical wiring, consistency of voltage in the area, and usage of current on the same circuit in the particular practice. Almost all machines used for small animals have a line voltage check device. Some have a meter and a dial to adjust line voltage and do not permit exposure until the voltage is manually adjusted. Other machines have an automatic line voltage adjustment. Almost all equipment in small animal practice uses 120 volts (i.e., right out of the socket).

FILM PROCESSING

Manual Processing

Film developing is a chemical process and is therefore dependent on both time and temperature.

Advantages and Disadvantages

- Advantages
  - Less expensive setup costs than those of automatic processor. Average setup cost is $300 to $1000.
  - No special electrical or structural changes are necessary for the darkroom.
- Disadvantages
  - Valuable technician time to develop films and maintain chemical baths (i.e., increased labor costs).
  - Quality is not consistent, due to human error, compared with automatic processors.
  - Longer time to prepare diagnostic films compared with automatic processors.

Accessories

- Developing tanks
- Two stirring paddles
- Two thermometers
- Film developing hangers of different sizes
- Chemicals
- Adjustable mixing valve for measuring water temperature
- Timer
- Dust-free drying cabinet or area

Darkroom Safelight

Darkroom safelights must produce enough illumination in the darkroom so that a person can see to process radiographic film (load and unload cassettes) without unwanted density (fog) to the film. Safelights utilize a wavelength of light different from that to which the film is sensitive. A Wratten 6B filter is adequate for blue-sensitive film. A GBX-2 filter is employed with green-sensitive or both green- and blue-sensitive films. Usually, 15-watt bulbs are used with safelights. The safelight is about 4 feet away from the film-handling area. No system is 100% safe; therefore, expose the film no longer than necessary.

Radiograph Labeling

- A radiograph is a legal document and must therefore have permanent labeling. On the label, include the hospital or veterinarian's name, the date the radiograph was taken, and the owner's name or animal's file number. Label the radiograph with right or left, dorsoventral/ventrodorsal (DV/VD), time marker on contrast studies, and Mitchell marker, when a horizontal beam is used. Basic types of permanent marking systems are available:
  - Lead letters and numbers in a holder with the hospital or veterinarian's name, placed on the cassette during exposure.
  - Radiopaque marking tape (lead-impregnated tape). Information may be written on the tape and the tape is placed on the cassette before exposure.
  - A darkroom printer transfers data from a card to the corner of the x-ray film that was shielded from radiation during exposure. This system requires cassettes with special windows. The film is removed from the cassette, and the corner of the film where it was blocked from light exposure is imprinted by exposing the patient information on a 5 × 7 inch card onto the film.

Silver Recovery

Recover silver from fixer solutions by either manual or automatic systems. Fixer solutions may be sold to companies for silver recovery. Alternatively, you may purchase a system (metallic replacement process, electrolytic recovery, or chemical precipitation) for silver recovery in your practice. Exposed developed and undeveloped film may also be sold for silver recovery. Usually, the supplier of the x-ray films or processing solutions can be consulted to determine if silver recovery is feasible and who to contact.

Procedure for Manual Film Processing

- Check temperatures, turn off room lights, use safelights, and agitate (mix) solutions well.
- Place the film on development hangers, making sure all four corners are attached.
- Set and start time, depending on the temperature in the developing tank.
- Place the hanger with the film into the developing tank. Rap hard against the tank wall to dislodge air bubbles. Agitate by pulling film out of the developer, and let the developer drain to one lower corner. Return film to the developer. Repeat agitation every minute. Manufacturers recommend a specific temperature for the developed solution that they produce, usually 68°F (20°C). Adjust for change in temperature (increased temperature, decreased time and vice versa). The chemical manufacturer can provide a time temperature development chart.

Example

60°F (15.5°C)	8.5 min
65°F (18.3°C)	6.0 min
68°F (20.0°C)	5.0 min
70°F (21.1°C)	4.5 min
75°F (23.8°C)	3.5 min

- At the end of the developing time, remove the hanger from the developer and drain over the rinse tank. Agitate film in rinse water for 30 seconds.
- Place the hanger with film in fixer at the end of the developing time.
- Set the timer. Fixer time equals twice the development time.
- Agitate film every 2–3 minutes while in the fixer.
- At the end of fixation time, remove film from fixer and drain.
- Place the hanger in wash water at the end of fixer time.
- Agitate after 2–3 minutes.
- Wash for 15–30 minutes, depending on water flow and temperature in wash tank.
- Provide no less than four water changes per hour in the wash tank.
- At the end of the wash, remove from water and drain.
- Place film in a drier cabinet or hang up to dry.

Automatic Processing

- Processors are a good investment for most veterinary practices. New, small, tabletop models are priced from $3500. Most of these processors develop an excellent quality film in 90–210 seconds. They can use cold water for processing; therefore, no special needs exist for plumbing. They are also easy to maintain.

▼ *Key Point* If your small animal practice is processing 7 to 10 films a day, consider an automatic processor.

- Advantages
  - Highly repeatable results
  - Short waiting time for diagnostic films
  - Ability to process large quantity of films quickly and accurately
  - Good quality control
  - Smaller darkroom necessary
- Disadvantages
  - Machine is expensive.
  - Darkroom structural changes are expensive.
  - Needs daily and weekly maintenance.
  - Repairs can be expensive.
- Equipment includes processor, safelight, water for processing, chemicals, sponges to clean rollers of processor, and processor cleaning solution.
- Tabletop film processors are easy to install (no special plumbing or wiring). Different models process films as fast as 90 seconds or as long as 3½ minutes. Most are made for easy care and cleaning. They are relatively inexpensive (from $3000–$7000).
- Large, hard-wired, 90-second film processors need special plumbing and electrical wiring, but they are able to process many films. They need special cleaning and repairs and are expensive ($15,000–$25,000).
- The more a processor is used, the fewer problems it will have. It is made to be used on a 24-hour basis. Chemical buildup on rollers can cause film artifacts. Rollers age and crack, if oxidized chemicals are left on them.
- Clean processors often.
  - All processors need cleaning daily when not in use. Take out the rollers and wash down with a sponge and water. Dry and replace rollers. Clean chemical tanks. Once a month, clean with processor cleaning solution. Cleaning a processor takes about 15 minutes a day but saves in wasted film and time.
- Consider purchasing a processor with a standby mechanism. This function helps to conserve water, energy, and chemicals.
- Automatic processor companies are listed in Table 4–4.

Darkroom

Recommendations

- *Darkroom location.* Locate the darkroom close to water and drains for plumbing purposes, and close to radiographic area to reduce unnecessary walking and to increase efficiency.
- *Darkroom layout* (Figs. 4–1 and 4–2). Darkrooms do not have to take up much room but are at least 6 × 8 feet. Many darkrooms are located where a bathroom might have been. This eliminates the process of bringing in new plumbing and electrical outlets. Try to include a sink for cleaning up and processor maintenance. Keep wet and dry areas separate to eliminate contamination of screens and unexposed film by chemicals. Always have good ventilation to keep heat, humidity, and chemical fumes from destroying film and to reduce exposure of personnel to chemical fumes. Paint all walls white to reflect light from the safelights and for a brighter working environ-

Table 4–4. AUTOMATIC PROCESSOR COMPANIES

AFP Imaging Corp. 250 Clearbrook Rd. Elmsford, NY 10523 800-592-6666	JNO. V. Doehren Co. 1450 N. McLean Blvd. Elgin, IL 60123 708-931-0075
Agfa Gavert Corp. 2803 Butterfield Rd. Suite 200 Oak Brook, IL 60521 414-274-9116	Konica Medical Corporation 411 Newark Pompton Turnpike Wayne, NJ 07470 201-633-1500
All Pro Imaging Corp. 70 Cantiague Rock Rd. P.O. Box 870 Hicksville, NY 11802 516-433-7676	Kramex Corp. 481 Sylvan St. Saddlebrook, NJ 07662 201-845-5156
Eastman Kodak Company Health Sciences Division Rochester, NY 14650 800-926-1519	Picker International, Inc. 595 Miner Rd. Highland Heights, OH 44143 216-473-3000
Fischer Industries Inc. 2630 Kaneville Ct. Geneva, IL 60134 708-232-2803	

ment. Use an adequate number and type of safelights. Make sure all the safelights are 40 inches from the working area to prevent film fogging.

TECHNIQUE CHARTS

- Have a working knowledge of equipment (tube rating charts and anode cooling curves). A constant focal film distance is recommended. The same film, screens, and darkroom technique are used, as described previously.
- The technique chart is set up to take radiographs of normal animals. Different animals may have the same lateral thoracic measurement but different body types (obese, emaciated). The emaciated animal may be overexposed with the technique from the chart; therefore, you need to decrease the exposure (kVp). The obese animal may be underexposed following the chart technique; therefore, you have to increase the exposure (kVp).
  - The technique may need to be increased (2–30%) for numerous reasons (e.g., obesity, pregnancy, ascites, pleural effusion, disease processes that increase lung opacity (such as pneumonia and atelectasis) and for positive contrast studies.
  - The technique may need to be decreased (2–30%) for numerous reasons, including emaciation, pneumothorax, emphysema, gastric dilatation, and volvulus.

▼ *Key Point* Always select the shortest possible exposure times. This entails the highest mA value to achieve the shortest exposure times.

Technique Chart (Grid) (Fig. 4–3)
Thorax Grid

1. Use a dog of average size and body condition for all measurements.
2. Take a lateral measurement across the chest at the widest point.
3. Find that measurement on your technique chart.
4. Underneath this lateral measurement, set your kVp at 95—a value in the middle of the ideal kVp parameters for a thorax.
5. Fill out your chart according to the kVp per cm increments.
6. Once the kVp values have been assigned, take three chest films at different mAs values. You may begin with 0.8, 1.6, and 3.2 for a rare earth system, and 5, 10, and 20 mAs for calcium tungstate, for example. Select the mAs value at 95 kVp that provides you with the best technique.

Abdomen Grid

1. Follow the first four steps under Thorax Grid.
2. Set your kVp at 85.
3. Fill out the chart according to the kVp per cm increments.
4. Double the mAs value used in the thorax technique.

Spine Grid

1. Follow the first four steps under Thorax Grid.
2. Set your kVp at 65.
3. Fill out the chart according to the kVp per cm increments.
4. Set the mAs value four times that used for the abdomen. This setting also works for femur, humerus, shoulder, and pelvis.

Technique Chart (Tabletop Without Grid) (Fig. 4–4)
Thorax, Abdomen, and Spine

1. On the grid chart for thorax, abdomen, and spine, find the last kVp setting for 11 cm.
2. Decrease the kVp as the thickness decreases. For example, if 74 kVp is at 11 cm, use 72 kVp at 10 cm, 70 kVp at 9 cm, and so forth.
3. Adjust the mAs by reducing to half (possibly more dependent on type of grid) the mAs value for the base techniques for the thorax, abdomen, and spine. If films are still overexposed, reduce the mAs in half again.

Extremity (see Fig. 4–4)

1. Measure a normal dog carpus. The average is 4–5 cm.
2. Underneath that measurement, set your kVp at 60 (a value in the middle of your ideal kVp parameters for extremities).
3. Fill out the chart, according to the kVp per cm increments.
4. Take films at three different mAs values (0.8, 1.6, and 3.2 with rare earth; and 5, 10, and 20 with cal-

Manual Processing Darkroom Layout

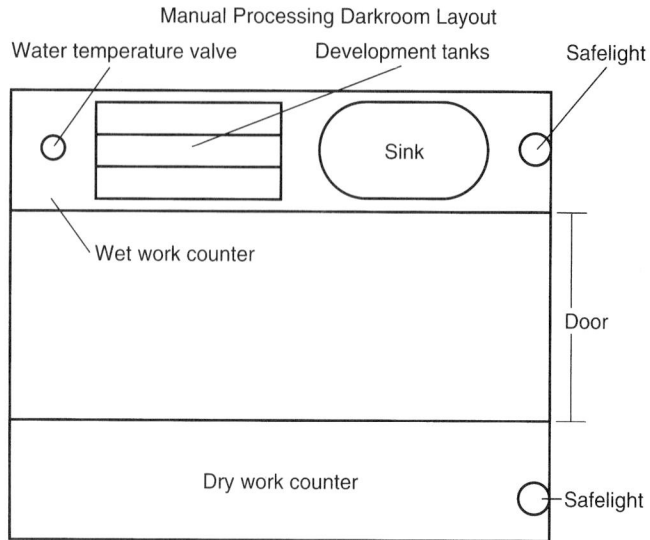

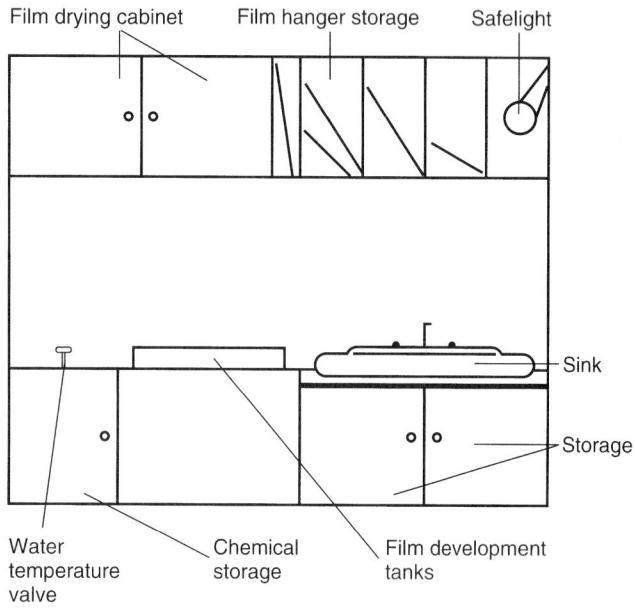

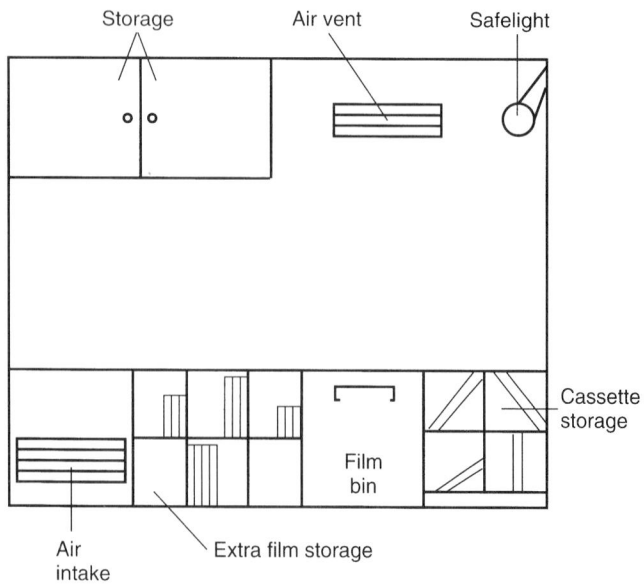

Figure 4–1. Floor plan for a darkroom using manual (wet tank) processing.

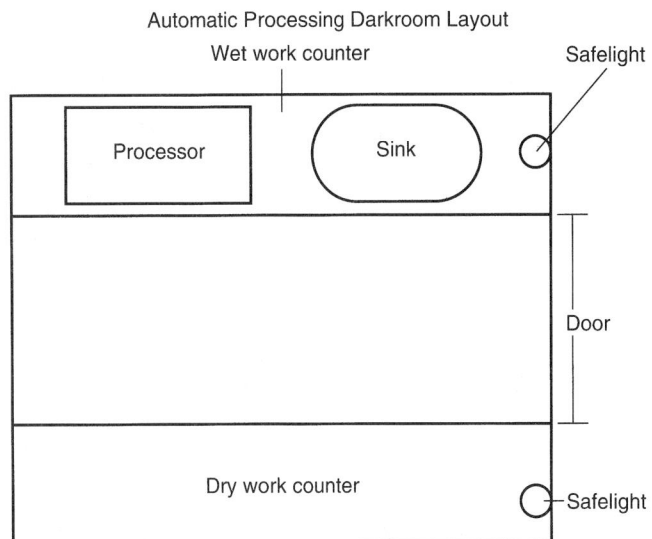

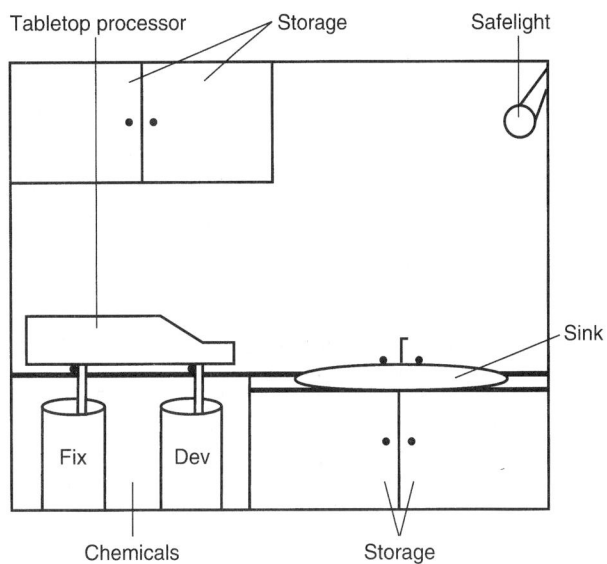

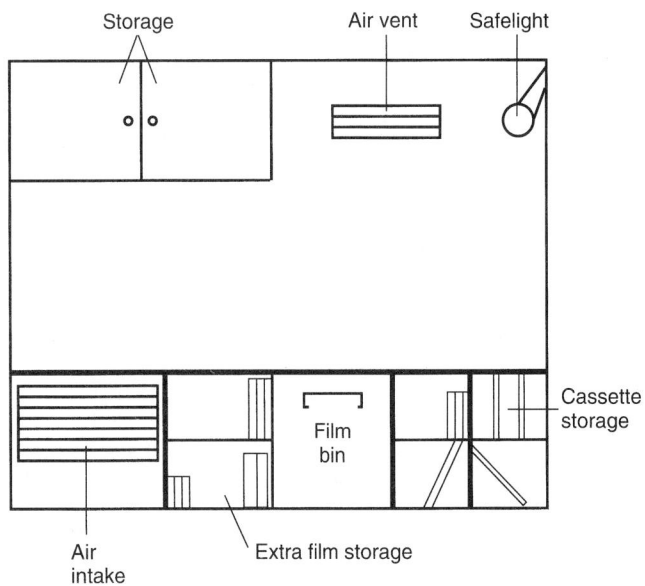

Figure 4–2. Floor plan for a darkroom using automatic processing.

Making a Technique Chart (Grid)

Ideal Parameters	kVp per cm Increments	Appreciable Difference
Thorax — 90 to 100 kVP Abdomen — 80 to 90 kVp Spine Skull — 60 to 80 kVp Pelvis Extremities — 50 to 70 kVp	40 to 80 range = 2 kVp per cm 80 to 100 kVp range = 3 kVp per cm ≥100 kVp = 4 kVp per cm **Chart Factors** Thorax___mAs___kVp base technique Abdomen - 2 X thoracic mAs, minus 10 kVp Spine - 4X abdomen mAs, minus 20 kVp	Amount of kVp change necessary to see a change in technique per kVp range 40 - 60 kVp = 2 - 4 kVp 60 - 80 kVp = 4 - 6 kVp 80 - 100 kVp = 6 - 8 kVp ≥100 kVp = 10 - 12 kVp

Thorax

11	12	13	14	15	16	17	18	19	20	21	22	23	24	25	26	27	28	29	30	cm
																				kVp
																				mAs

Abdomen

11	12	13	14	15	16	17	18	19	20	21	22	23	24	25	26	27	28	29	30	cm
																					kVp
																					mAs

**Spine
Skull
Pelvis**

11	12	13	14	15	16	17	18	19	20	21	22	23	24	25	26	27	28	29	30	cm
																					kVp
																					mAs

Figure 4–3. Technique chart to use with a grid.

cium tungstate). Continue selecting mAs values until an appropriate exposure has been made. Your table-top extremity chart is now complete. Employ this chart for all extremities distal to and including the elbow and stifle.

Nonscreen Film Technique Chart (Fig. 4–5)

- For the nonscreen film technique chart, the mAs in your technique chart may vary up or down from the example shown in Figure 4–5.

Figure 4–4. Technique chart. For tabletop exposures, take the Buckey grid technique and reduce mAs by 50–75%. Continue kVp down from Buckey chart.

POSITIONING AND TECHNIQUE

Measuring for Radiographic Studies

- Measure all animals standing.
- Measurements for thorax, abdomen, and thoracolumbar spine are all taken at the same place on the animal. Observe the back of the animal from above, looking for the widest point across the ribs and take a lateral measurement. The DV/VD measurement is

Table Top Technique Chart
(Without Grid)

Thorax ___ mAs

1	2	3	4	5	6	7	8	9	10	cm
										kVp

Abdomen ___ mAs

1	2	3	4	5	6	7	8	9	10	cm
										kVp

Spine
Skull
Pelvis ___ mAs

1	2	3	4	5	6	7	8	9	10	cm
										kVp

Extremities ___ mAs

1	2	3	4	5	6	7	8	9	10	cm
										kVp

Nasal, Dental, and High Detail Studies

Figure 4–5. Technique chart to use with non-screen film. Use a lateral measurement across the skull to set technique. Always use 50 kVp for the best contrast.

1	2	3	4	5	6	7	8	9	10	11	cm
50	100	125	150	200	250	300	350	400	450	500	mAs

made at the same point. The widest point is usually over the thoracolumbar junction.

- Measure the pelvis across the wings of the ilium. This is a very accessible area to measure, giving highly repeatable results.
- Measure extremities at the widest point.
- Make sure all personnel measure all areas at the same point, or the technique will vary from one study to the next.

Thorax

Obtain thoracic films at full inspiration. Include from the diaphragm to the thoracic inlet. In a large dog, this may take two radiographs for both lateral and DV/VD views. Short exposure times of ⅟60 second or less compensate for cardiac and respiratory motion. High kVp, low mAs technique increases latitude (increased shades of gray).

- For the lateral (right or left) measurement, elevate the sternum to the same plane as the spine. Pull the animal's legs cranially to reduce soft tissue over the cranial thorax. Include the sternum, and take the radiograph during peak inspiration (Fig. 4–6).
- For the DV/VD view, the sternum is superimposed over the spine. Center the beam at the caudal border of the scapula; center the beam on the spine. Take the radiograph during peak inspiration. VD radiographs are preferable to DV for evaluation of the accessory lung lobe and the caudal mediastinum. DV radiographs are preferred if evaluation of the caudal pulmonary vessels is important. The dog's disposition, clinical status (e.g., heart failure, pulmonary edema, pleural effusion), or position of previous radiographs help choose between VD and DV thoracic radiographs (Fig. 4–7).

- Take both right and left lateral views of the thorax with a VD/DV view to evaluate for pulmonary metastases or nongeneralized disease.

Abdomen

Withhold food for at least 12 hours for optimal abdominal radiographs. Encourage the animal to defecate and urinate before being radiographed. Radiographs include the diaphragm to the pelvic canal, and for large breed dogs, this may require two 14 × 17 inch films, for both the lateral and VD/DV views. Measure over the widest portion of the abdomen (costal arch). Use ⅟40 second or less exposure time to reduce motion; use a kVp in the 70–90 range for maximum latitude.

- For a lateral (right or left) radiograph, pull the legs caudally but not enough to stretch the abdominal musculature taut. Place the edge of the cassette 1–2 inches cranial to the xiphoid and the cranial edge of the acetabulum. Palpate the greater trochanter. Take the radiograph at peak expiration (Fig. 4–8).
- The VD/DV is the same as that for the lateral abdomen (Fig. 4–9).
- Use the horizontal beam to check for free abdominal air. Place the animal in left lateral recumbency for 10 minutes before radiography. Air is demonstrated around the right liver lobes. The technique is similar to the vertical beam technique in that distance remains at 40 inches. Remember to reduce the mAs if a grid is not used.

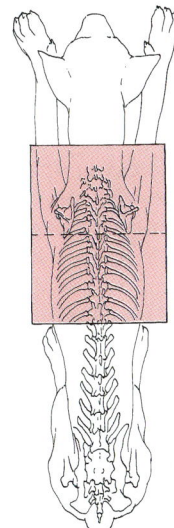

Figure 4–6. Positioning for lateral thoracic radiograph.

Center beam over caudal scapula

Sternum

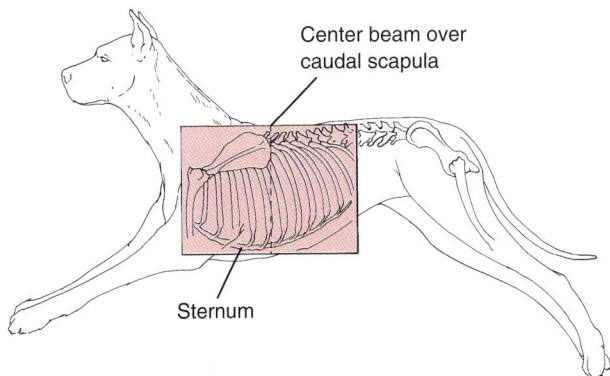

Figure 4–7. Positioning for dorsoventral (DV) or ventrodorsal (VD) thoracic radiograph.

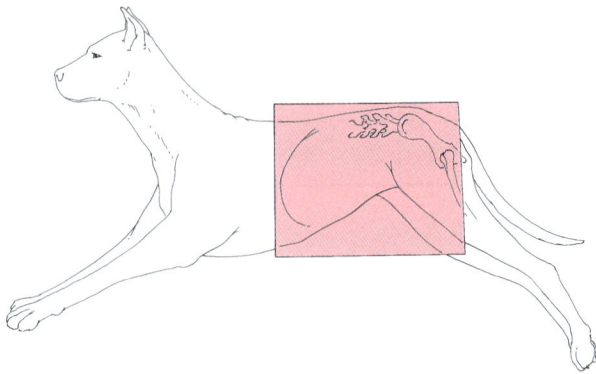

Figure 4–8. Positioning for lateral abdominal radiograph.

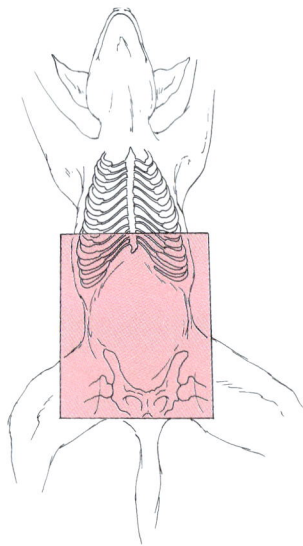

Figure 4–9. Positioning for ventrodorsal (VD) abdominal radiograph.

- A wooden spoon can be used to compress the abdomen for separation of structures. The spoon can separate the colon from the urinary bladder to demonstrate the uterus, for example. Remember to reduce the kVp, because you are decreasing the thickness of the tissue being radiographed.

Extremities

For radiography of the extremities, the animal needs a clean, dry haircoat. Remove splints and bandages if possible. Place the limb to be radiographed closest to the film. Employ a high mAs and low kVp (50–70) technique to produce high-contrast radiographs. Collimate closely. Use tabletop (nongrid) techniques on parts less than 10 cm thick. Administer anesthesia or tranquilizers whenever possible. Use positioning devices. Measure the part to be radiographed over the thickest area. If the part thickness varies greatly, two exposures (e.g., lateral pelvis and femur) may be necessary. In the case of moderate variation, choose the greater measurement to set the exposure and "hot light" the slightly overexposed areas when reading the film. When long bones are being radiographed, include the joints proximal and distal.

▼ *Key Point* Never hesitate to make a film of the opposite limb for comparison.

Scapula and Shoulder Joint

Caudocranial. The animal is in dorsal recumbency, with the sternum rotated away from the side being radiographed. The leg is fully extended. Center the x-ray beam at the mid-scapula. For the shoulder joint, center the beam at the point of flexion for the joint.

Mediolateral (ML). The animal is in lateral recumbency, with the down side to be radiographed. Extend the leg about 45° from the vertebral column. Flex the opposite leg and place over the thorax. Pull the head and neck back so that the cervical spine and trachea are not overlapping the joint space.

Humerus

Caudocranial. The animal is in dorsal recumbency, with the legs extended. Rotate the sternum away from the side being radiographed. Center the x-ray beam at the mid-humerus. The radiograph includes both the shoulder and elbow joints.

Mediolateral. Place the animal in a position similar to that for the ML view of the scapula and the shoulder joint. Center the x-ray beam at the mid-humerus. The radiograph includes both the shoulder and elbow joints.

Elbow Joint

Craniocaudal. The animal is in sternal recumbency, with the elbow joint in full extension. If the elbow cannot be completely extended, angle the x-ray beam 10° to 20°, craniodistal to caudoproximal.

Mediolateral. The animal is in lateral recumbency, with the elbow slightly flexed. Pull the opposite leg caudally. Center the beam on the palpable medial epicondyle. The elbow is in extreme flexion, if identification of the anconeal process is of importance.

Craniolateral-Caudomedial Oblique. This aids in imaging of the lateral aspect of the medial coronoid.

Antebrachium

Craniocaudal. Place the animal in sternal recumbency. Extend the leg and position the elbow for a true craniocaudal projection. The film includes both elbow and carpus.

Mediolateral. The animal is in lateral recumbency, with the leg in the neutral position. Move the opposite limb caudally; center the beam on the midshaft radius. It may be easier to obtain the radiograph if the elbow is slightly flexed. Include the elbow and carpal joint on the film.

Carpus/Metacarpus

Dorsopalmar (DP). By convention, positional terms change from cranial and caudal to dorsal and palmar distal to the radius. Place the animal in sternal recumbency, with the extremity extended. Allow the elbow to abduct slightly so that the carpus is in true DP view. Center the x-ray beam on the carpus or metacarpus.

Mediolateral. Place the animal in lateral recumbency, with the affected leg down. Slightly flex the carpus; center the x-ray beam on the carpus. A lateral view of the metacarpus is often unrewarding.

Oblique Views. Place the animal in sternal recumbency, with the carpus/metacarpus in DP. Rotate the extremity 45° in both directions for the two oblique views (dorsolateral to palmar medial oblique and dorsomedial to palmar lateral oblique).

Digits

Dorsopalmar. Place the paw flat against the cassette.

Mediolateral. Place the animal in lateral recumbency. Pull the specific digit to be examined dorsally with tape.

Pelvis

Tranquilization may be necessary for routine VD and lateral radiographs. General anesthesia is recommended for Orthopedic Foundation for Animals (OFA) or Penn-Hip hip dysplasia films.

Ventrodorsal Extended Hip. The animal is in dorsal recumbency, with the legs extended. The pelvis is straight; the femurs are parallel and as close to the cassette as possible. Patellae are superimposed over the distal femurs. Center the x-ray beam on the hip joints. Include the stifles on the radiographs. Legs are the same distance apart as the acetabula.

Lateral. The animal is in lateral recumbency, with the dependent leg pulled cranially. Elevate the nondependent leg with a foam block parallel to the tabletop.

Lateral Oblique. Place the animal in lateral recumbency. Place a foam wedge to elevate the dorsal aspect of the pelvis approximately 20°. Push the upper leg proximally to rotate.

Ventrodorsal Flexed Hip (Frogleg Position). Place the animal in dorsal recumbency, and flex and abduct the femurs so that the stifles are lateral to the abdomen. Place the femurs at an angle of 45° to the spine.

Femur

Craniocaudal. Place the animal in dorsal recumbency or in the erect sitting position, with the leg extended. Center the x-ray beam at mid-femur. Include the hip and stifle on the radiograph. Measure at the proximal femur.

Mediolateral. Place the animal in lateral recumbency with the leg to be examined on the cassette. Abduct the opposite leg and rotate out of the x-ray beam's path. Center the x-ray beam at mid-femur. Include the hip and stifle on the film.

Stifle

Caudocranial. Place the animal in ventral recumbency with the leg to be examined pulled caudally into maximum extension. In large dogs, angle the x-ray beam 15° caudodistal to cranioproximal. Center the x-ray beam at the joint space.

Mediolateral. Position the animal as for the mediolateral femur view, with the x-ray beam centered on the joint space. Usually, the tarsus is away from the cassette so you need to place a foam wedge under the hip and femur.

Tibia/Fibula

Caudocranial. Position the animal as for the caudocranial stifle view. The x-ray beam remains vertical and centered at the mid-tibia. Include stifle and tarsus on the film.

Mediolateral. Place the animal in lateral recumbency with the tibia and fibula included on the film.

Tarsus

Dorsoplantar. Place the animal in dorsal recumbency. Extend the leg, and center the x-ray beam at the proximal intertarsal joint.

Mediolateral. Place the patient in lateral recumbency. Slightly flex the tarsocrural joint. Center the x-ray beam at the proximal intertarsal joint.

Oblique (45°). Dorsolateral to palmar medial oblique (DLPMO) and dorsomedial to palmar lateral (DMPLO) oblique. Position the animal in dorsal recumbency, then rotate 45° in each direction (lateral and medial) for the two oblique views.

Metatarsus/Digits

Position the animal as for the metacarpus and digits of the forelimbs.

Spinal Positioning and Technique—General Principles

- Materials needed include sandbags, foam wedges, markers (right and left), and a Plexiglas trough to aid in positioning the animal without anyone in the room.
- Use general anesthesia or heavy sedation in all but the most subdued animals. Exceptions are suspected fracture, congenital malformation with instability, and other diseases in which the animal's condition or protective mechanisms that have maintained stability will be compromised.
- Short-scale, high-contrast (high mAs, low kVp) technique provides good detail. Use a grid and collimate to include only the spine.
- At least two radiographic views of the area of interest are needed: lateral and ventrodorsal. Specific situations occur in which the VD projection in the noncontrast study provides the most useful view for the diagnosis. These include (1) a productive or destructive lesion that involves the transverse vertebral process of the lumbar segments or the costovertebral articulations; (2) a destructive process that involves the dorsal articular processes caudal to the anticlinal vertebral segment; (3) a malalignment characterized by lateral shifting of the vertebral segments; and (4) a rotation of the vertebral segments that is easier to detect on the VD view because of the abnormal appearance of the prominent oval shadow cast by the dorsal spinous process.

Table 4–5. SPINAL SURVEY STUDIES

	Centering	
Study	Lateral	Ventrodorsal
Cervical spine	C3-4	C3-4
	C6–T1	(X-ray beam angled 15° ventrocaudal to dorsocranial)
Occipitoatlantoaxial	C1	C1
(Rostrocaudal open mouth	C1 flexion	
to visualize the dens)	C1 oblique	
Thoracic spine	T6-7	T6-7
Thoracolumbar spine	T6-7	T6-7
	T12-13	T12-13
	L3-4	L3-4
Lumbar spine	L3-4	L3-4
	LS	
Lumbosacral spine	LS flexion	LS
	LS extension	
Post-trauma	Center on area of suspected lesion	Cross-table–horizontal beam
		Center on area of suspected lesion

LS, lumbosacral.

- In the average-size dog, five vertebral segments can be adequately evaluated per film. Because of the divergence of the x-ray beam, all areas of interest have to be centered to evaluate intervertebral disc spaces.

▼ *Key Point* Poor patient positioning and poor radiographic quality commonly occur when animals are not anesthetized or heavily sedated for spinal films. Many radiographic lesions can be obscured by poor technique. Conversely, a normal structure can be falsely identified as a lesion.

- Ideal spinal survey studies are listed in Table 4–5.

Cervical Spine

Cervical Spine, Lateral View. For radiography, the spine must be parallel to the cassette. In many cases, support the center of the neck with radiolucent positioning blocks (sponges). Place the head in a normal position (neither flexed nor extended) relative to the neck. The head must be lateral because it controls the position of the proximal neck. Pull the front legs back over the thorax to allow thinning of the tissues over the caudal neck. The thorax must be in the accurate lateral position because it controls the position of the caudal neck. Extending the entire neck may help open up the caudal cervical disc spaces. Include both occipital and cervicothoracic areas on the radiograph.

Ventrodorsal View. The spine is not parallel to the cassette because of the anatomic variation between the head and thorax. The spine inclines away from the cassette at the thorax. Place the head in normal position (hard palate and dorsal nose at 60° angle to the cassette). If the head is in a true VD position, an undesirable arch is produced in the cervical spine. The midplane of the head and thorax must be perpendicular to the cassette. Tilting the x-ray tube ventrocaudal to dor-

socranial at approximately 10° to 20° permits imaging of the intervertebral disc spaces.

Thoracolumbar Spine

Thoracolumbar Spine, Lateral View. The midplane of the entire body must be parallel to the cassette. Most animals must have the sternum elevated for good lateral views of the spine. Pull the front legs cranially and the rear legs caudally to straighten the spine. Extending the entire neck may help open up the cranial thoracic disc spaces.

Ventrodorsal View. The midplane of the entire spine must be perpendicular to the cassette. When the dorsal spines are prominent as in thin animals, radiolucent positioning blocks may be beneficial. The body may be held by placing tension on the legs.

Skull Radiograph

- General anesthesia or deep tranquilization of the patient is essential, if not specifically contraindicated by the patient's physical condition, in order to obtain radiographs of good diagnostic quality.

▼ *Key Point* The lack of proper patient restraint is the most common cause of skull radiographs of nondiagnostic quality.

- The highest resolution (detail) radiographic image of the skull is produced with a nonscreen film or an ultradetail film/screen combination. Nonscreen film necessitates a 10- to 20-fold increase in mAs compared with film in par speed screen cassettes.
- The positioning of the patient and the number of projections needed for a complete study depend upon the area of the skull being evaluated. A minimum of two views is necessary.

Routine Skull. Lateral and DV views are used.

Nasal Cavity and Paranasal Sinuses. Lateral, DV occlusal (Fig. 4–10); VD open mouth (Fig. 4–11) (extraoral film); frontal (primary beam parallel to the hard palate) (Fig. 4–12); and lateral oblique (Fig. 4–13) (right and left) to evaluate small frontal sinuses.

Dental Arches. Maxillary—right and left lateral obliques (20° to 30°) (Fig. 4–14); VD open mouth (extraoral film); and DV occlusal. Mandibular—right and left lateral oblique (20° to 30°) open mouth (Fig. 4–15); and VD occlusal (Fig. 4–16).

Bisecting Angle Technique. Project the central beam perpendicular to an imaginary plane that bisects the angle formed by the long axis of the tooth (or teeth) and the plane of the film (Fig. 4–17).

Tympanic Bullae (Middle Ears). DV; open mouth frontal. The primary beam bisects the angle of the opened temporomandibular joint (TMJ) (Fig. 4–18); lateral oblique (Fig. 4–19) (30° by 30°) right and left. Palpate the jugular processes; when these processes are oblique, the bullae will also be properly oblique.

Foramen Magnum. Rostrodorsal-caudoventral oblique (fronto-occipital). The central beam passes between the eyes and exits through the foramen magnum (Fig. 4–20).

Temporomandibular Joint. DV, open mouth frontal (see Fig. 4–18). The primary beam bisects the angle of the opened TMJ; lateral oblique (20° to 30°) right and left (see Fig. 4–13).

Mandible. DV, lateral, and lateral oblique (right and left).

Maxilla. DV occlusal, VD open mouth, lateral, and lateral oblique (right and left).

Zygomatic Bone and Orbit. DV, lateral, lateral obliques (right and left), frontal, and VD open mouth.

CONTRAST STUDIES

Contrast Medium

- Positive contrast medium—iodine (ionic, nonionic), barium (liquid, paste) (Table 4–6).
- Negative contrast medium—room air, CO_2, nitrous oxide.

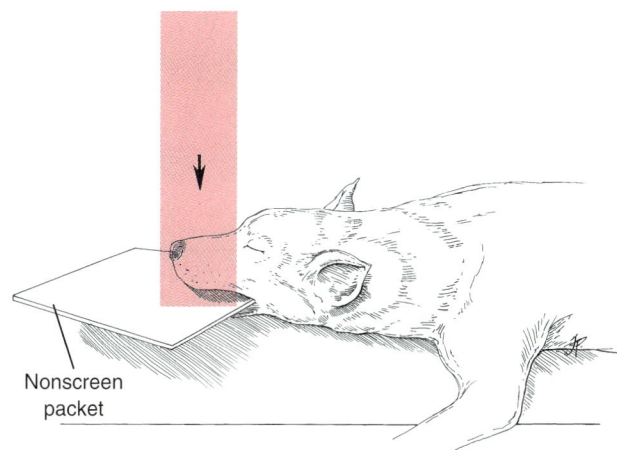

Figure 4–10. Positioning for dorsoventral (DV) occlusal (intraoral) radiograph of the skull.

Nonscreen packet

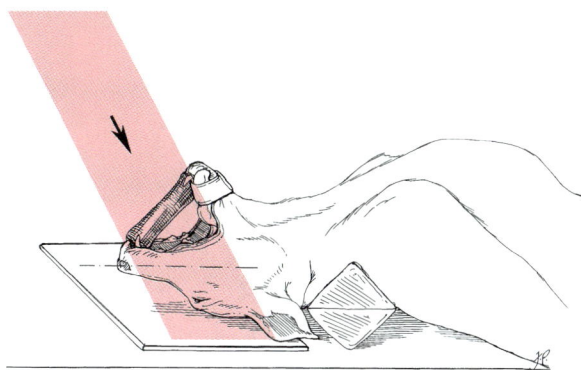

Figure 4–11. Positioning for the ventrodorsal (20° to 30° tube angle), open-mouth view of the skull.

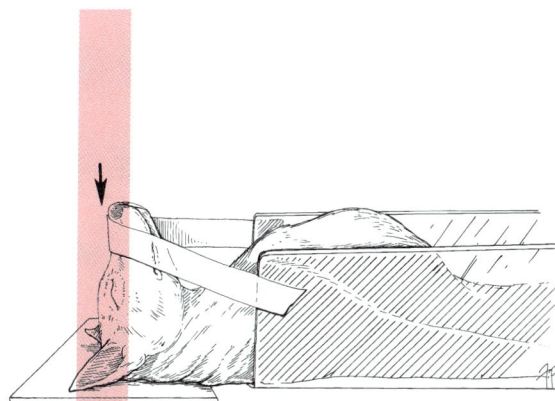

Figure 4–12. Positioning for the rostrocaudal (frontal) view of the skull.

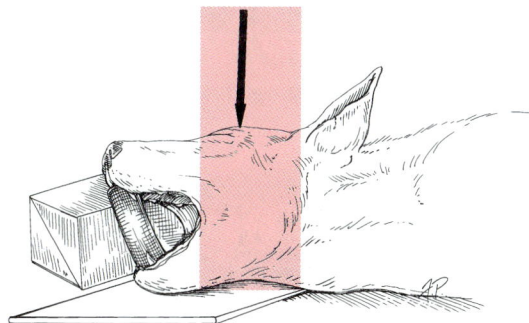

Figure 4–13. Positioning for the open-mouth lateral oblique (20° to 30°) view of the frontal sinuses.

Excretory Urogram/Intravenous Pyelogram/Intravenous Urogram

- A well-prepared animal is important for this contrast study (excretory urogram [EU], intravenous pyelogram [IVP], and intravenous urogram [IVU] are synonymous terms). Withhold food for 12–24 hours. Give enemas the night before and at least 2 hours before the study. Determine renal function (blood urea nitrogen and serum creatinine) before initiating the study.

▼ *Key Point* Always take scout films before doing contrast studies of the urinary tract.

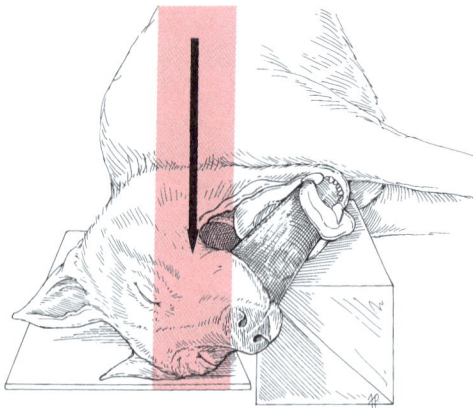

Figure 4–14. Positioning for the open-mouth lateral oblique (20° to 30°) view of the maxilla.

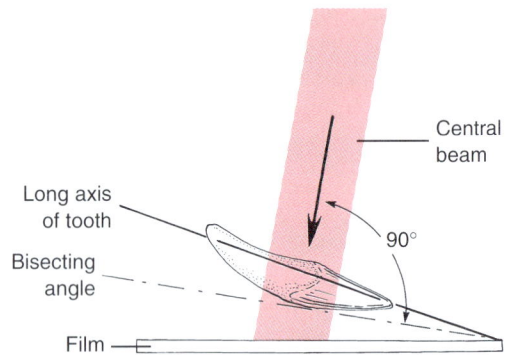

Figure 4–17. Bisecting angle technique for radiographing the teeth.

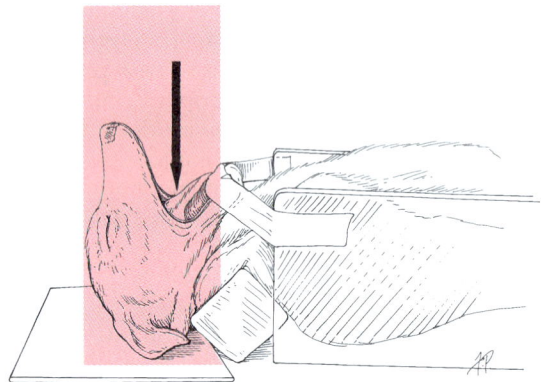

Figure 4–15. Positioning for the open-mouth lateral oblique (20° to 30°) view of the mandible.

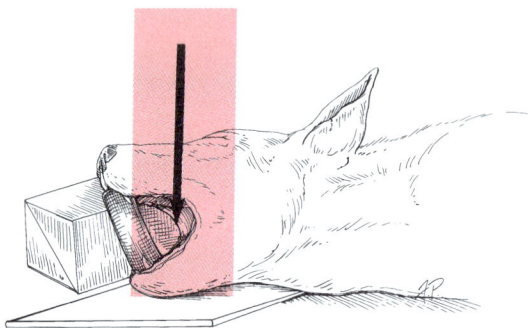

Figure 4–18. Positioning for the open-mouth rostrocaudal (basilar) view.

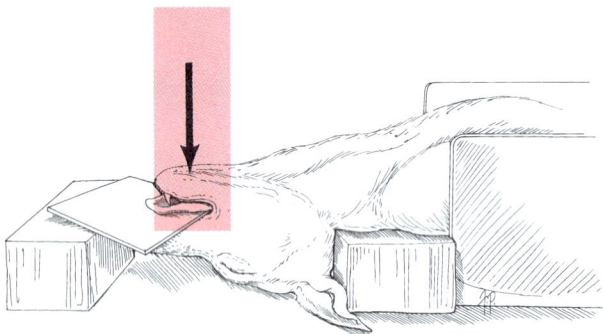

Figure 4–16. Positioning for the ventrodorsal (VD) occlusal (intraoral) view of the mandible.

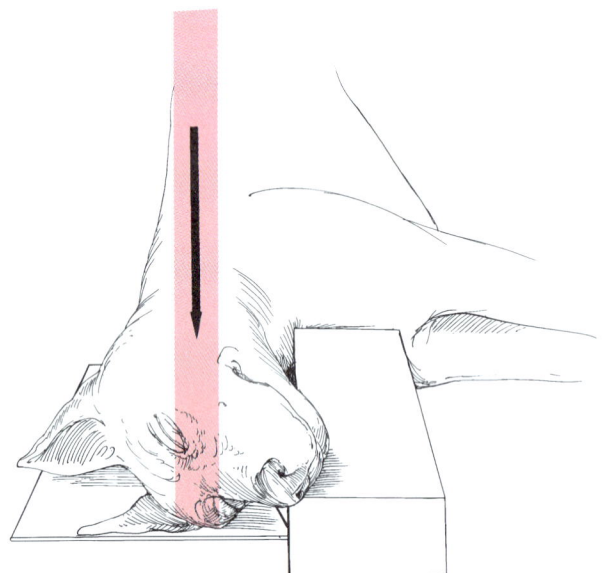

Figure 4–19. Positioning for the lateral oblique (30° nose elevated, then 30° oblique) view of tympanic bullae.

- The primary contraindication in animals is dehydration. Contrast medium is hypertonic and will compromise an already unstable patient. Make sure the patient is properly hydrated prior to EU. Contraindicated in people with diabetes mellitus, multiple myeloma, heart failure, and known hypersensitivity to the contrast medium.
- Use water-soluble, iodinated ionic contrast media (Renografin, Conray, Hypaque, Renovist). Dosage is 2 ml/kg IV (approximately 300–400 mg/ml iodine), not to exceed 90 ml or 35 g of iodine. For animals with impaired renal function, the dosage may need to be doubled (4 ml/kg). Place an indwelling catheter, to help avoid perivascular injections, and to allow IV access if complications occur. Give bolus as fast as possible.
- Increase radiographic technique 5–10% over scout films. Keep the kVp at approximately 70 to produce

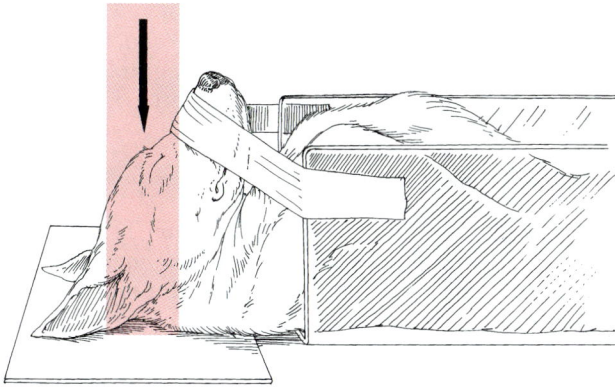

Figure 4–20. Positioning for the rostrodorsal-caudoventral (fronto-occipital) view of the skull.

better differentiation between kidney and contrast medium.

Technique

1. Immediate postinjection VD film demonstrates nephrographic phase.
2. VD/lateral films at 5 minutes.
3. In some cases, if there is poor filling of the renal pelvis, at 10–20 minutes following contrast administration, place an abdominal wrap between the blad-

der and kidney to compress the ureters, causing the pelvis and diverticula of the kidney to completely distend for better evaluation. This is contraindicated in cases of severely diseased bladder walls or mass lesions, in which it may cause rupture.

4. VD/lateral films at 15 minutes. for evaluation of the pyelographic stage.
5. VD/lateral films at 30 minutes.
6. Remove the compression wrap and take lateral and VD radiographs.
7. Modify this technique as needed for the suspected disease entity. For example, to evaluate for ectopic ureters, take oblique films at 15–20 minutes. A pneumocystogram may also be helpful for identifying the distal ureters and vesicoureteral junctions.

- Complications include perivascular injection, which can be treated by instillation of saline into tissues to dilute; nausea/vomiting; adverse systemic (anaphylactoid) reaction; and contrast-induced renal failure. The study may be nondiagnostic when the kidneys become bright (contrast enhanced) and remain that way, but there is no opacification of the collecting system, ureters, or bladder. Be careful in VD positioning to avoid aspiration.

Cystography

- Equipment
  - Contrast medium: For negative contrast, use nitrous oxide, room air, or CO_2; for positive contrast, use water-soluble iodinated ionic contrast medium (not barium).
  - Catheters: Foley, tom cat, male dog, or metal female catheters
  - Sterile lubricant gel
  - Three-way stopcock
- Contrast studies
  - Negative-contrast cystogram (pneumocystogram)
  - Positive-contrast cystogram (technique of choice for identifying urinary bladder location and tears)
  - Double-contrast cystogram (superior for demonstrating lesions involving the urinary bladder wall and intraluminal filling defects)

Technique

1. Withhold food for 12–24 hours.
2. Administer warm-water cleansing enemas the night before and 3–4 hours before the procedure.
3. Sedation or tranquilization may be necessary for catheterization, especially in cats and female dogs.
4. A small amount of lidocaine (1 ml mixed with 2 ml of sterile saline) infused into the urinary bladder before the contrast agent may reduce urinary bladder spasm.
5. Place the catheter tip within the bladder neck.
6. Empty the urinary bladder.
7. Infuse the contrast medium (1–7 ml, depending on animal's size), rotate the patient, and massage the bladder to distribute contrast medium and coat entire mucosal surface.
8. Slowly infuse negative-contrast material. Complete distention is desirable and can be judged by palpa-

---

Table 4–6. RADIOGRAPHIC CONTRAST AGENTS

Barium Product	
Brand Names	**Manufacturers**
Esophotrast (barium paste)	Barnes-Hind Barium Products (Sunnyvale, CA)
E-Z-Paste (esophageal cream)	E-Z-EM, Inc. (Westbury, NY)
Barosperse (esophageal cream)	Mallinckrodt (St. Louis, MO)
Liqui-Jug (barium suspension)	E-Z-EM, Inc. (Westbury, NY)
Liquid Polibar (barium suspension)	E-Z-EM, Inc. (Westbury, NY)
E-Z-Jug (barium suspension)	E-Z-EM, Inc. (Westbury, NY)
Novopaque	Lafayette Pharmacal (Lafayette, IN)

Iodinated Gastrointestinal Contrast Agent	
Gastrografin	Squibb Diagnostics (New Brunswick, NJ)
Omnipaque (iohexol)	Winthrop Labs (New York, NY)

Iodinated Contrast Agent	
Renovist, Renovist II, Renografin 60 or 76	Squibb Diagnostics (New Brunswick, NJ)
Hypaque-M 75% or 90%	Winthrop Labs (New York, NY)
Conray, Conray 30 or 400	Mallinckrodt (St. Louis, MO)

Myelographic Contrast Agent	
Omnipaque (iohexol)	Winthrop Labs (New York, NY)
Isovue (iopamidol)	Squibb Diagnostics (New Brunswick, NJ)

tion, back pressure felt on syringe plunger, or reflux of gas around catheter.

9. Use scout film technique for negative-contrast study and increase technique by 10% for positive-contrast study.
10. Take a lateral, two lateral obliques, and a VD radiograph to examine the bladder full on double-contrast cystograms. Only lateral and VD views are necessary for positive-contrast cystograms.
11. Evacuate contrast material from the bladder after the study.

- Complications
  - Fatal air embolism (rare cases). An increased risk exists with ulcerative or erosive cystitis. CO_2 is more soluble than room air in blood and thus less likely to cause this problem. Air embolism occurs immediately after the administration of negative-contrast medium. Place the animal in left lateral recumbency, and lower the head to maintain normal blood circulation through the heart. The air is trapped in the right ventricle.
  - Iatrogenic trauma (hematuria, bacterial contamination, cystitis, rupture)

Urethrography

- Retrograde positive-contrast study of the urethra using iodine.
- Equipment includes catheter (Foley, metal, male dog), sterile gel, lidocaine, and water-soluble iodinated contrast medium.

Technique

1. Evacuate the colon with an enema prior to the study; take scout films before the study to evaluate technique and preparation.
2. Pass a urinary catheter into the distal urethra. Inflate the balloon if a Foley catheter is used (in distal urethra for female dogs or cats and just proximal to the os penis in male dogs when possible).
3. Administer 2–5 ml of lidocaine before injecting contrast material to reduce urethral spasm.
4. Position male dogs with their legs drawn cranially.
5. Administer 10–20 ml contrast medium for male dogs and 5–10 ml for female dogs and cats. Inject as a bolus and take radiographs during the last few milliliters of injection.
6. A lateral radiograph may be sufficient, but subsequent lateral and VD oblique views may be helpful.

- Complications include iatrogenic trauma and bacterial contamination.

Esophagography

Technique

1. Take survey cervical and thoracic radiographs.
2. Position animal in lateral recumbency.
3. Administer contrast medium (see Table 4–6) (barium sulfate suspension, Esophotrast, barium burger) slowly into the buccal pouch.
4. Dose is variable (5–20 ml); use enough to induce swallowing and coat esophagus.

5. Obtain radiographs following swallows. The lateral view is most informative; a right ventral oblique view may also be helpful. Follow-up radiographs may be helpful if a bolus of contrast material is retained within the esophagus.

- Complications
  - Aspiration
  - Leakage of barium into mediastinum. Low osmolality, nonionic iodinated contrast medium (iohexol) may be indicated if perforation is suspected.

Gastrography

▼ **Key Point** Prior to contrast studies of the gastrointestinal tract, discontinue all drugs that may influence motility.

Technique

1. Fast patient 12–24 hours before the study.
2. Give cleansing enema the night before and 3–4 hours before the study, especially if complete upper gastrointestinal study is to be done.
3. Take plain films prior to the study. Then pass a stomach tube for administration of contrast medium.
4. Obtain negative-contrast gastrogram (pneumogastrogram) by administering 6–16 ml of room air per kg body weight via stomach tube. Immediately take four views (right and left lateral, VD, and DV). This is often valuable in the diagnosis of radiolucent foreign bodies.
5. Obtain positive-contrast gastrogram using barium (suspension, 30% weight/volume) at a dose of 6–12 ml/kg (see Table 4–6). Administer via a stomach tube, and take films immediately (right and left lateral, VD, and DV). Use this procedure to document gastric displacement, certain gastric foreign bodies, and gastric perforation. Barium begins leaving the stomach within 5–15 minutes. The stomach is emptied by 30–60 minutes in cats and 1–2 hours in dogs.
6. A double-contrast gastrogram can be done as a separate study or during an upper gastrointestinal study. Give barium, 60% weight/volume at a dose of 1.5–3 ml/kg, and insufflate with room air at 10 ml/kg. Immediately take DV, VD, and right and left lateral films. This study is indicated in cases of suspected gastric wall and mucosal lesions.

Upper Gastrointestinal Study

- Contrast medium
  - Use barium suspension, 30–60% weight/volume, for routine studies (see Table 4–6). Dose is 8–16 ml/kg.
  - Use iodinated contrast (ionic and nonionic) agents (see Table 4–6) with suspected perforation, for quick determination of small intestine patency and location, and when endoscopy is planned immediately following the contrast study.
- For restraint in canines use acepromazine and in felines use ketamine/acepromazine preparations. See

Chapter 2 for dosages. These sedatives have less effect on motility than do many others.

- Preparation requires a 12–24 hour fast, and an enema the night before and 3–4 hours before the study.

Technique

1. Take survey radiographs (right lateral [RL] and VD).
2. Immediately after administration of barium take right and left lateral and DV and VD views. Obtain right lateral and VD radiographs at 15, 30, and 60 minutes. Be consistent unless a lesion is identified that is better evaluated by repositioning the animal. Then, proceed at hourly intervals until the contrast material reaches the colon.
3. Modify this protocol for each individual depending on the suspected disease entity or the lesions visualized during the procedure.
4. Expected transit time to the colon is 3–4 hours for dogs and 1 hour for cats.

- Complications
  - Aspiration of barium with or without gastric contents.
  - Leakage of barium indicates a gastrointestinal (GI) perforation, which is a surgical emergency. Barium itself induces a chemical peritonitis that may make treatment of GI perforation more difficult.

▼ *Key Point* Whenever GI perforation is suspected, use nonionic iodinated contrast medium (e.g., iohexol) instead of barium.

Myelography

- Myelography is the radiographic evaluation of the spinal cord by injection of a positive-contrast agent into the subarachnoid space.
- Indications
  - To evaluate transverse myelopathy.
  - To determine nature, location, and extent of a lesion prior to surgery.
  - To identify multiple lesions when one lesion might be masked by another and therefore not detected clinically.
- Contraindications
  - Diffuse myelopathy that is not amenable to surgery.
  - Meningitis, which may be aggravated by contrast medium.
  - Myelography is not indicated when survey radiographs and clinical signs are adequate for diagnosis.
- Contrast medium (see Table 4–6).
  - Dose for cisternal tap—cervical study (0.2–0.3 ml/kg); thoracolumbar study (0.45 ml/kg).
  - Dose for lumbar tap—cervical study (0.45 ml/kg); thoracolumbar study (0.3 ml/kg).

▼ *Key Point* Always obtain survey spinal radiographs prior to myelography.

Basic Technique

1. Give general anesthesia.
2. Perform sterile preparation of the puncture site.
3. Take cerebrospinal fluid (CSF) collection and analysis, if deemed necessary.

Cisternal Tap Procedure

1. Position the animal in lateral recumbency.
2. Place the nose parallel to the tabletop and perpendicular to the spine.
3. Use a 20- or 22-gauge, 1.5–2.5 inch spinal needle with the bevel directed caudally.
4. Insert the needle on the dorsal midline, between the occipital protuberance and wings of the atlas.
5. Direct the needle toward the mandible.
6. If the needle hits bone, move the needle cranially or caudally until it falls into the atlanto-occipital (AO) space.
7. Remove the stylet and check for CSF flow often while advancing the needle.
8. Inject contrast material slowly after seeing CSF in the needle. Prior to injection, collect a specimen if CSF for later analysis is indicated.
9. Elevate the head for 5 minutes before taking radiographs.
10. Take lateral and VD radiographs (also VD oblique if necessary). Remove the endotracheal tube, if necessary, for the VD radiograph.

Lumbar Tap Procedure

1. Position the animal in lateral or sternal recumbency, and flex the rear legs to help open the interarcuate spaces.
2. Use a 20- or 22-gauge, 1.5–3.5 inch spinal needle.
3. Insert the needle through the L5-6 interarcuate space for small dogs and cats and L4-5 for large dogs. Place the needle on the dorsal midline just lateral to the dorsal spinous processes of L6 at a 50° to 60° angle, in a cranioventral direction toward the interarcuate space at L5-6. In cats, insert the needle off the cranial edge of the L6 dorsal spinous process perpendicular to the long axis of the spine. Direct the needle ventrally through the interarcuate space.
4. Inject in either the dorsal or ventral subarachnoid space. Always check for CSF flow prior to injection; however, it is not always obtained. Increase the likelihood of obtaining CSF by elevating the head and shoulders before placing the needle.
5. Perform a small test injection (0.25–0.50 ml) followed by a radiograph to check needle placement.
6. Slowly inject total dosage. Take radiograph views based on localization determined by neurologic examination.

- Complications
  - Seizures (incidence is reduced with new contrast agents, e.g., iohexol)
  - Exacerbation of clinical signs
  - Hyperesthesia
  - Apnea during injection

Extradural   Intradural   Intramedullary
Extramedullary

Lateral

Ventrodorsal

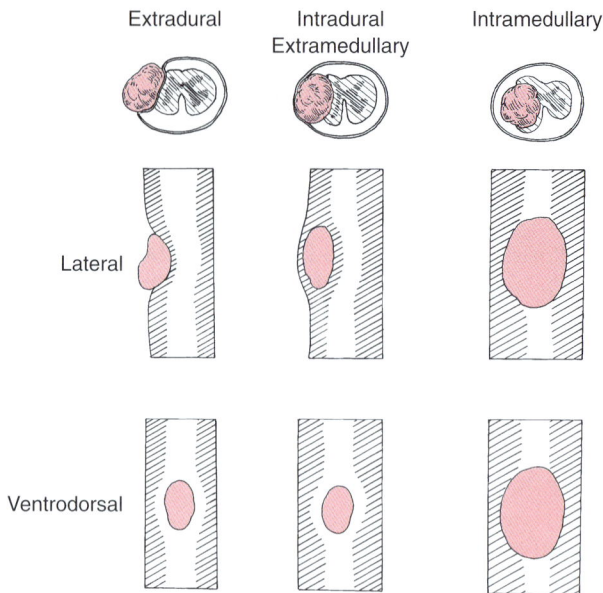

Figure 4–21. Radiographic patterns of myelographic lesions.

- Epidural injection will not have a negative impact on the health of the animal but negatively affects the quality of the myelogram.
- Central canal filling occurs when the needle is placed through the center of the cord. It usually appears thin on radiograph and sharply defined in the normal animal.
- *Interpretation.* Lesions are divided into three categories (Fig. 4–21).
1. Extradural, characterized by
   a. Displacement of the spinal cord.
   b. Narrowing or compression of the subarachnoid space.
   c. Deviation of the subarachnoid space.
   d. Spinal cord may appear wide on opposite view.
2. Intradural-extramedullary, characterized by
   a. Filling defect within the subarachnoid space ("golf tee" sign).
   b. Extradural or intramedullary component may be associated.
3. Intramedullary, characterized by
   a. Spinal cord widening in all views.

RADIATION SAFETY

Basic Radiation Safety

The objectives of radiation safety are to obtain the maximum amount of diagnostic information while keeping the radiation exposure to personnel and animals to a minimum.

▼ *Key Point* The responsibility for radiation safety lies solely with the owners of the practice.

Radiation protection in veterinary medicine is the subject of the National Council on Radiation Protection and Measurements (NCRP) Report No. 36 entitled *Radiation*

*Protection in Veterinary Medicine.** This report specifically outlines when radiation protection surveys are made. The report makes recommendations concerning tube housing, aluminum filtration, collimation types, and centering devices. A special section discusses radiography with portable and mobile diagnostic equipment. All practices need a copy of this report. Other NCRP reports that may be pertinent are No. 116, which discusses protection devices and provides recommendations for the maximum permissible dose (MPD), and No. 35, which discusses dental applications of diagnostic radiology.

The MPD was established to keep the radiation exposure of workers below a level at which adverse effects might be observed during a lifetime and to minimize the incidence of genetic effects in the entire population. The MPD does not apply to animal patients, to radiation emitted from natural background sources, or to radiation therapy. The actual risk to an individual exposed to MPD is small, but the risk is directly proportional to the received dosage. Therefore, radiation exposure must be kept as low as possible. Radiation can cause both tissue and genetic damage. The effects of radiation can be demonstrated in a short time, or they can be cumulative and not observed for a long time.

Federal regulations regarding use of x-ray equipment and radiation protection are published in the Code of Federal Regulations, available at university and public libraries. Individual states publish radiation control regulations that are reprinted from the state codes. These regulations include information concerning the licensing of x-ray machines, the licensing fee, and the procedure to be followed in obtaining licensing. The goal in diagnostic radiology is to obtain radiographs with minimum exposure to both patient and personnel.

Maximum Permissible Dose

The MPD is currently 5 rem per year.

▼ *Key Point* Be familiar with federal, state, and local regulations regarding use of x-ray equipment and radiation safety.

Reducing Exposure

Three methods reduce radiation exposure: (1) increased distance between the individual and the radiation source, (2) decreased duration of exposure, and (3) protective barriers between the individual and the radiation source.

- Limiting radiation exposure
  - Limit the number of individuals within the room where the procedure is taking place. Use positioning devices, such as sandbags, sponges, tape, and Plexiglas trough. Use a chemical restraint whenever possible.

▼ *Key Point* When you must be present within the radiographic room during film taking, always wear protective clothing.

*A copy of this report may be obtained from NCRP Publications, P.O. Box 30175, Washington, D.C., 20014

- Protective lead apparel includes apron, gloves, thyroid shield, and protective goggles. Lead apparel is usually 0.5-mm lead equivalent. Hang aprons up to prevent the lead from cracking. Store gloves so that liners can dry. Check all protective clothing at least twice a year for cracks and tears. Place the items on a film cassette and radiograph them at an exposure of approximately 85 kVp.

▼ *Key Point* Never permit any portion of the body to be within the primary beam, even if covered with protective clothing.

- Never hand-hold any x-ray tube. All x-ray tubes leak radiation from the housing.
- Use a shielding device whenever possible to protect all or part of your body. Lead glass may be part of this shield so that you may continue to see the patient. Lead-impregnated acrylic or plastic panels may be hung from the ceiling to give added protection.*
- When using a horizontal x-ray beam never position any part of your body behind the cassette.
- Use collimation. An unexposed border on the radiograph demonstrates that the primary beam did not exceed the size of the cassette (film). This practice helps reduce scatter radiation by decreasing the interaction between the primary beam and tissue, therefore increasing radiographic quality. Check the collimator light for accuracy; replace the bulb as needed.
- Use fast film, fast rare-earth screens, and high kVp techniques to lower the exposure factors and the amount of radiation produced.
- Use a 2.0-mm aluminum filter installed at the tube housing port to remove the softer (less energetic) radiation portion of the x-ray beam. This aids in the reduction of scatter radiation and exposure to the patient.
- Individuals within the room should always stand as far away from the radiation source as possible. If you double the distance from the source of radiation, you decrease your exposure level by a factor of 4 (inverse square law).
- All personnel working with radiation are required to wear a film badge or some other method of monitoring the amount of exposure, if they have the potential to receive greater than ¼ MPD. Remember that wearing the device does not protect the individual, but it serves as a reminder of working in a potentially hazardous environment. For a monitoring device to be most helpful in determining exposure to radiation, wear it consistently in the same location on the body outside the apron at the neck. Film badges register when exposed to heat, light, water, or pressure. They can be purchased through companies listed in Table 4–7.

▼ *Key Point* Never permit anyone under the age of 18 or a pregnant woman in the room during a diagnostic procedure.

---

*Available through Nuclear Associates, 100 Voice Rd., Carle Place, NY, 11514.

Table 4–7. SOURCES OF FILM BADGES

Landauer Inc.
2 Science Rd.
Glenwood, IL 60425
708-755-7000

Teledyne Brown Engineering
50 Van Buren Ave.
Westwood, NJ 07675
201-664-7070

- Rotate personnel, thus reducing the amount of exposure to each.
- Do not direct the x-ray beam into adjacent rooms that may be occupied.
- Use a gonadal shield for the patient.
- Always plan radiographic procedures (e.g., proper position and technique), thus reducing the number of films needed, which ultimately reduces the exposure to patient and personnel.

Clinic Construction

- Check with your state's health department (radiation protection division) for the latest laws on radiation safety and clinic construction.
- Register your x-ray machine with the state.
- Many states are now conducting "surprise spot checks" of x-ray machines and radiographic records. Maintain film and technique logs for complete records (Figs. 4–22 and 4–23).
- If constructing a new clinic, a drawing of the layout must be sent to the state radiation protection department. This drawing indicates the location of the x-ray machine and demonstrates how the space in the room where the x-ray machine is located will be used. The use of the adjoining rooms and an estimate of the degree of traffic in these areas are determined. The radiation safety department then sends a computerized layout of wall, ceiling, and floor materials to be used in certain areas of your clinic.

RADIOGRAPHIC INTERPRETATION

Radiology is a valuable adjunctive diagnostic tool. Do not interpret radiographs without considering the history, clinical signs, physical examination findings, and laboratory data. Radiographic signs are rarely pathognomonic; therefore, a specific diagnosis is seldom possible.

$$\begin{array}{c} \text{History} \\ \text{Physical exam} \\ \text{Lab findings} \end{array} + \begin{array}{c} \text{X-ray} \\ \text{signs} \end{array} = \begin{array}{c} \text{Differential} \\ \text{list} \end{array}$$

From the differential list additional tests can be done to help formulate a definitive diagnosis.

Radiology Log and Film Inventory

Date	Client Name	Type of Study Performed	Film Size and Number of Films			
			8×10	10×12 24×30	11×14 30×35	14×17 35×43

Figure 4–22. Film usage and inventory log.

Name _____

Clinic number _____

Species _____ Breed _____

Sex _____ Date of Birth _____

Radiology Technique Log

Date	Exam	Patient Thickness	Views Taken	mAs	kVp	Tabletop/ Grid	Film size	Screen	Notes

Figure 4–23. Radiology technique log.

$$\begin{array}{c}\text{Differential}\\\text{list}\end{array} + \begin{array}{c}\text{Contrast studies}\\\text{Ultrasound}\\\text{Lab data}\\\text{Biopsy, fine-needle}\\\text{aspirate, or surgery}\end{array} = \begin{array}{c}\text{Definitive}\\\text{diagnosis}\end{array}$$

- Successful interpretation of radiographs depends on many factors.

▼ **Key Point** The most important factor in the successful interpretation of radiographs is the quality of the radiographs being examined.

- At least two views at right angles to each other are needed. The use of right or left lateral radiographs is based on the preference of the individual reading the radiographs. The same holds true for VD and DV views, but be consistent.

- Maximize viewing conditions.
  - Dark, quiet room.
  - At least two view boxes to evaluate two views simultaneously.
  - Always place the film on the view boxes such that the anatomic structures are in the same position and direction: DV/VD radiograph with the animal's right to your left; lateral radiograph with the head to your left.
  - Have a shielded high-intensity (hot) lamp available.
  - Read films slowly and thoroughly.
  - Always have radiology and anatomy texts nearby.
- Evaluate the radiographs using a systematic approach. Evaluate the entire film before concentrating on obvious lesions.
  - Use an area method, evaluating the radiograph either peripheral to center, or center to peripheral.
  - Use an organ system method. Evaluate all parts of a system before examining the next system.
  - However you choose to evaluate films, be consistent from case to case.
- Knowledge of normal radiographic anatomy is essential.
- Descriptions of radiographic pathology involve the following:
  - Knowledge of normal topographic anatomy is a priority. Some organs, particularly in the abdomen, are nearly always seen, some organs are almost never seen or seen only when abnormal, and some organs are typically only partially seen. Because these organs are not always seen, one is still aware of where they are normally located. Always be able to describe the location of the lesion based on what it is near or adjacent to or what is ventral, dorsal, lateral, medial, axial, abaxial, cranial, caudal, or rostral. Describe the effect the lesion is having on surrounding structures.

Radiographic Signs

Radiopacity—Various radiographic opacities are due to the differential absorption of x-rays. The opacity of surrounding material also influences the observed opacity of a structure. The five radiopacities in decreasing order are those of metal, bone, soft tissue (fluid), fat, and gas. Metal is the only one that is not a biologic opacity.

Geometry—Size, shape, position, margination, and number.

Function—Excretion (intravenous urography), motility (upper gastrointestinal), patency, and integrity. Evaluation of function often requires contrast medium and multiple films.

ULTRASOUND

Ultrasound is rapidly becoming an accepted imaging modality in small animal practice. New and used equip-ment is available at reasonable prices, and usefulness has increased to include ophthalmic, cardiac, abdominal, and reproductive disease diagnosis. It is a safe, non-invasive diagnostic technique that provides information about the internal architecture of organs within the abdomen and thorax. Functional information can also be obtained with echocardiography. Ultrasound is not meant to replace diagnostic radiography, but to complement it. Ultrasound is operator-dependent. The quality of the image and the information gained are directly related to the ability of the person doing the study.

Equipment

The major components of the diagnostic ultrasound imaging system are pulser, transducer, receiver, memory, and display. Electrical pulses are produced by the pulser and these drive the transducer. The transducer produces ultrasound pulses for each electrical pulse it receives. The transducer also produces electrical pulses for each ultrasound pulse (reflection) it receives from tissues. The electrical pulses go to the receiver, where they are converted to information that the memory can utilize. Information from the memory drives the display, which produces an image.

Suppliers of ultrasound equipment are listed in Table 4–8.

Machines

- Questions to consider before purchasing or leasing ultrasound equipment:
  - What kind of scanning will I be doing (e.g., heart, abdomen, real-time, B mode, M mode)?
  - How large or small are my patients?
  - Is someone in the practice willing to accept primary responsibility for learning and doing the procedures?
  - How much money can I invest?
- Two types of real-time scanners
  - Linear array scanner produces a rectangular image and can be used to evaluate broad areas, where no bony or gas-filled structures interfere. These scanners are usually less expensive. New machines start at $7500 to $10,000; used at $2000 to $3000). The major drawback is the transducer contact zone, which makes intercostal and subcostal (heart, liver, biliary tract, and right kidney) imaging difficult.
  - Sector scanner produces a pie-shaped image. A smaller contact zone is used, which makes intercostal and subcostal imaging less difficult.

Mechanical—In a mechanical (sector) scanner the sound wave is focused a certain distance from the transducer (focal point). The sound wave is within focus for some distance on both sides of the focal point (focal zone). Resolution is best within this fixed focal zone. The scanner contains moving parts.

Electronic—These are linear or sector scanners with no moving parts; therefore, they are more durable than mechanical scanners. The beam is formed by adding together many small beams from an array of small

Table 4–8. ULTRASOUND COMPANIES

Advanced Technology Laboratories
22100 Bothell Highway S.E.
Bothell, WA 98041-3003
800-982-2011

Aloka
10 Fairfield Blvd
Wallingford CT 06492-7502
800-442-5652

Alliance Medical U.S.A.
112 N. Bridge St.
Smithville, MO 64089
888-689-3070

Classic Medical Supply
19900 Mona Road, Ste. 105
Tequesta, FL 33469
800-722-6838

Hitachi Medical Corp.
660 White Plains Rd.
Tarrytown, NY 10591
800-366-0198

Jorgensen Laboratories Inc
1450 N. Van Buren Ave.
Loveland, CO 80538
970-669-2500

Medelex Inc.
732 N. Pastoria Ave.
Sunnydale, CA 94086
800-644-0692

Products Group International
447 Main St.
P.O. Box 1807
Lyons, CO 80504
800-336-5299

Toshiba
Sound Technologies
5062 San Jacinto Cr.
Fallbrook, CA 92028
800-268-5354

Universal Medical Systems, Inc.
299 Adams St.
Bedford Hills, NY 10507
914-666-6200

crystals. The scanner has variable (dynamic) focusing. The focal zone therefore can be placed anywhere in the image depth.

- Image display
  - M-mode (motion-mode): Documents motion, especially that of the heart (echocardiography). A thin ultrasound beam is directed into the heart, is reflected back, and then is shown on the screen as numerous moving lines. Motion is indicated along the side, and time along the bottom of the screen.
  - B-mode (brightness-mode): Echoes are displayed as dots. The brightness of the dot changes with the amplitude of reflection. The larger the reflection, the brighter the dot—no reflection, black dot. The location of the dot corresponds to the location of the reflector in the body.
  - Real-time: The image is continually updated during the entire examination. This permits direct ob-

servation of moving structures (e.g., heart, bowel peristalsis).
- New versus used equipment

New equipment purchase is ideal because some companies offer training (in-house or continuing education course) and a year-long warranty with service and parts (in-house service or another unit is made available while your unit is serviced by the company). Manufacturer-reconditioned units may provide a year-long or shorter warranty. The major disadvantage of new equipment obviously is the higher cost.

A great deal of used equipment is available owing to the advent of newer technology. Older, used, outdated equipment is being replaced with new equipment based on new technology. The price of old equipment is very attractive, sometimes as low as $1000. Although initial cost is low, some significant expense may be required, including service, maintenance, transducers, and accessories. If the appropriate frequency transducers do not come with the unit (often only 2 and 3 mHz transducers come with units that were used on human patients), the cost can increase three to four times to purchase 5 and 7.5 mHz transducers.

Transducers

- Transducers are available in a variety of frequencies (2–10 mHz). Low-frequency transducers provide greater depth of penetration, but because of large wavelength, resolution is poorer. High-frequency transducers provide excellent resolution, but the beam is rapidly attenuated in tissue. They are therefore used to evaluate superficial tissues.
- Use as high a frequency transducer as possible to maximize resolution but still allow penetration to the depth needed.
- For transducer uses, see Table 4–9.

Ancillary Equipment

This may include a guided biopsy attachment for the transducer, calipers, screen-labeling device, and M-mode/B-mode split screen. Portability of the machine must also be considered.

Ultrasonographic Accessories

- Positioners
  - V-trough is easily constructed from wood or Plexiglas.
  - Surgical table can be formed into a V-trough.

Table 4–9. TRANSDUCER SELECTION

Transducer Type	Use
7.5 mHz	Eye, feline heart and abdomen, small canine abdomen (<25 lb), testicles
5.0 mHz	Medium-size canine (<55 lb) heart and abdomen
3.5 mHz	Very large breed canine heart and abdomen

- Cardiac table (wood or Plexiglas) with holes so that the transducers may be brought up under the recumbent patient. Lateral recumbency causes the heart to lay against the chest wall, providing an ultrasonographic window to the heart.
- Standoff pad
  - Commercially available pad. A water balloon or breast implant can also be employed.
  - Place between the transducer and the skin.
  - This pad provides an offset that serves to back the transducer away from the skin, moving the superficial structure to be imaged within the focal zone of the transducer.
- Coupling gel is necessary to transmit sound from the transducer through the skin.
  - Numerous brands are commercially available.
  - Water-soluble, hypoallergenic gel is available.

Image Storing

There are various methods of preserving the image for inclusion in the animal's medical record:

- Polaroid camera.
- Heat-sensitive, thermal-paper recorder (Sony, Mitsubishi); costs start at $1200.
- Multiformat camera can record multiple images on x-ray film. These are very expensive, however.
- Videotape; images are recorded allowing evaluation by others at a later time.

Ultrasound Technique

- Patient preparation
  - Tranquilization is usually not required, but the patient must always be adequately restrained.
  - The most common problem in obtaining good-quality images is poor transducer skin contact. Clip the hair over the area to be imaged with a #40 blade. Hair tends to trap air, acting as a barrier to the ultrasound. Clean the exposed skin to remove dirt, oil, and debris prior to applying the coupling gel to help achieve the best image.
- Patient positioning
  - Most abdominal imaging is done from the ventral surface. Alternate scanning planes from lateral and lateral intercostal can be chosen to avoid gas. When gas is a problem, gentle abdominal pressure from the transducer usually displaces it.
  - The heart is imaged through the intercostal spaces, usually while the animal is in lateral recumbency.
- Ultrasound image
  - It is a two-dimensional representation of a three-dimensional object.
  - Ultrasound reflects the anatomy tomographically (cross-sectionally).
  - Ultrasound permits identification of internal organ architecture.
- Image viewing
  - Abdomen (Figs. 4–24 and 4–25)
  - Cardiac
  - Longitudinal scan—cardiac base to the right.

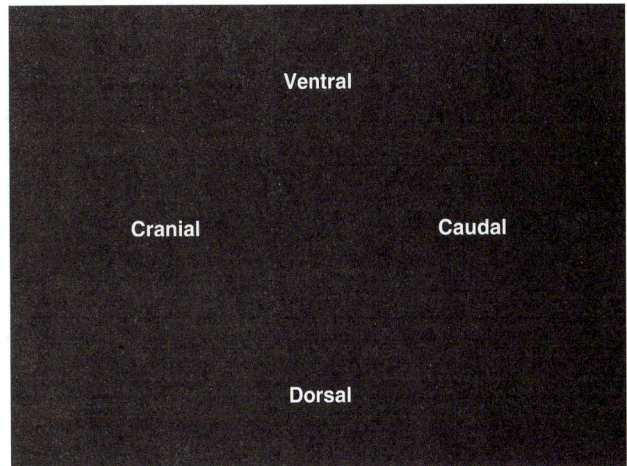

Figure 4–24. Viewing a longitudinal (sagittal) ultrasound image.

- Transverse scan—pulmonary valve (outflow tract) on the right of the screen.

Principles of Interpretation

Ultrasound Terminology

Anechoic—Area void of echoes (seen as black).

Hypoechoic—Lower level of echogenicity (darker) than adjacent structures.

Hyperechoic—Higher level of echogenicity (brighter) than adjacent structures.

Isoechoic—Level of echogenicity similar to adjacent structures.

Complexly echogenic—Area of multiple echogenicities.

Ultrasonographic barriers—Highly reflective or absorptive interfaces within the body that cause an almost complete attenuation of the sound beam. Examples include bone, mineral, and air. This barrier results in an absence of echoes deep to the interface (acoustic shadow).

Ultrasonographic windows—Soft tissue organs adjacent to the body wall used to help avoid gas or bone and to facilitate deeper imaging. Examples include imaging

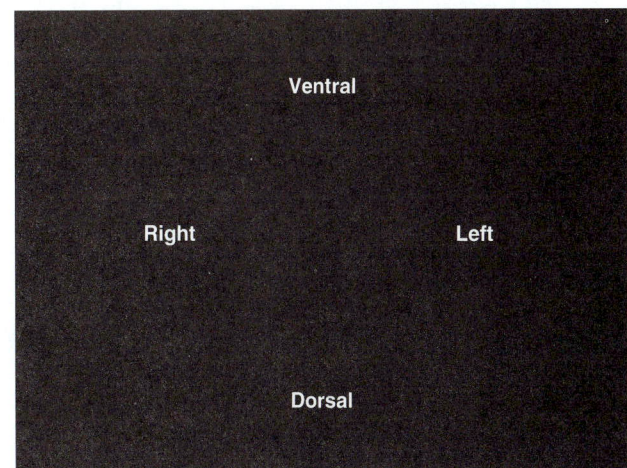

Figure 4–25. Viewing a transverse (axial) ultrasound image.

through the spleen on the left lateral abdominal wall to identify the left kidney and imaging through the urinary bladder to identify the area where sublumbar lymph nodes are found.

Acoustic enhancement (through transmission)—Sound passes through an anechoic structure with little attenuation and emerges with more intensity than expected in surrounding echogenic areas. This occurrence is expected deep to fluid-filled structures (e.g., gallbladder, hepatic cyst).

Organ Echogenicity

- Rank of abdominal parenchymal organs from least to most echogenic:
  - Renal medulla
  - Renal cortex
  - Liver
  - Spleen
  - Prostate
  - Renal sinus

Ultrasound Use

See respective chapters for ultrasound use in specific diseases. See Table 4–10 for an overview of ultrasound in various organs.

Interventional Ultrasound

- Uses
  - Ultrasound-guided needle biopsy for histopathology and culture.
  - Ultrasound-guided fine-needle aspirate (FNA) for cytology and culture.
  - Cystocentesis to obtain urine (small bladder, difficult animals).
  - Gallbladder aspirate for culture and cholangiography.
  - Abscess diagnosis and drainage.
  - Cyst diagnosis and drainage.
  - Renal pyelocentesis.
- Equipment
  - Real-time B-mode scanner.
  - Transducer biopsy guide.
  - Needles, syringe, slides, culture medium, formalin containers.
  - Sterile glove or transducer cover.
  - Sterile ultrasound gel.
  - Sedatives, lidocaine.
- Patient preparation
  - Complete an abdominal ultrasound examination.
  - Choose the site for FNA biopsy.
  - FNA—Rarely need sedation; sterile preparation of skin and transducer sterile glove cover.
  - Tissue biopsy—Sedation and/or local anesthesia; general anesthesia is sometimes necessary; surgical preparation of skin and transducer.
  - Sterile glove cover.
  - Determine packed cell volume (PCV); total plasma protein, activated clotting time, and platelet count.
  - Check +/− prothrombin time, partial thromboplastin time.

Table 4–10. ULTRASOUND USES

	Pathology	Usefulness
Heart	Wall thickness	+++
	Wall motion	+++
	Valve morphology	+++
	Valve motion	+++
	Mass lesion	+++
	Pericardial disease	+++
Thoracic area (extracardiac)	Pleural effusion	+++
	Pleural masses	+++
	Pulmonary masses*	+++
	Diaphragmatic hernia	++
	Mediastinal disease	+
Peritoneal cavity	Effusion	+++
	Carcinomatosis	+
	Lymphadenopathy	+++
Liver	Diffuse disease†	+/++
	Neoplasia	++/+++
	Abscess	++/+++
	Biliary disease	++/+++
	Portacaval shunt	+/++
	Nodular hyperplasia	+/++
Kidney	Hydronephrosis	+++
	Pyelonephritis	+/++
	Parenchymal disease‡	++
	Calculi	++/+++
	Perirenal disease	+++
	Neoplasia	+++
Urinary bladder	Calculi	+++
	Cystitis	+/++
	Neoplasia	+++
Adrenal gland	Hyperplasia	+/++
	Neoplasia	+++
Gastrointestinal system	Enteritis	+
	Obstruction	++/+++
	Intussusception	+++
	Foreign body	++/+++
	Neoplasia	++/+++
Pancreas	Pancreatitis	+/++
	Pseudocyst	++
	Neoplasia	++/+++
Reproductive tract	Ovary	+
	Testicular neoplasia	+++
	Peritesticular lesions	+++
	Pregnancy	+++
Prostate	Infection	++
	Paraprostatic cyst	+++
	Neoplasia	++
Eye	Detached retina	+++
	Retrobulbar mass	+/++

*If mass contacts thoracic wall.
†Lipidosis, steroid hepatopathy, suppurative hepatitis (dependent on severity of disease).
‡Glomerulonephritis, amyloidosis, ethylene glycol toxicity, renal dysplasia (dependent on severity of disease).
+++, good; ++, fair; +, poor.

- Monitor patient closely for signs of internal hemorrhage for 3–4 hours following biopsy.
- Methods
  - Guided—Transducer has an attachable biopsy guide. Ultrasound machine has biopsy capabilities (software). Biopsy guide maintains needle in the

scanning plane so that the entire procedure can be seen.

- Directed—Image the organ or lesion of interest. Determine the location, entrance angle, and depth. Obtain biopsy or aspirate blindly without ultrasound observation. More dependent on sonographer's experience. Biopsy guide and biopsy-capable machine are not necessary.
- Free hand—Localize biopsy site with transducer perpendicular to the skin. Place the needle with the other hand into the scanning plane to the desired depth. Biopsy procedure can be observed with real-time and is more dependent on sonographer's experience. Biopsy guide and biopsy-capable machine are not necessary.
- Complications—Very low incidence with all procedures.
  - Peritonitis
  - Hemorrhage
  - Tumor spread to local tissues

SUPPLEMENTAL READINGS

Barber DL, Lewis RE: Guidelines for Radiology Service in Veterinary Medicine. Schaumberg, IL: American Veterinary Medical Association, 1982.

Kleine LJ, Warren RG: Mosby's Fundamentals of Animal Health Technology: Small Animal Radiology. St. Louis: CV Mosby, 1983.

Morgan JP, Silverman S: Techniques of Veterinary Radiography, 3rd Ed. Davis, CA: Veterinary Radiology Associates, 1984.

NCRP Report No. 36: Radiation Protection in Veterinary Medicine. Recommendations of the National Council on Radiation Protection and Measurements. NCRP Publications, P.O. Box 30175, Washington, D.C. 20014.

Ticer JW: Radiographic Technique in Veterinary Practice, 2nd Ed. Philadelphia: WB Saunders, 1984.

5 Fluid Therapy for Dogs and Cats

Dennis J. Chew / Shane W. Bateman

Fluid therapy is one of the most important therapeutic measures in seriously ill animals. The effective administration of fluids requires an understanding of fluid and electrolyte dynamics in both healthy and sick animals.

Answer these questions to decide when fluid therapy is needed:

- Does a serious deficit or excess of water exist?
- Are there serious electrolyte disturbances (excesses or deficits)?
- Is there a serious disturbance in acid-base balance?
- Is there a serious disturbance in oncotic pressure or excessive protein loss?
- Is there an immediate need for full nutritional support with calories and protein?

Answer these questions to provide appropriate fluid therapy:

- By what route will fluids be given?
- How fast will fluids be given?
- What volume of fluids will be given?
- Which types of fluids will be given?
- Which, if any, supplements will be added to commercially available fluids?

INDICATIONS FOR FLUID THERAPY

- Most commonly for the correction of dehydration, hypokalemia, and metabolic acidosis.
- Less commonly for the specific correction of hypernatremia, hyponatremia, hypomagnesemia, hyperkalemia, decreased oncotic pressure, metabolic alkalosis, hypocalcemia, and hypercalcemia.
- For parenteral nutrition (see Chap. 3).

DISTRIBUTION OF BODY WATER AND ELECTROLYTES

Water

Total body water (TBW) represents 50–70% of body weight in adults. Usually 60% is chosen arbitrarily as an average figure.

- Two thirds of TBW is within cells (intracellular), or 40% of body weight.
- One third of TBW is extracellular fluid (ECF), or 20% of body weight.

- Interstitial water composes 15% of body weight.
- Intravascular water composes 5% of body weight.

Electrolytes

- Sodium and chloride exist in high concentration in serum ECF and in low concentration within cells.
- Potassium, magnesium, and phosphorus exist in high concentration within cells and low concentration in serum ECF.

MAINTENANCE REQUIREMENTS

Maintenance is defined as the volume of fluid (ml) and amount of electrolyte (mEq or mg) that must be taken in on a daily basis to keep the volume of TBW and electrolyte content normal. Obligate losses of water and electrolytes occur daily as a consequence of normal metabolism. Water taken into the body in all its forms equals water loss in healthy animals. Figure 5–1 shows the specific maintenance requirements of electrolytes and water in caged dogs and cats that have normal food intake.

- Water can be taken in by drinking, combined mechanically with food, or derived from food metabolism or tissue breakdown. Water is lost from the body through evaporation during breathing, from feces, and from urine. Obligatory loss of electrolytes occurs in fecal water and in urine, but the overall loss of electrolytes is less in proportion than is the loss of water.
- Normal losses of water contain sodium and osmole concentrations less than those of extracellular fluid; consequently, they are hypotonic (hypo-osmolal). Normal daily losses of water contain relatively more potassium than does the concentration of extracellular fluid.
- Maintenance volume varies with the size of the animal. Large patients (with low mass:body surface area ratios) require less fluid per kilogram on an individual basis than small animals (with high mass:body surface area ratios) (Table 5–1).
- Maintenance volume is composed of two subcomponents:
  - *Insensible loss* (not readily measured losses from respiratory evaporation and passage of normal feces) is estimated at 10 ml/lb/day (22 ml/kg/day) in

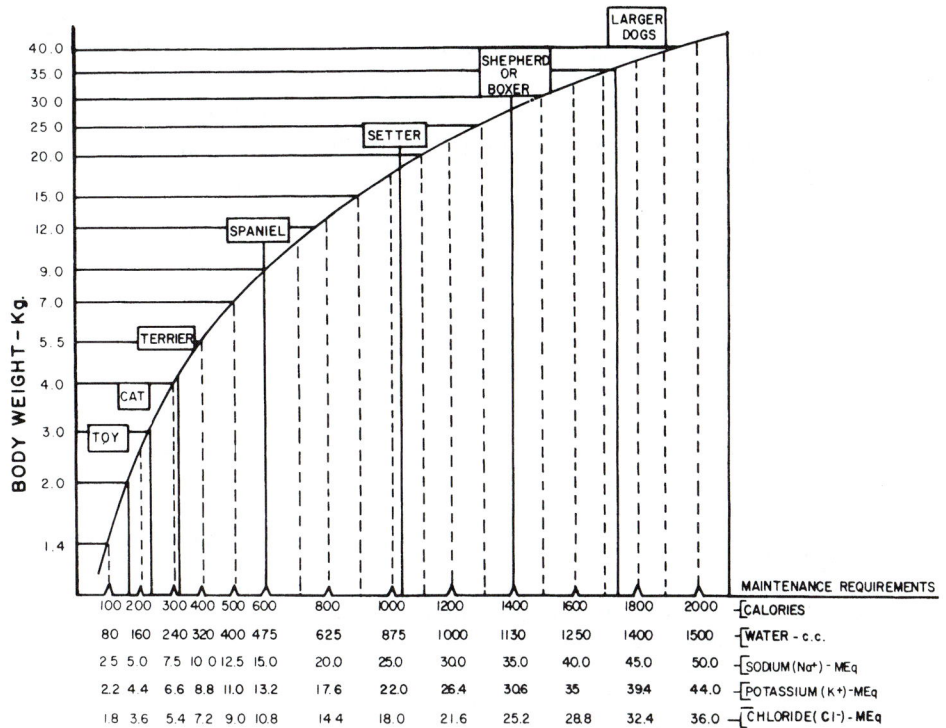

Figure 5–1. Maintenance fluid and electrolyte requirements of caged normal dogs and cats. (Finco, after Harrison JB: J Am Anim Hosp Assoc 8:179, 1972.)

Table 5–1. DAILY WATER REQUIREMENTS FOR DOGS

Body Weight (kg)	Total Water/Day (ml)	ml/kg
1	140	140
2	232	116
3	312	104
4	385	96
5	453	91
6	518	86
7	580	83
8	639	80
9	696	77
10	752	75
11	806	73
12	859	71
13	911	70
14	961	68
15	1011	67
16	1060	66
17	1108	65
18	1155	64
19	1201	63
20	1247	62
25	1468	59
30	1677	56
35	1876	54
40	2068	52
45	2254	50
50	2434	49
60	2781	46
70	3112	44
80	3431	43
90	3739	41
100	4038	40

From Ross L: Fluid therapy for acute and chronic renal failure. Vet Clin North Am 19:343, 1989.

normal animals. This can increase during febrile states, panting, and high environmental temperatures.

- *Sensible loss* (readily measured as urine production) is approximately 10 to 20 ml/lb/day (22 to 44 ml/kg/day) in normal animals.

- Urine output can decrease dramatically in acute intrinsic renal failure (oliguria/anuria); during urinary obstruction (anuria); and during severe dehydration (oliguria). Urine output can increase dramatically in polyuric renal failure and postobstructive diuresis.

▼ *Key Point* Lactated Ringer's and 0.9% sodium chloride solutions are *not* maintenance solutions because they contain too much sodium and chloride, are too high in osmolality, and do not contain enough potassium.

- 0.45% Sodium chloride in water or in 2.5% dextrose better approximates a maintenance solution for sodium and chloride content as well as for osmolality but does not contain adequate potassium. This does become an adequate maintenance solution when potassium is added to result in 20 to 30 mEq/L of potassium. Normosol-M (Abbott Laboratories) and Plasma-Lyte 56 (Baxter Healthcare) are commercial solutions that are formulated with 5% dextrose, increased potassium, lowered sodium, and a bicarbonate precursor that is suitable for maintenance.

▼ *Key Point* Maintenance fluids are low in sodium, chloride, and osmolality and high in potassium compared with normal plasma.

- Urine volume production dramatically decreases in animals that do not eat because of the associated decrease in solutes demanding renal excretion. Consequently, the maintenance fluid volume requirement during anorexia often is less than half of what is calculated by traditonal methods.

▼ *Key Point* Calculations for maintenance fluid volume often are erroneously high in patients who are not eating.

DEHYDRATION (REPLACEMENT NEEDS)

Dehydration exists when TBW decreases to less than normal.

- Technically, dehydration refers to loss of pure water. Clinical fluid loss usually is accompanied by some loss of electrolytes.
- Acute fluid and electrolyte loss in a disease process is initially from intravascular fluid.
- Compensatory shifts of water and electrolytes from intracellular and interstitial compartments subsequently occur. The magnitude of these shifts depends on the tonicity and hydrostatic pressure of the remaining extracellular fluid. Consequently, dehydration can occur to different degrees in the various compartments.

Causes of Dehydration

Decreased Water Intake (hypodipsia, adipsia)

- Lack of food intake also decreases available water (water from oxidation and that which is physically present within the food).
- Appetite and thirst centers may be depressed in systemically ill animals.
- Accidental or deliberate deprivation of adequate water and food.

Increased Water Loss

- Urinary (polyuria)—*common*
- Gastrointestinal (vomiting, diarrhea)—*common*
- Respiratory (fever, panting)
- Skin (burns, large wounds)
- Excessive salivation
- Peritoneal dialysis

▼ *Key Point* Fluid losses from the urinary and gastrointestinal tracts most frequently result in dehydration.

Characterization of Dehydration (Type)

Disease processes can display a range of fluid and electrolyte loss combinations, from mostly water loss (hypotonic loss) to water loss with significant quantities of accompanying electrolytes (isotonic or hypertonic). Evaluate the tonicity and sodium concentrations of the ECF in a dehydrated patient because this gives clues to the nature of the fluid that was lost and helps determine the type of fluid to be given as replacement during treatment. The type of dehydration is defined based on the serum sodium concentration at the time of dehydration.

- *Isotonic dehydration* is the type that occurs most commonly and is defined by finding a normal serum sodium concentration (145–157 mEq/L) in the presence of dehydration. Isotonic dehydration occurs from loss of water and electrolytes in proportion to those found in normal serum (isotonic loss).
- *Hypertonic dehydration* is the next most common type and is defined by an elevated serum sodium concentration (158 mEq/L or greater) with dehydration. Hypertonic dehydration occurs as a consequence of predominantly water loss—or water lost in excess of solute found in normal serum (hypotonic loss).
- *Hypotonic dehydration* is the least common type and is defined by a low serum sodium concentration (143 mEq/L or less) with dehydration. Hypotonic dehydration theoretically occurs as solute is lost in excess of the concentration in normal serum (hypertonic loss). This probably is not the most significant mechanism, however. More likely is the loss of isotonic fluid. With continued intake and absorption of hypotonic fluids (such as drinking of water), the remaining extracellular sodium concentration is diluted to below normal.

Detection of Dehydration

Clinical tools to detect dehydration are limited in both sensitivity and specificity. No single test or procedure accurately assesses the magnitude of dehydration. Integration of historical findings, physical examination abnormalities, and laboratory measurements is necessary to determine dehydration. Dehydration is not detectable by clinical means until at least 4 to 5% of body weight in water has been lost. An acute loss of greater than 12% body weight in water is considered life-threatening (Table 5–2).

History

History often leads the clinician to suspect dehydration and to assess its magnitude more accurately. Question the owner about volume of water intake (adipsia, hypodipsia, polydipsia, or normal). Because the volume of water intake may, in part, be a function stimulated by food intake, note also the presence or absence of anorexia. Abnormal losses of body fluid may be determined from the owner's answers to questions about vomiting, diarrhea, polyuria, panting, excessive salivation, and other bodily discharge. The duration of these historical signs and the magnitude of losses affect the severity of dehydration.

Physical Examination

Physical examination provides general guidelines for detecting dehydration but is subjective (see Table 5–2). Signs of listlessness and depression may occur from dehydration but may be partially attributable to underlying disease or concomitant electrolyte and acid-base ab-

Table 5–2. PERCENTAGES OF DETECTABLE DEHYDRATION

Dehydration	Signs
<5%	Not detectable; history may suggest dehydration.
5%	Subtle loss of skin elasticity.
6–8%	Definite delay in return of skin to normal position, eyes may be sunken in orbits, slightly prolonged capillary refill time, mucous membranes may be dry.
10–12%	Tented skin stands in place, prolonged capillary refill time, eyes sunken in orbits, dry mucous membranes, signs of shock (increased heart rate, weak pulses) may be observed.
12–15%	Signs of shock, collapse, and severe depression; death imminent.

normalities. As dehydration becomes more severe, decreased skin turgor, sunken eyes, dryness of mucous membranes, tachycardia, diminished capillary refill, and signs of shock may occur. An accurate recent body weight, when available, can be used as a baseline. The change in body weight can be an indicator of change in body water.

▼ *Key Point* An acute increase or decrease in an animal's body weight often reflects acute gain or loss of body water. This change is the most sensitive clinical tool for assessment of dehydration and rehydration. An acute loss or gain of 1 lb is the equivalent of 500 ml of fluid (1 kg = 1000 ml).

Skin Turgor

Skin turgor assessment during physical examination is important for estimating the percentage of body weight loss due to dehydration. Skin turgor is evaluated by determining the time required for skin, gently lifted away from the body, to return to its original position. This is referred to as the skin pinch. Normal skin pliability (turgor) depends on hydration of the tissues in the area tested. Choose skin from the trunk as a test area. Avoid dependent areas and skin from the neck. Normal skin returns immediately to its initial position when lifted a short distance and released. Dehydrated skin shows varying degrees of slow return to the original position. As dehydration becomes progressive, the time required for return of the pinched skin to its initial position becomes greater. The clinician assigns increasing percentages of dehydration to abnormal skin turgor of increasing severity (see Table 5–2).

Artifactual Findings

• Many artifacts confuse interpretation of skin turgor. Skin turgor of obese animals may appear normal despite dehydration, owing to the large amounts of subcutaneous fat. The skin of an emaciated animal with normal hydration may fail to return to its normal position owing to a lack of subcutaneous fat and elastic tissue. Consequently, underestimating dehydration in obese animals and overestimating dehydration in

emaciated animals occur. Avoid cervical skin as a test area because redundant skin in this area confuses the results. Skin turgor changes in long-haired animals are more difficult to detect than those in short-haired animals. Differences in turgor assessment can occur in the same animal when standing and when recumbent.

▼ *Key Point* Dehydration may be as little as 5% of body weight loss in lean dogs and as much as 10% or more in obese dogs before loss of skin turgor is detectable.

• Other physical examination artifacts include dry mucous membranes that may occur in animals that pant continually and in those given anticholinergics. Sunken eyes may be seen in catabolic diseases in which tissue behind the globe is reduced or atrophy of the muscles of mastication has occurred.

▼ *Key Point* Assessment of fluid, electrolyte, and acid-base status frequently is in error if the history and physical examination only are available for interpretation. The more seriously ill an animal, the more important it is to evaluate laboratory data.

Laboratory Evaluations
Hematocrit and Plasma Protein

These simple laboratory tests are helpful in evaluation of intravascular hydration. Packed cell volume (PCV) recorded in % and total plasma protein (TPP) in g/dl can be determined rapidly and inexpensively using a refractometer and microhematocrit. These two tests require only a few drops of blood that can be taken by capillary action from a 25-gauge venipuncture. Total plasma protein concentration may be more helpful in the detection of dehydration than is PCV. Increased TPP and PCV provide documentation for intravascular dehydration. Simultaneous evaluation of PCV and TPP is recommended to minimize interpretation errors due to preexisting anemia or hypoproteinemia. Additional data are obtained when PCV and TPP are followed serially because increasing values identify progressive dehydration.

Urinalysis

Urinalysis (UA) is important in all cases of suspected dehydration. An elevated specific gravity (SG) represents the healthy kidney's response to decreased perfusion. The finding of dilute urine (<1.030 SG) from a dehydrated animal immediately incriminates the kidneys as a major cause of, or contributor to, the dehydration.

Serum Biochemistry

No test accurately documents the volume of fluid loss, but serum electrolyte evaluation helps to characterize the nature of the fluid that was lost.

Blood Gases

Abnormalities in blood gas values may appear in dehydrated animals because of the loss or gain of certain body fluids, the activity of the underlying disease process itself, or the decreased perfusion of major organ systems.

▼ *Key Point* Animals may be severely dehydrated yet exhibit little or no serum biochemical abnormalities. Likewise, the PCV/TPP findings also can be normal in the presence of dehydration.

Natural History of the Specific Disease

Dehydration is anticipated in sick animals with certain disease syndromes known to predispose them to dehydration, regardless of physical examination or laboratory findings. For example, a collapsed diabetic animal is very likely to be dehydrated, as is the animal with advanced chronic renal failure or upper bowel obstruction.

Correction (Replacement) of Dehydration

- *Volume of fluid* to be replaced is calculated as follows, based on assessed % of dehydration and the patient's current body weight:
  - % dehydration × weight (kg) = liters of fluid to be replaced
  - % dehydration × weight (lb) × 500 = milliliters of fluid to be replaced
  - Alternatively, if a known recent body weight is available for comparison, replace 500 ml of fluid for every pound (1 L/kg) of acute body weight loss.
- *Type of fluid* that is chosen to accomplish this rehydration is based primarily on the serum sodium, chloride, and potassium concentrations, as well as acid-base disorders.

▼ *Key Point* Initial replacement with adequate fluid volume is usually more important than specific therapy for the electrolyte disorders.

- Return to the patient both the volume and quality (type) of fluid that has been lost or continues to be lost from the body. Base volume on measurement of the losses or, more commonly, on estimates. Base the quality of the fluid on the actual measurements of the losses or, more commonly, on the known biologic behavior of the specific disease that is causing the fluid losses.

▼ *Key Point* Choose a fluid type or add supplements to stock fluids so that electrolytes deficient in the plasma or body are administered and those that are excessive in the plasma are avoided.

CONTEMPORARY LOSSES

These are fluid losses greater than the normal loss from insensible and sensible mechanisms. Usually volumes of fluid loss from vomitus and diarrhea are estimated. When the ongoing losses are excessive urinary losses, temporary urethral catheter collection may give the clinician a better idea as to their magnitude.

The total volume for 24-hour infusion (replacement plus maintenance) can be calculated individually (Figure 5–2).

TYPES AND SELECTION OF FLUIDS

Table 5–3 lists a variety of available fluids and their composition.

Crystalloid Solutions

Crystalloid fluids contain no large macromolecules, allowing them to redistribute quickly from the vascular space to the interstitial and intracellular fluid spaces. Thus, their greatest benefit is for rehydration or replacement of prior fluid loss. Expansion of the vascular fluid space does occur initially, but with time, redistribution minimizes this effect.

Fluid Osmolality

Crystalloid fluids can be classified according to osmolality by comparison to the animal's normal serum osmolality of approximately 300 mOsm/kg. Osmolality of commercial fluids is determined largely by sodium and glucose concentrations. Fluids with osmolality less than

_____ ml = **Rehydration** = % dehydration × weight (lb) × 500
= % dehydration × weight (kg) × 1000

+

_____ ml = **Sensible** = 10 to 20 ml/lb/day or measured
= 22 to 44 ml/kg/day or measured

+

_____ ml = **Insensible** = 10 ml/lb/day
= 22 ml/kg/day

+

_____ ml = **Contemporary losses** = estimated or measured

_____ ml = **Total 24-hour needs**

Figure 5–2. Summation of individual components of fluid needs. Individual calculation of fluid volume needs, as listed, increases the likelihood of a more accurate fluid volume administration.

Table 5–3. COMPOSITION OF SOLUTIONS USED IN FLUID THERAPY

	Glucose* (g/L)	Na+ (mEq/L)	Cl− (mEq/L)	K+ (mEq/L)	Ca2+ (mEq/L)	Mg2+ (mEq/L)	Buffer† (mEq/L)	Osmolality (mOsm/L)	pH
Dextrose and Electrolyte Solution Composition									
5% dextrose	50	0	0	0	0	0	0	252	4.0
2.5% dextrose in 0.45% NaCl	25	77	77	0	0	0	0	280	4.5
5% dextrose in 0.45% NaCl	50	77	77	0	0	0	0	406	4.0
5% dextrose in 0.9% NaCl	50	154	154	0	0	0	0	560	4.0
0.45% NaCl	0	77	77	0	0	0	0	154	5.0
0.9% NaCl	0	154	154	0	0	0	0	308	5.0
3% NaCl	0	513	513	0	0	0	0	1026	5.0
Ringer's solution	0	147.5	156	4	4.5	0	0	310	5.5
Ringer's lactated solution	0	130	109	4	3	0	23(L)	272	6.5
2.5% dextrose in Ringer's lactated solution	25	130	109	4	3	0	28(L)	398	5.0
5% dextrose in Ringer's lactated solution	50	130	109	4	3	0	28(L)	524	5.0
Normosol-R§	0	140	98	5	0	3	27(A)	296	5.5
Plasma-Lyte 148‡	0	140	98	5	0	3	27(A)	294	5.5
Normosol-M in 5% dextrose§	50	40	40	16	5	3	16(A)	363	5.5
Plasma-Lyte 56 in 5% dextrose‡	50	40	40	13	0	3	16(A)	363	5.5
Plasma	1	145	105	5	5	3	24(B)	300	7.4
Additive Solutions									
20% mannitol	200(M)	0	0	0	0	0	0	1099	
7.5% NaHCO₃	0	893(B)	0	0	0	0	893(B)	1786	
8.4% NaHCO₃	0	1000(B)	0	0	0	0	1000(B)	2000	
10% CaCl₂	0	0	2720	0	1360	0	0	4080	
14.9% KCl	0	0	2000	2000	0	0	0	4000	
50% dextrose	500	0	0	0	0	0	0	2780	4.2
50% MgSO₄	0	0	0	0	0	4060	0	8120	

*All glucose, with one exception: M, mannitol.
†Buffers used: A, acetate; B, bicarbonate; L, lactate.
‡Baxter Healthcare.
§Abbott Laboratories.
From Chew DJ, DiBartola SP: Manual of Small Animal Nephrology and Urology. New York, Churchill Livingstone, 1986, pp 308–309.

300 are hypotonic (e.g., 0.45% saline in water), those greater than 300 are hypertonic (e.g., 5.0% dextrose in 0.9% NaCl), whereas those near 300 (e.g., Ringer's solution, Plasma-Lyte 148, Normosol-R) are isotonic. Physiologic saline (0.9% NaCl) at 308 mOsm/kg is also within the isotonic range. Lactated Ringer's solution often is referred to as an isotonic solution in some species, but at 272 mOsm/kg, it is mildly hypotonic for small animals.

▼ *Key Point* Serum sodium concentration is an indicator of tonicity and provides the basis for initial choice of fluid treatment. If no laboratory measurements are available, correct dehydration using isotonic balanced solutions.

Replacement Versus Maintenance

Crystalloid fluids also can be classified by their intended function for maintenance or replacement.

Replacement Fluids

Replacement fluids must be formulated for specific electrolyte or alkali deficits. Additives such as potassium chloride, magnesium sulfate, calcium chloride, or sodium bicarbonate often are added to commercially available solutions, but this varies greatly with the disease process and the patient's laboratory measurements. Replacement fluids usually are ideally suited to replenish fluid losses and resulting dehydration.

Maintenance Fluids

- *Maintenance fluids* are polyelectrolyte solutions that differ greatly from serum because they are lower in sodium and contain additional potassium and glucose. Although at administration they are isotonic, after the glucose is metabolized, their end effect is hypotonic. This class of fluids is intended for use in patients who have been rehydrated and simply are being maintained on IV fluids during hospitalization.

- The amount of energy provided by the glucose in these fluids is insufficient to meet patient needs, and utilization of specialized parenteral fluid solutions is much better suited for nutritional support. Introducing enteral nutrition in ill patients early in the course of hospitalization (when appropriate) also minimizes the need to switch to maintenance-type solutions after rehydration of the patient has been accomplished. Maintenance fluid and electrolyte needs often can be met with nutritional support rather than through maintenance crystalloid administration.
- Patients with intact renin-angiotensin-aldosterone axes should be able to excrete the sodium load present in replacement colloids if these fluids are used for a short-term basis after rehydration is accomplished. Maintenance crystalloid solutions are ideally suited for treatment of patients with congestive heart failure or advanced liver disease who cannot tolerate the sodium load present in replacement solutions or in patients with true water loss and hypernatremia.

Colloid Solutions

Colloid solutions differ from crystalloids because they contain large macromolecules (natural or synthetic). These molecules, because of their size, do not readily pass through the normal endothelium, thus giving them oncotic pressure effects. This allows them to affect water movement to and from the vascular and interstitial fluid spaces. Depending on the clinical situation, colloid molecules exert most of their effect in the intravascular space, making them less well suited for replacement of extravascular fluid losses and ideal for reexpansion of hypovolemia in the vascular space.

Natural Colloids

Natural colloids are produced by the body, harvested from volunteer donors, and stored for later use. This group of fluids includes the blood transfusion components, which possess albumin and other plasma proteins (whole blood, plasma). Indications for use of blood component therapy are covered elsewhere (see Chap. 20).

In human medicine, 5% and 25% concentrated albumin products also are manufactured. Unconcentrated natural colloids do not expand the vascular space, except by the volume administered. Concentrated natural colloids can expand the vascular space by up to five times (25% albumin) their volume, owing to their impressive oncotic pressure. Concentrated human albumin products have been used with success in canine patients, but their use carries the risk of adverse reaction.

Synthetic Colloids

The commercially available synthetic colloids, which currently are finding more frequent use in small animal medicine, are all complex polysaccharide molecules. The complex behavior and pharmacokinetics of these molecules do not allow accurate prediction of actual biologic behavior. As a result, the dose and duration of administration of these solutions vary with individual preference and patient characteristics and requirements. In addition, availability of these products in some countries is limited.

Synthetic colloids rarely should be used by themselves but are useful adjuncts to standard crystalloid fluid therapy in several well-defined situations. The synthetic colloids all have the capability of expanding the vascular volume because of their oncotic pressure effects. In most situations, this results in an average increase of 1.3 to 1.5 times the volume administered depending on the specific colloid used, dose, rapidity of administration, and the clinical situation. This effect must be kept in mind when calculating dosages of accompanying crystalloid fluids.

- Patients with hypoproteinemia and lowered oncotic pressure are likely to benefit from continuous infusions of hydroxyethyl starch (hetastarch or pentastarch) at doses of 20 ml/kg/24 hours (cats—10 ml/kg/24 hours) or more if needed.
- Hypovolemic patients, with concurrent lung or brain injury, who are at risk of worsened edema with crystalloid resuscitation, also may benefit from utilization of hydroxyethyl starches to reduce the total volume of resuscitation fluid. In these patients, colloids should be administered in 5-ml/kg (cats—2.5 ml/kg) boluses over 15 minutes, while monitoring cardiovascular parameters. Repetitive doses should be titrated to a stable cardiovascular endpoint. Total doses should not exceed 20 ml/kg/24 hours (cats—10 ml/kg) unless life-threatening consequences override these recommendations.
- Patients with diffuse vascular injury to the pulmonary vasculature and who are at risk for noncardiogenic pulmonary edema may be very sensitive to sudden elevations in intravascular volume. Thus, if increased oncotic pressure is desirable, continuous infusion rather than bolus administration of colloids is recommended.
- Synthetic colloids should be used with caution and at very reduced dosage rates in patients with congestive heart failure and in those with renal origin oliguria/anuria because rapid volume expansion could be detrimental.
- Of the three synthetic colloids mentioned, dextran 70 has the most potential to interfere with hemostasis. Although clotting times become elevated with use of the hydroxyethyl starches, clinically apparent hemostatic abnormalities typically are not encountered if the recommended dosages are used.
- Dextran 70 also carries a small risk of anaphylactic reaction, whereas reactions to administration of hydroxyethyl starches have not been reported. Consequently, and as a result of the decreasing cost differential between dextrans and hydroxyethyl starch, dextrans are being used with less frequency.

▼ *Key Point* As colloids become more economically available, consider their use during low-volume resuscitation and low oncotic pressure disorders.

Fluids to be Kept on Hand

- Clinical correction of most fluid problems can be accomplished by maintaining only a few stock solutions, usually lactated Ringer's solution (LRS), Plasma-Lyte 148 (P-148), or Normosol-R; 0.9% sodium chloride; and 5% dextrose in water.
- It is convenient, although not essential, to have 0.45% dextrose in 2.5% sodium chloride available for use in patients who cannot tolerate high sodium loads, as mentioned previously.
  - Alternatively, mixing equal portions of 0.9% sodium chloride with 5% dextrose in water provides the same solution.
- In addition, it may be useful to have one synthetic colloid solution available for use. The type will depend on availability, price, and types of patients commonly seen.
- These stock solutions are modified as needed with potassium, magnesium, glucose, or bicarbonate supplements (see subsequent discussion).
- An alkalinizing basic electrolyte solution (LRS, P-148, Normosol-R) is chosen most often as a "physiologic" solution that is similar in composition to normal plasma with the exception of protein. This solution is usually the fluid of choice until data about electrolyte, osmolality, and acid-base status are available.
  - Solutions that contain acetate as a bicarbonate precursor may be superior to lactate in critical care situations. Acetate is converted to bicarbonate by muscle, whereas lactate requires the liver to make this conversion. Additionally, acetate-based fluids are safer than lactate-based solutions for infusion during blood transfusions.
- The 0.9% sodium chloride or Ringer's solution is chosen when "extra" sodium or chloride is needed to maintain volume expansion or when the correction of metabolic alkalosis is needed.
- Low sodium fluids (0.45% saline in 2.5% dextrose, Plasma Lyte 56, Normosol-M, or 5% dextrose in water) are chosen when treating sodium-intolerant patients or patients with a water deficit (hypernatremia), or for maintenance.
- Synthetic colloids should be administered in conjunction with crystalloids when there is lowered oncotic pressure, or rapid (and low-volume) intravascular expansion is desired.

SUPPLEMENTATION OF PARENTERAL FLUIDS

After sodium, consideration of potassium is most important. Hypokalemia is commonly noted in hospitalized animals, particularly those with prolonged anorexia and those receiving potassium-deficient fluids. Other supplements can include alkali, magnesium, dextrose, phosphate, calcium, and vitamins.

Potassium Supplementation

Potassium supplementation usually is provided as potassium chloride, although potassium phosphate is given under unusual conditions. It is most common to use commercially available sterile vials with 2 mEq/ml of potassium for addition to fluids. Potassium supplementation to fluids is indicated when the serum potassium concentration is less than 3.5 mEq/L.

- The modified Sliding Scale of Scott (Table 5–4) recommends adding potassium chloride to maintenance fluid volumes proportional to the degree of hypokalemia—the lower the potassium concentration, the greater the amount of potassium added to the fluids. Supplemented fluids provide 28, 40, 60, or 80 mEq/L of potassium. An exact number of milliequivalents for supplementation is not calculated using this method. Potassium supplementation employing this scale can be started during correction of dehydration if fluids are distributed evenly throughout the day.
- Alternatively, a fixed concentration of potassium from 20 to 30 mEq/L can be given in maintenance fluids and is particularly helpful when frequent monitoring of serum potassium concentration is not possible. This concentration corresponds to the lower end of the Sliding Scale of Scott. Potassium to 35 mEq/L can be given in subcutaneous fluids without irritation to local tissues.
- Potassium supplementation still may be indicated when the concentration is from 3.5 to 4.5 mEq/L, especially if ventricular arrhythmias are present. This supplementation can prevent hypokalemia during fluid treatment and also can help replenish the total body potassium deficit that is not yet reflected by the serum potassium concentration.

Table 5–4. MODIFIED SLIDING SCALE OF SCOTT*

Serum K+ (mEq/L)	mEq K+ (To Add to 250 ml Fluid)	mEq K+ (To Add to 1 L Fluid)	Maximum Infusion Rate of IV Fluids (0.5 mEq/kg/hr)
<2.0	20	80	6
2.1–2.5	15	60	8
2.6–3.0	10	40	12
3.1–3.5	7	28	18
>3.5–<5.0	5	20	25

*For dogs or cats with hypokalemia or for those with potassium depletion and normal serum potassium levels. Infuse in maintenance volume of fluids.

- When managing arrhythmias, high normal levels of potassium (>4.0 mmol/L) are helpful because they reduce membrane hyperpolarization caused by low serum potassium levels.
- Maintenance needs for potassium in healthy dogs and cats are shown in Figure 5–1, but enhanced loss through urination during fluid administration can be expected.

▼ *Key Point* Potassium is added at approximately 20 to 30 mEq/L for maintenance fluids when serum potassium concentration is from 3.5 to 4.5 mEq/L.

- Caution is used whenever potassium-enriched fluids are infused. The rate of potassium infusion is usually more important than the total number of milliequivalents. Do not exceed 0.5 mEq/kg/hr to reduce any possibility of development of hyperkalemia and cardiotoxicity.
  - Animals with alkalosis and potassium translocation may not require vigorous potassium supplementation, if the alkalosis can be corrected rapidly. Potassium can rapidly return from the cells to the extracellular water.
  - Animals with severe emaciation have reduced lean body mass available for potassium uptake and are less vigorously supplemented with potassium in the fluid.
  - Reduced renal function and azotemia can lead to potassium retention and hyperkalemia during infusion of potassium-supplemented fluids, particularly if oliguria is present. Less vigorous potassium supplementation and careful monitoring are indicated in this situation.
- Potassium chloride supplementation increases the osmolality of fluids, particularly when high concentrations are provided. For example, potassium supplementation at 40 mEq/L increases the osmolality of the fluid by 80 mOsm/kg, 40 osmoles each from potassium and chloride. If the infused potassium and chloride enter the cells or are excreted, the transient increase in serum osmolality is of little concern.

▼ *Key Point* Although potassium supplementation is often beneficial, too much can result in death due to hyperkalemia. Do not supplement potassium supplementation at higher concentrations unless the serum concentration can be measured at least once daily. Electrocardiographic monitoring may be needed during supplementation of fluids with potassium in animals that are at risk for development of hyperkalemia.

Alkali Supplementation

- Addition of alkali to fluids sometimes is needed for partial correction of metabolic acidosis. It usually is not necessary or desirable to correct metabolic acidosis to normal by supplementation alone.
- Add sodium bicarbonate to fluids when alkali replacement is needed quickly. Do not rely on acetate or lactate at concentrations in commercially available solutions to correct severe metabolic acidosis. Lactate and acetate require metabolic conversion to bicarbonate before they can contribute to the correction of acidosis.

▼ *Key Point* Do not add sodium bicarbonate to fluids that contain calcium (LRS) because calcium precipitate may occur.

- Calculate the alkali replacement from either the bicarbonate value reported on the blood gas analysis or the total CO_2 value on the serum biochemical profile. Total CO_2 (mEq/L) can be substituted for bicarbonate in these calculations because it is usually only 1 to 2 mEq/L different.
  - Assume that normal HCO_3 is 24 mEq/L.
  - Subtract the patient's HCO_3 value from 24. This equals the HCO_3 deficit in mEq/L.
  - HCO_3 deficit $\times$ 0.6 $\times$ body weight (kg) = "missing" mEq bicarbonate from total body water at the time of sampling.
- Administer total replacement mEq over several hours of the day. It may take as long as 18 hours for administered bicarbonate to equilibrate inside cells. It is sometimes desirable, with severe metabolic acidosis, to administer ¼ to ½ of the calculated dose as a slow intravenous (IV) bolus injection and to add the remainder to fluids for 24-hour infusion.
- HCO_3 deficit $\times$ 0.3 $\times$ body weight (kg) = "missing" mEq bicarbonate from extracellular water at the time of sampling. Use this formula when (1) multiple injections of bicarbonate are likely to be needed during severe metabolic acidosis, (2) ongoing addition of acid or loss of alkali is anticipated, and (3) access to multiple HCO_3 measurements is possible.
- Without access to blood gas analysis or total CO_2, it is difficult to ascertain the magnitude of need. If the suspicion and clinical diagnosis for metabolic acidosis are high, bicarbonate may be administered empirically. Estimated at mild acidosis, give 3 mEq/kg bicarbonate in fluids for 24 hours. Estimated at moderate acidosis, give 6 mEq/kg bicarbonate in fluids for 24 hours. Estimated at severe acidosis, give 9 mEq/kg bicarbonate in fluids for 24 hours.
- In crisis situations that require bicarbonate, administer 1 to 2 mEq/kg of sodium bicarbonate as an IV slow bolus injection and reevaluate.
- Along with the bicarbonate, sodium is administered that can result in hypernatremia, hyperosmolality, hypertension, overhydration, and volume overload if not excreted.
- Overtreatment with alkali also can result in alkalosis, paradoxical cerebrospinal fluid (CSF) acidosis, ionized calcium shifts, and seizures. In critical care situations, intracellular acidosis can be worsened in poorly functioning myocardial cells and can lead to cardiac arrest.

Magnesium Supplementation

Magnesium recently has emerged as an important but seldom considered ion. It is a metabolic cofactor in hundreds of metabolic functions, most importantly as a cofactor in the sodium-potassium pump (Na^+, K^+-ATPase). Deficiencies in magnesium thus can lead to potassium wastage from the body. Hypokalemia and hypomagnesemia often are found together in many ill or dehydrated patients. Magnesium is lost with other electrolytes when urinary and gastrointestinal losses result in dehydration. Inadequate intake in anorexic patients exacerbates hypomagnesemia.

- Because magnesium is primarily an intracellular ion, serum measurements often are not reflective of total body stores. Low serum magnesium is generally reflective of low total body magnesium status, but decreased serum magnesium is often a late finding. Ion-specific electrodes are more sensitive for detecting hypomagnesemia but are not in common use.
- In patients with documented hypokalemia, and especially hypokalemia that seems to be resistant to supplementation efforts, consider magnesium supplementation. Do not use magnesium supplementation in oliguric patients because urine is the primary route of excretion of excessive amounts.
- The dose of magnesium supplementation is 2.5 to 5 mg/kg/hour, which can be added to most commercially available fluid types. Magnesium sulfate and magnesium chloride are the commonly available sources of magnesium. Magnesium sulfate is preferred to prevent excessive chloride administration. Magnesium supplementation can be extremely helpful in achieving and maintaining high normal levels of potassium when treating cardiac arrhythmias.

▼ *Key Point* Magnesium depletion is an underrecognized phenomenon that can have clinical consequences. Magnesium supplementation should be considered in patients with polyionic depletions (hypokalemia, hypocalcemia, and hyponatremia) and especially in those with refractory ventricular arrhythmias.

Dextrose Supplementation

If supplementation with dextrose is necessary, use 50% dextrose to vary the % dextrose in the final solution.

- To increase the dextrose concentration by 2.5%, add 25 g of dextrose, or 50 ml of 50% dextrose, to each liter. Long-term supplementation of dextrose through a peripheral vein should not exceed 5%, as the hypertonicity can induce significant phlebitis.
- Indications include hypoglycemia due to sepsis, insulin overdose, insulinoma, liver disease, and others. Dextrose supplementation at less than 10% concentration is not, however, effective as a source of calories in anorectic animals.

Vitamin Supplementation

The need for vitamins during parenteral fluid therapy in cats or dogs is not proved. It is plausible, however, that vitamins may be beneficial.

- Water-soluble vitamins can be added conservatively to parenteral fluids without known harm and may replenish rapidly depleted stores. Add 0.5 to 1.0 ml of water-soluble multi-vitamins to each liter of fluids to provide needed vitamins and to prevent thiamine deficiency.
- Dogs or cats in polyuric renal failure may benefit from water-soluble vitamins in parenteral fluids to replenish the urinary losses of these vitamins.
- Thiamine deficiency can be of clinical concern in cats and can develop during anorexia while on fluids, as thiamine is not stored for long periods. Initial signs of thiamine deficiency include anorexia, vomiting, and ataxia that can progress to dilated pupils and tonic ventroflexion of the neck, which often is confused with seizures. True seizures also can occur. Death is usually within 24 hours of convulsions, if the pet is not treated.

Calcium Supplementation

Calcium gluconate and calcium chloride can be supplemented in replacement and maintenance fluids for correction of symptomatic hypocalcemia. This is discussed in detail in Chapter 30. Calcium is not added to fluids containing lactate or acetate because precipitates may occur.

Phosphorus Supplementation

- Hypophosphatemia is present when the serum concentration is <2.5 mg/dl. Mild hypophosphatemia (2.0–2.5 mg/dl) is common and often transient. Mild to moderate hypophosphatemia often resolves quickly during the therapy directed at the underlying cause, without the need for phosphate supplementation.
- Severe hypophosphatemia (<1.5 mg/dl) is uncommon but can be life-threatening, particularly when less than 1.0 mg/dl; thus, treat by supplementing IV fluids with phosphate salts.

▼ *Key Point* Clinically significant hypophosphatemia is most likely to be observed in patients with diabetic ketoacidosis 12 to 48 hours after initiation of insulin therapy, or in patients in whom enteral nutrition is initiated after periods of anorexia. Specific treatment with phosphate salts may be required.

- When necessary, add supplemental sodium phosphate and potassium phosphate to replacement and maintenance fluids to correct symptomatic or severe hypophosphatemia. Do not add phosphate salts to fluids that contain calcium.
- Treat only when the hypophosphatemia is severe and its likely cause is ongoing. Oversupplementation can cause hyperphosphatemia, hypocalcemia, tetany/seizures, soft-tissue mineralization, hyperkalemia (if using potassium phosphate), and hypernatremia (if using sodium phosphate). Discontinue supplementation once the serum phosphorus concentration increases to >2.0 mg/dl.
- The IV dosage for phosphate supplementation is 0.01 to 0.03 mmol phosphate/kg/hr for 3 to 6 hours. A dosage of 2.5 mg/kg phosphate over 6 hours also has been suggested as a starting point. Patients with severe

hypophosphatemia may require prolonged supplementation or higher dosages (0.06–0.12 mmol/kg/hr). The most commonly used phosphate preparations provide 3.0 mmol/ml. For example, sodium phosphate provides 3.0 mmol/ml and 93.0 mg/ml phosphorus and 4.0 mEq/ml sodium.

GENERAL GUIDELINES FOR FLUID SELECTION

Serum Sodium Level as a Guide

Elevated Serum Sodium

If the serum sodium concentration is elevated, the animal has hypertonic dehydration and needs more water than salt for replacement (hypotonic fluid). Choose fluids that are effectively hypotonic (5% dextrose in water, 0.45% NaCl in 2.5% dextrose). Dextrose solutions in a 2.5 to 5% concentration are considered to be effectively hypotonic because of the rapid dextrose metabolism that removes its contribution to osmolality. The magnitude of the elevation in serum sodium and the patient's clinical status determine whether dextrose in water or dextrose in some concentration of saline is administered. Lowering of severe hyperosmolality and hypernatremia too rapidly can be detrimental, particularly to the brain. Do not use pure water without some electrolyte or glucose to add osmolality as severe problems with hemolysis and rapid change in serum osmolality can occur.

Normal Serum Sodium

If the serum sodium concentration is normal, the animal has isotonic dehydration and needs replacement fluids that are near-normal in serum sodium concentration and osmolality. Lactated Ringer's solution, Plasma-Lyte 148, Normosol-R, or 0.9% sodium chloride is an appropriate selection.

Decreased Serum Sodium

If the serum sodium concentration is low, the animal has hypotonic dehydration and needs additional sodium relative to water. Hypertonic fluid infusion is indicated theoretically but clinically is not chosen, unless the hyponatremia and hypo-osmolality are very severe and symptomatic. Isotonic fluids usually are chosen for replacement because the kidneys must excrete unnecessary water and reclaim needed sodium.

Fluid Selection for Shock

Choose 0.9% saline, LRS, Plasma-Lyte 148, or Normosol-R for rapid infusion to animals in shock until vascular volume is stabilized. Utilization of synthetic colloids is also appropriate for rapid reexpansion of the vascular space, especially in trauma patients with potential for brain or lung injury. For a complete discussion of shock therapy, see Chapter 72.

Fluid Composition

Further selection of fluid type requires laboratory measurement of albumin, total protein, potassium, chlo-

ride, magnesium, calcium, phosphorus, and blood gas values. When the serum concentration of an electrolyte is elevated, choose a fluid for infusion that lacks or is low in that electrolyte concentration. When the serum concentration of an electrolyte is low, choose a fluid for infusion that contains a high concentration of that electrolyte or provide supplementation of that electrolyte to the fluid. In some instances, supplemental electrolyte can be given to prevent deficits, as previously mentioned for potassium. Final osmolality of fluids for infusion is evaluated after supplementation of base solutions to ensure that they are appropriate because supplementation of base solutions often results in unappreciated hyperosmolality.

- Selection of fluid type can be confusing because clinical problems dictate that disparate fluid types should be chosen (e.g., use of acidifying solutions (0.9% NaCl) when the patient is severely acidemic (because high sodium content of this fluid is desirable). Thus, in these situations, identify the most severe problem and choose fluid based on this; then address secondary concerns as the primary problems are corrected. Fluid therapy is often dynamic and requires adjusting fluid type/additives frequently over the course of therapy.

Preservatives

Fluids containing preservatives of any kind are never used for administration to cats, puppies, or small dogs because of the likelihood of severe toxic reactions.

- Benzoic acid derivatives are found commonly in fluids for their antibacterial and antifungal effects, but cats are extremely susceptible to the toxic effects from these compounds even at low doses. Benzyl alcohol at 0.9% commonly is added to multiple dose vials of sodium chloride for injection.
- Clinical signs of toxicity are mostly neurologic and include changes in behavior: apprehension; aggression; hyperexcitability (to light and sound); salivation; marked ataxia; fasciculations of the muscles of the head and ears; widely dilated, nonresponsive pupils; seizures; and coma. Death follows. Immature animals may be at increased risk.

ROUTES OF ADMINISTRATION FOR PARENTERAL FLUIDS

The route of fluid therapy depends on the nature of the clinical disorder, its severity, and its onset (acute or chronic); the nature and magnitude of ongoing losses; and the composition of fluids to be given. The availability of personnel and equipment for monitoring during IV therapy also influences the decision to choose the parenteral route.

Subcutaneous Route

Subcutaneous (SC) administration of fluids is common in dogs and cats. Choose either isotonic or mildly hypotonic fluids to enhance absorption.

▼ *Key Point* Do not give 5% dextrose in water as an isotonic solution subcutaneously in cases of severe dehydration. Delayed absorption, with consequent equilibration of ECF electrolytes into the pocket of pooled, nonabsorbed subcutaneous fluid may occur.

Absorption of subcutaneous fluid is unreliable in conditions characterized by peripheral vasoconstriction (e.g., shock, severe dehydration, hypothermia). Never rely on this route for the emergency replacement of fluid in critically ill or severely dehydrated patients. Minimal dehydration may be corrected by this route, or dehydration in the anorexic animal may be prevented. In general, treat the critically ill or severely dehydrated animal initially with IV fluids.

The volume of fluid that can be administered subcutaneously is limited by the individual's skin elasticity. Animals differ in their ability to tolerate the infused load comfortably. Choose the site of the SC infusions somewhere on the trunk so that the fluid does not gravitate into the limbs. Avoid areas with surgical wounds because fluid may dissect the healing tissues.

Subcutaneous infusions may be given under gravitational forces through IV administration tubing or direct injection from a large-volume hypodermic syringe.

Intravenous Route

▼ *Key Point* Use IV fluid administration whenever accurate delivery of fluid volume and potent pharmacotherapeutic agents is required.

Give hypotonic, isotonic, and hypertonic fluids by the IV route as the need arises. Rapid infusions of fluid volume may be readily accomplished by this route.

Vein Selection

- The jugular vein and cephalic vein are most commonly chosen for indwelling IV catheterization. The lateral saphenous and femoral veins also may be used.
- The jugular vein in cats and small dogs is preferred for ease and convenience.
- The jugular vein is preferred in serious diseases, regardless of patient size.
  - Advantages of the jugular vein include the ability to measure central venous pressure (CVP) (see Chap. 3), to use large-bore catheters for more rapid infusions, to administer hypertonic solutions and other irritating drugs owing to greater dilutional effects from greater blood flow, and to obtain serial blood samples easily from the IV line. Use care to avoid clotting within the line.
  - The prime disadvantage of using peripheral veins is that the limb position often changes the rate of fluid infusion owing to partial or complete occlusion of the indwelling catheter when gravity flow is used. When fluid pumps are utilized, this effect is minimized.
- In cats and small dogs, 20- to 22-gauge catheters are often used; 14- to 20-gauge catheters generally are

used in larger animals. Short large-bore catheters or two catheters may be of value in emergency situations in facilitating rapid fluid administration. Clinician preference determines the type of catheter.

Intravenous Catheter Care

- Always perform aseptic catheter placement. This includes wide clipping of hair surrounding the vein and surgical scrub. After securing the catheter in the vein, place a gauze sponge with an antimicrobial cream over the puncture site.
- Catheter complications include thrombophlebitis, thromboembolism, bacteremia, and bacterial endocarditis, and catheter-fragment foreign body.
- To minimize problems:
  - Place the catheter aseptically.
  - Check the catheter site once to twice daily. If no redness, swelling, pain, or patient discomfort when injecting are present, catheters may be left in place longer than 48 to 72 hours.
  - Monitor the patient for fever, leukocytosis, and heart murmurs.
  - Keep the catheter site clean.
  - When the catheter is not in use, prevent clotting with heparinized saline (0.9% saline with 2 to 3 units heparin/ml).

Intraperitoneal Fluid Administration

- Severely anemic puppies and kittens may be transfused by this route when a vein cannot be catheterized (see Chap. 20 for details of blood transfusion).
- This route may be considered for rewarming very hypothermic animals or for cooling hyperthermic patients.
- Use isotonic to mildly hypotonic fluids for rehydration. The intravenous route is preferred when possible.

Intraosseous Route

- This route provides rapid access to circulation when venous catheterization is not successful or possible. Consider this route especially in puppies and kittens and in emergent situations when immediate IV access is difficult.
- Blood and crystalloid solutions can be infused safely.
- Bone marrow of femur, tibia, or humerus is catheterized with a bone-marrow or spinal needle and secured in place.

RATE OF FLUID INFUSION

The rate of fluid administration depends on the extent and rapidity of the fluid loss, the status of the patient, and the composition of the fluid to be infused. Rapid or extensive fluid losses demand rapid replacement. In chronic disorders, it is not always necessary to replace the dehydration deficit rapidly. Some clinicians prefer to calculate the dehydration deficit, add it to the daily maintenance requirements, and distribute this fluid load over 24 hours. Others prefer to replace the dehydration deficit over the first few hours (referred to as "front-end loading"). Deficit replacement of 75 to 80% on the first day and the remaining 25% deficit the second day is preferred by some clinicians. However, dehydration usually can be corrected safely within 24 hours in most cases. Table 5–5 lists the components of a complete prescription for fluid therapy (also see Fig. 5–3).

Maximum Hourly Infusion Rate

- Maximal infusion rates may be necessary in the treatment of shock or severe dehydration. Isotonic fluid of 1 blood volume/hr (40 ml/lb/hr or 90 ml/kg/hr for a dog; 30 ml/lb/hr or 66 ml/kg/hr for a cat) is recommended as the maximal rate of IV fluid infusion without CVP monitoring.
- Measure urine output during rapid fluid infusion as a guide to organ perfusion. In the case of persistent oliguria, be careful about maximal fluid infusion and monitor CVP to avoid overhydration (see Chaps. 3 and 72 for CVP).
- The rate of IV fluid infusion is important when considering potassium-rich fluids and those containing a large quantity of alkali. See previous discussion, Supplementation of Parenteral Fluids and Table 5–4.

24-Hour Infusion Rate

- In less critical conditions, distribute fluids evenly throughout the day. Physiologically, this technique may be advantageous because it allows more time for adequate equilibration of water and electrolytes between the body compartments. Ideally, a constant or continuous infusion of IV fluids over a 24-hour period accomplishes this. This ideal situation may not be possible if very small volumes of fluid are being infused or if 24-hour monitoring of the IV lines is unavailable.
  - Front-end loading of fluids to correct dehydration can be given over a 4- to 8-hour period when an animal's clinical condition dictates a more rapid correction of dehydration. Maintenance and contemporary losses then can be accomplished by infusion evenly over the remaining hours of the day.
- When fluid infusion can be observed for only part of the day, 24-hour needs are distributed over the number of hours that someone can watch the drip. The catheter then is flushed with heparinized saline to maintain patency until the infusion resumes. If severe dehydration has been corrected, additional fluids can be given subcutaneously until the IV drip can be restarted the next day.

Drip Rate

- The rate of infusion for the total 24-hour volume of fluid is specified as to the required number of milliliters per hour and the number of drops per minute to ensure accurate delivery of prescribed fluids.
- Intravenous administration sets are available in standard "macrodrip" volume of 10, 15, or 20 drops/ml. Pediatric administration sets also are available in the "minidrip" volume of 60 drops/ml. Patient size and volume of fluid to be infused determine the choice between the minidrip and macrodrip systems. The minidrip administration set is most suitable for cats and small dogs because it allows a simpler quantitation of small volumes of fluid for infusion.

Table 5–5. TOTAL FLUID PRESCRIPTION

1. Type of fluid to be infused (choose one):
   _____ Lactated Ringer's solution
   _____ 0.9% Sodium chloride in water
   _____ 0.45% Sodium chloride in 2.5% dextrose in water
   _____ 5% Dextrose in water
2. Supplements and amounts to be added to the fluid:

Sodium chloride	_____
Potassium chloride	_____
Sodium bicarbonate	_____
Glucose (dextrose)	_____
Calcium (gluconate)	_____
Phosphate	_____
Magnesium	_____
Other (specify _____)	_____

3. 24-hr fluid volume: _____ ml
4. Route of infusion: _____
5. Rate of fluid administration: _____ ml/24 hr
   _____ ml/hr
   _____ ml/min
   _____ drops/sec

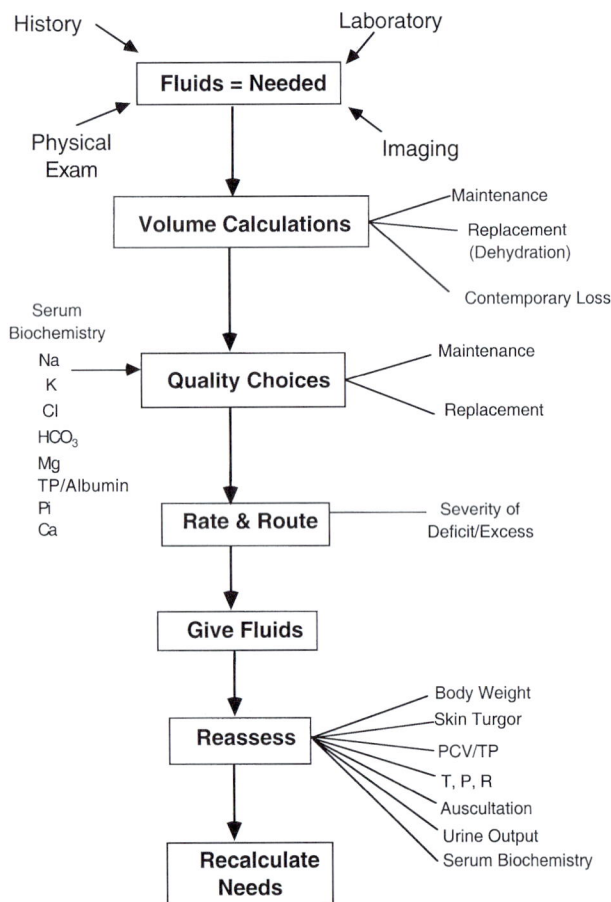

Figure 5–3. General assessment/decision tree—fluid therapy.

- Once the drip set has been adjusted to the desired rate, mark the IV bottle or bag with adhesive tape as subsequently indicated to monitor the hourly volume of fluids received. This practice allows adjustment for individual variations (e.g., animal changing position of the limb that contains the catheter).
- For small dogs and cats, consider the use of a Buretrol (Baxter Healthcare) or a similar device to accurately premeasure the fluids to be administered over the next few hours. Fluids from the reservoir bag are used periodically to reload the Buretrol device. This method minimizes the chance of overhydration because it allows more accurate delivery of small volumes.

Urine Output to Determine Fluid Input

- In dehydrated animals with either severe oliguria or diuresis, measurement of urine output may be helpful for accurately matching the needs of the animal with the fluid therapy ("ins and outs"). Without this system, a tendency exists to overestimate the actual fluid needs in an oliguric animal, resulting in overhydration, and to underestimate the fluid needs in a diuretic animal, resulting in failure to correct the dehydration.
- Replace previously calculated dehydration needs first and then proceed with the "ins and outs." In this technique, divide the day into six 4-hour intervals. The hour interval can vary and is chosen based on the severity of the condition (i.e., ranging from every hour to every 6 or 8 hours, as the need dictates). Determine the fluid needs for this interval, summating both calculated insensible (10 ml/lb or 22 ml/kg divided by 6, if 4-hour intervals are used) losses and measured sensible (urine-volume) losses. The measured volume of sensible losses from the previous 4-hour period is given back to the patient in the next 4-hour period.
- Carry this procedure out in identical fashion for an additional three or more time periods. This type of close attention to fluid volume administration is of benefit in the initial management of critically ill animals, particularly when CVP and renal status are uncertain.

Infusion Pumps

Infusion pumps provide an extremely accurate means of administering IV fluids.

- Enter ml/hr or drops/min depending on the type of machine.
- Most pumps are equipped with alarm systems if fluid flow is interrupted.
- A disadvantage is that new pumps are expensive. Refurbished used machines may be surprisingly affordable, however.
- Infusion pumps are especially useful for small dogs, cats, and animals receiving fluids supplemented with potassium or drugs for constant-rate infusion.

MONITORING EFFICACY OF FLUID THERAPY

Perform a physical examination several times daily during the initial fluid management to document rehydration, prevent overhydration, and detect contemporary fluid loss. The indicators of successful fluid therapy are normalization of skin turgor, moistening of mucous membranes, strengthening of pulses, increasing of perfusion (decreasing of refill time), and increasing of alertness. Table 5–6 provides guidelines for the database required to adequately assess the success of fluid therapy. Table 5–7 lists the possible reasons why dehydration has not been adequately corrected.

Body Weight

Increased body weight occurs during successful rehydration. An acute gain or loss of 1 lb suggests an increase or a decrease of 500 ml body water (or a 1 kg change in body weight is equivalent to 1000 ml). An anorexic animal, however, loses 0.1 to 0.3 kg body weight/day/1000 calories of the daily requirement, owing to tissue catabolism. Determine and record body weight accurately at least once daily.

Hematocrit and Plasma Protein

Follow packed cell volume (PCV) and total plasma protein (TPP) serially during fluid therapy. Decreases in both PCV and TPP suggest successful intravascular rehydration.

Table 5–6. DATABASES BEFORE AND DURING FLUID ADMINISTRATION

Minimum database (mild illness and dehydration)
  Body weight
  Packed cell volume (PCV); total plasma protein (TPP)
  Urine specific gravity
Extended database (severe dehydration with collapse)
  All the above, plus the following values:
    Serum sodium, potassium, and chloride
    Total Mg, total Ca, P
    Blood urea nitrogen (BUN) or serum creatinine
    Bicarbonate (total CO_2 from profile)
    Electrocardiogram
Advanced database (shock, oliguria; heart failure)
  All the above, plus the following values:
    Central venous pressure (CVP)
    Blood gas analysis (venous and arterial)
    Ionized calcium, ionized magnesium

Table 5–7. POSSIBLE CAUSES OF FAILURE TO ADEQUATELY CORRECT DEHYDRATION

Error in mathematic calculations
Error in assessment of initial degree of dehydration
Larger contemporary losses than expected
Too-rapid infusion resulting in diuresis and loss of fluid from body
Mechanical dysfunction of IV catheter or infusion system;
  calculated volume not infused
Increased sensible loss not appreciated (fever, panting, polyuria)

Central Venous Pressure

In difficult cases, particularly those animals with renal or heart failure, monitor the CVP to minimize the chances of overloading the heart and causing pulmonary edema when administering fluids rapidly (see Chap. 3 for CVP measurement technique).

- Monitor the CVP with a jugular catheter, the tip of which is level with the right atrium. Normal CVP is 0 to 10 cm H_2O.
- A sudden increase in CVP during fluid therapy indicates the inability of the cardiovascular system to accommodate the rate of fluid administration. Reduce the rate of administration accordingly. Signs of overhydration, unfortunately, still can occur even without a change in CVP.

Electrolyte and Acid-Base Status

Closely monitor all animals receiving fluid therapy. Determine the serial serum electrolyte and acid-base values in severely dehydrated animals receiving fluid therapy. Ideally, animals that had serum electrolyte deficiency or excess show improvement toward normal values after appropriate therapy. Follow the electrolyte determinations in those cases that had initially normal values to detect the possible consequences of volume expansion and changes in the underlying disease process.

▼ *Key Point* Successful fluid therapy ultimately depends on the clinician's ability to detect and correct the underlying cause for the loss of fluid, loss or retention of electrolytes, and acid-base disturbances. Identifying and stopping the ongoing fluid losses are particularly important.

OVERHYDRATION

Overhydration rarely occurs as a spontaneous disorder—it usually is iatrogenic after fluid treatments. Inability to excrete free water, as can occur in a variety of renal diseases and in congestive heart failure, predisposes the patient to overhydration.

Physical Examination

Body weight continues to increase above and beyond that expected to accomplish rehydration. Central venous pressure progressively increases during advanced overhydration. Decreased volume of urinations may be noticed, or the bladder may remain small during fluid administration. A gelatinous feel to the subcutaneous tissues may precede the development of obvious peripheral edema. Pulmonary edema, manifested as lung crackles and tachypnea, may be detected. Vomiting, diarrhea, serous discharge from the nose and eyes, and chemosis can develop during overhydration. Venous overdistention also may be noted.

Laboratory and Radiographic Findings

- Progressive decreases in PCV and total protein may be found.
- Radiographs may reveal increased lung density, indicating pulmonary edema. Cardiac enlargement may be noted if congestive heart failure is imminent.

Treatment

Immediate correction may be difficult when renal and cardiac function is impaired. Stop all IV infusions and give furosemide at 2 to 4 mg/kg IV. Give another dose of furosemide but double the dose if no diuresis occurs within 15 minutes. Morphine is considered as a treatment to increase compliance of pulmonary vessels, but this effect is controversial. Peritoneal dialysis with hypertonic dialysate can be considered for acute volume overload rescue, as can therapeutic phlebotomy.

Chapter

6 Feline Leukemia Virus

Robert G. Sherding

ETIOLOGY AND PATHOBIOLOGY

Feline leukemia virus (FeLV) is a horizontally transmitted retrovirus that is a major cause of morbidity and mortality in domestic cats. In a nationwide survey of 27,976 cats in 1990–1991, 13.3% of cats were positive for FeLV. Mostly high-risk cats were surveyed, such as sick cats or healthy cats exposed to other cats outdoors. Other surveys have found the prevalence to be 30% in cats living in an infected household or cattery, 1% to 3% in healthy free-roaming cats, and less than 1% in healthy indoor cats and cats in purebred catteries. The prevalence is declining.

Structure of the Virus

Certain structural components of the FeLV virion have clinical implications.

- *Core*—contains RNA and reverse transcriptase, an enzyme that allows insertion of FeLV into the DNA genome of an infected cell.
- *Core Proteins*—the protein designated p27 is detected as FeLV antigen by conventional FeLV diagnostic tests.
- *Envelope Glycoproteins* (gp70)—consist of subgroup antigens A, B, C, or combinations of these. They determine infectivity, host range, and pathogenicity. They also elicit the protective host neutralizing antibody response that occurs on natural exposure or vaccination.
- *Envelope Protein* (p15e)—a mediator of FeLV-related immunodeficiency.

Sequential Phases of FeLV Infection

- Transmission
  - Primarily through intimate oronasal contact with infectious saliva.
  - Transplacental transmission can occur, but milk-borne infection in nursing kittens is more common.
  - FeLV is readily inactivated and the virus survives no more than 24 to 48 hours in the environment.
- After the initial stages of replication within oronasal and then systemic lymphoid tissues, FeLV infects bone marrow cells. This appears to be a pivotal phase in the pathogenesis and outcome of infection because persistent viremia subsequently develops if FeLV overwhelms the host immune response, whereas transient infection and recovery occur if the immune response is successful.
- Cats that develop persistent viremia shed virus in most body secretions, especially saliva, and thus they are contagious to other cats.

Host Immune Response

Immunity to FeLV is the collective result of humoral antibody, cell-mediated immune mechanisms, complement, and interferon. Humoral antibody responses have been characterized as follows:

- Antiviral response is mediated by neutralizing antibody directed against FeLV envelope antigens.
- Antitumor response is mediated by anti-FOCMA (*fe*line *o*ncornavirus *c*ell *m*embrane–associated *a*ntigen)

antibody directed against FeLV-associated antigen (FOCMA) on the surface of FeLV-induced neoplastic cells.

Outcome of FeLV Exposure and Categories of Infection

The outcome of FeLV exposure is variable and can be categorized into three groups (Table 6–1):

Group 1 (Uninfected)

Group 1 contains 28% of exposed cats that do not get infected, either because of an inherent resistance to infection or because of insufficient exposure.

Group 2 (Persistently Infected)

Group 2 contains 10-30% of exposed cats that develop progressive infection with persistent viremia. This leads to FeLV-related disease after a variable disease-free interval. In a study that followed healthy FeLV-positive cats, the mortality rate was 33% at 6 months, 63% at 2 years, and 83% at 3.5 years.

Group 3 (Transiently Infected)

Group 3 contains 42% of exposed cats that develop a transient replicating infection that subsequently is rejected by the immune system.

- Replicating FeLV usually is eliminated 4 to 6 weeks after exposure, sometimes after a transient viremia lasting 1 to 5 weeks.
- These nonviremic cats that have "recovered" from transient infection usually become latent carriers of FeLV for a variable period of time. In latent FeLV infection, nonreplicating FeLV provirus remains dormant within the DNA genome of certain bone marrow and lymphoid cells. Latency can be detected only by specialized cell culture techniques or polymerase chain reaction assay in research laboratories.

▼ *Key Point* Latent FeLV infection cannot be detected by conventional FeLV diagnostic tests.

- In most transiently infected cats, the latent stage of infection eventually is eliminated uneventfully as part of the normal recovery process. This usually occurs within 6 to 9 months of exposure but sometimes can take a year or more.
- In some cats with latent FeLV (less than 10% of exposed cats), latency persists indefinitely.
- Clinical significance of latency
  - Minimal risk of developing FeLV-related disease
  - Minimal risk of contagiousness to other cats by contact transmission
  - Rare possibility of recrudescence (e.g., steroid-induced) of active replicating FeLV and viremia
  - Occasional infection by latent FeLV-infected queens of kittens in utero or during nursing through local mammary excretion of FeLV

MANIFESTATIONS AND CLINICAL SIGNS

The clinical manifestations of FeLV are attributable to the oncogenic, cytopathic, and immunosuppressive effects of the virus. FeLV-induced neoplasia can be lymphoid or myeloid. Degenerative and cytopathic effects on various cells include bone marrow cells (anemia, neutropenia, thrombocytopenia), lymphocytes (T-lymphocyte depletion, lymphoid atrophy, lymphoid hyperplasia), intestinal cells (enteritis), and the fetus and placenta (abortion, stillbirth). The immunosuppressive effects of FeLV cause profound immunodeficiency, resulting in susceptibility to a wide variety of opportunistic infections. In addition, FeLV-related immune dysfunction can cause immune-mediated and autoimmune diseases.

Lymphoproliferative Neoplasms

Both lymphoma and lymphoid leukemias are associated with FeLV infection. For general information regarding lymphoma, see Chapter 25; for treatment of lymphoma (i.e., chemotherapy), see Chapter 24.

- Alimentary lymphoma
  - Mesenteric lymph nodes—palpable enlargement
  - Stomach—vomiting, anorexia, and weight loss
  - Intestine—diffuse infiltration and thickening of the intestinal wall (diarrhea and weight loss) or palpable intestinal mass (obstruction)
  - Liver—diffuse hepatomegaly or nodular tumor masses within the liver (icterus, weight loss, vomiting, abnormal liver tests)
  - Spleen—diffuse splenomegaly

▼ *Key Point* Cats with gastrointestinal lymphoma are much older (mean age, 8 years) than cats with other

Table 6–1. CATEGORIES OF INFECTION AFTER FeLV EXPOSURE

Category of Infection	Percent (%) of Exposed Cats	Consequences
Noninfected	28	Uninfected due to insufficient exposure (may or may not be susceptible)
Persistent infection	10–30	High risk of mortality due to immunosuppression, anemia, lymphoma, and other FeLV-related diseases
Transient infection extinguished	30–35	Transient latency followed by recovery; immune to FeLV infection
Sustained latent infection	5–10	Usually asymptomatic and noncontagious; rarely, any one of the following can occur: recrudescence, in utero transmission to unborn kittens, milkborne transmission to kittens

FeLV, feline leukemia virus.

forms of lymphoma, and up to 75% have negative results on FeLV blood tests. This is the most common form of lymphoma in many areas.

- Mediastinal lymphoma (cranial mediastinal mass due to lymphoma of thymus or mediastinal nodes)
  - Pleural effusion (dyspnea)
  - Tracheal compression (dyspnea, cough)
  - Esophageal compression (dysphagia, regurgitation)
  - Sympathetic trunk impingement (Horner's syndrome)
  - Decreased cranial thoracic compressibility
  - Mass palpable at thoracic inlet (rare)
- Multicentric lymphoma
  - Generalized involvement of external and internal lymph nodes along with various other sites
  - Liver, spleen, kidneys, and other visceral organs
- Renal lymphoma
  - Signs—nonspecific (early), renal failure, and uremia (late)
  - Kidneys palpably enlarged and nodular ("lumpy")
- Ocular lymphoma
  - Retrobulbar mass—mimics retrobulbar abscess
  - Third eyelid mass—mimics "cherry eye"
  - Corneal infiltration—mimics eosinophilic keratitis
  - Uveal infiltration and hemorrhage—mimics anterior uveitis or choroiditis
- Nervous system lymphoma
  - Brain: seizures, ataxia, blindness, behavior aberrations, motor deficits, and cranial nerve signs
  - Spinal cord: paresis or paralysis
- Cutaneous lymphoma: multiple firm, nonpainful cutaneous nodules
- Lymphoid leukemia—primary bone marrow involvement with circulating neoplastic cells
- Others: lung, heart, urinary bladder, and nasal

Myeloproliferative Disorders

This is a group of neoplastic or neoplastic-like diseases characterized by the proliferation of one or more cell lines in the bone marrow at the expense and to the eventual exclusion of other marrow cells. The abnormal cells often are found in the peripheral blood as well as in the bone marrow, and their identification provides the diagnosis. These disorders are classified on the basis of the cellular origin of the abnormal cells.

- Nonspecific signs—anorexia, depression, and weight loss
- Progressive, unresponsive anemia and thrombocytopenia
- Diffuse hepatomegaly (icterus), splenomegaly, and lymphadenopathy from extramedullary hematopoiesis and/or neoplastic infiltration

FeLV-Related Anemia

Anemia may occur as the sole primary manifestation of FeLV as well as being present with many other FeLV-related diseases.

- Nonregenerative anemia: usually resulting from destruction, suppression, or abnormal maturation of erythrocyte precursors in bone marrow

- Other mechanisms: immune-mediated hemolysis, opportunistic *Hemobartonella* or *Ehrlichia* infection, bleeding from thrombocytopenia, and neoplastic or myelodysplastic bone marrow
- Clinical signs: listlessness, weakness, tachypnea, mucous membrane pallor, anemic murmur, splenomegaly, retinal hemorrhages, and pica
- Laboratory signs
  - Severe nonregenerative anemia (hematocrit may be <10%)
  - Erythrocyte macrocytosis
  - Leukopenia or thrombocytopenia—may accompany anemia
  - Bone marrow cytology—normal, hypocellular, aplastic, hypercellular, neoplastic, or dysplastic
- Treatment: blood transfusions and general supportive care (median survival in 49 treated cases was 4 months)

FeLV-Related Neutrophil Disorders

Neutrophils and myeloid precursors usually are infected in FeLV viremia.

- FeLV-induced neutropenia can be transient (for first 3–5 weeks of bone marrow infection with FeLV), persistent, or cyclic (10–14 days). Signs include chronic or recurrent bacterial infections and sepsis.
- Neutropenia can be a preneoplastic change that eventually develops into a myeloproliferative disorder.
- Myeloblastopenia (panleukopenia-like syndrome) is characterized by profound panleukopenia (WBC count = 300–3000/µl) and acute enterocolitis with fever, vomiting, and bloody diarrhea. Intestinal epithelial cells are infected heavily with FeLV.

FeLV-Related Platelet Disorders

Platelets and megakaryocytes usually are infected in FeLV viremia. Manifestations include:

- Thrombocytopenia
- Macroplatelets—abnormally large platelets with bizarre shapes occurring commonly in viremic cats, especially those with severe anemia (may be miscounted as RBCs by electronic counters)
- Platelet dysfunction (subclinical)

FeLV-Induced Immunodeficiency

FeLV causes profound lymphoid atrophy and suppression of the cat's immune system (especially T-lymphocytes), thereby increasing susceptibility to all types of infections, especially chronic or recurrent ones. This is the most important overall consequence of FeLV infection in many cats. Fever is often a presenting sign, along with signs of various opportunistic infections. Some examples follow.

- Viral—feline infectious peritonitis, herpesvirus
- Fungal—*Cryptococcus, Aspergillus, Candida*
- Rickettsial—*Haemobartonella*
- Protozoal—*Toxoplasma, Cryptosporidium*

- Bacterial
  - Oral—gingivitis, periodontitis, stomatitis
  - Respiratory infections—rhinitis, sinusitis, pneumonia, pyothorax
  - Enteritis—*Salmonella, Campylobacter,* diarrhea of undetermined cause
  - Cutaneous—pyoderma, nonhealing sores, abscesses, draining fistulas
  - Septicemia

Distinctive Peripheral Lymph Node Hyperplasia

- There is marked symmetric enlargement of peripheral and visceral lymph nodes (especially mandibular nodes), up to three times normal size.
- Primarily affects young adult cats (6 months to 2 years of age): 50% are asymptomatic and 50% have fever, anorexia, and depression.
- Outcome: some cases resolve in 2 to 4 weeks (with corticosteroids, cyclophosphamide, vincristine); some recur; and some evolve into lymphoma months to years later.

Immune-Mediated Disorders

Several immune-mediated disorders have been associated with FeLV infection:

- Immune complex glomerulonephritis
- Chronic progressive polyarthritis
- Immune-mediated hemolytic anemia
- Immune-mediated thrombocytopenia
- Pemphigus-like mucocutaneous disorders
- Systemic lupus erythematosus–like syndrome

The exact role of FeLV in these disorders is not fully understood, but it presumably involves viral antigen-antibody complexes or FeLV-induced disruption of immune regulation.

Infertility, Stillbirths, Abortions, and "Fading Kittens"

In FeLV-infected female cats, any of the following can occur: infertility, fetal resorption, abortion, stillbirth, "fading kitten syndrome" (viremic kittens), or milk-borne transmission to nursing kittens.

Miscellaneous

A role for FeLV in the following disorders has been suggested but unproved: chronic enteritis, seborrheic dermatitis, eosinophilic granuloma complex, cutaneous horns, multicentric osteochondromas, olfactory neuroblastoma, anisocoria, and degenerative myelopathy.

DIAGNOSIS

Diagnostic testing for FeLV infection has become one of the most frequently performed procedures in veterinary practice. FeLV tests are used to diagnose FeLV-related illnesses, to screen for subclinical infection in cats presented for FeLV vaccination, and to identify and eliminate FeLV infections in catteries. FeLV tests are available on a mail-in basis through commercial laboratories; however, simple diagnostic kits that allow the rapid in-office testing of blood, saliva, or tears for the presence of FeLV are used routinely by most veterinarians.

Overview of Diagnostic Tests for FeLV

Two tests available for routine clinical diagnosis of FeLV infection are the immunofluorescent antibody (IFA) test and the enzyme-linked immunosorbent assay (ELISA). Both tests detect FeLV group-specific core antigens (p27). The IFA test requires a specialized commercial or university laboratory and uses a smear of peripheral blood or bone marrow. The ELISA test can be performed on blood, saliva, or tears using any of several in-office test kits or an outside commercial laboratory. Guidelines for interpretation of IFA and ELISA test results are presented in Table 6–2.

In addition to the IFA and ELISA tests, some research laboratories can assay tissues and body fluids for FeLV by virus isolation (VI) as the "gold standard" for detection of FeLV infection. This assay is not, however, routinely available for clinical use. The bone marrow reactivation test detects latent (dormant, nonreplicating) FeLV infection in cultured bone marrow cells but also is available only for research applications.

IFA Test

The IFA test indicates cell-associated viremia by detecting FeLV antigen in circulating neutrophils and platelets on smears of peripheral blood or in bone marrow cells. The IFA test is very specific for FeLV and is often regarded as the best clinical test for confirming FeLV viremia. See Table 6–2 for IFA interpretation.

- Positive IFA results indicate an advanced stage of FeLV infection and is highly correlated (98%) with virus isolation assays. It also is correlated with persistent viremia because 90% to 96% of IFA-positive cats remain persistently infected. Healthy IFA-positive cats can be retested monthly for 3 months to differentiate transient and persistent infection with reasonable certainty. This is because transient FeLV-positive infections sometimes can last for up to, but very rarely longer than, 3 months. Thus, if a positive IFA test result remains positive for greater than 3 months, the infection is considered to be persistent, whereas if the result becomes negative within 3 months, the infection was transient.
- False-positive IFA results are very rare but can occur from improperly made blood smears that are too thick and cause nonspecific binding of the conjugate. Platelet clumping and eosinophilia also can cause rare false-positive results.
- False-negative IFA results may occur in neutropenia/thrombocytopenia and in early infections because the test result usually does not become positive until FeLV infects and replicates in the bone marrow. A false-negative IFA test result rarely may occur in low-level infections because the test is less sensitive than the ELISA test.

Table 6–2. INTERPRETATION OF FeLV TEST RESULTS

Test	Result	Interpretations to Be Considered
IFA	Positive	Persistent viremia (95%)
		Transient viremia (5%)
		False-positive (rare in experienced laboratories): due to thick smear, clumped platelets, eosinophilia
IFA	Negative	Nonexposed/noninfected
		Prior transient infection; now recovered (uninfected/immune)
		Prior transient infection; now latent (nonreplicating) infection
		Early infection too soon to detect (may be ELISA-positive)
		Compartmentalized ELISA-positive infection
		ELISA-positive infection with replication of antigens but not whole virus
		False-negative: due to inadequate neutrophils and platelets on the slide (neutropenia/thrombocytopenia)
ELISA	Positive	Persistent viremia (also IFA-positive)
		Transient viremia (also IFA-positive)
		Antigenemia without cell-associated viremia (IFA-negative)
		False-positive due to laboratory error (IFA-negative) (see Table 6–4)
ELISA	Negative	Nonexposed/noninfected
		Prior transient infection; now recovered (uninfected/immune)
		Prior transient infection; now latent (nonreplicating) infection
		Very early subclinical infection, too early to detect

FeLV, feline leukemia virus; IFA, immunofluorescent antibody; ELISA, enzyme-linked immunosorbent assay.

Table 6–3. ELISA TEST KITS FOR IN-OFFICE FeLV DIAGNOSIS

Test Kit	Manufacturer	Format
UNI-TEC FeLV	Synbiotics	Membrane filter
VIRACHEK/FeLV	Synbiotics	Microwell
ASSURE/FeLV	Synbiotics	Wand/tube (tests saliva)
Witness FeLV	Synbiotics	Membrane device
ICT Gold FeLV	Synbiotics	Membrane device
Snap-FeLV	IDEXX	Membrane filter (also tests saliva and tears)
Snap-Combo FeLV/FIV	IDEXX	Membrane filter (also tests for FIV)
Probe FeLV	IDEXX	Programmed, self-contained membrane filter device
Petchek FeLV	IDEXX	Microwell

ELISA, enzyme-linked immunosorbent assay; FeLV, feline leukemia virus; FIV, feline immunodeficiency virus.

brane filter–type ELISA systems are designed to reduce the risk of nonspecific false-positive reactions by providing flow-through design to facilitate thorough washing, individualization of test units to prevent splashing of reagents between specimens, a prefilter to filter out interfering biologic debris, and easy-to-interpret colorimetric results on a white background. Also, positive and negative controls are built in for each patient specimen so that false-positive and false-negative reactions can be detected readily as such.

Positive ELISA

A positive ELISA result indicates viremia (or antigenemia). In general, serum ELISA test results tend to become positive earlier after exposure to FeLV than IFA test results, and ELISA tests are more sensitive than the IFA test. After recent FeLV exposure, serum ELISA test results become positive 1 to 2 weeks earlier than saliva or tear ELISA test results. For additional reasons, ELISA tests on saliva and tears do not detect as many FeLV infections as serum ELISA tests. Healthy ELISA-positive cats should be retested at monthly intervals for 3 months to determine whether the infection is transient or persistent.

False-positive ELISA

False-positive ELISA titers sometimes occur, especially with the microwell format, primarily because of technical errors discussed in the next section.

False-negative ELISA

False-negative ELISA results are unlikely because of the inherently high sensitivity of this test.

ELISA Test

The ELISA test is used most commonly for routine screening for FeLV infection and can be performed on serum, plasma, whole blood, saliva, or tears. There are two formats for the ELISA test: the microwell ELISA and the membrane filter ELISA. Modifications of these are also available for testing saliva and tears. Each of these formats is available in test kit form for in-office testing (Table 6–3), and most provide results in less than 10 minutes. In addition, many commercial laboratories offer FeLV ELISA testing on mail-in specimens. See Table 6–2 for ELISA interpretation.

Microwell ELISA Format

The antibody-antigen-antibody sandwich ELISA reaction takes place on the inner surface of antibody-coated microwells. The microwell units are grouped for batch testing. Microwell-type ELISA test systems are the most susceptible to the various technical errors and pitfalls that cause false-positive results (see section on Discordancy).

Membrane Filter ELISA Format

The ELISA reaction takes place on antibody-coated dots on a pad or flow-through membrane. The mem-

Interpretation of Discordant Test Results

▼ *Key Point* The ELISA for FeLV is more sensitive and can detect infection earlier than the IFA test; however, false-positive results are more frequent with the ELISA. False-positive results are rare with the IFA test, and it has better correlation with persistent infection.

A major issue in FeLV testing is the fact that there is a considerable problem of discrepancy between ELISA and IFA test results. The agreement between a negative ELISA test and a negative IFA test is nearly 100%. The problem of discordancy primarily involves cats that test ELISA-positive but IFA-negative. Some reports suggest a discordancy rate of 30% or higher; however, in recent years, technical improvements in the ELISA systems have reduced this to less than 10%. There are legitimate biologic explanations for a small degree of discordancy, but the principal cause of discordancy is false-positive ELISA results due to technical laboratory errors, especially with microwell test systems.

Biologic Factors That Cause Discordancy

Biologic factors can cause discordancy, but collectively, these should not cause more than 5% to 10% of ELISA-positive cats to test IFA-negative.

- There is a brief period of a few weeks during early infection when FeLV antigens are detectable in the serum (ELISA-positive) but FeLV is not yet replicating in the bone marrow, so that blood cells do not yet contain virus (IFA-negative).
- The ELISA test is also more sensitive and thus may detect low-level infections that the IFA test may miss; however, this is probably uncommon because there is 98% correlation between IFA test and virus isolation results.
- Persistent antigenemia (ELISA-positive) with a negative IFA test may occur when there is sequestration of FeLV infection with replication in sites other than bone marrow, or when there is replication of FeLV antigens but not whole virus. These cats have persistent discordancy even on repeat testing, but they usually do not shed virus and are not likely to be contagious to other cats.

Technical Pitfalls and Laboratory Errors That Cause Discordancy

The most frequent cause of discordancy is false-positive ELISA results due to technical error in the performance of the ELISA procedures, especially as performed using the microwell ELISA kits by inexperienced or improperly trained personnel (Table 6–4).

- The most common problem is false-positive reactions owing to the presence of residual conjugate in the microwell after washing. This can be caused by insufficient washing, splashing of conjugate between wells during the procedure, or nonspecific binding of conjugate to microdefects in the plastic microwells (or

Table 6–4. CAUSES OF FALSE-POSITIVE RESULTS ON FeLV MICROWELL ELISA TESTS

Residual conjugate remaining in the wells due to inadequate washing.
Splashing of conjugate between wells.
Nonspecific binding of conjugate to plastic defects.
Cell debris (e.g., saliva, hemolyzed serum) or fibrin that sticks to the well and traps conjugate.
Presence of enzymes or other bioactive materials in the sample.
Presence of cross-reacting antimouse antibodies in the sample.
Interfering antibodies in patient serum induced by recent vaccination.
Misinterpretation of a weak positive reaction as a true positive result.

FeLV, feline leukemia virus; ELISA, enzyme-linked immunosorbent assay.

binding of conjugate to chew marks in the plastic device used for saliva testing).
- Biologic material in the sample may cause false-positive reactions. Cell debris and fibrin in the sample may stick to the microwell and trap conjugate. This is more likely to occur with saliva, tears, whole blood, or hemolyzed sera. Also, enzymes or other bioactive materials may react nonspecifically with the conjugate to produce the color change reaction.
- A false-positive ELISA reaction occasionally may be caused by antimouse antibodies in the patient specimen that cross-react with the murine-derived monoclonal antibody used as a reagent in the test system. Less than 1% of the cat population has interfering antimouse antibodies, and most test kits correct for this.

Recommendations for FeLV Testing

▼ *Key Point* To reduce false-positive ELISA test results, analyze nonhemolyzed serum rather than whole blood, saliva, or tears, and use a membrane filter test rather than a microwell test.

- Because saliva and tear ELISA tests only detect 80% to 90% of infected cats, do not use these to determine infection in individual cats. These tests can be used for mass screening of a group of cats to determine whether FeLV is endemic and for detection of cats that are actively shedding virus.
- Use only ELISA antibody reagents that are monoclonal to provide optimal specificity and to reduce nonspecific false-positive reactions. All the currently available ELISA test kits use monoclonal antibody reagents.
- Experience and meticulous technique are required to obtain accurate results with in-office microwell ELISA tests. Only under these circumstances is a microwell ELISA test kit an acceptable choice for routine FeLV screening. For most in-office testing situations, use an individual membrane filter ELISA device rather than a microwell system because they are less susceptible to technical error and have built-in positive and negative controls for each test. Alternatively, send specimens to a commercial laboratory for FeLV testing.

- To reduce false-positive results with microwell ELISA tests, perform thorough washing steps and avoid splashing of reagents between microwells.
- For diagnosis of a clinically ill cat, use a combination ELISA test because the clinical manifestations of FeLV and feline immunodeficiency virus (FIV) are often indistinguishable and these kits test for both of these viruses simultaneously.
- Interpret weak positive ELISA reactions as suspicious rather than definitive and repeat the test (consider repeating using a different ELISA method, an IFA test, or an outside laboratory).
- In a healthy cat, always confirm an ELISA-positive test result by retesting in 4 to 6 weeks and perhaps again at 3 months to distinguish transient from persistent infection and to rule out laboratory error. For retesting, consider using the IFA test as the confirmatory test, because it correlates better with persistent infection and is less susceptible to false-positive results.

PCR Testing

Detection of FeLV by PCR testing of blood correlates well with ELISA results and has no significant advantage over conventional ELISA tests. PCR may be a more sensitive method for detecting FeLV in biopsy specimens.

Antibody Tests

Serum antibody assays are of limited usefulness in the diagnosis or clinical evaluation of FeLV infection. They merely indicate prior exposure to FeLV through infection or vaccination but do not confirm current active infection. Vaccine-induced antibody titers have not correlated well with level of protection.

TREATMENT

There is as yet no proven effective treatment for FeLV, but research and therapeutic trials are in progress using various immune modulator and antiviral drugs.

Supportive care, such as antibiotics for secondary bacterial infections, fluid therapy, and nutritional support, may prolong survival in selected patients. Untreated lymphoma is usually fatal within 1 to 2 months, but anticancer chemotherapy (see Chaps. 24 and 25) can induce remission in many cats. The prognosis for cats with FeLV-related nonregenerative anemia and myeloproliferative disease is poor, although blood transfusions may prolong survival.

- Biologic response modifiers include nonspecific immune modulators and stimulants. Preliminary results in limited trials with the following agents have been encouraging, but inconclusive (however, treated cats usually remain FeLV-positive): staphylococcal protein A (SPA), *Propionibacterium acnes* (ImmunoRegulin, ImmunoVet), low-dose oral human alpha-interferon (Roferon-A; Roche), and acemannan (Carrisyn; Carrington Laboratories). Of these, the author prefers low-dose oral interferon (diluted to 30 µ/ml and given at 30 µ PO q24h for 7 days on alternate weeks).
- Antiviral drugs, such as suramin, zidovudine (AZT), and PMEA have been used in treating FeLV, but are not effective enough to recommend or are too toxic for cats. Future prototypes developed for treatment of human retrovirus infections likely will be explored in cats with FeLV.
- Extracorporeal immunoadsorption for removal of immune complexes has been limited to research.
- Bone marrow transplantation after whole-body irradiation also has been limited to research.

PREVENTION AND CONTROL

Because of the devastating consequences of FeLV infection and its prevalence in the cat population, prevention is of vital importance. Preventive measures include vaccination of individual cats to reduce susceptibility, restriction of free roaming outdoors to reduce exposure, and control measures to reduce spread of FeLV in catteries.

Vaccination

The effectiveness of FeLV vaccination and the methods used to demonstrate efficacy are controversial and unresolved issues, in part because most of the available efficacy data have been generated by manufacturers rather than by unbiased researchers. The currently available FeLV vaccine products and their various features are summarized in Table 6–5.

Administration

- All FeLV vaccines are given by subcutaneous or intramuscular injection beginning at 8 to 10 weeks of age or older; a second dose is given 2 to 4 weeks later, followed by an annual booster.
- FeLV testing at or before first vaccination is highly recommended but does not need to be strictly mandatory. There is no proven beneficial or detrimental effect from vaccinating a cat for FeLV that already is infected.

Safety

- Acute side effects are infrequent and include transient listlessness, fever, and injection site pain. Acute hypersensitivity (face and paw edema, vomiting, diarrhea, collapse) occurs rarely. These effects are attributable mostly to adjuvants.
- Inflammatory nodules occasionally develop at the vaccination site which can become vaccine-associated sarcomas in some cats weeks to years later (incidence: 1 per 10,000 vaccines).

Biopsy vaccination site lesions if they persist more than 3 months, are larger than 2 cm, or increase in size after one month post-injection.

Table 6–5. FEATURES OF COMMERCIALLY AVAILABLE FELINE LEUKEMIA VIRUS (FeLV) VACCINES

	Leukocell 2 (Pfizer)	VacSyn/FeLV (Synbiotics)	Fel-O-Vax Lv-K (Fort Dodge)	GenetiVac FeLV (Schering Plough)	Fevaxyn-FeLV (Schering Plough)	RM Leucat (Merial)
Released	1989 (1985)	1989	1989	1990	1991	1989
Type*	Inactivated subunits	Inactivated whole virus	Inactivated whole virus	Recombinant gp70 subunit	Inactivated whole virus	Inactivated whole virus
Adjuvant†	Yes	No	Yes	Yes	Yes	No
Subgroups‡	A, B, C	A, B, C	A	A (subunit)	A, B	A, B, C
Anti-FOCMA§	Yes	Yes	No	No	No	Yes
First Dose¶	Age ≥9 wk	Age ≥9 wk	Age ≥10 wk	Age ≥8 wk	Age ≥9 wk	Age ≥9 wk
Second Dose	3–4 wk later	2–3 wk later	3–4 wk later	2–3 wk later	3–4 wk later	2–3 wk later
Booster	Annually	Annually	Annually	Annually	Annually	Annually
Reactions‖	2.0%	0.01%	6.0%	6.2%	1.4%	0.02%
Resist Infection**						
Vaccinates	72% (18/25)	91% (40/44)	91% (82/90)	85% (17/20)	91% (80/88)	91%
Controls	40% (4/10)	15% (3/20)	7% (4/58)	30% (6/20)	18% (4/22)	15%
Efficacy††	53%	89%	90%	79%	89%	89%

FOCMA, feline oncornavirus-associated cell membrane antigen.

*Leukocell 2 is derived from Leukocell, which was released in 1985 as the first FeLV vaccine.

†All FeLV vaccines use one or two adjuvants for enhanced immunogenicity, with the exception of VacSyn/FeLV, which contains a high antigenic mass. Most vaccine reactions are attributable to the adjuvants.

‡Natural FeLV infections usually involve subgroup A envelope glycoprotein alone or in combination with B or C. Immunity elicited by a vaccine containing type A envelope antigen should be sufficient, but some vaccines also contain types B and C.

§Only Leukocell 2, as labeled, has demonstrated that it induces protective levels of anti-FOCMA antibody that protect against lymphoma.

¶For all vaccines, dosages of 1 ml are given subcutaneously as scheduled. FeLV vaccine can be given simultaneously with other multivalent cat vaccines without interference.

‖Side effects are usually mild and consist of transient listlessness, fever, or injection site pain. Acute hypersensitivity reactions (facial and paw edema, vomiting, diarrhea, acute collapse) are seen rarely. FeLV vaccinations cause occasional nodules and soreness at the injection site and have been associated with subsequent development of injection site sarcomas.

**Challenge data cannot be compared because of differences in age of cats, strain of FeLV, route of infection, dose of inoculum, and protocol for postchallenge testing as related to definition of protection and persistence.

††Efficacy is a calculation that takes into account the infection rate in vaccinates versus unvaccinated controls as follows:

$$\text{efficacy} = \frac{(\text{incidence of infection in controls as \%}) - (\text{incidence of infection in vaccinates as \%})}{(\text{incidence of infection in controls as \%})}$$

- For cats at risk of exposure, the benefits of FeLV vaccination far outweigh the risk of injection site sarcoma.

Efficacy

▼ *Key Point* Based on currently available information, there is insufficient evidence for recommending one vaccine product rather than another. Therefore, it is not justified to switch from one vaccine to another solely on the basis of manufacturers' claims.

- In general, vaccinated cats that are exposed to FeLV often develop transient viremia and sometimes latent infection despite vaccination; however, most vaccinated cats apparently are protected against persistent viremia and therefore against FeLV-related disease.
- Latent infections in exposed vaccinated cats are less frequent and usually do not persist, compared with unvaccinated cats. However, this benefit of vaccination may be overemphasized because the clinical significance of latent infections is probably minimal anyway, as discussed at the beginning of this chapter.
- One vaccine (Leukocell 2) also is claimed by the manufacturer to protect against lymphoma because it elicits an anti-FOCMA antibody response.
- The major difficulty with comparing manufacturer efficacy data (i.e., percentage of cats protected after laboratory challenge) is the variation in challenge methods used for each vaccine:
  - Different routes ("natural" oronasal challenge vs. injection)
  - Different FeLV strains (various field isolates vs. vaccine-derived strains)
  - Different definitions of "persistent" infection in postchallenge follow-up (e.g., positive by ELISA vs. IFA testing vs. VI, and positive at time intervals after challenge that vary from 4 to 12 weeks or more)
- As a general guideline for discussing vaccination expectations with animal owners, expect 70% to 90% of vaccinated cats to be protected against persistent FeLV infection. This expectation may need to be modified as further efficacy data become available.

▼ *Key Point* All available vaccines produce less than 100% protection against FeLV; therefore, even though vaccination may reduce the risk of FeLV infection, effective prevention also requires measures that reduce the risk of exposure.

Control in the Cattery or Multicat Household

Control in FeLV-Positive Catteries

The following "test and removal program" is recommended.

- Test all cats on the premises for FeLV (expect to find up to 30% persistently infected), and remove or strictly isolate all confirmed FeLV-positive cats.
- Quarantine the cattery so that there is no movement of new cats into the cattery.
- Vaccinate the remaining FeLV-negative cats.
- Clean and disinfect (especially food and water dishes)—FeLV is susceptible to most detergents and disinfectants and survives only a few hours outside the host when allowed to dry.
- Retest all cats every 1 to 3 months and continue to remove any confirmed FeLV-positive cats.
- Once all cats on the premises have had negative results on two successive testings 3 months apart, the cattery is considered "FeLV free."
- Then isolate all new incoming cats and test as described in the following section.

Control in FeLV-Negative Catteries

The following precautions should be taken for incoming cats.

- Obtain incoming cats from a source with a negative FeLV history.
- Screen incoming cats with ELISA; if test results are negative, vaccinate cats and then hold them in isolation for 3 months (in case they are incubating FeLV).

- After a second negative ELISA result at the end of the 3-month quarantine, the cat can join the cattery.
- ELISA-positive titers generally should be confirmed by IFA testing or by a repeat ELISA; however, in cattery situations, ideally the safest course is to reject any ELISA-positive cat from the cattery as "suspicious."

SUPPLEMENTAL READINGS

Cotter SM: Feline viral neoplasia. *In* Greene CE (ed.): Infectious Diseases of the Dog and Cat (2nd Ed.). Philadelphia: WB Saunders, 1998, p 71.

Essex M, Sliski AH, Cotter SM, et al: Immunosurveillance of naturally occurring feline leukemia. Science 190:790, 1975.

Hardy WD Jr, Hess PW, MacEwen EG, et al: Biology of feline leukemia virus in the natural environment. Cancer Res 36:582, 1976.

Hawkins EC, Johnson L, Pedersen NC, Winston S: Use of tears for diagnosis of feline leukemia virus infection. J Am Vet Med Assoc 188:1031, 1986.

Jarrett O, Golder MC, Stewart MF: Detection of transient and persistent feline leukaemia virus infections. Vet Rec 110:225, 1982.

Jarrett O, Golder MC, Weijer K: A comparison of three methods of feline leukaemia virus diagnosis. Vet Rec 110:325, 1982.

Lewis MG, Wright KA, Lafrado LJ, et al: Saliva as a source of FeLV antigen for diagnosis of disease. J Clin Microbiol 25:1320, 1987.

Lopez NA, Jacobson RH, Scarlett JM, et al: Sensitivity and specificity of blood test kits for feline leukemia virus antigen. J Am Vet Med Assoc 195:747, 1989.

Lutz H, Jarrett O: Detection of feline leukemia virus infection in saliva. J Clin Microbiol 25:827, 1987.

Lutz H, Pedersen NC, Harris CW, et al: Detection of feline leukemia virus infection. Feline Pract 10:13, 1980.

McClelland AJ, Hardy WD Jr, Zuckermann EE: Prognosis of healthy feline leukemia virus infected cats. Dev Cancer Res 4:121, 1980.

Pacitti AM: The risk of transmission of FeLV from latently infected cats. *In* Kirk RW, ed.: *Current Veterinary Therapy X.* Philadelphia: WB Saunders, 1989, p 526.

Pedersen NC: The clinical significance of latent feline leukemia virus infection in cats. Feline Pract 14:32, 1984.

Rojko JL, Hardy WD Jr: Feline leukemia virus and other retroviruses. *In:* Sherding RG (ed): The Cat: Diseases and Clinical Management. (2nd Ed.). Philadelphia: WB Saunders, 1994, p 263.

Feline Immunodeficiency Virus

Robert G. Sherding

ETIOLOGY

Feline immunodeficiency virus (FIV) is a member of the lentivirus subfamily of retroviruses.

- FIV has tropism for lymphocytes, macrophages, salivary glands, and the CNS.
- FIV primarily infects and gradually destroys selected populations of T-lymphocytes. After a prolonged, asymptomatic latent period that can extend for years, the progressive loss of T-lymphocytes results in an immunodeficiency syndrome characterized by chronic and recurrent infections. FIV infection is lifelong and eventually fatal.
- FIV originally was isolated in 1986 from a cattery in northern California; however, retrospective assay of stored cat sera has shown that FIV has been widespread in the world's cat population since at least the 1960s.
- Susceptible species include the domestic cat, the lion, the tiger, the jaguar, the snow leopard, the panther, and the bobcat.
- Various FIV subtypes have been identified based on differences in the envelope gene. Subtypes vary in geographic distribution and influence cell tropism and pathogenicity.

Epidemiology

- Geographic distribution: FIV has been found worldwide and throughout North America. In a 1991 nationwide survey of 27,976 high-risk cats presenting to veterinarians, 7.4% overall were infected with FIV, compared with 13.3% infected with feline leukemia virus (FeLV) and 1.5% coinfected with both (data from IDEXX, Inc.).
  - Of symptomatic cats, 11.6% were infected.
  - Of asymptomatic cats, 4.0% were infected.
  - Of low-risk cats living indoors in single-cat households, 1.4% were infected.
  - Of cats in purebred catteries, less than 1% were infected.
- High-risk/high-incidence situations
  - Free-roaming outdoor pet or stray cats or cats exposed to outdoor cats
  - Cats living in large multicat households that frequently introduce new cats
  - Seroprevalence in countries such as Japan and Italy with many free-roaming cats is 25 to 30%.
- Low-risk/low-incidence situations
  - Indoor pet cats in single-cat households
  - Cats in closed, well-controlled catteries (incidence in purebred cats is low)
- *Sex distribution:* male cats outnumber females three to one (see section on transmission).
- *Age distribution:* FIV affects cats of all ages (reported range is 2 months–18 years); however, the incidence increases with age, and FIV is most prevalent in cats 5 years of age and older.

▼ *Key Point* Because of an extended asymptomatic latent period that is typical for lentiviruses, most FIV-infected cats that have clinical signs are older than 6 years of age.

Transmission

- FIV is shed in saliva and transmitted primarily through direct bite-wound inoculation during territorial fights (hence the higher incidence in males). Experimentally, a single tooth puncture from an FIV-infected cat is an efficient method of transmitting FIV.

▼ *Key Point* Biting is the principal mode of FIV transmission. The highest risk for FIV is found in intact male cats that are allowed to roam freely outdoors, such that bite-wound transmission can occur during territorial disputes.

- Experimentally, acute, and chronically infected queens may transmit FIV to kittens in utero (congenital infection) and through infected milk (lactogenic infection). These are considered to be minor modes of transmission under natural conditions.
- FIV has been transmitted experimentally by oral, vaginal, and rectal inoculation and through artificial insemination; however, these routes are unlikely to be important under natural conditions.
- Transmission through intimate contact during cohabitation is unlikely but not impossible. In a study that confined FIV-positive and -negative cats together in the same cages for 2 years, only 1 of the 20 nega-

tive sentinel cats became infected. Contact transmission has occurred on rare occasions in catteries, but the route or mechanism is unknown.

Public Health Risks

FIV is a feline-specific virus and there is no evidence that it causes human infection. However, FIV-infected cats may harbor other pathogens because of their immunosuppression that can infect humans who are immunocompromised.

CLINICAL SIGNS

Acute Primary Phase of Infection

This stage begins 4 to 6 weeks postexposure; effects are transient and usually go unnoticed.

- Transient fever
- Neutropenia and lymphopenia
- Generalized lymphadenopathy characterized by follicular hyperplasia and plasmacytic infiltration
- Occasional complications: sepsis, cellulitis, pustular facial dermatitis, anemia, diarrhea, and stomatitis

Asymptomatic Latent Phase of Infection

There is a prolonged latency of variable duration that may last years before signs of immunodeficiency occur.

Chronic Terminal Phase of Infection

Advanced FIV infection is characterized by an acquired immunodeficiency syndrome of chronic, recurrent opportunistic infections with waxing and waning signs that progressively worsen over months to years and may involve any combination of the following manifestations.

General Manifestations

- Progressive weight loss and debilitation ("chronic wasting")
- Chronic recurrent bacterial infections that may resolve partially with antibiotics but recur
- Recurrent fevers of unknown origin
- Generalized lymphadenopathy
- Polyclonal hypergammaglobulinemia
- Persistent or recurrent anemia or leukopenia (neutropenia, lymphopenia) or thrombocytopenia

Chronic or Recurrent Bacterial Infections

- Oral cavity (most common)—stomatitis, gingivitis, periodontitis (suppurative or plasmacytic)
- Respiratory—purulent rhinitis and conjunctivitis; pneumonia
- Intestinal—acute or chronic diarrhea due to enterocolitis that can be ulcerative, necrotizing, or pyogranulomatous

- Cutaneous—pustular dermatitis, abscesses, purulent otitis
- Urinary—recurrent urinary tract infections (cystitis, pyelonephritis)

Specific Opportunistic Infections

- Viruses—calcivirus, herpesvirus, poxvirus, papillomavirus
- Chlamydia
- Bacteria—*Staphylococcus, Pseudomonas,* mycobacteria, *Yersinia, Mycoplasma*
- Fungi—*Candida, Cryptococcus, Aspergillus,* ringworm
- Rickettsia—*Hemobartonella*
- Protozoa—*Toxoplasma, Giardia,* cryptosporidia, coccidia
- Parasites—generalized *Demodex, Notoedres*

Encephalopathy

- Signs—behavioral changes, dementia, disrupted sleep pattern, compulsive wandering, licking motions, facial twitching, seizures
- Pathogenesis—direct effect of FIV on the central nervous system

Neoplasia

- FIV-infected cats have a higher than expected incidence of lymphoid and myeloproliferative neoplasia.
- Various other neoplasms occur sporadically
- This is likely the result of impaired immune surveillance function rather than a direct cause and effect of FIV.

Other Associated Manifestations

- Ocular—anterior uveitis, glaucoma, pars planitis, retinal hemorrhages, retinal degeneration
- Lymphocytic polymyositis
- Chronic renal failure

DIAGNOSIS

The diagnosis of FIV usually is based on the demonstration of anti-FIV serum antibodies using one of three formats: ELISA, IFA, or Western blot. Polymerase chain reaction (PCR) and virus isolation are used in research but are not available for clinical use.

▼ *Key Point* Because FIV antibodies indicate prior exposure and infection, and because FIV infection is lifelong, a confirmed positive FIV antibody test result means that the virus is present in the cat and will remain so for life.

ELISA Test for FIV Antibody

- The ELISA test is used as in-office screening for serum antibodies against FIV.
  - CITE-FIV and Snap-FeLV/FIV (IDEXX)
  - ELISA and IFA also are available from many commercial laboratories on a mail-in basis.

- Seroconversion usually occurs 2 to 4 weeks postexposure but occasionally takes up to 8 weeks.
- Accuracy is >99%; thus, it is the first choice for testing ill high-risk cats.
  - False-positives—0.5% nonspecific reactions (can be higher because of operator error); because of this, in low-risk asymptomatic cats, confirm ELISA positives with an IFA test or ideally by Western blot.
  - False-negative results can occur in the early stages of acute infection before seroconversion has occurred or rarely in the terminal stages of immunodeficiency when antibody levels may be depressed.
- Passively acquired maternal antibodies can cause positive test results in uninfected kittens up to 6 months of age; therefore, reevaluate all positive kittens at 6 months of age to determine their true status.

IFA Test for FIV Antibody

- Available on a mail-in basis from a few commercial laboratories
- Accuracy comparable to in-office ELISA tests

Western Blot Test

- Detects antibodies against specific viral proteins; considered to be the "gold standard" for confirming ELISA-positive results.
- Available in research and commercial laboratories.

Assays to Detect Virus

- Virus isolation, PCR, and antigen ELISA tests can detect FIV, but these tests are only available in research labs.
- Advantages—enables detection of cats in the early preseroconversion stage of infection and of cats in the terminal stages of infection when antigen levels may be high and antibody levels are depressed.

Virus Isolation

- Researchers can isolate FIV from blood, tissues, or body fluids of infected cats.

TREATMENT

▼ *Key Point* Even though FIV is incurable, asymptomatic cats can live for years before developing clinical signs, and symptomatic cats often can be sustained for many months with the judicious use of antibiotics to control secondary infections combined with supportive care.

Specific Antiviral Therapy

- No specific treatment for FIV effectively eliminates the infections; once a cat is infected with FIV, it is infected for life.
- Current and future antiretroviral therapies developed for human immunodeficiency virus (HIV) may or may not be applicable to FIV. Some anti-HIV drugs have been tried and are too toxic in cats. Oth-

ers are being evaluated. Treatment of FIV-infected cats with the nucleoside analogue, azidothymidine (AZT), at 15 mg/kg, PO or SC, q12h, has produced improved immunologic status and regression of stomatitis. AZT can cause Heinz body anemia; thus, treated cats shoud have their CBC monitored.

General Supportive Therapy

- Cats ill with FIV-related bacterial infections sometimes may respond dramatically to antibiotics. Treat each infection episode as it arises, using culture and sensitivity guidance whenever possible.
- Treat stomatitis with metronidazole (10mg/kg PO q12h) and clindamycin (12.5 mg/kg PO q12h), bovine lactoferrin (40 mg/kg topically q24h), or prednisone (5 mg/cat PO q12h). Full mouth dental extraction is required in refractory cases.
- Use fluid therapy and nutritional support as indicated by the patient's needs.
- Prevent exposure to other infectious diseases because of lowered resistance.
- Continue vaccinations in cats at risk of exposure (in early phases, FIV-positive cats respond), but killed products are preferred.
- Avoid use of griseofulvin (dermatophyte drug) because FIV-seropositive cats have an increased risk of griseofulvin-induced neutropenia.
- In the terminal stages of FIV, the prognosis for response to treatment is poor, as indicated by persistent anemia or leukopenia, severe weight loss, or central nervous system signs.
- In one study, the mortality rate for FIV-positive cats at 6 months postdiagnosis was 15%.

PREVENTION

Isolate Infected Cats

Keep infected cats isolated from uninfected cats until more is known about cat-to-cat contact transmission (nonbite transmission is considered very rare; see section on Transmission).

Prevent Exposure

- Advise owners not to allow cats to roam free.
- Recommend neutering of male cats (to reduce roaming/fighting).

▼ *Key Point* The best prevention for FIV is not to allow cats to roam freely outdoors.

Vaccination

Vaccination against FIV is not yet available; however, efforts to develop an effective vaccine are under way.

SUPPLEMENTAL READINGS

Sellon RK: Feline immunodeficiency virus infection. In Greene CE (ed): Infectious Diseases of the Dog and Cat (2nd Ed). Philadelphia: WB Saunders, 1998, p 84.

8 Feline Infectious Peritonitis

Robert G. Sherding

The spectrum of clinical signs associated with coronavirus infections in cats ranges from asymptomatic to diarrhea to feline infectious peritonitis (FIP). FIP is a progressive, fatal systemic disease of cats caused by feline coronavirus. Despite its name, the lesions of FIP are not restricted to the peritoneum, and there are effusive and noneffusive forms of the disease. Lesions result from an immune-mediated arthus-like response to macrophages infected with coronavirus. Macrophages replicate the virus and carry it to target tissues such as peritoneum, pleura, uvea, meninges, and ependyma.

ETIOLOGY

FIP Coronavirus

- FIP-producing strains of coronavirus (FIPV) have a tropism for macrophages and are antigenically indistinguishable from ubiquitous feline enteric coronaviruses (FECV) that only replicate in intestinal epithelial cells (see Chap. 12). FIPV is apparently a mutant of FECV, and in most cases the mutation takes place during replication within the intestinal tract of cats that go on to develop FIP. So far, mutations of the 3c and 7b genes have been identified in FIPV isolates.
- Coronaviruses of pigs, dogs, and humans are closely related to FCoV and can also infect cats.
- FIP virus (FIPV) causes systemic infection of the macrophage system and induces severe, widespread immune complex-mediated vasculitis with necrosis and pyogranulomatous inflammation.
- Antibodies to coronavirus sensitize cats to FIP, and humoral antibodies play a major role in pathogenesis of the disease.

Epidemiology

- FIPV is distributed worldwide in domestic cats.
- FIPV affects exotic Felidae, including the lion, the cougar, the cheetah, the jaguar, the leopard, the bobcat, the sand cat, the caracal, the serval, and the lynx.

Transmission

- FIPV is excreted in oral and respiratory secretions, feces, and possibly urine. Chronic FCoV carriers can shed virus in the feces for at least 10 months.
- Infection occurs by ingestion (feco-oral) and possibly by inhalation under conditions of close contact.
- Evidence suggests that FIPV may survive for up to 7 weeks in the environment in dried form; thus, fomite transmission is also a possibility.

Risk Factors

- Young age (most kittens become infected before 4 months of age, and FIP most often occurs between 6 months and 2 years of age, but cats of any age can be affected)
- Genetic susceptibility plays a role in purebred cats.
- Group confinement (multicat households, purebred catteries)
- Concurrent viral infection with feline leukemia virus (FeLV) or feline immunodeficiency virus (FIV)

CLINICAL SIGNS

Cats with FIP often present initially with nonspecific and nonlocalizing signs, such as fever, anorexia, inactivity, weight loss, vomiting, diarrhea, dehydration, and pallor (anemia). As the disease advances, nonspecific signs progress and the clinical signs are dominated by body cavity effusions in the "wet" form of the disease or by organ-specific findings in the noneffusive, or "dry," form (Table 8–1). Some cats manifest features of both forms of the disease.

▼ *Key Point* Chronic fluctuating fever that is unresponsive to antibiotics is the most frequent early sign of FIP.

Incubation and Clinical Course

- The natural incubation period is extremely variable, usually ranging from a few days to a few weeks, but some cats may remain coronavirus carriers for several months to years before developing clinical signs.
- The onset of clinical signs is often insidious, although FIP sometimes can develop very suddenly, especially in young kittens.
- Once viral dissemination occurs and clinical illness develops, the disease is almost always progressive and fatal. However, there is considerable variation in the duration of clinical illness before death; 3 to 6 weeks is typical, but prolonged illness exceeding 6 months can occur, as can intermittent illness punctuated by periods of remission.

Table 8–1. CLINICAL SITUATIONS IN WHICH THE DIAGNOSIS OF FIP SHOULD BE CONSIDERED

Nonspecific Signs

Chronic unresponsive fever of unknown origin
Unexplained anorexia, depression, and weight loss
Reproductive failure or neonatal kitten mortality

Effusion Signs

Fluid distension of the abdomen
Scrotal swelling
Dyspnea due to pleural effusion

Organ-Specific Signs

Enlarged, firm, irregular kidneys
Icterus or hepatomegaly
Neurologic signs (multifocal and progressive)
Uveitis (iridocyclitis; chorioretinitis)
Splenomegaly
Mesenteric lymphadenopathy
Segmental ileo-ceco-colonic pyogranulomatous mass
Granulomatous interstitial pneumonitis

Laboratory Findings

Nonregenerative anemia
Neutrophilic leukocytosis or leukopenia
Elevated serum protein (hyperglobulinemia)
Elevated serum liver enzymes and bilirubin (also bilirubinuria)
Azotemia of primary renal origin
Proteinuria of renal origin
Pyogranulomatous or fibrinous body cavity fluid (nonseptic exudate)
Elevated CSF protein and leukocytes (neutrophils)

FIP, feline infectious peritonitis; CSF, cerebrospinal fluid.

- For effusive FIP, the clinical course is usually acute.
- For noneffusive FIP the course is often slow, insidious, and smoldering.
- Cats with only ocular involvement sometimes survive for a year or more.

Effusive (Wet) Form of FIP

▼ *Key Point* In the effusive, or wet, form of FIP, 85% of infected cats have inflammatory effusion in the abdominal cavity and 35% have effusion in the thoracic cavity.

Abdominal Effusion (Peritonitis)

- There is progressive, nonpainful distension of the abdomen with fluid.
- Effusion is detected by palpation and percussion of a fluid wave. In the early stages, a small amount of abdominal fluid may be detected by palpation of intestinal loops that feel excessively slippery, as though the serosal surfaces are highly lubricated. Pain on palpation is rare.
- Scrotal swelling may occur in intact males as a direct extension of the abdominal effusive process into the testicular tunics.
- Extension of the peritoneal inflammation may involve the gastrointestinal tract (vomiting, diarrhea), hepatobiliary system (jaundice), or pancreas (vomiting due to pancreatitis).

- Adhesions may organize the mesentery and omentum into an irregular, firm mass that is palpable in the cranioventral abdomen.
- Abdominal effusion is confirmed by radiography or abdominocentesis, and fluid analysis is usually strongly indicative of FIP (see section on Diagnosis).

Thoracic Effusion (Pleuritis)

- Dyspnea and exercise intolerance are the major presenting signs because lung expansion is restricted by compression from fluid in the pleural space.
- The animal may prefer a sitting or sternal recumbent posture to facilitate breathing. Increased respiratory distress may occur with exercise, with physical restraint in the hospital, or with repositioning in lateral recumbency (orthopnea).
- Muffled heart and lung sounds may be found on auscultation, and dullness and a horizontal fluid line may be found on thoracic percussion.
- Pericardial effusion (fibrinous pericarditis) may accompany pleural FIP and is detectable by echocardiography, but only rarely is this extensive enough to cause cardiac tamponade.
- Thoracic effusion is confirmed by radiography or thoracocentesis (see Chap. 80). Fluid analysis is usually strongly indicative of FIP (see section on Diagnosis).

Noneffusive (Dry) Form of FIP

▼ *Key Point* The noneffusive, or dry, form of FIP is characterized by multifocal pyogranulomatous inflammation and necrotizing vasculitis in various organs, such as the abdominal viscera (liver, spleen, kidneys), the eyes, the central nervous system (CNS), and the lungs.

Pyogranulomas may be seen as multiple gray-white nodular masses of variable size on the surface and within the parenchyma of affected organs. Effusion is usually minimal or absent. The specific organs affected and the degree of resulting organ failure determine the presenting clinical signs.

Kidney Involvement

- Pyogranulomatous nephritis—kidneys become palpably enlarged, firm, and irregular ("lumpy") owing to the presence of granulomas scattered over the surface and extending into the renal cortex.
- Occasionally, when renal involvement is extensive, signs of renal failure (e.g., polyuria-polydipsia) and azotemia (elevated BUN [blood urea nitrogen] and serum creatinine levels) may develop.
- Proteinuria is probably the most consistent laboratory finding in renal FIP. In addition, subclinical immune complex glomerulonephritis may develop in cats with any of the other effusive and noneffusive forms of FIP.

Liver Involvement

- Pyogranulomatous hepatitis (hepatomegaly, jaundice, and nonspecific signs of hepatic failure) may occur.

- The most consistent laboratory abnormalities are bilirubinuria and hyperbilirubinemia. Mild to moderate elevations of serum liver enzymes (alanine aminotransferase, alkaline phosphatase) and serum bile acids also may occur.

Involvement of Other Abdominal Organs

- Granulomatous lesions may cause palpable enlargement of the visceral lymph nodes, spleen, or omentum.
- Pyogranulomatous enterocolitis may cause diarrhea and diffuse or masslike intestinal thickening, especially in the ileo-ceco-colonic region.
- Pancreatic involvement, although uncommon, has been associated with diabetes mellitus.

Eye Involvement

- Ocular lesions of FIP are usually bilateral and affect the vascular tunic or uvea (uveitis). Lesions may or may not impair vision.
- Manifestations of exudative anterior uveitis (iridocyclitis) may include miosis, aqueous flare, hypopyon ("mutton-fat" deposits of cells and fibrin), hyphema, keratic fibrinocellular precipitates, anterior chamber adhesions (synechia), and edema and deep neovascularization of the cornea.
- Chorioretinitis from posterior uveal involvement is detected by ophthalmoscopic examination and may include perivascular cuffing, exudative retinal detachment, and retinal hemorrhages.

Nervous System Involvement

- Multifocal pyogranulomatous meningoencephalitis may occur. In one report, 29% of all cats with FIP developed neurologic signs. The relentless progression and multifocal nature of the signs are characteristic features of neural FIP.
- The neuroanatomic distribution of the lesions determines clinical signs; some of the most common are posterior paresis, ataxia, tremors, vestibular dysfunction, seizures, hyperesthesia, and personality changes.
- Neuropathies occasionally involve the cranial nerves (e.g., trigeminal or facial) or peripheral nerves (e.g., brachial or sciatic).
- Some cats with neural FIP develop secondary hydrocephalus when the inflammatory process obstructs the flow of cerebrospinal fluid (CSF).
- The diagnosis of neural FIP depends on CSF analysis (see section on Diagnosis). CT or MRI scans identify the presence of obstructive hydrocephalus in many cases. Electroencephalography may show nonspecific changes.

Lung Involvement

- Granulomatous pneumonia usually is clinically silent and is discovered at necropsy, although occasionally a persistent cough is manifested.
- On thoracic radiographs, pyogranulomatous pneumonia may be detected as diffuse, poorly defined, patchy nodular densities within the pulmonary interstitium.

Table 8–2. DIAGNOSIS OF FELINE INFECTIOUS PERITONITIS (FIP)

Parameter or Procedure	Findings Suggestive of FIP
Age	6 mo to 2 yr; or >10 yr
Habitat	Cattery or multicat household
Signs (see Table 8–1)	Fever (unresponsive)
	Effusion (abdominal; thoracic)
	Liver disease
	Renal disease (with renomegaly)
	Ocular disease (uveitis)
	CNS disease (multifocal)
Clinical course	Progressive
Complete blood count	Nonregenerative anemia
	Neutrophilia or neutropenia; left shift
	Lymphopenia
	Neutrophil inclusions (immune complexes?)
Plasma proteins	Hyperglobulinemia (polyclonal: gamma, alpha$_2$, beta)
	Hyperfibrinogenemia (400–700 mg/dl)
Serum chemistries	Abnormal liver tests (increased ALT, ALP, bile acids, bilirubin)
	Azotemia (increased BUN, creatinine)
Urinalysis	Proteinuria; bilirubinuria
Radiography and ultrasonography	Effusions (abdominal, thoracic)
	Organomegaly (liver, kidney)
	Organ infiltration (lung)
CT and MRI scans	Hydrocephalus; ependymitis
Fluid analysis of effusion	
Appearance	Yellow, clear, sticky, foamy, fibrinous
Protein	4–10 g/dl (gamma globulin >32%, albumin <48%, A/G ratio <0.81)
Leukocytes	1000–20,000 cells/μl
Cytology	Pyogranulomatous exudate
Cerebrospinal fluid analysis	
Protein	50–350 mg/dl
Leukocytes	100–10,000 cells/μl (neutrophils >mononuclear)
Serology	High CV-Ab titer (see text)
PCR	FIP virus genome (in tissue effusion)
Histopathology	Vasculitis and pyogranulomatous inflammation

CNS, central nervous system; ALT, alanine transaminase; ALP, alkaline phosphatase; BUN, blood urea nitrogen; CT, computed tomography; CV-Ab, coronaviral antibody; MRI, magnetic resonance imaging; PCR, polymerase chain reaction.

Reproductive Involvement

- FIP virus is a suspected but unconfirmed factor in cattery reproductive problems such as infertility, fetal resorptions, abortions, stillbirths, congenital malformations, and birth of weak or "fading" kittens.

DIAGNOSIS

FIP usually is suspected and diagnosed on the basis of clinical signs (see Table 8–1) and potential for exposure in conjunction with supportive findings on various laboratory evaluations (hematology, serum chemistry, cytology, serology), radiography, and biopsy (summarized in Table 8–2).

▼ *Key Point* Clinical signs and results of laboratory evaluations in cats with FIP generally are not specific for the disease; however, collectively these may provide strong circumstantial evidence for a diagnosis of FIP.

Hematology and Serum Protein Electrophoresis

Hematology and serum protein electrophoresis assays reveal nonspecific abnormalities in most cats with FIP, reflecting the inflammatory and immune responses (see Table 8–2).

Serum Chemistry Profile and Urinalysis

These tests are useful in noneffusive FIP involving abdominal viscera to indicate liver, kidney, or pancreatic involvement (see Table 8–2).

Radiography and Ultrasonography

Radiography is useful mostly to confirm the presence of body cavity effusion (abdominal, pleural), organ enlargement (kidney, liver), or organ infiltration (lung). Affected abdominal organs and lymph nodes also can be imaged by ultrasonography.

Fluid Analysis of Abdominal or Thoracic Effusions

The distinctive characteristics of the fluid strongly support a diagnosis of effusive FIP.

- The fluid appears pale yellow to golden in color and nearly translucent because of its relatively low cell count (usually 1000 to 20,000 nucleated cells/µl).
- The fluid may seem tenacious or sticky and may contain flecks, strands, or clots of fibrin.
- The fluid is foamy because of its high protein concentration, which can approach that of plasma, usually ranging from 4 to 10 g/dl. Considering the high protein content of FIP fluid, the nucleated cell count is disproportionately low relative to that found in other types of exudate.
- When necessary, protein electrophoresis of the fluid may help to establish the diagnosis of FIP based on the following criteria: a gamma globulin content that is at least 32% of the fluid protein, an albumin that is less than 48% of the fluid protein, and an albumin-to-globulin ratio (A/G) that is less than 0.8.
- The cytologic pattern of FIP fluid is a nonseptic exudate, often called pyogranulomatous, because it is characterized by a predominance of well-preserved (nondegenerate) neutrophils and macrophages, but it also includes variable numbers of plasma cells and lymphocytes.
- Coronavirus can be detected in effusions by PCR (see PCR section).

Analysis of CSF or Aqueous Humor of the Eye

These laboratory tests are valuable in evaluating cats with neural or ocular FIP. Both the protein concentration and leukocyte count (especially neutrophils) are increased consistently in the CSF of cats with neural FIP and in the aqueous humor of cats with intraocular FIP. (see Table 8–2). These fluids can also be evaluated for the presence of anti-FCoV antibodies (see Serology) and coronaviral nucleic acid (see PCR section).

CT and MRI Imaging of the CNS

In cats with neural FIP, secondary obstructive hydrocephalus is a common finding on CT and MRI scans. The combination of elevated CSF protein, increased CSF leukocytes (especially neutrophils), and hydrocephalus in a cat with progressive neurologic disease is highly suggestive of FIP.

Coronaviral Serology

Detection of feline coronaviral antibody (FCoV-Ab) is informative, but the conventional methodology does not provide a definitive diagnosis because it does not differentiate FIP from non-FIP coronaviral (CV) infections or distinguish between carrier and active infection. Antibodies to all the related coronaviruses cross-react on this test, creating a problem in interpretation. Most cats that have positive titers do not develop FIP. Approximately one-third of seropositive cats excrete virus.

Many labs measure coronavirus titers; however, methodology and titer values that indicate a "strong positive" vary with the lab. FCoV-Ab also can be measured in effusions, CSF, and aqueous; however, this has no advantage over serum and interpretation is similar to serum titers

Causes of a Positive FCoV-Ab Titer

(This test is not sufficiently *specific* to be used as a definitive diagnostic test.) A positive titer does not equate with a diagnosis of FIP.

- Active FIPV infection causing disease
- Asymptomatic carrier of FCoV
- Recovery from prior exposure to FCoV
- Antibody response to FIP vaccination (postvaccinal titers in most cases will be negative or low)
- Seroconversion to other coronaviruses
- False-positive as a result of recent vaccination

Causes of a False-Negative FCoV-Ab Titer

This test is not sufficiently *sensitive* to be used as a definitive diagnostic test. A negative titer does not entirely rule out FIP.

- Laboratory error or insensitive assay system
- Low antibody level resulting from:
  - Peracute infection
  - Drop in level in terminal stages of infection
  - Consumption of antibody in immune complexes

▼ *Key Point* Use the feline coronoviral antibody titer as a diagnostic aid for FIP rather than as a definitive diagnostic test. Interpret a positive titer to indicate that FIP is *possible* (low titer) or *probable* (high or rising titer), when accompanied by supportive clinical findings, and interpret a negative titer to indicate that FIP is *unlikely*.

Competitive ELISA Snap Test

The FIP-Snap Test (IDEXX) is designed for rapid in-office serologic diagnosis; however, experience has shown that it correlates poorly with conventional serologic tests and with clinical indicators of FIP.

ELISA Test for 7b Protein

An ELISA-based serologic test for detection of antibody to the gene 7b protein is being marketed by Antech as an "FIP-specific test". However, mutation of this gene is no longer considered specific for FIPV; thus, more data is needed to substantiate the accuracy of this test.

Polymerase Chain Reaction (PCR)

Coronaviral genome can be detected by PCR in fluids, tissue, or serum. Detecting FCoV in serum by PCR is often unsuccessful (low sensitivity) and until the exact molecular markers that distinguish FIPV from FECV are known, specificity is uncertain. Thus, in its current form, PCR offers little or no advantage over serology.

Histopathology and Tissue Analysis

- Biopsy of affected tissues is a valuable diagnostic procedure in some cats because the FIP lesions of vasculitis and pyogranulomatous inflammation are fairly distinctive.
- Coronavirus can be identified in tissue specimens by PCR, immunofluorescent antibody, and immunohistochemistry techniques.

TREATMENT

There is currently no known cure for FIP, nor has any treatment protocol been effective in prolonging life or consistently inducing remission in cats with the disease. Palliative treatment seems beneficial in some cats, but the response rate is low. Although there are occasional spontaneous remissions in cats that are affected only mildly or in those with only ocular involvement, these are rare.

▼ *Key Point* Once a cat develops clinical illness due to FIP, the disease is nearly always fatal, regardless of treatment.

Palliative Chemotherapy

Temporary remissions occasionally occur with chemotherapy protocols combined with intensive supportive and nursing care. Unfortunately, even with aggressive therapy in well-selected cases, a beneficial response occurs in less than 10% of treated cats.

- Chemotherapy protocols combine a high dosage of corticosteroid with a cytotoxic alkylating agent such as chlorambucil, cyclophosphamide, or mephalan (Table 8–3).

Table 8–3. PALLIATIVE TREATMENT OF FIP

Mode of Therapy	Specific Treatment Measures*
Supportive treatment	Parenteral fluid therapy to maintain hydration
	Nutritional therapy via tube feeding—nasogastric, gastrostomy, or esophagostomy (see Chap. 3)
	Body cavity drainage as needed—especially thoracentesis to relieve dyspnea
	Blood transfusions—as needed for severe nonregenerative anemia
	Antibiotics—for control of complicating bacterial infections
Anti-inflammatory-immunosuppressive†	Prednisone—2–4 mg/kg, q24h, PO **plus‡**
	Chlorambucil (Leukeran)—20 mg/M^2, PO, q 2–3 wk **or**
	Cyclophosphamide (Cytoxan)—50 mg/M^2 q 48 h, or 200–300 mg/M^2 q 2–3 wk; PO **or**
	Melphalan (Alkeran)—2 mg/M^2 (¼ of 2-mg tablet), PO, q 48 h
Topical ophthalmic (for uveitis)	Prednisone acetate 1%—2–3 drops/eye q 6 h
	Atropine 1%—1–3 drops/eye up to q 6 h to maintain mydriasis
Low-dose oral interferon	Interferon-α$_2$ (Roferon A; Roche)—dilute to 30 u/ml and give 30 u PO q24h for 7 days on alternating weeks

*Cats most likely to respond are in good physical condition and have good appetite, with absence of central nervous system signs, anemia, and feline leukemia virus (FeLV) infection.

†For conversion of body weight to body surface area (M^2), refer to conversion tables.

‡Choose only *one* of the three.

- Corticosteroids and cytotoxic drugs have no effect on the virus itself, but by virtue of their antiinflammatory and immunosuppressive effects, they are aimed at controlling the secondary immune-mediated inflammatory reactions that occur in the disease.
- Corticosteroids and cytotoxic drugs may adversely affect cellular immunity mediated by T-lymphocytes and macrophages and thereby have the potential to promote the viral infection.
- The principal side effects of cytotoxic drugs are anorexia and bone marrow suppression; thus, hemograms should be monitored periodically (see Chap. 24 for more details on effects of these drugs).
- Persistent drug-induced anorexia is a frequent problem when these drugs are given daily. An alternative is pulse administration, using a large dose of the drug once every 2 to 3 weeks. In this way, a few days after each dose the appetite usually rebounds and is maintained between treatment cycles.
- Regardless of the regimen chosen, if no response is noted within the first 2 to 4 weeks, consider the chemotherapy ineffective, and either modify or discontinue it. If a positive response does occur, con-

tinue the treatment for a minimum of 3 months and possibly indefinitely.

Treatment of Ocular FIP

- For anterior uveitis, use topical ophthalmic corticosteroids and topical atropine for mydriasis (see Table 8–3 and Chap. 155).
- Subconjunctival or retrobulbar injections of long-acting corticosteroids are recommended by some clinicians.

Supportive Treatment

These measures may improve quality of life and possibly survival time.

- Intermittent body cavity drainage (in effusive cases)
- Parenteral fluid therapy
- Nutritional support (via nasogastric, esophagostomy, or gastrostomy tube-feeding techniques; see Chap. 3) (there is no evidence that megadoses of vitamins are beneficial in FIP)
- Blood transfusion (for severe nonregenerative anemia)
- Antibiotics (if secondary bacterial infections are suspected)

Oral Interferon

Low-dose oral interferon has been used empirically (see Table 8–3) to slow disease progression and improve appetite and well-being, especially in cats with dry FIP. Side effects are minimal.

PREVENTION

Vaccination

Description of FIP Vaccine

A modified-live, temperature-sensitive strain of FIPV became available in 1991 as an intranasal (IN) vaccine (Primucell FIP; Pfizer Animal Health).

- It replicates locally in the nasopharynx, but not systemically because of temperature sensitivity.
- It stimulates local nasal and gut mucosal immunity, salivary immunoglobulin A (IgA) antibody, and cell-mediated immunity (CMI). However, it does not protect against enteric infection.
- It does not appear to sensitize animals to FIP (minimal antibody-dependent enhancement).
- It cross-protects against multiple strains of FIPV.

Recommendations for Use of FIP Vaccine

- Give 2 doses of 0.5 ml each, intranasally, 3 to 4 weeks apart, at 16 weeks of age or older.
- Revaccinate annually (or perhaps every 6 to 9 months in high-risk situations).

Vaccine Efficacy

- Survival in various trials conducted by the manufacturer was 71% to 85% in vaccinates versus 17% to 20% in nonvaccinates when challenged within 6 months or less of vaccination.
- Limited studies since release have shown efficacy ranging from minimal to moderate. Experience in the field has been mixed.
- A pitfall is the lack of proven efficacy in kittens <16 weeks of age, because under many circumstances kittens first become infected with FCoV between 6 and 16 weeks old.

Vaccine Safety

- Based on data from the manufacturer, no serious adverse effects or sensitization (enhanced susceptibility to FIP) were noted. Several million doses have been used in the field with minimal adverse effects being reported.
- There is no interference with simultaneous vaccination with FeLV, panleukopenia, and respiratory agents.
- Side effects in field trials included sneezing and sniffling in a small percentage of cats.

Recommendations for Control of FIP in Cattery Situations

- Isolate cats with signs of FIP.
- Control FeLV in the cattery by vaccination, testing, and removal (see Chap. 6).
- Only seronegative cats should have entry to a coronavirus-free cattery.
- Use only proven queens in breeding programs; do not breed queens that have a previous history of producing sick or FIP-infected kittens.
- Queens should give birth and nurse kittens in isolation from other cats. Kittens from seropositive queens should be weaned early and isolated from their queen at 4–6 weeks of age.
- Use good husbandry (e.g., good hygiene and feeding practices, avoid overcrowding, limit feco-oral contamination).

SUPPLEMENTAL READINGS

Addie DD, Jarrett O: Feline coronavirus infection. In Greene CE (ed): Infectious Diseases of the Dog and Cat. (2nd Ed). Philadelphia: WB Saunders, 1998, p 58.

Pedersen NC: Feline infectious peritonitis. In Pedersen NC: Feline Infectious Diseases. Goleta, CA: American Veterinary Publications, 1988, p 45.

Shelley SM, Scarlett-Kranz J, Blue JT: Protein electrophoresis on effusions from cats as a diagnostic test for feline infectious peritonitis. J Am Anim Hosp Assoc 24:495, 1988.

Weiss RC: Feline infectious peritonitis and other coronaviruses. In Sherding RG (ed): The Cat, Diseases and Clinical Management. (2nd Ed). New York: Churchill Livingstone, 1994, p 449.

Feline Infectious Respiratory Disease

Robert G. Sherding

ETIOLOGY

The major causes of infectious upper respiratory disease in cats are two highly contagious viruses: feline herpesvirus-1 (FHV-1), also known as feline viral rhinotracheitis (FVR), and feline calicivirus (FCV). The clinical signs of infection with these two viruses overlap and are often indistinguishable; thus, they often are grouped together and referred to as the infectious respiratory disease complex or upper respiratory infection (URI) of cats.

A feline strain of *Chlamydia psittaci* is a nonviral cause of mild upper respiratory signs in cats that often is grouped in this disease complex with FHV and FCV; however, its predominant manifestation is persistent conjunctivitis.

Other potential respiratory pathogens, include reovirus, *Mycoplasma* spp, and *Bordetella bronchiseptica*.

Transmission

Young kittens, unvaccinated cats, and cats confined in animal shelters, catteries, or multicat households have the greatest risk of infection. Direct contact and fomites are the most important means of infection.

- *Direct contact:* oral, nasal, and ocular discharges are infective.
- *Fomites:* contaminated cages, examination tables, food and water dishes, and human hands and clothing can transmit these infectious agents.
  - FHV—susceptible to drying and most disinfectants; survives 18 to 24 hours outside the host.
  - FCV—very resistant virus; average survival outside the cat is 8 to 10 days; preferred disinfectant is 1:32 solution of sodium hypochlorite bleach.
  - Chlamydia—survives for several days in conjunctival discharges; inactivated by lipid solvents, detergents, and 1:1000 quaternary ammonium.
- *Aerosol:* sneezing and coughing can propel virus up to 4 feet into the air.

Subclinical Carriers as Reservoirs of Infection

Most cats (up to 80%) that recover from FHV and FCV infection remain subclinical carriers for months to years. Persistently infected or latent subclinical carriers perpetuate these viruses within the cat population and serve as the principal source for outbreaks in catteries,

multicat households, research colonies, veterinary hospitals, and shelters.

FHV

Recovered carriers shed virus intermittently coinciding with reactivation of latent virus infection by stress, parturition, lactation, or glucocorticoids. Episodes of shedding generally persist for 2 weeks and can be accompanied by recrudescence of mild clinical signs.

▼ *Key Point* Shedding of FHV often is triggered by lactation in carrier queens at the time when kittens are losing passive maternal immunity (5–7 weeks) and becoming susceptible. This is an important source of upper respiratory infection in young kittens.

FCV

Recovered carriers shed virus from the oropharynx continuously for many months, or even years, and can infect other cats. Isolation rates of FCV from healthy cat populations are 8% for pet cats, 25% for show cats, and 40% for colony cats.

Chlamydia and Bordetella

- Chlamydia is primarily shed from conjunctival secretions, and prolonged shedding up to 18 months has been documented after experimental infections.
- *Bordetella bronchiseptica* can be isolated from many healthy cats, indicating a widespread subclinical carrier state. Prolonged oronasal shedding for at least 19 weeks after experimental infection has been documented.

CLINICAL SIGNS

Typical signs of feline URI include anorexia, depression, fever, and naso-ocular discharge. Other signs specific to each etiologic agent are detailed in the following sections. The onset is often acute, and the signs are more severe in young kittens. Illness in previously-vaccinated cats tends to be less severe. Clinical disease is usually self-limiting within 5 to 7 days. (See Table 9–1 for a summary of the clinical manifestations of FHV and FCV.)

Table 9–1. CLINICAL MANIFESTATIONS OF FELINE VIRAL RESPIRATORY DISEASE

Manifestation	Feline Herpesvirus (FHV-1)	Feline Calicivirus (FCV)
Incubation	3–5 days	1–3 days
Duration	5–10 days (or more)	5–7 days
Anorexia and depression	Severe and frequent	Mild and inconsistent
Fever	Frequent	Inconsistent (diphasic)
Nasal signs	Sneezing—severe	Sneezing—mild
	Discharge—marked	Discharge—mild or absent
	Ulcerated nares	Ulcerated tip of nose
	Turbinate necrosis	
	Sequela—chronic rhinosinusitis	
Ocular signs	Conjunctivitis—severe (serous to mucopurulent discharge, chemosis, photophobia)	Conjunctivitis—mild
	Ulcerative keratitis	
	Panophthalmitis (neonates)	
	Sequela—sicca ("dry eye")	
Oral signs	Hypersalivation; rare ulcers	Frequent oral ulcers (tongue, palate)
		Sequela—chronic stomatitis-gingivitis and faucitis
Pulmonary signs	Rare bacterial pneumonia	Occasional viral pneumonia
Other signs	Abortion	Limping syndrome (arthritis, arthralgia, myalgia)
	Peracute neonatal death (hepatic necrosis)	Interdigital paw ulcers
		Enteritis (diarrhea and vomiting)
Postrecovery shedding	Intermittent (after stress)	Persistent

Feline Herpesvirus

- Herpesvirus has an affinity for conjunctival, nasal, and upper airway (laryngotracheal) epithelium. Necrosis at these sites causes rhinitis, tracheitis, laryngitis, and conjunctivitis. Osteolytic damage to turbinate bones can be permanent.
- Signs include sneezing, serous to mucopurulent naso-ocular discharge, cough, hypersalivation, and loss of voice.
- Corneal involvement causes keratitis or herpetic ulcers. Ulcers can have a punctate, oval, or branching (dendritic) pattern (see Chap. 153).
- Infection during pregnancy may result in abortion or in a severe generalized form of infection in newborn kittens, characterized by fatal encephalitis or focal necrotizing hepatitis.
- Secondary bacterial complication of the lesions may worsen and prolong FHV disease. Bacterial pneumonia is a serious complication in young kittens.

Feline Calicivirus

- Calicivirus has an affinity for oropharyngeal epithelium and alveolar pneumocytes of the lung.
- Infection is manifested most often as oral ulceration (tongue, palate, fauces), mild rhinitis (sneezing), and conjunctivitis, or viral interstitial pneumonia, depending on the strain of FCV. In some cats, the tip of the nose may be ulcerated and crusted.
- One FCV isolate reportedly causes consistent footpad and interdigital ulcers along with oral ulcers ("paw and mouth disease").
- FCV has been frequently isolated from cats with chronic ulcerative or proliferative lymphocytic

gingivitis/stomatitis, and faucitis. This may be a hypersensitivity response to persistent FCV infection, but its role in chronic oral disease is uncertain.
- A strain of FCV has been described that causes acute synovitis, fever, and joint pain (myalgia and arthralgia) without noticeable respiratory signs.
- FCV has been isolated from the intestines and feces of cats with acute and chronic enteritis.

Feline Chlamydiosis

- Ocular signs predominate, such as acute or chronic mucopurulent conjunctivitis that can begin unilaterally and later become bilateral (see Chap. 152).
- Mild nasal discharge, sneezing, and coughing can occur.
- Very mild subclinical pneumonia can occur but usually is only detectable histologically.

Feline Bordetellosis

- *B. bronchiseptica* may be a primary (rare) or secondary (occasional) respiratory pathogen, especially in kittens.
- Outbreaks of fatal bronchopneumonia have been attributed to *B. bronchiseptica;* however, experimental infections are characterized by fever, sneezing, and nasal discharge of less than 10 days in duration. Coughing is an inconsistent sign.

DIAGNOSIS

For individually infected cats, a diagnosis of "viral respiratory disease" or URI based on clinical signs and likelihood of exposure is adequate for patient management. Virology and molecular testing are the only means of definitive diagnosis, and availability of these is limited to selected reference and research laboratories (such as state animal diagnostic laboratories and colleges of veterinary medicine). These specialized diagnostic procedures should, however, be considered for evaluation of disease outbreaks in groups of cats.

▼ *Key Point* Severe naso-ocular signs are most consistent with FHV infection. Corneal ulceration is indicative of FHV, whereas oral ulceration is more likely with FCV. Persistent conjunctivitis is the predominant sign in chlamydiosis.

Routine Laboratory Diagnostics

Complete blood count (CBC), serum chemistries, and urinalysis are usually normal except in severe infections complicated by bacteria, in which a neutrophilic leukocytosis may be found on the CBC.

Tests for Immunodeficiency Syndromes

Persistent or recurrent signs of upper respiratory infection often develop in immunodeficient cats. Evaluate cats for underlying infections of feline immunodeficiency virus (FIV antibody test; see Chap. 7) and feline leukemia virus (FeLV antigen test; see Chap. 6) in the following situations:

- Cats with recurrent episodes of infectious respiratory disease
- Vaccinated adult cats with unusually severe signs
- Cats that have signs that linger beyond 2 weeks in duration

Detection of Inclusion Bodies

- **FHV:** intranuclear inclusions can occasionally be identified in conjunctival biopsies (H&E stain)
- **Chlamydia:** intracytoplasmic inclusions can be identified in some cases in scrapings of conjunctival epithelium (Diff-Quik stain), mostly during the first 2 weeks of infection

Chlamydia ELISA Kits

- Commercially available ELISA-based tests are available at many labs for testing conjunctival scrapings for chlamydia antigen.
- These tests have low sensitivity (many false negatives) and moderate to high specificity.

Direct Immunofluorescence

- Smears of nasal mucosa or conjunctiva are used to detect virus-infected cells.
- Test for FHV.

Virus Isolation

- This uses cell culture of swabs from oropharynx, nasal cavity, or conjunctiva.
- This is a good test for FCV; an acceptable test for FHV.

Culture

- For *B. bronchiseptica,* nasal, pharyngeal, or bronchial washing specimens can be cultured on selective media. For transport, use charcoal Amies transport medium (Beckton-Dickenson).
- For chlamydia, submit conjunctival swabs in chlamydia transport media for cell culture.

Polymerase Chain Reaction (PCR)

- PCR techniques can be used to identify FHV, FCV, and chlamydia in conjunctival, corneal, and nasopharyngeal mucosal specimens.
- PCR is not yet widely available, but it may become the future diagnostic method of choice. For PCR testing, place conjunctival swabs or scrapings in 1 ml of phosphate-buffered saline (PBS), freeze at $-20°C$, and submit for analysis.

Serology

- Serology is generally not very helpful because most cats have vaccine-induced antibody titers.
- A rising neutralizing antibody titer in serum from convalescent animal indicates a presumptive diagnosis of FCV.

TREATMENT

Viral respiratory disease is self-limiting in most cats within 5 to 7 days. Treatment is mainly supportive in nature, although in the future effective antiviral drugs may be developed. Hospitalize only cats that require parenteral fluid therapy, oxygen therapy, or intensive nutritional support therapy.

▼ *Key Point* Treat infectious respiratory disease in cats on an outpatient basis whenever possible to prevent cross-infection of other hospitalized cats.

Outpatient Treatment

Select from the following list the combination of treatments that are most applicable to the patient's manifestations.

- Clean discharge from eyes and nares as needed.
- Support nutrition and fluid intake:
  - Advise owners to offer a variety of flavorful, aromatic foods and broths to encourage continued intake of food and fluids. Soft or liquefied foods may be better tolerated in cats with inflammation of the oral cavity and pharynx.
  - Teach owners coax-feeding and syringe-feeding techniques.
  - Supplement inappetant cats with potassium (Tumil-K; Kaon) and vitamin B complex.
  - Diazepam (Valium: 0.1–0.2 mg/kg, IV) or oxazepam (Serax, Wyeth, 2.5 mg total dose, PO once or twice daily) as appetite stimulants just before feeding may overcome anorexia.

- Provide rest and warm ambient temperature (inhibits FHV replication).
- Prevent inspissation of respiratory secretions:
  - Promote airway humidification (humidifier or vaporizer).
  - Prevent dehydration (prescribe oral fluids or subcutaneous administration of isotonic electrolyte solution as needed).
- Promote nasal decongestion:
  - Prevent inspissation of secretions (see above).
  - Oxymetazoline 0.25% nasal spray (Afrin; Schering), every 12 hours, may be used but is not well tolerated by most cats.
- Irrigate necrotic oral lesions with 0.2% chlorhexidine solution (Nolvadent).
- Control secondary infections with antibiotics:
  - For secondary bacterial infection—doxycycline, amoxicillin, ampicillin, cephalosporins
  - For chlamydia or Bordetella—doxycycline (5 mg/kg PO q12h)
- Treat ocular lesions with topical eye medications (see Chaps. 152 and 153).
  - Triple antibiotic ophthalmic ointment for bacterial complications
  - Tetracycline ophthalmic ointment for chlamydia (continue for 4 weeks)
  - Antivirals can be applied topically every 6 hours for herpetic ulcers; however, reserve these for severe or refractory corneal lesions because they are very expensive and often irritating. Anti-herpetic ophthalmic products include trifluridine (Viroptic, Burroughs Wellcome); idoxuridine (Stoxil, Smith Kline; Dendrid, Alcon; Herplex, Allergan); and vidarabine (Vira-A, Parke Davis).

In-Hospital Treatment

In severe cases, hospitalization may be required for additional therapy.

- For prolonged anorexia: enteral hyperalimentation for nutritional support (via esophagostomy, gastrostomy, or nasogastric intubation; see Chap. 3)
- For moderate to severe dehydration: parenteral fluid therapy (see Chap. 5)
- For pneumonia and hypoxemia: oxygen via nasal catheter (see Chap. 3) or oxygen cage

Treatment of Latent FHV

- Preliminary evidence suggests that daily supplementation of L-lysine (250 mg PO once daily with food) may reduce replication and shedding of FHV in cats with chronic latent infection.
  - Empirically, low-dose oral or IN interferon (human IFN-α_2; Roferon A) at 30 U/da on alternate weeks has been suggested for immunomodulation of cats with chronic persistent nasal signs associated with FHV.

Sequelae

- Subclinical viral carriers (see section on Etiology)
  - Cattery problem
  - FHV recrudescence

- Chronic rhinitis/sinusitis and nasal obstruction can occur after FHV infection (sometimes called "chronic snuffler"). Potential causes might include:
  - Permanent turbinate damage resulting from necrosis, ulceration, and osteolysis
  - Bacterial sinusitis
  - Nasopharyngeal stenosis
  - Persistent local FHV infection
- Chronic ocular discharge
  - Bacterial or chlamydial follicular conjunctivitis (see Chap. 152)
  - Tear duct blockage/infection (dacryocystitis) (see Chap. 158)
  - Keratoconjunctivitis sicca (FHV) (see Chap. 158)
- Corneal sequestrum has been linked to FHV based on PCR findings (see Chap. 153).
- Chronic lymphoplasmacytic stomatitis, gingivitis, and faucitis have been attributed to chronic FCV infection (see Chap. 84).

PREVENTION

For prevention of infectious respiratory disease in the individual cat, vaccination is available for FHV, FCV, chlamydia, and Bordetella. For prevention of spread of disease in groups of cats confined together, additional control measures are indicated.

Vaccination

General Considerations

- Local immunity plays an important role in protection.
- FCV vaccine strains do not cross-protect equally well against all isolates.
- Duration of immunity for FHV and FCV vaccination is probably at least 3 years based on persistence of antibody titers, duration of anamnestic antibody response, and greater than 50% efficacy in cats experimentally challenged 7.5 years after receiving killed virus vaccine.
- Protocol: incorporate FHV and FCV into all routine feline vaccination programs. Initially give kittens at least two doses 3 weeks apart (usually 9 and 12 weeks of age), revaccinate one year later, and then revaccinate every 3 years thereafter except in cats in high-risk situations which are revaccinated annually.
- Chlamydia and Bordetella vaccines are optional and reserved primarily for high-risk cats. Vaccine efficacy is not as well established as it is for FHV and FCV vaccines. Duration of immunity has not yet been demonstrated to exceed 1 year; thus, annual revaccination is recommended.

▼ **Key Point** Immunization protects against clinical illness but not infection. It does not prevent or eliminate chronic viral carrier states or virus shedding.

Injectable Vaccine

Modified live virus (MLV), inactivated virus (killed), and genetically engineered (recombinant) vaccines are available.

- *Advantages:* fewer side effects and less chance of producing carriers than with intranasal vaccine.
- *Disadvantages:* slow onset of protection; humoral immunity not as effective as local immunity; adjuvant-related adverse effects (e.g., injection site sarcoma) with killed vaccines; transient febrile limping (arthralgia) syndrome with MLV vaccines.
- *Caution:* oronasal exposure to injectable MLV vaccine by inadvertent aerosolization or spilling on the haircoat occasionally can cause sneezing and oronasal ulcers.

Intranasal Vaccine (MLV)

- *Advantages:* more rapid (2–4 days) and possibly more reliable protection through local immunity; avoids adjuvant-related adverse effects
- *Disadvantage:* mild postvaccinal sneezing and naso-ocular discharge in some cats

Control Measures in Catteries
General Considerations

- FHV and FCV are perpetuated in catteries by virus that is shed from subclinical carriers and spread by aerosol, contact, and fomite transmission.
- When introducing a new cat, there is always a risk that the incoming cat is a subclinical carrier that can be the source for an outbreak.
- In endemic catteries, kittens lose their maternal immunity at 5 to 7 weeks and often become infected by virus shed from their own lactating dam.

▼ *Key Point* Subclinical shedders of respiratory viruses are prevalent. Cats that are free of signs of disease are not necessarily free of infection, even if they have been well vaccinated.

Recommendations

- Vaccinate all cats routinely.
- Avoid incoming cats from infected sources.
- Vaccinate (IN) and then isolate all incoming cats for 3 weeks:
  - To protect the incoming cat from viruses in the cattery
  - To protect the cattery from a new cat that might be in a state of virus incubation or stress-induced shedding of FHV

- For rapid onset of immunity in outbreak situations, use intranasal vaccine.
- In endemic breeding catteries with infection problems in kittens at 5 to 7 weeks of age:
  - Vaccinate queens before breeding (and possibly during pregnancy 3 to 4 weeks before queening, but only with inactivated vaccine, to enhance passive maternal antibody levels in kittens.
  - Move queens into isolation 3 weeks before term to prevent exposure of newborn kittens to carriers in the colony.
  - Wean kittens early at 4 to 5 weeks of age and raise them in isolation to reduce risk of acquiring infection from a carrier queen.
  - Use intranasal vaccine in kittens because it can induce local protection rapidly despite the presence of interfering maternal antibody.
- Identify and treat cats that have chronic chlamydial conjunctivitis and treat with oral doxycycline and topical tetracycline opthalmic ointment.
- In housing facilities for cats, avoid overcrowding, provide adequate ventilation (10 or more air changes per hour), maintain a warm nonfluctuating temperature, control humidity at approximately 50%, and provide separate cages with solid partitions and separate food and water dishes.
- Prevent fomite transmission by disinfecting cages (1:32 sodium hypochlorite bleach solution) and by minimizing cross-contamination by personnel.

SUPPLEMENTAL READINGS

Elston T, Rodan I, Flemming D, et al: 1998 Report of the American Association of Feline Practioners and Academy of Feline Medicine Advisory Panel on Feline Vaccines. J Am Vet Med Assoc 212:227, 1998.

Ford RB, Levy JK: Infectious diseases of the respiratory tract. *In* Sherding RG (ed): The Cat: Diseases and Clinical Management (2nd ed). New York: Churchill Livingstone, 1994, p 489.

Gaskell R, Dawson S: Feline respiratory disease. *In* Green CE (ed): Infectious Diseases of the Dog and Cat (2nd ed.), Philadelphia: WB Saunders, 1998, p. 97.

Scott FW: Feline respiratory viral infections. *In* Scott FW (ed): Infectious Diseases. New York: Churchill Livingstone, 1986, p 155.

Scott FW, Geissinger C: Duration of immunity in cats vaccinated with an inactivated feline panleukopenia, herpesvirus, and calicivirus vaccine. Feline Pract 25:12, 1997.

Scott FW, Geissinger CM: Long-term immunity in cats vaccinated with an inactivated trivalent vaccine. Am J Vet Res 60:652, 1999.

10 Canine Infectious Tracheobronchitis (Kennel Cough Complex)

Robert G. Sherding

Kennel cough complex (KCC) refers to a collection of highly contagious infectious diseases of the canine respiratory tract that cause tracheobronchitis and acute onset of a paroxysmal hacking cough lasting several days to a few weeks.

ETIOLOGY

The most frequent isolates in KCC are parainfluenza virus and *Bordetella bronchiseptica*. Clinical respiratory disease has also been associated with *B. bronchiseptica* infections in cats (see Chap. 9).

Incriminated Etiologic Agents

- *B. bronchiseptica*
- Canine parainfluenza virus (CPIV)
- Canine adenovirus, types 1 and 2 (CAV-1, CAV-2)
- Canine herpesvirus
- Canine reoviruses, types 1, 2, and 3
- Mycoplasmas and ureaplasmas

Transmission

▼ *Key Point* Kennel cough is highly contagious via aerosol spread (cough, sneezing); therefore, it is common wherever dogs are housed or confined together (e.g., boarding kennels, animal shelters, pet shops, veterinary hospitals, and research facilities).

- These agents also can be transmitted by fomites (e.g., personnel, cages, food and water bowls).
- Incubation period is usually 5 to 7 days (range of 3–10 days).

Pathogenesis

- Mixed infections are common and have a synergistic effect in producing clinical disease. Individually, these infectious agents cause mild self-limiting disease or are harbored in the airways of asymptomatic carriers.
- The primary target of these agents is the upper airway epithelium. The result is epithelial injury, acute inflammation, and dysfunction of the airway cilia.

▼ *Key Point* In young puppies and immunocompromised animals, secondary bacterial invasion of the lower respiratory tract may cause life-threatening pneumonia.

CLINICAL SIGNS

Mild Form

- The mild form of KCC is the most common. The highest incidence is in summer and fall.
- There is an acute onset of a dry-sounding, hacking cough due to tracheobronchitis. Even though the cough is often described as dry, KCC is characterized by production of increased mucus.

▼ *Key Point* Episodes of paroxysmal cough often are followed by gagging or retching motions that may be mistaken by the owner for vomiting or choking.

- Cough may be high-pitched because of laryngitis and swollen vocal folds.
- Cough may be more frequent during exercise, excitement, or changes in temperature and humidity of inspired air.
- Cough is easily elicited on tracheal palpation or by pulling on the collar.
- Mild, serous naso-ocular discharge is seen occasionally.
- Typically, the dog continues to eat, remains active and alert, and is nonfebrile.
- Clinical course is usually 7 to 14 days.

Severe Form

- The severe form of KCC is less common and is usually the result of mixed infections in very young or unvaccinated puppies, especially from pet shop and animal shelter environments. Complicating bacterial bronchopneumonia seems to be the determinant of severity and sometimes can be fatal.
- Productive cough may be present because of tracheobronchitis plus bronchopneumonia.
- Anorexia, depression, and fever may be present.

- Naso-ocular discharge may be present (serous or mucopurulent rhinitis and conjunctivitis).
- The severe form is difficult to distinguish from canine distemper.

DIAGNOSIS

KCC usually is diagnosed on circumstantial evidence of clinical signs and exposure history. A recent history of exposure to other dogs, especially under kennel conditions, is typical but not found in all cases. Hemograms, radiographs, and airway cytologies are usually unremarkable or reveal nonspecific findings.

Hemogram

- *Mild form:* usually normal or stress response (mature neutrophilia, lymphopenia)
- *Severe form:* neutrophilic leukocytosis with a left shift associated with complicating pneumonia

Thoracic Radiography

- *Mild form:* usually normal; a mild increase in interstitial lung density occasionally seen
- *Severe form:* interstitial and alveolar pattern with lobar consolidation associated with complicating bronchopneumonia

Airway Cytology

- Evaluation of airway cytology is optional in mild cases. Specimens can be obtained by transtracheal aspiration, endotracheal tube lavage, or bronchoscopic lavage or swab (see Chap. 74.).
- Findings include increased mucus, mucopurulent exudate, and sometimes bacteria.

Cultures

- Nasal swabs or tracheobronchial specimens can be cultured for *Bordetella* and mycoplasma.

▼ *Key Point* Nasal swabs for isolation of *Bordetella* are an effective alternative to tracheobronchial cultures.

- Isolation of *Bordetella* or mycoplasma allows only presumptive diagnosis because many asymptomatic dogs harbor these organisms in the respiratory tract.

Virology

- Virus isolation can identify CPIV and CAV from nasopharyngeal or tracheal swabs, but this is impractical for clinical use.
- Serology (paired acute and convalescent titers) can demonstrate viral exposure, but is rarely used.

TREATMENT

Because many of the principles of treatment for bronchitis and bacterial pneumonia can be applied to dogs with KCC, refer also to Chapters 78 and 79.

General Guidelines

- *For mild form:* Because this form is typically self-limiting in 7 to 14 days, dogs with mild signs do not necessarily require specific therapy.
- *For severe form:* Because lower respiratory tract involvement can be fatal, treat aggressively for bacterial bronchopneumonia (see Chap. 79). Avoid antitussives.
- *For cough that persists for more than 14 days:* Consider causes other than KCC and evaluate further with thoracic radiographs, hemogram, airway cytology and culture, and other diagnostics, as appropriate.
- *For all suspected KCC:* Treat on an outpatient basis whenever possible to prevent transmission to other hospitalized animals.

Antibiotics

- In mild self-limiting KCC, antibiotics are optional. For treatment of suspected or confirmed *Bordetella* infection, use amoxicillin-clavulanate (12.5–25 mg/kg PO q12h) or doxycycline (3–5 mg/kg PO q12h) for 10–14 days. For treatment of mycoplasmas, use doxycycline.
- For severe KCC complicated by bronchopneumonia or for refractory *Bordetella* infection, choose antibiotics based on culture and susceptibility testing whenever possible.

▼ *Key Point* Nebulization of antibiotics may be more effective than systemic use against *Bordetella* because the bacteria attach to the cilia on the mucosal surface and are hard to reach with systemic antibiotics.

- For refractory *Bordetella* infection, nebulize gentamicin (Gentocin, Schering-Plough), 50 mg diluted in 2 to 3 ml saline, by DeVilbiss jet nebulizer for 10 minutes, every 12 hours for 3 to 5 days.

Bronchodilators

- *Rationale:* Use these to reverse reflex bronchoconstriction triggered by airway irritation, thereby reducing discomfort and cough.
- *Examples:* theophylline, aminophylline, albuterol, and terbutaline (see Chap. 78 for dosages)

Antitussives

- *Rationale:* In diseases with a productive cough, it usually is recommended to avoid antitussives, but in uncomplicated KCC (no fever or evidence of bronchopneumonia), the cough can be such a nuisance and source of discomfort for owner and patient that antitussives may be required for relief.

- *Examples:* Hydrocodone (0.22 mg/kg PO q6–12h), and butorphanol (0.55–1.1 mg/kg PO q6–12h). Over-the-counter cough medicines are generally ineffective for treating KCC.

Corticosteroids

- Use anti-inflammatory dosages of corticosteroids (prednisolone 0.25–0.5 mg/kg PO q12h) as needed to control refractory cough in uncomplicated KCC.

Supportive Care

- Provide adequate fluid intake, airway humidification, nutritional support, and rest.

PREVENTION

Routine vaccination protocols for all dogs usually incorporate adenovirus and parainfluenza virus. In areas where KCC is common and in dogs exposed frequently to other dogs, a *Bordetella* vaccination also is indicated.

Vaccination

Both injectable and intranasal (IN) vaccines are available for parainfluenza virus and *Bordetella*. IN vaccines have the advantages of greater protection through local immunity, protection after one dose, more rapid onset of protection, and no interference from maternal antibody allowing use in puppies as young as 2 weeks of age. Side effects of IN vaccines may include nasal discharge, sneezing, and cough.

Adenovirus

- Injectable vaccines containing either CAV-1 or CAV-2 will cross-protect for both.

Parainfluenza Virus

- Injectable—protects against disease but not infection (therefore, this may not curtail spread from carriers to susceptible dogs in a kennel outbreak)
- Intranasal—protects against disease and infection

Bordetella

- Injectable (bacterin)
- Intranasal (live avirulent *Bordetella*)—more consistent protection than injectable (stimulates local immunity)

Kennel Prevention

- Avoid overcrowded, high-density confinement.
- Isolate infected (coughing) animals. In recovered animals, KCC viruses may be shed for 1 to 2 weeks, and *Bordetella* and mycoplasmas for 3 months or longer.
- Use caretaker hygiene to prevent fomite spread.
- Ensure proper kennel ventilation (at least 12 air changes per hour; 15–20 is best).
- Use disinfectants such as sodium hypochlorite (Clorox), chlorhexidine (Nolvasan), and benzalkonium-Cl (Roccal-D).

PUBLIC HEALTH CONSIDERATIONS

Humans are susceptible to *B. bronchiseptica*, especially if immunocompromised; however, the risk of acquiring infection from an infected pet is considered small.

SUPPLEMENTAL READINGS

Appel MJG: Canine infectious tracheobronchitis (kennel cough): A status report. Compend Contin Educ Pract Vet 3:70, 1981.

Bemis DA, *Bordetella* and *Mycoplasma* respiratory infections in dogs and cats. Vet Clin North Am Small Anim Pract 22:1173, 1992.

Dhein CR, Gorham JR: Canine respiratory infections. In: Scott FW, ed.: Contemporary Issues in Small Animal Practice. Infectious Diseases. New York: Churchill Livingstone, 1986, p 177.

Ford RB, Vaden SL: Canine infectious tracheobronchitis. In: Greene CE ed.: Infectious Diseases of the Dog and Cat. 2nd Ed. Philadelphia: WB Saunders, 1998, p 33.

Roudebush P, Fales W: Antibacterial susceptibility of *Bordetella bronchiseptica* isolates from small companion animals with respiratory disease. J Am Anim Hosp Assoc 17:793, 1981.

11 Canine Distemper

Robert G. Sherding

Canine distemper is a severe, highly contagious multisystemic viral disease of dogs and other carnivores, seen worldwide.

ETIOLOGY

Canine distemper virus (CDV) is a morbillivirus of the family Paramyxoviridae. It is closely related to measles virus.

Epidemiology

- *Distribution:* Enzootic worldwide
- *Incidence:* All ages affected; however, incidence is highest in unvaccinated puppies that are exposed after loss of maternal immunity (2–6 months of age)
- *Host range:* Domestic dogs and many wild carnivores, including
  - Canidae family—fox, dingo, coyote, wolf, jackal
  - Mustelidae family—ferret, mink, weasel, marten, skunk, badger, otter
  - Procyonidae family—raccoon, kinkajou, coati
  - Felidae—cheetah, lion, jaguar, margay, ocelot
  - Others—bear, panda, hyena, mongoose

Transmission

- Infected animals shed virus in all body secretions and excretions.
- The primary source of exposure is aerosol.
- The greatest opportunity for spread occurs where dogs are kept in groups (e.g., pet shops, kennels, animal shelters, research colonies).
- Transplacental transmission is a rare source of distemper in young pups (4–6 weeks of age).
- Viral shedding usually ceases 1 to 2 weeks after recovery; therefore, "carrier state" transmission is not a big problem. However, shedding for 60 to 90 days has been reported.
- The virus is labile in the environment, usually surviving only a few hours and no more than a few days outside of the host. It is readily destroyed by drying and by most disinfectants.

Pathogenesis

Stages of Infection

- *Day 1*: Airborne exposure leads to infection of tissue macrophages of the upper respiratory tract.

- *Days 2 to 4*: Infection spreads to local lymphoid tissues of the tonsils, retropharyngeal lymph nodes, and bronchial lymph nodes.
- *Days 4 to 6*: Widespread infection of systemic lymphoid tissues involves the liver, spleen, abdominal lymph nodes, and lamina propria of the gastrointestinal tract. This corresponds to a transient fever spike and the onset of lymphopenia caused by viral damage to T and B lymphoid cells.
- *Days 6 to 9*: Viremia occurs.
- *Days 8 and 9*: Virus is disseminated to epithelial tissues (epitheliotropism) and the central nervous system (CNS) (neurotropism).
- *Days 9 to 14*: The subsequent outcome varies depending on the host's immune response and can include recovery, severe multisystemic clinical disease, or CNS localization.

Host Immune Response

- If the immune response is rapid and effective, the infection is subclinical with complete recovery and elimination of the virus without clinical illness (by day 14 post infection). It is estimated that more than 50% of CDV infections are subclinical.
- If the immune response fails to develop by days 9 to 14 the outcome is rapid, widespread dissemination of the virus to the epithelial tissues such as the respiratory and gastrointestinal tracts and to the CNS (acute encephalomyelitis), resulting in multisystemic signs, a second fever spike, and a high mortality rate.
- If the immune response is sluggish or partial, multisystemic signs are prevented, CNS localization can result in chronic encephalomyelitis with delayed onset of neurologic signs.
- Role of immunosuppression: CDV causes widespread lymphoid damage, impaired B- and T-cell–mediated immunity, circulating lymphopenia, and thymic atrophy.

CLINICAL SIGNS

Clinical signs are multisystemic and extremely variable. The mortality rate can vary from 0 to 100% depending on the virulence of the CDV strain and the age and immune status of the host.

General (Systemic)

- Malaise: anorexia, depression, and dehydration
- Fever of 103° to 105°F (39.5°–41°C): diphasic (signs usually coincide with the second fever spike)

Respiratory System

- Rhinitis and conjunctivitis—serous to mucopurulent naso-ocular discharge
- Pneumonia
  - Initially—interstitial pneumonia (primary viral effect)
  - Later—bronchopneumonia (secondary bacterial infection)
  - Signs—productive cough, dyspnea, and auscultation abnormalities

Gastrointestinal System

- Vomiting and diarrhea

Eye

- Keratoconjunctivitis (serous to mucopurulent ocular discharge)
- Chorioretinitis (ophthalmoscopic lesions)
- Optic neuritis (blindness)

Nervous System

▼ *Key Point* Any region of the CNS can be affected by CDV. Diffuse or multifocal CNS involvement is typical. CNS signs tend to be progressive and can occur during, after, or in the absence of multisystemic illness.

Acute encephalomyelitis predominantly destroys gray matter (neurons), whereas subacute or chronic nonsuppurative encephalomyelitis predominantly affects white matter (demyelination). CNS signs can occur simultaneously with other multisystemic signs or can be delayed in onset until 1 to 3 weeks after apparent recovery from systemic illness. In some dogs, CNS involvement can occur as the only apparent manifestation of infection. (For additional details concerning the neurologic manifestations of CDV, see Chap. 145.)

- Acute encephalitis: generalized seizures, so-called "chewing-gum" seizures, pacing, circling, behavior changes
- Midbrain, cerebellar, and vestibular: ataxia and other disturbances of gait
- Spinal cord: disturbances of gait, abnormal spinal reflexes, paresis, and abnormal proprioception
- Peripheral and cranial neuropathies (including optic neuritis)
- Myoclonus: rhythmic, repetitive, motor movements or muscle twitches

Miscellaneous

- Dental enamel hypoplasia (pitted teeth) can result from infection before eruption of the permanent teeth.
- Hyperkeratosis of foot pads (hard pad disease)
- Abdominal pustular dermatitis
- Viral cardiomyopathy has been observed in neonatal (<7 days old) infections.
- Young growing large-breed dogs can develop metaphyseal osteosclerosis of the long bones.

DIAGNOSIS

▼ *Key Point* A presumptive diagnosis of distemper can be based on typical clinical signs in a young dog (2–6 months) that has a history of inadequate vaccinations and possibility of exposure to the virus.

In suspected cases of distemper, a complete blood count to assess leukocyte responses and thoracic radiographs to assess pneumonia are useful. In dogs presenting with neurologic disease suspected to be due to CDV, routine cerebrospinal fluid (CSF) analysis helps to distinguish CDV infection from other diseases. The presence of CDV-specific antibody in CSF can confirm the diagnosis but requires a special laboratory. Virology techniques can help to substantiate a diagnosis of distemper; however, this usually is not practical or necessary in most clinical situations, and false-negative results are common.

Hematology

- Lymphopenia (beginning with the initial fever spike)
- Neutrophilic leukocytosis occurs later (associated with secondary bacterial complications such as pneumonia).
- Distemper inclusions may rarely be found in circulating lymphocytes, monocytes, neutrophils, and erythrocytes.

Thoracic Radiography

- Interstitial pneumonia (early)
- Alveolar pattern and lobar consolidation with secondary bacterial bronchopneumonia (later)

CSF Analysis

- CSF may have increased protein and cell count (mostly lymphocytes), but normal findings do not rule out CDV (see Chaps. 144 and 145).
- The presence of CDV-specific antibody in CSF is diagnostic of CDV, but it is not present in all cases and specialized laboratory procedures are required.

Virology

- Intracytoplasmic viral inclusion bodies can sometimes be detected in peripheral blood cells (lymphocytes), epithelial cells (cytology specimens), or biopsies.
- Viral antigen can be identified by immunofluorescence in cells from blood, CSF, cytology specimens (e.g., conjunctival scraping, tracheobronchial aspirate), or frozen tissue specimens.

- Virus isolation (difficult and expensive) is best done on postmortem tissues.
- For any of these virologic procedures, negative test results do not rule out CDV.

Serology

- A single positive immunoglobulin G (IgG) titer is worthless because it does not distinguish current infection from past vaccination or exposure.
- The demonstration of a rising serum neutralizing antibody titer or a CDV-specific IgM titer is suggestive but not diagnostic of recent CDV infection.

TREATMENT

There is no effective antiviral treatment for CDV; therefore, treatment is supportive and symptomatic. Whenever possible, treat distemper on an outpatient basis to prevent aerosol exposure of other hospitalized animals.

Symptomatic Treatment

- Give broad-spectrum antibiotics (e.g., ampicillin, amoxicillin-clavulanate, or cephalosporins) for secondary bacterial infection, especially pneumonia (see Chap. 79)
- Provide humidification of airways
- For cough, give expectorants and bronchodilators and perform chest coupage (see Chaps. 78 and 79).
- For vomiting and diarrhea, restrict food intake and administer antiemetics (see Chap. 87) and antidiarrheals (see Chap. 89).
- For seizures, give a single dose of dexamethasone (1–2 mg/kg IV) for CNS edema and administer anticonvulsants such as phenobarbital and diazepam (see Chap. 146).
- Provide general supportive care, such as eyes and nose kept clear of discharges; nutritional support; and adequate fluid intake or parenteral fluid therapy

Prognosis

- Mortality rate varies but is highest in young puppies and when there is severe fulminant multisystemic disease or progressive neurologic disease.
- The neurologic deficits caused by CDV are often irreversible. It is justified to recommend euthanasia for patients with progressive neurologic signs that are severe and incapacitating.

▼ *Key Point* Do not be too optimistic with the owner, even with mild cases of distemper. The disease is often progressive despite therapy; some animals seem to recover, and then the symptoms exacerbate or incapacitating neurologic disease develops.

Client Education

- Discuss the multiplicity of signs that may be observed.
- Advise owners to isolate their animal from others to prevent contagion.

- Educate the client as to proper immunization procedures for future reference.
- Institute routine disinfection procedures and recommend at least a 1-week waiting period before bringing another dog onto the premises.

PREVENTION

Passive Maternal Antibody (Ab)

- The neonatal pup acquires passive immunity against CDV from its dam; most of this maternal-derived Ab comes from colostrum absorbed during nursing in the first few hours after birth.
- Maternal Ab gradually disappears, but it protects most pups until after weaning. Maternal Ab in the pup generally falls below protective levels sometime between 8 and 14 weeks of age.
- While present, maternal Ab also interferes with the response to vaccination; therefore, a series of vaccinations are given at 3- to 4-week intervals between 6 and 16 weeks of age. Vaccination can break through maternal Ab interference by 12 weeks of age in most puppies.

Vaccination

- Attenuated (modified live) CDV vaccine is nearly 100% protective; however, vaccine-induced encephalitis occasionally occurs 7 to 15 days after vaccination in very young puppies or in dogs that are severely ill, stressed, or immunocompromised. In these situations, consider using the recombinant canarypox-vectored distemper vaccine produced by Merial for its minimal risk of causing postvaccinal disease.
- Measles virus vaccine is not as protective as CDV vaccine, but it partially protects pups in the face of interfering maternal Ab so long as the level of Ab is not too high.

▼ *Key Point* For puppies 6 to 10 weeks of age, when a combined distemper-measles vaccine is given, the measles fraction can overcome maternal Ab interference if present and induce partial protection; however, if maternal Ab is minimal, the distemper fraction can induce complete protection.

- For puppies that received colostrum, vaccinate initially at 6 to 8 weeks of age and repeat every 3 to 4 weeks until 14 to 16 weeks of age. For the first vaccination in this series, consider using a combined distemper-measles vaccine.
- For colostrum-deprived puppies, vaccinate initially at 4 weeks of age and give a second dose 2 to 4 weeks later. Do not use modified live virus (MLV) distemper vaccine in pups younger than 3 to 4 weeks of age because of the risk of postvaccinal encephalitis. Safer alternatives for very young puppies are monovalent measles vaccine or recombinant canarypox-vectored distemper vaccine.
- For initial immunization of dogs older than 16 weeks of age, vaccinate twice, 2 to 4 weeks apart.

- Postvaccinal encephalitis has occurred occasionally after MLV distemper vaccination, primarily in neonatal puppies (<4 weeks of age); in severely ill stressed, or immunocompromised dogs; or in very young puppies infected with parvovirus.

▼ *Key Point* Immunity from distemper vaccination is solid and prolonged, but not necessarily lifelong. Vaccination boosters are recommended every 1 to 3 years depending on level of exposure risk.

SUPPLEMENTAL READINGS

Greene CE, Appel MJ: Canine distemper. In: Greene CE, ed.: Infectious Diseases of the Dog and Cat. 2nd Ed. Philadelphia: WB Saunders, 1998, p 9.

12 Intestinal Viruses

Robert G. Sherding

Parvoviruses, coronaviruses, rotaviruses, and possibly astroviruses have been established as causes of viral enteritis and diarrhea in dogs and cats and are discussed in this chapter. In addition to these, numerous other viruses of uncertain enteropathogenicity have been discovered in canine and feline feces by virus isolation or electron microscopy. Examples in dogs are astrovirus, herpesvirus, enteroviruses, calicivirus, parainfluenza viruses, adenovirus, and picornavirus; viruses identified in cats include astrovirus, calicivirus, picorna-like virus, reovirus, torovirus-like virus, and toga-like virus. In addition, the intestine may be involved as part of generalized viral infections in disorders such as canine distemper (see Chap. 11), feline leukemia virus (see Chap. 6), feline immunodeficiency virus (see Chap. 7), and feline infectious peritonitis (see Chap. 8).

CANINE PARVOVIRUS

Etiology

Canine parvovirus type 2 (CPV-2) causes an acute, highly contagious enteritis of dogs that has been prevalent worldwide since the late 1970s. Since 1980 variants designated CPV-2a and CPV-2b have evolved, the latter now being the predominant strain in North America.

▼ **Key Point** CPV has an affinity for the rapidly dividing cells of the intestine, bone marrow, and lymphoid tissues and thus causes intestinal crypt necrosis, severe diarrhea, leukopenia, and lymphoid depletion.

Transmission

CPV infection occurs by the fecal-oral route. During acute illness, and for about 1 to 2 weeks thereafter, massive amounts of parvovirus (over 1 billion virions per gram of feces) are shed in feces of infected dogs. Because the virus can survive and remain infectious for many months in the environment, fomites and environmental contamination play a major role in transmission.

Incubation

Signs of enteric disease usually begin 4–7 days after exposure, coincident with localization of virus in the mitotically active zones of intestinal crypt epithelia.

Age Incidence

Dogs of any age can be infected, but the incidence of clinical disease is almost entirely in puppies between weaning and 6 months of age. Puppies younger than 6 weeks of age generally are protected by passive maternal immunity, whereas most mature animals have been immunized or have seroconverted from subclinical infection.

Breed Incidence

Certain breeds appear to be at higher risk for parvovirus infection and susceptible to a more severe form of the disease. These include rottweilers, Doberman pinschers, pit bull terriers, german shepherds, and Labrador retrievers. The biologic basis for these breed susceptibilities is unknown.

Clinical Signs

- Parvovirus causes anorexia, depression, fever, vomiting, intractable fluid diarrhea (can be profuse and hemorrhagic), and rapidly progressive dehydration.
- Hypothermia, icterus, or hemorrhagic diathesis (disseminated intravascular coagulation) may develop terminally in those with bacterial sepsis or endotoxemia.
- Death may occur in severe cases, particularly in very young puppies and in the highly susceptible breeds, and is usually attributable to dehydration, electrolyte imbalances, endotoxic shock, or overwhelming bacterial sepsis related to leukopenia. Septic puppies often develop hypoglycemia
- The severity of clinical illness may be increased by factors such as stress, overcrowded or unsanitary kennel conditions, secondary bacterial infection, and concurrent diseases such as canine distemper, coronavirus, salmonellosis, campylobacteriosis, and intestinal parasitism.
- In nonimmunized mature dogs, mild or inapparent infections that result in seroconversion without clinical signs are probably common.
- In utero or postnatal infection can cause acute neonatal myocarditis. Because most dams are now immune and passively transfer immunity to their puppies, this form of perinatal parvoviral infection is practically nonexistent. Signs of parvoviral myocarditis include dyspnea due to acute heart failure, sudden death due to arrhythmias, and sometimes delayed-onset chronic congestive heart failure due to chronic myocardial fibrosis.

Diagnosis

Suspect parvovirus infection in young dogs that have an abrupt onset of vomiting and diarrhea, especially if associated with severe depression, fever, or leukopenia, or if these signs follow potential exposure to infected dogs or fomites.

▼ *Key Point* Because of the difficulty in breaking through maternal antibody interference with vaccination in young puppies, prior vaccination does not necessarily exclude parvoviral infection, especially in puppies 6 to 20 weeks of age.

Hematology

- A complete blood count (CBC) is particularly useful because in most dogs with parvoviral enteritis, severe leukopenia due to lymphopenia and granulocytopenia develops, often with a total of only 500 to 2000 leukocytes/µl, and occasionally even less. Depletion of circulating mature neutrophils is caused by extensive loss of neutrophils through the damaged intestinal mucosa coupled with impaired myelopoiesis caused by bone marrow disruption from the virus. The severity of the leukopenia is generally proportional to the severity of the clinical illness, and a rebound neutrophilia is a useful indicator of impending recovery.
- The hematocrit is variable. The PCV is often normal but can be moderately decreased in some dogs because of intestinal hemorrhage (especially noticeable after rehydration), whereas in other dogs PCV can be elevated because of dehydration (hemoconcentration).

Serum Chemistries

Abnormal serum chemistries are variable and nonspecific, such as electrolyte imbalances (most frequently hypokalemia), prerenal azotemia, and increased bilirubin and liver enzymes (ALT and ALP).

Abdominal Radiography

Gas and fluid distention of the gastrointestinal tract due to ileus are frequent radiographic findings in parvoviral enteritis and must be differentiated from small intestinal obstruction (e.g., foreign body or intussusception). Carefully palpate the abdomen to help rule out mechanical obstruction. Barium contrast radiography often reveals mucosal irregularity (corrugation or scalloping) and prolonged transit time.

Serology

- Determination of an anti-CPV antibody in serum is not sufficient for diagnosis because up to 95% of dogs in the population have seroconverted from prior vaccination or exposure.
- Specific IgM analysis by indirect fluorescent antibody (IFA) test or a 2-mercaptoethanol procedure provides serologic evidence of recent infection because IgM is found only in the first few weeks after infection.

Virology

▼ *Key Point* Definitive diagnosis of parvoviral enteritis requires demonstration of active excretion of virus or viral antigen in the feces because massive quantities of virus are shed during the acute illness.

- The most practical method for detecting parvovirus in the feces is an in-office enzyme-linked immunosorbent assay (ELISA) (CITE-Parvo Test, IDEXX; Assure-parvovirus, Symbiotics). Positive results are a reliable indicator of active fecal excretion of CPV-2. Occasionally, false-negative results occur. Attenuated vaccines may cause a false-positive result for 5–12 days postvaccination.
- Other methods for detecting fecal excretion of parvovirus, such as hemagglutination, latex agglutination, electron microscopy, and virus isolation, are less practical for routine clinical use because they require an outside diagnostic laboratory.

Necropsy

Necropsy diagnosis of parvovirus is based on identification of the characteristic intestinal lesions: necrosis of the rapidly proliferating intestinal crypt cells with secondary villous collapse and dilatation of the crypts with necrotic debris. Myeloid degeneration and widespread lymphoid depletion also are seen. Parvovirus can be demonstrated in frozen tissue samples by immunofluorescent and in fixed specimens by PCR.

Treatment

Because the treatment of parvovirus is mainly supportive and similar to what would be used in most animals with severe gastroenteritis, institute therapy whether or not definitive tests are done or while awaiting the return of results.

Fluid Therapy

▼ *Key Point* The cornerstone of treatment of CPV infection is rehydration and correction of electrolyte imbalances.

See Chapter 5 for specific guidelines and procedures for fluid and electrolyte therapy. Continue fluid therapy until vomiting ceases and oral intake resumes.

- In severe cases, intravenous fluid and electrolyte replacement is preferred (e.g., lactated Ringer's supplemented with potassium at 20–40 mEq/L). Correct dehydration over the first 24 hrs and continue with maintenance fluids plus replacement of ongoing losses. Two to three times normal maintenance levels are often required.
- Infuse colloid solution (Hetastarch or Dextran-70) at 10–20 ml/kg, IV, if infusion of balanced crystalloid solution does not restore hemodynamic stability.
- Dextrose also may be added to IV fluids at a 2.5% solution to control complicating hypoglycemia of

sepsis. Monitor serum glucose and increase to 5% if needed to maintain serum glucose at 120–160 mg/dl.
- Avoid administration of fluids by the subcutaneous route in dogs with severe leukopenia because there is a high incidence of secondary infection, cellulitis, and skin necrosis at administration sites.
- Monitor fluid therapy by tracking body weight, physical parameters, urine output, estimates of ongoing fluid losses (vomitus, diarrhea), and hematocrit and total plasma protein.

Antibiotics

Antibiotics are indicated to control potentially life-threatening bacterial sepsis. Initially, administer antibiotics parenterally, such as cefazolin in mild cases, or ampicillin combined with gentamicin or amikacin in dogs that are severely leukopenic. If an aminoglycoside is used, maintain hydration to prevent nephrotoxicity and monitor the urine daily for casts and proteinuria as early indicators of nephrotoxicosis.

Dietary Restriction

Give nothing per os (fluid needs are met by IV infusion) until vomiting has ceased for at least 24 hours and diarrhea has subsided and is free of gross hemorrhage. This can take 3 to 5 days in severe cases. When feeding is resumed, give small frequent feedings of a bland digestible diet, such as a commercial GI diet or cooked skinless chicken and rice, until gastrointestinal function appears to have recovered. The transition back to regular feeding should be gradual.

Antiemetics

For frequent or persistent vomiting associated with delayed gastric emptying that sometimes occurs in parvoviral infection, administer metoclopramide (Reglan; A.H. Robins) at 0.5 mg/kg, every 8 hours, SC, or most effectively as a continuous infusion of 1 to 2 mg/kg every 24 hours diluted in IV fluids. For gastritis, control of gastric acid secretion with an H_2 receptor blocker (see Chap. 87 for products and dosages) is often helpful as well. If these are unsuccessful in controlling vomiting, consider using a broad-spectrum phenothiazine antiemetic (e.g., chlorpromazine; see Chap. 87), but not until dehydration has been corrected because phenothiazines have a hypotensive effect. For persistent vomiting that is refractory to treatment, give odansetron (Zofran; 0.1–0.2 mg/kg slow IV, q6–12h), a serotonin-antagonist antiemetic.

Antidiarrheals

Parvoviral diarrhea is usually self-limiting, and treatment to control diarrhea usually is not needed as long as fluid needs are met; however, when diarrhea is profuse and persistent, administer loperamide (Imodium; 0.2 mg/kg, q8h, PO) (see Chap. 89).

Infusion of Whole Blood or Plasma

Occasionally infusion of blood or plasma (5–10 ml/kg, IV) is necessary for treatment of severe blood loss anemia or hypoproteinemia.

Other Treatments

- Dexamethasone (2–4 mg/kg IV, one dose)—to treat septic shock
- Flunixin meglumine (Banamine)—alternative to steroid as a single injection to treat septic shock. Beware of gastric ulceration; do not give repeated doses or combine with corticosteroids
- Antiendotoxin hyperimmune serum (Septi-serum; Immvac)—to bind and neutralize endotoxin; efficacy is not yet established.
- Recombinant human granulocyte colony-stimulating factor—has been used to treat neutropenia, but one study failed to show any beneficial effects in parvoviral neutropenia.

Prognosis and Complications

▼ *Key Point* Most dogs with CPV enteritis recover if treated appropriately to control dehydration and sepsis.

Once an animal survives the first 3 to 4 days of illness, recovery usually occurs rapidly.

- Some animals, however, succumb to bacterial sepsis and endotoxemia resulting from the leukopenia, immunosuppression, and breakdown of the intestinal mucosal barrier caused by CPV. In general, the younger the animal, the higher the mortality rate.
- Other complications may include hypoglycemia (probably secondary to sepsis), hypoproteinemia, anemia, intussusception, liver disease, central nervous system signs (likely due to concomitant canine distemper), and numerous secondary bacterial infections, such as endocarditis, thrombophlebitis, pneumonia (caused by aspiration in some dogs), urinary tract infection, injection site abscesses, and intestinal salmonellosis and campylobacteriosis.

Prevention: Reducing Exposure

- Dogs with CPV infection shed massive amounts of virus in the feces during their illness. These, as well as the fomites and premises that they contaminate, are highly infectious for other dogs. Thus, instruct the owner of a CPV-infected dog to keep the dog isolated from other dogs until at least 1 week after full recovery.

▼ *Key Point* Elimination of CPV from infected premises is difficult because the virus is so resistant; however, disinfection with a 1:32 dilution of sodium hypochlorite bleach is effective.

- CPV is ubiquitous, and because it is so stable outside of the animal and easily transmitted by fomites, prevention of exposure is almost impossible. Nevertheless, until vaccinations are complete, keep young puppies isolated as much as possible from other animals and from potentially infected premises.

Prevention: Vaccination

Vaccination is the only realistic and effective means of prevention and control of parvovirus infection.

Maternal Antibody Interference

Although widespread vaccination against parvovirus has markedly reduced the incidence of the disease in North America, parvoviral enteritis continues to be a problem in puppies as they are nearing the end of their maternal antibody protection between 6 and 20 weeks of age. This is so despite vaccination because of a period of susceptibility when maternal antibodies are too low to protect but at the same time high enough to interfere with the response to vaccination.

▼ *Key Point* In puppies from dams with high CPV titers, maternally derived antibody can persist at interfering levels for up to 18 weeks or more; thus, vaccination may not be able to break through this maternal antibody interference until as late as 18 weeks of age.

- In the first weeks of life, maternal antibody protects the puppy from infection, but at the same time it also interferes with active immunization.
- As the level of this maternal antibody gradually declines, there is a period of 2 to 4 weeks in which all puppies are refractory to vaccination but susceptible to infection if exposed.
- Almost all apparent "vaccination failures" in puppies probably result from exposure to infection during this critical period of susceptibility.
- Because the age at which pups can respond to vaccination for CPV is unpredictable, the most effective protocols use a series of vaccinations.
- Attenuated live CPV-2 vaccines that are "potentiated" (i.e., contain a high titer of a highly immunogenic strain of virus) are most effective at breaking through maternal antibody interference at a young age.

Recommendations for Routine Vaccination

- Advantages of attenuated or modified live virus (MLV) CPV-2 vaccines over inactivated (killed) vaccines:
  - Better magnitude of protection
  - More rapid onset of protection (as early as 1–3 days)
  - Longer duration of protection ($\geq$2 years)
  - Better able to break through maternal antibody interference
  - Prevention of shedding of virulent CPV if exposed (killed vaccines protect only against clinical disease but do not prevent subclinical infection or shedding)

▼ *Key Point* Commercially available CPV-2 vaccines effectively cross-protect against all known field strains of CPV, including the newer so-called variant strains.

- In puppies, begin vaccination series at 6 to 8 weeks of age and vaccinate every 3 to 4 weeks until at least 12 weeks of age using high-titer attenuated live CPV-2 vaccines (e.g., at 6, 9, and 12 weeks of age; plus an additional dose at 15–16 wks in high-risk breeds), or until at least 20 weeks with other unpotentiated vaccines (e.g., at 8, 12, 16, and 20 weeks). Do not space vaccinations less than 2 weeks apart because interference from shorter intervals can impair vaccine efficacy.
- In unvaccinated dogs 16 weeks of age or older, give two doses of vaccine 2 to 4 weeks apart.
- Concurrent administration of MLV CPV and distemper vaccines is considered to be safe; however, some have recommended in puppies less than 9 weeks of age the use of measles instead of MLV distemper vaccine to prevent the rare occurrence of distemper vaccine–induced encephalitis.
- Annual revaccination is currently recommended; however, duration of immunity probably is much longer than 12 months in mature dogs and less frequent boosters may be appropriate.
- Females should be revaccinated 2 weeks before breeding so that high maternal antibody titers are transferred to puppies.
- Use inactivated instead of MLV CPV vaccine in pregnant animals and in puppies less than 5 weeks of age (e.g., early vaccination in colostrum-deprived pups).

CANINE CORONAVIRUS

Etiology

Canine coronaviral enteritis is an acute contagious disease of dogs caused by an epitheliotropic virus that preferentially invades the enterocytes of the villous tips. The resulting villous destruction, atrophy, and fusion cause diarrhea of variable severity.

- The clinical importance of canine coronavirus (CCV) as a cause of enteritis is considered relatively minor.

▼ *Key Point* Most CCV infections are subclinical, although occasional epizootics of severe enteritis have occurred, primarily associated with kennels and dog shows.

- CCV is shed subclinically for months postinfection from dogs and spreads rapidly by fecal-oral transmission.

Clinical Signs

- Most dogs infected with CCV are asymptomatic, but some manifest an acute onset of anorexia and depression followed by vomiting and diarrhea. The character of the diarrhea varies from soft to watery and sometimes contains mucus and fresh red blood.

- Most dogs infected with CCV are afebrile. The signs are mild and easily confused with various other non-specific causes of mild diarrhea of brief duration.

Diagnosis

Consider coronaviral enteritis in dogs with an acute onset of signs of gastroenteritis, especially if other dogs on the premises are affected. Because coronaviral enteritis is usually nonfatal and the only treatment is supportive, definitive laboratory confirmation is not needed for effective case management except to document an epizootic outbreak. Coronaviral enteritis should, however, be distinguished from the more severe multisystemic parvoviral infection.

▼ **Key Point** In contrast to CPV infection, fever, leukopenia, hematochezia, and fatalities are not typical of coronaviral enteritis.

- Routine hematology, serum chemistries, and abdominal radiography are usually normal.
- Definitive diagnosis requires laboratory detection of CCV in feces by electron microscopy (EM), virus isolation, or PCR during the acute illness. Fecal examination by EM requires fresh feces (specimens can be kept refrigerated but not frozen). Both false-positive and false-negative results are a problem with EM because of misidentification of fecal particles. Virus isolation and PCR are preformed in research labs and are not readily available to the clinician.

▼ **Key Point** The mere identification of CCV in a dog's feces is not proof that it is the cause of diarrhea or illness because CCV is shed in the feces of many healthy dogs.

- Serology can provide only a retrospective diagnosis via demonstration of a fourfold or greater rise in serum antibody titer in paired sera (at the time of illness and 2–6 weeks later).

Treatment

Coronaviral enteritis is treated like any other acute diarrhea with fluid therapy and symptomatic treatment such as dietary restriction (see Chap. 89). Most dogs recover rapidly, although some have persistent diarrhea for 3 to 4 weeks. Fatalities have been reported, especially in neonates, but are considered rare.

Prevention

Vaccination for CCV is an optional part of the routine vaccination program for most dogs. Consider vaccinating dogs with a high risk of exposure, such as show and field trial dogs and kenneled (boarded) dogs.

- Killed (inactivated) and attenuated live CCV vaccines are commercially available; however, the efficacy

(completeness and duration of immunity) and justification for use of these products are controversial. In general, immunity to coronaviruses is brief and is mediated by local (IgA) immunity rather than the serum antibodies that would result from a parenteral vaccine. Parenteral vaccination does not prevent CCV infection, but it may reduce intestinal replication of virus and minimize clinical signs.

- Administer two doses of CCV vaccine at 2- to 3-week intervals and revaccinate annually.

CANINE ROTAVIRUS

Etiology

Rotaviruses have been recognized as one of the most important causes of neonatal diarrhea in humans and many other species of mammals and birds, but canine isolates appear to be involved rarely in causing diarrhea or clinical illness in dogs.

▼ **Key Point** Rotavirus has not been shown to be an enteropathogen of major clinical importance in the dog.

- The high incidence of antirotavirus antibodies in surveys of normal dogs (as high as 79%) indicates that most dogs experience rotavirus infection without showing signs.
- Transmission is by the fecal-oral route.
- Rotaviruses replicate exclusively in the mature enterocytes of the villous tip, causing blunted villi that are populated mainly with immature secretory cells from the crypts.

Clinical Signs

In adult dogs, rotaviral infection is usually subclinical, but clinical signs of acute enteritis occasionally are seen in young puppies.

- The diarrhea, which may be watery to mucoid, is usually self-limiting and of brief duration, although rare fatalities attributable to dehydration have been reported.
- Experimental inoculation of neonatal (2 days old) gnotobiotic puppies with canine rotavirus results in diarrhea and mild to moderate villous atrophy; however, deprivation of colostrum predisposes to much more severe diarrhea.
- It has been almost impossible to produce signs of rotavirus infection experimentally in dogs older than 6 months of age.

Diagnosis

Active rotavirus infection can be established by detection of virus in feces by commercial ELISA test kits, electron microscopy, or virus isolation.

Treatment

Rotaviral enteritis is treated like other types of acute diarrhea (see Chap. 89), with emphasis on supportive measures such as fluid therapy and dietary restriction. Most animals recover uneventfully with minimal treatment.

Prevention

There is currently no vaccine available for canine rotavirus. In neonates, the only group significantly threatened by rotavirus infection, the best protection is to ensure nursing of colostral antibodies in the first hours after birth.

FELINE PANLEUKOPENIA VIRUS

Etiology

Feline panleukopenia virus (FPV) is a severe, highly contagious parvoviral infection of cats. Panleukopenia currently is relatively rare because of effective control with vaccinations. Occasional infections are seen in unvaccinated kittens, especially those from shelters, farms, and urban stray populations.

- FPV can infect all species of Felidae as well as raccoon, coatimundi, and mink.
- FPV is shed in all body excretions for up to 6 weeks, especially feces.
- FPV is very resistant to inactivation but can be inactivated with a 1:32 dilution of sodium hypochlorite bleach.
- FPV is ubiquitous in the environment, where it can survive readily for more than 1 year and can be transmitted by oropharyngeal contact with contaminated fomites.
- FPV has a predilection for rapidly dividing cells, particularly the following:
  - Intestinal crypt epithelium, resulting in acute enteritis
  - Hemopoietic tissue, resulting in panleukopenia
  - Lymphoid tissues, resulting in lymphoid depletion
  - In utero fetus, resulting in fetal death or cerebellar hypoplasia

Clinical Signs

Subclinical Infection of Adult Cats

Infection in susceptible adult cats is usually subclinical. The generalized form can occur rarely.

Generalized Infection of Kittens

The incidence and mortality rate are highest in young kittens. Clinical features are similar to those of canine parvoviral enteritis: anorexia, depression, high fever 104° to 106°F (40°–41°C), persistent vomiting, diarrhea, and progressive dehydration. Vomitus is usually a bile-stained fluid, and feces may be watery, mucoid, or bloody. Intestinal loops may be palpably thickened and firm (rope-like), fluid-filled, and painful. There is increased susceptibility to bacterial sepsis and endotoxemia.

Perinatal Infection of Neonates

In utero infection of the fetus at the end of gestation or of the neonate in the first 2 weeks after birth may permanently damage the central nervous system and cause cerebellar hypoplasia. Affected kittens show nonprogressive signs of ataxia, hypermetria, falling to the side, broad-based stance, and intention tremors (see Chaps. 144 and 145). At the same time, FPV also may invade the thymus of neonates, causing thymic atrophy and early neonatal mortality (fading kitten syndrome), and it may invade the retina, causing retinal dysplasia.

In Utero Infection of the Fetus

The only manifestation of infection in the pregnant cat may be transplacental infection of the developing embryo or fetus, leading to early embryonic resorption (infertility), fetal death, fetal mummification, abortion, and stillbirth.

Diagnosis

Feline panleukopenia usually is diagnosed presumptively on the basis of clinical signs of acute gastroenteritis in a young susceptible (unvaccinated) cat with systemic involvement and profound panleukopenia.

▼ *Key Point* Profound leukopenia (total leukocyte count often <500/μl) is a consistent feature of feline panleukopenia and usually lasts 2 to 4 days before rebounding as recovery occurs. The degree of leukopenia is proportional to the severity of clinical illness.

- Serum chemistry abnormalities are nonspecific and occur inconsistently but can include electrolyte imbalances (especially hypokalemia), prerenal azotemia, and increased bilirubin and liver enzymes.
- If leukopenia persists for more than 5 days or is accompanied by severe nonregenerative anemia, consider the panleukopenia-like syndrome that is associated with feline leukemia virus infection (see Chap. 6). Other panleukopenia "look-alike" diseases include acute salmonellosis, acute bacterial sepsis with endotoxemia, and gastrointestinal foreign body with perforation and peritonitis (e.g., linear foreign body).
- Serologic diagnosis (paired neutralizing antibody titers), PCR, and virus isolation have been used in research but are rarely applicable to clinical practice.
- Necropsy diagnosis is based on lesions of severe necrosis of intestinal crypts.

Treatment

- The treatment for feline panleukopenia is similar to that for canine parvoviral enteritis, mainly nonspecific supportive treatment such as rehydration, parenteral antibiotics, antiemetics, good nursing care, and restriction of dietary intake. Correction of severe dehydration is most important, and the parenteral route is best (see Chap. 5).
- In young kittens with panleukopenia, the mortality rate is high (50–90%). A guarded prognosis is justified until impending recovery is indicated by cessation of vomiting and diarrhea, return of appetite to

normal, return of body temperature to normal, and rebound leukocytosis. However, complications, such as hypothermia and shock (endotoxemia), jaundice, secondary bacterial or mycotic infection, and disseminated intravascular coagulation usually indicate a fatal outcome.

Prevention

▼ *Key Point* Vaccination is highly effective for prevention of feline panleukopenia.

- Both attenuated (live) and inactivated (killed) vaccines are effective, but attenuated vaccination elicits a more effective and rapid onset of protection. This can be an important consideration in high-risk environments such as shelters, where cats are housed in groups. Parenteral and intranasal vaccines are available
- In kittens, vaccination usually can overcome maternal antibody interference by about 12 weeks of age.
- For routine vaccination: vaccinate at 8 to 9 weeks of age, then repeat every 2 to 4 weeks until 12 to 14 weeks of age for a total of at least 2 doses.
- Annual revaccination is recommended by manufacturers, but is not essential. Antibody titers and resistance to challenge persist for at least 3 to 4 years or more; thus, after the kitten series, a booster one year later and then every 3 years should be adequate.

▼ *Key Point* Use only inactivated panleukopenia vaccine in pregnant cats and in kittens younger than 4 weeks of age. MLV vaccine given perinatally can infect the unborn fetus or the neonatal cerebellum.

FELINE ENTERIC CORONAVIRUS

Etiology

Feline enteric coronavirus (FECV), appears to be ubiquitous in the cat population. Like enteric coronaviruses of other species, FECV invades the epithelium of the villous tip, resulting in villous atrophy. A mutant variant of this virus causes feline infectious peritonitis (see Chap. 8)

▼ *Key Point* FECV is shed in the feces of many normal cats, and a high percentage of cats are seropositive, indicating that inapparent infection is extremely prevalent.

Clinical Signs

- In young kittens, especially those 4 to 12 weeks of age, FECV can cause an acute but mild enteritis with diarrhea. Feces are soft to fluid and sometimes contain excess mucus and fresh red blood.
- Diarrhea may be accompanied by vomiting, low-grade fever, anorexia, and lethargy.
- Clinical signs are usually mild and self-limiting within 2 to 4 days. Fatalities are rare but have been reported.

Diagnosis

Serology can identify a convalescent rise in coronaviral antibody titer. This is more important because of the confusion it causes in serologic diagnosis for FIP (see Chap. 8) than as a diagnostic aid for enteric disease. Research facilities can use electron microscopy to identify coronaviral particles in fresh feces (specimens can be refrigerated but not frozen), but misidentification causes false-positive and false-negative results. PCR can also be used.

Treatment

Coronaviral enteritis is treated like any other acute diarrhea (see Chap. 89), with emphasis on supportive measures such as fluid therapy and dietary restriction. Most animals recover uneventfully.

Prevention

This virus appears to be practically ubiquitous and spreads very efficiently through catteries; thus, prevention may not be practical. The intranasal FIP vaccine does not appear to prevent intestinal replication of feline coronavirus (see Chap. 8).

FELINE ROTAVIRUS

Etiology

As in the canine, rotavirus has been isolated from both normal and diarrheic feces of cats, especially kittens, but its enteropathogenic significance currently is unclear. Infection is restricted to the gastrointestinal mucosa. Subclinical infection in mature animals is probably frequent, as indicated by surveys that found antibodies to rotavirus in 26 of 94 clinically healthy British cats and 23 of 50 cats in Louisiana.

Clinical Signs

Subclinical infection is probably the rule; the exceptions are neonates and cats in which mild, nonspecific diarrhea of brief (1–2 days) duration occasionally develops.

Diagnosis

As in dogs, feline rotavirus can be detected in feces by EM, PCR, or ELISA.

Treatment

Rotaviral enteritis is treated like any other acute diarrhea (see Chap. 89), with emphasis on supportive measures such as fluid therapy and dietary restriction. Most animals recover uneventfully with minimal or no treatment.

Prevention

Vaccines are unavailable for rotavirus. Because natural immunity is short-lived, vaccination is unlikely to be warranted.

FELINE ASTROVIRUS

Etiology

Very little is known concerning this viral agent, but a few reports have identified astroviruses in the feces of cats with diarrhea, and mild diarrhea was reproduced experimentally in kittens. A survey of British cats determined a seroprevalence of less than 10%. Astrovirus infections in other species are limited to infection of the mature villous epithelial cells of the intestinal mucosa. Transmission is by the fecal-oral route.

Clinical Signs

Feline astrovirus appears to cause mild, nonspecific diarrhea 4 to 14 days in duration. Transient low-grade fever, depression, and inappetance also may occur, but affected cats remain otherwise well. Astrovirus was implicated in a diarrhea outbreak in a cattery. As with other enteropathogenic viruses, kittens are most likely to be affected.

Diagnosis

Feline astrovirus is detected in feces by EM or PCR. Some cats shed the virus asymptomatically. Serum antibody to astrovirus has been identified in cats, but its significance is unknown.

Treatment

Diarrhea caused by astrovirus is treated like any other acute diarrhea (see Chapter 89), with emphasis on supportive measures such as fluid therapy and dietary restriction. Most animals recover uneventfully with minimal or no treatment.

Prevention

No preventive measures are available.

SUPPLEMENTAL READING

Greene CE, Scott FW: Feline panleukopenia. In: Greene CE (ed): Infectious Diseases of the Dog and Cat (2nd Ed). Philadelphia: WB Saunders, 1998, p 52.

Hoskins JD: Canine viral enteritis. In: Greene, CE (ed): Infectious Diseases of the Dog and Cat (2nd Ed). Philadelphia: WB Saunders, 1998, p 40.

Chapter 13

Rabies and Pseudorabies

Robert G. Sherding

RABIES

Etiology

- Rabies virus is a rhabdovirus (genus *Lyssavirus*) that can infect virtually all warm-blooded animals. It primarily attacks the nervous system and is shed in saliva.
- Rabies is most important as a cause of highly fatal encephalitis in humans. The incidence of human rabies in the United States is very low, and several countries are now classified as rabies-free.
- Rabies is transmitted in saliva from the bite of an infected animal. For both humans and domestic animals, the usual source is the bite of a rabid wild animal, most commonly a skunk, raccoon, bat, or fox. Some animals can shed rabies virus for prolonged periods in their saliva without evidence of clinical signs.
- Rabies virus is very labile outside the host; it is inactivated by many disinfectants.

▼ *Key Point* Rabies is rare in dogs and cats in the United States; however, cats are more susceptible, and the incidence in cats is higher than in dogs. Wild animals are the principal reservoir of infection.

Pathogenesis

Rabies virus is transmitted in saliva into a deep bite wound, where it enters the peripheral nervous tissue and spreads retrograde (centripetally) along peripheral nerves to the spinal cord and brain. Centrifugal spread then occurs along peripheral nerves from the brain to other tissues, such as the salivary glands. The incubation period before central nervous system (CNS) signs occur is extremely variable, but is usually 2 to 8 weeks. Incubation periods up to 24 weeks have been reported in dogs and cats. Virus shedding in saliva begins a short time (usually less than 10 days) before neurologic signs appear and continues until the animal dies.

Clinical Signs

The clinical course of rabies, although variable, is divided classically into three phases: the prodromal, furious, and paralytic phases. Death usually occurs within 3 to 7 days from the onset of signs; however, some animals develop atypical rabies and do not progress through these stages.

Prodromal Phase (2–3 Days)

This phase often passes unnoticed, but there may be subtle signs of erratic behavior, fever, slow corneal and palpebral reflexes, and chewing at the bite site.

Furious Phase (2–4 Days)

Initially the forebrain region of the CNS is invaded, resulting in signs of erratic and unusual behavior such as irritability, restlessness, barking, episodic aggression, vicious attacks on inanimate objects, pica, unexplained roaming, and abnormal sexual behavior. Ataxia, disorientation, and seizures may develop.

Paralytic Phase (2–4 Days)

Progressive lower motor neuron paralysis develops, causing signs of ascending paresis or paralysis of the limbs (often affecting a bitten extremity first), or signs of cranial nerve paralysis, such as laryngeal paralysis (change in bark, dyspnea), pharyngeal paralysis (drooling, dysphagia), and masticatory paralysis (dropped jaw). These are followed by depression, coma, and death from respiratory paralysis.

Atypical Rabies

Some animals develop subclinical, chronic, or recovered infections rather than the typical furious and paralytic forms.

Diagnosis

▼ *Key Point* Early laboratory confirmation of animal rabies is essential so that exposed humans can receive proper prophylaxis as early as possible.

Antemortem tests for rabies are too unreliable to be recommended; thus, always use evaluation of pathologic specimens for diagnosis. For laboratory analysis of brain and salivary tissue for the presence of rabies virus or antigen, submit the animal's head chilled on wet ice in a leakproof container, along with appropriate information and biohazard labeling. Specimens can be stored by refrigeration but not freezing, because thawing will ruin the specimen for subsequent virus detection.

Direct Fluorescent Antibody (DFA) Test

This is the test of choice used by most laboratories for rapid, reliable confirmation of rabies antigen in tissues. Brain tissue is used for routine postmortem testing. The DFA procedure also can be used for antemortem detection of rabies antigen in skin biopsies; however, a high percentage of false-negative results limits its usefulness.

Histopathology

This older, less sensitive test detects intracytoplasmic neuronal inclusions (Negri bodies), which are found in 75% of rabid dogs but rarely in cats.

Mouse Inoculation Test

This is a confirmatory test in which DFA-positive brain suspensions are inoculated intracerebrally into mice; the mice then are sacrificed and their brains examined by DFA testing 5 to 6 days postinoculation.

Tissue Culture Inoculation Test

This test is similar to the mouse inoculation test, except that cell cultures are inoculated and are examined by DFA testing 24 to 72 hours later.

Monoclonal Antibody Techniques

These techniques are used to identify antigenic variants of rabies virus and to differentiate vaccine virus strains from wild-type strains in DFA-positive brains.

Molecular Techniques

Rabies virus genomic RNA can be detected in brain tissue using molecular techniques such as polymerase chain reaction (PCR) and hybridization techniques. These are generally reserved for specimens with questionable DFA results.

Treatment

Rabies is almost always fatal in domestic animals. Because of the extreme public health danger, all animals suspected of rabies are either quarantined or euthanized, and local health department authorities must be notified.

Prevention in Dogs and Cats

▼ *Key Point* For rabies prevention and vaccination, follow the guidelines in the Compendium of Animal Rabies Control, published annually by the National Association of State Public Health Veterinarians.

- Vaccinate all dogs, cats, and ferrets against rabies according to local public health regulations.
  - Vaccinate at 2 or 3 months of age, 1 year later, and then every 1 or 3 years, depending on the product recommendations.

- Side effects: Adjuvants may cause local soreness, lameness, fever, lethargy, palpable inflammatory nodules, and rarely, injection site sarcomas in cats. The neurologic complications of earlier attenuated, modified live virus (MLV) vaccines are no longer a problem because only inactivated and recombinant vaccines are currently available in the United States.
- Do not vaccinate wild animals against rabies, even if they are kept as pets.
- Prevent pets from having contact with wild animals.
- Report all human and animal exposures to the local public health authorities. Recommendations for dogs and cats exposed to rabies (bitten by a known rabid animal or a wild animal that is unavailable for testing) are as follows:
  - In a previously vaccinated dog or cat, revaccinate immediately and keep under the owner's control and observation for 45 days.
  - In an unvaccinated dog or cat, euthanize immediately for examination of tissues. If euthanasia is refused by the owner, strict quarantine without human or animal contact is required for 6 months, with vaccination 1 month before release.

Prevention in Humans

Approximately 15% of humans untreated after a bite from a known rabid animal become infected. Once signs develop in a human, rabies is almost always fatal.

- For pre-exposure prevention in high-risk situations (e.g., veterinarians and their employees), immunization with human diploid cell vaccine (HDCV) or another vaccine approved by the Food and Drug Administration is recommended.

▼ *Key Point* Immediately notify local public health authorities when an animal bite to a human has occurred or whenever there is the possibility of contact with a rabid animal.

- Recommendations for humans bitten by animals:
  - Instruct owners that they must confine and observe for 10 days healthy pets that have bitten a human. During confinement, such animals must be isolated from contact with other animals and confined in an escape-proof enclosure or building except for leash walking under owner control. Any signs of illness in the confined animal must be reported to local public health authorities.
  - Regard wild animals and stray or unwanted dogs and cats that have bitten a human as potentially rabid and euthanize for examination of tissues.
  - Vigorously cleanse the wounds of an exposed human with copious amounts of soap and water to reduce virus in the wound. Ethanol (70%) or benzalkonium chloride (1–4%) are rabicidal. Depending on the circumstances, public health authorities decide immediately whether postexposure prophylaxis is indicated. Previously immunized humans receive two doses of vaccine (on days 0 and 3), whereas nonimmunized humans are

given rabies immune globulin and five doses of vaccine (on days 0, 3, 7, 14, and 28).

PSEUDORABIES

Etiology

Pseudorabies is a herpesvirus that predominantly infects pigs (also called Aujeszky's disease and mad itch). Most mammals are susceptible (but not humans) and infections are seen sporadically in dogs and cats in areas where the disease is enzootic in pigs. Pseudorabies in dogs and cats is almost always a direct result of ingestion of contaminated raw pork. The virus invades nerve endings in the pharynx and travels by way of nerve fibers to the brain, where it causes fulminant panencephalitis.

Clinical Signs

Pseudorabies in dogs and cats causes an acute disease that is almost always fatal within 3 to 5 days of exposure. Initial signs may include depression and inactivity or anxiety and restlessness. The most characteristic sign (but not seen in every case) is intense pruritus, especially involving the head and neck regions, that leads to excoriation and self-mutilation. Other signs may include fever, diarrhea, vomiting, copious hypersalivation, various cranial neuropathies, ataxia, and seizures. Progressive depression, dyspnea, coma, and death follow shortly thereafter; the duration of signs before death usually is only 36 to 48 hours.

▼ *Key Point* Suspect pseudorabies in a dog or cat with acute onset of violent, frantic scratching and self-mutilation around the face, head, neck, and ears, especially if there is a history of exposure to pigs or of ingestion of raw pork in an endemic area.

Diagnosis

- It is virtually impossible to make a definitive antemortem diagnosis of pseudorabies in dogs and cats. Routine hematologic and serum chemistry evaluations are normal. Cerebrospinal fluid may show nonspecific increases in protein and mononuclear cells suggestive of viral encephalitis. Serologic tests used in pigs are not diagnostically useful in dogs and cats.
- Postmortem diagnosis is based on specialized testing of brain tissue for virus using immunofluorescent, virus isolation, animal inoculation, or molecular techniques.

Treatment

No effective treatment is known.

Prevention

Pseudorabies can be prevented effectively in endemic areas by avoiding contact with pigs and by never feeding raw pork. An effective vaccine is not yet available.

SUPPLEMENTAL READINGS

Greene CE, Dreesen DW: Rabies. In: Greene CE, ed.: Infectious Diseases of the Dog and Cat. 2nd Ed. Philadelphia: WB Saunders, 1998, p 114.

Vandevelde M: Pseudorabies. In: Greene CE, ed.: Infectious Diseases of the Dog and Cat. 2nd Ed. Philadelphia: WB Saunders, 1998, p 126.

Miscellaneous Viral Diseases

Robert G. Sherding

INFECTIOUS CANINE HEPATITIS

Etiology

Infectious canine hepatitis (ICH) is caused by canine adenovirus type 1 (CAV-1), a virus related to but distinct from CAV-2 that causes infectious tracheobronchitis (kennel cough).

Incidence

Dogs, foxes, coyotes, other canids, and bears are susceptible to CAV-1. Because of widespread use of vaccination, canine ICH is rare and seen almost exclusively in unvaccinated dogs. Wild canids remain a reservoir of infection.

Transmission

CAV-1 is acquired through oronasal exposure. It is found in all tissues and is shed in all secretions during acute infection. It also is shed for at least 6 to 9 months in the urine after recovery. It is highly resistant to inactivation and disinfection, thus enabling spread by fomites and ectoparasites.

Pathogenesis

After oronasal exposure, CAV-1 causes viremia and disseminates to all tissues, especially targeting hepatocytes and endothelial cells. Hepatocyte injury results in acute hepatic necrosis or chronic hepatitis.

Endothelial injury can affect any tissue, but CAV-1 is noted particularly for its effects on corneal endothelium (corneal edema, anterior uveitis), renal glomeruli (glomerulonephritis), and vascular endothelium (disseminated intravascular coagulopathy [DIC]).

Clinical Signs

Peracute Infection

Acutely ill dogs become moribund and die within hours.

Acute Infection

A 5- to 7-day course is characterized by fever 103° to 106°F (39.5°–41°C), vomiting, diarrhea, abdominal pain, tonsillitis-pharyngitis, cervical lymphadenopathy and edema, cough (pneumonitis), and hemorrhagic diathesis (petechiae and ecchymoses, epistaxis, melena). Central nervous system (CNS) signs (disorientation, depression, stupor, coma, and seizures) may occur as a result of hepatic encephalopathy, hypoglycemia, or nonsuppurative encephalitis.

Ocular Infection

Ocular signs, occurring with acute infection or following recovery from inapparent infection, include corneal edema (cloudy cornea, also called "hepatitis blue eye") and anterior uveitis (blepharospasm, flare, miosis, and complicating glaucoma).

Chronic Active Hepatitis

In infected dogs with partial immunity, a persistent hepatic infection that causes chronic hepatitis and hepatic fibrosis may develop.

Diagnosis

Suspect ICH based on clinical signs in an unvaccinated dog, especially if younger than 1 year old.

Routine Laboratory Evaluations

ICH may cause neutropenia/lymphopenia (early), neutrophilic leukocytosis (later), increased alanine transaminase (ALT) and alkaline phosphatase (ALP) levels, thrombocytopenia and coagulation abnormalities typical of DIC (see Chap. 21), proteinuria, and occasionally hypoglycemia. The abdomen may contain a nonseptic exudate.

Definitive Diagnosis

Although definitive diagnosis is not essential for successful treatment, ICH can be confirmed by serologic testing, virus isolation, immunofluorescent studies, or histopathology (centrolobular hepatic necrosis with intranuclear viral inclusions).

Treatment

Treatment is supportive until recovery from the acute stage of infection and hepatocellular regeneration can occur. This usually requires parenteral fluid therapy using potassium and dextrose-supplemented solutions (see Chap. 5), treatment for DIC using fresh plasma or whole blood transfusion (see Chap. 21), treatment for hepatic encephalopathy (see Chap. 91), and antibiotics for secondary bacterial complications such as pneumonia or pyelonephritis.

Prevention

Vaccination has been highly effective for preventing CAV-1 infection.

- Modified live virus (MLV) CAV-1 or CAV-2 vaccines can induce effective immunity against ICH. Unlike CAV-2, CAV-1 vaccine viruses can localize in the kidney and produce mild nephritis and urine shedding of virus or they may localize in the eyes and produce anterior uveitis (in approximately 0.4% of vaccinates). The cloudy cornea usually is transient but sometimes is irreversible.
- Administer at least two doses, 3 to 4 weeks apart at 8 to 10 weeks and at 12 to 14 weeks of age. This usually is combined with canine distemper vaccinations (see Chap. 11). Annual revaccination is recommended, although initial immunization likely persists much longer than 1 year, perhaps for life. Therefore, consider extending the revaccination interval to 2 to 3 years in dogs with low exposure risk.

CANINE ACIDOPHIL CELL HEPATITIS

Etiology

A transmissible form of hepatitis has been described in dogs in Great Britain. Although the etiologic agent has not been identified, evidence strongly suggests that it is a virus and that it is distinct from CAV-1 and CAV-2.

Clinical Signs

Clinical forms of the disease, which may represent stages of progression, include acute hepatitis, chronic persistent hepatitis, cirrhosis, and occasionally hepatocellular carcinoma. Early signs, such as anorexia, vomiting, and occasional fever, are nonspecific. Later signs reflect progressive hepatic failure (ascites, hepatic encephalopathy).

Diagnosis

Laboratory findings are nonspecific and typical of those found in other types of acute and chronic liver disease. Increased serum ALT and ALP activities are the most consistent abnormalities. Diagnosis depends on liver biopsy to identify hepatitis associated with characteristic acidophil cells.

Treatment and Prevention

Specific measures for treatment and prevention are unknown; however, supportive treatment for liver failure in general and specific treatment used in other forms of hepatitis and cirrhosis may be applicable (refer to Chap. 91).

CANINE HERPESVIRUS

Etiology

Canine herpesvirus (CHV) infects only canids. Its biologic behavior is similar to herpesviruses of other species, and it is inactivated relatively easily outside the host.

Incidence

CHV is widespread in the canine population; however, it causes clinical disease almost exclusively in newborn puppies during the first month of life.

Transmission

Perinatal infection can be acquired before, at, or soon after birth via in utero transmission; during passage through the birth canal; or by direct oronasal contact with infected littermates, the dam's infectious oronasal secretions, or fomites. Respiratory and venereal transmission may occur in adults.

Clinical Signs

Whether signs occur and what they are depend on the animal's age at exposure.

Prenatal Infection

Fetal resorption, abortion, or stillbirth occur rarely.

Neonatal Infection

Infection before 1 to 2 weeks of age leads to viremia and virus dissemination to all tissues, resulting in a fatal generalized form of disease. The susceptibility to this form of CHV is related to the narrow temperature range of 35° to 36°C needed for optimal growth of CHV, which coincides with the body temperature often found in neonates in the first week of life.

- Neonatal infection is characterized by multifocal lesions of necrosis and hemorrhage (DIC) in many organs, including the kidneys, adrenal glands, liver, spleen, gastrointestinal (GI) tract, lungs, and the CNS.
- Signs include depression, refusal to nurse, incessant crying, subnormal body temperature, yellow-green diarrhea, abdominal pain, nasal discharge, petechial hemorrhages on mucosal surfaces, skin papules, and CNS signs (coma, opisthotonus, and seizures). Death usually occurs within 24 to 48 hours.
- This form occurs in puppies born to a seronegative dam. Subsequent litters produced by the dam rarely are infected because of protective maternal immunity.

Adult and Older Puppy Infections

Marked resistance to CHV develops abruptly in animals after 1 to 2 weeks of age because of effects of higher body temperature and better immune function; thus, infection beyond 2 weeks of age results only in mild or inapparent infection that is confined to the respiratory and genital tracts.

- Transient, mild respiratory, and conjunctival signs with episodic shedding can occur.
- A possible manifestation is vaginitis/balanoposthitis. This is characterized by lymphofollicular lesions of the genital mucosa with or without mild hyperemia and discharge. Local genital infection may be a source of venereal transmission between adult animals and of vaginal transmission to neonates during birth.

Diagnosis

- *For infected neonates*: The age of onset and clinical signs are fairly characteristic. Virus isolation is confirmatory. Positive serologic titers (virus neutralizing antibody) in the dam and surviving pups provides additional presumptive evidence. Necropsy lesions are usually diagnostic.
- *For adult carriers*: Virus isolation from the oropharynx or genital lesions confirms the diagnosis.

Treatment

There is no effective treatment for CHV. Treatment of the neonatal form probably is not warranted because it is almost always fatal, and the few puppies that do recover often have irreversible neurologic sequelae (e.g., cerebellar dysfunction).

Prevention

An effective vaccine for CHV is unavailable.

- In breeding kennels, promote proper husbandry practices and maintain warm ambient temperatures for neonates.
- In kennels with CHV problems:
  - Isolate infected bitches and their litters.
  - Disinfect the premises (CHV is susceptible to most detergents and disinfectants).
  - Administer hyperimmune antiserum (harvested from bitches that recently have produced CHV-infected litters), 1 to 2 ml, intraperitoneally, for prophylaxis in unaffected newborn puppies, including healthy-appearing members of an infected litter.

CANINE VIRAL PAPILLOMATOSIS

Etiology

The canine papillomavirus causes mucocutaneous tumors that are benign and self-limiting. Virus-induced papillomas are multiple (often 50–100 separate tumor nodules) and occur in young dogs, in contrast to noninfectious papillomas, which are solitary and usually affect older dogs. Transmission appears to be by direct viral contact with oral mucosa. The incubation period is 1 to 2 months.

Clinical Signs

The three forms of infectious papillomatosis in dogs are oral, ocular, and cutaneous.

- Oral papillomatosis is by far the most common form and usually affects dogs younger than 2 years of age. Lesions begin as smooth, white mucosal elevations that develop into cauliflower-like warts on the lip margins, oral mucosa, tongue, palate, pharynx, and epiglottis. They usually increase in number and size for 4 to 6 weeks and then begin to regress. Common presenting signs are halitosis, ptyalism, reluctance to eat, and oral bleeding.
- Ocular papillomatosis is uncommon; it affects dogs 6 months to 4 years of age and is characterized by papillomas on the conjunctiva, cornea, and eyelid margins.
- Cutaneous papillomatosis is rare (see Chap. 28).

Diagnosis

The history and physical appearance of the lesions are adequate for diagnosis of oral and cutaneous papillomatosis. In the ocular form of the disease, confirmatory excisional biopsy is advisable to exclude other ocular tumors that may have a similar physical appearance. Specialized techniques can be used to identify the presence of papillomavirus in tumor tissue.

Treatment

- For the oral form, treatment is not necessary because viral oral papillomas usually regress spontaneously within 3 months once immunity develops. There have been rare reports of failure to regress for more than 2 years.
- Removal by surgical excision, cryosurgery, or electrosurgery is indicated for ocular papillomas and for oral lesions that interfere with eating or that bleed and discharge excessively. Submit tissues for biopsy to confirm the diagnosis. Removal of some of the tumors often triggers regression of the remaining ones.
- When regression fails to occur, remission can be induced in some dogs with weekly single-agent chemotherapy using vincristine or cyclophosphamide at the usual antitumor doses (see Chap. 24).
- Recovered animals and dogs older than 2 years of age usually are immune to papillomatosis.

FELINE VIRAL PAPILLOMATOSIS

An uncharacterized papillomavirus has been identified in a few cats with papillomas. Feline papillomas are located on the head, neck, dorsal thorax, and abdomen. They appear as slightly raised verrucous plaques rather than typical warts. Most affected cats have been on immunosuppressive drugs or infected with feline immunodeficiency virus. The diagnosis is based on tumor histopathology and immunohistochemistry or electron microscopy to document the presence of papillomavirus. Treatment has not been evaluated.

FELINE POXVIRUS

Etiology

Cowpox virus (*Orthopoxvirus*) causes disease in cats more often than in any other species, including cows, but has been recognized only in Europe. The disease is characterized by widespread skin lesions with occasional systemic involvement. The source of infection is contact with rodents, mainly through contaminated skin wounds. Cats have also been infected with *Parapoxvirus* and uncharacterized poxviruses.

Clinical Signs

- The initial inoculation site or skin wound (usually a bite wound on the head, neck, or forelimb) is called the primary lesion.
- Then, 1 to 3 weeks later, after a period of viremia and sometimes mild systemic signs (low fever, anorexia, depression, and mild upper respiratory signs), widespread secondary pox lesions develop. These lesions begin as multiple, small (1 mm) skin nodules that progress and increase in number over 2 to 4 days to become well-circumscribed ulcers covered with scabs. Most cats have more than ten of these pox lesions. Buccal ulcers are seen occasionally.
- The scabs dry and fall off in 4 to 6 weeks, revealing underlying healing skin. Some lesions result in permanent bald patches.
- The disease is worsened by immunosuppressive conditions, such as feline leukemia or feline immunodeficiency virus infection or glucocorticoid therapy. Rarely, fatalities occur because of secondary bacterial infection.

Diagnosis

- Suspect feline poxvirus in rural cats that hunt rodents in endemic areas, expecially cats with typical secondary pox lesions after a recent history of a primary skin wound lesion.
- Confirm by detection of virus (preferred method) in the scabs by electron microscopy or by virus isolation, detection of poxvirus-specific antibody by serologic methods, or detection of the characteristic histopathologic abnormalities in skin biopsies.

Treatment

There is no specific treatment for poxvirus infections, but the disease is self-limiting, and skin lesions regress in 4 to 6 weeks. Antibiotics and topical cleansing help to control secondary bacterial infection of skin lesions, but take proper precautions (e.g., wear rubber gloves when handling cats) because cowpox virus is potentially transmissible to humans as a zoonotic disease. Corticosteroids are contraindicated.

SUPPLEMENTAL READINGS

Infectious Canine Hepatitis

Greene CE: Infectious canine hepatitis and canine acidophil cell hepatitis. In: Greene CE, ed.: Infectious Diseases of the Dog and Cat. 2nd Ed. Philadelphia: WB Saunders, 1998, p 22.

Polzin DJ: Infectious canine hepatitis. In: Barlough JE, ed.: Manual of Small Animal Infectious Diseases. New York: Churchill Livingstone, 1988, p 11.

Canine Herpesvirus

Barlough JE, Carmichael LE: Canine herpesvirus. In: Barlough JE, ed.: Manual of Small Animal Infectious Diseases. New York: Churchill Livingstone, 1988, p 19.

Carmichael LE, Greene CE: Canine herpesvirus infection. In: Greene CE, ed.: Infectious Diseases of the Dog and Cat. 2nd Ed. Philadelphia: WB Saunders, 1998, p 28.

Canine Viral Papillomatosis

Calvert CA: Canine viral papillomatosis. In: Greene CE, ed.: Infectious Diseases of the Dog and Cat. 2nd Ed. Philadelphia: WB Saunders, 1998, p 49.

Rosenthal RC: Canine viral papillomatosis. In: Barlough JE, ed.: Manual of Small Animal Infectious Diseases. New York: Churchill Livingstone, 1988, p 7.

Feline Viral Papillomatosis

Egberink HF, Horzinek MC: Feline viral papillomatosis. In: Greene CE, ed.: Infectious Diseases of the Dog and Cat. 2nd Ed. Philadelphia: WB Saunders, 1998, p 113.

Feline Poxvirus

Bennett M, Gaskell RM, Baxby D: Feline poxvirus infection. In: Greene CE, ed.: Infectious Diseases of the Dog and Cat. 2nd Ed. Philadelphia: WB Saunders, 1998, p 110.

Rickettsial Diseases

C. Guillermo Couto

Rickettsial diseases are common in dogs but rare in cats, with the exception of hemobartonellosis. Most rickettsial diseases in dogs are tick-borne, with the exception of salmon poisoning. The mode of transmission of hemobartonellosis in cats has not yet been elucidated. Because these diseases are acute in endemic areas, there is a higher prevalence during (or after) warm weather, when ticks are more prevalent.

The clinical course of rickettsial diseases can be acute (e.g., Rocky Mountain spotted fever, ehrlichiosis, hemobartonellosis) or subacute to chronic (e.g., ehrlichiosis, salmon poisoning). Most rickettsial infections respond to tetracycline, doxycycline, or chloramphenicol. Multisystemic rickettsial diseases are discussed in this chapter. The hemotropic rickettsia-like mycoplasmal agent *Hemobartonella* is discussed in Chapter 20.

CANINE EHRLICHIOSIS

Canine ehrlichiosis is a relatively common tick-borne rickettsial disease of dogs. Synonyms used in the literature for this disorder include tracker dog disease, tropical canine pancytopenia, canine hemorrhagic fever, and canine typhus. It is distributed worldwide and achieved prominence during the Vietnam war, when a large proportion of military dogs contracted this disease. Because of its chronic and insidious nature, ehrlichiosis is prevalent year-round, rather than only during the warm months of the year. Most available information pertains to *Ehrlichia canis* infection in dogs, and this is the emphasis of the following discussion.

Etiology
Etiologic Agents

- *Ehrlichia canis* (canine monocytic ehrlichiosis)
- *Ehrlichia platys* (canine cyclic thrombocytopenia)
- *Ehrlichia ewingii* (canine granulocytic ehrlichiosis)
- *Ehrlichia equi* (equine granulocytic ehrlichiosis)
- Experimentally, inoculation of *Ehrlichia risticii* (Potomac horse fever agent) can induce mild clinical or subclinical disease in dogs and cats.

Transmission

- The vector and reservoir for *E. canis* is the common brown dog tick *(Rhipicephalus sanguineus)*, which can transmit organisms for at least 5 months postengorge-

ment. Ehrlichiosis, as well as other rickettsial diseases, also can be transmitted iatrogenically through contaminated blood transfusions.
- The incubation period is 7 to 21 days.
- The organism is transmitted through tick bites. Ticks ingest the organism from an infected host.

Pathogenesis
Acute Phase

This phase of ehrlichiosis is variable in duration (2–4 weeks) and severity (from mild to severe). The organism replicates in mononuclear cells, mainly in the mononuclear phagocytic system (MPS) (in lymph nodes, spleen, liver, and bone marrow), resulting in hyperplasia of this cell line and organomegaly (lymphadenopathy, splenomegaly, and hepatomegaly). Thrombocytopenia due to peripheral destruction of platelets with or without anemia and leukopenia (or leukocytosis) is common during this phase.

Subclinical Phase

This phase may last for weeks to months and is characterized by persistence of the organism after apparent recovery from the acute phase. Dogs may eliminate the organism during this phase, or infection may progress to the chronic phase.

Chronic Phase

This phase occurs when the immune response is ineffective and the organism cannot be eliminated. The result is chronic vague illness, weight loss, and bone marrow dysfunction.

▼ *Key Point* In nonendemic areas, canine ehrlichiosis is usually chronic.

Clinical Signs and Laboratory Abnormalities

Clinical signs vary in the different phases of the disease.

Acute Phase

- Clinical signs and physical examination findings mainly are the result of widespread lymphoreticular hyperplasia and hematologic abnormalities. Therefore, fever, generalized lymphadenopathy, splenomegaly, hepatomegaly, dyspnea or exercise intolerance due to pneumonitis, neurologic signs due to meningoencephalitis, anterior uveitis and chorio-retinitis, and petechiae and ecchymoses due to thrombocytopenia or thrombocytopathia dominate the clinical presentation. Antibody titers may be negative during this phase because it takes up to 3 weeks to develop a significant titer.

- Hematologic and biochemical abnormalities include thrombocytopenia, mild to severe anemia, leukopenia or leukocytosis, hypercellular bone marrow cytology, mild hyperglobulinemia, and mild elevation of serum liver enzyme activities.

Subclinical Phase

- Patients are asymptomatic. Mild hematologic and biochemical abnormalities may be identified.

Chronic Phase

- Clinical signs can be mild or severe, develop 1 to 4 months after inoculation of the organism, and reflect the lymphoreticular hyperplasia and hematologic abnormalities. Any of the following may be observed: weight loss, pyrexia, spontaneous bleeding, pallor due to anemia, generalized lymphadenopathy, hepatosplenomegaly, anterior and/or posterior uveitis, neurologic signs caused by meningoencephalomyelitis, polyarthritis, and intermittent limb edema.
- Hematologic and biochemical abnormalities usually are pronounced and include nonregenerative anemia, thrombocytopenia, leukopenia, or all three (pancytopenia) due to bone marrow hypoplasia; bone marrow and splenic plasmacytosis; lymphocytosis (occasionally composed of large granular lymphocytes); hyperglobulinemia caused by polyclonal (or less often monoclonal) gammopathy; hypoalbuminemia; and proteinuria.

▼ **Key Point** Clinical signs, physical findings, and laboratory abnormalities in dogs with chronic ehrlichiosis may resemble multiple myeloma or chronic lymphocytic leukemia.

Diagnosis

- Identification of the organisms (morulae) in fine-needle aspiration cytology of the spleen, lymph nodes, and lungs, in cerebrospinal fluid and joint fluid leukocytes or in peripheral blood leukocytes, is confirmatory but time-consuming and difficult. Plasmacytosis also is frequently prominent in these cytologic specimens.
- The indirect fluorescent antibody test (IFA) for *E. canis* is highly sensitive and is the usual method of diagnosis of canine ehrlichiosis. Titers greater than 1:10 are considered diagnostic. Diagnostic titers may not be detected until 2 to 3 weeks postinoculation. There is often antigenic cross-reactivity between *E. canis* and other *Ehrlichia* spp. and *Neorickettsia helminthoeca*. As with some other infectious diseases, high titers do not confer protection against reinfection. Titers may persist for up to 9 to 12 months after treatment or recovery.

- Polymerase chain reaction (PCR) and Western immunoblotting can be used to diagnose ehrlichiosis in dogs with negative serology and to distinguish *E. canis* from *E. ewingii* and other *Ehrlichia* spp.; however, these techniques are not yet readily available for routine clinical use.

Treatment

- Doxycycline is the drug of choice for treating ehrlichiosis at a dosage of 2.5 to 5 mg/kg PO every 12 to 24 hours for 10 to 14 days. Alternatively, tetracycline can be used at a dosage of 22 mg/kg PO every 8 hours for 14 to 21 days, and should be administered on an empty stomach. Chloramphenicol is also effective, but it is not recommended in dogs with cytopenias. Enrofloxacin was not effective in eliminating infection in experimental dogs.
- Imidocarb dipropionate (Imizol), an anticholinesterase parasympathomimetic, administered at a dosage of 5 mg/kg, IM or SC, repeated in 14 days, has been effective in dogs with refractory ehrlichiosis and in dogs with mixed infections of *E. canis* and *Babesia canis*.
- Institute supportive therapy (blood or blood products, fluids) as deemed necessary (see Chapter 20 for discussion of blood transfusion).

Prognosis

The prognosis for canine ehrlichiosis is excellent with appropriate treatment, unless the bone marrow is severely hypoplastic. Clinical response usually begins within 48 hours after initiation of doxycycline, but in the chronic form may take up to 3 to 4 weeks. The chronic form of the disease appears to be more severe in German shepherd dogs and Doberman pinschers.

Prevention

Tick control constitutes the mainstay of prevention for ehrlichiosis. In addition, low doses of doxycycline (2 mg/kg PO q24h) or tetracycline (6.6 mg/kg PO q24h) may be used in endemic areas during tick season.

INFECTIOUS CYCLIC THROMBOCYTOPENIA

Ehrlichia platys causes infectious cyclic thrombocytopenia, in which thrombocytopenia develops at 1- to 2-week intervals in asymptomatic dogs. It is confined mainly to the Gulf Coast states. The diagnosis usually is based on serology for *E. platys* (by IFA testing). The organisms can be identified within platelets in Giemsa-stained blood smears as blue inclusions; however, this method of diagnosis is unreliable because organisms are present in low numbers. See Chapter 20 for a discussion of the differential diagnosis of thrombocytopenia. Doxycycline or tetracycline at the dosages used for *E. canis* (see preceding section) is effective for treating *E. platys*.

FELINE EHRLICHIOSIS

Etiology

Cats can be infected naturally with one or more species of *Ehrlichia* based on serologic evidence and the finding of *Ehrlichia*-like organisms within mononuclear cells and sometimes neutrophils of cats with illness resembling canine ehrlichiosis.

Transmission

The source of infection in cats is unknown, but transmission involving arthropods or mice is postulated.

Pathogenesis

Morulae of *Ehrlichia*-like organisms have been found in mononuclear cells and to a lesser extent in neutrophils, suggesting a pathogenesis comparable to canine monocytic and granulocytic forms of ehrlichiosis (see previous section, Canine Ehrlichiosis).

Clinical Signs and Laboratory Abnormalities

- Most affected cats are older than 2 years of age. The most frequent clinical signs are fever, lethargy, inappetance, weight loss, pallor, hyperesthesia, and joint pain. Splenomegaly, lymphadenopathy, and dyspnea due to interstitial pneumonitis also have been observed. Some cats have had concurrent infections with retroviruses or *Hemobartonella.*
- Laboratory abnormalities can include nonregenerative anemia, leukocytosis or leukopenia, thrombocytopenia, and hyperglobulinemia (polyclonal gammopathy).

Diagnosis

- Investigators using serologic tests similar to those used to diagnose canine ehrlichiosis have found positive titers for antibodies to *E. canis, E. risticii,* or both in cats. However, positive serologic test results also have been found in healthy cats; thus, the diagnosis should not be based on serologic tests alone. Also take into account the clinical signs, laboratory findings, and responsiveness to doxycycline or tetracycline.
- *Ehrlichia* morulae sometimes can be identified in mononuclear cells in cytologic specimens.

Treatment

Cats with *Ehrlichia* infection have responded to doxycycline (5–10 mg/kg PO q12h for 21 days), tetracycline (20 mg/kg PO q8h for 21 days), or imidocarb dipropionate (give 5 mg/kg IM once and repeat in 14 days).

ROCKY MOUNTAIN SPOTTED FEVER

This tick-borne disease is most prevalent in the east coast, midwest, and plains regions, and it represents the most important rickettsial disease in humans. Because of its acute nature, most cases occur during tick season, between April 1 and September 1.

Etiology

Agent

Rocky Mountain spotted fever (RMSF) is caused by *Rickettsia rickettsii.*

Transmission

- The recognized vectors for *R. rickettsii* are the American dog tick *(Dermacentor variabilis),* found primarily east of the Great Plains and in parts of the west coast, and the wood tick *(Dermacentor andersoni),* found in an area from the Rocky Mountains to the Cascades. These are three-host ticks; the permanent hosts are humans, dogs, and cats, and the reservoirs are rodents and dogs.
- Ticks usually acquire the organism through feeding on infected animals, although vertical transmission in ticks also can occur.
- Ticks usually do not infect the hosts until they have been attached for a minimum of 5 to 20 hours. This disease also can be transmitted iatrogenically through blood transfusions.

Pathogenesis

- Once inoculated into the host via a tick bite, the organism quickly invades and replicates in vascular endothelial cells, resulting in widespread necrotizing vasculitis, platelet aggregation, disseminated intravascular coagulation (DIC), and organ damage (e.g., skin, brain, heart, and kidneys).
- The incubation period varies from 2 to 14 days.

Clinical Signs and Laboratory Abnormalities

Natural and experimental infection can lead to either *subclinical* or *acute* manifestations of this disease.

Subclinical Stage

In the subclinical stages, dogs are usually asymptomatic, but mild laboratory abnormalities such as mild thrombocytopenia may be detected.

Acute Stage

Most dogs with acute RMSF present between April and September. The clinical signs and laboratory abnormalities are variable in severity, and, if the disease is untreated, last from 2 to 4 weeks. Because of the acute course, ticks are found commonly on the dog (or were recently removed by the owner).

- Common clinical signs and physical examination findings in dogs with acute RMSF include anorexia, fever, neurologic signs (e.g., altered mental status, vestibular signs), myalgia/arthralgia, generalized lymphadenopathy, edema of the face and limbs, and dyspnea or exercise intolerance due to pneumonitis. The rash, petechiae, and ecchymoses commonly seen in humans (which confer the name to this disease) are seen in only 20% or less of affected dogs. Cardiac arrhythmias (due to myocarditis) also can occur and may result in sudden death.

- The hematologic and biochemical abnormalities in dogs with RMSF include leukocytosis with left shift and monocytosis, mild anemia, thrombocytopenia, evidence of DIC (see Chapter 21), increased serum liver enzyme activities, azotemia, hypercholesterol-emia, hyponatremia, hypochloremia, and metabolic acidosis.

Diagnosis

- Serum titers usually do not rise until after 2 to 3 weeks following inoculation, which may be later than the onset of clinical signs. Therefore, obtain paired serum samples in patients with acute signs of disease.
- The prevalence of seropositivity is higher than the prevalence of the disease and must be considered when interpreting titers. High titers can persist for up to 1 year after successful treatment or recovery from the disease, which also must be considered.
- Several serologic tests are available for the diagnosis of RMSF, including microindirect fluorescence antibody (micro-IF), immunofluorescence, and ELISA tests. Of these, the micro-IF test is most commonly used in dogs. Titers greater than or equal to 1:128 usually are considered diagnostic; however, a fourfold rise in titer comparing a sample obtained during acute disease with a convalescent sample is required to establish a definitive diagnosis.
- IgM titers (indicative of recent infection) also can be detected by a modified micro-IF technique.
- The direct immunofluorescence test detects rickettsial antigens in fresh or paraffin-embedded tissues, especially skin. This test is diagnostic as early as 3 to 4 days postinoculation and can be performed on skin biopsies obtained with local anesthetic and a biopsy punch. A positive result is highly specific for RMSF; however, false-negative results occur in up to 30% to 40% of cases (low sensitivity).

Treatment

- Doxycycline is the drug of choice for treating dogs with RMSF, at a dosage of 5 mg/kg, PO or IV, q12 hours for 7 to 10 days. Tetracycline can also be used at a dosage of 22 mg/kg PO q 8 hours for 10 to 14 days, and should be administered on an empty stomach. Enrofloxacin (at a dosage of 3 mg/kg, SC or PO, q12 hours) and chloramphenicol (at a dosage of 15 to 25 mg/kg, PO, IM, or IV, q8 hours) are also effective in dogs with RMSF.
- Initiate supportive therapy as needed.

▼ **Key Point** Dogs with acute onset of neurologic signs, pyrexia, and other systemic signs in areas endemic for RMSF should be treated with IV doxycycline until a definitive diagnosis can be established.

Prognosis

- The prognosis is good when treatment is instituted promptly. Responses occur within hours of initiating

appropriate drug administration. Mortality is high if treatment is delayed until the disease is advanced or if an ineffective antibiotic is used.

- Dogs with severe CNS signs may die within hours of instituting treatment.

Prevention

- Prevention requires strict tick and rodent control.

SALMON POISONING DISEASE

Salmon poisoning disease is a rickettsial infection of dogs in the Pacific Northwest that has a high morbidity and mortality. It is transmitted by helminths rather than ticks.

Etiology

Etiologic Agent

- *Neorickettsia helminthoeca* (closely related to *Ehrlichia* spp.)
- Elokomin fluke fever agent (likely another strain of *N. helminthoeca*)

Transmission

Dogs acquire salmon disease after ingesting raw salmon (or related fish) that contain the metacercariae of the fluke *Nanophyetus salmincola* infected with *Neorickettsia helminthoeca* or the Elokomin fluke fever agent. These flukes require three hosts to complete a life cycle: a snail, a fish (salmonid), and a fish-eating mammal or bird.

Pathogenesis

- Five to 7 days after a dog ingests contaminated fish, the fluke matures and attaches to the intestinal epithelium of the dog, inoculating the organism. After infecting the intestinal epithelium, the organisms disseminate to the MPS organs (e.g., lymph nodes, spleen, liver), and to other areas such as the CNS and the lungs.
- The incubation period ranges from 5 to 21 days.
- Cats are not susceptible to salmon poisoning disease.

Clinical Signs and Laboratory Abnormalities

- Clinical signs and physical examination findings in dogs with acute salmon poisoning include fever (104°–107.6°F) followed by hypothermia, anorexia, persistent diarrhea (usually hemorrhagic), vomiting, profound weight loss, mild serous naso-ocular discharge, and generalized lymphadenopathy, which can be marked. These signs are easily confused with canine parvovirus infection.
- Laboratory abnormalities are nonspecific, but leukocytosis or leukopenia, thrombocytopenia, elevated serum alkaline phosphatase, and hypoalbuminemia are common findings.

Diagnosis

- Operculated fluke eggs are found on direct fecal smears or by standard sugar flotation or fecal washing-sedimentation techniques; however, the presence of trematode infection does not confirm rickettsial infection.

- Giemsa-stained fine-needle aspirates of enlarged lymph nodes usually reveal a reactive lymph node hyperplasia with intracytoplasmic rickettsial bodies (pleomorphic, coccobacillary, purple-staining) in macrophages.

Treatment

- Give doxycycline or tetracycline as described for canine ehrlichiosis and RMSF. Because of the severe vomiting and diarrhea that occur in this disease, begin with parenteral oxytetracycline (7 mg/kg IV q8h) for the first 3 to 5 days.
- Give praziquantel (Droncit), at one dose of 10 to 30 mg/kg, PO or SC, to eliminate the fluke.
- Use supportive treatment (e.g., fluid therapy, antiemetics, antidiarrheals, nutritional support) as needed.
- The prognosis is good with appropriate treatment.

Prevention

- To prevent the disease, keep dogs from feeding on raw infected fish.
- Freezing or thoroughly cooking fish destroys the metacercariae and the rickettsiae.

HEMOBARTONELLOSIS

Hemobartonella felis and *H. canis* are primarily hemotropic agents formerly classified as rickettsia and now considered to be mycoplasma, based on genetic evidence. Feline hemobartonellosis is characterized mainly by hemolytic anemia, and canine infections are usually subclinical. Hemobartonellosis in cats is discussed in Chapter 20.

SUPPLEMENTAL READING

Breitschwerdt EB: Tick-transmitted diseases. Proc Ninth Annual Vet Med Forum, ACVIM, New Orleans, 1991, pp 137–142.

Gorham JR, Foreyt WJ: Salmon poisoning disease. In: Greene CE (ed): Infectious Diseases of the Dog and Cat. Philadelphia: WB Saunders, 1998, pp 135–138.

Greene CE, Breitschwerdt EB: Rocky Mountain spotted fever, Q fever and typhus. In: Greene CE (ed): Infectious Diseases of the Dog and Cat. Philadelphia: WB Saunders, 1998, pp 155–165.

Greene CE, Burgdorfer W, Cavagnolo R, et al: Rocky Mountain spotted fever in dogs and its differentiation from canine ehrlichiosis. J Am Vet Med Assoc 186:465, 1985.

Iqbal Z, Chaichanasiriwithaya W, Rikihisa Y: Comparison of PCR with other tests for early diagnosis of canine ehrlichiosis. J Clin Microbiol 32:1658, 1994.

Lappin MR: Feline ehrlichiosis. In: Greene CE (ed): Infectious Diseases of the Dog and Cat. Philadelphia: WB Saunders, 1998, pp 149–154.

Neer TM: Canine monocytic and granulocytic ehrlichiosis. In: Greene CE (ed): Infectious Diseases of the Dog and Cat. Philadelphia: WB Saunders, 1998, pp 139–146.

Troy GC, Vulgamott JC, Turnwald GH: Canine ehrlichiosis: A retrospective study of 30 naturally occurring cases. J Am Anim Hosp Assoc 16:181, 1980.

16 Lyme Borreliosis

Paul A. Manley

Lyme borreliosis is a polysystemic tick-borne disease caused by the spirochete *Borrelia burgdorferi*. The disease has been associated with polyarthritis in dogs, cattle, horses, and humans. In Wisconsin, Minnesota, and northeastern coastal states, borreliosis is transmitted to animals and people by the bite of the deer tick, which acts as a host of the spirochete. *Borrelia* species belong to the eubacterial phylum of spirochetes (as do *Leptospira* and *Treponema*). *B. burgdorferi* is easy to isolate from ticks but is difficult to isolate from clinically affected patients. The outer membrane of the spirochete can undergo antigenic variation during the course of infection, which may limit the effectiveness of a vaccine.

ETIOLOGY

In the northeast, southeast, and midwest regions of the United States, *Borrelia burgdorferi* is carried by the deer tick, *Ixodes scapularis,* formerly designated *I. dammini*. In California and other western states, *I. pacificus* is believed to be the carrier. Other species of *Ixodes* ticks are involved in Europe and Asia. Other species of ticks, including *Amblyomma americanum* and *Dermacentor variabilis* (the dog tick), and insects such as horse flies, deer flies, and mosquitoes, can carry *B. burgdorferi;* however, only ticks have been linked with disease transmission. The route of infection is via the bite of an infected tick. Infection requires 48 hours of tick attachment.

Borreliosis commonly affects hunting dogs, but they are incidental hosts. Deer support the adult population of *I. dammini* but are not believed to become infected by the spirochete. Mice are the main reservoirs of borreliosis because they maintain the larval and nymphal stages of *I. dammini* and can become infected with the spirochete. Birds may be important reservoirs because they have the ability to transmit ticks and spirochetes over long distances.

CLINICAL SIGNS

- Polyarthritis is the most common clinical sign reported in dogs. The chronic nonerosive arthritis is usually subclinical but may be septic or immune-mediated because of the presence of the spirochete in the synovium and/or synovial fluid.

- Systemic signs include anorexia, weight loss, lethargy, lymphadenopathy, and fever; however, the animal may show no systemic signs other than lameness. In experimental infections, these clinical signs develop 2 to 5 months after tick exposure.
- Acute progressive renal failure and protein-losing glomerulonephropathy have been associated with Lyme borreliosis in dogs, especially Labrador and golden retrievers.
- Rheumatoid arthritis, meningitis, and myocarditis have also been reported in association with *Borrelia* infection in dogs.
- Naturally-occurring clinical disease is not well-documented in cats; however, many healthy cats are seropositive for *Borrelia* infection and experimentally infected cats develop polyarthritis, pneumonitis, lymphadenopathy, and CNS inflammation.

DIAGNOSIS

History

- Lameness can be acute or chronic and progressive.
- Often systemic signs may be traced to exposure of the animal to a wooded environment or a tick-infested area.

Physical Examination

- The seroprevalence of *Borrelia* antibodies is much greater than the prevalence of clinical disease attributable to Lyme borreliosis; thus, the disease is overdiagnosed on the basis of antibody titers alone.
- Swelling of one or more joints may be evident.
- There may be signs of considerable pain on palpation of the joints with no evidence of joint instability.

Laboratory Evaluation

- Whole-cell immunofluorescent antibody (IFA) tests and enzyme-linked immunosorbent assays (ELISA) are the most available diagnostic tests; serum titers less than 1:128 are negative; 1:128 to 1:256 are low positive; 1:512 or greater are highly positive.
  - In an endemic area, a positive titer can be an incidental finding.
- False-negative antibody titer results are rare; however, positive titers can be the result of prior infection, prior vaccination, or nonspecific reactivity to

other noncausative organisms and inflammatory conditions.

- Results are inconsistent between different commercial laboratories.
- Evaluate animals with a negative titer and clinical signs suggesting borreliosis for immune-mediated causes of polyarthritis (see Chap. 143); retest in 1 month for Lyme disease.
- Animals with a high titer and no clinical signs suggesting disease may have been exposed recently to *B. burgdorferi*. Retest in 1 month; a rising titer indicates active infection.
- Joint fluid analysis for titers may help to establish a diagnosis; also, joint fluid cytology of dogs with Lyme disease may show neutrophilic inflammation.
- Confirmatory tests can include immunoblot (Western blot), ELISA based on novel protein antigens, polymerase chain reaction, and culture; however, these procedures are not yet routinely available and adequately validated.

Radiographic Evaluation

Radiographically, there is evidence of joint effusion but usually little or no evidence of degenerative joint disease.

TREATMENT

- Treat all dogs that have clinical signs suggestive of borreliosis and a positive titer with antibiotics for 14 to 30 days. Appropriate choices are doxycycline (10 mg/kg q12h), and cephalexin or amoxicillin (22 mg/kg q8h). Treat refactory infections with a third-generation cephalosporin or azithromycin (5mg/kg q12h).
- Animals with active infection should show a rapid response to antibiotic therapy, especially early infections. If the therapy is effective, retest in 1 to 3 months to confirm the diagnosis (rising titer).
- If the initial response to therapy is poor, consider alternative antibiotics and other diagnoses.
- Prolonged antibiotic therapy (weeks to months) sometimes is required for animals with chronic established infections.

PREVENTION

Vaccination

- Killed whole-cell bacterin and recombinant protein vaccine products are marketed for immunizing dogs against Lyme borreliosis.

- Documentation of efficacy of these vaccines is limited and a disadvantage of vaccination is that it causes false-positive serologic tests for months to years later. Therefore, do not recommend Lyme vaccination routinely for all dogs. Reserve vaccination as an elective procedure for high-risk dogs (outdoor, hunting, and field trial dogs) in tick-infested areas with a high prevalence of borreliosis.

Vector Control

- For effective prevention of borreliosis in both dogs and cats in areas of high prevalence, routinely apply topical fipronil (Frontline Top Spot; Merial) once monthly according to label directions.
- Reduce the risk of exposure of animals by limiting access to tick-infested areas.
- Periodically check animals for ticks and promptly remove them to decrease exposure to *B. burgdorferi*.

PUBLIC HEALTH

- Human Lyme disease begins as an annular, nonpruritic, erythematous skin lesion several days following a tick bite and progresses to fever, flulike symptoms, polyarthritis, meningitis, myocarditis, and uveitis.
- Human infections have been reported in nearly all states; however, 85% of cases occur in the northeastern United States.
- Dogs and cats do not pose a risk of direct horizontal transmission to humans; however, they may serve as a minor source of infected ticks.
- Transmission requires prolonged tick attachment (48 hours); therefore, measures that reduce tick exposure are the best means of preventing human infection. In tick-infested areas, the tick repellant diethyltoluamide (DEET) is recommended for exposed skin.

SUPPLEMENTAL READINGS

Greene CE, Appel MJG, Straubinger RK: Lyme borreliosis. In Green CE (ed): Infectious Diseases of the Dog and Cat (2nd ed). Philadelphia, W.B. Saunders, 1998, p. 282.

Leptospirosis, Brucellosis, and Other Bacterial Infectious Diseases

Robert G. Sherding

A large diversity of bacteria can infect dogs and cats. This discussion focuses on leptospirosis and brucellosis. Other infectious diseases caused by bacteria are summarized in Table 17–1, and most are described in the respective organ-system chapters. Borreliosis (Lyme disease) is mainly a joint disease (see Chap. 16); brucellosis is mainly a cause of impaired reproductive function (see Chap. 114). *Bordetella bronchiseptica* is associated with the canine infectious tracheobronchitis complex (see Chap. 10), and tetanus causes severe neuromuscular dysfunction (see Chap. 147). Salmonellosis, campylobacteriosis, yersiniosis, and Tyzzer disease primarily involve the intestinal tract (see Chap. 89). Actinomycosis and nocardiosis are causes of pyothorax (see Chap. 80) and chronic skin disease (see Chap. 35). Mycobacterial infections are associated with chronic skin disease (see Chap. 36).

LEPTOSPIROSIS

Etiology

Leptospirosis is caused by serovars of *Leptospira interrogans*, a filamentous, motile spirochete that infects most wild and domestic animals, including humans. Several serovars infect dogs and cats, but clinical disease occurs only in dogs. The serovars that are associated with canine leptospirosis include *L. icterohaemorrhagiae, L. canicola, L. grippotyphosa, L. pomona,* and *L. bratislava.*

Transmission

Infection is spread by recovered animals that shed organisms in their urine for months to years after infection. Exposure usually occurs by mucocutaneous contact with leptospires in the environment (contaminated water, food, bedding, soil, vegetation, or fomites). The organisms penetrate mucosa or abraded skin. In addition, transplacental, venereal, and bite-wound transmission can occur. Wild animal and rodent populations are reservoirs for leptospirosis.

Pathogenesis

Leptospiremia occurs 4 to 12 days postinfection. The primary targets in leptospirosis are the kidneys and the liver. Fever and disseminated intra-vascular coagulation (DIC) may result from acute endothelial injury.

- *Leptospira* replicates in renal tubule epithelium and can cause acute injury and renal failure (especially *L. canicola*). Renal colonization and urine shedding are prolonged, even for months after recovery.
- *Leptospira* can injure hepatocytes, resulting in acute hepatic necrosis (especially *L. icterohaemorrhagiae*), icterus, hepatic fibrosis, and occasionally chronic active hepatitis (reported with *L. grippotyphosa*).
- Infection typically is subclinical in vaccinated (immune) and adult dogs and in all cats.

Clinical Signs

- Systemic signs of illness: fever, depression, anorexia, vomiting, reluctance to move (due to generalized muscle pain, renal pain, or meningitis), dehydration, and congested mucous membranes; vascular collapse and peracute death in some animals
- Acute renal failure, usually with oliguria or anuria, or subacute renal failure with polyuria (see Chap. 97)
- Acute hepatic failure, usually with icterus and DIC (see Chap. 91)
- Signs of DIC: widespread petechial and ecchymotic hemorrhages, melena, hematemesis, and epistaxis
- Occasional manifestations: abortion or stillbirths, uveitis, meningitis, acute interstitial pneumonitis (cough, dyspnea), or chronic hepatitis and hepatic fibrosis (signs of liver failure; e.g., cachexia, ascites, jaundice, or hepatic encephalopathy).

Diagnosis
Complete Blood Count (CBC)

- Leukopenia (early)
- Neutrophilia with left shift (at usual time of presentation)
- Thrombocytopenia and abnormal hemostasis reflecting DIC (see Chap. 21)

Urinalysis

- Proteinuria, pyuria, cylindruria, bilirubinuria, glucosuria, and isosthenuria

Table 17–1. BACTERIAL INFECTIOUS DISEASES OF DOGS AND CATS

Disease	Etiology (Source)	Clinical Signs	Diagnosis	Treatment
Leptospirosis	*Leptospira interrogans* (serovars: *L. canicola, L.icterohaemorrhagiae, L. grippotyphosa*) (urine shedding)	Acute renal failure, acute hepatic failure, anorexia, depression, fever, myalgia, DIC	Serology (MA, ELISA)	Penicillin, ampicillin, or amoxicillin, followed by doxycycline
Borreliosis (Lyme disease)	*Borrelia burgdorferi* (tick-borne)	Fever, polyarthritis (shifting lameness)	Serology (IFA, ELISA)	Tetracycline or doxycycline
Brucellosis	*Brucella canis* (semen, vaginal discharges, urine)	Male: infertility, orchiepididymitis, scrotitis Female: infertility, abortion Male and female: lymphadenopathy	Serology (slide test, tube test, AGID) Blood culture	Minocycline or doxycycline plus dihydrostreptomycin or gentamicin; spay/castrate
Bordetellosis (kennel cough)	*Bordetella bronchiseptica* (respiratory secretions)	Acute tracheobronchitis (cough); rhinitis	Culture (airways)	Amoxicillin-clavulanate or doxycycline
Tetanus	*Clostridium tetani* (wound contamination)	Muscle rigidity, stiffness, tetanic spasms (neurotoxin-induced)	Clinical signs	Tetanus antitoxin; penicillin G or metronidazole; sedatives
Campylobacteriosis	*Campylobacter jejuni* (feces)	Watery mucoid diarrhea or subclinical carrier	Fecal culture, fecal microscopy	Erythromycin, neomycin, clindamycin, or fluoroquinolone
Salmonellosis	*Salmonella typhimurium, S. enteritidis* (feces)	Acute gastroenteritis: fever, vomiting, diarrhea, bacteremia; subclinical carrier	Fecal culture	Enrofloxacin, trimethoprim sulfa, or chloramphenicol
Yersiniosis	*Yersinia enterocolitica* (human feces)	Diarrhea (rare) or subclinical carrier	Fecal culture	Cephalosporins, tetracyclines, etc.
Tyzzer disease	*Clostridium piliforme* (rodent feces)	Acute hepatic necrosis, necrotizing ileocolitis	Necropsy lesions, cell culture isolation	None (100% fatality)
Plague	*Yersinia pestis* (rodent fleas and rodent ingestion)	Cat: lymph node abscess, high fever, fatal septicemia Dog: mild fever or no signs	Lymph node cytology, culture, and IFA; serology; PCR	Gentamicin, enrofloxacin, doxycycline; chloramphenicol or tetracycline; flea control
Tularemia	*Francisella tularensis* (tick-borne; ingestion of rabbits or rodents)	Fever, lymphadenopathy, draining abscesses, fatal bacteremia	Serology (agglutinating antibody titer), culture	Streptomycin, gentamicin, fluoroquinolones, doxycycline
Actinomycosis	*Actinomyces* spp (oral flora migration, bitewounds)	Subcutaneous abscesses, draining fistulous tracts, pyothorax, osteomyelitis	Cytology (gram-positive filamentous rods), culture of exudate	Penicillin; debride wounds; drain and lavage pyothorax
Nocardiosis	*Nocardia spp* (soil via wounds, plant awns, inhalation)	Subcutaneous abscesses, draining fistulous tracts, pyothorax, pneumonia	Cytology (gram-positive filamentous rods), histopathology, culture of exudate	Sulfa drugs; debride wounds; drain and lavage pyothorax
Tuberculosis	*Mycobacterium tuberculosis, M. bovis, M. avium* (Dog: inhalation) (Cat: ingestion, e.g., milk)	Dog: granulomatous pneumonia, hilar lymphadenopathy Cat: granulomatous enteritis, mesenteric lymphadenopathy	Cytology (acid-fast bacteria); intradermal skin test (dogs only); culture (difficult)	Not recommended because of public health concerns and refractoriness
Feline leprosy	*M. lepraemurium* (contact with rats)	Ulcerating cutaneous nodules	Cytology or biopsy (acid-fast bacteria); PCR	Surgical excision; clofazimine or dapsone (toxic)
Atypical mycobacteriosis	*M. fortuitum, M. chelonei, M. smegmatis,* (skin contact with contaminated soil and water)	Spreading subcutaneous fistulous tracts	Cytology or biopsy (acid-fast bacteria)	Enrofloxacin, clarithromycin *(M. cheloni)*, and so on
Bartonellosis	*Bartonella henselae* (cat); *B. vinsonii* (dog)	Cat: subclinical, transient fever; dog: endocarditis; human: cat scratch fever, etc	Blood culture, serology (IFA), PCR	Enrofloxacin, doxycycline, rifampin

DIC, disseminated intravascular coagulation; MA, microscopic agglutination; ELISA, enzyme-linked immunosorbent assay; IFA, indirect fluorescent antibody; AGID, agar-gel immunodiffusion; PCR, polymerase chain reaction.

Serum Chemistries

- Azotemia—increased blood urea nitrogen (BUN), serum creatinine, and serum phosphorus
- Elevated serum concentrations of liver enzymes (ALT, AST, ALP), bilirubin, and bile acids
- Electrolyte imbalances reflecting renal and gastrointestinal effects

Serology

- Microscopic agglutination (MA) test
  - Titer becomes positive after 1 week, peaks at 3 to 4 weeks, and remains positive for months both after natural infection and after vaccination.
  - To confirm current infection (vs. previous infection or vaccination), a rising titer must be demonstrated. The titer during acute illness should increase fourfold when repeated during convalescence.
  - Because the timing of the titer peak varies, take a convalescent titer 2 to 3 weeks postinfection and another 1 to 2 weeks later.
  - Although single titers are never diagnostic of current infection, titers 1:300 or greater are suggestive and titers 1:1000 or greater are highly indicative of leptospirosis. However, booster vaccines given in the preceding 2 to 3 months can produce titers that overlap with these values.
  - The lab report will indicate titers for the various serovars tested. The highest titer is assumed to be the infecting serovar and other serovars with lower titers are considered to represent crossreactivity.
- Combined IgM-IgG enzyme-linked immunosorbent assay (ELISA) titers
  - IgM titer becomes positive within the first week of infection (before MA) and persists for 2 weeks.
  - IgG titer becomes positive 2 to 3 weeks after infection and persists for months.
  - Although not as available as the MA test, these help to differentiate current infection from previous infection or vaccination.

▼ *Key Point* Leptospira organisms are fastidious, slow-growing, and difficult to culture, and they are difficult to identify in fluids or tissues; thus, serology in conjunction with clinical signs is the most practical means of diagnosis.

- *Polymerase Chain Reaction (PCR) Test*

Genetic detection methods such as PCR have been used to detect Leptospira organisms in blood and urine; however, these tests are not yet available except in research labs.

Treatment

- Institute general therapy for dehydration (see Chap. 5), acute renal failure (see Chap. 97), acute hepatic failure (see Chap. 91), and DIC (see Chap. 21), as described in the appropriate chapters of this book. Anuria and fulminant DIC are life-threatening complications of leptospirosis that need immediate attention.

▼ *Key Point* The antibiotic of choice for eliminating leptospiremia is penicillin and for eliminating leptospiruria is doxycycline.

- *For leptospiremia:* initially give penicillin G (25,000–40,000 units/kg IV, q12h) or ampicillin (22 mg/kg IV, q6–8h). Once vomiting resolves, switch to amoxicillin (22 mg/kg PO, q8–12h) and continue treatment for 2 weeks.
- *For leptospiruria:* to eliminate the carrier state after treatment with a penicillin derivative, give doxycycline (5 mg/kg PO q12h) for 2 weeks.
- Leptospirosis is zoonotic; thus, recommend precautions and proper hygiene, especially regarding exposure to contaminated urine. Use iodophor disinfectants.

Prevention

Because prevention of exposure is not a realistic expectation, routine vaccination for leptospirosis is recommended. Vaccination helps reduce the incidence and severity of leptospirosis, but it does not prevent subclinical infection or urine shedding.

- Bivalent *Leptospira* bacterin (*L. canicola* and *L. icterohaemorrhagiae*) is a component of most polyvalent canine vaccines (included with canine distemper virus, parvovirus, and adenovirus) used for routine vaccination programs. Bivalent vaccine does not crossprotect against other serovars; consequently, these currently account for an increasing proportion of infections in dogs.
- Vaccinate dogs at 9, 12, and 15 weeks of age. At least three doses are required for primary immunization. Annual revaccination is recommended, but because the duration of immunity averages 6 to 8 months, dogs in endemic areas or high-risk situations may need biannual vaccination.
- Newer, improved vaccines derived from *Leptospira* outer membrane antigens may become available, with the following advantages over existing bacterins:
  - May contain up to 5 different serovar antigens
  - Protection against subclinical infection and shedding
  - More rapid onset of protection
  - Fewer doses required for primary immunization
  - Fewer allergic reactions

CANINE BRUCELLOSIS

Etiology

Canine brucellosis is caused by *Brucella canis*, a gram-negative aerobic coccobacillus.

Transmission

B. canis is found in semen (venereal), vaginal discharges (at estrus, breeding, and postabortion), aborted fetal tissues, and urine. Infection occurs by penetration of oronasal, conjunctival, and genital mucous membranes by the organisms.

Pathogenesis

Brucellosis is characterized by a prolonged leukocyte-associated bacteremia that lasts 6 to 24 months.

- *Brucella* organisms most often localize in:
  - The lymphoid and mononuclear phagocyte systems (lymphoreticular hyperplasia)
  - The prostate and testes of the male (orchiepididymitis, infertility)
  - The gravid uterus of the female (infertility, abortion)
- Rarely, the eye (anterior uveitis), kidney (glomerulonephritis), or intervertebral discs (discospondylitis) are involved.

Clinical Signs

Most infected animals have no overt clinical signs. Generalized lymphadenopathy, splenomegaly, and poor reproductive performance are the principal manifestations. Fever and systemic illness are rare.

- In males: infertility and physical findings of scrotal swelling, scrotal dermatitis, enlarged epididymis (epididymitis), and testicular atrophy
- In females: abortion of dead, partially autolyzed fetuses at 45 to 59 days of gestation without any other signs of illness; persistent discharge for 1 to 6 weeks after abortion; and failure to conceive (because of early fetal resorption)

Diagnosis

▼ *Key Point* Suspect brucellosis in any bitch that aborts 2 weeks before term.

- Routine CBC, urinalysis, and serum chemistries are normal except for occasional hyperglobulinemia.
- Lymph node cytology reveals nonspecific reactive hyperplasia.
- Semen abnormalities—more than 80% of sperm are morphologically abnormal, with increased leukocytes, and aspermia in the chronic stages.

Serology

Because other bacteria elicit antibodies that cross-react with *B. canis*, false-positive results are a problem. Hemolysis (hemoglobin) also causes false-positive results. False-negative titers can result from sequestration of infection or recent antibiotics. It can take 4 weeks to seroconvert; thus, when screening dogs for entry into a breeding kennel, a negative test result on day 1 and again after 4 weeks is required.

- Rapid slide agglutination test (D-Tec CB; Synbiotics) is an in-office screening test to detect suspects that need further testing. This test has accurate negative predictive value, but false-positive titers are common. Some 99% of negatives are true negatives, whereas only one half to two thirds of positives are confirmed to be truly infected.
- Tube agglutination and agar gel immunodiffusion (AGID) tests are available at commercial and state diagnostic laboratories. These titers are more specific for brucellosis but are not definitive (titers 1:50–1:100 are suspicious; titers ≥1:200 are highly suggestive).
- *Indicate fluorescent antibody test* available at diagnostic labs; may be less sensitive than agglutination tests.
- *ELISA* is very specific, but may be less sensitive than agglutination tests.
- *Cytoplasmic Antigen AGID* is the most specific confirmatory test for serologic diagnosis.

Bacterial Culture

- A positive blood culture is based on the characteristically prolonged bacteremia of brucellosis. Urine, semen, vaginal discharges, and aborted fetal tissues also can be cultured for *Brucella* organisms.

▼ *Key Point* Although a single high titer usually is indicative of active brucellosis, a positive blood culture is the gold standard for definitive diagnosis and should be used whenever possible for confirmation.

Treatment

- *Brucella* organisms are refractory to antibiotics and very difficult to eradicate (because of intracellular location and, in males, because of poor penetration of the blood-prostate barrier). Bacteremia can recur months after cessation of treatment; thus, eliminate infected dogs from breeding programs.
- The recommended antibiotic regimen is: minocycline (12.5 mg/kg, PO, q12h for 4 weeks) combined with dihydrostreptomycin (10 mg/kg, IM, q12h for 2 weeks on weeks #1 and #4); however, dihydrostreptomycin is no longer available. Gentamicin can be substituted for the dihydrostreptomycin, but is less effective, and doxycycline (5–10 mg/kg, PO, q12h) is an alternative to minocycline. Eradication of *Brucella* with antibiotics is difficult and highly unpredictable. Single antibiotic therapy is not effective.
- Recommend castration or ovariohysterectomy of infected animals
- Recommend caution for people in contact with *Brucella*-positive dogs because there have been rare instances of human infection. Canine brucellosis is regarded as a low-level public health risk.

Prevention

- Test all breeding stock for *Brucella* two times at a 4-week interval before entry into a breeding program and, ideally, test before each breeding in females and once or twice yearly in males.
- Eliminate infected dogs from breeding kennels.

SUPPLEMENTAL READINGS

Leptospirosis

Greene CE, Miller MA, Brown CE: Leptospirosis. In: Greene CE (ed): Infectious Diseases of the Dog and Cat (2nd Ed). Philadelphia: WB Saunders, 1998, p 273.
Rentko VT, Clark N, Ross LA, et al: Canine leptospirosis: a retrospective study of 17 cases. J Vet Inter Med 6:235, 1992.

Canine Brucellosis

Carmichael LE, Greene CE: Canine brucellosis. In: Greene CE (ed): Infectious Diseases of the Dog and Cat (2nd Ed). Philadelphia: WB Saunders, 1998, p 248.
Pollock RVH, Carmichael LE: Canine brucellosis. In: Barlough JE, (ed): Manual of Small Animal Infectious Diseases. New York: Churchill Livingstone, 1988, p 183.

Borreliosis

Greene CE, Appel MJG, Straubinger RK: Lyme borreliosis. In: Greene CE (ed): Infectious Diseases of the Dog and Cat (2nd Ed). Philadelphia: WB Saunders, 1998, p 282.

Tetanus

Greene CE: Tetanus. In: Greene CE (ed): Infectious Diseases of the Dog and Cat (2nd Ed). Philadelphia: WB Saunders, 1998, p 267.

Salmonellosis, Campylobacteriosis, Yersiniosis, Tyzzer Disease

Fox JG, Greene CE, Jones BR: Enteric bacterial infections. In: Greene CE (ed): Infectious Diseases of the Dog and Cat (2nd Ed). Philadelphia: WB Saunders, 1998, p 226.

Feline Plague

Macy DW, Plague. In: Greene CE (ed): Infectious Diseases of the Dog and Cat (2nd Ed). Philadelphia: WB Saunders, 1998, p 295.

Tularemia

Kaufman AF: Tularemia. In: Greene CE (ed): Infectious Diseases of the Dog and Cat (2nd Ed). Philadelphia: WB Saunders, 1998, p 300.

Mycobacterial Infections

Greene CE, Gunn-Moore DA, Lewis DT, Kunkle GA: Mycobacterial infections. In: Greene CE (ed): Infectious Diseases of the Dog and Cat (2nd Ed). Philadelphia: WB Saunders, 1998, p 313.
Wilkinson GT: Mycobacterial infections. In: Barlough JE (ed): Manual of Small Animal Infectious Diseases. New York: Churchill Livingstone, 1988, p 213.

Actinomycosis and Nocardiosis

Edwards DF: Actinomycosis and nocardiosis. In: Greene CE (ed): Infectious Diseases of the Dog and Cat (2nd Ed). Philadelphia: WB Saunders, 1998, p 303.
Love DN: Actinomycosis and nocardiosis. In: Barlough JE (ed): Manual of Small Animal Infectious Diseases. New York: Churchill Livingstone, 1988, p 203.

18   Systemic Mycoses

Robert G. Sherding

The four major deep systemic mycoses of dogs and cats are histoplasmosis, blastomycosis, coccidioidomycosis, and cryptococcosis. These are discussed in this chapter. Other fungi that usually affect individual organs are discussed in the appropriate organ-system chapters; for example, intestinal pythiosis is described in Chapter 89; nasal aspergillosis and penicilliosis are described in Chapter 79; and several cutaneous fungi are discussed in Chapters 35 and 37.

▼ *Key Point* Histoplasmosis, blastomycosis, and coccidioidomycosis are endemic to defined regions of North America (Fig. 18–1).

HISTOPLASMOSIS

Etiology

- The cause of histoplasmosis, *Histoplasma capsulatum*, is a dimorphic soilborne fungus found in many temperate and subtropical regions of the world. In North America, the disease is most prevalent in the river valley regions of the central United States, especially in areas bordering the Mississippi River and its tributaries (see Fig. 18–1).
- At ambient temperatures, soil enriched by decomposing nitrogenous matter (e.g., feces of birds or bats) provides an ideal growth medium for the mycelial phase of *Histoplasma*. The principal route of infection is by inhalation of airborne spores and mycelial fragments in windblown soil; however, intestinal infection via ingestion also may occur. At body temperature (37°C), *Histoplasma* organisms transform into a yeast phase that causes intracellular infection of macrophages.
- Histoplasmosis primarily invades the lung and cells of the mononuclear phagocyte system, but widespread hemolymphatic dissemination to virtually any tissue or organ system can occur.
- The outcome of exposure is influenced by level of exposure, age (clinical disease is most common in young animals <4 years of age), breed (highest incidence in sporting and hound breeds, perhaps because of higher exposure risk), immunosuppressive factors (corticosteroids may enhance dissemination), and host cell–mediated immunity. Inapparent infections without evidence of clinical disease are common.

Clinical Signs

Benign Asymptomatic Pulmonary Form

The benign form is an inapparent, self-limiting infection confined to the respiratory tract and is the most common outcome of natural infection. It is recognized radiographically as multiple, discrete, calcified interstitial foci (inactive encapsulated or healed lesions) and sometimes as calcified tracheobronchial lymph nodes.

Acute Pulmonary Form

The acute pulmonary form of histoplasmosis is characterized by severe fulminant granulomatous pneumonia with signs of cough, dyspnea, fever, and severe malaise. The radiographic findings are pronounced diffuse linear or nodular pulmonary interstitial infiltrates, often with patchy coalescing densities and moderately enlarged tracheobronchial lymph nodes.

Chronic Pulmonary Form

Chronic histoplasmosis is more common than the acute form and is characterized by chronic granulomatous pneumonia (diffuse or multifocal) with marked tracheobronchial lymphadenopathy that causes extrinsic airway compression. Clinical signs include chronic cough and mild dyspnea with variable weight loss and fever. Radiographically, massive enlargement of the tracheobronchial lymph nodes and variable linear or nodular interstitial infiltrates are seen.

Intestinal Form

Intestinal histoplasmosis is the most common extrapulmonary form in dogs and may represent dissemination or primary infection by ingestion. The colon, the small intestine, or a combination of both can be affected by extensive granulomatous thickening of the bowel wall and mucosal ulceration, often accompanied by mesenteric and visceral lymphadenopathy. Intractable diarrhea and progressive weight loss are the most consistent clinical signs.

- Granulomatous colitis—bloody-mucoid large bowel diarrhea and tenesmus (when the rectum is involved, mucosal proliferations may be detected by digital palpation of the rectum)

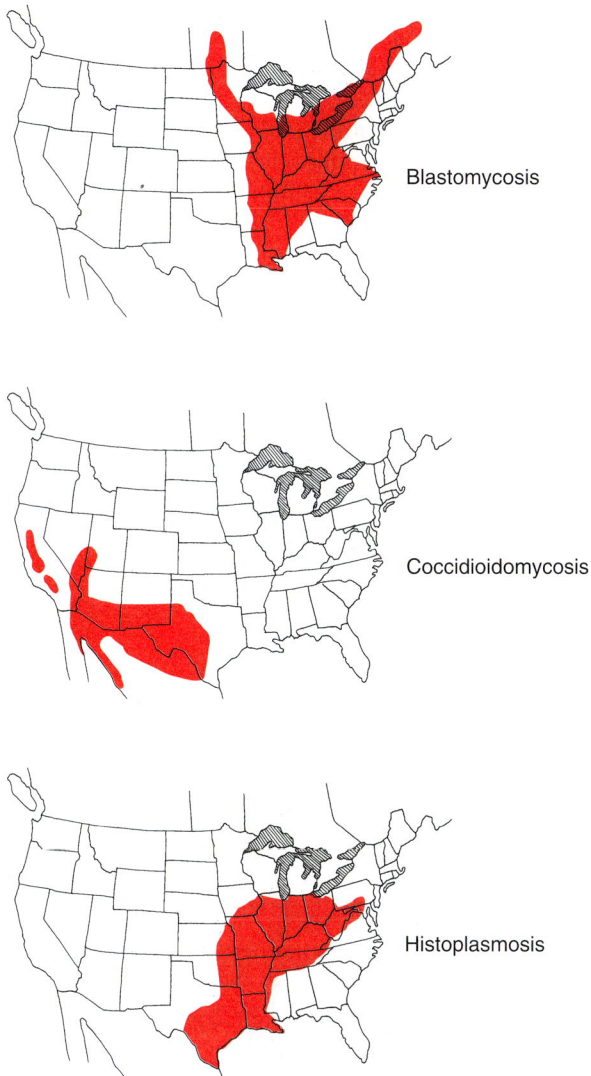

Figure 18–1. Geographic distribution of blastomycosis, coccidioidomycosis, and histoplasmosis in North America.

- Granulomatous enteritis—voluminous watery small bowel diarrhea, malabsorption, cachexia, protein-losing enteropathy, and palpably thickened intestines
- Other signs—fever, pallor, inappetance, vomiting, lethargy, and abdominal effusion

Other Extrapulmonary Disseminated Forms

Extrapulmonary dissemination may produce a diversity of acute or chronic manifestations, with or without clinical evidence of accompanying pulmonary involvement. Most cats develop these disseminated forms of histoplasmosis. The macrophage-monocyte system is a common site of dissemination. Manifestations can include any of the following:

- Liver—hepatomegaly, icterus, ascites
- Spleen—splenomegaly
- Lymph nodes—peripheral or abdominal lymphadenopathy
- Bone marrow—anemia

- Peritoneum—omental masses, mesenteric adhesions, nodular or granular serosal surfaces
- Eyes—exudative anterior uveitis, multifocal granulomatous chorioretinitis, optic neuritis
- Central nervous system—ataxia, seizures
- Skin—fistulous tracts that drain pus, skin and subcutaneous nodules that may be ulcerated
- Bone—lameness associated with proliferative or lytic bony lesions
- Oral cavity—ulcers

Diagnosis

Histoplasmosis should be suspected on the basis of clinical signs in animals from endemic areas. The results of routine laboratory evaluations are variable and nonspecific. Radiographic findings in the pulmonary form are often highly suggestive of histoplasmosis. Serology provides a presumptive diagnosis, but identification of the *Histoplasma* organisms is necessary for definitive diagnosis.

Hematology

- Normocytic-normochromic nonregenerative anemia
  - Can be the result of chronic inflammation, dissemination of *Histoplasma* into the bone marrow, intestinal blood loss, or hemolysis.
- Neutrophilic leukocytosis or neutropenia with left shift and monocytosis, occasionally pancytopenia in cats
  - *Histoplasma* organisms may be seen within circulating monocytes or neutrophils on routine blood smears, especially if 1000 cells are examined in differential cell counts or if buffy coat smears are examined.
- Thrombocytopenia
  - Usually mild and subclinical; however, platelet counts of less than 50,000/μl are seen occasionally in association with macroplatelets in the circulation and increased megakaryocytes in the bone marrow, suggesting platelet consumption or destruction.

Chemistry Evaluations

- Hypoalbuminemia, with or without concomitant hyperglobulinemia (in intestinal and disseminated forms)
  - Usually mild, but may be pronounced in dogs with severe protein-losing enteropathy (PLE).
- Elevated serum liver enzymes and bilirubin (with hepatic dissemination)
- Abnormal intestinal function tests in diffuse small intestinal disease
  - Increased fecal alpha-1-antitrypsin (PLE)
  - Impaired xylose absorption
  - Increased fecal fat
  - Decreased serum levels of folate and cobalamin

Radiography and Ultrasonography

- Thoracic radiography (in the pulmonary form of histoplasmosis)
  - Linear or nodular ("miliary") interstitial pulmonary infiltrates

- Hilar density around the tracheal bifurcation due to tracheobronchial lymphadenopathy
- Coalescing patchy alveolar infiltrates, calcified pulmonary interstitial nodules (healed lesions), and calcified tracheobronchial lymph nodes
- Contrast barium radiography (in the intestinal form of histoplasmosis)
  - Irregularity of the intestinal mucosa and thickening of the bowel wall, which are nonspecific indicators of a diffuse infiltrative lesion
- Other radiographic findings (depending on sites of dissemination)
  - Hepatosplenomegaly
  - Abdominal or thoracic effusions
  - Osteolytic and periosteal proliferative bone lesions
- Ultrasonography may show hepatic nodularity and hyperechogenicity

Serology

- Tests that detect anti-*Histoplasma* antibodies are not sufficiently reliable for definitive diagnosis; thus, every effort should be made to confirm infections through identification of the *Histoplasma* organisms.
- A complement fixation titer of 1 : 16 or greater or a positive agar-gel immunodiffusion (AGID) (precipitin) test is considered suggestive of histoplasmosis.
- Unfortunately, these tests often yield false-negative results in animals with histoplasmosis. Prior exposure may cause a false-positive result. In addition, other mycotic infections (e.g., blastomycosis) may cross-react on serodiagnostic tests for histoplasmosis, and anticomplementary sera may make complement fixation unusable in some animals.

▼ *Key Point* Definitive diagnosis of histoplasmosis requires identification of *Histoplasma* organisms in cytology, biopsy, or culture specimens.

Cytology

Exfoliative and fine-needle aspiration cytology generally are the most practical and high-yield methods for definitive diagnosis of histoplasmosis. Wright, Giemsa, or Diff-Quik stains (American Scientific Products, McGraw Park, IL) are ideal for identification of *Histoplasma* in cytology preparations. The organisms are found most often intracellularly within the cytoplasm of macrophages as round to oval bodies, 2 to 4 μm in size, surrounded by a characteristic clear halo or "pseudocapsule" that results from shrinkage during staining. Sources of cytologic specimens with potential diagnostic benefit depend on sites of involvement.

- Respiratory tract—bronchoscopic alveolar lavage, transtracheal washing, endotrachial washing, fine-needle lung aspirate
- Intestinal tract—smears of rectal mucosal scrapings, impression smears of endoscopic biopsies, and fine-needle aspirates of abdominal lymph nodes or intestinal masses
  - Consider endoscopy of the colon and duodenum for the collection of diagnostic cytology or biopsy

specimens. Histoplasmosis lesions appear endoscopically as areas of irregular mucosal thickening and proliferation that produce a corrugated or cobblestone appearance, with or without mucosal hemorrhage and ulceration.
- Liver, spleen, or lymph node aspirates
- Abdominal or thoracic effusions
- Bone marrow aspirates and buffy coat smears of peripheral blood
- Skin lesion impression smears
- Oculocentesis

Histopathology

Biopsies of affected tissues reveal granulomatous inflammation, but organisms are usually sparse and difficult to see with H&E stain. Detection of organisms in biopsies may be facilitated by use of special fungal stains such as periodic acid–Schiff (PAS), Grocott-Gomori methenamine silver nitrate, or Gridley.

Culture

Any of the specimens aforementioned for cytologic or biopsy identification of *Histoplasma* also can be used to culture the fungi in Sabouraud's media; however, these fungi are difficult to isolate in culture and require 10 to 14 days for growth. Culture media with mycelial growth is potentially infectious for humans; thus, avoid in-clinic culturing.

Treatment

Oral itraconazole is the treatment of choice for histoplasmosis. Treat for at least 2 months beyond clinical resolution. Treatment regimens and prevention are discussed at the end of this chapter.

BLASTOMYCOSIS

Etiology

- *Blastomyces dermatitidis* is a dimorphic soilborne fungus with a geographic distribution (see Fig. 18–1) similar to that of *Histoplasma*. The organisms reside in sandy, acidic soil near water. Most infected dogs live within 400m of water.
- Inhalation of soilborne spores is the primary route of infection and leads to mycotic pneumonia. In addition, focal skin infection sometimes occurs from direct cutaneous inoculation. Extrapulmonary dissemination is very common in blastomycosis.
- Dogs are considered highly susceptible to blastomycosis, and the canine infection rate in endemic areas is ten times the human infection rate. Infection in cats is uncommon.

Clinical Signs

Young (<5 years) male large-breed dogs are infected most frequently probably because of increased exposure through outdoor activities. Nonspecific signs of fever, anorexia, weight loss, and depression are common. Signs may be acute (days) or chronic (weeks to months).

Pulmonary Form

Lung lesions are present in 85% of cases. Cough and dyspnea are typical presenting signs. Respiratory manifestations may include (in decreasing order of frequency):

- Acute or chronic interstitial pyogranulomatous pneumonia, usually involving all lung lobes diffusely, sometimes focally
- Tracheobronchial lymphadenopathy
- Pleural effusion

Extrapulmonary Disseminated Form

Blastomycosis very commonly disseminates, especially to the skin (40% of cases), eyes (40% of cases), peripheral lymph nodes (50–60%), and, to a lesser extent, to the bone, central nervous system (CNS), male genitalia, oral cavity, and nasal cavity.

- Cutaneous blastomycosis may be manifested as fistulas that drain pus or bloody fluid, circumscribed raised ulcerating pyogranulomas, deep abscesses, paronychia, and regional lymphadenopathy.
- Ocular involvement may include anterior uveitis, chorioretinitis, retinal detachment or panophthalmitis.
- Fungal osteomyelitis is manifested as lameness and adjacent soft tissue swelling, usually in the distal limbs.
- CNS involvement may cause seizures, dementia, blindness, or ataxia.
- Granulomatous orchitis and prostatitis occur in 11% of infected male dogs.

Diagnosis

Hematology

Typical findings are a regenerative neutrophilic leukocytosis, mild nonregenerative anemia, monocytosis, and lymphopenia.

Thoracic Radiography

Radiography generally reveals a nodular (usually miliary) or diffuse pulmonary interstitial infiltrate and occasionally a moderate tracheobronchial lymphadenopathy. Less frequent findings include alveolar infiltrates, lobar consolidation, focal solitary nodules, pleural effusion, and cavitary lesions.

Serology

Serology provides a presumptive diagnosis of blastomycosis based on a positive AGID test (90% reliable) or a complement fixation titer of 1:32 or greater (less reliable than AGID).

Cytology, Biopsy, and Culture

Identification of *Blastomyces* organisms by one of these methods is required for definitive diagnosis. The source of specimens and method of procurement depend on sites of involvement.

- *Blastomyces* in tissues appears as an extracellular yeast (5–20 μm) with broad-based budding and a prominent, double-refractile cell wall. Any routine cytology stain can be used.
- Cytologies most often diagnostic for blastomycosis include pulmonary cytology (transtracheal washing, bronchoalveolar lavage, fine-needle lung aspirate), skin impression smears, and lymph node aspirates; however, any affected tissue can be sampled. Occasionally organisms are seen in fluid specimens such as urine, cerebrospinal fluid, or pleural effusion. Specimens for culture can be collected in a similar manner as for histoplasmosis. Do not use in-clinic culturing because mycelial growth poses a risk of human infection.

▼ *Key Point* Because *Blastomyces* yeast bodies are usually plentiful and easily identified in lesions, cytologies are the initial diagnostic tests of choice because of ease and rapidity of results.

- In blastomycosis lesions, fungal organisms are generally more prevalent and easily identified than in histoplasmosis lesions, and the inflammation is more pyogranulomatous (macrophages and nondegenerate neutrophils) than granulomatous.

Treatment

Oral itraconazole is the treatment of choice for blastomycosis. Details of treatment regimens and prevention are discussed at the end of this chapter.

COCCIDIOIDOMYCOSIS

Etiology

- *Coccidioides immitis* is a soilborne fungus distributed geographically to the dry, desert-like regions of the southwestern United States (see Fig. 18–1). In the soil, *Coccidioides* grow as mycelia that form arthrospores.
- Infection occurs by inhalation of these soilborne and windblown arthrospores. Cutaneous inoculation may occur, but rarely. In body tissues, *Coccidioides* form large spherules (20–100 μm) that release hundreds of endospores.

Clinical Signs

Self-limiting Inapparent Form

Subclinical pulmonary infection is most common.

Pulmonary Form

Pulmonary coccidioidomycosis is characterized by acute or chronic granulomatous pneumonia and tracheobronchial lymphadenopathy with signs of cough, fever, malaise, and occasionally dyspnea.

Extrapulmonary Disseminated Form

This form is usually chronic (months to years) and may involve the bones and joints (mostly osteoproliferative bone reaction, causing lameness and painful swelling), abdominal viscera (spleen, liver, lymph nodes, omentum, kidneys), heart and pericardium (myocarditis, pericarditis, congestive heart failure), eyes (uveitis), CNS, male genitalia, and skin (usually ulcerated nodules and fistulas over bone lesions). Bone involvement is most common in dogs, whereas skin lesions are the predominant finding in cats.

Diagnosis

Hematology and Serum Chemistry

Findings may include a variable leukocytosis, monocytosis, and nonregenerative anemia. Hyperglobulinemia and hypoalbuminemia can develop with chronicity.

Radiography

Granulomatous pneumonia and hilar lymphadenopathy are similar to that described for histoplasmosis. Occasionally, evidence of pericardial disease or congestive heart failure is identified. Dissemination to bone is common, especially to the distal aspects of long bones, and it results in multifocal osteoproliferative lesions on radiographs.

Serology

A fairly reliable presumptive diagnosis can be made on the basis of detection of antibodies against *Coccidioides*. The tube precipitin test, which detects the early IgM response, and the complement fixation test, which detects the later and sustained IgG response are the traditional serologic tests. Newer tests use immunodiffusion (AGID) or ELISA methods for detecting Coccidioides-specific IgM and IgG.

- The IgM response becomes positive 2 weeks post exposure and persists for 4–6 weeks. IgM also may be detected at the time of dissemination or recrudescence in association with high IgG levels.
- High IgG titers (≥1:64) usually indicate severe pulmonary or disseminated disease.

Cytology, Biopsy, and Culture

Definitive diagnosis depends on identifying the organisms (spherules) in affected tissues, using cytology or biopsy. However, spherules may be difficult to find in some cases. Lesions show pyogranulomatous inflammation. Cultures are not recommended.

Treatment

Coccidioidomycosis usually is treated with one of the oral azole drugs (ketoconazole, itraconazole, or fluconazole) for a minimum of 8 to 12 months, and sometimes indefinitely, using the regimens described in the last section of this chapter. Amphotericin B is not quite as effective but can be used in animals that do not tolerate oral azole drugs.

CRYPTOCOCCOSIS

Etiology

- *Cryptococcus neoformans* is found in many geographic regions. Infection is acquired from inhalation of soil-borne organisms or, usually in urban areas, from inhalation of organisms found in pigeon excreta.
- The organisms are budding yeasts (4–7 μm) that possess a prominent polysaccharide capsule. This thick capsule is essential to the pathogenicity of this fungus because it inhibits plasma cell function, phagocytosis, leukocyte migration, and complement. The capsule also allows the organisms to stand out in stained cytology preparations for easy identification and is the basis for the cryptococcal capsular antigen diagnostic test.

Clinical Signs

▼ *Key Point* In cats, *Cryptococcus* has a predilection for the nasal cavity, where the airborne organisms initially deposit, accounting for the chronic granulomatous rhinitis and sinusitis seen in at least 80% of cats with the disease.

In contrast to cats, clinically evident nasal disease is rare in dogs with cryptococcosis; instead, CNS and eye involvement are the predominant findings. Surprisingly, lung involvement is evident clinically only rarely; yet 50% of dogs and cats have lung lesions at necropsy. Fever occurs in less than 25% of the cases; in fact, temperatures exceeding 37°C inhibit *Cryptococcus*.

Nasal Form

The principal signs of nasal involvement are unilateral or bilateral mucopurulent or bloody nasal discharge, sneezing, sniffling, deformity of overlying nasal bones, and mucinous nasal granuloma mass lesions at the nostril.

Extrarespiratory Disseminated Form

The preferred sites for dissemination are the CNS (cats, 25%; dogs, >75%), eyes (cats, 25%; dogs, >60%), and skin (cats, 40%; dogs, 20%).

- CNS involvement from hematogenous spread or local extension through the cribriform plate results in diffuse or mass-like granulomatous meningoencephalitis or myelitis. Signs may include seizures, circling, head-pressing, blindness, dementia, ataxia, paresis, and cranial nerve (CN) deficits (e.g., CN II, VII, VIII).
- Eye involvement may include granulomatous (exudative) chorioretinitis, anterior uveitis, and optic neuritis.
- Skin involvement usually manifests as firm nodules that rapidly enlarge and then ulcerate and ooze, mostly in the head area and often near the nostrils.
- Other dissemination sites may include peripheral lymph nodes (especially the submandibulars), pharynx and oral cavity, kidneys (30% of animals have renal granulomas at necropsy), liver, spleen, heart, and skeletal muscle.

Diagnosis

Hematology

Findings are often normal, except for occasional neutrophilia or eosinophilia.

Radiography

Nasal radiographs may indicate nasal bone lysis or expansion, turbinate destruction, or an abnormal soft tissue density within the nasal cavity or frontal sinus.

Serology

Serologic testing provides a presumptive diagnosis based on detection of capsular antigen in serum, cerebrospinal fluid (CSF), or urine using latex agglutination or ELISA. False-negative results may occur, especially in nondisseminated disease. False positive results can occur in patients treated recently with hetastarch and in CSF contaminated with talc particles from latex gloves.

Cytology, Biopsy, and Culture

Definitive diagnosis requires identification of the organisms in cytologies (e.g., nasal exudate, CSF, skin exudate or impressions, lymph node aspirates, urine, oculocentesis) using Gram's, PAS, new methylene blue, or India ink stains or in biopsies using mucicarmine, H&E, PAS, or silver stains. *Cryptococcus* also can be cultured from similar specimens on Sabouraud's media.

Treatment

Treat cryptococcosis with oral itraconazole or fluconazole for at least 2 months beyond clinical resolution, which usually ranges from 6 to 10 months (mean, 8.5 months). Details are provided in the following section.

TREATMENT OF SYSTEMIC MYCOSES

General Principles of Treatment

- The oral azoles, such as fluconazole, ketoconazole, and itraconazole, are currently the first-choice antifungal drugs for single-agent treatment. Itraconazole and fluconazole are more effective than ketoconazole because of better absorption, greater potency, quicker onset of action, longer duration of action, and less toxicity. Ketoconazole is less expensive and used primarily when cost is a limiting factor.
- Fluconazole penetrates the eyes and CNS better than other azoles and is preferred, especially in cryptococcosis.
- The major disadvantages of amphotericin B are that it must be given parenterally and that it is frequently nephrotoxic. Nevertheless, amphotericin B can be combined with an azole drug for the initial treatment of advanced or rapidly progressing infections because of its more rapid onset of antifungal activity and because combination antifungal therapy may be more effective than either drug alone.

▼ *Key Point* Regardless of the treatment regimen, the unpredictable response in the disseminated forms of mycotic disease should dictate a guarded prognosis, especially if the CNS is involved.

Ketoconazole

Ketoconazole is used orally to treat histoplasmosis, blastomycosis, and coccidioidomycosis. It is less effective against *Cryptococcus*. Ketoconazole is not usually effective against ocular and CNS mycoses.

Pharmacology

- Ketoconazole depends on hepatobiliary metabolism and excretion, and it is distributed widely except in the CNS, eye, and testes.
- Acidity is required for optimal absorption of azole drugs, especially ketoconazole; thus, avoid concurrent use of antacids or drugs such as H_2 blockers that inhibit gastric acid secretion. Bioavailability is increased and nausea and vomiting are minimized when azole drugs are given with food.

▼ *Key Point* Azole drugs inhibit the biosynthesis of ergosterol in the fungal cell membrane. Because the onset of this fungistatic effect may be delayed for 1 to 2 weeks after therapy is initiated, the clinical response to azoles may be slow.

Induction Therapy

The usual oral dosage of ketoconazole for induction therapy in both dogs and cats ranges from 10 to 30 mg/kg/day. Divide this total daily dose into two or three doses for better gastrointestinal tolerance.

- For dogs—use the higher end of this range (20–30 mg/kg/day).
- For cats—start at the lower end of this dosage range (10–20 mg/kg/day, or a total dose of 50 mg once daily) because cats generally are more susceptible to the side effects of ketoconazole. If tolerance is still a problem in a cat, administer a dosage of 20 mg/kg on alternate days.

Maintenance Therapy

- Continue ketoconazole for at least 2 months beyond full clinical remission. The total duration of therapy is usually at least 4 to 6 months (8–12 months or longer in coccidioidomycosis).
- Because ketoconazole is a fungistatic drug, the duration of therapy is variable and relapses have occurred up to 1 year after therapy was discontinued. If recrudescence occurs, reinstitute a full course of ketoconazole or switch to another drug.

Combination Therapy

For initial treatment of advanced or rapidly progressing disseminated infections, use amphotericin B in combination with ketoconazole for the first few weeks or use itraconazole.

▼ *Key Point* If there is CNS, ocular, or genital involvement, ketoconazole is ineffective, and fluconazole or itraconazole should be used. Fluconazole has the highest penetration of these tissues. Recommend castration of dogs with mycotic orchitis or prostatitis, such as occurs in blastomycosis.

Side Effects

- The most common immediate side effects of ketoconazole are anorexia, vomiting, and diarrhea. These usually can be minimized by dividing the daily doses and administering them with food.
- Longer-term side effects may include hepatotoxicity (hepatomegaly, elevated serum liver enzymes, icterus), weight loss, and haircoat changes (lightening of color, alopecia). Because of hepatic effects, it is advisable to monitor serum liver enzymes monthly during treatment. The liver, gastrointestinal, and haircoat reactions are usually reversible with reduction in dosage.
- Ketoconazole inhibits adrenal and testicular steroidogenesis. In dogs, but not cats, ketoconazole diminishes serum testosterone and cortisol while increasing serum progesterone. Ketoconazole is embryotoxic and teratogenic and thus should not be used in pregnant animals.

Itraconazole

Itraconazole is the initial treatment of choice for histoplasmosis, blastomycosis, and cryptococcosis. Itraconazole is a newer generation azole drug that is more effective than ketoconazole with fewer side effects.

- Dogs—give 5mg/kg q12–24h PO, or 10 mg/kg/ q24h for dogs with CNS involvement.
- Cats—give 10 mg/kg q12–24h PO, or 20 mg/kg q24h.
- As with ketoconazole, consider combining amphotericin B with itraconazole as initial therapy in animals with rapidly progressive, life-threatening systemic mycotic infection.
- Adverse effects: Although itraconazole may cause anorexia and hepatotoxicity, it has fewer liver and gastrointestinal side effects than ketoconazole, and it does not appear to inhibit adrenal and testicular steroidogenesis.
- If hepatotoxicity occurs, stop treatment until appetite returns and liver enzymes decrease below 100 U/L, then reinstitute treatment at one-half dose and monitor serum liver enzymes every 2 weeks.
- An occasional side effect noted in treated animals is vasculitis, which produces ulcerative skin lesions and limb edema. This adverse reaction appears to be dose-dependent and reversible.

Fluconazole

The major advantage of fluconazole over other azoles is its much better penetration of the CNS in fungal meningitis; a disadvantage is that it is expensive. It is most often indicated for refractory mycotic disease with CNS or ocular involvement, especially cryptococcosis.

- Dosage—give 2.5–5.0 mg/kg q12–24h PO or IV. Use twice the recommended daily dosage for the first day as a loading dose. For CNS involvement in cats, give 10–15 mg/kg q12–24h or 50–100 mg total dose q12h.

Treat for 2 months beyond remission (usually 4–6 months total).

Amphotericin B

As a single drug, amphotericin B is most effective for treatment of blastomycosis and histoplasmosis. It is moderately effective for cryptococcosis and coccidioidomycosis. In severe cases of blastomycosis and histoplasmosis, combine amphotericin B with an azole for an initial 2- to 4-week induction phase of therapy and then follow up with the azole for several months of maintenance.

Pharmacology

- Amphotericin B (Fungizone; Squibb) is a polyene antibiotic for IV use that has both fungicidal and fungistatic actions. It binds to ergosterol in fungal cell membranes, thereby causing cell membrane damage and leakage of cell contents.
- Amphotericin B distributes well into most tissues, except for the CNS and the eye.
- Disadvantages are that it must be given parenterally and it frequently causes nephrotoxicity.
- Amphotericin B is available in its conventional deoxycholate form and as three newer lipid-complex formulations, including liposome-encapsulated, colloidal dispersion, and lipid complexed. The lipid-complexed amphotericin B formulations are supposed to be less nephrotoxic, thereby allowing use of higher dosages.

Dosage and Administration

Amphotericin B Deoxycholate

- *In dogs*, administer amphotericin B at a dose of 0.25–0.5 mg/kg, IV, on alternate days for 3 days per week, such as a Monday-Wednesday-Friday schedule, until a total cumulative dose of 8–12 mg/kg is received (6–12 wks).
- *In cats*, use a lower dosage of 0.15 to 0.25 mg/kg, IV, because of greater sensitivity to the toxic effects of the drug, and administer on a Mon-Wed-Fri schedule until a total cumulative dose of 4–6 mg/kg is received (6–12 wks).
- *Subcutaneous protocol:* A daily dose of 0.5–0.8 mg/kg is added to 400 ml (cats) or 500 ml (dogs) of 0.45% saline with 2.5% dextrose solution, then given SC two to three times weekly (q48h) until a total cumulative dose of 8–26 mg/kg is received (3–10 weeks).
- *In advanced, life-threatening or resistant fungal disease,* use a high-dose protocol of 1.0 mg/kg every other day. This increases the risk of nephrotoxicity.

Lipid–Complexed Amphotericin B

- Give 1.0 mg/kg IV on alternate days for 3 days per week until a total cumulative dose of 12 mg/kg is received (4 weeks). Higher individual doses up to 2.5 mg/kg IV and a longer duration of therapy can be used in refractory cases.

Renoprotective Measures

These measures are aimed at enhancing renal blood flow and glomerular filtration rate to reduce nephrotoxicity (see section on Side Effects), although efficacy has not been well documented. One or more of these may be used.

- Hydrate the patient before treatment.
- Dilute amphotericin in 5% dextrose solution, and administer as a slow (10 minute)bolus in 10–60 ml of dextrose solution or administrater by the slow IV infusion method over a period of 2 to 6 hours in 300–500 ml of dextrose solution.
  - Concurrently administer mannitol, 0.5 to 1.0 g/kg, IV
  - Saline loading to promote a sodium diuresis— 0.9% sodium chloride solution, 50 ml/kg, IV, given over a period of 1 to 3 hours before amphotericin or concurrently using a different vein to avoid amphotericin precipitation
  - Furosemide (Lasix), 2 mg/kg, IV after prior hydration

Side Effects

The major side effect of amphotericin B is nephrotoxicity. Other side effects in dogs and cats include transient fever of 24 to 36 hours in duration after the first dose, anorexia, nausea/vomiting, thrombophlebitis (local irritant effect), and perivascular irritation if extravasated.

- Nephrotoxicity is caused by a combination of reduced renal blood flow (arteriolar vasoconstriction) and direct renal tubular injury. Although there is considerable individual variation in susceptibility to nephrotoxicity, most animals treated with amphotericin B show some degree of renal dysfunction.
- Urinalysis and renal function (serum creatinine, BUN) should be evaluated before initiating amphotericin therapy and should be monitored frequently during treatment (once or twice weekly). In general, the earliest evidence of a renal effect is decreased urine specific gravity. This is followed by abnormal numbers of renal cells and casts in the urine sediment, and eventually azotemia may develop.

▼ *Key Point* If BUN exceeds 50 mg/dl or serum creatinine exceeds 2.5 mg/dl during amphotericin therapy, treatment should be suspended until BUN/creatinine levels return to normal. Azotemia in most cases is reversible when the drug is discontinued.

Flucytosine and Amphotericin Combination

Flucytosine (5-FC) (Ancobon; Roche) is an antimitotic, antifungal drug used in conjunction with amphotericin B for treatment of cryptococcosis. It is especially useful when there is CNS involvement, because 5-FC attains 60% to 80% of serum concentration in CSF.

- Use 5-FC only in combination with amphotericin B because fungal resistance develops rapidly if it is used alone.

Dosage

- Give 5-FC at 50 mg/kg, PO, q8h, or 75 mg/kg, PO, q12h.
- Give amphotericin B concurrently.

Lufenuron

Lufenuron (Program; Novartis) is a chitin synthesis inhibitor licensed for monthly flea control. Lufenuron may be effective for treatment of coccidioidomycosis at 5 mg/kg PO daily for 4 months or more.

Side Effects

The toxicity of 5-FC is hepatic and hematologic (leukopenia, thrombocytopenia).

PREVENTION

Because the principal source of systemic mycotic infection is windblown fungal elements from the soil, there is no practical means of prevention in endemic areas. High concentrations of *Histoplasma* can be found in chicken excreta, and of *Cryptococcus* in pigeon excreta; thus, exposure to these sources should be avoided. Animal-to-animal transmission of these mycotic infections is not likely. Although humans can be infected from the same environmental sources as animals, animal-to-human transmission is very rare. Vaccination for these mycoses is not available.

SUPPLEMENTAL READING

Armstrong PJ, DiBartola SP: Canine coccidioidomycosis: A literature review and report of 8 cases. J Am Anim Hosp Assoc 19:937, 1983.

Clinkenbeard KD, Wolf AM, Cowell RL, Tyler RL: Canine disseminated histoplasmosis. Comp Cont Educ 11:1347, 1989.

Greene CE, Watson ADJ: Antifungal chemotherapy. In: Green CE (ed): Infectious Diseases of the Dog and Cat (2nd Ed). Philadelphia: WB Saunders, 1998, p 357.

Jacobs GJ, Medleau L: Cryptococcosis. In: Green CE (ed): Infectious Diseases of the Dog and Cat (2nd Ed). Philadelphia: WB Saunders, 1998, p 383.

Legendre AM: Systemic mycotic infections. In: Sherding RG (ed): The Cat: Diseases and Clinical Management. New York: Churchill Livingstone, 1994, p 553.

Legendre AM: Blastomycosis. In: Green CE (ed): Infectious Diseases of the Dog and Cat (2nd Ed). Philadelphia: WB Saunders, 1998, p 371.

Medleau L: Imidazoles and triazoles. In: Kirk RW (ed): Current Veterinary Therapy X. Philadelphia: WB Saunders, 1989, p 577.

Mitchell M, Stark DR: Disseminated canine histoplasmosis: A clinical survey of 24 cases in Texas. Can Vet J 21:95, 1980.

Stickle JE, Hribernik TN: Clinicopathological observations in disseminated histoplasmosis in dogs. J Am Anim Hosp Assoc 14:105, 1978.

Wolf AM, Belden MN: Feline histoplasmosis: A literature review and retrospective review of 20 new cases. J Am Anim Hosp Assoc 20:995, 1984.

Wolf AM, Troy GC: Deep mycotic diseases. In: Ettinger SJ (ed): Textbook of Veterinary Internal Medicine. Philadelphia: WB Saunders, 1989, p 341.

19 Toxoplasmosis, Neosporosis, and Other Multisystemic Protozoal Infections

Robert G. Sherding

The protozoa that infect dogs and cats can be classified broadly into two categories: those that primarily live in the intestinal tract and those that disseminate and cause multisystemic disease. Enteric protozoal infections include intestinal coccidiosis, giardiasis, trichomoniasis, amebiasis, and balantidiasis; these are discussed in Chapter 89.

Toxoplasmosis, the most important multisystemic protozoal infectious disease in North America, is described in detail in this chapter, along with neosporosis. Several other multisystemic protozoal infections are important in tropical and subtropical regions of the world but are relatively uncommon in the United States. These are summarized in Table 19–1 at the end of this chapter and include diseases transmitted by insect vectors, such as leishmaniasis, trypanosomiasis (Chagas disease), hepatozoonosis, babesiosis, and cytauxzoonosis, and others that are transmitted without vectors, including encephalitozoonosis, acanthamebiasis, and pneumocystosis. Protozoa that parasitize erythrocytes, such as *Babesia* spp and *Cytauxzoon felis,* are discussed in Chapter 20.

TOXOPLASMOSIS

Etiology

Toxoplasma gondii is an obligate intracellular protozoan parasite. The feline species is the definitive host for this coccidia, but most warm-blooded animals can be infected as intermediate hosts, including dogs and humans. Serologic surveys in the United States estimate that 30% of cats and 25% to 50% of humans have been infected.

Routes of Transmission

Ingestion of Infected Animal Tissues

The ingestion of meat (carnivorism) that contains *Toxoplasma* cysts is the primary source of infection in cats. This includes uncooked meat (or meat scraps scavenged from garbage) or hunted prey (mice, birds). Ingestion of raw or undercooked meat also is an important source of toxoplasmosis in dogs and humans.

Ingestion of tachyzoites in raw milk, especially from goats, can be a source of infection.

Ingestion of Oocysts Shed in Cat Feces

Food, water, and soil contaminated with sporulated *Toxoplasma* oocysts are potentially important sources of infection for intermediate hosts such as humans, dogs, food-producing animals, and rodents. This is a relatively minor source of infection in the primary host, the cat. Oocysts can be transported by cockroaches, flies, and earthworms.

Congenital (Transplacental) Infection

When a pregnant animal or human becomes infected during gestation, *Toxoplasma* can cross the placenta and infect the unborn fetus. For this reason, toxoplasmosis has major public health significance in humans. In dogs and cats, congenital toxoplasmosis is uncommon, but it can be a cause of abortion, stillbirth, or neonatal mortality.

Stages of Infection

Fecal Oocyst Stage of Infection (Sporozoite Stage)

In cats that ingest infected meat from an intermediate host, the encysted *Toxoplasma* are liberated by the host's digestive enzymes and invade the intestinal epithelial cells. Multiplication within the intestinal epithelium results in fecal excretion of millions of oocysts beginning 3 to 10 days after exposure and continuing for 1 to 2 weeks. Infection by oocyst ingestion is a less important source in cats, but when it does occur, subsequent shedding of oocysts is delayed for 3 weeks or more and is much less pronounced. As excreted, oocysts are oval-shaped, 10×12 μm in size, and unsporulated (uninfective). To become infectious, excreted oocysts first must sporulate, which takes 1 to 5 days. These sporulated oocysts can remain infectious in the environment for months, and in soil for longer than 1 year. Clinical signs, if they occur at all, usually do not develop until the period of oocyst shedding is over.

▼ *Key Point* Fecal excretion of *Toxoplasma* oocysts, which can contaminate soil, water, and food and infect other animals, occurs only in the definitive host, the cat.

Acute Tissue Stage of Infection (Tachyzoite Stage)

Simultaneous with intestinal multiplication in cats or after infection by ingestion or transplacental transfer in any species, *Toxoplasma* invades extraintestinal tissues via blood and lymph. Almost any cell in any tissue can be parasitized by these rapidly multiplying tachyzoite forms. The tachyzoites eventually rupture and destroy the cell, releasing organisms to infect new cells and thereby producing foci of necrosis and inflammation. In a small percentage of animals, these lesions become extensive enough to cause overt clinical disease, with the signs dependent on which tissues are affected most severely. In most animals, however, the rapid multiplication stage is brief, and, as immunity develops and before signs occur, aggregates of these organisms encyst and become dormant.

Chronic Tissue Encystment Stage of Infection (Bradyzoite Stage)

Coincident with the onset of immunity, slowly multiplying bradyzoite forms develop and form large (10–50 μm) tissue cysts, especially in muscle, brain, and visceral tissues. There is minimal host response to these cysts, and they can persist in this dormant form for the life of the chronic carrier animal. They usually do not cause any clinical signs except in the rare instances when they rupture within the central nervous system (CNS) or eye or when the infection reactivates to an acute stage because of immunosuppression.

▼ *Key Point* In carnivores such as the cat, the principal source of infection is ingestion of *Toxoplasma* in the cyst stage, which is found in the meat of chronically infected food-producing animals, small mammals, and birds.

Clinical Signs

Clinical toxoplasmosis is recognized more frequently in cats than in dogs, but the spectrum of signs is similar for both species.

- Nonspecific signs of anorexia, depression, and fever (often >104°F and unresponsive to antibiotics) are common.
- Other signs are determined mostly by the site and extent of injury from extraintestinal dissemination. The most commonly affected organs are lung, eyes, brain, liver, and skeletal muscle.
- Clinical signs can occur at the time of initial infection (acute or primary toxoplasmosis) or from reactivation of encysted infection (chronic or secondary toxoplasmosis) caused by an underlying immunosuppressive condition.
- Clinical toxoplasmosis is most severe and usually fatal in neonatal kittens infected transplacentally.

▼ *Key Point* Most animals with toxoplasmosis are asymptomatic and have only serologic evidence of infection. It is estimated that up to 30% of cats in the United States have *Toxoplasma* antibodies, with the highest prevalence in free-roaming and feral cats that hunt for their food.

Ocular Signs

Uveitis (iridocyclitis, chorioretinitis) is one of the most common forms and can cause aqueous flare, keratic precipitates, hypopyon, glaucoma, lens luxation, retinal detachment, or fundic lesions (see Chaps. 155 and 157).

Respiratory Signs

Acute necrotizing pneumonia is common and can cause progressive dyspnea.

Neuromuscular Signs

- Encephalomyelitis can cause seizures, ataxia, tremors, paresis/paralysis, and cranial nerve deficits, depending on location of the lesions within the CNS.
- Myositis can cause hyperesthesia, stiff gait, and muscle atrophy.

Hepatic and Digestive Tract Signs

- Hepatitis and cholangiohepatitis can cause anorexia, vomiting, diarrhea, jaundice, and ascites.
- Pancreatitis can cause anorexia, vomiting, abdominal pain, and jaundice.
- Enterocolitis can cause vomiting and diarrhea.
- Mesenteric lymphadenitis can cause palpable abdominal lymph nodes.

Cardiac Signs

Myocarditis can cause cardiac arrhythmias or heart failure.

Reproductive Signs

Transplacental infection can cause birth of stillborn kittens or kittens that die of neonatal toxoplasmosis of the lung, liver, and CNS.

Diagnosis

▼ *Key Point* Because toxoplasmosis often is an opportunistic disease associated with immunosuppression, consider underlying factors such as feline immunodeficiency virus, feline leukemia virus, feline infectious peritonitis, hemobartonellosis, canine distemper, and glucocorticoid or antitumor therapy.

Hematology and Serum Chemistries

- Any of the forms can cause leukopenia with degenerative left shift (in acute disease) or neutrophilic leukocytosis. Nonregenerative anemia, lymphocytosis, and eosinophilia also can occur.
- Hepatitis can cause elevated serum bilirubin, liver enzymes, and bile acids.
- Pancreatitis can cause elevated serum amylase, lipase, or trypsin-like immunoreactivity.

- Myositis can cause elevated muscle enzymes (e.g., CK, AST).

Radiography

- The pulmonary form can cause generalized coalescing, patchy alveolar and interstitial pulmonary infiltrates, and mild pleural effusion.
- Abdominal forms can cause abdominal effusion and hepatomegaly.

Cerebrospinal Fluid (CSF) Analysis

- CSF protein may be normal or increased to 149 mg/dl.
- CSF nucleated cell count is usually mildly increased (maximum in one report was 28 cells/ml) with a predominance of lymphocytes.
- *Toxoplasma* antibodies can be measured in CSF (see under Serology).

Serology

For the most complete assessment of disease activity, evaluate immunoglobulin (Ig) M, IgG, and antigen simultaneously on a single serum sample.*

IgM Titer

IgM titers are determined by enzyme-linked immunosorbent assay (ELISA).

- IgM titer rises initially at 1 to 2 weeks after exposure (coincides with usual onset of signs) and persists for less than 12 weeks in most cats, thereby paralleling disease activity.
- *Interpretation:* IgM titer of 1:256 or greater suggests active or recent infection.
- A prolonged positive IgM titer may be associated with reactivation of chronic infection or delayed antibody class shift from IgM to IgG caused by concurrent feline immunodeficiency virus infection or glucocorticoid therapy.

▼ *Key Point* The serum IgM *Toxoplasma* antibody titer is the serologic test of choice for diagnosis of active or recent infection.

IgG Titer

Various serologic methods may be used to measure IgG titers.

- IgG titer rises initially at 2 to 4 weeks after exposure and usually persists for more than 1 year; thus, a single positive IgG titer does not distinguish previous infection from current active infection.
- *Interpretation:* A fourfold rise in the IgG titer in paired specimens over a 2- to 3-week period is indicative of active infection. Both must be measured together in the same test run on the same day to avoid variation.

*Available at Veterinary Diagnostic Laboratory, College of Veterinary Medicine, Colorado State University, Fort Collins, CO 80523 (Tel. 970-491-1281); and at Infectious Disease Laboratory, College of Veterinary Medicine, University of Georgia, Athens, GA 30602 (Tel. 706-542-5812).

- Polymerase chain reaction (PCR) has been evaluated on a limited number of cats for diagnosis of toxoplasmosis.

▼ *Key Point* A single high serum IgG *Toxoplasma* antibody titer is NOT diagnostic of active infection, no matter how high the titer level.

Antibody Titers in CSF and Aqueous Humor

- To evaluate local production of *Toxoplasma*-specific antibodies in animals with encephalitis or uveitis, measure *Toxoplasma* IgM and IgG titers in CSF or aqueous humor, respectively.
- Simultaneously measure *Toxoplasma* serum titers and compare with serum and CSF or aqueous titers of another agent (e.g., calicivirus [FCV] in cats) in order to distinguish true local production of *Toxoplasma* antibodies from passive vascular barrier leakage. Local production and a diagnosis of toxoplasmosis is indicated by a coefficient greater than 1 and especially when greater than 8, calculated as:

$$\frac{\text{Toxo CSF titer}}{\text{Toxo serum titer}} \times \frac{\text{FCV (or other agent) serum titer}}{\text{FCV (or other agent) CSF titer}}$$

Toxoplasma *Antigen Detection*

- Antigen testing becomes positive initially 1 to 4 weeks after exposure and then remains intermittently positive for up to 1 year. This does not distinguish active from past infection and thus has no advantage over antibody titers.

Identification of Toxoplasma Organisms

Detection of Tachyzoites

- Characteristic intracellular inclusions can be identified in aspirate and impression smear cytologies stained routinely or in biopsies.
- Specimens to consider include lung bronchoalveolar lavage [BAL], liver, lymph nodes, body cavity fluids, and cerebrospinal fluid.
- *Disadvantage:* Tachyzoites are often sparse and difficult to find; thus, sensitivity of detection is generally low. However, in experimentally infected cats BAL was an effective method of diagnosis.

Detection of Oocysts in Feces

- The best method for detection is Sheather's sugar centrifugation-flotation:
  - Sheather's solution: 500 g table sugar, 320 ml distilled water, and 6.5 g phenol crystals melted in hot water bath.
  - Make a fecal suspension with 5–10 grams of feces and water, then centrifuge 1 part fecal suspension with 2 parts Sheather's solution for 10 minutes at 1000 g and examine 1–2 drops from the meniscus.
- *Disadvantages:* Oocysts are small, easily overlooked, and morphologically indistinguishable from certain other coccidia (*Hammondia* spp, *Besnoitia* spp) without specialized animal inoculation studies. The

period of oocyst shedding does not usually coincide with when clinical signs occur.

- Nevertheless, assume coccidian oocysts 10 × 12 μm in size in feline feces to be *Toxoplasma* until proved otherwise.

▼ *Key Point* Detection of fecal oocysts is not a reliable diagnostic test for toxoplasmosis because oocyst shedding occurs only briefly and usually ends before clinical signs begin.

Treatment

Although it is estimated that approximately 60% of animals with clinical illness due to toxoplasmosis recover with treatment, no therapy is consistently effective; thus, the prognosis is guarded. Mortality rate is highest in neonates and in animals that are severely immunosuppressed. Antitoxoplasma drugs include clindamycin, sulfonamides, pyrimethamine, trimethoprim-sulfa, doxycycline, and newer macrolides (azithromycin, clarithromycin).

▼ *Key Point* Clindamycin is the treatment of choice for toxoplasmosis.

Clindamycin

- *Dosage:* Antirobe (Upjohn), 25 to 50 mg/kg per day, divided into two or three doses, PO or IM, for at least 2 weeks beyond remission (2–4 weeks).
- *Actions:* inhibits replication of *Toxoplasma;* effective for treatment of clinical disease and for reducing oocyst shedding; penetrates the blood-brain and blood-eye barriers.
- *Side effects:* anorexia, vomiting, and diarrhea; these are dose-dependent and can be controlled by discontinuing treatment for 24 hours, then reinstituting at a lower dosage.

Adjunct Therapy for Uveitis

- 1% prednisone drops, topically, every 6 to 8 hours for 2 weeks

Prevention

▼ *Key Point* The question often is raised, how dangerous is a healthy pet cat with a positive *Toxoplasma* antibody titer? Because oocyst shedding is usually over by the time the titer rises and because reinfection of an immune cat usually results in little or no shedding, a cat with a positive titer poses less of a danger to its owner than an antibody-negative (nonimmune) cat.

Prevention in Cats

- Do not feed cats raw meat, viscera, or bones, or allow them to scavenge these from garbage.
- Do not allow cats to ingest raw (unpasteurized) milk, especially from goats.
- Do not allow cats to roam free where they can hunt prey (mice, birds) for food.

- Do not allow cats to eat mechanical vectors (cockroaches, flies, earthworms).

Prevention in Humans

▼ *Key Point* Pregnant women and severely immunocompromised people should avoid contact with soil, cat feces or litter, and raw meat.

- Do not eat raw or undercooked meat (cook meat to 150°F to kill *Toxoplasma*).
- Wash hands and all materials (e.g., cutting boards, sink tops, knives) that come in contact with raw meat.
- Boil water before drinking if the source is questionable.
- Empty litter box daily (24 hours or more are required for fecal oocysts to sporulate and become infectious) and disinfect with boiling or scalding water.
- Wear gloves when gardening; wash garden vegetables thoroughly before eating in case soil is contaminated with *Toxoplasma* oocysts.
- Keep sandboxes covered when not in use so that cats cannot defecate in them.
- Control the stray cat population to reduce oocyst contamination of the environment (cats that defecate in the soil are likely to be the same cats that must hunt for their food and thereby have a high risk of infection).
- To reduce entry of *Toxoplasma* into the food chain, prevent cats from roaming where food-producing animals and their food are kept.

▼ *Key Point* Because of the way cats defecate, bury their feces, and keep their haircoats clean, transmission of *Toxoplasma* oocysts to humans by touching and caring for a pet cat is unlikely.

NEOSPOROSIS

Etiology

Neospora caninum is a coccidian parasite that resembles *Toxoplasma* in tissues. Its full life cycle is not known. Oral transmission through carnivorousness can occur; however, transplacental transmission is considered to be the predominant route. Natural infections have been seen in dogs, and cats have been infected experimentally. The definitive host is probably the dog and other infected animals (especially cattle) are intermediate hosts.

Clinical Signs

Multifocal, progressive neuromuscular signs predominate as a result of nonsuppurative encephalomyelitis, polyradiculoneuritis, and fibrosing polymyositis. These signs can include ascending paralysis, stiffness, muscle atrophy and contracture, and dysphagia. Phlebitis and dermatitis also have been seen.

- Less common manifestations include myocarditis (arrhythmias), pneumonia (fever, dyspnea, cough), ulcerative/pruritic dermatitis, chorioretinitis, and multifocal intra-abdominal dissemination (hepatitis, pancreatitis).

- Neospora also may cause in utero or neonatal puppy mortality.

Diagnosis

- Muscle involvement may cause increased serum levels of muscle enzymes (CK, AST) and abnormal electromyographic findings (see Chap. 149).
- Cerebrospinal fluid (CSF) shows a moderately increased protein (20–150 mg/dl) and increased leukocytes (10–100 cells/μl) composed of a mixture of small and large mononuclear cells and neutrophils.
- *Neospora* does not cross-react on serologic tests for *Toxoplasma*.
- A presumptive diagnosis can be based on indirect FA or ELISA serum antibody titers of greater than 200. *Neospora* organisms may be detected in CSF or biopsies of infected tissues.

Treatment and Prevention

Information on effective treatment or prevention is limited. In vitro assays have shown similar drug susceptibility patterns as Toxoplasma; thus, treat with clindamycin as for toxoplasmosis, either alone or in combination with trimethoprim-sulfonamide (15–20 mg/kg PO q12h) or pyrimethamine (1 mg/kg PO q24h) and sulfonamide (15–30 mg/kg PO q12h).

- Neospora infection has a large economic impact in cattle as a cause of abortion. Prevent contamination with dog feces of food and water for cattle.

OTHER PROTOZOAL INFECTIONS

Other multisystemic protozoal infections are summarized in Table 19–1.

SUPPLEMENTAL READINGS

Toxoplasmosis and Neosporosis

Dubey JP, Carpenter JL: Histologically confirmed clinical toxoplasmosis in cats: 100 cases (1952–1990). J Am Vet Med Assoc 203:1556, 1993.

Dubey JP: Toxoplasmosis and other coccidial infections. In: Sherding RG (ed): The Cat: Diseases and Clinical Management. (2nd ed). New York: Churchill Livingstone, 1994, p 565.

Dubey JP, Greene CE, Lappin MR: Toxoplasmosis and neosporosis. In: Greene CE (ed): Infectious Diseases of the Dog and Cat. (2nd ed). Philadelphia: WB Saunders, 1998, p 493.

Lappin MR, Greene CE, Prestwood AK, et al: Diagnosis of recent *Toxoplasma gondii* infection in cats by the use of an enzyme-linked immunosorbent assay for immunoglobulin M. Am J Vet Res 50:1580, 1989.

Lappin MR, Greene CE, Winston S, et al: Clinical feline toxoplasmosis: Serologic diagnosis and therapeutic management of 15 cases. J Vet Intern Med 3:139, 1989.

Leishmaniasis

Slappendel RJ, Ferrer L: Leishmaniasis. In: Greene CE (ed): Infectious Diseases of the Dog and Cat. (2nd ed). Philadelphia: WB Saunders, 1998, p 450.

Trypanosomiasis (Chagas Disease)

Barr SC: American trypanosomiasis. In: Greene CE (ed): Infectious Diseases of the Dog and Cat. (2nd ed). Philadelphia: WB Saunders, 1998, p 445.

Meurs KM, Anthony MA, Slater M, Miller MW: Chronic *Trypanosoma cruzi* infection in dogs: 11 cases (1987–1996). J Am Vet Med Assoc 213:497, 1998.

Hepatozoonosis

Craig TM: Hepatozoonosis. In: Greene CE (ed): Infectious Diseases of the Dog and Cat. (2nd ed). Philadelphia: WB Saunders, 1998, p 458.

Babesiosis

Tobada J: Babesiosis. In: Greene CE (ed): Infectious Diseases of the Dog and Cat. (2nd ed). Philadelphia: WB Saunders, 1998, p 473.

Cytauxzoonosis

Kier AB, Greene CE: Cytauxzoonosis. In: Greene CE (ed): Infectious Diseases of the Dog and Cat. (2nd ed). Philadelphia: WB Saunders, 1998, p 470.

Wagner JE, Kier AB: Cytauxzoonosis. In: Barlough JE (ed): Manual of Small Animal Infectious Diseases. New York: Churchill Livingstone, 1988, p 391.

Encephalitozoonosis

Didier PJ, Didier ES, Snowden K, Shadduck JA: Encephalitozoonosis. In: Greene CE (ed): Infectious Diseases of the Dog and Cat. (2nd ed). Philadelphia: WB Saunders, 1998, p 495.

Acanthamebiasis

Greene CE: Acanthamebiasis. In: Greene CE (ed): Infectious Diseases of the Dog and Cat. (2nd ed). Philadelphia: WB Saunders, 1998, p 491.

Pneumocystosis

Greene CE, Chandler FW: Pneumocystosis. In: Greene CE (ed): Infectious Diseases of the Dog and Cat. (2nd ed). Philadelphia: WB Saunders, 1998, p 524.

Table 19–1. SYSTEMIC PROTOZOAN INFECTIONS OF THE DOG AND CAT

Diseases	Etiology (Source)	Endemic Locations	Clinical Signs	Diagnosis	Treatment
Leishmaniasis	*Leishmania* spp (sandfly vector; bloodborne)	Southwest U.S. (rarely: Texas, Oklahoma), Mediterranean region, Central and South America, Asia, Africa	*Disease primarily in dogs:* Chronic diffuse skin hyperkeratosis (dry scaling), dry brittle haircoat, skin nodules, mucocutaneous ulcers, fever, muscle atrophy, weakness, cachexia, anorexia, inactivity, vomiting, diarrhea, lymphadenopathy, splenomegaly, uveitis, conjunctivitis, bleeding (epistaxis, melena), immune disease (glomerulonephritis, systemic lupus, hemolytic anemia, polyarthritis).	*General:* Endemic region, hyperglobulinemia, hypoalbuminemia, proteinuria, azotemia, elevated serum liver enzymes, anemia, positive autoimmune tests (Coombs test, antinuclear antibody, LE cell test). *Specific:* —Identify organisms by cytology (lymph node, bone marrow, spleen, liver). —PCR test. —Serology: not as sensitive or specific.	*Caution:* Zoonotic with public health risks. *Investigational per CDC:* —Meglumine antimonate (Glucantime; Rhône-Merieux):100 mg/kg; IV, SC, q24h for 1 mo. —Sodium stibogluconate (Pentostam; Glaxo Wellcome): 30–50 mg/kg; IV, SC, q24h for 1 mo. —Allopurinol: 6–8 mg/kg; PO, q8h *Prognosis:* Fair to good for remission but guarded to poor for cure.
American trypanosomiasis (Chagas disease)	*Trypanosoma cruzi* (reduviid "kissing" bug vector; bloodborne)	Southern U.S. (rarely), Central and South America	*Disease primarily in dogs:* Acute myocarditis (fever, weakness, sudden collapse, fatal tachyarrhythmias); chronic cardiomyopathy (after 1–3 years—heart failure, ascites, pleural effusion, edema); lymphadenopathy, splenomegaly, meningoencephalitis.	*General:* Endemic region, abnormal cardiac evaluations (radiographic, electrocardiographic, echocardiographic). *Specific:* —Identify organisms in blood (direct or buffy coat smear) or lymph node aspirates. —Serology: positive in active or past infection.	*Caution:* Zoonotic with public health risks. *Investigational per CDC:* —Nifurtimox (Lampit; Bayer): 2–7 mg/kg, PO,q6h for 3–5 mo. —Benznidazole: 5 mg/kg, PO, q24h for >2 mo. *Prognosis:* Poor.
Hepatozoonosis	*Hepatozoon canis* (tickborne)	U.S. (Texas, Oklahoma, Louisiana), Brazil, Europe, Asia, Africa	*Disease primarily in dogs:* Episodic fever, cachexia, chronic myositis and periosteal bone proliferation (reluctance to move, generalized muscle pain and atrophy), bloody diarrhea, nasoocular discharge.	*General:* Endemic region, mild anemia, neutrophilic leukocytosis, widespread periosteal bone proliferation. *Specific:* Identify organisms in blood smear (in WBC) or in muscle biopsy (most reliable test).	*Palliative:* aspirin. *Efficacy unproven:* —Diminazene aceturate (Berenil 10%; Ganaseg), 3.5 mg/kg, IM, once. —Imidocarb dipropionate, (Imizol; Glaxo Wellcome), 5–6 mg/kg, SC/IM, once. —Primaquine phosphate, 0.5 mg/kg, SC, once. —Toltrazuril (Baycox; Bayer) 5mg/kg, PO, q12h for 5 days *Prognosis:* Poor (response but no cure). *Table continued on following page*

Table 19–1. SYSTEMIC PROTOZOAN INFECTIONS OF THE DOG AND CAT *CONTINUED*

Diseases	Etiology (Source)	Endemic Locations	Clinical Signs	Diagnosis	Treatment
Babesiosis	*Babesia* spp. (tick vector; bloodborne)	*Dog: B. canis, B. gibsoni* (U.S. and worldwide) *Cat: B. felis,* etc. (Africa, Asia, South America)	Hemolytic anemia (pallor, depression, weakness, jaundice, hemoglobinuria, fever, splenomegaly), weight loss, subclinical carrier.	*General:* Regenerative anemia (often Coombs' positive), thrombocytopenia. *Specific:* —Identify organisms in Giemsa-stained smears of capillary blood (from ear or toenail) or splenic aspirate. —Serology: IFA titer >1:80 is positive.	*Dogs:* —Diminazene aceturate (Berenil 10%; Ganaseg), 3.5 mg/kg, IM, once, then repeat in 14 days. —Phenamidine isethionate (Oxopirvedene, Merial), 15 mg/kg, SC, q24h × 2 days. —Imidocarb dipropionate (Imizol; Glaxo Wellcome), 5 mg/kg, SC or IM, once. *Cats:* —Primaquine phosphate, 0.5 mg/kg, IM, once. *Prognosis:* Good but relapses are common.
Cytauxzoonosis	*Cytauxzoon felis* (tick vector; bloodborne)	U.S. (south central and southeastern states)	*Disease in cats only:* Anorexia, depression, high fever, anemia, jaundice, congestion and edema of lungs, spleen, liver, shock, death in less than 1 week.	*General:* free-roaming in a wooded area. *Specific:* Indentify organism in blood smear (ring-shaped RBC inclusions) or cytology of bone marrow, lymph node, or spleen.	—Imidocarb dipropionate (Imizol) 5mg/kg, IM, 2 doses 14 days apart. —Diminazene aceturate (Berenil) 2 mg/kg, IM, 2 doses 7 days apart. *Prognosis:* Poor.
Encephalitozoonosis	*Encephalitozoon cuniculi* (oronasal exposure to urine spores or ingestion of infected tissues)	U.S. (rarely), Europe, South Africa	*Neonatal disease in kennels:* stunted growth, acute nephritis (renal failure) and encephalitis (depression, muscle spasms, ataxia, seizures, blindness, aggression, paralysis).	*General:* Nonregenerative anemia, azotemia, pyuria, hematuria, elevated CSF protein and mononuclear cells. *Specific:* —Identify spores in gramstained urine sediment. —Serology: IFA or ELISA —PCR	No treatment known.
Acanthamebiasis	*Acanthamoeba* spp (water, sewage, soil)	U.S. (very rare; epizootics seen in greyhounds)	*Disease in dogs only:* Pneumonia (fever, cough, dyspnea, nasoocular discharge), encephalitis (ataxia, seizures); mimics canine distemper.	Leukopenia; no diagnostic test available (identify organisms in lung biopsies).	No established treatment protocol. Trimethoprim-sulfonamide: 30 mg/kg, PO, q12h
Pneumocystosis	*Pneumocystis carinii* (airborne)	Worldwide (very rare)	*Disease in dogs only:* Acute or chronic pneumonia in immunocompromised dogs (nonfebrile, exercise intolerance, dyspnea, mild cough, weight loss).	*General:* Neutrophilic leukocytosis, diffuse radiographic alveolar and interstitial lung densities. *Specific:* Identify organisms in lung cytology or biopsies (Giemsa and methenamine silver stains).	Trimethoprim-sulfa, 15 mg/kg, PO, q8h for 3 wks. Pentamidine isethionate (Lomidine; Merial): 4 mg/kg; IV or IM; q24hr for 3 wks *Prognosis:* Fair to guarded.

LE, lupus erythematosus; PCR, polymerase chain reaction; IFA, indirect fluorescent antibody; ELISA, enzyme-linked immunosorbent assay; WBC, white blood cell; RBC, red blood cell; CDC, Centers for Disease Control and Prevention.

3 Hematology/Oncology

Rodney L. Page

Chapter 20 Erythrocytes, Leukocytes, and Platelets

Rose E. Raskin

ERYTHROCYTE DISORDERS

Anemia—Overview

Anemia is characterized by a reduction in the number of erythrocytes or in hemoglobin content or in both. It is one of the most frequent hematologic abnormalities encountered in practice. Anemia is not a disease, but rather the reflection of a disease state. Causes of anemia may be divided into three general categories: blood loss, hemolysis, and decreased erythrocyte production.

▼ *Key Point* Determine the cause of the anemia before giving supportive treatment.

Clinical Signs

- The patient may present with lethargy, weakness, anorexia, heart murmur, dyspnea, and pale or icteric mucous membranes.
- Occasionally, the animal may appear normal, but routine blood evaluation before an elective surgical procedure may uncover the abnormality.
- Sedentary animals, especially cats, often have moderate anemias that go unnoticed for long periods.
- Splenomegaly frequently accompanies anemia as a response to increased extravascular hemolysis or extramedullary hematopoiesis.

General Diagnostic Considerations

Several tests can be used to document and characterize the anemia morphologically or by etiology.

History and Physical Examination

These should determine the following:
- Occurrence of trauma or surgery
- Drug, chemical, or toxin exposure
- Underlying infectious, parasitic, or neoplastic disease
- Duration of disease, sites of blood loss, and presence of organomegaly

Complete Blood Count (Table 20–1)

- Packed cell volume (PCV) is the most accurate and least expensive method of documenting anemia. Spin hematocrit tubes 5 minutes at 12,000 to 15,000 × G. Evaluate plasma color after centrifugation.
- Determine plasma protein or total solids by refractometer.
- Erythrocyte count usually is performed by an automated cell counter. This value is necessary for calculation of the erythrocyte indices.
- Hemoglobin concentration (Hgb) is determined most accurately by the cyanmethemoglobin method, using a colorimeter or spectrophotometer. Artifactual increases may occur with gross lipemia or an excessive number of Heinz bodies, both of which produce light interference.

Table 20–1. HEMATOLOGY REFERENCE RANGES FOR DOGS AND CATS*

Parameter	Canine	Feline
PCV (%)	37–54	30–47
Hgb (g/dl)	13–19	9–15
Erythrocyte ($\times 10^6/\mu$l)	5.4–7.8	5.8–10.7
MCV (fl)	64–74	41–51
MCH (pg)	22–27	13–18
MCHC (g/dl)	34–36	31–35
Reticulocytes ($\times 10^3/\mu$l)	<80	<30 Aggregate <500 Punctate
Platelets ($\times 10^3/\mu$l)	160–430	300–800
WBC (/μl)	6,000–17,000	5,500–19,500
Segmented neutrophils (/μl)	3,000–11,500	2,500–12,500
Band neutrophils (/μl)	0–300	0–300
Lymphocytes (/μl)	1,000–4,800	1,500–7,500
Monocytes (/μl)	150–1350	0–850
Eosinophils (/μl)	100–1250	0–1500
Basophils (/μl)	<100	<100
Plasma protein (g/dl)	6.0–7.8	6.2–8.0
Fibrinogen (mg/dl)	100–400	100–300

PCV, packed cell volume; Hgb, hemoglobin; MCV, mean corpuscular volume; MCH, mean corpuscular hemoglobin; MCHC, mean corpuscular hemoglobin concentration; WBC, white blood cell.

*These values are only meant as a guide; individual laboratories may vary in their ranges, depending on instrumentation and regional differences.

Source: University of Florida, Veterinary Clinical Pathology Laboratory.

- Mean corpuscular volume (MCV) may be determined directly by the automated cell counters or calculated as follows:

$$MCV \text{ (femtoliters)} = \frac{PCV \times 10}{\text{erythrocyte}(10^6/\mu l)}$$

The MCV reflects erythrocyte size and may be categorized as *macrocytic,* suggesting increased red cell turnover; as *microcytic,* suggesting defective cell growth; or as *normocytic* (unchanging cell size). Note that the Japanese Akita normally has microcytic erythrocytes.

- Other erythrocyte indices (mean corpuscular hemoglobin [MCH]; mean corpuscular hemoglobin concentration [MCHC]) help to classify the types of anemia into *normochromic* and *hypochromic.* Decreased levels reflect the presence of reticulocytes or abnormal hemoglobinization. Increased levels occur artifactually from hemolysis.
- Blood smear evaluation involves quantitation of changes in size *(anisocytosis),* shape *(poikilocytosis),* and color *(polychromasia).* The presence of immature nucleated forms and basophilic stippling often signal abnormal erythropoiesis or defective circulation of erythrocyte precursors. Infectious parasites and Heinz bodies often require careful examination of the smear.

▼ *Key Point* The most important part of the complete blood count (CBC) is an evaluation of the blood smear for morphologic abnormalities.

Reticulocyte Count

- This is the most accurate method to evaluate regeneration. Counts are recommended when PCV falls below 30% in dogs and 20% in cats.
- Incubate equal volumes of blood and 0.5% new methylene blue stain together for 15 to 20 minutes; then make a routine blood smear and count the number of aggregate and punctate forms per 1000 erythrocytes. Absolute numbers of reticulocytes per microliter are calculated by the following formula:

Absolute reticulocytes per microliter
$$= \frac{\% \text{ reticulocyte percentage} \times \text{erythrocyte}/\mu l}{100}$$

- Dogs normally have 0 to 1% reticulocytes (0–80,000/μl). In healthy cats, aggregated reticulocytes range from 0 to 0.4% (0–30,000/μl) and punctate reticulocytes are less than 5% (<500,000/μl). Aggregate reticulocytes represent the most active or recent form of regeneration in the dog and cat. Punctate reticulocytes in cats, which do not stain as polychromatophilic cells, represent regenerative attempts that occurred 2 to 4 weeks previously.
- By using the PCV instead of the erythrocyte count, a corrected reticulocyte percentage may be calculated as:

Corrected % reticulocytes
$$= \% \text{ reticulocytes} \times \frac{\text{patient's PCV}}{\text{normal PCV}}$$

Normal PCV is considered 45% for dogs and 35% for cats. A corrected percent reticulocyte value greater than 1% indicates increased RBC regeneration. Once initiated at the bone marrow level, regeneration may take at least 3 days before reticulocytes appear in the circulation.

Fecal Examination and Urinalysis

- These tests are performed to determine sources of blood loss and function of the kidney.

Biochemical Profile

- Biochemical profiles may reveal organic disease that can affect the ability to regenerate erythrocytes.

Bone Marrow Evaluation

- This is necessary whenever regenerative attempts appear diminished. Hemolytic conditions do not warrant marrow examination unless the response is less than normally expected. Results always must be compared with a recent CBC to determine the current status of regeneration.

▼ *Key Point* Bone marrow evaluation is best performed when both aspirate and core biopsies are taken together because each provides different information.

- This is a sterile procedure often performed with only local anesthesia; however, mild tranquilization or general anesthesia may be used if necessary.
- Sites frequently used in dogs include the dorsal ilium, humerus (best for obese animals), and femur (small dogs or puppies). Sites frequently used in cats include the femur, transilial, and dorsal ilium.
- *Aspiration biopsy* (special needles required*) is performed as follows:
    - Pass the needle with the stylet a few millimeters into the bone until it is firmly embedded.
    - Place a 12-ml syringe coated with 5% ethylenediaminetetraacetic acid (EDTA) solution onto the biopsy needle and collect 1 to 2 ml of bloody material.
    - Place the marrow material on a plastic Petri dish and pick up the glistening particles with a microhematocrit tube.
    - Gently blow this material out of the tube onto a glass slide.
    - Make a squash preparation by laying a second slide on the first and drawing them apart.
- *Core biopsy* (special needle required†) is performed using the following procedure:
    - Pass the needle with stylet through the skin and subcutaneous tissues.
    - Remove the stylet while advancing the needle 0.5 to 1.5 cm into the bone, depending on the size of the animal.
    - Twist the instrument sharply to cut the sample and withdraw the needle slowly.
    - Remove the core sample and roll it onto a glass slide for cytologic examination; then place the sample in 10% buffered formalin for histologic fixation.

Principles of Transfusion Therapy

Therapy depends on the etiology of the anemia. Rapid decreases in PCV warrant replacement of whole blood. However, slow daily decreases in PCV of 1 to 3% may not cause clinical signs of dyspnea or weakness.

Crossmatching

- Perform crossmatching before transfusion. The procedure, which involves collection of erythrocytes and serum or plasma from the donor and the patient, is as follows:
    - Wash erythrocytes and pellet three times in 0.9% saline.
    - Make a 4% cell suspension by adding 4.8 ml of saline to 0.2 ml of cells.
    - Measure compatibility between donor and patient optimally at three temperatures: 37°C, 20°C, and 4°C.

▼ *Key Point* Perform crossmatching prior to all blood transfusions to prevent incompatibility reactions.

---

*Illinois sternal disposable needle, 15 to 18 gauge, 1 to 2 inches long; Allegiance Healthcare, McGaw Park, IL.

†Jamshidi aspiration/biopsy disposable needle, 11–13 gauge, 2–4″ long; Allegiance Healthcare, McGaw Park, IL.

- Donors are incompatible if any agglutination or hemolysis occurs in the major crossmatch. The types of crossmatch are defined as:
    - *Major:* 100 μl donor cells + 100 μl patient serum/plasma
    - *Minor:* 100 μl patient cells + 100 μl donor serum/plasma
    - *Donor or patient controls:* 100 μl of donor or patient cells to 100 μl of donor or patient serum/plasma, respectively
- Under emergency conditions, donors may be used if mild agglutination occurs in the minor crossmatch. The crossmatching procedure is as follows:
    - After 15 minutes of incubation, centrifuge tubes at 280 × G for 1 minute.
    - Note any hemolysis in supernatant and gross agglutination of resuspended cells.
    - Place a small drop on glass slide and examine for microscopic agglutination.

Whole Blood Transfusion

- In dogs, this procedure is best performed using animals negative for DEA-1 and DEA-7 blood types. Although most cats have type A blood, it is best to crossmatch blood, because as little as 1 ml of mismatched blood can cause a fatal transfusion reaction in cats.
- Estimated dosage is 10 to 20 ml/kg in dogs or cats, with a maximum of 40 ml in an adult cat. A more specific guideline for the amount of donor blood in anticoagulant (ml) is:

$$kg \times 80 \ (dog) \ or \ 60 \ (cat) \times [desired \ PCV - patient \ PCV] \div donor \ PCV$$

- When performing whole blood transfusion, use appropriate filters and administration sets to retain clotted blood or debris.
- Warm blood before administration.
- For the first 30 minutes, keep initial rate of administration slow (0.25 ml/kg) to observe any incompatibility reactions (recommended rate of whole blood infusion in general is 10 ml/kg/hour). The rate of infusion depends on the hydration status of the patient.
- Evaluate hematocrit before and after transfusion:
    - To document relative improvement
    - To screen for hemolysis as an indicator of incompatibility.

Blood component therapy is described in Chapter 21.

Blood Loss Anemia

Large volumes of blood must be lost before appreciable changes occur in the numbers of erythrocytes or PCV. The immediate loss of blood results in little or no change to the PCV, owing to the concurrent loss of erythrocytes and plasma fluids. Over the course of several hours to days, redistribution of fluids occurs, resulting in a lowered PCV and plasma protein. Depending on the amount of blood lost and the time period over which it is lost, regenerative responses may range from moderate to extremely weak. Chronic blood loss causes decreased iron stores, resulting in decreased erythrocyte production.

Etiology

Causes of blood loss include

- Trauma
- Surgery
- External and internal parasitism
- Gastric ulcers
- Tumors of the gastrointestinal and urinary systems
- Splenic rupture
- Coagulation abnormalities

Treatment

Administer crossmatched whole blood for *acute* hemorrhage when the PCV drops to 20 to 25% in the dog or cat. Also consider autotransfusion if hemorrhage has occurred recently in a body cavity, and the blood is not contaminated with bacteria or neoplastic cells.

Hemolytic Anemia

A variety of causes are associated with hemolytic loss of erythrocytes. The net effect often is a very strong to moderate regenerative response (Fig. 20–1). However, in some cases, the anemia may occur so rapidly that the animal may have too little time to mount a regenerative response by the time the condition is recognized. A period of 2 to 3 days is necessary for erythrocyte maturation, once the stimulation from hypoxia or severe erythrocyte depletion has occurred. Depending on the severity or acuteness of the destruction and the conjugating ability of the liver, icterus may or may not

be present. Plasma protein concentrations usually are normal.

Causes of hemolytic anemia include congenital abnormalities, immune-mediated destruction, infections, chemical or toxic agents, mechanical fragmentation, and hypophosphatemia.

Congenital Erythrocyte Abnormalities

Pyruvate Kinase Deficiency

Pyruvate kinase deficiency is an erythrocyte enzyme deficiency associated with an autosomal recessive inheritance. During anaerobic glycolysis, pyruvate kinase is necessary for the production of adenosine triphosphate (ATP), which erythrocytes need to maintain their integrity and viability. The condition has been documented in several dog breeds, including the basenji, the beagle, the West Highland white terrier, and the Cairn terrier, in addition to Abyssinian cats. Young animals usually present with anemia, exercise intolerance, tachycardia, and splenomegaly. The outcome of the disease is usually death by 4 years of age. Myelofibrosis and osteosclerosis may occur, resulting in reduced hematopoiesis. Frequent erythrocyte destruction may lead to hemosiderosis and failure of organs such as the liver. Diagnosis of the disease is suggested clinically by the presence of an intense reticulocytosis (15–50%) along with frequent nucleated red cells in a young dog. Echinocytosis or erythrocytes with sharp projections unrelated to crenation may be seen in circulation. A genetic diagnostic test for pyruvate kinase deficiency is currently available for basenji dogs. Definitive diagnosis for other breeds requires a special erythrocyte assay for the enzyme.

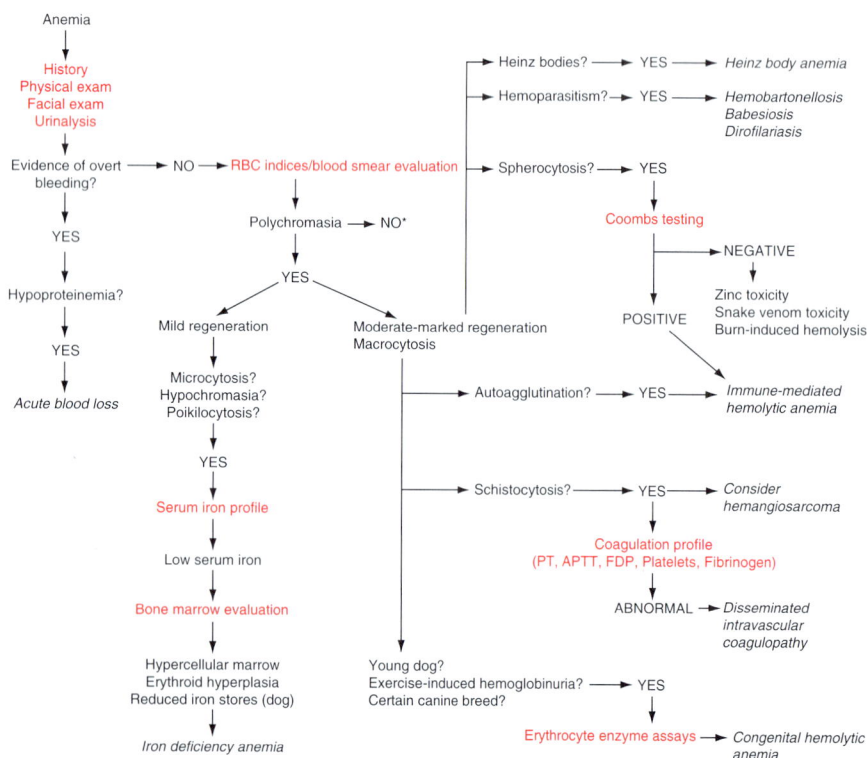

Figure 20–1. Diagnostic approach to common regenerative anemias in dogs and cats *See Figures 20–2 and 20–3. (PT, prothrombin time; APTT, activated partial thromboplastin time; FDP, fibrin degradation products).

Phosphofructokinase Deficiency

Phosphofructokinase deficiency has been identified in English Springer and American Cocker spaniel dogs as an autosomal recessive inheritance. This glycolytic enzyme deficiency causes a decrease in 2,3-diphospho-glycerate (2,3-DPG) concentration, resulting in an increase in intracellular pH. Erythrocytes from affected animals are especially fragile under alkaline conditions. Intravascular hemolysis may occur during hyperventilation-induced alkalemia, resulting in periodic bouts of hemoglobinuria and sometimes bilirubinuria. A constant state of hypoxia is produced by the low levels of 2,3-DPG, with subsequent increased oxygen binding to hemoglobin. The result is persistent reticulocytosis (10–30%) even though the PCV is normal or mildly decreased, except during hemolytic episodes. Clinical signs may involve lethargy, pale or icteric mucous membranes, mild hepatosplenomegaly, myopathy, and fever. Dogs may have a normal life span if properly managed. The enzyme deficiency is diagnosed by specialized erythrocyte assays in homozygous and heterozygous animals. A molecular diagnostic test recently has been developed to screen affected animals of any age.

Hereditary Stomatocytosis

Hereditary stomatocytosis is an autosomal recessive trait in Alaskan malamutes associated with chondrodysplasia. The defect may involve abnormalities of the cell membrane or of ion transport leading to increased water content and a larger cell size (96 fl). Dwarfism is recognized clinically, and there is a mild hemolytic anemia and slight reticulocytosis (2%). Erythrocyte numbers are reduced, but the PCV remains normal because of enlarged erythrocytes. Morphologically, some erythrocytes appear to have a slit- or mouth-like area of central pallor.

Feline Porphyria

Feline porphyria is an infrequent inheritable trait that results in an enzyme deficiency affecting heme synthesis. Clinical signs include pink urine, pinkish-brown teeth, and severe anemia resulting from the deposition of red nonheme pigments and the lysis of erythrocytes when exposed to sunlight. Discolored teeth often fluoresce red under ultraviolet light. Skin photosensitization can occur; therefore, exposure to sunlight should be avoided. The disease can be prevented by not breeding carrier animals.

Hereditary Nonspherocytic Hemolytic Anemia

Hereditary nonspherocytic hemolytic anemia is recognized in two breeds: poodles and beagles. Poodles develop an autosomal dominant condition that resembles pyruvate kinase deficiency, but decreases in this enzyme are not demonstrable. Affected animals have a persistent macrocytic hypochromic anemia (PCV of 13–31%) with moderate reticulocytosis. It is clinically evident by 1 year of age and fatal by 3 years of age. Myelofibrosis, osteosclerosis, and hemosiderosis are present at death. In beagles, the condition presents with chronic anemia and moderate reticulocytosis. The mode of inheritance is likely autosomal recessive. The disease is less severe in beagles than in poodles, and the disorder can remain subclinical for up to 4 years in affected dogs. In both breeds, erythrocytes are morphologically normal and enzyme activities are not affected. The short erythrocyte life span in beagles may be caused by an unidentified membrane abnormality.

Immune-Mediated Hemolytic Anemia

See the chapter on systemic immune-mediated disease (Chap. 22).

Infectious Causes of Hemolysis

Haemobartonellosis

Haemobartonellosis is caused by a mycoplasmal organism that infects the erythrocytes of dogs *(Hamobartonella canis)* and cats *(H. felis)*. It can be transmitted by ticks and fleas, or by queens to their newborn kittens in the absence of blood-sucking arthropods. Splenectomy (especially in the dog), immunosuppression caused by glucocorticoid therapy, or stress in cats with latent *H. felis* infection predispose to the development of clinical disease in the animal infected by the organism.

Clinical signs include those generally observed with anemia. Weight loss may occur if the anemia develops slowly, whereas acute, severe anemia produces sudden depression and icterus. Splenomegaly often is noted.

Laboratory findings generally reflect a strong regenerative response in the CBC. The absence of marked anisocytosis or polychromasia in confirmed cases of feline haemobartonellosis may suggest peracute infections with too little time to respond or concurrent infection with feline leukemia virus (FeLV) or feline immunodeficiency virus (FIV). Thin smears, made directly without anticoagulant, assist in finding the epicellular organisms. Blood films should be well stained without precipitate to minimize any confusion in identifying the parasite. Cats often have coccoid or ring shapes, whereas dogs mostly have linear chain forms. A positive Coombs test result may be associated with feline haemobartonellosis, presumably because of erythrocyte membrane alteration.

Treatment involves blood transfusion if the anemia is severe. Prednisolone (2 mg/kg, PO, every 12 hours) may be necessary initially to suppress the severe immune-mediated destruction of erythrocytes. Doxycycline is the treatment of choice at a dosage of 5 mg/kg PO q12h for dogs and 1–3 mg/kg PO q12h for cats, continued for 3 weeks. Tetracyclines can be given at a dose of 22 mg/kg PO every 8 hours for 3 weeks. Cats who recover may become latent carriers.

Babesiosis

Babesiosis is a tick-borne protozoal disease affecting erythrocytes of dogs *(Babesia canis, B. gibsoni)*. *Babesia felis* has not been reported in North American cats. Clinical signs of the acute disease include splenomegaly, icterus, anemia, thrombocytopenia, hemoglobinuria, and fever. It is common in kennel conditions and is associated especially with greyhounds.

Diagnosis is made by examination of a blood smear. A clear, teardrop-shaped organism in erythrocytes, sometimes seen in pairs, is the most common form that occurs in animals in the United States. An indirect fluorescent antibody (IFA) serum test is available. Concurrent infections with *Ehrlichia canis* may occur.

Treatment involves diminazene aceturate (Berenil, Hoechst) (3.5 mg/kg IM given once), imidocarb dipropionate 12% (Imizol, Mallinckrodt Veterinary, Inc.) (5 mg/kg IM given once), or phenamidine isethionate (15 mg/kg SC q24h for 2 days). These drugs are not approved for use in the United States and may be difficult to obtain.

Leptospirosis

Leptospirosis usually is associated with kidney disease (*Leptospira canicola*) or hemolysis, icterus, and coagulopathies (*L. icterohaemorrhagiae*). Toxins released from proliferating organisms interfere with cellular metabolism and damage cells. Clinical signs involve fever, anorexia, vomiting, depression initially, followed by icterus, mucosal hemorrhages, hemoglobinuria, and urinary inflammation. Diagnosis is based on demonstration of leptospires in the urine by darkfield microscopy or in the liver and kidney by histologic examination. Serologic testing of paired samples is also available. Treatment requires supportive care and antibiotics (see Chapter 17).

Chemical or Toxic Injury of Erythrocytes

Heinz Body Anemia

Heinz body anemia is produced by oxidant agents that cause precipitation of hemoglobin. Accelerated red cell destruction involves intravascular fragmentation or extravascular phagocytosis by the spleen. Chemicals, drugs, or plants associated with Heinz body formation include acetaminophen, methylene blue, onions, vitamin K_3, DL-methionine, zinc, topical benzocaine (e.g., Cetacaine) sprayed on the larynx to aid intubation, and propylene glycol. Heinz body formation in cats also has been associated with ketoacidosis in diabetic cats, hyperthyroidism, and lymphoma. Cats are predisposed to oxidant damage because of their hemoglobin structure.

Clinical signs occur acutely, such as depression, hemoglobinemia, hemoglobinuria, moderate to severe anemia, and occasional icterus.

Diagnosis is made by observation of a single, large, pale staining area in erythrocytes of Romanowsky-stained blood smears. They also may appear as a single blunt projection by the Heinz body bulging from the membrane surface. These structures appear as a dark blue spots when stained with new methylene blue in a direct wet mount procedure or after incubation of the stain with the blood. Erythrocyte refractile bodies are similar to Heinz bodies but are smaller, infrequent, and present in normal cats. Contrast these to many large Heinz bodies with signs of a regenerative response.

Treatment primarily involves removal of the source of oxidant. Emetics can be used if recent ingestion has occurred. Give blood transfusions or other forms of supportive care, as indicated. For acetaminophen-induced toxicity, give acetylcysteine (Mucomyst, Roxane Laboratories), 140 mg/kg of a 5% solution diluted with saline given IV as a loading dose; then give 70 mg/kg of a 5% solution every 4 hours for three to five treatments.

Snake Venom Toxicity

Snake venom toxicity has been recognized as a cause of hemolysis. Toxins, such as those produced from coral snakes, may be associated with spherocyte formation, in addition to neurologic and coagulation abnormalities. Diagnosis is based on the presence of a regenerative anemia and a bite wound with a history supporting recent exposure to a snake. For both coral snake and rattlesnake envenomation in dogs, a transient erythrocyte shape change of echinocytosis has been observed. Treatment involves use of a specific venom antidote and supportive care.

Zinc Toxicity

Zinc toxicity can produce intravascular hemolysis in dogs. Sources of the zinc include ingestion of galvanized wire or kennel cage nuts and pennies produced since 1983. Diagnosis involves presence of a regenerative anemia and proof of zinc exposure. Spherocytosis and Heinz bodies have been noted in some cases on blood smear evaluation. Radiograph the abdomen to identify metallic foreign bodies in the gastrointestinal tract and remove the source of zinc via surgery or endoscopy.

Mechanical Fragmentation of Erythrocytes

Heartworm Disease

Dirofilariasis may produce anemia after intravascular hemolysis as large numbers of adult heartworms (*Dirofilaria immitis*) obstruct blood flow, causing turbulence that mechanically disrupts erythrocytes. Clinical signs reflect the organs affected, such as the lungs, liver, or kidneys. A postcaval syndrome results from obstruction of the caudal vena cava causing, in addition to hepatic failure, erythrocyte fragmentation (schizocytosis), hemoglobinemia, and hemoglobinuria. Definitive diagnosis is based on detection of circulating microfilaria in the blood or on serologic detection of circulating antigens or antibodies (see Chapter 68).

Disseminated Intravascular Coagulopathy

Disseminated intravascular coagulopathy may cause a microangiopathic hemolytic anemia because of fibrin deposition that results from damage to small blood vessels. Mechanical fragmentation of erythrocytes appears in blood smears as schizocytes or spherocytes. The etiology involves a variety of conditions, such as neoplasia, infections, necrosis, toxins, and immune complex formation. These can lead to massive tissue destruction and activation of clotting pathways. Diagnosis is based on consumption of platelets (thrombocytopenia), reductions in clotting factors (prolonged prothrombin time [PT] and activated partial thromboplastin time

[APTT], hypofibrinogenemia), and increased amounts of fibrin degradation products. Treatment is aimed at the inciting condition (see Chapter 21).

Hypophosphatemia

Cases of feline diabetes mellitus and hepatic lipidosis have been associated with hypophosphatemia-induced hemolysis. Heinz body formation may play a role in the development of hemolytic anemia in these cases.

Nonregenerative Anemia

Nonregenerative anemia generally is related to direct toxicity of erythroid precursors in the bone marrow or secondary suppression of erythropoiesis (Fig. 20–2). Often neutrophils and platelets also are affected (Fig. 20–3). Reduction in erythrocytes, leukocytes, and platelets in circulation is termed *pancytopenia*. The term *aplastic anemia* is used to describe bone marrow failure involving the three cell lines that leads to peripheral pancytopenia. The bone marrow in this condition is severely hypoplastic, with total or near complete replacement of hematopoietic elements by adipose tissue. In contrast, crowding from abnormal cellular infiltrates can suppress hematopoiesis, producing *myelophthisis*. Chronic, nonregenerative anemias may not require blood transfusion until the PCV falls below 15% in the dog and 12% in the cat.

Causes of nonregenerative anemia include infectious agents, nutritional disturbances, organic disease, endocrine abnormalities, toxic agents, myelophthisis, irradiation, and immune-mediated destruction.

Infectious Agents

Feline Leukemia Virus (FeLV)

FeLV-associated anemia is usually normochromic and normocytic to macrocytic. Most cases are nonregenerative and related to suppression or destruction of erythroid progenitor cells. In addition, the virus affects the stromal microenvironment of the bone marrow coincidental with the development of anemia. Approximately 10% of the cases are hemolytic with regeneration related to immune destruction of erythrocytes.

Diagnosis is based on positive enzyme-linked immunosorbent assay (ELISA) or IFA test results. Bone marrow aspirate smears or core biopsy sections indicate decreased cellularity with increased fat infiltration when the infection is not associated with a proliferative leukemia.

Treatment varies depending on concurrent conditions such as neoplasia, haemobartonellosis, FIV, or feline infectious peritonitis (FIP). Supportive care, in the form of blood transfusions (see Principles of Transfusion section), antibiotics, appetite stimulants, and anabolic steroids, are often necessary (see Chapter 6).

Other Viruses

Other viruses, such as FIP, FIV, feline panleukopenia, canine parvovirus, and canine distemper, have been associated with suppression of erythropoiesis. The anemia is often mild to moderate and nonresponsive. Other cell lines, such as granulocytes or lymphocytes, are affected more severely. Diagnosis usually is determined by exposure history, clinical signs, virologic/serologic tests, characteristic histopathologic lesions, and identification of viral particles or inclusions within affected cells. In canine distemper, erythrocytes or leukocytes may contain one or more pale blue spots in the cytoplasm with Romanowsky-type stains. However, these inclusions stain a deep purple color with Diff-Quik.

Ehrlichiosis

Ehrlichiosis is a rickettsial disease caused by *Ehrlichia* spp. and transmitted by ticks. In dogs, it produces thrombocytopenia and a mild to moderate anemia as the most frequent hematologic abnormalities. Leukopenia and pancytopenia are less frequent findings and often occur late in the disease with monocytic ehrlichiosis. Diagnosis is based on positive or rising serum titers. Intracytoplasmic morulae are found infrequently in mononuclear cells or granulocytes, during the acute stage of the disease. Bone marrow, at this time, is often normocellular to hypercellular with increased numbers of megakaryocytes and plasma cells. Hyperglobulinemia, commonly as a polyclonal gammopathy or occasionally as a monoclonal gammopathy, often is noted. In the chronic or late stages of monocytic ehrlichiosis, bone marrow cellularity decreases severely, with fat replacing hematopoietic elements. Clinical ehrlichiosis in the cat may present as vague illness with nonregenerative anemia, fever, weight loss, lymphadenopathy, and hyperglobulinemia. Treatment is similar in both dog and cat, involving doxycycline (see Chapter 15).

Leishmaniasis

Leishmaniasis is an infrequent protozoal disease in dogs caused by *Leishmania* spp. The parasite, transmitted by sandflies, produces visceral or cutaneous manifestations. History usually indicates travel outside the United States to Greece, Spain, or Italy. An endemic focus in Oklahoma has been reported, as well as a research colony in Ohio. Clinical signs, which develop over months, include anorexia, weight loss, lymphadenopathy, and ulcerative dermatitis. Diagnosis often is made by cytology or histopathology. Organisms are present in macrophages of the bone marrow, lymph nodes, spleen, and liver. Serology and tissue culture are additional diagnostic aids. A mild to moderate normocytic, normochromic anemia may occur. Hyperglobulinemia presents rarely as a monoclonal gammopathy and accompanies the plasmacytosis found in tissues. The disease is zoonotic, and infected dogs can serve as a reservoir for human infection. Euthanasia should be considered. Treatment involves antimony compounds (as listed in Table 19–1 in Chapter 19), although these drugs may be difficult to obtain.

Cytauxzoonosis

Cytauxzoonosis is a highly fatal protozoal disease caused by *Cytauxzoon felis.* It is a tick-borne infection, most prevalent in the wooded areas of the southern United States. The bobcat is the natural reservoir host.

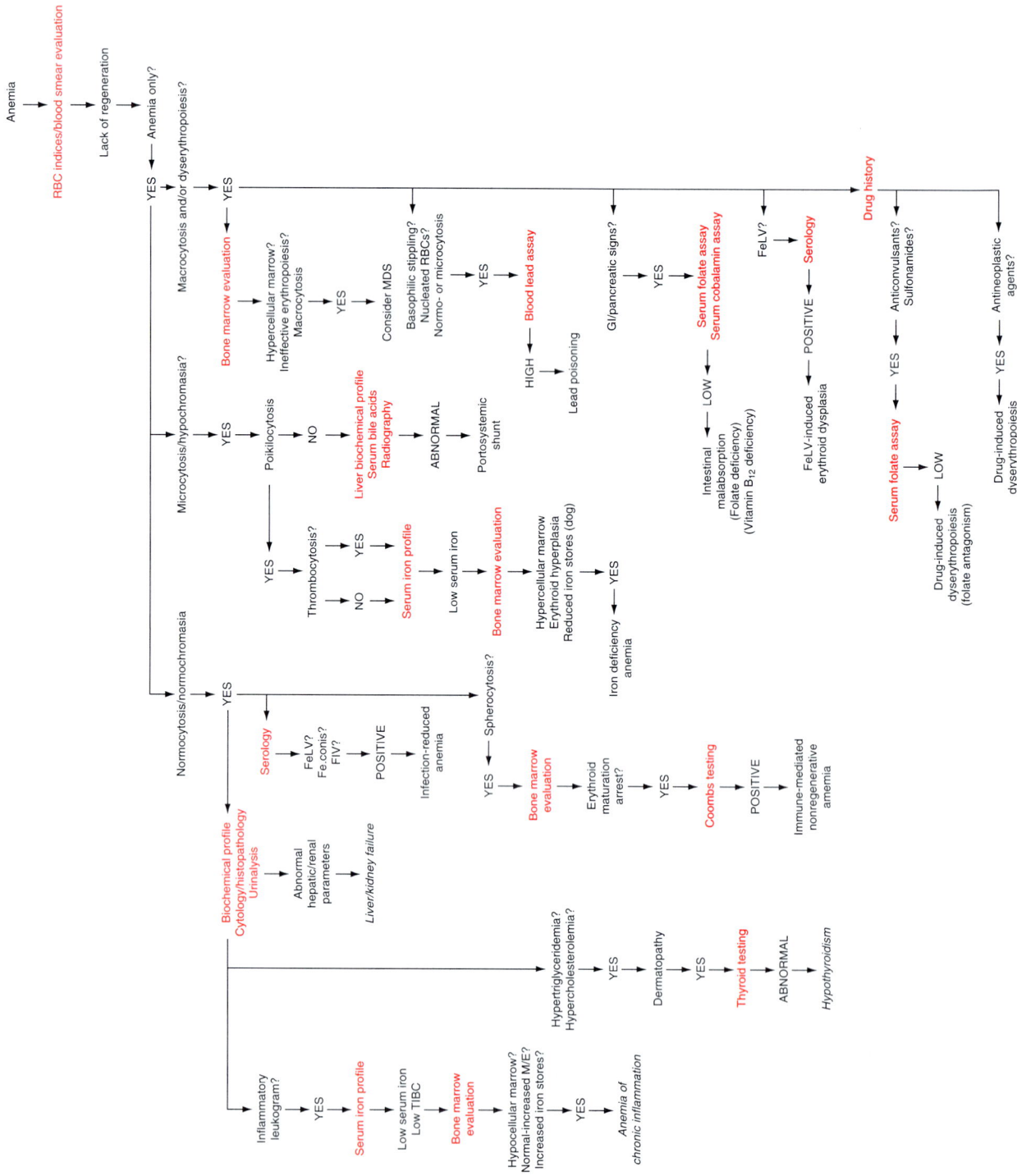

Figure 20-2. Diagnostic approach to common nonregenerative anemias in dogs and cats when only the erythrocyte line is involved. (TIBC, total iron-binding capacity; M/E, myeloid-to-erythroid ratio; FeLV, feline leukemia virus; FIV, feline immunodeficiency virus; MDS, myelodysplastic syndrome).

Anemia

↓

RBC indices
Blood smear evaluation

↓

Lack of regeneration?

↓

Cytopenia of >1 cell line? ⟶ YES ⟶ Further cytologic evaluation ⟶ Erythrocyte piroplasms?
                                                                      Tissue schizonts?

                               Bone marrow evaluation   ↓

⟶ Hypocellular?   YES

       ↓   ↓

      YES ⟶ History ⟶ Antibiotics?   Feline cytauxzoonosis
                        Anti-inflammatory drugs?
                        Estrogen-like compounds?
                        Antineoplastic agents?

                                        ↓

                                       YES ⟶ Drug-induced aplastic anemia

                        ⟶ Irradiation? ⟶ YES ⟶ Radiation-induced aplastic anemia

           ⟶ Serology ⟶ FeLV?
                         FIV?
                         Ehrlichia canis?
                         Canine distemper?

                              ↓

                         POSITIVE ⟶ Infection-induced aplastic anemia

           ⟶ Surgery/histopathology ⟶ Ovarian/testicular neoplasia?

⟶ Myelophthisis?   YES ⟶ Estrogen-induced aplastic anemia

       ↓

      YES ⟶ Fibrosis? ⟶ YES ⟶ Myelofibrosis
          ⟶ Necrosis? ⟶ YES ⟶ Myelonecrosis
          ⟶ Neoplasia? ⟶ YES ⟶ Primary leukemia
                                Metastatic malignancy

⟶ Dysplastic and/or hypercellular?

       ↓

      YES ⟶ Serology ⟶ FeLV?
                        FIV?
                        Ehrlichia canis?
                        RMSF?

                             ↓

                        POSITIVE ⟶ Infection-induced anemia

          ⟶ Serum folate assay
             Serum cobalamin assay

                     ↓

                    LOW ⟶ Folate deficiency
                          Vitamin B_{12} deficiency

          ⟶ Blast cell count

            ↓   ↓

           <30%   ≥30%

            ↓   ↓

           MDS   AML
           CML

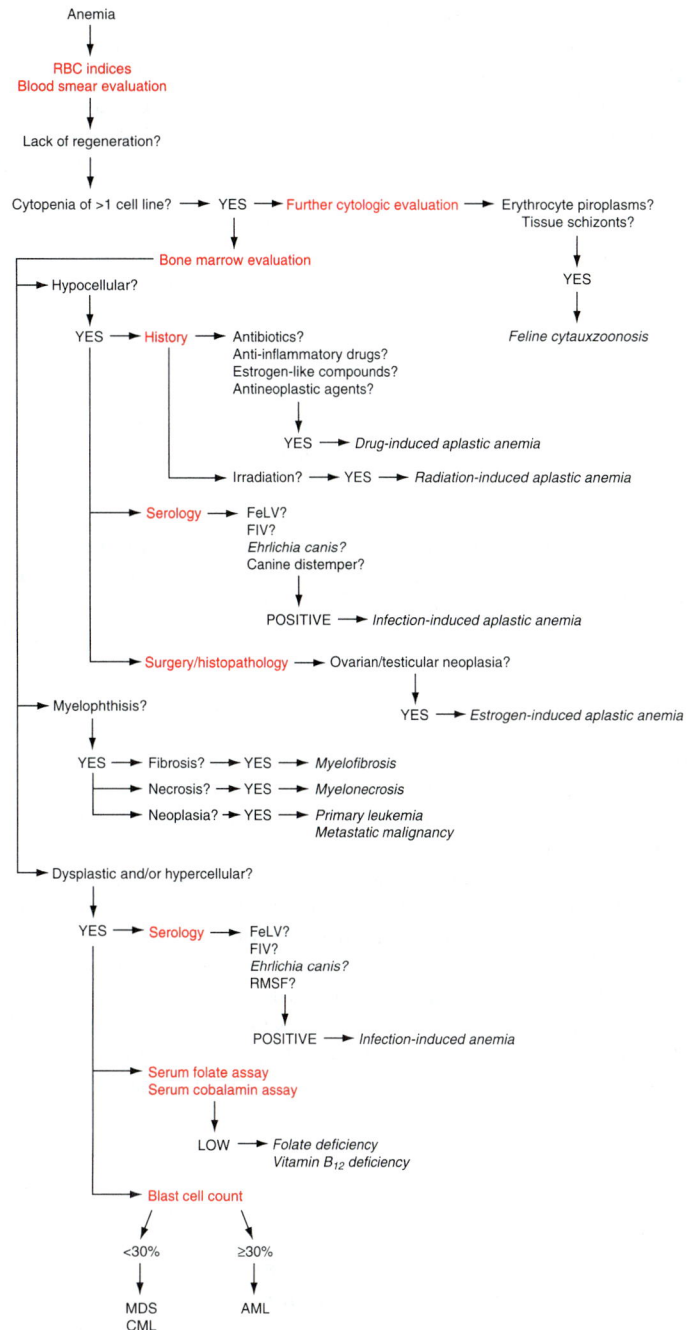

Figure 20–3. Diagnostic approach to common nonregenerative anemias in dogs and cats when pancytopenia is present. (FeLV, feline leukemia virus; FIV, feline immunodeficiency virus; RMSF, Rocky Mountain spotted fever, MDS, myelodysplastic syndrome; CML, chronic myeloid leukemia; AML, acute myeloid leukemia).

Initial clinical signs include anorexia, dehydration, and lethargy, with gradual development of fever. This progresses rapidly to icterus, moderate anemia, leukopenia, thrombocytopenia, and splenomegaly. Cats usually die within a week after clinical signs are recognized. Diagnosis generally is made postmortem by histologic identification of large schizonts in endothelial cells of the lungs, liver, bone marrow, or spleen. Terminally, blood films may contain small (1–2 μm in diameter) ring or "safety pin" structures within erythrocytes. Treatment is usually unsuccessful despite the use of antibiotics and supportive care. Most reported cases have been fatal, except one recent case of survival that demonstrated a regenerative erythrocyte response following fluid and antibiotic therapy.

Nutritional Deficiencies

Iron Deficiency

Iron deficiency produces a poorly regenerative anemia caused by deficient hemoglobin synthesis. It occurs with increased iron utilization, such as during growth or pregnancy, from decreased intestinal absorption of iron, and most commonly, when iron stores are reduced through hemorrhage or blood loss. Etiologies for this include neoplasia with tissue necrosis, trauma, internal or external parasites (hookworms, fleas), coagulopathies, and various gastrointestinal diseases that cause hematemesis, melena, or hematochezia.

Diagnosis is based on history and low serum iron levels. Erythrocytes in blood smears may appear normal in size but lighter in color, with increased central pallor (hypochromasia). Electronic cell counters report an MCV of less than 60 fl (microcytosis) in dogs. Poikilocytosis may be prominent in the form of schistocytes, keratocytes, codocytes, and elliptocytes. Thrombocytosis occurs in 50% of canine cases. Iron profiles have normal to increased level of transferrin (total iron-binding capacity) and decreased serum iron level (in cats < 60 μg/dl; in dogs < 80 μg/dl). Percent saturation of transferrin in iron deficient animals is often less than 19% (normal is about 33%). Bone marrow examination is necessary to determine iron storage amounts, especially in the dog. It is less helpful in the cat, which typically lacks stainable iron in the bone marrow. Aspirate and core biopsies of the bone marrow indicate hypercellularity with marked erythroid proliferation.

Treatment involves iron supplementation after correction of the inciting cause. Ferrous sulfate is given at a rate of 4 to 6 mg of iron/kg/day orally in divided doses. Therapy is continued for several weeks to months until the PCV and MCV return to normal.

Cobalamin Deficiency

Cobalamin (vitamin B$_{12}$) deficiency may occur through acquired disorders such as small intestinal disease, exocrine pancreatic insufficiency, or bacterial overgrowth in dogs. Selective malabsorption of vitamin B$_{12}$ has been described in giant schnauzers having an autosomal mode of inheritance. Clinical signs include weight loss, decreased appetite, and failure to thrive at 3 months of age. Laboratory findings involve chronic normocytic, normochromic, nonregenerative anemia with occasional erythroid dysplasia in peripheral blood or bone marrow. Serum cobalamin levels can be measured to determine affected animals (see Chapter 89). Resolution of clinical and hematologic effects occurs with parenteral administration of cobalamin (initially 1 mg IM daily).

Folate Deficiency

Folate deficiency may produce macrocytic anemia in animals with neoplasia, intestinal malabsorption, liver disease, dietary imbalance, and severe anorexia or starvation. Drugs such as anticonvulsants (phenobarbital, primidone), sulfonamides (sulfasalazine, trimethoprim-sulfadiazine) and antineoplastic agents (methotrexate) may act as folate antagonists by impairing its absorption or production. Diagnosis is based on a history of drug exposure or concurrent disease. Serum folate levels can be measured (see Chapter 89) to confirm the deficiency. The hemogram may indicate a normochromic anemia with macrocytosis and megaloblastic changes in erythroid precursors. Treatment is aimed at the inciting cause along with oral folate supplementation (5 mg/day in dogs; 2.5 mg/day in cats).

Chronic Inflammation

Anemia of chronic inflammation is a frequent cause of nonregenerative anemia. The mechanism may involve increased macrophage activity with cytokine release leading to decreased erythropoiesis, reduced iron availability through sequestration in macrophages, and decreased RBC survival. Primary infections and neoplasia are most often responsible for chronic inflammation. The animal may present with prolonged anorexia, weight loss, and weakness. Other clinical signs reflect the actual source of chronic inflammation or organ systems affected. Laboratory findings indicate a normocytic, normochromic anemia, inflammatory leukogram, low serum iron, low total iron-binding capacity, and increased bone marrow stores of iron. The bone marrow is usually hypocellular with a normal to increased myeloid-to-erythroid ratio. Treatment depends on the original cause. Iron supplementation does not effectively reverse this form of anemia.

Organic Disease

Kidney Disease

Chronic kidney disease may be associated with normocytic, normochromic nonregenerative anemia. The mechanisms involved include reduced erythropoiesis, decreased erythrocyte survival, and blood loss. Diagnosis of renal failure involves the presence of azotemia and an abnormal urinalysis. For pathogenesis, diagnosis, and treatment, see Chapter 97.

Liver Disease

Chronic liver disease may be associated with normocytic nonregenerative anemia. Pathogenetic mechanisms include concurrent inflammation with iron sequestration, reduced erythropoiesis, and decreased erythrocyte survival. Blood loss may occur from coagulopathies related to decreased synthesis of clotting factors. Portosystemic shunts may develop erythrocyte microcytosis, with or without anemia, possibly related to a relative decrease in iron availability. Laboratory findings suggestive of hepatic disease include elevated serum liver enzymes (ALT, SAP, GGT), increased serum bile acid levels, hypoalbuminemia, and hyperbilirubinemia. Blood smears often reveal poikilocytosis (acanthocytes, budding fragmentation). Liver disease is discussed in Chapter 91.

Endocrine Disease

Hypothyroidism

Hypothyroidism may present with mild anemia in one third of the cases. Pathogenetic mechanisms include reduced tissue oxygen demand and depressed erythropoiesis at the stem cell level. Diagnosis is based on history, dermatologic signs, and hormone assay results (see Chapter 29).

Hyperestrogenism

Hyperestrogenism is associated with endogenous production by tumors (e.g., testicular Sertoli cell or ovarian granulosa cell) or exogenous administration of estrogenic compounds. The mechanism of reduced erythropoiesis is thought to occur at the level of DNA transcription. Moderate to severe anemia may be accompanied by thrombocytopenia and leukopenia. Diagnosis of an estrogen-producing tumor may be confirmed by surgical removal with subsequent recovery of the cell lines. Supportive care, such as blood transfusion and anabolic steroids, may be necessary.

Hypoadrenocorticism

Hypoadrenocorticism may be a cause of nonregenerative anemia in a small percentage of cases. The anemia usually is discovered after fluid replacement for volume deficits associated with the disease (see Chapter 31).

Drug and Toxin-Induced Disease

Drugs

Drugs (e.g., estrogens, phenylbutazone, antineoplastic agents, thiacetarsamide, quinidine, meclofenamic acid, and trimethoprim sulfadiazine) are associated with reduced erythropoiesis and aplastic anemia in dogs. An idiosyncratic toxicosis caused by griseofulvin administration resulting in a nonregenerative pancytopenia has been reported in a cat.

Exogenous estrogens are toxic in the dog, depending on the dose given and age of the animal (worse in older dogs). Initially, anemia and thrombocytopenia occur along with leukocytosis, which is an inflammatory neutrophilia. Later, pancytopenia develops. After drug cessation, recovery begins in 1 month, starting with leukocytosis and followed by the return of the other cell lines.

Chloramphenicol administration in cats causes a dose-dependent, reversible marrow suppression involving the erythroid series primarily. Dogs are much less sensitive to chloramphenicol.

Treatment for drug-induced aplastic anemia often includes supportive care, such as blood transfusions (see Principles of Transfusion Therapy), anabolic steroids, and antibiotics in severe cases, once the drug has been stopped.

Lead Toxicity

Lead poisoning causes a mild anemia in some cases, possibly because of increased erythrocyte fragility and abnormal erythropoiesis. Lead primarily affects heme synthesis, causing defective maturation. Other clinical signs involve GI and neurologic disturbances.

Diagnosis often is based on a history of exposure to lead in paint or automobile batteries. Heparinized blood samples are used to determine lead levels. Affected animals have levels greater than 0.06 mg/dl. The hemogram strongly suggests lead poisoning when large numbers of nucleated erythrocytes are present with a normal or slightly decreased PCV. The anemia is often normocytic and normochromic but may be microcytic and hypochromic. Basophilic stippling is best seen with Romanowsky-stained blood films prepared without EDTA anticoagulant. Polychromasia generally is rare. Bone marrow aspirates or core biopsies are characterized by maturation arrest at the metarubricyte stage.

Treatment in dogs and cats involves calcium EDTA (100 mg/kg) diluted to 10 mg/ml in 5% dextrose and given SC, in four divided doses, daily for 5 days.

Myelophthisis

Neoplasia

Neoplasia of the bone marrow can occur with primary hemolymphatic tumors or metastatic tumors. Mild infiltrates or focal lesions within the bone marrow produce minimal peripheral blood changes. Cytopenias occur if the involvement is diffuse and severe. Approximately 57% of dogs with multicentric lymphoma have metastasis to the bone marrow at the time of diagnosis. Only half of these have evidence of abnormal cells in circulation. Diagnosis requires bone marrow examination by both aspirate and core biopsies (see discussion of Leukemic Disorders).

Myelofibrosis

Myelofibrosis usually occurs as a result of marrow damage produced by inflammation, necrosis, neoplasia, and toxic agents and may be seen in the terminal stages of pyruvate kinase deficiency. Pancytopenia is observed in severe cases along with poikilocytosis in the form of dacryocytes and schistocytes. Bone marrow aspiration attempts usually produce "dry taps" (i.e., blood alone without marrow particles). Bone marrow core biopsy is diagnostic. Myelofibrosis also is associated with myelodysplastic syndrome and acute myelogenous leukemia in cats (see discussion of Dysplastic and Leukemic Disorders). Supportive care, including antibiotics, blood transfusions, anabolic steroids, and glucocorticoids, often is required in severe cases. Myelofibrosis may be reversible under some conditions.

Myelonecrosis

Myelonecrosis is an uncommon cause of nonregenerative anemia. It often is associated with neoplasia but may be related to infections or toxic agents. The mechanism likely involves occlusion of microcirculation or direct injury to endothelium. Diagnosis is based on bone marrow examination. Aspirate biopsies may contain peripheral blood, degenerative cells, increased macrophage activity, and amorphous stringy material representing necrotic bone marrow particles. Focal to diffuse regions of necrosis appear on histologic sections of bone marrow. Treatment includes removal of the inciting cause along with supportive care. Prognosis is often poor.

Osteopetrosis

Osteopetrosis is an uncommon inheritable condition affecting the normal development of bone. It causes obliteration of the marrow cavities by bone and may be associated with refractory anemia or pancytopenia in immature or young adult dogs. Clinical signs usually are related to anemia. Diagnosis is established by the inability to obtain bone marrow material on aspiration and by distinctive radiographic findings. Increased bone density is present and cortices are thickened, leaving a narrow medullary region. Histologic examination of medullary bone reveals thickened trabeculae, reduced marrow cavities, and an absence of osteoclasts. Despite supportive care, the prognosis is poor.

Irradiation

Irradiation acts as a local cytotoxic agent for cancer therapy. It also is used to treat hemolymphatic malignancies and genetic defects before bone marrow transplantation. High doses produce irreversible pancytopenia and aplastic bone marrow. Supportive care (e.g., blood transfusions, antibiotics, and immunosuppressive drugs) often is given after transplantation.

Immune-Mediated Destruction (Pure Erythrocyte Aplasia)

This uncommon condition is characterized by severe reduction of erythroid stem cells without affecting granulocytic or megakaryocytic lines. Both congenital and acquired forms have been reported in dogs. The myeloid-to-erythroid ratio is usually 10:1 to 20:1. Coombs testing has been positive in a few dogs. The mechanism is considered to be immune-mediated because the disease often responds to prednisolone and/or cyclophosphamide therapy (see Chapter 22).

Polycythemia

Relative Polycythemia

Increase in erythrocytes (erythrocytosis) in relative polycythemia generally is related to fluid depletion (e.g., dehydration or hemoconcentration). However, excitement or fear may cause splenic contraction and a transient rise in PCV. Greyhounds normally have a high PCV of 60%. Clinical signs include dark red mucous membranes with slow capillary refill time. Diagnosis is based on a history of stress or fluid loss, elevated PCV, and increased erythrocyte and plasma protein concentrations. The erythrogram returns to normal after fluid replacement. If splenic contraction is suspected, the PCV should be retaken after the patient has relaxed.

Absolute Polycythemia

The erythrocytosis in absolute polycythemia may be primary or secondary, with a sustained increase in the circulating erythrocyte mass, based on erythropoietin production.

Primary erythrocytosis, or polycythemia vera, has low serum erythropoietin that suggests that the increased erythrocyte numbers are derived from an intrinsic stem cell defect (see section on Leukemic Disorders).

Secondary erythrocytosis involves overproduction of erythropoietin. Causes of secondary erythrocytosis include hypoxia (e.g., caused by high altitude, chronic pulmonary disease, or cardiac disease with right-to-left shunting), tumors that produce erythropoietin (e.g., renal lymphoma, renal carcinoma, and renal fibrosarcoma), and renal disease (e.g., pyelonephritis). Diagnosis of hypoxia is based on history and evidence of lung disease or right-to-left shunting heart disease. Renal disease, benign or malignant, can be excluded by urinalysis, radiography, ultrasonography, or biopsy. Serum erythropoietin levels currently are measured by radioimmunoassay and ELISA methods. Treatment of secondary erythrocytosis often involves removal of the inciting cause (e.g., nephrectomy).

Methemoglobinemia

Methemoglobinemia occurs from the oxidation of iron in hemoglobin. This form of oxidized hemoglobin is unable to bind and carry oxygen, producing a state of relative hypoxia. Clinically, the mucous membranes appear blue-gray or cyanotic if methemoglobin levels exceed 30%. The patient is often dyspneic, weak, and ataxic.

The appearance of dark red or chocolate-colored blood, even after exposure to air, is diagnostic for the condition. The color change, from dark to bright red in normal blood, is readily visible by a spot test on filter paper. The blood of affected animals shows no such color change if the methemoglobin content exceeds 15%. Severe disease is produced from oxidant drugs and chemicals, similar to those mentioned in the previous section on Heinz body formation. Both conditions present together, but methemoglobinemia tends to occur before Heinz bodies appear. Several breeds of dog and a domestic short-haired cat were reported to have a rare enzyme (NADH-methemoglobin reductase) deficiency with a mild to moderate form of the disease. Quantitative measurement of methemoglobin content is performed by spectrophotometry at specialized laboratories.

Treatment is similar to Heinz body anemia. In addition, methylene blue, if carefully administered, has been used to treat the condition caused by oxidant drugs. A dose of 1 mg/kg IV given as a 1% solution is recommended for small animals. Caution is necessary to avoid potentiating a hemolytic crisis. Therapy usually is not required for animals with the reductase enzyme deficiency.

▼ *Key Point* A mild secondary polycythemia may develop in animals with methemoglobin reductase deficiency.

LEUKOCYTE DISORDERS

Congenital Disorders

Pelger-Huët Anomaly

Pelger-Huët anomaly is an inherited disorder in dogs and cats involving granulocyte maturation. Leukocyte function in dogs is not impaired, and there is no predisposition to infection or immunodeficiency. Chondrodysplasia has been recognized in a cat with a homozygous form of this disorder. Diagnosis is based on the appearance of mature leukocytes in blood that have nuclei with condensed, coarse, and patchy chromatin-lacking segmentation. The nuclear shapes often resemble those of bands, metamyelocytes, and myelocytes. The cytoplasm undergoes normal maturation. Abnormalities frequently are found during routine preoperative screening and may be mistaken as a severe left shift. Inflammatory conditions should be ruled out. No treatment is necessary.

Feline Chédiak-Higashi Syndrome

This is a rare, inheritable disorder seen in blue-smoke Persian cats with yellow eye color. Pathogenesis involves abnormal and enlarged lysosomal granule formation in granulocytes and monocytes. Affected cats may be photophobic with cataract formation. There is increased bleeding time because of platelet granule defects. With Romanowsky stains, neutrophils contain characteristic large, pink to magenta cytoplasmic inclusions that stain positive with peroxidase and Sudan black B. These cats do not exhibit an increased susceptibility to infection.

Lysosomal Storage Diseases

Mucopolysaccharidosis (MPS) and gangliosidosis are inheritable lysosomal storage diseases reported in cats and dogs caused by an enzyme deficiency. MPS Types VI and VII have been reported in cats and dogs and present with skeletal and ocular lesions. In cats with GM_2-gangliosidosis, neurologic deficits and corneal opacification are displayed. In all these diseases, neutrophils may contain coarse, red-purple granules when stained with Wright-Giemsa or toluidine blue. Cells must be distinguished from toxic neutrophils. A urine spot test is used to screen for glycosaminoglycans, whereas a cell enzyme activity test is diagnostic. Experimentally, bone marrow transplantation has been used to treat some of these disorders. Affected animals should not be bred.

Other lysosomal storage diseases in dogs and cats that present with progressive neurologic dysfunction or skeletal lesions involve a distinctive lymphocyte morphologic abnormality. Affected lymphocytes have multiple punctate cytoplasmic vacuoles on blood films. These vacuoles should not be confused with the artifactual changes seen with prolonged storage of blood in EDTA. The specific lysosomal storage diseases that may display lymphocyte vacuolation include GM_1 and GM_2-gangliosidosis, Neimann-Pick disease, α-mannosidosis, MPS (Types I, VI, and VII), and α-fucosidosis. These different diseases may be distinguished by special tests for enzyme activity from blood and/or affected tissues.

Abnormal Granulation Syndrome in Birman Cats

This is a genetic anomaly recognized in Birman cats without associated clinical disease. Diagnosis is based on the presence of fine, pinkish-purple granules within the cytoplasm of neutrophils. These lysosomal granules have normal morphology, and neutrophil function is unaffected.

Neutrophilia

Neutrophilia is defined as more than 11,500 neutrophils/μl in the dog and more than 12,500 neutrophils/μl in the cat.

Physiologic

Epinephrine release as the result of stress, fear, or strenuous muscular exertion causes demargination of leukocytes, producing a rapid rise in neutrophils and lymphocytes. Within 30 minutes, the cell counts return to normal. The effect is more common and greater in cats than in dogs.

Corticosteroid-Induced

Neutrophilia may be related to exogenous administration or endogenous release of glucocorticoids. Cells are released from marginating pools and bone marrow storage pools. The magnitude and duration of the effect depends on the type of corticosteroid given. Diagnosis is determined by the history and by the presence of concurrent lymphopenia, eosinopenia, or monocytosis, without a left shift. Neutrophil hypersegmentation is common because of a prolonged life span.

Inflammatory

Evidence of inflammation is an increase in nonsegmented forms of neutrophils, termed a *left shift*. Etiology involves infectious or noninfectious sources.

- Infectious agents include bacteria, systemic fungi, protozoa, or rickettsiae (see Infectious Diseases chapters).
- Noninfectious conditions involve tissue necrosis, such as necrotizing pancreatitis, neoplasia, thrombosis, and burns.
- Certain malignancies (e.g., metastatic fibrosarcoma or renal tubular carcinoma) are reported to induce a leukemoid response, presumably as a paraneoplastic disorder, rather than from tissue necrosis alone. Leukemoid counts range from 50,000 to 100,000 leukocytes/μl with a left shift back to bands, metamyelocytes, and myelocytes.
- This extreme degree of leukocytosis also is observed with severe abscessation (e.g., pyometra).
- Immune-mediated reactions, such as systemic lupus erythematosus, can result in a left shift with neutrophilia.
- A granulocytopathy syndrome involving Irish setters is a congenital cause of inflammatory neutrophilia. Neutrophils appear morphologically normal but have impaired bactericidal activity related to a deficiency of adhesion proteins. Affected dogs have recurrent bacterial infections with extreme leukocytosis that can mimic chronic granulocytic leukemia (see section on Leukemic Disorders).

Diagnosis of inflammatory neutrophilia is based on a careful history and a CBC evaluation. A regenerative left shift requires a simultaneous neutrophilia. A left shift without neutrophilia is considered degenerative, especially if there is neutropenia or if more nonsegmented forms are present compared with mature neutrophils. In addition to a significant shift toward immaturity (bands > 1000/μl), neutrophils may exhibit toxicity. Toxins released from bacteria are mostly responsible for the focal or diffuse cytoplasmic basophilia and vacuolation found in mature or immature neutrophils. Antibiotic responsiveness suggests a bacterial cause. Tests for specific infectious agents and immune-mediated disorders may be indicated. Treatment depends on the inciting cause.

▼ *Key Point* Animals possessing neutrophil function defects present with neutrophilia and persistent and recurrent infections.

Neoplastic

See discussion on Leukemic Disorders.

Neutropenia

Neutropenia is defined as less than 3000 neutrophils/μl in the dog and less than 2500 neutrophils/μl in the cat.

Congenital

Cyclic neutropenia or cyclic hematopoiesis is an inherited disorder of gray collies. It is characterized by periodic fluctuations in neutrophils and, to a lesser extent in monocytes, platelets, and reticulocytes, as a result of the intrinsic bone marrow stem cell defect. Neutropenic cycles recur at 12-day intervals. Clinical signs during neutropenic episodes include lethargy, pyrexia, anorexia, arthritis, keratitis, and respiratory or GI infections. Diagnosis is based on history, clinical signs, and cyclic decreases in cell counts. Carrier animals can be determined only by test mating. Antibiotics and supportive care are necessary during neutropenic cycles. Most affected dogs die within 6 months, after chronic recurrent infections. Experimental treatments involve bone marrow transplantation and administration of lithium carbonate (21–26 mg/kg/day) or recombinant canine granulocyte-colony stimulating factor (5 μg/kg/day).

Infectious

Consumption of neutrophils during severe systemic inflammation often produces neutropenia with an increase of immature forms, termed a *degenerative left shift*. Gram-negative bacteria usually are involved, as with septicemia, severe enteritis, or other severe bacterial infections. Systemic mycoses and protozoal infections (e.g., *Toxoplasma*) also can cause neutropenia. Reduced granulopoiesis may be associated with such viruses as FeLV, feline panleukopenia virus, and canine parvovirus. FeLV is associated with a cyclic neutropenia that may respond to lithium and prednisone. *Ehrlichia canis* also may cause bone marrow suppression (see Infectious Diseases section). Diagnosis of infectious causes is based on the history, CBC, and bone marrow findings, in addition to specific serologic or bacterial culture results. Neutropenia without a marked left shift may indicate peracute consumption without adequate time for bone marrow response. The lack of a left shift, if persistent, suggests an absolute reduction of neutrophilic precursors or myeloid hypoplasia of the bone marrow. Treatment is directed at the inciting cause.

Toxic

Drugs that cause neutropenia due to myelotoxicity include estrogens, chloramphenicol, trimethoprim-sulfadiazine, griseofulvin, and cancer chemotherapeutic agents (see discussion of Nonregenerative Anemia). Antineoplastic agents that can cause neutropenia include cyclophosphamide, chlorambucil, busulfan, melphalan, cisplatin, cytosine arabinoside, methotrexate, mitoxantrone, doxorubicin, and hydroxyurea.

Cephalosporins and nonsteroidal anti-inflammatory drugs occasionally have been associated with myelotoxicity. Endotoxins from gram-negative sepsis produce a transient neutropenia. Mechanisms involve a shift of neutrophils from the circulation to the marginating pools and a shortened circulating half-life (normal is approximately 5.5–7.5 hours). Treatment requires cessation of the drug and supportive care, particularly antibiotics. The use of recombinant canine granulocyte colony-stimulating factor has shown promise in reducing the severity of drug-induced myelosuppression.

Immune-Mediated

Destruction of antibody-coated neutrophils by macrophages is a mechanism of neutropenia considered to occur in animals, but it has not been well documented. As in immune-mediated hemolysis, the disorder may involve antibody directed against surface antigens of the cell itself, or antibody directed toward drug antigens attached to neutrophils. Drugs responsible for suspected immune-mediated blood cell destruction include antithyroid drugs (e.g., thiouracil, methimazole) and cephalosporins. Definitive diagnosis requires detection of antineutrophil antibodies on the cells or in serum; however, such assays are not currently available for clinical usage. The bone marrow is expected to show myeloid hyperplasia, with a marked decrease in late-stage forms. In one suspected case in a dog, immunosuppressive doses of prednisone produced a positive response.

Myelophthisis

See discussion of Nonregenerative Anemia.

Irradiation

See discussion of Nonregenerative Anemia.

Monocytosis

Corticosteroid-Induced

Monocytosis, particularly in the dog, can be induced by glucocorticoid administration. Diagnosis is based on the history, but when it is unavailable, the presence of concurrent lymphopenia, eosinopenia, and mature neutrophilia should suggest the effects of corticosteroids.

Inflammatory

Acute and chronic inflammatory diseases that cause a high demand for macrophages may produce monocytosis. These include immune-mediated disorders, tissue necrosis, foreign body reactions, and mycobacterial or fungal infections. Diagnosis is based on the history, physical examination, immunologic testing, cytology, and histopathology.

Neoplastic

See discussion of Leukemic Disorders.

Eosinophilia

Parasitic

Peripheral eosinophilia may result from infiltration of the skin, respiratory tract, and alimentary tract by such parasites as *Ancylostoma* spp, *Trichuris vulpis, Toxocara canis, Dirofilaria immitis, Dipetalonema reconditum,* lung-worms (*Aelurostrongylus abstrusus, Capillaria* spp., *Filaroides* spp.), and *Paragonimus kellicotti.* Definitive diagnosis of parasitism is determined by positive fecal examinations, tracheobronchial washes, thoracic radiographs, and heartworm serologic or concentration techniques.

Allergic/Inflammatory

Hypersensitivity reactions can occur owing to the effects of fleas, food, grasses, and nonspecific allergens. The production of IgE causes mast cell degranulation and release of chemical mediators that attract eosinophils. The skin, respiratory, GI, and genitourinary systems often are affected. Eosinophilic granuloma is a localized infiltration of the dermis by eosinophils that occurs in the oral cavity or skin of dogs and cats (see Chapter 48). The history, physical examination, skin or food testing, and tracheobronchial lavage help to locate the type of allergen and the system most affected. In the case of eosinophilic granuloma, impression smears and histopathology may be diagnostic. Peripheral eosinophilia commonly is found in these conditions. Treatment usually involves elimination of the allergen, along with antihistamine and glucocorticoid administration.

Paraneoplastic Syndrome

Tumor-associated eosinophilia has been reported in dogs with fibrosarcoma, anaplastic mammary carcinoma, and mast cell tumors. In cats, mast cell tumors and lymphoma are the neoplasms most commonly associated with eosinophilia. Diagnosis depends on normalization or reduction of the eosinophil count in response to removal of the tumor.

Hypereosinophilic Syndrome in Cats

Hypereosinophilic syndrome is an uncommon form of peripheral eosinophilia accompanied by severe infiltration of eosinophils into many organs, often including the GI tract (see Chap. 89), liver, spleen, lymph nodes, and lung. It resembles a leukemia of well-differentiated eosinophils resulting from an apparent involvement of the bone marrow. The cause is idiopathic and difficult to separate from eosinophilic leukemia. Clinical signs may include anorexia, weight loss, fever, vomiting, diarrhea, and lymphadenopathy. Death results from organ dysfunction caused by tissue infiltration.

Neoplastic

See discussion of Leukemic Disorders.

Eosinopenia

Endogenous release or exogenous administration of corticosteroids produces eosinopenia within a few hours. Levels will normalize in 1 day after a single dose is given. Mechanisms implicated are enhanced margination, decreased bone marrow release, and reduced bone marrow production. Absolute reductions in eosinophils or relative decreases from a previous eosinophilia suggest the effects of glucocorticoids. Elevated cortisol levels and an endocrine dermatopathy support hyperadrenocorticism (see Chapter 31).

Basophilia

Parasitic

Heartworm infection, including occult disease, is a frequent cause of basophilia in dogs and cats. Dogs with hookworms also may have basophilia. Diagnosis often involves concurrent eosinophilia and positive proof of parasitic infestation. Basophil granules in dogs and cats normally stain poorly. The cells frequently are mistaken for toxic neutrophils in dogs or faded eosinophils in cats.

Allergic

Hypersensitivity reactions cause IgE production in such organs as the skin and lungs. The immune response leads to increased numbers of mast cells and basophils.

Lipid Metabolism

An association between basophilia without eosinophilia and lipemia is thought to be related to deficiency of heparin, which is found in basophils and is needed to activate lipoprotein lipase. This enzyme is necessary to clear lipemia. This has been associated with hypothyroidism but is observed infrequently.

Systemic Mastocytosis

Basophilia was found in 5 of 16 dogs with systemic mastocytosis. It also occurs in cats with splenic mastocytoma.

Neoplastic

See discussion on Leukemic Disorders.

Lymphocytosis

Epinephrine-Induced

A transient rise in lymphocytes occurs with severe exertion or physiologic stress. This is especially significant in the young cat. Transient lymphocytosis that normalizes after a short time suggests epinephrine effects on the leukogram.

Infectious

Lymphocytosis may be the result of antigen stimulation caused by FeLV, *Ehrlichia canis, Rickettsia rickettsii,* and systemic fungi. In particular, lymphocytosis involving granular lymphocytes has been associated with *E. canis* infection in dogs. Modified live vaccines also may produce lymphocytosis, along with the morphologic appearance of reactivity, about 1 week postimmunization. Slightly enlarged lymphocytes with deeply basophilic cytoplasm resembling plasma cells support the diagnosis of reactivity from antigen stimulation. Hyperglobulinemia due to a polyclonal gammopathy and plasma cell infiltration of tissues also may occur.

Neoplastic

Lymphocytosis resulting from metastatic lymphoma occurs in 20% of dogs and cats with lymphoma. Acute or chronic lymphoid leukemia often is characterized by lymphocytosis and atypical or immature lymphoid cells. However, rare blast cells may be found in nonneoplastic conditions such as immune-mediated hemolytic anemia and canine ehrlichiosis. Persistent hematologic abnormalities must be present to consider neoplasia and should be evaluated further with bone marrow aspiration and core biopsies (see Chapter 25).

Lymphopenia

Corticosteroid-Induced

Endogenous or exogenous corticosteroids produce an absolute lymphopenia or a normal value reduced from a previous lymphocytosis. It is transient because cell counts return to normal within 1 to 3 days after drug withdrawal. Lymphopenia also may relate to redistribution of lymphocytes to other tissues (see discussion of Neutrophilia). Lymphopenia often accompanies the stress of many acute diseases.

Infectious

Viral agents, such as canine distemper virus, FeLV, FIV, and canine or feline parvoviruses, may cause lymphopenia because of direct lymphocytolysis or lymphoid tissue destruction.

Lymphatic Damage

Rupture or malformation of lymphatic vessels (e.g., chylothorax or protein-losing enteropathy from lymphangiectasia) can cause lymphopenia because of a loss of lymph fluid into the pleural cavity or gut lumen, preventing recirculation (see Chapter 80, Pleural Effusion; Chapter 89, Diseases of the Intestines). Destruction of normal lymph node architecture or blockage of lymph drainage, as in lymphoma, may also lead to lymphopenia (see Chapter 25).

Congenital

Combined immunodeficiency of T and B lymphocytes occurs in bassett hounds. It is associated with severe bacterial infections within the first few weeks of life. Diagnosis is based on the presence of low immunoglobulin levels, depressed T-cell function, and histologic evidence of lymphoid cell depletion, as well as peripheral lymphopenia. Supportive therapy with antibiotics is suggested, but death may occur in severe cases.

Mastocytosis or Mastocythemia

See Chapter 26.

PLATELET DISORDERS

Thrombocytopenia

Platelets may be decreased in number through immune-mediated injury, increased consumption or utilization, sequestration, and decreased production.

Overview
Clinical Signs

- Petechial or ecchymotic hemorrhages involving the mucous membranes or skin are common manifestations of thrombocytopenia.
- Epistaxis, melena, hematuria, hyphema, or prolonged bleeding from venipuncture sites or wounds often occur.
- Evidence of inciting conditions, such as infection, neoplasia, or splenomegaly, may be present.

General Diagnostic Considerations

- The history should determine the occurrence of trauma, surgery, drug or toxin exposure, and neoplasia, as well as the time period involved.
- Physical examination discloses sites of hemorrhage, presence of hepatosplenomegaly, and concurrent infections or neoplasia.
- Use CBC to screen for hematologic abnormalities including the adequacy of the platelet numbers.
- Perform platelet counts on fresh samples (within 1–2 hours). Thrombocytopenia is considered to be less than 100,000 platelets/μl. However, clinical signs of bleeding are not expected until there are less than 20,000 platelets/μl.
- Include both aspirate and core biopsies in bone marrow evaluation to check for adequate megakaryocyte numbers.
- Perform clotting profile, including fibrinogen, prothrombin time (PT), and activated partial thromboplastin (APTT) or activated clotting time (ACT), to help rule out other coagulopathies (as described in Chapter 21). ACT may be slightly prolonged if platelet counts are less than 10,000/μl.
- Perform a von Willebrand factor assay if the breed and clinical signs suggest a deficiency (see Chapter 21).
- Bleeding time, a platelet function test, may be prolonged because of low platelet numbers.

▼ **Key Point** Examine the blood smear carefully, especially at the feathered edge, before a diagnosis of thrombocytopenia is made.

Treatment

Supportive therapy may include fresh blood transfusions (administered within 8 hours of collection) if both platelets and erythrocyte numbers are low. If only platelets are needed, administer platelet-rich plasma (see Chapter 21).

Immune-Mediated Platelet Injury

This is one of the most frequent and important causes of thrombocytopenia manifested by clinically significant bleeding (see Chapter 22).

Increased Platelet Consumption or Utilization

Infectious Agents

Thrombocytopenia produced by such agents as *Ehrlichia canis, E. ewingii,* and *E. equi* presumably is the result of increased consumption and the presence of antiplatelet antibodies. Bone marrow evaluation during the acute course of *E. canis* infection indicates megakaryocytic hyperplasia. The diagnosis of ehrlichiosis is based on a history of tick exposure and positive serologic testing (see Chapter 15). *E. platys* produces a cyclic thrombocytopenia occurring in 2-week cycles that may be diagnosed by direct observation of morula within platelets or by an indirect immunofluorescence antibody test.

Modified Live Virus Vaccination

Canine distemper virus vaccine may induce thrombocytopenia within 1 week postvaccination. The effect is transient but may persist for as long as 3 weeks. It is rarely of clinical significance unless surgery is performed during the platelet count nadir.

Hemorrhage

Bleeding can consume platelets. Consumption of platelets may occur through hemorrhage alone or in association with bacterial or viral infections that produce inflammation. Endotoxemia from gram-negative bacteria leads to endothelial damage and platelet activation. Diagnosis is based on history, physical examination, cytology, histopathology, and culture techniques. Treatment is aimed at the inciting agent. Whole blood or platelet transfusions may be necessary if thrombocytopenia is severe.

Disseminated Intravascular Coagulation

This condition leads to increased consumption of platelets as well as clotting factors. It is associated most often with infections, neoplasia, heartworm disease, pancreatitis, and shock. Clinical signs involve petechial and ecchymotic hemorrhages. Organ dysfunction usually reflects the effects of the primary disease. Diagnosis is based on the findings in tests of coagulation, including hypofibrinogenemia, prolonged PT and APTT, increased fibrin degradation products, and decreased antithrombin III activity. Microthrombi formation is found on histopathology. Treatment is aimed at the inciting or underlying cause when possible. Supportive care, including fluids, is necessary to prevent shock. Replacement of platelets and coagulation factors using fresh plasma usually is indicated. Heparin rarely is effective, especially if the hemorrhagic stage already has occurred (see Chapter 21).

Sequestration

Splenomegaly

The spleen normally stores approximately one third of the body's platelets. With enlargement of the spleen from any cause, there is an increase in blood volume that sequesters more platelets within endothelial passages, resulting in thrombocytopenia. Physical examination of an enlarged spleen without evidence of other conditions that induce thrombocytopenia supports the diagnosis. It is usually of little clinical significance if associated with benign enlargements of the spleen (see Chapter 23).

Decreased Platelet Production

Congenital Thrombocytopenia

Cyclic hematopoiesis in gray collie dogs may exhibit thrombocytopenia of a cyclic nature (see discussion of Neutropenia).

Infectious Agents

Canine distemper virus, parvoviruses, FeLV, and *Ehrlichia canis* may be associated with reduced thrombopoiesis. Approximately 20% of animals with ehrlichiosis have megakaryocytic hypoplasia of the bone marrow, especially in the late stages of the disease.

Drug-Induced

Causes of drug-induced thrombocytopenia are similar to those that produce aplastic anemia. (see section on Nonregenerative Anemia). Antineoplastic agents such as cisplatin, cyclophosphamide, chlorambucil, doxorubicin, and hydroxyurea produce significant thrombocytopenia.

Myelophthisic Thrombocytopenia

See discussion on Nonregenerative Anemia.

▼ *Key Point* Thrombocytopenia associated with neoplasia occurs through several mechanisms including hemorrhage, microangiopathy, disseminated intravascular coagulation, myelophthisis, immune-mediated destruction, and chemotherapeutic drugs.

Thrombocytosis

Physiologic

Increased numbers of platelets are released from the spleen as a result of epinephrine release or during heavy exercise. Pulmonary stores of platelets also may be released during exercise. This is transient and of no clinical significance.

Reactive

Conditions associated with reactive or regenerative thrombocytosis include acute blood loss, iron deficiency anemia, trauma, surgery, inflammation, splenectomy, hyperadrenocorticism, and neoplasia. Tumors that may cause thrombocytosis are mast cell tumor, hemangiosarcoma, osteosarcoma, lymphocytic and myeloid leukemias, and some carcinomas. Vincristine administration produces increased thrombopoiesis and cytoplasmic fragmentation of megakaryocytes because of a reduced maturation time. There are no clinical signs directly related to transiently elevated platelet counts. Diagnosis is supported by history, physical examination, platelet count greater than $600,000/\mu l$ (dog) or greater than $800,000/\mu l$ (cat), and mild to moderate megakaryocytic bone marrow hyperplasia without evidence of circulating megakaryoblasts. Pseudohyperkalemia can occur because of leakage of potassium from clotted platelets. Therefore, plasma is preferred for measurement of potassium levels in thrombocytotic samples. Treatment depends on the inciting cause.

Neoplastic

See discussion on Leukemic Disorders.

DYSPLASTIC DISORDERS

Congenital

An inherited disorder of toy and miniature poodles is associated with abnormal morphology of erythrocytes and their precursors. Affected animals present with no clinical signs of anemia, and the dysplastic findings are usually incidental. Diagnosis is based on the breed and on findings of a normal hematocrit, presence of macrocytosis (MCV > 80 fl), megaloblastosis in the blood and bone marrow, and absence of polychromasia or reticulocytosis. An asynchrony in maturation between the nucleus and cytoplasm characterizes the RBC abnormalities. Neutrophil hypersegmentation and giantism also may occur but are less common. The condition persists and is not responsive to folate or cobalamin. Megaplatelets as an inherited disorder have been reported in Cavalier King Charles spaniel dogs without hemorrhages or clinical signs.

Infectious

Abnormal morphology of erythroid, granulocytic, and megakaryocytic lines occurs in cats infected with either FeLV or FIV. Macrocytosis, megaloblastosis, neutrophil giantism, hypersegmentation, and dwarf megakaryocyte formation characterize the dysplastic changes found as a result of viral effects on nuclear development. Peripheral cytopenias arise from abnormal maturation of affected cell lines. Clinical signs often include concurrent bacterial or protozoal infections, neoplasia, and chronic wasting. Definitive diagnosis requires serologic testing. Treatment is supportive in nature. The median survival is 12 weeks.

Drug-Induced

Dyserythropoiesis characterized by macrocytosis, megaloblastoid changes, nuclear fragmentation, sideroblastosis, and siderocytosis may occur in animals treated with azathioprine, cyclophosphamide, cytosine arabinoside, vincristine, or chloramphenicol. Diagnosis is based on blood and bone marrow samples taken during routine posttreatment hematologic evaluations. These changes are not associated with folate deficiency. Normal morphology of hematopoietic cells returns several days after cessation of drug therapy.

Nutritional

Erythroid dysplastic changes and neutrophil hypersegmentation may occur in giant schnauzers with an inherited selective malabsorption of vitamin B_{12} (in this chapter, under Nonregenerative Anemia). A macrocytic nonregenerative anemia is found in acquired folate deficiencies such as intestinal malabsorption, neoplasia, liver disease, dietary imbalance, and severe starvation. In addition, drugs such as anticonvulsants, antibiotics, and antineoplastic agents that inhibit folate metabolism produce megaloblastic changes in erythroid precursors (see discussion on Nonregenerative Anemia).

Myelodysplastic Syndrome

Myelodysplastic syndrome is characterized by persistent peripheral cytopenias in one or more hematopoietic cell lines together with features of abnormal maturation. This condition often precedes an overt leukemia by several weeks to months. Cats affected usually are seropositive for FeLV. Clinical signs involve chronic infections, lethargy due to anemia, and hemorrhage.

Despite the cytopenias, the bone marrow is usually hypercellular, with a mild increase in numbers of myeloblasts (<30% of all nucleated cells). Dysplastic changes in the blood or bone marrow include macrocytosis, megaloblastosis, nuclear fragmentation, abnormal cytoplasmic granulation, neutrophil hypersegmentation or hyposegmentation, micromegakaryocyte or macrothrombocyte formation, and cell giantism.

Because the condition may persist for long periods of time without major clinical disease, treatment is usually supportive, including antibiotics and blood transfusions as needed. Antineoplastic agents, such as low-dose cytosine arabinoside, have been used to induce normal maturation and prevent conversion to a malignant state. Results with these agents have been mixed and therefore cannot be recommended as treatment. Dyserythropoiesis in dogs may respond to prednisone and recombinant human erythropoietin (100 U/kg SC q48h for 10 days).

LEUKEMIC DISORDERS

Lymphoid Leukemia

See Chapter 25.

Myeloid (Nonlymphoid) Leukemia

The etiology for this group of leukemias is generally unknown, although they often are associated with viral infection (e.g., FeLV), immunologic dysfunction, or irradiation. Clinical signs include pale mucous membranes (except in polycythemia vera), fever, lethargy, weight loss, chronic infections, hepatosplenomegaly, mild lymphadenopathy, and hemorrhagic tendencies.

Myeloid leukemias are suggested by the history (e.g., FeLV infection), clinical signs of unexplained or frequent infections, and hematologic abnormalities that affect multiple cell lines. Definitive diagnosis is made from bone marrow aspirate and core examinations. Acute myeloid leukemia involves subtypes M_1–M_7, which have blast cells in the bone marrow equal to or exceeding 30% of nonerythroid cells. In general, survival involves weeks to months for patients with acute myeloid leukemia. Chronic myeloid leukemia subtypes have increased numbers of blast cells but these account for less than 30% of nonerythroid cells of the bone marrow. A longer survival of months to years is expected for patients with chronic myeloid leukemia. Cytochemical staining of blast cells from blood and bone marrow smears may be performed on unfixed slides submitted to special laboratories to determine the cell type primarily involved.

Treatment generally consists of supportive care (e.g., antibiotics, blood transfusions, and fluids). Antineoplastic agents, including corticosteroids, cytosine arabinoside, chlorambucil, busulfan, and hydroxyurea, have been used with limited success. Bone marrow transplantation has been attempted in the cat but is cost prohibitive for clinical application.

Acute Myeloblastic Leukemia (M_1, M_2)

Acute myeloblastic leukemia (AML) is relatively common among leukemias and often is associated with FeLV in cats. It is characterized by a high percentage of myeloblasts in the bone marrow ($\geq$30% of nonerythroid cells). These cells have pale basophilic cytoplasm that may contain several small red granules. Nuclei are round, with prominent nucleoli. Intermediate- and late-stage forms of neutrophils are present to a variable degree. The CBC often indicates a severe nonregenerative anemia and thrombocytopenia. Total leukocyte counts usually are elevated. Cytochemical staining of blast cells is variably positive for peroxidase, Sudan black B, chloroacetate esterase, leukocyte alkaline phosphatase, and acid phosphatase. Rebounding from neutropenia, such as that following feline panleukopenia infection, can cause the blood to appear neoplastic because of the presence of large numbers of myeloblasts. Persistent hematologic abnormalities must occur to confirm leukemia.

Chronic Granulocytic (Neutrophilic) Leukemia

This disorder is characterized by a low percentage of myeloblasts in the bone marrow ($<$30% of all nucleated cells), with increased numbers of early forms such as progranulocytes to metamyelocytes in the blood and bone marrow. Leukocytes often are elevated markedly (40,000–200,000/μl). Anemia is mild to moderate, and platelet counts are variable. The elevated leukocyte count distinguishes this condition from myelodysplastic syndrome because both conditions have a similar bone marrow presentation. Marrow myeloid-to-erythroid ratio is 4:1 to 25:1. This form of leukemia must be differentiated from leukemoid reactions caused by highly suppurative infections such as pyometra (see section on Neutrophilia). Death often occurs months after detection and may be associated with a blast cell crisis, severe anemia, and thrombocytopenia.

Eosinophilic Leukemia

This type of leukemia is rare, but it has been documented in the cat associated with FeLV infection and in the dog. It is characterized by a high eosinophil count (often $>$ 50,000/μl) with a shift toward immaturity. A moderate anemia may be present. It may be difficult to differentiate this malignancy from reactive hypereosinophilic conditions (e.g., allergies, parasitism, eosinophilic inflammatory diseases, mast cell tumors, and certain lymphomas; see discussion of Eosinophilia). Leukemic eosinophils spread from the bone marrow and infiltrate other tissues, such as the lymph nodes, liver, and spleen.

Basophilic Leukemia

This disorder is rare, and most cases have been reported in the dog. It has been associated with thrombocytosis and anemia. Cytochemical staining with omega-exonuclease is helpful in identifying basophil precursors when cytoplasmic granulation is inapparent. Mature and immature basophils are increased in the blood or bone marrow, and tissue infiltration may occur. Basophilic leukemia must be differentiated from mast cell leukemia. Treatment is suggested using hydroxyurea (Hydrea, Squibb) at 50 mg/kg/day in dogs for 3 days a week until cell counts are reduced sufficiently. Survival has been reported up to 21 months.

Acute Monocytic Leukemia (M_5)

This condition has been reported in both dogs and cats. It is characterized by moderate to marked increases of monoblasts in the bone marrow, which are $\geq$30% of nonerythroid cells. These cells have basophilic cytoplasm that lacks any obvious granulation. Nuclei exhibit extreme irregularity, which gives the cell a folded appearance. Nucleoli are usually prominent. Cytochemical staining of the blast cells is generally positive for nonspecific esterases and acid phosphatase.

Acute Myelomonocytic Leukemia (M_4)

This is a common form of myeloid leukemia in dogs and cats. It involves the common stem cell for both granulocytes and monocytes. Cytochemical staining suggests the presence of both monoblasts and myeloblasts. The two blast cell types together are $\geq$ 30% of nonerythroid cells in the bone marrow.

Erythroleukemia (M_6)

Erythroleukemia incorporates the varied manifestations of erythroid leukemic cells. Rubriblasts may predominate or accompany neoplastic myeloblasts. Dysplastic changes are frequently prominent, such as megaloblastosis, neutrophil giantism, or hypersegmentation. Normochromic macrocytes and nucleated erythrocytes are found in the blood, without regenerative signs of polychromasia or reticulocytosis. Over time, this form of leukemia may change in appearance and progress to involve predominantly granulocytic precursors. It frequently is associated with FeLV infection in cats.

Polycythemia Vera

Polycythemia vera occurs rarely in dogs and cats. Clinical signs differ from other myeloid leukemias because they relate to increased erythrocyte mass and blood hyperviscosity. Mucous membranes are dark red because of hematocrits of 65% to 82%. Splenomegaly usually is not present. Polyuria, polydipsia, hemorrhage, and neurologic disorders occur in 50% of canine cases.

Diagnosis requires ruling out other causes of erythrocytosis (see discussion of Polycythemia). Arterial blood gas evaluations are normal, with no evidence of hypoxia. Erythropoietin levels are absent or reduced when measured at specialized laboratories. Leukocyte and platelet counts are normal to mildly elevated. Bone marrow examination indicates hyperplasia of the erythroid line, with normal morphology and maturation. Myeloblasts make up less than 30% of nucleated cells.

Treatment consists of phlebotomy for immediate relief (10–20 ml/kg/day). Survival of at least 1.5 years is possible with hydroxyurea given at 30 mg/kg/day for 1 week, then 15 mg/kg once daily until remission; then taper to lowest effective frequency of administration based on monitoring hematocrit. Monitor cats more closely because of greater risk of myelotoxicity. Radiophosphorus ^{32}P (2.4–3.3 mCi/m^2) has been used with encouraging results.

Megakaryoblastic Leukemia (M$_7$)

This is a rare type of leukemia reported in dogs and cats. It may be associated with irradiation in the dog. Laboratory findings indicate severe nonregenerative anemia, leukopenia, and often thrombocytopenia, although platelet counts are variable. Megakaryoblasts may appear in the circulation, and platelet morphology is often bizarre, characterized by giantism and abnormal granulation. Hemolymphatic organs usually are infiltrated by the neoplastic population, which rules out a benign proliferation. Immunocytochemical stains are used to determine the megakaryocytic origin of the blast cells.

Primary Thrombocythemia

Primary, or essential, thrombocythemia is a rare neoplastic proliferation of platelets reported in the dog and cat. It is not related to transient or reactive increases (see section on Thrombocytosis). Clinical signs include splenomegaly and platelet function abnormalities, such as spontaneous bleeding and thromboembolism. Platelet counts are persistently greater than 600,000/μl, usually >1 million/μl. Neutrophilia or basophilia also may be present. Treatment may include melphalan (2–4 mg/m^2), hydroxyurea (500 mg/m^2), or radiophosphorus ^{32}P (2.4–3.5 mCi/m^2). Therapy produces a survival of up to 32 months. Transformation to chronic myelogenous leukemia has been reported.

SUPPLEMENTAL READINGS

Boudreaux MK: Platelets and coagulation. Vet Clin North Am 26:1065, 1996.

Fox LE, Ford S, Alleman AR, et al.: Aplastic anemia associated with prolonged high-dose trimethoprim-sulfadiazine administration in two dogs. Vet Clin Pathol 22:89, 1993.

Greene CE, Watson ADJ: Antiprotozoal chemotherapy. *In* Greene CE, ed.: Infectious Diseases of the Dog and Cat, 2nd ed. Philadelphia: WB Saunders, 1998, pp 441–444.

Grindem CB, Breitschwerdt EB, Corbett WT, et al: Thrombocytopenia associated with neoplasia in dogs. J Vet Intern Med 8:400, 1994.

Harvey JW: Congenital erythrocyte enzyme deficiencies. Vet Clin North Am 26:1003, 1996

Hasler AH, Giger U: Serum erythropoietin values in polycythemic cats. J Am Anim Hosp Assoc 32:294, 1996.

Jain NC: The leukemias. *In* Jain NC, ed.: Essentials of Veterinary Hematology. Philadelphia: Lea & Febiger, 1993, pp 319–348.

Raskin RE: Myelopoiesis and myeloproliferative disorders. Vet Clin North Am 26:1023, 1996.

Walker DB, Cowell RL: Survival of a domestic cat with naturally acquired cytauxzoonosis. J Am Vet Med Assoc 206:1363, 1995.

Weiser MG, Thrall MA, Fulton R, et al: Granular lymphocytosis and hyperproteinemia in dogs with chronic ehrlichiosis. J Am Anim Hosp Assoc 27:84, 1991.

21 Coagulation Diseases

Marjory Brooks

Coagulation disorders are a group of bleeding diatheses caused by dysfunction of the clotting cascade and subsequent failure of fibrin clot formation. Included in this discussion of coagulation disorders are von Willebrand disease and disseminated intravascular coagulation. Common bleeding diatheses that are not coagulation disorders include thrombocytopenia and acquired platelet dysfunction (platelet disorders are discussed in Chapter 20). Differentiate patients affected with coagulation disorders from those with bleeding due to damaged or diseased blood vessels.

ETIOLOGY

Categories of bleeding disorders are listed in Table 21–1 and include coagulation factor deficiencies, von Willebrand disease, and disseminated intravascular coagulation.

Coagulation Factor Deficiencies

Acquired Deficiencies

Acquired deficiencies of functional coagulation factors are common disorders and are caused by decreased production of coagulation factors or inactivation of existing factors.

Production Defect

Most coagulation factors are proteins synthesized in the liver. Clinically significant reduction in these factors most often accompanies acute fulminant necrosis, chronic cirrhosis, and portosystemic shunting diseases; each of these causes severe liver failure and marked reduction in functional hepatic mass.

Inactive Factors

Vitamin K Deficiency
- The prothrombin group of coagulation factors (Factors II, VII, IX, X) require vitamin K for activation.
  - The most common vitamin K deficiency state in small animal medicine occurs after ingestion of anticoagulant rodenticides, which deplete body stores of vitamin K. Potency and duration of effect vary for different poisons.
  - Posthepatic biliary obstruction and infiltrative

bowel disease also can cause vitamin K deficiency by reducing its intestinal absorption.
- Occasionally, bleeding due to vitamin K deficiency is seen in neonatal puppies. Typically, these puppies are born prematurely or are delivered by cesarean section.

Heparin
- Heparin inhibits coagulation factor function by greatly enhancing activity of antithrombin III, a natural plasma anticoagulant.
  - Bleeding due to iatrogenic factor inactivation results from overdose of heparin for treatment of thrombotic disorders or excessive heparinization of transfused blood products.
  - Release of heparin from mast cell tumor granules often causes local tissue hemorrhage and edema. In rare cases, massive degranulation of disseminated tumor causes systemic anticoagulation.

Inherited Factor Deficiencies

Inherited factor deficiencies are caused by mutations in genes coding for specific, individual coagulation proteins. These defects are most common in certain lines of purebred dogs and cats and usually are perpetuated when asymptomatic carriers are bred. They also may arise by new, spontaneous mutations in previously unaffected families of purebred or mixed-breed animals. Inheritance patterns vary for different individual factor deficiencies.

X-linked Traits

Hemophilia is the most common severe coagulation factor deficiency and is inherited as an X-linked recessive trait. Spontaneous mutations causing hemophilia arise frequently in dogs and cats.

- Males inheriting one abnormal gene from their mother express the trait, whereas females inheriting one abnormal gene from either parent are asymptomatic carriers.
- Mutations in the factor VIII gene cause hemophilia A and arise about three times as often as those in the factor IX gene. Hemophilia B is a specific deficiency of factor IX.
- German shepherds, especially those with European dogs in their pedigree, have the highest prevalence of canine hemophilia A.

Table 21–1. CLASSIFICATION AND CAUSES OF COAGULATION DISORDERS

Category	Cause
Coagulation factor deficiency	
Acquired (multiple) factor deficiencies	Decreased factor production
	Liver failure (acute necrosis, chronic cirrhosis, portosystemic shunts)
	Decreased factor activation
	Vitamin K deficiency (anticoagulant rodenticide toxicity, biliary obstruction, malabsorption, neonatal)
	Heparin excess (iatrogenic, mast cell tumor)
Inherited (single) factor deficiency	X-linked traits—males affected
	Hemophilia A—factor VIII deficiency (most common defect in dogs and cats; German shepherd breed has highest prevalence)
	Hemophilia B—Factor IX deficiency (Airedale, Bichon, many breeds and mixed-breed dogs, cats)
	Autosomal traits—males and females affected
	Dysfibrinogenemia—uncommon (borzoi, French bulldog)
	Prothrombin deficiency—uncommon (boxer, English cocker)
	Factor VII deficiency—mild bleeding (beagle)
	Factor X deficiency—severe bleeding (American cocker)
	Factor XI deficiency—severe bleeding (English springer spaniel, Kerry blue terrier)
	Factor XII deficiency—no abnormal bleeding (common in domestic shorthaired cats)
von Willebrand disease	Inherited form—autosomal trait
	Variable severity in affected dogs, high prevalence (Doberman pinscher, golden retriever, standard poodle, Corgi, Akita, others)
	Severe bleeding in affected dogs (Scottie, Sheltie, German shorthaired pointer, Chesapeake retriever)
	Acquired form—bleeding associated with systemic disease
	Endocrinopathy (thyroid insufficiency, cortisol insufficiency, estrus, parturition)
	Infection (viral, bacterial, postvaccinal)
	Drug therapy (sulfa-trimethoprim, nonsteroidal anti-inflammatory drugs)
Disseminated intravascular coagulation	Factor depletion and systemic fibrinolysis
	Neoplasia (hemangiosarcoma, prostatic and mammary carcinoma, lymphoid tumors)
	Sepsis
	Intravascular hemolysis
	Severe tissue injury (burns, crush wounds)

Autosomal Traits

Males and females express these traits with equal frequency.

- Clinically significant bleeding disorders due to inherited deficiencies of factors XI, X, VII, II, and fibrinogen have been described.
- Factor XII deficiency is common in cats but does not cause abnormal hemostasis.

von Willebrand Disease

Von Willebrand (vWD) disease is the most common inherited bleeding disorder in dogs. Bleeding in affected individuals is caused by deficiency or dysfunction of von Willebrand factor (vWF), a plasma protein critical for normal platelet function in the primary phase of hemostasis.

- The trait is autosomal; both males and females can transmit and/or express vWD.
- Apparent acquired forms of vWD are seen where individuals first exhibit signs of abnormal hemostasis as adults. In these cases, concurrent infection, hormonal fluctuation, or endocrinopathy (especially thyroid insufficiency) often is present when bleeding diathesis is expressed.
- Breeds with highest prevalence of the vWD trait include Doberman pinscher, Scottish terrier, Shetland sheepdog, golden retriever, Pembroke Welsh corgi, and standard poodle.

Disseminated Intravascular Coagulation

Disseminated intravascular coagulation (DIC) is a dynamic disease process caused by systemic activation of the coagulation cascade with loss of localized clot formation and a secondary diffuse activation of the fibrinolytic system.

- Disorders that trigger the DIC process cause widespread damage to vascular tissue, platelet aggregation and consumption, or intravascular release of tissue factor.
- Clinically, DIC most often accompanies severe systemic diseases such as sepsis, neoplasia (especially hemangiosarcoma, lymphoma, prostatic and mammary carcinoma), burn or crush wounds, and intravascular hemolysis.
- Bleeding occurs in association with DIC because coagulation factors are depleted and the fibrinolytic pathway degrades clots before vessel repair is complete. Systemic fibrinolysis causes an increase in plasma fibrin degradation products, which inhibit coagulation factor function. Thrombocytopenia and platelet dysfunction often accompany DIC and further exacerbate bleeding.

CLINICAL SIGNS

Coagulation disorders are characterized by spontaneous hemorrhage and/or excessive bleeding after surgery or trauma. Hemorrhage into the central nervous system (CNS) may cause acute onset of neurologic dysfunction or sudden death. Thrombocytopenia (see Chapter 20), not coagulation disorder, is by far the most common cause of petechiae in small animals. Hemorrhagic macules, papules, and ecchymoses are lesions most characteristic of primary or secondary vasculitic diseases and rarely are caused by coagulopathy.

- **Coagulation factor deficiencies** tend to cause spontaneous bleeding into the chest, abdomen, or muscles, and subcutaneous hematoma formation.
- **von Willebrand disease** is associated most often with spontaneous hemorrhage from mucosal surfaces of oral and nasal cavities, or intestinal and genitourinary tracts.
- **Bleeding in association with DIC** is usually severe and occurs from mucosal surfaces and into body cavities; in addition, signs of the underlying disease are usually present.
- **Bleeding from venipuncture sites** most often accompanies severe deficiencies of multiple coagulation factors or fulminant DIC. Absence of this sign does not rule out a clinically significant coagulation disorder.

DIAGNOSIS

▼ *Key Point* The first consideration when evaluating bleeding patients is to differentiate blood loss due to injury of a single or local group of blood vessels from a systemic bleeding diathesis. This distinction is usually apparent after thorough history, physical examination, and evaluation of quick assessment tests.

History

The history should include specific questions to identify previous episodes of spontaneous bleeding or excessive hemorrhage after surgery or trauma.

- Gingival bleeding from tooth eruption and bleeding from docking or dewclaw removal are common signs of inherited coagulation factor deficiency and vWD. Conversely, history of severe trauma or invasive surgical procedure without excessive hemorrhage rules out an inherited hemostatic defect.
- Patients with histories of hepatic disease or disorders associated with DIC are at risk for acquired coagulation defects and should be further evaluated before invasive procedures.

Physical Examination

Physical examination should define as thoroughly as possible the nature, severity, and precise anatomic source of hemorrhage. In patients with a single obvious site of external blood loss, ophthalmoscopy, digital anorectal examination, careful auscultation, and joint palpation may identify additional sites of hemorrhage that would be suggestive of coagulation disorder.

Radiographic Examination

Radiography of the thorax and abdomen can detect fluid densities indicative of bleeding in pleural, peritoneal, or retroperitoneal spaces. Intrapulmonary hemorrhage causes an alveolar pattern on thoracic films. Epistaxis, hematuria, and gastrointestinal hemorrhage may be difficult to differentiate as being signs of local vessel trauma versus signs of systemic coagulation disorder. Contrast radiography, ultrasonography, and computed tomography (CT) scan can noninvasively identify erosive, infiltrative, or mass lesions causing vessel damage. CT scan is especially useful for evaluating the nasal cavity to identify focal lesions early in the disease process before they extend into the CNS.

Quick Assessment Tests

Quick assessment tests (QATs) are useful for identifying hemostatic defects and evaluating hemostatic function prior to performing invasive procedures. Table 21–2 presents additional diagnostic ruleouts and procedures, based on results of QATs, for differentiating coagulation disorders from other hemostatic defects. Table 21–3 lists expected results of the following QATs for categories of common coagulation disorders.

Slide Estimate of Platelet Number

Thrombocytopenia can be ruled out if examination of a stained blood film under oil immersion reveals at least 7–10 platelets per field for dogs and 10–15 platelets per field for cats.

Activated Clotting Time (ACT)

Most of the common acquired and inherited coagulation factor deficiencies can be detected by prolongation of ACT, a functional test of the intrinsic clotting system.

- Procedure
  - Collect 2 ml of whole blood directly into a test tube, maintain the needle (Vacutainer, Becton-Dickinson) in the vein, remove the first tube, and replace it with a second evacuated tube containing siliceous earth (Vacutainer, Becton-Dickinson) to withdraw a second 2-ml sample.
  - Warm the evacuated tube to 37°C before sampling.
  - Immediately after blood collection, gently invert the second tube several times to mix blood with siliceous activator, and then place it in a heating block calibrated at 37°C.
  - After incubation for 45 seconds, remove the tube from the block at 5- to 10-second intervals, gently tilt it, and evaluate for clot formation.
- ACT is the time elapsed from sampling to clot formation.
- Normal range of canine ACT is 60–120 seconds; feline range is 60–70 seconds.

Table 21–2. DIAGNOSTIC CHECKLISTS BASED ON RESULTS OF QUICK ASSESSMENT TESTS (QATs)

QAT	Result/Interpretation	Checklist
Platelet estimate	Low/thrombocytopenia	See Chapter 20
Bleeding time	Prolonged/defect of primary hemostasis	History (drug exposure, familial bleeding) CBC/metabolic profile Radiography vWF:Ag Thyroid function Fibrin split product titer Platelet aggregometry
Activated clotting time	Prolonged/defect of intrinsic coagulation system	History (toxin exposure, familial bleeding) Coagulation screening assays Coagulation factor analysis CBC/metabolic profile Liver function Radiography Fibrin split product titer Response to vitamin K therapy

CBC, complete blood count; vWF:Ag, von Willebrand factor antigen.

- ACT may be technically difficult to perform in cats and small dogs.
- Sampling from the jugular vein is not recommended in patients with severe hemorrhagic disorders because iatrogenic hematoma formation and subsequent upper respiratory obstruction might occur.

Bleeding Time Tests

Bleeding time tests are in vivo measures of hemostatic function performed by making a standard wound and timing the interval to cessation of blood flow. These tests should be performed only on patients with platelet counts greater than 100,000/ul because significant thrombocytopenia prolongs bleeding time.

Table 21–3. EXPECTED RESULTS OF QUICK ASSESSMENT TESTS (QATs) FOR COAGULATION DISORDERS

| Category | Tests | | | |
	Platelet Count	ACT	TBT	BMBT
Coagulation factor deficiency				
Acquired deficiencies	N	A	A	N
Inherited deficiencies				
Hemophilia (A and B)	N	A	A	N
Dysfibrinogenemia, Prothrombin, Factor X, XI deficiencies	N	A	A	N
Factor VII deficiency	N	N	N	N
Factor XII deficiency	N	A	N	N
vWD (inherited and acquired)	N	N	A	A
DIC (hemorrhagic phase)	A	A	A	N/A

ACT, activated clotting time; TBT, toenail bleeding time; BMBT, buccal mucosal bleeding time; vWD, von Willebrand disease; DIC, disseminated intravascular coagulation; N, normal; A, abnormal.

Buccal Mucosa Bleeding Time (BMBT) Test

- Procedure:
  - Evert the lip and then hold it in place with gauze that encircles the muzzle and causes the buccal veins to engorge slightly.
  - Use a template device (Simplate II, Organon Teknika) to make two parallel incisions in mucosa of the upper lip.
  - Collect hemorrhage from the wounds on filter paper applied underneath, but not directly to bleeding sites.
- BMBT is the average time elapsed from triggering the device until blood stops flowing from both incisions.
- Normal BMBT is 2 to 4 minutes for dogs and cats.
- BMBT is prolonged in patients with acquired and inherited platelet dysfunction and vWD but is normal for patients with coagulation factor deficiencies and in some patients with DIC.
- Cats require sedation for BMBT testing, but many dogs tolerate this procedure without chemical restraint.

Toenail Bleeding Time (TBT) Test

- Procedure:
  - Using a guillotine-type toenail clipper, make a clean transection at the tip of the nail cuticle.
  - Allow blood to flow freely from the injury.
- The time from transection until blood ceases to flow is the TBT.
- Normal TBT is 5 to 6 minutes; accuracy depends on technique and immobilization of the patient's digit during the procedure.
- TBT is less specific than BMBT and is prolonged for patients with clinically significant coagulation factor deficiencies, vWD, platelet dysfunction, and bleeding due to DIC.
- The TBT test is best performed on sedated or anesthetized patients.

Table 21–4. COAGULATION FACTORS OF THE INTRINSIC, EXTRINSIC, AND COMMON PATHWAYS

Intrinsic	Extrinsic	Common
High molecular weight kininogen	Tissue factor	Factor X
Prekallikrein	Factor VII	Factor V
Factor XII		Factor II (prothrombin)
Factor XI		Factor I (fibrinogen)
Factor IX		
Factor VIII		

Definitive Tests

Definitive tests to diagnose coagulation disorders depend on correct sampling technique and test systems that are validated specifically for canine and feline patients. Table 21–4 lists coagulation factors of the intrinsic, extrinsic, and common pathways, a classification system useful for in vitro diagnosis of bleeding disorders.

Table 21–5 presents expected results of diagnostic tests for categories of common coagulation disorders.

Coagulation Screening Assays

These tests measure the time, in seconds, for in vitro fibrin clot formation. Prolongation of screening assay times beyond the laboratory's normal range, or greater than 5–7 seconds from a control of the same species is indicative of coagulation factor deficiency or inhibition.

- *Activated partial thromboplastin time (aPTT)* is sensitive to deficiencies of intrinsic and common coagulation pathways.
- *Prothrombin time (PT)* detects deficiencies in extrinsic and common pathways.
- *Fibrinogen* concentration (mg/dl) is a quantitative measure of plasma fibrinogen.
- *Thrombin clotting time (TCT)* detects both deficiency and dysfunction of fibrinogen.
- Based on the pattern of abnormalities detected in coagulation screening assays, individual clotting factor analyses identify specific single or multiple coagulation factor deficiencies.

Table 21–5. DEFINITIVE DIAGNOSTIC TESTS FOR COAGULATION DISORDERS

Category	Tests	Results
Coagulation factor deficiency		
Acquired deficiencies		
Liver failure	APTT, PT, TCT	Prolonged
	Fibrinogen*	Low
	Factor analysis	Low activity most factors, variable activity—factor VIII
Vitamin K deficiency	APTT, PT	Prolonged
	TCT, fibrinogen	Normal
	Factor analysis	Low activity—factors II, VII, IX, X
Heparin excess	APTT, PT	Prolonged
	TCT	Marked prolongation
	Fibrinogen	Normal
Inherited deficiencies		
Hemophilia	APTT	Prolonged
	PT, TCT, fibrinogen	Normal
	Factor analysis	Low activity—factor VIII (hemophilia A) or factor IX (hemophilia B)
Dysfibrinogenemia	APTT, PT, TCT	Prolonged
	Fibrinogen	Low
Prothrombin deficiency or factor X deficiency	APTT, PT	Prolonged
	TCT, fibrinogen	Normal
	Factor analysis	Low activity—factor II or X
Factor VII deficiency	PT	Prolonged
	APTT, TCT, fibrinogen	Normal
	Factor analysis	Low activity—factor VII
Factor XI or XII deficiency	APTT	Marked prolongation
	PT, TCT, fibrinogen	Normal
	Factor analysis	Low activity—factor XI or XII
vWD (acquired and inherited)	Bleeding time	Prolonged
	vWF:Ag	Low
	vWF cofactor, multimers	Abnormal
DIC (hemorrhagic phase)	APTT, PT, TCT	Prolonged
	Fibrinogen, ATIII	Low
	Platelet count	Progressive decrease
	Fibrin split products†	Positive titer
	Red cell morphology	Schistocytes

APTT, activated partial thromboplastin time; PT, prothrombin time; TCT, thrombin clotting time; vWF:Ag, von Willebrand factor antigen; vWD, von Willebrand disease; DIC, disseminated vascular coagulation; ATIII, antithrombin III.
*Normal fibrinogen concentration is 150–475 mg/dl for dogs and 100–200 mg/dl for cats.
†Normal fibrin split product concentration is <5 μg/ml.

Specific vWF Assays

Specific tests must be performed to establish diagnosis of vWD. Clotting time tests, coagulation assays, and platelet count do not detect abnormal vWF.

- Measurement of vWF antigen (vWF:Ag) is the most commonly used quantitative vWF assay.
- Patients with vWF below the normal range (established at each testing laboratory) are considered at risk for carrying and/or expressing the vWD trait.
- In addition to low plasma vWF, affected individuals have abnormal in vivo bleeding time.

Diagnosis of DIC

Definitive diagnosis of DIC cannot be based on any one diagnostic test but depends on a combination of clinical signs and laboratory abnormalities. The DIC process is dynamic, and an early thrombotic or procoagulant phase is followed by later signs of hemorrhage as the disease progresses. Serial evaluations are useful to monitor response to therapy and determine prognosis.

- The presence of serum or plasma fibrin degradation products (FDPs) or fibrin split products (FSPs), especially in increasing titers, is compatible with ongoing systemic fibrinolysis usually caused by DIC.
- Additional findings, characteristic of the hemorrhagic phase of DIC, include:
  - Falling platelet count
  - Low concentration of plasma fibrinogen and antithrombin III
  - Prolongation of all coagulation screening assays (aPTT, PT, TCT)
  - Presence of schistocytes on stained peripheral blood smears
- Elevated values of plasma soluble fibrin monomer, D-dimer, and thrombin-antithrombin complex are specific indicators of a prothrombotic or procoagu-

lant state, and reduced levels of plasminogen concentration indicate accelerated fibrinolysis. Assays to detect these plasma proteins are being developed and validated for use in dogs and cats to better define DIC and determine optimal treatment.

TREATMENT

▼ *Key Point* Successful management of patients with coagulation disorders requires establishing an accurate diagnosis, and then administering appropriate transfusion and nontransfusion support. Pretreatment samples are invaluable for establishing definitive diagnosis early in the course of disease.

Transfusion Therapy

Transfusion therapy to supply active factors is required for patients with severe, inherited coagulation factor deficiencies, patients with inherited vWD, and patients with acquired disorders that are not responsive to correction of an underlying disease process. Table 21–6 lists blood product(s) and dosages for treating specific coagulation disorders (see Chapter 20 for a description of crossmatching protocol).

- Transfusion of whole blood, administered within 4 to 6 hours of collection, supplies active coagulation factors and vWF, as well as red blood cells (RBCs).
- Transfusion of plasma products (fresh plasma, fresh frozen plasma, plasma concentrate), rather than whole blood, reduces the risk of immunologic transfusion reactions, most importantly RBC sensitization. Plasma components also can be transfused preoperatively and repeatedly in 1 day without causing volume overload.
- Stored whole blood and packed red cells do not contain replacement levels of coagulation factors or vWF, but the administration of red cells is indicated for pa-

Table 21–6. GUIDELINES FOR TRANSFUSION*

Product	Volume	Frequency	Indications
Fresh whole blood† Packed red cells	12–20 ml/kg 6–10 ml/kg	q24h q12–24h	Signs of anemia accompanying: coagulation factor deficiencies von Willebrand disease disseminated intravascular coagulation
Fresh plasma† Fresh frozen plasma‡	6–12 ml/kg	q8–12h	Coagulation factor deficiencies von Willebrand disease Disseminated intravascular coagulation
Plasma cryoprecipitate§	1 unit‖/10 kg	q4–12h (as needed)	Hemophilia A (factor VIII deficiency) Fibrinogen deficiency von Willebrand disease
Cryosupernatant§	6–12 ml/kg	q8–12h	Hemophilia B (factor IX deficiency) Factor VII, X, or XI deficiency Vitamin K deficiency

*Transfuse at a rate of 1–2 ml/min for cats and puppies, 3–6 ml/min for adult dogs.
†Collected in citrate anticoagulant, transfused within 4–6 hours of collection.
‡Frozen within 4–6 hours of collection, stored below −20° C.
§Prepared from fresh frozen plasma.
‖1 unit = cryoprecipitate produced from 200 ml of fresh, frozen plasma.

tients having signs of acute or chronic blood loss anemia. Packed cells, in combination with an appropriate plasma product are the therapeutic equivalent of fresh whole blood. The use of blood components, rather than fresh whole blood, provides a more convenient, rapid, and often safer means of transfusion support.

- Routine pretreatment with antihistamine or corticosteroid before transfusion of any blood product is not recommended. Acute immune reactions directed against RBCs can be prevented in cats by using donors that are blood type and crossmatch compatible with the recipient. Anti-RBC reactions are prevented in dogs by using type compatible or "universal donor" type dogs. Dogs negative for dog erythrocyte antigen (DEA) 1 (1.1 and 1.2) and negative for DEA 7 are unlikely to sensitize recipients and can be considered universal donors.
- Cross-species transfusions of any blood product are contraindicated because fatal anaphylaxis can result.

Nursing Care

Nursing care practices that reduce hemorrhage include:

- Confinement to limit activity
- Feeding soft food
- Avoidance of neck leads and IM injections
- Use of peripheral veins for sampling or IV catheter placement

Do not give platelet inhibitory drugs, including sulfas and nonsteroidal anti-inflammatory agents.

Wound Management

Good management reduces the need for transfusion in some patients with coagulation disorders and mucosal or cutaneous hemorrhage. The best treatment, for even small wounds, is usually suture and/or pressure bandages. Application of tissue adhesive (Vetbond, 3M Co.) to focal areas of bleeding also can limit local blood loss.

Drug Therapy

Vitamin K Therapy

Vitamin K therapy improves hemostasis only in vitamin K–deficient patients. It often is initiated pending test results, but maintenance of vitamin K therapy is not indicated when diagnosis of inherited factor deficiency, nonobstructive liver disease, vWD, or DIC is made. Anticoagulant rodenticide toxicities are the most common cause of vitamin K deficiency in dogs and cats. Vitamin K reverses the anticoagulant effect of rodenticides over a period of 24 to 48 hours from initiation of therapy.

Treatment for Warfarin Toxicity

Warfarin is a relatively short-acting poison, and treatment for a total of 1 week usually is adequate. Standard treatment is as follows:

- Administer an initial dose of vitamin K_1 (Aqua-Mephyton, Merck, Sharp, Dohme), 2.2 mg/kg SC.

- Follow with a dose of 1.1 mg/kg SC, q12h, until active bleeding subsides.
- Then substitute an oral preparation (Mephyton) at the same twice-daily dosage.

Treatment for Long-Acting Rodenticides

To treat toxicity from second-generation or long-acting rodenticides (diphacinone, pindone, bromadiolone, and brodifacoum):

- Transfusion is indicated for patients having severe anemia, pulmonary or CNS hemorrhage at presentation (see Table 21–6).
- Initiate parenteral vitamin K_1 as for warfarin (2.2 mg/kg SC).
- Administer vitamin K_1 at 1.1 mg/kg SC, q12h until the hematocrit value stabilizes and active bleeding subsides.
- Maintain oral vitamin K_1 at 1.1 mg/kg PO, q12h for a total of 2 weeks.
- Taper the maintenance dose by one-half every 2 weeks during treatment.
- To prevent relapse, continue therapy for 4 to 6 weeks.

▼ *Key Point* Subcutaneous injection of vitamin K is the preferred parenteral route of administration because intravenous vitamin K can cause anaphylaxis, and hematomas may form at intramuscular injection sites. Vitamin K_3 (Synkayvite) is not effective for treating rodenticide toxicity because of its delayed onset of action.

Hormonal Therapy

Hormonal therapy may reverse bleeding resulting from acquired vWD in association with endocrine disorders.

Thyroxin

Thyroid insufficiency (see Chapter 29) is common in many of the breeds that have a high prevalence of the vWD trait.

- Treat responsive animals with L-thyroxine at a dosage of 0.02 mg/kg q12h PO. Hemostasis improves within 24 to 48 hours of initiating therapy. Maintenance of thyroid hormone therapy may prevent subsequent bleeding episodes.
- Because not all patients respond, assess bleeding time and clinical status after thyroid hormone supplementation to determine whether hemostasis has improved.

Desmopressin Acetate

Desmopressin acetate (DDAVP, USV Pharmaceutical), a vasopressin analogue, has shown efficacy in transiently improving hemostasis in some dogs affected with vWD.

- Its activity probably is the result of release of vWF from intracellular stores and its effectiveness depends on the patient's ability to produce functional vWF protein.

- Duration of action, after a dose of 1 µg/kg SC, is 3 to 4 hours; repeated dosage within 24 hours does not prolong response time.
- Demonstrate correction of abnormal bleeding time before undertaking invasive procedures because all patients do not respond.

Heparin Therapy

- Heparin therapy (100 units/kg q6–8h SC) is useful in managing some cases of DIC, when ongoing systemic coagulation is causing signs of vessel thrombosis or embolism. Remember that heparin can exacerbate bleeding by inhibiting platelet and coagulation factor function.
- Transfusion therapy with fresh blood or blood products to replace active coagulation factors, antithrombin III, and platelets is more likely than heparin therapy to benefit patients presenting with severe hemorrhage in association with DIC.

▼ *Key Point* The critical factor for successfully managing all patients with DIC is identification and correction of the underlying disorder.

SUPPLEMENTAL READING

Brooks MB: Emergency management of canine von Willebrand disease. Proceedings of the American College of Veterinary Internal Medicine, 14th Annual Forum 1996, pp 34–36.

Brooks M, Catalfamo J: Buccal mucosa bleeding time is prolonged in canine models of primary hemostatic disorders. Thromb Haemost 70:777, 1993.

Dodds WJ: Bleeding disorders. In: Morgan RV, ed: Handbook of Small Animal Practice. New York: Churchill Livingstone, 1988, pp 773–785.

Kristensen AT, Feldman BF: General principles of small animal blood component administration. In: Feldman BF, Kristensen AT (eds): Veterinary Clinics of North America: Canine and Feline Transfusion Medicine. Philadelphia: WB Saunders, 1995, pp 1277–1290.

Laneveschi A, Kramer JW, Greene S, Meyers KM: Evaluation of chromogenic substrate assays for fibrinolytic analytes in dogs. Am J Vet Res 57:1124, 1996.

Madewell BR: Sample preparation for the laboratory. In: Kirk RW, ed: Current Veterinary Therapy X. Philadelphia: WB Saunders, 1989, pp 410–419.

Wardrop KJ: Medical indications for plasma therapy. Proceedings of the American College of Veterinary Internal Medicine, 14th Annual Forum 1996, pp 31–33.

Systemic Immune-Mediated Diseases

James P. Thompson

Numerous immune-mediated or immune-associated diseases have been identified in dogs and cats. Management of these diseases focuses mainly on the recognition of the disease and appropriate immunosuppressive chemotherapy. This chapter focuses on the recognition and management of immune-mediated hemolytic anemia, immune-mediated thrombocytopenia, and systemic lupus erythematosus as frequently observed systemic abnormalities of the immune system. Organ-specific immune-mediated diseases are discussed in the respective organ system sections of this book; notably, pemphigus and other cutaneous immune disorders are discussed in Chapter 43, rheumatoid and immune polyarthropathies in the Orthopedic section, and immune-mediated neuromuscular disorders in the Neurology section.

IMMUNE-MEDIATED HEMOLYTIC ANEMIA

The major clinical concern in immune-mediated hemolytic anemia (IMHA) is accelerated erythrocyte destruction resulting from antibodies attached to the erythrocyte surface. Antibody-coated erythrocytes are destroyed by one of two basic mechanisms: extravascular phagocytosis or intravascular hemolysis.

Extravascular phagocytosis is the most common form of IMHA. Phagocytosis occurs primarily in the spleen and liver. Typically, IgG-coated erythrocytes are removed by the spleen, and IgM-coated erythrocytes are trapped by the liver; erythrocytes initially trapped by the liver can be released and subsequently removed by the spleen. For additional description of the spleen's role in this process, see Chapter 23.

Intravascular hemolysis is the result of antibody-induced complement activation. This class of IMHA generally is associated with IgM antibodies or very high concentrations of serum IgG.

Etiology

▼ *Key Point* IMHA is caused by a type II hypersensitivity (cytotoxic) immune response characterized by antibody molecules directed against red blood cell surface antigens.

- Antibody may be directed against unaltered endogenous erythrocyte membrane antigens (primary au-toimmune hemolytic anemia) or to exogenous antigens (secondary IMHA).
- The specific etiology of IMHA usually goes unrecognized. Occasionally the clinician can associate a drug with the onset of clinical and hematologic signs. Most cases of IMHA are classified as idiopathic until detailed studies of erythrocyte membrane antigens and antibody against these antigens are performed.
- A familial predisposition exists in dogs that implies a potential underlying genetic predilection. All breeds of dogs are susceptible, but poodles, Old English sheepdogs, Irish setters, and cocker spaniels are predisposed. Affected dogs usually are between 2 and 8 years of age. Female dogs appear to be affected three to four times more frequently than male dogs.

▼ *Key Point* Approximately one-half to three-fourths of IMHA in cats is associated with feline leukemia virus infection. Other feline diseases associated with IMHA include hemobartonellosis and lymphoma. No breed or sex predilection has been observed.

Clinical Signs

- Patients usually are presented for vague primary complaints that may include sensitivity to cold, anorexia, listlessness, weakness, and depression.
- Gastrointestinal disturbances manifested by pica, vomiting, and diarrhea may be observed.
- Patients occasionally are presented with the primary complaint of icterus.

Diagnosis

Physical Examination

The physical examination typically reveals pale mucous membranes, tachycardia, and tachypnea. A systolic heart murmur may be auscultated because of decreased blood viscosity. If extravascular hemolysis is the prominent mechanism of erythrocyte destruction, hepatomegaly and splenomegaly may be present. If the major mechanism of erythrocyte destruction is intravascular hemolysis, icterus and fever may be observed. Peripheral lymphadenopathy also may be noted.

Complete Blood Count (CBC)

- The most important aspect of the hemogram is the erythron response, which typically indicates a regenerative anemia that is characterized by macrocytosis. The presence of spherocytes (small globular erythrocytes without central pallor) in the absence of schistocytes (erythrocyte fragments) is nearly pathognomonic for IMHA.

- The CBC frequently demonstrates a leukocytosis characterized by an absolute neutrophilia and left shift; total leukocyte counts as high as $60,000/\mu l$ blood with 4000 metamyelocytes have been observed.
- The plasma fibrinogen concentration usually is elevated.
- If hemolysis is present in the patient's blood specimen, consider a diagnosis of intravascular lysis; be careful, however, to rule out lipemia-induced or sampling technique–induced in vitro hemolysis.

Serum Biochemistry Profile

- This assay generally is unrewarding.
- Serum lactic dehydrogenase activity usually is elevated as a result of enzyme release from damaged erythrocytes.
- Serum alanine and aspartate aminotransferase and alkaline phosphatase activities may be elevated.
- In extensive extravascular and intravascular hemolysis, hyperbilirubinemia is present, but the clinician probably already knows this, based on the presence of icterus.

Urinalysis

- Urinalysis is useful to document the presence of hemoglobinuria or bilirubinuria; remember that any amount of bilirubinuria in cats is abnormal, whereas dogs may exhibit detectable levels in the absence of disease.
- Excessive proteinuria may indicate extensive glomerular damage resulting from immune-complex deposition associated with intravascular lysis of circulating erythrocytes.
- Cylindruria (the presence of excessive numbers of casts in the urine) suggests tubular damage. If an active urine sediment is present, as evidenced by an excessive number of casts and inflammatory cells, adequate fluid intake is critical to ensure appropriate blood flow to the damaged kidney.

Antierythrocyte Antibody Detection

▼ *Key Point* Definitive diagnosis is made by detecting antibody molecules or complement on the surface of circulating erythrocytes.

Direct Agglutination Test

Attempt to demonstrate the presence of antibody-coated erythrocytes by performing the direct agglutination test.

- Place a drop of anticoagulated whole blood on a microscope slide and mix with the blood one drop of physiologic saline. The one drop of added saline is to reduce the plasma protein concentration by half and prevent rouleau formation; the reduction of antibody concentration by half generally does not reduce the concentration of antibody significantly to prevent agglutination of erythrocytes. If sufficient antibody molecules are present, agglutination is observed.

Direct Coombs Test

This test is used to identify antibodies bound to circulating erythrocytes when the concentration of antibody molecules is too low to cause direct agglutination. It should be performed in cases that demonstrate anemia in the absence of direct agglutination.

▼ *Key Point* Draw blood for Coombs testing before transfusion.

The Coombs reagents must be species specific. These reagents usually recognize IgG, IgM, and C3b; C3b is the membrane-bound protein-split product deposited on the erythrocyte surface from the third component of the complement cascade. Antibody or complement bound to the erythrocyte surface then is detected by cross-linking these molecules with species-specific reagents directed at these molecules.

In the interpretation of Coombs test results, the causes of false-positive and false-negative results must be understood.

- A *false-positive test* can be seen most frequently in cases in which:
  - Patients have received a prior erythrocyte transfusion
  - There is nonspecific adsorption of serum immunoglobulins onto the surface of damaged erythrocytes, such as occurs in disseminated intravascular coagulation (DIC)
- A *false-negative test* is caused most frequently by:
  - Poor laboratory technique
  - Insufficient antibody on the red blood cell (RBC) membrane to permit detection with the Coombs test

In the absence of a positive Coombs test result, the clinician is justified in making a diagnosis of immune-mediated hemolytic anemia only when underlying infection, neoplasia, and erythrocyte enzyme deficiencies have been eliminated.

Concurrent Diseases

Disorders that may accompany IMHA include immune-mediated thrombocytopenia and/or systemic lupus erythematosus; both of these are discussed later in this chapter. In all cases of IMHA, perform an absolute platelet count and submit serum for an indirect fluorescent antinuclear antibody (IFAA) test. In patients with a reduced platelet count and hypofibrinogenemia, rule out disseminated intravascular coagulation as an underlying etiology for the thrombocytopenia (see Chapter 20).

Treatment

The therapeutic goals are to prevent further destruction of erythrocytes, to prevent formation of antierythrocyte antibody, and to maintain tissue oxygenation. The erythron mass ideally returns to normal, although a mildly decreased packed cell volume (PCV) still can be compatible with a good quality of life.

Control of Erythrocyte Destruction

Treatment to reduce erythrocyte destruction focuses on:

- Reducing Fc receptors (immunoglobulin-binding receptors) on neutrophils, monocytes, and macrophages to prevent phagocytosis of antibody-coated erythrocytes.
- Preventing continued formation of antierythrocyte antibody.

Glucocorticoids

To reduce Fc receptors on phagocytic cells, treat with glucocorticoids.

- Parenterally administered dexamethasone (0.1–0.2 mg/kg q12h IV) is preferred by many clinicians for initial in-hospital treatment.
- Then use oral prednisone or prednisolone (1 mg/kg q12h PO) for follow-up maintenance; 3 to 6 months usually is required.
- To prevent glucocorticoid-induced gastric ulceration, consider using concomitant cimetidine (Tagamet, SmithKline); (5–10 mg/kg q6–12h IV or PO) or other measures described in Chapter 87 to control gastric acid and its effects.

Danazol

Consider concomitant danazol (Danocrine, Winthrop) therapy (5 mg/kg q12h PO).

- Danazol is a synthetic androgen.
- It suppresses the pituitary-ovarian axis by inhibiting the output of pituitary gonadotropins.
- It also reduces Fc receptors on phagocytic cells.
- The drug is expensive and has been associated with liver enzyme elevation.
- Clinicians should be aware that insulin requirements in diabetic patients may increase and that danazol may enhance the anticoagulant effects of warfarin because of decreased procoagulant factor synthesis in the liver.

Cyclophosphamide

Consider the use of cyclophosphamide to prevent antierythrocyte antibody formation. This is accomplished to some degree through the use of glucocorticoids; however, consider using a more potent humoral immune suppressive agent such as cyclophosphamide (Cytoxan, Bristol-Myers) along with glucocorticoids and danazol in patients that exhibit direct autoagglutination of blood or in patients with intravascular erythrocyte lysis. These patients generally have high concentrations of serum antibody and a poorer prognosis; thus, more aggressive attempts to prevent antibody formation are indicated. As a side effect, cyclophosphamide can decrease the peripheral platelet count, which potentially can lead to a bleeding diathesis. The presence of preexisting thrombocytopenia should be noted, and consideration should be given to the risk-benefit ratio of using cyclophosphamide; do not give cyclophosphamide if the platelet count is less than $30,000/\mu l$. Patients with severe gastrointestinal irritation manifested by vomiting and/or diarrhea also probably should not receive cyclophosphamide because it can inhibit epithelialization of the gastrointestinal tract and predispose to bleeding.

Cyclophosphamide is given by one of two methods:

- Single IV bolus at a dosage of 100–200 mg/m² (see Table 24–4 in Chapter 24, for conversion of body weight in pounds or kilograms to surface area in square meters)
- Oral dosage:
  - For dogs—50 mg/m² every other day
  - For cats—200 mg/m² q2wk

IV administration generally is used in dogs and cats that require a blood transfusion and have direct autoagglutination or intravascular erythrocyte lysis. The drug inhibits an immune response to the transfused blood as well as to the patient's own erythrocytes. Do not give cyclophosphamide IV more frequently than once every 2 weeks.

Oral administration is used in dogs that are refractory to glucocorticoid and danazol therapy or in dogs that have direct agglutination or intravascular hemolysis but do not require immediate blood transfusion.

▼ **Key Point** Cyclophosphamide may suppress reticulocytosis and may cause thrombocytopenia, although its greatest effect is on lymphocytes and immune function. If reticulocytopenia or severe thrombocytopenia develops, discontinue cyclophosphamide therapy. Patients with nonregenerative immune-mediated hemolytic anemia present a therapeutic dilemma.

Antibody serum levels are not reduced immediately after the administration of cyclophosphamide. Circulating antibodies must decline by normal antibody catabolism of roughly 3 weeks according to serum half-life clearance. In immune-mediated erythrocyte destruction, the half-life of antibody with specificity for circulating erythrocytes may be shorter because of adsorption onto circulating erythrocytes. Nevertheless, it likely will require 1 to 2 weeks before any significant benefit from cyclophosphamide is appreciated.

Cyclosporine

Cyclosporine (Sandimmune, Sandoz) is a cyclic peptide composed of 11 amino acids and has been used successfully in IMHA management. Its immunosuppressive effects result from inhibiting the synthesis of interleukin-2 and other T-lymphocyte cytokines. The mechanism of action involves a selective inhibition of cytokine gene transcription. This selective inhibition prevents helper T cells from interacting with the natural and specific immune systems resulting in reduced inflammation and elimination of specific immune responses. In autoimmune and immune-mediated diseases, this reaction can lead to reduced tissue destruction. Although cyclosporine has revolutionized organ transplantation, its efficacy in the treatment of autoimmune and immune-mediated diseases remains largely unknown. In the treatment of IMHA, cyclosporine is combined with the use of a glucocorticoid.

- Cyclosporine (10 mg/kg q24h PO) is administered for 5 consecutive days followed by 2 days without treatment. After the first week, the dose is decreased (5 mg/kg q24h PO) and is administered in an identical treatment scheme. The treatment then is continued using this administration scheme until disease resolution is obtained.
- After disease resolution, cyclosporine is discontinued, but maintenance therapy with a glucocorticoid is recommended.

Blood Transfusion

Transfusions should be given only if necessary because the procedure may accelerate or precipitate a hemolytic crisis. When transfusion is necessary, use cross-matched blood. In addition, consider administering cyclophosphamide to decrease the potential for an antibody response to the transfusion. If a second blood transfusion is required and more than 7 days have elapsed, a primary immune response to the previously transfused blood may have occurred, and reevaluation of a blood crossmatch is imperative.

Other Therapies

Plasmapheresis

Plasmapheresis is the removal of plasma (and antibodies) from withdrawn blood and retransfusion of the blood cells. It is performed to decrease the amount of circulating antibody with erythrocyte specificity. This results in a decreased rate of autologous destruction.

Splenectomy

This procedure must be approached with caution because an enlarged spleen may represent a source of significant extramedullary hematopoiesis. Before recommending splenectomy, evaluate a bone marrow aspirate to document significant erythroid hyperplasia. Also, consider performing fine-needle aspiration cytology of the enlarged spleen to document significant erythrophagocytosis. If significant erythrophagocytosis is present, splenectomy not only prevents this phenomenon, but also removes a likely source of significant antibody production. (See also Chapter 23 for a discussion of the spleen's role in this disease and for a description of splenectomy.)

Prognosis

The prognosis is guarded in the presence of severe hepatic disease or renal disease and when IMHA is associated with immune-mediated thrombocytopenia and/or systemic lupus erythematosus. Patients with intravascular hemolysis and direct agglutination have the poorest

prognosis and highest death rate. Mortality occurs in approximately 30% to 40% of all patients despite appropriate clinical management. Complications can include DIC, acute thromboembolism, sepsis, renal failure, and persistent hemolysis despite therapy.

IMMUNE-MEDIATED THROMBOCYTOPENIA

Decreased circulating platelets are presumed the result of increased antibody-mediated and complement-mediated thrombocyte phagocytosis within the spleen, liver, and bone marrow or secondary to decreased platelet production after destruction of megakaryocytes within the bone marrow. Immune-mediated thrombocytopenia (IMT) may occur as a single disease entity or may occur in association with other immune-mediated disease. The simultaneous occurrence of IMT and hemolytic anemia is known as Evans syndrome. Other immune-mediated diseases that may occur concurrently with IMT include systemic lupus erythematosus and rheumatoid arthritis.

Etiology

▼ *Key Point* Similar to IMHA, IMT is an example of a type II or cytotoxic hypersensitivity.

- Antibody may be directed against endogenous or exogenous thrombocyte surface antigens. The specific etiology usually is unidentified. However, certain drugs have been shown to create a hapten-platelet antigen complex and induce an antibody response; sulfadiazine and propylthiouracil, a drug used to treat hyperthyroidism in cats, have been associated with acquired IMT.
- The disease is observed commonly in dogs and rarely in cats. The average age of afflicted dogs is 5 to 6 years. Female dogs are affected nearly twice as frequently as males. Miniature poodles, toy poodles, and Old English sheepdogs may be predisposed.

Clinical Signs

Patients usually are presented for the primary complaint of bleeding. Bleeding most often is manifested by mucous membrane petechiation, dermal ecchymosis, and melena. Epistaxis, hyphema, hematemesis, and hematuria are observed less frequently. Lethargy and weakness also may be reported.

▼ *Key Point* Bleeding may be related not only to the absolute platelet numbers but also to the rate of platelet decline, the stability of capillary endothelial membranes, and the incidence of traumatic events.

Diagnosis

▼ *Key Point* The diagnosis of IMT generally is made by eliminating other causes of thrombocytopenia. Diagnostic tests exist that demonstrate platelet-specific antibody or antibody-coated megakaryocytes, but clinical signs and patient response to treatment generally are considered diagnostic.

Physical Examination

The physical examination most commonly reveals signs related to bleeding, especially mucous membrane petechiation, dermal ecchymosis and petechiation, and melena. Funduscopic examination may show retinal hemorrhage. Splenomegaly and/or hepatomegaly may be found on abdominal palpation. Tachycardia, tachypnea, and physiologic heart murmur may be noted, depending on the extent of blood loss. Some animals are febrile.

Complete Blood Count

The CBC must, by definition, demonstrate a thrombocytopenia, which in most animals with IMT is severe. Often there are less than 30,000 platelets/μl in patients with overt bleeding. Blood smears typically exhibit very few platelets; however, both microthrombocytes and macrothrombocytes usually are seen. Many animals demonstrate anemia and hypoproteinemia if bleeding has occurred. If the bleeding episode has been recent, the anemia is normocytic and normochromic and lacks signs of regeneration. If an episode of significant bleeding occurred more than 3 or 4 days before analysis, then a macrocytic, hypochromic anemia with reticulocytosis may be observed. Prolonged bleeding can cause an iron-deficient, microcytic hypochromic anemia.

Serum Biochemistry Profile

This typically is normal.

Urinalysis

Urinalysis may demonstrate proteinuria as the result of antigen-antibody complex deposition within the glomerulus and complement-induced glomerulitis. Hematuria is observed only rarely.

Coagulography

A coagulogram can rule out intrinsic and extrinsic coagulation system defects (see Chapter 21) as a cause of excessive bleeding with secondary platelet consumption.

Bone Marrow Cytology

Perform this procedure to document megakaryocytic response to the peripheral thrombocytopenia. In IMT, the megakaryocytes generally are increased with a predominance of immature forms. Only occasionally, when antibodies are directed against the megakaryocytes themselves, are the megakaryocytes decreased. Ehrlichiosis and hyperestrogenemia are other differential diagnoses associated with megakaryocytic hypoplasia.

Platelet Factor-3 Test

This test has been used to detect serum antibody with specificity against platelets. However, 30% to 70% of an-

imals suspected of having IMT do not exhibit a positive test result. The major pitfall associated with the platelet factor-3 test is that it uses platelets collected from a healthy dog rather than platelets collected from the patient. When patient serum is mixed with normal platelets, the assumption is made that the specific platelet antigen to which the serum antibody is directed will be present on the platelets collected from the healthy dog. This assumption may not necessarily be true and probably explains many of the observed false-negative test results.

Bone Marrow Direct Fluorescent Antibody (DFA) Test

The DFA test may be used to detect antibody bound to megakaryocytes; however, this test is technically demanding, subjective, and not routinely performed.

Treatment

▼ *Key Point* Treatment objectives are to resolve and prevent bleeding, reduce platelet destruction, and increase platelet release from megakaryocytes in selected patients.

Reduce Platelet Destruction

This is accomplished by the combined use of glucocorticoids and danazol (Danocrine, Winthrop). Glucocorticoids are the mainstay of therapy. Dexamethasone may be more effective than prednisone or prednisolone.

- Give *dexamethasone* (0.1–0.2 mg/kg q12h IV) for the first day followed by *prednisone or prednisolone* (1 mg/kg q12h PO).
- It is strongly advised that patients also receive *cimetidine* (5–10 mg/kg q6–12h IV or PO) or another H$_2$-blocker to control acid secretion in an attempt to prevent glucocorticoid-associated gastric ulceration.
- *Danazol* (5 mg/kg q12h PO) is used concurrently with the glucocorticoids as an additional aid to prevent platelet phagocytosis (see Immune-Mediated Hemolytic Anemia).

Increase Platelet Release

Platelet release from the bone marrow is increased by administration of *vincristine* (Oncovin, Lilly) (0.025 mg/kg IV) not more frequently than once weekly. Adequate bone marrow megakaryocytes must be present for vincristine to induce platelet release.

Blood and Plasma Transfusion

Use blood and platelet-rich plasma transfusions to support tissue oxygenation and to assist hemostasis, respectively. These transfusions will not restore the platelet count to normal; however, one clinical study suggests that dogs that receive a platelet-rich transfusion may be less likely to exhibit relapsing thrombocytopenia. Compatible erythrocytes as determined by major cross-match analysis should be used for whole blood transfusions (see Chapter 20).

Other Therapies

Splenectomy

Reserve splenectomy for patients that exhibit refractory IMT.

- This therapy is based on the assumption that the spleen is responsible for persistent platelet destruction and that removal of the spleen will:
  - Remove macrophages responsible for platelet ingestion
  - Remove a large source of plasma cells manufacturing platelet-specific antibody
- Perform splenectomy when splenomegaly is present and is not due to significant extramedullary hematopoiesis.
- Evaluate bone marrow cytology and document the presence of bone marrow megakaryocytic hyperplasia.

After splenectomy, up to 50% of dogs exhibit platelet counts greater than 200,000/μl and do not require medical therapy to maintain a normal platelet count. The remaining dogs may exhibit recurring thrombocytopenia (details of splenectomy are described in Chapter 23).

Vincristine-Loaded Platelet Transfusion

This complicated procedure is reserved for patients with refractory IMT. The rationale is that in vitro incubation of platelets with vincristine results in the binding of vincristine to tubulin within the platelet cytoplasm. After IV injection, macrophages of the reticuloendothelial system ingest the vincristine-loaded platelets and are destroyed. The major pitfall of this technique may be related to natural macrophage turnover. Repetitive treatment may be necessary and is technically difficult.

Prognosis

The prognosis for IMT is good. Approximately 40% to 50% of dogs experience only a single thrombocytopenic episode that responds to treatment within 2 to 7 days. Patient signalment, severity of initial thrombocytopenia, and the time required to achieve a platelet count of greater than 50,000/μl cannot identify dogs that will exhibit relapsing thrombocytopenia. Therefore, periodic monitoring is essential. Environmental stress and/or hormonal imbalance may precipitate relapses. Consider ovariohysterectomy for intact females after correction of the thrombocytopenia and bleeding abnormalities. Approximately 20% of patients die, usually as the result of severe intestinal hemorrhage.

SYSTEMIC LUPUS ERYTHEMATOSUS

Systemic lupus erythematosus (SLE) is characterized by its ability to affect numerous organ systems. SLE has been called "the great imitator." A wide variety of clinical presentations occur. Tissue inflammation is induced by circulating, soluble antigen-antibody complexes that diffuse into vascular endothelial spaces, activate the complement cascade, and facilitate the perivascular accumulation of inflammatory cells. The inflammation may result in acute necrotizing vasculitis with progressive fibrinoid deposition and sclerosis. Deposition of immune complexes within the renal glomerulus leads to membranous glomerulitis. Diffusion of immune complexes into joints results in polyarthritis.

Etiology

▼ **Key Point** SLE is an example of type III hypersensitivity caused by circulating antigen-antibody complexes. Occasional concurrent type II hypersensitivity occurs as a result of antibodies that bind surface antigens on erythrocytes, platelets, and leukocytes.

- The etiology is unknown.
- A familial tendency exists; however, no defined inheritance pattern has been documented. Shetland sheepdogs, collies, Afghan hounds, beagles, Irish setters, Old English sheepdogs, poodles, and German shepherds may be over-represented.
- The mean age of afflicted dogs is approximately 6 years. There is no sex predilection.

Clinical Signs

- The onset of signs may be acute or insidious. Signs may wax and wane for a considerable time before presentation.
- The most common reason for clinical presentation is a gait abnormality manifested by stilted movement or shifting leg lameness. This abnormality may be the result of polyarthritis (see Chapter 143) or polymyositis (see Chapter 149). Approximately 75% of dogs exhibit polyarthritis at some time during the progression of the disease.
- The animal may be presented for the complaint of focal or diffuse skin lesions that can affect virtually any body area (see Chapter 43).
- Nonspecific complaints include malaise, anorexia, and weakness.

Diagnosis

The diagnosis of SLE is based on clinical assessment and evaluation of laboratory tests.

▼ **Key Point** One specific diagnostic test for SLE does not exist. The diagnosis of SLE is based on documentation of (1) two major signs and a positive serologic test or (2) one major sign, two minor signs, and a positive serologic test. SLE is considered probable when there are (1) one major sign and positive serology or (2) two major signs and negative serology.

Clinical findings are separated into major and minor signs:

- Major signs include nonerosive polyarthritis, polymyositis, bullous dermatitis, proteinuria, and immune-mediated hemolytic anemia, thrombocytopenia, and leukopenia.

- Minor signs consist of fever of unknown origin, oral ulceration, pleuritis, myocarditis, pericarditis, peripheral lymphadenopathy, dementia, and seizures.

Physical Examination

Identify major and minor signs in the physical examination. The joints may be distended and painful; muscle pain and/or diffuse muscle wasting may be evident; and cutaneous lesions may be noted. Cutaneous manifestations, seen in nearly 50% of dogs, may include a symmetric or focal distribution of lesions affecting any body part. Mucocutaneous junctions and the oral cavity commonly are affected. The lesions may exhibit ulceration, erythema, crusting, oozing, and alopecia. Cellulitis, furunculosis, scarring, and leukoderma may be observed. Pyrexia and peripheral lymphadenopathy may be noted.

Complete Blood Count

The CBC may exhibit evidence of immune-mediated hemolytic anemia, thrombocytopenia, or leukopenia if a concurrent type II hypersensitivity to these cells exists. If a regenerative anemia is present without evidence of detectable blood loss or autoagglutination, perform a direct Coombs test. The PCV may be less than 20%.

- If a nonregenerative anemia exists, evaluate bone marrow cytology.
- If the hemogram demonstrates thrombocytopenia and/or leukopenia, follow up with bone marrow evaluation.
- If the hemogram demonstrates a nonregenerative anemia, thrombocytopenia, and leukopenia, and the bone marrow is nonregenerative:
  - Submit a serum sample for an *Ehrlichia canis* titer (see Chapter 15).
  - Treat with tetracycline (20 mg/kg q8h PO) or doxycycline (5 mg/kg q12h PO) pending serology results.
- In the absence of immune-mediated anemia, thrombocytopenia, or leukopenia, the hemogram usually demonstrates:
  - Leukocytosis characterized by neutrophilia and monocytosis
  - Increased plasma fibrinogen
  - Elevated plasma proteins compatible with chronic inflammation

Serum Biochemistry Profile

Results are not specific for SLE; however, assessment of serum albumin, globulin, urea nitrogen, creatinine, and muscle enzyme concentrations is important.

- If hypoalbuminemia, azotemia, or creatinemia exist, evaluate with urinalysis.
- If serum aspartate aminotransferase activity is elevated above alanine aminotransferase activity:
  - Suspect muscle inflammation
  - Assess serum creatine phosphokinase activity
  or

- Obtain a muscle biopsy, particularly if muscle pain and/or atrophy exists.
- If serum globulin levels are significantly increased, perform serum electrophoresis to document polyclonal gammopathy compatible with lupus erythematosus.

Urinalysis

Urinalysis may reveal proteinuria with or without casts. As many as 50% of cases exhibit evidence of glomerulitis as detected by the presence of proteinuria. Proteinuria can be quantitated in a 24-hour urine collection or assessed as the ratio of urine protein concentration to urine creatinine concentration (see Chapter 97).

▼ *Key Point* Absence of proteinuria does not rule out SLE.

Arthrocentesis

Perform *arthrocentesis* in patients that exhibit distended joints or lameness potentially related to arthritis. Cytologic analysis should reveal an increased cell count composed predominantly of nondegenerated neutrophils and some mononuclear cells and characterized by decreased synovial fluid viscosity, and absence of bacteria.

Radiography

Radiograph affected joints to document a nonerosive arthropathy.

Serologic Tests

Serologic tests that aid in the diagnosis of SLE include the indirect fluorescent antinuclear antibody (IFAA) test and the lupus erythematosus (LE) cell test. False-negative results may occur after recent glucocorticoid therapy, and false-positive titers may occur in other chronic inflammatory diseases, such as bacterial endocarditis.

IFAA Test

This indirect immunofluorescent test documents the presence of serum antibodies with specificity for nuclear antigens. It may be more sensitive than the LE cell test.

LE Cell Test

This test detects the presence of antinuclear antibodies in plasma by documenting phagocytized antibody-coated nuclear material within neutrophils and macrophages. Neutrophils or macrophages with phagocytized antibody-coated nuclear material are referred to as LE cells. This is a cytologic test that requires documentation of the number of LE cells seen on a buffy coat smear.

Treatment

The goal of treatment is to reduce tissue inflammation. It also is important to manage associated organ failure, avoid bacterial infections, and treat any identified infections specifically and aggressively.

The *reduction of tissue inflammation* usually is achieved through the use of prednisone or prednisolone (1–3 mg/kg q12h PO) until clinical improvement is observed. If improvement is not noted within 10 days, then concurrently administer:

- For dogs—azathioprine (Imuran, Burroughs Wellcome) (2 mg/kg q24h PO) for 10 days
- For cats—chlorambucil (Leukeran, Burroughs Wellcome) (0.25–0.5 mg/kg q48–72h PO)
- Alternatively, consider cyclosporine (Sandimmune, Sandoz) administration (10 mg/kg q24h PO) as described for immune-mediated hemolytic anemia.

Once clinical remission has been achieved, decrease drug dosage to the lowest possible amount that clinically controls the disease. Aspirin (dogs, 10–25 mg/kg q8h PO; cats, 10–40 mg/kg q72h PO) may provide additional analgesic, antipyretic, and anti-inflammatory relief. Remember that aspirin therapy is contraindicated in the presence of thrombocytopenia and gastrointestinal ulceration. Treatment likely will need to be continued indefinitely; however, after remission for 6 to 8 weeks, a trial period without treatment can be tried.

▼ *Key Point* SLE is associated with excess production of a wide variety of anticytoplasmic and antinuclear antibodies. Therapy with immunosuppressive agents such as glucocorticoids, azathioprine, and chlorambucil may reduce serum concentrations of these antibodies; however, serum antinuclear antibody titers usually remain high during periods of clinical disease remission.

Prognosis

The prognosis is guarded. Approximately 40% of dogs die within 1 year of diagnosis. Severe organ dysfunction makes the prognosis worse. The presence of severe infection warrants a grave prognosis. Patients often die of bronchopneumonia, septicemia, and steroid-induced pancreatitis.

SUPPLEMENTAL READINGS

Bucheler J, Cotter SM: Canine immune-mediated hemolytic anemia. In: Bonagura JD, ed: Kirk's Current Veterinary Therapy XII. Small Animal Practice. Philadelphia: WB Saunders, 1995, p 152.

Jans HE, Armstrong PJ, Price GS: Therapy of immune-mediated thrombocytopenia: A retrospective study of 15 dogs. J Vet Intern Med 4:4, 1990.

Klag AR, Giger U, Shofer FS: Idiopathic immune-mediated hemolytic anemia in dogs: 42 cases (1986–1990). J Am Vet Med Assoc 202:783, 1993.

Lewis RM, Picut CA: Veterinary Clinical Immunology: From Classroom to Clinics. Philadelphia: Lea & Febiger, 1989.

Thompson JP: Disorders of the immune system. In: Sherding RG, ed: The Cat: Diseases and Clinical Management. 2nd ed. New York: Churchill Livingstone, 1994, p 647.

Thompson JP: Immunologic diseases. In: Ettinger SJ, Feldman EC, eds: Textbook of Veterinary Internal Medicine. 4th ed. Philadelphia: WB Saunders, 1995, p 2002.

Weiser MG: Diagnosis of immunohemolytic disease. Semin Vet Med Surg Small Anim 7:311, 1992.

Williams DA, Maggio-Price L: Canine idiopathic thrombocytopenia: Clinical observations and long-term follow-up in 54 cases. J Am Vet Med Assoc 185:660, 1984.

23 Diseases of the Spleen

Margaret C. McEntee / Rodney L. Page

The spleen has many important functions. However, most of its functions can be taken over by other tissues such that it is not essential to life. The spleen is commonly an active or passive participant in a number of disease processes. As a part of the mononuclear phagocyte (reticuloendothelial) system, the spleen functions to filter and phagocytize cells (e.g., senescent red blood cells) and particles (e.g., bacteria). The spleen has an important role in a number of infectious diseases through phagocytosis, antibody production, and modulation of hemoparasitic infections. The spleen has a significant storage capacity. Splenic contraction occurs in response to stress (exercise, blood loss, excitement) with a resultant rise in blood volume.

Splenic disorders usually are identified by a change in shape, size, and function of the spleen. Symmetric or asymmetric enlargement of the spleen generally can be detected on physical examination or radiographic evaluation. Other signs (weakness, pallor, coagulation abnormalities) are related to, or are a function of, the underlying disease process.

Base therapeutic decisions on accurate clinical diagnosis. Splenectomy, for instance, may result in increased morbidity and mortality, and therefore should be performed only when necessary.

ANATOMY/HISTOLOGY

There are four main components to the spleen: the fibromuscular capsule, white pulp, marginal zone, and red pulp. The most significant difference between the canine and feline spleen is that the canine spleen is considered to be a sinusal spleen as opposed to the nonsinusal spleen in the cat. Blood cells in the canine spleen extravasate by moving between adjacent endothelial cells to obtain entrance to the red pulp sinus. Large gaps are present in the feline spleen between adjacent endothelial cells, allowing cells to move through without deformation of cell shape. As a result, the feline spleen has decreased pitting function (see later) compared with the canine spleen.

Fibromuscular Capsule

The capsule surrounds the spleen and branches to form trabeculae. The smooth muscle component allows for contraction and distention of the spleen.

White Pulp

The white pulp consists of lymphocytes and reticuloendothelial (RE) cells distributed along arterial vessels that form cylindrical structures called periarterial lymphatic sheaths rich in T-lymphocytes. B-lymphocytes are located in nodules along these sheaths and represent areas of B-lymphocyte proliferation and antibody production. As a result of blood flow dynamics, plasma is delivered to the white pulp while erythrocytes continue into the marginal zone. Soluble antigens are delivered to the white pulp for immune recognition and processing.

Marginal Zone

The marginal zone is not well developed in the dog and cat. It separates the white pulp from the red pulp. In other species, macrophages that have a phagocytic function are present as blood is filtered through this region.

Red Pulp

The red pulp consists primarily of venous sinuses, a reticulum filled with macrophages, and blood. As the arteries enter the red pulp, they lose the periarterial lymphatic sheath and are surrounded by a dense sheath of reticulum and macrophages called the periarteriolar macrophage sheath (also known as ellipsoids). Endothelial cells in the terminal arterial capillaries are separated by gaps. Particles, cells, and plasma pass through the gaps into the periarteriolar macrophage sheath, which is the major site for clearance of blood-borne particles. The red pulp is the site for culling abnormal blood cells and processing of particulate antigens for presentation to the white pulp, where an immune response is mounted.

PHYSIOLOGY/FUNCTIONS

Hematopoiesis

The spleen is a hematopoietic organ during fetal development, but the *normal* adult spleen in the dog and cat has no hematopoietic activity. The red pulp retains the ability for extramedullary hematopoiesis on demand.

Reservoir Function

Normally, 90% of the red cells pass quickly through the spleen while 9%, representing approximately 50% of the total number of red cells in the spleen at one time, take 7 to 8 minutes to move through the red pulp, and the remaining 1% have a transit time of 1 hour. The latter two components with slower transit times constitute the splenic reservoir. The blood storage capacity of the feline spleen is less than that of the canine spleen. In anesthetized dogs, the distended spleen may contain up to 30% of the red cell mass. With contraction, the packed cell volume (PCV) may increase 10% to 20% in dogs and cats.

Filtering Functions

Within the red pulp, active phagocytic cells deplete oxygen and glucose, which stresses erythrocyte metabolism and results in decreased red blood cell (RBC) deformability. These events, coupled with the slow blood flow, aid in removal of abnormal or senescent RBCs. Reticulocytes (immature erythrocytes that contain RNA) typically are sequestered in the spleen for remodeling and then released as mature erythrocytes.

Pitting is the removal of cytoplasmic inclusions that occurs because inclusions cause the RBCs to be less deformable. This occurs within the spleen, resulting in the removal of mitochondria, Howell-Jolly bodies, Heinz bodies, intracellular organisms, and nuclei. Pitting does not occur in the cat because of larger apertures in the walls of the pulp venule.

Immunologic Functions

Phagocytosis

The slow circulation in the spleen enhances contact time, and hence phagocytosis of microorganisms. The liver is more effective at removing blood-borne bacteria in the presence of specific antibacterial antibody because of its larger size and greater blood flow. In the absence of a significant amount of specific antibody, the spleen becomes crucial for removal of bacteria.

RBCs acquire surface immunoglobulins as part of the aging process. Splenic macrophages remove the portion of the erythrocyte membrane coated with IgG, resulting in a spherocyte. Spherocytes are less deformable and hence are culled.

The spleen plays an important role in protection against RBC parasites such as *Hemobartonella* and *Babesia* because of its pitting function.

Antibody Synthesis

Antigen processing occurs as a result of contact between splenic macrophages and blood. The splenic macrophages present the antigens to the immunocompetent cells of the spleen, resulting in B-lymphocyte proliferation and humoral antibody production. Evidence suggests that in asplenic patients, early events in antibody production are normal but the role of the spleen in augmenting stimulated lymphocyte subpopulations is compromised.

Cellular Immunity

Studies suggest that the spleen may play a role in T-cell activities and in providing host defense against solid tumor cells.

Miscellaneous Functions

Other functions of the spleen include:

- Storage and activation of factor VIII coagulant activity and factor VIII antigen
- Regulation of the formation, liberation, and degradation of angiotensin-converting enzyme
- Modulation of plasma norepinephrine levels and/or renal PGE2 activity
- Iron storage and recycling of iron to the bone marrow
- Platelet storage (up to 30% of platelets) and release on sympathetic stimulation and epinephrine release

ETIOLOGY/PATHOGENESIS

Splenic disorders can be separated into two categories: localized or asymmetric splenomegaly (e.g., discrete splenic mass) and generalized or symmetrical splenomegaly.

Causes of localized splenomegaly (Table 23–1) include:

- Primary or metastatic neoplasia
- Nodular hyperplasia
- Hematoma
- Abscess

Generalized splenomegaly (Table 23–2) may result from:

- Inflammatory/infectious diseases
- Hyperplastic splenomegaly
- Congestive splenomegaly
- Infiltrative diseases including both neoplastic and non-neoplastic diseases

Splenic masses are more common in dogs, whereas generalized splenomegaly is more common in cats.

Localized Splenomegaly

Neoplasia

Hemangiomas and hemangiosarcomas are the most common neoplastic splenic masses and are very common in the dog but rare in the cat. Other primary

Table 23–1. LOCALIZED SPLENOMEGALY

Non-Neoplastic	Neoplastic
Nodular hyperplasia	Primary
Hematoma	Hemangiosarcoma
Abscess	Hemangioma
	Sarcoma
	Secondary

Table 23–2. GENERALIZED SPLENOMEGALY

Infectious	Hyperplastic	Congestive	Infiltrative
Bacterial	Immune-mediated	Pharmacologic	Neoplastic
Septicemia	Autoimmune hemolytic anemia	Portal hypertension	Lymphoma
Toxoplasmosis	Immune-mediated thrombocytopenia	Splenic torsion	Leukemia
Salmonellosis	Systemic lupus erythematosus		Mastocytosis
Viral	Hypersplenism		Malignant histiocytosis
Infectious canine hepatitis	Primary (idiopathic)		Multiple myeloma
Feline infectious peritonitis	Secondary		Non-neoplastic
Mycotic			Extramedullary hematopoiesis
Blastomycosis			Hypereosinophilic syndrome
Histoplasmosis			Amyloidosis
Parasitic			
Hemobartonellosis			
Rickettsial			
Ehrlichiosis			
Rocky Mountain spotted fever			

neoplastic splenic masses include fibrosarcoma, leiomyosarcoma, leiomyoma, osteosarcoma, undifferentiated sarcoma, chondrosarcoma, rhabdomyosarcoma, myxosarcoma, liposarcoma, myelolipoma, fibrous histiocytoma, lipoma, mesenchymoma, and occasionally lymphoma. Metastasis to the spleen may occur from a number of sites.

Nodular Hyperplasia

Splenic nodular hyperplasia can be single or multiple nodules that are benign accumulations of lymphoid cells.

Trauma

Trauma can result in subcapsular hematoma formation, causing a mass effect in the spleen. Usually, no underlying cause can be identified. Splenic hematomas cannot be distinguished from hemangioma/hemangiosarcoma on the basis of size or shape; thus, histopathology is required to make the diagnosis. Trauma may result in splenic rupture potentially requiring surgical intervention.

Splenic trauma also can lead to splenosis, which is the dissemination of splenic tissue into the abdominal cavity (and potentially into the thoracic cavity if there is also a diaphragmatic tear) and the subsequent development of daughter spleens.

Abscess

Splenic abscesses can form from hematogenous spread of microorganisms but are very rare in the dog and cat. Splenic abscess has been associated with cholangiohepatitis in cats.

Generalized Splenomegaly

Inflammatory/Infectious Disease

A wide range of infectious diseases can result in diffuse splenomegaly. A partial list of the disorders that may be associated with splenomegaly is provided in Table 23–2 (please refer to the various chapters in this book on infectious diseases for details concerning these disorders). The various types can be classified on the basis of the primary type of cellular infiltrate.

Hyperplastic Splenomegaly

This type of splenomegaly occurs as a result of hyperplasia of the REs and lymphoid components of the spleen in response to blood-borne antigens and to RBC destruction (e.g., immune-mediated hemolytic anemia).

Congestive Splenomegaly

Splenic enlargement resulting from congestion can occur through a number of different mechanisms. Splenic distension occurs as a result of smooth muscle relaxation in the splenic capsule and trabeculae with the use of tranquilizers (e.g., phenothiazine) and barbiturates. Portal hypertension secondary to right-sided congestive heart failure, caudal vena cava obstruction, and intrahepatic obstruction may cause splenic congestion. Splenic torsion alone or in conjunction with gastric dilatation-volvulus can cause splenomegaly.

Infiltrative Diseases

Neoplastic Infiltration

This is one of the most common causes of splenomegaly. Splenomegaly is common in patients with acute and chronic leukemias (more common in the acute form). In leukemic patients, splenic enlargement primarily is caused by the presence of neoplastic lymphocytes of hematogenous origin, but extramedullary hematopoiesis (EMH) also may play a role. Other neoplastic conditions that result in diffuse splenomegaly in dogs and cats include systemic mastocytosis (most notably in cats), lymphoma, multiple myeloma, and malignant histiocytosis (dogs).

Non-neoplastic Infiltration

EMH is relatively common in dogs. RBC destruction, severe splenic or extrasplenic inflammation, immune-mediated thrombocytopenia, neoplastic infiltration of the spleen, bone marrow hypoplasia, and splenic congestion can stimulate EMH.

Hypereosinophilic syndrome of cats can lead to infiltration of the spleen with mature eosinophils (see Chapter 20). This syndrome is characterized by a peripheral blood eosinophilia, bone marrow hyperplasia of the eosinophil precursors, and multiple organ infiltration by mature eosinophils. Splenic amyloidosis can cause splenomegaly but is relatively rare.

Hypersplenism

Hypersplenism, strictly defined, is characterized by:

- Cytopenia(s)
- Bone marrow hyperplasia of the affected cell line or a normocellular bone marrow
- Splenomegaly
- Resolution of the cytopenia in response to splenectomy

Hypersplenism results mainly from the filtering and phagocytic functions of the spleen.

- *Primary hypersplenism* occurs when the splenic dysfunction is idiopathic.
- In *secondary hypersplenism,* an underlying disease process is identified that has resulted in splenomegaly.

Hyposplenism

Hyposplenism, or decreased splenic function, can occur secondary to a wide range of disease processes. A number of hematologic changes are recognized in association with hyposplenism, including reticulocytosis, acanthocytes, and Howell-Jolly bodies. These changes are the same as those seen in splenectomized animals.

CLINICAL SIGNS

Clinical signs of splenic disease typically are nonspecific and are more likely to be related to the underlying disease process than to enlargement of the spleen. Clinical signs include anorexia, weight loss, weakness, abdominal distension, vomiting, diarrhea, and polyuria/polydipsia.

DIAGNOSIS

History

The history can aid in identifying patients with certain types of splenic disease. For example, patients presenting with a relatively acute onset of abdominal distension and retching may have splenic torsion in conjunction with gastric dilatation-volvulus. Periodic weakness or collapse, particularly in certain breeds (e.g., German shepherds), raises the suspicion of splenic hemangiosarcoma with intermittent hemorrhage. A history of tick exposure in patients with splenomegaly can aid in the diagnosis of Rocky Mountain spotted fever and

erhlichiosis. Owners may report enlarged lymph nodes in patients with lymphoma. A history of drug exposure in a patient with a bleeding disorder may indicate drug-induced immune-mediated thrombocytopenia.

Physical Examination

The spleen is located in the left cranial abdominal quadrant and typically is oriented dorsoventrally. The dorsal extremity of the spleen is relatively fixed near the midline ventral to the left crus of the diaphragm, but the remainder of the spleen is otherwise freely movable and can be oriented longitudinally along the left flank. The normal spleen is palpable in many dogs and cats. A palpable spleen may be normal, particularly in German shepherds.

Splenomegaly (diffuse or localized) often can be detected with careful abdominal palpation. Raising the animal's front quarters during abdominal palpation can aid in identification of an enlarged spleen by shifting the abdominal contents caudally. Position of the spleen and ease of identification can vary, depending on such factors as breed conformation, presence of ingesta in the stomach, and whether the patient is overweight. If splenic enlargement has been identified, exercise caution because it is possible to rupture the spleen, especially with splenic hemangiosarcoma.

Splenomegaly is not always evident on physical examination. Additional tools such as abdominal radiography or ultrasound may be necessary to identify an enlarged spleen.

Other physical examination findings may include abdominal distension, peritoneal effusion, pain on palpation of the abdomen, petechiae, ecchymoses, pale mucous membranes, and fever.

Palpate peripheral lymph nodes because peripheral lymphadenopathy can occur in conjunction with splenomegaly in a number of different systemic disorders, including infectious (e.g., salmonellosis) and neoplastic diseases (e.g., lymphoma).

Minimum Data Base

The hemogram is the most helpful in diagnosing splenic disorders. Changes in the hemogram essentially are a result of either hyposplenism or hypersplenism. Perform a biochemical profile and urinalysis as well as a complete blood cell count (CBC) on all patients with splenic disease.

Hypersplenism is not as common as hyposplenism. Changes seen with hypersplenism include regenerative anemia, neutropenia, thrombocytopenia, and other cytopenias. Abnormalities associated with hyposplenism include target cells, acanthocytes, Howell-Jolly bodies, nucleated RBCs, an increased percentage of reticulocytes, and thrombocytosis. Similar changes can be seen in splenectomized patients.

Spherocytes commonly are found in patients with autoimmune hemolytic anemia. If thrombocytopenia is the only hematologic abnormality detected, consider immune-mediated thrombocytopenia (see Chapter 22).

A coagulation panel may aid in the identification of acute or chronic disseminated intravascular coagulation, which can occur in a subset of patients with splenic disease. It also is recommended before fine-needle aspiration cytology to identify patients at increased risk of hemorrhage resulting from aspiration of the spleen.

Biochemical abnormalities are more likely to reflect the primary disease process than to result from splenic enlargement. Hemoglobinemia and resultant hemoglobinuria commonly are identified in dogs with splenic torsion.

Abdominal Radiography

Abdominal radiography, ultrasonography, and other imaging modalities such as computed tomography and magnetic resonance imaging provide information about splenic anatomy but not about function. Obtain radiographs before tranquilization or anesthesia because these can cause splenomegaly.

In dorsoventral (or ventrodorsal) radiographic views of the abdomen, the spleen normally is seen between the gastric fundus and the left kidney. It is more variable in position and size in lateral radiographs.

Abdominal radiographs may be useful:

- To confirm splenic enlargement and indicate whether the enlargement is localized or generalized
- To identify concurrent problems such as gastric dilatation-volvulus (GDV), hepatomegaly, abdominal lymph node enlargement, and peritoneal effusion

Abdominal Ultrasonography

Ultrasound procedures (see Chapter 4 for a general description) can be helpful in many situations, including:

- Identification of a focal mass, multiple masses, or diffuse splenomegaly
- Evaluation of patients with ascites due to congestion or peritoneal effusion due to splenic rupture, when there is a loss of abdominal detail on survey radiographs
- Evaluation of the parenchyma of the spleen
- Assessment of the splenic vasculature, especially in dogs with splenic torsion
- Aid in guiding fine-needle aspiration and biopsy of the spleen

Fine-Needle Aspiration Cytology

Fine-needle aspiration cytology is a valuable tool that can aid in the selection of patients for exploratory surgery, splenic biopsy, and splenectomy. Conversely, it can help identify those patients that would not benefit from splenectomy.

The procedure includes the following steps:

- Place the patient in right lateral or dorsal recumbency.
- Restraint or mild sedation usually is sufficient. Avoid general anesthesia because splenic congestion can result in hemodiluted samples.
- Clip and prepare the site sterilely. Manually localize and stabilize the spleen.

- Use a 22- or 25-gauge needle 1 to 1½ inches long.
- After the procedure, observe the patient for 3–6 hours for evidence of hemorrhage.

▼ *Key Point* Fine-needle aspiration cytology is an easy and safe procedure that can aid in the diagnosis of splenic disease in more than 50% of animals.

Aspiration cytology is contraindicated in patients with large cavitary lesions, which may rupture during aspiration. In patients with splenic hemangiosarcoma, aspiration can result in seeding of the tumor along the tract, as well as splenic rupture and seeding of the abdominal cavity. Thrombocytopenia is *not* considered a contraindication for this procedure.

Potential complications include splenic rupture, hemorrhage, damage to other abdominal organs, peritonitis, and abdominal seeding of a splenic neoplasm. In two reports describing the use of this technique in a total of 63 patients, no complications were encountered.

Splenic Function Studies

Nuclear imaging studies employ ^{51}Cr-labeled heat-damaged red cells or 99mTc sulfur colloid, which are cleared by the spleen and provide a measure of splenic function. The procedure has limited availability for veterinary patients.

Hematologic changes evident on a routine hemogram, such as Howell-Jolly bodies, nucleated RBCs, and acanthocytes may be indicative of functional hyposplenism. Hematology is the primary means of evaluating splenic function in cats and dogs with splenic disorders.

Miscellaneous Tests
Bone Marrow Aspiration Cytology

Bone marrow aspiration cytology or a core bone marrow biopsy is indicated in patients with splenomegaly and cytopenia(s) (see Chapter 20 for details on bone marrow biopsy technique). Splenic enlargement may reflect an underlying bone marrow hypoplasia or aplasia. The spleen is capable of supplementing the hematopoietic function of the bone marrow when necessary. Splenectomy may be contraindicated in a patient with splenomegaly due to EMH secondary to bone marrow hypoplasia or aplasia. Bone marrow aspiration cytology may be supportive of (e.g., ehrlichiosis) or diagnostic for (e.g., lymphoma) the underlying disease process.

Lymph Node Aspiration Cytology

Lymph node aspiration cytology or biopsy is indicated in patients with peripheral lymphadenopathy. Marked peripheral lymphadenopathy typically is associated with lymphoma. Mild or moderate peripheral lymph node enlargement can be seen in a number of different diseases, including infectious and immune-mediated disorders.

Serologic Tests

Serologic tests for specific infectious and immune diseases can be performed. Rickettsial titers for ehrlichiosis, Coombs test for immune-mediated hemolytic anemia, and antinuclear antibody testing for systemic lupus erythematosus may be indicated for some patients. Test cats that present with splenomegaly for feline leukemia virus and feline immunodeficiency virus. The diagnosis of immune-mediated thrombocytopenia usually is made by elimination of other causes of thrombocytopenia (see Chapter 22). There are specific tests for immune-mediated thrombocytopenia, but they are not readily available. Blood cultures as well as cultures of other fluids (e.g., urine) or sites may be indicated in patients suspected of having diseases such as bacterial endocarditis, diskospondylitis, or septicemia.

Other Tests

A buffy coat examination to check for circulating mast cells is indicated in cats that present for splenomegaly and are suspected of having systemic mastocytosis.

Thoracic radiographs are important in patients with suspected neoplastic disease (e.g., splenic hemangiosarcoma to check for pulmonary metastasis) and may be helpful in a subset of patients with infectious diseases (e.g., blastomycosis).

TREATMENT

Splenectomy

Splenectomy is indicated for patients with splenic rupture, splenic torsion, or splenic masses, and in symptomatic patients.

Splenectomy in cats with systemic mastocytosis can significantly prolong life expectancy even if mast cells are present in the peripheral circulation.

Because of the potential for splenic rupture and death in patients with hemangiosarcoma, splenectomy is recommended. These patients typically are not cured by surgery and usually have evidence of recurrence within 4 months.

Adjuvant chemotherapy is indicated for splenic hemangiosarcoma but has been shown to be beneficial only in dogs with no or minimal gross evidence of spread at the time of splenectomy (Table 23–3). Doxorubicin alone (30 mg/m^2 IV every 3 weeks) has been shown to be of benefit in dogs with splenic hemangiosarcoma and results in similar survival times to combination chemotherapy protocols with fewer complications. All the various histopathologic types of splenic sarcomas (nonangiomatous/nonlymphomatous) warrant a poor prognosis and are associated with a high rate of metastasis. Adjuvant chemotherapy probably is warranted postoperatively for patients with nonangiomatous/nonlymphomatous splenic sarcomas, although limited information is available on the efficacy of therapy.

Splenectomy is contraindicated in patients with immune-mediated hemolytic anemia or thrombocytopenia, unless other forms of treatment have failed; in most patients with lymphoma or leukemia when there is splenic involvement (splenomegaly); and in patients with bone marrow hypoplasia or aplasia because the spleen is the major hematopoietic organ in these patients.

Comment: Splenectomy may be a therapeutic option in selected patients with lymphoma and leukemia.

In humans with non-Hodgkin's lymphoma, the indications for splenectomy are massive splenomegaly, hypersplenism syndrome, and autoimmune complications.

▼ **Key Point** Generalized splenomegaly often is not a surgical disease. Attempt to diagnose and treat the underlying disorder before performing a splenectomy.

Technique

Partial Splenectomy

1. Prepare the ventral abdomen for aseptic surgery.
2. Make a ventral midline abdominal incision from the xyphoid to 2–4 cm cranial to the pubis, or more caudally if necessary.
3. Place a Balfour retractor to expose the abdominal viscera.

Table 23–3. TREATMENT PROTOCOLS FOR HEMANGIOSARCOMA IN THE DOG

VAC Protocol 1

Day 1: doxorubicin,* 30 mg/m^2 IV; premedication-diphenhydramine, 0.5 mg/lb IV (maximum of 40 mg); cyclophosphamide† (CTX), 100–150 mg/m^2 IV
Day 7: vincristine‡, 0.7 mg/m^2 IV
Day 15: vincristine, 0.7 mg/m^2 IV
Day 21: repeat protocol
Prophylactic oral antibiotic therapy is recommended, such as trimethoprim-sulfonamide (Tribrissen), 15 mg/lb q12h for 14 days starting on day 1.

VAC Protocol 2

Day 1: doxorubicin and diphenhydramine, as above; vincristine 0.7 mg/m^2 IV
Day 7: CTX, 50 mg/m^2 PO SID for 4 days
Day 15: CTX, 50 mg/m^2 PO SID for 4 days
Day 21: repeat protocol
This protocol can be used for patients that are unable to visit the veterinarian weekly for treatment.

VAC = vincristine-Adriamycin-cyclophosphamide.

*Doxorubicin (Adriamycin; Pharmacia-Upjohn, Valhalla, NY) is potentially cardiotoxic. Evaluate an ECG and echocardiography (m-mode) before therapy. Repeat the cardiac evaluation at treatment number 4 or 5. The maximum amount of doxorubicin that should be administered over a course of treatment is 180 mg/m^2 or 6 dosages. If the patient develops a murmur or, more importantly, an arrhythmia, discontinue therapy.

†Cyclophosphamide (Cytoxan; Mead-Johnson, Evansville, IN) can cause hemorrhagic cystitis. If it occurs, discontinue cyclophosphamide immediately and usually limit therapy to oral antibiotics and corticosteroids. Resolution of signs occurs within days to 8 weeks later.

‡Oncovin (Eli Lilly, Indianapolis, IN) Evaluate a CBC before each chemotherapy treatment to check for bone marrow suppression, and periodically evaluate a metabolic panel to monitor for evidence of nephrotoxicity secondary to the doxorubicin.

Monitor patient progress monthly (radiographic evaluation as well as abdominal ultrasonography). Allow completion of 2 to 3 courses of treatment before making a decision about response to therapy.

4. Examine the spleen and other abdominal organs for evidence of abnormalities.
5. Gently pull the spleen out of the abdominal cavity.
6. Doubly ligate the splenic branches of the splenic artery and vein to the affected area of the spleen with absorbable suture. Divide the vessels between the ligatures.
7. Place two noncrushing clamps (e.g., Doyen) on the spleen between the healthy and diseased areas.
8. Divide between the clamps and remove the splenic tissue.
9. Oversew the splenic capsule on the remaining spleen (3-0 or 4-0 polydioxanone (PDS), simple continuous suture).

Total Splenectomy

1.–5. Same as for Partial Splenectomy.
6. Doubly ligate all the splenic branches of the splenic artery and vein with absorbable suture. Ligate the vessels close to the hilus of the spleen. Usually, two or three vessels can be included in each ligature. If possible, preserve the left gastroepiploic artery and vein (Fig. 23–1); this may not be possible when removing large splenic tumors.
7. Divide each vessel between the ligatures and remove the spleen.

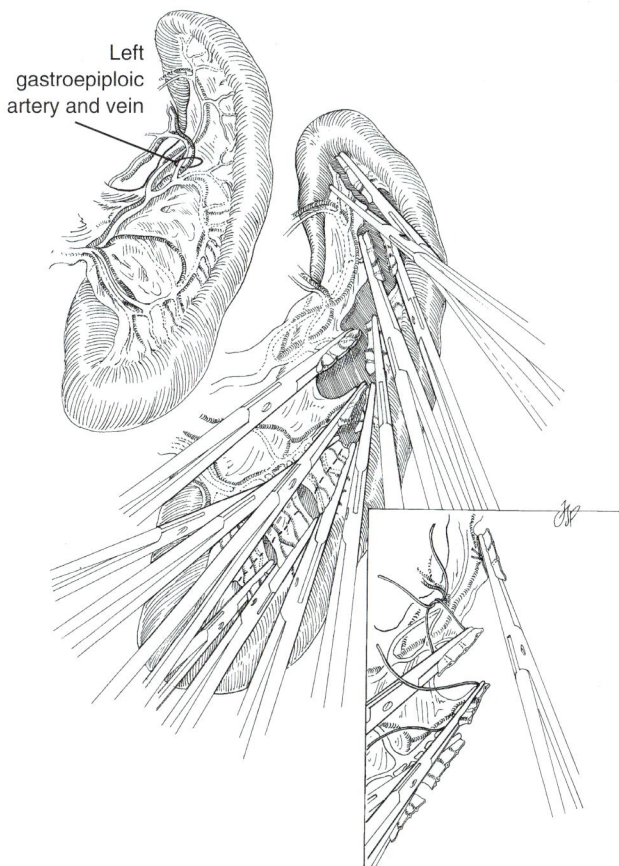

Figure 23–1. General procedure for total splenectomy. See text for details.

8. An alternative and more rapid procedure for total splenectomy is to place vascular clamps across the vessels before ligation. Include two or three of the vessels in each clamp. Divide the vessels between each pair of clamps and then place the next pair of clamps (see Fig. 23–1). After all vessels have been clamped and divided, remove the spleen. Ligate all vessels with absorbable sutures.
9. When splenic torsion is present, do not untwist the spleen because release of tissue breakdown products and bacteria may result. Ligate the entire vascular pedicle with two or three absorbable ligatures. Consider placing a transfixing ligature in large dogs. Place two clamps across the vascular pedicle, divide between them, and remove the spleen. Remove the remaining clamp and check the pedicle for hemorrhage.
10. Check the vessels for hemorrhage. Close the abdomen in a routine fashion.

Postoperative Care and Complications

- The gross appearance of the spleen cannot be used to differentiate hematoma, hemangioma, and hemangiosarcoma. A histopathologic diagnosis is crucial for determining postoperative treatment and prognosis.
- Postsplenectomy sepsis is a serious complication in humans and can be fatal. Although this is a rare complication in dogs and cats, partial splenectomy or splenic biopsy may be advisable in certain animals. Partial splenectomy is a viable option for those animals with localized masses unless malignancy is suspected.
- Other possible complications of splenectomy include exacerbation of certain diseases such as hemobartonellosis and babesiosis in animals that are latent carriers and cytopenia(s) in patients with EMH secondary to a primary bone marrow disorder.

Treatment of the Underlying Disease Process

- Treat infectious diseases with appropriate antibiotic therapy and supportive care.
- Treat immune-mediated diseases (immune-mediated hemolytic anemia, immune-mediated thrombocytopenia) as follows:
  - Use immunosuppressive doses of corticosteroids and other drugs as necessary (e.g., cyclophosphamide). Splenectomy may allow dose reduction of immunosuppressive drugs in patients requiring continuous or long-term therapy and should be considered in recurrent or resistant cases.
  - Use blood component therapy, if indicated (as described in Chapters 20 and 21).

Additional Therapy

Chemotherapy alone or in conjunction with the necessary supportive care is recommended for patients with acute and chronic leukemia and lymphosarcoma (see Chapter 25); and for dogs with systemic mastocytosis (see Chapter 26) and hemangiosarcoma.

Left gastroepiploic artery and vein

Treatment of Dogs with Hemangiosarcoma

For general recommendations, see Table 23–3. Evaluation should include a complete blood count (CBC), including a coagulation panel, if indicated, thoracic and abdominal radiographs, and cardiac and abdominal ultrasonography if available.

Perform splenectomy in dogs with splenic hemangiosarcoma. Splenectomy decreases the tumor burden and eliminates the risk of splenic rupture. Splenic rupture can occur as part of the natural progression of the disease, as a result of trauma (including abdominal palpation), or after initiation of chemotherapy in those tumors that respond to chemotherapy.

SUPPLEMENTAL READINGS

Couto CG, Hammer AS: Diseases of the lymph nodes and the spleen. In: Ettinger SJ, Feldman EC (eds): Textbook of Veterinary Internal Medicine. Philadelphia: WB Saunders, 1995, p 1930.

Day MJ, Lucke VM, Pearson H: A review of pathological diagnoses made from 87 canine splenic biopsies. J Small Anim Pract 36:426, 1995.

Johnson KA, Powers BE, Withrow SJ, et al: Predictors of neoplasia and survival after splenectomy. J Vet Intern Med 3:160, 1989.

Marino DJ, Matthiesen DT, Fox PR, Lesser MB, Stamoulis ME: Ventricular arrhythmias in dogs undergoing splenectomy: A prospective study. Vet Surg 23:101, 1994.

Neer TM: Clinical approach to splenomegaly in dogs and cats. Comp Contin Educ 18:35, 1996.

O'Keefe DA, Couto CG: Fine-needle aspiration of the spleen as an aid in the diagnosis of splenomegaly. J Vet Intern Med 1:102, 1987.

Prymak C, McKee LJ, Goldschmidt MH, Glickman LT: Epidemiologic, clinical, pathologic, prognostic characteristics of splenic hemangiosarcoma and splenic hematoma in dogs: 217 cases (1985). J Am Vet Med Assoc 193:706, 1988.

Richardson EF, Brown NO: Hematological and biochemical changes and results of aerobic bacteriological culturing in dogs undergoing splenectomy. J Am Anim Hosp Assoc 32:199, 1996.

Spangler WL, Culbertson MR: Prevalence, type and importance of splenic diseases in dogs: 1,480 cases (1985–1989). J Am Vet Med Assoc 200:829, 1992.

Spangler WL, Culbertson MR: Prevalence and type of splenic diseases in cats: 455 cases (1985–1991). J Am Vet Med Assoc 201:773, 1992.

Spangler WL, Culbertson MR, Kass PH: Primary mesenchymal (nonangiomatous/nonlymphomatous) neoplasms occurring in the canine spleen: Anatomic classification, immunohistochemistry, and mitotic activity correlated with patient survival. Vet Pathol 31:37, 1994.

Waldron DR, Robertson J: Partial splenectomy in the dog: A comparison of stapling and ligation techniques. J Am Anim Hosp Assoc 31:343, 1995.

Weinstein MJ, Carpenter JL, Schunk JM: Nonangiogenic and nonlymphomatous sarcomas of the canine spleen: 57 cases (1975–1987). J Am Vet Med Assoc 195:784, 1989.

Wrigley RH, Konde LJ, Park RD, Lebel JL: Ultrasonographic features of splenic lymphosarcoma in dogs. J Am Vet Med Assoc 193:1565, 1988.

Principles of Oncology

Stephen D. Gilson / Rodney L. Page

Cancer management in animals has evolved considerably over the past 2 decades as the result of several significant factors. Improved health care of animals has increased the age distribution of pets and hence the likelihood of developing cancer; clients are more aware of aggressive treatment choices; and there have been significant improvements in treatment success. There remains some controversy and confusion over the best course of treatment for many tumor types, and more studies are needed to provide the necessary data, but clinicians can use a generic framework for evaluation and treatment management of many tumor types. This chapter provides an outline useful for clinical management of an animal with cancer.

INITIAL CLINICAL PRESENTATION

Signalment

Many neoplasms more commonly affect animals of a certain age, sex, or breed, and such knowledge often aids diagnosis. Table 24–1 is a partial list of specific breeds and characteristics of dogs and cats predisposed to certain types of neoplasia.

History

The onset and duration of a mass, growth rate, presence of other masses, paraneoplastic signs, and prior treatments further help narrow diagnostic and treatment options and define the behavioral characteristics of a neoplasm.

Physical Examination

Examination is used to define the extent of tumor burden and identify concurrent diseases that may limit treatment or affect survival. Tumor characteristics such as *size* (measure with calipers to determine objectively), *location* (e.g., oral melanoma is more malignant than cutaneous melanoma), *invasiveness* (is mass fixed to adjacent tissue), and presence of *ulceration* or *necrosis* of the tumor are important to determine tumor behavior and plan adequately an appropriate biopsy and treatment regimen. Regional lymph nodes are evaluated for size, consistency, and fixation to adjacent tissues. To complete the clinical evaluation, a list of differential diagnoses are made and a diagnostic and staging plan are determined.

Client Counseling

A diagnosis of cancer can evoke considerable emotional response from owners. For many clients, the diagnosis implies pain, discomfort, and impending death of their pet. Proper counseling on the part of the veterinarian should include the following:

- Listen to the needs of the client and mutually determine a set of realistic goals for treatment.
- Explain treatment procedures, discussing risks, benefits, toxicity, and costs. It is helpful to provide written material for home review of information.
- Provide a realistic and *unbiased* view of all treatment options available and the animal's likely prognosis.
- Beware of the tendency for clinicians untrained in oncology to prematurely recommend euthanasia.
- Consider consultation with or referral to a specialist when appropriate.

DIAGNOSIS

Laboratory Evaluation

Assess general health status to identify concurrent disease or paraneoplastic syndromes that may adversely affect prognosis and limit or alter therapy. After a thorough physical examination, perform screening laboratory evaluations, including a complete blood count, serum biochemistry panel, and urinalysis. Perform other special laboratory tests as indicated to aid diagnosis (e.g., FeLV, FIV, bone marrow aspirate, adrenal function tests).

Diagnostic Imaging

- Obtain survey radiographs to detect metastases (thorax, abdomen, or skeletal), to evaluate orthopedic soundness before amputation or limb-sparing surgery for dogs with osteosarcoma, and to determine bone margins of oral or nasal masses.
- Contrast radiography is helpful for defining the extent of disease in hollow viscera.
- Computed tomography and magnetic resonance imaging are useful to delineate deep masses of the coelom and axial skeleton.
- Ultrasound is most useful to image abdominal viscera. It can determine accurately the parenchymal nature of a mass and tumor proximity to large ves-

Table 24-1. SOME FACTORS PREDISPOSING DOGS AND CATS TO SPECIFIC NEOPLASMS	
Factor	**Predilection For**
Age	
Histiocytoma	Young dogs
Viral papilloma	Young dogs
Sex	
Malignant melanoma	Males
Perianal adenoma	Males
Adrenal tumor	Females
Meningiomas	Females (dog), males (cat)
Color	
Squamous cell carcinoma	Nonpigmented regions
Malignant melanoma	Darkly pigmented regions
Breed	
Skin tumors	Basset, boxer, bull mastiff, Scottish terrier, Weimaraner
Mast cell tumor	Brachycephalic breeds
Bone tumors	Large/giant breeds
Thyroid tumor	Boxer, beagle, golden retriever
Hemangiosarcoma	Golden retriever, German shepherd

sels, and evaluate for intra-abdominal metastases to lymph nodes or organs.

Cytology

Cytology is useful to evaluate fine-needle aspirates of masses and lymph nodes, bone marrow aspirates, and buffy coat and peripheral blood smear preparations. It can provide rapid and inexpensive diagnosis and staging information. Do not overinterpret cytologic preparations. Base treatment decisions on cytologic diagnosis only when a definitive diagnosis can be made by a pathologist, as with lymphoma and mast cell tumors. Although a diagnosis may be accomplished with cytologic preparations, histologic assessment is often helpful to determine prognosis (i.e., grade of malignancy).

Biopsy

Many techniques are available for tumor biopsy. The method selected should procure safely and simply an adequate tissue sample to provide a proper diagnosis without compromising treatment.

General Considerations

- In general, larger tissue samples are more likely to provide an accurate diagnosis. Avoid traumatic tissue handling, electrocoagulation, and other tissue damage to provide a histologically useful sample.
- Fix tissue samples for routine histopathologic analysis in 10% buffered formalin (10:1 formalin to tissue ratio). For electron microscopy, fix samples in glutaraldehyde solution.
- Obtain samples for culture or other special analyses at the same time to avoid a second biopsy procedure if histologic analysis identifies an inflammatory or other nonneoplastic process.

- Include a complete history and description of the clinical and surgical findings with the biopsy specimen submission.
- If unsure of the most appropriate biopsy technique, consult a specialist or refer before biopsy.

Excisional Biopsy

- Complete removal of a tumor and submission for histologic diagnosis is most useful for cutaneous, mammary, central nervous system, and easily resectable masses found during laparotomy or thoracotomy.
- Ideally, an excisable mass is small and freely movable without significant adjacent tissue invasion.
- The mass must be excised with a histologically confirmed complete resection margin of normal tissue. Use suture tags to identify areas of possible inadequate resection that require closer histologic scrutiny.

Nonexcisional Biopsy

- Remove only a portion of a tumor (e.g., cutting needle, endoscopic, punch, or incisional biopsy) when definitive diagnosis or grading would influence treatment decisions.
- Take deep biopsies of superficial ulcerated masses to avoid sampling only overlying necrotic debris on the surface.
- Incisional and needle biopsy tracts are considered contaminated by tumor cells and must be completely within the future field of surgical resection or radiation treatment.
- Ideal histologic samples contain a margin of normal and neoplastic tissue. This allows assessment of tumor invasiveness, and margins are frequently the site of greatest tumor cell activity. Biopsy at the margin is often undesirable, however, because it disrupts the natural tumor margin and effectively extends it. This necessitates a wider resection or larger radiation field for definitive treatment.

▼ *Key Point* Improper biopsy technique can significantly alter treatment, increase treatment morbidity, and sometimes adversely affect prognosis.

Evaluation of Pathology Reports

The pathology report should include:

- Histologic diagnosis and, where appropriate, histologic grade (e.g., mast cell tumor, soft tissue sarcoma)
- Complete description of cellular characteristics and degree of anaplasia
- Mitotic index
- Identification of lymphatic or vascular invasion
- Evaluation of resection margins

If aspects of the report are questionable or do not match your clinical judgment, always discuss the results with the pathologist.

Tumor Staging

Accurate staging requires understanding the biologic behavior of different tumor types combined with the results of a thorough diagnostic workup based on this expected behavior. Tumor staging is used to:

- Determine the extent of neoplastic disease
- Provide a framework for rational treatment planning
- Facilitate communication between clinicians
- Allow for uniform comparison and evaluation of treatment results
- Aid in prognostication

Several staging systems are available. Most are based on assessment of local, regional, and distant disease involvement. Some systems include other factors, such as presence or absence of clinical signs (e.g., lymphomas), tumor histologic grade (e.g., mast cell tumors), or tumor location (e.g., squamous cell carcinoma of mouth, tonsil, pinna, digit). The TNM staging system devised by the World Health Organization is the standard system for most tumors in veterinary medicine. Table 24–2 describes this staging scheme and gives an example. Staging systems should be revised as new prognostic information is acquired.

Table 24–2. WORLD HEALTH ORGANIZATION TNM CLASSIFICATION OF TUMORS

T = Tumor Size or Extent
T_1–T_4 represent specific size categories designated for each tumor type and define the extent of local tumor involvement.

N = Lymph Node Involvement
N_1–N_3 ($\pm$ a, b) describes regional lymph node characteristics for presence or absence of neoplasia, number and location of enlarged lymph nodes, and occurrence of adjacent tissue adhesion.

M = Metastasis
M_0 or M_1 indicates absence or presence of distant metastasis.

Example—TNM Classification of Tumors of the Oral Cavity in Dogs or Cats:
T: Primary Tumor
  T_{is} = Preinvasive tumor (in situ)
  T_0 = No evidence of tumor
  T_1 = Tumor < 2 cm diameter
  T_2 = Tumor 2–4 cm diameter
  T_3 = Tumor 3 cm diameter
      subclassification of a (no bone invasion) or b (bone invasion) can be added.
N: Nodes
  N_0 = No evidence of lymph node enlargement
  N_1 = Movable ipsilateral nodes enlarged
  N_2 = Movable contralateral/bilateral nodes enlarged
  N_3 = Fixed nodes
M: Metastasis
  M_0 = No metastasis
  M_1 = Metastasis detected

Example of Stage Grouping for Oral Tumors:

Stage	T	N	M
I	T_1	N_0, N_{1a}, N_{2a}	M_0
II	T_2	N_0, N_{1a}, N_{2a}	M_0
III	T_3	N_0, N_{1a}, N_{2a}	M_0
	Any T	N_{1b}	M_0
IV	Any T	N_{2b}, N_3	M_0
	Any T	Any N	M_1

From Owen LN: Classification of Tumours in Domestic Animals. Geneva: WHO, 1980.

PRINCIPLES OF THERAPY

Rational treatment planning requires an accurate diagnosis, complete staging, and knowledge of expected tumor behavior with regard to local growth and propensity for developing regional and distant metastases. Many treatment options are available for the management of cancer, and each has its advantages and disadvantages. Clinicians must recognize the strengths and shortcomings of each treatment modality and apply therapy toward efficacious treatment of each aspect of expected tumor behavior (i.e., local, regional, and distant disease). Currently, multidisciplinary treatment is employed most commonly to maximize treatment results while minimizing related toxicity. Combinations of surgery, chemotherapy, and radiation often can more effectively eradicate cancer, especially multifocal cancer, than any one modality alone. The goal of treatment is to maintain the highest quality of life for the longest period of time.

▼ *Key Point* The probability of long-term tumor control is greatest when aggressive therapy is instituted early, before the tumor is disturbed by previous failed therapeutic attempts.

Surgery

Surgery is primarily useful for localized neoplasms. In select cases, en bloc dissection of regional lymph nodes and the primary mass is used for treatment of regional disease, and surgery can be useful for treatment of metastatic disease that is slow-growing or causing clinical morbidity.

Applications

Surgery is and will remain for the near future the most widely applied modality for cancer control. Surgery can be used for prevention (e.g., ovariohysterectomy before 2.5 years of age), diagnosis (see section on Biopsy), staging (see section on Staging), and treatment (cure or palliation). Surgery also is used for treatment of oncologic emergencies (e.g., obstruction or perforation) and for complications related to chemotherapy or radiotherapy (e.g., drug extravasation, radionecrosis).

Principles of Surgery

Special technique is used to prevent surgical spread of cancer cells and to ensure complete tumor resection.

▼ *Key Point* Aggressive initial surgical management of neoplasia may be the most important principle for improved cancer control. The best chance for complete resection and cure is with the first surgery.

- Decide resection margins in advance of the surgery based on tumor type, expected behavior, extent of local invasion, and the barrier provided by surrounding tissues (Fig. 24–1). Vascular-poor, collagen-rich tissue (e.g., cartilage, fascia) are most impermeable

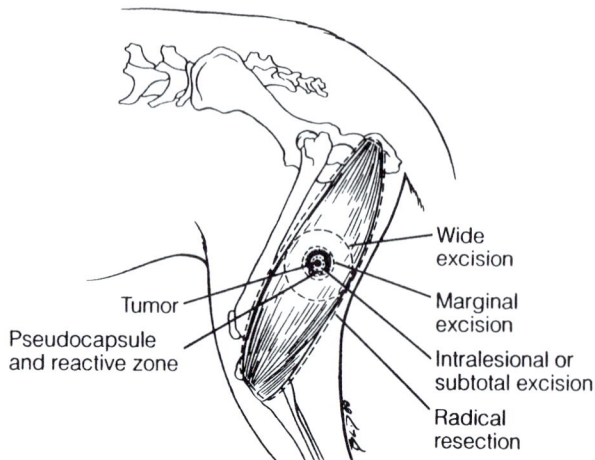

Figure 24–1. Surgical options for removal of a neoplasm. Wide excision or a more radical, compartmental resection is recommended for tumors that are not superficial or are infiltrative. Additional therapy may be indicated from histologic evaluation of tumor specimen. (Reprinted with permission from Gilson SD, Stone EA: Compend Contin Educ Pract Vet 12:1047, 1990.)

to tumor invasion. Other tissues (e.g., fat, subcutaneous tissue) provide less of a barrier.

- Resect all neoplastic tissue, leaving the wound open to heal if necessary. If uncertain about achieving complete resection or wound closure, consider referral to a specialist.
- Protect healthy tissues from tumor cell contamination by use of barrier drapes and laparotomy sponges. Employ glove, instrument, and drape changes as necessary to prevent seeding. Copious lavage of surface wounds also may reduce the likelihood of residual tumor.
- Minimize tumor manipulation. Handle tumors by placing stay sutures in normal margin tissues.
- Ligate vascular and lymphatic vessels early and always before severing, to prevent shedding of tumor emboli.
- Fulgurate or electrocoagulate any exposed tumor surfaces.
- When en bloc resection is performed, maintain adequate margins and dissect from the most peripheral affected lymph node toward the primary mass.
- When postoperative radiotherapy is used, all surgically exposed tissues plus a margin of normal tissue are irradiated. Position tissue grafts, flaps, and drains to minimize treatment fields.
- Submit all resected specimens for histologic analysis and evaluation of margins.

▼ *Key Point* A pseudocapsule made up of compressed cancer cells surrounds most tumors. Although seemingly a convenient plane for dissection, it is not a true capsule and provides no barrier to tumor invasion. A properly excised tumor is encased completely in an envelope of normal tissue.

Sources of Failure

Treatment failures result from surgery-related morbidity and mortality, local or regional tumor recurrence, and tumor seeding or metastatic disease. Most failures can be minimized by use of proper surgical technique and appropriate patient selection.

Chemotherapy

Chemotherapy is most useful for regional and disseminated neoplasms. It is used primarily for palliation; few cures are achieved. Some cancer types are notably chemosensitive. Lymphoid neoplasias and transmissible venereal tumors often are treated effectively; most other nonlymphoid tumors are only moderately sensitive. Chemotherapy is useful, however, for treatment of many tumor types as an adjunct therapy to other treatments or for palliation. Table 24–3 lists the most common neoplastic agents used in veterinary medicine. Indications and major toxicity also are listed. Table 24–4 is a conversion schedule for estimating body surface area for dogs and cats based on body weight. Cytotoxic agents must be used safely to avoid exposure to health care workers. General guidelines for handling cytotoxic agents are given in Table 24–5.

Applications

Most chemotherapeutic agents are administered intravenously. This is convenient and relatively noninvasive. Chemotherapy also is given by intraarterial or intracavitary routes to increase tumor/drug exposure. Drugs can be given before (neoadjuvant) or after surgery (adjuvant); the optimal sequence for most tumors is not yet known.

Advantages of Neoadjuvant Chemotherapy

- Reduced tumor size necessitating less surgery or radiotherapy
- Tumor vasculature is not altered by surgery or radiation, ensuring more uniform delivery of drug
- Drug therapy can be evaluated by monitoring tumor response

Advantages of Adjuvant Chemotherapy

- Resection of primary mass decreases the tumor burden; chemotherapy is more effective against a small tumor burden.
- Recruitment of dormant tumors cells into a more chemosensitive cell cycle phase increases tumor susceptibility to cytotoxic agents.

A preplanned protocol, regardless of sequence, is important for proper management of tumors that are likely to recur after single-modality treatment. Chemotherapy must be used appropriately to maximize treatment results and minimize toxicity.

Principles of Chemotherapy

- Use only drugs with documented activity against the specific tumor type.
- Administer all drugs at maximum tolerated doses and intervals.
- Some protocols are administered in two phases: an initial phase of intensive therapy (*induction*), followed

Table 24–3. COMMON CHEMOTHERAPEUTIC AGENTS USED IN VETERINARY MEDICINE

	Indication	Recommended Dosages	Toxicity
Alkylating Agents			
Cyclophosphamide (Cytoxan; Mead-Johnson)	Lymphoproliferative disorders, mast cell tumors, hemangiosarcoma, miscellaneous carcinomas	50 mg/m^2 PO q48 hr 50 mg/m^2 PO q24h for 4d weekly 100–300 mg/m^2 IV q3wk	BM, GI, hemorrhagic cystitis
Chlorambucil (Leukeran; Burroughs-Wellcome)	Lymphoproliferative disease, macroglobulinemia	2–4 mg/m^2 q24–48h	BM
Melphalan (Alkeran; Burroughs-Wellcome)	Multiple myeloma	2–4 mg/m^2 PO q24–48h	BM
Cisplatin (Platinol; Bristol)	Osteosarcoma, transitional cell carcinoma, squamous cell carcinoma	50–70 mg/m^2 IV q3wk (vigorous hydration)	BM, GI, renal; do not use in cats
Carboplatin (Paraplatin; Bristol)	Similar to cisplatin	250–300 mg/m^2 IV q3wk	BM, GI
Antimetabolites			
Methotrexate (Lederle)	Lymphoproliferative disorders	2.5 mg/m^2 PO q24h 15–20 mg/m^2 IV q3wk	BM, GI, renal
5-Fluorouracil (Roche)	Gastrointestinal and hepatic carcinoma	150–200 mg/m^2 IV q7d	BM, GI, CNS; do not use in cats
Cytosine Arabinoside (Cytosar-U; Upjohn)	Lymphoproliferative disorders, myeloproliferative disorders	100 mg/m^2 IV or SC for 4 days q3–4wk	BM, GI
Plant Alkaloids			
Vincristine (Oncovin; Eli Lilly)	Lymphoproliferative disorders, mast cell tumors, sarcomas, carcinomas	0.5–0.7 mg/m^2 IV q7d	GI, peripheral neuropathy; vesicant
Antibiotics			
Doxorubicin (Adriamycin; Adria Labs.)	Lymphoproliferative disorders, soft tissue sarcoma, carcinomas	20–25 mg/m^2 IV q3wk for dogs ≤ l0 kg and cats; 30 mg/m^2 IV q3wk for dogs > 10 kg; maximum cumulative dose = 180–240 mg/m^2	BM, GI, cardiac; severe vesicant; urticaria, alopecia
Mitoxantrone (Novantrone; Lederle)	Lymphoproliferative disorders	5–6 mg/m^2 q3wk	BM
Hormones			
Prednisone	Lymphoproliferative disorders, mast cell tumors, brain tumors	20–50 mg/m^2 q24–48h as needed	Iatrogenic Cushing's syndrome, GI
Miscellaneous			
L-Asparaginase (Elspar; Merck, Sharp & Dohme)	Lymphoproliferative disorders	10,000–30,000 IU/m^2 IM, SC, or IP as needed (pretreat with antihistamines, steroids)	Anaphylaxis, pancreatitis, coagulopathy

m^2, body surface area in square meters (see Table 24–4); PO, per os; IV, intravenously; IM, intramuscularly; SC, subcutaneously; IP, intraperitoneally; BM, bone marrow; GI, gastrointestinal; CNS, central nervous system.

by a period of less frequent drug administration (*maintenance*).

- Combination chemotherapy using agents with different mechanisms of action and no overlap in toxicity results in enhanced cancer cell destruction, reduced induction of drug resistance, and reduced toxicity.
- Continue chemotherapy past the time of complete remission because microscopic tumor remains after clinically detectable tumor has resolved.

Sources of Failure

Treatment failures result from excessive chemotherapy-related side effects (e.g., renal, hepatic, or myocardial toxicity; sepsis) or from progressive tumor growth because of intrinsic or acquired drug resistance. Intrinsic resistance results from molecular or biological adaptations within cancer cells that provide mechanisms for circumventing drug effects. The larger a tumor is, the more likely the existence of resistant cells. Clinically detectable tumors are likely to have multiple resistant cell lines.

Intrinsic Drug Resistance

Causes of intrinsic resistance include

- Inherent genetic mechanisms of cell protection
- Sanctuary sites (site where cells are protected, such as CNS)
- Tumor cell dormancy, or insensitivity to specific action of a drug
- Insufficient drug delivery

Table 24–4. CONVERSION FROM BODY WEIGHT (KG) TO BODY SURFACE AREA IN SQUARE METERS (M²) FOR DOGS*

kg	m²	kg	m²
0.5	0.06	29.0	0.94
1.0	0.10	30.0	0.96
2.0	0.15	31.0	0.99
3.0	0.20	32.0	1.01
4.0	0.25	33.0	1.03
5.0	0.29	34.0	1.05
6.0	0.33	35.0	1.07
7.0	0.36	36.0	1.09
8.0	0.40	37.0	1.11
9.0	0.43	38.0	1.13
10.0	0.46	39.0	1.15
11.0	0.49	40.0	1.17
12.0	0.52	41.0	1.19
13.0	0.55	42.0	1.21
14.0	0.58	43.0	1.23
15.0	0.60	44.0	1.25
16.0	0.63	45.0	1.26
17.0	0.66	46.0	1.28
18.0	0.69	47.0	1.30
19.0	0.71	48.0	1.32
20.0	0.74	49.0	1.34
21.0	0.76	50.0	1.36
22.0	0.78	51.0	1.38
23.0	0.81	52.0	1.40
24.0	0.83	53.0	1.41
25.0	0.85	54.0	1.43
26.0	0.88	55.0	1.45
27.0	0.90	56.0	1.47
28.0	0.92	57.0	1.48

*Specific values can be calculated using the following formula:

$$\text{Body surface area (m}^2) = \frac{(k) \times (Wt)^{2/3}}{10^4}$$

where (k) = 10.1 for dogs and 10.0 for cats.

Acquired Drug Resistance

- Acquired resistance arises from selection pressure induced by sublethal drug doses.
- Acquired resistance occurs when cancer cells survive long enough to:
  - Develop alternate metabolic pathways
  - Change drug transport mechanisms
  - Initiate cellular repair
  - Inhibit drug activation

Pleiotropic Drug Resistance

Resistance can develop to a single drug, a group of drugs, or many classes of drugs (pleiotropic resistance). Pleiotropic resistance is associated most commonly with the anthracyclines and vinca alkaloids.

Radiotherapy

Radiotherapy is primarily useful for local and regional neoplasia (Table 24–6). In selected cases, it is used for palliation of painful disseminated tumors.

Applications

Radiotherapy is administered as a single modality or is combined with surgery, chemotherapy, or hyperthermia. It can be administered:

Table 24–5. PRACTICAL RECOMMENDATIONS FOR SAFE HANDLING OF CYTOTOXIC ANTINEOPLASTIC AGENTS

1. Designate a specific hospital location for drug handling (reconstitution, preparation, disposal).
2. Use an absorbent, disposable, plastic-backed sheet to cover work surface; change regularly.
3. Wear latex nonpermeable gloves when handling all cytotoxic agents.
4. Reduce exposed skin surfaces by wearing laboratory coats, gowns, and other protective wear. Wear particulate respiratory filtration masks to prevent inhalation of aerosolized drug particles.
5. Reconstitute all materials carefully and safely, avoiding potential contamination of materials or aerosolization.
6. Clean reconstituted material of any contamination and properly mark and date it.
7. Dispose of contaminated materials in leak-proof, puncture-resistant containers. Proper disposal by health regulatory officials is necessary.
8. Wash hands thoroughly after removing gloves.

- As the initial form of therapy (neoadjuvant radiotherapy)
- Concurrent with other therapies (intraoperative radiation, concurrent chemotherapy or hyperthermia)
- As postoperative therapy (adjuvant radiotherapy)

Advantages of Neoadjuvant Radiotherapy

- Reduced tumor size, requiring less surgery and increasing the effectiveness of adjuvant chemotherapy
- Tumor vasculature is unaltered, decreasing local tumor hypoxia
- Viability of any surgically disseminated tumor cells is decreased
- Peripheral subclinical disease is eliminated

Table 24–6. RELATIVE RADIATION SENSITIVITY OF SELECTED CANINE TUMORS

Tumor Type	Site	Radiation Response
Squamous carcinoma	Gingiva	Good
	External nose	Poor
	Tonsil	Fair–poor
	Nasal cavity	Fair–poor
Malignant melanoma	Oral	Fair
Acanthomatous epulis	Gingiva	Excellent
Fibrosarcoma	Nasal cavity	Fair–good
Chondrosarcoma	Nasal cavity	Fair–good
Adenocarcinoma	Nasal cavity	Fair–good
Transmissible venereal tumor	Variable (usually penis and vulva)	Excellent
Soft tissue sarcoma	Peripheral	Poor–good
Mast cell tumor	Cutaneous	Fair–excellent
Perianal adenoma	Perianal	Excellent
Meningioma	Brain	Fair–good
Osteosarcoma	Any site	Fair (palliation only)
Solitary lymphoproliferative disease	Any site	Excellent

Advantages of Concurrent Therapy

- Improved radiation effectiveness by hyperthermia or chemotherapy-induced radiosensitization
- Decreased radiation toxicity to normal tissues with intraoperative radiation

Advantages of Adjuvant Radiation

- Improved effectiveness of radiation against smaller tumor burden
- More accurate radiotherapy planning based on information gained from surgery
- No delays in other therapy from radiation-related complications

Principles of Radiotherapy

- Irradiate all potentially affected tissues (such as regional lymph nodes and the tumor itself) and a margin of normal tissue.
- Radiation is more effective against a small tumor burden and well-oxygenated tumor cells.
- Higher energy radiation sources (linear accelerator, cobalt therapy), result in deeper, more uniform radiation penetration and greater sparing of skin and superficial tissues.
- Frequent small doses of radiation (e.g., < 3 Gy daily or every other day) are preferable to allow for reoxygenation of tumor cells, repair of normal cells, and decreased late effects of radiation toxicity.
- Damage to normal tissue is minimized by judicious treatment planning and use of multiple treatment ports and shrinking field techniques.
- Administer radiation doses to the maximum dose tolerated by adjacent normal tissues. Radiation-induced tissue changes are permanent; however, reirradiation of recurrent tumors is possible in some situations.
- Radiation-induced normal tissue effects may be classified as *acute,* occurring during the last portion of therapy or in the first few weeks after irradiation (e.g., mucositis, moist desquamation, hair loss, tissue inflammation), or *late,* occurring many months or years after treatment (e.g., contraction and fibrosis, tissue necrosis, cataract formation).
- After treatment, tumor volume may not change and biopsy samples can show the presence of nonviable neoplastic cells. Only gross evidence of active tumor growth indicates tumor recurrence.

Sources of Failure

Treatment failures result from radiation-related toxicity to normal tissues and from tumor- or treatment-related factors. Meticulous technique and use of advanced radiotherapy planning technology minimize these errors.

Tumor-Related Factors

- Histologic tumor type (some tumor cells are inherently more radioresistant)
- Tumor volume (larger volume increases the likelihood of radioresistant cells and tumor hypoxia)

Treatment-Related Factors

- Inadequate radiation dose
- Geographic miss (i.e., portion of tumor outside the treatment field)

Miscellaneous Therapy

Hyperthermia

Heat is an effective adjunct therapy because it enhances the cytotoxic effect of radiation and many chemotherapy agents. Hyperthermia is induced locally by ultrasound or radiowaves or implemented as whole body hyperthermia induced by a humidified chamber or radiant heat device.

Immunotherapy

Immunotherapy has emerged with renewed potential. Because neoplastic cells may be immunologically different from healthy cells, selective or nonselective induction of the host immune system by various biologic response modifiers (e.g., bacterial agents, interferons, monoclonal antibodies, lymphokines) may enhance elimination of tumor cells. Immunotherapy appears to have the greatest potential as an adjunct to other therapies to eliminate microscopic residual tumor.

Photodynamic Therapy

Many tumor cells selectively accumulate certain systemically administered photoactive chemicals. Tumors then are exposed to light of selected wavelengths (laser light), and the photoactive substances become cytotoxic. Various photoactive drugs and light sources currently are being tested. Early results indicate that photodynamic therapy may be useful for treatment of localized solid tumors.

Post-Treatment Monitoring

Patient monitoring after therapy is important to assess toxicity, adjust subsequent treatment, and monitor tumor response.

- Reevaluate animals at regular intervals (e.g., 1, 2, 3, 5, 7, 9, and 12 months, and so on).
- Tailor follow-up diagnostic tests to each patient and the particular stage and expected behavior of their tumor.
- The goal of follow-up evaluation is to detect tumor recurrence or metastasis at the earliest possible time and to maximize the response to additional alternate therapies if clinically chosen.

ADJUNCT CLINICAL CONSIDERATIONS

Nutritional Management

Many animals with cancer have alterations of metabolism that result in malnutrition. When severe, these alterations result in the clinical syndrome of *cancer cachexia.* Malnutrition impairs the immune system, inhibits wound healing and normal cell repair, and increases treatment morbidity and mortality.

- Factors contributing to malnutrition include:
  - Anorexia
  - Decreased nutrient intake
  - Metabolic or digestive abnormalities that cause inefficient or inappropriate use of nutrients
  - Treatment-related factors such as therapy-induced nausea and vomiting
- Proposed mechanisms of cachexia include:
  - Tumor-produced anorexigenic substances
  - Alterations in brain neurotransmitter and anabolic hormone function
- Treatment is directed toward early elimination of the cachexia syndrome (by elimination of neoplasia) and supportive care to minimize its effects during the interim. Nutritional support is provided by enteral or parenteral feeding (see Chap. 3), and should be provided when patients do not eat for more than 5 days or have greater than 10% acute loss of body weight. Laboratory parameters indicative of malnutrition include hypoalbuminemia, lymphopenia, and anemia.

Pain Management

Clinical management of pain in cancer patients is an important aspect of care to reduce morbidity and improve the quality of life.

- Pain can be:
  - Acute or chronic
  - Treatment- or tumor-related
  - Visceral, somatic, or neurogenic in origin
- Pain can contribute significantly to development of inappetence, weight loss, reduced mobility, depression, and poor interaction with the owner. Presence of pain is determined by changes, often subtle, in normal behavior patterns.
- The severity is determined and a treatment protocol implemented to provide adequate analgesia with minimal sedation and other side effects. Prevention or early treatment of pain is more effective than trying to resolve established significant or chronic pain signs. Therapy is by use of local or regional anesthesia, or with systemic treatment using transdermal delivery of narcotic-based pain medication, or parenterally administered nonsteroidal anti-inflammatory agents, and narcotics (see Chap. 2). Continual reassessment and modification of therapy is conducted.

Euthanasia

When treatment options fail and an animal's disease is progressing, consideration of euthanasia is appropriate. Encourage owners in advance to establish limits for their pet's level of deterioration. When the decision for euthanasia is reached by an owner, it should be supported by the veterinarian; for many owners, euthanasia is the last humane "treatment" they can give to their pet. Review the details of the euthanasia process in advance with owners and options for them to remain present or not. For clients having difficulty coping, provide assistance to help them find bereavement counseling. Condolence cards, telephone calls, or other forms of communication afterward are useful to provide closure. A positive experience with the euthanasia process often leaves clients with a positive feeling about the whole cancer treatment process.

SUPPLEMENTAL READINGS

Gillette EL (guest editor): Radiation oncology. Semin Vet Med Surg 10:127, 1995.

Gilson SD: Surgical oncology. Vet Clin North Am Small Anim Pract 25:1, 1995.

MacEwen EG, Helfand SC: Immunology and biologic therapy of cancer. In: Withrow SJ, MacEwen EG (eds): Small Animal Clinical Oncology 2nd ed. Philadelphia: WB Saunders, 1996, pp 99–116.

Ogilvie GK: Chemotherapy. In: Withrow SJ, MacEwen EG (eds): Small Animal Clinical Oncology. 2nd ed. Philadelphia: WB Saunders, 1996, pp 70–86.

Swanson LV: Potential hazards associated with low dose exposure to antineoplastic agents: Part I. Compend Contin Educ Pract Vet 10:293, 1988.

Swanson LV: Potential hazards associated with low dose exposure to antineoplastic agents: Part II. Compend Contin Educ Pract Vet 10:615, 1988.

25 Lymphoid Neoplasia

David M. Vail / Gregory K. Ogilvie

Lymphoproliferative disorders are characterized by neoplasia involving cells or cell lines of lymphoid origin, including lymphoma, lymphoid leukemia, and multiple myeloma/plasmacytoma. Because of differences in diagnosis, therapy, and prognosis among these conditions, they are discussed here as separate entities.

LYMPHOMA

Lymphoma (lymphosarcoma) is defined as a lymphoid neoplasm primarily affecting lymph nodes or other solid visceral organs such as the liver or spleen. It is the most common of the lymphoproliferative disorders in small animals. Middle-aged to older dogs primarily are affected, without sex predilection. Although lymphoma can occur in any purebred or mixed breed dog, it may be more prevalent in golden retrievers, German shepherds, boxers, poodles, bassets, and St. Bernards.

No breed predilection exists for cats; however, several reports have observed a 1.5:1 male-to-female ratio. Cats that are FeLV antigenemic tend to be younger (median age 3–5 years) than FeLV-negative cats (median age 7–10 years).

Etiology

Retrovirus

A retroviral etiology for certain forms of lymphoma has been demonstrated in a variety of species, including cats, chickens, and humans. In the cat, direct evidence exists for FeLV-induced lymphoma and indirect evidence exists for feline immunodeficiency virus (FIV)-lymphoma. Before 1985, most cats with lymphoma (>70%) were FeLV antigenemic. Since then, the general availability of FeLV vaccination and testing has increased and FeLV-positive cats currently make up a minority of lymphoma cases (<25%). Whether this is due directly to vaccination or whether FeLV antigen testing before vaccination has allowed separation of potentially infective cats from the susceptible population is unclear. In either situation, the result is a reduction in the number of FeLV-associated lymphomas. Conclusive evidence of a viral etiology is not yet established in the dog.

Genetic

A genetic predisposition for the development of certain forms of lymphoma may exist.

Carcinogenic Agents

Exposure to chemical, physical, and viral carcinogens may play a role in the development of many tumor types.

Classification and Clinical Signs

Traditionally, lymphoma is classified based on anatomic site. Clinical signs vary with the sites involved. In cats, the frequency of anatomic forms associated with FeLV antigenemia (i.e., mediastinal and multicentric forms) has declined along with the declining frequency of FeLV-associated lymphomas. Whereas these sites made up the bulk of cases observed in cats before 1985, they are now in the minority. Currently, the alimentary form, which only rarely is associated with FeLV antigenemia, makes up the bulk of lymphomas in cats. Other less common forms occurring in cats include renal, hepatic, and miscellaneous extranodal sites.

World Health Organization (WHO) clinical staging of lymphoma also can be used to classify the extent of the disease (Table 25–1).

Multicentric Lymphoma

This is the most common form in the dog. It usually manifests as increased lymph node size with nonspecific signs such as inappetence, weight loss, polyuria/polydypsia, and lethargy. Hepatic and splenic involvement, manifested as diffuse organ enlargement, also is common in multicentric lymphoma.

Alimentary Lymphoma

This type of lymphoma often is associated with vomiting, diarrhea, and nonspecific signs such as weight loss and lethargy.

Mediastinal Lymphoma

This form of lymphoma often causes respiratory signs secondary to pleural effusion, the mass effect of the tu-

Table 25–1. WORLD HEALTH ORGANIZATION CLINICAL STAGING FOR LYMPHOMA*

Stage†	Criteria
I	Involvement limited to single lymph node or lymphoid tissue in a single organ (excluding bone marrow)
II	Involvement of many lymph nodes in regional area (with or without tonsils)
III	Generalized lymph node involvement
IV	Liver and/or spleen involvement (with or without stage III)
V	Manifestations in blood and involvement of bone marrow and/or other organ systems (with or without stages I to IV)

*Reprinted with permission from World Health Organization: Owen LN: *TNM Classification of Tumors in Domestic Animals.* Geneva: WHO, 1980.

†Each stage is subclassified into: (a) without systemic signs and (b) with systemic signs.

mor, or precaval syndrome (i.e., facial and forelimb edema caused by reduced venous and/or lymphatic drainage). Approximately 40% to 50% of mediastinal lymphomas in the dog are associated with hypercalcemia, which can cause polyuria/polydipsia, anorexia, and weakness.

Cutaneous Lymphoma

Cutaneous lymphoma involves single or multiple skin lesions that can vary greatly in appearance. It may mimic other skin disorders such as seborrhea, pemphigus, and pyoderma. The cutaneous lesions can begin as a mild eczematous pruritic plaque and progress to nodular tumors. Approximately half of the reported cases of cutaneous lymphoma are pruritic.

Extranodal Forms

Miscellaneous extranodal forms of lymphoma include lymphoma of the eyes, central nervous system (CNS), bones, heart, kidneys, urinary bladder, and nasal cavity. Their presentations vary with respect to the site of involvement.

Classification by Immunophenotype

Lymphomas also can be classified by immunophenotype—that is, whether they are of B-lymphocyte or T-lymphocyte origin. Most (70–80%) lymphomas in dogs are composed of B-cells. T-cell origin lymphoma in dogs is associated more commonly with hypercalcemia and cranial mediastinal involvement. In cats, most FeLV-associated lymphomas are T-cell in origin. Alimentary lymphoma, the most common form in cats, tends to be B-cell in origin.

Diagnosis

The diagnosis of lymphoma is based on a complete history, physical examination, tissue diagnosis, and clinical staging. Clinical staging should include a complete blood count (CBC), platelet count, bone marrow aspi-

ration or core biopsy, biochemistry profile, and thoracic and abdominal radiographs.

History

The history should include an evaluation of past and present water intake and urination frequency because they may reflect hypercalcemia and subsequent renal disease.

Physical Examination

Perform a complete physical examination for all animals with lymphoma.

- Palpate all lymph nodes (including rectal palpation of sublumbar nodes) and abdominal viscera.
- Because bone marrow involvement can result in hematologic abnormalities, closely examine mucous membranes for signs of pallor or petechiae.
- Visceral involvement can lead to organ failure; therefore, look for any physical signs that may be indicative of liver or kidney disease (e.g., icterus, uremic ulcers).
- Ophthalmic abnormalities are present in more than one-third of dogs with lymphoma and include uveitis, hemorrhage, and ocular infiltration. Therefore, optic and fundic examinations should be conducted.

▼ *Key Point* Canine lymphoma usually is a disease of middle-aged and older animals; thus, it is essential to perform a complete examination to identify concomitant problems in other systems.

Laboratory Evaluations

Hematologic Abnormalities

- Hematologic abnormalities occur in most dogs and cats with multicentric lymphoma. Common abnormalities, in decreasing frequency, include atypical immature lymphocytes in the circulation, thrombocytopenia, eosinopenia, anemia, and nucleated erythrocytes.
- The anemia is usually that of chronic disease (normocytic, normochromic, and nonregenerative); however, a small percentage of animals have indices compatible with blood loss or hemolysis. FeLV-positive cats are more likely to be anemic than cats that are not infected.
- Bone marrow aspirate or core biopsy may reveal an altered bone marrow myeloid:erythroid ratio and bone marrow infiltration with neoplastic lymphocytes.

Biochemical Abnormalities

▼ *Key Point* Serum calcium is elevated in 15% to 20% of dogs with lymphoma. The likelihood of hypercalcemia is greatest in dogs with the mediastinal form.

- Paraneoplastic hypercalcemia (i.e., elevated serum calcium) may serve as a marker for response to therapy; however, it is more clinically significant as a cause of hypercalcemic nephropathy, a potentially irreversible cause of renal failure (see Chapter 97).

- Elevations in blood urea nitrogen and serum creatinine may result from neoplastic infiltration of the kidneys, hypercalcemic nephrosis, or dehydration.
- Increased serum concentration of liver enzymes or bilirubin may indicate neoplastic infiltration of the liver.
- Abnormally elevated serum globulins may be noted in some B-cell lymphomas.

FeLV Status

Approximately 80% of cats with mediastinal and multicentric lymphoma are FeLV-positive, in contrast to 50% with renal lymphoma, 5–10% with alimentary lymphoma, and a minority with cutaneous forms.

Radiography and Ultrasonography

Radiography and ultrasonography (see Chapter 4), although not diagnostic for lymphoma, are often useful for staging or determining the extent of disease.

- Half of all dogs with lymphoma have evidence of enlarged sternal and sublumbar lymph nodes, spleen, and liver.
- Thoracic radiographs are important for identification of thoracic masses that are due to mediastinal lymphoma and are recommended for any dog with hypercalcemia of unknown etiology.
- Contrast studies of the upper GI tract are abnormal in most animals with GI lymphoma.

Histopathology and Cytology

Histopathologic and cytologic evaluation of affected tissues is necessary for confirmation of lymphoma.

- Fine-needle aspiration cytology of lymph nodes, visceral organs, and other involved sites can be suggestive of neoplastic disease; however, conclusive histologic diagnosis is recommended.

▼ *Key Point* In the cytologic evaluation of lymph nodes in cats, neoplastic involvement is difficult to distinguish from benign lymphadenopathy syndromes. For this reason, only histopathologic examination is definitive.

- Avoid sampling lymph nodes draining reactive areas of the body (e.g., submandibular lymph nodes in the presence of periodontal disease) because reactive lymphoid hyperplasia can mask (or mimic) the true neoplastic condition.
- In addition to confirming a diagnosis of lymphoma, histologic and cytologic samples can be analyzed by various immunohistochemical and histochemical techniques to determine immunophenotype (B- vs. T-cell), tumor proliferation rates, and histologic subtype (high-, intermediate-, or low-grade tumors). The availability of such analysis is growing; however, at present only immunophenotype is consistently predictive of prognosis in dogs.

Additional Diagnostic Tests

Additional tests may be necessary to confirm the diagnosis of the extranodal forms of lymphoma.

- Stage the disease by performing a CBC, bone marrow evaluation, and thoracic and abdominal radiography. Staging is important in animals with extranodal lymphoma to ensure that the disease is not a sequela of the more common multicentric forms and to determine whether the disease is localized to the extranodal site.
- Perform exploratory laparotomy and full-thickness biopsy or fine-needle aspiration to diagnose most cases of alimentary lymphoma. Endoscopic biopsies of the mucosa may be too superficial to diagnose GI lymphoma because lymphoma usually originates in the submucosa. In addition, GI lymphoma often is accompanied by lymphocytic/plasmacytic mucosal infiltrations that may be misdiagnosed as a benign condition. However, improved endoscopic sampling techniques may reduce the likelihood of misdiagnosis.
- Cytological evaluation of cerebrospinal fluid (CSF) may be helpful in the diagnosis of CNS lymphoma in the dog, but CSF is rarely abnormal in feline spinal lymphoma because the tumor is usually extradural. Computed tomography and myelography may be helpful.

Differential Diagnosis

The differential diagnosis (DDx) varies with the anatomic form of the disease.

- *DDx for lymphadenopathies* includes infectious diseases (e.g., bacterial, viral, rickettsial, parasitic, and fungal; see Section 2, Infectious Diseases), immune-mediated diseases (e.g., systemic lupus erythematosus; see Chapter 22), and other types of metastatic neoplasia.
- *DDx for alimentary lymphoma* includes lymphocytic/plasmacytic enteritis, other types of intestinal neoplasia, granulomatous and infiltrative bowel disease, and hypereosinophilic syndrome (see Chapter 89).
- *DDx for mediastinal lymphoma* includes ectopic thyroid tumors, heart base tumors, thymoma, and pulmonary lymphomatoid granulomatosis.
- *DDx for cutaneous lymphoma* includes pyoderma, immune-mediated and parasitic skin disorders, and other neoplastic dermatopathies.

Treatment

Lymphoma is the most chemoresponsive malignancy encountered in veterinary medicine. Most dogs and cats with lymphoma have multisystemic disease and therefore require systemic chemotherapy to improve quality of life and survival time. Untreated, dogs and cats with malignant lymphoma live an average of only 4 to 6 weeks once a diagnosis has been made. With chemotherapy, 75% to 90% of dogs and cats go into remission and survive an average of 6–12 months with an excellent quality of life. With more elaborate combination protocols, approximately 25% of patients survive beyond 2 years. Cures are still uncommon. Cost is within the financial reach of many clients, especially with the advent of generic brands of cytotoxic drugs.

Many combination chemotherapy protocols have an "induction" period designed to place a dog or cat into a remission, followed by a less intensive "maintenance" treatment period intended to sustain a remission. The first remission is generally the longest. Second and third remissions are possible, although shorter.

Complete remission is more difficult to achieve in cats; however, if a remission can be achieved and maintained for approximately 6 months, cats are more likely to experience prolonged survivals compared with dogs. Cats are generally more resistant to the adverse effects of chemotherapy than dogs. The exception to this rule is cats treated with doxorubicin. Although dogs may receive doxorubicin every 21 days at a dosage of 30 mg/m^2, cats appear to be more sensitive to the drug and therefore are treated at a dosage of 25 mg/m^2 (or 1 mg/kg) given every 21 days.

Future goals are to increase the remission time while decreasing cost, toxicity, and time involved to treat the patient. Controversy exists within the veterinary community about (1) the benefit of single versus combination chemotherapy, (2) the role of immunotherapeutics, and (3) protocols that offer prolonged maintenance therapy (e.g., CVP maintenance for 2–3 years) versus shorter, intermittent protocols. Current data suggest that intensive "up front" therapy to induce a sound remission is as effective as standard less intense protocols with continuously administered maintenance therapy for most cats and dogs. Additional studies are essential to determine which patients need long-term maintenance therapy.

Criteria for Choosing Chemotherapy

When choosing a chemotherapy protocol, several points must be discussed with the pet owner.

- *Cost:* Many chemotherapeutic agents are generally affordable. The additional cost of blood work, office visits, and catheters, and the potential cost of treating toxicity also must be considered. Combination chemotherapy protocols, although often more effective, are also more expensive.
- *Time:* Time commitments can be more important than the cost of the therapy. Generally, the more elaborate the protocol, the more time invested in the care of the patient.
- *Efficacy:* As a general rule, the more complex the protocol, the longer the duration of remission and survival time. Conversely, single-agent chemotherapy is generally less effective than combination chemotherapy.
- *Toxicity:* The toxicity of most protocols is designed to be acceptable to the general public; however, the potential risks and benefits of each protocol must be discussed with each owner. Complex protocols increase the potential for toxicity and increase the importance of client education.
- *Experience of the attending clinician:* The successful application of any chemotherapy treatment requires experience and confidence because the effective dosage is very near the toxic dosage.

Chemotherapy Protocols

Several chemotherapy protocols for dogs and cats have been published (Table 25–2); this reflects the fact that cures are still uncommon and several investigators are continually attempting to improve on previous outcomes. The protocol used in individual cases ultimately rests on the client and veterinarian's choice based on the aforementioned points. However, the presence of doxorubicin in any protocol appears to be a key ingredient with respect to durability of response in both cats and dogs and should be offered. Listing dosage and timing of all available protocols is beyond the scope of

---

Table 25–2. EFFICACY OF CHEMOTHERAPY FOR THE TREATMENT OF LYMPHOMA*

Drug	Species	No. of Animals	Overall Response Rate (%)	Complete Response Rate (%)	Median Response Duration (Days)
Single-Agent Therapy					
Mitoxantrone	Dogs, cats	44	41	30	127
Epirubicin	Dogs	35	82	74	143
Idarubicin	Cats	13	—	—	—
Actinomycin D	Dogs, cats	12	85	70	42
Doxorubicin	Dogs	21	85	76	190
Combination Therapy					
LVPCD	Dogs	55	91	84	252
CVP	Dogs	—	89	75	180
CVPD	Dogs	46	87	83	210
VLCM	Dogs	147	94	—	140
VLCMP	Cats	103	82	62	—
CVP	Cats	38	94	79	321
VCM	Cats	62	—	52	112

L, L-asparaginase; V, vincristine; P, prednisone; C, cyclophosphamide; D, doxorubicin; M, methotrexate.
*From: Ogilvie GK: Chemotherapy. In: Withrow SJ, MacEwen EG (eds): Small Animal Clinical Oncology. Philadelphia: WB Saunders, 1996, p 73, with permission.

Table 25–3. CVP CHEMOTHERAPY PROTOCOL FOR DOGS AND CATS

Drug	Dose (mg/m²)	Weeks 1	2	3	4	5	6	7	8	9	10	11	12	13	52 Wks
Cyclophosphamide	250 PO	X			X			X			X			X	X
Vincristine	0.75 IV	X	X	X	X			X			X			X	X
Prednisone*	30 PO	>	>	>	>		>		>		>		>		>

*Prednisone is given daily for the first 21 days, then every other day thereafter. Note that maintenance is continued on a 3-week schedule for at least 1 year.

this chapter; therefore, the authors have chosen to elaborate on four protocols of varying cost, time commitment, and effectiveness; doxorubicin alone in dogs, cyclophosphamide-vincristine-prednisone (CVP) in dogs and cats, CVP plus doxorubicin in cats, and the University of Wisconsin-Madison protocol for dogs.

Doxorubicin

Doxorubicin is one of the most effective single-agent treatments for lymphoma in dogs. Of the dogs treated with doxorubicin (30 mg/m² IV q21d for 5–6 total treatments), 80% to 90% have a complete or partial remission. The duration of remission varies depending on the published report but is approximately 6–9 months.

Cyclophosphamide-Vincristine-Prednisone

The CVP protocol (Table 25–3) is effective for inducing a remission in 75% of dogs with lymphoma. A median duration of remission of 6 months is commonly seen. Approximately 20% of the dogs treated with the CVP regimen are in remission at 1 year.

In one study, 79% of cats with lymphoma treated with CVP achieved a complete remission, whereas only 29% of cats treated for lymphoblastic leukemia achieved a complete remission. Cats with lymphoma treated with CVP had a shorter remission time (64% achieved a complete remission, median remission 5 months) but proportionately more long-term survivors than dogs. Cats with renal lymphoma tend to have recurrence of tumor in the brain; therefore, cytosine arabinoside frequently is recommended as additional therapy.

CVP with Doxorubicin

Cats treated initially with CVP for the first 4 weeks to induce a remission and then switched to doxorubicin chemotherapy (1 mg/kg q21d for 5–8 dosages beginning 21 days after the second treatment with cyclophosphamide) had a longer remission and survival time compared with cats treated with CVP only.

University of Wisconsin-Madison Protocol

For the dog, the longest remission and survival times have been reported with the UW-Madison protocol noted in Table 25–4. This protocol is complex but gratifying because of consistently improved responses.

Prednisone Only

When more aggressive or expensive chemotherapy is declined by clients, an inexpensive, although only transiently effective, alternative is prednisone alone. With prednisone therapy, the average dog or cat lives 2 months. One-third of dogs and cats treated with prednisone go into complete remission, one-third go into partial remission, and one-third do not respond at all. Similar responses are seen in cats. Dogs and cats that receive high-dose prednisone for a significant period (>1–2 weeks) before traditional chemotherapy is initiated may develop resistance to the cytotoxic effects of other chemotherapy agents.

Chemotherapy in the Presence of Cytopenia

Drug therapy for multicentric lymphoma may have to be altered in the presence of thrombocytopenia

Table 25–4. UNIVERSITY OF WISCONSIN-MADISON CANINE LYMPHOMA PROTOCOL

Cycle 1 Induction
Week 1: Vincristine 0.7 mg/m² IV; L-asparaginase 400 IU/kg IM; and once daily prednisone, 2 mg/kg PO
Week 2: Cyclophosphamide, 200 mg/m² IV, and once daily prednisone, 1.5 mg/kg PO
Week 3: Vincristine, 0.7 mg/m² IV, and once daily prednisone, 1.0 mg/kg PO
Week 4: Doxorubicin, 30 mg/m² IV, and once daily prednisone, 0.5 mg/kg PO
Week 6: Vincristine, 0.7 mg/m² IV
Week 7: Cyclophosphamide, 200 mg/m² IV
Week 8: Vincristine, 0.7 mg/m² IV
Week 9: Doxorubicin, 30 mg/m² IV

Cycle 2
If in complete remission at week 9, continue treatment at 2-week intervals alternating vincristine 0.7 mg/m² IV, chlorambucil (Leukeran) 1.4 mg/kg PO, vincristine 0.7 mg/m², and methotrexate 0.8 mg/kg IV. Doxorubicin 30 mg/m² is substituted for every second methotrexate treatment. This cycle continues through week 25.

Cycle 3
If in complete remission at week 25, continue treatment sequence outlined in Cycle 2, but now at 3-week intervals. This cycle continues through week 51.

Cycle 4
If in complete remission at week 51, continue with treatment sequence outlined in Cycle 2, but now at 4-week intervals. Doxorubicin is no longer substituted for methotrexate. All treatment is discontinued at week 156.

($< 75,000/\mu l$) and neutropenia ($< 2000/\mu l$). Chemotherapeutic regimens that tend to spare bone marrow and are usually safe in the presence of low white blood cell (WBC) and platelet counts include prednisone, L-asparaginase, and vincristine. If myelosuppression is attributed to chemotherapy, discontinue treatment for 5–7 days and repeat the CBC and platelet count. When the platelet and WBC counts have rebounded, reinstitute therapy at a decreased dose or frequency. However, if the neutropenia and/or thrombocytopenia is secondary to myelophthisis (i.e., tumor infiltration into bone marrow) aggressive chemotherapy may be required despite the cytopenia, to allow normalization of marrow cellular constituents.

Extranodal Lymphoma Therapy

Therapy unique to extranodal lymphoma depends on the site of involvement and the extent of disease. Extranodal lymphoma that is determined, after thorough staging, to be a local disease can be treated locally (e.g., excisional surgery, radiotherapy) without the necessity for systemic chemotherapy. Diligent reevaluation schedules should be followed to identify recurrence or systemic spread of disease. Systemic chemotherapy should be initiated once systemic involvement has been documented.

Therapy for CNS lymphoma is dependent on location, the capacity of drugs to cross the blood-brain barrier, and the presence of disease outside the CNS. Surgical intervention can be used for diagnosis or removal of accessible CNS tumors, but usually this is not feasible or practical. More commonly, surgery is combined with adjuvant chemotherapy or radiotherapy. Of the chemotherapeutic agents commonly used in veterinary medicine, only prednisone and cytosine arabinoside consistently cross the blood-brain barrier in therapeutic concentrations. Radiotherapy also has been used successfully for the treatment of CNS lymphoma.

Cutaneous Lymphoma Therapy

Cutaneous lymphoma, if solitary and confined, can be treated with local radiotherapy or surgery; however, the likelihood of ultimate systemic spread is high. Generalized, cutaneous lymphoma tends to be less responsive to chemotherapy than multicentric lymphoma, and clinical signs can wax and wane considerably over time. Oral *cis*-retinoic acid therapy has proven effective in approximately 30% to 40% of dogs with cutaneous lymphoma, although long-term survival is uncommon.

Innovative Therapies

Innovative therapies for lymphoma that are being evaluated include:

- Immunotherapy in combination with traditional chemotherapy
  - Nonspecific immunostimulants, such as levamisole, and various bacterial extracts have not been efficacious.
  - Tumor cell vaccines derived from the host's own tumor and the use of specific monoclonal antibod-

ies presently are undergoing evaluation. Trials using monoclonal antibody against some canine lymphomas (MAB 231) showed early promise when used in dogs after chemotherapy-induced remission.
  - Antibody-targeted chemotherapeutics involving the linkage of a monoclonal antibody that recognizes some canine lymphomas with doxorubicin are presently under investigation.
- Total body irradiation (TBI) in combination with bone marrow transplant (BMT) techniques; these procedures may become available to the practitioner on a referral basis in the near future.
- Dose intensification and the compression of the total length of treatment are also under scrutiny at several institutions.

Therapy for Hypercalcemia

Treatment of hypercalcemia secondary to lymphoma is accomplished best by attaining tumor remission. If necessary, diuresis with high sodium crystalloids (0.9% NaCl) delivered at twice the maintenance rate (see Chap. 30) alone or in combination with furosemide (Lasix) (2 mg/kg IV) is usually successful. The addition of prednisone also decreases serum calcium levels; however, this should be initiated only after a histologic or cytologic diagnosis.

Prognosis

Prognostic Indicators for Dogs with Lymphoma

- WHO clinical stage V (see Table 25–1) is associated with shorter survival times, especially when the bone marrow involvement results in significant cytopenias.
- WHO substage b (i.e., presenting ill, with significant clinical signs) is strongly predictive of shorter remission and survival times.
- The presence of a T-cell origin lymphoma is strongly predictive of shorter remission and survival times.
- In some reports, but not all, female dogs have significantly longer remission and survival times than males.
- Proliferation indices (i.e., potential doubling time, argyrophilic nucleolar organizer region frequency) may influence prognosis.
- Hypercalcemia and mediastinal involvement have been reported to worsen prognosis; however, this has been shown to be due to their T-cell association rather than a direct effect.
- Anatomic site of involvement can have prognostic significance. Alimentary, disseminated cutaneous, and leukemic forms have a poorer prognosis than multicentric forms.

Prognostic Indicators for Cats with Lymphoma

- Higher clinical stage is associated with lower remission rates and survival times (approximately 90% complete remission rate in stage I vs. 50% in stage III or higher)
- FeLV status is strongly predictive of remission and survival times. FeLV-antigenemic cats and the anatomic

forms of lymphoma associated with them (mediastinal, multicentric) have a poorer prognosis than FeLV-negative cats (most often alimentary form).

- Leukemia, anemia, neutropenia, and sepsis all have a negative impact on response to therapy and survival times.
- Clinical substage b (i.e., presenting ill, with significant clinical signs) is predictive of shorter remission and survival times.
- Response to therapy is strongly predictive of outcome. Cats that achieve a complete remission early in their treatment often go on to have a prolonged and durable remission. This indicator cannot be assessed before therapy, however, and therefore is not clinically useful at initial diagnosis.

LYMPHOID LEUKEMIA

Leukemia is defined as the proliferation of neoplastic cells in the bone marrow; such cells may or may not be circulating in the peripheral blood. There are two major categories of lymphoid leukemia: acute lymphoblastic leukemia and chronic lymphocytic leukemia. Both forms are relatively rare in dogs; however, they may constitute up to one-third of feline lymphoid neoplasms.

Acute Lymphoblastic Leukemia

Acute lymphoblastic leukemia (ALL) is defined as an abnormal proliferation of morphologically immature lymphoblasts in the bone marrow or peripheral blood. This form of leukemia is rapidly progressive and responds poorly to therapy.

Epidemiology and Clinical Signs

- No sex, breed, or weight predilection exists. Most affected dogs are of late middle age; the mean age in cats with ALL tends to be younger, owing to an association with FeLV.
- Clinical signs can include fever, generalized or abdominal pain, anorexia, splenomegaly, and pale mucous membranes.
- Anemia occurs in nearly half of ALL patients, and one-fourth are thrombocytopenic.
- Most cats with ALL are FeLV-positive.

Diagnosis

- Diagnosis depends on documentation of abnormal lymphocytes in the bone marrow or peripheral blood.
- The presence of 30% or more abnormal cells in the bone marrow is diagnostic.
- Most patients have absolute leukocytosis with circulating abnormal lymphocytes; 10% are classified as having aleukemic leukemia (bone marrow involvement without peripheral blood involvement).
- In some forms, the neoplastic lymphoid cells are very undifferentiated, making special histochemical stains necessary to differentiate them from other forms of leukemia and myeloproliferative conditions.

- ALL may be clinically differentiated from late stages of lymphoma by:
  - The more acute progression of ALL
  - Less likelihood of lymphadenopathy (<50%)
  - Poor response to therapy
  - Shorter survival times

Treatment and Prognosis

- A poor prognosis resulting from a meager response to therapy generally is the rule.
- Because of severe bone marrow infiltration in ALL, chemotherapeutic agents that have a relatively low degree of bone marrow toxicity may be necessary in cases of severe neutropenia (<2000/µl) or thrombocytopenia (<50,000/µl). A combination of vincristine, prednisone, and L-asparaginase can be used in those cases with severe neutropenia and thrombocytopenia. The dosage regimens are the same as those described for lymphoma. If, however, neutrophil and platelet numbers do not rise within 1–2 weeks after initiation of therapy, more aggressive chemotherapy may be required despite the cytopenia to "clear" the bone marrow of tumor cells and allow normalization of marrow constituents. Strict attention to treatment of secondary infection is mandatory.

Chronic Lymphocytic Leukemia

Chronic lymphocytic leukemia (CLL) is defined as an abnormal proliferation of morphologically mature lymphocytes in the bone marrow or peripheral blood. It occurs primarily in older dogs and cats.

Clinical Signs

- Presenting complaints for the most part are nonspecific and include lethargy, inappetence, polyuria/polydipsia, bleeding diathesis, intermittent lameness, and episodes of collapse.
- Two-thirds of dogs have lymphadenopathy and splenomegaly; pale mucous membranes and fever are common.

Hematologic Abnormalities

- Most animals are anemic (normocytic, normochromic, and nonregenerative), and approximately half are thrombocytopenic.
- One-third of dogs are hyperproteinemic, and 50% have monoclonal gammopathies on serum electrophoresis, often with Bence Jones proteins in the urine, indicative of a B-cell origin.
- All reported cases in cats are FeLV-negative.

Treatment and Prognosis

- Therapy for CLL is recommended only if the patient is symptomatic or if anemia, hyperglobulinemia, splenomegaly, or lymphadenopathy is present.
- The prognosis for CLL is much better than that for ALL. Most dogs respond well to therapy, and quality of life is good.

- Prednisone and chlorambucil are the drugs most commonly used, and nearly 75% of animals respond, with median survivals of nearly 1 year.
- Chlorambucil (Leukeran), 20 mg/m^2 PO, given every 1 to 2 weeks, or 6 mg/m^2 daily, has provided excellent results.

PLASMA CELL NEOPLASMS

There are three primary clinical forms of plasma cell neoplasms: multiple myeloma (MM), solitary plasmacytoma of bone, and extramedullary plasmacytoma. MM is the most common form; the other two occur rarely. Plasma cell neoplasms are extremely rare in cats.

Multiple Myeloma

Epidemiology and Clinical Signs

- MM occurs primarily in aged dogs and has no sex predilection. German shepherd dogs may be at greater risk.
- Clinical signs include nonspecific anorexia, listlessness, and polyuria/polydipsia.
- Most dogs present with lameness secondary to paresis or pain.
- Bleeding diathesis (epistaxis or gingival bleeding) secondary to hyperviscosity syndrome or thrombocytopenia develops in approximately 50% of affected dogs.

Hematologic Abnormalities

- Three-fourths of animals with MM have associated monoclonal gammopathy, either the IgG or IgA subtype. A rare IgM-secreting primary macroglobulinemia (Waldenström's disease) also exists.
- Light-chain (Bence Jones) proteins may be detectable in the urine. These proteins cannot be detected by routine urine dipstick analysis and require phoretic technique to be identified.
- Dogs with MM often have nonregenerative, normocytic/normochromic anemia. Approximately 30% are thrombocytopenic, and 10% have circulating abnormal plasmacytes.
- Approximately 15% to 20% of MM patients are hypercalcemic secondary to bone resorption caused by osteoclast-activating factors or other substances released by the tumor.

Diagnosis

Diagnosis involves identification of the following triad of abnormalities:

- Bone marrow plasmacytosis (>20–30% plasma cells).
- Radiographic evidence of osteolytic bone lesions; often observed in dorsal spinous vertebral processes. Approximately 50% of dogs with multiple myeloma have radiographic evidence of bone lesions, whereas skeletal lesions are rare in cats with multiple myeloma.
- Serum or urine myeloma proteins, as revealed by immunoelectrophoresis.

Histological confirmation may be necessary for those cases that do not meet all three criteria.

Differential Diagnosis (DDx)

- DDx for monoclonal gammopathy includes ehrlichiosis (see Chapter 15) and benign hypergammaglobulinemia syndrome, which has been described in the dog.
- DDx for plasmacytosis includes carcinomas, connective tissue disorders, liver disease, hypersensitivity states, and infections, especially ehrlichiosis (see Chapter 15).

Treatment and Prognosis

- The short-term prognosis for MM in dogs is normally good, and long-term remissions are the rule. In cats, the prognosis is poor, and durable remissions after therapy are the exception.
- Extensive bone lesions, light chain proteinuria, hypercalcemia, and anemia have been reported to be negative prognostic indicators.
- Combination chemotherapy using melphalan (Alkeran; Burroughs Wellcome) (0.1 mg/kg daily for 10 days; then every other day) and prednisone (0.5 mg/kg q24h for 10 days, then every other day) has resulted in published remission rates of 90% and median survival times of 540 days in dogs.
- Serum protein levels should normalize within 2 to 3 months.
- Fractures accompanying MM can be treated by surgical reduction in combination with chemotherapy or radiotherapy. Healing normally accompanies remission of the MM; however, it may take many months and may not be complete.
- Rescue therapy is not well documented once remission is lost. Doxorubicin, vincristine, and dexamethasone combinations appear to work well in humans and may be of benefit in dogs.

Solitary Plasmacytoma of Bone

Solitary plasmacytoma of bone is rare. It usually is not accompanied by a secretory protein but tends to progress to systemic MM. Localized lesions can be treated with surgery or radiotherapy; however, careful clinical staging and a strict reevaluation schedule should be established because of the propensity for the development of systemic disease. Melphalan and prednisone are initiated once systemic involvement is documented.

Extramedullary Plasmacytoma

Two general categories of extramedullary plasmacytoma (EMP) exist, each with a very different biological behavior.

- Solitary cutaneous and oral EMP is a benign condition in dogs that is curable with complete surgical excision or local radiotherapy.
- Conversely, gastrointestinal EMP in the dog tends to behave in a malignant fashion. It rarely is associated with monoclonal gammopathies. Thorough staging

(e.g., bone marrow) is necessary to ensure that the disease is localized initially. If that is the case, local excision can be attempted. The likelihood of eventual systemic spread is high, and once documented, combination chemotherapy is initiated.

SUPPLEMENTAL READINGS

Cotter SM: Treatment of lymphoma and leukemia with cyclophosphamide, vincristine and prednisone: I, Treatment of dogs. J Am Anim Hosp Assoc 19:159, 1983.

Cotter SM: Treatment of lymphoma and leukemia with cyclophosphamide, vincristine and prednisone: III, Treatment of cats. J Am Anim Hosp Assoc 19:166, 1983.

Cotter SM, Goldstein MA: Comparison of two protocols for maintenance of remission in dogs with lymphoma. J Am Anim Hosp Assoc 23:495, 1987.

Hahn KA, Hahn EA: Pirubicin (4'-epi-doxorubicin) chemotherapy. In: Kirk RW, Bonagura JD (eds): Current Veterinary Therapy XI. Philadelphia: WB Saunders, 1992, pp 393–395.

Hammer A, Couto G, Ayl R, et al: Treatment of tumor bearing dogs and cats with actinomycin D. J Vet Intern Med 8:236, 1994.

Jeglum KA, Wheat A, Young K: Chemotherapy for lymphoma in 75 cats. J Am Vet Med Assoc 190:174, 1987.

Keller ET, MacEwen EG, Rosenthal RC, et al: Evaluation of prognostic factors and sequential combination chemotherapy for canine lymphoma. J Am Vet Med Assoc 7:289, 1992.

MacEwen EG, Brown NO, Patnaik AK, et al: Cyclic combination chemotherapy for canine lymphosarcoma. J Am Vet Med Assoc 178:564, 1987.

Matus RE: Chemotherapy of lymphoma and leukemia. In: Kirk RW (ed): Current Veterinary Therapy X. Philadelphia: WB Saunders, 1989, pp 482–489.

Mooney SC, Hayes AA, MacEwen EG: Treatment and prognostic factors in cats: 103 cases (1977–1981). J Am Vet Med Assoc 194:696, 1989.

Moore AS, Cotter SM, Ruslander D, et al: Interim analysis of the toxicosis and efficacy associated with idarubicin administration in cats with malignant tumors. Proceedings of the 11th Annual Conference of the Veterinary Cancer Society, 1991, pp 102–103.

Ogilvie GK, Obradovich JE, Elmslie RE, et al: Efficacy of mitoxantrone to dogs with malignant tumors. J Am Vet Med Assoc 198:1613, 1991.

Postorino NC, Susaneck SJ, Withrow SJ, et al: Single agent therapy with Adriamycin for canine lymphosarcoma. J Am Anim Hosp Assoc 25:221, 1989.

26 Soft Tissue Sarcomas and Mast Cell Tumors

Joanne C. Graham / Deborah A. O'Keefe

SOFT TISSUE SARCOMAS

Soft tissue sarcomas are tumors that arise from mesodermal tissue. They make up 14% to 17% of all malignancies in the dog and approximately 7% to 9% in the cat. These tumors are nonepithelial and extraskeletal and may arise from fibrous tissue, adipose tissue, muscle, and synovial tissue, as well as from blood and lymph vessels. Schwannomas, or neurofibrosarcomas, arise from primitive ectodermal tissues but are included in the soft tissue sarcoma category because of similarities in location, clinical presentation, and clinical behavior. Soft tissue sarcomas are classified histologically according to the specific tissue of origin. However, some tumors are so undifferentiated that this classification is difficult. These tumors are appropriately named undifferentiated sarcomas.

Etiology

The etiology of most soft tissue sarcomas remains unknown. Several causes and predisposing factors have been suggested. These include: genetic predisposition, viral agents, chemical carcinogens, ionizing radiation, foreign body implantation, trauma, and vaccination (in cats).

Genetic Predisposition

This is suspected to play a role in tumor development because certain breeds of dogs have a higher incidence of sarcomas. These breeds include boxers, German shepherds, Great Danes, Saint Bernards, golden retrievers, and basset hounds.

Viral Agents

Viruses have been implicated as causes of sarcoma development in rodents, poultry, nonhuman primates, and cats. Feline sarcoma viruses (FeSVs) are replication-defective variants of the feline leukemia virus (FeLV) (see Chap. 6). These retroviruses induce formation of multicentric fibrosarcomas in young cats. In contrast, solitary fibrosarcomas found in older cats usually are not associated with FeSV.

Chemical Carcinogens

Chemical carcinogens and environmental contaminants have been shown to induce sarcomas in rodents and humans. Although this has not been documented in dogs and cats, it likely occurs.

Ionizing Radiation

X-rays, gamma rays, and particulate radiation have been shown to cause sarcoma development. In dogs, sarcomas have been reported after orthovoltage radiotherapy of acanthomatous epulides.

Foreign Implants

Implants, particularly metallic orthopedic implants, are known to cause sarcoma development at the implant site. It is believed that this is the result of a foreign body reaction in the tissues rather than a direct carcinogenic effect of the implant. Most of these tumors are osteosarcomas, although fibrosarcomas and undifferentiated sarcomas have been reported.

Trauma

Both single and chronic traumatic episodes have been associated with intraocular sarcomas in the cat.

Vaccination

Recently, the development of certain soft tissue sarcomas in cats has been associated with the administration of killed vaccines (FeLV and rabies). The exact incidence is unknown but may be greater than 1 in 10,000 vaccinated cats. The mechanism behind vaccine-associated sarcoma development is under investigation.

Biologic Behavior

In general, soft tissue sarcomas are locally invasive and infiltrative along fascial planes, resulting in poorly defined tumor margins. They are often slow to metastasize, but when they do, it is via hematogenous spread to the lungs and liver. A brief description of the various soft tissue sarcomas follows.

Liposarcoma

Malignant tumor of adipocytes

- Rare in dogs and cats
- Invasive and aggressive
- Commonly occurs on the ventrum

- Metastasis is uncommon
- "Infiltrative lipomas," believed by some to be well differentiated liposarcomas, frequently occur on extremities

Hemangiopericytoma

Tumor of pericytes, spindle-shaped, contractile cells that surround precapillary arterioles

- Common in dogs (German shepherds at risk)
- Slow-growing
- Encapsulated appearance but quite infiltrative, and recurrence after excision is common
- Frequently occurs on extremities
- Metastasis is rare and is slow growing

Fibrosarcoma

Tumor of fibrocytes

- Common in dogs and cats
- Locally invasive, slow growing
- No site predilection
- Metastasis is rare

▼ **Key Point** Multicentric fibrosarcomas of young cats (younger than 5 years) may be caused by FeSV. These cats are always FeLV positive.

Hemangiosarcoma

Tumor of blood vessel endothelium (see also Chap. 23)

- Common in dogs (German shepherds at risk); rare in cats
- Very invasive, rapid-growing
- Spleen, heart, skin are common sites
- Metastasis is common

Schwannoma/Neurofibrosarcoma

Tumor of the nerve sheath or Schwann cell

- Relatively uncommon in dogs and cats
- Invasive, slow-growing
- Frequently occurs in the brachial or lumbosacral plexuses
- Progressive lameness is possible
- Metastasis is rare

Myxosarcoma

Fibrosarcoma-like tumor with a mucinous matrix

- Rare in dogs and cats
- Infiltrative
- No site predilection
- Metastasis is uncommon

Rhabdomyosarcoma

Tumor of striated muscle

- Uncommon in dogs and cats
- Infiltrative
- Heart, bladder, appendicular muscles are possible sites

- Metastasis is possible
- Botryoid rhabdomyosarcomas (grape-like appearance) found in the bladders of young large-breed dogs

Leiomyosarcoma

Tumor of smooth muscle

- Rare in dogs and cats
- Solitary, infiltrative, slow-growing
- Spleen, liver, gastrointestinal, and genitourinary tracts are the most common sites
- Metastasis is possible (common in dogs with liver tumors)
- GI obstructive signs or perforation are possible effects

Synovial Cell Sarcoma

Tumor of periarticular mesenchymal tissue, *not* the synovial membrane

- Uncommon in dogs, few reports in cats
- Large-breed dogs at risk
- Aggressive tumor
- Bones on both sides of major joints are commonly involved
- Metastasis is possible (22% at time of diagnosis)

Lymphangiosarcoma

Tumor of lymphatic endothelial vessels

- Rare in dogs and cats
- May be invasive
- Metastasis is rare
- Draining tracts on skin are possible presenting sign

Malignant Fibrous Histiocytoma

Tumor containing a mixture of fibroblast-like cells and histiocyte-like cells

- Uncommon in dogs and cats
- Invasive (may cause bone lysis)
- Usually found in subcutaneous tissue
- Metastasis is rare

Vaccine-Associated Sarcomas

Most are fibrosarcomas, but rhabdomyosarcomas, chondrosarcomas, osteosarcomas, malignant fibrous histiocytomas, and undifferentiated sarcomas are also reported

- Cats only
- Aggressive tumors
- Cervical/interscapular area and hindlimbs are the most common sites
- Metastasis is possible.

Clinical Signs

Clinical signs depend on the location, size, and degree of invasiveness of the tumor as well as on the presence and degree of metastatic disease.

- Soft tissue sarcomas are more common in older animals (mean age 9 years).

- Because of the widespread distribution of mesodermal tissues in the body, soft tissue sarcomas may occur in almost any anatomic location, including the abdomen.
- Tumors may become quite large before any clinical signs are apparent. They often are noticed first by the owner, either by observation or while handling the animal.
- Certain types of sarcoma may invade bone, causing lameness, or may obstruct lymphatics, causing edema.
- Gastrointestinal leiomyosarcomas may cause signs of obstruction (vomiting) or melena.
- Smooth muscle sarcomas of the bladder may cause hematuria or dysuria.
- Hemangiosarcomas may cause a variety of clinical signs, including collapse due to tumor rupture and hemorrhage.
- Vaccine-associated sarcomas are located in vaccine injection sites.

Diagnosis

The goals of diagnosis are to identify the histologic type of the primary tumor, to delineate the extent of the tumor, and to determine whether metastatic disease is present. Although history, physical examination, laboratory evaluation, and diagnostic imaging provide valuable information, the only way to obtain a definitive diagnosis is through biopsy and histopathologic evaluation of the tumor.

History

The history helps to determine how long the mass has been present and the rate of growth. Also important is information regarding exposure to carcinogens, recent vaccination, and past traumatic incidents. Concurrent systemic disturbances provide insight as to the possible presence of metastatic disease or paraneoplastic syndromes.

Physical Examination

Perform a thorough examination to determine the number of masses and their physical characteristics. In general, benign neoplasms are well delineated, slow-growing, and freely movable. They seldom are ulcerated or inflamed. Malignant tumors are often rapid-growing, fixed masses with ill-defined borders. However, some sarcomas are slow-growing and appear well demarcated. The appearance of these masses can be misleading and should not preclude biopsy.

A careful search may reveal evidence of metastasis. Palpate the regional lymph nodes for size and mobility. Look for hepatomegaly, splenomegaly, and increased respiratory sounds or dyspnea as signs of systemic involvement.

Clinical Pathology

Studies such as a complete blood count (CBC), platelet count, serum biochemical profile, and urinalysis often are unremarkable; however, they should be evaluated in animals with soft tissue sarcomas because they may suggest the presence of metastatic disease, paraneoplastic syndromes, or other concurrent disease. The values obtained also provide a baseline for future therapy. Abnormalities may include:

- Anemia of chronic inflammatory disease
- Leukocytosis
- Thrombocytopenia (may be associated with disseminated intravascular coagulation)
- Hypoglycemia
- Increased serum concentrations of alanine transferase (ALT), alkaline phosphatase (ALP), and gamma-glutamyl transpeptidase (GGT)

Diagnostic Imaging
Radiography

- Radiograph the mass to aid in determining the extent of the sarcoma.
- Radiograph the thorax and abdomen to help identify metastatic disease.
- Dystrophic calcification caused by some anaplastic sarcomas may be seen on the radiograph.

Ultrasonography

Use this technique to help determine the character, consistency, and extent of the mass. Ultrasound procedures are especially useful in the examination of abdominal masses.

Computed Tomography (CT)

This modality, when available, is particularly useful in precise localization of a mass.

Biopsy

Biopsy is essential to obtain a definitive diagnosis. (See Chapter 24 for details on the principles of tumor biopsy.)

- Plan carefully to ensure that a representative sample of the mass is obtained.
- Submit all biopsies for histopathologic evaluation.

Several methods for biopsy are available:

Fine-Needle Aspiration Biopsy

- For fine-needle aspiration (FNA), use a 22- or 25-gauge needle and a 12-ml syringe.
- Because soft tissue sarcomas do not exfoliate well, FNA is limited in value.
- FNA, however, is useful in the diagnosis of lipomas, lymphomas, and inflammatory masses that may appear similar to soft tissue sarcomas.

Needle Punch Biopsy

- For needle punch biopsy (NPB), use a Franklin modified Vim-Silverman needle (V. Mueller Co., Chicago, IL) or Tru-Cut biopsy needle (Travenol Labs., Deerfield, IL).

- NPB is useful for externally palpable masses.
- A larger sample of tissue can be obtained than with FNA.
- NPB usually can be performed using local anesthesia.

Incisional Biopsy

- Incisional biopsies yield an even larger sample than NBP biopsies.
- Plan the biopsy site so that it can be excised later when definitive resection is done.
- Include some normal tissue in the sample when possible.

Excisional Biopsy

- Excisional biopsies are indicated when knowledge of the histologic type of the tumor does not change the treatment and/or total excision is no more invasive than other types of biopsy.

Clinical Staging

An attempt should be made to stage all soft tissue sarcomas. Clinical staging is based on the classification system developed by the World Health Organization (WHO) (Table 26–1).

Treatment

The goal of treatment is to remove the primary tumor in its entirety, when possible, and to treat microscopic disease and metastasis. In the case of benign and some malignant tumors, surgical resection can be curative. In animals with nonresectable malignant tumors, attempts are made to prolong survival time while providing a good quality of life.

Surgery

Surgical excision remains the mainstay of therapy for soft tissue sarcomas. However, many of these tumors recur because of inadequate resection. Well-planned, aggressive initial surgery has the greatest likelihood of success.

▼ *Key Point* Excise soft tissue sarcomas with 3-cm margins in all planes.

- Remove overlying subcutaneous tissues and skin as well as underlying tissues to which the mass is fixed. (In some cases, limb amputation is indicated.)
- Include all previous biopsy sites in the excision.
- Remove the tumor intact to prevent seeding of normal tissue with malignant cells.
- Have the specimen margins histologically evaluated for completeness of excision.
- Do not remove regional lymph nodes unless they are involved.
- Also resect any solitary metastatic pulmonary nodules.

Radiation Therapy

Soft tissue sarcomas are reported to be less radioresponsive than carcinomas. However, radiation therapy alone has been reported to achieve up to 67% tumor control for approximately 1 year. Radiation therapy is used more frequently to reduce tumor volume preoperatively or to irradiate incompletely excised tumor fields.

Repeat irradiation of previously irradiated tumors is possible. A 38% local control rate 1 year after repeat irradiation has been reported. Unfortunately, if the regrowth of tumors is within 4 to 5 months of the first treatment, the chance of complications resulting from additional radiation therapy is much higher.

Hyperthermia

Hyperthermia involves the use of electromagnetic radiation or ultrasound to heat tissues. Hyperthermia is cytotoxic when used alone; however, the best results are seen when it is used as a combined modality with radiation or chemotherapy. A 91% response rate has been reported in dogs with hemangiopericytomas treated using orthovoltage irradiation in combination with hyperthermia.

Chemotherapy

Chemotherapy has been used with variable success to treat soft tissue sarcomas. Agents most often used are vincristine, doxorubicin, cyclophosphamide, mitoxantrone, dacarbazine, and carboplatin. Commonly used protocols are outlined in Table 26–2. Combination protocols that include doxorubicin are most effective. In dogs, response rates vary from 35% to 75%, depending on the tumor type and protocol used. One study of 13 cats with various tumors including sarcomas reported a 61% partial response rate using vincristine, cyclophosphamide, and methotrexate.

Table 26–1. WORLD HEALTH ORGANIZATION (WHO) CLINICAL STAGING SYSTEM FOR CANINE SOFT TISSUE SARCOMAS

T: Primary Tumor	N: Regional Lymph Node	M: Distant Metastasis
T_0—no evidence	N_0—no evidence	M_0—no evidence
T_1—tumor < 2 cm	N_1—movable ipsilateral	M_1—metastasis present
T_2—tumor > 2 cm and < 5 cm; minimal invasion	N_2—movable contralateral	
	N_3—fixed	
T_3—tumor > 5 cm	a—metastasis absent	
T_4—very invasive	b—metastasis present	

Stage

I	$T_1N_0M_0$, $T_2N_0M_0$
II	$T_1N_1M_0$, $T_2N_1M_0$
III	$T_1N_{2,3}M_0$, $T_2N_{2,3}M_0$, $T_3N_{0-3}M_0$, $T_4N_{0-3}M_0$, any N_b
IV	any M_1

From Owen, LN: Classification of Tumours in Domestic Animals. Geneva, Switzerland: World Health Organization, 1980.

Table 26–2. CHEMOTHERAPEUTIC PROTOCOLS FOR SOFT TISSUE SARCOMAS*

Drug (Trade Name)	Manufacturer	Dosage	Route	Day
Doxorubicin				
Doxorubicin (Adriamycin)	Adria Labs/Generic	30 mg/m^2 (dogs > 10 kg)	IV	1
		1–1.25 mg/kg (cats and dogs < 10 kg)		
Repeat cycle every 21 days for 4–6 treatments; do not exceed a cumulative dose of 240 mg/m^2				
Mitoxantrone				
Mitoxantrone (Novantrone)	Lederle	5–6 mg/m^2 (dogs)	IV	1
		6.5 mg/m^2 (cats)		
Repeat cycle every 21 days for 4–6 treatments				
AC Protocol				
Doxorubicin		As above	IV	1
Cyclophosphamide (Cytoxan)	Bristol-Myers	100–150 mg/m^2	IV	1
		or 50 mg/m^2	PO	3–6
Repeat cycle every 21 days for 4–6 treatments				
VAC Protocol (dogs only)				
Vincristine (Oncovin)	Eli Lilly/Generic	0.7 mg/m^2	IV	8 and 15
Doxorubicin		As above	IV	1
Cyclophosphamide		As above	IV	1
			or PO	3–6
Repeat cycle every 21 days for 4–6 treatments; very myelosuppressive protocol—may need prophylactic antibiotics				
ADIC Protocol (dogs only)				
Doxorubicin		As above	IV	1
Dacarbazine (DTIC)	Miles Lab.	800–1000 mg/m^2	IV	1
		or 200 mg/m^2	IV	2–5
Repeat cycle every 21 days for 4–6 treatments				

*Caution: The use of chemotherapeutics requires careful handling and knowledge of potential toxicities.

Biologic Therapy

Acemannan, a polysaccharide derived from the aloe vera plant, may enhance immune system function. Intraperitoneal and intratumoral injections of acemannan in dogs and cats with fibrosarcoma caused tumor necrosis and shrinkage, allowing the tumors to be excised surgically. Acemannan is best used before surgery or radiation.

MAST CELL TUMORS

Mast cell tumors (MCTs) compose approximately 7% to 20% of cutaneous neoplasms in the dog and 15% in the cat. MCTs may develop in almost any location but are found most commonly in the skin and subcutaneous tissues of the dog and in the skin, spleen, liver, and visceral lymphatics of the cat. Mast cells are a normal component of the immune system and are important in the inflammatory response to tissue trauma. Cytoplasmic granules found in mast cells contain biologically active substances such as heparin, histamine, platelet-activating factor, and eosinophilic chemotactic factor. The quantity and type of granules in MCTs depends on the degree of differentiation. Well-differentiated tumors contain more heparin than undifferentiated tumors, which have a higher histamine content.

Etiology

The cause of MCTs is unknown; however, breed predisposition, chronic inflammation, and viruses may play a role.

Breed Predisposition

Boxers, Boston terriers, English bulldogs, and English bull terriers are at risk. However, MCTs in boxers are more likely to be well differentiated and may have a more favorable prognosis. Siamese cats younger than 4 years of age have been reported to have a higher incidence of cutaneous histiocytic-like MCTs.

Chronic Inflammation

Chronic inflammatory sites in the dog have been reported to give rise to MCTs.

Viruses

The speculation that viruses may have a role in MCTs stems from experimental studies in which dogs developed MCTs after being given injections of cell-free tumor extracts.

Biologic Behavior

▼ **Key Point** Because it is often difficult to histologically differentiate benign from malignant tumors, all MCTs should be considered potentially malignant.

In the Dog

- Approximately 50% of MCTs are malignant.
- Tumor location and rate of growth may help predict biologic behavior:
  - Tumors in preputial, inguinal, and perineal areas may be more aggressive.
  - Slow-growing localized MCTs may have a better prognosis. (In one study, tumors that were present

for 28 weeks or longer before removal had a more favorable prognosis.)

- Regional lymph nodes, the spleen, and the liver are the most common sites of metastasis.
- Bone marrow involvement can occur.
- Pulmonary metastasis is uncommon.

In the Cat

Controversy exists about location and biologic behavior of MCTs in cats.

Older literature suggests that:

- Half of all MCTs arise from the skin and half from viscera.
- Most MCTs in cats are malignant.

Recent literature reports that:

- A higher percentage of MCTs may arise from the skin.
- Most MCTs do not display malignant behavior.
  - In particular, histiocytic MCTs seen in young Siamese cats have a benign course, often regressing spontaneously.

Clinical Signs

Clinical signs depend on the location and size of the tumor as well as on secondary systemic complications caused by the MCT.

- In the dog, most MCTs are observed as solitary masses in the skin of the trunk and perineal area (50%), followed by the extremities (40%), and the head and neck (10%).
- In the cat:
  - 40% to 60% of cutaneous MCTs are solitary masses on the head and neck.
  - Visceral MCTs arise in the spleen, small intestine, liver, and visceral lymphatics.
  - Cats with visceral MCTs may present with anorexia, vomiting, or diarrhea.
- Dermal MCTs are usually well-defined, raised masses that can be hairless, ulcerated, and erythematous.
  - Dermal MCTs may be diffuse, erythematous thickenings in the skin.
  - Subcutaneous MCTs may resemble lipomas.
- Mechanical manipulation of MCTs may cause degranulation, resulting in erythema and wheal formation (Darier's sign).

▼ *Key Point* Gastroduodenal ulcers have been reported in up to 80% of dogs with MCTs and are thought to be related to histamine release. These animals may have anorexia, vomiting, diarrhea, and melena.

- Heparin and proteolytic enzyme release by MCTs at the time of surgery may prolong coagulation times and delay wound healing.

Diagnosis

History, physical examination, clinical pathology, tumor and bone marrow cytology, and radiography are

Table 26–3. WORLD HEALTH ORGANIZATION (WHO) CLINICAL STAGING SYSTEM FOR CANINE MAST CELL TUMORS

Stage:

I	One dermal tumor without regional lymph node involvement
II	One dermal tumor with regional lymph node involvement
III	Multiple dermal tumors or a large infiltrative tumor with or without regional lymph node involvement
IV	Any tumor with distant metastasis, or recurrence with metastasis

Stages are subdivided into:
  (a) Without systemic signs
  (b) With systemic signs

useful in the diagnosis and staging of MCTs. An attempt should be made to stage all MCTs because the stage affects prognosis and therapeutic decisions. A classification system for staging has been developed by the WHO (Table 26–3).

History

The history can determine the length of time the mass has been present and the rate of growth.

Physical Examination

A thorough examination can detect the location and number of masses. Palpate carefully for hepatomegaly, splenomegaly, and lymph node enlargement as signs of metastasis.

Clinical Pathology

Routine laboratory evaluations may be unremarkable. Examine a CBC and a buffy coat smear for evidence of systemic dissemination. Circulating mast cells, eosinophilia, and basophilia are more common in the dog than in the cat. Microcytic-hypochromic anemia may suggest gastrointestinal hemorrhage.

Bone Marrow Aspiration

This is a more sensitive indicator of bone marrow involvement than a buffy coat smear. The presence of greater than 10 mast cells per 1000 nucleated cells is abnormal.

Radiography and Ultrasonography

Perform abdominal radiography or ultrasonography to detect hepatomegaly, splenomegaly, and sublumbar lymph node enlargement. A fine-needle aspirate of enlarged organs can be helpful to confirm metastatic MCT. Thoracic radiographs are seldom helpful.

Biopsy

Fine-Needle Aspiration

MCTs usually can be diagnosed by fine-needle aspiration. Aspirates generally contain mast cells, eosinophils, and fibroblasts.

Histopathology

Histopathology is important to evaluate completeness of excision and histologic grade.

Grading of Tumors

The most widely used grading system (Patnaik, et al., 1984) assigns grades I, II, and III to well-, moderately, and poorly differentiated tumors, respectively (based on histopathologic appearance).

The histologic grade affects prognosis:

- Low-grade tumors are less likely to recur or metastasize.
- Dogs with low-grade tumors have increased survival times.

Treatment of Canine Cutaneous Mast Cell Tumors

Treatment of MCTs may include surgery, radiation therapy, chemotherapy, or some combination of the three. The type of treatment instituted depends primarily on the histologic grade and clinical stage of the tumor. A summary of current treatment recommendations for dogs is given in Table 26–4.

Surgery

Wide surgical excision is the treatment of choice for canine MCTs; however, approximately 50% of tumors may recur.

▼ **Key Point** Although they appear to be discrete masses, MCTs usually extend deep into surrounding tissues, making wide surgical excision imperative.

- Administer an antihistamine (e.g., Benadryl, Parke-Davis; 2 mg/kg IV) just before surgery to decrease the effects of histamine release from the tumor.
- Excise the mass with 3-cm margins on all sides.
- Have the specimen margins histologically evaluated for completeness of excision.
- If the tumor extends to the margins, plan a second, wider excision (if possible).
- Remove regional lymph nodes if tumor is present.
- If tumors are excised incompletely or are nonresectable, proceed with radiation therapy and/or chemotherapy.

Radiation Therapy

Radiation therapy alone or in combination with other treatment modalities may be used to treat incompletely excised or nonresectable MCTs.

- Give a total dosage of 40–48 Gy over a period of 3 to 4 weeks.
- One-year control rates range from 48% to 78%.
- Irradiate involved regional lymph nodes, if necessary.

Chemotherapy

Chemotherapy is recommended for systemic mastocytosis, nonresectable or incompletely excised tumors, and grade III tumors. Glucocorticoids commonly are used to produce partial or complete remissions in dogs.

- Prednisone and prednisolone are most commonly used for oral therapy (see Table 26–4 for dosage). Unfortunately, they are effective in less than 25% of dogs when used alone.
- Intralesional triamcinolone (1 mg/cm of tumor diameter once every 14 days) may be used; however, side effects are more common with this route.
- Combination therapy using cyclophosphamide, vinblastine, and prednisone has been reported to cause remissions in dogs refractory to glucocorticoids.
- Discontinue therapy in animals that remain tumor-free after 6 months.

Ancillary Drug Therapy

Dogs and cats with systemic mastocytosis or gastroduodenal hemorrhage should receive ancillary drug therapy.

- Use H_2-antagonists to reduce gastric acid secretion and help decrease the incidence and severity of gastrointestinal ulcers in MCT patients. Administer:
  - Cimetidine (Tagamet), 5–10 mg/kg PO q8h
  or
  - Ranitidine (Zantac), 1–2 mg/kg PO q12h (see Chap. 87).
- When an active gastrointestinal ulcer is suspected in an animal with MCT, also administer:
  - Sucralfate (Carafate), 250–1000 mg PO q6–8h (see Chap. 87 for use and actions)

Table 26–4. THERAPY OF CANINE MAST CELL TUMORS

WHO Stage	Patnaik Grade	Recommended Therapy

I	I and II	Surgical excision
		    Complete: observation
		    Incomplete: wider excision or
		        radiation therapy

I	III	Surgical excision
		    Complete: prednisone*
		    Incomplete: wider excision and
		        prednisone* or radiation and
		        prednisone*

II	I–III	Surgical excision
		    Complete: prednisone*
		    Incomplete: Wider excision and
		        prednisone* or radiation and
		        prednisone* or prednisone* alone

III and IV		Local therapy if possible plus one of the
		    following:
		    Prednisone*
		    CVP† chemotherapy
		    Vinblastine 2 mg/m²/IV weekly

*Prednisone: 40 mg/m², PO, sid for 1 week; then 20 mg/m² sid for 3 weeks; then 20 mg/m² every other day for 3 weeks; then reduce the dose by 50% every 3 weeks.

†CVP: Cyclophosphamide (Cytoxan; Bristol-Myers) 50 mg/m² PO every other day or 4 days a week; vinblastine (Velban; Eli Lilly) 2 mg/m² IV once a week; prednisone 20–40 mg/m² PO every other day.

Treatment of Feline Mast Cell Tumors

Cutaneous

- Wide surgical excision is the treatment of choice.
- Chemotherapy and radiotherapy have not been well evaluated but may be helpful in recurrent or metastatic tumors.

Visceral

- Splenectomy may ameliorate clinical signs in cats with splenic MCTs even when other organs are involved.
- Treat intestinal MCTs by wide surgical excision (5- to 10-cm margins).
- Chemotherapy has not been evaluated critically; however, prednisone alone or in combination with vincristine and cyclophosphamide does not appear to prolong survival times.

SUPPLEMENTAL READINGS

Soft Tissue Sarcomas

Brown NO, Hayes AA, Mooney S: Combined modality therapy in the treatment of solid tumors in cats. J Am Anim Hosp Assoc 16:719, 1980.

Dubielzig RR: Ocular sarcoma following trauma in three cats. J Am Vet Med Assoc 184:578, 1984.

Helfand SC: Chemotherapy for nonresectable and metastatic soft tissue tumors. Columbus, OH; Proceedings Kal Kan Symposium, 1986.

King GK, Yates KM, Greenlee PG, et al.: The effect of acemannan immunostimulant in combination with surgery and radiation therapy on spontaneous canine and feline fibrosarcomas. J Am Anim Hosp Assoc 31:439, 1995.

Madewell BR, Theilen GH: Tumors of the skin and subcutaneous tissues. In: Theilen GH, Madewell BR (eds): Veterinary Cancer Medicine. Philadelphia: Lea & Febiger, 1987, p 233.

Owen LN (ed): TNM Classification of Tumors in Domestic Animals. 1st ed. Geneva: World Health Organization, 1980.

Priester WA, McKay FA: The Occurrence of Tumors in Domestic Animals. National Cancer Institute Monograph 54. Bethesda: U.S. Dept. of Health and Human Services, 1980.

Richardson RC, Anderson VL, Voorhees WD, et al.: Irradiation-hyperthermia in canine hemangiopericytomas: Large animal model for therapeutic response. J Natl Cancer Inst 73:1187, 1984.

Thrall DE, Gillette EL: Soft-tissue sarcomas. Semin Vet Med Surg (Small Anim) 10:173, 1995.

Thrall DE, Goldschmidt MH, Biery DN: Malignant tumor formation at the site of previously irradiated acanthomatous epulides in four dogs. J Am Vet Med Assoc 178:127, 1981.

Turrel JM, Theon AP: Re-irradiation of tumors in cats and dogs. J Am Vet Med Assoc 193:465, 1988.

White AS: Clinical Diagnosis and Management of Soft Tissue Sarcomas. In: Gorman ND (ed): Oncology: Contemporary Issues in Small Animal Practice. New York: Churchill Livingstone, 1986, p 243.

Withrow SJ, MacEwen EG: Small Animal Clinical Oncology. 2nd ed. Philadelphia: WB Saunders Co, 1996.

Mast Cell Tumors

Bostock DE: The prognosis following surgical removal of mastocytomas in dogs. J Small Anim Pract 14:27, 1973.

Buerger RG, Scott DW: Cutaneous mast cell neoplasia in cats: 14 cases (1975–1985). J Am Vet Med Assoc 190:1440, 1987.

Guerre R, Millet P, Groulade P: Systemic mastocytosis in a cat: Remission after splenectomy. J Small Anim Pract 20:769, 1979.

Holzinger EA: Feline cutaneous mastocytomas. Cornell Vet 63:87, 1973.

Macy DW: Canine and feline mast cell tumors: Biologic behavior, diagnosis, and therapy. Semin Vet Med Surg (Small Anim) 1:72, 1986.

Macy DW, MacEwen EG: Mast cell tumors. In: Withrow SJ, MacEwen EG (eds): Clinical Veterinary Oncology. Philadelphia: JB Lippincott, 1989, p 156.

Madewell BR, Theilen GH: Tumors of the skin and subcutaneous tissues. In: Theilen GH, Madewell BR (eds): Veterinary Cancer Medicine. Philadelphia: Lea & Febiger, 1987, p 233.

O'Keefe DA: Canine mast cell tumors. Vet Clin North Am 20:4, 1990.

Owen LN (ed): TNM Classification of Tumors in Domestic Animals. 1st Ed. Geneva: World Health Organization, 1980.

Patnaik AK, Ehler WJ, MacEwen EG: Canine cutaneous mast cell tumor: Morphologic grading and survival time in 83 dogs. Vet Pathol 21:469, 1984.

Turrel JM, Kitchell BE, Miller LM, Theon A: Prognostic factors for radiation treatment of mast cell tumor in 85 dogs. J Am Vet Med Assoc 193:936, 1988.

Wilcock BP, Yager JA, Zink MC: The morphology and behavior of feline cutaneous mastocytomas. Vet Pathol 23:320, 1986.

27 Mammary Gland Neoplasia

Elizabeth Arnold Stone

Mammary gland neoplasia is a disease of older female dogs and cats. Canine mammary gland tumors (MGTs) are the most common tumors in the bitch. In female cats, only cutaneous tumors and lymphomas are more common than MGTs. Mammary gland tumors are very rare in male dogs and cats.

ETIOLOGY

- The cause of mammary gland neoplasia is unknown.
- Although virus-like particles have been identified in feline and canine MGTs, their role as a causative agent has not been established.
- About 50% of canine mammary carcinomas have estrogen and progesterone receptors. The levels of receptors are much lower than levels found in normal glands or benign MGTs. Only benign and well-differentiated adenocarcinomas appear to be hormonally sensitive in bitches.
- Regular administration of progestogens for estrus prevention or as treatment for dermatologic problems increases the risk of MGTs in dogs and cats.
- Dogs with benign MGTs have more than a threefold risk of subsequently developing a mammary malignancy of a different cell type.

▼ *Key Point* Approximately 50% of MGTs in dogs are malignant. In cats, 86% of MGTs are malignant.

CLINICAL SIGNS

- A mass or swelling develops in the ventral thoracic or abdominal region. The mass is usually part of the mammae but may appear distant to the mammary gland.
- Metastatic lesions in the lungs may cause dyspnea.

DIAGNOSIS

The diagnostic plan is directed toward determining the extent of the disease and establishing the stage.

Signalment

Dogs

- In dogs, the risk of developing MGTs increases markedly after about 6 years of age.

- Greatest frequency of canine MGTs is reported in sporting breeds (pointers, retrievers, English setters, spaniels), poodles, Boston terriers, and dachshunds.

Cats

- Feline carcinomas occur most often in cats 8 to 12 years of age.
- In cats, 99% of MGTs occur in intact females.
- Siamese cats are reported to have twice the risk of developing mammary carcinoma as all other breeds combined.

History

- The owner may have noticed the tumor, or it may have been an incidental finding during a routine physical examination.
- The owner may have delayed seeking veterinary assistance. Average time from owner observation of mammary masses in cats to presentation to a veterinarian is 5 months.

Physical Examination

- In dogs, MGTs develop most frequently in the caudal mammary glands.
- Depending on the time of recognition, the tumors may be small and movable, lobular and firm, fixed to the body wall, and ulcerated.
- Dogs with inflammatory carcinoma have diffusely swollen glands with poor demarcation between normal and abnormal tissue, which may be confused with mastitis. However, in mastitis, the swelling is more localized and occurs after estrus, whelping, or false pregnancy.
- In young intact female cats, mammary hypertrophy can be mistaken for MGT. Mammary hypertrophy resulting from either endogenous or exogenous progesterone stimulation can be differentiated readily by the case history, and if necessary, histologic examination.
- In cats, infiltrated lymphatics may look like linear beads.
- Axillary and inguinal lymph nodes may be enlarged.
- Carefully examine dogs for evidence of lameness and bony swelling. If these signs are present, radiograph the affected area and obtain a nuclear bone scan, if possible.

Radiography

- Radiograph the thorax to look for metastasis; 25% to 50% of malignant MGTs in dogs have metastasized before surgery.
- If caudal glands are involved, radiograph or use ultrasonography of the abdomen to evaluate the iliac lymph nodes.

Histologic Evaluation

- Do not routinely perform aspiration or biopsy of mammary masses if surgical excision is contemplated. Most MGTs are difficult to classify based on cytologic diagnosis. Cytologic examination may be useful, however, to differentiate inflammatory carcinoma from mastitis in dogs and mammary hypertrophy from mammary carcinoma in cats.
- Aspirate skin masses on the ventral abdomen that are not associated with the mammary glands to determine whether they are mast cell tumors. Lymph node metastasis worsens the prognosis; therefore, aspirate enlarged inguinal or axillary lymph nodes.
- The histopathologic diagnosis does not alter current treatment recommendations for MGTs (except for inflammatory carcinoma, as explained in Contraindications). Although about 50% of MGTs are benign, many dogs have multiple tumors, often of different histologic types, both benign and malignant.
- The definitive diagnosis of MGT is based on histologic examination of each mass. Thus, surgical excision is performed for both diagnostic and therapeutic purposes. A wide excision is essential to ensure complete removal of the tumor cells (see Chapter 24).

Other Diagnostic Tests

If the animal is to undergo surgery, perform a CBC, biochemical profile, and urinalysis. These animals are usually older and may have concurrent diseases that require further evaluation.

If there is evidence of pleural fluid on thoracic radiographs, aspirate the thorax and examine the fluid microscopically.

TREATMENT–SURGICAL

The primary treatment objective is to excise the cancerous tissue while maintaining the animal's quality of life.

Preoperative Considerations

Indications

Surgical excision of noninvasive mammary gland carcinoma is beneficial in dogs. Surgical excision:

- Allows a histologic diagnosis
- Can modify disease progression
- Can improve quality of life
- Can be curative

Contraindications

Dogs with inflammatory carcinomas usually die soon after the diagnosis is made because the tumor is extremely aggressive and readily metastasizes. Treatment should be palliative, using antiinflammatory drugs and antibiotics. Surgery is not recommended for these animals because:

- It is impossible to remove all affected tissues.
- Disseminated intravascular coagulation often is induced.

The following discussion excludes inflammatory carcinoma.

▼ **Key Point** No particular surgical procedure (i.e., radical *vs.* simple mastectomy) has been shown to be more effective than others for dogs with MGTs.

Resection Margins

Determine resection margins before surgery. Dissect only healthy tissues during surgery; do not disrupt the tumor itself. The margins should be at least 1 cm from the neoplastic tissue.

Gland Excision in Dogs

Past recommendations have suggested regional mastectomy for MGTs in dogs (i.e., remove glands 4 and 5 for tumors in 4 or 5; remove glands 1, 2, and 3 for tumors in 1, 2, and 3). These recommendations were based on the lymphatic drainage in normal dogs. However, space-occupying masses disrupt normal drainage and open new channels between other glands.

Thus, in dogs the number of excised glands is based on having adequate resection margins of normal tissue around the tumor.

Gland Excision in Cats

In cats, removal of all glands on an affected side decreases local recurrence compared with a lumpectomy. However, this may not prolong survival time.

Other Recommendations

- If the tumor has invaded the subcutaneous tissue beneath the gland, include the ventral fascia of the underlying muscle in the excision.
- If the tumor has invaded the body wall, remove a wide section of body wall *en bloc* with the tumor.
- Remove the inguinal lymph nodes routinely during mastectomy of gland 5.
- Axillary nodes usually are not removed with gland 1 unless there is palpable or cytologic evidence of abnormality.

Surgical Procedures

Lumpectomy

Removal of tumor and 1 cm of normal tissue, without removal of surrounding gland *(lumpectomy)* is adequate if the tumor is small (<5 mm), circumscribed, and noninvasive.

Simple Mastectomy

In many instances, it is easier to remove the entire mammary gland *(simple mastectomy)* and avoid the problems of milk and lymph leakage into the wound.

Regional Mastectomy

When the incision must extend into the adjacent gland or glands to obtain adequate margins, the adjacent gland or glands are also removed *(regional mastectomy)*. Consider the blood supply to individual mammary glands when planning and executing the mastectomy (Fig. 27–1). When two or more glands are neoplastic, choose the most efficient approach. Involvement of two or three adjacent glands necessitates a regional mastectomy.

Complete Unilateral Mastectomy

When multiple glands contain tumors, all the ipsilateral glands and intervening tissue are removed *(complete unilateral mastectomy)*, rather than excising each gland separately and leaving tissue between glands.

Removal of Tumors in Contralateral Glands

Tumors in contralateral glands may be excised by bilateral simple, regional, or complete mastectomy. The limiting factor is the amount of skin that will be available after excision for closure. In relatively flat-chested dogs, such as Yorkshire terriers or Pekingese, and in cats, bilateral complete mastectomy is possible.

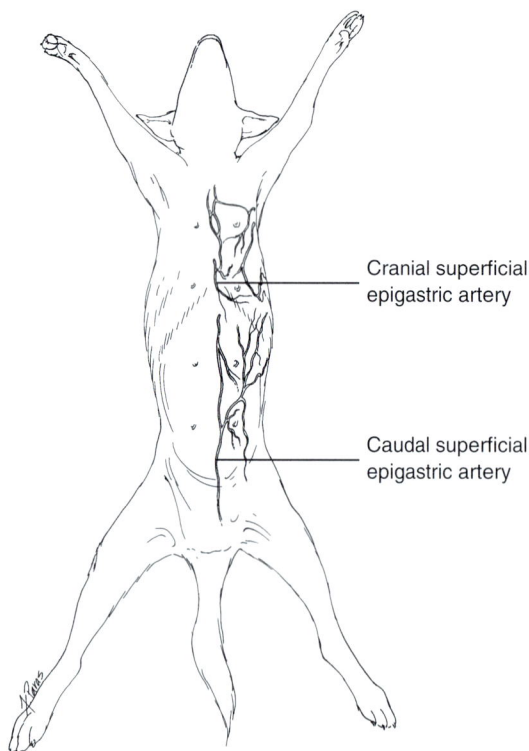

Cranial superficial epigastric artery

Caudal superficial epigastric artery

Figure 27–1. The blood supply to the individual mammary glands is considered in the planning and during the execution of the mastectomy.

In a deep-chested dog, such as an Irish setter or a pointer, often it is not possible to excise contralateral cranial glands with adequate margins of healthy tissue and still be able to close the skin. In this type of dog, perform a staged bilateral mastectomy. Operate on one side and then, after 2 to 4 weeks, operate on the other side.

Technique

1. Prepare the affected mammary glands and surrounding skin for aseptic surgery.
2. After skin and subcutaneous tissues are incised, suture drapes or towels to the normal wound edges to protect the skin from tumor implantation.
3. Place stay sutures in the margin tissues.
4. Using blunt and sharp dissection, remove the mammary glands and underlying subcutaneous tissue. Avoid handling the tumor with instruments or fingers.
5. Use meticulous hemostasis with electrocautery and vessel ligation.
6. Rinse the wound with 0.5–1 L of warm saline solution to remove exfoliated tumor cells.
7. Replace contaminated gloves and surgical instruments before beginning skin closure.
8. Meticulously close the subcutaneous tissues to relieve tension across the incision and prevent problems associated with surgical dead space.
9. Close skin routinely.
10. Consider a light bandage on the incision after extensive mastectomy to protect from trauma.

Ovariohysterectomy

Ovariohysterectomy performed at the time of tumor excision has not been shown to alter prognosis. Ovariohysterectomy does result in atrophy of the remaining glands, which may make it easier to detect new tumors. However, with aggressive MGTs, death from metastatic disease may occur before new tumors become problematic. If an ovariohysterectomy is planned during the same surgery, it should be done before the mastectomy to avoid seeding the abdomen with tumor cells. If the MGT extends across the midline, perform the mastectomy first, lavage the area, and use new gloves and instruments for the ovariohysterectomy.

Biopsy Evaluation

Because multiple tumor types can be present within one mass and each mass may be different, submit all excised tissue for histopathologic examination. Mark the edges of the tissue with suture material or India ink so that the pathologist can maintain proper orientation.

TREATMENT–MEDICAL

Chemotherapy

Successful chemotherapy for canine mammary carcinoma has not been reported. Cyclophosphamide and doxorubicin may induce short-term partial or complete response in cats with metastatic or nonresectable local disease. However, these drugs cause severe anorexia and mild myelosuppression. The value of these drugs as an adjunct to surgical excision is not known.

Anti-Estrogen Therapy

A response of MGTs to anti-estrogen therapy (e.g., tamoxifen) has not been proven. Estrogenic side effects (e.g., vaginal bleeding, vulval swelling, attractiveness to male dogs) are common.

Biologic Response Modifiers

Biologic response modifiers such as levamisole and bacille Calmette-Guérin (BCG) have not been proven successful.

PROGNOSIS

Client education regarding therapy for MGTs is complicated by the variable prognoses reported in the literature.

Cancer mortality rate after excision of nonmetastatic carcinomas was reported as 27%. Most cancer deaths occurred within the first postoperative year. Cancer mortality for dogs with invasive carcinomas or carcinomas with distant metastasis was 80%. The recurrence rate was higher in dogs with grossly invasive carcinomas (44%) than in dogs with benign and noninvasive carcinomas (12%).

Other studies have shown that:

- Dogs with tumors < 3 cm in diameter have a better prognosis than dogs with tumors > 3 cm in diameter.
- The presence of multiple tumors does not seem to change the prognosis in dogs.
- The prognosis in dogs worsens with increasing age.
- Mammary gland sarcoma and inflammatory carcinoma have a very poor prognosis.
- Cats with mammary carcinoma treated by surgical excision have an average survival of 7.7 months.
- Cats with tumors < 2 cm have less local recurrence and increased survival times compared with cats with tumors > 2–3 cm.
- Survival may be decreased in cats with multiple tumors.

- In the future, cell analysis, including S-phase rate or DNA ploidy measurements, may provide useful preoperative prognostic information.

PREVENTION

▼ *Key Point* The risk of MGT is almost completely eliminated in dogs that are spayed before their first estrus.

Ovariohysterectomy has a sparing effect on the development of MGT in dogs if done before the fourth estrus or before 2.5 years of age. In dogs spayed at any age, risk of MGT is reduced if dogs were thin at 9–12 months of age.

Spayed cats have 0.6% the risk for developing mammary carcinoma compared with intact cats.

SUPPLEMENTAL READINGS

Allen SW, Mahaffey EA: Canine mammary neoplasia: Prognostic indicators and response to surgical therapy. J Am Anim Hosp Assoc 25:540, 1989.

Donnay I, Rauis J, Devleeschouwer N, et al.: Comparison of estrogen and progesterone receptor expression in normal and tumor mammary tissues from dogs. Am J Vet Res 56:1188, 1995.

Gilbertson SR, Kurzman ID, Zachrau RE, et al.: Canine mammary epithelial neoplasms: Biologic implications of morphologic characteristics assessed in 232 dogs. Vet Pathol 20:127, 1983.

Hellman E, Bergström R, Holmberg L, et al.: Prognostic factors in canine mammary tumors: A multivariate study of 202 consecutive cases. Vet Pathol 30:20, 1993.

Kurzman ID, Gilbertson SR: Prognostic factors in canine mammary tumors. Semin Vet Med Surg 1:25, 1986.

MacEwen EG, Hayes AA, Harvey HJ, et al.: Prognostic factors for feline mammary tumors. J Am Vet Med Assoc 185:201, 1984.

Morris JS, Dobson JM, Bostock DE: Use of tamoxifen in the control of canine mammary neoplasia. Vet Rec 133:539, 1993.

Moulton JE: Tumors of the mammary gland. In Moulton JE (ed): Tumors in Domestic Animals. Berkeley: University of California Press, 1990, p 518.

Rutteman GR, Misdorp W: Hormonal background of canine and feline mammary tumors. J Reprod Fertil Suppl 47:483, 1993.

Sonnenschein EG, Glickman LT, Goldschmidt MH, et al.: Body conformation, diet, and risk of breast cancer in pet dogs: A case-control study. Am J Epidemiol 133:694, 1991.

Weijer K, Hart AAM: Prognostic factors in feline mammary carcinoma. J Nat Cancer Inst 70:709, 1983.

28 Tumors of the Skin and Subcutaneous Tissues

Janet L. Peterson / C. Guillermo Couto

The skin and subcutis are the most common sites of neoplasia in the dog, accounting for approximately 30–40% of all tumors. In the cat, only 20% of all tumors originate in the skin and subcutis, making it the second most common site of origin. Most canine skin tumors are benign, whereas most feline skin tumors are malignant. Owners often discover skin tumors while petting or grooming their animals.

▼ *Key Point* Skin tumors should not be ignored. Advising owners to "watch" the tumor rather than to seek a diagnosis could be life-threatening to their dog or cat.

The most common skin tumors in the dog are shown in Table 28–1; those in the cat are shown in Table 28–2. Dog breeds at an increased risk for skin tumors include the bassett hound, boxer, bull mastiff, Scottish terrier, and Weimaraner; there is no apparent breed predilection in the cat. In general, skin and subcutaneous tumors are more common in older dogs and cats. Common tumors in younger dogs are shown in Table 28–3. The etiology of most canine and feline tumors is unknown; however, some tumors have been associated with defined etiologic agents, such as those listed in Table 28–4.

Physical examination may assist the clinician in formulating a list of potential tumors in the small animal patient. A basic working knowledge of the anatomic location and tissue of origin of various tumors can assist the clinician in making educated decisions. Additionally, perform fine-needle aspiration to help make a definitive diagnosis without requiring an incisional or excisional biopsy.

CLASSIFICATION

Skin tumors can be classified by tissue of origin (Table 28–5), anatomic location (Table 28–6), and stratum of origin (Table 28–7). Miscellaneous tumors affecting the skin are listed in Table 28–8.

DIAGNOSIS

General Principles

- Diagnosis and characterization of a skin mass is important for several reasons. Knowledge of the tumor type before surgical excision allows the clinician

Table 28–1. MOST COMMON CANINE SKIN AND SUBCUTANEOUS TUMORS

Lipomas
Mast cell tumors
Histiocytomas
Sebaceous gland adenomas

Table 28–2. MOST COMMON FELINE SKIN AND SUBCUTANEOUS TUMORS

Basal cell tumors
Squamous cell carcinomas
Fibrosarcomas
Mast cell tumors

Table 28–3. MOST COMMON SKIN AND SUBCUTANEOUS TUMORS IN YOUNG DOGS

Histiocytoma
Transmissible venereal tumors
Viral papillomas

Table 28–4. ETIOLOGIC AGENTS

Etiology	Tumor Associations
Viruses	Canine squamous papilloma
	Warts
	Feline sarcoma virus–associated multiple fibrosarcomas
Solar and ionizing radiation	Squamous cell carcinoma
Hormones	Perianal adenoma
Thermal injuries	Squamous cell carcinoma
	Mast cell tumor
Genetic factors	Various tumors
Immunologic compromise	Feline lymphoma
Age	Many tumors

Table 28–5. CLASSIFICATION OF SKIN TUMORS BY TISSUE OF ORIGIN

Epithelial Neoplasia
Papilloma
Sebaceous adenoma/hyperplasia/adenocarcinoma
Perianal adenoma/hyperplasia/adenocarcinoma
Basal cell tumor
Ceruminous gland adenoma/adenocarcinoma
Squamous cell carcinoma
Apocrine gland adenocarcinoma
Intracutaneous cornifying epithelioma (keratoacanthoma)
Dermoid/epidermal inclusion cyst

Mesenchymal Neoplasia
Lipoma/infiltrative lipoma/liposarcoma
Fibrosarcoma
Nerve sheath tumor
Hemangiosarcoma
Hemangiopericytoma
Histiocytoma
Mast cell tumor
Extramedullary plasmacytoma

Melanoma

Table 28–7. CLASSIFICATION OF SKIN TUMORS BY STRATUM OF ORIGIN

Dermoepidermal
Basal cell tumor
Squamous cell carcinoma
Sebaceous adenoma/hyperplasia
Mast cell tumor
Perianal adenoma
Malignant melanoma
Ceruminous gland adenocarcinoma
Lymphoma
Transmissible venereal tumor
Hemangioma/hemangiosarcoma
Cysts

Subcutaneous
Mast cell tumor
Hemangiopericytoma
Lipoma
Hemangiosarcoma
Nerve sheath tumor
Fibrosarcoma

(1) to plan an appropriate surgical approach (e.g., in a mast cell tumor that requires 3-cm margins beyond the tumor edges), (2) to consider radiation therapy (e.g., nonresectable mast cell tumors), or (3) to institute medical treatment (e.g., vincristine chemotherapy is usually curative for transmissible venereal tumors).

Table 28–6. CLASSIFICATION OF SKIN TUMORS BY ANATOMIC LOCATION

Head and neck
Basal cell tumor
Squamous cell carcinoma
Sebaceous adenoma
Papilloma
Histiocytoma
Mast cell tumor (primarily in cats)
Ceruminous gland adenoma/adenocarcinoma
Hemangiosarcoma

Extremities
Mast cell tumor
Hemangiopericytoma
Squamous cell carcinoma (nail bed)
Malignant melanoma (nail bed)
Nerve sheath tumor
Synovial cell sarcoma
Hemangiosarcoma

Trunk
Mast cell tumor
Lipoma
Sebaceous gland adenoma
Fibrosarcoma
Nerve sheath tumor
Hemangiosarcoma

Perineum/Genitals
Mast cell tumor
Perianal adenoma
Transmissible venereal tumor
Perianal adenocarcinoma
Anal sac (apocrine gland) adenocarcinoma

- To detect the presence of metastatic disease before surgery, evaluate every enlarged regional lymph node cytologically (fine-needle aspiration) or histologically. Additionally, consider lymph node excisional biopsy at surgery for more accurate staging.
- Perform thoracic radiographs (3 views) on all animals with suspected (or confirmed) malignant tumors with potential for pulmonary metastases. Perform abdominal radiography and/or abdominal ultrasonography in those cases in which dissemination to the abdominal organs or cavity or multicentricity is suspected (e.g., mast cell tumor, hemangiosarcoma). Evaluate skeletal structures on thoracic and abdominal radiographs for metastatic disease.

▼ *Key Point* Diagnosis and staging of a skin tumor before surgery are critical to ensure complete excision and to determine appropriate additional treatment.

Fine-Needle Aspiration Cytology
Equipment

- Aspiration Handle (Cook, Veterinary Division)
- 12- or 20-ml syringe
- 22- or 25-gauge needle
- Glass cover slips or glass slides
- Diff-Quick or Wright-Giemsa stain

Table 28–8. MISCELLANEOUS TUMORS AFFECTING THE SKIN

Intracutaneous cornifying epithelioma (keratoacanthoma)
Trichoepithelioma and pilomatrixoma (tumors of the hair follicles)
Epidermal inclusion cyst (epidermoid, epidermoid cyst)
Dermoid cyst

Technique

- Isolate and hold the mass firmly while inserting the needle into it.
- Apply negative pressure (10–20 ml) to the syringe to obtain cells.
- Release the negative pressure before withdrawing the needle from the mass.
- Remove the needle from the syringe and fill the syringe with air.
- Replace the needle and expel the contents (within the hub of the needle) onto the glass slide or coverslip.
- Prepare the smear by placing the two slides or coverslips together and pulling them apart in a parallel motion ("horizontal pull-apart" technique).
- An alternative technique is to insert the needle without a syringe into the mass ("pass-through" technique)

The contents of the needle are expelled using a syringe and prepared as aforementioned.

Cytologic Classification of Neoplasia

Cytology can be used to classify masses as neoplastic or nonneoplastic. If the mass is not neoplastic, then the decision must be made as to whether it is inflammatory or noninflammatory. Masses also can be classified as mixed, as in the case of a neoplastic mass with a necrotic center and associated inflammation. Infectious agents also may be identified cytologically (e.g., bacteria, fungi, protozoa).

Cytologic examination may allow classification of tumors into one of three categories: epithelial, mesenchymal, or round cell neoplasm (includes epithelial, mesenchymal, and melanocytic tumors).

Epithelial Tumors

Epithelial cells cluster because of desmosomes. Aspiration cytology reveals round to polygonal cells with basophilic cytoplasm (with and without vacuoles) and cell-to-cell association. The latter may be absent in squamous cell carcinomas.

Mesenchymal Tumors

Mesenchymal tumors arise from connective tissue, including fibrous tissue, muscle, fat, and blood vessels. They do not exfoliate well on fine-needle aspiration; however, when they do exfoliate, they appear as individual cells or in small groups of cells, with a spindle to polygonal shape.

Round Cell Tumors

On fine-needle aspiration, round cell tumors tend to exfoliate as single cells. Transmissible venereal tumors usually clump, however. The cells have distinct cell membranes like epithelial cells. Some cells may have cytoplasmic granules (i.e., mast cells, melanoma cells, large granular lymphocytes).

Round cell tumors include lymphoma, melanoma, histiocytoma, transmissible venereal tumor, mast cell tumor, and plasma cell tumor. Additionally, squamous cell carcinomas and basal cell tumors can resemble round cell tumors cytologically.

Incisional Biopsy

Punch Biopsy

The skin punch biopsy using the Baker biopsy punch is a relatively simple technique for obtaining a sample of superficial masses. The advantage of skin punch biopsies is that they can be done using only local anesthetic and can be accomplished in a short time. See Chapter 49 for skin biopsy technique.

Needle Biopsy

Tru-cut or spring-loaded needle biopsies can be used to obtain representative samples of larger or subcutaneous masses using only local anesthesia.

Wedge Biopsy

A routine surgical procedure is used to obtain a "wedge" biopsy (see Chapter 24).

Excisional Biopsy

Excisional biopsy implies that all or most of the tumor or mass is removed and submitted for histopathologic examination. This approach is indicated for small, easily excisable masses. Margins of excised tissue should be at least 1 cm in all cases. All excised tumors must be fixed properly. Label each tumor by location if there are multiple tumors, and finally, send all tumors to a qualified veterinary pathologist for examination. Principles of surgical biopsy of tumors are described in Chapter 24.

▼ *Key Point* Perform histopathologic examinations on all excised skin masses, no matter how "benign" they appear. Appropriate treatment necessitates a definitive diagnosis.

Staging

Clinical staging is helpful to characterize the extent of the disease. Obtain thoracic radiographs (left and right lateral and ventrodorsal views) when malignancy is suspected. Perform abdominal radiography or ultrasonography for tumors such as cutaneous hemangiosarcoma and mast cell tumor to evaluate for splenic and hepatic involvement (metastases or primary tumor).

SELECTED TUMORS OF THE SKIN AND SUBCUTANEOUS TISSUE

Epithelial Neoplasia

Papilloma

Origin and Etiology

Papillomas (squamous papillomas, squamous cell papillomatosis, warts, cutaneous papillomatosis) originate from the squamous epithelium. Papillomas have a DNA viral etiology in puppies, but the etiology is unknown in older dogs.

Description

Papillomas may appear as cauliflower or wart-like growths that are usually well-encapsulated. They can be sessile or pedunculated and may bleed if traumatized. They can occur as a single tumor (usually nonviral etiology) or as multiple tumors (usually viral etiology) in the skin, mucous membranes, or mucocutaneous regions.

Epidemiology and Biological Behavior

Papillomas are common in dogs but rare in cats. The virally induced papillomas found in young dogs often appear as multiple or occasionally single masses on the head, eyelids, feet, or mouth. These tumors are contagious to other dogs and have an incubation period of approximately 30 days. In older dogs, nonviral papillomas tend to appear as solitary dermoepidermal masses. Some papillomas in older dogs can transform into squamous cell carcinomas.

Treatment

Papillomas tend to regress spontaneously in younger dogs (usually within 1–2 months) and therefore do not require treatment. Surgically remove viral papillomas that do not regress and nonviral papillomas that cause a clinical problem.

Sebaceous Gland Tumors

Origin and Etiology

Sebaceous gland adenoma, hyperplasia, and adenocarcinoma originate from the epithelium of the sebaceous glands.

Description

These tumors are common in dogs (especially spaniels) and rare in cats. Hyperplasia usually appears as pink, smooth, lobulated wart-like growths that are firm, dermoepidermal, well-circumscribed masses with an alopecic surface. They may be pigmented and can occur anywhere on the body. These tumors are frequently multiple. They often appear as bleeding and ulcerated masses. Sebaceous gland adenocarcinoma is poorly circumscribed, large, invasive, and frequently ulcerated. These are extremely rare.

Cytology

Cytologic examination of sebaceous gland hyperplasia reveals mature secretory epithelial cells, frequently with a "signet-ring appearance" because of the accumulation of secretions within the cell. Sebaceous adenocarcinoma cells exhibit typical features of malignancy.

Epidemiology and Biological Behavior

Sebaceous gland hyperplasias can occur as single tumors; however, they frequently tend to occur in multiple sites. They occur in older female dogs, especially poodles and cocker spaniels. When metastases from sebaceous gland adenocarcinomas occur, they generally spread to the regional lymph nodes and subsequently to the lungs.

Treatment

Surgical excision of sebaceous gland hyperplasia lesions may not be necessary unless they occur in an area that is easily traumatized. Perform wide surgical excision on all sebaceous adenocarcinomas. Adjunct treatment with radiotherapy and/or FAC protocol (5-fluorouracil, doxorubicin [Adriamycin], and cyclophosphamide) (Appendix I) may be beneficial.

Perianal Tumors

Origin and Etiology

Perianal adenomas, hyperplasia, and adenocarcinomas originate from the perianal (hepatoid) glands. These are sebaceous glands that encircle the anus of the dog and also are located in the skin of the tail, prepuce, thigh, and over the dorsum of the back. The growth and maintenance of these cells are dependent on the presence of testosterone.

Description

Perianal adenoma and hyperplasia can occur as solitary or multiple nodules. These are most common in *older* intact male dogs, and their behavior is usually benign. They can be found wherever perianal glands are located (see Origin and Etiology), but they are most common in the perineal region. Perianal adenocarcinomas are frequently larger, ulcerative, and invasive.

Cytology

Cytologic examination usually reveals large hepatoid cells. It is impossible to differentiate perianal adenoma from hyperplasia. Malignancy can be difficult to assess solely on the basis of cytology.

Epidemiology and Biological Behavior

Perianal adenocarcinomas metastasize to the local lymphatics, especially the iliac lymph nodes, and to the lungs. These tumors occur primarily in male dogs.

Treatment

Perianal adenoma and hyperplasia usually regress with castration because of their testosterone dependency. Castration therefore is recommended for all dogs in which perianal adenoma or hyperplasia constitutes a problem. Perform aggressive surgical excision on all resectable perianal adenocarcinomas and those perianal adenomas that fail to respond to castration. Other treatment options are radiation therapy or chemotherapy using carboplatin, mitoxantrone, VAC (vincristine, doxorubicin [Adriamycin], and cyclophosphamide), or FAC protocols (see Appendix I).

Basal Cell Tumors

Origin and Etiology

Basal cell tumors (basal cell carcinoma, basal cell epithelioma) originate from the basal cells of the epidermis and adnexa.

Description

Basal cell tumors commonly occur as solitary nodules. They can be sessile or pedunculated, firm, and well demarcated from the underlying tissues. These tumors frequently are pigmented, contain cystic spaces, and occasionally are ulcerated (in cats). Basal cell tumors tend to be found more frequently on the head, neck, and shoulder of the dog. They commonly are found almost anywhere in the cat, in which they represent the most common skin tumor.

Cytology

Cells may be arranged in cords or pallisades. "Pallisading" clusters and uniform nuclei generally are seen on cytologic examination. The cells usually appear malignant on cytologic and histopathologic examination.

Epidemiology and Biological Behavior

Basal cell tumors are common in older dogs and cats. Cocker spaniels and poodles may be at increased risk for these tumors. The tumors usually are benign and may have been present from months to years before diagnosis. When these tumors are identified histologically as basal cell carcinoma, this is generally a reliable diagnosis, and their behavior must be considered very aggressive.

Treatment

Wide surgical excision is the treatment of choice for basal cell tumors. Complete excision is curative. Nonresectable or invasive tumors can be treated successfully with radiation therapy and/or chemotherapy.

Ceruminous Gland Tumors

Origin and Etiology

Ceruminous gland adenomas and adenocarcinomas originate from the epithelium of the ceruminous glands in the ear canal.

Description

They are usually brown tumors associated with cerumen production, which may resemble chronic otitis. Ceruminous gland adenomas are small, pedunculated masses that frequently are located near the tympanic membrane and extend exteriorly. Adenocarcinomas are similar to adenomas; however, they are frequently invasive.

Cytology

Cytologic examination reveals mature or immature (ceruminous gland adenocarcinoma) secretory cells with epithelial characteristics.

Epidemiology and Biological Behavior

This is the most common external ear tumor in older dogs and cats but appears to be more common in cats.

Treatment

Total ear canal resection may be necessary to completely excise these tumors (see Chap. 56). Surgical removal may be sufficient in animals with ceruminous gland adenomas; however, external beam irradiation is recommended strongly for dogs and cats with ceruminous gland adenocarcinomas with incomplete resection after an aggressive ear canal ablation and for recurrent or nonexcisable adenomas. Chemotherapy also may be considered for patients with incomplete tumor resection or metastases, using protocols that contain cisplatin, carboplatin, mitoxantrone, and doxorubicin.

Squamous Cell Carcinoma

Origin and Etiology

Squamous cell carcinoma may occur secondary to ultraviolet light exposure in cats and dogs with hypopigmented areas. It originates from stratified squamous epithelium. The cell of origin is the keratinocyte.

Description

These tumors frequently appear as ulcerated, necrotic, nonhealing lesions. Common sites in dogs include the ventral abdomen, digits (especially nail bed), limbs, scrotum, lips, and nose. In the cat, they include the ear pinnae, lips, nose, and eyelids. Proliferative tumors may resemble a red firm plaque or a cauliflower-like lesion. Digital squamous cell carcinoma can be proliferative, ulcerative, locally aggressive, and erosive. It also can appear as a nonhealing wound. Multiple nailbed squamous cell carcinomas have been observed in black dogs.

Cytology

These epithelial cells are polygonal and may keratinize as they mature. Typical epithelial cells mixed with keratinizing cells frequently are noted. Aging squamous epithelial cells tend to be more angular or polyhedral, with a pyknotic nucleus and bluer cytoplasm. Abundant neutrophils and other inflammatory cells frequently are observed.

Epidemiology and Biological Behavior

These tumors occur more frequently in cats, especially in white cats or in those with hypopigmented areas that are more likely to be exposed to sunlight, especially ear tips and nose. Dogs have an increased frequency of these tumors in the ventral abdomen (especially), trunk, scrotum, and lips. They are locally invasive with late metastases to the local lymph nodes and lungs.

Treatment

Complete surgical excision is recommended for squamous cell carcinomas if they are in an easily accessible location. Complete pinna resection is advised for tumors of the ear (see Chap. 56) and digital amputation for squamous cell carcinoma of the digit (see Chap. 133). Consider radiation therapy and photodynamic therapy for dogs and cats with nonresectable or incompletely excised squamous cell carcinomas. Consider chemotherapy for nonresectable or metastatic tumors, using cisplatin, carboplatin, bleomycin, mitoxantrone, and doxorubicin.

Anal Sac or Apocrine Gland Adenocarcinoma
Origin and Etiology

Apocrine gland adenocarcinomas are derived from the apocrine glands that empty into the anal sac.

Description

These tumors can vary from very small masses that can be located only after careful rectal and perirectal palpation to large masses protruding from the rectum. They may cause ulceration of the overlying skin.

Cytology

Cytologic examination reveals large cells with abundant cytoplasm and eccentric round nuclei.

Epidemiology and Biological Behavior

Apocrine gland adenocarcinomas are most commonly found in older female dogs. Hypercalcemia is frequently associated with these tumors (see Chap. 30). Metastases are common (90% of cases) and most frequently spread to the regional (i.e., iliac) lymph nodes.

Treatment

Surgical excision offers the best option for a cure. Chemotherapy also may be considered, using melphalan, FAC, carboplatin, and mitoxantrone (see Appendix I). Hypercalcemia generally resolves after remission of this tumor.

Intracutaneous Cornifying Epithelioma (Keratoacanthoma)
Origin and Etiology

This tumor is derived from the superficial epithelium between hair follicles.

Description

Intracutaneous cornifying epitheliomas may be located on the skin of the neck, the dorsal thorax, the legs, and occasionally on the ventral abdomen. A toothpaste-like material may be expressed from these masses.

Cytology

Cytologic evaluation may reveal keratin associated with inflammatory cells.

Epidemiology and Biological Behavior

These are benign tumors that can occur in a solitary form in many breeds of dogs and in a multicentric form in Norwegian elkhound and keeshond dogs.

Treatment

Surgical excision is the treatment of choice, although it may not be required. Consider retinoid therapy for the multicentric form.

Dermoid and Epidermal Inclusion Cyst
Origin and Etiology

Dermoid and epidermal inclusion cysts originate from the dermis and epidermis. Epidermal inclusion cysts are frequently secondary to an occluded hair follicle, whereas dermoid cysts may be developmental defects.

Description

Dermoid cysts contain epidermal appendages, hair, and sebaceous and sweat gland secretions, in addition to the keratin that is in the epidermal inclusion cysts. A semisolid material frequently is contained within these cysts.

Cytology

A clear-to-brown fluid frequently is obtained for cytologic examination.

Epidemiology and Biological Behavior

These are benign tumors.

Treatment

Surgical excision is the treatment of choice, although it is not always required.

Mesenchymal Neoplasia
Lipomas and Liposarcomas
Origin/Etiology

Lipomas, infiltrative lipomas, and liposarcomas originate from adipocytes or fat cells.

Description

Lipomas can occur either as single or multiple masses and are located over the thorax, sternum, abdomen, and proximal limbs of dogs. These masses are usually subcutaneous; well-circumscribed, although not necessarily well encapsulated; fluctuant; soft; and sometimes multilobulated. Infiltrative lipomas infiltrate the deep tissue and are extremely difficult to excise. Liposarcomas are uncommon and usually solitary tumors that tend to be very infiltrative, firm, and poorly circumscribed.

Cytology

Fatty-appearing material usually is present on the slide before staining. Most cells from aspirates of lipomas are "washed off" by the methanol in the fixative. Occasionally, oily material with few intact adipocytes or fatty cells remains on the slide or cover slip. Cytology of liposarcoma reveals immature mesenchymal cells with vacuoles and round, indented nuclei. Variation in cell size is common, and occasionally, multinucleation is noted.

▼ *Key Point* Evaluate all "lipomas" cytologically because they are indistinguishable from mast cell tumors in physical appearance and clinical presentation.

Epidemiology and Biological Behavior

Lipomas are benign tumors that appear to be more common in older spayed female dogs. They are the most common mesenchymal tumor in the dog but are extremely rare in the cat. Infiltrative lipomas are also benign; however, because of their highly infiltrative nature, they may require extensive surgical excision, including amputation of the affected limb. Liposarcomas are extremely rare tumors in both dogs and cats, but are found most often in dogs older than 10 years of age. They are locally invasive and may metastasize to the lungs and/or liver.

Treatment

It may or may not be necessary to remove lipomas, depending on their size, location, and owner preference. If surgery is considered, remove these lipomas while they are small and before they become too large and difficult to resect. Treat infiltrative lipomas with aggressive surgery and radiation therapy if indicated. Treat all liposarcomas with complete surgical excision.

Fibrosarcoma

Origin and Etiology

These tumors typically originate in the subcutaneous fibrous connective tissue from fibrocytes or fibroblasts. In cats, fibrosarcomas present in association with feline sarcoma virus/feline leukemia virus, as vaccine-associated sarcomas, and as those nonretrovirus-induced. Retrovirus-induced fibrosarcomas occur in young cats, are rare, and do not respond to any form of treatment (see Chap. 6). Fibrosarcomas generally occur on the head, trunk, or limbs. There is a strong association between the administration of inactivated vaccines (e.g., feline leukemia virus, rabies, and certain herpescalici-panleukopenia [FVRCP] vaccines) and subsequent development of soft tissue sarcomas (primarily fibrosarcomas) at the vaccination site.

Description

Fibrosarcomas can occur as solitary or multiple masses. They are frequently firm, lobulated, and infiltrative into underlying tissues.

Cytology

Cytology reveals typical spindle or mesenchymal cells, although cells from these tumors tend not to exfoliate well.

Epidemiology and Biological Behavior

Most fibrosarcomas occur in older dogs and cats (i.e., nonretrovirally induced). Fibrosarcomas that are associated with feline sarcoma virus tend to occur in younger cats and are multiple. Vaccine-associated fibrosarcomas have an overall prevalence of between 1 and 3 cases per 10,000 vaccinated cats. Other types of fibrosarcoma are very locally invasive but usually metastasize late in their course (less than 10% of cats and dogs with solitary fibrosarcoma have metastases at presentation).

Treatment

Wide and deep surgical excision is recommended, although this can be difficult because of the invasive nature of this tumor. Histological evaluation of margins is very important because complete excision is usually curative. Consider surgical amputation in patients with tumors on the extremities.

Response to chemotherapy is variable. Histologically, poorly differentiated fibrosarcomas and fibrosarcomas with giant cells in cats appear to be more responsive to chemotherapy. Chemotherapy protocols include VAC (cats, dogs; see Appendix I) and A-DIC (doxorubicin and dacarbazine [DTIC]) (dogs; see Appendix I). Other treatment options include radiation therapy and hyperthermia.

Nerve Sheath Tumors

Neurofibromas, neurofibrosarcomas, schwannomas, and neurolemmomas are discussed in Chapter 148.

Hemangiosarcomas

Origin and Etiology

These tumors (also known as malignant hemangioendotheliomas and angiosarcomas) originate from the vascular endothelium.

Description

Hemangiosarcomas generally are solitary masses found on the limbs, flank, or neck. They can occur in the skin and/or subcutaneous tissue. Those in the subcutaneous tissue also may infiltrate the underlying muscle. Hemangiosarcoma must be differentiated from hemangioma.

Cytology

Cytology reveals spindle-shaped or polygonal cells with large nuclei and a lacy chromatin pattern; one or more nucleoli; and a bluish, usually vacuolated cytoplasm. Hemangiosarcomas also can exfoliate cells in sheets similar to those of epithelial cells.

Epidemiology and Biological Behavior

Hemangiosarcomas of the skin can be either primary or metastatic. Hemangiosarcomas are much more common in dogs, especially German shepherds and golden retrievers, than in cats. The prognoses of these tumors are variable depending on location. Those patients in which the tumor is confined to the dermis have an excellent prognosis, whereas if the tumor involves the subcutaneous tissue, the prognosis is poor. Muscular involvement warrants a guarded prognosis.

Treatment

Perform complete surgical excision when feasible. Chemotherapy probably is not necessary for those tumors involving only the dermis, whereas those involving the subcutaneous tissue with or without muscular involvement probably require chemotherapy using the VAC protocol (see Appendix I).

Hemangiopericytoma

See Chapter 26.

Histiocytoma

Origin and Etiology

The origin of canine cutaneous histiocytomas is the monocyte-macrophage cells in the skin.

Description

This is a dermoepidermal tumor frequently located on the head and neck, and less commonly on the extremities. They are round, alopecic, sometimes pink or erythematous, and they occasionally ulcerate. Because of their gross appearance, they also are referred to as "button tumors."

Cytology

Cytology reveals a round cell tumor with a moderate amount of cytoplasm and, possibly, an eccentrically located nucleus. Histiocytomas also tend to be highly pleomorphic and moderately vacuolated. Lymphocytes are abundant. These tumors can appear inflammatory.

Epidemiology and Biological Behavior

These tumors generally exhibit benign behavior and are found mostly in young dogs (approximately 1–3 years). Histiocytomas usually regress spontaneously within 4 to 8 weeks of diagnosis. This tumor does not occur in cats.

Treatment

Observation alone may be appropriate in most of these tumors because the majority regress with age. Perform surgical excision if this tumor does not regress in a reasonable period of time, in older dogs, for cosmetic reasons, and finally, to avoid an erroneous diagnosis and further growth of the tumor.

Mast Cell Tumor

Mastocytoma, mast cell sarcoma, and mastocytosis are discussed in Chapter 26.

Extramedullary Plasmacytoma

See Chapter 25.

Cutaneous Lymphoma

Dermal lymphoma, mycosis fungoides, and histiocytic lymphoma are discussed in Chapter 25.

Transmissible Venereal Tumor

Origin and Etiology

Transmissible venereal tumors frequently are transmitted at coitus or through close contact. The cell of origin is considered to be from the monocyte-macrophage system. See also Chapters 108 and 112.

Description

Transmissible venereal tumors tend to occur on the external genitalia and the face and frequently appear as ulcerated, solitary or multiple, friable, cauliflower-like masses.

Cytology

Cytology reveals round-to-ovoid cells with round nuclei and numerous mitotic figures. The cytoplasm is blue or transparent, contains distinct clear vacuoles, and is surrounded by a distinct cell membrane.

Epidemiology and Biological Behavior

This tumor tends to be transmitted by coitus, licking, biting, and scratching. It occurs more frequently in areas where dogs are free-roaming. No breed or sex predilections have been observed. These tumors have a low metastatic potential.

Treatment

Transmissible venereal tumors can be cured with vincristine chemotherapy (see Appendix I), surgery, and/or radiation therapy.

Malignant Fibrous Histiocytoma (Extraskeletal Giant Cell Tumors)

See Chapter 26.

Melanocytic Tumors (Melanomas)

Origin and Etiology

Melanomas originate from melanocytes (melanin-producing cells) or melanoblasts, which are cells of neuroectodermal origin.

Description

These are typically brown-to-black pigmented nodules (although they may be nonpigmented) that occur more frequently on the face, the trunk, the feet, mucocutaneous regions, and the nailbed.

Cytology

Cytologic examination may reveal cells that vary from round to spindle-shaped. They frequently contain brown to black granules.

Epidemiology and Biological Behavior

Melanomas are considerably more common in dogs than in cats. Tumors originating in the skin tend to be benign, whereas tumors of the mucocutaneous regions (e.g., oral cavity, nailbeds) tend to be malignant.

Treatment

Local recurrence and distant metastases are very common. Surgery is the treatment of choice. Results of chemotherapy have been unrewarding; however, DTIC, carboplatin, and cisplatin may be the drugs of choice (see Appendix I). Palliative radiation therapy may be another option in some cases.

SELECTED REFERENCES

Holzworth J: Diseases of the Cat. Philadelphia: WB Saunders Company, 1987.

Ogilvie GH, Moore AS: Managing the Veterinary Cancer Patient. Trenton: Veterinary Learning Systems, 1995.

Theilen GH, Madewell BR: Veterinary Cancer Medicine. Philadelphia: Lea and Febiger, 1987.

Withrow SJ, MacEwen EG: Clinical Veterinary Oncology. Philadelphia: WB Saunders Company, 1996.

Appendix I: Chemotherapy Protocols

Soft Tissue Sarcoma

1. *ADIC protocol (dogs)*
   Doxorubicin (Adriamycin): 30 mg/m^2 BSA, IV, q3 weeks
   DTIC (Dacarbazine): 1000 mg/m^2 BSA, IV drip for 6–8 hours; repeat q3 weeks
2. *VAC protocol (21-day cycle) (dogs)*
   Vincristine (Oncovin): 0.75 mg/m^2 BSA, IV, days 8, 15
   Doxorubicin (Adriamycin): 30 mg/m^2 BSA, IV, day 1 (dogs)
   Cyclophosphamide (Cytoxan): 100–200 mg/m^2 BSA, IV, day 1
   Tribrissen: 14 mg/kg, PO, q12h
3. *VAC protocol (21-day cycle) (cats)*
   Vincristine (Oncovin): 0.5 mg/m^2 BSA, IV, days 8, 15
   Doxorubicin (Adriamycin): 20 mg/m^2 BSA, IV, day 1
   Cyclophosphamide (Cytoxan): 100–200 mg/m^2 BSA, IV, day 10
   Tribrissen: 14 mg/kg, PO, q12h

Carcinoma—Dog

1. *CMF protocol*
   5-Fluorouracil (5-FU): 150 mg/m^2 BSA, IV, once a week
   Cyclophosphamide (Cytoxan): 50 mg/m^2 BSA, PO, 4 days a week or qod
   Methotrexate: 2.5 mg/m^2 BSA, PO, 2 or 3 times a week
2. *VAF protocol*
   Vincristine (Oncovin): 0.75 mg/m^2 BSA, IV, days 8, 15
   Doxorubicin (Adriamycin): 30 mg/m^2 BSA, IV, day 1
   5-Fluorouracil (5-FU): 150 mg/m^2 BSA, IV, days 1, 8, 15
3. *VAC protocol*
4. *Cisplatin (Platinol):* 50–70 mg/m^2 BSA, IV drip, 3 weeks; prior intensive diuresis is required
5. *FAC protocol*
   5-Fluorouracil (5-FU): 150 mg/m^2 BSA, IV, days 8, 15
   Doxorubicin (Adriamycin): 30 mg/m^2 BSA, IV, day 1
   Cyclophosphamide (Cytoxan): 100–200 mg/m^2 BSA, IV, day 1
   Tribrissen: 14 mg/kg, PO, BID
6. *Carboplatin (Paraplatin):* 300 mg/m^2 BSA, IV, q21d
7. *Mitoxantrone (Novantrone):* 6 mg/m^2 BSA, IV, q21d

Carcinoma—Feline

1. *Vincristine (Oncovin)/Cyclophosphamide (Cytoxan)*
   Vincristine (Oncovin): 0.5 mg/m^2 BSA, IV, once a week
   Cyclophosphamide (Cytoxan): 50 mg/m^2 BSA, PO, 4 days a week or qod
2. *As above, plus methotrexate:* 2.5 mg/m^2 BSA, PO, 2 or 3 times a week
3. *VAC protocol (28-day cycle)*
4. *Mitoxantrone (Novantrone)/Cytoxan Protocol (21-day cycle)*
   Mitoxantrone: 3–5 mg/m^2, IV over 45 minutes, day 1
   Cyclophosphamide (Cytoxan): 200–300 mg/m^2 BSA, PO, day 15
5. *Carboplatin (Paraplatin):* 150–250 mg/m^2 BSA, IV, q21d
6. *Mitoxantrone (Novantrone):* 6.5 mg/m^2 BSA, IV, q21d

Transmissible Venereal Tumor

Vincristine (Oncovin): 0.5 mg/m^2 BSA, IV, once weekly until and at least 1 week beyond resolution of the tumor

Anal Sac or Apocrine Gland Adenocarcinoma

1. *FAC protocol*
2. *Melphalan (Alkeran)*
   Melphalan (Alkeran): 2 mg/m^2 BSA, PO, q24h × 1 week; then qod, i.e., 6–8 mg/m^2 PO q24h × 5 days; repeat q3 weeks
3. *Carboplatin (Paraplatin):* 300 mg/m^2 BSA, IV, q21d
4. *Mitoxantrone (Novantrone):* 6.0 mg/m^2 BSA, IV, q21d

Extramedullary Plasmacytoma

Melphalan (Alkeran): 2 mg/m^2 BSA, PO, q24h × 1 week; then qod

4 Endocrine and Metabolic Disorders

Mark E. Peterson

Chapter

29 Diseases of the Thyroid Gland

David L. Panciera / Mark E. Peterson / Stephen J. Birchard

HYPOTHYROIDISM IN DOGS

Hypothyroidism is a common, multisystemic disease in dogs. Thyroid hormone deficiency affects virtually all body systems, resulting in a wide array of clinical signs. It occurs predominantly in middle-aged, pure-breed dogs, including the golden retriever, Doberman pinscher, Irish setter, boxer, miniature schnauzer, dachshund, and cocker spaniel. There is no strong sex predilection.

Etiology

Primary Hypothyroidism

Primary hypothyroidism, resulting from gradual destruction of the thyroid gland, is responsible for over 95% of cases.

- *Lymphocytic thyroiditis.*
  - Immune-mediated destruction.
  - Circulating antithyroglobulin antibodies are present in most cases.
  - Lymphocytic infiltrate in thyroid gland.
- *Idiopathic thyroid gland atrophy.*
  - Replacement of thyroid parenchyma by adipose tissue without inflammation.
  - Cause is unknown.
  - Not associated with antithyroglobulin antibodies.

- Uncommon causes of primary hypothyroidism include congenital types (e.g., dyshormonogenesis, thyroid dysgenesis), replacement of thyroid gland parenchyma by nonfunctional neoplastic tissue, surgical thyroidectomy, and radioiodine treatment.

Secondary (Pituitary) Hypothyroidism

Secondary (pituitary) hypothyroidism is caused by impaired secretion of thyroid-stimulating hormone (TSH). This etiology accounts for less than 5% of cases.

- *Pituitary tumors.* Destruction of normal pituitary thyrotrophs by neoplastic invasion.
- *Cystic Rathke pouch.* This form occurs in German shepherd pituitary dwarfs and is associated with concurrent hormone deficiencies including growth hormone deficiency, hypoadrenocorticism, and hypogonadism (see also Chap. 34).

Tertiary (Hypothalamic) Hypothyroidism

Tertiary (hypothalamic) hypothyroidism resulting from deficient production or release of thyrotropin-releasing hormone (TRH) has not yet been documented in dogs.

▼ *Key Point* The majority of hypothyroid dogs have primary disease due to lymphocytic thyroiditis or atrophy.

Table 29–1. CLINICAL SIGNS AND LABORATORY FINDINGS IN DOGS WITH HYPOTHYROIDISM

Common Findings	Uncommon Findings
Dermatologic abnormalities	Neuropathy
Seborrhea	Vestibular
Alopecia	Facial
Pyoderma	Generalized
Myxedema	Laryngeal paralysis
Obesity	Myopathy
Lethargy	Megaesophagus
Weakness/exercise intolerance	Central nervous system abnor-
Low-voltage ECG complexes	malities
Bradycardia	Dwarfism
Hypercholesterolemia	Reproductive abnormalities
Nonregenerative anemia	(anestrus)
	Insulin-resistant diabetes mellitus
	Ocular abnormalities
	Myxedema stupor or coma

ECG, electrocardiographic.

Clinical Signs

The clinical signs of hypothyroidism are insidious in onset because of the gradual destruction of the thyroid gland. Signs are diverse and range from mild to severe (Table 29–1).

General Appearance and Behavior

- Weight gain (mild to marked obesity).
- Lethargy, dullness, exercise intolerance.
- Cold intolerance, hypothermia (uncommon).

Integument

- Excessive scaling and dry haircoat are often the earliest changes.
- Excessive shedding.
- Alopecia.
  - Often begins on the tail and neck (areas of friction).
  - May progress to bilaterally symmetric truncal alopecia sparing the head and extremities.
- Cutaneous hyperpigmentation.
- Recurrent otitis externa or pyoderma.
- Myxedema: Thickening of the skin, especially facial, secondary to glycosaminoglycan accumulation, leading to a "tragic" facial expression.
- Pruritus is not present except when associated with secondary pyoderma, seborrhea, or *Malassezia* infection.

Nervous System and Muscle

- Peripheral neuropathy.
  - Generalized neuropathy can cause weakness, ataxia, and abnormal proprioception.
  - Vestibular neuropathy.
  - Facial neuropathy, often concurrent with vestibular signs.
  - Unilateral forelimb lameness with pain in the glenohumeral joint.

- Megaesophagus is very rare, and may occur secondary to myopathy, neuropathy, or concurrent myasthenia gravis.
- Nonspecific weakness and exercise intolerance may be caused by myopathy or mild neuropathy.
- Behavioral abnormalities including aggression have been reported with hypothyroidism.

Cardiovascular System

- Bradycardia, apex beat and pulses weak.
- Decreased amplitude of R wave, first-degree atrioventricular block.
- Atrial fibrillation may occur rarely in dogs with hypothyroidism.
- Decreased myocardial contractility (mild and subclinical).

Reproductive System

- No clinically significant effects on male reproduction.
- Anestrus, infertility, and abortion are possible in females.
- Inappropriate galactorrhea in intact females.

Eyes

- Ocular manifestations of hypothyroidism are rare and appear to be associated with hyperlipidemia.
  - Corneal lipid deposits.
  - Chronic uveitis.

Bleeding Disorders

- Recent evidence suggests that hypothyroidism does not alter von Willebrand factor concentrations or bleeding time in dogs.
- Thyroid hormone supplementation in hypothyroid dogs is associated with a decrease in von Willebrand factor.
- There is no evidence that thyroid hormone administration increases von Willebrand factor in dogs with congenital von Willebrand disease.

Congenital Hypothyroidism

- Lethargy, mental dullness, weak nursing, constipation.
- Disproportionate dwarfism, broad skull, macroglossia, delayed dental eruption, hypothermia, distended abdomen, retention of puppy haircoat, dry skin, gait abnormalities.
- Some abnormalities (e.g., short stature, osteoarthritis, impaired mental function) may persist despite treatment.

Myxedema Stupor and Coma

- Most severe and rarest form of hypothyroidism.
- Stupor or coma, hypothermia without shivering, bradycardia, hypotension, hypoventilation, in addition to the more common signs of hypothyroidism.
- Hypercholesterolemia, hyponatremia, hypoglycemia, high creatine kinase level.

▼ *Key Point* Dogs may develop various clinical signs of hypothyroidism. Although one sign may predominate, cutaneous abnormalities, lethargy, and/or weight gain are present in most cases.

Diagnosis

Because of the diverse clinical signs and difficulty in interpreting thyroid function tests, hypothyroidism is often diagnosed inappropriately. Many nonthyroidal factors can influence thyroid function tests, resulting in low serum thyroid hormone concentrations in euthyroid dogs. Diagnosis is dependent on both compatible clinical signs and abnormal thyroid function tests, not either alone.

Screening Laboratory Tests

- Complete blood count shows normocytic, normochromic anemia in 30% of cases.
- Serum biochemical analysis shows hypercholesterolemia in 75% of cases. Hypertriglyceridemia is also common.

Basal Total Thyroid Hormone Concentration (T_4 and T_3)

- Normal serum thyroxine (T_4) concentration rarely occurs in the hypothyroid dog.
- Serum triiodothyronine (T_3) concentration is unreliable in the diagnosis of hypothyroidism since it is often within the reference range in hypothyroid dogs.
- Serum T_4 is often below normal in euthyroid dogs for the following reasons:
  - Normal daily fluctuation results in low serum T_4 in 50% of dogs on repeated sampling.
  - Breed differences result in low serum T_4 in greyhounds, deerhounds, Alaskan sled dogs, and probably other breeds.
  - Nonthyroidal illness (e.g., hyperadrenocorticism, renal disease, neoplasia) causes a decrease in total T_4 and T_3.
  - Administration of various drugs, including glucocorticoids, sulfonamides, anticonvulsants, nonsteroidal anti-inflammatory drugs, and radiocontrast agents, lowers serum T_4 and T_3.

▼ *Key Point* Low total T_4 concentration is almost always present in hypothyroidism. If total T_4 is normal, hypothyroidism is very unlikely.

Free Thyroxine Concentration

- Free T_4 is the portion of T_4 that is not bound to plasma carrier proteins (normally 0.1% of total T_4).
- Free T_4 is not affected by most nonthyroidal illnesses and drugs.
- Equilibrium dialysis is the only reliable method for measurement of free T_4 in dogs with nonthyroidal illness. Free T_4 by equilibrium dialysis is the most accurate single test for diagnosing hypothyroidism.

Serum Endogenous Canine Thyroid-Stimulating Hormone Concentration

- Serum TSH concentration is increased in most cases of primary hypothyroidism due to loss of negative feedback of T_4 and T_3 on the pituitary gland.
- High serum TSH and low serum T_4 or free T_4 are diagnostic of hypothyroidism.
- Serum TSH concentration is normal in 20–40% of hypothyroid dogs.
- Serum TSH concentration may be increased in euthyroid dogs with nonthyroidal illness.

Thyroid-Stimulating Hormone Stimulation Test

- The most reliable method of confirming the diagnosis of hypothyroidism in dogs is by demonstrating a low resting T_4 that fails to increase following TSH administration.
- Test protocol: Collect blood for measurement of serum T_4 before and 6 hours after intravenous (IV) administration of 0.1 unit/kg bovine TSH.
- TSH is difficult to obtain and expensive, making this test impractical in most cases.

Thyrotropin-Releasing Hormone Stimulation Test

- TRH administration results in a small and inconsistent increase in serum T_4 and free T_4 in dogs, making this test inadequate for routine use.
- Measurement of serum TSH after TRH administration may prove useful in the diagnosis of hypothyroidism, although preliminary studies have been disappointing.

Antithyroglobulin Antibodies

- Autoimmune thyroiditis is associated with serum antibodies directed against thyroglobulin.
- These antibodies can be present in normal dogs and dogs with other endocrine diseases, and their association with thyroiditis has not been proved.
- This assay has been proposed as a method to identify dogs affected with autoimmune thyroid disease prior to development of hypothyroidism to help plan breeding.

Thyroid Hormone Autoantibodies

- Antibodies occasionally form against T_3 and T_4 that interfere with radioimmunoassay of these hormones.
- These antibodies cause a false increase in T_3 or T_4 in most assays, with apparent elevation of the hormone into the hyperthyroid range.
- Dogs with thyroid hormone autoantibodies may or may not have signs of hypothyroidism.
- Measurement of free T_4 by equilibrium dialysis is not affected by T_4 autoantibodies.

Thyroid Biopsy

- Biopsy is an effective method of diagnosing lymphocytic thyroiditis, but assessment of thyroid function from a biopsy may be difficult because an incisional biopsy sample may not be representative of the entire thyroid gland.

▼ *Key Point* The most reliable method of confirming a diagnosis of hypothyroidism in a dog with compatible clinical signs is the demonstration of decreased serum total T_4 or free T_4 by equilibrium dialysis combined with elevated serum endogenous TSH.

Treatment

Treatment of dogs with hypothyroidism consists of daily administration of thyroid hormone. Response to treatment is usually noted within 1–2 weeks with an increase in activity and improvement in attitude. Weight loss and neurologic abnormalities usually begin to resolve within 1–4 weeks of initiating treatment, whereas dermatologic changes may require 4–6 weeks to improve and months to completely resolve. Failure to respond within 6–8 weeks of initiating treatment should prompt reevaluation of the diagnosis and reasons for possible therapeutic failure.

Synthetic L-Thyroxine

Synthetic L-thyroxine (L-T_4) is the treatment of choice in all cases of hypothyroidism. Synthetic L-triiodothyronine (L-T_3), combinations of synthetic L-T_4 and L-T_3, and desiccated thyroid gland preparations or extracts are not indicated in the treatment of canine hypothyroidism.

- The initial dosage of L-T_4 is 0.022 mg/kg q12h PO.
- Decrease the dosage slightly in dogs over 30 kg.
- Reevaluate after 6–8 weeks of treatment by examining for resolution of clinical signs and measuring serum T_4 and T_3.
- A serum T_4 concentration collected 4–6 hours after pill administration should be near the upper limit or slightly above the reference range; T_3 concentration may be low despite normal or high T_4.
- If signs of hyperthyroidism occur, such as polyuria, polydipsia, tachycardia, weight loss, diarrhea, or tachycardia, measure serum T_4 and T_3, and reduce the dosage based on this evaluation.
- Treatment for myxedema stupor and coma consists of IV administration of L-T_4 (0.66 mg/kg), passive warming, judicious fluid therapy, glucocorticoid supplementation, and mechanical ventilation if necessary. The prognosis is guarded.

HYPOTHYROIDISM IN CATS

▼ *Key Point* Spontaneous hypothyroidism is extremely uncommon in cats.

Most clinical cases of feline hypothyroidism occur as a result of treatment for hyperthyroidism—also a rare occurrence. Noniatrogenic feline hypothyroidism has been reported primarily in kittens with dwarfism. Cretinism is the most common cause of endocrine congenital dwarfism in cats (growth hormone deficiency has not been reported in cats). Adult onset spontaneous hypothyroidism has been proven in only 1 cat.

Etiology

- *Congenital hypothyroidism* is associated with thyroid gland atrophy or defective thyroid hormone biosynthesis. In many kittens, this may go undetected and may result in early death.
- *Primary iatrogenic hypothyroidism* results from surgical removal of thyroid glands or their destruction by radioactive iodine in the treatment of feline hyperthyroidism.

Clinical Signs

Congenital Hypothyroidism

- Disproportionate dwarfism (stunted growth of long bones, enlarged head).
- Lethargy and mental dullness.
- Hypothermia.
- Bradycardia.
- Bilaterally symmetric alopecia does *not* occur.

Primary Iatrogenic Hypothyroidism

- History of treatment for hyperthyroidism.
- Lethargy.
- Seborrhea sicca, dry haircoat.
- Obesity is common.
- Bilaterally symmetric alopecia does *not* occur.

Diagnosis

- Strong index of suspicion based on history and clinical signs.
- Confirmed by finding subnormal resting serum T_4 concentration that fails to increase 4–6 hours after IV administration of TSH (see Hypothyroidism in Dogs).
- Can also be confirmed by finding low serum concentrations of total T_4 and free T_4 (see Hypothyroidism in Dogs).
- Determination of serum TSH concentration is not generally useful in diagnosis of hypothyroidism in cats, inasmuch as most available TSH assays do not measure feline TSH.

Treatment

- Treatment for congenital cretinism is not very rewarding because growth abnormalities and mental deficiencies may not be reversible.
- Treatment for iatrogenic hypothyroidism involves daily T_4 supplementation.
  - The initial dosage of T_4 is 0.01–0.02 mg/kg (10–20 μg/kg) per day PO.
  - Adjust the dosage based on resolution of clinical signs and on postpill serum T_4 concentrations.

HYPERTHYROIDISM IN CATS

Feline hyperthyroidism, a multisystemic metabolic disorder resulting from excessive circulating concentrations of thyroid hormone, is the most common endocrinopathy of middle-aged and older cats. There is no breed or sex predilection. The clinical signs of the disease are the result of increased basal metabolic rate and the body's inability to meet excessive metabolic demands.

Etiology

Adenomatous Hyperplasia

Functional adenomatous hyperplasia of one or both lobes of the thyroid gland, causing high circulating concentrations of T_4 and T_3, is the most common cause. Both lobes are enlarged in approximately 70% of cases. The pathogenesis of this adenomatous hyperplasia is unknown.

- In cats, the disease most closely resembles toxic nodular goiter in human patients, which is caused by hyperfunctioning adenomatous thyroid nodules.
- Hyperthyroidism in cats is not analogous to the autoimmune disorder Graves disease, the most common form of hyperthyroidism in human patients.

Thyroid Carcinoma

Thyroid carcinoma occurs in only 1–2% of cats with hyperthyroidism.

Clinical Signs

All of the clinical manifestations of hyperthyroidism are due to the effects of excessive thyroid hormone. These effects are generally stimulatory. They cause increased heat production and heightened protein, carbohydrate, and lipid metabolism in virtually all body systems and tissues. Clinical signs can range from mild to severe (Table 29–2).

▼ *Key Point* The classic clinical signs of feline hyperthyroidism include weight loss despite an increase in appetite.

Table 29–2. FREQUENCY OF HISTORICAL AND CLINICAL SIGNS IN CATS WITH HYPERTHYROIDISM

Clinical Finding	Percent of Cats
Weight loss	95–98%
Hyperactivity/difficult to examine	70–80%
Polyphagia	65–75%
Tachycardia	55–65%
Polyuria/polydipsia	45–55%
Cardiac murmur	20–55%
Vomiting	33–50%
Diarrhea	30–45%
Increased fecal volume	10–30%
Decreased appetite	20–30%
Lethargy	15–25%
Polypnea (panting)	15–30%
Muscle weakness	15–20%
Muscle tremor	15–30%
Congestive heart failure	10–15%
Dyspnea	10–15%

General Appearance and Behavior

- Weight loss.
- Restlessness, hyperexcitability, difficult to examine.
- Impaired stress tolerance. The hyperthyroid cat is prone to respiratory distress and weakness when stressed. Cardiac arrhythmias or arrest can occur in extreme cases.
- Unkempt haircoat, excessive shedding and matting of hair, especially in longhaired cats.

Thyroid Gland

- Enlargement of one or both lobes of the thyroid gland is palpable in >90% of cats with hyperthyroidism. To palpate the thyroid gland, extend the cat's neck and tilt the head back slightly. Using the thumb and forefinger, gently palpate the tissues on either side of the trachea, starting at the larynx and moving caudally to the thoracic inlet.
- A small percentage of cats have intrathoracic thyroid nodules. These nodules evade palpation.

Nervous System and Muscle

- Hyperactivity.
- Weakness and increased fatigability.

Gastrointestinal System

- Increased appetite is due to increased energy utilization and high metabolic demands. The increased caloric intake observed in most cats is, however, inadequate to compensate for increased demand.
- Decreased appetite. Approximately 5% of cats with hyperthyroidism experience periods of decreased appetite. The cause is unclear but usually is associated with concurrent disease (e.g., renal or cardiac disease).
- Vomiting, often secondary to rapid polyphagia, occurs shortly after eating.
- Diarrhea and increased volume and frequency of defecation are due to polyphagia, intestinal hypermotility, and decreased fat absorption.

Renal System

- Polyuria and polydipsia. Thyroid hormones may have a diuretic action. Alternatively, a hypothalamic disturbance associated with hyperthyroidism might cause primary polydipsia, with secondary renal medullary solute washout.

Respiratory System

- Dyspnea, panting, and hyperventilation at rest are attributable to any of the following: respiratory muscle weakness, increased tissue carbon dioxide production and inability to meet tissue oxygen demand, and/or congestive heart failure (see subsequent discussion).

Cardiovascular System

- Tachycardia, systolic murmurs, gallop rhythm, and arrhythmias may be attributable to the catecholamine-like effects of thyroid hormone and increased tissue oxygen demand, or they may be associated with other signs of congestive heart failure (CHF) secondary to hyperthyroidism.

- Signs of CHF (e.g., dyspnea, muffled heart sounds, tachycardia, ascites) may develop, especially in cats with severe or advanced hyperthyroidism. Electrocardiographic and echocardiographic findings are often suggestive of hypertrophic, or, much less commonly, dilative cardiomyopathy. Hyperthyroidism results in a high-output cardiac state in which vascular resistance is low and cardiac output is high due to increased tissue metabolism and oxygen requirements. The cardiac compensatory mechanisms are dilation (in response to volume overload) and hypertrophy (in response to dilation). There also appears to be a direct myopathic effect of thyroid hormones on cardiac muscle.

Apathetic Hyperthyroidism

- In about 5% of cats with hyperthyroidism the predominant clinical signs are depression, lethargy, anorexia, and weakness rather than the hyperexcitability, restlessness, and polyphagia observed in 95% of cases.
- Weight loss and cardiac abnormalities are common findings in these cats.
- In most of these cats, a severe concurrent disease is also present, including CHF, renal failure, or cancer.

Diagnosis

The diagnosis of hyperthyroidism in cats is made on the basis of clinical signs; palpable goiter (thyroid enlargement); and, except in cases of occult hyperthyroidism (see subsequent discussion), high serum T_4 concentrations. Serum T_3 concentrations are less useful in the diagnosis of hyperthyroidism in cats.

The differential diagnoses for cats with clinical signs of hyperthyroidism include diabetes mellitus, renal disease, gastrointestinal lymphoma, and chronic inflammatory bowel disease. Cardiac manifestations of hyperthyroidism can be confused with cardiomyopathy. Hyperthyroid cats with high serum liver enzyme levels can be difficult to distinguish from cats with primary liver disease.

Screening Laboratory Tests

- Complete blood count
  - Mature leukocytosis and eosinopenia are common findings.
  - A slight elevation in packed cell volume is found in more than half of cats with hyperthyroidism. Macrocytic erythrocytes may cause an elevated mean corpuscular volume.
- Serum biochemical analysis
  - High alanine aminotransferase, aspartate aminotransferase, and alkaline phosphatase activity occur singly or in combination in 50–75% of cats with hyperthyroidism.

Thyroid Hormone Measurement

- High resting serum concentrations of T_4 and, less reliably, T_3 are the biochemical hallmark of hyperthyroidism in the majority of cats with the disease.
- Some cats (10–20%) maintain normal serum T_3 concentration despite elevation in T_4. These cats generally have milder disease; serum T_3 concentration in these cats is expected to increase eventually.
- Thyroid hormone concentrations in some cats are subject to a degree of fluctuation. In cats with mild disease, serum T_4 concentrations have been shown to fluctuate in and out of the normal range. The finding of a single normal serum T_4 concentration in a cat with clinical signs of hyperthyroidism does not rule out the diagnosis of this disease, especially if an enlarged thyroid can be palpated.
- Severe concurrent, systemic nonthyroidal illness (e.g., primary hepatic disease, renal disease, diabetes mellitus) can cause serum thyroid hormone concentrations to decrease. Because nonthyroidal illness is expected to reduce the serum thyroid hormone concentration into the subnormal range in a euthyroid cat, concomitant hyperthyroidism should be suspected in any middle-aged to old cat with high-normal serum T_4 concentration in the face of severe nonthyroidal illness, especially if clinical signs of hyperthyroidism are also present.

▼ **Key Point** In most cats with hyperthyroidism, the diagnosis can be confirmed by a high serum T_4 concentration alone.

Thyroid Radionuclide Uptake and Imaging

- Increased thyroidal uptake of radioiodine after the administration of a small tracer dose of radionuclide is a characteristic finding in cats with hyperthyroidism. However, the relative lack of nuclear medicine facilities available to small animal practitioners limits the usefulness of this diagnostic modality.
- Thyroid imaging (scanning) can be performed using either radioiodine or pertechnetate and is useful in delineating hyperfunctioning thyroid tissue. This technique is a helpful adjunct in the diagnosis of hyperthyroidism in cats and provides valuable preoperative information. The disadvantage is that nuclear medicine facilities are required.

Diagnosis of Occult Hyperthyroidism

Some cats with early or mild hyperthyroidism have high-normal resting serum T_4 concentration despite clinical signs of thyrotoxicosis. This condition is referred to as occult hyperthyroidism.

Basal Thyroid Hormone Determinations

If a high-normal serum T_4 concentration is found in a cat suspected of having hyperthyroidism, repeat the measurement a few weeks later. Fluctuation of thyroid hormone concentration in and out of the normal range has been documented in cats with early, mild hyperthyroidism.

Determination of Free Thyroxine by Dialysis

Determination of the serum concentration of free T_4 by dialysis (Free T_4 kit, Nichols Institute) is useful in the diagnosis of hyperthyroidism in cats, especially in those cats with clinical signs of the disease and a palpable thyroid nodule in which the basal total T_4 value is normal or only slightly elevated. In these cats with mild or occult hyperthyroidism, the free T_4 value is usually clearly elevated.

Cats with nonthyroidal disease usually maintain normal free T_4 concentrations; however, a false-positive elevation of free T_4 concentration also occurs in 5–10% of these sick cats without hyperthyroidism. Based on reported clinical studies, the following recommendations can be made regarding the use of free T_4 as a diagnostic test to identify cats with mild hyperthyroidism:

- Free T_4 by dialysis is a useful diagnostic test for hyperthyroidism and eliminates the need for provocative testing (T_3 suppression test or TRH stimulation test; see following section) in most cases. However, in order to interpret the test result, the cat *must* have clinical signs (i.e., weight loss despite a good appetite) and physical exam findings (i.e., a palpable thyroid nodule) that are consistent with hyperthyroidism.
- Always measure free T_4 in conjunction with a total T_4 determination. In cats with occult hyperthyroidism, the total T_4 concentration is expected to be in the mid to high end of the reference range limits (i.e., 2.5–4.0 μg/dl; 25 to 50 nmol/L).
- Never use free T_4 alone as the sole screening test for hyperthyroidism because high free T_4 concentrations also occasionally are found in cats with nonthyroidal diseases that do not have hyperthyroidism. The reason for high free T_4 concentrations in these cats with nonthyroidal disease is unclear, but almost all of these cats have serum total T_4 concentrations that are below or at the low end of the reference range.
- If a high free T_4 concentration is found in a cat without classic clinical signs of hyperthyroidism, and especially if a thyroid nodule cannot be palpated, repeat the tests (total and free T_4 determinations) in 2–4 weeks. Alternatively, use one of the provocative tests (T_3 suppression or TRH stimulation; see following section) to confirm hyperthyroidism.

Triiodothyronine Suppression Test

Administration of exogenous T_3 causes suppression of pituitary TSH secretion and a subsequent drop in thyroidal T_4 secretion in the normal cat. In cats with autonomously hyperfunctioning thyroid adenomas, TSH secretion has been chronically suppressed and exogenous T_3 administration does not appreciably affect the pituitary-thyroid axis. The protocol for the T_3 suppression test is as follows:

- Collect a blood sample for T_4 and T_3 measurements.
- Administer oral T_3 (liothyronine: Cytomel, Smith-Kline Beecham) starting the next morning at a dosage of 25 μg/cat q8h for 2 days.

- On the morning of the third day, give the cat a final 25-μg dose of T_3 before returning to the veterinarian for blood sampling.
- Measure serum T_4 and T_3 in the same assay run on both basal and postexogenous T_3 blood samples.
- In cats with hyperthyroidism, minimal, if any, suppression of serum T_4 occurs. A rise in serum T_3 concentration confirms owner compliance in administering the drug to the cat.

Thyrotropin-Releasing Hormone Stimulation Test

Administration of TRH stimulates pituitary TSH secretion and produces a subsequent rise in thyroidal T_4 secretion in the normal cat. In cats with autonomously hyperfunctioning thyroid adenomas, TSH secretion has been chronically suppressed and exogenous TRH administration does not appreciably effect the pituitary-thyroid axis. The protocol for the TRH stimulation test is as follows:

- Collect a blood sample for serum T_4 measurement.
- Administer TRH at a dosage of 0.1 mg/kg IV.
- Collect another blood sample for serum T_4 measurement 4 hours later.
- Although the effects are transient, TRH administration causes hypersalivation, tachypnea, and vomiting in most cats. However, this test is less time-consuming than the T_3 suppression test and does not rely on owner compliance.
- Interpretation:
  - Administration of TRH to normal cats and cats with nonthyroidal disease causes a twofold or greater increase in serum T_4 concentrations at 4 hours.
  - In contrast, serum T_4 concentration in cats with mild hyperthyroidism generally increases little, if at all, after administration of TRH.

Treatment

Treatment of hyperthyroidism in cats is usually rewarding and is aimed at reducing circulating concentrations of thyroid hormone. This is accomplished by blocking production of thyroid hormone from the thyroid gland or by destruction or removal of hyperfunctioning adenomatous thyroid tissue. Antithyroid drugs can be used effectively to block thyroid hormone synthesis but are not curative. Adenomatous thyroid tissue can be removed by surgical thyroidectomy or destroyed by radioiodine therapy. On return to euthyroidism, the clinical manifestations of thyrotoxicosis, including cardiac abnormalities, generally resolve completely. Azotemia may occur following treatment of hyperthyroidism by any method due to normalization of renal blood flow.

Antithyroid Drugs (Methimazole)

- Methimazole (Tapazole, Lilly) and propylthiouracil (PTU) are the two thiourylene antithyroid drugs available in the United States. Both are supplied in oral tablet form and act by inhibiting synthesis of thyroid hormones.
- Do not use PTU in cats. This drug produces a high incidence of mild to serious adverse effects including

anorexia, vomiting, lethargy, immune-mediated hemolytic anemia, thrombocytopenia, and development of serum antinuclear antibodies in both normal and hyperthyroid cats.

- Methimazole is better tolerated and safer than PTU in the cat and can be considered the antithyroid drug of choice for hyperthyroidism.

- Initially, administer methimazole at a dose of 5–15 mg/day PO, depending on the severity of the hyperthyroid state. Ideally, the methimazole dose is divided q8h–q12h. Some cats have been effectively managed by giving methimazole once a day.

- Perform complete blood counts, including platelet count, and serum T_4 determinations every 2 weeks during the first 3 months of drug therapy.

- Increase or decrease the daily drug dosage by 2.5–5 mg and continue further testing at 2- to 3-week intervals until the lowest daily dose is found that effectively maintains serum T_4 concentrations within the low-normal range.

- Mild clinical side effects associated with methimazole treatment are relatively common (approximately 15% of cats) and include anorexia, vomiting, and lethargy. Self-induced excoriations of the face and neck also may develop in a few cats within the first few weeks of therapy.

- A variety of hematologic abnormalities may develop in cats during treatment with methimazole. Those abnormalities that do not appear to be associated with any adverse clinical effects include eosinophilia, lymphocytosis, and transient leukopenia with normal differential count. More serious hematologic reactions that develop in a few cats treated with methimazole include severe thrombocytopenia, agranulocytosis (panleukopenia), and hemolytic anemia.

- If serious hematologic reactions develop during methimazole therapy, stop the drug and give supportive care. These adverse reactions should resolve within 5 days after the methimazole is withdrawn. Most life-threatening side effects usually develop quickly after beginning the drug again. If they occur, consider alternative therapy with surgery or radioiodine.

- Long-term antithyroid drug treatment has some advantages over surgery and radioiodine, including absence of certain complications such as postsurgical hypoparathyroidism. Unlike surgery and radioiodine, antithyroid drug therapy requires no advanced skills, training, or special licensing, and is a practical treatment choice for most practitioners.

▼ *Key Point* Daily antithyroid drugs can block T_4 secretion and control hyperthyroidism, but surgery or radioiodine can cure the disorder.

Alternative Drugs (Ipodate)

- Ipodate (Oragrafin Calcium granules, Squibb Diagnostics), a cholecystographic agent, is a feasible alternative to methimazole for medical treatment of some cats with hyperthyroidism, particularly those that cannot tolerate methimazole and are not candidates for surgery or radiotherapy.

- The drug's mechanism of action is inhibition of outer-ring 5′-deiodination of T_4 to the more active T_3, as well as some direct inhibitory effects on thyroid hormone secretion. Therefore, ipodate induces a rapid, marked decrease in serum T_3 concentration. Serum T_4 concentration usually does not change.

- Initial dosage of ipodate is 100 mg q24h PO. Monitor the drug's effects on clinical signs, body weight, heart rate, and serum T_3 concentrations. Increase the dosage of ipodate to 150–200 mg/day if serum T_3 remains high or a good clinical response is not observed at the lower dose.

- Adverse clinical signs attributable to ipodate treatment are uncommon.

- Cats with severe hyperthyroidism are less likely to respond to ipodate than are cats with mild or moderate disease. Cats in which serum T_3 concentration does not normalize are unlikely to have an adequate improvement in clinical signs.

Surgical Thyroidectomy

See under Thyroidectomy.
- Usually successful.
- Preoperative thyroid nuclear imaging is useful if available.
- The modified extracapsular method is most effective for removal of all diseased tissue.

▼ *Key Point* Use methimazole for 2–4 weeks preoperatively (if possible) to restore euthyroidism and to reduce the anesthetic and surgical risks, especially in cats with severe hyperthyroidism.

- Monitor for postoperative hypocalcemia secondary to removal or damage of parathyroid glands (only a risk following bilateral thyroidectomy).
- Postoperative laryngeal paralysis due to recurrent laryngeal nerve damage occurs uncommonly.
- After bilateral thyroidectomy, serum T_4 concentration is often below normal, but thyroid hormone supplementation is rarely needed longer than 2–3 months. Permanent, surgically induced hypothyroidism in cats is rare. Long-term T_4 replacement is needed only in those cats that develop clinical signs of hypothyroidism (e.g., lethargy, weight gain, dermatopathy) or azotemia together with persistently low serum T_4 concentrations.

Radioactive Iodine (^{131}I) Therapy

- Usually successful.
- No preoperative medication or anesthesia is needed.
- Lowest incidence of side effects of any treatment modality.
- Requires adherence to strict radiation safety regulations.
- Treatment protocols vary depending on facility used and severity of disease.
- Main disadvantage is long hospitalization time required (generally 1–2 weeks).
- Often expensive.

THYROID NEOPLASIA IN DOGS

Unlike thyroid tumors found in the cat, the majority of thyroid neoplasms in dogs do not secrete excessive thyroid hormone. Less than 20% of these tumors are associated with hyperthyroidism. Because these tumors can destroy normal thyroid parenchyma, hypothyroidism sometimes occurs.

▼ *Key Point* Most canine thyroid tumors, unlike feline thyroid tumors, are large, invasive carcinomas.

About 90% of thyroid tumors in dogs are malignant. Local invasion into the larynx; trachea; cervical muscles, vessels, and nerves; and esophagus frequently occurs. Distant metastasis, especially to the lungs, occurs in 60–80% of cases. The prognosis associated with most of these tumors is poor.

Clinical Signs

See Table 29–3.

Nonthyrotoxic Thyroid Tumors

Clinical signs are related to structural damage to the cervical area and metastatic disease.

- A palpable cervical mass (goiter) is often hard and attached to surrounding soft tissues and irregular in shape.
- Respiratory distress, cough.
- Vomiting.
- Dysphagia.
- Anorexia.
- Weight loss.

Hyperfunctional Thyroid Tumors

See Hyperthyroidism in Cats for explanation of similar signs.

- A palpable cervical mass (goiter) is often hard and attached to surrounding soft tissues and irregular in shape.
- Polydipsia, polyuria (common).
- Weight loss.
- Polyphagia.
- Heat and stress intolerance.
- Nervousness, hyperexcitability.
- Diarrhea, increased volume of feces.
- Tremors.

▼ *Key Point* In dogs, most thyroid tumors that result in hyperthyroidism are malignant (carcinoma). Polydipsia and polyuria are very prominent clinical signs.

Diagnosis

Thyroid carcinoma is suspected in any dog with a ventral cervical mass.

- *Thyroid gland biopsy* is mandatory for the diagnosis of thyroid carcinoma.

Table 29–3. INCIDENCE OF CLINICAL SIGNS IN DOGS WITH THYROID TUMOR

Sign	Percent of Cases
Nontoxic (euthyroid or hypothyroid) thyroid tumor	
Goiter (enlarged thyroid gland)	100%
Respiratory distress/cough	30%
Metastases to lung or lymph nodes	35%
Vomiting	10%
Dysphagia	10%
Anorexia	10%
Weight loss	5%
Hyperfunctional (hyperthyroid) thyroid tumor	
Goiter	100%
Polydipsia and polyuria	95%
Weight loss	80%
Weakness and fatigue	75%
Polyphagia	70%
Heat intolerance	60%
Nervousness	50%
Hyperdefecation/diarrhea	30%
Tremor	20%

- *Screening laboratory tests* are indicated.
- *Thoracic radiography* is an essential part of the diagnostic workup because pulmonary metastasis occurs commonly.
- *Serum thyroid hormone concentrations* are indicated when clinical signs suggest hyperthyroidism or hypothyroidism.
- *Thyroid imaging (thyroid scan)* can be useful in determining the size and location of neoplastic thyroid tissue.

Treatment

The prognosis for a dog with thyroid carcinoma depends on the developmental stage, size and palpable characteristics of the tumor. Small, movable tumors that have not metastasized can sometimes be cured by surgical excision. For dogs with more invasive or metastatic tumors, the prognosis is usually poor and treatment is rarely curative regardless of the modality.

Surgery

See under Thyroidectomy.

- Thyroidectomy can be a difficult procedure.
- Complete excision of a thyroid carcinoma is uncommon.

Chemotherapy

- Doxorubicin 30 mg/m^2 body surface area (for conversion table, see Chap. 24), IV, every 3 weeks for five treatments.
- A potentially limiting long-term side effect of doxorubicin is congestive cardiomyopathy.
- Combination treatment with doxorubicin and cyclophosphamide has been used with varying degrees of success and with less cardiac toxicity.

External Beam (Cobalt) Irradiation

- Useful adjunct therapy for thyroid carcinoma.
- Combination of surgical debulking followed by external irradiation may be considered in those cases in which most of the tumor was resected.

Radioactive Iodine

- Administration of large doses of ^{131}I (10–100 mCi) can temporarily control hyperfunctional thyroid carcinoma and can lead to palliation of clinical signs of hyperthyroidism. However, this treatment will most likely fail to control metastatic growth.
- Radioiodine does not work well in dogs with nontoxic thyroid tumors that have a low degree of radioiodine uptake.

THYROIDECTOMY

Thyroidectomy in dogs and cats is usually performed to treat neoplasia of the gland. Biopsy is occasionally performed but not as commonly as the complete removal of one or both lobes. A thorough understanding of thyroid anatomy and physiology is necessary before performing surgery.

Anatomy

Thyroid

- The thyroid gland consists of two lobes located just caudal to the larynx.
- The normal gland is a pale tan color and approximately 1–1.5 cm in length.
- Blood supply is via the cranial thyroid artery (branch of the common carotid artery (Fig. 29–1). The caudal thyroid artery is absent in cats. Venous drainage is via cranial and caudal thyroid veins.
- The thyroid gland has a distinct but thin capsule.

Parathyroid

- Two parathyroid glands are associated with each thyroid lobe: one intracapsular (internal) and one ex-

tracapsular (external). The extracapsular parathyroid gland is usually located at the cranial pole of the thyroid.
- The parathyroid is usually off-white and can be confused with fat; the gland is usually 2–5 mm in length.
- Blood supply to the parathyroid glands is also from the cranial thyroid artery.
- Only one functional parathyroid gland is required for normocalcemia.

Thyroidectomy in the Cat

Preoperative Considerations

- If available, review the thyroid radionuclide scan to determine the extent of the disease (e.g., Is the tumor unilateral or bilateral? Are ectopic tumors present?).
- Hyperthyroidism is a multisystemic disease that can be associated with anesthetic and surgical complications.
- In addition to establishing euthyroidism with antithyroid drugs (see earlier in this chapter), correct dehydration preoperatively if necessary.
- Obtain thoracic radiographs to evaluate the heart's size and the presence of any pulmonary problems or mediastinal masses.
- Anesthesia (see Chap. 2 for drug dosages and other specifics).
  - Premedicate with acepromazine. Avoid anticholinergics, such as atropine and glycopyrrolate.
  - Induce with a thiobarbiturate IV.
  - Maintain anesthesia with isoflurane and oxygen via a cuffed endotracheal tube.
  - Closely monitor the electrocardiogram for arrhythmias.
  - Have propranolol (Inderal, Wyeth-Ayerst) ready in the event that premature ventricular contractions develop. Dilute to make a solution of 0.1 mg/ml and give 0.01 mg IV slowly (over 3–5 minutes).

Surgical Procedure

Objectives

1. Remove all abnormal thyroid tissue.
2. Maintain meticulous hemostasis.
3. Preserve at least one of the parathyroid glands.
4. Avoid injury to the recurrent laryngeal nerves.

Equipment

1. Standard surgical pack
2. Bipolar cautery
3. Tenotomy scissors
4. Sterile cotton-tipped applicators
5. Gelfoam

Technique

1. Place the cat in dorsal recumbency with the front legs tied caudally and the neck slightly hyperextended over a rolled towel.
2. Prepare the ventral cervical region from caudal mandibles to manubrium for aseptic surgery.

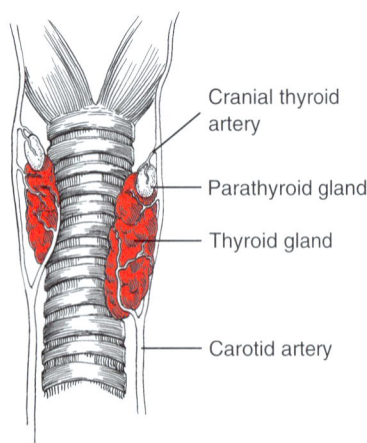

Cranial thyroid artery

Parathyroid gland

Thyroid gland

Carotid artery

Figure 29–1.   Gross appearance of bilateral thyroid tumors in a cat.

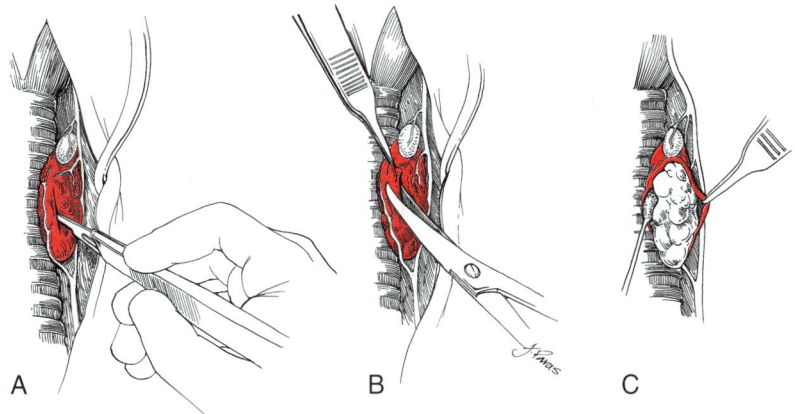

Figure 29-2. Intracapsular dissection for removal of a thyroid tumor in a cat. Make a nick incision *(A)* in a relatively avascular area of the thyroid capsule and extend the incision with scissors *(B)*. Bluntly remove the gland from the capsule using a sterile cotton-tipped applicator *(C)*. Ligate or cauterize blood vessels as necessary.

3. Incise the skin on the ventral cervical midline from larynx to manubrium.
4. Separate the paired sternohyoideus and sternothyroideus muscles and retract the muscles with self-retaining retractors.
5. Carefully examine both thyroid lobes. Remove the affected lobes. If doubt exists as to involvement of a lobe, remove it because microscopic adenomatous hyperplasia may be present.
6. Attempt to identify the parathyroid glands.
7. Ligate the caudal thyroid vein and grasp the caudal aspect of the capsule.
8. Perform dissection as shown in Figures 29-2 and 29-3. Use the intracapsular technique if the parathyroid glands are not visible (see Fig. 29-2). When implementing the intracapsular technique, be sure to remove all remnants of thyroid tissue that may remain attached to the capsule. Use the extracapsular technique if the parathyroid glands are visible and can be easily separated from the thyroid (see Fig. 29-3). If a parathyroid gland is accidentally removed, place it in a small incision in one of the sternohyoideus muscles. Maintain meticulous hemosta-

sis with judicious use of bipolar cautery and small pieces of Gelfoam.
9. Routinely close muscle, subcutaneous tissue, and skin. This is the same as that in the dog, as discussed in the section that follows.

Postoperative Care and Complications

- Monitor for hypothermia, hemorrhage at the incision site, and hypocalcemia.
- Hypoparathyroidism
  - Rare with careful surgical technique (5% incidence of hypocalcemic tetany).
  - Check serum calcium concentrations for 48 hours postoperatively or longer if the concentration is dropping.
  - Monitor for tetany if calcium concentration is dropping.
  - Treatment of hypoparathyroidism is described in Chapter 30.
- Thyroid hormone replacement (see previous discussion on iatrogenic feline hypothyroidism).
- Relapse of hyperthyroidism is rare (10% incidence, 2-3 years postoperatively) but does occur, probably because of the incomplete removal of adenomatous tissue. Treat by surgical removal of remaining thyroid tissue. The incidence of hypoparathyroidism is higher than with the first surgery.

Thyroidectomy in the Dog
Preoperative Considerations

- Accurate preoperative diagnosis is important. Carefully palpate the tumor. Small, movable tumors are usually amenable to surgical resection. Fine-needle aspirate or tissue biopsy of the thyroid tumor helps establish the type of tumor.

▼ *Key Point* Biopsy of thyroid tumors in the dog can result in significant hemorrhage. Observe the patient closely after biopsy.

- Cervical radiographs may be helpful to determine tracheal displacement or tumor calcification. Thoracic radiographs are mandatory to rule out pulmonary metastasis or other cardiopulmonary disorder.

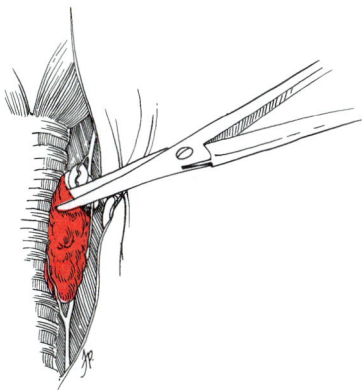

Figure 29-3. Extracapsular dissection for removal of a thyroid lobe in a cat. Incise the thyroid capsule immediately adjacent to the parathyroid gland. Carefully cauterize capsular blood vessels, if necessary. Bluntly separate the thyroid gland from the parathyroid gland using a sterile cotton-tipped applicator. After ligating or cauterizing blood vessels as necessary, remove the thyroid gland and its capsule.

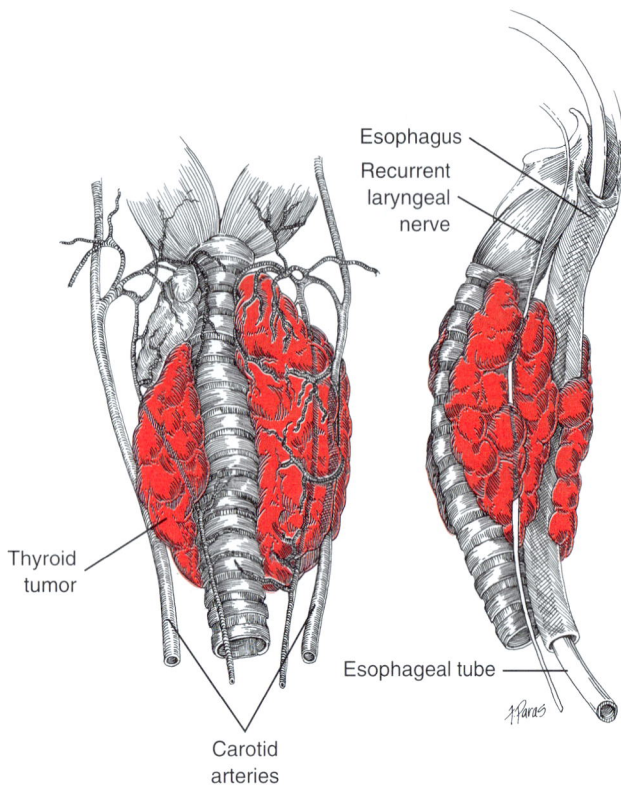

Figure 29–4. Gross appearance of an invasive thyroid carcinoma in a dog.

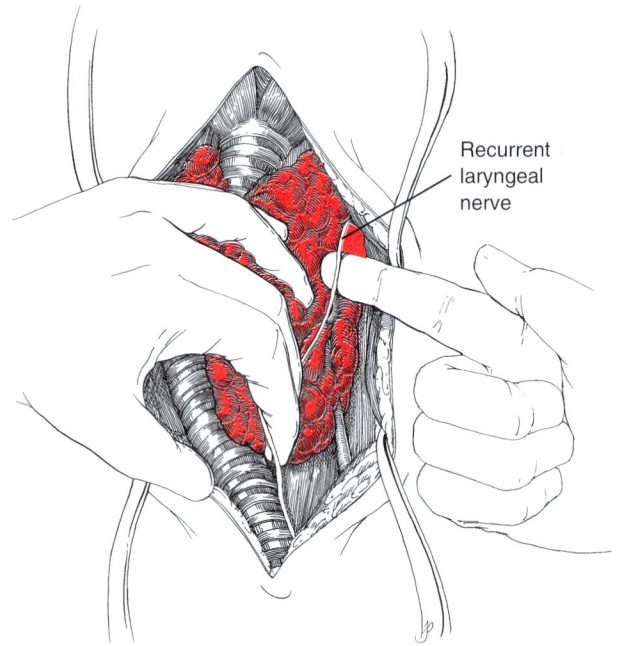

Figure 29–5. Remove canine thyroid tumors with a combination of blunt and sharp dissection. Finger dissection of the tumor and surrounding structures may be necessary for large invasive tumors. Be careful when handling the recurrent laryngeal nerve to avoid the possibility of postoperative laryngeal paralysis.

Surgical Procedure

Objectives

1. Completely remove or debulk the thyroid mass.
2. Preserve at least one parathyroid gland.
3. Minimize blood loss.
4. Preserve recurrent laryngeal nerves.

Equipment

1. Standard general surgical pack and sutures
2. Gelpi or Weitlaner retractors
3. Army-Navy retractors
4. Penrose drains

Technique

1. Patient preparation and surgical approach are the same as those described for the cat.
2. Dissection
   a. These tumors are very vascular, and dissection is difficult.
   b. Avoid injury to the esophagus, carotid artery, jugular vein, vagosympathetic trunk, and recurrent laryngeal nerve (Fig. 29–4).
   c. A stomach tube or small endotracheal tube in the esophagus helps identify this structure.
   d. Ligate or cauterize the extensive vascular network and carefully dissect out the tumor (Fig. 29–5).
   e. If possible, identify and preserve the parathyroid glands. With large malignant tumors, this may be impossible.
   f. If complete removal is impossible, debulk the mass, leaving the portion closest to the larynx intact to preserve the parathyroid glands.
3. Closure
   a. Place Penrose drains if significant dead space results from tumor removal. Have the drains exit through separate stab incisions in the caudal, ventral neck.
   b. Close the muscle routinely with simple continuous, absorbable suture; the subcutaneous tissue with simple continuous, absorbable suture; and the skin with simple interrupted, nonabsorbable suture.

Postoperative Care and Complications

Short-Term

- Closely monitor for hemorrhage or seroma formation.
- Check serum calcium concentrations at least 2–4 days postoperatively if a bilateral thyroidectomy was performed. Monitor the calcium concentrations longer if decreasing.
  - Treat hypoparathyroidism if necessary, according to the guidelines in Chapter 30.
- Check serum T_3 and T_4 levels if bilateral thyroidectomy is performed.
  - Treat hypothyroidism if present (see previous discussion of hypothyroidism).

Long-Term

- Reevaluate the dog frequently (every 3 months) for recurrence of the primary tumor and metastasis.

- Consider postoperative chemotherapy or radiotherapy if the tumor was malignant (see previous discussion on treatment of thyroid tumors and Chap. 24 on chemotherapy).

SUPPLEMENTAL READINGS

Birchard SJ, Peterson ME, Jacobson A: Surgical treatment of feline hyperthyroidism: Results of 85 cases. J Am Anim Hosp Assoc 20:705, 1984.

Chastain CB, Panciera DL: Hypothyroid diseases. *In* Ettinger SJ, Feldman EC, eds.: Textbook of Veterinary Internal Medicine, 4th Ed. Philadelphia: WB Saunders, 1995, pp 1487–1500.

Feldman EC, Nelson RW: Hypothyroidism. *In* Feldman EC, Nelson RW: Canine and Feline Endocrinology and Reproduction, 2nd Ed. Philadelphia: WB Saunders, 1996, pp 68–117.

Ferguson DC: Update on diagnosis of canine hypothyroidism. Vet Clin North Am 24:515, 1994.

Harari J, Patterson JS, Rosenthal RC: Clinical and pathologic features of thyroid tumors in 26 dogs. J Am Vet Med Assoc 188:1160, 1986.

Jaggy A, Oliver JE, Ferguson DC, et al: Neurological manifestations of hypothyroidism: A retrospective study of 29 dogs. J Vet Intern Med 8:328, 1994.

Murray LAS, Peterson ME: Ipodate treatment of hyperthyroidism in cats. J Am Vet Med Assoc 211:63, 1997.

Panciera DL: A retrospective study of 66 cases of canine hypothyroidism. J Am Vet Med Assoc 204:761, 1994.

Panciera DL, Johnson GS: Plasma von Willebrand factor antigen concentration and buccal mucosal bleeding time in dogs with experimental hypothyroidism. J Vet Intern Med 10:60, 1996.

Peterson ME: Hyperthyroid diseases. *In* Ettinger SJ, Feldman EC, eds. Textbook of Veterinary Internal Medicine: Diseases of the Dog and Cat. Philadelphia: WB Saunders, 1995, pp 1466–1487.

Peterson ME, Becker DV: Radioiodine treatment of 524 cats with hyperthyroidism. J Am Vet Med Assoc 207:1422, 1995.

Peterson ME, Broussard JD, Gamble DA: Use of the thyrotropin releasing hormone stimulation test to diagnose mild hyperthyroidism in cats. J Vet Intern Med 8:279, 1994.

Peterson ME, Graves TK, Gamble DA: Triiodothyronine (T$_3$) suppression test: An aid in the diagnosis of mild hyperthyroidism in cats. J Vet Intern Med 4:233, 1990.

Peterson ME, Kintzer PP, Cavanagh PG, et al.: Feline hyperthyroidism: Pretreatment clinical and laboratory evaluation of 131 cases. J Am Vet Med Assoc 183:103, 1983.

Peterson ME, Kintzer PP, Hurvitz AI: Methimazole treatment of 262 cats with hyperthyroidism. J Vet Intern Med 2:150, 1988.

Peterson ME, Kintzer PP, Becker DV, Hurley JM: Radioactive iodine treatment of a functional thyroid carcinoma producing hyperthyroidism in a dog. J Vet Intern Med 3:20, 1989.

Peterson ME: Feline hypothyroidism. *In* Kirk RW, Bonagura JD, eds.: Current Veterinary Therapy X. Philadelphia: WB Saunders, 1989, p 1000.

Refsal KR, Nachreiner RF: Monitoring thyroid hormone replacement therapy. *In* Bonagura JD, ed.: Kirk's Current Veterinary Therapy, 12th Ed. Philadelphia: WB Saunders, 1995, pp 364–368.

Rijnberk A, Leav I: Thyroid tumors. *In* Kirk RW, ed.: Current Veterinary Therapy X. Philadelphia: WB Saunders, 1977, p 1020.

Welches CD, Scavelli TD, Matthiesen DT, Peterson ME: Occurrence of problems after three techniques of bilateral thyroidectomy in cats. Vet Surg 18:392, 1989.

30 Diseases of the Parathyroid Gland and Calcium Metabolism

Marcia Carothers / Dennis Chew / Tom Van Gundy

NORMAL CALCIUM METABOLISM

The calcium ion is a major component of bone and is very important in many biologic processes such as muscle contraction, blood coagulation, neural excitability, membrane permeability, and enzyme activity. Although calcium is the most abundant electrolyte in the body, most of this ion is present in the skeleton and is not available for immediate use.

Distribution

There are three major fractions of serum calcium: protein-bound, ionized (or free), and complex-bound calcium.

Protein-Bound Calcium. This fraction accounts for approximately 40% of the total serum calcium concentration. Albumin is the primary protein bound to calcium; this binding increases as the pH increases and decreases as the pH decreases.

Ionized or Free Calcium. This is the biologically active form of calcium and makes up approximately 50% of the total serum calcium concentration.

Complex-Bound Calcium. Complex-bound calcium composes approximately 10% of the total serum calcium concentration. This form is bound to anions such as lactates, bicarbonates, citrates, and sulfates.

▼ *Key Point* The partitioning of calcium is influenced by the amount of calcium entering and leaving the extracellular fluid, the quantity of protein available for binding, the amount of complexes available for binding, and the acid-base status.

Regulation of Calcium

Calcium levels are regulated primarily through the actions of three hormones: parathyroid hormone (PTH), calcitonin, and vitamin D.

Parathyroid Hormone

PTH is produced by the chief cells of the parathyroid glands and is the principal hormone that controls minute-to-minute regulation of serum calcium concentration. Secretion of this hormone is stimulated by hypocalcemia. Hydroxylation of 25-hydroxycholecalciferol to 1,25-dihydroxycholecalciferol and other vitamin D metabolites is partially regulated by PTH. The major target organs are bone and kidneys.

- *Bone*—PTH mobilizes calcium from the skeletal reserves to the extracellular fluid.
- *Kidney*—PTH has a direct effect on renal tubular function, leading to decreased phosphate resorption and phosphaturia and increased resorption of calcium.

▼ *Key Point* The net effect of PTH is to increase serum calcium and decrease serum phosphorus concentrations.

Calcitonin

This polypeptide is secreted by the C (parafollicular) cells of the thyroid glands. The rate of secretion increases with increased calcium concentration. Bone and kidneys are the major target organs.

- *Bone*—Calcitonin blocks bone resorption by inhibiting the release of calcium and phosphorus from bone.
- *Kidney*—Calcitonin decreases the resorption of phosphorus and calcium.

▼ *Key Point* The net effect of calcitonin is to decrease the serum calcium and phosphorus concentrations.

Vitamin D

Vitamin D (ergosterol and cholecalciferol) primarily affects bone, intestines, and kidneys following activation to $1,25(OH)_2$ vitamin D (calcitriol). Small amounts of 1,25-dihydroxycholecalciferol (the active metabolite of vitamin D) are necessary for the PTH effect on bone (permissive effect).

- *Bone*—Calcitriol stimulates osteoclastic calcium mobilization and resorption of bone.
- *Intestine*—Calcitriol increases calcium, phosphorus, and magnesium absorption.
- *Kidney*—Calcitriol increases renal tubular resorption of calcium and phosphorus.

▼ *Key Point* The net effect of calcitriol is to increase both serum calcium and phosphorus concentrations.

Table 30–1. ROUTINE LABORATORY AND SERUM HORMONE ASSAY RESULTS OF CALCIUM METABOLISM IN DISEASE STATES ASSOCIATED WITH HYPERCALCEMIA AND HYPOCALCEMIA

Disorder	Total Calcium	Ionized Calcium	Phosphorus	Creatinine	PTH	Calcitriol	25(OH)-D	PTHrP
Primary hyperparathyroidism	↑	↑	−, ↓	−, ↑	↑	−, ↑	−	−
Secondary hyperparathyroidism								
Nutritional	↓, −	↓, −	↑, −	−	↑	↓, −	−	−
Renal, chronic	−	−, ↓	↑, −	↑	↑	↓, −	−	−
Renal, chronic	↓	↓	↑, −	↑	↑	↓, −	−	−
Renal, chronic	↑	↓, −, ↑	↑, −	↑	↑	↓, −	−	−
Renal, acute	↓, −	↓, −	↑, −	↑	↑	↓, −	−	−
Malignancy-associated hypercalcemia								
Humoral	↑	↑	−, ↓	−	↓, −	↓, −, ↑	−	↑
Local osteolytic	↑	↑	↑, −	−	↓	↓	−	−
Elevations in vitamin D metabolites								
Cholecalciferol toxicity	↑	↑	↑, −	−, ↑	↓	−, ↑	↑↑	−
Lymphosarcoma	↑	↑	−, ↓	−	↓	↑	−	↑
Granulomatous inflammation	↑	↑	−, ↑	−	↓	↑	−	−
Addison disease	↑	−, ↑	−, ↑	↑, −	↓	−	−	−
Dehydration	↑	↑, −	−	−, ↑	↓	−	−	−
Primary hypoparathyroidism	↓	↓	↑, −	−	↓	−, ↓	−	−
Hypoalbuminemia	↓	−, ↓	−	−	−	−	−	−
Hypovitaminosis D	↓	↓	−	−	−, ↑	↓	↓	−
Eclampsia	↓	↓	−, ↓	−	↑	↑	−	−

Key: ↑, high concentration; ↓, low concentration; −, normal or no change.

From: Chew DJ, Nagode LA, Rosol TJ, et al: Utility of diagnostic assays in the evaluation of hypercalcemia and hypocalcemia: Parathyroid hormone, vitamin D metabolites, parathyroid hormone–related protein, and ionized calcium. In Bonagura JD, Kirk RW, eds: Kirk's Current Veterinary Therapy XII. Philadelphia: WB Saunders, 1995, p. 379.

DIAGNOSTIC TESTS OF CALCIUM METABOLISM

Measurement of total calcium, ionized calcium, and hormones of calcium metabolism aid in the diagnosis of calcium disorders (see Table 30–1).

Total Serum Calcium

Total serum calcium concentration is part of most routine serum profile evaluations.

Colorimetric Method. Colorimetric measurements of serum calcium are subject to spurious elevation of calcium if lipemia or hemolysis is present.

Potentiometry. This ion-selective method has the advantage of measuring total and ionized calcium concentrations. However, this technique requires special handling of the sample to maintain anaerobic conditions.

Corrected Total Calcium Values. These are calculated to adjust for abnormalities in serum protein or albumin concentrations. The following formulas are helpful guidelines for interpreting serum calcium under conditions of hypoproteinemia or hypoalbuminemia, but they have not been verified using ionized calcium measurements. These formulas are based on a linear relationship between calcium and albumin (i.e., as albumin increases or decreases, so does total calcium concentration). The linear relationship is not seen in the cat, suggesting that these formulas are invalid for this species.

$$\text{Corrected total Ca (mg/dl)} = \text{Serum total Ca (mg/dl)} - \text{Serum albumin (g/dl)} + 3.5$$

or

$$\text{Corrected total Ca (mg/dl)} = \text{Serum total Ca (mg/dl)} - 0.4\,[\text{Serum total protein (g/dl)}] + 3.3$$

Ionized Calcium Concentration

- Ion-selective methods are more readily available in some laboratories. Special handling of the serum or heparinized plasma sample is necessary to prevent lowering of ionized calcium due to pH increases. Serum samples appear to be stable for 72 hours at 4°C if handled anaerobically.
- A hand-held analyzer (I-STAT, Heska Corp., Fort Collins, Colorado) is now available for cage-side analyses. Use whole blood or heparinized whole blood samples to obtain not only ionized calcium concentrations but also sodium, potassium, chloride, pH, PO_2, and packed cell volume evaluations. A venous sample from a free-flowing vessel (e.g., jugular vein) provides an accurate ionized calcium concentration.

Parathyroid Hormone

- The PTH molecule is composed of three portions (amino-terminus, mid-molecule, and carboxy-terminus). The amino-terminus is the biologically active portion of the molecule. All three portions can be assayed, and a two-site assay has been developed to detect both the amino-terminus and carboxy-terminus (intact PTH).

- PTH fragments are excreted by the kidneys. In animals with renal failure, elevations of the inactive fragments may overrepresent the amount of intact, active PTH. Therefore, use only intact molecule or amino-terminus assays in animals with renal disease or failure.

Parathyroid Hormone–Related Protein

Parathyroid hormone–related protein (PTH-rP) is a hormone isolated from some malignant neoplasms in animals with hypercalcemia. This hormone can bind to PTH receptors in the kidneys and bone and result in humoral hypercalcemia of malignancy (HHM). A protease inhibitor (aprotinin) is necessary to prevent degradation of the molecule. Amino-terminus and two-site assays are useful in dogs and cats with HHM.

Vitamin D Metabolites

25-Hydroxycholecalciferol (Calcidiol). This steroid can be assayed by radioimmunoassay and competitive protein-binding techniques. There is no species difference with this steroid, and the assays are useful in both dogs and cats. Samples should be protected from light because vitamin D metabolites are light-sensitive.

1,25-Dihydroxycholecalciferol (Calcitriol). This vitamin D metabolite is the most active metabolite and circulates in low concentrations. A radioreceptor assay has been developed to measure this; however, owing to the expense of the kit, the test is not readily available.

HYPERCALCEMIA

The definition of hypercalcemia is a fasting serum total calcium concentration >12.0 mg/dl in dogs and >11.0 mg/dl in cats. Young dogs may have a mild hypercalcemia (usually <13.0 mg/dl) related to skeletal growth. Lipemic and/or hemolyzed blood samples may result in spurious elevations of calcium; interpret with caution.

Etiology

See Table 30–2 for a list of hypercalcemia-related conditions.

Clinical Signs

Clinical signs in hypercalcemia depend on the magnitude of the calcium elevation, how quickly the hypercalcemia developed, and the duration of the hypercalcemia. Serum total calcium concentrations of <15 mg/dl may not be associated with systemic signs; however, serum concentrations of >18 mg/dl are often associated with severe life-threatening signs. Abnormalities in sodium and potassium may magnify clinical signs of hypercalcemia because of their effects on cell membrane permeability, particularly in nerve and muscle. Soft tissue mineralization may occur with prolonged hypercalcemia when the product of calcium (mg/dl) times phosphorus (mg/dl) equals 70.

Table 30–2. CONDITIONS ASSOCIATED WITH HYPERCALCEMIA

Nonpathologic Conditions
Lipemia
Nonfasted serum samples
Young growing dogs
Laboratory error or improper handling of sample

Transient Conditions
Hemoconcentration
Hyperproteinemia

Pathologic Conditions
Malignancy-associated hypercalcemia
   Lymphoma
   Adenocarcinoma of the apocrine glands of the anal sac
   Multiple myeloma
   Metastatic bone tumors
   Miscellaneous tumors (lymphocytic leukemia, mammary carcinoma, fibrosarcoma, pancreatic adenocarcinoma, testicular interstitial cell tumor, lung carcinoma, squamous cell carcinoma, thyroid adenocarcinoma, and osteosarcoma)
Hypoadrenocorticism
Renal failure
Hypervitaminosis D
   Cholecalciferol (rodenticide) toxicity
   Iatrogenic—dietary supplementation
   Houseplants (*Cestrum diurnum*, day-blooming jessamine, *Solanum malocoxylon*, *Triestum flavescens*)
   Granulomatous disease—blastomycosis
Primary hyperparathyroidism
Bone lesions—sepsis, disuse osteoporosis
Severe hypothermia

- Polydipsia and polyuria are the most common signs of hypercalcemia, owing to direct stimulation of the thirst center and a decreased ability of the kidneys to concentrate the urine.
- Anorexia, vomiting, and constipation can result from decreased excitability of gastrointestinal smooth muscle.
- Generalized weakness may develop from decreased muscle excitability.
- Depression, muscle twitching, and seizures can occur as neurologic manifestations.
- Cardiac arrhythmias can develop from direct effects on the myocardium or secondary to cardiac mineralization.

Diagnostic Evaluation

Abnormalities depend on the underlying cause, severity, and duration of the hypercalcemia (see later under Conditions Associated with Hypercalcemia).

History and Physical Examination. A complete history and thorough physical examination are essential to the diagnosis of the cause of the hypercalcemia.

Laboratory Tests. Tests such as serum calcium assay, complete blood count (CBC), and serum chemistry profile can aid in the diagnosis (see previous section, Diagnostic Tests of Calcium Metabolism).

Radiography. Soft tissue mineralization of the kidneys, heart, lungs, stomach, and other tissues may be detected radiographically.

Electrocardiography. Prolongation of the PR interval, shortening of the QT interval, and cardiac arrhyth-

Table 30–3. TREATMENT OF HYPERCALCEMIA

Treatment	Dose	Indications	Comments
Volume Expansion			
SC saline (0.9%)*	75–100 ml/kg/day	Mild hypercalcemia	Contraindicated if peripheral edema is present
IV saline (0.9%)*	100–125 ml/kg/day	Moderate to severe hypercalcemia	Contraindicated in congestive heart failure and hypertension
Diuretics			
Furosemide (Lasix, Hoechst Marion Roussel)	2–4 mg/kg initially q12h, then q8h IV, SC, or PO	Moderate to severe hypercalcemia	Volume expansion necessary prior to use of this drug
Alkalinizing Agent			
Sodium bicarbonate	1 mEq/kg IV slow bolus; may continue at $0.3 \times$ base deficit $\times$ kg per day	Severe hypercalcemia	Requires close monitoring
Glucocorticoids			
Prednisone	1–2.2 mg/kg q12h PO, SC, or IV	Moderate to severe hypercalcemia	Do not use these drugs prior to identification of etiology; may make definitive diagnosis difficult
Dexamethasone (Azium, Schering Plough)	0.1–0.22 mg/kg q12h IV or SC		
Bone Resorption Inhibitors			
Calcitonin (Calcimar, Rhone-Poulenc-Rorer)	4–6 IU/kg SC initially q12h, then q8h	Hypervitaminosis D toxicity	Response may be short-lived; vomiting may occur
Bisphosphonates			
Etidronate (Didronel, Norwich Eaton)	5–10 mg/kg daily to q12h	Moderate to severe hypercalcemia	Expensive, use in dogs limited
Pamidronate (Aredia, Novartis)	1.3 mg/kg IV in 150 ml of 0.9% NaCl q7days prn	Chronic, moderate to severe hypercalcemia	Successful in dogs with experimental vitamin D_3 toxicosis
Clodronate	20–25 mg IV over 4 hr	Chronic, moderate to severe hypercalcemia	Successful in some dogs with lymphoma and vitamin D_3 toxicosis
Mithramycin (plicamycin) (Mithracin, Miles)	25 µg/kg IV in D_5W over 2–4h q2–4 wk	Severe, refractory hypercalcemia	Limited use in dogs and cats; nephrotoxicity, hepatotoxicity
Miscellaneous			
EDTA	25–75 mg/kg/hr	Severe, refractory hypercalcemia	Nephrotoxic
Peritoneal dialysis	Low calcium dialysate	Severe, refractory hypercalcemia	Short duration of response; use in hypercalcemia not reported

*Potassium supplementation is necessary. Add 5–40 mEq KCl/L, depending on serum potassium concentration (see Chap. 5).

mias (ventricular fibrillation) may develop with severe hypercalcemia.

Principles of Treatment of Hypercalcemia

The definitive treatment of hypercalcemia is treating or removing the underlying cause. Unfortunately, the etiology may not be apparent, and supportive measures must be taken to decrease the serum calcium concentration (see Table 30–3 for specific drugs and dosage recommendations). Supportive measures may include the following.

Volume Expansion. Volume expansion with intravenous (IV) 0.9% NaCl solution decreases hemoconcentration and encourages renal calcium loss by improving glomerular filtration rate and sodium excretion, which results in less calcium resorption.

Loop Diuretics. Diuretics such as furosemide increase calcium excretion; however, high doses may be needed (see Table 30–3). Diuretic use in a dehydrated patient is contraindicated because volume contraction and further hemoconcentration may worsen the hypercalcemia. Thiazide diuretics, which decrease calcium excretion by the kidneys, are contraindicated.

Sodium Bicarbonate. Sodium bicarbonate given as an IV bolus or as a continuous infusion has been shown to decrease serum total calcium concentration. Although the magnitude of calcium reduction is mild, alkalosis also favors the shift of ionized calcium to protein-bound calcium. Sodium bicarbonate therapy is more beneficial when combined with other treatments.

Glucocorticoids. Glucocorticoids decrease bone resorption of calcium, decrease intestinal calcium absorption, and increase renal calcium excretion, leading to a substantial decrease in serum calcium concentration in animals with hypercalcemia secondary to lymphoma, myeloma, hypervitaminosis D, and hypoadrenocorticism.

▼ *Key Point* The use of glucocorticoids before determining the etiology of hypercalcemia may make definitive diagnosis difficult.

Calcitonin. Calcitonin has been reported as an antidote to cholecalciferol toxicity by the manufacturer of a cholecalciferol-based rodenticide. For calcitonin to decrease serum calcium requires multiple injections per day. Long-term side effects include anorexia and vomiting. Diminished effectiveness of calcitonin treatment in lowering serum calcium may occur over time. Use calcitonin when other treatments have not adequately lowered serum calcium.

Bisphosphonates (Diphosphonates). These compounds inhibit osteoclastic bone resorption, but reports of their use in veterinary medicine have been limited. Etidronate (Didronel, Norwich Eaton) has been used with some success as an oral agent for long-term control of hypercalcemia. Intermittent IV injections of pamidronate (Aredia, Novartis) have recently shown promise for control of vitamin D_3–induced hypercalcemia in dogs. A single IV infusion of clodronate given over 4 hours was effective in decreasing serum calcium within 48 hours in some dogs with lymphoma or vitamin D_3 toxicosis.

Mithramycin. This drug is a potent inhibitor of osteoclastic bone resorption; however, mithramycin has been associated with many serious side effects, such as thrombocytopenia, hepatic necrosis, renal necrosis, and hypocalcemia.

EDTA. Ethylene diaminetetra-acetic acid reduces the ionized fraction of calcium by chelating calcium, which is then excreted by the kidneys. Since EDTA is nephrotoxic, use only for severe refractory hypercalcemia.

Peritoneal Dialysis. Consider this procedure, using a calcium-free dialysate, as a last resort when other methods fail to decrease serum calcium concentration.

CONDITIONS ASSOCIATED WITH HYPERCALCEMIA

Important conditions are discussed here. For a complete list of hypercalcemia-related conditions, see Table 30–2.

Hypercalcemia Associated with Malignancy

▼ *Key Point* Malignancy-associated hypercalcemia is the most common cause of persistent hypercalcemia in dogs and cats.

Hypercalcemia primarily results from increased osteoclastic bone resorption and increased renal tubular resorption. Rarely, increased intestinal absorption also may play a role. Factors that may be produced by tumors and result in humoral hypercalcemia of malignancy include PTH, PTH-related protein, transforming growth factor, 1,25-dihydroxycholecalciferol, prostaglandin E_2, osteoclast-activating factor, and other cytokines (interleukin-1, interleukin-2, and gamma-interferon).

▼ *Key Point* In dogs, lymphoma, adenocarcinoma of the apocrine glands of the anal sac, and multiple myeloma are the most common tumors associated with hypercalcemia.

Lymphoma

- Lymphoma is the most common tumor associated with hypercalcemia in the dog (see Chap. 25). Of dogs with lymphoma, 10–40% have been reported to have concurrent hypercalcemia, and a large number of these have the mediastinal form of lymphoma. Although detectable lymphadenopathy usually is present, hypercalcemia may be the first abnormality noted.
- A thorough physical examination, together with thoracic and abdominal radiography, abdominal ultrasonography, multiple lymph node aspirates or biopsies, and multiple bone marrow aspirates or core biopsies may be necessary to make the diagnosis.
- Treatment with corticosteroids decreases the serum calcium; however, their lympholytic effect makes subsequent identification of lymphoma very difficult. Animals with hypercalcemic lymphomas have a shorter survival time with chemotherapy than those with normocalcemic lymphomas. The return of hypercalcemia may precede clinical evidence of tumor regrowth in animals undergoing chemotherapy.

Apocrine Gland Adenocarcinoma of the Anal Sac

- This tumor usually occurs in older female dogs, with hypercalcemia developing in approximately 90% of cases. Humoral mechanisms are most likely responsible for the hypercalcemia, as a PTH-like protein has been identified from tumor tissue in dogs. The tumor is usually malignant and has metastasized to regional lymph nodes at the time of diagnosis.
- Surgical resection is associated with reduction of serum calcium (see Chap. 95 for description of surgery). Failure to remove all of the tumor or recurrence of the tumor usually results in the return of hypercalcemia. Despite surgical excision, radiation, and various chemotherapy protocols, the tumor usually recurs, and reported survival times range from 2–21 months.

Multiple Myeloma

- Multiple myeloma in dogs has been associated with hypercalcemia in 10–15% of cases. Humoral factors as well as direct lysis of bone may account for the increased serum calcium.
- Long-term survival has been reported following treatment of multiple myeloma with chemotherapy (see Chap. 25), but associated hypercalcemia, light chain proteinuria, and extensive bony lesions are associated with a shorter survival time.

Hypoadrenocorticism

- Approximately 20% of dogs with hypoadrenocorticism (Addison disease) have mild hypercalcemia (<15 mg/dl).

- Multiple factors that may result in the hypercalcemia include increase in calcium citrate (complex calcium), hemoconcentration (relative increase), increase in renal resorption of calcium, and increased affinity of serum proteins for calcium. Although total serum calcium concentrations may be increased, the ionized fraction usually is normal.
- Resolution of the hypercalcemia occurs quickly with therapy for hypoadrenocorticism (see Chap. 31).

Renal Failure

Chronic renal failure is associated with hypercalcemia of unknown pathogenesis in 10–15% of dogs and cats. Familial renal disease may be associated more often with hypercalcemia than are other forms of chronic renal failure. Hypercalcemia may be present in acute renal failure during the polyuric phase of recovery.

▼ *Key Point* If serum phosphorus is low or normal, it is not likely that renal failure is the cause of hypercalcemia.

Hypervitaminosis D

▼ *Key Point* Hypercalcemia can be associated with hyperphosphatemia in hypervitaminosis D in the absence of renal failure.

Rodenticides Containing Cholecalciferol

Cholecalciferol-based rodenticides (Quintox, Bell Labs; Rampage, Ceva; Rat-Be-Gone, Ortho) have gained popularity over anticoagulant rodenticides because, unlike anticoagulant rodenticides, there is no rodenticide resistance, and there is no secondary toxicity to species that ingest poisoned rodents. Although one manufacturer (Bell Labs) reports the median lethal dose (LD_{50}) to be 88 mg/kg, toxicity in dogs and cats has been seen with much lower doses (<10 mg/kg). Duration of the effect may last for weeks.

Clinical Manifestations

- Clinical signs are vague and related to hypercalcemia (see previous discussion of clinical signs under Hypercalcemia).
- Hypercalcemia is often severe (serum calcium 15–20 mg/dl) and accompanied by hyperphosphatemia at initial presentation.
- Azotemia may occur several days after ingestion, secondary to renal damage from hypercalcemia.

Goals of Treatment

- Decrease cholecalciferol absorption in the gastrointestinal tract.
- Correct the fluid and electrolyte imbalances.
- Reduce the hypercalcemia.
- Treat miscellaneous complications such as seizures and cardiac arrhythmias.

Treatment

- A low calcium diet (e.g., low protein diets from Hill's, Waltham, Purina, and others) and restriction of milk products.
- Phosphate binders that do not contain calcium (e.g., aluminum hydroxide, Amphojel, Wyeth-Ayerst; 10–30 mg/kg q8h PO with meals), which may be helpful in decreasing the calcium:phosphorus product.
- In severe cases of hypercalcemia, aggressive treatment with IV fluids, furosemide, prednisone, and/or calcitonin (see Table 30–3) may be necessary for several weeks.
- Recent studies suggest that intermittent IV pamidronate may be useful in dogs and may be superior to calcitonin as ancillary treatment.
- Because of the prolonged half-life of 25-hydroxycholecalciferol, monitor serum calcium, phosphorus, and creatinine weekly for 4–6 weeks. If aggressive therapy is maintained for several weeks, complete recovery is usually achieved.

Iatrogenic Vitamin D Intoxication

- Iatrogenic vitamin D intoxication has been reported following the administration of vitamin D products and dietary supplements. Use of ergocalciferol (vitamin D_2) may cause hypercalcemia because its slow onset of action and prolonged duration make it difficult to dose correctly.
- Treatment is directed at discontinuing the supplement or decreasing the dose of vitamin D (see discussion of surgery of the parathyroid gland under Parathyroidectomy, Postoperative Care and Complications section).

Houseplants

Houseplants such as *Cestrum diurnum* (the day-blooming jessamine), *Solanum malacoxylon,* and *Triestum flavescens* contain a substance similar to calcitriol that may cause hypercalcemia when ingested.

Granulomatous Diseases

Granulomatous disorders such as systemic fungal diseases and tuberculosis are rare causes of hypercalcemia in dogs. Serum calcium concentrations return to normal with treatment (e.g., antifungal drugs, surgical removal).

Primary Hyperparathyroidism

Primary hyperparathyroidism results from excessive secretion of PTH by one or more abnormal parathyroid glands. This disease has been reported sporadically in dogs and cats and is characterized by persistent and long-standing hypercalcemia.

Etiology

- Solitary parathyroid adenoma.
- Parathyroid carcinoma (infrequent).
- Parathyroid hyperplasia of one or all four glands (rare).

- Gross enlargement may not be present.
- The diagnosis is made based on microscopic abnormalities.
- Hereditary neonatal parathyroid hyperplasia has been reported in two German shepherd puppies.

Signalment

- Middle-aged or older animals are at risk:
  - Dogs from 5–13 years, mean age 10 years
  - Cats from 8–15 years, mean 12.9 years
- There is no sex predilection in dogs; however, there may be increased risk in female cats.
- No breed predilection has been noted, but the keeshond, German shepherd, and Norwegian elkhound are overrepresented, and several reported cats were Siamese.

Clinical Signs

- Anorexia, lethargy, and depression are the most common signs, but many animals may be asymptomatic.
- Polydipsia and polyuria are usually present.
- Constipation, weakness, shivering, twitching, vomiting, stiff gait, and facial swelling are less often reported.

Physical Examination

- In dogs, the physical examination is usually normal.
- In cats, 50% may have palpable cervical masses.

Diagnosis

Laboratory Tests
- Hypercalcemia, normal to low serum phosphorus, and decreased urine specific gravity are the most consistent findings.
- Azotemia and increased serum alkaline phosphatase and alanine aminotransferase activity may be present in some patients with moderate hypercalcemia.
- If renal failure is present, the serum phosphorus may be increased above normal.
- A high normal or increased PTH concentration (based on comparison with normal values for a validated immunoassay) in hypercalcemic animals with normal renal function is suggestive of primary hyperparathyroidism.

Hematology. The hemogram is usually unremarkable.

Radiography. Radiographs are generally normal but may reveal generalized osteopenia, increased bone resorption typically at the subperiosteal surfaces, and cyst-like areas in bone.

Ultrasonography. Ultrasound may identify the enlarged parathyroid gland and determine whether it is internal or external to the thyroid gland.

Exploratory Surgery. Consider exploratory surgery of the cervical region for diagnosis if no other cause of hypercalcemia can be determined.

- If a parathyroid nodule is not identified, give an IV infusion of methylene blue (3 mg/kg) to aid in the identification of parathyroid tumors. Although complications are uncommon with this technique, hemolysis, acute renal failure, and death have been reported.
- Negative findings may be due to ectopic PTH production (e.g., parathyroid adenoma in the cranial mediastinum or the unlikely event of a nonparathyroid tumor producing PTH).

Treatment

Treatment of primary hyperparathyroidism is surgical excision of the parathyroid adenoma. Before surgery, attempt to decrease the hypercalcemia with IV fluids (saline) and furosemide (see Table 30–3; see also Parathyroidectomy section).

HYPOCALCEMIA

Hypocalcemia is defined as a serum total calcium concentration < 8.5–9.0 mg/dl. Normal serum calcium concentration in older dogs may be slightly lower than that in middle-aged dogs.

Etiology

Various causes of hypocalcemia are listed in Table 30–4. Hypoalbuminemia is the most common cause of a low serum total calcium; however, it is of no clinical consequence because only the protein-bound fraction is affected. A mildly decreased serum calcium without signs of hypocalcemia can be seen in various systemic conditions such as renal failure, pancreatitis, and intestinal malabsorption. In the section that follows, conditions associated with symptomatic hypocalcemia are discussed.

Table 30–4. CONDITIONS ASSOCIATED WITH HYPOCALCEMIA

Causes of Severe Symptomatic Hypocalcemia
Puerperal tetany/eclampsia
Hypoparathyroidism
  Spontaneous (lymphocytic parathyroiditis)
  Iatrogenic secondary to bilateral thyroidectomy
  Postoperative secondary to removal of parathyroid adenoma/
    carcinoma
Phosphate enemas (acute hyperphosphatemia causes reciprocal
  calcium decrease)

Causes of Mild Asymptomatic Hypocalcemia
Hypoalbuminemia (most frequent cause of hypocalcemia)
Primary renal disease (see Chap. 97)
  Chronic renal failure
  Acute renal failure (urethral obstruction, ethylene glycol
    toxicity)
Pancreatitis (see Chap. 93)
Intestinal malabsorption syndromes (see Chap. 89)
Chelating agents that bind calcium (EDTA, citrates, oxalates,
  phosphates)
Rhabdomyolysis due to soft tissue trauma
Nutritional secondary hyperparathyroidism
Dilutional with infusion of calcium-free fluids
Laboratory error/artifact
Idiopathic (unexplained)

Clinical Signs

The severity of clinical signs may not always be commensurate with the degree of hypocalcemia. Concurrent acid-base disorders, other electrolyte imbalances, and ionized calcium concentration play a role in the development of clinical signs that are often episodic.

- Tremors, twitching, tetany, muscle spasms, and gait changes (stiffness and ataxia) result from increased neuromuscular excitability. Occasionally generalized seizure activity may be seen.
- Behavior changes (restlessness, aggression, panting, hypersensitivity to stimuli, and disorientation) are frequent.
- Bradycardia, hyperthermia, polyuria, polydipsia, and vomiting are sometimes seen.

Diagnostic Evaluation

History and Physical Examination. A complete history and a thorough physical examination can aid in the diagnosis of the underlying cause of the hypocalcemia.

Routine Laboratory Tests. Evaluate a serum calcium level (total and ionized if possible), CBC, and serum chemistry profile.

Electrocardiography. Prolongation of QT interval and ventricular premature contractions may be seen on electrocardiogram (ECG).

See specific diseases discussed later for other diagnostic tests.

Principles of Treatment of Hypocalcemia

The definitive treatment for hypocalcemia is to eliminate the underlying cause. Administer the following supportive measures to restore normocalcemia pending the diagnosis (Table 30–5).

Parenteral Calcium. This may be necessary in patients with active tetany, hyperthermia, and seizures.

- Calcium gluconate and calcium chloride usually are given by slow IV administration.
- Signs of toxicity from injection of too much calcium too fast include bradycardia and shortening of the QT interval.
- Calcium can also be diluted in saline and given as a continuous IV drip to maintain normal serum calcium concentrations (see Table 30–5).
- Calcium gluconate (diluted 1:1 with saline) may be given subcutaneously.

Oral Calcium. Oral calcium supplementation may be beneficial.

Table 30–5. TREATMENT OF HYPOCALCEMIA

Parenteral Calcium*

Drug	Preparation	Available Calcium	Dose	Comment
Calcium gluconate	10% solution	9.3 mg Ca/ml	Slow IV to effect (0.5–1.5 ml/kg IV) then 5–15 mg/kg/hr IV or 1–2 ml/kg diluted 1:1 with saline SC q8h	Stop if bradycardia or shortened QT interval occurs; infusion to maintain normal Ca may be given SC
Calcium chloride	10% solution	27.2 mg Ca/ml	5–15 mg/kg/hr IV	Give only IV, as extremely caustic perivascularly

Oral Calcium†

Drug	Preparation	Available Calcium (%)	Dose	Comment
Calcium carbonate	Many sizes	40% (tab.)	25–50 mg/kg/day	Most common calcium supplement
Calcium lactate	Tablets (325, 650 mg)	13%	25–50 mg/kg/day	
Calcium chloride	Powder	27.2%	25–50 mg/kg/day	
Calcium gluconate	Tablets (many sizes)	10%	25–50 mg/kg/day	May cause gastric irritation

Vitamin D

Preparation	Daily Dose	Time for Maximal Effect to Occur	Time for Toxicity Effect to Resolve
Vitamin D$_2$ (ergocalciferol)	Initial: 4000–6000 U/kg/day Maintenance: 1000–2000 U/kg once daily to once weekly	5–21 days	1–18 weeks
Dihydrotachysterol	Initial: 0.02–0.03 mg/kg/day Maintenance: 0.01–0.02 mg/kg q 24–48h	1–7 days	1–3 weeks
1,25-Dihydroxyvitamin D$_3$ (calcitriol)	20–30 ng/kg/day divided bid loading dose for 3–4 days, then 10–20 ng/kg/day as maintenance	1–4 days	2–14 days

*Do not mix calcium solution with bicarbonate-containing fluids because precipitation may occur.
†Calculate dose based on elemental calcium content.

- The daily requirements are 1–4 g for dogs and 0.5–1 g for cats.
- Base the dose of calcium on the amount of elemental calcium in the product.

Vitamin D. Vitamin D supplementation usually is necessary to increase calcium absorption in the intestines.

▼ *Key Point* Calcitriol is the vitamin D compound of choice for chronic maintenance treatment of symptomatic hypocalcemia.

- Several forms of vitamin D are available, and the response and duration of action of these drugs depend on the form used.
- Iatrogenic hypercalcemia is a common complication of treatment with cholecalciferol, ergocalciferol, and dihydrotachysterol. Treatment with calcitriol is rarely associated with hypercalcemia.

CONDITIONS ASSOCIATED WITH HYPOCALCEMIA

Puerperal Tetany (Eclampsia)

Puerperal tetany or eclampsia occurs in lactating bitches and queens as a result of calcium loss into the milk and poor dietary calcium intake (see Table 30–4). In nonlactating animals, this condition may be associated with high calcium supplementation resulting in suppression of PTH secretion and increasing calcitonin secretion. These changes decrease the osteoclast pool and availability of bone calcium.

Clinical Signs

- Small bitches with large litters are most often affected; puerperal tetany is rare in large dogs and cats.
- Onset of signs is acute, occurring most often 2–4 weeks post partum.
- Tetany, tremors, twitches, and seizures are common.
- Hyperthermia may occur in severe cases.
- Panting and restlessness may be early signs.

Diagnosis

Diagnosis is made based on history, clinical signs, hypocalcemia (total serum calcium usually < 7 mg/dl), and response to treatment.

Treatment

- Immediately give an IV infusion of calcium (slow IV administration to effect; then 5–15 mg/kg/h of elemental calcium; see Table 30–5).
- Supplement oral calcium (25–50 mg/kg/day of elemental calcium) for the remainder of lactation.
- Supplement vitamin D if serum calcium concentration remains low.
- If tetany recurs during the same lactation, wean the litter from the bitch.

Hypoparathyroidism

The marked hypocalcemia seen in hypoparathyroidism results from a deficiency in PTH. Hypoparathyroidism in dogs and cats may be spontaneous or iatrogenic.

Etiology

Spontaneous Hypoparathyroidism. Spontaneous hypoparathyroidism occurs uncommonly in dogs and cats. Lymphocytic parathyroiditis and atrophy are the most common causes and presumably are autoimmune. Agenesis occurs very rarely.

Iatrogenic Hypoparathyroidism. This form may occur after bilateral thyroidectomy (see Chap. 29) or parathyroidectomy for parathyroid adenoma/carcinoma and hyperplasia due to atrophy of the remaining glands. Normal function of the glands usually returns in 4–6 weeks.

Signalment

- In dogs the mean age is 6 years, although a wide age range (6 weeks to 12 years) has been reported. In cats, young to middle-aged patients are reported.
- Females are more commonly reported in dogs, but four of the five reported feline cases were males.
- Canine breeds predisposed to developing hypoparathyroidism include toy poodles, miniature schnauzers, Labrador retrievers, German shepherds, and terriers.

Clinical Signs

- Signs are usually episodic and most often include:
  - Nervousness, tremor, and twitching.
  - Rigid limb extension, stiff gait, and muscle spasms.
- Other signs include:
  - Ataxia, panting, and episodic weakness.
  - Facial rubbing, biting at feet, and aggression.
  - Polydipsia and polyuria.
  - Vomiting and diarrhea.
  - Weight loss, anorexia, depression, and listlessness.

Physical Examination

- Neuromuscular findings—extensor rigidity, muscle fasciculations, and seizures.
- Cardiac findings—tachycardia, paroxysmal tachyarrhythmias, and weak pulses.
- Cataracts—small punctate to linear (reported in a few dogs and cats).

Diagnosis

- Hypocalcemia is usually < 6 mg/dl.
- Hyperphosphatemia is usually present.
- ECG findings include prolongation of QT and ST segments, deep wide T waves, and tachyarrhythmias.
- Absolute PTH concentrations are low compared with normal values for validated immunoassay. Relative PTH concentrations may appear to be within the normal range but are inappropriately low in the presence of hypocalcemia.

- Parathyroid biopsy confirms lymphocytic parathyroiditis.

Treatment

Restore serum calcium level to the low end of the normal range. Avoid elevating calcium levels above this in order to prevent calcium-induced renal damage due to the lack of PTH (see Table 30–5 for dosages) and resultant hypercalciuria.

- If hypocalcemic tetany or seizures are present, immediately administer calcium IV.
- For maintenance of normocalcemia, supplement oral calcium and vitamin D compounds.

Hypercalcemia. Hypercalcemia is a common complication of vitamin D therapy and may be delayed and prolonged depending on the type of vitamin D supplementation used. Monitor serum calcium concentrations weekly at first, and then monthly when serum calcium has stabilized at the desired level. If hypercalcemia does occur as a complication of treatment, manage as discussed previously under Hypercalcemia. Discontinue calcium supplementation and use vitamin D alone at a lower dosage for maintenance.

Postoperative Hypoparathyroidism. Supplement calcium and vitamin D compounds postoperatively (see Table 30–5). If serum calcium concentrations remain normal, discontinue calcium supplementation and then gradually decrease and finally discontinue vitamin D. Evaluate serum calcium weekly for 1 month. If hypocalcemia returns, reinstitute vitamin D and calcium supplementation. Occasionally, permanent supplementation is necessary.

PARATHYROIDECTOMY

Parathyroidectomy is the treatment of choice for primary hyperparathyroidism caused by benign functional adenomas of the parathyroid gland in dogs. Functional adenocarcinomas are very rare. Parathyroidectomy is an infrequent procedure because primary hyperparathyroidism is uncommon in dogs and extremely rare in cats.

Anatomy. Familiarity with normal thyroid and parathyroid anatomy is essential before surgery (see Chap. 29).

Preoperative Considerations

- Always submit all excised parathyroid gland tissue for histopathology to confirm the diagnosis.
- Ectopic parathyroid gland adenomas are uncommon but may be present in the cranial mediastinum or near the base of the heart.
- Identification of parathyroid adenomas can be enhanced with preoperative IV infusion of methylene blue (3 mg/kg). However, this has been associated with severe hemolysis and fatal acute renal failure in some cases; thus, administer methylene blue with caution and only if a PTH adenoma is highly suspected but not identified during exploratory surgery.
- If the animal is hypercalcemic, attempt to decrease serum calcium levels (see Table 30–3) preoperatively to reduce risks of anesthesia and surgery if possible.

Surgical Procedure

Objectives

- Explore the thyroid and parathyroid region.
- Remove the parathyroid adenoma.
- Maintain meticulous hemostasis.

Equipment

- Standard general surgical pack and suture
- Self-retaining retractors (e.g., Gelpi)
- Magnifying loop (optional)

Technique

1. Place the dog in dorsal recumbency with the forelimbs tied caudally and the neck hyperextended with a rolled towel.
2. Prepare the ventral cervical region from caudal mandible to manubrium for aseptic surgery.
3. Incise the skin on the ventral midline from larynx to manubrium.
4. Separate the paired sternohyoideus and sternothyroideus muscles.
5. Exploration
   a. Identify all four parathyroid glands if possible. The nonadenomatous glands are often atrophied and difficult to identify.
   b. Parathyroid adenomas are firm, whitish solid structures 4–20 mm in diameter.
   c. If an enlarged parathyroid gland is cystic, it is probably not a neoplasm but an incidental congenital cyst.
   d. If a readily identifiable mass is not found in the thyroid area, explore the accessible region along the trachea to the base of the neck and cranial mediastinum.
   e. Avoid injury to the carotid sheath structures and recurrent laryngeal nerves.
6. Dissection of the mass
   a. Perform complete excision of the mass, using appropriate blunt and sharp dissection. Remove the associated thyroid lobe if necessary.
   b. Carefully examine the surgical field for evidence of residual hemorrhage prior to closure.
7. Routinely close the muscle (simple continuous absorbable suture), subcutaneous tissue (simple continuous absorbable suture), and skin (simple interrupted nonabsorbable monofilament suture).

Postoperative Care and Complications

- Monitor for hypothermia, hemorrhage at the incision site, and hypocalcemia.
- Postoperative hypocalcemia
  - Return of serum calcium concentrations to normal or subnormal values indicates successful parathyroidectomy.

▼ *Key Point* Most dogs exhibit hypocalcemia within 48 hours of tumor removal. Suspect severe hypocalcemia in those patients with long-standing hypercalcemia and those in which hypercalcemia preoperatively was not severe.

- Check serum calcium concentrations 1 and 2 days postoperatively. Frequent evaluation of calcium concentration is indicated if a hypocalcemic trend is noted.
- Monitor for muscle tremors, excitement, and tetany if calcium concentrations are decreasing.
- Treat hypocalcemia according to guidelines in the Hypocalcemia section of this chapter.
- Hypocalcemia without clinical signs usually does not require treatment unless the total serum calcium is < 6 mg/dl.
- Use weekly evaluation of serum calcium concentrations as the basis for modifying therapy with vitamin D compounds and calcium.
  - Gradually decrease dosages to maintain low-normal serum calcium levels until the atrophied parathyroid glands begin to function normally.
- Hypercalcemia may result from replacement therapy and should be avoided if possible.

Prognosis

The prognosis is good if the tumor is found and excised. Preexisting hypercalcemia-mediated renal dysfunction may be irreversible.

SUPPLEMENTAL READINGS

Berger B, Feldman EC: Primary hyperparathyroidism in dogs: 21 cases (1976–1986). J Am Vet Med Assoc 191:350, 1987.

Chew DJ, Nagode LA, Carothers MA, et al.: Disorders of calcium: Hypercalcemia and hypocalcemia. *In* DiBartola SP, ed.: Fluid Therapy in Small Animal Practice. Philadelphia: WB Saunders, 1992, p 116.

Chew DJ, Nagode LA, Rosol TJ, et al.: Utility of diagnostic assays in the evaluation of hypercalcemia and hypocalcemia: Parathyroid hormone, Vitamin D metabolites, parathyroid hormone–related protein, and ionized calcium. *In* Bonagura JD, Kirk RW, eds.: Kirk's Current Veterinary Therapy XII. Philadelphia: WB Saunders, 1995, p 378.

Feldman EC, Nelson RW: The parathyroid gland. *In* Feldman EC, Nelson RW, eds.: Canine and Feline Endocrinology and Reproduction. Philadelphia: WB Saunders, 1996, p 454.

Meuten DJ, Armstrong PJ: Parathyroid disease and calcium metabolism. *In* Ettinger SJ, ed.: Textbook of Veterinary Internal Medicine: Diseases of the Dog and Cat. Philadelphia: WB Saunders, 1989, p 1610.

Nesbitt T, Crowe SW, Aronsohn M: The parathyroid. *In* Slatter DH, ed.: Textbook of Small Animal Surgery. Philadelphia: WB Saunders, 1985, p 1874.

Petrie G: Management of hypercalcemia using dichloromethylene bisphosphonate (clodronate). Paper presented at the 6th Annual Congress of the European Society of Veterinary Internal Medicine, 1996, p 80.

Rumbeiha WK, Kruger J, Fitzgerald S, et al.: The use of pamidronate disodium for treatment of vitamin D_3 toxicosis in dogs. Paper presented at the 40th Annual Meeting of the American Association of Veterinary Laboratory Diagnosticians, Louisville, Kentucky, October 17–24, 1997, p 71.

Diseases of the Adrenal Gland

Peter P. Kintzer / Mark E. Peterson / Holly S. Mullen

HYPOADRENOCORTICISM IN DOGS AND CATS

Hypoadrenocorticism is an endocrinopathy characterized by a deficiency of glucocorticoid and/or mineralocorticoid secretion from the adrenal cortex. Spontaneous hypoadrenocorticism is uncommon in dogs and is rare in cats.

Etiology

Primary Adrenocortical Insufficiency

Primary adrenocortical insufficiency (Addison disease) is the result of atrophy or destruction of all layers of the adrenal cortex, usually resulting in glucocorticoid and mineralocorticoid deficiency. Potential causes include:

- Idiopathic (probably immune-mediated).
- Iatrogenic, which can result from mitotane therapy of hyperadrenocorticism in dogs. Mineralocorticoid concentrations remain normal in most dogs and the glucocorticoid deficiency is usually transient (weeks to months). However, permanent iatrogenic Addison disease can occur.
- Granulomatous (fungal) adrenalitis, neoplasia, hemorrhage (very rare).

Secondary Hypoadrenocorticism

Secondary hypoadrenocorticism is due to deficient pituitary adrenocorticotropic hormone (ACTH) secretion resulting in inadequate glucocorticoid production; mineralocorticoid secretion is preserved. Potential causes include:

- Abrupt withdrawal of long-term and/or high-dose glucocorticoid administration.
- Megestrol acetate (Ovaban, Schering Plough) therapy in cats.
- Lesions of the hypothalamus or pituitary gland (e.g., tumors).
- Idiopathic ACTH deficiency (rare).

Signalment

- *Age:* Most dogs and cats are young to middle-aged, but can range in age from 6 months to over 10 years.
- *Breed:* In dogs, any breed can be affected, but Great Danes, Portuguese water dogs, rottweilers, Standard poodles, West Highland white terriers, and Wheaton

terriers appear to be at an increased risk of developing naturally occurring primary hypoadrenocorticism. No breed predilection has been reported in cats.
- *Sex:* Female dogs appear to be at an increased risk of developing naturally occurring primary hypoadrenocorticism (71% females in one recent study). No sex predilection has been reported in cats.

Clinical Signs

No historical or clinical finding or set of clinical signs is pathognomonic for hypoadrenocorticism, and most clinical signs occur frequently in various other more common disorders. The severity and duration of clinical signs vary greatly among patients.

Acute Hypoadrenocorticism

- History consistent with chronic hypoadrenocorticism preceding the acute addisonian crisis.
- Weakness and depression progressing to collapse.
- Slow capillary refill time, weak pulses progressing to hypovolemic shock.
- Bradycardia and hypothermia.
- Cardiac arrhythmias (secondary to electrolyte abnormalities, acidosis, azotemia, and poor perfusion).

Chronic Hypoadrenocorticism

- Anorexia, vomiting, and diarrhea.
- Muscle weakness, lethargy, and depression.
- Weight loss, dehydration, shaking, polydipsia, polyuria, melena, abdominal pain, and hair loss may be present.
- Waxing and waning course.
- Previous response of clinical signs to administration of fluids and/or glucocorticoids.
- Exacerbation of clinical signs associated with "stress."

Diagnosis

History and Clinical Signs

A high index of suspicion is necessary because both history and clinical signs are nonspecific and seen with many other more common disorders such as:

- Gastrointestinal disorders.
- Primary renal failure.
- Other causes of acute collapse or episodic weakness (cardiovascular disease, neuromuscular disease, and metabolic disorders).

Hemogram

- Absolute eosinophilia and lymphocytosis are present in some cases.
- High hematocrit and total plasma protein may occur secondary to dehydration.
- Mild anemia is present in some cases.

Serum Biochemical and Electrolyte Abnormalities

▼ *Key Point* Hyperkalemia and hyponatremia are seen in the vast majority of animals with primary hypoadrenocorticism, but do not rely on these abnormalities for definitive diagnosis.

- Serum electrolyte concentrations.
  - *Hyperkalemia* and an Na^+/K^+ ratio of less than 27 is present in 95% of cases of primary hypoadrenocorticism.
  - Occasionally, primary hypoadrenocorticism may be associated with normal serum electrolyte concentrations (atypical primary hypoadrenocorticism). Several determinations may be necessary to demonstrate the typical electrolyte abnormalities in some animals with primary hypoadrenocorticism.
  - Iatrogenic hypoadrenocorticism caused by mitotane or ketoconazole therapy usually is associated with normal serum electrolyte concentrations.
  - Secondary hypoadrenocorticism is usually associated with normal serum electrolyte concentrations, but hyponatremia can occur.
- *Azotemia* is common (>80%) in primary hypoadrenocorticism and may also occur in secondary hypoadrenocorticism.
- *Hypercalcemia* is seen in 30% of affected dogs and cats, possibly due to decreased renal calcium excretion.
- *Hypoglycemia* (rare) may occur secondary to decreased gluconeogenesis and glycogenolysis.
- *Metabolic acidosis* is not uncommon, especially in an addisonian crisis.

Urine Specific Gravity

Urine specific gravity is below 1.030 in over half of cases despite prerenal azotemia. This decreased urine concentrating ability is probably due to medullary washout secondary to renal sodium wasting and decreased medullary blood flow.

Electrocardiographic Abnormalities

Electrocardiographic (ECG) changes are primarily attributable to hyperkalemia. Although electrocardiography can be of value in estimating the degree of hyperkalemia, these ECG abnormalities may correlate poorly with serum potassium concentrations because of the effects other serum electrolyte abnormalities, metabolic acidosis, and impaired tissue perfusion have on the cardiac conduction system.

- Widening and flattening of P waves, increased duration of the PR interval.
- Increased T-wave amplitude.
- Decreased amplitude and prolongation of QRS complexes.
- Bradycardia.
- Sinoatrial standstill (absence of P waves).
- Ventricular premature contractions, atrial fibrillation, and heart block.

Radiographic Findings

- Microcardia, microhepatica, and hypoperfusion of lungs (as manifestations of hypovolemia).
- Megaesophagus (rare).

ACTH Stimulation Test

Definitive diagnosis of hypoadrenocorticism requires demonstration of inadequate adrenal reserve by use of the ACTH stimulation test. This test measures the relative "thickness" of the adrenal cortex.

Intravenous Procedure

- In dogs, obtain a plasma or serum sample for cortisol determination before and 1 hour after IV injection of 250 µg of the synthetic ACTH, cosyntropin (Cortrosyn, Organon Pharmaceuticals). Lower doses of synthetic ACTH based on body weight (5 µg/kg IV) have also been described.
- In cats, obtain a plasma or serum sample for cortisol determination before and 1 hour after IV administration of 125 µg of cosyntropin.

Intramuscular Procedures

- Alternatively, in dogs, obtain a plasma or serum sample for cortisol analysis before and 2 hours after IM injection of 2.2 units/kg ACTH gel (Acthar Gel, Rhone Poulenc).
- In cats, obtain a plasma or serum sample for cortisol determination before and 1 and 2 hours after IM injection of 2.2 units/kg ACTH gel (Acthar Gel, Rhone Poulenc).
- Some formulations of ACTH gel appear to lack biologic activity in some dogs and cats (e.g., ACTH repository corticotropin injection, Austin).

Interpretation

- Dogs and cats with hypoadrenocorticism show a blunted or absent cortisol response to ACTH administration.
- *Primary hypoadrenocorticism:* Basal and post-ACTH cortisol concentrations are usually <1 µg/dl (<30 nmol/L).
- *Secondary hypoadrenocorticism:* The serum cortisol response to exogenous ACTH is blunted; however, post-ACTH concentrations of cortisol may be as high as 3.0 µg/dl (85 nmol/L) in some cases.
- False elevations of cortisol concentrations may occur after administration of prednisone, prednisolone, cortisone, or fludrocortisone because these cross-react on the cortisol radioimmunoassay. Discontinue these drugs 24–48 hours prior to the test.

- Dexamethasone and desoxycorticosterone pivalate (DOCP) do not interfere with the cortisol assay (see Treatment section); however, dexamethasone is a potent steroid and suppresses the pituitary adrenal axis.

Plasma Concentration of ACTH

Plasma concentration of ACTH is high (>500 pg/ml) in dogs and cats with primary hypoadrenocorticism and very low or undetectable with secondary hypoadrenocorticism. This assay is available on a mail-in basis from the Endocrine Diagnostic Laboratory of the Michigan State University College of Veterinary Medicine.

Treatment

▼ *Key Point* Collect proper blood and urine samples and perform necessary diagnostic testing before instituting therapy.

The ACTH stimulation test (preferably using synthetic ACTH administered IV) can be performed simultaneously with initial therapy if dexamethasone is used for glucocorticoid replacement because it does not interfere with the cortisol assay.

Acute Hypoadrenocorticism

This is a medical emergency requiring immediate intervention.

- Correct hypotension and hypovolemia.
- Improve vascular integrity.
- Provide an immediate source of rapid-acting glucocorticoid.
- Correct electrolyte imbalance and acidosis.
- Following stabilization of the acute addisonian crisis, institute long-term mineralocorticoid and glucocorticoid replacement therapy as described for treatment of Chronic Hypoadrenocorticism.

Hypovolemia and Hyponatremia

- Infuse 0.9% NaCl solution at 60–80 ml/kg/hr IV over the first 1–2 hours; then gradually reduce the rate to maintenance requirement, depending on patient response. Monitor urine output.
- Administer dexamethasone sodium phosphate, 2–4 mg/kg IV, or prednisolone sodium succinate, 15–20 mg/kg IV. Repeat in 2–6 hours as needed. Glucocorticoid supplementation is gradually tapered to a maintenance dose of prednisone (0.2 mg/kg/day) over the following 3–5 days as the patient's condition improves.

Hyperkalemia

- Hyperkalemia associated with hypoadrenocorticism can often be successfully treated with parenteral fluid therapy (0.9% NaCl solution) only.
- For severe hyperkalemia causing life-threatening bradyarrhythmias and sinoatrial standstill, more aggressive therapy is indicated. Administer short-acting insulin (e.g., regular insulin) and dextrose IV (first choice), sodium bicarbonate, or calcium salts.

- A rapid-acting parenteral mineralocorticoid formulation is no longer available. However, begin oral supplementation with fludrocortisone (Florinef, Squibb) immediately if the animal is not vomiting.

Acidosis

- Correct mild to moderate acidosis with parenteral fluid therapy (0.9% NaCl solution).
- Treat severe acidosis (pH < 7.1) with serum bicarbonate. Give 25% of the calculated bicarbonate deficit over the first 6–8 hours of therapy if serum bicarbonate concentration is <12 mEq/L. It is unusual for additional bicarbonate administration to be needed.
- Correction of acidosis also drives extracellular potassium into cells, thereby reducing hyperkalemia.

Other Supportive Care As Needed

- Correct hypothermia.
- Treat symptomatic hypoglycemia with a slow IV bolus of 1.5 ml/kg of 50% dextrose.

Chronic Hypoadrenocorticism

Animals with chronic disease generally do not require aggressive therapy; however, parenteral fluid therapy and parenteral glucocorticoid supplementation may initially be indicated in some cases. Dogs and cats with primary hypoadrenocorticism require lifelong glucocorticoid and mineralocorticoid replacement therapy and sometimes addition of salt to the diet. Animals with documented secondary hypoadrenocorticism require glucocorticoid replacement only.

Hypovolemia

- Give 0.9% NaCl solution, 60–80 ml/kg/day IV, for initial correction of hypovolemia.
- Decrease fluid volume over 48–96 hours based on return of clinical and laboratory parameters to normal.

Mineralocorticoid Supplementation

Use one of the following treatment protocols:

- *Fludrocortisone acetate* (Florinef, Squibb).
  - Give an initial dosage of 0.01 to 0.02 mg/kg/day PO.
  - Monitor serum electrolytes, blood urea nitrogen (BUN), and creatinine every 1–2 weeks until stabilized in the normal range; then reevaluate every 3–4 months.
  - Adjust dose by 0.05–0.1 mg/day based on serum electrolyte concentrations.
  - Average dose to control the disease is 0.02–0.03 mg/kg/day; very few animals can be controlled on less than 0.01 mg/kg/day.
  - Side effects include polyuria, polydipsia, polyphagia, and weight gain.
  - Development of side effects, relative resistance to the drug, or financial considerations may necessitate a change to DOCP.
- *Desoxycorticosterone pivalate* (DOCP), (Percorten–V, Ciba-Geigy Animal Health).

- DOCP is a long-acting injectable mineralocorticoid; give initially at 2.2 mg/kg IM or SQ, every 4 weeks. A dosage interval of 3–4 weeks is effective in most cases.
- Percorten–V was recently approved by the FDA for treatment of primary hypoadrenocorticism in dogs.
- Monitor serum electrolytes, BUN, and creatinine every 1–2 weeks until stabilized in the normal range to ensure an appropriate dose and duration of action; then reevaluate every 3–6 months during long-term therapy.
- Less than 10% of dogs require a dosage >2.2 mg/kg. Dosages <2.2 mg/kg may be sufficient in some cases. If financial constraints are present, gradually reduce to the lowest effective dose while monitoring serum electrolyte concentrations.
- Side effects are rare.

Glucocorticoid Supplementation

Many patients require glucocorticoid supplementation in addition to mineralocorticoid therapy to prevent signs of glucocorticoid deficiency or to control persistent mild azotemia. Use one of the following:

- Prednisone or prednisolone, 0.2 mg/kg/day PO.
- Cortisone acetate, 1 mg/kg/day PO.
- Give 2- to 10-fold higher glucocorticoid doses for brief periods of stress, surgery, or illness.

Sodium Chloride Therapy

- NaCl, 1–5 g daily, may be beneficial in some patients to help normalize serum sodium concentration.
- NaCl supplementation may have a sparing effect on the required fludrocortisone dose in occasional dogs.

HYPERADRENOCORTICISM IN DOGS

Spontaneous hyperadrenocorticism (Cushing syndrome) is a collection of clinical and biochemical abnormalities caused by chronic overproduction of cortisol by the adrenal cortices.

Etiology

Hyperadrenocorticism can be pituitary-dependent, secondary to cortisol-secreting adrenocortical neoplasia, or iatrogenic.

Pituitary-Dependent Hyperadrenocorticism

This is the most common cause of naturally occurring hyperadrenocorticism in dogs, accounting for 85% of cases. The excessive secretion of ACTH from pituitary corticotroph hyperplasia, microadenoma, macroadenoma, or (very rarely) adenocarcinoma results in bilateral adrenocortical hyperplasia.

Cortisol-Secreting Adrenocortical Tumors

These tumors are responsible for approximately 15% of dogs with spontaneous Cushing syndrome. About half of adrenocortical tumors are benign and half are malignant.

Iatrogenic Hyperadrenocorticism

Excessive or prolonged administration of corticosteroids can cause iatrogenic hyperadrenocorticism.

- Clinical signs and physical examination findings are similar to those seen in the natural disease.
- Endogenous ACTH production is suppressed resulting in atrophy of the adrenal cortices.

Signalment

- *Age:* Spontaneous hyperadrenocorticism is primarily a disease of middle-aged to older dogs, but can be seen in dogs ranging from 6 months to 20 years of age.
- *Breed:* All breeds can be affected. Poodles, dachshunds, Boston terriers, and boxers appear to be at greater risk of developing pituitary-dependent hyperadrenocorticism. Adrenal tumors are more common in larger dogs (>20 kg).
- *Sex:* No sex predilection is seen in dogs with pituitary-dependent hyperadrenocorticism. In contrast, two-thirds of dogs with adrenal tumors are female.

Clinical Signs

▼ *Key Point* Dogs with hyperadrenocorticism usually develop clinical signs that reflect dysfunction of many organ systems, although in some dogs only one or a few clinical signs may predominate.

General Appearance

- Pendulous, distended, or "pot-bellied" abdomen.
- Haircoat changes reflecting hair loss.
- Muscle atrophy and weakness.

Integument

- Hair loss ranging from a thinning of the coat to bilaterally symmetric alopecia.
- Thin hypotonic skin susceptible to bruising.
- Hyperpigmentation.
- Seborrheic changes.
- Secondary pyoderma and *Malassezia* dermatitis.

Urinary and Reproductive Systems

- Polyuria and polydipsia are seen in up to 90% of dogs with hyperadrenocorticism. Glucocorticoids decrease the renal tubular reabsorption of water by increasing the glomerular filtration rate and renal blood flow and by inhibiting the action of antidiuretic hormone (ADH) at the tubular levels.
- Urinary tract infection can occur secondary to the immunosuppressive effects of cortisol excess. The typical signs of pollakiuria, hematuria, and stranguria may be minimal in some dogs as a result of the anti-inflammatory action of cortisol.
- Glomerulopathy and associated proteinuria may occur.

- Testicular atrophy and female infertility (anestrus) can occur, secondary to low concentrations of pituitary follicle-stimulating hormone (FSH) and luteinizing hormone (LH) caused by negative feedback from high circulating cortisol concentrations.

Respiratory System

- Excessive panting is quite common and is attributed to decreased pulmonary compliance, respiratory muscle weakness, pulmonary hypertension, or the direct effects of cortisol on the respiratory center.
- Pulmonary thromboembolic disease, a rare complication of hyperadrenocorticism, can cause moderate to severe respiratory distress, and sometimes is fatal.

Endocrine System

- Some dogs with hyperadrenocorticism develop diabetes mellitus and the associated clinical signs of polyuria, polydipsia, weight loss, and polyphagia.
- The hallmark of steroid-induced diabetes is the development of insulin resistance, defined clinically as persistent hyperglycemia despite insulin doses of >2.5 U/kg per injection.
- Cortisol antagonizes the actions of insulin by interfering with its action at the cellular level (receptor and postreceptor effects).
- Hypertension may occur.

Central Nervous System and Neuromuscular System

- Lethargy is the most common CNS disturbance. Lethargy may be associated with high concentrations of ACTH or the effects of excessive cortisol on cerebral enzymes and on neurotransmitter synthesis.
- CNS signs of circling, seizures, behavior change, and depression to obtundation may be caused by the local compressive effects of a large, expanding pituitary tumor.
- Muscle weakness is quite common and results from muscle wasting secondary to the catabolic effects of glucocorticoid excess.

Gastrointestinal System

- Polyphagia is common.
- Hepatomegaly is often detected.
- Pancreatitis secondary to excess cortisol levels is occasionally seen.

Diagnosis
History

Common owner complaints include polyuria and polydipsia, polyphagia, hair loss, weight gain, lethargy, and weakness. Determine recent corticosteroid administration (including eye, ear, and topical preparations).

Physical Examination

Perform a careful examination to determine the clinical signs listed above.

▼ *Key Point* The most important diagnostic procedures for hyperadrenocorticism are a careful and complete history and physical examination.

Routine Laboratory Testing

- The hemogram may reveal a stress leukogram and mild erythrocytosis.
- Up to 85% of dogs with hyperadrenocorticism have high serum alkaline phosphatase activity, composed primarily of the steroid-induced isoenzyme.
- Elevated serum cholesterol concentration is common.
- Increased serum alanine aminotransferase (ALT) and aspartate aminotransferase (AST) concentrations are common.
- Mild hyperglycemia is common. Overt diabetes mellitus (glucose >250 mg/dl) occurs in 10% of dogs with untreated hyperadrenocorticism.
- Urinalysis often reveals a low specific gravity (<1.020).
- Proteinuria is occasionally seen. A urine protein to creatinine ratio >3.0 is usually due to glomerular disease or urinary tract infection.

Radiography

- Hepatomegaly is common.
- Approximately one-third of adrenal tumors are mineralized and, therefore, detectable on abdominal radiographs.
- Mineralization of bronchial walls is a frequent incidental finding.
- Pulmonary metastasis is rarely detected in some dogs with adrenal carcinoma.

Ultrasonography

Ultrasonography is more sensitive than radiography for imaging the adrenal glands and is a recommended part of the workup of all dogs with hyperadrenocorticism. This is a very user-dependent technique.

- Bilateral adrenomegaly is found in most dogs with pituitary-dependent hyperadrenocorticism.
- An adrenal mass is usually readily identified in dogs with adrenal neoplasia. The contralateral adrenal is atrophied and unlikely to be found. Bilateral adrenal tumors are very rare.
- In dogs with adrenal neoplasia, evaluate the liver for metastasis and the caudal vena cava for tumor thrombus.

Computed Tomography and Magnetic Resonance Imaging

- Pituitary tumors >1 cm in diameter (macroadenomas or macroadenocarcinomas) are relatively easy to define with these imaging techniques.
- Pituitary microadenomas may be identified if they are ideally positioned or approach 1 cm in diameter. MRI is more sensitive than CT for imaging pituitary microadenomas.
- CT and MRI are the most accurate and reliable meth-

ods for imaging the adrenal glands followed by diagnostic ultrasonography and then plain radiography. With CT or MRI, the location of the adrenal tumor and evidence of metastasis can be identified in most dogs.

Pituitary-Adrenal Function Tests

Basal Serum Cortisol Concentrations

Basal serum (or plasma) cortisol concentrations cannot be used to diagnose hyperadrenocorticism because of significant overlap among dogs with hyperadrenocorticism, dogs with nonadrenal illness, and normal dogs.

ACTH Stimulation Test

This is an adrenal function test that measures the relative "thickness" of the adrenal cortex. Therefore, the ACTH stimulation test is the best test to differentiate spontaneous from iatrogenic hyperadrenocorticism.

- *Procedure*
  - Obtain a plasma or serum sample for cortisol determination before and 1 hour after IV injection of 250 μg of synthetic ACTH, cosyntropin (Cortrosyn, Organon Pharmaceuticals). Lower doses of synthetic ACTH based on body weight (5 μg/kg IV) have also been described. Once reconstituted, the ACTH solution is stable for 3 months.
  - Alternatively, obtain a plasma or serum sample for cortisol analysis before and 2 hours after intramuscular (IM) injection of 2.2 units/kg of ACTH gel (Acthar Gel, Rhone Poulenc). Some formulations of ACTH gel appear to lack biologic activity in some dogs (e.g., ACTH repository corticotropin injection, Austin).
- *Interpretation*
  - Of the dogs with pituitary-dependent hyperadrenocorticism, 85–90% demonstrate an exaggerated cortisol response to exogenous ACTH. A post-ACTH cortisol concentration >20 μg/dl (>550 nmol/L) is consistent with hyperadrenocorticism.
  - Approximately 50% of dogs with adrenocortical tumors show an exaggerated cortisol response, whereas the remainder have a normal response. Some dogs with adrenal carcinoma have extremely high post-ACTH cortisol concentrations (>50 μg/dl or >1500 nmol/L).
  - Dogs with iatrogenic hyperadrenocorticism have a "blunted" or no response to ACTH administration.

Low-Dose Dexamethasone Suppression Test

This test is also useful in confirming the diagnosis of hyperadrenocorticism. The overall sensitivity of this test is 90–95%; in most dogs, this test does not differentiate pituitary-dependent hyperadrenocorticism from cortisol-secreting adrenal neoplasia.

- *Procedure*
  - Collect plasma or serum samples for cortisol determination before and 4 and 8 hours after IV or IM administration of 0.015 mg/kg dexamethasone (Azium, Schering Plough).

- *Interpretation*
  - In normal dogs, serum cortisol concentrations are suppressed below 1 μg/dl (30 nmol/L) by 4 hours after administration of dexamethasone and remain suppressed at 8 hours. In contrast, cortisol concentrations in most dogs with hyperadrenocorticism remain above 1 μg/dl (30 nmol/L) during the 8-hour test period.
  - Approximately 25% of dogs with pituitary-dependent hyperadrenocorticism show a pattern of "escape" from suppression; serum cortisol concentrations fall below 1 μg/dl (30 nmol/L) by 4 hours after administration of dexamethasone and rise above 1 μg/dl (30 nmol/L) by the eighth hour of the test, a pattern diagnostic for pituitary-dependent hyperadrenocorticism.

Urinary Cortisol to Creatinine Ratio

This is a convenient screening test for hyperadrenocorticism. A normal value virtually excludes a diagnosis of hyperadrenocorticism. A positive result must be confirmed with an ACTH stimulation test or a low-dose dexamethasone suppression test.

- *Procedure*
  - Submit a single morning urine sample to the laboratory for measurement of urine cortisol and urine creatinine concentrations. Ideally, the sample should be collected at home by the owner rather than by catheterization or cytocentesis in the hospital.
- *Interpretation*
  - When urine cortisol is expressed as nmol/L and creatinine is expressed as mmol/L, a ratio >30 is consistent with hyperadrenocorticism in most laboratories.

▼ *Key Point* All pituitary-adrenal function tests used to diagnose hyperadrenocorticism commonly show false-positive results in dogs with nonadrenal disease. Whenever possible pituitary-adrenal function testing should be postponed until the nonadrenal disease has been resolved.

Endogenous Plasma ACTH Concentration

This test reliably distinguishes pituitary-dependent hyperadrenocorticism from adrenocortical tumors.

- *Procedure*
  - Collect blood in an EDTA tube, centrifuge immediately, and remove the plasma. The addition of aprotinin to EDTA tubes allows for routine handling of ACTH samples and shipment using cold packs (instead of dry ice). Contact the appropriate reference laboratory (e.g., Endocrine Diagnostic Laboratory of the Michigan State University College of Veterinary Medicine) for detailed instructions.
- *Interpretation*
  - Dogs with pituitary-dependent hyperadrenocorticism have a normal to high ACTH concentration (>40 pg/ml).

- Dogs with adrenal tumors have low or undetectable plasma concentration of ACTH (<20 pg/ml).

High-Dose Dexamethasone Suppression Test

This test is used to differentiate dogs with pituitary-dependent hyperadrenocorticism from those with adrenocortical neoplasia. The test is easily performed in practice.

- *Procedure*
  - Collect a serum or plasma sample for cortisol determination before and 4 and 8 hours after IV or IM injection of 0.1–1.0 mg/kg of dexamethasone.
  - In dogs with pituitary-dependent hyperadrenocorticism, the degree of cortisol suppression tends to be greater after administration of the 1.0 mg/kg dose.
- *Interpretation*
  - Dogs with adrenal tumors do not show feedback suppression of cortisol after administration of a high dose of dexamethasone, with serum cortisol concentrations remaining >1.5 µg/dl (>40 nmol/L) during the testing period. Suppression of serum cortisol concentration to <1.5 µg/dl excludes an adrenal tumor.
  - In dogs with pituitary-dependent hyperadrenocorticism, approximately 80% demonstrate suppression of cortisol (<1.5 µg/dl or <40 nmol/L) after administration of a high dose of dexamethasone.
  - The remaining 20% of dogs with pituitary-dependent hyperadrenocorticism fail to demonstrate adequate cortisol suppression (i.e., all cortisol values remain >1.5 µg/dl or >40 nmol/L). Additional testing is necessary to distinguish these dogs from those with an adrenal tumor. Many dogs with non-suppressible pituitary-dependent hyperadrenocorticism have large pituitary tumors.

Treatment

Medical Management of Pituitary-Dependent Hyperadrenocorticism Using Mitotane

Mitotane (o,p'DDD; Lysodren, Bristol-Myers Squibb) is the drug most frequently used in the treatment of hyperadrenocorticism in dogs. Mitotane causes selective necrosis of the zona fasciculata and zone reticularis of the adrenal cortex. The administration protocol for mitotane involves an initial induction phase that uses a daily dosage for induction of remission (loading dosage), followed by a maintenance phase that uses a dosage given once or twice weekly (maintenance dosage).

Induction Phase

- The *initial loading dosage* of mitotane is 30–50 mg/kg/day, given once daily or divided q12h PO, for 7–10 days. Mitotane absorption is enhanced by food (especially fat) and, therefore, should be given with a meal.
- *Concurrent glucocorticoid supplementation* with oral prednisone or prednisolone (0.15–0.25 mg/kg/day,

up to a maximum daily dose of 5 mg/day/dog) can be used to mitigate the adverse effects associated with serum cortisol concentrations falling rapidly into the normal or subnormal range during this initial treatment. The major disadvantage of providing glucocorticoid is that it may not be possible to know if overdosage has occurred, since clinical signs of glucocorticoid deficiency may not develop.
- Common side effects during the induction phase of therapy (the loading period) include lethargy, vomiting, anorexia, weakness, and diarrhea. If adverse effects occur during initial therapy, discontinue mitotane and give glucocorticoids until the dog can be evaluated. Monitor the dog's appetite closely during the induction period, and if anorexia develops, discontinue mitotane and evaluate by ACTH stimulation test.
- Monitor therapy with the ACTH stimulation test. Perform this test at the end of the 10-day induction phase, or sooner if adverse effects develop.

▼ *Key Point* The goal of therapy is to achieve subclinical hypoadrenocorticism, whereby both basal and post-ACTH cortisol concentrations are within the normal basal (or resting) cortisol range (1–5 µg/dl or 30–150 nmol/L for most laboratories).

- If basal and post-ACTH concentrations fall below the normal basal range (<1 µg/dl or <30 nmol/L), temporarily suspend mitotane administration and supplement glucocorticoids as needed until circulating cortisol concentrations normalize. Cortisol concentrations generally return to the normal range within 2–4 weeks, but occasionally take several weeks.
- If basal or post-ACTH cortisol concentrations are above the normal resting range, continue daily mitotane treatment and repeat ACTH stimulation tests at 5–10 day intervals until serum cortisol concentrations fall within the normal resting range.

Maintenance Phase

- When desired cortisol concentrations are documented by ACTH stimulation testing, continue mitotane at a *maintenance dosage* of 50 mg/kg weekly in 2–3 divided doses. Lifelong maintenance therapy is needed to maintain remission of the disease.
- If adverse side effects occur during maintenance therapy, discontinue mitotane and supplement glucocorticoids until the dog can be evaluated by serum electrolyte determinations and an ACTH stimulation test. In most dogs with iatrogenic hypoadrenocorticism (but normal serum electrolytes), maintenance mitotane can be resumed 2–6 weeks later, when serum cortisol concentrations have returned into the normal resting range. About 20–25% of dogs experience side effects, usually mild, at some point during induction or maintenance mitotane therapy.
- About 5% of dogs develop iatrogenic hypoadrenocorticism with associated hyponatremia and hyperkalemia. These dogs generally require lifelong sup-

plementation with mineralocorticoids, i.e., fludro-cortisone acetate or DOCP (see Hypoadrenocorticism).

- Nearly 50% of dogs with hyperadrenocorticism have a relapse of disease within the first 12 months of maintenance therapy. These cases require reinduction with daily doses of mitotane for 7–10 days, followed by a higher maintenance dosage (weekly dosage usually increased by 50%).
- To ensure continued control and prevent serious relapse during mitotane treatment, repeat ACTH stimulation testing after 3 and 6 months of maintenance treatment and every 6 months thereafter. Relapse of hyperadrenocorticism can thereby usually be detected before recurrence of clinical signs is evident.

Medical Management of Hyperadrenocorticism Using Ketoconazole

- Ketoconazole (Nizoral, Janssen) reversibly inhibits adrenal steroidogenesis through enzymatic blockade.
- The initial dosage of ketoconazole is 10 mg/kg q12h PO.
- Assess adrenal reserve with an ACTH stimulation test after 7–10 days of therapy.
- The goal of therapy is to achieve subclinical hypoadrenocorticism, whereby both basal and post-ACTH cortisol concentrations are within the normal basal cortisol range (1–5 μg/dl or 25–150 nmol/L for most laboratories).
- The dosage of ketoconazole can be increased (up to 20 mg/kg q12h) if necessary.
- Once adequate control is achieved, lifelong twice-daily therapy is required to maintain remission of the hyperadrenocorticism.
- Adverse effects include anorexia, vomiting, diarrhea, lethargy, and idiosyncratic hepatopathy.
- The major problems of ketoconazole compared with mitotane include its high cost, the necessity for lifelong twice-daily administration, and reported lack of efficacy in some cases (up to 50% in some reports).

Medical Management of Pituitary-Dependent Hyperadrenocorticism Using L-Deprenyl

- L-Deprenyl (selegiline HCl; Anipryl, Pfizer) is a selective, monoamine oxidase type B inhibitor that decreases pituitary ACTH secretion by increasing dopaminergic tone to the hypothalamic-pituitary axis, with a resultant fall in serum cortisol concentrations.
- Initiate L-deprenyl therapy at a dosage of 1 mg/kg PO daily. If an inadequate response is seen after 2 months of therapy, increase the dose to 2 mg/kg/day. Should this dose also prove ineffective, use alternative therapy. If effective, continue daily therapy for the remainder of the dog's life.
- The drug is indicated for the treatment of uncomplicated cases of pituitary-dependent hyperadrenocorticism. L-Deprenyl is not recommended for treatment in dogs with concurrent diabetes mellitus, pancreatitis, heart failure, renal disease, or other severe illness,

and it is not effective for the treatment of cortisol-secreting adrenocortical neoplasia.

- The manufacturer's multicenter trial reported that 75–80% of dogs had a good response to therapy as assessed by resolution of clinical signs and monthly low-dose dexamethasone suppression testing. Other investigators have reported lower efficacy rates (≤50% in some studies).
- The current label recommendation is to evaluate the efficacy of L-deprenyl therapy based solely on resolution of clinical signs of hyperadrenocorticism. It seems prudent, however, to monitor low-dose dexamethasone suppression tests every 4–6 weeks to evaluate for normalization (or improvement) of the pituitary-adrenal axis in dogs receiving the drug. The ACTH stimulation test is not indicated for assessing the response to treatment with L-deprenyl.
- Adverse effects such as anorexia, lethargy, vomiting, and diarrhea are uncommon (<5% of dogs) and usually mild.
- Do not administer L-deprenyl concurrently with other monoamine oxidase inhibitors, opioids, or tricyclic antidepressants (e.g., fluoxetine), as significant adverse drug interactions have been reported in humans.
- Drawbacks of L-deprenyl therapy include the need for lifelong daily administration and the expense of the medication.

Radiation Therapy in the Treatment of Pituitary-Dependent Hyperadrenocorticism

- Radiation therapy may be useful in dogs with hyperadrenocorticism caused by a pituitary macroadenoma or macrocarcinoma.
- Deliver the total dose of radiation in fractions over a period of 4–6 weeks. Complications appear to be minimal in most cases.
- The primary prognostic factor is the severity of neurologic signs. Dogs with a pituitary macroadenoma and severe neurologic signs have a grave prognosis.
- The disadvantages of radiation therapy include its high cost and limited availability.
- Plasma ACTH and serum cortisol concentrations may take weeks to months to normalize. In the interim, medical management of the hyperadrenocorticism may be necessary.

▼ **Key Point** Advances in diagnostic imaging (CT and MRI) have enabled the antemortem diagnosis of pituitary macroadenomas. Treatment of pituitary tumors may be attempted with radiotherapy, especially if a diagnosis of macroadenoma can be made before the onset of profound neurologic signs.

Surgical Management of Adrenocortical Tumors

See the section on Adrenalectomy.

Medical Management of Adrenocortical Tumors with Mitotane

- Mitotane is an effective and relatively safe treatment alternative for most dogs with adrenal tumors. Mitotane therapy has been successful for over 24 months in some dogs with adrenocortical adenomas and carcinomas. In general, higher dosages of mitotane are required than for treatment of dogs with pituitary-dependent hyperadrenocorticism. Only 15–20% of dogs with adrenal tumors respond to the standard treatment protocol used in dogs with pituitary-dependent hyperadrenocorticism.

▼ *Key Point* In dogs with adrenal tumors, mitotane is used as a true chemotherapeutic agent with the goal of destroying all functional, neoplastic adrenocortical tissue. Therefore, both the serum basal and post-ACTH cortisol concentrations should be low to undetectable (<1 μg/dl or <30 nmol/L). The induction of overt hypoadrenocorticism may improve the long-term prognosis, but mitotane toxicity (from the high doses of mitotane needed) prevents this approach in many dogs.

- *Indications* for mitotane therapy of adrenal tumors
  - Gross metastatic disease evident prior to surgery.
  - Unresectable or incompletely resectable tumor.
  - Residual disease after adrenalectomy as detected by ACTH stimulation testing.
  - Unacceptable anesthetic or surgical risks to the patient.
  - Refusal of surgery by the client.
- *Procedure*
  - Initiate mitotane therapy at a daily dosage of 50–75 mg/kg/day and repeat ACTH stimulation testing every 10–14 days to evaluate adrenal reserve. Administer a glucocorticoid (e.g., prednisone or prednisolone, 0.2 mg/kg/day PO) throughout the period of mitotane administration to help prevent adverse effects secondary to hypoadrenocorticism.
  - Continue daily mitotane at this dosage or increase it (based on ACTH stimulation test results) until desired cortisol levels are reached or drug intolerance develops. Dogs with adrenal tumors often require a cumulative mitotane induction dose up to 10 times higher than dogs with pituitary-dependent hyperadrenocorticism (due to a longer period of daily mitotane administration).
  - Once serum cortisol concentrations are undetectable to low, start maintenance therapy at 75–100 mg/kg weekly in divided doses. Continue daily glucocorticoid supplementation. Perform an ACTH stimulation test in 1 month to ensure continued suppression of serum cortisol concentrations.
  - Dogs with adrenal tumors typically require higher maintenance dosages of mitotane than dogs with pituitary-dependent hyperadrenocorticism; about 25% need a maintenance dosage >150 mg/kg weekly. Relapses are not uncommon.
  - Although not correlated with tumor response in all dogs, cortisol determinations are a practical and relatively reliable means of monitoring therapy. They should be performed 1 month after any change in mitotane dosage and every 3–6 months during long-term therapy. Periodic ultrasono-

graphic evaluation is also useful for evaluating tumor response.

- *Common side effects* include anorexia, weakness, vomiting, diarrhea, and lethargy and are seen in up to 60% of cases. Adverse effects may be due to development of hypoadrenocorticism, but in approximately 50% of dogs the side effects appear to result from a direct drug toxicity. If adverse reactions occur, stop the drug and evaluate the dog as soon as possible to exclude glucocorticoid and mineralocorticoid deficiency. If a direct drug toxicity is occurring, start mitotane again later at a 25–50% lower dosage. Reinstitution of the higher maintenance dosage can be attempted later but usually results in recurrence of adverse effects. Complete glucocorticoid and mineralocorticoid deficiency (Addison disease) has been reported in a few cases.

Patient Monitoring

Mitotane overdosage and underdosage can complicate therapy; long-term monitoring is therefore necessary. Instruct owners to observe for recurrence of symptoms, especially polyuria and polydipsia. Perform an ACTH stimulation test every 3–6 months to assess adrenal reserve and to guide mitotane dosage adjustments.

The prognosis for hyperadrenocorticism is always guarded because of the many complications associated with the disease. Dogs that succumb to such complications usually do so within the first 3–6 months after diagnosis. Dogs that survive this period typically die of other geriatric disorders unrelated to hyperadrenocorticism. The average life span after diagnosis is 2 years. Complications include:

- Thromboembolism.
- Infection.
- Hypertension.
- Congestive heart failure.
- Recurrence of clinical signs.
- Progression of CNS signs (expanding pituitary tumor).
- Glomerulopathy.
- Pancreatitis.

HYPERADRENOCORTICISM IN CATS

Etiology

Hyperadrenocorticism in cats can be due to pituitary-dependent disease, adrenocortical neoplasia, or iatrogenic disease. Hyperadrenocorticism is uncommon in cats.

- *Pituitary-dependent hyperadrenocorticism* is the most common cause of the naturally occurring disorder in cats, accounting for 80% of the cases.
- *Cortisol-secreting adrenocortical neoplasia* is present in approximately 20% of cats with spontaneous hyperadrenocorticism. About one-third of adrenal tumors in cats are malignant.
- *Iatrogenic hyperadrenocorticism* can occur in cats, despite the relative resistance of cats to the effects of glucocorticoids when compared with dogs.

Signalment

- *Age:* Spontaneous hyperadrenocorticism is a disease of middle-aged to older cats (range, 5–16 years).
- *Breed:* No breed predilection.
- *Sex:* Sixty percent of reported cases have been female.

Clinical Signs

General Appearance

- Pendulous, distended, or "pot-bellied" abdomen.
- Bilaterally symmetric alopecia with dull, dry, haircoat and scaling (seborrhea sicca).
- Thin skin.
- Muscle atrophy.

Endocrine and Urinary System

- *Polyuria, polydipsia* and *polyphagia.* In contrast to dogs with hyperadrenocorticism, polyuria and polydipsia in affected cats appear to be secondary to concurrent diabetes mellitus in the vast majority of cases.
- Glucose intolerance and insulin resistance are common.

▼ *Key Point* The majority of cats (almost 80%) with hyperadrenocorticism have concurrent diabetes mellitus.

Diagnosis

History

Common reported signs include polyuria and polydipsia, pot-bellied appearance, thin skin, bilateral alopecia, lethargy, and weakness. Determine if exogenous glucocorticoids have recently been given.

Physical Examination

Many of the clinical signs listed above may be noted. Other findings may include hepatomegaly, obesity or weight loss, and fragile tearing skin.

Routine Laboratory Testing

- Hyperglycemia and glycosuria are seen in up to 90% of cats.
- Hypercholesterolemia and elevated serum ALT activity are common.
- Leukocytosis, eosinopenia, and lymphopenia may be noted.

▼ *Key Point* In contrast to the disease in dogs, elevated serum alkaline phosphatase is *not* a consistent finding in cats with hyperadrenocorticism.

Pituitary-Adrenal Function Tests

ACTH Stimulation Test

This is a valuable screening test for hyperadrenocorticism in cats.

- *Procedure*
  - Collect a plasma or serum sample for cortisol analysis before and at 60 and 120 minutes after IM injection of 2.2 units/kg ACTH gel (Acthar Gel, Rhone Poulenc). The maximal rise in cortisol concentration occurs at 2 hours in 60% of normal cats, whereas the remaining cats peak at 1 hour after ACTH injection.
  - Alternatively, collect a plasma or serum sample before and 60 minutes after IV administration of 0.125 mg of synthetic ACTH (cosyntropin; Cortrosyn, Organon Pharmaceuticals).
- *Interpretation*
  - Approximately 66% of cats with naturally occurring hyperadrenocorticism show a high-normal or exaggerated cortisol response to exogenous ACTH.
  - Cats with iatrogenic hyperadrenocorticism show a "blunted" or no response to ACTH.
  - The ACTH stimulation test does not differentiate pituitary-dependent hyperadrenocorticism from a functional adrenal tumor.

Low-Dose Dexamethasone Suppression Test

- Suppression of serum cortisol concentration (<1.5 μg/dl; <40 nmol/L) 8 hours after administration of a low dose of dexamethasone (0.01–0.015 mg/kg IV) excludes a diagnosis of hyperadrenocorticism.
- However, cats with nonadrenal illness (e.g., diabetes mellitus) frequently demonstrate inadequate suppression, as do cats with hyperadrenocorticism. Because of these frequent false-positive results (low specificity), this test is not recommended as the sole diagnostic test for hyperadrenocorticism in cats.

High-Dose Dexamethasone Suppression Test

- *Procedure:* Collect plasma or serum samples for cortisol analysis before and at 4 and 8 hours after IV administration of 0.1 mg/kg dexamethasone.
- This test is useful in distinguishing normal cats or cats with nonadrenal disease from cats with hyperadrenocorticism.
- In contrast to most dogs with pituitary-dependent hyperadrenocorticism, 75% of cats with pituitary-dependent disease fail to show adequate cortisol suppression after high-dose dexamethasone suppression testing.
- All cats with adrenal-dependent hyperadrenocorticism fail to show adequate cortisol suppression after high-dose dexamethasone suppression testing.
- Therefore, this test cannot readily distinguish pituitary-dependent hyperadrenocorticism and adrenal tumor in cats.
- Due to the potential for false-negative results in cats with pituitary-dependent hyperadrenocorticism, do not exclude the diagnosis on the basis of a single normal result, especially if clinical signs or imaging studies support the diagnosis.

▼ *Key Point* The low-dose dexamethasone suppression test has not been well standardized in the cat.

The high-dose dexamethasone test (0.1 mg/kg IV) appears to be the preferred method of screening for hyperadrenocorticism in cats at this time.

Urine Cortisol to Creatinine Ratio

- This may be a useful screening test for hyperadrenocorticism in cats. A normal result makes a diagnosis of hyperadrenocorticism very unlikely.
- As in dogs, a positive test must be interpreted cautiously due to the low specificity of the test, and the diagnosis should be confirmed with an ACTH stimulation or a dexamethasone suppression test.

Plasma ACTH Concentration

- Endogenous plasma ACTH concentration can be used to distinguish pituitary-dependent hyperadrenocorticism from adrenocortical tumors in cats. Cats with pituitary-dependent hyperadrenocorticism have a normal to high ACTH concentration (>40 pg/ml).
- Cats with cortisol-secreting adrenal tumors have a low plasma concentration of ACTH (<20 pg/ml).

Imaging Studies

- *Radiography.* Radiography has limited value in determining the etiology of hyperadrenocorticism in cats unless an obvious adrenal mass is apparent.
- *Ultrasonography.* Ultrasonography can be a sensitive means for evaluating the adrenal glands of cats with hyperadrenocorticism. Bilateral adrenal enlargement is seen in most cats with pituitary-dependent hyperadrenocorticism and a unilateral adrenal mass is seen in almost all cats with adrenal neoplasia.
- *CT and MRI.* CT and MRI scans can be useful and sensitive for determining the cause of hyperadrenocorticism; however, they require anesthesia and have limited availability.

Treatment

Medical Treatment

- *Mitotane (Lysodren, Bristol-Myers Squibb)* has been safely administered to cats with hyperadrenocorticism at dosages comparable to those given dogs. However, it has not been effective in controlling the disorder in most reported cases, and some cats tolerate the drug poorly.
- *Ketoconazole* does not reliably decrease serum cortisol concentrations in cats with hyperadrenocorticism. Two of four cats with pituitary-dependent hyperadrenocorticism given 10–20 mg/kg daily showed some improvement, whereas two cats with adrenal neoplasia failed to show significant improvement.
- *Metyrapone,* an enzyme inhibitor that blocks adrenal synthesis of glucocorticoids, has been used with mixed results in treating cats with hyperadrenocorticism at dosages ranging from 200–500 mg daily. Some cats showed clinical improvement without significant side effects.
- *L-Deprenyl,* as used for the treatment of dogs with pituitary-dependent hyperadrenocorticism, is not yet established as a safe and effective treatment for cats.

Surgical Treatment

In cats with adrenal tumors, perform unilateral adrenalectomy as the treatment of choice (see under Adrenalectomy). Bilateral adrenalectomy remains a viable and probably the most successful treatment for pituitary-dependent hyperadrenocorticism in cats.

Radiation Therapy

This has been partially successful in a few cats with pituitary-dependent hyperadrenocorticism. It is the treatment of choice in cats with large pituitary tumors. Concurrent medical management may be necessary for a few to several months.

▼ *Key Point* Adrenalectomy appears to be the most successful means of treating hyperadrenocorticism in cats. To date, medical therapy has not been consistently successful.

PHEOCHROMOCYTOMA

Etiology

Pheochromocytoma is a rare catecholamine-producing neuroectodermal tumor derived from chromaffin cells of the adrenal medulla. About half of reported pheochromocytomas in dogs have been malignant. Reported metastatic sites include lungs, liver, bone, kidney, and lymph nodes. Concurrent pheochromocytoma and adrenocortical neoplasia has been reported.

Signalment

- Pheochromocytoma generally occurs in older dogs.
- There is no breed or sex predilection.

Clinical Signs

▼ *Key Point* Most pheochromocytomas are not detected antemortem and are incidental findings at necropsy because of vague, episodic clinical signs.

- Clinical signs develop either as a result of the space-occupying nature of the adrenal tumor and its metastasis, or as a result of excessive secretion of catecholamines with resultant systemic hypertension and other manifestations.
- Weakness, lethargy, anorexia, vomiting, weight loss, polyuria, polydipsia, restlessness, and excessive panting are the most frequent signs, but these occur in less than 50% of affected dogs.
- Other less common signs may include diarrhea, cough, dyspnea, hind leg edema, abdominal distention, acute blindness, epistaxis, anxiety, shaking, ataxia, seizures, cyanosis, pacing, and adipsia.

Diagnosis

History, Physical Examination, and Routine Laboratory Testing

- History and clinical findings are typically vague and nonspecific (e.g., lethargy and tachypnea).

- Duration of signs varies from days to years.
- An abdominal mass can be palpated in about 10% of dogs with pheochromocytoma.
- Routine laboratory findings are usually not helpful.
- ECG abnormalities may include sinus tachycardia, arrhythmias, and evidence of cardiac chamber enlargement.

Radiography and Other Imaging Techniques

- Abdominal radiographs reveal a cranial abdominal mass in the region of the adrenal gland in up to one-third of dogs with pheochromocytoma. Ten percent of tumors show evidence of mineralization.
- Specialized imaging techniques such as ultrasonography, computed tomography, and MRI are more sensitive than radiography and are very useful for detecting and staging pheochromocytomas.
- Echocardiography may demonstrate left ventricular hypertrophy.

Arterial Blood Pressure

Up to 50% of dogs with pheochromocytoma are hypertensive. Catecholamine secretion, and therefore hypertension, tends to be episodic.

Biochemical and Pharmacologic Tests

Measurement of urinary and resting plasma catecholamine concentrations, the clonidine suppression test, and the phentolamine test can be used to demonstrate excessive production of catecholamines (epinephrine and norepinephrine) or their metabolites. Unfortunately, the limited availability, technical difficulty, and expense of these tests severely limits routine use of these in veterinary medicine.

▼ *Key Point* The antemortem diagnosis of pheochromocytoma in dogs must usually rely on surgical exploration and biopsy.

Treatment

- Adrenalectomy is the treatment of choice for pheochromocytoma (see following discussion under Adrenalectomy).
- Medical therapy is indicated preoperatively (to control hypertension and to help prevent cardiac arrhythmias before and during surgery), as well as for long-term treatment of inoperable and incompletely resected tumors.
- Treat severe hypertension with phenoxybenzamine (0.2–1.5 mg/kg q12h PO) or prazosin (0.5–2.0 mg/kg q12h PO).
- Administer beta blockers such as propanolol or atenolol if necessary to control tachycardia or arrhythmias, but do not use these without concurrent alpha blockade.
- Chemotherapy and radiation therapy have been employed in humans with pheochromocytoma, but the use of these modalities has not been reported in dogs or cats.

ADRENALECTOMY

Adrenalectomy usually is performed for treatment of hyperadrenocorticism in the dog and cat. Unilateral adrenalectomy is done primarily for removal of adrenal neoplasia (adenoma, adenocarcinoma, or pheochromocytoma). Bilateral adrenalectomy is less commonly used for bilateral adrenocortical hyperplasia. The anatomy and surgical and medical management for adrenalectomy is the same in the dog and cat. Adrenalectomy is performed infrequently in cats owing to the low incidence of hyperadrenocorticism and adrenal neoplasia.

Surgical Anatomy of the Adrenal Gland

- The adrenal glands are paired, flattened, bilobed glands located retroperitoneally and craniomedial to the kidneys (Fig. 31–1).
- The right adrenal gland lies at about the level of the last thoracic to the first lumbar vertebrae.
- The capsule of the right adrenal gland may be contiguous with the tunica externa of the caudal vena cava.
- The left adrenal gland is slightly caudal to the right and is separated from the caudal vena cava by a layer of fat.
- Adrenal size is breed-dependent. In dogs, the average size is 22 mm long, 10 mm wide, and 4 mm thick.
- The adrenal glands are well vascularized by branches of the renal, accessory renal, phrenic, cranial abdominal, phrenicoabdominal, and lumbar arteries.
- Venous drainage is through the left and right adrenal and the phrenicoabdominal veins.
- The phrenicoabdominal artery crosses the dorsal surface of the adrenal glands; the phrenicoabdomi-

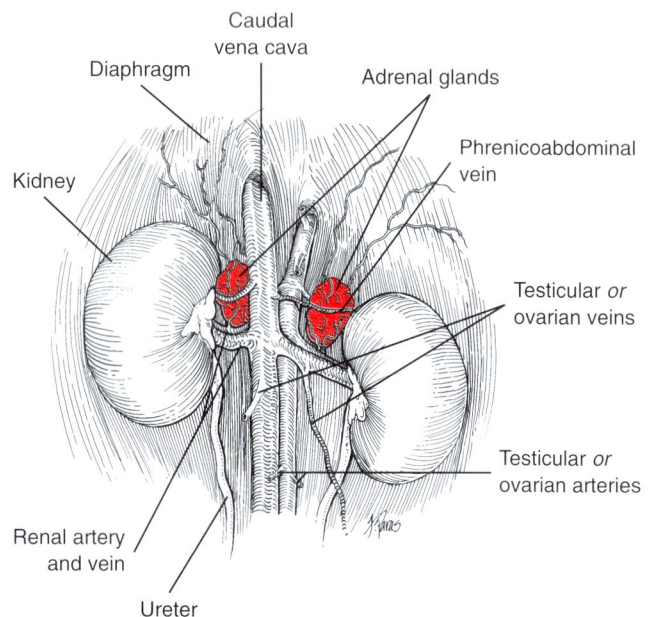

Figure 31–1. Anatomy of the adrenal glands from the ventral midline abdominal approach.

nal vein courses across the ventral surface. These paired vessels are the largest supplying the adrenal glands.

Preoperative Considerations

- Obtain a minimum database consisting of complete blood count, serum chemistry profile, and thoracic radiographs.
- Abdominal radiographs may help localize a unilateral adrenal mass, especially if the tumor is mineralized.
- Ultrasonography is also very helpful in identifying a mass and determining if invasion of the vena cava has occurred.
- Correct any fluid and electrolyte abnormalities.
- Treat arrhythmias and hypertension that may accompany pheochromocytoma (see next section).

Anesthesia and Perioperative Care

For Hyperadrenocorticism

- Induce and maintain anesthesia following standard procedures.
- Isoflurane is preferred over halothane, as it does not sensitize the myocardium to catecholamines.
- Administer a broad-spectrum bactericidal antibiotic by IV bolus 30 minutes before surgery.
- Supplement corticosteroids in the form of dexamethasone (0.1–0.2 mg/kg IV) immediately before the onset of surgery, at the completion of the surgical procedure, and then every 6 to 8 hours during the immediate postoperative period (24–48 hours).

For Pheochromocytoma

- Avoid premedication with atropine because of the potential for severe tachycardia.

▼ *Key Point* Dogs with pheochromocytoma produce high circulating concentrations of the catecholamines epinephrine and norepinephrine, which may cause profound arrhythmias.

- Induce anesthesia with thiopental (6–10 mg/kg IV) or oxymorphone (0.1–0.3 mg/kg IV) and glycopyrrolate, or proprofol (3–5 mg/kg).
- Isoflurane is the inhalant agent of choice for dogs with pheochromocytoma.
- Administer methoxyflurane (rather than halothane) if isoflurane is not available.
- Administer fluids and antibiotics as for hyperadrenocorticism.
- Closely monitor blood pressure and ECG.
- To manage ventricular arrhythmias, give either lidocaine (1 mg/kg IV) or propranolol (0.1–0.3 mg/kg IV).
- Treat hypertensive episodes with phentolamine (alpha blocker) (0.02–0.1 mg/kg IV), repeated as needed.
- Manage hypotension with vigorous IV fluid administration.

Surgical Procedure

Objectives

- Handle tissue gently, especially tumor tissue.

▼ *Key Point* Surgical handling of a pheochromocytoma may precipitate catecholamine release and hypertension. Profound hypotension may rapidly occur following tumor removal.

- Use meticulous hemostasis to minimize blood loss.
- Avoid trauma to the caudal vena cava.
- Close the linea alba with a nonabsorbable suture material.

▼ *Key Point* Animals with hyperadrenocorticism are prone to delayed healing and incisional infection because of cortisol inhibition of fibroblast proliferation and collagen synthesis.

Equipment

- Standard general surgical pack and suture
- Balfour retractors
- Bipolar cautery
- Sterile cotton-tipped applicator sticks
- Hemostatic clips
- Gelfoam

Technique

1. Make a ventral midline abdominal incision, extending from the xiphoid to about 2 cm caudal to the umbilicus. This may be combined with a paracostal incision (Fig. 31–2).
   a. Alternatively, use a retroperitoneal approach (Fig. 31–3). This provides good exposure of the

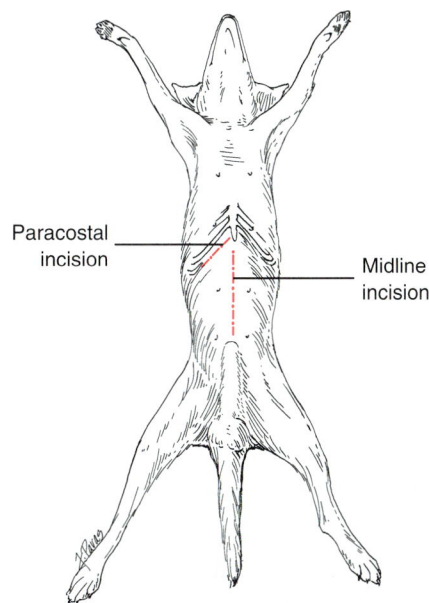

Figure 31–2. Incision for the ventral midline approach may be extended paracostally for better exposure of the adrenal gland.

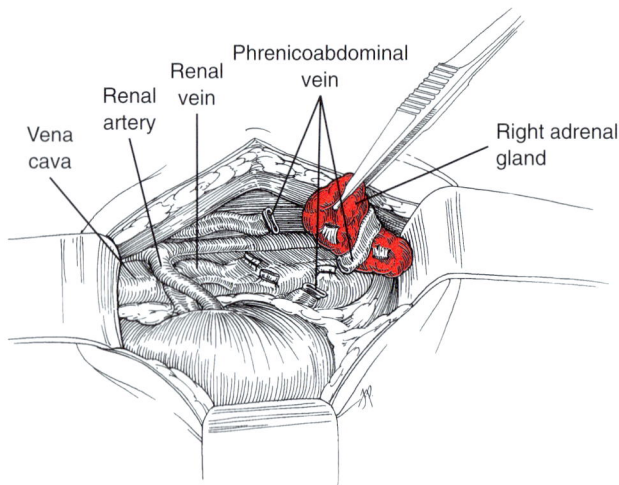

Figure 31–3. Surgical anatomy of the right adrenal gland and its associated vascular structures as viewed from the retroperitoneal approach.

ipsilateral gland but must be performed bilaterally if bilateral adrenalectomy is required.

2. Expose the affected gland(s) and isolate with moistened laparotomy sponges.
3. Perform gentle dissection with cotton-tipped applicator sticks, especially when separating the gland from the vena cava.
4. Ligate the phrenicoabdominal artery and vein and any other vascular structures serving the adrenal gland. Hemostatic vascular clips are very helpful for this.

▼ *Key Point* Identify and preserve the renal artery and vein, which may lie close to the adrenal glands.

5. Completely resect all abnormal tissue, including the adrenal capsule, and tumor thrombus in the vena cava, if possible.
6. Prior to closure, carefully check the surgical field for hemorrhage.
7. Inspect the abdominal viscera, especially the liver, for metastatic disease, and biopsy any suspicious lesions.
8. Perform a routine, three-layer abdominal closure using nonabsorbable suture material to close the linea alba.

Postoperative Care
Unilateral Adrenalectomy for Adrenocortical Tumor

- Supplement glucocorticoids starting at 24–48 hours after surgery with prednisone (0.5 mg/kg q12h PO for 3 days, then taper the dosage over 10–14 days to 0.2 mg/kg q24h PO) until the contralateral adrenal gland is functioning normally.
- Perform an ACTH stimulation test on the first postoperative day and at 2–4 week intervals following surgery until adrenal reserve normalizes.
- The remaining adrenal gland usually functions normally within 2 months following surgery.

Unilateral Adrenalectomy for Pheochromocytoma

Function of the contralateral gland is not suppressed; therefore, there is no need for postoperative glucocorticoid or mineralocorticoid supplementation.

Bilateral Adrenalectomy

- Supplement glucocorticoids (prednisone, 0.2 mg/kg q24h PO).
- Supplement mineralocorticoid (fludrocortisone acetate or DOCP) as described in the preceding section on hypoadrenocorticism.
- Check serum electrolytes periodically to adjust the dosages of mineralocorticoid replacement therapy.

Complications

Complications may include:

- Hemorrhage.
- Cardiac arrest and/or arrhythmias.
- Fluid and electrolyte abnormalities.
- Pulmonary artery thrombosis.
- Pancreatitis.
- Acute renal failure.
- Pneumonia.
- Adrenal insufficiency.

Prognosis
Unilateral Adrenocortical Tumor

- Good if the tumor is benign.
- Fair if the tumor is malignant but completely resected.
- Extremely poor for invasive adenocarcinoma.

Unilateral Pheochromocytoma

- Excellent prognosis for benign tumor.
- About 50% of pheochromocytomas are malignant and metastatic at the time of surgery, indicating a grave prognosis.

Bilateral Adrenal Hyperplasia

- Fair to good prognosis; however, medical therapy is preferred over surgery for this lesion in dogs.
- Metastatic disease is not a problem; however, regulating the iatrogenic hypoadrenocorticism created by bilateral adrenalectomy may be difficult.

SUPPLEMENTAL READINGS

Barthez PY, Marks SL, Woo J, et al.: Pheochromocytoma in dogs: 61 cases (1984–1995). J Vet Intern Med 11:272, 1997.
Barthez PY, Nyland TG, Feldman EC: Ultrasonographic evaluation of the adrenal glands in dogs. J Am Vet Med Assoc 207:1180, 1995.
Duesberg C, Peterson ME: Adrenal disorders in cats. Vet Clin North Am Small Anim Pract 27:321, 1997.
Duesberg CA, Nelson RW, Feldman EC, et al.: Adrenalectomy for treatment of hyperadrenocorticism in cats: 10 cases (1988–1992). J Am Vet Med Assoc 207:1066, 1995.
Enns SG, Johnston DE, Eigenmann JE, Goldschmidt MH: Adrenalectomy in the management of canine hyperadrenocorticism. J Am Anim Hosp Assoc 23:557, 1987.

Feldman EC, Nelson RW, Feldman MS: Use of low- and high-dose dexamethasone tests for distinguishing pituitary-dependent from adrenal tumor hyperadrenocorticism in dogs. J Am Vet Med Assoc 209:772, 1996.

Gilson SD, Withrow SJ, Wheeler SL, Twedt DC: Pheochromocytoma in 50 dogs. J Vet Intern Med 8:228, 1994.

Grooters AM, Biller DS, Theisen SK, Miyabayashi T: Ultrasonographic characteristics of the adrenal glands in dogs with pituitary-dependent hyperadrenocorticism: Comparison with normal dogs. J Vet Intern Med 10:110, 1996.

Kintzer PP, Peterson ME: Mitotane treatment of 32 dogs with cortisol-secreting adrenocortical neoplasms. J Am Vet Med Assoc 205:54, 1994.

Kintzer PP, Peterson ME: Mitotane (o,p′-DDD) treatment of 200 dogs with pituitary-dependent hyperadrenocorticism. J Vet Intern Med 5:182, 1991.

Kintzer PP, Peterson ME: Treatment and long-term follow-up of 205 dogs with hypoadrenocorticism. J Vet Intern Med 11:43, 1997.

Melián C, Peterson ME: Diagnosis and treatment of naturally occurring hypoadrenocorticism in 42 dogs. J Small Anim Pract 37:268, 1996.

Peterson ME: Considerations and complications in anesthesia with pathophysiologic changes in the endocrine system. *In* Short CE, ed. Principles and Practice of Veterinary Anesthesiology. Philadelphia: Williams & Wilkins, 1987, p 251.

Peterson ME, Greco DS, Orth DN: Primary hypoadrenocorticism in ten cats. J Vet Intern Med 3:55, 1989.

Peterson ME, Kintzer PP: Pretreatment clinical and laboratory findings in dogs with hypoadrenocorticism: 225 cases (1979–1993). J Am Vet Med Assoc 208:85, 1996.

Peterson ME, Kintzer PP: Medical treatment of pituitary-dependent hyperadrenocorticism: Mitotane. Vet Clin North Am Small Anim Pract 27:255, 1997.

van Sluijs FJ, Sjollema BE, Voorhout G, et al.: Results of adrenalectomy in 36 dogs with hyperadrenocorticism caused by adrenocortical tumour. Vet Q 17:113, 1995.

Widmer WR, Guptill L: Imaging techniques for facilitating diagnosis of hyperadrenocorticism in dogs and cats. J Am Vet Med Assoc 206:1857, 1995.

32 Diabetes Mellitus

Deborah S. Greco

ETIOLOGY

Type 1 Diabetes Mellitus

- Insulin-dependent diabetes mellitus (IDDM), also referred to as type 1 diabetes, is a diabetic state in which endogenous insulin secretion is never sufficient to prevent ketone production.
- Insulin secretion may be reduced or absent and the diabetic state is readily corrected by exogenous insulin.

Type 2 Diabetes Mellitus

- Non–insulin-dependent diabetes mellitus (NIDDM), also referred to as type 2 diabetes, is a diabetic state in which insulin secretion is usually sufficient to prevent ketosis but not enough to prevent hyperglycemia.
- Insulin secretion may be high, low, or normal but is insufficient to overcome insulin resistance in peripheral tissues.
- The metabolic hallmarks of type 2 diabetes are impaired insulin secretion, increased hepatic glucose output, and insulin resistance (Fig. 32–1).
- In cats and in humans with type 2 diabetes, insulin secretion secondary to a glucose load is impaired. The early phase of insulin secretion is delayed or absent and the second phase of insulin secretion is delayed but exaggerated.
- Amyloid deposition in the pancreatic islets may be the cause of impaired insulin secretion in cats.
- Obesity is a risk factor in type 2 diabetes because it causes insulin resistance.

▼ *Key Point* Most dogs suffer from type 1 diabetes, or IDDM. Most cats probably suffer from type 2 (NIDDM) diabetes; however, by the time a diagnosis of diabetes is confirmed in many cats with NIDDM, they have become insulin-dependent.

Type 3 Diabetes Mellitus

- Type 3, or secondary, diabetes mellitus is the result of another primary disease or drug therapy that produces insulin resistance (e.g., hyperadrenocorticism, hyperthyroidism, acromegaly, progestational drugs) or destroys pancreatic tissue (pancreatitis). Sec-

ondary diabetes is common in both dogs (pancreatitis) and cats (drugs, endocrinopathies, pancreatitis).

PATHOPHYSIOLOGY

Uncomplicated Diabetes Mellitus

- In animals with uncomplicated diabetes mellitus, hyperglycemia results from impaired glucose utilization, increased gluconeogenesis, and increased hepatic glycogenolysis.
- Decreased peripheral utilization of glucose leads to hyperglycemia followed by osmotic diuresis. This causes the classic clinical signs of polyuria with compensatory polydipsia and progressive dehydration.
- Impaired glucose utilization by the hypothalamic satiety center combined with loss of calories in the form of glycosuria results in polyphagia and weight loss, respectively.
- Insulin is anabolic; therefore, insulin deficiency leads to protein catabolism and contributes to weight loss and muscle atrophy.
- As a consequence of protein catabolism, amino acids are used by the liver to promote gluconeogenesis and contribute to hyperglycemia.
- With insulin deficiency, the hormone-sensitive lipase system, which is normally suppressed by insulin, becomes activated. The unrestrained lipolytic activity of hormone-sensitive lipase contributes to weight loss in a previously obese or overweight animal.

Complicated (Ketoacidotic) Diabetes Mellitus

▼ *Key Point* Diabetic ketoacidosis (DKA) is the culmination of IDDM that results in unrestrained ketone body formation in the liver, metabolic acidosis, severe dehydration, shock, and possibly death.

- With time, uncomplicated diabetes mellitus may progress to complicated or ketoacidotic diabetes. In these animals, insulin deficiency causes abnormal lipid metabolism in the liver such that nonesterified fatty acids are converted to acetyl coenzyme A (acetyl-CoA) rather than being incorporated into triglycerides.
  - Acetyl-CoA accumulates in the liver and is converted into acetoacetyl-CoA and then ultimately to acetoacetic acid.

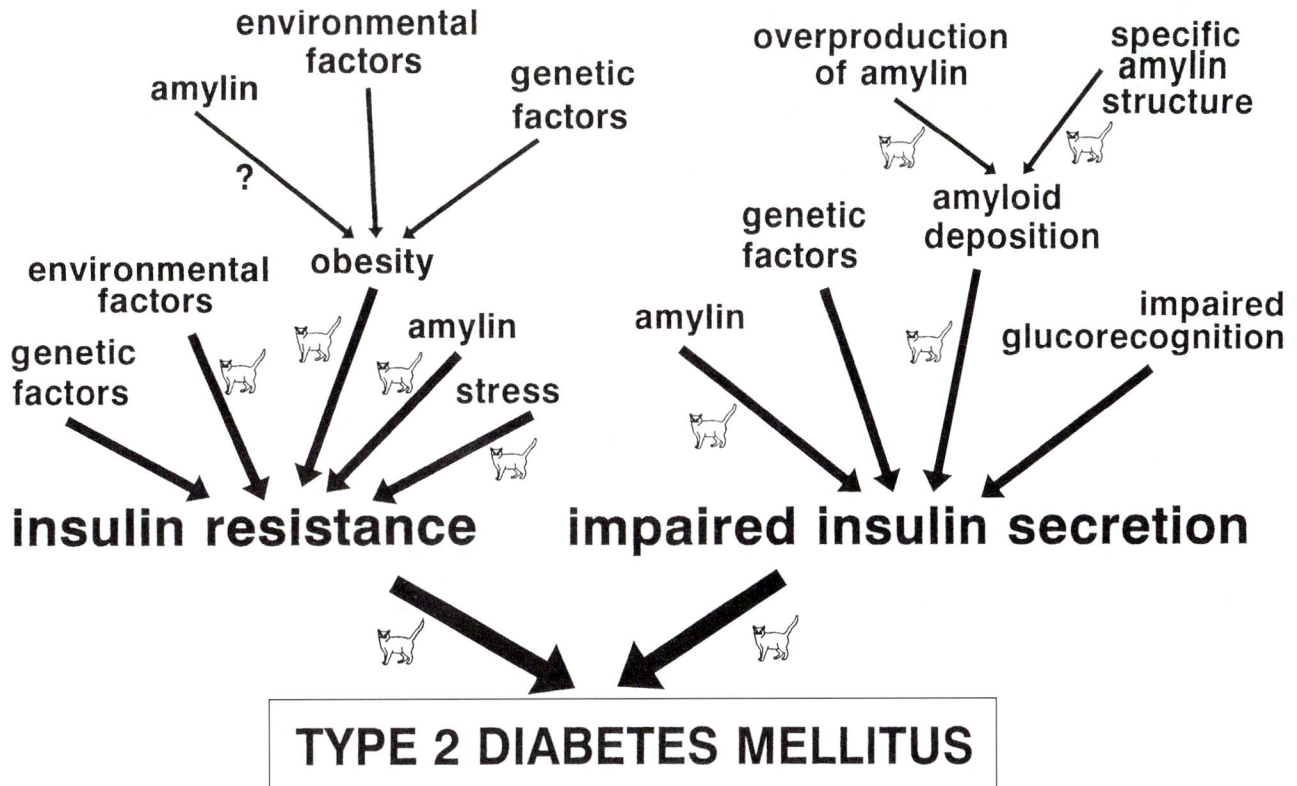

Figure 32-1. Summary of the pathophysiologic factors contributing to hyperglycemia in non–insulin-dependent (type 2) diabetes mellitus. (From Lutz TA, Rand JS: Pathogenesis of feline diabetes mellitus. Vet Clin North Am Small Anim Pract 25:544, 1995; with permission.)

- Finally, the liver starts to generate ketones including acetoacetic acid, beta-hydroxybutyrate, and acetone.
- As insulin deficiency culminates in DKA, accumulation of ketones and lactic acid in the blood and loss of electrolytes and water in the urine results in profound dehydration, hypovolemia, metabolic acidosis, and shock.
  - Ketonuria and osmotic diuresis caused by glycosuria result in sodium and potassium loss in the urine and exacerbation of hypovolemia and dehydration.
  - Nausea, anorexia, and vomiting, caused by stimulation of the chemoreceptor trigger zone via ketonemia and hyperglycemia, contribute to the dehydration caused by osmotic diuresis.
  - Dehydration and shock lead to prerenal azotemia and a decline in the glomerular filtration rate. Declining GFR leads to further accumulation of glucose and ketones in the blood.
- Stress hormones such as cortisol and epinephrine contribute to the hyperglycemia in a vicious cycle.
- Eventually severe dehydration may result in hyperviscosity, thromboembolism, severe metabolic acidosis, renal failure, and finally death.

CLINICAL SIGNS

Uncomplicated Diabetes Mellitus

- Most diabetic animals have the classic clinical signs of polyuria and polydipsia.
- Weight loss is more common in dogs than in cats.
- Acute onset of blindness caused by bilateral cataract formation is a common presenting complaint of diabetes mellitus in dogs.
- Cats may present with chronic complications of diabetes, such as gait abnormalities resulting from diabetic neuropathy, or chronic gastrointestinal signs such as vomiting, diarrhea, and anorexia.

Complicated (Ketoacidotic) Diabetes

- Depression, vomiting, anorexia, and weakness are the most common clinical signs of ketoacidosis in dogs and cats.
- Animals with DKA often present in shock.
- Physical examination findings may include depression, tachypnea, dehydration, weakness, vomiting, and occasionally, a strong acetone odor on the breath.

- Cats may present recumbent or comatose, which may be a manifestation of severe ketoacidosis or mixed ketotic hyperosmolar syndrome.
- Approximately one-third of diabetic cats with ketosis exhibit icterus at presentation. Icterus may be a result of associated hemolysis, hepatic lipidosis, or acute pancreatitis.

DIAGNOSIS

Base the diagnosis of diabetes mellitus on typical clinical signs and evidence of fasting hyperglycemia and glycosuria.

Clinicopathologic Findings in Uncomplicated Diabetes Mellitus

- Fasting hyperglycemia.
- Hypercholesterolemia.
- High serum activity of liver enzymes (alkaline phosphatase, alanine aminotransferase).
- Glycosuria.

Clinicopathologic Findings in Diabetic Ketoacidosis

Findings in DKA may include all of the above findings plus the following:

- Azotemia.
- Hyponatremia.
- Hyperkalemia.
- Ketonemia and ketonuria.

Diagnostic Pitfalls

- With regard to fasting hyperglycemia, many cats are susceptible to "stress-induced" hyperglycemia in which the serum glucose concentrations may approach 300–400 mg/dl.
- Renal glycosuria may be found in animals with renal tubular disease and occasionally with stress-induced hyperglycemia.
- It may be difficult to differentiate early type 2 diabetes in cats from stress-induced hyperglycemia, because cats with early NIDDM are often asymptomatic.

Glycosylated Proteins

Glycosylated proteins, such as glycosylated hemoglobin and fructosamine, may aid in the diagnosis of early type 2 diabetes in cats.

Glycosylated Hemoglobin

- Glycosylated hemoglobin is formed by an irreversible, nonenzymatic binding of glucose to hemoglobin. As plasma glucose concentrations increase, hemoglobin glycosylation increases proportionately.

Fructosamine

- Serum fructosamine is formed by glycosylation of serum protein such as albumin. The concentration of fructosamine in serum is directly related to blood glucose concentration.
- Serum fructosamine measurement may be beneficial in differentiating early or subclinical diabetes mellitus in the cat from stress-induced hyperglycemia.

TREATMENT OF DIABETIC KETOACIDOSIS

Treatment of diabetic ketoacidosis, as outlined in Table 32–1, includes the following steps in order of importance:

Step 1. Fluid therapy using 0.9% saline initially, followed by 2.5% or 5% dextrose as serum glucose declines.
Step 2. Insulin therapy (low-dose intramuscular [IM] or intravenous [IV]).
Step 3. Electrolyte supplementation (potassium, phosphorus, magnesium).
Step 4. Treatment of metabolic acidosis.

Fluid Therapy

- Use 0.9% NaCl supplemented with potassium as the fluid therapy of choice when insulin therapy is initiated (see Table 32–1).
- Administer fluid therapy using a large central venous catheter, as animals in DKA are severely dehydrated and require rapid fluid administration; central venous pressure may also be monitored via a jugular catheter to avoid overhydration.
- Base the fluid administration rate on the severity of dehydration, maintenance requirements, continuing losses (vomiting and diarrhea), and the presence of concurrent disease (e.g., congestive heart failure; see Chap. 5).

Insulin Therapy

Initiate insulin therapy as soon as possible using either IV insulin or low-dose IM methods. Administer IV insulin via a separate peripheral catheter using the guidelines in Table 32–1.

- The species of origin of regular insulin (beef, pork, or human) does not affect response; however, the type of insulin given is very important. Use only regular insulin because it has a rapid onset and short duration of action and it can be given intravenously. Never give lente, ultralente, or NPH insulin IV.
- Dilute regular insulin at a dosage of 2.2 U/kg in dogs or 1.1 U/kg in cats in 250 ml of saline.
- Allow approximately 50 ml of fluid and insulin mixture to flow through the IV drip set and discard it, because insulin binds to the plastic tubing.
- With IV insulin administration, blood glucose decreases to below 250 mg/dl by approximately 10 hours in dogs and after about 16 hours in cats.
- Once euglycemia has been achieved, maintain the animal on subcutaneous (SC) regular insulin (0.1–0.4 U/kg q4–6h SC) until it starts to eat and/or the ketosis has resolved.
- For the transition from hospital to home maintenance insulin therapy, use a low dose (1–2 U) of

Table 32–1. STEPWISE TREATMENT OF DIABETIC KETOACIDOSIS

Step One: Fluids

a. Place an IV catheter, preferably central venous.
b. Fluid rate: Estimate dehydration deficit (%) × body weight (kg) × 1000 ml = no. of ml to rehydrate.
   Estimate maintenance needs: 2 ml/kg/hr × no. of hr required to rehydrate (in 24 hr).
   Estimate losses (vomiting, diarrhea).
   Dehydration deficit + maintenance + losses = no. of ml of fluid/24 hr = hourly fluid rate
c. Fluid composition

Blood Glucose (mg/dl)	Fluids	Rate	Route	Monitor	Frequency
>250	0.9% saline	Up to 45 (cat) and 90 (dog) ml/kg/hr to rehydrate	IV	PCV, TS, Na, K, osmolality	q4h
200–250	0.45% saline plus 2.5% dextrose	Up to 90 ml/kg/hr to rehydrate	IV	PCV, TS, Na, K, osmolality	q4h
150–200	0.45% saline plus 2.5% dextrose	Up to 90 ml/kg/hr to rehydrate	IV	CVP, urine output	q2h
100–150	0.45% saline plus 2.5% dextrose	Up to 90 ml/kg/hr to rehydrate	IV	CVP, urine output	q2h
<100	0.45% saline plus 5% dextrose	Up to 90 ml/kg/hr to rehydrate	IV	CVP, urine output	q2h

Step Two: Insulin

Intravenous (regular only), mixed in 250 ml of 0.9% NaCl; discard 50 ml through IV tubing.

Blood Glucose (mg/dl)	Rate	Route	Dose (U/kg)	Monitor	Frequency
Intravenous (Regular Only)					
>250	10 ml/hr	IV	1.1 (cats), 2.2 (dogs)	Blood glucose	q1–2h
200–250	7 ml/hr	IV	1.1 (cats), 2.2 (dogs)	Blood glucose	q1–2h
150–200	5 ml/hr	IV	1.1 (cats), 2.2 (dogs)	Blood glucose	q1h
100–150	5 ml/hr	IV	1.1 (cats), 2.2 (dogs)	Blood glucose	q1h
<100	Stop IV, begin insulin q4h	SC	0.1	Blood glucose	q4h
Intramuscular (Regular Only)					
>250	Initial dose	IM	0.2	Blood glucose	Hourly
	q1h	IM	0.1	Blood glucose	Hourly
<250	q4–6h	IM	0.1	Blood glucose	q4–6h
	q6–8h	SC	0.1–0.4	Blood glucose	q6–8h

Step Three: Electrolytes

Concentration	Amount (mEq/L) Added to 1 L of Fluids	Maximum Rate (ml/kg/hr)
Potassium (mEq/L)		
3.6–5.0	20	26
2.6–3.5	40	12
2.1–2.5	60	9
<2.0	80	7
Phosphorus (mg/dl)		
1–2	0.03 mmol phosphate/kg/hr	Monitor serum phosphorus q6h
<1.0	0.1 mmol phosphate/kg/hr	Monitor serum phosphorus q6h
Magnesium (mg/dl)		
<1.2	0.75–1 mEq/kg/day constant rate infusion; use MgCl or MgSO$_4$	Use 5% dextrose: magnesium is incompatible with calcium-containing and NaHCO$_3$ solutions

Step Four: Acid-Base Balance

pH	Bicarbonate Concentration	Dose of Bicarbonate (ml)	Rate
<7.1	<12 mEq/L	IV = 0.1 × body weight (kg) × (4 − HCO$_3$ [mEq/L])	Over 2 hr

CVP, central venous pressure; IM, intramuscular; IV, intravenous; PCV, packed cell volume; SC, subcutaneous; TS, total solids.
From Greco DS: Endocrine pancreatic emergencies. Comp Cont Educ Pract 19:23, 1997; with permission.

regular insulin combined with intermediate- or long-acting maintenance insulin at the recommended dosages (see Treatment of Uncomplicated Diabetes).

Electrolyte Supplementation

Potassium

- Supplement potassium as soon as insulin therapy is initiated (see Table 32–1).
- Although serum potassium may be normal or elevated in ketoacidosis, the animal actually suffers from total body depletion of potassium. Correction of the metabolic acidosis tends to drive potassium intracellularly in exchange for hydrogen ions. Insulin facilitates this exchange and the net effect is a dramatic decrease in serum potassium, which must be attenuated with appropriate potassium supplementation in fluids.

Magnesium

- Refractory hypokalemia may be complicated by hypomagnesemia. Supplementation of magnesium along with potassium as outlined in Table 32–1 may be indicated in cats or dogs with hypokalemia that is unresponsive to potassium chloride supplementation in fluids.

Phosphorus

- Serum and tissue phosphorus may also be depleted during a ketoacidotic crisis; thus, supplement one-third of the potassium dose as potassium phosphate (see Table 32–1), particularly in small dogs and cats who are most susceptible to hemolysis caused by hypophosphatemia.
- Use caution, as oversupplementation of phosphorus can result in metastatic calcification and hypocalcemia.

▼ *Key Point* In cats suffering from ketoacidosis, hemolysis may be caused by hypophosphatemia and/or Heinz body anemia.

Bicarbonate Therapy

- Bicarbonate therapy may be necessary in some patients with blood pH <7.1 or if serum HCO_3 is less than 12 mEq/L.
- Bicarbonate dosages are given in Table 32–1. Use caution, because metabolic alkalosis may be difficult to reverse.

TREATMENT OF UNCOMPLICATED DIABETES

Diet

The goals of dietary therapy in diabetes mellitus for both cats and dogs are to provide sufficient calories to maintain ideal body weight and correct obesity or emaciation, to minimize postprandial hyperglycemia, and to facilitate ideal absorption of glucose by timing meals to coincide with insulin administration.

- Maintain caloric intake at 60–70 Kcal/kg/day for smaller dogs and cats and 50–60 Kcal/kg/day for larger dogs.
- Reduce the body weight of obese animals gradually over a period of 2–4 months by feeding 60–70% of the calculated caloric requirements for ideal body weight.
- Feed underweight animals a high caloric density food based on caloric intake for optimum body weight. Once ideal body weight is reached, switch the animal to a high fiber diet. Table 32–2 lists the fiber and caloric content of various pet foods.

Table 32–2. MACRONUTRIENT CONTENT OF SELECTED AVAILABLE DOG FOODS

Diet	Food Form	% Nutrient (Dry Matter Basis)			
		Protein	Fat	Digestible Carbohydrate	Fiber
Theradiet Reducing*	Canned	27	7	24	29
Prescription Diet r/d†	Canned	26	7	36	21
Prescription Diet w/d†	Canned	16	12	56	13
Science Diet Maintenance Light†	Canned	17	10	61	8
Cycle 3 Light‡	Canned	19	9	53	8
Prescription Diet r/d†	Dry	25	7	39	22
Prescription Diet w/d†	Dry	17	7	54	16
Science Diet Maintenance Light†	Dry	17	7	57	14
Theradiet Reducing*	Dry	26	7	43	14
Purina Dog Chow–Low Calorie Formula§	Dry	16	6	~60	11
Fit N Trim§	Dry	17	9	61	9
Cycle 3 Light‡	Dry	19	9	53	5

*Theradiet, Sanofi Sante Animale, Victoriaville, Quebec.
†Hill's Pet Products, Topeka, KS.
‡Gaines Division, General Foods Corporation, White Plains, NJ.
§Ralston Purina Company, St. Louis, MO.
From Ihle SL: Nutritional therapy for diabetes mellitus. Vet Clin North Am Small Anim Pract 25:593, 1995.

▼ *Key Point* Increased dietary fiber improves glycemic control by slowing glucose absorption from the intestinal tract, reducing postprandial hyperglycemia, and controlling obesity.

- Adjust the feeding schedule to the timing of insulin therapy. If oral hypoglycemic agents are being used, the animal may have access to the required amount of food during the day. This is especially true for cats that eat by "nibbling" throughout the day.

▼ *Key Point* Feeding multiple small meals throughout the day or allowing the animal to "nibble" throughout the day minimizes postprandial hyperglycemia.

Exercise

- Keep the exercise level constant in a diabetic animal. Instruct the owner to walk the dog daily and avoid intermittent episodes of strenuous exercise, such as racing or hiking.
- Increasing exercise in an obese diabetic animal reduces insulin resistance and improves glycemic control.

Insulin Therapy

Insulin Source (Species of Origin)

- *Human recombinant insulin* is the most available insulin preparation on the market and is perfectly acceptable as insulin therapy for all dogs and most cats.
- *Porcine insulin* is identical to canine insulin in its amino acid structure and human insulin is very similar to canine insulin.
- *Beef insulin* is most similar to cat insulin, differing by only one amino acid in the A chain.

Insulin Preparations (Duration of Action)

Insulin preparations may be short-acting (regular insulin), intermediate-acting (Lente, NPH), or long-acting (Ultralente, protamine zinc insulin [PZI]).

NPH and Protamine Zinc Insulin

- NPH and PZI insulins are made by adding protamine in increasing concentrations to retard insulin absorption.
- PZI was discontinued as a human preparation in 1991 and has just recently become available again to veterinarians.

Semilente, Lente, and Ultralente

- Lente preparations control absorption by regulating the size of the insulin crystals.
- Semilente is composed of small zinc-insulin crystals, and Ultralente is composed of large zinc-insulin crystals that are more slowly absorbed.
- Lente insulin is a mixture of 30% prompt zinc-insulin suspension (Semilente) and 70% extended zinc-insulin (Ultralente).
- Lente insulin, because of the small zinc-insulin crys-

tal component, may be used to attenuate postprandial hyperglycemia.

Insulin Concentration

- Insulin is commercially available in 40, 100, and 500 units per milliliter concentrations, which are designated U-40, U-100, and U-500, respectively. One unit of insulin is approximately equivalent to 36 μg. PZI insulin is manufactured in U-40 concentration only.
- Regardless of the concentration of insulin used for therapy, it is absolutely essential that owners purchase the appropriate syringe for the concentration of insulin. U-100 insulin syringes are manufactured in low-dose (0.3 ml, 0.5 ml) and 1-ml capacities; U-40 syringes are available only in 1-ml capacity.
- In cats and small dogs (<10 kg), use low-dose (0.3 or 0.5 ml) syringes. These syringes are designed to accurately draw up a small dosage of U-100 insulin without the need for dilution.
- All insulin syringes are packaged with a 26- or 27-gauge injection needle.

Insulin Dosage (Table 32–3)

- Intermediate-acting insulin tends to be more bioavailable and, therefore, more potent. For this reason, dose intermediate-acting insulin (NPH, Lente) at the lower end of the range.
- In dogs, if intermediate-acting insulin is administered twice daily, use an initial dosage of 0.4–0.5 U/kg q12h SC (see Table 32–3).
- In cats, use an initial insulin dosage range of 0.2–0.5 U/kg for intermediate-acting insulin (NPH, Lente). The author prefers NPH twice daily in cats over Lente insulin.
- PZI insulin is available as a beef-pork product. Ultralente is available only as human recombinant insulin. Use an initial dosage range of 0.5–0.7 U/kg once or twice daily for long-acting insulin such as PZI or Ultralente.

Frequency of Insulin Administration (see Table 32–3)

- In order to mimic the physiologic release of insulin, ideally insulin should be given with each meal. The author recommends feeding the animal and injecting the insulin at the same time.
- If the animal does not eat, reduce the insulin dosage (usually by one-half) or skip the insulin entirely and determine the cause of the anorexia.

Adjusting Insulin Dose

- In dogs, make adjustments to insulin dosage in increments of 0.5–3 U/dog (depending on the size of the dog).
- In cats, make adjustments to insulin dosage in increments of 0.5 U/cat.
- Once adequate insulin therapy has been established, reassess diabetic control every 3–6 months as described in the following section.

Table 32–3. INITIAL INSULIN REGIMENS FOR DIABETIC DOGS AND CATS

Insulin Type	Initial Dose	Frequency of Dosing	Feeding Schedule	Insulin Adjustment	Frequency of Adjustment
Dogs					

Lente
  Humulin-L (Lilly),
  Novolin-L (Novo Nordisk)
	0.5 U/kg	q12h	q12h	0.5–3 U/dog	q5–7d

NPH
  Humulin-N (Lilly),
  Novolin-N (Novo Nordisk)
	0.5 U/kg	q12h	q12h	0.5–3 U/dog	q5–7d

Ultralente
  Humulin-U (Lilly)
	0.7 U/kg	q24h	$\frac{2}{3}$ morning;
			  $\frac{1}{3}$ evening
				1–4 U/dog	q5–7d

Cats					
NPH NPH (Novo Nordisk)	0.2–0.5 U/kg	q12h	Throughout day	0.5 U/cat	q5–7d

Lente
  Humulin-L (Lilly),
  Novolin-L (Novo Nordisk)
	0.2–0.5 U/kg	q12h	Throughout day	0.5–1 U/cat	q5–7d

Ultralente Humulin-U (Lilly)	1–3 U/cat	q12–24h	Throughout day	0.5 U/cat	q5–7d

Protamine zinc insulin
  Protamine analine zinc
    (Anthony)
	1–3 U/cat	q24h	Throughout day	0.5 U/cat	q5–7d

Modified from Greco DS, Broussard JD, Peterson ME: Insulin therapy. Vet Clin North Am Small Anim Pract 25:684, 1995; with permission.

Monitoring Insulin Therapy

Home Monitoring

- Instruct the client to monitor the insulin effect and overall control of hyperglycemia by noting changes in appetite, attitude, body condition, polydipsia, polyuria, and urine glucose and ketone concentrations.
- Initially monitor urine glucose and ketones daily (morning). Urine glucose should decrease to trace or 1+ with appropriate therapy. Decrease urine monitoring to once weekly or biweekly in well-regulated diabetic animals.
- Consistently high urine glucose readings coupled with uncontrolled clinical signs, such as polyuria/polydipsia, indicate that the insulin dose may be inadequate.
- Consistently negative readings on urine glucose may indicate that insulin dosages are either adequate or excessive.
- In dogs, collect urine with a long-handled cup holding device (males) or a flat pie tin (females). Collect cat urine by placing a small amount of litter in the pan, by placing plastic wrap over litter, or by using a nonabsorbent litter substitute (e.g., aquarium gravel).

Blood Glucose Curves

Evaluate insulin therapy once weekly for the first month and as needed thereafter by serial blood glucose curves (blood glucose, 100–250 mg/dl), assessment of body weight, and resolution of clinical signs.

Procedure for Blood Glucose Curve

1. Collect initial blood sample.
2. Feed usual amount and type of food.
3. Feed and give insulin at the usual time.
4. Watch the owner administer the insulin.
5. Assess the owner's injection technique.
6. Collect serial blood samples at 2-hour intervals for 12 hours.

Ideal Blood Glucose Curve

The ideal blood glucose curve is characterized by three features (Fig. 32–2): the glucose nadir, the timing of the nadir, and the glucose differential.

- The ideal blood glucose curve has a glucose nadir (lowest blood glucose concentration on the curve) between 80 and 120 mg/dl.
- The time of the glucose nadir indicates peak insulin action. The nadir should occur approximately halfway through the dosing interval. For example, if insulin is being given every 12 hours, the nadir should occur 5–6 hours after the dose.
- The glucose differential is the difference between the glucose nadir and the blood glucose concentration prior to the next insulin dose.
  - Aim for a glucose differential of <100 mg/dl in dogs without cataracts and <150 mg/dl in dogs with cataracts.
  - Cats generally have a higher glucose differential; however, aim for <200–250 mg/dl.
- The duration of insulin action is related to both the time of the glucose nadir and the absolute concentration of the glucose nadir. Insulin duration cannot be determined unless the target glucose nadir concentration (80–120 mg/dl) has been achieved. If the glucose nadir occurs approximately halfway through the dosing interval, the duration of action of insulin should be adequate.

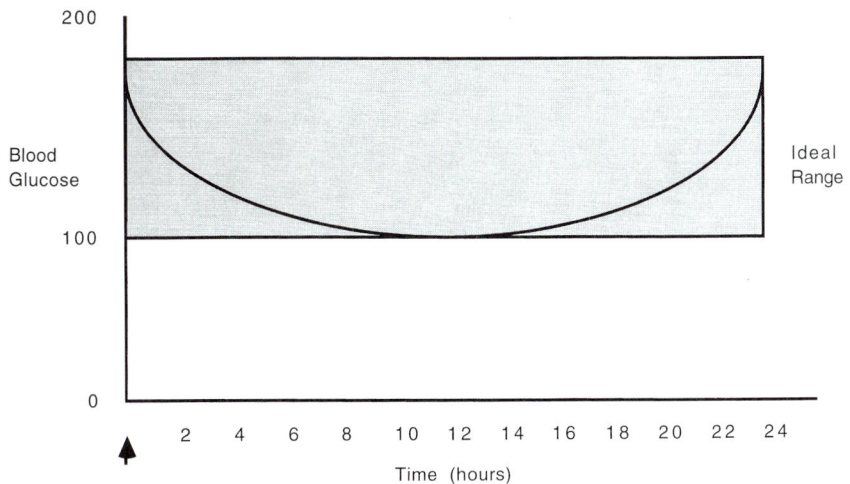

Figure 32–2. Ideal blood glucose curve for an animal on once-daily insulin therapy (*arrow* indicates insulin injection). (From Miller E: Long-term monitoring of the diabetic dog and cat: Clinical signs, serial blood glucose determinations, urine glucose, and glycated blood proteins. Vet Clin North Am Small Anim Pract 25:573, 1995; with permission.)

Problems Identified on the Blood Glucose Curve

It is rare to obtain a perfect glucose curve. Several possible outcomes of blood glucose monitoring are illustrated in Figure 32–3. Generally, blood glucose curve problems can be differentiated by the characteristics of the curve and the insulin dosage (per dosing interval).

- If the patient is receiving >2.2 U/kg of insulin per dose, evaluate for causes of insulin resistance, such as hyperthyroidism, hyperadrenocorticism, acromegaly, estrus, drug therapy, and infections. The approach to insulin resistance is outlined in Tables 32–4 and 32–5.
- If the animal is receiving <2.2 U/kg per dose, the blood glucose curve may indicate one of the following (see Fig. 32–3):
  - Insufficient dosage of insulin. Corrective action—increase the insulin dose.
  - Short duration of action of insulin. Corrective action—change to a longer-acting insulin or twice-daily insulin regimen.
  - Insulin-induced hypoglycemic hyperglycemia (Somogyi effect). Corrective action—reduce insulin dosage by 25%.
  - Insulin overlap. Corrective action—change to a shorter-duration insulin.
  - Prolonged insulin action. Corrective action—change to an insulin mixture of 30% regular and 70% NPH.
- Causes of hyperglycemia and hypoglycemia in diabetic dogs and cats are listed in Table 32–6.

Fructosamine and Glycosylated Hemoglobin

Monitor long-term insulin therapy by serum fructosamine or glycosylated hemoglobin concentrations. These glycosylated blood proteins are indicative of mean glucose concentrations in serum over an extended period of time.

- Glycosylated blood proteins are particularly useful for monitoring diabetic cats that may be stressed by hospitalization and venipunctures for serial blood glucose curves.
- As plasma glucose concentrations increase, hemoglobin glycosylation increases proportionately. Similarly, serum fructosamine is formed by glycosylation of serum protein such as albumin; thus, serum concentration of fructosamine is also directly related to blood glucose concentration.
- Because of the shorter life span of albumin compared with hemoglobin, fructosamine concentrations reflect more recent (1–3 weeks) changes in serum glucose concentrations.
- In general, fructosamine and glycosylated hemoglobin concentrations that lie within reference range limits indicate good to excellent diabetic control, whereas slightly increased levels indicate fair to good control, and very high levels indicate poor glycemic control. Relative changes in serum concentrations may be more helpful than absolute values in some cases.

Hypoglycemia

- Clinical signs of hypoglycemia in diabetic animals are associated with epinephrine excess, which is released to counter the hypoglycemia. Nervousness, anxiety, vocalization, muscle tremors, ataxia, and pupillary dilatation should alert the owner to the possibility of hypoglycemia. Have the owner offer food to the animal, then bring it in for reevaluation.
- Late in the course of hypoglycemic shock the animal may become recumbent, or comatose, or may have a seizure.
- If access to a vein is not readily available or if the owner is administering therapy, 50% dextrose solution, Karo syrup, or pancake syrup may be applied to the mucous membranes of the mouth using a large syringe. Caution the owner to pour the syrup on the gums from a reasonable distance from the animal's teeth to prevent accidental injury from biting. Have the owner transport the animal to a veterinarian as soon as possible.
- In a veterinary facility, treat hypoglycemia by slow IV bolus of 50% dextrose (0.5 g/kg diluted 1:4) followed by continuous infusion of 5% dextrose until the animal can be fed.
- Many animals that experience insulin overdose suffer cerebral edema and temporary blindness or behavior

Unregulated Diabetic Patient
(persistent PU/PD, polyphagia, and weight loss)

Management errors ➝ Yes ➝ Correct
(improper injection technique, outdated insulin, improper storage of insulin, etc.)

No

Insulin dose > 2.2 U/kg

Rapid metabolism
Antibody formation
Hyperthyroidism

Insulin antagonism
Hyperadrenocorticism
Exogenous steroids
Progestogen therapy
Unspayed bitch
Bacterial infection
Hypothyroidism
Acromegaly
Hyperandrogenemia
Pheochromocytoma
Hyperglucagonemia

Insulin dose < 2.2 U/kg

Serial blood glucose monitoring

Nadir too high

Increase dose

Short duration of action

Change to twice daily
or longer acting insulin

Insulin-induced hyperglycemia

Reduce dose

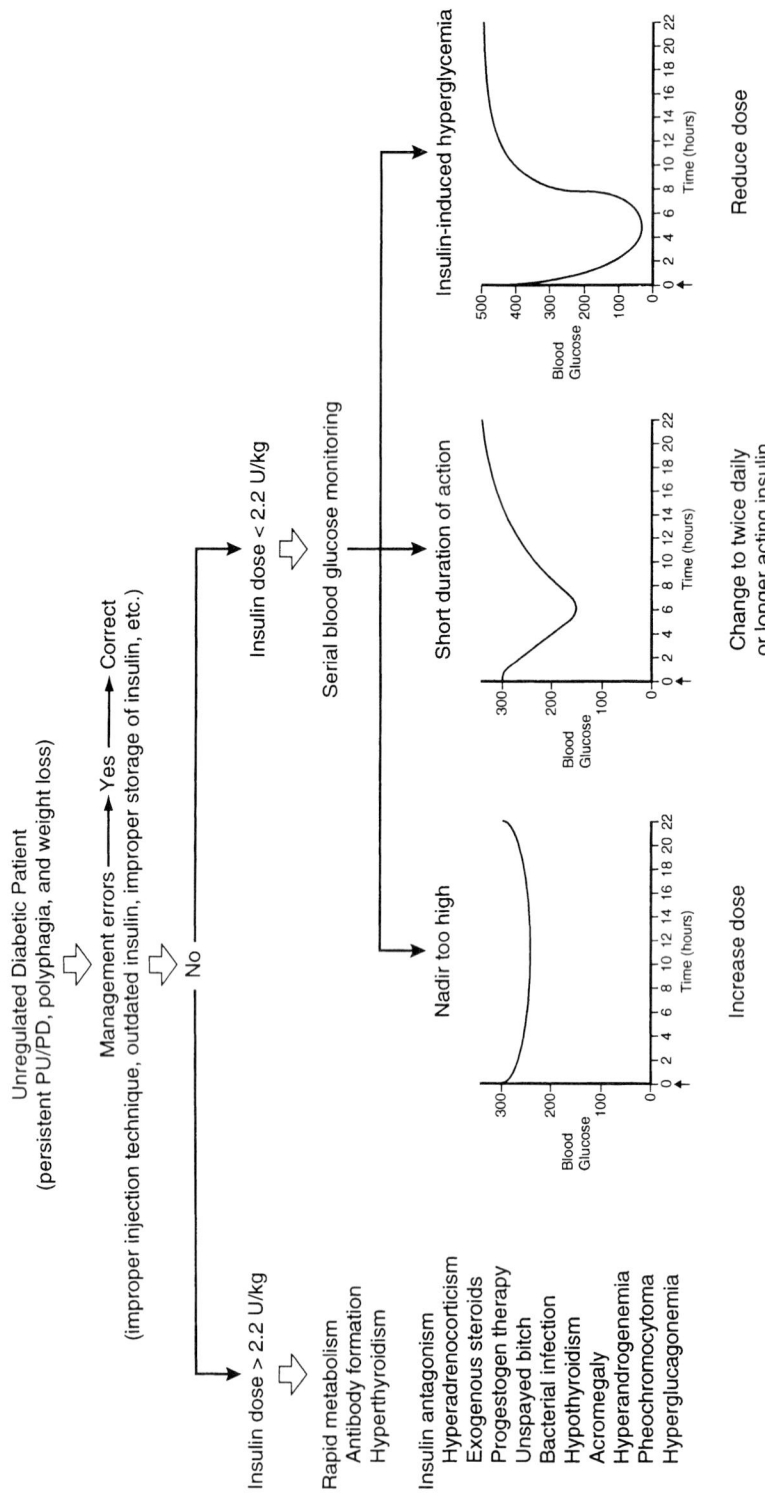

Figure 32–3. Algorithm for the unregulated diabetic dog or cat. (From Miller E: Long-term monitoring of the diabetic dog and cat: Clinical signs, serial blood glucose determinations, urine glucose, and glycated blood proteins. Vet Clin North Am Small Anim Pract 25:582, 1995; with permission.)

Table 32–4. RECOMMENDED STEPS IN THE WORKUP FOR THE DIAGNOSIS AND TREATMENT OF INSULIN RESISTANCE IN CATS

Steps	Causes of Insulin Resistance	Procedure or Test	Treatment
Step 1	Glucocorticoids or megestrol acetate administration	History	Discontinue use of drugs
Step 2	Obesity	Physical examination, weight	Diet change (low calorie, high fiber)
Step 3	Poor absorption of subcutaneous insulin (long-acting preparation)	Evaluate response to change in insulin type; evaluate serum glucose response to regular insulin administered IV or IM	Change from long-acting insulin to insulin with shorter duration of action; use insulin mixtures (e.g., NPH/regular)
Step 4	Infection, ketoacidosis, or concurrent disease	CBC; serum chemistry profile; urinalysis; urine culture; radiographs; abdominal ultrasound	Appropriate antibiotics; correct ketoacidosis or underlying illness
Step 5	Hyperthyroidism	Serum T$_4$ concentration	Antithyroid drugs; thyroidectomy; radioiodine
Step 6	Cushing syndrome	Review clinical signs and physical examination; ACTH stimulation and dexamethasone suppression tests; CT scan	Adrenalectomy, pituitary (cobalt) radiation therapy
Step 7	Acromegaly	Review clinical signs and physical examination; CT scan; measure serum insulin-like growth factor concentration	Pituitary (cobalt) radiation therapy
Step 8	Insulin antibodies	Measure serum insulin concentration 24 hr after last insulin injection; insulin antibody titers (not widely available)	Switch to human insulin (or beef insulin, if available)
Step 9	Clinically undefined insulin resistance	All of the above procedures and tests	Raise insulin dose; change to insulin with shorter duration of action; mix NPH/regular insulin

ACTH, adrenocorticotropic hormone; CBC, complete blood count; CT, computed tomography; IM, intramuscularly; IV, intravenously; T$_4$, thyroxine.

From Peterson ME: Diagnosis and management of insulin resistance in dogs and cats with diabetes mellitus. Vet Clin North Am Small Anim Pract 25:705, 1995.

changes; often these signs are temporary and resolve after several weeks or months.

▼ *Key Point* Endogenous glucose stores may have been depleted by the insulin overdose and it may take several days for hyperglycemia to recur. In these cases, discontinue insulin therapy until hyperglycemia recurs.

TREATMENT OF TYPE 2 (NON–INSULIN-DEPENDENT) DIABETES

Type 2 diabetes can be treated through diet, exercise, oral hypoglycemic drugs, insulin, or any combination of the aforementioned. Appropriate diet and exercise are described under Treatment of Uncomplicated Diabetes.

▼ *Key Point* Treatment of type 2 diabetes is aimed at decreasing hepatic glucose output and glucose absorption from the intestine, increasing peripheral insulin sensitivity, and increasing insulin secretion from the pancreas.

Oral Hypoglycemic Drugs

Overview

- Human diabetics can be divided into three therapeutic categories according to beta cell function:

  1. Those who require exogenous insulin to control hyperglycemia.

Table 32–5. RECOMMENDED STEPS IN THE WORKUP FOR THE DIAGNOSIS AND TREATMENT OF INSULIN RESISTANCE IN DOGS

Steps	Causes of Insulin Resistance	Procedure or Test	Treatment
Step 1	Glucocorticoids or megestrol acetate administration	History	Discontinue use of drugs
Step 2	Diestrus/acromegaly	History (intact female; last estrus); serum progesterone concentration	Ovariohysterectomy
Step 3	Obesity	Physical examination, weight	Diet change (low calorie, high fiber)
Step 4	Poor absorption of subcutaneous insulin (long-acting preparation)	Evaluate response to change in insulin type; evaluate serum glucose response to regular insulin administered IV or IM	Change to insulin with shorter duration of action; use insulin mixtures (NPH/regular)
Step 5	Infection, ketoacidosis, or concurrent disease	CBC; serum chemistry profile; urinalysis; urine culture, radiographs; abdominal ultrasound	Appropriate antibiotics; correct ketoacidosis or underlying illness
Step 6	Cushing syndrome	Review clinical signs and physical examination; ACTH stimulation and dexamethasone suppression tests; CT scan	Mitotane; pituitary (cobalt) radiation therapy; unilateral adrenalectomy for adrenal tumor
Step 7	Hyperlipidemia	Review signalment (Schnauzer); measure serum cholesterol and triglycerides	Low-fat diet; lipid drugs
Step 8	Hypothyroidism	Serum T_4, free T_4, and cTSH concentrations	Thyroid hormone (L-thyroxine) replacement therapy
Step 9	Insulin antibodies	Measure serum insulin concentration 24 hr after last insulin injection; insulin antibody titers (not widely available)	Switch to human or pork insulin
Step 10	Clinically undefined insulin resistance	All of the above procedures and tests	Raise insulin dose; change to insulin with shorter duration of action; mix NPH/regular insulin

ACTH, adrenocorticotropic hormone; CBC, complete blood count; CT, computed tomography; cTSH, canine thyroid-stimulating hormone; IM, intramuscularly; IV, intravenously; T_4, thyroxine; TRH, thyroid-releasing hormone; TSH, thyroid-stimulating hormone.

From Peterson ME: Diagnosis and management of insulin resistance in dogs and cats with diabetes mellitus. Vet Clin North Am Small Anim Pract 25:706, 1995.

2. Those who require only dietary therapy because of sufficient pancreatic islet cell function and insulin sensitivity to maintain relatively normal glucose levels.
3. Those who have sufficient pancreatic islet cell function and insulin sensitivity to respond to oral hypoglycemic drugs.

- In cats, differentiation among these categories is almost impossible before treatment; therefore, use the *response* to oral hypoglycemic agents as a guide to whether the cat can be managed with oral hypoglycemic agents.
- Oral hypoglycemic agents include the following (Table 32–7):

- Sulfonylureas (e.g., glipizide, glyburide, glimepiride).
- Biguanides (e.g., metformin).
- Thiazolidinediones (e.g., troglitazone).
- Alpha-glucosidase inhibitors (e.g., acarbose).
- Transition metals (e.g., chromium, vanadium).
- Most of the oral hypoglycemic agents work by increasing insulin secretion, decreasing insulin resistance, decreasing glucose absorption, decreasing hepatic glucose production, or a combination of these (Fig. 32–4).

▼ *Key Point* Indications for oral hypoglycemic therapy in diabetic cats include normal or increased body

Table 32–6. CAUSES OF HYPERGLYCEMIA AND HYPOGLYCEMIA IN DIABETIC DOGS AND CATS

Causes of Hyperglycemia in Diabetic Cats and Dogs
Insufficient insulin dosage
Insufficient duration of insulin action
Outdated, inactive insulin
Owner administration problems
Overfeeding
Stress
Insulin resistance caused by Cushing syndrome, infections, drugs, thyroid disease, pancreatitis, acromegaly

Causes of Hypoglycemia in Diabetic Cats and Dogs
Insulin overdose
Concentrated insulin (old)
Overlap of insulin action
Transient diabetes
Somogyi effect
Anorexia caused by oral disease, ketosis
Maldigestion caused by exocrine pancreatic insufficiency, bacterial overgrowth
Malabsorption caused by inflammatory bowel disease, lymphangiectasia, lymphoma, and so forth.

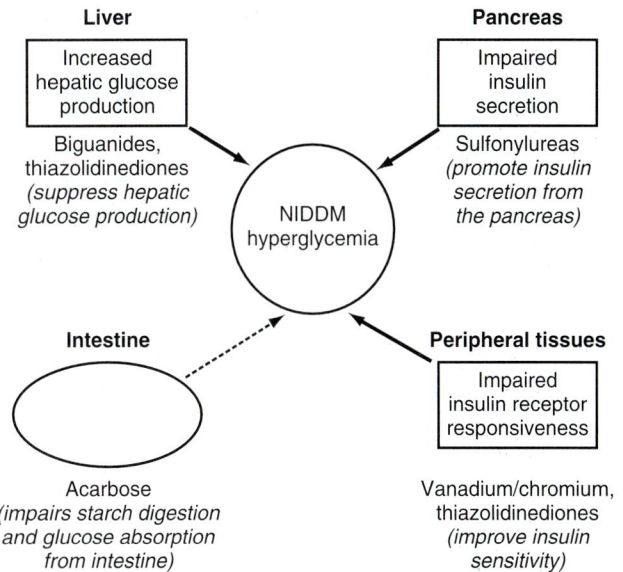

Figure 32–4. Mechanisms of action of oral hypoglycemic agents in the treatment of non–insulin-dependent (type 2) diabetes mellitus.

weight, lack of ketones, probable type 2 diabetes with no underlying disease (pancreatitis, pancreatic tumor), and the owner's willingness to administer oral medication rather than an injection.

Sulfonylureas (e.g., Glipizide)

- The mechanism of action of the *sulfonylureas* is to increase insulin secretion and improve insulin resistance; however, these agents also cause an increase in hepatic gluconeogenesis. This leads to delayed hyperinsulinemia, weight gain, and atherosclerosis in humans treated with sulfonylureas.

- *Glipizide* (Glucotrol, Roerig), a sulfonylurea drug, has been used to successfully treat type 2 diabetes in cats at a dosage of 2.5–5 mg q12h PO with food (high fiber diet). An outline for monitoring and managing cats undergoing glipizide therapy is shown in Figure 32–5.

- Side effects of sulfonylureas include severe hypoglycemia (rare in cats), cholestatic hepatitis, and vomiting. Gastrointestinal side effects, which occur in about 15% of cats treated with glipizide, resolve when the drug is administered with food.

Table 32–7. ORAL HYPOGLYCEMIC DRUGS USED IN THE TREATMENT OF TYPE 2 DIABETES (NIDDM) IN HUMANS AND CATS

Drug (Trade Name)	Dose	Frequency	Side Effects	Mechanism of Action
Glipizide (Glucotrol, Pfizer)	2.5–5 mg/cat	q8–12h, PO	Hepatotoxicity, hypoglycemia, vomiting	Increases insulin secretion and sensitivity
Glimepiride (Amaryl, Hoechst-Marion Roussel)	1–4 mg (humans); 1 mg/cat	q24h (humans); q24h (cat)	Same as above but lower incidence	Same as above
Metformin (Glucophage, Bristol-Myers Squibb)	500–750 mg (humans); unknown (cat)	q12h (humans); unknown (cat)	Anorexia, vomiting	Inhibits hepatic glucose production
Precose (Acarbose, Bayer)	50 mg (humans); 12.5–25 mg (cat)	q8–12h with meals	Flatulence, soft stool	Alpha-glucosidase inhibitor, impairs glucose absorption from gut
Troglitazone (Rezulin, Parke-Davis)	200–400 mg (humans); unknown (cat)	q24h	Mild decreases in WBC, platelet, and Hb counts	Increases insulin receptor sensitivity
Chromium	200 µg/cat	q24h	Unknown	Increases insulin receptor sensitivity
Vanadium	200–400 µg/cat	q24h in food or water	Anorexia, vomiting	Increases insulin receptor sensitivity

Hb, hemoglobin; WBC, white blood cell count.

Initiate Glipizide 5 mg Orally Twice a Day and Diet

Blood Glucose > 200 mg/dL   Blood Glucose < 200 mg/dL

Symptomatic   Discontinue glipizide and recheck blood glucose in 1–2 weeks, then monitor every 2–4 weeks

Yes   No   Glucose > 200 mg/dL   Glucose < 200 mg/dL

Insulin   Continue glipizide if stable   Reinstitute glipizide   Continue diet

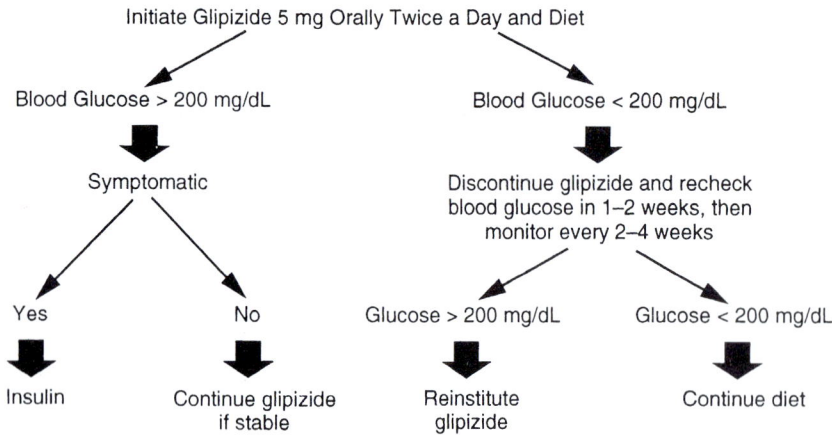

Figure 32–5. Possible clinical consequences of glipizide treatment. (From Ford SL: NIDDM in the cat: Treatment with the oral hypoglycemic medication, glipizide. Vet Clin North Am Small Anim Pract 25:611, 1995; with permission.)

Biguanides (e.g., Metformin)

- *Metformin* belongs to the biguanide group of oral hypoglycemic agents, which work by *inhibiting* hepatic glucose release and by improving peripheral insulin sensitivity.
- One advantage of the biguanides is that they do not promote insulin release; therefore, there is little potential for the development of hypoglycemia when metformin is used as a sole agent.
- Side effects of the biguanides include lactic acidosis and gastrointestinal signs such as nausea and diarrhea.
- Contraindications for metformin therapy in humans and presumably in cats include concurrent renal disease, liver dysfunction, and cardiac disease.

Alpha-Glucosidase Inhibitors (e.g., Acarbose)

- *Acarbose,* an alpha-glucosidase inhibitor, impairs glucose absorption from the intestine by decreasing fiber digestion and hence glucose production from food sources.
- Acarbose is used as initial therapy in obese prediabetic patients suffering from insulin resistance or as adjunct therapy with sulfonylureas or insulin to enhance the hypoglycemic effect in patients with overt diabetes mellitus.
- One advantage of acarbose is that it is not absorbed systemically and may be used in conjunction with other oral hypoglycemics.
- Side effects of acarbose include flatulence, loose stool, and overt diarrhea at high dosages.
- Acarbose is not indicated in patients of low or normal body weight because of the negative effects on nutrition.

Thiazolidinediones (e.g., Troglitazone)

- The thiazolidinedione compounds facilitate insulin-dependent glucose disposal and inhibition of hepatic glucose output via attenuation of gluconeogenesis and activation of glycolysis. In addition, the thiazolidinediones have been shown to have beneficial effects on lipid disturbances in type 2 diabetes.
- *Troglitazone* is the thiazolidinedione compound that has progressed to clinical development for use in humans with type 2 diabetes. In fact, some authors have suggested that use of this drug early in the course of type 2 diabetes may prevent development of overt diabetes.
- Initial studies using troglitazone for the treatment of feline type 2 diabetes have been disappointing.

Transition Metals: Vanadium and Chromium

- *Vanadium* and *chromium* are transition elements that have been shown to have extensive insulin-like properties. Oral vanadium and chromium cause a marked and sustained improvement in glucose homeostasis in type 2 diabetes by exerting an insulin-like effect on peripheral tissues; furthermore, vanadium prevents the exhaustion of insulin stores in the pancreas. Unlike insulin, vanadium does not lower blood glucose concentrations in normal animals.
- Low doses of oral vanadium decrease blood glucose and serum fructosamine concentrations and alleviate the signs of diabetes (polydipsia, polyuria) in cats with *early* type 2 diabetes mellitus.
- Side effects of oral vanadium include anorexia and vomiting.

Insulin and Oral Hypoglycemics

- Changes from insulin to oral hypoglycemic agents or vice versa may be necessary in some diabetic cats. If a cat is particularly sensitive to insulin or exhibits transient diabetes because of reversal of "glucose toxicity," consider a change to an oral hypoglycemic.
- If a cat is being managed with oral hypoglycemic agents and ketosis develops, switch the cat to insulin therapy.
- Agents that impair glucose absorption from the intestine (acarbose) or increase insulin sensitivity (vanadium, metformin, troglitazone) may be combined with insulin to improve glucose control.
- In the case of "brittle diabetics" in which small incremental changes in insulin dose may precipitate hypoglycemia, addition of a drug that enhances the action of insulin may lead to a reduction in the insulin dosage required to attain euglycemia.

- In humans, acarbose, chromium, vanadium, and metformin are commonly used in conjunction with insulin or with other oral hypoglycemics (sulfonylureas) that cause insulin release.
- Use caution when combining an oral hypoglycemic agent with insulin, as hypoglycemic reactions may occur.

Monitoring Oral Hypoglycemic Therapy

- It appears that methods of assessing *long-term* glycemic control are better indicators of response to therapy with oral hypoglycemics than are spot glucose determinations or blood glucose curves. Monitor resolution of clinical signs and serum fructosamine concentrations in cats undergoing oral hypoglycemic therapy.
- For clinical signs, body weight should increase or remain stable and polydipsia and polyuria should resolve with effective oral hypoglycemic therapy.
- Normal fructosamine concentrations are consistent with moderate to good long-term control of hyperglycemia. Relative improvement of serum fructosamine may be more important than absolute fructosamine values.

PREVENTION

- In humans, and presumably in cats, obesity management may be helpful in preventing development of type 2 diabetes mellitus.
- In dogs and cats, prevention of secondary forms of diabetes is possible by limiting the use of diabetogenic drugs such as glucocorticoids, progestational compounds, and somatotropin.
- Similarly, prevention and treatment of underlying disease is the mainstay of prevention of secondary diabetes resulting from hyperthyroidism, hyperadrenocorticism, or acromegaly.

SUPPLEMENTAL READINGS

Feldman EC, Nelson RW: Canine and Feline Endocrinology and Reproduction, 2nd Ed. Philadelphia: WB Saunders, 1996.

Genuth S: Classification and diagnosis of diabetes mellitus. Med Clin North Am 66:1191, 1982.

Greco DS, Peterson ME, eds.: Diabetes mellitus. Vet Clin North Am Small Anim Pract 25, 1995.

Jackson RA, Hawa MI, Jaspan JB, et al.: Mechanism of metformin action in non-insulin dependent diabetes. Diabetes 36:632, 1987.

Nelson RW: Diabetes mellitus. In Ettinger SJ, Feldman EC, eds.: Textbook of Veterinary Internal Medicine, 4th Ed. Philadephia: WB Saunders, 1995, p 1510.

O'Brien TD, Butler PC, Westermark P, Johnson KH: Islet amyloid polypeptide: A review of its biology and potential roles in the pathogenesis of diabetes mellitus. Vet Pathol 30:317, 1993.

Peterson ME: Endocrine diseases. In Sherding RG, ed.: The Cat, Diseases and Clinical Management, 2nd Ed. New York: Churchill Livingstone, 1994, p 1465.

Saltiel AR, Olefsky JM: Thiazolidinediones in the treatment of insulin resistance and type II diabetes. Diabetes 45:1661, 1996

Shechter Y. Shisheva A: Vanadium salts and the future treatment of diabetes. Endeavour 17:27, 1993.

Wallace MS, Peterson ME, Nichols CE: Absorption kinetics of regular, isophane and protamine zinc insulin in normal cats. Domest Anim Endocrinol 7:509, 1990.

33 Pancreatic Beta Cell Neoplasia

Richard W. Nelson / S. Kathleen Salisbury

Tumors of the beta cells of the pancreatic islets are functional tumors that secrete excessive amounts of insulin independent of normal regulatory mechanisms. Hyperinsulinism causes hypoglycemia and corresponding clinical signs. Consider beta cell neoplasia in the differential diagnosis of hypoglycemia in middle-aged and older dogs.

ETIOLOGY

- Insulin-secreting tumors are almost always malignant.
- Metastatic sites include the lymphatics and lymph nodes (duodenal, mesenteric, hepatic, splenic), liver, mesentery, and omentum.
- The hyperinsulinemia caused by beta cell tumors interferes with glucose homeostasis by decreasing the rate of glucose release from the liver and by increasing the uptake of glucose by insulin-sensitive tissues.
  - The net effect is hypoglycemia and secretion of the diabetogenic hormones (most notably glucagon and epinephrine).
  - The clinical signs of hypoglycemia result from neuroglycopenia and stimulation of the sympathoadrenal system.

CLINICAL SIGNS

- The most common clinical signs include seizures, weakness, collapse, and ataxia (Table 33–1).
- Clinical signs are usually present for 1–6 months before presentation to the veterinarian.
- Clinical signs tend to be episodic and often develop during fasting, exercise, excitement, and eating.

DIAGNOSIS

▼ *Key Point* The diagnosis of an insulin-secreting beta cell tumor requires initial confirmation of hypoglycemia and then documentation of inappropriate insulin secretion.

Signalment

The signalment (i.e., older dog), normal physical examination, and lack of abnormalities other than hypo-glycemia on hemogram, serum biochemical panel, and urinalysis strongly suggest beta cell neoplasia as the cause of the hypoglycemia (Table 33–2).

- Insulin-secreting tumors typically occur in the middle-aged or older dog, with an age range of 6–14 years.
- There is no apparent sex or breed predilection, although the Labrador retriever, German shepherd, Irish setter, golden retriever, collie, fox terrier, and standard poodle are commonly affected in our hospital.
- Islet cell neoplasia is rare in cats.

Physical Examination

The physical examination of dogs with insulin-secreting tumors is surprisingly unremarkable.

- Weight gain is evident in some dogs and is probably a result of the potent anabolic effects of insulin.
- Peripheral neuropathies have been reported in dogs with insulin-secreting tumors and may be manifested as proprioception deficits, depressed reflexes, and muscle atrophy.

Laboratory Studies

- The only consistent abnormality found on the hemogram, biochemical panel, and urinalysis is hypoglycemia.
- Hypoalbuminemia, hypophosphatemia, hypokalemia, and an increase in alkaline phosphatase and alanine aminotransferase have been reported, but these findings are considered nonspecific and not helpful in achieving a definitive diagnosis.
- A correlation has not been found between liver enzyme elevations and metastasis of the pancreatic tumor to the liver.

Blood Glucose Assay

- Dogs with insulin-secreting tumors occasionally may have a normal blood glucose concentration on random testing. Such a finding does not eliminate intermittent hypoglycemia as a cause of episodic weakness or seizure activity.
- To identify hypoglycemia, fast the animal and evaluate the blood glucose hourly.
- A fast of 8 hours or less is successful in demonstrating hypoglycemia in most dogs with insulin-secreting tumors; occasionally longer fasts are required.

Table 33–1. CLINICAL SIGNS ASSOCIATED WITH BETA CELL NEOPLASIA IN THE DOG

Seizures	Muscle fasciculations
Weakness	Bizarre behavior
Collapse	Lethargy
Ataxia	Weight gain
Posterior paresis	Polyphagia

Table 33–2. DIFFERENTIAL DIAGNOSIS FOR HYPOGLYCEMIA

Beta cell neoplasia
Nonpancreatic neoplasia
    Hepatocellular carcinoma, hepatoma
    Leiomyosarcoma, leiomyoma
    Hemangiosarcoma
Hepatopathy
    Vascular shunts
    Chronic fibrosis, cirrhosis
    Hepatic necrosis
Sepsis
Hypoadrenocorticism
Toy-breed puppy
Chronic renal failure
Glycogen storage disorder
Polycythemia
Starvation
Artifact

Ultrasonography

Abdominal ultrasonography can be used to identify a mass in the region of the pancreas and to assess for potential metastatic lesions in the liver and surrounding structures; however, negative findings do not rule out an insulin-secreting tumor.

Insulin Secretion Measurement

Confirmation of an insulin-secreting neoplasm requires documentation of inappropriate insulin secretion during hypoglycemia. Measuring serum insulin concentration when the blood glucose is <60 mg/dl (<40 mg/dl using glucose reagent strips) usually establishes the diagnosis. A 4–8 hour fast may be required to obtain this level of hypoglycemia, but when the blood glucose concentration falls to <60 mg/dl, the simultaneous blood insulin concentration is interpreted as follows:

- Blood insulin is above normal (>120 pmol/L): an insulin-secreting neoplasm is likely.
- Blood insulin is in the high-normal range (60–120 pmol/L): an insulin-secreting tumor remains possible.
- Blood insulin is in the low-normal range (30–60 pmol/L): an insulin-secreting tumor has not been confirmed.
  - Low-normal blood insulin may be found with hypoglycemia associated with non–islet cell tumors as well as insulin-secreting tumors.
  - Blood insulin in the low-normal range in a dog with hypoglycemia is an indication for further diagnostics, including repeating the blood glucose and insulin determinations.
- Blood insulin is in the below-normal range (<30 pmol/L): insulinopenia has been documented, and an insulin-secreting tumor has been ruled out.

MEDICAL TREATMENT FOR ACUTE HYPOGLYCEMIC CRISIS

The acute onset of clinical signs of hypoglycemia (see Table 33–1) typically occurs in the dog in the home environment or immediately postoperatively in the dog with an inoperable tumor or metastases. Therapy depends on the severity of clinical signs and the location of the dog or cat (i.e., home or hospital).

- In the hospital, administer 50% dextrose solution (2–15 ml) slowly IV until clinical signs are controlled.

- If the dog is home, instruct the owner to rub a sugar-containing solution (e.g., Karo syrup) on the buccal mucosa until clinical signs are controlled.
- Dogs and cats with hypoglycemia should respond to the administration of glucose in 30–120 seconds.

▼ *Key Point* Avoid overstimulation of the tumor when administering dextrose IV. Overstimulation of the tumor can result in excessive release of insulin into the circulation and cause severe rebound hypoglycemia. A vicious cycle that is difficult to break may ultimately result in persistent seizures and eventually death.

- The goal of therapy is to control the clinical signs, not correct hypoglycemia, through the judicious administration of dextrose.
- Administer small amounts of dextrose slowly rather than large boluses rapidly to minimize stimulation of the tumor.
- Avoid administering excessive amounts of dextrose.

Seizures

If intractable seizures due to hypoglycemia develop:

- Discontinue bolus injections of dextrose.
- Begin continuous IV infusion of 2.5–5.0% dextrose solution at 1½–2 times the maintenance rate (90–120 ml/kg/24 hr).
- Add dexamethasone, 0.5–1.0 mg/kg, to the IV fluids and administer over a period of 6 hours.
- Administer the somatostatin analog SMS 201-995 (octreotide [Sandostatin, Sandoz]), 10–40 µg q8–12h SC, to decrease insulin secretion by the tumor.
- Aggressive anticonvulsant therapy or pentobarbital anesthesia, as described in Chapter 146, for control of intractable seizures may be necessary to gain time until the aforementioned therapy becomes effective.

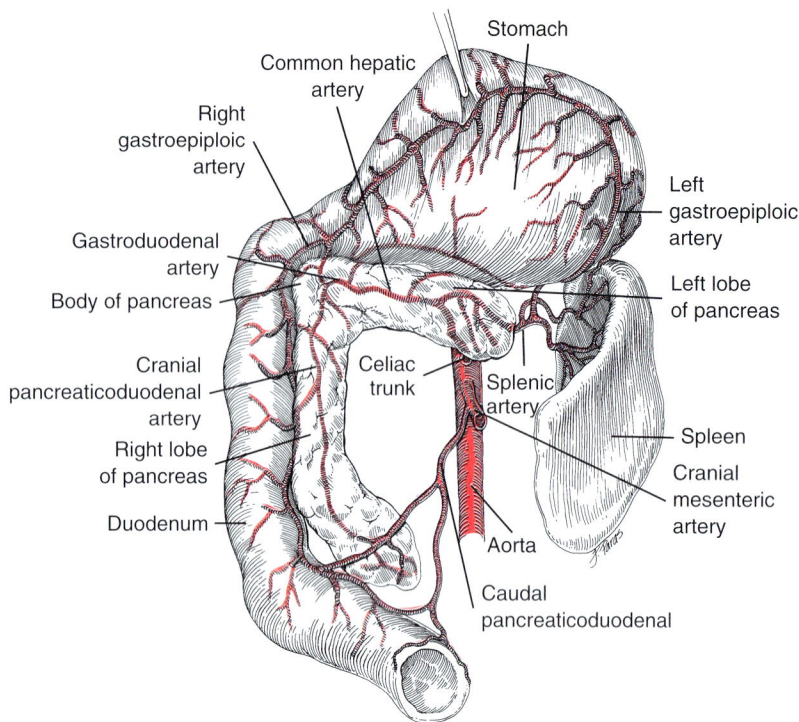

Figure 33–1. Anatomy and blood supply of the right and left lobes of the pancreas.

SURGICAL TREATMENT

Surgical Anatomy

The pancreas consists of the right and left lobes, and the body.

Right Lobe. The right lobe is located in the mesoduodenum adjacent to the descending duodenum. The proximal portion of the right lobe is intimately associated with the duodenum (Fig. 33–1). The cranial and caudal pancreaticoduodenal arteries supply the right lobe of the pancreas and the duodenum. Damage to the pancreaticoduodenal vessels may result in avascular necrosis of the duodenum.

Left Lobe. The left lobe is located caudodorsal to the stomach in the deep leaf of the greater omentum. It is exposed by reflecting the greater omentum, spleen, and stomach cranially and retracting the transverse colon caudally. This lobe of the pancreas is supplied by branches of the gastroduodenal, common hepatic, and splenic arteries.

Body of the Pancreas. The body of the pancreas is located at the cranial duodenal flexure and is in close proximity to the pylorus and common bile duct. The portal vein crosses the dorsal portion of the body.

Lymphatics. Lymphatics from the pancreas drain into the duodenal, hepatic, splenic, and mesenteric lymph nodes.

Pancreatic Ducts. Excretory ducts of the pancreas exit the pancreatic parenchyma in the area of the body to enter the duodenum. There are usually two, which intercommunicate within the gland. There are several variations in the anatomy of the pancreatic ducts:

- In the dog, most commonly the pancreatic duct enters the duodenum with the common bile duct at the major duodenal papilla approximately 5 cm distal to the pylorus. The accessory pancreatic duct, which is the main pancreatic duct, enters the duodenum at the minor duodenal papilla approximately 8 cm distal to the pylorus (Fig. 33–2).
- In the cat, the pancreatic duct is the main excretory duct; the accessory duct often is absent.

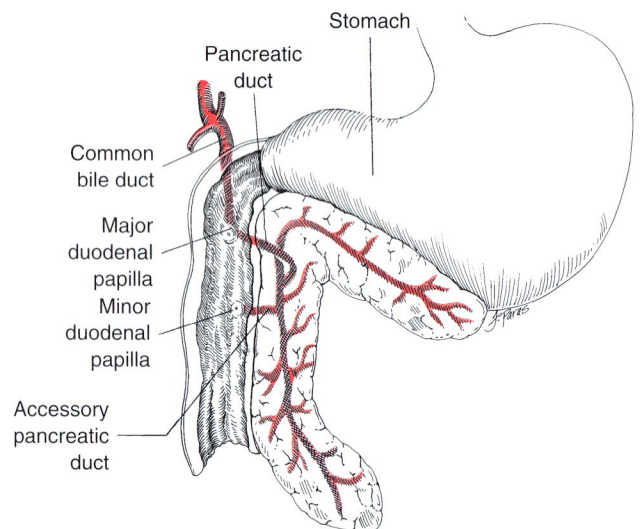

Figure 33–2. Anatomy of the pancreatic ducts in relationship to the duodenum.

Preoperative Considerations

- To minimize hypoglycemia during the preoperative period, feed the animal frequent small meals and, if necessary, give prednisone, 0.25–0.5 mg/kg q12h PO.
- Fluid therapy prior to and during surgery is important to maintain systemic blood pressure and pancreatic perfusion, thereby minimizing the development of pancreatitis.

▼ *Key Point* On the *day of surgery,* administer a balanced electrolyte solution containing 5% dextrose IV at 1½–2 times daily maintenance requirements. *Intraoperatively,* administer this same solution at a rate of 8–16 ml/kg/hr.

Surgical Procedure

The objectives of exploratory celiotomy are to:

- Confirm a neoplasm.
- Define the clinical stage of the tumor.
- Remove the primary pancreatic tumor and any metastatic lesions (see the following section). Although this may not effect a cure, it usually reduces clinical signs and may facilitate medical management.

Identification of Neoplastic Tissue

Islet cell tumors occur with approximately equal frequency in all areas of the pancreas. Although single lesions are most common, multiple lesions in nonadjacent areas of the pancreas have been reported in about 15% of cases. Diffuse involvement of the pancreas without a discrete mass also has been reported.

Using Visual Examination and Palpation

Technique

1. Approach the abdomen via a ventral midline incision from the xiphoid to the pubis.
2. Examine the entire pancreas visually and by careful palpation.
   a. Islet cell tumors are usually firmer than the surrounding tissue.
   b. Islet cell tumors may be small and sandwiched between pancreatic lobules so that they are not readily visible.

Using Methylene Blue Intravenous Infusion

The following technique to facilitate tumor identification utilizes IV infusion of methylene blue. It should be considered only if a mass cannot be identified at surgery.

Technique

1. Surgically expose the pancreas as described previously.
2. Administer methylene blue as an IV infusion in normal isotonic saline solution to a total dose of 3 mg/kg body weight. Begin the infusion 30 minutes before the pancreas is exposed.
3. Methylene blue is concentrated by the endocrine pancreas and intensely stains hyperfunctional areas.
   a. Normal pancreatic endocrine tissue is stained a dusky slate blue.
   b. Hyperfunctional tissue is stained more intensely (often a reddish blue).
4. Potential complications include hemolytic anemia and acute renal failure postoperatively.

Removal of Neoplastic Tissue

Technique

1. Remove abnormal pancreatic masses by partial pancreatectomy or by local excision. Make a wide excision and handle the pancreas very gently to avoid inducing pancreatitis.
2. Remove tumors located in the left lobe or the distal portion of the right lobe by partial pancreatectomy (Fig. 33–3).
   a. Divide the mesentery surrounding the affected lobe and ligate and divide the appropriate vessels (see Fig. 33–3A).
   b. Incise the mesentery covering both surfaces of the pancreas at the level of transection of the lobe.
   c. Remove the lobe at least 1–2 cm proximal to the tumor.
   d. Bluntly separate the lobules using a mosquito hemostat, dissecting alternately from each side of the gland (see Fig. 33–3B).
   e. Isolate the main duct, ligate with a monofilament synthetic suture material, and transect it (see Fig. 33–3C).
3. When the tumor is located in the proximal portion of the right lobe or the body, local excision of the tumor, including at least 1–2 cm margins of normal-appearing pancreatic tissue, is the preferred technique because of the vascular and ductal anatomy of the area.
   a. Gently separate the pancreatic lobules by blunt dissection with a mosquito hemostat. Cauterize small vessels and ligate and divide larger vessels.
   b. Preserve the pancreaticoduodenal vessels supplying the duodenum. Avoid damaging the pancreatic ducts and the common bile duct.
4. Explore the entire abdomen for evidence of metastatic disease. The most common sites of metastasis are the liver and regional lymph nodes (duodenal, hepatic, splenic, greater mesenteric).

▼ *Key Point* Metastatic disease is common; approximately 45% of cases have identifiable metastasis to the liver or regional lymph nodes at the time of surgery.

   a. Resect all enlarged lymph nodes and suspicious hepatic lesions if possible and submit them for histopathologic examination.
   b. Biopsy lesions that cannot be completely excised.

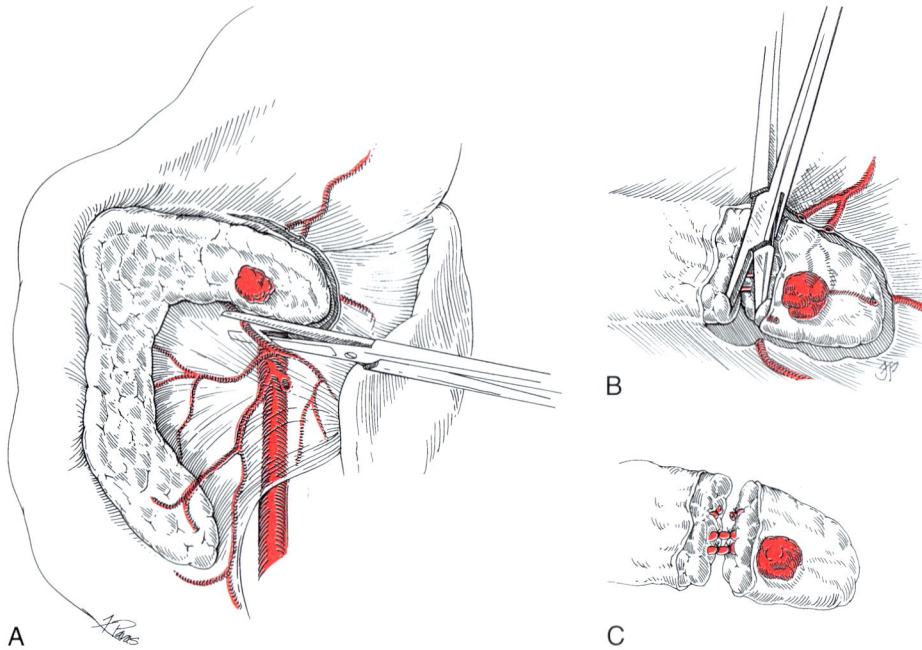

Figure 33–3. *A–C*, Schematic of partial pancreatectomy procedure. See text for details.

▼ *Key Point* Many dogs with metastases of islet cell neoplasms can be managed medically for longer than a year.

5. Thoroughly lavage the abdomen prior to closure with warm, sterile isotonic saline to dilute any pancreatic secretions that may have been released during surgical manipulation of the pancreas.
6. Close the abdomen routinely.

Postoperative Care and Complications

Postoperative Care

- Give nothing by mouth for 48 hours.
- Administer a balanced electrolyte solution IV containing 5% dextrose at 1½–2 times daily maintenance requirements (90–120 ml/kg/24 hr).
  - Monitor blood glucose concentration at least twice daily.
  - Discontinue the dextrose infusion if hyperglycemia (>150 mg/dl) develops.
- If vomiting does not occur, offer small amounts of water after 48 hours and then small amounts of a bland, easily digestible diet (e.g., rice and cottage cheese) after 72 hours.
- If the dog tolerates a bland diet well, resume the normal diet in 5–7 days.

Complications

- Hyperglycemia may occur following surgery due to inadequate insulin secretion by atrophied non-neoplastic beta cells. This often resolves within a few days.
  - If hyperglycemia and glycosuria persist for several days following surgery, initiate insulin therapy (see Chap. 32).

- Diabetes mellitus is usually transient and resolves within a few weeks to several months.
- Periodically, discontinue insulin therapy on a trial basis to determine if endogenous insulin production is resuming.
- If hypoglycemia does not resolve postoperatively or if it recurs following resection of an islet cell tumor, assume metastatic disease to be present and institute medical therapy for chronic hypoglycemia, as described in the following section.
- Other potential postoperative complications include pancreatitis, duodenal necrosis (from vascular compromise), and central nervous system dysfunction secondary to prolonged hypoglycemia.

MEDICAL TREATMENT FOR CHRONIC HYPOGLYCEMIA

Initiate palliative medical management for chronic hypoglycemia when an exploratory celiotomy is refused by the owner or when an inoperable tumor or metastases result in recurrence of clinical signs.

The goals of chronic palliative therapy are to:

- Reduce the frequency and severity of clinical signs.
- Prevent an acute hypoglycemic crisis through dietary management and nonspecific antihormonal therapy.

Antihormonal therapy minimizes hypoglycemia by:

- Increasing absorption of glucose from the intestinal tract.
- Increasing hepatic gluconeogenesis and glycogenolysis.
- Inhibiting the synthesis, secretion, or peripheral cellular actions of insulin.

Diet and Exercise Recommendations

- Feed frequent small meals to provide a constant source of calories, which may prevent or reduce the number of hypoglycemic episodes.
- Use a diet that is high in proteins, fats, and complex carbohydrates.
- If commercial pet food is used, recommend a combination of canned and dry food, fed in 3–6 small meals daily.
- Avoid simple sugars (including soft moist foods) except as needed to treat signs of hypoglycemia.
- Limit exercise to short walks on a leash.

Glucocorticoid Therapy

Goal of Therapy

Initiate glucocorticoids when dietary manipulations are no longer effective in preventing signs of hypoglycemia.

Mechanisms

Glucocorticoids antagonize the actions of insulin at the cellular level, stimulate hepatic glycogenolysis, and provide the necessary substrates for hepatic gluconeogenesis.

Dosage

- Administer prednisone at an initial dosage of 0.5 mg/kg/day given in divided doses.
- Increase the dosage as needed to control clinical signs of hypoglycemia up to a maximal daily dose of 4–6 mg/kg/day.
- Signs of iatrogenic hypercortisolism ultimately limit the amount of prednisone that is administered.

Diazoxide Therapy

Mechanism

Diazoxide (Proglycem, Schering Plough) is a benzothiadiazide diuretic that inhibits insulin secretion, stimulates hepatic gluconeogenesis and glycogenolysis, and inhibits tissue use of glucose. The net effect is hyperglycemia.

Goal of Therapy

The goal of diazoxide therapy is to establish a dosage in which hypoglycemia and its clinical signs are reduced or absent, while avoiding hyperglycemia (>180 mg/dl) and its associated clinical signs.

Dosage

- Administer diazoxide at an initial dosage of 10 mg/kg q12h PO.
- Gradually increase the dose as needed to control signs of hypoglycemia, but do not exceed 60 mg/kg/day.

Side Effects

- The most common adverse reactions to diazoxide are anorexia and vomiting. Minimize these by adminis-

tering diazoxide with a meal or temporarily decreasing the dosage.
- Other potential complications include diarrhea, tachycardia, bone marrow suppression, aplastic anemia, thrombocytopenia, diabetes mellitus, sodium and fluid retention, and cataracts.

Somatostatin Analog (SMS 201-995) Therapy

- SMS 201-995 (octreotide [Sandostatin, Sandoz]) is an analog of somatostatin that inhibits the secretion of insulin by normal and neoplastic beta cells.
- The responsiveness of insulin-secreting tumors to the suppressive effects of SMS 201-995 is variable, being dependent on membrane receptors for somatostatin on the tumor cells.
- The dosage is 10–40 µg q8–12h SC.
- Adverse reactions have not been seen at these dosages.

PROGNOSIS

The long-term prognosis for survival is guarded to poor because of the malignant nature of insulin-secreting tumors and the often extended period of time (months) before a diagnosis is established.

- The mean survival time for dogs treated medically is approximately 12 months from the onset of clinical signs of hypoglycemia.
- The ability of surgery to improve the prognosis depends on the clinical stage of the disease, most notably the presence or absence of metastasis.

A multiuniversity study (Caywood and coworkers, 1988) involving a total of 73 dogs with insulin-secreting neoplasia found:

- Fifty percent of dogs with a solitary tumor and no visible metastases at the time of surgery were free of hypoglycemia 14 months after surgery.
- Less than 20% of dogs with visible metastasis were disease-free at 14 months.
- Eighty percent of dogs with a solitary mass were dead 24 months from the time of diagnosis.
- Approximately 50% of dogs with metastasis to the liver (the most common site) were dead by 6 months and all were dead by 18 months from the time of diagnosis.

SUPPLEMENTAL READINGS

Breitschwerdt EB, Loar AS, Hribernik TN, et al.: Hypoglycemia in four dogs with sepsis. J Am Vet Med Assoc 178:1072, 1981.

Caywood DD, Klausner JS, O'Leary TP, et al.: Pancreatic insulin-secreting neoplasms: Clinical, diagnostic, and prognostic features in 73 dogs. J Am Anim Hosp Assoc 24:577, 1988.

Feldman EC, Nelson RW: Canine and Feline Endocrinology and Reproduction. Philadelphia: WB Saunders, 1996, p 422.

Fingeroth JM, Smeak DD: Intravenous methylene blue infusion for intraoperative identification of pancreatic islet-cell tumors in dogs. Part II: Clinical trial and results in four dogs. J Am Anim Hosp Assoc 24:175, 1988.

Leifer CE, Peterson ME, Matus RE, et al.: Hypoglycemia associated with nonislet cell tumor in 13 dogs. J Am Vet Med Assoc 186:53, 1985.

Leifer CE, Peterson ME, Matus RE: Insulin-secreting tumor: Diagnosis and medical and surgical management in 55 dogs. J Am Vet Med Assoc 188:60, 1986.

Mehlhaff CJ, Peterson ME, Patnaik AK, et al.: Insulin-producing islet cell neoplasms: Surgical considerations and general management in 35 dogs. J Am Anim Hosp Assoc 21:607, 1985.

Nelson RW: Textbook of Veterinary Internal Medicine. Philadelphia: WB Saunders, 1995, p 1501.

34 Diseases of the Hypothalamus and Pituitary

John F. Randolph / Rhett Nichols / Mark E. Peterson

NORMAL ANATOMY AND PHYSIOLOGY

The *pituitary* gland (hypophysis) consists of the neurohypophysis surrounded by the adenohypophysis.

Neurohypophysis

The neurohypophysis, also called the *pars nervosa* and *infundibulum* (Fig. 34–1), extends ventrally from the hypothalamus.

- It is composed of nerve tracts terminating from nuclei within the hypothalamus.
- Antidiuretic hormone (ADH, vasopressin) and oxytocin, produced by the supraoptic and paraventricular hypothalamic nuclei, travel down the axons to be stored in and secreted from the neurohypophysis.

Adenohypophysis

The adenohypophysis is an embryonic outgrowth of the pharynx connected to the hypothalamus by a vascular network that allows humoral control of adenohypophyseal secretions by the hypothalamus.

- In response to the neurotransmitters, specialized neurosecretory cells within the hypothalamus release factors that control production and secretion of hormones from the adenohypophysis (Table 34–1).
- Hormones produced by target endocrine organs in response to specific adenohypophyseal hormones exert a negative feedback (or feedback inhibition) on further elaboration of the hypothalamo-hypophyseal hormones.
  - Because growth hormone (GH), prolactin, and melanocyte-stimulating hormone (MSH) do not have target endocrine organs to participate in negative feedback controls, releasing and inhibiting factors from the hypothalamus control production of these hormones (see Table 34–1).
- The adenohypophysis is subdivided into the pars distalis, pars tuberalis, and pars intermedia (see Fig. 34–1).
  - The pars intermedia, unlike the pars distalis, does not have an extensive blood supply contiguous with the hypothalamus. The cells of the pars intermedia appear to release their hormones in response to dopaminergic and serotonergic innervation.

Adenohypophyseal Cells

These are classified by staining properties of their secretory granules.

- Immunohistochemical staining identifies the specific hormone content of the cells.
- Hematoxylin and eosin staining identifies adenohypophyseal cells as:
  - Acidophils: Somatotrophs and lactotrophs.
  - Basophils: Gonadotrophs, corticotrophs, and thyrotrophs.
  - Chromophobes (cells that do not stain selectively): Degranulated, undifferentiated, or actively synthesizing cells (some investigators consider chromophobes to include corticotrophs).

Alternative Nomenclature

Alternatively, the pituitary gland is composed of the anterior lobe and posterior lobe, with the two lobes separated by the hypophyseal cleft (the residual lumen of

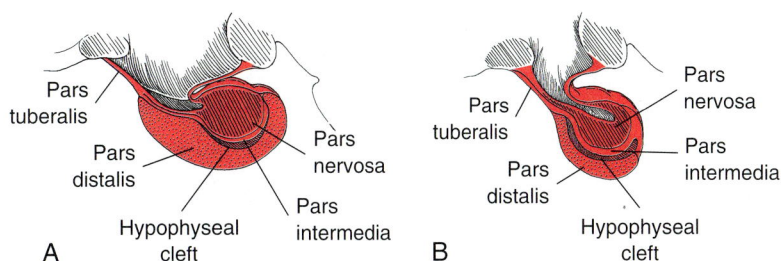

Figure 34–1. Schematic diagram of a mid-sagittal section through the pituitary gland of a normal dog (A) and cat (B). (Modified from Dellmann HD, Brown DM: Textbook of Veterinary Histology, 3rd Ed. Philadelphia: Lea & Febiger, 1987.)

Table 34–1. ADENOHYPOPHYSEAL HORMONES AND THEIR REGULATORY HYPOTHALAMIC HORMONES

Adenohypophyseal Hormone	Hypothalamic Hormone
Thyroid-stimulating hormone (TSH)	Thyrotropin-releasing hormone (TRH)
Adrenocorticotropic hormone (ACTH)	Corticotropin-releasing hormone (CRH)
Growth hormone (GH, somatotropin)	GH-releasing hormone (GHRH, somatocrinin)
	GH-release-inhibiting hormone (somatostatin)
Follicle-stimulating hormone (FSH)	Gonadotropin-releasing hormone (GnRH)
Luteinizing hormone (LH)	Gonadotropin-releasing hormone (GnRH)
Prolactin (lactotropic hormone [LTH])	Prolactin-releasing factor
	Prolactin inhibitor (dopamine)
Melanocyte-stimulating hormone (MSH)	MSH-releasing hormone (MSH-RH)
	MSH-release-inhibiting hormone (MSH-RIH)

Rathke's pouch) (see Fig. 34–1). The terms anterior and posterior, although anatomically correct for the human pituitary, are not accurate when used to describe the lobes of the feline or canine pituitary gland.

- Anterior lobe: Pars tuberalis (glandular pituitary stalk) and the pars distalis.
- Posterior lobe: Pars nervosa and pars intermedia.

DISEASES OF PITUITARY HORMONE EXCESS

Growth Hormone–Secreting Pituitary Hyperplasia/Neoplasia: Acromegaly

Excess production of GH causes overgrowth of bone, connective tissue, and viscera. If GH oversecretion (hypersomatotropism) occurs after closure of the epiphyses, acromegaly develops. In acromegaly, only the membranous bones (e.g., nose, mandible, and portions of the vertebrae) increase in length, because the long bones cannot grow longitudinally once the epiphyses close.

Growth hormone exerts both direct and indirect effects on the body. The indirect actions of GH, mediated by somatomedin C (also known as insulin-like growth factor I [IGF-I]), are anabolic and include increased protein synthesis and soft tissue and skeletal growth. In contrast, the direct effects of GH are predominantly catabolic (e.g., lipolysis and restricted cellular glucose transport).

Etiology

- *In dogs:* Endogenous (diestrus) or exogenous progestogens may cause acromegaly by inducing hyperplasia and hypertrophy of the GH-secreting somatotrophs of the pituitary. However, recent work suggests that progestogen-induced GH excess originates from hyperplastic ductular epithelium of the mammary glands of dogs.
- *In cats:* The major cause of acromegaly is a GH-secreting tumor of the pituitary gland.

▼ *Key Point* Acromegaly in dogs is caused by progestogens. Feline acromegaly develops from a GH-secreting pituitary tumor.

Clinical Signs

Signalment

- *Age:* Middle to old age.
- *Breed:* No breed predilection.
- *Sex:* Most acromegalic cats are male, whereas acromegalic dogs are female.

General Appearance

▼ *Key Point* The clinical features of acromegaly develop so insidiously that they are frequently overlooked.

- Large paws.
- Soft tissue swelling of the head and neck with prominent skin folds.
- Prognathism due to mandibular enlargement.
- Widened interdental spaces.
- Macroglossia.
- Increase in body size and weight; sometimes, weight loss.
- Pot-bellied appearance.
- Long, thick, or coarse haircoat.
- Rapid growth of toenails.

Respiratory System

- *In dogs:* Excessive panting, exercise intolerance, and inspiratory stridor develop because oropharyngeal soft tissue proliferation compresses the upper airway.
- *In cats:* Dyspnea as a result of pulmonary edema or pleural effusion from GH-induced cardiac failure.

Cardiovascular System

In cats, cardiac involvement includes:

- Systolic murmur (64%).
- Cardiomegaly (86%).
- Congestive heart failure (43%) characterized by pulmonary edema, pleural effusion, or ascites.

Endocrine System

▼ *Key Point* Some dogs and most cats with acromegaly have insulin-resistant diabetes mellitus.

- Diabetes mellitus and its accompanying clinical signs of polyuria, polydipsia, and polyphagia develop because GH restricts cellular glucose transport. Insulin resistance results, and large doses of insulin (>2.2 U/kg/day) are frequently needed to control the hyperglycemia.
- In acromegalic cats, the growth-promoting effects of GH lead to enlargement of endocrine glands (thyroid, parathyroid, adrenal), but the function of these glands remains normal.
- In contrast, dogs in which acromegaly is caused by chronic administration of progestogens have subnormal basal cortisol concentrations. The glucocorticoid-like activity of these progestogens probably suppresses adrenocorticotropic hormone (ACTH) secretion and causes secondary hypoadrenocorticism.

Skeletal System

- Spondylosis deformans.
- Hyperostosis of the skull.
- Mandibular enlargement (prognathism).
- Arthropathy: Excess GH causes proliferation of cartilage and soft tissue, resulting in widening of the joint space. Some cats develop degenerative arthropathy with time. Acromegalic dogs seem less likely to develop joint problems.

Nervous System

- Growth of the pituitary tumor in feline acromegaly may impinge on brain tissue, causing circling, seizures, or behavioral changes.

Urinary System

- GH excess causes renal hypertrophy and increased glomerular filtration rate and renal plasma flow.
- Renal failure develops in about 50% of acromegalic cats. The kidneys of these cats have mesangial thickening of the glomeruli that may result from the glomerulosclerosis associated with unregulated diabetes mellitus and GH-mediated glomerular hyperfiltration.

Reproductive System

- Dogs with progesterone-induced acromegaly may develop pyometra, mucometra, and mammary gland nodules.

Diagnosis

▼ **Key Point** Suspect acromegaly in female dogs receiving progestogens and in intact female dogs that develop diabetes mellitus or laryngeal stridor due to soft tissue overgrowth. Suspect acromegaly in all cats with insulin-resistant diabetes mellitus.

Physical Examination

Look for the clinical signs listed previously. To confirm enlargement of the head and paws, redundant skin folds, and prognathism, compare the animal's appearance with earlier photographs of the animal, if possible.

Routine Laboratory Tests

- Severe hyperglycemia and glucosuria are found in most cats and some dogs with acromegaly. Despite the poorly regulated diabetic state of most acromegalic cats and the enhancement of ketogenesis by GH, ketosis rarely develops.
- Less frequently, increases in cholesterol, alanine aminotransferase (ALT), and serum alkaline phosphatase (ALP) may be caused by the diabetic state. However, in many acromegalic dogs without diabetes, ALP activity is increased.
- Mild to moderate hyperproteinemia occurs in 50% of acromegalic cats, but the serum protein electrophoretic pattern is normal.
- Hyperphosphatemia may occur secondary to increased renal tubular reabsorption of phosphorus by GH.
- There may be stress leukogram, anemia (in dogs, the cause is uncertain), or mild erythrocytosis (in cats, due to GH-stimulated erythropoiesis).
- Acromegalic cats that develop renal failure have persistent proteinuria (100–300 mg/dl) with dilute urine specific gravity (1.015–1.025).

Radiography

Examine for:

- Visceral enlargement (cardiomegaly, hepatomegaly, renomegaly).
- Soft tissue proliferation (oropharyngeal region, head, limbs).
- Bony changes (spondylosis, hyperostosis of the calvarium, periarticular periosteal reaction).
- Left ventricular and septal hypertrophy in acromegalic cats with cardiomegaly (by echocardiogram).

Other Diagnostic Imaging

- Magnetic resonance imaging (MRI) and computed tomography (CT) are helpful in identifying a possible pituitary tumor.

Growth Hormone Determination

Increased circulating GH concentrations confirm a diagnosis of acromegaly. However, GH concentrations may be normal in some acromegalic patients and may be increased in a variety of other diseases.

- Increased GH concentration in the presence of profound hyperglycemia supports a diagnosis of acromegaly because hyperglycemia would normally be expected to suppress GH secretion.
- Alternatively, an integrated 24-hour GH concentration determined by frequent sampling throughout the day may be more indicative of GH hypersecretion than solitary determinations.
- Validated GH radioimmunoassays are not widely available for the dog or cat. Utrecht University in the Netherlands measures canine and feline GH concen-

trations in plasma. However, until such assays are routinely obtainable, diagnose acromegaly presumptively as follows.

- Base a presumptive diagnosis of *feline acromegaly* on:
  - Clinical and laboratory features characteristic of acromegaly.
  - Radiographic documentation of a pituitary mass.
  - Normal results on thyroid and adrenal testing.
- Base a presumptive diagnosis of *canine acromegaly* on:
  - Characteristic clinical and laboratory findings.
  - Exposure to a progestogen source and improvement in clinical signs following removal of that progestogen source.
  - No evidence of spontaneous hyperadrenocorticism on adrenal testing.
- Determination of somatomedin C (IGF-I) gives an indirect indication of GH concentration. Increased somatomedin C concentrations develop in acromegalic dogs and, seemingly, in acromegalic cats. A validated assay is available at the Endocrine Diagnostic Laboratory of Michigan State University (Telephone: 517-353-0621).

Treatment of Progesterone-Induced Acromegaly

Treat progesterone-induced acromegaly by ovariohysterectomy or discontinuation of progestogen drugs. The soft tissue overgrowth and respiratory stridor resolve; however, the skeletal changes persist. The insulin requirement for GH-induced diabetes mellitus also declines, but the reversibility of the diabetes depends on the insulin reserve of the pancreatic beta islet cells.

Treatment of Growth Hormone–Secreting Pituitary Tumors

Manage these tumors by surgery, radiation, or drug therapy.

Surgery

- Acromegaly attributable to a GH-secreting pituitary tumor has not yet been corrected by surgery.
- Because surgical excision of the tumor probably necessitates a hypophysectomy, expect deficiencies of pituitary hormones postoperatively.
- Before surgery, precisely localize the pituitary tumor by CT or MRI because neoplastic extension into the hypothalamus precludes surgery.
- Trans-sphenoidal cryotherapy of a pituitary tumor in an acromegalic cat has been performed.

Radiation

The results of *cobalt irradiation* of pituitary tumors (total dose of 4800 cGy divided equally in 12 treatments during 4 weeks) in acromegalic cats have been variable. In one report involving two cats, no effect was seen on tumor size or GH concentration in one cat; in the other cat, the tumor shrunk with subsequent reduction in GH concentration. These changes developed within 2 months of radiation treatment but lasted for only 6 months before relapse. In another report, two of three acromegalic cats treated by irradiation had long-term remission (16 and 28 months).

Pharmacologic Management

This includes dopamine agonists and long-acting somatostatin analogs.

- *Dopamine agonists.* Bromocriptine lowers GH concentrations in many acromegalic humans, but its effect on GH concentrations in acromegalic cats is unknown.
- *Long-acting somatostatin analogs.* Analogs such as SMS 201-995 (octreotide) inhibit GH secretion in most humans with acromegaly. However, subcutaneous doses of octreotide, ranging from 10–200 µg/day, did not reduce GH concentrations in four acromegalic cats.

Management of Concurrent Growth Hormone–Induced Conditions

Provide symptomatic treatment of GH-related disorders in the initial management of acromegalic dogs and the long-term care of acromegalic cats.

- Congestive heart failure in some acromegalic cats initially responds to furosemide treatment (see Chap. 64 for more details on treatment of congestive heart failure).
- Inspiratory stridor in acromegalic dogs partially responds to cage rest, cooling, and oxygen therapy.
- The diabetes mellitus of feline acromegaly generally is refractory and requires insulin (NPH, protamine zinc insulin, or Ultralente) twice daily. In some cats, combinations of short-acting insulin (Regular insulin) with NPH insulin may help control hyperglycemia (see Chap. 32 for more details on management of diabetes mellitus).

Prevention

- No preventive measures currently are known to avoid the development of GH-secreting pituitary tumors in cats.
- Prevent acromegaly in dogs by ovariohysterectomy of nonbreeding females and judicious use of progestogen drugs.

ACTH-Secreting Pituitary Hyperplasia/Neoplasia: Cushing Disease

Hyperplasia or neoplasia of the pituitary corticotrophs with resultant oversecretion of ACTH is the major cause of hyperadrenocorticism (Cushing disease) in the dog and cat. Excess ACTH may originate from the corticotrophs in either the pars distalis or the pars intermedia. Clinical signs, diagnostic testing, and treatment of Cushing disease are discussed in Chapter 31.

DISEASES OF PITUITARY HORMONE DEFICIENCY

Hypopituitary Dwarfism: Growth Hormone Deficiency

Etiology

- In German shepherds and Carelian bear dogs, hypopituitary dwarfism is inherited as an autosomal recessive trait, and is associated with cystic distention of the craniopharyngeal duct (Rathke's pouch).

- It is not known whether expansion of the pituitary cyst destroys adjacent adenohypophyseal tissue or whether a primary defect in differentiation and secretory capability of the adenohypophyseal cells creates the cyst.
- Weimaraners develop GH deficiency in association with thymic abnormalities.

Clinical Signs

Signalment

- *Age:* Young animals are affected. Discrepancies in growth compared with littermates are apparent at 6–8 weeks of age.
- *Breed:* This is an autosomal recessive trait in the German shepherd and Carelian bear dog.
- *Sex:* There is no sex predilection.

General Appearance

- Growth retardation is characterized by proportionately stunted short stature. Affected German shepherd dogs usually fail to exceed 13.5 kg in body weight or 47.5 cm in shoulder height by 1 year of age.
- The hair is soft and woolly, with retention of secondary (lanugo) hairs and lack of primary (guard) hairs. Progressive, bilaterally symmetric truncal alopecia develops with age.
- Dental eruption may be delayed.

Concurrent Deficiencies of Other Pituitary Hormones

- Thyroid-stimulating hormone deficiency (secondary hypothyroidism; see Chap. 29).
- ACTH deficiency (secondary hypoadrenocorticism; see Chap. 31).
- Follicle-stimulating hormone/luteinizing hormone deficiency (secondary hypogonadism).

Diagnosis

Differentiate hypopituitary dwarfism from other causes of growth retardation (Fig. 34–2).

History

- Identify breed predisposition and postnatal onset of growth problems (see Fig. 34–2).

Physical Examination

- The puppy is proportionately stunted.
- The haircoat initially remains as the animal matures, but truncal alopecia eventually develops.
- Additional clinical features characteristic of hypothyroidism, hypoadrenocorticism, or hypogonadism depend on the extent of hypophyseal involvement.

Routine Laboratory Tests

- Hematologic, serum biochemical, and urinalysis results usually are normal for immature dogs. Hypophosphatemia may result from lack of GH-mediated renal tubular reabsorption of phosphorus.

Radiographic Abnormalities

- Delayed closure of the epiphyses.
- Delayed dental eruption.
- Delayed or incomplete calcification of the os penis.

Growth Hormone Determination

- Basal GH concentrations do not differentiate normal dogs from dogs with GH deficiency.
- GH stimulation tests classically have been used to evaluate pituitary GH secretory capability.
- Measure circulating GH concentrations in fasted dogs before and 5, 15, 30, 45, 60, and 90 minutes after intravenous administration of
  - 0.1 or 0.3 mg of xylazine/kg (Rompun, Haver), or

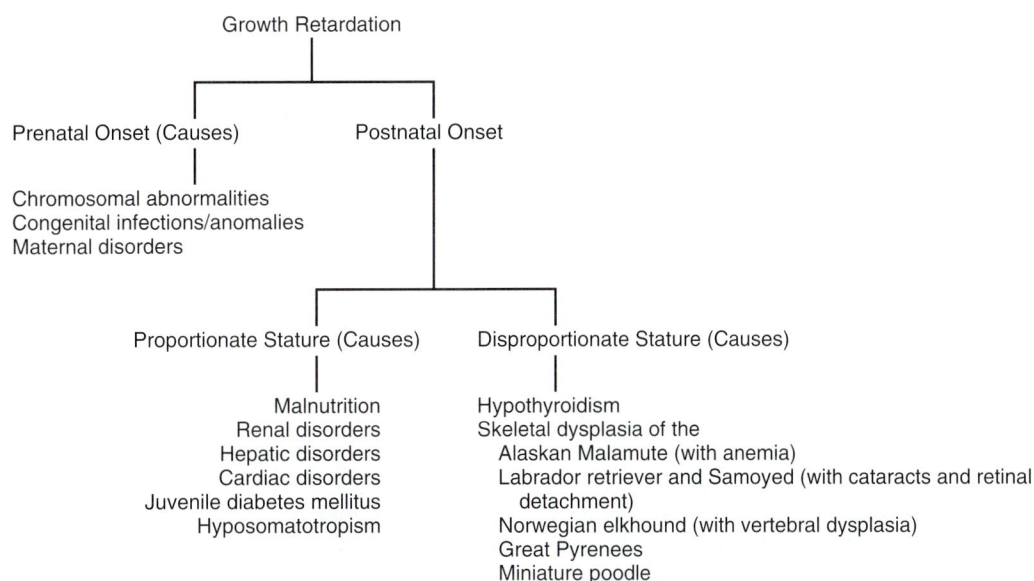

```
                        Growth Retardation
                               |
          ┌────────────────────┴────────────────────┐
   Prenatal Onset (Causes)                   Postnatal Onset

   Chromosomal abnormalities
   Congenital infections/anomalies
   Maternal disorders

                    ┌──────────────────────┴──────────────────────┐
          Proportionate Stature (Causes)        Disproportionate Stature (Causes)
                     |                                     |
               Malnutrition                        Hypothyroidism
               Renal disorders                     Skeletal dysplasia of the
               Hepatic disorders                     Alaskan Malamute (with anemia)
               Cardiac disorders                     Labrador retriever and Samoyed (with cataracts and retinal
               Juvenile diabetes mellitus              detachment)
               Hyposomatotropism                     Norwegian elkhound (with vertebral dysplasia)
                                                     Great Pyrenees
                                                     Miniature poodle
```

Figure 34–2. Classification of growth retardation by onset of growth problems and stature of dog.

- 3 or 10 µg of clonidine/kg (Catapres, Boehringer Ingelheim), or
- 1 µg of human GH-releasing hormone (hGHRH)/kg (Geref, Serono Laboratories).
- Interpretation
  - In normal dogs, circulating GH concentrations increase within 30 minutes of xylazine, clonidine, or GHRH administration and then decline by 60–90 minutes.
  - In dogs with hypopituitary dwarfism, no substantial increase in GH concentration develops after pharmacologic stimulation.
- In some children with GH neurosecretory dysfunction, GH response to pharmacologic stimulation is normal; nevertheless, spontaneous physiologic pulsatile GH secretion is decreased, as determined by 24-hour blood sample monitoring. A similar disorder may account for the delayed growth reported in a litter of German shepherds.

Somatomedin C Measurement

Currently, validated GH radioimmunoassays are not routinely available for the dog, except at Utrecht University, the Netherlands. However, measurement of serum somatomedin C, produced in response to GH, gives an indirect indication of GH concentration. This assay is available at the Endocrine Diagnostic Laboratory of Michigan State University.

- In GH-deficient German shepherds with pituitary dwarfism, somatomedin C concentrations are subnormal.
- Somatomedin C concentrations in related but clinically unaffected dogs that are presumably heterozygous for the dwarf trait are intermediate between the somatomedin C concentrations found in normal German shepherds and those obtained in dwarf German shepherds.

Other Endocrine Tests

- Investigate for secondary hypothyroidism associated with hypopituitary dwarfism (see Chap. 29) and for secondary hypoadrenocorticism associated with hypopituitary dwarfism (see Chap. 31).

Skin Biopsy

- In canine GH deficiency, nonspecific histologic skin changes (atrophy of hair follicles, epidermis, and sebaceous glands) are similar to those seen in other canine endocrinopathies; however, a decreased number of elastin fibers is present in the dermis.

Treatment
Growth Hormone Replacement Therapy

- Current guidelines recommend bovine or porcine GH preparations subcutaneously at 0.1 IU/kg three times weekly for 4–8 weeks. Historically, GH replacement for the dog has been difficult to obtain and expensive. With the recent development of biosynthetic bovine GH (Posilac, Monsanto), an inexpensive source of GH seemed readily available. Unfortunately, this product, designed for use in cattle, cannot be formulated for the dog's smaller dose requirement and is not approved for use in dogs.
- Biosynthetic human GH appears to induce antibody formation in dogs that interferes with its effectiveness, and similar immunogenicity problems may be associated with bovine GH administration to dogs. Porcine GH, similar immunologically to canine GH, is available through Dr. A. F. Parlow, Pituitary Hormones and Antisera Center, Harbor-UCLA Medical Center, Torrance, California.
- No increase in size occurs if dogs are treated after epiphyseal closure.
- Because GH is diabetogenic, monitor blood glucose concentrations during treatment.

Thyroid Hormone or Glucocorticoid Replacement Therapy

- Initiate therapy if concurrent hypothyroidism or hypoadrenocorticism exists (see Chaps. 29 and 31).

Prevention

Because hypopituitary dwarfism is inherited in an autosomal recessive manner in German shepherd and Carelian bear dogs, genetic counseling may help eliminate this disease. Identify possible heterozygotes by somatomedin C assay, and eliminate these carrier animals from breeding programs.

Central Diabetes Insipidus: Antidiuretic Hormone Deficiency

Diabetes insipidus (DI) is a disorder of water metabolism characterized by polyuria and polydipsia. It is caused by defective secretion or synthesis of ADH (central DI) or the inability of the renal tubule to respond to this hormone (nephrogenic DI). Deficiency of ADH or renal insensitivity to ADH can be partial or complete.

Etiology

Central DI (also called neurogenic DI) is an uncommon condition that results from disorders that disrupt the ADH-producing hypothalamic neurohypophyseal neurons.

- Idiopathic.
- Central nervous system (CNS) trauma.
- CNS neoplasia.
- CNS inflammation.
- Congenital anomalies.

Clinical Signs
Signalment

- *Age* is variable, depending on the cause.
  - Idiopathic and trauma-induced DI have no specific age predilection.
  - Animals with suspected congenital DI are <1 year of age.

- Animals with DI caused by CNS neoplasia are usually middle-aged to older.
- *Breed:* No predilection.
- *Sex:* No predisposition.

Polyuria and Polydipsia

- ADH acts on the distal tubules and collecting ducts of the kidneys to allow increased water reabsorption.
- Lack of ADH or ADH receptors, interference with the ability of ADH to bind to its receptors, or medullary washout (which often occurs to some degree in polyuric disorders) results in water diuresis.
- This primary polyuria results in volume contraction and subsequent compensatory polydipsia.

Diagnosis

The diagnosis of DI requires its differentiation from other, more common causes of polyuria and polydipsia such as primary renal disease, diabetes mellitus, pyometra, feline hyperthyroidism, and canine hyperadrenocorticism.

History

- Profound polyuria and polydipsia (>100 ml/kg/day; normal is approximately 40–70 ml/kg/day) are found.

Physical Examination

Findings are usually normal with the following exceptions:

- Weight loss (if the animal is preoccupied with drinking).
- Dehydration (if water is withheld).
- Neurologic signs (e.g., disorientation, seizures, blindness) may develop in animals with pituitary or hypothalamic neoplasia or trauma.

Routine Laboratory Tests

- Hematologic and serum biochemical results are usually normal, or consistent with mild dehydration (mild increases in packed cell volume and serum concentrations of total protein and sodium).

▼ *Key Point* Urine dipstick and sediment evaluations are normal, but urine specific gravity (USG) is persistently in the range of 1.000–1.007 in the dog, and 1.008–1.012 in the cat.

- Animals with partial deficiencies in ADH may produce more concentrated urine. Urine culture is negative.

Radiography

- Findings usually are normal.

Other Diagnostic Imaging

- MRI and CT can aid in identifying a pituitary or hypothalamic lesion.

Water Deprivation Tests

These tests are designed to determine whether endogenous ADH is released in response to dehydration, and whether the kidneys can respond to ADH. Minimal increases in plasma osmolality should stimulate release of ADH.

▼ *Key Point* Water deprivation tests are contraindicated in animals that are already dehydrated (since the stimulus for ADH release already exists) or in the presence of other laboratory abnormalities such as azotemia or hypercalcemia.

Because water deprivation causes dehydration, these tests are potentially dangerous and can result in acute renal failure, neurologic complications, and death. For this reason, perform routine laboratory testing consisting of a complete blood count, serum biochemical profile, and complete urinalysis to rule out disorders that may decompensate following dehydration (e.g., pyometra, pyelonephritis, renal insufficiency, and hypercalcemia).

Abrupt Water Deprivation Test
- Procedure: See Table 34–2.
- Interpretation: When deprived of water, normal animals can concentrate the USG to 1.075 in cats and 1.045 in dogs. Nevertheless, a USG of 1.025 is generally considered an adequate response to water deprivation. Failure to concentrate to this degree in the absence of renal disease or other laboratory abnormalities indicates that the animal has central or nephrogenic DI and/or medullary washout (Fig. 34–3).

Gradual Water Deprivation Test
- Indication: Patients with medullary washout do not concentrate their urine following an abrupt water deprivation test. Gradual reduction in water intake, however, does allow them to reestablish the medullary gradient.
- Procedure: See Table 34–2.
- Interpretation: Failure to concentrate urine in the absence of renal disease or other laboratory abnormalities indicates that the animal has central or nephrogenic DI (see Fig. 34–3).

Antidiuretic Hormone Response Test

If the animal fails to concentrate urine adequately following water deprivation, perform an ADH response test. The test evaluates the ability of the renal tubule to respond to exogenous ADH and concentrate urine in the face of dehydration.

- Procedure:
  - Immediately following either an abrupt or gradual water deprivation test, administer aqueous vasopressin (Pitressin, Parke-Davis) 0.5 unit/kg (maximum dose, 5 units) IM.
  - Withhold all water and food during the test.
  - Empty the urinary bladder and measure USG (and osmolality if possible) at 30, 60, 90, and 120 minutes after vasopressin injection.
  - The animal may drink once the test is completed.

Table 34–2. PROCEDURES FOR ABRUPT AND GRADUAL WATER DEPRIVATION TESTS

Abrupt Water Deprivation Test	Gradual Water Deprivation Test
Empty urinary bladder and measure urine specific gravity (and urine osmolality if possible).	Quantitate daily unrestricted water consumption.
Weigh animal.	Measure urine specific gravity and weigh animal.
Withhold food and water.	Reduce water intake by 5% daily (to not less than 66 ml/kg/day).
	Feed normally.
Every 2–4 hours, reweigh animal, empty urinary bladder, and measure urine specific gravity (and urine osmolality if possible).	Weigh animal and measure urine specific gravity daily.
Use the criteria below as end points.	Use the criteria below as end points.

Stop the test when any of the following occur:
1. The animal loses more than 5% of its body weight.
2. The animal is clinically dehydrated or ill.
3. The urine specific gravity exceeds 1.025.

- Interpretation: Failure to concentrate urine with water deprivation followed by a rise in USG >1.025 after ADH administration is diagnostic of central DI (see Fig. 34–3); an inability to concentrate urine after the ADH response test is suggestive of nephrogenic DI or uncorrected medullary washout (see Fig. 34–3).

Therapeutic Antidiuretic Hormone Trial

As an alternative to the water deprivation test or ADH response test following water deprivation, perform a closely monitored therapeutic trial with desmopressin acetate (DDAVP, Rhone-Poulenc Rorer).

▼ *Key Point* Prior to performing a therapeutic ADH trial, rule out all common causes of polyuria and polydipsia, thus limiting the differential diagnosis to central DI or nephrogenic DI.

- Procedure: Administer the intranasal preparation of DDAVP in the conjunctival sac (1 to 4 drops q12h) for 3 to 5 days.

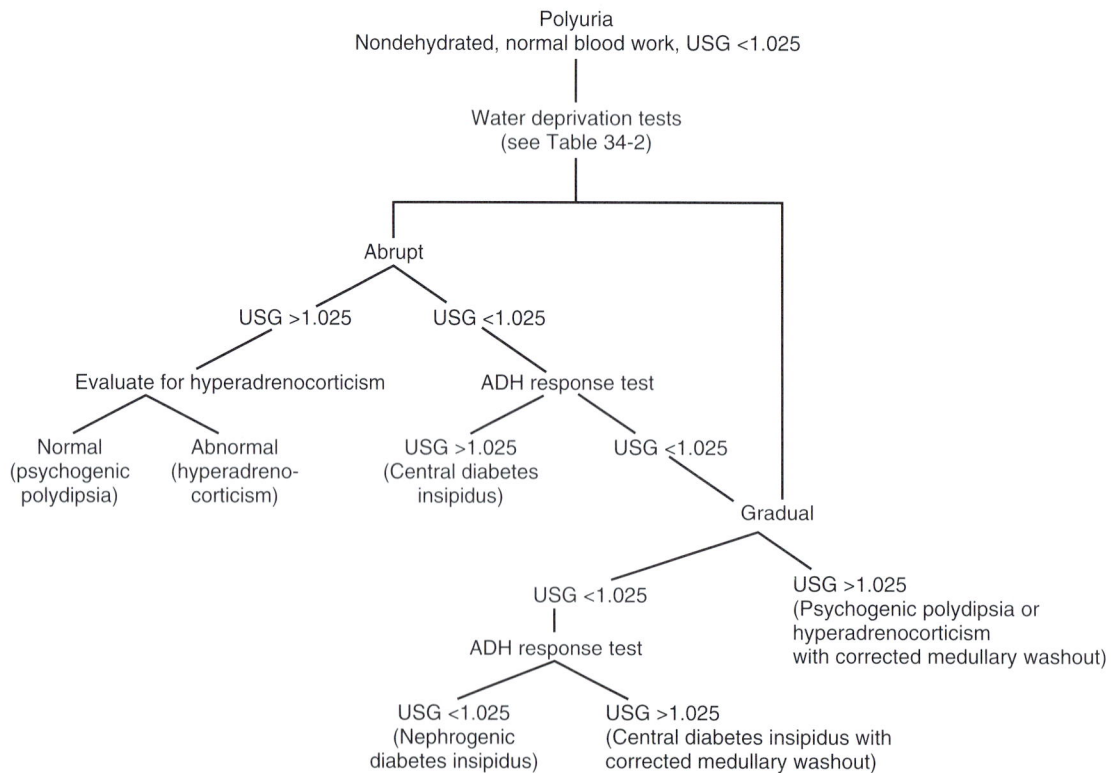

Figure 34–3. Algorithm for evaluation of an animal with polyuria/polydipsia. ADH, antidiuretic hormone; USG, urine specific gravity.

- Interpretation: A dramatic reduction in water intake (greater than 50%) during the treatment period would strongly suggest a diagnosis of central DI. When polyuria is due to other causes, the decrease is seldom more than 30%.

Treatment

Antidiuretic Hormone Replacement Therapy

- Desmopressin acetate (DDAVP, Rhone-Poulenc Rorer), a synthetic analog of ADH, is the drug of choice for the treatment of central DI in dogs and cats.
- Repositol ADH (vasopressin tannate in oil), once the only long-acting ADH preparation available, is no longer manufactured.
- DDAVP is available as an aqueous solution (100 μg/ml) intended for intranasal use, and as oral tablets (0.1 mg and 0.2 mg).
- The intranasal form of DDAVP is also effective when applied topically in the conjunctival sac (1–4 drops q12–24h) or injected subcutaneously (2–5 μg q12–24h). The oral form of DDAVP (DDAVP tablets, 0.1 mg) is equivalent to approximately 1 drop (4 μg) of intranasal DDAVP.
- Adjust the daily dose to control polyuria and polydipsia.
- The major disadvantage of this treatment is expense.

Nonhormonal Therapy

- *Hydrochlorothiazide* (Hydrodiuril, Merck, Sharp, & Dohme) may reduce the polyuria of DI, but it is never as effective as ADH replacement. Thiazide diuretics reduce total body sodium by an initial natriuresis, resulting in decreased extracellular fluid volume and reduced glomerular filtration rate. These changes cause increased fluid reabsorption in the proximal renal tubule and reduce urine output.
  - Administer hydrochlorothiazide at a dose of 2–4 mg/kg q12h PO.
  - Restrict salt intake to potentiate the drug's effectiveness.
  - Because hypokalemia may develop with thiazide diuretic therapy, monitor serum electrolyte concentrations during treatment.
- *Chlorpropamide* (Diabinese, Pfizer) is an oral hypoglycemic agent that potentiates the action of ADH on the renal distal tubules and collecting ducts. Because chlorpropamide requires some ADH to be effective, it reduces only the polyuria in animals with partial ADH deficiency.
  - Administer chlorpropamide at a dose of 10–40 mg/kg/day.
  - Monitor blood glucose concentrations during treatment.

Secondary (Pituitary) or Tertiary (Hypothalamic) Hypoadrenocorticism: ACTH or Corticotropin-Releasing Hormone Deficiency

See Chapter 31.

Secondary (Pituitary) or Tertiary (Hypothalamic) Hypothyroidism: Thyroid-Stimulating Hormone or Thyrotropin-Releasing Hormone Deficiency

See Chapter 29.

MISCELLANEOUS DISORDERS

Adipsia/Hypodipsia

Adipsia/hypodipsia is absent or reduced thirst. Normally with water loss, mild increases in plasma osmolality stimulate osmoreceptors in the hypothalamus to increase water consumption and ADH secretion. However, even with maximal ADH secretion, hyperosmolality (specifically hypernatremia) escalates unless the thirst mechanism is intact. With adipsia or hypodipsia, hypernatremia develops with resultant dehydrating effects on the cells of the CNS. It is usually unclear whether the defect in thirst in affected animals is due to an increased osmoreceptor threshold (reset setpoint) or to structural lesions in the thirst center of the hypothalamus.

Etiology

- Idiopathic.
- Hypothalamic dysplasia/congenital anomalies.
- Hypothalamic degeneration.
- Hypothalamic inflammation, neoplasia, or trauma.

Clinical Signs

- Signalment
  - *Age:* Young (usually <1 year) in idiopathic and congenital forms of the disorder.
  - *Sex:* Female predisposition in the miniature schnauzer.
  - *Breed:* Miniature schnauzer.
- Depression/stupor/coma.
- Personality change.
- Disorientation.
- Anorexia.
- Weakness/lethargy.
- Irritability/seizures.

Because hypothalamic conditions associated with adipsia/hypodipsia may cause neurologic signs regardless of the sodium concentration, the relative contribution of hypernatremia to the CNS signs can be assessed once a normal sodium concentration is restored.

Diagnosis

History

- Adipsia/hypodipsia has occurred despite free access to water, and the clinical signs listed previously are present.

Physical Examination

- There is evidence of dehydration and signs of altered mentation.

Routine Laboratory Tests

Hematologic, serum biochemical, and urinalysis results are consistent with dehydration:

- Hypernatremia (profound).
- Hyperosmolality (profound).
- Hyperchloremia.
- Azotemia (mild).
- Hyperalbuminemia (mild).
- Hypersthenuria.

Radiography

- Findings usually are normal.

Other Diagnostic Imaging

- MRI and CT can sometimes identify a hypothalamic lesion; however, studies have been normal in adipsic miniature schnauzers.

Treatment

The brain attempts to adapt to the hyperosmolar state by increasing its cellular osmolality with sodium, potassium, amino acids, and unidentified solutes (idiogenic osmoles). If plasma hyperosmolality is corrected too rapidly, the brain cells continue to be hyperosmolar relative to the plasma, and cerebral edema may develop.

▼ *Key Point* Rapid correction of chronic hyperosmolar states may lead to cerebral edema.

Initial Therapy

- For initial management of the normotensive animal in order to correct hypernatremia without lowering serum osmolality too rapidly, administer a sodium-restricted isotonic fluid IV (D_5W or 0.45% NaCl with 2.5% dextrose) to correct the animal's water deficit. Alternatively, if the animal is cooperative, administer oral fluids to correct the water deficit.
- Calculate the animal's water deficit based on the serum sodium concentration or osmolality and a normal total body weight of water of 60%:

$$\text{Water deficit (liters)} = 0.6 \times \text{body weight (kg)} \times \left(1 - \frac{\text{Normal sodium (mEq/L)}}{\text{Patient's sodium (mEq/L)}}\right)$$

- Replace the water deficit to lower serum sodium concentration by 0.5 mEq/L/hr. Generally, this rule translates to replacing the calculated water deficit during a period of 3 days.
- Add maintenance fluid requirement (60 ml/kg/day) with isotonic polyionic solution to the daily infusion.
- If the animal is hypotensive, reestablish tissue perfusion with isotonic saline or Ringer's solution before using sodium-restricted fluids. The osmolality of these solutions is still less than the patient's serum osmolality, so some reduction in serum sodium concentration and osmolality may occur.

Maintenance Therapy

- For chronic management once the animal is eating, mix maintenance daily water intake (50–60 ml/kg/day) with food.

SUPPLEMENTAL READINGS

Crawford MA, Kittleson MD, Fink GD: Hypernatremia and adipsia in a dog. J Am Vet Med Assoc 184:818, 1984.

Eigenmann JE: Pituitary-hypothalamic diseases. *In* Ettinger SJ, ed.: Textbook of Veterinary Internal Medicine. Philadelphia: WB Saunders, 1989, p 1579.

Feldman EC, Nelson RW, eds.: Canine and Feline Endocrinology and Reproduction. Philadelphia: WB Saunders, 1996.

Goossens MMC, Feldman EC, Nelson RW, et al.: Cobalt 60 irradiation of pituitary gland tumors in three cats with acromegaly. J Am Vet Med Assoc 213:374, 1998.

Nichols R, Hohenhaus AE: Use of the vasopressin analogue desmopressin for polyuria and bleeding disorders. J Am Vet Med Assoc 205:168, 1994.

Peterson ME, Randolph JF, Mooney CT: Endocrine diseases. *In* Sherding RG, ed.: The Cat: Diseases and Clinical Management. New York: Churchill Livingstone, 1994, p 1403.

Peterson ME, Taylor RS, Greco DS, et al.: Acromegaly in fourteen cats. J Vet Intern Med 4:192, 1990.

Randolph JF, Miller CL, Cummings JF, et al.: Delayed growth in two German shepherd dog littermates with normal serum concentrations of growth hormone, thyroxine, and cortisol. J Am Vet Med Assoc 196:77, 1990.

Selman PJ, Mol JA, Rutteman GR, et al.: Progestin-induced growth hormone excess in the dog originates in the mammary gland. Endocrinology 134:287, 1994.

5 Skin and Ear Diseases

Richard K. Anderson

35 Pyoderma

Edmund J. Rosser, Jr.

Pyoderma refers to any pyogenic infection of the skin and is most commonly used in reference to bacterial skin infections. However, fungal organisms (especially yeast) have also been recognized as potentially significant opportunists in the development of surface pyoderma in the dog. Pyoderma is a very common problem in clinical practice.

- Bacterial skin infection may be primary, which by definition is a skin infection that does not recur after the appropriate treatment. These infections are most likely the result of a transient and nonrecurrent insult to the skin.
- Secondary pyodermas are much more common and are associated with a persistent or recurrent underlying problem that alters the skin's resistance to infection. Until the underlying problem is identified, the infection usually responds only temporarily to therapy and subsequently recurs.
- Pyodermas are caused by bacterial colonization or invasion of the skin by coagulase-positive staphylococci, usually *Staphylococcus intermedius*. Invariably this is the initiating organism. In chronic, recurrent, or deep pyodermas, secondary bacterial invaders may be present, especially *Pseudomonas* spp., *Proteus* spp., and *Escherichia coli*.

SURFACE PYODERMAS

Surface pyoderma is a bacterial colonization of the surface of the epidermis only, without invasion into the stratum corneum or hair follicles. The two types are acute moist dermatitis ("hot spot") and skin fold pyoderma.

Acute Moist Dermatitis (Hot Spot)

Etiology

Self-trauma to the skin, due to an underlying pruritic or painful process, can result in a focal surface pyoderma referred to as acute moist dermatitis (hot spot). Underlying conditions that may be associated with the development of hot spots are listed in Table 35–1.

Table 35–1. CONDITIONS THAT MAY BE ASSOCIATED WITH HOT SPOTS

Disease Category	Examples
Allergic skin diseases	Flea allergy dermatitis
	Atopy
	Food allergy
	Allergic contact dermatitis
	Staphylococcal hypersensitivity
Ectoparasites	Canine scabies
	Cheyletiellosis
Otitis externa	Allergic otitis externa
	Ceruminous otitis externa
Environmental causes	Irritant contact dermatitis
	Poor grooming
	Burs or plant awns in the skin or hair coat
Musculoskeletal disorders	Hip dysplasia
	Degenerative joint disease
	Arthritis and other arthropathies
Anal sac problems	Impacted anal sacs
	Anal sacculitis

From Rosser EJ, Sams A: Pruritus. *In* Allen DG, ed.: Small Animal Medicine. Philadelphia: JB Lippincott, 1991, p 704.

Clinical Signs

- Acute moist dermatitis (hot spot) is usually a single alopecic lesion that is circumscribed, erythematous, thickened, and erosive. A thin exudative film occurs over the surface, and peripheral hairs are matted onto the lesion. The lesion develops subsequent to the dog's chewing and licking at a focal area of pruritus or pain, and develops within a matter of hours. The lesion is usually painful.
- Thick-coated, longhaired breeds are most commonly affected.
- Lesions that appear clinically similar to an acute moist dermatitis, but develop in the absence of a history of self-trauma, are often associated with a deeper bacterial folliculitis and/or furunculosis and are most commonly observed on the side of the face, or cheek region. The breeds more commonly affected by this deeper form of an acute moist dermatitis are golden retrievers, Saint Bernards, bouviers, and Newfoundlands.

Diagnosis

▼ *Key Point* Diagnose acute moist dermatitis by the history of self-trauma to the skin, acute onset, rapid development of the lesion (within hours), and the typical appearance of the lesion on physical exam.

- History includes questioning the owner about any pruritic skin disease, painful process, or environmental irritant that might indicate the reason for the dog's self-trauma of the area (Table 35–1). In instances of recurrent hot spot formation, identify the underlying problem to prevent any further recurrences.
- Biopsy lesions that appear clinically similar to an acute moist dermatitis, that develop in the absence of a history of self-trauma, and that respond poorly or are nonresponsive to initial treatment. This is to determine if the lesion is associated with a deeper bacterial folliculitis and/or furunculosis, which requires a more aggressive treatment regimen.

Treatment

Whenever an underlying disease process can be identified, institute the specific treatment recommended for that disease as well as the treatment necessary for the hot spot. One objective of treatment is to clip and clean the lesion to facilitate better aeration and to allow better contact and penetration of topical agents.

Topical Therapy

- First gently clip and thoroughly cleanse the area with an antiseptic shampoo, such as povidone-iodine (Betadine, Purdue Frederick) or chlorhexidine (Hexadene, Allerderm/Virbac; Nolvasan, Fort Dodge; ChlorhexiDerm, DVM Pharmaceuticals). Because the lesion is often very painful, this step may require sedation or general anesthesia.
- Dry the lesion by applying an astringent, such as Burow's solution (Domboro powder and water;

Bayer) or hamamelis extract (DermaCool with Lidocaine, Allerderm/Virbac), then apply an antibiotic/steroid cream such as Panalog Cream (Solvay), q12h, for 5–10 days.

Systemic Therapy

- Corticosteroids are indicated in the treatment of hot spots because the lesion is often painful or pruritic and because the most common underlying causes are allergic skin diseases. Begin treatment with a short-acting, injectable form of prednisolone, such as prednisolone phosphate in aqueous suspension at 0.5 mg/kg IM. The next day administer oral prednisolone at 0.5 mg/kg q12h for 5–7 days, then 0.5 mg/kg q24h for the next 5–7 days.
- Systemic antibiotics are also indicated in cases in which a deep folliculitis and/or furunculosis is suspected, or has been confirmed after histopathologic examination of a skin biopsy (see discussion of treatment under Deep Pyodermas).

Prevention

- In instances of recurrent hot spot formation, the underlying disease problem must be identified to prevent any further recurrence of the lesions.

Skin Fold Pyoderma

Etiology

- Deep skin folds, where the skin rubs against itself causing irritation, can result in a surface pyoderma referred to as a skin fold pyoderma (intertrigo). These skin folds create a moist, dark, and warm environment with poor air circulation that promotes subsequent bacterial *(S. intermedius)* or yeast *(Malassezia pachydermatis)* overgrowth and inflammation.
- Pyoderma can occur in any skin fold in any breed of dog, but intertrigo is most commonly associated with the skin folds in certain breeds of dogs. Table 35–2 lists the anatomic sites of the more common skin fold pyodermas and their breed predispositions, and includes lip fold, facial fold, vulvar fold, tail fold, body fold, and leg fold pyodermas.

Clinical Signs

- Skin fold pyoderma is characterized by inflammation and mild exudation. This pyoderma is best identified by simply widening the skin fold. The area is often noted to be malodorous.
- The animal is usually rubbing, licking, or biting excessively at the area. Evidence may exist of excoriation, alopecia, and erythema around the skin fold region.

Diagnosis

▼ *Key Point* Skin fold pyodermas are usually diagnosed by close inspection of the skin fold and demonstration of inflammation, mild exudation, and malodor from within the fold.

Table 35–2. SKIN FOLD PYODERMAS

Anatomic Site	Breed Predisposition	Comments
Lip fold	Cocker spaniel Springer spaniel Saint Bernard Irish setter	Lower lip fold Halitosis
Facial fold	Brachycephalic types Shar-Pei	Between nose and eyes Lateral facial region
Body fold	Shar-Pei	Also any breed with pendulous mammary glands Obese patients
Vulvar fold	None	Obese females Juvenile vulva Spayed early in life
Leg fold	Chondrodystrophic types (bassethound, dachshund)	Obese patients
Tail fold	Bulldog Boston terrier Pug	"Corkscrew tails" Anal odor

Treatment

The objectives of treatment are to cleanse and disinfect the skin fold region using agents that will dry the area and prevent recurrence of pyoderma. Topical therapy is usually adequate to control the problem.

- First gently expose and cleanse the skin fold with a benzoyl peroxide shampoo (OxyDex Shampoo, DVM Pharmaceuticals; Pyoben Shampoo, Allerderm/Virbac).
- Dry the area manually and apply a topical mild astringent, such as Burow's solution (Domboro powder and water; Bayer).
- Follow with a twice-daily application of a benzoyl peroxide–containing gel (OxyDex Gel, DVM Pharmaceuticals; Pyoben Gel, Allerderm/Virbac) into the skin fold region for 10–14 days.
- In cases involving a more severe inflammatory response, treat for the first 2–3 days with twice-daily applications of an antibiotic/steroid cream (Panalog Cream, Solvay) into the skin fold region. Once the inflammation has subsided, institute the benzoyl peroxide gel.

Prevention

Topical Therapy. Because the skin folds that develop pyoderma are usually deep, owing to a given breed characteristic, this condition tends to be a low-grade, recurrent problem. Once the infection has been treated as recommended, use the benzoyl peroxide gel as needed to prevent recurrence. This measure may require application ranging from daily, to once or twice weekly.

Corrective Surgery. When a more permanent solution to the problem is desired, remove the skin fold using cosmetic surgery techniques (see Chap. 50).

SUPERFICIAL PYODERMAS

- Superficial pyoderma is a bacterial invasion of the epidermis that can manifest itself in one of two ways. The bacteria can penetrate the stratum corneum with the subsequent formation of subcorneal pustules and is referred to as impetigo (puppy pyoderma). Second, the bacteria can invade the opening of the hair follicle causing inflammation and is referred to as folliculitis.
- Coagulase-positive staphylococci are the most common pathogens involved in a superficial pyoderma. *S. intermedius* is most frequently isolated.

Impetigo

Etiology

Impetigo is most often observed in young dogs before puberty. The condition can result from certain contributing factors, such as poor nutrition, dirty environment, and ectoparasite or endoparasite infection.

Clinical Signs

- Impetigo occurs as pustules in the inguinal and ventral abdominal regions. Occasionally, pustules are noted in the axillary region.
- The pustules do not involve hair follicles (i.e., no hair shafts protrude through the center of the pustule). Minimal erythema is noted, and the patient is usually nonpruritic.
- Impetigo is often an incidental finding during the physical examination of a recently acquired puppy.

Diagnosis

▼ *Key Point* Impetigo is usually diagnosed in young dogs before puberty by observing nonfollicular pustules in the inguinal and ventral abdominal regions with minimal erythema and absence of pruritus.

- *History.* Ask the owner about the animal's previous and current nutrition and housing environment.
- *Physical examination.* See Clinical Signs section.
- *Cytologic examination.* Stained contents of an intact pustule most often reveal neutrophils and cocci.
- *Skin scrapings.* Examine routine skin scrapings for ectoparasites such as *Demodex canis*, *Sarcoptes scabiei* and *Cheyletiella* spp.
- *Bacterial culture.* This is rarely necessary, but if done, *S. intermedius* is usually isolated.
- *Skin biopsy.* This is rarely necessary to establish the diagnosis of impetigo. Histopathology indicates subcorneal pustules containing neutrophils and cocci.
- Evaluate the puppy for intestinal parasites.

Treatment

▼ *Key Point* Objectives include identifying contributing factors for superficial pyoderma and correcting

Table 35–3. SYSTEMIC ANTIBIOTICS RECOMMENDED FOR STAPHYLOCOCCAL PYODERMAS

Antibiotic	Recommended Oral Dosage
Oxacillin	22 mg/kg q8h
Erythromycin	11 mg/kg q8h
Cephalexin	22 mg/kg q8h, or 33 mg/kg q12h
Cefadroxil	22 mg/kg q8–12h
Trimethoprim/sulfadiazine	30 mg/kg q12h
Ormetroprim/sulfadimethoxine	55 mg/kg on day 1, then 27.5 mg/kg q24h
Amoxicillin/clavulanate	14 mg/kg q12h

these as an adjunct to specific treatment. Improve the nutritional status and the housing environment and treat any endoparasite or ectoparasite infections.

Topical Therapy. Topical therapy is usually all that is required for this superficial staphylococcal infection, once any predisposing factors have been eliminated. Bathe the dog with a benzoyl peroxide shampoo (Oxy-Dex Shampoo, DVM Pharmaceuticals; Pyoben Shampoo, Allerderm/Virbac) two to three times weekly for 2–3 weeks.

Antibiotics. Systemic antibiotic therapy is rarely needed in impetigo. However, when topical therapy fails to resolve the pyoderma, add a systemic antibiotic to the topical therapy protocol. Table 35–3 lists the more commonly provided antibiotics and their recommended dosages for staphylococcal pyodermas in the dog.

Superficial Folliculitis

Etiology

- Superficial folliculitis induced by coagulase-positive staphylococci occurs occasionally as a primary problem.
- Secondary superficial folliculitis is much more common and is associated with a persistent or recurrent underlying problem that alters the skin's resistance to infection. Until the underlying problem is identified, the infection usually responds only temporarily to therapy and subsequently recurs (see the discussion under Recurrent Superficial and Deep Pyodermas).

Clinical Signs

- Superficial folliculitis initially appears similar to impetigo, with pustules in the inguinal and ventral abdominal regions. However, pustules often extend to the axillary region and the ventrolateral thorax.
- The pustules are oriented around the hair follicle (i.e., hair shafts protrude through the center of the pustule). The base of the pustule is often erythematous, and the patient is usually pruritic.

- Other lesions may include papules, crusts, and epidermal collarettes.
- When the truncal skin is affected, the haircoat often takes on a "moth-eaten" appearance.

Diagnosis

▼ *Key Point* Superficial folliculitis is usually diagnosed by observing pustules around hair follicles in the inguinal, ventral abdominal, and axillary regions. The base of the pustule is erythematous and the patient is usually pruritic.

- *History.* Superficial folliculitis is often secondary to an underlying disease problem. Question the owner about the effect of antibiotic therapy alone on the disease problem. This is a very important diagnostic tool in the systematic approach to a patient with a recurrent pyoderma. See also the discussion under Recurrent Superficial and Deep Pyodermas.
- *Physical examination.* See Clinical Signs section.
- *Cytologic examination.* The contents of an intact pustule usually reveal neutrophils and cocci.
- *Skin scrapings.* These are routinely examined for the presence of ectoparasites, such as *D. canis, S. scabiei,* and *Cheyletiella* spp.
- *Bacterial culture and sensitivity tests.* These are indicated in cases of recurrent superficial folliculitis to evaluate for resistent bacteria. Cultures usually reveal *S. intermedius.* The sensitivity results are used as a guideline for antibiotic selection.
- *Fungal culture.* Submit a sample of the hairs from follicular pustules for a fungal culture in cases that are nonresponsive to appropriate antibacterial therapy. In some instances, a folliculitis due to a dermatophyte infection can appear clinically indistinguishable from a folliculitis caused by bacteria.
- *Skin biopsy.* Typical findings include folliculitis or perifolliculitis, with coccoid bacteria within the hair follicle. Folliculitis due to a dermatophyte infection would reveal the presence of spores or hyphae within the hair follicle.

Treatment

▼ *Key Point* Be certain that an appropriate antibiotic for staphylococci has been selected (see Table 35–3) and that the duration of therapy has been adequate. The treatment required for folliculitis is generally more vigorous than that required for impetigo. In recurrent cases, define the underlying disease process and initiate a systematic approach to the disease. See the discussion under Recurrent Superficial and Deep Pyodermas.

Topical Therapy. This includes twice-weekly bathing with a benzoyl peroxide shampoo (OxyDex Shampoo, DVM Pharmaceuticals; Pyoben Shampoo, Allerderm/Virbac) for 3 weeks.

Antibiotics. Systemic antibiotic therapy can be initially selected on an empiric basis, choosing an antibiotic effective against coagulase-positive staphylococci (see Table 35–3). Treat for a minimum of 21 consecutive days, and for at least 7 days beyond apparent clinical cure.

DEEP PYODERMAS (DEEP FOLLICULITIS AND FURUNCULOSIS)

A deep pyoderma is a bacterial skin infection that extends beyond the epidermis and into the dermis and occasionally into the subcutaneous tissues. Although there are many possible forms of deep pyoderma, this discussion is limited to the most common form, deep folliculitis and furunculosis.

- The disease begins as a superficial folliculitis, then extends deeper into the hair follicle causing a deep folliculitis.
- This inflammatory process often results in a furunculosis, which is the destruction of the hair follicle wall and the release of the bacteria, hair shaft material, and follicular keratins into the surrounding dermis and occasionally the subcutaneous tissues.
- Subsequently, the bacteria can produce septicemia and/or bacteremia, and the released hair shafts and follicular keratins induce a foreign body and pyogranulomatous inflammatory reaction in the dermis.

Etiology

- Coagulase-positive staphylococci are the most common pathogens initially involved in deep pyoderma. *S. intermedius* is the most frequently isolated.
- In contrast to a superficial pyoderma, secondary invasion with other bacteria often occurs with *Pseudomonas* spp., *Proteus* spp., and *E. coli*.
- Deep pyoderma is rarely a primary disease process and is invariably related to some other underlying problem.

Clinical Signs

- Deep folliculitis and furunculosis initially begin as superficial folliculitis. See discussion of clinical signs under Superficial Pyodermas, and see Superficial Folliculitis.
- When deep folliculitis and furunculosis develop, the papules and pustules become larger and nodular on palpation. Exudation and crust formation follow. Draining tracts may develop. Hemorrhagic bullae may also be noted.
- In addition to the inguinal, ventral abdominal, and axillary regions, the pressure and wear areas of the body can also be affected. The disease may become generalized.
- The lesions are painful and/or pruritic.
- Peripheral lymphadenopathy is a common finding. Signs of systemic illness may be present (anorexia, depression, weight loss). The patient may also be febrile, an indication of bacteremia and/or septicemia.
- A specific form of deep pyoderma can occur in German shepherd dogs (so called "German shepherd dog pyoderma"), which is often related to multiple underlying problems in the affected patient.

Diagnosis

▼ *Key Point* Deep folliculitis and furunculosis are usually diagnosed by observing papules and pustules that become nodular on palpation, with exudation, crust formation, and draining tracts.

History and Physical Examination

Deep folliculitis and furunculosis are invariably secondary to an underlying disease process. Question the owner about the effect of antibiotics alone on the disease, as this is a very important diagnostic tool in the systematic approach to a patient with recurrent pyoderma. See discussion under Recurrent Superficial and Deep Pyodermas. Physical exam findings are described earlier under Superficial Pyoderma and Superficial Folliculitis.

Laboratory Tests

Cytologic Examination. Pustules, exudates, and draining tracts usually reveal neutrophils, macrophages, cocci, and rods.

Skin Scrapings. Evaluate for *D. canis* mites, a common ectoparasitic cause of deep pyoderma.

Bacterial Culture. Perform both aerobic and anaerobic bacterial culture and sensitivity tests in all cases of deep pyoderma. This form of pyoderma is capable of causing bacteremia and/or septicemia resulting in a life-threatening situation.

Fungal Culture. Do this in cases of deep pyodermas that are refractory to antibiotic therapy. Fungi are another possible cause of a deep folliculitis and furunculosis. Fungal diseases to consider include sporotrichosis, blastomycosis, coccidioidomycosis, aspergillosis, histoplasmosis, and cryptococcosis.

Skin Biopsy. This usually reveals deep folliculitis, perifolliculitis, and furunculosis. Bacterial or fungal organisms may or may not be identified on special staining.

Blood Culture. Do this when bacterial sepsis is suspected in patients with a fever and evidence of systemic illness.

Treatment

▼ *Key Point* Be certain that an appropriate antibiotic has been selected to eliminate the organism causing the deep pyoderma. Choose the antibiotic based on the results of bacterial culture and sensitivity tests. In general, treatment is more vigorous than that for superficial folliculitis. In recurrent cases, define the underlying disease process and initiate a systematic approach. See the discussion under Recurrent Superficial and Deep Pyodermas.

Topical Therapy

- Clip the hair around the affected areas. In cases of generalized deep pyoderma in long-coated breeds of dogs, clip the entire body.

- Initially bathe the patient twice daily (preferably in a whirlpool bath) using a povidone-iodine preparation (Betadine Whirlpool Concentrate, Purdue-Frederick) for the first 1–2 weeks of treatment. As the patient responds to treatment and the lesions have dried and begun to heal, change the treatment to once- to twice-weekly bathing with a benzoyl peroxide shampoo (OxyDex Shampoo, DVM Pharmaceuticals; Pyoben Shampoo, Allerderm/Virbac) for the next 4–8 weeks.

Systemic Antibiotics

Systemic antibiotic selection is always based on the results of a bacterial culture and sensitivity tests in cases of deep pyoderma. Use the appropriate dosage (Table 35–3). Treat for approximately 6–8 consecutive weeks. Severe cases of deep pyoderma may require a longer treatment regimen. Treat for at least 2 weeks beyond the complete clinical remission of the infection.

RECURRENT SUPERFICIAL AND DEEP PYODERMAS

Antibiotic-responsive but recurrent pyoderma is often a very frustrating problem in clinical practice. This section stresses the need to evaluate the patient with this problem for some of the more common, underlying diseases associated with recurrent pyoderma.

Etiologic and Predisposing Conditions

Inadequate Treatment

- Inappropriate antibiotic selection or inadequate duration of therapy can be simple reasons for the development of recurrent pyoderma.
- Long-term glucocorticoid use can predispose the patient to recurrent pyoderma and cause varying degrees of iatrogenic Cushing disease. Most patients with a pyoderma are pruritic; therefore, glucocorticoids are often used as adjuncts to the antibiotic therapy. This treatment may be acceptable on a first-time basis; however, discontinue glucocorticoids once it becomes apparent that the pyoderma is a recurrent problem. By treating the pruritic patient that has a pyoderma with antibiotics only, very important information can be learned. This can help guide the clinician to the underlying disease condition. See section on Diagnosis for guidelines on the use of antibiotics and response to therapy as a diagnostic tool.

▼ *Key Point* The following discussion of common underlying diseases resulting in recurrent pyoderma requires that the patient has first been placed on a prolonged antibiotic treatment protocol, as discussed under the Diagnosis section. Therefore, the observations being made are those that are noted after the pyoderma has been symptomatically put into remission.

Allergic Skin Disease

Flea Allergy Dermatitis. Patients with flea allergy dermatitis have pruritus that persists after resolution of the pyoderma and that primarily affects the caudal third of the body. Most patients initially have the problem in warmer weather only. For further discussion, see Chapter 40.

Atopy. Patients with atopic dermatitis (atopy) have pruritus that persists after resolution of the pyoderma and that affects various combinations of the following areas of the body: face, ears, axillae, inguinal region, proximal cranial foreleg region, and feet. Most patients initially have the problem in warmer weather only. For further discussion, see Chapter 41.

Food Allergy. Patients with food allergy have pruritus that persists after resolution of the pyoderma and that affects various combinations of the following areas of the body: face, ears, axillae, inguinal region, proximal cranial foreleg region, and feet. All patients have a nonseasonal (i.e., year-round) problem from the onset. For further discussion, see Chapter 42.

Parasitic Skin Disease

Demodicosis. Patients with demodicosis may or may not be pruritic, once the pyoderma has resolved. As previously stated, all patients with pyoderma require that several deep skin scrapings be performed, because demodicosis is a common cause of recurrent pyoderma that can be easily diagnosed. For further discussion, see Chapter 38.

Scabies. Patients with sarcoptic mange have pruritus that persists after resolution of the pyoderma and that initially affects the ear, elbow, and hock regions. All patients have a nonseasonal (i.e., year-round) problem from the onset. For further discussion, see Chapter 39.

Keratinization Disorders

Patients with keratinization abnormalities may be pruritic, once the pyoderma has resolved. The lesions that persist are suggestive of a keratinization (seborrheic) abnormality. For further discussion, see Chapter 44.

Endocrine Skin Diseases

Patients with hypothyroidism and hyperadrenocorticism (Cushing disease) are nonpruritic, once the pyoderma has resolved. The patient is evaluated by history and physical examination for evidence suggestive of these metabolic diseases. For further discussion see Chapters 29 and 31.

Staphylococcal Hypersensitivity

Patients with staphylococcal hypersensitivity exhibit a temporary resolution of both the pyoderma and the pruritus on antibiotic treatment alone. Staphylococcal hypersensitivity as a primary disease is one of the more controversial topics in veterinary dermatology. In this disease the staphylococcal infection alone, without any underlying disease, is the cause of the pruritus (i.e., a primary pruritic pyoderma). This disease is best diagnosed by exclusion of other underlying causes for a recurrent pyoderma. Therefore, all of the underlying diseases discussed up to this point must first be systematically ruled out before one can establish the diagnosis of a primary staphylococcal hypersensitivity.

Immunodeficiency

Immunodeficiency disorders as the primary cause for a recurrent pyoderma are extremely rare. Disorders to consider are cell-mediated immunity disorders, such as T-lymphocyte deficiency, and humoral immunity disorders, such as IgA deficiency.

Clinical Signs

See discussions of the clinical signs under Superficial Pyoderma, Superficial Folliculitis, and Deep Pyodermas elsewhere in this chapter.

Diagnosis

- First consider the procedures recommended elsewhere in this chapter for the diagnosis of superficial pyoderma, superficial folliculitis, and deep pyoderma.
- Use antibiotics as a diagnostic tool. Use antibiotics along with antibacterial shampoo therapy without any antipruritic drugs, especially glucocorticoids. Treat in this manner for 3 weeks and then reexamine. If the patient is still pruritic, note the distribution pattern and question the owner as to whether the condition was initially a predominantly warm-weather seasonal problem or a nonseasonal problem. For common underlying pruritic skin diseases, refer to the section on Etiologic and Predisposing Conditions. If the lesions and pruritus have both resolved on antibiotics alone, continue the antibiotic treatment for a total of 8 consecutive weeks. In some instances, this treatment results in a permanent resolution of the pyoderma. If the pyoderma recurs after stopping antibiotic therapy, evaluate the animal for underlying endocrine disease, staphylococcal hypersensitivity, and immunodeficiency disorders.
- For the specific testing procedures to diagnose the various underlying disease problems, please refer to the appropriate chapters in this book, as recommended under the section on Etiologic and Predisposing Conditions.
- Specific tests for primary immunodeficiency disorders are not readily available and are usually only offered by veterinary university laboratory services. Testing procedures to consider are the mitogen stimulation test for evaluation of lymphocyte function and measurement of serum IgA levels as an indirect evaluation for a secretory IgA disorder.

Treatment
General Principles

- Specific treatment of identifiable underlying diseases is essential for the resolution of an antibiotic-responsive but recurrent pyoderma.

Table 35–4. STAPHAGE LYSATE INJECTION PROTOCOL*

Week	Volume (ml)
1	0.25
2	0.50
3	0.75
4	1.00

*Follow this protocol with 1–2 ml every 3–21 days as needed to prevent recurrence of the pyoderma. Administer injections subcutaneously.
From Rosser EJ, Sams A: Papular/pustular, vesicular/bullous, and erosive/ulcerative dermatoses. In Allen DG, ed.: Small Animal Medicine. Philadelphia: JB Lippincott, 1991, p 719.

- Topical therapy is discussed under the treatment sections for Superficial Pyoderma, Superficial Folliculitis, and Deep Pyodermas.
- Systemic therapy is discussed under the treatment sections for Superficial Pyoderma, Superficial Folliculitis, and Deep Pyodermas.

Immunomodulators

- Immunomodulating drug therapy is indicated in cases of primary staphylococcal hypersensitivity and primary immunodeficiency disorders. Many treatment alternatives are available, but the author's preference is to use a staphylococcal bacterin (Staphage Lysate, Delmont Labs). See Table 35–4 for the recommended Staphage Lysate injection protocol.
- Remember that the patient is also given an appropriate systemic antibiotic for the first 4–8 weeks of treatment.

Maintenance Antibiotics

- In instances in which an underlying disease process cannot be identified (so-called "idiopathic chronic recurrent pyoderma"), consider a maintenance antibiotic treatment protocol.
- Before this recommendation is offered, make the owner aware of the possible risk for resistant bacterial infections, either in the skin or elsewhere in the body.
- There are several protocols, but the author's preference is use of the antibiotic on a continuous basis at a suboptimal dose. As an example, if the initial appropriate dose of the antibiotic is 500 mg q8h, give the antibiotic at that dosage until clinical remission of the pyoderma has been reestablished. Then gradually decrease the dosage over several weeks to 500 mg q12h, and finally to 250–500 mg q24–48h.
- Bactericidal antibiotics with a low potential for development of resistance and minimal side effects have been most effective, such as oxacillin or cephalexin. In cases of a relapse of the pyoderma, perform bacterial culture and sensitivity to examine for possible bacterial resistance to the antibiotic.

SUPPLEMENTAL READINGS

DeBoer DJ: Strategies for management of recurrent pyoderma in dogs. Vet Clin North Am 20:1509, 1990.

Kwochka KW: Recurrent pyoderma. *In* Griffin CE, MacDonald JM, Kwochka KW, eds.: Current Veterinary Dermatology. St Louis: CV Mosby, 1993, pp 3–21.

Rosser EJ: German shepherd dog pyoderma: A prospective study of 12 dogs. J Am Anim Hosp Assoc 33:355, 1997.

Rosser EJ, Sams A: Papular/pustular, vesicular/bullous, and erosive/ulcerative dermatoses. *In* Allen DG, ed.: Small Animal Medicine. Philadelphia: JB Lippincott, 1991, pp 711–732.

Rosser EJ, Sams A: Pruritus. *In* Allen DG, ed.: Small Animal Medicine. Philadelphia: JB Lippincott, 1991, pp 689–710.

Scott DW, Miller WH, Griffin CE: Muller and Kirk's Small Animal Dermatology, 5th Ed. Philadelphia: WB Saunders, 1995, pp 279–328.

36 Mycobacteriosis

Alan C. Mundell

Although a variety of mycobacterial organisms can cause sporadic disease in human beings and in animals, feline leprosy and atypical mycobacteria are the principal mycobacterial organisms seen in small animal practice that produce skin lesions. All mycobacterial organisms contain a lipid-rich cell wall that inhibits host defense mechanisms and imparts a characteristic staining property in the laboratory. This staining property involves the retention of carbolfuchsin after acid and alcohol decolorization. Thus, mycobacteria are classified as acid-fast staining organisms.

FELINE LEPROSY

Feline leprosy is a mycobacterial disease of cats that was first recognized in Australia during the early 1960s. The condition has since been identified in New Zealand, Great Britain, France, the Netherlands, and the west coast of the United States and Canada. The disease is usually confined to cats living in port cities and coastal areas. Feline leprosy has no breed or sex predilection. However, onset is usually between 2 and 5 years of age.

Etiology

- The cause of feline leprosy is *Mycobacterium lepraemurium,* the rat leprosy organism. Although the rat leprosy organism had been suspected for many years, it was only in the 1980s that sophisticated culture techniques and biochemical analysis could identify *M. lepraemurium* as the etiologic agent.
- The mode of transmission is unknown. However, rat bites, insect vectors, and aerosolization of contaminated nasal secretions are proposed methods of transmission.
- In experimental infections, the incubation period is 2 to 18 months.

Clinical Signs

- These consist of skin lesions that range from solitary to multiple, intradermal to subcutaneous, nodular to plaque-like, and haired to ulcerated. Fistulization and exudation are uncommon.
- Although skin lesions may occur anywhere on the body, head and limbs are frequent sites. Additionally, lesions may occur on the lips, gums, tongue, and nasal mucosa. Regional lymph nodes may be enlarged with lymphoid hyperplasia and infiltration of epithelioid cells and macrophages. The feline leprosy organism is occasionally isolated from these lymph nodes.
- Rarely the condition disseminates to spleen, bone marrow, liver, kidney, lung, or adjacent muscle. Cats with disseminated disease usually show signs of systemic illness, not seen in cats with localized infection.

Diagnosis

- The diagnosis is achieved primarily through histologic evaluation in conjunction with compatible history, physical examination, cytology, culture, and laboratory animal inoculation findings.
- The differential diagnosis for feline leprosy includes atypical mycobacteriosis, tuberculosis, foreign body dermatitis, deep mycotic infections, mycetomas, dermatophyte pseudomycetomas, chronic bacterial infections, eosinophilic granuloma complex, and neoplasia.
- *History* must be compatible with feline leprosy. The cat will typically be young to middle-aged, allowed to roam, and living in a cool, moist, coastal climate.
- *Physical examination* findings usually reveal lesions that are firm and indolent and lack exudation or fistulization. Lesions are frequently solitary or regionally grouped. Affected cats appear clinically healthy and oblivious to the disease. However, they should be evaluated for underlying immunosuppressive diseases, including feline leukemia and feline immunodeficiency viruses (see Chaps. 6 and 7).
- *Cytology* of lesional impression smears consists of mixed inflammatory cells with macrophages and histiocytes containing variable numbers of acid-fast bacilli. Ziehl-Neelsen and a modified Fite's stain are the acid-fast stains most commonly used.
- *Biopsy* specimens of lesions are fixed in 10% buffered formalin and evaluated histologically, using both hematoxylin-eosin and acid-fast stains (Ziehl-Neelsen and modified Fite's). The histology is somewhat analogous to that of human leprosy with the presence of both tuberculoid and lepromatous forms. The tuberculoid form consists primarily of nonencapsulated epithelioid granulomas that are interspersed with neutrophils and surrounded by a zone of lymphocytes. Low numbers of organisms are associated with this tuberculoid pattern. The lepromatous form is composed of sheets of large foamy macrophages that

contain large numbers of acid-fast bacilli. In human beings, the lepromatous form indicates a more immunocompromised host and thus imparts a poorer prognosis. In cats, however, this correlation remains to be demonstrated. One major histologic difference between human and feline leprosy is the lack of consistent cutaneous nerve infiltration by the feline leprosy organism.

▼ *Key Point* Culture of the feline leprosy mycobacterium is difficult to obtain because the organism fails to grow on blood agar and standard mycobacterial media (Löwenstein-Jensen and Stonebrink).

A 1% Ogawa egg yolk medium can be used to grow the organism when incubated under precise temperature and CO_2 conditions. Most commercial laboratories do not perform Ogawa egg yolk medium cultures. However, tissue maceration cultures (obtained via sterile biopsies) incubated on blood agar and routine mycobacterial media can help differentiate feline leprosy mycobacteria from atypical or tuberculosis-causing mycobacteria.

- *Laboratory animal inoculation* is used primarily in research to propagate and investigate the feline leprosy organism. This procedure is of greatest value when differentiating feline leprosy from tuberculosis. Only tuberculosis-producing mycobacteria routinely kill guinea pigs within 6–8 weeks after inoculation.

Treatment

- *Treatment* may not be necessary when lesions are small, unobtrusive, and likely to be self-limiting. However, this strategy is seldom effective and is recommended only for lesions that appear to be resolving spontaneously at the time of diagnosis.

▼ *Key Point* Surgical excision is the treatment of choice when lesions are limited in number and wide surgical margins can be obtained. However, disease recurrence is common and may require additional surgical intervention and/or medical management.

- *Medical management* has been attempted using a variety of drugs that have shown efficacy in treating human leprosy. Dapsone and rifampin were the first human antileprosy drugs investigated. Unfortunately, in the cat, toxicity to these drugs is common and efficacy is variable. Another common human antileprosy drug, clofazimine (Lamprene, Ciba-Geigy), has been more effective. Clofazimine is an iminophenazine dye with antimycobacterial properties that is suspended in olive oil and packaged in 50- and 100-mg capsules. Although the pharmacokinetics of clofazimine in the cat are unknown, a dosage of 2–3 mg/kg q24h PO, for 6–12 weeks past complete clinical resolution appears to be very effective. At this dosage minimal side effects are noted. Higher dosages may produce transient elevations in liver enzyme levels. To obtain the proper feline dose, the capsule is punc-

tured and the contents proportioned. Wear latex gloves to prevent staining of hands. Clofazimine is not approved by the United States Food and Drug Administration (FDA) for animal use.

Prevention

- This is probably best achieved by confining cats to an exclusively indoor environment. Because of the rare and sporadic nature of the disease, it is unlikely that this measure is necessary.
- Avoidance of immunosuppressive drugs while disease is active may help prevent exacerbation.

ATYPICAL MYCOBACTERIOSIS

Nontuberculous, nonlepromatous mycobacteria are classified as atypical or opportunistic. Runyon placed these mycobacteria into four groups, depending on laboratory culture properties. Almost all dog and cat atypical mycobacterial skin infections belong to the rapid-growing group IV. These saprophytic, facultative pathogens are ubiquitous in nature and are typically isolated from water and moist soil. Atypical mycobacteriosis is more prevalent in cats than in dogs, with no apparent age, breed, or sex predilection.

Etiology

Mycobacterium fortuitum-chelonei complex, Mycobacterium phlei, Mycobacterium thermoresistible, Mycobacterium xenopi, and *Mycobacterium smegmatis* have produced skin lesions in dogs and cats. In the United States, *M. fortuitum-chelonei* is responsible for most atypical mycobacterial infections. Skin infection follows contamination of traumatized skin, especially bite wounds and deep scratches.

Clinical Signs

- These consist of dermal to subcutaneous soft nodules that tend to ulcerate and drain a serous to seropurulent discharge. Tissue grains are not present. Unlike feline leprosy, fistulization and exudation are classically observed. Lesions can occur anywhere on the body; however, flank and inguinal regions are common locations.
- Except for regionalized lymphadenopathy, clinical signs of systemic disease are uncommon, even when lesions are extensive.

Diagnosis

- Perform bacterial culture and histologic evaluation of lesions. The differential diagnosis for cutaneous atypical mycobacteriosis is extensive and includes feline leprosy (in cats only), tuberculosis, foreign body dermatitis, deep mycotic infections, mycetomas, dermatophyte pseudomycetomas, chronic bacterial infections, generalized demodicosis (in dogs primarily), sterile nodular panniculitis, pansteatitis, eosinophilic granuloma complex, and neoplasia.

▼ *Key Point* Atypical mycobacterial organisms are difficult to isolate. In all suspected cases perform cultures, biopsies, and cytologic examination of lesional exudates.

- *History* must be compatible with cutaneous atypical mycobacteriosis. A history of trauma to the involved skin site weeks to months before the onset of lesions is not uncommon.
- *Physical examination* findings reveal soft nodules that fistulate and drain. Lesions are typically nonpainful, and the animal otherwise appears healthy.
- *Cytology* of lesional impression smears and smears of biopsy tissue consists of mixed inflammatory cells and, occasionally, acid-fast bacilli. Cytologic evaluation frequently fails to confirm acid-fast organisms. Ziehl-Neelsen and modified Fite's stain are the acid-fast stains most commonly used.
- *Handle biopsy* samples of lesions similar to those in feline leprosy except that special techniques, such as snap (instant) freezing the formalin-fixed tissue before staining or rapid Ziehl-Neelsen staining, may be necessary to reveal the organisms. Characteristically, fewer acid-fast bacilli are observed in atypical mycobacteriosis than in feline leprosy. Nodular pyogranulomatous dermatitis along with panniculitis is the common histologic pattern. If organisms are found they are usually located within extracellular lipid vacuoles that are ringed by neutrophils. Besides the paucity of organisms, atypical mycobacteriosis also differs from feline leprosy by the extracellular location of the organisms.
- *Culture* consists of growing the organism on standard mycobacterial media (Löwenstein-Jensen and Stonebrink) as well as on blood agar. Use sterile swab and biopsy techniques to obtain cultures. Notify the laboratory that atypical mycobacteriosis is suspected so that appropriate cultures are performed. Runyon group IV mycobacteria are called rapid growers because colonies appear within 7 days after media inoculation. In contrast, most other mycobacteria are either difficult to culture or require weeks to months to grow.
- *Laboratory animal inoculation* is seldom performed. If cultures fail to identify the mycobacterial organism and the possibility of tuberculosis exists, perform guinea pig inoculation.

Treatment

These options vary greatly because reported cases are too infrequent to establish a preferred therapeutic protocol.

▼ *Key Point* Most reports of successful disease management are anecdotal or involve low numbers of cases. Because the condition naturally waxes and wanes with occasional prolonged periods of remission, the success of all treatment options must be carefully assessed. Clinical remission may be more easily achieved in the dog than in the cat.

- An approach of no therapy may be taken if the disease involves a reasonably small area and the condition does not bother the animal or owner. When owners are unwilling to commit to a prolonged course of therapy, allowing the disease to naturally undergo its cycle may be a viable alternative. In time, the skin lesions may become more extensive; however, the disease rarely becomes systemic.
- *Surgical excision* is most successful for small, simply excised lesions. Obtain wide surgical margins. Unfortunately, surgical site dehiscence is common.

▼ *Key Point* Surgically debulking the lesions while treating the animal with a prolonged course of an appropriate antibiotic may provide a prolonged remission. Surgical excision may be more effective when managing canine lesions.

- *Medical management* has been attempted using a variety of drugs. Table 36–1 provides the dosages of the more effective agents. Most of these drugs are not approved by the FDA for use in dogs or cats. In vitro sensitivity testing may be helpful when selecting a therapeutic agent. However, the clinical response is frequently less than what the sensitivity test suggests. In general, medication is administered for 2–6 months past clinical cure. If the medication is effective in achieving clinical remission but the lesions return after discontinuing the medication, prolonged or indefinite therapy may be needed. Closely monitor the animal for adverse side effects. This monitoring typically requires periodic blood and urine laboratory evaluation, especially for drugs with known potential toxicities (e.g., aminoglycosides with nephrotoxicity and ototoxicity). It is beyond the scope of this chapter to discuss drug toxicities and the monitoring procedures. However, this information is available in current human and veterinary

Table 36–1. SELECTED DRUGS FOR TREATMENT OF CUTANEOUS ATYPICAL MYCOBACTERIOSIS

Treatment	Product (Manufacturer)	Dosage
Clofazimine	Lamprene (Ciba-Geigy)	8–12 mg/kg PO q24h
Enrofloxacin*	Baytril (Bayer)	2.5–5 mg/kg PO q12h
Doxycycline	Vibramycin (Pfizer)	2.5–5 mg/kg PO q12h
Amikacin	Amiglyde-V (Fort Dodge)	5–7 mg/kg SC, IM q12h
Kanamycin	Kantrim (Fort Dodge)	5–7 mg/kg SC, IM q12h
Gentamicin	Gentocin (Schering-Plough)	2 mg/kg SC, IM q12h

*An adjunctive transdermal route of drug delivery has also been used by mixing a 1:1 solution of 2.27% enrofloxacin in 90% dimethyl sulfoxide. A dose of 1 ml is applied to affected areas.

pharmacology textbooks. A thorough understanding of all drugs administered increases the safety of the therapeutic protocol.

Prevention

- This is best achieved by decreasing the likelihood of traumatic injury to the skin and subcutaneous tissue. If animals are allowed to roam freely, confining them to house or yard may decrease the likelihood of trauma. However, because of the rare and sporadic nature of the disease, these measures are probably unnecessary.
- Avoidance of immunosuppressive drugs may help prevent exacerbation or recurrence of atypical mycobacteriosis.

SUPPLEMENTAL READINGS

Kunkle GA: Feline leprosy. *In* Greene CE, ed.: Infectious Diseases of the Dog and Cat. Philadelphia: WB Saunders, 1990, p 567.

Kunkle GA: Atypical mycobacterial infections. *In* Greene CE, ed.: Infectious Diseases of the Dog and Cat. Philadelphia: WB Saunders, 1990, p 569.

Mundell AC: New therapeutic agents in veterinary dermatology. Vet Clin North Am Small Anim Pract 20:1544, 1990.

Scott DW, Miller WH, Griffin CE: Small Animal Dermatology. Philadelphia: WB Saunders, 1995, p 312.

White PD: Enrofloxacin-responsive cutaneous atypical mycobacterial infection in two cats. Proceedings of the Annual Meeting of the American Academy of Veterinary Dermatology, 7th Annual Meeting, Phoenix, Arizona, 1991, p 95.

White SD: Cutaneous mycobacteriosis. *In* Kirk RW, ed.: Current Veterinary Therapy IX: Small Animal Practice. Philadelphia: WB Saunders, 1986, p 529.

37 Dermatophytosis

Karin Muth Beale

Dermatophytosis is an infection of keratinized tissues usually caused by one of three species of dermatophytes: *Microsporum, Trichophyton,* and *Epidermophyton.* These organisms are keratinophilic and invade and live within the keratinized hair, nail, or skin. The majority of infections in dogs and cats are caused by three species of dermatophytes: *Microsporum canis, Microsporum gypseum,* and *Trichophyton mentagrophytes.* Other fungi are uncommon causes of dermatophytosis in pets. Dermatophytes are classified into groups based on their natural habitat as geophilic, zoophilic, or anthropophilic. Geophilic dermatophytes naturally inhabit the soil, zoophilic species are adapted to animals, and humans are the hosts for anthropophilic species. As a general rule, geophilic and anthropophilic dermatophytes tend to produce many more inflammatory lesions in animals than do the more host-adapted species.

ETIOLOGY

Microsporum gypseum

M. gypseum is a geophilic dermatophyte that normally inhabits the soil and decomposes keratinaceous debris. However, this organism is the second most common cause of dermatophytosis in dogs in the United States, and it occasionally infects cats. *M. gypseum* is most commonly isolated from animals that spend much time outdoors. Because the organism is not specifically adapted to living on animals, it tends to incite inflammation. Lesions are commonly seen in areas with significant soil contact, such as the feet and muzzle.

Microsporum canis

This zoophilic dermatophyte is responsible for the majority of the clinical cases of dermatophytosis in dogs. *M. canis* is the cause of approximately 98% of the cases of feline dermatophytosis. It was previously thought that cats served as the reservoir for *M. canis;* however, recent studies show that it is rarely isolated from healthy pet cats. The isolation of *M. canis* from a dog or cat is a significant finding, and the condition requires treatment.

Trichophyton mentagrophytes

This zoophilic dermatophyte is the third most common cause of dermatophytosis in dogs and less commonly affects cats. *T. mentagrophytes* is the most common cause of dermatophytosis in rodents and rabbits. Pet rodents or rabbits should be considered as possible reservoirs of infection. Wild rodents are commonly infected, and the infections may be clinically inapparent. Cats that hunt may be predisposed to acquiring infection with this type of dermatophyte.

Anthropophilic Dermatophytes

Anthropophilic dermatophytes such as *Microsporum audouini* rarely affect pets but can cause intensely inflamed lesions in animals. Zoophilic species of dermatophytes other than *M. canis* and *T. mentagrophytes,* such as *Trichophyton equinum, Trichophyton verrucosum,* and *Microsporum nanum,* may cause dermatophytosis in dogs or cats; however, such animals usually are in contact with livestock that are natural reservoirs or hosts for those organisms.

CLINICAL SIGNS

Canine Dermatophytosis

- Canine dermatophytosis is characterized by alopecia and scaling. Usually there are focal to multifocal circumscribed affected patches of skin.
- Hair loss, broken hairs, scaling, pustules, papules, exudation, crusting, and hyperpigmentation may be seen. Pruritus is variable.
- The classic lesion is a circular area of alopecia and scaling with central healing; however, the lesions may be irregular in appearance.
- Several factors influence the severity of the lesions. Young and immunocompromised animals tend to develop more extensive lesions that take longer to resolve than do those of healthy adult animals. This is because the ability to mount an effective inflammatory response is necessary to eliminate the infection. Additionally, the pathogenicity and the species of dermatophyte affect the degree of inflammatory response.

Kerion

A kerion is a round, raised, nodular lesion that results when follicular rupture, furunculosis, and pyogranulomatous inflammation occur with a dermatophyte infection.

- Kerions are most commonly seen in dogs on the limbs and face.
- The etiology usually is *M. gypseum.*
- These lesions often are secondarily infected with *Staphylococcus intermedius.*

Generalized Dermatophytosis

Generalized dermatophytosis is uncommon in the dog and is usually caused by *M. gypseum* or *T. mentagrophytes.*

- Characteristic findings are widespread alopecia and seborrhea with or without pruritus.
- Other lesions, similar to those of focal dermatophytosis, may also be present.
- Generalized dermatophytosis in adult dogs is often associated with immunosuppression or systemic disease.

Feline Dermatophytosis

▼ *Key Point* Feline dermatophytosis can occur in many different clinical forms. Consider dermatophytosis in the differential diagnosis of most feline dermatoses.

Classic Ringworm

Ringworm lesions may be present in cats; however, the circular lesions of alopecia and scaling with central healing are much less common in cats than in dogs. Cats may have what appears to be a localized infection, when in reality the infection is generalized. This is especially true of longhaired cats.

Subclinical Infection

Adult cats may have subclinical dermatophyte infections. These cats may have minimal (e.g., a minor degree of scaling or a few broken hairs) or no apparent clinical lesions. These cats serve as an important reservoir in the spread of dermatophytosis, and culture is necessary to identify affected cats.

Miliary Dermatitis

In cats, dermatophytosis may occur as a *miliary dermatitis* that may or may not be pruritic (see Chap. 48).

Symmetric Alopecia

Symmetric alopecia may be caused by dermatophytosis in cats. Excessive grooming as a result of pruritus, combined with follicular inflammation, can lead to excessive hair loss in some cats.

Pseudomycetoma

- Pseudomycetoma (Majocchi granuloma) is a form of granulomatous dermatitis in the cat caused by a dermatophyte, usually *M. canis.*
- This type of lesion is most common in Persian cats.
- In this lesion the fungus is sequestered in the dermis but does not proliferate; a nodular, ulcerating dermatitis is the result.

- Affected cats usually have generalized dermatophytosis.

Onychomycosis

- This dermatophyte infection of the nails is seen in both dogs and cats.
- The lesions usually are caused by *T. mentagrophytes* in dogs, and *M. canis* in cats.
- The nails are dry, cracked, brittle, and frequently deformed.
- Onychomycosis very rarely affects all four feet.
- Usually there is a concurrent infection with inflammation of the nail fold, and the pads may be affected as well.

DIAGNOSIS

▼ *Key Point* False-positive diagnosis of dermatophytosis in animals with circular lesions of alopecia is common. Follicular infections with *Demodex* and *Staphylococcus* organisms produce similar lesions.

- Do not diagnose dermatophytosis solely on the basis of clinical signs. Because of the numerous clinical conditions in dogs and cats that can mimic dermatophytosis, it is necessary to perform specific diagnostic procedures to obtain a definitive diagnosis.
- Canine dermatophytosis
  - In the dog, the most common cause of circular alopecia is staphylococcal folliculitis (see Chap. 35), followed by localized demodicosis (see Chap. 38).
  - Follicular infections with different organisms share common reaction patterns of papules, pustules, alopecia, scaling, and crusting.
  - Use diagnostic tests such as skin scrapings, bacterial cultures, and skin biopsies to rule out some of the more common causes of focal alopecia in dogs.
  - Consider dermatophytosis in the differential diagnosis of a generalized scaling, crusting, alopecic dermatosis. A number of different conditions can cause a generalized dermatitis similar to that seen in generalized dermatophytosis in the dog (Table 37–1).
  - The differential diagnosis for kerions and pseudomycetomas includes the various causes of nodular dermatitides, such as cutaneous neoplasms, staphylococcal furunculosis, and acral lick dermatitis (see Table 37–1). Kerions are generally found as raised, pink, solitary lesions with a predilection for the face, mimicking histiocytomas.
- Feline dermatophytosis
  - The list of disorders to be considered in the differential diagnosis of feline dermatophytosis is extensive and includes all causes of miliary dermatitis and symmetric alopecia (see Chaps. 47 and 48).

History

An accurate history can provide useful information regarding the possible source of infection.

Table 37–1. DIFFERENTIAL DIAGNOSIS FOR DERMATOPHYTOSIS IN DOGS

Focal to Multifocal Dermatophytosis

Demodicosis
Staphylococcal folliculitis
Dermatophilosis
Abrasions
Pemphigus foliaceus/erythematosus
Zinc-responsive dermatosis

Generalized Dermatophytosis

Demodicosis
Staphylococcal folliculitis
Dermatophilosis
Pemphigus foliaceus
Cheyletiellosis
Sebaceous adenitis
Primary keratinization defects
Secondary keratinization abnormalities (allergic dermatoses, endocrinopathies, nutritional deficiencies, etc.)
Mycosis fungoides (epidermotropic lymphoma)

Kerions

Histiocytoma, mast cell tumor, other neoplasms
Staphylococcal furunculosis
Demodicosis and furunculosis
Acral lick dermatitis
Foreign bodies
Subcutaneous mycoses
Actinomycotic infections
Mycobacterial infections

Onychomycosis/Nail Fold Dermatophytosis

Staphylococcal onychitis
Demodicosis
Zinc-responsive dermatosis
Pemphigus vulgaris/foliaceus
Symmetric lupoid onychodystrophy

- Obtain an accurate drug history.
- Try to determine whether the animal has had any abnormalities suggestive of systemic disease, particularly older animals.

Physical Examination

- Look for signs suggestive of dermatophytosis.
- Thoroughly examine adult animals with widespread lesions, especially dogs, for signs of systemic disease such as hyperadrenocorticism.

Wood's Light Examination

- Use the Wood's light to screen for dermatophytosis. The light emitted may cause fluorescence of hairs infected with *M. canis*.
- Be wary of false-positive results. Scale, ointments, creams, and bacterial folliculitis may all fluoresce under the light; however, they do not give the typical apple-green fluorescence of the hair shaft seen with *M. canis* infection.
- Hairs may remain fluorescent after an *M. canis* infection has resolved. Therefore, positive fluorescence alone should not be used to confirm infection or monitor therapy.

▼ *Key Point* Hairs infected with *M. gypseum* and *T. mentagrophytes* do not fluoresce an apple-green color under Wood's light, and less than 50% of *M. canis*–infected hairs fluoresce. Use the Wood's light only as a screening tool, not as a confirmatory diagnostic test.

Direct Microscopic Examination of Hair

Direct microscopic examination can provide a diagnosis of dermatophytosis within minutes if affected hairs are properly examined.

- Selection of the sample to be examined is critical.
  - Pluck hair from areas of active inflammation.
  - Broken or frayed hairs are ideal.
  - If there was fluorescence with Wood's light examination, select those individual hairs that fluoresced.
- Place the hairs to be examined on a glass slide.
  - Clear the sample to facilitate observation of spores and hyphae (Table 37–2).
  - When the specimen has been cleared, scan the slide using low magnification (10×) for abnormal hairs. Look for hairs that are frayed, swollen, and pale.
  - When you have located the hair, examine it at a higher magnification (20–40×).
- The presence of ectothrix spores surrounding the hair and of hyphae within the hair shaft is diagnostic for dermatophytosis.
  - Ectothrix spores appear as round-to-oval, greenish, translucent beads (Fig. 37–1).

This technique requires some practice. A negative direct microscopic examination does not rule out dermatophytosis.

▼ *Key Point* Avoid false-positive diagnoses based on direct examination. Dermatophytes do not produce

Table 37–2. CLEARING AGENTS USED FOR MICROSCOPIC EXAMINATION OF SPECIMENS OF HAIR

Agent	Instructions
10–20% KOH	Place several drops on the slide, apply a coverslip, and allow the slide to clear for 30 min before examining.
10–20% KOH	Follow the same procedure as above, but gently heat the slide for 15 sec, allow it to cool, and then examine it.
2 parts KOH, 1 part DMSO	Place several drops on the slide, apply a coverslip, and allow it to clear for 5 min before examining.
Chlorphenolac (50 g chloral hydrate, 25 ml liquid phenol, and 25 ml liquid lactic acid)	Place several drops on the slide, apply a coverslip, and examine immediately.

DMSO, dimethyl sulfoxide; KOH, potassium chloride.

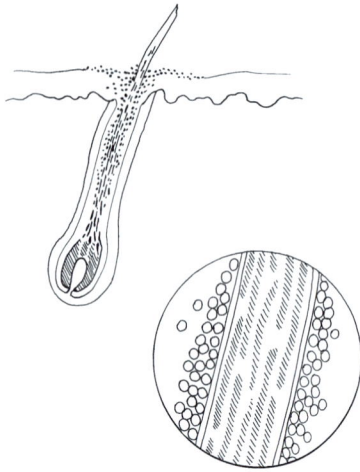

Figure 37–1.   Arthrospores can be visualized outside infected hair shafts (ectothrix) in animals. Fungal hyphae may be seen within infected hair shafts *(inset).*

macroconidia in the tissue. Nonpathogenic fungal conidia and plant pollen are frequently mistaken for dermatophytes; these structures are darkly pigmented whereas dermatophytes are not.

Fungal Culture

▼ *Key Point* Fungal culture is the most reliable and definitive method of identifying infected animals; it is the only method of identifying the species of fungi and should be performed in all suspected cases of dermatophytosis.

The ideal culture media for dermatophytes is dermatophyte test media (DTM), which is composed of Sabouraud's agar, antimicrobials to inhibit bacterial and fungal saprophyte growth, and phenol red as a pH indicator. DTM is available in screw-cap containers or in plates with DTM on one side and plain Sabouraud's agar on the other. The plates are preferred over the tubes because it is easier to obtain samples from the plates for species identification. Plain Sabouraud's agar is better for evaluating colony morphology because DTM may suppress the formation of conidia and alter colony coloration.

Technique

1. Specimen collection of hair involves three steps:
   a. Clip hairs to 0.5 cm in an area of active inflammation; areas of broken, stubbly hairs of positive Wood's light fluorescence are ideal.
   b. Lightly swab the area with alcohol and allow to air-dry.
   c. Gently remove the clipped hairs from the follicles; hemostats are ideal for this purpose.
2. Place hairs on the media (not deeply embedded).
3. In cases of onychomycosis, clip the proximal nail into small pieces for culture.
4. Place the sample (hairs or nail particles) in a dark environment, protected from ultraviolet light and desiccation. Do not close the container tightly.

5. Observe the sample daily for colony growth and for a color change in the media.
6. As a general rule, dermatophytes turn DTM red simultaneously with colony growth, whereas saprophytes generally do not turn the media red until after a week or so of growth.
7. Fungal colonies that are darkly pigmented (blue, green, black, or a combination) are *not* dermatophytes.

▼ *Key Point* Some species of fungi other than dermatophytes may turn the DTM media red within the first 7–10 days; therefore, microscopic examination of the mycelia is necessary to identify the fungus definitively as a dermatophyte.

Identification of Subclinically Infected Cats

- Identification of the dermatophytosis in the asymptomatic cat can be accomplished using a toothbrush technique. Vigorously brush the cat over the entire body with a new toothbrush.
- Gently place the collected hairs and scale onto the fungal culture media.

Identification of Dermatophyte Species from a Fungal Colony

The colony morphology in combination with the characteristic microscopic morphology allows identification of the dermatophyte species causing the infection (Table 37–3). The easiest and most practical method of observing microscopic morphology is the "acetate tape" method:

- Gently touch a 2-cm strip of clear acetate tape to the surface of a mature culture colony (>5 days). A colony on plain Sabouraud's agar is preferable, if available.
- Then place the tape over a glass slide with a drop of lactophenol cotton blue or new methylene blue stain.
- Observe the slide microscopically for identification of dermatophyte species by conidia formation (Fig. 37–2).

Biopsy and Histopathology

Generally it is not necessary to biopsy skin for identification of a dermatophyte infection. However, dermatophytes may be visible in hematoxylin-eosin (H & E)–stained sections and are readily detected with periodic acid–Schiff (PAS) and Gomori methenamine silver (GMS) stains. In cases of suspected dermatophyte onychomycosis, the nail itself may be submitted in 10% formalin for histopathologic evaluation.

TREATMENT

▼ *Key Point* Dermatophytosis is a zoonotic disease, and children and immunocompromised individuals are at increased risk; therefore, minimize exposure of people and other animals to the affected animal.

Table 37–3. COLONY AND MICROSCOPIC MORPHOLOGY OF DERMATOPHYTE CULTURES ON SABOURAUD'S DEXTROSE AGAR

Organism	Colony Morphology	Microscopic Morphology*
Microsporum canis	The surface is cottony to woolly and white. The reverse side is yellow-orange.	Abundant spindle-shaped macroconidia with thick, spiny walls and a terminal knob are present. Six or more cells are found in the macroconidia. One-celled microconidia are uncommon.
Microsporum gypseum	The surface is flat, granular, and light tan to cinnamon in color with white mycelia. The reverse side is pale yellow to tan.	Abundant spindle-shaped macroconidia with no terminal knobs are present. Macroconidia contain up to six cells. Microconidia are uncommon.
Trichophyton mentagrophytes	The surface usually is cream-colored and powdery. The reverse side is tan to brown, or red.	Some strains produce spiral hyphae. Microconidia are numerous and often are arranged in grape-like clusters along the hyphae. Macroconidia are uncommon; if present, they are slender and cigar-shaped with smooth thin walls.

*See Figure 37–2.

Dermatophyte infections are usually self-limiting; however, plan treatment with the goals of eliminating the infection in the animal and preventing the spread of infectious materials to other pets or people in the household (Table 37–4).

Always treat cats with dermatophytosis with systemic antifungal therapy. Dogs with localized lesions of dermatophytosis may be treated with topical therapy only; however, treat dogs with kerions, onychomycosis, or multiple/generalized lesions with systemic antifungal therapy.

Topical Therapy

Topical Shampoo and Dip Therapy

- Topical shampoos and dips as the sole treatment for dermatophytosis are ineffective in resolving infection. Topically treated animals are not culture-negative any sooner than untreated animals.

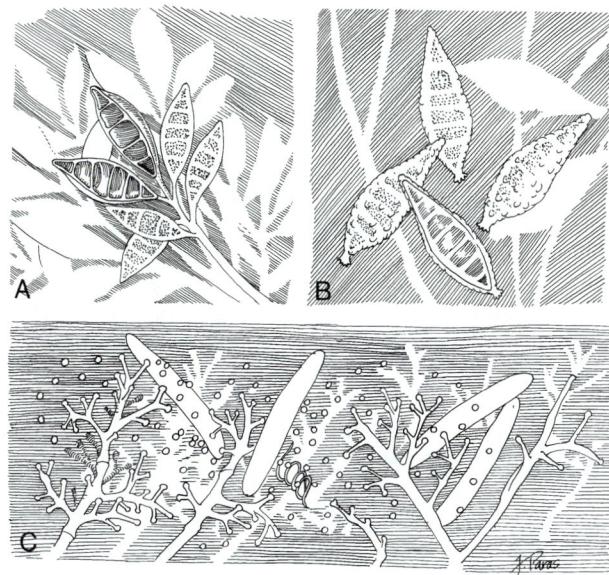

Figure 37–2. Identification of dermatophyte species from mature fungal colonies is possible by microscopically examining the conidia morphology: *A, Microsporum gypseum; B, Microsporum canis; C, Trichophyton mentagrophytes.*

- Shampoo therapy may actually spread the lesions through mechanical trauma.
- Topical therapy may have value in limiting environmental contamination by killing spores on the haircoat that would otherwise be shed into the pet's environment.
- Limited topical therapies have shown usefulness in killing spores on the haircoat. Useful treatments include lime sulfur (1:16), enilconazole (bottle dilution), and miconazole shampoo. Enilconazole is not approved for use in dogs and cats in the United States.
  - Because shampooing may spread the lesions through mechanical trauma, it would appear that the most effective topical whole-body therapy approved for use in the United States is lime sulfur. The lime sulfur should be applied as a rinse, and gently sponged or patted (not rubbed) onto the animal.
  - If lime sulfur is used on a cat, an elizabethan collar should be worn after dipping to prevent ingestion of the substance.

Local Topical Therapy

- Localized topical therapy with creams and ointments seems to have limited value. Restrict use to localized lesions in dogs. This form of therapy may not speed resolution of the lesion, but it may help prevent dissemination of infective materials.
- Creams and ointments are not recommended for cats with dermatophytosis.

Clipping the Haircoat

- A close shave of the whole body or infected area is no longer recommended, as mechanical trauma may actually help spread the lesions. Gently cutting the hairs around a lesion may help prevent spread of infected hairs into the environment.
- Hairs that are cut should be collected with a vacuum system while the cutting is being performed to prevent spread of these infected hairs. The vacuum bag should be disposed of immediately.

Systemic Therapy

- Systemic antifungal therapy (see Table 37–4) is the only therapy demonstrated to improve cure rate

Table 37–4. SYSTEMIC ANTIFUNGAL THERAPY FOR TREATMENT OF DERMATOPHYTOSIS

Agent	Brand Name (Manufacturer)	Application	Comments	Side Effects
Griseofulvin-microsize	Fulvicin U/F (Schering) Grifulvin V (Ortho)	25–50 mg/kg q24h	Available as tablets, pediatric suspension	Nausea, vomiting, diarrhea, idiosyncratic myelotoxicity, ataxia
Griseofulvin-ultramicrosize	Gris-PEG (Dorsey)	5–10 mg/kg q24h	Available as tablets	Nausea, vomiting, diarrhea, idiosyncratic myelotoxicity, ataxia
Ketoconazole	Nizoral (Janssen)	10 mg/kg q24h	Available as tablets; administer the dose divided q12h if nausea or anorexia occurs Not recommended for cats	Gastric irritation, anorexia, hepatotoxicity, idiosyncratic lightening of haircoat, teratogenicity
Itraconazole	Sporanox (Janssen)	10 mg/kg q24h	Available as capsules	Teratogenicity

(time until a negative fungal culture is obtained) in cats with dermatophytosis. This is also the only effective therapy in dogs with generalized or multifocal dermatophytosis, kerions, or onychomycosis.

- There are three systemic therapies for the treatment of dermatophytosis: griseofulvin, ketoconazole, and itraconazole.

Griseofulvin

▼ **Key Point** Griseofulvin, a fungistatic antimicrobial, is the drug of choice for treating dermatophytosis, unless contraindicated (e.g., pregnancy, feline immunodeficiency virus).

Absorption of the drug is enhanced when it is given with a fatty meal. Griseofulvin is available in microsize and ultramicrosize formulations in polyethylene glycol to enhance absorption so that lower doses can be used.

- Never administer griseofulvin, which is a teratogen, to pregnant animals.
- Common side effects include anorexia, vomiting, and diarrhea.
- Less common side effects, which appear to be idiosyncratic, include pyrexia, icterus, ataxia, angioedema, and myelosuppression.
- During therapy, monitor purebred cats, which may be predisposed to develop myelosuppression.
- Do not treat cats infected with feline immunodeficiency virus (FIV) with griseofulvin, as they are very susceptible to toxicity from this drug.

Ketoconazole

Ketoconazole is a fungistatic imidazole derivative with broad-spectrum antifungal activity against both superficial and deep mycotic infections. Use for dogs with griseofulvin-resistant dermatophytosis and for dogs that cannot tolerate griseofulvin therapy. For further information concerning usage and side effects of ketoconazole, see Chapter 18.

Ketoconazole may not be effective against certain strains of *M. canis*.

- Because nausea and anorexia are frequently encountered in cats when using ketoconazole, and because *M. canis* may be resistant, do not use.

Itraconazole

Itraconazole is a triazole that is effective for the treatment of dermatophytosis.

- Itraconazole is better tolerated by cats than ketoconazole. Use in cats that have griseofulvin-resistant infections, or that do not tolerate griseofulvin.
- Itraconazole is the drug of choice in FIV-positive cats.
- It is also effective in dogs; however, the expense of the drug may preclude its use in many cases.
- Itraconazole is teratogenic at high doses; therefore, do not use it in pregnant animals.

Antifungal Vaccines

There is a commercially available, killed–*M. canis* vaccine. The product insert claims its use is as an "aid in the prevention and treatment of clinical signs of disease caused by *Microsporum canis*." The vaccine is intended as an adjuvant to traditional therapy, not a replacement. The insert also states that "vaccination has not been demonstrated to eliminate *M. canis* organisms from infected cats." Studies by the manufacturer indicate that there is a decrease in clinical signs in affected vaccinated cats compared with unvaccinated cats. However, there is no data to suggest that a cure is obtained faster when using this product, or that this vaccine helps to prevent infection in challenged animals.

MONITORING THERAPY

Animals may appear clinically normal long before they are actually cured or culture-negative. Animals should be reassessed frequently to monitor response to therapy and to assess the need for modifications in therapy.

- Check animals on treatment at least every 3–4 weeks. Monitor for medication side effects.

- After 5–6 weeks of systemic therapy, check fungal cultures every 1–2 weeks.
- Do not discontinue therapy until two negative cultures have been obtained.

PREVENTION

When planning and carrying out preventive measures, remember that dermatophyte spores can remain viable in the environment for several years.

Current Recommendations for Disinfection

The purpose of environmental disinfection is to prevent reinfection of the pet, and to prevent infection of other household members. Unfortunately, many of the disinfectants that are currently in use today are not effective at killing dermatophyte spores. Evaluation of several different disinfectants found that only concentrated bleach and 1% formalin were 100% effective in killing spores. These products are not acceptable for routine environmental disinfection.

- Thoroughly vacuum floors, carpeting, and furniture to remove infected hairs. Dispose of vacuum bag after each use.
- Clean surfaces that will not be damaged by the solution with a 1:10 dilution of bleach (NaOCl).
- Dispose of all grooming equipment.
- Wash hands thoroughly after handling infected animals.

Identification of the Source of Exposure

- Examine other animals in the household.
- Specific dermatophyte species that are cultured can provide helpful clues. For example, if *T. mentagrophytes* is isolated from a dog that spends most of the time indoors and there is a pet rodent in the household, brush culture the rodent for the presence of dermatophytes.
- Treat all infected animals in the household.

Preventive Measures in a Cattery

- Identify all infected animals. For best results, use the toothbrush technique described previously.
- Separate infected from culture-negative animals.
- Treat infected cats until tests are culture-negative before reintroducing them to the general cat population.
- Disinfect cages on a regular basis and vacuum and disinfect air vents.
- Never use the same grooming equipment on both infected and culture-negative cats.
- Place all new animals brought into a cattery in isolation until culture-negative results have been obtained.

SUPPLEMENTAL READINGS

Foil CS: Dermatophytosis. *In* Greene CE, ed.: Clinical Microbiology and Infectious Diseases of the Dog and Cat, 2nd ed. Philadelphia: WB Saunders, 1990, p 362.

Moriello KA: Management of dermatophyte infections in catteries and multiple-cat households. Vet Clin North Am Small Anim Pract 20:1457, 1990.

38 Demodicosis

Alan C. Mundell

Demodicosis refers to the inflammatory parasitic skin disease of dogs and cats caused by an abnormal proliferation of a mite from the genus *Demodex*. The mites are considered part of the normal skin fauna when present in low numbers. The disease state, demodicosis, is most frequently recognized in the dog. When generalized and chronic, demodicosis is a frustrating and difficult condition to treat.

ETIOLOGY

Canine Demodicosis

Canine demodicosis occurs when there is an overpopulation of the mite *Demodex canis* (Fig. 38–1) on the skin. The mite is a normal inhabitant of the hair follicle and occasionally of the sebaceous gland. Although it is not known what allows the mites to proliferate by the thousands, genetic and/or immunologic abnormalities are suspected. It has been shown that some dogs with generalized demodicosis have decreased levels of interleukin-2 production and interleukin-2 receptor expression which may represent a poor Th1 helper T-cell response relative to Th2 helper T-cell response.

- The entire *life cycle* of the mite is spent on the host and consists of four major stages: egg, larva, nymph (several stages), and adult. The life cycle is believed to take between 20 and 35 days to complete.
- *Transmission* occurs during the first few days of life by direct contact from dam to pup.

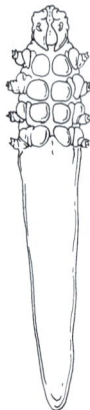

Figure 38–1. *Demodex canis.*

- The mites are not considered to be contagious to normal healthy adult dogs. Thus, demodicosis is most likely a dysfunction of the dog, not an increase in virulence of the mite.
- A second species of *Demodex* has been found on the dog. Little is known about the life cycle or clinical importance of this unnamed mite. When observed, the mite is shorter and wider than *D. canis*, and frequently found in conjunction with *D. canis* demodicosis.

Feline Demodicosis

Two species of *Demodex* mite cause disease in cats.

- *Demodex cati* was the mite species first recognized. *D. cati* resembles *D. canis* in appearance, cutaneous habitat, and life cycle. The life cycle of this mite is believed to be completed in 18–24 days.
- The second type of *Demodex* mite is unnamed. This mite has a shorter and wider abdomen than *D. cati* and resembles the hamster mite, *Demodex criceti*. Little is known about its life cycle. This unnamed *Demodex* species resides in pits in the stratum corneum, not in hair follicles or sebaceous glands.

CLINICAL SIGNS

Localized Demodicosis

Canine

- Canine localized demodicosis typically occurs in dogs less than 1 year of age. There is no breed or sex predilection.
- The lesions are commonly observed on the head and extremities.
- Alopecia is the most consistent finding with variable degrees of erythema, scale, hyperpigmentation, comedo formation, pyoderma, and pruritus.
- It is estimated that in approximately 10% of dogs with localized demodicosis, the condition eventually becomes generalized.

Feline

- Feline demodicosis (localized or generalized) has no breed or sex predilection. However, most cases occur in older cats.

- Localized demodicosis in the cat usually appears as a focal area of alopecia on the face or ears.
- As with canine localized demodicosis, the degree of erythema, scale, hyperpigmentation, comedo formation, and pruritus is variable. Secondary pyodermas are rare.

Generalized Demodicosis

Canine

- Generalized demodicosis in the dog frequently is categorized according to the age of initial disease onset (juvenile or adult). Although both types have identical clinical signs, the distinction is the result of differences in predisposing factors and prognosis.
  - Adult-onset generalized demodicosis has a more guarded prognosis because of the increased probability of serious predisposing conditions.
  - The prognosis for dogs less than 1 year of age with generalized demodicosis is more favorable because spontaneous cures are not uncommon.
- Clinical signs of generalized demodicosis consist of large, multifocal to regional areas of alopecia. These areas typically have scaling, crusting, erythema, comedo formation, hyperpigmentation, and pyoderma.
  - If the pyoderma is deep, lymphadenopathy and cutaneous drainage tracts with hemorrhagic to purulent exudates may be present.
- Occasionally, cellulitis occurs.

Feline

Generalized demodicosis in the cat may produce a variety of clinical signs.

- Lesions range from large areas of patchy alopecia with variable amounts of erythema, scale, crusts, and hyperpigmentation to regional miliary dermatitis.
- Secondary pyodermas are rare.
- When pruritic, the intensity of the itch is usually mild. Intense pruritus is rarely observed.

Pododemodicosis/Otodemodicosis

Canine

In the dog, pododemodicosis may be exclusively confined to the feet or may be present in conjunction with more generalized disease. A similar situation exists with otodemodicosis in the external ear canal. The reason for addressing these areas separately is because of the increased treatment difficulty and the more guarded prognosis when these areas are involved.

- Pododemodicosis
  - This may manifest as mild erythematous alopecia of the paws with variable degrees of scaling and crusting.
  - However, in chronic and/or severe infestations the interdigital, nail fold, and palmar areas frequently are swollen with crusted papules, nodules, pustules, vesicles, drainage tracts, and scar tissue formation.

- Otodemodicosis
  - The usual clinical signs are ceruminous otitis externa with erythema and swelling.
  - When untreated, the otitis externa may become purulent and/or proliferative.
  - Canine otodemodicosis as a solitary condition is rarely identified.

Feline

- Pododemodicosis in the cat is not usually a distinct clinical entity but a manifestation of a more generalized condition.
  - The lesions are not as severe as typically seen in canine pododemodicosis.
  - Partial alopecia with variable degrees of erythema, scale, crusts, and pruritus are the usual clinical signs.
- In feline otodemodicosis, a ceruminous otitis externa is the most common clinical sign. The external ear infestation may be the only indication of demodicosis, or it may be a part of a more generalized disease.

DIAGNOSIS

▼ *Key Point* Demodicosis usually is diagnosed from skin scrapings. Obtain skin scrapings of all animals with alopecia, pyoderma, and keratinization disorders.

History

The history can help to identify possible predisposing causes.

- Suspect canine demodicosis if there is a familial history of demodicosis and the clinical signs are compatible.
- Question owners about potentially taxing events or conditions that could decompensate the animal's ability to control the proliferation of the mite. Predisposing events or conditions may include:
  - Stress, poor nutrition, trauma, separation anxiety, and chronic fatigue.
  - Estrus, parturition, and lactation.
  - Parasitism, rapid growth, vaccinations, adverse environmental temperatures, and debilitating disease.
- Older dogs and cats frequently have an underlying internal disease or neoplastic condition that predisposes them to develop demodicosis. The underlying conditions may be incipient at the time of diagnosis and may require months, possibly years, to be recognized.
- The use of immunosuppressive agents such as corticosteroids, antineoplastic drugs, or antilymphocyte antibodies can induce or exacerbate localized or generalized demodicosis.

Physical Examination

Perform a thorough physical examination to identify predisposing factors and/or diseases.

Laboratory Tests

Use laboratory tests to screen for predisposing diseases, especially when canine generalized demodicosis and feline demodicosis (localized or generalized) are present.

- Serum biochemical profile, urinalysis, and complete blood cell count (CBC) are the basic screening tests.
- Additionally, test all cats for feline leukemia virus (FeLV) and feline immunodeficiency virus (FIV) (see Chaps. 6 and 7).
- If the history, physical examination, and screening laboratory tests indicate endocrine or possible internal organ dysfunction, perform more specific tests (e.g., testing for hyperadrenocorticism [see Chap. 31]).

Skin Scrapings

This is the primary method for diagnosing demodicosis.

Procedure

- Clip hair over area to be scraped.
- Squeeze skin gently to facilitate mite collection.
- Scrape skin using a dull #10 surgical blade moistened with mineral oil.
  - Stroke the skin in the direction of hair growth until capillary bleeding occurs.
  - Place debris on a glass slide containing one drop of mineral oil.

▼ *Key Point* Obtain multiple skin scrapings.

Examination of Scrapings

Examine the slide under low-power magnification ($40\times$ and $100\times$).

- Because *Demodex* mites are normal skin inhabitants, finding one mite does not confirm demodicosis; however, it does increase the suspicion of demodicosis. Therefore, following such a finding, perform multiple deep-skin scrapings.
- Use skin scrapings to monitor the response to therapy by assessing the ratio of live to dead mites and the ratio of adult to immature forms.
  - If there is an increase in live mites or immature forms, mite resistance to therapy may be occurring.

Skin Biopsies

- Use skin biopsies when demodicosis is suspected but mites cannot be identified in routine skin scrapings (see Chap. 49 for skin biopsy technique). This occasionally occurs in chronically affected areas (especially feet) where scar tissue impedes proper scraping.

- Biopsies may be necessary to diagnose demodicosis in Chinese Shar Pei dogs.

Ear Swabs and Ear Curettes

Use ear swabs and curettes to obtain otic debris for mite evaluation.

TREATMENT

▼ *Key Point* *Never* use corticosteroids in dogs or cats with demodicosis. If possible, avoid the use of all immunosuppressive agents.

The ideal therapeutic agent for the treatment of canine and feline demodicosis should be safe, highly effective, easy to administer, reasonably priced, and approved by the United States Food and Drug Administration (FDA). Unfortunately such a drug does not exist.

The only FDA-approved agent for the treatment of canine generalized demodicosis is amitraz (Mitaban, Pharmacia and Upjohn). This drug, which can be moderately effective when used as labeled, is discussed in detail further on. No FDA-approved treatment is available for feline demodicosis. Therefore,

- Consider the risk-benefit ratio when recommending therapies not approved by the FDA.
- Advise clients of all treatment options and success and risks of each.
- Obtain written client consent when using treatments not approved by the FDA.

Localized Demodicosis

Canine

- Localized demodicosis in the dog usually is a self-limiting condition, especially in dogs less than 18 months of age. Thus, the primary goal is to identify and eliminate predisposing causes.
- Spontaneous remission typically occurs within 2 months. If lesions persist or if owners insist on treatment, use topical agents.
- Treat lesions topically once daily until skin scrapings are negative with 1% rotenone ointment (Goodwinol, Goodwinol Products) and benzoyl peroxide shampoos or gels (Oxydex, DVM Pharmaceuticals; Pyoben, Allerderm).
- Rotenone ointments and benzoyl peroxide gels can be irritating, especially because they are not rinsed off. Use these agents with caution when treating periocular lesions; ocular irritation can be severe.
- Although therapies designed to treat generalized demodicosis (e.g., amitraz) are effective for localized demodicosis, they are best reserved for the generalized condition.
- Limiting the use of more potent acaricidal agents helps decrease the potential for developing acaricide resistance. This ensures peak acaricidal performance for when the agent is needed most.

Feline

Treat localized demodicosis in the cat in a manner similar to that for canine localized demodicosis. Although localized lesions can spontaneously regress, many progress and become generalized. In cats, the rotenone and benzoyl peroxide agents used to treat canine localized demodicosis are less effective and more irritating. Although feline localized demodicosis, like canine localized demodicosis, has been treated successfully with the drug amitraz (see further on), its use is discouraged for the reasons previously stated.

Canine Generalized Demodicosis

Besides the FDA-approved protocol for using amitraz (see later) for canine generalized demodicosis, several moderately effective treatments are available.

- Common to all protocols is the need to identify and correct predisposing factors.
- Additionally, treat all secondary pyodermas with appropriate antibiotic and topical therapy (see Chap. 35). If a deep pyoderma is present, base antibiotic selection on bacterial culture and sensitivity results (see Chap. 35).

Amitraz—FDA-Approved Protocol

This drug is a formamidine acaricidal compound that inhibits monoamine oxidase. However, the precise acaricidal mechanism of action is unknown.

Procedure

- Closely clip all medium- to long-haired dogs. Repeat monthly or as necessary.
- Bathe the animal with a benzoyl peroxide shampoo.
- Allow the shampoo to remain on the dog for 10 minutes before rinsing.
- Completely dry the dog before proceeding with amitraz rinses.

▼ *Key Point* Do not apply amitraz to dogs with extensive open lesions (deep pyodermas with drainage tracts). Postpone application until antibiotics and shampoo therapy improve these lesions.

- Prepare a fresh 0.025% amitraz solution (one vial of Mitaban per 2 gallons of water) and sponge on the dog. Sponging procedure should last at least 10 minutes.
  - While the dog is being sponged, soak the feet in the mixture.
- Apply amitraz solution in well-ventilated areas, taking strict protective measures to avoid human exposure.
- Keep the animal dry (including feet) until the next amitraz application (2 weeks later).
- Continue amitraz applications every 2 weeks until no viable mites are found after at least two successive treatments.

Results

- Reported long-term cure rates (no mites identified for more than 1 year) are variable (20–99%). However, a well-controlled study found only a 53% long-term cure rate.
- The percentage of dogs in which mite populations are adequately controlled is much higher. These dogs remain asymptomatic while receiving maintenance applications.

Side Effects

- A variety of adverse side effects have been reported; the most common are mild transient sedation, pruritus, and/or gastrointestinal disturbances.
- The manufacturer (Upjohn) believes that the drug temporarily alters the dog's homeostatic maintenance abilities. Therefore, avoid placing the dog in stressful situations for at least 24 hours after dipping. Avoid use of anesthetics and sedatives for at least 48 hours before and after dipping.
- Many side effects have been associated with amitraz's alpha$_2$-adrenergic stimulatory property.
- Do not use amitraz with other monoamine oxidase inhibitors (e.g., hydroxyzine HCl).
- Experimentally, these side effects have been reversed using xylazine reversal doses of yohimbine (0.11 mg/kg) (Yobine, Lloyd Labs). In the dog, yohimbine is FDA-approved only as an intravenous xylazine reversing agent.

Amitraz Weekly Rinses

(Protocol Not Approved by FDA)

- Apply amitraz as previously outlined, except at a once-weekly rate.
- Continue acaricidal rinses for 2–6 weeks after multiple negative skin scrapings.
- Long-term cure rates for this protocol are believed to be 60–70%.

Amitraz Daily Half-Body (Alternating) Rinses

This protocol is not approved by the FDA or the Environmental Protection Agency (EPA).

Procedure

- Prepare 0.125% amitraz solution from a 12.5% amitraz solution (1 ml of Taktic [Hoechst-Roussel], in 100 ml of water).
- Clip the dog and treat pyodermas as previously discussed. Bathe dogs with concurrent keratinization disorders once weekly with appropriate shampoos.
- Using a sponge, rub 0.125% amitraz solution daily onto one-half of the dog's body. Alternate the treated and untreated halves daily. Air-dry the dog.
- Treat dogs with pododermatitis with daily foot soaks using the 0.125% amitraz solution.
- All dogs receive otic treatments (1.5 ml Taktic in 8.5 ml of mineral oil q3–7d) unless otic irritation develops.

- During the first week of therapy hospitalize and monitor the dog for adverse side effects.
- Continue therapy for 2 weeks after multiple skin scrapings are negative.

Results

The reported cure rate with this protocol is 79% of the dogs treated. This includes a 75% resolution rate in dogs previously found to be unresponsive to standard whole-body biweekly, weekly, or twice-weekly amitraz dips.

Side Effects

- The incidence of adverse side effects is reportedly less than 6%, including mild transient sedation that spontaneously resolves without a change in therapy.
- Extreme caution must be used with this procedure in order to prevent adverse side effects in humans.

▼ *Key Point* The EPA considers it a violation of federal law to use a registered pesticide that is inconsistent with its labeling. Thus, always try conventional amitraz protocols before resorting to daily applications.

Daily Oral Milbemycin Oxime

(Protocol Not Approved by FDA)

Milbemycin oxime (Interceptor, Ciba-Geigy) is a macrolide antibiotic derived from the fermentation of *Streptomyces hygroscopicus*. The drug is presently approved by the FDA as a once-monthly heartworm preventive agent for dogs. The precise mechanism of action against the *Demodex* mite currently is unknown.

The protocol described here is based on research conducted by W. Miller and D. Scott at Cornell University. Dogs treated in their studies were heartworm-negative adult dogs with generalized demodicosis. All dogs were in reasonably good health with no identifiable predisposing factors. Concurrent pyodermas were treated with oral antibiotics; benzoyl peroxide shampoo baths and amitraz rinses were not used during the clinical trial.

- A variety of dosages were tested; the dosage of 2 mg/kg q24h PO for 1–2 months past the point of negative skin scrapings appeared to be the most effective.
- The only adverse side effect was ataxia in small dogs receiving daily milbemycin doses of greater than 2.5 mg/kg. The ataxia disappeared quickly following discontinuation of the medication.
- A cure rate of approximately 60% was noted for dosages of 1 mg/kg q24h PO, whereas an 85% cure rate was noted when 2 mg/kg q24h PO was used.

Daily Oral Ivermectin

(Protocol Not Approved by FDA)

Ivermectin (Ivomec or Eqvalan, Merial) is a fermentation product of the actinomycete, *Streptomyces avermitilis*. The precise mechanism of action against the *Demodex* mite is unknown. However, in other parasites it stimulates the release of the inhibitory neurotransmitter γ-aminobutyric acid, resulting in hyperpolarization of the postsynaptic membrane, paralysis, and death of the parasite. The drug is presently approved by the FDA as a once-monthly heartworm preventive agent for dogs and as a systemic parasiticide for horses, cattle, and hogs.

- Administer 300–600 μg/kg q24h PO for 1 month past the point of negative skin scrapings. Clinical trials indicate the higher dosage is more effective.
- Long-term cure rates have been reported to be 83% when the 600 μg/kg dosage was used, but only 48% when 400 μg/kg was used. In addition, when lower dosages were successful they usually required a more prolonged course of treatment.
- Adverse side effects include loss of appetite, increased salivation, confusion, ataxia, weakness, coma, and death, and the higher the dosage the greater the chance of these adverse effects. Side effects can occur following the administration of a single dose or after months of therapy. Many veterinary dermatologists recommend a gradual increasing dosage protocol, such as 100 μg/kg q24h PO for 5 days, then 200 μg/kg q24h for 5 days, etc., until the 600 μg/kg maximal dose is reached, and this dose is continued for 1 month past the point of negative skin scrapings.

▼ *Key Point* Because of a greater risk of severe idiosyncratic reactions, ivermectin should not be used to treat collies, Shetland sheepdogs, Old English sheepdogs, Australian shepherds, or other herding breeds and their crosses.

Feline Generalized Demodicosis

- Identify and treat any underlying abnormalities. Generalized demodicosis in the cat is a potential marker for internal disease.
- Clip all medium- to long-haired cats before topical therapy.
- Because there are no FDA-approved treatments for generalized (and localized) demodicosis in cats and because cats are very sensitive to many insecticides, always try the most benign therapy first.
  - Presently, this consists of topical 2–3% lime sulfur (Lym Dyp, DVM Pharmaceuticals) applied once weekly for 2–4 weeks past the point of negative skin scrapings.

Amitraz Rinse

(Protocol Not Approved by FDA)

- A potentially more effective, but also potentially more hazardous, treatment involves a weekly topical application of a 0.0125% amitraz solution.
- Continue the rinses for at least 2 weeks past the point of negative skin scrapings.
- Common side effects include mild sedation, anorexia, diarrhea, ptyalism, and abnormal behavior. These side effects are usually mild and transient.

- However, if side effects are severe, an experimental (not approved by FDA) dose of yohimbine (0.11 mg/kg IV) may resolve the clinical signs.

Pododemodicosis/Otodemodicosis

Canine

In the dog, pododemodicosis and otodemodicosis are usually associated with more generalized disease; therefore, treat these demodicoses as previously discussed. However, because of the difficulty in treating these areas, the following additional measures (not approved by FDA) often are required.

- Treat affected feet daily or q48h using either standard aqueous dilutions of amitraz (0.025%) or amitraz mixed with mineral oil (1 ml of Mitaban/15–30 ml of mineral oil). (*Caution:* amitraz/mineral oil treatments can be messy!)
- Treat otodemodicosis with amitraz in mineral oil (as described) administered q2–7d (see also previous discussion of amitraz daily half-body rinses under Canine General Demodicosis).
- If irritation develops, discontinue medication or increase the treatment interval.

Feline

Pododemodicosis and otodemodicosis in the cat, like their canine counterparts, usually are associated with more regional or generalized conditions.

- Feline pododemodicosis usually is not a distinct entity and does not require special management.
- Feline otodemodicosis may appear as a distinct condition and may be treated similarly to canine otodemodicosis.
- Discontinue therapy when no mites are found on ear swabbing or when it is no longer necessary to treat the more generalized condition. Additionally, discontinue if irritation develops.

▼ *Key Point* Check with current state and federal laws when using insecticides in an extra-labeled manner.

PREVENTION

▼ *Key Point* Advise all owners of dogs with generalized demodicosis to have them neutered. This prevents the stresses associated with breeding and the transmission of a heritable trait.

A key to prevention of demodicosis in pets is to identify and eliminate all potential predisposing factors. If possible, avoid all future use of any immunosuppressive agent.

SUPPLEMENTAL READINGS

Kwochka KW: Canine Demodicosis. *In* Kirk RW, ed.: Current Veterinary Therapy IX: Small Animal Practice. Philadelphia: WB Saunders, 1986, p 531.

Lemarié SL, Horohov DW: Evaluation of interleukin-2 production and interleukin-2 receptor expression in dogs with generalized demodicosis. Vet Derm 7:213, 1996.

Medleau L: Recently described feline dermatoses. Vet Clin North Am Small Anim Pract 20:1626, 1990.

Medleau L, Ristic Z, McElveen D: Daily ivermectin for the treatment of generalized demodicosis in dogs. Vet Derm 7:209, 1996.

Medleau L, Willemse T: Efficacy of daily amitraz therapy for generalized demodicosis in dogs: Two independent studies. Proceedings of the 7th Annual Meeting of the American Academy of Veterinary Dermatology, 1991, p 41.

Miller WH: Treatment of generalized demodicosis in dogs. *In* Bonagura JD, ed.: Current Veterinary Therapy XII: Small Animal Practice. Philadelphia: WB Saunders, 1995, p 625.

Scott DW, Miller WH, Griffin CE: Small Animal Dermatology. Philadelphia: WB Saunders, 1995, p 417.

39 Scabies, Notoedric Mange, and Cheyletiellosis

Richard K. Anderson

Scabies, notoedric mange, and cheyletiellosis are parasitic dermatoses caused by acarine mites living on or within the skin of the host animal. The resultant lesions may be due to mechanical damage from the burrowing mite, pruritogenic substances secreted by the mite, or a hypersensitivity reaction developed against one or more extracellular products of the mite. Variability of clinical manifestations of these parasitic dermatoses probably reflects variations in the duration and intensity of the hypersensitivity reaction and in the capacity of the host to limit parasite multiplication.

Exposure to these mites and the corresponding incidence of parasitic dermatoses are closely related to environmental factors, especially animal contact and the presence of endemic areas. Although the causative mites are not completely host-specific, they do exhibit host preference. They also have zoonotic potential for causing dermatoses in humans.

SCABIES

Etiology

- Scabies (sarcoptic mange) is an intensely pruritic papulocrustous dermatosis of dogs caused by the epidermal mite *Sarcoptes scabiei* var. *canis* (Fig. 39–1). Although fairly host-specific, the mite can affect cats, fox, and humans. In cats an underlying disease (i.e., feline immunodeficiency virus infection) is likely.
- The adult mite is microscopic (200–400 μm), roughly circular in shape, and characterized by two pairs of short legs anteriorly, which bear long unjointed stalks with suckers, and two pairs of rudimentary legs posteriorly that do not extend beyond the border of the body.
- The parasite completes its life cycle (egg-larva-nymph-adult) in 17–21 days in tunnels and molting pockets in the stratum corneum.
  - Although the parasite is susceptible to high temperature and drying, it can live in the environment for up to 21 days.
- Scabies is highly contagious and is primarily transmitted by close contact, but grooming instruments and kennels may be point sources of infection for other animals.

- The incubation period is highly variable and is dependent on the number of mites present and the time required for the development of hypersensitivity to the mite. The use of systemic corticosteroids appears to allow the mite population to increase more rapidly.
- Dermatologic changes are often completely out of proportion to the number of mites present, suggesting that hypersensitivity plays an important role in the course of the disease.

Clinical Signs

▼ *Key Point* Scabies is manifested primarily by intense pruritus that usually is minimally responsive to corticosteroids. Even during the physical examination, the dog scratches and chews at itself.

- The typical distribution pattern involves the ventral portion of the chest, the lateral aspect of the elbow and hock, and the margin of the pinna.

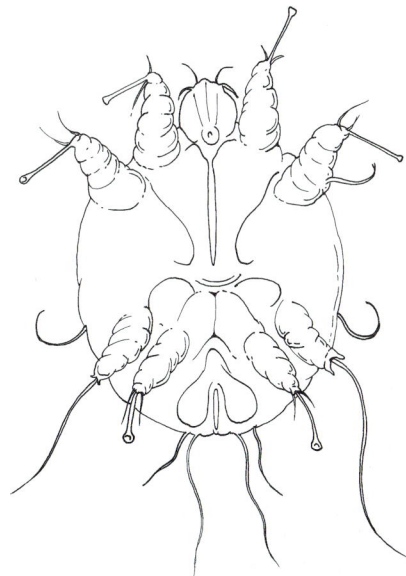

Figure 39–1. *Sarcoptes scabiei.*

- Early lesions are characterized by a polymorphous eruption with erythematous macules and papules, patchy alopecia, and small hemorrhagic crusts. The intense and constant scratching rapidly produces extensive excoriations, thick yellow crusts, and more generalized alopecia.
- Some dogs just scratch incessantly and have few, if any, lesions other than mild erythema and occasional excoriations.

Diagnosis

- Suspect scabies based on
  - History of rapid onset of intense pruritus and rapid progression of lesions with inconsistent response to corticosteroids.
  - Potential exposure of the affected dog to other animals, especially fox.
  - Pruritic dermatitis involving dogs and humans in contact with the affected dogs.
  - Nature and distribution of cutaneous lesions as described.
- Perform superficial skin scrapings from nonexcoriated areas, with emphasis on the ears, elbows, hocks, and ventral thorax.
  - Even with multiple scrapings the mite is often difficult to find; often only the large oval eggs or small foci of brown fecal pellets can be found, but these are of diagnostic significance.

▼ *Key Point* Failure to find the mite should not eliminate the diagnosis of scabies. Always use trial therapy if the diagnosis remains in question and the degree of suspicion is high enough to justify its use.

- An enzyme-linked immunosorbent assay for IgG antibodies to *Sarcoptes* mite antigens has been reported to have diagnostic sensitivity and specificity of up to 92% and 96%, respectively. When commercially available, it could prove to have diagnostic value. Keep in mind that the house dust mite, which is a common allergen in atopic dogs, shares some antigens with *S. scabiei.*
- Differential diagnosis includes any pruritic skin disease, especially allergic and other parasitic dermatoses.

Treatment

▼ *Key Point* The emergence of resistant strains of the *Sarcoptes* organism and the array of commercial products available make selection of parasiticides difficult. Products highly efficacious in one geographic location may be ineffective in another.

- When scale and crusts are present, bathe with keratolytic shampoos before dipping.
- Dips known to be effective include
  - Amitraz (Mitaban, Upjohn), applied three times at 2-week intervals (not approved for this use by the United States Food and Drug Administration [FDA])

  - Lime sulfur, 4% solution, applied weekly for 6 treatments or for 2 weeks past clinical remission; this is the safest dip for young animals or sick and debilitated patients.
- Ivermectin (Ivomec injection for cattle, Merck Ag Vet) is very effective at 0.3 mg/kg PO or SC three times at 1–2 week intervals.
  - It is not approved by the FDA for use in dogs at this dosage. Do not administer to collies, collie crosses, Shetland sheepdogs, Old English sheepdogs, or Australian shepherds.
  - Evaluate the animal's heartworm status before drug administration.
  - Adverse reactions to ivermectin may include tremors, ataxia, mydriasis, stupor, coma, and death. As there is no known antidote for ivermectin toxicity, only supportive therapy (fluids, parenteral nutrition) is available.
- Milbemycin (Interceptor, Novartis) is also a very effective systemic treatment, especially in breeds of dogs in which ivermectin is contraindicated, at 2 mg/kg PO three times at 1-week intervals (not approved for this use by the FDA).
- Treat all dogs in contact with the patient or on the premises.
- Although the mites die after a few days when off the host, clean up the environment and use one application of a parasiticide such as malathion when there are a number of animals affected (e.g., a kennel or pet shop).

NOTOEDRIC MANGE

Etiology

- Notoedric mange (feline scabies) is an intensely pruritic, crusting dermatosis of cats caused by the sarcoptiform mite, *Notoedres cati* (Fig. 39–2). The mite may also infest dogs, fox, and rabbits and may cause transient lesions in humans.
- Although rarely seen today, notoedric mange may be endemic in a few localities.
- *N. cati* is a burrowing mite very similar to *S. scabiei* in both morphology and life cycle. *N. cati* is smaller

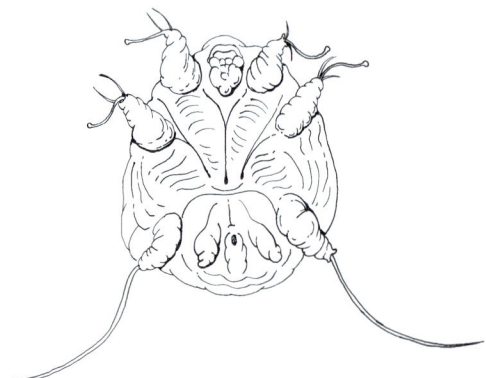

Figure 39–2. *Notoedres cati.*

than *S. scabiei* and has a dorsal anus in contrast to the terminal anus of *S. scabiei*.

- Notoedric mange is highly contagious, usually by direct contact. The mite can survive off the host for only a few days.
- Although characteristically a disease of adult cats, notoedric mange may present as a fulminating dermatitis in kittens.
- Usually, large numbers of mites are found on affected animals; however, allergic disease associated with very few mites may be more frequent than realized.

Clinical Signs

- Lesions appear first on the margin of the pinna but spread rapidly to the face and neck. Occasionally, lesions can be found on the feet and perineum.
- Initially there is a papular eruption, but the skin soon becomes thickened with dry, adherent crusts.
- Intense pruritus results in self-induced alopecia, erythema, and excoriations.

Diagnosis

- The intense pruritus and distribution of lesions are diagnostic features.

▼ *Key Point* As opposed to dogs with canine scabies, cats with feline scabies have large numbers of mites that are easily found on skin scrapings. The best areas to scrape are the ears and face. Use trial therapy only if the diagnosis remains in question and the degree of suspicion is high enough to justify its use.

Differential diagnoses include food hypersensitivity, *Otodectes* infestation, atopy, dermatophytosis, cheyletiellosis, pemphigus foliaceus or erythematosus, systemic lupus erythematosus, and fight wounds.

Treatment

- Bathe the cat with a keratolytic shampoo before dipping.
- Dips that may be effective include
  - Lime sulfur, 2% solution, applied weekly for 6 weeks; this is the safest dip for young kittens or sick and debilitated animals.
  - Amitraz (Mitaban, Upjohn), 0.025% solution, applied once and repeated in 2 weeks (not approved for cats by the FDA).
  - An elizabethan collar should be worn after dipping to prevent ingestion of the substance.
- Ivermectin (Ivomec injection for cattle, Merck Ag Vet) is effective at 0.3 mg/kg PO or SC, given three times at 2-week intervals (not approved for cats by the FDA).
- Treat other animals in the household concurrently.
- Because the mite does not persist for long off the host, a single thorough cleaning of the environment suffices. Use one application of a parasiticide such as malathion in a cattery where multiple animals are infested with the mite.

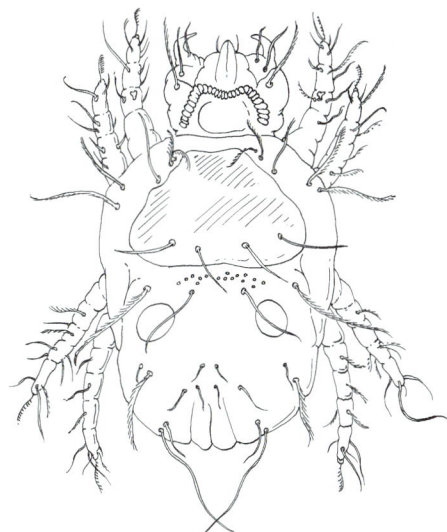

Figure 39–3.   *Cheyletiella yasguri.*

CHEYLETIELLOSIS

Etiology

- Cheyletiellosis (*Cheyletiella* dermatitis) is a dorsally distributed papulocrustous or scaling dermatosis caused by the surface mite, *Cheyletiella yasguri* (dog, Fig. 39–3), *C. blakei* (cat), and *C. parasitovorax* (rabbit).
- The three species of mites may go freely to various host species including humans. The disease may not be as uncommon as previously thought.
- *Cheyletiella* species are comparatively large (500 μm), saddle-shaped mites that can be identified by their prominent hook-like accessory mouthparts. All four pairs of legs extend beyond the body margin and bear combs terminally.
- The life cycle (egg-larva-nymph-adult) is spent entirely on the host and is completed in approximately 3–5 weeks. Eggs are cemented to hairs.
- The mites are surface dwellers that feed on epidermal debris, but periodically pierce the skin feeding on tissue fluids. Female mites may live free of their hosts for as long as 10 days.
- Cheyletiellosis is highly contagious. Indirect transmission via fomites may be as important as direct transmission. Eggs attached to hair shed into the environment may be an important source for reinfestation.
- In some animals, the intensity of the pruritus and dermatologic changes are out of proportion to the number of mites present, suggesting the development of a hypersensitivity to the mite.

Clinical Signs

- The lesions elicited by the mite are characterized primarily by a scaling and crusting exfoliative or papular dermatitis with dandruff-like flakes in the haircoat. Cats may have a papulocrustous eruption (miliary dermatitis).

- Dorsal truncal distribution is typical, although generalized distribution may occur.
- Pruritus is highly variable, ranging from completely absent to intense.
- Asymptomatic carriers may exist.

▼ *Key Point* The most common clinical presentation of cheyletiellosis is a puppy or kitten recently acquired from a pet shop, kennel, or cattery with a variably pruritic, dorsal scaling or papulocrustous dermatosis.

Diagnosis

The variability in clinical presentation along with the difficulty in finding the mite can make cheyletiellosis a challenging condition to diagnose.

- Suspect cheyletiellosis based on
  - Nature and distribution of the cutaneous lesions, as previously described
  - Exposure of the patient to other animals
  - Involvement of in-contact animals and humans; clinical signs in human contacts are often characteristic (pruritic papules with central necrosis) and may be the only evidence that the animal in the household is infested.
- Techniques used to demonstrate the mite or its eggs include
  - Direct examination of the surface of the skin and haircoat for "crawling white scales" with a magnifying lens
  - Superficial skin scrapings
  - Acetate (Scotch) tape impression smears of the affected areas
  - Collection of epidermal debris with a flea comb followed by 10% potassium hydroxide (KOH) digestion and centrifugation with a saturated sugar solution
  - Fecal flotation

▼ *Key Point* The most effective diagnostic techniques for cheyletiellosis are the acetate tape impression smears and the collection of epidermal debris with a flea comb.

- In some cases, the mite or its eggs cannot be demonstrated, and diagnosis thus depends on the response to a therapeutic trial.
- Differential diagnoses include other mite infestations, pediculosis, flea bite hypersensitivity, food hypersensitivity, all of the causes of seborrhea, and all of the causes of miliary dermatitis in the cat.

Treatment

▼ *Key Point* Although *Cheyletiella* mites appear to be susceptible to most insecticides, they may be extremely difficult to eradicate. Treatment of the patient, all in-contact animals, and the premises is mandatory.

- Bathe the animal with an antiseborrheic shampoo to remove crusts and scales before dipping.
- Treat dogs, cats, or rabbits with pyrethrins or 2% lime sulfur dips; place an elizabethan collar on cats after dipping to prevent ingestion of the substance. Organophosphates, carbamates, or amitraz (not approved for this use by the FDA) are also effective for use on dogs. Repeat treatments every second week for 6–8 weeks.
- Ivermectin (Ivomec injection for cattle; Merck Ag Vet), 0.3 mg/kg PO or SC, given three times at 2-week intervals is effective in dogs, cats, and rabbits (not approved for this use by the FDA).
  - Evaluate the dog's heartworm status before administration.
  - Do not administer to collies, collie crosses, Shetland sheepdogs, Old English sheepdogs, or Australian shepherds.
- Clean and spray animal's quarters and bedding with a residual insecticide appropriate for killing adult fleas. Professional exterminators may be required.

SUPPLEMENTAL READINGS

Bornstein S, Thebo P, Zakrisson G: Evaluation of an enzyme-linked immunosorbent assay (ELISA) for the serological diagnosis of canine sarcoptic mange. Vet Derm 7:21, 1996.

Griffin CE: Scabies. *In* Griffin CE, Kwochka DW, MacDonald JM, eds.: Current Veterinary Dermatology. St. Louis: Mosby–Year Book, 1993, pp 85–89.

Moriello KA: Treatment of *Sarcoptes* and *Cheyletiella* infestations. *In* Kirk RW, Bonagura JD, eds.: Current Veterinary Therapy XI: Small Animal Practice. Philadelphia: WB Saunders, 1992, p 558.

Moriello KA: Cheyletiellosis. *In* Griffin CE, Kwochka KW, MacDonald JM, eds.: Current Veterinary Dermatology. St. Louis: Mosby–Year Book, 1993, pp 90–95.

Paradis M: Ivermectin in small animal dermatology. *In* Kirk RW ed.: Current Veterinary Therapy X: Small Animal Practice. Philadelphia: WB Saunders, 1989, p 560.

Scott DW, Miller WH, Griffin CE: Small Animal Dermatology. Philadelphia: WB Saunders, 1995, p 441.

40 Flea Allergy Dermatitis

Craig E. Griffin

Flea allergy dermatitis (FAD) is a hypersensitivity reaction to one or more components of flea saliva. Several types of hypersensitivities, such as cutaneous basophil hypersensitivity, immunoglobulin E (IgE)–mediated immediate hypersensitivity, late-onset IgE reaction, and delayed-type hypersensitivity, can occur alone or in combination. The hypersensitivity reactions cause inflammation and pruritus, which induce most of the lesions.

In most geographic areas, FAD is the most common cause of skin disease. During the summer it is often the most common disease seen by the small animal practitioner.

ETIOLOGY

- *Ctenocephalides felis* is the species that usually infests both dogs and cats.
- *Pulex irritans* and less commonly *Ctenocephalides canis* may be responsible in some areas.

CLINICAL SIGNS

- *Primary lesions*
  - *Pruritus* is the primary clinical sign observed by the owner and can be manifested as chewing (as if eating corn on the cob), rubbing, rolling, or scratching. Cats may groom excessively or pull out their hair. Severe chewing may lead to excessive wear of the incisor and canine teeth.
  - *Papules* and *erythematous macules* also usually are present.
- *Secondary lesions* result from the chronic inflammation and pruritus-induced trauma. Alopecia, broken hairs, dry hair, scaling, hyperpigmentation, and lichenification may occur.
- *Pattern of involvement* most often includes tail base and dorsal lumbar region. The caudal thighs, groin, and abdomen frequently are affected, although less severely than the dorsal lumbar region. In chronic and severe cases, there is extension of the lesions cranially.

▼ *Key Point* Pinnal or facial involvement in the dog is not typical of FAD and suggests other concurrent allergic diseases.

- *Cats with FAD* commonly have miliary crusts in the cervical as well as dorsal lumbar region. Lesions may be limited to the abdomen and groin or cervical area.
- *Secondary problems* that may occur often represent focal sites of infection, foci of severe trauma possibly from the itch-scratch cycle, or a different pathologic reaction. Acute moist dermatitis (hot spots), acral pruritic nodules, eosinophilic plaques, and eosinophilic granulomas may be seen in dogs and cats.
- *Superficial or deep pyoderma* may develop, especially in animals repeatedly treated with corticosteroids. Animals with superficial pyoderma will present with pustules, crusted papules, or circular spreading rings of crust over erythematous erosions, lichenified plaques, or papules.

DIAGNOSIS

▼ *Key Point* Flea allergy dermatitis is diagnosed in pruritic animals with typical patterns of involvement and evidence of fleas. Always consider the presence of coexistent allergies. Frequently they are overlooked.

History

Identify typical patterns of involvement and seasonality compatible with fleas. A history of otitis externa suggests that other or concurrent allergies are present. Obtain information regarding the number and type of pets, housing and type of floor covering, possible sources of exposure to fleas, current pesticide use, and client concerns regarding the use of pesticides.

Physical Examination

The following procedures may be useful:

- Examine for fleas or flea dirt in longhaired animals by brushing the pet over white paper; in shorthaired animals flea combing may be helpful.
- Closely examine areas of involvement typical for other allergies (see Chaps. 41 and 42) for evidence of coexisting disease.
- Closely examine the dorsal lumbar area for papules, which are the primary lesions seen in canine FAD.

- Carefully palpate the skin in cats; this is important because the typical small crusted papules (miliary crusts) often are more easily felt than seen.
- Shave the haircoat to allow closer observation of the lesions.
- Examine for lymphadenopathy in cats, a common finding in chronic FAD.

Dermatopathology

- Dermatopathology is not specific but may be suggestive of or compatible with FAD.
- A superficial mixed perivascular dermatitis with eosinophils is typical in FAD.

Intradermal Testing

Intradermal testing with 1/1000 wt/vol flea antigen (Greer) has been documented as a reliable test for diagnosing FAD.

- Positive reactions may occur in 15 minutes (immediate), 6–8 hours (late onset), or 24–48 hours (delayed).
- A positive test indicates that flea hypersensitivity is present, but it does not document that all clinical signs are related to fleas.
- A negative test at all observation times usually indicates (>90%) that flea allergy is not present.
- False-negative results may occur if glucocorticoids and antihistamines are not properly withdrawn before testing.

In Vitro Testing

The radioallergosorbent test (RAST) and the enzyme-linked immunosorbent assay (ELISA) have not been documented to be as accurate as intradermal testing (see Chaps. 41 and 42).

False-negative results are the most common problem, but false-positive results may also occur in RAST and ELISA.

Response to Therapy

A favorable response following parasiticidal therapy directed against fleas is helpful in making a diagnosis of FAD. It does not eliminate the diagnosis of coexisting diseases.

▼ *Key Point* The most definitive diagnosis requires a positive intradermal test, the presence of fleas, and a complete response to effective flea control.

TREATMENT

FAD is best treated by eliminating exposure to the flea allergen (effective flea control). When a complete flea control program is used, more than 90% of cases can be controlled without additional treatment. Raising the allergic and pruritic thresholds by treating coexistent problems also may be helpful. In cases in which adequate flea control cannot be achieved, blocking the allergic reaction with systemic therapy is required.

Decrease Allergic Load (Flea Control)

Complete flea control requires treating the affected pet, other pets in the same environment, and the pet's environment. In severely infested environments, effective control may take 4–8 weeks to achieve. Client compliance and proper application of insecticides is required. Once flea control is achieved, clients may find that only one or two aspects of flea control are required for maintenance.

▼ *Key Point* Failure to obtain client compliance and improper application of parasiticidal agents are the major reasons for poor response of FAD patients to flea control.

Environmental Treatment

Because the majority of flea eggs, larvae, and pupae are located in the environment, it is essential to treat environmental areas.

Indoors. Treatment of indoor areas is critical when the affected animal spends most of the time indoors. This is the habitat that can be controlled most effectively.

- Lufenuron (Program, Novartis Animal Health) at 10 mg/kg q30 days in dogs and 30 mg/kg q30 days in cats is valuable in keeping flea infestations from becoming reestablished. However, this systemic therapy is not rapidly effective in decreasing the environmental burden and works best following initial use of traditional environmental parasiticides. It is very helpful as adjunctive therapy.
- For topical adulticide therapy of all dogs and cats in a closed environment, use fipronil (Frontline, Merial) or imidacloprid (Advantage, Bayer). These new topical adulticides along with lufenuron are especially effective in eliminating fleas from a closed environment.
- In houses in which floors are primarily carpeted, electrostatically charged sodium polyborate powder (Rx for Fleas) is most effective, lasting up to 1 year. It is also safe, with no reported toxicity.
- Monthly spraying of all floor surfaces and furniture that pets have access to with chlorpyrifos, permethrin, or pyrethrin in conjunction with a growth hormone regulator (methoprene, pyriproxyfen) is advisable. Effective products include Siphotrol Plus II House Treatment (Vet-Kem), Ectogard House and Carpet Spray (Tech America), and Impass Complete Premise Spray (Coopers).
  - If pyrethrin alone is used, weekly spraying for the first 3 weeks is necessary.

▼ *Key Point* Be careful when using organophosphates in an environment in which cats are present. Some cats are very sensitive and may have problems with toxicity even after a single application.

- Microencapsulation technology makes possible less frequent application of parasiticides without the need for a growth hormone regulator (Sectrol Pet and House Flea Spray, 3M; Duratrol Premise Spray, 3M).
- Treat linoleum and tile floors by frequent mopping with routine disinfectants.

Outdoors. Treat outdoor pens and similar enclosures weekly for 3 weeks and then monthly. A liquid application of chlorpyrifos, permethrin, or diazinon is preferred. Although helpful in long-term control, granular and microencapsulated insecticides have been less beneficial for obtaining initial control.

- The insect growth regulator pyriproxyfen is photostable and therefore a useful adjunct to outdoor therapy when used with adulticides.

Unaffected Pets

Treat unaffected animals in the same environment with adulticidal and/or insect development inhibitor flea products that lack flea repellent effects.

- Regular use of the topical adulticides fipronil or imidacloprid or lufenuron helps to prevent unaffected animals from contributing to reintroduction of fleas into the home environment.
- Weekly or bimonthly dips with chlorpyrifos (Duratrol Dip, 3M) or permethrin (Expar Dip, Coopers; Permectrin, Bioceutic) products are effective.

▼ *Key Point* Do not use permethrin dips on cats because toxicity may result, and use only permethrin sprays that are approved for cats.

- In cases in which dips cannot be used, use sprays or foams containing pyrethrins and/or permethrin at the maximal approved frequency.
- Use an approved flea collar on cats that cannot be treated with dips, sprays, or foams.

Affected Pets

Treat affected animals with an adulticidal product and repellents as frequently as allowed for these products.

- The new topical adulticides fipronil and imidacloprid have been shown to be efficacious for treating flea allergy dermatitis in dogs and cats, even when environmental treatment is not done. Fipronil in the spray formulation appears to be more efficacious than the spot application and is preferred for the affected pet if client compliance is not a problem.
- Do not apply alcohol-containing products frequently because of their drying effect.
- Combination of weekly dips (see earlier) and sprays (DuoCide L.A., Allerderm/Virbac; Synerkyl Spray, DVM Pharmaceuticals; Sectrol Pet and Household Spray and Sectrol Flea Foam, 3M) between dips is most effective.
- Use water-based pyrethrin and/or permethrin sprays (DuoCide L.A., Allerderm/Virbac) that contain a repellent. Apply daily if approved for such use.

- If used in conjunction with a dip, a light mist on the surface of the coat is all that is required.
- If used alone, apply the spray to the skin surface (not just the hair).
- Avoid using systemic parasiticidal agents because flea bites are required for their effectiveness; however, their use is preferable to no treatment.

Increase Allergic/Pruritic Threshold

- Control *concurrent allergic diseases* such as atopy and food allergy.
- Treat *secondary pyoderma*, which often increases pruritus, with systemic antibiotics (see Chap. 35).
- Eliminate *dry skin* by use of baths, moisturizing sprays or rinses, and fatty acid supplements.
- Remove other *irritants or allergens on the skin surface,* which may aggravate inflamed skin, by frequently bathing the animal. Use this option cautiously so that it will not hinder the effectiveness of the topically applied adulticides, such as fipronil and imidacloprid.

Block Allergic Reactions

A variety of systemic drugs may be used to alter the allergic reaction. This approach is often used at the beginning of the flea control program and to break the itch-scratch cycle. Resort to long-term use of systemic drugs only when clients cannot effectively control fleas. This most often occurs with outdoor/roaming pets, especially cats.

Systemic Glucocorticoids

Systemic glucocorticoids usually are required. Prednisone or prednisolone, 1–2 mg/kg PO q12–24h, is initially used to stop the pruritus associated with FAD.

- Use either oral triamcinolone acetonide (Vetalog, Solvay), 0.25–0.5 mg/kg q12–24h, or methylprednisolone (Medrol, Upjohn), 0.8–1.6 mg/kg q12–24h if polyuria, polydipsia, or polyphagia associated with prednisone or prednisolone is unacceptable to the client.
- When pruritus is controlled, change to an alternate-day program and then taper to the lowest effective dose.

Antihistamines

Antihistamines are infrequently effective for FAD. They may be used in conjunction with glucocorticoids and have a synergistic effect that makes possible a reduction in the glucocorticoid dose.

- Diphenhydramine HCl, 2 mg/kg PO q8h; hydroxyzine HCl, 2 mg/kg PO q8h; doxepin HCl, 1–2 mg/kg PO q12h; or clemastine, 0.05–0.1 mg/kg q12h PO, may be useful in dogs.
- Chlorpheniramine may be helpful in dogs at a total dose of 2–6 mg PO q8–12h. It is especially useful in cats at a total dose of 2 mg PO q12h.

Fatty Acid Supplements

Fatty acid supplements (DVM Derm Caps, DVM Pharmaceuticals) alone rarely control FAD. However, they may be helpful in controlling concurrent atopy, alleviating dry skin, and modulating the production of inflammatory mediators. These effects may raise the pruritic/allergic threshold and have a synergistic effect with other treatments, allowing a reduction in the glucocorticoid dose.

Hyposensitization

Hyposensitization used with standard protocols has not been shown to be efficacious. However, hyposensitization used alone has been reported to be an effective control in individual cases. It is not considered cost-effective for most clients, considering the low percentage of efficacy.

PREVENTION

- Prevention is achieved by long-term continuation of a flea control program. Long-term treatment may not have to be as complete or as frequent as the initial treatment program.

▼ *Key Point* The topical adulticides fipronil or imidacloprid, with or without lufenuron, appear to be most effective for long-term control.

- Another option is to use prevention by anticipating increases in flea population and increasing the use of parasiticidal therapy just before the onset of environmental conditions favoring these increases.
- Work is in progress to develop a vaccine against FAD.

SUPPLEMENTAL READINGS

Bevier-Tournay DE: Fleas and flea control. *In* Kirk RW, ed.: Current Veterinary Therapy X. Philadelphia: WB Saunders, 1989, p 586.

Kwochka KW: Fleas and related disease. Vet Clin North Am 17:1235, 1987.

MacDonald JM, Miller TA: Parasiticide therapy in small animal dermatology. *In* Kirk RW, ed: Current Veterinary Therapy IX. Philadelphia: WB Saunders, 1986, p 571.

Schick MP, Schick RO: Understanding and implementing safe and effective flea control. J Am Anim Hosp Assoc 22:421, 1986.

41 Atopy

Patricia D. White

Canine atopy is an inherited tendency to develop IgE antibodies to environmental allergens (molds; grass, tree, and weed pollens; epidermal agents; house dust; insects; house dust mites). Although popular theory states that canine atopy develops subsequent to sensitization to environmental allergens via the respiratory tract, the ventral, pedal, and facial distribution of cutaneous lesions strongly suggests that percutaneous exposure may also play a role in the development of clinical signs. This disease comprises a significant proportion of canine dermatologic complaints and has been estimated to involve 3–15% of the canine population.

Feline atopy is believed to be a type I hypersensitivity reaction to environmental allergens. There are ample examples of cutaneous and respiratory hypersensitivity reactions in cats caused by exposure to aeroallergens in support of this theory, but there is no evidence to support an inherited predisposition to atopy in this species. Feline atopy may cause a variety of focal and diffuse dermatologic clinical signs including miliary dermatitis, eosinophilic granuloma, eosinophilic ulcer, eosinophilic plaque, and symmetric alopecia.

ETIOLOGY

Pathogenesis

- Atopy classically is described as an *IgE-mediated type I hypersensitivity reaction*. Once contact is made, the allergen is processed by tissue macrophages into a form which can be presented with the assistance of T helper lymphocytes to B lymphocytes. The B cells then produce allergen-specific IgE antibodies and memory cells. The IgE antibodies affix to tissue mast cells and basophils. On reexposure, allergens bind the surface IgE molecules. Cross-linking of two IgE antibodies results in degranulation of the mast cell and the release of preformed inflammatory mediators, and stimulation of the arachidonic acid cascade. The combination of preformed and arachidonic acid–derived inflammatory mediators (leukotrienes, prostaglandins, and hydroxy fatty acids) results in inflammation (erythema, edema, pruritus).
- A reaginic antibody similar to canine IgE has been identified in cats, but its relationship to atopy is unknown.

Incidence

▼ *Key Point* Atopy is the second most common allergic skin disorder in dogs and cats, second only to flea allergy dermatitis.

- Age of onset in dogs is between 1 and 3 years. The disease usually starts as a seasonally pruritic dermatosis with the signs peaking in the summer and fall. The problem may become nonseasonal.
- Both sexes are represented, although female dogs may have a slightly higher incidence of occurrence.
- Breeds predisposed to developing atopy include Cairn, West Highland white, and wire-haired fox terriers; Lhasa apsos; golden and Labrador retrievers; boxers; bulldogs; dalmatians; English and Irish setters; and Chinese Shar-Peis. The disease also occurs in other breeds and in mixed-breed dogs.
- Because atopy in cats is diagnosed less frequently than in dogs, trends in age, breed, and sex are not appreciated.

CLINICAL SIGNS

Pruritus

Pruritus is the hallmark of atopy in both dogs and cats.

- Pruritus is the only sign early in the disease, and skin lesions may be absent. An itch-scratch-itch cycle is established leading to self-trauma that may be severe.
- In dogs, as the disease progresses, face rubbing, foot licking or chewing, and scratching lead to erythema, alopecia, edema, lichenification, and hyperpigmentation of the periocular, perilabial, interdigital, ventral, axillary, and antebrachial regions of the body.
- Acral lick granulomas are commonly seen in some breeds, such as the Doberman pinscher and dalmatian, and reflect focally intense pruritus and severe self-trauma.

Other Signs in Dogs

Otitis Externa. Otitis may accompany the other clinical signs or may be the sole presenting complaint (see Chap. 55).

- A pruritic and erythematous pinna and ear canal in the early stages of the disease eventually become complicated by secondary yeast or bacterial infection that presents as a brown waxy or purulent exudate. The otitis may be unilateral or bilateral.

Pyoderma. *Superficial bacterial infection* is the most common but frequently overlooked problem accompanying canine atopy.

- The self-trauma caused by pruritus encourages the establishment of pathogenic staphylococcal bacteria, leading to pyoderma.
- Staphylococcal antigens are capable of eliciting a toxic, inflammatory, or antigenic effect on epidermal and dermal tissues, resulting in cutaneous damage with release of proteolytic enzymes and inflammatory mediators. Because pyoderma may be intensely pruritic, the presence of this condition in an animal with atopy worsens the existing pruritus (see Chap. 35).

Seborrheic Dermatitis. Dermatitis characterized by flaky skin and a dry or greasy haircoat often occurs in conjunction with the pruritus and pyoderma.

Other Signs in Cats

- Cats commonly present with a *head and neck pruritus* or *ventral abdominal dermatitis with alopecia*.
- Clinical signs also include one or a combination of the following:
  - Mild to severe symmetric alopecia without dermatitis
  - Focal or diffuse miliary dermatitis (see Chap. 48).
  - Eosinophilic plaques, ulcers, and granulomas (see Chap. 48).
  - Generalized seborrhea

DIAGNOSIS

▼ *Key Point* Base the diagnosis of atopy on history, clinical signs, elimination or control of other causes of pruritic dermatitis, and results of appropriate diagnostic tests. Age of onset, season of occurrence, breed, and response to therapy provide adequate information to make a tentative diagnosis.

History

A thorough and complete history is mandatory; look for a seasonal pattern of occurrence that may progress to a nonseasonal problem.

Physical Examination

The typical distribution of skin lesions corresponds to the severity of pruritus.

- Of affected animals, 60–70% have visible skin lesions including erythema, papules, scale, alopecia, hyperpigmentation, and lichenification involving the face, ears, feet, axille, flexor and extensor surfaces of joints, groin, and abdomen.
- Reddish brown discoloration (saliva staining) of the hair in dogs, and bilaterally symmetric or ventral abdominal alopecia in cats are changes associated with licking and chewing.

Differential Diagnosis

- The signalment, history, and clinical signs enable the clinician to develop a list of differential diagnoses. In the differential diagnosis* consider:
  - Food, contact, and flea allergies
  - Superficial pyoderma
  - Scabies, notoedric mange (feline scabies)
  - *Malassezia* dermatitis
  - Demodicosis
  - Dermatophytosis
  - Intestinal parasite hypersensitivity (rare)
- In every case:
  - Take skin scrapings for sarcoptiform and demodectic mange mites. Perform culture for dermatophytes and a fecal examination for parasites.
- Screen for flea exposure because about 80% of atopic dogs also are allergic to fleas.
  - Use a flea comb to check for fleas, flea eggs, and flea feces.
  - If there is evidence of fleas, treat the affected animal, all other pets, and their environment.

▼ *Key Point* Eliminate or control fleas prior to evaluating and treating atopy, which can be time-consuming and expensive.

- In nonseasonally pruritic animals, institute a hypoallergenic food trial.

Specific Diagnostic Tests

Intradermal Allergy Testing

Intradermal allergy testing (IDAT) is a sensitive in vivo method of identifying clinically relevant allergens. Perform the test by injecting individual allergens intradermally and measuring the magnitude of a classic "wheal and flare" response. Accurate interpretation of IDAT is directly related to the skill and experience of the individual performing the test and reading the results.

- Select IDAT in cases in which:
  - The animal's allergy season lasts longer than 3 months.
  - Medical therapy no longer controls the symptoms.
  - Avoidance of the allergens is not possible.
  - The animal is young and would have long-term benefits from immunotherapy.
- Consider the *cost* of allergens and supplies and the time involved in test kit preparation before choosing to perform IDAT. This test must be performed an average of two to three times weekly to ensure accuracy and consistency of test results and their interpretation.
- To maximize the information gained from IDAT, withdraw anti-inflammatory drugs, which are the

---

*Consult the appropriate chapters for details regarding diagnosis of these conditions.

most common cause of false-negative results, for an appropriate period before performing IDAT. Withdrawal time depends on the drug, carrier vehicle, route of administration, and duration of therapy. The following are minimal withdrawal times.

- Discontinue topical drugs containing glucocorticoids (including otic and ophthalmic) and short-acting systemic glucocorticoids (prednisone and prednisolone) for a *minimum* of 3 weeks before IDAT. Longer-acting corticosteroids require a withdrawal time of 6–8 weeks (dexamethasone, triamcinolone acetonide) to 12 weeks (methylprednisolone acetate).
- Discontinue antihistamines for at least 2 weeks.
- Although other nonsteroidal anti-inflammatory drugs (NSAIDs) have not been critically evaluated, these products theoretically may depress the response to intradermal allergens by affecting the production of inflammatory mediators. Therefore, discontinue these drugs for 2 weeks before skin testing.
- Essential fatty acid supplements do not appear to affect IDAT results; thus withdrawal is not necessary.
- Other causes of false-negative results include outdated allergens, too little allergen, subcutaneous injections, endogenous glucocorticoid release, off-season testing, and anergy.

▼ *Key Point* The best time of year to test a dog or cat with seasonal allergies is at the end of the season and after clinical signs have declined. Animals with nonseasonal allergies may need to be tested twice a year at opposite seasons.

- Perform a histamine response test before testing or before referring for IDAT.
  - As a pretest, inject intradermally 0.1 ml of 1:100,000 histamine phosphate as the positive control and 0.1 ml of saline as the negative control before performing the full skin test.
  - Read the test 10–15 minutes after making the injections.
  - A red, firm wheal approximately 15 mm in diameter or four times the size of the saline control bleb is an adequate positive response to histamine.
- Some dogs may be tested with manual restraint, but endogenous glucocorticoid release may affect the results. Xylazine HCl (Rompun, Bayer) is the sedative of choice and will not interfere with the results.
  - Give atropine sulfate at 0.02–0.04 mg/kg IM or SC, 15 minutes before administering the xylazine (0.2–0.4 mg/kg IV). The two drugs may also be mixed in the same syringe and given together slowly IV.
  - Other anesthetics and tranquilizers may cause false-negative results.
- Cats may best be tested with chemical restraint in lateral recumbency. Ketamine HCl (5–10 mg/kg IM) is the sedative of choice for cats.
- Use the same antigens in cats as used in the canine test. Read test sites within 10 minutes because the reactions are less indurated, are less erythematous, and dissipate more quickly than in dogs. Experience is vital in performing and interpreting the results in cats.
- Results of IDAT should correlate with clinical history in order to be diagnostic. See Halliwell and Gorman (1989) for a complete discussion of interpreting test results.

In Vitro Allergy Tests

In vitro allergy tests may be helpful when IDAT is not an option because of lack of availability, drug interference, or poor condition of the skin. The radioallergosorbent test (RAST) and the enzyme-linked immunosorbent assay (ELISA) are commercially available in vitro diagnostic tests offered by numerous diagnostic laboratories. A third method uses a liquid phase immuno-enzymatic assay.

These tests detect circulating antigen-specific IgE antibodies in serum. All results are based on a reference standard since there is no commercial source of purified canine IgE. These tests may not be valid for diagnosing feline atopy because feline IgE has only recently been identified experimentally.

Mechanism. The RAST and ELISA are based on incubation of the patient's antibody-laden serum with a substrate containing antigen.

- After incubation, the substrate is rinsed to remove unbound antibody.
- Anti-canine IgE labeled with a radioisotope (RAST) or an enzyme (ELISA) is then added to detect the antigen-antibody complexes formed during the incubation period.
- After several additional washings, the number of complexes is evaluated by a gamma counter to measure the amount of radioactivity (RAST) or a spectrophotometer to measure the degree of color change (ELISA).
- These values are compared with a standard curve from positive control counts to arrive at a semiquantitative measurement of antigen-specific IgE antibodies.

Advantages
- The RAST and ELISA have the following reported benefits:
  - Only 3–5 ml of serum is necessary.
  - Antihistamines and other NSAIDs need not be discontinued.
  - Sedation is not required.
  - Dogs with severely affected skin may be evaluated.
  - Whether residual effects from long-term or concurrent use of corticosteroids can affect test results is controversial.

Accuracy
- Agreement between these tests and IDAT results varies with the allergen (e.g., ragweed, 82%; dandelion, 12%).
- Reproducibility has been shown to be 79.3% for the RAST and 93.1% for the ELISA.
- A correlation between relative antibody levels and clinical hypersensitivity has not been determined.

- In vitro allergy tests have been linked with frequent false-positive results (i.e., normal dogs identified as atopic). False-positive results are thought to be due to high levels of circulating endoparasitic or ectoparasitic IgE antibodies.
- Results of serologic testing and formulation of an allergy vaccine should correlate with the clinical history. Success with desensitization depends on the clinician's ability to accurately interpret the results of either IDAT or in vitro allergy test and to select appropriate antigens for inclusion in a vaccine. Response to hyposensitization based on serologic test results is reportedly comparable to that seen with IDAT results.

TREATMENT

General Treatment Principles

▼ *Key Point* When planning management of atopy, consider concurrent dermatologic abnormalities, length of allergy season, severity of clinical signs, and response to medical therapy. Strict avoidance or elimination of the allergen is the most effective long-term therapeutic approach but is seldom practical or feasible. Consequently, use immunotherapy and medical management to develop a protocol that is tailor-made to fit the individual animal's specific needs.

Pruritic Threshold and Summation of Effects

Understanding and control of these two conceptual phenomena that occur with clinical atopy determine the degree of success of medical therapy.

- The *pruritic threshold* is an individually determined point at which pruritic stimuli will cause an individual to scratch.
- A *summation of effects* occurs when a single stimulus is not sufficient to push the patient over its pruritic threshold, but when a second or third pruritic stimulus is added, pruritus occurs.
  - For example, a dog with atopy remains asymptomatic until xerosis (dry skin) or pyoderma (each potentially pruritic alone) provides the additional stimulus to exceed the pruritic threshold.
  - Treating the pyoderma or dry skin makes the animal asymptomatic again.
- One goal of therapy is to eliminate all factors that lower the pruritic threshold and result in clinical disease. Other dermatologic conditions such as xerosis, pyoderma, and external parasites should be controlled before attempting to treat the allergy.

Concurrent Pyoderma

Concurrent *superficial pyoderma* is the most commonly overlooked cause of pruritus in allergic dogs.

- Pyoderma typically is characterized clinically by follicular papular and pustular eruptions, serous crusts, epidermal collarettes, and patchy alopecia (for a detailed discussion of pyoderma, see Chap. 35).

Concurrent Malassezia Infection

Malassezia pachydermatis, a unipolar budding yeast found in small numbers on normal skin, may cause clinical disease in some dogs and cats as a result of overgrowth. Environmental and patient factors that support the development of clinical disease include increased heat and humidity, abnormal or suppressed immunity, allergies, keratinization disorders, and pyoderma. Treatment of a concurrent pyoderma may result in its resolution, but yeast infections may need to be treated specifically with topical and/or systemic antifungal therapy.

- Infections may be localized or generalized and are characterized by erythema, dry scaly or greasy brown malodorous seborrhea, and intense pruritus.
- In dogs, intertriginous areas such as the ventral neck, tail, facial folds or axillae and the nail beds are commonly affected. Face rubbing, foot licking, and scooting the perineum can be frenzied. Alopecia, hyperpigmentation, and lichenification can develop quickly. In cats, the face, ear canals, interdigital skin, and nail beds are commonly affected.
- Diagnosis is based on finding yeast organisms on cytologic evaluation of material collected from the affected skin.
- Appropriate antifungal topical therapy requires 10- to 15-minute contact time and may include:
  - Chlorhexidine shampoo 1–2% (ChlorhexiDerm [2 and 4%], DVM Pharmaceuticals; Hexadene [3%], Allerderm/Virbac; Sebattex [2%], EVSCO Pharmaceuticals)
  - Benzoyl peroxide (OxyDex and SulfOxydex, DVM Pharmaceuticals; Pyoben, Allerderm/Virbac)
  - Selenium sulfide (Selsun Blue [1%], Ross; Seleen [2.5%], Ceva)
  - Miconazole shampoo (Dermazole—2% miconazole and 0.5% chlorhexidine, Allerderm/Virbac; Miconazole 2%, EVSCO Pharmaceuticals); or ketoconazole (Nizoral, Janssen)
  - Medicated rinses after the shampoo may prolong the therapeutic effect. Rinses include enilconazole (Imaverol, Janssen); acetic acid (white vinegar) and water at a 1:1 or 1:2 ratio; and lime sulfur (LymDyp, DVM Pharmaceuticals).
- Systemic therapy may include ketoconazole (Nizoral, Janssen) at 5–10 mg/kg q12–24h PO for 30 days or itraconazole (Sporanox, Janssen) at 5 mg/kg q24h PO.
- Focal lesions may respond to antifungal creams or lotions containing miconazole (Conofite lotion/cream, Pitman-Moore) or clotrimazole (Lotrimin, Schering Plough).
- Identify and treat the underlying disease. Treat concurrent pyoderma with oral antibiotics and antibacterial shampoo therapy.

Immunotherapy with Hyposensitization

▼ *Key Point* Hyposensitization is the treatment of choice for animals that exhibit signs for longer than 3–4 months, remain uncomfortable with symptomatic therapy, or cannot tolerate corticosteroids.

Medical management, especially with corticosteroids, generally provides immediate relief and is best for short-term use. However, because of the potential for long-term negative systemic side effects as well as the need for higher dosages over time, consider hyposensitization for optimal management of the disease in both dogs and cats. Ideally, the goal of therapy is to increase the patient's ability to tolerate environmental allergens without clinical signs. Realistically, immunotherapy usually allows a significant reduction in symptomatic medical therapy and, occasionally, its elimination. The goal of therapy is to control signs with the minimum amount of medication.

- Of treated dogs, 60–85% are reported to show 50% improvement or better with hyposensitization. Response to therapy may be equivalent with either IDAT or serologic test–based vaccines.
- Most allergy vaccines are made from alum-precipitated or aqueous extracts. Response to both types of vaccines has been similar. Aqueous extracts are more popular in the United States.
  - Alum-precipitated extracts are more expensive than aqueous extracts but are associated with fewer adverse reactions and allow longer intervals between injections.
  - Aqueous extracts are less expensive but must be administered more frequently.
- An allergy vaccine is made for the individual patient based on either serologic or intradermal test results. In addition, selection of antigens is based on the presence of allergens in the environment and a strong correlation of clinical signs with the pollination season.
- No more than 10 antigens are placed in one vaccine, and the maximum amount of antigen should not exceed 20,000 protein nitrogen units (PNU) per milliliter. Although there is no single standard vaccine protocol, all require an initial loading period followed by a maintenance dosage. Once the maintenance dosage is reached, it is repeated every 1–3 weeks and continued year-round.
- Side effects associated with vaccines include postinjection pruritus, pain, urticaria, and occasionally vomiting or diarrhea. Severe anaphylaxis is rare.
- Response to therapy varies with each animal and usually takes several months. Approximately 25% show some improvement in 3 months, another 50% in 6 months, and the remaining 25% in 6–12 months.
  - Continue therapy for at least 12 months before deciding on efficacy.
  - Make sure that other causes of pruritus or dermatitis (e.g., fleas, pyoderma, *Malassezia*, dry skin, food allergy) are not the cause of a perceived failure.

- Signs may return or worsen during the allergy season. The frequency of allergen injections may need to be increased during this period.
  - Antihistamines or alternate-day short-acting glucocorticoids may be added to the immunotherapy as needed. Antihistamines should be added early in the allergy season and continued throughout.
- Evaluate animals that show an initial response but relapse for other causes of pruritus (summation of effects).
  - A second test may be required to identify allergens that were missed because of the time of year when the first test was performed or because the animal has developed sensitivity to new allergens.

Medical Therapy

Medical therapy is the most common approach to management of atopy in both dogs and cats. Choose this protocol when an owner does not wish a full diagnostic workup, when the allergy season is short, or when an animal is too old to fully benefit from hyposensitization.

Medical therapy may also be adjunctive to hyposensitization. Use antihistamines, glucocorticoids, NSAIDs, essential fatty acid (EFA) supplements, and topical shampoo therapy to help control the signs of atopy. Design the therapeutic protocol to fit the animal's specific needs.

Antihistamines

Antihistamines alone control pruritus in approximately 20–40% of purely atopic dogs and are the drugs of choice for symptomatic therapy. The magnitude of response varies individually. If antihistamines are unable to control all the signs, they are at least "steroid sparing," allowing a lower dosage of glucocorticoids to be used.

▼ *Key Point* Identify and control other cutaneous diseases such as flea allergy, food allergy, xerosis, superficial pyoderma, and *Malassezia* infection because antihistamines are rarely effective when these conditions are present.

- Antihistamines are used to provide anti-inflammatory and antipruritic benefit through blockage of H_1 receptors. Some antihistamines also have antianxiety, analgesic, or sedative effects that add to patient comfort (Table 41–1).
- Doxepin HCl and amitriptyline HCl are tricyclic antidepressant drugs with potent antihistamine effects. These are often tried when the animal fails to respond to chlorpheniramine or diphenhydramine, or when there is a "behavioral component" to self-trauma (pruritus).
- Adverse side effects of antihistamines include sedation, hyperexcitability, and anticholinergic reactions.
- It is helpful to prescribe a 2-week course for each of three different antihistamines representing different classes and then choose the one most effective for maintenance therapy.

Table 41–1. ANTIHISTAMINES USED COMMONLY FOR PRURITUS

Class	Antihistamine	Brand Name	Recommended Oral Dosage Canine	Feline
Alkylamine	Chlorpheniramine maleate	Chlor-Trimeton (various)	0.4 mg/kg q8–12h	2–4 mg/cat q12h
Ethanolamine	Diphenhydramine HCl	Benadryl (various)	2.2 mg/kg q8–12h	—
Piperazine	Hydroxyzine HCl	Atarax (various)	2.2 mg/kg q8–12h	10 mg/cat q12h
Piperidine	Cyproheptadine	Periactin (various)	0.5–1.0 mg/kg q12h	—
Tricyclic antidepressant	Doxepin HCl	Sinequan (various)	2.2 mg/kg q8–12h	—
Tricyclic antidepressant	Amitriptyline HCl	Elavil	2.2 mg/kg q8–12h	10 mg/cat q12h
Unclassified	Terfenadine	Seldane	5–10 mg/kg q12h	—
Ethanolamine	Clemastine fumarate	Tavist	0.05 mg/kg q12h	—

- Antihistamines in combination with allergen avoidance, immunotherapy, EFA supplements, or NSAIDs may render the animal asymptomatic.

Systemic Glucocorticoids

- These drugs are very effective in controlling pruritus; however, use them as exclusive therapy only in seasonally (<3 months in duration) allergic animals.
- Glucocorticoids are valuable as adjunctive therapy; their use along with antihistamines, EFA supplements, or immunotherapy allows smaller quantities to be given less frequently.
- Although they are the most rapidly effective of anti-inflammatory drugs, they are also associated with the worst side effects.
- Principles for the use of systemic glucocorticoids include
  - Establish the cause of pruritus and provide specific treatment.
  - Eliminate contributory processes such as pyoderma, *Malassezia* infection, fleas, or dry skin.
  - Educate the owner and minimize risk to the patient.
  - Use the lowest dose of an oral short-acting glucocorticoid on an alternate-day basis when possible.
  - Combine alternative therapy (antihistamines, EFAs, etc.) with glucocorticoids to achieve the lowest dosage possible.
  - Strive to manage the disease without steroids.
- Never use glucocorticoids when concurrent pyoderma is present.

Mechanism of Action
- Glucocorticoids decrease inflammation and pruritus by the following mechanisms:
  - Inhibiting chemotaxis of inflammatory cells.
  - Inhibiting normal function of lymphocytes and macrophages.
  - Stabilizing cellular membranes and thereby preventing mast cell degranulation and the release of intracellular and membrane-associated inflammatory mediators.
  - Inhibiting vasodilation and the resulting erythema and edema.
- Low-dose alternate-day therapy provides the antipruritic effects without interfering significantly with the hypothalamic-pituitary-adrenal (HPA) axis or the normal immune response.
- Anti-inflammatory dosages do not interfere with antibody production or antigen-antibody interaction.
- Once the corticosteroid is discontinued, the inflammatory processes proceed uninhibited. Symptoms return and are often more severe than before therapy.

Side Effects
Side effects are numerous and reflect individual sensitivity as well as formulation, dosage, and duration of therapy.

- A *stress leukogram* (leukocytosis with neutropenia, eosinopenia, monocytosis) and increased serum alkaline phosphatase is seen in almost every case. Some animals also show an increase in serum alanine aminotransferase, glucose, and cholesterol.
- *Polyuria, polydipsia, polyphagia, and weight gain* are commonly observed with the short-acting oral glucocorticoids (prednisolone and prednisone).
- Occasionally an animal will become *anorectic*, with evidence of *weight loss and muscle wasting*. Panting, muscle weakness, exercise intolerance, hepatomegaly, and pancreatitis also may occur.
- All glucocorticoids *suppress the HPA axis*. With repositol glucocorticoids, this suppression lasts longer than the anti-inflammatory effects. Slowly withdraw long-acting glucocorticoids that have been administered for an extended period of time, because treated animals are functionally addisonian and will not have the reserve necessary to respond to stress. Alternate-day prednisone and prednisolone prevent this phenomenon.
- Some animals demonstrate bizarre *behavior changes* even with low dosages of glucocorticoids; these are eliminated on discontinuance of the drug.
- *Dermatologic changes* observed in both dogs and cats that are associated with glucocorticoids include xerosis, comedone formation (dogs), loss of skin tone and elasticity, epidermal and dermal atrophy, bruising, and calcinosis cutis (dogs).
- *Suppression of immune and inflammatory responses* may result in of pyoderma, demodicosis, or dermatophyte infection.

▼ *Key Point* When previously well-controlled animals become acutely pruritic or develop a nonpruritic pustular dermatosis, take skin scrapings, fungal culture, and culture of an intact pustule for bacteria. Positive results dictate weaning from the corticosteroid, appropriate treatment of the infection, and the use of an alternative symptomatic therapeutic protocol.

Dosage and Formulation

- The dosage and formulation of a glucocorticoid determines whether it will have antipruritic, anti-inflammatory, or immunosuppressive effects.
  - Classified as *short-acting glucocorticoids,* prednisone and prednisolone are anti-inflammatory when given at an initial dosage of 2.2 mg/kg q12h PO to cats, and 0.5 mg/kg q12h PO to dogs. Antipruritic effects are seen with 0.1–0.25 mg/kg q12h PO in the dog and with 0.5 mg/kg q12h PO in the cat.
  - An anti-inflammatory dosage of an *intermediate-acting glucocorticoid* such as triamcinolone (Vetalog, Solvay) at 0.25 mg/kg q24h PO for 5 days, then q48–72h PO is appropriate for managing atopic animals with a limited season.
  - An alternative approach is to give a single dose of triamcinolone at 0.25 mg/kg IM to dogs and 1 mg/kg IM to cats; the antipruritic effect may last up to six weeks.
  - An anti-inflammatory dosage of dexamethasone is 0.2–0.4 mg/kg q24h IM.
  - *Long-acting glucocorticoids* continue to suppress the HPA axis long after the antipruritic effects have waned and are not recommended for maintenance therapy.
- *Course of therapy.* Initiate a short-acting glucocorticoid at an anti-inflammatory dose, q12h for 5 days, reduce to q24h for 5 days, and then administer q48h for 2 weeks.
- If the animal remains asymptomatic, further reduce the dosage to the lowest possible level that controls pruritus. Continue this dose throughout the allergy season.
- Methylprednisolone acetate (Depo-Medrol, Upjohn) is a potent *ultra-long-acting glucocorticoid.*
  - This glucocorticoid is of questionable value in canine atopy and is restricted to dogs with very short (<3 months) allergy seasons whose symptoms can be managed with one or two injections. Never administer it more frequently than every 8 weeks in dogs.
  - Methylprednisolone acetate (4.4 mg/kg IM) is frequently chosen for the pruritic cat. Do not administer it more frequently than every 8 weeks in cats.

Topical Glucocorticoids

Use these agents to treat focal areas of inflammation. The potency of the preparation is determined by the specific steroid and its concentration, the carrier vehicle (lotion, cream, or ointment), and the method of application. The more occlusive the vehicle, the more potent the product. Ointments are more occlusive than creams; creams are more occlusive than lotions.

- Remember that dry lesions should be moistened so a more occlusive dressing can be used. Moist lesions must be allowed to dry.
- Side effects may be local (poor wound healing, cutaneous atrophy, or pigmentary changes) or systemic (iatrogenic hyperadrenocorticism, folliculitis), depending on the potency of the product and how much is systemically absorbed.
- Control the dermatitis using a potent fluorinated steroid such as amcinonide (Cyclocort, Lederle) for the first several days. Then switch to the lowest-potency topical steroid that will control the dermatitis over the long term (0.5–1.0% hydrocortisone cream).
- Where large areas of the body are affected, medicated shampoos (Cortisoothe, Allerderm) containing 1% hydrocortisone provide temporary relief. Leave-on rinses (ResiCort, Allerderm) have a more prolonged effect than shampoos and are applied after a medicated shampoo.

Essential Fatty Acids

The essential fatty acids (EFAs), which comprise linoleic acid (LA), alpha linolenic acid (ALA), and arachidonic acid (AA), are long-chain omega-3 (ALA) and omega-6 (LA and AA) polyunsaturated fatty acids that are incorporated into all cellular membranes. They are required for all cellular membrane structure and function, cannot be synthesized de novo, and therefore must be provided in the diet. AA also is the substrate for inflammatory mediators called eicosanoids (leukotrienes, prostaglandins, hydroxy fatty acids). Certain dietary EFAs exhibit anti-inflammatory properties by competing with AA.

- EFA supplements marketed for use in cutaneous inflammatory skin disease contain a combination of gamma linolenic acid (GLA, from evening primrose oil), eicosapentaenoic acid (EPA, from fish oil), and linoleic acid (LA, from vegetable oil).

▼ *Key Point* The two most important "anti-inflammatory" EFAs are GLA and EPA because they both compete with AA for cellular binding sites and for the enzymes that make eicosanoids.

- Administration of GLA alone and in combination with EPA has resulted in improvement in redness, scale, and pruritus associated with inflammatory skin diseases. Clinical improvement is speculated to be associated with simultaneous changes in tissue eicosanoids and fatty acids. Studies indicate that optimal biochemical effects are not seen until 6–12 weeks of therapy. Optimal clinical improvement is not seen until 8–12 weeks of therapy.
- EFA veterinary products are numerous. Results are variable in the improvement of pruritus, erythema, and coat condition when used alone.

- The amount and ratio of specific fatty acids in veterinary products vary considerably. Atopic dermatitis with pruritus responds best to products that contain GLA and EPA with minimal or no LA.
- Because a variety of proteolytic enzymes and inflammatory mediators are involved in the pathogenesis of allergic dermatitis in dogs and cats, results from EFA supplementation range from zero to marked improvement. Realistically, expect a mild to moderate improvement in clinical signs when administering EFA supplements alone.
- Synergistic effects are achieved when used with antihistamines or glucocorticoids. Administer at twice the manufacturer's recommended dosage q12h for a minimum of 8 weeks before assessing response.

Nonsteroidal Anti-Inflammatory Agents

- Aspirin (10 mg/kg q12h PO with food) is occasionally beneficial in dogs and provides temporary relief from pruritus and inflammation, especially during periods of glucocorticoid withdrawal (usually 1–2 weeks) prior to skin testing.
- Anorexia, vomiting, melena, or evidence of abnormal bleeding signals the need to discontinue the drug.
- Do not use NSAIDs of any kind in cats and do not use ibuprofen and acetaminophen in dogs.

Supportive Topical Therapy

This is one of the most beneficial forms of adjunctive therapy.

- The broad range of products available allows the therapy to be fairly specific for the dermatologic problem.
- As the condition improves, modify topical therapy accordingly.
- Disadvantages:
  - It is time-consuming for the owner.
  - The patient must be fairly cooperative.
  - The immediate benefits (reduction in pruritus) are usually short-lived.

Shampoo Therapy. Shampoo therapy is helpful in the atopic animal to remove dirt and antigenic debris, to rehydrate a dry stratum corneum, and to provide the soothing effects of hydrotherapy.

▼ *Key Point* Contact time for shampoo therapy should be at least 10 minutes. Less time results in the removal of surface oils without the benefit of rehydrating the stratum corneum.

- *Antibacterial shampoos* include benzoyl peroxide (Pyoben, Allerderm; OxyDex and Sulf-OxyDex, DVM Pharmaceuticals; Benzoyl Plus, EVSCO Pharmaceuticals); chlorhexidine (Nolvasan, Fort Dodge; ChlorhexiDerm, DVM Pharmaceuticals; Sebahex, EVSCO Pharmaceuticals), and ethyl lactate (Etiderm, Allerderm). Benzoyl peroxide shampoos have the added benefit of follicular flushing and antipruritic activity but can be very drying. Use a humectant or bath oil rinse after bathing to diminish this side effect.
- *Antiseborrheic shampoos* containing 2% sulfur and 2% salicylic acid (SebaLyt, DVM Pharmaceuticals; SeboRx, DVM Pharmaceuticals; Sebolux, Allerderm) have mild antipruritic and antibacterial properties in addition to their ability to reduce the production of epidermal scale.
  - Tar shampoos, which usually are formulated with sulfur and salicylic acid, provide the additional benefit of strong degreasing activity but tend to be irritating.
  - Do not use tar products on cats.

Cool Water Soaks. These are excellent for managing acute exacerbations of local and generalized pruritus.

- An astringent such as aluminum acetate (Domeboro, Bayer) may be added to the water (one tablet or packet per pint of water) and will decrease the redness and swelling associated with inflammation.
- Colloidal oatmeal products (Epi-Soothe Bath Treatment, Allerderm; Aveeno, Rydelle Labs) added to the cool water or used in a shampoo (Epi-Soothe, Allerderm/Virbac) will reduce the redness, swelling, and pruritus for several hours after application.

Humectants. Humectants (Humilac, Allerderm/Virbac; Micro Pearls Humectant Spray, EVSCO Pharmaceuticals) and bath oils (HyLyt*efa, DVM Pharmaceuticals; Sesame Oil Rinse, Veterinary Prescription; Alpha Keri Bath Oil, Westwood) help raise the pruritic threshold by relieving dry skin conditions.

- The most beneficial effects are seen when applied after the stratum corneum has been hydrated (i.e., after a bath).
- The most even distribution is achieved when the product (2–5 capfuls) is added to 1–2 quarts of water and used as a rinse after the bath.

SUPPLEMENTAL READINGS

Bevier D: Long-term management of atopic disease in the dog. Vet Clin North Am 20:1487, 1990.

Griffin C: RAST and ELISA testing in canine atopy. *In* Kirk RW, ed.: Current Veterinary Therapy X. Philadelphia: WB Saunders, 1989, p 592.

Griffin CE: Canine atopic disease. *In* Griffin CE, Kwochka KW, MacDonald JM, eds.: Current Veterinary Dermatology: The Science and Art of Therapy. St. Louis: Mosby–Year Book, 1993, pp 3–21.

Halliwell REW, Gorman NT: Veterinary Clinical Immunology. Philadelphia: WB Saunders, 1989, p 232.

Sousa CA, Norton AL: Advances in methodology for diagnosis of allergic skin disease. Vet Clin North Am 20:1419, 1990.

Willemse TA: Atopic dermatitis. *In* Nesbitt GH, ed.: Contemporary Issues in Small Animal Practice: Dermatology. New York: Churchill Livingstone, 1987, p 57.

Willemse TA, Van Den Brom WE, Rijnberk A: Effect of hyposensitization on atopic dermatitis in dogs. J Am Vet Med Assoc 184:1277, 1984.

42 Food Hypersensitivity

Stephen D. White

Adverse reactions to foods have been well documented in small animals. The terms "food allergy" and "food hypersensitivity" have been used interchangeably in the human and veterinary medical literature to describe symptoms induced by food ingestion in which there are demonstrable or highly suspected immunologic reactions. The terms "food intolerance" and occasionally "food sensitivity" have been used when an immunologic etiology is unlikely or has not been established. Although the causes of abnormal reactions to ingested foods have not always been well established in small animals, food hypersensitivity and food allergy are the terms commonly used. The author prefers the former as being more accurate in describing an abnormal response of the immune system. For discussion of inhalant allergies, see Chapter 41.

ETIOLOGY

The exact mechanisms of food hypersensitivity have not been delineated in dogs and cats. Reactions to food have been noted in dogs and cats that could be termed immediate (i.e., hypersensitivity type I, occurring within minutes to hours after ingestion) or delayed (i.e., type IV, occurring within hours to days of ingestion).

- Food contaminants such as pathogenic bacteria and toxins, food additives such as tartrazines, and vasoactive amines such as tyramine in cheese have all been implicated or suspected as mimicking food hypersensitivity in humans. Their importance in small animals is unknown.
- Suspected or confirmed dietary allergens are numerous in the literature. Confirmed allergens include beef, soy, dairy products, and cereal as the most common allergens in dogs and beef, milk, and fish as the most common in cats. Other allergens reported include cheese, chicken, chicken eggs, lamb, and chocolate.
  - The author has identified fish as an offending allergen in 50% of cats with food hypersensitivity.
  - The vast array of foodstuffs used in commercial pet foods, as well as variable processing methods, probably accounts for the large numbers of allergens reported.

CLINICAL SIGNS

▼ *Key Point* Although the age of onset is variable, predisposition is noted for young dogs (≤1 year of age). Owners seldom relate the onset of clinical signs to any change in diet.

No sex predilections have been noted in dogs or cats with food hypersensitivity. Terriers and Siamese cats may be predisposed. Clinical signs are variable.

- Pruritus is the most common sign in dogs; rarely, nonpruritic animals are reported. The pruritus is often distributed similar to that in inhalant allergies (i.e., feet, ears, face, and axillae). Cutaneous lesions noted in dogs include papules, erythema, epidermal collarettes, pododermatitis, seborrhea, and otitis externa.
- In cats with food hypersensitivity, clinical signs include generalized pruritus, miliary dermatitis, facial and head pruritus, pruritic angioedema-urticaria, eosinophilic plaque, eosinophilic ulcer, and erythema.
- Gastrointestinal signs (vomiting, diarrhea) have also been noted (see Chaps. 87 and 89). These may be more common than previously thought. Dogs in particular may show signs suggestive of colitis. In cats, food hypersensitivity has been manifested as lymphocytic-plasmacytic colitis.
- Neurologic signs (epileptiform seizures, malaise) and respiratory distress (asthma-like syndromes) occasionally have been reported.
- Multiple organ involvement is uncommon.

DIAGNOSIS

- Suspect food hypersensitivity in the following situations:
  - Nonseasonal occurrence of pruritic skin lesions.
  - Lack of response to steroidal or other anti-inflammatory drugs in dogs and cats, although efficacy of corticosteroids in controlling pruritus does not rule out a diagnosis of food hypersensitivity.
  - Lack of response to progestational drugs in cats.

Laboratory Findings

There are no consistent laboratory findings in small animals with food hypersensitivity. Peripheral eosinophilia may or may not be present. Histopathologic findings are nondiagnostic, usually characterized by a perivascular dermatitis, with neutrophils or mononuclear cells predominating and variable secondary suppurative changes. Tissue eosinophilia is uncommon but has been reported.

Intradermal Skin Testing

Intradermal skin testing with food extracts usually has been unrewarding in humans and small animals, possibly owing to changes in composition of the allergen with digestion or to improper dilution of the test allergen.

Serologic Diagnostic Tests

Serologic diagnostics using the radioallergosorbent test (RAST) or the enzyme-linked immunosorbent assay (ELISA) for reaginic antibodies in humans correlate with history and provocative exposure tests in over 50% of cases reported. However, the data from two studies, one utilizing RAST (White and Mason, 1990) and one utilizing the ELISA test (Jeffers et al., 1991), have shown that these tests are of no value in small animals.

▼ *Key Point* The most valid and most often recommended method for diagnosis of food hypersensitivity is the restricted ("hypoallergenic") test diet.

Hypoallergenic Test Diet

- Feed the pet a diet with a limited number of foodstuffs. It is important to select foods that the animal has not been fed previously. The author currently uses a 1:1 mix of pinto beans and potatoes for dogs. If the dog refuses to eat this diet, tuna fish packed in water, using enough to flavor the potatoes, is used. Dogs that live in households with cats may already have been exposed to fish through their ingestion of cat food or cat feces.
- For cats, one can use lamb-based baby food, provided it is not flavored with onion powder, and there is thus no concern of inducing a Heinz-body hemolytic anemia. Other single protein sources (such as turkey or rabbit) also can be used. If the cat will not eat such a diet, one of several commercially prepared foods may be fed. Of the latter, the author has the most experience in using a lamb-based food (Prescription Diet Feline d/d, Hill's Pet Products) or a rabbit-, lamb-, duck- or venison-based food (Innovative Veterinary Diets).
- Hypoallergenic diets should be free of colorings, preservatives, and flavorings. Do not give palatable medications, such as certain heartworm preventatives (substitute another type of heartworm preventative for the duration of the diet), and omit all vitamin and mineral supplements.
- Commercially prepared pet foods, including diets containing no preservatives and diets marketed as

"natural," are *not* adequate test diets. These products do not meet the criteria for a true restricted test diet because of the many foodstuffs they contain and the processing of these ingredients.
- Clinical signs may recur when animals are switched from the home-prepared test diet to the aforementioned commercially prepared limited-antigen diets.
- Occasionally, an animal may be presented to the clinician with pruritus so severe that administration of oral corticosteroids is justified while the diet is in progress.
  - Administer prednisone or prednisolone, 0.5–1.0 mg/kg PO q24h for 10 days, and then stop.
  - Continue the diet for a minimum of 2 weeks beyond discontinuation of the medication in order to properly evaluate response to diet.
  - Apply the same guidelines when giving antibiotics to animals with secondary pyoderma.

Results

- Clinical improvement is observed in most animals within 24 hours to 3 weeks after starting the diet.
- In the author's experience, 8 weeks is a reasonable length of time in which to expect some improvement. Improvement is best defined as a reduction of pruritus (or other clinical signs if pruritus is absent).
- If only partial improvement is noted, the diet may not have been given long enough for full effectiveness.
- Alternatively, evaluate the restricted diet's content and consider a change (e.g., substitute potatoes for rice).
- Consider other, concurrent hypersensitivities, such as fleas and inhalant allergens.

TREATMENT

Once improvement is noted, several treatment alternatives are open to the clinician.

- Ideally, challenge the animal with its original diet in order to substantiate the diagnosis. This is particularly important when the clinical improvement noted has been seen over the course of a change in season. This could have resulted in a decreased exposure to environmental aeroallergens (such as pollens) which may have led to improvement in an atopic pet, rather than improvement from the change in diet. A relapse in the condition is usually seen within 72 hours but may take as long as 2 weeks, particularly when a hypersensitivity to cereals is involved. Add individual foodstuffs to the restricted diet at 5- to 10-day intervals until a balanced diet is achieved or the offending allergen(s) is discovered.
- Many owners are unwilling to exacerbate a clinically improved animal or separate out various components of foods to determine potential allergens and are more interested in achieving a balanced, less expensive diet as soon as possible.
- Once the diagnosis of food hypersensitivity is confirmed, the pet's diet may be changed to one of the

commercially available limited-allergen diets. In cats, the author uses those diets previously mentioned (see Hypoallergenic Test Diet). In dogs, the author has the most experience using a fish-based food (Response Formula FP, Iams Company) or a rabbit-, lamb-, duck- or venison-based food (IVD, Innovative Veterinary Diets). If the new diet is not tolerated, most animals show a recurrence of clinical signs within 72 hours, although a few pets may take longer.

- If the animal cannot tolerate a commercial diet, use a home-prepared diet consisting of a protein and carbohydrate source supplemented with vitamins, minerals, and, for cats, 60–100 mg of taurine daily. Supplementation with 0.5 teaspoon of clam juice per day, recommended by some, is *not* adequate taurine supplementation. For further information on additive-free supplements for homemade hypoallergenic diets, the reader is referred to the article by Roudebush and Cowell (1992).

SUPPLEMENTAL READINGS

Carlotti DN, Remy I, Prost C: Food allergy in dogs and cats: A review and report of 43 cases. Vet Derm 1:55, 1990.

Guaguère E: Food intolerance in cats with cutaneous manifestations: A review of 17 cases. Eur J Comp Anim Pract 5:27, 1995.

Harvey RG: Food allergy and dietary intolerance in dogs: A report of 25 cases. J Small Anim Pract 34:175, 1993.

Jeffers JG, Meyer EK, Sosis EJ: Responses of dogs with food allergies to single ingredient dietary provocation. J Am Vet Med Assoc 209:608, 1996.

Jeffers JG, Shanley KJ, Meyer EK: Diagnostic testing for canine food hypersensitivity. J Am Vet Med Assoc 198:245, 1991.

Patterson S: Food hypersensitivity in 20 dogs with skin and gastrointestinal signs. J Small Anim Pract 36:529, 1995.

Rosser EJ: Diagnosis of food allergy in dogs. J Am Vet Med Assoc 203:259, 1993.

Rosser EJ: Food allergy in the cat: A prospective study of 13 cats. *In* Ihrke PJ, Mason IS, White SD, eds.: Advances in Veterinary Dermatology, Vol 2. Oxford, England: Pergamon Press, 1993, pp 33–39.

Rosser EJ, White SD: Diet and the skin in companion animals. *In* Kwochka KW, von Tscharner C, Willemse T, eds: Advances in Veterinary Dermatology, Vol 3. Oxford, England: Pergamon Press, 1998.

Roudebush P, Cowell CS: Results of a hypoallergenic diet survey of veterinarians of North America with a nutritional evaluation of homemade diet prescriptions. Vet Derm 3:23, 1992.

White SD: Food allergy in dogs. Compend Contin Educ 20:261 1998.

White SD: Food hypersensitivity in 30 dogs. J Am Vet Med Assoc 188:695, 1986.

White SD, Mason IS: Proceedings of the Dietary Allergy Workshop. *In* Von Tscharner C, Halliwell REW, eds.: Advances in Veterinary Dermatology, Vol I. London: Baillière Tindall, 1990, p 404.

White SD, Sequoia D: Food hypersensitivity in cats: 14 cases (1982–1987). J Am Vet Med Assoc 194:692, 1989.

43   Immune-Mediated Dermatoses

Karen Helton-Rhodes

Immune-mediated dermatoses are a relatively uncommon group of diseases in domestic animals. This group may be divided into autoimmune and immune-mediated categories according to immunopathogenesis.

- Autoimmune diseases, which include the pemphigus complex, bullous pemphigoid, and Vogt-Koyanagi-Harada syndrome, are characterized by a specific antibody- or cell-mediated immune response produced and directed against a normal component of the skin or body.
- Systemic lupus erythematosus and cutaneous (discoid) lupus erythematosus are examples of immune-mediated dermatoses in which antigen-antibody complexes are formed and then deposited in various locations (vessel walls, glomeruli of the kidney, or basement membrane zone of the skin) (see Chap. 26). This deposition of immune complexes may then trigger an inflammatory response that results in tissue destruction.
- Vasculitis may be placed in the autoimmune or the immune-mediated category, depending on the underlying etiology (see Chap. 46).

PEMPHIGUS COMPLEX

The pemphigus complex of diseases includes pemphigus foliaceus (the most common of this group), pemphigus erythematosus, pemphigus vulgaris, and pemphigus vegetans.

▼ **Key Point** Pemphigus foliaceus is the most common autoimmune skin disorder in dogs and cats.

- Pemphigus erythematosus is considered a variant of pemphigus foliaceus. It may have clinical and histopathologic features of lupus erythematosus and is therefore considered a "crossover" between the pemphigus and lupus erythematosus complexes.
- Pemphigus vegetans is an extremely rare variant of pemphigus vulgaris that is distinguished clinically from the other autoimmune diseases by the production of lesions that are vegetative (i.e., proliferative) rather than pustular or ulcerative.

Etiology

The exact cause or stimulant of the production of the pemphigus antibody is unknown.

- Some investigators believe that a virus spread by an insect vector may be the initial stimulus. This theory gains support from an endemic form of pemphigus (fogo selvagem) in humans in South America.
- Genetic factors may be equally important.
- In humans, once formed, the antibody binds with components found in the core of the desmosome (desmoglein I or plakoglobin). Desmosomes function as attachment areas between keratinocytes of the skin. This binding stimulates plasminogen activators, i.e., serine proteases, which subsequently cause the conversion of plasminogen to plasmin.
  - The production of plasmin causes the disruption of the desmosome attachments and therefore a loss of keratinocyte adhesion. This loss of adhesion between adjacent cells is called acantholysis, and the individual cells are termed acantholytic cells.
- All of the diseases in the pemphigus complex appear to have the same immunopathogenesis, but the location of the bulla or separation within the epidermis differs (e.g., pemphigus foliaceus has a more superficial bulla than pemphigus vulgaris).

Clinical Signs

Pemphigus Foliaceus

- Breeds that are predisposed include Akitas, chow chows, bearded collies, dachshunds, Doberman pinschers, schipperkes, and rottweilers.
- Lesions consist of erythematous macules that progress rapidly to a pustular phase and then appear as a dry, yellow crust. These lesions may be limited to the pinnal, perioral, periocular, dorsal muzzle, nasal planum, and/or nail bed regions or they may be generalized.
- Animals may present with marked hyperkeratosis (scaling) of the footpads with or without nail bed involvement. The nails usually are normal.
- Cats commonly exhibit a marked paronychia that appears as a thick "cheesy" core of exudate when the nails are extruded manually.
- Mucocutaneous and oral lesions are rare.
- Pruritus is variable.

Pemphigus Erythematosus

- Pemphigus erythematosus is a rarely recognized variant of pemphigus foliaceus.
- Collies appear to be at risk.

- Lesions are similar to those of pemphigus foliaceus but are limited to the face.
- Some animals may show depigmentation of the planum nasale.

Pemphigus Vulgaris

- Lesions are characterized as vesicobullous eruptions that rapidly ulcerate, leaving thick crusts.
- Lesions may be primarily mucocutaneous in location or generalized.
- Onychomadesis (loss or shedding of the nails) and footpad ulcerations are common.
- Ulceration of the oral cavity may be an initial presenting sign in over 50% of cases.
- Pruritus and pain are variable.

Pemphigus Vegetans

- Pemphigus vegetans is an extremely rare variant of pemphigus vulgaris.
- Lesions usually are generalized rather than mucocutaneous.
- Lesions are vegetative (proliferative) or verrucous (wart-like).

Diagnosis

▼ *Key Point* Histopathologic examination of skin biopsies gives the most valuable diagnostic information. Obtain at least three biopsies of the freshest pustules, vesicles, or bullae or from the edge of an ulcerated lesion.

Pemphigus Foliaceus

- Direct smear of an intact pustule or surface beneath a thick crust reveals numerous acantholytic cells.
- Complete blood count (CBC), serum biochemical profile, and urinalysis are nondiagnostic.
- Antinuclear antibody (ANA) tests are negative.

▼ *Key Point* False-positive ANA titers may be seen in animals with pemphigus, rheumatoid arthritis, idiopathic thrombocytopenia, autoimmune hemolytic anemia, thyroiditis, endocarditis, cancer, hepatotoxicity, feline leukemia, feline infectious peritonitis, dirofilariasis, demodicosis, and flea allergy dermatitis, and even may be seen in clinically normal animals.

- Histopathologic findings include subcorneal and/or intragranular pustules with acantholytic cells.
- Direct immunofluorescent antibody (IFA) tests and direct immunoperoxidase staining (IPS) tests are positive, with intercellular staining of immunoglobulin and/or complement in the upper one-third of the epidermis.

▼ *Key Point* Indirect pemphigus titers using serum are unreliable in dogs and cats.

▼ *Key Point* IFA is positive in only 50% of autoimmune cases, whereas IPS is very sensitive and is positive in 95% of confirmed cases. However, IPS is not very specific; positive results are obtained in 73% of animals with pyoderma, 67% with dermatophytes, 50% with demodicosis, and 100% with scabies. Also, IPS is positive with the immunoreactant IgG in an intercellular pattern in biopsies obtained from normal canine planum nasale and footpads. IFA is positive with the immunoreactant immunoglobulin M (IgM) in a basement membrane zone pattern in 75% of normal canine nasal biopsies and 45% of biopsies of normal footpads, thus yielding false-positive results.

Pemphigus Erythematosus

- Direct smears are similar to those of pemphigus foliaceus.
- CBC, serum biochemical profile, and urinalysis are nondiagnostic.
- ANA tests are positive, with low titers, in 50% of cases.
- Histopathologic findings include subcorneal and/or intragranular pustules, hydropic degeneration of the basal cell layer, and dyskeratotic cells.
- IFA and IPS are positive (see preceding Key Point), with staining in the intercellular pattern with or without concurrent staining in the basement membrane zone.

Pemphigus Vulgaris

- Direct smears are similar to those of pemphigus foliaceus.
- CBC, serum biochemical profile, and urinalysis are nondiagnostic.
- ANA tests are negative.
- Histopathologic findings include suprabasilar pustules with acantholysis.
- IFA and IPS are positive (see preceding Key Point), with intercellular deposition of immunoglobulin or complement in the lower one-third of the epidermis.

Pemphigus Vegetans

- Direct smears are similar to those of pemphigus foliaceus.
- CBC, serum biochemical profile, and urinalysis are nondiagnostic.
- ANA tests are negative.
- Histopathologic findings include intraepidermal acantholytic eosinophilic microabscesses with significant surface crusting and verrucous vegetations and papillomatous proliferations.
- IFA and IPS are positive (see preceding Key Point), with an intercellular staining pattern.

Treatment

General Considerations

Management is similar for each of the diseases in the pemphigus complex.

▼ *Key Point* The goal in treating autoimmune skin diseases is to keep the condition in satisfactory remission on a "safe" dose of medication. It is better for the animal to have a few lesions present on low-dose alternate-day steroids than for the animal to have normal skin on high doses of daily steroids.

- For initial therapy choose prednisone. If the response is poor, add a chemotherapeutic agent such as azathioprine to the protocol.
- For more rapid and complete resolution of clinical signs with less resistance to therapy, start with a regimen of prednisone and an adjunctive chemotherapeutic drug.
- Maintain medications at a high dose until clinical signs have resolved at least 75–85%, then gradually decrease dosages while monitoring the animal for exacerbation of disease.
- Taper either the prednisone or the chemotherapeutic agent first, depending on side effects noted.
- Another option is to alternate the dosage decreases of the two medications until there is complete remission and therapy is no longer necessary or until the minimum dosage of drug needed to control the disease is found.
- Initially, monitor CBC and platelet count every 2 weeks. After the disease is controlled and the level of medication is being tapered, gradually decrease the frequency of monitoring to every 1–2 months.

Therapeutic Protocols

Prednisone as a Single Therapeutic Agent

- Prednisone, 2–4 mg/kg PO divided q12h (dogs) or 2–6 mg/kg, PO divided q12h (cats)
- Use in conjunction with over-the-counter sunscreens and topical steroids.
- Treatment of choice for pemphigus erythematosus

Prednisone with Azathioprine

- Prednisone, 2–4 mg/kg PO divided q12h in combination with azathioprine (Imuran, Burroughs-Wellcome), 1–2 mg/kg PO q24–48h (dogs)
- Treatment of choice for pemphigus foliaceus, pemphigus vulgaris, and pemphigus vegetans
- Side effects of azathioprine include vomiting, diarrhea, pancreatitis, dermatitis, anemia, bone marrow suppression, and hepatotoxicity.
- Monitor CBC and platelet count every 2 weeks.

▼ *Key Point* Do not use azathioprine in cats because of idiosyncratic reactions characterized by severe, nonresponsive leukopenia and thrombocytopenia.

Prednisone with Chlorambucil

- Prednisone, 2–4 mg/kg PO divided q12h in combination with chlorambucil (Leukeran, Burroughs-Wellcome), 0.2 mg/kg PO q24–48h
- Treatment of choice for pemphigus complex in small dogs and all cats
- Toxicity from this protocol is mild and includes vomiting, anorexia, and diarrhea (usually resolves when the dose is changed from a daily to an alternate-day regimen) and a mild, gradual, and rapidly reversible myelosuppressive effect.
- Monitor CBC and platelet count every 2 weeks.

Gold Therapy

- Aurothioglucose (gold salts) (Solganal, Schering), 1 mg/kg IM once weekly, until remission is achieved (usually 6–8 weeks); then every 2 weeks for 6 months; then monthly as a maintenance regimen
- Prednisone, 2 mg/kg PO divided q12h, also may be needed until remission is achieved.
- Gold therapy is suitable for both dogs and cats; however, results appear to be much better in cats.
- Auranofin (Ridaura, SmithKline Beecham), an oral form of gold salts, has been tried in a limited number of cases but needs further investigation for use in dogs and cats.
- Side effects include thrombocytopenia, aplastic anemia, toxic epidermal necrolysis, stomatitis, nephrotic syndrome, hepatotoxicity, dermatitis, and pancreatitis. Eosinophilia may herald toxicity.
- Monitor CBC, platelet count, and urinalysis every 2 weeks during the first 3 months of treatment and serum chemistry values monthly.

BULLOUS PEMPHIGOID

Etiology

The immunopathogenesis of bullous pemphigoid involves antibody production directed against the hemidesmosomes located in the lamina lucida region of the basement membrane zone of the skin. The complement cascade is then activated, causing the release of components C3a and C5a, which triggers mast cell degranulation. Mast cell mediators attract inflammatory cells that release lysosomal enzymes, resulting in tissue destruction and subepidermal blisters.

Clinical Signs

- Bullous pemphigoid is a relatively uncommon autoimmune dermatosis.
- Collies, Doberman pinschers, and Shetland sheepdogs may be predisposed.
- Clinical signs and lesions mimic those of pemphigus vulgaris.
- Vesicles and bullae of bullous pemphigoid are more stable than those seen with pemphigus; this is most likely due to the depth of the lesion.
- Oral cavity lesions are common and occur in 80% of cases, but they are not usually the initial presenting clinical sign. Cutaneous or mucocutaneous vesicobullous lesions generally precede oral cavity involvement.
- Pruritus and pain are variable.

Diagnosis

- Direct smears are negative for acantholytic cells because this disease does not affect intercellular adhesion.

- CBC, serum biochemical profile, and urinalysis are nondiagnostic.
- ANA is negative.
- Histopathologic findings include a subepidermal cleft or bulla with a lichenoid infiltrate of neutrophils and/or eosinophils.
- IFA and IPS are positive, with a linear band of staining along the basement membrane zone.

Treatment

Therapeutic options for bullous pemphigoid are the same as those available for the pemphigus complex.

VOGT-KOYANAGI-HARADA SYNDROME

Etiology

The exact immunopathogenesis of Vogt-Koyanagi-Harada (VKH) syndrome is unknown. In humans, circulating lymphocytes from patients with VKH syndrome show significant cytotoxic activity against P-36 human melanoma cells. The factors responsible for the cellular hyperactivity against melanin-containing cells have not been determined. Deficiency of T-suppressor cells, viral inducement of immunologic abnormality, and genetic factors have all been implicated.

Clinical Signs

- Akitas, Samoyeds, and Siberian huskies appear to be predisposed.
- In humans, three phases have been recognized:
  - *Meningoencephalitic phase*—fever, malaise, headache, nausea, vomiting, and tinnitus
  - *Ophthalmic phase*—photophobia, uveitis, blindness
  - *Dermatologic phase*—leukoderma (acquired lack of skin pigment) and leukotrichia (acquired lack of hair pigment)
- Dogs appear to exhibit primarily the ophthalmic and dermatologic phases.
- Dermatologic lesions (leukoderma, leukotrichia) affect primarily the nose, lips, footpads, eyelids, and anus.
- Erosions and ulcerations may or may not be present in conjunction with leukoderma.

Diagnosis

- Direct smears are negative.
- CBC, serum biochemical profile, and urinalysis are nondiagnostic.
- ANA is negative.
- Histopathologic findings include a histiocytic interface dermatitis with pigmentary incontinence (histiocytes contain fine melanin granules).
- IFA and IPS are negative.

Treatment

- Treatment is similar to that for the pemphigus complex.

- VKH syndrome is very difficult to control and usually requires high levels of prednisone and azathioprine.
- Ocular changes usually dictate the therapeutic course. For treatment of uveitis, see Chapter 155.

LUPUS ERYTHEMATOSUS COMPLEX

Etiology

The exact immunopathogenesis of systemic lupus erythematosus (SLE) and discoid (cutaneous) lupus erythematosus (DLE) is unknown. Antigen-antibody complexes are produced and subsequently lodge in small vessels and the basement membrane zone of the skin (SLE and DLE) and in various organ systems (SLE). Genetic factors, T-cell defects, B-cell hyperactivity, hormonal alterations, and viral inducement of antigen-antibody complex formation have all been implicated. (See Chapter 22 for more information about SLE.)

Clinical Signs

Discoid Lupus Erythematosus

- Collies, Shetland sheepdogs, German shepherds, and Siberian huskies are predisposed.
- There are no internal manifestations of disease except in very rare "potential" crossover cases that, in time, become more consistent with SLE.
- The initial lesion is an area of depigmentation or erythema that slowly progresses to erosions, ulcers, and crusts.
- The planum nasale is the area most commonly affected, although lesions have been noted on the eyelids, lips, footpads, and concave surface of the pinnae and in the oral cavity.
- Profuse hemorrhage may occur following minor trauma to the planum nasale.
- Sunlight exacerbates the lesions and may play a role in the pathogenesis of DLE.

Systemic Lupus Erythematosus

- Collies and Shetland sheepdogs are predisposed.
- SLE is a multiorgan disease with dermatologic manifestations in 32–54% of cases.
- Cutaneous signs associated with SLE include ulcerative stomatitis, seborrhea, mucocutaneous ulceration, footpad ulceration, panniculitis (lupus profundus), urticaria, and purpura.
- Noncutaneous signs of SLE (see Chap. 22) include polyarthritis, fever, glomerulonephritis, hemolytic anemia, thrombocytopenia, polymyositis, neurologic signs, pleuritis, myocarditis, and lymphadenopathy.

Diagnosis

Discoid Lupus Erythematosus

- Direct smears are nondiagnostic.
- CBC, serum biochemical profile, and urinalysis are nondiagnostic.

- ANA is positive in 5% of cases of DLE (may indicate those animals with the potential for conversion to SLE that therefore should be closely monitored).
- Histopathologic findings include a lichenoid interface dermatitis composed primarily of lymphocytes and plasma cells, thickened basement membrane zone, hydropic degeneration of the basal cell layer, apoptotic keratinocytes in the lower layers of the epidermis, pigmentary incontinence, and an excess of dermal mucin.
- IFA and IPS are positive, with a granular or rough band of immunoglobulin and/or complement deposited at the basement membrane zone.

Systemic Lupus Erythematosus

- Direct smears are nondiagnostic.
- CBC, serum biochemical profile, and urinalysis may show a variety of abnormalities, depending on the noncutaneous organs involved (see Chap. 22).
- ANA is positive in 85–90% of cases.
  - The negative titers in 10–15% of ANA tests may be a laboratory "fault" because of the current inability of most laboratories to test for extractable nuclear antigens.
- The lupus erythematosus cell preparation is unreliable and not routinely used in veterinary medicine.
- Histopathologic findings include epidermal and dermal lesions similar to those seen in DLE and also may include leukocytoclastic vasculitis and mononuclear panniculitis.
- IFA and IPS are positive, with a band of staining at the basement membrane zone of the skin and involved dermal and subcutaneous vessels.

Treatment

Discoid Lupus Erythematosus

- Administer *prednisone:* 2 mg/kg PO divided q12h.
- Apply *topical corticosteroids* to the planum nasale. This may be the only form of corticosteroid needed to treat and control mild cases.
- Apply *topical sunscreens* to the planum nasale during periods of sun exposure.
- Administer vitamin E 400 IU PO q12h. Give 2 hours before or after a meal.
  - Vitamin E has a 30–60 day lag phase, and therapy usually is maintained for the life of the dog.
  - No side effects have been reported in dogs. Problems noted in humans include thrombophlebitis, hypertension, fatigue, cardiac disease, and diabetes mellitus.
- Tetracycline and niacinamide in combination may be effective. In dogs over 10 kg, the initial dosage is 500 mg of each drug PO q8h, and in dogs under 10 kg, the dosage is 250 mg of each drug PO q8h. Once response is noted, the dosage can be decreased to q12h and then to q24h. Side effects include anorexia, vomiting, and diarrhea.
- Severe cases of DLE may require the use of *azathioprine,* as described earlier in the treatment of the pemphigus complex (see Prednisone with Azathioprine under Therapeutic Protocols).

Systemic Lupus Erythematosus

- Use *prednisone* and *azathioprine* combination therapy as described for the treatment of the pemphigus complex.
- *Gold salts are contraindicated* because of the potential for both the drug and the disease to produce glomerulonephritis.
- In severe cases of anemia and thrombocytopenia, *splenectomy* may be indicated (see Chap. 23).

VASCULITIS

Etiology

Most of the recognized vasculitic syndromes are caused by deposition of immune complexes within vessel walls. Complement components are then activated and act as chemoattractants for neutrophils. Neutrophils infiltrate the vessel wall and release lysosomal enzymes such as elastase and collagenase, which damage the vessel wall. Thrombosis, occlusion, hemorrhage, and necrosis may develop. Blood flow turbulence and hydrostatic tension may also play a role in the immunopathogenesis of vasculitis.

Inciting causes of vasculitis are varied and include allergic diseases, bacterial and viral infections, drug reactions, chemicals, neoplasia, SLE, rickettsial diseases, polyarteritis nodosa, rheumatoid arthritis, and cold hemagglutinin disease. (See Chapter 69 for more information on vasculitis.)

Clinical Signs

- Vasculitis is a polysystemic disease.
- Dermatologic signs include petechiae, ecchymoses, hemorrhagic bullae, ulcerations, urticaria, and edema.
- Noncutaneous signs are similar to those described for SLE.

Diagnosis

- Direct smears are nondiagnostic.
- Diascopy, the application of a glass slide pressed to an erythematous lesion, may help rule out vascular fragility. The lesion clears if the erythema is due to vascular dilatation but remains if hemorrhage or vascular leakage has occurred.
- CBC, serum biochemical profile, and urinalysis changes are dependent on the underlying etiology and on the target organ system.
- ANA is negative unless SLE is the underlying cause of the vasculitis.
- Histopathologic findings include leukocytoclastic vasculitis, fibrinoid degeneration of vessel walls, thrombosis, and endothelial swelling.
- IFA and IPS may be positive in early lesions, with immunoglobulin and complement detected in and around vessel walls. Affected animals have high levels

of circulating immune complexes and low levels of complement.

Treatment

- Treatment is similar to that described for the pemphigus complex.
- Do not use steroids if there is an infectious etiology.
- Sulfone therapy (dapsone, Jacobus), 1 mg/kg PO q24h, may be used in cases of idiopathic neutrophilic vasculitis.

SUPPLEMENTAL READINGS

Crawford MA, Foil CS: Vasculitis: Clinical syndromes in small animals. Compend Contin Educ 11:400, 1989.

Rosenkrantz W: Immunomodulating drugs in dermatology. *In* Kirk RW, ed.: Current Veterinary Therapy X. Philadelphia: WB Saunders, 1989, p 570.

Scott DW, Miller WH Jr, Griffin CE: Muller and Kirk's Small Animal Dermatology, 5th Ed. Philadelphia: WB Saunders, 1995, p 484.

44 Keratinization Defects

Kenneth W. Kwochka

Primary defects of keratinization are dermatoses that are manifested clinically by localized or generalized excess scale formation. The scale may be formed from the interfollicular epidermis or may emanate from hair follicles as comedones and follicular casts. Histologically, the most striking abnormalities involve the keratinizing structures of the body including the epidermis, hair follicle outer root sheath, and hair cuticle.

▼ *Key Point* Cutaneous scaling of dogs is a very common clinical sign. In most cases, it is not due to a primary keratinization defect but is secondary to other dermatologic diseases. Conditions causing secondary scaling include demodicosis, scabies, cheyletiellosis, atopy, food allergy, flea allergy, pyoderma, dermatophytosis, hypothyroidism, hyperadrenocorticism, sex hormone abnormalities, pemphigus foliaceus, mycosis fungoides, and environmental influences. A primary keratinization defect is never diagnosed until the secondary causes of scaling have first been considered.

ETIOLOGY

For most of the diseases classified as primary keratinization defects, the pathophysiology is unknown. For others, the cause is known and the primary pathophysiology involves a defect in the keratinizing epithelium or the cutaneous glandular function.

- *Primary idiopathic seborrhea* is the most common chronic keratinization disorder in dogs. Predisposed breeds include cocker spaniels, English springer spaniels, West Highland white terriers, basset hounds, Irish setters, German shepherds, dachshunds, Doberman pinschers, Chinese Shar Peis, and Labrador retrievers. In cocker spaniels and Irish setters, at least part of the pathophysiology of scale formation involves hyperproliferation of basal epidermal keratinocytes.
- *Vitamin A–responsive dermatosis* is a rare, nutritionally responsive scaling disorder primarily in cocker spaniels. Similar syndromes have been reported in other breeds, including miniature schnauzers, Labrador retrievers, and Chinese Shar Peis in Europe. This condition is not a systemic vitamin A deficiency but probably represents a local deficiency in

the epidermis, a problem with uptake in the skin, a disorder of cutaneous utilization, or a positive pharmacologic effect of high doses on the epidermis.
- *Zinc-responsive dermatosis* is a rare, nutritionally responsive scaling disease of several breeds of dogs, especially Alaskan malamutes and Siberian huskies. The incidence of this disease seems to be decreasing.
- *Epidermal dysplasia* is an extremely severe keratinization disorder reported only in West Highland white terriers. It appears to be a genetic keratinization abnormality, although the actual mode of inheritance and pathophysiology are unknown.
- *Lichenoid-psoriasiform dermatosis* is an extremely rare, probably inherited, keratinization defect. It has been reported only in English springer spaniels.
- *Schnauzer comedo syndrome* is a follicular keratinization defect of miniature schnauzers characterized clinically by multiple comedones along the dorsal midline of the back. It is probably genetic because of the exclusive occurrence in miniature schnauzers. There may be a developmental defect in the hair follicle leading to abnormal keratinization, comedo formation, follicular plugging and dilation, and secondary bacterial folliculitis.
- *Ichthyosis* is an extremely rare congenital keratinization defect of dogs, especially terriers, characterized by very severe scaling of the skin and footpads. The canine disease seems to most closely resemble lamellar ichthyosis seen in children. Ichthyosis may be an autosomal recessive trait in dogs, as it is in humans, although the exact genetics have not been studied.
- *Sebaceous adenitis* is an inflammatory disease process directed against the sebaceous glands of the skin. Predisposed breeds include standard poodles, Akitas, Samoyeds, and Vizslas. The pathophysiology is unknown but may include an inherited defect of sebaceous gland development, an immune-mediated sebaceous gland destruction, a primary follicular keratinization defect with obstruction of sebaceous ducts and inflammation, and an abnormality in lipid metabolism affecting sebaceous secretions and keratinization.
- *Idiopathic nasodigital hyperkeratosis* is a primary keratinization disorder characterized by excess keratin accumulation on the planum nasale, footpads, or both. It is most commonly seen in cocker spaniels and English springer spaniels, although any breed may be affected.

- *Canine ear margin dermatosis* is a rare idiopathic keratinization defect, which affects only the pinnae of the ears in a bilaterally symmetric pattern. This dermatosis occurs primarily in dachshunds.
- *Canine acne* is a fairly common disorder of follicular keratinization resulting in comedones and secondary bacterial folliculitis and furunculosis. It is seen most commonly in short-coated breeds, especially English bulldogs, boxers, Doberman pinschers, and Great Danes. Canine acne may be due to abnormalities in sebaceous secretions that result in altered follicular keratinization, comedo formation, and secondary bacterial folliculitis. The organisms most commonly isolated are *Staphylococcus intermedius* and *Staphylococcus aureus*.

CLINICAL SIGNS

Disorders of keratinization are characterized clinically by mild-to-severe dry, waxy, or greasy scales. Some degree of "seborrheic odor" is associated with the skin condition. Because hair follicles and glandular structures may also be involved, it is not unusual to see comedones and follicular casts. *Comedones* are blackheads resulting from dilation of hair follicles with keratin plugs. *Follicular casts* are tightly adherent scale around hair shafts. Common secondary findings include alopecia, inflammation, crusts, pruritus with secondary excoriations, yeast dermatitis, and pyoderma.

▼ *Key Point* Primary keratinization defects are usually hereditary and appear during the first 2 to 3 years of life. A breed incidence for these disorders is known. An observant owner usually indicates that the scaling was present before the development of secondary signs.

- *Primary idiopathic seborrhea* causes clinical signs ranging from dry scaling to greasy scaling, to scaling and greasiness with inflammation and pruritus, and any combination of these abnormalities on the same animal.
  - *Seborrhea sicca* describes the dry scaling of several breeds with primary idiopathic seborrhea. These animals have dull, dry haircoats with focal to diffuse accumulations of white to gray nonadherent scales. Breeds affected with this form of idiopathic seborrhea include Doberman pinschers, Irish setters, German shepherds, and dachshunds.
  - *Seborrhea oleosa* is reserved for primary idiopathic seborrheic breeds with greasy skin and haircoat. These dogs have greasy, brownish yellow clumps of lipid material that adhere to the skin and hair. The material on the hair shafts has been described as "nit-like." Concurrent ceruminous otitis is common. One of the most common owner complaints with this form is a severe rancid odor associated with secondary infections. The breeds most predisposed to this form include cocker spaniels, English springer spaniels, basset hounds, West Highland

white terriers, Chinese Shar Peis, and Labrador retrievers.
  - *Seborrheic dermatitis* is a more severe variant of seborrhea oleosa. The clinical lesions are as described for seborrhea oleosa, but additionally there is significant cutaneous inflammation, bacterial folliculitis, pruritus, and multifocal plaques of hyperkeratotic material with inflammation. The most common areas of the body involved are the external ear canals, ear pinnae, ventral neck, chest, axillae, and inguinal and perineal areas. Secondary skin infections are very common with seborrheic dermatitis.
- *Vitamin A–responsive dermatosis* has clinical signs consisting of refractory generalized scaling, dry haircoat with easy epilation, prominent comedones, and hyperkeratotic plaques with large "fronds" of keratinous material protruding from the follicular ostia. The plaques are usually on the ventral and lateral thorax and abdomen, but the neck and face may also be involved. Other clinical features include a rancid odor from the skin, ceruminous otitis externa, and varying degrees of pruritus.
- *Zinc-responsive dermatosis* is typically divided into the following two clinical syndromes:
  - *Zinc-responsive dermatosis of Siberian huskies and Alaskan malamutes* is the first syndrome. It is also reported in Doberman pinschers and Great Danes.

    Alaskan malamutes have a genetic defect affecting zinc absorption from the intestines. Thus, the condition may occur even while the dog is on a well-balanced commercial diet.

    Zinc-responsive dermatosis may be precipitated by stress, estrus, and gastrointestinal disorders affecting absorption.

    Diets high in calcium and phytate (plant-derived protein) may also precipitate the disorder by binding zinc in the gastrointestinal tract.

    A condition resembling zinc-responsive dermatosis has been described in dogs fed nutritionally incomplete generic dog food.

    Lesions usually develop in dogs before puberty or in young adulthood. They include alopecia, erythema, scaling, and crusting involving the face, head, scrotum, and legs. Lesions often encircle the mouth, chin, eyes, ears, prepuce, and vulva. Thick crusts may be found on the elbows and other pressure points of the body. The footpads may be hyperkeratotic. The haircoat is generally dull and dry.
  - *Zinc-responsive dermatosis of rapidly growing puppies* on zinc-deficient diets or oversupplemented vitamins and minerals, especially calcium, is the second syndrome. It is also seen with diets high in phytate.

    Commonly affected breeds include Great Danes, Doberman pinschers, beagles, German shepherds, German shorthaired pointers, Labrador retrievers, and Rhodesian ridgebacks.

    In addition to the scaling and crusting, the dogs have secondary infections, lymphadenopathy, depression, and anorexia. The most obvious cutaneous lesions involve the head, elbows, other joints, and footpads.

- *Epidermal dysplasia* of West Highland white terriers develops in either sex, usually during the first year of life.
  - Clinical signs begin with erythema and pruritus of the ventrum and extremities. These rapidly progress to a generalized disorder ("armadillo disease") with severe erythema and pruritus, alopecia, hyperpigmentation, lichenification, lymphadenopathy, greasy skin and haircoat, rancid odor, ceruminous otitis, and secondary bacterial infection.
  - Some of the dogs have secondary *Malassezia pachydermatis* colonization of the surface and infundibular keratin, which may contribute to the severity of the disease.

▼ *Key Point* Secondary staphylococcal and *Malassezia* infection may be associated with any of the primary and secondary causes of scaling. Always look for the presence of bacteria and yeast with skin cytologic examination.

- *Lichenoid-psoriasiform dermatosis* of English springer spaniels has clinical signs including nonpruritic, erythematous, lichenoid papules and plaques involving the pinnae, external ear canal, preauricular and periorbital skin, lips, prepuce, and inguinal region. Chronic cases have papillomatous-type lesions, which may involve the face, ventral trunk, and perineum. A more generalized distribution of greasy scales and crusts may also be present.
- *Schnauzer comedo syndrome* usually develops in young adult dogs. Clinical signs include crusted, papular comedones (blackheads) along the dorsal midline of the back, from the neck to the tail.
  - In the early stages and in mild cases, the lesions are difficult to visualize through the haircoat but are more easily palpated as "bumps" down the back.
  - Animals with advanced disease frequently have secondary bacterial folliculitis and, rarely, furunculosis. The lesions may be accompanied by pruritus and pain. The infection leads to alopecia, with a "moth-eaten" appearance to the coat. The condition is chronic—for the life of the dog. Dogs with advanced disease should be evaluated for hypothyroidism and hyperadrenocorticism.
- *Ichthyosis* is reported most commonly in terriers and terrier crosses. In most cases, the entire body is covered with tightly adherent fine white scales. Some may appear as feathered keratinous projections. Extensive alopecia, hyperpigmentation, and lichenification may occur. Large quantities of waxy adherent scales may also be produced, especially in the flexural creases and intertriginous regions. Severe footpad hyperkeratosis may be present with the margins more severely involved.
- *Sebaceous adenitis* has two different clinical presentations related to coat length as follows:
  - Long-coated breeds, such as standard poodles, Akitas, and Samoyeds, have *nonpruritic patchy or symmetric alopecia* with excess scale formation and dull brittle hairs. Specific areas include the dorsal planum of the nose, top of the head, dorsal neck and trunk, tail, and pinnae. Advanced lesions include tightly adherent silver-white scales, follicular casts, matted hair, and secondary bacterial folliculitis.
  - Short-coated breeds, such as Vizslas, have *circular areas of alopecia and scaling* of the head, ears, trunk, and extremities. These areas may enlarge and eventually coalesce into serpiginous patterns or diffuse alopecia.
- *Idiopathic nasodigital hyperkeratosis* may have focal or diffuse lesions characterized by tightly adherent, thick accumulations of keratin on the nasal planum, footpads, or both. This material is usually extremely dry and may be accompanied by cracks, fissures, erosions, and ulcers. Severe footpad involvement may result in pain and lameness.
- *Canine ear margin dermatosis* has greasy plugs adhering tightly to the skin surface and hair shafts on the pinnal margins. Alopecia may develop with time. Pruritus is usually absent. In severe, untreated cases a progression to ulceration and necrosis has been reported that is due to thrombosis of capillaries that supply blood to the pinnal margins. This condition may result in severe scarring and fissures.
- *Acne* lesions include comedones, papules, pustules, and furuncles of the chin, lips, and muzzle. In some cases, lesions are mild and inapparent to the owner. In others, severe cellulitis with multiple draining tracts and pain occurs. In most dogs, spontaneous resolution takes place after sexual maturity. However, in the short-coated breeds, it may be a recurrent problem for the life of the animal, especially if not treated correctly when young.

DIAGNOSIS

▼ *Key Point* No specific laboratory test exists for a definitive diagnosis of a primary keratinization disorder. A combination of factors is used, including age of onset, breed, history, diagnostic elimination of the more common secondary causes of scaling, findings on histologic examination of skin biopsies, and response to therapy.

▼ *Key Point* Skin biopsy (see Chap. 49) is the most important diagnostic tool for primary keratinization defects. Biopsy results not only help to make a definitive diagnosis but also help to rule out dermatoses associated with secondary scaling. Take several biopsies from lesions of various ages. Send samples to a veterinary pathologist who specializes in dermatopathology.

- A definitive diagnosis of *primary idiopathic seborrhea* requires a number of different supporting factors, including age of onset, breed, history, diagnostic elimination of secondary causes of scaling, and findings on histopathologic examination of skin biopsy specimens.

- The most important aspect of the diagnostic plan is a full investigation for secondary causes of scaling. The primary differentials are allergic dermatitis, scabies, dermatophytosis, demodicosis, bacterial folliculitis, hypothyroidism, and vitamin A–responsive dermatosis.
- Biopsy samples are usually characterized by orthokeratotic and parakeratotic hyperkeratosis, follicular hyperkeratosis, and dyskeratosis. Often, the follicular abnormalities are more impressive than are the changes in the surface epidermis.

- *Vitamin A–responsive dermatosis* is characterized clinically by an early age of onset of refractory generalized scaling with hyperkeratotic plaques in cocker spaniels.
  - A firmer diagnosis can be made with skin biopsy findings consisting of marked follicular hyperkeratosis and very distended follicular ostia, mild orthokeratotic hyperkeratosis of the epidermis, and mild irregular epidermal hyperplasia.
  - Even with classic clinical and histologic findings, a definitive diagnosis can be confirmed only by response to supplementation with vitamin A alcohol-retinol.
  - The major diagnostic differentials for this condition include primary idiopathic seborrhea, zinc-responsive dermatosis, generic dog food dermatosis, sebaceous adenitis, and superficial necrolytic dermatitis.

- *Zinc-responsive dermatosis* is characterized clinically by early age of onset, dietary history, breed, and physical examination findings.
  - A firmer diagnosis is made with skin biopsy findings consisting of a marked diffuse surface and follicular parakeratotic hyperkeratosis and a hyperplastic superficial dermatitis.
  - A definitive diagnosis can be confirmed only by response to dietary zinc supplementation.
  - Important diagnostic differentials for this syndrome include demodicosis, dermatophytosis, pemphigus foliaceus, generic dog food dermatosis, and superficial necrolytic dermatitis.

- *Epidermal dysplasia* is characterized clinically by early age of onset of severe ventral erythema and pruritus rapidly progressing to chronic lesions in a West Highland white terrier.
  - A firmer diagnosis is made with skin biopsy findings consisting of a hyperplastic perivascular dermatitis with epidermal abnormalities, including hyperchromasia, excessive keratinocyte mitosis, crowding of basilar keratinocytes, epidermal "buds," loss of epidermal cell polarity, and parakeratosis. Budding yeast organisms and gram-positive cocci may also be found in surface and infundibular keratin.
  - The principal diagnostic challenge in these dogs is to determine if the condition is caused by epidermal dysplasia, some other pruritic skin disease, or their combination.
  - Primary diagnostic differentials that must be con-

sidered include atopy, food allergy dermatitis, scabies, and primary idiopathic seborrhea. Evaluate all of these by appropriate testing or response to therapy in the diagnostic workup.
  - A definitive diagnosis of epidermal dysplasia can be made only with characteristic clinical and histologic findings and after these other diagnostic differentials have been eliminated.
  - Another challenge is to determine how much the secondary bacterial infection or the *Malassezia* colonization is contributing to the severity of the clinical condition. This can be assessed only by evaluating response after treatment with appropriate topical and systemic antimicrobial agents.

- *Lichenoid-psoriasiform dermatosis* is characterized clinically by the early age of onset of refractory plaque-like lesions involving the face, ears, and ventrum in an English springer spaniel.
  - Perform skin scrapings and fungal culture to rule out the diagnoses of demodicosis and dermatophytosis.
  - The definitive diagnosis is based on skin biopsy findings. Histologic examination reveals a lichenoid dermatitis (i.e., a band of mononuclear cells in the superficial dermis) with psoriasiform epidermal hyperplasia, intraepidermal microabscesses, and Munro microabscesses. Advanced lesions may show papillated epidermal hyperplasia and papillomatosis.

- *Schnauzer comedo syndrome* is characterized clinically by dorsal follicular comedones in a miniature schnauzer.
  - The diagnosis is confirmed by skin biopsy showing dilated hair follicles filled with keratinous debris. Dilated or cystic sebaceous or apocrine glands, folliculitis, perifolliculitis, or furunculosis may be found.
  - Diagnostic differentials include demodicosis, dermatophytosis, and bacterial folliculitis.
  - Obtain a complete drug history in miniature schnauzers with comedo syndrome. Glucocorticoids are comedogenic, and long-term administration may precipitate or worsen the condition. I have also seen older miniature schnauzers with endogenous Cushing disease and hypothyroidism develop dorsal comedones.

- *Canine ichthyosis* is characterized clinically by congenital, severe cutaneous scaling and footpad hyperkeratosis in terriers.
  - Histologic findings confirm the diagnosis. They include increased mitotic activity in the basal keratinocytes, a prominent stratum granulosum, a severe laminated orthokeratotic hyperkeratosis, vacuolated keratinocytes in the superficial epidermis, and a follicular hyperkeratosis and plugging.
  - Because of the congenital nature of this disorder, it is rarely confused diagnostically with other keratinization defects. However, if its presence at birth cannot be firmly established, the diagnostic differentials include zinc-responsive dermatosis, nasodigital hyperkeratosis, primary idiopathic seborrhea, canine distemper virus, pemphigus foliaceus,

lupus erythematosus, hypothyroidism, generic dog food dermatosis, and superficial necrolytic dermatitis.

- A tentative clinical diagnosis of *sebaceous adenitis* is made based on breed, history, and clinical findings.
  - The definitive diagnosis is based on skin biopsy findings, including nodular granulomatous to pyogranulomatous inflammation at the level of the sebaceous glands.
  - Ask the pathologist to perform special stains for bacteria and fungi. Perform cultures for bacteria and fungi.
  - Advanced lesions are characterized histologically by a complete loss of sebaceous glands with periadnexal fibrosis.
- *Idiopathic nasodigital hyperkeratosis* is diagnosed by finding nasal and/or digital hyperkeratosis without evidence of other concurrent diseases.
  - All diseases that may cause the lesions must be considered. Unfortunately, the list is long, and includes canine distemper virus, pemphigus foliaceus, pemphigus erythematosus, lupus erythematosus, nasal solar dermatitis, hypothyroidism, zinc-responsive dermatosis, generic dog food dermatosis, and superficial necrolytic dermatitis. Pemphigus foliaceus and lupus erythematosus are the most common causes of nasal and digital hyperkeratosis.
  - Perform extensive diagnostic tests only when the condition is severe or when the clinical signs suggest that one of the other more serious diseases listed previously is present. Idiopathic nasodigital hyperkeratosis is merely cosmetic for most dogs and requires neither extensive diagnostic workup nor treatment.
  - When warranted, a complete diagnostic evaluation requires a good history; complete blood count (CBC); serum biochemical profile; thyroid evaluation with baseline thyroxine and a thyroid-stimulating hormone level; biopsy for histologic evaluation; and antinuclear antibody test.
  - Biopsy for direct immunofluorescence testing is valuable when taken from fresh lesions on other parts of the body. Skin from the nose and footpads commonly shows false-positive reactions.
  - Histopathologic findings are most helpful in ruling out the diagnostic differentials. Abnormalities for idiopathic nasodigital hyperkeratosis are nonspecific and consist of irregular epidermal hyperplasia with severe orthokeratotic and parakeratotic hyperkeratosis.
- *Canine ear margin dermatosis* is tentatively diagnosed in the early stages when only scale is present by breed and clinical signs alone.
  - Perform skin scrapings and fungal culture to rule out the diagnoses of scabies (a consideration only if pruritus is present), demodicosis, and dermatophytosis.
  - Skin biopsy findings reveal prominent orthokeratotic and parakeratotic hyperkeratosis. However, biopsy is unnecessary and the ear margin is a difficult part of the body from which to remove tissue.

- The differential diagnosis is more extensive when the condition has progressed to ulceration and necrosis and includes lupus erythematosus, pemphigus complex, cutaneous vasculitis, dermatomyositis, cold agglutinin disease, frostbite, drug reactions, and lymphoreticular neoplasms.

  Diagnostic procedures to differentiate these diseases include CBC, serum biochemical profile, urinalysis, skin biopsy for routine histologic examination and direct immunofluorescence, Coombs testing, and antinuclear antibody testing.
- Skin biopsy specimens reveal necrosis and ulceration. Some sections may demonstrate vascular thrombosis. However, the changes are rather nonspecific and may be seen with many of the diagnostic differentials. Therefore, all of the aforementioned diagnostic tests are recommended to eliminate the differentials and to establish a definitive diagnosis of canine ear margin dermatosis.
- *Canine acne* is tentatively diagnosed by the history, age, and breed and the clinical appearance of the lesions.
  - Differential diagnoses include demodicosis, dermatophytosis, and bacterial folliculitis.
  - Perform skin scrapings and fungal culture in all cases.
  - Cytologic examination of pustular contents or exudate from furuncles confirm the presence or absence of suppurative inflammation and cocci. Consider culture and susceptibility testing in cases of deep infection, when a systemic antibiotic is to be selected.
  - Skin biopsy findings provide a definitive diagnosis but are rarely needed.

TREATMENT

▼ *Key Point* After a definitive diagnosis of a primary keratinization defect is established, warn owners that the condition is most likely controllable but not curable. Some type of topical and systemic treatment will probably be needed for the remainder of the patient's life.

Most of the primary keratinization disorders are treated with various combinations of topical antiseborrheic agents in shampoo formulations and systemic retinoids (i.e., vitamin A or its metabolites).

- As in most primary keratinization disorders, the treatment goal in *primary idiopathic seborrhea* is to control scale formation, not cure the disease.
  - Moisturize the skin and haircoat when dry scaling is present. This task is accomplished with twice-weekly moisturizing hypoallergenic shampoos (HyLyt*efa, DVM Pharmaceuticals; Allergroom, Allerderm/Virbac) and frequent moisturizing rinses (HyLyt*efa Bath Oil Coat Conditioner, DVM Pharmaceuticals; Humilac, Allerderm/Virbac).
  - When dry scaling is severe and some keratolytic activity is needed, the treatment usually consists of sulfur and salicylic acid shampoos (SebaLyt, DVM

Pharmaceuticals; Sebolux, Allerderm/Virbac) followed by moisturizing rinses.

- Dietary supplementation with essential fatty acids (DVM DermCaps, DVM Pharmaceuticals) may also be beneficial.
- Use keratolytic and keratoplastic degreasing shampoos to control the scale and odor associated with seborrhea oleosa. Effective topical agents include coal tar (Clear Tar, Veterinary Prescription; NuSal-T, DVM Pharmaceuticals; T-Lux, Allerderm/Virbac; LyTar, DVM Pharmaceuticals; Allerseb-T, Allerderm/Virbac), benzoyl peroxide (OxyDex, DVM Pharmaceuticals; Sulf OxyDex, DVM Pharmaceuticals; Pyoben, Allerderm/Virbac), and selenium sulfide (Selsun Blue, Ross).
- The synthetic retinoid etretinate (Tegison, Roche) has been effective for idiopathic seborrhea in cocker spaniels, springer spaniels, Irish setters, golden retrievers, and mixed-breed dogs at 1 mg/kg PO q24h. Response is seen within 2 months and consists of decreased scale, odor, and pruritus, and softening and thinning of seborrheic plaques. Some dogs have been maintained without signs of toxicity over several months on alternate-day therapy.

▼ *Key Point* The synthetic retinoids are associated with teratogenicity. Do not use in breeding animals, and warn clients about the serious potential risks from accidental human ingestion. Other potential side effects include keratoconjunctivitis sicca; pain in legs and joints; and mild elevations in cholesterol, triglycerides, and liver enzyme levels. These are usually reversible on discontinuation of therapy or lowering the dosage.

- Calcitriol (Rocalcitrol, Roche) has been effective for idiopathic seborrhea in cocker spaniels at 10 ng/kg PO q24h. Give the medication as far removed as possible from the main meal of the day to decrease the possibility of hypercalcemia. Response is seen within 2–3 months. Treatment should be continued for life with monitoring of calcium and parathyroid hormone levels.
- Use systemic antibiotics for patients with secondary bacterial folliculitis and yeast dermatitis.
- A 7–10 day course of prednisone or prednisolone at an anti-inflammatory dose may occasionally be needed during periods of severe inflammation and pruritus in dogs with seborrheic dermatitis.
- Treat patients with *vitamin A–responsive dermatosis* with 625–800 IU/kg PO q24h of vitamin A alcohol (retinol).
  - Improvement is seen within 4–6 weeks, complete remission is obtained by 10 weeks, and treatment is needed for life.
  - Retinol at this dosage is well tolerated in dogs; therefore, no clinicopathologic monitoring is necessary.
  - Keratolytic shampoos containing benzoyl peroxide have excellent follicular flushing activity. Twice-weekly treatment helps remove keratinous debris from follicles and hastens recovery.

- Treatment of *zinc-responsive dermatosis* depends on the specific syndrome.
  - The first syndrome of zinc-responsive dermatosis usually responds to zinc sulfate at 10 mg/kg PO q24h or divided q12h with food. An alternative is zinc methionine at 2 mg/kg PO q24h. Correct any dietary imbalances (e.g., high calcium and phytate, generic diets). Symptoms resolve rapidly, but lifetime therapy is usually needed. Zinc may cause vomiting, in which case lower the dose and give the medication with food.
  - The second syndrome in puppies usually responds over time to dietary corrections alone. However, recovery may be hastened by supplementation as discussed for the first syndrome. Some puppies may need supplementation until maturity.
- *Epidermal dysplasia* is generally nonresponsive to medical therapy. The prognosis is poor, especially if the condition is chronic and severe secondary changes have occurred.
  - Two forms of therapy offer hope in at least some of these dogs. First, in patients with secondary *M. pachydermatis* colonization, there may be significant improvement in pruritus and skin condition with ketoconazole (Nizoral, Janssen), 5–10 mg/kg PO q12–24h, or itraconazole (Sporonox, Janssen), 5 mg/kg PO q24h, and twice-weekly application of a topical antifungal shampoo.

    Over time, the yeast colonization will return secondary to the keratinization defect. However, this problem can sometimes be controlled with maintenance ketoconazole or itraconazole given once or twice per week.
  - Second, in some cases seen very early in the course of the disease and before chronic cutaneous changes occur, a dramatic response to immunosuppressive levels of short-acting glucocorticoids may occur.

    Administer prednisone or prednisolone at 1.1 to 2.2 mg/kg PO q12h until the condition is controlled. Follow by a very gradual decrease in the dosage to alternate-day therapy for long-term maintenance. Some patients experience relapse, whereas others remain in long-term remission. Before such therapy is used, evaluate the patient for allergies and explain to the owner the side effects of long-term steroid administration.
- *Lichenoid-psoriasiform dermatosis* is a waxing and waning dermatitis. Response is minimal to medical therapy.
  - Antibiotics, especially cephalexin, may be helpful when secondary pyoderma is present.
  - Prednisone at 2.2 mg/kg PO q24h has improved lesions in some cases but has not resulted in complete remission.
- The majority of cases of *schnauzer comedo syndrome* can be controlled with periodic application of benzoyl peroxide shampoos (OxyDex, DVM Pharmaceuticals; Pyoben, Allerderm/Virbac) to flush follicles and control secondary bacterial folliculitis.
  - A combination benzoyl peroxide and sulfur shampoo (Sulf OxyDex, DVM Pharmaceuticals) is espe-

cially effective because of an enhanced keratolytic activity.

- Benzoyl peroxide gels (OxyDex Gel, DVM Pharmaceuticals; Pyoben Gel, Allerderm/Virbac) are helpful to remove tightly adherent comedones.
- Gentle agitation with a mildly abrasive sponge (Buff-Puff, Johnson & Johnson) helps to mechanically remove adherent comedones.
- Systemic antibiotics for a minimum of 3 weeks are indicated to control secondary staphylococcal folliculitis.
- If there is no response to topical therapy, the synthetic retinoid isotretinoin (Accutane, Roche), 1–2 mg/kg PO q24h, has been very effective. Rapid response is seen within 3–4 weeks. After lesions resolve, most dogs can be maintained in remission without signs of toxicity on alternate-day therapy.

- The long-term prognosis for *ichthyosis* is poor because of the severity of the scale formation and because of the continual therapy that will be needed for the entire life of the patient.
  - Topical therapy is helpful, including warm water soaks to help remove scales, antiseborrheic shampoos (SebaLyt, DVM Pharmaceuticals; Sebolux, Allerderm/Virbac), antiseborrheic gels (KeraSolv, DVM Pharmaceuticals; Retin-A, Ortho) for locally severe lesions, lactic acid as a total body rinse or spray (Humilac, Allerderm/Virbac; Micro Pearls Humectant Spray, Evsco Pharmaceuticals), and a combination rinse of 75% propylene glycol and 25% humectants (Humilac, Allerderm/Virbac). Topical therapy other than shampoos is used twice daily until the scale and odor are controlled and then is used as often as necessary for maintenance.
  - Excellent results have been obtained with isotretinoin (Accutane, Roche) at 1–2 mg/kg PO q24h, and etretinate (Tegison, Roche) at 1–2 mg/kg PO q24h. Remission is usually within 8–12 weeks, although some dogs take up to 6 months. Some dogs can be maintained on alternate-day therapy.

- Response to therapy for *sebaceous adenitis* depends on the stage and severity of the disease.
  - Immunosuppressive dosages of glucocorticoids may be effective very early in the course of the disease when severe inflammation is present.
  - Isotretinoin (Accutane, Roche) at 1 mg/kg PO q12–24h may be effective in refractory cases, especially in short-coated breeds. After remission is obtained, the goal is to gradually decrease the dosage to 1 mg/kg PO q48h.
  - Etretinate (Tegison, Roche) at 1–2 mg/kg PO q24h is effective and may be useful, especially in long-coated breeds.
  - Cyclosporine (Sandimmune, Sandoz) has also been used in refractory cases at 5 mg/kg PO q12h.
  - Topical therapy with sprays or rinses consisting of 75% propylene glycol and 25% humectants (Humilac, Allerderm/Virbac) is helpful when applied once daily.
  - Other therapy consists of essential fatty acid dietary supplements, antiseborrheic shampoos and emollients, antibiotics, and antibacterial and follicular flushing shampoos.

- Medical treatment of *idiopathic nasodigital hyperkeratosis* includes hydration of the hyperkeratotic tissue by water soakings or wet dressings followed by application of petrolatum jelly as an occlusive agent to help seal moisture into the stratum corneum.
  - Although simple hydration may be adequate for mild lesions, more severe hyperkeratosis requires a topical agent with keratolytic activity. A gel containing salicylic acid, lactic acid, and urea (KeraSolv Gel, DVM Pharmaceuticals) is helpful, as is topical 0.025% or 0.01% tretinoin gel (Retin-A, Ortho). The gel is used q12h until the condition is controlled, followed by application as needed for long-term maintenance. Irritation may be a problem, especially with tretinoin.
  - Corticosteroid and antibiotic ointments, creams, or gels may be needed when severe inflammation or secondary infection is present.
  - When very severe projections of keratin are present, especially on footpads and causing lameness, they may be surgically removed by trimming the dead tissue with scissors.

- The mild scaling form of *ear margin dermatosis* is usually controllable but rarely curable with topical therapy.
  - Periodic use of an antiseborrheic shampoo to remove the scales and waxy accumulations is all that is needed to control the mild form of the condition. Helpful agents include sulfur and salicylic acid (SebaLyt, DVM Pharmaceuticals; Sebolux, Allerderm/Virbac) and benzoyl peroxide (OxyDex, DVM Pharmaceuticals; Sulf OxyDex, DVM Pharmaceuticals; Pyoben, Allerderm/Virbac).
  - A topical glucocorticoid cream, such as 1% hydrocortisone, may be needed in severe unresponsive cases or in those with severe inflammation.
  - The advanced ulcerative and necrotic stage is resistant to medical therapy. However, the condition can usually be cured by surgical removal of the affected ear margin.

    Remove tissue well into the normal portion of the pinna. This can be done to both pinnae, resulting in a symmetric and cosmetically acceptable outcome.

    The full list of differential diagnoses for this condition is considered before such aggressive surgery. The procedure is not effective if the ulceration is due to autoimmune disease, vasculitis, or dermatomyositis.

- Mild cases of *canine acne* need no treatment and spontaneously resolve with sexual maturity. Aggressive topical therapy may actually worsen the condition by mechanical trauma of inflamed hair follicles.
  - For the more severely affected patient, treatment includes benzoyl peroxide shampoos (OxyDex, DVM Pharmaceuticals; Sulf OxyDex, DVM Pharmaceuticals; Pyoben, Allerderm/Virbac) and gels (OxyDex Gel, DVM Pharmaceuticals; Pyoben Gel, Allerderm/Virbac). These are applied twice daily until control is noted and then as needed for main-

tenance. Benzoyl peroxide is effective because of its follicular flushing and antimicrobial activity. It may cause cutaneous irritation in some animals.

- The most effective topical antibiotic for control of the secondary infection associated with canine acne is mupirocin (Bactoderm, Pfizer).

  This antibiotic has excellent activity against gram-positive cocci, is bactericidal, works well at an acid pH, is not systemically absorbed, and is not chemically related to other antibiotics. It penetrates well into granulomatous deep pyoderma lesions and, therefore, works well when furuncles and draining tracts have developed on the chin.

  Mupirocin is applied q12h. Consider alternating it with benzoyl peroxide for the follicular flushing activity offered by that agent.

- In recurrent cases or in those with deep infections, systemic antibiotics and warm water soaks are necessary.

- Short-term glucocorticoids, such as prednisone or prednisolone at 1.1 mg/kg PO q24h, help reduce inflammation associated with foreign body granulomas secondary to ingrown hairs or keratin debris. This results in a more rapid response, but administer the steroids for only 7–10 days, while continuing the antibiotics for much longer until the chin pyoderma has resolved.

- Cases refractory to more conventional therapy may benefit from topical tretinoin (Retin-A, Ortho), q12h, or systemic isotretinoin (Accutane, Roche) at 1–2 mg/kg PO q24h.

SUPPLEMENTAL READINGS

August JR, Chickering WR, Rikihisa Y: Congenital ichthyosis in a dog: Comparison with the human ichthyosiform dermatoses. Compend Contin Educ Pract Vet 10:40, 1988.

Gross TL, Halliwell RE, McDougal BJ, et al.: Psoriasiform lichenoid dermatitis in the springer spaniel. Vet Pathol 23:76, 1986.

Ihrke PJ, Goldschmidt MH: Vitamin A–responsive dermatosis in the dog. J Am Vet Med Assoc 182:687, 1983.

Kunkle GA: Zinc-responsive dermatoses in dogs. In Kirk RW, ed.: Current Veterinary Therapy VII. Philadelphia: WB Saunders, 1980, p 472.

Mason KV, Halliwell RE, McDougal BJ: Characterization of lichenoid-psoriasiform dermatosis of springer spaniels. J Am Vet Med Assoc 189:897, 1986.

Power HT, Ihrke PJ: Synthetic retinoids in veterinary dermatology. Vet Clin North Am 20:1525, 1990.

Scott DW, Miller WH: Epidermal dysplasia and Malassezia pachydermatis infection in West Highland white terriers. Vet Dermatol 1:25, 1989.

45 Growth Hormone–Responsive Alopecia and Sex Hormone–Associated Dermatoses

Lynn P. Schmeitzel

Growth hormone (GH)–responsive alopecia is an acquired symmetric alopecia of adult dogs that responds to growth hormone supplementation. The Pomeranian, poodle, chow chow, Samoyed, keeshond, and American water spaniel breeds are most frequently affected.

Sex hormone (SH)–associated dermatoses are skin diseases in any age, sex, or breed of dog that are caused by sex hormone imbalances or that respond to sex hormone treatment. A variety of organ systems, including the skin, may be clinically affected.

GH-responsive alopecia and SH-associated dermatoses are less common than dermatoses caused by hypothyroidism and hyperadrenocorticism (see Chaps. 29 and 31). However, these syndromes should be considered as differential diagnoses for suspected endocrine dermatoses of dogs.

ETIOLOGY

The cause of GH-responsive alopecia and of many of the naturally occurring suspected SH-associated dermatoses is unknown. Imbalances in growth hormone, estrogen, progesterone, and androgens often are suspected, although proof may be lacking. Imbalances in more than one of these hormones may be observed in the same dog.

Growth Hormone

- GH, also called somatotropin, is secreted by the pituitary gland.
- GH has anabolic effects on tissues that are directly mediated by the hormone and indirectly mediated by somatomedins, which are insulin-like growth factors produced in response to GH.
- In pituitary dwarfism, absolute GH deficiency causes alopecia and decreased elastin fiber content in the skin.
- Although some cases of GH-responsive alopecia are GH-deficient, a large number (up to 30%) have normal GH function tests, suggesting another etiology.
- Adrenal and gonadal sex hormone imbalances have also been observed in some dogs affected with GH-

deficient alopecia. (See Chap. 34 for further discussion of pituitary diseases.)

Estrogens

- Estrogens, including 17β-estradiol, estrone, and estriol, are produced by the ovaries, testes, and adrenal cortex and by peripheral conversion of androgens.
- Estrogens increase or decrease epidermal thickness, cause hyperpigmentation and sebaceous gland atrophy, decrease hair growth, increase dermal thickness, and decrease subcutaneous fat thickness.
- Hypoestrogenism and hyperestrogenism have been associated with clinical signs.
- Exogenous estrogen administration by any route may cause signs of hyperestrogenism in dogs.

Androgens

- Androgens, including dehydroepiandrosterone (and its sulfated conjugate), androstenedione, testosterone, and dihydrotestosterone, are produced by the ovaries, testes, and adrenal cortex and by peripheral conversion of weaker androgens to more potent androgens.
- Androgens increase epidermal thickness, pigmentation, sebum production, and dermal thickness and have variable effects on hair growth.
- In cases of GH-responsive alopecia, response to castration in the chow chow and other breeds and the presence of elevated serum androgen concentrations of adrenal origin in the Pomeranian breed suggest that this syndrome may be associated with androgenic hormone imbalance.

Progesterone

- Progesterone is produced by the ovaries, testes, and adrenal cortex and is a precursor hormone for both androgens and estrogens.
- Progesterone has androgenic, synandrogenic, and antiandrogenic effects.
- Relatively little is known regarding the effects of progesterone on the skin, although hyperprogesteronemia has been observed in dogs with testicular tumors and GH-responsive alopecia.

Photoperiod

- The photoperiod regulates pineal gland hormone release.
- A reduction in the photoperiod increases pineal hormone release, suppresses hypothalamic-pituitary gonadotropin release, and reduces sex hormone concentration.
- Abnormal release of these hormones associated with changes in the photoperiod may cause seasonal flank alopecia.

CLINICAL SIGNS

Skin

- *Alopecia* is bilateral and symmetric and involves the neck, trunk, caudal thighs, pinnae, and tail while sparing the head and distal legs.
  - In SH-associated dermatoses the alopecia may begin in the perineum and flank regions.
  - Bilateral flank alopecia may develop on a seasonal basis: fall/winter in males and spring/summer in spayed females.
  - Some dogs develop complete alopecia of the affected areas; other dogs lose their guard (primary) hairs and retain their undercoat (secondary) hairs.
  - Hair remaining in the affected areas is often dry and brittle, and epilates easily. Hair on the head and distal legs is usually normal in amount and texture.
  - Presence of disease may not be known until the dog is clipped and the hair fails to regrow.
  - In some dogs the first clinical sign is a failure to shed in the spring.
  - Postpartum telogen defluxion is a "normal" generalized alopecia that develops about 6–8 weeks after whelping in certain bitches.
- *Hyperpigmentation* usually develops after the alopecia and may be very intense, especially in GH-responsive alopecia.
- *Coat color changes* are observed mostly in darker-haired dogs. Their coats may fade and develop a reddish tint.
- *Skin* may be thinner, normal, or thicker.
- *Linear preputial dermatosis* is a well-demarcated area of erythema or hyperpigmentation on the ventral aspect of the prepuce and may be observed in dogs with testicular neoplasms.
- *Pruritus* is usually minimal or absent unless a secondary pyoderma or seborrhea is present also. Rarely, a hormonal "hypersensitivity" with intense pruritus may occur that disappears with neutering.
- *Perianal adenomas* and *tail gland hyperplasia* have been associated with hyperandrogenism of gonadal or adrenal origin.

Reproductive Disorders

Reproductive abnormalities may or may not be observed in SH-associated dermatoses.

- *Gynecomastia* may be present in both sexes affected with SH-associated dermatosis. The nipples and/or mammary glands are enlarged, and a small amount of secretion may be expressed from the nipples.
- *Feminization* is usually associated with hyperestrogenism. Affected males may lack libido, have a pendulous prepuce, and attract other male dogs. Affected females often have an enlarged clitoris and vulva.
- *Infantile vulva and mammary glands* may be observed in hypoestrogenism.
- *Testicular abnormalities* often are observed in intact male dogs with sex hormone imbalances.
  - A testicle may be enlarged because of a testicular tumor, and the opposite testicle will atrophy if the tumor is producing estrogen or estrogen-like hormone.
  - Some dogs have atrophy of both testicles.
  - Some are cases of unilateral or bilateral cryptorchidism.
- *Prostatic hyperplasia* may be associated with hyperandrogenism or hyperestrogenism (due to squamous metaplasia of the gland).
- *Irregular heat cycles, pseudocyesis,* and *pyometra* may be associated with hair loss in the intact bitch.
- *Libido* may be increased or decreased in the male dog. Some females may develop nymphomania or excessive mounting of other female dogs. Increased aggression may develop concurrently with increased libido, primarily when hyperandrogenism is present.
- *Vaginal hyperplasia-prolapse* may be observed in hyperestrogenism.

Other Clinical Signs

- Urinary incontinence in the spayed female may be associated with hypoestrogenism.
- Bone marrow suppression may be associated with hyperestrogenism.

DIAGNOSIS

▼ *Key Point* Before making a diagnosis of GH-responsive alopecia or SH-associated dermatosis, rule out hypothyroidism and hyperadrenocorticism with appropriate function tests (as described in Chaps. 29 and 31).

Signalment

GH-Responsive Alopecia. This syndrome usually develops in young adult dogs of the Pomeranian, chow chow, poodle, Samoyed, keeshond, and American water spaniel breeds near the onset of puberty, although any age may be affected.

SH-Associated Dermatoses. These may develop in any age, sex, or breed of dog.

- Castration-responsive dermatosis (woolly syndrome) has been described in Siberian huskies, Alaskan malamutes, and keeshonds.
- Seasonal flank alopecia occurs in intact and castrated male Airedale terriers, English bulldogs, and boxers; and in spayed female English bulldogs, boxers, miniature schnauzers, and miniature poodles.

History

Identify any reproductive abnormalities or behavior changes and their association with the development of skin lesions.

Physical Examination

- Evaluate the skin for secondary seborrhea and pyoderma and for perianal adenomas.
- Evaluate the testicles, vulva, nipples, and mammary glands for asymmetry, enlargement, or atrophy. Squeeze the nipples to determine if a secretion can be expressed.
- Palpate the abdomen for an enlarged uterus (pyometra) or abdominal mass (from ovarian tumor or from testicular tumor in a cryptorchid animal).
- Palpate the prostate for enlargement.
- Examine the mucous membranes for color (paleness) and petechiae.
- Palpate sublumbar lymph nodes for enlargement.

Laboratory Tests

Serum Biochemical Profile, Urinalysis, Complete Blood Count (CBC), and Platelet Count

- Perform these tests in dogs with bilateral symmetric alopecia to identify abnormalities indicating other potential causes such as hypothyroidism (see Chap. 29) and hyperadrenocorticism (see Chap. 31), or to identify severe metabolic derangements causing telogen/anagen defluxion.
- A CBC and platelet count may reveal anemia, leukopenia, and thrombocytopenia in dogs with hyperestrogenism.

Skin Scrapings and Fungal Cultures

Use these tests to rule out demodicosis and dermatophytosis as causes of the alopecia.

Preputial or Vaginal Cytology

Cytologic examination can reveal cornified cells with pyknotic or absent nuclei in dogs with hyperestrogenism.

Skin Biopsy

- See Chapter 49 for technique.
- Perform a skin biopsy to confirm the presence of an endocrinopathy, such as orthokeratotic hyperkeratosis, follicular keratosis and dilatation, telogenization of hair follicles (follicular atrophy), epidermal melanosis, epidermal atrophy, and sebaceous gland atrophy.
- Histologically, some cases of hyperestrogenism may have a superficial perivascular dermatitis (spongiotic or hyperplastic) instead of an endocrinopathy.
- Skin biopsy can also identify a secondary pyoderma.

Radiography

- Perform abdominal radiography and ultrasonography to identify intra-abdominal testicular and ovarian masses and sublumbar lymphadenopathy, indicating possible metastasis.
- Use thoracic radiography to identify ovarian and testicular tumor metastases.

Endocrine Function Tests

- Perform thyroid function tests before evaluating sex hormones in most cases (see Chap. 29).
- Adrenal function tests:
  - Perform a low-dose dexamethasone suppression test before evaluating sex hormones in most cases to rule out hypercortisolemia (see Chap. 31).
  - Perform an adrenocorticotropic hormone (ACTH) stimulation test to evaluate adrenal gland production of sex hormones and their precursor hormones. Send samples to the University of Tennessee College of Veterinary Medicine (contact author for details) for testing.
- Baseline sex hormones
  - Most laboratories can evaluate 17β-estradiol, progesterone, and testosterone.
  - Results may be "normal" in SH-associated dermatoses because many sex hormones are not routinely measured (e.g., dihydrotestosterone, estrone, estriol, biosynthetic precursors).
- GH function tests are not yet available commercially.

Laparoscopy or Exploratory Surgery

Surgery may be necessary to identify ovarian cysts and tumors in females and cryptorchid testicular tumors in males.

TREATMENT

GH-responsive alopecia may respond to neutering, sex hormone alterations, or GH supplementation. SH-associated dermatoses may respond to neutering or sex hormone alterations. If response is not observed with one therapeutic modality, switch to another.

▼ **Key Point** Neutering is the treatment of choice in intact animals affected with GH-responsive alopecia or SH-associated dermatoses.

Sex Hormone Supplementation

Diethylstilbestrol (DES)

- Give DES 0.1 mg up to 1.0 mg total dose PO q24h for 3 weeks; stop for 1 week; then repeat the 3-week treatment.
- Observe for response in 3 months.
- After response is achieved, continue the same dose once or twice weekly for maintenance.
- If estrogen therapy causes signs of estrus, reduce the dose by one-half.

▼ **Key Point** Caution: Estrogen therapy may cause fatal bone marrow suppression manifested by anemia, leukopenia, and thrombocytopenia. This is most likely after repositol injections of estradiol cyclopropionate. Perform weekly CBC and platelet counts while dogs are on daily DES therapy.

Methyltestosterone (Android, ICN Pharmaceuticals) or Fluoxymestrone (Halotestin, Upjohn)

- Give either of these androgens at 1.0 mg/kg up to 30 mg total dose PO q48h for 3 months.
- After response is achieved, continue the same dose once or twice weekly for maintenance.
- Possible side effects include aggressive behavior, hepatotoxicity, prostatic hypertrophy, and perianal gland hypertrophy.

Growth Hormone Supplementation

- Use GH only after neutering and sex hormone supplementation have been tried and shown to be ineffective.
- This product is available on a very limited basis, although bovine somatotropin may become readily available in the future.
- Give 0.1 IU/kg SC three times per week for 4–6 weeks.
- Observe for response in 4–6 weeks after completion of therapy.
- Remission of clinical signs after discontinuing GH varies from 6 months to greater than 3 years.
- Review the effects of GH excess (acromegaly) in Chapter 34.

▼ *Key Point* Growth hormone is diabetogenic, and dogs treated with GH may develop transient or permanent diabetes mellitus. Measure fasting blood glucose levels before and weekly during GH supplementation. Discontinue supplementation if hyperglycemia persists.

Other Therapies

Megestrol acetate (Ovaban, Schering-Plough) may be effective for its antiandrogen effects. Mitotane (Lysodren, Bristol Laboratories) can be used in dogs with excessive adrenal gland production of sex hormones (see Chap. 31).

SUPPLEMENTAL READINGS

Lothrop CD Jr: Pathophysiology of canine growth hormone-responsive alopecia. Compend Contin Educ 10:1346, 1988.

Miller WH Jr: Sex hormone-related dermatoses in dogs. *In* Kirk RW, ed.: *Current Veterinary Therapy X.* Philadelphia: WB Saunders, 1989, p 595.

Schmeitzel LP: Sex hormone-related and growth hormone-related alopecias. Vet Clin North Am Small Anim Pract 20:1579, 1990.

Schmeitzel LP, Lothrop CD Jr: Hormonal abnormalities in Pomeranians with normal coat and in Pomeranians with growth hormone-responsive dermatosis. J Am Vet Med Assoc 197:1333, 1990.

Scott DW: Seasonal flank alopecia in ovariohysterectomized dogs. Cornell Vet 80:187, 1990.

46 Necrotizing Skin Diseases

Gail A. Kunkle

Necrotizing dermatitis refers to those skin conditions in which there is death of tissue. With many cases of necrotizing dermatitis, ulceration is the visible clinical sign and it occurs when there is cell death, especially within the epidermis and including the hair follicle. In other necrotizing skin diseases, the tissue destruction may arise in the dermis or even from compromise of deeper vessels. In these cases the first clinical signs may be discoloration, swelling, or coldness to the skin followed later by cutaneous ulceration. Causes of necrotizing skin disease are categorized in Table 46–1.

▼ *Key Point* Dependent on the depth of necrosis or the percentage of surface area which is ulcerated, necrotizing dermatoses can be life-threatening.

CLINICAL SIGNS

Necrotizing skin diseases are characterized clinically by well-defined areas of devitalized skin, which may vary from pinpoint in size to involvement of a large portion of the skin surface. The area may be discolored, ranging from dark red to purple to yellow to black. There may be swelling and even gas production within the tissues. Common sequelae are systemic signs of toxicity.

PRINCIPLES OF DIAGNOSIS

Significant necrosis of the skin is a dermatologic emergency and may result in death; thus initiate the diagnostic approach to necrotizing skin disease as quickly as possible. Early identification of an underlying cause and specific treatment generally allows a better clinical outcome. The approach should be as thorough as possible to increase the chance of a definitive diagnosis.

▼ *Key Point* Diagnosis is best made by routine histopathology from representative primary cutaneous lesions and/or tissue samples adjacent to necrosis, in conjunction with a careful history and thorough physical examination.

History

- Identify or exclude several of the potential etiologies of necrotizing dermatoses.

- Record a thorough drug history and take note of environmental factors.
- Record a careful timetable of events in addition to the owner's description of the earliest cutaneous lesions and their temporal relationship to any noted systemic signs.

Physical Examination

- Thoroughly examine all of the skin, including the inside of the ears, the oral cavity, and haired as well as nonhaired skin.
- Note any primary lesions.
- Look for secondary lesions and for evidence of how they may have developed.
- Palpate all peripheral lymph nodes for enlargement.
- Take the body temperature.
- Perform a general physical examination, including examination of the eyes, auscultation of the thorax and palpation of the abdomen, to evaluate for systemic signs.

Serum Biochemical Profile, Urinalysis, and Complete Blood Count

- Evaluate these in animals with systemic signs such as anorexia, fever, and depression.
- Use these as baseline information when progressive disease is suspected.

Tests for Systemic Immune-Mediated Diseases

- Perform antinuclear antibody (ANA) testing of serum to assess the presence or absence of antibodies directed against multiple nuclear antigens.
- Other immune tests such as Coombs testing and cryoglobulin identification may be indicated in cases in which specific diseases are suspected.
- See Chapter 22 for further discussion of testing for systemic immune-mediated diseases.

Skin Biopsy

- Skin biopsy is an important diagnostic tool in necrotizing skin diseases (see Chap. 49).
- Collect lesions that are primary eruptions and/or skin immediately adjacent to necrotic skin.
- Use formalin as a fixative and try to take representative tissue samples from various types of lesions. A pathologist familiar with dermatopathology often can determine if systemic or topical disease is present.

Table 46–1. CLASSIFICATION AND CAUSES OF NECROTIZING DERMATOSES

Category	Cause
Immune-mediated	Systemic lupus erythematosus (see Chap. 43) Bullous pemphigoid (see Chap. 43) Pemphigus complex (see Chap. 43) Cold agglutinin disease Vasculitis
Vasculitis	Sepsis Immune-mediated Systemic infectious disease Drug-induced Hypersensitivity Focal (rabies vaccination) Neoplasia Idiopathic
Neoplasia	Squamous cell carcinoma (see Chap. 28) Mast cell (see Chap. 26) Lymphoma (see Chap. 25) Other tumors (see Chap. 28)
Drug-induced	Antibiotics Biologicals Barbiturates Phenylbutazone Gold salts
Toxic epidermal necrolysis/ erythema multiforme	Drug-induced Systemic disease Neoplasia Idiopathic
Environmental	Contact irritant Snake bite Spider bite Radiation Burns Frostbite Decubitus ulcers
Infectious	Bacterial cellulitis (see Chap. 35) Deep fungal infection (see Chap. 18)
Vascular compromise	Thrombovascular necrosis Mechanical occlusion Diabetes mellitus (see Chap. 32)
Necrolytic migratory erythema	Hepatopathy/cirrhosis (see Chap. 91) Diabetes/glucagonoma

- Most pathologists now use formalin-fixed tissue for immunoperoxidase staining for the presence of antibody. However, absence of antibody does not rule out autoimmunity as a cause.

Skin and Blood Cultures

- Evaluate the patient for infection by culturing the skin for bacterial and fungal agents.
- For systemic diseases, blood cultures may be indicated.

Other Diagnostic Evaluations

- Evaluate rickettsial serum titers and other disease-specific hematologic tests as indicated.
- Perform liver function tests to assess a suspected case of necrolytic migratory erythema.

- Radiography and ultrasonography are useful if cutaneous lesions are suspected to be secondary to malignancy or systemic disease.
- In rare cases, response to therapy, or removal of a suspected inciting drug confirms the diagnosis.

PRINCIPLES OF TREATMENT

▼ **Key Point** Therapy is most effective when a specific etiology is identified; treatment can then be focused on the elimination or modification of the underlying cause.

Cutaneous necrosis is best managed aggressively with treatment directed against a definitive cause. If there is a possibility that drugs are implicated, discontinue all drugs until establishing a definitive or probable diagnosis. Secondary infection is likely and best treated with a broad-spectrum antibiotic (preferably one that the patient has not previously received). Toxins associated with tissue necrosis can have systemic effects; therefore, debride tissues and flush frequently with sterile saline. When the cause cannot be identified, supportive care is the mainstay of treatment. Hydration and provision of a high-quality protein diet are important aspects of therapy.

SPECIFIC NECROTIZING DERMATOSES

Immune-Mediated Dermatoses

- Immune-mediated dermatoses are one of the more common categories of necrotizing skin diseases. Autoimmune diseases that affect the skin include systemic diseases, such as systemic lupus erythematosus, cold agglutinin disease, and immune-mediated vasculitis, and the more cutaneous conditions of bullous pemphigoid and pemphigus complex. These are discussed elsewhere (see Chap. 43).
- Immune-mediated dermatoses usually cause rather acute lesions that may include vesicles, bullae, ulcers, hemorrhagic nodules, and erosions. The mucocutaneous junctions may be involved. The animal is generally middle-aged or older and may have systemic signs. See Chapter 43 for discussion of autoimmune diseases.
- Treatment depends on the type of immune-mediated disease, the severity, and the extent of lesions. Initially, give systemic corticosteroids at immunosuppressive dosages (prednisone or prednisolone at 2.2–4.4 mg/kg q12–24h PO for dogs; approximately twice that dosage for cats). Other immunosuppressive drugs such as azathioprine (Imuran, Burroughs-Wellcome), cyclophosphamide (Cytoxan, Bristol-Myer), and chlorambucil (Leukeran, Burroughs-Wellcome) may be necessary in severe or refractory cases.

Vasculitis

- Vasculitis is an inflammatory process that occurs in blood vessels and can result in necrosis of the vessels and subsequent death of the adjacent tissue. In addition to vasculitis secondary to immune complex deposition within vessel walls, there are several other known causes of vasculitis.

- Necrotizing vasculitis can be seen with a variety of infections caused by bacteria, viruses, disseminated fungi, and tickborne organisms such as *Rickettsia rickettsii*.
- Specific drugs can induce lesions of vasculitis in animals; the antifungal drug, itraconazole, at a dosage of 5 mg/kg q12h PO has been observed to cause vasculitides in some dogs.
- Allergic vasculitis, which is leukocytoclastic, has been noted in the skin of animals in association with drug administration, especially antibiotics.
- Focal cutaneous vasculitis has been reported at the site of rabies vaccination.
- Neoplasia can result in vessel wall necrosis through production of toxins.
- Unfortunately, a specific cause of vasculitis cannot be identified in a significant number of cases.
- Vasculitis signs usually consist of necrosis and ulceration. These commonly occur on the pressure points, foot pads, pinnae, and extremities. Mucocutaneous ulcerations may be present as well as fever, lymphadenopathy, anorexia, and depression. Signs may be chronic and gradual in onset, or they may be acute.
- Vascultitis is best managed by treatment of the underlying disease.
  - If immune complexes are being deposited in vessel walls, give immunosuppressive corticosteroids or other drugs.
  - If sepsis or generalized bacterial, fungal, or rickettsial disease is identified, treat the infectious agent.
  - If the vasculitis is drug-induced, discontinue the offending drug immediately. Corticosteroids at anti-inflammatory dosages (prednisone or prednisolone, 1.1 mg/kg q12–24h PO) are advocated by some for the management of drug-induced vascultitis.
  - In idiopathic and hypersensitivity-induced vasculitis, corticosteroids may be beneficial. Some cases are self-limiting. In others, dapsone (Avlosulfone, Jacobus) has induced remission. The initial dosage of dapsone is 1 mg/kg q8–12h PO; when the disease is controlled, gradually reduce the dosage. Potential side effects of dapsone include leukopenia, thrombocytopenia, and hepatotoxicity; thus, use dapsone with caution.

Neoplasia-Related Skin Necrosis

- Neoplasia can cause skin necrosis and cutaneous ulceration through a variety of mechanisms. As mentioned previously, neoplasia can cause vasculitis. Through release of necrosis factors generated by tumor cells, there may be local death of tissues. Also, the encroaching growth of a rapidly advancing lesion may cause circulatory compromise leading to cutaneous tissue necrosis. There are many neoplastic conditions that may result in dermal necrosis, including cutaneous lymphoma.

- Clinical signs depend on the type and location of the tumor as well as the stage of the disease. In epidermotropic lymphoma and in some cases of cutaneous lymphoma, ulceration and necrosis of the tissues at the mucocutaneous junctions and inside the oral cavity may be seen with or without well-defined tumors. In other cases of cutaneous lymphoma, multifocal cutaneous necrotic lesions may occur without mucocutaneous lesions.

- Neoplasia treatment depends on the type of tumor, its potential for metastasis, and its biologic behavior. Surgical resection is indicated for solitary lesions. Treatment of other tumors should be based on current recommendations for the individual type of neoplasia.

Drug-Induced Necrosis

- Drug-induced necrosis of the skin followed by ulceration may occur with various drugs. Hypersensitivity may be responsible in many of these cases but proving this can be difficult. Vesiculobullous drug eruptions may precede ulceration, and purpura may occur before there is apparent tissue death.

- Drug-induced necrosis of the skin can cause a wide variety of clinical signs and can mimic almost any condition.
  - When this is due to a systemically administered drug, the cutaneous lesions frequently start out focally but rapidly may become generalized. *Fixed drug eruption* is an exception to this because it always occurs in the same local area on subsequent exposures. Fixed drug reaction can result in focal ulceration. Most drug eruptions begin with generalized erythroderma or erythematous macules, followed by vesiculation and then necrosis or ulceration of the skin. Historically these eruptions may occur during the first exposure to a drug. If they occur with first exposure, they do not usually develop clinically until after 5–7 days of drug administration.
  - Drug reactions to topically applied drugs can occur if the animal has an idiosyncratic reaction or more often if prior exposure has induced hypersensitivity. Contact allergic dermatitis can be the result of a topical drug, and extensive ulceration can occur, especially if the diagnosis is not made early.

- For treatment of drug-induced necrosis, discontinue the offending drug immediately. If the adverse effects resolve and are known to be dosage-dependent, resume therapy at a much lower dosage if the primary disease mandates continuation of the drug. In most instances, it is preferable to substitute a different drug and to avoid giving the suspect drug to the animal in the future. The efficacy of corticosteroids, both at immunosuppressive and at anti-inflammatory levels, for drug reactions are highly controversial. Assess each case individually for potential advantages and disadvantages.

Toxic Epidermal Necrolysis and Erythema Multiforme

Toxic epidermal necrolysis (TEN) and erythema multiforme (EM) are commonly caused by drugs. Although they may have similar etiologies, the histopathology and clinical course of TEN and EM are quite separate. These conditions also may be the result of systemic diseases such as cholangiohepatitis, hepatic necrosis, and endocarditis. Drugs that have been implicated in TEN and EM in dogs and cats include levamisole, penicillins, cephalosporins, sulfonamides, gold salts, 5-fluorocytosine, and antiserum.

Toxic Epidermal Necrolysis

- Toxic epidermal necrolysis (TEN) may mimic EM in its early signs, but it is a much more serious disease. Eventually full-thickness necrosis and sloughing of the skin occur, often involving large areas of skin. The clinical appearance can mimic a burn. There may be a positive Nikolsky sign in which normal-appearing skin can be slid away from the underlying dermis with firm manual pressure.

▼ *Key Point* Because of the extensiveness of TEN, it is crucial to pursue an early diagnosis and to eliminate the inciting cause as quickly as possible while providing aggressive supportive therapy.

- Toxic epidermal necrolysis represents a true dermatologic emergency. Immediately discontinue any suspect drugs and search for systemic disease or neoplasia. Once full-thickness necrosis of the skin begins, start aggressive supportive care with intravenous (IV) fluids such as lactated Ringer's solution to replace estimated fluid loss. Keep affected tissues clean and debrided; and cover with a topical cream such as silver sulfadiazine (Silvadene, Marion) to decrease evaporation from large denuded areas. Corticosteroids (prednisone or prednisolone, 2.2–4.4 mg/kg q12h PO initially, and then reduce) are recommended, especially early in the course of the disease.
- The prognosis is guarded, and in spite of removal of the causative agent or disease, TEN can continue to progress and may be fatal.

Erythema Multiforme

- Erythema multiforme (EM) tends to be less severe than TEN. Multifocal lesions may appear papular, macular, vesicular, bullous, or target-like, with central areas of redness surrounded by an erythematous ring. The patient may show systemic signs of malaise and fever, and cutaneous lesions usually progress to multifocal ulcerations.
- Erythema multiforme is treated by discontinuation of any potential causative drugs as soon as possible and giving supportive care. Symptoms may continue for several days past withdrawal of the offending agent, and pain and scarring may occur.
- The prognosis for survival is better if the primary causative condition is not life-threatening.

Environmental Injury of the Skin

Environmental factors are frequently causative factors in necrosis and ulceration of the skin. The clinical signs of environmental injuries of the skin vary depending on the specific etiology.

Contact Irritant Chemicals

- Contact irritant chemicals can caustically burn or necrose the skin after topical exposure. The list of primary irritants is extensive and includes soaps, detergents, insecticidal sprays, fertilizers, and caustics such as strong acids or alkalies.
- Lesions of cutaneous necrosis can occur wherever the skin was exposed to the irritant. Usually the feet, scrotum, and ventral abdomen are involved if the animal walked or lay down on the causative agent. The muzzle or oral cavity may be involved if the animal tried to remove the compound by licking.
- Treatment requires removal of the irritant followed by supportive care.

Snake Bite

- Snakes, including pit vipers (copperhead, cottonmouth, and rattlesnake) and coral snakes, produce venoms that alter the integrity of blood vessels, blood cells, and coagulation; affect the nervous system; and result in necrosis at the site of envenomation.
- Snake bites most frequently occur during the spring and summer in rural regions with a large indigenous population of venomous snakes. The face and extremities are the common sites of involvement. Initial cutaneous lesions begin with localized soft tissue swelling that spreads rapidly. Local hemorrhage occurs, followed by necrosis of tissue and sloughing.
- Treatment of snake bite varies with the severity of the clinical signs, location of the bite, and length of time since the bite. Initially, immobilize the lesion and keep the patient quiet. Application of tourniquets is controversial, as is glucocorticoid therapy. When polyvalent antivenom (Antivenin, Fort Dodge) is indicated, give one vial slowly IV as soon as possible after the bite and repeat injections as necessary. Monitor the patient closely for anaphylaxis. Broad-spectrum antibiotics are generally indicated because both anaerobic and aerobic infections are often sequelae to the bite. Keep the lesions clean and debride wounds regularly.

Spider Bite

- Spiders (e.g., brown recluse) cause necrotizing skin lesions by injection of a potent dermonecrotic toxin into the tissue when they bite. The enzymes in the venom and the immunologic response of the host both play a role in dictating the clinical response.
- Bite wounds from the brown spider and the brown recluse spider contain potent dermonecrotic toxins. Excise the bite wound if the lesion is identified early as a spider bite of these types. Corticosteroids and antivenom do not appear to reduce local necrosis.
- When systemic signs are present, corticosteroids

combined with supportive care are beneficial. Intravascular hemolysis and renal failure are possible sequelae.

Radiation Injury

- Radiation injuries may be acute or chronic, and necrosis and ulceration of the tissue can occur days to weeks after exposure.
- Radiation injury occurs in the anatomic area previously exposed to radiation. The clinical signs include erythema of the skin, moist desquamation, pigmentation or change in hair color, and loss of hair.
- Treat acute radiation damage with gentle topical cleansing, followed by topical creams. Use medications to control pain as needed.
- Chronic radiation injury and areas of cutaneous atrophy caused by acute damage later necrose and slough. This condition usually is progressive. Supportive care is the primary treatment.

Burn Injury

- Burn injuries can result from heat, sun, flames, scalding liquids, friction, and electricity. The history usually identifies the source of injury.
- Burns can cause significant necrosis and loss of skin. Depending on the depth of the burn, necrosis may involve only the epidermis or may extend deeper into the tissues. Clinical signs usually include pain, erythema, and eschar formation on full-thickness burns. Deeper burns may result in shock, electrolyte and protein disturbances, and life-threatening secondary bacterial infection.
- Treat burns according to their depth (partial- or full-thickness) and extent over the body. Apply intensive and aggressive topical therapy in severe cases. Give medications such as morphine to control pain. Cleanse, debride, and cover burns with an antibacterial cream (e.g., Silvadene, Marion). Fluid replacement and protein supplementation are important. Because secondary bacterial (e.g., *Pseudomonas*) infection is common, systemic broad-spectrum antimicrobial drug therapy is essential. Skin grafts may be necessary for extensive full-thickness burns.
- The prognosis depends on the extent of surface area involved.

Frostbite

- Frostbite occurs when exposure to environmental cold results in vasoconstriction so severe that the effects are not totally reversible on rewarming of the tissues.
- Frostbite most often results in necrosis and sloughing of the tips of the ears or tail. In the dog, the scrotum can also be affected. Debilitated animals are more susceptible because of immobility and poor circulation.
- Frostbite-affected animals usually are presented long after the damage has occurred, and supportive care with debridement is necessary. In early cases, rapidly rewarm the tissues in water heated to 40°–42°C.

Whirlpool therapy can be helpful. Medication for pain may be necessary. If self-trauma can be minimized, the lesions are best left uncovered. Systemic antibiotics are necessary to manage secondary infection.

Decubitus Ulcers

- Decubitus ulcers are a form of vascular compromise related to environmental conditions, characterized by loss of soft tissue cushion over bony prominences.
- Decubitus ulcers usually are secondary to pressure necrosis in recumbent animals. Pressure points, especially stifles, elbows, hocks and hips, are common sites. These lesions are well demarcated, with full-thickness necrosis usually extending to the underlying musculature.
- Decubitus ulcers are best treated by making the patient ambulatory, but if this is not possible, then supportive care is required. Clean and rotate the patient often. Soft bedding or a water mattress is useful. Ulcerated areas need to be kept free of fecal and urine contamination. If possible, cover affected areas with clean dressings. A wide variety of agents are available for topical use. In some cases, surgical debridement and reconstruction are indicated.

Infection-Induced Necrosis

- Infection from deep bacterial or fungal invasion can lead to local areas of cellulitis or abscessation and subsequent necrosis. Embedded foreign bodies may result in central necrosis of the tissue due to release of neutrophilic enzymes. The lesion ruptures and drains externally at the most necrotic site.
- Infection can also cause sepsis and vasculitis resulting in necrolytic dermatitis.
- Treat by administering systemic antimicrobial agents against the offending etiologic agent, based on culture and sensitivity testing. Establish and maintain local drainage.

Vascular Compromise

- Vascular compromise can occur whenever there is interruption of the normal circulation to an area of tissue. This is involved in many of the aforementioned conditions and can be the result of a thrombus, vasculopathy, or mechanical or pressure constriction (e.g., elastic bands).
- Vascular compromise can lead to sloughing or ulcerated lesions. In mechanical occlusion of the circulation, the necrotic lesion is distal or beneath the obstruction. For example, an elastic band tightened around the tail over time causes underlying tissue death and sloughing of the distal tail.
- There is a unique thrombovascular problem in some dachshunds that affects the dependent portion of the aural pinnae.
- In diabetes mellitus, vasculopathies may occur rarely in the extremities of dogs and cats. In these cases a chronic ulcerated lesion on an extremity usually fails to heal even with symptomatic treatment.

- Vascular compromise should be treated based on the etiology and the location of the necrosis. In thrombovascular necrosis of the ears, the therapy of choice is resection of all affected tissue. When mechanical occlusion causes incomplete circulation to the tissue, the mechanical device must be removed. In diabetes mellitus, the optimal approach to the vasculopathy is to carefully monitor and control the diabetes.

Necrolytic Migratory Erythema

- Necrolytic migratory erythema (*superficial necrolytic dermatitis, hepatocutaneous syndrome*) can occur secondary to cirrhosis or diabetes mellitus, but the exact metabolic etiology is still undefined.
- This generally involves ulceration of the mucocutaneous junctions, face, foot pads, and extremities. Extensive crusts are often present over the ulcerated areas.

- The prognosis for successful treatment is poor. Most cases do not respond to long-term dietary manipulation or supportive care, but some cases have a tendency to wax and wane over months. Many of these dogs have very painful feet which may lead to euthanasia.

SUPPLEMENTAL READINGS

Moriello K: Ulcerative Skin Lesions. *In* Moriello K, Mason I, eds.: Handbook of Small Animal Dermatology. Oxford: Pergamon (Elsevier) 1995, pp 105–117, 183–192.

Scott DW, Miller WHM, Griffin C: Small Animal Dermatology. Philadelphia: WB Saunders, 1995, pp 590–606, 872–876.

47 Feline Symmetric Alopecia

Vicki J. Scheidt

Alopecia is defined as the absence of hair from skin areas where it normally is present. In order to properly define the clinical problem and formulate an appropriate differential diagnosis, it is helpful to further categorize alopecia based on the degree (partial or complete), duration (permanent or transient), and distribution (generalized, localized, or regional) of the hair loss. Alopecia in the cat, whether symmetric or asymmetric, may be associated with varying degrees of pruritus and skin reactivity depending on the underlying disease. Note the degree, distribution, and relationship of the pruritus and skin lesions with the alopecia.

NORMAL SHEDDING OF HAIR

In animals, the haircoat aids in thermal regulation, protects the skin, and has important aesthetic qualities. Cats are fastidious and spend a great deal of time grooming their coats. Normal grooming behavior aids in hair removal and normal shedding. However, when grooming becomes excessive, it may accentuate hair damage and skin disease.

Hair follicles have specific cycles of growth (anagen) and rest (telogen) that are primarily stimulated by changes in the photoperiod and to a lesser extent by temperature. From winter to late spring in temperate climates, minimal hair growth occurs and the thick winter coat is shed. Therefore, cats who live outside in colder climates may shed excessively in late spring and develop a transient thinning of the coat (hypotrichosis). Secondary hairs undergo a growth phase in the fall and winter that results in the thick, heavy coat needed for colder temperatures. Seasonal changes are less dramatic in tropical regions or in environments with artificial lighting (e.g., cats confined indoors). Under these conditions, a small amount of hair loss occurs continuously.

ETIOLOGY OF ALOPECIA

Multiple factors play a role in normal hair follicle development and growth (Table 47–1). Absence or changes in one or more of the factors can alter the normal hair growth process and result in alopecia. The underlying causes of feline symmetric alopecia can vary depending on the area or region of the body affected. This review focuses on the causes of symmetric alopecia that are pri-

marily confined to the trunk (dorsum, perineum, caudal thighs, flanks, ventral abdomen, and thorax). The underlying causes of feline symmetric alopecia affecting the trunk region have been classified into those that are associated with self-trauma or pruritus (e.g., licking or scratching) and those that are nonpruritic (Table 47–2).

▼ *Key Point* Determine whether pruritus and concurrent skin inflammation are present when formulating a differential diagnosis for symmetric alopecia in the cat.

Psychogenic Alopecia

This condition is often an enigma. Alopecia develops because the cat excessively licks, bites, or pulls out hair from those areas normally groomed (perineum, ventral abdomen, flank). The etiology or predisposing factor may be due to a primary disease, such as impacted anal glands or cystitis, or to a pruritic skin disease, such as inhalant, food, or flea allergy. However, in most cases a stressful event such as moving to a new surrounding, being hospitalized or boarded, loss of a favorite companion, or the introduction of a new pet or person (baby) into the environment precipitates the disease. Psychogenic alopecia is most common in nervous or "high-strung" cats, such as Siamese, Abyssinian, or black-colored cats. Typically, the areas affected are regions the cat can easily lick, such as the dorsal lumbosacral region, tail, medial and caudal thighs, ventral abdomen, flanks, and perineum. Partial to complete alopecia and stubbled hairs are observed, and concurrent skin changes (e.g., erythema, erosions, exudation, and crusting) are rare.

Feline Endocrine Alopecia

This is a disease of unknown cause. It is presumed to result from hormonal imbalances or deficiencies based on the positive response observed following treatment with specific hormones. The condition is characterized by nonpruritic, symmetric hair loss on the perineum, ventral abdomen, and caudal or medial thighs. Although the alopecia may spread to the flanks, lateral thorax, and proximal tail, the dorsum is usually spared. A thinning of the hair, rather than complete baldness, with normal, noninflamed skin is the classic presentation. Feline endocrine alopecia primarily affects neutered females and males. However, this syndrome

Table 47–1. INTERNAL AND EXTERNAL FACTORS INFLUENCING HAIR FOLLICLE GROWTH AND DEVELOPMENT

Internal Factors	*External Factors*
Genetic	Nutritional
Hormonal	Infectious
Immunologic	Bacterial
Neoplastic	Fungal (dermatophytes)
Stress	Parasitic
	Physical (traumatic)
	Chemical (toxins, drug therapy)

has been reported in intact cats. Significant controversy exists regarding the relationship of hypothyroidism to feline endocrine alopecia. Affected cats usually have normal baseline serum thyroxine (T_4) levels; however, serum T_4 levels at 6 hours following stimulation with thyroid-stimulating hormone (TSH) have been low as compared with TSH stimulation results in normal cats. These findings suggest that some cats with feline endocrine alopecia may have a low thyroid reserve. Feline hyperadrenocorticism is rare; however, natural-occurring and iatrogenic Cushing disease can produce symmetric alopecia of the trunk or pinnae associated with thin hypotonic skin.

Flea Infestation

When associated with mild pruritus and minimal dermatitis, fleas can cause a symmetric alopecia of the dorsum, proximal tail, flanks, perineum, and ventral abdomen. Fleas and/or their feces are usually present on examination. Although a similar presentation can be seen in cats with flea bite allergy, flea-allergic cats are much more pruritic and typically have concurrent skin lesions (miliary dermatitis) along the dorsum, tail base, and ventral abdomen (see Chap. 40).

Food Allergy

Food allergy in cats is associated with nonseasonal pruritus and a variety of clinical presentations, including symmetric alopecia. The skin lesions and severe pruritus may be generalized or confined to the face and

Table 47–2. UNDERLYING CAUSES OF FELINE SYMMETRIC ALOPECIA OF THE TRUNK

Pruritic (Self-Inflicted)	*Nonpruritic*
Psychogenic alopecia	Feline endocrine alopecia
Allergic dermatoses	Sex hormone–related
Food allergy	Hypothyroidism
Atopy	Hyperadrenocorticism
Flea allergy	Systemic disease
Demodicosis	Diabetes mellitus
Dermatophytosis	Renal disease
Otodectic mange	FeLV-FIV
	Telogen effluvium
	Demodicosis
	Dermatophytosis

FeLV, feline leukemia virus; FIV, feline immunodeficiency virus.

ears, or trunk. Alopecia, whether diffuse or symmetric, results from excessive pruritus triggered by an allergic reaction to specific food items ingested (see Chap. 42). Stubbled or broken hairs, with or without concurrent focal erythema, papules, and crusting (miliary dermatitis), are usually present.

Feline Atopy

Atopy in cats may be associated with seasonal or nonseasonal alopecia and pruritus (see Chap. 41). Similar to that seen in feline food allergy, the alopecia is secondary to pruritus and associated with broken or stubbled hairs and concurrent skin lesions. The alopecia may be generalized, or confined to the head and neck or distal extremities.

Dermatophytosis

This is a common cause of localized or generalized alopecia in cats (see Chap. 37). Fungal organisms invade the hair shaft and grow downward but do not penetrate the mitotic region of the hair. Alopecia is not permanent unless the follicle is destroyed by secondary inflammation. A wide spectrum of clinical presentations can be seen with feline dermatophytosis, including the asymptomatic carrier state, particularly in long-haired cats. Classically, the alopecia is focal to diffuse with small numbers of fractured or stubbled hairs and mild epidermal erythema and scaling. The majority of dermatophyte infections (98%) in cats are caused by the zoophilic fungus *Microsporum canis*.

Demodicosis

Demodicosis is a rare cause of alopecia in cats (see Chap. 38). The pathogenesis of feline demodicosis is reported to be similar to that described in the dog and caused by either *Demodex cati* or a recently described and unnamed *Demodex* species. *D. cati* is a normal inhabitant of feline skin, which under favorable conditions proliferates in hair follicles. Lesions consist of focal to diffuse alopecia, erythema, scaling, and crusts that may be localized and self-limiting or generalized. In some cases, these lesions may mimic feline endocrine alopecia. Generalized demodicosis in the cat is usually associated with an underlying immunosuppressive disease, such as feline leukemia virus (FeLV), feline immunodeficiency virus (FIV), or diabetes mellitus. A pruritic, symmetric alopecia of the trunk caused by an unnamed *Demodex* species has been described in cats.

Otodectic Mange

Otodectes mites are the most common cause of otitis externa in cats (see Chap. 55). Otodectic mites can live on the skin surface and infrequently cause a symmetric alopecia over the lower back and tail base. Concurrent otitis externa may or may not be present. The degree of pruritus is variable.

Telogen Effluvium

This is a syndrome in which the anagen cycle is shortened and a wave of hairs simultaneously enter the resting phase. Conditions associated with physiologic stress (e.g., fever, shock, pregnancy and lactation, malnutrition, adverse drug reactions, or a severe debilitating disease) can precipitate rapid shedding in animals. The resultant alopecia can be partial to complete, localized or generalized, and usually is nonpruritic. Affected hairs are easily epilated by friction or grooming.

Systemic Disease

Diffuse, symmetric or asymmetric hair loss in the cat can be caused by systemic disease. Hair follicles are sensitive to pathologic and physiologic changes resulting from systemic diseases, such as end-stage kidney disease, chronic hepatitis, diabetes mellitus, and viral infections (FeLV, FIV). The degree of pruritus and skin lesions associated with the alopecia is variable.

CLINICAL SIGNS

- Feline symmetric alopecia is either pruritic (a direct result of the cat excessively licking or pulling the hair out) or nonpruritic (hair follicles fall out independently). The finding of stubbled or broken hairs suggests self-trauma. However, invasion of organisms, such as dermatophytes, into the hair shaft can also produce fractured or stubbled hairs.
- Excoriations, erosions, and/or ulcerations in conjunction with stubbled hairs usually imply that the hair loss and skin changes are self-inflicted. These lesions, however, may also be secondary manifestations of a primary vesicular or bullous disease.
- Easy epilation of hair from the skin implies that the follicle is in the resting stage. However, hairs frequently epilate easily when a cat is stressed or debilitated.
- Cats who are nervous, poorly adjusted, or high-strung are more likely to develop excessive grooming behavior (e.g., psychogenic alopecia) and subsequent alopecia.
- Pruritic or self-inflicted alopecia that is responsive to systemic corticosteroid therapy suggests an underlying allergic or parasitic etiology. Alopecia that is responsive to systemic progestational therapy, however, may have a hormonal, an allergic, or a psychogenic basis.
- Systemic signs (e.g., anorexia, vomiting, weight loss, polydipsia, polyphagia, or polyuria) may be present when the alopecia is associated with either a primary systemic disease (e.g., renal disease, diabetes mellitus) or a secondary hormonal imbalance (e.g., iatrogenic Cushing disease).

DIAGNOSIS

▼ *Key Point* Feline symmetric alopecia can be classified as either pruritic or nonpruritic based on the history and gross appearance of the haircoat and skin. The goal of diagnostic evaluations is to identify the underlying disease. When self-induced alopecia is suspected but not supported by history and physical findings, preventing the cat from licking the body, using an Elizabethan collar continually for 4–6 weeks, is often conclusive. In such cases, obtain baseline diagnostic tests first (e.g., skin scrapings, fungal culture).

History

Evaluate for pruritus, the general psychological state of the cat, environmental changes that preceded the alopecia, past and current hormonal status of the cat, concurrent systemic signs, and possible nutritional or therapy-related causes.

Physical Examination

Perform a thorough examination of the integument and all internal organ systems.

- Examine hair shafts and follicles from affected areas, grossly and microscopically, for structural abnormalities (e.g., fractures, bulges, constrictions). Telogen hairs plucked from the skin have a fusiform appearance and a dry, white, club-shaped root on gross or microscopic examination. In contrast, growing or anagen hairs have a blunt end that is glistening, pigmented, and surrounded by a root sheath.
- Examine the skin in both alopecic and normal areas for primary (erythema, papules) and secondary (crusts, scale, hyperpigmentation) lesions. Note the thickness and elasticity of the skin.
- Search for external parasites (fleas, flea dirt).
- Note abnormalities in other organ systems.

Diagnostic Tests

Tests for Mites

- Perform *skin scrapings* to rule out feline demodicosis, *Otodectes cyanotis*, or other external mite infestations.
- Collect *ear smears* from cats with concurrent otitis externa or those with a history of recurrent otodectic mange (ear mites).

Tests for Dermatophytes

- Perform *fungal culture* to identify a dermatophyte infection. Examine affected hairs with an ultraviolet light (Wood's lamp). Approximately 50% of the cases of *M. canis* fluoresce. Use hairs that fluoresce an apple-green color, both for culturing and for microscopic examination for fungal spores or hyphae, using a clearing agent (KOH). Refer to Chapter 37 for details concerning the diagnosis of dermatophytosis.

Allergy Testing

- Institute an *elimination diet* trial (see Chap. 42), using rice and lamb baby food or rabbit meat, in cats with a history of symmetric alopecia and nonseasonal pruritus that is partially or completely responsive to systemic corticosteroids. The diagnosis of food allergy is confirmed with amelioration of the pruritus and/or excessive licking during a 4- to 6-week diet trial and recurrence of signs following provocative exposure to the original diet or offending antigen.

- Perform *intradermal skin testing or in vitro allergy testing* for flea and environmental allergens in cats with a history of seasonal (spring to fall) and nonseasonal pruritus that is responsive to systemic corticosteroid therapy. Correlate positive reactions with the history of allergen exposure and seasonality.

Skin Biopsy

- *Skin biopsy* of affected and unaffected areas is helpful in evaluating the growing stages of hair follicles and in identifying any concurrent follicular inflammation—whether infectious, parasitic, or allergic. (See Chapter 49 for skin biopsy technique.)

Endocrine Tests

- Obtain *baseline serum thyroid hormone* levels or perform a *TSH stimulation test* in cats with nonpruritic alopecia and histopathologic findings consistent with an endocrine-based alopecia. A TSH stimulation test is superior to serum baseline T_4 levels for diagnosing hypothyroidism in the dog and cat and is the test of choice (see Chap. 29).
- Perform an *adrenocorticotropic hormone (ACTH) stimulation test* in cats with nonpruritic alopecia and concurrent polyuria, polydipsia, polyphagia, lethargy, pendulous abdomen, and/or thin, easily torn skin to rule out iatrogenic or naturally occurring hyperadrenocorticism (see Chap. 31).

Laboratory Tests

- Perform a *complete blood count, serum biochemical profile, and urinalysis* in cats with symmetric alopecia and concurrent systemic signs (e.g., fever, depression, anorexia, polyuria-polydipsia) to identify any underlying primary disease (e.g., diabetes mellitus) or adverse reaction to previous therapy (e.g., iatrogenic Cushing disease resulting from prolonged systemic corticosteroid or progestational therapy).
- The finding of peripheral eosinophilia in a cat with seasonal or nonseasonal pruritus and/or licking is suggestive of an allergic or parasitic dermatitis.
- Perform *FeLV and FIV tests* in cats with generalized demodicosis, nonhealing skin infections, or protracted systemic signs (see Chaps. 6 and 7).

TREATMENT

Feline symmetric alopecia is often managed with "scientific neglect" during the early stages when hair loss is mild and pruritus is absent. However, if the alopecia progresses or is observed to be self-inflicted, pursue an underlying cause and prescribe appropriate treatment. Determine from the onset whether the hair loss is due to self-inflicted behavior (licking, chewing, hair pulling) or to an underlying, nonpruritic disease (hormonal, systemic disease). Many cats are "closet lickers"; therefore, the owners may not observe excessive licking or chewing. In such cases, applying an Elizabethan collar on the cat for 3–4 weeks can be very helpful in iden-

tifying whether or not the cat is actually licking the hair out. Chronic cases of symmetric alopecia that are associated with secondary skin changes and pruritus often require symptomatic treatment with anti-inflammatory agents during the initial stages of the diagnostic workup. Avoid prolonged corticosteroid therapy until the primary etiology has been identified and appropriately treated.

Anti-Inflammatory Therapy

Use anti-inflammatory drugs in cats with symmetric alopecia and concurrent pruritus who are suspected of having an underlying allergic disease (e.g., food allergy, atopy, or flea allergy). Short-term treatment with systemic antihistamines or corticosteroids may be used during the initial stages until the causative allergen is identified (diet trial, intradermal or serum allergy testing) and is eliminated or appropriately controlled (hypoallergenic diet, hyposensitization, flea control).

Systemic Antihistamines

Compared with systemic corticosteroid use, systemic antihistamine use is generally not as effective in controlling pruritus in cats. Chlorpheniramine maleate, given at 2 mg/cat q12h PO, can be an effective treatment in cats with pruritus of an unknown or idiopathic nature. The author has found hydroxyzine hydrochloride, given at 10 mg/cat q12h PO, to be effective for control of pruritus in cats with feline atopy.

Fatty Acid Supplements

DVM Derm Caps (DVM Pharmaceuticals), 0.11 ml/kg q24h PO, are occasionally effective in controlling pruritus in cats when given alone or in combination with an antihistamine (chlorpheniramine, hydroxyzine). However, 4–8 weeks may be required before improvement is noted.

Systemic Corticosteroids

Corticosteroids are very effective in the management of pruritus in cats. Cats require much higher doses than dogs to suppress or control pruritus of an allergic nature. Compared with other species, cats appear to be more resistant to the harmful side effects of systemic corticosteroid therapy and development of iatrogenic Cushing disease. Administer prednisolone or prednisone at 2 mg/kg q24h PO for 7–14 days; then decrease to an alternate-day schedule and gradually taper to the lowest effective dose. Methylprednisolone acetate (Depo-Medrol, Upjohn) given at 4–5 mg/kg or 20 mg/cat SC is also effective when administered every 2–3 weeks. The total treatment period, when giving repeated corticosteroid injections (Depo-Medrol) every 2–3 weeks, should not exceed 3 months.

Systemic Progestational Compounds

These compounds have been used for years to treat various feline skin diseases, including symmetric alopecia, both pruritic (e.g., atopy, psychogenic alopecia) and nonpruritic (e.g., feline endocrine alopecia). In cats, progestational compounds such as megestrol acetate

(Ovaban, Schering-Plough) are immunosuppressive and have potent anti-inflammatory activity. They exhibit a wide spectrum of actions and side effects. Serious side effects in the cat include decreased spermatogenesis, pyometra, mammary gland fibroadenomatous hyperplasia in both male and female intact and neutered animals, permanent or transient diabetes mellitus, adrenocortical suppression, and various behavioral abnormalities (e.g., polyphagia with subsequent weight gain, polyuria, polydipsia, and lethargy). The oral dosage in cats is variable and starts with an induction dose of 2.5–5 mg per cat q24h for 5 days, decreases to every other day, and is tapered to 2.5–5 mg every 5–7 days for 1–2 months.

▼ *Key Point* Progestational compounds are not approved for use in cats. Because of this and their numerous side effects, they are administered only as the last choice.

Hormonal Therapy

Hormonal therapy has been successfully used in the cat to treat nonpruritic, symmetric alopecia that is associated with normal-appearing skin and classified as endocrine in origin (see Chap. 45). Although various hormones have been effective in the treatment of feline endocrine alopecia, relapses are common and intermittent lifelong therapy is often necessary.

Combined Estrogen and Testosterone

These have been used successfully in both neutered male and female cats with feline endocrine alopecia. Repositol testosterone (12.5 mg/cat) and repositol diethylstilbestrol (0.625 mg/cat) are given IM separately or in combination. Although hair regrowth is usually present by 6 weeks, relapses are common. Side effects, including signs of estrus in females, aggressive behavior or urine spraying in males, and hepatobiliary disease in both, have been reported following androgen and/or estrogen therapy.

Thyroid Hormone

Supplemental thyroid hormone has been found to be effective in cats with feline endocrine alopecia, despite normal serum baseline thyroid levels. Sodium levothyroxine is effective at 0.05–0.1 mg q12–24h PO. Sodium liothyroxine (Tertroxin, Glaxo) given at 50 µg q12h PO has been reported to produce complete hair regrowth in 73% of cats treated (Thoday, 1989).

Progestational Compounds

These compounds can be effective in the management of feline endocrine alopecia. Megestrol acetate (2.5–5.0 mg/cat PO once every other day for 1–2 months) is preferred over repositol progesterone due to potential side effects of the latter in cats.

Adrenalectomy

Either unilateral or bilateral adrenalectomy is the treatment of choice for naturally occurring hyperadrenocorticism in the cat (see Chap. 31). Discontinue and avoid future treatment with systemic corticosteroids and progestational compounds in cats with iatrogenic hyperadrenocorticism.

Antianxiety Drugs and Tranquilizers

These drugs can be used in conjunction with behavior modification to treat cats with stress-induced symmetric alopecia or psychogenic alopecia. Because response to systemic antianxiety medication is variable in cats and requires much patience and effort on the part of the owner, identification and removal (if possible) of the predisposing cause is crucial. Use diazepam, phenobarbital, or megestrol acetate as adjunctive therapy to behavioral modification. The main goal is to calm the cat and eventually discontinue the antianxiety medication.

- *Diazepam* (Valium, Roche) given at 1–2 mg/cat q24h PO for 4–8 weeks has a calming effect and is effective in some cases.
- *Phenobarbital* given orally at 2–5 mg/kg q12h PO is effective. However, adjustment of the dosage may be required.
- *Megestrol acetate* acts directly on the limbic system and behavior center, transforming the high-strung cat into a very euphoric, affectionate animal. The dosage is 2.5–5.0 mg/cat q24h PO for 5 days; then treat every other day for 2 weeks, tapered to twice a week for a total treatment period of 2–3 months.

Specific Therapy
Hypoallergenic Diet

Feed a hypoallergenic diet to cats with symmetric alopecia caused by a dietary allergy (see Chap. 42). Home-cooked diets containing lamb or rabbit meat, vegetable baby food, and cooked rice can be fed. Many cats are finicky eaters and will not eat home-cooked diets. Pureeing the foods often increases the palatability of home-cooked diets. Use a daily multiple mineral-vitamin supplement when home-cooked diets are used for a prolonged period. The author has found several commercial diets to be well tolerated by food-allergic cats including canned Response Formula LB/Feline (Eukanuba Veterinary Diets) and canned or dry Limited Diets Feline/venison and potato (Innovative Veterinary Diets).

Hyposensitization

Hyposensitization has been reported to be an effective treatment for feline atopy (see Chap. 41). In a recent study, Halliwell found an improvement of at least 50% in 42 cats with various dermatologic manifestations of feline atopy following desensitization. The percent of response for each dermatologic manifestation varied, ranging from 60–94%.

Flea Control

Flea control is a critical part of the management of feline flea allergy and infestation. Currently, there are several topical and/or systemic products available for use in cats and dogs which are so effective that environmental treatment is often not necessary (see Chap. 40).

Lufeneron (Program, Novartis), given orally at 10–15 mg/kg once a month, prevents the synthesis of chitin which is needed for normal flea development. Eggs laid by fleas that feed on treated cats or dogs fail to hatch and new larvae fail to molt. It has no affect on adult fleas. In contrast, topical solutions containing either imidacloprid (Advantage, Bayer) or fipronil (Frontline Top Spot, Rhone Merieux), when applied once a month to the skin surface, kill adult fleas before they have a chance to lay eggs, eliminating the need for concurrent environmental flea treatment. Hyposensitization, using commercial flea antigens, has not been effective for treatment of flea allergy in the cat.

Antifungal Therapy

Clinical management of feline dermatophytosis includes clipping and cleansing of the affected areas, generalized topical antifungal therapy, isolation and appropriate sanitation, and systemic antifungal therapy (griseofulvin, ketoconazole, itraconazole) in severe generalized cases. Refer to Chapter 37 for details concerning the treatment of feline dermatophytosis.

Miticidal Therapy

- Apply miticidal solutions containing 2% lime sulfur (DVM Pharmaceuticals) or 0.025% amitraz (Mitaban, Upjohn) weekly for 4–6 weeks to treat symmetric alopecia caused by *D. cati* or other *Demodex* species. However, amitraz has not been approved for use in cats (see Chap. 38).

- Treat symmetric alopecia caused by otodectic mange with topical or systemic ivermectin (Ivomec, MSD Agvet) at 0.2–0.4 mg/kg PO or SC weekly for 4–6 weeks. Because of the contagious nature of *O. cyanotis*, both the affected cat and all contact animals are treated for 4–6 weeks with a miticidal otic preparation or ivermectin.

SUPPLEMENTAL READINGS

Halliwell REW: Efficacy of hyposensitization in feline allergic diseases based upon results of in vitro testing for allergen-specific immunoglobulin E. J Am Anim Hosp Assoc 33:282, 1997.

Kirk RW: Feline alopecia. *In* Kirk RW, ed.: Current Veterinary Therapy VII. Philadelphia: WB Saunders, 1980, p 490.

Miller WH, Scott DW: Efficacy of chlorpheniramine maleate for management of pruritus in cats. J Am Vet Med Assoc 197:67, 1990.

Muller GH, Kirk RW, Scott DW: Small Animal Dermatology, 4th Ed. Philadelphia: WB Saunders, 1989, p 701.

Scott DW: Feline dermatology, 1900–1978: A monograph. J Am Anim Hosp Assoc 16:334, 1980.

Scott DW: Feline dermatology, 1979–1982: Introspective retrospections. J Am Anim Hosp Assoc 20:537, 1984.

Scott DW, Miller WH, Griffin CE: Muller and Kirk's Small Animal Dermatology, 5th Ed. Philadelphia: WB Saunders, 1995.

Thoday KL: Differential diagnosis of symmetric alopecia in the cat. *In* Kirk RW, ed.: Current Veterinary Therapy IX. Philadelphia: WB Saunders, 1986, p 545.

Thoday KL: Aspects of feline symmetric alopecia (abstract). First World Congress of Veterinary Dermatology, Dijon, France, September 1989.

48 Miliary Dermatitis and Eosinophilic Granuloma Complex

Wayne S. Rosenkrantz

Miliary dermatitis (MD) and eosinophilic granuloma complex (EGC) are extremely common cutaneous reaction patterns in the cat. The term *miliary* is a descriptive one, and it implies that the papules and crusts characteristic of the syndrome resemble millet seeds. The term *eosinophilic granuloma* is also descriptive of a group of lesions affecting the skin and oral cavity of the cat. The three clinical histologic syndromes included in this complex are eosinophilic ulcer, eosinophilic plaque, and eosinophilic (collagenolytic) granuloma.

ETIOLOGY

▼ *Key Point* Miliary dermatitis and eosinophilic granuloma complex are neither final diagnoses nor pathognomonic for any one disease. Many etiologies exist for both reaction patterns. The ability to control or cure chronic or recurrent cases is dependent on pursuing the underlying cause. The two conditions share similar etiologies and therefore are discussed together in this chapter.

Underlying causes or predisposing factors for MD and EGC (Table 48–1) include (1) allergies, (2) parasites, (3) infectious diseases, and (4) miscellaneous conditions.

Allergies

Allergies to biting insects (e.g., fleas, mosquitos and flies), foods, inhalants, and contact substances have been associated with MD in the cat. With the exception of contact allergies, all of these reactions have also been associated with EGC. In particular, flea and other biting insect hypersensitivities have been emphasized as etiologies in EGC.

Parasites

Parasites, such as fleas, *Cheyletiella*, *Notoedres*, chiggers, *Otodectes*, lice, cat fur mites, and endoparasites, have been associated with MD. Fleas have also been implicated in EGC as a cause of a hypersensitivity reaction. These parasites also produce lesions in MD by way of a hypersensitivity reaction. Refer to the respective chapters concerning these various parasites for additional information.

Infectious Diseases

Infectious causes for both entities include bacterial infections and dermatophytosis. In EGC, viral infections are an additional consideration.

- The most common bacteria isolated in both entities include *Staphylococcus*, β-hemolytic *Streptococcus*, *Pasteurella*, and *Bacteroides* species. Positive clinical response to a variety of antibiotics in both MD and EGC gives support to a bacterial etiology.
- The major dermatophyte species isolated from cats is *Microsporum canis* (see Chap. 37). This dermatophyte can produce MD, but it can also be found on cats without MD. This dermatophyte is rarely isolated from EGC lesions, and its significance in this complex is questionable.

Miscellaneous Causes

Miscellaneous conditions causing MD include genetic factors, immune-mediated diseases, drug reactions, nutritional factors, epitheliotropic lymphoma, and idiopathic causes. Genetic factors, immune-mediated disease, and idiopathic causes have received attention as etiologies in EGC.

- *Hereditary (genetic) factors* have been implicated based on reports of offspring from affected cats, which have developed similar MD or EGC lesions.
- *Immune-mediated disorders*, such as pemphigus foliaceus, can produce MD-like lesions. Immune-mediated disease has not received much consideration in EGC, although antiepithelial antibodies (IgG) have been documented in cats with eosinophilic ulcers.
- *Drug reactions* can mimic any skin disease. Cases of drug-induced MD lesions have been seen but are rare. Drug-induced EGC lesions are questionable; however, some of the dorsal cervical eosinophilic ulcerative lesions can be due to injection site reactions.
- *Nutritional factors* related to fatty acid or biotin deficiencies have been reported in the older literature as causes of MD. Such deficiencies are unlikely in cats on commercial well-balanced diets.
- *Cutaneous neoplasms* (squamous cell carcinoma, mast cell tumor, lymphoma) can mimic MD and/or EGC.
- *Idiopathic* cases exist in both MD and EGC. Such cases most likely reflect the inability to identify one of the

TABLE 48–1. ETIOLOGIES OF MILIARY DERMATITIS AND EOSINOPHILIC GRANULOMA COMPLEX

	Miliary Dermatitis	Eosinophilic Granuloma Complex
Allergies		
Flea allergy	++++	++++
Mosquito and biting fly hypersensitivity	+	+++
Food allergy	+++	+++
Atopy	+++	+++
Contact allergy	+	
Parasitic Diseases		
Fleas	+++	++
Cheyletiella	++	
Notoedres	++	
Chiggers (trombiculiasis)	++	
Otodectes	++	
Lice (pediculosis)	++	
Demodicosis	+	
Cat fur mite	+	
Endoparasites	+	
Infectious Diseases		
Bacterial	+++	+++
Dermatophytosis	+++	+
Viral		+
Miscellaneous Conditions		
Genetic	+	++
Immune-mediated diseases	+	+
Drug reactions	+	
Nutritional	+	
Neoplasia	+	++
Idiopathic causes	+++	+++

+, Rare cause of syndrome; ++, uncommon cause of syndrome; +++, frequent cause of syndrome; ++++, major cause of syndrome.

aforementioned diseases. Undefined allergic reactions may account for a number of these idiopathic cases.

CLINICAL SIGNS

Miliary Dermatitis

- The lesions of MD are usually small erythematous papules (1–2 mm) that develop into crusts. Secondary lesions result from self-trauma and produce alopecia, erosions, excoriations, and acute pyotraumatic dermatitis. The distribution can be localized to a specific area or generalized. The dorsal lumbosacral, cervical, and inguinal areas are the most common sites affected.
- Additional physical signs that may be noted in MD include the following:
  - Peripheral lymphadenopathy of the inguinal lymph nodes
  - Personality changes such as depression and hiding
  - Pain or twitching over affected sites
  - Concurrent lesions of EGC

Eosinophilic Granuloma Complex

The lesions of EGC are variable and are classified into three types.

- *Eosinophilic ulcer* (indolent, rodent, and lip ulcer) is a well-circumscribed, red-brown to yellow, ulcerated lesion most commonly found on the upper lip of the cat. The lesions are generally nonpainful and nonpruritic.
- *Eosinophilic plaque* is a well-circumscribed, raised exudative lesion that is highly pruritic and generally found on the abdomen or inguinal region. This lesion is the most common form of EGC in cats with concurrent MD.
- *Eosinophilic collagenolytic granuloma* is seen primarily in young cats and is a well-circumscribed, raised, erythematous to yellow linear, papular, or nodular lesion. It is most commonly found in a linear pattern (linear granuloma) over the caudal thighs and in a nodular pattern on the lower lip and in the oral cavity. Other sites include the bridge of the nose, chin, lips, pinnae, footpads, paws, and perianal region.

DIAGNOSIS

History

History helps identify seasonal allergies, such as flea and other insect hypersensitivities, atopy, and chiggers. A history of pruritus with MD lesions is more typical of parasitic and allergic hypersensitivity disorders.

Physical Examination

Physical examination can also help narrow the differential diagnosis in both MD and EGC.

Miliary Dermatitis

The distribution of MD lesions favors some etiologies over others:

- Dorsal distribution (especially the lumbosacral area) favors flea hypersensitivity. Cheyletiellosis can also have a dorsal distribution.
- When the head and neck are affected consider notoedric mange, otodectic mange, food allergy, atopy, pyoderma, or pemphigus.

Eosinophilic Granuloma Complex

The distribution of EGC lesions is less helpful in limiting the differential diagnoses.

- Nasal and pinnal forms of eosinophilic collagenolytic granuloma tend to support the diagnosis of insect bite reactions (i.e., mosquito and black fly).
- Eosinophilic plaques on the abdomen and inguinal region suggest the diagnosis of flea hypersensitivity.
- Pruritic cervical EGC lesions are more commonly seen in food allergy, atopy, bacterial infection, or possible injection site reactions.

Minimum Database

- *Skin scrapings, Scotch tape preparations,* and *combings of hair and dander* for fleas and mites are very important in the initial MD diagnostic evaluation.
- *Skin cytology* can be of value to determine the presence of infectious organisms and inflammatory cells. Skin cytologic specimens are obtained by fine needle aspirate of the lesion or by touching a glass slide to the lesion. Tissue eosinophilia suggests the diagnosis of parasitic and allergic disorders.
- *Dermatophyte culture* is the best way to rule out a dermatophyte as the cause of MD (see Chap. 37).

Bacterial Culture

Bacterial culture and sensitivity tests, performed on a skin biopsy sample, can give additional information on etiology and choice of correct antibiotic for therapy.

Routine Blood Tests

- *Complete blood counts* may reveal peripheral eosinophilia associated with parasitic and allergic disorders, especially flea allergy. Peripheral eosinophilia tends to be seen in most cases of eosinophilic plaque and in many cases of eosinophilic collagenolytic granuloma, especially with oral lesions.
- *Serum biochemical analysis* helps rule out other concurrent medical problems. *Viral testing* for feline leukemia virus and feline immunodeficiency virus are recommended in recurrent cases of MD and EGC (see Chaps. 6 and 7). Results of both chemistry and viral screens will influence treatment and prognosis.

Skin Biopsy

Dermatopathology is one of the most important diagnostic tests performed. Findings may support the clinical assessment, suggest additional diagnoses, or provide a specific diagnosis. With EGC, specific histologic patterns have been associated with the three clinical entities.

- *Eosinophilic ulcer* is usually characterized by a chronic ulcerative suppurative dermatitis. In some cases histopathology may reveal an eosinophilic collagenolytic dermatitis with palisading granulomatous inflammation.
- *Eosinophilic plaque* is characterized by marked intercellular edema (spongiotic dermatitis) and tissue eosinophilia. This is similar to what is seen histologically in some MD lesions.
- *Eosinophilic collagenolytic granuloma* is characterized by eosinophilic collagenolytic dermatitis with palisading granulomatous inflammation.

Allergy Testing

- A *food elimination diet* is the only way to accurately rule out food allergy (see Chap. 42). Such a diet consists of a protein source that the cat does not or has not eaten routinely. The common choice is lamb baby food, but ham baby food, home-cooked chicken, turkey, fish, rabbit, and other protein sources have been provided successfully (see Chap. 42). If baby food is used, feed a product that does not contain onion powder (i.e., Beechnut) to avoid potential for Heinz body anemia. The diet is fed strictly for 6–8 weeks.
- *Intradermal allergy testing* helps rule out the diagnoses of insect and inhaled allergies. Allergy testing in the cat is difficult to perform and interpret. Testing is, therefore, best done by an experienced veterinary allergist (see Chap. 41).
- *In vitro allergy testing* has improved significantly in the cat. The author has had results comparable to skin testing using a liquid-phase enzymoimmunometric assay (VARL; Pasadena, CA) for selecting antigens for hyposensitization.

TREATMENT

▼ *Key Point* Many forms of therapy have been described for both MD and EGC. The best long-term management is achieved when a definitive diagnosis of the underlying cause has been established and specific therapy for that disease is prescribed.

Corticosteroid Therapy

This therapy can be tried in first-time cases of MD and EGC. In chronic recurrent cases, alternative therapy is given, based on information from an appropriate workup. Even with proper workup, refractory allergies or idiopathic cases of both MD and EGC may require long-term corticosteroid therapy. A variety of corticosteroids can be tried.

- Methylprednisolone acetate (Depo-Medrol, Upjohn) at 4 mg/kg IM is a commonly used, and often efficacious, long-acting injectable corticosteroid. Cases of refractory EGC may need three injections at 2-week intervals. In general, after remission, do not use methylprednisolone acetate more often than every 3 months.
- As an alternative to methylprednisolone acetate, give anti-inflammatory doses of prednisone at 2.2 mg/kg PO q24h for resolution of lesions. Decrease the dose to 1–2 mg/kg PO q48h for maintenance.
- Some cases can be successfully managed with initial injections of methylprednisolone acetate and then maintained with oral prednisone at 1–2 mg/kg PO q48h.
- Other oral corticosteroids can be tried in refractory cases. Use triamcinolone at 0.4–0.6 mg/kg PO q24h, then tapering to 0.2–0.3 mg/kg PO q48h–72h for maintenance; or dexamethasone at 0.25–0.5 mg PO q24h, then tapering to 0.25–0.125 mg q48h–72h for maintenance.
- Use intralesional triamcinolone (Vetalog, Squibb) in refractory EGC lesions at a dose of 1–4 mg injected intralesionally.

Antihistamine Therapy

Antihistamines can be tried in atopy, flea allergy, and idiopathic MD and EGC: chlorpheniramine at 2–4 mg PO q12h; amitriptyline at 10 mg PO q12–24h; or hydroxyzine HCl at 10 mg PO q12h. Chlorpheniramine appears to be more effective and has fewer sedative or excitatory side effects.

Food Allergy Management

After determining that a cat has a food allergy, manage with a balanced home-cooked diet or a commercial diet that is tolerated (see Chap. 42).

Hyposensitization Therapy

Hyposensitization, based on in vitro or in vivo testing, is becoming more promising in cases of EGC and MD in which atopy is the underlying cause. In a limited number of cases antigen injections can manage recurrent EGC and MD lesions (see Chap. 41). Flea hyposensitization has had little benefit in controlling flea allergy in the cat. Protocols are similar to those in dogs.

Parasiticidal Therapy

Because parasites directly or indirectly, via a hypersensitivity reaction, contribute to the lesions in MD and EGC, the control of parasites on the pet and in the environment is extremely important. Flea control is described in Chapter 40. Treatment of *Notoedres* and *Cheyletiella* is described in Chapter 39.

Antimicrobial Therapy

Use antibiotic therapy for primary or secondary infections in both MD and EGC. Initially, select antibiotics empirically based on cytologic findings. In chronic cases, culture and sensitivity results are employed. Antibiotics for empiric therapy include trimethoprim-potentiated sulfas, 30 mg/kg PO q12h; cefadroxil (Cefa-Tabs, Fort Dodge), 20 mg/kg PO q12h; amoxicillin-clavulanate (Clavamox, SmithKline Beecham), 12–15 mg/kg PO q12h; or enrofloxacin (Baytril, Bayer), 5 mg/kg PO q24h. Continue treatment for a minimum of 2 weeks and 10 days past clinical cure. Therapy for dermatophytosis is described in detail in Chapter 37.

Immunomodulating Therapy

Drugs that either stimulate or suppress the immune response have been tried with EGC. Chlorambucil (Leukeran, Burroughs Wellcome), 0.1–0.2 mg/kg PO q48h or aurothioglucose (Solganal, Schering-Plough), 2 mg/kg IM weekly, may be used in refractory EGC. Both drugs have long lag phases before response is seen and can create side effects (e.g., bone marrow suppression) which should be monitored. Interferon (Roferon, Hoffman La Roche) has also been tried in refractory EGC cases at a dose of 30 IU/cat, PO once daily for 7 days on a one-week-on/one-week-off schedule, with limited success.

Progestational Therapy

Progestational compounds have been advocated for treating both MD and EGC. Most veterinary dermatologists do not use or recommend these products because of their potential for severe side effects. They are not approved for use in cats. With the effectiveness of other forms of therapy, progestational drug therapy is undesirable.

SUPPLEMENTAL READING

Rosenkrantz W: Eosinophilic granuloma confusion. *In* August JR, ed.: Consultations in Feline Internal Medicine. Philadelphia: WB Saunders, 1990, pp 121–124.

Rosenkrantz W: Feline eosinophilic granuloma complex. *In* Griffin CE, Kwochka KW, MacDonald JM, eds.: Current Veterinary Dermatology. St. Louis: Mosby–Year Book, 1993, pp 319–324.

49 Skin Biopsy

Robert O. Schick / Mary P. Schick

BIOPSY SELECTION

- Properly selected, collected, and processed skin biopsies are likely to provide the definitive diagnosis and prognosis for many skin diseases. Skin biopsy samples are valuable in determining the malignancy of neoplastic skin lesions as well as their invasive nature.
- Biopsy "fresh" vesicles, bullae, or pustules that are less than 24 hours old. Skin lesions, such as nonhealing wounds, pigmented lesions, and purpura, and those of infiltrative diseases, such as discoid or systemic lupus erythematosus and amyloidosis, are best biopsied within 1 month of detection.

▼ *Key Point* Biopsy of primary and fresh skin lesions is most likely to yield a definitive diagnosis. Certain types of skin lesions yield less valuable information, because of altered histology, including chronic, traumatized, previously treated, or old lesions.

EQUIPMENT

- Use a cold sterilization tray filled with an appropriate antiseptic solution holding the various instruments for easy accessibility.
- Use the following instruments to handle the delicate skin specimens:
  - Scissors (straight or curved iris)
  - Fine eye forceps
  - Curved hemostats
  - Needle holder
  - Suture scissors
  - Scalpel blades (# 11 or # 15)
  - Scalpel handle
  - Black indelible-ink pen (Sharpie, Sanford Corp.)
- Obtain disposable skin punch biopsies (Baker's Biopsy Punch, Key Pharmaceutical) primarily of 4 and 6 mm (Fig. 49–1).

▼ *Key Point* To obtain the best skin punch biopsy, do not reuse the disposable punches.

- Lidocaine 2% (Lidocaine 2%, Butler Company) or lidocaine HCl 1% solution with epinephrine 1:100,000 (Xylocaine 1%, Antra Pharmaceutical Products) are the local anesthetics of choice.

BIOPSY PROCEDURES

Scalpel Wedge Biopsy

The scalpel is most commonly used to perform excisional biopsies, especially subcutaneous ones that are not amenable to punch biopsies.

- Indications
  - To obtain a large sample or an entire lesion.
  - To provide lesional, transitional, and normal tissue for histopathologic viewing.
  - To excise deep lesions or neoplasms. The lower dermis or subcutaneous fat provides characteristic histologic features for orientation.

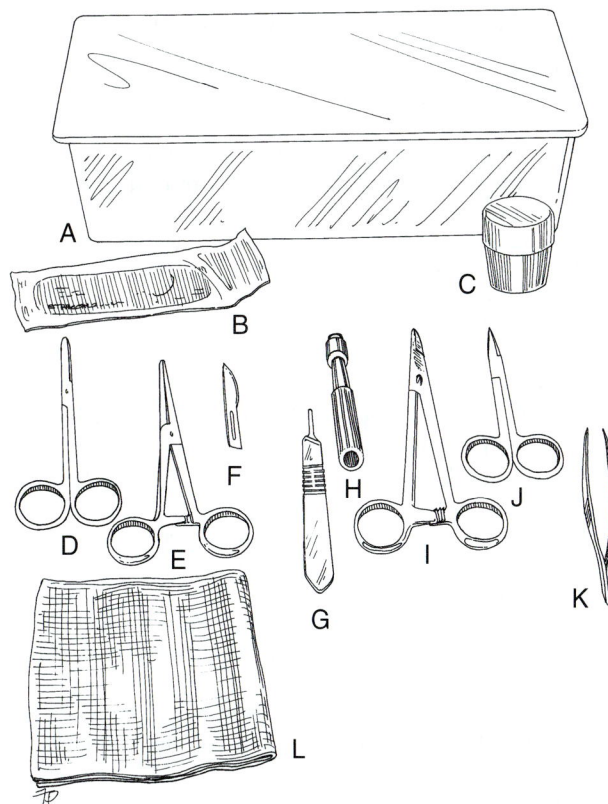

Figure 49–1. Skin punch biopsy instruments. *A*, Cold sterilization boat; *B*, suture material; *C*, formalin specimen container; *D*, suture scissors; *E*, straight hemostat; *F*, scalpel blade; *G*, scalpel blade handle; *H*, biopsy punch; *I*, needle holder; *J*, iris scissors; *K*, tissue forceps; and *L*, gauze sponge.

- To excise an entire neoplasm along with adjacent normal tissue to assess histologically for depth and width of neoplastic cell infiltration.
- Advantages
  - Total removal of solitary neoplasm may be possible.
  - Fragile bullous or vesicular lesions and subcutaneous fat are easily obtained intact.
  - Specimen preparation on the long axis may provide a microscopic histologic view of the abnormal tissue, transitional zone, and normal tissue boundaries, so that a prognosis as well as a diagnosis may be obtained.
- Disadvantages
  - Pain to the animal and extensive time may be involved in removal.
  - General anesthesia may be required.
  - Large defects may not allow for cosmetic closure.

Technique

1. Use local or general anesthesia, depending on the size and location of the lesion.
2. Hold the scalpel perpendicularly or slightly angled with respect to the lesion to allow for the best cosmetic closure. Undermine the adjacent subcutaneous tissues to loosen the skin for best closure.

Punch Biopsy

This is the most commonly used technique to obtain skin specimens for histologic examination.

- Indications
  - For collection of abnormal tissue for histologic examination
  - For biopsy of samples from neoplasms
  - For biopsy of samples from early bullous, vesicular, or pustular lesions

▼ *Key Point* Take multiple biopsy samples to obtain optimal histologic examination of the various stages of a particular skin disease.

- Advantages
  - This relatively easy and fast procedure usually provides the definitive diagnosis of skin disease.
  - A minimal number of sutures is required to close the skin defect.
  - Minimal cosmetic defects are created by the procedure.
- Disadvantages
  - Subcutaneous fat may be lost during the biopsy procedure precluding its histopathologic examination.
  - Multiple skin biopsy samples may be necessary for adequate representation of the disease process.

Technique

Consider general anesthesia for the biopsy of skin lesions that have definite or suspected subcutaneous involvement as well as those in sensitive areas: pedicular, perioral, periauricular, perianal, and so forth.

1. Clip hair at the biopsy site. No cleansing or other topical preparations are advised.
2. To ensure accurate biopsy of anesthetized lesions, mark the biopsy site with an indelible-ink pen.
3. Use a 25-gauge needle and 1-cc syringe to inject 0.5 to 1.0 cc of lidocaine or lidocaine with epinephrine SC at the site to be biopsied.
4. Biopsy the lesion skin approximately 5 minutes after anesthetizing.
5. Obtain the biopsy specimens entirely within lesion boundaries.
6. Rotate the 4-mm or 6-mm disposable biopsy punch (sizes preferred by most veterinary pathologists) in one direction through the skin and into the subcutis.
7. Gently remove the resultant core of skin with a pair of fine eye forceps and iris scissors.
8. The 25-gauge needle employed to inject local anesthetic can also elevate the biopsy sample.
9. Impale the subcutaneous fat with the needle, and lift to allow for cutting underneath.
10. Quickly transfer the specimens into the fixative solution.
11. Suture the biopsy sites if needed. This may not be necessary for 4-mm defects, but use one to two sutures for 6-mm defects.

Shave Biopsy

- Indications
  - The shave biopsy is used in human medicine when a skin disease process is suspected to be limited to the epidermis or upper dermis. In veterinary medicine, there are fewer applications.
- Advantages
  - A very fast procedure
  - Some superficial lesions (e.g., papillomas and skin tags) may be totally removed and submitted for histopathologic examination.
  - No suturing is needed.
  - Minimal to no scarring occurs afterward, because the lower dermis is left intact.
- Disadvantages
  - Can be used only to diagnose benign and extremely superficial lesions.
  - Cannot be used to determine the depth of neoplastic infiltration. Only benign superficial neoplasms can be diagnosed.

Technique

1. Local anesthesia is optional, depending on the lesion's size and location.
2. The skin is raised as a fold. The scalpel blade is held parallel to the skin surface.
3. The scalpel is then used to cut across the lesion.
4. After the shave biopsy, use curettage or electrodesiccation to remove deeper aspects of the lesion.

Curettage

This is the least satisfactory method of collecting skin specimens for histopathologic examination. It is unavoidable that scanty, superficial, fragmented, and distorted skin specimens are collected. If this technique is attempted, make a single firm stroke across the lesion to obtain the best specimen.

HANDLING FORMALIN-FIXED SKIN BIOPSY SPECIMENS

- Bisect all nodules that might have an infectious etiology.
- Submit half the nodule for histopathology; submit the other half in a sterile container for bacterial and fungal cultures.
- After removing the skin specimen, quickly roll the core sample or blot the wedge sample on bibulous (absorbent lint-free) paper to remove excess blood. Gently press the skin specimen subcutaneous side down onto a piece of a wooden tongue depressor.
- The specimen is now in correct anatomic orientation and is floated upside-down or immersed in 10% phosphate-buffered formalin fixative for routine histopathologic examination.
- The fixative volume is 10 times the sample volume to ensure proper fixation.
- Slice large specimens, such as wedge biopsy samples, to limit thickness to 2 cm regardless of area.
- Keep the freshly formalin-fixed specimens at room temperature for at least 6 hours before shipping in the extreme cold of winter.
- Avoid freezing of formalin-fixed biopsy tissue.
- Enclose a brief but detailed summary of the patient's clinical history and lesions with the specimens.

▼ *Key Point* Decide on any special histopathology studies before immersing tissue into formalin. Formalin may ruin the sample for these purposes.

▼ *Key Point* Submit specimens to a veterinary pathologist with training in dermatopathology.

HANDLING MICHEL'S MEDIA-FIXED SKIN BIOPSY SPECIMENS

- Immunologic abnormalities of the skin, especially of connective tissue and in bullous diseases, may result in deposition of immunoglobulin, complement, and fibrin. These depositions in the skin may be detected by direct immunofluorescent microscopy.
- When submitting skin specimens for direct immunofluorescence, use the same biopsy procedures as those done for formalin fixation.

▼ *Key Point* Take the Michel's media samples before the samples for routine histopathology. Formalin residue on the instruments can lead to false-negative direct immunofluorescence results.

- Michel's transport media and fixative maintain skin specimens indefinitely at room temperature.
- Skin punch biopsies of 4 mm allow for the best penetration of the fixative.
- Negative immunofluorescence test results do not eliminate the diagnosis of an autoimmune disease. This test is positive in only 50% of autoimmune skin diseases.
- Positive immunofluorescence test results do not always confirm autoimmune disease. The test results may be positive in many infectious and inflammatory dermatoses and in some normal dogs and cats.

▼ *Key Point* Save the Michel's media-fixed specimens at the hospital. Do not submit them for direct immunofluorescence until the results of the routine histopathologic examination of the formalin-fixed specimens indicate changes consistent with autoimmune skin disease.

SUPPLEMENTAL READINGS

Fitzpatrick TB, Eisen A, Wolff KA, et al.: Dermatology in General Medicine, 3rd Ed. New York: McGraw-Hill, 1987, p 47.

Ihrke PJ, Gross TL: The skin biopsy: maximizing benefits. Scientific Proceedings of the American Animal Hospital Association, San Francisco, 1988, p 299.

Lever WF, Schaumburg-Lever G: Introduction. *In* Pedersen DD, ed.: Histopathology of the Skin. Philadelphia: JB Lippincott, 1983, p 1.

50 Surgery of Intertriginous Dermatoses

Jamie R. Bellah

Intertriginous dermatoses are surface pyodermas that are associated with skin folds. Chronic skin apposition results in friction, minor trauma, and poor air circulation along with a moist environment conducive to colonization and infection by bacteria and yeasts.

▼ *Key Point* Inflammation and exudate associated with pyoderma cause pain, pruritus, and malodor. Conservative treatment is only palliative. Resolution of these conditions can be accomplished only by surgery.

ETIOLOGY

Normal skin defense mechanisms are as follows:

- Intact epidermis and stratum corneum
- Sebum that contains antibacterial and antifungal fatty acids
- Skin microflora that may secrete antibiotic-like substances

Skin fold pyoderma is classified as a surface pyoderma. (See Chapter 35 for a complete discussion of pyoderma.)

- Bacteria and yeasts remain on top of the skin.
- Warm, moist environment within recess of the skin fold allows colonization by *Staphylococcus intermedius* or *Malassezia pachydermatis*.
- Other infecting organisms include *Streptococcus, Escherichia coli, Pseudomonas, Proteus,* and *Candida*.
- Surface bacteria and yeasts act on trapped secretions and sebum, producing breakdown products that are irritating and odoriferous.
- Superficial skin erosions and inflammation result.
- Self-trauma and obesity tend to worsen the condition.

Locations, characteristics, and breeds associated with intertriginous dermatoses include the following:

Facial or Nasal Fold
- Frequently associated with secondary ulcerative keratitis
- Brachycephalic breeds: Pekingese, English bulldog, pug, French bulldog, Boston terrier
- Persian cats

Lip Fold
- Common in dogs with excessive mandibular labial tissue, such as spaniels, Saint Bernard, Irish setter, Newfoundland, Golden retriever, Labrador retriever
- Redundant lip fold is usually located behind the mandibular canine tooth.
- Can be bilateral.
- Causes severe halitosis.
- May occur after partial mandibulectomy or maxillectomy if a skin fold is created during wound closure.

Body Fold
- Usually affects obese or Chinese Shar Pei dogs.
- With Shar Pei puppies, body folds become less redundant with growth but persist on the head and face.
- May occur in female dogs or cats along the abdominal midline if mammary glands or body fat creates a skin fold.
- Moist seborrhea predisposes the animal to body fold pyoderma.

Vulvar Fold
- Most common in older, obese, spayed female dogs and rarely cats.
- Seen in younger dogs with infantile vulvas.
- Accumulation of urine and vaginal secretions occur.
- Animal may have a secondary urinary tract infection.

Tail Fold ("Screw Tail")
- Common in English bulldog, pug, Boston terrier, and schipperke breeds.
- Also seen in Manx cats.
- Caused by redundant skin around the tail and the corkscrew conformation of the terminal coccygeal vertebrae.
- A full-thickness ulcer may be present in the skin under the ventrally deviating tail. Such a condition can be very painful and uncomfortable for affected dogs.
- Contamination by fecal flora causes fulminating pyoderma.
- Self-trauma and scooting exacerbate the condition.

PREOPERATIVE CONSIDERATIONS

- Conservative treatment, including clipping hair from the skin fold, cleansing with dilute antibacterial solutions, medicated soaps, antiseborrheic shampoos, astringents, and topical and systemic antibiotics, is palliative only.

- Medical treatment may be advisable before surgery in some animals to lessen the amount of wound exudate and to lower bacterial numbers at the time of surgery. (See Chapter 35.)
- In the presence of severe infection (i.e., tail fold pyoderma), administer a preoperative antimicrobial to prevent a postoperative wound infection.
- When show animals are affected, counsel the owner with regard to the expected postoperative appearance and consult breed requirements for show.

SURGICAL PROCEDURES

Objectives

- En bloc excision of the skin fold and associated pyoderma.
- Resolution of wound infection.

Equipment

- Standard general surgical pack.
- Suture material appropriate for infected wounds.
- Bone-holding forceps aid manipulation of the tail during caudectomy for screw tail.
- Bone-cutting forceps or Gigli saw for caudectomy.
- Penrose drains.

Technique

1. *Facial or nasal fold excision*
   a. Position the animal in ventral recumbency
   b. Protect the eyes with an ophthalmic ointment during preparation and surgery.
   c. Clip hair from the facial skin folds and ventral eyelids sufficient to drape an appropriate margin around the fold to be excised.
   d. Plan the boundaries of the incision so that removal of too much skin is avoided. Skin is needed for closure without tension (Fig. 50–1A).
   e. With two paired incisions, excise enough of the facial fold to alleviate the recess created by the fold and to eliminate any chance of hair contacting the eye.

▼ *Key Point* Stay at least 1 cm from the medial canthus of the eye, and avoid lacrimal structures and large vessels in the region.

   f. Undermine skin edges gently and carefully, if required.
   g. Close in two layers using fine (3-0 or 4-0) absorbable suture for subcutaneous tissue and fine monofilament suture for skin closure (Fig. 50–1B).
   h. Cut the suture ends short so that they do not contact the cornea.
2. *Lip fold excision* (cheiloplasty)
   a. Position the animal in dorsal recumbency.

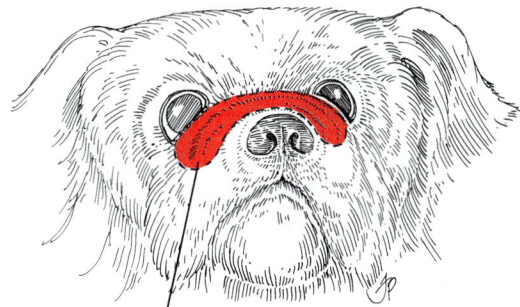

A   Area to be removed

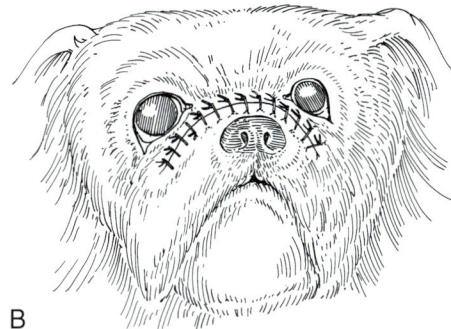

B

Figure 50–1. Facial fold excision. *A,* Incision boundaries are planned so that enough skin for closure without tension remains. *B,* Final suture pattern.

   b. Clip and prepare the skin over the mandible from its rostral tip to the mandibular angle (Fig. 50–2A).
   c. Make an elliptical incision around the lip fold, and remove the entire fold and infected region (Fig. 50–2B).
   d. It is very rare that the mucosal surface of the lip needs to be incised.
   e. Try to avoid incising the underlying muscles of the lip.
   f. Close the incision in two layers using fine absorbable suture for subcutaneous tissue and fine nonabsorbable suture for skin (Fig. 50–2C).

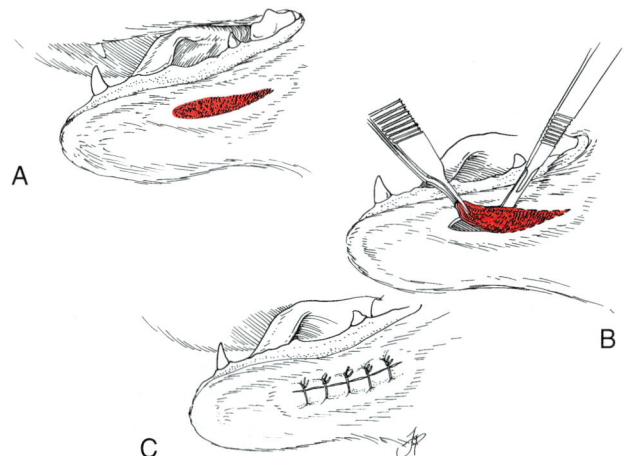

Figure 50–2. Lip fold excision (cheiloplasty). *A,* Preparation of skin. *B,* Excision of fold. *C,* Closure pattern.

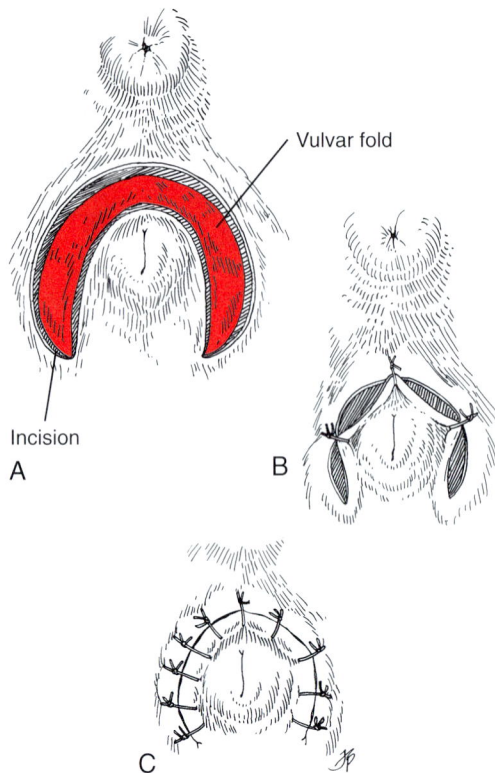

Figure 50–3. Vulvar fold excision (episioplasty). *A,* Incision pattern around base of vulvar fold. *B,* Simple sutures approximate wound margin. *C,* Suture pattern.

g. Close the buccal mucosa, if incised, with fine interrupted absorbable sutures.

3. *Body fold excision*
   a. Position the dog so that optimal access to the body fold to be removed is accomplished.
   b. Prepare the skin wide enough so the fold can be excised in its entirety.
   c. Make two incisions parallel to the fold near its base being certain to leave sufficient skin for closure.
   d. Closure is done in two layers using fine absorbable suture for subcutaneous tissues and interrupted nonabsorbable sutures for skin apposition.
   e. Mastectomy (see Chap. 27) may be required to resolve body fold pyoderma that has resulted from rolls of abdominal fat or from pendulous mammary tissue.

4. *Vulvar fold excision* (episioplasty)
   a. Place the animal in ventral recumbency with the perineal region at the end of the table. If the rear legs are draped over the end of the table be sure to pad them sufficiently.
   b. Place a pursestring suture around the anus.
   c. Prepare the perivulvar region for aseptic surgery.
   d. Make an elliptical incision around the base of the vulvar fold, then undermine and remove the incised area of skin (Fig. 50–3*A*).
   e. Place simple interrupted cuticular sutures equidistant from one another around the incision to approximate the wound margins (Fig.

50–3*B*). This step helps to determine if adequate skin and subcutaneous fat have been removed.
   f. Close the skin in two layers using fine absorbable suture for subcutaneous tissue and fine nonabsorbable sutures for skin (Fig. 50–3*C*).
   g. Remove the pursestring suture.

5. *Tail fold excision and caudectomy*
   a. Place the animal in ventral recumbency with the perineum facing the end of the table. A frogleg position is used for this procedure.
   b. Place a pursestring suture around the anus.
   c. Clip the entire perineum and tailhead region.
   d. It is difficult to clip hair from the fold region adequately, therefore give a prophylactic antimicrobial drug before and during surgery.
   e. Make an incision around the tail and tail fold. Skin dorsal to the tail may be preserved and aids in cosmetic skin closure (Fig. 50–4*A*).
   f. Attempt to dissect around the tail and skin fold without penetrating the fold.
   g. Sometimes, because ventral deviation of the tail causes full-thickness erosion through the skin and en bloc excision cannot be performed, layered debridement must be done.
   h. Manipulate the tail using bone-holding forceps (Fig. 50–4*B*).

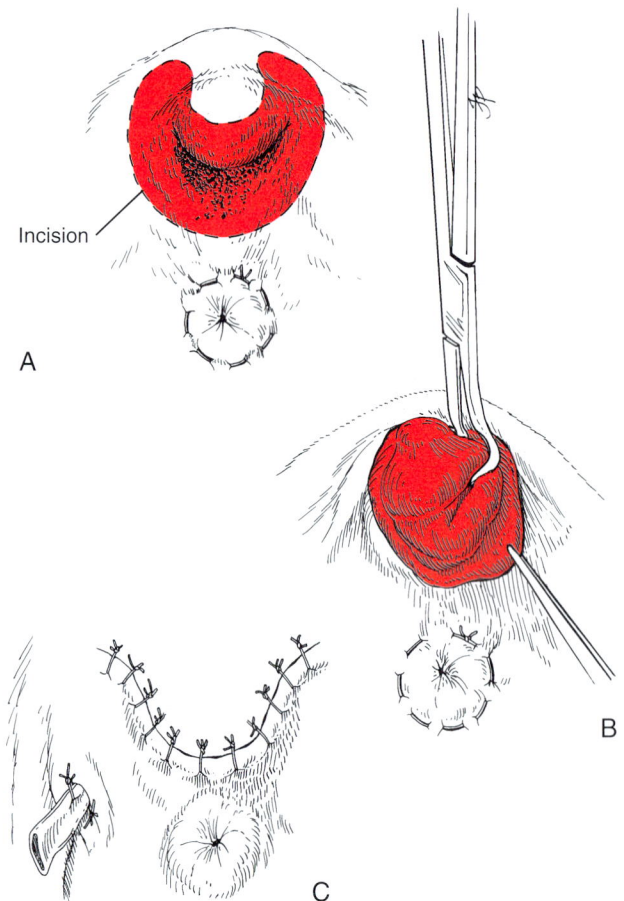

Figure 50–4. Tail-fold excision and caudectomy. *A,* Place a pursestring suture around the anus, and incise the tail-fold region as shown. *B,* Manipulate tail with tail-holding forceps. *C,* Wound closure pattern and drain.

i. Incise coccygeal and levator ani muscular attachments.

j. Using a Gigli wire or bone-cutting forceps, transect the tail rostral to its ventral deviation.

▼ **Key Point** Be careful during transection of the tail not to traumatize the rectum, which is just ventral to the tail base.

k. Liberally flush the surgical site with sterile saline.

l. Use several interrupted absorbable sutures to close dead space.

m. Place Penrose drains at this time, if necessary.

n. Close the wound in two layers, using fine absorbable sutures for subcutaneous tissues and fine nonabsorbable sutures for skin apposition (Fig. 50–4C).

o. Remove the pursestring suture.

POSTOPERATIVE CARE AND COMPLICATIONS

Postoperative Care

- Prevent self-trauma (elizabethan collar).
- Antimicrobial therapy may be given, based on culture and sensitivity testing if deemed necessary.

- Keep oral incisions free of food and saliva.
- Keep perineal incisions clean, and remove fecal contamination.
- Remove Penrose drains in 3–5 days.

Complications

- Self-trauma
- Wound infection
- Dehiscence
- Ectropion (aggressive facial fold removal)
- Insufficient skin fold removal (relapse of pyoderma)

SUPPLEMENTAL READINGS

Krahwinkel DJ Jr: Correction of specific skin defects. *In* Swaim SF, ed.: Surgery of Traumatized Skin: Management and Reconstruction in the Dog and Cat. Philadelphia: WB Saunders, 1980.

Krahwinkel DJ, Bone DL: Surgical management of specific skin disorders. *In* Slatter DH, ed.: Textbook of Small Animal Surgery. Philadelphia: WB Saunders, 1985, p 501.

McLoughlin M: Surgical management of skin fold pyoderma. *In* Bojrab MJ, ed.: Current Techniques in Small Animal Surgery, 2nd Ed. Philadelphia: WB Saunders, 1990, p 489.

Scott DW, Miller WH, Griffin CE: Small Animal Dermatology. Philadelphia: WB Saunders, 1995, p 885.

51 Management of the Traumatic Wound by Primary Closure

Steven F. Swaim

Following proper initial management of a traumatic wound by debridement and lavage, the wound may be closed. Sufficient viable tissue must be present to allow closure without excessive tension. Wounds may be closed by primary closure, delayed primary closure, or secondary closure. See Chapter 52 for a discussion of open wound management.

ANATOMY

- Dogs and cats have abundant skin on the trunk and neck but a sparsity of skin on the distal limbs and tail.
- Direct cutaneous vessels run parallel to the skin surface and supply the subdermal plexus of the skin. See Chapter 53 for more details regarding blood supply to the skin.
- Some areas of the body have panniculus musculature underlying the skin. The skin's blood supply runs both superficial and deep to this musculature.
- Other areas of the body have loose areolar fascia deep to the dermis in which vasculature is located, and in other areas the skin is closely associated with underlying fascia.

PREOPERATIVE CONSIDERATIONS

▼ *Key Point* If a traumatically induced wound is to be closed, it is imperative that the tissues be viable and clean enough that wound healing can progress uneventfully. Perform adequate debridement and lavage.

- Perform a thorough physical examination and appropriate diagnostic tests on all traumatized animals to rule out associated injuries.
- Perform primary closure when:
  - The animal is in good condition.
  - A short time (6–12 hours) has elapsed since injury.
  - Minimal contamination and tissue trauma have occurred.
  - Adequate debridement and lavage have been done.
- Perform delayed primary closure when:
  - Wounds show evidence of heavy contamination, purulent exudate, residual necrotic or question-able tissue, edema, erythema at the wound margins, lymphangitis, and skin tension.
  - Local infection has been controlled by debridement, lavage, topical and/or systemic antibiotics, and appropriate bandages. This control is usually 3–5 days after infliction.
- Perform a secondary closure when:
  - The wound is in the reparative stage of healing at presentation, with a healthy bed of granulation tissue and evidence of epithelialization.
  - The wound has disrupted and has subsequently developed a healthy bed of granulation tissue.
  - It has been necessary to leave the wound open for longer than 5 days to control infection (see Preoperative Considerations, Delayed primary closure, Local infection control).

SURGICAL PROCEDURES

Primary or Delayed Primary Closure *Without* Tension

Objectives

- Close the wound.
- Provide drainage if necessary.

Equipment

- Standard general surgical pack
- Undyed polyglactin 910, dyed or undyed polydioxanone, 3-0 (Vicryl or PDS II; Ethicon, Somerville, NJ.) and polypropylene or nylon, 2-0 and 3-0 (Prolene or Ethilon, Ethicon, Somerville, NJ.)
- Wound lavage solution of 0.05% chlorhexidine diacetate or gluconate (Nolvasan Solution, Fort Dodge, IA. or ChlorhexiDerm Disinfectant, DVM Pharmaceuticals, Miami, FL.)

Technique

1. Pack the wound with sterile surgical sponges moistened with physiologic saline, or fill it with sterile water-soluble lubricant (K-Y Jelly, Johnson & Johnson, New Brunswick, NJ.) or water-soluble lubricant that contains chlorhexidine gluconate (Surgilube, E. Fougera & Co., Mellville, NY.)

2. Prepare the area around the wound for aseptic surgery.
3. Remove the wound packing or sterile lubricant.
4. Lavage the wound frequently during surgery along with removal of devitalized tissue and debris as indicated.
5. Use as few simple interrupted absorbable sutures as necessary to close dead space in deep layers of the wound.
6. Be careful not to include major vessels or nerves in the sutures.
7. Place a Penrose drain if there is any possibility of residual dead space and/or wound drainage.
8. Place a simple continuous suture in the subcutaneous tissue at the wound edge using absorbable suture material.
9. Close the skin with nonabsorbable simple interrupted sutures.

Postoperative Care and Complications

- Postoperative care
  - Place absorbent surgical sponges over the suture line, with extra sponges over the drain.
  - Apply an absorbent secondary wrap to the area, followed by an outer wrap of porous adhesive tape.
  - Change the bandage every second or third day if there is no concern about possible complications. Change the bandage daily if there is concern about possible complication and/or a drain has been placed. The amount and nature of drainage should be assessed at each bandage change.
  - Remove the drain and discontinue bandaging when the drainage becomes minimal and is the same in quantity at successive bandage changes.
  - Remove the skin sutures 7–10 days postoperatively.
- Complications
  Hematoma, seroma, or infection may result from improper wound evaluation, debridement, lavage, closure, or drain management.

Primary, Delayed Primary, or Secondary Closure *With* Tension

Objectives

- Close the wound.
- Relieve tension on the wound closure.
- Provide drainage if necessary.

Equipment

- See equipment under Primary or Delayed Primary Closure *Without* Tension.

Technique

1. The general techniques for closure of wounds with tension are the same as those for primary or delayed primary closure without tension (see previous section), with the exception of suture pattern (see tension-relieving suture patterns discussed subsequently).
2. Wounds that are in the reparative stage of healing with healthy granulation tissue and epithelialization.

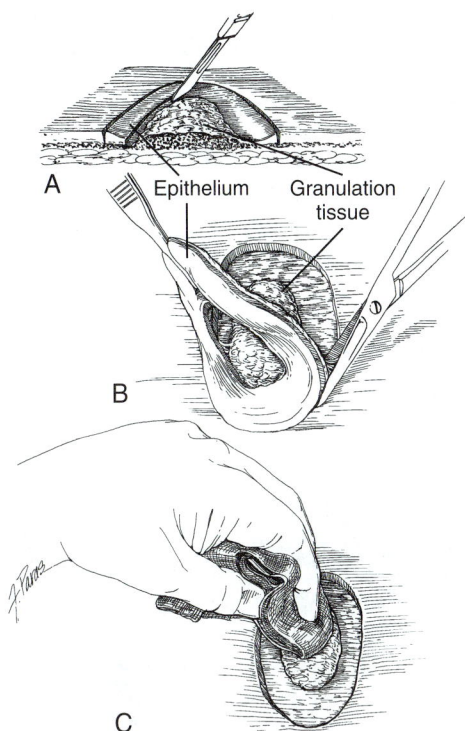

Figure 51–1. Preparation of a wound in the reparative stage of healing for secondary closure. *A,* Incising the epithelium. *B,* Removing the epithelium. *C,* Cleaning the surface of the healthy granulation tissue.

  a. Excise epithelium from the edge of the wound, leaving healthy granulation tissue in the center.
  b. Gently clean the surface of the granulation tissue with 0.05% chlorhexidine solution (Fig. 51–1).
3. Gently undermine the skin surrounding the wound.
  a. Undermine bluntly, using Metzenbaum scissors, leaving some loose areolar connective tissue on the dermis or undermine beneath any panniculus musculature that is present.
  b. Undermine sharply with scissors or scalpel blade in areas where skin is closely associated with the underlying fascia.

▼ *Key Point* Leave large identifiable blood vessels (i.e., direct cutaneous blood vessels) intact when undermining. Use good judgment when manipulating recently traumatized skin to avoid added insult to skin vasculature, which could result in skin slough.

4. One of the following tension-relieving suture patterns may be used to close the wound.
  a. Place "walking" sutures (my choice for closing wounds under tension) with absorbable material in staggered parallel rows, beginning just in front of the plane where undermining stopped. Place a simple continuous subcuticular absorbable suture along the wound edge before skin closure with nonabsorbable simple interrupted sutures (Fig. 51–2).

b. Place an absorbable intradermal continuous horizontal mattress suture to appose the skin edges. This can be reinforced with nonabsorbable simple interrupted skin sutures (Fig. 51–3).

c. Place nonabsorbable vertical mattress sutures near the wound edge over segments of Penrose drain. Use simple interrupted nonabsorbable sutures to appose skin edges (Fig. 51–4).

d. Place nonabsorbable "far-near-near-far" or "far-far-near-near" sutures in the order of their names to act as apposition and tension sutures (Fig. 51–5).

e. Preplace nonabsorbable stent sutures deep to the wound tissues prior to closure of the wound. These sutures are then tied over a roll of surgical

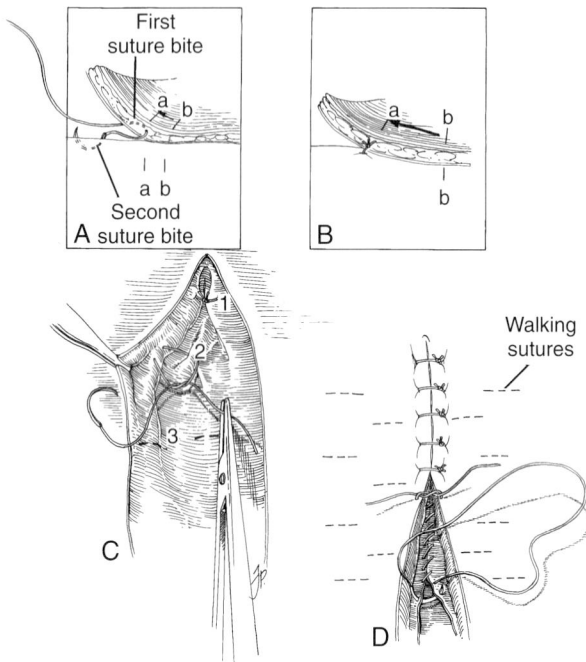

Figure 51–2. "Walking" sutures. *A,* Placing first and second suture bites. Segment of skin to be stretched (a to b). *B,* Tying a "walking" suture advances the skin toward the center of the wound (a to b increased). *C,* "Walking" sutures placed in rows. 1, Walking suture tied; 2, placing a walking suture; 3, areas where bites will be taken for a walking suture *(broken lines)*. *D,* Placing a simple continuous subcuticular suture along the wound edge, and simple interrupted skin apposition sutures. Broken lines are buried walking sutures. (After Swaim SF: The repair of the skin: Techniques of plastic and reconstructive surgery. *In* Bedford PGC, ed.: Atlas of Canine Surgical Techniques. Oxford: Blackwell Scientific Publications, 1984, p 49; and Swaim SF, Henderson RA: Small Animal Wound Management, 2nd Ed. Baltimore: Williams & Wilkins, 1997, p 154.)

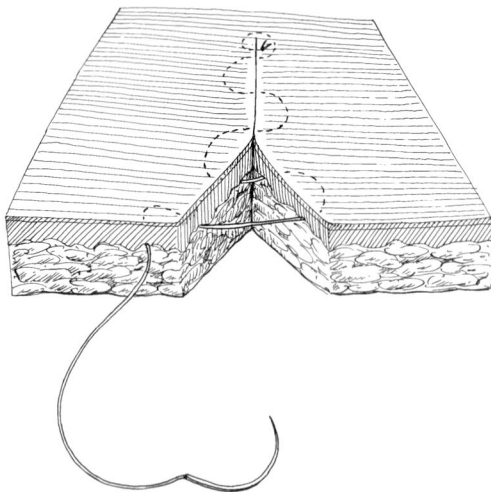

Figure 51–4. Vertical mattress tension sutures. *A,* Vertical mattress sutures placed over Penrose drains. *B,* Simple interrupted skin apposition sutures used with tension sutures.

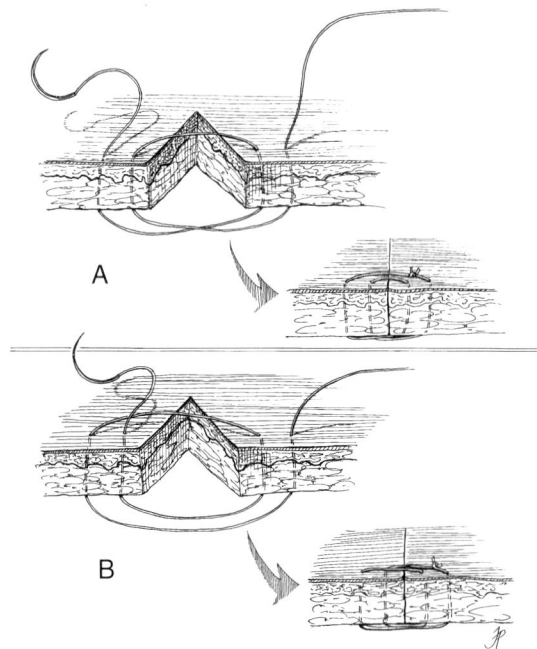

Figure 51–3. Intradermal sutures. Using 3-0 or smaller absorbable suture material in a continuous pattern, place intradermal sutures with each bite being passed horizontally. (Redrawn from Scardino MS, Swaim SF, Henderson RA, Wilson ER: Enhancing wound closure on the limbs. Compend Contin Educ 18:919, 1996.)

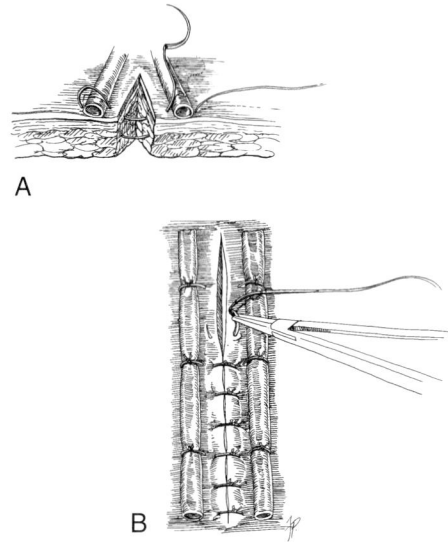

Figure 51–5. Combination apposition and tension sutures. *A,* "Far-near-near-far" sutures. *B,* "Far-far-near-near" sutures. (After Swaim SF, Henderson RA: Small Animal Wound Management, 2nd Ed. Baltimore: Williams & Wilkins, 1997, p 165.)

sponges or a rolled towel to act as a tension suture as well as to obliterate dead space (Fig. 51–6).

f. Place nonabsorbable Lembert sutures in the skin adjacent to the wound the day before surgery. The sutures are tied under tension. The following day, the presutures are removed and the wound is closed using the prestretched skin (Fig. 51–7).

g. On wounds that cannot quite be closed, or to help prevent further wound edge retraction, place a monofilament nonabsorbable intradermal continuous horizontal mattress suture. The ends are left untied and a button and two fishing weights (split shot) are placed on each end of the suture. Traction is placed on each free suture end daily to advance the edges toward each other. Two new split shots are placed on the suture adjacent to the button after each tightening to hold the edges under tension and advance them toward the wound center (Fig. 51–8).

5. Use one of the following relaxing incisions for additional tension release.

a. Make unilateral or bilateral bipedicle flaps when undermining does not provide enough relaxation for wound closure. Make an incision parallel to the wound's long axis but slightly curved toward the wound, with the width of the created flaps being equal to the wound width. Use absorbable walking sutures to advance and tack the flaps in place and a regular or tension-relieving suture pattern to suture the skin. Close the defects that resulted from moving the flaps (Fig. 51–9). Make unilateral or bilateral simple relaxing incisions as in creating a bipedicle flap. Move the flaps and suture in place as with bipedicle flaps. Do not close the defects that remain from

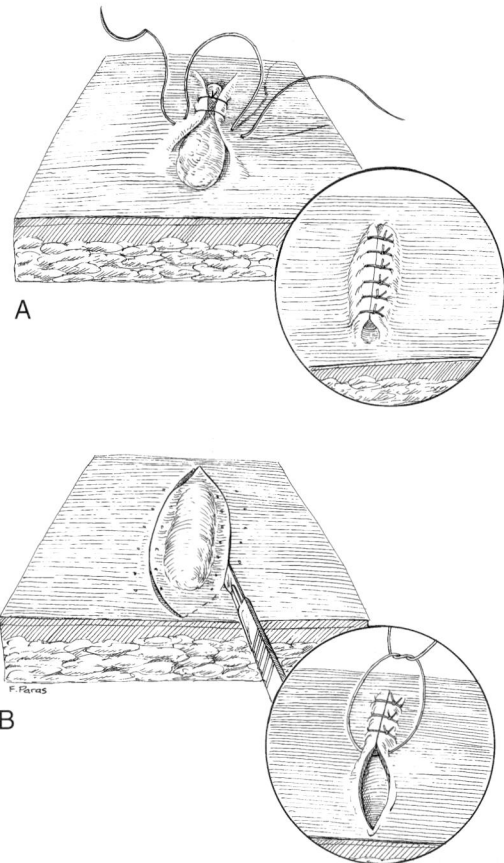

A

B

Figure 51–7. Presutures. *A,* The day before surgery, suture the skin adjacent to the lesion over the lesion using a Lembert suture pattern. *B,* The following day, remove the presutures and excise the lesion. *Inset,* Close the resulting defect or wound using the stretched skin made available by the presutures. (Redrawn from Scardino MS, Swaim SF, Henderson RA, Wilson ER: Enhancing wound closure on the limbs. Compend Contin Educ 18:919, 1996.)

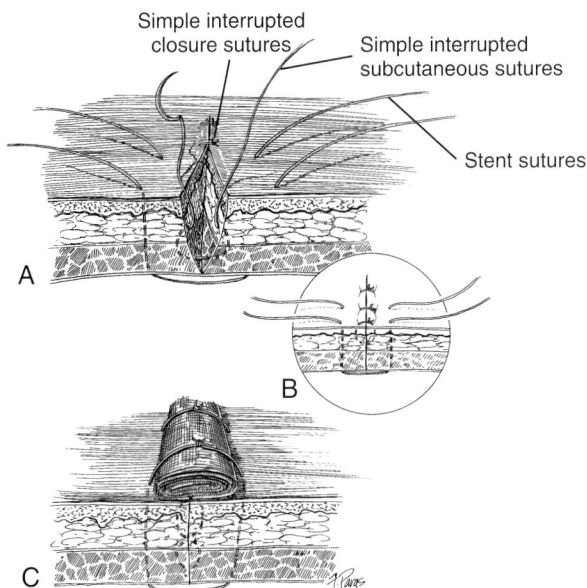

Simple interrupted closure sutures

Simple interrupted subcutaneous sutures

Stent sutures

A

B

C

Figure 51–6. Stent sutures. *A,* Preplace stent sutures deep to the wound tissues. *B,* Wound tissues are closed. *C,* Tie stent sutures over a roll of gauze or rolled towel.

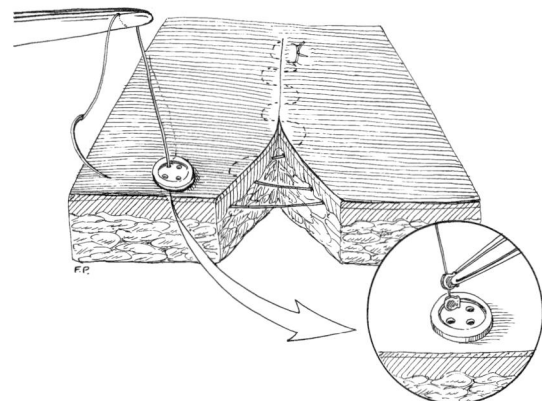

Figure 51–8. A half-buried horizontal mattress suture starts the suture at one end. Then advance the suture as an intradermal horizontal mattress suture with each bite slightly advanced. On the final bite, pass the needle through the entire thickness of the skin and through a hole in a sterile button. After the wound edges are advanced as far as possible, use two split shots to hold the suture tight (see *inset*). (Redrawn from Scardino MS, Swaim SF, Henderson RA, Wilson ER: Enhancing wound closure on the limbs. Compend Contin Educ 18:919, 1996.)

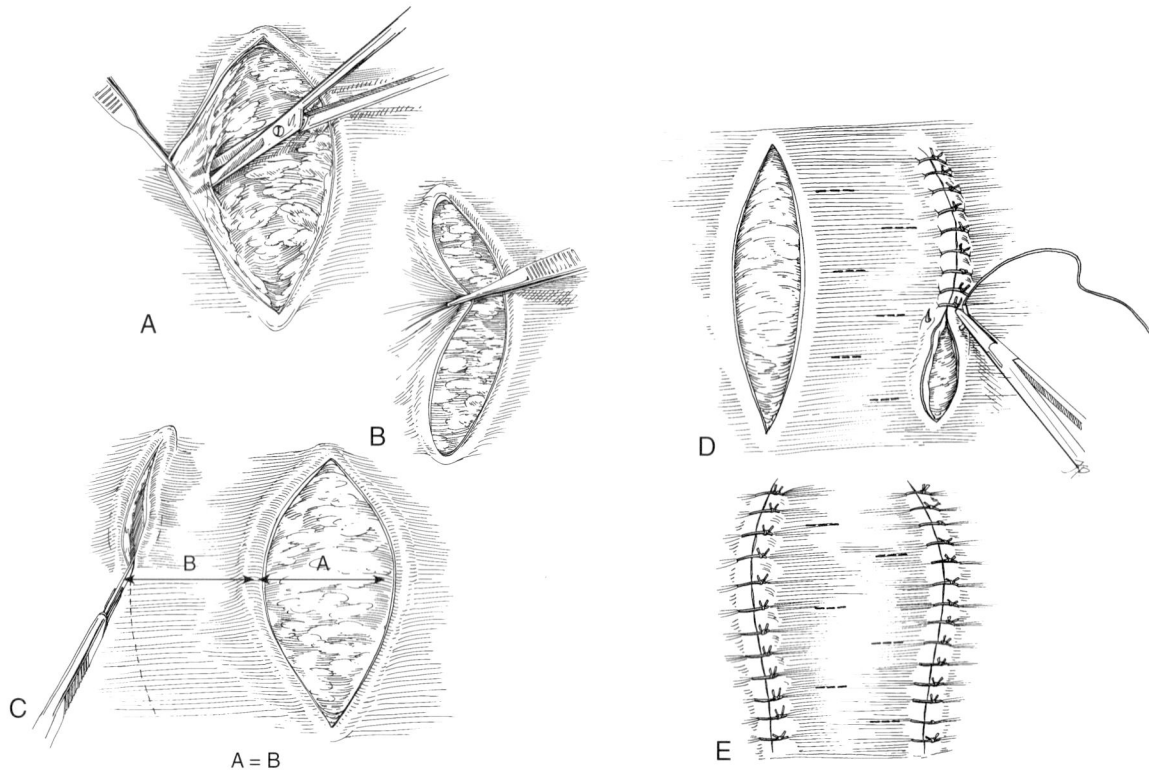

Figure 51–9.   Unilateral bipedicle flap. *A,* Undermining the skin on the side of defect from which the flap will come. *B,* Checking to see if undermining provided sufficient skin for wound closure. *C,* Making an incision to create a bipedicle flap. Wound and flap width are equal (A = B). *D,* Flap being sutured into position after walking sutures have advanced it *(broken lines)*. *E,* Donor site sutured. (After Swaim SF, Henderson RA: Small Animal Wound Management. 2nd Ed. Philadelphia: Williams & Wilkins, 1997, p 176.)

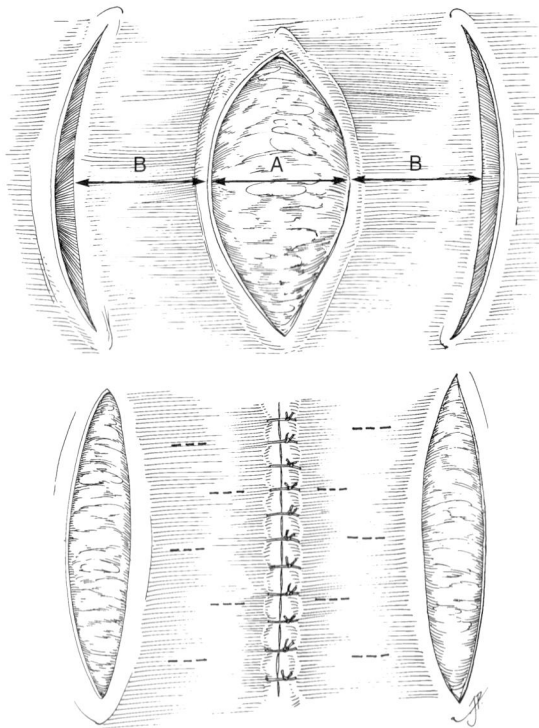

Figure 51–10.   Bilateral simple relaxing incisions. *Top,* One bipedicle flap has been created on each side of the wound, with flaps equal in width to the defect width (A = B). *Bottom,* After undermining and moving the flaps with walking sutures *(broken lines)* to close the wound, leave the relaxing incision defects to heal as open wounds. (After Swaim SF, Henderson RA: Small Animal Wound Management. 2nd Ed. Philadelphia: Williams & Wilkins, 1997, p 177.)

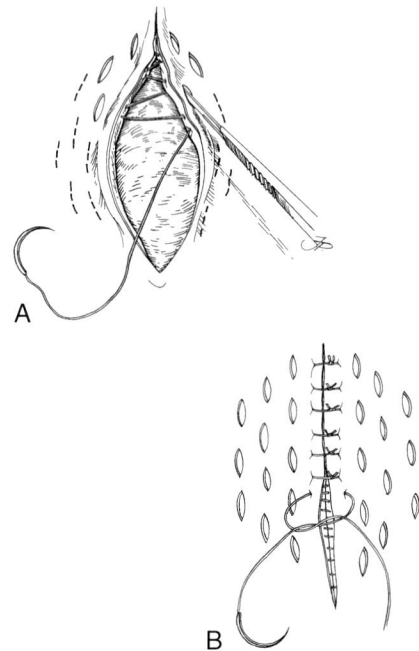

Figure 51–11.   Multiple punctate relaxing incisions. *A,* Make parallel staggered rows of incisions as needed on both sides of a wound while a simple continuous intradermal suture is placed and tightened. *B,* Final wound apposition with simple interrupted sutures. (After Swaim SF, Henderson RA: Small Animal Wound Management. 2nd Ed. Philadelphia: Williams & Wilkins, 1997, pp 189–190.)

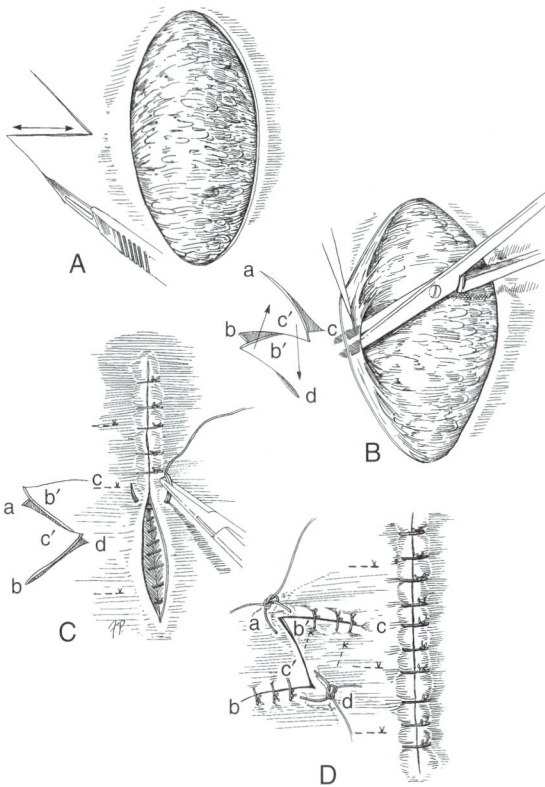

Figure 51–12. Z-plasty as a relaxing incision for wound closure. *A,* Make a 60° equal-angle, equal-limb-length Z-plasty designed adjacent to a wound, with the central limb in the direction relaxation is needed. *B,* Z-plasty has been cut. Undermine Z-plasty flaps and adjacent skin (*arrows* indicate Z-plasty flap transposition). *C,* Closure of the defect with automatic transposition of Z-plasty flaps. *D,* Suturing the Z-plasty flaps into their new positions. (After Swaim SF, Henderson RA: Small Animal Wound Management. 2nd Ed. Philadelphia: Williams & Wilkins, 1997, p 186.)

moving the flaps but leave them to heal as open wounds (Fig. 51–10).

b. Make multiple, punctate, relaxing incisions 1 cm long and 0.5 cm apart in parallel, staggered rows bilaterally, as needed to allow wound closure as a simple continuous intradermal absorbable suture is placed and tightened. Final skin apposition is with simple interrupted, nonabsorbable sutures (Fig. 51–11).

c. Design and incise a 60° equal angle, equal limb-length Z-plasty adjacent to the wound with the central limb of the Z in the direction in which relaxation is needed. After undermining the skin edges and Z-plasty flaps, close the wound using regular or tension sutures. Suture the Z-plasty flaps into their new positions (Fig. 51–12).

d. Make a V-shaped incision adjacent to the wound with the point of the V away from the wound. After undermining the resulting skin flap, use absorbable walking sutures to advance and tack the flap in place. A regular or tension suture pattern is used to suture the original skin defect. Close the V with simple interrupted nonabsorbable sutures, beginning at the ends. When tension develops, close the remainder of the defect, beginning at the point of the V to form a Y-shaped suture line (Fig. 51–13).

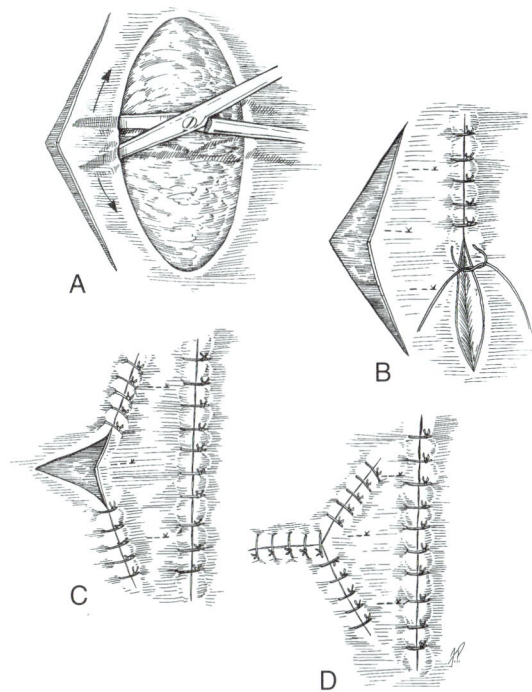

Figure 51–13. V-to-Y plasty relaxing incision. *A,* Make a V-shaped incision adjacent to the defect with point of the V away from the defect. Undermine skin between the defect and incision. *B,* Closure of the defect with walking sutures holding the flap in position (*broken lines*). *C,* Closure of the V-shaped incision beginning at the ends. *D,* Closure of the stem of the Y. (After Swaim SF, Henderson RA: Small Animal Wound Management. 2nd Ed. Philadelphia: Williams & Wilkins, 1997, pp 181–182.)

6. Drains to prevent dead space are generally not needed in wounds sutured under tension, especially if open relaxing incisions have been made.

Postoperative Care and Complications

Postoperative Care

- Bandaging is similar to that for postoperative care of wounds closed without tension. Do not remove "walking" sutures and absorbable intradermal continuous horizontal mattress sutures. Remove vertical mattress tension sutures after 3–4 days. Remove "far-near-near-far" and "far-far-near-near" sutures at about 10 days. Remove stent sutures after 7–10 days, and remove presutures within 24 hours after their placement. The adjustable horizontal mattress suture (see Fig. 51–8) may be left in place and tightened daily for several days to a week.
- Prevent self-mutilation of wounds with Elizabethan collar or other device, if necessary.

Complications

- When vertical mattress tension sutures are applied, there may be areas of pressure necrosis of the skin near the wound edge under the Penrose drain segments.
- Simple relaxing incisions may result in a wound equal in size to the closed wound.
- Large and numerous multiple punctate relaxing incisions may result in good tension relief but may

jeopardize the blood supply to the skin between incisions with a resultant slough.

- Skin closed too tightly around a limb may result in a "biologic tourniquet," with edema and hypothermia distal to the closure site. Skin closed too tightly around the thorax may result in impaired respiration. Consider suture removal to release the tension in such cases.

SUPPLEMENTAL READINGS

Bigbie R, Shealy P, Moll D, Gragg D: Presuturing as an aid in the closure of skin defects created by surgical excision. Proc Am Assoc Equine Pract 36:613, 1990.

Laing MD, Briggs P, Heckler FR, Futrell J: Presuturing—A new technique for closing large skin defects: Clinical and experimental studies. Plast Reconstr Surg 81:694, 1988.

Lee AH, Swaim SF, Henderson RA: Surgical drainage. Compend Contin Educ 8:94, 1986.

Lee AH, Swaim SF: Granulation tissue and how to take advantage of it in management of open wounds. Compend Contin Educ Pract Vet 10:163, 1987.

Pavletic MM: Undermining for repair of large skin defects in small animals. Mod Vet Pract 67:13, 1986.

Pavletic MM: Atlas of Small Animal Reconstructive Surgery. Philadelphia: JB Lippincott, 1993, pp 146–182.

Scardino MS, Swaim SF, Henderson RA, Wilson ER: Enhancing wound closure on the limbs. Compend Contin Educ 18:919, 1996.

Swaim SF: Management of skin tension in dermal surgery. Compend Contin Educ 2:758, 1980.

Swaim SF, Henderson RA: Small Animal Wound Management, 2nd Ed. Baltimore: Williams & Wilkins, 1997, pp 143–190.

Tobin GR: Closure of contaminated wounds: Biologic and technical considerations. Surg Clin North Am 64:639, 1984.

Vig MM: Management of integumentary wounds of extremities in dogs: An experimental study. J Am Anim Hosp Assoc 21:187, 1985.

Vig MM: Management of experimental wounds of the extremities in dogs with Z-plasty. J Am Anim Hosp Assoc 28:553, 1992.

52   Management of the Open Wound

David Knapp

Open wound management is a method of treatment which should be considered when immediate primary wound closure may not be possible. Understanding the advantages and indications for open wound management requires a basic knowledge of wound healing and experience gained through clinical application. For more comprehensive descriptions of basic wound healing, see other texts. The following material is focused on traumatic wounds but may be applied to defects created by surgical excision of tumors, restrictive scar tissue, or dysfunctional tissues or masses. Reconstruction of open wounds using skin flaps or grafts is discussed in Chapter 53.

CAUSES OF OPEN WOUNDS

- Vehicular trauma resulting in lacerations and/or degloving injuries
- Bite wounds
- Gunshot or stab injuries
- Skin loss due to abscesses or embolic vascular events
- Burns resulting from thermal, electrical, chemical, and radiation injury
- Large defects resulting from surgical excision of lesions, especially tumors

PREOPERATIVE CONSIDERATIONS

Indications

Consider leaving a wound open as a method of treatment in the following situations:

- Grossly contaminated wounds.
- Wounds with established infections.
- Wounds with large skin losses or excessive tissue trauma.
- Wounds with inadequate adjacent tissue available for closure.
- Wounds that have failed previous closures.
- Temporary wound management while awaiting results of orthopedic or neurologic diagnostics.
- Temporary wound management before grafting techniques, the use of skin expanders or skin stretchers, or while awaiting microscopic examination of wound margins following tumor excision.

Advantages of Open Wound Management

- Provides ability for continual debridement through surgical, mechanical, or chemical means.
- Provides for optimal wound drainage when compared with primary closure combined with other methods of drainage.
- Provides ability for daily wound lavage when indicated.
- Provides for daily wound inspection to evaluate progress and to adjust treatment as indicated.

Disadvantages of Open Wound Management

- Labor-intensive, requiring more time and effort on the part of the veterinarian and owner.
- More expensive due to hospitalization and repeated bandage changes, often requiring anesthesia or sedation and tranquilization.
- The wound must be protected from further injury caused by exposure or self-mutilation.
- Increased risk of nosocomial or ascending infection.
- Protein loss from large wounds with excessive drainage.

INITIAL WOUND MANAGEMENT

Patient Evaluation

- Evaluate and treat as needed for concurrent life-threatening injuries, particularly hypovolemic shock, thoracic and/or abdominal trauma, and cerebral edema or hemorrhage.
- Evaluate for concurrent orthopedic or neurologic trauma (e.g., fractures, ligamentous or tendinous injuries, spinal cord injuries, or peripheral nerve damage).
- Evaluate wounds involving the extremities for vascular, orthopedic, and neurologic involvement.

▼ *Key Point* Vascular compromise may lead to loss of the limb; therefore, tissues distal to the wound should be carefully assessed. Several days may be required to fully appreciate the extent of vascular injuries.

- *Orthopedic.* Orthopedic injuries are common and may be located at the wound site or distant from the open defect. Evaluate for fractures and ligamentous injuries in all cases of trauma-related wounds. Carefully palpate the long bones and joints for pain and stability and obtain radiographs when indicated.

- *Neurologic.* Assess neurologic injury through deep and superficial pain perception and motor function. It is uncommon for limb function to be severely compromised as a result of an injury to the lower portions of an extremity.

Initial Wound Evaluation

- Analgesic or anesthetic drugs (if necessary) aid in the evaluation and treatment of the wound, especially if extensive debridement and lavage are required. Administer postoperative analgesia, intravenously at first, as needed to facilitate management of the patient during recovery and further wound assessment.
- Use sterile gloves to help prevent further bacterial invasion.
- Consider the following during the initial evaluation:
  - The extent of tissue damage to both soft and osseous structures.
  - The degree of contamination or probability of existing infection.
  - The feasibility of successful primary closure.
  - If a limb is involved, the feasibility of the leg becoming functional again.
  - The anticipated time required as well as the expense to the owner.
- Obtain bacterial cultures in advance of wound debridement and lavage.

Clipping and General Cleaning

Protect the wound from loose debris and hair during the initial preparation and clipping of the adjacent area. Use a sterile water-soluble gel, sterile towel clamps, or sutures to provide an economical and efficient temporary closure. Clip a generous margin surrounding a truncal wound or the expected bandaged portion of a limb and scrub with an antiseptic soap or solution.

Cleansing the Wound

Lavage Solution

The ideal lavage solution is sterile, nonirritating, noncytotoxic, normothermic, and isotonic. Of available solutions, warmed sterile saline best meets these criteria.

- The use of antibiotic or antiseptic solutions for wound lavage is controversial. There is evidence for both beneficial and detrimental effects. Controversy exists between in vitro versus in vivo studies and the antibacterial versus the cytotoxic effects of varying concentrations of chlorhexidine and povidone-iodine solutions. Use a 0.5–1.0% chlorhexidine solution due to its broad-spectrum and extended residual activity.
- Tap water is an economical alternative to other commonly used sterile solutions, even though it does not

meet all criteria for an ideal lavage solution. When large volumes are anticipated, tap water may be the most practical irrigation solution.

- Effective lavage often depends more on the copious volume of fluid rather than the contents of the solution.

Lavage Delivery Systems

Delivery systems are categorized based on pressures at which the lavage solution is applied to the wound.

- *High-pressure systems* (e.g., Water Pik) deliver solutions at pressures near 60 psi. Advantages are their ability to dislodge debris and bacteria. A potential disadvantage is the possibility of driving bacteria into tissues near wound margins resulting in microabscessation.
- *Medium-pressure systems* deliver solutions at pressures near 7–8 psi, which has been shown to be effective in dislodging foreign material and bacteria without risk of driving bacteria into the wound. Such a system can be developed by using a 35-ml syringe and an 18-gauge needle.
- *Low-pressure systems* are ineffective at dislodging bacteria and debris. Such systems are a syringe without a needle, a bulb syringe, and tap water.
- Removal of lavage solution from the wound by suction, gauze sponges, or gravity avoids dilution of opsonins necessary for phagocytosis.

Debridement

▼ *Key Point* Surgical debridement is the most effective method for removal of dead or devitalized tissue.

- Inspect and palpate questionable tissues to determine tissue viability. Signs suggestive of nonviable tissues include the following:
  - Black, bluish-black, or a shiny white discoloration (especially if there is a distinct demarcation between abnormal and normal color).
  - Texture is leathery to touch or skin is very thin.
  - Skin temperature is cool.
  - Hair is easily epilated.
- Reddish discoloration or severe edema is not necessarily indicative of nonviable tissues.
- During the surgical debridement it is best to maintain a conservative approach, leaving critical tissues of questionable viability while surgically excising only confirmed nonviable tissues.
- Daily mechanical debridement may be accomplished when the primary layer of the bandage is removed.
- Chemical debridement is an enzymatic removal of devitalized tissue, while selectively sparing viable structures. Such treatments may be irritating to the healing wound bed.

Bandaging

Bandages used in the management of open wounds are composed of primary, secondary, and tertiary layers. If immobilization or support is indicated, splints of metal, plastic, or fiberglass may be incorporated between the secondary and tertiary layers.

Primary Contact Layer

The primary or contact bandage layer may be adherent or nonadherent.

Adherent Dressings

- Adherent dressings are defined by their condition on application and removal and can be classified as wet-to-wet, wet-to-dry, and dry-to-dry. Wet dressings aid in the movement of viscous exudate away from the wound and into the secondary layer, while dry dressings adhere to necrotic tissue and debris, producing mechanical debridement when removed.
- *Wet-to-dry dressings* are the most frequently employed method in the early management of wounds. They allow for effective removal of exudate and mechanical debridement. To apply a wet-to-dry dressing, soak sterile cotton gauze sponges in sterile saline or antiseptic solution, hand squeeze to remove excess solution, and place the sponges in contact with the wound bed, being sure to pack all recesses of the wound. Remove the dressings at 12- to 24-hour intervals, permitting the gauze to dry and adhere to necrotic tissue and debris which provides mechanical debridement on removal. Continue wet-to-dry dressings only as long as mechanical debridement or excessive viscous exudate removal are necessary.
- *Wet-to-wet dressings* are used for wounds requiring removal of viscous exudate but no necrotic tissue or debris. Place sterile cotton gauze sponges soaked in sterile saline or another lavage solution in contact with the wound bed. The secondary layer is a nonabsorbent material which aids in maintaining a wet primary dressing.
- *Dry-to-dry dressings* are used on wounds with no exudate or a very serous exudate but which do require mechanical debridement of necrotic tissue and debris. Place dry sterile cotton gauze sponges in contact with the wound bed. An absorbent secondary layer is not necessary with this method.

Nonadherent Dressings

- Nonadherent dressings are used in the management of newly formed granulation tissue where minimal disruption of the wound bed is desirable. They are commonly used following the methods previously described or for surgically created wounds not amenable to primary closure.
- *Semiocclusive nonadherent dressings* are composed of man-made materials such as polyester films (Telfa pads) or gauze sponges with a layer of a petrolatum-based product (Adaptic, Johnson & Johnson).
- *Occlusive nonadherent dressings* (e.g., Ulcer Dressing, Johnson & Johnson) do not allow for absorption of wound exudate, and therefore are used in nonexudative wounds and are left in place for longer periods of time.

- Occlusive dressings speed reepithelialization of partial-thickness defects. Constituents of occlusive dressings include polyethylene, polyurethane, hydrocolloids, and hydrogels.

Secondary Layer

- The secondary layer of the bandage functions as the absorptive constituent, drawing fluid away from the wound and then acting as a reservoir for wound exudate or the absorbed lavage solution.
- This layer is often composed of cotton pads or layers of rolled cotton.

Tertiary Layer

- The tertiary layer functions to hold the other layers of the bandage in place and is a layer of rolled gauze covered with adhesive tape or self-adherent tape (e.g., Vetwrap, 3M).
- Wounds over areas of increased motion or on limbs with concurrent orthopedic injuries may require splints incorporated into the tertiary layers for support or immobilization.

Tie-Over Bandage

- If the area of the wound is not amenable to standard bandaging techniques (e.g., over the shoulder, hip, or axilla), a tie-over bandage may be used to secure the primary and secondary layers to the wound bed.
- To make a tie-over bandage, place 6 to 8 "eyelet" sutures around the wound (Fig. 52–1). Lace umbilical tape through these sutures to hold the layers of the bandage in place (Figs. 52–2 and 52–3).

Antibiotics

- Antibiotic therapy, whether applied topically or given systemically as a prophylactic measure, is controver-

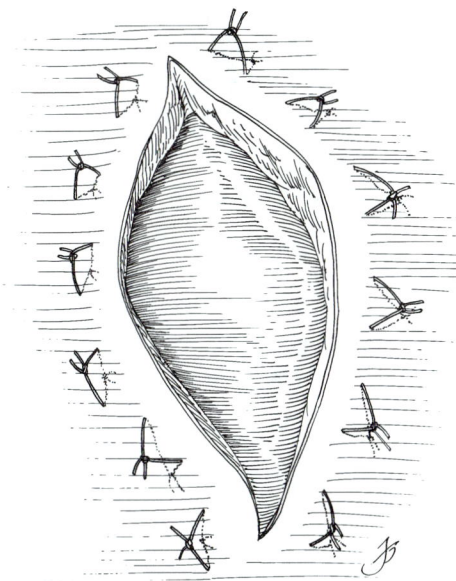

Figure 52–1. Place eyelets for a tie-over dressing around the wound using large suture material.

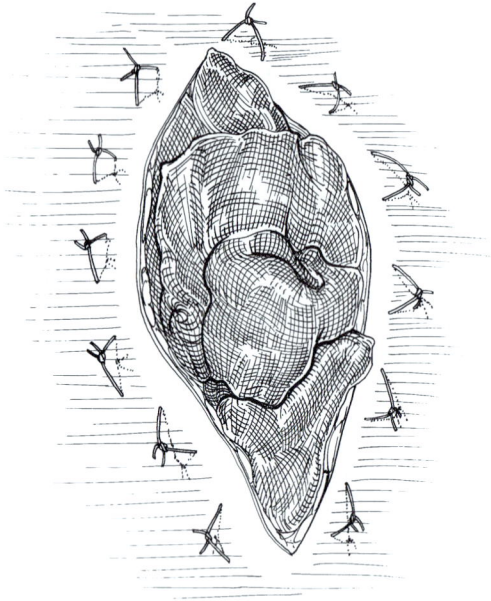

Figure 52–2.   Place appropriate primary and secondary bandage layers over the wound.

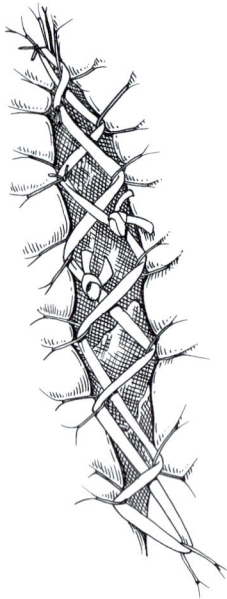

Figure 52–3.   Lace sterile gauze or umbilical tape over the layers.

sial. If an established infection exists, topical therapy is often all that is necessary.

▼ *Key Point* Control of infection is most effective through good open wound management, especially copious lavage and frequent bandage changes.

- Whenever possible, select antibiotics based on culture and sensitivity results. Use a broad-spectrum antibiotic while awaiting culture and sensitivity results.

- Use a combination of IV beta-lactam (e.g., cephalosporin) and aminoglycoside (e.g., gentamicin) antibiotics if septicemia is suspected.

DAILY WOUND MANAGEMENT

Frequency

- The timing of bandage changes is influenced by the need for debridement, the amount of exudate from the wound bed, and manageability of the patient.
- Early in wound management, change bandages on a daily or twice-daily schedule. Wounds with healthy granulation tissue may be inspected and rebandaged every other or every several days.
- The volume of wound exudate or nature of the exudate in the bandage is often the guide to frequency of bandage changes. If wound drainage increases, then more frequent bandage changes and a change of primary layer may be indicated.

Analgesia

- Animals with extensive wounds often require analgesics or anesthetics at the time of bandage changes. Once granulation tissue begins to form, this may no longer be needed.

Debridement

- During the early management of wounds, intermittent surgical debridement is the best means of removing necrotic tissue and debris.
- Surgical debridement is complemented by the use of mechanical debridement through regular bandage changes.

Lavage

- Daily wound lavage aids in dislodgement of bacteria, removal of debris, dilution of exudates, and promotion of drainage.
- Whirlpool baths may benefit animals with extensive truncal wounds. If such treatments are instituted, monitor closely for any signs of wound infection.

Bacterial Cultures

- With daily bandage changes and wound inspections the nature of the wound bed and exudate may be monitored. If during these inspections a change in the wound is noted and infection is suspected, submit wound swab samples or debrided tissue for culture and sensitivity.

Rebandaging

- As wound healing progresses to healthy granulation tissue, change the type of dressing from adherent to nonadherent and decrease the frequency of bandage changes.
- In cases of infection or deterioration of the wound, a change from a nonadherent to an adherent dressing may be necessary.

WOUND CLOSURE

Subsequent closure of open wounds can be accomplished nonsurgically by natural second intention healing, or surgically by delayed primary closure or secondary closure. Surgical methods of closure are described in Chapter 51. Consider surgical closure of open wounds once healthy granulation tissue is apparent. Epithelialization often coincides with granulation tissue. In most cases this tissue provides adequate blood supply with little risk of infection.

Second Intention Healing

Second intention healing is the body's natural method of wound closure and is the progressive formation of granulation tissue followed by wound contraction and epithelialization.

Advantages

- Additional surgery may be avoided.
- Less expensive than other closure options.
- In cases in which no tension is involved, the wound is covered with full-thickness, normal-appearing skin if contraction is complete.

Disadvantages

- Contracture and disfigurement from excessive contraction and scar tissue formation. If a joint is involved, decreased range of motion may result.

- With incomplete wound contraction, the epithelium may not cover the remaining defect.
- If the wound defect is large, the epithelium covering the defect is often fragile, easily disrupted, and has a poor aesthetic appearance.

SUPPLEMENTAL READINGS

Bauer MS, Aiken S: The healing of open wounds. Semin Vet Med Surg 4:268, 1989.

Lee AH, Swaim SF: Granulation tissue: How to take advantage of it in management of open wounds. Comp Cont Ed 10:163, 1988.

Pavletic MM: Atlas of Small Animal Reconstructive Surgery. Philadelphia: JB Lippincott, 1993.

Pavletic MM: The integument. In Slatter D, ed.: Textbook of Small Animal Surgery, 2nd Ed. Philadelphia: WB Saunders, 1993, pp 260–268.

Pope ER: Skin healing. In Bojrab MJ, ed.: Disease Mechanisms in Small Animal Surgery, 2nd Ed. Philadelphia: Lea & Febiger, 1993, pp 151–155.

Swaim SF: Surgery of Traumatized Skin: Management and Reconstruction in the Dog and Cat. Philadelphia: WB Saunders, 1980.

Waldron DR, Trevor P: Management of superficial skin wounds. In Slatter D, ed.: Textbook of Small Animal Surgery, 2nd Ed. Philadelphia: WB Saunders, 1993, pp 269–280.

Selected Skin Graft and Reconstructive Techniques

Stephen J. Birchard / Daniel D. Smeak

Large skin wounds can occur (1) from trauma directly to the skin or to its blood supply; (2) secondary to necrotizing skin diseases (see Chap. 46); and (3) after en bloc removal of large skin, subcutaneous, or body wall neoplasms. Most open wounds eventually heal by the formation of granulation tissue, wound contraction, and epithelialization. Skin flaps or grafts are indicated when wound healing is not progressing. Full-thickness skin is necessary to prevent problems caused by repeated trauma (e.g., in the dorsum of the leg or paw). Skin reconstruction is also necessary if the open wound is so large it will cause significant patient morbidity or wound contracture is likely to cause a significant problem (e.g., the wound is over a joint). Skin flaps are usually preferred over skin grafts because they are simpler to perform and have a higher success rate. However, if sufficient skin is not available adjacent to the wound, consider a skin graft.

Consider several factors before performing skin flaps or skin grafts, such as viability of adjacent tissue, systemic illness that may affect wound healing, function of the affected area of the body, tolerance of the wound by the animal, feasibility of long-term bandaging of the affected part, desired cosmetic result, and cost to the owner. Thoroughly discuss these factors with the owner prior to performing any of these procedures.

This chapter describes practical methods of reconstructing skin using skin flaps and grafts. More complicated methods of skin grafting that require specialized skill or equipment, such as using a dermatome for split-thickness skin grafts, or tube grafts, are not discussed in this chapter. Primary closure of skin wounds is reviewed in Chapter 51, and open wound management in Chapter 52.

SURGICAL ANATOMY

Skin

The skin is composed of the epidermis and dermis.

- Structures that compose the skin adnexa, hair follicles, sweat glands, and sebaceous glands are located in the dermis.
- Besides adnexa, the dermis is composed of fibroblasts, collagen fibers, and various other structures, such as blood vessels, nerves, tissue cells, and fluid.

Subcutaneous Tissue

The subcutaneous tissue is mainly composed of loose connective tissue, including elastic fibers, fat, blood vessels, and nerves.

Cutaneous Muscles

- Thin, superficial muscles, collectively called the panniculus muscle, lie within the subcutis in certain body regions in both dogs and cats. Examples are the platysma muscle in the neck and the cutaneus trunci muscle in the trunk.
- Preservation of these muscles is a very important principle in the formation of viable skin flaps for reconstruction.

Blood Supply to the Skin

- Deep or subdermal plexus
  - This plexus is the major source of blood supply to the skin and of most importance to the surgeon.

▼ *Key Point* When creating skin flaps in dogs and cats, preserve the deep vascular plexus.

- In regions where cutaneous musculature is present, this vascular network is present on the superficial and deep layers of the muscle. Dissection beneath this thin muscle layer is critical to flap survival.
- Direct cutaneous arteries are present in several areas of the body. They arise from deep vessels that course superficially and run parallel to the skin. These direct cutaneous arteries communicate with the deep vascular plexus.
- Middle and superficial plexuses complete the layers of vascular network to the skin.

SKIN FLAPS

Skin flaps are a means of reconstructing open wounds by rotating or advancing adjacent or regional skin to allow wound closure. Blood vessels supplying these flaps are maintained. Therefore, skin flaps do not require a bed of granulation tissue for their blood supply and nutrition. Skin flaps can be classified according to their blood supply, such as *random subdermal flaps* versus *axial pattern flaps*, or according to their location with respect to the recipient bed, such as *local flaps* versus *distant flaps*.

Random Subdermal Flaps

Random subdermal skin flaps are those constructed with skin that does not contain a direct cutaneous artery. Viability of these skin flaps is dependent on the availability of local blood vessels. To help prevent avascular necrosis of the flap, make the flap base slightly wider than the flap body. Random subdermal skin flaps can be further classified as *advancement flaps*, *rotation flaps*, and *transposition flaps*, depending on how the flap is moved to the defect; *single pedicle* and *bipedicle flaps*, depending on how the flap is attached to the body; and *direct distant flaps*, depending on use for extremity skin defects.

- Advancement refers to how the flap is moved to the wound. These are usually rectangular flaps. Simple advancement flaps are undermined and pulled (horizontally or vertically) directly to the wound (Fig. 53–1).
- A transposition flap is constructed immediately adjacent to the wound, and is rotated (clockwise or counterclockwise) to cover the wound (Fig. 53–2).
- A rotation flap is a semicircular flap that rotates into an adjacent recipient bed. Single or paired flaps can be employed to close triangular defects (Fig. 53–3); no secondary defect is created with this flap.
- Direct distant flaps include thoracic or abdominal single pedicle or bipedicle direct distant flaps that can be used as a method for transferring skin to the distal extremities.
  - Single pedicle: Attached to the body only at one end (Fig. 53–4*A, C*). The pedicle provides the vascular attachment to the flap.
  - Bipedicle: Attached to the body at both ends (Fig. 53–4*B*).
  - These flaps are transferred from a distance to the recipient defect. The lesion is advanced to the flap rather than the flap being transferred to the lesion as in construction of advancement flaps.

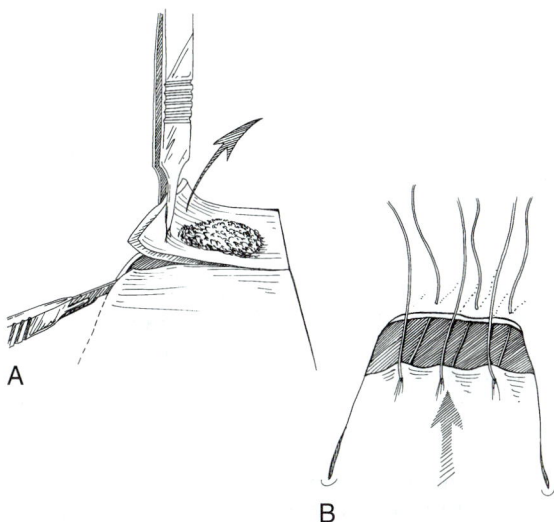

Figure 53–1. Simple advancement flap. Make the initial incisions *(A)*, then deeply undermine the flap and advance to the defect *(B)*.

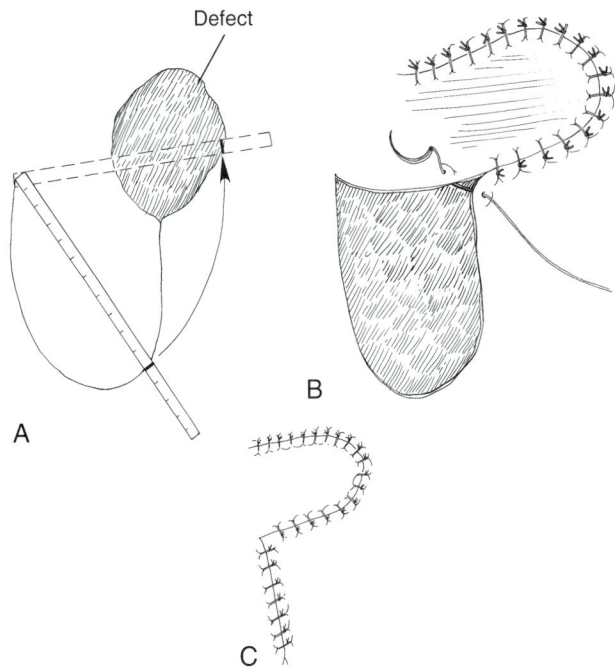

Figure 53–2. Transposition flap. After measuring the length of flap needed, make the incisions and rotate the flap to the defect. Suture the flap first and then close the remaining defect.

- Forelimb defects are more often reconstructed using this technique than are rear limb defects.

Indications

Advancement, Rotation, and Transposition Flaps

- For large skin wounds that are located in areas with adjacent loose, redundant skin (e.g., neck, flank, dorsal trunk) that allow formation and closure of defects remaining after flap transfer without tension.
- As a general rule, do not consider these flaps for denuded areas distal to the stifle, elbow, or tail head.

Direct Distant Pedicle Flaps

- For large wounds of the distal extremities in which local skin is not available or would be closed under excessive tension.
- These flaps are usually made from skin over the lateral thoracic or abdominal wall. The leg is attached to the side of the animal's body for a period of time while healing of the pedicle to the extremity wound progresses. The pedicle is removed from the thorax or abdomen and the leg returned to its normal position.
- These flaps are very successful, but patient tolerance is variable.

Preoperative Considerations

- Carefully plan the surgical procedure. Review vascular anatomy of the region. The size, location, shape, and condition of the wound dictate the type of flap.
- Check the looseness and pliability of the skin adjacent to the lesion or wound to determine feasibility of the intended skin flap.

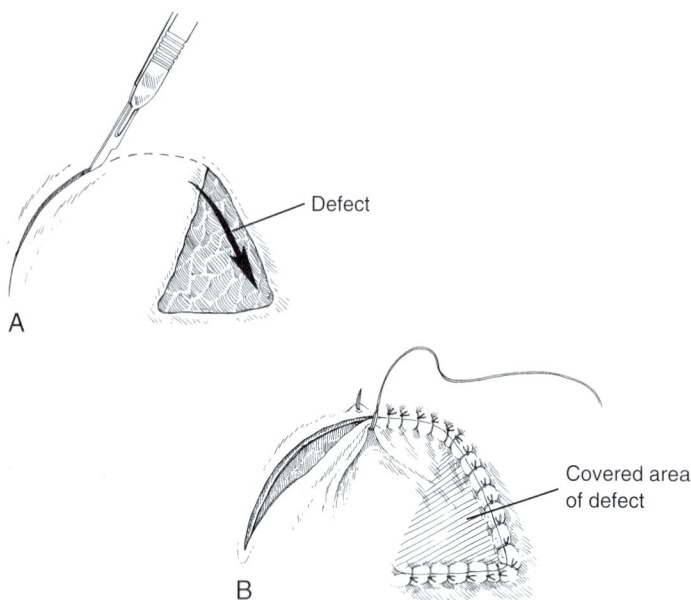

Figure 53–3. Create a curved incision in a stepwise fashion to close a triangular wound.

- Consider administration of prophylactic antibiotics, given intravenously at induction of anesthesia, if significant contamination of the surgical site is possible.
- Prepare the recipient bed preoperatively to ensure that the area is free of infection, foreign material, and necrotic tissue.

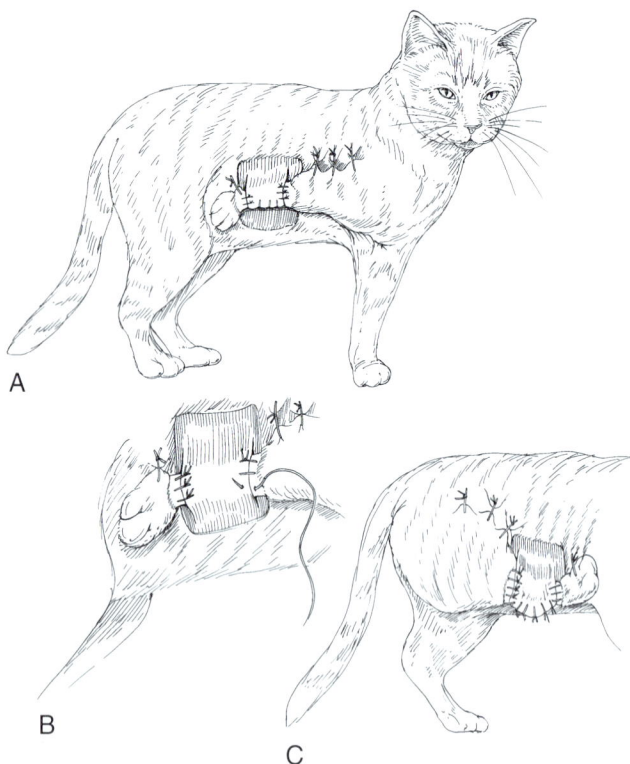

Figure 53–4. Direct distant flap. Make the skin flap using the lateral thoracic or abdominal skin. Suture the flap to the limb defect. This flap can have a single *(A)* or double *(B)* pedicle. Secure the limb to the lateral body wall with skin sutures placed between the leg and the body wall *(C)*. Place a padded bandage around the body to help stabilize the elevated limb.

- Distant flap technique requires two surgical procedures to complete. The owner is made fully aware of the costs involved, the inconvenience of bandage management, and the problems related to the prolonged immobilization period. Hair direction and cosmetic problems are more common with distant compared with local flap techniques.

▼ *Key Point* Consider the mobility of the extremity that contains the defect when determining the location and type of direct distant flap. Evaluate the size and temperament of the patient. Smaller animals with calm dispositions seem to tolerate this technique best.

Surgical Procedure

Objectives

- To provide full-thickness reconstruction of a large skin wound.
- To avoid tension along the suture line.
- To create flaps that maintain viability and provide satisfactory cosmesis.

Equipment

- Standard surgical pack and suture.
- Measuring device to plan length and width of flaps.
- Sterile marking pen to draw incisions (optional). Sterile methylene blue and a cotton-tipped applicator can be effective as a marker.
- A piece of sterile double-knit cloth can be used as a pattern for designing flaps intraoperatively.
- Penrose drains (¼–½ inch).

Technique

Advancement or Transposition Flaps

1. Carefully position the patient to free up any available skin in the region and to reduce tension while the flap is being sutured.

2. Aseptically prepare a liberal amount of skin in the region of the proposed flap and donor sites.

3. Remove epithelialized portions of the granulation bed by sharp dissection. Attachments of skin at the margin of the granulation bed are undermined to free up the bordering skin.

4. Gently manipulate the skin margins surrounding the defect to ascertain the availability of adjacent local skin.

5. Optimally, the donor area has enough skin available to elevate a flap without leaving a secondary defect that cannot be closed primarily.

6. If possible, avoid choosing a donor area that may be subject to excessive motion or tension.

7. Choose the type of flap depending on the availability of skin, shape and location of the defect, and size of the area to be covered.

8. It is better to create two adjacent short flaps rather than one long flap, which has a greater risk of necrosis from inadequate blood supply.

9. Try to design the flap so that the base is slightly wider than the width to avoid inadvertently devascularizing the flap.

10. Design the flap to fill the defect without tension.

11. Create the flap by sharply incising along the preplanned donor skin margins.

12. Use stay sutures or fine skin hooks when elevating the flap to avoid causing excessive damage.

▼ *Key Point* The depth of flap undermining is very important to preserve the deep vascular plexus under the panniculus muscle group. Be especially careful when undermining in the region of the base of the flap to avoid interrupting critical direct cutaneous vessel branches.

13. Transfer the skin flap to the defect (see Figs. 53–1 and 53–2).

14. Consider placing a Penrose drain in large dead space areas (under flaps and donor areas) if the condition of the tissues warrants it. Exit the drain in a ventral-dependent area of the wound away from the primary suture line.

15. Meticulously close subcutaneous tissues with fine (4-0 to 5-0), simple interrupted, absorbable suture material to evenly distribute skin tension.

16. Use fine (4-0) monofilament nonabsorbable suture material placed in a simple interrupted pattern to close the skin. Skin staples may also be used. This allows for individual control of suture tension. If fluid accumulation develops in the dead space, simple removal of one or two skin sutures in a gravity-dependent area often allows adequate drainage.

Technique

Direct Distant Flap (Single or Double Pedicle)

1. Aseptically prepare the entire limb and lateral thoracic wall, for a forelimb defect, or abdominal wall, for a rear limb defect. When preparing a bipedicle flap, meticulously clip and clean the portion of paw or limb that will be in contact with the subcutaneous tissue.

2. Position the affected limb in the most comfortable angle possible to locate the donor area (see Fig. 53–4).

3. Attempt to construct the flap so that any movement of the limb will pull the flap onto the defect rather than away from it.

4. Create a bipedicle flap if the defect is large or nearly circumferential (Fig. 53–4B), or a single pedicle flap if the defect is less than 180° circumferential (Fig. 53–4A, C), using the principles described previously in the section on advancement flap technique.

5. After creating a single pedicle flap, a skin defect remains that must be closed. Use advancement or rotation flaps to close this defect.

6. Place the limb through the bipedicle flap or adjacent to the single pedicle flap.

7. Suture as much of the flap to the defect margins as possible.

8. Small Penrose drains may be placed to drain fluids that may accumulate under the flap or limb.

9. Large (2-0 to 0) suture material can be selected to help tack the skin of the limb to the thoracic wall skin in several areas to help immobilize the limb.

▼ *Key Point* Complete immobilization of the limb is mandatory for at least 14 days to ensure adequate vascularization of the flap from the wound bed.

10. Design a bandage for immobilization that will remain in place for the full 2 weeks but will still allow the flap area to be monitored and separately rebandaged.

11. If the flap appears healthy, sharply incise the pedicles from the donor area. Suture the remaining free skin margins to the defect to complete the transfer.

Axial Pattern Flaps

Axial pattern flaps are those skin flaps that are developed using a major direct cutaneous artery as the primary blood supply. Considerably more flexibility in the length and mobility of these flaps is possible compared with random skin flaps. These flaps can be made with long vascular pedicles to transfer skin to more remote areas of the body, because of the direct cutaneous artery allowing an adequate perfusion of a large area of tissue. Axial pattern flaps are created in a one-step procedure, as compared with direct distant flaps.

Axial pattern flaps can be based on many direct cutaneous arteries, such as the caudal superficial epigastric, the cervical cutaneous branch of the omocervical, the thoracodorsal, the deep circumflex iliac, and the genicular branch of the saphenous artery. The caudal superficial epigastric axial pattern flap is commonly selected for large defects of the proximal thigh and flank. Only this technique is described here. However, other axial pattern flaps as listed previously can be created using similar principles and are described in veterinary surgical textbooks (see Pavletic, 1998).

Indications

- Similar to those for random subdermal flaps except that axial pattern flaps are used when the skin defect is very large or when the donor skin needs to be transferred over a large distance to the recipient site.
- A major direct cutaneous artery and vein must be in the region of the skin defect for this technique to be indicated.

Preoperative Considerations

- Same as those for random subdermal flaps, plus the following:
  - Carefully plan the design of the flap.
  - Consider how the resultant defect of the donor area will be closed.
  - Be sure the skin and the direct cutaneous artery that will be used for the flap are viable.

Surgical Procedure

Objectives

- Same as those for random skin flaps, plus:
  - Preserve viability of the direct cutaneous artery by avoiding excessive surgical trauma to the tissue.

Equipment

- Same as that for random skin flaps.

Technique

Caudal Superficial Epigastric Axial Pattern Flap
1. Use preparation and tissue handling principles as described for advancement or rotation flaps.
2. Be particularly careful when positioning the patient so that the vascular pedicle will not become distorted before planning the incisions.
3. Incisions are created as shown in Figure 53–5.
4. The entire mammary chain up to the cranial thoracic gland can be included in this flap.
5. Deeply undermine the flap just superficial to the abdominal fascia.
6. Dissect very carefully around the origin of the direct cutaneous vessel to avoid inadvertent damage to this vessel, which is vital to the survival of the flap.
7. Avoid creating a kink or excess tension in the base of the flap, which could obstruct blood flow.
8. Drain the dead space if needed.
9. Suture the flap to the defect, as described for the other flap techniques.

Postoperative Care and Complications

All Flap Types

- Restrict exercise until suture removal.
- Apply an Elizabethan collar before the patient is recovered from anesthesia and leave on the animal until the flaps are completely healed.
- Change wound dressings as necessary.

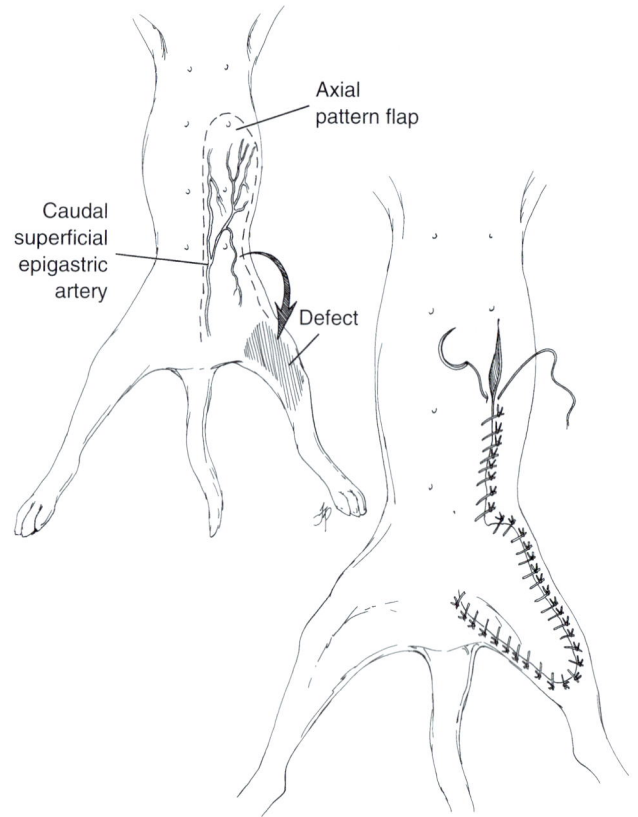

Figure 53–5. Example of an axial pattern flap. This flap is based on a direct cutaneous artery—the caudal superficial epigastric artery. Design the flap around this artery and deeply undermine the skin and mammary tissue. Rotate the flap and suture to the defect.

- Immobilize the limb for at least 14 days for direct distant flap techniques.
- Major complications resulting from skin flaps include local problems, such as partial or total ischemia of the flap, infection, seroma, and dehiscence of the flap or donor suture line.
- Dehiscence of donor site incisions is usually due to excessive skin tension. If dehiscence occurs, allow these areas to heal by second intention. Excise ischemic areas of flaps when these areas are clearly demarcated.

FREE SKIN GRAFTS

Free skin grafts involve complete removal of skin from one area of the body and implantation to another. These grafts are completely separated from their blood supply, and they are dependent on the wound bed for viability. For the first 3 or 4 days after grafting, the skin graft obtains its nutrition from the wound bed by diffusion, a process called imbibition. During this process, the graft acts like a sponge, soaking up fluid and oxygen from the granulation tissue of the wound. This is a very delicate process that is easily disrupted by complicating factors, such as excessive movement of the wound, seroma formation, and infection. During this initial phase of healing, the graft usually looks its worst, appearing congested and sometimes purple. After a few days, this appearance dramatically improves if the graft "takes."

After the first 3–4 days, viability of the graft depends on ingrowth of capillaries from the wound bed into the graft (i.e., inosculation). These are very fragile structures and are easily damaged by trauma (such as licking of the graft), excessive motion, and infection. Once this blood supply becomes well-established, viability of the graft is maintained.

Skin grafts vary in their final cosmetic result. The best cosmesis is obtained from a full-thickness skin graft, because this allows hair to form over the area. However, full-thickness grafts are the most difficult to establish, because they are thicker than split-thickness grafts. This greater thickness makes the initial process of imbibition more difficult, resulting in a higher incidence of graft failure.

Pinch Skin Grafts

Pinch skin grafting is performed by simply harvesting small (2–3 mm) sections of full-thickness skin and placing them into the wound granulation bed. They are not difficult to perform and are highly successful. However, the major disadvantage of pinch grafts is the final cosmetic result. Uniform full-thickness skin does not form over the wound with pinch grafts; therefore, very little hair grows over the area.

Preoperative Considerations

- Determine the desired result of the graft. If a high degree of success and rapid epithelialization of the wound are desired, consider pinch grafts. If complete regrowth of hair and excellent cosmesis are necessary, employ a different skin graft method, such as mesh graft. If the recipient site is over a joint or area that is frequently traumatized, full-thickness grafts may be needed and pinch grafts may not be satisfactory.

▼ *Key Point* Maximize the chances of graft "take" by properly preparing the wound bed before grafting.

Use standard techniques of wound debridement, lavage, and bandaging (see Chapter 52) for several days prior to grafting to establish a healthy bed of granulation tissue. Postpone the graft procedure if any evidence of infection is present.

Surgical Technique

Objectives

- To establish epithelial coverage of an open wound.
- To atraumatically harvest small plugs of skin from an area of redundant skin.
- To implant these plugs of skin into an area of healthy granulation tissue to promote healing.

Equipment

- Same as for skin flaps, plus:
  - Several #15 scalpel blades
  - Skin biopsy punch (optional)

Technique

1. Aseptically prepare the wound bed and the harvest site.
2. Gently pick up the skin with thumb forceps or stay suture and excise a 1-mm piece of skin, using the #15 scalpel blade. Be careful not to include subcutaneous tissue with the skin pinch.
3. Alternatively, harvest the skin using a skin biopsy punch. Place the punch at the same angle as the hair follicle during harvesting.
4. Trim subcutaneous tissue from the bottom of the pinch of skin.
5. Place the skin pinch or punch in a saline-moistened surgical sponge.
6. Make a "vest pocket" stab incision in the granulation tissue with a #15 scalpel blade (Fig. 53–6).
7. Slide the skin pinch into the incision in the granulation tissue (Fig. 53–6). Be sure the epithelial side of the pinch is facing out.
8. Repeat this process as many times as necessary to have skin pinches covering the wound at about 1–2 cm apart.
9. Place a nonadherent dressing over the wound. The primary layer of the dressing can be petrolatum-impregnated gauze or Telfa strips with a thin layer of triple antibiotic ointment (Bacitracin-Neomycin-Polymyxin, Pharmaderm).
10. Let the donor sites heal by second intention.

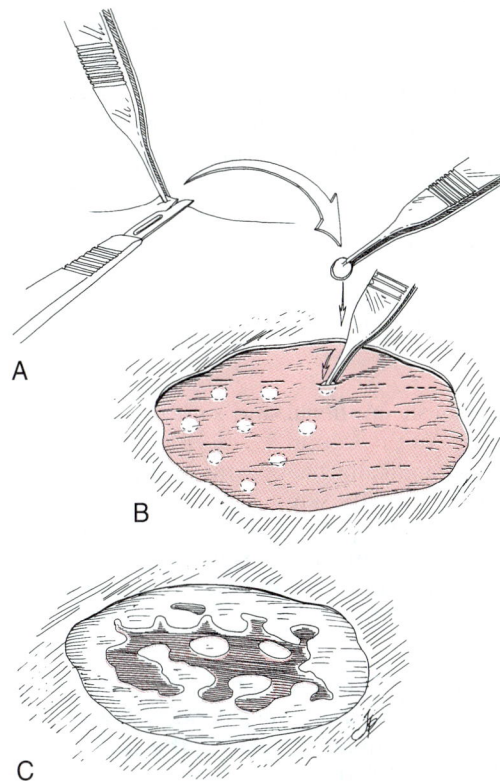

Figure 53–6. Pinch skin graft. Obtain small pinches of skin using a scalpel. *(A),* Make small "vest-pocket" incisions in the granulation bed, and slide skin pinches into these incisions with the epidermal side facing out. *(B),* Pinches can be approximately 1 to 2 cm apart. Wound will be filled in by epidermal growth from the pinch grafts *(C).*

Postoperative Care and Complications

- Restrict exercise to leash walking only.
- Change the wound dressing every day for the first 5–7 days, then every 2–3 days if wound healing is progressing normally.
- Keep the wound dressed until it is completely covered with epithelium.
- If necessary, place an Elizabethan collar on the animal to prevent licking of the wound.
- Potential complications include dislodgement of the pinch grafts due to self-trauma or excessive motion and poor cosmetic result due to sparsity of hair formation.

Mesh Skin Grafts

Mesh skin grafts are usually full-thickness skin grafts that are harvested, stripped of subcutaneous tissue, and "meshed" by making multiple scalpel cuts in them. The purposes of making holes in the graft are to increase coverage of the wound by the graft and to allow escape of fluid from underneath the graft. Mesh grafts provide better cosmesis than pinch grafts. The healed wound has some hair coverage although it may not be as much as on the surrounding skin, depending on how much the mesh is expanded.

Mesh grafts are fairly simple to perform and require no special equipment. Although reportedly effective in both dogs and cats, our results have been very good in cats (nearly 100% success), but only fair in dogs (approximately 50–60%).

Preoperative Considerations

- These are the same as those for pinch grafts.
- Consider giving a prophylactic systemic antibiotic (beginning preoperatively) to help prevent infection of the graft.
- Do not perform the procedure if any evidence of infection is present in either the donor or recipient sites.

Surgical Procedure

Objectives

- To establish epithelial and some full-thickness skin coverage of the wound.
- To atraumatically harvest the donor skin from an area of redundant skin.
- To meticulously prepare the graft for implantation by removing all subcutaneous fat and creating a mesh by making multiple small holes in the skin.

Equipment

- Same as for pinch grafts, plus:
  - A sterile board (plastic, wood, or cardboard) for stretching out and preparing the graft.
  - #11 scalpel blade.

Technique

1. Aseptically prepare the donor and recipient sites.
2. Estimate the size of the wound by measuring or cutting out a template using sterile drape material.
3. Sharply excise the donor skin from an area of redundant skin (e.g., dorsum of the neck and lateral flank area).
4. Avoid excising the subcutaneous tissues.
5. Note the direction of hair growth in the harvested skin.
6. Place multiple stay sutures at the edge of the harvested skin.
7. Place the skin on a sterile board (epidermal side down), and stretch it out using the stay sutures (Fig. 53–7).
8. Carefully dissect all remaining subcutaneous fat from the skin using sharp dissection (Fig. 53–7A).
9. Lavage the skin frequently with sterile saline.
10. Make multiple full-thickness holes, approximately ½ cm in length and ½–1 cm apart (Fig. 53–7B).
11. Place the mesh graft on the wound.
12. Position the graft so that the hair growth will be in the same direction as that of the adjacent hair.
13. Suture the graft to the surrounding skin (Fig. 53–7C).

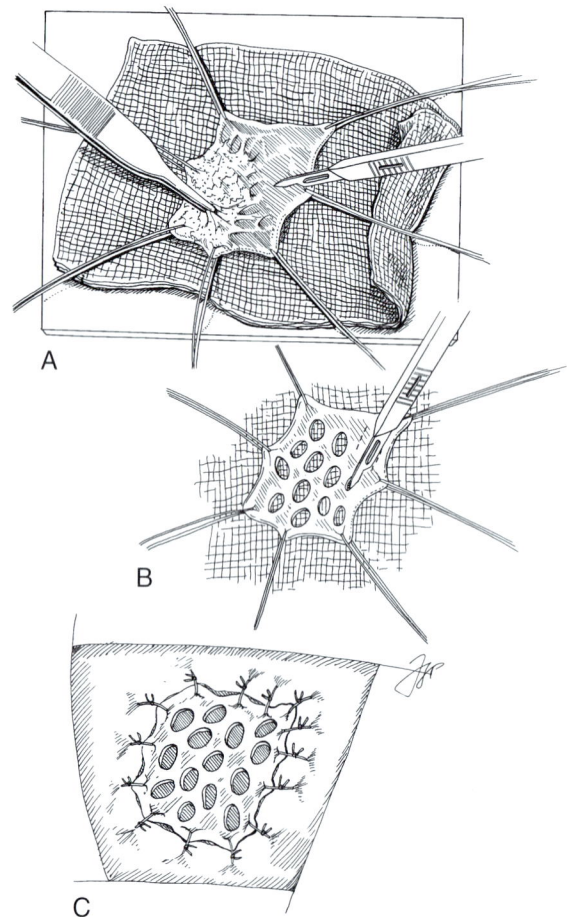

Figure 53–7. Mesh skin graft. Harvest skin and stretch it out on a sterile board using stay sutures and meticulously remove all subcutaneous fat (A). Make multiple slits in the graft using a scalpel (B). Suture the graft, with the epidermal side facing out, to the granulation bed (C).

14. Suture the graft under slight tension so that the mesh expands and the granulation tissue can be seen through the graft (Fig. 53–7*C*).

15. Place additional tacking sutures from the center of the graft to the granulation bed to prevent movement of the graft and separation of the graft from the wound bed.

16. Cover the wound with a nonadherent dressing (see the description under pinch grafts).

Change the dressing as needed to prevent desiccation of the primary layer and adherence to the graft.

▼ *Key Point* When changing the dressing, be very careful to prevent separation of the graft from the underlying granulation tissue.

Postoperative Care and Complications

* Same as for pinch grafts, plus:
  * Prevent desiccation of the graft by applying small amounts of triple antibiotic ointment or sterile petrolatum directly on the skin graft.

* Immobilize the limb if grafting over a joint (e.g., elbow, carpus, stifle, hock) to prevent excessive movement of the graft.
* The major complication is failure of the graft to heal due to infection, excessive motion, or lack of adherence of the graft to the underlying granulation tissue.

SUPPLEMENTAL READINGS

Pavletic MM: Pedicle grafts. *In* Slatter DH, ed.: Textbook of Small Animal Surgery. Philadelphia: WB Saunders, 1985, p 458.

Pavletic MM: Skin-grafting and reconstruction techniques. *In* Bojrab MJ, ed.: Current Techniques in Small Animal Surgery, 4th Ed. Philadelphia: Lea & Febiger, 1998, p 585.

Swaim SF: Skin grafts. *In* Slatter DH, ed.: Textbook of Small Animal Surgery. Philadelphia: WB Saunders, 1985, p 486.

54 Diseases of the Pinna

Mary P. Schick / Robert O. Schick

The pinna of the ear is a relatively common site for numerous dermatologic diseases. Distinct underlying etiologies exist for most pinnal diseases, even though clinically they may appear similar (Table 54–1). Careful differentiation is paramount in obtaining a definitive diagnosis and successful treatment.

Pinnal dermatoses may be primary or secondary. Primary pinnal dermatoses are defined as those limited to or those that arise on the pinnae before affecting other body areas. Secondary pinnal dermatoses involve the pinnae along with other body lesions. Factors that must be considered in the diagnosis of either primary or secondary diseases include self-trauma, sun exposure, and age, breed, and sex of the animal.

In all patients with pinnal disease, definitive diagnosis, prognosis, and therapeutic protocol depend on a thorough history, complete physical examination, and several routine baseline diagnostic aids. The patient history determines the duration and progression of the pinnal lesions, development of similar lesions on other body areas, and concurrent systemic signs. Previous medications and treatment response are also important factors. The physical examination assesses the site and extent of disease. Determine whether the haired or nonhaired areas of the pinnae are affected.

▼ *Key Point* Certain diseases, such as demodectic mange, dermatophytosis, and bacterial pyoderma, are usually restricted to hair follicle invasion.

A routine minimum database allows for a definitive diagnosis (Table 54–2). The database may detect other organ system involvement and provides a baseline evaluation of organ system function for future reference, before initiation of medication.

Histopathologic examination of lesions provides valuable information in the diagnosis of pinnal disease. Obtain the pinnal biopsy specimen with extreme care. A permanent scarring defect may result as a complication of pinnal biopsy. For skin biopsy techniques, see Chapter 49.

▼ *Key Point* Histopathologic examination and possibly immunofluorescence testing enable differentiation of pinnal diseases that are clinically similar.

Consider more specific laboratory evaluations, including hormonal assays, food restriction diets, intradermal allergy tests, and direct immunofluorescence tests of skin biopsy specimens, to obtain a definitive diagnosis.

INFLAMMATORY DISEASES OF THE PINNA

Most pinnal skin diseases are characterized by erythema. Pinnal erythema is frequently followed by secondary scaling and alopecia. In this discussion, the most common etiologies of pinnal erythema are presented.

Atopy, Contact Dermatitis, and Food Hypersensitivity

Clinical Signs

These particular diseases may affect both pinnae solely or concurrently with other body areas. Atopy and food hypersensitivity (see Chaps. 41 and 42, respectively) appear clinically as diffuse erythema and accompanying edema or urticarial lesions of the concave and/or convex surfaces of the pinna. Contact allergies usually occur nonseasonally on surfaces of the pinna that touch the offending agent. Initially, in any of these three allergic diseases, the animal may exhibit flare-ups of erythema and accompanying pruritus that may appear and remit spontaneously. With time, an initial seasonal pattern of erythema and pruritus may become year-long with atopy. Chronic trauma of the pinna may cause alopecia, excoriation, fibrosis, and secondary infection.

Diagnosis

- The differential diagnoses of these allergic pinnal dermatoses include pruritic otitis externa secondary to mange mite infestation, foreign body embedment (e.g., grass awns), and bacterial folliculitis.
- Diagnosis of atopy and food hypersensitivity is made by obtaining the minimum database for pinnal dermatoses in addition to special food restriction diets and intradermal allergy testing (see Chaps. 41 and 42).

Treatment

- Ideally, if identifiable offending allergens are eliminated from the animal's environment, signs of allergy disappear. On removal of the allergen in con-

Table 54–1. DIFFERENTIAL DIAGNOSES OF PINNAL DISEASES BASED ON CLINICAL PRESENTATION

Clinical Manifestation	Differential Diagnoses
Macules/papules	Parasitic dermatoses/hypersensitivities
	Bacterial folliculitis
	Drug eruption
	Food allergy
	Dermatophytosis
	Lupus erythematosus
Nodules	Neoplasia
	Eosinophilic granuloma complex
	Sterile granuloma/pyogranuloma
	Mycoses
Vesicles	Pemphigus/pemphigoid
	Dermatomyositis
	Lupus erythematosus
Pustules	Pemphigus/pemphigoid
	Dermatomyositis
	Lupus erythematosus
	Demodectic mange
	Drug eruption
	Dermatophytosis
	Bacterial folliculitis
	Eosinophilic folliculitis
Alopecia (focal)	Bacterial folliculitis
	Drug eruption
	Dermatophytosis
	Demodectic mange
	Dermatomyositis
	Alopecia areata
	Sex hormone imbalance
	Periodic alopecia
	Notoedric mange (feline)
Hyperpigmentation	Hypothyroidism
	Sex hormone imbalance
	Hyperadrenocorticism
	Growth hormone responsive
Induration	Juvenile cellulitis
	Neoplasia
	Urticaria
	Feline relapsing polychondritis
Erosions/ulcers	Parasitic infestation
	Dermatomyositis
	Vasculitis
	Dermatophytosis
	Pemphigus/pemphigoid
	Toxic epidermal necrolysis
Exfoliation	Pemphigus
	Cutaneous lymphoma
	Ichthyosis
	Hepatocutaneous syndrome
Plaques	Lichenoid psoriasiform dermatosis
	Lichenoid dermatosis
	Zinc-responsive dermatosis
	Cutaneous lymphomas

Table 54–2. MINIMUM DATABASE FOR PINNAL DERMATOSES

Otoscopic examination
Microscopic examination
  Skin scrapings for mites and fungi
  Cytology (impression smears)
  Mineral oil ear swab for mites
Culture for bacteria and fungi
Skin biopsy
  Histopathologic examination
  Immunofluorescence testing (if indicated)
Blood analysis
  Complete blood count, serum biochemical profile, endocrine screen (if indicated)
Urinalysis

(0.25–0.5 mg/kg q12h PO), then taper to alternate days or as infrequently as possible. Antibiotic therapy may be instituted as necessary to control secondary bacterial infections.

▼ *Key Point* Contact and food hypersensitivity in animals responds unpredictably to systemic corticosteroid therapy. Atopic animals usually respond well, at least initially.

Feline Solar Dermatitis

Clinical Signs

- Chronic sun exposure of white-haired pinnae and other white-haired facial areas of cats may cause feline solar dermatitis. This syndrome also occurs in dogs but less frequently.
- The clinical signs of pinnal erythema and scaling (solar dermatitis) are considered precancerous and herald malignant transformation into carcinoma in situ. Squamous cell carcinoma is usually locally invasive, and with time, the pinna becomes progressively edematous, ulcerated, hemorrhagic, and deformed (fissuring, curling, and finally obliteration).

Diagnosis

- Differential diagnoses include feline scabies, frostbite, trauma, pemphigus complex, systemic lupus erythematosus, and other cutaneous neoplasias.
- Definitive diagnosis requires skin biopsy. Extensive pinnal involvement necessitates submandibular lymph node biopsy to assess for metastasis.

Treatment

- Solar dermatitis may be responsive to supportive therapy. Reduce the animal's sun exposure as much as possible.
- Apply topical sunscreen cream on the ears as necessary. Do not use a para-aminobenzoic acid–based product because this is a contact sensitizing agent.
- Treatment of squamous cell carcinoma is most amenable to pinnal resection or amputation depending on the extent of neoplasia. The CO_2 laser has been used safely and effectively to resect pinnal and

---

tact allergic animals, the improvement in clinical signs is dramatic. In most situations of atopy the allergens (as identified by intradermal skin testing) are not easily removed. Hyposensitization of the animal to the various inhalant allergens is the treatment of choice (see Chap. 41).

- Pinnal pruritus secondary to atopy may be controlled initially by topical and/or systemic corticosteroids. Administer anti-inflammatory doses of prednisone

facial squamous cell carcinoma in cats. Laser surgery affords the most cosmetically favorable results when compared with conventional surgery.

Dermatophytosis

Clinical Signs

Superficial fungal infections (see Chap. 37) of the pinnae in dogs and cats are most commonly caused by *Microsporum canis*. Initially, minimal to marked erythema is present. Infected hair follicles and interfollicular epidermis become inflamed, and focal to multiple areas of alopecia and scaling occur secondarily.

Diagnosis

Diagnostic aids include skin scrapings (to detect fungal arthrospores microscopically), fungal culture, and skin biopsy. Once the definitive diagnosis of dermatophytosis is made, brush the remainder of the animal's body with a sterile toothbrush. Submit this sample for fungal culture.

Treatment

- Treatment includes clipping the pinna and whole body if necessary (depending on the toothbrush sample's culture results), topical dips in lime sulfur (LymDyp, DVM Pharmaceuticals) weekly for a minimum of 8 weeks, and daily topical applications of antifungal creams (Conofite, Pitman-Moore). Institute an oral griseofulvin (Gris-Peg, Dorsey) regimen for 6–8 weeks for each infected and in-contact animal if the disease is extensive on the body, especially in Persian cats. For further information on treatment of generalized dermatophytosis, see Chapter 37.

Demodicosis

Clinical Signs

Demodicosis of the pinna may occur in dogs and cats (see Chap. 38). The clinical picture of infestation is similar to that of dermatophytosis because of the mite's predilection to inhabit hair follicles. Erythema, scaling, and alopecia are common clinical signs.

Diagnosis

Obtain multiple skin scrapings of the pinnae and other body areas to determine the extent of infestation. Perform laboratory testing of blood to detect underlying systemic abnormalities.

Treatment

Clip the pinnal and other body hair as necessary. Apply whole body dips or localized therapy using the appropriate agents as described in Chap. 38.

Juvenile Cellulitis (Juvenile Moist Pyoderma, Puppy Strangles)

Clinical Signs

The pinnae are usually affected bilaterally. Golden retrievers, dachshunds, and Gordon setters appear to be predisposed. Any number of puppies in a litter may be affected, and puppies between 4 and 16 weeks of age are most commonly affected. Diffuse erythema and edema of the pinna progress rapidly to pustular, erosive-to-ulcerative, exudative dermatitis. Other facial areas and submandibular lymph nodes may become involved and exude pus. This disease is considered to be a sterile inflammatory process of unknown etiology (see Chap. 35 for more information on pyoderma).

Diagnosis

Obtain the minimum database using appropriate aids to make a definitive diagnosis.

Treatment

- Treat the lesions topically with astringent soaks (Domeboro, Bayer). Give prednisone 1.0 mg/kg PO q12h until the disease is inactive (usually 2–3 weeks), then taper the dosage. Also administer an oral bactericidal antibiotic. Refer also to Chapter 35.

SCALING AND CRUSTING PINNAL DISEASES

Differential diagnoses of pinnal lesions of this type include fly strike and canine breed–specific epidermal keratinization defects.

Fly Strike

Clinical Signs

This is a summer-fall disease of dogs that are confined primarily outdoors. *Stomoxys calcitrans* is the most common species of biting blood-feeding flies. Others incriminated are *Culicoides* spp. and *Simulium* spp. that cause erythematous, papular pinnal lesions. Affected dogs exhibit head shaking and ear scratching in response to the extremely irritating fly bites. Secondary excoriation, exudation, and hemorrhage appear on the ear tips of erect-eared dogs and at the proximal fold of the pinna of pendulous-eared dogs. Other facial areas may be involved as well.

Diagnosis

- Differential diagnoses include sarcoptic mange, otodectic mange, atopy, vasculitis, and systemic lupus erythematosus.
- Obtain the minimum database using appropriate aids to make the definitive diagnosis (see Table 54–2).

Treatment

Treat the problem in a two-step approach.
- First, eradicate the flies or reduce exposure in the dog's immediate environment.
- Second, apply topical fly repellent (Skin So Soft, Avon Products) and/or insecticides onto the entire body of the dog with more on the head areas.
- Apply topical antibiotic-corticosteroid ointments (Panalog, Solvay) to the affected pinna to decrease inflammation and secondary bacterial infection and to provide a mechanical barrier against flies.

Ear Margin Seborrhea

Clinical Signs

Keratinization disorders of the pinna occur most commonly in pendulous-eared breeds of dogs, such as cocker spaniels and dachshunds (see Chap. 44 for a complete discussion of seborrhea). Clinical signs include scaling, crusting, and alopecic areas on the margins, especially severe on the apex of the pinna. Pinnal hair becomes embedded with scale crusts in a waxy exudate.

Diagnosis

- Differential diagnoses include zinc-responsive dermatosis, dermatophytosis, pemphigus complex, sarcoptic mange, systemic lupus erythematosus, ichthyosis, and vasculitis. Obtain the minimum database to make the definitive diagnosis (see Table 54–2).

Treatment

- While awaiting biopsy results, initiate supportive therapies: antiseborrheic shampoo and application of follicular flushing agents that contain benzoyl peroxide (Pyoben Gel, Allerderm).
- Topical corticosteroid cream or synthetic vitamin A gel (Retin-A Gel, Ortho) may be effective long-term therapy for idiopathic keratinization defects. For additional information, refer to Chapter 44.

Otodectic Mange

Clinical Signs

Initially, *Otodectes cyanotis* may infest the external ear canal and cause pruritic otitis externa in dogs and cats. Hypersensitivity to *Otodectes* mites results in severe self-trauma to the pinna, even though the number of mites may be small. Erythema, papules, excoriations, and alopecia are initial signs that progress into edema, exudation, fissuring, crusting, and scabbing.

Diagnosis

- Differential diagnoses include other mange mites and parasitic infestations.
- Obtain the appropriate minimum database to make the definitive diagnosis (see Table 54–2).

Treatment

- Treat all infested and in-contact animals with weekly pyrethrin-based shampoos for 4 weeks and/or weekly applications of pyrethrin-based flea powder to the entire body for 4 weeks.
- Concurrently, initiate local therapy using one of the numerous mineral oil–based acaricidal ear preparations (Tresaderm, Merck; Mitox, SmithKline Beecham). Drops are applied daily to the external ear canal and pinna as directed by the manufacturer.

Sarcoptic and Notoedric Mange

Clinical Signs

These particular mange mites are usually host-specific (*Sarcoptes scabiei* var. *canis* in dogs; *Notoedres cati* in cats)

(see also Chap. 39). Dogs and cats that become infested with these mites develop similar clinical signs of intense pruritus and yellow crusting. The pinnal margins as well as the ventrum, elbows, and hocks of dogs and the head and neck areas of cats are the most common areas of involvement.

Diagnosis

- Diagnosis is made through identification of the mites by microscopic examination of skin scrapings.
- If scabies is suspected but no mites are found, perform a diagnostic and therapeutic miticidal trial. A good dramatic response is considered as evidence of a positive diagnosis.
- Parasitic infestations, such as those caused by stick-tight fleas or ticks, may cause similar clinical signs. Such parasites are readily identified on the pinnae. Other differential diagnoses include allergic dermatoses, seborrheic dermatitis, dermatophytosis, pemphigus foliaceus, and systemic lupus erythematosus.

Treatment

For the treatment of sarcoptic and notoedric mange, refer to Chapter 39.

PUSTULAR PINNAL DISEASES

Clinical Signs

- Primary pustular lesions may or may not be observed on the pinna owing to their fragility. Secondary crusting and scaling are usually seen.

Diagnosis

- Common differential diagnoses include pemphigus foliaceus and demodicosis.
- Rare pustular dermatoses include subcorneal pustular dermatosis and linear IgA dermatosis.
- Primary bacterial pyodermas do not commonly affect solely the pinna.
- Obtain the minimum database to rule in or out the various differential diagnoses.

Treatment

- The choice of treatment protocol must be made prudently and is predicated on the results of histopathologic examination of pustular pinnal lesions. Once the diagnosis is made, refer to the pertinent chapter for treatment recommendations.

NODULAR PINNAL DISEASES

Clinical Signs

Most nodular diseases of the pinna are neoplastic (see Chap. 28 for a complete discussion of cutaneous neoplasia). In addition to squamous cell carcinoma, as previously discussed, other neoplasms with predilections for the pinnae include basal cell carcinomas, histiocytomas, mast cell tumors, fibrosarcomas, and benign se-baceous adenomas (hyperplasia). Other papular-to-nodular lesions located on the concave aspect of the feline pinna may include linear granulomas (see Chap. 48) and deep mycotic infections (see Chap. 18).

Diagnosis

Perform a skin biopsy for histopathologic examination to make the definitive diagnosis.

Treatment

Surgical resection is the treatment of choice for most neoplasms. CO_2 laser surgery allows for the most precise removal of nodular neoplasms with minimal to no cosmetic defects. If conventional surgery is used, care must be taken not to create undue cosmetic defects in this sensitive area. Other types of nodular diseases are treated according to their definitive diagnoses.

NONINFLAMMATORY PINNAL DISEASES

Pattern/Endocrine Alopecia

Male Dachshund

- The male dachshund may develop a nonpruritic bilateral noninflammatory pinnal alopecia at approximately 1 year of age. The condition is probably hereditary and slowly progresses to complete pinnal baldness within several years. Owners may not notice slowly progressing alopecia until the dog is of middle age.
- No specific treatment exists for alopecia of hereditary origin.

Female Dachshund

- Spayed female dachshunds may develop pinnal alopecia associated with hypoestrogenemia and concurrently involving the perineum, ventral abdomen, and ventral neck areas. Differential diagnoses include demodectic mange, dermatophytosis, and endocrine disease. The diagnosis is determined by obtaining the minimum database for pinnal dermatoses along with special hormonal assays, if needed. Administer estrogen replacement in female dogs with hypoestrogenemia.

Cats

- In cats, hyperadrenocorticism can cause pinnal alopecia and fragile, atrophic skin.

▼ *Key Point* One of the hallmarks of iatrogenic hyperadrenocorticism in cats is an obvious medial curling of the tips of the pinnae.

- Obtain the minimum database for pinnal dermatoses and perform specific adrenal function tests to diagnose this disease.
- Treat pituitary-dependent hyperadrenocorticism in cats carefully with ortho, para-dichlorodiphenyl-dichlorethane (o,p'-DDD; Lysodren, Bristol-Myer) as described in Chapter 31. Lysodren is a chlorinated hydrocarbon and potentially toxic to cats.

Some Siamese cats and some miniature poodles develop spontaneous, periodic, bilateral pinnal alopecia of unknown origin. In these specific breeds, alopecia may last for several months and hair then regrows without treatment.

For additional information regarding nonpruritic alopecia, refer to Chapters 45 and 47 and other appropriate chapters in the endocrine section of this book.

Alopecia Areata

Clinical Signs

Alopecia areata is a rare condition that may occur with focal or multifocal areas of alopecia at the pinnal base and on the head of dogs and cats.

Diagnosis

The diagnosis is based on physical findings and histopathology.

Treatment

Although corticosteroids are recommended in treating human patients, the response in animals is variable. Some animals spontaneously regrow hair within 6 months to 2 years.

Melanoderma and Alopecia of Yorkshire Terriers

Clinical Signs

This dermatosis is of unknown etiology. The disease is seen primarily in young Yorkshire terriers and may be inherited. There is no sex predilection. Affected dogs develop symmetric alopecia and marked hyperpigmentation of the pinnae and bridge of the nose and, occasionally, of the feet and tail. The lesions are nonpruritic and nonpainful.

Diagnosis

Diagnosis is made based on clinical signs and histopathology.

Treatment

Therapy is supportive and nonspecific.

MISCELLANEOUS PINNAL DISEASES

Ear Margin Necrosis

- A variety of etiologies may produce this lesion, including vasculitis, cold agglutinin disease, frostbite, and squamous cell carcinoma.
- Necrosis of the pinnae was reported to occur in cats that had ingested spoiled scallops and in cats with various severe systemic disorders such as disseminated intravascular coagulation.

- Treatment depends on the definitive diagnosis obtained from the minimum database for pinnal dermatoses (see Table 54–2).

Sterile Eosinophilic Pinnal Folliculitis

- This is an idiopathic, nonseasonal, bilaterally symmetric alopecia with follicular papules and pustules. Affected animals are otherwise healthy.
- Make the diagnosis by biopsy of the affected pinnae.
- This disorder is chronic and requires long-term topical and/or systemic corticosteroid maintenance therapy.
- We have diagnosed a similar condition in two young cats less than 1 year of age. In each cat, the cause was ruled idiopathic and remitted spontaneously within 1 month of diagnosis and without recrudescence.

Cold Agglutinin Disease

- This rare immune-mediated disorder occurs in animals when the IgM class of autoantibodies reacts with erythrocytes at temperatures below $32°C$.
- Exposure to cold temperature results in pinnal erythema of the apex margin which progresses to ulceration and necrosis. Usually, all body extremities are affected.
- A positive Coombs test result for IgM at $4°C$ confirms the diagnosis. Underlying neoplastic or infectious diseases must be identified and treated aggressively.
- Treat idiopathic cold agglutinin disease with immunosuppressive dosages of corticosteroids and elimination of exposure to cold temperatures. Refer to Chapter 43 for more information on immune-mediated dermatoses and Chapter 22 for information on systemic immune-mediated diseases.

Trauma

- Traumatic damage may affect the epidermis, dermal vasculature, and underlying cartilage of the pinna. Mange mite infestations of the pinna, puncture wounds, lacerations, and secondary bacterial infections may incite pinnal pruritus and subsequent self-trauma.
  - *Aural hematomas* may appear as fluctuant-to-firm pinnal swellings as a result of trauma to pinnal vasculature.
  - *Ear fissures* are the result of chronic active trauma to the ears from scratching or shaking the head. These fissures usually enlarge and hemorrhage. Underlying factors include parasitic infestations and otitis externa. Treatment consists of surgical resection of the distal pinna just proximal to the edge of the fissures. Bandage the ear across the head to prevent the trauma caused by postoperative head shaking.
  - *Pinnal lacerations* are managed as described for other wounds in Chapters 51 to 53. Principles of pinnal surgery are discussed in Chapter 56.

SUPPLEMENTAL READINGS

Griffin CE: Diseases of the pinnae. The 1986 Scientific Proceedings of the American Animal Hospital Association, 1988, p 198.

Scheidt VJ: Dermatoses of the pinnae. *In* Kirk RW, ed.: Current Veterinary Therapy X: Small Animal Practice. Philadelphia: WB Saunders, 1989, pp 621.

Scott DW, Miller WH Jr, Griffen CE: Muller and Kirk's Small Animal Dermatology, 5th Ed. Philadelphia: WB Saunders, 1995, pp 720, 824, 956.

55 Otitis Externa

James O. Noxon

Otitis externa is an inflammation of the soft tissue components of the external auditory meatus. This condition is one of the most common and frustrating problems encountered in small animal practice. Otitis externa can be a primary or secondary disease process.

▼ *Key Point* Otitis externa is often a clinical manifestation of a generalized dermatologic condition.

The cause of otitis externa in a patient may be multifactorial, making the diagnosis and treatment difficult.

ETIOLOGY

Primary Factors

- Primary factors are those conditions or disorders that initiate the inflammatory process within the ear canal.
- Examples include parasites *(Otodectes cynotis);* allergies (food, atopy, contact); foreign bodies (grass awns, foxtails); keratinization disorders (seborrhea); and, less frequently, trauma, autoimmune disease, sebaceous adenitis, and zinc-responsive dermatosis.
- Primary factors may initially induce disease outside the external ear canal. Otitis externa may be an extension of a pinnal disorder (see Chap. 54), otitis media, or otitis interna (see Chap. 57).

Predisposing Factors

- Predisposing factors facilitate the inflammation by permitting an environment conducive to survival of perpetuating factors.
- Examples include conformation of the ear canal (long canal with a deep vertical component), moisture in the canal, hair in the ears (e.g., in poodles and terriers), breed predisposition (e.g., Chinese Shar Pei, stenotic canals), immunodeficiency syndromes, endocrine imbalances, iatrogenic ear trauma (e.g., hair removal and cleaning with cotton-tipped applicators), and obstructive disease (e.g., cancer, polyps, and hyperplasia).

Perpetuating Factors

- Perpetuating factors sustain and aggravate the inflammatory process.
- Mechanisms include occlusion of the canal, which prevents drying or proper application of medication; secretion of irritating factors; alterations in pH of the canal; and formation of a focus of infection (otitis media).
- Examples include bacterial infections *(Staphylococcus intermedius, Proteus mirabilis, Pseudomonas aeruginosa, Corynebacterium* spp., and *Escherichia coli),* and yeast infection *(Malassezia pachydermatis).* Otitis media serves as a source of infectious agents, and chronic hyperplastic changes of the ear canal may obstruct the canal.

▼ *Key Point* Medication may also act as a perpetuating factor (or a primary factor) of otitis externa, by causing secondary contact irritation or allergy (e.g., neomycin and topical anesthetics) or by leaving residue in the canal (e.g., oil-based preparation).

CLINICAL SIGNS

Signs Directly Related to Ear Involvement

- Head shaking
- Scratching and rubbing of the ears
- Pain around the ears or head (manifested as crying or whining)
- Malodor
- Behavioral changes
  - Pets may become irritable and aggressive toward family members as a result of ear pain.
  - Licking of ears by *other* pets in the household may indicate malodor and an inflammatory process.
- The pet's loss of hearing, although difficult to document, is a common owner's complaint.

Signs Reflecting an Underlying (Predisposing) Dermatologic Disorder

- Face rubbing, sneezing, foot licking, anal scooting, and generalized scratching suggest underlying allergic disease.
- Severe pruritus may incriminate parasitic (scabies, *Notoedres* mange) or allergic (flea allergy dermatitis) causes.
- Scaling and crusting may indicate seborrheic disease or sebaceous adenitis as a primary disease.
- Recurrent bacterial dermatitis suggests an endocrine imbalance or immunologic insufficiency.
- Accompanying alopecia may reflect various factors.

- Bilaterally symmetric alopecia with easily epilated hair is a feature of endocrine disease.
- Focal alopecia or alopecia characterized by broken or fragmented hairs may indicate trauma (pruritus) or infectious (bacterial, fungal) disease.

Signs of Accompanying Otitis Media and Otitis Interna

Refer to Chapter 57.

DIAGNOSIS

Diagnostic procedures are directed toward identifying primary factors (initiating factors), predisposing factors, and perpetuating factors. All etiologic factors must be considered for successful long-term management of the patient.

History

- History is used to detect evidence of allergies (seasonality), parasites (possible exposure), and environmental factors of concern.
- Determine the frequency of ear problems and the response to previous treatment, which may give important clues about the pathologic processes.

Physical Examination

- Physical evaluation includes palpation of the external ear canals, smelling of the ears, and careful examination of the skin over the entire body for evidence of systemic disease.
- Examine for vestibular and cranial nerve abnormalities that could indicate otitis media and otitis interna (see Chap. 57).

Otoscopic Examination (see Chap. 1)

- For equipment, a standard otoscope is generally adequate; however, a video otoscope (Vetscope; MedRx, Inc.) or pediatric endoscope can be used for enhanced imaging and specialty applications.
- Evaluate for the size of the ear canals; the presence of parasites, exudate, hair, or foreign material; the color of the epithelium; the presence of ulcers or masses; and the appearance and integrity of the tympanic membrane.
- Sedation of the animal may be necessary.
  - Topical anesthesia with 1–2% lidocaine HCl, 0.5% proparacaine, or other similar agents may be sufficient.
  - General anesthesia is indicated for removal of most foreign objects; for biopsy; and for thorough evaluation of the horizontal ear canal, in some patients.
- Avoid trauma to the ear canal by advancing the otoscope cone only while directly visualizing the canal.
- Otoscopic abnormalities:
  - Erythema (reddened epithelium)
  - Exudation: dark, dry, granular exudate is found with ear mite infection; moist, yellow, odoriferous exudate is often a sign of bacterial infection; brown

and waxy exudate is consistent with yeast infection and overgrowth; and yellow, waxy-to-oily exudate is found with keratinization disorders.
- Hyperplasia (lichenification, hyperpigmentation) is a sign associated with chronicity. Surgical management may be necessary in patients with severe hyperplasia (occlusion).
- Ulceration suggests more severe disease and indicates a need for aggressive treatment.

▼ *Key Point* *Cytology* is a rapid, inexpensive diagnostic procedure that is indicated in all cases of otitis externa.

Cytology

- Cytology often provides an indication for the best initial treatment plan.
- Use a cotton-tipped applicator to swab the external canal as deeply as possible without packing exudate farther into the ear canal. Remove and gently roll the applicator on a clean glass slide.
- Examine slides prior to staining or after adding mineral oil to look for external parasites. Stain with a modified Wright-Giemsa preparation (Diff-Quik; American Scientific Products).
- Examine for parasites, cellular components, and infectious agents (bacteria, yeast, fungi). Notice whether infectious agents are present within inflammatory cells or free in the exudate.

Culture and Susceptibility Testing

- Bacterial culture of the external ear canal is recommended when:
  - Cytologic examination of exudate from the external ear canal shows a uniform population of gram-negative bacteria
  - Inflammatory cells (e.g., neutrophils) are found on cytologic examination of exudate from the ear canal
  - A bacterial infection continues to be present (as demonstrated by cytologic examination of smears from the ear canal) despite empiric antimicrobial treatment.
- In animals with chronic otitis externa, otitis media may also be present even when the tympanic membrane is intact. Thus, bacterial culture of the middle ear by myringotomy may be indicated (see Chap. 57).

Biopsy

- Biopsy is indicated when abnormal growths are detected.
- Biopsy instruments, designed for endoscopic procedures, are useful to collect a small tissue sample from the ear canal.
- Excisional biopsy of lesions is preferred whenever possible.

Radiography

- Radiography is occasionally indicated (especially in severe or chronic otitis) to evaluate the patency of the ear canal, to detect the presence of otitis media and otitis interna, and to determine the extent of involvement of surrounding structures.

Other Tests

- Miscellaneous diagnostic tests are helpful to identify predisposing and primary factors. See respective chapters for details on these tests. Tests frequently recommended include hematology, serum biochemistry profiles, urinalysis, thyroid function tests, adrenal function tests, intradermal skin tests, in vitro allergy tests, skin scrapings, fungal cultures, and dietary trials.

TREATMENT

The initial treatment of otitis externa is directed toward control of the active inflammatory process, because this aspect of the disease is of immediate concern to the client and patient. After the perpetuating factors are controlled, treatment is directed toward removing the underlying predisposing factors and the disease processes.

Successful long-term management of otitis externa requires identification and treatment of perpetuating factors, predisposing factors, and primary etiologic factors.

Principles of Medical Treatment

- Most commercial ear preparations contain multiple therapeutic agents. Select otic preparations carefully for the desired active agents (Table 55–1).

▼ *Key Point* Do not apply cleansing agents, parasiticides, ceruminolytic/keratolytic agents, disinfectants, ototoxic antimicrobials, or oil-based medications into the ear canal of animals in which the tympanic membrane is ruptured.

- Choose the delivery vehicle for medication carefully.
  - Lotions and solutions are more easily applied deep in the external canal.
  - Oil-based medications are useful to treat dry, scaly lesions, such as those of seborrhea sicca.
  - Creams, pastes, and powders are difficult to apply deep in the external ear canal and may leave a residue. These formulations are rarely indicated in the treatment of otitis externa in dogs and cats.
- Apply topical otic medications liberally to ensure delivery of adequate amounts of medication to the deeper aspects of the canal.
- Gently massage the external canal to help to deliver medications deep into the horizontal canal.

Cleaning the External Canal

▼ *Key Point* The initial objective of medical management of otitis externa is to clean and dry the external canal. This process makes the environment less favorable for sustained microbiologic growth and reduces the inflammatory process in most patients.

Table 55–1. ACTIVE INGREDIENTS COMMONLY PRESENT IN OTIC PREPARATIONS

Ceruminolytic
  Hexamethyltetracosane
  Docusate sodium (dioctyl sodium sulfosuccinate, DSS)
  Squalane

Keratolytic
  Carbamide peroxide
  Benzoic acid
  Salicylic acid
  Sulfur
  Resorcinol

Antifungal
  Nystatin
  Thiabendazole
  Miconazole
  Clotrimazole
  Cuprimyxin

Antibacterial
  Chloramphenicol
  Colistin
  Neomycin B sulfate
  Gentamicin
  Polymyxin B
  Penicillin G
  Bacitracin
  Sulfacetamide
  Sulfur

Anti-inflammatory
Glucocorticoids
  Hydrocortisone
  Prednisolone
  Isoflupredone acetate
  Triamcinolone acetonide
  Dexamethasone
  Fluocinolone acetonide
Dimethyl sulfoxide

Antiparasitic
  Pyrethrins
  Thiabendazole
  Carbaryl
  Rotenone

Topical Anesthetic
  Tetracaine
  Lidocaine

- Supplies and equipment include ear-cleansing solutions, bulb or injection syringe, ear curette, and cotton balls. A water propulsion device may be helpful, if used on low settings.
- Several commercially available irrigating solutions are effective for routine cleansing of the external ear canal (Table 55–2).
- Owners of pets with chronic otitis externa, especially ceruminous otitis externa, should be taught the proper ear-cleansing technique that facilitates long-term management of their pet's condition (Table 55–3).
- Ceruminolytic agents may be applied in cases of severe, exudative otitis to facilitate removal of the wax; they are most effective when applied to the external canal for 15 minutes before flushing. Ceruminolytic agents are contraindicated when the tympanic membrane is not intact.

Table 55–2. COMMERCIAL PREPARATIONS USEFUL IN CLEANING AND DRYING THE EXTERNAL EAR CANAL*

Category	Product	Active Ingredients
Cleansing/Flushing Solutions	Oti-Clens (SmithKline)	Propylene glycol
		Malic acid
		Benzoic acid
	Epi-Otic Cleanser (Allerderm)	Lactic acid
		Salicylic acid
		Propylene glycol
		Docusate sodium
	Betadine solution (Purdue Fredrick)	Povidone-iodine
	Xenodine (Solvay)	Polyhydroxydine solution
Drying Solutions	ClearX Drying Solution (DVM Pharmaceuticals)	Acetic acid
		Sulfur
		Hydrocortisone acetate
	Bur-Otic (Allerderm)	Burow's solution
		Acetic acid
		Propylene glycol
	Panodry (Solvay)	Boric acid
		Isopropyl alcohol

*Commercial otic medications generally have more than one function. Products listed are examples—many other effective medications are commercially available.

- Deep and thorough cleansing of the ear canal often requires the patient to be placed under a general anesthetic. Alternatively, the ear canal can be flushed with warm isotonic saline and suctioned with a soft rubber feeding tube to remove debris dislodged during the flushing.
- Use warm 0.9% saline to flush the ear canal when the integrity of the tympanic membrane is unknown.
- Use the ear curette carefully to remove impacted debris and wax. General anesthesia is recommended.

Table 55–3. EAR CLEANSING TECHNIQUE

Several commercial ear cleansing solutions are suitable for this procedure (see Table 55–2). Isotonic (0.9% saline is also an effective cleanser and is recommended for ear cleansing if the integrity of the ear canal is unknown.

1. Using a bulb syringe or injection syringe (without a needle), fill the entire ear canal with the desired cleansing solution.
   a. Do not force the solution into the ear canal under pressure.
   b. Fill the entire canal, so that the solution is overflowing from the external ear canal.
2. Place a clean, dry cotton ball into the opening of the external ear canal.
3. Gently massage the external canal using a circular motion in an attempt to pull cleansing solution up from the canal into the cotton ball.
4. Replace the cotton ball periodically to absorb the solution and to remove exudate.
5. Repeat the process as many times as needed to ensure cleansing of the canal. The amount of exudate removed during the massaging process should decrease with each rinsing.
6. Remove any excess fluid (not removed by the cotton balls) with a bulb syringe or cotton-tipped applicator. If clients are using this procedure, they may dry the visible portions of the ear canal with a cotton ball or cotton-tipped applicator.
7. Infuse a drying solution into the ear canal.

Drying the External Canal

- Several commercial drying solutions are available (see Table 55–2). Active ingredients include acetic acid, sulfur, boric acid, alcohol, benzoic acid, and others.
- Infusion of solutions containing alcohol can result in severe discomfort (stinging sensation) to the patient and are avoided when the external ear canal is ulcerated.

Specific Topical Therapy

Topical Anti-inflammatory Agents

▼ *Key Point* Glucocorticoids applied to the external canal are significantly absorbed and may affect the hypothalamic-pituitary-adrenal axis.

- Otic glucocorticoid administration may interfere with diagnostic procedures, such as intradermal skin tests, adrenal function tests, thyroid function tests, and routine hematologic and biochemical tests (e.g., serum alkaline phosphatase activity).
- Use the least potent glucocorticoid necessary to accomplish the desired effect.
- Most preparations also contain antiparasitic and/or antimicrobial agents.

Topical Antibacterial Agents

- Base choice on cytologic findings or culture and susceptibility results.
- Medications include aminoglycosides, polymyxin B sulfate, chloramphenicol, chlorhexidine, iodophors, propylene glycol, and silver sulfadiazine cream (1%) (Silvadene, Marion).

- TRIS-EDTA alone or added to antimicrobials increases the sensitivity of resistant *Pseudomonas* spp. to several antibiotics.
- Other antibiotic preparations, available as otic or ophthalmic preparations for humans, may be applied to the external ear canal. Examples include colistin sulfate (Coly-Mycin Otic, Parke-Davis) and tobramycin (Tobrex Ophthalmic Solution, Alcon).

Topical Antifungal Agents

- Clotrimazole (Lotrimin, Schering) is effective against *Malassezia* spp. yeast.
- Miconazole lotion (Conofite, Pitman-Moore) may be used in the external canal to control yeast or fungal infections (contains alcohol and may be irritating).
- Chlorhexidine
- Povidone-iodine
- Cuprimyxin cream
- Silver sulfadiazine cream (1% Silvadene, Marion) may be diluted with sterile saline or water (1 part cream to 9 parts saline or water) and infused into the ear twice daily as effective treatment against *Malassezia pachydermatis*.

Topical Antiparasitic Agents

- Preparations containing pyrethrins, carbaryl, thiabendazole, and rotenone are effective against ear mites.
- Apply these preparations to the external ear canal regularly (every day or every other day) for 3 weeks.
- Apply a topical parasiticide (i.e., preparations used for adult fleas) to the skin over the remainder of the animal once weekly during the treatment period.

Acidifiers

- Acidifiers, such as acetic acid and benzoic acid, are somewhat helpful in controlling yeast and bacterial infections.

Systemic Therapy

Glucocorticoids

- Systemic glucocorticoids may help alleviate the pain and inflammation of otitis externa.
- Administer a single injection of short-acting glucocorticoid (Meticorten, Schering) or prednisone (1.1 mg/kg PO q24h) for 5–7 days.
- Short-term glucocorticoid therapy is occasionally useful to reduce the inflammation in an ear. This allows a thorough otoscopic examination of the external canal. Administer the glucocorticoid as described previously, and perform the otic examination 24–48 hours later.
- Long-term glucocorticoid therapy may be indicated in a patient with an allergic disease.

Antimicrobial and Antiparasitic Therapy

- Systemic antimicrobial therapy is indicated in a patient with bacterial otitis externa when the tympanic membrane is ruptured (see Chap. 57), the epithelium of the canal is ulcerated, or inflammatory cells containing bacteria are found during cytologic examination.
- Systemic antifungal therapy is rarely necessary but is indicated in patients with severe recurrent yeast infections, in patients that are difficult to medicate topically, or in patients with otitis externa that is caused by a systemic mycotic agent (e.g., *Cryptococcus* spp.). Ketoconazole (10 mg/kg PO q24h) is effective against *Malassezia pachydermatis* infection or overgrowth in dogs and cats.
- Ivermectin (300 µg/kg PO) is reported to be effective against ear mite infections in dogs and cats. Treatment may be necessary weekly for 3 to 4 doses to eliminate infection. Do not administer this to collies and collie-mix breed dogs or to known heartworm-infected animals, because treatment of these breeds or in these circumstances may result in profound adverse reactions.

PREVENTION

- *Behavioral modification* is directed toward decreasing activities that predispose the animal to otitis, such as swimming, running through the woods and fields, and so forth.
- *Regular medical care* may decrease the recurrence of otitis externa in predisposed patients.
  - Thoroughly clean and dry ears after swimming.
  - Regularly clean ears of pets with seborrheic disorders.
  - A topical medication containing an astringent such as boric acid or Burow's solution may be infused into the ears of patients who swim to help keep the ears dry and make the local environment less favorable for bacterial and yeast infections.

▼ *Key Point* Remove hair only when indicated by the patient's history. Hair clipping or plucking is not recommended as part of routine ear care in most animals, because the irritation associated with these procedures may predispose them to otitis externa.

- *Surgical management* of otitis externa is indicated to correct conformational defects that predispose an animal to inflammatory disease and to improve ventilation and drainage in affected ears (see Chap. 56).

SUPPLEMENTAL READINGS

August JR: Otitis externa: A disease of multifactorial etiology. Vet Clin North Am 18:731, 1988.

Chester DK: Medical management of otitis externa. Vet Clin North Am 18:799, 1988.

Cole LK, Kwochka KW, Kowalski JJ, Hillier A: Microbial flora and antimicrobial susceptibility patterns of isolated pathogens from the horizontal ear canal and middle ear in dogs with otitis media. J Am Vet Med Assoc 212:534, 1998.

Macy DW: Diseases of the ear. *In* Ettinger SJ, ed.: Textbook of Veterinary Internal Medicine. Philadelphia: WB Saunders, 1989, p 246.

Wilke JR: Otopharmacology. Vet Clin North Am 18:783, 1988.

56 Surgery of the External Ear Canal and Pinna

Daniel D. Smeak

External ear canal surgery is performed to provide exposure and drainage for the vertical and horizontal ear canal or to remove irreversibly infected tissue or neoplasia. Procedures for the external ear canal include lateral ear canal resection, vertical ear canal ablation, and total ear canal ablation. Drainage of auricular hematoma is the most common surgical procedure of the pinna; this is discussed later in this chapter.

Success of ear surgery relies on an:

- Accurate diagnosis
- Appreciation of the severity and extent of the disease
- Appropriate postoperative medical treatment of the local disease and any underlying systemic skin disease

▼ *Key Point* As a general rule, surgical intervention is considered when appropriate medical treatment for otitis externa fails.

As ear disease progresses, more extensive surgery is required to relieve clinical signs. Frequency and severity of complications, however, also increase as the surgery becomes more extensive.

GENERAL SURGICAL INDICATIONS

- For ear disease that fails to respond to appropriate medical treatment
- For relapse of clinical signs after initial response to medical therapy
- For extensive irreversible changes of cartilage and/or epithelium
- For a predisposing factor causing the ear condition (congenital or acquired malformation, stenosis or atresia of the ear canal, or neoplasia)

▼ *Key Point* External ear surgery rarely is indicated in the cat except for traumatic or neoplastic conditions. Inflammatory polyps extending into the external ear canal usually do not require external ear surgery for removal. See middle ear surgery (see Chapter 58) for further information.

ANATOMY

Understanding the anatomy of the ear and related structures is critical to successful ear surgery. The surgeon must identify and preserve several key structures, especially during horizontal canal dissection.

External Ear Canal

- The normal external ear canal (Figs. 56–1 and 56–2) is a pliable cartilaginous tube lined by glandular epithelium, extending from the base of the pinna to the tympanic membrane.
- The normal canal is between 5 and 10 cm long and narrows to between 4 and 7 mm in diameter, proximally.

Vertical Ear Canal

- From the external opening (aditus), the vertical canal (auricular cartilage) runs ventrally and slightly rostrally, before bending toward the skull to form the shorter horizontal canal.

Horizontal Ear Canal

- The horizontal canal consists of a circular (annular) cartilage extending from the ligamentous attachment to the auricular cartilage medially to the short osseous ear canal (projection of the petrous temporal bone). The canal ends at the tympanic membrane.

Important Local Structures

Glands (Fig. 56–2B)

- The V-shaped parotid salivary gland overlays the ventrolateral aspect of the vertical ear canal and extends ventral to the distal aspect of the horizontal ear canal.

Blood Vessels (Fig. 56–2B)

- Blood supply to the ear is via the great auricular artery, arising from the external carotid artery located medial to the parotid gland and ventral to the osseous bulla.
- Small branches of the great auricular and maxillary arteries run dorsally, parallel to the long axis of the pinna, and medial to the pinna cartilage.

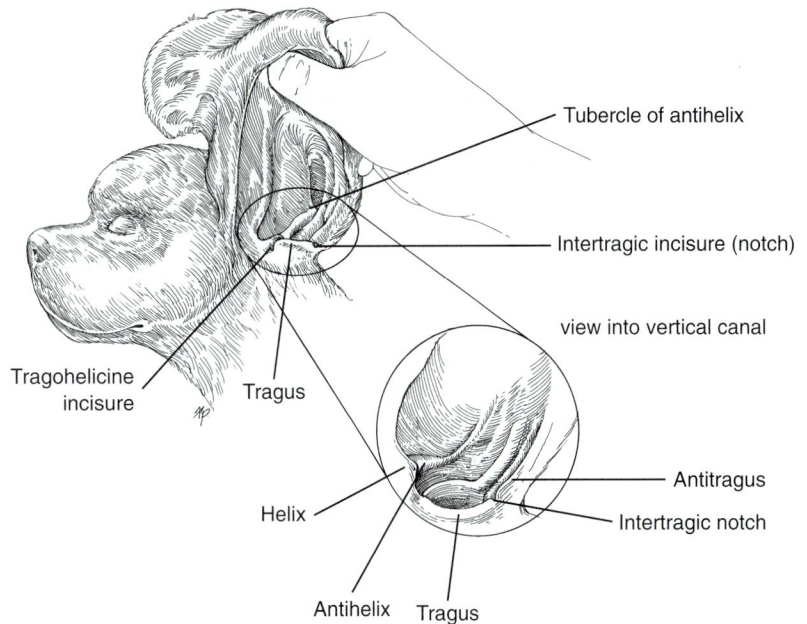

Figure 56–1. Anatomy of the external aditus of the ear.

Nerves (Fig. 56–2B)

- The facial nerve arises from the stylomastoid foramen located just caudal to the osseous ear canal.
- The nerve courses rostroventrally directly under the horizontal ear canal.
- Terminal branches of the facial and auriculotemporal branch of the mandibular portion of the trigeminal nerve are located just cranial to the ear canal.

PREOPERATIVE CONSIDERATIONS

An accurate preoperative diagnosis along with determination of the extent of disease is important when choosing the surgical procedure.

The ear canal is difficult to prepare aseptically, and contamination is inevitable during surgery.

Administer a broad-spectrum, bactericidal, IV antibiotic (optimally based on preoperative culture and susceptibility) before and during surgery so that adequate blood levels are maintained in tissues during dissection.

Ear Palpation

- Sharp pain elicited on deep palpation of the external ear canal usually indicates middle ear infection.
- Palpation of severely thickened and firm ear canal tissue indicates that irreversible changes have occurred.

Dermatologic Examination

- Perform a complete dermatologic examination and obtain appropriate tests to determine whether primary systemic skin disease (e.g., hypothyroidism, atopy) is present.

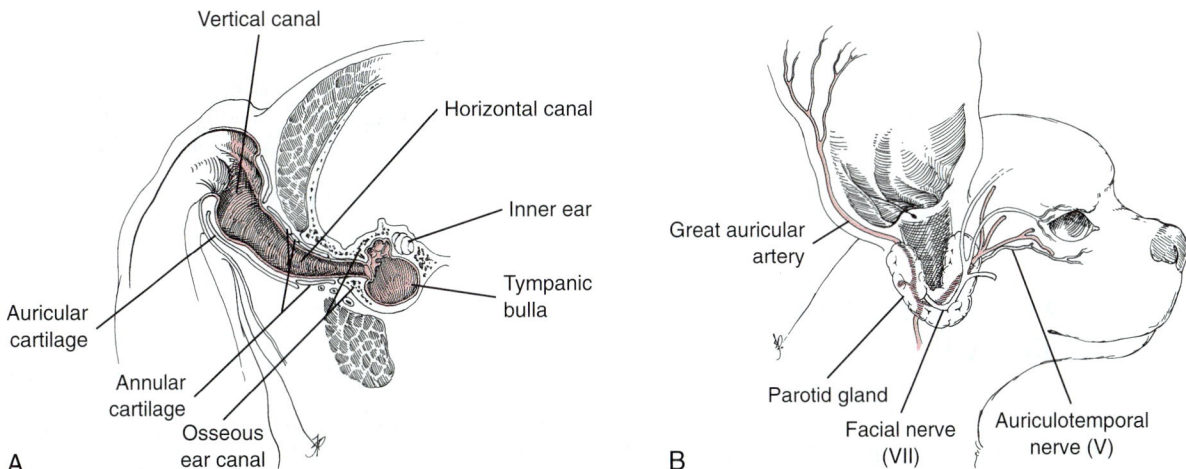

Figure 56–2. Important anatomic structures of the external ear canal. *A,* Transverse section of the head showing ear canal regions and middle ear and inner ear structures. *B,* Location of branches of the external carotid artery in relation to the ear canal and middle ear, and important neural structures in the external ear canal region.

Neurologic Examination

- Perform a neurologic examination, especially in chronic cases of otitis externa, to evaluate for facial nerve involvement (e.g., hemifacial spasm and slow or absent palpebral reflex) and involvement of inner ear structures (e.g., nystagmus and circling).
- Evaluate the patient's ability to hear and alert the owner to any problems before contemplating bilateral ear canal ablation.

Radiographic Examination

- Ventrodorsal skull radiograph is the view of choice to evaluate horizontal canal diameter and to determine whether the walls of the canal have undergone irreversible calcification.

▼ *Key Point* Evaluate for middle ear involvement (Chap. 57) before deciding on the surgical procedure.

- Open-mouth radiography of the bulla is the view of choice to evaluate for middle ear involvement (see Chap. 4).

▼ *Key Point* Lack of osseous changes on bulla radiographs does not rule out otitis media.

- Bulla osteitis takes months to form after deep-seated infection. Changes are often very subtle, and evaluation of fluid density within the bulla also is not an accurate method of diagnosis.

Otoscopic Examination

- Perform a thorough ear cleansing after obtaining the appropriate diagnostic specimens for culture and susceptibility, cytology, and biopsy (see Chap. 55).
- Otoscopic examination is the most important diagnostic modality to evaluate the severity and extent of disease and tympanic membrane rupture.

▼ *Key Point* A thorough otoscopic examination for planning surgical strategy usually requires general anesthesia.

Staging of Neoplastic Disease

- Perform regional lymph node aspiration, cytology, biopsy, and thoracic radiography if neoplasia is suspected in the underlying ear disease.

LATERAL EAR CANAL RESECTION—ZEPPS MODIFICATION (LECR)

Objectives

- To expose the medial portion of the vertical canal and horizontal ear canal. Exposure enhances medical treatment of otitis externa and changes local ear conditions favoring drainage.

- Ventilation of the area improves the local environment by decreasing moisture, humidity, and temperature in the ear canal.
- To resect the lateral portion of the vertical ear canal to remove tumors or to relieve congenital or acquired nonproliferative vertical canal stenosis that is restricting ear drainage and interfering with medical treatment.

▼ *Key Point* Do not perform LECR if the horizontal or vertical ear canal is hyperplastic and filled with proliferative tissue. Likewise, LECR is contraindicated if medically uncontrolled primary skin disease (e.g., seborrhea) is present because progressive ear disease would be expected in the remaining section of the ear canal.

Equipment

- Standard general surgical pack and suture
- Heavy serrated straight Mayo scissors

Technique (Fig. 56–3)

1. Place the animal in lateral recumbency with the head positioned, aseptically prepared, and draped so that the ear region, including the pinna, is exposed and all anatomic relationships are identifiable.
2. Use forceps to determine vertical canal depth and position of the horizontal canal.
3. Incise the lateral portion of the vertical ear canal and reflect ventrally.
4. Preserve the proximal portion of the lateral canal flap for a "drain board."
5. Begin closure at the base of the flap, then appose the distal flap to the skin. Appose the remaining ear epithelium and skin so that no cartilage is exposed.

Postoperative Care and Complications

- Continue systemic antibiotics until the incisions are healed and the ear discharge has stopped.
- Continue appropriate topical medical treatment and ear cleansing (see Chap. 55) until no signs of ear infection are present.
- Place an Elizabethan collar to prevent self-inflicted trauma to the wound until suture removal.
- If wound dehiscence occurs, let it heal by second intention closure.
- Remove sutures in 14 days.
- Continue treatment of primary skin disorders as required.

Prognosis

- Prognosis for control of ear disease is good provided that:
  - Surgery is performed correctly and for the right indication.
  - No middle ear disease is present.
  - Postoperative medical management of otitis externa is appropriate.

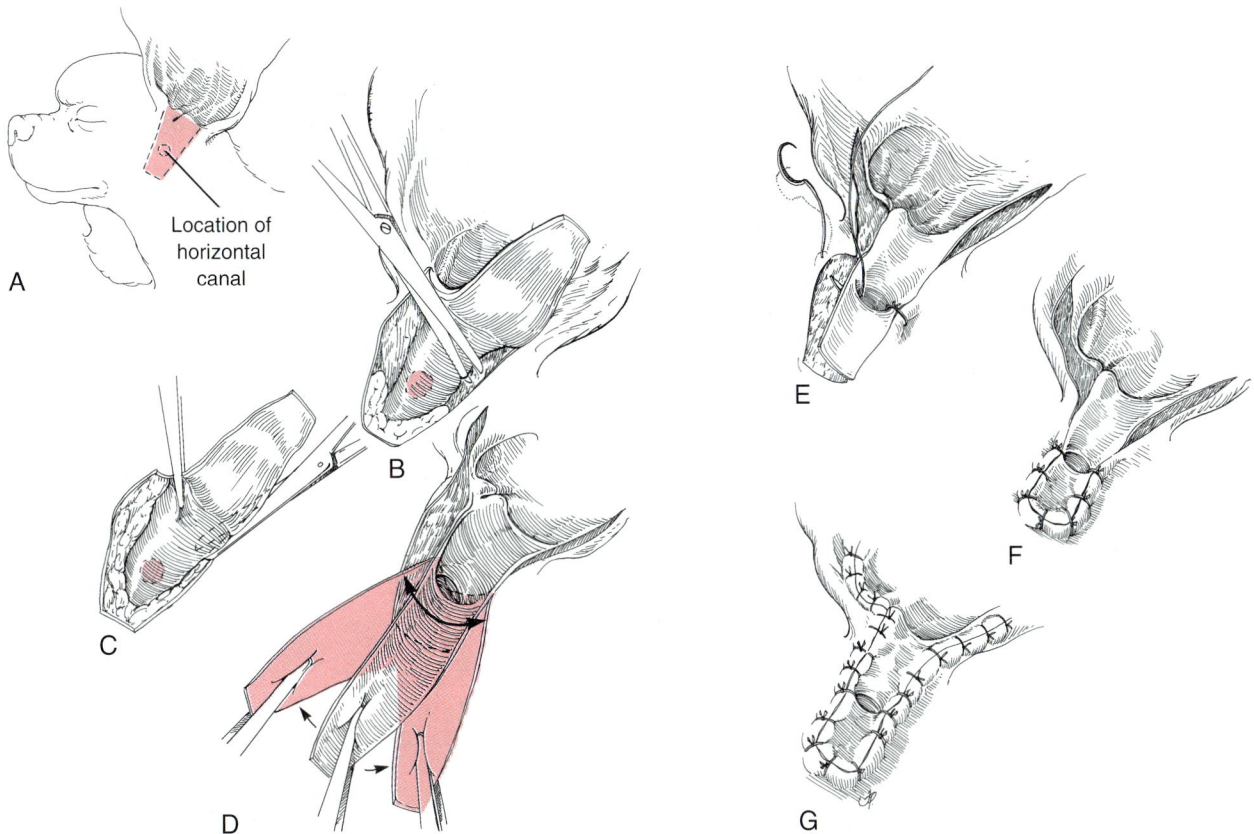

Figure 56–3. Lateral ear canal resection technique. *A,* Two skin incisions are extended parallel to each other from the intertragic notch and tragohelicine notch, tapering down to a distance of 1.5 to 2 cm between the incisions, about 1.5 to 2.5 cm (depending on the size of the animal) ventral to the horizontal ear canal. A transverse incision joins the two vertical incisions. Undermine the skin flap dorsally up to the margin of the aditus.

B, Incise through the subcutaneous tissue to the level of the vertical ear cartilage. Expose the entire lateral aspect of the vertical ear canal by blunt and sharp dissection of the subcutaneous tissue in a rostral and caudal direction and parotid gland ventrally.

C, Place an Allis tissue forceps on the tragus, and apply dorsal traction so that the vertical ear canal can be seen from the dorsal aspect of the head. With scissors, make two incisions through the vertical ear canal on the rostrolateral and caudolateral margins while maintaining dorsal traction. Extend the rostral and caudal incisions ventrally in an alternating fashion until the floor of the horizontal canal is reached. The vertical canal essentially is divided into lateral and medial halves.

D, Extend incisions medially toward the head until the horizontal canal is fully exposed after the lateral wall is reflected ventrally. The base of the lateral wall flap should approximate the width of the horizontal canal. More cartilage can be removed from the remaining ear canal as necessary to fully expose the remaining vertical canal. Manipulate the flap rostrally and caudally until the horizontal canal is held open as wide as possible.

E, Remove the skin flap and all but the proximal portion of the lateral wall. The 1.5- to 2-cm cartilage (drain board) flap remaining is modified to lie flat and fit the skin defect ventral to the horizontal ear canal.

F, Begin closure by placing simple interrupted 3-0 to 4-0 monofilament nonabsorbable sutures from the caudal and rostral margins of the proximal most aspect of the drain board to the skin. Throughout closure, place sutures through ear canal epithelium and cartilage first and then to skin to aid in skin coverage of cartilage.

G, Appose the remaining portion of the flap to the skin with simple interrupted sutures so that the flap is flat against the head. Place additional sutures so that the skin and ear canal epithelium edges are apposed but not crushed.

- Up to 35% of LECRs fail because the aforementioned considerations are not met.

VERTICAL EAR CANAL ABLATION (VECA)

This technique combines some of the advantages of the LECR (maintenance of horizontal canal drainage) and total ear canal ablation (removal of chronically infected vertical canal tissue).

▼ *Key Point* VECA is contraindicated if irreversible hyperplastic thickening or neoplasia is present in the horizontal canal.

In my experience, if chronic hyperplastic tissue is present in the vertical canal, it usually extends into the horizontal canal. Therefore, this procedure is not commonly indicated, but VECA may be an alternative method for those patients requiring LECR. Some clinicians believe that VECA may be performed in dogs with end-stage inflammatory ear disease. Owners need to be aware that clinical signs may improve, but continued ear cleaning may be needed after surgery.

Objectives

- To remove the vertical ear canal and preserve the horizontal canal.
- To provide drainage for the horizontal canal.

Equipment

- Same as that for LECR.

Technique (Fig. 56–4)

1. Patient positioning, skin preparation, and vertical ear canal exposure are the same as those described for LECR.
2. Isolate the entire vertical ear canal and resect distal to the annular cartilage.
3. Incise the remaining section of the ear canal to create a dorsal and ventral flap.
4. Appose the skin to ear epithelium.
5. The closure forms a T-shape.

Postoperative Care and Complications

- Similar to those of lateral ear canal resection.
- This procedure affects ear carriage; LECR rarely does.

Prognosis

Prognosis is good provided the procedure is performed for the correct indications. In a large retrospective study of 75 dogs undergoing VECA, 72 were asymptomatic within 12 weeks postoperatively.

TOTAL EAR CANAL ABLATION (TECA)

Total ear canal ablation is a salvage procedure that involves removal of the entire vertical and horizontal ear canal cartilage and epithelium. If severe horizontal canal disease is present, only TECA is successful in eliminating the associated clinical signs.

▼ *Key Point* Neglected chronic otitis externa results in extensive chronic inflammatory changes in periannular tissue. These greatly increase the risk of iatrogenic complications associated with difficult ear canal dissection.

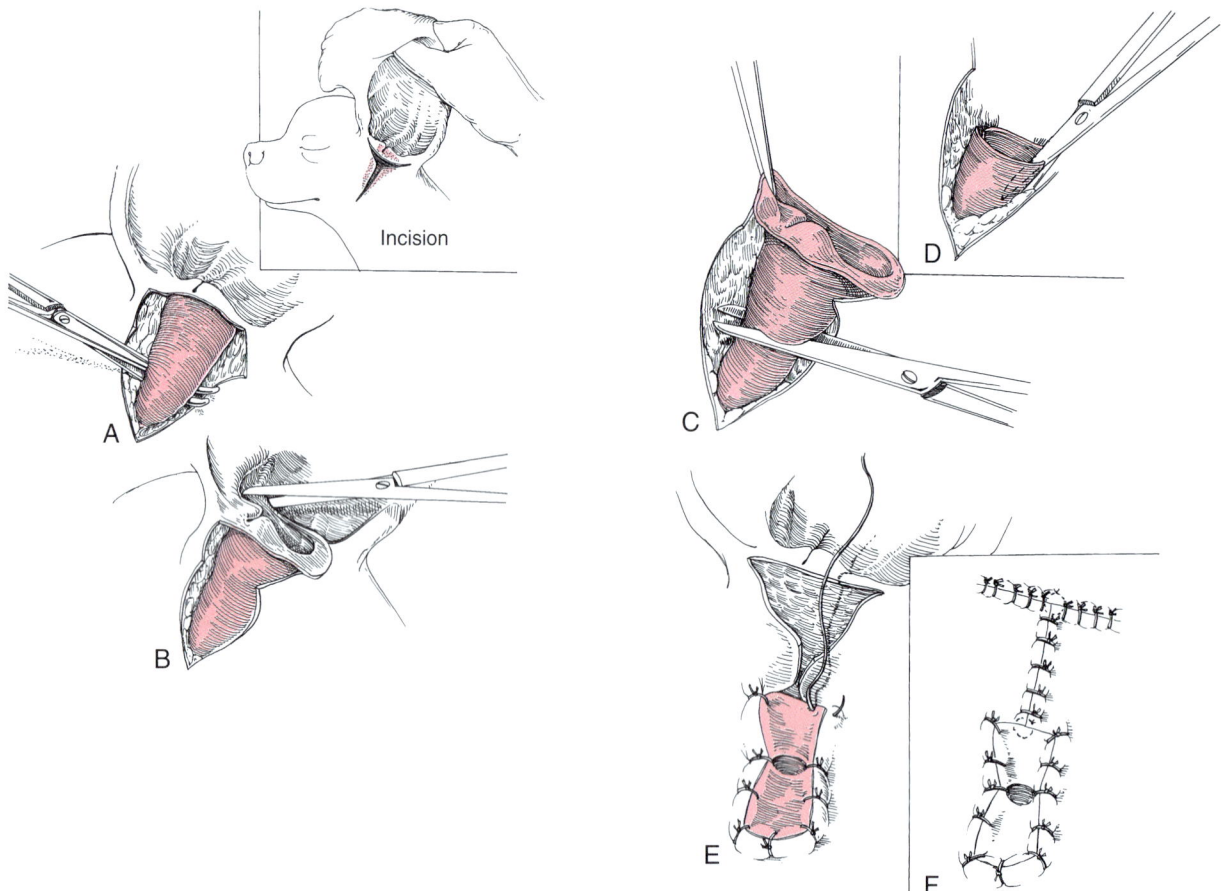

Figure 56–4.   Vertical ear canal ablation technique. Begin with T-shaped skin incision over the ear canal.

A, Continue blunt dissection medially until the entire vertical canal is isolated and freed up. Dissect just underneath the cartilage to avoid damaging vascular supply to the pinna.

B, Cut the auricular cartilage with heavy straight Mayo scissors, removing all affected tissue on the dorsal aspect of the medial vertical canal and pinna. This step allows complete mobilization of the vertical canal, which remains attached only at its proximal aspect.

C, Remove the vertical canal approximately 1 to 2 cm distal to the annular cartilage junction.

D, Incise remaining vertical canal rostrally and caudally, if necessary, to fully expose the horizontal ear canal.

E, Suture the ventral flap to the skin in a fashion similar to that in lateral ear resection.

F, Suture the dorsal flap to appose the cut edges of the canal and skin with simple interrupted 3-0 to 4-0 monofilament nonabsorbable material. Remaining skin is apposed to form a T-shaped closure.

Objective

- To remove the entire external ear canal without trauma to the facial nerve.
- To provide access to the tympanic bulla to observe for evidence of infection or other disease.

Indications

- Severe ear trauma that cannot be managed adequately with reconstruction.
- Congenital or acquired deformity affecting the horizontal ear canal.
- Irreversible hyperplastic and proliferative ear disease or neoplasia extending into the horizontal canal.
- Persistent otitis externa after LECR or VECA. If signs stem from middle ear infection, drainage of the middle ear is all that may be required, provided the horizontal ear canal is not affected irreversibly.

▼ *Key Point* TECA alone is contraindicated when middle ear infection is present because it eliminates a drainage exit for the tympanic cavity. The auditory tube cannot be relied on to drain thickened exudates within the middle ear. In these common instances, TECA can be performed successfully if a means of tympanic bulla drainage also is provided.

Equipment

- Standard general surgical pack and suture
- Gelpi or Weitlaner self-retaining retractors
- Senn retractors
- Heavy serrated Mayo scissors
- Suction apparatus and Frazier suction tip
- Electrocoagulation unit and sterile electrode
- Lempert and Cleveland bone rongeurs
- Straight Simon and Daubenspeck curettes
- Penrose drains (¼ inch)

Technique (Fig. 56–5)

1. Use the same positioning, skin preparation, and draping as for LECR.
2. Make a T-shaped skin incision to expose the ear canal.
3. Reflect loose connective tissue from the vertical ear canal.
4. Isolate the vertical and horizontal canal by blunt and sharp dissection. Maintain dissection immediately adjacent to the ear canal cartilage. Occasionally, the facial nerve is found embedded in the annular cartilage.
5. Careful dissection along the stylomastoid foramen isolates the origin of the nerve.
6. Carefully dissect the nerve out along its course adjacent to the horizontal canal.
7. In some patients with chronic proliferative otitis externa, a greenish-brown epithelial pouch forms between the tympanic bulla and the annular cartilage. This epithelium extends lateral and ventral to the tympanic bulla. Removal of this tissue is critical to the success of the surgery because chronic fistulation occurs if it is not removed fully. Use hemostatic forceps to grasp the edges of the pouch and, with traction, bluntly dissect the pouch out without injuring major local vessels and nerves.
8. Sharply amputate the annular cartilage from the petrous temporal bone, excise the ear canal, and submit it for biopsy.
9. Carefully remove the secretory epithelial lining of the short osseous external auditory canal by curettage. Submit this lining for culture and susceptibility.
10. Examine the middle ear for exudates and chronic thickened epithelium. If no changes are evident, place a Penrose drain within the dead space remaining where the ear canal was removed, exiting ventral to the T-shaped incision.
11. Place a percutaneous suture through the dorsal end of the Penrose tube to prevent premature dislodgement.
12. If middle ear infection or hyperplastic epithelium is present, remove the ventral and lateral aspect of the bulla with rongeurs.
13. Remove all epithelium and debris with irrigation and curettage.
14. Avoid inner ear structures on the craniodorsal aspect of the bulla.
15. To permit drainage in severely affected ears, leave the entire wound open to heal by second intention, and irrigate the middle ear through the wound.
16. Place subcutaneous and skin sutures to form a T-shaped wound.

Postoperative Care

- Examine the wound for evidence of fluid accumulation or ensuing infection.
  - Rebandage daily until drainage stops.
  - If acute postoperative infection occurs, open the wound for drainage.
  - Flush and bandage the open wound daily.
- Administer systemic antibiotics based on susceptibility testing and potential for causing ototoxicity for a minimum of 3 to 4 weeks, if otitis media is present (see Chap. 57).
- If facial nerve injury has occurred, place eye lubricants (e.g., Hypotears, Cibavision) in the affected eye q6h, especially if the dog has decreased tear production or has an exophthalmic conformation.
- Remove skin sutures in 14 days.
- Remove Penrose tubes when drainage has decreased significantly. Generally, this is in 3 to 4 days.
- Patients with established severe otitis media may require extensive postoperative wound management.
- If the surgical wound is left open, irrigate it once or twice daily with 25 ml lukewarm (1:100) diluted povidone-iodine (Betadine) solution and saline (or TRIS-EDTA if *Pseudomonas* sp. is isolated) for 5 to 10 days.

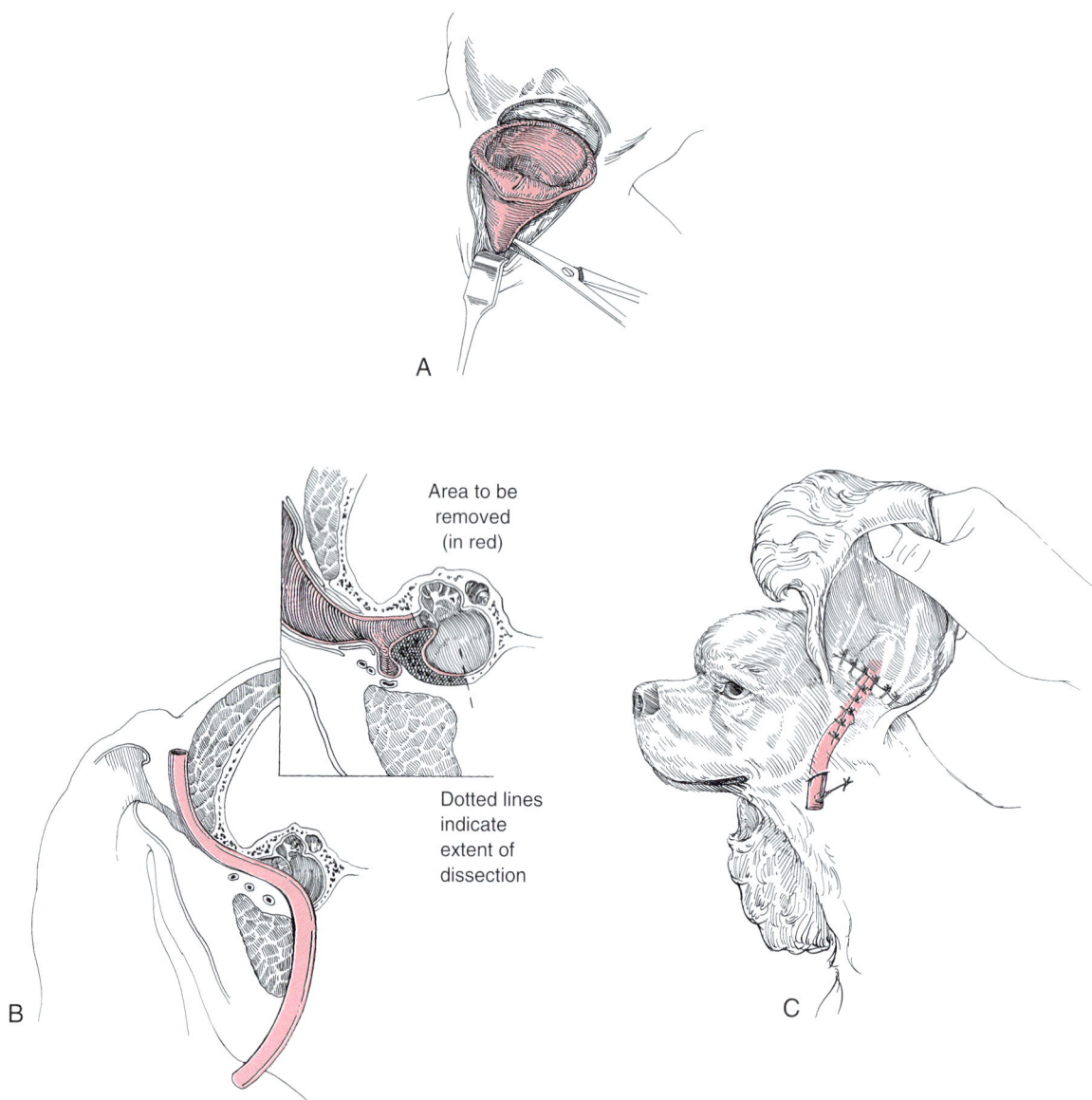

Figure 56–5.   Total ear canal ablation technique.

Make a horizontal incision parallel and just below the upper edge of the tragus between the tragohelicine and intertragic notches (also see Fig. 56–4B inset). Make a vertical incision perpendicular from the midpoint of the horizontal incision to a point just ventral to the horizontal canal, forming a T-shaped incision. The two triangular skin flaps are undermined and retracted, exposing the lateral aspect of the ear canal. After hemostasis is achieved, bluntly dissect the vertical canal free from the surrounding tissues, avoiding the auricular vessels located medial to the canal (A).

Use heavy serrated Mayo scissors to cut the medial aspect of the proximal vertical ear canal connecting the ends of the original horizontal incision. Removal of wedge-shaped portions of skin from the rostral and caudal vertical skin margins and retention of as much of the normal medial vertical canal as possible encourages ear support in cats and dogs with erect ears (see Fig. 56–4B).

The parotid gland is retracted ventrally. By a combination of blunt and sharp dissection, isolate the horizontal canal to the level of the tympanic bulla. While maintaining meticulous hemostasis, dissection continues as close to the cartilage as possible, carefully exposing and retracting the facial nerve away from the line of dissection. Excise the ear canal and remove epithelium from osseous ear canal.

B, Transverse section of head shows common location of epithelial pouch between annular cartilage and petrous temporal bone. If otitis media is present, a lateral bulla osteotomy is performed to expose the bulla for curettage and to improve ventral drainage. Crosshatching indicates area of resection of the lateral and ventral osseous bulla. Be sure all exudate and tissue are moved from the tympanic cavity. A Penrose drain exits ventral to the skin incision.

C, Completed ear ablation showing placement of drainage system and skin closure.

Complications

▼ *Key Point* Owner education is critical before attempting TECA because the following serious and long-standing complications are possible.

- Acute pharyngeal edema and upper airway obstruction.

- Acute postoperative wound infection (up to 40% of patients).
- Facial nerve damage (usually temporary; but permanent paralysis occurs in <10% of patients).
- Transient hypoglossal nerve dysfunction (rare and usually temporary).
- Chronic fistulation from unresolved middle ear infection or retained ear canal epithelium may occur

up to 1 to 2 years after surgery ($< 10\%$ of patients). Perform middle ear exploration and complete removal of epithelial remnants, and administer systemic antibiotic therapy for 4 to 6 weeks.

- If inner ear signs are present before surgery, their exacerbation is common after surgery. Neurologic signs usually improve over time if otitis media is controlled, but minor signs usually persist indefinitely.
- Horner's syndrome (usually temporary) if middle ear surgery also is performed, especially in cats.
- Dogs undergoing bilateral TECA generally hear about as well as they did before surgery.
- Like VECA, this procedure affects ear carriage.

Prognosis

Long-term follow-up for dogs undergoing TECA shows improvement in clinical signs in up to 90% of patients and shows the same or worse in 10%. Poor results usually are caused by persistent infection from unresolved middle ear infection or retained infected epithelial tissue. A total of 25 of 26 owners of dogs undergoing TECA with long-term follow-up indicated satisfaction with the procedure and improvement in their dogs' demeanor.

AURICULAR HEMATOMA

Auricular or aural hematoma is an accumulation of blood within the cartilage of the pinna, usually caused by violent head shaking or scratching. The blood collection usually is confined to the concave surface of the pinna. This injury is seen most often in pendulous-eared dogs but occasionally is seen in erect-eared dogs and, less frequently, in cats.

▼ *Key Point* Auricular hematomas occur secondary to inflammatory conditions of the pinna or external ear canal, such as foreign bodies, atopy, food allergy, bacterial infection, yeast infection, and ear mites. Indentify the underlying cause of the irritation, if possible, to avoid further injury and recurrence.

Anatomy

The major blood supply to the pinna is derived from branches of the external carotid artery and internal maxillary vein. The great auricular arteries and veins arborize and course longitudinally along the long axis on the convex side of the pinna. Mattress pattern sutures placed in the ear are oriented parallel to these vessels to avoid interrupting the blood supply to the pinna.

Preoperative Considerations

- The first objective for management of auricular hematoma is to identify the source of the ear irritation.
- Perform a thorough otoscopic examination to identify abnormalities within the ear canal.
- Obtain complete history and perform a dermatologic examination, particularly when no obvious

cause of the irritation is uncovered during otoscopic examination.
- Rule out the diagnosis of atopy or other systemic manifestation of skin disease.

▼ *Key Point* Drain auricular hematomas as soon as possible because delay often leads to enlargement and extension throughout the pinna. With time, fibrous organization of the hematomas eventually leads to a permanently thickened, cauliflower-like ear.

- If the cosmetic appearance of the pinna is of secondary importance to the owner, the incision and drainage technique is the most consistently successful. I prefer this technique for more chronic hematomas because it allows for thorough debridement of organized clots.
- A more cosmetic and less time-consuming technique is the drainage-only procedure. Use this technique only in hematomas with fluid consistency (acute cases) and, preferably, those located toward the distal aspect of the pinna. Owners must understand that recurrence develops more often with drainage only compared with incision and suture. Simple aspiration alone is not a good option because of a high rate of hematoma recurrence.

Surgical Procedure
Objectives

- To treat the source of irritation
- To drain the hematoma
- To maintain apposition of cartilage surfaces for an adequate time to prevent recurrence

Equipment

- Standard general instrument pack
- Penrose drain, ¼ inch (if drain-only technique is planned)
- Skin biopsy punch (3.5 or 5 mm) for alternative punch technique

Technique
Incision, Drainage, and Bandage

1. Clip both sides of the pinna and prepare the ear for aseptic surgery. Place sterile 4 × 4 sponges in the ear canal to soak up blood from the hematoma.
2. Incise the hematoma with a #10 blade in a linear fashion on the concave side no closer than 1 cm from the margin of the pinna.
3. Make this incision along the long axis of the pinna extending the length of the hematoma. Removal of a strip of skin to widen the incision and permit drainage is not necessary.
4. Explore the hematoma and remove any fibrin tags or blood clots.
5. Place 1-cm–wide mattress sutures (3-0 or 4-0 monofilament nonabsorbable material) parallel to and no closer than 0.5 cm from the incision.

6. Hold the incised edges of the skin 2 to 3 mm apart when placing the first row of sutures. Sutures need not penetrate both skin surfaces because this creates another source of irritation and entry way for contamination.
7. Pass the needle carefully from the concave surface of the pinna, catching both cartilage planes.
8. Place the remaining mattress sutures in a staggered fashion 1 cm apart until the entire dead space area is obliterated.
9. Tie sutures with just enough tension to appose cartilage surfaces.

Alternative Technique Using Biopsy Punch and Suture
(Fig. 56–6)

1. For acute hematomas, this technique creates a cosmetic result with minimal recurrence problems.
2. Prepare pinna for surgery as described for incision and drainage technique.
3. Punch staggered holes over hematoma on concave pinna surface.
4. Tack skin adjacent to punch holes to underlying cartilage.
5. Bandaging usually is not necessary.

Drainage Only

1. Aseptically prepare the skin on the concave surface of the pinna only. Do not clip the convex, haired surface because this creates more inflammation, which could lead to continual head shaking or scratching. Place 4 × 4 sponges in the ear canal to soak up blood from the hematoma.
2. Make a small (0.5- to 1-cm) incision extending into the hematoma at its most proximal and distal extent on the pinna.
3. Remove all fluid and fibrin tags with mosquito hemostats and digital expression.
4. Place a drain (¼-inch Penrose or sterilized IV extension tubing) through the dead space and exiting both stab wounds.
5. Suture the drain to the skin near the stab incisions with a loose nonabsorbable suture.

Postoperative Considerations

- After treatment of the hematoma by the incision method, bandage the affected ear over the top of the head in pendulous-eared dogs. Bandage erect ears in an upright position.
  - Leave the ear canal exposed in each method to permit cleansing and medication as needed.
  - Leave the bandages on for at least 10 days and change as needed.
  - Remove sutures in 3 weeks (incision or punch method).
- No bandages are used for the drainage-only method or punch method unless the patient continues violent or persistent head shaking.
  - Use an Elizabethan collar to reduce the incidence of self-trauma in all cases.
  - Leave drains in place for 3 to 4 weeks.

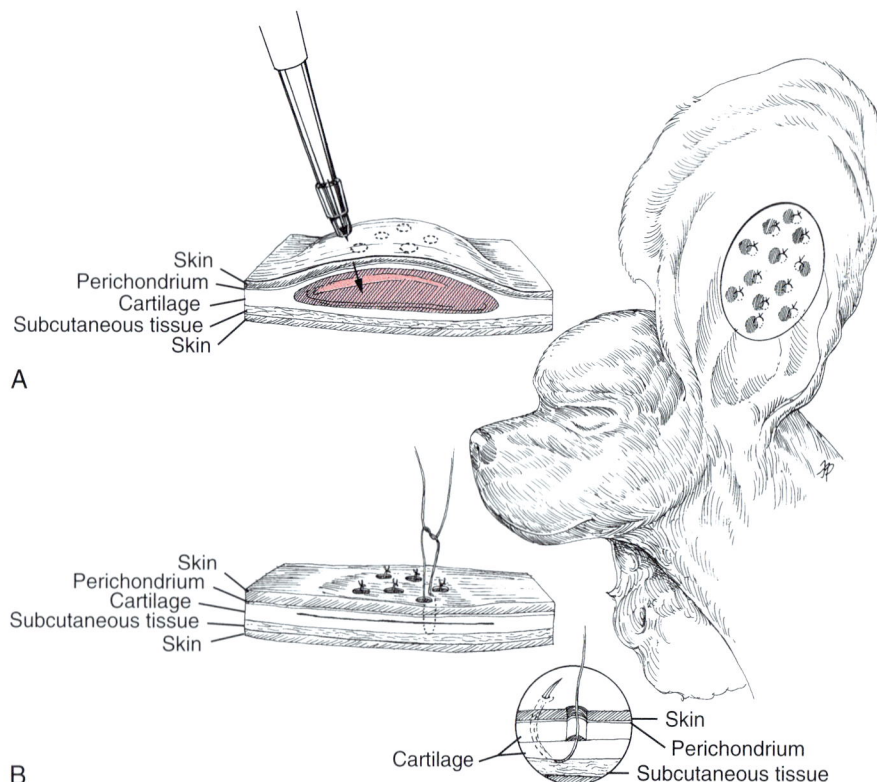

Figure 56–6. Concave surface of the pinna. Shaded area indicates hematoma location. Create staggered (3.5 or 5 mm) punch biopsies approximately 1 to 1.5 cm apart over the hematoma. Use 4-0 filament nonabsorbable sutures to tack through each punch into underlying cartilage to adjacent skin edge for dead space obliteration.

- Instruct the owners to watch for signs of infection and to milk out any fluid that may accumulate within the hematoma during this time.
- Instruct the owners about the proper treatment of the primary source of the ear irritation.
- The appearance of the ear after surgery is related to the drainage technique and to the chronicity of the hematoma. Inadequate drainage or continued inflammation results in a permanently thickened pinna.
  - Make no guarantees to the owners regarding the final cosmetic appearance of the ear and the impossibility of recurrence, because these are often unpredictable.
- Re-evaluate the patient weekly after drainage to determine the response to primary treatment and any problem related to wound management.

SUPPLEMENTAL READINGS

Beckman SL, Henry WB, Cechner P: Total ear canal ablation combining bulla osteotomy and curettage in dogs with chronic otitis externa and media. J Am Vet Med Assoc 196:84, 1990.

Gregory CR, Vasseur PB: Clinical results of lateral ear canal resection in dogs. J Am Vet Med Assoc 182:1087, 1983.

Krahwinkel DJ: External ear canal. In: Slatter DH (ed): Textbook of Small Animal Surgery. 2nd ed. Philadelphia: WB Saunders, 1993, p 1560.

Harvey CE: Ear canal disease in the dog. J Am Vet Med Assoc 177:136, 1980.

Krahwinkel DJ, Pardo AD, Sims MH, Bubb WJ: Effect of total ablation of the external acoustic meatus and bulla osteotomy on auditory function in dogs. J Am Vet Med Assoc 202:949, 1993.

Siemering GH: Resection of the vertical ear canal for treatment of chronic otitis externa. J Am Anim Hosp Assoc 16:753, 1980.

Smeak DD: Total Ear Canal Ablation. In: Bojrab MJ (ed): Current Techniques in Small Animal Surgery. Philadelphia: Lea & Febiger, 1990, p 140.

Smeak DD, Crocker CB, Birchard SJ: Treatment of recurrent otitis media that developed after total ear canal ablation and lateral bulla osteotomy in dogs: Nine cases (1986–1994). J Am Vet Med Assoc 209:937, 1996.

Smeak DD, DeHoff WD: Total ear canal ablation. Clinical results in the dog and cat. Vet Surg 15:161, 1986.

Wooley RE, Jones MS, Gilbert JP, Shotts EB: *In vitro* action of combinations of antimicrobial agents and EDTA-tromethamine on *Pseudomonas aeruginosa.* Am J Vet Res 44:1521, 1983.

57 Otitis Media and Otitis Interna

Linda G. Shell

Otitis media—Inflammation of the middle ear structures, which include the tympanic membrane, tympanic cavity, auditory or eustachian tube, three auditory ossicles, and tympanic nerve (a small branch of the facial nerve).

Otitis media is most often a sequela to otitis externa, having an incidence rate of 16% in early cases of otitis externa to 50% or more in chronic cases. For a complete discussion of otitis externa, see Chapter 55.

▼ *Key Point* Otitis media should always be suspected in cases of chronic or recurrent external ear canal disease.

Occasionally, otitis media may result from extension of a pharyngeal infection via the auditory tube or from hematogenous spread of pathogens to the middle ear.

Otitis interna—Inflammation of the inner ear structures, which include the cochlea, vestibule, and semicircular canals. The most likely route of infection to the inner ear is an extension of otitis media. Hematogenous spread has occasionally been observed.

ETIOLOGY

Causes of middle ear inflammation include (1) bacteria, (2) yeasts and fungi, (3) parasites, (4) foreign bodies, (5) trauma, (6) polyps, and (7) neoplasms.

- *Bacteria* are the most common causes of otitis media. *Staphylococcus* and *Streptococcus* spp. are among the most frequently isolated organisms, but they have also been isolated from the middle ears of healthy dogs. This makes their role as the primary inducers of inflammation questionable. Other bacteria that have been isolated from cases of otitis media include *Proteus, Pseudomonas, Escherichia coli,* and *Clostridium* spp. Recent evidence suggests that the bacteria causing otitis media are frequently different from those causing otitis externa in the same patient. Although it is not known what organisms are most commonly involved in otitis interna, it is presumed that they are the same as those in otitis media.
- *Yeasts and fungi* are uncommon causes of otitis media and interna. *Malassezia pachydermatis, Aspergillus* spp., and *Candida* spp. are among those most frequently mentioned. *Paecilomyces* is a rare cause.

- *Parasites,* such as the mite *Otodectes cynotis,* occasionally contribute to the rupture of the tympanic membrane and the subsequent signs of otitis media and interna, especially in cats.
- *Foreign bodies,* such as plant awns, are more common in the western United States and are suspect when clinical signs are unilateral.
- *Trauma* is an uncommon cause of otitis media and interna.
- *Polyps* can occur in the middle ear cavity or auditory tube of cats. Some polyps push through the tympanic membrane and can be observed in the external ear canal.
- *Neoplasms* can initiate inflammation because of their expansive or invasive growth. Squamous cell carcinoma, fibrosarcoma, and lymphoma have been reported to affect the middle ear, and neurofibrosarcoma, meningioma, and carcinoma have been reported to affect the inner ear.

CLINICAL SIGNS

Otitis Media

- Many clinical signs of otitis externa (see Chap. 55) are common with otitis media, because otitis media is frequently a sequela to chronic otitis externa. Unrecognized otitis media is an important cause of recurrent or chronic otitis externa.
- Signs include head shaking, pawing, or rubbing the affected ear, discharge from the external ear canal, and increased sensitivity or pain when the head is touched or the mouth is opened.
- Depression, anorexia, and fever are uncommon signs.
- Injury to the facial nerve, as it courses near the middle ear, produces drooping of the upper lip or ear, drooling of saliva, and decreased or absent palpebral reflex.
- Horner's syndrome may be present if injury occurs to the sympathetic nerve fibers that course near the middle ear. Ipsilateral miosis, ptosis, enophthalmos, and protruding nictitans may be observed. Other causes of Horner's syndrome are discussed in Chapter 160.
- Keratitis sicca, characterized by reduced tear production and mucopurulent ocular exudate, may occur if the parasympathetic nerves that innervate the tear

glands are injured (see Chap. 158). These nerve fibers course with the facial nerve.

Otitis Interna

- Head tilt, circling, leaning, or rolling to the affected side are observed with unilateral inner ear inflammation.
- Spontaneous horizontal or rotary nystagmus may be prominent. The fast phase of the nystagmus is away from the side of the lesion.
- Ataxia of limbs is present, yet the animal can usually ambulate and perform postural reactions with no decrease in strength.
- Vomiting may occasionally occur because of the vestibular connections to the emetic center in the brain stem.
- Hearing loss is not usually detected clinically unless bilateral inflammation is present.
- Signs of bilateral otitis interna include wide head excursions, little or no spontaneous nystagmus, absent or poor oculocephalic response, and ataxia of all limbs. An erect tail and a crouched posture are frequently observed in cats.
- Occasionally, bacterial migration from the inner ear to the brain stem occurs, producing severe depression, loss of limb strength and conscious proprioception, and possibly other cranial nerve deficits.

DIAGNOSIS

History and Physical Examination

- *History* identifies the clinical signs and any predispositions to external ear disease.
- *Physical examination* may detect systemic signs of disease or localized infections that suggest hematogenous spread of pathogens to the middle or inner ears.
  - Palpate the temporomandibular joints for irregularities, swelling, or pain.
  - Examine the pharynx for signs of inflammation or masses that could have spread to or from the middle ear via the auditory tube.
  - *Otoscopic examination* (see Chap. 1) detects signs of otitis externa; ruptured, bulging, or discolored tympanic membrane; or obstruction of the ear canal (Table 57–1). Ulcerations, masses, exudate, or hyperplastic tissue often hamper exposure of the tympanic membrane. Lavage of the ear canal with warm normal saline may help remove exudate and debris.

▼ *Key Point* In many cases heavy sedation or general anesthesia is necessary to thoroughly examine the external ear canal and the tympanic membrane.

  - *Neurologic examination* detects signs of Horner's syndrome and/or facial nerve dysfunction, which may be observed with middle ear disease. Signs of vestibular dysfunction support inner ear disease. See Chapter 145 for a discussion of the differential diagnosis of vestibular and cranial nerve disorders.

Table 57–1. CHARACTERISTICS OF NORMAL AND ABNORMAL TYMPANIC MEMBRANES

Characteristic	Normal	Abnormal
Transparency	Translucent	Cloudy Opaque
Luster	Glistening	Dull
Color	Pearl-gray	Blue: intratympanic hemorrhage Red: acute otitis media White: purulent material Amber: serous exudate
Tension	Slightly concave	Bulging: material accumulated behind tympanum
Vessels	Radiating	Obscured or torn

▼ *Key Point* Peripheral vestibular signs, which occur with otitis interna, must be distinguished from central vestibular signs, which occur with brain stem disease (Table 57–2).

- The *Schirmer tear test* evaluates the integrity of the parasympathetic nerve fibers (cranial nerve VII) to the eye.

Cytology and Culture

- *Cytologic examination* of exudate may help to identify an etiologic agent. Take samples before flushing or cleaning of the ear canal.
- *Culture and sensitivity* are also helpful to identify an etiologic agent and appropriate antibiotic therapy. Take samples before cleaning the ear canal. Obtain culture samples from both the middle ear and external ear canal.

Myringotomy

- *Myringotomy* is done if the tympanic membrane is bulging or discolored, or if chronic otitis externa is present (see Chap. 58).
- Under general anesthesia, use a 20-gauge, 3.5-inch spinal needle or blunt probe and direct it through a clean otoscope cone to perforate the tympanic membrane caudal to the malleus. The tip should be directed ventrally to avoid the auditory ossicles and chorda tympani nerve which are located dorsally.
- Using a syringe attached to the needle, aspirate fluid or material and evaluate by cytology and culture. The small hole in the tympanic membrane usually seals over rapidly.

Radiography

- Obtain ventrodorsal, oblique lateral, and open mouth views. General anesthesia is necessary for proper positioning.
- A soft tissue density in the normally air-filled tympanic cavity suggests fluid, granulation tissue, or neoplasia.

Table 57–2. VESTIBULAR SIGNS ASSOCIATED WITH INNER EAR VS. BRAIN STEM LOCATIONS

Sign	Inner Ear	Brain Stem
Head tilt	Present	Present
Circling	Present	Present
Falling, rolling	Present	Present
Positional strabismus	Present	Present
Nystagmus	Usually spontaneous and type (horizontal, rotary) does not vary with position of head	Usually not spontaneous but found with changes in head position; type (horizontal, rotary, vertical) varies with head position
Conscious proprioception	Normal	Delayed or absent
Horner's syndrome	May be present	Usually absent
Cranial nerve deficits	VII	V, VI, VII
Gait changes	Mild to severe ataxia	Ataxia and weakness
Postural reactions (e.g., hopping, hemiwalking, wheelbarrowing)	Normal if examined slowly	Weak or absent
Cerebellar signs (hypermetria, head intention tremors)	Absent	May be present

- Destruction of the bulla may be seen with osteomyelitis or neoplasia.
- Changes may not be present for several weeks in acute cases of otitis media.
- Chronic cases may show only sclerosis or thickening of the normally fine outline of the bulla.

▼ *Key Point* Absence of radiographic signs of otitis media does not rule out the disease.

TREATMENT

Otitis Media

The goals of treatment of otitis media are to remove infected, inflammatory, or foreign material from the bulla and to provide ventilation and drainage. These goals are accomplished with medical and/or surgical intervention, depending on the chronicity and results of otoscopic and radiographic evaluations. For details of treating the external ear canal (otitis externa) medically, see Chapter 55, and surgically, see Chapter 56. Surgery for otitis media and interna is discussed in Chapter 58.

Ear Canal Lavage and Myringotomy

- *Flushing* the ear canal with warm isotonic saline helps eliminate debris and aids visualization of the tympanic membrane.
  - Use a water-propulsion dental device (Water Pik), suction system, or bulb syringe very carefully.
  - Always dry the ear canal after flushing by gentle aspiration, low-vacuum suction, or Otic Domeboro solution (Miles Pharmaceuticals).
- *Myringotomy* is indicated if the tympanic membrane is intact but discolored and bulging, or if chronic otitis is present (see Diagnosis and Chap. 58).
  - A myringotomy allows for samples to be obtained for culture and cytology and allows for some drainage from the middle ear cavity to relieve pain and pressure.
  - Gently flush the middle ear cavity with several milliliters of warm normal saline through the myringotomy perforation; follow by aspirating the saline. Use a 12-gauge, 3.5-inch cannula to enlarge the opening if necessary.

Systemic Antibiotics

- If there is no radiographic evidence of fluid or material within the bulla, use systemic antibiotics for 3–6 weeks.
- If a culture cannot be obtained, administer broad-spectrum antibiotics, such as chloramphenicol, 25–50 mg/kg PO q6–8h; a cephalosporin (e.g., cefadroxil, 20 mg/kg PO q12h; cephalexin, 10–30 mg/kg PO, SQ, IM, or IV q8h); trimethoprim-sulfa, 15–30 mg/kg PO q12h; or a quinolone (e.g., enrofloxacin, orbifloxacin, difloxacin). Do not use trimethoprim-sulfa if keratitis sicca is present or if tear production is decreased.
- If little or no response occurs with systemic antibiotic treatment, repeat radiographs of the bulla. Exploratory bulla surgery may be necessary (see Chap. 58).
- If otoscopic or radiographic evaluations support the presence of fluid or material within the middle ear cavity, systemic antibiotics are indicated. However, surgery is frequently necessary to allow for proper drainage (see Chap. 58).

Topical Therapeutic Agents

- Use cautiously if the tympanic membrane is not intact, because many drugs have the potential to cause ototoxicity characterized by acute deafness or vestibular signs.
- Ototoxic agents include aminoglycosides (gentamicin, neomycin), chloramphenicol, iodine, iodophors, and chlorhexidine.

Other

- Use *artificial tears* as described in Chapter 158, if keratitis sicca is present.
- Consider *surgery* if there is radiographic evidence of fluid or material in the tympanic bulla or poor response to medical treatment (see Chap. 58).

▼ *Key Point* Reevaluate the ear canal 1 week after beginning treatment and every 2 weeks afterward, until the problem is resolved. Repeat flushing may be needed.

Otitis Interna

- Treat underlying otitis externa and media if present.
- If only otitis interna is present, use systemic antibiotics as outlined for otitis media.
- If the signs do not abate in 1–3 weeks, repeat the bulla radiographs to evaluate the possibility of otitis media acting as a nidus of infection that may require surgical intervention.

SUPPLEMENTAL READINGS

Cole LK, Kwochka KW, Kowalski JJ, et al.: Microbial flora and antimicrobial susceptibility patterns of isolated pathogens from the horizontal ear canal and middle ear in dogs with otitis media. J Am Vet Med Assoc 212:534, 1998.

Denny HR: The results of surgical treatment of otitis media and interna in the dog. J Small Animal Pract 14:585, 1973.

Remedios AM, Fowler JD, Pharr JW: A comparison of radiographic versus surgical diagnosis of otitis media. J Am Anim Hosp Assoc 27:183, 1991.

Shell LG: Otitis media and otitis interna. Vet Clin North Am Small Anim Pract 18:885, 1988.

Spreull JSA: Tympanotomy, bulla osteotomy and vestibular osteotomy. *In* Bojrab MJ, ed.: Current Techniques in Small Animal Surgery. Philadelphia: Lea & Febiger, 1975, p 71.

58 Surgery for Otitis Media and Otitis Interna

Harry W. Boothe

Selection of a surgical procedure to treat otitis media and interna is based on duration of clinical signs, response to previous treatment, status of the external ear canal, and the surgeon's familiarity with related anatomy and technique. Surgical options for treating otitis media and interna include myringotomy, lateral bulla osteotomy, and ventral bulla osteotomy. Nasopharyngeal polyps are most appropriately excised using a bulla osteotomy in combination with other excision techniques. Potential complications of bulla osteotomy surgery include facial nerve injury, Horner's syndrome (ptosis, miosis, enophthalmos, nictitating membrane protrusion), and vestibular signs. See Chapter 57 for diagnosis and medical treatment of otitis media and interna.

ANATOMY

- The tympanic membrane slopes downward, forward, and inward—toward the middle ear cavity. The membrane is composed of a larger, more peripherally located pars tensa and a smaller, triangular-shaped pars flaccida.
- The air-filled tympanic cavity constitutes the major portion of the middle ear and is connected to the nasopharynx by the auditory tube.
- Structures located within the dorsal aspect of the tympanic cavity include the three auditory ossicles, associated muscles and ligaments, and tympanic nerve.

▼ *Key Point* The feline tympanic cavity is divided into a larger ventromedial and a smaller dorsolateral compartment by a nearly complete thin bony septum.

- Surgically important structures near the tympanic bulla are the facial nerve (ventrolaterally), the carotid artery (medially), and the hypoglossal nerve (ventrally).

MYRINGOTOMY

Preoperative Considerations

- Thorough cleansing of the external ear canal is indicated to enable the myringotomy to be performed under the guidance of otoscopic monitoring.
- Myringotomy can be performed alone or in combination with bulla osteotomy.

Surgical Procedure

Objectives

- Drain and flush material from within the tympanic cavity.
- Obtain specimens for microbiologic and cytologic sampling.
- Instill medication into the tympanic cavity.

Equipment

- 3/32-inch Steinmann pin.
- Open-end 3.5 Fr. feline urethral catheter.
- Warm physiologic saline solution and 12-ml syringe.

Technique

1. Position the patient in lateral recumbency and clean the ear canal.
2. Incise the caudoventral aspect of the tympanic membrane under otoscopic guidance with the Steinmann pin.
3. Insert the end of the feline urethral catheter into the tympanic cavity and aspirate material from the middle ear cavity.
4. Collect samples for microbiologic and cytologic analysis (see Chap. 57).
5. Gently flush the tympanic cavity with warm saline solution until the washings are clear. Aspirate fluid from the middle ear cavity.
6. Instill a nonototoxic antibiotic (avoid aminoglycosides) into the tympanic cavity.

Postoperative Care and Complications

Short-Term

- Administer systemic antibiotics based on culture and susceptibility results for at least 3 weeks.
- Potential short-term complications are usually limited to transient vestibular signs and/or Horner's syndrome.

Long-Term

- Minimal long-term drainage results from uncomplicated myringotomy.
- With successful resolution of otitis media, healing of the tympanic membrane occurs in approximately 50% of the animals.
- Recurrence of otitis media is a potential long-term complication.

Prognosis

- Myringotomy is more likely to resolve otitis media if it is performed early in the course of the disease.

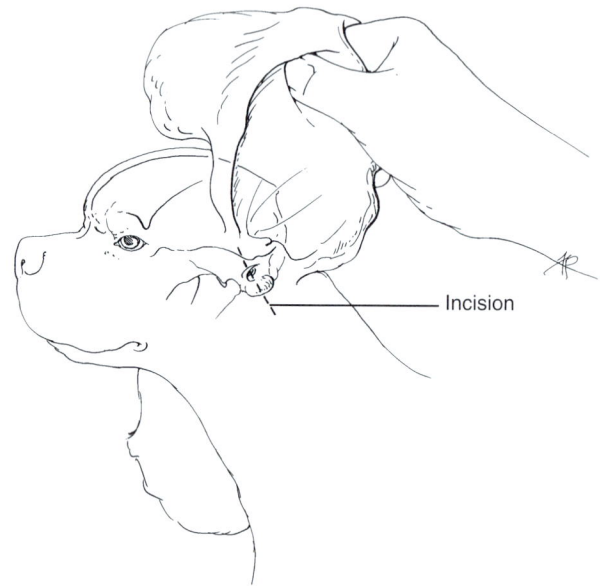

Figure 58–1. Skin incision for performing a lateral bulla osteotomy without total ear canal ablation.

LATERAL BULLA OSTEOTOMY

Preoperative Considerations

- Determine the condition of the external ear canal.
- Evaluate the radiographic appearance of the tympanic bulla and the microbiologic status of the middle ear before lateral bulla osteotomy.
- Lateral bulla osteotomy is simplest when performed in conjunction with a total ear canal ablation. If the external ear canal is normal or only mildly affected by infection, bulla osteotomy can be performed via a lateral (without ear canal ablation) or ventral approach. The ventral approach technique is preferred by most surgeons.
- Assess the integrity of the facial nerve preoperatively.

Surgical Procedure

Objectives

- Provide access to the tympanic cavity for diagnostic intervention.
- Provide drainage and access to the middle ear cavity for therapeutic intervention (e.g., flush, curettage, and resection of abnormal tissue).

Equipment

- Standard general surgery pack and suture
- Periosteal elevator, Steinmann pin, hand chuck, and rongeurs
- Warm saline solution and tubing for flushing the tympanic cavity

Technique for Lateral Bulla Osteotomy Without Total Ear Canal Ablation

1. Position the patient in lateral recumbency, and prepare the lateral aspect of the head and neck.

2. Incise the skin over the vertical ear canal to a point ventral to the horizontal ear canal (Fig. 58–1).
3. Bluntly dissect between the parotid salivary gland and the ventral aspect of the horizontal ear canal to reveal the facial nerve.
4. Retract the facial nerve ventrocaudally near its exit from the stylomastoid foramen.
5. Elevate the soft tissue overlying the lateral aspect of the osseous bulla using a periosteal elevator.
6. Enter the tympanic cavity ventral to the horizontal ear canal with the Steinmann pin and hand chuck.
7. Enlarge the osteotomy site ventrally with rongeurs.
8. Obtain microbiologic samples, and flush the middle ear cavity using warm saline solution. If curettage is performed, avoid traumatizing the inner ear structures on the dorsomedial aspect of the bulla.
9. Instill a nonototoxic antibiotic into the tympanic cavity.
10. Place and secure a drain tube into the tympanic cavity by suturing it to the adjacent soft tissue with fine absorbable suture material.
11. Routinely close the subcutaneous tissue (simple interrupted, absorbable suture) and the skin (simple interrupted, nonabsorbable suture).
12. Position the drain tube so that it exits the skin adjacent to the primary incision.

Technique for Lateral Bulla Osteotomy with Total Ear Canal Ablation

1. Position the patient in lateral recumbency, and prepare the lateral aspect of the head and neck, including the external ear canal.
2. Incise the skin over the vertical ear canal, and perform a total ear canal ablation (see Chap. 56).

3. Reflect the soft tissue from the lateral aspect of the tympanic bulla, insert the rongeur tips into the external auditory meatus, and remove the ventral aspect of the bony auditory meatus.
4. Extend the osteotomy site as far ventrally into the middle ear cavity as possible, and flush the cavity with warm saline solution. Use a bone curette to carefully remove epithelium and debris from the bulla.
5. Place a drain tube to exit the ventral aspect of the bulla osteotomy site and skin adjacent to the primary incision.

Postoperative Care and Complications

Short-Term

- Prevent self-inflicted trauma to the drain tube by using an Elizabethan collar or similar device.
- Facial nerve damage, manifested by inability to close the eye and by drooping of the upper lip on the ipsilateral side, may be observed.

▼ *Key Point* Administer eye lubricant (artificial tears) to animals with facial nerve damage to prevent corneal ulceration.

- Remove the drain tube when drainage has decreased significantly, generally within 3–4 days.
- Continue an appropriate systemic antibiotic for at least 3 weeks.

Prognosis

- Extent of response to bulla osteotomy tends to be incomplete in long-standing cases of otitis media and interna.
- Immediate response following bulla osteotomy indicates a more favorable prognosis.

VENTRAL BULLA OSTEOTOMY

Preoperative Considerations

- See Preoperative Considerations under Lateral Bulla Osteotomy.
- Radiographically assess the density of the tympanic bulla to assist in the initial osteotomy procedure.

Surgical Procedure

Objectives

- See Objectives under Lateral Bulla Osteotomy.
- To establish ventral drainage of the middle ear cavity.

Equipment

- See Equipment for Lateral Bulla Osteotomy Without Total Ear Canal Ablation.

Technique

1. Position the patient in dorsal recumbency, and prepare the ventral cervical region from the mid-mandibular area to the wings of the atlas.

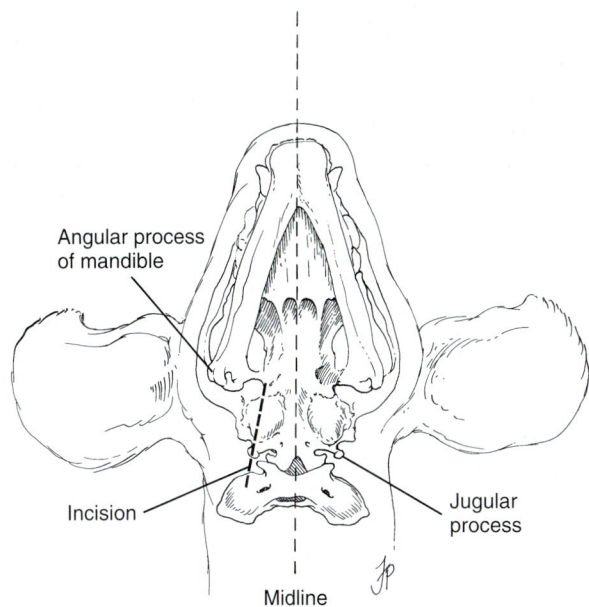

Figure 58–2. Skin incision for ventral bulla osteotomy.

2. Incise the skin just off the midline between the level of the angular process of the mandible and the wings of the atlas (Fig. 58–2).
3. Bluntly dissect between the digastricus muscle and the hyoglossal and styloglossal muscles. The hypoglossal nerve on the lateral aspect of the hyoglossal muscle helps verify the proper dissection plane.
4. Carefully retract the adjacent musculature to reveal the rounded tympanic bulla between the more angular jugular process of the skull (caudal) and the angular process of the mandible (rostrolateral).
5. Reflect the thin jugulohyoideus muscle that covers the osseous bulla in the dog.
6. Accurately locate the bulla before proceeding with the osteotomy. Penetrate the ventral aspect of the tympanic bulla with a Steinmann pin in a hand chuck, and enlarge the osteotomy site using rongeurs (Fig. 58–3). In cats, fenestrate the septum to fully expose the tympanic cavity.

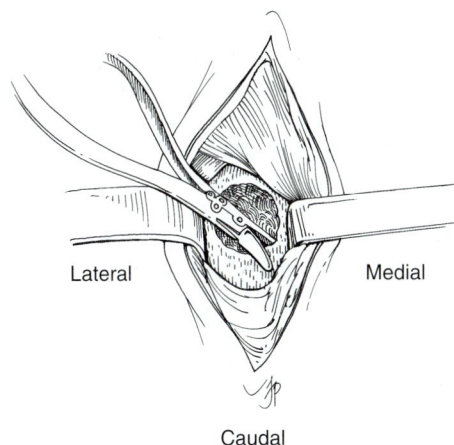

Figure 58–3. Osteotomy technique.

7. Flush the middle ear cavity with warm saline solution, and place a drain to exit the ventral cervical skin through a separate skin incision. The dorsal aspect of the drain may also be positioned to exit the external ear canal.

8. Routinely close the subcutaneous tissue (simple interrupted, absorbable suture) and the skin (simple interrupted, nonabsorbable suture).

Postoperative Care and Complications

- See Postoperative Care and Complications under Lateral Bulla Osteotomy.

SURGICAL MANAGEMENT OF NASOPHARYNGEAL POLYPS

Preoperative Considerations

- Carefully inspect the nasopharynx by rostrally displacing the soft palate to assess the size of the nasopharyngeal mass.
- Radiographically assess the tympanic bulla to determine the potential involvement of the middle ear cavity.

Surgical Procedure

Objectives

- Excision of the mass using both an oral approach and a ventral bulla osteotomy.
- To remove the mass from the nasopharynx or ear canal using a simple traction technique, while carefully excising polypoid tissue from the tympanic cavity via a ventral bulla osteotomy.

Equipment

- See Equipment for Lateral Bulla Osteotomy Without Total Ear Canal Ablation.

Technique

1. Position the cat in dorsal recumbency and prepare the ventral cervical region from the mid-mandibular area to the wings of the atlas. Perform the procedure with the cat's mouth held open.

2. Displace the soft palate rostrally using a soft tissue retractor to provide adequate exposure of the mass.

3. Apply traction to the mass to remove the pharyngeal component of the polyp.

4. Perform a ventral bulla osteotomy, as previously described, and excise tissue proliferations within the tympanic cavity using careful curettage. Perform a bilateral bulla osteotomy if it is unclear which middle ear is involved.

5. Examine the ipsilateral ear canal, and excise any polypoid tissue.

Postoperative Care and Complications

Short-Term

- Temporary Horner's syndrome of 1–2 weeks' duration is common following curettage of the middle ear cavity.
- See short-term complications following lateral bulla osteotomy.

Long-Term

- Recurrence of the polyp is possible, although less likely, following both excision by traction and ventral bulla osteotomy than following excision by traction alone.
- Disruption of the otic ossicles from trauma to the dorsal aspect of the tympanic cavity results in hearing loss.

Prognosis

- The long-term outlook following removal of nasopharyngeal polyps using both the traction excision and ventral bulla osteotomy techniques is good. Recurrence is uncommon.

SUPPLEMENTAL READINGS

Boothe HW Jr: Ventral bulla osteotomy: Dog and cat. *In* Bojrab MJ, ed.: Current Techniques in Small Animal Surgery, 4th Ed. Philadelphia: Lea & Febiger, 1998, p 109.

Evans HE, Christensen GC: Miller's Anatomy of the Dog. Philadelphia: WB Saunders, 1979, p 1062.

Howard PE, Neer TM, Miller JS: Otitis media. Part II. Surgical considerations. Compend Contin Educ Pract Vet 5:18, 1983.

Kapatkin AS, Matthiesen DT, Noone KE, et al.: Results of surgery and long-term follow-up in 31 cats with nasopharyngeal polyps. J Am Anim Hosp Assoc 26:387, 1990.

Little CJL, Lane JG: The surgical anatomy of the feline bulla tympanica. J Small Anim Pract 27:371, 1986.

McAnulty JF, Hattel A, Harvey CE: Wound healing and brain stem auditory evoked potentials after experimental total ear canal ablation with lateral bulla osteotomy in dogs. Vet Surg 24:1, 1995.

McAnulty JF, Hattel A, Harvey CE: Wound healing and brain stem auditory evoked potentials after experimental ventral tympanic bulla osteotomy in dogs. Vet Surg 24:9, 1995.

Sharp NJH: Chronic otitis externa and otitis media treated by total ear canal ablation and ventral bulla osteotomy in thirteen dogs. Vet Surg 19:162, 1990.

Smeak DD, Kerpsack SJ: Total ear canal ablation and lateral bulla osteotomy for management of end stage otitis. Semin Vet Med Surg (Small Anim) 8:30, 1993.

Trevor PB, Martin RA: Tympanic bulla osteotomy for treatment of middle-ear disease in cats: 19 cases (1984–1991). J Am Vet Med Assoc 202:123, 1993.

6 Cardiopulmonary System

John D. Bonagura

59 Auscultation and Physical Diagnosis

Robert L. Hamlin

Physical examination follows the obtaining of a complete history and the consideration of the signalment. Diagnosis, or at the very least a number of plausible diagnoses, may be made in many instances by history and signalment; however, following a thorough physical examination, a single, "most likely" diagnosis can be made with reasonable assurance in most patients with cardiac problems. Physical examination is performed best in a systematic manner, initially conducting those portions that are least likely to aggravate or to cause discomfort to the patient. Physical examination of the cardiovascular system can be separated into four steps: *inspection, palpation, percussion,* and *auscultation.* What separates the physical examination from the remainder of the cardiac examination is the close relationship between the veterinarian and the patient, and, with the exception of the stethoscope, the absence of elaborate instrumentation (e.g., radiography, echocardiography.

INSPECTION

Inspection of the patient is conducted as one obtains the history. It should be performed while the animal enters the room; while the pet stands, sits, or walks; while the owner supports the pet; and while the pet stands alone.

Condition, Attitude, and Posture

- *Body condition* of the patient is classified according to the degree of fat.
  - Normal overweight animals usually are not ill from heart failure but may manifest signs caused by pul-

monary disease (e.g., chronic lung disease, pulmonary fibrosis).
  - Animals with moderate to long-standing heart failure are often thin to cachectic.
- *Attitude* of an animal with heart failure is usually depressed.
- *Posture* of animals with heart failure is often:
  - Standing—reluctant to lay down—with thoracic limbs abducted and neck extended to ease ventilation.
  - Swayback with the tail between the legs because of muscular weakness occasionally caused by digitalis toxicity from either administering too much drug or from impaired renal excretion due either to dehydration or primary renal disease.
    Swayback can also result from electrolyte imbalance—in particular hypokalemia—caused by prolonged or excessive use of diuretics without consumption of sufficient electrolytes.
  - Dogs with cardiomyopathy often have weakness of skeletal muscles and dogs with heart failure are often exhausted owing to the work of breathing.

Mucous Membrane Color

- Mucous membranes may be cyanotic in late stages of heart failure or in puppies or very young dogs with tetralogy of Fallot or other congenital heart defects with right-to-left intracardiac shunts (see Chap. 70).
- Cyanosis occurs much more commonly in all stages of pulmonary diseases.
- Mucous membranes may be dark red in stages just prior to frank cyanosis.

- Mucous membranes may be pale with concomitant anemia or low cardiac output but without pulmonary congestion (e.g., low output heart failure, severe aortic stenosis).

Abdominal Distention and Edema

- Abdominal distention may be a result of gas in the gastrointestinal (GI) tract from aerophagia associated with chronic obstructive pulmonary disease (COPD) or pulmonary failure (PF), or from primary GI disease.
- Ascites and enlargement of abdominal organs may indicate venous hypertension or passive congestion due to right-sided heart failure.
- Primary disease of abdominal organs (e.g., neoplasia) can also cause abdominal distention.
- Pitting edema of the limbs, brisket, and prepuce can be caused by right-sided heart failure.

▼ *Key Point* Subcutaneous edema in the absence of ascites or jugular distention argues *against* a diagnosis of congestive heart failure.

Pattern of Ventilation

Pattern of ventilation is extremely important. Characterize the rate and depth of breathing, and identify dyspnea.

- *Rate of breaths per minute* should be between 12 and 20 for dogs and 20 and 40 for cats, but may increase from excitement, fever, anxiety, warm environment, COPD/PF, left-sided heart failure, or pulmonary injury.
- *Depth of ventilation* is difficult to quantify, but hyperpnea (increased depth) is often a sign of blood gas derangement (e.g., response to metabolic acidosis). It is not often observed in heart disease except with severe pulmonary edema.
- *Dyspnea* (labored ventilation) may occur as increased rate and/or depth of ventilation or merely as increased effort. With dyspnea one observes
  - Bulging eyes.
  - Flaring nares.
  - Outward motion of thoracic limbs.
  - Reluctance to lay down.
  - Abdominal "pumping."
  - Extension of neck and open mouth breathing.

Cough

Cough is a sign of both heart and lung disease. It may be characterized as follows.

- Hacking, honking, brassy cough indicates disease of the large airways, such as tracheobronchial collapse (see Chap. 77), compression of the left mainstem bronchus due to mitral regurgitation or generalized cardiomegaly, tracheobronchitis, or bronchopulmonary parasitism. This type of cough is seldom due to injury of the parenchyma of the lung (e.g., edema, pneumonia).
- Subtle or "half-hearted" cough may be caused by pulmonary edema, pneumonia, or diaphragmatic hernia.

- So-called moist or truly productive coughs usually indicate an exudative process; however, in *late stages of left-sided congestive heart failure* it is common to have serosanguineous pulmonary edema fluid gush from the nares and/or mouth.)

Jugular Vein Evaluation

Analysis of the *jugular* vein (Fig. 59–1) is simpler if the hair is clipped from around the jugular furrow or if it is moistened with 70% alcohol.

- A firm, distended jugular vein that collapses briefly immediately after the second heart sound is consistent with pericardial tamponade, such as that observed in dogs with hemorrhage in the pericardial sac due to a bleeding neoplasm or hemorrhage from a rupture of the left atrium with severe mitral regurgitation. Constrictive pericarditis (see Chap. 67) and COPD/PF can also cause these jugular vein changes.
- Vigorous pulsation of the jugular vein
  - Jugular venous pulses ("cannon *a* waves") occurring more than 120/min with the ventricular rate very slow (usually below 60/min) indicates third degree (complete) or high-grade second-degree atrioventricular block.

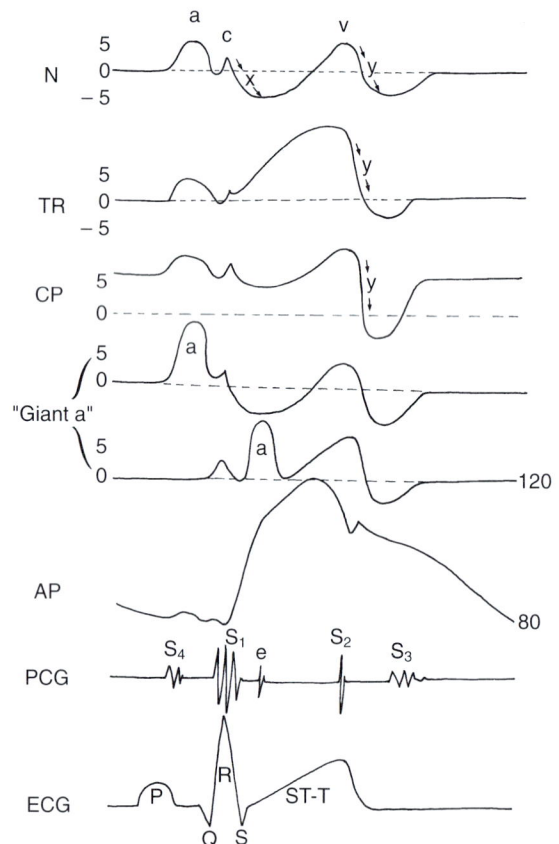

Figure 59–1. Analysis of venous pulses. A normal pulse is shown for reference (N), as are systemic arterial pressure (AP), phonocardiogram (PCG), and electrocardiogram (ECG). Abnormal pulses shown are those produced by tricuspid regurgitation (TR) and constrictive pericarditis (CP); also shown are two types of cannon, or giant, *a* waves.

- If cannon *a* waves occur between the first and second heart sounds it indicates regurgitation of blood from the right ventricle to the right atrium during tricuspid regurgitation.
- If cannon *a* waves occur just before the first heart sound it may rarely indicate tricuspid stenosis or possibly stiffness of the ventricles (e.g., pulmonic stenosis).
- Hepatojugular reflux
  - Pushing on the abdomen of a standing dog displaces the liver dorsad and "milks" blood from the liver to the right side of the heart. If the right ventricle cannot pump the extra venous return through the lungs or if right ventricular filling is restricted owing to pericardial tamponade or constriction, the extra venous return "wells up" in the jugular vein, producing added distention, which is a positive hepatojugular sign.
  - The jugular vein normally collapses totally when the long axis of the torso makes a head-up tilt at an angle of 45° with the horizontal.
  - If the jugular vein does not collapse, the venous pressure may be elevated owing to heart failure, COPD/PF, or ventricular filling restriction due to pericardial disease.
  - The jugular vein also normally collapses during inspiration and immediately after the second heart sound.

Miscellaneous

- Inspect the pharynx and mouth to identify: tonsillitis, pharyngitis, elongated soft palate, neoplasia, or periodontal disease.
- Watch the animal walk to identify and to quantify:
  - Exercise intolerance from heart failure or COPD.
  - Weakness due to heart failure or severe aortic stenosis.
  - Neuromuscular or skeletal disease.

PALPATION

Thorax

- Technique
  - Performed with the animal standing and being held by an assistant with the assistant's hands cupped around the neck.
  - The palpator stands at the side or back of the animal.
  - The palpator places his or her hands in the axilla and slides them caudad stopping at:
  1. The second to third intercostal space.
  2. The fourth to sixth intercostal spaces.
  3. Just caudad to the rib cage.
  4. All points on the abdomen.
  5. The femoral arteries.
- Determine where the heart "thumps" most vigorously on the thoracic wall. The point of maximal impulse is normally at the fifth intercostal space two to three fingerbreadths from the left sternal border *and* at the right third intercostal space near the right ster-

nal border. Cardiomegaly or space-occupying intrathoracic masses may displace this impulse.
- Classify heart sounds according to:
  - Intensity (see Auscultation).
  - A "booming" S_1 heart sound indicates forceful contraction, short atrioventricular conduction (PQ interval), or skinny thorax, or it may be detected in dogs with advanced mitral regurgitation.
  - A "soft" S_1 heart sound indicates weak ventricle, long atrioventricular conduction (PQ interval), obesity, hyperinflation of lungs, pleural effusion, or pneumothorax.
  - Frequency—to assess autonomic tone and heart rhythm.
  - Regularity—to detect arrhythmias.
  - Presence of a thrill—palpable manifestation of a murmur. This indicates a murmur of at least grade V or VI.
- Palpate for abnormal breath sounds:
  - "Snoring" of sonorous rhonchi (rattling sounds).
  - "Honks" of tracheal wall vibrations due to collapse.
  - "Tight" crackles or rales.

Abdomen

- Gently palpate under caudal ribs to identify hepatomegaly.
- Palpate abdomen for ascites, organomegaly, or neoplasia.

Femoral Pulses

- Palpate femoral arteries for pulse rate, which is relatively independent of body size.

Heart Rates	Dog	Cat
Quiet (asleep)	50–90	90–120
During examination	80–160	140–220
Exercise	230	230

- Force (Table 59–1 and Fig. 59–1).
- Rhythm
  - Respiratory sinus arrhythmia—average rate is usually as described previously for sleep. The rate speeds up during inspiration but seldom more than three or, at most, four heartbeats during an inspiration. More than four beats during inspiration may indicate abnormal ventilation caused by chronic pulmonary disease. Pulse rate slows during exhalation, occasionally to as low as 30 beats/min but only very briefly.
  - Atrial fibrillation or frequent short bursts of supraventricular or ventricular tachycardia are characterized by rapid pulse rate; irregularly irregular rhythm (i.e., *not* in sync with ventilation); variable intensity; and *pulse deficit*—fewer femoral pulses than heartbeats.
  - Occasionally supraventricular or ventricular premature beats occur singly and are characterized by apparent single skipped pulses followed by a pulse stronger than usual.

Table 59–1. TYPICAL SYSTEMIC ARTERIAL* PULSES FOR ANIMALS WITH VARYING PHYSIOLOGIC AND/OR PATHOLOGIC STATES

	Character	Pressure Systolic/ Diastolic	Pressure Differential	Rate	Pulse Character
Normal animal	Normal	120/80	40	Normal	N
Patent ductus arteriosus (PDA) or aortic regurgitation (AR)	Bounding	160/40	120	Increased	PDA, AR
Aortic stenosis (AS) or early heart failure (HF)	Weak	90/60	30	Increased	AS, HF
Mitral regurgitation (MR), ventricular septal defect (VSD), late heart failure (HF), or hyperkinetic ventricle (HK)	Sharp, brief	120/80	40	Rapid	MR, VSD, HF, HK

*For example, femoral artery.

- Weak pulses are found in:
  - Heart failure.
  - Aortic stenosis.
  - Dilated cardiomyopathy.
- Extremely bounding (water-hammer) pulses are found in:
  - Patent ductus arteriosus.
  - Aortic regurgitation.
  - Complete heart block with very slow ventricular rate.
- Regularly irregular pulses in sync with respirations are found with sinus arrhythmia.
- "Skipped" beats (when combined with cardiac auscultation) are found with single premature depolarizations.
- Rapid and irregularly irregular pulses are found with atrial fibrillation or with supraventricular or ventricular tachycardias in brief bursts. However, they are not rapid in large-breed dogs with hypothyroidism or preserved myocardial function, or in dogs with relatively slow-conducting atrioventricular nodes approaching complete heart block.
- Absent pulses are found in cats with aortic embolism due to cardiomyopathy or endocarditis.

PERCUSSION

This is the technique (Fig. 59–2) of thumping on the thorax and/or abdomen to determine the relative density of structures underneath the points of percussion (see also Chap. 82).

Types of percussion notes and their meanings are as follows:

- *Hyper-resonant notes* sound like a tympany drum and indicate a normal lung or a gas-filled structure (e.g., pneumothorax, hyperinflated lung, gas-filled stomach) underneath. Hyper-resonant sounds may be illustrated by drinking a can of carbonated beverage, jumping up and down for 15 seconds, and then thumping on the left side of your abdomen just over your stomach.

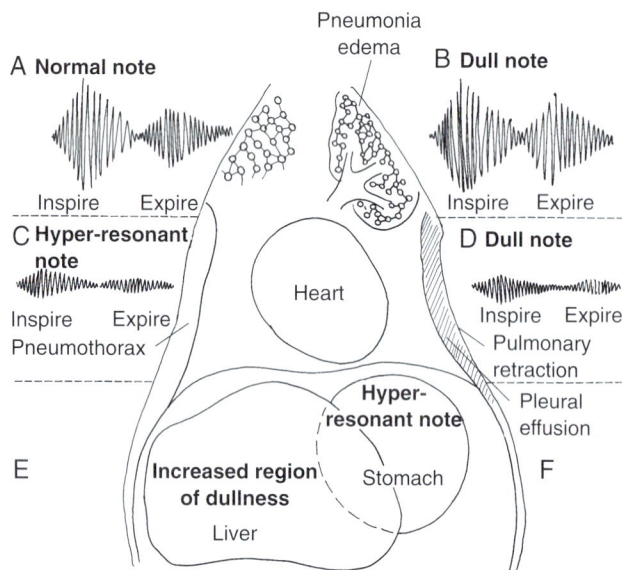

Figure 59–2. Schematic diagram of thorax and cranial portion of the abdomen viewed from the ventral aspect. *A* indicates the normal breath sounds and percussion. *B* shows a dull percussion note and louder than expected inspiratory and expiratory sounds due to pneumonia or edema. *C* represents the hyper-resonant percussion note and diminished breath sounds caused by pneumothorax, as illustrated by air between the thoracic wall and collapsed lung. *D* demonstrates a dull percussion note and diminished breath sounds due to pleural effusion, shown as density between thoracic wall and lungs. *E* indicates dull percussion notes because of an enlarged, dense liver. *F* is a hyper-resonant percussion note caused by gas in the stomach.

- *Dull notes* sound "dead," like thumping one's skull, and indicate a dense, usually water-filled structure (e.g., pneumonia, pleural effusion, pulmonary edema, consolidation) underneath. The normal notes of percussion may be learned by percussing thoraces from many normal male and female animals of varying ages and body conformations. Regions of cardiac dullness are less obvious in quadrupeds than in primates, but large pulmonary lesions or pleural effusion may be detected effectively by percussion.
- See Figure 59–2, which integrates the findings of percussion and auscultation for the differential diagnoses of
  - Edema/pneumonia.
  - Pneumothorax.
  - Pleural effusion.
  - Consolidation/neoplasia.
  - COPD/pulmonary fibrosis.

AUSCULTATION

- Definition: Listening to heart and breath sounds, usually with the aid of a stethoscope.
- Methods:
  - The best environment is a quiet room.
  - The animal is standing and restrained by an assistant standing to the front of the patient and holding the mouth closed to discourage panting.
  - The auscultator is to the back or side of the patient and keeps a hand or arm between the pet's mouth and his or her face.
- Stethoscope
  - Preferably use a stethoscope with ear pieces large enough to occlude most of the external acoustic meatus but not so large as to be airtight. The internal canal of the ear piece must be clean, and the outside sanitized if used by more than one person.
  - Two tubes of commercial stethoscope tubing extend from ear pieces to chest piece.

- The chest piece has a hard rubber or plastic diaphragm for characterizing high-pitched sounds and a deep trumpet bell for relatively low-pitched sounds.
- Areas of auscultation are shown in Figures 59–3 and 59–4.

ABNORMALITIES OF AUSCULTATION, PERCUSSION, AND PALPATION

Findings in Respiratory Disease

Normal

(See Fig. 59–2 for normal and abnormal breath sounds and percussion.)

- Normal vesicular breath sounds are heard with sounds of inspiration being louder than sounds of expiration.
- The percussion note of normal resonance is not too dull and not too resonant.

▼ *Key Point* In order to know what normal is, you must auscultate and percuss hundreds of normal animals of various ages, breeds, and conformations.

Pulmonary Edema and/or Pneumonia (see Chap. 79)

- Breath sounds are termed bronchial or bronchovesicular, i.e., sounds are louder in both inspiration and expiration but are much louder and higher pitched during expiration. The increased intensity arises from these sounds being "made" normally at larger airways but being transmitted better than usual via water-logged parenchyma.
- Percussion note is dull because of fluid-filled parenchyma.

Pneumothorax (see Chap. 82)

- All breath sounds are softer than normal because the free air space between the stethoscope chest piece

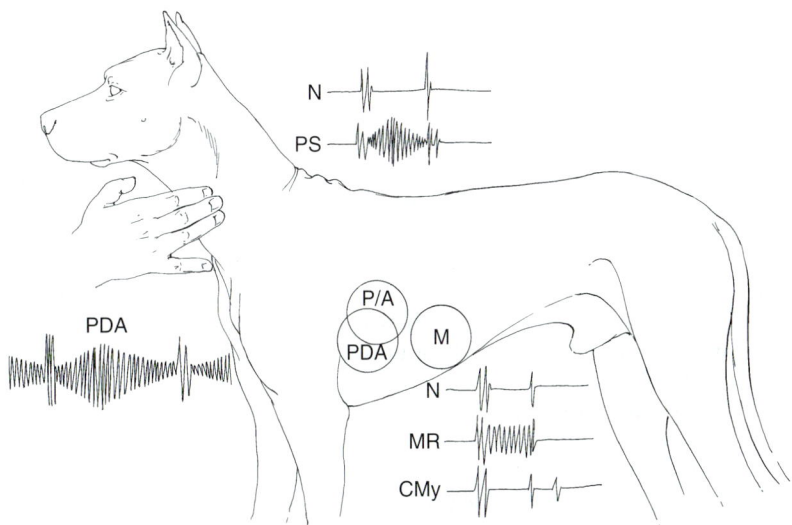

Figure 59–3. Regions where murmurs are heard best on the left hemithorax. Diagrams of murmurs typical of specific defects are shown. Normal (N) heart sounds are indicated above the murmurs of pulmonic stenosis (PS) and mitral regurgitation (MR). The diastolic gallop heard with dilated cardiomyopathy (CMy) is shown below the murmur for mitral regurgitation. PDA is the continuous murmur of patent ductus arteriosus. P/A is the ejection murmur of pulmonic stenosis or aortic stenosis. (Note: Loud murmurs of aortic stenosis may be heard equally on the right base as well.) M demonstrates systolic regurgitant murmur of mitral regurgitation.

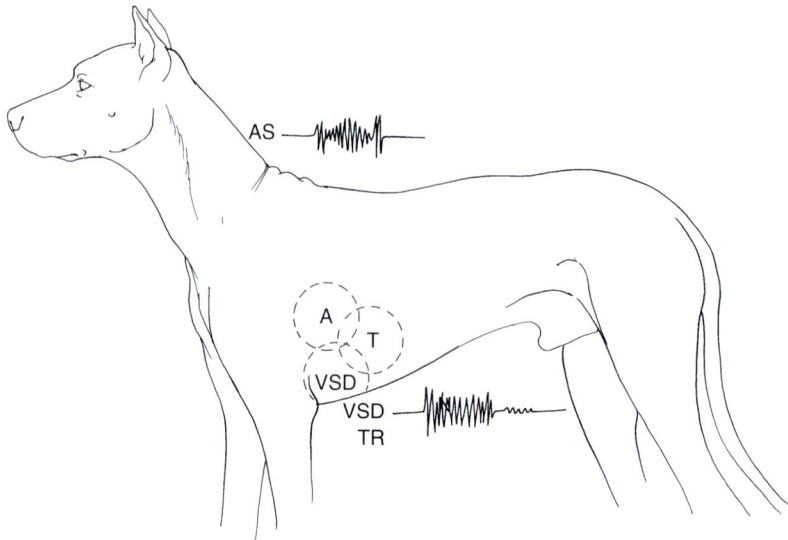

Figure 59–4. Left lateral view demonstrating where murmurs are heard best on the right hemithorax. A is the systolic ejection murmur of aortic stenosis (AS) and may be equally loud at left and right hemithorax. Systolic regurgitant murmur of ventricular septal defect (VSD) is heard best at the right sternal border. A soft diastolic murmur may also be heard from concurrent aortic regurgitation or increased flow across the mitral valve. T indicates where the systolic murmur of tricuspid regurgitation (TR) is heard best.

and the lung insulates against the transmission of sound.

- Percussion note is hyper-resonant (i.e., sounds like thumping on a tympany drum) because the thoracic wall acts like a drumhead stretched over an air-filled chamber underneath.

Pleural Effusion (see Chap. 80)

- All breath sounds are softer than normal because free liquid between pulmonary parenchyma and chest wall reflects sound away from its pathway to the stethoscope chest piece.
- Percussion note is dull because the water-filled cavity vibrates at high frequency and low amplitude and is dampened rapidly.
- Pulmonary retraction is an indention of the thoracic wall caused by fatigue of muscles of ventilation. Regions of the thoracic wall affected must generate greatest tension during ventilation and do not have assistance from thoracic limbs. Pulmonary retraction produces an "hourglass" configuration to the thorax in the dorsoventral radiograph.

Abdominal Percussion

- *Hepatic enlargement* generates a dull note over a larger area than expected because the liver is an exceptionally dense structure.
- *Bloated (air-filled) stomach* is distended and generates a hyper-resonant percussion note because skin serves as the head of the drum and the gas in the stomach serves as the air-filled kettle of the drum. The abdomen bloated with gas produces an exceptional hourglass configuration with pulmonary retractions. It can be differentiated from organomegaly and/or ascites by the following:
  - It is tympanic (hyper-resonance).
  - It comes and goes quickly.
  - Air is often in the esophagus.

Auscultatory Findings in Heart Disease

Left Hemithorax (see Fig. 59–3)

Mitral Valve Region

- This region is also known as the left apical region and is at the left fifth intercostal space near approximately two to three fingerbreadths from the left sternal border.
- Normally, S_1 is louder, longer in duration, and lower pitched than S_2. S_1 is mimicked as a "lub"; S_2 is mimicked as a "dup."
- The murmur of mitral regurgitation extends from S_1 to, and often through, S_2.

▼ *Key Point* The intensity of the murmurs of mitral and tricuspid regurgitation does *not* consistently correlate with the severity of the regurgitation and is influenced profoundly by the force of contraction of the ventricle.

- In dogs and cats with dilated cardiomyopathy, there is often an S_3 gallop producing a set of sounds like lub-dup-uh.

Pulmonary Artery Region

- This is normally where S_2 is heard the loudest.
- The murmur of pulmonic stenosis (see Chap. 70) is heard loudest here. It is usually very loud and radiated dorsad; it is short in duration and very rough.
- There is often a pronounced splitting of S_2 caused by the pulmonic valve closing later than the aortic valve—this is particularly pronounced during inspiration.
- The murmur of aortic stenosis (see Chap. 70) is heard equally loudly here and at the same position on the right hemithorax.

▼ *Key Point* The intensity of murmurs of pulmonic and aortic stenoses correlates well with the severity of the stenosis.

Patent Ductus Arteriosus Region

The continuous murmur of the patent ductus arteriosus (PDA) is heard the loudest in the PDA region. With this murmur, S_2 may not be heard because the murmur of blood rushing through the PDA is loudest during the time S_2 is generated. See Chapters 70 and 71 for more on PDA.

Right Hemithorax

- At the region of the right fourth intercostal space at the sternal border, S_1 is louder than S_2. The systolic murmur of ventricular septal defect is heard best here and is louder during exhalation.
- At the region of the right fifth intercostal space above the costochondral junction the systolic murmur of tricuspid regurgitation is heard best and is louder during inspiration.
- At the region of the right base the systolic murmur of aortic stenosis is almost as loud as at the left base and is louder during exhalation than during inhalation.

60 Cardiovascular Radiography

Wendy Myer / John D. Bonagura

Thoracic radiography is useful in the recognition and assessment of cardiovascular diseases. When combined with the results of the clinical examination, thoracic radiographs may contribute to the specific cardiac diagnosis, verify the presence of congestive heart failure (CHF), and assist in the differential diagnosis of respiratory signs such as coughing and dyspnea. Analysis of thoracic radiographs, including vascular patterns, is discussed in detail in Chapter 75. This chapter describes specific aspects of radiography useful in cardiac diagnosis.

▼ *Key Point* The importance of the technical quality of thoracic radiographs is often underestimated. A poor radiograph with inadequate penetration or poor patient positioning may be misleading and worse than no radiograph at all.

This can be avoided by addressing the following technical aspects prior to radiographic evaluation for cardiac disease.

GENERAL PRINCIPLES

Obtaining the Radiograph

- Two views, a lateral projection and either a dorsoventral (DV) or ventrodorsal (VD) projection, are needed for complete thoracic evaluation.
  - Cardiomegaly may be suspected on one view but may not be confirmed on the complementary projection.
  - The caudal lobar pulmonary arteries are best seen using DV projection.
- Radiographic technique (see Chap. 4):
  - Take films at the peak of inspiration.
  - Expiratory films are ineffective for evaluating the lung parenchyma for pulmonary edema.
  - A long-scale (high-kVp, low-mAs) technique is most helpful for assessing thoracic disease. Underexposure mimics pulmonary disease by increasing apparent pulmonary density, whereas overexposure leads to an underestimation of the severity of pulmonary changes.
- Patient positioning:
  - Rotation often accentuates normal structures such as the main pulmonary artery on the VD projection or the left atrium or right ventricle on the lateral projection.

- False apex shifting due to patient rotation on the VD projection may cause overestimation of ventricular size.

Interpreting the Radiograph

Once an adequately positioned and exposed radiograph has been obtained, attempt to answer the following general questions during the radiographic assessment of cardiac disease.

- Is cardiomegaly present or absent? If present, is this cardiac enlargement mild, moderate, or severe?
  - Species and conformational variations are important in this assessment (e.g., barrel-chested dogs normally have wider and more rounded hearts, and the cardiac size appears large relative to the thoracic volume, whereas deep-chested dogs have a narrower, more vertically oriented heart shadow).
  - It may be useful to calculate a vertebral heart score in dogs, particularly in cases of equivocal cardiomegaly. This score can be useful in toy breed dogs, which often appear to have cardiomegaly by subjective evaluation.
- Which specific cardiac chambers are abnormal? Is more than one cardiac chamber affected? Is the abnormality restricted to one side of the heart or is it generalized?
  - Enlargement of one ventricle may cause the heart to rotate, leading to overestimation of the size of other cardiac chambers (e.g., right ventricular enlargement causes the apex to shift toward the left thoracic wall on the VD projection, mimicking left ventricular enlargement).
- Is the cardiac apex in its normal position? If not, is this shift due to poor patient positioning?
- Are the great vessels (aorta and main pulmonary artery) normal or abnormal in appearance?
- Are the pulmonary vessels normal, small, or enlarged (see Chap. 75)? Are the changes restricted to the arteries (e.g., heartworm), veins (e.g., venous congestion), or are both altered in size (e.g., pulmonary under- or overcirculation or pulmonary hypertension from left-sided heart failure)?
- Is the radiographic opacity of the lung normal, decreased, or increased? Are areas of increased opacity generalized or focal? If diffuse, what is the distribution of the pulmonary infiltrates (generalized, dorsal-caudal, or cranial-ventral)? See Chapter 75 for

more information on radiography of the respiratory tract.

- Is there evidence of pleural effusion?
  - This may be indicative of biventricular or severe right-sided CHF or may be noncardiogenic in origin.
  - Thoracocentesis is necessary to determine the type of fluid present (see Chap. 80).
  - The cardiac silhouette is more obscured on a DV projection than on a VD projection in the presence of a mild to moderate amount of pleural fluid due to the effect of gravity on fluid distribution.
  - Patient stress may preclude a complete radiographic examination initially, but further films may be possible following thoracocentesis. These radiographs should be made with the patient in the same position as the original examination, as this allows a more accurate comparison of residual fluid volume.
- Are the diaphragm and extrathoracic structures normal? If not, are the changes most likely congenital (e.g., peritoneopericardial hernia) or acquired (e.g., rib fractures indicating recent thoracic trauma)?

CARDIAC EVALUATION: NORMAL FINDINGS

Lateral View (Fig. 60–1)

Dogs

- The cardiac outline is roughly tear-shaped.
- Orientation—approximately a 45° angle with the sternum (varies with breed).
- Location—extends from the third to sixth ribs, and the heart and diaphragm usually touch or overlap.
- Size—ventricles occupy approximately three intercostal spaces and using the vertebral score method, 8.5–10.6 (mean, 9.7) vertebral bodies (T4) in dogs, and 8.5–9.0 in cats.

- Cardiac borders represent:
  - Cranial—right ventricle and auricle (rounded border).
  - Caudal—left ventricle and atrium (straight border).
  - Dorsal—both atria, pulmonary arteries, both venae cavae, and aorta.
- Quadrants: The cardiac silhouette can be divided into sections on the lateral radiograph by drawing a line from the tracheal bifurcation to the apex parallel to the cardiac axis and a second horizontal line at the level of the vena cava.
  - Atria are dorsal to the horizontal line.
  - Ventricles are ventral to the horizontal line.
  - Right-sided heart structures make up the cranial three-fifths of the heart shadow.
  - Left-sided heart structures make up the caudal two-fifths of the heart shadow.

Cats

- The cardiac outline is more elongated and elliptical than in the dog.
- Orientation is more variable than in the dog, with a more horizontal major cardiac axis.
- Location—the heart and diaphragm are separated by one to two intercostal spaces.
- Size—the ventricles occupy approximately 2–2.5 intercostal spaces and the heart extends about two-thirds of the ventrodorsal height of the thorax.
- Cardiac borders are similar to those in the dog.

Ventrodorsal or Dorsoventral Views (Fig. 60–2)

Dogs

- The cardiac outline has a curved right border and a straight left border.
- Orientation—the apex is slightly to the left of midline, approximately at a 30° angle with the spine.

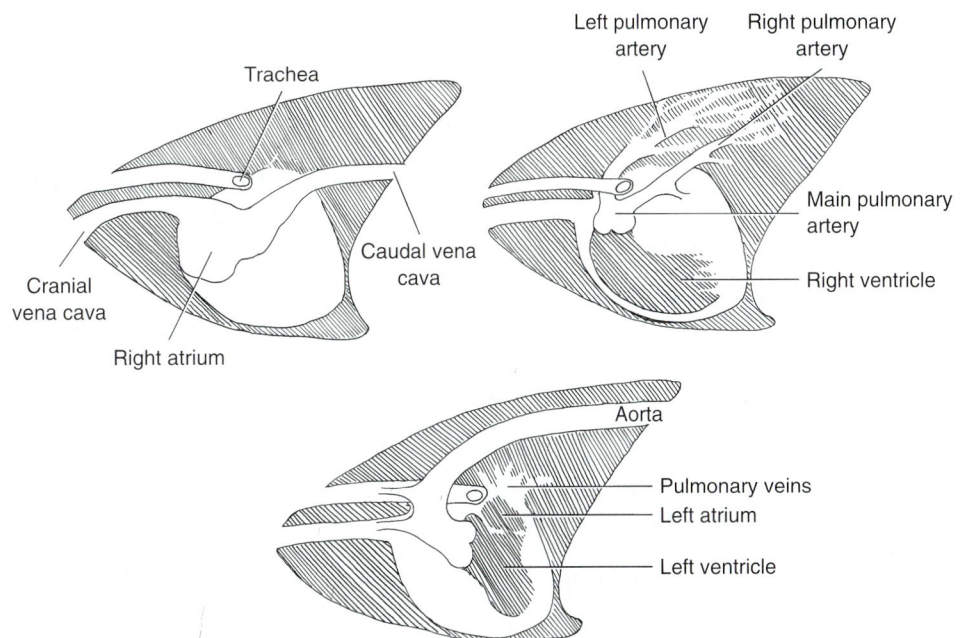

Figure 60–1. Three lateral views of the normal heart showing chamber location.

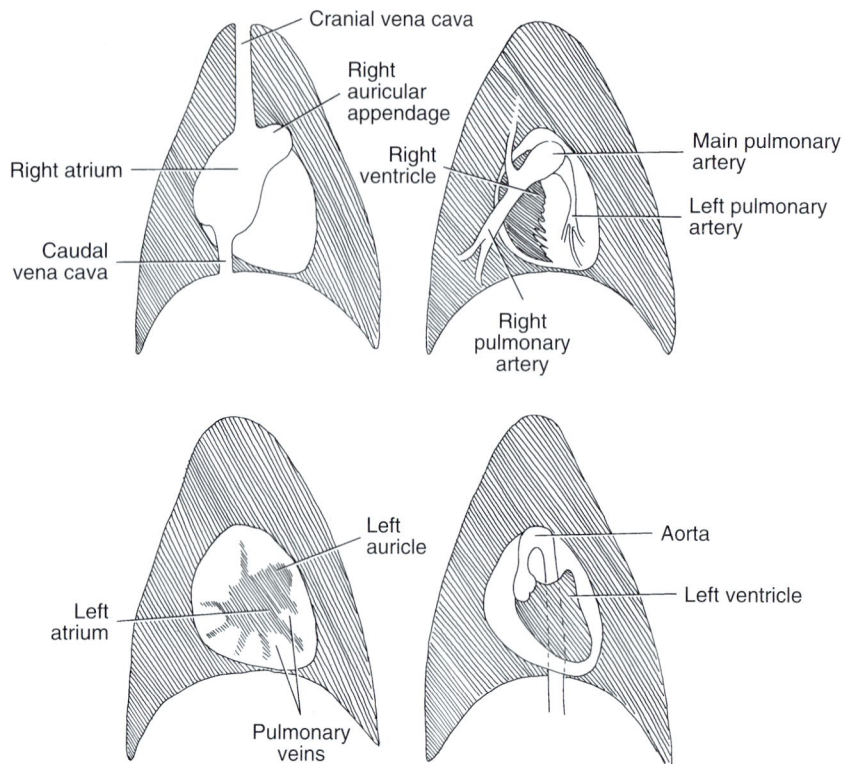

Figure 60–2. Four ventrodorsal views of the normal heart showing chamber location.

- Location—extends from the third to the eighth vertebrae, often touching the diaphragm.
- Size—the cardiac-thoracic index (ratio) is about 60–65% of the thorax as measured from right to left.
- Cardiac borders (using the clock face analogy):
  - 11 to 1 o'clock—aortic arch
  - 1 to 2 o'clock—main pulmonary artery
  - 2 to 3 o'clock—left auricular appendage
  - 3 to 6 o'clock—left ventricle
  - 6 to 11 o'clock—right ventricle
  - 9 to 11 o'clock—right atrium

Cats

- The cardiac outline is slightly more elongated than in the dog.
- Orientation—the apex is at or slightly to the left of midline.
- Location—the heart and diaphragm are separated by one to two intercostal spaces.
- Cardiac borders are similar to those in the dog, except that the main pulmonary artery does not usually contribute to the 1 to 2 o'clock border.

Pulmonary Arteries and Veins

- Lateral view—the artery (A) is dorsal to the bronchus (B) and vein (V) (A-B-V from dorsal to ventral).
- VD or DV views:
  - Arteries are lateral to the bronchus and vein.
  - Arteries originate cranial to the carina.
  - Veins terminate in the left atrium caudal to the carina (veins are ventral and central).
- Size:
  - Arteries and veins are approximately equal in size.

- Normal vessel to rib ratio (compare with proximal one-third of fourth rib) is 0.75–0.8 (with a wide range of 0.5–1.25).
- The arteries and veins appear larger on DV views because of magnification.
- Margination:
  - Vessels are best seen on the lateral view as they extend into the cranial lobes.
  - Vessels in the lung farthest from the cassette are magnified.
- Arteries are more dense than veins, slightly curved, and have dichotomous branching (branches of equal size).
- Veins are less visible, are straighter and blunter than arteries, and have branches of unequal size.

RADIOGRAPHIC SIGNS OF CARDIOVASCULAR DISEASE

Right Atrial Enlargement

The right atrium (RA) is the most difficult chamber to detect radiographically (Fig. 60–3).

Lateral View

- RA enlargement usually is not seen on this view.
- Loss or filling in of the normal concave angle between the ventral edge of the cranial mediastinum and the cardiac silhouette (the cranial "waist") may be seen due to bulging of the right auricular appendage. In some cases the cranial waist may become accentuated due to discrete auricular enlargement.

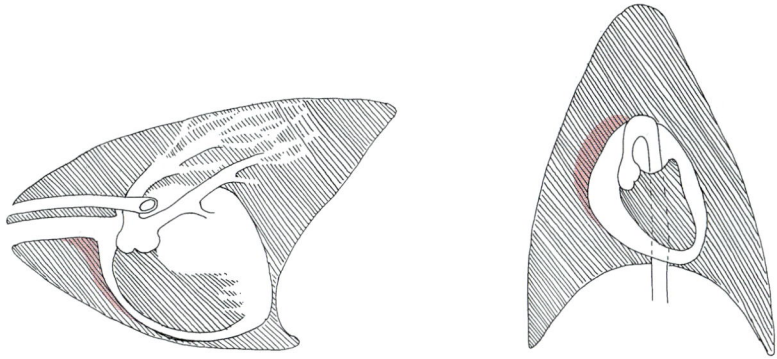

Figure 60-3. Radiographic appearance of right atrial enlargement. The red areas denote the abnormal region.

Dorsoventral or Ventrodorsal Views

- Bulging of the cranial right heart border (9 to 11 o'clock) is typical of RA dilation.
- RA dilation is often masked by concurrent right ventricular enlargement.

Causes

- Atrial septal defect (ASD).
- Pulmonic stenosis.
- Tricuspid regurgitation.
- RA tumors.
- Atrial fibrillation.
- Advanced heartworm disease.
- Pulmonary hypertension (including cor pulmonale).
- Primary right atrial or ventricular myocardial disease.
- Chronic bradycardia.
- Tricuspid stenosis (congenital).

Right Ventricular Enlargement (Fig. 60–4)

Lateral View

- Increased overall width of the heart.
- Rounding of the cranial heart border.
- Elevation of the cardiac apex and caudal vena cava.
- In severe right ventricular (RV) enlargement, elevation of the trachea cranial to the carina and some degree of cardiac elongation.

Dorsoventral or Ventrodorsal View

- Rounding of the right heart border (6 to 11 o'clock).

- "Reversed D" appearance if the main pulmonary artery is also dilated.
- Increased overall width of the heart.
- Decreased distance between the right side of the heart and thoracic wall or shifting of the apex to the left side.

Causes

- Pulmonic stenosis.
- Tricuspid regurgitation.
- Pulmonary hypertension of any cause (e.g., heartworm disease, cor pulmonale, congenital disease with Eisenmenger reaction, pulmonary thromboembolism).
- Tetralogy of Fallot.
- ASD.
- Some ventricular septal defects (VSDs).
- Primary right ventricular cardiomyopathy.
- Chagas disease.
- Chronic bradycardia.
- High-output heart failure (moderate to severe anemia, hyperthyroidism, arteriovenous fistula).

Left Atrial Enlargement (Fig. 60–5)

Lateral View

- Elevation of the distal end of the trachea with dorsal displacement and compression of the left main stem bronchus between the left atrium and descending aorta.
- Bulging of the caudal-dorsal heart border (dorsal to the caudal vena cava).
- Filling in and loss of the normal caudal indentation

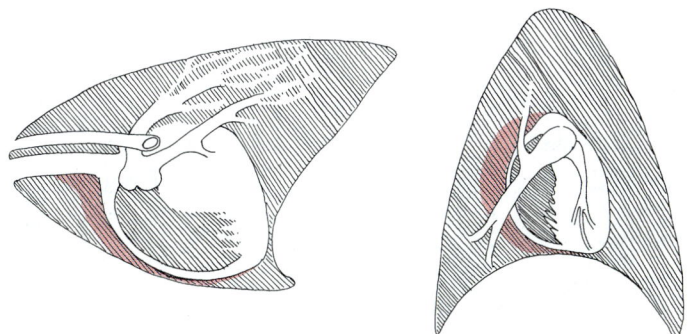

Figure 60-4. Radiographic appearance of right atrial and ventricular enlargement. The red region denotes the abnormality.

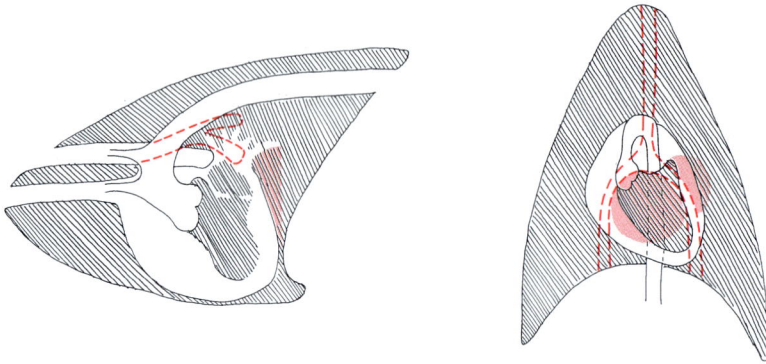

Figure 60–5. Radiographic appearance of left atrial enlargement. The red region denotes the abnormality. (Dotted red lines outline the trachea and mainstem bronchi.)

of the cardiac border (the caudal waist); or, with marked dilation, accentuation of the caudal waist as the atrium projects caudodorsally.

Dorsoventral or Ventrodorsal View

- The left atrium proper is a midline structure and does not normally contribute to the heart border on this view.
- There is displacement and separation of the main stem bronchi as they approach the cranial border of the left atrium and bifurcate around this chamber (producing a "bow-legged cowboy" appearance to the bronchial tree).
- On a well-exposed DV view, the enlarged atrium may be seen as a round, soft tissue mass summated on the caudal heart border.
- Left auricular dilation is seen in dogs as bulging of the left heart border at 2 to 3 o'clock, and in cats as a bulge from 1 to 3 o'clock.

Causes

- Mitral regurgitation (MR).
- Patent ductus arteriosus (PDA).
- Ventricular septal defect.
- Cardiomyopathy (all forms).
- Mitral dysplasia (causing MR ± mitral stenosis).
- Hyperthyroidism.
- Hypertensive heart disease.
- Left-sided CHF from any cause.

Left Ventricular Enlargement (Fig. 60–6)

Lateral View

- Elongation of the cardiac silhouette and possibly widening of the silhouette.
- Rounding of the caudal heart border.
- Elevation of the carina and distal end of the trachea (causing the trachea to more closely parallel the spine than the sternum; this finding depends on chest conformation and breed).

Dorsoventral or Ventrodorsal View

- Elongation, rounding, and expansion of the left heart border.
- Rounding of the cardiac apex.
- Decreased distance between the left heart border and thoracic wall, or shifting of the cardiac apex to the right (especially common in cats).

Causes

- Mitral regurgitation.
- Patent ductus arteriosus.
- Ventricular septal defect.
- Aortic stenosis.
- Aortic regurgitation (e.g., bacterial endocarditis).
- Cardiomyopathy of any cause.
- Hyperthyroidism.
- Hypertensive heart disease.
- High-output heart failure (moderate to severe anemia, arteriovenous fistula).

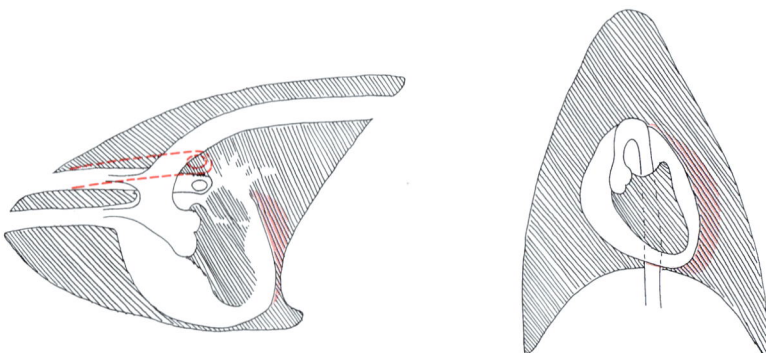

Figure 60–6. Radiographic appearance of left ventricular (with or without atrial) enlargement. The red region denotes the abnormality. (Dotted red lines outline the trachea.)

Generalized (Biventricular) Cardiac Enlargement

- This is a relatively common feature of many cardiac disorders.
- It usually is difficult to determine which ventricle is most enlarged on survey films alone; therefore, ancillary studies such as echocardiography are extremely helpful in assessing chamber size and ventricular function.
- The heart appears generally rounded, and usually there is increased sternal contact on the lateral view.

Causes

- Chronic valvular heart disease (mitral and tricuspid regurgitation).
- Left-sided heart failure (any cause) with secondary pulmonary hypertension.
- Ventricular septal defect.
- Dilated cardiomyopathy.
- Mild to moderate pericardial effusion (mimics cardiomegaly).
- High-output heart failure (moderate to severe anemia, arteriovenous fistula, hyperthyroidism).
- Overinfusion of intravenous fluids.

Microcardia

- A generalized decrease in cardiac size is most often associated with plasma volume contraction, shock, or trauma.
- Decreased cardiac size allows the heart to shift off the midline when the patient is in lateral recumbency, making the heart appear elevated from the sternum similar to the radiographic appearance of pneumothorax.
- Pulmonary circulation often appears diminished.

Causes

- Hypovolemic shock.
- Addison's disease.
- Hemorrhage.
- Protracted vomiting/diarrhea.
- Obstructive hepatic circulation (cirrhosis, caudal vena cava obstruction).

Aortic Enlargement (Fig. 60–7)

- The direction of bulging depends on the underlying etiology.
  - Patent ductus arteriosus—some cranial bulging of the aortic arch is seen, but the most pronounced bulging is toward the left side at the site of the patent ductus ("ductus bump"). This is seen on the DV or VD view.
  - Aortic stenosis—there is dilation of the ascending aorta (cranioventrally) and aortic arch (cranially) caused by poststenotic turbulence; a similar feature is observed with tetralogy of Fallot and pulmonary atresia due to increased aortic blood flow (right-to-left shunt) and dextropositioned aorta.
- Persistent right fourth aortic arch—on the VD or DV view, the aorta may descend to the right side (mirror-image arch) instead of left of midline.
- Dilation and tortuosity of the ascending aorta, arch, or descending aorta may be observed in cats with hyperthyroidism or systemic hypertension, or as an incidental senile change in aged cats.

Pulmonary Artery

Enlargement of the main pulmonary artery leads to bulging of the left cranial cardiac border at 1 o'clock (DV or VD view) in the dog (usually not evident in cats).

Causes

- Increased blood flow (PDA, VSD, ASD).
- Poststenotic dilation (pulmonic stenosis).
- Pulmonary hypertension (heartworm disease, severe pulmonary thromboembolism, or related to congenital pulmonary vascular disease).

Pulmonary Vascularity (Fig. 60–8)

- Assessment of pulmonary vascularity requires judgment and evaluation of other cardiac structures. General guidelines include:
  - Lateral view: Evaluate vessels as they extend into the cranial lobes. The lobar artery is dorsal to the bronchus and vein. Peripheral vascular markings normally are prominent in deep-chested dogs and in many cats (following full inspiration).

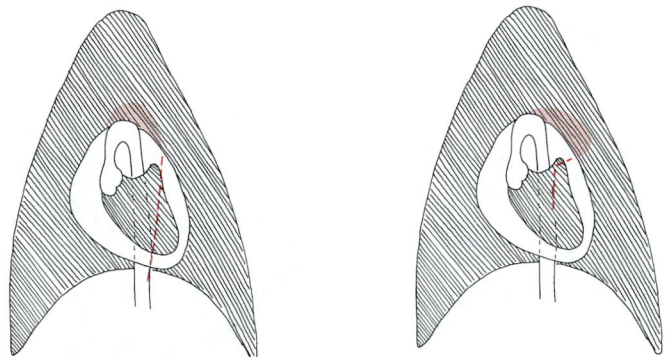

Figure 60–7. Radiographic appearance of aortic enlargement. *Left,* Aortic stenosis. *Right,* Patent ductus arteriosus.

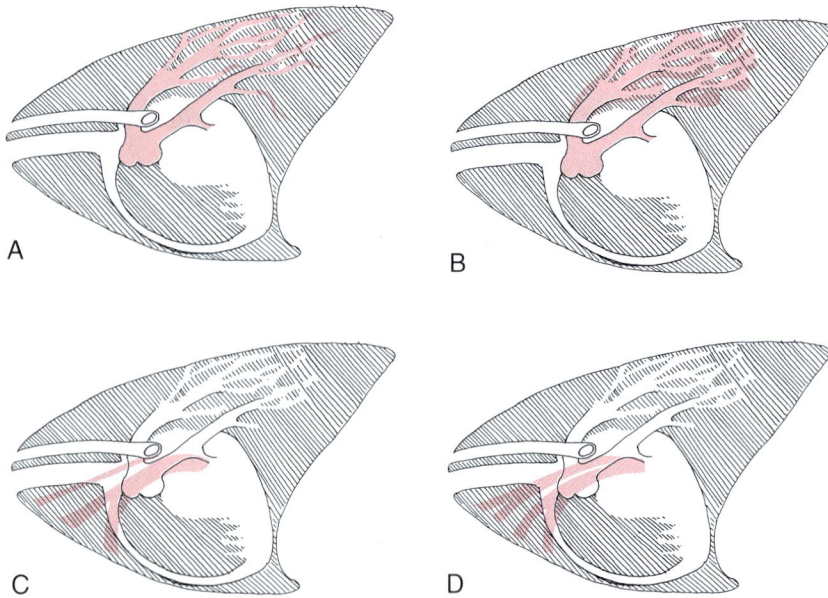

Figure 60–8. Radiographic appearance of pulmonic circulatory disorders. *A,* Normal pulmonary circulation. *B,* Pulmonary arterial hypertension caused by heartworm disease. *C,* Effects of venous congestion due to mitral insufficiency. *D,* Signs of pulmonary overcirculation caused by left-to-right shunt or pulmonary hypertension due to left-sided congestive heart failure.

- DV or VD view: Evaluate vessels as they extend beyond the heart border. The lobar artery is lateral to the bronchus and vein.
- The normal artery and vein should be equal in size and average 75% of the width of the proximal one-third of the rib at the same level (fourth rib on the lateral view). Also, the vessels should not exceed the width of the ninth rib at the point of intersection.
- Decreased vascular markings are typical of under-circulation due to right-to-left cardiac shunts (e.g., tetralogy of Fallot), low cardiac output (e.g., tricuspid regurgitation, cardiac tamponade), or plasma volume contraction (e.g., shock).

Causes

- Overcirculation (increased flow due to left-to-right shunts such as patent ductus arteriosus, ventricular and atrial septal defects, or hyperdynamic circulation as with severe anemia or thyrotoxicosis) leads to dilation of both pulmonary arteries and veins. Enhanced vascularity in the peripheral lung fields also may be evident.
- Pulmonary arterial and venous hypertension causes widening of the affected vessels. Left-sided CHF

causes pulmonary venous hypertension. Pulmonary arterial hypertension is caused by heartworm disease, pulmonary embolism, Eisenmenger reaction, and left-sided CHF. When arterial hypertension is caused by left-sided CHF, pulmonary venous distention also is prominent.

Congestive Heart Failure

- Cardiomegaly is expected, particularly atrial enlargement (Fig. 60–9).
- Increased pulmonary venous size indicates elevated pulmonary venous pressure ("congestion" or "venous hypertension"). Secondary pulmonary arterial hypertension may be observed as well.

Left-Sided Congestive Heart Failure

- Left-sided CHF is characterized by increased pulmonary density.
- Initially, perivascular interstitial densities that blur vascular margins are seen. These progress to a diffuse interstitial density and airway cuffing with ensuing alveolar flooding.
- Alveolar patterns are recognized as fluffy, coalescing densities with increased air-filled bronchi contrasted

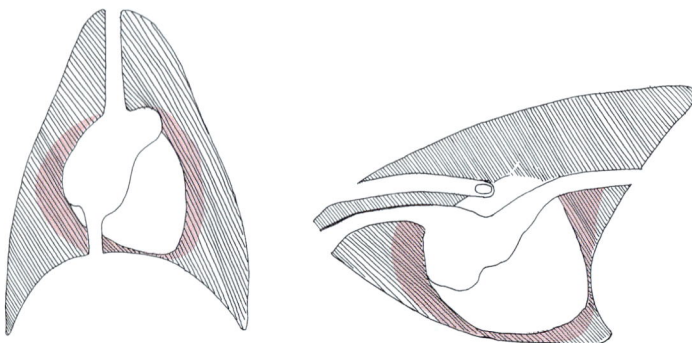

Figure 60–9. Radiographic appearance of generalized cardiomegaly. The red regions denote the abnormalities.

with the fluid-filled lung (air bronchogram sign). Fluid density structures such as the heart and diaphragm may be obscured (border effacement).

- Distribution of cardiac edema is usually perihilar, dorsal, and bilateral; however, right-sided prominence is common in severe edema due to different lymphatic drainage between the right and left lung. Diffuse or dependent infiltrates may be observed in fulminant cardiogenic edema.
- Expect mobilization of alveolar edema within 48–72 hours following aggressive therapy for CHF (see Chap. 64). Radiographic changes often lag behind clinical improvement or deterioration by 12–18 hours. Failure to resolve increased pulmonary densities following appropriate treatment should prompt a reconsideration of the diagnosis of cardiogenic lung edema.
- Development of pleural fissure lines and pleural effusion is usually a sign of biventricular CHF. Severe pleural effusion often indicates right ventricular decompensation associated with pulmonary hypertension secondary to left-sided disease. Cardiac tamponade is another cause of pleural effusion.

▼ *Key Point* Chronic left-sided CHF can be characterized by recurrent, labile pulmonary infiltrate (edema) or by a static, fine, interstitial lung density that may represent congestion-induced pulmonary fibrosis. Alveolar infiltrates are unlikely unless therapy is suspended or there is acute deterioration in heart function (e.g., ruptured mitral chorda tendinea or atrial fibrillation).

RADIOGRAPHIC FINDINGS IN SPECIFIC DISEASES

The radiographic features of many cardiac disorders are described in detail in other chapters in Section 6. Table 60–1 summarizes typical features of common conditions. Some clinical pointers are offered in the following sections.

Valvular Heart Disease (see Chap. 65.)

- The degree of atrial dilation seen radiographically usually corresponds to the severity of chronic valvular regurgitation; however, in acute heart failure or with a ruptured chorda tendinea, left atrial enlargement may not be marked.
- Chronic regurgitation allows the atrium to expand and increase its compliance; therefore, severe cardiomegaly can develop prior to onset of CHF.
- Compression of the left main stem bronchus by the enlarged left atrium may persist following resolution of lung edema. This finding is often associated with recurrent coughing.

Cardiomyopathy (see Chap. 66)

Hypertrophic Cardiomyopathy

Hypertrophic cardiomyopathy is now the most common cause of CHF in cats. The radiographic features

are variable, and heart size can change dramatically following diuretic therapy. Other cardiomyopathies, severe anemia, or advanced hyperthyroid heart disease can produce similar radiographic features.

- Dilation of the left atrium or auricle is the most consistent feature, and left auricular enlargement may produce a "valentine-shaped heart" on the VD projection.
- LV hypertrophy is concentric, but often leads to elongation of the heart.
- Pulmonary edema can be widespread or patchy, and distributed ventrally (dependent), dorsad, or generalized.
- Pleural effusion develops in chronic cases secondary to pulmonary hypertension and biventricular CHF.

Dilated Cardiomyopathy

Dilated cardiomyopathy is characterized by biventricular dilation and often a rounded cardiac silhouette.

- A globoid appearance may mimic the changes seen with pericardial effusion; however, pulmonary venous congestion is usually evident with cardiomyopathy but absent in pericardial effusion.
- Left-sided or biventricular heart failure may develop.

▼ *Key Point* The radiographic features of dilated cardiomyopathy cannot be reliably distinguished from those of chronic atrioventricular valve regurgitation. Echocardiography is required.

Pericardial Disease

- The radiographic appearance depends on the degree of pericardial effusion. When there is only a small amount of fluid, the heart may appear normal or minimally enlarged.
- Progressive pericardial effusion causes the heart to appear globular in shape on both views ("pumpkin heart").
- Pleural effusion may be evident, as well as hepatomegaly and ascites, when there is concurrent CHF.
- Pulmonary vascularity, when evident, is often diminished.
- Acute pericardial effusion in dogs with chronic mitral valve disease may indicate left atrial rupture.
- Heart base tumors are often associated with some degree of pericardial effusion. A bulge may be noted near the aortic arch, heart base, or within the cranial mediastinum.

Peritoneopericardial Hernia

Peritoneopericardial hernia, very common in cats, leads to some features of pericardial effusion. Other signs include:
- The heart shadow cannot be separated from the diaphragm.
- Gas-filled loops of bowel within the pericardial shadow may be seen (more common in dogs).
- Fat density (omentum) may be noted in the caudal ventral pericardial space (especially in cats).

Table 60–1. TYPICAL RADIOGRAPHIC FEATURES OF HEART DISEASE

Disorder	LV	LA	Ao	RV	RA	MPA	Pulmonary Circulation	Additional Findings
Patent ductus arteriosus	+	+	+ Desc Ao	0*	0		+ Artery + Vein	Left-sided CHF
Ventricular septal defect	+	+	0	+†	0†	+	+ Artery + Vein	Left-sided CHF
Atrial septal defect	0	0‡	0	+	+	+	+ Artery + Vein	Right-sided CHF
Mitral regurgitation	+	+	0	+†	0	0	+ Vein 0/+ Artery†	Left-sided CHF
Tricuspid regurgitation	0	0	0	+	+	0	0	Dilated vena cava Right-sided CHF
Aortic stenosis	+	0/+	+ Asc Ao	0	0	0	0/+ Vein 0/+ Artery†	Left-sided CHF
Pulmonic stenosis	0	0	0	+	+	+	0/− Artery 0/− Vein	Right-sided CHF
Tetralogy of Fallot	0	0	+§	+	+	‖	− Artery − Vein	
Dilated cardiomyopathy	+	+	0	+	+	0	+ Vein 0/+ Artery	Biventricular CHF
Hypertrophic cardiomyopathy	+	+	0	0/+†	0/+†	0	+ Vein 0/+ Artery†	Left-sided or biventricular CHF
Restrictive cardiomyopathy	+	+	0	+	+	−	+ Vein 0/− Artery†	Variable findings
Pericardial effusion	+	+	0	+	+	0	0/− Artery 0/− Vein	Possible mass lesion
Hyperthyroidism	+	+	+	+	+	0	0/+ Artery 0/+ Vein	Dilated or tortuous aorta
Pulmonary hypertension	0/+¶	0/+¶	0	+	+	+	−/0/+ Artery −/0/+ Vein¶,#	Lungs may be abnormal or undercirculated
Heartworm disease	0	0	0	+	+	+	+ Artery 0 Vein	Pulmonary infiltrate

*Although the RV may appear enlarged, the echocardiograph demonstrates that LV dilatation accounts for ventricular enlargement; in the rare case of reversed patent ductus arteriosus, the radiograph resembles that of pulmonary hypertension.

†Right-sided cardiomegaly develops if there is pulmonary hypertension due to increased pulmonary flow, increased pulmonary vascular resistance, or both. Otherwise, right-sided cardiomegaly is variable.

‡In the typical ostium secundum (high) atrial septal defect (ASD), blood flows immediately into the RA and the LA doesn't enlarge substantially. In cases of primum ASD with concurrent ventricular septal defect, or mitral dysplasia (endocardial cushion defect), LA dilation also develops.

§The aorta is dextropositioned and receives the most blood flow; this causes widening of the ventrocranial mediastinum on the lateral projection.

‖The pulmonary artery is not dilated because blood preferentially shunts across the ventricular septal defect into the aorta.

¶In cases of pulmonary hypertension secondary to left-sided CHF, left-sided heart structures are enlarged.

#In cases of pulmonary hypertension secondary to left-sided CHF, pulmonary venous distention is also present; in pulmonary hypertension caused by pulmonary vascular disease (e.g., reversed patent ductus arteriosus, primary pulmonary hypertension), peripheral pulmonary vascularity is decreased, whereas central lobar vessels are dilated from pressure.

Ao, aorta; CHF, congestive heart failure; LA, left atrium; LV, left ventricle; MPA, main pulmonary artery; RA, right atrium; RV, right ventricle; 0, no change; +, enlarged or increased; −, decreased; desc, descending; asc, ascending.

- A persistent mesothelial remnant is evident ventral to and parallel to the caudal vena cava (which is displaced dorsally).
- The entry of the caudal pulmonary veins into the left atrium is abnormal (displaced cranially on the lateral view).
- There may be pectus excavatum or an absence or malformation of the last sternebra.

SUPPLEMENTAL READING

Suter PF: Thoracic Radiography: A Text Atlas of Thoracic Diseases of the Dog and Cat. Wettswil, Switzerland: Peter F. Suter, 1984, pp 351–516.

61 Electrocardiography

Francis W. K. Smith, Jr. / Larry Patrick Tilley / Michael S. Miller

Electrocardiography is the graphic representation of the electrical activity of the heart. Electrocardiograms (ECGs) are easy to perform and readily available to practicing veterinarians. There are numerous indications for performing ECGs. This test provides a wealth of information that is useful in the diagnosis and management of cardiac and systemic disturbances.

GENERAL PRINCIPLES OF ELECTROCARDIOGRAPHY

Indications for Performing Electrocardiography

- To diagnose an arrhythmia detected on physical examination (auscultation, arterial pulse deficits, palpable precordial heart beat irregularities, or abnormal jugular venous pulsations).
  - The ECG is the most sensitive test for the diagnosis of arrhythmias and for monitoring the effect of antiarrhythmic therapy.

▼ *Key Point* Perform an ECG on all animals with tachycardia or bradycardia and on all cats with any irregularity in rhythm. Perform an ECG on any dog with an irregularity in rhythm that is related to a pulse deficit or is not related to phases of respiration.

- To rule out arrhythmias or conduction disturbances in patients with a history of syncope, seizures, or exercise intolerance.
- To monitor effectiveness of antiarrhythmic therapy.
- To assess cardiac size in patients with known or suspected cardiac disease.
  - The ECG is not a very sensitive indicator of heart size. A heart enlargement pattern on the ECG usually correlates with cardiac chamber enlargement or hypertrophy. The more criteria for heart enlargement that are present in a patient, the more likely the heart is enlarged. Most dogs with normal hearts will not exhibit heart enlargement patterns on ECGs.

▼ *Key Point* A normal ECG does not rule out a diagnosis of heart enlargement. Thoracic radiographs and echocardiography are more sensitive tests for evaluating heart size.

- To help individualize and monitor therapy in patients with heart failure.
  - The diagnosis of congestive heart failure (CHF) cannot be made based on an ECG alone.

▼ *Key Point* An arrhythmia or a heart enlargement pattern supports the diagnosis of heart disease but does not confirm CHF. Obtain thoracic radiographs along with an ECG in a patient suspected of having CHF. The ECG is useful in patients with heart failure for the diagnosis and treatment of associated arrhythmias.

- To evaluate patients with suspected digoxin or other cardiac drug toxicity.
- To screen for electrolyte disturbances, especially hyperkalemia, hypercalcemia, and hypocalcemia.
- To look for evidence to support a diagnosis of pericardial effusion, hypothyroidism, hyperthyroidism, or hypoadrenocorticism (Addison's disease).

Technique for Recording an ECG

- For accurate measurements, place the patient in right lateral recumbency.

▼ *Key Point* If the animal is dyspneic or if restraint would be dangerous to the patient, obtain a rhythm strip with the animal supported in any comfortable position.

- Wet the skin with alcohol or ECG electrode gel and attach the electrodes just above the elbows and stifles.
- Hold the upper limbs perpendicular to the long axis of the patient and parallel to the floor. If the thoracic limbs are not parallel, the mean electrical axis will be altered.
- Record approximately three to four complexes in each of the six limb leads and then record a long lead II strip for rhythm evaluation. Push the standard calibration button at the beginning and end of each recording.
- Chest leads can be obtained using the V lead electrode, while keeping the limb leads attached. See Table 61–1 for electrode placement.
  - Chest leads are not necessary for all patients. However, they may be quite useful when the ECG complexes in the limb leads are small and difficult to evaluate. Often, P waves that cannot be seen in the limb leads become apparent on a chest lead.

Table 61–1. ELECTRODE PLACEMENT

Chest Lead	Placement of the V Lead
CV_5RL (rV_2)	Fifth intercostal space on the right side near the sternum
CV_6LL (V_2)	Sixth intercostal space on the left side near the sternum
CV_6LU (V_4)	Sixth intercostal space on the left side at the costochondral junction
V_{10}	Over the dorsal spine of the seventh thoracic vertebra

- Evaluation of chest leads may also be helpful in evaluating heart enlargement patterns.
- The chest leads most commonly used in veterinary patients are CV_5RL (rV_2), CV_6LL (V_2), CV_6LU (V_4), and V_{10}.

Normal Cardiac Conduction

The ECG records the electrical activity of the heart. Electrical impulses originate in specialized pacemaker tissue in the sinus node of the right atrium. The impulse rapidly traverses the atrium, causing atrial contraction and then slows, as it passes through the atrioventricular (AV) node located at the proximal portion of the interventricular septum. Electrical activity then rapidly passes through the bundle of His, the anterior and posterior branches of the left bundle branch, the right bundle branch, and the terminal Purkinje fibers. This causes activation of the interventricular septum and the left and right ventricular myocardium (Fig. 61–1).

Components of the Electrocardiographic Tracing

(Fig. 61–2)

- P wave indicates atrial depolarization.
- P-R interval indicates time for conduction of the impulse from the sinoauricular (SA) node to the AV

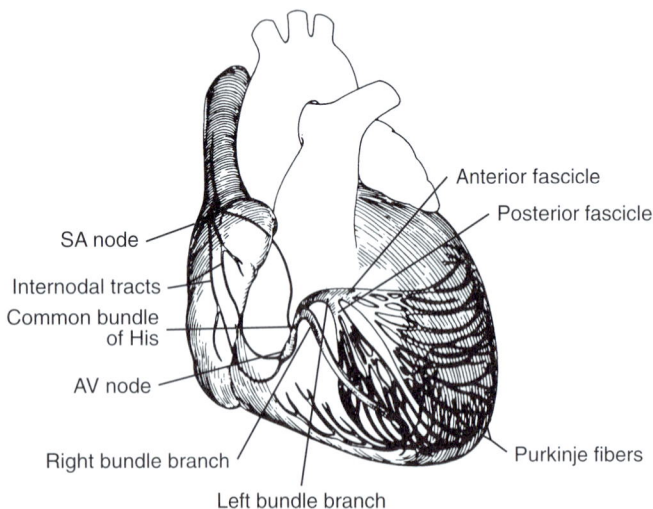

Figure 61–1. Normal conduction pathway in the heart. (From De Sanctis RW: Disturbances in cardiac rhythm and conduction. *In* Rubenstein R, ed.: Scientific American Medicine, section 1, subsection VI. © 1991 Scientific American, Inc. All rights reserved.)

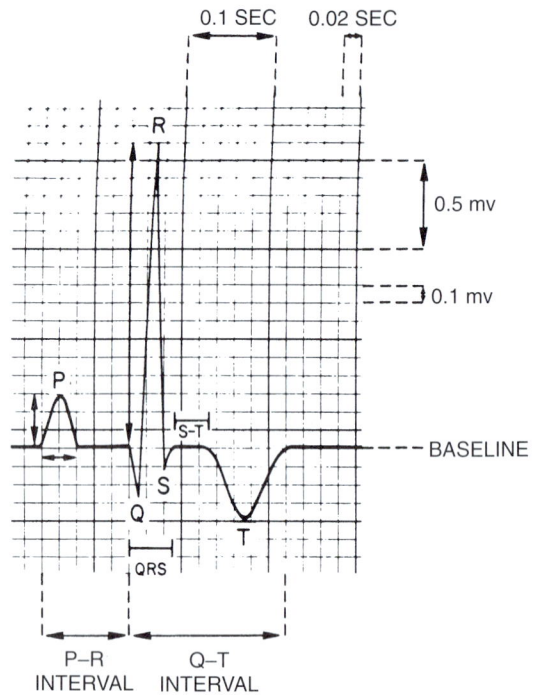

Figure 61–2. Normal electrocardiogram with components labeled. (From Tilley LP: Essentials of Canine and Feline Electrocardiography, 3rd Ed. Philadelphia: Lea & Febiger, 1992.)

node and delay of the impulse in the AV node, His bundle, bundle branches, and Purkinje system.
- QRS complex indicates ventricular myocardium depolarization.
- Q wave (lead II) is associated with depolarization of the interventricular septum.
- R wave (lead II) is associated with depolarization of the left ventricle.
- S wave (lead II), when present, is associated with depolarization of the right ventricle.
- T wave indicates ventricular repolarization.
- Q-T interval indicates an approximate interval of ventricular systole.

How to Evaluate the Electrocardiogram

- Always evaluate the ECG from left to right.
- Identify and label the ECG waveforms (P–QRS–T).
- Calculate the approximate heart rate (HR) by counting the number of R-R intervals in 3 seconds (two sets of time markers at 50 mm/sec) and multiplying by 20.
- Determine the mean electrical axis:
  - One of the easiest ways to approximate the axis is to identify the isoelectric lead (sum of the positive and negative deflections of the QRS complex closest to zero).
  - Determine the perpendicular lead, and evaluate that lead to see if the complexes are positive or negative.
  - The axis is in the direction of the main deflection of the perpendicular lead (see Fig. 61–3 for an example).

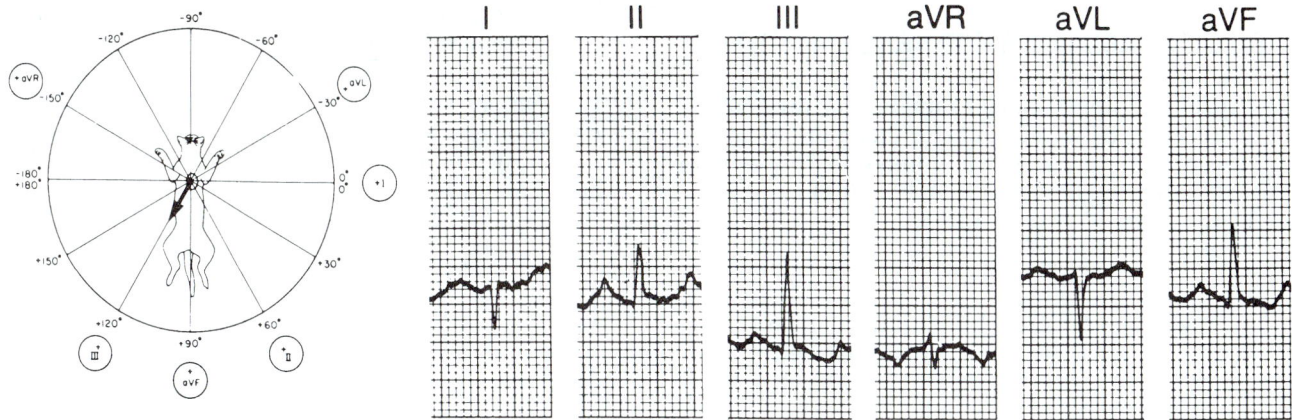

Figure 61–3. Electrocardiogram from a cat. Lead aVR is isoelectric. Lead III is perpendicular to aVR. The QRS deflection in lead III is positive, making the axis +120. If lead III had been negative, the axis would have been −60. (From Tilley LP: Essentials of Canine and Feline Electrocardiography, 3rd Ed. Philadelphia: Lea & Febiger, 1992.)

- If all leads are isoelectric, an axis cannot be determined in the frontal plane.
- Determine the rhythm.
  - A sinus rhythm has near constant P-R and R-R intervals.
  - A sinus arrhythmia has a near constant P-R interval, but the R-R interval varies, usually with the phase of respiration. For a more detailed discussion of arrhythmia evaluation, refer to Chapter 62.
- Measure the height and width of the complexes.
- Determine the P-R and Q-T intervals and evaluate the S-T segment.
- Compare the heart rate, rhythm, and sizes of the complexes to the normal values (Table 61–2).

Table 61–2. NORMAL CANINE AND FELINE ELECTROCARDIOGRAM VALUES*

	Canine	Feline
Heart rate (HR)	Puppy: up to 220 bpm Toy breeds: up to 180 bpm Standard: 70–160 bpm Giant breeds: 60–140 bpm	120–240 bpm
Rhythm	Sinus rhythm Sinus arrhythmia Wandering pacemaker	Sinus rhythm
P wave		
Height	Maximum: 0.4 mV	Maximum: 0.2 mV
Width	Maximum: 0.04 sec (giant breeds 0.05 sec)	Maximum: 0.04 seconds
P-R interval	0.06–0.13 sec (>0.13 sec in giant breeds)	0.05–0.09 sec
QRS		
Height	Small breeds: 2.5 mV maximum Large breeds: 3.0 mV maximum†	Maximum: 0.9 mV
Width	Small breeds: 0.05 sec maximum Large breeds: 0.06 sec maximum	Maximum: 0.04 sec
S-T segment		
Depression	No more than 0.2 mV	None
Elevation	No more than 0.15 mV	None
Q-T interval	0.15–0.25 sec at normal HR	0.12–0.18 sec at normal HR
T waves	May be positive, negative, or biphasic Amplitude range ± 0.05–1.0 mV in any lead	Usually positive and <0.3 mV
Electrical axis	+40° to +100°	0° to ± 160°
Chest leads		
CV₅RL (rV₂)	T positive; R <3.0 mV	
CV₆LL (V₂)	S <0.8 mV; R <3.0 mV	R <1.0 mV
CV₆LU (V₄)	S <0.7 mV; R <3.0 mV	R <1.0 mV
V₁₀	QRS negative; T negative except in Chihuahua	T negative; R wave/Q wave <1

*Measurements are made in lead II unless otherwise stated.
†Not valid for thin, deep-chested dogs <2 years of age.
bpm, beats per minute; HR, heart rate.

ELECTROCARDIOGRAPHIC ABNORMALITIES

Electrocardiographic abnormalities can be divided into those involving heart rate and rhythm and those involving the configuration of the complexes. This chapter discusses abnormalities involving the ECG complexes. Arrhythmias are discussed in Chapter 62.

Intraventricular Conduction Disturbances

- The right bundle branch is thinner and therefore more susceptible to injury than the left bundle branch.
- Injury to more than one bundle branch may result in first-, second-, or third-degree AV block.
- A bundle branch block does not cause hemodynamic changes and therefore does not warrant therapy.
- Rate-related bundle branch blocks can occur intermittently in association with either bradycardia or tachycardia. The right bundle branch cells have a longer refractory period than the left bundle branch cells. This makes the right bundle more sensitive to abrupt changes in the heart rate.

Right Bundle Branch Block (Fig. 61–4)

- ECG characteristics of RBBB include:
  - QRS width greater than 0.07 second (dog) or 0.06 second (cat)
  - Right axis deviation
  - Wide S waves in leads I, II, III, aVF, and lower left precordial leads, such as CV_6LL and CV_6LU
  - W-shaped pattern in V_{10}
  - Terminal QRS complex positive in aVR, aVL and M-shaped in CV_5RL
- Incomplete RBBB may be present if the aforementioned criteria are present but complexes are of normal width.
  - Differentiate from left posterior fascicular block.
- Differentiate RBBB from right ventricular enlargement by radiographs or echocardiography. Right ventricular enlargement and RBBB can occur together.
- RBBB has been associated with the following conditions: congenital malformations, cardiac surgery, cardiac needle puncture or cardiac arrest, cardiac neoplasia, trauma, *Trypanosoma cruzi* infection (dog), cardiomyopathy, hyperkalemia (cat), acute ventricular dilation, balloon valvuloplasty, and doxorubicin cardiotoxicity. RBBB may be an incidental finding in patients without apparent cardiac disease (e.g., beagles).

Left Bundle Branch Block (Fig. 61–5)

- ECG characteristics of LBBB include:
  - QRS width greater than 0.07 second (dog) or 0.06 second (cat)
  - QRS positive in leads I, II, III, aVF, CV_6LL, and CV_6LU
  - QRS negative in leads aVR, aVL, and CV_5RL
  - Absent or small Q wave in leads I, CV_6LL, and CV_6LU (dog)
  - Q wave absent in leads I and CV_6LU (cat)
- LBBB indicates greater cardiac damage than RBBB—often cardiomyopathy
- Differentiate LBBB from left ventricular enlargement by radiographs or echocardiography. Left ventricular enlargement and LBBB also can occur together.
- LBBB is most often associated with the following conditions:
  - In dogs—cardiomyopathy, cardiac needle puncture, subaortic stenosis, and doxorubicin cardiotoxicity.
  - In cats—uncommon but associated with hypertrophic cardiomyopathy.

Left Anterior Fascicular Block (Fig. 61–6)

- ECG characteristics of LAFB include:
  - QRS width normal
  - Left axis deviation (dog < +40°, cat <0°)
  - Small Q and tall R in leads I and aVL (small Q not essential)
  - Deep S wave in leads II, III, and aVF (exceeding the R wave)
- Associated conditions include hypertrophic cardiomyopathy, causes of left ventricular hypertrophy, hyperkalemia, ischemic cardiomyopathy, and cardiac surgery.

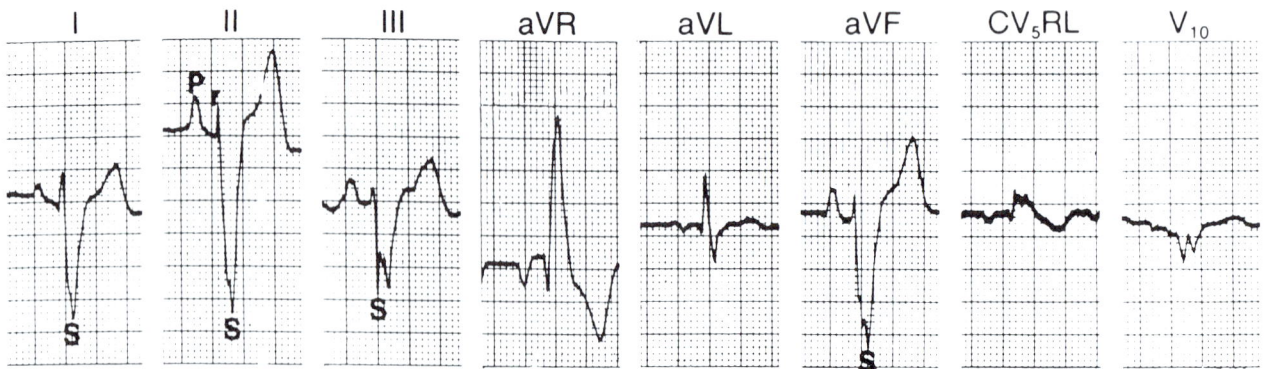

Figure 61–4. Example of right bundle branch block in the dog. Note the right axis (−110); the wide S wave in leads I, II, III, and aVF; and the M-shaped CV_5RL and W-shaped V_{10}. (From Tilley LP: Essentials of Canine and Feline Electrocardiography, 3rd Ed. Philadelphia: Lea & Febiger, 1992.)

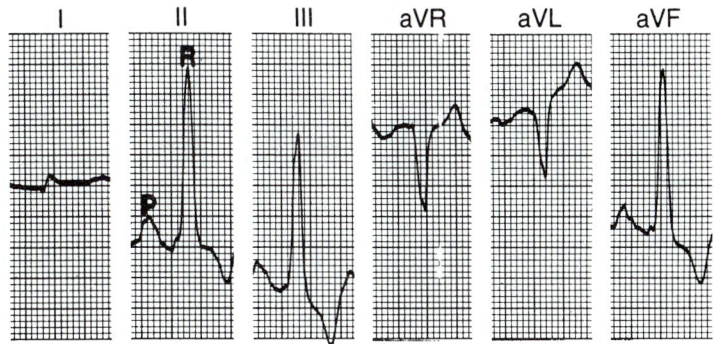

Figure 61–5. Left bundle branch block in a dog. Note the wide QRS complexes (0.08 sec). This electrocardiogram could also be consistent with left ventricular enlargement. (From Tilley LP: Essentials of Canine and Feline Electrocardiography, 3rd Ed. Philadelphia: Lea & Febiger, 1992.)

- Differentiate from left ventricular enlargement, altered position of the heart within the thorax, hyperkalemia, and ventricular preexcitation.

Left Anterior Fascicular Block and Right Bundle Branch Block (Fig. 61–7)

- ECG characteristics include:
  - QRS width greater than 0.07 second (dog) or 0.06 second (cat)
  - Left axis deviation
  - S waves deep and wide in leads I, II, III, aVF, and CV_6LU
  - Small Q and tall R in leads I and aVL
  - M-shaped QRS in lead CV_5RL
- Associated conditions: Same as for LAFB

Aberrant Conduction

- A premature beat is conducted through a bundle branch that is in an absolute or a relative refractory period.

- More common at slower heart rates or during sudden changes in R-R intervals. Aberrant complexes usually have an RBBB pattern, because of the longer refractory period of the right bundle branch cells.
- Aberrant beats are frequently confused with ventricular premature complexes (VPCs).
  - Look for P waves to differentiate the two.
  - An aberrantly conducted beat will have an associated P wave with a normal or slightly prolonged P-R interval.
  - VPCs do not have associated P waves with consistent P-R intervals. Refer to Chapter 62 for further discussion.

Preexcitation

Anatomy. In some patients, accessory pathways exist that allow electrical impulses to bypass the AV node and go directly to the bundle of His or ventricular myocardium. Electrical impulses in these patients simultaneously go through the AV node. The bundles of Kent

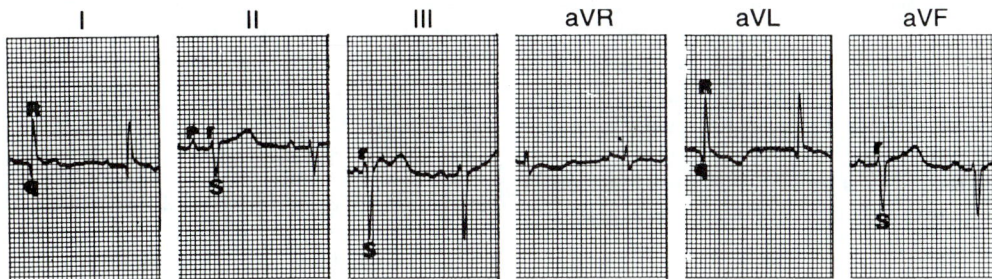

Figure 61–6. Left anterior fascicular block in a cat with hypertrophic cardiomyopathy. (From Tilley LP: Feline electrocardiography. Vet Clin North Am 7:257, 1977.)

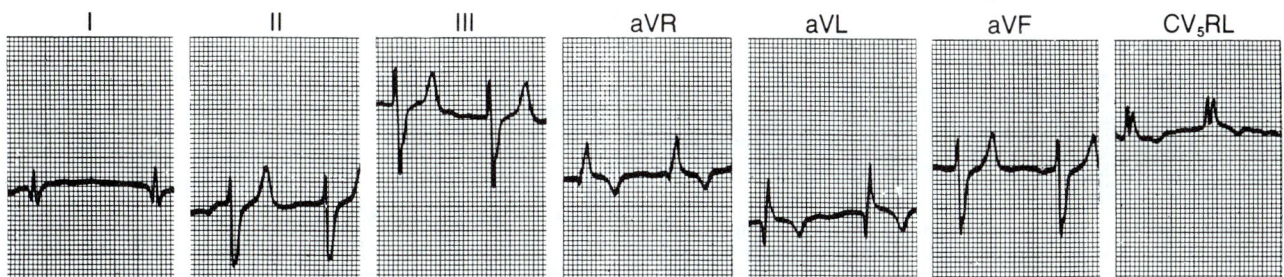

Figure 61–7. Left anterior fascicular block and right bundle branch block in a cat with hypertrophic cardiomyopathy. (From Tilley LP: Essentials of Canine and Feline Electrocardiography, 3rd Ed. Philadelphia: Lea & Febiger, 1992.)

ATRIUM

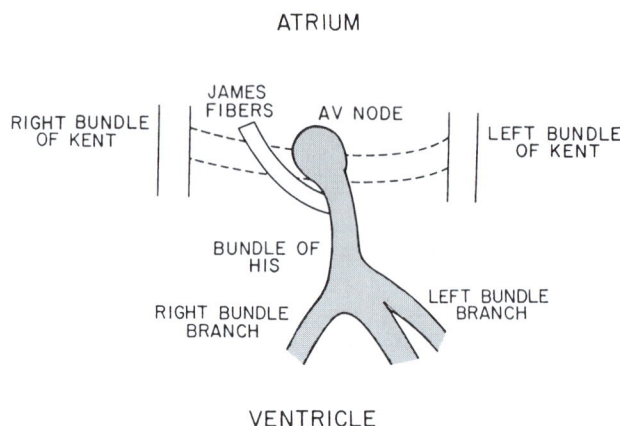

Figure 61–8.   Anatomy of accessory pathways. (From Tilley LP: Essentials of Canine and Feline Electrocardiography, 3rd Ed. Philadelphia: Lea & Febiger, 1992.)

allow direct atrioventricular conduction. The James fibers bypass the AV node and connect to the bundle of His (Fig. 61–8).

ECG Characteristics. Electrical conduction through these accessory pathways is faster than through the AV node, resulting in a shortened P-R interval. If impulses are conducted over the bundles of Kent, the QRS complexes will be of longer duration and a delta wave will usually be present at the beginning of the complex (Fig. 61–9). The delta wave indicates the direct depolarization of the ventricular myocardium via the bypass tract. If the preexcitation impulse is conducted by the James fibers, the P-R interval will be of short duration but the QRS complexes will be of normal duration with no delta waves. This finding is due to the impulses bypassing the AV node but still activating the ventricles through the bundle of His, the bundle branches, and the Purkinje system. P waves are normal, and a 1:1 relationship exists between P waves and QRS complexes. In most patients, no clinical signs are seen with this conduction disturbance. However, reentrant supraventricular tachycardia can develop in association with preexcitation. These are discussed in Chapter 62.

Associated Conditions. Preexcitation is often noted as a congenital finding without other evidence of or-

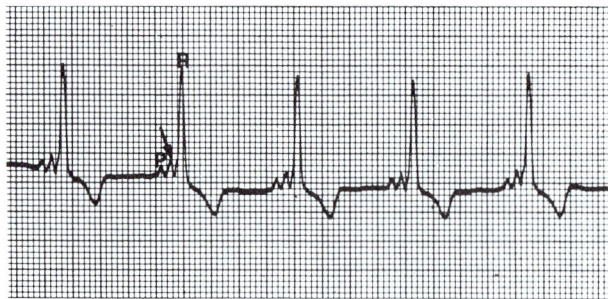

Figure 61–9.   A dog with ventricular preexcitation and a history of syncope. The arrow points out the delta wave. (From Tilley LP: Essentials of Canine and Feline Electrocardiography, 3rd Ed. Philadelphia: Lea & Febiger, 1992.)

ganic heart disease. Preexcitation may be seen in conjunction with other congenital cardiac diseases, such as atrial septal defect. In cats, preexcitation has been associated with hypertrophic cardiomyopathy.

Abnormalities of the QRS Complexes

Electrical Alternans (Fig. 61–10)

- Electrical alternans is a pattern of alternating configurations of the ECG complexes. The most common pattern is a variation in the height (taller to shorter) of the QRS complexes.
- Electrical alternans can be associated with a large pericardial effusion, supraventricular tachycardia, and alternating bundle branch block.
- Tachypnea (e.g., pleural effusion) can cause "pseudo-alternans" when cardiac and respiratory rates are synchronized.
- Electrical alternans is not present in all cases of pericardial effusion.

Small Complexes

Low amplitude complexes (R wave amplitude < 0.5 mV in lead II in dogs) may be a normal variant and may be associated with pericardial effusion, pleural effusion, pulmonary edema, hypothyroidism, obesity, pneumothorax, and hypoalbuminemia, and any cause of severe myocardial damage and loss of cardiac muscle mass.

Abnormalities of the S-T Segment

S-T Elevation

- S-T elevation (dog > 0.15 mV in lead II, III, or aVF or those leads with dominant R waves) is seen with myocardial hypoxia, pericarditis, pericardial effusion, and digitalis toxicity.
- Transmural myocardial infarction causes S-T segment elevation in leads overlying the infarcted myocardium.

S-T Depression

- S-T depression (dog >0.2 mV in lead II, III, aVF, or those leads with dominant R waves) is seen with myocardial hypoxia, hyperkalemia or hypokalemia, and digitalis toxicity.
- Subendocardial myocardial ischemia causes S-T segment depression in leads overlying the ischemic and infarcted myocardium.
- Pseudodepression due to prominent T_a waves (atrial repolarization) caused by atrial disease or tachycardia also causes S-T segment depression.

Other S-T Changes

- S-T segment changes can occur secondary to bundle branch blocks, myocardial hypertrophy, and ventricular premature complexes. The changes in the S-T segment are in the opposite direction from the main QRS deflection. The S-T segment change in these

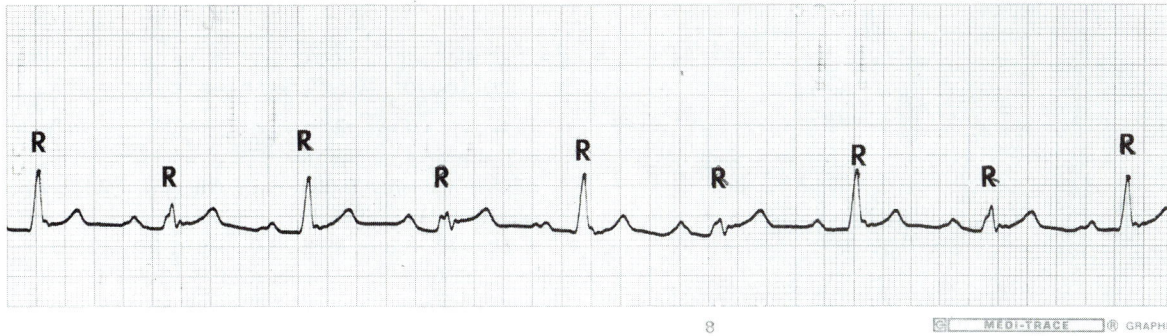

Figure 61–10. Electrical alternans in a dog with pericardial effusion.

conditions is often one of slurring or coving of the S wave into the T wave.

- Artifact related to baseline motion.
- Normal variant.

Abnormalities of the Q-T Interval

- Q-T interval changes are relatively nonspecific. The Q-T interval is inversely related to the heart rate, being shorter with more rapid heart rates. As a general rule, the Q-T interval should be less than half the preceding R-R interval.
- Q-T prolongation is associated with hypokalemia, hypocalcemia, hypothermia, quinidine administration, intraventricular conduction disturbance (associated with prolongation of the QRS complex), bradycardia, ethylene glycol toxicity, strenuous exercise, and central nervous system disturbance.
- Q-T interval narrowing is associated with hypercalcemia, hyperkalemia, and digitalis administration.

Abnormalities Involving the T Waves

- T-wave changes are relatively nonspecific. In general, the T wave should not be more than one-fourth the height of the associated R wave (Q or S wave, if either is larger than R), or more than 1.0 mV in any lead.
- In most leads, normal T waves may be positive, negative, or biphasic.
- Polarity should be consistent on serial electrocardiograms if HR is constant. T waves should be positive in CV_5RL in dogs greater than 2 months of age and negative in V_{10}, except in the Chihuahua.
- *Large T waves* can be seen with myocardial hypoxia, intraventricular conduction disturbance, ventricular enlargement, hypothermia, and in animals with heart disease and bradycardia.
- *Large and sharply pointed* (positive or negative) T waves are associated with hyperkalemia.
- *Small biphasic T waves* can be seen with hypokalemia.
- *Nonspecific T-wave changes* can be seen secondary to metabolic disturbances (hypoglycemia, anemia, shock, fever), drug toxicities (digitalis, quinidine, procainamide), and neurologic disease.
- *T wave alternans* (alternating positive and negative T waves) has been reported secondary to hypocal-

cemia, high levels of circulating catecholamines, and sudden increases in sympathetic tone.

Electrolyte Disturbances

The ECG is not very sensitive or specific in diagnosing systemic disturbances. However, it can be useful as a rapid screening test for certain electrolyte disturbances (predominantly moderate to severe hyperkalemia).

Hyperkalemia

ECG changes vary with the degree of hyperkalemia.

- The earliest change is the development of sharply pointed (spiked) T waves (Fig. 61–11), followed by a reduction in the height of the P waves and prolongation of the P-R interval. Changes in the P waves are most consistently observed in dogs and cats.
- The QRS complexes then start to widen, and the P waves disappear (atrial standstill).
- The QRS complexes become progressively wider and more bizarre in shape, and cardiac arrest or ventricular fibrillation follows.
- AV block and escape beats may also be seen with hyperkalemia.

Hypokalemia

- Q-T prolongation may develop along with prominent U waves. A U wave is a repolarization deflection of the Purkinje fibers that occurs after the T wave; however, U waves are uncommon in animals.

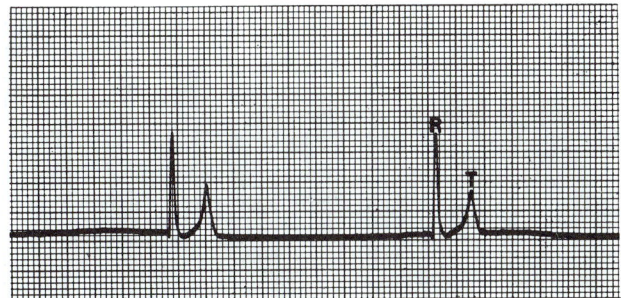

Figure 61–11. Atrial standstill and tall spiked T waves in a dog with severe hyperkalemia associated with Addison's disease.

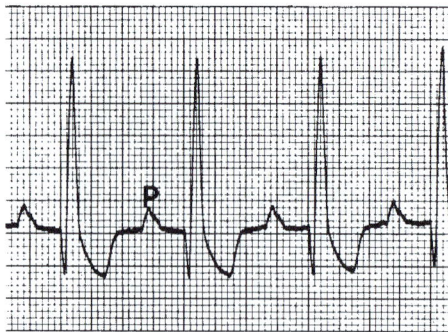

Figure 61–12. Wide and notched P waves in a dog with left atrial enlargement secondary to degenerative mitral valve disease. (From Tilley LP: Essentials of Canine and Feline Electrocardiography, 3rd Ed. Philadelphia: Lea & Febiger, 1992.)

- T waves may be small and notched.
- The S-T segment becomes progressively depressed.
- P-R prolongation and an increase in the height and width of the P and QRS complexes may be seen.

Hypercalcemia

- Q-T interval may be shortened.
- S-T segment shortening and depression have been reported.

Hypocalcemia

- Q-T prolongation develops.
- Duration of S-T segment correlates with the severity of hypocalcemia.
- T wave alternans has been reported.
- Deep wide T waves, tachycardia, and tall R waves may be present.

Heart Enlargement Patterns

Left Atrial Enlargement

Left atrial enlargement is characterized by wider than normal P waves in lead II (Fig. 61–12).

- Dog and cat P greater than 0.04 second (>0.05 second in giant breed dogs)

Left Ventricular Enlargement

Left ventricular enlargement is characterized by one or more of the following (Fig. 61–13):

- Left axis orientation (dog < +40°; cat <0°)
- S-T slurring or coving
- QRS duration > 0.06 second (dog) or 0.04 second (cat)
- Tall R waves
  - *Dog:* R greater than 3.0 mV in leads II, aVF, V_6LU (V_4), CV_6LL (V_2), and CV_5RL (rV_2). R greater than 1.5 mV in lead I. Sum of R-wave amplitude in leads I and aVF greater than 4.0 mV.
  - *Cat:* R > 1.0 mV in CV_6LU (V_4). R > 0.9 mV in Lead II or aVF. R wave/Q wave > 1.0 in V_{10}.

Right Atrial Enlargement

Right atrial enlargement is characterized by taller than normal P waves in lead II (Fig. 61–14).

- *Dog:* P > 0.4 mV (or prolonged P wave in some dogs).
- *Cat:* P > 0.2 mV (may also indicate left atrial enlargement).

Right Ventricular Enlargement

Right ventricular enlargement is characterized by one or more of the following (Fig. 61–15):

- Right axis orientation (dog > +100°; cat > +160°)
- S wave in leads I, II, III, and aVF
- S wave in lead I greater than 0.05 mV (dog)
- Chest leads
  - *Dog:* CV_6LL (V_2): S greater than 0.8 mV; CV_6LU (V_4): S greater than 0.7 mV; R:S ratio less than 0.87; V_{10}: T positive (except Chihuahua) and W-shaped QRS complex.
  - *Cat:* Prominent S waves in CV_6LL (V_2) and CV_6LU (V_4); T positive in V_{10}.

SPECIAL DIAGNOSTIC PROCEDURES

Postexercise Electrocardiography

Patients with suspected cardiac disease or arrhythmia, based on auscultation or history of syncope or exercise intolerance, may have normal resting ECGs. Sometimes, an arrhythmia can be documented by repeating

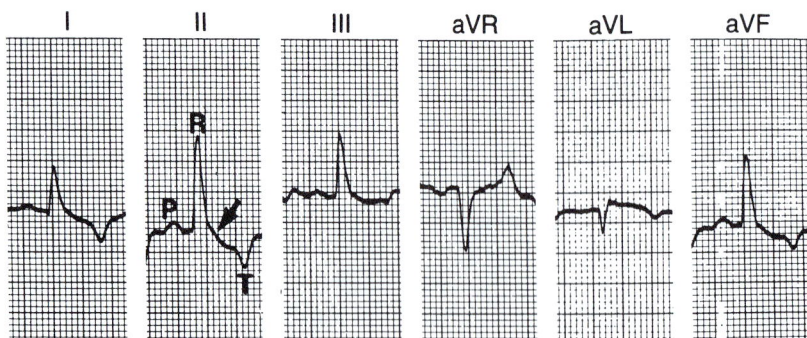

Figure 61–13. Tall and wide QRS complexes and S-T slurring *(arrow)* indicate left ventricular enlargement in this cat with hypertrophic cardiomyopathy. (From Tilley LP: Essentials of Canine and Feline Electrocardiography, 3rd Ed. Philadelphia: Lea & Febiger, 1992.)

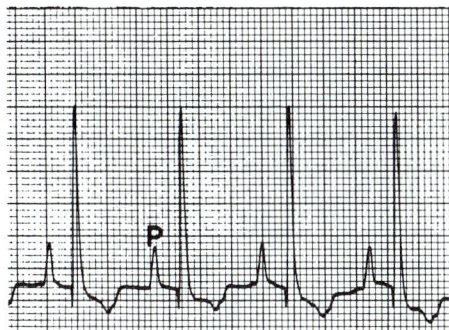

Figure 61–14. Tall P waves suggestive of right atrial enlargement. (From Tilley LP: *Essentials of Canine and Feline Electrocardiography*, 3rd Ed. Philadelphia: Lea & Febiger, 1992.)

an ECG after vigorous exercise. T-wave changes or S-T segment abnormalities may become apparent following exercise, suggesting underlying myocardial disease.

Vagal Maneuvers

Indications

- Vagal maneuvers are useful in evaluating supraventricular tachycardias and may terminate reentrant supraventricular tachycardia.
- Vagal maneuvers may also help evaluate baroreceptor and sinus node functions, or "uncover" atrial flutter when there is regular AV conduction.

Technique

- While running a lead II rhythm strip, vigorously massage the carotid sinuses that are located under the mandible in the jugular furrow.

- If this maneuver does not break the tachycardia, apply ocular pressure.
- If still unsuccessful, apply ocular pressure along with carotid sinus massage.

Interpretation

- If a supraventricular tachycardia breaks abruptly and the rhythm remains normal for at least a short time after stopping the vagal maneuver, the arrhythmia was probably reentrant atrial (supraventricular) tachycardia.
- If the rate gradually slows during the vagal maneuver and then speeds up again after the vagal maneuver, the rhythm is probably sinus tachycardia.
- If multiple P waves (>300/minute) are observed, related to vagal-induced AV block, either atrial tachycardia or flutter is likely.
- If there is no change during the vagal maneuver, no conclusion can be made regarding the nature of the supraventricular tachycardia.
- Another area in which a vagal maneuver may be helpful is in trying to rule out bradyarrhythmia as a cause of syncope. If the vagal maneuver results in prolonged periods of sinus arrest or produces AV block, this supports sinus or AV nodal disease as a cause of syncope.

Holter Monitoring

Holter monitors provide a 24-hour ECG recording (Fig. 61–16). They are ideal for identifying intermittent arrhythmias, determining the frequency and severity of arrhythmias, and monitoring the efficacy of antiarrhythmic drug therapy. Perform Holter monitoring in

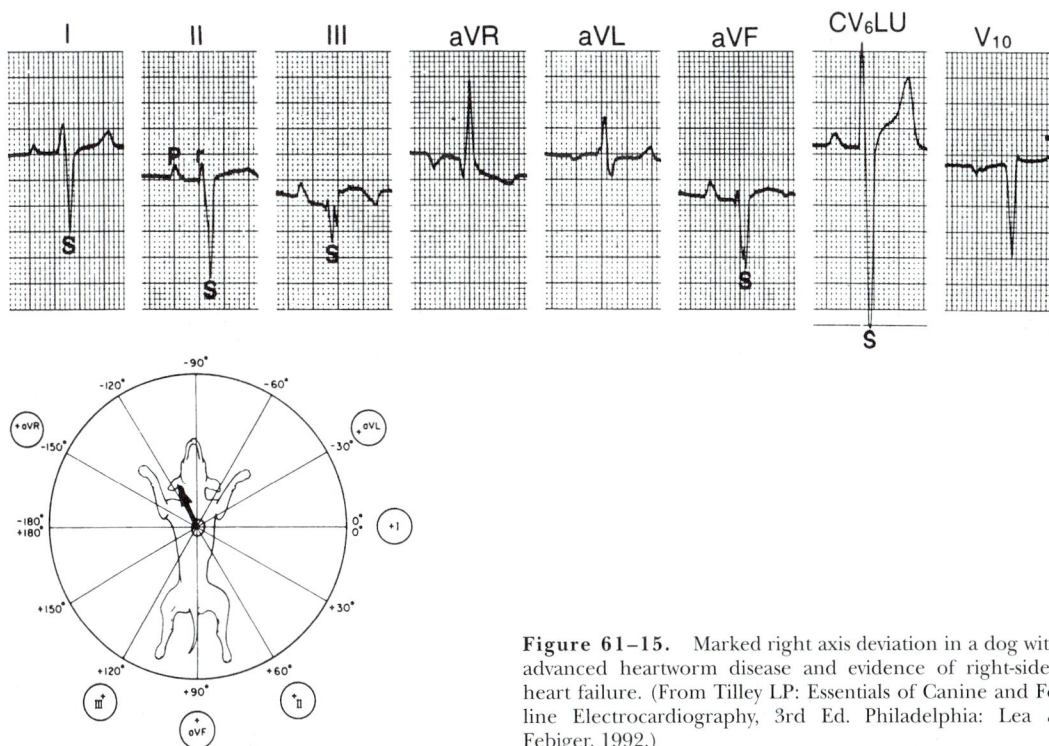

Figure 61–15. Marked right axis deviation in a dog with advanced heartworm disease and evidence of right-sided heart failure. (From Tilley LP: *Essentials of Canine and Feline Electrocardiography*, 3rd Ed. Philadelphia: Lea & Febiger, 1992.)

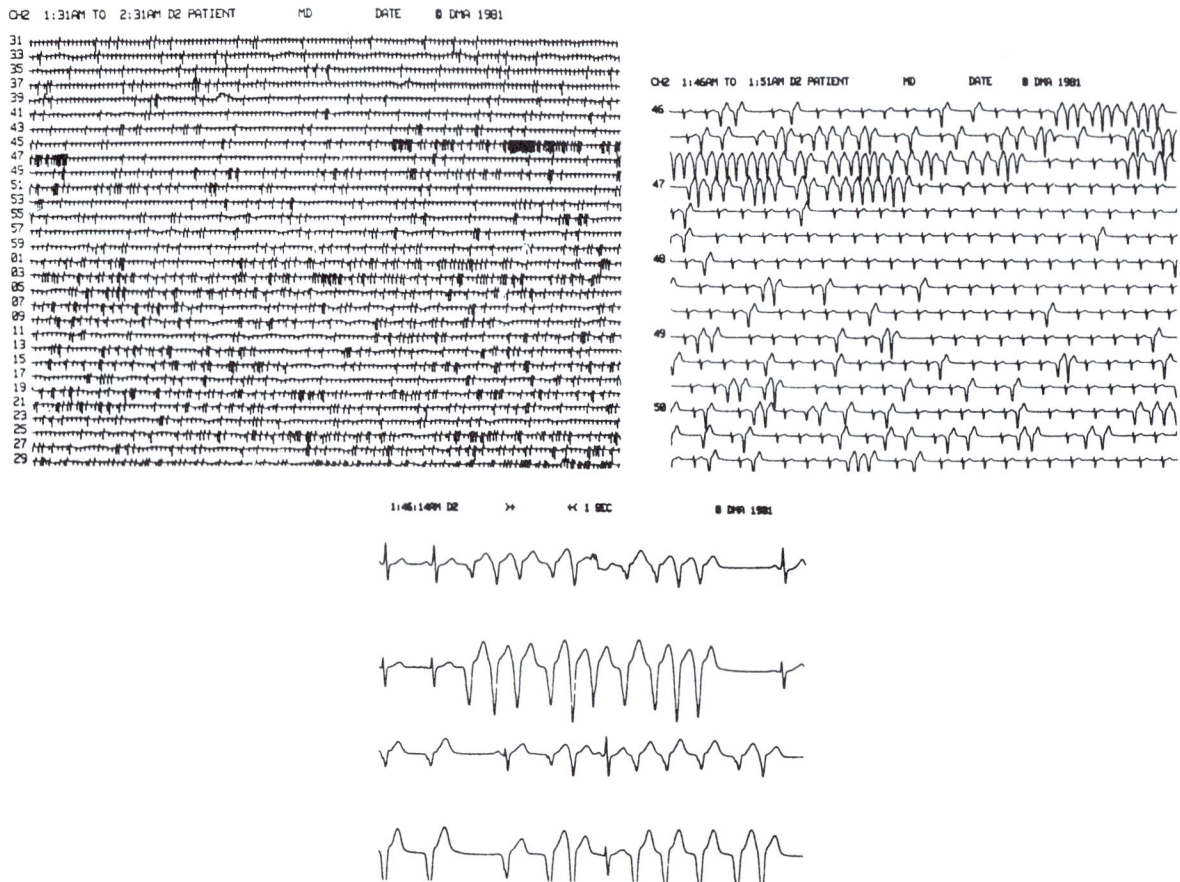

Figure 61–16. Printouts of three displayed time segments from a 24-hour electrocardiographic (ECG) recording (Holter monitoring). The period of ventricular tachycardia can be easily recognized and correlated with the times of occurrence by referring to the digital time entries displayed adjacent to the ECG data. Detected ventricular ectopic activity can be efficiently enlarged, especially on the 15-second time segment for complete analysis and documentation. (From Tilley LP: Essentials of Canine and Feline Electrocardiography, 3rd Ed. Philadelphia: Lea & Febiger, 1992.)

patients with syncope in which routine ECGs and laboratory evaluation do not confirm a diagnosis. If arrhythmias are identified on Holter monitoring of a patient with a history of syncope, they may be the cause of the collapsing episodes. Holter monitoring is offered by some veterinary cardiologists, transtelephonic ECG services, and sometimes can be arranged through a local medical cardiologist. Have Holter recordings reviewed by a veterinary cardiologist, as technicians trained to read human Holter studies often overinterpret atrial premature complexes on canine ECGs.

▼ *Key Point* One cannot be certain that an arrhythmia identified on a Holter recording of an animal with syncope is the cause of the animal's problem, unless the animal has a syncopal episode or related clinical signs at the same time the arrhythmia is recorded.

Event Recorders

Event or loop recorders are the best diagnostic tool for identifying arrhythmias as the cause of syncope. These are small ECG recorders that can easily be worn by even small dogs and cats. These units record a continuous 5-minute loop of ECG. After the veterinarian attaches the

system, the animal is sent home. When the animal has an event (e.g., syncope, collapse, or seizure) the owner pushes a button to activate the memory feature, which preserves the ECG in memory for a preprogrammed time before, during, and following the event. After the recording is made, it can be transmitted transtelephonically for printing the ECG and interpretation.

Lidocaine Response Test

Patients with sustained, wide complex tachycardia (ventricular tachycardia or atrial tachycardia with a bundle branch block) may be administered lidocaine (2–4 mg/kg IV) to help establish a diagnosis and to terminate the arrhythmia, if it is a lidocaine-responsive ventricular tachycardia. Occasionally, an atrial tachycardia will break following the administration of lidocaine.

Atropine Response Test

Patients with symptomatic bradyarrhythmia may be administered atropine (0.05 mg/kg IM or SC) and undergo an ECG 30 minutes later. This test is helpful in determining the role of vagal tone in the bradyarrhythmia and whether or not oral anticholinergic drugs (e.g., propantheline bromide) might alleviate symptoms associated with the bradycardia, particularly if pacing is not an option.

SUPPLEMENTAL READINGS

Bonagura JD: Cardiovascular diseases. *In* Sherding RG, ed.: The Cat, Diseases and Clinical Management. New York: Churchill Livingstone, 1989, p 649.

Edwards NJ: Bolton's Handbook of Canine and Feline Electrocardiography, 2nd Ed. Philadelphia: WB Saunders, 1987.

Ettinger SJ, Suter PF: Canine Cardiology. Philadelphia: WB Saunders, 1970, p 102.

Harpster NK: The cardiovascular system. *In* Holzworth J, ed.: Diseases of the Cat: Medicine and Surgery. Philadelphia: WB Saunders, 1987, p 820.

Miller MS, Tilley LP, Smith FWK Jr, Fox PR: Electrocardiography. *In* Fox PR, Sisson D, eds.: Canine and Feline Cardiology, 2nd Ed. Philadelphia: WB Saunders, in press.

Tilley LP: Essentials of Canine and Feline Electrocardiography, 3rd Ed. Philadelphia: Lea & Febiger, 1992.

62 Disorders of Cardiac Rhythm

Michael S. Miller / Larry Patrick Tilley / Francis W. K. Smith, Jr.

Cardiac arrhythmias include disorders of cardiac impulse formation, conduction, rate, and regularity. Terms such as dysrhythmia and ectopia also are used to identify arrhythmias. Cardiac arrhythmias can be benign and clinically insignificant, or they can cause clinical signs. They can even progress to malignant arrhythmias that lead to heart failure or sudden death.

Causes of cardiac arrhythmias include heart disease and disorders involving the autonomic nervous system, endocrine system, electrolytes, and other body systems. Cardiac arrhythmias are diagnosed and classified electrocardiographically; see Chapter 61 for additional pertinent information.

ETIOLOGY

- Cardiac arrhythmias are classified in Table 62–1. They occur with congenital or acquired cardiac disease or systemic disorders (Table 62–2).
- Cardiac pathology does not necessarily correlate with the type and severity of arrhythmias.
- Arrhythmia variation in animals with cardiac or systemic disorders may be explained by the complex interactions among cardiac cell transmembrane potentials, the autonomic nervous system, and body fluids.

MECHANISM

- The normal cardiac impulse is generated automatically in the sinus node and is spread through the atria rapidly and sequentially via the His bundle, the bundle branches, and the intraventricular conduction system to the ventricular myocardium.
- The normal atrioventricular (AV) node serves as a bridge between the atria and the ventricles and slows the cardiac impulse prior to rapid impulse conduction through the ventricles.
- Reentry, a common arrhythmia mechanism, typically is caused by functional dissociation of cardiac tissue, unidirectional block in one pathway, and slowed conduction in the other pathway. The impulse then returns to the origination point by retrograde conduction through the unidirectionally blocked pathway.
- Triggered activity is caused by early or late after-depolarizations.

DIAGNOSTIC APPROACH

Systematic Evaluation of the Electrocardiographic Strip (See Chap. 61)

- Is sinus rhythm or an arrhythmia present?
- Is the heart rate rapid, slow, or normal?
- Are P waves present?
  - *Yes.* Do the P (atria) waves occur at regular or irregular intervals? What is the height, width, direction?
  - *No.* What reason or abnormality explains the absence of the P wave? Is the P wave superimposed on a portion of the QRS complex, S-T segment, or T wave? Is the arrhythmia atrial standstill, atrial fibrillation, atrial flutter, AV junctional escape rhythm, or atrial tachycardia?
- Do the QRS (ventricular) complexes occur with regularity and uniformity? What is their morphology? If

Table 62–1. CLASSIFICATION OF CARDIAC ARRHYTHMIAS

Supraventricular Rhythms
Sinus rhythm
Sinus arrhythmia
Sinus bradycardia
Sinus tachycardia
Atrial premature complexes
Sinus block and/or arrest
Atrial tachycardia
Atrial/supraventricular tachycardia (reentrant)
Atrial flutter
Atrial fibrillation
Atrioventricular junctional rhythm

Ventricular Rhythms
Ventricular escape (rhythm)
Ventricular premature complexes
Idioventricular tachycardia
Ventricular tachycardia
Ventricular asystole
Ventricular fibrillation

Conduction Disorders
Atrial standstill
First-degree AV block
Second-degree AV block
Complete (third-degree) AV block

Arrhythmias and Conduction Disturbances
Sick sinus syndrome
Ventricular preexcitation and the Wolff-Parkinson-White syndrome

Table 62–2. CAUSES OF CARDIAC ARRHYTHMIAS

Cardiac

Dogs
Heredity (genetics not documented in all cases)
    Doberman (His bundle degeneration)
    English springer spaniel (persistent atrial standstill)
    Miniature schnauzer, dachshund, cocker spaniel, West Highland
       white terrier (sick sinus syndrome)
    Pug, Dalmatian (sinus node disease)
    Pug (stenosis and degeneration of the His bundle)
    Wolff-Parkinson-White syndrome
    Golden retriever (Duchenne muscular dystrophy)
    German shepherd (ventricular tachyarrhythmia)
Atrial and/or ventricular arrhythmias
    Atrial enlargement, secondary to congenital defects or acquired
       disease
    Cardiomyopathy
    Congenital heart disease
    Congestive heart failure
    Mitral valve disease (congenital and acquired)
    Myocarditis, endocarditis
    Myocardial ischemia
    Trauma
    Drugs
Conduction system disease
    Acquired sinus and AV node disease (sick sinus syndrome)
    Cardiomyopathy
    Neoplasia
    Surgical damage to conduction tissue
    Trauma
    Vascular (e.g., microscopic intramural myocardial infarction)
    Ventricular septal defect and other congenital defects
    Infection (Lyme disease)
    Drugs
    Degeneration

Cats
Heredity (rare)
    Wolff-Parkinson-White syndrome
Atrial and ventricular arrhythmias
    Cardiac enlargement secondary to congenital heart defects
    Cardiomyopathy
    Neoplasia
    Trauma
    Systemic diseases
Conduction system disease
    Cardiomyopathy
    Neoplasia
    Idiopathic fibrosis in older cats

Noncardiac

Dogs and Cats
Acidosis or alkalosis
Autonomic nervous system imbalance (parasympathetic or sympa-
    thetic); central nervous system (pain, excitement, fear); respira-
    tory, gastrointestinal, organic brain disease
Drug toxicity (e.g., digitalis, preoperative sedatives, anesthetic agents,
    catecholamines, antiarrhythmic agents, bronchodilators)
Electrolyte disorders (hyperkalemia, hypercalcemia, hypokalemia,
    hypocalcemia, hypomagnesemia)
Endocrinopathies (hypothyroidism, hyperthyroidism, Addison's
    disease, pheochromocytoma)
Hypothermia
Hypovolemia
Hypoxia, anemia
Mechanical stimulation (cardiac catheterization, intravenous
    catheter)
Neoplasia
Shock
Toxemia, sepsis
Trauma

Adapted from Miller MS, Tilley LP: Treatment of arrhythmias and conduction disturbances. *In* Miller MS, Tilley LP, eds.: Manual of Canine and Feline Cardiology. Philadelphia: WB Saunders, 1995, with permission.

wide and bizarre, is this due to a ventricular arrhythmia or caused by a premature atrial impulse that is aberrantly conducted, or is bundle branch block evident?
- What is the relationship between the P waves and the QRS complexes? Is the relationship consistent?
- If AV dissociation is present, from where does the QRS complex evolve? Are AV junctional and/or Purkinje or idioventricular foci involved?

Questions to Be Answered in the Interpretation of Cardiac Arrhythmia

- What is the possible mechanism for the arrhythmia?
- Is it atrial, AV junctional, or ventricular in origin?
- Is there a conduction abnormality?
- What is the severity and frequency of the arrhythmia?

SUPRAVENTRICULAR RHYTHMS

Sinus Rhythm

Definition

- Impulses originate in the sinus node.
- The rhythm is regular with less than a 10% variation in the R-R interval.
- There is a normal P wave for each QRS complex, with a constant P-R interval.
- The heart rate is 60–180 beats per minute (bpm) in dogs and 120–240 bpm in cats.

Etiology and Clinical Significance

- Sinus rhythm is a normal resting rhythm in dogs and cats and requires no therapy.
- Animals with symptomatic cardiac disease or noncardiac disease may show a sinus rhythm.

Sinus Arrhythmia

Definition

- Impulses originate in the sinus node.
- The rhythm is irregular with more than a 10% variation in the R-R interval.
- There is a normal P wave for each QRS complex, with a constant P-R interval.
- A wandering pacemaker (change in morphology of the P wave due to a change in pacemaker location or conduction) is often present.
- Heart rates are similar to sinus rhythm.

Etiology and Clinical Significance

- Sinus arrhythmia is a normal rhythm variation in the resting dog, often correlated with varying levels of sinus node vagal tone, which changes with respiration (decreased vagal tone and increased heart rate during inspiration).
- Sinus arrhythmia is unusual in cats.
- Pronounced sinus arrhythmia occurs in the normal resting dog and in dogs and cats with respiratory disease.

Treatment

- No treatment is required unless there is symptomatic bradycardia, in which case anticholinergics may be helpful.

Sinus Bradycardia

Definition

- Impulses originate in the sinus node, but at a slower than normal frequency.
- The rhythm is regular.
- There is a normal P wave for each QRS complex, with a constant P-R interval.
- The heart rate is < 70 bpm in dogs (< 60 bpm in giant breeds) and < 120 bpm in cats.

Etiology and Clinical Significance

- Sinus bradycardia may be a normal physiologic rhythm variation resulting from high levels of resting vagal tone.
- Hypothyroidism, sinus node disease (sick sinus syndrome), and hypothermia are pathologic causes of sinus bradycardia.
- Drugs that can cause a sinus bradycardia include acepromazine, xylazine, other alpha$_2$-agonists (e.g., medetomidine), digoxin, propranolol, diltiazem, pilocarpine, and general anesthetics.
- Animals with sinus bradycardia are often asymptomatic.
- Clinical signs of weakness, lethargy, and syncope may accompany sinus bradycardia.

Treatment

- Asymptomatic dogs or cats require no specific therapy.
- When correlated with signs of weakness or syncope an atropine response test should be performed (0.04 mg/kg IM) followed by an electrocardiogram (ECG) in 15–30 minutes.
  - If there is an increase in the cardiac rate following atropine administration, the animal may benefit from oral anticholinergic agents (Table 62–3).
  - A poor clinical response to atropine suggests the need for a temporary or permanent cardiac pacemaker.

- Congestive heart failure (CHF) may also develop, in which case consider diuretics and vasodilators as adjunctive treatment. Digitalis may exacerbate the sinus arrest in these cases. Hypotension may develop from vasodilator therapy.

Sinus Block and/or Sinus Arrest (Fig. 62–1)

Definition

- A primary disorder of the sinus node resulting in lack of generation of the cardiac impulse or its poor propagation across surrounding tissue.
- It is not possible to distinguish between sinus block and sinus arrest in dogs because of the normal variation in the R-R interval (sinus arrhythmia).
- The heart rate is variable and is often correlated with a bradycardia or slow sinus arrhythmia.
- The rhythm is regularly irregular or irregular with pauses.
- There is a normal P wave for each QRS complex with a pause equal to or greater than two times the normal R-R interval.
- The P wave may vary in shape if a concurrent wandering pacemaker is present.

Etiology and Clinical Significance

- Sinus arrest may be consistent with an increase in vagal tone (e.g., ocular pressure, irritation of the vagus nerve, brachycephalic breeds).
- Diseases of the atria including fibrosis, cardiomyopathy, and neoplasia, and drug toxicity (e.g., digitalis, propranolol, quinidine, xylazine, and acepromazine) may result in sinus arrest.
- Sinus arrest is one of the arrhythmias in the sick sinus syndrome.

Electrocardiographic Differentials

- Sinus block and/or sinus arrest can be confused with marked sinus arrhythmia and sinus bradycardia and nonconducted atrial premature complexes (APCs).

Treatment

- Treat the same as sinus bradycardia.

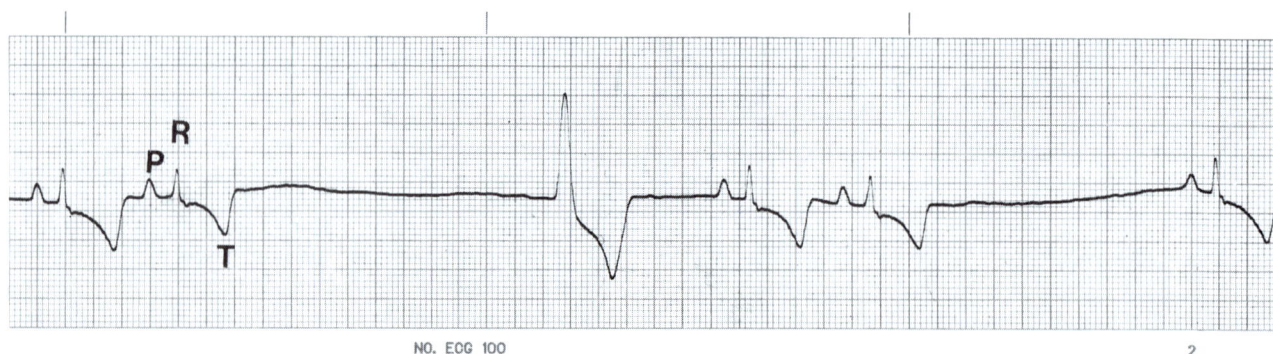

Figure 62–1.   Sinus block and/or arrest with a ventricular escape beat in a dog. (Lead II rhythm strip, paper speed 50 mm/sec; 1 cm = 1 mV.)

Table 62–3. COMMON ANTIARRHYTHMIC DRUGS

Generic Drug (Trade Name)	Formulation	Indications	Dosage for Dogs (D) and Cats (C)	Comments
Atenolol (Tenormin)	Tab: 25, 50, 100 mg	Atrial and ventricular arrhythmias, hypertrophic cardiomyopathy, hypertension	D: 0.25–1.0 mg/kg q12h–q24h PO C: 6.25 mg q12h	Less bronchoconstriction, vasoconstriction, and interference with insulin therapy than with propranolol Taper dose when discontinuing therapy Decrease dose with renal disease
Atropine sulfate*	Inj: 0.1, 0.4, 0.5 mg/ml	Sinus bradycardia, AV block, SSS	D: 0.02 mg/kg IV; 0.045 mg/kg q6h–q8h IM, SC C: Same as D	May transiently worsen bradyarrhythmia More potent chronotropic effects than glycopyrrolate
Digitoxin* (Crystodigin)	Tab: 0.05, 0.1 mg	Supraventricular arrhythmias, myocardial failure	D: 0.033 mg/kg PO; small dogs q8h; large dogs q12h C: None	GI side effects less common than with digoxin Dose based on total body weight Toxicity potentiated by hypokalemia, hyponatremia, hypercalcemia, thyroid disorders, hypoxia Preferred to digoxin in renal failure
Digoxin* (Cardoxin, Lanoxin)	Tab: 0.125, 0.25, 0.5 mg Inj: 0.25 mg/ml Elixir: 0.05 mg/ml, 0.15 mg/ml Cap: 0.05, 0.1, 0.2 mg	Supraventricular arrhythmias, myocardial failure	D: 0.22 mg/m² q12h PO; 0.0055–0.01 mg/kg q12h PO; 0.01 mg/kg IV in divided dose 2 hr apart C: 0.01 mg/kg every otherday (Tab preferred); 0.007 mg/kg every other day (with furosemide and aspirin)	Toxicity potentiated by hypokalemia, hyponatremia, hypercalcemia, thyroid disorders, hypoxia Base dose on lean body weight; reduce dose 10–15% with elixirs Therapeutic range 1–2.4 ng/ml; 8 hr after dose Rapid digitalization not recommended except in emergency Reduce dose 50% with quinidine
Diltiazem (Cardizem)	Tab: 30, 60, 90, 120 mg	Supraventricular arrhythmias, hypertrophic cardiomyopathy, hypertension	D: 0.5–1.5 mg/kg q8h PO (titrate up to effect) C: 0.5–2.5 mg/kg q8h PO	Less myocardial depression than verapamil
Dobutamine HCl (Dobutrex)	Inj: 12.5 mg/ml	Short-term management of severe myocardial failure and bradyarrhythmias not responsive to atropine	D: 5–20 μg/kg/min (titrate up to effect); administer in D_5W C: 2–5 μg/kg/min (titrate up to effect); administer in D_5W	Monitor ECG, BP, and pulse quality Preferable to dopamine in CHF but more expensive Inotropic effect is dose dependent Less arrhythmogenic than most other catecholamines Intermittent use may result in sustained improvement
Epinephrine* (Adrenalin)	Inj: 1:1000 conc (1 mg/ml) 1:10000 conc (0.1 mg/ml)	Cardiac arrest	D: 0.02–0.2 mg/kg q3–5 min IV; double dose for IT administration C: Same as D	Monitor with ECG Higher dose may be more effective but more likely to induce ventricular fibrillation Expand volume with fluids to prevent hypotension
Esmolol (Brevibloc) Isoproterenol* (Isuprel)	10 mg/ml Inj: 1:5000 (0.2 mg/ml)	Supraventricular tachycardia Short-term management of sinus bradycardia, AV block, SSS	0.05–0.1 mg/kg slow IV bolus D: 0.04–0.09 μg/kg/min IV; 0.1–0.2 mg q4–6h IM, SC C: Same as D	Maximum cumulative dosage: 0.5 mg/kg
Lidocaine* (Xylocaine)	Inj: 5, 10, 15, 20 mg/ml (without epinephrine)	Ventricular arrhythmias	D: 2–8 mg/kg slowly IV in 2 mg/kg boluses followed by IV drip at 30–80 μg/kg/min CRI C: 0.25–1 mg/kg IV over 5 min	Drug of choice for initial control of ventricular tachycardia in dogs Use with caution in cats Effects increased by high potassium and decreased by low potassium Seizures controlled with diazepam Do not use formulations with epinephrine for arrhythmia control
Mexiletine (Mexitil)	Cap: 150, 200, 250 mg	Ventricular arrhythmias	D: 5–8 mg/kg q8h PO C: None	Reduce dose with liver disease Administer with food to reduce GI side effects Side effects: Proarrhythmia, AV block, sinus bradycardia, tremors, ataxia, vomiting, drowsiness Contraindications: Heart block (2nd or 3rd degree), SSS Precautions: Liver disease, CHF, respiratory depression Drug interactions: Blood levels increased by cimetidine and beta-blockers; synergism with other class I agents and beta-blockers; decreased effects with barbiturates, increased theophylline levels, possible proarrhythmia with theophylline

Table continued on following page

Table 62–3. COMMON ANTIARRHYTHMIC DRUGS *CONTINUED*

Generic Drug (Trade Name)	Formulation	Indications	Dosage for Dogs (D) and Cats (C)	Comments
Procainamide* (Procan SR, Pronestyl)	Cap: 250, 375, 500 mg Tab: 250, 375, 500 mg Tab SR: 500, 750, 1000 mg Inj: 100, 500 mg/ml	Ventricular and supraventricular arrhythmias, WPW syndrome	D: 8–20 mg/kg q6h IM (SR, q8h) 2 mg/kg IV over 3–5 min up to total dose of 20 mg/kg; 20–50 μg/kg/min CRI C: 3–8 mg/kg q8h IM or PO	Beware of hypotension with q6h dosage (switch to q8h) Effects increased by high potassium and decreased by low potassium Monitor ECG; 25% prolongation of QRS is sign of toxicity Fewer GI and CV side effects than quinidine Use with caution in cats Reduce dose with severe renal disease Can cause hair discoloration
Propantheline bromide* (Pro-Banthine)	Tab: 7.5, 15 mg	Sinus bradycardia, AV block, SSS	D: small: 7.5 mg q8h PO; medium: 15 mg q8h PO; large: 30 mg q8h PO C: 7.5 mg sid–tid PO	
Propranolol* (Inderal)	Tab: 10, 20, 40, 60, 80, 90 mg Inj: 1 mg/ml	Atrial and ventricular arrhythmias, hypertrophic cardiomyopathy, hypertension, thyrotoxicosis	D: 0.2–1.0 mg/kg q8h PO; 0.02–0.06 mg/kg slowly IV C: <4.5 kg—2.5–5 mg q8–12h PO; >4.5 kg—5 mg q8–12h PO; 0.02–0.06 mg/kg IV slowly	Nonselective blocker Start with low dose and titrate to effect Taper dose when discontinuing therapy
Quinidine gluconate* (Quinaglute Dura-Tabs)	Tab: 324 mg Inj: 80 mg/ml	Ventricular and supraventricular arrhythmias, WPW syndrome, conversion of atrial fibrillation	D: 8–20 mg/kg q6h PO, IM; 8–20 mg/kg q8h PO with SR products; 5–10 mg/kg IV very slowly C: None	Decrease digoxin dose 50% with quinidine Effects increased by high potassium and decreased by low potassium Monitor ECG: 25% prolongation of QRS is sign of toxicity Has vagolytic, negative inotropic, and vasodilating properties Hypotension is frequent with IV administration Reduce dose in CHF, hepatic disease, and hypoalbuminemia
Sotalol (Betapace)	Tab: 80, 160, 240 mg	Ventricular arrhythmias	D: 1–2 mg/kg q12h PO C: None	Beta-blocking (class 2) effects in addition to class 3 antiarrhythmic effects; reduce dose with renal disease Side effects: Proarrhythmia, GI disturbances Contraindications: Sinus bradycardia, 2nd degree or complete AV block, uncontrolled CHF Precautions: COPD Drug interactions: Class Ia (quinidine, procainamide), class 2 and class 3 antiarrhythmics are not recommended as concomitant therapy; increased incidence of proarrhythmia with digoxin; use with caution with calcium blockers, as may have additive depressant effect on AV conduction and myocardial contractility; avoid other drugs that prolong QT interval (e.g., terfenadine, astemizole, phenothiazines, class Ia antiarrhythmics)
Tocainide (Tonocard)	Tab: 400, 600 mg	Ventricular arrhythmias	D: 10–20 mg/kg q8h PO C: None	Oral analog of lidocaine Giving with food may decrease GI upset or neurologic side effects
Verapamil* (Calan, Isoptin)	Tab: 80, 120, 240 mg Inj: 2.5 mg/ml	Supraventricular arrhythmias, hypertrophic cardiomyopathy	D: 0.05–0.2 mg/kg IV slowly (5–10 min) in boluses of 0.05 mg/kg; 1–3 mg/kg q6–8h PO C: Same as D	Can cause ocular lesions Diltiazem is safer alternative in heart failure Potent vasodilator and negative inotrope

*Available in generic preparation.

AV, atrioventricular; BP, blood pressure; Cap, capsule; CHF, congestive heart failure; conc, concentration; COPD, chronic obstructive pulmonary disease; CRI, constant rate infusion; CV, cardiovascular; ECG, electrocardiogram; GI, gastrointestinal; Inj, injectable; IT, intrathecal; IV, intravenous; SR, slow release; SSS, sick sinus syndrome; Tab, tablet.

Sinus Tachycardia

Definition

- Impulses originate in the sinus node, but at a faster than normal frequency.
- The rhythm is regular.
- There are normal P waves for each QRS complex.
- The heart rate is > 140 bpm in the giant breeds, 180 bpm in toy-breed dogs, and 240 bpm in cats.

Etiology and Clinical Significance

- Sinus tachycardia may be a normal physiologic rhythm resulting from high sympathetic tone occurring with exercise or excitement.
- Sinus tachycardia may also occur with conditions such as stress, anxiety, pain, shock, fever, anemia, congestive heart failure, hyperthyroidism, and pheochromocytoma.
- Drugs (e.g., atropine, sympathomimetic agents, ketamine, diazepam, and light anesthesia) also can cause sinus tachycardia.

Electrocardiographic Differentials

- Other supraventricular tachyarrhythmias confused with sinus tachycardia include paroxysmal (atrial or AV junctional) tachycardia, atrial flutter with 2:1 AV block, and ventricular tachycardia when sinus tachycardia is associated with wide QRS complexes.
- A vagal maneuver (e.g., carotid sinus or ocular stimulation for 5–10 seconds) may result in a transient, gradual slowing of the sinus tachycardia.

Treatment

- Identify and treat the underlying cause of the sinus tachycardia.
- Antiarrhythmic drugs are seldom required.
- Administer atenolol (6.25 mg q12–24h PO) or propranolol (2.5 mg q8–12h PO) to hyperthyroid cats with intractable tachycardia (i.e., unresponsive to antithyroid medication).
- Administer digitalis for sinus tachycardia in congestive heart failure. Digoxin will reestablish normal baroreceptor function and lessen sympathetic tone.

Atrial Premature Complexes (Fig. 62–2)

Definition

- Impulses originate from an atrial focus, often other than the sinus node.
- The rhythm is irregular and the heart rate varies with the sinus node rate.
- There is usually an abnormal P′ wave (premature P wave) followed by a normal QRS complex. The P′-R interval of the APC may vary from the sinus rhythm P-R interval. The P′ wave may have various morphologies and may be fused with the T wave of the preceding beat.
- The P′ wave may occur so early in the cardiac cycle that the AV conduction system will be refractory, and the impulse will not be conducted to the ventricles (e.g., APC with physiologic AV block).
- The pause following the APC is often less than fully compensatory, because of premature depolarization and resetting of the sinus node. Full compensatory pause occurs when the R wave–to–R wave interval surrounding the APC is equal to two normal R-R intervals.
- The QRS complex is usually normal, but the intraventricular conduction system may be, in a relative or absolute refractory period, causing a bizarre (abnormal shape or direction) QRS complex. This abnormality is termed an APC with aberrant ventricular conduction.

Etiology and Clinical Significance

- APCs often indicate underlying cardiac disease (e.g., chronic valvular fibrosis, cardiomyopathy, congenital defect, cor pulmonale).
- Other causes include electrolyte disturbances, thyrotoxicosis, hypoxia, anemia, drug toxicity (e.g., digitalis, dobutamine, dopamine), toxemia, and increased sympathetic tone.

Electrocardiographic Differentials

- Sinus rhythm with APCs may be confused with marked sinus arrhythmia and ventricular premature complexes (VPCs) during auscultation, and with VPCs on the ECG, when APCs are conducted with aberrant ventricular conduction.

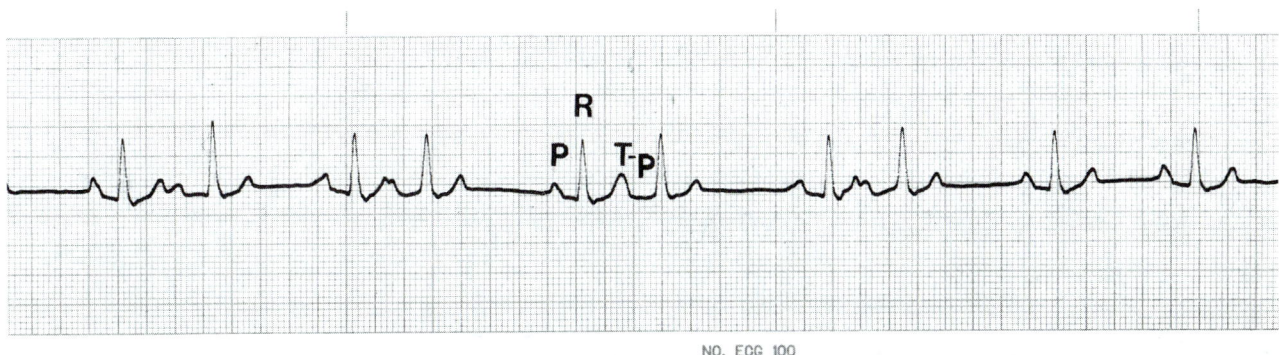

NO. ECG 100

Figure 62–2. Atrial premature complexes in a dog. (Lead II rhythm strip, paper speed 50 mm/sec; 1 cm = 1 mV.)

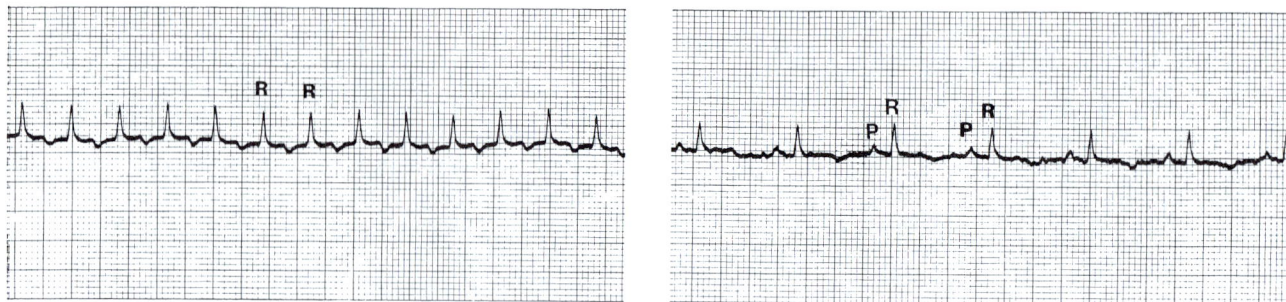

Figure 62–3. Paroxysmal atrial tachycardia *(left)* and after termination by a vagal maneuver *(right)* in a cat. (Lead II rhythm strip, paper speed 50 mm/sec; 1 cm = 1 mV.)

- A P′ wave preceding the abnormal QRS complex and a similarity of the initial deflection of the QRS complex compared with a preceding normal beat supports the diagnosis of aberrant conduction.

Treatment

- Infrequent APCs may be a normal variation and do not require treatment.
- If this arrhythmia is associated with congestive heart failure, treat the arrhythmia with digoxin.
- If the APCs are associated with poor hemodynamic status without myocardial failure, prescribe digoxin, diltiazem, or a beta-blocker (e.g., propranolol or atenolol; see Table 62–3).

Atrial Tachycardia (Figs. 62–3 and 62–4)

Definition

- Atrial tachycardia indicates rapid, abnormal impulses originating from an atrial site other than the sinus node.
- The atrium and/or AV junctional areas may be involved in a reentrant circuit that allows the impulse to restimulate the atrium as well as to pass to the ventricles. (A vagal maneuver may abolish this arrhythmia.)
- An abnormal automatic focus in the atrium may also be responsible for this arrhythmia (a vagal maneuver will cause AV block but not abolish the atrial tachycardia).

- The heart rate is > 140–180 bpm in dogs, > 240 bpm in cats and often approaches 300 bpm.
- The rhythm is usually regular but may be slightly irregular.
- There is a P′ wave for each QRS complex, although the P′ wave is usually of different morphology than the sinus P wave. The P-R interval is constant.
- The P′ wave may not be evident because it may be fused with the preceding T wave or occur simultaneously with the preceding QRS complex.
- The QRS complex may also be of different morphology because of aberrant ventricular conduction.
- An irregular R-R interval may be caused by concurrent AV block or by multifocal atrial tachycardia (P′ waves varying in shape; firing of two or more ectopic atrial foci).

Etiology and Clinical Significance

- Atrial tachycardia suggests severe myocardial or conduction system disease.
- This arrhythmia also may be secondary to digitalis toxicity or may occur under general anesthesia.
- Systemic disease that results in autonomic nervous systemic abnormalities also may be a cause.
- In cats, this arrhythmia is correlated with cardiomyopathy and hyperthyroidism.

Differential Diagnosis

- Atrial tachycardia can be confused with sinus tachycardia, AV junctional tachycardia, and atrial flutter.

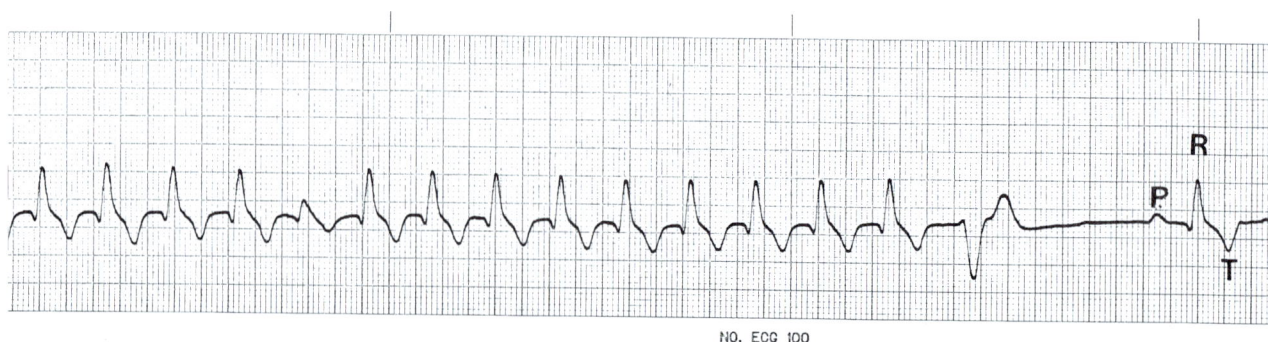

Figure 62–4. Paroxysmal atrial tachycardia terminated after a ventricular premature complex in a dog. (Lead II rhythm strip, paper speed 50 mm/sec; 1 cm = 1 mV.)

- A vagal maneuver may abruptly terminate AV nodal reentry or cause transient AV block with atrial tachycardia or atrial flutter (P waves or flutter waves can then be identified on the baseline).

Treatment

- Sustained (nonparoxysmal) atrial tachycardia often is associated with weakness, hypotension, congestive heart failure, and syncope and requires immediate therapy.
- A vagal maneuver (ocular pressure or carotid sinus pressure; see Chap. 61) may terminate a reentrant atrial tachycardia.
- If congestive heart failure is present, administer digitalis for the arrhythmia. Intravenous (IV) digoxin, given cautiously, may slow the ventricular response and improve the clinical status (see Table 62–3).
- If digoxin is ineffective, intravenous adenosine, verapamil, diltiazem, esmolol, or propranolol may convert supraventricular tachycardia (or atrial tachycardia) to sinus rhythm or slow the ventricular response rate. Use propranolol and verapamil with caution because they may depress cardiac contractility and exacerbate congestive heart failure.
- For atrial tachycardia without congestive heart failure, initiate therapy with adenosine, verapamil, a beta-blocker (e.g., esmolol, atenolol, or propranolol), or diltiazem.
- Intramuscular (IM) quinidine gluconate also has been used to convert atrial tachycardia to normal sinus rhythm in dogs with refractory atrial tachycardia.
- Reserve electrical cardioversion for refractory cases, to be administered only by an experienced veterinary cardiologist possessing the proper equipment.

Atrial Fibrillation (Fig. 62–5)

Definition

- A high number of disorganized atrial impulses, caused by a disorder of reentry within the atria, bombard the AV node, leading to an irregular rhythm.
- Many of these impulses approach the AV node in a refractory period and are not conducted to the ventricles, or they affect the conduction of subsequent impulses (concealed conduction).
- The heart rate is usually rapid (often > 180 bpm in dogs, and > 240 bpm in cats), and the rhythm is irregular.

▼ *Key Point* The lack of P waves and an irregularly irregular rhythm on all ECG leads and an arterial pulse deficit are the hallmarks of atrial fibrillation.

- No P waves are seen, but there are normally shaped QRS complexes. Instead of P waves, small or large oscillations (f waves) are present.
- There may be some variation and widening of the QRS complexes due to aberrant ventricular conduction or bundle branch block.

Etiology and Clinical Significance

- Atrial fibrillation commonly occurs in patients with cardiomyopathy, advanced chronic valvular heart disease, pericarditis, and progressive congenital heart disease.
- Other etiologies include severe ischemia or shock (gastric dilatation-volvulus, after cardiac arrest), atrial tumor (hemangiosarcoma), and electrolyte disturbances (hyperkalemia).
- Loss of atrial contraction decreases the stroke volume and cardiac output. The rapid ventricular rate also results in poor cardiac output.
- Slow atrial fibrillation (< 100 bpm) may signify drug toxicity (e.g., digitalis), concurrent AV block, or low sympathetic tone (most often observed in giant-breed dogs without CHF, often Irish wolfhounds).

Differential Diagnosis

- Atrial fibrillation can be confused with frequent APCs, AV junctional tachycardia with AV block, atrial tachycardia with AV block, and atrial flutter with AV block.
- Atrial flutter usually shows a regular R-R interval, and the atrial oscillations (F waves) are larger than f waves.

Treatment

- Give digoxin (see Table 62–3) to slow the ventricular response. Rarely, a sinus rhythm will return.
- After approximately 3–7 days, if the ventricular rate is not controlled, add a beta-blocker such as propranolol (begin with 0.2 mg/kg q8h) or a calcium channel antagonist such as diltiazem (begin with 0.5 mg/kg q8h) and increase the dose slowly until the resting ventricular rate is adequately controlled (<140–160 bpm).

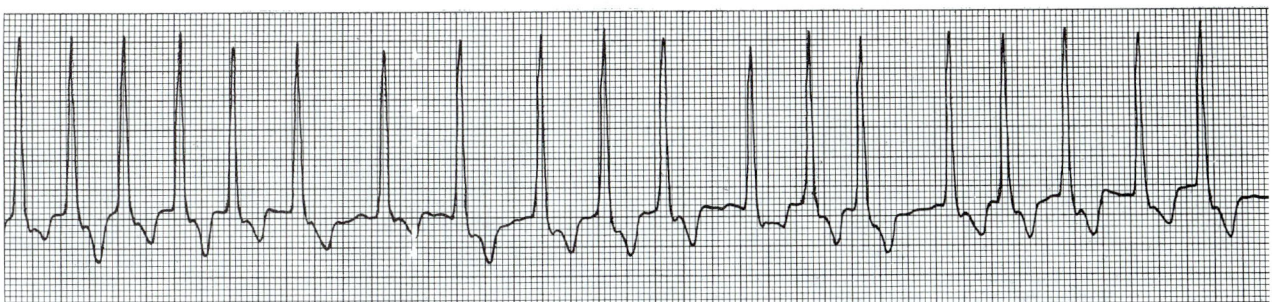

Figure 62–5. Atrial fibrillation in a dog. (Lead II rhythm strip, paper speed 50 mm/sec; 1 cm = 1 mV.)

- Although it is unusual to convert atrial fibrillation to normal sinus rhythm in dogs, the antiarrhythmic drug quinidine or calcium channel blockers (verapamil, diltiazem) may be useful for this purpose provided the dog is not in heart failure. A normal-sized heart, recent onset of atrial fibrillation, and lack of CHF favor the use of quinidine. Use quinidine with caution because it may increase the ventricular response rate.
- Electrical cardioversion is rarely if ever done in dogs (consult a specialist).

Atrioventricular Junctional Rhythm

Definition

- Impulses are generated in the AV junctional tissue and spread backward (retrograde) through the atrium and forward (antegrade) to the ventricles.
- The heart rate varies with the mechanism; that is, a passive escape rhythm (60 bpm) versus an enhanced AV junctional rhythm (>60 bpm but <100 bpm) versus a junctional tachycardia (>100 bpm in the dog).
- The rhythm usually is regular.
- The negative P′ wave may occur before, during, or after the normal QRS complex. The P′-R or R-P′ interval is constant.
- The P′ wave location depends on the area of impulse generation and relative speed of retrograde conduction through the atrium compared with antegrade conduction through the AV node, His bundle, and ventricular conduction system.

Etiology and Clinical Significance

- Digitalis toxicity may cause an AV junctional rhythm. When abnormally rapid, this arrhythmia is difficult to distinguish from atrial tachycardia.
- An AV junctional escape rhythm may occur in patients with depressed sinus node function, as in the sick sinus syndrome.
- Myocarditis may be associated with an enhanced AV junctional rhythm or AV junctional tachycardia.

Differential Diagnosis

- AV junctional rhythm can be confused with atrial standstill and slow atrial fibrillation.

Treatment

- Usually no treatment is needed and the rhythm reverts spontaneously.
- If weakness or syncope is associated with a slow AV junctional rhythm, atropine, dobutamine, or isoproterenol may be used in an attempt to accelerate the sinus node in order to help regain function as the primary pacemaker.
- Oral anticholinergic agents also may be useful for chronic therapy.
- If CHF is present with an enhanced AV junctional rhythm, administer digitalis.

VENTRICULAR RHYTHMS

Ventricular Premature Complexes (Figs. 62–6 to 62–8)

Definition

- Ectopic impulses originate from a focus below the AV node and AV junction.
- The heart rate is variable, depending on the frequency of ventricular premature complexes (VPCs); the rhythm is irregular.
- VPCs are usually related (coupled) to normal beats. If a VPC is not coupled to a normal beat, the origination site is referred to as a parasystolic focus.
- Usually there is a full compensatory pause following a VPC.
- Interpolated VPCs occur between normal beats and are not usually followed by a full compensatory pause.
- P waves that are seen are normal in shape, but are not associated with the QRS complex of the VPCs. The QRS complex often is wide and bizarre.
- If the major deflection of the QRS complex is negative in lead II, the ectopic focus likely is in the left ventricle; if the major deflection is positive in lead II, the ectopic focus probably is in the right ventricle.

Etiology and Clinical Significance

- The ventricular arrhythmia may be due to cardiac disease (e.g., congestive heart failure, myocarditis, endocarditis; see Table 62–2).

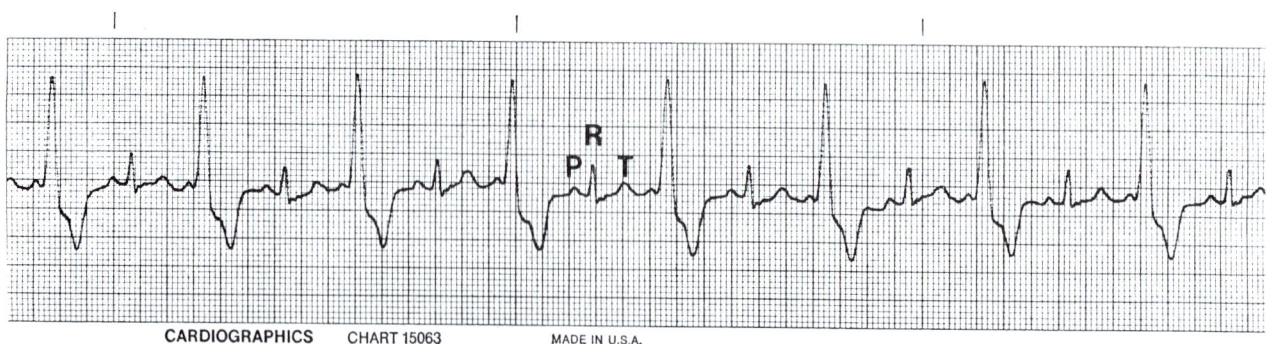

Figure 62–6. Ventricular premature complexes in a cat. (Lead II rhythm strip, paper speed 50 mm/sec; 1 cm = 1 mV.)

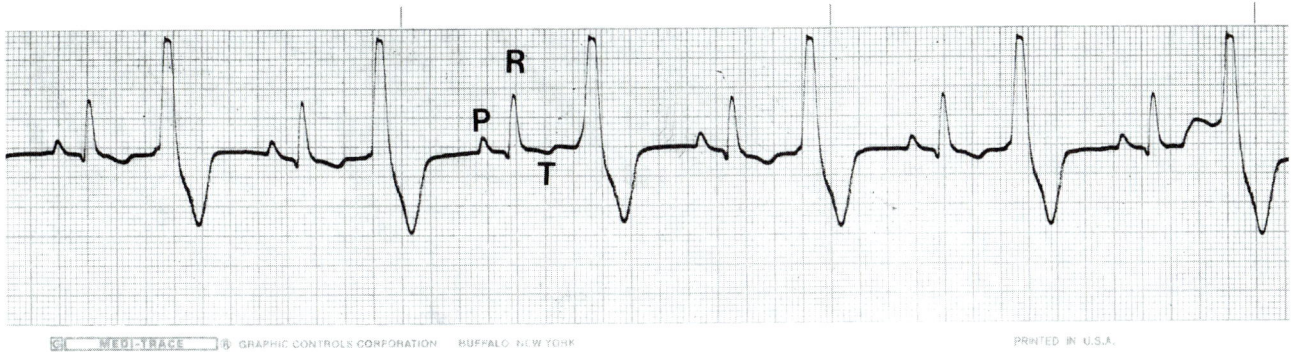

Figure 62–7. Ventricular premature complexes in a dog. (Lead II rhythm strip, paper speed 50 mm/sec; 1 cm = 1 mV.)

- Secondary causes of VPCs include trauma, electrolyte disturbances, autonomic changes, hypoxia, systemic infections, ischemia, and drug toxicosis.
- Frequent VPCs or VPCs occurring during the preceding Q-T interval may be electrically unstable (depending on underlying heart disease) and may progress to ventricular tachycardia and/or fibrillation and sudden death.
- A 24-hour tape-recorded (Holter) ECG may be necessary to assess the severity of a ventricular arrhythmia (see Chap. 61; Fig. 61–16).

Differential Diagnosis

- VPCs can be confused with atrial premature complexes with aberrant ventricular conduction and right or left bundle branch block.

Treatment

- VPCs do not generally require antiarrhythmic therapy.
- Consider antiarrhythmic therapy for:
  - Frequent *symptomatic* VPCs (>20–30/minute).
  - Repetitive complexes or runs of VPCs at very rapid rates (e.g., >180/minute), especially if causing signs or hypotension.
  - Multifocal QRS configurations (not a definite indication).
  - R on T phenomena (vulnerable period for development of ventricular fibrillation), in which the VPC occurs during the Q-T interval of the previous complex.

- Associated clinical signs of poor cardiac output (e.g., weakness, dyspnea, syncope) are probably the clearest indication for therapy.
- Do not treat ventricular escape complexes (similar to VPC configuration but at the end of pauses) because they represent a safety mechanism for maintaining cardiac output.
- Antiarrhythmic drugs commonly used to control VPCs include intravenous lidocaine and parenteral or oral procainamide, quinidine, tocainide, propranolol, atenolol, sotalol, and mexiletine (see Table 62–3 for dosages).

Ventricular Tachycardia (Figs. 62–8, 62–9, and 62–10)

Definition

- Impulses are repetitively generated (greater than three VPCs in a row) from one or more ventricular foci.
- This arrhythmia may be paroxysmal or sustained.
- The rate usually is >100 bpm in dogs, and >150 bpm in cats.
- Once established, the rhythm is regular unless the arrhythmia is intermittent or variable exit block (Purkinje cells to ventricular myocardium) is present.
- The P waves that are seen are normal in shape but have no fixed relationship to wide and bizarre QRS complexes.
- A sustained ventricular rhythm slower than the above rates is termed an idioventricular rhythm.

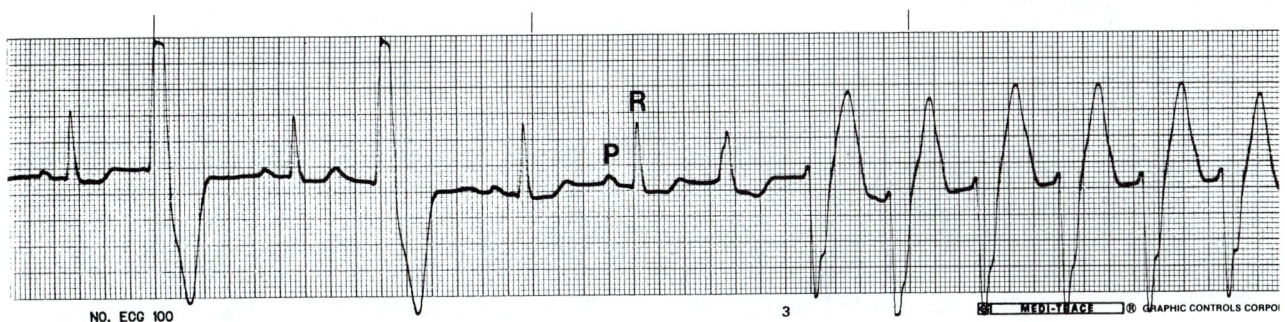

Figure 62–8. Sinus rhythm with ventricular premature complexes (right ventricular foci) and paroxysmal ventricular tachycardia (left ventricular foci) in a dog. (Lead II rhythm strip, paper speed 50 mm/sec; 1 cm = 1 mV.)

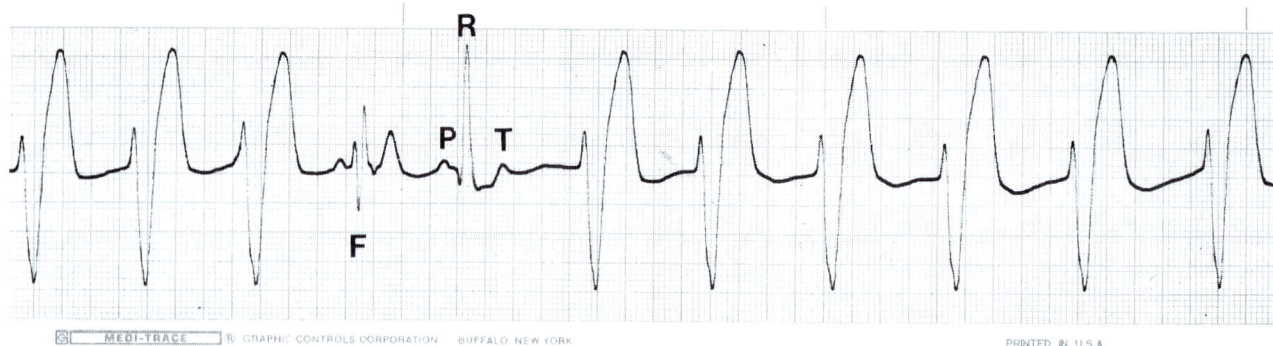

Figure 62–9. Paroxysmal ventricular tachycardia (showing fusion beat [F] in a dog. (Lead II rhythm strip, paper speed 50 mm/sec; 1 cm = 1 mV.)

Etiology and Clinical Significance

▼ *Key Point* Ventricular tachycardia can be well-tolerated or represent a life-threatening arrhythmia that, if sustained, may lead to hypotension, myocardial ischemia, syncope or seizures, shock, and sudden death. Each case must be individually evaluated.

- Some patients with ventricular tachycardia show no clinical signs, especially if there is no underlying primary cardiac disease.
- All etiologies of VPCs (e.g., primary and secondary cardiac disease; see Table 62–2) may lead to a ventricular tachycardia; however, not all are dangerous to the patient.

Differential Diagnosis

- Ventricular tachycardia can be confused with sinus tachycardia, atrial tachycardia, or atrial fibrillation with a conduction disturbance (e.g., left or right bundle branch block).

Treatment

- Antiarrhythmic therapy is required for some patients with sustained ventricular rhythms. Exceptions include patients with:
  - Complete heart block in which the ventricular rhythm may be an escape mechanism.
  - "Slow" ventricular rhythms (also called idioventricular tachycardias in which the ectopic rate is <180

bpm, does not cause hypotension, and the rhythm alternates with the sinus rhythm).
- Correct severe acid-base or electrolyte disturbances, such as hypomagnesemia, hypokalemia or hyperkalemia, which may respond to specific electrolyte or fluid therapy. Hypomagnesemia can cause or potentiate ventricular tachycardia. Magnesium chloride (1–2 mg/kg/min for 20–30 minutes) can also exert a primary antiarrhythmic effect.

▼ *Key Point* Cats with ventricular tachycardia associated with hypokalemia may respond to simple KCl therapy (IV in fluids; oral; see Chap. 5).

- Lidocaine hydrochloride without epinephrine (2–3 mg/kg) via slow IV administration is the initial preferred treatment in the dog.
  - This drug may also be used in the cat (initial bolus of 0.25 mg/kg slow IV); beware of seizures.
  - Administer diazepam IV for seizures.
  - Hypotension or sinus arrest also may occur if the bolus is administered too rapidly.
- If necessary, repeat the lidocaine bolus several times at 10-minute intervals, although the higher dosages will increase the incidence of toxicity.
- The maximum total dose for dogs is 8 mg/kg over 10–15 minutes. Seizures and vomiting may occur in dogs at toxic doses.
- The therapeutic effect of lidocaine is short-term, and repeat boluses or constant-rate infusion may be required for a sustained antiarrhythmic effect. To

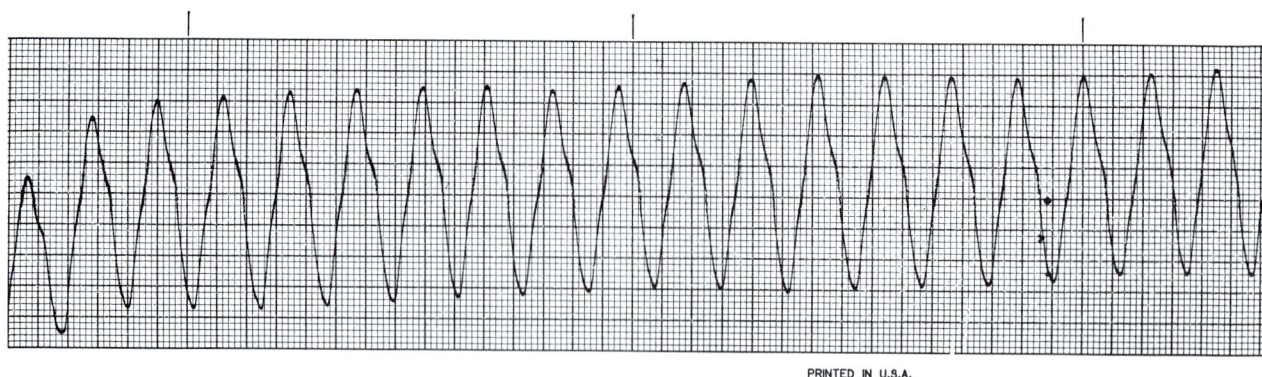

Figure 62–10. Ventricular tachycardia-flutter in a dog. (Lead II rhythm strip, paper speed 50 mm/sec; 1 cm = 1 mV.)

calculate the amount of lidocaine to be added to IV fluids over 6 hours, use the following equation:

BW kg × 30–80 µg/kg/min × 0.36 = lidocaine in mg

- When the arrhythmia is controlled with lidocaine, initiate intramuscular or oral therapy with procainamide, quinidine, mexiletine, or tocainide (see Table 62–3), and slowly reduce the lidocaine infusion over a 24- to 48-hour period.
  - Treat hypokalemia, hypomagnesemia, and acidosis because they may cause therapeutic failure.
- When lidocaine therapy is not indicated or practical, give quinidine gluconate or procainamide IM to provide initial control of ventricular tachycardia.
- Prolonged therapy may be continued with oral quinidine or procainamide at appropriate doses. Other antiarrhythmic drugs that may be useful include propranolol, atenolol, mexiletine, sotalol, tocainide, and phenytoin (for digoxin toxicity).
- Reserve electrical cardioversion for refractory ventricular tachycardia. An experienced cardiologist and proper equipment are necessary.
- If the arrhythmia worsens, consider antiarrhythmic drug toxicity (proarrhythmia) as the cause rather than worsening disease.
  - Multiform ventricular tachycardia (torsades de pointes) due to procainamide or quinidine toxicity may be a life-threatening complication of antiarrhythmic medication.
  - Treat this arrhythmic complication with drug withdrawal, bicarbonate, and isoproterenol or dopamine.
- If the arrhythmia is well controlled, consider discontinuing the antiarrhythmic agent after a 2- to 3-week period. This may avoid complications of long-term therapy and the expense of antiarrhythmic drugs. Evaluate the ECG before each decrease in dosage, or within 1 week after stopping the medication.
- In cases of refractory or recurrent ventricular tachycardia, consult a cardiologist.

Ventricular Fibrillation (Fig. 62–11)

Definition

- Cardiac impulses are generated and propagated in the ventricles in a chaotic, asynchronous manner.

- The heart rate is rapid and disorganized.
- The rhythm is irregular.
- There are no P waves present and there are no recognizable QRS complexes. There are continuous positive and negative oscillations that are chaotic and bizarre. The oscillations may be large (coarse) or small (fine).

Etiology and Clinical Significance

▼ *Key Point* The most common arrhythmia associated with cardiac arrest is ventricular fibrillation.

- There is no effective cardiac output.
- Conditions such as myocardial ischemia, electrolyte imbalance, autonomic nervous system imbalance, hypoxia, hypothermia, slow conduction, increased automaticity, drug toxicity, and unstable ventricular arrhythmias cause electrical instability and trigger ventricular fibrillation.
- Ventricular fibrillation is associated with a very grave prognosis.

Differential Diagnosis

- Differentiate ECG artifact (e.g., 60-cycle electrical interference, respiratory movement, use of electrocautery during surgery) from ventricular fibrillation. A palpable arterial pulse and rhythmic precordial heart beat rule out ventricular fibrillation.

Treatment

- Perform cardiopulmonary resuscitation (CPR) immediately (see Chap. 73).
- Electrical defibrillation is mandatory.
- Intracardiac lidocaine occasionally is successful in converting ventricular fibrillation to normal sinus rhythm.
- Open-chest cardiac massage may be effective in converting ventricular fibrillation to normal sinus rhythm if no defibrillation equipment is available (particularly in the cat). External blows to the chest (thump-version) are less effective.

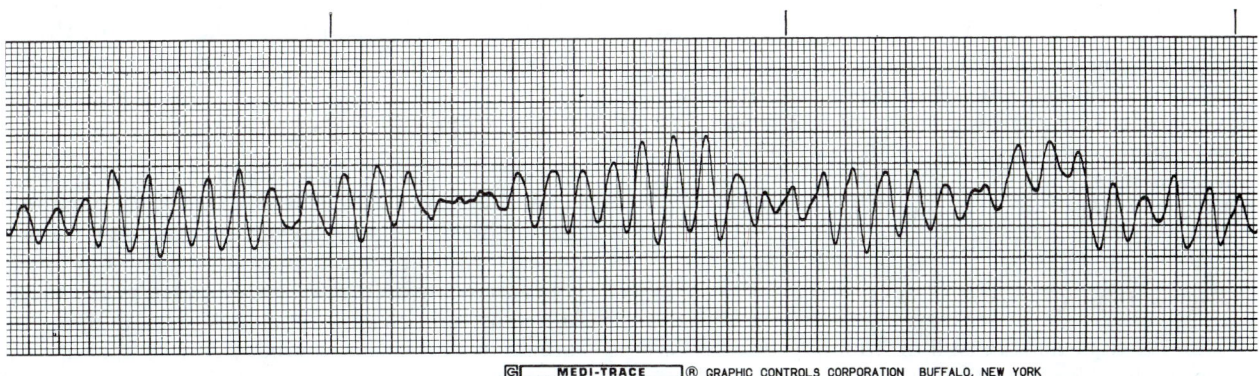

MEDI-TRACE ® GRAPHIC CONTROLS CORPORATION BUFFALO, NEW YORK

Figure 62–11. Ventricular fibrillation in a dog. (Lead II rhythm strip, paper speed 50 mm/sec; 1 cm = 1 mV.)

Ventricular Asystole

Definition

- No impulses are generated from atrial, junctional, or ventricular pacemakers.
- There is no cardiac rate or ventricular rhythm.
- No QRS complexes are seen.

Etiology and Clinical Significance

- Ventricular asystole is associated with cardiac arrest and if left untreated is a lethal arrhythmia.

Differential Diagnosis

- Differentiate ECG artifact (e.g., electrocardiograph is not on a proper lead or is connected improperly) from ventricular asystole.

Treatment

- Perform CPR immediately (see Chap. 73).
- Epinephrine, along with CPR, may be lifesaving.

CONDUCTION DISORDERS

Atrial Standstill

Definition

- Impulses are not generated in the sinus node and are poorly conducted or nonconducted through the atrial tissues.
- The heart rate is <60 bpm in dogs and <160 bpm in cats.
- No P waves are seen, and the QRS complexes are normal or bizarre depending on the intraventricular conduction. The S-T segment may be elevated or depressed. The T wave may be tall due to shortened repolarization (see Chap. 61; Fig. 61–11).
- The rhythm may be regular or irregular.

Etiology and Clinical Significance

▼ *Key Point* Atrial standstill is a life-threatening abnormality when associated with hyperkalemia (hypoadrenocorticism, acute renal failure, urinary obstruction, and diabetic ketoacidosis).

- Persistent atrial standstill occurs in English springer spaniels (may be correlated with a muscular dystrophy, as in humans) and other breeds and develops occasionally in cats with dilated cardiomyopathy in which there is degeneration and fibrosis of the atrial myocardial cells.
- There is cardiac enlargement, but electrolytes are normal with persistent atrial standstill.

Differential Diagnosis

- Differentiate atrial standstill on multiple lead ECGs from AV junctional rhythm, idioventricular rhythm, and atrial fibrillation with complete heart block.

Treatment

- If hyperkalemia is present, perform emergency therapy to dilute and transfer extracellular potassium into the cells, thereby restoring normokalemia.
- Administer 0.9% saline, 40–90 ml/kg/hr, until hyperkalemia and hypovolemia are corrected.
- In addition, administer 2 mEq/kg of sodium bicarbonate slowly IV. This may restore more narrow QRS complexes and increase myocardial contractility; repeat the dose if needed within 15–30 minutes; beware of paradoxical cerebral acidosis.
- As an alternative therapy to sodium bicarbonate, administer 0.5 U/kg of regular insulin coupled with 2 g of dextrose (in a 5–10% dextrose drip) per unit of insulin, slowly IV.
- For life-threatening conditions, give calcium gluconate (1 ml of 10% solution/10 kg BW, slowly IV) to counteract the cardiotoxic effects of hyperkalemia.
- If hypoadrenocorticism is the cause of hyperkalemia, mineralocorticoid and glucocorticoid replacement is necessary (see Chap. 31).
- In the English springer spaniel with symptomatic atrial standstill, a permanent cardiac pacemaker is required. Consult a cardiologist.

Incomplete (First- and Second-Degree) Atrioventricular Block

Definition

- The cardiac impulse is delayed or intermittently blocked in the region of the AV node or AV junction.
- The heart rate is variable, depending on the rate of the sinus node pacemaker and the AV conduction sequence.
- The rhythm usually is regular in first-degree AV block (unless other arrhythmias are present) and irregular in second-degree AV block.
- *First-degree AV block* shows a prolonged but constant P-R interval (AV conduction) with normal P wave and QRS complexes at a 1:1 ratio.
- *Second-degree AV block* has normal P wave and QRS complexes with a constant P-R interval and with intermittent P waves not followed by QRS complexes.
- In *Mobitz type I (Wenckebach) AV block*, the P-R interval is gradually prolonged before a dropped ventricular beat occurs. The rhythm is regularly irregular.
- In *Mobitz type II AV block*, a consistent P-R interval occurs prior to a dropped ventricular beat. The rhythm often is irregular.

Etiology and Clinical Significance

- First-degree and Mobitz type I second-degree AV blocks often are caused by an increase in vagal tone (e.g., in brachycephalic breeds and in patients with respiratory, gastrointestinal, or neurologic disease), digitalis, and sedatives (e.g., xylazine and acepromazine).
- Antiarrhythmic drugs (beta-blockers, quinidine, procainamide, diltiazem, digoxin, and verapamil) and AV nodal disease are associated with these types of AV block.

- Physiologic AV block may occur following ectopic beats or atrial tachyarrhythmias that occur during the AV node's absolute or relative refractory periods (will slow down or block impulse).
- Mobitz type II AV block is a more advanced degree of block occurring in the AV junction, His bundle, or below. It may progress to complete heart block. Causes include:
  - Idiopathic fibrosis (older dogs and cats), hereditary stenosis of the His bundle in the Pug and Doberman pinscher, and hypertrophic cardiomyopathy in dogs and cats.
  - Neoplastic infiltration secondary to metastatic neoplasia.
  - Profound electrolyte disorders.
  - Infection (e.g., Lyme disease).
- The development of clinical signs (e.g., weakness, syncope, congestive heart failure) depends on the degree of AV block, ventricular rate, and ventricular function.
- In cats there may be abrupt fluctuation between incomplete and complete AV block. Older cats (>12 years) may tolerate second- and third-degree AV block very well, and these bradyarrhythmias may be incidental findings.

Differential Diagnosis

- Differentiate complete AV block from advanced second-degree AV block on the ECG.

Treatment

- Treatment usually is not required for Mobitz type I AV block. If the block is related to drug toxicity, stop the drug or lower the dosage.
- Therapy for Mobitz type II AV block depends on the clinical signs. If the cardiac rate is slow and weakness or syncope is evident, begin therapy with atropine, dobutamine, isoproterenol, or a temporary or permanent cardiac pacemaker.

Complete (Third-Degree) AV Block (Fig. 62–12)
Definition

- The cardiac impulse is completely blocked in the region of the AV junction and/or the His bundle.
- The atrial rate (P-P interval) is within normal limits, and there is a slow idioventricular escape rhythm.

The rhythm is usually regular. In dogs, an idioventricular escape rhythm has a rate of 40–60 bpm.
- An enhanced AV junctional or idioventricular rhythm (AV dissociation) has a more rapid rate, with the ventricular rate approaching the atrial rate.
- The P wave is completely dissociated from the QRS complex.
- The P-R interval is variable, and usually there are many P waves with few QRS complexes.
- The morphology of the QRS complexes varies depending on the origin of the ventricular escape rhythm.

Etiology and Clinical Significance

- Complete AV block often is associated with the clinical signs of weakness, syncope, and congestive heart failure.

Differential Diagnosis

- Differentiate complete AV block on the ECG from advanced second-degree AV block, atrial standstill, and ventricular tachycardia (idioventricular rhythm).

Treatment

- A permanent cardiac pacemaker is the only consistently effective long-term treatment in symptomatic animals.
- Drugs that may be useful for short-term stabilization and treatment include atropine, isoproterenol, dobutamine, and corticosteroids (anti-inflammatory). An IV dobutamine or isoproterenol infusion may be useful for increasing the rate of the ventricular escape rhythm during required surgical procedures.
- In situations in which pacemaker implantation is not an option, oral therapy with methylxanthines (e.g., theophylline, aminophylline) or sympathomimetics (e.g., albuterol, terbutaline) may accelerate the ventricular escape rhythm.

Intraventricular Conduction Disturbances

Right bundle branch block (RBBB), left bundle branch block, left anterior fascicular block (LAFB), and combined RBBB-LAFB are described and illustrated electrocardiographically in Chapter 61.

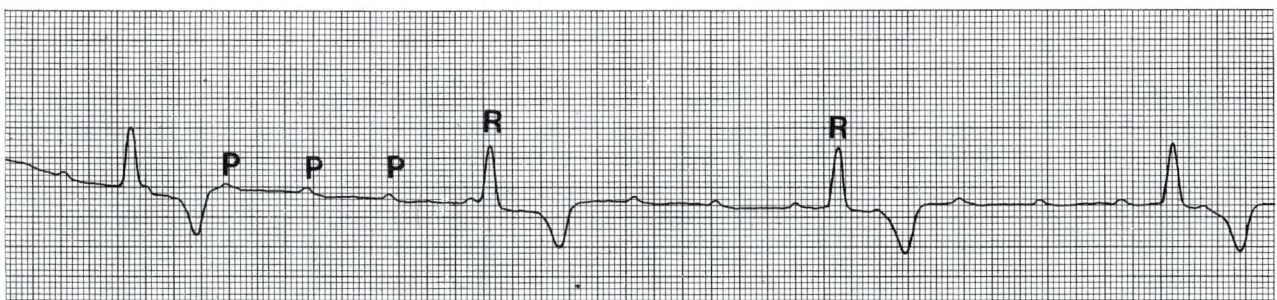

Figure 62–12. Complete (third-degree) atrioventricular block in a cat. (Lead II rhythm strip, paper speed 50 mm/sec; 1 cm = 1 mV.)

OTHER ARRHYTHMIAS AND CONDUCTION DISTURBANCES

Sick Sinus Syndrome

Definition

- In SSS, cardiac impulses are generated in the sinus node at a slower than normal rate or are blocked from exiting the sinus node.
- The atria and AV node may also be involved, resulting in an atrial tachyarrhythmia (e.g., atrial tachycardia, flutter, or fibrillation).
- A bradycardia-tachycardia syndrome may occur, with alternating periods of slow and rapid heart rates.
- There is a normal P wave for each QRS complex. The P-R interval is constant unless the bradyarrhythmia-tachyarrhythmia syndrome is present.

Differential Diagnosis

- Differentiate the multiple ECG abnormalities included in SSS from isolated sinus bradycardia, sinus block and/or arrest, and atrial tachycardia due to other causes. A poor (blunted) response to atropine (<50% increase in heart rate) supports the diagnosis of SSS.

Etiology and Clinical Significance

- SSS occurs predominantly in geriatric, small-breed females. Miniature schnauzers, cocker spaniels, West Highland white terriers, and dachshunds are over-represented.
- Clinical signs of SSS are variable but often include weakness and syncope.

Treatment

- If the animal is asymptomatic, no therapy is required.
- Anticholinergic drugs are rarely successful in symptomatic dogs.
- In animals with bradycardia-tachycardia syndrome, an artificial ventricular-demand pacemaker may be required for long-term control of bradyarrhythmias, and digoxin, propranolol, or diltiazem may control the tachyarrhythmia; do not use these drugs unless a pacemaker is implanted.

Ventricular Preexcitation and Wolff-Parkinson-White Syndrome

Definition

- In ventricular preexcitation the cardiac impulses are generated in the sinus node but spread to the ventricle via an anomalous conduction pathway as well as the AV node. (See Chapter 61 for additional information.)
- In WPW syndrome, a premature impulse finds the bypass pathway or AV node in its refractory period, allowing the development of a macro-reentry circuit that contributes to a tachycardia.

- During ventricular preexcitation, the cardiac rate and rhythm are normal. In the WPW syndrome, the rate may be very rapid (e.g., 300 bpm).
- The P waves are normal in ventricular preexcitation and are unrecognizable in WPW syndrome.
- The QRS complex is widened with notching of the R wave (delta wave) in ventricular preexcitation (see Chap. 61; Fig. 61–9). In WPW syndrome, the QRS complex may be normal, wide, or bizarre, depending on the circuit of the atrial tachycardia.
- The P-R interval is short in ventricular preexcitation. In WPW syndrome, often there is a P wave for every QRS complex (1:1 conduction).
- A short P-R interval may be correlated with a normal QRS complex if the anomalous pathway bypasses the AV node to the area of the His bundle (Lown-Ganong-Levine syndrome in humans).

Etiology and Clinical Significance

- Ventricular preexcitation and WPW syndrome may be a congenital problem in the dog or cat that occurs with or without other congenital heart defects (e.g., atrial septal defect, valvular dysplasia, hypertrophic cardiomyopathy).

Differential Diagnosis

- Differentiate the tachycardia of WPW syndrome from AV junctional tachycardia, atrial tachycardia, and ventricular tachycardia.

Treatment

- Ventricular preexcitation without tachycardia requires no therapy.
- In animals with WPW syndrome, control and/or convert the sustained tachycardia with a vagal maneuver (e.g., ocular or carotid sinus pressure), with drugs such as verapamil and adenosine, or with DC shock.

THERAPEUTIC PRINCIPLES

- Determine a precise diagnosis for the arrhythmia.
- Mechanisms for arrhythmias include isolated or concurrent disorders in impulse generation (automaticity), conduction (block or reentry), and triggered activity. These are often impossible to determine with certainty.
- Eliminate noncardiac causes (e.g., acid-base and electrolyte abnormalities, hypothermia, hypovo-lemia, hypoxemia, anemia, infections, and other systemic problems) before using an antiarrhythmic drug.
- Stop other drug therapy if it may be the cause of the arrhythmia (e.g., digitalis, xylazine, acepromazine).
- Treat heart failure if present.
- Drug therapy for cardiac arrhythmias is intended to prevent clinical signs such as weakness, syncope, seizures, personality changes, and congestive heart failure. Also, drug therapy may decrease electrical instability and the likelihood of progression to a lethal arrhythmia (e.g., ventricular fibrillation).

- Select the antiarrhythmic drug best suited to the underlying cause of the arrhythmia (e.g., digoxin plus a beta-blocker or calcium channel blocker for atrial fibrillation, lidocaine to terminate ventricular arrhythmias). See Chapter 63 for description of the various antiarrhythmic cardiac drugs and refer to Table 62–3 for dosages.
- Be aware of synergistic effects of antiarrhythmic drugs (e.g., digoxin and propranolol may additively delay AV conduction) and antagonistic effects (e.g., quinidine may cause serum digoxin levels to rise, increasing the possibility of digoxin toxicity).
- Refractory arrhythmias may require a combination of antiarrhythmic agents, although these may increase the possibility of drug-related toxicity (e.g., digoxin and diltiazem or propranolol, procainamide and propranolol).
- Be aware that some arrhythmias may require antiarrhythmic drugs in addition to other therapeutic modalities (e.g., for SSS with bradyarrhythmia-tachyarrhythmias, a pacemaker for the bradyarrhythmia and an antiarrhythmic drug for the tachyarrhythmia).

- Be aware of the proarrhythmic potential of antiarrhythmic drugs. Digoxin can cause any arrhythmia and conduction disturbance. Monitor ECGs frequently.

SUPPLEMENTAL READINGS

Kittleson MD, Kienle RD: Small Animal Cardiovascular Medicine. St. Louis, Mosby, 1998, p. 502.

Miller MS: Quicksands of Electrocardiography. Annual Proceedings, Am Coll Vet Intern Med 1991, p 707.

Miller MS, Calvert CA: Special tests to diagnose arrhythmias. In Tilley LP, ed.: Essentials of Canine and Feline Electrocardiography, 3rd Ed. Baltimore: Williams & Wilkins, 1992.

Miller MS, Tilley CP: Treatment of arrhythmias and conduction disturbances. *In* Miller MS, Tilley LP, eds.: Manual of Canine and Feline Cardiology. Philadelphia: WB Saunders, 1995, p 371.

Miller MS, Tilley LP, Smith FWK, Fox PR: Electrocardiography. *In* Fox PR, Sisson DD, Moise NS (eds): Canine and Feline Cardiology, 2nd Ed. Philadelphia: WB Saunders, 1999.

Strickland KN: Advances in antiarrhythmic therapy. Vet Clin North Am 28:502, 1998.

Tilley LP: Essentials of Canine and Feline Electrocardiography, 3rd Ed. Baltimore: Williams & Wilkins, 1992.

William W. Muir, III / John D. Bonagura

To effectively use drugs that affect the heart and circulation, the clinician must understand the pathophysiology of the disease and appreciate the relevant pharmacology of the drugs prescribed (Table 63–1). The purpose of this chapter is to review aspects of cardiovascular pharmacology that are particularly applicable to small animal veterinary practice. Specific drugs and recommended dosages are listed in Table 63–2. Drugs used in management of cardiopulmonary-cerebral recuscitation are discussed in Chapter 73. Management of shock and cardiovascular collapse is found in Chapter 72.

DRUGS USED TO TREAT HEART FAILURE

Congestive heart failure (CHF) is a clinical syndrome involving cardiac, hemodynamic, neurohormonal, and renal dysfunction and is associated with impaired exercise capacity, edema, and high mortality. CHF develops when the heart is unable to fill or pump normally and thereby maintain adequate cardiac output, arterial blood pressure, tissue perfusion, and exercise capacity. Heart failure is triggered by a restricted cardiac output stemming from myocardial failure, valvular diseases, arrhythmias, or restriction of cardiac filling (e.g., pericardial diseases or severe ventricular hypertrophy). Heightened neurohormonal activity is an important com- ponent of the heart failure syndrome, and it is charac-terized by activation of *vasoconstricting* and *sodium-retaining* systems and inhibition of vasodilator and sodium-excreting systems. Renal retention of sodium and water can be profound in CHF, and fluid accumulation is a characteristic of chronic heart disease. These compensations become *mal*adaptive, causing clinical signs of CHF and also leading to myocardial injury. Pharmacologic and dietary treatments represent attempts to control the compensatory mechanisms activated to maintain blood pressure in animals with failing hearts. The ultimate goal of therapy, whether definitive or palliative, is to improve the quality of life and prolong life.

Drugs are used in the treatment of heart failure to alter the determinants of ventricular performance: inotropism, venous pressure and preload, and arterial resistance and afterload. Some drugs also may improve the diastolic (lusitropic) function of the heart. Others help to regulate heart rate and rhythm. Some of the most suc-cessful agents for prolonging survival in CHF attenuate vasoconstricting systems, which are injurious to the heart muscle and potentiate signs of CHF (e.g., angiotensin inhibitors, beta blockers). Because most causes of heart disease are not amenable to specific treatment, the clinician must be adept at administering symptomatic therapy for heart failure. The clinical pharmacology of three groups of drugs used for treatment of CHF—the diuretics, positive inotropic drugs, and vasodilator drugs—are summarized in the following sections.

Diuretics

▼ *Key Point* Diuretics inhibit reabsorption of sodium, water, and other electrolytes in the renal tubules and play a crucial role in the therapy of *congestive* heart failure.

With contraction of the vascular volume, venous and capillary hydrostatic pressures are lowered. This decreases formation of edema and effusions.

- Diuresis also reduces cardiac dimensions (preload) and, in cardiac dilatation, has the potential to reduce systolic wall tension (afterload) and decrease mitral regurgitation (by reducing the size of the regurgitant orifice).
- Perivascular edema may diminish the responsiveness of blood vessels to vasodilator drug therapy. Diuretic therapy may improve vascular responsiveness in CHF.
- Diuretics typically are classified by renal tubular site of action. The diuretics most often used in treatment of cardiovascular (CV) diseases include loop diuretics, thiazide diuretics, and potassium-sparing diuretics.

Clinical Pharmacology
Loop Diuretics

- The loop diuretics—furosemide, bumetanide, and torsemide—are potent drugs that inhibit active ion and water transport in the thick ascending portion of Henle's loop. Loop diuretics block the sodium-potassium-chloride co-transporter and promote a marked diuresis of chloride, sodium, potassium, hydrogen ion, and free-water. Furosemide (Lasix) is the diuretic most frequently used in clinical practice.

Table 63–1. EXAMPLES OF COMMONLY USED CARDIOVASCULAR DRUGS

Type of Drug	Drugs	Principle Effects	Examples of Use
Positive inotropic drugs	Digitalis glycosides (digoxin, digitoxin)	Positive inotropic drug, neurotropic drug (increases vagal tone), slows heart rate	CHF due to dilated cardiomyopathy, chronic valvular disease, atrial fibrillation
	Dobutamine, dopamine	Positive inotropic drug	Cardiogenic shock, severe CHF
	Amrinone	Positive inotropic drug/vasodilator	Cardiogenic shock, severe CHF
Diuretics	Furosemide	Diuretic	Pulmonary edema, ascites, pleural effusion
	Hydrochlorothiazide and spironolactone	Combination diuretic, blocks aldosterone, retains potassium	Refractory ascites or pleural effusion due to CHF
Vasodilator therapy	Hydralazine	Systemic arteriolar vasodilator, decreases left ventricular afterload, reduces mitral regurgitation	Mitral regurgitation, pulmonary edema, concurrent systemic hypertension
	Nitroglycerin ointment	Systemic venodilator, pools blood in systemic veins	Pulmonary edema, left-sided CHF
	Enalapril, lisinopril, benazepril	Angiotensin-converting enzyme inhibitors, vasodilators, decrease aldosterone	Chronic CHF due to cardiomyopathy or valvular heart disease
	Sodium nitroprusside	Direct arteriolar and venodilator	Emergency Rx of pulmonary edema
Calcium channel antagonists	Diltiazem	Decreases AV nodal conduction, improves ventricular relaxation, arterial vasodilator	Atrial fibrillation, hypertrophic cardiomyopathy
	Verapamil	Decreases AV nodal conduction	Acute therapy of supraventricular tachycardia
	Amlodipine	Arterial vasodilator	Systemic hypertension
Beta-blockers	Propranolol, atenolol, nadolol, metoprolol, carvedilol	Decreases heart rate, slows AV nodal conduction, decreases outflow obstruction	Hypertrophic cardiomyopathy, atrial fibrillation, antiarrhythmic therapy
Antiarrhythmic drugs	Lidocaine, procainamide, quinidine, mexiletine, sotalol, amiodarone	Antiarrhythmic drugs	Cardiac arrhythmias

AV, atrioventricular; CHF, congestive heart failure.

Table 63-2. CARDIOPULMONARY DRUGS—APPROXIMATE DOSAGES IN DOGS AND CATS

Drug	Preparation(s)	Usual Dose*
Amlodipine	Norvasc: 2.5-mg tablet	Cat: ¼–½ tablet 12–24h for hypertension
Aminone	Inocor: 5 mg/ml (20-ml vials)	1–3 mg/kg, IV followed by 30–100 µg/kg/min infusion
Atenolol	Tenormin: 25, 50 mg tablets	Dog: 6.25–25 mg q12h Cat: 6.25–12.5 mg daily
Atropine USP	USP: 0.4 and 0.5 mg/ml for injection	0.01–0.04 mg/kg, IV, IM, SQ
Benazepril HCl	Lotensin: 5-, 10-, 20-, 40-mg tablets	Dog: 0.5 mg/kg 12–24h Cat: 0.25–0.5 mg/kg q24h
Butorphanol	Torbutrol 0.5 mg/ml; 1-, 5-, 10-mg tablets	Dog: 0.5 mg/kg PO q6–12h as an antitussive Dog: 0.4 mg/kg IM mixed with acepromazine as a sedative
Captopril	Capoten: 12.5, 25, 50 mg tablets	Dog, cat: 0.5–2.0 (to 3.0) mg/kg orally q8h
Digoxin	Lanoxin, Cardoxin, digoxin USP: 0.125-, 0.25-, 0.5-mg tablets; 0.05-mg/ml and 0.15-mg/ml elixirs; 0.25-mg/ml Lanoxin for injection	Dog: 0.0055–0.0075 mg/kg q12h Cat: using a 0.125-mg tablet of Lanoxin—¼ tablet qod to qd
Dihydrocodone	Hycodan 5-mg tablets	Dog: 2.5–5 mg q8–24h for cough
Diltiazem	Cardizem: 30-, 60-, 90-, 120-mg tablets; Dilacor XR (Rhone-Poulenc Rorer) 120-, 180-, 240-mg capsules; Cardizem CD (Marion Merrell Dow) 120-, 180-, 240-mg capsules	Dog: 0.5–1.3 mg/kg orally q8h Cat: 0.5–2.0 mg/kg q8–12h for standard cardizem Dilacor—½ of a 60-mg pellet [taken from the 240-mg capsule] q12–24h; or long-acting forms (Cardizem CD) must be compounded
Dobutamine	Dobutrex: 250-mg (20 ml) vial for injection	Dog: 2.5 to 20 µg/kg/min, constant rate IV infusion. Cat: 2.5 to 10 µg/kg/min CRI
Dopamine	Intropin, dopamine USP: 200-mg, 400-mg, and 800-mg vials for injection	2–10 µg/kg/min, constant rate IV infusion
Enalapril	Enacard, Vasotec: 1.25-, 2.5-, 5-, 10-, 20-mg tablets	Dog: 0.5 mg/kg orally q12–24h Cat: 0.25–0.5 mg/kg orally qd
Epinephrine	Adrenaline, USP: 1:10,000 (0.1 mg/ml) and 1:1000 (1 mg/ml)	IV dose: 0.05–0.2 mg/kg
Esmolol	Brevibloc: 100 mg/ml–10 ml vial	Dog, cat: 50–150 mcg/kg/min after initial loading dose of 200 µg/kg administered over 1 min
Furosemide	Lasix: 12.5-, 50- [Vet] mg, 20-, 40-, 50- [Vet], 80-mg tablets; 1% syrup (10 mg/ml)	Dog: 2–6 mg/kg repeated q8–12h as needed (IV, IM, SQ, oral) Cat: 1–4 mg/kg repeated q12h as needed (IV, IM, SQ, oral)
Hydralazine	Apresoline: 10, 25-, 50-mg tablets	Dog: 1–2 mg/kg orally q12h (initial dose 0.5 mg/kg, titrate to effect or 1 mg/kg q12h)
Hydrochlorothiazide/ spironolactone	HydroDIURIL, USP: 25-, 50-mg tablets; Aldactazide: 25 mg hydrochlorothiazide combined with 25 mg spironolactone	Dog, cat: 2–4 mg/kg once or twice daily (of either HCT or combined product
Isosorbide dinitrate	Sorbitrate oral tabs, Isordil: 5-, 10-mg tablets	Dog: 2.5–5 mg orally q12h

Lidocaine	Xylocaine, lidocaine USP: 2% (20 mg/ml) for injection (without epinephrine)	Dog: 2 mg/kg [IV] up to 8 mg/kg over a 10-min period; 25–75 μg (occasionally up to 100) kg/min constant rate IV infusion Cat: 0.25–0.75 mg/kg [IV] over a 3–5-min period
Lisinopril	Prinivil (Merck & Co.) 2.5-, 5-, 10-, 20-, 40-mg tablets (unscored)	Dog: 0.25–0.5 mg/kg q12–24h
Magnesium	20% MgCl₂⁻ contains 1.97 mEq of Mg⁺⁺ per ml	0.75–1 mEq/kg/24h IV (50% of dose can be given in 2–4 hours if necessary)
Mexiletine	Mexitil: 150, 200, 250-mg capsules	Dog: 5–8 mg/kg orally q8h
Morphine sulfate	USP: 15 mg/ml (5–15 mg/ml)	Dog: 0.1–0.25 mg/kg, IV, IM
Nitroglycerin ointment (2%)	Nitrol, Nitro-Bid, Nitrostat: one inch = 15 mg NTG; Minitran transdermal patches 2.5, 5, 10, 15 mg/24 hr	Dog: 4–12 mg (up to 15 mg) topically q12h CAT: 2–4 mg topically q12h (doses approximate)
Procainamide	Pronestyl (-SR), Procan SR: capsules and tablets (SR): 250, 375, 500 mg	Dog: 2 mg/kg (IV) up to a maximum total dose of 20 mg/kg over a 30-min period; 25–40 μg/kg/min IV infusion; 8–20 mg/kg, IM q4–6h or orally q6h Cat: 3–8 mg/kg, IM or PO q6–8h
Propranolol	Inderal (-LA), USP: 1-mg ampule for injection; 10-, 20-, 40-, 60-, 80-mg tablets; Inderal LA capsules—60, 80, 120, 160 mg	Dog: 0.2–1.0 mg/kg orally q8h Cat: 2.5–5.0 mg orally tid; IV dose: 60 μg/kg over 5–10 min
Tocainide	Tonocard: 400-, 600-mg tablets	Dog: 10–20 mg/kg q8h
Quinidine	Quinidine gluconate (80 mg/ml for injection), Quinidex (sulfate—sustained release) and Quinora (sulfate) 300-mg tablets [=250 mg Q-base], Quinaglute (gluconate) 324 mg [= 202 mg Q-base]	Dog: 6–20 mg/kg IM, q6h; 6–20 mg/kg orally q6–8h (Note: "base-equivalent" of quinidine varies with the quinidine salt.)
Sotalol	Betapace (Berlex) 80 mg/160 mg; 240 mg all scored	Dog: 40–80 mg q12h (large breeds only)
Sodium bicarbonate	Sodium bicarbonate USP: 8.4% (= 1 mEq/ml of NaHCO₃)	0.5–1 mEq/kg IV or as guided by blood gas analysis
Theophylline and related salts	Theophylline USP, Theo-Dur, Slo-phyllin; Choledyl (oxtriphylline); amino-phylline: 100-, 200-, [300-, 400]-mg tablets; aminophylline 250-mg/10 ml vials	Dog: 10–20 mg/kg orally q8h; 6–10 mg/kg IV slowly Cat: 6–10 mg/kg orally q12h
Verapamil	Isoptin 5-, 10-mg ampules for injection; Isoptin, Calan 40-, 80-, 120-mg tablets	Dog: 0.05 mg/kg, IV every 10–30 min to a maximum cumulative dose of 0.15 mg/kg
Warfarin	Coumadin 1-, 2-mg scored tablets	Cat: 0.5 mg initial dose; titrate dose to an international normalized ratio (INR)

*Check dosing information and standard textbooks for specific dosing recommendations; advise owners that most cardiovascular drugs are used extralabel. Recommendations are based on current recommendations.

- A loop diuretic is delivered by renal blood flow, actively secreted into the proximal tubules, and then carried in the filtrate to the loop of Henle. High doses of a loop diuretic may be needed to attain an effect if renal perfusion is poor, as occurs with cardiogenic shock and some forms of primary renal disease.
  - Loop diuretics have a rapid onset of effect (generally within 30 min) and a shorter duration of effect than do the thiazides. In some animals, this relatively brief effect may be negated by compensatory renal retention of sodium and increased thirst. This can be overcome by more frequent dosing (2–3 times daily).
  - When administered chronically as monotherapy for CHF, the renin-angiotensin-aldosterone system is activated consequent to volume contraction. For this reason, furosemide typically is prescribed with an inhibitor of the angiotensin-converting enzyme (ACE), such as enalapril.
  - IV administration of furosemide may release atrial naturetic peptide and prostaglandins. This may explain the venodilator effect that has been reported and may act to pool blood away from the heart and pulmonary veins.
  - In advanced CHF, the distal convoluted tubules may overcome the effects of furosemide by increasing reabsorption of sodium and water distal to the site of furosemide action.
  - In advanced right-sided CHF, reduced oral bioavailability of furosemide may diminish the efficacy of diuretic therapy.

Thiazide Diuretics

- Thiazide diuretics act primarily on the proximal tubule and prevent sodium, chloride, and water reabsorption. Both chlorothiazide and hydrochlorothiazide can be used in small animals.
  - The thiazides are effective and well-tolerated diuretics in the dog and cat. Thiazides exert a relatively long duration of action. Given orally q12–24h.
  - Thiazides may be combined with a potassium-sparing diuretic to minimize potassium loss during diuresis.
  - When combined with a loop diuretic, solute and water reabsorption is blocked at sequential sites along the nephron. This type of treatment represents aggressive therapy for refractory CHF.

Potassium-Sparing Diuretics

- Potassium-sparing diuretics include spironolactone, triamterene, and amiloride. These drugs reduce distal tubule potassium loss.
  - These drugs are weak diuretics when administered as monotherapy and typically are administered either in combination with a thiazide diuretic or a loop diuretic.
  - Spironolactone is a competitive inhibitor of aldosterone and blocks aldosterone effects in the kidney (sodium retention/potassium loss) and in the myocardium (aldosterone-induced myocardial fibrosis).

- As a general rule, do not give potassium supplementation in association with potassium-sparing diuretics. Combination therapy may lead to hyperkalemia. Potassium-sparing diuretics should be used cautiously with ACE inhibitors, such as enalapril, which also act to conserve potassium.

Indications for Diuretic Therapy

- Indications of diuretic therapy include management of life-threatening pulmonary edema caused by left-sided CHF or noncardiogenic mechanisms. Diuretics also are used as adjunctive therapy of pleural effusion (with thoracocentesis) when caused by CHF.
- In right-sided CHF with ascites (or peripheral edema), diuretics reduce the tendency toward abnormal fluid accumulation by lowering venous and capillary pressures and preventing further sodium retention.
- Chronic use of diuretics is based on the concept that CHF is associated with chronic activation of harmful sodium- and water-retaining mechanisms.
- Diuretic drugs are occasionally used in the control of systemic hypertension. Reduced preload decreases cardiac output and arterial blood pressure.

▼ *Key Point* Diuretic therapy is the most important treatment for life-threatening pulmonary edema caused by congestive heart failure.

Contraindications for Diuretic Therapy

- Do not use diuretics in animals with heart failure without overt edema or congestion.
- Treat pericardial effusion and constrictive pericardial disease by other methods because diuresis simply reduces ventricular filling and cardiac output.
- Hyponatremia (unless caused by CHF) is a contraindication.
- Low cardiac output states, unrelated to CHF, are contraindications. These include: shock, hypoadrenocorticism (Addison's disease), states of dehydration, and prerenal azotemia. Any diuretic, especially when given in combination therapy, can cause volume contraction, reduced cardiac output, hypotension, decreased renal perfusion, and progressive or acute renal failure.
- Low serum potassium is a relative contraindication because loop and thiazide diuretics may aggravate hypokalemia. Hypokalemic, nonrespiratory acidosis is a contraindication.

Administration

- Furosemide is used most often for hospital and home treatment of CHF. Administer furosemide (or other loop diuretics) by parenteral (IV, IM, SQ) routes in patients with overt edema or fluid accumulation. This is best accomplished in the hospital. The precise dose and dosing interval depends on the severity of CHF and response to prior treatments.

- After initial diuresis, lower the dose and begin oral dosing if possible. When changing to oral therapy, increase the dose by up to 50% because oral bioavailability or potency is seldom as high.
  - Occasionally, the diuretic can be discontinued after establishment of other treatments for heart failure; however, this is the exception, not the rule. Often the dose can be reduced in cats with acute CHF caused by hypertrophic cardiomyopathy.
  - Minimize adverse effects by intermittent administration (i.e., every other day); however, daily dosing promotes more stable hemodynamics and is needed in advanced CHF.
  - In severe, chronic CHF in dogs, a loop diuretic typically is needed q8–12h.
  - Oral furosemide may be ineffective in advanced left- or right-sided CHF or in patients that are volume depleted, requiring other treatment strategies to mobilize edema fluid (see Chap. 64). Combining a loop diuretic with an osmotic diuretic (mannitol) or a potassium-sparing diuretic (spironolactone, amiloride, or hydrochloro-thiazide plus spironolactone) may be helpful in some dogs with refractory fluid accumulation. These are given once or twice daily in conjunction with bid–tid furosemide. Consider administration of an inotrope (dobutamine) to improve renal blood flow.
- There is a critical balance between excessive venous pressure (promoting edema) and inadequate venous pressure that reduces cardiac filling and cardiac output. A number of methods can be used to monitor the home diuretic dosage.
  - Inquire about objective signs of fluid retention (weight, ability to rest and sleep, coughing, exercise tolerance, muscle strength).
- Examine the patient for fluid accumulation (by physical examination and radiography).
- Estimate and observe the jugular venous pressure.
- Identify *excessive* diuretic therapy by periodically measuring arterial blood pressure, renal function (serum BUN, creatinine), and serum electrolytes (especially potassium).

Toxicity

Toxicity includes hemodynamic consequences of volume depletion, disorders related to electrolyte disturbances, and effects that are additive to other drugs.

- Diuretics are well tolerated by most patients provided that water is not withheld and the animal is eating and drinking. Excessive plasma volume contraction reduces cardiac filling, preload, cardiac output, and blood pressure and activates renin-angiotensin-aldosterone and related systems. Diuretics also can impair cardiac filling in conditions characterized by diastolic dysfunction, as with feline hypertrophic cardiomyopathy.
- Hypotension—including symptomatic orthostatic hypotension—may occur owing to diuretic therapy.
- Diuretic therapy can cause prerenal azotemia. Combination diuretic therapy, leading to sequential nephron blockade, can induce sudden and marked volume depletion and acute renal failure.
- Electrolyte disturbances secondary to diuretic therapy are common and range from mild to severe.
  - Mild hypochloremia is the most frequently encountered abnormality associated with treatment with a loop diuretic. Loss of chloride, in excess of sodium, predisposes to metabolic alkalosis. This is further potentiated in states of potassium depletion.
  - Hypokalemia is a more serious adverse effect; however, in current practice, most small animals treated for chronic CHF also receive an ACE inhibitor, which helps conserve potassium.
    - When present, hypokalemia and hypomagnesemia (another consequence of diuretic treatment) predispose to muscle weakness, cardiac arrhythmias (increases membrane excitability), nonrespiratory (metabolic) alkalosis, and digoxin toxicosis.
    - Hypokalemia from diuretic therapy is especially common after vigorous parenteral diuretic therapy. Marked hypokalemia is more likely to develop in cats.
- Treat diuretic complications by reducing the diuretic dosage and, if necessary, infusing fluid therapy (5% dextrose in water or 0.45 NaCl/2.5% dextrose *plus* potassium chloride at 10–20 mEq KCl per 500 ml crystalloid fluid).

Drug Interactions

- Arterial blood pressure also may decrease from the combined effects of diuretic therapy and vasodilator therapy.
- Acute renal failure is a recognized complication of combination treatment with ACE inhibitors in volume-depleted animals.
- Patients with diuretic toxicity are at risk for digoxin toxicosis because azotemia reduces the renal clearance of digoxin.
- Potassium-sparing diuretics, when combined with oral potassium supplements or an ACE inhibitor, can predispose to hyperkalemia, although this is rarely serious enough to require treatment.
- Nonsteroidal antiinflammatory drugs decrease the renal and systemic response to diuretics by interfering with the production of prostaglandins (PGE_2).

Positive Inotropic Drugs

Positive inotropic drugs increase the force of myocardial contraction by increasing calcium influx into myocytes or by sensitizing the contractile apparatus to intracellular calcium concentrations. These drugs generally can be grouped by mechanism of action into (1) digitalis glycosides, (2) catecholamines, and (3) phosphodiesterase inhibitors. Ventricular stroke volume, cardiac output, and tissue (myocardial, splanchnic, renal) perfusion may increase as a consequence of positive inotropic therapy. Additional hemodynamic effects occur as a consequence of vascular, autonomic, or extracardiac effects.

Digoxin

Clinical Pharmacology

- Digoxin is the most widely used of the digitalis glycosides in heart failure and is prescribed for its effects on myocardial contractility, heart rate, and autonomic balance.
- Digitalis glycosides inhibit membrane Na-K ATPase and the Na-K pump. This effect increases the intracellular sodium concentration, which activates another membrane pump that exchanges sodium for extracellular calcium. This leads to increased concentrations of intracellular calcium and a modest positive inotropic effect.
- Digitalis also enhances baroreceptor responsiveness, sensitizing the receptors to prevailing arterial blood pressure. This effect is most prominent in CHF and leads to withdrawal of sympathetic tone and increased vagal tone to the heart. There is also some evidence of reduced renin release related to reduced sympathetic nervous system (SNS) tone and to inhibition of the renal sodium pump.
- Reductions in SNS drive and inhibition of the renin angiotensin system may lead to modest peripheral vasodilation, offsetting the slight direct constrictive effects of digitalis glycosides on vascular tone.
- Digoxin exerts electrophysiologic effects and antiarrhythmic actions indirectly through alterations in autonomic efferent activities. There are also some poorly characterized direct electrophysiologic effects on cardiac cell membranes.
  - Sinus node discharge rate and atrioventricular (AV) nodal conduction are depressed as a result of increasing vagal tone and withdrawal of sympathetic activity. Resting sinus tachycardia, which commonly develops in CHF, may abate with the use of digitalis.
  - Increased vagal tone may suppress atrial ectopic activity, but this effect is inconsistent. When either atrial flutter or fibrillation is present, digoxin, by depressing AV conduction, generally slows the ventricular rate (although the atrial rhythm disturbance usually persists). This effect on ventricular rate is most evident at rest. Digoxin often is combined with a beta blocker or a calcium channel blocker for control of heart rate in atrial fibrillation. The combination therapy more effectively limits the number of atrial fibrillatory impulses that traverse the AV node to enter the ventricles.

▼ *Key Point* To achieve better heart rate control in atrial fibrillation during periods of exercise or stress, combine digoxin with a beta blocker or a calcium channel antagonist.

  - The effect of digoxin on junctional or ventricular arrhythmias is typically neutral or negative. However, at toxic concentrations, digoxin activates the area postrema of the brain and SNS tone is augmented creating a proarrhythmic effect. Furthermore, enhancement of calcium currents in cardiac cells (oscillatory potentials) may promote junctional or ventricular ectopic rhythms.

- Pharmacokinetics and metabolism of digoxin:
  - Digoxin can be administered by IV (rarely) or oral routes. After oral administration, digoxin is absorbed relatively well, although antacids, kaolin-pectin, malabsorption states, and food may interfere variably with gastrointestinal absorption.
  - Digoxin elixirs are prepared in an alcohol base and are somewhat better absorbed than tablets (e.g., 85% vs. 65–75% bioavailability). However, the adverse taste is often a limiting factor (especially in cats).
  - The elimination half-life of digoxin is related to renal function, and in the dog is approximately 24–30 hours. Elimination is protracted in the cat, and the half-life can be more than 48 hours in some animals.
    - Because digoxin elimination is via glomerular filtration, use the drug cautiously, if at all, in azotemic (renal failure) animals.
    - In contrast to digoxin, another cardiac glycoside, digitoxin, is rapidly eliminated by the canine liver, leading to a longer half-life partially due to enterohepatic cycling. This is the main reason that digitoxin has been recommended for use in dogs with concurrent CHF and renal impairment. However, digitoxin is highly protein bound (> 90%), should be administered q8h, and does not come in a convenient canine dosing size. Thus, despite theoretical benefit, this glycoside is currently used rarely.

Indications

- Digitalization is indicated for treatment of dogs, cats, and ferrets with CHF caused by dilated cardiomyopathy, advanced chronic valvular disease, and restrictive cardiomyopathy (cats).
- Digoxin is prescribed for control of ventricular rate response in patients with atrial fibrillation (AF).
- Digoxin may be of value in some cases of severe CHF related to congenital heart disease or heartworm disease.
- Digitalization may be of value for reasons other than the mild positive inotropic effect exerted by this compound. Enhanced baroreceptor sensitivity slows resting heart rate and may yield more appropriate baroreceptor responses. In this regard, it may diminish syncopal episodes in some dogs with heart failure when orthostatic hypotension is involved.

Contraindications

- Digoxin is *contraindicated* in situations of predominant diastolic heart failure, such as that caused by pericardial diseases and hypertrophic cardiomyopathy (unless there is concurrent atrial fibrillation).
- Digoxin is not indicated in subclinical valvular heart disease.
- Digoxin should be *withheld* in moderate to severe renal failure because renal elimination of digoxin may be impaired.
- Hypokalemia and possibly hypomagnesemia predispose to digitalis intoxication. Administration of digoxin to animals with hypokalemia may promote the

development of serious atrial or ventricular ectopic rhythms.

- Digitalis glycosides are contraindicated in the presence of complex or repetitive ventricular ectopic complexes.
- With infrequent or occasional ventricular premature complexes, give digoxin cautiously, if at all. Ectopic activity can become more frequent because digitalis can precipitate abnormal cellular automaticity. Conversely, a potential benefit on ventricular arrhythmias may occur if myocardial blood flow improves, if heart rate slows, or if renal perfusion normalizes acid-base status and electrolytes.
- Electrocardiographic evidence of AV nodal disease is a relative contraindication to digitalization because high-grade or complete AV block may result. In such cases, be sure to perform serial electrocardiograms and monitor electrolyte status.
- Digitalis is contraindicated in ventricular pre-excitation syndromes (e.g., Wolff-Parkinson-White) because it may "force" premature atrial impulses away from the AV node and down the accessory pathway and into the ventricle. Should atrial fibrillation develop, such a pathway may cause dangerously rapid activation of the ventricles.

Administration

- Digoxin therapy must be individually tailored to each patient and generally is administered orally. There is a low toxic:therapeutic ratio; choose the daily dosage carefully with attention to patient variables, including cardiac rate and rhythm, renal function, electrolyte status (especially potassium), and concurrent medications. The safest approach is to choose a dose at the lower end of the dosage range (e.g., 0.005 mg/kg q12h in dogs) and adjust the daily dose if signs of toxicity occur after 1 or 2 weeks.
- Digoxin is most useful for chronic therapy of CHF and has little role in the hospital management of acute CHF in dogs and cats unless it is complicated by atrial fibrillation.
- In most instances, digitalization is accomplished by daily administration of a maintenance dose. In dogs, give the drug q2h; in cats, give the drug once every other day. Attainment of steady-state plasma concentrations generally requires about 5 to 7 days of consistent dosing in dogs.
- There is little need for a loading dose except for animals with atrial fibrillation with circulatory collapse, severe CHF, or high resting ventricular rate response (e.g. > 225/min in the dog). A loading dose can be calculated by doubling the maintenance dose for the first 24 hours.
- An effective dosage is one that provides modest benefit without signs of toxicosis.
  - Effective digitalization is accompanied by subtle diuresis (due to increased cardiac output and renal perfusion) and generally mild improvement in the clinical signs of CHF.
  - Electrocardiographic changes are variable but include: slowing of resting heart rate, ST-T changes

in the ECG change, reduction of ectopic atrial depolarizations, and prolongation of the P-R interval. These are often subtle findings at best and are not reliable measures of a therapeutic dosage.

- The superior way to monitor treatment is to first interview the animal's owner about attitude, appetite, and adverse effects (such as vomiting or diarrhea) and to record "trough" serum digoxin levels, measured by radioimmunoassay (RIA) and available through most commercial laboratories. As expected from its protein binding, therapeutic blood levels of digitoxin (15–35 ng/ml) are markedly greater than for digoxin (approximately 0.8–2.0 ng/ml, usually aiming for 0.9–1.2 ng/ml at trough). Once steady state has been obtained (typically 7 days after beginning therapy), measure a serum digoxin level, adjust the dose to attain the target trough concentration, and periodically reevaluate the serum digoxin (e.g., every 3–6 months or if problems develop).

Toxicity

- Digitalis intoxication is relatively common in clinical practice. Toxicosis is enhanced by hypokalemia, hypomagnesemia, or by drugs that interact and increase serum concentrations. Measure a serum concentration of digitalis to ensure that the signs are related to excessive dosing.
- Mild clinical signs of toxicity include depression, anorexia, borborygmus, and diarrhea; treat by skipping 2 to 4 doses, then restarting therapy at a lower dose (50–75% of the original dose).
- Management of serious toxicity (continual emesis, anorexia, collapse, serious arrhythmias) requires hospitalization and additional treatments.
  - Withdraw digoxin for 2 to 4 days, and obtain appropriate laboratory data (serum digoxin, potassium, BUN, or creatinine).

▼ **Key Point** Record an electrocardiogram (ECG) because digitalis intoxication can cause virtually any cardiac arrhythmia. Sinus bradycardia, atrioventricular block, junctional tachycardia, and ventricular bigeminy are most common during digitalis toxicosis. Although AV block may be self-limiting, ventricular tachycardia may require treatment with lidocaine, potassium chloride, and magnesium chloride infusions.

- Administer supportive therapy including antiemetics, if needed, and intravenous crystalloids (with attention to respiratory rate). Infuse 0.45% saline solution in 2.5% dextrose or a 5% dextrose-in-water solution, supplemented with KCl (at least 6–12 mEq/250 ml) to slowly rehydrate the patient and replace potassium loss without delivering intolerable sodium loads. Fluid volumes of 20–40 ml/kg/day are typical. Continue low-dose diuretic therapy (0.5–1 mg/kg furosemide bid) to prevent sodium retention and pulmonary edema. In cats, lactated Ringer's solution may be needed to prevent hyponatremia. Continue other treatments (e.g., ACE inhibitors) are continued unless there is overt hypotension.

- Once the patient is stabilized, the need for digoxin is reassessed, and if necessary, prescribe a recalculated dosage and monitor serum concentrations more frequently.

Drug Interactions

Be cognizant of drug interactions or confounding drug effects with digoxin.

- Calcium channel blockers may increase the serum concentration of digoxin about twofold. This is common with verapamil and variable with diltiazem.
- Antiarrhythmic drugs (quinidine, amiodarone, propafenone) may increase the serum digoxin level. Quinidine displaces digoxin from muscle-binding sites, reduces its renal clearance, and can exaggerate digitalis proarrhythmic effects.
- Diuretics or furosemide and ACE inhibitors can promote digitalis intoxication by reducing renal blood flow and glomerular filtration pressure.

Catecholamines: Dobutamine and Dopamine

Severe or refractory CHF may require aggressive therapy to increase cardiac output, improve renal perfusion, and maintain a critical arterial blood pressure. This is especially true in advanced myocardial failure, as typified by dilated cardiomyopathy wherein the triad of low cardiac output, pulmonary edema, and systemic arterial hypotension may be encountered. In these instances, a 24- to 72-hour infusion of the norepinephrine precursor, dopamine, or the synthetic catecholamine, dobutamine, can significantly improve cardiac performance and help stabilize the patient. Unlike catecholamines that are predominantly alpha-adrenergic (such as phenylephrine) or beta-adrenergic agonists (such as isoproterenol), both dobutamine and dopamine demonstrate combined beta-adrenergic and alpha-adrenergic agonist effects.

Clinical Pharmacology

- Beta receptor stimulation increases contractility (inotropy), heart rate (chronotropy), and conduction velocity (dromotropy). In healthy myocardium, myocardial relaxation (lusitropy) also is enhanced. Myocardial cell membranes contain predominantly β-1 receptors; however, there are also β-2 receptors. Vasodilation is the consequence of extrasynaptic β-2 receptor stimulation in blood vessels.
- Alpha-adrenergic effects are mediated by different intracellular pathways but also result in increased calcium influx and enhanced contractility. Peripheral vascular effects are opposite, however, with alpha-stimulation leading to dose-dependent vasoconstriction.
- Both dobutamine and dopamine drugs are potent inotropic agents when compared with digitalis glycosides.
- Dobutamine produces a slightly less chronotropic effect than dopamine for a given inotropic effect. This is one reason that dobutamine is preferred in CHF.

- Vascular effects are also different between dobutamine and dopamine.
  - The combined vascular effect of dobutamine (both α-1 and β-2 agonist) at low to moderate doses results in a relatively balanced peripheral effect; accordingly, arterial vasoconstriction may not occur. At higher doses, alpha effects are initiated in the vasculature, leading to vasoconstriction.
  - Dopamine produces similar direct effects to dobutamine and also stimulates release of endogenous norepinephrine. At equally inotropic dosages, dopamine tends to cause more vasoconstriction (α-1 effect). At lower doses (less than 5 μg/kg/min), dopamine may activate dopaminergic receptors that lead to vasodilation and increased mesenteric and renal blood flow. At higher doses, alpha-adrenergic effects predominate.
- These drugs are metabolized rapidly, and the effects are short-lived (minutes) after cessation of an infusion.
- Downregulation of beta receptors may require progressively higher doses to achieve a constant CV effect.

Indications for Catecholamines

- The major indication for catecholamine therapy of CHF is treatment of severe myocardial failure with pulmonary edema and hypotension, often referred to as *cardiogenic shock*. Despite downregulation of beta receptors that occurs in severe heart failure (due to chronic sympathetic activation), catecholamines are usually effective treatment.
- There are also wide applications for catecholamine infusions in critical care medicine and anesthesia, including inhalation anesthetic overdose.

Contraindications for Catecholamines

- Systemic hypertension.
- Uncontrolled tachyarrhythmia. For example, in dogs with atrial fibrillation, catecholamines increase the ventricular rate unless the AV node is blocked partially with digoxin or with a calcium channel blocker such as diltiazem.
- Ventricular ectopia is a relative contraindication. Ventricular tachycardia is a contraindication and first must be suppressed (e.g., with lidocaine) before infusion of a catecholamine.
- Beta-adrenergic blockers—the effects are antagonistic (unless trying to overcome beta blocker toxicosis).
- Moderate to severe hypokalemia—beta-adrenergic stimulation may reduce serum potassium.

Administration and Monitoring

- Give dobutamine and dopamine by IV infusion (typically mixed in 5% dextrose solution or in 45% NaCl in 2.5% dextrose solution) and administer as a constant rate IV infusion using an infusion pump. Potassium chloride (at least 8–12 mEq/250 ml fluid) can be added to the solution.

- Because dopamine has more prominent vasoconstricting effects on blood vessels and beta effects on the heart rate, use dobutamine in patients with CHF.
- Both short-term benefits (patient stabilized and released from hospital) and long-term benefits (lasting weeks) may accrue from a 2- to 3-day infusion of dobutamine.
- The typical infusion starts at 2.5 µg/kg/min and is increased to 5 µg/kg/min after 30 minutes. The initial dose should be low; increase the drug infusion rate as needed. The final infusion dose is typically between 2–10 µg/kg/min) lasting for 24–48 hours. Doses as high as 15–20 µg/kg/min have been used infrequently.
- The therapeutic benefit of catecholamines is obvious: improved pulse pressure, increased arterial blood pressure, better color, and increased urinary output. Thus, these drugs are relatively easy to use if the clinician monitors clinical parameters, blood pressure, and ECG.
- Although cardiac output and arterial blood pressure increase during catecholamine infusions, venous pressures—and the tendency toward pulmonary edema—may not be reduced significantly. Thus, additional therapy (diuretics, venodilators) is needed to treat patients with low cardiac output and pulmonary edema.

Toxicity

- The toxicity of catecholamines is an extension of sympathomimetic effects of beta- and alpha-adrenergic stimulation and include tachycardia, stimulation of ectopic complexes, and hypertension. Increased ventricular load is undesirable in patients with left-sided CHF. Treat severe beta-adrenergic toxicity by discontinuing the drug and administering the ultrashort beta-blocking drug esmolol.
- Central nervous system (CNS) side effects may develop, including vomiting and seizures (especially in cats).
- Precipitation of severe ventricular arrhythmias including ventricular fibrillation.

Drug Interactions

- The combination of diuretic therapy and catecholamine infusion may lead to hypokalemia.
- Combination therapy of digoxin and catecholamines may predispose patients to ventricular ectopic rhythms.

Phosphodiesterase Inhibitors

These drugs enhance calcium influx, leading to marked increases in contractility. Additionally, phosphodiesterase inhibition in arterioles causes vasodilation, which reduces afterload on the left ventricle. A number of these *inodilator* compounds have been developed for oral or IV administration. These include the bipyridine analogs, *amrinone, milrinone,* and *pimobendan.* The latter also "sensitizes" the contractile apparatus to the effects of intracellular calcium. The net pharmacologic effects of these drugs include increased myocardial contractility, arteriolar vasodilation, reduced ventricular afterload, and the logical consequence of augmented ventricular stroke volume. Currently, these drugs are used infrequently in veterinary practice; however, pimobendan may be released for veterinary use in Europe.

- Each of these inodilators are potent positive inotropic drugs. Intravenous amrinone or milrinone may be considered as expensive alternatives to dobutamine in the hospital management of severe CHF. These drugs are metabolized in the liver.
- A potential advantage of the bipyridine analogs is the peripheral vasodilation that may reduce mitral regurgitant fraction in dogs with CHF from mitral valve disease.
- Heart rate and atrioventricular conduction are not depressed. Digoxin or a calcium channel blocker (diltiazem) is needed to control heart rate if there is concurrent atrial fibrillation.
- Like other potent inotropic agents, there is a potential induction of ventricular ectopic rhythms.
  - Other toxicities include: vomiting, diarrhea, hypotension from vasodilation, and blood dyscrasias (e.g., thrombocytopenia).
- Contraindications include preexistent ventricular ectopia and situations that might be worsened by arteriolar vasodilation (fixed and dynamic ventricular outflow tract obstruction, hypotension, cardiac tamponade).
- Although current results are encouraging, more clinical information is needed before these drugs can be recommended on a routine basis (Table 63–2).

Vasodilators

Congestive heart failure is characterized by increased activity of vasoconstrictor systems and inhibition of vasodilators. This activation is important in terms of both hemodynamics and survival of the patient. Inhibiting vasoconstricting systems in CHF can benefit the animal both in terms of clinical signs of CHF and long-term survival. A heterogeneous group of drugs, loosely termed "vasodilators" can be used in the management of CHF. Most of these drugs originally were developed to treat systemic hypertension (see Chap. 69), and they are still useful for this purpose.

- The ventricular stroke volume is affected by the inherent contractility (inotropism) of the muscle, the ventricular preload (filling), and the ventricular afterload. Afterload can be considered the tension in the ventricular wall required to open the semilunar valve and eject blood against the arterial impedance. Increasing afterload has a *negative* effect on ventricular stroke volume. Moreover, afterload (tension), heart rate, and the level of myocardial inotropism determine myocardial oxygen demand. Another related issue is the concept of *afterload or ventriculoarterial coupling mismatch,* whereby the *failing* left ventricle is less able to work against even a normal arterial blood pressure.

▼ *Key Point* High vascular resistance can contribute to increased impedance to ejection of blood, reducing stroke volume and increasing mitral regurgitant volume. This can be reversed partially by lowering the blood pressure with an arteriolar vasodilator.

- Antagonizing vasodilator systems, especially sympathetic activity and the renin-angiotensin system, are associated with increased survival time in dogs with CHF.

Clinical Pharmacology of Vasodilator Drugs

- Vascular smooth muscle in blood vessels constrict in response to an increase in intracellular calcium. A number of vasoconstrictor and vasodilator systems are found in both vascular endothelium and in smooth muscle cells of blood vessels.
- Vasodilator drugs impair one or more of the vasoconstrictor mechanisms or activate a vasodilator system. These mechanisms/vasodilators include:
  - Vascular endothelium and vascular smooth muscle (via generation of nitric oxide [NO]). Examples include nitrates such as nitroglycerine ointment and sodium nitroprusside.
  - Channels that control calcium influx into vascular smooth muscle. Examples include calcium channel blockers amlodipine and diltiazem.
  - Vascular smooth muscle using undefined mechanisms (possibly by altering potassium channels). Hydralazine is a commonly used "direct" acting arterial vasodilator.
  - Adrenergic receptors and intracellular messaging system. The alpha-adrenergic blocker prazosin and the combination beta-alpha-adrenergic blocker drug carvedilol work via this mechanism.
  - Angiotensin II (AT-II) receptors (receptor subtype-1, also impact calcium influx). Inhibitors of the ACE prevent conversion of angiotensin I to angiotensin II. Drugs ending in -pril, such as enalapril, are ACE inhibitors. Newer drugs, such as losartan, directly block AT-II receptors on vascular smooth muscle.
  - Intracellular messengers (e.g., cAMP) that modulate signaling and calcium flux. These include the inodilators and phosphodiesterase inhibitors, such as amrinone, milrinone, and pimobendan.
- Vasodilator effects are much more pronounced on *systemic* versus pulmonary vessels. Drugs can be categorized further by major site of action as *venodilators*, arterial *vasodilators*, or *balanced* vasodilators.
- The hemodynamic effects of venodilation include:
  - Dilation of systemic veins and increases in systemic venous capacitance.
  - Redistributed pulmonary blood to dilated systemic veins.
  - Lowered ventricular end-diastolic pressures and venous pressures.

- Dilation of coronary arteries and increased ventricular diastolic compliance.
- Reduced myocardial oxygen demand.

▼ *Key Point* The desired effects of venodilators are reduction in the high venous and ventricular end-diastolic pressures typical of CHF. This decreases formation of edema and decreases cardiac size and the mitral-regurgitant orifice. In this capacity, venodilator effects are additive to diuretics.

- The hemodynamic effects of arterial vasodilation in CHF include:
  - Reduced systolic and diastolic arterial blood pressure and left ventricular afterload.
  - Increased stroke volume.
  - Reduced myocardial tension and myocardial oxygen consumption.
  - Decreased mitral regurgitant fraction. This can be explained by earlier opening of the aortic valve; shorter time available for "isolated regurgitation"; and reduction in the pressure gradient between the left ventricle and left atrium during systole. Arteriolar vasodilation increases forward stroke volume, and indirectly, can reduce pulmonary venous pressure by decreasing mitral regurgitant fraction.
  - In left-to-right cardiac shunts, a reduction of systemic blood pressure reduces the pressure gradient for left-to-right shunting, decreasing shunt fraction.
- The ACE inhibitors have been proven in canine veterinary trials (enalapril and benazepril) to reduce clinical signs (hemodynamic benefit) and to increase survival. The latter effect may stem in part from a protective effect on the myocardium.
- Increases in tissue perfusion develop in response to vasodilator therapy. Chronic treatment with some vasodilator drugs (e.g., ACE inhibitors) is associated with improved exercise tolerance.

Indications for Vasodilator Therapy

- Systemic hypertension and hypertensive heart disease. In severe systemic hypertension, aggressive vasodilation may be needed to protect target organs (eyes, brain, kidneys, heart) from further injury.
- Pulmonary edema from left sided CHF (in combination with other therapy)
- Chronic CHF (typically an ACE inhibitor)
- Hemodynamically significant mitral regurgitation
- Left-to-right cardiac shunt leading to CHF
- Aortic regurgitation (use vasodilators with caution)

Contraindications for Vasodilator Therapy

- Systemic hypotension
- Isolated diastolic hypotension (e.g., from severe aortic regurgitation)
- Shock
- Hyperkalemia (ACE inhibitors)
- Relative contraindication: fixed heart rate (e.g., sinus node disease or atrioventricular blocks) wherein reflex tachycardia cannot be activated in response to hypotension

▼ *Key Point* The major risk of arterial vasodilation is systemic hypotension.

Administration of Specific Vasodilators

Angiotensin-Converting Enzyme (ACE) Inhibitors

- *ACE inhibitors* include captopril, enalapril, benazepril, and lisinopril as well as other drugs with the suffix "pril." These vasodilators are used for long-term (home) management of canine and feline CHF.
  - These drugs inhibit the conversion of angiotensin I to angiotensin II and they also reduce the degradation of kinins (which act as venodilators). They are considered "balanced" vasodilators. Administration of enalapril or benazepril therapy, added to background treatments of digoxin and furosemide, can prolong a dog's life and reduce clinical signs of heart disease.
  - Because concentrations of aldosterone also fall, sodium retention is decreased, an effect that may help prevent edema and ascites.
  - Of potentially great importance are the benefits derived from reduction in myocardial cell injury and fibrosis caused by heightened activities of the renin-angiotensin system (RAS) and aldosterone. Of the vasodilators commonly used, only the ACE inhibitors have been shown to reduce this cellular injury; other vasodilator drugs do not. This may be an important aspect in the long-term survival of patients with CHF due to myocardial disease.
  - ACE inhibitors are administered orally. The dose and frequency of administration required to inhibit 90% or more of ACE activity varies among the drugs and depends in part on the metabolism of active metabolites from "pro-drugs" (e.g., enalapril). Captopril is associated with anorexia, must be given 3 times a day and rarely is used. Administer enalapril and benazepril once or twice daily. The latter drug is excreted by both renal and hepatic mechanisms, whereas enalapril and lisinopril are primarily dependent on and affected by renal elimination.
  - Begin enalapril and benazepril in dogs with CHF at 0.5 mg/kg PO once daily. In cats with CHF, the initial dose is 0.25 to 0.5 PO mg/kg once daily. Increase to 0.5 mg/kg PO q12h if needed. Occasionally, this dose is exceeded in dogs with advanced CHF.
  - Monitor ACE inhibitor therapy in CHF by periodic measurement of blood pressure (target systolic pressure is 90–120 mm Hg) and serum biochemistries. Adjust the dose (increase blood urea nitrogen or creatinine) if signs of CHF are progressive or adverse effects are evident.
  - ACE inhibitors are also a reasonable first-line treatment of canine hypertension, especially when related to glomerular disease. In contrast, calcium channel blockers such as amlodipine are preferable first-line antihypertensive drugs in cats.
  - Among the major potential adverse effects of ACE inhibitors are hypotension and acute renal failure (the combination of hypotension and vasodilation

of the renal efferent arteriole can markedly decrease intraglomerular filtration pressure). Other concerns include the possibility of neutropenia, hyperkalemia (from decreased aldosterone; avoid KCl supplement or potassium-sparing diuretics), and protracted anorexia that may require discontinuation of the drug. Humans rarely experience laryngeal edema that can cause recurrent cough or dyspnea (this may be a factor in some dogs).

Hydralazine

- *Hydralazine* is a direct-acting arteriolar (precapillary resistance vessel) dilator that is effective after oral administration. Approximately 90% of the peak effect on blood pressure is obtained about 2 hours after oral administration. Duration of action is between 6 to 12 hours in the dog. The drug generally is given twice a day. Hydralazine is metabolized by the liver, but elimination is influenced by renal excretion.
  - Hydralazine is used most often to decrease regurgitant fraction in dogs with mitral regurgitation and is a valuable drug for the initial hospital treatment of life-threatening pulmonary edema due to valvular heart disease. Hydralazine (or amlodipine) can be add-on therapy in the management of refractory pulmonary edema in dogs that have failed to respond to treatment with digoxin, a diuretic, and an ACE inhibitor.
  - Effects on the pulmonary circulation are much less prominent (other than the indirect effects produced by increasing left heart output and reducing mitral regurgitant fraction) and severe hypotension may be produced when administered to some dogs with high systemic or pulmonary vascular resistance (e.g., heartworm disease).
  - Hydralazine is best given by titration initiated in the hospital. Initial doses of approximately 1 mg/kg can be increased to obtain a systolic arterial pressure of 85 to 90 mm Hg. A dose of 0.8 to 2 mg/kg typically is required.
  - Adverse effects include hypotension with reflex tachycardia, and activation of the renin-angiotensin system (due to hypotension). Anorexia is a common and limiting adverse effect in small-breed dogs.

Sodium Nitroprusside, Nitroglycerin

- *Sodium nitroprusside, nitroglycerin* (transdermal ointment or patch, transmucosal spray, and intravenous injection) and *isosorbide dinitrate* are vasodilators that, when metabolized in the blood vessel wall, generate nitric oxide, a potent vasodilator. Intravenous preparations are balanced vasodilators affecting both arteries and veins (unless there is reflex arterial vasoconstriction from hypotension). Topical nitrates and oral medications such as isosorbide dinitrate have greater effects on systemic venous smooth muscle and are considered venodilators. These drugs are metabolized by the liver.
  - The most common use of nitrates is for management of acute pulmonary edema (to lower venous

pressure and preload). The preparation selected depends on severity of CHF. Nitroglycerin 2% paste often is used in conjunction with furosemide for management of mild to moderate cardiogenic pulmonary edema. In life-threatening pulmonary edema, the addition of a potent arteriolar dilator may be beneficial, and sodium nitroprusside may be preferred. Some veterinarians prescribe oral or topical nitrates for long-term (bid) treatment of CHF.

- Nitroprusside is a potent antihypertensive of value in management of severe complicated systemic hypertension (e.g., with retinal detachment or stroke).
- Nitrate tolerance develops with repeated or constant administration; thus, intermittent use of topical nitrates (q8–12 h) is recommended.
- The principal adverse effects of nitrates are an excessive reduction in preload or decrease in systemic arterial blood pressure, as described previously. Cyanide is generated by metabolism of sodium nitroprusside, but this is not likely to be important when the infusion is limited to 48 hours or less.

Calcium Channel Blockers

- *Calcium channel blockers* have diverse clinical uses as arterial vasodilators and antiarrhythmics, and for the treatment of diastolic function. These drugs are described subsequently in greater detail (see Calcium Channel Blockers section). Their major use is for control of systemic hypertension (amlodipine). When used as antiarrhythmics (diltiazem, verapamil) or the treatment of diastolic dysfunction of the left ventricle (diltiazem), consider the vasodilator effects.

Toxicity

- Vasodilation reduces blood pressure. This is well tolerated when the decline is modest (e.g., systolic pressure still > 85 mm Hg). Weakness, depression, excessive sleeping, shivering, orthostatic hypotension, syncope, and reflex tachycardia are potential consequences of excessive vasodilation. Monitor blood pressure and question clients about these signs during follow-up examinations.
- Additionally, some drugs (e.g., hydralazine) are more likely than others to cause reflex sinus tachycardia and activation of the renin-angiotensin-aldosterone system in response to a sudden lowering of blood pressure. This makes some vasodilators acceptable for short-term or hospital use but less desirable for long-term therapy of CHF.
- Venodilation reduces venous return unless the initial venous pressures are quite high, in which case venous return may not be seriously compromised. However, at lower venous pressures, cardiac output can fall from decreased venous return and reduced ventricular preload.
- Acute renal failure is a complication of ACE inhibitors, especially in volume-depleted patients or when combined with diuretics.
- Other adverse effects are listed under specific vasodilator drugs (see subsequent sections).

CALCIUM CHANNEL BLOCKERS

The calcium channel antagonists are a diverse group of drugs with the common ability of blocking the entry of calcium ions into cardiac muscle, specialized cardiac nodal tissues, and vascular smooth muscle. Drugs in this group have variable effects on vascular smooth muscle, with the dihydropyridine (DHP or nifedipine-like) group of calcium antagonists predominantly affecting vascular rather than cardiac calcium channels. Other calcium channel blockers—diltiazem and verapamil—are principally used for their effects.

Clinical Pharmacology of Calcium Channel Blockers

- Cardiac effects of diltiazem and verapamil are related to blockade of L-calcium slow channels, which modulate calcium influx into cardiac cells. The physiologic consequences can be explained by the reduced entry of calcium into myocytes or specialized tissues.
  - Calcium channel antagonists may be useful for improving ventricular filling, although the precise mechanism of benefit is not certain and may be related to indirect effects (reflex sympathetic activity; improved coronary perfusion). This potential for positive lusitrophy is the reason that diltiazem is prescribed for cats with hypertrophic cardiomyopathy.
  - Both diltiazem and verapamil impair slow channel (calcium dependent) depolarization and recovery in the sinoatrial (SA) node and the AV node. As a result of slowing of AV nodal conduction, decreases in ventricular rate (response) can be expected in patients with arrhythmias (see section on antiarrhythmics) in response to atrial fibrillation or flutter. Occasionally these drugs actually convert atrial tachyarrhythmias to sinus rhythm.
  - Because these two drugs produce negative inotropic effects, they must be used with caution (e.g., graded doses) in patients with heart failure.
  - Coronary vasodilation is an expected result of calcium channel blocker therapy.
- Vascular effects of the calcium channel blockers, especially the DHP group, are related to impaired calcium entry into vascular smooth muscle with resultant vasodilation. Drugs such as amlodipine and felodipine are used most often for this purpose. Diltiazem has more "balanced" cardiac and vascular effects. The DHPs (drugs ending in "pine") are used to treat hypertension (via arterial vasodilation) or reduce left ventricular afterload in CHF. Coronary artery perfusion (via vasodilation) is an anticipated effect of arterial vasodilation.
- Metabolism occurs in the liver; accordingly, these drugs must be used cautiously in liver failure. Metabolites (generally inactive) often are excreted by renal mechanisms or via the gut.

Indications for Calcium Channel Blockers

- The DHPs (amlodipine) are useful for management of systemic arterial hypertension. Amlodipine therapy is highly effective in cats at doses of 0.625–1.25 mg PO q12–24h. Amlodipine also is used in dogs for management of hypertension at an initial dose of 0.05–0.1 mg/kg daily. The elimination half-life in healthy dogs is quite long.

- Diltiazem is used in feline hypertrophic cardiomyopathy to improve diastolic function and is especially likely to be used in cats with diastolic dysfunction sufficient to cause left-sided congestive heart failure.
- Amlodipine may be used to unload the left ventricle in dogs with severe CHF and mitral regurgitation, especially when a dog is intolerant to hydralazine.
- Uses of diltiazem and verapamil for arrhythmias are summarized in a subsequent section (see Antiarrhythmic Drugs). These drugs are used primarily for suppression of supraventricular tachyarrhythmias, blocking of reentrant supraventricular tachycardia, or control of heart rate during atrial flutter and fibrillation.

Contraindications for Calcium Channel Blockers

- Hypotension or shock because blood pressure may decrease.
- Left ventricular outflow tract obstruction (relative contraindication).
- Sinus node disease because severe sinus bradycardia or arrest can occur (especially with verapamil and diltiazem).
- Preexistent AV block because calcium currents are responsible for AV nodal cell depolarization, and excessive doses in healthy animals can lead to AV block.
- Untreated systolic heart failure because myocardial contractility is further depressed; when used in careful, graded doses (titrating the dose up), calcium channel blockers can be used in animals with congestive heart failure.
- Calcium channel blockers must be used *with caution* with digoxin or beta blockers because each can depress the SA node and the AV node.

Administration

- Begin managing feline hypertrophic cardiomyopathy by administering 30 mg of a long-acting diltiazem preparation once daily (see Chap. 66). Twice-daily dosing is tolerated by some cats. Precise dosing is difficult to monitor, but signs of anorexia, depression, or bradycardia (heart rate [HR] < 140 beats/min) should prompt dose reduction.
- Begin amlodipine treatment of systemic hypertension with a 0.625-mg oral dose (¼ tablet of a 2.5-mg tablet) in cats. If the blood pressure does not decline sufficiently, gradually increase the dose (to ½ tablet q12–24h). The end point of dosing is sufficient control of hypertension (see Chap. 69).
- Antiarrhythmic treatment is described subsequently.

Toxicity

- Depression of the sinus node, causing sinus bradycardia
- Depression of the atrioventricular node, causing AV block

- Depression of myocardial contractility, decreasing stroke volume and cardiac output
- Excessive vasodilation, causing systemic hypotension
- Skin rashes, anorexia (diltiazem in cats)

Drug Interactions

- Verapamil and possibly diltiazem increase the serum digoxin concentration.
- Cimetidine may decrease clearance of calcium channel blockers (e.g., amlodipine), increasing the plasma concentration of the drug.
- The negative inotropic effect of a beta blocker and calcium channel blockers make concurrent use difficult and generally inadvisable.
- The DHPs should not be used in hypertrophic obstructive cardiomyopathy of cats because the peripheral vasodilation may lead to increased dynamic obstruction following the reduction in LV load.

BETA-ADRENERGIC BLOCKERS

Sympathetic tone is generally elevated in patients with cardiovascular diseases and can be injurious to the heart, worsen preexisting cardiac conditions, contribute to high blood pressure, and produce cardiac arrhythmias. The effects of neuronal and vascular-borne sympathetic activators can be blocked in part by drugs that occupy beta-adrenergic receptors (beta blockers). Beta blockers are used in a variety of CV diseases. Some conditions that may be responsive to beta blockade include hypertrophic cardiomyopathy, systemic hypertension, atrial arrhythmias, ventricular arrhythmias, and hyperthyroid heart disease.

Clinical Pharmacology

- IV or oral administration of drugs that block beta adrenoceptors to depress the sinoatrial and AV nodes, slows the heart rate in patients that are in sinus rhythm and the ventricular rate in patients that have atrial flutter or fibrillation. Myocardial inotropism, heart rate, and wall tension (and therefore myocardial oxygen consumption) decrease. Blood pressure usually decreases. Sympathetic triggering of renin release is impaired. These effects depend in part on prevailing sympathetic nervous system activity.
- Beta blockers vary with respect to: receptor selectivity (beta$_1$ vs. beta$_2$ receptors), lipophilicity (most are dependent on liver metabolism), and intrinsic sympathomimetic activity (ISA). Of the dozens of beta blockers available, the following are used in small animal practice.
  - *Propranolol* is the prototypical beta-adrenergic (beta$_1$ and beta$_2$) blocker. It lacks ISA, is metabolized by the liver, and has a 4- to 6-hour duration of action.
  - *Atenolol* produces longer duration of effect and is relatively beta$_1$ specific. Twice-daily administration is satisfactory, and in some cats, once-daily administration controls heart rate for up to 20 hours.

- *Carvedilol* is a new beta/alpha blocker that may be useful for heart failure caused by cardiomyopathy. Clinical studies in dogs or cats are lacking.
- *Esmolol* is an ultrashort-acting IV beta blocker useful when sudden beta blockade is needed, or when the effect of beta blockade needs to be examined in a critically ill patient. It is hydrolyzed by plasma esterases within minutes of administration.

Indications for Beta Blockers

- Use beta blockers in the management of feline hypertrophic cardiomyopathy. Salutary effects include: slowing of sinus rate with increased time for ventricular filling, slowing of AV nodal conduction, decreasing myocardial oxygen consumption, reduction of dynamic (muscular) left ventricular outflow obstruction, and nonspecific antiarrhythmic activity. There is also "cardioprotection" from stress-induced surges of sympathetic activity.
- Hyperthyroid heart disease and other conditions of heightened sympathetic activity, including theobromine toxicosis (chocolate poisoning) and pheochromocytoma.
- Beta-adrenergic blockers also have been used to palliate tetralogy of Fallot and pulmonic stenosis (to reduce dynamic right ventricular outflow obstruction).
- Atenolol often is prescribed, empirically, for cardioprotection (myocardial ischemia with ST-segment changes, arrhythmias, and sudden death) in dogs with congenital subaortic stenosis.
- Beta blockers stabilize cardiac membranes in vitro; however, their major *antiarrhythmic effects* depend on blocking sympathetic effects on the heart. Arrhythmias can be precipitated or aggravated by sympathetic tone, and beta blockers are considered "broad-spectrum" antiarrhythmics. They are frequently prescribed for control of heart rate, atrial and ventricular premature complexes and for heart rate control in supraventricular tachycardias, including atrial tachycardia and atrial fibrillation.
- Beta blockers may be effective as *antihypertensive* drugs when administered as co-therapy with other vasodilator drugs in refractory hypertension.
- Chronic sympathetic stimulation in patients with CHF causes a reduction in myocardial beta receptors (downregulation). Beta blockers may permit some degree of upregulation of these receptors because beta receptor numbers and sensitivity increase in an attempt to overcome beta-blocking effects. This may make the heart more responsive to sympathetic stimulation or catecholamines in periods of stress such as exercise. Human and research studies suggest that judicious doses of beta blockers can protect the myocardium in CHF, and over time, improve myocardial function (ejection fraction) in dilated cardiomyopathy. Combination beta/alpha blockers—such as carvedilol—have the advantage of reducing left ventricular afterload (reduced ABP by alpha-adrenergic blockade). This may protect the failing ventricle from the initial negative inotropic effects of beta blockade.

- Beta blockers (timolol) are contained in some topical medications used to treat glaucoma.

Contraindications for Beta Blockers

- Untreated or severe congestive heart failure
- Hypotension
- Sinus node disease or sinus bradycardia
- Atrioventricular nodal disease or AV block

Administration

- The dosages of beta blockers are empiric and have been developed largely from limited pharmacokinetic studies and clinical experience. Titrate dosages to the desired effect. The ECG can be examined to determine the effects of intravenously administered drugs on heart rate and rhythm. Because one obvious effect of beta blockade is slowing of heart rate, this variable can be easily monitored in the hospital and at home. For example, a cat receiving a beta blocker with a heart rate of < 150 beats/min is probably demonstrating effects of blockade. Measure blood pressure periodically.
- The duration of drug effect may be prolonged in cats because metabolites of beta blockers may be active.
- Pharmacokinetic studies of beta blockers in dogs with spontaneous CV diseases are unavailable. In healthy dogs, most orally administered propranolol is removed from the circulation by the liver before reaching the systemic circulation (first-pass effect). Thus, oral doses are much higher than IV dosages.

Toxity

- Most of the antiarrhythmic drugs, with the possible exception of the beta blockers, have the potential to induce ventricular arrhythmias (proarrhythmic effect). This is especially likely with drugs in class IA, IC and III and may be heralded by prolongation of the QRS and QT intervals with eventual development of polymorphic ventricular tachycardia or ventricular fibrillation.
- Neurotoxicity can occur with lidocaine and mexiletine. Signs include CNS excitation then depression, nervousness, vomiting, twitching, and generalized convulsion; serious complications are controlled with diazepam.
- Gastrointestinal side effects can develop with many antiarrhythmic drugs, especially quinidine.
- Hematologic, immune-mediated, and dermatologic problems are recognized with procainamide therapy.
- Hypotension related to depression of myocardial function and/or peripheral vasodilation is possible during therapy with most antiarrhythmic drugs. Drug dose, route of administration, and type of drug influence the effects on myocardial and vascular function. In general, the beta blockers, calcium channel blockers, and sotalol produce the most cardiac depression; lidocaine and mexiletine the least; and quinidine and procainamide intermediate.
- Depression of the sinus node, causing sinus bradycardia, and the AV node, leading to atrioventricular block, is possible with most antiarrhythmic drugs. In

particular, the beta blockers and calcium channel blockers depress these tissues.

- Ophthalmic and renal side effects have made to-cainide an uncommonly used drug.
- Amiodarone has a long list of potential and serious adverse effects (see PDR before prescribing).

Drug Interactions

- Beta blockers and calcium channel blockers combine to depress cardiac tissues, reduce heart rate, and decrease contractility.
- Lipophilic beta blockers (e.g., propranolol) are highly dependent on liver blood flow, and elimination can be impaired by cimetidine.

ANTIARRHYTHMIC DRUGS

Antiarrhythmic drugs are used to treat disorders of heart rate and rhythm. Effective use of any antiarrhythmic drug depends on accurate interpretation of the ECG experience. Furthermore, efficacy is dependent on the cause of the arrhythmia and the extracellular potassium and magnesium concentrations. Hypokalemia and hypomagnesemia can decrease or nullify the beneficial effects of many antiarrhythmic drugs. Established drugs, including lidocaine, procainamide, mexiletine, diltiazem, and the beta blockers are used most often in clinical practice. Increasingly newer drugs such as sotalol are prescribed. Antiarrhythmic therapy has been tempered by an appreciation that in some cases, treatment may have no impact on mortality, that the cost and adverse effects of drug therapy are significant. Some antiarrhythmic drugs not only affect cardiac tissues but can cause vasodilation. CV effects may be related to changes in the autonomic nervous system. Specific treatment plans are discussed elsewhere in this section (see Chap. 62).

Clinical Pharmacology

- Antiarrhythmic drugs can be classified based on their electrophysiologic characteristics; however, no classification system is ideal. Therapeutic and toxic concentrations can produce markedly different cardiac electrophysiologic effects.
  - Class I—Membrane stabilizers or drugs that reduce the rate of transmembrane Na^+ influx by blocking the rapid sodium channel. These drugs generally decrease the rate of depolarization, slow conduction, and increase the effective refractory period of cardiac cells.
    - *IA drugs* (e.g., quinidine and procainamide) lengthen the action potential duration and the refractory period and reduce automaticity.
    - *IB drugs* (e.g., lidocaine and mexiletine) shorten the action potential duration but increase the refractory period. These drugs decrease automaticity of cardiac tissues. Refractoriness is prolonged minimally. Lidocaine reduces disparities in action potential duration in ischemic tissue, making it suitable for pre-

venting re-entrant ventricular arrhythmias in the setting of myocardial ischemia.
  - *IC drugs* (e.g., propafenone) have little effect on action potential duration but slow conduction in cardiac tissues, exerting a profound effect on the fast sodium channel. This slows conduction in the His-Purkinje system but has an unusual effect of shortening the action potential of Purkinje cells. Propafenone can exert proarrhythmic effects in patients with arrhythmias and severe cardiomyopathy.
- Class II—Beta adrenoceptor blockers include drugs such as propranolol and esmolol (see previous section). Beta blockers decrease sinus node rate, slow AV nodal conduction, and reduce arrhythmias related to high sympathetic tone.
- Class III—These drugs are antifibrillatory and prolong action potential duration and cell refractoriness. They produce minimal effects on automaticity or conduction velocity. Included are drugs such as amiodarone and combination drugs such as sotalol (also a beta blocker).
- Class IV—These drugs are calcium channel blockers such as verapamil and diltiazem (see previous section) and act to *block the movement of Ca^{++} ions across the slow calcium-dependent channel*. These drugs decrease heart rate, slow AV nodal conduction, and demonstrate some other variable antiarrhythmic effects.

Quinidine and Procainamide

- *Quinidine* and *procainamide* are class 1A antiarrhythmic drugs that have been used extensively in dogs but currently are prescribed less commonly. Quinidine and procainamide represent broad-spectrum antiarrhythmic agents with potential value for the treatment of atrial fibrillation, suppression of atrial, junctional, and ventricular premature complexes, and control of atrial and ventricular tachycardias. The short elimination half-lives of 4–6 hours for quinidine and 2–4 hours for procainamide in the dog necessitate frequent administration of these drugs. Sustained-release oral preparations of these drugs are available that sustain reasonable plasma concentrations with tid to qid dosing.
  - Quinidine metabolism and excretion are hepatic. Autonomic effects are important, with a pronounced vagolytic effect as well as the potential to block alpha-adrenergic receptors and decrease blood pressure. These autonomic effects can enhance conduction of atrial impulses across the AV node, causing a more rapid ventricular rate before conversion of an atrial tachyarrhythmia to sinus rhythm. This effect can be blunted by prior digitalization to slow AV conduction.
  - Quinidine usually is administered by the IM or oral route in the dog.
  - Procainamide is quite similar to quinidine in its electrophysiologic actions; however, it is not an alpha blocker and has minimal anticholinergic effects. Procainamide is particularly versatile because

it can be given IV, IM, or SQ, and orally. It has been used infrequently in cats.

Lidocaine

- *Lidocaine, mexiletine,* and *tocainide* are class 1B drugs. Lidocaine is the more widely used IV agent and mexiletine the most often prescribed oral 1B drug. Drugs in this class are potentially neuroexcitatory and should be used only with caution, if at all, in cats.
  - Lidocaine has a very rapid onset of action; it is metabolized quickly by the liver (1–3 hours). Intravenous boluses must be repeated (every 10–20 minutes) or supplemented with a constant-rate IV infusion. Effectiveness of therapy depends on the extracellular K^+, which must be maintained in the normal range.
  - Initial administration of lidocaine as a bolus (or loading infusion), followed by simultaneous use of smaller boluses with constant intravenous infusion, is the usual method for controlling acute ventricular tachycardia in the dog.
  - Lidocaine is relatively easy to administer and, compared with other antiarrhythmics, has minimal adverse hemodynamic effects. Lidocaine may be followed by treatment with mexiletine or can be combined with procainamide or quinidine.
  - Lidocaine is used infrequently in species other than the dog because the cat and horse are more sensitive to the neuroexcitatory effects. Give lidocaine to these species slowly and at lower dosages.
  - Mexiletine, like lidocaine, is used to suppress ventricular arrhythmias. It can be given orally. The drug usually is combined with a beta blocker for chronic management of severe ventricular arrhythmias in the dog.

Propafenone

- Class IC drugs such as *propafenone* are not used often because the potential for proarrhythmia is great. Of the available agents, only propafenone (Rythmol) is used occasionally for refractory arrhythmias in dogs.

Beta Blockers

- *Beta-adrenergic blockers* such as propranolol have been described previously. These are broad-spectrum antiarrhythmic drugs useful for suppressing atrial premature complexes and atrial tachycardias; depressing AV nodal conduction and decreasing the ventricular rate response to atrial flutter or fibrillation; and treating severe sinus tachycardia in thyrotoxicosis.
  - Beta blockers can be added to a class I antiarrhythmic drug when ventricular arrhythmia control cannot be attained with one drug and sometimes can be useful as monotherapy for partial control of complex or repetitive arrhythmias. Use IV cautiously owing to negative inotropic effects.
  - Ultrashort-acting IV beta blockade (esmolol) or graded IV doses (propranolol) can be used to control arrhythmias in the critical care setting.

Sotalol, Amiodarone, and Bretylium

- *Sotalol, amiodarone* and *bretylium* are not prescribed often, although sotalol is gaining favor for control of serious ventricular arrhythmias in dogs. Sotalol and amiodarone have dose-related class III activity and beta-blocking effects (sotalol much greater than amiodarone). Bretylium can be administered to prevent recurrent ventricular fibrillation but rarely is used in veterinary practice.
  - Amiodarone demonstrates a prolonged duration of action (days) due to an extremely long elimination half-life with hepatic metabolism.
  - Myocardial contractility is depressed by these drugs so that use in CHF is only with caution. Prolongation of the QT interval related to prolongation of the action potential can lead to torsade de pointes, a particularly malignant form of polymorphic ventricular tachycardia. This proarrhythmic effect, other side effects, and costs limit the usefulness of these drugs.

Calcium Channel Blockers

- The pharmacology of the *calcium antagonists,* including verapamil and diltiazem, has been discussed previously. Antiarrhythmic activities are related to impaired calcium influx into myocytes and specialized tissues. Adenosine (Adenocard) is an unrelated drug that profoundly depresses calcium currents in AV nodal tissues and may be useful for acute therapy of supraventricular tachycardia or for helping to distinguish SVT with bundle branch block from a ventricular tachycardia. It rarely is used in veterinary practice and requires close patient monitoring and higher dosing than for human beings.
  - Each of these drugs have profoundly negative effects on AV nodal conduction and can effectively slow the ventricular rate response in atrial flutter or fibrillation. Infrequently, there is conversion to normal sinus rhythm.
  - Calcium channel blockers can convert AV nodal reentrant tachycardia (circuit tachycardias that use the AV node as part of the loop).

Indications for Antiarrhythmic Drugs

- Indications for treatment of arrhythmias with antiarrhythmic drugs include the potential to: reduce clinical signs (such as syncope); reduce the risk of sudden cardiac death (e.g., from ventricular fibrillation); or improve the hemodynamics (e.g., atrial fibrillation with rapid ventricular rate).
- Sinus rhythm disturbances:
  - Sinus tachycardia is rarely an indication for treatment. The underlying condition should be controlled (e.g., pain, hypotension, anxiety, fever hypokalemia).
  - Sinus bradycardia and periods of sinus arrest usually are treated, when required to prevent hypotension and low cardiac output, by addressing the underlying condition and administering vagolytic

drugs such as atropine or glycopyrrolate or sympathomimetic drugs such as dopamine or dobutamine). Chronic sinus brady-arrhythmias are treated by cardiac pacing.

- Atrial rhythm disturbances:
  - Premature atrial complexes and paroxysmal atrial tachycardia are managed by treating CHF when present and then prescribing digoxin, a beta blocker, diltiazem, or a combination of two drugs. Less often, drugs such as sotalol, amiodarone, or procainamide are prescribed to prevent paroxysmal atrial fibrillation.
  - Sustained atrial tachyarrhythmias such as ectopic atrial tachycardia, atrial flutter, or atrial fibrillation usually are managed with digoxin combined with diltiazem or a beta blocker. This therapy may either suppress the rhythm or slow AV nodal conduction to prevent an excessive ventricular rate response. Uncommonly, drugs such as quinidine, procainamide, injectable diltiazem or verapamil, or adenosine are used to convert these rhythms in the hospital.
  - Re-entrant supraventricular tachycardias that use the atrium as part of the circuit usually are treated initially with verapamil or diltiazem.
- Ventricular rhythm disturbances:
  - Lidocaine and procainamide are the usual intravenous agents of choice for control of severe ventricular tachycardia in hospitalized dogs. Beta blockers are used in cats.
  - For recurrent ventricular arrhythmias that require therapy, the clinician may consider monotherapy with a beta blocker, combination therapy of a beta blocker with mexiletine or procainamide, or treatment with sotalol.

Contraindications for Antiarrhythmic Drugs

- The major contraindication to antiarrhythmic therapy is treatment of a rhythm disturbance that is not a risk for ventricular fibrillation or hemodynamic compromise.
- Atrioventricular block is generally a contraindication to antiarrhythmic treatment because of the risk of suppressing escape pacemaker activity.
- Drugs with potential for marked neuroexcitatory activity (lidocaine, mexiletine) generally are contraindicated in cats.

Toxicity

- Because of their antiadrenergic actions, beta blockers can demonstrate potent negative inotropic and chronotropic effects. *Doses must be titrated* to effect while observing for adverse signs that include: bradycardia, hypotension, AV block, precipitation or worsening of heart failure or impairment of renal function.

▼ *Key Point* Beta Blockers must be given very cautiously in CHF because of the negative inotropic effect (first control CHF, then titrate the dose from a low starting dose).

- As a result of B_2 bronchoconstrictive actions, nonspecific beta blockers(propranolol) are contraindicated in bronchial disease or asthma. For a similar reason, these drugs are relatively contraindicated in arterial thrombosis (may block collateral vessel receptors).
- Beta blockade can interfere with beta-adrenergic responsiveness to the effects of low blood sugar (anxiety, tachycardia) in patients with diabetes mellitus.

Administration

- The indication for therapy should be clear and drug selection appropriate to the rhythm disturbance. ECG documentation is needed to ensure the rhythm diagnosis and to assess response to treatment. Ambulatory (Holter) ECG recordings are especially valuable in this regard.
- Choose the drug dosage based on established guidelines (Table 63–1) and response to therapy.
- Plasma concentrations of some drugs can be obtained at commercial laboratories. Procainamide, for example, is a relatively easy drug to monitor. Therapeutic (trough) concentrations are typically 5–10 µg/ml in the dog but occasionally are higher.
- Inform the animal's owner about adverse effects and the need to report them.
- Be aware of common and infrequent adverse effects. This information is found in most reference textbooks and in the PDR.
- Duration of therapy depends on the rhythm and cause. For specifics, see Chapter 62.

Drug Interactions

- Both propranolol and cimetidine reduce liver blood flow and delay excretion of lidocaine. CHF, hypotension, and halothane anesthesia may reduce lidocaine clearance.

SUPPLEMENTAL READINGS

Hardman JG, Limbird LE, Molinoff PB, Ruddon RW, Gilman AG (eds): Goodman & Gilman's The Pharmacological Basis of Therapeutics. 9th ed. New York: McGraw-Hill, 1996.

Opie LH: Drugs for the Heart. 4th ed. Philadelphia: WB Saunders, 1995.

Plumb DC: Veterinary Drug Handbook. 2nd ed. Ames: Iowa State University Press, 1995

OVERVIEW OF HEART FAILURE

- Heart failure is a state wherein the cardiac output is inadequate to meet the perfusion needs of the metabolizing tissues and exercise capacity is limited. Venous filling pressures are normal to increased in heart failure; the initial decrease in cardiac output is attributable to systolic and often to diastolic dysfunction of the heart.

- Heart failure is characterized by cardiac, hemodynamic (pressure/flow/resistance), renal, and neurohormonal abnormalities. The morbidity and mortality of heart failure is related in large measure to cardiac, systemic, and local tissue "compensations" that develop in response to limited cardiac output.

- *Cardiac output* is a function of the ventricular systolic function (stroke volume) and the heart rate (and cardiac rhythm).

  - Systolic cardiac function depends first on ventricular diastolic function because this directly affects cardiac filling (*preload*).

  - Myocardial *contractility* is the second determinant because stroke volume increases with increasing inotropism.

  - The load against which the left and right ventricles must work (*afterload*) is reflected in the systolic ventricular *wall tension* that must be generated (this tension is related in part to blood pressure and ration of ventricular diameter to wall thickness). Afterload represents a negative determinant of ventricular function inasmuch as increasing afterload reduces stroke volume.

  - A fourth issue affecting stroke volume is *valvular function* because valve incompetency or stenosis can negatively affect stroke volume. The method of classifying the *pathophysiologic basis* of heart failure centers on the *mechanisms of ventricular dysfunction*.

CAUSES OF HEART FAILURE

Identifying the cause and classifying the pathophysiologic basis of cardiac failure allows the clinician to direct appropriate therapy and render a more accurate prognosis. Anatomic and physiologic disorders responsible for heart failure in dogs and cats are summarized in Table 64–1. Most of these disorders can be classified in one of the following categories.

- *Contractility (inotropic or myocardial) failure* of the heart muscle—These conditions (e.g., dilated cardiomyopathy) are characterized by inherent loss of myocardial contractility and decreased ventricular ejection fraction (stroke volume/end diastolic volume) despite a normal or increased ventricular preload.

- *Systolic hemodynamic overload* of the ventricle—With *volume* overload (e.g., mitral regurgitation, patent ductus arteriosus), the total ventricular stroke volume is increased for each heartbeat; with *pressure* overload (e.g., subvalvular aortic stenosis, heartworm disease), the stroke volume must be ejected at a higher than normal ventricular pressure. Myocardial contractility is well preserved for some time in these conditions but eventually may deteriorate, producing the "cardiomyopathy of overload."

- *Diastolic dysfunction* or *compliance failure* of the ventricle(s)—These conditions primarily affect cardiac filling (e.g., pericardial disease, hypertrophic cardiomyopathy, restrictive cardiomyopathy) and impair systolic function only indirectly (by reducing preload). It also should be appreciated that many conditions characterized by marked ventricular dilation, hypertrophy, or fibrosis also reduce ventricular compliance or increase chamber stiffness.

- *Arrhythmia or conduction disturbance* of the heart—These disorders can lead to heart failure (e.g., relentless ventricular tachycardia, complete atrioventricular (AV) block) or precipitate heart failure in a previously compensated patient (e.g., atrial fibrillation).

COMPENSATORY MECHANISMS EVOKED IN HEART FAILURE

The onset of a cardiac lesion does not immediately trigger heart failure. The hemodynamic changes in cardiac output or blood pressure trigger compensatory responses. Blood pressure can be maintained through alterations in the neuroendocrine system, kidney, and heart. In general, heart failure is associated with heightened activity of vasoconstrictor systems, attenuation of vasodilator systems, and increased activity of tissue mediators of muscle hypertrophy and fibrosis. The well-compensated cardiac patient often can maintain cardiac output and blood pressure within the normal range at rest (basal state) by activating compensatory mechanisms.

Table 64–1. CAUSES OF HEART DISEASE AND HEART FAILURE IN DOGS AND CATS

Valvular (Endocardial) Diseases

Chronic valvular heart disease in dogs (mitral and tricuspid valve endocardiosis)—most common cause of heart disease in the dog; never a substantiated report of chronic valvular disease in cats

Bacterial endocarditis—usually a multisystemic disorder with fever, polyarthritis, and immune-mediated findings (*Note:* There is no evidence that endocarditis leads to chronic valvular heart disease in dogs, nor is there any evidence [despite popular belief] that areas of inflammation [e.g., dental or periodontal disease] lead to chronic valvular disease.)

Congenital valve malformation (pulmonic stenosis, [sub]aortic stenosis, mitral and tricuspid valve dysplasia)

Abnormality of the support apparatus causing AV valvular insufficiency—rupture of mitral chorda tendinea in dogs (MR much greater than TR); ventricular dilation or hypertrophy (MR or TR); dynamic left ventricular outflow tract obstruction (MR)

Myocardial Diseases

Dilated cardiomyopathy (myocardial failure unrelated to structural lesions of the heart valves or coronary arteries)

Idiopathic dilated cardiomyopathy (dog and cat)—DCM in dogs is second most common cause of CHF

Taurine deficiency (cat, cocker spaniels, small breeds, ?Golden retrievers, ?other breeds)

Systemic or myocardial levo-carnitine deficiency (boxer dogs, spaniels, ?other breeds—overall significance of L-carnitine deficiency in the pathogenesis of DCM is certain)

Feline hypertrophic cardiomyopathy—LV hypertrophy unrelated to endocrine disease, hypertension, or congenital disease

Idiopathic (probably genetic)—most important cause of symptomatic heart disease in cats

Canine HCM is rare

Feline restrictive (intermediate) cardiomyopathy, also called feline endomyocardial fibrosis

Thyrotoxicosis from thyroid tumor (cats); iatrogenic from high-level thyroid supplementation (dogs)

Anemia (high-output heart failure) observed in cats >>> dogs

Hypertensive heart disease (e.g., primary (idiopathic or "essential" or secondary to renal disease or Cushing's disease)

Myocarditis (e.g., sepsis, parvovirus infection, ?borreliosis)—quite uncommon

Congenital defects of the cardiac septae—atrial septal defect, ventricular septal defect, cor triatriatum dexter

Myocardial degeneration and fibrosis (usually affects one or both atria leading to progressive atrial dilation or often loss of sinus or atrial electrical activity, so-called silent atrium or silent atria syndromes of dogs and cats); ± ventricular involvement

Myocardial trauma

Myocardial infiltration—neoplastic (e.g., lymphosarcoma)

Acute myocardial infarction is a rare observation in dogs, although transient myocardial ischemia often causes arrhythmias

Pericardial Diseases

Cardiac tamponade from pericardial effusion

Idiopathic pericardial hemorrhage or pericarditis—most common cause of pericardial effusion in dogs < 8 years of age

Infective pericarditis—not common but does occur in dogs and cats (always consider FB in cases of septic pericarditis)

Cardiac, intrapericardial, or heart neoplasia

Causing pericardial effusion (from bleeding = hemorrhagic fluid; or obstruction of lymphatic drainage = transudate)

Constrictive pericardial disease—typically constrictive-effusive disease in dogs (i.e., thickened pericardium + fluid)

Electrical Disturbances—Cardiac Arrhythmias

Atrial arrhythmias (e.g., atrial tachycardia, flutter, and fibrillation)

Junctional (nodal) tachycardia

Re-entrant supraventricular tachycardia

Ventricular tachycardia

Bradyarrhythmias—persistent sinus bradycardia or arrest (with escape rhythm), silent atrium (persistent atrial standstill), high-grade second-degree or third-degree (complete) atrioventricular block

Vascular Diseases (Congenital or Acquired)

Extracardiac shunts—patent ductus arteriosus, congenital or acquired arteriovenous fistula

Pulmonary vascular disease leading to pulmonary hypertension and cor pulmonale, including dirofilariasis, pulmonary thromboembolism, pulmonary hypertension related to chronic left heart failure, and idiopathic pulmonary hypertension

---

MR, mitral regurgitation; TR, tricuspid regurgitation; DCM, dilated cardiomyopathy; CHF, congestive heart failure; LV, left ventricular; HCM, hypertrophic cardiomyopathy; FB, foreign body.

- Initial signs of cardiac failure may only become evident with exercise.
- Compensatory mechanisms, although initially beneficial, can injure the patient in the long term. Many of the clinical signs of congestive heart failure (CHF) are attributed to progressive decline in cardiac function with increased activity of these "compensatory" responses.
- Excessive neurohormonal and renal compensatory responses contribute to the genesis of CHF, organ and tissue injury, morbidity, and cardiac-related death.
- Therapy of heart failure involves modulating these compensatory mechanisms with the aim toward minimizing clinical signs of CHF and prolonging life.

Activation of the Sympathetic Nervous System

- Heart failure is associated with increased activity of the sympathetic nervous system (SNS), increased circulating concentrations of norepinephrine, and increased activity of the sympathetic modulating hormone, angiotensin II.
- High sympathetic activity is associated with increased mortality. Blocking B_1/B_2 cardiac receptors chronically has been associated with less cardiac dilation, preserved myocardial function, and increased survival in CHF in people and in canine models of myocardial failure. For this reason, some clinicians have recommended adding a beta blocker when treating CHF or atrial fibrillation caused by dilated cardiomyopathy

(although clinical studies are needed to examine this approach). It should be stressed, however, that acute or high-dose beta blockade may be harmful to the cardiac patient because sympathetic support of the failing myocardium (both inotropic and chronotropic) is suppressed.

- Downregulation of myocardial beta receptors is characteristic of chronic CHF and may impair the ability of the heart to respond appropriately to stress (such as exercise) with a sympathetic-mediated increase in heart rate and ventricular stroke volume. There is some evidence that downregulation can be prevented in part with low doses of beta-adrenergic blockers.
- Other issues of relevance to SNS activation include: precipitation of ventricular and atrial arrhythmias; persistent tachycardia, including a rapid ventricular rate response to atrial fibrillation; and increased myocardial cell injury and myocardial fibrosis.

Activation of Vasoconstricting and Sodium-Retaining Mechanisms

Mechanisms of vasoconstriction involved include enhanced *sympathetic* nervous system activity, activation of the *renin-angiotensin-aldosterone* system (RAAS), release of *arginine vasopressin* (ADH), and increased relative activity of *local vasoconstrictor* systems (e.g., endothelin). Constriction of systemic *veins* acts to increase venous pressures and filling of the heart.

- Increased vascular resistance supports mean arterial blood pressure (ABP) and the perfusion of the cerebral and coronary circulations; however, *blood flow is redistributed* and perfusion of less vital regional circulations is decreased. Reduced perfusion can impair tissue function. For example, a hallmark feature of CHF is reduced exercise capacity of skeletal muscle contributing to *exercise intolerance.*
- Systemic vasoconstriction also *increases left ventricular afterload*. The failing ventricle is especially sensitive to afterload. Greater ventricular wall tension may be required to overcome systemic vascular resistance and aortic impedance; thus, the stroke volume may decrease. This situation has been termed "afterload mismatch" by Ross.
- Systemic vasoconstriction can *worsen mitral regurgitation* by raising diastolic arterial pressure and prolonging the onset of aortic valve opening. Lowering the ABP actually decreases the mitral regurgitation (MR) fraction.
- Modulating "excessive" arterial vasoconstriction with vasodilator drugs can be beneficial to the heart failure patient, with maintenance of a systolic blood pressure of 90 to 120 mm Hg a clinically reasonable target.
- Activity of the RAAS occurs with progressive heart failure. This and related vasoconstrictor/sodium-retaining systems eventually overwhelm vasodilator/naturetic hormones (e.g., atrial naturetic peptide).
- Mediators of arterial vasoconstriction—especially angiotensin II and norepinephrine—*may injure the myocardium.* Angiotensin II is a growth promoter and increases hypertrophy and fibrosis (these tissue effects are potentiated by the hormone *aldosterone,* which is a component of both systemic and tissue renin-angiotensin-aldosterone systems).

- Inhibition of the renin-angiotensin-aldosterone system with drugs that include angiotensin-converting enzyme (ACE) inhibitors ("-prils") or aldosterone antagonists (spironolactone) may be especially beneficial and increase survival related to protective effects on the myocardium.
- The kidney behaves in cardiac failure as it does in hypovolemia, reabsorbing sodium and water in excess of "normal." This retention increases plasma volume, venous pressures, ventricular filling, and heart size. Ultimately, this fluid retention contributes to the development of pulmonary edema or body cavity effusions.
- Mechanisms that may contribute to sodium and water retention by the kidney include increased sympathetic activity (releases renin and can alter renal blood flow), angiotensin II, aldosterone, antidiuretic hormone, and progressive insensitivity to atrial naturetic peptide. Strict sodium restriction (e.g., feeding only a heart diet) also can activate the RAAS.
- The most deleterious effects of fluid retention are the excessive elevation of venous/capillary pressures and the formation of *edema or effusions.*
- Venous hypertension and elevated capillary hydrostatic pressure develop foremost in those vascular beds behind the failing side of the heart. This is related to: (1) the increased plasma volume caused by sodium and water retention, (2) abnormal pumping function of the ventricle (systolic failure), (3) impairment of ventricular filling (diastolic failure), or (4) (most often) a combination of these factors.
- This combination of insufficient cardiac function *(backward failure)* coupled with renal retention of sodium and water volume *(forward failure)* produces the edematous state referred to as *congestive heart failure* (CHF).
- Chronic right-sided or biventricular heart failure can be associated with the retention of large volumes of fluid. Because the pulmonary circulation can store less blood than the systemic circulation, acute pulmonary congestion can develop if the left ventricle suddenly fails to clear venous return from the lungs. Thus, in left-sided CHF, chronic fluid retention may not be an essential component to the development of pulmonary edema.
- Successful therapy of CHF generally includes administration of diuretic drugs that contract the plasma volume and lower venous pressures while counteracting further renal reabsorption of sodium and water. Restriction of dietary sodium is another commonly used approach to limit sodium retention.

Cardiac Hypertrophy and Dilation

- Cardiac muscle hypertrophy develops in response to either volume or pressure work (common in dogs) or as an idiopathic or genetically programmed process (hypertrophic cardiomyopathy—rare in dogs). Ventricular hypertrophy serves to normalize systolic wall stress (and hence afterload) and often maintains a normal forward stroke volume, even in the face of increased cardiac work.

- Ventricular dilation helps to maintain stroke volume in the face of progressive myocardial failure (e.g., dilated cardiomyopathy) or volume overload (e.g., mitral regurgitation); however, dilation increases wall stress and ventricular afterload.
- Distortion of ventricular geometry frequently leads to atrioventricular valvular regurgitation.
- Hypertrophy in some conditions often is associated with increased myocardial fibrosis.
- Myocardial injury and fibrosis may be limited by treatment with an angiotensin inhibitor, spironolactone (inhibitor of aldosterone), or perhaps a beta blocker.

HEMODYNAMIC ABNORMALITIES AND CLINICAL SIGNS OF CONGESTIVE HEART FAILURE

Clinical signs of heart failure are related largely to abnormalities of hemodynamics and fluid dynamics in the microcirculation.

Cardiac Output

- Basal cardiac output (CO) is not a sensitive indicator of heart function because compensatory mechanisms can maintain the resting CO within the normal range for quite some time.
- The CO in response to exercise is inadequate in heart failure, and in advanced heart failure, the resting CO may be low, contributing to exercise intolerance and organ hypoperfusion.

Systemic Arterial Blood Pressure

- Blood pressure in CHF is generally normal despite a limitation of CO. This is explained by the compensatory mechanisms of cardiac dilation and hypertrophy, tachycardia, and *increased systemic vascular resistance* mediated by peripheral vasoconstriction.
- Arterial hypotension can be measured in severe heart failure (e.g., from dilated cardiomyopathy) or after the administration of high doses of diuretics (which reduce plasma volume) or vasodilator drugs (which mitigate vasoconstriction).
- ABP is measured readily with a Doppler flow detector or through oscillometric techniques.

Pulmonary Arterial Blood Pressure

- Pulmonary hypertension develops in response to left-sided heart failure (pressure "backup") and in some dogs as a consequence of increased pulmonary vascular resistance.
- Significant pulmonary hypertension (often exceeding 50 mm Hg), without radiographic evidence of pulmonary edema, is observed in some dogs with chronic left-sided CHF. This situation probably represents a primary increase in *pulmonary vascular resistance* of undetermined mechanisms.
- Pulmonary hypertension, when severe, can lead to secondary right-sided CHF.
- High pulmonary vascular resistance is also the mechanism for right-sided CHF that develops secondary to canine heartworm disease.

Systemic Venous Pressure (Central Venous Pressure)

- The central venous pressure (CVP) often is increased in CHF because of venoconstriction, fluid retention, and increased plasma volume. The CVP is especially high when there is right—as opposed to left—ventricular failure because systemic venous pressure depends not only on plasma volume but on the ability of the right ventricle to accept and pump the venous return.
- An elevated CVP also impairs the drainage of lymph from the thoracic duct into the systemic venous circulation. This is the probable mechanism for chylothorax secondary to severe right-sided CHF. The CVP (mm Hg or cm of H_2O) can be measured with a jugular venous catheter, but it is more practical simply to estimate pressure by inspection and gentle digital palpation of the jugular veins.

Pulmonary Venous Pressure

- The pulmonary venous and capillary pressures are elevated in left-sided CHF, but they cannot be measured noninvasively.
- CVP does *not* predict wedge pressure.

Microcirculation

- Abnormalities in the microcirculation explain the development of edema and cavity effusions.
- Once the venous system draining a capillary bed becomes hypertensive, the *capillary hydrostatic pressure* also increases. This enhances ultrafiltration across the capillary wall and predisposes to edema.
- A concurrent increase in lymphatic drainage provides a margin of safety against fluid accumulation, but once the lymph system is overwhelmed, interstitial pulmonary edema develops. Acute elevations of hydrostatic pressure are more likely to precipitate alveolar pulmonary edema.
- Elevated pressure in the systemic capillaries of the liver leads to increased ultrafiltration across this organ, promoting ascites.
- Elevated capillary pressures in the skin cause subcutaneous edema, although this is not common in small animals unless there is concurrent hypoproteinemia.
- Pleural effusion can be caused by elevation of capillary pressures along the parietal pleural surface (right-sided venous drainage) or visceral pleural surface (left-sided drainage). Biventricular CHF is the most common cause of pleural effusion because there is increased formation of thoracic lymph and

impaired drainage owing to elevated right atrial pressures.

Clinical Signs of Heart Failure

Heart failure typically is described as "left-" or "right"-sided. This designation, although useful, neglects the fact that left and right ventricular outputs must be equal and that biventricular failure is common. Right-sided cardiac disorders such as tricuspid regurgitation or pulmonary hypertension cause weakness and syncope by decreasing right ventricular, and consequently left ventricular, stroke volume. Similarly, left ventricular failure with pulmonary venous hypertension can cause the right ventricle to fail by increasing pulmonary venous pressure and elevating the right ventricular pressure required for pulmonary arterial perfusion.

- Clinical manifestations of left ventricular failure include the following:
  - Exertional weakness, tiring, pallor, and syncope
  - Oliguria and prerenal azotemia due to reduced renal blood flow
  - Cardiac arrhythmias (possibly from myocardial ischemia)
  - Pulmonary edema with tachypnea, "dyspnea," orthopnea, lung crackles, hemoptysis, and cyanosis
  - Coughing from pulmonary edema or airway compression
  - Pleural effusion (a sign of left-sided, biventricular, or severe right-sided CHF)

▼ *Key Point* Marked left atrial enlargement can lead to bronchial compression and attendant cough—this is a sign of heart disease but not necessarily heart failure because the cough can develop before pulmonary edema and persist after successful therapy of pulmonary edema.

- Clinical manifestations of right ventricular failure include:
  - Exertional weakness, tiring, pallor, and syncope
  - Systemic venous congestion with jugular venous distention and elevated CVP
  - Enlargement (congestion) of the liver and sometimes the spleen
  - Accumulation of fluid in extravascular spaces, including:
    - Small to moderate pericardial effusion (although at times it can be moderate to large)
    - Pleural effusion leading to atelectasis, tachypnea, respiratory distress, and cyanosis
    - Peritoneal effusion (ascites)
    - Subcutaneous edema (uncommon in small animals)
    - Jugular venous distension and pulsations

▼ *Key Point* The diagnosis of right-sided CHF is likely when the jugular venous pressure is elevated, when cardiac auscultation is abnormal, and when there is hepatomegaly and abnormal fluid accumulation.

Functional Class of Heart Disease

It is common to speak in terms of "functional" classes of heart disease. These classes, often used in clinical studies and in therapy recommendations, are extrapolated from the New York Heart Association criteria for human patients and are based on symptoms, signs, and exercise capacity.

- Class I—objective signs of heart disease, but no clinical evidence of cardiac failure;
- Class II—objective signs of heart disease and clinical evidence of cardiac failure with exertion or vigorous activity;
- Class III—objective signs of cardiac failure with minimal activity or periodically while at rest (e.g., nocturnal orthopnea);
- Class IV—objective signs of cardiac failure at rest.

From a more practical standpoint, veterinary patients are better described as having heart failure that is:

- Without clinical signs of heart failure (similar to class I)
- Mild to moderate CHF (classes II and III)—the animal has obvious exercise limitations or has intermittent or progressive clinical signs of heart failure (coughing, tachypnea)
- Severe CHF (class IV)—left, right or biventricular CHF is obvious in the resting animal.

Other Clinical Findings in Congestive Heart Failure

- Most cases of heart failure are associated with some *abnormality of auscultation;* for example, murmur, gallop, arrhythmia, or muffled heart sounds.
- Respiratory auscultation may be abnormal; for example, tachypnea, loud bronchial sounds, crackles (small airway dysfunction), wheezes (from airway narrowing), or muffled sounds (pleural effusion).
- *Cardiac cachexia,* manifested as poor appetite, and substantial loss of muscle mass is prominent in some patients, especially giant breed dogs with dilated cardiomyopathy. The proposed causes are numerous.
- *Fever* or a history of fever is important in cases of bacterial endocarditis.

ESTABLISHING THE CAUSE OF HEART FAILURE

Cardiac Diagnoses

The clinician should strive to make three types of diagnoses—etiologic, anatomic, and physiologic.

- The *relative prevalence of these lesions* depends on the type of practice and geographic location. The most common causes of CHF in dogs are mitral and tricuspid valve endocardiosis, dilated cardiomyopathy, pericardial effusion, advanced heartworm disease, and untreated congenital heart disease (HD). Endocarditis is considered only when there are multisystemic signs (fever, polyarthritis). Arrhythmias are common and often complicate the aforementioned diseases. In cats, heart failure almost always is caused by a form of cardiomyopathy, by advanced hyperthyroid heart disease, or by untreated congenital heart disease (see Cardiomyopathy in this section).

- The clinical diagnosis of right-sided CHF is often a *physical diagnosis*. Diagnosis of left-sided CHF usually *requires ancillary tests* to rule out other causes of respiratory disease. Determination of the exact cause of CHF requires a more complete database, identifying radiographic, electrocardiographic, echocardiographic, and laboratory abnormalities.
- The precise abnormalities encountered in the dog with heart failure depend on the cause of heart disease and the severity of the condition. The usual cardiac "database" includes the signalment and client history, results of cardiac auscultation and physical examination, blood pressure, thoracic radiographs, electrocardiogram, and routine blood tests. An echocardiogram can be very helpful for determining the cause of heart failure. The following are points relevant to cardiac diagnosis. Results of diagnostic tests in specific disorders are described elsewhere in this section.

Radiography

Cardiomegaly (ventricular/atrial), systemic or pulmonary venous dilation, and abnormal fluid accumulation in the lung (pulmonary interstitial or alveolar edema) or pleural space (pleural effusion) are expected radiographic features in virtually all cases of CHF.

- Clinical signs of coughing very often are the result of *left mainstem bronchus compression* in dogs with MR. Often there is no other radiographic or auscultatory evidence of pulmonary edema. This finding is best appreciated on the lateral projection.
- The clinician must remember that dogs with chronic respiratory disease, but without CHF, often have cardiomegaly (cor pulmonale, pericardial fat, poor chest expansion that mimics cardiomegaly).

Electrocardiography

The electrocardiogram (ECG) is usually abnormal in CHF and may contribute to the differential diagnosis (e.g., increased voltage or widened QRS complexes would be expected with dilated cardiomyopathy, whereas attenuated QRS complexes are typical of pericardial effusion).

- Arrhythmias are common in heart failure but also can develop in noncardiac conditions such as systemic infections, metabolic diseases, and electrolyte imbalances.
- Some arrhythmias, like atrial fibrillation, are very characteristic of advanced heart disease and are likely to be associated with CHF.

▼ *Key Point* A normal or equivocal ECG *does not* rule out CHF.

Echocardiography

This specialized imaging technique is very helpful in establishing the cause of CHF. Characteristic features of common causes of heart failure include:

- Mitral valve endocardiosis—thickened valves, dilated left (± right) heart chambers, hypercontractile left ventricle.
- Dilated cardiomyopathy—dilated cardiac chambers with a hypocontractile left ventricle.
- Hypertrophic cardiomyopathy (or hyperthyroidism)—thickened, well-contracting left ventricle walls with left atrial dilation.
- Restrictive cardiomyopathy—dilated left and right atria, dilation of basilar left ventricle, variable hypertrophy of papillary muscles and left ventricular (LV) wall, prominent subendocardial echoes or midventricular bands, marginal shortening fraction.
- Pericardial effusion—an echo-free pericardial space is evident. Compression of the right heart chambers occurs in cases of cardiac tamponade. Cardiac or intrapericardial masses may be evident as well.
- Heartworm disease—right-sided dilation, dilated pulmonary arteries, and shifting of the septum into the left ventricle; may see parasites in pulmonary artery (PA).
- Congenital heart disease—the cardiac malformation and associated flow disturbances are evident with echo and Doppler studies; in general, these cases are best evaluated by a cardiologist.

Hematologic Tests

Hematologic tests (CBC, biochemical profile, serum thyroxin) and urinalysis are indicated to evaluate metabolic function and may provide pointers regarding the underlying disease.

- Common abnormalities observed in CHF are prerenal azotemia, mild to moderate hypoproteinemia, and mild to moderate elevations in liver enzymes.
- Hyponatremia is a feature of very advanced CHF (free-water retention). Hypokalemia is a common complication of diuretic therapy and anorexia.
- Specialized tests such as plasma taurine concentration and blood cultures may be indicated in some patients.
- Tests for *heartworm* microfilaria or serologic tests for heartworm antigens are appropriate in cases of right-sided CHF.
- If the patient is taking digoxin, a serum digoxin concentration should be measured (see below).

TREATMENT OF CONGESTIVE HEART FAILURE

Overview of Congestive Heart Failure Therapy

Treatment of CHF can be classified roughly into symptomatic and specific therapies. Treatments also can be categorized as more appropriate for *urgent* or *hospital care*, with others typical of *chronic home care* administered by the client.

- Symptomatic medical therapy includes reducing activity and anxiety, improving blood and tissue oxygenation, decreasing edema and effusions, supporting cardiac output, and controlling cardiac arrhythmias.
- Specific treatment includes measures that either correct or address the underlying anatomic or pathophysiologic disorder.
- Goals CHF therapy are substantial improvement in quality of life and duration of life for our patients and accompanying client satisfaction.

Drug and Dietary Therapy of Heart Failure

The clinical pharmacology of drugs used to treat heart failure is described elsewhere in this section and is not repeated here (see Chapter 63). Most drugs used to treat CHF are classified as diuretics, positive inotropic drugs, and vasodilator drugs.

Diuretics

Diuretics are given for two main reasons: (1) to diurese edematous patients or those with substantial body cavity effusions while in the hospital (using injectable agents); and (2) to prevent the chronic sodium and water retention that accompany most cases of chronic CHF. Furosemide should be administered to patients with respiratory distress due to pulmonary edema before performance of diagnostic studies.

- Furosemide is the most commonly used diuretic in the treatment of heart failure. Furosemide acts by inhibiting the cotransporter of chloride in Henle's loop and leads to loss of chloride, sodium, water, and potassium in the urine. The drug must be delivered by renal blood flow to be effective.
- Reduced renal blood flow (e.g., CHF), renal failure, and hypoproteinemia can negatively affect delivery of furosemide to the proximal tubule (where it must be actively secreted and carried in the filtrate to Henle's loop). For that reason, an initial, high-dose treatment, parenterally (at least 4–6 mg/kg, IV or IM) is recommended in life-threatening CHF to facilitate delivery of sufficient drug to the renal tubules. Once diuresis has ensued, the dose is reduced (1–2 mg/kg).
- A diuresis should be evident or the bladder palpably enlarged from baseline within 30–45 minutes of initial parenteral dosing of furosemide; if not, repeat or increase the dose and re-administer. After the onset of diuresis, the dosage is lowered and the interval increased to minimize dehydration and electrolyte depletion.
- Malabsorption or decreased delivery of furosemide seems to be important in severe right-sided CHF, and the ascites often responds better to intermittent dosing with subcutaneous furosemide (Lasix) in the home environment (substitute an oral dose with the SC dose 3 times weekly, then try to decrease the use).
- Combination diuretic therapy (furosemide + thiazide + spironolactone) is one strategy for unresponsive pulmonary edema or ascites. Administer furosemide alone at least twice daily and with the other diuretic once or twice daily.

- Preparations include proprietary (Lasix) and generic forms—12.5- and 50-mg tablets (veterinary), 20-, 40-, 80-mg tablets (human); injectable 5% solution (50 mg/ml); syrup (10 mg/ml).
- The usual dose range for furosemide is 1–4 mg/kg, IV, IM, or SC once to three times daily, as needed; oral furosemide is approximately 50% less potent (because there is less absorption or renal delivery) when compared with parenteral furosemide.
- The loop diuretic *bumetanide* (Bumex) may be substituted for furosemide; bumetanide is dosed at approximately $\frac{1}{40}$ of the furosemide dose. Another new loop diuretic, *torsemide*, recently has been released. The advantage of these diuretics over furosemide in clinical situations is not yet evident.
- *Thiazide* diuretics such as hydrochlorothiazide (HCT) sometimes are used alone or in combination with furosemide for management of fluid retention in CHF. Thiazides inhibit sodium, chloride, and water reabsorption in the distal tubule and the connecting segment. When used in combination with furosemide, these agents can prevent some of the distal sodium reabsorption that escapes the effects of the loop diuretics. HCT often is formulated with the diuretic spironolactone (which antagonizes aldosterone) or triamterene (to spare potassium) and increase the diuretic effect. The 50-mg tablet combination HCT + spironolactone at 2–4 mg/kg (of the combined 25 mg/25 mg product) may be useful.
- Chronic use of diuretics commonly leads to mild volume depletion (possibly leading to azotemia), hypochloremia with metabolic alkalosis, and potentially hypokalemia (although this is blunted by adequate food intake and by ACE inhibitors). Magnesium depletion also may develop, although the overall importance of this is uncertain. Combination diuretic therapy, even with potassium-sparing agents, can lead to profound hypokalemia and hyponatremia (follow ABP and serum biochemistries).

Positive Inotropic Drugs

Inotropic drugs are prescribed to improve ventricular performance and increase stroke volume. Potent injectable drugs such as dobutamine and dopamine are used in hospital treatment of life-threatening CHF. Digoxin, a modest inotropic drug that also induces secondary autonomic effects on the heart, is used for some forms of chronic CHF and to control heart rate in atrial fibrillation.

- *Digitalis glycosides*, principally digoxin, are used in the chronic management of CHF. Digitalis glycosides also sensitize baroreceptors, leading to a withdrawal of harmful sympathetic activity and increased vagal efferent tone. This can slow the resting sinus node rate and also decrease the ventricular rate response to atrial fibrillation. Digoxin is used almost exclusively in veterinary practice.
- *Indications for digoxin therapy:*
  - Digoxin is administered to virtually all small animal patients with dilated cardiomyopathy or atrial fibrillation.

- In patients with atrial fibrillation, digoxin is administered both to increase myocardial contractility and to slow AV nodal conduction, yielding a slower ventricular rate response.
- Dogs with advanced CHF caused by chronic valvular disease or congenital heart diseases, unless there is a contraindication (usual contraindications are: complex ventricular arrhythmias, moderate to severe renal failure, known individual hypersensitivity), are treated with digoxin.
- Digoxin plays a *minor* role in the acute hospital therapy of CHF, unless it is complicated by atrial fibrillation (in which case digoxin should be started immediately).
- Digitalis generally is *not* prescribed for diastolic problems such as pericardial disease or hypertrophic cardiomyopathy.

- Digoxin is contraindicated in the setting of complex ventricular arrhythmias and must be used with care in the setting of ventricular extrasystoles because it may or may not worsen the arrhythmia.
- Digoxin is excreted by the kidneys. The elimination half-life is long in the dog (about 24 hours). Hypokalemia, verapamil, ± diltiazem, and quinidine can elevate serum digoxin concentration.
- Preparations include Lanoxin tablets (0.125, 0.25 mg) and Lanoxin pediatric elixir (0.05 mg per ml) and Cardoxin elixirs (0.05 or 0.15 mg/ml). Usual total daily dose for the dog is 0.01 to 0.015 mg/kg, with the daily dose divided twice daily (0.005–0.0075 mg/kg bid). When splitting pills, it may not be possible to give two equal doses (e.g. ½ of a 0.125-mg tablet in the AM and ¼ of a 0.125-mg tablet in the PM). A loading dose (twice the calculated maintenance dose for 2–3 treatments) can be administered to patients in atrial fibrillation if the initial resting ventricular rate response exceeds 220/min, and Doberman pinschers often are well digitalized with 0.125 mg of Lanoxin twice daily.

▼ *Key Point* Be conservative in dosing digoxin. One always can increase the dose. Larger dogs seldom tolerate > 0.01 mg/kg per day.

- Common *adverse effects* of digoxin include anorexia, depression, vomiting, borborygmus, and diarrhea. Increased calcium influx or excessive vagal tone can lead to cardiac arrhythmias (junctional rhythms, ventricular extrasystoles, sinus bradycardia, AV block). Virtually any arrhythmia can develop with digitalis excess.
- *Monitor digitalis therapy* by history, heart rate, ± ECG, and trough serum digoxin levels (sample blood 10–12 hours postdosing; the therapeutic goal for a trough measurement is 0.8–1.2 ng/ml. *Note:* this is lower than previously recommended). The ECG is over-rated for monitoring (unless there are new arrhythmias), and the serum digoxin concentration is significantly underused in monitoring digoxin therapy.
- *Dobutamine HCl* (Dobutrex) is an injectable catecholamine (synthetic analogue of dopamine) with beta- and alpha-adrenergic agonist properties. The principal *indication* is treatment of cardiogenic shock in dogs such as Doberman pinschers or other large-breed dogs with life-threatening CHF due to dilated cardiomyopathy (DCM). Not all cases of DCM require such aggressive treatment.
  - Dobutamine (2.5–10 µg/kg/min constant rate infusion) improves the clinical signs of cardiogenic shock (i.e., severe CHF plus hypotension). The clinical signs of cardiogenic shock include dyspnea from pulmonary edema, hypothermia, muscle weakness, mucous membrane pallor (intense vasoconstriction), depression, and low mixed venous PO_2 (which indicates increased tissue extraction of oxygen).
  - Therapeutic effects of dobutamine include increased cardiac output, elevated ABP, increased tissue perfusion (color and refill time), increasing body temperature, and improvement in attitude and strength.
  - Adverse effects include tachycardia, excessive vasoconstriction, and induction of extrasystoles. Seizure activity is observed infrequently.
  - The dose is adjusted based on clinical response and blood pressure (measure with Dinamap or Parks Doppler flow meter and manometer cuff) and by observing for adverse effects.
  - The usual infusion is continued for 24 to 48 hours; higher doses may be tolerated and required with progressive downregulation of myocardial beta adrenoreceptors.
- *Dopamine HCl* has similar effects to dobutamine but with greater alpha-adrenergic vasoconstriction and tachycardia for equal inotropic doses; therefore, dobutamine is preferred in CHF. One potential benefit of dopamine is improved renal perfusion and urinary output via dopaminergic receptor activation (renal vasodilation and less reabsorption of sodium in renal tubules). However, most dogs with CHF experience diuresis during dobutamine and furosemide therapy.

Vasodilator drugs are used in both acute and chronic heart failure. This group includes a variety of agents capable of unloading the ventricles, reducing mitral regurgitant fraction, decreasing ventricular filling pressures, and antagonizing the RAAS. Direct acting drugs such as nitrates, hydralazine, and sodium nitroprusside are used in hospital management of CHF. ACE inhibitors such as enalapril and benazepril are used most often for chronic treatment of CHF in dogs and increasingly in cats.

- *Nitroglycerin ointment* (Nitrol, Nitro-bid, Nitrostat, and others) or (2.5 or 5 mg) patch:
  - Topical nitrates work through nitric oxide (NO) mediated vasodilation.
  - These drugs are mostly venodilators (unless given IV or at high doses) and may be effective in reducing venous pressure by allowing translocation of pulmonary venous blood secondary to nitrate-induced pooling in systemic veins. They have not been studied critically in animals.

- Nitrate tolerance develops if they are given too frequently.
- Indications for nitrate therapy include hospital therapy of pulmonary edema and home use in dogs with nocturnal dyspnea (apply at bedtime) or in difficult to medicate dogs that tolerate topical therapy (NTG 2% ointment = approximately 15 mg/inch; approximate dose: feline = ¼ inch cutaneously q12–24h; canine = ½ to 1½ inches cutaneously, q12–24h).
- *Sodium nitroprusside* (Nipride) is a potent dilator of systemic arterial and venous smooth muscle (probably generating NO). Reduced mitral regurgitation (MR fraction), decreased LV afterload (increasing forward flow), and reduced venous pressure (from venous pooling) are beneficial effects of this potent drug.
  - Nitroprusside is used principally for hospital treatment of life-threatening pulmonary edema caused by cardiomyopathy or mitral valvular disease
  - Nitroprusside is given when initial doses of furosemide and nitroglycerine fail to provide relief from pulmonary edema or when pulmonary edema is so fulminant that the patient is expectorating bloody froth.
  - When used in patients with dilated cardiomyopathy, dobutamine should be infused at the same time to prevent hypotension. Initial nitroprusside doses of 1–2 μg/kg/min for 24 hours are generally well tolerated. The infusion rate can be increased to 10 μg/kg/min; however, doses > 2.5 μg/kg/min are uncommonly required. Avoid use for more than 36 to 48 hours. Wean the patient from the drug over a 4- to 6-hour period.
  - Frequent monitoring of arterial blood pressure is *essential* when using this drug.
- *Hydralazine* (Apresoline—10- and 25-mg tablets: 0.5–2 mg/kg orally q12h).
  - Hydralazine acts directly on vascular smooth muscle to induce vasodilation in systemic arterioles.
  - Hydralazine is administered by mouth and has a significant vasodilating effect within 2 hours, reaching a near peak effect within 3–5 hours postadministration. The drug can cause substantial hypotension. It is more predictable and potent an arteriolar vasodilator than the ACE inhibitors.
  - By decreasing systolic and diastolic arterial blood pressure, left ventricular afterload decreases and the aortic valve can be opened "earlier" in systole. The results are reduced mitral regurgitant fraction and increased stroke volume and cardiac output.
  - *Indications:* Hydralazine is most useful for acute treatment of severe pulmonary edema associated with mitral regurgitation, particularly after rupture of a chorda tendinea. It also can be prescribed for end-stage left-sided CHF due to dilated cardiomyopathy.
  - Combination treatment with oxygen, furosemide, nitroglycerine, and hydralazine is very effective for *emergency management of acute pulmonary edema due to mitral disease;* the hydralazine-nitrate combination has benefits that are similar—although not as rapid-acting—to those of nitroprusside.
  - Hydralazine also can be used in combination with an ACE inhibitor in treatment of *refractory* coughing or pulmonary edema caused by mitral regurgitation or DCM plus MR. Combined vasodilator therapy should be initiated in the hospital with arterial blood pressure monitoring.
  - *Adverse effects:* Anorexia (especially in small dogs); hypotension (as with any vasodilator); reflex sinus tachycardia (compensating for the hypotension); and activation of the RAAS (thus, it is less preferred for long-term use unless an ACE inhibitor also is prescribed).
- *Angiotensin-converting enzyme inhibitors* (ACEIs) There are numerous ACEI drugs (ACEI = _____ + pril). The ACE inhibitors exert their therapeutic action through inhibition of the RAAS, blocking the conversion of angiotensin I (AT-I) to AT-II by inhibiting the converting enzyme. Onset of vasodilation is not as abrupt or as marked as with hydralazine or nitroprusside; however, these drugs are arterial vasodilators (via inhibition of AT-II receptors) and also venodilators (presumably by preventing the degradation of venodilator kinins) while exerting measurable effects on blood pressure and afterload.
  - *Captopril* (Capoten—12.5- and 25-mg tablets: 0.5–2 mg/kg, orally q8h.) The prototype ACEI currently is used less often because of possible problems with anorexia and the need for q8h dosing.
  - *Enalapril* (Enacard; Cardiovet—veterinary 1.25-, 2.5-, 5-, 10-mg tablets; Vasotec—human; 2.5-, 5-, 10-,and 20-mg tablets: 0.25–0.5 mg/kg, orally q12–24h) is the most commonly used ACEI drug and the only agent licensed for veterinary use in North America.
  - *Lisinopril*—Prinivil (Merck & Co.) 2.5-, 5-, 10-, 20-, 40-mg tablets (unscored) also may be considered (0.25–0.5 mg/kg once daily). Although not approved for animal use, it is of lower cost for equivalent ACE inhibition.
  - *Benazepril* (Lotensin) is the newest and equally effective ACEI used in clinical veterinary practice based on European studies (0.5 mg/kg qd–q12h). It is approved in Europe but has extra-label use in North America. The hepatic elimination of this drug is considered a potential (although unproven) benefit in patients with renal failure.
  - As a group, these drugs are very useful for long-term management of CHF due to dilated cardiomyopathy and other causes of CHF, and they improve survival in canine CHF, perhaps related to effects on tissues (e.g. less myocardial injury and fibrosis from angiotensin and aldosterone) or tempering effects on the sympathetic nervous system. In dogs with chronic valvular disease and CHF, the ACEI drugs appear beneficial although perhaps not as much as for dogs with DCM. The ACEI drugs are the current vasodilator drugs of choice for management of *chronic* CHF.
    - The initiation of ACEI therapy should be considered in the following situations:
    - In patients with CHF that requires hospitalization—after the initial stabilization (see treatment plans section)

- In DCM—at the first identification of the condition (even if asymptomatic)
- In canine mitral valve disease—there is no clear indication of benefit from early intervention, although many cardiologists prescribe an ACEI when there is definite evidence of left heart volume overload on radiographs; others wait until the onset of overt CHF
- In canine mitral valve disease complicated by systemic hypertension—antihypertensive therapy is also beneficial to the heart and should reduce MR volume

- *Adverse effects*—beware of hypotension and acute renal failure. These problems can be minimized by lowering the dosage of diuretic by 25–50% after initial diuresis has been completed, and/or beginning with a low dose (e.g. 0.25 mg/kg enalapril once daily) and increasing the dosage after a 2-week period. Serious electrolyte disturbances are less common, and anorexia is not important unless you are prescribing captopril.

▼ *Key Point* Angiotensin-converting enzyme inhibitors reduce clinical signs and prolong life in dogs with heart failure caused by dilated cardiomyopathy or chronic valvular disease.

- *Antiarrhythmic drugs* including beta blockers, calcium channel blockers, mexiletine, and sotalol are prescribed when necessary, such as in atrial fibrillation or in severe, recurrent ventricular tachycardia. A specific use of the calcium channel blocker diltiazem is in the treatment of CHF caused by hypertrophic cardiomyopathy in cats (see Chapter 66).
- *Sedation* may be indicated in CHF to reduce activity and anxiety and to allow further therapy to be administered with a minimum of stress.
  - Morphine sulfate is a relatively safe sedative for dogs with CHF, administered to dogs at 0.1 mg/kg, IM or SC. Morphine also decentralizes blood volume, probably by hepatic venoconstriction, and may partially relieve pulmonary edema. Morphine can release histamine, cause emesis (and bradycardia), and depress respiration.
  - If morphine is unavailable, acepromazine (0.025 mg/kg) can be mixed in a syringe with buprenorphine (Buprenix 0.01 mg/kg) or butorphanol (0.2–0.4 mg/kg butorphanol) and administered IM. Although less desirable than morphine, these combinations appear to be safe for most dogs, and the acepromazine (0.1 mg/kg IM) with butorphanol (0.25 mg/kg IM) mixture is preferred in cats.
- *Sodium-restricted diet* is recommended once substantial CHF has developed to minimize sodium retention by the kidney. Such restriction is inadvisable in asymptomatic heart disease because low sodium diets can activate the renin-angiotensin-aldosterone system. The addition of other factors such as fish oils to reduce the negative activity of cytokines are under investigation.
- *Nutriceuticals* often are considered in treatment of canine and feline dilated cardiomyopathy. These dietary supplements are thought to increase inotropic activity of the muscle in animals either deficient for these "micronutrient" compounds or those affected with L-carnitine transport disorders.
  - *Taurine*—Plasma taurine concentrations have been demonstrated to be reduced in some cases of DCM. Certain breeds appear to be "at risk" (cocker spaniels, small canine breeds, ± other canine breeds). Affected animals may respond to dietary supplementation with taurine; generally, 500 mg–1000 mg q12h for dogs) or taurine + L-carnitine. When suspected, taurine deficiency can be documented with blood or plasma samples, typically sent to the laboratories at the University of California, Davis.
  - *Levo-carnitine*—L-carnitine, which is needed for fatty acid transport across mitochondrial membrane, sometimes is recommended in the treatment of canine DCM. Doses ranging from 1 to 3 g PO q8–12h (or more) may be useful in some dogs with DCM, although it is difficult to determine which animals are deficient or which may benefit from supplementation. Some boxer dogs and some cocker spaniels with DCM have been reported to respond. Other cases have been less consistent. Assay of L-carnitine activity must be done in special metabolism laboratories (and myocardial levels can be low even when plasma concentrations are normal). Clients are advised to purchase this compound from health food stores to partially control the prohibitive cost of medical grade L-carnitine.
  - *Co-enzyme Q$_{10}$,*—There are *no* published data indicating efficacy after supplementation of this ubiquitous cellular coenzyme in spontaneous canine heart disease; thus, it is difficult to advocate its use at this time.
  - Use of the "nutriceuticals" is largely empiric unless a deficiency is documented.

Key questions to ask regarding cardiac drug or dietary therapy include:

- What kind of drug is this? What are the principal drug effects and mechanisms of action?
- What is the indication for the drug?
- What are nonindications or contraindications?
- How will the drug be administered? How will I determine the initial dose?
- Which co-therapy will be used?
- How will the drug be eliminated? Why might it accumulate? Are there any drug interactions?
- How do I know if I am prescribing enough (i.e., the correct dose)?
- How will I know if I am giving too much?

Other Treatments

- *Thoracocentesis* should be performed with the patient in sternal recumbency when there is a large pleural effusion leading to tachypnea or dyspnea.
- *Abdominocentesis* should only be done to relieve tense ascites, and most of the fluid volume should be left in the patient.
- *Pericardiocentesis* is the treatment of choice for stabilization of the patient with cardiac tamponade and CHF caused by pericardial effusion.

- *Oxygen therapy*—animals in severe congestive heart failure are placed at rest in an oxygen-enriched environment (40–60% O_2). If an oxygen cage or nasal oxygen is unavailable, a cool, well-ventilated area is chosen.
- *Ventilator therapy* is needed to prevent or treat respiratory arrest in some dogs. The work of breathing can be so great as to lead to respiratory muscle fatigue, progressive hypoxemia and hypercarbia, and sudden ventilatory failure (a common cause of death in CHF). Some cats with severe edema due to hypertrophic cardiomyopathy benefit from 4 to 8 hours of ventilatory support and then can be weaned.

Hospital Therapy of Congestive Heart Failure—Urgent Treatment Plans

A number of medical "treatment plans" have proven useful in the acute management of CHF. Medical therapy is appropriate initial management of virtually all causes of congestive heart failure unless the condition is pericardial effusion with tamponade (in which case the treatment is pericardiocentesis).

- Caveats:
  - Handle the patient gently.
  - Do not position the patient on its back for radiographs.
  - If you believe there is a large pleural effusion, perform thoracocentesis (even with a small needle to rule it out).
  - Provide oxygen by face mask, cage, or tent if the patient will tolerate it. If not, use the airflow of a fan to the face.
  - If marked anxiety or frantic behavior is evident, sedate the patient (see above).
  - Tabulate and trend important vital signs: temperature, respiratory rate and depth, breath sounds, heart rate, heart rhythm, membrane color and refill time, pulse strength, attitude, and noninvasive arterial blood pressure.

FON—Furosemide, Oxygen, and Nitroglycerin Ointment

- This form of therapy is applicable to most cases of CHF, regardless of cause, and is useful when the clinician suspects CHF but is uncertain of the underlying cause (e.g., dilated cardiomyopathy vs. chronic valvular heart disease; hypertrophic vs. restrictive cardiomyopathy).
- Diuresis is initiated, the tendency toward edema is decreased, and PO_2 is increased, promoting better tissue oxygenation.
- Record and trend vital signs (see Caveats).
- Most mild cases of CHF respond nicely to this treatment.
- After 24–48 hours of therapy, and after completion of the diagnostic workup, begin oral home therapy (see home therapy section).

FON-H—Furosemide, Oxygen, Nitroglycerin Ointment, and Oral Hydralazine

- This form of therapy is applicable to most cases of *severe* left-sided CHF in dogs with mitral valve disease.

Clinical markers include nasal frothing or hemoptysis, severe respiratory distress, lack of response to simple FON, or a "white-out" lung of fulminant pulmonary edema (careful: distinguish diffuse edema from pleural effusion, which is treated by thoracocentesis).

- Most of these dogs have normal ABP (especially after cage rest and FON) and can tolerate the afterload-reducing effects of hydralazine.
- Mitral regurgitant volume can be reduced significantly (by 50% in some cases), helping to lower left atrial and pulmonary venous pressures.
- First administer furosemide, oxygen, and nitroglycerin ointment. Allow the patient 15–30 minutes at rest to stabilize.
- Measure the ABP. Record and trend vital signs (see Caveats).
- Administer hydralazine. The dose of hydralazine can be titrated to clinical effect and ABP. The initial dose is approximately 1 mg/kg PO. The target systolic arterial blood pressure is 90 to 100 mm Hg. If after 3 hours, the ABP is still greater than 120 mm Hg and the dog is still dyspneic, administer another 0.5 to 1 mg/kg PO.
- Most dogs with severe pulmonary edema due to MR respond to this therapy.
- After 24 to 48 hours, FON-H can be stopped and chronic home therapy can be initiated (see home therapy section).
- *Note:* An alternative to FON-H is to substitute sodium nitroprusside for the nitrate ointment and hydralazine. Frequent ABP monitoring is required.

FON-D—Furosemide, Oxygen, Nitroglycerin Ointment, and Dobutamine

- This form of therapy is applicable to cases of cardiogenic shock (pulmonary edema or pleural effusion with hypotension), and other forms of CHF with low cardiac output. Dilated cardiomyopathy dogs (often Doberman pinschers) are typical.
- First administer furosemide, oxygen, and nitroglycerin ointment. Allow the patient 15–30 minutes at rest to stabilize, and prepare dobutamine solution.
- Prepare the dobutamine solution in 500 ml of 5% dextrose in water with 8 mEq of KCl added per 500 ml. Prepare a stock solution of dobutamine for dogs as follows:
  - Hang a bottle of 500 ml D5W, attach appropriate infusion set for accurate control, and flush the line.
  - Add KCl 8 mEq per 500 ml.
  - Add 250 mg of dobutamine to 500 ml of 5% dextrose solution (approximate concentration = 500 μg/ml).
  - Attach the infusion line to an infusion pump, and prime the line with dobutamine solution.

Use the following guide for a *5-μg/kg/min infusion rate.* Adjust the rate as needed.

- Place an IV; measure baseline variables of ABP, heart rate, rectal temperature, breath sounds, color, and refill time.

Weight (kg)	μg/min	μg Needed per Hour	ml of Fluid Per Hour* for a 5-μg/kg/min Infusion
10	50	3000	6
20	100	6000	12
30	150	9000	18
40	200	12,000	24
50	250	15,000	30
60	300	18,000	36

*Adjust as needed for 2.5-, 5-, 7.5-, or 10-μg/kg/min infusion.

- Attach an ECG monitor if available.
- Connect the infusion line to the patient and begin the infusion at 2.5 μg/kg/min; after 30 minutes, consider increasing to 5 μg/kg/min.
- Remeasure the clinical variables. Record and trend vital signs (see Caveats).
- Therapeutic effects of dobutamine include increased cardiac output, elevated ABP, increased tissue perfusion (better color and shorter refill time, stronger pulse), increasing body temperature, and improvement in attitude and strength. Adverse effects include increasing heart rate, excessive vasoconstriction, and induction of extrasystoles. Seizure activity is observed infrequently.
- If benefit is obtained, continue the infusion for 24 to 48 hours.
- Many dogs with cardiogenic shock respond to this therapy. Once ABP is greater than 90 mm Hg, oral therapy with enalapril (0.25 mg/kg bid) can be initiated (see later).
- Withhold digoxin for the first 24 hours unless there is atrial fibrillation, in which case initiate therapy with oral loading doses (see earlier).
- Avoid beta blockers during dobutamine therapy (agonist: antagonist)
- After 48 hours of therapy, reduce the dobutamine rate by 50% each 2 hours, then stop.
- If you cannot wean the patient from dobutamine, up the infusion rate and either increase the enalapril (to 0.5 mg/kg PO bid) or initiate hydralazine (0.5–1 mg/kg PO bid).
- After 24–72 hours of hospital therapy, and after completion of the diagnostic workup, begin oral home therapy (see home therapy section).

FON-T—Furosemide, Oxygen, Nitroglycerin Ointment, and Thoracocentesis

- This form of therapy is applicable to cases of CHF dominated by a large pleural effusion. Substantial pleural effusions often develop in dogs with DCM and atrial fibrillation.
- First, administer furosemide, oxygen, and nitroglycerin ointment.
- Administer a sedative if needed.
- Prepare needed materials (e.g., clippers, skin preparation materials, large syringes, 3-way stopcock, butterfly or needle or thoracocentesis catheter, sample tube for cytology ± extension tubing ± lidocaine with a syringe, with a 25-gauge needle for local infiltration).

- Place the patient in sternal recumbency with gentle restraint. Clip a suitable intercostal space, relatively ventral in location, perform a quick preparation, give a local block (optional), and perform thoracocentesis. If there is an inadequate response to unilateral centesis, repeat over the other hemithorax.
- If hypotension is present, consider starting dobutamine (see earlier).
- If DCM or restrictive CM are present and you are not using dobutamine, begin digoxin.
- Record and trend vital signs (see Caveats)
- After 24–48 hours of therapy, and following completion of the diagnostic workup, begin oral home therapy (see home therapy section).

FON-Dig—Furosemide, Oxygen, Nitroglycerin Ointment, and Digoxin

- This form of therapy is applicable to cases of CHF in which atrial fibrillation is present at admission. In general, Lanoxin or Cardoxin (brands of digoxin) are not indicated until the initial therapy of CHF has resulted in less tissue hypoxia. However, in the setting of atrial fibrillation, digoxin should be initiated to slow the ventricular rate response.
- First, administer furosemide, oxygen, and nitroglycerin ointment; perform thoracocentesis if indicated (see earlier).
- Record vital signs (see Caveats).
- Confirm the rhythm diagnosis with an ECG.
- Administer digoxin. Usual total daily dose for the dog is 0.01–0.015 mg/kg, with the daily dose divided q12h (0.005–0.0075 mg/kg q12h). When splitting pills, it may not be possible to give two equal doses (e.g. ½ of a 0.125-mg tablet in the AM and ¼ of a 0.125-mg tablet in the PM). An oral loading dose (twice the calculated maintenance dose for 2 to 3 treatments) is administered to patients in atrial fibrillation if the initial resting ventricular rate response exceeds 220/min with the dog at cage rest.
- After 24 hours, if there has been satisfactory control of CHF, add either a beta blocker or a calcium channel antagonist (diltiazem). Initial dose of propranolol is 0.2 mg/kg PO q8h; it can be increased in 0.1–0.2-mg/kg increments every day to a maximum dose of 0.6 mg/kg PO q8h. Alternative: diltiazem (Cardizem) 0.5 mg/kg PO q8h; daily dose can be increased in 0.25-mg/kg increments up to 1.25 mg/kg PO q8h.
- After 48–72 hours of hospital therapy, and after completion of the diagnostic workup, begin oral home therapy for CHF (see home therapy section).

FON-A—Furosemide, Oxygen, Nitroglycerin Ointment, and Antiarrhythmic Therapy for Ventricular Tachycardia (VT)

- This form of therapy is applicable to cases of CHF in which ventricular tachycardia—either sustained or recurrent—is present at admission. In general, positive inotropic drugs, including digoxin and dobutamine, are contraindicated in the setting of complex ventricular arrhythmias. If needed, the arrhythmia first must be controlled medically with an antiarrhythmic drug.
- First, administer furosemide, oxygen, and nitroglycerin ointment; perform thoracocentesis if indicated (see earlier).
- Record vital signs (see Caveats).
- Confirm the rhythm diagnosis with an ECG.
- Obtain blood for a serum potassium and possibly a serum magnesium.
- For sustained VT, administer lidocaine (2 mg/kg/min bolus; repeat up to 8 mg/kg total dose over 10 min); if successful, start constant rate infusion at 50–70 μg/kg/min. Avoid beta blockers and cimetidine (reduce hepatic clearance of lidocaine).
- Alternative to lidocaine—procainamide 2 mg/kg/min; up to 15 mg/kg cumulative dose over 30–40 min; use caution in CHF because ABP may fall. If effective, begin SC or IM procainamide (10–20 mg/kg, q6–8h) or IV infusion at 25–40 μg/kg/min.
- If this fails, consider magnesium infusion. First be certain you are not dealing with a bundle branch block, which can resemble VT. Magnesium is dosed using 20% MgCl$_2$ solution, which contains approximately 2 mEq of Mg^{++}/mL; the usual dosage is 0.75–1 mEq/kg/24h IV (50% of dose can be given in 2–4 hours if necessary).
- If this fails, consult a cardiologist.

Chronic Home Therapy of CHF

A variety of drugs are available to treat chronic CHF and diseases of the heart. Following are some typical treatment plans for common canine conditions. Treatment of CHF in cats is outlined elsewhere in this section (see Cardiomyopathy).

Chronic Mitral Valve Regurgitation

Chronic mitral valve disease often leads to left-sided CHF and left mainstem bronchial compression. A typical treatment plan includes dietary sodium restriction, a diuretic (furosemide), and an ACE inhibitor (e.g., enalapril). Digoxin is recommended by many cardiologists if there is no contraindication (moderate to severe azotemia or complex ventricular arrhythmia).

- In very advanced cases of left-sided CHF, in which pulmonary edema is becoming refractory to increasing diuretic doses, both enalapril and hydralazine (starting at 0.5–1.0 mg/kg q12h) are prescribed (with maintenance doses of furosemide and digoxin). One must monitor blood pressure when using combination vasodilator therapy. Amlodipine (0.05–0.1 mg/kg PO daily) is an alternative to hydralazine.
- Cough suppressants (hydrocodone) may be beneficial for coughing secondary to bronchial compression, but the clinician first should ensure that effective treatment of pulmonary edema has occurred.
- Ensure that the patient is not hypertensive (e.g., from chronic renal disease). If so, work to decrease the systolic ABP to less than 140 mm Hg or even lower (100–120 mm Hg range).

Chronic Right-Sided CHF

Predominant right-sided CHF can be related to chronic mitral valve regurgitation complicated by pulmonary hypertension and tricuspid regurgitation (common in slowly progressive mitral regurgitation); congenital heart disease (e.g., tricuspid valve malformation or pulmonary stenosis); primary right-sided cardiomyopathy (RV cardiomyopathy, silent atrium), or pulmonary hypertension (idiopathic, from *severe* chronic pulmonary disease, or from dirofilariasis). Although some dogs with DCM present with predominately right-sided CHF, most have biventricular failure (see later).

- Treatment of predominant right-sided CHF involves the following: rest (helps to mobilize ascites); thoracocentesis if indicated for a large pleural effusion, partial abdominocentesis to relieve a very tense ascites; stricter dietary sodium limitation (e.g., a low sodium prescription diet); digoxin if there is no contraindication, high-dose furosemide and low-dose enalapril (0.125–0.25 mg/kg q12h, initially with an eye to increasing the dose to 0.5 mg/kg PO q12h if systolic ABP is sustained at 90 mm Hg or greater).
- Vasodilators must be used carefully to prevent hypotension. If the CHF is isolated to the right side only (no left atrial enlargement as with congenital tricuspid valve malformation or primary right-sided myocardial disease), digoxin, furosemide, sodium restriction, and low-dose ACEI are initial treatments.
- Subcutaneous furosemide or alternating diuretics (hydrochlorothiazide-spironolactone) may be useful but should be monitored carefully with serum biochemistries and blood pressure determinations.

Dilated Cardiomyopathy

This disorder often presents with left-sided or biventricular CHF. After hospital stabilization, treatment includes daily digoxin, furosemide, enalapril, and dietary sodium restriction, supplemented with fish oils.

- Some dogs with substantial MR (and marked left atrial dilation) respond better to once or twice daily enalapril or lisinopril (0.25–0.5 mg/kg) plus twice-daily hydralazine or amlodipine.
- Antiarrhythmic drugs are often necessary for control of heart rate in atrial fibrillation (add diltiazem or a beta blocker) or for control of recurrent or complex ventricular tachycardia (procainamide, sotalol, or mexiletine).

- Some patients may respond to supplementation with taurine or L-carnitine (see Nutriceuticals). We recommend evaluating taurine concentrations in spaniel breeds, small dogs with DCM (not valvular disease), and boxer dogs with overt DCM, and in atypical breeds (e.g., golden retrievers with DCM). The use of carnitine is problematic, but one should discuss the pros and cons with owners for their decision.

Heartworm Disease

Treatment of heartworm disease that is complicated by right-sided CHF requires careful use of cardiac drugs. The patient first is stabilized with strict cage rest, furosemide, and dietary sodium restriction.

- A short anti-inflammatory dose of prednisolone (0.5–1.0 mg/kg daily in divided doses) may be helpful if there is active pulmonary parenchymal disease (evaluate radiograph) because reduction of infiltrate may improve ventilation-perfusion inequalities.
- The merits of aspirin (3–5 mg/kg q12h) to reduce pulmonary vascular reaction are debated, and it definitely should not be prescribed as co-therapy with prednisone or prednisolone.
- Oxygen therapy (24–48 h) also may reduce PA pressures by raising the alveolar pO_2, causing arterial vasodilatation.
- When these treatments (including parenteral furosemide) fail to control ascites, hydrochlorothiazide-spironolactone is added once daily and a cautious maintenance dose of digoxin is administered. Should this fail, enalapril 0.25 mg/kg—every day for 2 weeks, then twice daily thereafter—is tried.
- After 2 to 4 weeks of good quality stabilization, adulticide therapy is instituted with melarsomine using the two treatment phase approach.

FOLLOW-UP EVALUATION

The initial examination usually is scheduled about 1 week to 10 days after release from the hospital and should coincide with a trough level for measurement of digoxin concentration.

The Medical History

Question the owner about current medication (exact dosage and frequency) and response to medication and ask questions that might indicate the presence of drug toxicosis (e.g., appetite, emesis, depression, or weakness after vasodilator therapy). Politely but persistently ensure medication compliance. Ask owners to carry medications with them to ensure proper labeling and pill numbers.

- Ascertain activity level and exercise capacity.
- Question the owner about ability to sleep and rest without orthopnea, respiratory rate, and coughing.
- Confirm diet, treats, and fluid intake and availability.
- Ask about the general attitude of the patient and the owner's attitude toward the situation and their sense of the animal's overall well-being.

Examination

- Record heart and respiratory rate, temperature, and body weight (noting change since last visit).
- Carefully examine the patient, directing special emphasis to the heart rate and rhythm, arterial pulse, jugular venous pressure, mucous membranes, heart sounds, breath sounds and pattern of ventilation, liver size, abdominal girth and cavity, and hydration.

Diagnostic Studies

Consider obtaining the following studies (depending on the circumstances):

- Arterial blood pressure (to monitor vasodilator therapy and diuretic therapy); target systolic pressures should be between 90 and 120 mm Hg.
- Chest radiographic films (for assessment of heart and lungs, especially if the patient is coughing or tachypneic or if there is evidence of a pleural fluid line)
- Serum biochemistries (particularly BUN/creatinine, electrolytes, total protein, and albumin); deterioration in renal function may be related to excessive diuretic therapy or ACE inhibitor therapy.
- Serum digoxin/digitoxin concentration—if currently receiving this medication; this is the optimal method to screen for digitalis intoxication or inadequate dosage.
- ECG (for arrhythmias detected during auscultation, when changes are noted in the cardiac rhythm, for ECG evidence of drug toxicosis).

From these results, place the patient into a current functional class (mild, moderate, severe heart disease) and determine the trend of heart disease. Identify risks or complicating factors that might cause cardiac decompensation (see following section); correct these if possible.

Problems that Complicate CHF

Heart failure may worsen for a variety of reasons including:

- Progression of valvular disease or myocardial dysfunction with enhanced neurohormonal compensation
- Insufficient or inappropriate therapy for stage of disease
- Poor client compliance
- Inadequate follow-up
- Drugs exerting negative inotropic effects (beta blockers, calcium channel blockers, antiarrhythmic drugs)
- Development of atrial fibrillation or other sustained arrhythmias
- Rupture of a chorda tendinea
- Ruptured left atrium with cardiac tamponade (in dogs with severe mitral regurgitation)
- Excessive exercise
- Hyperthyroidism (usually iatrogenic in dogs)
- Anemia (increases cardiac workload)
- Infections—especially with fever (increases cardiac workload)

- Excessive sodium intake (e.g., ingestion of processed meats)
- Compulsive drinking
- Systemic hypertension (e.g., idiopathic or from chronic renal disease)
- Environmental stress (heat, high humidity)

Nonspecific Clinical Problems

The patient may become depressed, anorectic, or weak because of:

- Iatrogenic causes—excessive or inappropriate drug therapy causing hypotension, dehydration, renal failure
- Overt drug toxicosis (e.g., digitalis)
- Multiorgan failure, especially renal failure or liver disease
- Infections
- Arrhythmias
- Neoplasia
- Poor acceptance of dietary changes
- Changes in owner's attitudes/behavior
- Progression of CHF with pleural effusion

Prognosis

The *prognosis* of CHF depends on the cause, severity, and care received. Many dogs survive more than 1 year after the first signs of CHF. The prognosis for DCM always is more guarded, especially in Doberman pinscher dogs. Once CHF has progressed to severe ("functional class IV") failure, the outlook generally is guarded to poor, and a 3- to 9-month prognosis is typical.

- There are no critical studies that prospectively examine prognostic criteria across all groups. The multi-center enalapril (North America) and benazepril (Europe) studies clearly indicate improved survival and reduction of clinical signs in canine CHF caused by DCM or chronic valvular disease when an ACE inhibitor is added to background therapy of furosemide ± digoxin.
- Most clients can make decisions about timing euthanasia by considering their perception of clinical signs (coughing, difficulty of ventilation, exercise capacity); quality of life (interest, attitude, appetite); and medication and veterinary issues (adverse effects, compliance with care, cost of treatment, and evaluation).

SUPPLEMENTAL READINGS

Keene BW, Rush JE: Therapy of heart failure. In: Ettinger SJ, Feldman EC (eds): Textbook of Veterinary Internal Medicine. 4th ed. Philadelphia: WB Saunders, 1995, pp 867–892.

Knight DH: Pathophysiology of heart failure and clinical evaluation of cardiac function. In: Ettinger SJ, Feldman EC (eds): Textbook of Veterinary Internal Medicine. 4th ed. Philadelphia: WB Saunders, 1995, pp 844–867.

McCall D, Rahimtoola SH (eds): Heart Failure. New York: Chapman and Hall, 1995.

Sisson D: Evidence for or against the efficacy of afterload reducers for management of heart failure in dogs. Vet Clin North Am Small Anim Pract 21:945, 1991.

Woodfield JA, Bauer TG, Ettinger SJ, et al: Controlled clinical evaluation of enalapril in dogs with heart-failure: Results of the Cooperative Veterinary Enalapril Study Group. J Vet Intern Med 9:243, 1995.

Woodfield JA, Bauer TG, Rush JE, et al: Acute and short-term hemodynamic, echocardiographic, and clinical effects of enalapril maleate in dogs with naturally acquired heart-failure: Results of the Invasive Multicenter Prospective Veterinary Evaluation of Enalapril Study. J Vet Intern Med 9:234, 1995.

65 Valvular Heart Disease

John D. Bonagura / David Sisson

VALVE FUNCTION AND DYSFUNCTION

The Cardiac Valves

The heart contains four valves:

- The *mitral* or left atrioventricular (AV) valve
- The *tricuspid* or right AV valve
- The *aortic* or left semilunar valve
- The *pulmonic* or right semilunar valve

Structure

The semilunar valves consist of three individual leaflets that are closed during ventricular diastole and open during ventricular systole. The left and right AV valves consist of two major leaflets ("tricuspid" is a misnomer in dogs and cats), which are attached, via the chordae tendineae, to the papillary muscles (2 for the mitral, 3–5 for the tricuspid). The base of each AV valve is supported by a valve annulus that is well defined for the mitral and poorly defined for the tricuspid valve. The AV valves are open during diastole and closed during systole.

Normal Function

The heart valves serve as one-way passages for blood and prevent retrograde (regurgitant) flow. The cardiac valves open and close in a cyclical pattern that is dictated by changes in pressure within the cardiac chambers and great vessels. Competent cardiac valves permit the development of high ventricular pressures during systole and facilitate the maintenance of low ventricular pressure during diastole. Vibrations attending closure of the AV and semilunar valves are manifested as the first and second heart sounds and herald the onset of ventricular systole and ventricular diastole, respectively.

Valve Dysfunction

Cardiac valves may be dysfunctional as a consequence of developmental or acquired heart disease. General patterns of disease include:

- Obstruction to flow, termed *valvular stenosis*
- Incompetent closure allowing *valvular regurgitation* (= insufficiency)

Valvular stenosis is almost always a congenital abnormality in animals. Valvular regurgitation may result from congenital malformation or acquired diseases. Common anatomic and functional causes of AV valvular regurgitation are listed in Table 65–1.

▼ *Key Point* Because the AV valve consists of multiple anatomic components, disease of any portion of the apparatus, or geometric changes in the ventricle, can lead to AV valvular regurgitation.

Table 65–1. CAUSES OF ATRIOVENTRICULAR VALVULAR REGURGITATION*

Mitral valve dysplasia (MR)
Tricuspid valve dysplasia (TR)
Myxomatous valvular disease (endocardiosis causing MR, TR)
Bacterial endocarditis (MR)
Ruptured chordae tendineae (MR)
Avulsion of the papillary muscle (MR, TR)
Transmural myocardial infarction (MR)
Causes of ventricular or atrial dilation
    Patent ductus arteriosus (MR)
    Ventricular septal defect/endocardial cushion defect (MR, TR)†
    Atrial septal defect (TR)
    Aortic regurgitation (MR)
    Pulmonary regurgitation (must be severe to cause TR)
    Myocarditis—for example, parvovirus, Chagas disease (MR, TR)
    Dilated cardiomyopathy (MR, TR)
    Intermediate/restrictive cardiomyopathy (MR, TR)
    Atrial muscular dystrophy—"silent atrium" (TR)
    Right ventricular cardiomyopathy—RV dysplasia (TR)
    Hyperdynamic circulation—AV fistula, anemia, hyperthyroidism (MR, TR)
    Chronic bradyarrhythmia—for example, complete AV block (MR, TR)
    Pulmonary hypertension, including heartworm disease and chronic left-sided congestive heart failure (TR)
Causes of left ventricular hypertrophy (causing MR)
    Subaortic stenosis
    Hypertrophic cardiomyopathy
    Systemic hypertension—for example, chronic renal disease
    Hyperthyroidism
    Acromegaly
Causes of right ventricular hypertrophy (causing TR)
    Pulmonic stenosis
    Pulmonary hypertension
Cardiac arrhythmias preventing synchronous closure of AV valves—for example, ventricular premature beats

---

MR, mitral regurgitation; TR, tricuspid regurgitation.

*While this list is extensive, note that the most common causes of atrioventricular (AV) regurgitation are AV dysplasia, myxomatous degeneration, cardiomyopathy (any form), endocarditis, and hyperthyroidism (cats).

†May include mitral cleft or other AV valve malformation.

Cardiac Murmurs

The hallmark clinical finding in valvular heart disease is a cardiac murmur. Murmurs are produced by high velocity and turbulent blood flow across the valve as the blood moves from a higher to a lower pressure chamber or vessel. With few exceptions, the absence of a cardiac murmur virtually excludes the presence of clinically significant valvular disease (see Chap. 59).

- Semilunar valve stenosis or AV valve insufficiency can lead to systolic murmurs. Stenotic valves also may be incompetent, causing diastolic murmurs.
- Cardiac murmurs may *not* be evident in the following situations:
  - Trivial valve regurgitation or stenosis (Note, however, that trivial stenosis may be relevant in breeding soundness examinations—for example, in dogs with subaortic stenosis.)
  - Dynamic ventricular outflow tract obstruction in cats with hypertrophic cardiomyopathy or in dogs with subtle mitral valve malformation. Murmurs are often labile in this situation
  - Massive, "wide-open" AV valve regurgitation, in which the atrium and ventricle act as a common chamber and there is no pressure difference across the valve
  - Animals with very low cardiac outputs
  - Heart sounds muffled by lung sounds, pleural or pericardial fluid, or pneumothorax

VALVULAR DISEASES OF CLINICAL IMPORTANCE

Endocardiosis

Endocardiosis occurs primarily in dogs. It also is known as chronic "myxomatous" valvular heart disease or chronic mitral and tricuspid valvular fibrosis.

▼ *Key Point* Endocardiosis, a degenerative disorder, is the most important cause of heart disease in veterinary medicine.

Congenital Aortic Stenosis

This lesion usually is a *subvalvular* fibrous obstruction that may extend to the valves proper (see Chap. 70, for a discussion of congenital valvular disorders).

Congenital Pulmonic Stenosis

A variety of anatomic lesions may contribute to narrowing of the right ventricular outflow tract.

Congenital Mitral and Tricuspid Valve Dysplasia

Anomalies of the chordae tendineae, papillary muscles, or valve cusps can lead to incompetency of the valves and in some cases to stenosis, as well.

Infective (Bacterial) Endocarditis

This condition almost always involves the left-sided heart valves in dogs and cats. Destruction of valve tissue commonly results in valvular insufficiency, and large vegetation(s) may obstruct the valve less often.

AV Valvular Regurgitation Due to Cardiomegaly

Valvular regurgitation may develop secondary to *ventricular dilation or hypertrophy,* which in turn results from a variety of causes (see Table 65–1).

CHRONIC VALVULAR HEART DISEASE (ENDOCARDIOSIS) IN DOGS

Chronic valvular heart disease is a degenerative disorder of unknown cause affecting the subendocardial portions of the valve leaflets, primarily in middle-aged and older dogs. It is not a consequence of endocarditis, nor is it a sequela to oral disease or infection. The AV valves are principally involved, with the mitral valve affected in nearly 100% of cases, the tricuspid in 34%, and the aortic valve in 3% of cases.

Pathology

- The valve leaflets typically are thickened and distorted by nodular changes in the free edge and base of the valve. The valve surface glistens and the endocardium is intact, distinguishing this degenerative change from endocarditis.
- The chordae are thickened near the valve attachment, and *chordal stretch* or *rupture* may be observed.
- Focal subendocardial *myocardial fibrosis* may be evident, especially involving the papillary muscles.
- Secondary *dilation of the left atrium and ventricle* develops. Ventricular hypertrophy is of the eccentric type (with dilation of the ventricle), except when concurrent disorders (e.g., systemic hypertension from renal disease) stimulate the development of concentric hypertrophy (muscle wall thickening). The mitral valve annulus dilates as the ventricular dimensions increase.
- Endocardial sclerosis develops in the left atrium secondary to mechanical irritation from regurgitant streams of blood. These "jet lesions" consist of fibrous and elastic tissue and smooth muscle. Fresh or healed linear left atrial tears commonly are found at necropsy, but rupture of the left atrium with pericardial tamponade rarely is encountered.
- The right ventricle can be dilated because of concomitant tricuspid regurgitation or from pulmonary hypertension caused by chronic left ventricular failure.
- In some dogs, *arteriosclerosis* (hyalinization) of the small intramural myocardial arterioles is present. Adjacent to these diseased vessels are focal areas of myocardial necrosis and fibrosis.

Pathophysiology

Endocardiosis represents a progressive process and does not cause detectable signs during the period of early structural changes. Progressive valvular distortion leads to detectable valvular insufficiency; however, heart failure does not develop in all animals. The entire process can

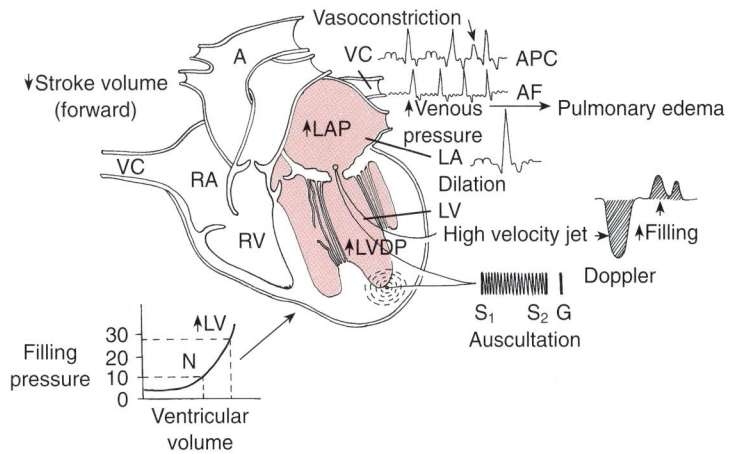

Figure 65–1. Diagrammatic representation of mitral regurgitation. Consult the text for an explanation of abbreviations and symbols.

take many years, although some breeds (e.g., Cavalier King Charles spaniel) are affected relatively early in life and may have a rapid progression to heart failure.

Mitral regurgitation (MR) can cause left ventricular volume overload and left heart failure and predispose to cardiac arrhythmias (Fig. 65–1).

▼ *Key Point* Mitral valve disease is the most important cause of heart murmurs and left-sided congestive heart failure (CHF) in mature dogs.

Mitral Regurgitant Volume

Total left ventricular (LV) stroke volume often is greatly increased, but a large proportion of LV output can be regurgitated into the left atrium. Therefore, the ability to eject blood in a forward direction is limited.

Left-Sided Cardiomegaly

Chronic mitral insufficiency increases left atrial (LA) volume and pressure, causing LA dilatation. The increased atrial pressure increases LV filling, causing ventricular diastolic volume overload. Eccentric hypertrophy with dilatation of the left ventricular chamber ensues.

Pulmonary Venous Hypertension

LA and pulmonary venous (PV) pressures increase for a number of reasons:

- Progressive MR increases LA pressure, initially during systole. If the regurgitant volume increases gradually, LA compliance increases, and the condition is well tolerated. This explains why many dogs have severe cardiomegaly but minimal clinical signs. If the regurgitant volume is very large, or if regurgitation develops suddenly (e.g., chordal rupture), the limits of atrial distensibility are exceeded and mean LA and PV pressures increase, leading to pulmonary edema.
- The dilated left ventricle may become stiffer than normal, offering increased resistance to filling. This results in higher LV diastolic pressure, which is transmitted to the left atrium and pulmonary veins.
- Reduced forward output may lead to retention of sodium and water by the kidneys (see Chap. 64).

Pulmonary Edema

Elevation of PV pressures can lead to elevated pulmonary capillary pressure and pulmonary edema. Clinical consequences include tachypnea, hypoxemia, coughing, and exercise intolerance.

Bronchial Compression

The left main-stem bronchus can become trapped between the pulsating aorta and the enlarging atrium. During systole, the bronchus is compressed by combined expansion of the aorta and the left atrium. As a result, exertional coughing and wheezing may occur even in the absence of lung edema.

Pulmonary Dysfunction

Chronic passive congestion of the lung causes ventilation perfusion inequalities (leading to hypoxemia) and, with chronicity, also can induce pulmonary fibrosis, which increases lung stiffness and the work of breathing.

Myocardial Failure

Chronic volume work by the left ventricle can cause biochemical and structural changes in the myocardium that lead to reduced LV contractility and cardiac muscle failure ("cardiomyopathy of overload"). This is especially likely in larger dogs. However, CHF often is manifest before substantial myocardial failure.

Low Cardiac Output

If forward stroke volume is inadequate, signs of low output (weakness, exertional or cough-related syncope, and prerenal azotemia) may develop. Low output signs are often the result of the concurrent development of pulmonary hypertension, tricuspid regurgitation, and right-sided CHF.

Right Ventricular (RV) Failure

Left heart failure with secondary pulmonary hypertension combines with tricuspid regurgitation to cause RV dilation. RV failure may ensue, as evidenced by hepatomegaly and ascites. Low output signs often are exacerbated by severe right-sided CHF; however, pulmonary edema may resolve spontaneously as blood flow to the left heart decreases.

Cardiac Arrhythmias

Arrhythmias are common and can further decrease cardiac output (see Chap. 62).

- Atrial arrhythmias are triggered by dilation of the atria. Atrial premature complexes (APCs) frequently are recorded on the electrocardiogram (ECG). Atrial tachycardia and atrial fibrillation are evident in some cases.
- Ventricular premature complexes (VPCs) develop in some dogs, but sustained ventricular tachycardia appears to be less common than in dogs with dilated cardiomyopathy.
- Iatrogenic arrhythmias (e.g., sinus bradycardia, AV block, APCs, and VPCs) may be precipitated by digitalis intoxication or diuretic-induced hypokalemia.

Ruptured Chordae Tendineae

This condition commonly is observed during echocardiographic examination of dogs with advanced MR. Depending on the location of the chordal rupture, the added hemodynamic burden may be reasonably well tolerated, or severe CHF may supervene.

Left Atrial Rupture

Rupture of the left atrium, although uncommon, can cause acute cardiac tamponade, cardiogenic shock, and sudden death.

▼ *Key Point* Rupture of the mitral valve chordae tendineae, the development of sustained atrial tachyarrhythmias, and LA rupture are important diagnostic considerations when rapid hemodynamic deterioration occurs in dogs with chronic MR. Appropriate therapeutic intervention can stabilize many of these patients, allowing sufficient time for further compensation.

Clinical Signs and Diagnosis

Signalment

Endocardiosis is most common in toy and small breeds of dogs (e.g., poodle, Yorkshire terrier, Cavalier King Charles spaniel, schnauzer, cocker spaniel). Some breeds, particularly the spaniels, German shepherds, and Afghan hounds, are prone to both valvular degeneration and dilated cardiomyopathy. Endocardiosis is an incidental finding in many aged dogs.

▼ *Key Point* Occasionally, CHF from primary valvular disease develops in large-breed dogs, but dilated cardiomyopathy is a more important cause of CHF in these dogs.

History

The presenting complaints typically are those attributable to bronchial compression, pulmonary congestion, or low cardiac output and include cough, tachypnea, tiring, and syncope. Weight loss is a frequent but subtle finding. Unless there are other metabolic problems, such as hyperadrenocorticism, few dogs with overt CHF are obese. The opposite is true in dogs with chronic respiratory disease. In general, the clinical signs gradually become more severe, reflecting the progressive nature of the disease. Syncope may be related to one or more of the following problems:

- Cough-syncope—fainting after vigorous coughing caused by decreased venous return or transient bradyarrhythmias.
- Paroxysmal atrial or ventricular tachyarrhythmias that may be induced by exercise or excitement.
- Orthostatic hypotension—sudden weakness after rising may be related to abnormal baroreceptor activity.
- Insufficient forward flow from severe MR or from pulmonary hypertension, typically observed at the onset of exercise or with excitement.
- Neurocardiogenic syncope represents another reason for exercise-induced syncope.
- Iatrogenic—hypotension secondary to diuretics, vasodilators, or angiotensin-converting enzyme inhibitors (ACEIs).

Physical Examination

Auscultation

As the disease progresses, the left apical systolic murmur of mitral insufficiency generally increases in intensity, and the duration increases from early systole to midsystole extending throughout systole (holosystolic). The murmur of MR radiates in the direction of the regurgitant jet, typically dorsal to the mitral valve on the left hemithorax, but usually to the right hemithorax as well. The intensity of the first heart sound also increases with worsening disease.

▼ *Key Point* A systolic murmur heard best over the (palpable) left apex almost always is caused by MR. The murmur may radiate widely.

- A short systolic murmur usually indicates early disease but also may be heard in dogs with peracute CHF. The murmur of MR usually evolves from a soft decrescendo to a loud holosystolic murmur over a period of months to years.
- Left apical midsystolic clicks often are detected in asymptomatic dogs and may be confused with a ventricular gallop. They may indicate chordal laxity and valve prolapse.
- A ventricular gallop (third heart sound) after the murmur of MR may be heard at the left apex in some dogs with CHF. This sound often resolves after successful therapy.
- Cardiac arrhythmias and pulse deficits may be detected.

Precordial Palpation

The point of the left apical impulse shifts caudoventrally as the left ventricle enlarges. A precordial thrill reflecting valvular incompetency may be palpable over the left apex or tricuspid valve area.

Arterial Pulse

The arterial pulse is variable and depends on forward stroke volume, cardiac rhythm, and current therapy. Heart rate typically is increased when CHF is evident.

▼ *Key Point* Pronounced sinus arrhythmia is atypical in dogs with untreated CHF caused by mitral valve disease but is common in patients with primary respiratory disease.

Pulmonary Auscultation

As lung congestion develops, ventilation and lung sounds become abnormal. Inspiratory crackles and cyanosis may be detectable. Wheezes, representing "cardiac asthma" from peribronchial edema (cuffing) or left main-stem bronchial compression may be noted. Pleural effusion may cause muffling of heart sounds.

Right-Sided CHF

If the right heart fails, jugular venous pressure and liver size increase. Ascites is typical of advanced right-sided CHF. Pleural effusion usually indicates biventricular CHF. Occasionally, a dog is presented with predominant signs of RV failure due to pulmonary hypertension and severe tricuspid regurgitation (TR). Consider heartworm disease, pericardial effusion, dilated cardiomyopathy, and atrial muscular dystrophy/myocarditis in the differential diagnosis.

▼ *Key Point* When there is pleural effusion and no venous distention, ascites, or atrial fibrillation, consider noncardiac causes for the effusion.

Imaging—Radiography and Echocardiography

(See also Chap. 60)

- Progressive cardiomegaly is detected with left-sided heart enlargement predominating. Cardiac widening and LA enlargement typically are the first abnormalities detected. A vertebral heart score (comparison of length and width of cardiac silhouette to the length of the fourth thoracic vertebra) >10.8 is good evidence of volume overload. As the disease progresses, LV elongation, left main-stem bronchial compression, and pulmonary venous distention are observed.
- Left-sided CHF causes radiographic abnormalities that include increased lung density (interstitial and alveolar infiltrates) in the perihilar lung zones. These infiltrates characteristically are dorsal and bilaterally symmetric. However, owing to differences in pulmonary lymphatic drainage, edema may be worse in the right caudal lobe. Pleural effusion and ascites are present with right-sided or biventricular failure and commonly occur in association with atrial fibrillation.
- Echocardiographic findings include cardiomegaly, thickened AV valves, and variable changes in LV shortening fraction. Valve prolapse may be observed. In many cases, ventricular contractility appears normal to increased because the LV ejects a large por-

tion of the total stroke volume backward into the low-resistance left atrium. The shortening fraction is rarely below the lower limits of normal reference values, helping to distinguish this condition from dilated cardiomyopathy. Ruptured chordae tendineae frequently are observed. Doppler studies can demonstrate mitral and tricuspid regurgitant flow and often Doppler evidence of pulmonary hypertension. Often, aortic regurgitation (that is silent to auscultation) is evident as well.

Electrocardiography

- The ECG can be normal and does not rule out a diagnosis of CHF due to endocardiosis. Heart rate and rhythm usually are normal until significant cardiomegaly or CHF develops.
- Arrhythmias become common as the disease progresses. Sinus tachycardia, supraventricular premature beats, paroxysmal or sustained atrial or supraventricular tachycardia, atrial fibrillation, and VPCs may be recorded (see Chap. 62).
- Cardiac enlargement often causes widening of the P wave (P mitrale) as well as increased amplitude. LV enlargement is suggested by increased voltages in leads II, III, and aV$_F$, widening of the QRS complex, and slurring or coving of the ST segment (see Chap. 62). Left axis deviation is uncommon.
- A tape-recorded, 24-hour ECG (Holter recording) or an event monitor ECG is helpful for evaluating dogs with syncope and for determining the need for and response to antiarrhythmic therapy.

Clinical Laboratory Tests

Laboratory changes that accompany advancing endocardiosis typically reflect the hemodynamic changes and renal responses that develop in dogs with CHF. Laboratory studies help to identify complications caused by extracardiac diseases (e.g., Cushing's disease, renal failure) and drug therapy (e.g., diuretics).

- Significant pulmonary edema or tissue hypoperfusion causes arterial hypoxemia (decreased PaO$_2$), and the associated increase in ventilatory effort can cause respiratory alkalosis.
- Mild to moderate increases in blood urea nitrogen (BUN), serum creatinine, and phosphorus are detected in many dogs with endocardiosis as a result of chronic renal disease, decreased cardiac output, or hypotensive drug therapy. Diuretic therapy prevents use of urine specific gravity as a measure of interstitial-tubular function.
- Poor hepatic perfusion and hepatic congestion may cause mild to moderate elevations of serum alanine aminotransferase (ALT) and aspartate aminotransferase (AST). Persistently elevated liver enzymes usually indicate a noncardiac disorder of the liver, particularly when such changes are marked.
- Serum electrolyte abnormalities are uncommon. Hyponatremia sometimes is detected in dogs with severe biventricular heart failure, especially in those with marked ascites and polydipsia, and is a poor prognostic sign.

- Hypochloremia and hypokalemia are usually iatrogenic as a result of diuretic therapy and anorexia.

Differential Diagnosis

The differential diagnosis of valvular heart disease includes the following:

Systolic Murmurs

For the systolic murmurs of MR or TR, consider the possibilities outlined in Table 65–1. The most important considerations in the diagnosis of MR and *left-sided CHF* are dilated cardiomyopathy and congenital AV valve malformations (especially in young to middle-aged large-breed dogs) and bacterial endocarditis.

- The typical age, breeds, and clinical presentation make the diagnosis of endocardiosis straightforward in most cases.
- The echocardiogram is useful for distinguishing endocardiosis from congenital valve malformation or dilated cardiomyopathy.
- Endocarditis is associated with other clinical findings. Physical, radiographic, and echocardiographic features of healed mitral endocarditis may be difficult to distinguish from myxomatous changes.

Respiratory Disease

Because of similar signs, respiratory disease and CHF can be difficult to distinguish.

- When signs of tachypnea, cough, and dyspnea are present, consider tracheal collapse (especially in toy breeds), primary bronchial collapse, chronic bronchitis, pulmonary fibrosis, and other primary pulmonary disorders (e.g., pneumonia, neoplasia, allergic pulmonary disease, heartworm disease, and noncardiac causes of pleural effusions).
- CHF is commonly misdiagnosed in patients with chronic respiratory disease because these dogs often have cough, shortness of breath, and pulmonary crackles (which can be misinterpreted as "wet lungs," as opposed to small airway dysfunction).
  - The heart often appears enlarged in respiratory disease owing to inadequate expansion of the thorax, pericardial fat, or cor pulmonale (right heart enlargement secondary to chronic lung disease).
- Seek to identify positive findings of heart disease, such as murmur, arrhythmias, abnormal ECG, cardiomegaly (vertebral heart score > 10.8) with left atrial enlargement, and radiographic signs of pulmonary venous hypertension and edema. Do not consider endocardiosis in the diagnosis unless the definitive murmur of MR is evident.
- If CHF is a possibility, consider a trial course of furosemide (2 mg/kg, q12h) for 5 to 7 days. Anticipate a good response in cases of left-sided CHF. Some patients with chronic lung disease also respond partially to diuretics (mechanism uncertain).
- Pulmonary crackles without a murmur, a history of untreated, chronic (> 6 months) cough, right heart enlargement, and marked sinus arrhythmia are more typical of chronic respiratory disease than of chronic

CHF. Thoracic radiography, airway cytology and culture, and bronchoscopy can usually establish the cause as respiratory.

Treatment

Use combination drug therapy in the management of heart failure and respiratory complications caused by chronic mitral valvular disease. Surgical replacement of a cardiac valve is rare in veterinary practice. Use medical therapy to control CHF, mitigate neurohormonal activation, reduce mitral regurgitant fraction, prolong life, and control clinical signs. Diuretics, ACE inhibitors, direct vasodilators, digoxin, pulmonary medications, and dietary measures may be prescribed at various times during the course of the disease. Although ventricular arrhythmias are not common in chronic valvular disease, atrial arrhythmias are a frequent complication and may require control. This is especially true of atrial fibrillation, which must be managed with digoxin combined with either a beta blocker or calcium channel blocker (see Chap. 62). The clinical pharmacology of these cardiac medications is reviewed in Chap. 63 in this section. Specific management strategies for the hospital and home treatment of heart failure are summarized in Chap. 64 in this section. The following is a summary of general therapeutic approaches.

The Asymptomatic Dog

- The ideal approach to the management of the asymptomatic dog has not been determined. Clinical trials currently are evaluating potential benefits of ACE inhibitors (enalapril, benazepril) or neutral endopeptidase inhibitors on the progression of heart disease.
- Some clinicians withhold all therapy until there are objective signs of CHF. Others prefer to prescribe an ACE inhibitor, empirically, if there is evidence of significant cardiomegaly (e.g., a vertebral heart score exceeding 10.8) or when progression of cardiomegaly is clearly evident on serial radiographs (taken every 3–6 months). Most clinicians choose enalapril (0.5 mg per kg PO once daily) for empirical treatment.
- There is no evidence that early enforcement of a sodium-restricted diet is of benefit; in fact, current data suggest that this practice may be harmful because rigid salt restriction activates the renin-angiotensin-aldosterone system.

Coughing in the Dog with Mitral Regurgitation

- A harsh cough is often the initial clinical sign of advanced MR.
  - Coughing is a frequent complication of left bronchial compression, a condition that often precedes the onset of overt pulmonary edema. This form of the "cardiac cough" is similar to that caused by primary airway diseases, including tracheal collapse and chronic bronchitis.
  - Often there is no clear-cut clinical or radiographic evidence of pulmonary edema in the dog with a mitral murmur and cough. Many dogs exercise

well (except for an exertional cough) and sleep comfortably without tachypnea. It is unlikely that these dogs have overt CHF unless transient bouts of pulmonary edema develop with exertion.

- The best therapeutic approach to bronchial compression is unresolved.
  - One approach is prescription of an ACE inhibitor, possibly combined with a once-a-day diuretic. Such therapy can decrease cardiac size and blood pressure, which in turn may decrease regurgitant fraction. This therapy also is likely to mitigate transient, exercise-induced pulmonary edema and to delay the onset of CHF.
  - If the cough continues, medications effective for primary airway disease may be helpful. This can include a cough suppressant (butorphanol 0.55 mg/kg PO q8–12h, or hydrocodone 0.22 mg/kg PO, q8–12h) and possibly a brief course of prednisolone (0.5 mg/kg daily for 5–7 days) to reduce inflammation. An empiric course of a theophylline salt can be tried (10–20 mg/kg of a sustained release preparation, PO, q12h). This should be discontinued if a clear response is not evident within 2 weeks.

Hospital Treatment of Left-Sided CHF

- Once CHF has developed, the initial course of management is based on the severity of clinical signs of pulmonary edema. Initial therapy generally includes cage rest, oxygen if required, and furosemide (2–4 mg/kg, q6–q12h, IV or IM). Some clinicians also add nitroglycerin paste (½ to 1½ inches cutaneously q8–12h) as a venodilator. Others administer aminophylline (10 mg/kg q8h) if there is a concern about bronchospasm. The efficacy of bronchodilators has not been established, and they may induce tachycardia or anxiety in some dogs.
- Life-threatening pulmonary edema requires more aggressive treatment (see Chap. 64). In addition to oxygen and high-dose IV furosemide, consider treatment with a direct arterial vasodilator, hydralazine (1–2 mg/kg PO), or IV administration of sodium nitroprusside (1–5 μg/kg/min).
  - The dose of these vasodilators should be titrated to a systolic arterial blood pressure of 85–95 mm of mercury. Aggressive afterload reduction significantly decreases the mitral regurgitant fraction. Such therapy is especially important in cases of peracute regurgitation caused by ruptured mitral valve chordae tendinea.
- Some patients in severe CHF exhibit marked anxiety and air hunger. Treatment with morphine may be useful if it does not induce vomiting (morphine: 0.1 mg/kg: administer 25% IM; administer the balance SC 15 minutes later). Alternatively, consider subcutaneous administration of acepromazine (0.025 mg/kg) mixed with buprenorphine (0.005 mg/kg).

Home Therapy of Left-Sided CHF

- Chronic therapy of heart failure caused by mitral valvular disease includes a maintenance dose of furosemide (2–6 mg/kg q8–24h), an ACE inhibitor

such as enalapril or benazepril (0.5 mg/kg PO q12–24h), and dietary sodium restriction. Titrate the daily doses of furosemide and the ACE inhibitor to clinical signs, objective measures of fluid accumulation, arterial blood pressure (to maintain a systolic pressure of 90–120 mm Hg), and renal function. Reduce dosages if hypotension or progressive azotemia develops.

- Digoxin also is prescribed by many cardiologists. Use an initial conservative dose (0.005 mg/kg q12h), and adjust based on serum digoxin concentrations (target is 0.8–1.2 ng/ml at a 10–12 hour trough). The use of digoxin in dogs with sinus rhythm always has been controversial in this disease; however, we usually prescribe digoxin when there is objective evidence of CHF and provided there are no contraindications (such as moderate to severe azotemia, complex ventricular ectopia).
  - Atrial fibrillation or frequent atrial ectopics represent clear indications for digitalization. Once CHF is controlled and digoxin has been initiated, co-therapy with a beta blocker or diltiazem may be required to attain better rate control (see Chap. 62).

▼ *Key Point* Combination therapy is preferred in the management of CHF. Monotherapy with a diuretic or a diuretic and sodium-restricted diet is no longer considered appropriate treatment for most dogs because volume depletion activates the renin-angiotensin-aldosterone system.

- Treat progressive or refractory pulmonary edema first by optimizing current therapy. Should q12h ACE inhibitor therapy and q8h doses of furosemide fail to control this problem, consider either another vasodilator or a second diuretic.
  - Combination therapy with an ACE inhibitor and hydralazine (0.5–1 mg/kg PO q12h) or amlodipine (0.05–0.1 mg/kg PO q24h daily) can more effectively reduce mitral regurgitant fraction. Such treatments are best initiated in the hospital, where arterial blood pressure can be monitored frequently. Most dogs can tolerate a systolic blood pressure as low as 80–85 mm Hg without overt clinical signs of hypotension.
  - An alternative approach is the addition of another diuretic, which is described in a following section.

Other Respiratory Complications in Advanced MR

- It is not uncommon for a nonresponsive cough to persist in animals with otherwise-controlled CHF. Bronchial compression or intercurrent airway disease may be the culprit in many of these cases. Provided there is no radiographic evidence of pulmonary edema, it is reasonable to continue the current cardiac medications and to add a cough suppressant, such as hydrocodone or butorphanol, or even a brief course of prednisolone, to control the cough.
- In other dogs, signs develop that suggest accelerated pulmonary fibrosis, perhaps from recurrent pulmonary congestion.

- These dogs have exercise intolerance, some may faint, and some are persistently tachypneic but generally sleep well without any resting dyspnea.
- Auscultation reveals diffuse inspiratory crackles that might be easily confused with those caused by pulmonary edema. There is often hypoxemia. Radiography indicates "clear" lung fields or minimal interstitial density despite marked cardiomegaly. Many of these dogs have Doppler evidence of pulmonary hypertension.
  - Do not overinterpret the crackles as evidence of edema because increasing the drug doses is not likely to improve the respiratory signs and may predispose the animal to syncope by reducing blood pressure.
- Other reasons for persistent respiratory signs in dogs with MR include tracheal collapse, chronic bronchitis, pulmonary neoplasia, pneumonia, and recurrent pulmonary thromboembolism. Pleural effusions—both of cardiac and noncardiac etiologies—also can lead to respiratory distress. These problems are discussed elsewhere in this section of cardiopulmonary disorders.

Treatment of Right-Sided Congestive Heart Failure

- Right-sided CHF with ascites or biventricular CHF with pleural effusion is more likely to occur in dogs in which pulmonary hypertension, tricuspid regurgitation, atrial fibrillation, or some combination of these problems develops. Pulmonary hypertension occurs consequent to chronic elevation in left atrial pressure or secondary to pulmonary vascular narrowing (that accompanies chronic MR or develops independently from primary lung disease).
- When right-sided CHF dominates the clinical picture, it is not uncommon to notice a reduction of dyspnea and an increase in exercise intolerance. The magnitude of ascites and prominence of the jugular venous pulse can be dramatic. Radiography often demonstrates minimal pulmonary edema, whereas Doppler echocardiography may show signs of pulmonary hypertension, such as high-velocity tricuspid regurgitation.
- Management of dogs with a prominent component of right-sided CHF includes treatment with an ACE inhibitor (q12h), digoxin (to achieve therapeutic concentrations), furosemide (q8h), and a restricted sodium diet. Should these methods fail, then consider other strategies. Initially, the dog may be hospitalized, treated with subcutaneous furosemide (or other loop diuretic), and receive judicious paracentesis for tense ascites (removing between ¼ to ½ of the fluid accumulation). Treat atrial fibrillation if present. Two or 3 days of enforced cage rest and parenteral diuretic therapy may alleviate most of the retained fluid. At that point, treatment strategies can include any (or all) or the following:
  - Markedly increasing the oral dose of furosemide to effect (because poor absorption of the medication may be partially responsible for the refractory ascites).
  - Using flexible subcutaneous diuretic dosing (having the client substitute a subcutaneous dose of furosemide for the usual oral dose). This is scheduled on some regular basis (e.g., every Monday, Wednesday, and Friday).
  - Adding spironolactone (2 mg/kg PO q12h) or another potassium-sparing diuretic to the regimen.
  - Adding hydrochlorothiazide and spironolactone (2–4 mg/kg PO q12h of the combined product) to the regimen. This approach is especially aggressive because sodium reabsorption is blocked at sequential points along the nephron. Accordingly, the potential for volume depletion and electrolyte disturbances is high and must be monitored carefully (reevaluate the patient, blood pressure, and serum biochemistries at 3 days, 7 days, and 14 days after starting this treatment).
- Pleural effusion in valvular heart disease is generally a poor prognostic sign. Assuming it is not secondary to a malignancy, treatment of pleural effusion is as discussed previously for progressive ascites. Periodic thoracocentesis may be required.

Patient Follow-Up

Follow-up examinations and complications are described elsewhere in this section (see Chap. 64).

Prognosis

The prognosis for longevity is variable. Dogs with heart murmurs but without clinical signs of heart disease may survive for many years and often succumb from a noncardiac disorder. Clinical signs associated with bronchial compression indicate that sufficient volume overload has developed to compress the airways, but this alone is not an indication of CHF. Once *overt* pulmonary edema or ascites develops, the prognosis for life becomes guarded. Assuming initial stabilization is successful, a survival range of between 3 months and 2 years should be discussed with the client. With good veterinary and home care, most dogs live for 9 to 12 months before spontaneous death or euthanasia. Treatment with an ACE inhibitor prolongs life and reduces clinical signs responsible for hospital visits. This is especially likely if "full" doses are used (e.g., 0.5 mg/kg q12h of enalapril or benazepril).

INFECTIVE (BACTERIAL) ENDOCARDITIS

Bacterial endocarditis (BE) is an infection of the valvular or mural endocardium. The mitral and aortic valves are the most common sites of cardiac infection in dogs and cats. Establishment of a cardiac infection requires a portal of bacterial entry into the circulation, subsequent bacteremia, and colonization of the endocardium. Because of the nature of the injury and the host's response to infection, a multisystemic disorder often develops. Acute and chronic forms of BE are recognized in dogs and cats.

Etiology

- A diverse group of pathogenic bacteria have been identified in dogs and cats with endocarditis, including streptococci, staphylococci, corynebacteria, *Escherichia coli*, *Enterobacter aerogenes*, and *Pseudomonas*, *Pasteurella*, *Erysipelothrix*, and *Bartonella* spp. Many of these bacteria are normal inhabitants of the skin, oral cavity, and respiratory and intestinal tracts.
- Bacteria can gain access to the circulation via external wounds, established infections, and a variety of surgical procedures and invasive medical interventions; however, in many cases, there is no evidence of these sources. Endocarditis also may be a sequela to septic arthritis, osteomyelitis, infected catheters, and other infections.
- Immunosuppressive drugs (e.g., corticosteroids, anticancer chemotherapy) also predispose to infection.
- Injudicious use of antibiotics may predispose to infection by resistant or virulent organisms.

Pathogenesis

- The pathogenesis of infective endocarditis involves entry of bacteria into the circulation and invasion of the valve endocardium by direct extension from the bloodstream.
  - Virulent bacteria may attach themselves to the valve surface and aggressively ulcerate the endocardium and invade the valve stroma.
  - Previously diseased valves are believed to be more susceptible, particularly when the endocardium is disrupted. Dogs with subaortic stenosis are at increased risk for endocarditis, presumably because of jet lesions on the aortic valve. Conversely, in dogs with endocardiosis, in which the endocardium usually is not eroded, BE rarely develops.
  - Some forms of endocarditis are associated with high titers of agglutinating antibodies that cause clumping of bacteria, thereby increasing the size of the infectious inoculum.
- Collagen is exposed when microorganisms colonize and ulcerate the endocardium, causing platelet aggregation and the local accumulation of fibrin.
  - Vegetations resembling thrombi form on the valve surface. These vary in color from yellowish red to gray and are covered by a thin layer of clotted blood.
  - Lesions usually are localized to the valve but can extend to the mural endocardium, chordae tendineae (causing rupture), or sinuses of Valsalva (this may hasten the spread of septic foci via the coronary arteries to the myocardium).
- Chronic valvular infections are established when layers of fibrin are deposited repeatedly at the site of infection, "protecting" the bacterial colonies from host responses and from many antibacterial agents.
- Deformation of the valve usually results in *valvular insufficiency*. Exuberant vegetation may form in such a way as to produce valve stenosis, but this is less common.
- Parts of the vegetation may break off, seeding the various tributaries of the systemic circulation, including the coronary arteries.
- Intermittent bacteremia causes persistent or recurrent fever.
- Thromboemboli, which can be septic or "bland" (aseptic), are shed from the infected valve.
- Formation of immune complexes is an important host response; these may be filtered into the joints, kidneys, or other tissues, attract complement and leukocytes, and cause inflammation in these tissues.

Pathophysiology

The clinical signs of infective endocarditis result from cardiac injury, bacteremia and sepsis, thromboembolic complications, and immune-mediated processes (Fig. 65–2).

Cardiac Injury

A variety of cardiac manifestations are possible, including:

- Mitral and aortic valvular insufficiency
- Valvular stenosis (less common)
- Coronary occlusion with myocardial infarction
- Secondary myocardial invasion, causing myocarditis or myocardial abscessation
- Pericarditis
- Left-sided CHF (from valvular injury)
- Arrhythmia
  - Arrhythmias may be related to endomyocarditis, "toxemia," or extension of aortic root abscesses into the conduction system, causing AV block.

Bacteremia and Metastatic Infection

- Bacteremia causes fever, shivering, malaise, and anorexia.
- Other tissues may be seeded, resulting in brain abscesses, splenitis, osteomyelitis, septic arthritis, pyelonephritis, or other remote infections.
- In advanced cases, it is difficult to distinguish a primary infection (portal of entry) from a metastatic infection.
- Bacteremia and sepsis may be associated with disseminated intravascular coagulopathy (DIC) and lead to death from septic shock or organ failure.

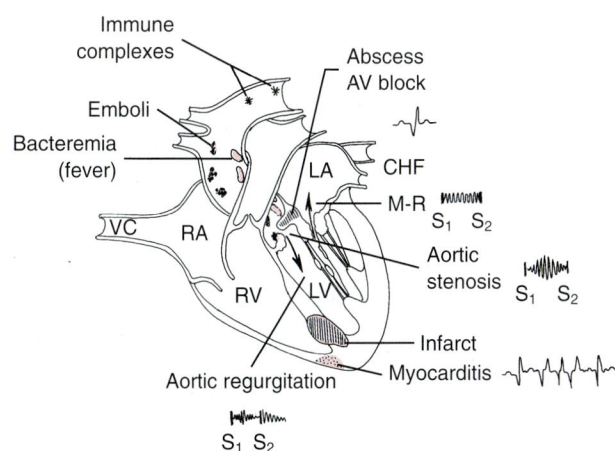

Figure 65–2. Diagrammatic representation of endocarditis. Consult the text for an explanation of abbreviations and symbols.

Immune-Mediated Disease

Immune complexes may form and be trapped in many organs or tissues, with the following effects:

- The kidneys, leading to glomerulonephritis
- The brain and meninges, causing meningoencephalitis
- The joints, causing polyarthritis
- The skeletal muscles, causing myositis and myalgia
- The small blood vessels, leading to vasculitis, thrombosis, hemorrhages, or disseminated coagulopathy
- The eye, leading to chorioretinitis

▼ *Key Point* Do not confuse the clinical findings seen in endocarditis of recurrent fever, multisystemic involvement, polyarthritis, and disseminated intravascular coagulation (DIC) with those of primary immunologic or neoplastic diseases; such an assumption may prompt inappropriate therapy with corticosteroids.

Thromboembolic Complications

Septic or bland (sterile) thrombi derived from the vegetation may be carried to distant tissues. Consequences include:

- Myocardial infarction and myocarditis
- Renal infarcts, abscess, pyelonephritis, and glomerulonephritis
- Stroke, meningitis, and encephalitis
- Bone infarcts and osteomyelitis
- Vascular obstruction including aortic-iliac occlusion
- Splenic infarcts
- Intestinal ischemia

Because of the low incidence of right-sided endocarditis in small animals, pulmonary embolism and pneumonia are rare. The notable exceptions are BE secondary to infection from patent ductus arteriosus surgery, and infection of a transvenous pacing lead.

Clinical Signs and Diagnosis

Signalment

Endocarditis is more common in certain large-breed male dogs (e.g., German shepherds) and in dogs with congenital subaortic stenosis.

History

- The history may suggest previous or concurrent infection (especially of the skin, oral cavity, gut, bone, or urogenital tract).
- Certain diagnostic and therapeutic procedures predispose to BE by causing bacteremia (e.g., endoscopy, colonoscopy, dental extractions).
- Persistent use of corticosteroids or antineoplastic drugs or improper use of antibiotics may predispose to BE.

Physical Examination

Physical examination findings may include:

- Antibiotic-responsive fever, depression, anorexia, and shaking "chills."
- Polyarthritis (shifting lameness) with or without joint effusion and myalgia.
- Signs of vasculitis with hemorrhages (skin, eye, mucous membranes).
- Multifocal neurological deficits from meningitis or encephalitis.
- Signs of cardiac injury:
  - A cardiac murmur, particularly a "new" or changing murmur, often is detected.
  - BE destroys portions of the valve; therefore, regurgitant murmurs (MR, aortic regurgitation) usually are present in dogs and cats with BE. A systolic ejection murmur often accompanies the diastolic murmur of aortic insufficiency due to increased LV stroke volume. Large vegetation(s) on the valves also may contribute to valve stenosis murmurs.
  - The pulse pressure increases with aortic insufficiency, which causes hyperkinetic femoral pulses with rapid run-off of diastolic pressure. Always consider BE when aortic regurgitation, which is uncommon in mature animals, is present.
  - Signs of overt left-sided CHF or arrhythmias (especially ventricular premature complexes) may develop from cardiac injury.

Laboratory Studies

Complete Blood Count (CBC)

Mild anemia and leukocytosis with neutrophilia and monocytosis may be present; red blood cell (RBC) fragments may suggest vasculitis (see Chap. 69) or DIC.

Serum Biochemistries

These may reflect organ injury from infection, thrombosis, infarction, or poor perfusion from heart failure.

Autoimmunity Tests

Tests such as lupus erythematosus (LE) preparation and antinuclear antibody (ANA) assays can be positive in patients with BE.

Blood Cultures

Two or more positive blood cultures, obtained from a patient with compatible clinical signs, strongly suggest BE.

- Cultures are most rewarding if taken near febrile bouts when the animal is not receiving antibiotics. Cultures may be positive before, during, or after bouts of fever.
- Serial positive blood samples, taken 1 to 2 hours apart from different sites, help to rule out the possibility of skin contamination. (Aseptically prepare the skin before obtaining the sample.)
- Transfer sufficient blood (5–10 ml) into special broth media tubes (usual blood:medium ratio of 1:10). Aerobic and anaerobic culture and sensitivity are indicated. Special antibiotic adsorbing media are available for patients who have received antibiotic therapy. Some microorganisms are difficult to culture (e.g., *Bartonella* spp.).

- Consider culturing the catheter tip in patients suspected of being infected by an IV catheter.

Urinalysis

Hematuria, proteinuria, pyuria, or casts may be shown if pyelonephritis or glomerulitis is present. Culture the urine if there are any abnormalities, but do not automatically assume that organisms cultured from urine are responsible for the cardiac infection.

Cardiac Studies

Cardiac studies may substantiate the diagnosis and indicate the degree of cardiac injury. Serial studies after successful therapy are useful.

- Radiographs may indicate cardiomegaly, valve calcification (from chronic BE), CHF, or (rarely) embolic pneumonia.
- Electrocardiograms can be normal, but they may indicate chamber enlargement or arrhythmias (most often ventricular premature contractions).
  - ST-T changes, indicating ischemia or infarction, may be present (check precordial leads for these).
  - AV block in endocarditis likely indicates aortic valve involvement with a perivalvular inflammation affecting the bundle of His.
- Echocardiography is useful, especially for prognosis.
  - Routine 2-D or M-mode echocardiography may demonstrate a vegetation (oscillating thrombus) and signs of hemodynamic overload (cardiomegaly). A negative examination result does not rule out BE.
  - However, echocardiography cannot always differentiate mitral BE from advanced mitral endocardiosis.
  - Doppler studies can document both abnormal valvular regurgitation and stenosis.
- Progressive cardiomegaly demonstrated by echocardiography or radiography indicates clinically significant valvular injury and regurgitation and a poor prognosis.

Other Studies

Other studies may be abnormal depending on the organ involved. *Cerebrospinal fluid (CSF)* and *joint fluid* cytology and culture may show evidence of septic or aseptic (immune complex) suppurative inflammation.

Treatment

Consider the following principles:

- Use bactericidal antibiotics. Because the bacteria are sequestered within the vegetation, normal defense and healing processes (e.g., granulation) are impeded.
- Because the drug must penetrate fibrin, do not use most sulfa drugs.
- Long-term (2–3 months) therapy is needed to ensure sterilization of the vegetation.

- Ideally, use IV therapy to obtain the highest possible plasma concentrations (this is sometimes impractical).
- Guide antibiotic therapy by monitoring blood cultures. It is appropriate to delay therapy for 2 to 4 hours while blood cultures are being obtained, unless the patient is demonstrating signs of septic shock.
- Empirical therapy for BE often includes the following drugs:
  - Penicillins (high doses) are safe and useful for streptococcal infections.
  - Aminoglycosides, combined with a synthetic penicillin or cephalosporin, provide wider antimicrobial coverage. Use of these drugs requires good patient hydration and careful monitoring for nephrotoxicity.
  - A patient with renal failure may be treated with a newer-generation cephalosporin (e.g., moxalactam) in lieu of an aminoglycoside.
- Treat for at least 4 weeks (at least 10–14 days when using an aminoglycoside, with continuation of the penicillin or cephalosporin for the full 4 weeks). Some cardiologists recommend treatment for 6–8 weeks. Repeat blood cultures following discontinuation of therapy or if fever should recur.
- If left-sided CHF develops, treat according to guidelines in Chapter 64. Vasodilator therapy is contraindicated for dogs with septic shock.
- Use prophylactic antibiotics if the patient undergoes any procedure that may cause bacteremia. (The general subject of prophylactic therapy of BE is unresolved, and no firm recommendations can be made.)

Prognosis

The prognosis is guarded.

- Acute, ulcerative BE may cause dramatic clinical signs but, if promptly treated, may leave only mild cardiac dysfunction.
- Chronic BE with severe valvular destruction is more difficult to treat because severe CHF may develop.
- Echocardiographic evidence of diffuse, large vegetative lesions and documentation of volume overload imply a poor prognosis. The likelihood of CHF is high in these instances.

SUPPLEMENTAL READING

Beardow AW, Buchanan JW: Chronic mitral valve disease in Cavalier King Charles spaniels: 95 cases (1987–1991). J Am Vet Med Assoc 203:1023, 1993.

Buchanan JW, Bucheler J: Vertebral scale system to measure canine heart size in radiographs. J Am Vet Med Assoc 206:194, 1995.

Elwood CM, Cobb MA, Stepien RL: Clinical and echocardiographic findings in 10 dogs with vegetative bacterial-endocarditis. J Small Anim Pract 34:420, 1993.

Woodfield JA, Sisson D: Infective endocarditis. In: Ettinger SJ (ed): Textbook of Veterinary Internal Medicine, 3rd ed. Philadelphia: WB Saunders, 1989, pp 1151–1162.

66 Cardiomyopathy

John D. Bonagura / Linda B. Lehmkuhl

DEFINITIONS

- The ventricles react to increases in volume and pressure by myocardial dilatation and hypertrophy. These responses commonly are observed with valvular heart disease, cardiac shunts, thyrotoxicosis, chronic anemia, and arterial hypertension.
- Myocardial failure can develop secondary to increased workload, a process termed the *cardiomyopathy of overload*.
- Chronic tachyarrhythmias, especially ventricular tachycardia, can lead to a reversible loss of myocardial contractility.
- "Cardiomyopathy" usually pertains to a myocardial disease that cannot be explained by congenital or acquired cardiac or coronary artery lesions. When myocardial disease develops secondary to a systemic disorder, the term "secondary cardiomyopathy" sometimes is used.
- Cardiomyopathies often are classified by the postmortem anatomic appearance of the left ventricle (LV) and by the echocardiographic features of the ventricular anatomy and function. For a classification of myocardial disorders, see Table 66–1.

Dilated Cardiomyopathy

- *Dilated (congestive) cardiomyopathy* (DCM) is characterized by dilatation of all cardiac chambers, decreased myocardial contractility, and decreased LV ejection fraction (EF), an index of left ventricular systolic function

  (EF = stroke volume divided by end-diastolic volume)

  DCM is recognized in many species, particularly the dog and, to a lesser degree, the cat and ferret.
  DCM may be the end result of diverse processes that affect myocardial cell function, including deficiency of metabolic substrates (e.g., taurine, L-carnitine, selenium); myocarditis with necrosis of myocytes (e.g., parvovirus infection); global myocardial ischemia; or toxic injury to myocytes (e.g., doxorubicin, monensin) (see Table 66–1).
  Many cases of DCM in the dog are considered to be idiopathic or genetic predispositions.

- *Hypertrophic cardiomyopathy* (HCM) occurs primarily in cats and is characterized by *idiopathic* left ventricular observed hypertrophy. Ventricular hypertrophy decreases ventricular relaxation and compliance, causing ventricular dysfunction primarily during diastole. When HCM occurs in dogs, it may lead to sudden cardiac death.

  The LV ejection fraction is usually high. The hypertrophy may be symmetric (LV wall = LV septal thickness), asymmetric (interventricular septum to LV > 1.3:1), or localized to areas of the LV free wall or interventricular septum (IVS).

  Hypertrophic obstructive cardiomyopathy describes the situation of myocardial hypertrophy associated with dynamic (i.e., not fixed) left ventricular outflow obstruction. Midsystolic pressure gradients develop in the left ventricular outflow tract (between the IVS and the anterior mitral leaflet), causing dynamic subaortic stenosis.

  Although LV anatomy may appear similar, established causes of LV hypertrophy (e.g., aortic stenosis, systemic hypertension, and hyperthyroidism) should not be designated HCM. These conditions are managed differently and demonstrate a different natural history.

Restrictive Cardiomyopathy

- *Restrictive cardiomyopathy* (RCM, also called "intermediate" cardiomyopathy or endomyocardial fibrosis) is a poorly defined condition affecting the cat. The LV is characterized by (1) variable degrees of dilation and hypertrophy with mild-to-moderate depression of EF ("intermediate" between HCM and DCM) and (2) multifocal or diffuse myocardial fibrosis (thought to restrict ventricular filling; hence, "restrictive"). There almost always is marked left atrial dilation because the left atrium must empty into a restricted, noncompliant LV.

Myocarditis

- *Myocarditis* is inflammation of the myocardium. There are many potential causes of myocarditis (see Table 66–1).

  Idiopathic nonsuppurative myocarditis also may accompany the various forms of cardiomyopathy (CM) previously described.

Table 66–1. CAUSES OF CARDIOMYOPATHY (CM)

Disorder*	Feline	Canine
Myocarditis		
Noninfective	Idiopathic Thymoma (immune-mediated)	Idiopathic Boxer dog† English bulldog Trauma
Infective	Toxoplasmosis Feline infectious peritonitis?	Bacterial Parvovirus Distemper virus Systemic mycoses Lyme carditis *(Borrelia)* Chagas disease *(Trypanosoma cruzi)*

Dilated CM (DCM) (also see infective
and noninfective myocarditis because
DCM can develop secondary to
severe inflammatory disease)
	Taurine deficiency
	Idiopathic
	Potassium iodide toxicity
	Hyperthyroidism
	Sustained ventricular or supraventricular
	tachycardia
	Chronic hypokalemia (causes taurine
	deficiency?)
		Idiopathic†
		Carnitine deficiency
		Breed-"specific" DCM†
		  Doberman pinscher
		  Boxer dog
		  Cocker spaniel
		  "Giant" purebred dogs
		  Springer spaniel muscular dystrophy
		Doxorubicin toxicity
		Global ischemia?

Hypertrophic CM Left ventricular concentric hypertrophy	Idiopathic† (familial?) Acromegaly (rare) Hypertension† Hyperthyroidism†	Idiopathic
Restrictive-intermediate CM	Idiopathic*	
Cardiotoxicity	Sodium iodide	Catecholamines Brain-heart syndrome Doxorubicin *Digitalis purpurea* (foxglove) and *Strophanthus* spp. Toad *(Bufo)* toxicity Chocolate toxicity

*Both primary (idiopathic) and secondary causes of cardiomyopathy are considered here.
†Most important types.

Potential sequelae of myocarditis include myocardial fibrosis, decreased myocyte contractility, and DCM.

▼ **Key Point** Cardiomyopathies can cause congestive heart failure (CHF), cardiac arrhythmias, sudden death, and systemic arterial embolism (in cats). Effective therapy of cardiomyopathy requires an accurate morphologic diagnosis.

See Table 66–2.

HYPERTROPHIC CARDIOMYOPATHY IN THE CAT

Etiology

- The cause of HCM (Fig. 66–1) is unknown. A genetic basis is strongly suspected in cats, which is similar to humans.

Pathology

- Left ventricular concentric hypertrophy is found and includes the papillary muscles and the IVS and results

in decreased LV chamber volume. Hypertrophy is either symmetric, asymmetric, or localized. Focal areas of LV myocardial fibrosis are common.
- In older cats, a localized hypertrophy of the subaortic ventricular septum often is observed.
- A dilated and hypertrophied left atrium (LA) may be seen.

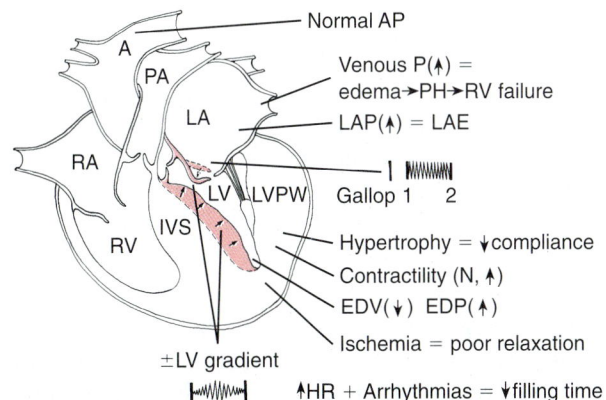

Figure 66–1. Diagrammatic representation of hypertrophic cardiomyopathy. Explanation of the abbreviations can be found in the text.

Table 66–2. DIFFERENTIAL DIAGNOSIS OF FELINE CARDIOMYOPATHY AND HEART FAILURE*

Other Causes of Dyspnea/Tachypnea
Airway obstruction
  Nasopharyngeal polyp
  Laryngeal paresis
  Tracheal or esophageal foreign body, neoplasm, granuloma, abscess
  Mediastinal masses
    Lymphosarcoma or thymoma
Primary bronchopulmonary disease
  Bronchial asthma/bronchitis
  Lungworms and lung flukes
  Pneumonia (viral, bacterial, fungal, toxoplasmic)
  Neoplasia
  Aspiration
Pulmonary vascular disease/embolism
  Heartworms/spontaneous worm death
Noncardiogenic pulmonary edema
  Electrocution
  Trauma (shock lung)
  Anaphylaxis
Trauma
  Diaphragmatic hernia
  Pulmonary hemorrhage/edema
  Pneumothorax
  Hemothorax
Pleural effusion
  Pyothorax
  Hemothorax
  Feline infectious peritonitis (FIP)
  Lymphosarcoma-associated effusion
  Chylothorax
Hyperthermia/fever
Anemia
Methemoglobinemia
  Acetaminophen toxicity
  Cetacaine
Abnormal ventilatory pattern
  Metabolic acidosis
  Central nervous system disease

Other Causes of Acute Lameness/Paresis/Gait Abnormality
Musculoskeletal pain or injury
Bite wounds
Hypokalemia (weakness)
Peripheral neuropathy
  Related to diabetes mellitus

Spinal cord disease
  Injury
  Neoplasia
  FIP infection
  Extradural mass/granuloma
Urinary obstruction
  Causing abdominal pain and reluctance to move

Other Causes of Cardiac Murmurs/Gallops/Arrhythmias/ Cardiomegaly
Congenital heart disease
  Especially septal defects and mitral valve dysplasia
Congenital peritoneopericardial-diaphragmatic hernia
Bacterial endocarditis
Pericarditis
  FIP infection
  Idiopathic
  Bacterial
  Neoplastic
    Lymphosarcoma
    Mesothelioma
Cardiac neoplasia
  Lymphosarcoma
Cor pulmonale
  Heartworms
  Severe chronic respiratory disease
Chronic degenerative valvular disease (mitral, aortic)?
Dilation of the aortic root with aortic regurgitation
Cardiac arrhythmias (primary electrical disturbances)
  Chronic bradyarrhythmias
    Atrioventricular block in aged cats
  Tachyarrhythmias and premature complexes
  Sedatives, tranquilizers, anesthetic drugs
Chronic or severe anemia
Hyperthyroidism
Acromegaly
Systemic hypertension
  Chronic renal disease
  Hyperthyroidism
  Idiopathic
Electrolyte abnormalities
  Hyperkalemia
    Urinary obstruction
  Hypokalemia
    Renal disease

*The most common clinical presentations of feline cardiomyopathy are dyspnea from congestive heart failure, rear-limb paresis from aortic thromboembolism, and inactivity. The veterinarian often detects a murmur, gallop rhythm, arrhythmia, or cardiomegaly during examination.

- There may be evidence of thrombosis, such as a left atrial mural thrombus or systemic arterial thromboembolism—usually lodged in the terminal aorta.
- Pulmonary edema and pleural effusion due to CHF are frequent findings.
- Intramural coronary artery sclerosis, myocyte disarray, and interstitial fibrosis are commonly observed histologic lesions in the LV.
- Occasionally there is enlargement of the right ventricle (RV) secondary to pulmonary hypertension.

Pathophysiology

- The hypertrophic LV is less distensible (decreased compliance), and the hypertrophied myocardium may not relax normally (decreased lusitropy). Papillary muscle hypertrophy further encroaches on the LV lumen. These abnormalities result in a decreased LV end-diastolic volume (EDV) and high ventricular filling pressures.
  - Cardiac output (CO) can be maintained by increased sympathetic activity, vigorous ventricular contraction, high LV ejection fraction, and increased heart rate (HR); however, these responses can be deleterious (see subsequent discussion).
  - Anesthetics may precipitate LV failure.
- LV filling requires higher than normal venous and atrial pressures, causing the LA to dilate. This predisposes the cat to elevated pulmonary venous pressure and to pulmonary edema.
  - Affected cats can be poorly tolerant of infusions of crystalloid and of blood.
  - Diuretic drugs, such as furosemide, are highly effective in decreasing venous pressure and treating pulmonary edema, but excessive diuresis can decrease the ventricular preload and cardiac output.

- A vigorous atrial contraction (atrial "kick") from LA hypertrophy assists LV filling and helps maintain CO. Loss of LA contraction due to development of atrial fibrillation (AF)—a potential complication of severe atrial dilation—can be disastrous.
- Mitral regurgitation (MR) develops in many cats because of the geometric changes in the ventricle, the altered papillary muscle support, or the abnormal anterior mitral leaflet movement during midsystole (see subsequent discussion). Large regurgitant volumes increase left atrial pressure (LAP) further.
- Tachycardia caused by stress (e.g., hospitalization), pain (e.g., due to aortic thrombus), arrhythmias (e.g., atrial fibrillation), or drugs (e.g., ketamine HCl) is poorly tolerated. Even sinus tachycardia does the following:
  - Shortens ventricular filling and coronary artery perfusion times while increasing the myocardial oxygen consumption
  - Promotes myocardial ischemia or limits oxygen delivery, which further impairs myocardial relaxation and LV compliance
- In cases of "obstructive" cardiomyopathy, intraventricular pressure gradients develop during systole. This finding is associated with movement of the anterior mitral leaflet toward the ventricular septum (systolic anterior motion of the mitral valve) and with mitral-septal contact.
  - Mitral regurgitation develops.
  - Increased LV pressure contributes to further subendocardial ischemia.
  - Reducing systolic anterior motion can decrease mitral regurgitation (see the discussion of therapy for HCM).
- Chronic increases of LA and pulmonary venous pressures can lead to pulmonary hypertension, right ventricular overload, and biventricular CHF with pleural effusion.
- Hemodynamic abnormalities include high pulmonary capillary wedge pressures, elevated LV end-diastolic pressure, and a prominent left atrial "a" wave. Pulmonary hypertension may be present, especially in cats with CHF. Intraventricular systolic gradients can be measured in hypertrophic "obstructive" CM.

Clinical Signs

Signalment

- Mean age is 6 to 9 years, with a wide range of 6 months to 13 years. Male cats are affected more commonly. Persian cats, Maine coon cats, and ragdoll cats are among the breeds genetically predisposed to HCM. HCM may be more common in urban areas.

History

- The cat may or may not be symptomatic.
  - Most affected cats seem normal, and HCM is identified during the course of a routine physical examination and auscultation.
  - Nonspecific signs of disease include anorexia, depression, inactivity, and reluctance to move.
  - Respiratory distress or tachypnea commonly is observed and is caused by pulmonary edema or

pleural effusion. Cough is unusual in cats with CM. Some cats vomit or retch, but the mechanism is unknown.
- Thromboemboli can cause paralysis, especially of the rear limbs and, less often, the right forelimb. The cat may present to the veterinarian because of relentless crying secondary to pain from an aortic embolism.
- Syncope is observed infrequently but can occur.
- Most owners do not notice significant premonitory signs of CHF because of the fastidious nature of the cat. Cats can appear normal until they undergo some stressful event.

Physical Examination

- Arterial pulse (AP) is normal unless there is an aortic embolus or a cardiac arrhythmia. Arterial blood pressure is normal.
- Jugular venous pressure/pulses may be elevated if there is pulmonary hypertension (PH) or biventricular CHF.
- Cardiac auscultation is often abnormal.
  Mitral regurgitation is evident in many cats as a systolic murmur heard best over the left apex/left sternal border. The left apical impulse is typically strong.
  A murmur due to ventricular outflow obstruction is thought to be uncommon; however, mitral septal contact predisposes to mitral regurgitation. This murmur can be quite labile and may disappear if the cat is calm and the heart rate is relatively slow.
  An atrial gallop (S_4), due to reduced ventricular relaxation, is common.
  Sinus rhythm or sinus tachycardia is typical. Premature atrial or ventricular complexes or AF may be detected infrequently.
- Respiratory distress, sternal recumbency, open-mouth breathing, and cyanosis are potential signs of CHF. Auscultation of pulmonary crackles and wheezes suggests pulmonary edema due to left-sided CHF. Pleural effusion, subsequent to biventricular failure, is indicated by muffled heart and breath sounds and dull thoracic percussion ventrally.
- Clinical signs of aortic embolism may be detected (see subsequent discussion).
- Hepatomegaly is likely if there is biventricular CHF. The kidneys may be painful or "pitted" on palpation if current or prior renal thromboembolization has occurred.

Diagnosis

- A presumptive diagnosis of HCM is made by recognizing signs of heart disease from history and physical examination, by identifying left-sided cardiomegaly from radiography or electrocardiogram (ECG), and by ruling out other known causes of LV hypertrophy, such as the following disorders:
  - *Hyperthyroidism* is common in cats older than 7 years (see subsequent discussion of hyperthyroid heart disease in this chapter).

- *Systemic hypertension* is particularly common in cats with chronic renal disease but also may be idiopathic. This is an important diagnosis to rule out. Although hypertensive heart disease does not cause heart failure or thromboembolic complications, it can lead to serious ocular, neurologic, or renal injury. Hypertension is discussed elsewhere in this section (see Chap. 69).
- Rule out *acromegaly* in cats with diabetes mellitus or facial deformity (see Chap. 34).
- Consider *congenital aortic stenosis* or *mitral dysplasia* in young cats or in cats with a long history of cardiac murmur.
- Echocardiography is required for definitive diagnosis.

Radiography

- Concentric LV hypertrophy and secondary left auricular dilation with shifting of the apex to the midline cause a typical "valentine"-shaped cardiac silhouette on the ventrodorsal view in many cases (see Chap. 60). Elongation of the heart shadow is also typical.
- Radiographic signs of left-sided heart failure include pulmonary venous dilation, pulmonary edema, and pulmonary arterial (PA) enlargement, with or without pleural effusion. Although classic cardiogenic perihilar infiltrates may be present, diffuse or dependent pulmonary edema is not uncommon.

▼ **Key Point** The radiographic features of the different forms of feline cardiomyopathy overlap; thus, a definitive anatomic diagnosis of HCM is not possible from survey radiograph films.

Echocardiography

- Two-dimensional (2-D) echocardiography is the method of choice for the noninvasive diagnosis of HCM and other forms of cardiomyopathy. Anatomic abnormalities can be identified, including increased wall thickness, mitral septal contact, and increased left atrial size. Ventricular shortening fraction and EF are usually greater than normal. Small pericardial effusions are common.
- Doppler studies can document valvular regurgitation, left ventricular outflow obstruction, and diastolic dysfunction.

Electrocardiography

- Sinus rhythm or sinus tachycardia is typical, but premature complexes and atrial arrhythmias, including AF, occasionally are observed. Ventricular pre-excitation also has been reported.
- Increased P-wave amplitude (> 0.25 mV) or duration (> 0.035 sec) suggests left atrial enlargement (LAE).
- Left axis deviation secondary to LV hypertrophy or left anterior fascicular block is characteristic of HCM and perhaps related to lesions in the left bundle branch. A normal axis with increased voltage of R waves in leads II and aV_F (> 0.7 mV) is another common abnormality that suggests LV hypertrophy.

Laboratory Abnormalities

- Laboratory abnormalities encountered in cats with HCM are quite variable but may include the following:
  - Azotemia secondary to CHF, aortic thrombosis, renal embolization, or dehydration.
  - Serum skeletal muscle enzyme levels, such as creatine kinase and aspartate aminotransferase (AST), are elevated in cats with aortic thrombosis. Elevated levels of alanine aminotransferase (ALT) are also common with thrombosis, and these may reflect leakage from hepatocellular injury or a skeletal muscle isoenzyme.
  - Laboratory abnormalities compatible with disseminated intravascular coagulation (DIC) are common in cats with thrombosis.
  - Pleural effusion is typically a modified transudate. Sometimes a chylous effusion is present.

Treatment

Drugs Used in the Management of Feline Hypertrophic Cardiomyopathy

Treatment of cats with HCM may include various combinations of furosemide, calcium channel blockers, beta-adrenergic blockers, angiotensin-converting enzyme (ACE) inhibitors, and drugs that impair coagulation. There are no large, sufficiently controlled studies to indicate a superior treatment for asymptomatic disease, for recurrent bouts of CHF, or for thromboembolic episodes. Prevention of arterial thromboembolism is a persistent problem. Following is a discussion of the relevant clinical pharmacology of these drugs as it pertains to feline HCM.

Beta Blockers

Propranolol (2.5–7.5 mg, PO q8h) or atenolol (12.5 mg qd or q12h) is used most often to block the adverse effects of sympathetic stimulation of the heart. Once-daily atenolol (can begin with 6.25 mg daily for the first week then increase to 12.5 mg q12–24h) often controls heart rate (HR) in cats at less than 150 bpm for almost 24 hours, although pharmacokinetic studies suggest that twice-daily treatment may be better.

- Beta blockers prevent sinus tachycardia and prolong diastole, increasing time for both coronary perfusion and ventricular filling. Myocardial oxygen demand is reduced through decreases in heart rate, contractility, and blood pressure.
- Beta blockade is especially helpful for reducing dynamic left ventricular outflow obstruction (gradients). The murmur of mitral regurgitation—when caused by dynamic systolic anterior motion of the valve—may partially abate with beta blockade.
- The net effect of beta blockade on diastolic function in cats with HCM is unknown. The direct effect on myocardial relaxation is unfavorable; however, indirect effects, such as reduced myocardial oxygen demand, decreases in intraventricular gradients, and prolongation of diastole, also should benefit diastolic function.

- Adverse effects in cats include severe sinus bradycardia (examination HR < 100 beats/min), depression, and precipitation of CHF in cats with reduced myocardial contractility or those dependent on heart rate for cardiac output. Bronchospasm is a risk, especially in cats with chronic airway disease.
- Owing to the nonspecific blocking effects of propranolol, do not use in cats with uncontrolled pulmonary edema or in cats with arterial thromboembolism until collateral circulation has been restored.

Diltiazem

The calcium channel antagonist diltiazem is a popular drug for chronic management of HCM. Calcium channel blockers are thought to improve left ventricular relaxation. The precise mechanism for this benefit has not been elucidated. Indirect effects, by reducing blood pressure and reflexively increasing sympathetic tone, could be involved. Alternatively, myocardial perfusion may increase with diltiazem because the drug is a coronary vasodilator and also can decrease resting heart rate (although in most cats, HR is reduced far less effectively than with a beta blocker).

- Overall, diltiazem should reduce myocardial oxygen demand by decreasing heart rate, contractility, and blood pressure.
- Effects on reducing dynamic outflow tract gradients have been disappointing at the doses commonly used.
- Although the chronic administration of diltiazem has been reported to decrease LV hypertrophy in cats with *very severe* HCM, we have not been impressed with consistent regression, especially in mild to moderate cases of HCM, even after prolonged therapy with diltiazem.
- Overall, we prefer diltiazem when a cat has *already experienced* CHF or when a cat has moderate to severe LV hypertrophy and left atrial dilation as demonstrated by echocardiography.
- Diltiazem is also reasonable therapy for the cat with HCM and concurrent atrial fibrillation.
- Preparations of diltiazem vary and include: (1) diltiazem (30-mg tablet; ¼ tablet PO q8h); (2) Dilacor XR brand of diltiazem (open the 240 mg Dilacor capsule to reveal 4 60-mg tablets that can be split in half with a pill cutter to yield 8 30-mg pellets; the dose is 30 mg q12–24h); or (3) Cardizem CD (120-, 180-, 240-mg capsules; compounded to provide 30 mg q24h).
- Anorexia, skin reactions and erythema/edema have been observed in some cats receiving this drug. Depression, weakness, and hypotension may indicate sinus bradycardia, AV block, or arterial vasodilation from too high a dose or sensitivity to the drug (e.g., in older cats with inherent AV conduction disease).
- A *combination* of atenolol and diltiazem may be considered in cats with HCM and dynamic LV outflow tract obstruction (30 mg Dilacor in PM; 6.25–12.5 mg atenolol in AM); however, monitor heart rate and blood pressure with this combination therapy because of the combined effect of these drugs on heart rate, contractility, and blood pressure.

Furosemide

Furosemide—administered by a parenteral route—is the treatment of choice for cats with pulmonary edema (1–2 mg/kg IV, IM, or SC q8–12h for 24–48 hrs).

- Oral therapy is prescribed for home care of cats that have experienced pulmonary edema; however, the maintenance dosage often is titrated down to a relatively low 1–2 mg/kg every second to third day. This can be accomplished over a period of 2 to 3 weeks. In many cases, furosemide can be discontinued completely. Conversely, doses of 2 mg/kg, q8–12h, or higher, may be needed to treat progressive pulmonary edema or pleural effusion.
- Dietary sodium restriction can be combined with furosemide, but many cats will not eat a new diet.
- Azotemia, hypokalemia, and hyponatremia are very common in cats taking furosemide on a daily basis. Mild to moderate azotemia (e.g., BUN 30–90 mg/dl) is not necessarily an indication to alter furosemide therapy in a cat with persistent fluid accumulation because the edema is likely to worsen if furosemide is decreased. In contrast, reduce the dose of furosemide in the cat with azotemia and a completely "clear" chest cavity to prevent unneeded volume contraction.

Angiotensin-Converting Enzyme (ACE) Inhibitors

Consider ACE inhibitors such as enalapril (Enacard) and benazepril (Lotensin) for recurrent or progressive pulmonary edema or pleural effusions.

- An initial dosage of 0.25 to 0.5 mg/kg q24h is usually well tolerated. If necessary, the dosage can be increased over a 2- to 4-week period to 0.5 mg/kg q12h, provided hypotension and moderate to severe azotemia are avoided.
- Whether ACE inhibitors reduce myocardial hypertrophy in this disease is unknown, but clinically these drugs seem to benefit the fluid accumulation of CHF.

Nitroglycerin

Nitroglycerin ointment (1/4″ topically once or twice daily) can be used for hospital management of CHF and also can be prescribed for home use, particularly if the cat experiences bouts of dyspnea or if the client has trouble medicating their pet.

Digoxin

Digoxin is used in cats with HCM very infrequently, and there are no data supporting use of cardiac glycosides in this disease. The principle indications for digoxin in feline HCM are atrial fibrillation (along with diltiazem or a beta blocker) or progressive left ventricular systolic failure and cardiac dilation seen on echocardiography. These problems are occasional consequences of long-standing feline HCM.

- Digoxin is eliminated by renal mechanisms and the elimination $T_{1/2}$ is very long, even in healthy cats (often 2–3 days).

- Digitalize cats at a dose of ¼ of a 0.125 mg Lanoxin tablet every 48 hours. Measure a serum digoxin concentration about 14 days later with the blood sample drawn 10–12h after treatment.
- A trough serum concentration between 1 and 2 ng/ml is the therapeutic goal.

Anticoagulant Drug Therapy

Anticoagulant drug therapy is discussed in the Complications of Feline Cardiomyopathy section.

Specific Treatment Plans for Feline Hypertrophic Cardiomyopathy

Asymptomatic Cats

There are no data that indicate any substantial benefits of therapy in asymptomatic cats with HCM. However, with marked left ventricular hypertrophy, especially with concurrent left atrial dilation, there must be a concern for the presence of substantial diastolic dysfunction or mitral regurgitation. These cats are at greater risk for CHF or arterial thromboembolism.

- More problematic are cats with asymptomatic or mild HCM (diastolic wall diameter between 6 and 7.5 mm) and with normal left atrial size. These cats could go untreated because many show little progression of disease at follow-up. However, because it is difficult to predict what will happen to an individual cat, empiric therapy frequently is offered.
- A previously asymptomatic cat may feel worse on therapy (especially with high doses of diltiazem). Occasionally, owners remark that a cat with HCM seems more active when treated with a beta blocker or diltiazem. Whether this is a placebo effect or a real benefit has not been studied.
- Thus, in the asymptomatic cat, consider prescribing no therapy, a beta-adrenergic blocker, or diltiazem.
  - We prescribe atenolol for cats with mild to moderate HCM, especially if there is evidence of moderate to severe left ventricular outflow tract (LVOT) obstruction.
  - We prefer to use diltiazem in cats with moderate to severe left atrial enlargement or with severe LV hypertrophy (e.g., LV wall > 8–9 mm). If there is also substantial LVOT obstruction, we add atenolol (6.25–12.5 mg daily) after 2 weeks of treatment with Dilacor (30 mg per day).
- Anticoagulant therapy also may be recommended.
- Repeat thoracic radiographs every 6 to 12 months. Repeat echocardiogram in 3 months and 9 to 12 months after initial diagnosis. Thereafter, evaluate the stable cat every 6 to 12 months. In many cases, the disease is quite static, and there is little justification for excessive reevaluation after 1 year follow-up.

Cats with Congestive Heart Failure

Management of Acute Heart Failure. Initial efforts are directed at improving tissue hypoxia, relieving stress, and reducing the venous and pulmonary capillary pressures.

- Perform thoracocentesis if there is a large pleural effusion. Place the cat at rest, give oxygen (40–50%) by cage oxygenator, and sedate if necessary (butorphanol, 002 mg/kg, mixed with acepromazine, 0.05 to 0.1 mg/kg, subcutaneously; beware of hypothermia).
- Administer furosemide (2–4 mg/kg IV, IM) until diuresis occurs, and then reduce the dose (to 1 mg/kg q8–12h).
- Administer nitroglycerin (2%) ointment (¼″, applied cutaneously, q12h) also when there is moderate-to-severe pulmonary edema.
- Administer parenteral furosemide, oxygen, and nitroglycerin for 24 to 48 hours. Subsequently, stop oxygen and nitrate paste, and lower the dosage of furosemide and titrate to the severity of pulmonary edema or pleural effusion.
- Hypokalemia and prerenal azotemia develop in many cats during this intense therapy. Mild cases need not be treated, but if the cat refuses to eat and drink after 24 to 36 hours of therapy, administer judicious fluid therapy (e.g. 20 ml/kg/day) and potassium supplementation (IV or oral).

Management of Chronic Congestive Heart Failure

- Prescribe furosemide, diltiazem, and a treatment to prevent thromboemboli.
- Should furosemide dosage requirement exceed more than 1 mg/kg daily, add enalapril at an initial dose of 0.25 mg/kg q24h for 2 weeks, with an intent to increase the dose to 0.5 mg/kg q24h if blood pressure, renal function, and serum electrolytes remain at reasonable levels.
- Perform periodic reevaluation (at 1 week, 4 weeks, and then at least every 3 to 6 months for 2 years). This should include history and physical examination, blood pressure measurement, thoracic radiographs, serum biochemical profile, and a "recheck" echocardiogram. The exact timing of specific examinations depends on clinical circumstances and economic considerations.

Prognosis

- Longevity in asymptomatic cats with mild left ventricular hypertrophy (LVH) can be great, often exceeding 5 years.
- Progressive LA dilation is a poor prognostic sign and portends development of CHF or thromboembolism.
- Prognosis after onset of CHF is variable. Many cats live for more than 2 years after a documented bout of pulmonary edema. With progressive heart disease, CHF episodes become worse. Development of thromboembolic complications, pleural effusion, or atrial fibrillation in cats with long-standing HCM are poor prognostic indicators (see subsequent discussion of the complications of cardiomyopathy).
- Regression of HCM occurs sporadically and without an obvious association to any therapy.

DILATED CARDIOMYOPATHY (DCM) IN THE CAT

Etiology

▼ *Key Point* Most cases of DCM (Fig. 66–2) in the cat have developed secondary to a dietary deficiency in taurine. This form of feline DCM is reversible.

- Metabolic differences also may occur among cats in their ability to use taurine. Exclusive feeding of single diets or genetic factors may help to explain the predominance of DCM observed in some breeds (Burmese, Abyssinian). Some cats with DCM have normal plasma and whole blood taurine levels, and the condition may represent a different process, such as postmyocarditis DCM.

Pathology

- Lesions that often are observed in advanced cases include dilatation of all cardiac chambers, particularly the LV and LA chambers, a subjectively "flabby" myocardium, atrophied papillary muscles, increased heart weight compatible with eccentric hypertrophy, and left atrial and systemic arterial thrombi.
- Histologic lesions are nonspecific and include focal endocardial fibrosis, muscle cell degeneration and necrosis, and separation of cells by edematous extracellular ground substance or connective tissue.

Pathophysiology

- Myocardial inotropism is markedly depressed, leading to ventricular myocardial failure.
- LV ejection fraction is depressed, and stroke volume and cardiac output are limited.
- Neurohumoral compensations lead to sympathetic activation and to renal retention of sodium and water (see discussion of heart failure, Chap. 64).
- The ventricles progressively dilate in most cases.
- Diastolic function also is compromised, owing to ventricular dilatation and fibrosis. Ventricular diastolic pressures increase.

- Atrioventricular (AV) valve annulus dilatation and altered papillary muscle function lead to mitral regurgitation (MR) and tricuspid regurgitation (TR).
- Ventricular dilatation and failure, valvular regurgitation, and renal sodium and water retention combine to increase atrial and venous pressures.
- CHF ensues and usually is characterized by biventricular failure.

Clinical Signs

- Cats of any age can be affected, with both males and females affected in approximately equal numbers. Burmese, Abyssinian, and Siamese cats are over-represented in some reports.
- Historical abnormalities are identical to those described for feline HCM. Dietary history is important. Some cats eat only a single commercial diet. In particular, "off-brand" diets often are suspected as potentially deficient in taurine. Most feline diets have been sufficiently supplemented with taurine.

Physical Examination

- Arterial pulse is usually hypokinetic, and it may be absent if there is aortic embolus or irregular if a cardiac arrhythmia is present. Arterial blood pressure can be very low.
- Jugular venous distention is usually present if there is CHF.
- Cardiac auscultation/palpation is usually abnormal.
    Heart sounds are soft, even in the absence of pleural effusion, suggesting decreased contractility. The left apical impulse is typically weak.
    A ventricular gallop (S₃) or summation gallop (S₃ and S₄) is typically present as a result of ventricular dilation and reduced ventricular compliance.
    Sinus tachycardia, sinus bradycardia, or arrhythmias may be detected. Sinus bradycardia may indicate severe hypotension or cardiogenic shock.
    Mitral regurgitation or tricuspid regurgitation murmurs are common.
- Hypotension, hypothermia, severe depression, weakness, pallor, and slow capillary refill time (from vasoconstriction) are evidence of cardiogenic shock.

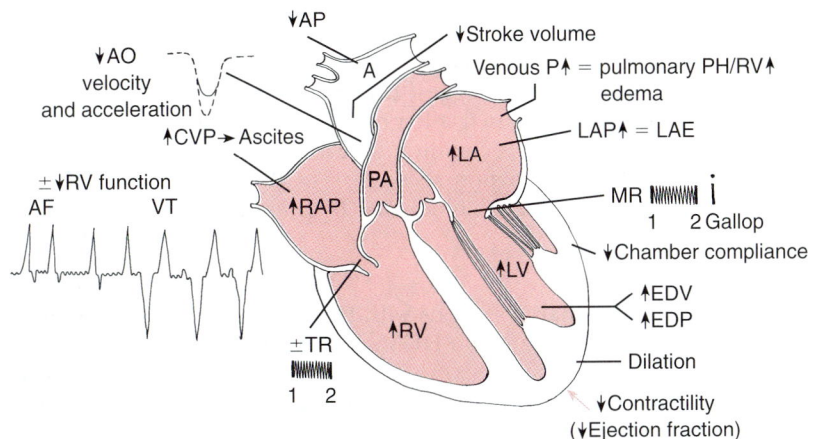

Figure 66–2. Diagrammatic representation of dilated cardiomyopathy. Explanation of the abbreviations can be found in the text.

- Examination of the ocular fundus may reveal abnormal hyper-reflective areas of retinal degeneration adjacent to the optic disc, which are typical of taurine deficiency.
- Other respiratory, abdominal, and physical findings—including those of aortic thrombosis—are similar to those described for feline HCM.

Diagnosis

- Make a presumptive diagnosis of feline DCM by considering the breed and dietary history, clinical signs, and exclusion of other causes.
- Differential diagnosis includes other types of LV cardiomyopathy, right ventricular cardiomyopathy, persistent atrial standstill, chronic hyperthyroid heart disease, heart failure secondary to anemia, pericardial effusion, atrial septal defect, and chronic bradycardia (e.g., 3° AV block).
- Definitive diagnosis of feline DCM requires echocardiography. Confirm taurine deficiency as the cause of DCM by measuring the plasma or whole blood taurine concentration and monitoring the response to supplementation.

Radiography

- Generalized cardiomegaly is evident with rounding of the cardiac apex. The valentine-shaped heart (ventrodorsal view) is far less common than in HCM.
  - The heart may not appear substantially enlarged after volume contraction with diuretic drugs.
  - Pleural effusion is typical; however, some cats manifest radiographic signs of pulmonary edema only.

Echocardiography

- Echocardiography is the diagnostic procedure of choice for DCM. Anatomic abnormalities can be identified. End-systolic dimension is increased because of low LV shortening fraction, which is often between 5% and 20%. Normal shortening fraction is more than 35%. Doppler studies can document valvular regurgitation and low aortic outflow velocity.

Electrocardiography

- A variety of arrhythmias are possible. Sinus bradycardia is not uncommon. Sinus arrest and junctional (nodal) rhythms may be observed.
- P waves that are increased in amplitude (> 0.25 mV) or duration (> 0.035 sec) suggest LA enlargement.
- A normal axis with increased voltage R waves in leads II and aV_F (> 0.7 mV) is common and indicates LV dilation. Right axis deviation secondary to RV dilation or right bundle branch block may be present.

Laboratory Abnormalities

- Laboratory abnormalities in cats with DCM are similar to those found in cats with HCM, with the following exceptions:
  - Plasma or whole blood taurine concentration may be below the reference range for the laboratory. Both plasma and whole blood levels are helpful;

however, some evidence suggests that taurine concentration in whole blood is a better diagnostic index of taurine status. Contact the laboratory regarding handling and interpretation.
- Cats with persistent hypokalemia may be predisposed to taurine depletion.
- Occasionally, a form of DCM develops in cats with hyperthyroidism; therefore, measure serum thyroxine (T_4) in cats older than 7 years of age. Hyperthyroidism also can complicate DCM and precipitate CHF.
- Moderate-to-severe anemia (packed cell volume $<$ 18%) can precipitate CHF owing to increased cardiac output demands.

Treatment

- Assess the degree of functional impairment: asymptomatic, CHF (left ventricular or biventricular), arrhythmia, thrombosis, renal failure, and shock. Recognize that cardiogenic shock requires aggressive therapy to prevent death from hypoxia and hypotension. After the initial therapy for severe CHF, prescribe maintenance therapy.
- For the acutely symptomatic patient with CHF:
  - Minimize stress but avoid sedatives.
  - Administer oxygen (40–60%).
  - For pulmonary edema or pleural effusion, administer furosemide (Lasix, Hoerst) initially at 2 mg/kg IM or IV, and then 0.5 to 1.0 mg/kg q8–12h over the first 24 hours of therapy. In addition, apply 2% topical nitroglycerin ointment (Nitrol; Nitrobid) cutaneously. The usual dose is ¼ inch, q8–12h.
  - Using a 21- or 23-gauge butterfly needle, aseptically drain each hemithorax as required to relieve pleural effusion.

▼ **Key Point** Thoracocentesis is essential for the management of large pleural effusions in cats with DCM.

- Prevent heat loss by placing the cat in a warm environment.
- Place an IV catheter, and administer warmed IV or SC fluids only after lung edema is controlled or pleural effusion is aspirated. Use 0.45% NaCl in 2.5% dextrose solution IV or lactated Ringer's solution SC, with 8 mEq KCl per 250 ml fluid, if the cat is not oliguric or hyperkalemic. The usual rate of infusion is 20–40 ml/kg over 24 hours, provided that the effusion has been drained and diuresis has been attained.
- Treat cardiogenic shock by infusion of dobutamine (Dobutrex, Lilly, 2–5 µg/kg/min) or dopamine (Intropin, Armour, 2–5 µg/kg/min) for up to 36 hours. Alternatively, use the inotropic-dilator amrinone (Inocor, Winthrop) at the labeled human dose. Titrate the infusion to a dose sufficient to increase the systolic blood pressure to 90–100 mm Hg.
- For therapy of thromboembolism see the subsequent discussion of the complications of cardiomyopathy.
- For long-term therapy of feline DCM
  - Prescribe aspirin or warfarin as described under "Complications of Feline Cardiomyopathy."

- Titrate furosemide to prevent recurrent pulmonary edema and pleural effusion as described for HCM. Daily furosemide is required unless the cat has taurine-responsive CHF (see subsequent discussion).
- Recommend a diet supplemented with taurine (most name-brand commercial diets).
- Prescribe enalapril or benazepril (Vasotec, Merck) for cats, with an initial dosage of 0.25 mg/kg, PO, q24h. Aim to increase the dosage to 0.5 mg/kg PO q12h over the next 2 weeks (unless hypotension or acute renal failure occur).
- Prescribe digoxin (Lanoxin, Burroughs-Wellcome; or Cardoxin, Evsco) at a dosage of 0.01 mg/kg, q48h for elixirs; *or* one-fourth of a 0.125-mg digoxin tablet, q48h. Avoid digoxin if the serum creatinine level remains higher than 2.5 mg/dl.
- Beta-adrenergic blockers and calcium channel blockers typically are not prescribed because of the negative inotropic effects of these drugs.
- DCM secondary to taurine deficiency (i.e., low plasma levels) still occurs sporadically. Most cats with DCM have normal plasma taurine levels. Nonetheless, after a plasma or whole blood sample for taurine concentration has been obtained, it is prudent to treat *all* cats with DCM with taurine (250 mg, PO, q12h) for at least 12 weeks.

DCM is reversible after 4 to 6 weeks of taurine supplementation in cats with taurine-induced DCM.

In cats with taurine-deficiency DCM, therapy for CHF may be gradually withdrawn after 4 to 6 weeks if there is radiographic and echocardiographic documentation of improved myocardial function.

Periodically evaluate plasma and whole blood taurine concentrations.

Follow-Up and Prognosis

- Monitor cats with CHF caused by DCM for progressive CHF (pulmonary edema, pleural effusion) or for complications of therapy (hypotension, progressive azotemia, electrolyte disturbances). Initially, examine the cat once weekly for a month, thereafter, every month until it is stable, then the intervals are increased.
- Prognosis for taurine deficiency DCM is favorable provided that the cat does not die of CHF during the first 4 to 6 weeks of therapy. Prognosis for cats with CHF but with normal taurine blood concentration is guarded. Prognosis for cats in cardiogenic shock is very poor. Prognosis for cats with shock and aortic thromboembolism is grave.

RESTRICTIVE (INTERMEDIATE) CARDIOMYOPATHY IN THE CAT

Etiology

- RCM (Fig. 66–3) is a poorly defined condition of unknown cause. The most likely etiologies are antecedent myocarditis with healing by fibrosis or HCM complicated by repeated myocardial infarctions.

- Cats with RCM have clinical and functional disorders that are similar to those in cats with both HCM and DCM.
- Most cats with RCM have normal plasma taurine levels.

Pathology

- A variety of necropsy lesions have been observed in cats demonstrating clinical features of RCM. LV endomyocardial fibrosis is the prominent lesion, and this may be patchy, multifocal, or diffuse in distribution. Extensive endocardial fibrotic scarring may be observed, and when extreme it can affect the mitral valve apparatus, lead to mid-ventricular constriction or stenosis, or obliterate the left ventricular apex.
- The most striking finding is left atrial or biatrial dilation and hypertrophy.
- The left ventricle may be hypertrophied, dilated, or normal in size. Often there is regional thinning of the LV free wall or LV apex interspersed with focal or regional wall hypertrophy. Prominent papillary muscle hypertrophy or fibrosis is evident in some cats.
- Myocardial infarction has been recognized, most often at the LV apex or free wall.
- Systemic thromboemboli are common, and left atrial and ventricular mural thrombi may be observed.
- Histologic lesions include endocardial thickening, endomyocardial fibrosis, myocardial interstitial fibrosis, myocyte hypertrophy, and focal myocytolysis and necrosis. Arteriosclerosis of intramural coronary arteries may be recognized.

Pathophysiology

The pathophysiology of RCM in the cat is unresolved, but the following points merit consideration.

- Echocardiography generally demonstrates a low normal to mildly reduced shortening fraction (EF). Regional left ventricular wall dysfunction may be observed, characterized by diminished free wall systolic thickening and excursion.
- Doppler studies may demonstrate mitral insufficiency, but the regurgitation is usually mild. Because the abnormalities of myocardial and mitral valve function do not sufficiently explain the marked LA dilation characteristic of this disease, impaired LV distensibility is assumed to be the principal disorder.

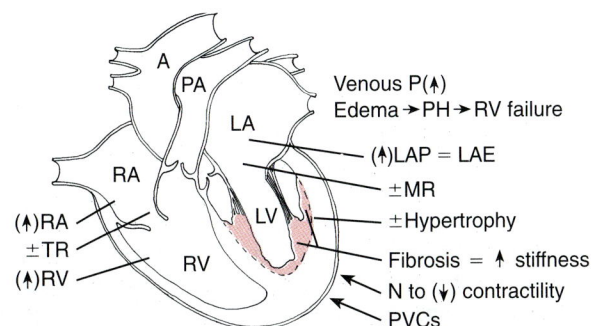

Figure 66–3. Diagrammatic representation of restrictive cardiomyopathy. Explanation of the abbreviations can be found in the text.

Myocardial or endomyocardial fibrosis is the most likely explanation for this diastolic dysfunction.

- If present, myocardial ischemia, relaxation abnormalities, cardiac arrhythmias, or ventricular dilation could further impair ventricular diastolic function.
- Progressive increases of LA pressure develop to fill the stiff left ventricle and thereby predispose the cat to elevated pulmonary venous pressure and pulmonary edema. The marked LA dilation and fibrosis may increase the resistance to RV ejection. These factors probably lead to chronic pulmonary hypertension and cause the progressive enlargement of the right side of the heart and contribute to the elevated central venous pressure that is often observed in advanced cases.
- Pulmonary edema, pleural effusion, and hepatic congestion are typical manifestations of CHF.
- Stasis of blood in a dilated left atrium predisposes affected cats to atrial thrombi and systemic thromboembolism.

Clinical Signs

- Most cats with RCM are middle-aged or older, although young cats also have been recognized with this condition. There is no known breed predisposition.
- Clinical signs of RCM are similar to those of other heart diseases in cats.
  - The most frequently observed historic problems are tachypnea and respiratory distress caused by CHF. Sudden paresis, most often affecting the rear limbs, is typical of thromboembolic occlusion of the terminal aorta. Clients also may report decreased activity or exercise capacity, malaise, weight loss, or inappetence.
  - Stress, fever, moderate-to-severe anemia, thyrotoxicosis, anesthesia, or fluid therapy may precipitate CHF. Some affected cats appear normal to the client; however, cardiac auscultation or thoracic radiography may indicate heart disease.

Physical Examination

- Examination of the cat with RCM can reveal a variety of physical manifestations.
  - The most consistent auscultatory finding is a gallop sound, indicative of ventricular diastolic dysfunction. A soft to moderately loud systolic murmur of mitral or tricuspid regurgitation may be detected near the left or right sternal borders, but a murmur is not a consistent finding. Premature ventricular or atrial beats may be heard, leading to an irregular rhythm and arterial pulse.
  - The femoral pulse is otherwise normal or slightly reduced in amplitude. Blood pressure is usually normal.
  - Pulmonary edema or pleural effusion is manifested as tachypnea and respiratory distress. Palpable hepatomegaly, pleural effusion, and elevated jugular venous pressure are suggestive of concurrent RV failure. Thoracic auscultation is variable,

but careful auscultation may reveal loud bronchial sounds, fine crackles, or a pleural fluid line.
- Signs of aortic thromboembolism may be evident.

Diagnosis

- Presumptive diagnosis is made based on age, clinical signs, auscultation, and radiography. Definitive diagnosis requires echocardiography performed by an experienced examiner. The differential diagnosis of RCM includes those aforementioned for feline DCM.

Radiography

- Radiographic findings are characterized by LA dilatation and cardiac elongation that is typical of LV enlargement. A bulging left auricular border typifies the dorsoventral and ventrodorsal views. The cardiac apex can be pointed or rounded.
- Some cats manifest astounding LA enlargement that, on the lateral projection, can be seen to separate the mainstem bronchi and create a convex dorsocaudal border.
- Generalized cardiomegaly is observed in some cats, whereas other cats demonstrate a "valentine-shaped" heart reminiscent of HCM.
- Pulmonary hypertension may be evident radiographically as dilation of both lobar arteries and veins.
- Interstitial and alveolar infiltrates indicative of pulmonary edema or bilateral pleural effusions indicate CHF.

Electrocardiography

- The electrocardiogram is frequently abnormal in cats with RCM. Ventricular enlargement and myocardial disease can be manifested as any of the following abnormalities: widened QRS complexes (>0.04 sec); increased amplitude R-waves (>0.7 mV) in leads II, aV_F, or III; intraventricular conduction disturbances including splintered R-waves, right axis deviation, or left bundle branch block; and ventricular extrasystoles.
- Atrial enlargement is characterized by widened (>0.035 sec) or tall (>0.2 mV) P-waves, atrial ectopic rhythms, or atrial fibrillation.

Echocardiography

▼ *Key Point* The most characteristic feature of RCM is marked LA or biatrial dilation.

- The left ventricle, in typical cases of RCM, is neither as hypertrophied nor as dynamic as that observed in most cases of HCM. In contrast to cats with DCM, ventricular shortening fraction is either normal or just mildly reduced (generally $> 25\%$) and the mitral opening to septal distance is minimally increased. However, marked regional wall dysfunction may be noted, most often affecting segments of the LV free wall.
- Two-dimensional echo examination often reveals a ventricle that is mildly dilated (>18 mm end-diastolic dimension) just below the mitral valve; yet, apically

the left ventricle may appear hypertrophied and the papillary muscles thick or rigid. Discrete thinned areas of ventricular atrophy, infarction, or scar may be imaged. Subendocardial, hyperechoic wall segments probably denote fibrosis or endomyocardial plaques. In extreme cases, fibrous tissue bands may bridge the septum or partially obliterate the apical LV cavity. The right ventricle often is dilated in symptomatic cats but otherwise is devoid of structural lesions.

- LA or LV mural thrombi are observed infrequently.
- Doppler studies can indicate AV valve regurgitation, but it is not often severe. Doppler evidence of restrictive physiology may be noted if the heart rate is not too high.
- Mild-to-moderate pericardial effusion is common but decreases markedly after successful treatment of heart failure.

Laboratory Abnormalities

- Clinical laboratory studies of cats with RCM are not specific, and most abnormalities are attributable to CHF, diuretic therapy, or thromboembolism.
- Measure plasma or whole blood taurine because decreased concentrations have been noted in some cats and could contribute to reduced myocardial contractility. When plasma taurine concentration is low, re-explore the dietary history.
- Analysis of pleural fluid indicates a transudate, modified transudate, or chyle.

Therapy

Hospital Management

- When pleural effusion is present and sufficient to cause atelectasis, perform thoracocentesis while the cat rests in sternal recumbency. Submit a sample of the effusate for chemical and cytologic analysis.
- Pulmonary edema can be severe in some cats with RCM. Initial therapy includes supplemental oxygen, furosemide (2–4 mg/kg IM or IV q8h), and 2% transdermal nitroglycerin paste (¼ inch, topically q12h). Once diuresis has been observed, decrease the diuretic dose (1–2 mg/kg, SC q8–12h).
- Supportive treatment: (1) prevent hypothermia, (2) provide good nursing care, and (3) treat dehydration. After initial diuresis, give the cat fresh water ad libitum. Should water be refused or continual weight loss occur, give maintenance IV or subcutaneous fluids (40–50 ml/kg/24h of 0.45% NaCl/2.5% dextrose solution; add 8–12 mEq KCl per 500 ml fluid). In cats with aortic thrombosis, monitor both serum potassium and renal function at least daily and more often if reperfusion is observed. Consider liquid nutritional support (eg. Jevity; Ross Labs) given by an indwelling nasogastric tube if anorexia persists; however, most cats begin to eat after effective resolution of CHF.

Management of Chronic Congestive Heart Failure

- Prescribe combination therapy of furosemide, digoxin, and enalapril (see Feline Hypertrophic Cardiomyopathy for information about using these drugs in cats). Dispense a sodium-restricted diet if it is eaten.
- The daily furosemide dosage depends on the severity of fluid accumulation and must be individualized. Initial doses between 1–2 mg/kg q12h are reasonable; however, doses as high as 4 mg/kg q8h have been tolerated. Monitor efficacy of diuretic therapy using respiratory rate, level of activity, and the chest radiograph. Overzealous diuresis can be detected by periodic measurement of blood pressure, serum BUN, creatinine, and electrolytes. Mild azotemia is often the necessary price of effective diuretic therapy in cats.
- Digitalization is accomplished at a dose of ¼ of a 0.125-mg Lanoxin tablet every 48 hours. Measure serum digoxin concentration 10 to 14 days later, with the blood sample drawn 10–12 hours post-treatment. A serum concentration falling between 1 and 2 ng/ml is the therapeutic goal.
- Prescribe the ACE inhibitor enalapril at 0.25 mg/kg, PO, q24h, and increase the dose over the next 2 weeks to 0.5 mg/kg PO, q12h, if tolerated. Monitor enalapril therapy by measuring indirect arterial blood pressure and with periodic monitoring of renal function and serum sodium and potassium. If systolic blood pressure is below 90 mm Hg, reduce the dose of enalapril, furosemide, or both by 33 to 50%. Give aspirin (1 baby aspirin q3d) or warfarin (0.5 mg daily) to inhibit thrombogenesis. Administer warfarin in cats with prior thromboemboli or those with LA internal dimension exceeding 20 mm and spontaneous echocardiographic contrast observed therein.
- The value of other treatments in RCM is unresolved. The calcium channel antagonist diltiazem often is prescribed to improve diastolic function and coronary perfusion in feline HCM. Whether such treatment is useful in the RCM heart with extensive fibrosis is uncertain. Diltiazem or a beta blocker is indicated in cases of RCM complicated by atrial fibrillation because either drug can slow the rapid ventricular rate response that develops with this arrhythmia. Treatment of very frequent and recurrent ventricular extrasystoles or ventricular tachycardia in cats with RCM is problematic. Treatments are reserved for symptomatic (i.e., syncopal) patients or those with sustained ventricular arrhythmias. Consult with a specialist.
- Occasional ventricular extrasystoles are relatively common in this condition and are not treated.

Follow-Up and Prognosis

- Initial follow-up is similar to that described for feline DCM. Because cats with RCM can have very severe CHF, reevaluate frequently until the patient is stable.
- The long-term prognosis of RCM is guarded and quite variable. Many cats have been managed successfully for CHF for more than 1 year. Unfortunately, relentless CHF, refractory pleural effusion, or systemic thromboembolism presents formidable obstacles to long-term survival.

COMPLICATIONS OF FELINE CARDIOMYOPATHY

Systemic Thromboembolism

- *Systemic thromboembolism* (TE) is common in all forms of cardiomyopathy. Thrombi are believed to form in the left atrium. When a thrombus breaks free from the atrial wall, an embolus is formed. Small emboli may terminate in the coronary circulation or cranial aortic branch vessels. Large thrombi are swept around the arch to the iliac arteries, causing acute rearlimb paresis, and severe anxiety and pain. The stress and associated tachycardia may precipitate CHF. Less common thromboembolic syndromes include acute (typically right) foreleg paresis, acute renal failure due to suprarenal or renal thrombus, or colic related to gut ischemia. Cats with renal thrombosis or mesenteric ischemia may display *severe* abdominal pain. Cerebral thromboemboli are probably more common than realized and cause strokelike attacks that are usually self-limiting.

Clinical Signs

- The typical aortic "saddle thrombus" is wedged in the external iliac arteries and the common origin of the internal iliac arteries. Clinical signs are explained by vascular, neurologic, and skeletal muscle dysfunction.
  - Vascular. Loss of femoral pulse and coccygeal pulse (via rectal examination); cool, pale limbs; and absence of bleeding from cut nail beds.
  - Neurologic. Lower motor neuron paresis is usually present, and the cat may be paralyzed. Involvement may be unilateral or bilateral. The tail may or may not be involved. Severe ischemic neuropathy is characterized by paralysis, areflexia, and loss of deep pain.
  - Musculoskeletal. Muscle contracture (gastrocnemius, semitendinosus, quadriceps), muscle pain, and eventual muscle necrosis characterized by persistent blue discoloration and progressive softness with edema.

    Skeletal muscle enzymes (creatine kinase [CK], AST) leak into the serum, and levels are severely elevated severely.

    Serum ALT levels also may be elevated. The source of this enzyme (from the liver or from a massive skeletal muscle necrosis) is uncertain.

    Although enzyme concentrations are increased within hours of the insult and ischemic myopathy develops almost immediately, it may take 3 to 10 days for severe skeletal muscle injury to be evident clinically. Fever may develop 3 to 14 days after the insult.

Laboratory Abnormalities

- Laboratory abnormalities depend on the site of obstruction and severity of tissue injury.
  - Elevated serum CK, AST, and ALT may be seen.

- Hyperkalemia often develops from reperfusion of injured and necrotic tissues after spontaneous, drug-induced, or surgical revascularization.
- Metabolic acidosis is not uncommon.
- Laboratory test findings of disseminated intravascular coagulopathy are common and may contribute to bleeding in other organs.
- Renal infarction or suprarenal thrombosis is associated with elevated BUN and serum creatinine concentrations.
- Leucocytosis with a left shift usually occurs after 2 to 5 days.

Diagnosis

- In most cats, the diagnosis of TE is made from the history and physical examination. Markedly elevated skeletal muscle enzyme concentrations support the diagnosis. Angiography almost never is required for diagnosis and may be a dangerous added stress in the clinical setting of acute embolism with uncontrolled CHF. Abdominal ultrasound examination may successfully delineate the thrombus.
  - Differential diagnosis includes bacterial endocarditis of the aortic or mitral valve; tumor infiltration of the pelvic canal or iliac arteries; missile-like foreign body (pellet), which is very rare; and trauma to the caudal abdomen.
  - Advise the client that arterial TE in the cat almost always is associated with underlying heart disease. This concern may limit the use of anesthesia and surgery for treatment of this condition.

Treatment

General therapy applicable for all cats includes the following:

- Administer *analgesics* for this painful condition, such as butorphanol (Torbugesic, Fort Dodge), 0.2–0.4 mg/kg, IV, SC, IM but not in rear limbs. Alternatively, use buprenorphine (Buprenex, Norwich Eaton) 0.01–0.02 mg/kg, IM. If combined with a tranquilizer (acepromazine, 0.1–0.2 mg/kg IM or SC), expect substantial sedation, which may be beneficial.
- Prevent hypothermia, but do not subject the limbs to external temperatures exceeding normal body temperature.
- Sodium bicarbonate can be administered for presumed metabolic acidosis (1 mEq/kg, slowly IV over 15 minutes, and repeat thereafter if required based on ECG monitoring and measurement of blood gas and serum potassium values).
- Administer maintenance fluid therapy (as for feline DCM) to prevent acute renal failure and hyperkalemia. Delay this treatment until CHF is controlled. Ensure urine output and potassium excretion with furosemide 1 mg/kg q12h. Measure serum potassium at least every 24 hours for the first 3 days.

Determine the baseline clotting times for monitoring anticoagulant therapy (e.g., partial thromboplastin time, prothrombin time, and activated clotting time or international normalization ratio [INR] (see Chap. 21).

Drugs Used for Treatment and Prevention of Thromboembolism

A number of drugs can be prescribed in an attempt to induce clot lysis or minimize the chance of future arterial thromboembolism.

- Thrombolytic therapy with either streptokinase or tissue plasminogen activator is expensive and very difficult to control. To be effective, thrombolytic therapy must be administered within a few hours of the thromboembolic event and there may be severe complications from this therapy, including fatal hyperkalemia from rapid reperfusion of muscles. Currently, there is little enthusiasm for thrombolysis in cats. Consult a specialist before embarking on such therapy.
- Sodium heparin can be administered to prevent further thrombosis (initial dose 200–300 IU/kg, administered IV, then 150–200 IU/kg SC, q8h for 72 hrs). We combine the general measures described in the previous section with at least 72 hours of heparin therapy in the treatment of cats with aortic thromboembolism.
- Prevention of further thrombosis should be a therapeutic goal for treatment of cats that previously have experienced thromboemboli or for cats at high risk for these events. *Relative risk* can be assessed by examining the left atrium by thoracic radiography and echocardiography. When the LA diameter exceeds 20 mm or when echogenic "smoke" (a specific type of density) is observed in the left atrium, the risk of embolism is high. Prior emboli, atrial fibrillation, and low cardiac output states represent additional major risk factors. There are no prospective studies demonstrating efficacy of any preventive treatment. Empirically two treatment approaches have evolved—namely, aspirin (1 baby aspirin or ¼ of an adult aspirin q3d) or warfarin (Coumadin, starting at ½ of a 1-mg tablet daily).
  - *Aspirin* may inhibit platelet function in some cats. The dose is probably critical, but good guidelines are lacking. Anorexia, vomiting, and gastric erosions are potential complications of therapy. This method of prevention is losing favor; however, it may be the only reasonable approach in some cases and is much safer than warfarin. In cats at relatively low risk for left atrial thrombi, we prescribe either aspirin or no anticoagulant therapy.
  - *Warfarin (Coumadin)* represents a more aggressive approach to prevention of thrombotic complications in cats with cardiomyopathy. We typically reserve warfarin for cats with a prior TE event, or when smoke is identified in a grossly dilated left atrium.
    - Monitor warfarin treatment by serial measurements of the prothrombin time or the international normalization ratio (INR) as described subsequently. If the client cannot comply with regular monitoring, use aspirin.

- Because warfarin initially enhances coagulation, give cotherapy with heparin (100 IU/kg, SC) for the first 48 to 72 hours.
- Do not use warfarin with aspirin. Consider drug interactions (see the *Physicians' Desk Reference* (PDR), Dupont Pharmaceuticals).
- Should bleeding occur at any site (have owners check litter box), immediately discontinue therapy and reestablish the INR at 2.0 to 3.0.

Monitoring Anticoagulant Therapy

- As a minimum, obtain a baseline one-stage prothrombin time (PT) and reevaluate every 24–48 hours while the cat is receiving heparin. The usual therapeutic goal is prolongation of the PT two to three times over the baseline value.
- The INR may be a superior method for evaluation of heparin or warfarin anticoagulant therapy. The $INR = (\text{patient PT} \div \text{control population PT})^{ISI}$ where ISI = international sensitivity index of the thromboplastin used in the PT assay.
  - The validity of using this approach in cats has not been determined completely but merits consideration.

Because of the complexity of monitoring anticoagulant therapy, consult a specialist.

- An INR of 2.0 to 3.0 (blood drawn about 2 hours after dosage) is considered "therapeutic." (Note: to obtain an *INR between 2.0 and 3.0*, the PT ratio must be between 2.0 and 3.0 when the ISI equals 1.0; between 1.6 and 2.2 when the ISI equals 1.4; between 1.5 and 1.8 when the ISI equals 1.8; between 1.4 and 1.6 when the ISI equals 2.3; or between 1.3 and 1.5 when the ISI equals 2.8. For more details see: Coumadin in the *PDR*).
- When warfarin is used for long-term prevention of thromboembolism, the INR should be measured periodically; for example, weekly for a month, then every other month.

Natural History and Prognosis

▼ *Key Point* Provided that the cat with TE does not die in the hospital of CHF, arrhythmia, or reperfusion hyperkalemia, a significant percentage (40–50%) develop spontaneous revascularization of the limbs and progressive improvement in motor function over the next 2 to 4 weeks.

- Function returns, progressing from proximal to distal.
  - It is not always possible to predict the outcome based on initial evaluation. Some cats with severe embolism improve dramatically.
  - Unfortunately, such severe skeletal muscle necrosis and ischemic neuropathy develop in some cats that the limb atrophies and becomes a fibrotic and useless appendage.
  - Gangrene also may develop and is considered in any cat with a soft, edematous limb and progressive, antibiotic-resistant fever. Sepsis is another potential complication.

- Amputation of such severely affected limbs may be required 1 to 4 weeks after the initial insult (see Chap. 135). Some cats do well after amputation.
- Recurrent arterial TE can occur in some cats. In some cases, a rapid return to limb function ensues, perhaps related to development of collateral vessels. Other cats die or are euthanatized because of severe tissue injury or client-related concerns.

Atrial Fibrillation

- *Atrial fibrillation* (AF) is infrequent in cats but is most common with hypertrophic and restrictive forms of feline CM. This condition is disastrous in cats with stiff ventricles because the atrial contribution to filling is lost.
  - Paroxysmal AF develops in some cats. This may convert to sinus rhythm spontaneously or after therapy with a calcium channel blocker.
  - For persistent or chronic AF, administer digoxin (see discussion of feline DCM) along with diltiazem (see discussion of feline HCM). The goal is control of ventricular rate response to less than 200/minute. Titrate diltiazem dose to the desired heart rate. In emergencies, give diltiazem or verapamil (0.05 mg/kg) IV by slow bolus.
  - Pleural effusion often develops in cats with AF, and thoracocentesis may be required.

Pleural Effusion

- *Pleural effusion* is a consequence of left-sided, right-sided, or biventricular CHF.
- *Chylothorax* secondary to CHF is not uncommon and can be controlled only when the underlying cardiac condition can be managed. The following are considered in treatment:
  - Optimize furosemide therapy (1–3 mg/kg, q8–12h), ensuring that serum creatinine concentration does not exceed 2.5 mg/dl and serum potassium concentration does not decrease. Consider intermittent SC dosing by the client to ensure maximum effect.
  - Prescribe enalapril as described for RCM. Monitor serum creatinine levels and blood pressure periodically.
  - For cats with HCM, prescribe diltiazem to improve diastolic function (see discussion of feline HCM).
  - Should atrial fibrillation supervene, control the ventricular rate response (see preceding discussion of atrial fibrillation).
  - Instruct the client to feed the patient a sodium-restricted diet.
  - Perform thoracocentesis to relieve moderate to severe effusions.

MYOCARDITIS

Etiology

- Inflammation of the myocardium may develop secondary to infectious agents (see Table 66–1) or in association with cardiomyopathy (e.g., feline cardiomyopathy and boxer dog cardiomyopathy), trauma, ischemic injury, or toxicity. It also can be idiopathic. Myocarditis eventually may cause DCM and may be the underlying cause of "idiopathic" DCM or RCM in some animals.

Pathology

- Myocarditis is classified histologically based on the predominant cellular infiltrate, which varies depending on the cause and duration. The heart can respond to injury in a limited number of ways, so that most inflammations are nonsuppurative (consisting of mononuclear cells, predominantly lymphocytic-plasmacytic), granulomatous, suppurative, or, rarely, eosinophilic. Infective agents may or may not be present.
  - A variable, predominantly nonsuppurative endomyocarditis has been observed in most forms of feline CM. Inflammation often involves the conduction system and may explain the conduction disturbances that occur in some cats with CM.
  - Diffuse or multifocal, nonsuppurative myocarditis has been found at necropsy in a number of cats that died of CHF.
  - CHF due to acute necrotizing myocarditis can be fatal in litters of pups infected neonatally by parvovirus (see Chap. 12).
  - Boxer dogs with "boxer myocarditis" may have nonsuppurative myocarditis that is associated with malignant ventricular arrhythmias (see subsequent discussion of canine dilated cardiomyopathy).
  - In the southwestern United States, dogs with Chagas disease develop granulomatous myocarditis that can cause heart failure, arrhythmias, or AV conduction block.
- Myocardial degeneration and necrosis are consequences of myocarditis. Advanced stages have significant subendocardial infiltrate, with macrophages and histiocytes accompanying the predominant inflammatory cells. The myocardium is replaced by granulation tissue consisting of histiocytes, Anitschkow's cells, hemorrhage, and inflammatory cells. In chronic myocarditis, fibrosis may be the principal lesion and may be evidenced grossly at necropsy as a white, unraised discoloration of the myocardium.

Clinical Signs

- When myocarditis causes decreased myocardial contractility, either exercise intolerance or overt CHF may develop (e.g., necrotizing myocarditis caused by parvovirus in pups leads to death from pulmonary edema). Clinical features in this situation are virtually identical to those in DCM of the cat or dog.
- Most often, myocarditis becomes evident because cardiac arrhythmias develop.
  - Clinical signs can include weakness and syncope, CHF, abnormal heart sounds and pulses, and sudden death.
  - Ventricular premature complexes and ventricular tachycardia are associated most commonly with myocarditis; however, atrial arrhythmias and AV block also can occur.

- Healed myocarditis may resolve as endomyocardial fibrosis or restrictive cardiomyopathy.
- Myocarditis associated with trauma or with infectious agents (e.g., *Trypanosoma*, *Borrelia*) may be unrecognized if other clinical signs dominate.

Diagnosis

- Clinical recognition of myocarditis may not be easy because no test specifically confirms a diagnosis of myocardial inflammation other than biopsy. Transvenous endomyocardial biopsy can be done with little risk; however, it requires special equipment and training and rarely is done.
- Laboratory diagnosis of myocarditis—elevated myocardial fractions of the serum muscle enzymes (creatine kinase, lactic dehydrogenase [LDH], and AST)—is suggestive of myocarditis, but these isoenzyme fractions must be measured in a laboratory using human standards. There is little laboratory experience interpreting these test results in animals.

Treatment

- Management of myocarditis or secondary myocardial injury has the following objectives:
  - Treatment of the primary cause, if it can be identified.
  - Treatment of cardiac arrhythmias (see Disorders of Cardiac Rhythm, Chap. 62, in this section).
  - Treatment of CHF when present (see Heart Failure, Chap. 64, in this section).
  - The role of corticosteroids in the treatment of certain types of myocarditis remains uncertain.

DILATED CARDIOMYOPATHY IN DOGS

Etiology

- DCM is common in dogs. The causes are unknown; however, a number of explanations have been proposed (see Table 66–1).
  - DCM occurs after a presumed change in the myocardium induced by inflammation, toxins, lack of essential cellular nutrients, or inborn errors of myocardial metabolism.

    The underlying cause of DCM is unknown in most cases. Because it is most common in certain large and "giant" breeds and in a number of spaniel breeds, a genetic or familial link is likely. *Giant breed cardiomyopathy* is considered synonymous with DCM.

    Keene's group has demonstrated a deficiency of L-carnitine (used for fatty acid energy metabolism in the mitochondria) in a number of dogs with DCM. Partial reversal of DCM is observed in a small percentage of dogs given L-carnitine supplementation.

    Kittleson's group has found plasma taurine levels to be low in some American cocker spaniels; however, when all breeds are considered, taurine deficiency is sporadic and not pivotal to the pathogenesis of DCM in the dog.

Toxic injury to the myocardium can lead to DCM. This may occur with long-term administration of doxorubicin (Adriamycin), an anticancer chemotherapeutic.
- Although myocytes cannot undergo hyperplasia, myocardial cell proteins and myosin enzymes frequently turn over in the heart. A change in their structure or function leads to a loss of myocardial cell contractility. Thus, DCM can develop slowly or somewhat rapidly.

Pathology

- Dilation of all the cardiac chambers is accompanied by mild-to-moderate (eccentric) hypertrophy. The papillary muscles may appear flattened and atrophic.
- Mild-to-moderate myxomatous valvular changes also can be present (AV valve endocardiosis), but these are not the primary lesions of this condition.
- Lesions of CHF include serous cavity effusions, hepatomegaly, and pulmonary edema.
- Histologic lesions are minimal in most cases and may include the following: congestion, mononuclear and occasional neutrophilic infiltration, hemorrhage, necrosis, fibrosis (possibly resolved inflammation or the result of myocyte degeneration), and fatty change. Histologic lesions do *not* satisfactorily explain the pathogenesis of DCM.

Pathophysiology

- Similar to feline DCM, this condition in the dog represents principally a "systolic dysfunction" syndrome due to myocardial failure. The LV ejection fraction is decreased.
- The AV valve annulus dilatation or the geometric changes in the papillary muscles often result in mitral and tricuspid valvular insufficiency.
- Lord also has demonstrated decreases in ventricular diastolic compliance probably secondary to fibrosis and marked dilation of the ventricle.
- Arrhythmias are common. *Atrial fibrillation* and *ventricular tachycardia* are the most important because these tachyarrhythmias further depress ventricular function in the following ways:
  - Tachycardia decreases coronary perfusion time while myocardial oxygen consumption increases.
  - Ventricular filling time is erratic and shortened.
  - With AF, the normal atrial "kick" is lost, which further decreases ventricular preload, especially at rapid ventricular heart rates.
  - Ventricular tachycardia activates the ventricle abnormally, causing a less forceful beat. Moreover, the heart is made less electrically stable, and ventricular premature beats may progress suddenly to a fatal rhythm, that is, ventricular fibrillation or cardiac arrest.
  - Decreased cardiac output triggers renal and neurohormonal compensatory mechanisms, contributing to venous congestion and LV or biventricular CHF.
  - Acute and severe ventricular arrhythmias may cause sudden death before or after the onset of CHF.

Clinical Signs

- "Giant" breeds, other large dogs (>15 kg), and spaniel breeds, particularly springer and cocker spaniels, are predisposed. A male predominance is reported in most surveys. The affected dogs are often relatively young, with many between 2 and 5 years of age.
- Dogs with "occult" DCM are healthy and are diagnosed incidentally when discovery of a murmur or an arrhythmia, or client demand, prompts an echocardiogram. Symptomatic dogs usually are presented for signs referable to progressive heart disease, CHF, or cardiac arrhythmia, including the following:
  - Exercise intolerance, lethargy, and tiring.
  - Respiratory problems, such as tachypnea, dyspnea, orthopnea, or coughing.
  - Fulminant pulmonary edema may cause hemoptysis, which is particularly common in the Doberman pinschers.
  - Weight loss is often dramatic and may occur quickly (e.g., 2–4 wks). This sign probably represents cardiac cachexia.
  - Abdominal distension (from ascites)
  - Sudden weakness or syncope (from an arrhythmia).

▼ *Key Point* The two major clinical syndromes of DCM in the dog are CHF and paroxysmal or sustained cardiac arrhythmia. Often, these two problems occur together.

Physical Examination

- Weight loss, poor body condition, and depression
- Slow capillary refill time due to reduced cardiac output and peripheral vasoconstriction.
- Pulse abnormalities, including (1) hypokinetic pulses due to decreased stroke volume or cardiac arrhythmias; (2) rapid, erratic pulse with pulse deficits suggesting atrial fibrillation or ventricular arrhythmias; and (3) alternating intensity pulse (pulsus alternans), indicating severe myocardial failure or bigeminal arrhythmia.
- Arterial blood pressure can be normal or decreased.
- Prominent jugular pulses and increased jugular venous pressures usually indicate right-sided CHF.
- Abnormalities of cardiac auscultation may include the following: (1) soft first sound, which signifies myocardial failure; (2) ventricular (S_3) or summation ($S_3 + S_4$) gallop (the gallop is easiest to detect when the dog is in sinus rhythm and may diminish after successful therapy of CHF); (3) left or right apical systolic murmurs of mitral or tricuspid regurgitation (when compared with the murmurs commonly detected with canine endocardiosis, the murmurs of DCM are typically less intense—usually grade 2 to 4/6); or (4) auscultory evidence of cardiac arrhythmia, which is typical.

  Rapid, irregular, chaotic, variable intensity heart sounds typify atrial fibrillation, which is the *most common arrhythmia* in dogs with CHF.

Premature beats may be heard, suggesting atrial or ventricular ectopia.

Periods of rapid, regular rhythm with variable intensity (or split) sounds that start and stop abruptly typify paroxysmal ventricular tachycardia.

- Respiratory examination in symptomatic dogs usually reveals signs of left-sided or biventricular CHF: (1) tachypnea and dyspnea are common because of pulmonary edema or pleural effusion; (2) inspiratory pulmonary crackles suggest pulmonary edema; and (3) inspiratory dyspnea with muffled heart and breath sounds (and dull percussion) ventrally suggest pleural effusion.
- Hepatomegaly with or without ascites indicates right-sided CHF.
- Signs of cardiogenic shock are evident in some dogs. Doberman pinschers are particularly prone to this syndrome. Clinical findings include severe pulmonary edema, weakness, depression, hypothermia, hypotension, and mucous membrane pallor.

Diagnosis

- A presumptive diagnosis of DCM is not difficult to make because most large and giant breeds with CHF have DCM. Many dogs with DCM are relatively young.
  - Congenital heart disease usually can be eliminated from the differential diagnosis by noting the lack of prior clinical signs or indicators of congenital heart disease (no murmur).
  - Differentiate DCM from heartworm disease, bacterial endocarditis, cardiac tumors, and pericardial disease.
  - Some breeds—spaniels, standard Schnauzers, Afghan hounds, German shepherds—are at risk for both DCM and endocardiosis. Echocardiography may be required to determine whether one or both conditions are present.

▼ *Key Point* Definitive diagnosis of DCM is made by echocardiography. The low LV shortening fraction and absence of other structural cardiac lesions are characteristic.

- Dogs with primary tachyarrhythmias (e.g., atrial tachycardia, ventricular tachycardia) may appear to have DCM; however, after successful resolution of the arrhythmia, LV function returns to normal. This is not the case with idiopathic DCM.

Radiography

- Advanced DCM is characterized by generalized cardiomegaly and radiographic signs of CHF. Dilation of the LV and LA are most evident in some dogs.
  - Of note is the Doberman pinscher breed, in which marked dilatation of the left atrium with pulmonary edema is often the principal finding.
  - Pulmonary venous congestion is a feature of DCM before the onset of lung edema.

- Pulmonary edema can be severe and diffuse, particularly in Doberman pinschers and in dogs that suddenly develop atrial fibrillation.
- Pleural effusion is common.

Echocardiography

Echocardiography is the current clinical "gold standard" for diagnosis of DCM. The cardinal findings are LV and atrial dilatation with depressed myocardial systolic function (fractional shortening is low, <25% and usually <15% in symptomatic dogs). Right-sided chambers frequently are dilated. Doppler studies can document mitral or tricuspid regurgitation, diastolic dysfunction, and decreased aortic ejection velocity typical of myocardial failure.

The echocardiographic diagnosis of "occult" DCM is not always straightforward, and the evaluation may benefit from specialty consultation.

Electrocardiography

- The ECG is abnormal in most dogs with DCM. Common abnormalities include one or more of the following:
  - Tachycardia due to sinus or atrial tachycardia, atrial fibrillation, or ventricular tachycardia.
  - Isolated atrial or ventricular premature complexes (PVCs) may be observed. These can be the earliest detectable sign of DCM in some asymptomatic dogs.
  - Ventricular tachycardia is very common in Doberman pinschers and in boxer dogs with cardiomyopathy.

    Harpster's classification of "boxer cardiomyopathy" is based on ECG and clinical criteria:

    I—Asymptomatic with isolated PVCs; the echocardiogram is usually normal.

    II—Symptomatic (weakness, syncope) due to periods of sustained ventricular tachycardia; the echocardiogram is often normal. Types I and II represent forms of "arrhythmogenic" cardiomyopathy.

    III—Symptomatic for CHF with concurrent atrial or ventricular arrhythmias. This last group is virtually indistinguishable from giant breed DCM and is treated in the same manner.

    The best method by which to evaluate the severity and therapy of ventricular arrhythmias in DCM is with ambulatory (Holter) monitoring.

▼ *Key Point* Atrial fibrillation is the most common arrhythmia associated with CHF in giant breeds.

- P-waves often are prolonged (>0.04 sec), indicating atrial dilatation.
- QRS prolongation (>0.06 sec) or increased QRS voltages suggests ventricular LV dilatation.

  A widened QRS with a slurred R-wave descent (leads II and aVF), associated with *ST-T slurring*, strongly suggests myocardial disease.

  Left (more common) or right bundle branch block may occur (see Chap. 62).

- The ST-T segment may be depressed secondary to myocardial ischemia.
- Low QRS voltages suggest pleural effusion, concurrent hypothyroidism, or breed variation (e.g., many boxers have small QRS complexes).

Laboratory Abnormalities

- Routine hematologic and urinalysis findings are usually normal unless altered by severe heart failure, therapy for heart failure, or concurrent disease.
  - Prerenal azotemia, generally mild, occurs in about 25% of cases.
  - Mild hypoproteinemia is observed in about 25% of cases.
  - Hypokalemia, hypochloremia, and metabolic alkalosis can be observed after vigorous diuretic therapy.
  - Hyponatremia is usually a sign of severe heart failure and an indication for aggressive medical therapy.
  - Hypothyroidism may be present in some dogs as a complicating disease, but overall prevalence is quite low.
  - Low plasma taurine concentration is found in some American cocker spaniels, small breeds, and some golden retrievers.
  - Low plasma or myocardial L-carnitine concentrations are found in some dogs with DCM, but these tests are not readily available.
  - Pleural effusions and ascitic fluid typically are found to be transudates or modified transudates and, rarely, chylous.

Treatment

- See Chap. 64 for treatment of acute CHF, cardiogenic shock, and chronic CHF. General principles of therapy include administration of positive inotropic drugs, diuretics, and ACE inhibitors/vasodilators. Control cardiac arrhythmias. Exercise restriction and sodium restriction are also appropriate.
- Prescribe digoxin (Lanoxin, Burroughs Wellcome, or Cardoxin, Evsco) at an initial dosage of 0.005 to 0.007 mg/kg, PO, q12h.
  - Digoxin increases myocardial contractility and improves baroreceptor activity to slow heart rate.
  - For atrial fibrillation, initiate therapy with digoxin to help slow ventricular rate response. An oral loading dose (twice the daily maintenance dose) can be used for the first 24 hours (see Chap. 64).
  - Digoxin therapy, alone or in combination with a beta blocker or calcium channel blocker, typically does not lead to conversion to normal sinus rhythm. However, combination therapy more effectively slows the ventricular rate response (see the following discussion).
  - Doberman pinschers are very sensitive to digoxin. Usual *total daily dosage* in this breed is 0.25 to 0.375 mg.
  - Use digoxin cautiously, if at all, for complex ventricular arrhythmias.

- Administer furosemide parenterally (2–4 mg/kg, q8h) to mobilize edema and ascites. A switch to oral dosage then is initiated, titrated to the patient's response.
- Initial vasodilator therapy for pulmonary edema can include nitroglycerin ointment, which can be discontinued in 24 to 48 hours. Begin an ACE inhibitor (enalapril, benazepril, or lisinopril) at 0.5 mg daily PO. Increase the dosage in 1 or 2 weeks to 0.5 mg/kg, q12h. If a dog with DCM also has severe mitral regurgitation, a combination of hydralazine (Apresoline; CIBA), 0.5–1.0 mg/kg PO q12h and enalapril (0.5 mg/kg q12h) may be most effective.
- The use of nutriceuticals is controversial. Consider oral supplementation with taurine (500 mg, q12h) in American cocker spaniels with DCM, particularly if a low plasma taurine level has been documented. Oral administration of L-carnitine (50–100 mg/kg, q8h) may be helpful in dogs with deficiency of L-carnitine; however, no readily available method exists for assessing myocardial carnitine, and L-carnitine supplementation is very expensive. Consequently, we do not routinely prescribe this drug unless we document low plasma or myocardial L-carnitine concentration and the client understands the empirical and costly nature of the treatment. (Note: Do not use D-carnitine.)
- Drugs to slow heart rate. Successful therapy of CHF, combined with digitalization, should slow the resting heart rate in a dog with DCM and underlying sinus mechanism. Persistent sinus tachycardia may indicate arterial hypotension, excessive drug dosages (e.g., diuretic, vasodilator), or presence of an ectopic atrial (not sinus) tachycardia.
  - The tachycardia associated with *atrial fibrillation* generally does not respond to simple therapy with digoxin. To decrease the resting heart rate, either a calcium channel blocker or a beta blocker is added to therapy after digoxin has been administered for at least 24 to 36 hours.
  - Judicious use of diltiazem (Cardizem; Marion), beginning at 0.5 mg/kg, PO, q8h, and increasing the dosage over 48 to 72 hours to 1.0 to 1.5 mg/kg, q8h, usually reduces the ventricular rate response.
  - Alternatively, use a beta blocker, such as propranolol (Inderal, Wyeth-Ayerst) or atenolol (Tenormin, Stuart), to slow rate response. Begin propranolol at 0.2 mg/kg, PO, q8h, and increase over 72 hours up to 0.6 mg/kg, q8h. The initial dosage of atenolol for a giant breed dog with CHF is 6.25, PO, q12h.
  - Diltiazem and beta blockers are negative inotropic drugs. Use with caution only after initial stabilization of CHF. Titrate the doses to obtain a resting ventricular rate of 120 to 160 beats/minute. Both drugs can worsen CHF.
  - The aforementioned therapy merely controls the ventricular rate by depressing AV nodal conduction. It generally does not convert the rhythm from atrial fibrillation to sinus rhythm.
  - Electrical cardioversion is not likely to yield a permanent conversion in dogs with DCM and CHF and is not recommended.

- Ventricular arrhythmias. When sustained or recurrent ventricular tachycardia or frequent or multiform PVCs are present, prescribe either procainamide, mexiletine, or sotalol (see Chaps. 62 and 63).
  - Antiarrhythmic drug therapy is best monitored by 24-hour ECG analysis (Holter monitor) because antiarrhythmic drugs can promote arrhythmias (leading to ventricular fibrillation), suppress escape rhythms during cardiac arrest (ventricular standstill), and depress myocardial inotropism.
  - Abrupt symptoms of low output and cardiac syncope in dogs with documented ventricular arrhythmias are indications for antiarrhythmic therapy, provided that drug-induced hypotension is excluded as the cause.
- Concurrent medications
  - L-Thyroxine. Give L-thyroxine to dogs with documented hypothyroidism at the lowest possible dose needed to prevent signs of hypothyroidism. Avoid higher doses commonly used for dermatologic manifestations (e.g., 0.1 mg/10 kg q12h) to circumvent taxing the circulatory system or inducing tachycardia or atrial arrhythmias. Dosages of 0.05 mg/10 kg daily are reasonable. When initiating therapy with thyroid hormone, gradually increase the dose every 2 to 3 weeks until the target dosage is attained.
  - Anti-inflammatory drugs. Dogs with musculoskeletal disorders that require either nonsteroidal anti-inflammatory drugs (NSAIDs) or corticosteroids can receive these medications; however, the potential for gastrointestinal ulceration may be higher than usual. Aspirin inhibits vasodilatory prostaglandins, which may be a problem in severe CHF. Glucocorticoids are unlikely to cause sodium retention in dogs and can be prescribed along with cardiac medications.
  - Occasionally, an H$_2$-blocker improves appetite in anorexic dogs with CHF. The course of this empirical therapy should be short (<3 wks).

Prognosis

- The prognosis of symptomatic DCM with CHF, atrial fibrillation, or recurrent ventricular tachycardia is guarded. With excellent home care and regular veterinary attention, most dogs live for 6 to 12 months after the initial onset of CHF or syncope. Experience with Doberman pinschers is most unfavorable, and those presented in cardiogenic shock, even when stabilized, often die or are euthanized within 3 to 6 months, or sooner. Some breeds—Irish wolfhound, Saint Bernard, Great Dane, cocker spaniels—seem to stabilize after 1 to 2 months of therapy and may have a good quality of life for extended periods, often more than 1 year.
  - The echocardiogram findings have minimal prognostic value in dogs with CHF, and repeated studies are unnecessary to guide therapy.
  - Clients must be made aware of the possibility of sudden death in these dogs. Recurrent ventricular

arrhythmias increase the possibility of sudden arrhythmic death, even when CHF is controlled.
- Intractable CHF, unresponsive to the most aggressive therapy, is an indication for euthanasia.

HYPERTHYROID HEART DISEASE

Etiology

- Hyperthyroid heart disease develops most often in older (>8 years) cats due to thyroid adenoma (see Chap. 29). Iatrogenic hyperthyroidism (from oversupplementation) or spontaneous hyperthyroidism (from a functional tumor) is diagnosed occasionally in the dog. Iatrogenic hyperthyroidism is becoming more prevalent as older, large-breed dogs are prescribed increasingly higher doses of L-thyroxine (0.1 mg/10 kg bid).

Pathology

- Spontaneous hyperthyroidism in the cat leads to myocardial hypertrophy and dilatation. Marked increases in ventricular mass can develop over a matter of weeks.

Pathophysiology

- The noncardiac effects of thyrotoxicosis are described in Chapter 29. Most cats with hyperthyroid heart disease manifest increased cardiac demand from the hypermetabolic state, peripheral vasodilation, systemic hypertension, and the direct effects of thyroid hormone on the heart.
  - Most cats have a hypertrophied, hyperdynamic left ventricle. Myocardial failure that resembles DCM develops in a minority.
  - The cardiac lesions, both functional and anatomical, are largely reversible with appropriate therapy.

Clinical Signs

History and Physical Examination

- The clinical signs of hyperthyroidism are described elsewhere (see Chap. 29). Cardiac manifestations include tachycardia, arrhythmias, and systolic murmurs and/or gallop rhythm. Biventricular CHF may develop.
- Most commonly, a systolic murmur of mitral regurgitation or a systolic flow murmur along the cranial sternal border is detected. Less often, a murmur compatible with tricuspid regurgitation is heard.
- The heart rate may be very high, often more than 250 beats/minute.
- CHF is not common but when present generally is characterized by development of pleural effusion.
- Systemic hypertension may be present.

Diagnosis

Radiography

- Cardiac elongation, typical of LV enlargement, and left auricular enlargement are typical; right-sided heart enlargement is variable. The aorta may be dilated, especially the ascending aorta and aortic arch (possibly an age-related change or caused by increased cardiac output or systemic hypertension).
- Pulmonary edema and pleural effusion are uncommon.

Electrocardiography

- Increased voltages typical of ventricular enlargement are common.
- Axis deviations and conduction blocks, left anterior fascicular block and right bundle branch block, may be detected.
- AV block, when present, is an incidental finding of senile degeneration of the conduction system, which is not uncommon in aged cats.
- Sinus tachycardia and atrial and ventricular premature beats are common.

Echocardiography

- The left ventricle is dilated and hyperkinetic; the LV wall and interventricular septum are hypertrophied; the left atrium and right atrium are dilated; and the aorta is increased in diameter.
- In cats with CHF, the right-sided chambers are markedly dilated.
- Doppler studies show AV valve regurgitation and turbulence in the ascending aorta.

Laboratory Abnormalities

- Laboratory studies are typical of hyperthyroidism (increased thyroxin, elevated liver enzyme levels) and make the diagnosis of hyperthyroid heart disease a straightforward one in most cases. A radionuclide scan is needed for diagnosis in some cats. Failure of cardiac disease to regress (or stop progressing) after appropriate therapy prompts the reconsideration of the diagnosis (e.g., could there also be idiopathic cardiomyopathy?). Measure blood taurine levels in cats with CHF and decreased myocardial function.

Treatment

- Hyperthyroid heart disease usually responds to control of hyperthyroidism with antithyroid medication (e.g., methimazole [Tapazole] 2.5–5 mg, PO, q8–12h), surgery, or radioactive iodine treatment, as described in Chapter 29.
  - Prognosis is good unless CHF has developed. In this case, prognosis is guarded, but therapy can be successful and ventricular function may improve over time.
  - Cats with severe depression of shortening fraction may die of CHF.
  - When CHF develops, administer furosemide (Lasix; 1–2 mg/kg, q12h) and enalapril (Enacard; 0.25 mg/kg, PO, q12h) and recommend rest.
  - Perform thoracocentesis for initial stabilization.

- Prescribe methimazole; treat medically for 2 to 4 weeks until CHF is stabilized.
  - At that time, radioactive iodine therapy or surgery can be considered (see Chap. 29).
- Prescribe atenolol (6.25–12.5 mg q12–24h) for cats that cannot be treated by conventional methods or those being given methimazole in which hepatotoxicity develops.

SUPPLEMENTAL READINGS

Fox PR, Sisson DD, Moise NS: Canine and Feline Cardiology. Philadelphia, WB Saunders, 1999.

Harpster NK, Baty CJ: Warfarin therapy of the cat at risk of thromboembolism. In: Bonagura JD (ed): Kirk's Current Veterinary Therapy XIII. Philadelphia: WB Saunders, 1995, pp 868–873.

67 Pericardial Diseases and Cardiac Neoplasia

John R. Reed / Steven E. Crow

The parietal pericardium is a strong, flask-shaped sac that surrounds and attaches via the visceral pericardium to the heart and its major arteries. Under normal conditions, the pericardium serves to protect the heart and major vessels. When diseased, however, it can cause life-threatening restriction of ventricular function. If pericardial disease remains unrecognized, signs of heart failure and potentially death will ensue.

▼ *Key Point* Pericardial disease is one of the most common causes of right-sided heart failure in the dog.

Clinically significant pericardial disease is uncommon in cats. The most common causes of pericardial dysfunction are the acquired disorders (Table 67–1).

ETIOLOGY

Congenital Disorders

- *Pericardial defects* are rare and clinically insignificant.
- *Peritoneopericardial diaphragmatic hernia* (PPDH) may be recognized in patients ranging from 4 weeks to 15 years of age. The majority of cases are diagnosed within the first year of life. Of reported cases, 58% occur in males. Evidence suggests that Weimaraners may be predisposed. This condition is common in cats, and is often an incidental finding in this species.
- *Pericardial cysts* are uncommon but clinically significant. These cysts may result from incarceration of the omentum. This defect is manifested clinically in relatively young patients. Affected patients may develop pericardial effusion.

Acquired Disorders

▼ *Key Point* Pericardial effusion is the most common type of pericardial disease.

Pericardial Effusion

Insignificant amounts of pericardial effusion develop in patients with many forms of heart disease and with certain metabolic disorders. Cats with untreated heart failure occasionally develop moderate pericardial effusion.

Clinically significant effusion is typically exudative or hemorrhagic. It may be idiopathic or caused by hemangiosarcoma, heart base tumor, mesothelioma, ruptured left atrium due to chronic mitral regurgitation, or infection. Hemorrhagic effusion is more commonly diagnosed in large-breed dogs older than 6 years of age. The German shepherd and golden retriever appear to be commonly affected breeds. Small breeds (e.g., dachshund) are predisposed to ruptured left atria. Pericardial effusion in a large-breed dog has approximately a 50% chance of being caused by idiopathic or neoplastic conditions. Clinically significant pericardial effusion in cats is usually due to infectious or neoplastic causes.

Constrictive Pericarditis

Constrictive pericarditis is not as common as pericardial effusion. It primarily occurs in large-breed dogs and causes compression and/or restriction to myocardial diastolic filling. The causes are listed in Table 67–1.

CLINICAL SIGNS

Cardiac Displacement

- In PPDH the degree of herniation can be variable. Clinical signs often occur acutely. Clinical signs may be absent, and the hernia diagnosed as an incidental finding. A large hernia tends to displace the heart dorsolaterally and cranially. The clinician may hear heart sounds in unlikely locations.
- Gastrointestinal signs (vomiting, diarrhea, colic, anorexia, weight loss) are the most common presenting signs.
- Respiratory signs (dyspnea, cough, wheeze) are the second most common.
- Pericardial effusion (no matter what the cause) does not cause cardiac displacement.
- Some forms of constrictive pericarditis (e.g., infection) and pericardial mass lesions commonly impinge on the right side of the heart.

Pathophysiology

- The principal hemodynamic effect of pericardial disease is a decrease in ventricular diastolic compliance. As a result, end-diastolic pressure increases and end-

Table 67–1. CAUSES OF PERICARDIAL DISEASE IN THE DOG AND CAT

Congenital Disorders
Peritoneopericardial diaphragmatic hernia (PPDH)
Pericardial cyst

Acquired Disorders
Pericardial effusions
   Transudates*
     Congestive heart failure
     PPDH
     Hypoalbuminemia
     Heart base tumors
   Exudates
     Infection (bacterial, fungal)
     Sterile uremic
     Feline infectious peritonitis
   Hemorrhagic
     Neoplasia (hemangiosarcoma, heart base tumor,
       mesothelioma, carcinoma, lymphoma)
     Trauma
     Cardiac rupture (left atrial tear)
     Infection (bacterial)
     Idiopathic
Constrictive pericardial diseases
   Infection (fungal, bacterial)
   Neoplasia
   Pericardial foreign body
   Idiopathic
Pericardial mass lesions
   Pericardial abscess
   Pericardial cyst

*Conditions that rarely cause significant cardiac compression.

diastolic volume decreases (Fig. 67–1). Decreased cardiac output, renal retention of sodium and water, and increased venous pressure cause right-sided heart failure (pleural effusion, ascites).

- As the diastolic pressures of all chambers rise, signs of cardiac tamponade occur and cardiogenic shock may develop. Obvious signs of left-sided heart failure are absent. Systolic function including contractility is usually normal.
- Acute intrapericardial hemorrhage can suddenly increase intrapericardial pressure leading to cardiac

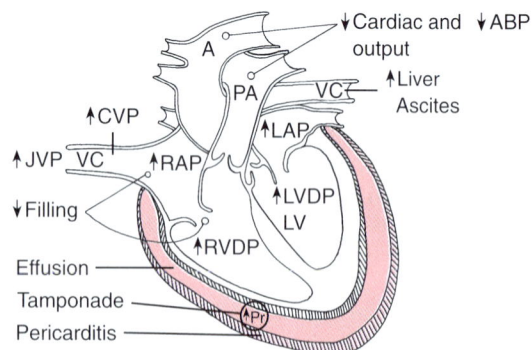

Figure 67–1. Diagrammatic representation of pericardial effusion. See text for explanation. A, aorta; ABP, arterial blood pressure; CVP, central venous pressure; JVP, jugular venous pressure; LAP, left atrial pressure; LV, left ventricle; LVDP, left ventricular diastolic pressure; PA, pulmonary artery; Pr, pressure; RAP, right atrial pressure; RVDP, right ventricular diastolic pressure; VC, vena cava.

tamponade, hypotension, and syncope but without obvious signs of congestive heart failure.

- PPDH infrequently causes diastolic impairment.
- Systolic dysfunction rarely occurs in pericardial diseases.
  - Hemangiosarcoma can impair cardiac function via metastasis throughout the myocardium. Systolic function is reduced via destruction of muscle and arrhythmias. In some cases, this tumor may grow into the chambers of the right side of the heart, impairing inflow and outflow.
  - Infrequently, cardiac tamponade is associated with apparent cardiac "stunning" characterized by transient (1- to 2-week) depression of systolic function.
  - Some heart-based tumors reduce cardiac function by infiltration of myocardium and through induction of severe arrhythmias.
  - Pericardial mass lesions may impinge on the right ventricle to the point of significantly reducing inflow and outflow.

DIAGNOSIS

Physical Examination

- Increased respiratory effort may be seen in all cases of pericardial disease.
- In effusive and constrictive pericardial diseases, the femoral arterial pulse may be weak and/or pulsus paradoxus (an exaggerated increase and decrease in arterial pulse pressure during expiration and inspiration) may occur.
- Jugular venous distention indicates systemic venous hypertension and is frequently seen in pericardial disease.

▼ *Key Point* Ascites and pleural effusion are very common findings in pericardial disease. Systemic venous hypertension and fluid retention cause right-sided heart failure.

- Auscultation
  - In PPDH, heart sounds can be displaced cranially, laterally, and/or dorsally.
  - With pericardial effusion, heart sounds are often muffled; however, in small dogs and cats heart sounds may be normal. Arrhythmias sometimes are present.
  - In constrictive pericarditis, heart sounds are usually diminished. A pericardial friction rub is very rare.
  - Pericardial masses may cause displaced heart sounds.
- Fever is commonly seen in pericardial diseases of infectious origin.

Electrocardiogram

- The ECG may be normal or demonstrate an axis deviation in PPDH.
- Pericardial effusion
  - In dogs, the QRS amplitudes are often, but not al-

ways, diminished to less than 1.0 mV in all leads. ECGs in cats are normal.
- Nonspecific ST-segment changes or ST-segment elevation are uncommon.
- Electrical alternans occurs in approximately 50% of dogs with high-volume effusion. This finding has not been reported in cats.
- Myocardial infiltration or ischemia sometimes produces supraventricular and ventricular arrhythmias.
- Constrictive pericardial disease
  - Diminished QRS voltages are typical.
  - Increased P-wave duration (>0.45 second).
- Cardiac rhythm is usually normal in pericardial disease. Supraventricular arrhythmias are sometimes noted. Atrial fibrillation is occasionally observed.

Thoracic Radiographs

Peritoneopericardial Diaphragmatic Hernia

In PPDH, radiographic findings are variable and dependent on the volume and contents of the hernia. Some common features are as follows:

- Border effacement of the diaphragm and heart.
- A very enlarged, elongated, or spherical cardiac silhouette.
- Gas patterns within the cardiac silhouette.
- A double-density cardiac shadow due to omental fat, liver, or spleen with craniodorsal displacement of the heart (Fig. 67–2).
- Deformities of the sternum (e.g., pectus excavatum).
- When barium is given, it may outline the stomach or intestines if they are displaced into the pericardial sac.

Pericardial Effusion

- With pericardial effusion, a rounded cardiac silhouette in both views is a common feature. Small effusions may cause only mild changes in the size and shape of the cardiac silhouette, whereas large effusions may cause marked enlargement of the cardiac silhouette.

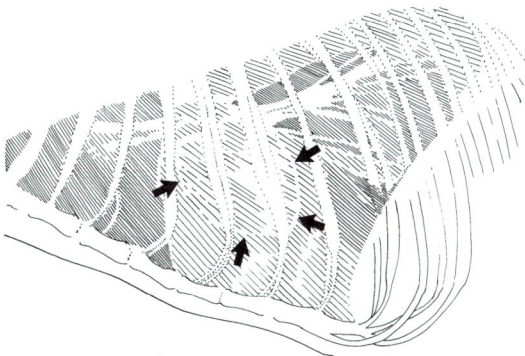

Figure 67–2. Representation of the enlarged cardiac silhouette and double-density cardiac shadow caused by omental fat in a patient with peritoneopericardial diaphragmatic hernia. Arrows indicate the edge of the heart.

- Pleural effusion or enlarged caudal vena cava are frequent findings. In animals with pleural effusions, adequate pleural fluid drainage must be accomplished before the cardiac silhouette can be seen.
- A cardiac silhouette that is enlarged and has the same shape as it had before enlargement is typical of a left atrial tear. The left atrium is usually prominent.
- Tracheal elevation or deviation can indicate a heart base tumor.
- Pulmonary metastatic lesions are suggestive of a right atrial hemangiosarcoma.
- Pneumopericardiography is useful when echocardiography is unavailable. Mass lesions may be outlined at the heart base, over the right atrium, or within the pericardial space itself.
- In affected cats, the cardiac silhouette varies in shape. Sometimes the silhouette appears rounded and is suggestive of pericardial effusion. Frequently the cardiac silhouette has a normal morphology, yet it is enlarged. In these situations, it is difficult to differentiate pericardial effusion from other feline cardiac diseases.

Constrictive Pericardial Disease

- Radiographic findings of constrictive pericardial disease are subtle and may include mild to moderate cardiac enlargement, rounding of the right side of the heart in one or both views, enlarged caudal vena cava, and pleural effusion.

Echocardiography

- PPDH can be detected routinely when the liver and omentum are displaced forward into the pericardial sac. When the intestines are displaced forward, a poorer quality image may result because of intraluminal gas.

▼ *Key Point* Echocardiography is the most sensitive procedure for documenting pericardial effusion and for detecting pericardial and cardiac masses.

- Effusion causes a hypoechoic space (fluid) surrounding all four chambers of the heart.
- Compression of the right side of the heart is indicative of cardiac tamponade.
- Congenital pericardial cysts are seen near the apex. These cysts are attached to the pericardium and not the heart.
- Hemangiosarcoma lesions are seen at the junction between the right atrium and ventricle. Sometimes this tumor grows inward, causing partial obstruction to inflow into the right ventricle.
- Heart base tumors are observed adjacent to the ascending aorta.
- Pericardial abscesses impinge on the right ventricle. Right ventricular collapse can be observed.
- Echocardiography is less reliable in determining constrictive pericardial disease. Sometimes pericardial thickening or loculated effusion can be observed. A number of subtle Doppler echocardiographic findings point to the diagnosis. Consider referral for advanced ultrasound studies.

Magnetic Resonance Imaging

MRI is a nonivasive imaging technique (see Chap. 4) that is useful for identifying cardiac tumors associated with pericardial effusion and for determining whether tumors are operable.

Hemodynamic Studies

- Elevated central venous pressure (usually >12 cm H_2O) is typical of pericardial disease that is severe enough to cause heart failure.
- Cardiac catheterization may be necessary for the diagnosis of constrictive and effusive-constrictive pericardial disease. The normal pressure differences between cardiac chambers are lost and end-diastolic pressures equilibrate throughout the heart.

Routine Laboratory Analysis

- Mild elevations of liver enzyme levels are commonly seen when signs of right-sided heart failure (ascites) are present.
- Normal to low-normal serum protein concentrations may be present in effusive and constrictive pericardial disease.
- Anemia with nucleated red blood cells can be seen with hemangiosarcoma.
- Infectious pericarditis or pericardial abscesses can cause leukocytosis with a left shift.

Pericardial Fluid Analysis

Pericardial fluid analysis yields variable diagnostic results.

- Purulent, serosanguineous, chylous, and transudative effusions are easy to identify.
- It is very difficult to differentiate between idiopathic and neoplastic effusion, because both are serosanguineous.
- It is also difficult to differentiate cytologically between neoplastic cells and reactive mesothelial cells (Table 67–2).
- It is not uncommon for infectious pericardial effusions to be serosanguineous in the dog.
- Heart base tumors occasionally cause a clear transudative effusion related to obstruction of lymphatic drainage.

Table 67–2. CLASSIFICATION OF HEMORRHAGIC PERICARDIAL EFFUSIONS

	Idiopathic	Hemangio-sarcoma	Heart Base Tumor
Protein	0.9–5.7 g/dL	3.0–6.0 g/dL	1.3–3.0 g/dL
Red blood cell count (RBC)	0.01–8.75 $\times 10^6/\mu L$	0.13–12.5 $\times 10^6/\mu L$	0.89–4.1 $\times 10^6/\mu L$
Nucleated RBC	1.1–18.0 $\times 10^3/\mu L$	1.8–30.9 $\times 10^3/\mu L$	0.9–4.6 $\times 10^3/\mu L$
Mesothelial cells*	Reactive	Reactive	Less reactive

*Reactive mesothelial cells are easily misinterpreted as neoplastic cells.

TREATMENT

Pericardiocentesis

- Use pericardiocentesis—*not* medical therapy—to treat patients with pericardial effusion. Use diuretics in low doses only *after* pericardiocentesis, and only briefly, to assist in diuresis of retained fluid. Digoxin and angiotensin-converting enzyme (ACE) inhibitors are contraindicated.

▼ *Key Point* Pericardiocentesis is the treatment of choice to relieve cardiac compression due to pericardial effusion.

- A needle, or an over-the-needle catheter, is directed into the pleural space between the right fourth or fifth intercostal space, at the level of the costal chondral junction and into the pericardial space.
- Aspirate as much of the pericardial fluid as possible.
- In idiopathic pericardial effusion, repeat pericardial taps as needed. Approximately 50% of idiopathic cases have return of the effusion and may require subtotal pericardiectomy. Corticosteroid therapy has not been shown to be of benefit in preventing this recurrence.
- In neoplastic effusions, repeated taps, thoracoscopy-guided pericardial window, or surgery are necessary to relieve cardiac tamponade.
- For hemangiosarcoma the prognosis is poor; however, options are repeated pericardial taps, a pericardial window, and surgery/chemotherapy (see Chap. 26). Euthanasia must be considered eventually because of the aggressive nature of this form of cancer.
- Infectious pericarditis can sometimes be treated by placing an indwelling catheter for drainage and infusion of antibiotics or other antimicrobials directly into the pericardial space.

Surgery

Peritoneopericardial Diaphragmatic Hernia

Dogs with PPDH require surgical correction (see Chap. 82).

- Even if the hernia is small and contains only fat, there is a potential risk for a hernia of abdominal viscera in the future.
- The hernia should be surgically corrected in young cats, but judgment is needed prior to embarking on unnecessary surgery in older cats.

Pericardial Cysts and Abscesses

Pericardial cysts and abscesses require thoracotomy or sternotomy (see Chap. 83). The incision site depends on the location of the abnormal structure. These structures generally are found on the right side of the heart.

Recurrent Idiopathic Pericardial Effusion and Pericarditis

- Subtotal pericardiectomy is recommended for treatment of recurrent idiopathic pericardial effusion; for management of infective pericarditis of any cause; or to treat or palliate neoplasm-related pericardial effusion.

- Constrictive pericarditis requires surgery.
  - Pericardiectomy is curative when the parietal pericardium only is affected. A favorable prognosis exists under these circumstances.
  - When epicardial fibrosis is present, epicardial stripping is required. This is a very difficult, high-risk procedure.
  - Patients with constrictive pericarditis have high rates of postoperative complications (pulmonary embolization).
  - Resolution of ascites often takes 2–3 days after surgery.

Technique for Pericardiectomy

1. Perform either a right-sided or left-sided thoracotomy or a sternotomy (see Chap. 83). Perform a subtotal pericardiectomy ventral to the phrenic nerve.
2. Identify the phrenic nerves on the dorsal right and left sides of the pericardial sac.
3. After placing pericardial stay sutures make a stab incision 1 cm ventral to the nerve.
4. Remove pericardial fluid via suction.
5. Incise the pericardium circumferentially using scissors. Avoid trauma to the myocardium.
6. Control hemorrhage via electrocautery (avoid touching the heart).
7. Place a chest tube.
8. Close the thoracotomy or sternotomy routinely.
9. Always perform histopathologic evaluation of the pericardium to rule out neoplasia (e.g., mesothelioma).

Heart Base Tumors

When heart base tumors have been determined by echocardiography or by MRI to be small and not invading major vessels, the tumor may be surgically removed.

- For better access to the tumor perform a sternotomy.
- Several hours of very delicate and intense surgery are necessary to remove these tumors.
- Also perform a pericardiectomy.
- In the rare situation in which the tumor is completely resectable a good prognosis may be warranted. These tumors are slow-growing and rarely metastasize.
- When heart base tumors are inoperable, continued pericardiocentesis or pericardiectomy is necessary. Even though the tumor increases in size, many patients live 1–2 years after pericardiectomy.

Right Atrial Hemangiosarcoma

A small, suspected hemangiosarcoma requires immediate attention. Perform a right-sided thoracotomy (see following section on removal of atrial tumors).

- Examine the lungs for possible metastasis.
- Remove the right atrial lesion if it is both small and easily isolated. Submit the tissue for histopathologic evaluation.

- An alternative to open thoracotomy for pericardiectomy is thoracoscopy. However, specialized equipment and expertise are needed for this technique.

Technique for Removal of Atrial Appendage Tumors

1. Double-clamp the atrial appendage with Satinsky clamps proximal to the tumor.
2. Incise the tissue between the clamps, and remove the tumor.
3. Oversew the appendage over the clamp using 4-0 polypropylene (Prolene, Ethicon; Summervilles, NJ) with simple continuous sutures. Carefully remove the clamps, and place a second simple continuous suture layer. Place additional sutures at areas of bleeding.
4. Alternatively, use surgical staples (TA, US Surgical; Norwalk, CT) to close the atrial tissue prior to tumor removal.
5. Place an indwelling chest tube, and close the incision routinely.
- Once healing has occurred, initiate chemotherapy (see Chap. 24). In the majority of cases, by the time a suspected hemangiosarcoma lesion is seen, it has already metastasized; thus, the prognosis is very poor.

Chemotherapy

Experience in the chemical treatment of cardiac and pericardial neoplasms is limited, with only a few cases reported. Consequently, recommendations are based on theoretic considerations and reports from cases in human medicine. Consult an oncologist.

Although a complete cure cannot be expected using chemotherapy for any of these neoplasms, some prolongation of life is possible for animals with hemangiosarcomas but less so for those with mesotheliomas. Chemotherapy may "stem the tide" in pericardial neoplasia, temporarily improving the quality of the animal's life, with dramatic results in the occasional case.

Hemangiosarcoma

Hemangiosarcoma is a rapidly metastasizing malignant neoplasm. Assume that metastasis has probably occurred, even if no gross evidence of distant disease exists.

- Initiate aggressive chemotherapy following diagnosis, especially when surgery appears to have rendered the patient free of gross tumor.
- Combination chemotherapy regimens, such as vincristine/Adriamycin/cyclophosphamide (VAC) or Adriamycin/dacarbazine (ADIC) (Table 67–3), have been advocated. Objective responses have been reported using several of these agents singly or in combination.
- The therapy regimens are generally well tolerated by dogs if cardiac and renal function are not severely compromised. The major toxicity of both combinations is myelosuppression. Monitor blood counts every 7–14 days to detect neutropenia. Occasionally, thrombocytopenia may require the temporary discontinuation of chemotherapy.

Table 67–3. CHEMOTHERAPY FOR CARDIAC AND PERICARDIAL NEOPLASMS

Single Agents		
Cyclophosphamide	50 mg/m^2	PO every other day
(Cytoxan)	250 mg/m^2	IV every 14 days
Melphalan (Alkeran)	2 mg/m^2	PO daily
Thiotepa	7.5–15 mg	IC every 7–14 days
Cisplatin	50–70 mg/m^2	IV every 21–28 days
Combination Protocols		
VAC (21-day cycle)		
Vincristine	0.6 mg/m^2	IV on day 8 and day 15
(Oncovin)		
Adriamycin	30 mg/m^2	IV on day 1
Cyclophosphamide	100–200 mg/m^2	IV on day 1
ADIC		
Adriamycin	30 mg/m^2	IV every 21 days
DTIC	1000 mg/m^2	IV every 21 days

IC, intracavitary; IV, intravenously; PO, orally; VAC, vincristine-Adriamycin/cyclophosphamide; ADIC, Adriamycin/dacarbazine; DTIC, dacarbazine. See also Chapter 24, and consult an oncologist.

- Repeat radiographs and/or ultrasound examinations regularly (every 3 weeks) to monitor the response to chemotherapy.

Heart Base Tumors

Heart base tumors tend to be slow-growing, invasive neoplasms with minimal metastatic potential.

- Aggressive chemotherapy is rarely indicated because of the relatively small growth fraction (percentage of dividing cells) characteristic of these well-differentiated neoplasms.
- Chemotherapy may be advisable when surgical resection is impossible. Cyclophosphamide and melphalan are good therapy choices because they can be administered orally. Observe the animal carefully for sterile hemorrhagic cystitis when providing cyclophosphamide, especially with prolonged therapy. Other drugs to be considered include vincristine and dactinomycin.

Pericardial Mesothelioma

Mesothelioma is typically a rapidly progressive neoplasm that spreads to adjacent tissues, primarily by transcoelomic implantation. It is one of the most treatment-resistant malignancies in human beings. Anecdotal reports in the veterinary literature suggest a similar behavior for this neoplasm in dogs.

- Systemic chemotherapy is largely ineffective.
- Intrathoracic instillation of triethylenethiophosphoramide (thiotepa) or cisplatin has been advocated following pericardiectomy for the management of malignant effusion caused by mesothelioma.
- Treatment with radioactive phosphorus (^{32}P) has occasionally controlled the severity of effusions caused by mesothelioma.

SUPPLEMENTAL READINGS

Bonagura JD, Pipers FS: Echocardiographic features of pericardial effusion in dogs. J Am Vet Med Assoc 179:49, 1981.

Evans SM, Biery DN: Congenital peritoneopericardial diaphragmatic hernia in the dog and cat: A literature review and 17 additional case histories. Vet Radiol 21:108, 1980.

Miller MW, Sisson DD: Pericardial disorders. *In* Ettinger SJ, Feldman EC, eds.: Textbook of Veterinary Internal Medicine, 4th Ed. Philadelphia: WB Saunders, 1995.

Reed JR: Pericardial diseases. *In* Fox PR, ed.: Canine and Feline Cardiology. New York: Churchill Livingstone, 1988.

Richter K, Jackson J, Hart JR: Thoracoscopic pericardiectomy in 12 dogs. Proceedings of the American College of Veterinary Internal Medicine, 14th Annual Veterinary Medical Forum, May 1996.

Sutter PF: Thoracic radiography. *In* Sutter PF, ed.: A Text Atlas of Thoracic Diseases of the Dog and Cat. Wettswill, Switzerland, 1984.

Thomas WP, Sisson D, Bauer TG, Reed JR: Detection of cardiac masses in dogs by two-dimensional echocardiography. Vet Radiol 25:65, 1984.

Wagner SD, Breznock EM: Surgical management of pericardial and intramyocardial diseases including chemodectomas. *In* Bojrab MJ, ed.: Current Techniques in Small Animal Surgery, 2nd Ed. Philadelphia: Lea & Febiger, 1983.

68 Heartworm Disease

Clay A. Calvert / Clarence A. Rawlings / John McCall

Heartworm disease is a common problem in many areas of the world, particularly in tropical and subtropical regions. The disease has been endemic along the southeast Atlantic and Gulf coasts of the United States as far west as Texas for more than 50 years. Heartworm infection has spread north and west to most areas of the United States, but the prevalence is still low at high elevations and in most northern states. Endemic foci frequently occur in regions with otherwise low prevalences. It is difficult to eliminate heartworms from a region once they have been established; therefore, all dogs should be tested regularly, and veterinarians should be alert for dogs immigrating from endemic regions.

ETIOLOGY AND PATHOGENESIS

Heartworm infection is produced by the parasite *Dirofilaria immitis* and is transmitted to dogs by many species of mosquitos. Infection rates vary among cats in endemic regions but are usually 10% or less than that of dogs within the same enzootic region.

Life Cycle in Dogs

- Female mosquitos are the intermediate hosts and acquire the first-stage larvae (microfilariae) during feeding on infected dogs.
  - Larvae develop within the mosquito to the third stage in 2–2.5 weeks
  - Third-stage larvae (L_3) infect the dog via the bite wound created during the feeding of the mosquito. In the United States, transmission is unlikely to occur during the dry cold months of the year, even in the southeastern region.
- Larvae migrate through the subcutaneous tissues and vascular adventitial tissues for approximately 100 days.
  - During this time, two molts occur.
  - Young adults (fifth-stage, or L_5, larvae) enter the vascular system at 3–3.5 months postinfection.
  - Young adult *Dirofilaria immitis* worms are in the small pulmonary arteries at 5–6 months postinfection.

▼ *Key Point* Patent infection, as evidenced by microfilaremia, occurs approximately 6 months after transmission from the mosquito.

- Microfilarial concentrations increase for the next 6 months, plateau for several months, and then decrease if further infection does not occur.
- Microfilaria-specific antibody-mediated, occult infections occur in the presence of persistent host antibody excess. Antibody-dependent leukocyte adhesion entraps microfilariae in the pulmonary microcirculation.
  - Between 10% and 67% of all heartworm infections are occult.
  - In most endemic regions, the incidence of occult infections is approximately 20% to 25% of all heartworm infections.
- Microfilaria-leukocyte (neutrophils and eosinophils) complexes are engulfed by phagocytic cells of the mononuclear phagocyte system, resulting in granulomatous inflammation.
  - Predominately eosinophilic inflammation, with minimal granulomatous inflammation, produces allergic pneumonitis.
  - Progressive granulomatous inflammation occasionally leads to pulmonary eosinophilic granulomatosis.
- Other causes of occult infections include unisex infections, drug-induced suppression of microfilaremia associated with monthly heartworm prophylaxis, and high-dose (>200 µg/kg) ivermectin administration.

Life Cycle in Cats

The cat is relatively resistant to infection, requiring a greater L_3 innoculum. Some cats appear to be immune. Consequently, the infection rate in unprotected cats is likely to range from one-fifth to one-tenth that of unprotected dogs in an endemic area. Some mosquito species, as intermediate hosts, do not like to feed on cats. The number of infective larvae that mature are fewer than in dogs, and the pre-patent period is usually longer.

Epizootiology

Prevalence

Heartworm infection is most common in tropical and subtropical climates.

- Infection rates in dogs approach 50% along the Atlantic and Gulf coasts as far inland as 150 miles.
- Most unprotected dogs in highly endemic regions become infected.

- The prevalence in cats varies by geographic region:
  - Much lower than dogs in some areas.
  - Similar to dogs in some areas.
  - The incidence is probably higher than suspected.

Signalment

- Male dogs are infected more often probably because of increased outdoor exposure.

▼ *Key Point* Dogs housed outdoors have a four- to fivefold increased risk of heartworm infection when compared to indoor dogs.

- Large and medium-sized dogs are infected more often probably because of increased outdoor exposure as compared with toy and miniature breeds.
- Infection is diagnosed most often in dogs 4 to 7 years of age. In highly endemic regions, it is common in younger dogs.

Pathogenesis

Disease onset and severity largely reflects the number of adult heartworms, which can vary from 1 to more than 250 in a single dog. In infected cats, the average number of adult worms is three. Acute dyspnea and even sudden death are more common in cats despite the low worm burden.

Worm Location

- Until the adult worm burden exceeds 50 in a 25-kg dog, nearly all worms are located in the pulmonary arteries.
- Worm burdens of approximately 75 are associated with worms located in the right atrium.
- The vena cava syndrome typically is associated with worm burdens of 100 or more.

Response to Live Worms

- Pulmonary arterial endothelial damage and subsequent myointimal proliferation most often affects the caudal and intermediate lung lobes.
- Pulmonary lobar arterial enlargement, tortuosity, and obstruction of smaller branches begin within a few weeks of worm arrival.
- Intrapulmonary blood flow is obstructed as the disease progresses, and blood is diverted to less severely affected lobes.
- Small downstream arterioles become damaged and leak plasma and inflammatory cells into the surrounding lung parenchyma. This causes interstitial and alveolar lung disease with potential signs of fever, coughing, leukocytosis, and dyspnea.

Response to Dead Worms

The most severe disease is seen in response to dead worm fragments that are swept into small arterioles.

- Worm death may be spontaneous or may result from arsenical drugs.

- Pulmonary vascular compliance and blood flow become severely impaired, resulting in pulmonary hypertension and increased right ventricular afterload.
- Parenchymal lung disease (infarction and consolidation) occurs secondary to pulmonary arterial thromboembolism and increased vascular permeability.

CLINICAL SIGNS

The clinical signs associated with heartworm infection reflect the adult worm burden, duration of infection, and host-parasite interaction. Respiratory signs are often prominent.

Clinical Signs in Dogs

- Exercise intolerance, coughing, dyspnea, and respiratory crackles occur in dogs with moderate and advanced heartworm disease.
- Hemoptysis occurs in severe disease associated with pulmonary thromboembolism and pulmonary hypertension. It can be seen before but occurs more often after adulticide treatment.
- Acute dyspnea and increased pulmonary alveolar densities may develop secondary to spontaneous worm death.

Syncope

Syncope is associated with severe pulmonary arterial disease and pulmonary hypertension.

Elevated Central Venous Pressure

Signs of elevated central venous pressure indicate severe pulmonary hypertension with incipient to advanced right-sided congestive heart failure (CHF). Clinical signs include prominent jugular pulse, distended jugular veins, hepatomegaly, and ascites.

Hemoglobinuria

Hemoglobinuria commonly occurs in association with the vena cava syndrome (i.e., acute hemolytic crisis caused by obstruction of the vena cava with adult worms) and occasionally when severe pulmonary arterial disease results in fragmentation hemolysis due to fibrin-thrombus formation or disseminated intravascular coagulation (DIC). Thrombocytopenia is usually a consequence of these complications.

Nephrotic Syndrome

This syndrome occasionally occurs as the result of severe glomerular disease manifested as amyloidosis or immune complex glomerulonephritis (see Chap. 97). Manifestations can include proteinuria, hypoalbuminemia, hypercholesterolemia, azotemia, peripheral edema, or ascites.

Clinical Signs in Cats

Clinical signs of heartworm infection in cats are somewhat different than in dogs.

- *Respiratory signs*
  - Coughing in cats usually is associated with allergic or parasitic lung diseases; heartworm disease represents one cause.
  - Asthmatic signs are a common manifestation and often occur when young adult worms (4–7 months old) have reached the heart.
  - Dyspnea.
- *Vomiting* (intermittent) is a common sign (approximately 20%) and occurs sporadically. It often is not associated with eating, but vomitus may include food. Mucus and bile are often the major components of the vomitus Vomiting and coughing in the same cat should increase the index of suspicion.
- *Sudden death* related to spontaneous worm death and thromboembolism is more common in cats than in dogs.
- *Neurologic signs* including seizures may be observed, especially with aberrant worm migration.

DIAGNOSIS

The diagnosis of heartworm infection is based on a positive immunodiagnostic test and/or the presence of microfilariae in the peripheral blood in dogs with or without clinical or radiographic findings consistent with the disease. Testing puppies younger than 6 months of age is not indicated. Affected cats are usually negative for microfilariae but may have characteristic radiographs and a positive enzyme-linked immunosorbent assay (ELISA) test for either heartworm antigen or antibody.

History

The history in dogs with heartworm infection varies considerably.

- Most heartworm-infected dogs have not received prophylactic therapy.
- Some dogs are totally without signs; others have unexplained tachypnea, exercise intolerance, or cough.
- Signs consistent with pulmonary hypertension with or without overt right-sided CHF are associated with severe heartworm disease.
- Coughing, emesis, and sudden dyspnea are typical signs in cats.

Physical Examination

- Findings vary from clinically normal to signs of right-sided CHF (see Chap. 64).
- Pulmonary crackles, rhonchi, and loud bronchial sounds may be auscultated.
- Signs of pulmonary hypertension and cardiac decompensation may be evident.

Laboratory Studies

Standard laboratory studies vary, depending on the patient's age, clinical signs, and preference of individual clinicians.

- The minimum pretreatment database for all dogs suspected of having heartworm infection includes packed cell volume (PCV), blood urea nitrogen (BUN), urine specific gravity, and heartworm antigen test.
- Middle-aged and older dogs and dogs with moderate to severe signs, occult infections, infection of unknown duration, and concomitant problems should have a more extensive database.
  - Include a complete blood count (CBC), platelet count, serum biochemistry profile, and urinalysis.
  - We recommend thoracic radiographs because they reveal more about disease severity than any other single test.
- Cats always require thoracic radiographs. Fecal studies for lungworms, cardiac ultrasound, and/or a nonselective angiogram often are needed for diagnosis. A tracheal or bronchial wash can rule out other lung diseases.

Screening

Screening for heartworm infection usually is done in the spring in cooler climates to maximize the likelihood of detecting infections acquired in the previous year. In hotter climates where the transmission season is longer than 6 months, infections may be acquired as late as November and early December, and these infections are not detectable until May or June. Antigen testing is the preferred method for dogs. Antibody testing, followed by antigen testing when the antibody test is positive, is appropriate for cats.

Immunodiagnostic Tests

These tests must be performed in strict compliance with the manufacturer's instructions. False-positive test results are usually the result of poor technique.

- Immunodiagnostic testing currently is the recommended screening procedure.
  - The absence of circulating microfilariae in infected dogs is common (10–50%), and they rarely are detected in infected cats.
  - In some highly endemic regions, such as Hawaii, as many as 50% of infected dogs lack circulating microfilariae.

Heartworm Antigen Tests

- Serodiagnosis of adult heartworm antigens in dogs is accomplished readily by ELISA, colloidal gold, and agglutination tests. A number of very specific and sensitive tests are available.
- The particular test employed is influenced by the number of tests performed daily, the amount of whole blood or serum required, and the speed of results.
  - Some tests, such as Dirochek (Synbiotics), are very efficient for testing multiple samples simultaneously.
  - Some tests require more serum than others.
  - The so-called stat tests provide quick results while the client waits.
- Weakly positive test results should be verified either by repeating the test, preferably using a different

antigen test, or by microfilarial tests or thoracic radiographs.

- All immunodiagnostic tests are semiquantitative because rapid and strong positive test results are thought to be related to higher antigen concentrations.
  - The greater the antigen concentration, the greater the worm burden.
  - Alternative adulticide treatment protocols for heavy worm burdens may be warranted.
- Immunodiagnostic tests are the tests of choice in dogs receiving chronic preventive therapy with ivermectin, milbemycin, or moxidectin.
- In cats, antigen tests are specific but less sensitive, and false-negative results are common. False-negative test results are explained by typically low worm burden, single-sex infections, and infection with young worms.

Heartworm Antibody Tests

Heartworm-associated antibody tests (Animal Diagnostics, St. Louis, MO, and Heska Corporation, Ft. Collins, CO) are useful to rule out infections in cats.

- Often performed in combination with an antigen test.
- A negative test result weighs heavily against the diagnosis.
- A strongly positive test result indicates preadult infection, live adult infection, or persistent antibodies after adult heartworm death. An antigen test or other studies are needed to confirm the diagnosis.
- Intermediate titers should be repeated in 1 month, if necessary. Also, other tests that may support a diagnosis should be evaluated—thoracic radiographs, serum globulins (hyperglobulinemia), CBC (eosinophilia, basophilia), and echocardiogram.

Microfilaria Detection

- In dogs, the incidence of occult (microfilaremic) infections is greater than the incidence of false-negative antigen test results.
- Annual microfilarial detection tests are recommended for dogs receiving diethylcarbamazine prophylaxis.
- Microfilarial detection tests are indicated for heartworm antigen-positive dogs.
  - Evaluate a direct blood smear immediately after procurement of a diagnostic blood sample. If the direct smear is negative, a concentration test is indicated.
  - The Knott test (a centrifugal, concentration test) or a filter test (e.g., Difil Test, Evsco) is acceptable for the detection of microfilariae. Each methodology has advantages and disadvantages, but efficacy is similar.

Radiography
Pulmonary Arterial Disease

- The degree of caudal lobar arterial disease is best assessed by the dorsoventral projection.

- The caudal lobar arteries, especially the right, are the first to enlarge and typically are the most severely diseased. The diameters of the caudal lobar arteries should not exceed that of the ninth rib at the point of their superimposition.
- Tortuosity and pruning of the arteries (the latter due to thromboembolism) are best seen on the dorsoventral projection; the caudal lobar vessels are the most severely affected.
- The cranial lobar arteries are best evaluated on the lateral projection; their diameters should not exceed that of the proximal portions of the fourth rib. In cats, nonselective angiograms delineate these vessels more clearly.
- Nonselective angiography may be diagnostic in cats with heartworm disease and is useful in suspected cases when the ELISA antigen test is negative.
  - Not required if the heartworm antibody test is negative
  - Not required if worms are identified by echocardiography

▼ **Key Point** Thoracic radiography is the most important diagnostic test for determining the severity of heartworm disease.

Parenchymal Lung Disease

- Parenchymal lung disease results from the pulmonary arteriolar thromboembolism with leakage of plasma and inflammatory cells into the adjacent tissues.
- Severity varies; disease is most prevalent in the caudal and intermediate lung lobes and is most concentrated surrounding the lobar arteries.

Allergic Pneumonitis

- It is associated with occult infections, eosinophilia, coughing, and dyspnea.
  - This incidence is 10% to 20% of occult infections.
  - This mixed diffuse interstitial-alveolar lung disease is best visualized in the caudal lobes.
- It often occurs with minimal pulmonary arterial enlargement.
- It may be mistaken, radiographically, for left-sided CHF (pulmonary edema) or blastomycosis.
- It responds rapidly to antiinflammatory dosages of corticosteroids continued for 3 to 7 days.
  - Begin adulticide treatment soon after clinical and radiographic signs subside.

Feline Asthma-Like Syndrome

- Coughing, wheezing, and dyspnea are consistent with feline heartworm infection.
- Radiographic picture resembles feline asthma.
- Typically occurs 3–5 months postinoculation of L_3.
- May be associated with eosinophilia or basophilia.

Clinical Pathology

No abnormal test results are pathognomonic for heartworm infection.

Complete Blood Count

- *Eosinophilia and basophilia* are the most common abnormalities in dogs.
  - Eosinophilia is more common; the highest eosinophil and basophil counts tend to occur in occult infections.
  - *Dipetalonema reconditum* infections produce eosinophilia equal to or greater than that associated with heartworm disease.
- *Neutrophilic leukocytosis,* often with a left shift, occurs with pulmonary thromboembolism.
- *Thrombocytopenia* commonly is associated with severe pulmonary arterial and parenchymal lung disease.
  - Activated clotting time is increased marginally to moderately in many cases.
  - DIC develops in some animals with severe thromboembolic disease.
- *Hemoglobinuria,* usually accompanied by thrombocytopenia, is seen with the vena cava syndrome and with severe pulmonary thromboembolic disease.
  - Heparin, 75–200 U/kg q8hr SC, usually reduces hemoglobinuria due to severe lung disease.

Serum Biochemistries and Urinalysis

- *Azotemia* may occur in dogs with complicated infections.
  - Prerenal azotemia can be caused by dehydration or right-sided CHF.
  - Primary azotemia can result from glomerulopathies, including immune complex disease and amyloidosis.
- *Increased serum hepatic enzyme levels* may occur; however, increases up to 10-fold do not affect treatment, complications, or survival.
- *Hepatic insufficiency,* evidenced by increased serum bile acid levels, can occur, but mild to moderate increases do not alter the treatment protocol.
- *Proteinuria* is common and is most pronounced in patients with severe infections or renal amyloidosis.
  - Nephrotic syndrome is a contraindication to treatment.
  - In the absence of hypoalbuminemia, most cases of proteinuria resolve after effective heartworm treatment.
- *Hypoalbuminemia* occurs in some dogs with severe infections; hyperglobulinemia is common in dogs and cats with chronic heartworm disease.
  - Loss of albumin into the third space occurs with right-sided CHF and is complicated by hepatic insufficiency, intestinal congestion, and free-water retention.
  - Proteinuria, when severe, produces hypoalbuminemia.

Electrocardiography

Electrocardiography (ECG) is sometimes helpful in animals with severe heartworm disease, especially for evaluation of arrhythmias; however, it is not a sensitive test for identification of mild-to-moderate hypertrophy.

- A right ventricular hypertrophy pattern is common in dogs with severe pulmonary hypertension and is found in 90% of dogs with overt right-sided CHF (ascites). However, significant pulmonary hypertension may exist in the absence of ECG abnormalities.
- Occasionally, cardiac rhythm disturbances occur in dogs with severe infections. Atrial fibrillation is the most common arrhythmia, especially in larger breeds.

Ultrasonography

- Evidence of right ventricular and pulmonary artery enlargement can be detected by M-mode and two-dimensional (2-D) echocardiography in patients with moderate to severe pulmonary hypertension.
- Occasionally, worms may be detected in the right ventricle and the main pulmonary artery during 2-D ultrasonography.
- Ultrasonography is particularly useful in cats in which the diagnosis of infection is often difficult, and worms are more likely to be found in the heart or proximal pulmonary arteries.
- Echocardiography is the test of choice for diagnosis of caval syndrome (mass of worms is found in the tricuspid valve orifice).

CLASSIFICATION OF HEARTWORM DISEASE SEVERITY

Severity of heartworm disease is determined by worm burden, duration of infection, and host responses to the worms. Most severe pulmonary complication are associated with occult infections. Four classes are defined to customize Immiticide treatment.

- Class 1: Asymptomatic or mild clinical signs.
- Class 2: Moderate clinical and radiographic abnormalities.
- Class 3: Severe clinical and radiographic abnormalities, including right-sided CHF.
- Class 4: Caval syndrome.

TREATMENT

The goal of treatment is to kill all adult heartworms with an adulticide and all microfilariae with a microfilaricide, and to accomplish this with minimal drug toxicity and a tolerable degree of pulmonary thromboembolism from the dying worms.

Patient Selection

Although most heartworm-infected dogs can be treated successfully, there are exceptions. Most clinicians consider the mortality associated with thiacetarsamide therapy in cats unacceptably high, and a safe and effective regimen for melarsomine dihydrochloride is not yet established; consequently, adulticide therapy seldom is recommended for cats.

Contraindications to Adulticide Treatment

- Hepatic failure
- Nephrotic syndrome
- Advanced renal failure
- Combination of right-sided CHF and severe renal azotemia
- Concomitant life-threatening disorders

Treatment of Old Dogs

- Experience is limited in the treatment of very old dogs. Heartworm disease may be nonprogressive in old dogs that have chronic infections with low worm burdens.
  - Low antigen level is seen.
  - Monthly administration of ivermectin (Heartgard Plus, Meriel) at the standard prophylactic dosage (see Prevention section) will gradually kill adult worms in 16 to 20 months.

Treatment of Cats

- Treat pulmonary signs in cats with prednisolone (1.0–2.0 mg/kg, daily for 10 days; then taper the dose to prevent signs of disease). Do not use aspirin in cats; thiacetarsamide is used only as a last resort, and melarsomine dihydrochloride should not be used until a safe and effective dosage and treatment schedule for cats has been determined.

Adulticide Therapy

The approved available adulticidal agent is melarsomine dihydrochloride (Immiticide; Meriel). Thiacetarsamide sodium (Caparsolate) is not currently available and is not recommended by the authors. The following regimens have proved effective in dogs (see *Aspirin*, this chapter.)

- Immiticide is the treatment of choice.
  - Highly efficacious
  - Reasonably good therapeutic index
  - Easy to administer

Standard Immiticide Protocol

The manufacturer recommends that Class 1 and Class 2 heartworm infections be treated by the standard Immiticide protocol.

- 2.5 mg/kg Immiticide injected IM twice, 24 hours apart.
- The two doses contain 0.75 mg/kg of total arsenic compared with 1.56 mg/kg of total arsenic administered by the standard four doses of Caparsolate. This lower arsenic dosage results in increased heartworm kill, as compared with Caparsolate, because more unbound arsenic is available for worm uptake, and lethal concentrations are maintained for a longer time period.
- Two injections (separated by 24 hours) are given into the epaxial musculature at the level of the third to fifth lumbar vertebrae. One injection is given on each side of the dorsal midline.
- The appropriate volume of the reconstituted drug is aspirated into a syringe, and then a new needle is placed on the syringe.
- For dogs weighing more than 10 kg, a 1½-inch 22-gauge needle is used, and for smaller dogs, a 1-inch 23-gauge needle is used.
- The injection should be completed before the needle is withdrawn, and finger pressure should be applied over the needle tract during and for a short time after withdrawal.

Alternate Immiticide Protocol

Class 3 infections, pound dogs, and dogs with high antigen concentrations should be treated by the alternate Immiticide protocol. Some clinicians prefer to treat all infections using the alternate protocol.

- There is concern that the high kill rate associated with the standard Immiticide protocol provokes more frequent or more severe post-treatment pulmonary thromboembolism. Such concern is based, up to this point in time, on anecdotal experiences, not on controlled studies.
- A single, initial injection (2.5 mg/kg) is used.
- Fifty percent of adult worms are killed; therefore, postadulticide thromboembolic complications are reduced.
- Two follow-up injections, each at the same rate as the previously administered injection, at a 24-hour interval, are administered after 1 to 2 months. Post-treatment thromboembolism reoccurs, but the severity is reduced because fewer worms are present.
- The extra 1 to 2 months required for maximum worm kill do not appear to be detrimental.
- Current data indicate that 100% of male and 98% of female worms are killed.

▼ *Key Point* Use the alternate Immiticide protocol to treat dogs with Class 3 infections, pound dogs, and those with high antigen concentrations.

Treatment of Class 3 Heartworm Disease

Severe pulmonary arterial disease occurs in 10% of infected dogs in highly endemic regions. Infections are often occult. There are at least four treatment options.

- Option 1 is recommended for dogs that do not require continuous supplemental oxygen therapy, are eating, and have normal or pale pink mucosal color.
- Options 2, 3, or 4 are recommended for hemodynamically unstable dogs that require oxygen support, are anorectic, and have very pale, grey, or cyanotic mucosal color.

Option 1

Use the alternate Immiticide protocol (see Adulticide Therapy section). Supportive therapy, such as judicious fluid administration, low-salt diet, and diuretics or short-term corticosteroids may be indicated.

Option 2

Forceps extraction of adult worms from the pulmonary arteries.

- Only for patients with many worms in the right heart and pulmonary arteries.
  - High antigen concentration.
  - Ultrasound confirmation of high worm burden.
- Requires fluoroscopy and a long, flexible, alligator forceps that is introduced into the right jugular vein via a surgical approach and manipulated through the heart into the pulmonary arteries. Numerous passages to grasp and remove worms are required.
- This procedure is highly effective in experienced hands.
- Treat with an adulticide to kill remaining worms after the patient has stabilized, if worms remain, based on:
  - Ultrasound detection.
  - Positive antigen test result after 3–4 months.
- Follow with microfilaricide therapy when appropriate.

Option 3

Cage confinement and aspirin in conjunction with the alternate Immiticide protocol (see Adulticide Therapy section).

- Place patient in cage confinement for 1 to 3 weeks before, during, and for 3 weeks after adulticide therapy. This may be the important component of treatment.
- Begin Immiticide therapy after 3 weeks of cage confinement.
- Give aspirin (5 mg/kg daily) throughout the treatment period, beginning 1 to 3 weeks before adulticide therapy and continuing 3 weeks after the second course of treatment.
  - Gastrointestinal (GI) bleeding is possible.
  - Monitor the hematocrit.
  - Although efficacy is unproven, consider GI protection with an H_2 blocker and/or sucralfate.
- Prescribe a diuretic and low-salt diet for patients with concomitant, overt right-sided CHF.
- If the patient lives long enough to complete the treatment, the survival rate is 70% to 80%, compared with 40% to 50% in patients given standard treatment.
- This option is time consuming, labor intensive, and expensive.

Option 4

Cage confinement and heparin in conjunction with the alternate Immiticide protocol (see Adulticide Therapy section).

- Place patient in cage confinement for 1 week before, during, and for 3 weeks after the second adulticide treatment.

- Give heparin (75 units/kg, SC, q8hr) for 1 week before, during, and for 3 weeks after the second course of Immiticide treatment.
- Prescribe a low-salt diet and diuretic for patients with concomitant, overt right-sided CHF.
- Survival rate is at least 70% to 80% if the patient lives long enough to complete the treatment.
- This option is time consuming, labor intensive, and expensive.

Side Effects and Efficacy

- Mild myositis of 1 to 3 days' duration often is observed after Immiticide injections. Approximately one-third of treated dogs experience some swelling, and a sterile seroma occurs uncommonly.
- Hepatic and renal toxicity associated with Immiticide is uncommon; toxic doses produce pulmonary edema in dogs and cats.
- Immiticide (2 doses) kills a greater percentage of adult and immature heartworms (90%) as compared with those killed by 4 doses of Caparsolate (30–86%).
  - Confirmation of efficacy can be established at 4 months after Immiticide injection by antigen testing.
  - At least 80% seroconversion occurs with Immiticide compared with 67% seroconversion with Caparsolate.
  - Mean antigen concentration is reduced to 1% of pretreatment levels, indicating nearly complete elimination of worms, whereas antigen levels are reduced to 10% of pretreatment levels 4 months after Caparsolate treatment.

Postadulticide Complications

Strict patient confinement is essential for 4 to 6 weeks post-treatment.

- Thromboembolic complications may occur from several days to 4 or even 6 weeks postadulticide.
- Most complications occur between 1 to 3 weeks postadulticide.
- Most severe reactions occur in dogs with Class 3 infections and those associated with high antigen concentrations.
  - Coughing, gagging, lethargy, anorexia, tachypnea, dyspnea, syncope, hemoptysis, and fever are common.
  - Thrombocytopenia, inflammatory leukogram, and prolonged activated clotting time often are observed.
  - Radiographic evidence of parenchymal lung disease is usual.

Drug Storage

- Immiticide is purchased as a lyophilized powder that does not require refrigeration and has a shelf life of at least 2 years.
  - Reconstituted drug must be kept refrigerated. The potential for loss of potency during prolonged storage has not been investigated.

Treatment of Vena Cava Syndrome

Vena cava syndrome (Class 4) is uncommon except in highly endemic regions. It is associated with large numbers of worms in the right heart and vena cava. It is seen most often in the late spring and early summer in young dogs that have received a heavy L_3 inoculation over a short time period the previous year.

- Acute cardiovascular collapse and shock occur.
  - It is rapidly lethal unless surgical treatment is provided quickly.
  - Clinical signs variably include a systolic heart murmur, gallop heart rhythm, and hemoglobinuria.
  - Echocardiography is diagnostic.
- Surgical retrieval of the worms is the only recommended acute treatment.
  - Use minimal sedation
  - Administer local anesthesia and perform surgical cutdown on the right jugular vein
  - Introduce and advance a long alligator forceps to to the heart base and retrieve as many worms as possible during multiple passages
  - This is highly effective but experience is required for optimal results
- Provide supportive care for 1–3 weeks.
- Adulticide treatment then is administered to eliminate remaining worms.

Microfilaricide Therapy

Always complete adulticide treatment before initiating microfilaricide therapy, which is recommended 4 weeks postadulticide.

- Attempts to eliminate microfilariae before completion of adulticide treatment are only partially effective.
- Adverse reactions to microfilaricide treatment are either toxic or microfilaricidal in origin.
  - Because of the high therapeutic indices of these drugs, toxic reactions should not occur at recommended dosages.
  - Some collies react to microfilaricidal doses of either ivermectin or milbemycin oxime.
- Rapid death of high numbers of microfilariae may produce adverse effects.
  - Less than 10% incidence
  - Usually mild
  - Cardiovascular shock is uncommon and responds to fluids and corticosteroids, if detected early in its course.
  - Decreased appetite and lethargy may be observed for 1–2 days in any dog.

▼ **Key Point** Ivermectin and milbemycin oxime are the most effective microfilaricidal drugs; they are associated with the fewest complications and are the easiest to use. Treatment recommendations are based on published research because neither drug is FDA approved for use as a microfilaricide. Their use for this purpose is considered the standard of practice.

Ivermectin (Ivomec; MSD Agvet)

- Administer 50 µg/kg as a 1:9 dilution (1 ml Ivomec added to 9 ml of water or propylene glycol) at a dosage of 1 ml/20 kg PO at 4 weeks postadulticidal therapy.
  - Diluted drug must be used immediately, not stored.
- To maintain dosage accuracy in small dogs, Heartgard brand of ivermectin is recommended at the aforementioned dosage.
- Safe for use in collies at the recommended preventive dosage.
- Administer the drug in the morning and observe the patient throughout the day for signs of toxicity, such as vomiting, depression, diarrhea, and shock. If cardiovascular instability is suspected, give IV lactated Ringer's solution (20 ml/kg), with a soluble corticosteroid (dexamethasone SP, 2 mg/kg, IV).
- Perform a microfilarial concentration test in 3 weeks. If the test is positive, two options are available.
  - If few microfilariae are detected, macrolide prophylaxis may be initiated, and the remaining microfilariae will disappear over a period of 6–8 months.
  - The other option is to repeat the ivermectin protocol; then repeat the microfilarial concentration test in 3 weeks. Positive results in this test indicate that persistent adult worms are likely present, requiring repetition of the adulticide phase of therapy.
- If the test is negative, begin prophylactic therapy (see discussion on heartworm prevention).

Milbemycin Oxime (Interceptor)

- Administer at 0.5 mg/kg.
- Follow the same treatment and follow-up guidelines as for ivermectin.

Therapy Variations
Occult Infections

Microfilaricide therapy is not indicated in the absence of microfilaremia.

Microfilariae: To Treat or Not to Treat

Some veterinarians do not administer a microfilaricide.

- There is an absence of proven pathologic changes associated with microfilariae.
- With the advent of highly sensitive antigen tests, it is no longer necessary to document the persistent elimination of microfilariae to confirm the elimination of adult worms.
- Macrolide prophylaxis eliminates microfilariae in 6–8 months.
- There is fear of adverse reaction in collies.
- However, it must be appreciated that microfilaremic dogs are reservoirs of heartworm infection until the microfilariae disappear.

When to Start Prophylaxis

Prophylaxis usually is initiated 3–4 weeks after adulticide treatment of occult infections or immediately after elimination of microfilariae.

- If Immiticide is used as the adulticide, a window of opportunity for reinfection is closed because this drug is also larvacidal.
- The "reach-back" effect of Heartgard also closes the window of reinfection for up to 4 months previously as long as the drug is administered every month for at least 1 year.

Confirmation of Adulticide Efficacy

Four months after adulticide treatment, an antigen test should be performed.

- A strongly positive test result indicates that live heartworms remain.
  - It most often is associated with Caparsolate treatment and is rare with Immiticide.
  - Retreatment is recommended, and Immiticide is the drug of choice.
- A weakly positive test result may be the result of a few persisting live worms.
  - Wait 1 additional month and retest.
  - Whether to retreat is controversial. If Immiticide was the adulticide that was administered, very few worms are likely to have survived. Retreatment may not be necessary. For Class 3 infections, for infections with an initially high antigen concentration, if clinical signs persist, and for performance dogs, retreatment is recommended.

Adjuncts in Adulticide Therapy

Aspirin

- Reduces pulmonary arterial lesions and improves intrapulmonary blood flow.
- For Class 3 disease only, we recommend prescribing 5 mg/kg, q24h, PO, beginning 7 to 21 days before adulticide therapy, during, and continuing for 21 days after.
- Combine with strict cage confinement.
- Avoid the combination of aspirin and glucocorticoids (increased risk of serious gastrointestinal ulceration).

Heparin

- Can be used for Class 3 infections instead of aspirin.
- 75 units/kg, SC q8h, for 1 week before, during, and for 21 days after adulticide treatment.
- Combine with strict cage confinement.

Corticosteroids

- Reduces parenchymal disease in the lungs but promotes thrombosis and reduces pulmonary arterial blood flow if used for longer than 10 to 14 consecutive days.
- Do not use routinely but only as needed to control sequelae (see the following discussion).

Oxygen

- The only effective means of dilating the pulmonary arteries.
- For Class 3 infections associated with dyspnea, orthopnea, or congestive heart failure.
- Administer intranasally or by oxygen cage.

TREATMENT OF SEQUELAE

Occult Heartworm Allergic Pneumonitis

This complication occurs in 10% to 20% of patients with occult infections.

- Clinical signs include dyspnea, coughing, respiratory crackles, and exercise intolerance.
- Thoracic radiographs reveal diffuse interstitial-alveolar infiltrates.
- Eosinophilia is common, and in tracheal lavage cytology eosinophils usually predominate.
- The syndrome responds well to oral prednisone (1–2 mg/kg, q24h for several days). Stop prednisone therapy after 3–7 days and begin adulticide therapy.

Pulmonary Eosinophilic Granulomatosis

This uncommon complication of occult heartworm disease probably results from the granulomatous inflammation known to be associated with occult infections. The reaction in some cases is progressive and assumes a neoplastic-like behavior.

- Clinical signs are coughing and dyspnea.
- Eosinophilia and basophilia are common findings, and hyperglobulinemia may occur.
- Pleural effusion (eosinophilic) occurs occasionally.
- Intrathoracic lymphadenopathy is always present.
- Multiple pulmonary nodules develop simultaneously and sequentially, grow at variable rates, and are 1–10 cm in diameter or larger.
- The trachea, liver, spleen, kidneys, abdominal lymph nodes, and intestines sometimes are infiltrated with eosinophils and eosinophilic granulomas.
- Combination chemotherapy is recommended:
  - Prednisone (50 mg/m^2 q24h) plus azathioprine (Imuran) (50 mg/m^2, q24h PO for 7–10 days; then alternate days).
- Therapy usually results initially in partial or complete remission, but relapse is common even with continued aggressive therapy or when drug dosages are reduced.
- The duration of therapy is indefinite, and the prognosis is poor.
- Consider lung lobectomy for focal lesions.

Thromboembolic Lung Disease

This common sequela of moderate to severe pulmonary arterial disease can occur before adulticide therapy (especially in cats) but is most common 7–21 days after adulticide therapy. In dogs:

- Clinical signs include coughing, dyspnea, fever, and occasionally hemoptysis.

- A regenerative leukocytosis with thrombocytopenia usually is present.
- Thoracic radiographs reveal severe pulmonary arterial disease with periarterial parenchymal disease of variable severity.
- The following therapy usually is successful:
  - Initiate cage confinement for 5–10 days.
  - Administer prednisone (1.0 mg/kg, q24h for 3–10 days).
  - Use intranasal or cage-administered oxygen for dyspneic patients.

PREVENTION

A microfilarial examination is indicated before the initiation of any preventative. A microfilarial examination always is indicated before initiation of diethylcarbamazine and before each restarting of diethylcarbamazine. Prevention should be in place whenever the average daily temperature exceeds approximately 57°F. Year-round prevention usually is practiced in hotter climates, even though transmission is less likely in December and January in the continental United States.

- Start as early as 6–8 weeks of age.
  - In cooler climates, start puppies on prophylaxis as soon after 6–8 weeks of age as dictated by seasonal risk.
- Macrolides (ivermectin, milbemycin) should be started within 1 month of the transmission season. These drugs kill migrating larvae during the first 6–8 weeks after L_3 inoculation.
- Milbemycin is a potent microfilaricide at the preventative dosage.
  - Test for microfilariae before prescribing.
  - Adverse reactions can occur if the microfilarial count is high.
- Successful prophylaxis is confirmed by a negative antigen test result 1 year after initiation.
- Macrolides are safe for collies when prescribed according to the label.
- After adulticide treatment of infected dogs, preventive treatment should be initiated 1 month later.
  - 1 month after the second injection of the standard Immiticide protocol
  - 1 month after the last treatment of the alternate Immiticide protocol

▼ *Key Point* In all studies to date, owner administration compliance has been poor.

Ivermectin

Ivermectin (Heartgard; MSD Ag Vet), 6–12 μg/kg given monthly, is an effective preventive drug. A chewable formulation of Ivermectin plus pyrantel pamoate (Heartgard Plus) is an effective heartworm preventive that also controls ascarid and hookworm infections.

- Drug reactions are rare at the recommended dosage.
- Chronic administration of ivermectin suppresses microfilariae in heartworm-positive dogs.
- If initiated within 4 months of L_3 inoculation and continued for at least 1 year, the likelihood of developing infection is reduced by at least 98%.
- Heartgard Plus kills adult heartworms slowly over a 16- to 20-month period.
- A dose of 24 μg/kg administered monthly is an effective heartworm prophylaxis in cats, and it removes and controls hookworms in this host.

Milbemycin Oxime

Milbemycin (Interceptor; Ciba-Geigy), 0.5–0.99 mg/kg, is an effective once-a-month preventive agent for heartworm disease in dogs and cats.

- It is not as effective as ivermectin at preventing the maturation of larvae when monthly administration is started 4 months postinoculation.
- It also controls hookworms, roundworm, and whipworm infestations.

Moxidectin

Moxidectin (Fort Dodge/American Cyanamid), 1–3 μg/kg, is an effective once-a-month heartworm preventive.

▼ *Key Point* All macrolide preventive drugs kill microfilariae; for this reason, chronic dosing with ivermectin or milbemycin leads to "occult" nonmicrofilaremic status in infected dogs.

Diethylcarbamazine

Diethylcarbamazine (2.5–3.0 mg/kg, PO) given daily is an effective prophylactic drug. If the owner skips more than 2 days of treatment, do not reinstitute preventive treatment before performing a microfilarial concentration test.

▼ *Key Point* Never initiate diethylcarbamazine treatment in microfilaremic dogs because an anaphylactoid reaction may develop.

- Duration of efficacy is short because the drug appears to affect the L_3–L_4 (larval) molt 9–12 days postinfection.
- Begin therapy before the mosquito season and continue for 2 months after the first frost (or year-round in regions that have mosquitos all year).
- All diethylcarbamazine products are equally effective.
- Combination diethylcarbamazine and oxibendazole (Filaribits Plus; Pfizer) is a popular product in regions where intestinal helminths are prevalent. An occasional side effect of oxibendazole is characterized by increased liver enzyme activity, icterus, and hepatic insufficiency, which is usually reversible after drug discontinuation.

Retesting Dogs Receiving Macrolide Prophylaxis

Macrolide prophylactic drugs are highly efficacious, and therefore annual retesting often is not performed; however, we recommend retesting.

- Owner compliance has been proven to be poor in all regions examined.
- Inadequate dosing is likely in growing puppies.

SUPPLEMENTAL READINGS

Calvert CA, Rawlings CA, McCall JW: Feline heartworm disease. In Sherding RG (ed): The Cat: Diseases and Clinical Management. New York: Churchill Livingstone, 1994, p 623.

Calvert CA, Rawlings CA: Canine heartworm disease. In Fox PR (ed): Canine and Feline Cardiology. New York: Churchill Livingstone, 1997.

Hribernik TN: Canine and feline heartworm disease. In Kirk RW (ed): Current Veterinary Therapy, X. Philadelphia: WB Saunders, 1989, p 263.

Rawlings CA, Calvert CA: Heartworm disease. In: Ettinger SJ (ed): Textbook of Veterinary Internal Medicine. Philadelphia: WB Saunders, 1995, p 1046.

69 Vascular Diseases

John D. Bonagura / Rebecca L. Stepien

Lesions of the blood vessels are quite common in small animals. In many instances, the vascular endothelium or vessel wall represents the target tissue of a multisystemic disease. In other situations, vascular disease impairs organ function by affecting tissue perfusion or venous return.

This chapter considers some of the more important disorders of the vascular system in small animals. Both systemic hypertension and pulmonary hypertension represent emerging disorders of clinical importance. Systemic arterial thrombosis and arterial embolism can produce devastating clinical conditions that suddenly impact organ or tissue function. Pulmonary thromboembolism is recognized as a complication of a number of diverse diseases. Additional vascular disorders of clinical importance include vasculitis, arteriosclerosis, atherosclerosis, vascular neoplasia, and arteriovenous fistula.

SYSTEMIC HYPERTENSION

Factors Affecting Blood Pressure

Systemic arterial hypertension can be defined as an increase in systolic or diastolic arterial blood pressure (ABP). Hypertension is identified by measurement of the ABP. In most cases, this is done noninvasively, using either a Doppler flow technique or an oscillometric method. The following aspects of ABP tracings are pertinent to assessment and measurement.

Systolic Pressure

- Peak ABP depends on the prior diastolic pressure, the ventricular stroke volume, and the compliance of the arterial system (especially the aorta). Consider pressures exceeding > 160 mm Hg suspicious and values persistently greater than 180 mm Hg abnormal, provided that the animal is quiet, does not have tachycardia, and is not struggling.
- A potential reason for isolated systolic hypertension in cats is the aortic increase in rigidity associated with age-related aortic dilation.
- Similarly, systemic illnesses associated with increased sympathetic nervous system activity (e.g., hyperthyroidism) may be associated with increased stroke volume and systolic hypertension.

Diastolic Pressure

Diastolic pressure is the minimum arterial blood pressure.

- Diastolic ABP depends on systemic vascular resistance, cardiac output, and heart rate. Vasodilation associated with systemic diseases or therapies (e.g., anemia, hyperthyroidism, or arterial vasodilator therapy) often lowers diastolic pressure.
- Diastolic pressure is more difficult to estimate with the Doppler method, but it is possible to gauge an approximate diastolic pressure. Consider diastolic pressures exceeding 100 to 110 mm Hg to be high, assuming that the animal is not excited during the recording. Begin treatment if values exceed 120 mm Hg.
- The arterial *pulse pressure* is the difference between systolic and diastolic ABP.

Mean Arterial Blood Pressure

- The mean arterial pressure is the geometric mean of pressure during the cardiac cycle and is closer to the diastolic than the systolic reading. To estimate mean ABP, calculate the pulse pressure, divide this by ⅓, and then add the result to the diastolic pressure.
- Oscillometric ABP devices measure this variable by detecting maximum oscillations in the blood vessel wall that correspond to the mean ABP.

CLINICAL FEATURES OF SYSTEMIC HYPERTENSION

Be familiar with the causes and clinical associations related to systemic hypertension because some disorders are treatable and may minimize the need for antihypertensive therapy. Hypertension is idiopathic, or "essential," in some dogs and cats.

Etiology

A variety of clinical disorders have been associated with increases in ABP in dogs and cats. The precise mechanisms underlying hypertension in animals are not well understood except in experimental cases. Inability to regulate plasma volume (e.g., renal disease, hyperadrenocorticism), excessive adrenergic activity (e.g., pheochromocytoma), increased cardiac output (e.g., hyperthyroidism), and activation of the reninangiotensin system are likely mechanisms. Common clinical associations include:

- Renal disease (particularly glomerular disease)
- Hyperadrenocorticism—both Cushing's disease (glucocorticoid excess) and Conn's disease in cats (mineralocorticoid excess)
- Pheochromocytoma (catecholamine-producing tumor of the adrenal medulla)
- Hyperthyroidism
- Drugs (e.g., alpha-adrenergic agonists causing vasoconstriction)
- Central nervous system (CNS) disorders
- Idiopathic or "essential" hypertension

Clinical Signs of Hypertension

Injury to blood vessels or direct transmission of pressure across the microcirculation is responsible for many of the clinical signs of hypertension. Additionally, the left ventricle must hypertrophy to maintain an increase in pressure work. Other clinical signs are attributed to the underlying disease responsible for elevated ABP. The eyes, brain, heart, and kidneys are the main *target organs* of systemic hypertension.

- Retinal edema or hemorrhage and retinal detachments causing blindness. Sudden blindness also may develop due to intraocular hemorrhage and hyphema.
- Cerebral or brainstem vascular injury leading to edema or hemorrhage. Clinical signs include abnormal mentation, neurologic deficits, head tilt, seizures, and coma.
- A systolic cardiac murmur or atrial (S_4) gallop sound may indicate hypertensive heart disease. Left ventricular hypertrophy and cardiomegaly are the markers for chronic hypertension and can be identified by an echocardiogram (most sensitive), electrocardiogram, or thoracic radiograph (least sensitive). A systolic heart murmur may represent mitral regurgitation or flow into a dilated aorta. Chronic systemic hypertension can lead to aortic dilatation even in relatively young animals. Coronary arteries also are injured from high arterial pressures. Heart failure stemming from hypertensive heart disease is exceedingly rare; however, distinguish the condition from primary hypertrophic cardiomyopathy in cats. In dogs with chronic mitral valve disease, systemic hypertension increases the load on the left ventricle and increases the regurgitant volume.
- Abnormal renal contour or size, proteinuria, and mild-to-moderate azotemia often are found in hypertensive animals. Not only can renal disease be the trigger of systemic hypertension, but elevated ABP causes further injury to glomerular vessels and damages renal tissues.
- Epistaxis or bleeding from other sites also has been reported with hypertension, especially the labile hypertension of pheochromocytoma.

Diagnosis of Systemic Hypertension

Diagnosis of hypertension requires measurement of ABP using either an arterial puncture or an indirect determination that uses a reliable technology. Both oscillometric methods and Doppler flow methods have been used successfully for measuring ABP in dogs. Systolic ABP is slightly underestimated by this technique. Cats are difficult to evaluate noninvasively, but systolic pressures can be readily determined using Doppler flowmeter and occlusion cuff. Care must be taken to consider normal variation in excited animals. Slight differences between front and back limbs are normal in many animals, and the cuff size (diameter) is critical to prevent overestimation (too small a cuff) or underestimation (too wide a cuff). Because technical details are very important in establishing a correct diagnosis, consider the following pointers.

Technique for Measuring Blood Pressure

- Understand your unit and how it works.
- Practice on numerous animals of different sizes. Practice improves skill and confidence. Train others to measure ABP and compare results. When using Doppler methods, learn to evenly decrease the pressure in the cuff and manometer.
- Have a supply of different-sized pediatric cuffs (e.g., #1 through #6 pediatric cuffs, Critikon). Have a nonelastic, self-adhesive tape available to place around the cuff to prevent slippage (e.g., VetWrap). Do not allow the airlines to kink.
- Measure the limb and use an appropriate sized cuff. The cuff must compress the limb evenly and occlude the artery with the approximate pressure recorded by the manometer. Use the smallest cuff appropriate for the size. Cuff diameter should be 40% of the limb circumference in dogs and between 30% and 40% of the limb circumference in cats. There is often a 10- to 15-mm Hg difference between next sized cuffs.
- Place the cuff around the distal radius over a cylindrical portion of the limb. Secure the cuff and attach it to the manometer.
- Place the patient in either lateral or sternal recumbency on a *padded table*, in a *quiet room*, with *calm people*. Gently restrain the patient, and give the pet time to acclimatize to the environment.
- Measure heart rate (HR). If it is high (e.g., > 160 in a dog; > 240 in a cat), try to help the animal relax before proceeding.
- Consider the site of measurement relative to heart level (gravitational effects are minimal in most recumbent animals but could be considerable in a standing dog).
- Inflate the cuff one or two times, slowly and gently, and allow the animal to experience what will happen during measurement. Then record the pressure. With a Doppler method, place the crystal palmar and just distal to the large carpal pad. Repeat the measurement two more times noting values and HR.
- If using an automated device, measure at the tail base, antebrachium, or metatarsus. Place the two cuff

lines on either side of the artery. Measure HR with a stethoscope because it should correspond almost exactly with the automated monitor. If it does not, do not accept the displayed values.

- If the pressure is high, try the next sized larger cuff that will more easily compress the artery. If ABP is still high, the measurement is probably accurate.
- Interpret the findings of elevated pressure in conjunction with other clinical findings. In animals with ocular, renal, CNS, or cardiac disease, an elevated ABP measurement probably represents a true finding of hypertension. If other clinical findings are negative, measure the pressure at another time or day. Be sure of the diagnosis of "hypertension" before initiating drug therapy.
- If the ABP value is "low"—systolic pressure < 90 mm Hg—try the next smaller cuff. If still low, go to the hind limb to verify the low value. If the animal is not symptomatic, interpret the clinical situation and determine the most likely cause.

When evaluating the hypertensive patient, look for underlying causes. At a minimum, diagnostics include renal/adrenal (e.g., serum biochemistries, urinalysis, abdominal ultrasound, and possibly adrenal function tests). Perform thyroid evaluation in older cats.

TREATMENT OF HYPERTENSION

General Points

- Large studies of therapeutic efficacy in animals are unavailable. Treat the underlying problem (e.g., hyperthyroidism, hyperadrenocorticism) whenever possible.
- Modest dietary sodium restriction is reasonable, provided that the diet is eaten and caloric intake maintained. However, attempting to control significant hypertension by diet alone is ill advised; diet should be viewed as an adjunct to antihypertensive drug therapy.
- Blood pressure can be lowered pharmacologically by reducing cardiac output or dilating systemic arterioles. Therapy of systemic hypertension usually involves a stepwise approach, starting with a moderate dosage of one drug, increasing the dose to the desired effect as needed, or adding other drugs if required. Consider possible drug interactions when prescribing multiple drugs.

▼ *Key Point* Manage severe hypertension (e.g., ABP > 250 mm Hg), or hypertension in a symptomatic patient (retinal detachment, acute blindness, progressive CNS signs), aggressively. Treat with a diuretic plus a direct vasodilator (amlodipine in cats; hydralazine or nitroprusside in dogs). When the patient is not symptomatic, treat more conservatively. A variety of drugs can be prescribed for treatment of hypertension, discussion of which follows.

Calcium Channel Blockers

- Most clinicians initiate treatment of systemic hypertension in cats with the vasodilator, calcium-channel antagonist amlodipine besylate (Norvasc). This is effective and well-tolerated therapy based on a number of small, but convincing, clinical studies.
- The starting dose in cats is ¼ of a 2.5-mg tablet PO once daily. In some cases, higher doses, up to 1.25 mg PO q12h, may be needed. Unless urgent control of ABP is needed, increase the dose gradually, over several weeks. Amlodipine has a relatively slow onset and prolonged duration of action.
- Amlodipine monotherapy works better than either an angiotensin-converting enzyme (ACE) inhibitor or a beta blocker in cats.
- Amlodipine also can be used in dogs at an initial dose of 0.1 mg/kg PO q12–24h. Response is variable in dogs.

Angiotensin-Converting Enzyme Inhibitors

- Dogs often are treated initially with an ACE inhibitor (benazepril 0.5 mg/kg q12–24h or enalapril at the same dose). This is particularly reasonable therapy in dogs with glomerular disease (see Chap. 97).
- An ACE inhibitor also can be added to a calcium channel blocker in dogs or cats. In dogs with both mitral regurgitation and systemic hypertension, initiate therapy with an ACE inhibitor, even if the hypertension is mild and the dog asymptomatic. If this approach fails, add either a diuretic or amlodipine.

Diuretics

- Diuretics decrease cardiac filling and cardiac output and lower ABP.
- However, diuretic monotherapy is rarely successful, and the resulting volume contraction can worsen azotemia and activate the renin-angiotensin system.
- Diuretics are more appropriate as adjunctive therapy in urgent hypertensive situations or in unresponsive cases.
- A loop diuretic such as furosemide (1–3 mg/kg q12–24h) or a hydrochlorothiazide-spironolactone combination (2–4 mg/kg of the combined product q12–24h) can be used.

Beta-Adrenergic Blockers

- Beta blockers (propranolol 0.5–1.0 mg/kg q8h or atenolol 1–2 mg/kg PO q12–24h) decrease heart rate, cardiac output, and plasma renin activity and are useful as cotherapy in unresponsive cases of hypertension.
- Consider a beta blocker for initial management of hypertension caused by hyperthyroidism.

Other Drugs

- The direct-acting arterial vasodilator drug *hydralazine* (1–2 mg/kg q12h) combined with a diuretic is good *emergency* therapy for dogs or even cats with recent retinal detachments, although amlodipine still works well in cats for both acute and chronic treatment of hypertension.

- A 1- to 5-μg/kg/min infusion of *sodium nitroprusside* represents aggressive antihypertensive therapy.
- The alpha-adrenergic blocker *prazosin* is not used often because the drug is inconvenient to dose, but it can be effective in dogs unresponsive to other medications.

Follow-Up

- Reevaluate blood pressure regularly to ensure efficacy and prevent further organ injury.
- Signs of hypotension (weakness, depression, syncope, acute renal failure) must be anticipated and treated by reducing medication dosages.
- Because there are no large prospective studies to guide therapy, treat each patient individually.

ARTERIAL THROMBOSIS AND EMBOLISM

General Concepts

- *Thrombosis* refers to a blood clot within a blood vessel. Thrombi are capable of obstructing blood flow. *Embolism* is the sudden occlusion of an artery that occurs when a thrombus (or other substance) is carried from one point to another by the vascular system.
- Thrombosis may be initiated by different mechanisms.
  - Stasis of blood and activation of clotting factors cause systemic venous thrombosis (red thrombus). Deficiencies of plasma antithrombin III appear to predispose to venous thrombosis.
  - A systemic arterial thrombus typically starts with activation and aggregation of platelets (white thrombus). Arterial thrombosis frequently is initiated by injury to vascular endothelium or atrial endocardium.
- A thrombus can dislodge from the site of formation, producing a *thromboembolus*. Systemic thromboemboli are carried from the left side of the heart to the termination of an artery in the systemic circulation. Systemic venous thrombi can dislodge and travel with venous return across the right side of the heart and into the pulmonary arteries.
- A thrombus or embolus may obstruct blood flow. Consequences of vascular obstruction include *ischemia, infarction,* and *necrosis* of tissues nourished by that vessel and associated inflammatory reactions.
- Thrombus formation in a systemic vein or right side of the heart may obstruct systemic venous flow or be carried to the lungs, causing a *pulmonary embolism.*

Etiology

A number of clinical disorders are associated with the development of thrombi or emboli.

- Systemic arterial thrombi/emboli include:
  - Feline cardiomyopathy (thrombi form in the dilated left atrium)
  - Inflammation of the vessel wall (arteritis or vasculitis)
  - Bacterial endocarditis (thrombi can be shed from the vegetation)
  - Degenerative arterial disease (e.g., atherosclerosis)
  - Missile-like shotgun pellets that directly penetrate the vascular system
  - Aberrant filarial parasites in systemic arteries (*Dirofilaria immitis*)
  - Torsion of a vascular pedicle (e.g., splenic torsion, mesenteric torsion)
  - Cartilaginous embolism of the spinal cord vessels
  - Direct trauma or iatrogenic injury to arterial blood vessels
  - Disseminated intravascular coagulopathy
  - Polycythemia
  - Invasive neoplasia (e.g., pheochromocytoma)
- Systemic venous or pulmonary arterial thrombi/emboli include:
  - Hypercoagulable states, including those related to deficiency of antithrombin III (e.g., renal amyloidosis), immune-mediated hemolytic anemia, and Cushing's disease
  - Venous stasis
  - Venous inflammation (phlebitis) or obstruction (thrombophlebitis)
  - Physical injury to a vein (e.g., trauma, IV catheter)
  - Chemical injury to a vein (e.g., chemotherapy, thiacetarsamide)
  - Verminous pulmonary arteritis (e.g., heartworm disease)
  - Heartworm embolus from adulticide therapy (dogs) or spontaneous worm death (cats)
  - Fat emboli (from long bone fractures)
  - Air emboli (from procedures such as cystography or cryosurgery)
  - Retrograde venous embolus of the spinal cord

Pathophysiology

The pathogenesis of clinical signs depends on the acuteness of injury, location of vascular obstruction, magnitude of thrombosis, collateral circulation, the tissue affected, and inflammatory mediators.

- *Pathological consequences* of ischemia or infarction of the systemic circulation include:
  - *Limbs*—Muscle ischemia, rhabdomyocytolysis, peripheral neuropathy
  - *Bone*—Infarcts and zones of bone necrosis
  - *Myocardium*—Myocardial ischemia or infarction, arrhythmias, abnormal ventricular wall motion, and ventricular failure
  - *Spinal cord*—Neuronal degeneration, ischemic or hemorrhagic necrosis

- *Brain*—Ischemia-induced neuronal damage, edema, cell necrosis, hemorrhagic necrosis
- *Kidney, adrenal gland, liver, spleen, or gut*—Infarcts, hemorrhages, and parenchymal necrosis may occur with subsequent organ dysfunction
- *Skin*—Infarcts or cutaneous hemorrhages
- *Pathological consequences* of ischemia or infarction of the systemic venous or pulmonary circulation include:
  - *Systemic veins*—Obstruction of venous return, elevation of venous and capillary pressures, and edema of dependent tissues are seen.
  - *Lung*—Pulmonary embolism and pulmonary parenchymal injury leading to ventilation:perfusion inequality in the lung. A massive pulmonary embolus can obstruct the left or right pulmonary artery, severely limit cardiac output, and lead to hypotension, myocardial ischemia, and cardiac arrest. Embolization of smaller pulmonary vessels can cause pulmonary infarction and also initiate the release of vasoactive chemicals that cause lung edema and inflammation. Recurrent pulmonary thromboembolism reduces vascular cross-sectional area, increases pulmonary vascular resistance, and predisposes patients to pulmonary hypertension.

Clinical Signs

The clinical diagnosis of thrombosis or embolism requires a high level of suspicion. A sudden onset of clinical signs is typical of some conditions. The clinician must be mindful that many conditions predispose the animal to thrombosis or embolism. The physical examination and laboratory signs of embolism depend on the vessels involved. Abnormalities range from subtle to obvious. Following are typical findings of various thrombotic or embolic diseases:

- *Limbs*—Sudden onset of limb weakness or paresis. The affected limb is pale, cold, and pulseless. Signs of ischemic lower motor neuron sensory and motor neuropathy and ischemic myopathy (pain, muscle contracture, elevated serum muscle enzymes) are present. Bone infarcts may be associated with diffuse or shifting lameness or pain.
- *Myocardium*—Ischemia causes discomfort and anxiety. There are electrocardiogram (ECG) abnormalities (ST-T segment deviation, infarction patterns, ventricular arrhythmias). Laboratory abnormalities include elevation of cardiac muscle enzymes (myocardial-MB-band of creatine kinase [CK]), and echocardiographic abnormalities, such as regional ventricular wall hypokinesis.
- *Spinal cord*—Rapidly progressive segmental spinal cord disease is the typical feature. Signs depend on the level and extent of cord injury.
- *Brain*—Ischemic neuropathy or "stroke" with neurologic deficits or seizures.
- *Thrombosis of renal, adrenal gland, splenic, or splanchnic vessels*—Renal or severe abdominal pain and colic. Serum biochemical abnormalities may reflect end-organ injury, such as azotemia or an Addisonian crisis of hypoadrenocorticism. Splenic and hepatic in-

farcts are difficult to diagnose unless they are detectable by ultrasonography.
- *Skin*—Cutaneous hemorrhages, petecchiae, or ecchymosis may be evident.
- *Systemic venous thrombosis*—Cutaneous veins are swollen and may be "knobby," do not collapse, and may be warm and painful (thrombophlebitis). There is usually subcutaneous edema in the tissues drained by the venous system. Deep venous thrombosis involving the external iliac veins may lead to bilateral limb edema. Bilateral jugular thrombosis can lead to intermandibular edema. Thrombosis of the cranial vena cava can cause intermandibular and "brisket" edema, pleural effusion, or chylothorax. Any systemic venous thrombus can predispose patients to pulmonary thromboembolism.
- *Pulmonary thromboembolism*—Pulmonary thromboembolism can lead to numerous clinical syndromes that vary in severity and acuteness, including:
  - Shock, hypotension, or sudden death due to massive pulmonary thromboembolism, air embolism, or a heartworm embolus.
  - Acute dyspnea syndrome with marked increases in alveolar lung density in cats due to spontaneous heartworm death.
  - Tachypnea, dyspnea, and hypoxemia with increased interstitial/alveolar infiltrates, subpleural infiltrates, and localized pleural effusion due to distal pulmonary thromboemboli.
  - Pulmonary hypertension resulting in acute onset of tricuspid insufficiency and/or right-sided congestive heart failure due to loss of pulmonary vascular area.

Diagnostic and Laboratory Studies

Laboratory studies can be useful in confirming the diagnosis of thrombosis or embolism. Appropriate laboratory studies vary with the suspected cause and tissues injured. Specialists should be consulted regarding specialized radiographic, ultrasonic, angiographic, radionuclide (perfusion studies), and clinical laboratory tests. These studies may demonstrate the thrombus or changes attributable to decreased blood flow, organ ischemia, or tissue necrosis.

- Diagnosis of cutaneous, superficial venous, and appendicular thrombosis/embolism usually can be made from physical examination. Iliac arterial thrombosis in cats leads to marked elevations in skeletal muscle enzymes (CK, aspartate transaminase [AST]) and also to increases in serum alanine transaminase (ALT) (which also may be released with massive muscle injury). Duplex Doppler ultrasound can be used to examine vessel lumen and blood flow.
- Diagnosis of embolism to the central nervous system is based on history, exclusion of other CNS disorders, and imaging studies such as computed tomography (CT) scan or magnetic resonance imaging (MRI).
- Myocardial infarction is diagnosed by characteristic ECG changes, by elevations of specific cardiac muscle isoenzymes, or by echocardiographic wall motion studies.

- Diagnosis of abdominal thrombosis or embolism may be difficult and require surgical exploration in the case of an acute abdomen. Ultrasound with Doppler studies may be useful in some cases.
- Suspect pulmonary thromboembolism from the history, clinical signs, and thoracic radiographs. Large proximal thrombi and heartworms often can be identified on ultrasonography. Distal thrombi must be diagnosed from radionuclide scans or angiography.

Treatment

- Principles of therapy for thrombosis and thromboembolism include prevention of further thrombosis, treatment of the underlying disorder, removal or disintegration of the clot when possible, and supportive care to damaged tissues. Unfortunately, thrombolytic therapy with either streptokinase or tissue plasminogen activator has not been evaluated adequately in veterinary medicine. Although potentially effective in clot lysis, the adverse effects (including severe reperfusion hyperkalemia) are serious, and the mortality associated with therapy is very high. For these reasons, use of these drugs is not recommended. Consult a specialist before embarking on thrombolytic therapy.

Heparin

- *Heparin sodium* (or *potassium heparin*) often is prescribed for hospitalized patients to reduce the expansion of existing clots and to prevent new thrombus formation.
  - Recommended doses vary widely, ranging from 10–75 IU/kg SC q8h for "prevention" or treatment of disseminated intravascular coagulation (DIC), to 200–300 IU/kg SC q8h for cases of established thrombosis (e.g., deep venous thrombosis, bilateral jugular thrombosis, pulmonary thromboemboli, iliac thromboembolism in cats).
  - The authors usually administer an initial IV dose of 200–300 IU/kg IV, followed by 150–200 IU/kg SC q8h. Obtain a baseline clotting profile and adjust the dose to maintain the activated partial thromboplastin time (aPTT) or prothrombin time at approximately 2 to 2½ times baseline; alternatively, the international normalization ratio (INR) prothrombin time can be prolonged to a value of 2.0 to 3.0.

Aspirin

- *Aspirin* has been recommended for the prevention of arterial thromboembolism but probably has little, if any, role in the therapy of established thrombotic disease.
  - Doses of aspirin are empirical, and there are doubts regarding efficacy. Commonly used doses in dogs with heartworm disease are 10 mg/kg divided q12h.
  - In cats with cardiomyopathy, the usual dose is one child's aspirin (about 100 mg) every third day.

- Gastric ulceration is a concern. Do not use aspirin with other anticoagulants because of the risk of bleeding.

Warfarin

- *Warfarin* (Coumadin, 1-mg tablets) is used increasingly in home care to prevent further thromboses in dogs with recurrent pulmonary thromboembolism or deep venous thrombosis and in cats with cardiomyopathy.
  - There is more experience using warfarin in the cardiomyopathic cat that either has survived an embolic episode or is at high risk for future thromboembolism. An initial dose of ½ of a 1-mg tablet PO daily is recommended. Ideally, first heparinize the cat at 100 IU/kg q8h for 24 hours, and continue heparin for the first 48 hours of therapy.
  - The initial dose of warfarin in dogs is unresolved and usually is extrapolated from doses used in human patients. The INR should be prolonged to a value of 2.0 to 3.0.

Surgery

- *Surgical intervention* is recommended infrequently in the management of vascular thrombosis. Some blood vessels are simply inaccessible. Surgery in cats with iliac thrombosis due to cardiomyopathy is complicated by the risk of anesthesia, development of DIC, and the severe reperfusion hyperkalemia that can develop (see Chap. 66). Surgically remove an aortic thrombus in cases of suprarenal aortic thrombosis. Monitor ECG and serum potassium carefully intra- and postoperatively. Other indications for surgery include multiple splenic thromboses, suspected bowel infarction or volvulus, and bleeding/thrombosis with associated mechanical compression (e.g., extradural bleeding). The use of embolectomy (Fogarty) catheters has not been evaluated satisfactorily in animals, but this technique often is limited by the small size of many veterinary patients.
- Treat thrombophlebitis of superficial veins by removal of any catheters from the affected vein or limb, hot-packing of the area, antibiotic therapy, and gentle wrapping of the limb to reduce edema and self-trauma. If there is a concern about extension of the thrombus centrally, examine the vessel should be examined using Duplex Doppler ultrasound. Therapy with heparin, or even warfarin, as aforementioned, also can be used.
  - Treat chemical phlebitis (e.g., thiacetarsamide) with topical dimethyl sulfoxide (DMSO) and a corticosteroid ointment (q8–12h) with concurrent administration of prednisolone (0.5 mg/kg PO or SC q12h).

VASCULITIS

Arteritis

Arteritis (i.e., inflammation involving arterioles or arteries) can be caused by infection with various microorganisms and is often a component of *multisystemic infections,* including infectious canine hepatitis, (see Chap. 14), infectious feline peritonitis (FIP) (see Chap. 8), and Rocky Mountain spotted fever (see Chap. 15). Immune-mediated arteritis is believed to be important in FIP, systemic lupus erythematosus, idiopathic vasculitis in Akita, spitz, and Doberman pinscher dogs, and some drug reactions. Cutaneous manifestations of vasculitis are discussed in other chapters in this text.

Clinical Signs

Clinical signs are related to inflammatory mediators, increased vascular permeability, and interruption of the vascular endothelial lining and include

- Fever
- Subcutaneous edema
- Cutaneous hemorrhages
- Coagulation disorders including thrombocytopenia and disseminated intravascular coagulopathy that develop secondary to vasculitis
- Thrombosis and ischemic injury (see previous discussion of thrombosis)

Vasculitis Syndromes

Specific clinical vasculitis syndromes commonly seen in cats and dogs include

- FIP (Chap. 8)
- Verminous arteritis associated with dirofilariasis and angiostrongyliasis (damage occurring primarily within the pulmonary arteries; angiostrongyliasis is uncommon in the United States).
- *Rocky Mountain spotted fever,* which is a tick-borne infection caused by *Rickettsia rickettsii* that affects dogs and human beings (see Chap. 15). Invasion of vascular endothelial cells causes vasculitis with mononuclear inflammation, microscopic thrombosis, and microinfarction. Thrombocytopenia is common.
  - Multiple organs are affected, including the heart (myocarditis and arrhythmias), brain (stupor, coma), blood (thrombocytopenia, neutropenia), and skin (edema, rash).
  - Fever is common, and death may occur.
  - Blood from affected dogs has public health significance (contagion).
  - Diagnosis is made by clinical and laboratory signs and serology.
- *Uremic vasculitis,* which causes myoarteritis of small arteries, particularly in the stomach. This condition leads to hemorrhage and necrosis, predisposing to uremic gastritis and gastrointestinal ulceration and melena.

Treatment

- Treatment depends on the underlying cause.
- Management of FIP (see Chap. 8), systemic lupus erythematosus and immune-mediated vasculitis (see Chap. 22), and spotted fever (see Chap. 15) are discussed elsewhere in this text.
- Immunosuppressive doses of glucocorticoids are indicated for the management of some vasculitides.

- Thrombotic complications may require prophylactic heparin (10–100 IU/kg, q8h SC).

ARTERIOSCLEROSIS

Arteriosclerosis is a chronic arterial metamorphosis characterized by loss of elasticity, luminal narrowing, and proliferative and degenerative lesions of the intima and media. *Atherosclerosis* pertains to the arteriosclerotic state that also includes fatty degenerative changes in the arterial wall. This is the typical underlying lesion of coronary artery disease in human patients.

- Coronary arteriosclerosis, prominent in older dogs with endocardiosis, has been related to small and microscopic areas of myocardial fibrosis. Presumably this is due to ischemic necrosis and infarction of myocytes secondary to reduced perfusion.
- Similar lesions also have been observed in dogs with congenital subaortic stenosis, in dogs with diabetes mellitus, and in cats with hypertrophic cardiomyopathy.
- Naturally occurring atherosclerosis occurs in severe canine hypothyroidism (see Chap. 29) when serum cholesterol concentrations are very high (generally >750 mg/dl).
- In canine and feline patients, clinically important hyaline arteriosclerosis is primarily related to the coronary vasculature. The overall clinical significance of arterial degenerative changes in animals is relatively small compared with that in human beings.

Diagnosis

The diagnosis of arteriosclerosis is difficult. Suspect this condition in patients with severe hypercholesterolemia and in association with the aforementioned cardiac disorders.

- Small-vessel (intramural) arteriosclerosis may contribute to the morbidity of other cardiac disorders by causing ischemia-induced arrhythmias (e.g., premature ventricular contractions) or increased myocardial stiffness (e.g., hypertrophic cardiomyopathy, subaortic stenosis).
- Suspect acute myocardial infarction due to extramural coronary thrombosis in dogs with respiratory distress, ventricular arrhythmias, and severe ST-T segment changes on the ECG (particularly ST-T segment elevation). Diagnosis is presumptive because coronary angiography and myocardial enzyme analysis are rarely performed in animals.
- In the differential diagnosis of extramural coronary artery obstruction or thrombosis, rule out embolic complications of bacterial endocarditis.

Treatment

Management includes treatment of the underlying disease and the complications of ischemia (e.g., ventricular antiarrhythmic therapy).

- In cases of presumed myocardial infarction, administer oxygen and nitroglycerin ointment (see Chap. 63) empirically.
- Beta blockers (e.g., propranolol, 0.4–1.0 mg/kg, q8h PO), by decreasing myocardial oxygen consumption, may be cardioprotective in animals with multifocal small vessel coronary arteriosclerosis.
- Calcium channel blockers (e.g., diltiazem, 0.5–2.0 mg/kg, q8h PO) may act as a coronary vasodilator and prevent coronary vascular spasms (see discussion of feline hypertrophic cardiomyopathy).

VASCULAR NEOPLASIA

Etiology

Vascular tumors can be primary or metastatic. The endocardium and vascular elements of the heart also may become neoplastic.

- *Primary* arterial and venous tumors are uncommon:
  - Aortic and carotid body tumors (chemodectomas) can act as space-occupying lesions in the thorax or about the ascending aorta.
  - Aortic body tumors are an important cause of hemorrhagic pericardial effusion in older brachycephalic dogs. These tumors also may be an incidental finding at necropsy (see Chap. 67).
- *Tumors from vascular elements* (e.g., hemangiosarcoma) and malignancies metastatic to blood vessels are described in detail in Chapter 26. Hemangiosarcoma is the most common intracardiac tumor. Multicentric involvement (e.g., liver, spleen, heart) is common. Pulmonary metastasis is frequent.
- *Extravascular neoplasms* may invade blood vessels; for example, obstruction of the caudal vena cava can develop secondary to ingrowth of a pheochromocytoma from the adrenal medulla (see Chap. 31).

Pathophysiology

- Tumor-related hemorrhage into the pericardial space can cause cardiac tamponade.
- Intraluminal obstruction to venous return (usually of the caudal vena cava) causes ascites. This is most common with hemangiosarcoma; however, other primary intracardiac tumors, such as myxoma and fibrosarcoma, can cause similar problems.

Clinical Signs

- Clinical signs of cardiac or vena caval neoplasia are usually those of right-sided CHF (hepatomegaly, ascites, pleural effusion).
- Compression of the cranial vena cava (e.g., from mediastinal lymphosarcoma) can cause intermandibular and ventrocervical subcutaneous edema.

Differential Diagnosis

- Differential diagnosis of caudal vena cava obstruction includes idiopathic sclerosis, neoplasia, kinking, or trauma of the caudal vena cava.

Imaging Studies

- Radiographic studies may demonstrate mass lesions; however, the cardiac silhouette may be radiographically normal when the obstruction is intraluminal. Nonselective angiography (peripheral venous injection) may demonstrate vascular obstruction or interruption.
- Ultrasound studies may demonstrate dilated hepatic veins typical of obstructed hepatic venous drainage or solid tissue mass lesions.
- Echocardiography can reveal intracardiac mass lesions.

Treatment

Therapy for vascular neoplasia is complicated and requires surgery, and possibly chemotherapy (see Chap. 24). Tranfer most patients to a referral hospital.

ARTERIOVENOUS FISTULA

An arteriovenous (AV) fistula is a congenital or acquired communication between artery and vein.

- Congenital lesions tend to be multiple and involve the limbs, whereas a post-traumatic fistula is usually a single direct connection associated with abnormal healing of the injured blood vessels.
- Declawing operations and tumors have been rarely associated with AV fistula formation in the feline paw.
- Thyroid carcinoma may lead to a cervical AV communication in dogs. AV fistulas have been reported secondary to other tumors.
- A hepatic AV fistula is a special type of congenital vascular malformation. This condition usually is associated with portal hypertension and ascites (see Chap. 92).

Clinical Signs

Clinical signs include local vascular changes (due to venous hypertension) and cardiac manifestations (due to increased cardiac output required to perfuse the shunt). Any combination of the following signs may be observed:

- Edema, pain, inability to use the limb, a warm or cool extremity, and abnormal tissue growth
- A continuous murmur (bruit) detectable over the affected area as blood shunts continuously through the fistula

▼ *Key Point* A positive Branham sign may be present in large AV shunts; slowing of the heart rate follows digital occlusion of the artery—the result of a sudden increase in arterial resistance and pressure.

- An overall increase in cardiac output (equal to the shunt flow), which may be manifested by tachycardia, cardiomegaly, and increased pulmonary vascularity
  - Increased cardiac work, cardiac dilation, renal retention of sodium and water, elevation of venous

filling pressures, and eventually, congestive heart failure can develop; this is particularly true of large shunts.

Diagnosis

Make the diagnosis by clinical signs, ultrasonography (including Doppler studies), and angiography. These studies generally require transfer of the patient to a referral hospital.

Treatment

- Ligation or removal of the shunt is the treatment of choice.
- The surgical approach usually is guided by imaging and vascular contrast studies.
- Other methods of vessel occlusion (e.g., catheter-delivered "umbrellas") have not been used routinely in veterinary practice.

Complications and Prognosis

- The prognosis is good for animals with acquired AV fistulas that are not associated with malignancy.

- Congenital AV fistulas may be problematic and difficult surgical procedures.
- Limb amputation may be necessary if the exact location of the shunt cannot be isolated and ligated or if the limb becomes devitalized.
- Management of hepatic AV fistulas may require partial hepatectomy of the involved lobe.

SUPPLEMENTAL READINGS

Fox PR: Peripheral vascular disease. *In* Ettinger SJ, Feldman E, eds.: Textbook of Veterinary Internal Medicine, 5th ed. Philadelphia: WB Saunders, in press.

Henik RA: Diagnosis and treatment of feline systemic hypertension. Compend Cont Educ Pract Vet 19:163, 1997.

Littman MP: Spontaneous systemic hypertension in 24 cats. J Vet Intern Med 8:79–86, 1994.

Olivier NB: Pathophysiology of arteriovenous fistulae. *In* Slatter DH, ed.: Textbook of Small Animal Surgery. Philadelphia: WB Saunders, 1985, p 1051.

Suter PF: Peripheral vascular disease. *In* Ettinger SJ, ed.: Textbook of Veterinary Internal Medicine, 3rd ed. Philadelphia: WB Saunders, 1989, p 1185.

70 Congenital Heart Disease

Matthew W. Miller / John D. Bonagura

ETIOLOGY

▼ *Key Point* Congenital heart disease (CHD) is the most common cause of cardiovascular disease in animals younger than 1 year of age.

- Common defects include patent ductus arteriosus (PDA); subvalvular aortic stenosis (SAS); pulmonic stenosis (PS); mitral and tricuspid dysplasia, causing insufficiency or stenosis of the valve; atrial and ventricular septal defects (ASD, VSD); and the tetralogy of Fallot. Congenital peritoneopericardial diaphragmatic hernia is a common defect of the diaphragm and pericardium (see Chap. 67).
- Signalment, physical examination, thoracic radiography, and electrocardiography often provide an accurate diagnosis. Definitive diagnosis of the type and severity of CHD often requires more sophisticated tests, including echocardiography and selective angiocardiography. Although the management of CHD is often interesting to the practicing veterinarian, one must consider the following points:
  - Some dogs with seemingly simple defects, such as PDA, may have complicating or concurrent conditions, such as myocardial failure, tricuspid dysplasia, PS, VSD, or subaortic stenosis. These complications are particularly common in larger breeds of dogs.
  - Most congenital heart defects have a genetic basis, but the mode of inheritance is rarely a simple mendelian pattern.
  - Mildly affected dogs, such as those with trivial subaortic stenosis, may be clinically normal; however, owners usually are advised not to breed these animals. Doppler or catheterization studies may be required to diagnose such conditions.
  - Young animals may appear to tolerate even severe congenital defects for many months or even a few years. Heart failure may develop suddenly and unexpectedly.
- When the veterinarian suspects CHD and clients are interested in optimal care, especially if cardiac surgery or interventional catheterization is a possibility, referral should not be delayed.

▼ *Key Point* After a tentative diagnosis of CHD, the best course of action for the patient is generally re-ferral to a cardiologist or a specialist with training and experience in the management of CHD.

- The balance of this chapter discusses the approach to recognition of cardiac malformations and an overview of the management options.

CLINICAL SIGNS

- Most animals with CHD are asymptomatic.
- Stunted growth
  - Most commonly associated with right-to-left shunts (cyanotic heart disease) or congestive heart failure (CHF).
  - Respiratory distress, exercise intolerance, and tachypnea are typical in cases of CHF or cyanotic heart disease (e.g., tetralogy of Fallot).
- Fainting and exertional collapse are signs of severe CHD and may be related to:
  - Right-to-left shunts (hypoxemia)
  - Paroxysmal arrhythmias
  - Ventricular outflow tract obstruction (e.g., aortic and pulmonic stenosis)
  - CHF
- Exercise intolerance is usually a sign of moderate-to-severe CHD.

DIAGNOSIS (Fig. 70–1)

Signalment

- Breed, age, and sex predilection are used in conjunction with physical examination findings to formulate an initial list of differential diagnoses (Table 70–1).

Physical Examination

In addition to complete physical examination, cardiac auscultation is the key to recognition of CHD.

Cardiac Murmurs

- May be absent in right-to-left shunting defects with polycythemia, with pulmonary or aortic atresia, large (unrestrictive) VSD, severe tricuspid dysplasia (especially in cats), or with severe pulmonary hypertension.

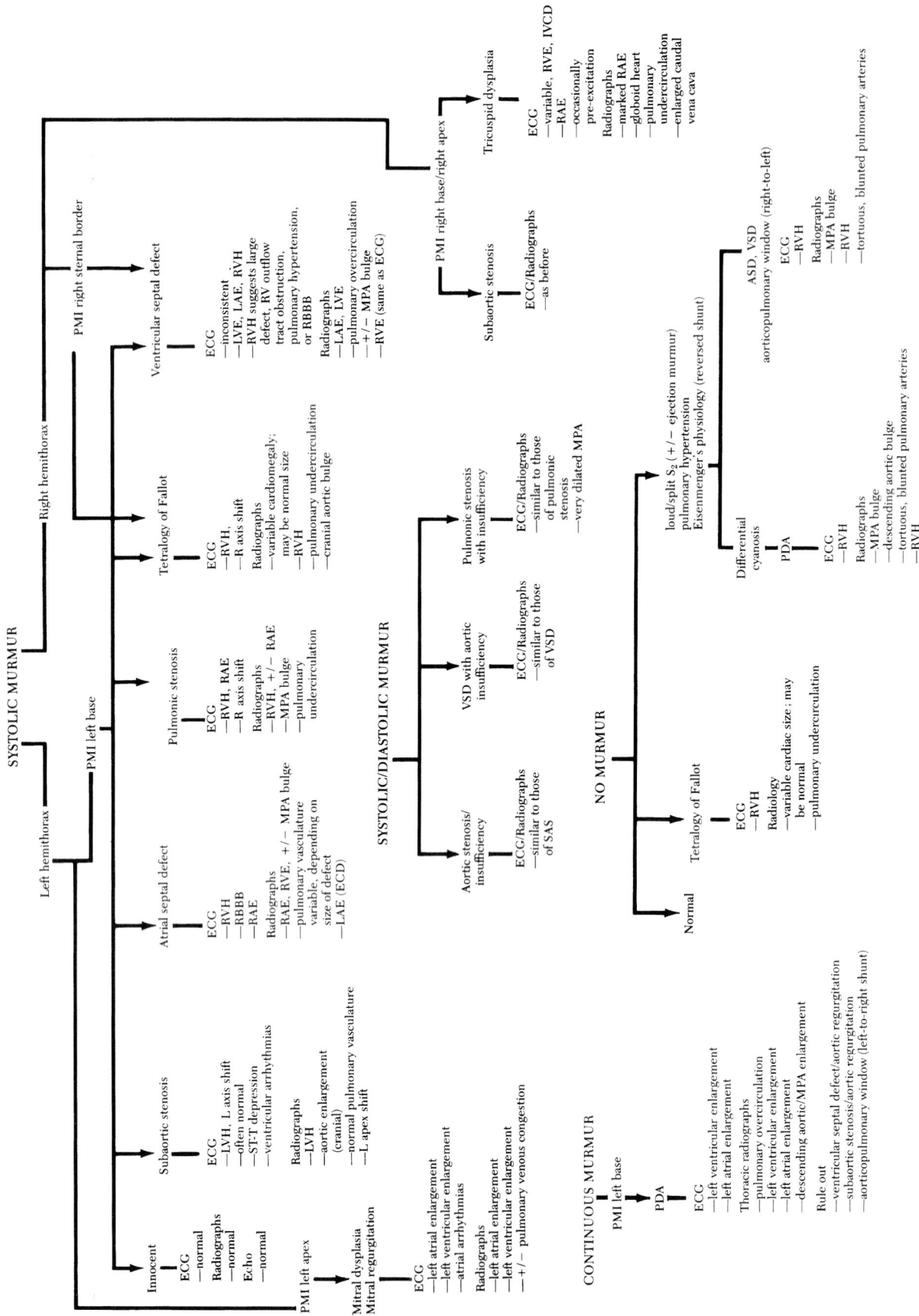

SYSTOLIC MURMUR

- **Left hemithorax**
  - **PMI left base**
    - **Innocent**
      - ECG —normal
      - Radiographs —normal
      - Echo —normal
    - **Subaortic stenosis**
      - ECG —LVH, L axis shift —often normal —ST-T depression —ventricular arrhythmias
      - Radiographs —LVH —aortic enlargement (cranial) —normal pulmonary vasculature —L apex shift
    - **Atrial septal defect**
      - ECG —RVH —RBBB —RAE
      - Radiographs —RAE, RVE, +/− MPA bulge —pulmonary vasculature variable, depending on size of defect —LAE (ECD)
    - **Pulmonic stenosis**
      - ECG —RVH, RAE —R axis shift
      - Radiographs —RVH, +/− RAE —MPA bulge —pulmonary undercirculation
    - **Tetralogy of Fallot**
      - ECG —RVH, —R axis shift
      - Radiographs —variable cardiomegaly; may be normal size —RVH —pulmonary undercirculation —cranial aortic bulge
  - **PMI left apex**
    - **Mitral dysplasia**
    - **Mitral regurgitation**
      - ECG —left atrial enlargement —left ventricular enlargement —atrial arrhythmias
      - Radiographs —left atrial enlargement —left ventricular enlargement —+/− pulmonary venous congestion
- **Right hemithorax**
  - **PMI right sternal border**
    - **Ventricular septal defect**
      - ECG —inconsistent —LVE, LAE, RVH —RVH suggests large defect, RV outflow tract obstruction, pulmonary hypertension, or RBBB
      - Radiographs —LAE, LVE —pulmonary overcirculation —+/− MPA bulge —RVE (same as ECG)
  - **PMI right base/right apex**
    - **Tricuspid dysplasia**
      - ECG —variable, RVE, IVCD —RAE —occasionally pre-excitation
      - Radiographs —marked RAE —globoid heart —pulmonary undercirculation —enlarged caudal vena cava
    - **Subaortic stenosis**
      - ECG/Radiographs —as before

SYSTOLIC/DIASTOLIC MURMUR

- **Aortic stenosis/insufficiency**
  - ECG/Radiographs —similar to those of SAS
- **VSD with aortic insufficiency**
  - ECG/Radiographs —similar to those of VSD
- **Pulmonic stenosis with insufficiency**
  - ECG/Radiographs —similar to those of pulmonic stenosis —very dilated MPA

NO MURMUR

- **Tetralogy of Fallot**
  - ECG —RVH
  - Radiology —variable cardiac size; may be normal —pulmonary undercirculation
- **Normal**
- **Differential cyanosis**
  - loud/split S_2 (+/− ejection murmur) pulmonary hypertension Eisenmenger's physiology (reversed shunt)
  - **ASD, VSD**
  - **aorticopulmonary window (right-to-left)**
    - ECG —RVH
    - Radiographs —MPA bulge —RVH —tortuous, blunted pulmonary arteries
  - **PDA**
    - ECG —RVH
    - Radiographs —MPA bulge —descending aortic bulge —tortuous, blunted pulmonary arteries —RVH

CONTINUOUS MURMUR

- **PMI left base**
  - **PDA**
    - ECG —left ventricular enlargement —left atrial enlargement
    - Thoracic radiographs —pulmonary overcirculation —left ventricular enlargement —left atrial enlargement —descending aortic/MPA enlargement
    - Rule out —ventricular septal defect/aortic regurgitation —subaortic stenosis/aortic regurgitation —aorticopulmonary window (left-to-right shunt)

Figure 70–1.   ASD, atrial septal defect; ECD, endocardial cushion defect; LAE, left atrial enlargement; LVE, left ventricular enlargement; LVH, left ventricular hypertrophy; MPA, main pulmonary artery; PDA, patent ductus arteriosus; PMI, point of maximal intensity; RAE, right atrial enlargement; RBBB, right bundle branch block; RV, right ventricle; RVE, right ventricular enlargement; RVH, right ventricular hypertrophy; SAS, subaortic stenosis; VSD, ventricular septal defect.

Table 70–1. BREED AND SEX PREDILECTIONS FOR CERTAIN CONGENITAL CARDIAC DEFECTS*

Defect	Predilection
Patent ductus arteriosus (PDA)	Poodle, Bichon friese, collie, Pomeranian, German shepherd, Shetland sheepdog, and many other breeds (female : male, 2.2 : 1)
Pulmonic stenosis (PS)	Beagle, bulldog, fox terrier, miniature schnauzer, Chihuahua, Samoyed, Labrador retriever
Subaortic stenosis (SAS)	Newfoundland, boxer, German shepherd, German shorthaired pointer, golden retriever, rottweiler, bull terrier
Ventricular septal defect (VSD)	English bulldog, springer spaniel
Atrial septal defect (ASD)	Samoyed, boxer, Doberman pinscher
Mitral dysplasia	Great Dane, German shepherd, bull terrier (male > female)
Tricuspid dysplasia	Great Dane, German shepherd, Weimaraner, Labrador retriever (male > female)
Tetralogy of Fallot	Keeshond, English bulldog

*Note: SAS, PDA, and PS are the most common defects in dogs. ASD/VSD and atrioventricular valve dysplasias are the most common defects in cats.

- May be characteristic of a particular cardiac defect (see Fig. 70–1). See the discussion of a cardiovascular examination in Chapter 59.
- May be soft and possible to confuse with an innocent murmur (e.g., mild subaortic stenosis).
- The intensity of the murmur does not correlate with the severity of the cardiac lesion except in ventricular outlet obstruction, in which louder and later peaking murmurs usually indicate a progressively tighter obstruction.

Precordial Palpation

Palpate the thorax over the heart.
- Apical impulse identifies the relative areas of the mitral and tricuspid valve sounds and murmurs and is thereby useful in localizing cardiac murmurs.
- Strong left apical impulse suggests left ventricular hypertrophy (e.g., aortic stenosis [AS]).
- Right-sided impulse equal to or greater than that on the left suggests right ventricular hypertrophy (e.g., PS).
- Precordial thrill is a vibration that identifies the point of maximum intensity (PMI) of a loud (grade V or VI/VI) murmur.

Arterial Pulse

- Pulses are often normal. Weak (hypokinetic) pulses suggest left ventricular outflow obstruction or cardiac failure.

- Bounding (hyperkinetic) pulses are most commonly associated with PDA or congenital aortic insufficiency.
- Severe right-sided lesions or CHF may be associated with weak arterial pulses.

Venous Pulses

- Distended or pulsating jugular vein suggests a right-sided heart lesion (e.g., PS, tricuspid dysplasia) or pulmonary hypertension.

Mucous Membranes

- Pink membranes are typical.
- Pallor with prolonged capillary refill time suggests cardiac failure or concurrent anemia.
- Cyanotic membranes may indicate pulmonary dysfunction, from left-sided CHF or pneumonia, or may suggest right-to-left shunting (tetralogy of Fallot, reversed ASD, VSD, PDA).
- Differential cyanosis—oral membranes pink, caudal membranes (vulva, prepuce) cyanotic—suggests a reversed PDA (i.e., blood flow from the pulmonary artery to the aorta).

Electrocardiography (See Chapter 61)

Especially valuable in CHD for diagnosis of cardiac chamber enlargement when there is moderate-to-severe cardiomegaly. The electrocardiogram is of little value in mild CHD (e.g., mild AS). Chamber enlargement patterns (canine) are as follows:
- Atrial enlargement patterns (P wave > 0.04 sec; > 0.4 mV) are relatively insensitive for predicting right vs. left atrial dilation.
- Left ventricular enlargement (R wave > 2.5–3.0 mV in lead II or left-axis deviation) occurs in PDA, VSD, mitral dysplasia, subaortic stenosis.
- Right ventricular hypertrophy (right-axis deviation with prominent S waves in leads I, II, III, AVF, and V_2 to V_6); ± widened QRS (right bundle branch blocks) occurs in PS, ASD, and VSD (some cases); tricuspid dysplasia; tetralogy of Fallot; and pulmonary hypertension associated with right-to-left shunts.

Thoracic Radiography (See Chapter 60)

Normal pups have a relatively dominant right ventricular shadow until approximately 8–12 weeks of age. Right-sided dilation often causes apical shifts, leading to overestimation of the left side of the heart. Radiographic interpretation focuses on the following (see Fig. 70–1 and the discussion of cardiac radiography in Chap. 60):
- Cardiac size and shape; specific chamber enlargement
- Great vessels (aorta, pulmonary artery)
- Pulmonary vascularity (overcirculation and undercirculation; left-sided CHF)

Echocardiography (Table 70–2)

- In certain defects, the anatomic abnormality may be visualized, for example, in ASD, VSD, and subaortic

Table 70–2. ECHOCARDIOGRAPHIC (DOPPLER) FEATURES OF SELECT CONGENITAL HEART DEFECTS

Defects	Echocardiographic (Doppler) Features
Patent ductus arteriosus (PDA)	Dilated left atrium, left ventricle, and pulmonary trunk; possible identification of PDA; turbulent flow in main pulmonary artery, with retrograde diastolic flow and increased transmitral and aortic flow velocities, reduced LV systolic myocardial function
Pulmonic stenosis (PS)	Right ventricular hypertrophy, right atrial and pulmonary artery enlargement, outflow tract obstruction, thickened valve leaflets, septal flattening and/or paradoxical septal motion, high-velocity flow (> 1.5 m/sec) across the pulmonic valve
Subaortic stenosis (SAS)	Left ventricular (LV) hypertrophy, dilated aorta, subvalvular narrowing, high-velocity flow (> 2.0 m/sec) across the aortic valve
Ventricular septal defect (VSD)	Variable chamber enlargement, most commonly left atrial and ventricular, possible identification of defect, right ventricular hypertrophy if pulmonary hypertension (PH) or very large defect, visualization of flow across defect, may be bidirectional; increased transmitral and PA flow velocity, right-to-left shunt in the case of PH (Doppler or bubble study).
Atrial septal defect (ASD)	Right atrial and ventricular enlargement, possible identification of defect, main pulmonary artery enlargement, flow across defect, increased velocity flow across tricuspid (diastole) and pulmonic (systole) valves
Mitral valve dysplasia	Left atrial and left ventricular enlargement, abnormal mitral valve anatomy, increased transmitral diastolic flow velocity, turbulent retrograde systolic transmitral flow
Tricuspid valve dysplasia	Right atrial and ventricular enlargement, abnormal tricuspid valve anatomy, increased transtricuspid diastolic flow velocity, turbulent retrograde systolic transtricuspid flow
Tetralogy of Fallot	Right ventricular hypertrophy, right ventricular outflow tract obstruction, identification of VSD, over-riding aorta, small left heart, contrast study indicating right-to-left shunting, septal flattening and flattening and/or paradoxical septal motion, right-to-left flow across VSD (Doppler or bubble study), decreased diastolic transmitral flow, possibly increased transaortic systolic flow, increased flow velocity across the pulmonic valve
Pulmonary hypertension (PH)	Right ventricular hypertrophy, right atrial enlargement, dilated main pulmonary artery, visualization of associated shunt, right-to-left shunt by Doppler or bubble study, increased flow *acceleration* across pulmonary valve

narrowing. A normal, two-dimensional echocardiographic study does not rule out the diagnosis of mild congenital heart disease. Doppler or cardiac catheterization studies may be needed to identify minor flow abnormalities in potential breeding animals.

- Determination of the degree of cardiac enlargement/hypertrophy is useful in assessing the overall significance of the lesion because mild lesions do not lead to substantial cardiomegaly.
- Saline injections (contrast echocardiography) into a peripheral vein readily demonstrate right-to-left shunting lesions.
- Doppler echocardiography is highly effective for noninvasive quantitation of the severity of the lesion and has supplanted cardiac catheterization for routine diagnosis. A complete Doppler study (with color flow imaging) can provide anatomic detail; blood flow information, including abnormally high velocity of flow; and intracardiac pressure estimates.

Cardiac Catheterization

- Useful when echocardiographic-Doppler study findings are equivocal or when therapeutic intervention is necessary. Of possible assistance when outlining the surgical anatomy.
- Usually necessitates referral to a cardiologist or a specialist with training and experience in the diagnosis and management of CHD.
- Can involve therapeutic manipulations in some cases (e.g., balloon valvulotomy for PS, balloon dilation for subaortic stenosis, and transcatheter coil occlusion of PDA).

TREATMENT

Definitive treatment of CHD usually requires cardiac surgery or interventional catheterization. In addition, complications such as CHF and arrhythmias may necessitate medical management.

Congestive Heart Failure

Treat the same as for left-sided CHF that is associated with acquired diseases (see Chap. 64).

- Digoxin (0.005–0.01 mg/kg, q12h, PO)
- Diuretics (furosemide [Lasix], 0.5–2.0 mg/kg, q12h, q8h PO)
- Vasodilators may control CHF and reduce left-to-right shunting (e.g., VSD). Enalapril (Enacard, 0.25–0.5 mg/kg, q12h PO) is given for CHF unless there is a left-to-right shunt. In this case, the lower dose of enalapril is provided, and hydralazine (0.5–2.0 mg/kg, q12h PO) or amlodipine (0.05–0.1 mg/kg q24h PO) is titrated to decrease shunting.
- Exercise limitation and moderate dietary sodium restriction are prescribed.
- Use direct-acting vasodilators with caution—if at all—in patients with subaortic stenosis (SAS).

Arrhythmias

See Chapter 62.

- Supraventricular (atrial tachycardia, flutter, fibrillation)
  - Digoxin (0.005–0.01 mg/kg, q12h, PO)
  - Atenolol (0.5–2.0 mg/kg q12–24h PO) or propranolol (0.2–0.8 mg/kg q8h, PO)

- Diltiazem (1.0–1.5 mg/kg, q8h, PO)
- Combinations of the aforementioned when necessary
- Ventricular tachycardia
  - Procainamide (5–20 mg/kg, IV or IM; 25–40 μg/kg/min constant rate infusion; 12–20 mg/kg, q8h to q6h, PO)
  - Mexiletine (Mexitil; 5–8 mg/kg q8h, PO)
  - Lidocaine (50–75 μg/kg/min constant rate infusion for intraoperative, perioperative control)
  - Atenolol (0.5–2.0 mg/kg q12–24h, PO) or equivalent beta blocker has been used for empirical prophylactic therapy in dogs with subaortic stenosis to prevent arrhythmias and sudden death.

Surgical Correction

Surgical management of cardiac defects must not be undertaken without proper training and experience in thoracic surgery (see Chap. 83).

Patent Ductus Arteriosus

- Surgical ligation is the therapy of choice and is associated with a perioperative mortality of < 5% at most institutions (see Chap. 71).
- Percutaneous transcatheter coil occlusion may soon supplant surgery at some institutions.

Ventricular and Atrial Septal Defects

- Definitive repair has been reported with varying degrees of success. Requires cardiopulmonary bypass.
- Pulmonary artery banding may reduce the left-to-right shunt in VSD and is useful for patients with CHF or for those developing pulmonary hypertension.

Pulmonic and Subaortic Stenosis

- Pulmonic stenosis
  - Patch graft, pulmonary valvulectomy, surgical or balloon valvuloplasty, or their combination, has been used.
- SAS
  - Balloon catheter dilation of the subvalvular stenosis has been associated with variable long-term success.
  - Open surgical resection of the stenotic lesion provides the best long-term success, but availability is severely limited. Requires cardiopulmonary bypass.

Tetralogy of Fallot

Palliative therapy for tetralogy of Fallot involves the creation of an extracardiac shunt between a systemic artery (aorta or subclavian) and the pulmonary artery to increase pulmonary circulation and left-sided venous return. This therapy may produce significant clinical improvement.

For polycythemia, phlebotomy with replacement of blood with isotonic saline may provide symptomatic improvement (see Chap. 20).

NATURAL HISTORY AND PROGNOSIS

Cardiac Shunts

- PDA has an excellent prognosis with surgery or transcatheter occlusion. Approximately 60% of pups die within 1 year without surgery. Prognosis with reversed PDA is poor, and surgery is contraindicated. Occasionally, dogs live beyond 5 years of age.
- Prognosis for small and restrictive VSD is good; however, large, unrestrictive VSD leads to CHF or pulmonary hypertension.
- ASD is similar to VSD.
- In endocardial cushion defect (ASD, VSD, AV valvular malformation), CHF is common.

Valvular Malformations

- In PS, the prognosis is good unless the obstruction is severe and the transvalve Doppler gradient exceeds 100 mm Hg, in which case CHF or sudden death is more likely to occur.
- Subaortic stenosis has a guarded to good prognosis unless the obstruction causes >100 mm Hg Doppler gradient, in which case CHF or sudden death may occur.
- Mitral and tricuspid valve dysplasia lesions are well tolerated if mild; however, severe stenosis or severe regurgitation often leads to CHF or atrial fibrillation.
- Aortic regurgitation can complicate VSD. Prognosis for severe aortic regurgitation is poor because CHF is likely to develop.

Tetralogy of Fallot

- Progressive hypoxemia, polycythemia, tachypnea, and exercise intolerance are typical, usually leading to sudden death.

Pulmonary Hypertension

- Pulmonary hypertension due to high vascular resistance may develop secondary to a left-to-right shunt. This condition usually occurs before 6 months of age. Prognosis is poor, and surgery is contraindicated. Polycythemia is controlled by intermittent phlebotomy. Medical therapy is ineffective.

SUPPLEMENTAL READINGS

Bonagura JD, Darke PGG: Congenital heart disease. In: Ettinger SJ, Feldman EC (eds): Textbook of Veterinary Internal Medicine, 4th ed. Philadelphia: WB Saunders, 1995.
Miller MW, Bonagura JD: Congenital heart disease. In: Kirk RW (ed): Current Veterinary Therapy X. Philadelphia: WB Saunders, 1989.

71 Surgical Correction of Patent Ductus Arteriosus

Eric R. Schertel

Ligation of the patent ductus arteriosus (PDA) in dogs and cats is a rewarding surgical procedure. When performed by an experienced surgeon, the combined operative/postoperative mortality rate is relatively low (8–10%) compared with surgery of other forms of congenital heart disease. The long-term prognosis after correction is excellent. However, like any thoracic or cardiovascular procedure, special attention to the details of anesthetic and surgical techniques is necessary for success. An accurate diagnosis is important, as is a thorough knowledge of the anatomy and physiology of the cardiovascular system.

ANATOMY AND PHYSIOLOGY

- The ductus arteriosus is a remnant of the left sixth aortic arch and connects the pulmonary artery and the descending aorta in the fetus and newborn. Its continued patency after birth results in left-to-right shunting of blood causing volume overload of the left atrium and ventricle. In severe cases, left ventricular failure may be present.
- The relationship of the descending aorta, main pulmonary artery, and right and left pulmonary arteries with the PDA must be appreciated (Fig. 71–1).
- The PDA may vary in size and shape but generally is approximately one-fifth to one-fourth the diameter of the aorta, or slightly smaller than the left main pulmonary artery. The PDA is usually short (0.5–1.0 cm), bridging the small distance between the aorta and pulmonary artery.
- The left vagus nerve lies over the ductus and is immediately underneath the visceral pleura. The recurrent laryngeal nerve arises from the vagus and courses caudal and medial to the PDA.
- Rarely, a persistent left cranial vena cava may be found coursing over the pulmonary artery. This does not pose a surgical problem in PDA ligation.

PREOPERATIVE AND PERIOPERATIVE CONSIDERATIONS

- Consult the chapter on congenital heart disease (see Chap. 70) for details of diagnosis and medical management.

- Institute conservative medical management before surgery when there is evidence of heart failure. More aggressive medical management may not benefit the patient as much as surgery.
- Mortality with surgery is higher when congestive heart failure (CHF), atrial fibrillation, or substantial myocardial failure is present. The mortality of nonsurgically managed PDA patients also is high. Thus, if conservative therapy for heart failure is not effective in 24–48 hours, surgery combined with intensive medical management is the appropriate course of action in most patients.
- Administer IV fluids only with care during anesthesia and surgery, especially in animals with heart failure.
- Perioperative mortality is 8–10% according to published reports.
- Perioperative complications occur in 10–15% of cases.

LIGATION OF THE PATENT DUCTUS ARTERIOSUS

Objectives

- Careful exposure and definition of the ductus arteriosus through a left fourth intercostal space thoracotomy. (The left fifth space may be indicated in cats.)
- Double ligation of the ductus without trauma to the vessels.

Equipment

- General surgery pack and standard suture, plus instruments required for thoracic surgery (see Chap. 83).
- Assorted sizes of right-angle forceps
- Vascular clamps, preferably pediatric/infant ductus clamps (three pairs)
- Multipurpose peripheral vascular clamps (two pairs)
- Suture; nonabsorbable, 5-0 or 6-0, on a cardiovascular needle

Technique

1. Use an appropriate anesthetic regimen based on the preoperative assessment of cardiac function

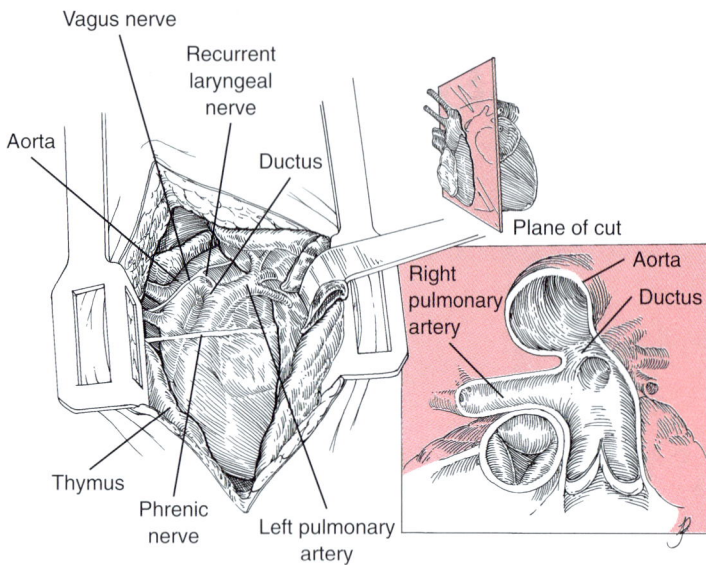

Figure 71–1. Retraction of the left cranial lobe of the lung allows exposure of the region of the ductus.

(see Chap. 2 for discussion of anesthesia techniques). Positive pressure ventilation is required during the majority of the procedure.

2. Place the patient in right lateral recumbency. Clip and aseptically prepare the left thorax from the cranial border of the scapula to rib 13, and from the dorsal to the ventral midline. Include the left shoulder and axilla, and extend past the elbow.

3. Perform a standard left fourth intercostal space thoracotomy (see Chap. 83).

4. Identify the region of the ductus following caudal retraction of the left cranial lung lobe (see Fig. 71–1). Retract the lobe with a moist sponge or laparotomy pad.

5. Elevate the vagus nerve and encircle with silk suture or umbilical tape for retraction to expose the PDA. Identify the location of the recurrent laryngeal nerve as it courses from the vagus to the caudal aspect of the ductus.

6. Palpate the thrill in the main pulmonary artery for reference.

7. Begin blunt and sharp dissection cranial and caudal to the PDA. Extend the dissection caudally between the aorta and left main pulmonary artery for a distance of at least 1.5–2 times the diameter of the ductus (Fig. 71–2, *top*). Extend the dissection cranioventrally between the aorta and main pulmonary artery a similar distance. The depth of the dissection should be at least equal to the width of the ductus (Fig. 71–2, *inset*). Dissection should be adjacent to the relatively thick-walled aorta.

8. Consider preparing the craniodorsal aspect of the aorta just distal to the left subclavian artery by reflecting the pleura and adjacent mediastinal tissues. This requires a small amount of time and ensures a clear path for clamp placement if hemorrhage control is necessary (see below).

9. The pericardium has a variable insertion at the level of the ductus. It may insert on the aortic side or on the main pulmonary artery side of the ductus. Thus, the ductus occasionally is within the peri-

cardium. In these circumstances, incise the pericardium at its insertion on the ductus or aorta.

10. Once the cranial and caudal aspects of the ductus are exposed, initiate blunt dissection behind the PDA using right-angle forceps (Fig. 71–2, *bottom*).

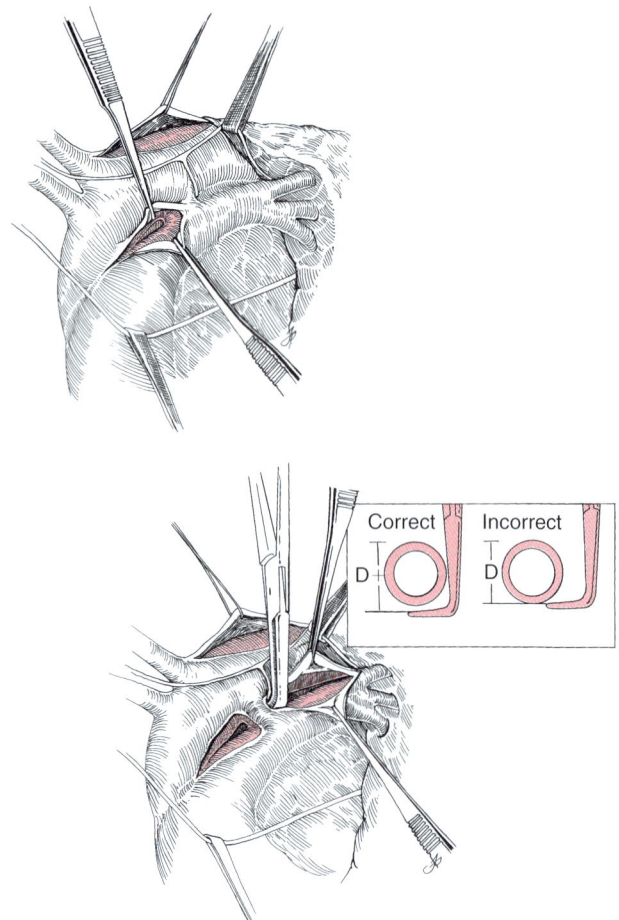

Figure 71–2. Exposure of the ductus. *Top,* Initial area of dissection. *Bottom,* Use of closed right-angle forceps to dissect the region behind the patent ductus arteriosus. See text for further details.

Take care to identify the depth of the ductus. Accomplish dissection behind the ductus by inserting closed forceps, spreading gently, and removing the forceps. Carry out dissection *adjacent* and *parallel* to the surface of the aorta.

11. The author prefers caudal to cranial dissection to avoid repeated work in the cranial aspect of the ductus. The vascular structures of the cranial region are under greater tension and are most prone to hemorrhage. However, minor medial dissection in this area often is necessary.

12. When the majority of the medial dissection is complete, gently separate the aorta and main pulmonary artery cranial to the ductus to allow identification of the tips of the right-angle forceps as they are passed from caudal to cranial. When the tips are visible, carefully incise the remaining *fascia* over the tips of the forceps with a # 15 blade. This is preferable to repeated efforts at pressing through this fascia.

▼ *Key Point* Do not cut any tissue unless it is certain that it is fascia and not vessel wall.

13. Individually pass two strands of 1-0 or 2-0 silk suture, depending on the size of the dog and the ductus (Fig. 71–3, *top*).

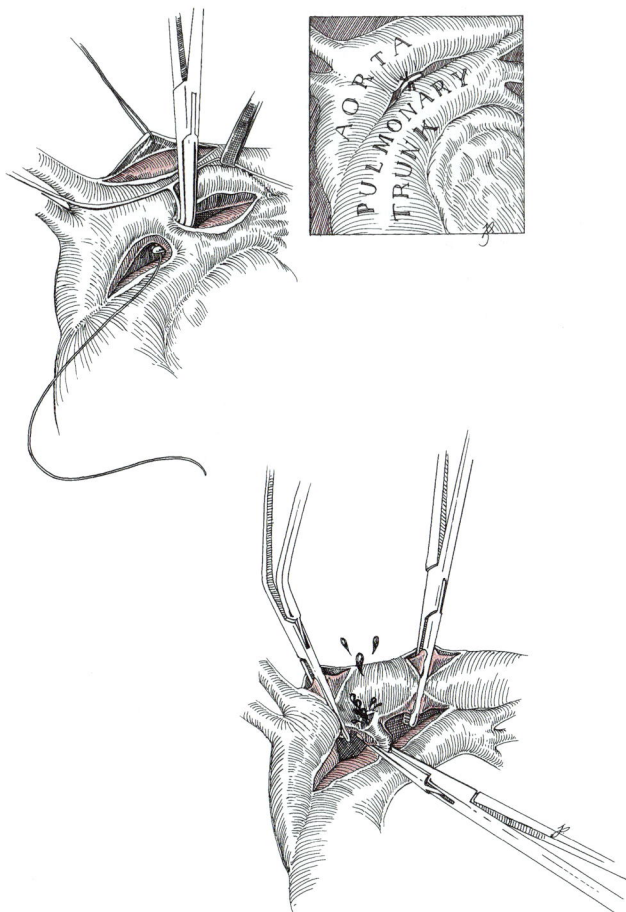

Figure 71–3. *Top,* Initial suture placement for double ligation of the ductus. *Bottom,* Procedure for controlling hemorrhage after ductus rupture.

14. Attenuate the ductus prior to ligation to observe the hemodynamic effects. If bradycardia is observed, atropine may be given. Double-ligate the ductus, aortic side first. Palpate the pulmonary artery again for ductal-related thrill or turbulence.

15. If hemorrhage is encountered from perivascular structures, control with pressure, ligation, or cautery. If the ductus ruptures and aggressive hemorrhage is encountered, first use digital pressure to control blood loss. Next, place vascular clamps on the aorta in the previously prepared region just caudal to the left subclavian artery and cranial to the ductus (Fig. 71–3, *bottom*). Also place clamps caudal to the ductus on the aorta and across the base of the ductal origin from the pulmonary artery. Identify the region of hemorrhage and suture with 5-0 or 6-0 nonabsorbable suture on a cardiovascular needle.

16. Subcutaneously tunnel a #5 or 8 Fr. red rubber tube from a small wound made caudal to the skin incision. Place the tube in the thorax through the thoracotomy. Close the thorax in a routine manner, incorporating the temporary thoracic tube (see Chap. 83).

17. After evacuating air and fluid from the thorax, remove the temporary thoracic tube. If hemorrhage or inadvertent lung injury occurs, place a standard indwelling thoracic tube (see Chap. 3).

POSTOPERATIVE CARE AND COMPLICATIONS

Short-Term

▼ *Key Point* Close postoperative monitoring in an intensive care setting is of the utmost importance.

- Monitor the following parameters/signs:
  - Mucous membrane color, capillary refill time, respiratory rate, blood pressure
  - Dyspnea, urine output
  - Recovery of body temperature, pulse, thoracic auscultation
- Analgesic therapy is indicated in animals with pain (see Chap. 83) for discussion of post-thoracotomy analgesics).
- Some surgeons treat routinely with furosemide (1–2 mg/kg) during the preoperative and immediate postoperative periods. This may be guided by the preoperative status, course of surgery, patient size, and operative fluid balance. If preoperative medical management was instituted, continue it postoperatively until clinical signs resolve.
- Perform frequent intermittent evacuation of the thorax (e.g., q2h) if a tube was left in place. Remove the thoracic tube when negative pressure is achieved or danger of hemorrhage has subsided.
- Limit fluid therapy but maintain a sterile intravenous catheter for 24 hours.
- Auscultate the heart postoperatively for persistent murmur. A systolic murmur of mitral insufficiency, caused by left ventricular dilation, may be present.

This murmur generally abates within 10 days. There should be no diastolic murmur if ligation was successful.

Long-Term

- Reevaluate heart sounds at 2 weeks when sutures are removed, at 6 months, and then yearly thereafter to detect the uncommon occurrence of recanalization.

- Recanalization of the PDA occurs rarely (1–2% of cases) and is treated by religation or division of the ductus and oversewing of the cut ends.
- PDA ligation has excellent long-term results if ligation is complete.

72 Shock

Eric R. Schertel

▼ **Key Point** Shock is the clinical state resulting from an inadequate supply of oxygen to the tissues or an inability of the tissues to utilize oxygen properly.

Shock involves numerous physiologic disturbances and pathologic changes that affect multiple organ systems in different ways. Veterinarians often are alerted to the presence of shock in their patients by the physical findings of depressed mentation, pale mucous membranes, tachycardia, and weak pulse pressure. These clinical signs are the manifestations of a complex process and do not represent the full extent of the problem. The objective of this chapter is to provide a simplified approach to the diagnosis, monitoring and treatment of shock. Information on the various manifestations, mechanisms, and temporal patterns of shock is beyond the scope of this book, but nonetheless is considered important to appropriate and successful therapy. Therapy for shock caused by acute heart failure is discussed in Chapter 64. See appropriate chapters for discussion of specific diseases that can cause shock.

ETIOLOGY AND CLASSIFICATION

Shock generally is classified by etiology because each cause of shock may produce distinct primary and secondary pathophysiologic changes and temporal patterns. Shock etiologies can be organized into those forms that result from:

- An abnormality or inadequacy of the vehicle of oxygen transport (blood)
- An abnormality of the transport system (cardiovascular system)

Hypovolemia and hypoxemia (anemic, hypoxic) are examples of the first category (Table 72–1). Diseases that disrupt the cardiovascular system and its control mechanisms (circulatory control mechanisms) also cause shock. The three important circulatory control mechanisms regulate:

- Blood pressure and blood flow distribution
- Blood volume distribution
- Cardiac function

Shock may develop from a disruption of one or more of these systems.

- Sepsis is an example of a condition in which shock is caused by a loss of control of blood flow distribution.
- Endotoxemia and gastric dilatation-volvulus also cause shock by interfering with the distribution of blood volume, but via different mechanisms.
- Heart failure creates shock due to inadequate cardiac function.

CLINICAL SIGNS

Mental Attitude. Depressed mentation often is the most apparent physical finding. This parameter is subjective and may be complicated by head injury.

- *Causes:* Decreased cerebral blood flow and oxygen delivery, circulating toxins, or head injury.

Arterial Pulse Pressure. A weak pulse is common but not necessary for shock to exist. The pulse feels weak at mean arterial pressures <60–70 mm Hg. Below 40 mm Hg, the pulse is not palpable.

- *Causes:* Low cardiac output or low peripheral vascular resistance.

Mucous Membrane Color. The color may be pale, gray (muddy), cyanotic, brick-red, or normal.

- *Causes:* Pale mucous membranes reflect hypovolemia or anemia. Gray or cyanotic mucous membranes generally indicate severe cardiovascular compromise or arterial hypoxemia. Brick-red mucous membranes are common in septic shock. Mucous membrane color may be normal.

Body/Extremity Temperature. Hypothermia (<99°F [<37.2°C]) and cold extremities are common. Patients that are septic may be hyperthermic (>103°F [>39.4°C]) with warm extremities.

- *Causes:* Decreased cardiac output, oxygen delivery, and ambient temperature. Cold extremities result from severe vasoconstriction. Hyperthermia results from the increased metabolic rate that commonly accompanies sepsis. Warm extremities reflect peripheral vasodilatation.

Capillary Refill Time. Capillary refill time typically is prolonged (>2 seconds), but may be normal.

- *Causes:* Prolonged capillary refill time reflects hypovolemia and poor peripheral blood flow.

Table 72–1. CLASSIFICATION AND COMMON ETIOLOGIES OF SHOCK

Shock Involving Normal Circulatory Control Mechanisms
Hypovolemia
Hypoxemia
  Anemia
  Hypoxia

Shock Involving Abnormal Circulatory Control Mechanisms
Blood flow maldistribution
  Sepsis
  Trauma—surgical and accidental
Blood volume maldistribution
  Endotoxemia
  Anesthesia
  Neurogenic shock
  Anaphylactic shock
  Gastric dilatation-volvulus
Impaired cardiac function
  Systolic functional failure
    Cardiomyopathy
    Valvular heart disease
    Myocardial ischemia
    Myocardial contusion
    Arrhythmias
  Diastolic functional failure
    Pericardial disease—tamponade
    Myocardial disease—decreased diastolic compliance

Heart Rate. Heart rate is commonly elevated; >140 beats per minute (bpm) in large-breed dogs, >160 bpm in small-breed dogs, and >180 bpm in cats. Begin monitoring with electrocardiography (ECG) if an irregular rhythm is detected.

- *Causes:* Hypotension, hypovolemia, pain, stress, and fever may cause tachycardia. Irregular rapid heart rhythms result from ventricular tachycardia and atrial tachyarrhythmias, including atrial fibrillation (see Chap. 62).

Respiratory Rate. Increased respiratory rate (tachypnea) is common, but may be due to excitement or fever.

- *Causes:* Hypoxemia, metabolic acidosis, pain, fever, and excitement.

Urine Output. Urine output is decreased (normal range is 1–2 ml/kg/hr).

- *Causes:* Urine formation virtually ceases when mean arterial pressure is <60 mm Hg. Blood pressure may be normal in mild to moderate hypovolemia.

MONITORING AND TREATMENT

Goals

The goal of management of the shock patient is to optimize the functions of the cardiovascular system. Employ monitoring techniques that provide accurate information about functional parameters, such as blood volume, cardiac output, arterial blood pressure, and oxygen delivery.

Cardiac output, arterial blood pressure, and oxygen delivery are dependent on blood volume. When blood volume is expanded these other parameters commonly return to normal.

▼ *Key Point* Blood volume is the most important parameter to optimize and monitor in shock patients.

Monitoring

Blood Volume

- Physical signs and findings do not accurately reflect blood volume.
- Central venous pressure (CVP) is the simplest measurement that reflects blood volume. It may be obtained via a jugular catheter positioned so that its tip is within the thorax (see Chap. 3). CVP is equivalent to right atrial pressure and reflects the function of the systemic circulation and the right heart (Fig. 72–1).
- CVP is easily measured by a water manometer attached to the jugular catheter (see Chap. 3).
- Normal CVP ranges from 0–5 cm H_2O. In shock, CVP usually is −3 to 2 cm H_2O but may be as low as −5 cm H_2O. The goal of fluid therapy in shock is to optimize blood volume by administering fluid in an amount that increases CVP to between 5 and 12 cm H_2O.
- Plasma proteins, particularly albumin, maintain plasma volume. Assess total plasma proteins prior to fluid therapy and frequently during treatment to ensure that values remain above 4.0 g/dl (albumin >1.5 g/dl).

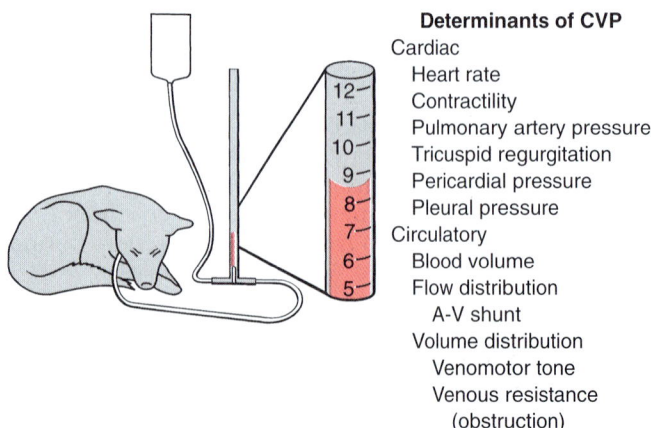

Determinants of CVP
Cardiac
  Heart rate
  Contractility
  Pulmonary artery pressure
  Tricuspid regurgitation
  Pericardial pressure
  Pleural pressure
Circulatory
  Blood volume
  Flow distribution
    A-V shunt
  Volume distribution
    Venomotor tone
    Venous resistance
      (obstruction)

Figure 72–1.   Determinants of central venous pressure (CVP).

Arterial Pressure

- Digital palpation may be used to assess mean arterial pressure (MAP). Strong pulse pressure usually reflects a MAP of >70 mm Hg. A weak pulse is detected when MAP is <70 mm Hg. When MAP is <40 mm Hg, the pulse is difficult or impossible to palpate.
- Arterial pressure also may be assessed using Doppler or oscillometric methods. These techniques are noninvasive and generally accurate, except when arterial pressure is low.

Cardiac Output

- Capillary refill time, body temperature, and mentation are the physical findings that best reflect cardiac output. However, these are not always accurate.
- Urine output is a good indicator of cardiac output. When cardiac output is reduced, sympathetic nervous system activity may maintain blood pressure within normal limits but may decrease renal blood flow. Consequently, urine output will be decreased (<1 ml/kg/hr). However, other causes of reduced urine formation must be considered.
- Cardiac rhythm influences cardiac output and can be monitored by ECG.

Oxygen Delivery

- Oxygen delivery is determined by cardiac output as assessed above; pulmonary function is assessed by arterial oxygen pressure (PaO_2) or oximetry; and hemoglobin is assessed by hematocrit.
- Mucous membrane color, mentation, body temperature, and respiratory rate are the physical findings that best reflect oxygen delivery.
- Obtain blood samples for hematocrit measurement prior to treatment for shock. Repeat measurements frequently during aggressive fluid therapy (e.g., q1–2h). Maintain hematocrit >20%; in severe shock, it should be >30%.

Treatment

Preliminary Measures

- Establish an airway and ventilate if necessary. Administer 100% oxygen via an endotracheal tube, mask, nasal tube, or tracheal catheter.
- To evaluate the patient for the cause of shock, obtain a history and perform a physical examination. The time allotted for these efforts depends on the condition of the patient.
- Place and secure a large-gauge intravenous (IV) catheter, preferably jugular. The jugular catheter should be long enough to reach the thoracic cavity.
  - Jugular catheterization has the advantages of allowing the use of a large-gauge catheter even in small patients, ease of placement, access for blood sampling, rapid fluid administration, CVP measurement, and catheter security. The major disadvantage is that jugular catheters are slightly more expensive.
- Obtain blood for storage in EDTA and clot tubes. Measure hematocrit and total protein, serum elec-

trolytes, serum creatinine, blood glucose, and a complete blood count.

Optimize Blood Volume

- Initially, administer sodium-rich isotonic crystalloid fluids (e.g., 0.9% NaCl, lactated Ringer's solution) at a rate of 60–90 ml/kg/hr (Table 72–2). To ensure effective plasma volume expansion, maintain the sodium concentration of the isotonic fluid at >130 mEq/L.
- Administration of 7% NaCl (hypertonic saline) is an alternative resuscitation regimen. Deliver the initial dosage of 4–6 ml/kg over 5–10 minutes (Table 72–3). The hypertonic saline may be combined with 6% dextran 70 and given at the same dosage. Supplement this form of initial treatment by giving isotonic crystalloid fluids at a minimum rate of 20 ml/kg/hr.
- The goal of the initial rapid rate of fluid administration is to establish a normal arterial pressure and optimize blood volume. An adequate arterial pressure is easily determined by palpation of pulse pressure. Physical signs, including pulse pressure, may be normal despite continuing tissue hypoxia and less than optimal or unstable blood volume.
- Blood volume is optimized when CVP is 5–12 cm H_2O.
- To treat hypoproteinemia, fresh or frozen plasma may be administered at a dosage of 10–20 ml/kg/day IV.
- Alternatively, synthetic colloids may be used to treat hypoproteinemia. Those useful in small animal patients include 6% dextran 70 and 6% hetastarch. The dosages are similar to those for plasma (10–20 ml/kg/day) and commonly are divided into 5–10 ml/kg slow IV infusions (over 10–20 minutes).
- Fresh or stored blood may be given to optimize blood volume if the hematocrit and total protein are decreased below acceptable levels. Blood collected from the abdominal or thoracic cavity may be autotransfused if other, more acceptable sources are unavailable. This blood must be free of bacterial and neoplastic contamination and should be administered via a blood administration set (including filter). Autotransfused blood will have decreased platelets, clotting factors, and fibrinogen concentration.

Optimize Blood Flow

- Cardiac output increases and is often optimized as a result of aggressive volume expansion.
- If volume expansion has increased the CVP to 5–12 cm H_2O but urine output and other physical signs reflecting cardiac output are not normalized, evaluate cardiac function with ECG.
- If the ECG is normal, administer a positive inotropic agent. Dobutamine (Dobutrex, Lilly) and dopamine (Intropin, DuPont) are inotropic drugs (see Chap. 63) that are commonly used to enhance cardiac function in shock.
  - Dobutamine produces dose-dependent increases in contractility when administered at a dosage of 2–15 µg/kg/min IV (Fig. 72–2).

Table 72–2. TREATMENT OF SHOCK

Therapeutic Goal	Therapy	Specific Objectives	Dosage Recommendations

Optimize blood volume	Crystalloids
	  Isotonic
	  Hypertonic
	Colloids
	Whole blood
		CVP 5–12 cm H_2O
		Wedge pressure 7–20 mm Hg
		Total protein >4.0 g/dl
		Albumin >1.5 g/dl
		Normal skin turgor
			Isotonic fluids: 0.9% NaCl or LRS; 60–90 ml/kg/hr to effect IV
			Hypertonic saline/dextran: 7% NaCl or 7% NaCl in 6% dextran 70, 4–6 ml/kg slowly IV
			Plasma: 10–20 ml/kg IV
			6% Dextran 70: 10–20 ml/kg/day IV
			6% Hetastarch: 10–20 ml/kg/day IV
			Whole blood: 20–30 ml/kg IV

Optimize blood flow	Fluids Inotropic agents	Urine output >1 ml/kg/hr CRT < 2 sec PvO_2 > 35 torr Cardiac index 150–200 ml/min/kg	See Optimize Blood Volume in text Dopamine: 2–10 μg/kg/min IV Dobutamine: 2–15 μg/kg/min IV
Optimize oxygen delivery and consumption	Fluids Whole blood Packed red cells O_2 supplementation Mechanical ventilation Respiratory care	PaO_2 > 70 torr PvO_2 > 35 torr Hct > 25 Pink mucous membranes Patient bright, alert, responsive	See Optimize Blood Volume in text Packed red cells: 10–20 ml/kg IV FIO_2: 40–100%

Optimize blood pressure	Fluids
	Vasopressors
		Arterial pressure:
		  Systolic, 100–160 mm Hg
		  Mean, 70–120 mm Hg
		  Diastolic, 50–100 mm Hg
		Strong pulse
			See Optimize Blood Volume in text
			Dopamine: 5–10 μg/kg/min IV
			Epinephrine: 0.1–0.3 μg/kg/min IV
			Phenylephrine: 0.01–0.1 μg/kg/min IV
			Methoxamine: 0.2 μg/kg IV

Optimize heart rate/rhythm	Fluids Antiarrhythmics	70–160 bpm Sinus rhythm	See Optimize Blood Volume in text Lidocaine: 1–2 mg/kg bolus IV, 25–75μg/kg/min IV Procainamide: 15–20 mg/kg IM
Correct acid-base imbalance	$NaHCO_3$	pH > 7.3 and < 7.5	Sodium bicarbonate: 0.5–5.0 mEq/kg IV or mEq = 0.3 × base deficit × kg
Optimize urine output	Fluids	1–2 ml/kg/hr urine production	Furosemide: 2–4 mg/kg IV Mannitol (20%): 1–2 g/kg IV
Control sepsis	Antibiotics Surgery Culture and sensitivity	Negative culture Wound/infection management	Cephalothin: 20 mg/kg IV q6h Ampicillin: 20 mg/kg IV q6h Gentamicin: 2 mg/kg IV q8h
Optimize blood glucose	Glucose Insulin	Blood glucose 60–120 mg/dl	Dextrose 5% in maintenance fluids Dextrose 50%: 0.5–2.0 g/kg/hr Insulin (regular): 0.5–2 units/kg q2–6h IV (if hyperglycemic)
Immune/inflammatory modulation	Corticosteroids	Same as Therapeutic Goal	Dexamethasone sodium phosphate: 1–2 mg/kg IV Prednisolone sodium succinate: 10–20 mg/kg IV

CRT, capillary refill time; CVP, central venous pressure; FIO_2, inspired oxygen fraction; Hct, hematocrit; LRS, lactated Ringer's solution; PaO_2, arterial oxygen partial pressure; PvO_2, venous oxygen partial pressure.

Table 72–3. HYPERTONIC SALINE AND SYNTHETIC COLLOID THERAPY*

	Sodium Chloride Solutions			Synthetic Colloids	
	3% NaCl	5% NaCl	7% NaCl	6% Dextran 70	6% Hetastarch
Approximate osmolality (mOsm/kg)	1000	1800	2400	N/A†	N/A
Maximum dosage range (ml/kg IV)	20	6–10	4–8	10–20	10–20
Maximum infusion rate (ml/kg/min IV)	2	1	1	1	1
Available products	3% NaCl	5% NaCl	7% NaCl	Gentran 70	Hespan
Manufacturers	Baxter, Kendall McGaw	Baxter, Abbott, Kendall McGaw	Butler	Baxter	DuPont

*Indications: hypovolemia, traumatic shock, endotoxemia, septicemia, gastric dilatation-volvulus. Contraindications: dehydration, hypernatremia, hyperosmolality, heart/renal failure.

†N/A: not applicable.

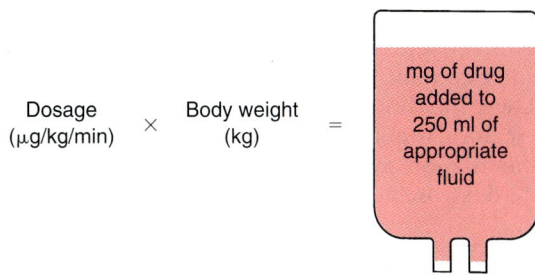

Figure 72–2. Simplified method of dosage formulation for continuous-infusion drugs. Once formulated, administer at 15 ml/hr or 1 drop/4 sec from a 60-drop/ml administration set to achieve desired dosage.

- Dopamine administered at dosages of 1–3 μg/kg/min IV improves renal and mesenteric blood flow. At dosages of 3–10 μg/kg/min IV, dopamine improves contractility and increases cardiac output and peripheral vascular resistance, causing renal and mesenteric arterial vasoconstriction.
- Cardiac arrhythmias may contribute to low cardiac output. Consider causes of arrhythmias (myocardial hypoxia, myocardial contusion, and electrolyte disturbances) and correct them if possible (see Chap. 62). Ventricular arrhythmias are the most common and may be treated with lidocaine administered IV at 1–2 mg/kg or as a continuous infusion of 25–75 μg/kg/min (see Chap. 63).

Optimize Blood Pressure

- Arterial blood pressure often is returned to normal by fluid therapy.

▼ **Key Point** When arterial blood pressure is <40 mm Hg (pulse weak or not palpable), increase blood pressure immediately.

- In cases of severe shock, epinephrine may be needed to increase peripheral vascular resistance and cardiac output until fluid therapy can be initiated and blood volume expanded.
  - The IV dosage of epinephrine for cardiac arrest is 0.02–0.2 mg/kg (0.02–0.2 ml/kg of 1:1000 dilution).
  - When the primary problem is severe hypotension, not cardiac arrest, administer epinephrine continuously at a dosage of 0.1–0.3 μg/kg/min IV (see Fig. 72–2).
  - Once blood volume is expanded and cardiac output and mean arterial pressure are restored, discontinue epinephrine.
- Use of an abdominal wrap or "belly band" to augment arterial blood pressure and to tamponade abdominal bleeding may be dangerous and is not recommended. Any increase in arterial resistance (arterial pressure) created by an abdominal wrap may be counteracted by obstruction of the vena cava and portal vein and by decreased venous return. Furthermore, the abdominal wrap may compromise respiratory function, exacerbate diaphragmatic hernia, and lead to hypotension when it is removed.
- Manage uncontrolled intra-abdominal hemorrhage by aggressive fluid replacement, and perform surgical exploration if the condition fails to stabilize.

Optimize Oxygen Delivery

- Optimal oxygen delivery is often attained by aggressive volume replacement.
- Hemodilution or pre-existing anemia may limit oxygen delivery. Red blood cell (RBC) replacement (whole blood, packed red cells) is necessary when hematocrit is <20%. Administer whole blood at a dosage of 20–30 ml/kg and packed RBCs at 10–20 ml/kg (see Chap. 20).
- Administration of corticosteroids (e.g., prednisolone sodium succinate, 10–20 mg/kg) before transfusion minimizes the risk of severe transfusion reaction and improves the RBC function of stored blood.
- Oxygen supplementation improves arterial blood oxygen content and may be administered via mask, nasal catheter, oxygen cage, or transtracheal catheter and is particularly crucial when the patient is anemic (see Chap. 3).
- In cases of severe lung injury, provide ventilatory assistance. This requires anesthetizing the patient and placement of an endotracheal tube. Alternatively, a tracheostomy may be performed (see Chap. 3).

Correction of Acid-Base and Electrolyte Disturbances

- The metabolic acidosis that results from shock that is mild or of short duration often can be managed effectively by fluid replacement therapy.
- The degree of metabolic acidosis that develops in shock depends on the severity and duration of the oxygen delivery deficit. If blood gas analysis can be performed, the milliequivalent (mEq) dosage of $NaHCO_3$ required to correct the acidosis may be calculated by the following formula:

$$NaHCO_3 \text{ (mEq)} = 0.3 \times \text{body weight (kg)} \times \text{base deficit}$$

- If blood gas analysis is not available, an estimate of the base deficit may be made based on the severity of the shock state and its duration. Mild, moderate, and severe shock may be treated with $NaHCO_3$ dosages of 1.0, 3.0, and 5.0 mEq/kg of body weight, respectively (see Chap. 5 for more information on treatment of acidosis).
- Hyperkalemia is the most common serum electrolyte concentration abnormality observed in shock. Hyperkalemia generally responds to aggressive volume replacement, increased urine output, and improvement of metabolic status. Glucose and $NaHCO_3$ infusions facilitate reduction of serum potassium concentration (see Chap. 5).
- Hypokalemia often occurs after aggressive volume replacement. Once maintenance fluids are started, they should contain 15–20 mEq/L of KCl (see Chap. 5).

Corticosteroid Therapy

- Corticosteroids may be of benefit in most forms of shock, but are not recommended for septic shock. Administer early in the course of therapy to derive maximum benefits.
- Use water-soluble drugs, including dexamethasone sodium phosphate (Azium-SP, Schering), 1–2 mg/kg IV, and prednisolone sodium succinate (Solu-Delta-Cortef, Upjohn), 10–20 mg/kg IV.

Miscellaneous Treatments

- Broad-spectrum antibiotics are indicated in most forms of severe shock, particularly septic shock.
- Surgical management of a septic focus should be performed as soon as cardiorespiratory stability is established.

- IV glucose can provide some of the caloric requirements of the shock patient. Maintenance fluids should contain 5% dextrose. This treatment is helpful over the short term, but supplies only a fraction of the caloric requirements. More complete caloric supplementation may be achieved by administration of 50% dextrose at an hourly dosage of 0.5–2.0 g/kg.

SUPPLEMENTAL READINGS

Schertel ER, Tobias TA: Hypertonic fluid therapy. *In* DiBartola SP, ed.: Fluid Therapy in Small Animal Practice. Philadelphia: WB Saunders, 1992, p 471.

Tobias TA, Schertel ER: Shock: Concepts and management. *In* DiBartola SP, ed.: Fluid Therapy in Small Animal Practice. Philadelphia: WB Saunders, 1992, p 436.

73 Cardiopulmonary Cerebral Resuscitation

William W. Muir, III

Resuscitation is the restoration of life after apparent death. Cardiopulmonary resuscitation (CPR) includes therapy to restore heart and lung function to normal. Most resuscitative techniques incorporate methods to maximize and maintain cerebral blood flow and clinicians have redefined CPR as cardiopulmonary cerebral resuscitation (CPCR). Preparedness and early recognition of the signs of sudden death are the major factors that determine long-term outcome (Tables 73–1 and 73–2).

CPCR is divided into three phases:

- *Phase 1,* basic life support (BLS), consists of establishing an airway (A), breathing (B), and circulatory support (C).

- *Phase 2,* advanced life support (ALS), incorporates the use of drugs (D), electrocardiography (E), and methods to convert ventricular fibrillation or asystole (F) to sinus rhythm.
- *Phase 3,* prolonged life support (PLS), includes measures that focus on treating the causes of cardiac arrest and deciding whether to continue resuscitative efforts. Gauging (G) (monitoring of patient trends), hypnogenesis (H) (use of sedation, anesthesia, and pain control), utilization of methods to restore cerebral function, and intensive care (I) oriented toward preventing multiorgan failure are also elements of PLS.

BASIC LIFE SUPPORT: AIRWAY, BREATHING, AND CIRCULATION

Airway

▼ *Key Point* Establishing a patent functional airway is the first step when performing CPCR.

Establishing an Airway

Mouth to Endotracheal Tube. To pass a cuffed endotracheal tube of appropriate size place the patient on the sternum, open the mouth widely, and maximally extend the head and neck. Expose the larynx (using a laryngoscope if necessary) and proceed with intubation.

Tracheotomy. A tracheotomy may be necessary in animals with upper airway obstruction, brachycephalic animals, or in dogs and cats that are successfully resuscitated, regain consciousness, and object to oral-tracheal intubation (This procedure is described in Chap. 3.)

Mouth to Muzzle. Tightly cup hands around the muzzle of small dogs and cats, or place mouth directly over the patient's muzzle. Blow exhaled air into the animal's lungs.

Mouth to Mask. A variety of masks have been developed for use in dogs and cats for the delivery of oxygen or inhaled anesthetics.

▼ *Key Point* Mouth to muzzle and mouth to mask methods do not secure the airway but may be useful when equipment is limited. Distention of the

---

Table 73–1. SIGNS OF CARDIOPULMONARY ARREST

Evaluations	Clinical Signs and Observations
Effort, rate, and rhythm of breathing	Dyspnea (abdominal breathing)
	Gasps (gurgling sounds)
	Tachypnea
	Bradypnea
	Altered patterns of breathing:
	Cheyne-Stokes
	Biot (periodic breathing)
	Agonal
Heart rate and rhythm	Tachycardia
	Bradycardia
	Irregular rhythm
Pulse	Peripheral arterial pulse is difficult or impossible to palpate at ABPs <50–60 mm Hg
Heart sounds	Heart sounds are inaudible at ABPs <50 mm Hg
Bleeding	Absence of bleeding
	Change in color of blood from red to blue during surgical procedure
Peripheral perfusion	Change in mucous membrane color:
	Pale or white
	Blue or cyanotic—5 g/dl of reduced Hb imparts bluish discoloration to mucous membranes regardless of Hb concentration; anemic animals (<5 dl Hb) do not demonstrate cyanosis
Pupils	Pupils dilate within 1–2 min after cardiac arrest
Mental state	Altered consciousness
	Coma

ABPs = arterial blood pressures; Hb = hemoglobin.

Table 73–2. ESSENTIAL EQUIPMENT TO PERFORM CPCR*

1. Assortment of cuffed endotracheal tubes with inside diameter of 2–15 mm
2. Oxygen supply source
   a. Small animal anesthetic machine
   b. Demand valve
   c. Oxygen hose to deliver nasal oxygen
   d. Respirator (pressure or volume cycled)
   e. Oxygen chamber
3. Fluid and drug administration equipment
   a. Assortment of intravenous needles and catheters
      (1) Needles—18–25 gauge
      (2) Over-the-needle or through-the-needle catheters—17–22 gauge
   b. Assortment of syringes—1, 3, 6, 12, and 60 ml
   c. Solution administration sets
      (1) Standard solution administration sets (10 drops/ml) for animals over 5 kg
      (2) Mini-drop solution administration sets (60 drops/ml) for animals <5 kg and to deliver drugs that must be administered by infusion
   d. Venous extension tubing to prolong the time until drug effect, by increasing distance between fluids and patient
   e. Three-way stopcocks and catheter plugs
4. Fluids
   a. Balanced electrolyte solutions to be administered IV in most emergency situations; rate of fluid administration is determined by circumstances (see text for dosages):
      (1) 20 ml/kg/hr during hypotension
      (2) 40 ml/kg/hr following acute cardiac arrest
      (3) 80 to 90 ml/kg/hr following circulatory failure due to hemorrhage
   b. Other solutions
      (1) 5% dextrose in water to supply volume and additional calories and dilute plasma potassium concentration
      (2) Normal saline (0.9% NaCl) to supply volume and dilute plasma potassium concentration
      (3) Colloid solutions (6% dextran 70; hetastarch) to supply volume and oncotic value
      (4) Mannitol (20% Osmotrol) to be used as an osmotic diuretic and as an oxygen free radical scavenger
   c. Special solutions
      (1) Hypertonic saline solutions (usually 3 or 7%) to restore vascular volume; the appropriate quantity of NaCl may be mixed in 6% dextran 70; 7% NaCl in 6% dextran 70 can be administered IV, 4 ml/kg, over 1–2 min
      (2) Blood substitute (Oxyglobin, Biopure), 10–30 ml/kg/hr IV, to maintain tissue oxygenation following acute hemorrhage or in severe anemia
5. Drugs (see text for dosages)
   a. Anticholinergics (atropine or glycopyrrolate)
   b. Epinephrine (1:1000 and 1:10,000)
   c. Dopamine or dobutamine
   d. Calcium chloride
   e. Lidocaine (2%)
   f. Injectable procainamide
   g. Glucocorticosteroids (dexamethasone, prednisolone sodium succinate)
   h. Furosemide
   i. Mannitol
   j. Diazepam, thiobarbiturate (thiopental), phenytoin
   k. Oxymorphone, other opioids
   l. Doxapram
6. Surgical instruments
   a. Scalpel and several #10 blades
   b. Mosquito and Kelly hemostats
   c. Rib retractors
   d. Thumb forceps
   e. Metzenbaum and Mayo scissors, needle holders
7. Bandage material (1, 2, and 4 inch)
   a. Sterile 4–inch × 4–inch gauze sponges
   b. Cotton bandage
   c. Elastic bandage
   d. Tape
8. Other equipment
   a. Clippers
   b. Leg splints (tongue depressors can be used in animals under 10 kg)
   c. Water circulating heating pad
   d. Electrocardiographic machine
   e. Electrical defibrillator
   f. Aspiration or suction device and tubing
   g. Assortment of suture material

*This material should be kept in one place, preferably on an emergency cart or in a large tool chest.

stomach with air may limit lung expansion and predisposes to regurgitation.

Proper Endotracheal Tube Placement

Correct placement of the endotracheal tube can be verified by:

- Direct observation of the tube positioned through the larynx (most reliable technique)
- Palpation of the endotracheal tube in the trachea
- The appearance of water vapor on clear endotracheal tubes
- The inability of the animal to vocalize
- Gas exiting the endotracheal tube during exhalation. This sign, which frequently is used clinically, should not be the only method used to ensure proper endotracheal tube placement.

Air or Oxygen Delivery Systems (Fig. 73–1, top)

- *Self-refilling bags* connected to oxygen (Ambu bag) can be used to provide an air or oxygen source during controlled breathing.

- *Demand valves,* which are oxygen-powered, manually triggered ventilatory devices, permit both the initiation and termination of ventilation.
- *Anesthetic machines* are the most readily available source of oxygen in most hospitals.
- *Automatic pressure- or volume-cycled ventilators* can be used to assist (control volume) or control (control rate and volume) breathing. Most ventilators do not function properly during thoracic compression.
- In *translaryngeal or tracheal insufflation* (see Fig. 73–1, *bottom*), place an over-the-needle catheter (Surflo, Terumo Medical Corp.) (17–14 gauge) in the trachea and attach to a three-way stopcock, venous extension tubing, and oxygen supply.

Breathing

A ventilator, delivering 50–100% oxygen, can be used to assist or control breathing. The resuscitator's exhaled air, which contains 16–18% oxygen, may be expelled into a properly placed endotracheal tube and is adequate for maintaining PaO$_2$ if large tidal volumes are used.

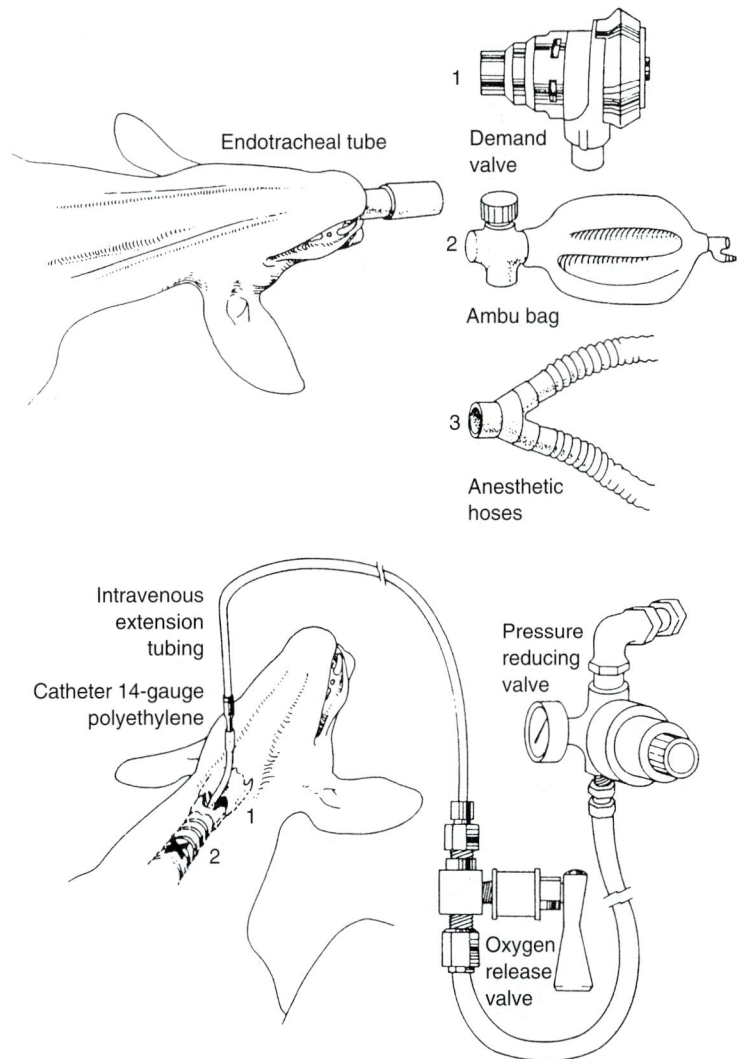

Figure 73–1. Methods of endotracheal oxygen administration *(top)*; transtracheal oxygen administration *(bottom)* via catheter placement through the cricothyroid notch (1) or between tracheal rings (2). (Modified from Sherding RG: Medical Emergencies. New York: Churchill Livingstone, 1985.)

Maximal oxygenation of arterial blood with minimal hemodynamic impairment can be obtained by:

- Providing a source of 100% oxygen
- Proper placement of an endotracheal tube
- Slow (1–2 sec) inflation of the lungs
- Providing adequate (14–20 ml/kg) tidal volume
- Providing adequate (25–30 cm H_2O) but not excessive inspiratory pressure
  - Inflation of the lung with an excessive volume of gas impairs venous return and cardiac output during closed chest CPCR. Therefore, be careful not to overinflate the lung.
- Sedation and/or anesthesia may be necessary to control ventilation in conscious or semiconscious patients (see Chap. 2) that resist placement of an endotracheal tube.
  - Diazepam, 0.2–0.5 mg/kg IV
  - Propofol, 4–6 mg/kg IV; 0.2–0.4 mg/kg/min
  - Isoflurane, 1–2%
- Positive end-expiratory pressure (PEEP; 5 cm H_2O) helps to prevent small airway closure, thereby improving gas exchange.

Circulation: Closed Chest Compression

The early re-establishment of normal or near-normal hemodynamics, particularly cerebral blood flow, is vital to long-term survival.

▼ *Key Point* External chest compression is effective in restoring blood flow to the systemic circulation and brain if proper techniques are utilized.

One-Rescuer CPCR with Intermittent Positive Pressure Ventilation (IPPV). Perform one-rescuer chest compression (80–100 compressions/min) by placing the animal in lateral recumbency and manually compressing the thorax from side to side, using the thumb and first two index fingers in animals less than 5 kg and the palms of the hands in larger animals (Fig. 73–2). Ventilate the lungs following every 15 chest compressions.

Two-Rescuer CPCR with IPPV. The technique for compressing the chest is identical to that in one-rescuer CPCR (see above). Ventilate intermittently without slowing the rate of chest compression (1 breath for each 15 chest compressions) or simultaneously with chest compression (SVC or simultaneous compression ventilation–CPCR). Take care not to overinflate the lungs (use <40 cm H_2O), in order to prevent or minimize pulmonary barotrauma and pneumothorax.

Three-Rescuer CPCR with IPPV and Abdominal Pressure. Applying steady or intermittent abdominal pressure during CPCR or SVC-CPCR may augment carotid arterial pressures and cerebral and myocardial blood flow.

- The palm of the hand (third rescuer) may be used to compress the abdomen against the backbone for periods of 5–10 seconds. Repeat this procedure 2–3 times per minute.
- An elastic bandage can be tightly wrapped around the rear legs to prevent venous pooling and promote venous return.

ADVANCED LIFE SUPPORT

The primary purpose of advanced life support techniques is to restore adequate spontaneous circulation. Open-chest CPCR is considered an advanced life support technique. Antiarrhythmic, inotropic, and antishock drugs (glucocorticosteroids, free radical scavengers) are used in conjunction with fluid therapy to restore supernormal hemodynamics.

Drug Therapy

Drugs and fluids are preferably administered intravenously (see Table 73–3 for dosages and side effects; also see Chap. 63 for additional details regarding the pharmacologic actions of cardiovascular and antiarrhythmic drugs). Place a large-bore catheter (18–14 gauge) in the cephalic or jugular vein. Placement of an IV catheter may require a "cutdown" or placement of an intraosseous needle (20 or 18 gauge), because the veins collapse shortly after cardiac arrest (see Chap. 3).

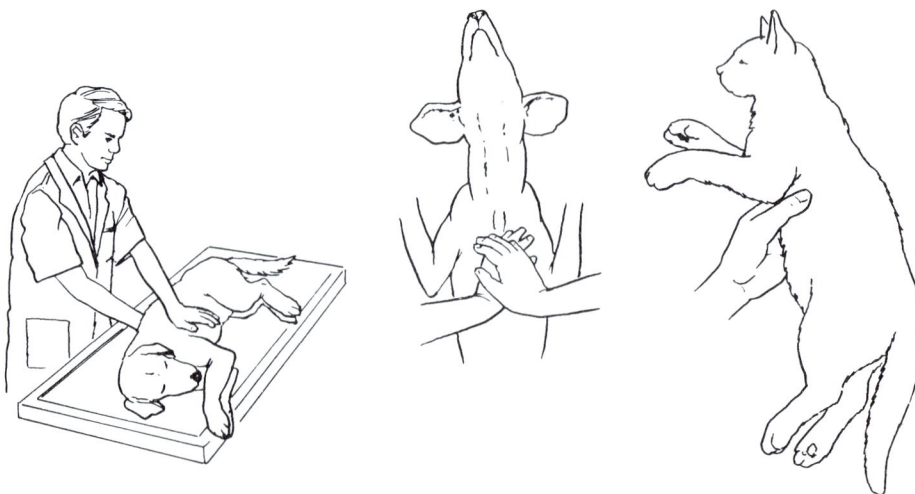

Figure 73–2. Chest compression in the dog *(left, middle)*; chest compression in the cat *(right)*.

Table 73–3. THERAPEUTIC MANAGEMENT OF PROBLEMS ASSOCIATED WITH CARDIAC ARREST

Problem	Treatment	Trade Name or Device	Dosage	Side Effects or Contraindications
Hypovolemia				
Fluid loss	Crystalloid	Lactated Ringer's solution	50–90 ml/kg/hr IV	Hypervolemia, pulmonary edema, hypoproteinemia
	Hypertonic saline (7%)		5 ml/kg IV	Hypokalemia, hypernatremia, acidosis, arrhythmias
Plasma loss	Colloid expanders	Gentran 70	10–20 ml/kg IV	Hypervolemia, pulmonary edema, allergic reactions
		Hetastarch	10–20 ml/kg IV	
Blood loss	Whole blood		10–40 ml/kg IV	Hypervolemia, allergic reactions
	Blood substitute	Oxyglobin	15–30 ml/kg IV	Hypervolemia, pulmonary edema
Hypotension	See Hypovolemia			
	Phenylephrine	Neo-Synephrine	10–50 µg/kg IV	Hypertension, tachycardia, arrhythmias
	Epinephrine	Adrenalin	3–5 µg/kg IV	
	Dopamine	Intropin	3–10 µg/kg/min IV	
	Dobutamine	Dobutrex	3–10 µg/kg/min IV	
Cardiac arrhythmias				
Bradycardia	Atropine	Atropine	0.01–0.02 mg/kg IV	Tachycardia
	Glycopyrrolate	Robinul	0.005–0.01 mg/kg IV	Tachycardia
Tachycardia	Propranolol	Inderal	0.05–0.01 mg/kg IV	Bradycardia, cardiac failure
Atrial arrhythmias	Quinidine	Quinidine gluconate	4–8 mg/kg/10 min IV	Hypotension
	Diltiazem	Cardizem	0.5–2.0 mg/kg PO q8h; 5–10 µg/kg/min	Hypotension, AV block
	Lidocaine	Xylocaine	2–4 mg/kg IV dogs; 1 mg/kg IV cats 40–60 µg/kg/min IV	CNS excitement
Ventricular arrhythmias	Procainamide	Pronestyl	6–20 mg/kg/10 min IV	Hypotension
	Calcium chloride		1 ml 10%/10 kg IV	
Acute heart failure	Epinephrine	Adrenalin	3–5 µg/kg IV	Hypertension, tachycardia, cardiac arrhythmias
	Dopamine	Intropin	3–10 µg/kg/min IV	
	Dobutamine	Dobutrex	3–10 µg/kg/min IV	
Respiratory failure				
Hypoxia	O₂ nasal catheter; oxygen cage		2–4 L/min	
	Ventilation		Tidal volume = 14 ml/kg	Decreased venous return, respiratory alkalosis
Hypercarbia	Doxapram	Dopram V	1–2 mg/kg	CNS excitement
	Ventilation		Tidal volume = 14 ml/kg	Decreased venous return, respiratory alkalosis
Dyspnea	Tracheostomy			
	Chest tube			
	Ventilation		Tidal volume = 14 ml/kg	Decreased venous return, respiratory alkalosis
Sepsis	Surgery (if indicated)			
	Gentamicin	Gentocin	1–3 mg/kg q6–8h IM, IV	Muscle weakness, renal toxicity
	Kanamycin	Kantrim	10 mg/kg q6h IM	Muscle weakness, renal toxicity
	Ampicillin	Omnipen	10 mg/kg q6h IV	
	Cephalothin	Keflin	20–30 mg/kg IV q6h	Phlebitis, myositis
Metabolic acidosis	Sodium lactate*		Bicarbonate dose = base deficit × 0.3 × wt (kg) or 0.5 mEq/kg/10 min IV to effect	Metabolic alkalosis, hyperosmolarity, CSF acidosis hyperkalemia, hypocalcemia
	Sodium acetate*			
	Sodium bicarbonate			
Hyperkalemia	Sodium bicarbonate		0.5–2.0 mg/kg IV	As above
	NaCl 0.9% solution		10–40 ml/kg/hr IV	Hypervolemia, hypoproteinemia
	Calcium gluconate		0.5 ml/kg of 10% solution IV	Tachycardia
	Hyperventilation		Tidal volume = 14 ml/kg	Decreased venous return, respiratory alkalosis
	Dextrose 50%		1–2 ml/kg IV	Hyperosmolarity
Hypoglycemia			0.5–1.0 g/kg/hr; 10% glucose	
Renal ischemia	Fluids	Lactated Ringer's solution	10–40 ml/kg/hr IV	Hypervolemia, hypoproteinemia, pulmonary edema

Table 73–3. THERAPEUTIC MANAGEMENT OF PROBLEMS ASSOCIATED WITH CARDIAC ARREST Continued

Problem	Treatment	Trade Name or Device	Dosage	Side Effects or Contraindications
Renal ischemia (*continued*)	Mannitol 20%	Osmitrol	0.5–2.0 g/kg IV	Hyperosmolality
	Furosemide	Lasix	1.0–2.0 mg/kg IM, IV	Decreased cardiac output
Hypothermia (<36°C)	Fluids	Lactated Ringer's solution	10–40 ml/kg/hr, warmed to 37°C	Hypervolemia, hypoproteinemia, pulmonary edema
	H$_2$O-filled heating pad		Warmed slowly to 38°C	
Disseminated intravascular coagulation	Correct hypotension	Lactated Ringer's solution	10–40 ml/kg/hr IV	Hypervolemia, hypoproteinemia, pulmonary edema
	Correct hypoxemia	Nasal catheter	2–4 L/min	
		Ventilation	Tidal volume = 14 ml/kg	Decreased venous return, respiratory alkalosis
	Correct acidosis	Sodium bicarbonate	0.5–1.0 mg/kg IV	
	Heparin		Dog: 500 U/kg SC q8h for 24 hr	Bleeding
			Cat: 250–400 U/kg SC q8h for 24 hr	
Cellular ischemia	Fluids	Lactated Ringer's solution	10–40 ml/kg/h IV	Hypervolemia, hypoproteinemia, pulmonary edema
	Mannitol	Osmitrol	0.5–2.0 g/kg IV	
	Oxygen	Nasal catheter	2–4 L/min	
	Dexamethasone sodium phosphate	Azium	4–6 mg/kg IV	
	Prednisolone sodium succinate	Solu-Delta-Cortef	>10 mg/kg IV	

Modified from Muir WW, Bonagura JD: Cardiovascular emergencies. *In* Sherding RG, ed.: Medical Emergencies. New York: Churchill Livingstone, 1985, p 52.
*Questionable efficacy during severe low-flow states.

Table 73–4. EMERGENCY DOSES OF EPINEPHRINE

Route	Dose	Comments
Intravenous		
Arrest/ventricular fibrillation	0.01–0.1 mg/kg	Dose determined by heart rate; begin at low dose
Bradycardia	0.01–0.1 mg/kg	
Intracardiac	0.01–0.02 mg/kg	Potentially arrhythmogenic
Intratracheal	0.05 mg/kg	Dilute with 0.9% NaCl (1 ml/5 kg body weight), ineffective during cardiac arrest/fibrillation

Epinephrine

▼ *Key Point* Epinephrine is the drug of choice for the treatment of cardiac arrest regardless of cause (Table 73–4).

- Large doses of epinephrine (0.2 mg/kg IV) produce dramatic increases in heart rate, arterial blood pressure, and cerebral blood flow in dogs and cats suffering from severe bradycardia (<30) with hypotension, but may induce ventricular arrhythmias and ventricular fibrillation in animals that are in sinus or idioventricular rhythms.
- Initial doses of 0.01 mg/kg IV are adequate in most patients with hypotension or bradycardia and may be adjusted upward according to the patient's response (see Table 73–4).

Lidocaine

Lidocaine is the first choice antiarrhythmic for the treatment of ventricular arrhythmias in dogs and cats.

- It is the drug of choice for the treatment of cardiac arrhythmias induced by catecholamines and digitalis glycosides, and ventricular arrhythmias produced by inhalation anesthetics (halothane) and thiobarbiturates.
- Initial IV bolus dosages should not exceed 4 mg/kg in dogs and 1.0 mg/kg in cats. A lidocaine infusion (40–60 μg/kg/min) produces a sustained antiarrhythmic effect. A solution containing 1 mg (1000 μg) of lidocaine per ml is made by mixing 25 ml of 2% lidocaine in 500 ml of lactated Ringer's solution (infuse 0.5 ml/10 kg/min).

▼ *Key Point* Lidocaine is relatively ineffective in hypokalemic patients and should never be administered to patients with complete (third-degree) AV block.

Procainamide

Procainamide is an antiarrhythmic drug used for acute therapy of ventricular arrhythmias (see Table 73–4).

- Dosages range from 6–20 mg/kg IV slowly, followed by an infusion of 40–60 μg/kg/min if necessary. Procainamide can also be administered IM, at a dose of 10–20 mg/kg.

Sodium Bicarbonate

Sodium bicarbonate administration helps to combat the development of metabolic acidosis and, more specifically, lactic acidosis produced by anaerobic metabolism secondary to circulatory arrest.

- The initial dose of sodium bicarbonate (1 mEq/kg IV) is not required until after 10–15 minutes of arrest and may be repeated (0.5 mEq/kg IV) every 10–15 minutes until resuscitative efforts are successful or terminated.

Anticholinergics

Atropine (0.01–0.02 mg/kg IV) or glycopyrrolate (0.005–0.01 mg/kg IV) is effective for the treatment of bradyarrhythmias (sinus bradycardia, high-grade second-degree and third-degree AV block) produced by increases in vagal tone.

▼ *Key Point* Do not administer anticholinergics unless indicated. Anticholinergics can produce sinus tachycardia and predispose to cardiac arrhythmias and ventricular fibrillation in hypotensive patients.

Calcium Chloride

Calcium chloride and calcium gluconate have the potential to increase the force of myocardial contraction and thereby increase cardiac output and peripheral blood flow.

- IV administration of calcium chloride (1 ml/10 kg of a 10% solution) is indicated for the treatment of hyperkalemia, hypocalcemia, and inhalation anesthetic or calcium antagonist (e.g., verapamil, diltiazem) overdose.
- Do not routinely use calcium during the initial phases of CPCR because calcium-mediated cardiac injury (calcium overload) can occur.

Isoproterenol

Isoproterenol is a mixed (β_1, β_2) beta-adrenoceptor agonist that produces marked increases in heart rate and the force of cardiac contraction. Concurrent vasodilation makes it a poor drug for CPCR.

- Isoproterenol is effective (5 μg/kg IV; 0.05–1 μg/kg/min) in some cases of bradycardia (e.g., third-degree atrioventricular block).

Parenteral Fluids

Fluid therapy is mandatory during cardiac arrest in order to treat the hypovolemia and hypotension and to establish diuresis. The basic principles of IV administration of drugs described previously also apply to parenteral fluid administration. See Chapter 5 for a comprehensive discussion of fluid therapy.

▼ *Key Point* Administer fluids cautiously with close monitoring in traumatized patients when there is a suspicion of ongoing hemorrhage. Rapid fluid administration may facilitate uncontrolled hemorrhage and pulmonary edema, and increase mortality.

Crystalloids

- A minimum of 10–15 ml/kg of crystalloids (e.g., lactated Ringer's solution) is needed to reverse the relative blood loss due to venous pooling and vasodilation caused by cardiac arrest.
- Replace blood loss by administering at least three times as much crystalloid as blood lost (3:1) and guide by changes in the packed cell volume (PCV), total protein concentration, and central venous pressure when appropriate.

▼ **Key Point** Do not dilute the PCV <20% or the total plasma protein <3.0 g/dl with crystalloids.

Colloids

Colloids (e.g., 6% dextran 70 [Gentran]; hetastarch) provide colloid osmotic pressure and produce marked improvement in cardiac output and arterial blood pressure while helping to prevent blood sludging and capillary microembolization.

- Colloids are relatively confined to the intravascular fluid compartment and are used to replace blood loss in a ratio of 1:1 (thereby producing less hemodilution than crystalloids). Colloids are administered up to 10 ml/kg IV to a total volume of 20 ml/kg.

Hypertonic Saline

- Hypertonic sodium chloride solutions (3% and 7%) are extremely effective in drawing interstitial fluid into the vascular compartment, thereby increasing cardiac output and arterial blood pressure and restoring peripheral perfusion following hemorrhage in dogs and cats.
- The effects of hypertonic saline solutions can be prolonged by mixing 7% hypertonic saline with 6% dextran 70 or hetastarch. A 7% solution of hypertonic saline in 6% dextran 70 is produced by adding 70 mg of sodium chloride to each ml of 6% dextran 70. The dose of 7% sodium chloride mixed with either colloid is 5 ml/kg IV.

Blood

- Blood replacement therapy is indicated whenever hemorrhage is severe (>25 ml/kg), the PCV is <20%, or the total plasma protein is <2.5 g/dl.
- Like colloids, blood replacement therapy is administered in a ratio of 1:1 with blood loss.

Blood Substitute

- The blood substitute Oxyglobin (Biopure) is an oxygen-carrying oncotic solution that does not require cross-matching and has a 2-year shelf life.
- Administer 15–30 ml/kg/hr IV, for tissue oxygenation that is equal to or better than that of blood.

Electrocardiography

Electrocardiography (ECG) can be used to detect changes in heart rate and rhythm, particularly asystole and ventricular fibrillation (Fig. 73–3; Table 73–5).

Treatment of Ventricular Fibrillation

▼ **Key Point** The only consistently effective method for treating ventricular fibrillation is electrical defibrillation.

- Both external and internal techniques for converting ventricular fibrillation to sinus rhythm are successful in healthy patients that unexpectedly develop ventricular fibrillation (Table 73–6).
- The prior administration of epinephrine and lidocaine helps to reduce the energy required for defibrillation and the possibility of postdefibrillation ventricular arrhythmias, respectively.
- Use extreme care to avoid electrical injury to personnel.

Open-Chest Cardiac Massage

Open-chest direct cardiac massage may be the only way to provide adequate coronary and systemic blood flow, particularly in barrel-chested dogs and animals with penetrating chest trauma, broken ribs, pneumothorax, hemothorax, pericardial effusion, or thoracic masses.

- Consider open-chest direct cardiac compression within the first 5 minutes if closed chest compressions and IV epinephrine are ineffective.

Technique

1. After minimal skin preparation, make a skin incision at the fourth or fifth intercostal space on the left side.
2. Make a small hole in the pericardium near the apex of the heart and reflect the pericardium dorsally.
3. Compress the heart between the thumb and forefingers or in the palm of the hand, concentrating effort on the left ventricle. The usual compression rate is 60–80/minute.
4. Administer epinephrine (5–10 µg/kg) into the apex of the heart (left ventricular chamber) to initiate or strengthen contractions. This technique can also be used during ventricular fibrillation prior to electrical defibrillation.

PROLONGED LIFE SUPPORT

Prolonged life support incorporates all the medical and surgical methods necessary to prevent central nervous system and multiple organ failure following cardiac arrest (Table 73–7).

▼ **Key Point** Adequate tissue oxygenation is vital to long-term survival. Patients may require supplemental oxygen (nasal or tracheal O_2; O_2 cage) for several days following successful resuscitation. Maintain PCV >20%.

Drug Therapy

Catecholamines

Dopamine and Dobutamine. These produce dose-dependent increases in cardiac output and peripheral perfusion.

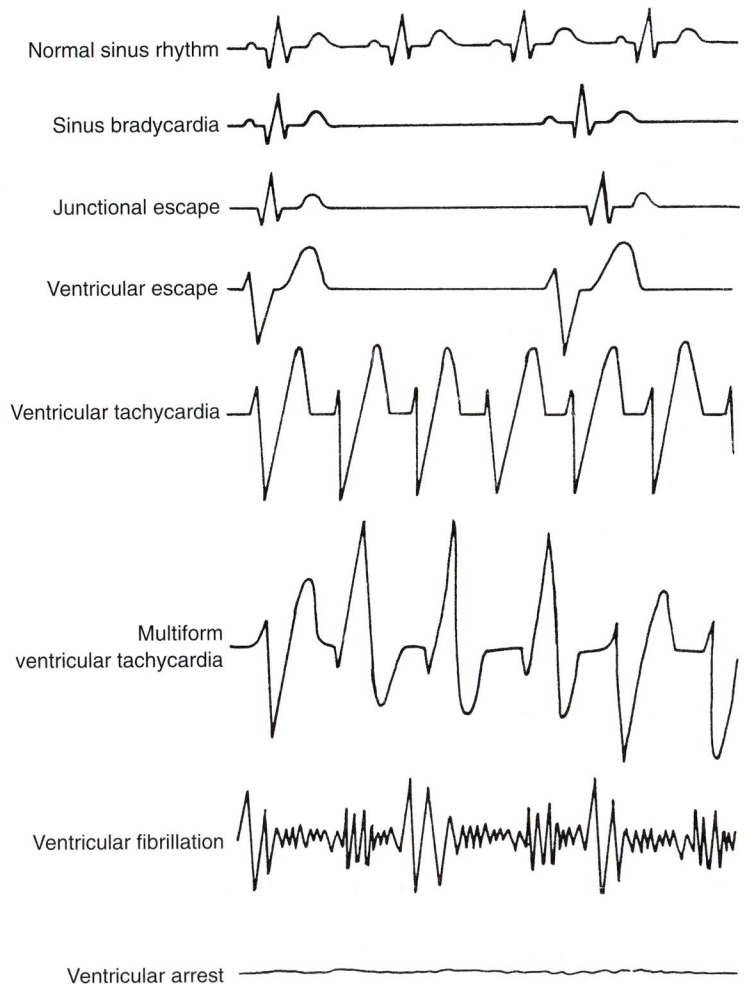

Figure 73–3. Significant cardiac rhythm patterns during cardiopulmonary cerebral resuscitation. (From Muir WW, Bonagura J: Cardiac emergencies. *In* Sherding R, ed.: Medical Emergencies. New York: Churchill Livingstone, 1985, pp 37–93.)

Table 73–5. DISTINGUISHING CHARACTERISTICS OF SEVERAL TYPES OF CARDIAC FAILURE AND ARREST

Cause	Peripheral Pulse	Auscultation of Heart Sounds	ECG	Visual Observation
Ventricular tachycardia	Weak, rapid, pulse deficit	Muffled; may be variable intensity	Wide QRS-T complexes; absence of P-QRS, large T wave relationship (see Fig. 73–3)	Disorganized, rapidly beating heart
Ventricular fibrillation	None	None	Absence of QRS-T complexes; fibrillation waves (see Fig. 73–3)	Fine to coarse rippling of ventricular myocardium
Bradycardia	Slow; may be irregular	Normal or muffled; infrequent	Infrequent or irregular P-QRS-T complexes; junctional or ventricular escape complexes (see Fig. 73–3)	Infrequent coordinated ventricular contractions
Ventricular asystole	None	None	Absence of QRS-T complexes; straight-line ECG	No cardiac improvement
Electromechanical dissociation	None	None	Normal or near-normal P-QRS-T complexes	Feeble or absent cardiac contractions

Modified from Muir WW, Bonagura JD: Cardiovascular emergencies. *In* Sherding RG, ed.: Medical Emergencies. New York: Churchill Livingstone, 1985, p 80.

Table 73–6. DEFIBRILLATION TECHNIQUES

Ventricular Tachycardia with Severe Hypotension or Ventricular Fibrillation

Direct current fibrillators: 0.5–2.0 ws/kg internal; 5–10 ws/kg
    external
    Small patient (<7 kg):
        5–15 ws internal
        50–100 ws external
    Large patient (>10 kg):
        20–80 ws internal
        100–400 ws external
Alternating current defibrillators
    Small patient:
        30–50 V internal
        50–100 V external
    Large patient:
        50–100 V internal
        150–250 V external

Unresponsive Ventricular Fibrillation

Evaluate ventilation
Evaluate chest or cardiac compression
Repeat epinephrine 0.02 mg/kg (see Table 73–4)
Repeat sodium bicarbonate administration every 10 min
Administer lidocaine
Repeat electrical defibrillation (direct current; see above)

Modified from Muir WW, Bonagura JD: Cardiovascular emergencies. *In* Sherding RG, ed.: Medical Emergencies. New York: Churchill Livingstone, 1985, p. 90.
ws = watt seconds; V = volts.

- The IV infusion rate varies from 1–5 μg/kg/min but may be increased to 15–20 μg/kg/min, depending on the patient's response.
- Administer dopamine to produce heart rates ranging from 120–160 beats/min. Administer dobutamine or dopamine to sustain systolic blood pressure (by Doppler) >100 mm Hg.

- Dobutamine is less likely to produce tachycardia than dopamine and is preferred in patients with preexisting sinus tachycardia or supraventricular arrhythmias.

Diuretics

Furosemide and Bumetanide. These highly potent loop diuretics are used to treat edema (e.g., pulmonary edema), promote diuresis, and "mobilize fluids."

- The dosage of furosemide is 1–2 mg/kg IV.
- The dosage for bumetanide is 0.005–0.01 mg/kg IV.

Mannitol. Mannitol (osmotherapy) produces an osmotic gradient that causes tissue dehydration and diuresis. Use mannitol (0.5–1.0 g/kg IV) if the period of cardiac arrest exceeds 3 minutes. This dose can be repeated at approximately 2–4 hours.

Glucocorticosteroids

Therapy with dexamethasone (Azium; 3–5 mg/kg IV) or prednisolone sodium succinate (Solu-Delta-Cortef; 10–20 mg/kg IV) has multiple benefits. These drugs can:

- Stabilize lysosomal membranes
- Reduce and prevent histamine release
- Protect against increases in capillary membrane permeability
- Cause vasodilation and inhibit phospholipase A_2 breakdown of arachidonic acid to prostaglandins and leukotrienes
- Impart a feeling of well-being

Calcium Entry Blockers

Calcium entry blockers, or calcium antagonists, are potentially beneficial in preventing reperfusion and re-

Table 73–7. BRAIN-ORIENTED RESUSCITATION

Problem	Therapy/Drug	Dose
Hypotension	Lactated Ringer's solution	35–70 ml/kg IV
	6% dextran 70	10 ml/kg IV
	7% NaCl	5 ml/kg IV
	7% NaCl in 6% dextran 70	5 ml/kg IV
	Dopamine	2–5 μg/kg/min IV
	Dobutamine	1–3 μg/kg/min IV
Seizures	Pentobarbital	1–3 mg/kg IV
	Thiopental	1–3 mg/kg IV
	Phenytoin	10–20 mg/kg IV
	Diazepam	0.1–0.2 mg/kg IV
Cerebral edema or increased intracranial pressure	Ventilation	$PaCO_2$ 25–35 mm Hg
	Oxygenation	PaO_2 60 mm Hg
	Furosemide	1 mg/kg IV
	Mannitol	0.5–1.0 g/kg IV
	Methylprednisolone sodium succinate	5–10 mg/kg IV
Cerebral vasospasm	Nimodipine	10 μg/kg IV
		10 μg/kg/min
	Diltiazem	2–3 mg/kg q8h PO; 1–5 μg/kg/min
Toxic cellular products*	Desferoxamine	25–50 mg/kg IV slowly
	Dimethyl sulfoxide	250–500 mg/kg IV
	Allopurinol	10 mg/kg PO

Modified from Muir WW: Brain hypoperfusion post-resuscitation. Vet Clin North Am [Small Anim Pract] 19:1151, 1989.
*These therapies await clinical verification of efficacy.

Airway
Breathing

Circulation

BASIC
LIFE
SUPPORT

Unwitnessed CPA
Patient evaluation
  Airway patency
  Breathing pattern
  Pupillary reflexes
  Color/refill
  Auscultation/percussion
  Heartbeats
  Arterial pulses

Witnessed CPA
  Airway/breathing — with oxygen
  Chest compression (80–100/min)
  IV fluids

Yes ⟶ Pulse or heartbeats present ⟶ No

Intubate and ventilate with oxygen (15 ml/kg; 10–15 breaths/min)
IV fluids (10–20 ml/kg IV)
Sodium bicarbonate (if necessary) 1.0 mEq/kg IV, 10 min
Evaluate heart rate and rythm

Intubate and ventilate with oxygen
Chest compression
Sodium bicarbonate (1.0 m/Eq/kg IV)
Epinephrine (0.01–0.02 mg/kg IV)
Lidocaine (1–4 mg/kg IV); (cats 0.5–1 mg/kg)
Spontaneous return of pulse

Yes — No

ECG Available **B**

A

ECG

Ventricular tachycardia
Antiarrhythmia
Lidocaine
  (1–4 mg/kg IV;
  cats 0.5–1 mg/kg;
  50 μg/kg/min)
Procainamide
  (6–20 mg/kg IV)

Bradycardia
  Glycopyrrolate
    (0.005 mg/kg IV)
  Epinephrine
    (0.01 mg/kg IV)
  Dopamine
    (1–5 mg/kg/min)

Normal rate
  Continue ventilation
  Reevaluate patient

⟶ Strong pulses
Good perfusion

Yes — No

Continue to ventilate
  until conscious
Treat for shock
Manage complications
Corticosteroids
  (10–15 mg/kg IV
  prednisolone sodium
  succinate)
Mannitol (1–2 g/kg IV)
Antibiotics
Supportive

Infusion of dopamine, dobutamine
  (1–5 mg/kg/min, IV)

ADVANCED
LIFE
SUPPORT

Evaluation of
cardiac rythm

Yes — No

Asystole
  Epinephrine
    (0.05 mg/kg IV)
  Electrical
  defibrillation
    (1–4 Ws/kg,
    internal)

Ventricular flutter
or fibrillation
  Electrical
  defibrillation
  Epinephrine
    (0.01–0.1
    mg/kg IV)

Electrical mechanical
dissociation
  Epinephrine
    (0.2 mg/kg IV)
  Dopamine
    (1–5 μg/kg/min)

No

Epinephrine, if no
response
  (0.01–0.1 mg/kg IV)
Defibrillation

Heartbeats present

Yes
Go to **A**

No

Open chest
Internal cardiac
  massage
Evaluate heart
  rate, rythm,
  color, tone
Go to **B**

PROLONGED
LIFE
SUPPORT

Therapy (see text)
Glucocorticosteroids (prednisolone sodium succinate, 10–15 mg/kg IV)
Diuretics (furosemide, 1–2 mg/kg IV)
Calcium entry blockers
  (diltiazem, 5–10 μg/kg/min for 10 min)

Free radical scavengers (mannitol, 1–2 g/kg IV)
Sedatives, anesthetics (diazepam, 3–10 mg/kg/min)
Antibiotics (gentamicin, 1–3 mg/kg IM q6 h)

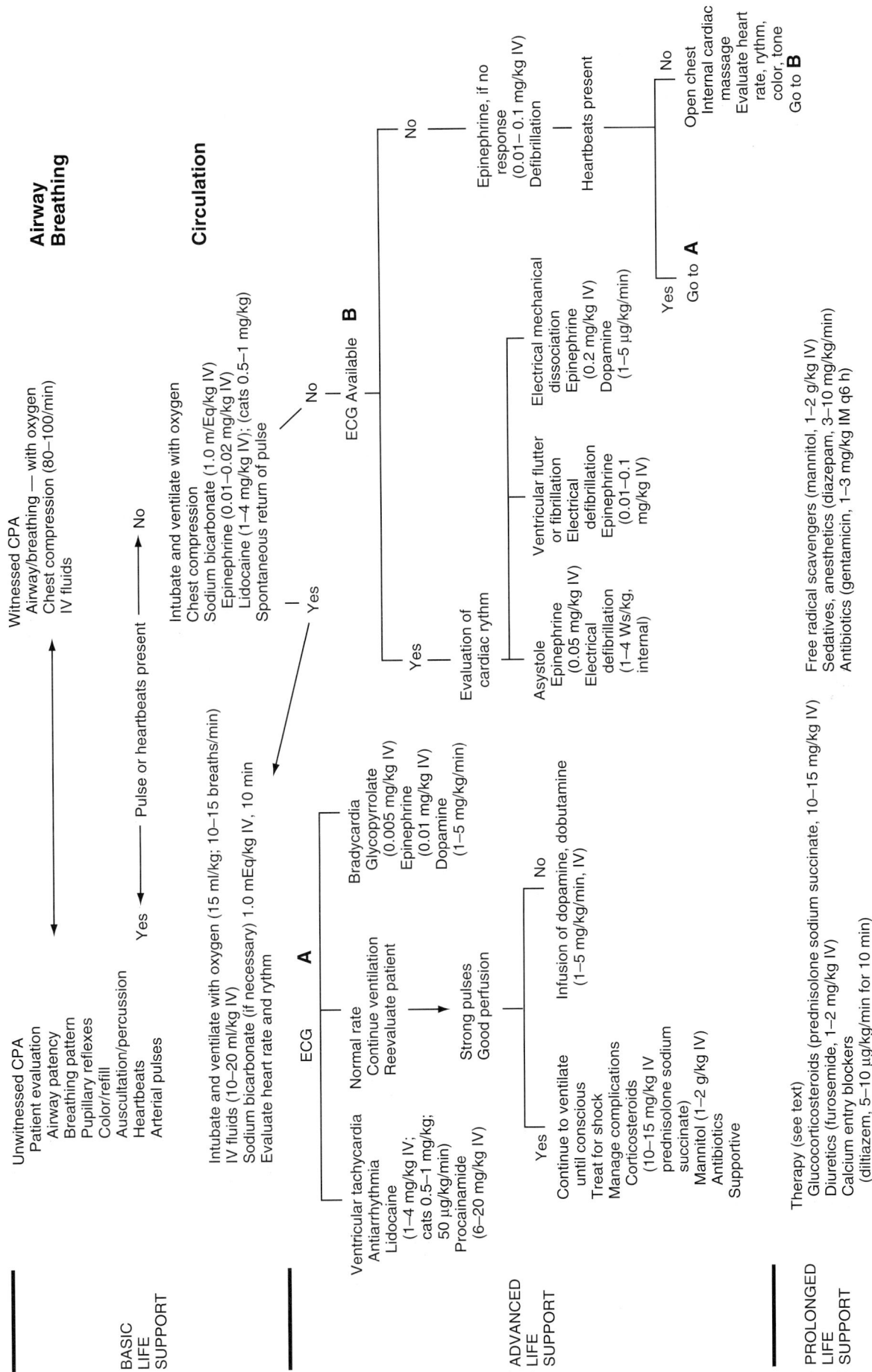

Figure 73-4. Flow chart for decision making during cardiopulmonary resuscitation. CPA: cardiopulmonary arrest

603

oxygenation injury, thereby limiting the detrimental effects of platelet aggregation, and the vasoactive and membrane damaging effects of prostaglandins and leukotrienes and other ischemia-induced (reperfusion injury) cascades.

- Diltiazem can be given at 0.5–2.0 mg/kg/q8h PO or 5–10 µg/kg/min IV for 10 minutes.
- Calcium solutions (chloride, gluconate) can be used to antagonize the negative inotropic actions of any of the calcium entry blockers.

Iron Chelators

Deferoxamine, a selective chelator of ferric iron, is potentially useful in preventing the deleterious effects of increases in intracellular free iron. Doses of 5–15 mg/kg IV, IM, or SQ have been used in experimental studies.

Free Radical Scavengers

Dimethyl sulfoxide (DMSO) (250–500 mg/kg, IV) and allopurinol (10 mg/kg, PO), are experimental drugs potentially useful as oxygen–free radical scavengers. Mannitol (see previous discussion) is also an oxygen–free radical scavenger.

Heparinization

The administration of 100 IU/kg SC q6–8h of heparin is of questionable value in the postarrest period (once hemorrhage has been controlled); it may limit the clotting cascade and microcirculatory plugging.

Sedation

- Dosages of pentobarbital (1–3 mg/kg IV) are adequate to reduce cerebral oxygen requirements and prevent seizures in most dogs and cats.
- Phenytoin, 15 mg/kg IV, may be used for the same purpose.
- Diazepam, 0.1–0.3 mg/kg IV, or an infusion, 2–10 µg/kg/min, is an excellent alternative to pentobarbital and produces less CNS depression.

Antibiotics

The choice of antibiotics is based on the potential for efficacy (see Table 73–3).

PREDICTING OUTCOME

- Rapid recovery of eye (corneal) reflexes, upper airway reflexes including swallowing and sneezing, and spontaneous breathing (lung inflation) are good prognostic signs.
- Continued unconsciousness, nonresponsive pupils, hypothermia, and progressive deterioration of responses to physical stimulation after initial partial recovery are poor prognostic signs.

A simple algorithm for CPCR is illustrated in Figure 73–4.

Diagnostic Methods in Respiratory Disease

Larry Berkwitt / James Prueter

UPPER RESPIRATORY TRACT

Nasal Cavity Diseases

Sneezing and nasal discharge are the principal clinical problems associated with nasal cavity and sinus diseases.

History

When taking the history, include:

- The chronology, progression, and duration of clinical signs, such as sneezing
- Type of nasal discharge
- Site of involvement (unilateral or bilateral)

Sneezing

- *Acute paroxysmal sneezing* typically is associated with viral rhinitis, nasal foreign body, allergic rhinitis, and trauma.
- *Chronic sneezing* suggests neoplasia, parasites, prolonged infection or inflammation (e.g., fungal rhinitis), long-term foreign body, or trauma with secondary infection or osteomyelitis.
- *Reversed sneezing* can be a sign of disease or inflammation in the nasopharynx.

Nasal Discharge

- Serous discharge typically is associated with acute foreign body, allergy, and viral infection.
- Mucopurulent and/or serosanguineous discharge typically is associated with viral infections (complicated by bacteria); bacterial, mycotic, and parasitic infections; long-term foreign body; neoplasia; and lymphocytic-plasmacytic inflammation.
- Hemorrhagic discharges suggest trauma, neoplasia, coagulopathy, and prolonged infection.
- Foodstuffs in the discharge suggest a communicating congenital defect (cleft palate) or acquired oro-nasal fistula.

Duration of Clinical Signs

- Sudden onset of signs suggests foreign body, viral infection, trauma, or coagulopathy.

- Chronic signs are associated with neoplasia, infection, foreign body, parasite infection, chronic inflammation, or congenital defect.

Site of Involvement

- Unilateral discharge suggests early neoplasia, foreign body, early infection, dental disease, or trauma.
- Bilateral discharge suggests chronic infection or inflammation, prolonged foreign body with resulting infection/osteomyelitis, advanced neoplasia, coagulopathy, pneumonia, parasites, allergy, or trauma.

Physical Examination

A complete physical examination includes a thorough evaluation of the oral cavity, mucous membranes, tonsils, hard and soft palate, retropharyngeal area, regional lymph nodes, and teeth. Sedation and/or anesthesia may be required. The use of dental mirrors and a spay hook or an endoscope (in the retroflexed position) for visualization above the soft palate also is often necessary.

- Look for swelling and asymmetry of the face, palate, or eyes (exophthalmos) that might suggest neoplasia, fungal infection, or trauma.
- Identify areas of pain that may localize the disorder.
- Evaluate for loss of patency of one or both nasal passages.
- Note ocular discharge that may be associated with nasolacrimal duct inflammation and/or obstruction secondary to inflammation or neoplasia.
- Identify cracked, loose, and infected teeth.

Complete Blood Count (CBC), Serum Chemical Profile, and Coagulation Screen

These evaluations are important when systemic diseases may be an underlying cause of signs. Although clotting disorders can cause epistaxis, it is usually associated with platelet disorders such as immune-mediated thrombocytopenia, von Willebrand's disease, thrombocytopathia, and ehrlichiosis.

Serology

- Serologic tests such as immunodiffusion and enzyme-linked immunosorbent assay (ELISA) for aspergillo-

605

sis and penicilliosis antibodies and for cryptococcal capsular antigen can be used for diagnosis of mycotic rhinitis. However, false-negative results are common, limiting the usefulness of serology.

- Cytology, culture, and biopsy are more reliable than serology for identifying nasal fungi.

Radiography

- General anesthesia is essential for proper positioning and for prevention of motion artifacts.
- Include the following radiographic views (see Chap. 4):
  - Open-mouth ventrodorsal
  - Intraoral (occlusal)
  - Rostral-caudal frontal skyline
  - Lateral
  - Oblique skull views, particularly if dental arcade problems are suspected.

Computed Tomography (CT) and Magnetic Resonance Imaging (MRI)

Use CT of the nasal cavity and skull to delineate the extent of masses and involvement of other cranial structures. Use MRI for better definition of brain involvement from invading nasal tumors.

Nasal Flushing for Cytology

Nasal cytologic evaluation is often of little or no value unless it is performed with aggressive nasal flushing or by rhinoscopic visualization with the animal under anesthesia.

- Perform aggressive nasal flushing with a polypropylene (rigid) male urinary catheter. Measure the length (nares to medial canthus) prior to insertion to avoid penetrating past the cribriform plate.
- Perform intermittent flushing and suctioning via syringe to obtain as much nasal fluid and/or tissue fragments as possible.
- Place gauze sponges in the nasal pharynx to catch any tissue that may be extracted during the flushing procedure.
- Submit samples for culture, cytology, and histopathology.
- Small clamshell forceps can be used to obtain biopsy samples with or without benefit of rhinoscopy.

Rhinoscopy

Rhinoscopic examination under anesthesia allows visualization, biopsy, and procurement of specimens for cytology and culture and sensitivity. Instrumentation can include any of the following:

- Otoscope with bright light source
- Arthroscope or otoscope with outer diameter of 1.9–5 mm
- Bronchoscope with outer diameter of 2.9–5 mm
- Flexible pediatric bronchoscope
- Flexible cytoscope or rhinoscope with outer diameter of 2 mm.

Surgery

- Exploratory rhinotomy with removal of a bone flap (see Chap. 76) provides complete exposure of the nasal cavity for biopsy, foreign body retrieval, culture, and debridement of diseased tissue.
- Drainage tubes can be placed at the time of surgery for treatment of bacterial and/or fungal infections.

Laryngeal Diseases

History

Clinical signs of laryngeal disease often are slowly progressive, and the owner may have noted them for an extended period of time. Laryngeal paralysis is common in a number of breeds (see Chap. 77).

- The owner may report hoarseness, progressive changes in voice, or complete loss of voice.
- Noisy respirations characterized by high-pitched inspiratory stridor or by mild, raspy, or fluid-sounding noise are common.
- Choking, gagging, and coughing may be observed, particularly while the animal is eating and/or drinking. This often worsens as the disease progresses.
- Exertional dyspnea, cyanosis, and syncope may be observed in patients with laryngeal obstruction (e.g., laryngeal collapse, paralysis, foreign body, or neoplasia).

Physical Findings

- The most frequent physical findings in laryngeal disease are inspiratory dyspnea and stridor. Auscultation can detect upper respiratory inspiratory stridor ("wheeze") or lower-pitched obstructive sounds centered over the larynx.
- Palpation of the laryngeal area may detect the site of pain, fractures, and subcutaneous emphysema in cases of trauma and asymmetry due to neoplasia, granulomas, laryngitis, or unilateral muscle atrophy.

Laryngoscopy/Bronchoscopy

- Perform direct visualization under a *light* plane of anesthesia for evaluation of pharyngeal structures, soft palate, and laryngeal motor function. Tiletamine HCl/zolazepam HCl (Telazol) can cause laryngeal paralysis, so another form of sedation should be used.
- Observe laryngeal (arytenoid) movement during both phases of respiration. Often asymmetry is observed between the left and right arytenoids and vocal folds.
- A bronchoscope allows the best evaluation of the pharynx and the subglottic area for masses, infiltrates (areas of discoloration), granulomas, and polyps.
- Aspiration or brush cytology and endoscopic biopsy may be performed at the time of examination, if appropriate.

Radiography

- A lateral radiograph of the larynx is rarely diagnostic but may demonstrate:
  - Dilated lateral saccules in cases of paralysis

- Soft tissue swelling and/or asymmetry caused by neoplasia or trauma
- Fractures, dislocations, or subcutaneous air caused by trauma
- Elongated soft palate
- Collapsed or ruptured trachea
- Thoracic radiographs may reveal chronic pulmonary or cardiac disease associated with upper respiratory diseases.

Electromyography

Abnormal electromyographic studies of the laryngeal muscles may be associated with neuromuscular, immune-mediated, and hypothyroid-related laryngeal disorders.

Thyroid Function Testing

Infrequently patients with acquired laryngeal paralysis may have subnormal levels of triiodothyronine (T_3) and thyroxine (T_4), as well as abnormal results of TSH assay and TSH stimulation tests (see Chap. 29).

Histopathology

Histopathology of any abnormal growth or mass is important in order to differentiate chronic granulomatous disease and neoplasia and may also be useful in a generalized case of polyneuropathy.

Tracheal Diseases (see also Chap. 77)

History

- Usually there is a chronic, unproductive, dry "honking" cough with intermittent attacks of dyspnea, particularly elicited with excitement, exercise, drinking, or eating, and tracheal pressure (e.g., digital pressure or collar).
- Dyspnea and occasionally cyanosis may be demonstrated.
  - Inspiratory dyspnea and stridor develop if the trachea collapses in the cervical area (extrathoracic).
  - Expiratory dyspnea is evident with intrathoracic collapse.
- Both phases of ventilation (although worse on expiration) are abnormal if the entire trachea is involved.

Physical Examination

- Tracheal palpation may demonstrate "sharp" edges or angles of the collapsible margins of the trachea.
- Cardiac examination is important to differentiate tracheal disease from primary heart disease and for evaluation of coexisting chronic heart disease (see Chap. 59).
- Auscultate the entire respiratory tract to localize primary abnormalities and to differentiate tracheal disease from lower respiratory tract disease (see Chap. 79).

Radiography

Radiographic examination (ventrodorsal and lateral views) is mandatory for routine evaluation of the cervical and thoracic trachea (see Chap. 75).

- Be careful in positioning to avoid artifactual deviations of the trachea.
- Attempt to obtain both inspiratory and expiratory films in order to identify an intermittently collapsing trachea or bronchus (this may be difficult or impossible in small-breed dogs).
- Survey radiography has limited sensitivity and specificity for diagnosis.
- Fluoroscopy or tracheoscopy is necessary to evaluate dynamic tracheal functions and intermittent tracheal collapse.

Transtracheal Wash

Perform the tracheal wash (via a sterile endotracheal tube) for cytology, fluid analysis, and microbiologic evaluations to identify initiating or complicating factors that may be important in the treatment regimens. See Bronchopulmonary and Pleural Space Disorders in this chapter for a description of this procedure.

Tracheoscopy

Tracheoscopy can be used to visualize the area of collapse. Extreme care must be taken because of the potential of worsening the collapse by trauma and iatrogenic irritation. Tracheoscopy is best utilized in uncertain diagnoses or in those cases in which there is concern for neoplasia, mass lesion, congenital defects, or concurrent mainstem bronchial collapse. See Bronchoscopy in the Bronchopulmonary section for further discussion of this procedure.

BRONCHOPULMONARY AND PLEURAL DISEASES

The diagnosis of diseases of the respiratory tract and pleural space depends on information obtained from a thorough history, a physical examination, and a series of ancillary tests that are well conceived and organized so as to limit the patient's discomfort and stress.

When evaluating the dyspneic patient, use sound clinical judgment in selecting tests that will aid in the diagnosis but will not place the patient in further respiratory distress. Often these patients must be stabilized, based on the physical examination, history, and a dorsoventral thoracic radiograph prior to performing other tests.

History

Coughing, tachypnea, dyspnea, and exercise intolerance are the principal signs associated with bronchopulmonary and pleural disease.

- Determine the patient's signalment, because certain breeds or age groups are more susceptible to particular diseases. For example, small and toy breed dogs are more susceptible than large-breed dogs to lower respiratory disease secondary to a collapsing trachea. Cocker spaniels are prone to chronic bronchitis.
- Note the client's complaint. Determine if the patient's problem is acute or chronic and if it is improving, unchanging, or progressive.

- When evaluating a cough, determine the time of day of the cough. Cardiac coughs are usually nocturnal, whereas an infectious cough will occur throughout the day.
  - Determine the quality of the cough, such as dry hacking (nonproductive) or moist (productive).
- Note prior medical and travel history.
  - It is imperative to know what medications have been given previously and what medical response was obtained.
  - Consider geographically distributed diseases (e.g., systemic mycoses) in pets that travel or have lived in various locations.
  - Determine the patient's recent exposure to other pets that might be a source of infectious disease (e.g., in a kennel or grooming situation).
- Note the patient's current medical history. Do not overlook routine history questions about water consumption, appetite, and eliminations, because this information can give insight into the diagnosis of systemic diseases.

Physical Examination

Perform a complete physical examination.

- It is important to evaluate each body system, because key diagnostic physical findings may be present and pulmonary complications of heart disease may be evident. For example:
  - A remote lesion such as a rectal carcinoma may be the source of metastases that cause dyspnea and abnormal lung sounds.
  - Skin lesions and lymphadenopathy suggest a diagnosis of blastomycosis in a coughing patient.
- Physical examination of the lower respiratory system and pleural space includes observation, auscultation, palpation, and percussion (see also Chap. 59).

Observation

Observe the patient's rate and pattern of breathing. Certain diseases cause inspiratory versus expiratory dyspnea.

- Note whether the patient is barrel-chested or overweight.
  - Barrel chest may indicate chronic obstructive pulmonary disease.
  - Pickwickian-type syndrome in obese animals may account for breathing problems.
- Slow, deep breathing with inspiratory difficulty can be due to large upper airway obstructive disease.
- Short, shallow breathing may be associated with restrictive disease.

Pulmonary Auscultation

Pulmonary sounds usually are classified as normal or vesicular, bronchial, or bronchovesicular. Adventitious sounds include crackles (rales), wheezes, stridor, rhonchi, and rubs.

- As air travels through the lung, it produces vesicular or bronchovesicular sounds. Depending on the medium through which the air travels (e.g., fluid or mucus) or if there are changes in diameter of diseased airways, the sound is modified (e.g., crackles, rhonchi, wheezes).
- Identification of crackles (small airway/parenchymal disease), rhonchi (airway disease or exudate), and wheezes (airway obstruction) indicates a need for additional diagnostic studies.

Percussion

The lungs and thoracic cavity emit a specific resonance when percussed by striking the second phalanx (p) of the middle finger positioned on the chest with the knuckle joint (p1–p2) fully extended.

- Dull resonance is associated with increased density (fluid or mass lesion) within the underlying pleural space or lung.
- Increased resonance (drum-like) is associated with increased air within the pleural space or lung.

As an example of incorporating all parts of the physical examination, consider the patient that has a mammary mass with louder or adventitious lung sounds on auscultation and dull percussion on the left side of the thoracic wall. This patient may have pleural effusion associated with metastatic disease. If dull percussion is present without lung sounds, suspect a consolidating mass lesion.

Thoracic Radiography (see also Chap. 75)

Standard radiographic views include inspiratory lateral and ventrodorsal views.

- To evaluate for metastatic lung disease a right and left lateral projection with the ventrodorsal view may be helpful.
- In a dyspneic animal, a single dorsoventral view is recommended to avoid unnecessary stress and to enable the clinician to initiate stabilizing therapy prior to further evaluation.

Evaluation

Good-quality radiographs are important because excess motion or underexposure may result in false information regarding the pulmonary interstitium (see Chap. 4). Expiratory films may cause the pulmonary interstitium to have an increased density that can be mistaken as abnormal.

To evaluate thoracic radiographs:

- Determine the type of radiographic infiltrative pattern present, such as interstitial, alveolar, bronchial, vascular, or combinations of these.
- Characterize the location of the infiltrate as localized or diffuse; cranial or caudal; and ventral, dorsal, or hilar.
- Pleural effusion is indicated by blunted costophrenic angles, pleural fissure lines, and ventral scalloping of the lungs on the lateral projection.

CBC

The CBC may be helpful in evaluation of respiratory disease. For example:

- Leukocytosis can indicate infection or inflammation.
- Polycythemia is associated with chronic hypoxemia.
- Eosinophilia may suggest a parasitic or allergic disease.
- Nucleated red blood cells may indicate acute hypoxemia.

Serum Chemistry Profile

No single segment of the standard automated serum chemistry profile is pathognomonic for respiratory system disease; however, this study is useful as a baseline to evaluate other organ systems. For example:

- If a patient has a localized anterior ventral alveolar infiltrate, calcification of the airways, neutrophilic leukocytosis, lymphopenia, and eosinopenia with elevated alkaline phosphatase and cholesterol levels, a tentative diagnosis of bacterial pneumonia secondary to hyperadrenocorticism might be made pending confirmatory tests.

Arterial Blood Gas (ABG) Analysis and Pulse Oximetry

The ABG specimen usually is drawn from the femoral artery or dorsal pedal artery or via an indwelling arterial catheter. ABG arterial analysis evaluates the patient's ability to oxygenate arterial blood. Alternatively, evaluate pulse oximetry.

- In the normal patient breathing room air, the partial pressure of oxygen is >95 mm Hg.
- When the level is <60 mm Hg, a severe degree of respiratory failure is present.
- Elevations in CO_2 indicate ventilatory failure and contribute to respiratory acidosis. If a patient has decreased PaO_2 and increased PCO_2 the prognosis is guarded to poor.
- Alveolar-arterial oxygen difference (A-aDO_2; normal 4–17 mm Hg) is a parameter of gas exchange efficiency calculated as $(150 - PaCO_2) - PaO_2$ when breathing room air at sea level, or using the standard full formula.

Serology

Specific serologic evaluations aid in the diagnosis of fungal, rickettsial, and immune-mediated disease as a possible cause of intrathoracic disorders.

Fecal Examination

To establish the diagnosis of parasitic lung disease, evaluate fecal specimens by direct smear, flotation, and sedimentation (available from commercial laboratories) techniques. Fecal sedimentation is important for detection of lungworm larvae (e.g., *Filaroides, Aelurostrongylus*) that can be overlooked if flotation is used.

Transtracheal Washing

Tracheal washing is a simple, inexpensive procedure in which warm sterile saline is instilled in the lower respiratory tract and then retrieved. Use this technique to obtain specimens for cytologic and microbiologic evaluation of the lower respiratory tract to aid in the diagnosis of bronchopulmonary disease.

Technique

1. In *dogs,* insert a long through-the-needle catheter (12 or 18 inches) percutaneously between the tracheal rings or through the cricothyroid membrane and then advance it into the lower airway.
2. In *cats,* use an open-end urinary catheter placed through a sterile endotracheal tube.
3. The catheters ideally should extend to the level of the tracheal bifurcation.
4. Inject warm sterile saline (6 ml in cats and small dogs; up to 20 ml in large dogs) through the catheter.
5. After instillation of the fluid, induce coughing by gently slapping the rib cage bilaterally.
6. Retrieve the fluid from the airway by aspiration.
7. Prepare samples of the lavage fluid for cytology, culture, and sensitivity testing.
8. Any fluid remaining in the airways is harmless because it is rapidly absorbed by the pulmonary lymphatics.

Bronchoalveolar Lavage and Bronchoscopy
Bronchoalveolar Lavage

This is an effective method for retrieving diagnostic material from the lung and is particularly useful in alveolar-interstitial lung diseases and in tachypnea/dyspnea when prominent cough is absent.

Technique

1. Advance a flexible fiberoptic bronchoscope into the bronchial tree.
2. Visually locate the diseased area and wedge the bronchoscope within the bronchus.
3. Instill 20–30 ml of warm saline (for a 15 kg dog) through the bronchoscope channel and then retrieve it. Thoracic coupage may facilitate fluid retrieval.
4. Prepare samples for cytology, quantitative cell counts, culture, and sensitivity testing.

Bronchoscopy

Bronchoscopy allows direct visualization of the lower airway to the level of the third, fourth, or fifth bronchial divisions, depending on the size of the patient and the length and diameter of the bronchoscope.

- Bronchoscopy is a valuable alternative when no diagnostic material is obtained using the tracheal wash procedure. This can occur because there is not enough cellular material present within the airway or because the catheter is too short to retrieve any material.
- Diseased areas can be directly visualized, and the exudate or tissue can be removed for cytology or histopathology.
- If there is no visible material present, bronchial brushing or bronchoalveolar lavage can retrieve cells that may aid in a diagnosis.

- Direct biopsy of visible lesions can be performed through the bronchoscope as well as transbronchial lung biopsy described as follows.

Lung Biopsy

When the cause of diffuse lung disease cannot be determined using one of the methods described previously, consider a lung biopsy. The types of lung biopsy procedures performed in small animals include:

- Fine-needle aspiration
- Bronchoscopy
- Ultrasound- or CT-guided biopsy
- Mini-thoracotomy
- Thoracoscopy (referral centers)

Fine-Needle Aspiration

The simplest, most cost-effective procedure is fine-needle aspiration. This is usually performed on diffuse or large superficial lesions within the parenchyma or pleural space.

Technique

1. Clip and surgically prepare the thoracic wall and instill a local anesthetic at the site.
2. Insert a 22-gauge needle with 12 ml syringe attached through the chest wall, staying on the cranial aspect of the rib in order to avoid the intercostal vessels.
3. Apply suction to obtain samples for cytologic evaluation and biopsy.

Bronchoscopic Biopsy

A lung biopsy can be obtained utilizing the bronchoscope. This method is used with deeper, more central lesions and ideally should be performed under fluoroscopy. The endoscopic biopsy forceps are passed through the bronchial wall into the pulmonary parenchyma.

Mini-Thoracotomy

The most invasive type of biopsy is performed via a mini-thoracotomy.

Technique

1. Make an incision 2–4 cm long between the ninth and tenth ribs.

2. Bring the lung tissue into the incision, place a ligature around the lung, and remove the sample.

Potential Risks of Biopsy

Because of the risk of hemorrhage and pneumothorax with all these procedures, postbiopsy monitoring is essential.

- Open-lung biopsy decreases the risk of pneumothorax because the biopsy site is visualized and all leakage can be controlled.
- In fine-needle aspiration, withdrawal of infectious material can contaminate the pleural space and cause pyothorax.

Thoracocentesis

The diagnosis of pleural effusion generally depends upon analysis of pleural fluid obtained by thoracocentesis (see Chap. 3). Thoracocentesis can also be therapeutically beneficial. Perform the procedure with minimal stress to the patient.

Electrocardiography and Ultrasonography

Often, it is difficult to determine whether a patient's problem is respiratory or cardiovascular.

- With pulmonary hypertension secondary to thoracic disease, the electrocardiogram may show P-pulmonale evidenced by p waves >0.4 mV and deep s waves in leads I, II, III, and aVF.
- Ultrasonography can identify specific cardiac abnormalities and masses within the mediastinum, pleural space, and pulmonary parenchyma (see Chaps. 4 and 75).

Other Specialized Diagnostic Tests

Other useful tests include thoracoscopy, bronchography, lymphangiographic studies for evaluation of chylothorax, computed tomography, magnetic resonance imaging, and vascular and radioisotopic studies to identify pulmonary thromboembolism. These procedures, if necessary, are performed at referral diagnostic centers.

75 Diagnostic Imaging in Respiratory Disease

Wendy Myer

INDICATIONS FOR RADIOGRAPHIC EVALUATION

Radiography is a widely available, rapidly performed, and noninvasive method for evaluating respiratory disease in small animals. It also has the advantage of allowing repeated evaluations of an animal. Although radiography is a sensitive method for detecting respiratory disease, changes are nonspecific, and similar radiographic patterns are seen in many different disease processes. Therefore, radiographic findings should be considered morphologic, rather than etiologic, in nature.

RADIOGRAPHIC ANATOMY

- Radiographic evaluation of the *upper airways* is best accomplished with the animal in lateral recumbency. The soft palate and epiglottis are well outlined by air within the oral and nasal pharynx. Mineralization of the laryngeal cartilages, including the epiglottis, is a common finding in dogs. The normal *larynx* is slightly wider than the *trachea;* the remainder of the trachea is uniform in diameter throughout its length.

▼ *Key Point* The normal trachea should be no smaller than three times the diameter of the proximal end of the third rib.

- The following structures should be visible on a normal thoracic radiograph: the cardiac silhouette, pulmonary arteries and veins, caudal vena cava, descending aorta, trachea, diaphragm, and (in young animals) the thymus.
- The following structures usually are *not* visible on a normal thoracic radiograph: the cranial vena cava, aortic arch, great vessels, esophagus, interlobar pleural fissures, bronchial walls (except in the hilar area), and the mediastinal, hilar, and sternal lymph nodes.
- Radiographically the *pulmonary vessels* account for the majority of the pulmonary pattern. The pulmonary arteries and veins are approximately equal in size.
  - On the lateral view the arteries are dorsal to the bronchi and veins; on the ventrodorsal (VD) view, the arteries are lateral to the veins (i.e., "veins are ventral and central").
  - On the lateral view the ratio of the cranial lobar vessels to the proximal one-third of the fourth rib should be approximately 0.75. Measure the vessels at the point where they cross the cardiac silhouette.
- The bronchi normally are thin-walled and seen clearly only in the hilar area. Their walls may appear as pairs of faint, soft tissue density lines running between and parallel to the vessels, and in cross section they are seen as small thin-walled doughnuts.

TECHNICAL CONSIDERATIONS

For a general discussion of radiographic equipment and techniques, see Chapter 4.

Inspiration Versus Expiration

▼ *Key Point* Obtain all thoracic radiographs at the height of inspiration. This allows the best evaluation of the lung and gives a more accurate assessment of cardiac size.

A poorly aerated lung will appear diffusely increased in density and may lead to an erroneous impression of pulmonary disease. Inspiratory and expiratory films obtained during the same examination may be used to demonstrate dynamic problems such as expiratory airway collapse and paralysis of the diaphragm.

Respiratory Motion

Failure to control respiratory motion is one of the major causes of nondiagnostic thoracic radiographs in small animals. Use of a low mAs technique helps to decrease exposure time and to minimize respiratory motion. In tachypneic animals, temporarily holding off or blowing into the animal's nose may briefly arrest respiratory motion.

Effect of Gravity on the Dependent Lung

When an animal is placed in lateral recumbency, the lung closest to the cassette becomes partially atelectatic and receives more blood and less air than normal. This decreases the air available to contrast normal or abnormal soft tissue density structures or areas of consolidation within the dependent lung. Therefore, masses that are seen on other thoracic views may seem to disappear when they are in the dependent portion of the lung. This is especially evident in the part of the lung adjacent to the heart or diaphragm. Thus, soft tissue density pulmonary structures are best seen radiographically when they are in the better aerated, *nondependent* portion of the lung. For this reason, both right and left lateral views are sometimes useful (e.g., for detecting early pulmonary metastases).

Follow-Up Studies

▼ *Key Point* When retaking radiographs for the purpose of following disease progression, use the same radiographic technique and positioning as in the initial examination to provide the most accurate comparison.

This is especially critical in animals with pneumonia, because pathologic changes in the dependent lung may not be well appreciated on the lateral view. Accurate assessment of pleural fluid volume is also difficult when comparing dorsoventral (DV) and VD projections even when the two radiographs are taken during the same examination.

RADIOGRAPHIC ABNORMALITIES OF THE NASAL CAVITY AND LARYNX

- Upper airway disease such as brachycephalic upper airway obstruction syndrome, laryngeal paralysis, and laryngospasm are best evaluated using visual examination externally or endoscopically. Laryngeal masses or foreign bodies may appear radiographically as soft tissue densities within the airway.
- The nasal passages are best evaluated using occlusal DV or open-mouth VD views of the maxilla. On these views the turbinates appear as thin, lacy mineralized structures surrounded by air.
- Rhinitis, foreign bodies, and nasal neoplasms may cause focal or diffuse increases in radiographic density of the nasal passages. Turbinate destruction is often present in animals with neoplasia or erosive rhinitis. Most cases of bacterial or foreign body rhinitis tend to primarily involve the middle and rostral portions of one or both nasal passages.
- Neoplastic processes often appear more destructive and primarily involve the caudal portion of the nasal passages.
- Despite these characteristics, a definitive diagnosis of nasal disease usually is not possible by radiography alone; thus, rhinoscopy with biopsy, cytology, and/or culture is often indicated as well.

RADIOGRAPHIC ABNORMALITIES OF THE TRACHEA (Fig. 75–1)

- *Tracheal hypoplasia* is manifested as a uniform decrease in tracheal diameter owing to decreased size

of the dorsal tracheal muscle. In severely affected animals, the tracheal diameter may be reduced to 50% of the laryngeal diameter. This condition is congenital and is most commonly seen in brachycephalic breeds, especially English bulldogs.

- *Tracheal edema* and *pseudomembranous tracheal inflammation* can also result in a diffuse decrease in tracheal diameter and must be considered in animals with an apparent decrease in tracheal diameter.
- *Tracheal perforation* usually occurs in the thoracic inlet portion of the trachea, and results in subcutaneous emphysema, pneumomediastinum, and/or pneumothorax.
- *Complete tracheal rupture* is uncommon and life-threatening. In addition to severe peritracheal air accumulation, discontinuity of the tracheal wall is seen with separation of tracheal rings. This is best assessed on the lateral view. This occurs most commonly in the cat just cranial to the heart base.
- *Focal tracheal stenosis* is manifested as a focal area of narrowed tracheal lumen. Tracheal perforation from a dog fight or prolonged intubation with an endotracheal tube with an overinflated cuff results in a stricture.
- *Tracheal collapse* appears as a focal or diffuse decrease in the dorsoventral diameter of the trachea. The collapse can be persistent or intermittent, occurring commonly during periods of excitement or coughing (see also Chap. 77).
- To adequately assess tracheal dynamics, obtain lateral thoracic radiographs at the peaks of inspiration and expiration. The extrathoracic (cervical and thoracic inlet) portion of the trachea collapses during inspiration, whereas the intrathoracic portion of the trachea collapses during expiration. In some dogs, the degenerative cartilaginous changes may extend into the mainstem bronchi, causing them to collapse severely during expiration.

▼ *Key Point* Superimposition of the esophagus over the dorsal aspect of the trachea is a common finding that may lead to the misdiagnosis of tracheal collapse in a normal dog. This appearance does not change during respiration; however, the tracheal diameter in an animal with true tracheal collapse

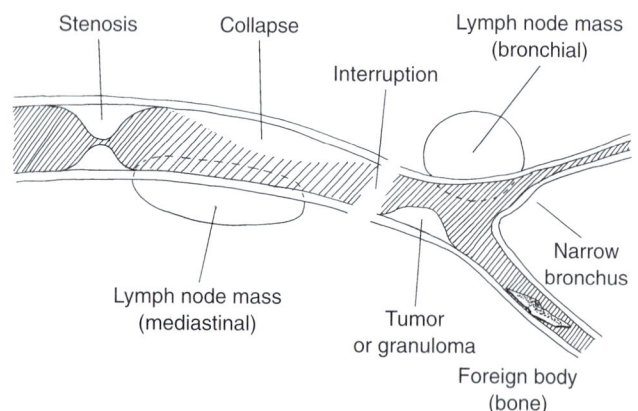

Figure 75–1. Schematic representation of various causes of tracheobronchial disease.

varies during the various phases of the respiratory cycle.

- *Tracheal masses* or *foreign bodies* appear as soft tissue or mineral-dense objects within the tracheal lumen. Small foreign bodies often pass into the bronchi, causing obstruction or pulmonary abscessation.
- *Exudate* within the trachea usually is not evident, because of the recumbent positioning used in small animals; however, it may be evident if horizontal beam films are obtained.

RADIOGRAPHIC ABNORMALITIES OF THE EXTRAPLEURAL SPACE

- The extrapleural space communicates with many of the fascial planes of the body via the thoracic inlet. It can be divided into two areas:
  - The potential space between the parietal pleura and the body wall
  - The potential space within the mediastinum
- Conditions affecting the extrapleural space include abscesses, hematomas, granulomas, and neoplasms.
- Radiographically, most extrapleural diseases appear as relatively spherical, smoothly marginated masses that have a convex surface facing the lung with tapered or concave cranial and caudal borders, and that do not involve the pleural space until late in the disease process.
- Mediastinal lymphadenopathy and rib tumors with secondary rib destruction are common extrapleural lesions.

Thoracic Lymph Nodes (Fig. 75–2)

▼ *Key Point* Thoracic lymph nodes are not seen radiographically in normal animals.

- The thoracic lymph nodes are located in three areas within the mediastinum:
  - Dorsal to the second sternebra (*sternal lymph nodes*)
  - In the dorsal portion of the cranial mediastinum (*mediastinal lymph nodes*)

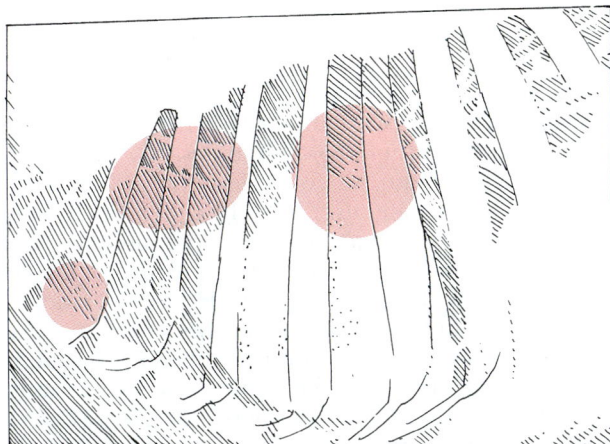

Figure 75–2. Location of thoracic lymph nodes.

- At the hilar area of the lung surrounding the bifurcation of the trachea (*tracheobronchial lymph nodes*)
- When any of these nodes are substantially enlarged, they will appear as soft tissue density masses in these locations, causing the mediastinum to appear widened on the VD view and often displacing the trachea.
- Enlargement of the tracheobronchial lymph nodes may compress the mainstem bronchi mimicking the radiographic appearance of left atrial enlargement on the VD view. However, on the lateral view the bronchi are displaced ventrally with a soft tissue mass seen dorsal to the bronchi.

Thymic or Cranial Mediastinal Lymphoma

- In the cat, this disorder frequently causes a large cranial thoracic mass (see Chap. 25).
- Radiographic signs include dorsal tracheal deviation, a variable amount of pleural fluid, and caudal displacement of the heart, cranial lung borders, and tracheal bifurcation. It is not uncommon for the tracheal bifurcation to be displaced to the level of the seventh or eighth ribs from its normal position at the fifth to sixth ribs.

Pneumomediastinum

- Pneumomediastinum (i.e., air within the mediastinum) may result from perforating injury of the esophagus, trachea, or bronchus near the hilus, usually in association with penetrating wounds of the cervical soft tissues or thoracic inlet.
- This condition allows radiographic identification of the normally invisible mediastinal structures such as the esophagus, cranial vena cava, and other mediastinal vessels.
- Because of its communication with the fascial planes of the body, extensive subcutaneous emphysema is a common complication of this condition.
- Pneumothorax may also occur secondary to pneumomediastinum; however, the reverse does not occur.

RADIOGRAPHIC ABNORMALITIES OF THE PLEURAL SPACE

The normal pleural space is not visible radiographically. Filling of this space with air (pneumothorax), fluid (hydrothorax), or viscera (diaphragmatic hernia) will cause the space to enlarge and become apparent radiographically.

Pneumothorax

In animals with pneumothorax, the pleural space appears widened and radiolucent, the lung appears smaller than normal and relatively radiopaque, and the heart appears elevated off the sternum on the recumbent lateral view, due to shifting of the heart off the midline. Pneumothorax may be classified as open or closed.

Open Pneumothorax

In open pneumothorax, there is a defect in the body wall and the pleural air comes from outside the chest cavity.

Closed Pneumothorax

In closed pneumothorax, there is a break in the visceral pleura and the pleural air comes from the lung (see Chap. 82).

Closed pneumothorax can be further subdivided into simple and tension forms.

Simple Closed Pneumothorax. This is caused by a puncture wound or laceration of the lung that allows free movement of air through the defect during both inspiration and expiration. There is rapid equilibration between the lung and pleural cavity, and the severity of the condition depends on the size of the injured area.

Tension Pneumothorax. This is due to a flaplike lesion that allows air to enter the pleural space during inspiration but closes and does not allow air to leave during expiration. Thus, pressure within the pleural space may continue to increase, and progressive pulmonary atelectasis and cardiovascular compromise may develop. This condition is a medical emergency. Radiographically, tension pneumothorax is characterized by flattening of the diaphragm, severe and progressive pulmonary atelectasis, and microcardia.

Hydrothorax

Hydrothorax is a nonspecific term that indicates filling of the pleural space with fluid. It is not possible to radiographically determine the type of effusion within the pleural space; thus, thoracocentesis (see Chap. 3) with fluid analysis (see Chap. 80) is necessary to reach a definitive diagnosis.

- Radiographically, the pleural space appears widened and radiopaque and the lung appears smaller and relatively radiolucent.
- The ease with which pleural fluid can be detected depends on the amount and distribution of the pleural fluid. Small amounts of fluid gravitate to the dependent portions of the thorax.
  - Thus, on the DV view the fluid may result in a diffuse haziness of the thorax and obscured outline of the cardiac apex.
  - On the lateral and VD views, the fluid is seen surrounding retracted lung borders, and the heart and diaphragm are obscured in areas where they contact fluid.

▼ *Key Point* If fluid accumulation is limited to one side of the thorax or if the caudal lobar edges are persistently rounded, consider the possibility of restrictive pleuritis due to chronic pyothorax or chylothorax.

Diaphragmatic Hernia

Most diaphragmatic hernias are traumatic in origin, although hiatal, peritoneal-pericardial, and mediastinal hernias also occur.

- The radiographic appearance of a diaphragmatic hernia varies, depending on the size and location of the defect and the amount of herniated viscera. The most obvious radiographic signs are discontinuity of the diaphragm and herniation of abdominal viscera into the thorax. The lungs, heart, and mediastinum often will be shifted cranially or laterally. The heart and part of the diaphragm adjacent to the hernia may be obscured owing to their contact with herniated viscera or with pleural fluid, which also may be present.
- Herniation of the liver through a small diaphragmatic rent may result in strangulation of a portion of liver with secondary pleural effusion. Cranial gastric displacement may be a helpful radiographic sign in these cases.
- Although gas is often present within herniated small bowel or stomach, administration of a small amount of barium (1.0 ml/kg) may be helpful to verify herniation of a portion of the gastrointestinal tract.
- Herniation of the stomach may result in acute gastric dilation and is a potential source of life-threatening cardiovascular compromise.

Positive-Contrast Peritonography

If the diagnosis of a diaphragmatic hernia is uncertain, abdominal ultrasound or positive-contrast peritonography may be helpful to assess diaphragmatic integrity. Prior to peritonography, remove pleural and abdominal fluid.

Procedure

- Administer 1–2 ml/kg of a sterile aqueous triiodinated contrast agent such as that used for intravenous (IV) urography (see Chap. 4). Warm the contrast agent to body temperature and mix with 0.1 ml/kg of lidocaine prior to intraperitoneal administration.
- Shave, surgically prepare, and locally anesthetize a small area just to the right of the umbilicus. Pass a needle-catheter combination, such as an Intrafusor (Abbott Laboratories) into the abdomen, avoiding trauma to the spleen, bladder, or bowel. Perform aspiration to verify that there has been no perforation of a hollow viscus or laceration of a blood vessel.
- Slowly introduce the warmed contrast agent/lidocaine mixture into the peritoneal cavity, remove the needle, and gently roll the animal to facilitate distribution of the contrast agent.
- Obtain radiographs immediately; if findings are inconclusive, repeat in 15–20 minutes.
- Optimally, obtain all four views of the abdomen (right and left laterals, DV, and VD). However, if the clinical state of the animal is compromised and only limited views can be taken, place the area of the suspected rent dependently (i.e., left lateral and DV views for a suspected ventral left-sided tear).
- In a normal animal the contrast material will coat the abdominal surface of the diaphragm. Discontinuity of this silhouette or extension of the contrast material into the thorax indicates a diaphragmatic tear.

RADIOGRAPHIC ABNORMALITIES IN PULMONARY DISEASE

Principles of Interpretation

A number of different methods have been used to describe the radiographic findings associated with pulmonary disease. One common technique uses a pattern approach that is based on the microscopic pathologic changes involved in the disease process.

▼ *Key Point* The radiographic patterns of pulmonary disease are alveolar, interstitial, bronchial, vascular, and mixed.

When making a radiographic differential diagnosis evaluate the extent of a lesion (diffuse or focal), the location of the lesion within the lung, and any associated abnormalities of other thoracic structures, such as the heart, large blood vessels, and thoracic wall. Two radiographic signs important in the evaluation of pulmonary disease are the *silhouette sign* and *summation.*

Silhouette Sign. The silhouette sign occurs when two objects of the same radiographic density contact one another and are oriented in such a way that there is a gradual rather than an abrupt change in thickness at their borders (Fig. 75–3, *left, top and bottom*).

- Radiographically these objects appear to blend together and the borders between them are obscured. Therefore, it is not possible to perceive where one object ends and the other begins.

- This sign is most commonly seen in the thorax when abnormal fluid density within the lung ("classic" silhouette sign) or pleural space (also called border effacement) contacts the heart or diaphragm, and the borders of these structures become indistinct.

Summation. The opposite effect occurs with summation (Fig. 75–3, *right, top and bottom*). Summation occurs when two objects are superimposed in such a way that there is an abrupt change in thickness at the border where these structures overlap or when they are separated by material of a different radiographic density.

- This occurs when a soft tissue density mass is within a well-aerated portion of lung and is superimposed over the heart or diaphragm. In this case the heart and mass are separated by air and the densities of the mass and the heart will be additive.

- Thus, the margin where the two objects overlap is enhanced and the mass appears denser than it actually is.

Alveolar Pattern

The alveolar pattern of pulmonary disease indicates decreased air within the lung as the result of alveolar collapse or filling of the alveolar air spaces with fluid or cellular debris. It is not possible to determine radiographically what type of fluid (especially if present only 1–2 days) is within the alveoli. Often there is a lag period, both at the beginning and at the end of a disease process, in which radiographic signs may not correlate with the severity of clinical signs; thus, the history, signalment,

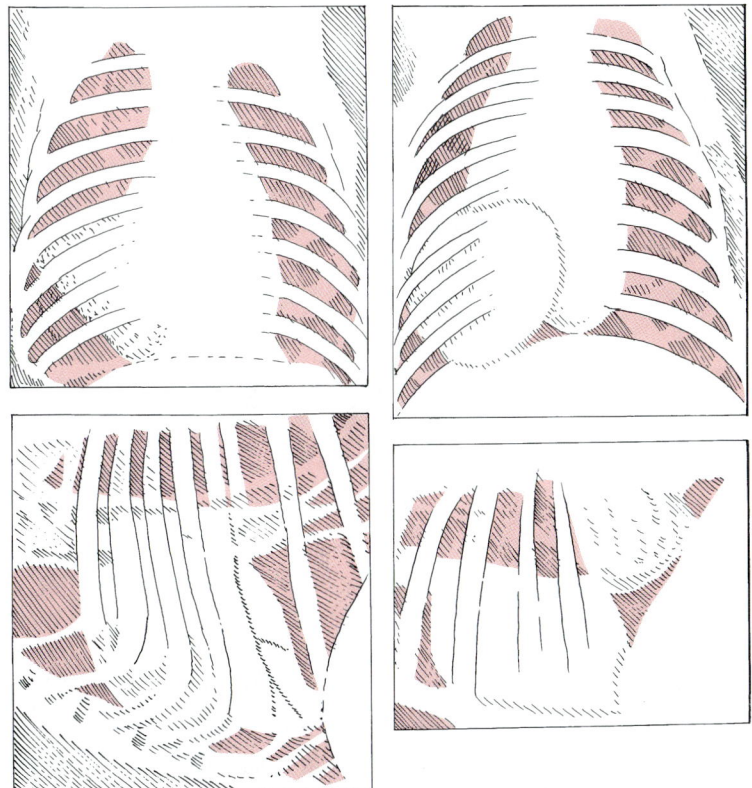

Figure 75–3. Representation of silhouette sign *(left, top and bottom)* and summation *(right, top and bottom).*

and other clinical information are extremely important in arriving at a definitive diagnosis.

Characteristics of Alveolar Disease

- Patchy, ill-defined areas of infiltration that fade into adjacent normal lung ("cotton candy" effect).
- The tendency for these lesions to coalesce, leading to lobar consolidation.
- Rapid progression or regression of the infiltrates.
- Air bronchograms and the silhouette sign.

Air Bronchogram. In an air bronchogram, the air within the bronchus provides excellent contrast with the fluid-filled lung, and the bronchus appears as a faint, gray, branching tube within the abnormally radiopaque lung (Fig. 75–4). The soft tissue density bronchial walls and pulmonary vessels within the affected portion of lung *are not seen* because of silhouetting of these structures by the infiltrated lung (these signs distinguish the alveolar from the bronchial pattern).

▼ *Key Point* The *air bronchogram sign* is one of the most reliable characteristics of alveolar disease. Air bronchograms are due to an air-filled bronchus within an area of fluid-filled alveoli.

Associated Disease Processes

Common disease processes that cause an alveolar pattern include bronchopneumonia, pulmonary edema, and pulmonary contusions. The distribution of the alveolar pattern in the lung may be helpful in the differential diagnosis of these conditions.

Bronchopneumonia

- Inhalation pneumonia and bronchopneumonia usually lead to focal or diffuse alveolar infiltration of the cranioventral portion of the lung. The right middle lobe is one of the most commonly affected lobes. Air bronchograms and lobar consolidation are common findings in patients with bronchopneumonia.

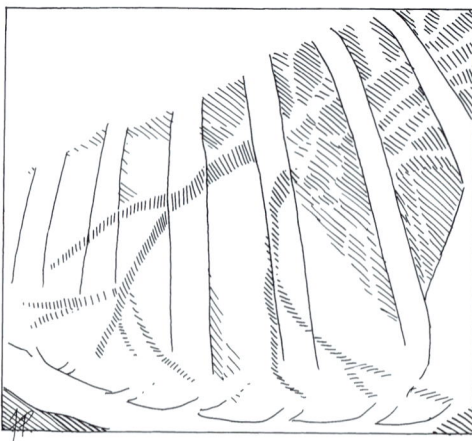

Figure 75–4. Alveolar lung consolidation with air bronchograms (shaded areas in ventral lung).

- In contrast, pneumonia due to hematogenous spread of bacteria, fungi, or other infectious agents often has a diffuse or dorsocaudal distribution.
- For further discussion of diagnosis and treatment of bronchopneumonia, see Chap. 79.

Pulmonary Edema

- Pulmonary edema, whether cardiogenic or noncardiogenic, usually has a dorsal or dorsocaudal distribution.
- Edema due to anaphylaxis, left-sided congestive heart failure, or electrocution usually is most dense in the hilar area of the lung.
- Air bronchograms may not be a consistent feature of cardiogenic edema secondary to mitral insufficiency, possibly because of the slow onset and chronic nature of this type of heart failure. Animals with acute onset of pulmonary edema from any cause are more likely to have air bronchograms because of the rapid accumulation of pulmonary fluid. Right caudal lobe predominance is observed in some cases of heart failure.
- Edema secondary to seizures or head trauma ("neurogenic") tends to affect the more peripheral portions of the caudal lobes.
- Acute upper airway obstruction is a relatively uncommon cause of pulmonary edema. When it occurs, it is often similar in distribution to cardiogenic edema.

Interstitial Pattern

The interstitium surrounds and supports the pulmonary vessels, lymphatics, bronchi, and alveoli; therefore, diseases of these structures may be reflected in the interstitium. The interstitial pattern can be subdivided into structured (nodular) and unstructured patterns.

Nodular Interstitial Pattern

The nodular interstitial pattern is one of the most common pulmonary patterns. The ease of detection of pulmonary nodules depends on the size and number of nodules, their distribution within the lung, and their margination and density. Soft tissue nodules <0.5 cm in diameter are extremely difficult to detect unless they are numerous, mineralized, or superimposed over soft tissue structures such as the heart or diaphragm.

Smooth Versus Indistinct Nodules

- Nodules with smooth, well-defined borders suggest a slowly progressive process with minimal involvement of the surrounding alveoli. Examples include primary and metastatic neoplasia and chronic (inactive) pulmonary granulomas and abscesses.
- An indistinct nodular margin suggests a more active process that extends into the adjacent alveoli or is causing associated edema. Highly aggressive neoplasms, active granulomas, and pulmonary abscesses often appear irregular or indistinct in margination.

Differentiating Nodules from Vessels

- On-end pulmonary vessels can be differentiated from nodules because they are:
  - More numerous in the hilar area.
  - Consistently more dense than the adjacent vasculature.
  - Associated with a longitudinal vessel of which they are a branch.
  - Progressively less numerous and smaller in the periphery of the lung.
- In contrast, tumor nodules are:
  - Randomly distributed throughout the lung (i.e., small nodules may be seen centrally and large nodules peripherally).
  - Often less dense or have the same density as the pulmonary vascular pattern.
  - Frequently cannot be associated with a vessel of similar or greater size.

Granulomas

- Granulomas, such as those secondary to *Paragonimus kellicotti* (see Chap. 79), may be solitary or multiple, cavitated, and may occur anywhere in the lung.
  - Radiographic appearance varies from lesions that are almost entirely cystic to those that are primarily granulomatous with only a small cystic cavity.
  - Spontaneous pneumothorax may occur secondary to rupture of air-filled cysts.
- Immune-mediated, eosinophilic, or lymphomatoid pulmonary granulomatosis is typically associated with hilar lymphadenopathy.

Neoplasia

- Primary lung tumors are relatively uncommon and are usually carcinomas.
  - Bronchogenic carcinoma is usually hilar in location and occurs most commonly as a large, irregularly marginated soft tissue mass in the caudal lobes, especially on the right side.
  - Cavitation is uncommon but may develop in large necrotic tumors. Intrapulmonary metastasis also may be seen.
  - Although pulmonary carcinomas commonly metastasize to hilar lymph nodes, these metastases generally are not large enough to be evident radiographically. (For further discussion of lung neoplasia, see Chap. 81).
- Metastatic neoplasia generally appears as multiple, variably sized nodules randomly distributed throughout the lung. When small, these nodules are occasionally confused with cross-sectional views of pulmonary vessels.

Unstructured Interstitial Pattern

This pattern is one of the most difficult to diagnose because it is commonly mimicked by poor radiographic technique. The lung generally appears denser than normal, with blurring of the vascular shadows (Fig. 75-5). Diseases causing diffuse unstructured interstitial

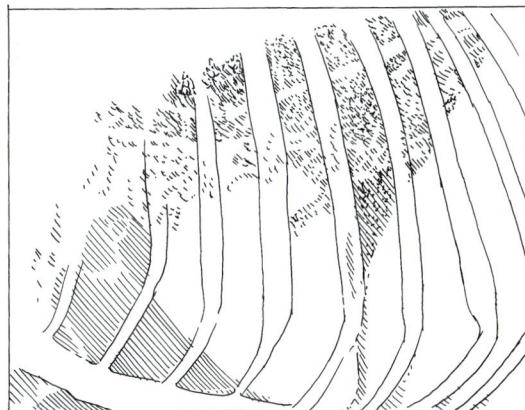

Figure 75-5.   Diffuse dorsal caudal interstitial pattern.

infiltration usually have a widespread or dorsocaudal distribution.

▼ *Key Point* The unstructured interstitial pattern must be differentiated from respiratory motion, poor inflation of the lung such as might occur in a recumbent or obese animal, and radiographic underexposure.

Pulmonary Edema

Pulmonary edema, both cardiogenic and noncardiogenic, usually appears initially as an interstitial pattern. As the disease progresses, fluid extends farther into the alveoli resulting in an alveolar pattern.

Interstitial Pneumonia

Interstitial pneumonia of fungal, parasitic, and especially viral etiology typically causes a diffuse increase in interstitial density of the dorsal and hilar lung areas. Secondary bacterial bronchopneumonia can simultaneously produce a mixed or alveolar infiltrate of the cranioventral portions of the lung.

Pulmonary Fibrosis

Lung fibrosis is a very common cause of diffuse interstitial density especially in older dogs.

Neoplasia

Most neoplastic processes of the lung tend to be nodular; however, in some neoplasms there is a less structured and more diffuse increase in interstitial pulmonary density. These neoplastic cells may reach the lung lymphogenously (e.g., pulmonary lymphoma) or hematogenously (e.g., the scirrhous form of mammary adenocarcinoma). Differentiation of this type of neoplastic infiltration from other causes of diffuse interstitial density is difficult.

- Clinically affected animals may present with a degree of respiratory distress disproportionate to the degree of pulmonary infiltration.
- Fine-needle aspiration of the lung, bronchoalveolar lavage, or lung biopsy may be needed for diagnosis.

Vascular Pattern

- The vascular pattern of pulmonary disease is primarily determined by the size of the pulmonary arteries and veins.
- As mentioned previously, the vessels are best appreciated on the lateral thoracic radiograph as they extend from the hilar area into the cranial lobes.
- On the DV and VD views they are seen just lateral to the spine.
- The arteries extend into the caudal lobes from their origin at the left cranial heart border, and the veins enter the left atrium at the caudal aspect of the heart.

Hypovascularity

This appears as a decrease in the size of both the arteries and veins and is associated with relative pulmonary underperfusion, which may be due to:

- Congenital shunting of blood in a right-to-left direction, as in tetralogy of Fallot.
- Acquired circulatory problems, such as acute blood loss, shock, and cardiac tamponade.

Hypervascularity

Hypervascularity can refer to enlargement of both the arteries and veins, the arteries alone (pulmonary arterial hypertension), or the veins alone (venous congestion).

- Enlargement of both the pulmonary arteries and veins usually is associated with overhydration with intravenous fluids or with some type of congenital cardiac left-to-right shunt, resulting in pulmonary overcirculation. Examples include patent ductus arteriosus and ventricular septal defects (see Chap. 70).
- High-output states such as hyperthyroidism also may produce prominent pulmonary vascularity.
- Severe left-sided heart failure due to cardiomyopathy or chronic mitral insufficiency with long-standing venous congestion and secondary pulmonary hypertension also may lead to enlarged arteries and veins.

Acquired Pulmonary Arterial Hypertension

- In the dog, this condition most commonly is the result of heartworm disease (see Chap. 68).
  - In early heartworm disease, there is right heart enlargement and a mild to moderate increase in interstitial pulmonary density in the dorsal lung fields.
  - As the condition progresses, the right ventricle becomes more rounded, giving a "reversed D" shape to the cardiac silhouette on the VD view, and the main pulmonary artery segment and peripheral pulmonary arteries become enlarged and tortuous (Fig. 75–6).

▼ *Key Point* Truncation or abrupt termination of the peripheral vessels, also called the "pruned tree" effect, is commonly seen in the caudal lobar vessels in advanced cases of heartworm disease.

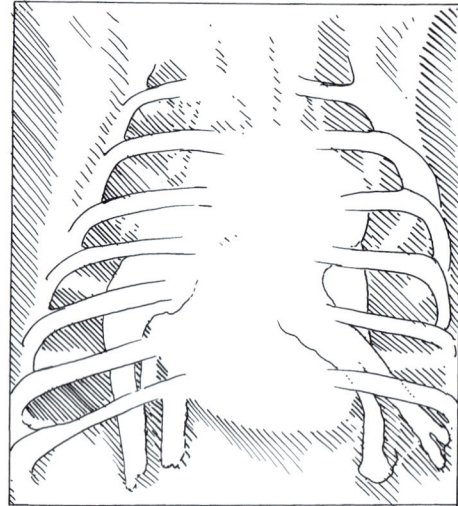

Figure 75–6. Radiographic appearance of heartworm disease. Note large, truncated lobar arteries.

- Focal areas of pulmonary infarction appear as patchy alveolar densities, primarily around the caudal lobar vessels.
- Pulmonary arterial hypertension also occurs in the cat and may be due to heartworm disease or aelurostrongylosis.

Venous Congestion

Venous congestion, characterized by enlarged pulmonary veins, usually is associated with left heart failure (see Chap. 64) from congenital or acquired cardiac disease.

- Early interstitial edema, which in the dog is usually restricted to the hilar area, causes a symmetric increase in interstitial density of the hilar area of the lung, with blurring of the veins on radiographs.
- As the pulmonary edema progresses, alveolar infiltrates become evident in the caudal lobes.
- In the cat, pulmonary edema is somewhat less predictable in its distribution and may appear more focal and asymmetric than that in the dog.

Bronchial Pattern

- Increased bronchial prominence in the dog may occur as a normal aging change or may be secondary to chronic bronchial inflammation.
- Radiographic changes in animals with acute bronchitis may be absent or restricted to pulmonary overinflation or air trapping.
- As the disease progresses, the bronchial walls tend to appear thickened. This often results in a relative decrease in luminal diameter and is best appreciated on cross-sectional views in which the bronchi appear as thick-walled "doughnuts" (Fig. 75–7).
- When viewed longitudinally, the bronchial walls appear as paired, nearly parallel linear densities or "tram lines" extending into the lung periphery.
- Bronchial mineralization is a common sequela of chronic bronchitis, especially in cases with an allergic or immune-mediated etiology.

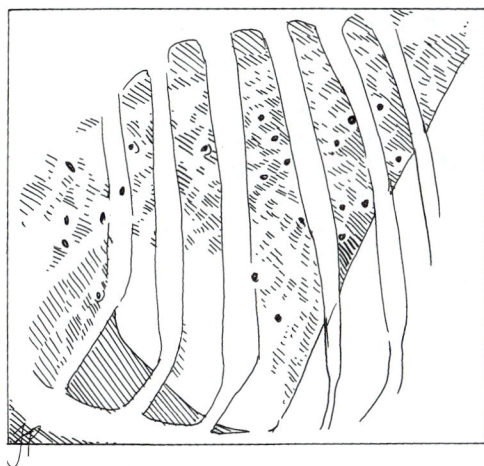

Figure 75–7.   Bronchial pattern.

Bronchial Prominence in Cats

This pattern in cats is most commonly associated with *bronchitis* or *feline asthma,* although infection with *Aelurostrongylus abstrus* may occasionally cause this appearance.

- Cats presenting with acute respiratory distress generally show evidence of thoracic overexpansion with a flattened diaphragm and a barrel-shaped thorax in addition to bronchial prominence.
- Asymptomatic animals may appear radiographically normal unless the disease is chronic and the animal has had several acute episodes of dyspnea.
- Some cats with chronic bronchitis have chronic consolidation or atelectasis of the right middle lung lobe, the result of mucus plugs in the middle lobe bronchus, chronic fibrosis, and volume loss in this lobe.

Bronchiectasis

Bronchiectasis, or irreversible bronchial dilatation, generally occurs secondary to chronic bronchial disease.

- It may be cylindrical or saccular, and on cross-sectional views the affected bronchi have prominent walls that appear relatively thin compared with the enlarged bronchial lumen.
- Animals with bronchiectasis are prone to secondary bronchopneumonia because of poor mucociliary pulmonary clearance.

Mixed Patterns

Although the pattern approach to pulmonary evaluation is helpful in arriving at a differential diagnosis, many disease processes result in a mixture of the aforementioned patterns. These patterns often vary depending on the stage of the disease process during which the animal is evaluated. Diseases commonly causing a mixed pattern include heartworm disease, heart failure, and pneumonia.

Increased Pulmonary Radiolucency

- Abnormal pulmonary radiolucency is probably easiest to recognize when it is focal.
- Thin-walled bullae or blebs often occur secondary to pulmonary trauma. They are generally subpleural in location and resolve spontaneously.
- Thicker-walled cavitary lesions may be the result of parasitic cysts (e.g., *Paragonimus kellicotti*), congenital bronchial cysts, cavitated abscesses, neoplasms, and granulomas. These may be single or multiple, and their location within the lung is variable.
- Horizontal beam radiographs may be helpful in determining if fluid or cellular debris is present in the "cystic" areas.

Emphysema. Emphysema may occur as a compensatory change following surgical removal of a lung lobe or volume loss in one of the lung lobes; it also can be the result of aging or of true histologic breakdown of the alveolar septae. True emphysema, as seen in humans, is relatively uncommon in dog and cats.

- True emphysema with rupture and confluence of alveoli must be differentiated from causes of reversible hyperinflation including asthma or tracheobronchial obstruction (e.g., foreign body).
- Radiographically, hyperinflation is recognized by:
  - Relative pulmonary hyperlucency.
  - Flattening of the diaphragm.
  - Increased separation of the heart and diaphragm.
  - Apparent decreased size of the pulmonary vessels.
  - A barrel-shaped chest.
  - Decreased differences in diaphragmatic excursion between inspiratory and expiratory films.
- Radiographic overexposure and severe hypovolemia (e.g., hypoadrenocorticism) are other causes of apparent pulmonary hyperlucency but usually are not accompanied by the other radiographic signs seen in generalized emphysema.

ALTERNATE IMAGING MODALITIES

Ultrasonographic Evaluation of the Lung and Mediastinum

- It is not possible to evaluate the normally aerated lung using ultrasonography, because of the large acoustic mismatch between air and soft tissue and the reflection of most of the ultrasound beam at the pleura-lung interface.
- Focal areas of pulmonary infiltration may be evaluated as long as they extend to the pulmonary periphery. Fine-needle aspiration of these areas also can be done for microscopic evaluation and culture (see Chap. 4).
- In animals with pleural effusion, the lung is displaced away from the body wall, allowing assessment of the character of the pleural fluid to determine if it is cellular or noncellular or contains fibrin.
- Large mediastinal masses also displace the lung, allowing assessment of whether these masses are single

or multiple; solid, vascular, or cystic; mineralized or nonmineralized; and whether the heart or great vessels are affected. These masses are usually imaged through the intercostal spaces or through the thoracic inlet.

- Thymomas, ectopic thyroid neoplasia, and lymphoma are among the mediastinal masses that can be evaluated and aspirated using ultrasonographic guidance.
- Ultrasonography can aid the diagnosis of diaphragmatic hernia.

Nuclear Medicine

- Nuclear medicine is rarely used for identification of pulmonary thromboembolism in animals and is mostly limited to referral centers.
- Perfusion-ventilation studies are commonly done in humans and were first used in dogs to evaluate the effects of heartworm disease.

- Special aerosol masks and trapping mechanisms are used to deliver the radioactivity for the ventilation portion of the study.
- The perfusion part of the study involves IV administration of technetium 99m macroaggregated albumin (MAA). Because this agent is trapped in the capillary network of the lung on the first pass following an IV injection, it can be used to detect areas of decreased pulmonary perfusion, as with pulmonary thromboembolism.

SUPPLEMENTAL READINGS

Suter PF: Thoracic Radiography: A Text Atlas of Thoracic Diseases of the Dog and Cat. Wettswil, Switzerland: P. F. Suter, 1984.

Thrall DE: Textbook of Veterinary Diagnostic Radiology. Philadelphia: WB Saunders, 1986.

76 Surgery of the Nasal Cavity and Sinuses

Cheryl S. Hedlund

Signs in dogs and cats with chronic nasal and paranasal sinus disease may include nasal discharge, epistaxis, sneezing, gagging, stertorous breathing, nasal discomfort, and nasal deformity. Causes of nasal cavity and paranasal sinus diseases can be difficult to identify, but most cases are traumatic, infectious, inflammatory, mechanical, or neoplastic in origin. Rhinotomy may be necessary to arrive at a definitive diagnosis and may facilitate treatment of the disease. Hemostatic abnormalities may lead to epistaxis.

ANATOMY

Nasal Cavity

- The nasal cavity extends from the nostrils to the nasopharyngeal meatus and is divided into two chambers by the nasal septum. The rostral portion of the nasal septum is cartilaginous and difficult to evaluate radiographically.
- The rostral nasal chambers are occupied by the dorsal and ventral nasal conchae (Fig. 76–1).
- The caudal nasal chamber is filled with ethmoidal conchae. The ethmoidal conchae extend into the frontal sinus, forming narrow communicating ostia between the frontal sinus and nasal cavity (see Fig. 76–1).
- In the cat, the nasal cavity is shorter, the ethmoidal conchae are larger, and the nasal conchae are smaller than in the dog.
- The cribriform plate is a sievelike partition between the nasal and cranial cavities (see Fig. 76–1). It articulates with the frontal bones dorsally and the presphenoid bones ventrally and laterally.
- The blood supply to the nasal cavity originates from the external carotid arteries via branches of the maxillary artery, including the sphenopalatine, ethmoid, greater palatine, dorsal nasal, lateral nasal, and maxillary labial arteries.

Paranasal Sinuses

- The paranasal sinuses enlarge with age and vary in size depending on the breed of the animal.
- The frontal sinus extends roughly from the medial canthus of the eyes to the temporal line. In dogs (but not in cats), it is divided into rostral, lateral, and me-

dial compartments (see Fig. 76–1). The frontal sinus varies more in size than other cavities in the skull. The lateral compartment is particularly large in dolichocephalic breeds. Brachycephalic breeds have small lateral compartments, and the medial compartment may be absent.
- The maxillary sinus or recess is found dorsal to the roots of the third and fourth premolars and medial to the infraorbital canal. The maxillary recess in the cat is very narrow.
- Cats have a small sphenoid sinus. Dogs do not have a sphenoid sinus.

PREOPERATIVE CONSIDERATIONS

Disease Conditions

- Signs of chronic nasal disease can include unilateral or bilateral nasal discharge, epistaxis, sneezing, nasal discomfort, gagging, reverse sneezing, stertorous breathing, ocular discharge, and facial or nasopharyngeal distortion. Neurologic signs are seen if the disease extends into the cranium.
- The most frequent causes of chronic nasal and paranasal sinus disease are neoplasms, infections, and foreign bodies.
- Other causes include parasites (*Pneumonyssus caninum, Linguatula serrata*), dental disease, trauma,

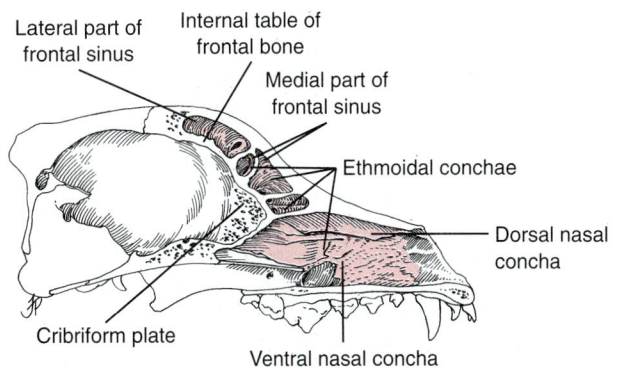

Figure 76–1. Sagittal section of the skull illustrating the anatomy of the nasal cavity and paranasal sinuses in relationship to the cranium. (Redrawn with permission from Evans HE, ed.: Miller's Anatomy of the Dog, 3rd Ed. Philadelphia: W.B. Saunders, 1992.)

lymphocytic-plasmocytic inflammation, and congenital anomalies. Nasal polyps, which are benign lesions, occur rarely.

Tumors

- Tumors of the nasal cavity and paranasal sinuses account for approximately 1% of all neoplasms in cats and dogs.
- Most intranasal tumors are diagnosed in older dogs and cats (>8–10 years) and in large-breed dogs.
- Tumors in the nasal cavity are usually found in the caudal third of the nasal passages.
- Most intranasal tumors are malignant (80%). Adenocarcinomas are most common, but squamous cell carcinoma, fibrosarcoma, chondrosarcoma, osteosarcoma, lymphosarcoma, hemangiosarcoma, undifferentiated sarcomas or carcinomas, and transmissible venereal tumors also occur.
- The prognosis for malignant nasal neoplasms is guarded because of rapid local invasion and recurrence after therapy. Typically, these tumors do not metastasize until late in the course of the disease.
- Therapies that may help control some tumors include radiotherapy, immunotherapy, cryotherapy, and chemotherapy (see Chap. 81). These modalities are sometimes combined with surgical debulking of the lesion.

Infections

- Infections, especially those caused by fungal organisms, frequently cause nasal and paranasal cavity disease.
- Systemic diseases such as distemper, feline upper respiratory viral infections, and Rocky Mountain spotted fever can also cause acute or chronic rhinitis.
- Primary bacterial rhinitis is uncommon and usually is associated with foreign bodies, immunosuppression (feline leukemia virus [FeLV], feline immunodeficiency virus [FIV]), or dental disease.

Fungal Rhinitis. The most commonly reported pathogenic fungi are *Aspergillus* and *Penicillium* species in dogs and *Cryptococcus neoformans* in cats. Other reported pathogens are *Rhinosporidium* and *Alternaria alternata*.

- Dogs with fungal rhinitis due to *Aspergillus* or *Penicillium* are usually young (1–7 years).
- Patients with fungal rhinitis generally do not have facial distortion but may exhibit ulceration of the nares and more nasal discomfort than dogs with nasal neoplasia.
- Treatment of fungal rhinitis is primarily medical, although surgery may be necessary for definitive diagnosis or creating ports for medical therapy.
- Medical therapy may be systemic (itraconazole, ketoconazole, thiabendazole), topical (enilconazole or clotrimazole administered directly into the nasal cavity), or both (see Chap. 79 for details).
  - If indicated, perform topical therapy by placing fenestrated balloon catheters via endoscopy or rhinoscopy, placing indwelling fenestrated tubes into the frontal sinuses and nasal cavity, or creating a nasal stoma for nasal irrigation or swabbing.

- Nasal rhinosporidiosis is treated by surgical excision of the lesion.

Diagnosis

Follow a standard protocol of evaluation, including a thorough history and physical examination, for all dogs and cats presenting with chronic nasal disease. Besides a complete blood count (CBC), serum chemistry profile, and urinalysis, consider a coagulation profile, radiography, enzyme-linked immunosorbent assay (ELISA) for FeLV and FIV in cats, computed tomography (CT) or MRI (magnetic resonance imaging), fungal serology, antegrade and retrograde rhinoscopy, and nasal biopsy.

History

The clinical history can provide important diagnostic clues.

- Suspect a destructive process if the discharge changes from unilateral to bilateral.
- Sneezing suggests involvement of the mid- and rostral nasal chambers.
- Gagging or reverse sneezing suggests nasopharyngeal involvement or postnasal drainage.
- A history of trauma or dental disease suggests an oronasal fistula.

Physical Examination

- Facial or palatal deformity suggests neoplasia.
- Mouth breathing indicates nasopharyngeal obstruction.
- An ocular discharge may indicate nasolacrimal duct erosion.
- Neurologic signs may indicate disease extension into the brain.

Laboratory Studies

- A CBC, serum chemistry profile, and urinalysis can assess the patient's overall status.
- A coagulation profile is indicated if exploratory rhinotomy is planned or if epistaxis is a major clinical sign.

Imaging Studies

Radiography

Obtain radiographs of the thorax in the conscious patient, and obtain radiographs of the nasal cavity and paranasal sinuses with the patient under general anesthesia.

- Include lateral, ventrodorsal, rostrocaudal, and rostroventral-caudodorsal open-mouth or occlusal radiographic views (see Chap. 4).
- The two most useful radiographic views are the ventrodorsal view of the maxilla using intraoral radiographic film and the rostrocaudal projection highlighting the frontal sinuses.

▼ *Key Point* To avoid iatrogenic fluid densities within the cavities, schedule radiography before performing any rhinoscopic, flush, or biopsy procedures.

CT or MRI

Although not widely available, CT or MRI should be performed when possible to localize lesions more accurately than is possible with radiography.

Rhinoscopy

Perform rhinoscopy in the anesthetized patient following skull radiography. The nasal mucosa is very sensitive to manipulation, and exposure can be obliterated by hemorrhage. Therefore, use gentle manipulation, lavage, and suction techniques.

- The rostral aspect of the nasal cavity may be seen with an otoscope, cystoscope, or small fiberoptic scope. A flexible pediatric bronchoscope or 2–3 mm diameter rigid telescope facilitates examination of the remainder of the cavity and allows retropharyngeal examination of the choanae for lodged foreign bodies, nasal mites, mucosal invasion (mycoses), or extruding nasal tumors.
- It may be impossible to perform a rhinoscopic examination on very small dogs and cats because of the size discrepancies between the scope and nasal passages. However, examine the pharynx and choanae in these animals.
- Use rhinoscopy to obtain specimens for biopsy, cytology, and culture.

Biopsy

- During the rhinoscopic procedure, lesions can be biopsied using endoscopic biopsy instruments. Biopsy the nasal mucosa even if no obvious lesions are found.

Other Diagnostic Procedures

- Perform *nasal flushing* or coring procedures with the patient still under anesthesia if endoscopic biopsy was not possible or successful.
  - In this procedure, slide a stiff plastic tube (e.g., the plastic cover of a Sovereign [Sherwood Medical, Ireland] indwelling catheter) vigorously in and out of the nasal passages (inserted through the nares and not extending beyond the medial canthus) while flushing and aspirating saline.
  - Premeasure the catheter to avoid trauma to or beyond the cribriform plate.
  - Collect the lavage fluid and debris and examine for tissue fragments.
- *Nasal swabs* for culture or cytologic evaluation are of limited value. Positive fungal cultures can be obtained in about 40% of normal dogs so diagnosis should also rely on identifying characteristic mucosal lesions grossly and on histopathology. Occasionally, cryptococcosis organisms are identified by examining a stained, direct smear.
- *Serologic evaluation* for *Aspergillus* and *Penicillium* species is useful, but false-positive results are possible. Latex agglutination test for *Cryptococcus neoformans* is useful in cats.
- Perform *rhinotomy* as a diagnostic procedure if a diagnosis is not achieved by other means.

Anesthesia

- Place a fentanyl patch 8–12 hours prior to surgery to enhance postoperative analgesia (*note:* prevent ingestion of the patch).
- Induce and maintain routine general anesthesia for diagnostic and surgical procedures (see Chap. 2).
- Prior to extubation examine and suction the nasopharyngeal area. Leave the endotracheal tube cuff partially inflated to prevent tracheal aspiration of blood clots, fluid, and debris.

SURGICAL PROCEDURES

Objectives

- Obtain sufficient tissue samples to achieve a definitive diagnosis for the patient's chronic rhinitis/sinusitis.
- Completely remove or debulk the lesion.
- Facilitate administration of adjuvant therapy.
- Minimize blood loss.
- Maintain a cosmetically acceptable appearance.

Equipment

- Standard general surgical pack and suture
- Umbilical tape, vascular tape (Vas-Tie, Sil-Med Corp., Taunton, MA), or bulldog vascular clamps for temporary carotid occlusion
- Periosteal elevator
- Oscillating saw, air drill, pins and pin chuck, and/or osteotome and mallet to create bone flap
- Gelpi retractor
- Bone curette, rasp, bur, rongeur, and trephine
- Fenestrated, indwelling tubes or balloon catheters to facilitate application of topical medications.
- Synthetic mesh to span the bony defect (usually not needed).

Temporary Bilateral Carotid Artery Occlusion

This procedure is performed prior to entry into the nasal cavity or paranasal sinuses if major surgery such as rhinotomy and turbinectomy is to be performed. Carotid artery occlusion decreases blood loss and improves exposure during rhinotomy. *Not all surgeons choose to use this technique.*

Technique

1. Place the dog in dorsal recumbency with the front legs secured caudally and a rolled towel placed under the neck.
2. Clip and aseptically prepare the ventral neck from the caudal aspect of the mandibles to the manubrium.
3. Incise the skin and subcutis on the ventral cervical midline from the larynx to the mid-trachea.
4. Separate the paired sternohyoideus muscles to expose the ventral trachea.
5. Bluntly dissect lateral to the trachea and palpate the carotid pulse.

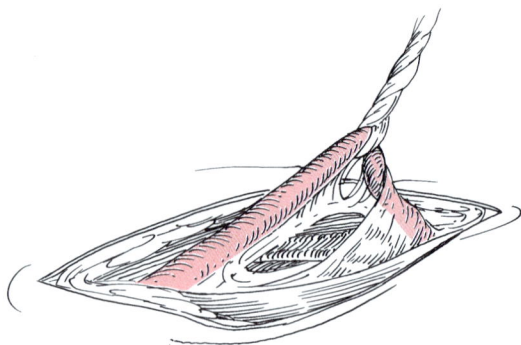

Figure 76–2. Exteriorize and incise the carotid sheath located lateral to the trachea, separate the common carotid artery *(top)* from the vagosympathetic trunk and internal jugular vein *(bottom)* and occlude.

6. Exteriorize the carotid sheath and separate the external carotid artery from the vagosympathetic trunk and internal jugular vein (Fig. 76–2).
7. Occlude the carotid artery with a vascular tie, umbilical tape, or vascular clamp (see Fig. 76–2).
8. Repeat the procedure on the opposite carotid.
9. Appose the separated sternohyoid muscles and skin in two layers with simple continuous suture patterns.
10. Cover the surgical site with sterile draping material and, if necessary, reposition the patient for rhinotomy.
11. Following rhinotomy, reexpose the carotids and release occlusion. Lavage the area and routinely close in three layers (muscle, subcutis, and skin).

Dorsal Rhinotomy

Following carotid occlusion, expose the nasal cavity and frontal sinuses for exploration and biopsy.

Technique

1. Position the patient in ventral recumbency.
2. Prepare the nasal and frontal sinus areas for aseptic surgery.
3. Incise the skin and subcutis along the dorsal midline (Fig. 76–3).
4. Elevate the dense fascia and periosteum with a periosteal elevator and retract these tissues laterally with Gelpi retractors.
5. Create a unilateral or bilateral bone flap with an oscillating saw or drill.
   a. Alternatively, make holes (drill or pin chuck) at the edges of the proposed bone flap and connect them with an osteotome and mallet.
   b. Another method is to make a hole into the nasal cavity with a trephine or pin and chuck; rongeur adjacent bone and discard.
   Expose the nasal cavity and the rostral portion of the frontal sinus for complete exploration (see Fig. 76–3).
6. Remove or debulk the lesion and involved turbinates, using forceps, Metzenbaum scissors, and/or a bone curette (Fig. 76–4). Save all tissues for culture and histologic evaluation.

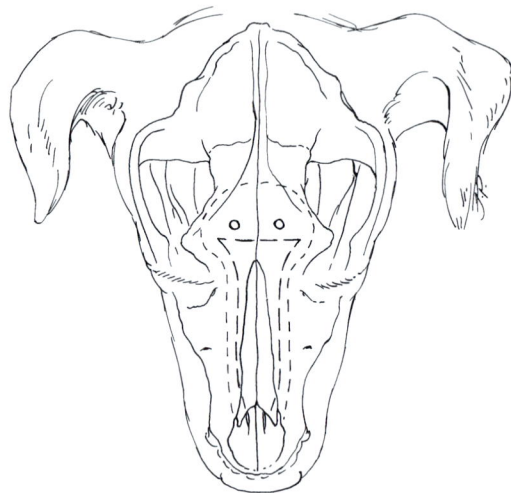

Figure 76–3. Dorsal rhinotomy. The outer dotted line delineates the approximate extent of the nasal cavity and frontal sinuses. The inner dashed lines delineate the bone flap for a unilateral or bilateral approach. The holes over the frontal sinuses indicate the site for insertion of drains. (Redrawn with permission from Bojrab MJ, ed.: Current Techniques in Small Animal Surgery, 3rd Ed. Philadelphia: Lea & Febiger, 1990.)

7. Remove exudate from the frontal sinus, curette the lining to remove all diseased tissue, and enlarge the ostia to facilitate drainage.
8. Lavage and suction the nasal cavity and sinuses thoroughly with copious amounts of saline to dislodge debris and blood clots.
9. If required for adjuvant therapy or to minimize subcutaneous emphysema, place a fenestrated, indwelling tube (e.g., Brunswick feeding tube) into the frontal sinus and extending into the nasal cavity.

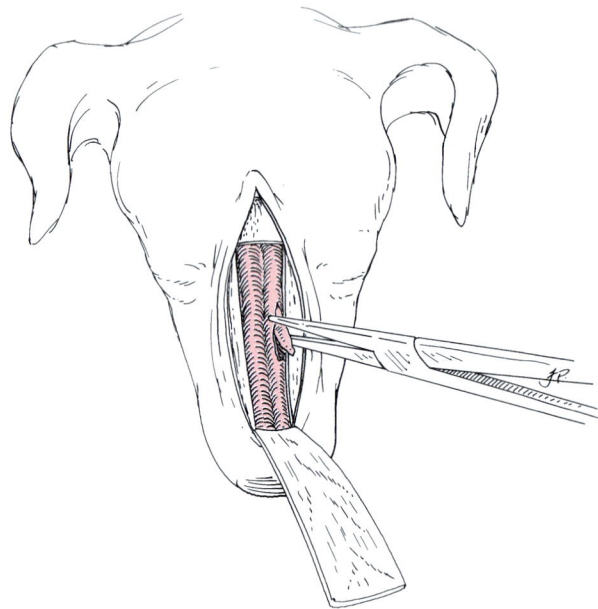

Figure 76–4. Reflect the bone flap rostrally or remove it. Perform turbinectomy using forceps, scissors, and curets. (Redrawn with permission from Bojrab MJ, ed.: Current Techniques in Small Animal Surgery, 3rd Ed. Philadelphia: Lea & Febiger, 1990.)

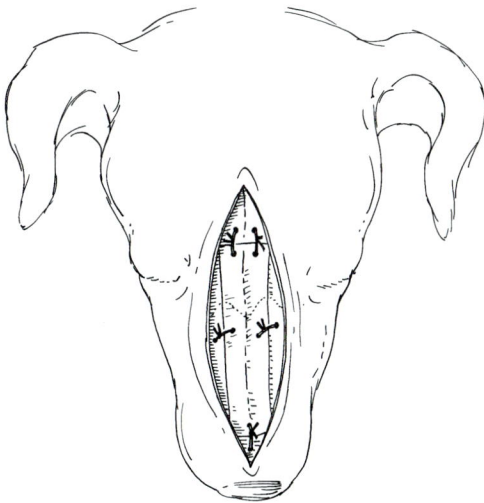

Figure 76–5. Replace the bone flap by placing sutures through holes drilled in the flap and margins of the defect. (Redrawn with permission from Bojrab MJ, ed.: Current Techniques in Small Animal Surgery, 3rd Ed. Philadelphia: Lea & Febiger, 1990.)

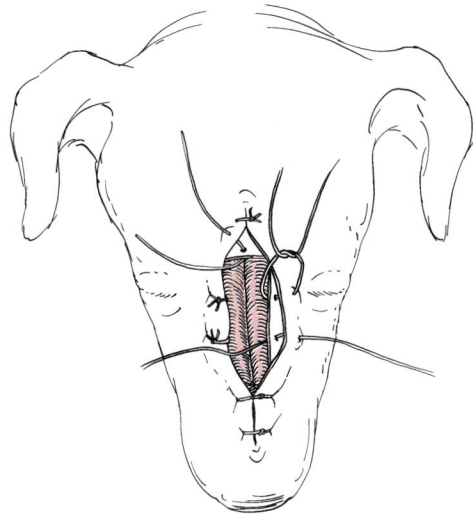

Figure 76–6. If a stoma following rhinotomy is desired, drill holes in the margins of the defect and pass sutures through these holes and the skin.

Create the opening in the frontal sinus with a trephine, drill, or intramedullary pin.

10. To replace the nondiseased bone flap, drill holes in the bone flap and rhinotomy margins and place nonmetallic sutures through adjacent holes to secure the flap (Fig. 76–5). Alternatively, discard the bone flap and proceed with soft tissue closure.

11. Close, using continuous suture patterns in the fascial and periosteal layer, subcutaneous tissues, and the skin. When the defect is large and cosmetic appearance is critical, implant a synthetic mesh (e.g., Marlex mesh) across the bony defect and secure with nonabsorbable, monofilament sutures.

12. The skin edges may be secured directly to the margins of the bony defect, creating a stoma into the nasal cavity to facilitate topical therapy or to prevent subcutaneous emphysema (Fig. 76–6).

13. If the stoma is small it may heal by second intention; otherwise, following conclusion of medical therapy, debride, undermine, and appose the skin edges.

14. Dogs tolerate rhinotomy very well. Aggressive rhinotomy in cats can be associated with a higher rate of morbidity and mortality.

Ventral Rhinotomy

The nasal cavity and nasopharynx can be explored using a ventral approach. With this technique, evaluation of the frontal sinuses is limited to the rostral half.

Technique

1. Position the patient in dorsal recumbency with the oral cavity exposed by hanging and securing the mandible in a wide, open-mouth position (Fig. 76–7).

2. Cleanse the oral cavity, dental arcade, and nasopharyngeal area with a mild antiseptic solution (dilute chlorhexidine or povidone-iodine).

3. Incise the mucoperiosteum of the hard palate on the midline from the level of the canine teeth caudally to the fourth premolar or continue through the mucosa of the soft palate if the lesion extends into the nasopharyngeal area (Fig. 76–8).
   a. Alternatively, use a U-shaped mucoperiosteal incision parallel to the dental arcade (Fig. 76–8).

4. Bilaterally reflect and retract the mucoperiosteum laterally.

5. Identify and preserve the major palatine arteries. They penetrate the hard palate near the caudal aspect of the fourth premolar and run parallel to the course of the dental arcade about midway between it and the midline of the hard palate (see Fig. 76–8).

6. Create a window into the nasal cavity by removing a flap of hard palate with an oscillating saw, air drill, or osteotome and mallet (Fig. 76–9). Enlarge the window with rongeurs, if necessary.

7. Remove the lesion and involved turbinates with forceps and curettage.

8. Lavage and suction blood clots and debris from the area with copious amounts of saline.

9. Replace or discard the bone flap as for dorsal rhinotomy.

10. Close the mucoperiosteum with simple interrupted sutures. If possible, close the soft palate incision in two or three layers (nasal mucosa, muscle and connective tissue, pharyngeal mucosa) (Fig. 76–10).

Frontal Sinus Procedures

Chronic rhinitis/sinusitis (especially in cats) generally recurs in a variable period of time with either of the following procedures.

Technique for Sinus Flushing

1. Insert indwelling tubes for repeated frontal sinus flushing by first trephining a hole into the sinus.

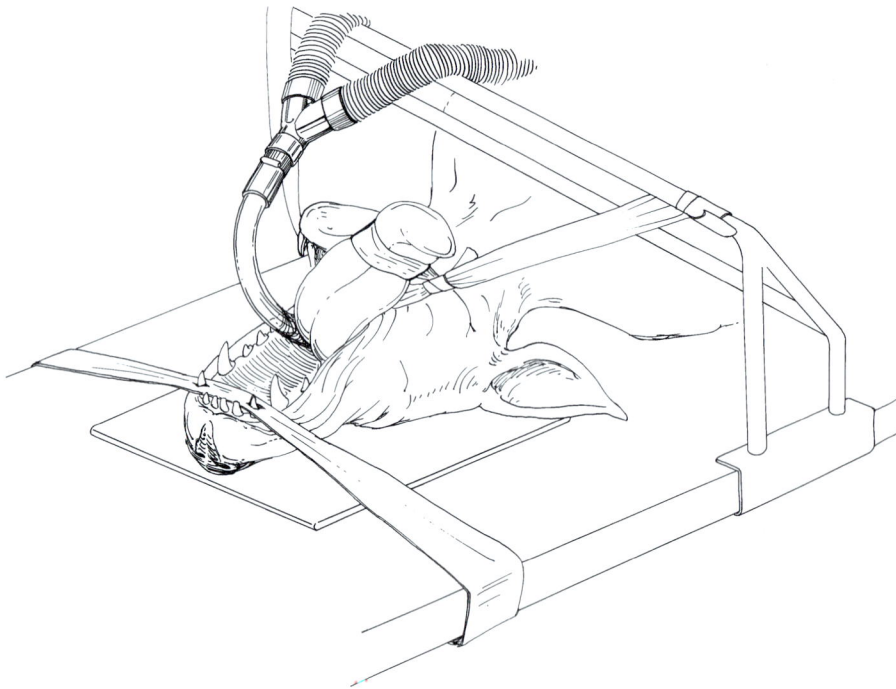

Figure 76–7. Positioning for ventral rhinotomy. (Redrawn with permission from Slatter DH, ed.: Textbook of Small Animal Surgery. Philadelphia: W. B. Saunders, 1985.)

2. Make an incision in the soft tissues and trephine a hole in the bone just lateral to the midline, on a line connecting the rostral margins of the supraorbital processes.
3. Collect biopsy and culture specimens.
4. Insert the fenestrated tube into the sinus and secure it to the skin (Fig. 76–11).
5. Following tube removal, allow the openings to heal by second intention.

Technique for Sinus Obliteration

1. Create a bone flap to expose the frontal sinuses and caudal nasal cavity.

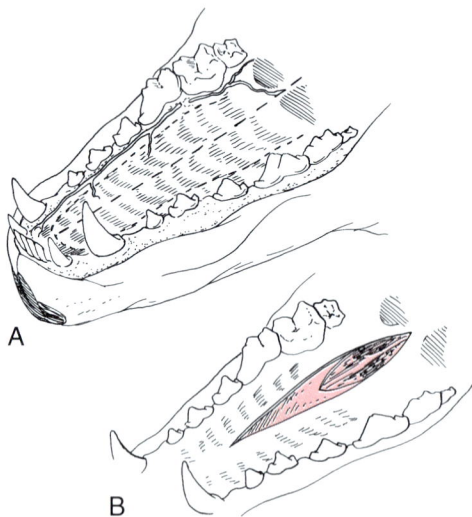

Figure 76–8. Ventral rhinotomy. Incise the mucoperiosteum on the midline or in the shape of a U, which parallels the dental arcade (A). The incision may extend into the soft palate to expose lesions extending into the nasopharynx (B).

2. Remove the compartment divisions and mucosal lining of the frontal sinus and aperture with a pneumatic bone bur.
3. Cover the aperture of the frontal sinus into the nasal cavity with a free fascial or muscle patch.
4. Lavage the area and fill the sinus with fat harvested from a secondary site (e.g., falciform ligament).
5. Close the periosteum, subcutaneous tissue, and skin.

POSTOPERATIVE CARE AND COMPLICATIONS

Patient Care

- Following rhinotomy, place the patient in a slightly head-down position and remove the endotracheal tube with the cuff slightly inflated to help remove fluid and debris.
- Give postoperative analgesics such as morphine (0.2–0.4 mg/kg IM or SC) or buprenorphine (Buprenex, Norwich Eaton), 0.005 mg/kg IM or IV, for the first 24 hours as needed.

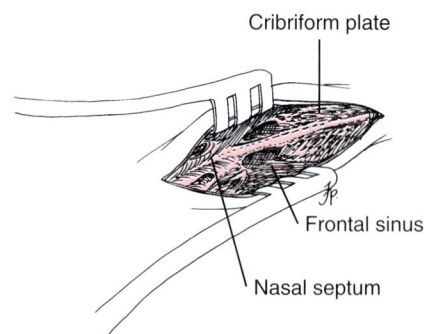

Cribriform plate
Frontal sinus
Nasal septum

Figure 76–9. Exposure using ventral rhinotomy: cribriform plate, frontal sinus, remnant of nasal septum. (Rostral is to the left.)

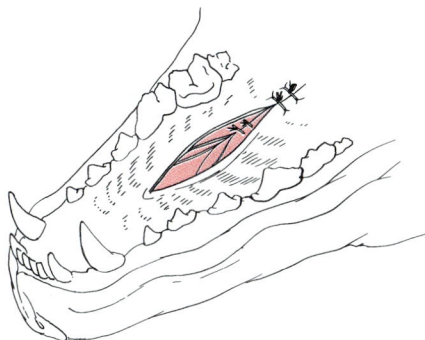

Figure 76–10. Following ventral rhinotomy appose the muco-periosteum with simple interrupted sutures. Appose the soft palate using two or three layers of simple interrupted or simple continuous sutures.

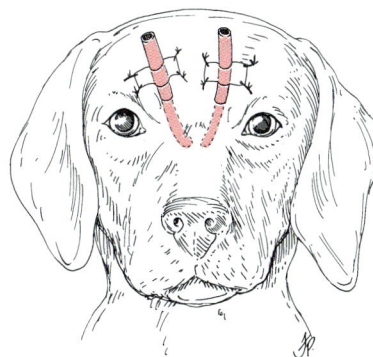

Figure 76–11. Position of tubes inserted into the frontal sinus and nasal cavity for topical treatment of chronic rhinitis and sinusitis. (Redrawn with permission from Slatter DH, ed.: Textbook of Small Animal Surgery. Philadelphia: W. B. Saunders, 1985.)

- Chewing on hard objects is forbidden if the bone flap from the hard palate is discarded.
- Prior to creating a nasal stoma, graphically describe to the client the postoperative appearance of the patient (optimally by viewing pictures of other patients). Many clients are initially reluctant to accept their pets' appearance following rhinostomy.
- Following rhinotomy, discharge patients from the hospital within 2–3 days unless complications or adjuvant therapy dictates longer hospitalization.

Complications

- Expect sneezing and mild epistaxis for several days.
- Breathing sounds are harsh and resonant, often sounding "hollow."
- Appetite may be depressed for several days. Give cats diazepam or oxazepam to stimulate appetite if necessary.
- A serous to serosanguineous nasal discharge occurs for several days to weeks, depending on the primary disease condition and the effectiveness of adjuvant therapy.
- Inward and outward movement of the skin flap may occur if the bone flap is discarded, but is usually temporary.
- Chronic rhinitis/sinusitis and its causative agents will persist or recur if rhinotomy and turbinectomy are performed without appropriate medical therapy (see Chap. 79). Exceptions may include nasal disease caused by foreign bodies or *Rhinosporidium* organisms.
- If carotid artery occlusion is not employed, blood loss during surgery may be excessive, requiring transfusions and vigorous fluid therapy.
- Indwelling catheters can be dislodged by the patient; therefore, some surgeons create temporary rhinostomies to facilitate topical therapy.
- Subcutaneous emphysema may occur. It is usually localized to the head and resorbs without treatment. If emphysema is excessive, place a tube in the frontal sinus to vent the air and aspirate subcutaneous air.

- Disease erosion of the cribriform plate or curettage may result in exposure of the brain and cerebral edema. Treat brain edema with rapid-acting water-soluble IV corticosteroids, osmotic agents (mannitol), hyperventilation, hyperbaric oxygen, calcium channel blockers, and antioxidants.
- Airway obstruction is rare but may occur due to failure to mouth-breath, mucosal edema, and anxiety. Sedate these animals and provide supplemental oxygen in a quiet cool environment. Give corticosteroids to reduce mucosal edema.
- Nasocutaneous or oronasal fistulas may form if healing is interrupted.
- Replaced bone flaps may sequestrate secondary to infection or radiation therapy.
- The chronic nasal discharge may persist because it is not possible to remove all diseased tissue during turbinectomy, and the epithelium may have undergone squamous metaplasia.

Prognosis

- Survival following various combinations of therapy for nasal neoplasms ranges from 4 to > 24 months.
- Fungal rhinitis is refractory to antifungal agents currently available in about 50% of the cases. Antifungal agents are usually given for 6–8 weeks.

SUPPLEMENTAL READINGS

Birchard SJ: A simplified method for rhinotomy and temporary rhinostomy in dogs and cats. J Am Anim Hosp Assoc 24:69, 1988.
Hedlund CS, Tangner CH, Elkins AD, Hobson HP: Temporary bilateral carotid artery occlusion during surgical exploration of the nasal cavity in the dog. Vet Surg 12:83, 1983.
Holmberg DL, Fries C, Cockshutt J, Van Pelt D: Ventral rhinotomy in the dog and cat. Vet Surg 18:446, 1989.
Pavletic MM, Clark GN: Open nasal cavity and frontal sinus treatment of chronic canine aspergillosis. Vet Surg 20:43, 1991.
Sharp NJH, McEntee M, Gilson S, Thrall D: Nasal cavity and frontal sinuses. Problems in Veterinary Medicine: Head and Neck Surgery 3:170, 1991.

Obstructive Upper Airway Disorders

Roger B. Fingland

Obstructive upper airway diseases typically are insidious in onset and result in progressively worsening respiratory stridor and dyspnea. The dimensions of the upper airway play a fundamental role in the efficiency of breathing and progression of disease. In narrowed regions of the upper airway, air velocity is higher and pressure is lower than elsewhere (Bernoulli effect), which tends to narrow susceptible regions of the upper airway still more.

ETIOLOGY

Congenital obstructive upper airway diseases are diagnosed so commonly in brachycephalic dogs that they are referred to collectively as the brachycephalic syndrome. Most other obstructive upper airway diseases are acquired and are diagnosed in middle-aged and older dogs. Obstructive upper airway diseases are diagnosed less frequently in cats.

Brachycephalic Syndrome. The brachycephalic syndrome consists of stenotic nares, elongated soft palate, and everted laryngeal saccules.

- *Tracheal hypoplasia* is a generalized narrowing of the tracheal lumen diameter diagnosed commonly in English bulldogs and, less commonly, in other brachycephalic breeds.
- *Stenotic nares* and elongated soft palate are congenital conditions diagnosed quite frequently in brachycephalic dogs.
- *Laryngeal saccule eversion* is a consequence of chronic upper airway obstruction.

Laryngeal Collapse. Laryngeal collapse is recognized most commonly in brachycephalic dogs with chronic obstructive upper respiratory disease (brachycephalic syndrome). Loss of the supporting function of the laryngeal cartilages results from pressure changes within the larynx induced by obstruction rostral to the rima glottidis. Laryngeal collapse is a progressive, end-stage disease.

Laryngeal Paralysis. This condition is seen primarily in old, large, and giant-breed dogs. Interruption of the innervation to the intrinsic muscles of the larynx, particularly the cricoarytenoideus dorsalis muscle, results in failure of the arytenoid cartilages and vocal folds to abduct during inspiration. The condition is congenital in the Bouvier des Flandres breed and is related to an inherited degenerative process in the nucleus ambiguus. Laryngeal paralysis also has been associated with hypothyroidism (see Chap. 29) and diffuse polyneuropathies in dogs (see Chap. 148). In many cases laryngeal paralysis is idiopathic.

Nasopharyngeal Polyps. These inflammatory masses arise from the epithelium of the nasopharynx, auditory canal, or tympanic cavity (see Chap. 58).

- Polyps commonly occur in cats and may be congenital in young cats.
- Masses that arise from or involve the nasopharynx result in upper airway obstruction. Although nasopharyngeal polyps are rare in dogs, upper airway obstruction related to soft tissue proliferation can develop in dogs with hyperprogesteronism secondary to drug administration or excessive hormone production in the bitch.

Tracheal Collapse. This condition is seen primarily in old toy-breed dogs. Occasionally it is diagnosed in young dogs and may be congenital.

- The etiology of tracheal collapse is not known, but most likely is multifactorial, and related to changes in air flow dynamics due to primary small airway or upper airway disease. Potential etiologic factors include:
  - Predisposition in small-breed dogs
  - Obesity
  - Degeneration of tracheal cartilages
  - Chronic bronchitis.

Tracheal Stenosis. Tracheal stenosis is usually a sequela of traumatic tracheal disruption. Animal bite wounds, traumatic intubation or extubation, and cervical gunshot wounds are common causes of tracheal injury.

Intraluminal Foreign Bodies. Tracheal foreign bodies rarely cause complete obstruction; large items usually are retained at the carina whereas small ones often pass into the bronchi, leading to bronchial obstruction and pneumonia.

Primary Tracheal Neoplasia. These tumors are uncommon in dogs and rare in cats.

- Primary tracheal tumors reported in dogs include osteosarcoma, osteochondroma, chondrosarcoma, leiomyoma, mast cell tumor, adenocarcinoma, and squamous cell carcinoma.
- Primary tracheal lymphoma and adenocarcinoma have been reported in cats.

Extraluminal Compression of the Trachea. Segmental tracheal stenosis can be caused by compression from extraluminal masses such as parasitic granulomas *(Oslerus [Filaroides] osleri)*, thyroid carcinoma (see Chap. 29), hilar lymphadenopathy (see Chap. 81), left atrial enlargement (see Chap. 60), mediastinal lymphoma (see Chap. 25), and mediastinal lipoma.

CLINICAL SIGNS

Stertor and Stridor. These signs of obstructive upper respiratory disease are so common in brachycephalic dogs that owners frequently do not recognize noisy breathing as abnormal.

- Stridor is a high-pitched inspiratory sound generated from obstruction of laryngeal air flow.
- Dogs with an elongated soft palate often have characteristic stertorous "gurgling" respiratory sounds that result from occlusion of the rima glottidis by the excessively long soft palate.
- Stridor and voice change are common in cats with nasopharyngeal polyps and in dogs with laryngeal paralysis.

Dyspnea. Dyspnea is observed in most animals with obstructive upper respiratory disease.

- Inspiratory dyspnea, expiratory dyspnea, or a combination may be present, depending on the location and severity of obstruction.
- Collapse of the cervical segment of the trachea results in primarily inspiratory dyspnea, whereas collapse of the thoracic segment of the trachea often is associated with expiratory dyspnea.
- Animals with fixed upper respiratory obstruction such as tracheal stenosis and laryngeal collapse usually are continually dyspneic. Dyspnea may be intermittent and exacerbated by exercise, stress, or high ambient temperature in dogs with tracheal collapse or laryngeal paralysis.

Cough. Coughing is common in dogs with tracheal collapse and, with less frequency, in dogs with tracheal stenosis or laryngeal paralysis.

- Approximately 50% of dogs with tracheal collapse have a characteristic "goose honk" cough associated with vibration in the collapsing segment. Other dogs with tracheal collapse do not have a characteristic cough, and some do not cough.
- Dogs with tracheal collapse rarely cough continuously. The cough may be intermittent, and paroxysms usually are exacerbated by stress, excitement, and mechanical stimulation of the trachea.

Decreased Exercise Tolerance. Occasionally, decreased exercise tolerance is observed in dogs with laryngeal paralysis, tracheal stenosis, or brachycephalic syndrome.

Voice Change. This may be an early clinical sign in dogs with laryngeal paralysis. It is also common in cats with nasopharyngeal polyps.

Hyperthermia. Symptoms of laryngeal paralysis frequently are not apparent until the animal is exposed to high ambient temperature; some dogs with laryngeal paralysis are presented with profound hyperthermia.

▼ *Key Point* Evaluate laryngeal function in large-breed dogs requiring treatment for hyperthermia.

Gagging. Occasionally, gagging is observed early in the course of obstructive upper airway diseases such as laryngeal paralysis and elongated soft palate.

Dysphagia. Dysphagia may occur in cats with nasopharyngeal polyps and, rarely, in dogs with laryngeal paralysis.

Syncope. Fainting associated with exercise (overexertion), excitement, or coughing spells occurs in some dogs with tracheal collapse.

DIAGNOSIS

History

- Animals in the early stages of obstructive upper airway disease typically are asymptomatic at rest.
- Excitement or stress leads to varying degrees of coughing, dyspnea, and stridor.
- Clinical signs may progress to constant, severe coughing and dyspnea.
- Some animals with severe obstructive upper respiratory disease are presented with a history of cyanosis or syncope.

General Physical Examination

The physical examination often is unremarkable in dogs with obstructive upper respiratory diseases.

- Distinct lateral tracheal borders may be identified on cervical palpation in dogs with tracheal collapse. Gentle tracheal palpation may cause paroxysms of coughing.
- An ear discharge occasionally is identified in cats with nasopharyngeal polyps. Otoscopic examination may reveal polypoid masses within the external ear canal.
- Stenosis of the external nares may be evident in brachycephalic dogs.

Oropharyngeal Examination

A thorough oropharyngeal examination under light general anesthesia is diagnostic for most obstructive upper airway diseases.

Brachycephalic Syndrome

- The soft palate overlaps the tip of the epiglottis.
- Everted laryngeal saccules are identified as oval mucosal masses projecting into the ventral rima glottidis, lateral to the vocal folds.
- Enlarged tonsils and edematous pharyngeal mucosa are common.

Laryngeal Paralysis

- Animals with laryngeal paralysis are unable to abduct the arytenoid cartilages and vocal folds during inspiration.

▼ **Key Point** Use *light* anesthesia for evaluation of laryngeal function. A surgical plane of anesthesia will obliterate normal laryngeal reflexes.

- Slight, asynchronous abduction of the arytenoids may be observed in some cases.
- The majority of dogs with laryngeal paralysis have bilateral dysfunction of the cricoarytenoideus dorsalis muscle. Unilateral laryngeal paralysis (hemiplegia) is identified infrequently, perhaps because animals with unilateral involvement remain asymptomatic.
- Laryngeal edema and inflammation also may be seen.
- Evaluate arytenoid abduction during inspiration. Don't be fooled by passive *expiratory* opening of the glottis and arytenoids.

Laryngeal Collapse

- The corniculate and cuneiform processes of the arytenoid cartilages are apposed or overlap, causing collapse of the airway.
- Abduction of the arytenoids is not observed.

Nasopharyngeal Polyp

- With the animal in dorsal recumbency, expose the polyp by gently retracting the soft palate ventrally and rostrally.

Radiography

Obtain radiographs of the pharyngeal, cervical, and thoracic regions.

- A soft tissue density cranial to the pharynx or increased radiodensity of one of the osseous bullae may be identified on skull radiographs of cats with nasopharyngeal polyps.
- The soft palate may appear thickened and lengthened in dogs with elongated soft palate. Normally, the soft palate does not extend beyond the tip of the epiglottis.
- Narrowing of the tracheal diameter may be evident on lateral cervical and thoracic radiographs in dogs with tracheal collapse. Collapse occurs most commonly at the thoracic inlet. Tracheal collapse is a dynamic disease, especially in the early stages. Obtain full inspiratory and expiratory views because the trachea may not be collapsed during all phases of respiration. A normal or near-normal tracheal diameter on plain film radiographs does not rule out tracheal collapse.
- Tracheal stenosis is identified on a lateral cervical or thoracic radiograph as a focal reduction of the tracheal lumen diameter. Radiographs usually are adequate to establish a diagnosis of tracheal stenosis, owing to the static nature of the condition.

- Aspiration pneumonia is an infrequent sequela of obstructive upper respiratory disease. Aspiration pneumonia typically is characterized by a mixed alveolar-interstitial density in the dependent portions of the cranial and middle lung lobes (see Chap. 79).

Fluoroscopy

Fluoroscopy allows continual assessment of the tracheal lumen diameter during all phases of the respiratory cycle. In dogs suspected of having tracheal collapse, evaluate the entire trachea and both mainstem bronchi during quiet respiration and induced coughing.

Tracheoscopy

Tracheoscopy is beneficial in assessing the location and severity of stenotic tracheal lesions. Perform tracheoscopy under general anesthesia and pay close attention to patient oxygenation.

TREATMENT

Brachycephalic Syndrome

Nasal Wedge Resection

Surgical Anatomy. In the dog, the nasal vestibule is occupied by the end of the ventral nasal concha, called the alar fold.

Preoperative Considerations
- Administer oxygen through a face mask for 3–5 minutes prior to induction (preoxygenation). Minimize stress to the patient.
- Consider temporary tracheostomy in brachycephalic dogs undergoing upper respiratory tract surgery.
- Rapid induction of anesthesia and control of the airway is essential. Mask induction is discouraged.
- A thorough evaluation of the upper airway is essential in animals with stenotic nares. Staphylectomy (soft palate excision) and laryngeal sacculectomy probably will be necessary.

Surgical Procedure
Objective. To increase the cross-sectional area of the nasal vestibule.

Equipment
- #15 or #11 blade
- 4-0 or 5-0 monofilament nylon or polypropylene suture material
- Standard minor surgery pack

Technique
1. Excise a vertical triangular or elliptical wedge of tissue extending from the wing of the nostril caudally to include part of the alar cartilage. The base of the wedge should include one-third to one-half of the free edge of the nostril (Fig. 77–1).
2. Close the incision with 4-0 or 5-0 nylon suture material in a simple interrupted pattern.

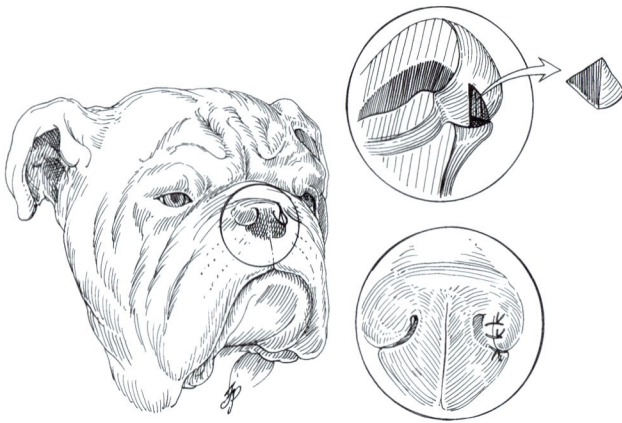

Figure 77–1. Wedge resection of the alar fold for stenotic nares.

3. If the cross-sectional area of the nasal vestibule has not been increased adequately, remove the sutures and excise more tissue.

Postoperative Care and Complications
- Carefully monitor the dog during recovery and for several hours after surgery.
- Incisional hemorrhage may occur but resolves with direct pressure.
- Signs of respiratory obstruction persist following nasal wedge resection if concurrent obstructive upper respiratory diseases have not been managed properly.

Staphylectomy (Correction of Elongated Soft Palate)

Surgical Anatomy
- The soft palate is a valve-like partition composed of mucosal and muscular layers.
- The free edge of the soft palate should appose or slightly overlap the epiglottis.

Preoperative Considerations. See preceding discussion under Nasal Wedge Resection.

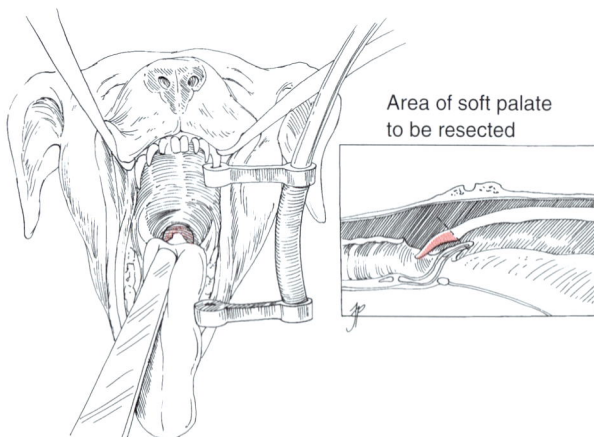

Figure 77–2. Staphylectomy for elongated soft palate. The area of soft palate to be resected is in red.

Surgical Procedure
Objectives
- To shorten the soft palate so that the free edge apposes or barely overlaps the epiglottis.
- To minimize pharyngeal and laryngeal edema by using an atraumatic technique.

Equipment
- Standard instrument pack and suture
- Babcock forceps

Technique (Fig. 77–2)
1. Position the dog in ventral recumbency with the mouth held open with an oral speculum or adhesive tape sling.
2. Determine the portion of the soft palate that is excessive by placing it adjacent to the epiglottis.
3. Place traction sutures of 4-0 absorbable suture material in the lateral aspect of the soft palate adjacent to the point at which the epiglottis touches the soft palate.
4. Grasp the center of the free border of the soft palate with Babcock forceps and retract it rostrally.
5. Incise approximately one-third the width of the soft palate with Metzenbaum scissors. Suture the incised mucosal edges with 4-0 absorbable suture material in a simple continuous pattern. The nasal mucosa tends to retract caudally.
6. Continue the "cut-and-sew" technique (Fig. 77–3) until the palate is resected and closure is complete.
7. Avoid using crushing clamps and electrocautery.

Postoperative Care and Complications
- Laryngeal edema is a common postoperative complication in brachycephalic dogs that have had surgery on the upper respiratory tract.
- At the conclusion of the surgical procedure administer a combination of prednisolone sodium succinate (2.5–5.0 mg/kg IV) and dexamethasone (0.5 mg/kg IV) or dexamethasone sodium phosphate alone (0.5 mg/kg IV), to reduce laryngeal edema.

▼ **Key Point** Excessive resection of the soft palate may allow aspiration of food postoperatively because the shortened palate is unable to close the nasopharynx during swallowing.

- Clinical signs may persist if resection of the palate was inadequate.

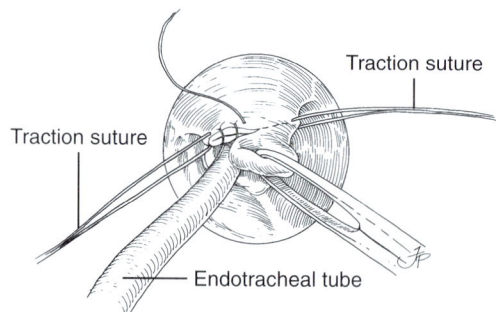

Figure 77–3. "Cut-and-sew" procedure for soft palate resection.

Laryngeal Sacculectomy

Surgical Anatomy. Laryngeal saccules are small, mucosa-lined outpouchings that lie lateral to the vestibular folds.

Preoperative Considerations. See discussion under Nasal Wedge Resection.

Surgical Procedure

Objective. To remove the everted laryngeal saccules and thereby relieve the obstruction.

Equipment
- Metzenbaum scissors
- Babcock or Allis tissue forceps

Technique
1. Position the dog in ventral recumbency with the mouth held open with an oral speculum or adhesive tape sling.
2. Grasp the saccule with Babcock or Allis tissue forceps and retract it rostrally.
3. Amputate the saccule at its base with Metzenbaum scissors.
4. Use direct pressure to control hemorrhage. The cuff of the endotracheal tube can be used to apply pressure.

Postoperative Care and Complications. See discussion under Staphylectomy.

Laryngeal Paralysis

Surgical Anatomy
- The larynx is supported by the cricoid and thyroid cartilages.
- Left and right arytenoid cartilages covered with mucous membrane are located at the rostral end of the larynx and form the dorsal part of the glottal cleft. The corniculate and cuneiform processes of the arytenoid cartilages project into the glottal cleft.
- The vocal folds form the ventral part of the glottal cleft.
- The cricoarytenoideus dorsalis muscles are innervated by the recurrent laryngeal nerves and are the only abductors of the arytenoid cartilages and vocal folds.

Preoperative Considerations
- Medical therapy for hyperthermic dogs in acute cyanotic crisis includes oxygen administration, alcohol or ice water baths, intravenous (IV) fluid therapy, and corticosteroids (prednisolone sodium succinate, 2.5–5.0 mg/kg IV, and dexamethasone, 0.5 mg/kg IV).
  - Sedation may be necessary (e.g., acepromazine) to calm hyperthermic animals.
  - Temporary tracheostomy (see Chap. 3) may be necessary for animals that do not respond to initial conservative treatment.
- Evaluate thyroid function (see Chap. 29).
- Preoxygenate the dog and gain control of the airway rapidly during induction of anesthesia (i.e., via tracheal intubation).
- Prepare for tracheostomy tube insertion.

Surgical Procedure: Arytenoid Lateralization

Objective. To increase the diameter of the rima glottidis by lateralizing the arytenoid cartilages, which is also known as a tie-back procedure.

Equipment
- Standard surgical pack and suture
- Narrow malleable retractors
- Gelpi or Weitlaner retractors

Arytenoid lateralization involves freeing the arytenoid cartilage from its cartilaginous attachments and placing a nonabsorbable suture to permanently abduct the cartilage, thus increasing the diameter of the rima glottidis. The procedure should be performed unilaterally. Unilateral lateralization usually is successful in alleviating clinical signs.

Advantages. Advantages of arytenoid lateralization over other techniques, such as arytenoidectomy, are:

- Intraoperative hemorrhage and postoperative edema are less compared with intraoral procedures.
- Postoperative laryngeal scar formation is uncommon.
- Voice change is minimal because a ventriculocordectomy is not performed.
- Temporary tracheostomy is seldom needed.

Technique
1. Prepare the ventral cervical region for aseptic surgery.
2. Place the dog in dorsal recumbency with the neck extended over a small rolled towel.
3. Make a paramedian incision adjacent to the larynx, approximately in the jugular furrow. If bilateral arytenoid lateralization is planned, make a ventral midline incision from 2 cm rostral to 2 cm caudal to the larynx.
4. Continue the incision through the superficial muscle and subcutaneous fat and identify the sternothyroideus, thyrohyoideus, cricopharyngeus, and thyropharyngeus muscles (Fig. 77–4).
5. Grasp the dorsal edge of the thyroid cartilage through the thyropharyngeus muscle. Rotate the thyroid cartilage ventrally.
6. Transect the thyropharyngeus muscle along the dorsal edge of the thyroid cartilage (Fig. 77–5).
7. Elevate the exposed dorsal edge of the thyroid cartilage and incise the articulation of the thyroid and cricoid cartilages. The intrinsic muscles of the larynx are exposed. Identify the cricoarytenoideus dorsalis muscle.
8. Transect the cricoarytenoideus dorsalis muscle near its insertion on the muscular process of the arytenoid cartilage (Fig. 77–6). Preserve a section of the muscle for histologic analysis.
9. Retract the remainder of the cricoarytenoideus dorsalis muscle rostrally and identify the cricoarytenoid articulation.
10. Separate the cricoarytenoid articulation with Mayo scissors.
11. Retract the arytenoid cartilage laterally.
12. Pass Mayo scissors between the arytenoid and cricoid cartilages and transect the arytenoid-

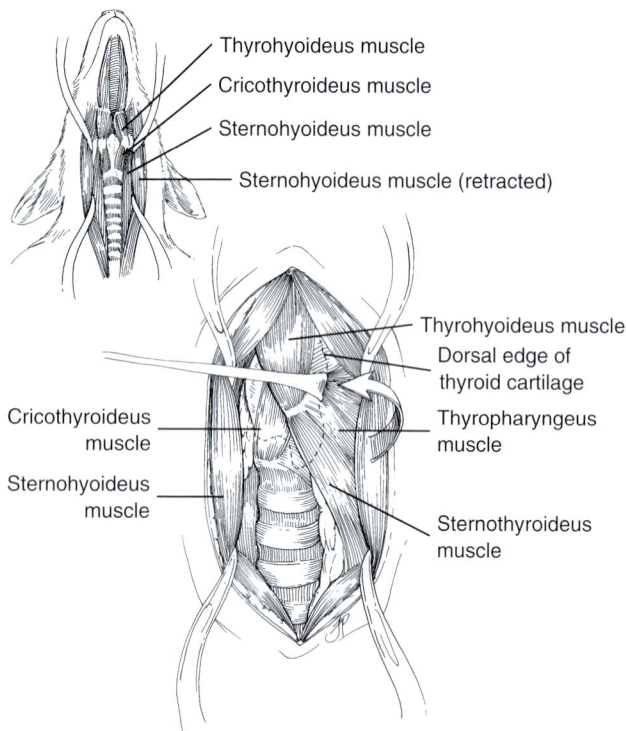

Figure 77–4. Arytenoid lateralization. Expose the surgical area and rotate the thyroid cartilage.

arytenoid articulation on the dorsal midline of the larynx. Avoid incising the laryngeal mucosa.

▼ *Key Point* Wound infection and postoperative stricture formation are more likely if the laryngeal mucosa is incised during this procedure.

13. Pass a monofilament nonabsorbable suture (0 nylon or polypropylene) from the muscular process of the arytenoid cartilage to the caudodorsal por-

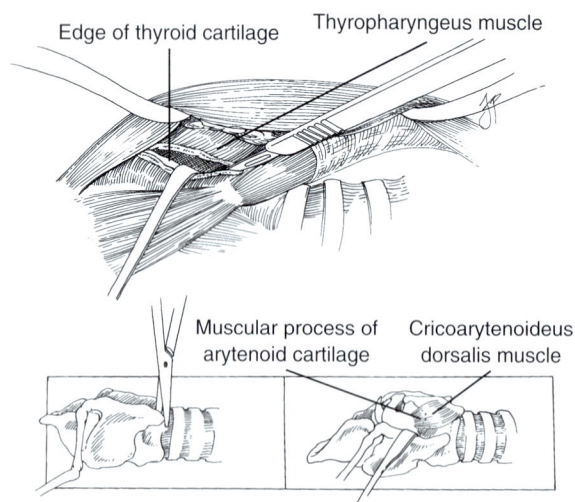

Figure 77–5. Arytenoid lateralization. Transect the thyropharyngeus muscle and expose the arytenoid cartilage. *Below left*, Transect the cricothyroid articulation; *below right*, expose the arytenoid cartilage by retracting the thyroid cartilage.

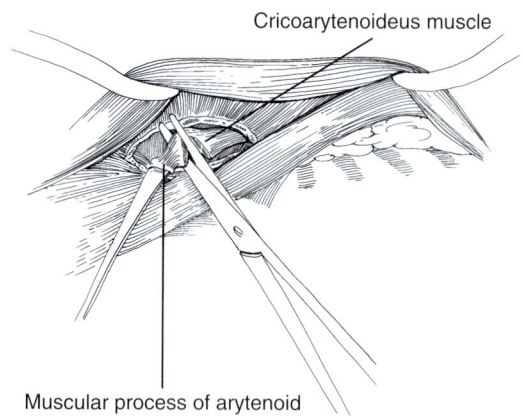

Figure 77–6. Arytenoid lateralization. Transect the cricoarytenoideus dorsalis muscle.

tion of the thyroid cartilage (Fig. 77–7). Alternatively, pass the suture from the muscular process of the arytenoid cartilage to the caudodorsal aspect of the cricoid cartilage (see inset in Fig. 77–7).

14. Temporarily extubate the patient and have an assistant perform an oral examination to evaluate the degree of arytenoid lateralization. Temporary extubation is not necessary if anesthetic gases are being delivered through an endotracheal tube passed through a temporary tracheostomy.

15. Tighten the suture as an assistant evaluates the position of the arytenoid cartilage. Knot the suture at the point of maximal abduction.

16. Replace the endotracheal tube if it was removed.

17. Close the thyropharyngeus muscle with 3-0 absorbable suture in a simple continuous pattern.

18. If indicated, perform the procedure on the contralateral side.

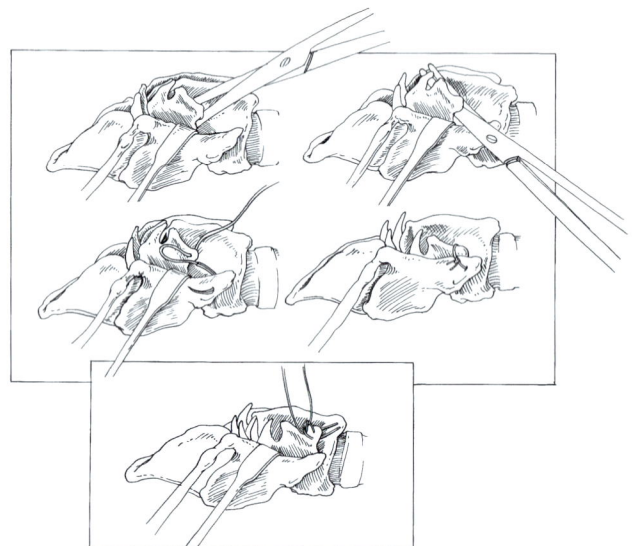

Figure 77–7. Arytenoid lateralization—suture adduction. *Top*, Transect the arytenoid-cricoid articulation *(left)*, then the arytenoid-arytenoid articulation carefully *(right)*, avoiding incising the laryngeal mucosa. Suture the muscular process of the arytenoid cartilage to the caudodorsal portion of the thyroid cartilage. *Inset*, In the alternative LaHue approach, suture from the muscular process of the arytenoid to the dorsocaudal aspect of the cricoid.

▼ *Key Point* If the diameter of the rima glottidis is not adequate following unilateral lateralization, perform the procedure on the contralateral side. Postoperative aspiration pneumonia is more likely after bilateral lateralization.

19. Close the subcutaneous and skin layers routinely.

Postoperative Care and Complications

- Laryngeal edema is a common sequela of laryngoplasty. Carefully monitor postoperative laryngoplasty patients that do not have a tracheostomy tube for signs of upper respiratory obstruction. Administer corticosteroids and supplemental oxygen if laryngeal edema develops. Be prepared for emergency tracheostomy.
- Manage tracheostomy tubes meticulously. Clean the tube as needed (at least every 2 hours). Double-cannula tracheostomy tubes are ideal (see Chap. 3).
- Laryngeal scar formation resulting in cranial glottic stenosis is a potential complication of arytenoidectomy, especially when excision of the vocal folds or arytenoid cartilages extends into the dorsal or ventral commissures; however, the lateralization procedure avoids this complication.
- Failure to open the rima glottidis adequately may result in recurrence or persistence of clinical signs after surgery.
  - Consider lateralization of the contralateral arytenoid cartilage if signs recur or persist after unilateral arytenoid lateralization.
  - Consider arytenoidectomy (Fig. 77–8) only as a last resort when bilateral lateralization fails.
- Bilateral arytenoidectomy or excision of excessive arytenoid tissue during partial arytenoidectomy may result in laryngeal dysfunction or excessive enlargement of the lumen characterized by episodes of aspiration pneumonia and gagging. Surgical amelioration of this condition is unlikely. Permanent tracheostomy can be performed as a salvage procedure.

Laryngeal Collapse

Treat the predisposing factors, such as stenotic nares, everted laryngeal saccules, and elongated soft palate. If clinical signs persist, reevaluate the respiratory tract. Persistence of clinical signs after appropriate surgical management of predisposing factors may necessitate a permanent tracheostomy.

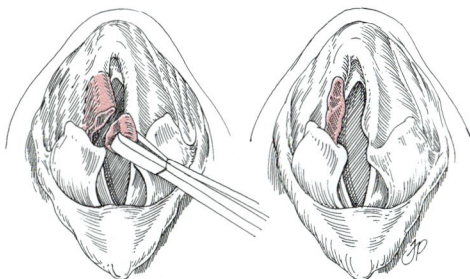

Figure 77–8. Partial arytenoidectomy for laryngeal paralysis.

Permanent Tracheostomy

Preoperative Considerations

- Permanent tracheostomy is a salvage procedure that usually is indicated for treatment of end-stage laryngeal disease. Permanent tracheostomy can be performed following laryngectomy for laryngeal neoplasia.
- Detailed client communication is vital prior to performing permanent tracheostomy. Explain the procedure, potential postoperative complications, and activity restrictions (see below).
- Make certain the segment of the trachea distal to the proposed tracheostomy site is normal. Tracheoscopy or fluoroscopy is preferable; however, inspiratory and expiratory cervical and thoracic radiographs may be adequate to evaluate the integrity of the distal trachea.
- Use an endotracheal tube with a high-volume, low-pressure cuff that has been checked for leaks. Place the cuff distal to the proposed tracheostomy site.

Surgical Procedure

Objective. To create a permanent stoma in the cervical segment of the trachea.

Equipment

- Standard surgical pack and suture
- Tracheostomy tube with a high-volume, low-pressure cuff (tube must be long enough to allow positioning of the cuff in the caudal cervical trachea)

Technique

1. Place the dog in dorsal recumbency with the neck extended over a rolled towel. Prepare the ventral cervical region for aseptic surgery.
2. Make a ventral cervical midline incision through the skin and subcutaneous tissues, beginning at the larynx and extending caudally approximately 10 cm. Center the incision over the proposed tracheostomy site.
3. Separate the paired sternohyoideus muscles, exposing the trachea.
4. Bluntly dissect the cervical fascia from the entire circumference of the trachea between the second and sixth tracheal cartilages.

▼ *Key Point* Identify and avoid the recurrent laryngeal nerves when dissecting the cervical fascia from the trachea.

5. Preplace two horizontal mattress sutures (2-0 polyglycolic) between the sternohyoideus muscles, passing *dorsal* to the trachea where the cervical fascia was dissected.
6. Tie the horizontal mattress sutures. This apposes the sternohyoideus muscles dorsal to the trachea, decreasing tension on the mucocutaneous anastomosis by deviating the trachea ventrally to the level of the skin.
7. Make a partial-thickness rectangular incision in the tracheal wall. Make the segment to be excised three tracheal cartilages long (include the third, fourth, and fifth cartilages) and approximately one-third

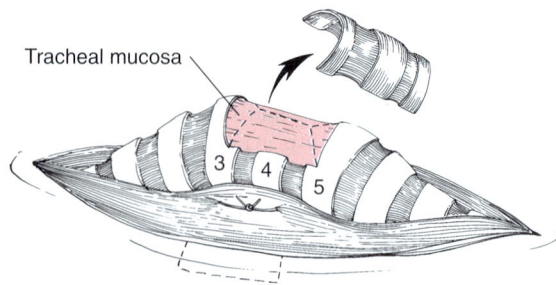

Figure 77–9. Permanent tracheostomy. Remove the segment of ventral trachea with remaining mucosa intact *(red)*. The dotted line indicates the area of mucosa and skin to be incised to complete the stoma.

the width of the tracheal circumference (Fig. 77–9).

▼ *Key Point* Do not make a full-thickness incision in the tracheal wall. Incise the tracheal wall to the level of the mucosa.

8. Bluntly elevate the tracheal cartilages and annular ligaments from the tracheal mucosa inside the boundaries of the rectangular incision. Remove the cartilages and annular ligaments, leaving the mucosa intact.

9. Excise a rectangular section of skin adjacent to the stoma bilaterally. Make each section equal to the length and approximately one-half the width of the tracheal stoma (Fig. 77–10).

10. Secure the skin to the trachea by placing simple interrupted sutures (2-0 polyglycolic) between the dermis (not the skin edge) and the fascia on the lateral aspect of the trachea.

11. Check the endotracheal tube position and make certain that the cuff is inflated. The cuff should be positioned approximately 2 cm distal to the stoma.

12. Incise the tracheal mucosa, as shown in Figure 77–10.

13. Place simple interrupted sutures (4-0 monofilament nylon) 2 mm apart between the skin and tracheal mucosa. Precise apposition is important.

▼ *Key Point* Make certain that there is no tension on the mucocutaneous sutures. Tension predisposes to dehiscence and stenosis.

14. Close the skin incision cranial and caudal to the stoma.

15. Gently suction the tracheal lumen proximal to the cuff to remove clotted blood.

Postoperative Care and Complications

- Clean the stoma every 4–6 hours for 48 hours after surgery. Cleaning is needed less frequently after 48 hours. Instruct the owner to clean the stoma once a day.
- Protect the stoma from self-trauma. Elizabethan collars are not recommended. Rarely, rear-limb hobbles are necessary to keep the animal from scratching the surgery site.
- Apply petroleum jelly to the skin around the stoma once a day for approximately 2 weeks to prevent irritation from dried secretions. This usually is not necessary after hair regrows. Avoid putting petroleum jelly in the stoma.
- Trim the hair around the stoma frequently.
- Dirty, dusty environments and swimming must be avoided.
- Skin fold occlusion of the stoma resulting in episodes of respiratory distress is the most common postoperative complication. Excision of redundant skin may be necessary, especially in brachycephalic breeds.
- Approximately 60% of dogs and cats are unable to bark or purr after permanent tracheostomy.
- All tracheostomies stenose approximately 20–40%. The degree of stenosis is variable and can be minimized by meticulous surgical technique.
- Closure of the stoma rarely is indicated. Closure is accomplished by resection of the stomal segment and primary anastomosis (see discussion under Tracheal Resection and Anastomosis).

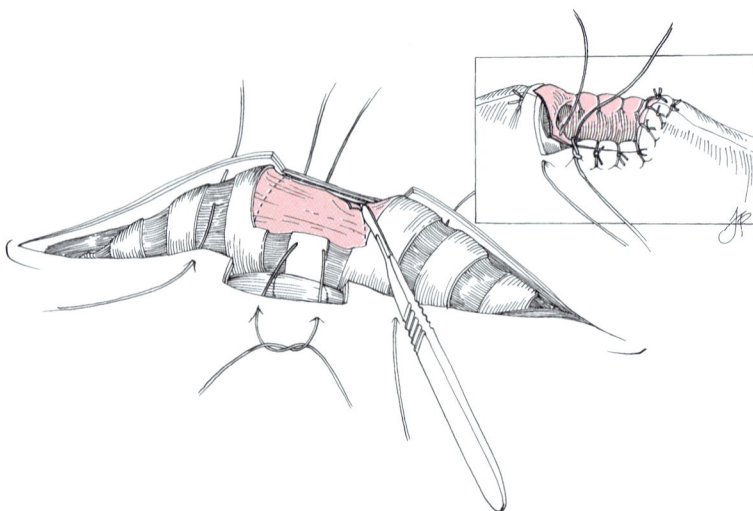

Figure 77–10. Permanent tracheostomy. After the mucosa is incised and reflected laterally, suture the skin directly to the peritracheal fascia and the annular ligament. Complete the stoma by closing the mucosa and skin with simple, interrupted sutures *(inset)*.

Nasopharyngeal Polyp

Surgical Anatomy

- The auditory (eustachian) tube extends from the nasal pharynx to the rostral portion of the tympanic cavity. The pharyngeal opening of the auditory tube is an oblique, slit-like opening that lies on the lateral wall of the nasal pharynx above the middle of the soft palate.
- The tympanic bulla is a smooth bulbous enlargement of the temporal bone, located between the retroarticular and jugular processes.

Preoperative Considerations

- Obtain skull radiographs preoperatively. Evaluate the tympanic bulla and petrous-temporal bones for evidence of middle ear infection, including osseous bulla thickening, increased density within the tympanic cavity, and sclerosis of the petrous-temporal bone.
- Be prepared to perform a ventral bulla osteotomy in cats with radiographic signs or clinical signs of otitis media.

Surgical Procedure

Objective. To remove the polyp from the pharynx and bulla.

Equipment

- Standard surgical pack and suture
- Atraumatic spay hook
- Allis tissue forceps
- Steinmann pin
- Rongeurs
- Curette

Technique

1. If a ventral bulla osteotomy is indicated, position the cat in dorsal recumbency and prepare the ventral cervical region for aseptic surgery.
2. Perform a ventral bulla osteotomy (see Chap. 58) on the side with radiographic evidence of otitis media. If the cat is affected bilaterally, perform the osteotomy on the side of origin of the polyp. If the side of origin cannot be determined, perform the osteotomy on the side with the most pronounced radiographic changes.
3. Expose both the dorsomedial and ventrolateral compartments of the tympanic cavity and carefully remove all inflammatory tissue. Submit tissues for histologic analysis. Avoid curettage of the dorsomedial aspect of the tympanic cavity.
4. Submit material from the bulla for bacterial culture and sensitivity testing.
5. Place a small rubber drain in the bulla that exits from an opening in the skin adjacent to the primary incision.
6. Place the cat in sternal recumbency with the mouth held open by a mouth speculum or adhesive tape sling.
7. Retract the soft palate cranially and ventrally with an atraumatic spay hook.
8. Grasp the nasopharyngeal polyp with an Allis tissue forceps and apply slow steady traction until the mass is removed. A long stalk should be attached at the base.
9. Submit the excised tissue for histologic evaluation.

Postoperative Care and Complications

- Observe for laryngeal edema.
- Horner syndrome is a common complication of bulla osteotomy in cats. Clinical signs typically resolve within 4 weeks.
- Leave the drain in the bulla osteotomy site for 3–5 days.
- Administer antibiotics based on results of culture and sensitivity testing.
- Nasopharyngeal polyps may recur as a result of incomplete excision of inflammatory tissue. Failure to perform a bulla osteotomy in cats with middle ear involvement is a common cause of recurrence.

Tracheal Collapse

Application of Extraluminal Prostheses

Surgical Anatomy

- Individual C-shaped cartilage rings provide structural rigidity for the trachea.
- The space left by failure of the cartilage rings to meet dorsally is spanned by the transversely oriented trachealis muscle and connective tissue, collectively referred to as the dorsal tracheal membrane.
- The left recurrent laryngeal nerve lies on the left lateral or dorsolateral aspect of the trachea.
- The trachea is supplied by the cranial thyroid, caudal thyroid, and bronchoesophageal arteries. These arteries are enmeshed in delicate sheets of connective tissue on the lateral aspects of the trachea called lateral pedicles. Small, transversely oriented branches penetrate between tracheal rings and arborize in the tracheal submucosa.

Preoperative Considerations

- Consider surgical management on initial presentation only in dogs that are experiencing life-threatening dyspnea or syncope. Treat other dogs medically (Table 77–1) for approximately 4 weeks before considering surgical management. Dogs with mild to moderate tracheal collapse that respond well to medical management may not require surgery.
- Perform a tracheal wash, preferably bronchoscopically, and submit samples for routine cytology and bacterial culture and sensitivity testing.
- Identify the location of collapse using radiography or bronchoscopy.
- Anesthesia (see Chapter 2 for details on drug dosages):
  - Choose an endotracheal tube that is long enough to reach the thoracic inlet. Test the cuff.
  - Premedicate with diazepam.
  - Administer a *light* dose of thiobarbiturate.

▼ *Key Point* Always evaluate laryngeal function in dogs with tracheal collapse.

- Induce anesthesia and rapidly gain control of the airway by passing an endotracheal tube.

Table 77–1. MEDICAL TREATMENT OF TRACHEAL COLLAPSE

Patient Management

Avoid airborne irritants or allergens.

Identify and then minimize exacerbating factors. Excitement, stress, extremes of air temperature and humidity should be avoided.

Control daily activity. Minimize fatigue, episodes of exercise-induced cough or dyspnea.

Provide nutritional counseling. Correct overweight body condition.

Schedule routine preventive dental care. Dental prophylaxis reduces bacterial contamination of the pharynx and upper airway.

Prevent dehydration. Adequate hydration maintains low viscosity of airway secretions and thereby promotes clearance.

Promote clearance of airway secretions. Liquefy secretions using humidifier/vaporizer treatments (probably more effective than expectorant drugs), and then facilitate their removal using physiotherapy (light exercise, coupage, or percussion).

Prevent infectious tracheobronchitis (kennel cough complex). Vaccination for parainfluenza, adenovirus, and *Bordetella* is preventive.

Drug Therapy

Antibiotics. If complicating bacterial airway infections are suspected, use amoxicillin-clavulanate cephalosporins, trimethoprim-sulfa, quinolones, or others as guided by tracheobronchial cultures; aerosol administration (gentamicin, 50 mg q12h for 5–7 days) may be more effective for eliminating *Bordetella* from the airways.

Reduce airway inflammation. Use an oral corticosteroid (prednisone, 1–2 mg/kg/day for 1–2 weeks; if improvement is noted, then continue with alternate-day maintenance.

Bronchodilator therapy. See Chapter 78 for table of drug dosages. Administer drugs such as aminophylline, theophylline, oxtriphylline, or terbutaline, although the reversibility of lower airway obstruction in canine bronchitis and tracheobronchitis may be limited.

Antitussive therapy. See Chapter 78 for table of drug dosages. Administer drugs such as hydrocodone to control cough that is distressful to the owner or that causes exhaustion or episodic collapse in the animal; use cautiously and only intermittently if possible, because suppression of the cough reflex may be detrimental to clearance of airway secretions in chronic bronchitis.

- Prepare for mechanical ventilation.
- Administer cefazolin (25 mg/kg IV) at induction of anesthesia and 2 hours after the first dose.

Surgical Procedure

Objective. To provide rigid support for the collapsed tracheal segment and maintain function of the mucociliary system.

Equipment

- Spiral- or ring-shaped prostheses made from the case and barrel of a 3-ml polypropylene syringe case (Fig. 77–11).
- 4-0 Polypropylene suture material with a tapercut needle.
- Standard instrument pack and suture
- Small Gelpi retractors

Technique

1. Place the dog in dorsal recumbency with the neck extended over a small rolled towel.
2. Prepare the ventral cervical region for aseptic surgery.
3. Incise the skin on the ventral cervical midline from the larynx to the manubrium.
4. Separate the paired sternohyoideus and sternothyroideus muscles on the midline and retract the

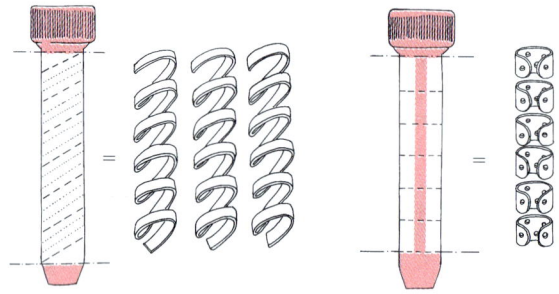

Figure 77–11. Extraluminal prosthesis. The barrel of a 3-cc polypropylene syringe case can be used to make spiral or ring-shaped tracheal prostheses.

muscles laterally with Gelpi retractors. Partially myotomize the sternocephalicus muscles at the manubrial attachment.

5. Identify the left recurrent laryngeal nerve.
6. Beginning approximately 2 cm caudal to the larynx and preserving the caudal thyroid artery, dissect the lateral pedicle from the left side of the trachea to the level of the thoracic inlet.
7. Make a 5-mm window in the right lateral pedicle 2 cm caudal to the larynx, preserving the caudal thyroid artery.
8. Place a right-angle forceps dorsal to the trachea through the window in the right lateral pedicle; grasp the spiral prosthesis and direct the prosthesis around the trachea.
9. Rotate the prosthesis onto the trachea, making a small window in the right lateral pedicle where the prosthesis passes around the right lateral aspect of the trachea. Place the prosthesis over the collapsed segment of the trachea (Fig. 77–12).
10. When applying total ring prostheses, simply make small windows through the right and left lateral pedicles to allow placement of the rings.
11. Deflate the endotracheal tube cuff and reposition the tube either cranial or caudal to the prosthesis. Reinflate the endotracheal tube cuff.
12. Suture the prosthesis to the trachea with 4-0 polypropylene suture material placed in simple interrupted fashion. Place a row of sutures laterally, ventrally, and dorsally, including the dorsal tracheal membrane. All sutures enter the tracheal lumen (Fig. 77–13).
13. Apply additional prostheses caudally as needed. Gentle cranial traction on the cervical trachea affords limited exposure to the segment of the trachea in the thoracic inlet.
14. Deflate the endotracheal tube cuff and gently move the tube in the trachea to ensure that sutures have not been placed through the endotracheal tube cuff. Reinflate the cuff.
15. Appose the sternocephalicus, sternohyoideus, and sternothyroideus muscles. Close the subcutaneous tissue and skin in a routine manner.
16. The intrathoracic segment of the trachea can be supported by performing a right third intercostal thoracotomy (see Chap. 83) and applying prostheses, as described above.

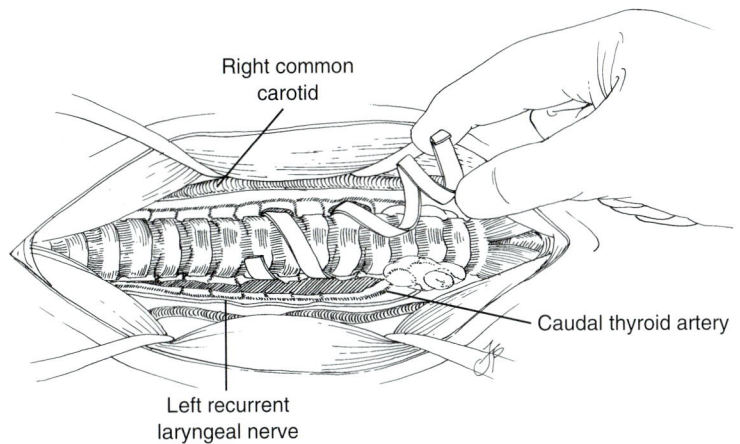

Figure 77-12. Extraluminal prosthesis. Rotate the prosthesis onto the trachea.

Postoperative Care and Complications

- Leave the endotracheal tube in place with the cuff inflated until the dog has a strong swallowing reflex. Deflate the cuff prior to removing the tube.
- Administer supplemental oxygen postoperatively as needed.
- Administer corticosteroids immediately postoperatively and at 6 hours postoperatively to minimize tracheal mucosal swelling (see discussion under Staphylectomy for drugs and dosages).
- Continue antibiotic therapy for 14 days after surgery.
- Continue antitussive and bronchodilator therapy as needed to control coughing (see Table 77-1).
- Observe the dog for subcutaneous emphysema and signs of tracheal obstruction for 5 days after surgery.
- Ischemic necrosis of the trachea resulting from dissection of the lateral pedicles occurs in a limited number of cases. Gentle tissue handling and minimizing dissection of the lateral pedicles reduces the incidence of this complication.

Tracheal Foreign Body Retrieval

Tracheal foreign bodies often can be removed with a fiberoptic endoscope. Various transendoscopic retrieval devices are available for flexible and rigid endoscopes.

Technique

General anesthesia is required for this procedure:

1. Attach a Y-shaped swivel adapter that has a self-sealing port for passage of the endoscope (Fiberoptic Scope/Suction Catheter Adapter with Swivel, Portex, Wilmington, DE) to the endotracheal tube. This allows simultaneous tracheoscopy and inhalation anesthesia in dogs intubated with a tube with an inner diameter > 7.5 mm.
2. Anesthetize small dogs and cats with an intravenous anesthetic and pass the endoscope directly into the trachea.
3. Place the animal in sternal recumbency with the head elevated.

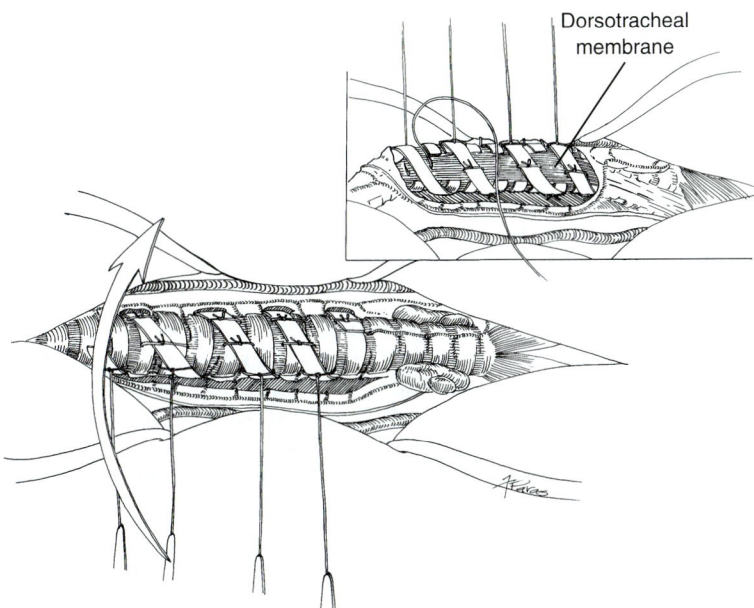

Figure 77-13. Extraluminal prosthesis. Suture the prosthesis to the trachea laterally, ventrally, and dorsally. All sutures enter the tracheal lumen.

4. Insert an oral speculum to prevent the animal from biting and damaging the endoscope.
5. Carefully insert the endoscope into the trachea. Examine the larynx, trachea, and bronchi and locate the foreign body.
6. Critically evaluate the type and position of the foreign body before attempting to remove it. Foreign bodies embedded in the tracheal mucosa or that have sharp edges may not be amenable to transendoscopic removal.
7. Pass the retrieval instrument through the operative port of the endoscope. Position the retrieval instrument either cranial (forceps) or caudal (basket device) to the foreign body.
8. Grasp the foreign body and *gently* retract the endoscope and foreign body together. Tracheotomy or tracheal resection and anastomosis may be necessary if the foreign body is firmly lodged in the trachea.

▼ *Key Point* Excessive traction on a foreign body firmly lodged in the trachea may cause severe tracheal trauma.

9. After the foreign body has been removed, replace the endoscope and perform a thorough, systematic inspection of all accessible parts of the trachea and bronchial tree.

Postoperative Care and Complications
- Complications are rare after transendoscopic removal of a tracheal foreign body.
- Moderate coughing from tracheal irritation is common but transient.
- If the foreign body was firmly lodged in the trachea and removal was difficult, closely monitor the animal for signs of tracheal trauma (e.g., subcutaneous emphysema) for 48–72 hours.

Segmental Stenosis

Tracheal Resection and Anastomosis

Tracheal resection and anastomosis is indicated for treatment of tracheal stricture, tracheal neoplasia, and, rarely, for removal of a tracheal foreign body. Meticulous surgical technique is imperative to minimize postanastomotic stenosis.

Surgical Anatomy
- Review surgical anatomy in the tracheal collapse section.
- The tracheal cartilages are joined ventrally and laterally by 1-mm wide fibroelastic bands called annular ligaments.

Preoperative Considerations
- Identify the extent of the stenotic lesion radiographically and/or endoscopically.
- Anesthesia:
  - Gain control of the airway by rapidly passing an endotracheal tube. Mask induction is not advisable.
  - Endotracheal intubation may be difficult or impossible when the cranial cervical segment of the trachea is stenotic. Be prepared to perform a tracheostomy for delivery of anesthetic gases.

- Administer cefazolin (25 mg/kg IV) at induction of anesthesia and 2 hours after the first dose.

Surgical Procedure
Objective. To remove the stenotic segment of the trachea and create an airtight anastomosis under minimal tension.

Equipment
- Standard surgical pack and suture
- Gelpi retractors
- 2-0 and 3-0 polypropylene suture material with a tapercut needle

Technique
Many techniques for tracheal resection and anastomosis have been described. The split-cartilage technique is ideal because the technique is easy to perform and results in more precise anatomic alignment with less luminal stenosis compared with other anastomotic techniques.

1. Patient positioning and surgical approach are the same as for application of tracheal prostheses.
2. Dissect the right and left lateral pedicles from the stenotic segment of the trachea.
3. Place stay sutures one cartilage cranial and one cartilage caudal to the stenotic segment to prevent retraction and facilitate manipulation of the incised ends.
4. Reposition the endotracheal tube so that the cuff is distal to the stenotic segment. Perform the resection and anastomosis over the endotracheal tube if possible. Do not manipulate the distal segment with the endotracheal tube cuff inflated.
5. Using a #10 blade, circumferentially split in half one tracheal cartilage at each end of the stenotic segment. Incise the stenotic segment longitudinally and remove it. Submit the diseased segment for histologic evaluation.
6. Preplace four to six simple interrupted tension-relieving sutures with 2-0 polypropylene suture material between the cranial and caudal tracheal segments. Pass each suture around the second or third tracheal cartilage cranial and caudal to the anastomotic site.
7. Bring the cranial and caudal segments into apposition by tying the tension sutures.
8. Place eight to 12 simple interrupted sutures, encompassing the split tracheal cartilage at the end of the cranial and caudal segment. Penetrate the tracheal lumen and tie knots on the outside of the trachea. Make certain that the edges of the dorsal tracheal membrane are apposed.

Postoperative Care and Complications
- Leave the endotracheal tube in place with the cuff inflated until the dog has a strong swallowing reflex. Deflate the cuff and then carefully remove the tube.
- Observe for signs of tracheal obstruction. Mucosal swelling rarely is a problem after resection and anastomosis.
- Discourage extension of the neck if the resected segment was large (i.e., more than five tracheal cartilages).

- Obtain cervical radiographs 1, 2, and 3 months after surgery. Follow-up tracheoscopy to assess healing is ideal.
- Postanastomotic stenosis is the most common complication. Excessive anastomotic tension usually is the cause. Complications such as air leakage, infection, mucostasis, and dehiscence occur rarely.

SUPPLEMENTAL READINGS

Buback JL, Boothe HW, Hobson HP: Surgical treatment of tracheal collapse in dogs: 90 cases (1983–1993). J Am Vet Med Assoc 208:380, 1996.

Evans HE: The Respiratory System. *In* Evans HE, Christensen GC, eds.: Miller's Anatomy of the Dog, 3rd Ed. Philadelphia: WB Saunders, 1993, p 463.

Fingland RB, DeHoff WD, Birchard SJ: Surgical management of cervical and thoracic tracheal collapse in dogs using extraluminal spiral prostheses. J Am Anim Hosp Assoc 23:501, 1987.

Hedlund CS: Surgical diseases of the trachea. Vet Clin North Am Small Anim Pract 17:301, 1987.

Rosin E, Greenwood K: Bilateral arytenoid cartilage lateralization for laryngeal paralysis in the dog. J Am Vet Med Assoc 180:515, 1982.

Bronchopulmonary Disease

Lynelle R. Johnson / Philip A. Padrid

Diseases of the tracheobronchial tree and pulmonary parenchyma are quite common in canine and feline patients. They are responsible for substantial morbidity in the pet animal population and occasional mortality. Because there are no easily performed tests of pulmonary function available in small animal practice, the true incidence of respiratory disease in dogs and cats is probably underestimated.

CLINICAL SIGNS

Coughing, dyspnea, and exercise intolerance are the presenting complaints most commonly seen in cats and dogs with diseases involving the respiratory tree. Early in the course of disease, disorders of the conducting airways primarily cause cough. In more severe and protracted cases, shortness of breath and decreased ability to exercise may become more evident. Parenchymal disorders can also lead to disordered breathing with exercise intolerance. In chronic airway or interstitial disease, complications such as syncope and cyanosis may also arise.

CAUSES IN DOGS

A wide variety of infectious, inflammatory, degenerative, and neoplastic diseases can cause clinical signs referable to the respiratory tract in dogs.

- The most common causes of clinical signs of respiratory disease in dogs are (1) tracheal collapse, (2) chronic bronchitis, and (3) pulmonary fibrosis. This is particularly true of small-breed dogs, including Yorkshire terriers and toy poodles. Clinical signs of cough and exercise intolerance are common to all three conditions. Isolated tracheal collapse may be distinguished by the observation of a high-pitched, honking cough, compared with the lower-pitched cough of chronic bronchitis or fibrosis. Additionally, in more severe cases tracheal collapse may result in inspiratory stridor. Pulmonary fibrosis is characterized by increased respiratory effort on *inspiration*, and this may be compared to the increase in *expiratory* effort seen in dogs with chronic bronchitis.
- Acute respiratory distress, characterized by extreme tachypnea, cyanosis, or collapse, may be observed in animals with decompensated chronic tracheobronchial or interstitial disease. This should be dis-

tinguished from other causes of acute respiratory signs such as pulmonary edema (cardiogenic and noncardiogenic), pulmonary thromboembolism, and disease of the pleural space (pneumothorax or pleural effusion).

CAUSES IN CATS

Cats may present with a history of acute or chronic respiratory disease. Cats with chronic respiratory disease often show acute signs of respiratory discomfort because they are easily stressed and undergo rapid physical decompensation.

- The most common cause of respiratory signs in cats is chronic bronchial disease, including chronic bronchitis and asthma. These airway disorders have many features that are similar to parallel disorders in people, including spontaneous airflow limitation, airway inflammation, and hyper-responsiveness.
- Cats are susceptible to pulmonary infection with bacteria. Interestingly, clinically significant and well-documented bacterial infection of feline airways is a relatively uncommon phenomenon. One exception to this is found in New Mexico, where cats can be infected with *Yersinia pestis,* the cause of bubonic and pneumonic plague.
- Other infectious agents to consider as causes of respiratory disease in cats include systemic mycoses (particularly blastomycosis and histoplasmosis), parasites (lungworm and heartworm), viruses (calicivirus, herpesvirus, feline infectious peritonitis), and protozoa (toxoplasmosis).
- Other differential diagnoses for cats with primarily dyspnea include pleural effusion (chylothorax, pyothorax, hydrothorax, hemothorax), pneumothorax, pulmonary thromboembolism, neoplasia, and cardiac failure. Additional causes of cough that should be considered are tracheobronchial foreign body and tracheal neoplasm.

TRACHEAL COLLAPSE

Etiology

- Hypocellular tracheal cartilage with deficient production of glycosaminoglycans and chondroitin sulfate has been found in some dogs with tracheal collapse. These metabolic deficiencies cause a reduction of bound water within tracheal cartilage and result in decreased turgidity of the ring structure. The abnormalities in chondrogenesis that result in tracheal collapse may be congenital or inherited, or may be related to dietary deficiencies.

- Tracheal injury can lead to static collapse of the airway in dorsoventral or lateral orientation.
- In cats, tracheal collapse has been associated with masses that obstruct the upper airway.

Pathophysiology

- Loss of structural support in the cartilage of the tracheal ring allows a reduction in luminal diameter during the lessening in airway pressure that occurs during inspiration.
- Dorsoventral collapse of the trachea typically occurs with prolapse of the dorsal tracheal membrane into the lumen. Long-term collapse results in lengthening and flattening of the tracheal ring. Reduction in the radius of the airway increases the resistance to airflow, which necessitates an increase in driving pressure to maintain normal air movement into and out of the lungs.
- Collapse may be cervical, intrathoracic, or may occur in both regions.
  - Cervical tracheal collapse occurs on inspiration. Normally, during inspiration a pressure drop occurs from the glottis into the lung as air flows into the alveoli. Dogs that lack rigidity in the trachea will experience collapse on inspiration. A larger pressure gradient develops in the cervical trachea when upper airway obstruction is present, and this increases the tendency to collapse. Prolapse of the dorsal tracheal membrane into the airway lumen accentuates mechanical trauma to the wall of the trachea, which leads to further mucosal irritation, inflammation, and cough.
  - Intrathoracic airway collapse or collapse of the mainstem bronchi is encountered on expiration when intrapleural pressures exceed intra-airway pressures, and poorly supported airways tend to close. Chronic bronchitis enhances the likelihood of collapse because of changes in the pressure gradients within the lung. In addition, generalized airway inflammation increases irritability and stimulates a cough, which can exacerbate signs related to tracheal collapse.

Clinical Signs

Signalment

- Small-breed dogs are typically affected with tracheal collapse. An increased incidence is suspected in the Yorkshire terrier, poodle, Pomeranian, and Chihuahua. Animals of any age may present with signs related to tracheal collapse.

History

- A long-term history of chronic, intermittent cough is typically reported with or without episodes of respiratory distress. These signs have often been present since the patient was much younger. It is important to emphasize that stress, heat, humidity, eating, drinking, or external pressure on the trachea can all trigger clinical signs of disease.
- The coughing and retching associated with tracheal collapse can be mistaken for vomiting. This occurs when swallowed mucus is expectorated during the cough. Owners may suspect a tracheal foreign body or "kennel cough."
- Paroxysms of coughing often occur and may lead to cough syncope.
- Animals with tracheal collapse have long periods of normalcy between episodes of apparent acute disease. Exacerbations of clinical signs may be associated with any additional respiratory-related complication including inflammation or infection (bronchitis or pneumonia), upper airway obstruction (laryngeal paralysis or everted saccules), or congestive heart failure.

Physical Examination

- Obesity is common in patients with tracheal collapse. Hepatomegaly has also been reported, which may be a result of fat deposition in the liver.
- On respiratory exam, dogs can appear normal at rest. Excitement induces a honking cough, and in more severe cases can result in airway obstruction and respiratory distress. Animals typically have marked tracheal sensitivity, and even gentle palpation can precipitate a crisis.
- Musical inspiratory noises are sometimes heard over the narrowed trachea in animals with cervical collapse. The presence of stridor indicates that concurrent laryngeal paralysis should be considered.
- An end-expiratory snap may be heard over the thorax with collapse of the mainstem bronchi or intrathoracic trachea.
- Auscultation of wheezes or crackles suggests the presence of concurrent bronchitis or interstitial fibrosis.

Diagnosis

The presence of a honking cough in a small-breed dog is often considered diagnostic of tracheal collapse. A full diagnostic workup should be offered in order to describe and treat all coincident disorders that complicate the clinical presentation.

Radiography

- Inspiratory and expiratory lateral views and a ventrodorsal view are recommended to evaluate tracheal luminal diameter, pulmonary infiltrates, and cardiac size.
  - The cervical trachea may be seen to collapse on inspiration.
  - The intrathoracic trachea or mainstem bronchus may collapse on expiration.
- The trachea can appear normal in greater than 50% of static films. Dynamic radiographs taken during

stimulation of a cough or fluoroscopy may be required to aid in the diagnosis.

Airway Sampling

Obtaining respiratory samples for cytology and culture helps rule out infectious or inflammatory conditions (pneumonia, bronchitis, or fibrosis), which can accentuate clinical signs. Bronchoscopy offers the most complete evaluation of the respiratory tract. Upper airway structure and function should be evaluated in all animals sedated for tracheal wash or bronchoscopy.

* Samples are evaluated for cytologic abnormalities that might suggest inflammation or infection. Bacterial culture and special culture for *Mycoplasma* spp. are recommended (see discussion under Chronic Bronchitis).

Transtracheal Wash

* Sedation and oral intubation are recommended when a tracheal wash is performed on a patient with tracheal collapse. A sterile endotracheal tube of small diameter should be used to avoid increasing tracheal irritation.
* After intubation, a sterile polypropylene urinary catheter or feeding tube is passed to the level of the carina (the fourth intercostal space), and sterile nonbacteriostatic saline is injected (4–5 ml) and then aspirated back into the syringe. A second and third aliquot may be instilled if the sample recovered is inadequate. Stimulating a cough and performing coupage during aspiration will increase the return of fluid. Only 1–2 ml of fluid are required for sample processing. Alternatively, culture can be performed with a guarded swab passed through the endotracheal tube. This system will not be contaminated by the tip of the tracheal tube.

Bronchoscopy

* When available, bronchoscopy is useful both for collection of airway samples and for grading the extent and severity of tracheal collapse. Bronchoscopy can confirm the presence of isolated cervical tracheal collapse, which would imply that surgical correction is possible.
* Bronchoalveolar lavage can be used to collect lower airway samples. The bronchoscope is gently wedged into a small airway, 10–20 ml of warmed saline are instilled, and gentle suction is applied to the syringe to regain the sample. At least two aliquots should be infused at each lavage site to obtain the most representative alveolar sample.

Treatment

General

* Weight loss is beneficial for most patients. Reducing the amount of fat on the thoracic cage improves chest wall compliance and decreases the work of breathing.
* Efforts should be made to limit exposure to environmental stressors such as high humidity and heat during exercise. Harnesses should be used in place of a collar.
* Sedatives may be required during periods of high stress. Acepromazine (0.05–0.25 mg/kg SC or IM) or butorphanol (0.05–0.2 mg/kg SC or IM) may be used alone or in combination. Dosages should be reduced substantially if the two drugs are used in combination.

Antitussives

Cough suppressants are essential in most cases of tracheal collapse in order to break the cycle of cough-induced airway injury. Over-the-counter dextromethorphan-containing compounds are occasionally efficacious. Narcotic agents such as hydrocodone (0.2 mg/kg PO q6–12h) or butorphanol (0.5–1.1 mg/kg PO q6–12h) are most often needed. The dosing regimen must be flexible enough to control cough without inducing excessive sedation.

Bronchodilators

* Dogs that have intrathoracic airway collapse and evidence of small airway disease may benefit from the use of bronchodilators (Table 78–1). These drugs act through dilating small airways, thus making it easier

Table 78–1. BRONCHODILATORS COMMONLY USED IN CANINE AND FELINE BRONCHOPULMONARY DISEASE

Drug	Dosage	Side Effects
Theophylline		
Theo-Dur tablets	dog: 20 mg/kg PO q12h* cat: 20 mg/kg PO q24h (PM)	Multiple drug interactions GI upset, tachycardia
Slo-bid Gyrocaps	dog: 25 mg/kg PO q12h cat: 25 mg/kg PO q24h (PM)	
Beta-Agonists		
Terbutaline	dog and cat: 0.01 mg/kg SC, IV dog: 0.625–5.0 mg/dog PO q12–24h cat: 0.625 mg/cat PO q24h	Tachycardia, hypotension
Albuterol	dog: 0.05 mg/kg PO q12h	Tachycardia, hypotension
Epinephrine	20 μg/kg IV, IM, SC, IT	Cardiac arrhythmias, hypertension, vasoconstriction

*Range 10–20 mg/kg bid

for air to flow out of the lungs and lessening the tendency for collapse in the large airways. Bronchodilators have no clinically significant effect on the large airways and do not result in an increased diameter in the tracheal lumen.

Anti-Inflammatory Drugs

- Chronic bronchitis is treated as described. Occasionally, tracheal inflammation may require a short course of therapy with glucocorticoids for resolution of airway injury. Five to 7 days of prednisone, 0.25–0.5 mg/kg q12–24h followed by rapid tapering of the dose, is usually sufficient to treat inflammation.

Antibiotics

- It is uncommon for clinically significant bacterial infection to complicate the course of tracheal collapse. When a bacterial infection is documented, the choice of antibiotics should be based on culture and sensitivity results. Before cultures become available, antibiotics with efficacy against oral bacteria, including *Mycoplasma* are recommended. Doxycycline and enrofloxacin both provide a good spectrum of activity and are efficacious against most of the bacteria typically encountered.

Surgery

- Surgical placement of tracheal ring prostheses has been successful in reducing clinical signs in dogs with focal cervical tracheal collapse. The surgery is technically demanding and is associated with occasionally serious complications. However, most owners report that the surgery is beneficial in improving the quality of life for their pet (see Chap. 77).

Prognosis

Dogs with tracheal collapse generally have irreversible disease. The goal of preventive and acute therapy is to minimize clinical signs, prevent worsening of bronchopulmonary disease, and improve the overall quality of life.

CHRONIC BRONCHITIS

Etiology

- The etiology of chronic bronchitis in the dog is unknown; however, it is likely that chronic mucosal irritation or immunologic stimulation is responsible for airway inflammation and clinical signs of disease. Smoking remains the major cause of chronic bronchitis in people.
- Congenital abnormalities such as immunoglobulin A (IgA) deficiency or ciliary dysfunction may provide an appropriate environment for chronic airway colonization by infectious agents resulting in long-term damage to the bronchi.
- Poor mucociliary clearance caused by ciliary dyskinesia, *Mycoplasma* infection, or exposure to smoke promotes trapping of secretions in the lower airway and may predispose to the development of recurrent airway infection or bronchial inflammation.

Pathophysiology

- Chronic airway inflammation results in characteristic changes in lower airway structure and function. Neutrophilic infiltration of the airway results in release of proteases and toxic oxidant species that damage the mucosa, stimulating a chronic cycle of injury and repair of the epithelium.
- Chronic bronchitis is characterized by hypertrophy and hyperplasia of mucous glands and goblet cells. These changes result in accumulation of mucus within the airway, which obstructs airflow and leads to clinical signs of cough and exercise intolerance.
- Histopathologic changes reported in dogs with chronic bronchitis include increased inflammatory cells in the lamina propria, goblet cell proliferation, enlargement of mucous glands, epithelial erosion with healing by basal cell proliferation, and squamous metaplasia. Mild emphysema, characterized by increased alveolar air space and loss of interalveolar septae, is occasionally seen.

Clinical Signs

Signalment

The classic signalment for the patient with chronic bronchitis is the small-breed dog; however, large breed dogs can also be affected. Usually the animal is middle aged to older, and often the patient is obese.

History

- The characteristic historical finding in chronic bronchitis is the presence of a chronic cough for at least 2 months' duration, in the absence of other disorders that can cause cough. An acute exacerbation of disease may cause the owner to seek veterinary attention. Often the dog has coughed for several years before being taken to the veterinarian.
- The cough associated with chronic bronchitis may be a dry hacking cough or may be reported as moist or harsh. Swallowing or licking the lips excessively after a cough suggests that the cough is productive.
- Exercise intolerance, fatigue, or increased panting may be reported in addition to the cough; however, typically the patient is not systemically ill. This characteristic helps distinguish chronic bronchitis from other causes of cough including pneumonia, congestive heart failure, thoracic neoplasia, or pyothorax.

Physical Examination

- Animals with chronic bronchitis are often overweight.
- Tracheal sensitivity is usually present but this is a nonspecific finding associated with airway inflammation. Concurrent tracheal collapse may be detected as the characteristic goose-honk cough or as a snapping

sound over the thoracic cage as the intrathoracic airways collapse on expiration.

- Adventitious lung sounds are often found in chronic bronchitic dogs with coarse, diffuse crackles reported most commonly. These crackles are typically harsher and louder than those associated with pulmonary edema or pneumonia.
- The presence of normal lung sounds does not rule out the diagnosis of chronic bronchitis. Stimulating a large inspiration by causing breath-holding or inducing a cough will increase the detection of abnormal lung sounds in a large number of cases. Expiratory crackles and wheezes are heard when air is forced through mucus-laden airways.
- Chronic bronchitis is classified as an obstructive airway disease that classically results in a slow, deep respiratory pattern in order to decrease the work of breathing. When observed carefully, animals severely affected by chronic bronchitis may show prolonged expiration with an expiratory push. These animals may also be intermittently cyanotic or syncopal. Dogs with chronic bronchitis may pant or appear short of breath when excited or agitated during an examination.
- Cardiac auscultation can reveal concurrent mitral valve insufficiency in many older, small-breed dogs. Heart rate may be helpful in ruling out congestive heart failure as a cause of cough, because animals in heart failure typically exhibit tachycardia. However, this may not be observed in dogs coughing from bronchial compression related to left atrial dilation. Dogs with respiratory disease usually have a normal to slow heart rate, and may show an exaggeration of sinus arrythmia due to increased vagal tone from pulmonary disease.

Diagnosis

The history of a long-term cough in an otherwise bright and healthy small-breed dog is suggestive of chronic bronchitis; however, it is a diagnosis of exclusion. Pneumonia and pulmonary neoplasia can cause similar signs. Also, small-breed dogs often have concurrent cardiopulmonary conditions such as tracheal collapse, bronchial collapse, bronchial compression, or heart failure. A complete diagnostic workup defines the role each condition might play in the generation of clinical signs. Laboratory evaluation (CBC, chemistry panel, urinalysis) should be done to evaluate systemic health; however, there are no typical abnormalities for chronic bronchitis. The diagnosis is based on the history, clinical findings, chest radiographs, airway sampling, and—if needed—bronchoscopy. Bacterial culture and cytologic findings rule out other pulmonary causes of cough.

Radiography

- It is not uncommon to find normal chest radiographs in a dog with chronic bronchitis, and this should not rule out the condition as a diagnosis.
- Classically, a generalized increase in interstitial or peribronchial infiltrates is reported in chronic bronchitis. This pattern is usually characterized by "doughnuts" (end-on bronchi) or "tram lines" (airways seen in longitudinal section), which represent airway walls thickened by inflammation. Often these radiographic findings are considered normal aging changes, but in the authors' opinion, when these abnormalities are detected in dogs radiographed for cough, they are an indicator of airway pathology.
- Alveolar infiltrates are not typically found in chronic bronchitis and would suggest that pneumonia or pulmonary edema should be considered as a diagnosis.
- Pulmonary infiltrates may be blurred by fat overlying the thoracic cage in obese animals. Obesity also leads to decreased thoracic compliance, which restricts expansion of the thorax and can lead to an apparent reduction in lung volume.
- Heart size can be difficult to interpret in patients with chronic bronchitis. True right-sided cardiomegaly may be seen in severely affected patients who develop pulmonary hypertension or cor pulmonale. However, many chondrodysplastic breeds will appear to have cardiomegaly due to breed conformation. Also, obesity can cause an enlarged cardiac silhouette as a result of intrapericardial deposition of fat.

Airway Sampling

It is necessary to characterize the cellular infiltrate in the airways and to rule out infectious causes of cough in order to provide optimal therapy. Samples may be obtained through endotracheal, transtracheal, or bronchoscopic methods.

Transtracheal Wash

- An endotracheal wash through an endotracheal tube may be performed as described under tracheal collapse.
- A transtracheal wash can be performed through the tracheal rings (as low on the trachea as possible), or through the cricothyroid ligament. A through-the-needle jugular catheter (19–21 gauge) is the most convenient apparatus to use for a transtracheal wash.
- A sterile preparation is performed in the site desired. Local anesthetic block can be achieved with subcutaneous infiltration with 2% lidocaine.
- The needle is placed between the rings, with the bevel of the needle pointing downward. When the trachea has been entered, a slight "pop" is felt and the animal will usually cough. The catheter is threaded through the needle to the level of the carina (the 4th intercostal space).
- The needle is withdrawn slightly from the neck and the guard secured over the needle-catheter junction.
- When performing a tracheal wash, the catheter should not be withdrawn back into the needle during any time in which the needle is present in the trachea. This would greatly increase the risk of shearing the catheter off into the airway.
- Tracheal wash is performed with one to three aliquots of 4–6 ml of sterile, nonbacteriostatic saline or lactated Ringer's solution. Stimulation of a cough or coupage of the chest during aspiration can enhance

recovery of fluid. Only 1–2 ml is necessary for sample processing.

Bronchoscopy

- Bronchoscopy is an extremely useful tool in the diagnosis of chronic bronchitis, particularly in cases that lack typical radiographic findings. It allows visualization of airway changes, localization of disease, collection of deeper and more specific airway samples, and characterization of dynamic changes in airway caliber, and provides the opportunity to identify and biopsy lesions.
- All dogs with chronic bronchitis have some degree of erythema and a roughened appearance to the airway. The majority have increased mucus in the airways. Animals with long-standing bronchitis can have nodular proliferations of fibrous tissue protruding into the airway. These nodules are usually of varying size and are found throughout the airway. In some cases these must be differentiated from the nodules produced by the parasite *Oslerus osleri*, which are typically found on the floor of the airway just cranial to the carina.
- Bronchoalveolar lavage is performed as described under tracheal collapse.

Tracheobronchial Cytology

- Healthy dogs have 5–6% neutrophils, 5–6% eosinophils, 5–6% lymphocytes, and 75–95% macrophages in bronchoalveolar lavage fluid. An increased number or percentage of neutrophils is seen in most dogs with chronic bronchitis. This is usually a reflection of inflammation within the airway and does not indicate a septic process. However, the presence of toxic neutrophils or intracellular bacteria indicates that infection is likely.
- A smaller percentage of patients will have a predominance of eosinophils in airway washings, which may be a reflection of the generalized immune response, or in some cases may suggest an allergic basis for disease, hypersensitivity response, or parasitic infection. Further workup should be considered in these patients (see Other Laboratory Tests).
- Activated or inactivated macrophages may comprise a percentage of the cells obtained from transtracheal wash if the wash fluid has encountered the alveolar space. Macrophages are usually the predominant cell in bronchoalveolar lavage fluid, even when neutrophil percentages are increased above normal because of bronchitis.
- Increased mucus may be seen in airway fluid and occasionally Curschmann's spirals are seen, which represent bronchial casts of airway mucus and chronic inflammation.
- A large number of epithelial cells on cytology suggests sloughing of the airway mucosa. Squamous metaplasia may also be noted.

Tracheobronchial Culture

- The trachea and lungs are not a sterile environment, and a variety of oral contaminants or commensal bacteria may be found in tracheal wash or bronchoalveolar lavage samples, despite careful attention to technique. Interpretation of positive culture results must take into account cytologic abnormalities.
  - The presence of oral contaminants on cytology, such as squamous cells or *Simonsiella* bacteria, makes a positive culture result of questionable importance (Table 78–2).
  - Identification of intracellular bacteria and toxic neutrophils supports the presence of true bacterial infection.
- Animals with chronic bronchitis may aspirate oral bacteria during episodes of coughing or panting. In some cases these bacteria may overwhelm host defenses. Previously stable bronchitic patients who develop an exacerbation of disease may be experiencing true bacterial infection.

Other Laboratory Tests

- Nonspecific abnormalities on the minimum database, such as a stress neutrophilia or eosinophilia, may be seen in animals with chronic bronchitis. The presence of neutrophilia with a left shift, neutropenia, or monocytosis indicates that other conditions such as pneumonia or bronchiectasis should be considered.
- Animals with eosinophilic airway washes should be screened for airway parasites and larval migration through appropriate fecal exams (see Chap. 74). Heartworm disease must be ruled out. Intradermal skin testing might be considered in select patients.
- An electrocardiogram often shows an exaggerated sinus arrythmia and may give an indication of right atrial enlargement ($P > 0.4$ mV) or infrequently of right-sided cardiomegaly (large S wave in leads I, II, III, aVF).
- Arterial blood gas analysis may exhibit mild to moderate hypoxemia. Hypercarbia is not detected unless respiratory failure ensues. In one study, nuclear ventilation scans confirmed the existence of patchy areas of deficient ventilation in dogs with chronic bronchitis.
- Tidal breathing flow volume loops in dogs with chronic bronchitis have shown reductions in expiratory flow and loop shapes similar to those seen in humans with chronic bronchitis.

Table 78–2. BACTERIA RETRIEVED FROM THE AIRWAYS OF HEALTHY DOGS AND CATS

Pasteurella spp.
Mycoplasma spp.
Streptococcus spp.
Staphylococcus spp.
Acinetobacter
Moraxella
Enterobacter
Pseudomonas spp.
Escherichia coli
Klebsiella spp.
Bordetella bronchiseptica

Treatment

General

- Obesity worsens clinical signs in dogs with chronic bronchitis by decreasing thoracic wall compliance, by increasing the work of breathing, and by increasing abdominal pressure on the diaphragm. Gradual weight loss should be stressed for all overweight animals.
- Gradually increasing amounts of exercise may be useful in encouraging weight loss. Animals with concurrent tracheal collapse or marked tracheal sensitivity may benefit from using a harness instead of a collar.
- Environmental stressors, such as cigarette smoke, dust, pollutants, heat, and low humidity should be avoided whenever possible.
- Some patients may benefit from intermittent airway humidification via steam inhalation or nebulization. Owners should be instructed to coupage the chest after nebulization or encourage gentle exercise in order to facilitate clearance of secretions.

Anti-Inflammatory Drugs

- Airway inflammation is the cause of clinical signs of chronic bronchitis. This can be ameliorated by treatment with glucocorticoids. It is essential that infectious diseases have been ruled out and that concurrent abnormalities, such as severe dental disease or congestive heart failure, have been successfully treated prior to initiation of anti-inflammatory treatment.
- Prednisone or prednisolone are generally safe and effective in dogs with uncomplicated bronchitis. The dosage regimen should be tailored to the individual, with the severity of signs, chronicity of infection, and systemic health playing a role in decisions regarding treatment.
  - Dogs often require initial dosages of glucocorticoids ranging from 0.5–1.0 mg/kg q12h for 5–7 days to induce remission of clinical signs. After this time, the dosage should be decreased by half every 5–7 days until the lowest possible dose is achieved. Long-term therapy (2–3 months) should be expected in most cases.
  - Alternate day use of steroids or possible discontinuation of medication should be the goal of therapy.
  - Animals that do not respond to steroids alone may benefit from addition of a bronchodilator (see Bronchodilators).
  - Exacerbation of disease in the early stages of treatment requires returning to the higher dose of glucocorticoid that controlled clinical signs. It is very common for dogs to suffer recurrence of clinical signs throughout life. Repeated episodes require additional workup when complicating infections or other cardiopulmonary diseases contribute to illness.
  - Failure to respond to glucocorticoids indicates that the diagnosis of chronic bronchitis should be reconsidered.

Bronchodilators

Bronchodilators may be helpful in reducing clinical signs in dogs with bronchitis that do not show complete response to glucocorticoids. Bronchoconstriction is probably not a common component of chronic bronchitis in the dog; however, bronchodilator therapy may provide a multitude of beneficial effects such as reducing airway inflammation, reducing dyspnea, and stimulating mucociliary clearance.

- The clinical effects of methylxanthine derivatives probably result from adenosine inhibition. Theophylline (Theo-Dur tablets, Key Pharmaceutical and Slo-bid Gyrocaps, Rhône-Poulenc Rorer) has been shown to achieve predictable plasma levels in dogs that approximate the human therapeutic range of 10–20 µg/ml (see Table 78–1).
- Adverse effects reported with use of methylxanthines include gastrointestinal signs, nervousness, and hyperexcitability.
  - Theophylline metabolism is affected by a multitude of factors, including fiber in the diet, smoke in the environment, congestive heart failure, and other factors. Drug therapy must be tailored to the individual because there is a wide variation in the dose that causes side effects. One of the authors (LJ) initiates therapy with half the recommended dosage then increases the dose if needed and if the dog tolerates the drug.
  - Enrofloxacin has been proven to inhibit metabolism of theophylline. Use of the two drugs concurrently may result in toxic plasma levels of theophylline. At least a 30% reduction in theophylline dose is recommended when enrofloxacin is required to treat coincident infection.
- Beta-2 agonists are likely to provide more profound bronchodilation than methylxanthine derivatives due to direct relaxant effects on airway smooth muscle.
  - Terbutaline and albuterol have been used successfully in cases of chronic bronchitis.

Antitussives

- Coughing serves an essential function in clearance of the viscid secretions associated with chronic bronchitis. However, chronic coughing can lead to repeated airway injury and may be responsible for syncopal events.
  - Cough suppressants have an important role in management of chronic bronchitis, after infection has been ruled out and after the majority of inflammation has resolved (see Tracheal Collapse).

Antibiotics

When infection has been documented through appropriate culturing technique, and cytologic findings confirm the likelihood of infection, antibiotic treatment is warranted. Infection is not a major component of the syndrome of chronic bronchitis; however, bronchitis does result in an abnormal environment in the airways and disrupts normal host defenses by altering mucociliary clearance and disrupting the mucosal barrier. Thus, every animal should be screened for concurrent infection.

- Antibiotics should be based on culture and sensitivity results in every case possible. Chosen drugs should have a broad spectrum of activity against bacteria commonly found in the conducting airways. They should be lipophilic in order to facilitate penetration of the airway, and they should be relatively free of side effects. When possible, the authors prefer chloramphenicol, doxycycline, or enrofloxacin.
- Infection plays a predominant role in cases that have concurrent bronchiectasis. In these patients, long-term antibiotic therapy is indicated.

Prognosis

- Owners should be informed that bronchitis is a chronic disease. The goals of therapy should be to (1) control the degree of inflammation present, (2) diagnose and treat infection when it occurs, (3) limit clinical signs, and (4) prevent worsening airway disease that might lead to debilitating sequellae such as bronchiectasis and cor pulmonale.

BRONCHIECTASIS

Etiology

- Bronchiectasis is characterized by irreversible dilatation of the airways with concurrent suppuration.
- Possible etiologies include chronic inflammation related to uncontrolled bronchitis, chronic infection due to unresolved pneumonia or a bronchial foreign body, or as a sequela to an airway insult such as smoke inhalation. Bronchiectasis can also be encountered in association with primary ciliary dyskinesia.

Pathophysiology

- Proteases and elastases released from neutrophils during a chronic inflammatory or infectious process destroy the support structure of the bronchial walls. The negative pressure in the surrounding pulmonary tissue pulls the airways open, resulting in dilatation.
- Dilated airways lack normal mucociliary clearance and trap secretions distally. Airflow is obstructed by airway secretions, and mucus-laden airways stimulate a productive cough. Chronic recurrent pneumonia can develop because the bronchial environment is primed for continual bacterial growth.
- Because bronchiectasis is difficult to recognize clinically, proper therapy is often delayed. As a result, it is common for airway changes to have progressed beyond the reversible stage by the time of diagnosis.

Clinical Signs

Signalment

- Bronchiectasis is a disease affecting dogs primarily; it is rarely documented pre- or postmortem in cats.

Cocker spaniels have an increased incidence of bronchiectasis.
- Patients with primary ciliary dyskinesia are typically younger, with a history of chronic airway infections. Other animals are generally older, with evidence of chronic pulmonary disease.

History

- A chronic, productive cough and recurrent pneumonia are the primary complaints noted. Failure to respond to standard therapy for pulmonary disease along with frequent and serious exacerbations of disease seem to be characteristics of patients with bronchiectasis.
- In some dogs, hemoptysis may be reported.

Physical Examination

- Animals often present with systemic signs resembling pneumonia with fever, anorexia, and tachypnea. A noxious oral odor may be noted.
- Lung sounds are generally abnormal. Loud bronchial noises are sometimes heard over dilated airways. Harsh and "moist" crackles can be ausculted throughout the mucus-filled air spaces. Tracheal sensitivity is usually marked and animals often expectorate and swallow mucus.

Diagnosis
Laboratory Evaluation

The CBC may show signs that reflect the chronic nature of the inflammatory process. Neutrophilic monocytosis, anemia, and hyperglobinemia may be present.

Radiography

- Radiography is insensitive for detecting dilatation of the airways. Bronchography was previously used in human medicine but has been replaced by thin-section computed tomography.
- Ventral consolidation of the lung is seen when airways are obstructed with mucus or purulent secretions. Dilated airways are more visible when a severe pneumonic infiltrate is present.

Bronchoscopy

In veterinary medicine, bronchoscopy can be very useful in documenting dilation of the airways. In addition, foreign bodies can be identified and removed, bacterial cultures can be obtained, and the extent of disease can be assessed.

- Bronchiectasis often results in reddening of the mucosa and a large amount of yellow to green viscid mucus.
- Bronchoalveolar lavage fluid is characterized by a preponderance of neutrophils. Cells should be assessed for the presence of intracellular bacteria. Blood-tinged fluid may be recovered or macrophages may contain hemosiderin as an indicator of previous alveolar hemorrhage.

- Both aerobic and anaerobic cultures should be obtained because suppuration can lead to an anaerobic environment. *Pseudomonas* is the most common pathogen isolated from humans with bronchiectasis. Occult infections may also occur, which can complicate decisions regarding therapy.

Other Laboratory Tests

- Electron microscopy on biopsies of ciliated airway epithelium (nasal or tracheal samples) can be used to document primary ciliary dyskinesia in suspected cases.

Treatment
General

- Antibiotics are the mainstay of therapy, and long-term or lifelong therapy may be required.
- Foreign body removal greatly assists in resolution of clinical signs of disease. However, focal bronchiectasis can result, which then serves as a source of chronic reinfection or recurrent signs. In these patients, lung lobectomy should be considered.
- Chest coupage and postural drainage assist in removal of secretions from the airway. Maintenance of systemic and airway hydration through oral intake, intravenous fluids, or nebulization should be used when necessary.
- Cough suppressants should be avoided in virtually every instance because failure to remove infectious and inflammatory secretions will perpetuate disease.

Antibiotics

- Antibiotics should be based on culture and sensitivity results. The occurrence of occult infection makes it difficult to choose specific therapy in some cases. In all animals, broad-spectrum antibiotics, which penetrate the pulmonary tissue, should be chosen. Fluoroquinolones are useful agents; however, resistance by streptococcal species poses a serious concern. Chloramphenicol, doxycycline, and clindamycin have been used with success.
- When long-term (6 months to lifelong) antibiotics are required, a monthly rotation of several drugs might be considered to avoid development of resistant species.

Prognosis

- Bronchiectasis associated with a foreign body may be partially resolved by retrieval of the material and with aggressive antibiotic treatment, but most cases of bronchiectasis are at continued risk for infection and worsening lung disease.

FELINE BRONCHIAL DISEASE

Etiology

- Feline bronchial disease appears to result from the initiation of an inflammatory process within the airways, which results in mucosal edema, smooth muscle hypertrophy, hypertrophy of mucous glands with increased bronchial mucus, and reversible bronchoconstriction.
- Triggers of the inflammatory condition have not been identified and it is likely that individual susceptibility to the induction of airway inflammation and hyper-responsiveness is quite variable.
- Environmental conditions or infectious agents have not been proven to cause bronchial disease; however, they may be responsible for exacerbation of preexisting disease.
- The lung worm *Aelurostrongylus abstrusus* has been proposed as one cause of hypersensitivity lung disease.

Pathophysiology

- Current research suggests that cats with bronchial disease have hyper-responsive airways, analogous to asthma in humans. Human atopic asthma is associated with an accumulation of inflammatory cells and mediators within the airway.
- Degranulation of mast cells with release of histamine and serotonin is associated with an acute inflammatory response within the airways. Release of inflammatory mediators aids in recruitment and activation of T lymphocytes and eosinophils.
- T lymphocytes contribute to airway inflammation through production of cytokines including interleukin-5, which enhances expression of leukocyte adhesion molecules and facilitates the ingress of eosinophils.
- The products of eosinophils are likely contributors to the pathology seen in feline bronchial disease. Major basic protein, eosinophil-derived cationic protein, eosinophil peroxidase, and eosinophil-derived neurotoxin are released from eosinophil granules. Major basic protein is particularly damaging to the airway, causing ciliostasis, epithelial cell death, and bronchoconstriction.
- Inflammatory injury to the mucosal lining exposes sensory endings in the lung, which results in enhanced neural responsiveness to noxious stimuli. Thus, inflammation leads to a perpetual state of airway hyperexcitability and potential hyper-responsiveness.

Clinical Signs

All ages of cats and both male and female cats are affected. There is a suggestion of an increased incidence and severity of disease in the Siamese cat.

History

- Cats with bronchial disease may have a long-term history of coughing, gagging, and decreased activity levels, suggesting chronic disease. Another subset of cats will develop respiratory distress and cyanosis acutely and require emergency care.
- Feline bronchial disease can be misdiagnosed as a vomiting disorder because cats tend to retch and bring up bronchial secretions during a cough.

- Occasionally owners will report noisy breathing or wheezing. Signs of upper respiratory tract infection often precede the onset of bronchial signs. This may be similar to viral-induced asthmatic symptoms in susceptible human patients.

Physical Examination

- Physical examination and thoracic auscultation are normal in some cats, whereas others exhibit adventitious lung sounds ranging from subtle wheezes to harsh crackles. Asthma is classified as an obstructive airway disease, and pulmonary function testing has shown prolonged expiratory times in most cats. This can be observed in some cats at rest; however, excitement induced in the exam room often leads to tachypnea or panting.
- Cats with bronchial disease usually have increased tracheal sensitivity, and post-tussive crackles can be auscultated.
- Decreased thoracic compliance may be detected due to hyperinflation of the lungs.
- Open-mouthed breathing with or without cyanosis occurs in some cats and represents a medical emergency.

Diagnosis

The history and physical examination are helpful in establishing a presumptive diagnosis of bronchial disease. The remainder of the diagnostic workup may elucidate a primary cause of underlying airway hyper-reactivity, such as lung worm infection, and it can rule out complicating conditions.

Laboratory Evaluation

- Peripheral eosinophilia may be present in cats with bronchial disease. When seen, it does not confirm an allergic basis of disease but may relate to the severity of disease. Neutrophilia and monocytosis reflect the chronicity of disease.
- Fecal examination, both routine float and Baermann examination, are useful in detecting parasitic infection. Heartworm testing should be considered in endemic areas when radiographs suggest pulmonary vascular disease.
- Hyperglobulinemia may be present but is not specific.

Radiography

- An interstitial peribronchial pattern with "doughnuts" and increased linear markings is considered classic for feline bronchial disease. Dyspneic animals may show hyperinflation of the lungs with caudal displacement of the diaphragm. Occasionally a larger airway retains a mucous plug, resulting in atelectasis of the lobe supplied by that bronchus. This most commonly occurs in the right middle lung lobe due to its dependent position; however, this is found in a minority (10%) of cats.
- Normal chest radiographs do *not* rule out the diagnosis of bronchial disease.

- An alveolar infiltrate is not generally consistent with bronchial disease. However, one author (PP) has treated six asthmatic cats with excessive bronchial mucus that caused patchy atelectasis mimicking alveolar infiltrates radiographically.

Airway Sampling

Evaluation of airway washings through transoral (endotracheal) wash is recommended for patients that are stable enough to undergo the procedure. Anesthetic protocols that include ketamine are generally safe and effective for the procedure.

Endotracheal Wash

- Cytologic findings in feline bronchial disease include eosinophilic, neutrophilic, and mixed inflammatory responses. Feline airways are very rich in eosinophils, and it is not uncommon for healthy cats to have greater than 25% eosinophils in an airway wash.
- Studies have reported that 25–42% of airway cultures are positive for bacteria or *Mycoplasma*. When cytologic findings suggest airway infection, these positive cultures likely represent true infection, but a large percentage of healthy cats have positive airway cultures. Also, bacteria may establish temporary residence in the respiratory tract of cats with bronchial disease during dyspneic episodes without causing true infection.

Bronchoscopy

- Cats with bronchial disease do not show mucosal changes as do dogs with chronic bronchitis. While bronchoscopy is useful for obtaining uncontaminated lower airway samples, it does not offer the amount of visual information that it does in the canine patient with chronic cough.

Other Laboratory Tests

Pulmonary function tests can be performed in certain referral institutions. Anesthesia is required for measurement of airway resistance and lung compliance. Cats with bronchial disease exhibit higher airway resistance due to bronchoconstriction. Administration of terbutaline decreases resistance in some cats indicating partial reversibility of smooth muscle contraction.

Treatment
Emergency Therapy

- Minimization of stress is one of the most important aspects in management of the acutely dyspneic cat. A quiet, cool environment with supplemental oxygen should be provided.
- Short-acting parenteral corticosteroids will often result in a rapid improvement in clinical signs (Table 78–3). The respiratory rate declines, expiratory effort lessens, cyanosis resolves, and the cat appears more comfortable.
- Cats often benefit from concurrent administration of a bronchodilator such as terbutaline, which is a

Table 78–3. ANTI-INFLAMMATORY AGENTS USED IN THE TREATMENT OF FELINE ASTHMA

Drug	Dosage	Mechanism of Action	Side Effects
Glucocorticoids: Prednisone or prednisolone Methylprednisolone acetate Prednisolone sodium succinate	1–2 mg/kg PO, IM q12–48h 10–20 mg/cat IM every 2–8 wk 50–100 mg/cat IV	Decrease influx of inflammatory cells, stabilize lysosomal membranes, decrease capillary permeability	Immunosuppression, diabetogenic effects
Cyproheptadine	1–2 mg/cat PO q12h	Blockade of serotonin receptor	Weight gain
Cyclosporine	10 mg/kg PO q12h (adjust dosage to produce trough levels in the blood >500 ng/ml)	T-cell inhibition	Nephrotoxicity, immunosuppression, gastrointestinal irritation

smooth muscle relaxant and generally provides rapid bronchodilation.

- Aminophylline is painful when administered by subcutaneous or intramuscular injection and can cause agitation when given intravenously. Its bronchodilatory effects are suspected to be relatively minimal, and other drugs are probably more useful in emergency situations.
- In cases of life-threatening bronchoconstriction, epinephrine can be administered cautiously if terbutaline is not available. Beta-2 agonist effects will produce reliable bronchodilation; however, cardiovascular stimulatory actions can cause side effects.

Chronic Management

- Anti-inflammatory agents are the mainstay of therapy. Oral or injectable corticosteroids are the most commonly used agents and are generally successful in alleviating clinical signs (see Table 78–3). Prednisolone is the preferred anti-inflammatory agent. High dosages (1–2 mg/kg PO q12h) are given initially and tapered weekly according to clinical response. Approximately 50% of cats can be stabilized and medication can be discontinued.
- Alternate anti-inflammatory agents used in animals that cannot tolerate corticosteroids include cyproheptadine, a serotonin blocker, which is effective in vitro, and cyclosporine, an inhibitor of T cells. Side effects associated with cyclosporine limit its use to severe and refractory cases.
- Bronchodilators may help control clinical signs and decrease the dosage of corticosteroids required. Terbutaline, a beta-agonist, and theophylline (Theo-Dur tablets, Key Pharmaceuticals; or Slo-bid Gyrocaps, Rhône-Poulenc Rorer), a methylxanthine derivative, can be used. Individual cats will react differently to the drugs available. If the initial response to terbutaline is not adequate or if pills can be given only once daily, a theophylline derivative should be substituted.
- Some cats suffer exacerbation of disease in dusty or polluted environments, in response to cigarette smoke, or when they encounter specific noxious elements or stressful situations. Recognition and elimination of these triggers can reduce the frequency of dyspneic attacks or coughing episodes.

Contraindications

- Cats have significant sympathetic innervation to the airway. Blockade of beta receptors with propranolol (a nonselective beta blocker) or atenolol (a selective beta-1 blocker) can result in bronchoconstriction and respiratory distress in cats with bronchial disease. These drugs should be avoided.
- Diuretics and anticholinergic agents should not be used. There are no primary indications for these classes of drugs, and they have the negative effects of dehydrating the mucus layer and increasing mucus trapping.

Prognosis

- Feline bronchial disease can be a chronic disorder and cats often exhibit either chronic persistent signs or recurrent episodes of clinical disease. Owners should be informed of this probability, encouraged to follow anti-inflammatory therapy closely, and asked to pursue regular communication with their veterinarian for follow-up care.

PULMONARY FIBROSIS

Etiology

- The etiopathogenesis of pulmonary fibrosis is unknown, and the origin of disease is most likely multifactorial. Hundreds of inhaled agents, drugs, chemicals, and chronic infection or inflammation have been shown to lead to pulmonary fibrosis in humans. It is likely that chronic exposure to any of these substances could lead to pulmonary fibrosis in dogs.
- Genetic factors may play a role in the development of pulmonary fibrosis since West Highland white terriers and other terrier breeds seem more likely to develop this condition.

Pathophysiology

- Exposure to a variety of insults can lead to the release of inflammatory mediators in the lung, which initiate a chronic progressive inflammatory disease in the interstitium. Accumulation of the inflammatory products and cellular components of neutrophils and macrophages causes thickening of the alveolar wall and destruction of alveolar architecture.

- The presence of cellular debris within the alveoli and the formation of enlarged, dysfunctional alveolar units result in mismatching of ventilation and perfusion with subsequent hypoxemia.
- Interstitial fibrosis results in a thickened barrier to diffusion for gas exchange. Diffusion impairment leads to hypoxemia during exercise and in severe cases can cause clinical signs at rest.
- Lung compliance is decreased by fibrosis causing increased work of breathing and tachypnea. End-stage restrictive lung disease develops.

Clinical Signs

Signalment

- Terrier-type dogs, particularly the West Highland white terrier, and perhaps other small-breed dogs seem to be at increased risk for development of pulmonary fibrosis. Males and females are equally affected, and while any age is susceptible, older animals tend to develop fibrosis more commonly because of prolonged exposure to inciting agents.

History

- The classic history in patients with pulmonary fibrosis is shortness of breath and exercise intolerance. Owners may attribute easy fatigability to advancing age and fail to recognize the presence of respiratory disease.
- Syncope may result from hypoxemia or pulmonary hypertension.
- Historically, the cough associated with pulmonary fibrosis is dry and nonproductive, and may be minimal, unless the dog's presentation is complicated by acute bronchitis.

Physical Examination

- Patients may appear relatively normal at rest, but develop shortness of breath and possibly cyanosis on exertion. On close observation, most animals have a more rapid, shallow respiration than normal individuals.
- The hallmark of pulmonary fibrosis is the presence of diffuse end-inspiratory crackles across the thorax.
- A wide range of findings is possible on pulmonary auscultation, ranging from normal breath sounds to fine ventral crackles, to diffuse "Velcro" crackles, which are audible without a stethoscope.
- In cases that have developed pulmonary hypertension, cardiac auscultation may reveal a prominent pulmonic component to the second heart sound, a split S_2, or a murmur of tricuspid regurgitation.

Diagnosis

Definitive diagnosis of pulmonary fibrosis requires an open-lung biopsy. However, exclusion of other diseases that result in dyspnea and crackles, along with the failure to respond to standard treatment for bronchitis, is suggestive of the diagnosis.

Radiography

- Radiographs may be remarkably normal, particularly in view of the degree of dyspnea present in the patient. Classically, a generalized, diffuse interstitial pattern is detected.
- True cardiomegaly in these patients is characterized by right-sided cardiomegaly, and this may be an indicator of pulmonary hypertension. Artifactual cardiomegaly can be present due to breed conformation, decreased inspiratory volume, or reduced lung expansion.

Airway Sampling

- Bronchoalveolar lavage will show an increase in the percentage of neutrophils, usually to greater than 25% (normal 5–6%). It is not possible to differentiate pulmonary fibrosis from chronic bronchitis based on cytologic findings alone; however, absence of increased bronchial mucus or anatomic changes at bronchoscopy argues against a diagnosis of chronic bronchitis.
- Cultures are usually negative unless infection complicates the disease.
- Histopathology shows thickening of alveolar walls with infiltration by plasma cells and lymphocytes. In later stages, increased fibroblasts and marked collagen deposition are seen. End-stage disease results in loss of alveolar spaces with dilatation of terminal bronchioles.

Other Laboratory Tests

- Arterial blood gas analysis may show extreme hypoxemia in certain cases or the animal may be normoxemic at rest.
- Doppler echocardiography may be used to document pulmonary hypertension when either tricuspid regurgitation or pulmonic insufficiency is present.

Treatment

General

- Exposure to identifiable inhaled or ingested risk factors should be minimized.
- Weight control is desirable to improve thoracic compliance.

Anti-Inflammatory Drugs

- Immunosuppressive doses of prednisone have shown some success in treatment of human patients with pulmonary fibrosis; however, the prognosis for dogs with pulmonary fibrosis is generally dismal. Animals that will benefit from steroid therapy should show a response after 2–3 weeks of treatment with prednisone or prednisolone at 1–2 mg/kg q12h. High-dose therapy may result in continued improvement over 1–2 months, but the risk of severe immunosuppression and other complications must be considered.
- Variable success has been found in human patients when cytotoxic agents are used alone or in combination with glucocorticoids. The risk of systemic side effects related to immunosuppression or myelosuppression

increases dramatically when cyclophosphamide is utilized.

Bronchodilators

- It is reasonable to consider a trial on bronchodilators for patients suspected of having pulmonary fibrosis. Theophylline or beta-2 agonists may reduce dyspnea and improve cardiac and respiratory muscle function in some patients.

Prognosis

- The prognosis for control of disease is guarded. Some animals can be made relatively comfortable for variable amounts of time, but respiratory distress typically worsens.
- Patients with pulmonary fibrosis are at risk for pulmonary hypertension and cor pulmonale.

PULMONARY INFILTRATES WITH EOSINOPHILS

Etiology

- Eosinophils accumulate in the canine airway in response to infection with heartworm, lungworms (*Filaroides hirthi, Capillaria aerophila*), or with parasitic bronchitis (*Oslerus osleri, Paragonimus kellicotti*). Larval migration can also result in an eosinophilic pulmonary infiltrate.
- Antigen-antibody reactions or a hypersensitivity response to inhaled or ingested allergen can trigger eosinophil chemotaxis and deposition in the airway.

Pathophysiology

- Eosinophils in the airway release effector molecules such as major basic protein and eosinophil-derived cationic protein, which normally act to kill parasites or to combat an immunologic insult. The products of eosinophils damage cells of the respiratory system, resulting in ciliary paralysis and erosion and sloughing of the mucosa.
- Eosinophils stimulate release of preformed mediators from mast cells such as histamine and serotonin, and increase circulating levels of leukotrienes and platelet activating factor. These substances increase the permeability of the epithelium, increase the secretion of mucus, and may also mediate smooth muscle contraction, causing bronchoconstriction.
- Eosinophil activation causes an increase in airway mucus, leading to increased resistance to air flow and subsequent hypoxemia.

Clinical Signs

History

- The most common clinical complaint is a cough that is nonresponsive to antibiotic treatment. Hemoptysis may be present with *Paragonimus* infection or from pulmonary hypertension. Dogs may be short of breath, febrile, anorexic, and exhibit exercise intolerance.

Physical Examination

- The animal may be bright and alert or show variable degrees of depression and weight loss. Occasionally, severe systemic signs are present.
- Loud bronchial noises can be heard along with diffuse coarse crackles. Marked tracheal sensitivity is typically present.

Diagnosis

Laboratory Evaluation

- The CBC often shows leukocytosis with eosinophilia and basophilia; however, peripheral eosinophil numbers may be normal despite significant pulmonary involvement.
- Heartworm disease must be ruled out with an occult heartworm test, and animals should have multiple fecal examinations (fecal flotation and Baermann examination) performed to detect possible lungworm infection.

Radiography

- Thoracic radiographs typically show a mixed infiltrative pattern with both interstitial and alveolar densities. Young animals with larval migration have primarily a caudodorsal distribution of infiltrates.
- *Paragonimus* infection may show the characteristic thick-walled cystic structures on radiographs. Occasionally, rupture of a cyst can lead to pneumothorax.

Airway Sampling

- Increased numbers of eosinophils are seen on cytology from tracheal wash fluid or on bronchoalveolar lavage. Cytology preparations should be carefully searched for parasite eggs and larvae.

Other Laboratory Tests

- Intradermal skin testing might be considered in an attempt to identify an offending allergen, but has never been well correlated to spontaneous canine lung diseases.

Treatment

- The primary treatment for eosinophilic infiltration of the airways or pulmonary parenchyma is based upon immunosuppression with glucocorticoids. Prednisone is used initially at 1 mg/kg q12h for 3–7 days. The dose is rapidly tapered as signs resolve and the drug can usually be discontinued in 2–4 weeks.
- Removal of an offending allergen can result in resolution of clinical signs, but most animals also require glucocorticoid therapy.
- Parasitic infections and larval migration should be treated with appropriate anthelmintics.

GRANULOMATOUS PULMONARY DISEASES

Etiology

- Granulomatous pulmonary disease is commonly seen with systemic fungal infections (histoplasmosis, blastomycosis, and coccidioidomycosis).

- Noninfectious granulomatous lung diseases are uncommonly encountered in the dog.
  - Eosinophilic pulmonary granulomatosis is a nodular lung disease that has been linked to occult heartworm infection in the majority of cases.
  - Pulmonary lymphomatoid granulomatosis has been described in dogs and is similar to a neoplastic condition in humans characterized by proliferation of T lymphocytes. Some animals with lymphomatoid granulomatosis have had a history of heartworm disease.

Pathophysiology

- Fungal elements typically incite a type IV hypersensitivity immune response with infiltration of macrophages and lymphocytes.
- Eosinophilic granulomatosis may be induced by an immune reaction to heartworm antigens, dirofilarial immune complexes, or other unidentified stimuli. Characteristics of type III and type IV hypersensitivity reactions are present, with proliferation of epithelioid cells, macrophages, and eosinophils within the parenchyma.
- The generation of lesions associated with lymphomatoid granulomatosis is also poorly understood, but probably represents a form of lymphoma. Histopathologic lesions are typically described as an angiocentric infiltrate of mononuclear cells, lymphocytes, plasma cells, mast cells, and occasionally eosinophils.

Clinical Signs

Signalment

Any age or breed of animal may develop granulomatous pulmonary disease, although young to middle-aged, large-breed dogs and young cats are more commonly affected.

History

- These diseases often result in a chronic course of disease with signs present from 1–12 months prior to diagnosis. Respiratory signs include a nonproductive cough, dyspnea, and exercise intolerance. These are found with systemic signs of disease such as fever, anorexia, and weight loss. A relentless course of disease is typical, and treatment with glucocorticoids results in worsening disease in the case of fungal disease or minimal improvement with granulomatous disease. These disorders are also nonresponsive to antibiotic treatment.

Physical Examination

- Systemic involvement is indicated by the generally debilitated state of the patient. Additional organs are often affected in cases with systemic mycoses (see Chap. 18) but not in primary granulomatous pulmonary diseases.
- Respiratory abnormalities include an elevated respiratory rate, increased tracheal sensitivity, harsh coarse crackles, and loud bronchial wheezing noises.

Diagnosis

Laboratory Evaluation

- The CBC typically shows a leukocytosis with variable degrees of neutrophilia, monocytosis, eosinophilia, or basophilia. Hyperglobulinemia may be present in association with chronic antigenic stimulation.
- Occult heartworm testing and fungal titers are recommended in suspected cases.

Radiography

- Fungal disease typically results in a nodular pattern on chest radiographs, with a homogeneous population of small or large nodules, depending on the type and duration of fungal infection.
- The presence of multiple pulmonary masses varying in size is suspicious for a granulomatous disease or metastatic neoplasia. Pulmonary masses ranging from 1–7 cm and lobar consolidation have been reported in eosinophilic and lymphomatoid granulomatosis.
- Hilar lymphadenopathy is present in virtually all granulomatous lung diseases and can be severe. Partial obstruction of a main stem bronchus often occurs due to enlargement of hilar nodes.

Airway Sampling

- Fungal elements can be seen on transtracheal wash, bronchoscopic-guided airway washing, or on fine-needle aspiration of the lung.
- Definitive diagnosis of nonfungal granulomatous disease is based on characteristic histopathologic findings from biopsy of a lung mass. Eosinophils are commonly encountered on cytology of eosinophilic granulomatosis and may also be seen in lymphomatoid granulomatosis.

Treatment

- Pulmonary mycosis should be treated as described (see Chap. 18).
- Therapy for eosinophilic or lymphomatoid granulomatosis should begin with treatment of heartworm disease, when present. Treatment for the granulomatous component of disease requires the use of immunosuppressive and cytotoxic drugs. Prednisone along with cyclophosphamide or cyclophosphamide/vincristine has been used with some success; however, prognosis is guarded for these conditions. A remission rate of less than 25% has been reported.

NONCARDIOGENIC PULMONARY EDEMA

Etiology

- Noncardiogenic pulmonary edema may be categorized as high-pressure edema or permeability edema. High-pressure edema may be more amenable to therapeutic intervention.
  - High-pressure edema results from overexpansion of the extracellular fluid volume by overzealous administration of fluids, from decreased oncotic

pressure, or in association with overcirculation, which may occur with pulmonary thromboembolism.

- Permeability edema can result from pulmonary insults such as aspiration of acidic GI contents, near drowning, and smoke inhalation, or from extrapulmonary insults such as pancreatitis, DIC, sepsis, and anaphylaxis.
- A combination of these two types of noncardiogenic pulmonary edema may result from electric cord shock, after upper airway obstruction, or in pulmonary edema, which can occur following rapid reexpansion of the lungs after a long period of atelectasis (i.e., with long-standing pleural effusion or chronic diaphragmatic hernia).

Pathophysiology

- Noncardiogenic pulmonary edema is not associated with primary cardiac insufficiency. In high-pressure edema, overexpansion of plasma volume or decreased oncotic pressure leads to fluid accumulation in the lung due to a disruption of Starling forces.
- Damage to the alveolocapillary membrane occurs in permeability edema, which causes protein-rich fluid to flood the alveoli. This results in refractory hypoxemia, decreased pulmonary compliance, and eventual hyaline membrane formation. In people, the severest form of this condition is known as acute (or adult) respiratory distress syndrome (ARDS).

Clinical Signs

- Dogs or cats with serious systemic illness that develop signs of dyspnea or tachypnea should be suspected of having noncardiogenic pulmonary edema or pulmonary thromboembolism. Typically, animals with noncardiogenic pulmonary edema are poorly responsive to conventional therapy.

History

The history usually reveals a serious illness, often multisystemic, acute, or chronic in nature, requiring significant supportive care. Noncardiogenic edema may be associated with chronic vomiting syndromes. Respiratory abnormalities noted include tachypnea, dyspnea, and cyanosis.

Physical Examination

- Thoracic auscultation reveals the fine crackles of pulmonary edema. Underlying lung disease may result in coarse crackles or absence of lung sounds due to lobar consolidation.
- The remainder of the physical examination will give clues to the inciting event, such as electric cord burns, peripheral edema, neurologic abnormalities, stridor, abnormal abdominal palpation, or other physical exam abnormalities.

Diagnosis

The history of a precipitating catastrophic event along with acute onset of respiratory distress is highly sugges-

tive of the diagnosis. Refractory hypoxemia despite aggressive supportive care increases the index of suspicion for noncardiogenic pulmonary edema.

Radiography

- Patchy alveolar densities are found, particularly in the periphery or caudodorsal lung lobes. The pattern of distribution helps distinguish this type of pulmonary edema from cardiogenic edema in the dog. Typically, with noncardiogenic pulmonary edema, the infiltrate is severe and bilateral rather than perihilar in distribution, and it fails to clear with diuretic therapy.
- Radiographic signs of aspiration pneumonia such as cranioventral alveolar infiltrates or consolidation of middle lung lobes may be present in some cases.

Other Laboratory Tests

- Arterial blood gas analysis is helpful in following the course of disease and in determining prognosis. Animals are hypoxemic, there is an increased alveolar to arterial gradient, and oxygen responsiveness is minimal.

Treatment

General

Aggressive therapy must be instituted to correct the primary disease. Acid-base imbalances and electrolyte abnormalities are identified and normalized early in the course of disease. Prognosis is guarded in most cases.

- In cases with high-pressure edema, intravenous fluid support is *discontinued* as soon as the problem is identified. Overhydration can usually be resolved with diuretic therapy. Oncotic pressure may be elevated transiently through infusion of plasma or dextrans, and this may clear the pulmonary infiltrate.
- Animals that develop noncardiogenic pulmonary edema due to increased permeability in the alveolocapillary membrane often have more severe derangements in gas exchange and are more difficult to stabilize.
  - Oxygen therapy must be instituted and ventilator therapy is usually required.
  - Intravenous fluids must be administered *very* cautiously to avoid alveolar flooding; generally fluid therapy will exacerbate the edema.
  - Diuretic therapy should be used cautiously because it can deplete intravascular fluid volume and lead to hypotensive shock while failing to clear pulmonary congestion.
  - There is no clear evidence that corticosteroids are efficacious in patients with noncardiogenic pulmonary edema. Steroids may be useful in rare cases of noncardiogenic pulmonary edema associated with shock or anaphylaxis.
  - Plasma infusion can be helpful by replacing proteins lost through the alveolocapillary membrane and maintaining oncotic pressure.
  - Positive inotropic support may be helpful in certain cases to maintain blood pressure, especially when fluid intake is restricted.

- Progressive respiratory distress, respiratory failure, or obvious fatigue should prompt intubation and ventilation.

SUPPLEMENTAL READING

Berry CR, Moore PF, Thomas WP, et al.: Pulmonary lymphomatoid granulomatosis in seven dogs (1976–1987). J Vet Int Med 4:157, 1990.

Buback JL, Boothe HW, Hobson HP: Surgical treatment of tracheal collapse in the dog: 90 cases (1983–1993). J Am Vet Med Assoc 208(3):380, 1996.

Calvert CA: Eosinophilic pulmonary granulomatosis, *In* Kirk RW, Bonagura JD, eds.: Current Veterinary Therapy XI Philadelphia: WB Saunders, 1992, p 813.

Drobatz KJ, Concannon K: Noncardiogenic pulmonary edema. Compen Contin Edu Pract Vet 16(3):333, 1994.

Dye JA, McKiernan BM, Rozanski EA, et al.: Bronchopulmonary disease in the cat: Historical, physical, radiographic, clinicopathologic, and pulmonary functional evaluation of 24 affected and 15 healthy cats. J Vet Int Med 10:385, 1996.

Moise SN, Wiedenkeller D, Yeager AE, et al.: Clinical, radiographic, and bronchial cytologic features of cats with bronchial disease: 65 cases (1980–1986). J Am Vet Med Assoc 194(10):1467, 1989.

Padrid PA, Hornof WA, Kurpershoek CJ, Cross CE: Canine chronic bronchitis, a pathophysiologic evaluation of 18 cases. J Vet Int Med 4:172, 1990.

Padrid PA, Feldman BF, Funk K, et al.: Cytologic, microbiologic, and biochemical analysis of bronchoalveolar lavage fluid obtained from 24 healthy cats. Am J Vet Res 52(8):1300, 1991.

79 Respiratory Infections

John D. Bonagura / Robert G. Sherding

- The respiratory system is a common portal of entry for infectious agents of all types. A large number of infectious agents have been identified as respiratory pathogens (Tables 79–1 and 79–2). The purpose of this chapter is to emphasize clinical aspects of common respiratory infections in dogs and cats. For details concerning specific infectious diseases, the reader is referred to Chapter 9 for respiratory virus and chlamydia infections of the cat, Chapter 10 for bordetella and viral tracheobronchitis of the dog, Chapter 11 for canine distemper, Chapter 18 for the systemic mycoses, and Chapter 19 for toxoplasmosis. Diagnostic procedures relevant for respiratory infections are summarized in Table 79–3 and are discussed in Chapters 74 and 75 in this section. Management of noninfective bronchopulmonary diseases and of chronic bronchitis in the dog and cat are described in Chapter 78. Management of pleural infections is described in Chapter 80.
- The nasal cavity, nasopharynx, larynx, and the trachea are normally inhabited by a variety of microorganisms. Aspirated bacteria from the upper respiratory tract intermittently populate the tracheal-bronchial tree. Thus the potential for *secondary* opportunistic infection is high when underlying pulmonary injury is present or when the host is immunologically compromised. In addition, the clinician can expect to culture microorganisms from the upper airways when performing diagnostic studies. These results must be interpreted with care.
- Many infectious agents are *primary* pathogens of the respiratory epithelium, pulmonary interstitium, or pleural space. This is particularly true of upper respiratory infections caused by viral agents or bacteria like *Bordetella bronchiseptica*.
- The respiratory system also may be involved in *multi-systemic* infections. This is common with the systemic mycoses, *Blastomyces dermatitidis* and *Histoplasma capsulatum*.
- It is helpful to identify the principal *anatomical site(s)* of infection, as many infectious agents produce a characteristic pattern of respiratory disease. This may help to direct the clinician toward specific diagnostic considerations. Good examples of localized respiratory disease are the viral upper respiratory infections of cats and canine infectious tracheobronchitis. Because clinicians generally speak in terms of the anatomic diagnosis—rhinitis, sinusitis, laryngitis, tracheitis, bronchitis, pneumonia, pleuritis, or mediastinitis—respiratory infections will be discussed using this classification (Tables 79–2 and 79–3).

▼ *Key Point* Because many respiratory infections are secondary to another condition, consider the possibility of *underlying* respiratory disease or the possibility of host immunosuppression.

Table 79–1. ETIOLOGIC CLASSIFICATION OF COMMON RESPIRATORY SYSTEM INFECTIONS

Viruses	Protozoa
Canine adenovirus-2, canine distemper virus, canine parainfluenza virus, feline calicivirus, feline infectious peritonitis coronavirus, herpesviruses (canine HV, feline rhinotracheitis virus), reoviruses	*Toxoplasma gondii, Leishmania donovani*
Rickettsia	**Fungi**
Ehrlichia canis, Rocky Mountain spotted fever, salmon poisoning disease	*Aspergillus* spp., *Blastomyces dermatitidis, Coccidioides immitis, Cryptococcus neoformans, Histoplasma capsulatum, Penicillium* spp., *Rhinosporidium seeberi,* various saprophytic fungi
Bacteria	**Nematodes/Trematode**
Gram-positive bacteria, gram-negative bacteria, anaerobic bacteria, *Actinomyces* spp., *Bordetella bronchiseptica, Chlamydia psittaci,* mycobacteria, *Mycoplasma* spp., *Nocardia asteroides*	*Aelurostrongylus abstrusus, Angiostrongylus vasorum, Capillaria aerophilia,* cuterebra and other grubs, *Dirofilaria immitis, Eucoleus boehmi,* gapeworm (*S. ierei*), *Osleri/Filaroides* spp.: *osleri, milksi, hirthi, Paragonimus kellicotti,* nasal mites (*P. caninum*)

Table 79–2. CLASSIFICATION OF COMMON RESPIRATORY INFECTIONS BY ANATOMIC LOCATION

Rhinitis and Sinusitis

Herpesvirus (rhinotracheitis) [F]†
Calicivirus [F]†‡
Chlamydia psittaci
Parainfluenza virus [C]†
Canine distemper virus [C]†‡
Adenovirus-2 [C]†‡
Salmon poisoning rickettsial agent [C]
Bordetella bronchiseptica [C,F]†‡
Secondary bacterial infection (find predisposing cause)
Aspergillus flavum [C]
Penicillium spp. [C]
Rhinosporidium seeberi [C]
Cryptococcus neoformans [F]
Cuterebra and other grubs
Pneumonyssus (Pneumonyssoides) caninum [C]
Eucoleus boehmi [C]

Tracheitis

Upper respiratory virus (see above)
Bordetella bronchiseptica [C]‡
Osleri (Filaroides) osleri [C]

Bronchopulmonary Infections§

Some upper respiratory viruses (see above)
FIV infection—can cause alveolitis in cats
Bacteria bronchopneumonia—both gram-positive and gram-negative infections
Bordetella bronchiseptica [C, F]
Gram-negative bacteria: *Escherichia coli, Klebsiella* spp., *Pseudomonas* spp., *Pasteurella* spp.
Gram-positive bacteria: *Streptococcus* spp., *Staphylococcus* spp.
Mycoplasma spp. [F>C]
Parasitic infections [F, C]
Aelurostrongylus abstrusus [F]
Paragonimus kellicotti [C, F]
Capillaria aerophilia [C, F]
Osleri (Filaroides) infection *(F. milksi, F. hirthi)* [C]
Aspergillosis (endobronchial infection)
Viral infections: feline calicivirus; canine distemper virus
Chlamydia psittaci [F]
Rickettsial infections *(Ehrlichia canis;* Rocky Mountain spotted fever) [C>>F]
Toxoplasma gondii [F>C]
Hematogenous bacterial infection
Nocardia spp., *Actinomyces,* anaerobes‖
Leishmania donovani [C]
Systemic mycoses: *Histoplasma encapsulatum, Blastomyces dermatitidis, Coccidioides immitis, Cryptococcus neoformans* [C>F]
Response to parasitic infection: migrating nematodes [C]
Dirofilaria immitis [C>F]
Lungworms and flukes [F, C]

Pleuritis and Pleuropneumonia

Feline infectious peritonitis
Anaerobic bacteria
Aerobic bacteria (*Pasteurella* spp., *E. coli,* etc.)
Nocardia asteroides
Actinomyces spp.
Blastomyces dermatitidis [C>>F]
Toxoplasma gondii [F>>C]

---

*This list is not comprehensive; important clinical conditions are indicated with the most commonly affected species designated as [C] = canine; [F] = feline.
†Infection commonly extends to the larynx and trachea.
‡Infection commonly extends to the bronchi and may cause pneumonia.
§Alveolar involvement may develop in some cases of interstitial pneumonia.
‖Pulmonary abscess, pleuropneumonia, and pyothorax may develop with these agents.

Table 79–3. DIAGNOSIS OF RESPIRATORY INFECTIONS

Nasal Cavity and Paranasal Sinuses

Signalment (age, breed, sex), vaccination status, history
Physical examination (emphasis: head, eyes, nose, oral cavity, regional lymph nodes, skin)
Auscultation
Serologic tests (aspergillosis, FeLV, FIV, and cryptococcus)
Skull, dental, and nasal radiographs
CT or MRI of the nasal cavity and paranasal sinuses
Examination of the teeth, oral cavity, oropharynx, and tonsils under anesthesia (inspection, palpation, examination with dental probes and mirrors)
Rhinoscopy (nasal cavity and retroflex rhinoscopy of the nasopharynx and posterior choanae)
Nasal culture (bacterial, fungal)
Aspiration biopsy/cytology (swab or nasal flush) of nasal exudate
Mucosal biopsy of the nasal cavity
Fine-needle aspiration biopsy/cytology of enlarged regional lymph nodes or mass lesions
Surgical exploration of the nasal cavity and paranasal sinuses for culture, biopsy, and debridement
Virology: Immunocytologic identification of viruses (e.g., immunofluorescence for canine distemper, feline herpes) and virus isolation (e.g., feline calicivirus)

Larynx

Visual examination of the larynx during light anesthesia
Radiography

Trachea

Radiography (cervical and thoracic)
Fluoroscopy
Tracheoscopy (endoscopy)
Cytologic examination of tracheal lesions (brush cytology of the tracheal mucosa)

Bronchopulmonary Diseases

History and physical examination (observation, auscultation, percussion of the thorax)
Thoracic radiography
Complete blood count
Heartworm (HW) tests (enzyme-linked immunosorbent assay [ELISA] antigen tests for dogs and cats, microfilaria tests for dogs, HW antibody test for cats)
Fecal examinations (flotation and Baermann sedimentation to detect lung parasites)
Serologic testing
    (e.g., immunodiffusion or other tests for systemic mycoses, IgM ELISA for toxoplasmosis)
Arterial blood gas
Pulse oximetry
Bronchoscopy
Culture of tracheobronchial secretions
    (transtracheal wash, endotracheal approach using a guarded culture swab, or aspiration through sterile tubing advanced through a sterilized endoscopic port)
Cytologic examination of the bronchi or lower airways
    Transtracheal wash of tracheobronchial secretions
    Endotracheal aspiration cytology
        Via a catheter placed in the trachea or bronchial tree
        Via an endotracheal tube (method sometimes used in cats and very small dogs)
    Brush cytology of the bronchial mucosa
    Bronchial aspiration cytology (selective, via a bronchoscope catheter)
    Bronchoalveolar lavage with a wedged bronchoscope
Fine-needle aspiration (FNA) of the lung or a mass lesion
Lung biopsy
Pulmonary function testing

Table 79–3. DIAGNOSIS OF RESPIRATORY INFECTIONS *(Continued)*

Diseases of the Pleural Space

History and physical examination (observation, auscultation, percussion of the thorax)
Thoracic radiography (pre- and post-thoracentesis)
Thoracentesis
Cytology of pleural effusate
Culture and sensitivity of pleural effusate
Serological testing when appropriate (FIV, FIP)
Biochemical tests (e.g., serum/pleural effusion triglyceride concentration)
Ultrasound examination
Computed tomography (CT) or magnetic resonance imaging (MRI) of thorax
Lymphangiography

Diseases of the Mediastinum

History and physical examination (observation, auscultation, percussion of the thorax)
Thoracic radiography
Ultrasound examination
CT or MRI of mediastinum
FNA of mediastinal masses
Barium swallow and esophagram
Tracheoscopy/bronchoscopy

- The subject of infectious disease is extensive. For more detailed information on specific infections, the reader is directed to other sources such as *Greene's Infectious Diseases of the Dog and Cat.*

RHINITIS AND SINUSITIS OF INFECTIOUS ETIOLOGY

Etiology

- Infections of the nasal cavity and nasal sinuses are not uncommon, especially those associated with acute, contagious viral infections in dogs and cats. Etiologic agents are summarized in Table 79–2.

History

- Cardinal signs of upper airway infection are sneezing, nasal discharge, and frequently a dry cough.
- Contagion is an issue with some causes of upper respiratory infections.
- Acute viral rhinitis is usually self-limiting within 1–2 weeks.
- Persistence of viral or bacterial rhinitis or sinusitis can occur in immunocompromised cats infected with feline leukemia virus (FeLV) or feline immunodeficiency virus (FIV). In addition, feline herpesvirus persists in a latent subclinical carrier form in recovered cats, and this occasionally recrudesces to result in episodic or persistent rhinitis.
- Primary bacterial rhinitis and sinusitis are uncommon (except with *Bordetella bronchiseptica*); however, secondary bacterial infection can develop as a sequel to mucosal injury or obstructed nasal passages caused by upper respiratory viral infection, foreign

body, periodontal disease and root abscesses, oral-nasal fistula or cleft palate, trauma (sequestrum), allergic rhinitis, lymphocytic-plasmacytic rhinitis, congenital ciliary dyskinesia (Kartagener's syndrome), polyps, neoplasia, and fungal infection.

- *B. bronchiseptica* infection can lead to significant rhinitis as well as tracheobronchitis.
- Chronic bronchitis or lobar pneumonia can predispose to sinusitis, and vice versa. It is likely that a sinubronchial route of migration reinforces each infection.
- Bacterial isolates in rhinitis/sinusitis are variable and typify bacteria normally encountered in the nasopharynx, including gram-positive, gram-negative, and anaerobic organisms.
- Fungal infection of the nasal cavity or sinuses (see Table 79–2) can also be associated with immunosuppression; however, this may be difficult to demonstrate in dogs. *Aspergillus flavus* for example is a normal inhabitant, but may invade respiratory epithelium in dogs with altered immunity or preexistent inflammation (e.g., lymphocytic-plasmacytic rhinitis, foreign body, or trauma).
- Nasal parasites, such as the nasal mite, *Pneumonyssus (Pneumonyssoides) caninum*, are not common but are a potentially treatable cause of upper nasal/pharyngeal signs.

Clinical Signs

- Sneezing, nasal discharge, and gagging or retching from postnasal drip are the typical signs of infectious rhinitis and sinusitis.
- Involvement of the ocular conjunctiva is not uncommon with contagious causes of rhinitis. Corneal involvement may suggest herpesvirus infection. Chorioretinitis may develop consequent to infectious canine distemper virus or cryptococcosis.
- Reversed sneezing may occur with nasopharyngeal irritation from any source.
- Cough may indicate postnasal drip with pharyngeal irritation or concurrent involvement of the larynx, trachea, or bronchial tree.
- Some dogs retch and expectorate secretions that have accumulated in the pharynx.
- A serous discharge is typical of acute viral disease, whereas mucopurulent nasal exudate suggests a bacterial or fungal component.
- Other clinical findings such as fever, enlargement of the tonsils, bony swelling, regional lymphadenopathy, oral ulceration, and ocular or neurological involvement may be evident depending on the underlying causes of disease.

Diagnosis

- The differential diagnosis of upper respiratory infections is expansive (Table 79–4). The age, vaccination status, history, and physical examination tend to focus the diagnostic considerations in most cases. The diagnostic studies chosen depend on the presumptive diagnosis and response to initial therapy (see Table 79–3). Primary infectious diseases and foreign bodies with secondary infection are the most impor-

Table 79–4. DIFFERENTIAL DIAGNOSIS OF UPPER AIRWAY INFECTIONS

Causes of Nasal Discharge

Infectious causes of nasal discharge in dogs and cats (see Table 79–2)
Inflammatory causes of nasal discharge
   Lymphocytic plasmacytic rhinitis
   Idiopathic, including "allergic" rhinitis
   Postinflammatory scars at posterior choanae
Congenital diseases predisposing to nasal discharge
   Ciliary dyskinesis
   Congenital—cleft palate
   Imperforate posterior choanae openings
   Immunodeficiency disease (IgA)
Physical disorders leading to nasal discharge
   Foreign body
   Acquired—oro-nasal defect
   Trauma leading to nasal bleeding or fracture/sequestrum
   Abnormal drainage from the nasal cavity due to inflammatory or congenital webs, tumors, or polyps
Neoplastic causes of nasal discharge

Dogs—Malignant Tumors

Adenocarcinoma (most common)
Chondrosarcoma
Fibrosarcoma
Mast cell tumor
Osteosarcoma
Squamous cell carcinoma
Transmissible venereal tumor

Cats—Malignant Tumors

Squamous cell carcinoma
Adenocarcinoma
Lymphoma

Benign Tumors (Dogs and Cats)

Polyps (more common in cats)
Adenoma
Fibroma

Causes of Epistaxis

Thrombocytopenia from any cause
Thrombocytopathia
Ehrlichiosis
Hyperglobulinemia or other hyperviscosity syndromes
Polycythemia (serous discharge or epistaxis)
Hypertension (including pheochromocytoma)
Coagulopathy with normal platelets (not typical; usually due to platelet problems)
Neoplasms
Foreign bodies
Violent sneezing from any cause
Some chronic infections

Table continued on following page

tant cause of rhinitis and sinusitis in younger dogs and cats. Older pets (older than 8 years of age) tend to be afflicted with nasal tumors complicated by secondary nasal infection.
- Radiographs generally demonstrate increased fluid density in the nasal cavity or sinuses; various degrees of bony destruction may be evident with chronic infection or with infection related to neoplasia.
- Idiopathic lymphocytic-plasmacytic inflammation in dogs, which might be allergic, may facilitate secondary

Table 79–4. DIFFERENTIAL DIAGNOSIS OF UPPER AIRWAY INFECTIONS *(Continued)*

Other Upper Airway Disorders

Inflammatory polyps
Disease of the tonsils
Laryngeal edema consequent to inflammation, trauma, or increased work of breathing
Unilateral or bilateral laryngeal paresis
Inflammatory nodules on the vocal folds
Eversion of the laryngeal saccules
Airway obstruction
Collapse of the glottic opening
Congenital tracheal lesions (segmental lesions)
Tracheal collapse
Relentless barking
Foreign body or foreign material
Swallowing disorders, esophageal masses or megaesophagus
Trauma leading to hematoma, edema, fracture, perforation, laceration, or disruption
Iatrogenic injury (traumatic intubation, excessive cuff inflation)
Mass lesions: granulomas, tumors, and neoplastic conditions

Other Respiratory Disorders

Mediastinal lymphadenopathy or heart base tumors causing airway compression
Primary bronchial collapse
Left main bronchus compression by an enlarged left atrium
Primary chronic bronchitis (noninfectious)
Heartworm disease
Lungworms
Pulmonary neoplasm
Granulomatous disease

---

mucosal invasion by bacteria or fungi. Biopsy is required for diagnosis.

- Infections caused by *Aspergillus* spp. and *Penicillium* spp. require histologic examination of nasal tissue sometimes with special staining (e.g., silver stains) to detect hyphae. A positive agar gel immunodiffusion (AGID) test may also be supportive of the diagnosis. Routine culture is nonspecific because these fungi can be normal inhabitants of the nasal cavity.

- Infection by *Cryptococcus neoformans* may be diagnosed by cytology of exudate (consider india ink staining) or in cats by the latex cryptococcal antigen test.

- High-quality rhinoscopy and radiography, and possible surgical exploration may be required to identify *Rhinosporidium* infection, foreign bodies, or mass lesions. A retroflexed bronchoscope or a dental mirror may be needed to identify lesions at the caudal choanae, including infection with some nasal mites.

▼ *Key Point* Because bacteria and fungi can normally be cultured from the nasal cavities, a careful exclusion of an underlying condition is essential and overinterpretations of positive cultures must be avoided.

Treatment

- Treatment of acute upper respiratory infection depends on the underlying condition. Supportive nursing care, maintenance of hydration, and prevention of secondary bacterial infections by administration of a broad-spectrum antibiotic (avoid tetracycline in puppies less than 8 weeks of age, enrofloxacin in growing animals, or chloramphenicol in cats). Ophthalmic medications may be needed.

- Dogs older than 8 months with bordetellosis may be treated with tetracycline; however, this brush-border inhabitant is difficult to eradicate with systemic antibiotics. Where *B. bronchiseptica* has been definitively diagnosed by culture, empirical therapy with nebulized gentamicin can be considered (for details, see Infectious Tracheobronchitis).

- Treat immunosuppressed patients with secondary bacterial rhinitis with broad-spectrum antibiotics when clinical signs worsen or if lower respiratory infection develops.

- A variety of treatments have been suggested for fungal rhinitis/sinusitis, and treatment can be complicated and, in many cases, unsuccessful. Surgical curettage and drainage tubes combined with medical therapy represent one method; medical therapy alone represents another approach. The clinician should consult detailed textbooks or current literature before embarking on any course of therapy for these serious conditions. The drugs used often have significant adverse effects—such as hepatotoxicity—which must be discussed with the client. With rhinosporidiosis, the "puff-ball granulomas" should be treated by surgical extraction.

- *Aspergillus flavus* and *Penicillium* spp. have been treated with a variety of medications.
  - Topical enilconazole (10 mg/kg, in 10 ml of solution divided between each nasal cavity). Nasal tubes are placed in the frontal sinus either surgically or by use of an endoscope to instill enilconazole. Treatment lasts 10–14 days.
  - Clotrimazole (1%) may be a better treatment, administered via feeding tubes. Tubes are inserted via the nostrils (nonsurgical) or the frontal sinuses (which requires surgery). Recent reports suggest that even one or two treatments (120 ml over a 1-hour infusion period) of clotrimazole may effectively treat nasal aspergillosis and provide sufficient penetration throughout the nasal cavities. However, some cases do not respond fully.
  - Oral itraconazole (Janssen)—another azole derivative—may be effective when given for an extended period of time at a dosage of 5 mg/kg PO q12h for 2–3 months.
  - Thiabendazole (Mintezol; Merck) is less effective (40–50% positive response) and is hepatotoxic, but can be administered at a dose of 10–20 mg/kg PO q12h with food (start at lower dose) for 6–8 weeks.
  - Ketoconazole (Nizoral, Janssen; 5–10 mg/kg PO q12h for 6–8 weeks) is about as effective as thiabendazole.

- *Cryptococcus neoformans* infection of the upper airways is treated with fluconazole, itraconazole, ketoconazole, or amphotericin B (alone or in combination with either ketoconazole or flucytosine). Fluconazole seems to be useful at 50 mg total dose per cat q24h for 2–4 months. Itraconazole at 5 mg/kg q12h may be an alternative and needs to be continued even after the control of nasal discharge. Occasionally, higher doses are needed.

INFECTIOUS TRACHEOBRONCHITIS

General Points

- Acute tracheobronchitis refers to an inflammation of the trachea and bronchial tree of recent onset and short duration.
- Canine infectious tracheobronchitis (ITB), also known as the kennel cough complex refers to a group of acute contagious infections in dogs that cause inflammation of the larynx, trachea, and bronchi.
- Feline upper respiratory infection (URI) complex refers to a group of acute contagious upper respiratory diseases in the cat that may also involve the trachea or bronchial tree. In some cases the lung is involved as well.
- The clinical signs of tracheobronchitis typically include a paroxysmal, harsh, dry cough that can last for days to weeks.
- The condition may be accompanied by other signs of upper respiratory infection such as nasal discharge and sneezing (which are typical in cats and may be noted in dogs with *Bordetella* infection). In many cases, signs are isolated to the tracheobronchial tree.
- Common canine infectious agents include *B. bronchiseptica*, canine parainfluenza virus, canine adenoviruses (types 1 and 2), canine distemper virus, canine reoviruses (types 1 and 2), and canine herpesvirus. *B. bronchiseptica* is the most common bacterial and canine parainfluenza virus and is the most common viral isolate noted in the dog with canine infectious tracheobronchitis (ITB). In cats, feline herpesvirus and calicivirus are considered the most common causes of contagious upper respiratory disease. Calicivirus is more likely to involve the lower airways. Mycoplasma infection and bordetellosis may also be in the differential diagnosis for lower airway disease in cats.
- Many of these infectious diseases are very contagious and associated with high-density populations. The infectious agents can be transmitted by aerosol or fomite. Incubation periods are typically between 3 and 10 days. Vaccinations confer partial to complete protection in most cats and dog.
- In addition to infectious (contagious) causes, other conditions may *predispose* to tracheobronchial infection or inflammation. Some of these include:
  - Abnormal local immunity
  - Boarding kennels/catteries
  - Ciliary dyskinesis (rare)
  - Contagious diseases
  - Debilitation/poor nutrition
  - Drying of the mucous membranes

- General anesthesia (intubation; aspiration)
- Poor vaccination history
- Recurrent or chronic bronchial disease
- Acute tracheobronchitis indicates an inflammatory reaction. The usual consequences of this inflammation are variable increases in tracheobronchial secretions and cough. If respiratory clearance mechanisms or immunity is insufficient, pneumonia may develop from the primary agent (e.g., bordetellosis) or from secondary bacterial invaders.

History

- Certain predisposing conditions may be pertinent (see above).
- Vaccination status and record of immunizations should be known. Vaccination does not confer complete immunity from contagious diseases.
- Recent exposure to other dogs such as at boarding kennel, veterinary hospital, animal shelter, pet shops, research facility, or other area of high animal density within 2–10 days is typical of infectious tracheobronchitis.
- Puppies and kittens often have more severe disease.
- Cough is the hallmark sign of tracheobronchitis.
- Cough of typical upper respiratory infection is usually loud, harsh, and "dry" and increases with activity or exercise (typical).
- Coughing that yields a high-pitched sound, such as a "goose honk"-type cough, is typically of tracheal origin; wheezing suggests bronchial involvement.
- Gagging (often interpreted by the owner as vomiting) is common in acute—as well as chronic—tracheobronchitis. A small amount of white mucus or foam may be expectorated at the conclusion of the cough. More often, any sputum or secretions are swallowed.
- Sneezing is typical in feline upper respiratory disease complex; dogs with concurrent naso-ocular discharge may sneeze as well (also consider distemper; bordetellosis).
- Complications of ITB
- Persistent anorexia, depression, and fever are not typical of uncomplicated ITB in dogs, and if present, thoracic radiographs and a more thorough workup should be completed.
- Anorexia may be observed in severe forms of upper airway infection in cats, especially with calicivirus-related oral ulcers or when there is marked airway exudate as with severe rhinotracheitis (herpesvirus).
- Clinical signs of pneumonia are an indication for additional tests.
- A clinical course of 7–14 days is typical of most self-limiting infectious conditions; chronicity suggests complications or a different disorder.

Physical Examination

- Fever is compatible with both acute contagious conditions as well as secondary bacterial pneumonia.
- Anorexia, depression, fever, and dehydration are more likely in severe forms of ITB with complicating

pneumonia or in particularly young or debilitated animals.

- Cough and gagging are induced typically by gentle palpation of the trachea.
- Respiratory distress is not anticipated in acute tracheobronchitis and should prompt further investigation.
- Examine the mouth, tonsils, and oropharynx for lesions or discharge.
- Ulcerative dermatitis of the face occurs in some cats with upper respiratory infection caused by herpesvirus infection.
- Serous nasal discharge is typical of viral infection; mucopurulent discharge suggests bordetellosis in dogs or secondary bacterial infection in dogs or cats.
- Ocular involvement (corneal ulcers or conjunctivitis) in cats is suggestive of herpesvirus infection (or possibly chlamydia or mycoplasma infections). Retinitis may be noted in dogs with distemper.
- Lymph nodes are usually normal, except for submandibular nodes when there is involvement of the upper respiratory tree. It should be remembered that it is normal for young animals to have prominent lymph nodes.
- Pulmonary auscultation should demonstrate primarily loud referred nasal or tracheal sounds. The detection of crackles, rhonchi, or expiratory wheezes should prompt further evaluation.

Diagnosis of Tracheobronchitis

- In general, one diagnoses feline upper respiratory infections and canine infectious tracheobronchitis from the history and physical examination. The long list of potential causes of signs of acute tracheobronchitis includes the conditions listed in the lower portion of Table 79–4.
- Some conditions (e.g., noninfective bronchitis, neoplasia) are more likely in mature animals and should be excluded initially by examination and thoracic radiography.
- The duration of signs and the response to supportive treatment will largely determine which diagnostic considerations are pursued. In classic "kennel cough" with no constitutional signs, diagnostic studies are generally negative and are not indicated. Poor responders should be worked up.

Diagnostic Tests

- The diagnosis of acute tracheobronchitis is based on history, physical examination, and clinical signs. Routine hematologic tests and radiographs are usually unremarkable; however, the client must understand that a number of other conditions can lead to similar clinical signs and be prepared to support further examinations if indicated. If the patient is very ill, or if the clinical course of expected improvement is not met, additional tests are indicated.
- Radiography of the thorax is probably the most indicated of studies and can be justified to rule out bronchial pneumonia and other causes of acute cough. The right middle lung lobe is predisposed to

infection in upper respiratory diseases and is best seen on a VD or DV projection.

- A CBC and serum chemistry panel (especially renal function, glucose) is appropriate for sick animals.
- Fecal flotation $+/-$ empiric deworming is recommended for puppies and kittens.
- If significant ocular signs such as photophobia or anisocoria are noted, cornea should be stained for ulcers.
- In previously untested cats, perform FeLV and FIV tests to screen for immunosuppressive diseases.
- Culture and cytology of the tracheobronchial airway secretions are indicated in unresponsive cases or those with confounding bacterial pneumonia. A transtracheal wash in cooperative dogs or an endotracheal wash in puppies or cats can be used to obtain a diagnostic sample.
- Other diagnostic tests may be considered in ruling out the differential diagnosis. These are indicated in Table 80–3.

Therapy of Infectious Tracheobronchitis

General Treatment Measures

- Initial therapy of infectious tracheobronchitis is supportive and includes
  - Limiting exercise and enforcing rest
  - Providing adequate fluid intake
  - Mobilizing secretions and reducing coughing in many dogs with tracheobronchitis by having the client provide humidified air
  - Replacing a restraint collar with a harness to decrease airway irritation
  - Avoiding environmental stresses including house dust, vapors, chemical fumes, and tobacco smoke
- The viral causes of these diseases are usually self-limiting, and often no treatment is necessary. This is especially true in mild, uncomplicated cases with minimal constitutional signs (i.e., those without fever, still eating, and not acting sick).

Cough Suppressants

Cough suppressants are appropriate for nonproductive coughs in dogs.

- The use of cough suppressants varies on a case-by-case basis but can be safely prescribed in cases of uncomplicated ITB. In dogs with nonbacterial ITB, breaking the cough cycle is an essential part of treatment. Cough suppressants are contraindicated in cases complicated by lobar pneumonia or if the cough is significantly productive. Of course, in cases of mild cough, a cough suppressant may not be required.
- Butorphanol (Torbutrol, Bristol) dosed at 0.5–1.1 mg/kg, orally q8–12h, can be prescribed as a modest antitussive in dogs with ITB. Some prefer to initiate therapy with an injection of butorphanol at the labeled dosage.
- More aggressive cough suppressants may be needed in some cases. Treatment of dogs with codeine-derivative cough suppressants like hydrocodone

(Tussionex, Fisons; Hycodan, Du Pont) at a total dose of 1.25–5 mg PO q8–12h is often most effective. Hycodan also comes as a liquid (usually 1 mg/ml) for dosing very small dogs. The dosage can gradually be reduced to the lowest effective dose. Sedation is a common side effect, but this may actually be beneficial if excitement or stress triggers coughing.

▼ **Key Point** Antimicrobial therapy is often recommended as empirical therapy in URI or ITB, but it is not known to shorten the duration of clinical signs or the transmissibility of infection.

Antimicrobial Therapy

- Antibiotics are recommended if the patient remains febrile, anorectic, or depressed; if there is a purulent nasal or ocular discharge; or should other evidence of a secondary bacterial infection develop. Radiographic evidence of bronchopneumonia is a definitive indication for antibiotic therapy of at least 2–3 weeks' duration. If signs of ITB develop in an older dog with severe periodontal or dental disease and high opportunity to inhale bacteria-laden particulate, then a course of antibiotics seems appropriate.
- Antibiotic choices include:
  - Tetracycline—22 mg/kg q8h PO for 14 days (*avoid* in puppies <8 weeks and in pregnant females).
  - Trimethoprim-sulfonamide (Tribrissen)—15 mg/kg q12h or 30 mg/kg q24h for 7–14 days.
  - Cefadroxil (Cefa-Tabs; Cefa-Drops)—22 mg/kg q12h PO.
  - Fluoroquinolones such as enrofloxacin (Baytril; 2.5 to 5 mg/kg q12h IM or 5 mg/kg q12–24h PO or orbifloxacin—see labeled dosing range) have a more broad antibacterial spectrum that includes *mycoplasma* (but not anaerobes); however, these drugs are too potent for routine cases except in cases of documented bacterial pneumonia (*avoid* in growing dogs, larger breeds especially should not be treated with fluoroquinolones—see package insert).
- Use culture and sensitivity obtained by transtracheal or endotracheal wash as a guide to antibiotic therapy in chronic situations or in animals with documented pneumonia.
  - Some dogs develop a recurrent bacterial bronchitis that responds very well to antibiotic treatment until a relapse occurs. Especially in younger dogs this may indicate a resistant or unusual microorganism (e.g., mycoplasma, bronchopulmonary aspergillosis in dogs that have received steroids), an anatomic lesion of a bronchus, an endobronchial foreign body, a lack of local immunity, or abnormal cilia (ciliary dyskinesis). Such animals might benefit from cultures and bronchoscopy, particularly if a single lung lobe remains infiltrated or pneumonic.
  - When *B. bronchiseptica* is cultured from a case of ITB, remember that antibiotics may not sufficiently contact this microorganism, which resides in the brush border of the airway mucosa. In difficult cases consider gentamicin nebulization, using an anesthetic face mask interfaced with a glass nebulizer (such as the Devilbiss model #40) and the oxygen output line of a gas anesthetic machine.
- Combine gentamicin (4–6 mg/kg) with 3–5 ml of saline in the nebulization pot, and use 1–3 L per minute of oxygen flow to nebulize the solution into the face mask until the reservoir is empty. Administer this therapy twice daily for 5 days.
- Current data indicate that gentamicin is not absorbed systemically from the lung.
- Ophthalmic complications in tracheobronchitis
  - In cases of ocular involvement of upper respiratory infection in cats, consider special ophthalmic medications.
  - *Avoid* topical steroids.
  - If there is corneal ulceration and the clinical diagnosis is herpesvirus, then either idoxuridine solution (Herplex, Allergan) or trifluridine (Viroptic, Burroughs Wellcome) can be prescribed, with the latter preferred unless there is irritation. For infections associated with just conjunctivitis but without corneal involvement, a tetracycline-polymyxin B or chloramphenicol ointment can be prescribed, both of which are effective against chlamydia and mycoplasma.
  - Mucopurulent exudate should be removed with warm compresses and eye wash.
- Corticosteroids
  - Prednisolone has been recommended for short-term administration at anti-inflammatory doses (0.25 to 0.5 mg/kg q12h) in uncomplicated ITB, but this therapy generally is *not* recommended because of the risk of secondary infection. Prednisolone is also not thought to decrease the disease duration and clearly predisposes to other infections. If used at all, it should be for no longer than 1 or 2 days.

Follow-up

- If there is no improvement, have the client return for a chest radiograph, CBC, and antibiotic therapy.

Prevention

Vaccination in dogs can be performed routinely with the following antigens: *B. bronchiseptica*, canine parainfluenza virus, canine adenovirus type 2, and canine distemper virus. Cats can be vaccinated against herpes-, calici-, and panleukopenia (parvo) viruses and bordetellosis. Vaccination does not appear to completely prevent infection or prevent local viral replication or development of a career state in cats.

BRONCHOPNEUMONIA

Etiology

- Pulmonary infections are common in dogs and in cats. Bacterial pneumonia is an important cause of morbidity and mortality in dogs and cats.

- Though numerous infectious agents (viruses, rickettsia, and systemic mycoses) can cause interstitial pneumonia, most cases of bronchopneumonia are bacterial in origin. Common microorganisms responsible for pneumonia are indicated in Table 79–2.
- The route of infection is typically inhalation.
- Hematogenous spread of bacterial pneumonia to the lungs is less common and can be very difficult to treat.
- The clinician should appreciate possible risk factors and predisposition for pneumonia, including
  - Contagious upper respiratory infection (e.g., infective tracheobronchitis after boarding)
  - Preexistent bronchopulmonary disease (including noninfectious bronchitis, lung contusion, heartworm disease, smoke inhalation, pulmonary atelectasis, thromboembolic disease)
  - Inhalation or aspiration of pharyngeal or gastric fluid or contents (due to anesthesia, swallowing disorders, megaesophagus, neuromuscular disease, laryngeal paralysis, posterior fossa lesion, stupor, vomiting, prolonged recumbency)
  - Oro-nasal sources of infection (sinusitis, dental disease)
  - Immunosuppression caused by another virus (FeLV, FIV, canine distemper, parvovirus) or disease (e.g., hyperadrenocorticism, diabetes mellitus, generalized demodecosis)
  - Immunosuppressive drug therapy (glucocorticoids, anticancer chemotherapy)
  - Abnormal respiratory defense mechanisms (Cushing's disease, chronic bronchitis, ciliary dyskinesia, neutrophil dysfunction syndromes)
  - Bronchial foreign body
  - Foreign body aspiration pneumonia (e.g., food, mineral oil in cats)
  - Debilitation, hospitalization, nosocomial infection
  - Indwelling intravenous catheter sepsis (hematogenous spread)
  - Contaminated endotracheal tube, tracheostomy tube, or bronchoscope
  - Aspiration or inhalation of liquid foreign material during diagnostic or therapeutic procedures (barium sulfate, medications, mineral oil, nutritional supplements)
  - Following thoracic surgery
- Prompt recognition and treatment of bronchopneumonia is important. It is equally important to identify the predisposing cause so that further episodes can be prevented or anticipated.

Clinical Signs

- The history often indicates a predisposing factor for bronchopneumonia.
- Tachypnea, respiratory distress, productive cough, and fever are typical findings.
- Constitutional signs—depression, anorexia, and listlessness—may be observed as the only features of disease.

- Mucopurulent nasal exudate may be present.
- Pulmonary adventitious sounds—especially rhonchi and crackles—may be ausculted; however, loud or asymmetric bronchial sounds can be the only auscultatory finding.

Diagnosis of Bacterial Bronchopneumonia

- Clinical signs, radiography, and the CBC are usually sufficient to make a presumptive diagnosis of bacterial pneumonia.
- Thoracic radiographs are key to the diagnosis of bronchopneumonia.
  - The typical findings are increased lung density that is most commonly alveolar in nature leading to border effacement (silhouetting) of the heart. The lobe may become consolidated, producing a fluid density lobar sign.
  - The right middle lung lobe is most prone to bacterial infection; the cranial lobes also are frequently involved. In contrast, dorso-caudal pulmonary infiltrates are very unlikely to be associated with bacterial infection of the lung with the rare exception of hematogenous pneumonia (from sepsis), which is diffuse, beginning as an interstitial pattern and progressing as an alveolar.
  - A cranioventral distribution of bacterial bronchopneumonia is typical.
  - With some foreign bodies, the intermediate lobe may be involved.
  - Lung consolidation may occur, leading to an eventual loss of air bronchograms except in the most proximal portion of the lobe.
- The radiographic differential diagnosis is also important.
  - Hilar or sternal lymphadenopathy is uncommon with bacterial infection.
  - Nodular densities are more typical of fungal disease, granulomatosis, or pulmonary neoplasia.
  - The combination of bronchopneumonia with concurrent septic pleural effusion (pyothorax) is very uncommon in dogs and cats. These findings are suggestive of an atypical infectious agent such as *Nocardia asteroides* or actinomycosis, presence of a foreign body, concurrent malignancy, or pulmonary embolus.
  - Pneumonia caused by viral, protozoal (e.g., toxoplasmosis), rickettsial, or fungal infection is typically interstitial in distribution. Fungal and *Toxoplasma* infections produce granulomatous lesions in the lung, and with systemic mycoses, hilar lymphadenopathy can be pronounced.
  - Esophageal air or dilatation may indicate simple air swallowing or a more serious condition such as megaesophagus or myasthenia gravis.
- Leukocytosis, left shift, and monocytosis are typical; however, the magnitude of change is not consistently related to the extent of infection. Overwhelming fulminant bacterial pneumonia may cause a neutropenia with degenerative left shift.

- Infected cats also may be FIV or FeLV positive. FIV infection has also been associated with nonbacterial alveolitis and interstitial pneumonia.
- Airway cytology and culture can confirm the diagnosis.
  - Transtracheal or endotracheal aspiration cytology demonstrates neutrophilic inflammation, often with degenerative PMNs and intracellular bacteria.
  - Cocci are usually streptococcus and rods are usually gram-negative bacteria.
  - The culture is typically positive for bacterial growth (see Tables 79–1 and 79–2).
  - Avoid percutaneous needle aspiration of the infected lung in order to prevent inoculation of the pleural space.
- The predisposing condition may be evident from the history, physical examination, neurological evaluation, radiographs, laboratory tests, or from special studies such as a barium swallow, acetylcholine receptor antibody titer, or bronchoscopic evaluation.

Treatment of Bacterial Bronchopneumonia

- Keep the patient well hydrated and warm. Fluid therapy is often required to prevent dehydration and inspissated respiratory secretions.
- Perform thoracic coupage 4–6 times daily. Once the patient feels better, brief walks, followed by coupage, help to mobilize tracheobronchial secretions.
- Airway humidification may assist in expectoration of secretions. Expectorants like guaifenesin are of uncertain merit and are not usually prescribed.
- Bronchodilator therapy (sustained release theophylline; Theo-Dur 10–20 mg/kg PO q12h for dogs) is not of proven efficacy but may reverse irritative bronchoconstriction and strengthen respiratory muscle effort in dyspneic animals.
- Cough suppressants are contraindicated in bronchopneumonia.
- Humidified oxygen should be administered to dyspneic, cyanotic, or hypoxemic animals.
- Antibiotics should be prescribed *for at least 3 weeks*. The duration of therapy may be longer pending clinical results and radiographs.
- Antibiotic choice should be based on culture and sensitivity (obtained by transtracheal washing) and with consideration of current or prior antibiotic therapy.
- Consider initially treating (while awaiting culture results) with an extended spectrum antibiotic such as cephalosporins, sulfadiazine-trimethoprim, fluoroquinolone (enrofloxacin or orbifloxacin), amoxicillin-clavulanic acid, tetracycline (dogs >8 weeks old), or chloramphenicol (if available, but not for cats).
- In life-threatening sepsis, the combination of intravenous cephalothin or cefazolin (20 mg/kg q8h) or ampicillin (20 mg/kg q8h) plus amikacin (15–20 mg/kg q24h) should be considered.
- Newer generation cephalosporins (e.g., moxalactam) are very expensive and usually reserved for resistant infections.

- Diffuse pulmonary infiltration in cats may be associated with mycoplasma or hematogenous bacterial infections. The quinolones, tetracyclines, and erythromycin have demonstrated activity against *Mycoplasma* spp.
- Management of bacterial pyothorax requires thoracostomy tube drainage and antibiotics. Because anaerobic organisms are commonly involved in pyothorax, treatment with penicillin (20,000–40,000 units/kg PO or IV q6–8h), alone or in combination with sulfadiazine-trimethoprim (Tribrissen 15 mg/kg PO q12h), or clindamycin (Antirobe, Upjohn, 5–10 mg/kg PO q12h) is recommended.

Follow-Up

- Thoracic radiographs should be obtained to ensure resolution of infection. Areas of lobar consolidation may take 2–6 weeks to become totally clear. Failure of steady clinical and radiographic improvement indicates a need to reevaluate the patient and to consider a tracheal wash or bronchoscopy with bronchial fluid aspiration.
- Recurrent pneumonia also is common, particularly in those animals with persistence of predisposing factors, including swallowing disorders, chemotherapy, ciliary dyskinesia, and acquired or congenital immune deficiencies. Infrequently, an unresponsive or refractory single lobe infection requires surgical lobectomy for resolution of the problem. Surgery is also indicated in cases of lung abscess or pneumonia due to a foreign body that cannot otherwise be retrieved.

RESPIRATORY PARASITES

Etiology

- A number of respiratory parasites have been identified in dogs and cats (see Table 79–1). The life cycle of some respiratory parasites is complex and involves intermediate and transport hosts. Some of the more important infections include:
- *Aelurostrongylus abstrusus* is a parasite of cats. This nematode requires a snail or slug as an intermediate host. Cats are often infected by eating transport hosts including birds, small mammals, and reptiles.
- *Paragonimus kellicotti* is a fluke parasitic to dogs and cats. Infection follows ingestion of an intermediate host (crayfish, aquatic snail) or a transport host (e.g., raccoon).
- *Capillaria aerophilia* is a nematode parasite of the dog and cat that has a direct life cycle. Pathogenic potential appears very low.
- *Crenosoma vulpis*, the fox lungworm, infrequently infects dogs.
- *Osleri/Filaroides* spp. are nematodes that invade the respiratory tract of the dog. Transmission is direct, often from bitch to pups. Three related species have been associated with respiratory disease, *O. osleri* (found in granulomas near the tracheal bifurcation),

F. milksi (a bronchopulmonary parasite), and *F. hirthi* (a lung parasite of importance to research colonies).

- *Dirofilaria immitis* infects the pulmonary arteries, causing secondary pulmonary injury (see Chap. 68).
- *Toxoplasma gondii* is a protozoan capable of multisystemic infection that is usually subclinical, but occasionally can cause pneumonia (see Chap. 19). Immunosuppression predisposes to toxoplasmosis.
- Parasites of the nasal cavity include cuterebra and other grubs, the microscopic nematode *Eucoleus boehmi*, nasal mite *Pneumonyssus (Pneumonyssoides) caninum,* and the gapeworm *(S. ierei).*

Clinical Signs

- Signs depend on the specific parasite, site and severity of infection, and the magnitude of the host reaction.
  - Mild cases are asymptomatic and only detected if ova are identified during routine fecal examination.
  - Clinically apparent infections occur most often in younger animals (<2 years) that are heavily infested.
  - Sneezing, nasal discharge, and reversed sneezing are signs of nasal mite infestation.
  - A chronic cough is typical of *O. osleri* infection.
  - Coughing is the most common sign of lower respiratory parasitic infections. Exercise intolerance and weight loss also may occur.
- Fever and tachypnea are typical of toxoplasmosis but not of other respiratory parasites. Multisystemic disease may be present in toxoplasma infection including neurological signs, anterior uveitis, chorioretinitis, and hepatitis.

Diagnosis

- Diagnosis of respiratory parasites is made following clinical examination, endoscopy, radiography, or identification of either ova or larvae in fecal samples or respiratory secretions.
- Eosinophilia is not uncommon in lungworm or fluke infections.
- Diagnosis of nasal mites or other nasal parasites is by direct visualization, often using a retroflexed bronchoscope. Diagnosis of *E. boehmi* requires mucosal biopsy.
- Diagnosis of *O. osleri* usually requires tracheoscopy, identification of nodules (which contain small, filamentous worms), or biopsy of a granuloma. There are no obvious radiographic changes unless soft tissue granulomas proximal to the carina are observed within the air-filled trachea. Occasionally, larvae may be obtained via tracheal washings.
- Radiographs are helpful in the recognition of advanced lungworm infections.
  - *Aerulostrongylus* causes an indistinct interstitial-nodular pattern in the lung. Distribution of infiltrates varies but caudal lung lobes are typically involved.

- *Paragonimus* generally causes a granulomatous interstitial reaction with appearance of air-filled cystic structures (especially in the dog).
- *Filaroides* infections can cause a diffuse interstitial infiltrate ranging from severe *(F. milksi)* to mild. *F. hirthi* seldom leads to clinical disease.
- *Toxoplasma* when manifested in the lung leads to a mixed interstitial-alveolar infiltrate.
- Fecal flotation can identify ova from some parasites (double-operculated *Capillaria* ova, single-operculated *Paragonimus* ova) or larvae of *Aelurostrongylus* or *Osleri/Filaroides* spp. Baermann fecal sedimentation techniques may be required to identify larvae.
- Transtracheal washing or aspirations of tracheobronchial secretions may demonstrate parasitic ova or larvae. In some cases, ova are scarce. An eosinophilic pulmonary infiltrate with accompanying neutrophilia is typical.
- Diagnosis of pulmonary toxoplasmosis depends on clinical signs and serological evaluation.

Treatment

- Treatment of respiratory parasites involves destroying the infective organism, reducing parenchymal reaction, and instructing the owner about the prevention of further infection. A number of drugs (at varying dosages) have demonstrated efficacy against respiratory parasites, though treatments for some parasites are difficult. Fenbendazole (Panacur) is generally the safest antiparasitic drug. In cases of severe eosinophilic pulmonary reaction, adjunctive therapy with prednisolone (0.5 mg/kg, orally, once or twice daily for 7–14 days) may be quite helpful.
- Nasal parasites are treated by manual removal of large parasites or by treatment with oral ivermectin (consult a parasitologist or specialist).
- Aelurostrongylosis is treated with fenbendazole (Panacur, 50 mg/kg, orally, once daily for 10 days).
- Paragonimiasis is treated with either fenbendazole (as above), praziquantel (Droncit, 25 mg/kg, orally, q8h for 2 days), or albendazole (25–50 mg/kg orally q12h for 10–20 days).
- *Filaroides* spp. are treated with fenbendazole, albendazole, or oral ivermectin (200 μg/kg/wk for 3 doses or 400 μg/kg once; do not administer to collies).
- Capillaria infection is often asymptomatic but can be treated as per *Filaroides* infection.
- The prognosis for recovery and elimination of signs is generally good unless severe granulomatous disease has developed, in which case, residual cough may occur.

ADDITIONAL READING

Angus JC, Jang SS, Hirsh DC: Microbiological study of transtracheal aspirates from dogs with suspected lower respiratory tract disease—264 cases (1989–1995). J Am Vet Med Assoc 210:55, 1997.
Bemis DA: Bordetella and mycoplasma respiratory-infections in dogs and cats. Vet Clin North Am Small Anim Pract 22:1173, 1992.

Drost WT, Berry CR, Breitschwerdt EB, et al.: Thoracic radiographic findings in dogs infected with rickettsia-rickettsii. Vet Radiol Ultrasound 38:260, 1997.

Ford RB: Role of Infectious Agents in Respiratory-Disease. Vet Clin North Am Small Anim Pract 23:17, 1993.

Gartrell CL, Ohandley PA, Perry RL: Canine nasal disease. 2. Comp Cont Educ Pract Vet 17:539, 1995.

Gartrell CL, Ohandley PA, Perry RL: Canine nasal disease. 1. Comp Cont Educ Pract Vet 17:323, 1995.

Hawkins EC: Radiographic findings in cats with intranasal neoplasia and chronic rhinitis—29 cases (1982–1988). J Am Vet Med Assoc 208:1299, 1996.

Hawkins EC, Denicola DB, Plier ML: Cytological analysis of bronchoalveolar lavage fluid in the diagnosis of spontaneous respiratory tract disease in dogs—A retrospective study. J Vet Intern Med 9:386, 1995.

Murphy ST, Ellison GW, Mckiernan BC, et al.: Pulmonary lobectomy in the management of pneumonia in dogs—59 cases (1972–1994). J Am Vet Med Assoc 210:235, 1997.

Richardson EF, Mathews KG: Distribution of topical agents in the frontal sinuses and nasal cavity of dogs—Comparison between current protocols for treatment of nasal aspergillosis and a new noninvasive technique. Vet Surg 24:476, 1995.

Schoning P, Dryden MW, Gabbert NH: Identification of a nasal nematode (Eucoleus boehmi) in greyhounds. Vet Res Commun 17:277, 1993.

Sharp NJH, Sullivan M, Harvey CE, et al.: Treatment of canine nasal aspergillosis with enilconazole. J Vet Intern Med 7:40, 1993.

Van Pelt DR, Lappin MR: Pathogenesis and treatment of feline rhinitis. Vet Clin North Am Small Anim Pract 24:807, 1994.

Van Pelt DR, McKiernan BC: Pathogenesis and treatment of canine rhinitis. Vet Clin North Am Small Anim Pract 24:789, 1994.

Wolf AM: Fungal diseases of the nasal cavity of the dog and cat. Vet Clin North Am Small Anim Pract 22:1119, 1992.

80 Pleural Effusion

Robert G. Sherding / Stephen J. Birchard

Pleural effusion is an abnormal accumulation of fluid within the pleural space and is a clinical manifestation of conditions such as pyothorax, feline infectious peritonitis, congestive heart failure, intrathoracic neoplasia (e.g., lymphoma, thymoma, pulmonary neoplasia, mesothelioma), chylothorax, heartworm disease, hemothorax, hypoalbuminemia, lung lobe torsion, and diaphragmatic hernia. Pleural effusion is usually suspected from clinical signs and physical findings and confirmed by thoracentesis or thoracic radiography.

ETIOLOGY

Pleural effusion occurs when one or, more often, a combination of the factors that determine pleural fluid dynamics are altered so as to increase fluid formation or decrease fluid absorption or both. For example, pleural effusion is often associated with congestive heart failure (CHF) because increased capillary hydrostatic pressure results in increased pleural fluid formation. Extreme hypoalbuminemia may lower systemic colloidal osmotic pressure sufficiently to cause increased formation and decreased absorption of pleural fluid. Inflammation of the pleura may increase the formation of pleural fluid because of increased blood flow (hydrostatic pressure) and permeability of the pleural capillaries along with increased intrapleural colloidal osmotic pressure due to a higher concentration of protein in the fluid. Pleural effusion may also result from lymphatic insufficiency caused by thoracic duct obstruction, intrathoracic neoplasia, pleural thickening, or lymphatic hypertension secondary to CHF. The major causes of pleural effusion in dogs and cats are listed in Table 80–1.

DIAGNOSIS

Suspect pleural effusion on the basis of clinical signs and physical findings. Confirm pleural effusion by thoracentesis (see Chap. 3) or thoracic radiography (see Chap. 75). The cause is often determined through analysis of pleural fluid obtained by thoracentesis, in conjunction with post-thoracentesis radiographs. Depending on the suspected etiology, consider other diagnostic procedures such as laboratory evaluations, cardiac evaluations, ultrasonography, and specialized imaging procedures (contrast radiography, scintigraphy, computed tomography [CT]). Rarely, exploratory thoracotomy is required for definitive diagnosis.

Clinical Signs

- Dyspnea and exercise intolerance (inactivity) are the most consistent presenting signs of pleural effusion. Dogs and cats generally accommodate to small to moderate increases in the volume of intrapleural fluid by gradually decreasing their level of activity. Thus the signs of early pleural effusion are subtle and often imperceptible to the owner. As the accumulation of intrapleural fluid becomes substantial, however, tachypnea and respiratory distress become apparent during mild exertion and eventually even at rest.
- To facilitate breathing, the animal may prefer a sitting or crouched sternal posture, with the head and neck extended and the elbows abducted away from the thorax. An anxious facial expression and open-mouth breathing with forceful abdominal efforts during inspiration may be observed. Cyanosis may be seen in severe cases.

▼ *Key Point* Any struggling or increased distress during examination procedures may worsen dyspnea and induce respiratory arrest because of limited respiratory reserve.

- Other clinical signs associated with pleural effusion depend on the underlying cause but may include anorexia, depression, weight loss, dehydration, pallor, fever, hypothermia, or cough. Cough in animals with pleural effusion may indicate tracheal compression by a mediastinal mass (lymphoma, thymoma), intrapulmonary involvement (e.g., lung tumor, pulmonary edema, heartworm disease, pneumonia), or pleuritis.

Physical Examination
Thoracic Auscultation and Percussion

- Auscultation generally reveals muffled or inaudible heart and lung sounds ventrally, while breath sounds are preserved dorsally.
- On percussion, pleural effusion causes the thorax to sound dull and hyporesonant, and a horizontal fluid line may be demonstrable.

Table 80–1. CAUSES OF PLEURAL EFFUSION AND CRITERIA FOR DIAGNOSIS

Causes of Pleural Effusion	Potential Distinguishing Radiographic Findings	Fluid Patterns	Other Diagnostics
Common Diseases			
Pyothorax	Effusion may be unilateral or encapsulated; rounded or collapsed lung lobes (constrictive pleuritis)	Septic exudate	CBC; fluid culture
Feline infectious peritonitis	Concurrent abdominal effusion in some cases; rounded or collapsed lung lobes (constrictive pleuritis)	Nonseptic exudate (pyogranulomatous)	Fluid protein electrophoresis; serology
Congestive heart failure	Cardiomegaly; pulmonary edema and venous congestion; dilated caudal vena cava; abdominal effusion (rare)	Pure transudate; modified transudate; chylous effusion	Echocardiography; electrocardiography; angiocardiography
Heartworms (dirofilariasis)	Prominent pulmonary arteries; right-sided heart enlargement	Modified transudate; chylous effusion	Heartworm tests; echocardiography
Mediastinal neoplasia (lymphoma, thymoma)	Mediastinal mass (widened mediastinum; dorsally displaced trachea, caudally displaced heart and carina, esophageal compression)	Neoplastic: modified transudate; nonseptic exudate; chylous effusion	Ultrasound; fine-needle aspiration cytology
Bronchopulmonary neoplasia (carcinoma)	Pulmonary mass or infiltration	Neoplastic (variable): modified transudate; nonseptic exudate; chylous effusion; hemorrhage	Ultrasound; fine-needle aspiration cytology; thoracotomy
Chylothorax	Rounded or collapsed lung lobes (constrictive pleuritis); effusion may be unilateral	Chylous effusion	Fluid triglyceride; lymphangiogram; evaluate for underlying causes
Uncommon Diseases			
Diaphragmatic hernia	Other signs of thoracic trauma; loss of diaphragm shadow; displaced abdominal organs; concurrent abdominal effusion	Modified transudate; nonseptic exudate	Ultrasound; contrast peritoneography
Hemothorax	Other signs of thoracic trauma	Hemorrhage	If nontraumatic: coagulation tests; evaluate for underlying causes
Lung lobe torsion	Opaque lung lobe (right middle or either cranial lobe)	Nonseptic exudate; hemorrhage	Ultrasound, bronchoscopy; thoracotomy
Hypoalbuminemia	Concurrent abdominal effusion	Pure transudate	Evaluate kidneys, liver, and GI tract
Mesothelioma	No distinguishing characteristics	Neoplastic (variable): modified transudate; nonseptic exudate	Ultrasound; fine-needle aspiration cytology; thoracotomy
Thymic branchial cyst	Mediastinal mass (similar appearance to mediastinal neoplasia)	Modified transudate; nonseptic exudate	Ultrasound; thoracotomy
Pancreatitis	Concurrent abdominal effusion	Nonseptic exudate	Abdominal ultrasound; serum trypsin assay
Pulmonary thromboembolism	Hypovascularity of lung; blunted pulmonary arteries; right-sided heart enlargement	Modified transudate; nonseptic exudate	Angiography; pulmonary perfusion scan

Other Physical Findings

- Fever suggests an inflammatory, infectious, or neoplastic process.
- Jugular venous distention or pulsations and auscultation of murmurs, gallops, and arrhythmias are signs suggestive of cardiogenic pleural effusion. Pleural effusion can be associated with congestive heart failure in cats with hyperthyroidism; thus, palpate the thyroid region for the presence of thyroid gland nodules or enlargement.

- Decreased compressibility of the cranial thorax is suggestive of a mediastinal mass, usually lymphoma or thymoma. Mediastinal lymphoma can also compress the esophagus, causing signs of dysphagia and regurgitation; it also can impinge on the sympathetic innervation of the eye, causing Horner syndrome.
- Animals with pleural effusion should also be thoroughly examined for evidence of a tumor in any location, since extrathoracic neoplasms may metastasize to the pleural cavity and cause pleural effusion (e.g., mammary adenocarcinoma).

- Ophthalmoscopy may reveal lesions of chorioretinitis in cats with feline infectious peritonitis (FIP).
- External signs of trauma may indicate hemothorax or diaphragmatic hernia.

Thoracic Radiography

Routine thoracic radiography is generally effective for confirming pleural effusion.

▼ *Key Point* If the animal is in extreme respiratory distress, perform pleural drainage to stabilize the patient before radiography. Otherwise, the stress of manipulation during radiography could prove fatal.

The radiographic signs of pleural effusion include separation of the lung lobes from the parietal pleura and sternum by extrapulmonary fluid density (i.e., compression of lung lobes by a pleural fluid density), fluid-filled interlobar fissures producing a scalloped appearance to the edges of the lungs, and obscuring of the cardiac and diaphragmatic shadows, which is referred to as the silhouette sign (see Chap. 75). There is also widening of the mediastinum and blunting or filling of the costophrenic angles by intrapleural fluid density on a ventrodorsal view. In addition, the various causes of pleural effusion may be associated with other radiographic findings of diagnostic significance (see Table 80–1).

- A rounded contour to the caudal lobar borders, often accompanied by atelectasis of the cranial and middle lobes, is suggestive of a chronic fibrosing reaction of the visceral pleura that is exerting a constrictive and restrictive effect on the lung lobes (especially in cats with chronic chylothorax). Atelectatic lobes may be mistaken for pulmonary masses, hilar masses, or lung lobe torsion.
- Although most pleural effusions are bilateral, unilateral effusion is seen occasionally. This is most suggestive of pyothorax because the natural walling-off response to septic suppuration can cause extensive pleural thickening, which may seal off the mediastinum and limit the effusion to one side. Pleural thickening associated with chylothorax can also result in unilateral effusion. In addition to pyothorax and chylothorax, unilateral effusion is occasionally observed in traumatic hemothorax, diaphragmatic hernia, pulmonary neoplasia, and lung lobe torsion.
- Pleural effusion is sometimes found in combination with ascites. Simultaneous pleural and peritoneal effusions (double effusion) occur most often in cats with FIP but also with severe hypoalbuminemia, diaphragmatic hernia, widely disseminated neoplasia, pancreatitis, and CHF.

▼ *Key Point* Since many intrathoracic structures are obscured by the presence of pleural effusion, obtain radiographs *after* removal of pleural fluid to facilitate visualization of such abnormalities as mediastinal mass, cardiomegaly, intrapulmonary lesions (masses, infiltrates, vascular changes), lung lobe torsion, or diaphragmatic hernia (see Table 80–1).

- Both right and left lateral radiographic views of the thorax may be indicated when a unilateral lesion is suspected (e.g., focal fluid accumulation, pulmonary mass or focal density, lung lobe torsion). Horizontal beam radiography (e.g., standing lateral view) can be used to confirm small-volume effusions, to demonstrate fluid encapsulation, and to facilitate visualization of thoracic structures by shifting fluid away from the structures of interest.

Thoracentesis and Fluid Analysis

In most animals with pleural effusion, the combination of radiographic findings and fluid analysis establishes the diagnosis or determines the direction for additional diagnostic evaluations. Drainage of the pleural fluid also provides therapeutic benefit and may be lifesaving.

Thoracentesis

- Thoracentesis is a safe and generally effective method for removal of fluid from the pleural space. See Chap. 3 for a description of thoracentesis technique.
- Following collection of diagnostic specimens, enough fluid should be aspirated to relieve respiratory distress. In some animals it may be difficult to obtain an adequate volume of fluid if the fluid is compartmentalized within the pleural space by adhesions or if it is viscid and full of fibrin or debris. In this case, or if repeated pleural drainage is anticipated, place a thoracostomy tube (see Chap. 3).

Pleural Fluid Analysis

Perform the following analyses on the pleural fluid.

- Cytologic examination of direct smears and centrifuged cell concentrate smears stained with routine hematologic stains. In scanty aspirates, smears for cytologic examination are the first priority
- Total nucleated cell count (differentiates transudates from exudates)
- Physical and biochemical characteristics, such as color, turbidity (correlates with nucleated cell count in nonchylous fluids), odor (foul odor suggests pyothorax), specific gravity and total protein concentration (differentiates transudates from exudates), viscosity and clot formation (indicates fibrinous exudate as in FIP), and presence of chylomicrons (tests for triglyceride indicate chylous effusion)
- Chemical analyses (not routine); e.g., pH (<6.9 in pyothorax), glucose (<10 mg/dl in pyothorax), lactic dehydrogenase (>200 IU/L in exudates), adenosine deaminase (elevated in inflammatory exudates), and fibronectin (elevated in neoplastic effusion)
- If infection is suspected, Gram stain, acid-fast stain, culture and sensitivity testing for aerobic and anaerobic bacteria, and, in some cases, culture for fungi
- If FIP is a possibility, set aside an aliquot of fluid in case protein electrophoresis and a polymerase chain reaction test are later warranted based on preliminary findings (see under Feline Infectious Peritonitis)

Classification of Pleural Fluid Patterns

On the basis of these analyses, pleural effusions are generally classified into one of several patterns: transudate, modified transudate, nonseptic exudate, septic exudate, chylous effusion, and hemorrhage (Table 80–2). In addition, any of these can be subcategorized as neoplastic versus non-neoplastic depending on whether or not neoplastic cells are present on cytologic evaluation. There can be considerable overlap between these various categories; nevertheless, they are helpful for understanding the pathogenesis and determining the cause of pleural effusions.

Transudate

Transudative effusions are generally associated with alteration of capillary hydrostatic pressure caused by CHF or decreased plasma colloidal osmotic pressure caused by hypoalbuminemia. The typical features of a pure transudate are low protein concentration and low cell count consisting predominantly of mesothelial cells; this is comparable to the characteristics of normal pleural fluid.

Modified Transudate

Long-standing transudative effusions often become modified transudates, as they acquire greater cellularity and protein content. Modified transudates and nonseptic exudates can be very similar.

Septic Exudate

Septic exudates are purulent effusions consisting of numerous degenerating neutrophils, usually in association with intra- and extracellular bacteria. The fluid usually has marked turbidity, high protein concentration, and a foul odor, whereas the color is variable. The presence of a septic exudate within the pleural space indicates septic pleuritis (pyothorax) and is an indication for culture and Gram stain of the effusion (see under Pyothorax).

Nonseptic Exudate

Disorders that cause lymphatic or venous obstruction, such as neoplasia, diaphragmatic hernia, lung lobe torsion, pulmonary infarction, and thymic branchial cysts may result in a nonseptic exudative effusion that is difficult to distinguish from a modified transudate. Some clinicians subclassify such effusions as obstructive effusions or, if neoplastic cells are evident cytologically, as neoplastic effusions.

- *Feline infectious peritonitis* causes a nonseptic pyogranulomatous exudate that has fairly distinctive characteristics—yellow and translucent in appearance with a viscous consistency, high protein concentration (approximating serum levels), high fibrin content, and low to moderate cellularity consisting mostly of nondegenerate neutrophils and macrophages (see under Feline Infectious Peritonitis; see also Chap. 8). If FIP is suspected, consider performing protein electrophoresis of the fluid. If gamma globulin is greater than 32% of the protein in effusates, FIP is strongly considered; conversely, if more than 48% of protein is albumin or if the albumin-to-globulin ratio is greater than 0.81, FIP is unlikely.
- *Eosinophilic effusion* (>10% eosinophils) can be either an exudate or modified transudate. The most frequent cause has been intrathoracic neoplasia (e.g., systemic mastocytosis, lymphoma). Eosinophilic pleural effusion has also been associated with heartworm disease, allergy, bronchointerstitial lung disease, eosinophilic granulomatosis, and trauma.

Chylous Effusion

Chylous effusions are caused by extravasation or leakage of intestinal lymph (chyle) from an obstructed or ruptured thoracic duct. Chylothorax in dogs and cats may be idiopathic or associated with trauma, thoracic lymphangiectasia, intrathoracic neoplasia, heart disease, heartworms, venous thrombosis, diaphragmatic hernia, and lung lobe torsion (see under Chylothorax). The milky white opaque fluid contains mostly lymphocytes accompanied by variable numbers of neutrophils, depending on the duration of the effusion and the extent of the resulting pleuritis (see Table 80–2). Chylous effusions are confirmed by the presence of chylomicrons, which can be demonstrated by the ether clearance test, by the presence of a cream layer on refrigeration, and microscopically by the presence of Sudanpositive orange fat droplets, but these are relatively insensitive methods.

Table 80–2. PLEURAL FLUID ANALYSIS PATTERNS*

Fluid Category	TP	WBC	Disease Associations
Transudate	<1.5	<1000	CHF (early), hypoproteinemia
Modified transudate	2.5–5	1000–7000	CHF, neoplasia (e.g., lymphoma), diaphragmatic hernia, pulmonary thromboembolism
Nonseptic exudate	3–6	5000–20,000	FIP, neoplasia, diaphragmatic hernia, lung lobe torsion, pancreatitis, pulmonary thromboembolism
Septic exudate	3–7	5000–300,000	Septic pleuritis (pyothorax)
Chylous effusion	2.5–6	1000–20,000	CHF, lymphoma, thoracic lymphangiectasia, heartworms, jugular vein thrombosis (catheter-induced), diaphragmatic hernia, lung lobe torsion
Hemorrhage	>3.0	5000–20,000	Trauma, coagulopathy, neoplasia, lung lobe torsion

*The six basic fluid patterns and their most frequent clinical associations are indicated. Any of these can be subcategorized as neoplastic versus non-neoplastic depending on whether neoplastic cells are present on cytologic evaluation.

▼ *Key Point* The most reliable test for chylous effusion is the comparison of the triglyceride and cholesterol concentrations measured simultaneously in the fluid and serum. Chylous effusion is characterized by a high triglyceride concentration (usually >300 mg/dl) compared with that of serum and a pleural fluid cholesterol-to-triglyceride ratio of less than 1. The fluid cholesterol concentration is less than or equal to that of serum.

Hemorrhagic Effusion

Hemorrhage into the pleural space may be associated with trauma, hemostatic abnormalities, or neoplasia. The physicochemical and cytologic features of the effusion are similar to those of defibrinated peripheral blood. The presence of erythrophagocytosis by macrophages confirms that the hemorrhage is not merely the result of a traumatic collection.

Laboratory Evaluations

Various laboratory evaluations may provide useful diagnostic information depending on the suspected underlying cause of pleural effusion.

- The complete blood count may reveal a neutrophilia with a left shift in pyothorax, FIP, lung lobe torsion, and neoplasia. Lymphopenia is common in animals with chylothorax, but it can also be a nonspecific manifestation of stress. Anemia and various other hematologic abnormalities may be associated with lymphoma and feline leukemia virus (FeLV).
- Serum protein determinations may reveal hypoalbuminemia, a cause of transudation, or hyperglobulinemia, a common finding in FIP and other conditions of chronic immune stimulation. Severe proteinuria would be expected on the urinalysis of a dog or cat with hypoalbuminemia and transudation associated with nephrotic syndrome.
- Diagnostic testing may be indicated for infectious and parasitic diseases that have been associated with pleural effusion, such as FeLV, feline immunodeficiency virus (FIV), FIP, heartworm disease, and aelurostrongylosis. Specific aspects of these various diagnostic tests are described in the appropriate chapters elsewhere in this book.
- In cats with cardiogenic pleural effusion, the serum concentrations of thyroxine and taurine may be indicated for the diagnosis of hyperthyroid cardiomyopathy and taurine-deficient cardiomyopathy, respectively (see Chap. 66).

Cardiac Evaluations

- Echocardiography is the most useful procedure for diagnosis of cardiogenic causes of pleural effusion such as cardiomyopathy (idiopathic, taurine deficiency, hyperthyroidism), pericardial diseases (pericarditis, neoplasia), congenital heart defects, and heartworm disease.
- Angiocardiography is also helpful for determining the underlying cardiac abnormality in selected cases

of cardiogenic pleural effusion. A detailed discussion of cardiac evaluation is found elsewhere in this book.

Ultrasonography

The inability of ultrasound to penetrate air-filled structures limits the diagnostic usefulness of ultrasound examination of the lungs; however, in animals with pleural effusion ultrasonography can provide meaningful information because the pleural fluid provides an "acoustic window" for transmission. Thoracic ultrasonography is possible when air-filled lung is collapsed, displaced (by fluid, mass, or herniated abdominal viscera), replaced (by neoplastic tissue), or consolidated. Because the presence of pleural fluid actually enhances ultrasound transmission, it is preferable to perform the procedure prior to evacuation of the pleural fluid.

- Pleural fluid usually appears as an anechoic or hypoechoic space between the thoracic wall or diaphragm and lung. The fluid in pyothorax and hemothorax may contain internal echoes.
- In addition to confirming pleural effusion, ultrasonography is helpful for the diagnosis of pulmonary, mediastinal, and pleural neoplasms; pulmonary abscesses associated with pyothorax; lung lobe torsion; cardiac abnormalities; and diaphragmatic hernia.
- Ultrasonography can also be used to guide needle placement accurately for fine-needle aspiration or biopsy of pleural, mediastinal, and pulmonary masses.

Specialized Imaging Techniques

Depending on the suspected etiology of the pleural effusion and the results of other diagnostic evaluations, specialized imaging techniques may be indicated, such as contrast radiographic procedures (contrast peritoneography for the diagnosis of diaphragmatic hernia, contrast lymphangiography for the diagnosis of chylothorax, contrast pleurography), lymphoscintigraphy, and CT.

Positive Contrast Peritoneography

When diaphragmatic hernia is suspected but cannot be confirmed on routine thoracic and abdominal radiographs, ultrasonography should be the next approach; however, if ultrasound is unavailable, positive contrast peritoneography is an alternative method for diagnosis of diaphragmatic hernia. Inject an aqueous contrast iodide (Renovist; 1 ml/kg) into the peritoneal cavity, and roll the animal from side to side for several minutes to distribute the contrast agent. Obtain radiographs to determine whether the contrast agent has entered the pleural space through a defect in the diaphragm.

Lymphangiography

Positive-contrast lymphangiography is used to evaluate the thoracic duct lymphatic channel in dogs and cats with unexplained chylous effusion. This is usually done by catheterizing an intestinal lymphatic just prior to, and in preparation for, surgical ligation of the thoracic duct to treat chylothorax (see Chap. 83 for a description of this procedure).

SPECIFIC DISEASES

Pyothorax (Septic Pleuritis)

Pyothorax is the accumulation of purulent exudate (pus) within the pleural space as a result of intrapleural bacterial infection (septic pleuritis) or, rarely, mycotic infection.

Etiology

Microorganisms

A diversity of microorganisms has been isolated from the pleural fluid of dogs and cats with pyothorax; mixed bacterial infections composed mostly of obligate and facultative anaerobes are found most consistently.

- In many cases, the infection consists entirely of anaerobic bacteria. The most frequent isolates are *Bacteroides* spp., *Clostridium* spp., *Peptostreptococcus* spp., *Fusobacterium* spp., *Pasteurella multocida*, and *Actinomyces* spp. The isolates from cats with pyothorax and their relative frequency closely resemble those found in subcutaneous cat bite abscesses and mirror the normal oropharyngeal flora of the cat.
- Other bacteria found sporadically include *Pseudomonas* spp., *Escherichia coli*, *Klebsiella* spp., *Proteus* spp., *Streptococcus* spp., *Staphylococcus* spp., *Corynebacterium pyogenes*, *Nocardia* spp., *Borrelia* spp., *Eubacterium* spp., and mycoplasmas.
- Fungi, such as *Cryptococcus neoformans*, *Blastomyces dermatitidis*, and *Candida albicans*, are rare causes.
- In addition, pleuritis has been reported as a rare manifestation of infection with *Aelurostrongylus abstrusus*, the feline lungworm.

Source of Infection

The source of infection is not identified in most dogs and cats with pyothorax. Microorganisms may potentially enter the pleural space through penetrating chest wounds (e.g., bite wounds), perforations of mediastinal structures (i.e., esophagus, trachea, bronchi), migrating pleural foreign bodies (e.g., grass awns), and direct extension from the lung in bacterial pneumonia (parapneumonic effusion). Mediastinitis, pleuritis, and pyothorax are frequent complications of esophageal perforation caused by esophageal foreign bodies, especially those with irregular sharp edges, such as plastic, glass, wood, and bone. Iatrogenic esophageal rupture can occur during endoscopic foreign body retrieval or during balloon dilation of esophageal strictures. Intrapleural infection can also result from hematogenous or lymphatic spread from distant infection sites.

Clinical Signs

Dyspnea is the most consistent sign of pyothorax. Cough is observed in some cases. In addition, nonspe-

cific systemic signs are common, including inactivity, exercise intolerance, fever, depression, anorexia, dehydration, weight loss, and pallor. Advanced cases may present in a moribund state with endotoxic shock and hypothermia.

Diagnosis

- Physical findings (auscultation and percussion) and radiographic findings in pyothorax are typical of pleural effusion. In some animals with pyothorax, the pleural fluid may become encapsulated or compartmentalized by fibrinous adhesions and fibrosis (walling-off process), producing radiographic signs of unilateral or nongravitating effusion and rounded lobar edges.
- The hematologic findings in pyothorax are typical of a serious septic inflammatory process and support the diagnosis. A neutrophilic leukocytosis with a left shift and with toxic-appearing neutrophils are found in most cases, while a neutropenia with a degenerative left shift may develop terminally. The hemogram also usually reveals a mild to moderate nonregenerative, normochromic, normocytic anemia of chronic infection.
- Confirm the diagnosis of pyothorax with pleural fluid analysis, which indicates septic inflammatory (purulent) exudate. The fluid is usually malodorous and cloudy or opaque, with color varying from red to brown to yellow. The fluid also may contain a flocculent sediment of fibrinous and cellular debris. The total protein concentration generally exceeds 4.5 g/dl and there are usually 50,000 to 100,000 or more nucleated cells/μl, consisting of mostly (greater than 85%) degenerating neutrophils. Cytologic examination usually reveals abundant intra- and extracellular bacteria.
- Culture the pleural fluid for confirmation of the diagnosis and for determination of optimal antibacterial therapy. In most cases, a mixed infection (see above under Etiology) involving primarily anaerobic bacteria is found. If only routine aerobic culture techniques are used, only the aerobic component of the infection will be identified, and because some dogs and cats with pyothorax have an exclusively anaerobic infection, there may be no growth at all. Thus, perform both aerobic and anaerobic cultures.
- Since retroviral status may influence prognosis, test cats with pyothorax for FeLV (see Chap. 6) and FIV (see Chap. 7).

Treatment

Treat pyothorax with systemic antibiotics and closed-chest drainage and lavage by means of an indwelling chest tube thoracostomy (see elsewhere for thoracic tube placement). The chest tube provides for repeated drainage and irrigation of the pleural space.

Antibiotics

Start antibiotic therapy intravenously and then continue orally at home for at least 4–6 weeks. Until the results of culture and sensitivity of the effusion are available, assume that a mixed anaerobic and aerobic infection is present (see above under Etiology). Most isolates are susceptible to antibiotics of the penicillin family, such as penicillin G, ampicillin, amoxicillin, or amoxicillin with clavulanate; thus, standard dosages of any one of these are a good initial choice (see Table 80–3), although approximately 20% of anaerobes may be resistant to the penicillin-ampicillin group. Other effective antibiotics for anaerobic infections include clindamycin and metronidazole (see Table 80–3). For gram-negative infections, add an aminoglycoside (gentamicin or amikacin), enrofloxacin, or trimethoprim-sulfadiazine. Trimethoprim-sulfadiazine is indicated for *Nocardia* spp.

Pleural Drainage and Lavage

Place a thoracic drain tube to drain purulent material from the pleural space and allow lavage of the pleural cavity. Although some animals with severe effusion may require continuous chest drainage, intermittent drainage is adequate for most patients.

- Perform lavage at least twice daily. The lavage solution should consist of a sterile isotonic saline or lactated Ringer's solution warmed to body temperature. Prior to each irrigation procedure, evacuate any fluid that has accumulated since the previous lavage and record the quantity. Warm the irrigation solution to body temperature and infuse 10 to 20 ml/kg body weight slowly over about 5 minutes through the chest tube. If respiratory distress occurs, stop the infusion.
- Leave the solution in the thorax for 5–10 minutes while the animal is gently rolled to enhance distribution; then aspirate as much as possible. A return of 75% or more of the irrigation solution is expected, which can sometimes be facilitated by repositioning the animal or rolling it from side to side during aspiration.
- If the animal is initially dehydrated, rehydration should be accomplished before, or simultaneous to, the first lavage; otherwise, much of the instilled fluid will be absorbed from the pleural space with very little returned on aspiration.
- Obtain samples of interlavage fluid for cytologic examination on a daily basis and examine for disappearance of microorganisms and degenerative neutrophils. Remove the chest tube once the interlavage pleural fluid becomes characteristic of a modified transudate (clear in appearance and free of microorganisms and degenerative neutrophils) and the quantity that accumulates is small and can be accounted for merely by the presence of the drain itself (i.e., up to 2–3 ml/kg/day). There should also be radiographic resolution of pleural effusion.
- The duration of the pleural drainage phase of therapy in most cases is 4–7 days. Monitor serum proteins and electrolytes (especially potassium) because depletion can occur with prolonged lavage. Evaluate thoracic radiographs about 1 week following tube removal to ensure resolution, and continue systemic antibiotics a minimum of 4–6 weeks.

Complications

Adverse sequelae to pyothorax may include restrictive pleuritis, pleural adhesion formation, and pulmonary abscessation. Occasionally, adhesions render closed-chest drainage and lavage ineffective. In such cases, perform a thoracotomy (see Chap. 83) to manually break down adhesions, drain pockets of exudate, remove debris, and place a drainage tube in the most favorable location for postoperative thoracic lavage. In addition, thoracotomy may be necessary if a migrating pleural foreign body is suspected.

Chylothorax
Etiology

Chylothorax results from the leakage or extravasation of chylomicron-laden intestinal lymph (chyle) into the pleural space from an obstructed, ruptured, or anomalous thoracic duct or its collateral branches. The cause

Table 80–3. USEFUL ANTIBIOTICS FOR TREATMENT OF PYOTHORAX

Antibiotic	Trade Name	Dosage	Indications
Penicillin G	many	20,000–40,000 U/kg q6–8h IV IM	anaerobes,* *Pasteurella, Actinomyces*
Ampicillin	Omnipen	20 mg/kg q6–8h IV IM SC	anaerobes,* *Pasteurella* and some other gram negatives
Amoxicillin	Amoxi-Tabs	20 mg/kg q8–12h PO	anaerobes,* *Pasteurella* and some other gram negatives
Amoxicillin/clavulanate	Clavamox	20 mg/kg cat q12h PO	anaerobes,† *Pasteurella* and many other gram negatives
Chloramphenicol	Chloromycetin	50 mg/cat q12h IV SC PO	anaerobes,† gram-positive and gram-negative aerobes
Clindamycin	Antirobe	10 mg/kg q12h PO	anaerobes†
Metronidazole	Flagyl	10–15 mg/kg q8–12h PO IV	anaerobes†
Enrofloxacin§	Baytril	5–10 mg/kg q12h IV SC PO	most gram-negative and gram-positive aerobes
Trimethoprim-sulfadiazine	Tribrissen	15 mg/kg q12h PO	*Nocardia*
Gentamicin‡	Gentocin	3 mg/kg q8h IV IM SC	gram negatives§
Amikacin‡	Amiglyde-V	10 mg/kg q8–12h IV IM SC	gram negatives§
Cefoxitin	Mefoxin	20–30 mg/kg q8h IV IM	anaerobes,† gram negatives
Ticarcillin	Ticar	30–50 mg/kg q6h IV IM	anaerobes,† gram negatives, *Pseudomonas*

*Excluding *Bacteroides fragilis*.

†Including most penicillin-resistant strains of *Bacteroides fragilis*.

‡Caution: uncorrected dehydration may potentiate aminoglycoside nephrotoxicity.

§Enrofloxacin and aminoglycosides are ineffective against anaerobes; thus, always use in combination with penicillin or other antibiotic with activity against anaerobes when treating pyothorax.

of chylothorax is frequently not apparent; however, chylous pleural effusions in dogs and cats have been associated with lymphangiectasia of intrathoracic lymphatics (resulting from obstruction of thoracic duct inflow into the cranial vena cava), traumatic rupture of the thoracic duct, intrathoracic neoplasia (mediastinal lymphoma, thymoma), heart disease (cardiomyopathy, heartworms, hyperthyroidism, pericarditis), diaphragmatic hernia, peritoneopericardial diaphragmatic hernia, lung lobe torsion, and vena caval thromboembolism (iatrogenic from indwelling jugular venous catheterization).

Clinical Signs

In addition to typical signs of pleural effusion, such as dyspnea and tachypnea, it is noteworthy that dogs and cats with chylothorax often present with coughing.

Diagnosis

- Confirmation that pleural fluid is chyle depends on demonstration of the presence of chylomicrons. The most reliable criteria for chyle are an increased concentration of triglyceride in the fluid compared with serum and a fluid cholesterol-to-triglyceride ratio of less than 1 (see under Classification of Pleural Fluid Patterns).
- In the veterinary literature, many milky effusions have been called pseudochylous (which implies lipid in the form of cholesterol and lecithin derived from degenerating cells) when, in fact, if triglyceride analysis had been performed, these effusions would probably have been true chyle.
- The predominant cell in chyle is usually the small lymphocyte. However, over time the irritant effect of chyle results in an influx of inflammatory cells, especially neutrophils.
- Once chylothorax is confirmed, use routine radiography and other clinical evaluations (e.g., ultrasonography, echocardiography, heartworm testing) to search for underlying causes, such as heart disease, heartworms, neoplasia, or diaphragmatic hernia.

Medical Treatment

- If an underlying cause is identified, treatment is directed toward the underlying primary disorder. In the rare case when there is a history of recent thoracic trauma, conservative medical management may be tried for a 2-week period in hopes of spontaneous healing of the injured lymphatic. This consists of (1) pleural drainage by either periodic thoracentesis or continuous chest tube drainage, and (2) decreasing thoracic duct flow by exercise restriction (cage rest).
- A fat-restricted diet supplemented with medium-chain triglycerides (MCTs) has been recommended in the past; however, this has not been effective clinically, and in normal dogs it has been shown experimentally that altering dietary fat content or using MCTs does not significantly affect thoracic duct lymph flow and that orally administered MCTs are carried in thoracic duct lymph.

Surgical Treatment

- If no underlying medically treatable cause of chylothorax is found, surgical intervention is indicated. The surgical approach to treatment of chylothorax involves ligation of the thoracic duct at the level of the diaphragm in association with evaluation of the thoracic duct and intrathoracic lymphatics by pre- and immediate postoperative contrast lymphangiography. Lymphangiography is performed by cannulating a mesenteric lymphatic via a flank abdominal approach. After delineating the thoracic duct and its branches with the dye study, the duct is ligated via a 10th intercostal space thoracotomy (right side in dogs, left side in cats). Ligate the duct as close to the diaphragm as possible, and be sure to occlude all branches. Postligation lymphangiography then confirms complete occlusion of the thoracic duct system. The details of these procedures are provided in Chapter 83.
- The reported success rate of this procedure varies from 20–60% in cats and 55–60% in dogs. Commercially available pump devices (e.g., Hakim-Cordis ventricular-peritoneal catheter, Cordis Corporation, Miami, FL; double-valve Denver peritoneal-venous catheter, Denver Biomaterials Inc., Evergreen, CO) are available for active pleuroperitoneal shunting of chylous effusion in refractory chylothorax. Disadvantages of shunt devices are that they are expensive, they are easily occluded, they require considerable owner compliance, and the complication rate is high.
- When chylothorax is unresponsive to thoracic duct ligation or shunt procedures, pleurodesis using intrapleural instillation of a sclerosing agent such as tetracycline or sterile talc may be palliative. Pleurodesis is intended to reduce or stop pleural effusion by causing diffuse adhesions between the parietal and visceral pleura. It is an effective technique in humans but has not been efficacious in dogs either with experimental or spontaneous effusion.

Complications

Chronic diffuse fibrosing pleuritis is a sequela of chylothorax that may cause constriction and collapse of lung lobes and restrict the expandability of the lungs. Radiographically, fibrosing pleuritis is indicated by rounded lung lobe borders and atelectasis of cranial or middle lobes. The atelectatic lobes may be mistaken for pulmonary masses, hilar masses, or lung lobe torsion. In order to avoid excessive pleural fibrosis, surgical intervention in animals with chylothorax, especially cats, should not be delayed. Surgical removal of the layer of fibrin and fibrotic reaction covering the visceral pleura, a process called decortication, is difficult in cats and usually results in significant laceration of underlying lung tissue that requires continuous pleural drainage for postoperative pneumothorax and effusion.

Feline Infectious Peritonitis
Etiology

Feline infectious peritonitis is a highly fatal chronic progressive coronaviral infection of cats characterized by widespread immune complex-mediated vasculitis and pyogranulomatous inflammation (see Chap. 8 for a comprehensive description of the disease). In the effusive form of FIP, exudative peritonitis or pleuritis may occur.

Clinical Signs

Pleural involvement is manifested as dyspnea and by other signs of pleural effusion, often accompanied by nonspecific signs such as anorexia, depression, fever, and pallor. Pericardial effusion due to fibrinous pericarditis may accompany pleural FIP and is detectable by echocardiography, but only rarely is this extensive enough to cause cardiac tamponade.

Diagnosis

- The diagnosis can usually be established by analysis of a specimen of pleural fluid obtained by thoracentesis. The fluid of FIP is a nonseptic exudate, often described as pyogranulomatous or fibrinous. It is typically pale yellow to golden in color, nearly translucent because of its relatively low cell count (usually 1000–10,000 nucleated cells/µl), and foamy because of its high protein content. The fluid of FIP may seem viscous, tenacious, and sticky, and it may contain flecks, strands, or clots of fibrin. The concentration of protein often approaches that of serum, ranging from 4–10 g/dl. Fluid protein electrophoresis is a reliable diagnostic indicator of FIP when gamma globulin composes more than 32% of the protein, albumin is less than 48% of the protein, and the albumin-to-globulin ratio is less than 0.81. A somewhat distinctive mixture of inflammatory cells characterizes the pyogranulomatous nature of FIP exudate, with nondegenerate neutrophils and macrophages predominating, but also including plasma cells and lymphocytes.
- Ancillary laboratory findings that may support the diagnosis of FIP include neutrophilic leukocytosis, neutropenia, lymphopenia, normocytic-normochromic nonregenerative anemia, and hyperglobulinemia.
- A high serum titer of anticoronaviral antibody indicates the possibility of FIP but is not a confirmatory test. A polymerase chain reaction (PCR) test for coronavirus in pleural fluid is a useful diagnostic aid (low sensitivity but high specificity) providing a validated assay is used.

Treatment

In general, the results of treatment of FIP have been disappointing, and the prognosis must be considered poor. Nevertheless, occasional remissions have been obtained with immunosuppressive therapy and with drainage of the intrapleural exudate (see Chap. 8).

Congestive Heart Failure
Etiology

Pleural effusion can be a manifestation of CHF in dogs and cats (Ch. 64). It is most commonly associated with cardiomyopathy (see Chap. 66), but also occurs with cardiac arrhythmias, congenital cardiac defects, peri-

cardial diseases, heartworm disease, and hyperthyroid cardiomyopathy. Although pleural effusion is considered primarily a sign of right-sided CHF, animals with severe or chronic left-sided failure also develop pleural effusion.

Clinical Signs

In animals with pleural effusion due to heart disease, presenting signs often include tachypnea, dyspnea, depression, inactivity, and weakness. Anorexia and vomiting may also be observed. Physical findings that may indicate a cardiogenic cause for pleural effusion include:

- Signs of low cardiac output, such as pallor, hypothermia, cold extremities and pinnae, and weak femoral pulses
- Jugular venous distention, jugular pulsation, or positive hepatojugular reflex
- Concurrent hepatomegaly (due to hepatic congestion) or ascites (although, unlike dogs, cats rarely develop significant ascites from CHF)
- Abnormalities of cardiac auscultation, such as murmurs, diastolic gallops, or arrhythmias
- Ophthalmoscopic lesions of taurine-deficient retinopathy in cats (see Chap. 157)
- A palpable thyroid nodule in hyperthyroid cats

Diagnosis

The diagnosis of cardiogenic pleural effusion can be difficult because the effusion may muffle the heart sounds on auscultation and obscure the cardiac silhouette on thoracic radiographs.

- Radiographic findings that suggest pleural effusion is associated with CHF include cardiomegaly, pulmonary infiltrates (edema), pulmonary venous distention, distended caudal vena cava, and hepatomegaly. In many cases, these findings are more apparent on radiographs taken after fluid has been drained from the pleural space.
- Pleural fluid analysis may determine the effusate to be a transudate, modified transudate, or chylous effusion, the predominant cells being erythrocytes, mesothelial cells, and small lymphocytes.
- Other methods of cardiac imaging, especially echocardiography and sometimes angiocardiography, may be necessary to confirm and assess cardiac disease. Cardiac arrhythmias and conduction disturbances are evaluated electrocardiographically.

Treatment

The treatment options for CHF as described in Chapter 64 are employed for control of cardiogenic pleural effusion.

Intrathoracic Neoplasia
Etiology

Intrathoracic neoplasia is one of the most common causes of pleural effusion in dogs and cats. Causes of neoplastic pleural effusion include mediastinal lymphoma and thymoma, primary and metastatic pulmonary neoplasia (see Chap. 81), and malignant pleural mesothelioma. The mechanism of pleural effusion in these conditions generally involves hemolymphatic obstruction.

Diagnosis

- Use radiography (both right and left lateral views) and ultrasonography to characterize or identify the location of an intrathoracic mass (see Chap. 75).
- The fluid can vary from modified transudate to nonseptic exudate to chylous effusion. Lymphoma is usually diagnosed cytologically. Confirmation of nonlymphomatous intrathoracic neoplasia can be a diagnostic challenge. Clumps of reactive mesothelial cells exfoliate into pleural effusions and are easily mistaken for neoplastic cells, especially carcinoma cells. Ideally, similar-appearing cells should be aspirated from pulmonary or intrathoracic masses before a definitive diagnosis of neoplasia is made. Conversely, many primary and metastatic tumors do not exfoliate cells into pleural fluid; thus, an absence of neoplastic cells in pleural effusion does not necessarily exclude neoplasia as the cause.

Treatment

Chemotherapy for mediastinal lymphoma is discussed in Chapter 25. The surgical aspects of intrathoracic neoplasia (thoracotomy, lobectomy) are discussed in Chapter 83.

Hemothorax

Etiology

- Hemothorax, the accumulation of blood within the pleural space, may be associated with any form of thoracic trauma that lacerates the lung parenchyma or ruptures intrathoracic vessels (see Chap. 82). It can also be caused by disorders of hemostasis (see Chap. 21) or by intrathoracic neoplasms that rupture or erode into vessels. Lung lobe torsion and pulmonary infarction are rare causes.
- The seriousness of hemothorax depends on the rate and volume of blood loss. Bleeding from the venous circulation or the low-pressure pulmonary arterial circulation is usually self-limiting, whereas bleeding from high-pressure systemic arteries, such as the intercostal or bronchoesophageal arteries, may be more severe. Hemorrhage due to injury of the heart or great vessels results in massive hemothorax that is rapidly fatal.
- The two major consequences of hemothorax are shock due to loss of circulating blood volume into the pleural space and ventilatory impairment due to fluid compression of the lung. As a general rule, in rapidly developing hemothorax, fatal circulatory failure (exsanguination) occurs before the volume of pleural fluid that accumulates is sufficient to cause serious respiratory compromise. However, blood or fluid replacement therapy in the presence of continued bleeding may lead to greater accumulation of intrapleural fluid, resulting in severe lung compression and ventilatory failure.

Clinical Signs

Clinical signs of hemothorax are attributed to shock and pleural effusion—dyspnea, tachypnea, weakness, pallor, and weak femoral pulses.

Diagnosis

- The heart and lung sounds are usually muffled, and percussion of the ventral thorax may be hyporesonant. In the trauma victim, this is distinguished from the hyperresonance of pneumothorax.
- Confirm intrapleural fluid radiographically.
- Definitive diagnosis is made by aspiration of defibrinated (nonclotting) blood from the pleural space. Blood clots rapidly (within 45 minutes) in the pleural space; thus, unless there is ongoing or very recent bleeding, the aspirated hemorrhagic effusion will not clot or contain platelets.

Treatment

The treatment of hemothorax involves treatment of shock with intravenous fluids or blood, as well as relief of respiratory distress via thoracentesis if necessary. See Chapter 82 for more details on treatment of hemothorax.

Lung Lobe Torsion

Etiology

Torsions of either the right middle lung lobe or the right or left cranial lung lobe have occasionally been found in dogs and cats with pleural effusions. The mechanism of lung lobe displacement that culminates in torsion is poorly understood. Lung lobe torsion can occur secondary to pleural effusion, or it can be the cause of a serosanguineous effusion.

Clinical Signs

The signs usually include dyspnea, tachypnea, depression, anorexia, and weight loss.

Diagnosis

- The diagnosis of lung lobe torsion is suggested by visualization of a consolidated cranial or middle lung lobe on post-thoracentesis radiographs. Radiographic differential diagnoses for lobar consolidation should include pneumonia, edema, hemorrhage, atelectasis, and neoplasia.
- The pleural fluid may be nonspecific (i.e., nonseptic exudate), or it may reflect the underlying disease state (i.e., chylous, septic, or neoplastic effusion).
- Ultrasonography is helpful for identifying lung lobe torsion in some animals with pleural effusion.
- Confirmation of lung lobe torsion can only be made by thoracotomy in many cases.

Treatment

The treatment is lung lobectomy of the affected lobe (see Chap. 83).

Thymic Branchial Cysts

Branchial cysts develop from vestiges of the fetal branchial arch system. These are rare, but when they develop in the thymus they produce an encapsulated, multilobulated, multicystic mass in the cranial mediastinum that compresses adjacent structures and usually causes pleural effusion. Pleural fluid is blood-tinged and characteristic of modified transudate (obstructive pattern) or nonseptic exudate. On the basis of their radiographic appearance, thymic branchial cysts must be differentiated from other cranial mediastinal masses such as lymphoma and thymoma (see under Intrathoracic Neoplasia). Because of their cystic nature, branchial cysts should be distinguishable from solid mediastinal masses by ultrasonography. Treat branchial cysts by surgical resection.

Diaphragmatic Hernia

Pleural effusion can be a complication of diaphragmatic hernia, especially when the liver or omentum is incarcerated in the hernia. The effusion can complicate the radiographic diagnosis of diaphragmatic hernia. The pleural fluid is usually a modified transudate, but in some cases it may be blood or chyle. Diaphragmatic hernia is discussed further in Chapter 82.

Pancreatitis-Associated Effusion

Mild transient pleural effusion has occasionally been associated with acute pancreatitis. Accompanying peritoneal effusion may also be present. Pleural effusion is a well-known complication of pancreatitis in humans; the pathogenesis is not fully understood, but it has been attributed to chemical pleuritis associated with toxins and activated pancreatic enzymes such as lipase reaching the pleural cavity via intercommunicating lymphatics. Generalized vascular injury and increased vascular permeability associated with acute pancreatitis may also play a role. The pleural effusion is usually a small volume and self-limiting with resolution of the pancreatitis; thus, no specific treatment is necessary. See Chapter 93 for further discussion of pancreatitis.

Pulmonary Thromboembolism

Pleural effusion can occur in association with pulmonary thromboembolism whenever it is extensive enough to produce infarction and ischemic necrosis of the lung and inflammation of adjacent pleura.

- Clinical signs are unresponsive dyspnea and signs of right-sided heart failure.
- Underlying causes of pulmonary thromboembolism include heartworm disease, pulmonary neoplasia, and hypercoagulability caused by septicemia, amyloidosis, hyperadrenocorticism, and immune-mediated hemolysis.
- The effusion is usually a modified transudate or nonseptic exudate, but secondary infection of the infarcted lung can result in a septic effusion.
- Radiographically, blunted pulmonary arteries, hypovascularity of the affected lung, and evidence of right-sided heart enlargement or failure suggest pulmonary thromboembolism; however, the diagnosis can be difficult to document because radiographic abnormalities may be absent or very subtle.
- Specialized procedures such as right ventricular and pulmonary artery pressure measurements, angiography, and radionuclide lung perfusion scan may be required for definitive diagnosis.
- Treatment is based on resolving the underlying cause of the thromboembolism, providing pleural drainage as needed, supplemental oxygen therapy, and control of secondary bacterial infection.

81 Respiratory Neoplasia

Marcia Carothers

Neoplasms of the respiratory tract are relatively uncommon in small animals, representing 4–5% of all neoplasms in the dog and cat. More than 80% of respiratory tract tumors are malignant. In addition to primary tumors affecting the respiratory tract, the lungs are common sites of metastatic neoplasia.

NEOPLASMS OF THE NASAL PASSAGES AND PARANASAL SINUSES

Neoplasms of the nasal cavity are more common in dogs than in cats and constitute approximately 75% of all respiratory tract tumors in dogs. The prevalence of sinonasal tumors has been reported to be 0.3–2.4% in dogs and 4.2% in cats. Approximately 80% of primary nasal tumors are malignant. Nasal tumors are more likely to originate in the caudal two-thirds of the nasal passages and often invade the sinuses. Local invasion of the surrounding tissues is typical of these tumors. Paraneoplastic syndromes are rare and include hypercalcemia (associated with an adenocarcinoma) and polycythemia (associated with fibrosarcoma).

Tumor Types

- Histologically, epithelial tumors are most common, representing 60–75% of all nasal tumors. Adenocarcinomas (31%), squamous cell carcinomas (28%), and chondrosarcomas (12%) occur most frequently. Benign tumors are rare.
- Although nasal tumors are locally invasive, approximately 40% have distant metastasis at the time of necropsy. Mesenchymal tumors have the lowest rate of metastasis and neuroendocrine tumors and esthesioneuroblastomas have the highest rate (80–100%). Brain, lymph nodes, lung and liver are the sites of metastasis.
- Table 81–1 lists tumors of the nasal passages and paranasal sinus occurring in dogs and cats.

▼ *Key Point* Malignant nasal tumors usually are locally invasive, with metastasis occurring late in the course of the disease.

Signalment

- Nasal tumors are more common in older animals. Mean ages range from 7–12 years in dogs, with chon-

drosarcomas having the lower mean (7 years) and neuroendocrine tumors having the higher mean (12 years). Cats have reported mean ages of 8–10 years.
- In one study (Patnaik, 1989), male canines had a slight sex predilection (1.8 : 1.0), while other studies report no significant sex predilection. Male cats appear to be at higher risk than female cats.
- Dolichocephalic and medium- to large-breed dogs are predisposed to developing nasal neoplasms. Canine breeds reported to be at high risk for the development of nasal neoplasms include the Airedale terrier, bassett hound, Old English sheepdog, Scottish terrier, collie, German shepherd, keeshond, and German short-haired pointer.

History

- The average duration of clinical signs prior to diagnosis is approximately 3 months.

Table 81–1. NEOPLASMS OF THE NASAL PASSAGES AND PARANASAL SINUSES*

Malignant Tumors in Dogs
Epithelial tumors
  Adenocarcinoma
  Squamous cell carcinoma
Mesenchymal tumors
  Chondrosarcoma
  Osteosarcoma
  Lymphoma
  Fibrosarcoma
  Fibrous histiocytoma
Miscellaneous tumors
  Neuroendocrine tumors
  Esthesioneuroblastoma
  Transmissible venereal tumor
  Mast cell tumor

Malignant Tumors in Cats
Squamous cell carcinoma
Adenocarcinoma
Lymphoma—usually feline leukemia virus (FeLV) negative
Undifferentiated carcinoma
Esthesioneuroblastoma
Fibrosarcoma

Benign Tumors in Dogs and Cats
Polyps (more common in cats)
Adenoma
Fibroma
Chondroma

*Listed in decreasing order of frequency.

- Sneezing, nasal discharge, epistaxis, and epiphora are the most common presenting signs.
- A partial response to antibiotic therapy can be observed initially; however, intermittent and progressive signs continue.

Clinical Signs

- *Unilateral or bilateral nasal discharge* (hemorrhagic, serohemorrhagic or mucopurulent) and/or ocular discharge are the most common signs noted.
- Sneezing, snoring, or reverse sneezing may also be reported by the owner.
- Facial deformity (i.e., exophthalmos and nasal swelling) is common in dogs with skeletal neoplasms and may occur late in the course of other types of nasal tumors.
- Seizures, blindness, and behavioral changes may result from invasion of the central nervous system (CNS) by direct extension. CNS involvement has been reported in 20% of cases and is more common in neuroendocrine tumors and esthesioneuroblastomas.

▼ *Key Point* Chronic nasal discharge unresponsive to antibiotic therapy is most likely caused by neoplasia.

Diagnosis

Imaging Studies

- Plain radiographs (occlusal dorsoventral, open-mouth ventrodorsal, lateral, frontal sinuses, and ventrodorsal views) may demonstrate loss of trabecular pattern, increase in soft tissue density, septal destruction, facial bone destruction, frontal sinus opacification, and/or periosteal bone formation (see Chaps. 4 and 75).
- Computed tomography (CT) or magnetic resonance imaging (MRI) are useful for evaluating the extent of the tumor and for planning radiation therapy.

Cytology and Histopathology Studies

Cytologic and/or histologic confirmation is diagnostic. Procedures (and their specific uses) include:

- *Rhinoscopy* (performed with cystoscope or arthroscope)—for viewing the tumor and acquiring tissue for cytology, histopathology, and culture. Retrograde rhinoscopy using a retroflexed endoscope or a dental mirror can demonstrate tumors extending caudal to the posterior choanae.
- *Nasal flushes*—for cytologic identification (see Chap. 76 for technique).
- *Blind biopsy procedures* using a biopsy needle, catheter, or polypropylene tube (covering of intravenous catheter)—to obtain diagnostic specimen for cytology-histopathology (see Chap. 76).

▼ *Key Point* Premeasure nasal biopsy devices to avoid penetration of the cribriform plate.

- *Rhinotomy and nasal exploratory surgery*—for direct exposure of the tumor and to obtain larger biopsy specimens.
- *Transnasal curettage* (through nostril)—to obtain tissue specimens for cytology and histopathology.

Treatment

Surgical Cytoreduction

Surgical cytoreduction alone or followed by radiation therapy has been reported, but is less favored based on current information.

- Rhinotomy (nasal flap) with curettage or turbinectomy is the most common procedure (see Chap. 76).
- Transnasal curettage using a uterine curette and suction may be less invasive.
- Survival times for animals treated with surgical cytoreduction alone are similar to that for untreated animals.
- Survival times may be improved in some cases with combination surgical cytoreduction and orthovoltage radiation therapy.

Radiation Therapy

In radiation therapy (orthovoltage, cesium, cobalt, or linear accelerator), the dose and fractionation of treatment is determined by tumor type and source of radiation (for specific recommendations, consult a radiologist or oncologist).

- Radiation therapy has been shown to increase survival times in dogs and cats with nasal tumors. Orthovoltage (due to low tissue penetration) is effective only when combined with surgical cytoreduction.
- Brachytherapy using iridium-192 has been used to treat nasal tumors with lower survival times (7.1 month median) compared with other forms of radiation therapy.

Complications

The following post-treatment complications have been reported:

- Rhinitis may be severe but usually subsides within 2 months.
- A slight nasal discharge and sneezing may persist.
- Ulcerative dermatitis usually occurs at the irradiated site but generally responds to topical therapy.
- Ocular complications of nasal radiation may include keratoconjunctivitis sicca, corneal ulcers, uveitis, retinal degeneration, and cataract formation.

Chemotherapy

Chemotherapy may be effective in certain tumor types (see Chap. 24 for discussion of chemotherapy).

- Combination drugs (doxorubicin, cyclophosphamide, vincristine, 5-fluorouracil) have been used to treat adenocarcinoma, lymphoma, and transmissible venereal tumor.

- Single-agent therapy with dactinomycin, doxorubicin, cisplatin, and mitoxantrone has had variable results.
- Myelosuppression, anorexia, vomiting, diarrhea, and lethargy may occur secondary to chemotherapy.

▼ *Key Point* To maximize survival times and reduce complications of radiotherapy, include CT or MRI with radiation therapy planning to provide optimal treatment fields and minimize exposure to normal tissues (i.e., eyes and brain).

Prognosis

Prognostic factors include histologic type and tumor size. Survival times of 3–5 months have been reported for animals with no treatment.

- Prognosis for nasal polyps is good, but recurrence is possible.
- Dogs with adenocarcinoma or sarcoma have longer median survival times than dogs with undifferentiated or squamous cell carcinoma.
- Larger and more extensive tumors have a poorer prognosis; however, animals with facial deformity may respond to radiation therapy as well as those with no deformity.
- In cats with nasal tumors, radiation therapy has had good results.

NEOPLASMS OF THE LARYNX

Table 81–2 lists the types of laryngeal neoplasms seen in dogs and cats. These tumors are uncommon and usually are locally invasive; however, distant metastasis has been reported.

Table 81–2. NEOPLASMS OF THE LARYNX

Primary Malignant Tumors in Dogs
Squamous cell carcinoma
Lymphoma
Osteosarcoma
Melanoma
Mast cell tumor
Adenocarcinoma
Chondrosarcoma

Metastatic Tumors in Dogs
Thyroid carcinoma
Lymphoma
Pharyngeal rhabdomyosarcoma

Primary Malignant Tumors in Cats
Lymphoma
Squamous cell carcinoma
Adenocarcinoma

Benign Tumors in Dogs and Cats (Uncommon)
Unilateral polyps, generally inflammatory in origin
Oncocytoma* and rhabdomyoma
Leiomyoma

*The second most common laryngeal tumor in dogs. See text for description.

Malignant neoplasms are more common than benign tumors. However, oncocytomas, which are usually benign, are the second most common laryngeal tumor in dogs. Oncocytes are epithelial cells sporadically present within the seromucinous glands of the upper airway. There is some speculation that oncocytomas may be a form of rhabdomyoma. Rhabdomyomas are large tumors in dogs that are minimally invasive.

Signalment

- Laryngeal tumors occur in middle-aged to older animals (5–15 years) with the exception of oncocytomas and rhabdomyomas, which occur in young to middle-aged dogs (2–8 years).
- Males appear to be at increased risk.

History

- *Noisy breathing* and *respiratory distress* are the most common complaints reported.
- *Exercise intolerance, change in voice,* and *loss of bark or purr* may be noted by the owner.

Clinical Signs

- *Inspiratory dyspnea* and *cyanosis* usually occur when the animal is stressed. *Laryngeal stridor* is common on inspiration.
- Coughing due to *aspiration pneumonia* may occur secondary to laryngeal dysfunction.
- Palpable laryngeal masses are uncommon except with rhabdomyomas.

▼ *Key Point* Inspiratory dyspnea is the most common sign of laryngeal obstructive disease. Neoplasia must be differentiated from laryngeal paralysis, foreign body, or other obstructive upper airway disorder via laryngoscopy.

Diagnosis

- The history and physical findings may suggest laryngeal disease.
- Radiography may demonstrate laryngeal distortion, increased soft tissue density of the larynx, and decreased laryngeal space.
- Laryngoscopic evaluation (using a laryngoscope or endoscope) may reveal a laryngeal swelling or mass.
- Biopsy and histopathology provide a definitive diagnosis. Biopsy with alligator biopsy forceps, needle biopsy instruments, or bronchoscopic biopsy forceps is usually successful in obtaining a diagnosis.

Treatment

Surgery

Surgical excision may be curative if the tumor is benign, but it only provides palliation for malignant disease. Complete laryngectomy with a permanent tracheostomy (see Chap. 77) has been done rarely in veterinary medicine because of associated complications.

Radiation Therapy

Radiation may be beneficial in the treatment of some laryngeal tumors (e.g., squamous cell carcinoma, mast cell tumor, lymphoma).

Chemotherapy

Chemotherapy for laryngeal tumors has been reported rarely.

- Lymphoma usually responds to combination chemotherapy (see Chap. 25), but little information is available concerning laryngeal lymphoma.
- Mast cell tumors, adenocarcinomas, and sarcomas may respond to chemotherapy (see Chaps. 24 and 26).

Prognosis

The prognosis for most laryngeal tumors is guarded because advanced disease usually is present at the time of diagnosis. However, if tumors are benign (e.g., polyps, oncocytomas, rhabdomyomas), the prognosis is good with surgical excision.

NEOPLASMS OF THE TRACHEA

Tracheal tumors are rare in dogs and cats. See Table 81–3 for common types of tumors.

Signalment

Young animals are at higher risk for osteochondroma.

▼ *Key Point* Tracheal tumors are rare; consider them malignant in older animals.

History

Exercise intolerance, panting, and *cough* may be present for weeks prior to presentation.

Clinical Signs

- *Cough,* usually nonproductive, is the most common sign.

Table 81–3. NEOPLASMS OF THE TRACHEA

Malignant Tumors in Dogs
Osteosarcoma
Chondrosarcoma
Lymphoma
Mast cell tumor
Adenocarcinoma

Malignant Tumors in Cats
Adenocarcinoma
Lymphoma
Squamous cell carcinoma

Benign Tumors in Dogs and Cats
Osteochondroma (dogs)
Leiomyoma
Polyps
Eosinophilic granuloma (cats)
Nodular amyloidosis (dogs)

- *Stridor,* usually inspiratory, may be noted during exercise or panting.
- Tumors located at the carina cause both inspiratory and expiratory respiratory distress.
- *Cyanosis, dyspnea,* and *collapse* may occur with severe obstruction.

Diagnosis

- *Radiography* may demonstrate a soft tissue density within the tracheal lumen or decrease in lumen size.
- *Bronchoscopy* may be needed to reveal a tracheal mass.
- *Biopsy* and *histopathology* are diagnostic.

Treatment

Surgical Excision

Surgery is the primary treatment for tracheal masses (see Chap. 77).

- Benign lesions may be cured with surgical resection.
- Tracheal resection and end-to-end anastomosis is usually the most appropriate surgical treatment (see Chap. 77).

Chemotherapy

Cyclophosphamide, vincristine, and prednisone can prolong survival in animals with lymphoma (see Chap. 25).

Prognosis

Benign tumors respond well to surgical excision. Little information regarding treatment and prognosis is available for most tracheal tumors.

NEOPLASMS OF THE LUNG

Primary pulmonary neoplasms represent approximately 1.2% and 0.5% of all tumors in the dog and cat, respectively. Primary lung tumors may metastasize to bronchial lymph nodes, lung, brain, bone, and pleura via lymphatics, airways, blood vessels, and transpleural spread.

Paraneoplastic syndromes may be associated with primary pulmonary neoplasms.

- Hypertrophic osteopathy is the most common paraneoplastic syndrome associated with large lung masses and has been reported in 3–15% of animals with pulmonary neoplasia.
- Other paraneoplastic syndromes include paraplegia and subclinical neuromyopathy, hypercalcemia, neutrophilic leukocytosis associated with metastatic fibrosarcoma, and secretion of adrenocorticotropic hormone resulting in clinical signs of hyperadrenocorticism.

▼ *Key Point* Pulmonary neoplasia is the most likely diagnosis in dogs with hypertrophic osteopathy.

Tumor Types (see Table 81–4)

Primary Pulmonary Neoplasms. Carcinomas are the most common primary lung tumors in dogs. In primary

Table 81–4. PULMONARY NEOPLASMS

Primary Tumors in Dogs
Carcinoma
  Bronchoalveolar adenocarcinoma (>70%)
  Epidermoid (squamous cell)
  Bronchogenic or bronchial gland
  Anaplastic or alveolar (small cell, large cell, adenomatous)
Sarcoma (uncommon)
  Lymphoma
  Fibrosarcoma
  Hemangiosarcoma
  Osteosarcoma
Miscellaneous
  Lymphomatoid granulomatosis
  Malignant histiocytosis (in Bernese mountain dogs)
Benign
  Adenoma
  Fibroma
Primary Tumors in Cats
Carcinoma
  Adenocarcinoma (papillary, bronchoalveolar)
  Epidermoid (squamous cell)
  Bronchial gland
Sarcoma (rare)
  Hemangiosarcoma
  Spindle cell
  Reticulum cell
Benign (rare)
  Bronchial adenoma
  Hemangioma
Metastatic Tumors in Dogs and Cats
Mammary carcinoma
Osteosarcoma
Thyroid carcinoma
Transitional cell carcinoma
Melanoma
Hemangiosarcoma
Squamous cell carcinoma

pulmonary adenocarcinomas and epidermoid carcinomas, 50% and 80%, respectively, have metastasized at the time of diagnosis.

Metastatic Pulmonary Neoplasms. These tumors are more common than primary pulmonary neoplasms. Metastasis occurs by spread of tumor emboli via lymphatics or blood vessels. Because of the capillary network in the lungs, these tumor emboli are trapped and may proliferate and form nodules. See Table 81–4 for a list of common metastatic tumors.

Signalment

- Pulmonary neoplasms occur in older animals (>10 years), except lymphomatoid granulomatosis, which occurs in young dogs (1–6 years).
- Most studies do not recognize a breed or sex predilection; however, boxers and Bernese mountain dogs have been reported to be at increased risk for primary lung tumors.
- Larger dogs (>10 kg) may be at increased risk.

History

History may vary depending on the tumor type, size, and doubling time. Many dogs are asymptomatic, and pulmonary nodules are discovered during a medical workup.

Clinical Signs

- Approximately 25% of dogs have no clinical abnormalities.
- *Cough* (harsh, nonproductive) is one of the most common presenting signs. The duration is usually chronic, and occasionally hemoptysis is also present.
- *Dyspnea, tachypnea,* and *cyanosis* may be present and associated with pleural effusion and/or diffuse disease.
- *Decreased exercise tolerance* is usually related to respiratory compromise.
- Less common signs include anorexia, fever, weight loss, dysphagia, vomiting, and regurgitation.
- *Lameness* may be associated with hypertrophic osteopathy or with skeletal muscle and/or bone metastasis. Cats may present with multiple digit swellings and lameness associated with metastasis from primary pulmonary tumors (adenocarcinomas and squamous cell carcinomas).

Diagnosis
Radiography

Routine thoracic radiographs usually establish the diagnosis of a mass lesion(s). However, approximately 11% of pulmonary neoplasms are missed on survey radiographs because of:

- Small size of the lesions (<5–10 mm).
- Lack of tumor contrast with pulmonary parenchyma or tumor site in a hidden location (e.g., the subpleural space or paraspinal recesses).
- Presence of pleural fluid.
- Atelectasis of one or more lung lobes.

▼ *Key Point* Some clinicians recommend evaluating three radiographic views (ventrodorsal, right, and left lateral) of the thorax when primary or metastatic pulmonary neoplasia is suspected.

Radiographic Pattern

The most common radiographic pattern seen in dogs and cats with metastatic neoplasms is that of circumscribed nodules. Patterns include:

- Solitary circumscribed nodule
- Multiple circumscribed nodules
- Interstitial disseminated reticulonodular pattern
- Mixed disseminated alveolar pattern
- Homogeneous lobar consolidation

Other Diagnostic Signs

- Radiographic changes associated with pulmonary tumors include pleural effusions, pleural thickening, and thoracic lymphadenopathy.
- Calcification and cavitation of masses have been associated with adenocarcinomas.
- The right side and caudal lung lobes are the most common locations of primary pulmonary neoplasms

in dogs. The left lung lobes are affected more often than the right side in cats.

Other Diagnostic Evaluations

- *Percutaneous transthoracic fine-needle aspiration or biopsy* for cytologic or histologic evaluation may provide a diagnosis in 50% of cases.
- *Cytologic evaluation* of tracheal wash fluid, bronchoalveolar lavage fluid, and pleural fluid may detect neoplastic cells in some cases.
- *Bronchoscopy* may be valuable in perihilar masses.
- *Exploratory thoracotomy* (see Chap. 83) and biopsy provide a definitive diagnosis and aid in staging the tumor. Lobectomy may be curative for an isolated mass lesion without lymphatic metastasis.
- *Thoracoscopy* may be used to obtain a diagnosis in the case of multiple pulmonary lesions.

Treatment

Surgical Excision

Surgical excision by lobectomy is the treatment of choice for solitary lung tumors (see Chap. 83).

- Obtain biopsy samples from regional lymph nodes when possible.
- Adjunctive chemotherapy may improve survival in some cases in which metastasis or local invasion is present.

▼ *Key Point* Always submit lung tumors for histopathologic evaluation to establish diagnosis and prognosis.

Chemotherapy

Chemotherapy may be beneficial in some tumors.

- Lymphomatoid granulomatosis may respond to combination chemotherapy with prednisone, vincristine, and cyclophosphamide (see Chap. 24 for dosages).
- Malignant histiocytosis in Bernese mountain dogs may respond to doxorubicin, cyclophosphamide, and vincristine (see Chap. 24 for dosages).
- Complete and partial responses have been reported in the treatment of metastatic neoplasms (hemangiosarcoma, thyroid carcinomas, squamous cell carcinoma, mammary adenocarcinomas) with doxorubicin, cyclophosphamide, and vincristine (see Chap. 24 for dosages).

Prognosis

- Factors that decrease survival time include large tumor burden, thoracic lymph node involvement, and other metastases. Absence of lymphatic invasion by the lung tumor has been associated with increased survival times.
- Small (<5 cm), solitary primary lung tumors without metastasis or malignant effusion are associated with prolonged survival (>1 year). Even large lobar masses can be removed successfully with a reasonable (>6 months) survival time, provided metastases have not yet developed.
- In cats, the prognosis is poor because >75% of primary lung tumors are inoperable at the time of diagnosis.
- Following treatment, monitor with routine thoracic radiographs every 1–3 months.

SUPPLEMENTAL READINGS

Adams WM, Withrow SJ, Walshaw R, et al: Radiotherapy of malignant nasal tumors in 67 dogs. J Am Vet Med Assoc 191:311, 1987.

Carlisle CH, Biery DN, Thrall DE: Tracheal and laryngeal tumors in the dog and cat: Literature review and 13 additional patients. Vet Radiol 32:229, 1991.

Carothers MA, Couto GC: Respiratory neoplasia. *In* Kirk RW, ed.: Current Veterinary Therapy X. Philadelphia: WB Saunders, 1989, p 399.

Evans SM, Goldschmidt M, McKee LJ, et al.: Prognostic factors and survival after radiotherapy for canine intranasal neoplasms: 70 cases (1974–1985). J Am Vet Med Assoc 194:1460, 1989.

Lang J, Wortman FA, Glickman LT, et al.: Sensitivity of radiographic detection of lung metastases in the dog. Vet Radiol 27:74, 1986.

Madewell BR, Priester WA, Gillette EL, Snyder SP: Neoplasms of the nasal passages and paranasal sinuses in domesticated animals as reported by 13 veterinary colleges. Am J Vet Res 37:851, 1976.

Madewell BR, Theilen GH: Tumors of the respiratory tract and thorax. *In* Theilen GH, Madewell BR, ed.: Veterinary Cancer Medicine. Philadelphia: Lea & Febiger, 1987, p 535.

May C, Newsholme SJ: Metastasis of feline pulmonary carcinoma as multiple digit swelling. J Small Anim Pract 30:302, 1989.

McEntee MC, Page RL, Heidner GL, et al.: A retrospective study of 27 dogs with intranasal neoplasms treated with cobalt radiation. Vet Radiol 32:135, 1991.

Mehlhaff CJ, Mooney BA: Primary pulmonary neoplasia in the dog and cat. Vet Clin North Am 15:1061, 1985.

Ogilvie GK, Haschek WM, Withrow SJ, et al.: Classification of primary lung tumors in dogs: 210 cases (1975–1985). J Am Vet Med Assoc 195:106, 1989.

Ogilvie GK, LaRue SM: Canine and feline nasal and paranasal sinus tumors. Vet Clin North Am 22:1133, 1992.

Ogilvie GK, Weigel RM, Haschek WM, et al.: Prognostic factors for tumor remission and survival in dogs after surgery for primary lung tumor: 76 cases (1975–1985). J Am Vet Med Assoc 195:106, 1989.

Patnaik AK: Canine sinonasal neoplasms: Clinicopathological study of 285 cases. J Am Anim Hosp Assoc 25:103, 1989.

Saik JE, Toll SL, Diters RW, Goldschmidt MH: Canine and feline laryngeal neoplasia: A 10-year survey. J Am Anim Hosp Assoc 22:359, 1986.

Thrall DE, Harvery CE: Radiotherapy of malignant nasal tumors in 21 dogs. J Am Vet Med Assoc 183:663, 1983.

Wheeldon EB, Suter PF, Jenkins T: Neoplasia of the larynx in the dog. J Am Vet Med Assoc 180:642, 1982.

Withrow SJ: Tumors of the respiratory system. *In* Withrow SJ, MacEwen EG, ed.: Clinical Veterinary Oncology. Philadelphia: JB Lippincott, 1989, p 215.

82 Thoracic Trauma

Dale E. Bjorling

Thoracic trauma in dogs and cats most often is the result of automobile accidents. The lack of apparent external injuries often is misleading; the diaphragm, thoracic wall, heart, or lungs may be severely damaged with little apparent damage to the overlying skin. Evaluate animals presented for treatment of thoracic trauma thoroughly but rapidly; if necessary, institute treatment prior to completing a full patient assessment. Animals with thoracic trauma may suffer concurrent abdominal injuries.

Surgical correction of injuries associated with thoracic trauma may be required on an emergency basis; however, in general veterinary practice it is preferable to avoid emergency surgery of animals suffering thoracic trauma unless absolutely necessary.

This chapter discusses the major disorders caused by thoracic trauma: pulmonary and myocardial contusions, pneumothorax, rib fractures and flail chest, hemothorax, and diaphragmatic hernia; see Chapter 80 for discussion of chylothorax.

Injuries to abdominal viscera are discussed in respective organ-system chapters.

ETIOLOGY

Blunt Trauma

- Blunt trauma to the thoracic cavity usually is the result of automobile accidents. It may also be the result of a kick by a human or farm animal (horse, cow), being struck by a heavy object, or falling from heights (e.g., falling from a window of high-rise buildings).
- The severity of injury depends on the mass of the object delivering the blow, the velocity of the object, and the area to which the blow is delivered. It has been shown experimentally that when a blow equivalent to that delivered by a car is administered to the thorax of anesthetized dogs, the thoracic viscera may be compressed until the opposing parietal pleural surfaces underlying the ribs may almost be brought into contact. The ribs of young animals are pliable and tend to fracture less often than those of older animals.
- Blunt trauma can cause pneumothorax, hemothorax, pulmonary contusions, fractured ribs, and any combination of these.

Penetrating Trauma

- Penetrating trauma usually is the result of a gunshot. It may also result from a sharp instrument (e.g., a knife, screwdriver, stick, arrow) or from deep bite wounds inflicted by a big dog on a smaller dog or cat.
- Consider the type of projectile, point of entry, and path of the penetrating object when attempting to diagnose thoracic trauma, even if wound entry is distant to the thoracic cavity. The path of a projectile may be altered if it strikes bony structures.
- It is often unclear whether thoracic injuries have resulted from penetrating wounds. Depending on the extent of injury, signs of cardiovascular collapse or respiratory distress may develop more slowly in patients suffering penetrating injuries of the thorax.

CLINICAL SIGNS

- *Tachypnea or dyspnea* (difficulty breathing) are typical presenting signs in dogs and cats that suffer thoracic trauma. The animal may have an anxious or distressed appearance. The owner may or may not have observed the injury. Clinical signs of thoracic trauma may be delayed in onset, especially those associated with diaphragmatic hernia.
- *Hypovolemic shock* may result from internal or external hemorrhage or accumulation of fluid within tissue spaces. An animal suffering from hypovolemic shock has an increased heart rate, weak peripheral arterial pulses, cold extremities, and pale mucous membranes, and often appears depressed or stuporous (see Chap. 72 for further discussion of shock).
- *Gastrointestinal signs* (diarrhea or vomiting due to obstruction) may be observed if a portion of the gastrointestinal tract has been displaced into the thoracic cavity through a diaphragmatic hernia. These signs are not commonly present immediately after the injury has occurred.

DIAGNOSIS

▼ *Key Point* Treatment of hypovolemic shock or other life-threatening disorders takes precedence over patient evaluation.

History

- Attempt to identify recent or past traumatic episodes.
- Question the owner regarding the onset and progression of the current clinical signs.
- Take the history while initial evaluation of vital signs is in progress so that life-threatening injuries (e.g., tension pneumothorax) can be detected and treated immediately.

Physical Examination

After initially determining the animal's vital signs (e.g., heart rate, respiratory rate, mucous membrane color and refill, temperature, level of consciousness), examine the respiratory system by:

- Observation (of breathing)
- Palpation
- Auscultation
- Percussion
- Radiography

Observation

- Observe the rate, depth, and effort of respirations.
- Rapidly developing dyspnea usually is the result of pneumothorax, pulmonary contusion, or hypovolemia.
- Rapid, shallow, choppy breathing can result from restriction of the thoracic wall because of painful rib fracture.
- Paradoxical motion of the chest wall is caused by collapse of a portion of the rib cage on inspiration when multiple rib fractures create an unstable flail chest wall.
- Decreased hemithorax movement (fixation) can be seen on the side into which abdominal viscera have herniated through a ruptured diaphragm.
- Herniation of the lung into the intercostal space countercurrent with each respiration indicates torn intercostal muscles.

Palpation

- Palpate the thoracic wall for rib fractures, unstable (flail) segments, hematomas (usually adjacent to rib fractures), subcutaneous emphysema (crepitus), intercostal muscle tears (usually under intact skin), and abnormal location of the cardiac apex beat (displaced by herniation of abdominal viscera).
- Also palpate the abdominal cavity for concurrent intra-abdominal injuries. The absence of viscera suggests their displacement into the thoracic cavity.

Auscultation

- Carefully auscultate the entire thoracic cavity to determine whether breath sounds can be identified throughout the thoracic cavity. The absence of respiratory sounds strongly suggests displacement of the lungs by air, fluid (e.g., blood), or abdominal viscera. Crackles suggest intrapulmonary fluid accumulation.
- Auscultate the heart as well. A change in the location or pitch of heart sounds suggests displacement of the heart by air, fluid, or viscera. Ventricular arrhythmias frequently occur as the result of traumatic myocarditis or myocardial ischemia; however, their onset is more frequently observed 24–48 hours after the traumatic episode.
- See also Chapter 59.

Percussion

- Perform percussion of the thoracic wall to determine increased or decreased resonance. By placing one hand flat on the thoracic wall and tapping the knuckle of the middle finger with a percussion hammer or the tips of the fingers of the opposite hand, a sound of consistent frequency is produced in normal animals.
- In animals with air or air-filled viscera underlying the thoracic wall, the pitch is deeper and more resonant, whereas the sound produced in animals with fluid or solid viscera immediately under the thoracic wall is dull and less resonant.
- Percussion aids detection of pneumothorax, pleural effusion (e.g., hemothorax, chylothorax), diaphragmatic hernia, and consolidation of lung lobes.
- Skilled use of this technique requires frequent practice on normal animals to allow a distinction between normal and abnormal sounds.
- See also Chapter 59.

Fractures

- Thoracic injuries may occur in more than 30% of dogs and cats sustaining traumatic fractures.
- Examine the animal for the presence of fractures; do not be distracted by the obvious presence of broken bones but continue searching for evidence of more serious internal injuries.
- If spinal fractures are suspected, handle the animal with great care until these have been stabilized or it is determined radiographically that the spine is intact.
- The presence of fractures suggests that trauma of sufficient force to inflict injury to the thorax and its contents has occurred. A survey of dogs injured in motor vehicle accidents found that over 50% of animals with intrathoracic injuries also had fractured bones.

Surface Wounds and Abrasions

- Clip hair from the thoracic wall area as necessary to identify abrasions, bruises, or wounds that may point to likely sites of intrathoracic injury.
- Open wounds that freely communicate with the pleural space can cause progressive pneumothorax; seal them immediately.

Thoracic Radiography

Take radiographs to evaluate the heart, lungs, pleural space, and thoracic wall (see Chaps. 60 and 75 for a discussion of thoracic radiography).

- It is sometimes advisable to delay thoracic radiography of the injured animal until after higher priority conditions such as shock have been stabilized by emergency treatment. Pulmonary contusion, characterized by hemorrhage and fluid accumulation within the lungs, may not reach its greatest extent for 6–12 hours and then often may not appear radiographically to be improved for 7–10 days after injury.

▼ *Key Point* The full severity of pulmonary contusions may not be apparent on thoracic radiographs made within 1–2 hours of injury.

- A narrowed cardiac silhouette may suggest hypovolemia.
- Evaluate the pleural space carefully for fluid, air or abdominal viscera, and evaluate the integrity of the diaphragmatic outline.
- Look for radiographic evidence of fracture or dislocation of skeletal structures and subcutaneous emphysema, which indicates leakage of air into the subcutaneous space from the environment, the thoracic cavity, or a major airway.
- Pneumomediastinum is seen as air outlining the mediastinal contents and is indicative of tracheobronchial rupture.
- If the animal's condition does not preclude this, obtain two radiographic projections.
- Often it is difficult to identify a diaphragmatic hernia on thoracic radiographs, particularly if obscured by accumulation of fluid within the pleural space. If a large quantity of pleural fluid is present, remove it and repeat the radiographs (see Chap. 75), or obtain an ultrasound examination, if readily available.
  - Observations suggesting a diaphragmatic hernia include cranial displacement of the stomach, loss of the caudal outline of the liver, and the presence of gas-filled viscous organs within the thoracic cavity.
  - If a diaphragmatic hernia is suspected but unconfirmed by plain radiographs, consider positive-contrast celiography or abdominal ultrasonography (see Chap. 4).

Thoracocentesis

If indicated, perform thoracocentesis to obtain a sample of pleural fluid or to drain air from the pleural space (see Chap. 3 for technique).

- Analyze the fluid for the presence and concentration of red blood cells (RBCs) and plasma protein. The fluid may be whole blood, or may be a combination of transudate, exudate, chyle, or blood, depending on the severity and duration of injury and the organs affected.
- Centrifuge an aliquot of the fluid and examine the cellular portion microscopically for degenerative neutrophils, bacteria, and organic matter (see Chap. 80). These findings may suggest a severe inflammatory process and possibly perforation of the esophagus or gastrointestinal tract.
- On rare occasions, the biliary tract may be ruptured in the presence of diaphragmatic hernia, and this can be identified by determining the concentration of bilirubin within pleural fluid.

Blood Samples

- Draw blood and store the sample in an anticoagulant and serum tube (preferably before initiating treatment).
- Although these samples may not be needed, often it is helpful to determine the biochemical status of the animal at the time of hospital admission when attempting to distinguish between preexistent disease and that which has developed acutely after injury. These same considerations apply to the collection and storage of urine samples.

Packed Cell Volume and Plasma Protein Concentration

- Determine the packed cell volume (PCV) and plasma protein concentration (PPC) as soon as possible after the initial examination.
- It is critical to record these values because the diagnosis of continuing hemorrhage often relies on the comparison of serial determinations of PCV and PPC.
- If hemorrhage is ongoing, these two values continue to decline at a similar rate. If, however, hemorrhage has ceased, it is not uncommon for the PPC to stabilize while the PCV continues to decline.
- The administration of intravenous (IV) fluids may further decrease these values; consider this fact when evaluating these parameters.

Arterial pH and Blood Gas Tensions

- These values give an indication of ventilatory function.
- Satisfactory oxygenation of the blood by the lungs requires adequate cardiac output, and decreased cardiac output caused by hypovolemic shock or depressed cardiac function may profoundly affect blood gas values.

Electrocardiography

- If available, obtain serial electrocardiographs (ECGs) to check for arrhythmias associated with myocardial injury.
- If ECG is not available, closely monitor the animal's heart rate and rhythm and the occurrence of pulse deficits.

TREATMENT

Modify treatment to suit the individual needs of each trauma patient. Place and maintain at least one IV catheter for administration of fluids and drugs early in the course of treatment. In severely traumatized animals, place two IV catheters (one may be a central venous line) to allow more rapid infusion of IV fluids.

When confronted with a seriously injured animal, often it is difficult to develop a logical, disciplined treatment plan. The ABC approach is a consistent, comprehensive plan for initial treatment of animals with thoracic trauma.

Airway, Breathing, and Circulation (ABC) Approach

Airway

Be sure that the animal has a patent airway.

- Remove debris from the trachea and bronchi by forceps or suction or by passing an endotracheal tube.
- If the pharynx, larynx or cranial portion of the trachea is severely damaged, consider performing a tracheostomy (see Chap. 3).

Breathing (Spontaneous or Assisted) and Oxygen Therapy

Restore thoracic wall integrity by sealing open ("sucking") chest wounds with an occlusive dressing and stabilizing flail segments so the animal can ventilate effectively. If the animal is not able to ventilate satisfactorily, institute assisted breathing.

- This requires an endotracheal or tracheostomy tube and may necessitate anesthetizing the animal or giving neuromuscular blocking drugs to paralyze the animal (see Chap. 2).
- Supplemental oxygen may be provided by an incubator or oxygen cage, face mask, nasal catheter (see Chap. 3), transtracheal cannula or catheter, or endotracheal or tracheostomy tube.
  - When supplemental oxygen is administered to the animal in such a manner that it does not pass through the nasal passages, prewarm and humidify the air.
- A transtracheal catheter may be placed using a large-gauge (12–18) jugular catheter passed between the rings of the trachea.
  - Secure the catheter to the skin and attach to the oxygen source. Deliver oxygen via the transtracheal catheter at an initial rate of 10–20 ml/kg/min.

Circulation

If myocardial function is satisfactory, administer IV fluids as needed to increase the circulating blood volume and cardiac output.

- In most cases of hypovolemic shock, administer a blood volume (90 ml/kg in dogs and 65 ml/kg in cats) as rapidly as gravity flow allows.
- In the presence of significant ongoing hemorrhage, fluid bags may be pressurized to increase the rate of administration.
- After the rapid infusion of a bolus of IV fluids equivalent to one blood volume, reassess the status of the patient and determine the need for ongoing fluid administration.
  - If signs of hypovolemic shock have abated and hemorrhage has ceased, continue to administer fluids at a rate of 30–50 ml/kg/24 hr (see Chap. 72).
  - If the animal's condition does not stabilize, continue rapid fluid administration.
- Auscultate the lungs for evidence of pulmonary edema and carefully monitor for other signs of edema (e.g., tachypnea, chemosis, tearing, tissue swelling, decreasing PCV and PPC).

- If necessary, monitor the central venous pressure (CVP) to determine the ability of the right side of the heart to eject the volume of blood presented to it (see Chap. 3 for CVP techniques). The relative change in CVP is more significant than the absolute value, and an increase of 7–10 cm H_2O indicates that the rate of fluid administration should be slowed.
- Because of the low oncotic pressure of the crystalloid fluid that may contribute to fluid loss into the tissue space, a general rule for replacement of blood loss by crystalloid fluids is:
  - For every 1 ml of blood lost, administer 3 ml of crystalloid fluid.

Pleural Space Drainage

- The pleural space may be drained intermittently by thoracocentesis using a hypodermic needle.
- If continuous or prolonged pleural drainage for removal of fluid or air is required, place a thoracostomy tube (see Chap. 3 for thoracic drainage techniques).
  - Attach thoracostomy tubes to a three-way stopcock to allow intermittent aspiration of the tube (e.g., q2–4h) or to a continuous suction device.
  - If continuous suction is used, carefully control the negative pressure; it should not be less than −5 to −10 cm H_2O.
- Alternatively, attach the thoracostomy tube to a Heimlich one-way flutter valve.
  - If using this valve, carefully monitor the animal for complications.
  - Be aware that if the valve becomes cracked or the valve's diaphragm becomes wet, the one-way function of the valve may be lost and severe pneumothorax may develop.
  - This valve is available in two sizes, and animals weighing <10 kg frequently may be incapable of activating the larger valve, resulting in continued accumulation of air within the thoracic cavity.
- If fluid or air cannot be aspirated from the thoracostomy tube, the pleural space may be completely evacuated or the tube may be obstructed by a fibrin clot or by the tube's bending on itself. Obtain thoracic radiographs and flush the tube with sterile saline to confirm patency.

Tube Removal. Remove the tube when it is no longer needed.

- The presence of the thoracostomy tube results in continued production of a small volume of fluid (at least 30–60 ml/24 hr in a dog weighing 25 kg).
- It also is possible that a small volume of air may continue to accumulate within the pleural space due to air migration along the external surface of the chest tube or through leaks in the tubing.
- Therefore, it is often not possible to wait until there is no air or fluid accumulation within the thorax to remove the thoracostomy tube, and the tube usually is removed when the volume of air and fluid has reached insignificant levels.

Treatment of Pneumothorax

Pneumothorax can be closed or open; in *closed* pneumothorax, the most common type, air escapes from the injured lung or airway into the pleural space; in *open* pneumothorax, air enters the pleural space through an open wound in the chest wall (e.g., bites, sharp objects, projectiles).

Simple Pneumothorax

Accumulation of air in the pleural space that is not progressive is termed simple pneumothorax and is a common complication of thoracic trauma.

- Conservative treatment with thoracic drainage and cage rest usually is adequate. The air leak usually seals itself within hours, and residual intrapleural air is reabsorbed within a few days.
- Occasionally, oxygen therapy may be needed as initial treatment in animals that are severely dyspneic on presentation until the pleural space can be evacuated.
- Simple pneumothorax frequently is accompanied by other thoracic problems, such as pulmonary contusions and rib fractures, which can combine to cause serious ventilatory problems.

Tension Pneumothorax

Laceration of the lung, bronchus, or trachea may result in tension pneumothorax, which is the progressive accumulation of air in the pleural space that results in positive intrapleural pressure.

- Animals with tension pneumothorax need immediate life-saving thoracic drainage via a thoracostomy tube to prevent lung collapse, decreased systemic venous return to the heart, and rapid death. This reestablishes negative intrapleural pressure and allows lung reexpansion.
- Intermittent thoracic drainage may not be adequate to allow proper ventilation, and continuous suction drainage frequently is necessary. In this case, connect the thoracic tube to a suction drainage unit such as Pleur-Evac (Deknatel Inc., Fall River, MA).
- Consider exploratory thoracotomy (see later discussion in this chapter; also see Chap. 83) if the patient's condition fails to stabilize.

Treatment of Pulmonary Contusions

A pulmonary contusion is analogous to a bruise, with disruption of the tissues and capillaries resulting in extravasation of blood and accumulation of fluid within the pulmonary parenchyma. As previously mentioned in the discussion of IV fluid administration, aggressive fluid therapy may result in fluid accumulation within the lungs. This most likely is the result of decreased plasma oncotic pressure. IV infusion of the equivalent of one blood volume of crystalloid fluids over the course of 1 hour does not increase the extent of experimentally created pulmonary contusions in dogs. It is unlikely that IV fluid administration will increase fluid accumulation within pulmonary contusions unless the

PPC is <3.0 g/dl or the plasma albumin concentration is <1.5 g/dl.

- Transfusions of plasma or whole blood or administration of colloid (hetastarch) help to maintain plasma oncotic pressure.
- Corticosteroids (2–4 mg/kg dexamethasone phosphate or 30 mg/kg methylprednisolone sodium succinate) may be useful in limiting the severity of pulmonary contusions if administered soon after injury.
- Diuretics have been recommended to remove excess water and limit the severity of contusions; however, diuretics may act to reduce total body fluid at a time when volume expansion is critical to resuscitate the patient.
- Administer antibiotics to animals with pulmonary contusions to minimize the potential for development of bacterial pneumonia (antibiotic therapy for patients with thoracic trauma is discussed at the end of this chapter).
- In animals that are recumbent, frequent repositioning may help to prevent hypostatic congestion, atelectasis, and pneumonia.
- Administer oxygen to treat or prevent hypoxemia.
- Bronchodilators (e.g., aminophylline, 6–10 mg/kg q8h PO, IM, or IV in dogs; 6.6 mg/kg q12h PO in cats) may improve ventilation by keeping airways open.
- Closely monitor animals with moderate to severe contusions. If deterioration of respiratory function continues despite the above-mentioned measures, positive-pressure assisted ventilation may be necessary.

Treatment of Myocardial Contusions

Administration of corticosteroids as described for treatment of pulmonary contusions may be beneficial in the treatment of myocardial contusions, but the efficacy of any form of treatment is uncertain.

- Monitor ventricular arrhythmias (see Chap. 62) that develop as a result of traumatic myocarditis by continuous ECG and treat initially with IV administration of lidocaine (2 mg/kg boluses to a maximum of 8 mg/kg/hr).
  - If lidocaine therapy is effective but a constant infusion is required, administer lidocaine at a rate of 50–80 μg/kg/min. Adjust the rate to achieve the desired effect.
- Procainamide may also be given (8–20 mg/kg q8h IM, 10–20 mg/kg q6h PO, or 20–50 mg/kg q8h extended release PO).

Treatment of Hemothorax

Hemothorax (blood accumulation in the pleural space) occurs secondary to any form of trauma that causes laceration of blood vessels, heart, lung, or thoracic wall (diseases other than trauma can cause hemothorax and are discussed in Chap. 80). Hemothorax causes two major problems: hypovolemic shock and impairment of ventilation. Massive hemorrhage from rupture of the heart or one of the great vessels usually causes rapid death.

- Treatment of traumatically induced hemothorax involves aggressive and rapid supportive care consisting of IV fluids and/or blood transfusions and pleural drainage (see Chap. 72 for details of treatment of hypovolemic shock).
- Consider autotransfusions for animals with significant hemothorax not complicated by an infectious or neoplastic process in the thorax.
  - Aseptically collect the blood via a chest tube and return to the patient using a blood administration set.
  - Closely monitor the patient's vital signs, PCV, and PPC.
- Consider exploratory thoracotomy for animals that fail to stabilize (see subsequent discussion in this chapter). However, surgical treatment of hemothorax may be unsuccessful because the source of hemorrhage is sometimes not identifiable.

Stabilization of Rib Fractures and Flail Chest

▼ *Key Point* Stabilization of rib fractures is required when a gross deformity has occurred, displacement of the fragments results in ongoing damage to the underlying viscera, or displacement or instability of the fragments interferes with ventilation (e.g., flail chest).

- Potential complications of rib fractures include:
  - Pneumothorax (from lung laceration by the sharp end of a fragment).
  - Pulmonary contusions.
  - Hemothorax (bleeding from torn intercostal vessels, lacerated lung, or exposed rib marrow cavity).
  - Unstable chest wall (flail chest).
- *Flail chest* occurs when two or more adjacent ribs are fractured or dislocated both dorsally and ventrally, resulting in the paradoxical movement of a segment of the thoracic wall during respiration. This may diminish lung volume and damage the underlying viscera as the flail segment is displaced during respiration.
- Rib fractures may be stabilized by open fixation using pins and wires.
- Alternatively, the ribs may be secured to an external frame by percutaneous placement of sutures around the ribs (this procedure has been used successfully to stabilize flail chest).
  - A frame made of malleable rodding used to construct splints is contoured to the normal curvature of the thoracic wall. Bars pass over the dorsal and ventral aspects of the flail segment. Place at least two sutures around the ribs of the flail segment, dorsally and ventrally, and tie to the frame to displace the flail segment in a lateral or outward direction (Fig. 82–1). Alternatively, tongue depressors, or other stiff materials of sufficient length to span the flail segment can be used to stabilize the damaged ribs.
  - Damage to the underlying lung tissue usually does not occur during passage of the suture needle around the rib because of the presence of pneumothorax. Minimize the risk of potential damage to

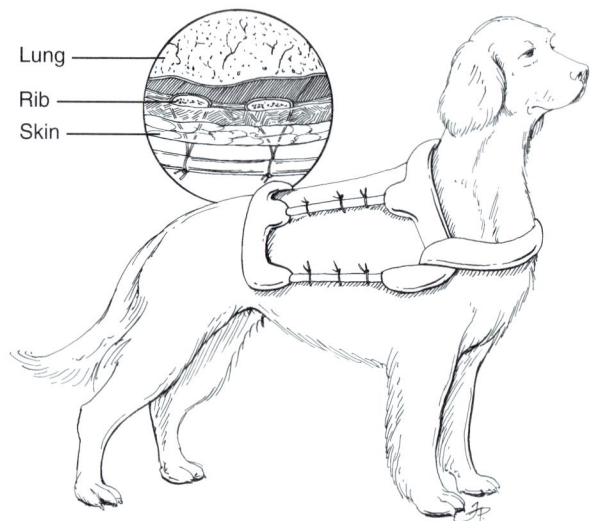

Figure 82–1. Fractured ribs can be secured to an external frame contoured to the body wall. Place sutures around the ribs dorsally and ventrally and tie them around the bars of the frame. (Redrawn from Bjorling DE, DeNovo RC, Kolata RJ: Flail chest: Review, clinical experience, and new method of stabilization. J Am Anim Hosp Assoc 18:269, 1982.)

the underlying lungs by grasping a rib with a towel forceps and retracting the flail segment laterally.
  - Keep the frame in place for at least 3 weeks.
- Do not apply tight bandages for stabilization of rib fractures, because this displaces the ribs medially, resulting in continued damage to the underlying viscera and healing of the ribs in such a position that lung volume is permanently decreased.
- Adjunctive therapy for rib fracture includes analgesia and intercostal nerve blocks to control pain (see Chap. 2), thereby promoting uninhibited cough and deeper, less restrictive breathing that helps to prevent hypoventilation, atelectasis, retained secretions, and pneumonia.

Treatment of Open Chest Wounds

- Immediate treatment of open chest wounds consists of minor cleansing of the wound and application of a bandage to restore continuity of the chest wall.
- Treat the resultant pneumothorax with thoracocentesis or chest tube.
- Allow small penetrating wounds to heal as an open wound (if air is not leaking into the pleural space), or they may be explored, debrided, and sutured. Surgically explore, debride, and close large open wounds of the thoracic wall.
- It may be necessary to remove ribs that are devoid of musculature and vascular supply.
  - Up to four adjacent ribs can be removed and the thoracic wall closed by apposing the remaining ribs.
  - Larger defects require the use of synthetic mesh (e.g., polypropylene) to compensate for the tissue lost.

Diaphragmatic Hernia Repair

Some hernias remain undetected for months or years before signs of pleural effusion, weight loss, gastrointestinal dysfunction, or jaundice occur (see Chap. 75 for radiographic diagnosis of diaphragmatic hernia).

- Minor perforations of the diaphragm usually seal without treatment.
- Surgically repair diaphragmatic defects (most can be closed by suture) that result in displacement of viscera into the thoracic cavity (see Technique). The liver, spleen, omentum, and gastrointestinal tract commonly are herniated.
- Timing of diaphragmatic hernia repair depends on the patient's condition.
  - It is preferable to delay diaphragmatic hernia repair until the patient has stabilized; however, if respiratory function cannot be stabilized despite aggressive supportive care, it may be necessary to repair the diaphragmatic hernia on an emergency basis.

▼ *Key Point* Acute dilatation of herniated stomach or strangulation of herniated bowel requires emergency correction of a diaphragmatic hernia.

Technique

1. Keep the animal on mechanical ventilation throughout the repair.
2. Approach the diaphragm through a ventral midline abdominal incision.
3. Initially it may be necessary to enlarge the diaphragmatic rent in order to reduce the herniated viscera. If so, make the incision ventrally to simplify repair.
4. In cases of chronic hernia, adhesions between viscera and diaphragm or lungs may be present. Break these down carefully.
5. Following reduction of displaced organs and examination of the lungs and pleural space, close the rent with synthetic absorbable or monofilament nonabsorbable suture (simple continuous or horizontal mattress pattern).
6. Begin with the most dorsal aspect of the hernia and work ventrally to close the repair.
7. Grasp large "bites" of the abdominal wall musculature or ribs when suturing diaphragm that has avulsed from the ventrolateral body wall. Identify and avoid the caudal vena cava.
8. If large portions of diaphragm have been destroyed, repair the defect with synthetic mesh or transposition of a transversus abdominis muscle flap.
9. Place a thoracostomy tube to remove air and fluid after surgery prior to closure of the diaphragmatic defect.

Postoperative Care and Complications

- Remove the thoracostomy tube when no longer needed.
- Advise the owner to limit the patient's activity for 2–4 weeks.
- Complications are rare and the prognosis usually is good.
- Reexpansion pulmonary edema rarely develops (more often in cats), and is characterized by fulminant pulmonary edema immediately after reexpansion of the lung lobes. Treat with diuretics and oxygen.

Exploratory Thoracotomy

Thoracotomy for treatment of ongoing hemorrhage or air leakage on an emergency basis is difficult and may be unrewarding. The animal is at significant risk due to the effects of anesthesia, and often it is difficult to identify and effectively treat the site of hemorrhage or air leakage.

- Before undertaking an exploratory thoracotomy, be sure that adequate equipment and personnel are available to successfully complete the procedure.
- Perform exploratory thoracotomy for treatment of traumatic injuries of the thoracic cavity only after aggressive medical therapy and tube drainage have failed to stabilize the animal's condition.
  - If the site of injury can be identified, a lateral thoracotomy approach may be used (see Chap. 83). Unfortunately, this rarely is possible.
  - A midsternal approach (splitting the sternum) allows exploration of both sides of the thorax (see Chap. 83).

Antibiotic Therapy

- Administer antibiotics to prevent:
  - Development of bacterial pneumonia resulting from traumatic injuries of the lungs.
  - Wound infection as a result of disruption of the thoracic wall.
- Initially give antibiotics intravenously to establish satisfactory tissue concentrations. This can be followed by oral administration of antibiotics.
- Prophylactic antibiotic treatment for pulmonary injuries should provide broad-spectrum antibacterial activity. A satisfactory combination is cephazolin (20 mg/kg q8h IM or IV) and gentamicin (2–4 mg/kg q12h or 4–8 mg/kg q24h SC, IM, or IV).
- Wound infections due to contamination of tissues with dirt most often are caused by gram-positive bacteria. Cephazolin or other cephalosporin antibiotics have good activity against the most common organisms involved.

SUPPLEMENTAL READINGS

Bjorling DE, DeNovo RC, Kolata RJ: Flail chest: Review and clinical experience. J Am Anim Hosp Assoc 18:269, 1982.

Buttrick ML, Riedesel DN, Selcer BA, Barstad RD: Hypoxemia in the acutely traumatized canine patient. J Vet Emerg Crit Care 2:73, 1993.

Cockshutt JR: Management of fracture-associated thoracic trauma. Vet Clin North Am Small Anim Pract 25:1031, 1995.

Griffon DJ, Walter PA, Wallace LJ: Thoracic injuries in cats with traumatic fractures. Vet Comp Orthop Traumatol 7:98, 1994.

Houlton JEF, Dyce J: Does fracture pattern influence thoracic trauma? Vet Comp Orthop Traumatol 5:90, 1992.

McAnulty JF: A simplified method for stabilization of flail chest injuries in small animals. J Am Anim Hosp Assoc 31:137, 1995.

Sweet DC, Walters DJ: Role of surgery in the management of dogs with pathologic conditions of the thorax. Part II. Compend Contin Ed Pract Vet 13:1671, 1991.

83 Principles of Thoracic Surgery

Stephen J. Birchard / Eric R. Schertel

Thoracic surgery frequently is performed in small animals, especially in referral centers. Thoracotomy is commonly performed to correct routine cardiovascular defects such as patent ductus arteriosus and to evaluate and correct respiratory diseases such as pulmonary neoplasia. Exploratory thoracotomy may be indicated to determine the extent of diseases such as neoplasia and diffuse infection and to obtain biopsies to help establish a definitive diagnosis. It is important to be well versed in the anatomy and physiology of the thoracic cavity and its major structures and to be familiar with the principles of anesthetic management of the thoracic surgery patient.

This chapter discusses the surgical anatomy and physiology of the thorax, thoracic surgical technique, and patient care before, during, and after thoracic surgery.

SURGICAL ANATOMY

Bony Structures

- The bony structures of the thorax usually consist of 13 pairs of ribs and costal cartilages, 13 vertebrae, and 8 sternebrae.
- The first nine ribs, called the sternal ribs, articulate with the sternum. The last four ribs are called the asternal ribs. The costal cartilages of ribs 10–12 make up the costal arch. The 13th pair of ribs are also called the floating ribs.
- The manubrium is the most cranial aspect of the sternum, and the xyphoid is located caudally. The xyphoid cartilage is the caudal extension of the xyphoid. Intersternebral cartilages are located between each sternebra. The sternebrae are very narrow structures, making midline division somewhat difficult. The sternebral midline is characterized by a slight bony ridge.

Soft Tissues

Muscles

- The external and internal intercostal muscles are located between each rib.
- Other surgically important muscles of the lateral thoracic wall are the serratus ventralis and serratus cranialis dorsalis, scalenus, and external abdominal oblique. The latissimus dorsi, a large fan-shaped muscle extending from the ribs to the forelimb, is the

first major muscle encountered during lateral thoracotomy.

Vessels and Nerves

- The intercostal arteries, veins, and nerves are located on the caudal aspect of each rib. The internal thoracic artery and veins run horizontally just lateral to the sternum, within the thorax.
- The cutaneous and muscular branches of the thoracodorsal artery are frequently encountered during lateral thoracotomy.

PREOPERATIVE CONSIDERATIONS

History, Physical Examination, and Diagnostic Tests

- Review the animal's history and perform a thorough physical examination.
  - Give special consideration to the patient's cardiopulmonary status (mucous membrane color and refill time, heart rate and rhythm, pulse rate and character, heart and lung sounds, ventilation, thoracic palpation and percussion).
- Review diagnostic tests already performed and repeat if necessary.
  - Evaluate thoracic radiographs to become familiar with the animal's disease and to plan the surgical approach.
  - Evaluate blood tests, such as complete blood count (CBC) and serum chemistry profile, to establish the patient's baseline before surgery. If the condition is severe, blood gas analysis may be helpful to further evaluate the patient's respiratory status.
  - Thoracic ultrasound may assist in planning the surgical approach. Advanced imaging (computed tomography, magnetic resonance imaging) may be of benefit in selected cases.

Preoperative Treatment and Stabilization

General Supportive Care

- Administer appropriate medical therapy that will stabilize the animal and reduce the level of anesthetic and surgical risk.
  - For example, if a dog with patent ductus arteriosus is in congestive heart failure, treat with the appro-

priate drugs to improve cardiopulmonary function before anesthesia and surgery.

- Correct fluid and electrolyte deficiencies.
- Maintain the animal's nutritional status. Consider placing a nasogastric, esophagostomy, or percutaneous endoscopic gastrostomy (PEG) tube if the animal will not eat and is becoming debilitated (see Chap. 3).
- Closely observe the patient's condition. The clinical states of animals with thoracic disease may change rapidly.

Thoracic Drainage

- If pleural fluid or air is present, tap the thorax before anesthesia to allow better ventilation.
- Place an indwelling thoracic drainage tube if fluid or air accumulation is recurrent (see Chap. 3).
  - Use intermittent or continuous suction drainage.
  - Quantify amount of fluid or air recovered to establish a baseline before surgery.

Oxygen

- Administer oxygen to severely dyspneic or cyanotic animals.
  - Place the animal in an oxygen cage at 40–50% concentration or place a nasal oxygen tube to raise the concentration of inspired oxygen (see Chap. 3).
- If possible, analyze blood gases before and after oxygen administration to establish its effectiveness. Pulse oximetry may be useful as well.

Prophylactic Antibiotics

- Use prophylactic antibiotics if the planned operation will be a clean-contaminated, contaminated, or "dirty" procedure.
- Thoracotomy to open and/or resect a portion of the respiratory tract is considered a clean-contaminated procedure. However, the authors use prophylactic antibiotics only if there is a strong suspicion that significant contamination of the surgical field will occur (e.g., foreign bodies, abscess, necrotic tumor, bacterial pneumonia). Thoracotomy for drainage and resection of the pericardium for pericarditis is an example of an indication for preoperative use of antibiotics.
- Administer the prophylactic antibiotic immediately before surgery to ensure sufficient blood concentrations of the drug at the time of surgery. Discontinue antibiotic administration 24–48 hours postoperatively unless evidence of infection is present.
- Choose an antibiotic that is effective against the suspected contaminant and that reaches therapeutic concentrations in the target tissues.

Blood

- Cardiac surgery or removal of large, vascular neoplasms may be associated with acute blood loss.
- Ensure that a blood donor or packed cells are available if significant blood loss is anticipated.

- Crossmatch or type the donor's blood if multiple transfusions are anticipated.

Client Communication

Risks

- Major cardiac and respiratory surgery is associated with a high incidence of morbidity and mortality.
- Review the incidence of complications and death associated with the planned procedure and discuss this information with the client.

Cost

Thoracic surgery and patient care may be quite expensive.

- Discuss the cost of preoperative diagnosis and therapy, anesthesia and surgery, and postoperative intensive care with the client.

ANESTHETIC CONSIDERATIONS

The general principles of anesthesia described in Chapter 2 apply to thoracic surgery patients. Special considerations for thoracic surgery patients are outlined in this section.

Premedication

- Avoid phenothiazines such as acepromazine because of possible side effects of hypotension and myocardial depression. However, at low doses (up to 0.1 mg/kg SC or IM), they may be beneficial for calming animals with respiratory compromise but normal cardiac function. Acepromazine can be combined with one of the opiates (e.g., butorphanol) as an effective preanesthetic treatment (see Chap. 2).
- Diazepam (Valium) is a safe drug that can be used as a premedicant (0.2 mg/kg IV). It has minimal effects on the cardiovascular and respiratory systems.
- Xylazine (Rompun, Miles) causes undesirable cardiac and respiratory depression, making it a poor choice for thoracic surgery.
- Avoid using anticholinergics (e.g., atropine) because they increase viscosity of respiratory secretions, can increase anatomic dead space, and may induce cardiac arrhythmias.

Induction

- Diazepam, 0.2 mg/kg IV, followed by administration of a thiobarbiturate (e.g., thiopental), 6–10 mg/kg IV, provides relatively safe and rapid, smooth induction that allows immediate intubation and control of ventilation.
- The combination of ketamine and diazepam (1:1 mixture; 1 ml of mixture/10 kg) also can be used for thoracic surgery patients. Hemodynamics are minimally compromised by this combination. However, ventilatory support may be necessary.
- Propofol is another alternative choice for induction of anesthesia. See Chapter 2 for indications and dosage.

Table 83–1. GENERAL GUIDELINES FOR CONTROLLED VENTILATION

Physiologic Parameter	Value
Respiratory	8–12 breaths/min
Tidal volume	15–20 ml/kg ideal body weight
Peak airway pressure	15–20 cm H_2O—closed
	20–30 cm H_2O—open
Inspiratory time	1–1.5 sec
Expiratory time	2–3 sec
Inspiratory:expiratory ratio	1:2–1:4

Modified from Faggella AM, Raffe MR: Anesthetic management of thoracotomy. Vet Clin North Am 17:480, 1987.

Maintenance

- Any of the commonly used inhalation anesthetics can be used successfully for thoracic procedures. Isoflurane is preferred because of less myocardial depression, although hypotension commonly occurs.
- Avoid nitrous oxide in patients with respiratory disease, pneumothorax, anemia, or hypoxia.
- Provide positive pressure ventilation by manual compression of the bag or with a mechanical ventilator (see Table 83–1 for ventilation guidelines).

▼ *Key Point* Adequate positive pressure ventilation in the thoracic surgery patient is essential for preventing hypoxia, respiratory acidosis, and atelectasis.

Fluids

- Thoracotomy diminishes the functional reserve of the heart by decreasing effective filling pressures. This may be compensated for, in part, by fluid therapy.
- Place one or two intravenous catheters for fluid administration.
- Administer balanced electrolyte solutions at a surgical maintenance rate of 10–20 ml/kg/hr.

Monitoring

Cardiovascular

- The standard methods of cardiovascular monitoring (e.g., heart rate, color, pulse quality, capillary refill) are very important, because alterations due to the disease or surgical manipulations are common.
- Monitoring with electrocardiography (ECG) is helpful to determine when and why cardiac problems arise.
- Blood pressure measurements obtained with an arterial catheter or a Doppler unit with a pneumatic cuff placed over an accessible artery (e.g., metatarsal artery) help determine circulatory status during the anesthetic period.

Respiratory

- Carefully monitor the respiratory rate and depth. In the patient with respiratory compromise, be especially aware of spontaneous respirations before thoracotomy and immediately after closure of the thorax.
- Monitor blood gas analysis or pulse oximetry to determine respiratory status; make necessary adjustments.

Other

- Use standard techniques for monitoring depth of anesthesia (see Chap. 2).
- Ensure good communication between anesthetist and surgeon, which is essential for a smooth and successful procedure. Indicate to the anesthetist when major manipulations of the heart and lungs are imminent, and point out when problems arise such as atelectasis due to inadequate ventilation, or acute blood loss. The anesthetist should keep the surgeon informed of the patient's overall status.

SURGICAL PROCEDURES

Instruments

A standard general pack is needed. See Table 83–2 for additional instruments that are particularly useful in thoracic surgery.

Lateral Thoracotomy

Indications

- This is the standard approach to most intrathoracic structures. See Table 83–3 for location of structures exposed through intercostal thoracotomy.

Table 83–2. SPECIAL INSTRUMENTS RECOMMENDED FOR THORACIC SURGERY

Scissors
Long-handled Metzenbaum
Potts

Needle Holders
Mayo-Hegar (long-handled)
DeBakey
French eye

Tissue Forceps
DeBakey general thoracic
DeBakey vascular

Other Forceps
Satinsky clamps
Angled or curved forceps
    Gallbladder
    Rumel thoracic and dissecting
    Mixter hemostatic, thoracic
    Lahey gall duct thoracic
Bronchus clamps
Vascular clamps

Retractors
Finochietto rib
Burford rib

Other
Rib approximator

Table 83–3. LOCATION OF THORACIC STRUCTURES VIA INTERCOSTAL THORACOTOMY

Thoracic Structure	Intercostal Space	
	Left	Right
Heart and pericardium	4, 5	4, 5
PDA, PRAA	4 (5)	
Pulmonic valve	4	
Trachea		3
Lungs	4–6	4–6
Cranial lobe	(4) 5	(4) 5
Intermediate lobe		5
Caudal lobe	5 (6)	5 (6)
Esophagus		
Cranial		3, 4
Caudal	7–10	7–10
Caudal vena cava	(6–7)	7–10
Diaphragm	7–10	7–10
Thoracic duct (caudal)		
Dog		8–10
Cat	8–10	

Modified from Orton C: Thoracic wall. *In* Slatter DH, ed.: Textbook of Small Animal Surgery. Philadelphia: WB Saunders, 1985, p 539.
PDA, patent ductus arteriosus; PRAA, persistent right aortic arch.

Objective

- To gain access to the right or left hemithorax for exposing the heart, lungs, or other structures.

Equipment

- See Table 83–2 for specific instruments useful in thoracic surgery.

Technique

1. Place the animal in lateral recumbency. Place a towel or small pillow under the thorax to slightly arch the contralateral thoracic wall, making the surgical approach easier. Prepare the lateral thorax for aseptic surgery.
2. Count the intercostal spaces to approximate the location of the incision.
3. Incise the skin, subcutaneous tissues, and cutaneous trunci muscle, from dorsal to ventral, from the costovertebral junction to the sternum.
4. Incise the latissimus dorsi muscle from ventral to dorsal (Fig. 83–1).
5. Re-count the intercostal spaces from cranial to caudal unless the incision is located in the caudal thorax.
6. Incise through the remainder of muscles: serratus ventralis (can be bluntly separated rather than incised), scalenus, external abdominal oblique, and external and internal intercostal (Fig. 83–2). Penetrate the pleura (instruct the anesthetist to stop positive pressure ventilation before introducing sharp instruments into the thorax), and incise the pleura dorsally and ventrally with Metzenbaum scissors. Avoid trauma to the internal thoracic artery when incising ventrally.

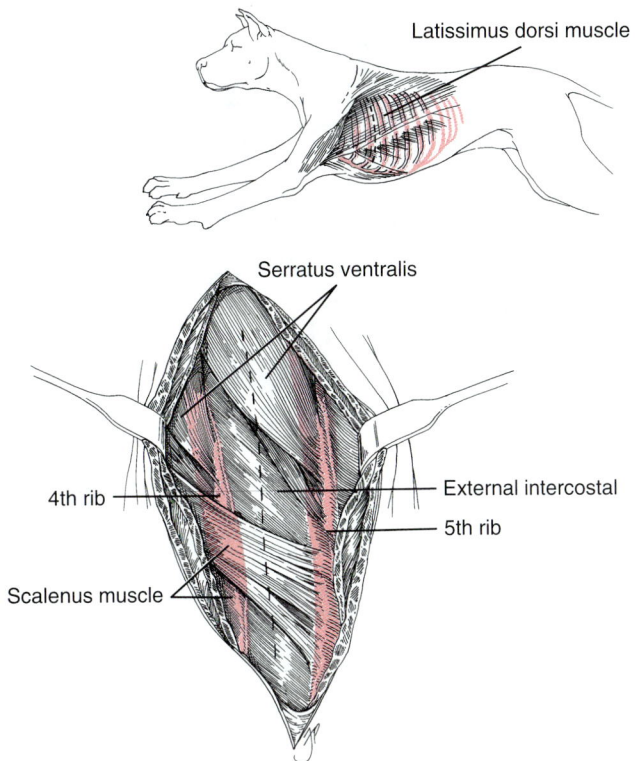

Figure 83–1. Thoracotomy technique. *Top,* Incise the skin at the intercostal space between ribs 4 and 5 *(dotted line)*. *Below,* Cut the latissimus dorsi muscle and retract to expose the serratus ventralis, dorsalis, scalenus, and external intercostal muscles.

7. Protect the ribs and muscle tissue with moistened sponges and insert a self-retaining rib retractor to expose the thoracic viscera (Fig. 83–3).
8. Closure
   a. Preplace a temporary or permanent thoracic drain tube.
   b. Perform an intercostal nerve block by injecting bupivacaine (Marcaine) adjacent to two rib heads on each side of the incision (administer a total dose of 1 mg/kg).
   c. Preplace several large (2-0, 0, or 1) absorbable sutures around the ribs. Hug the caudal rib during suture passage to avoid damage to the intercostal vessels and nerve.
   d. While an assistant approximates the ribs with one of the sutures, tie the rib sutures using a surgeon's knot (Fig. 83–4).
   e. Close the deep muscles in one layer (serratus, scalenus, external abdominal oblique, and intercostal muscles) in a simple continuous pattern.
   f. Close the latissimus dorsi muscle in a simple continuous pattern (Fig. 83–5).
   g. Close the cutaneous trunci muscle and subcutaneous tissues in the next layer in a simple continuous pattern; then close the skin routinely, using the pattern of your choice.
   h. Perform thoracocentesis using the thoracic tube to evacuate air or fluid.
   i. Place a light, loosely fitting bandage over the incision and thoracic tube.

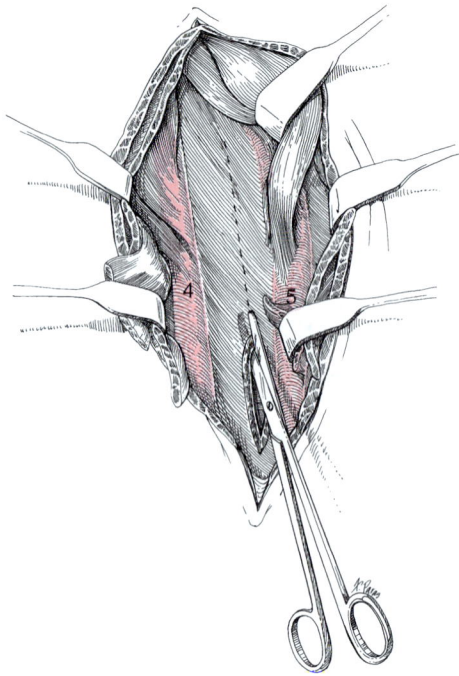

Figure 83–2. Cut or separate the serratus and scalenus muscles between ribs 4 and 5 so that an incision can be made in the intercostal muscles and the pleura.

Median Sternotomy

Median sternotomy is indicated when bilateral exposure of the thorax is necessary.

Examples are

- Multiple lung lesions
- Pericardectomy
- Mediastinal tumors (e.g., thymoma)
- Alternate approach to the pulmonic valve or for other cardiac procedures

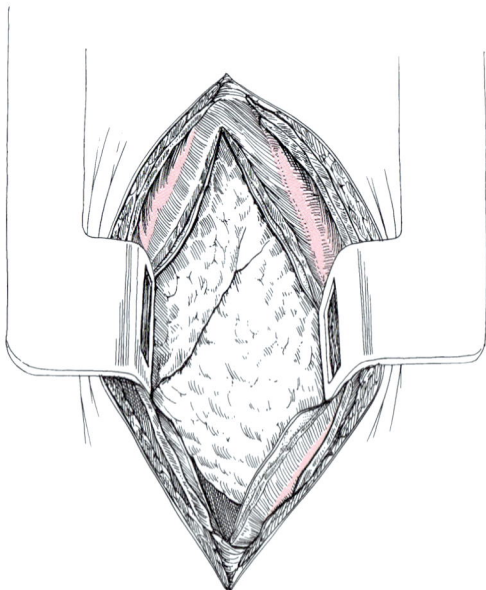

Figure 83–3. After the intercostal muscles and pleura are cut, retract the ribs to expose the lung.

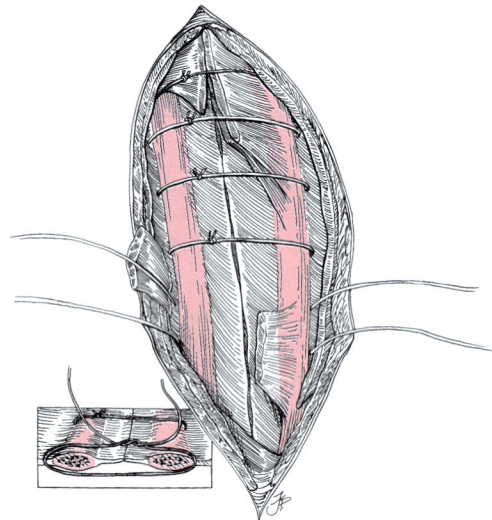

Figure 83–4. For lateral thoracotomy closure, place sutures around ribs 4 and 5 and secure each with a surgeon's knot.

- Hepatic surgery
- Complicated diaphragmatic hernia or other diaphragmatic surgery

Objective

- Bilateral exposure of the thorax

Equipment

- See Table 83–2 for special equipment needed for thoracic surgery
- Oscillating bone saw for medium to large dogs (an alternative is the Lebsche sternal knife; however, the saw is preferred)
- Osteotome and mallet
- Orthopedic wire (0.028–0.035 gauge) for medium to large dogs; wire cutters; wire-twisting instrument
- Electrocautery

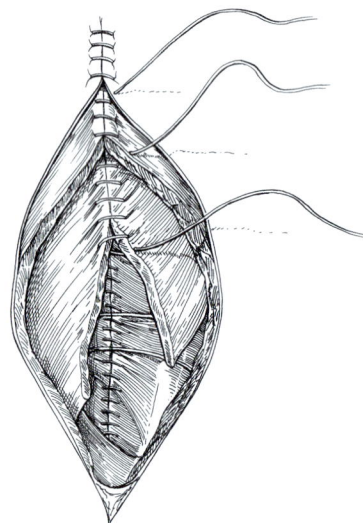

Figure 83–5. Close the latissimus dorsi muscle (simple continuous suture), the subcutaneous tissue (simple continuous suture), and the skin (simple continuous or interrupted suture).

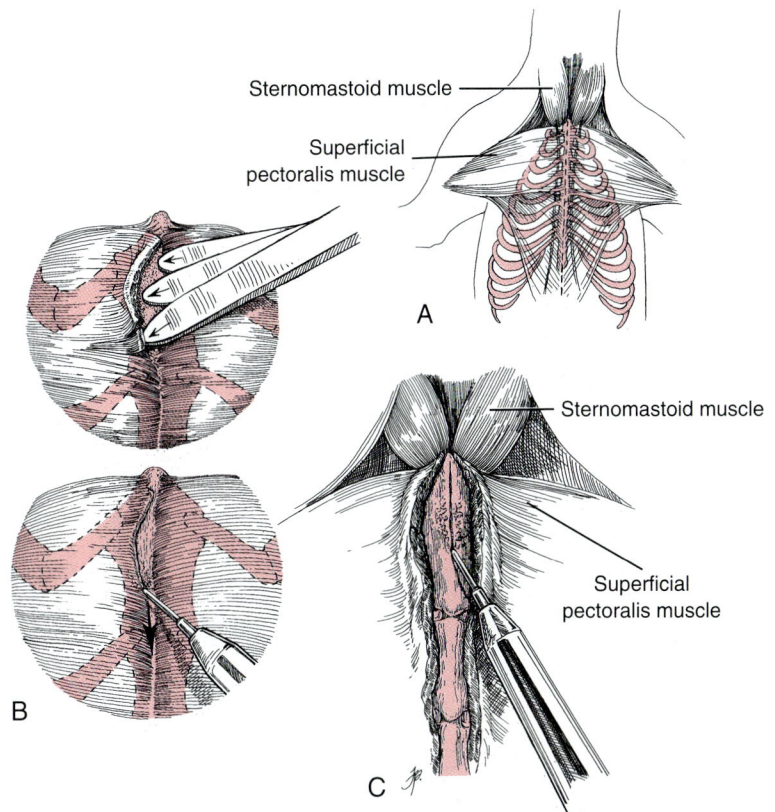

Figure 83–6. Technique for median sternotomy. *A,* Determine the middle of the sternum and associated muscle attachments; *B,* bluntly dissect muscle off the sternum (upper), or incise muscle attachments with electrocautery (lower); *C,* score the exposed periosteum on the midline.

Technique

1. Place the dog in dorsal recumbency.
2. Prepare the sternum and ventral half of the thorax for aseptic surgery.
3. Incise the skin and subcutaneous tissues from manubrium to xyphoid.
4. Divide the muscular attachments to the sternum along the thin, white fascial raphe to expose the sternum. This is best performed using electrocautery (Fig. 83–6).
5. Score the sternebrae on the ventral midline with a scalpel or electrocautery (see Fig. 83–6).
6. Cut two-thirds of the thickness of the sternebrae with the bone saw. Finish the cut with an osteotome and mallet, being careful not to injure the heart or internal thoracic vessels.

▼ *Key Point* When performing sternotomy, make the sternal cut exactly on the midline to facilitate secure closure with full cerclage wire.

7. If possible, leave at least one sternebra uncut (e.g., cranial or caudal extent) to counteract sheer forces on the sternum after closure.
8. Protect the sternum with moistened sponges and retract with a rib retractor.
9. Closure
   a. Place a temporary or permanent thoracic drain tube.
   b. Preplace cerclage wire or heavy suture (e.g., 0 or 1 polypropylene in a cat or small dog) around each sternebra, using hemostatic forceps (Fig. 83–7). Stay close to the bone to avoid the internal thoracic vessels. Tighten the wire, using wire-holding forceps.
   c. Close the muscle tissue, using an absorbable suture in a simple continuous pattern.
   d. Close the subcutaneous tissue and skin in a routine fashion.
   e. Perform thoracocentesis, using the thoracic tube to evacuate air and fluid.
   f. Loosely place a lightly padded bandage over the incision and thoracic tube.

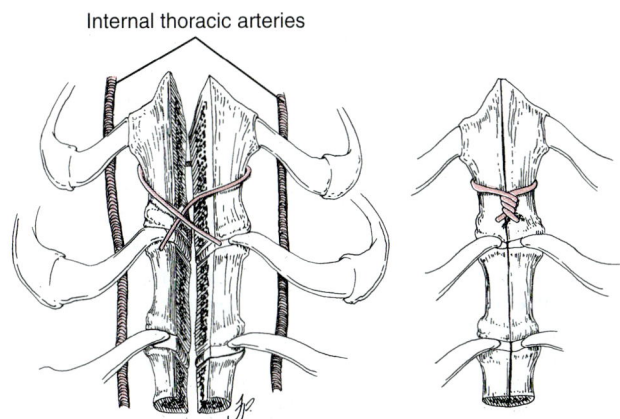

Figure 83–7. Close each sternebra with full cerclage wire twisted with a needle holder or wire twister.

Lung Lobectomy

Indications

- Neoplasia
- Abscesses or granuloma of the lung
- Lung lobe torsion or severe trauma
- Irreversible atelectasis
- Bronchoesophageal fistula
- Emphysematous bulla
- Refractory lobar pneumonia

Objectives

- Remove part or all of a lung lobe.
- Maintain good hemostasis, especially of the major pulmonary blood vessels.
- Establish an airtight seal of the bronchus.
- Leave adequate pulmonary tissue to avoid compromise of the patient's cardiopulmonary status.

Equipment

The same equipment used for lateral thoracotomy or median sternotomy plus

- Babcock tissue-holding forceps
- Small suture with swaged needle (e.g., 4-0 nylon or polypropylene)
- Tissue stapling device (TA30, 55, or 90 Thoracoabdominal Autosuture stapler; U.S. Surgical, Wallingford, Connecticut) (optional)

Technique

1. See preceding surgical techniques for description of approaches to the lung lobes.
2. Explore the thorax and determine the extent of disease and which lobes are involved.
3. Determine which bronchus or bronchi supply the affected lobe(s).
4. Mobilize the lobe.
   a. Caudal lung lobe—incise the pulmonary ligament that attaches the caudal aspect of the lobe to parietal pleura.
   b. Incise the pleural attachments between the affected lobe and adjacent lobes.
   c. Gently incise or dissect adhesions between the lobe and surrounding tissues (especially a problem in pulmonary neoplasia).
5. Partial lobectomy
   a. Place a noncrushing clamp (e.g., Satinsky) between the lesion and the hilus and incise distally to the clamp with scalpel or scissors.
   b. Close the remaining lobe with 4-0 or 5-0 nylon or polypropylene in a continuous horizontal mattress pattern. Oversew the incised tissue with a simple continuous pattern to prevent air leakage.
   c. Alternatively, place the Autosuture stapler between the lesion and the hilus. Staple the lung, incise distal to the stapler, and remove the diseased tissue.
   d. Check for hemostasis. Check for air leakage by flooding the lung incision with sterile saline, inflating the lung by positive pressure inspiration, and observing for bubbles. Place additional sutures if necessary to control leaks.
6. Complete lobectomy
   a. Dissect the pulmonary artery and vein free from the adjacent bronchus.
   b. Triple-ligate each vessel with silk or chromic catgut.
   c. Divide each vessel between the ligatures, leaving two ligatures with the animal.
   d. Place two clamps (e.g., Satinsky) across the bronchus and divide it between the clamps. Remove the lung lobe.
   e. Close the bronchus with monofilament nylon or polypropylene, using a horizontal mattress pattern followed by a simple continuous pattern.
   f. Alternatively, use the stapling device previously mentioned to close the hilar vessels and bronchus.

POSTOPERATIVE CARE AND COMPLICATIONS

Thoracic Tubes

- If a thoracic tube has been placed, leave it in as long as necessary, depending on the animal's condition and production of air or fluid (see Chap. 3 for details on thoracic tube management).
- In routine procedures in patients without recurrent pneumothorax or effusion, pull the tube as soon as negative pressure has been reestablished after completion of surgical closure.
- After major pulmonary resection, consider leaving a thoracic tube in place for a minimum of 24 hours even if no air or fluid is recovered. Otherwise, leave the tube in until insignificant amounts of air or fluids are being recovered (<2 ml/kg/day).
- Obtain thoracic radiographs prior to removal of the thoracic tube to ensure that there is no significant pleural air or fluid.

Pain

- Thoracic surgery is associated with postoperative pain that causes discomfort and can inhibit ventilation by making the animal reluctant to expand the thorax.
- Be careful when handling the animal, especially around the thoracotomy site. Unilateral forelimb lameness is common after lateral thoracotomy but should resolve within several days.
- Local analgesia can be used as a method of decreasing postoperative discomfort. See lateral thoracotomy closure earlier in this chapter for intercostal nerve block technique.
- Systemic analgesia can also be used for those animals exhibiting significant pain.
  - Administer morphine (0.2–0.4 mg/kg IM or SC), for 2–5 hours of analgesia. Respiratory depression or nausea may occur.
  - Other opioids that can be used are butorphanol (Torbutrol) (0.4 mg/kg IM), for 2–3 hours of analgesia, and buprenorphine (Buprenex) (.01–.03

mg/kg IM), for 4–8 hours of analgesia. A fentanyl patch is highly effective for longer (days) control of pain (see Chap. 2).

Pneumothorax

- Small amounts of residual air in the pleural space are common after thoracic surgery and rarely cause a clinical problem.
- Persistent postoperative pneumothorax can be a serious problem after surgery of the lung or airways if continuing leakage occurs at the site of incision or excision.
- If pneumothorax causes respiratory compromise and a thoracic tube is not already present, tap the animal's chest with a butterfly needle, syringe, and stopcock. Place a thoracic tube and consider performing thoracic radiography if improvement in the animal's condition does not occur or if the pneumothorax is recurrent. Evaluate the heart, lungs, pleural space, and location of the thoracic tube.

Hemothorax

- Postoperative hemothorax can occur after any thoracic surgery but is more common after major cardiac or vascular surgery, or after removal of large, highly vascular tumors. This can be a difficult complication to manage because reoperation does not usually reveal the source of bleeding.
- If large quantities of bloody fluid are aspirated from the thorax, obtain a packed cell volume (PCV) assay of the fluid. If the fluid is consistent with whole blood and the animal is losing considerable volume (i.e., clinical evidence of shock or PCV <20), use supportive care to replace volume (isotonic or hypertonic fluids). A steadily declining PCV in evacuated pleural fluid is a good indicator of pending hemostasis.
- Perform autotransfusion if the blood is not contaminated. Give whole blood from a donor dog if autotransfusion is not possible. (See Chapter 20 for more information on blood transfusions.)
- Monitor peripheral PCV and total protein until the animal's condition is stabilized.
- As a general rule, some surgeons recommend reexploration of the thorax if blood loss is > 2 ml/kg/hr for 3–4 hours and unresponsive to conservative therapy.

Ventricular Arrhythmias

- Cardiac arrhythmias are not uncommon and may develop 24–48 hours postoperatively (see Chap. 62).

Infection

- Postoperative infection after thoracotomy is uncommon but may occur if bacterial contamination occurs during the surgery or associated with the indwelling thoracic tube.
- Treat pleural infection with appropriate antibiotics (based on culture and sensitivity of the pleural fluid) and thoracic drainage (see Chap. 80). Rarely, thoracic lavage with fluids is necessary.

SUPPLEMENTAL READINGS

Evans HE, Christensen GC, eds.: Miller's Anatomy of the Dog, 3rd Ed. Philadelphia: WB Saunders, 1993, p 482.

Nelson AW: Lower respiratory system. *In* Slatter DH, ed.: Textbook of Small Animal Surgery. Philadelphia: WB Saunders, 1993, p 777.

7 Gastrointestinal Disorders

Susan E. Johnson

Chapter 84 Dentistry and Diseases of the Oropharynx

Sandra Manfra Marretta

Dental disease and diseases of the oropharynx are common in dogs and cats. These diseases can be divided into categories including oral surgical disease, periodontal disease, endodontic disease, orthodontic disease, stomatitis/gingivitis, neoplastic disease, and salivary gland disease. Neoplastic disease of the maxilla and mandible is discussed in Chapter 118.

ORAL SURGICAL DISEASE

The two major categories of oral surgical (non-neoplastic) disease are

- Diseases requiring dental extraction
- Oronasal fistulas and palatal defects that can be surgically corrected

Diseases Requiring Dental Extraction

Etiology

Dental diseases in which extraction is a treatment option include retained deciduous and supernumerary teeth, maloccluded teeth, advanced periodontal disease, fractured teeth, gross decay/erosions, diseased teeth in the fracture site of the mandible or maxilla, periapical abscess, impacted and deformed teeth, and teeth causing ophthalmic problems.

Clinical Signs

Common historical findings and signs of dental disease include changes in eating habits, halitosis, pawing at the mouth, abnormal salivation, oral hypersensitivity, facial swelling, oral hemorrhage, sneezing, nasal discharge, ophthalmic changes, and abnormal behavior.

Diagnosis and Indications for Extraction

The decision to perform dental extraction depends not only on the dental disease present but also on the client's ability and desire to pursue alternatives to extraction, such as periodontal, endodontic, and orthodontic therapy.

▼ *Key Point* If a client is unwilling to pursue alternatives for treatment of a painful tooth, then the tooth should be extracted.

Retained Deciduous and Supernumerary Teeth. Deciduous teeth are considered overly retained if they are firmly attached following the initial stage of eruption of the permanent tooth. Failure to extract deciduous teeth during this initial stage may result in malocclusion of the permanent teeth. Retained deciduous teeth and supernumerary teeth can be diagnosed as extra teeth present in the dental arcade. Deciduous teeth may be differentiated from supernumerary permanent teeth by their smaller crown size grossly and smaller root structure radiographically.

Maloccluded Teeth. Extraction may be required for maloccluded teeth that cause traumatic soft tissue occlusion or interfere with proper closing of the mouth. Orthodontic therapy is a viable alternative in these cases.

Advanced Periodontal Disease. Extremely mobile teeth caused by severe periodontal disease should be extracted. Other indications for extraction of teeth affected by periodontal disease include periodontal pockets extending to the apex of the tooth, pockets that reach the nasal cavity or maxillary sinus, and periapical abscess (discussed later).

Fractured Teeth. Extract fractured teeth with exposed pulp tissue if endodontic therapy is not an option. To diagnose pulpal exposure, place a dental explorer over the suspected exposure site. If the explorer penetrates into the tooth, the pulp is exposed.

Gross Decay/Dental Erosion. Gross decay, characterized by soft areas of demineralized enamel or dentin, is rare in dogs and cats. Dental erosive lesions or odontoclastic resorptive lesions are very common in cats.

- In dogs, gross decay, which usually occurs on the occlusal or biting surface of the maxillary first molar, and less frequently on the distal cusp of the mandibular first molar, can be identified with a dental explorer placed into the soft carious lesion. Penetration of the explorer into the soft demineralized enamel/dentin confirms gross decay. Radiographs of the affected tooth will show the extent of the lesion.
- Odontoclastic resorptive lesions are very common in cats. These defects are also called external root resorptions (ERRs) or neck lesions.
- ERRs often are extensive and painful and usually are covered by granulation tissue. Removal of the granulation tissue reveals the underlying erosive lesion.
  - Determine the extent of the erosion in the neck and crown of the tooth with a dental explorer.
  - Radiographs are imperative to determine the severity of root resorption, because minor erosions in the crown may be associated with major root resorption.
- Treat dental caries and external root resorptive lesions that extend into the pulp with extraction. Minor lesions can be restored with various dental restorative materials.

Diseased Teeth in a Mandible or Maxilla Fracture Site. Extract teeth in a fracture site that are severely affected with periodontal disease or that have fractured roots. If the fracture line in the jaw is located along the periodontal ligament and communicates with the apex of the tooth, the tooth is extracted. Careful gross assessment and radiographic examination of the fracture site can determine if an extraction is necessary.

Periapical Abscess. In small animals, a periapical abscess (infection around the apex of a tooth) usually is secondary to periodontal or endodontic disease and is characterized by acute, severe painful swelling in the area of the affected tooth. Periapical abscess may occur in a tooth that appears grossly normal. Concussive trauma without overt trauma to the tooth surface can cause pulpal necrosis with secondary periapical abscess.

- Carefully examine teeth in the area of acute facial swelling for deep periodontal pockets with a periodontal probe and for pulpal exposure with a dental explorer.

- Periapical lysis will be present around the apex of the affected root. Radiographs can confirm the diagnosis.
- Extraction of the affected tooth is recommended.

Impacted Teeth. Impacted (unerupted) teeth may cause nasal discharge, orthodontic problems, and bone loss.

- Dentigerous cysts may occur and can cause expansion of bone with subsequent facial asymmetry, extreme displacement of teeth, severe root resorption of adjacent teeth, and bone loss.
  - Dentigerous cysts may give rise to ameloblastomas.
- Radiography can diagnose impacted teeth. Perform extraction if they are causing problems and when associated with a dentigerous cyst. Remove the entire cyst lining to prevent recurrence of the cyst.

Deformed Teeth. Diagnose deformed teeth based on gross and radiographic appearance. Usually they result from trauma or fever that occurred during tooth development. Abnormalities in development of teeth occur rarely and include gemination of teeth, which results when a single tooth bud attempts to divide into two teeth.

- Diagnose minor dental deformities such as enamel hypoplasia based on the observation of symmetric defects and staining of enamel combined with a history of illness during tooth development. No treatment is required in these cases.
- Extract severely deformed teeth, secondary to dental trauma, that are causing pain.
- Gemination of the teeth usually requires no treatment. When a tooth has this developmental defect, perform dental radiography before extraction to determine the location of abnormal roots.

Ophthalmic Manifestations of Dental Disease. Tooth roots of the maxillary fourth premolar and first and second molars in dogs are in close proximity to the orbital floor and globe. Periodontal and endodontic disease of these teeth can result in ophthalmic signs, including orbital, periorbital, conjunctival, nasolacrimal, and neuro-ophthalmologic abnormalities.

- When signs of ophthalmic disease are suggestive of a primary dental disorder, do a complete oral examination under general anesthesia or sedation.
- Examine the maxillary teeth for fractures or deep periodontal pockets.
- Take dental radiographs of the maxillary teeth to check for periapical lysis.
- Extract teeth that are causing secondary ophthalmic disease.

Surgical Anatomy

Proper performance of dental extractions requires a thorough knowledge of dental formulas, dental root structure, and pericoronal and periradicular anatomy.

▼ *Key Point* Determine the number of roots in any tooth to be extracted to ensure that all roots are removed during extraction.

Table 84–1. DECIDUOUS AND PERMANENT DENTAL FORMULAS FOR DOGS AND CATS

Deciduous Dentition
Dog: 2(I3/3 C1/1 P3/3) = 28
Cat: 2(I3/3 C1/1 P3/2) = 26

Permanent Dentition
Dog: 2(I3/3 C1/1 P4/4 M2/3) = 42
Cat: 2(I3/3 C1/1 P3/2 M1/1) = 30

I, incisor; C, canine; P, premolar; M, molar.

- Deciduous and permanent dental formulas for dogs and cats are listed in Table 84–1.
- In both dogs and cats, all incisors and canines have only a single root. The dentition, including root structure, of dogs and cats is illustrated in Figures 84–1 and 84–2, respectively. Tooth roots for both species are listed in Table 84–2.
- Basic anatomic structures of the teeth and related areas are illustrated in Figure 84–3 and defined in Table 84–3.

Preoperative Considerations

- Before performing dental extractions, perform a thorough physical examination, standard laboratory tests including a complete blood count (CBC), serum biochemistry, and urinalysis.
- Perform appropriate radiographic procedures, based on the animal's clinical signs, physical examination findings, and age.
- Correct any underlying metabolic abnormalities such as dehydration, azotemia, electrolyte imbalances, hyperglycemia, and hypoglycemia.

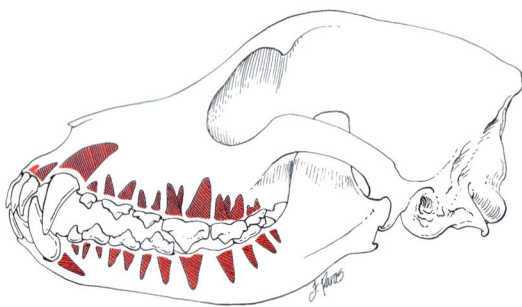

Figure 84–1. Dental root structure in the dog.

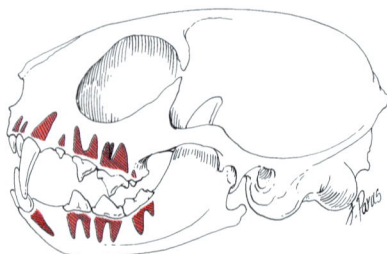

Figure 84–2. Dental root structure in the cat.

Table 84–2. TOOTH ROOTS IN DOGS AND CATS

Type of Tooth	No. of Roots
In Dogs	
Incisor	1
Canine	1
Maxillary (upper) cheek teeth:	
1st (1st P)	1
2nd and 3rd (2nd and 3rd P)	2
4th–6th (4th P; 1st and 2nd M)	3
Mandibular (lower) cheek teeth:	
1st and last (1st P; 3rd M)	1
2nd–6th (2nd–4th P; 1st and 2nd M)	2
In Cats	
Incisor	1
Canine	1
Maxillary (upper) cheek teeth:	
1st (2nd P)	1
3rd (4th P)	3
All others	2
Mandibular (lower) cheek teeth:	
All	2

P, premolar; M, molar.

Surgical Procedure

There are three basic types of extractions: simple, multirooted, and complicated surgical. See Tables 84–4 through 84–6 for equipment and materials recommended for all types of dental procedures.

Simple Extraction. Simple extraction refers to the extraction of a small single-rooted tooth such as an incisor.

Technique

1. Place an appropriate-size dental elevator in the gingival sulcus to sever the attachments of the gingiva around the tooth.
2. Advance the elevator apically (toward the apex or tip of the root) between the alveolar bone and root.
3. Rotate the elevator 90° and hold for 15-second intervals to tear the periodontal ligament (Fig. 84–4A).
4. Advance the elevator again apically, rotate it 90°, and hold for 15 seconds.
5. When the tooth is loose, place an appropriate-size dental extraction forcep on the crown near the gingival margin and rotate and remove the tooth from the alveolus (Fig. 84–4B).
6. Examine the tooth to confirm that the root has been removed completely.

Multirooted Extraction. Multirooted teeth such as premolars and molars are more difficult to extract than incisors. Often only one root is affected and the other root(s) are firmly attached to the alveolar bone. Furthermore, most roots are embedded in the alveolar bone at divergent angles, making removal of the intact tooth difficult.

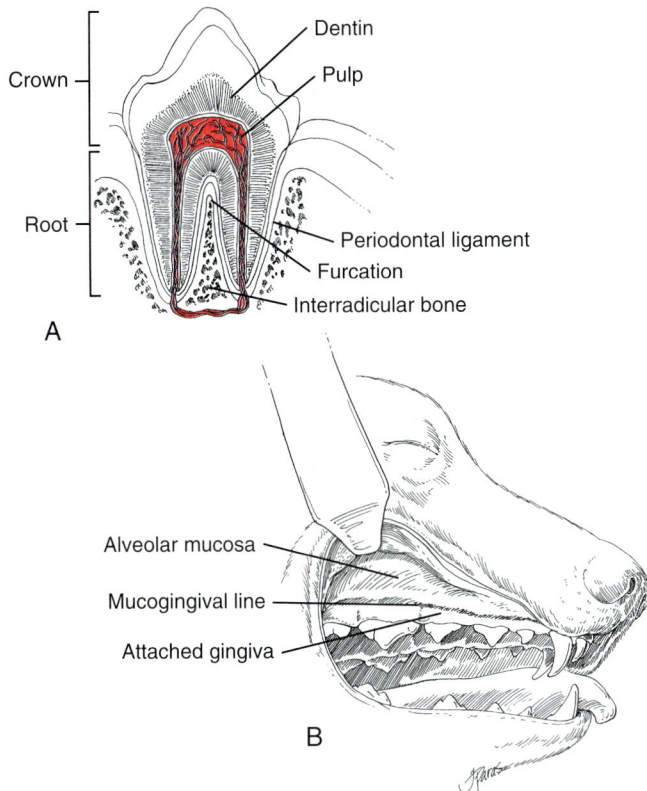

Figure 84–3. *A,* Anatomy of the tooth. *B,* Gingival anatomy.

▼ *Key Point* Sectioning of a multirooted tooth into two or three sections converts the procedure into multiple simple extractions. A high-speed handpiece or a low-speed electric handpiece with adequate irrigation can be used for sectioning teeth.

Technique

1. Locate the furcation with a dental elevator.
2. Place a tapered fissure bur (#701 in small animals

and #702 in larger animals) at the furcation and direct it through the crown (Fig. 84–5*A*).
3. Advance the elevator apically between two roots.
4. Rotate the elevator 90° and hold for 15 seconds to gently force the roots apart (Fig. 84–5*B*).

Table 84–4. DENTAL EQUIPMENT

Equipment	Applications
Portable electric dental drill with low-speed hand piece and prophy angle (VC-30, Henry Schein, Inc.; Port Washington, NY)	Sectioning teeth, removal of alveolar bone, polishing teeth
Mobile delivery system with high-speed handpiece, low-speed handpiece, water and air syringe (Vet-Base, Henry Schein, Inc.)	Sectioning teeth, removal of alveolar bone, polishing teeth, cavity and crown preparations
Piezoelectric scaler, electric or air driven (Spartan USA, Inc.; Fenton, MO)	Permits rapid, easy removal of dental calculus
Dental radiography unit (Minxray; Northbrook, IL)	Permits rapid, easy exposure of dental radiographs

---

Table 84–5. DENTAL INSTRUMENTATION

Instrumentation*	Applications
Oral Surgery	
Dental elevator (ST8/ST9)	Tears periodontal ligament during extraction
Extraction forceps (ST5/ST6)	Completes breakdown of periodontal ligament and removal of tooth from alveolus during extraction
Root tip pick (ST11)	Removal of small-breed deciduous teeth or broken root tips
Bone curette (ST10)	Debridement of alveolus following extraction
Periosteal elevator (ST7)	Elevation of mucoperiosteum during oronasal fistula repair and palatal surgery
Periodontic	
Periodontal probe/explorer (ST4)	Measurement of depth of periodontal pocket (probe); detection of pulpal exposures and carious lesions (explorer)
Hand scalers (ST2)	Subgingival scaling
Curette (Columbia #13/14)	Removal of accretions on the root surface and of granulation tissue from the pocket wall
Prophylaxis paste (Zircon F)	Polishing teeth following scaling
Endodontic	
Endodontic files (Hedstrom/K-Files)	Debridement of necrotic pulpal tissue from canal
Lentulo spiral filler	Placement of zinc oxide and eugenol in canal
10:1 Reduction gear (Contra Angle)	Attachment of lentulo spiral filler to low-speed handpiece
Root canal plugger	Compression of gutta percha into the apex

*Available from Henry Schein, Inc.; Port Washington, N.Y.

Table 84–3. BASIC ANATOMIC STRUCTURES OF THE DENTITION

Crown:	Portion of the tooth located in the oral cavity. It is covered by enamel.
Root:	Portion of the tooth that lies within the alveolar bone. It is covered by cementum.
Furcation:	The space between the roots of a multirooted tooth.
Periodontal ligament:	Ligament that attaches the root of the tooth to the alveolar bone.
Interradicular bone:	Bone located between the roots.
Buccal bone:	Bone located on the buccal, or cheek, side of the tooth root.
Attached gingiva:	Keratinized gingiva firmly attached to the underlying alveolar bone.
Alveolar mucosa:	Mucosa that is loosely attached to the underlying alveolar bone.
Mucogingival line:	Anatomic landmark that separates the attached gingiva from the alveolar mucosa.

Table 84–6. DENTAL MATERIALS

Material	Applications
Amalgam (Strat-O-Caps, Schein; Contour, Kerr)	Restorations following endodontic therapy or cavity preparation
Composite resins (Concise, 3M; Adaptic, Johnson & Johnson)	Aesthetic restorations following endodontic therapy or cavity preparation
Glass ionomers (Ketac-Bond, Espe-Premier)	Restoration of feline external root resorptive lesions
Endodontic sealers (zinc oxide–eugenol and AH-26, Henry Schein, Inc.)	Endodontic filling material
Calcium hydroxide paste (Dycal, Caulk)	Stimulates closure of an apex and reparative dentin formation following pulpotomies
Gutta percha	Fills the pulp canal following debridement during root canal therapy
Zinc phosphate cement	Used as base following the placement of endodontic filling material and prior to placement of final restorative material

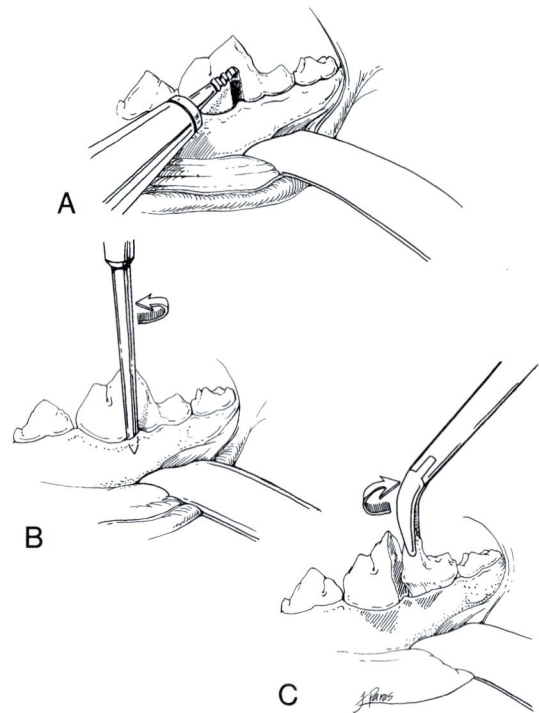

Figure 84–5. *A,* Tooth is sectioned with a tapered fissure bur. *B,* Elevator is rotated 90°. *C,* Extraction forceps is used to extract each root separately.

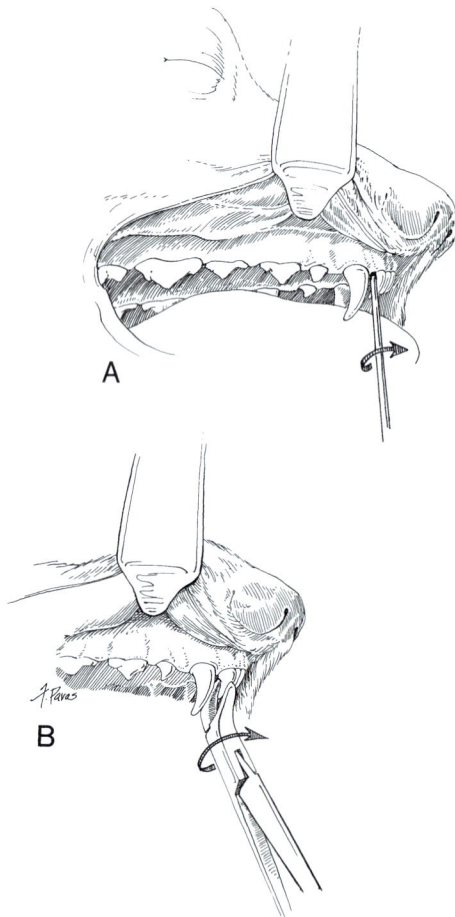

Figure 84–4. *A,* Dental elevator in gingival sulcus is rotated 90°. Tooth is rotated with extraction forceps.

5. Advance the elevator further apically, rotate it 90°, and hold for 15 seconds.
6. Place a dental extraction forceps on each crown segment and rotate to extract each root independently (Fig. 84–5C).

Complicated Surgical Extraction. This procedure involves the removal of teeth with large roots, such as the canine teeth in dogs, or large multirooted teeth, such as the mandibular first molars.

Technique

1. Reflect a mucoperiosteal flap to expose buccal alveolar bone overlying the root (Fig. 84–6A).
2. Remove the buccal alveolar bone overlying the root with a large round bur (Fig. 84–6B).
3. If the tooth is multirooted, section it with a #702 bur.
4. Elevate and extract the tooth.
5. Perform an alveoloplasty to remove the rough edges of the alveolus, using a large, round bur.
6. Curette and flush the alveolus.
7. Incise the deepest layer of the flap, the periosteal layer, over the entire width of the most dorsal aspect of the flap to prevent tension on the flap closure.
8. Replace and suture the mucoperiosteal flap to the adjacent gingiva with 2-0 or 3-0 chromic catgut suture in a simple interrupted pattern (Fig. 84–6C).

Postoperative Care and Complications

• Offer a soft diet for 3–10 days, depending on the number and complexity of dental extractions.

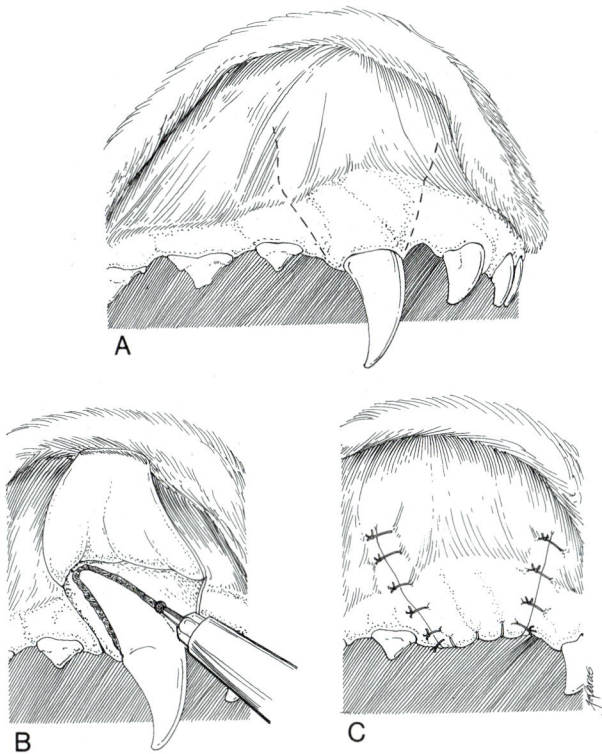

Figure 84–6. *A,* Proposed mucoperiosteal flap incision site for extraction of a maxillary canine tooth. *B,* Buccal alveolar bone is removed. *C,* Mucoperiosteal flap is replaced and sutured.

- Administer a broad-spectrum antibiotic (e.g., amoxicillin clavulanate) for 3–7 days when infection is present.

Hemorrhage. Hemorrhage is a common complication of dental extractions and usually is minor and can be easily controlled with a gauze sponge and digital pressure. Control persistent alveolar hemorrhage by suturing the gingiva over the alveolus, thereby permitting clot formation.

Broken Root Tips. Broken root tips are common when inappropriate dental extraction techniques are used. Various types of dental pathology such as odontoclastic resorptive lesions, dental caries, and ankylosis of the root to the alveolar bone may predispose to broken root tips.

▼ *Key Point* Always remove any tooth roots that break during extraction.

- Differentiate broken root tips from surrounding alveolar bone by the following features:
  - The tooth is whiter than the surrounding off-white bone.
  - The tooth is harder than the surrounding bone, as detected by a dental explorer.
  - The hard tissues of the tooth do not bleed.
- Remove root tips with a root tip pick or obliterate with an appropriate-size round bur (Fig. 84–7). Removal with a root tip pick is preferred because obliteration of roots with a bur may cause damage to underlying structures.

▼ *Key Point* Permanent teeth may be damaged during the extraction of deciduous teeth.

Damage to Permanent Teeth. Careful extraction of deciduous teeth can help minimize this complication. However, extraction of deciduous teeth before complete formation of the permanent crowns (especially at 8–12 weeks of age) can result in enamel hypocalcification, enamel hypoplasia, crown deformity, and eruption failure.

Misplaced Tooth or Root Tip. A tooth or root tip infrequently may be misplaced in the nasal cavity, maxillary sinus, or mandibular canal during an extraction. Advanced periodontal disease in combination with aggressive extraction techniques can force a tooth or root tip into the nasal cavity, maxillary sinus, or mandibular canal.

- Enlarge the defect in the floor of the extraction site to remove a misplaced tooth or root tip.

Iatrogenic Fractures. Severe periodontal disease, inappropriate extraction techniques, and metabolic bone disease in geriatric animals may be predisposing factors in iatrogenic mandibular fractures.

- Careful elevation of the tooth, digital support of the mandible during extraction, and a rotational movement with the dental extractor can help prevent iatrogenic mandibular fractures.

Osteomyelitis and Bony Sequestra. Osteomyelitis following extraction of teeth may be caused by retained tooth roots, exposed alveolar bone, and osseous necrosis. A bone sequestrum may develop when a segment of alveolar bone is fractured off during a dental extraction and left in the extraction site.

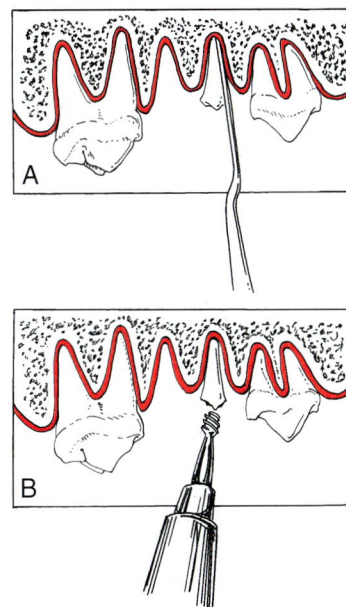

Figure 84–7. Elevation of root tip with root tip pick. *B,* Obliteration of root tip with round bur.

- Treat osteomyelitis and bony sequestra by removing retained tooth roots and bony sequestra and by curettage of necrotic bone to the level of healthy, bleeding bone.

Ophthalmic Complications of Dental Extractions. Inappropriate techniques during extraction of the maxillary fourth premolar and the first and second molars in dogs may result in severe ophthalmic complications caused by penetration of the elevator into the orbit or globe, causing orbital cellulitis, orbital abscess, or endophthalmitis.

- Prevent ophthalmic complications of dental extractions by using a finger stop near the tip of the elevator during extraction of the maxillary fourth premolar and the first and second molars to prevent deep penetration of the elevator into orbital tissues or the globe.

Oronasal Fistulas and Palatal Defects

Oronasal fistulas are abnormal communications between the oral and nasal cavity. Palatal defects may occur anywhere in the palate and result in a communication between the oral and nasal cavity or the oral cavity and the maxillary sinus.

Etiology

Palatal defects may be congenital or acquired.

Congenital Defects

Congenital palatal defects occur primarily in brachiocephalic breeds, miniature schnauzers, cocker spaniels, beagles, and cats. Congenital abnormalities of the primary palate (incisive bone) are referred to as a hare lip. These defects may occur concomitantly or independent of secondary palate (hard and soft palate) abnormalities.

Acquired Defects

- Acquired palatal defects are most frequently caused by a deep maxillary periodontal pocket that has progressed toward the apex of the tooth, resulting in lysis of the thin layer of bone that separates the palatal aspect of the root of the maxillary tooth and the nasal cavity or maxillary sinus.
- Acquired palatal defects that have etiologies other than dental disease usually are located in the hard palate and may be caused by various types of trauma including dog bites, blunt head trauma, electrical shock, gunshot wounds, foreign body penetration, and pressure necrosis. They also may occur as a complication of maxillectomy for oral neoplasia.

Clinical Signs

- Clinical signs associated with oronasal fistulas and palatal defects include unilateral or bilateral mucopurulent and occasionally hemorrhagic nasal discharge.
- Animals often are presented because of recurrent episodes of sneezing, especially after eating.

Diagnosis

- Identify defects in the hard palate by an oral examination.
- Perform thorough periodontal examination to identify oronasal and oroantral fistulas secondary to periodontal disease. This requires tranquilization or general anesthesia.
  - Insert a probe into the suspected periodontal pocket, which often is located on the palatal aspect of the maxillary canine tooth but may be located anywhere along the periodontal ligament of the maxillary cheek teeth.
  - If the probe penetrates easily into the nasal cavity or maxillary sinus, when the nose is tipped ventrally, immediate ipsilateral nasal hemorrhage confirms the presence of an oronasal or oroantral fistula.

Surgical Anatomy

▼ *Key Point* Oronasal fistulas are associated most frequently with defects in the area of the maxillary canine tooth.

The surgical anatomy varies with the location of the defect. The mucoperiosteal flap used in the repair of oronasal fistulas extends from the margins of the defect across the mucogingival line (the anatomic landmark separating the attached gingiva from the alveolar mucosa). Surgical techniques used to repair defects in the hard palate often require preservation of the palatine arteries, which arise approximately 1 cm palatal to the maxillary fourth premolar and course rostrally along the hard palate (Fig. 84–8).

Preoperative Considerations

▼ *Key Point* Tube- or bottle-feed animals with congenital hard palatal defects until they are 3 months of age to decrease the incidence of inhalation pneumonia.

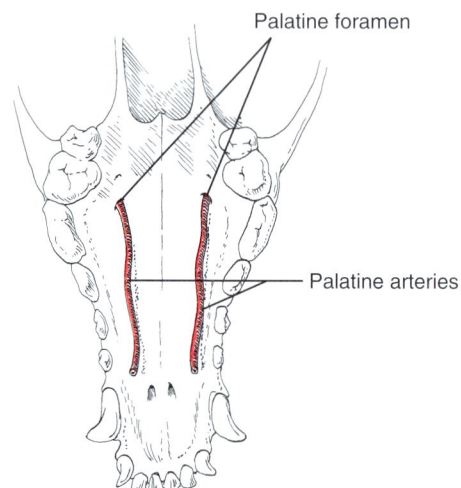

Figure 84–8.   Palatine arteries.

- Perform surgery when the animal is 3–4 months of age following thoracic radiography to check for pneumonia.
- Give animals with severe, purulent rhinitis or pneumonia antibiotics before surgery.

Surgical Procedure

Two techniques used frequently for the repair of oronasal fistulas include the single-layer and the double-layer mucoperiosteal flap. The overlapping flap technique is used frequently for the repair of hard palatal defects.

Single-Layer Mucoperiosteal Flap

Technique

1. Place the animal in lateral recumbency.
2. Debride the epithelial margin of the fistula with a #15 scalpel blade.
3. Make two divergent incisions in the mucosa, beginning at the mesial and distal aspects of the fistula and extending across the mucogingival line (Fig. 84–9A).
4. Using a periosteal elevator, gently raise the flap (Fig. 84–9B).

5. Reflect the flap apically and incise the deepest layer of the flap (the periosteal layer) the entire width of the flap at its most dorsal aspect (Fig. 84–9C).
6. If necessary, remove excess buccal bony plate with a rongeur or dental bur to permit tensionless apposition of tissues (Fig. 84–9D).
7. Before closure, remove all infected bone and soft tissue with a bone curette, and irrigate the surgical site with sterile saline.
8. Suture the flap to the palatal and gingival mucosa with 2-0 or 3-0 chromic catgut suture or PDS (polydioxanone) in a simple interrupted pattern (Fig. 84–9E).

Double-Layer Mucoperiosteal Flap. Use to repair large chronic or recurrent oronasal fistulas.

Technique

1. Debride the mesial, distal, and buccal epithelial margins of the fistula with a #15 blade. Do not debride the palatal epithelial margin.
2. Elevate an elliptical palatal mucoperiosteal flap with a periosteal elevator, preserving the lateral attachment of the base of the flap (Fig. 84–10A).
3. Fold over and suture the flap to the periosteum of the edge of the defect with 2-0 or 3-0 chromic catgut

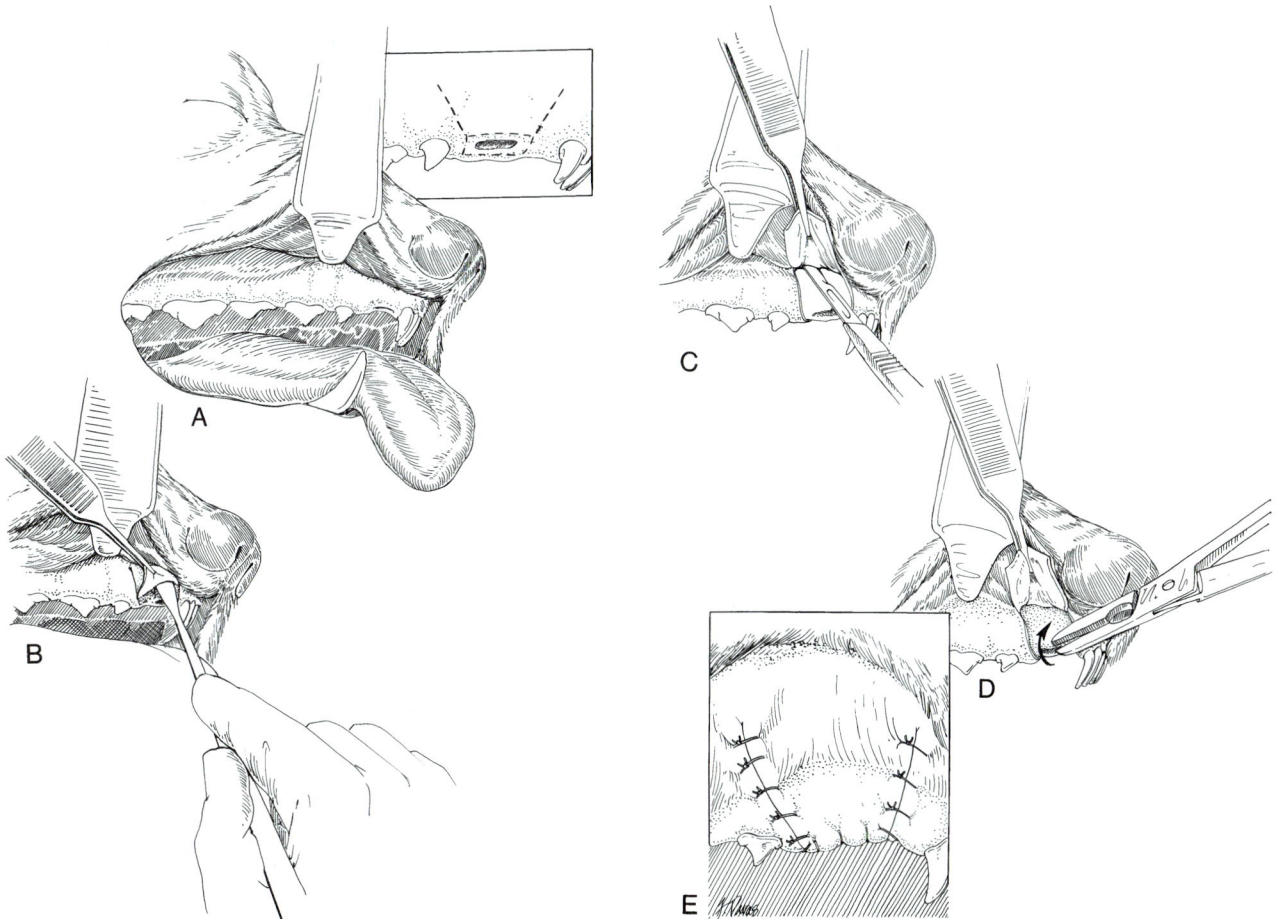

Figure 84–9. *A*, Proposed incision sites in mucosa for oronasal fistula repair. *B*, Elevation of mucoperiosteal flap. *C*, Incision of periosteal layer of flap. *D*, Removal of rough edges of buccal alveolar bone with rongeurs. *E*, Mucoperiosteal flap is replaced and sutured.

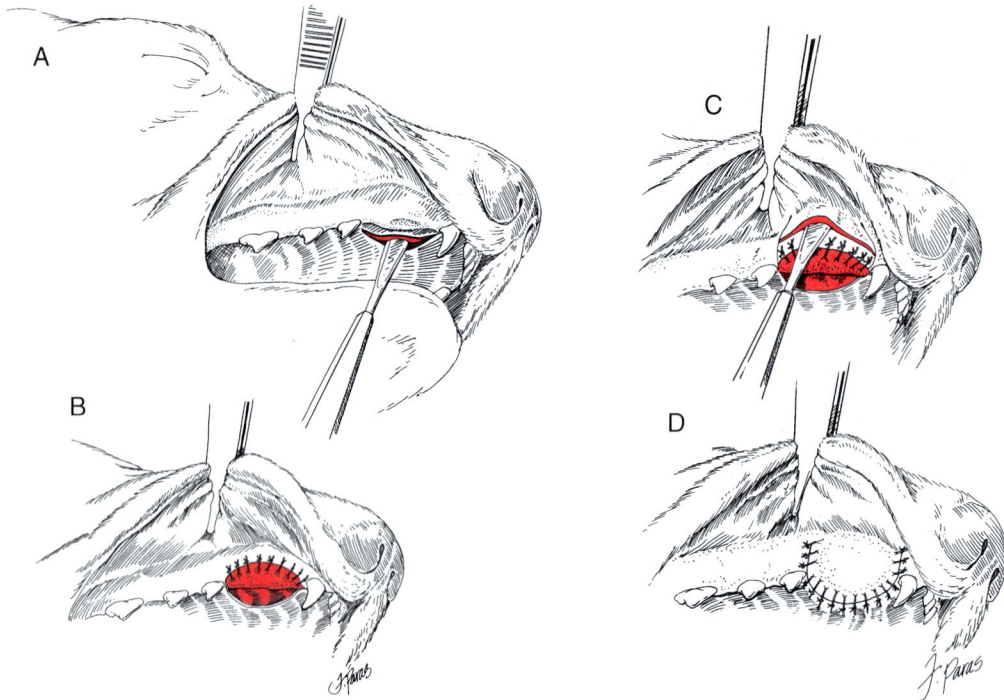

Figure 84–10. *A*, Periosteal elevation of palatal flap. *B*, Palatal flap is sutured to debrided edges of defect. *C*, Buccal mucoperiosteal flap is elevated and advanced palatally. *D*, Flap is sutured to palatal and gingival mucosa.

suture or PDS in a simple interrupted pattern (Fig. 84–10*B*).

4. Elevate a buccal mucoperiosteal flap from the lateral aspect of the oronasal fistula (see Fig. 84–9*C*).
5. Advance the buccal mucoperiosteal flap palatally to cover the inverted flap and the denuded palatine bone (Fig. 84–10*C*).
6. Suture the flap to the palatal and gingival mucosa with 2-0 or 3-0 chromic catgut suture or PDS in a simple interrupted pattern (Fig. 84–10*D*).

Overlapping Flap Technique. Use for repair of hard palatal defects, especially on the midline.

Technique

1. Make an incision the length of the palatal defect in the palatal mucosa just palatal to the maxillary dental arcade. The rostral and caudal aspects of these incisions are connected to the rostral and caudal aspects of the palatal defect (Fig. 84–11*A*).
2. Incise the opposite side of the palatal defect along the entire length of the defect and gently elevate with a periosteal elevator to create a recipient site for the mucoperiosteal flap. Carefully elevate the mucoperiosteal flap with a periosteal elevator, preserving the palatine artery (see Fig. 84–8) that arises

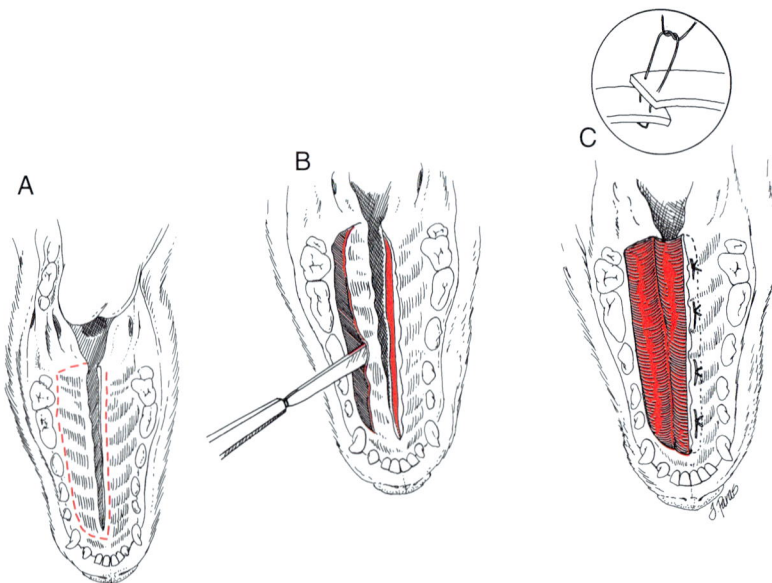

Figure 84–11. *A*, Palatal incisions to create flaps for overlapping flap technique. *B*, Periosteal elevation of flap. *C*, The larger flap is placed beneath the smaller flap and the flaps are sutured together.

approximately 1 cm palatal to the upper fourth premolar (Fig. 84–11*B*).

3. Hinge the mucoperiosteal flap at the end of the palatal defect and place beneath the mucosa on the other side of the defect.
4. Preplace 3-0 polyglactin 910 sutures in an interrupted horizontal mattress pattern through the recipient site and the flap.
5. Tie the sutures from caudal to rostral to complete the procedure (Fig. 84–11*C*).

Postoperative Care and Complications

- Feed a soft diet (gruel or liquid) for 2–3 weeks. For animals requiring complicated repair, consider using esophagostomy or gastrostomy tube feeding (see Chap. 3). Place Elizabethan collars on patients that paw at the oral cavity.
- In 3 weeks, reexamine the patient to assess the integrity of the repair.
  - If the repair is intact, gradually return to a normal diet over the next 1–2 weeks.
  - If the repair was unsuccessful, schedule a second operation in approximately 4 weeks.

PERIODONTAL DISEASE

▼ *Key Point* Periodontal disease is the most common cause of oral infection and tooth loss in dogs.

Periodontal disease occurs in two forms: gingivitis and periodontitis. Gingivitis is a reversible inflammation of the gingiva. Periodontitis involves deeper inflammation with loss of tooth support and permanent damage.

The purpose of periodontal therapy is to prevent gingivitis from progressing to periodontitis and to delay the progression of periodontitis once it is established.

Etiology

- Periodontal disease is initiated by an accumulation of large amounts of bacteria at the junction of the tooth and the gingiva. Prolonged retention of these bacteria results in a change of the predominant flora from gram-positive aerobic coccoid bacteria to more motile gram-negative anaerobic rod-shaped bacteria.
- Tissue destruction occurs secondary to inflammation, resulting in a loss of periodontal support. Over a period of time (usually years), the presence of plaque, calculus, and gingivitis results in loss of periodontal support.

Clinical Signs

- Common signs include mobile teeth, periodontal and periapical abscesses, facial swelling, periodontal pockets, nasal discharge, and oronasal and oroantral fistulas.
- Severe gingival sulcus hemorrhage, pathologic mandibular fractures, intranasal tooth migration, and osteomyelitis with or without bone sequestra develop uncommonly.

Diagnosis

The diagnosis of periodontal disease is based on a thorough oral and periodontal examination and dental radiography.

Gingivitis

- Animals with gingivitis have swollen gingival margins that bleed after the application of light pressure. Serous or purulent exudate may be produced from the gingival sulcus. Halitosis commonly is present.
- Examination with a periodontal probe is normal and there is no radiographic evidence of bone loss around the teeth.

Periodontitis

- Hyperplasia and gingival recession are seen, as well as severe gingival inflammation with various amounts of calculus and debris.
- Periodontal probing reveals periodontal pockets that can progress to tooth loss if untreated.
- Dental radiographs can identify bone loss, which most frequently is horizontal or parallel to the cemento-enamel junction (CEJ), which separates the crown from the root. Less frequently the bone loss is vertical or parallel to the long axis of the root.

Surgical Anatomy

The periodontal tissues are composed of the gingiva, cementum, periodontal ligament, and alveolar bone. An accurate estimate of the amount of support that has been lost around a tooth depends on the appropriate use of a periodontal probe and the recognition of a few anatomic landmarks.

- Locate the cemento-enamel junction that separates the anatomic crown from the anatomic root, 1–2 mm below the normal gingival margin (Fig. 84–12).
- The free gingival margin, an important anatomic landmark when assessing periodontal disease, is the highest point of gingival tissue that lies on the tooth. In normal tissues, the free gingival margin is just above the CEJ (see Fig. 84–12).

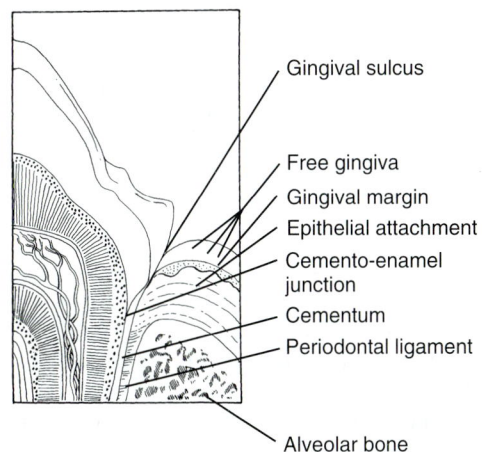

Figure 84–12. Normal periodontal anatomy.

Gingival sulcus
Free gingiva
Gingival margin
Epithelial attachment
Cemento-enamel junction
Cementum
Periodontal ligament
Alveolar bone

- When gingival recession is present, the free gingival margin is below the CEJ.
- In cases of gingival hyperplasia, it is >2 mm above the CEJ.
- Measure and record the depth of the pocket in millimeters. Also note the relationship of the free gingival margin to the CEJ. These values will adequately assess the level of attachment and thereby dictate the appropriate therapy.

Preoperative Considerations

- Prior to treatment, a thorough physical examination and clinical laboratory testing are recommended to rule out concurrent disease.
- In severe cases, administer perioperative broad-spectrum antibiotics (amoxicillin clavulanate). Initiate antibiotic therapy before the dental procedure so that adequate blood levels are present during the dental procedure.

Surgical Procedures

Several procedures are used to treat periodontal disease. These include scaling, root planing, subgingival curettage, polishing, gingivectomy, and open-flap curettage.

Dental Scaling

Dental scaling can be divided into two main categories: supragingival and subgingival.

Supragingival Scaling. This involves the removal of calculus located above the gingival margin. It is most easily performed with a power scaler.

Technique

1. A universal tip is most appropriate for use in small animals.
2. Place the side of the tip below the edge of the calculus and gently lift to remove calculus.
3. Move the tip gently across the surface of the tooth with a paint brush–type movement.
4. Continuously move the tip across the dentition during scaling; never hold it on one tooth continuously for more than 10–15 seconds.
5. Spray copiously with water to prevent overheating of the tooth and to wash away dislodged calculus.

Subgingival Scaling. Following supragingival scaling, perform subgingival scaling, root planing, and curettage with a power scaler designed for subgingival scaling, hand scalers, and curettes.

Technique

1. Use a power scaler such as a piezoelectric scaler subgingivally with a light touch, copious water spray, and constant motion to remove the major portion of subgingival calculus. Alternatively, hand scalers may be used.
2. With a hand instrument such as the Columbia 13/14 curette, complete the root cleaning. Place the curette at the bottom of the pocket, then engage the

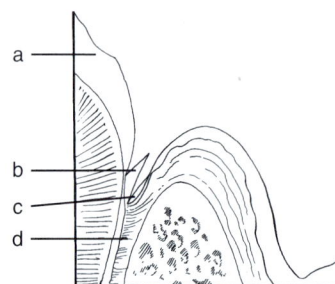

Figure 84–13. Cross section of curette placed beneath calculus for subgingival scaling: (a) enamel, (b) calculus, (c) curette in cross section, (d) periodontal ligament.

root with the edge of the curette and pull the curette coronally along the surface of the root (Fig. 84–13).
3. Continue subgingival scaling and root planing (scaling of the root) until the root is smooth and clean.
4. Following removal of subgingival calculus, record areas of pathologic deepening (>3 mm) on a dental chart.
5. Perform subgingival curettage by gently scraping the soft tissue lining of the pocket with a sharp curette until all epithelial and granulation tissue is removed.

Polishing Technique

1. Place a prophylaxis angle on a slow-speed handpiece. Fill the cup with medium-grit prophylaxis paste.
2. Rotate the cup over the entire exposed surface of the teeth, smoothing the surface of the enamel.
3. Rinse the teeth with forced air and water spray to remove any residual debris.

Gingivectomy

Gingivectomy is the resection of unsupported gingival tissue. This technique is used to eliminate periodontal pockets greater than 5 mm deep that are caused by horizontal bone loss. Gingivectomy is also used to remove hyperplastic gingival tissue and for harvesting gingival biopsies.

▼ *Key Point* Do not perform gingivectomy unless sufficient attached gingiva (>3 mm) can be retained following the procedure, because removal of tissue below this point may result in dehiscence of the gingiva.

Technique

1. With a periodontal probe, mark the depth of the periodontal pocket on the gingiva opposite the affected tooth (Fig. 84–14A).
2. Make a beveled incision in the gingiva, slightly apical to the pocket mark, to create a natural gingival contour to the gingiva following the gingivectomy (Fig. 84–14B). The incision can be made with a gingivectomy knife, scalpel blade, or electrosurgery tip. If electrosurgery is used, surgical cutting modes are recommended.

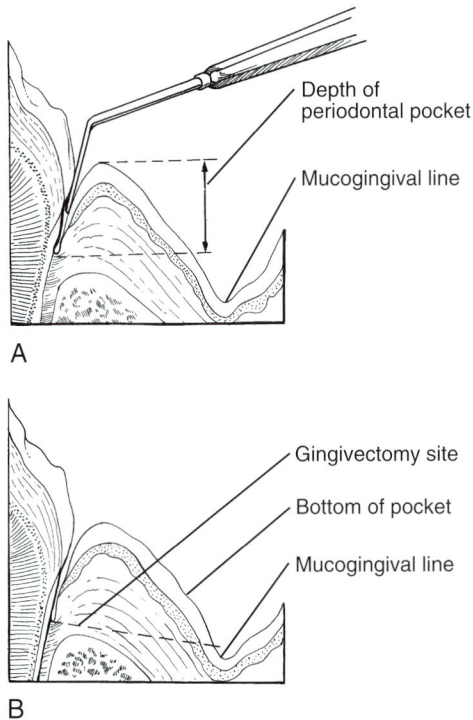

Figure 84–14. *A,* Periodontal probe measures pocket depth. *B,* Proposed gingivectomy site.

3. Following removal of excessive hyperplastic tissue and pocket elimination, scale and polish the exposed tooth surface.

Open-Flap Curettage

This technique is used to treat periodontal pockets that extend beneath the level of the alveolar crest. Open-flap curettage permits access to intrabony defects without loss of attached gingiva.

Technique

1. Make an incision with a #11 or #15 scalpel blade 1–2 mm from the tooth and directed toward the alveolar crest (Fig. 84–15*A*).
2. Make a scalloped incision on the buccal and lingual or palatal surfaces of the affected tooth, dipping interproximally (between the teeth) to preserve most of the gingival tissue.
3. Elevate the mucoperiosteal flaps 3–5 mm from the edge of the incision, using a sharp periosteal elevator (Fig. 84–15*B*).
4. Remove the collar of gingival tissue around the tooth with curettes.
5. Perform scaling and root planing on the exposed tooth surface.
6. Polish the tooth and liberally irrigate the area with sterile saline.
7. Reposition the flaps and hold in place with 4-0 chromic catgut sutures in a simple interrupted pattern, placed interdentally (Fig. 84–15*C*).

Postoperative Care and Complications

- To retard the recurrence of plaque and calculus accumulation, instruct the owner to irrigate the animal's mouth with a 0.2% chlorhexidine solution (Nolvadent; Fort Dodge, IA) for 2 weeks. Additionally, recommend daily toothbrushing with warm water, or C.E.T. toothpaste (VRx Products; Harbor City, CA).
- If significant stomatitis (discussed later in this chapter) or abscess secondary to periodontal disease occurs, give broad-spectrum antibiotics such as amoxicillin (10–20 mg/kg PO q12h) and metronidazole (15 mg/kg PO q12h) or amoxicillin clavulanate (14 mg/kg PO q12h).
- Reevaluate the animal in 2 weeks. Annual or semiannual scaling is recommended.
- Complications are minimal when procedures are properly performed.

▼*Key Point* Prolonged application of an ultrasonic tip to a tooth without adequate water spraying can result in pulpal necrosis.

- Failure to remove subgingival calculus adequately can result in progressive periodontal disease.
- Inadequate irrigation of the gingival sulcus following therapy can result in entrapment of debris subgingivally and subsequent periodontal abscess.

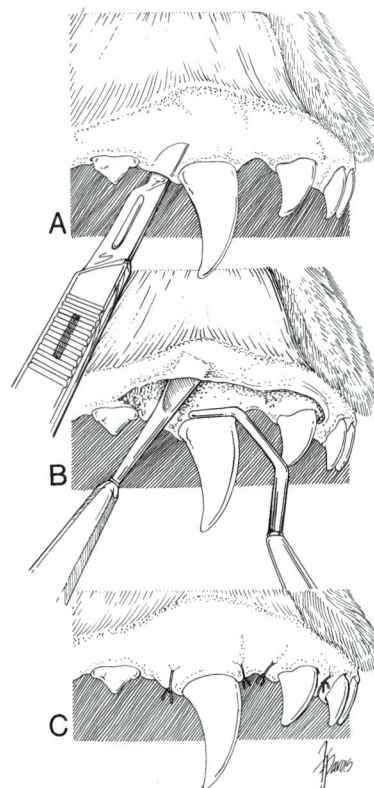

Figure 84–15. *A,* Open-flap curettage is initiated with an incision directed toward the alveolar crest. *B,* Mucoperiosteal flaps are elevated 3–5 mm to permit open curettage. *C,* The flaps are repositioned with 4-0 chromic sutures.

ENDODONTIC DISEASE

Endodontic disease refers to disease of the pulp (the inner aspect of the tooth). It occurs frequently in small animals and may cause significant pain. Pulp cap, pulpotomy, apexogenesis, apexification, and nonsurgical and surgical endodontic therapy can result in the resolution of endodontic disease and retention of a functional, painless tooth.

Etiology

- The most common cause of endodontic disease in small animals is a fractured tooth with pulpal exposure.
- Less common causes include rapid dental attrition (tooth wear), deep odontoclastic resorptive lesions in cats, deep caries, severe periodontal disease with secondary endodontic disease, and dental trauma with secondary internal pulpal hemorrhage or damage to the apical vessels.

Clinical Signs

Pulpal exposure can result in the progressive development of the following conditions:

- Bacterial pulpitis
- Pulp necrosis
- Apical granuloma
- Periapical abscess
- Acute alveolar periodontitis
- Osteomyelitis
- Sepsis

The time required for this progression varies from months to years. When a tooth is fractured and the pulp is exposed, the pulp will bleed.

▼ *Key Point* Pulpal exposure is extremely painful, and animals with a fractured tooth with pulpal exposure hypersalivate, are reluctant to eat, and exhibit other abnormal behaviors.

Over a period of several months, the pulp becomes necrotic and the animal no longer has signs of pain until an inflammatory reaction occurs around the apex of the tooth, at which time the pain recurs.

Diagnosis

The diagnosis is based on a thorough oral examination and dental radiography.

Physical Examination

- Differentiate teeth suspected of being diseased secondary to fractures from worn teeth. Worn teeth, or dental attrition, rarely result in pulpal exposure.
  - A dental explorer will penetrate into the pulp canal when the pulp is exposed.
  - When dental attrition is the cause of a shortened crown, the explorer will not penetrate the tooth but will be stopped by the reparative dentin, or "brown spot," that fills in the area of receded pulp.

- Evaluate the color of the tooth. A discolored tooth (red, purple, or gray) may be diseased.
- Percussion of a tooth with endodontic disease may be painful because of periapical inflammation.
- Soft tissue fistulas may occur secondary to endodontic disease. Usually they are located apical to the mucogingival line. When probed, they will be found to originate from the apex of an endodontically diseased tooth.
- Severe maxillary or mandibular swelling may be present with endodontic disease when the disease process has progressed to a periapical abscess or osteomyelitis.

Radiography

Perform dental radiography to delineate the endodontic system and confirm endodontic disease. Radiography reveals the stage of apical development.

- Chronic endodontically diseased teeth have an area of periapical lysis around one or more roots.
- When soft tissue fistulas are present, radiopaque material such as a gutta percha point may be placed into the fistula before radiography to confirm that the fistula arises from the apex of the affected tooth.

Surgical Anatomy

Surgical anatomy varies with each tooth. The endodontic system is divided into two parts: the pulp chamber and the pulp canal.

- The endodontic system generally follows the external anatomic contours of the tooth, including its root structure.
- The size of the endodontic system also varies with the age of the patient. Young animals have immature teeth with open apices. As the tooth develops, the apex is formed and, as the tooth matures, the dentinal layer thickens, resulting in a thinner endodontic system.

Preoperative Considerations

- Examine the teeth for concurrent periodontal disease with a periodontal probe.

▼ *Key Point* Teeth with combined periodontal and endodontic lesions have a poorer prognosis than teeth with only endodontic lesions.

Surgical Procedures

Numerous endodontic procedures are available (Table 84–7). The type selected depends on the status of the endodontic system and the following factors:

- Vital pulp versus nonvital pulp
- Mature versus immature tooth
- Closed versus opened apex
- Exposure time

Pulp Cap

This procedure is used when the pulp of a vital tooth is inadvertently exposed during a dental procedure.

Table 84–7. ENDODONTIC PROCEDURES RECOMMENDED FOR COMMON ENDODONTIC PROBLEMS

Procedure	Indication
Pulp cap	Vital tooth with iatrogenic pulpal exposure
Pulpotomy and apexogenesis	Vital immature tooth with open apex and traumatic pulpal exposure <5 days
Apexification	Immature nonvital tooth with open apex
Nonsurgical root canal	Nonvital mature tooth with closed apex
	Vital mature tooth with prolonged pulpal exposure
Surgical root canal	Nonvital mature tooth with apical lysis
	Unsuccessful nonsurgical root canal

Technique

1. Flush exposed pulp with sterile saline.
2. Control pulpal hemorrhage with a cotton pellet or paper point.
3. Apply calcium hydroxide powder (Schein) to the exposed pulp with a sterile amalgam carrier.
4. Apply a layer of hard-setting calcium hydroxide paste (Schein). In larger teeth, apply a cement base (Schein).
5. Apply a restoration material such as composite or amalgam.

Pulpotomy

This is similar to a pulp capping procedure, except that the coronal portion of the pulp is removed. Removal of this pulp is indicated in immature vital teeth that have extended pulpal exposure of up to 5 days, which results in coronal pulp contamination.

Technique

1. Remove the contaminated pulp with a sterile #2 or #3 round bur.
2. Place a sterile, moist cotton pellet over the pulp for 3–5 minutes to control hemorrhage.
3. Persistent hemorrhage for greater than 5 minutes may indicate an irreversibly affected pulp. Perform a more apical amputation to reach healthier tissue.
4. Apply calcium hydroxide powder to the pulp with a sterile amalgam carrier, and condense lightly with a sterile amalgam plugger to a thickness of 2–4 mm.
5. Apply a layer of firm-setting calcium hydroxide paste.
6. Place a permanent restorative material.

Apexogenesis

This endodontic procedure allows the root to continue to grow. Apexogenesis is useful in cases in which apical development and closure are not complete and the pulp is not irreversibly compromised. Maintenance of vitality of an immature tooth is desirable so that the tooth will continue to develop, resulting in a thicker dentinal layer and a formed apex.

Technique

Remove the involved or injured portion of the pulp and treat as described for pulpotomy.

Apexification

This procedure is used in the treatment of immature teeth in which there is an absence of vital tissue. Teeth in which early pulp death has occurred have large open apices, making root canal filling by nonsurgical techniques difficult. Apexification permits closure of the apex by cementum formation, which is stimulated by the application of calcium hydroxide.

Technique

1. Remove the necrotic contents of the immature root canal just short of the radiographic apex. During debridement, do not disrupt the root-forming tissues beyond the apex.
2. Irrigate the canal with sterile saline.
3. Carefully dry the canal with premeasured paper points to prevent penetration into the apical tissue, which can result in additional hemorrhage.
4. Mix calcium hydroxide powder and sterile saline to a thick consistency, place in the root canal with a sterile amalgam carrier, and condense with a sterile blunt plugger.
5. Place a layer of quick-setting calcium hydroxide paste.
6. Restore the access hole with composite or amalgam.
7. Replace the calcium hydroxide every 3–6 months until apexification is complete.
8. Following formation of the apex, perform a nonsurgical root canal procedure.

Nonsurgical (Conventional) Root Canal

This procedure is used to treat nonvital mature teeth with closed apices and vital mature teeth with pulpal exposure of greater than 8 hours.

▼ **Key Point** Nonsurgical root canal therapy is preferable to surgical treatment in most cases of endodontic disease because of its relative ease and speed of completion, noninvasive nature, and relative decreased cost.

Technique

1. Using an appropriate-size round bur, obtain access to the pulp at a point that will permit straight delivery of the files to the apex of the tooth (Fig. 84–16).
2. Begin debridement of the canal with a #15 file inserted to the apex of the tooth. Use a rubber stop to mark the length of the file, and insert all subsequent files to that depth.
3. Introduce progressively larger files into the canal. Flush the canal with 2.5% sodium hypochlorite solution before changing files.
4. Debridement is complete when white dentinal shavings are present on the file and there is no further bleeding from the canal.

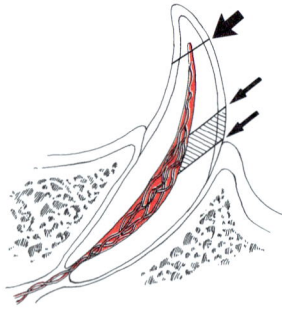

Figure 84–16. Large arrow points to fracture site; small arrows show straight access site to apex.

5. Dry the canal with paper points.
6. Transfer a mixture of zinc oxide–eugenol paste to the root canal with a slowly rotating spiral paste filler.
7. Fill the root canal.
   a. Cut a gutta percha point the same size as the largest file that reaches the apex to the appropriate length, and use a plugger to compress the gutta percha to the apex.
   b. An alternative technique for filling the canal is vertical condensation using hot gutta percha. In this technique small amounts of hot gutta percha (Successfil,) are placed on the end of a sterile file and rotated counterclockwise into the canal and then vertically condensed with the plugger. This process is repeated until the canal is adequately filled.
8. Remove any excess zinc oxide–eugenol paste from the access site.
9. Place an intermediate cement layer.
10. The access site is undercut with an inverted cone bur.
11. Apply restorative material (silver amalgam or composite) to the access site to complete the procedure.

Surgical (Nonconventional) Endodontic Therapy

This is the treatment of endodontic problems with an approach through oral soft tissue and bone rather than through the crown of the tooth. In a nonsurgical root canal procedure, the pulp canal is accessed by the crown only.

Indications for surgical endodontic therapy include

- Apical root resorption
- Incomplete root development
- Complications during conventional root canal therapy (broken files)
- Recurrent apical abscessation following nonsurgical root canal therapy (recurrent swelling over the apex of the tooth root or periapical draining fistulous tracts)
- Size, length, or curvature of the canal that makes instrumentation impossible

Technique

1. Perform a conventional root canal procedure before surgical endodontic therapy. Do not flush or fill the canal, if the apex is open, until the periapical tissues around the apex are packed off with cotton pellets.
2. An apical approach for most teeth is through a mucoperiosteal incision just apical to the mucogingival line. However, access to the apex of the mandibular canine is most easily gained through a cutaneous incision overlying the ventral border of the mandible.
3. Access to the apex is achieved by removing the alveolar bone overlying the apex with a #4 or #6 round bur.
4. Perform apical curettage to remove necrotic and fibrotic granulation tissue surrounding the periapical region.
5. Perform an apicoectomy (amputation of the apex of the tooth) using a #701 bur. The exposed face of the cut root tip is beveled at a 45° angle to increase exposure of the canal access site.
6. Flush the periapical region with sterile saline solution.
7. Pack the periapical region with #0 cotton pellets or a hemostatic agent to control hemorrhage.
8. Create an undercut in the root canal of the apex with a #33 inverted cone bur.
9. Place a 2–4 mm layer of zinc-free amalgam in the apical end of the canal, using a retrograde amalgam carrier, and condense the amalgam with a small amalgam plugger.
10. Before closure, remove all cotton pellets and flush the periapical region with sterile saline solution.
11. Reposition the mucoperiosteal flap and suture with 3-0 chromic catgut in a simple interrupted pattern. Procedures involving the mandibular canine teeth are closed with nonabsorbable suture material in the skin.

Postoperative Care and Complications

- Immediately following endodontic therapy, take a radiograph to document and assess the procedure.
- Administer a broad-spectrum antibiotic, such as amoxicillin clavulanate, for 1 week.
- Reexamine and radiograph the treated tooth 6 months postoperatively, and then annually, to evaluate the success of the endodontic therapy.

Intraoperative Complications

Intraoperative complications usually are associated with improper use of instrumentation or inappropriate technique. Examples are:

- Broken endodontic files lodged in the root canal
- Perforation of the root canal or pulpal floor

Postoperative Complications

Postoperative complications usually are associated with improper technique, inadequate apical seal, or inadequate follow-up.

- Vital endodontic procedures such as pulp cap, pulpotomy and apexogenesis require oral and radiographic reevaluations 3–6 months postoperatively and then annually. If there are persistent signs such as periapical swelling, periapical fistulas, painful tooth percussion, and progressive radiographic periapical lysis in teeth previously treated with vital endodontic techniques, repeat treatment with nonvital techniques.

- Nonvital techniques include apexification and nonsurgical and surgical root canal therapy.
  - Perform surgical root canal therapy on teeth unsuccessfully treated with apexification and nonsurgical root canal techniques.
  - If there is persistent endodontic pathology following surgical root canal therapy, retreatment or extraction is recommended.

ORTHODONTIC DISEASE

Orthodontic disease refers to malocclusions. Veterinary orthodontics involves the movement and repositioning of teeth to a more normal position.

▼ *Key Point* Veterinary orthodontic therapy is indicated to alleviate traumatic malocclusions that result in pain or in inability to function or eat; it should not be used to correct cosmetic or genetic dental alignment defects.

Etiology

The majority of malocclusions are genetic in origin. Previous trauma or an eruption pattern discrepancy resulting from retained deciduous teeth may also result in a malocclusion of the permanent dentition.

Clinical Signs

Clinical signs depend on the severity of the malocclusion.

- Animals with pronounced prognathic occlusion (mandibular teeth are rostral to their normal position in relation to the maxillary dentition) may be presented because of difficulty in prehending food. This condition is not severe enough to cause nutritional problems.
- Animals with brachygnathic occlusion (maxillary teeth are rostral to their normal position in relation to the mandibular dentition) may be presented because of drooling, but this is usually not severe.
- The majority of dental malocclusions are cosmetic and cause no clinically significant problems. However, animals with lingually displaced mandibular canines may have painful palatal defects caused by traumatic occlusion.
- A dental malocclusion in which one tooth traumatically occludes against another tooth can result in dental attrition of the affected teeth.

Diagnosis

The diagnosis is based on a thorough oral examination. Assess the following factors:

- *Incisor relationship:* The maxillary incisors should overlap the facial surface of the mandibular incisors.
- *Canine tooth relationship:* The lower canines should be centered between and not touching either the upper canine or the upper lateral incisor.
- *Lower fourth premolar:* The large cusp of the lower fourth premolar should be centered between the upper third and fourth premolar.
- *Interdigitation of other premolars:* The cusp tips of the upper premolars should interdigitate with the cusp tips of the lower premolars.
- *Premolar horizontal alignment:* The space between the upper and lower premolars should have good horizontal alignment.
- *Head symmetry:* The midlines of the maxillary and mandibular dental arches are centered over each other, and these must also be in alignment with the midplane of the head.

Deviations from these criteria for normal occlusion result in malocclusions of varying severities.

Surgical Anatomy and Orthodontic Principles

Tipping is the most common type of corrective movement used in veterinary orthodontics. A single force is applied to the crown of a tooth, resulting in a tipping action. During orthodontic movement, alveolar bone is *resorbed* (osteoclastic activity) on the side of the tooth with less tension on the periodontal ligament. Conversely, alveolar bone is *deposited* (osteoblastic activity) on the side of the tooth with more tension on the periodontal ligament.

Preoperative Considerations

Prior to correction of orthodontic defects, attempt to determine the etiology of the problem. Correction of genetically induced, cosmetic orthodontic defects is contraindicated. Attempt to correct orthodontic defects resulting in a traumatic occlusion. The timing of orthodontic movement is important.

▼ *Key Point* Delay orthodontic movement until the animal is 1–2 years of age unless simple, quick interceptive movements of the tooth can be achieved.

Surgical Procedures

▼ *Key Point* Extraction of overly retained deciduous teeth can prevent malocclusions of the permanent dentition.

Extraction of overly retained deciduous teeth is referred to as *interceptive orthodontics*. Extract a deciduous tooth that is still firmly attached when the permanent tooth starts to erupt to allow the permanent tooth to erupt in its normal position. Perform extraction carefully to avoid disruption of the permanent tooth.

Correction of Lingually Displaced Mandibular Canines. A technique that can be easily applied in one visit is the intraorally fabricated acrylic inclined plane.

Technique

1. Clean and polish the teeth.
2. Create a retaining wall around the proposed site of the inclined plane with modeling clay or dental wax and apply a thin layer of petroleum jelly to the rostral aspect of the palate.
3. Fabricate an acrylic incline plane in layers by adding powder and liquid components of the acrylic material until the splint is approximately 1-cm thick.
4. When the splint is hard, remove the retaining wall and create the appropriate inclined plane with an acrylic bur, so that when the lingually displaced mandibular canine hits the side of the acrylic splint it will be deflected labially into a normal position. The incline path for the affected tooth should be formed so that the sloping angle is approximately 60° toward its target site.
5. Add additional acrylic to create a band around the canine teeth to provide retention for the splint.

Postoperative Care and Complications

- Instruct the client to
  - Restrict the animal's chewing activities and to feed a soft diet.
  - Observe the orthodontic device daily, making sure that it is not displaced or causing excessive soft tissue trauma.
  - Gently clean the acrylic splint daily with a stream of water from a curve tip syringe.
- Leave the orthodontic appliance in place until the appropriate movement has been achieved. This usually takes about 6 weeks.
- Complications usually are caused by inappropriate techniques or inadequate postoperative care.
  - Misapplication of orthodontic forces can result in resorbed roots, devitalized teeth (necrotic pulp), avulsed teeth, periodontal pockets, gingivitis, and failure to achieve the desired orthodontic movement.

STOMATITIS/GINGIVITIS

Stomatitis/gingivitis is a common clinical problem. Always attempt to identify a specific underlying cause, because this can determine the therapeutic approach and prognosis. When a specific cause cannot be identified or specific therapy is not available, treatment is symptomatic and supportive. Chronic relapsing stomatitis can be particularly frustrating to manage.

Etiology

Causes of stomatitis/gingivitis are listed in Table 84–8. Many systemic diseases that cause stomatitis/gingivitis are discussed in detail elsewhere in this book, including viral upper respiratory infections of cats (see Chap. 9), feline leukemia virus (FeLV) (see Chap. 6), feline immunodeficiency virus (FIV) (see Chap. 7), renal failure (see Chap. 97), autoimmune diseases such as systemic lupus erythematosus (SLE) (see Chap. 22) and pemphigus (see Chap. 43), and eosinophilic granuloma complex (see Chap. 48).

Periodontal Disease

Periodontal disease is a common predisposing cause of stomatitis/gingivitis in dogs and cats (see previous discussion).

▼ **Key Point** In any animal with stomatitis/gingivitis, perform a complete periodontal examination and dental prophylaxis, including tooth extractions if necessary, to eliminate periodontal disease as a contributing factor.

Physical Injury

Foreign bodies (plant awns, sticks, bones), oral trauma, and thermal, electrical, and radiation burns can cause stomatitis/gingivitis. A history of exposure combined with the oral examination may be diagnostic.

- Plant awn stomatitis (bur tongue, vegetative stomatitis) occurs in outdoor dogs that groom burs from their coat or eat horse feces containing burs. The awns become embedded in the tongue and gingiva, causing glossitis, gingivitis, and gingival hyperplasia.
  - On oral examination, close inspection will reveal tiny plant spicules embedded in tissue, and plant material may be seen on biopsy.

Chemical Injury

Strong alkalis (lye solutions) and acids, petroleum distillates, and phenols can damage the oral cavity. In many cases, the specific agent is not identified and the diagnosis is based on circumstantial evidence. Concurrent esophageal and gastrointestinal mucosal injury supports the diagnosis of ingestion of a caustic substance.

Nocardia Infection

Nocardia spp. have been associated with severe halitosis, gingivitis, and oral ulcerations in dogs. In severe cases, necrosis and pseudomembranes are present. Lesions are most severe in periodontal areas. Rarely, mandibular lymph nodes and adjacent skin may be involved.

Oral Candidiasis

This uncommon cause of stomatitis is characterized by white plaques or pseudomembranes on the oral mucosa. Conditions that may predispose to candidal stomatitis include immunosuppression (including chemotherapy), systemic diseases, and long-term antibiotic therapy.

Necrotizing Ulcerative Stomatitis

This form of stomatitis is characterized by gingivitis, oral ulcerations, tissue necrosis, severe halitosis, and pain on eating. Numerous bacteria have been incriminated as contributing to this disorder, including spirochetes and fusiform bacilli.

Table 84–8. DIAGNOSIS AND TREATMENT OF STOMATITIS

Disorders	Diagnosis	Treatment*
Periodontal Disease	Oral exam, dental radiography	Dental prophylaxis, antibiotics
Physical Injury Foreign bodies (e.g., plant awns, sticks, bones, fiberglass); trauma; thermal, electrical, radiation burns	Exposure history, oral exam, tissue biopsy for microscopic agents	Remove foreign bodies; for plant awns, scrape with dry 4 inch × 4 inch sponge or scalpel blade Debride necrotic tissue
Chemical Injury Strong alkalis (lye solutions); acids; petroleum distillates; phenol	Exposure history, oral exam (lesions may extend into esophagus and GI tract)	Immediate therapy; rinse mouth with water Alkaline chemicals: flush with vinegar solution or citrus juice Acid chemicals: flush with bicarbonate solution
Drug- or Toxin-Induced Drug reaction; toxic epidermal necrolysis; heavy metal poisoning (thallium); *Dieffenbachia* (house plant) ingestion	Exposure history	Symptomatic therapy only
Infection Feline herpesvirus/calicivirus	History, physical exam (naso-ocular discharges, fever)	Symptomatic therapy only
Ulcerative necrotizing stomatitis	Oral exam, bacterial culture, impression smears for spirochetes	Treat with antibiotics for at least 3 wk
Candidiasis	Oral exam, fungal culture	Ketoconazole (Nizoral) 5–10 mg/kg PO q12h Nystatin 2% in Orabase applied topically
Nocardiosis	Oral exam, bacterial culture	Sulfadiazine, 80 mg/kg PO q8h
Immunodeficiency or Immunosuppression Feline leukemia virus (FeLV)	FeLV antigen test	Symptomatic therapy only
Feline immunodeficiency virus (FIV)	FIV antibody test	Same as above
Metabolic Disorders Renal failure	Creatinine, BUN, urinalysis	Correct or control underlying disorder
Diabetes mellitus	Blood and urine glucose	Same as above
Hypothyroidism	T_4, TSH stimulation tests	Same as above
Autoimmune Disorders Systemic LE; pemphigus complex; bullous pemphigoid	Physical exam (other mucocutaneous areas affected); biopsy (including IFA test); ANA and LE tests	Immunosuppressant therapy (e.g., glucocorticoids, azathioprine, cyclophosphamide, gold salts)
Neutropenia Cyclic neutropenia; agranulocytosis; leukemia	CBC, bone marrow aspiration	Symptomatic therapy only
Nutritional Deficiencies† Niacin deficiency (black tongue)	Diet history	Vitamin supplementation
Idiopathic Feline plasma cell stomatitis	Biopsy, total serum protein; protein electrophoresis; dental radiography	Symptomatic therapy including antibiotics and dental prophylaxis initially; other therapies include prednisolone, megestrol acetate, gold therapy and low-dose azathioprine; results are inconsistent Dental extractions in refractory cases
Eosinophilic granuloma complex	Physical exam (may have other dermatologic involvement); biopsy	Cats: methylprednisolone acetate (Depo-Medrol), 20 mg/cat SC q2wk for at least 30 days; alternate therapy for refractory cases includes megestrol acetate, surgery, cryosurgery, CO_2 laser, radiation therapy, levamisole, gold salts; correct underlying problem (flea control, hypoallergenic diet, hyposensitization) Dogs: Prednisolone, 0.5–1.0 mg/kg PO q12h for 7 days; then taper dose over 2–3 wk
Underlying Oral Neoplasia	Physical exam (enlarged regional lymph node with metastases); biopsy and needle aspirate of lesion and lymph nodes; thoracic and skull radiography	Treat underlying neoplasia (see text)

*Symptomatic therapy appropriate for all causes of stomatitis may include systemic, oral antibiotics, especially for severe gingivitis or necrotic oral ulcerations, such as amoxicillin (10–20 mg/kg q12h), metronidazole (25 mg/kg q12h), clindamycin (10 mg/kg q12h), and tetracycline (20 mg/kg q8h); oral rinses with 0.1–0.2% chlorhexidine or 1% hydrogen peroxide, 3–4 times daily; dental prophylaxis as needed; and soft food (canned or gruel).

†Rare in clinical practice.

ANA, antinuclear antibody; BUN, blood urea nitrogen; CBC, complete blood count; GI, gastrointestinal; IFA, indirect fluorescent antibody; LE, lupus erythematosus; T_4, thyroxine; TSH, thyroid-stimulating hormone.

Immunosuppression

Immunosuppression secondary to FeLV and FIV infection is an important predisposing cause of chronic stomatitis/gingivitis in cats.

▼*Key Point* Always test for FeLV and FIV in cats with chronic stomatitis/gingivitis.

Uremia

Uremia is a common cause of stomatitis and oral ulcerations. Urease-containing bacteria metabolize urea to ammonia, which is irritating to the oral mucosa. Dehydration and drying of the oral mucous membranes may contribute to the problem. In uremic animals, the rostral portion of the tongue may slough, possibly owing to uremic vasculitis and thrombosis.

Plasma Cell Stomatitis

Plasma cell stomatitis in cats is a disease of unknown etiology characterized by proliferative, often symmetric, hyperemic friable lesions at the glossopalatine arches or angles of the mouth, also called fauces. The condition is also called faucitis.

- Concurrent pharyngitis is common.
- Ulcerative gingivitis may occur. This condition is extremely painful and can cause difficulty on eating.
- Some cats have concurrent plasma cell pododermatitis.
- An association with chronic calicivirus infection has been found in some cases and supported by experimental and epidemiologic evidence.
- On biopsy, lesions are characterized by plasma cells infiltrated with lesser numbers of lymphocytes, neutrophils, and histiocytes.
- Hyperglobulinemia, characterized as a polyclonal gammopathy, is often present and probably indicates chronic immune stimulation. An immune-mediated basis for the disease is suspected.

▼*Key Point* Underlying dental disease, especially odontoclastic resorptive lesions, may be a contributing factor in plasma cell stomatitis of cats.

- Perform dental radiography to identify resorptive lesions, broken teeth, and retained roots. Some cases respond to extraction of adjacent teeth.
- FeLV and FIV infection does not appear to be a predisposing factor. Calicivirus infection has been identified in many cats by virus isolation.
- The disease is often refractory to medical treatment, and relapse is common after treatment is discontinued.
- Treatment of inflamed mucosa with a CO_2 laser may be beneficial.

Feline Eosinophilic Granuloma Complex

This disorder is an important cause of oral lesions in cats.

- Any of three forms (indolent ulcer, collagenolytic [linear] granuloma, and eosinophilic plaque) may occur in the oral cavity. The indolent ulcer involving the upper lips is most common.
- Differentiate lesions from squamous cell carcinoma.
- Oral lesions may coexist with dermatologic involvement. The disorder may be a hypersensitivity reaction associated with underlying atopy, food allergy, or flea bite hypersensitivity. Diagnosis and treatment are discussed in Chapter 48.

Canine Oral Eosinophilic Granuloma

This disorder occurs in all breeds of dogs, but especially in young Siberian huskies.

- The cause is unknown but a hypersensitivity reaction to an as yet unidentified antigen is suspected, based on the dramatic response that occurs with corticosteroid therapy. Spontaneous regression also may occur. Hereditary factors may play a role.
- Lesions are characterized by proliferative tissue with superficial ulcerations that occur primarily on the lateral and ventral surfaces of the tongue. Soft palate involvement may also occur.
- Peripheral eosinophilia is common. Histologically, the lesion appears identical to collagenolytic (linear) granuloma in cats. Degenerating collagen is surrounded by granulomatous inflammation with an eosinophilic component.
- Differentiate lesions from neoplasia (especially mast cell tumor), mycotic infections, and foreign body reaction.

Clinical Signs

Clinical signs of stomatitis/gingivitis include hypersalivation, drooling, halitosis, oral bleeding, reluctance to eat dry food, dysphagia, anorexia, and weight loss.

▼*Key Point* Chronic stomatitis/gingivitis can be extremely painful and can cause behavioral changes such as reclusive behavior, dropping food while eating, and running away from the food dish because of pain on eating.

Diagnosis

Base the overall strategy for diagnosis of stomatitis/gingivitis without an obvious underlying cause (e.g., foreign body) on the following measures:

- Rule out underlying systemic disorders with appropriate laboratory testing.
- Pursue specific diagnostics such as dental evaluation and oral biopsies and cultures.
- Perform dental prophylaxis (as needed) and initiate symptomatic therapy while awaiting test results (see Table 84–8).

History

- Obtain a complete history, with special emphasis on potential exposure to foreign bodies, chemicals, drugs, and toxins.

- Look for signs suggesting underlying systemic disease (see Table 84–8).

Physical and Oral Examinations

- Perform a general physical examination. In particular, evaluate for concurrent dermatologic lesions, especially at mucocutaneous junctions (e.g., nail beds, anus, vulva, prepuce) that suggest an underlying autoimmune disorder.
- Oculonasal discharges and fever in a cat supports the diagnosis of an underlying viral upper respiratory infection (see Chap. 9).
- Perform a complete oral examination, including periodontal evaluation, to identify and characterize the nature and extent of the lesions. This usually requires sedation or general anesthesia. A specific diagnosis can sometimes be made on oral examination (e.g., foreign body, periodontal disease).

Laboratory Evaluation

- Perform routine laboratory tests including a CBC, biochemical profile, and urinalysis to identify underlying systemic diseases such as renal failure (see Chap. 97) and diabetes mellitus (see Chap. 32).
- If general anesthesia is required for complete oral examination, obtain results of laboratory tests before anesthesia.
- Perform ancillary tests as suggested by specific historical and physical examination findings, such as FeLV and FIV tests in cats with chronic stomatitis/gingivitis, fine-needle aspiration of enlarged mandibular lymph nodes for suspected neoplasia, and antinuclear antibody (ANA) and lupus erythematosus (LE) tests for suspected SLE.
- Bacterial and fungal cultures of the oral cavity can be performed on scrapings, swabs, or pieces of tissue. Unfortunately, cultures are not usually helpful, owing to the large number of potentially pathogenic organisms present as normal flora. Exceptions include isolation of *Candida* and *Nocardia* organisms.
- If bacterial cultures yield a large growth of a single organism, antibiotic therapy based on sensitivity patterns may be warranted.
- Specialized laboratories can use virus isolation techniques to detect calicivirus infection, but the clinical significance of a positive result in cats with chronic stomatitis is poorly understood.

Radiography

- In animals with periodontal disease, radiograph involved areas to identify periodontal defects, retained root tips, and external root resorptive lesions, as discussed elsewhere in this chapter.
- Skull radiographs may show lysis of bone secondary to neoplastic disease.

Biopsy and Histopathologic Evaluation

Tissue biopsy is essential when evaluating chronic stomatitis, especially when proliferative lesions are present. Histopathology is useful to characterize the cellular response, identify specific causes, and differentiate neoplastic from non-neoplastic lesions.

- If autoimmune disease is suspected, evaluate oral and skin biopsies as described in Chapter 43.
- Cytology can be performed on impression smears of exudates or biopsied tissue and may be useful to diagnose underlying neoplasia (e.g., melanoma) and infection (e.g., *Nocardia* and *Candida* spp.).

Treatment

Treatment is based on the initiating cause. Whenever possible, institute specific therapy, such as removal of foreign bodies, immunosuppressive therapy for autoimmune diseases, corticosteroids for eosinophilic granuloma complex, sulfadiazine for nocardiosis, and ketoconazole for candidiasis (see Table 84–8). Symptomatic treatment of stomatitis usually is warranted, regardless of whether specific therapy is available.

- Because periodontal disease may be the underlying cause of stomatitis or, at the very least, an important contributing factor, perform thorough dental prophylaxis in all animals.
  - Apply a 0.1–0.2% chlorhexidine solution topically at the gingival margin once a day to retard plaque formation and provide local antibacterial activity.
  - Cleanse the oral cavity in animals with stomatitis with cotton-wrapped applicators soaked in saline or an oral rinse such as 0.1–0.2% chlorhexidine solution 3–4 times daily.
- Administer systemic antibiotics such as amoxicillin, metronidazole, clindamycin, amoxicillin clavulanate, and tetracycline to control secondary bacterial infections, particularly in cases of severe gingivitis or oral ulcerations (see Table 84–8).
- Initiate fluid therapy (see Chap. 5) and tube feeding (nasogastric, esophagostomy, or gastrostomy tube) as needed in animals with severe stomatitis/gingivitis that refuse food and water.
- Consider extraction of the teeth (at least of the premolars and molars) in animals with severe stomatitis/gingivitis that is refractory to medical management and for which extensive diagnostic tests do not reveal an underlying cause.
- Cats with plasma cell stomatitis/gingivitis/pharyngitis, in particular, may have an excellent response following extraction of all teeth or all teeth except the canine teeth when the inflammation is limited to areas around the teeth. Cats with severe pharyngeal or glossopalatine arch inflammation should be given a more guarded prognosis and may require continued medical management with antibiotics and corticosteroids or CO_2 laser treatment.

▼ *Key Point* Advise owners of animals with chronic nonresponsive stomatitis/gingivitis that long-term therapy may be necessary to control the problem.

- Reexamine animals with chronic stomatitis/gingivitis 2 weeks after initial therapy, and then every 1–3 months to assess and reevaluate response to treatment.

- In animals with chronic nonresponsive stomatitis/gingivitis treated with tooth extraction, thoroughly examine the oral cavity 1 month postoperatively to assess proper gingival healing. Take radiographs of regional areas of gingival hyperemia to reveal retained roots. Extraction of these roots permits normal gingival healing.

TONSILLITIS

Tonsillitis is seen occasionally in dogs and less frequently in cats.

▼ *Key Point* Tonsillitis usually occurs secondary to other diseases associated with chronic irritation or contamination of the pharynx.

Etiology

Disorders that predispose to tonsillitis (and pharyngitis) include chronic vomiting or regurgitation, chronic productive cough, and chronic contamination of the nasopharynx (e.g., severe periodontal disease, cleft palate, nasal disease with discharge). Primary tonsillitis is rare but may occur in young, small-breed dogs.

- The spectrum of bacteria cultured from dogs with pharyngitis/tonsillitis is similar to that cultured from the pharynx of healthy dogs, including *Escherichia coli,* and *Streptococcus, Staphylococcus, Pasteurella, Proteus, Pseudomonas,* and *Diplococcus* organisms.
- Group A *Streptococcus pyogenes,* the cause of "strep throat" in humans, does not cause signs of pharyngitis/tonsillitis in dogs and cats, and the prevalence of infection appears to be low. Dogs and cats can acquire a transient infection from close contact with infected humans; thus, they may serve as a reservoir for human reinfection. When recurrent group A *S. pyogenes* infection in humans in the household is a problem, treatment of pets as well as humans is warranted to prevent reinfection. In dogs and cats, effective antibiotics include penicillin, erythromycin, and chloramphenicol.

Clinical Signs

- Signs of tonsillitis include retching, cough, fever, anorexia, and lethargy.
- When tonsillitis is secondary to other disorders, signs of the primary disease overshadow those of the tonsillitis.

Diagnosis

- Base the diagnosis of tonsillitis on the gross appearance of the tonsils, which may be swollen and bright red with small hemorrhages or punctate white foci (abscesses). Concurrent pharyngitis is common.
- Attempt to identify important predisposing disorders (see Etiology) with a complete history, physical examination, and appropriate laboratory tests.
- Perform bacterial cultures in cases of primary tonsillitis refractory to routine antibiotic therapy.

- Differentiate chronic enlargement of the tonsils from underlying neoplasia (e.g., lymphoma, squamous cell carcinoma), which can be diagnosed by tonsillar biopsy.

Treatment

Secondary tonsillitis is usually resolved with identification and treatment of the predisposing disorder. When a predisposing disorder cannot be identified, administer a course of broad-spectrum antibiotics such as ampicillin or amoxicillin (10–20 mg/kg PO q8–12h) for 2 weeks. Tonsillectomy rarely is necessary.

TONSILLAR NEOPLASIA

Etiology

Squamous cell carcinoma and lymphoma are the most common tumors of the tonsil.

Clinical Signs

- Retching and coughing may occur owing to pharyngeal irritation by the mass.
- A cervical mass may be present as a result of metastasis to regional lymph nodes.

▼ *Key Point* Carefully examine the tonsils in all dogs with a cranial cervical mass.

Diagnosis

- Diagnosis is based on oral examination and biopsy (tonsillectomy) findings. The tonsils appear enlarged and inflamed, and may have an obvious irregular mass.
- Perform partial or complete tonsillectomy to obtain tissue for histopathology.

Technique

Tonsillectomy (Biopsy)

1. Place the animal in ventral recumbency. Place an oral speculum.
2. Grasp the tonsil with an Allis tissue forceps.
3. Cut the base of the tonsil with scissors or a tonsillectomy snare and remove the tissue.
4. Control hemorrhage with ligation of vessels, with electrocautery, or direct pressure, using a surgical sponge.
5. If a large defect remains, close the tissue using a continuous pattern with 3-0 chromic catgut.
6. Submit the tissue for histopathology.

Treatment

- For the management of tonsillar lymphoma see (Chap. 25).
- In animals with tonsillar squamous cell carcinoma, combination chemotherapy (doxorubicin and cisplatin) and radiation therapy have been reported to give the best results.

Prognosis

The prognosis is poor.

SALIVARY GLAND DISEASES

Diseases of the salivary glands that may be encountered include

- Mucoceles
- Fistulas
- Sialoadenitis
- Neoplasia

Etiology

Mucoceles. Salivary mucoceles, or sialoceles, result from damage to the duct or gland, with subsequent leakage of saliva into the tissues. Salivary mucoceles are lined with granulation tissue rather than epithelium. The sublingual and mandibular salivary glands are most commonly involved. The sites for mucoceles include cervical mucoceles, sublingual mucoceles (ranulas), and, less commonly, mucoceles of the pharyngeal and orbital region.

Fistulas. Salivary gland fistulas occur infrequently in small animals, and they are usually the result of trauma to the parotid salivary gland or duct.

Sialoadenitis. Sialoadenitis (an inflammatory reaction in the salivary glands) occurs infrequently in small animals. The zygomatic salivary gland is most commonly involved.

Neoplasia. Tumors of the salivary glands (e.g., adenocarcinoma) are rare. The parotid and submandibular salivary glands are most susceptible to tumor formation.

Clinical Signs

Clinical signs depend on the salivary gland affected and the type of disease present.

Mucoceles. Clinical signs depend on the location of the mucocele.

- Animals with cervical mucoceles usually are presented because of a soft, fluctuant nonpainful mass in the cervical area.
- Animals with a ranula often are presented because of abnormal tongue movements, reluctance to eat, dysphagia, and blood-tinged saliva.
- Animals with a pharyngeal mucocele usually are presented because of difficulty breathing or swallowing.
- Animals with zygomatic mucoceles usually have exophthalmos, divergent strabismus, and a fluctuant nonpainful swelling in the orbital area.

Fistulas

- Clinical signs include a small skin opening in an area overlying a salivary gland that drains serous fluid. The amount of drainage increases when the animal is eating.

Sialoadenitis

- *Zygomatic sialoadenitis*—exophthalmos, tearing, divergent strabismus, reluctance to eat, extreme pain on opening the mouth, inflammation of the oral mucosa near the papilla, and mucopurulent discharge from the duct
- *Parotid sialoadenitis*—a painful, warm, firm parotid salivary gland with mucopurulent discharge from the duct

Neoplasia

- Most dogs and cats with salivary gland tumors are presented because of an asymptomatic palpable mass in the region of a salivary gland.
- Associated clinical signs from enlargement, impingement on adjacent structures, and local infiltration can occur.

Diagnosis

The diagnosis of salivary gland disease is based on history, clinical signs, clinical pathologic findings, radiography, and histopathology.

- The diagnosis of mucoceles usually is based on palpation and aspiration of a clear or blood-tinged, viscid, mucinous fluid that is consistent with saliva.

▼ *Key Point* Perform aspiration of mucoceles under aseptic conditions to prevent infection of a mucocele.

Sialography also can be used; however, it is somewhat difficult to perform and is usually not necessary.

- Base the diagnosis of sialoadenitis on clinical signs, an elevated white blood cell count, and histopathology.
- Histopathology is necessary to diagnose salivary gland neoplasia. Thoracic radiography can evaluate for metastatic disease.

Surgical Anatomy

There are four pairs of major salivary glands in the dog and cat: parotid, mandibular, sublingual, and zygomatic (Fig. 84–17).

- The *parotid salivary gland* is located at the base of the auricular cartilage. The parotid duct is formed by two or three short radicles and passes lateral to the masseter muscle. It enters the oral cavity opposite the maxillary fourth premolar.
- The *mandibular salivary gland* is located at the junction of the maxillary and linguofacial veins. It is covered by a dense capsule. The mandibular duct leaves the medial surface of the gland and courses between the masseter muscle and mandible laterally and the digastricus muscle medially and then passes over the digastricus muscle and between the styloglossus muscle medially and the mylohyoides muscle laterally. The mandibular duct enters the mouth on a papilla lateral to the rostral end of the frenulum.
- The *sublingual salivary glands* consist of a caudal portion (monostomatic) located at the rostral pole of the mandibular gland and a rostral portion (polystomatic) that lies directly below the oral mucosa lateral to the tongue. The sublingual salivary duct origi-

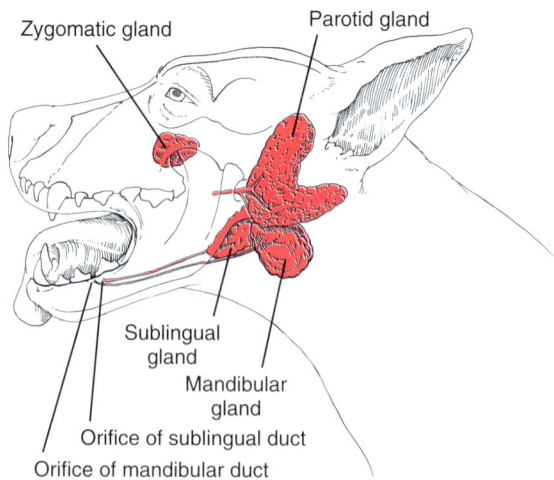

Figure 84–17. Salivary glands in the dog.

nates at the caudal portion of the gland and accompanies the mandibular duct to a common or separate opening on the papilla at the rostral end of the frenulum.

- The *zygomatic salivary glands* are located ventral to the zygomatic arch. The major zygomatic duct opens about 1 cm caudal to the parotid papilla on a ridge of mucosa.

Preoperative Considerations

- Prior to salivary gland surgery, perform a thorough physical examination and appropriate laboratory tests and radiographic procedures, based on the animal's clinical signs, physical examination findings, and age.
- Diagnosis of the type of salivary disease is necessary before surgical intervention.

▼ *Key Point* Surgery is not recommended for animals with sialoadenitis. Treat with systemic antibiotics, drainage of the abscess, and application of warm compresses.

Surgical Procedure

Several surgical procedures have been described in the treatment of salivary gland diseases, including

- Excision of the mandibular and sublingual salivary glands
- Marsupialization of ranulas
- Drainage and excision of the zygomatic salivary gland
- Management of pharyngeal mucoceles

Excision

The technique for surgical excision of the mandibular and sublingual salivary glands (Fig. 84–18) follows.

Technique

1. Determine the affected side by placing the animal in dorsal recumbency. The mucocele will gravitate to the affected side.

2. Place the animal in dorsolateral recumbency and routinely prepare the surgical site.
3. Make a skin incision from the junction of the maxillary and linguofacial veins to the angle of the mandible.
4. Locate the mandibular salivary gland and make an incision in the capsule.
5. Bluntly dissect the mandibular salivary gland from the capsule, ligating and severing the arteries and veins that enter the dorsomedial aspect of the gland.
6. Continue dissecting the sublingual gland rostrally between the masseter and digastricus muscles.
7. Clamp and ligate the glands and ducts as far rostrally as possible with a monofilament nonabsorbable suture.
8. Using a simple interrupted pattern, close the dead space with a few sutures in the capsule and deep tissue.

▼ *Key Point* To prevent the formation of seroma and provide drainage of the mucocele, place a Penrose drain from the site of the excised gland to the most ventral aspect of the mucocele.

9. Close the skin routinely.

Marsupialization (Surgical Management of Ranula)

Technique

1. Place the animal in lateral recumbency and routinely prepare the surgical site.
2. Incise the ranula longitudinally and remove the redundant portion of the mucosa.
3. Join the mucosal edges of the ranula to the adjacent oral mucosa with a few 4-0 chromic catgut sutures.

If the ranula recurs, removal of the mandibular-sublingual salivary gland complex is recommended.

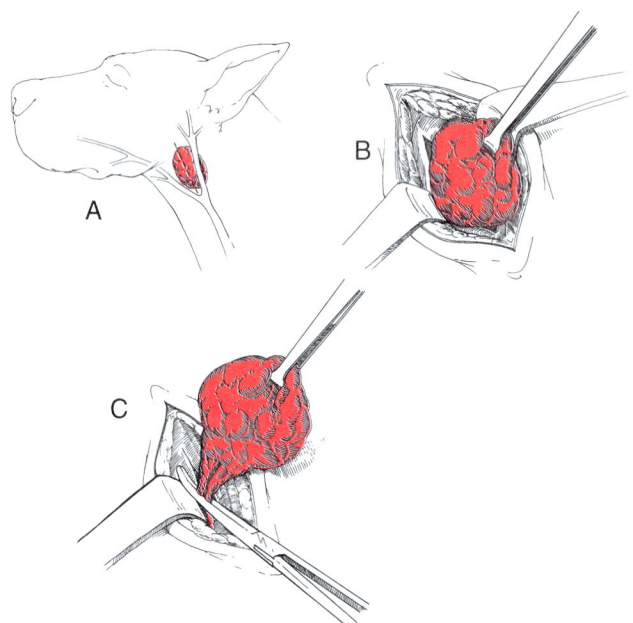

Figure 84–18. *A–C*, Surgical excision of the mandibular and sublingual salivary glands. See text for details.

Drainage of Zygomatic Salivary Gland (Treatment of Sialoadenitis)

Technique

1. Place the animal in lateral recumbency and swab the mucosa caudal to the maxillary second molar with dilute povidone-iodine (Betadine) solution.
2. Gently advance a small mosquito forceps through a small stab incision in the inflamed oral mucosa caudal to the last maxillary molar.
3. Use caution to prevent damage to the maxillary artery and nerve that course ventromedial to the orbit.

Surgical Excision of Zygomatic Salivary Gland (Treatment of Mucocele)

Technique

1. Place the animal in lateral recumbency and routinely prepare the surgical site.
2. Protect the animal's eyes from irritants with ophthalmic ointment.
3. Make an incision along the dorsal aspect of the zygomatic arch.
4. Reflect the periosteum of the zygomatic arch ventrally and retract the palpebral fascia dorsally.
5. Remove the dorsal aspect of the zygomatic arch, using rongeurs.
6. Retract the globe dorsally to expose the zygomatic salivary gland beneath the periorbital fat.
7. Retract the gland dorsally, ligate the vessels supplying the gland, and remove the gland.
8. Suture the palpebral fascia to the periosteum of the zygomatic arch, using absorbable sutures.
9. Close the subcutaneous tissues and skin routinely.

Management of Pharyngeal Mucoceles

- Treat by marsupialization or by excision of the entire mucocele.
- Remove the ipsilateral mandibular and sublingual salivary glands to prevent recurrence of the mucocele.

Postoperative Care and Complications

- Administer broad-spectrum antibiotics perioperatively.
- Feed a soft diet for 1 week postoperatively.

Complications

Complications vary according to the initial problem.

- *Salivary mucocele recurrence*—re-explore for residual salivary tissue. Ligation of the mandibular and sublingual salivary ducts with a nonabsorbable suture during the initial surgery will aid in the localization of residual salivary tissue. Removal of residual tissue is curative.
- *Sialoadenitis*—clinical response is good if drainage is adequate and appropriate antibiotics, based on bacterial culture and sensitivity testing, are given.
- *Neoplasia*—recurrence is possible. Postoperative adjuvant chemotherapy and/or radiation therapy may be beneficial in animals with salivary gland adenocarcinomas.

SUPPLEMENTAL READINGS

Harvey CE, Emily PP: Small Animal Dentistry. St. Louis: CV Mosby, 1993.

Holmstrom SE, Frost P, Eisner E: Veterinary Dental Techniques. Philadelphia: WB Saunders, 1998.

Knecht CD: Salivary glands. *In* Bojrab MJ, ed.: Current Techniques in Small Animal Surgery. 4th Ed. Williams and Wilkins, 1998, p183.

Manfra Marretta S: Maxillofacial surgery. Vet Clin North Am Small Anim Pract 28:1285, 1998.

Ramsey DT, Manfra Marretta S, Hamor RE, et al.: Ophthalmic manifestations and complications of dental disease in dogs and cats. J Am Anim Hosp Assoc 32:215, 1996.

Wiggs RB, Lobprise HB: Veterinary Dentistry Principles & Practice. Philadelphia: Lippincott-Raven, 1997.

Diseases of the Esophagus and Disorders of Swallowing

Susan E. Johnson / Robert G. Sherding

OVERVIEW

Etiology

Esophageal disease in dogs and cats can be classified as structural disorders (e.g., foreign body, stricture, vascular ring anomaly) and motility disorders (e.g., oropharyngeal dysphagia, megaesophagus). Motility disorders may be caused by primary neuromuscular disease of the esophagus or may be secondary to systemic neuromuscular disorders.

Clinical Signs

Clinical signs of esophageal disease include regurgitation, dysphagia, odynophagia (painful swallowing), ptyalism, and exaggerated swallowing. Weight loss, polyphagia, anorexia, cough, dyspnea, and fever also may be seen.

Regurgitation. Regurgitation is the passive expulsion of food or fluid from the esophagus and is influenced by mechanical events in the esophagus. The timing of regurgitation in relation to eating is determined by the location of esophageal dysfunction, degree of obstruction, and presence or absence of esophageal dilatation.

- Regurgitation immediately after eating is most likely to occur with proximal esophageal lesions or esophageal obstruction.
- Regurgitation may be unassociated with eating when the esophagus is dilated, because this provides a reservoir for food and fluid.
- Selective retention of fluids over solid food is more likely with partial obstruction.

▼ *Key Point* Differentiate regurgitation, which is the passive expulsion of esophageal contents, from vomiting, which is the centrally mediated reflex expulsion of contents from the stomach and duodenum.

- In contrast to regurgitation, vomiting is preceded by hypersalivation, retching, and abdominal contractions.

Dysphagia, Odynophagia, Ptyalism, and Exaggerated Swallowing. These signs are most likely to occur with oropharyngeal and proximal esophageal disorders.

Weight Loss. Weight loss occurs secondary to inadequate food intake and is related to the severity of esophageal dysfunction.

Polyphagia. Polyphagia occurs when an animal is otherwise healthy but is unable to retain ingested food owing to partial or complete esophageal obstruction (e.g., esophageal stricture).

Anorexia, Cough, Dyspnea, and Fever. These signs may be seen with secondary aspiration pneumonia, esophageal perforation, or bronchoesophageal fistula.

Diagnosis

The diagnosis of esophageal disease requires an accurate history, radiographic evaluation of the esophagus, and, in many cases, esophagoscopy.

▼ *Key Point* Aspiration pneumonia is a frequent and serious complication of esophageal disease that must be detected and treated appropriately (see Chap. 79).

Signalment

The signalment may suggest certain breed predispositions for esophageal disease (Table 85–1). The age at onset is also important because regurgitation caused by a vascular ring anomaly or congenital idiopathic megaesophagus usually begins at the time of weaning.

History

- Obtain a complete history with emphasis on exposure to foreign bodies or chemicals, recent anesthesia (reflux esophagitis, esophageal stricture), and systemic signs such as neurologic dysfunction or muscle weakness, atrophy, or pain (central nervous system [CNS] disease, generalized peripheral neuromuscular disorders).
- The onset and duration of clinical signs may provide important clues to the underlying disorder. For example:
  - When the onset of regurgitation is acute, consider an esophageal foreign body or caustic esophagitis.

Table 85–1. PROFILES FOR ESOPHAGEAL DISEASE BASED ON SIGNALMENT

Parameter	Clinical Association
Age	
Young	Vascular ring anomaly; idiopathic megaesophagus; foreign body
Mature	Esophageal neoplasia
Breed	
Boston terrier	Vascular ring anomaly (PRAA)
Bouvier	Dysphagia due to hereditary muscular dystrophy (oropharyngeal dysphagia and megaesophagus)
Cocker spaniel	Cricopharyngeal achalasia
Collie	Familial canine dermatomyositis (oropharyngeal dysphagia and megaesophagus)
English bulldog	Vascular ring anomaly (esophageal compression by left subclavian artery and brachiocephalic artery)
	Esophageal deviation cranial to the heart (normal variant)
German shepherd	Idiopathic megaesophagus
	Vascular ring anomaly (PRAA)
	Acquired myasthenia gravis
	Giant axonal neuropathy
Golden retriever	Idiopathic megaesophagus
	Acquired myasthenia gravis
Great Dane	Idiopathic megaesophagus
	Vascular ring anomaly (PRAA)
Greyhound	Idiopathic megaesophagus
Irish setter	Idiopathic megaesophagus
	Vascular ring anomaly (PRAA)
Jack Russell terrier	Congenital myasthenia gravis
Labrador retriever	Idiopathic megaesophagus
	Hereditary myopathy (megaesophagus)
Miniature schnauzer	Idiopathic megaesophagus
Newfoundland	Idiopathic megaesophagus
Rottweiler	Spinal muscular atrophy (megaesophagus)
Shar-Pei	Idiopathic megaesophagus
	Hiatal hernia
	Esophageal deviation cranial to the heart (mild regurgitation)
Smooth fox terrier	Congenital myasthenia gravis
Springer spaniel	Cricopharyngeal achalasia
	Polymyopathy (megaesophagus)
	Congenital myasthenia gravis
Wire-haired fox terrier	Idiopathic megaesophagus
Siamese cat	Idiopathic megaesophagus

PRAA, persistent right aortic arch.

- A long-standing history of regurgitation is consistent with disorders such as idiopathic megaesophagus, vascular ring anomaly, and esophageal neoplasia.
- Intermittent signs often are seen with hiatal hernia and secondary reflux esophagitis.
- If both regurgitation and vomiting occur, give special consideration to a hiatal hernia, gastroesophageal intussusception, or reflux esophagitis secondary to disorders causing chronic vomiting.

- In the southern United States, consider *Spirocerca lupi*–associated granuloma and neoplasia of the esophagus.

Physical Examination

Perform a complete physical examination.

- Palpate the cervical esophagus to detect masses and foreign bodies.
- Distention of the cervical esophagus may occur with mechanical obstruction or diffuse motility disorders and frequently can be induced in animals with megaesophagus by compressing the thorax while the nostrils are occluded.
- A mucopurulent nasal discharge, pulmonary crackles, and fever suggest secondary aspiration pneumonia.
- A rigid stance, in conjunction with fever and depression, may be seen with mediastinitis secondary to esophageal perforation.
- Weight loss and emaciation can be seen with severe, long-standing esophageal disease.
- Other physical findings depend on the underlying cause of esophageal disease and include:
  - Horner syndrome and noncompressible cranial thorax associated with a mediastinal mass
  - Muscle weakness, atrophy, or pain associated with generalized muscle disorders
  - Neurologic deficits associated with primary CNS disease and esophageal denervation
- Observe how the animal eats (using both dry and canned food) to detect abnormalities of prehension and swallowing (suggesting oropharyngeal dysphagia) and to confirm that regurgitation rather than vomiting is occurring.

Radiography

Radiography is the most important tool available for diagnosis of esophageal disease. Survey and contrast radiography provide adequate information to diagnose structural disorders. Esophageal motility disorders are best identified with fluoroscopy.

- Perform survey thoracic and cervical films to evaluate the entire esophagus. The esophagus is not normally visible unless it contains air, fluid, food, or foreign material. Evaluate thoracic radiographs for complications of esophageal disease such as aspiration pneumonia and esophageal perforation.
- Perform a contrast esophagram using barium sulfate paste or an aqueous organic iodine (see Chap. 4).

▼ *Key Point* If esophageal perforation is suspected, use a water-soluble nonionic iodinated contrast agent such as iohexol (Omnipaque, Nycomed) rather than barium when performing contrast esophagography, because it is readily absorbed and less irritating to periesophageal tissues.

- Esophageal motility disorders, especially those causing oropharyngeal dysphagia, are best evaluated with image-intensified fluoroscopy and rapid-sequence filming. Use of fluoroscopy is limited to universities and large referral centers because of the cost of equipment.

Endoscopy

Endoscopic evaluation of the esophagus is a unique, noninvasive method for diagnosis of esophageal disorders. The gross appearance of the mucosa can be assessed and tissue obtained for biopsy, cytology, and culture. In addition, esophageal foreign body removal or dilatation of esophageal strictures with endoscopy can be therapeutic. Either rigid or flexible endoscopes can be used for esophagoscopy.

- The normal esophagus of the fasted animal is usually empty or contains a minimal amount of clear fluid or foam.
- Under anesthesia, the normal esophagus becomes flaccid and dilated, which makes the lumen appear large when distended by air insufflation.
- The canine esophagus has longitudinal folds throughout. The feline esophagus has less prominent longitudinal folds in the proximal two-thirds, and a ring-like pattern of circular annular ridges in the distal one-third.
- Normal esophageal mucosa is smooth, glistening, and pale pink. Superficial submucosal vessels are more visible in the cat. Heavily pigmented dog breeds (e.g., Chow Chow, Shar-Pei) may have patchy pigmentation of the esophageal mucosa.
- The gastroesophageal sphincter is normally closed, forming a slit-like opening that is eccentrically located at the confluence of a rosette pattern of mucosal folds.

Esophageal Manometry

This modality evaluates intraluminal esophageal pressures and is useful for evaluation of esophageal motility disorders. Unfortunately, this procedure is infrequently performed in veterinary patients because of lack of availability of equipment and lack of patient cooperation.

Treatment

Treatment of esophageal disease is discussed under each specific disorder. General management of esophageal disease involves fluid therapy as needed (see Chap. 5), management of complications such as secondary aspiration pneumonia (see Chap. 79), and in severe cases, nutritional support by tube gastrostomy (see Chap. 3).

OROPHARYNGEAL DYSPHAGIA

Oropharyngeal dysphagia is defined as difficulty in moving a bolus of food or water from the oral cavity to the cervical esophagus. This disorder can be subclassified as oral dysphagia or pharyngeal dysphagia, based on the clinical findings (Table 85–2).

- *Oral dysphagia* involves difficulty with prehension or aboral transport of ingesta to the hypopharynx during bolus formation.
- *Pharyngeal dysphagia* is defined as interrupted transport of a bolus from the oropharynx through the cranial esophageal sphincter into the cervical esophagus. It includes disorders of the cranial esophageal sphincter (cricopharyngeus muscle) such as failure of the sphincter to open (cricopharyngeal achalasia), failure to close (cricopharyngeal chalasia), and lack of coordination between cranial esophageal sphincter relaxation and pharyngeal contraction during swallowing.

Etiology

Oropharyngeal dysphagia usually is caused by morphologic disease that interferes with normal prehension and swallowing (see Table 85–2). Functional oropharyngeal dysphagia is associated with neuromuscular disorders that affect the tongue, muscles of mastication, or the cranial nerves involved in voluntary and involuntary swallowing.

Clinical Signs

- Oral dysphagia is characterized by abnormalities of prehension and mastication. Weight loss is not a problem because animals compensate for their deficits and maintain food intake. Secondary aspiration pneumonia is uncommon because pharyngeal function is unaffected.
- Pharyngeal dysphagia is characterized by repeated unsuccessful attempts to swallow, with gagging, retching, and spitting out of saliva-covered food. Aspiration pneumonia is a common and serious complication. Weight loss is also common.
- Regurgitation may be a prominent clinical sign since many of the systemic neuromuscular disorders causing oropharyngeal dysfunction can also cause esophageal hypomotility (megaesophagus).
- When a neuromuscular disorder is the underlying cause of oropharyngeal dysphagia, generalized signs of muscle weakness, atrophy, and neurologic deficits are often present.

Diagnosis

The strategy for diagnosis of oropharyngeal dysphagia includes the following:

- Identify underlying morphologic disorders with a complete oropharyngeal and radiographic evaluation.
- Characterize functional dysphagia by the affected stage of swallowing.
- Pursue ancillary testing to identify underlying neuromuscular disorders that may be associated with functional dysphagia (see Table 85–2).

Signalment

The signalment may suggest certain breed predispositions for congenital neuromuscular disorders associated with oropharyngeal dysphagia (see Table 85–1).

Table 85–2. DIAGNOSIS OF OROPHARYNGEAL DYSPHAGIA*

	Anatomic Association	Clinical Findings	Etiology	Diagnosis	Treatment
Oral Dysphagia					
(Abnormalities of prehension and mastication)	Teeth, tongue, hard palate, bony structures, and TMJ	Difficulty prehending food or lapping water Excessive chewing and chomping Exaggerated head movements when eating Submerging muzzle to drink Dropping food from mouth Pawing at face Excessive salivation No weight loss or aspiration pneumonia	*Morphologic Disorders* Dental disease Oral foreign body Oral neoplasia Severe stomatitis Cleft palate Persistent frenulum Skeletal disorders (e.g., TMJ, craniomandibular osteopathy)	Oral exam, radiography Oral exam, radiography Oral exam, radiography, biopsy Oral exam, biopsy Oral exam Oral exam Oral exam, skull radiography	See Chapter 84 for treatment of morphologic disorders.
			Functional Disorders CNS disease or peripheral neuropathy (cranial nerves V, VII, XII)	Oral exam (atrophy or deviation of tongue secondary to denervation), neurologic exam, EMG, nerve biopsy, CSF tap, CT scan (see Chap. 144)	See Chapters 145 and 148.
			Neuromuscular disease (e.g., myasthenia gravis, botulism)	Neurologic exam, EMG with repetitive nerve stimulation, Tensilon test, ARA titer (see Chap. 149)	See Chapter 149.
			Myopathy or myositis (e.g., masticatory myositis, immune polymyositis, hypothyroidism)	EMG, muscle biopsy, CK, AST, ANA, LE, T_4 and TSH assay (see Chap. 149)	See Chapter 149.
Pharyngeal Dysphagia					
(Abnormalities of bolus transport from the oropharynx through the cranial esophageal sphincter)	Pharyngeal constrictor muscles, soft palate, cranial esophageal sphincter	Normal food and water uptake but repeated unsuccessful attempts to swallow Spitting out saliva-covered food Eating with head and neck tucked ventrally Pharyngeal food retention and pharyngitis Gagging, retching Regurgitation Nasal discharge Cough, fever (pneumonia)	*Morphologic Disorders* Inflammatory or neoplastic diseases of the pharynx, tonsils, or retropharyngeal lymph nodes Retropharyngeal foreign body or abscess Soft palate disorders (e.g., cleft soft palate or iatrogenic shortening) *Functional Disorders* CNS disease or peripheral neuropathy (cranial nerves V, VII, IX, X)	Oral exam, skull and pharyngeal radiography, biopsy of inflammatory or mass lesions, fine-needle aspiration of lymph nodes, endoscopy Oral exam, pharyngeal radiography, fine-needle aspiration, endoscopy Oral exam Neurologic exam, EMG, nerve biopsy, CSF tap, CT scan (see Chap. 144)	See Chapter 84 for treatment of morphologic disorders. See Chapters 145 and 148.

Table continued on following page

Table 85–2. DIAGNOSIS OF OROPHARYNGEAL DYSPHAGIA* *Continued*

	Anatomic Association	Clinical Findings	Etiology	Diagnosis	Treatment
Pharyngeal Dysphagia (*Continued*)					
			Functional Disorders (Continued)		
		Weight loss	Myopathy or myositis (e.g., immune polymyositis, hypothyroidism)	EMG, muscle biopsy, CK, AST, ANA, LE, T₄ and TSH assay (see Chap. 149)	See Chapter 149.
			Neuromuscular disease (e.g., myasthenia gravis, botulism)	Neurologic exam, EMG with repetitive nerve stimulation, Tensilon test, ARA titer (see Chap. 149)	See Chapter 149.
			Congenital cricopharyngeal achalasia	Barium swallow with fluoroscopy, response to myotomy	Cricopharyngeal myotomy (see Chap. 86)
			Cricopharyngeal dysphagia†	Barium swallow with fluoroscopy	Cricopharyngeal myotomy is contraindicated

*The type of dysphagia is first characterized as oral dysphagia versus pharyngeal dysphagia based on observing the animal eat (e.g., prehension of food and water, swallowing). Barium swallow with fluoroscopy is useful to characterize functional oropharyngeal dysphagia but is not indicated for evaluation of morphologic disorders.

†Includes failure of the cranial esophageal sphincter to close or lack of coordination between cranial esophageal sphincter opening and pharyngeal contraction.

ANA, antinuclear antibody; ARA, acetylcholine receptor antibody; AST, aspartate aminotransferase; CK, creatine kinase; CNS, central nervous system; CSF, cerebrospinal fluid; CT, computed tomography; EMG, electromyography; LE, lupus erythematosus; T₄, thyroxine; TMJ, temporomandibular joint; TSH, thyroid-stimulating hormone.

History

Obtain a complete history, including a description of eating and drinking. Evaluate for signs suggestive of aspiration pneumonia (cough, dyspnea, anorexia, depression) or a systemic neuromuscular disorder (weakness, muscle pain, gait abnormalities).

Physical Examination

Many of the morphologic diseases that cause dysphagia are detected initially by oropharyngeal examination. Tranquilization or general anesthesia may be required for a thorough oropharyngeal evaluation. A general physical and neurologic examination (see Chap. 144) is particularly important to identify focal and generalized neuromuscular abnormalities that may be associated with functional oropharyngeal dysphagia.

▼ *Key Point* Observation of the animal eating and drinking is an important extension of the physical examination to confirm that dysphagia is present and to characterize it as an oral or pharyngeal problem (see Table 85–2).

Radiography

- Perform survey radiographs of the skull and pharyngeal area to identify morphologic disorders such as a pharyngeal foreign body or retropharyngeal abscess that can cause oropharyngeal dysphagia.
- Perform thoracic radiographs to detect aspiration pneumonia and associated megaesophagus.

- A barium swallow with fluoroscopic examination is required for definitive characterization of functional swallowing abnormalities, and it is essential for the diagnosis of cricopharyngeal achalasia. Unfortunately, fluoroscopy is available only at large referral centers.

Ancillary Testing

Ancillary tests frequently indicated for further diagnosis of causes of functional oropharyngeal dysphagia include:

- Tensilon response test (edrophonium chloride [Tensilon, ICN Pharmaceuticals]), acetylcholine receptor antibody titer, and electromyography (EMG) for myasthenia gravis (see Chap. 149)
- EMG and muscle biopsy for polymyositis and polymyopathy (see Chap. 149)
- Cerebrospinal fluid (CSF) tap and computed tomography (CT) scan for primary CNS diseases (see Chap. 144).

Treatment

- The treatment and prognosis for oropharyngeal dysphagia depend on the underlying disorder (see Table 85–2).
- Supportive care is especially important with pharyngeal dysphagia. Detect and treat aspiration pneumonia (see Chap. 79) and provide appropriate nutritional support, including a gastrostomy tube in severely emaciated animals (see Chap. 3).

ESOPHAGEAL HYPOMOTILITY (MEGAESOPHAGUS)

Esophageal hypomotility refers to a decrease in esophageal tone or peristalsis that may be segmental or diffuse. The term *megaesophagus* commonly is used when a diffuse, severe motility disorder results in a large, flaccid esophagus. In most cases, the primary disturbance is an abnormality of the body of the esophagus rather than failure of the gastroesophageal sphincter to relax (achalasia), as occurs in humans. Clinical findings associated with megaesophagus reflect impaired esophageal transport with secondary complications such as weight loss and aspiration pneumonia.

Etiology

- Esophageal hypomotility disorders may be congenital or acquired. A familial predisposition for congenital idiopathic megaesophagus has been suggested for many breeds of dogs and Siamese cats (see Table 85–1). Breeding of affected animals is not recommended.
- Acquired megaesophagus may occur secondary to many disorders, especially diseases causing diffuse neuromuscular dysfunction (Table 85–3). However, in most cases, a cause is not identified and the diagnosis is idiopathic megaesophagus.
- The underlying pathophysiologic mechanism for idiopathic megaesophagus is unknown. Efferent neuromuscular pathways appear to be intact and a defective afferent component of the neural reflex is suspected. Mechanisms may be similar for both congenital and acquired idiopathic megaesophagus.

Clinical Signs

- The primary clinical sign is regurgitation, which may or may not be related to eating. In most cases, the more liquid the food, the less likely it is to be regurgitated. Weight loss and emaciation occur secondary to inadequate retention of food.
- Dyspnea, cough, and fever are indicative of secondary aspiration pneumonia, a common complication of megaesophagus.
- In cases in which megaesophagus is associated with an underlying disorder (see Table 85–3), additional clinical signs may be detected, including:
  - Generalized muscle weakness with myasthenia gravis, polymyositis, polymyopathy, or hypoadrenocorticism
  - Neurologic deficits with CNS disease or polyneuropathy
  - Generalized muscle atrophy or pain with polymyositis
  - Obesity and alopecia with hypothyroidism
  - Oropharyngeal dysphagia with generalized neuromuscular dysfunction.

Diagnosis

Idiopathic megaesophagus is a diagnosis of exclusion. Strategies for diagnosis of megaesophagus should include:

Table 85–3. CAUSES OF ESOPHAGEAL HYPOMOTILITY (MEGAESOPHAGUS)

Idiopathic

Congenital
Acquired

Central and Peripheral Neuropathies

CNS (caudal brain stem) disorders (e.g., distemper, trauma, neoplasia)
Immune polyneuritis
Polyradiculoneuritis (coonhound paralysis)
Bilateral vagal nerve damage (e.g., surgery, trauma, neoplasia)
Giant axonal neuropathy
Hereditary spinal muscular atrophy
Dysautonomia
Ganglioradiculitis

Neuromuscular Junctionopathies

Myasthenia gravis (congenital or acquired)
Botulism
Tick paralysis
Anticholinesterase toxicity

Myopathy or Myositis

Polymyositis (e.g., SLE, idiopathic, infectious)
Muscular dystrophy
Hereditary myopathy
Familial canine dermatomyositis
Glycogen storage disease type II
Trypanosomiasis

Miscellaneous

Hypothyroidism
Hypoadrenocorticism
Lead toxicity
Thallium toxicity
Acrylamide toxicity
Thymoma
Pituitary dwarfism
Esophagitis
Esophageal fistula
Tetanus
Gastric dilatation volvulus
Dystrophin deficiency

CNS, central nervous system; SLE, systemic lupus erythematosus.

- Confirmation of a persistently dilated esophagus
- Evaluation for underlying obstructive esophageal disease
- Evaluation for underlying causes of megaesophagus (see Table 85–3)

Signalment

The signalment is important since idiopathic megaesophagus is a common disorder in young animals with regurgitation and certain breeds are predisposed (see Table 85–1).

History

Obtain a complete history. In young animals with congenital idiopathic megaesophagus, regurgitation is often noted at weaning when solid food is first introduced. Multiple animals in a litter may be affected. Historical findings that indicate the need for a more complete evaluation for predisposing causes include systemic lethargy or weakness, concurrent oropharyngeal dysphagia, and neurologic abnormalities.

Physical Examination

The physical examination may be unremarkable except for weight loss.

- Distention of the cervical esophagus can be accentuated by compressing the thorax while the nostrils are occluded.
- A mucopurulent nasal discharge, pulmonary crackles, and fever suggest secondary aspiration pneumonia.
- Perform a complete neurologic examination with emphasis on cranial nerves IX (glossopharyngeal) and X (vagus).
- Evaluate all skeletal muscles (especially temporal and limb muscles) for weakness, atrophy, or pain.
- Additional physical examination findings are determined by the underlying cause (see Table 85–3).

Radiography

- Survey thoracic radiographs usually show distention of the entire intrathoracic esophagus with gas, fluid, or food. If hypomotility is mild, radiographs may be unremarkable. Evaluate for evidence of aspiration pneumonia.
- A barium esophagram can be useful to confirm persistent dilatation of the esophagus and to evaluate for possible mechanical obstruction at the gastroesophageal junction.
- Esophageal motility disorders are best evaluated with fluoroscopy, which provides a means of subjectively assessing the intensity and coordination of esophageal peristalsis and is the only modality that can detect subtle esophageal motility disorders.

Routine Laboratory Tests

Perform a minimum database of tests, including:

- *Biochemical profile* to screen for changes associated with underlying systemic disorders causing megaesophagus (e.g., hyponatremia and hyperkalemia with hypoadrenocorticism; hypercholesterolemia with hypothyroidism; increased creatine kinase [CK] and aspartate aminotransferase [AST] levels with polymyositis)
- *Complete blood count* (CBC) to detect a neutrophilia and left shift consistent with aspiration pneumonia
- *Acetylcholine receptor antibody titer* to evaluate for acquired myasthenia gravis (MG), even in the absence of generalized muscle weakness, because acquired focal MG may mimic idiopathic megaesophagus (see Chap. 149).

Other Tests

- Perform other tests as indicated by clinical and laboratory findings to detect underlying causes of megaesophagus, such as:
  - Adrenocorticotropic hormone (ACTH) stimulation test for hypoadrenocorticism

  - Thyroid-stimulating hormone (TSH) assay and thyroxine level for hypothyroidism
  - Antinuclear antibody (ANA) and lupus erythematosus (LE) tests for systemic LE
  - Blood lead assay for lead poisoning
  - Tensilon test for MG
  - EMG for polymyopathy, polymyositis, polyneuropathy, and MG
  - Muscle biopsy for polymyopathy and polymyositis
  - CSF tap for CNS disease (see Chap. 144)
- Transtracheal wash for cytology, and culture and sensitivity testing if aspiration pneumonia is suspected (see Chap. 79).

Esophagoscopy

Esophagoscopy is not routinely indicated for evaluation of megaesophagus unless obstructive disease of the gastroesophageal sphincter or reflux esophagitis is suspected. With idiopathic megaesophagus, the esophagus appears flaccid and dilated throughout its entire length and contains variable amounts of froth, fluid, or food. The esophageal mucosa is usually normal.

Esophageal Manometry

This is an extremely useful diagnostic tool to detect and characterize esophageal motility disorders in humans, but it is not widely used in veterinary medicine because of the expense and the lack of patient cooperation.

Treatment

▼ *Key Point* Treatment of megaesophagus is primarily supportive and symptomatic, unless a reversible underlying disorder can be identified.

- Offer frequent small meals with the animal in an upright position. Maintain the upright position for 10–15 minutes after eating, so that gravity can assist entry of food into the stomach. In most cases, the more liquid the diet, the easier it is to reach the stomach. However, different types of food should be given on a trial basis to identify those best tolerated.
- Place a gastrostomy tube for temporary nutritional support of animals with severe malnutrition (see Chap. 3).
- Give antibiotics for treatment of aspiration pneumonia, based on results of culture and sensitivity testing (see Chap. 79). Caution the owner that recurrent pneumonia is a common problem and that early detection and treatment are essential for long-term success.
- Treat the underlying disorder whenever possible (see Table 85–3).
- Prokinetic drugs do not appear to be useful in the management of idiopathic megaesophagus in dogs. Metoclopramide (Reglan, Robins) increases gastroesophageal sphincter pressure but has no effect on the body of the esophagus. Cisapride (Propulsid, Janssen) has anecdotally been associated with clinical improvement in some dogs with megaesophagus. In theory, cisapride should not improve esophageal peristalsis in dogs because it is a smooth muscle pro-

kinetic agent and the canine esophagus consists entirely of skeletal muscle. Cisapride also increases gastroesophageal sphincter pressure (as does metoclopramide), which may decrease esophageal clearance in dogs with idiopathic megaesophagus. In healthy experimental dogs, cisapride actually slowed the transit rate of a food bolus through the esophagus. Cisapride may be useful as a prokinetic agent in cats with motility disorders involving the distal esophagus because of the smooth muscle composition of this segment of the feline esophagus.

- Surgical myotomy of the gastroesophageal sphincter is not recommended because "achalasia" of the sphincter is not usually present.

Prognosis

- Some animals with congenital idiopathic megaesophagus may improve in time with diligent supportive care.
- Idiopathic acquired megaesophagus is usually irreversible. The animal may do well for months to years if the owner is dedicated to performing appropriate feeding procedures and if pneumonia is detected and treated early.
- Aspiration pneumonia and euthanasia are the most common causes of death in animals with megaesophagus.

ESOPHAGEAL FOREIGN BODY

Esophageal foreign bodies are common. They usually lodge at narrowed areas of the esophagus including the thoracic inlet, at the base of the heart, or at the hiatus of the diaphragm. The extent of secondary esophageal damage depends on the type of object, its size and shape, and the duration of time in contact with the mucosa. Complications of esophageal foreign body include esophagitis, esophageal perforation and mediastinitis, esophageal stricture, and, rarely, bronchoesophageal fistula.

Etiology

The most commonly encountered esophageal foreign bodies are bones. Other objects include needles, fishhooks, string, toys, and, in cats, vomited hairballs.

Clinical Signs

- Most dogs and cats with esophageal foreign bodies are presented for evaluation of acute onset of gagging, salivation, dysphagia, and regurgitation.
- If esophageal foreign bodies go undiagnosed initially, they may cause chronic regurgitation and dysphagia.

Diagnosis

History

Foreign body ingestion may be reported by the owner.

Physical Examination

- The physical examination often is normal except for dysphagia, ptyalism, or gagging and retching.
- Cervical esophageal foreign bodies may be palpable.
- Findings of depression, anorexia, fever, cough, and dyspnea may suggest secondary aspiration pneumonia or esophageal perforation. Cervical swelling may be palpated with foreign body–induced perforation of the cervical esophagus.

Radiography

- Thoracic and cervical radiographs usually are diagnostic for metal or bone foreign bodies. Evaluate thoracic radiographs for aspiration pneumonia. Findings of pneumomediastinum, pneumothorax, and mediastinal or pleural effusion suggest esophageal perforation.
- Contrast radiography may be necessary to identify radiolucent objects. Use iohexol (Omnipaque, Nycomed), a water-soluble nonionic iodinated contrast agent, rather than barium sulfate if perforation is a possibility (see Chap. 4).

Routine Laboratory Tests

A CBC, serum biochemical profile, and urinalysis may be indicated.

- Perform routine blood work before general anesthesia for foreign body removal, especially in older animals with possible concurrent systemic diseases (e.g., renal failure) that might warrant special anesthetic considerations.
- With secondary aspiration pneumonia or esophageal perforation, the CBC may indicate a neutrophilia and left shift.

Esophagoscopy

Esophagoscopy is indicated to confirm the diagnosis, remove the object, and assess secondary mucosal damage.

Treatment

Esophageal foreign bodies should be considered an emergency situation. Do not delay foreign body removal, as the likelihood of complications increases with time. Institute fluid therapy as needed to correct secondary fluid and electrolyte imbalances before general anesthesia.

▼ *Key Point* Endoscopic removal of esophageal foreign bodies usually is successful and should be attempted before surgery.

Technique for Foreign Body Removal

1. Perform esophagoscopy with the animal under general anesthesia.
2. Use a rigid or flexible endoscope with foreign body retrieval (grasping) instruments.

3. Grasp the object and attempt to dislodge it by gentle rotation. Perform all manipulations cautiously to prevent further mucosal damage or perforation.
4. If the object cannot be extracted orally without trauma, advance it into the stomach and remove it by gastrotomy. Gastrotomy is not required for bone foreign bodies, as they dissolve rapidly once reaching the stomach. In this situation, perform serial abdominal radiographs to confirm that the bone has dissolved and does not cause obstruction.
5. If a fishhook is embedded in the esophageal wall, use a rigid endoscope and pass rigid alligator forceps through the lumen of the endoscope to grasp the fishhook. Apply torque to the fishhook with the forceps to dislodge it from the wall. If the hook cannot be dislodged, perform surgery to expose the esophagus so that the barbs can be cut off the hook. Retrieve the remainder of the hook endoscopically.
6. Once the object is removed, assess the mucosa for hemorrhage, erosions, lacerations, and perforations.
7. Following an uncomplicated foreign body retrieval, withhold oral food and water for 24–48 hours and give parenteral fluids and parenteral broad-spectrum antibiotics such as ampicillin (22 mg/kg q8h SC, IM, or IV) if mild esophagitis is detected. (See elsewhere in this chapter for diagnosis and management of complications of esophageal foreign bodies such as esophagitis, esophageal perforation, and esophageal stricture.)
8. If the foreign body cannot be removed endoscopically and cannot be advanced into the stomach, an esophagotomy is indicated (see Chap. 86).
9. Surgical exploration is preferred over endoscopy when retrieving penetrating esophageal foreign bodies located at the heart base because of the risk of lacerating the aorta or pulmonary vessels.

Prognosis

The prognosis for recovery after endoscopic foreign body removal is excellent unless secondary complications occur. With perforation and mediastinitis, the prognosis is guarded.

ESOPHAGEAL PERFORATION

Perforation of the intrathoracic esophagus is more likely to be associated with significant morbidity than is perforation of the cervical esophagus.

Etiology

- *Esophageal foreign bodies* are the most common cause of esophageal perforation, especially objects with irregular or sharp edges, such as bones, and chronically lodged foreign bodies that cause secondary pressure necrosis.
- *Iatrogenic perforation* may occur during esophagoscopy for foreign body removal and during therapeutic dilatation of an esophageal stricture. Perforation may also be a sequela of esophageal surgery or laser treatment.

- *Penetrating injuries* of the cervical esophagus can be caused by bite wounds and gunshot injuries.

Clinical Signs

- Anorexia, depression, odynophagia, fever, and a rigid stance are seen with esophageal perforation.
- Cough and dyspnea may occur with perforation of the thoracic esophagus that leads to mediastinitis and pleuritis.

Diagnosis

History

Exposure to potential foreign bodies or trauma to the cervical esophagus may be elicited in the history.

Physical Examination

Findings suggesting perforation include depression, fever, and pain. With cervical perforations, there may be cervical swelling, cellulitis, and a draining fistula.

Routine Laboratory Tests

A CBC usually reveals neutrophilia and a left shift.

Radiography

- With esophageal perforation, thoracic radiography shows pneumomediastinum, pneumothorax, and mediastinal or pleural effusion.
- Perform a contrast esophagram using Omnipaque, a water-soluble nonionic iodinated contrast agent, to confirm perforation (see Chap. 4).

Esophagoscopy

Esophageal perforation may be detected by esophagoscopy as a deep laceration in the esophagus, or a defect in the thoracic esophagus that bubbles bloody fluid.

▼ *Key Point* If perforation is present or occurs during endoscopy, life-threatening tension pneumothorax may require immediate thoracentesis and chest tube placement (see Chap. 3).

Treatment

- If a small tear occurs secondary to a sharp foreign body or during endoscopic manipulations, conservative medical management may be sufficient.
- Give broad-spectrum antibiotics, fluid therapy, and nothing per os for 5–7 days; monitor closely for clinical deterioration.
- Consider nutritional support by tube gastrostomy or parenteral alimentation (see Chap. 3).
- Perform repeated thoracic radiographs (for thoracic perforations) on a daily basis to monitor response to therapy and to detect evidence of mediastinitis and pleuritis.
- If perforation is accompanied by fever, and mediastinitis or pleuritis, surgical exploration for primary repair is indicated (see Chap. 86).

ESOPHAGITIS

Etiology

- *Foreign bodies* are a common cause of esophagitis.
- *Chemical irritants or caustic substances* may cause esophagitis. Concurrent stomatitis (see Chap. 84) and gastritis (see Chap. 87) may occur.
- *Thermal injury* may occur with ingestion of food that has been heated to high temperature (e.g., in a microwave).
- *Gastroesophageal reflux* of gastric or duodenal contents is a common cause of esophagitis. Esophageal damage is attributed to mucosal contact with gastric acid, pepsin, bile acids, and trypsin. Predisposing factors that may contribute to reflux esophagitis include general anesthesia, use of a head-down tilt table for surgery, indwelling nasogastric tube or pharyngostomy tube, hiatal hernia, chronic vomiting, and delayed gastric emptying.
- Severe necrotizing pyogranulomatous esophagitis caused by *Pythium insidiosum* has been described in two dogs from the southern United States. Infection is believed to occur from the ingestion of zoospores in stagnant fresh water. Diagnosis is confirmed by demonstrating characteristic hyphae with Grocott's methenamine silver stain on an esophageal biopsy. Medical therapy of pythiosis is usually unsuccessful; however, itraconazole (10 mg/kg/day) has been effective in a few dogs with enteric pythiosis (see Chaps. 18 and 89).

Clinical Signs

- Signs of esophagitis are nonspecific for esophageal disease in general and include dysphagia, regurgitation, repeated swallowing, and excess salivation.
- Anorexia, depression, and fever suggest secondary aspiration pneumonia or perforation.
- Weight loss and dehydration may occur with chronic or severe esophagitis.
- With mild esophagitis, signs may be absent.

Diagnosis

History

Look for potential predisposing factors such as exposure to foreign bodies or caustic materials and recent general anesthesia.

Physical Examination

Oral ulcerations or stomatitis may be present if caustic injury occurred. Weight loss and dehydration may be detected when esophagitis is severe.

Radiography

- Survey radiographs usually are unremarkable. Occasionally, small amounts of gas may be seen in the esophagus and mild focal esophageal dilatation may occur secondary to delayed motility.
- Contrast studies often are normal. When esophagitis is severe, the mucosa may appear irregular. Segmental luminal narrowing can occur with involvement of the submucosa and tunica muscularis. This radiographic appearance can be difficult to distinguish from a fibrous stricture.

Endoscopy

Endoscopic evaluation of the esophageal mucosa is the most sensitive method for detecting esophagitis.

- Findings include mucosal erythema, hemorrhage, increased friability, erosions or ulcers, and in severe cases, pseudomembranes, indistensibility, and strictures.
- If gastroesophageal reflux is the cause of esophagitis, lesions are most severe in the distal esophagus, especially linear erythematous streaks and erosions, and the gastroesophageal junction may appear dilated.
- Reflux of gastric contents into the esophagus may be noted during endoscopy.

Treatment

Mild esophagitis frequently resolves without treatment and may not require additional therapy, especially when the cause (e.g., foreign body) can be easily resolved.

General Therapy

- Administer antibiotics (e.g., as ampicillin, amoxicillin, cephalosporins) routinely to prevent or control infection of the altered mucosa by oral bacteria.
- Maintain adequate nutrition in mild cases with frequent oral feeding of small portions of a nonabrasive, soft food. Place a gastrostomy tube in animals with severe esophagitis, prolonged anorexia, or inability to retain food.

Reflux Esophagitis

- Give metoclopramide (Reglan, Robins) or cisapride (Propulsid, Janssen) to decrease gastroesophageal reflux (by increasing gastroesophageal sphincter pressure) and promote gastric emptying (see Table 87–3 for drug dosage).
- Decrease acidity of refluxed gastric juice by giving an H_2-receptor blocker such as cimetidine (Tagamet, SmithKline Beecham), ranitidine (Zantac, Glaxo Wellcome), or famotidine (Pepcid, Merck) (see Table 87–3 for drug dosages). H_2-receptor blockers are preferable to antacids for control of acid secretion because of their potency and ease of administration.
- Sucralfate suspension is beneficial in the treatment of reflux esophagitis. Sucralfate (Carafate) is an aluminum salt that binds selectively to injured gastroesophageal mucosa and acts as an effective barrier against the damaging actions of acid, pepsin, and bile acids associated with reflux esophagitis (see Table 87–3 for drug dosage).
- Consider omeprazole (Prilosec), a proton pump inhibitor, for treatment of severe reflux esophagitis in dogs that is unresponsive to the previously described treatments (see Table 87–3 for drug dosage).

- Give prednisolone (0.5 mg/kg PO q12h) in animals with severe esophagitis to prevent healing by fibrosis and stricture formation. Be sure to control any infection (e.g., aspiration pneumonia) before starting corticosteroid therapy.

Prognosis

The prognosis is good for mild to moderate esophagitis and guarded or poor for severe esophagitis, especially when accompanied by perforation. Strictures may occur secondary to severe esophagitis (see later).

ESOPHAGEAL STRICTURE

An intramural esophageal stricture results when severe esophagitis involving the submucosa and tunica muscularis heals by fibrosis. Multiple strictures may occur secondary to diffuse esophagitis.

Etiology

- Esophageal stricture may occur secondary to severe esophagitis of any etiology.
- *Reflux esophagitis* associated with gastroesophageal reflux of gastric acid and enzymes during general anesthesia and *esophageal foreign bodies* are the most commonly recognized causes.
- Esophageal surgery may be complicated by healing with stricture formation.

Clinical Signs

- Clinical signs of regurgitation and dysphagia are attributable to esophageal obstruction.
- Regurgitation usually occurs immediately after eating. If the stricture is chronic, regurgitation may not be related to eating because esophageal distention cranial to the stricture acts as a food reservoir.
- A ravenous appetite is common because of inability to get food past the strictured area.

Diagnosis

History

Progressive dysphagia for solid foods with preferential retention of liquids is common. Clinical signs from a stricture usually occur 5–14 days after onset of esophageal injury and esophagitis.

Physical Examination

The physical examination is often unremarkable unless the stricture has been present for a long time, resulting in weight loss. Animals are often otherwise bright and alert.

Radiography

- Survey radiographs usually are normal unless the esophagus is distended with food or fluid proximal to the stricture. Evaluate for aspiration pneumonia.
- A contrast study of the esophagus using barium paste or barium mixed with food demonstrates the stric-

ture (see Chap. 4). Contrast radiography is useful to assess the number, location, and length of strictures.

Endoscopy

Endoscopy can diagnose an esophageal stricture and, at the same time, allow treatment of the stricture by bougienage or balloon dilatation.

At endoscopy, a stricture appears as a ring or ridge of white fibrous tissue which circumferentially narrows the esophageal lumen and fails to distend with insufflation. Multiple strictures are sometimes present, causing the tubular shape of the esophagus to be distorted and angulated. Esophagitis, erosions, and ulcers may also be detected.

Procedure
- If possible, pass the endoscope through the stricture to assess its length and to evaluate the esophagus distal to the strictured area.
- Perform a complete endoscopic examination of the esophagus and stomach to evaluate for severity of esophagitis and to identify potential underlying causes of esophagitis and stricture formation (e.g., foreign bodies, hiatal hernia/intussusception).
- If the endoscope cannot be passed through the stricture, contrast studies may be necessary (if not previously performed) for complete evaluation of number and length of strictures. Balloon dilatation of the stricture may allow subsequent passage of the endoscope.
- Mucosal biopsies of the strictured area may be warranted in some cases to rule out underlying neoplasia, especially when the stricture is associated with a mass effect or mucosal proliferations, or fails to respond to therapy.

Complications. Gastric overdistention can be a significant complication of endoscopy in animals with esophageal stricture; thus, use insufflation sparingly. If the stricture precludes passage of the endoscope into the stomach, air introduced during insufflation will pass through the stricture and accumulate in the stomach, and it cannot be suctioned off through the endoscope.

Treatment

Esophageal strictures can be managed surgically or endoscopically. Surgery may be indicated if the stricture is too small to pass a dilator or if inadequate dilatation is achieved after multiple attempts (see Chap. 86). Mechanical dilatation of the stricture is performed under general anesthesia with endoscopic visualization.

▼*Key Point* Conservative management of esophageal strictures with endoscopically guided balloon catheter dilatation or bougienage is preferable to surgery.

Bougienage

- A well-lubricated dilator, such as a bougie or tapered probe (or the endoscope itself), is passed through the stricture. Avoid excessive force because esophageal perforation is a life-threatening complication.

- Passage of progressively larger bougies results in stretching and dilatation of the stricture.
- The procedure is repeated at intervals of 5–7 days as needed to maintain clinical improvement.
- The total number of dilatations (3–10) is determined by the severity of the stricture and the clinical response.

Balloon Catheter Dilatation

This technique, which is the preferred method for dilatation of esophageal strictures, appears to be superior to bougienage because there is less likelihood of perforation, fewer repeated dilatations are required, and there is a longer response time between dilatations.

Balloon catheters (Rigiflex Dilator, Microvasive Inc., Milford, MA) used in dogs and cats have 10-mm, 15-mm, and 20-mm diameters and 8-cm length when inflated. These catheters can be passed through a 2.8-mm endoscopic biopsy channel, or they can be carefully passed adjacent to the endoscope using endoscopic or fluoroscopic guidance.

- Procedure—With the patient under anesthesia and using endoscopic guidance, insert the catheter with deflated balloon into the lumen of the stricture and center the balloon in the stricture. Distend the balloon with distilled water (or contrast material for fluoroscopy) to the pressure recommended by the manufacturer (usually 45–50 psi). Use a pressure gauge to avoid overdistention and inadvertent balloon rupture. Distend the balloon for 1–2 minutes, and then deflate it to evaluate the size of the stricture and the extent of secondary mucosal hemorrhage. The procedure can be repeated immediately using the next larger balloon.
  - Balloon dilatations are usually performed 2–5 times at intervals of 5–7 days.
- Give prednisolone, 0.5 mg/kg PO q12h for 10–14 days, to prevent further healing by fibrosis and stricture recurrence; taper dosage over the remaining period of time that the stricture requires dilatation.
- During the series of dilatation procedures and for 2–3 weeks after the last one, institute therapy as described under Esophagitis.
- An esophageal diameter of 1 cm is usually adequate for a cat or small dog to be maintained on canned food. Larger dogs may require an opening 1.5–2 cm in diameter.

ESOPHAGEAL DIVERTICULA

Etiology

- Esophageal diverticula are large pouch-like sacculations of the esophageal wall that may be congenital or acquired. They are rare in veterinary medicine. Diverticula most commonly affect the esophagus at the thoracic inlet or just cranial to the diaphragm.
- Acquired diverticula are classified as *pulsion* or *traction* diverticula. Pulsion diverticula are believed to occur because of increased intraluminal pressure secondary to obstruction or altered motility. They have been associated with foreign bodies, stricture, vascular ring anomalies, esophagitis, idiopathic megaesophagus, and hiatal hernia.
- Traction diverticula occur secondary to periesophageal inflammation that results in fibrosis and contraction, which pulls out the wall of the esophagus into a pouch.

Clinical Signs

- Large diverticula interfere with orderly movement of ingesta through the esophagus and cause clinical signs because they predispose to impaction with foreign bodies or food, which may lead to esophagitis and even perforation.
- Signs include regurgitation, distress after eating, anorexia, weight loss, intermittent thoracic or abdominal pain, and respiratory signs.
- Clinical signs may not occur with small diverticula.

Diagnosis

Radiography

- Thoracic radiography frequently reveals a gas- or food-filled mass in the area of the esophagus.
- A barium esophagram confirms that a pouch communicates with the esophageal lumen.

Endoscopy

- Esophagoscopy reveals a sac-like outpouching with variable esophagitis and accumulation of ingesta and fluid in the sac.
- Use caution to avoid perforation of diverticula.

Treatment

- Large diverticula require surgical resection (see Chap. 86).
- Small diverticula can be managed medically with upright feeding of frequent small meals of a soft food diet.
- Identify predisposing causes and treat when possible.

ESOPHAGEAL FISTULA

Esophagotracheal, esophagobronchial, and *esophagopulmonary fistulas* are patent communications between the esophagus and the respective airways. They occur rarely in dogs and cats. Of these, esophagobronchial (bronchoesophageal) fistulas are most commonly described. Clinical signs are related to contamination of the airways with esophageal secretions and food.

Etiology

Esophageal fistulas may be congenital or acquired. Acquired fistulas are most likely and are usually associated with esophageal foreign bodies, especially bones. Other causes include trauma, malignancy, and severe infection.

In most cases, a lodged esophageal foreign body is

suspected to cause esophageal wall necrosis with subsequent development of a fistula.

- Most esophagobronchial fistulas occur in the caudal esophagus, probably due to the close anatomic proximity of the caudal esophagus and bronchi in this region.
- Esophagobronchial fistulas commonly are accompanied by an esophageal diverticulum.
  - A traction diverticulum may develop secondary to periesophageal inflammation and fibrosis in the region of the fistula.
  - A pulsion diverticulum may develop secondary to lodging of a foreign body.
  - The diverticulum may occur first, and predispose to lodging of a foreign body and subsequent fistula formation.

Clinical Signs

- Clinical signs are primarily associated with the respiratory tract. Coughing, especially after drinking liquids, is a common presenting sign. Anorexia, fever, dyspnea, and weight loss are attributed to aspiration pneumonia.
- Signs of esophageal disease such as regurgitation, gagging, and retching may be seen but are not consistently described.
- Contamination of the airways can lead to recurrent localized bacterial pneumonia, pulmonary abscesses, and pleuritis.

Diagnosis

History

Suspect an esophageal fistula when there is a history of chronic cough, recurrent localized pneumonia, and signs of esophageal disease.

Physical Examination

Findings reflect the secondary pulmonary involvement and may include fever, pulmonary crackles, muffled heart sounds (pleural effusion), and weight loss.

Radiography

- Thoracic radiographic abnormalities are primarily indicative of pulmonary complications and include localized alveolar, bronchial, or interstitial patterns, pulmonary consolidation, and pleural effusion. Radiopaque esophageal foreign bodies may be identified. The caudal lung lobes are most commonly affected.
- A barium esophagram is required for definitive diagnosis. Contrast material will outline the communicating airway. Use a thin mixture of barium sulfate (20–30% wt/vol) to enhance filling of small fistulas.

▼ *Key Point* Do not use oral iodinated contrast material (e.g., Gastrografin, Squibb) because it is hypertonic and may cause pulmonary edema.

- Esophagoscopy and bronchoscopy can be performed, but a contrast study is more reliable in detecting fistulas.

Treatment

- Treatment of esophageal fistulas requires surgery for esophagotomy, foreign body removal, fistula resection, and lobectomy.
- Perform culture and sensitivity testing of involved tissues for appropriate antibiotic therapy.

Prognosis

If severe complications such as pneumonia, pulmonary abscesses, and pleuritis are present, the prognosis is poor.

VASCULAR RING ANOMALIES

Etiology

Vascular ring anomalies are congenital malformations of the great vessels and their branches that entrap the intrathoracic esophagus and cause clinical signs of esophageal obstruction.

Persistent Right Aortic Arch

This malformation accounts for 95% of vascular ring anomalies in dogs and cats. Persistent right aortic arch (PRAA) occurs when the embryonic right rather than the left fourth aortic arch becomes the functional adult aorta. The ductus arteriosus continues to develop from the left side, forming a band that crosses over the esophagus to connect the main pulmonary artery and the anomalous aorta (Fig. 85–1). Esophageal compression occurs by the aorta on the right, the ligamentum arteriosum (remnant of the ductus arteriosus) dorsolaterally on the left, the pulmonary trunk on the left, and the base of the heart ventrally.

PRAA appears to have a familial tendency, because certain breeds, especially German shepherds and Irish setters (see Table 85–1), appear to be predisposed and multiple animals in a litter may be affected. The mechanism of inheritance may involve single or multiple recessive genes. Breeding of affected animals is not recommended.

Other Anomalies

Other anomalies that have been described include double aortic arch, persistent right ductus arteriosus (with normal left aortic arch), aberrant left or right subclavian arteries, and (in English bulldogs) esophageal compression by the left subclavian and brachiocephalic arteries.

Clinical Signs

- Affected animals are usually presented for regurgitation of solid food that began at the time of weaning. Regurgitation of undigested food commonly occurs immediately after eating but is sometimes delayed, as

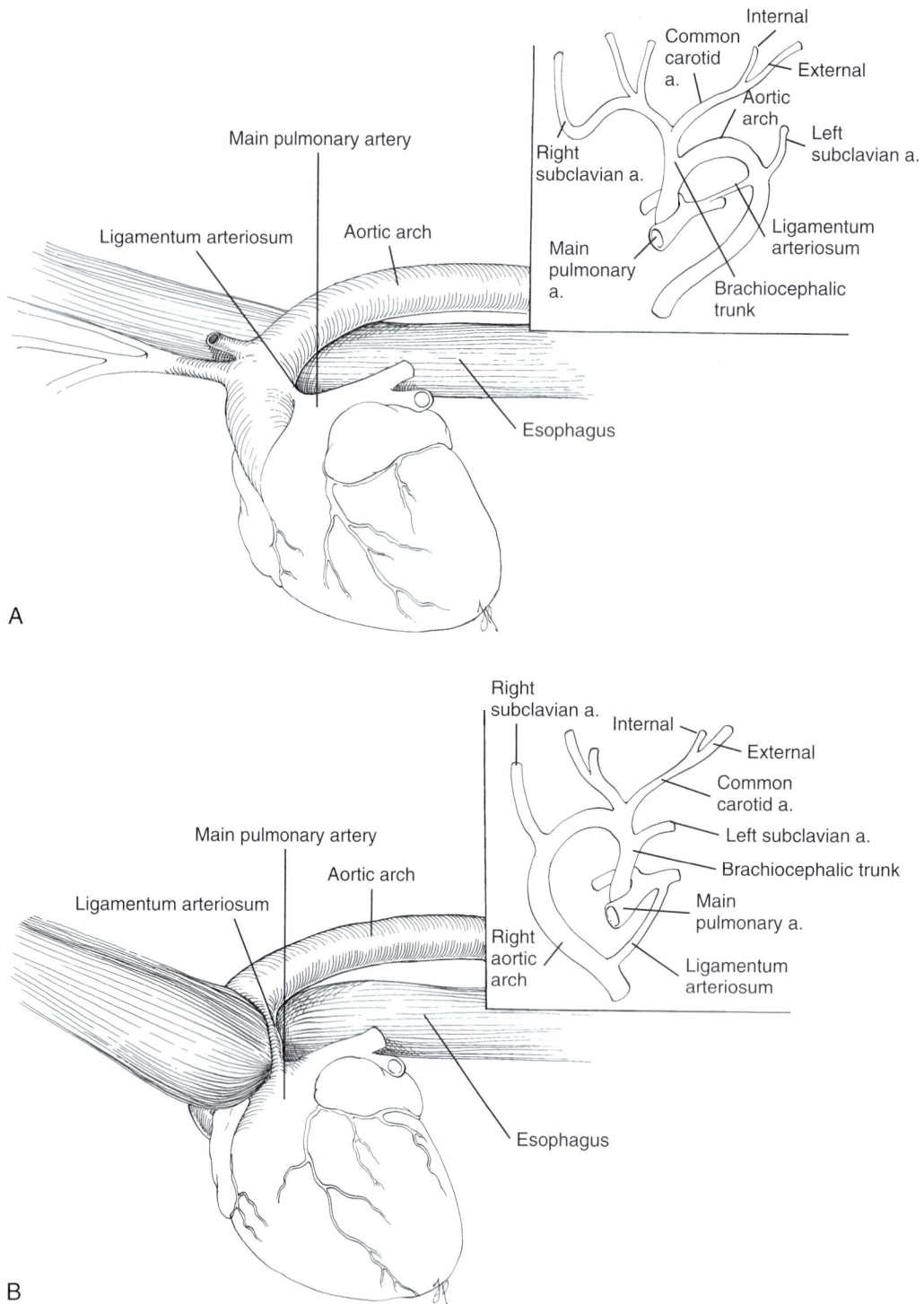

Figure 85–1. Persistent right aortic arch. *A,* Normal development of the aortic arch viewed from the animal's left side. Inset shows normal embryonic development of the great vessels from a dorsoventral view. *B,* When the embryonic right fourth aortic arch becomes the adult aorta, esophageal constriction occurs. Inset shows dorsoventral view of the vascular malformation.

ingesta is retained in a large esophageal pouch that develops cranial to the obstruction. Liquids and semisolid food are preferentially retained because they can pass through the constricted area.
- Weight loss or failure to gain weight despite a good appetite is common.
- Cough and dyspnea suggest aspiration pneumonia.

Diagnosis

Differentiate vascular ring anomalies from other causes of regurgitation in young animals such as congenital megaesophagus and, less frequently, esophageal foreign bodies. Diffuse esophageal hypomotility (megaesophagus) occasionally complicates vascular ring anomalies in dogs.

History

Regurgitation since weaning is very suggestive of a vascular ring anomaly. Most animals are presented by 6 months of age, although occasionally signs are mild and a diagnosis is not made until later in life.

Physical Examination

The cervical esophagus may be distended secondary to partial obstruction and development of a pouch. Cough, dyspnea, pulmonary crackles, and fever indicate aspiration pneumonia.

Radiography

- Survey thoracic radiographs often suggest a vascular ring anomaly. The dilated esophagus appears as a food- or fluid-filled density cranial to the heart, which tapers to normal at the base of the heart. In the ventrodorsal view of PRAA, the normal bulge of the aortic arch to the left is absent.
- Perform a barium esophagram (see Chap. 4) to confirm the location of esophageal obstruction and severity of esophageal distention. Differential diagnoses for this radiographic appearance include an intramural stricture, segmental motility disorder, or congenital diverticulum.
- Fluoroscopy is useful to evaluate generalized esophageal hypomotility.
- Angiography is seldom necessary but in selected cases can be used for definitive confirmation of the type and location of vascular ring anomaly prior to surgery.

Endoscopy

- Endoscopy can distinguish a mural lesion from extraluminal compression. In animals with PRAA, the indentation in the esophagus caused by external compression by the ligamentum arteriosum is visible. The cranial thoracic esophagus is usually dilated.
- Endoscopy is also helpful to rule out cranial esophageal foreign bodies or hairballs (especially) that become lodged secondary to the PRAA.

Treatment

- Definitive therapy for PRAA is surgical ligation and transection of the ligamentum arteriosum (see Chap. 86).
- If the animal is debilitated and malnourished, improve nutritional status before surgery. Give frequent elevated feedings of small amounts of a semimoist or liquid diet. If this diet is poorly tolerated, consider feeding through a gastrostomy tube (see Chap. 3).
- Control aspiration pneumonia with antibiotics before surgery (see Chap. 79).
- Significant clinical improvement usually occurs after surgery, although mild esophageal distention often persists, especially if a large cranial pouch was present.
- Manage as described for megaesophagus if regurgitation persists.

- Recovery of normal esophageal function is more likely if surgery is performed at an early age and esophageal dilatation is not severe.

HIATAL DISORDERS

Anatomic abnormalities of the hiatus include hiatal hernia and gastroesophageal intussusception (GEI).

- A *sliding* hiatal hernia is a protrusion of any structure (usually the distal esophagus and stomach) through the esophageal hiatus of the diaphragm into the thorax.
- A *paraesophageal* hiatal hernia involves displacement of a portion of the stomach through a diaphragmatic defect adjacent to the esophageal hiatus and is rare in veterinary medicine.

Differentiate hiatal hernia from GEI, in which the stomach (and occasionally other structures such as the spleen, proximal duodenum, pancreas, and omentum) invaginates or prolapses into the distal lumen of the esophagus. Hiatal hernias and GEI may be intermittent or persistent.

Etiology

Congenital or acquired enlargement of the esophageal hiatus or laxity of the surrounding ligaments may predispose to hiatal hernias and GEI.

- Most hiatal hernias are probably congenital, and Shar-Pei dogs appear to have an increased incidence.
- Acquired hiatal hernias may occur secondary to high positive intra-abdominal pressure (e.g., blunt abdominal trauma, vomiting) or very negative intrathoracic pressure associated with chronic upper airway obstruction (e.g., laryngeal disease).
- Reversible hiatal hernia and megaesophagus may be seen as a complication of tetanus in dogs.
- Young male dogs appear to be predisposed to GEI.
- Congenital idiopathic megaesophagus predisposes to GEI, presumably due to decreased esophageal motility and decreased gastroesophageal sphincter pressure.

Clinical Signs

- Small hiatal hernias or intussusceptions may not be associated with clinical signs. If the hernia or intussusception occurs intermittently, clinical signs also may be intermittent. Common signs include vomiting, regurgitation, hypersalivation, and weight loss. Dyspnea also is common and may be due to aspiration pneumonia or compression of the lungs secondary to large hernias.
- *Hiatal hernias*—signs are due primarily to impaired gastroesophageal sphincter function, which predisposes to gastroesophageal reflux and reflux esophagitis. If large portions of the stomach are displaced through the diaphragm, signs occur because of esophageal and gastric obstruction.
- *GEI*—GEI can cause both esophagitis and esophageal

obstruction. When a large portion of the stomach is intussuscepted, rapid clinical deterioration is evidenced by signs of dyspnea, hematemesis, profound depression, collapse, and sudden death.

Diagnosis

History

Regurgitation prior to the onset of GEI suggests that megaesophagus may be a predisposing factor. When GEI causes esophageal obstruction, the acuteness of onset and rapid progression to death often preclude an antemortem diagnosis.

Physical Examination

Findings often are unremarkable unless a large hernia or intussusception is causing esophageal obstruction. In this situation, dyspnea, collapse, and shock predominate.

Radiography

- Survey thoracic radiography may confirm both hiatal hernia and GEI if they are large and persistently present. A soft tissue and gas density mass (the stomach) can be seen in the caudal dorsal mediastinum. The normal gastric gas bubble usually seen in the cranial abdomen may be diminished in size.
- Perform a barium esophagram to confirm a hernia or GEI and to distinguish masses arising from other mediastinal structures or the esophagus. With a hiatal hernia, the gastroesophageal junction and gastric rugae are visible cranial to the diaphragm but the linear relationship between the esophagus and the stomach is preserved. Gastroesophageal reflux also may be demonstrated. With GEI, gastric rugae are seen within the esophageal lumen and esophageal obstruction is present.
- Hiatal hernias and GEI that are small and reduce spontaneously are a diagnostic challenge. Because of their intermittent nature, they may not be identified routinely on either survey or contrast radiographs. Application of pressure to the abdomen during radiography, especially fluoroscopy, may be useful for detection of small hernias and gastroesophageal reflux.

Endoscopy

Endoscopy can assess secondary reflux esophagitis and may confirm hiatal hernia or GEI.

- In hiatal hernia, findings include enlargement of the hiatal opening, cranial displacement and dilatation of the gastroesophageal sphincter, rugal folds of the stomach extending through the hiatus into the thoracic esophageal region as viewed from the esophageal and gastric retroflex positions, and evidence of reflux esophagitis.
- In GEI, the rugal folds of the invaginated stomach form a bulging mass in the lumen of the caudal thoracic esophagus.

Treatment

- Surgery is indicated for treatment of large hiatal hernias and intussusceptions (see Chap. 86). Emergency surgery is required for reduction of a large GEI, along with intensive fluid therapy for treatment of shock (see Chap. 72).
- Small intermittent hiatal hernias or intussusceptions do not usually require surgery. Medical management of reflux esophagitis (see earlier in this chapter) usually controls clinical signs. In refractory cases, consider other causes of regurgitation and vomiting before surgical intervention.

PERIESOPHAGEAL OBSTRUCTION

Etiology

- Mass lesions arising from the periesophageal tissues may cause signs of esophageal disease because of esophageal compression with partial or complete obstruction.
- Examples include thyroid tumors (cervical esophagus) or tumors arising from mediastinal structures (e.g., lymph node, thymus, heart base), lung tumors, and intrathoracic abscesses.

Clinical Signs

- Clinical signs associated with external compression of the esophagus by mass lesions (especially neoplasia) include chronic progressive regurgitation, dysphagia, and hypersalivation.
- Signs of esophageal disease may be overshadowed by signs reflecting involvement of other systems (e.g., pulmonary metastases, pleural and pericardial effusion), such as dyspnea, cough, and exercise intolerance.

Diagnosis

Radiography

- Survey thoracic radiographs usually identify an intrathoracic mass.
- If survey films are unremarkable, a barium esophagram is indicated to identify the location and severity of obstruction.

Endoscopy

Endoscopy determines the extent of esophageal obstruction and helps to characterize whether it is extra- or intramural. A stenotic region with normal-appearing mucosa is indicative of extramural compression by a periesophageal mass rather than stricture or primary neoplasia of the esophagus.

Biopsy

The diagnosis depends on identifying the cause of the offending mass lesion with fine-needle aspiration or biopsy via thoracotomy (see Chap. 83).

Treatment

Treatment and prognosis are determined by the underlying cause of esophageal compression.

ESOPHAGEAL NEOPLASIA

Etiology

Primary esophageal neoplasms are rare. Malignant tumors of the esophagus include squamous cell carcinoma, osteosarcoma, fibrosarcoma, and undifferentiated carcinoma. Metastatic tumors occasionally involve the esophagus but unless the tumor is large, clinical signs of esophageal disease are absent.

- Esophageal fibrosarcoma and osteosarcoma in dogs can develop after malignant transformation of esophageal granulomas associated with infection by the helminth parasite *Spirocerca lupi*. Infection with this parasite occurs in the southeastern United States. The life cycle involves a coprophagous beetle that is eaten by the dog or a transport host (mouse, chicken, bird, reptiles) that is subsequently eaten by the dog.
- Squamous cell carcinoma is the most commonly reported esophageal tumor in cats.
- The most common benign esophageal tumor is leiomyoma.

Clinical Signs

- Animals with esophageal neoplasia have signs of chronic regurgitation, dysphagia, and ptyalism that are slowly but relentlessly progressive.
- Anorexia, weight loss, and cachexia result from inability to retain food or are secondary to metastatic disease and the systemic effects of cancer.
- Signs associated with *S. lupi* infection are often subclinical until late in the disease and include anorexia, lethargy, regurgitation, and dyspnea (with large masses).

Diagnosis

History

Chronic progressive signs of obstructive esophageal disease in an older animal suggest esophageal neoplasia.

Physical Examination

- Findings may include weight loss and emaciation consistent with the secondary effects of chronic malnutrition.
- Cervical esophageal tumors may be palpable.
- Dyspnea may occur with a large intrathoracic mass or pulmonary metastatic disease.

Radiography

- Survey thoracic radiographs may be normal or may reveal a mass in the region of the esophagus. With partial to complete esophageal obstruction, the esophagus may be dilated proximal to the mass and contain air, fluid, or food.

- Evaluate the lungs for metastases.
- Spondylitis of the caudal thoracic vertebrae or hypertrophic osteopathy may be associated with *S. lupi* esophageal granulomas.
- A barium esophagram can confirm the presence of a mass or obstruction, characterize the mass as esophageal or periesophageal in origin, and evaluate the extent of esophageal wall involvement.

Endoscopy/Biopsy

Endoscopy and biopsy are required for definitive diagnosis of esophageal neoplasia.

- If esophageal sarcoma is caused by *S. lupi* infection, adult worms may be seen protruding into the lumen of the esophagus from the affected tissue. *S. lupi* eggs may be detected on fecal sedimentation.
- Squamous cell carcinoma usually appears as a proliferative mass with an irregular, friable, ulcerated surface and causing variable obstruction of the lumen.
- Obstruction may cause the esophagus to be dilated with ingesta or fluid proximal to the tumor site.

Treatment

- Successful treatment of esophageal neoplasia requires surgical resection of the tumor (see Chap. 86).
  - For best results, it is important to make an early diagnosis before metastasis or extensive esophageal involvement has occurred.
  - In many cases, the tumor is too extensive for complete surgical resection, and thus the prognosis is poor.
- Anthelmintic therapy for *S. lupi* infection includes:
  - Doramectin (Dectomax, Pfizer), which reportedly cured six dogs of spirocercosis at 200 µg/kg SC at 14-day intervals for three doses, or at 500 µg/kg PO daily for 6 weeks in refractory cases.
  - Disophenol as a single dose (10 mg/kg SC) that is repeated in 7 days if no improvement is noted; however, disophenol is no longer available.
  - Although unproved, fenbendazole (50 mg/kg PO) or ivermectin (200 µg/kg, single oral dose) may be effective against larvae.
  - Levamisole is not recommended because it sterilizes but does not kill adult *S. lupi* organisms.

SUPPLEMENTAL READINGS

Guilford WG, Strombeck DR: Diseases of Swallowing. *In* Guilford WG, Center SA, Strombeck DR, eds.: Strombeck's Small Animal Gastroenterology, 3rd Ed. Philadelphia: WB Saunders, 1996, p 211.

Johnson SE: Diseases of the esophagus. *In* Sherding RG, ed.: The Cat: Diseases and Clinical Management, Vol 2, 2nd Ed. New York: Churchill Livingstone, 1994, p 1153.

Sherding RG, Johnson SE, Tams TR: *In* Tams TR, ed.: Small Animal Endoscopy, 2nd Ed. St. Louis: Mosby, 1999, p 39.

Twedt DC: Diseases of the esophagus. *In* Ettinger SJ, ed.: Textbook of Veterinary Internal Medicine, Vol 2, 4th Ed. Philadelphia: WB Saunders, 1995, p 1124.

86 Surgery of the Esophagus

Ronald M. Bright

In general, the signs of esophageal disease are related to loss of function, to obstruction, or to inflammation of the esophagus and the surrounding structures. Surgery on the esophagus probably requires more skill and precision than any other portion of the alimentary tract. The esophagus is constantly moving, lacks a serosal layer, and does not have omentum to help seal small leaks. If suture line reinforcement is necessary, adjacent muscle, diaphragmatic tissue, or pericardium may be used. Extra-abdominal movement of omentum on a pedicle through a rent in the diaphragm can also be used for this purpose.

ANATOMY

Upper Esophageal Sphincter

The upper esophageal sphincter is located at the proximal end of the esophagus. There is no obvious thickening of the esophageal tissue.

- Sphincter function is performed primarily by the cricopharyngeal muscle.
- Innervation of the cricopharyngeal muscle is from branches of the glossopharyngeal and vagus nerves.
- The blood supply is derived primarily from branches of the cranial thyroid artery.

Lower Esophageal Sphincter

The distal 2 cm of the esophagus is located intra-abdominally below the diaphragm and is thought to have a slightly thickened inner circular muscle that acts as a sphincter.

- Sling fibers from the lesser curvature of the stomach may reinforce the sphincteric function.
- The pinchcock effect of the diaphragmatic hiatus is thought to assist in preventing gastroesophageal reflux.
- Innervation is primarily from the vagus.
- The major portion of the blood supply is derived from the esophageal branch of the left gastric artery.

Body of the Esophagus

- The esophagus has a cervical and thoracic portion.
- The esophagus has four layers—adventitia, muscularis (striated in the dog, smooth muscle in the cau-

dal one-third of the cat), a thin submucosal layer, and mucosa composed of stratified squamous epithelium.
- The blood supply is from the thyroid and esophageal branches of the carotid artery proximally; the bronchoesophageal artery supplies the thoracic and distal portion of the esophagus. A few branches from the left gastric artery are located just above and below the lower esophageal sphincter.

CRICOPHARYNGEAL ACHALASIA

This rare form of dysphagia is characterized by inadequate relaxation of the cricopharyngeal muscle and affects primarily young animals.

Preoperative Considerations

As described in Chapter 4, perform barium swallow fluoroscopy preoperatively to distinguish cricopharyngeal achalasia from other forms of oropharyngeal dysphagia and to evaluate motility of the body of the esophagus. Evaluate for aspiration pneumonia and treat accordingly.

Surgical Procedure (Cricopharyngeal Myectomy)
Objectives

- Surgically relieve the constriction by removing fibers of the cricopharyngeal muscle.
- Allow unobstructed movement of food from the pharynx to the esophagus while decreasing the incidence of aspiration pneumonia.

Equipment

- Standard surgical pack
- Gelpi or Weitlaner retractors
- Surgical suction and cautery

Technique

1. Place the animal in dorsal recumbency with the legs tied caudally.
2. Aseptically prepare the ventral portion of the neck, from the angle of the mandible to the manubrium.
3. Make a ventral midline cervical incision, starting just cranial to the larynx and extending caudally 15–20 cm.

4. Separate the sternohyoideus muscles to expose the trachea and cricothyroideus muscles.
5. Expose the dorsum of the trachea by rotating the larynx and trachea 180° in either direction. If working on the dog's right side, pull the trachea to the right.
6. Remove a thin layer of connective tissue, exposing the dorsal aspect of the cricopharyngeal musculature.
7. Incise the cricopharyngeal musculature on its midline. Gently elevate the muscle from the underlying esophagus with meticulous and careful blunt dissection. Consider placing an inflated Foley catheter or endotracheal tube in the esophagus to help delineate the structures.
8. Elevate the cricopharyngeal muscle laterally and then cranially to the thyropharyngeal muscles.
9. Cut the halves of the muscle belly along their lateral attachments and remove the muscle (Fig. 86–1).
10. Allow the larynx and trachea to return to their normal position, and appose the sternohyoideus muscle with a continuous suture, using 4-0 synthetic absorbable suture.

Postoperative Care and Complications

Short-Term

- Give blenderized food for 48 hours.
- Slowly return to normal diet over the next 48–72 hours.
- If *oral phase dysphagia* is present (see Chap. 85), there may not be any improvement seen following surgery.
- If *pharyngeal phase dysphagia* is present (see Chap. 85)

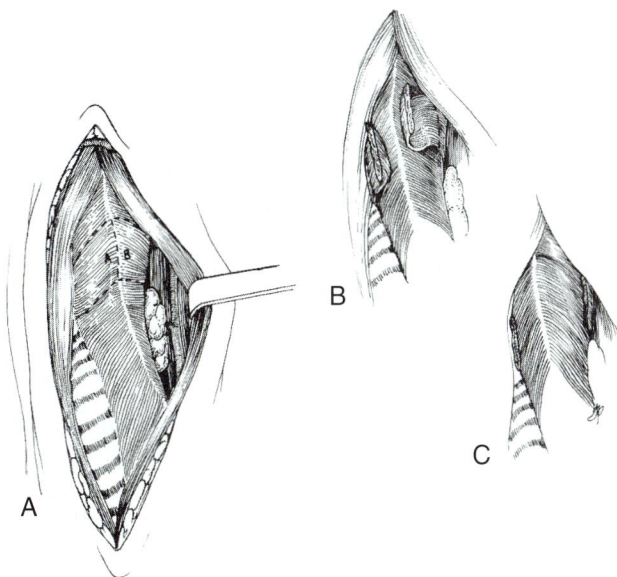

Figure 86–1. Myotomy of the cricopharyngeus muscle for cricopharyngeal achalasia. The cranial esophagus has been exposed via a ventral midline cervical approach. *A,* Rotate the esophagus so that the dorsal aspect is exposed and the cricopharyngeal muscles are seen. *B,* Initially incise on the midline (raphe) to separate the paired muscles. Use care not to perforate the esophagus. *C,* Make two longitudinal incisions laterally, one in each muscle belly, in the cricopharyngeal muscles. Remove each section of muscle.

concurrently, a cricopharyngeal myectomy may worsen the animal's signs and the aspiration pneumonia.
- Hypomotility of the proximal esophagus may interfere with a successful outcome. Food and liquids pass more easily through the cricopharyngeal sphincter, but decreased clearance by the esophagus enhances the likelihood of stasis and retrograde movement of material into the trachea. Aspiration pneumonia continues to be a problem.

Long-Term

- If concurrent disease is present, as previously described, feeding a gruel with the animal in a standing position may be necessary to prevent aspiration pneumonia and promote the passage of nutrients into the stomach.

Prognosis

- If there is no concurrent oropharyngeal or esophageal neuromuscular disorder, the prognosis is fair to good.

VASCULAR RING ANOMALY

Preoperative Considerations

- Any young dog or cat with regurgitation should be suspected of having a vascular ring anomaly.
- Most animals with a vascular ring anomaly are presented to the veterinarian at the age of 4–10 weeks. Rarely, an animal may reach adulthood before a vascular ring anomaly is diagnosed.
- Persistent right aortic arch (PRAA) accounts for 95% of vascular ring anomalies in dogs.
- Rule out other causes of megaesophagus.
- Confirm the diagnosis by contrast esophagography and endoscopy of the esophagus.
- Fluoroscopy can evaluate motility of the esophagus above and below the site of constriction.
- Evaluate the lungs radiographically for aspiration pneumonia. If necessary, institute antibiotic therapy several days preoperatively.
- Debilitated animals may benefit from hyperalimentation via a gastrostomy tube (see Chap. 3) for 7–10 days before surgery.

Surgical Procedure

Objectives

- Relieve the constricted portion of the esophagus caused by the vascular ring.
- Allow unobstructed passage of food to the stomach.
- Avoid perforation of the esophagus.

Equipment

- Finochietto rib retractors
- Suction and cautery
- Right-angle forceps
- DeBakey thumb forceps
- Foley catheter or balloon dilator

Technique

1. Place the animal in right lateral recumbency.
2. Aseptically prepare the left lateral thoracic wall from three intercostal spaces above to five spaces below the fourth intercostal space.
3. To approach the vascular ring, perform a thoracotomy through the fourth intercostal space (see Chap. 83 for thoracotomy technique).
4. Identify the ligamentum arteriosus, which is a constricting band encircling the esophagus. In a PRAA, the aorta is on the animal's right side and cannot be seen through a left thoracotomy (see Fig. 85–1).
5. If a PRAA is not the problem, consider vascular anomaly variations, including a left subclavian artery originating from the brachiocephalic trunk and, less commonly, a double aortic arch.
6. Double-ligate (e.g., with 3-0 or 4-0 silk) and divide the constricting vessel.
7. Gently dissect the mediastinum and adventitia away from the esophagus 1–2 cm above and below the constricted portion. Dissect any restricting bands of tissue away from the esophagus.

▼ **Key Point** The esophageal wall usually is very thin; use great care to avoid perforation during dissection.

8. Pass a large Foley catheter or balloon dilator into the esophagus per os to further expand the esophagus at the site of constriction.

Closure

1. Administer a long-acting local anesthetic agent (e.g., mepivacaine) caudal to the head of the rib above and below the thoracotomy incision.
2. Place a chest tube before closure.
3. Close the thoracotomy incision routinely (see Chap. 83).

Postoperative Care and Complications

Short-Term

- Evacuate the pleural cavity and administer mepivacaine through the indwelling chest tube to control pain as necessary postoperatively. The chest tube usually can be removed within 24 hours.
- Regurgitation may continue to be a problem early in the postoperative period. Feeding blenderized food with the animal in a standing position may be necessary because of concurrent esophageal hypomotility.

Long-Term

- Amelioration of signs followed by a return of regurgitation several weeks after surgery may signal extraluminal scar formation acting as a constricting band.
- Repeated endoscopic balloon dilatation (see Chap. 85) of these strictures sometimes ameliorates signs.
- An esophagoplasty or resection of the stenotic segment may be necessary.

Prognosis

- The prognosis is good in most animals. Animals with severe dilatation of the esophagus cranial to the obstruction have a poor prognosis.
- Although not well documented, it is believed that the younger the patient at the time of surgical correction, the better the prognosis.
- The prognosis is thought to be better in animals in which preoperative fluoroscopy shows:
  - Normal or near-normal motility of the esophagus above and below the constriction
  - Absence of severe esophageal dilatation cranial to the obstruction

ESOPHAGOTOMY

The most common indication for an esophagotomy is to remove a foreign body that could not be removed by intraluminal retrieval methods.

Preoperative Considerations

- Place a large-bore tube in the esophagus just before an esophagotomy to aspirate esophageal contents, act as a support while incising into the lumen of the esophagus, and help immobilize the esophagus.
- Treat concurrent aspiration pneumonia, aggressively before and after esophagotomy.
- Although surgery of the esophagus carries a low risk of postoperative infection, some contamination occurs. Perioperative antibiotics are recommended (given 30 minutes before surgery and repeated once or twice). The antibiotic chosen should be effective against gram-positive pathogens (e.g., a cephalosporin).

Surgical Procedure

Objectives

- Gain access to the lumen of the esophagus to assist in the removal of a foreign body.
- Make the incision over healthy esophageal tissue.
- Handle esophageal tissues gently to preserve blood supply and optimize healing.
- Establish a watertight seal with closure.

Equipment

- Standard general surgery pack and suction unit
- Laparotomy pads to isolate the esophagus and prevent contamination of the surrounding tissues
- Fine-tipped needle holders to assist in delicate placement of sutures during closure
- Long-handled Metzenbaum scissors for thoracic esophagus dissection
- DeBakey thumb forceps

Technique (Cervical)

1. Make a ventral midline cervical incision extending from the manubrium to the larynx.
2. Retract the trachea and carotid sheaths gently to the right side.

3. Isolate the esophagus from surrounding structures with moistened laparotomy pads.
4. Following the insertion of a large-bore orogastric tube, make an incision into the esophagus.

Closure

1. A two-layer closure is preferred:
   a. The first layer incorporates the submucosa and mucosa; use 3-0 or 4-0 monofilament nonabsorbable sutures with the knots tied in the lumen.
   b. The second layer incorporates the muscle and adventitia. Use an absorbable synthetic suture for this layer.
2. Alternatively, close both layers with a single interrupted appositional suture pattern. Place sutures 2–3 mm deep and at intervals of 2–3 mm.
3. Irrigate the surgical field with a copious amount of sterile saline.
4. If infection is present or tissue trauma excessive, use a closed drainage system with silicone tubing, for 3–5 days.

Technique (Cranial Thoracic)

1. To approach the cranial thoracic esophagus (T2–T6), perform a right-sided third or fourth intercostal space thoracotomy.
2. Retract the cranial and middle lung lobes caudally with moistened sponges.
3. If necessary, dissect the azygos vein free and ligate.
4. Dissect the mediastinal pleura overlapping the esophagus to just above and below the proposed site of esophagotomy.

▼ *Key Point* Avoid trauma to the vagal nerve trunks located laterally along the esophagus.

Technique (Caudal Thoracic)

1. Perform a right-sided seventh or eighth intercostal space thoracotomy to gain exposure to the caudal one-half of the thoracic esophagus.

Closure

1. Closure of an esophagotomy incision is similar to that described under Cervical Technique.
2. Place a chest tube before thoracotomy closure.

Postoperative Care and Complications

- Remove the chest tube 24–48 hours postoperatively unless esophageal perforation and mediastinitis were present.
- Withhold all food and water (NPO) and give intravenous fluid therapy for at least 48 hours.
  - If esophageal tissue was devitalized or compromised at the time of esophagotomy, it may be necessary to maintain the NPO period for several weeks.
  - Ideally, use a gastrostomy tube for nutritional support during the NPO period (see Chap. 3).
- For the next 5–7 days, feed a blenderized diet. Gradually return to a normal diet by postoperative day 10.

- If infection was present at the time of esophagotomy, submit a tissue sample for culture and sensitivity testing and initiate appropriate antimicrobial therapy.

Prognosis

- The prognosis is good if the tissue was viable at the time of esophagotomy.
- If perforation has already occurred and infection is present, the prognosis is poor.

ESOPHAGEAL RESECTION AND ANASTOMOSIS

Indications for resection and anastomosis include foreign bodies, esophageal strictures, neoplasia, and granulomas.

Preoperative Considerations

▼ *Key Point* Some type of nutritional support (e.g., via gastrostomy tube) for patients undergoing an esophageal resection and anastomosis should always be part of the preoperative treatment strategy.

- If the site of anastomosis is unhealthy or compromised, a reinforcement or grafting technique may be necessary.
- Many patients requiring esophageal resection are dehydrated and malnourished and may have aspiration pneumonia. Ideally, correct these conditions before resection and anastomosis.

Surgical Procedure

Approaches to the various parts of the esophagus are described under Esophagotomy. Closure following anastomosis and resection is described here.

Objectives

- Resect the lesion and reappose the esophagus under minimal tension.
- Restore esophageal continuity while minimizing the risk of early postoperative leakage or later stricture formation.

Equipment

- Similar to that for esophagotomy plus intestinal noncrushing forceps

Technique—Closure

1. A two-layer closure, using a simple interrupted appositional suture pattern, is preferred (Fig. 86–2).
   a. Use noncrushing forceps (or fingers) to occlude esophageal ends during closure.
   b. Use multiple stay sutures to maintain alignment of the tissues.
2. Close the contralateral adventitial and muscular layers, using 3-0 or 4-0 synthetic nonabsorbable sutures.

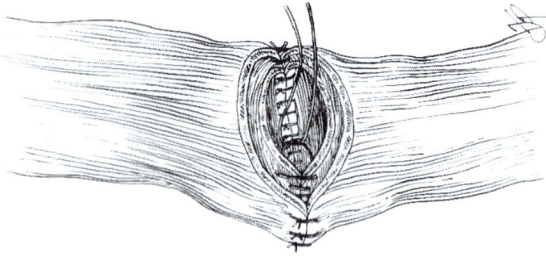

Figure 86–2. Esophageal resection and anastomosis. Close the esophageal layers in the following order: far wall, seromuscular layer; far wall, mucosal layer (knots in the lumen); near wall, mucosal layer (knots in the lumen); near wall, seromuscular layer.

3. Appose the contralateral mucosal-submucosal layers with 3-0 or 4-0 monofilament nonabsorbable sutures with the knot tied in the lumen; follow with closure of the ipsilateral mucosa-submucosa.
4. Close the ipsilateral superficial layers as in Step 2.
5. To relieve excessive tension across the suture line:
    a. A circular myotomy (including only the outer muscular layer) adjacent to the anastomosis can be performed. Injecting saline between the muscle layers helps to identify the outer layer.
    b. Mobilizing the stomach cranially through an enlarged hiatal opening can also help to reduce tension across the suture line.
6. If necessary, reinforce the sutures by bringing omentum on a pedicle through a small rent in the diaphragm or by using pericardial tissue or intercostal musculature.
7. Place a chest tube before thoracotomy closure.

Postoperative Care and Complications
Short-Term

▼ *Key Point* Bypass the esophageal anastomotic site and provide nutrition via gastrostomy tube for a minimum of 7 days.

- Monitor closely for fever, which often signals an infection secondary to leakage.
- Allow water consumption and return to oral feeding beginning on day 7. Retain the gastrostomy tube until normal food and water intake can be restored.

Long-Term

- Dysphagia or regurgitation occurring 3–6 weeks postoperatively probably indicates a stricture.
- Bougienage or balloon dilatation may be necessary to relieve the postoperative stricture (see Chap. 85 for discussion of esophageal stricture).

Prognosis

- Esophageal surgery of any kind carries a poorer prognosis than surgery on any other portion of the alimentary tract.
- If the anastomosis is done with precision and the tension across the suture line is minimal, fair to good results can be expected.

- Any compromise of the tissue at the anastomotic site carries a guarded to poor prognosis.

ESOPHAGOTRACHEAL/ESOPHAGOBRONCHIAL FISTULAS

Preoperative Considerations

- These fistulas usually are sequelae to a chronic foreign body.
- Most affected animals are high-risk patients because of severe bronchopneumonia.
- It may be necessary to sacrifice a lung lobe to achieve a cure.
- The use of gas anesthesia may cause the stomach to become overinflated if the endotracheal tube is located cranial to the fistula.

Surgical Procedure
Objectives

- Isolate the esophagus and the trachea or bronchus associated with the fistula.
- Close the abnormal communication between the alimentary and respiratory tracts.

Equipment

- General surgical pack
- Laparotomy pads
- Finochietto retractors
- TA stapler (U.S. Surgical Corporation, Norwalk, CT) (optional for lung lobectomy)
- Chest tube

Technique

1. If a lobectomy is contemplated, the approach is through the sixth or seventh intercostal space.
2. Isolate the esophagus and trachea or affected bronchus and dissect around the fistula. Obtain samples for culture and sensitivity testing.
3. Sever the fistula near its respiratory attachment; debride the opening and close using 3-0 or 4-0 nonabsorbable sutures.
4. If necessary, enlarge the opening to the esophagus to remove the foreign body if it is still present. The wound is then debrided and the esophageal defect closed in two layers as described previously under Esophagotomy.
5. Remove the affected lung if it is irreversibly damaged.
6. Place a chest tube before the thoracotomy closure.

Postoperative Care and Complications
Short-Term

- Treat concurrent pneumonia, emphysema, or septicemia aggressively, and administer a broad-spectrum antibiotic pending culture and sensitivity testing results.
- If empyema is present, consider leaving the chest tube in for an extended period of time for ongoing

evacuation of fluid from the pleural space (see Chap. 3).
- Maintain enteral feeding for an extended period of time via a tube gastrostomy to decrease the likelihood of leakage from the esophageal wound and allow healing of the esophagus.

Long-Term

- Stricture is always a potential sequela to esophageal surgery.

Prognosis

- In most cases, pulmonary involvement is significant, and the mortality rate is high.
- If the degree of pulmonary involvement and esophageal trauma is minimal, the prognosis is better.

ESOPHAGEAL DIVERTICULECTOMY

Preoperative Considerations

- Perioperative antibiotics are necessary to decrease the potentially deleterious effects of bacterial leakage.
- If regurgitation is severe, dehydration may occur; correct with fluid therapy before surgery.

Surgical Procedure

Objectives

- Resect the large diverticula and reconstruct the esophageal wall.
- Remove the primary cause of the diverticulum, including strictures or periesophageal adhesions.

Equipment

- General surgical pack
- Finochietto rib retractors
- Chest tube
- Noncrushing intestinal or vascular clamp

Technique

1. A left eighth intercostal space thoracotomy is used to approach most diverticula because of their epiphrenic location (just cranial to the diaphragm).
2. Isolate the diverticulum by blunt dissection down to its base.
3. Place a noncrushing clamp across the base of the diverticulum.
4. Excise the diverticulum below the clamp and close the esophagus in an open two-layer technique as described previously under Esophagotomy.
5. Place a chest tube before thoracotomy closure.

Postoperative Care and Complications

Short-Term

- Dietary restrictions are the same as those used following esophagotomy. A gastrostomy tube usually is not necessary.

- Monitor for elevated temperature and neutrophilia closely, because these suggest esophageal dehiscence and mediastinitis.
- Before discharge, perform contrast esophagography to evaluate esophageal motility.

Long-Term

- Stricture formation may be a sequela to extensive excision of the esophagus.
- Special dietary management may be necessary for the life of the animal if motility dysfunction remains.

Prognosis

- The prognosis is good if the underlying cause can be corrected.

ESOPHAGEAL STRICTURE REPAIR

Preoperative Considerations

▼ *Key Point* Attempt surgical correction of esophageal stricture only after bougienage or balloon dilatation (as described in Chap. 85) is unsuccessful.

- Cervical strictures carry less risk with surgical correction than do those involving the thoracic esophagus.
- Correction of fluid and electrolyte imbalances is imperative before any surgical procedure.

Surgical Procedure

Objectives

- Increase the size of the esophageal lumen by reconstructive procedures or resection.
- Resection of a lesion greater than 3 cm in length may require an esophageal lengthening procedure or a suture line reinforcement technique.

Equipment

- Standard general surgery pack
- Cervical location—Gelpi retractors; thoracic location—Finochietto retractors
- Chest tube (thoracic repair)
- Intestinal noncrushing clamps

Technique

Esophagoplasty

If the stricture is not too wide, a longitudinal full-thickness incision followed by a transverse closure (two-layer) may be adequate to increase lumen size. This is similar to Heineke-Mikulicz pyloroplasty (see Chap. 88).

Patch-Grafting Technique in Cervical Region

1. Resect a partial circumference stricture, leaving a defect.
2. Separate a belly of one of the paired sternohyoideus or sternocephalicus muscles from its attachment to the other belly and reflect it laterally.

3. Transpose the muscle to lie deeply against the esophageal defect. Suture the muscle to the edges of the defect. Be sure that the muscle fills the entire defect.
4. The muscle graft must be mobile enough and of sufficient width to prevent postoperative stricture.

Resection and Anastomosis

This is described previously under Esophageal Resection and Anastomosis.

Postoperative Care and Complications

Short-Term

- Monitor signs of infection that may suggest leakage from the surgical site; the more extensive the resection, the more likely that signs of early leakage will occur.
- Placement of a gastrostomy tube is probably necessary in most cases to prevent leakage and enhance esophageal healing.

Long-Term

- Stricture is likely to recur.
- Lifelong tube gastrostomy to bypass the stricture may be necessary if surgery fails and if the owner is willing to maintain nutrition by this method.

Prognosis

- The more extensive the surgery, the poorer the prognosis.
- Less aggressive procedures (e.g., esophagoplasty) carry a better prognosis.

HIATAL HERNIA

Preoperative Considerations

▼ *Key Point* The radiographic presence of a hiatal hernia does not by itself indicate the need for surgical repair.

- The reflux esophagitis that results from hiatal hernia can be managed successfully in most cases with medical therapy alone (see Chap. 85).
- Sphincter reinforcement procedures (e.g., fundoplication) probably are not indicated in most cases of hiatal hernia, because incompetence of the lower esophageal sphincter is seldom a factor in dogs and cats (in contrast to humans).
- Treat gastroesophageal intussusception using similar surgical techniques as described next.

Surgical Procedure

Objectives

- Restore the anatomic relationship of the stomach, diaphragm, and distal esophagus.
- Decrease the size of the enlarged hiatus.
- "Fix" the distal esophagus and stomach to structures below the diaphragm.

Equipment

- General surgery pack
- Abdominal self-retaining retractors
- 28 Fr. orogastric tube
- Malleable (ribbon) retractors

Technique

1. Place the animal in dorsal recumbency with the forelimbs gently drawn forward.
2. Aseptically prepare the ventral midline from the mid-sternum to 2–3 cm cranial to the pubis.
3. Pass a 28 Fr. orogastric tube into the stomach per os.
4. Incise the skin and underlying tissues from just below the xiphoid to several centimeters caudal to the umbilicus.
5. Cover the left side of the liver with a saline-soaked laparotomy pad and retract the liver to the right and caudally with a wide malleable retractor.
6. Evaluate the esophageal hiatus for size. Gently dissect the surrounding tissue to expose the margins of the hiatus. Identify and protect the vagus nerves.
7. While an assistant places caudal traction on the stomach, plicate the hiatus with 1-0 or 2-0 nonabsorbable sutures (Fig. 86–3).

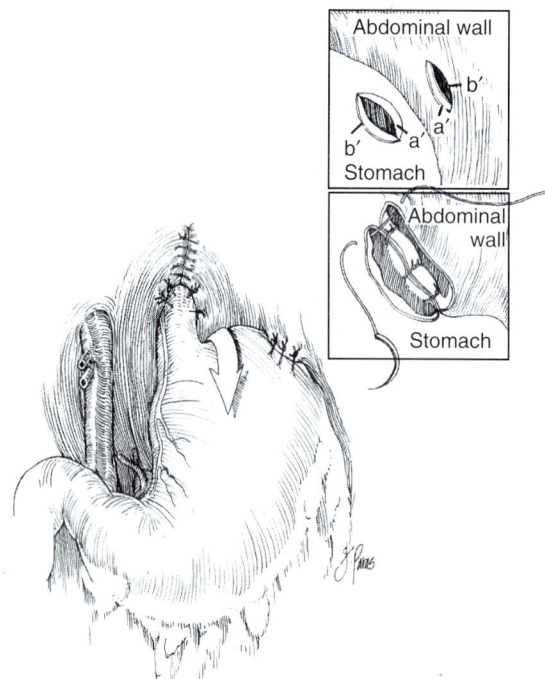

Figure 86–3. Hiatal plication for hiatal hernia. Place the stomach in its normal position and put slight caudal traction on the stomach to expose the distal esophagus and esophageal hiatus. Plicate the esophageal hiatus with nonabsorbable sutures, then perform an esophagopexy by placing sutures from the diaphragm to the esophageal wall, being careful not to penetrate the lumen and not to injure the vagus nerves. Perform a pexy of the fundus to the interior body wall (*insets*). Incise the seromuscular layer of the fundus and then incise the peritoneum and underlying muscle adjacent to the fundic incision. Suture the stomach wall to the body wall as shown.

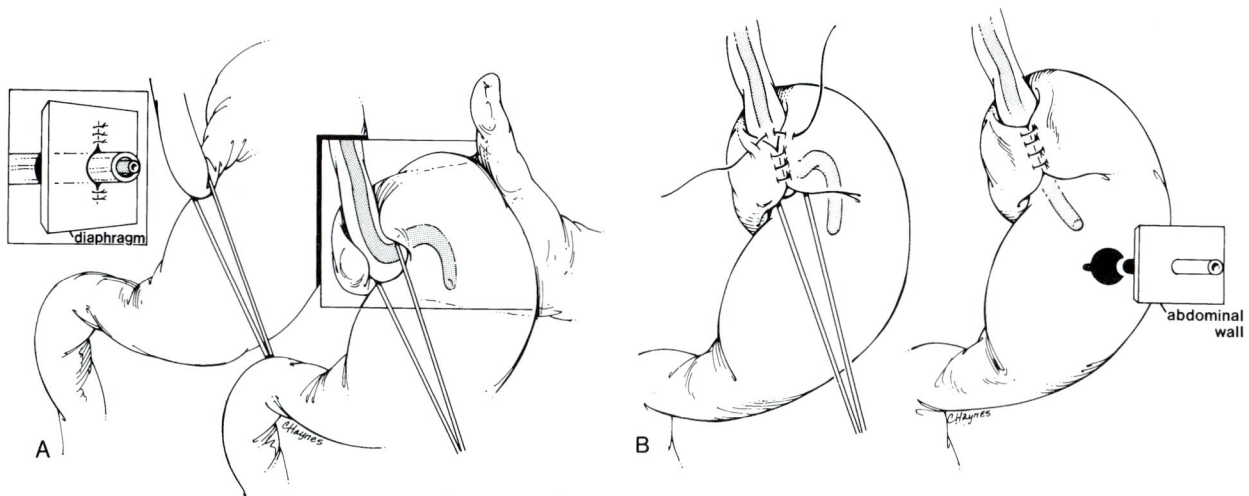

Figure 86–4.   Surgical treatment of hiatal hernia. *A,* Place traction on the distal esophagus and wrap the fundus around the esophagus. *B,* Plicate the fundus around the distal esophagus and place a tube gastrostomy.

8. When plication is completed, it should be possible to insert two fingers through the hiatus.
9. Perform esophagopexy by placing 2-0 nonabsorbable sutures between the diaphragm and the lateral aspect of the distal esophagus as it passes through the hiatus; incorporate the muscle layers of the esophagus (see Fig. 86–3).
10. Fix the fundus of the stomach to the left abdominal wall by performing an incisional gastropexy.
11. Make an incision 3–4 cm long through the serosa and muscular layers of the stomach. Make a similar incision in the peritoneum and transversalis musculature.
12. Appose the margins of the two surgical wounds, using 6–8 size 1-0 nonabsorbable sutures.

Postoperative Care and Complications

Short-Term

- Feed a gruel diet for 3–5 days. A return to a normal ration usually is possible thereafter.
- Some animals may need to be fed from an elevated position for an indefinite period of time.
- If severe esophagitis was present before surgery, continue medical therapy for reflux esophagitis (see Chap. 85) with a systemic antacid postoperatively.
  - Omeprazole (0.7 mg/kg PO once daily) is the preferred antacid. Ranitidine (2–4 mg/kg PO q8–12h) or cimetidine (5 mg/kg PO q8h) can be substituted.
  - Administer metoclopramide (0.2–0.4 mg/kg PO q8h) or cisapride (0.5–0.7 mg/kg PO q8h) to most patients for 2–3 weeks postoperatively.
- Some dysphagia is common for several days following surgery. However, unrelenting dysphagia suggests that the hiatus has been narrowed too much. Reoperation is necessary in those cases that do not respond to medical therapy and when there are signs of dysphagia beyond 1 week.

Long-Term

- Perform esophagography if signs of regurgitation continue in spite of surgery and follow-up medical therapy.
- If failure of the "pexy" procedure or if incompetence of the lower esophageal sphincter is suspected, surgical intervention is necessary.
  - If a sphincter-reinforcement procedure is indicated, perform the Nissen fundoplication (Fig. 86–4).

Prognosis

- The prognosis is good if aspiration pneumonia is controlled.
- Chronic reflux esophagitis associated with a hiatal hernia may cause various degrees of esophageal stricture. If the pathology is advanced to this degree, the prognosis is poor.

SUPPLEMENTAL READINGS

Cricopharyngeal Achalasia

Rosin E: Cricopharyngeal achalasia. *In* Bojrab MJ, ed.: Current Techniques in Small Animal Surgery I. Philadelphia: Lea & Febiger, 1975, p 190.
Shelton GD: Swallowing disorders in the dog. Comp Contin Educ Pract Vet 4:607, 1982.
Suter PF, Watrous BJ: Oropharyngeal dysphagias in the dog: A cineradiographic analysis of experimentally induced and spontaneously occurring swallowing disorders. Oral stage and pharyngeal stage dysphagia. Vet Radiol 21:24, 1980.

Vascular Ring Anomaly

DeHoff WD: Persistent right aortic arch. *In* Bojrab MJ, ed.: Current Techniques in Small Animal Surgery I. Philadelphia: Lea & Febiger, 1975, p 301.
Lawson DD, Purie HM: Conditions of the canine esophagus II: Vascular rings, achalasia, tumors, and perioesophageal lesions. J Small Anim Pract 7:117, 1966.

Shires PK, Liu W: Persistent right aortic arch in dogs: A long-term follow-up after surgical correction. J Am Anim Hosp Assoc 17:773, 1981.

Esophagotomy

Flanders JA: Problems and complications associated with esophageal surgery. *In* Matthesen DT, ed.: Problems in Veterinary Medicine: Gastrointestinal Surgical Problems, Vol. 1. Philadelphia: JB Lippincott, 1989.

Parker N, Caywood D: Surgical diseases of the esophagus. Vet Clin North Am 17:333, 1987.

Esophageal Resection and Anastomosis

Bright RM: Esophagus and stomach. *In* Harvey C, Newton C, Schwartz A, eds.: Small Animal Surgery. Philadelphia: JB Lippincott, 1990, p 323.

Flanders JA: Problems and complications associated with esophageal surgery. *In* Matthesen DT, ed.: Problems in Veterinary Medicine, Gastrointestinal Surgical Problems, Vol. 1. Philadelphia: JB Lippincott, 1989.

Esophagotracheal/Esophagobronchial Fistulas

Park RD: Bronchoesophageal fistula in the dog: Literature survey, case presentations, and radiographic manifestations. Comp Contin Educ Pract Vet 6:669, 1984.

vanEe R, Dodd VM, Pope E: Bronchoesophageal fistula and transient megaesophagus in a dog. J Am Vet Med Assoc 188:874, 1986.

Esophageal Diverticulectomy

Lantz GC, Bojrab MJ, Jones BD: Epiphrenic esophageal diverticulectomy. J Am Anim Hosp Assoc 12:629, 1976.

Esophageal Stricture Repair

Craig D, Todhunter R: Surgical repair of an esophageal stricture in a horse. Vet Surg 16:251, 1987.

Pearson H, Darke PG, Gibbs C, et al.: Reflux oesophagitis and stricture formation after anesthesia: A review of seven cases in dogs and cats. J Small Anim Pract 19:507, 1978.

Sooy TE, Adams W, Pitts RP, et al.: Balloon catheter dilatation of alimentary tract strictures in the dog and cat. Vet Radiol 28:131, 1987.

Hiatal Hernia

Bright RM, Sackman JE, DeNovo RC, et al.: Hiatal hernia in the dog and cat: A retrospective study of 16 cases. J Small Anim Pract 31:244, 1990.

Ellison GW, Lewis DD, Phillips L, et al.: Esophageal hiatal hernia in small animals: Literature review and a modified surgical technique. J Am Anim Hosp Assoc 23:391, 1987.

Prymak C, Saunders HM, Washabau RJ: Hiatal hernia repair by restoration and stabilization of normal anatomy: An evaluation in four dogs and one cat. Vet Surg 18:386, 1989.

87 Diseases of the Stomach

Susan E. Johnson / Robert G. Sherding / Ronald M. Bright

VOMITING

Vomiting is a common clinical sign associated with many gastrointestinal (GI) and nongastrointestinal (non-GI) disorders of dogs and cats. Vomiting is a central nervous system reflex that is integrated in the vomiting center of the brain stem. Afferent stimuli can originate from the cerebral cortex, chemoreceptor trigger zone, pharynx, peritoneum, or abdominal viscera. Vomiting must be differentiated from regurgitation, which is the passive expulsion of undigested food indicating a pharyngeal (swallowing) or esophageal disorder (see Chap. 85).

The metabolic consequences of vomiting vary, depending on the volume and composition of the expulsed fluid. Mild vomiting of short duration usually is not accompanied by overt fluid, electrolyte, or acid-base imbalances. Frequent or profuse vomiting can cause metabolic complications such as dehydration; electrolyte imbalances such as hypokalemia, hyponatremia, and hypochloremia; and acid-base imbalances such as metabolic acidosis or metabolic alkalosis. Metabolic alkalosis is most likely to occur in dogs and cats with vomiting secondary to pyloric obstruction. Other potential complications of vomiting include aspiration pneumonia and reflux esophagitis.

Etiology

Vomiting is a clinical sign, rather than a diagnosis, and can be associated with numerous GI and non-GI disorders (Table 87–1).

▼ *Key Point* Remember that non-GI disorders commonly cause vomiting; do not overlook these before evaluating for primary GI causes of vomiting.

Clinical Signs

- Vomiting frequently is preceded by nausea (evidenced by hypersalivation, licking of the lips, repeated swallowing), retching, and abdominal contractions.
- Vomitus consists of stomach and duodenal contents such as food, mucus, and foamy or bile-stained fluid with a neutral or acidic pH.
- The term *hematemesis* is used when vomitus contains blood flecks, blood clots, or brown coffee grounds–like material (digested blood).

- Vomitus may contain hair, plant material, or other ingested foreign material that can irritate the stomach.
- Vomiting of undigested or partially digested food more than 12 hours after eating suggests delayed gastric emptying (functional or mechanical).
- Projectile vomiting (the forceful ejection of vomitus from the mouth that may be expelled a considerable distance) usually indicates gastric or upper small bowel obstruction.
- Other clinical signs may be present depending on the underlying cause of vomiting and the presence of complications such as dehydration or electrolyte and acid-base imbalances.

Diagnosis

The diagnostic approach to vomiting is directed toward identifying the underlying disorder (see Table 87–1) and is influenced by whether vomiting is acute or chronic and by the associated historical and physical findings.

Acute Vomiting. Acute vomiting is a common problem in dogs and cats and may be caused by benign, self-limiting disorders such as acute gastritis or serious life-threatening diseases such as acute pancreatitis, intestinal obstruction, or acute renal or hepatic failure (see Table 87–1).

- Extensive diagnostic testing is not necessarily warranted in every dog or cat with acute vomiting, because nonspecific, self-limiting acute gastritis is a common cause of acute vomiting.
- Base the decision to perform further testing in an acutely vomiting dog or cat on historical and physical findings.
  - Further evaluation is usually warranted at initial presentation if abnormal physical findings such as fever, lethargy, depression, weakness, dehydration, or palpable abdominal abnormalities are detected.
  - A history of possible GI foreign body exposure may warrant abdominal radiographs even if the physical examination is normal.
- If the history and physical examination are unremarkable, further diagnostic evaluation may be postponed and symptomatic therapy given on an outpatient basis.
- If vomiting does not resolve in 2–3 days or if additional clinical signs develop, further evaluation is indicated.

Table 87–1. CAUSES OF VOMITING IN DOGS AND CATS

Acute Vomiting (<1 wk)	Chronic Vomiting (>1–2 wk)
Gastrointestinal Disorders	***Gastrointestinal Disorders***
Diet-related	Diet-related
Sudden diet change	Food intolerance
Food intolerance or allergy	Food allergy
Dietary indiscretion (e.g., garbage)	Chronic gastritis
Acute gastritis or enteritis	Lymphocytic-plasmacytic
Ingested bacterial enterotoxins	Eosinophilic
Foreign bodies (e.g., bones, plants, plastic, rocks, hairballs)	Granulomatous (e.g., pythiosis)
Ingested chemical irritants or toxins	Foreign bodies (including hairballs)
Drug-induced (e.g., aspirin and other NSAIDs, glucocorticoids, antineoplastics, erythromycin)	Parasites *(Ollulanus, Physaloptera)*
Viral enteritis (e.g., canine parvovirus, feline panleukopenia, canine distemper)	Reflux gastritis
Bacterial infection (e.g., *Helicobacter* spp.)	Hypertrophic gastropathy
Parasites (e.g., *Physaloptera*)	Gastrointestinal ulceration
Gastric or intestinal obstruction	Gastric neoplasia
Foreign bodies	Gastric outflow obstruction
Intestinal volvulus	Foreign bodies
Intestinal intussusception	Gastric neoplasia
Gastric dilatation-volvulus	Gastric polyps
	Hypertrophic gastropathy
Nongastrointestinal Disorders	Pyloric stenosis
Acute pancreatitis	Chronic gastritis
Acute renal failure	Granuloma (pythiosis)
Acute hepatic failure	External compression
Ketoacidotic diabetes mellitus	Partial gastric dilatation-volvulus
Pyometra	Gastric motility disorder
Prostatitis	Hiatal hernia
Peritonitis	Diaphragmatic hernia
Drug-induced (e.g., cardiac glycosides, narcotics, antineoplastics)	Chronic colitis
Sepsis	Obstipation
CNS disorders (inflammation, edema)	Partial distal intestinal obstruction
Motion sickness	
Vestibular disease	***Nongastrointestinal Disorders***
	Renal failure
	Hepatic disease
	Hypoadrenocorticism
	Hyperthyroidism (feline)
	Chronic pancreatitis (feline)
	Heartworm (feline)
	CNS disorders (e.g., inflammatory, neoplastic, visceral epilepsy)
	Lead toxicity

CNS, central nervous system; NSAIDs, nonsteroidal anti-inflammatory drugs.

Chronic Vomiting. Chronic or persistent vomiting is always an indication for further workup.

History

- Perform a complete history.
- Characterize vomiting as to duration, frequency, progression, relationship to eating, and other specific features (e.g., presence of hematemesis, foreign material, partially digested food).
- Determine if there are other associated clinical signs.
  - Is the appetite decreased or increased?

- Has there been weight loss?
- Has there been a change in attitude (depression)?
- Has there been any diarrhea?
- Is polyuria or polydipsia present?
- Is there a history of cough or dyspnea?
- Determine the past medical and worming history, vaccination status, diet, and if there has been any recent exposure to medications, toxins, plants, string or other foreign bodies, garbage, or other sick animals.

Physical Examination

- The physical examination is often unremarkable in animals with gastric disorders.
- Perform a complete oropharyngeal examination to detect a sublingual string foreign body (especially in cats).
- Palpate the GI tract for masses, foreign bodies, trichobezoars, thickenings, distention, plication, or pain.
- Evaluate for evidence of non-GI causes of vomiting (e.g., lumpy, enlarged, or small kidneys with renal failure; cranial abdominal pain and fever with pancreatitis; icterus or hepatomegaly with liver failure; palpable thyroid nodule with feline hyperthyroidism).
- Perform a digital rectal examination to evaluate the character of the feces (e.g., presence of melena, foreign material, blood, and mucus) and to obtain a sample for fecal evaluation.
- Evaluate for systemic effects or complications of vomiting (e.g., dehydration, weakness, cachexia).
- Findings that suggest potentially serious underlying disease include hematemesis, weakness, severe depression, anorexia, abdominal mass, fever, abdominal pain, abdominal distention, dehydration, and shock.

Laboratory Evaluation

- When further diagnostic testing is indicated, a stepwise strategy is recommended.
- Perform routine hematology, biochemistries (including serum amylase and lipase), urinalysis, survey abdominal radiographs, and miscellaneous ancillary tests, such as serum thyroxine (T_4) in cats greater than 6 years of age, feline leukemia virus (FeLV) antigen test, and feline immunodeficiency virus (FIV) antibody test, as indicated by the history and physical examination. These evaluations are necessary to rule out non-GI disorders that cause vomiting before evaluating for primary GI disorders with contrast radiology, endoscopy, or exploratory laparotomy.
- Routine blood tests are also helpful to detect and characterize metabolic complications of vomiting such as dehydration and electrolyte imbalances.
- Perform a fecal flotation test to diagnose GI parasitism, especially if vomiting is accompanied by diarrhea.
- Evaluate cats for heartworm disease in endemic areas, since vomiting is a frequent presenting sign in cats.

- Perform a fecal occult blood test to detect occult GI bleeding when blood loss is suspected but overt melena is absent.

Radiography

- Perform routine ventrodorsal and lateral abdominal radiographs to identify radiopaque foreign bodies, gastric or intestinal obstruction, and abdominal masses or abnormalities of the kidneys, liver, and pancreas.
- Perform contrast radiography to evaluate for GI causes of vomiting such as radiolucent foreign bodies, obstruction, and mural thickening or irregularity. Barium administered by stomach tube is usually recommended (see Chap. 4). Barium mixed with food may be better than liquid barium to detect a gastric retention disorder. Double air-barium contrast gastrography can also be performed.
  - Use aqueous iodide contrast (iohexol; Omnipaque, Nycomed) rather than barium if perforation is suspected.
  - Barium-impregnated plastic spheres (BIPS) are an alternative method of evaluating gastric emptying and GI transit times.
- Perform abdominal ultrasonography to evaluate for non-GI disorders associated with vomiting that are suspected based on initial blood test results (e.g., pancreatitis, hepatic or renal disease). Ultrasonography may also be helpful to evaluate for primary GI disorders such as intussusception, GI masses, and gastric outflow obstruction.

Endoscopy

Endoscopy of the stomach and proximal duodenum is a noninvasive technique for evaluation of primary upper GI disorders associated with vomiting. Endoscopy is used to visually examine the GI lumen, obtain biopsies, remove foreign bodies, and collect intraluminal juices.

- Endoscopy requires general anesthesia and a flexible fiberoptic endoscope. The most versatile endoscope for use in evaluating the GI tract of dogs and cats is one at least 100 cm long with a 7.9-mm diameter shaft, 2.0- to 2.8-mm biopsy channel, four-way angulation of the tip, and flush and suction capabilities.
- Routinely evaluate the esophagus, stomach, pylorus, and proximal duodenum. Perform mucosal biopsies in all cases because abnormal histologic findings may be present despite a normal gross appearance.

Laparotomy

- Exploratory laparotomy is sometimes indicated for diagnosis or treatment of primary GI disorders, especially when endoscopy is not available.
- Obtain full-thickness gastric and intestinal biopsies (see Chaps. 88 and 90).

Treatment

Treatment strategies in the vomiting animal are directed toward:

- Correction of the underlying cause of vomiting, whenever possible.
- Symptomatic and supportive therapy of vomiting and its metabolic complications.
- Surgery is indicated to remove large gastric foreign bodies, excise localized tumors and deep ulcers, and correct gastric outflow obstruction.

Fluid Therapy

- Give fluids parenterally because vomiting usually precludes adequate oral intake of fluid. Treat mild dehydration, in the absence of other systemic signs, with subcutaneous fluid administration. Intravenous fluid therapy is preferred for animals with moderate to severe dehydration. Daily fluid therapy requirements in the vomiting dog or cat depend on the degree of dehydration, ongoing fluid losses, and maintenance needs (see Chap. 5).
- Ideally, base the choice of replacement fluid on serum electrolyte concentrations and blood gas analysis, because the electrolyte and acid-base changes that occur secondary to vomiting may vary considerably. In the absence of such information, use a balanced electrolyte solution such as lactated Ringer's or 0.9% saline. Additional potassium supplementation (see Chap. 5) usually is necessary because hypokalemia is a common complication of vomiting.
- If metabolic acidosis is present, use an alkalinizing solution such as lactated Ringer's. Sodium bicarbonate administration is necessary only in the treatment of severe metabolic acidosis (pH < 7.1–7.2) (see Chap. 5).
- Hypochloremic metabolic alkalosis is most likely to occur with pyloric obstruction. Give 0.9% saline supplemented with potassium chloride.
- For a comprehensive discussion of fluid therapy, refer to Chapter 5.

Dietary Management of Acute Vomiting

- Restrict oral intake of food to minimize vomiting and further fluid loss. Withhold food for at least 12–24 hours.
- If vomiting resolves, offer a bland, digestible, moderately fat-restricted diet such as chicken and rice, low-fat cottage cheese and rice, or a commercially available veterinary diet that meets these requirements.
- After 2–3 days on the bland diet, gradually reintroduce the animal's routine diet over a period of 2–3 days.

Antiemetics

Antiemetics are used for symptomatic control of acute vomiting on a short-term basis or to control profuse vomiting that results in fluid, electrolyte, or acid-base imbalances.

Phenothiazines. Phenothiazine derivatives are broad-spectrum, central-acting antiemetics that inhibit the chemoreceptor trigger zone (CRTZ) at low doses and depress the vomiting center at higher doses. Phenothiazines, especially chlorpromazine (0.5 mg/kg SC, IM, or IV q6–8h, and prochlorperazine (0.5 mg/kg SC, IM, or IV q6–8h) are the most widely used antiemetics.

- Hypotension, a potentially serious side effect, is caused by alpha-adrenergic receptor blockade. Consequently, use phenothiazines cautiously in patients with preexisting dehydration.
- Sedation may occur because of concurrent tranquilizing properties; however, the dose required for antiemetic activity is lower than the sedative dose.
- Phenothiazine derivatives decrease seizure threshold and should not be used in animals with seizure disorders.
- Phenothiazine derivatives are the most effective central-acting antiemetic in cats, regardless of the underlying cause.

Metoclopramide. Metoclopramide (Reglan, Robins) (0.2–0.4 mg/kg PO, IM, or SC q8h; or 1–2 mg/kg q24h as a constant-rate IV infusion) possesses both central and peripheral antiemetic properties. Central effects are attributed to antidopaminergic activity at the CRTZ; the peripheral antiemetic effect is due to its stimulant effect on GI motility.

- Metoclopramide promotes gastric emptying by increasing the tone and amplitude of gastric contractions and relaxation of the pylorus (Fig. 87–1). Because gastric relaxation and retroperistalsis are key events preceding vomiting, their inhibition may account in part for the drug's peripheral antiemetic effect.
- Metoclopramide is used to control chemotherapy-induced nausea and vomiting.
- It is indicated for control of vomiting associated with parvoviral gastroenteritis because this disorder may be complicated by delayed gastric emptying.

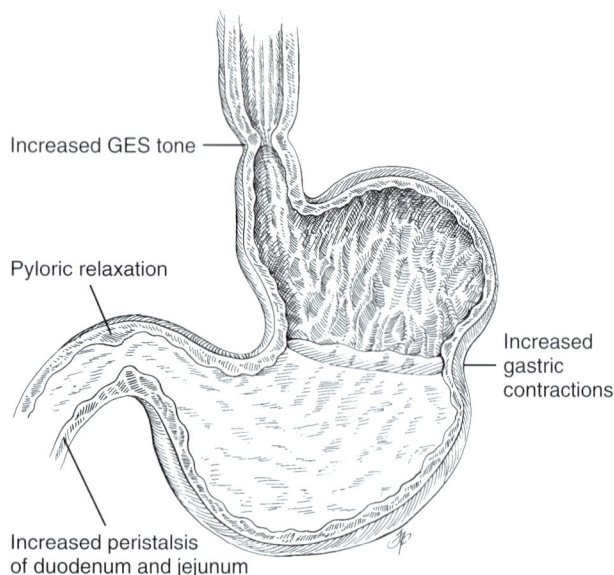

Figure 87–1. Effects of promotility agents such as cisapride and metoclopramide on the gastrointestinal tract. Promotility drugs increase gastroesophageal (GES) sphincter tone and promote gastric emptying by coordinating increased gastric contractions with pyloric relaxation and increased intestinal peristalsis.

- Metoclopramide may not be as useful a central-acting antiemetic in cats as in dogs because D_2 dopamine receptors are less important in mediating vomiting in cats.
- Metoclopramide should not be used in animals with seizures or those receiving phenothiazines, butyrophenones, narcotics, or anticholinergic drugs.
- Decrease the dose in renal failure.

Ondansetron. Ondansetron (Zofran, Cerenex Pharmaceuticals) (0.1–0.5 mg/kg IV, q6–12h or 0.5–1.0 mg/kg PO q6–12h) represents a new class of antiemetics known as 5-hydroxytryptamine type 3 (5-HT_3) serotonergic receptor antagonists. The site of antiemetic action is the CRTZ and vagal afferent neurons. It is especially effective for control of chemotherapy-induced vomiting in dogs, but is also useful to control vomiting associated with parvoviral enteritis and acute pancreatitis.

- Because it is expensive, ondansetron is not used as a first-choice general antiemetic.
- Little information is available on the use of ondansetron in cats.
- Side effects in dogs include sedation, lip licking, and head shaking.

Butorphanol. Butorphanol (Torbutrol, Fort Dodge), an opiate receptor antagonist, has antiemetic activity presumed to be due to decreased sensitivity of the vomiting center to chemical stimuli. It is effective in controlling vomiting in dogs treated with chemotherapy (Cisplatin) at a dose of 0.4 mg/kg IM.

- The only side effect is mild sedation.
- Concurrent analgesic effects may make it a good choice as an antiemetic in dogs with acute pancreatitis.
- Butorphanol can be given as a constant-rate IV infusion (0.1 mg/kg/hr) for control of vomiting in dogs.
- Antiemetic efficacy in cats is unknown.

Anticholinergic Drugs. Avoid the use of anticholinergic drugs such as isopropamide, atropine, and aminopentamide (Centrine, Fort Dodge) for routine symptomatic control of vomiting.

- Although anticholinergics may decrease peripheral afferent stimulation of the vomiting center by relieving GI smooth muscle spasms or inhibiting intestinal secretions, their side effects include xerostomia, mydriasis, tachycardia, urinary retention, ileus, and gastric retention.
- Because delayed gastric emptying caused by anticholinergics can in itself cause vomiting, these drugs should not be used any longer than 3 days in a vomiting patient.

ACUTE GASTRITIS

Acute gastritis is a common disease in dogs and cats. It is usually a mild, self-limiting condition that rarely warrants biopsy confirmation. Clinical diagnosis of acute gastritis often is made when acute vomiting occurs with-

Figure labels:
- Increased GES tone
- Pyloric relaxation
- Increased gastric contractions
- Increased peristalsis of duodenum and jejunum

out apparent cause and resolves on its own in 24–48 hours.

Etiology

There are numerous potential etiologies of acute gastritis (see Table 87–1), but the cause often is not determined. Possible causes include the following:

- *Dietary indiscretion* is frequently associated with acute gastritis and vomiting. Gastritis is most likely due to ingestion of rancid or spoiled foods that contain fermentation byproducts, bacterial enterotoxins, or mycotoxins.
- *Foreign body ingestion* (e.g., rocks, aluminum foil, small toys, food wrappings, or plastic) can cause mechanical irritation of the gastric mucosa.
- *Ingested plant material* including grass and house plants is a common cause of acute gastritis.
- *Chemical irritants or toxins* (e.g., fertilizers, herbicides, cleaning agents, heavy metals such as lead) can cause gastric irritation.
- *Drugs* (e.g., aspirin, nonsteroidal anti-inflammatory drugs, glucocorticoids) can cause acute gastritis which is frequently accompanied by erosions and ulceration.
- *Viral infections* such as canine parvovirus, feline panleukopenia, or canine distemper can cause lesions of gastritis in addition to more diffuse intestinal and systemic involvement.
- *Bacterial infections* causing gastritis are uncommon. Gastric spiral bacteria (*Helicobacter* spp.) may play a role in gastritis in some dogs and cats but can also be present in asymptomatic animals.
- *Parasitic infections* of the stomach are uncommon. *Physaloptera* spp. infect dogs and cats but the infection is not consistently associated with clinical signs. *Ollulanus tricuspis* is a cause of chronic gastritis in cats.
- *Systemic disorders* such as uremia, liver disease, neurologic disease, shock, stress, and sepsis may cause acute gastritis by altering the gastric mucosal barrier, mucosal blood flow, or gastric acidity.

Clinical Signs

- Acute onset of nausea and vomiting.
- Acute anorexia, lethargy, and diarrhea (from concurrent enteritis).

Diagnosis

Because acute gastritis is usually self-limiting, diagnostic evaluations are not usually warranted unless specific historical or physical findings suggest a more serious problem. Response to supportive therapy in 1–3 days indirectly supports the diagnosis of uncomplicated acute gastritis as the cause of vomiting.

History

- Acute vomiting in an otherwise healthy animal suggests the possibility of acute gastritis.
- Perform a detailed historical evaluation including recent exposure to drugs or other sick animals and the potential for dietary indiscretion.

Physical Examination

- The physical examination is usually unremarkable except for dehydration in severe cases.

Treatment

Identify and treat underlying causes when possible.

Dietary Restriction

- Withhold food for 12–24 hours.
- Reintroduce food when vomiting has ceased for longer than 24 hours. Offer a bland, digestible, moderately fat-restricted diet such as chicken and rice, low-fat cottage cheese and rice, or a commercially available veterinary diet that meets these requirements.
- After 2–3 days on the bland diet, gradually reintroduce the animal's routine diet over a period of 2–3 days.

Maintenance of Hydration

- For oral hydration, offer ice cubes, small amounts of water, or an oral glucose and electrolyte solution such as Pedialyte (Ross). Give at frequent intervals to provide daily maintenance requirements.
- Parenteral fluid therapy is indicated to treat dehydration (see previous discussion of fluid therapy in the vomiting patient and refer to Chap. 5).

Medical Therapy

- Consider using antiemetics for short-term symptomatic control of vomiting (see previous section, Antiemetics under Vomiting) and acid control therapy (see later section, Gastroduodenal Ulceration).
- If vomiting does not resolve in 1–3 days, pursue further diagnostic evaluation (see under Vomiting).

GASTRIC FOREIGN BODIES

Gastric foreign bodies are most common in dogs owing to their dietary habits and indiscriminant chewing behavior.

Etiology

- Gastric foreign bodies frequently seen in dogs include needles, coins, stones, sticks, peach pits, plastic, aluminum foil, cloth, rubber balls, and small toys.
- String and other linear foreign bodies are more likely in cats.
- Gastric foreign bodies cause clinical signs because of mechanical irritation (e.g., acute or chronic gastritis) or gastric outflow obstruction.

Clinical Signs

- Most dogs and cats with a gastric foreign body are presented for acute onset of vomiting. However, if the foreign body goes undiagnosed initially, chronic vomiting may be the primary complaint.

- Additional clinical signs may be seen if systemic absorption of a toxic component occurs. For example:
  - Zinc-induced hemolytic anemia has been described secondary to ingestion of zinc-containing nuts and bolts or pennies minted in 1983 or later.
  - Lead-containing foreign bodies may be associated with significant lead absorption and toxicity.
  - Neurologic signs due to absorption of aluminum also have been described.

Diagnosis

Consider gastric foreign bodies in all animals with acute vomiting and a history of chewing on foreign objects.

Physical Examination

- This is often unremarkable except when gastric foreign bodies are very large and palpable.

Radiography

- Abdominal radiographs can identify radiopaque objects (e.g., coins, needles, other metal objects), radiodense objects, and gastric outflow obstruction (gas-, fluid-, or food-distended stomach).
- A contrast gastrogram may be necessary to detect radiolucent gastric foreign bodies.

Endoscopy

- Endoscopy can confirm a suspected gastric foreign body and, more important, can remove most objects noninvasively. For this reason, endoscopy often is preferable to barium-contrast radiography, unless general anesthesia is contraindicated.

Treatment

When a gastric foreign body is identified radiographically, consider whether immediate removal is necessary.

- Remove the object promptly if it is large, sharp, or potentially toxic (e.g., pennies, nuts and bolts, lead objects) or if the animal is persistently vomiting, anorexic, or dehydrated.
- Small, nontoxic foreign bodies may pass through the GI tract uneventfully and thus can be managed conservatively if the animal is not symptomatic. Allow a period of 7–10 days while periodically repeating radiographs to monitor progress. If clinical signs develop, immediate removal is recommended.
- Bones are rapidly decalcified and softened, and do not require removal from the stomach.

Endoscopic Removal

Attempt endoscopic removal of gastric foreign bodies before gastrotomy, because most foreign bodies can be removed in this manner.

- Fast the animal 8–12 hours before anesthesia to be sure that the stomach is empty, because food can obscure the endoscopic view. Correct fluid, electrolyte, and acid-base imbalances before general anesthesia.

- Repeat abdominal radiographs immediately before induction of anesthesia to confirm that the object remains in the stomach. This avoids an unnecessary procedure if the object has already entered the intestinal tract and is beyond the reach of the endoscope.
- The key to removing foreign bodies endoscopically is to get a firm grip on the object, using a grasping forceps or a basket retrieval instrument.
  - Use forceps for retrieval of needles, coins, and small soft objects. To remove the foreign body, grasp the object, pull it up near the end of the endoscope, and remove the endoscope, instrument, and foreign body as one unit.
  - Use the basket for retrieval of small round objects such as marbles or stones that cannot be grasped with the forceps. Large smooth objects are also removed with a basket, but they can be especially difficult to maneuver back through the gastroesophageal sphincter (or upper esophageal sphincter).
  - Use an overtube (a plastic tube that fits over the shaft of the endoscope and can be advanced over the end of the endoscope) to protect the esophageal mucosa when sharp or pointed objects are withdrawn. An overtube is also useful to assist removal of objects through the gastroesophageal sphincter by maintaining sphincter dilatation.
- After removing the foreign body, perform a thorough examination of the stomach to look for other objects or mucosal lesions. This should be done even if only one object is seen radiographically, because radiolucent objects may not have been detected or multiple objects may have previously adhered to each other, appearing as one. If food obscures the endoscopic view, reposition the animal in the alternate lateral position or in ventral dorsal position.

Gastrotomy

If endoscopic equipment is unavailable or the object cannot be retrieved endoscopically, gastrotomy is indicated (see Chap. 88).

Postoperative Care and Complications

- Food and water can be given orally 12–24 hours after foreign body removal.
- If mucosal injury is severe, treat as for gastric ulcer (see next section).

GASTRODUODENAL ULCERATION

For the purposes of this discussion, gastroduodenal ulceration is defined as mucosal defects associated with bleeding, which includes petechiae, erosions, and ulcers. Clinical recognition of gastroduodenal ulceration as a complicating factor in many disorders is becoming more common, most likely due to the increased use of endoscopy.

Etiology

Many disorders have been associated with gastroduodenal ulceration (Table 87–2). Ulceration is more likely when two or more risk factors are present. General mechanisms of gastroduodenal ulceration include direct damage to the gastric mucosal barrier, increased gastric acid secretion, delayed gastric epithelial renewal, and decreased gastric mucosal blood flow.

Nonsteroidal Anti-Inflammatory Drugs (NSAIDs). NSAIDs (see Table 87–2) are frequent causes of gastric ulceration. These drugs inhibit prostaglandin synthesis, which decreases mucosal blood flow and alters gastric mucus production, thus predisposing to ulceration.

- Both gastric hemorrhage and large perforating ulcers may occur. A predilection for ulceration of the pyloroantral region has been recognized.
- Ulceration is most likely to occur when NSAIDs are given to animals with other risk factors (see Table 87–2).
- Dogs are more susceptible to the ulcerogenic effects of NSAIDs than are humans.
- Carprofen (Rimadyl, Pfizer), a recently marketed NSAID for use in dogs, is much less likely to cause GI bleeding. However, it should not be used in the presence of ulcers or inflammatory GI disease.

Glucocorticoids

- Glucocorticoid therapy has been associated with gastric erosions and bleeding but usually only when

Table 87–2. RISK FACTORS FOR GASTRODUODENAL ULCERATION

Drug-induced gastrointestinal damage
   Aspirin
   Flunixin meglumine
   Ibuprofen
   Indomethacin
   Meclofenamic acid
   Naproxen
   Phenylbutazone
   Piroxicam
   Sulindac
   Glucocorticoids
Infiltrative disease
   Gastric neoplasia
   Eosinophilic gastroenteritis
   Lymphocytic plasmacytic gastroenteritis
   Gastric pythiosis
Liver disease
Renal failure
Mast cell tumor
Spinal cord disease
Stress conditions
   Severe illness
   Major surgery
   Hypotension
   Trauma
   Shock
   Sepsis
Hypoadrenocorticism
Lead poisoning
Cyclic hematopoiesis (gray collies)
Duodenogastric reflux
Gastrinoma (Zollinger-Ellison syndrome)

combined with other risk factors for ulceration such as NSAIDs (see Table 87–2).

- Dexamethasone, especially at high doses, is more likely to cause GI bleeding than is prednisolone.

Hepatic Disease. Hepatic diseases of all types are commonly associated with ulceration. Potential mechanisms include decreased mucosal blood flow secondary to portal hypertension, decreased gastric epithelial cell turnover associated with negative nitrogen balance and hypoalbuminemia, increased gastric acid secretion due to impaired degradation of a secretagogue (possibly histamine), or stimulation of gastrin release by increased serum bile acids.

- Coexisting coagulopathies magnify GI blood loss.
- Duodenal ulceration is more common than gastric ulceration.

Renal Failure. Renal failure may be associated with GI hemorrhage and ulceration. Multiple factors probably contribute, including decreased mucosal blood flow due to diffuse vascular injury, gastroduodenal reflux, acidosis, and increased concentrations of gastrin with hypersecretion of gastric acid.

Gastritis. Eosinophilic gastritis, lymphocytic-plasmacytic gastritis, and granulomatous gastritis may be complicated by mucosal ulcerations.

Neoplasia. Gastric neoplasia, especially adenocarcinoma, frequently is associated with mucosal hemorrhage and erosions.

Mast Cell Tumors. These tumors can cause GI ulceration due to histamine-induced gastric acid hypersecretion.

- Perform a thorough search for cutaneous masses in all animals with GI bleeding and ulceration to identify a predisposing mast cell tumor.

Gastrinoma. This rare gastrin-producing tumor, arising from the amine precursor uptake and decarboxylation (APUD) cells of the pancreas, causes gastric acid hypersecretion and gastroduodenal ulceration.

- Suspect gastrinoma when ulceration is associated with gastric mucosal hypertrophy or when ulcers respond to medical management but relapse when therapy is discontinued and no underlying cause can be identified.
- Diagnosis is made by documenting hypergastrinemia and identifying the tumor on surgical exploration.
- Most pancreatic gastrinomas are small (<2 cm) and have metastasized to regional lymph nodes and liver at the time of diagnosis.
- Tumor cytoreduction may be a useful palliative procedure to temporarily control clinical signs along with medical therapy to control ulceration (see under Treatment).

Neurologic Disease. Neurologic disease can predispose to GI ulceration, especially in dogs with spinal cord disease that are receiving corticosteroids. Lower GI bleeding and hematochezia appear to be more common than upper GI bleeding in this setting. Colonic perforation, septic peritonitis, and sudden death have been described.

Stress Conditions. Severe illness, major surgery, trauma, shock, sepsis, and hypotension predispose to gastroduodenal bleeding and ulceration.

- Acutely ill, intensive-care patients are most at risk.
- Consider a presumptive diagnosis of gastroduodenal ulceration when vomiting or hematemesis occurs in this clinical setting.

Clinical Signs

- Signs include anorexia, vomiting, melena, abdominal pain, and weight loss. The vomitus may contain digested blood (coffee-grounds appearance) or fresh blood with clots. Overt hematemesis and melena may not be consistently observed by the owner. Weakness associated with blood loss anemia may occur.
- Ulcer perforation and septic peritonitis are suggested by acute onset of abdominal pain, depression, collapse, and shock.

Diagnosis

History

Perform a detailed history. Determine if any ulcerogenic drugs have been administered recently (see Table 87–2).

Physical Examination

- Palpate the abdomen for abdominal pain.
- Evaluate the mucous membranes for evidence of anemia.
- Perform a rectal examination to evaluate for melena.
- If hematemesis and melena are present, evaluate the skin and mucous membranes for hemorrhages, which may suggest that GI bleeding is secondary to a systemic abnormality of hemostasis.
- Perform a thorough examination for cutaneous masses that may be mast cell tumors.

Laboratory Evaluation

Complete Blood Count (CBC). Perform a CBC to assess for anemia.

- Acute GI bleeding is associated with a normocytic normochromic regenerative anemia, whereas chronic blood loss is characterized by iron deficiency and microcytic hypochromic anemia (see Chap. 20).
- With peracute GI bleeding, nonregenerative anemia may be detected initially until the bone marrow has adequate time to respond (3–5 days).
- Iron deficiency is further characterized by decreased serum iron concentration and decreased percent saturation.
- With active bleeding, anemia is accompanied by hypoproteinemia.
- A neutrophilia and left shift may be seen with severe inflammation and ulcer perforation.

Other Laboratory Tests
- Perform a biochemistry profile to identify underlying liver disease (see Chap. 91), renal failure (see Chap. 97), and hypoadrenocorticism (see Chap. 31). De-

creased total protein and albumin levels are common with blood loss, but liver disease, renal disease, and malnutrition also may contribute to these changes.
- Evaluate for dehydration and electrolyte imbalances secondary to vomiting.
- Perform blood gas analysis to assess acid-base imbalances.
- Perform a urinalysis to screen for underlying systemic disorders.
- If GI blood loss is suspected and the stool is grossly normal, perform a fecal occult blood test. Perform a fecal flotation to diagnose hookworm infection as a cause of GI blood loss.
- Screen for underlying bleeding disorders with evaluations such as one-stage prothrombin time, activated partial thromboplastin time, platelet count, fibrinogen, and fibrin degradation products (FDPs) (see Chap. 21).
- Perform fine-needle aspiration (or biopsy) of any cutaneous masses to diagnose mast cell tumor.
- If gastrinoma is suspected, evaluate a fasting serum gastrin concentration and measure gastrin after a provocative secretin injection.

Radiography

- Survey abdominal radiographs usually are unremarkable unless ulcer perforation results in pneumoperitoneum or peritoneal effusion (peritonitis).
- A GI contrast study usually outlines large ulcers but is an insensitive method for detecting small ulcers and erosions. If perforation is suspected, use a water-soluble nonionic iodide contrast agent, such as iohexol (Omnipaque, Nycomed) rather than barium.

Abdominocentesis

If ulcer perforation is suspected, perform abdominocentesis to detect septic peritonitis. Submit a sample for bacterial culture and antibiotic sensitivity testing.

Endoscopy

Endoscopy is indicated to characterize the location and severity of upper GI bleeding.

▼ **Key Point** Endoscopy is the most reliable procedure for detection of mucosal ulcers and erosions and is preferred over contrast radiography, unless general anesthesia is contraindicated.

- Concurrent gastric mucosal thickening or mass lesions suggest an underlying neoplastic or inflammatory disorder.
- Perform mucosal biopsies regardless of the gross appearance, to identify predisposing causes such as gastritis or gastric neoplasia.
- If perforation is suspected, perform exploratory laparotomy.

Laparotomy

Laparotomy can be used to diagnose and resect gastroduodenal ulcers.

- Evaluate other abdominal organs, including the kidneys and liver.
- Carefully examine the pancreas to identify gastrinoma nodules.

Treatment

The goals of management of gastroduodenal ulceration include the following:

- Eliminate or control predisposing factors (see Table 87–2).
- Correct fluid, electrolyte, and acid-base imbalances.
- Control any GI bleeding and correct resulting anemia. If the packed cell volume (PCV) is less than 15%, give a blood transfusion (see Chap. 20).
- Control gastric acid secretion (Fig. 87–2).
- Promote mucosal cytoprotection.

Agents That Control Gastric Acid Secretion

Antacids. Antacids can effectively neutralize gastric acid secretion; however, H₂ blockers are preferred because of their ease of administration and greater potency (Table 87–3).

H₂ Blockers. These drugs are most commonly used to control acid secretion. They inhibit basal, nocturnal, and meal-stimulated acid secretion by blocking the H₂ receptors on gastric parietal cells (see Fig. 87–2). H₂ blockers inhibit acid secretion stimulated by histamine but have less of an inhibitory effect against other secretagogues such as gastrin and acetylcholine. Several H₂ blockers (e.g., cimetidine, ranitidine, famotidine, nizatidine) are available that are equally effective but differ

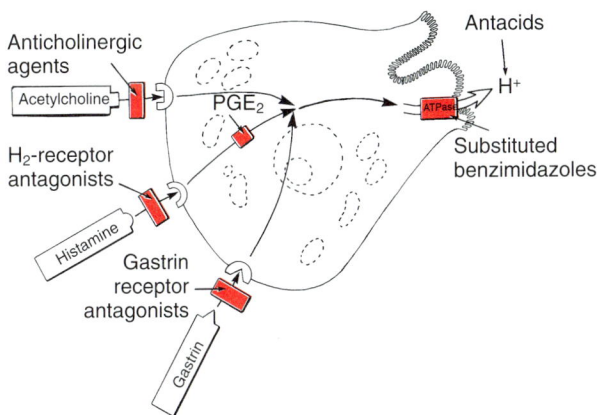

Figure 87–2. Representation of a gastric parietal cell showing the site of action of various therapeutic agents used to decrease gastric acidity. Acid secretion may occur via acetylcholine, histamine, or gastrin stimulation of their respective receptors. H₂-receptor antagonists (blockers) primarily inhibit histamine-induced acid secretion. Prostaglandin (PGE₂) analogs, such as misoprostol, inhibit acid secretion by blocking histamine-induced cyclic adenosine monophosphate production. Use of anticholinergic drugs to inhibit acid secretion is limited by systemic side effects. The gastrin receptor antagonist proglumide is given for experimental purposes only. Substituted benzimidazoles, such as omeprazole, have broad-spectrum antisecretory activity because they interrupt the final common pathway of acid secretion by inhibiting hydrogen potassium ATPase. Antacids neutralize luminal gastric acid.

in potency, frequency of administration, and potential to inhibit hepatic P-450 enzymes (see Table 87–3).

Omeprazole. Omeprazole (Prilosec, Astra Merck) is a potent inhibitor of gastric acid secretion that acts by inhibiting hydrogen potassium adenosine triphosphatase (ATPase) (the proton pump) of the gastric parietal cell (see Fig. 87–2). This drug has broad-spectrum antisecretory activity because the proton pump is the final common pathway for HCl production, regardless of initiating stimulus. Because of its long duration of action, omeprazole can be given on a once-daily basis (see Table 87–3). It is more expensive than the H₂ blockers but is indicated when ulcers do not respond to treatment with H₂ blockers and sucralfate. Omeprazole is more effective than cimetidine in treating aspirin-induced gastritis.

Agents That Promote Mucosal Cytoprotection

Sucralfate. Sucralfate (Carafate, Marion Merrell Dow) is an aluminum salt that selectively binds to injured gastroesophageal mucosa, forming a protective "bandage." Sucralfate neutralizes acid, inactivates pepsin, adsorbs bile acids and pancreatic enzymes, and stimulates local prostaglandins which are cytoprotective. It is a safe drug with minimal systemic absorption.

▼ *Key Point* For initial treatment of gastric ulcers and erosions, combine an H₂ blocker for acid control with sucralfate for mucosal cytoprotection.

Misoprostol. Misoprostol (Cytotec, Searle) is a synthetic prostaglandin analog that at low doses (3–5 µg/kg) is cytoprotective and at high doses (10 µg/kg) has antisecretory activity (see Fig. 87–2). The primary indication for use of misoprostol in dogs is to prevent NSAID-induced gastric injury. Once an NSAID-induced ulcer has occurred, omeprazole appears to be more effective for treatment of ulceration. Side effects of misoprostol (especially at the higher dose) include diarrhea and abortion (see Table 87–3).

Antibiotic Therapy

- Give systemic antibiotics when ulcer perforation is suspected or confirmed.
- Select the antibiotic based on results of culture and sensitivity testing of abdominal fluid or affected tissue.
- Give an aminoglycoside (e.g., amikacin) combined with a cephalosporin (e.g., cefazolin sodium) while awaiting culture results. Avoid aminoglycosides in the presence of renal insufficiency.

Laparotomy

Emergency exploratory laparotomy is indicated when perforation of a gastroduodenal ulcer is suspected or confirmed (see Chap. 96 for detailed description of treatment for peritonitis).

- Correct fluid, electrolyte, and acid-base imbalances as rapidly as possible before surgery.
- Treat shock as described in Chapter 72.

Table 87-3. DRUGS USED FOR TREATMENT OF GASTRIC DISEASE

	Product (Manufacturer)	Preparations	Dosage	Special Indications	Comments*
H₂ Receptor Blocker					
Cimetidine	Tagamet (SmithKline Beecham)	Liquid: 60 mg/ml Tabs: 100 mg (OTC), 200 mg, 300 mg, 400 mg, 800 mg Injectable: 150 mg/ml	5–10 mg/kg PO or IV q6–8h	Decreases gastric acid secretion	Inhibits hepatic P-450 drug metabolizing enzymes. Decrease the dose of the following drugs if used concurrently: lidocaine, propranolol, theophylline, diazepam, phenytoin, warfarin. Does not decrease hepatic blood flow. Simultaneous oral administration of cimetidine and sucralfate or cimetidine and metoclopramide is acceptable if using the higher dose range for cimetidine. Separate oral administration from antacids by ≥1 hr. Decrease dosage in renal failure
Ranitidine	Zantac (Glaxo Wellcome)	Liquid: 15 mg/ml Tabs: 75 mg (OTC) 150 mg, 300 mg Injectable: 25 mg/ml	2.0 mg/kg PO or IV q8–12h (dog); 2.5 mg/kg IV q12h or 3.5 mg/kg PO q12h (cat)	Decreases gastric acid secretion. Preferred over cimetidine when concurrently administering drugs dependent on hepatic metabolism.† Less frequent administration than cimetidine. Promotes gastric emptying	4–10 times as potent as cimetidine. Minimal inhibition of hepatic P-450 enzymes. No effect on hepatic blood flow. Separate oral administration from antacids by ≥1 hr. Decrease dose in renal failure. Stimulates GI motility (stomach, small intestine, colon) by inhibiting acetylcholinesterase activity
Ranitidine bismuth citrate	Tritec (Glaxo Wellcome)	Tabs: 400 mg (162 mg ranitidine, 128 mg bismuth, 110 mg citrate)	See ranitidine	Used for treatment of *Helicobacter* in combination with clarithromycin	
Famotidine	Pepcid (Merck)	Liquid: 8 mg/ml Tabs: 10 mg (OTC), 20 mg, 40 mg Injectable: 10 mg/ml	0.5–1.0 mg/kg PO or IV q12–24h	Decreases gastric acid secretion. Preferred over cimetidine when concurrently administering drugs dependent on hepatic metabolism.† Once-a-day dosing convenience	20–50 times as potent as cimetidine. No inhibition of hepatic drug metabolizing enzymes and no effect on hepatic blood flow. Decrease dose in renal failure
Nizatidine	Axid (Lilly)	Caps: 75 mg (OTC), 150 mg, 300 mg	2.5–5.0 mg/kg PO q24h	Decreases gastric acid secretion. Promotes gastric emptying. Once-a-day dosing	Similar potency as ranitidine. No effect on hepatic P-450 enzymes. Stimulates gastric emptying at antisecretory doses by inhibiting acetylcholinesterase activity, similar to ranitidine
Mucosal Protectant					
Sucralfate	Carafate (Hoechst Marion Roussel)	Tabs: 1 g Liquid: 1 g/10 ml	1 g: large dogs, 0.5 g: small dogs, 0.25 g: cats PO q8–12h	GI erosions or ulcers; NSAID-induced gastritis; reflux esophagitis (susp)	Safe local-acting drug. Potential for nonspecific binding with impaired absorption of simultaneously administered oral drugs. No effect (in dogs) on absorption of the following drugs: digoxin, quinidine, propranolol, aminophylline, diazepam, imipramine, and chlorpromazine. Minor effect on cimetidine absorption, not clinically significant at higher doses of cimetidine (and other H₂ blockers?). Separate phenytoin, tetracycline, and fluoroquinolone antibiotics from sucralfate by ≥2 hr. Antacids interfere with sucralfate binding; give antacids ≥30 min after sucralfate. Contains aluminum—use cautiously in renal failure. Side effect: constipation

Proton Pump Inhibitor

Omeprazole‡	Prilosec (Astra Merck)	Caps: 20 mg (delayed-release)	0.75–1.0 mg/kg PO q24h§ or 20 mg/day (1 cap) for animals >20 kg; 10 mg/day (½ cap) for animals >5 but <20 kg; 5 mg/day (¼ cap) for animals <5 kg	Severe GI ulceration, unresponsive to H₂ blockers; severe reflux esophagitis, unresponsive to metoclopramide and H₂ blockers; gastrinoma (Zollinger-Ellison syndrome)	Inhibits subset of hepatic P-450 drug metabolizing enzymes. Decrease the dose of concurrently administered diazepam and phenytoin but not theophylline or propranolol. 2–7 times as potent as cimetidine. No dose adjustment necessary in hepatic or renal failure. Sustained-release capsule (20 mg) limits dosing options§

Prostaglandin Analog

Misoprostol‡	Cytotec (Searle)	Tabs: 100 µg, 200 µg	3–5 µg/kg PO q6h	Prevention of NSAID-induced GI injury	Gastric mucosal cytoprotection at low doses, inhibits gastric acid secretion at higher doses. Side effects: diarrhea, abortion

Promotility Agent

Metoclopramide	Reglan (Robins)	Syrup: 1 mg/ml Tabs: 5 mg, 10 mg Injectable: 5 mg/ml	0.2–0.4 mg/kg PO, IM, or SC 30 min before eating, q8h or 1–2 mg/kg/24 h given in fluids as constant-rate infusion	Central antiemetic (CRTZ) for drug-induced vomiting, parvoviral enteritis, and uremic gastritis; promotility for reflux esophagitis, functional gastric emptying disorder, recurrent gastric hairballs, reflux gastritis, gastric stasis 2° to gastric surgery, ileus	Side effects: anxiety, agitation, tremors, twitching, constipation. Contraindicated in patients with mechanical gastric outflow obstruction or epilepsy. Should not be used in combination with phenothiazines, butyrophenones, or narcotics. Atropine or other anticholinergic drugs antagonize effects of metoclopramide. When oral metoclopramide is given simultaneously with oral cimetidine, decreased cimetidine absorption occurs. Probably not clinically significant if cimetidine given at higher dosage range. Decrease dose in renal failure. Metoclopramide is physically incompatible when mixed with cephalothin sodium, sodium bicarbonate, chloramphenicol sodium succinate, or tetracycline. Light sensitivity of metoclopramide occurs in dextrose solutions after 24 hr
Cisapride	Propulsid (Janssen)	Tabs: 10 mg, 20 mg Liquid: 1 mg/ml	0.25–0.5 mg/kg PO q8h (dogs); 1.0 mg/kg PO q8h or 1.5 mg/kg q12h (cats)	Same promotility indications as metoclopramide but has no central antiemetic effect; has effects on motility of distal small bowel and colon; megacolon in cats, idiopathic megaesophagus in cats (?)	Decrease dose in hepatic but not renal failure
Erythromycin	Many	Liquid: 25, 50, and 100 mg/ml Tabs: 250 mg, 333 mg, 500 mg Caps: 125 mg, 250 mg Injectable: 100 mg/ml	0.5–1.0 mg/kg PO q8h	Reflux esophagitis (cats); delayed gastric emptying; postoperative ileus (dogs)	Increases gastroesophageal sphincter pressure in cats. Promotes gastric emptying and small intestine transit by a motilin-like effect. Promotility effects occur at lower dose than the antimicrobial dose

Table continued on following page

Table 87-3. DRUGS USED FOR TREATMENT OF GASTRIC DISEASE *Continued*

Product (Manufacturer)	Preparations	Dosage	Special Indications	Comments*
Antacids				
Many available (OTC) Maalox (Al + Mg) Quick Dissolve Maalox (CaCO₃) Mylanta II (Al + Mg + simethicone) Amphojel (AlOH) Tums tabs (CaCO₃)	Tabs and liquid	1–2 tabs or 5–10 ml PO q4–6h	Safe and inexpensive treatment of GI ulceration	Potency varies between products. Crush tablets for maximum effectiveness. Difficult to administer in animals. Potential side effects: constipation (AlOH, CaCO₃), diarrhea (Mg salts), hypernatremia and alkalosis (NaHCO₃), hypercalcemia and acid rebound (CaCO₃), phosphate depletion (AlOH); impaired excretion of aluminum and magnesium in renal failure; nonspecific binding of concurrently administered drugs (e.g., cimetidine, ranitidine); interference with binding of sucralfate to GI ulcers

*All drugs that decrease gastric acidity could potentially decrease absorption of orally administered drugs that are weak bases (e.g., ketoconazole), and increase absorption of drugs that are weak acids (e.g., diazepam, aspirin, furosemide).
†Examples include lidocaine, propranolol, theophylline, diazepam, phenytoin, and warfarin.
‡Limited experience with use in cats.
§When dosages of less than 20 mg are used, repackage the enteric-coated granules in a gelatin capsule to avoid gastric acid degradation.
CRTZ, chemoreceptor trigger zone; GI, gastrointestinal; NSAID, nonsteroidal anti-inflammatory drug; OTC, over the counter (nonprescription); susp, suspension.

Prevention

- Avoid giving NSAIDs other than carprofen (Rimadyl, Pfizer) or aspirin to dogs and cats. Use recommended doses and monitor for occult bleeding, melena, or vomiting to detect early GI bleeding. Do not give glucocorticoids concurrently.
  - Misoprostol is the drug of choice to prevent NSAID-induced injury.
  - Omeprazole provides some protection against the development of aspirin-induced GI damage in dogs, but cimetidine appears to be ineffective.
- The use of an H_2 blocker or sucralfate to prevent ulceration in animals being given glucocorticoids is probably not warranted on a routine basis.
- In one study, cimetidine, sucralfate, or misoprostol did not alter the incidence of GI bleeding in dogs with spinal cord disease undergoing spinal surgery and treated with methylprednisolone sodium succinate.
  - Consider the use of these drugs if multiple risk factors are present or if any degree of GI bleeding would be poorly tolerated by the patient.

CHRONIC GASTRITIS

Chronic gastritis is a common cause of chronic and episodic vomiting in dogs and cats. Chronic gastritis is classified based on histologic features such as type of inflammatory infiltrate and the presence of fibrosis, atrophy, or mucosal hypertrophy. The most common histologic category is lymphocytic-plasmacytic gastritis, which is a nonspecific tissue reaction to many insults.

Etiology

Regardless of the initial insult, damage to the gastric mucosa allows back-diffusion of gastric acid, which, in turn, promotes further mucosal injury. Immune-mediated mechanisms may occur secondary to mucosal damage and further promote inflammation.

- The underlying etiology of chronic gastritis is seldom determined. Possible causes include all factors capable of causing acute gastritis (see Table 87–1) in which repeated or persistent exposure occurs.
- In cats, lymphocytic-plasmacytic gastritis is often accompanied by diffuse inflammatory bowel disease (see Chap. 89).
- Gastroduodenal ulcerations may be associated with secondary lymphocytic-plasmacytic gastritis that resolves after ulcer therapy. Conversely, lymphocytic-plasmacytic gastritis may be complicated by gastric erosions and ulcerations.
- The nematode parasite, *Physaloptera rara*, inhabits the stomach and duodenum of dogs and cats and is an infrequent cause of lymphocytic-plasmacytic gastritis and chronic intermittent vomiting. Embryonated eggs passed in the feces are ingested by an intermediate host (cockroach, cricket, or beetle) in which infected larvae develop. Infection occurs when a dog or cat ingests an intermediate or transport host (rodent or snake). The worm burden is low (usually one

to five worms). Diagnosis of *Physaloptera* spp. is difficult. Fecal flotation using either sodium dichromate or magnesium sulfate solution is often recommended but eggs may not be detected due to the small number of parasites, low fecundity of the female nematodes, and the presence of single sex infection. Diagnosis is usually made by endoscopic detection of the adult worms attached to the stomach mucosa.

- *Ollulanus tricuspis* is associated with chronic fibrosing gastritis in cats.
- Granulomatous gastritis occurs rarely and has been described in association with infection caused by *Pythium insidiosum.*
- Reflux gastritis (or bilious vomiting syndrome) refers to gastric mucosal damage caused by persistent enterogastric reflux of potentially damaging constituents such as bile and pancreatic enzymes. Inappropriate pyloric relaxation predisposes to excess reflux, and impaired gastric motility contributes to delay in clearing previously refluxed material from the stomach. Reflux gastritis is a poorly documented clinical entity in dogs.
- Gastric spiral bacteria (*Helicobacter* spp.) are a common finding in apparently healthy dogs and cats without clinical signs of gastrointestinal disease. *Helicobacter* spp. may play a role in chronic gastritis in some dogs and cats but there is little information on the relationship of *Helicobacter* to gastric disease in these species.
- Eosinophilic gastritis is discussed later in this chapter.

Clinical Signs

- Animals with *chronic gastritis* have intermittent vomiting, usually over a period of weeks to months. Vomiting is not consistently associated with eating. Hematemesis and melena may occur if gastritis is associated with mucosal erosions or ulcers.
- Other signs such as depression, anorexia, weight loss, and abdominal pain are present less frequently.
- Signs of *reflux gastritis* include nausea, vomiting of bile-stained fluid or foam early in the morning when the stomach is empty, and abdominal pain. Most animals are otherwise healthy and do not usually vomit any other time of day.

Diagnosis

Confirmation of chronic gastritis requires a gastric mucosal biopsy, obtained by endoscopy or laparotomy.

History

Obtain a complete history, emphasizing potential exposure to ingested drugs, foreign bodies, chemicals, irritants, and unusual diets (see Table 87–1).

- Response to previous therapy (e.g., a change in diet) may indirectly suggest a dietary intolerance or allergy.

Physical Examination

The physical examination often is unremarkable.

Laboratory Evaluation

- A CBC, biochemical profile, and urinalysis are indicated to exclude non-GI causes of vomiting and to characterize any fluid, electrolyte, or acid-base imbalances occurring secondary to vomiting.
- Test results usually are normal in animals with chronic gastritis unless vomiting is profuse, mucosal erosions or ulcers cause blood loss anemia, or inflammation of the antral and pyloric region results in gastric outflow obstruction.

Radiography

- Survey abdominal radiographs usually are unremarkable.
- Upper GI contrast studies may be normal or show thickening of gastric rugal folds, mucosal irregularity, mass lesions, or delayed gastric emptying. These findings are nonspecific, and gastric biopsy is required to distinguish chronic gastritis from other disorders such as gastric neoplasia.

Endoscopy

This is the diagnostic method of choice to obtain mucosal biopsies to confirm chronic gastritis.

- Endoscopically, the gastric mucosa may appear grossly normal or show thickened rugae, mucosal irregularity or friability, hemorrhage, ulceration, or firm areas of fibrosis.
- Severe chronic gastritis may have a diffuse nodular appearance that must be differentiated from gastric lymphoma.

▼ *Key Point* Always obtain biopsies because histologic changes in chronic gastritis may be present despite a normal endoscopic appearance.

- Carefully examine the entire gastric and proximal duodenal mucosa for adult *Physaloptera,* which appear as white, 1-cm-long nematodes that may be attached to the mucosa or living free on the mucosal surface. Often only one worm is present. Remove any worms observed by use of the grasping forceps.
- If *O. tricuspis* is suspected, aspirate gastric juice for microscopic examination for adult and larval forms.
- Gastric foreign bodies can be detected and removed.
- In patients with reflux gastritis, large amounts of bile-stained fluid may be present in the stomach and the pylorus may appear wide open.

Laparotomy

- Perform laparotomy to obtain full-thickness gastric biopsies and to correct associated gastric outflow obstruction.
- Full-thickness biopsy may be necessary to differentiate severe lymphocytic gastritis diagnosed by endoscopic biopsy from gastric lymphoma.

Treatment

Eliminate underlying causes of gastritis whenever possible. For example:

- Discontinue suspected drugs (e.g., aspirin).
- Remove gastric foreign bodies.
- Treat *Physaloptera* infections with fenbendazole (50 mg/kg/day PO for 3 days) or pyrantel pamoate (15 mg/kg PO initially and repeat in 2–3 weeks).
- Treat *O. tricuspis* infections with fenbendazole (50 mg/kg/day PO for 3 days) or pyrantel pamoate.
- Avoid further exposure to plants, chemicals, and other irritants.

In most cases, a specific cause of gastritis cannot be identified, and therefore specific therapy is unavailable.

Dietary Trials

- Perform dietary trials in all animals with chronic gastritis because dietary factors or antigens could be the inciting cause. Feed a controlled diet that is easily digestible, carbohydrate-based, and moderately fat-restricted. Give frequent small meals.
  - Commercial diets or homemade diets of boiled rice and cottage cheese can be used in dogs.
  - Homemade turkey-, lamb-, or chicken-based diets without additives or preservatives can also be tried for both dogs and cats.
  - Commercial or homemade hypoallergenic diets (single protein or novel protein source) can also be offered.
- Avoid high-fiber diets or feeding only one large meal per day.
- Perform dietary trials for at least 2–4 weeks before assessing response to therapy.
- If gastritis is mild, dietary modification may be all that is required to control clinical signs.
- Reflux gastritis often responds to frequent feedings or feeding a late bedtime meal. Food may be effective because it buffers refluxed duodenal contents and stimulates gastric motility. Metoclopramide (Reglan, Robins), discussed further on, also may be effective.

H₂ Blockers

Reduction of acid secretion with H_2 blockers (discussed previously) may be useful in animals with chronic gastritis even if gross mucosal erosions or ulcerations are absent (see Table 87–3). A 2-week trial is recommended, but long-term therapy may be required, depending on clinical response. Ranitidine and nizatidine also promote gastric emptying which may be useful for secondary motility disorders that may accompany chronic gastritis.

Anti-Inflammatory/Immunosuppressant Drugs

Prednisolone

- If no response is obtained with dietary control and H_2 blocker therapy, give prednisolone (1–2 mg/kg/day in divided doses) for a 2-week trial period.
- If remission occurs, taper this dose over a period of 6–8 weeks, and maintain alternate-day therapy using the lowest effective dose.

Azathioprine

- Azathioprine (Imuran, Glaxo/Wellcome), an immunosuppressive drug, may be useful for treatment of chronic gastritis in dogs and cats that have not responded to prednisolone or when glucocorticoid side effects are a problem.
- The initial dose for dogs is 2 mg/kg PO q24h. The dose can be tapered after a clinical response is obtained, usually by giving the same dose on an alternate-day basis.
- Administer a lower dose (0.3 mg/kg q48h PO) in cats.
- Because of azathioprine's ability to suppress the bone marrow, periodically monitor the CBC to detect neutropenia and thrombocytopenia.

Metoclopramide

- Secondary motility disorders may accompany chronic gastritis. If postprandial vomiting occurs, add metoclopramide to the above therapy (see Table 87–3; Fig. 87–1).

Antibacterial Drugs for *Helicobacter*

- Although the clinical significance of gastric spiral bacteria (*Helicobacter* spp.) in dogs and cats is not yet determined, treatment is sometimes empirically initiated when marked chronic gastritis is present and large numbers of spiral bacteria are detected on biopsy.
- Principles of therapy for *Helicobacter* spp. are extrapolated from human medicine.
- Antimicrobials effective against *Helicobacter* include amoxicillin, metronidazole, tetracyclines, bismuth, and clarithromycin.
- Traditional therapy consists of a combination of bismuth, metronidazole, and either amoxicillin or tetracycline. Multiple antibiotics are used because single antibiotic therapy is ineffective. Resistance to metronidazole commonly develops.
- Omeprazole or ranitidine have been used in combination with antibiotics to potentiate antimicrobial activity by increasing intragastric pH, resulting in high eradication rates (80–90%).
- Omeprazole plus amoxicillin given for 2 weeks is commonly used in humans but the cure rate is variable (46–80%).
- Ranitidine bismuth citrate (Tritec, Glaxo Wellcome) given for 4 weeks, plus clarithromycin given for the first 2 weeks, was 80% effective in eradicating *Helicobacter* in humans.
- Omeprazole, amoxicillin, and clarithromycin (5 mg/kg PO q12h) in combination appear to be approximately 95% effective in humans after only 1 week of therapy.

Prognosis

The prognosis for chronic gastritis is variable.

- If the underlying cause can be identified and corrected, the prognosis for recovery is good.
- In animals with idiopathic chronic gastritis, long-term dietary and medical management may be required.

EOSINOPHILIC GASTRITIS AND GRANULOMA

Eosinophilic gastritis is characterized by diffuse or focal infiltration of mature eosinophils into the mucosa, submucosa, or muscularis. Variable increases in lymphocytes, plasma cells, and neutrophils may also occur.

- Eosinophilic inflammation of the stomach in dogs occurs as two distinct pathologic entities:
  - Diffuse eosinophilic infiltration of the gastric mucosa and submucosa is most common and is usually associated with generalized eosinophilic gastroenterocolitis.
  - Single or multiple eosinophilic granulomatous lesions (scirrhous eosinophilic gastritis) with transmural eosinophilic inflammation, severe arteritis, and fibrosis occur less frequently.
- In cats, eosinophilic gastritis is usually a manifestation of inflammatory bowel disease which is similar to eosinophilic gastroenterocolitis in dogs. Rarely, eosinophilic gastroenteritis in cats is associated with hypereosinophilic syndrome (see Chap. 89).

Etiology

- The cause of eosinophilic gastritis or granuloma in dogs is unknown. The presence of increased numbers of circulating and tissue eosinophils suggests an allergic or immunologic hypersensitivity, possibly in response to dietary components or parasites.
- Food allergy or hypersensitivity has been proposed but not proven as a cause of eosinophilic gastritis in dogs.
- Microfilariae have been observed on histologic sections in a dog with diffuse eosinophilic gastritis.
- Eosinophilic gastroenteritis with multiple focal eosinophilic granulomas has been described in German shepherds with visceral larva migrans but is not an important clinical cause of eosinophilic gastroenteritis.

Clinical Signs

- Dogs with eosinophilic gastritis usually have signs of chronic vomiting, anorexia, and weight loss. Eosinophilic gastritis is more likely to be associated with mucosal ulceration and bleeding (suggested by hematemesis and melena) than are other types of chronic gastritis.
- Additional clinical signs may be present if gastritis is a component of diffuse eosinophilic gastroenterocolitis. Small intestinal involvement is characterized by malabsorption and voluminous watery diarrhea, whereas colonic or rectal involvement is characterized by bloody-mucoid diarrhea with tenesmus (see Chap. 89).

Diagnosis

History

- Determine previous diets and clinical response to dietary changes.

- A dramatic response to previous corticosteroid therapy is consistent with but not specific for eosinophilic gastritis.

Physical Examination

- Weight loss is common.
- Less common findings include pain on palpation of the stomach, or the stomach may feel diffusely rigid and firm. With large focal granulomas, a mass in the stomach wall may be palpated.
- Additional findings that indicate more extensive intestinal involvement include focal or diffuse thickening of the small intestine or colon or mesenteric lymphadenopathy.

Laboratory Evaluation

- A hemogram often reveals eosinophilia, but not in all cases.
- Gastric erosions and ulcerations can cause anemia and hypoproteinemia.
- Heartworm and fecal flotation tests are indicated to identify underlying parasitism.

Radiography and Ultrasonography

- Abdominal radiography is usually normal unless gastric outflow obstruction occurs secondary to transmural involvement or granuloma formation at the antral or pyloric region.
- Contrast radiography may demonstrate irregularity of the gastric mucosa or diffuse or focal thickening of the gastric wall.
- With concurrent intestinal involvement, associated radiographic changes may be identified.
- Abdominal ultrasonography may identify gastric wall thickness or enlarged mesenteric lymph nodes.

Endoscopy

- Visual endoscopic findings are nonspecific and may mimic other inflammatory and neoplastic diseases. The gross appearance may be normal in some cases.
- Involved areas of the stomach may appear diffusely thickened, with hemorrhages, erosions, or ulcers. Granulomas appear as focal mass lesions.
- Endoscopy is the preferred initial method for biopsy rather than laparotomy, unless mechanical obstruction requiring surgical decompression is present.
  - Obtain multiple biopsies from the stomach and duodenum.
  - Cytologic examination of mucosal biopsies reveals increased numbers of eosinophils.
- A disadvantage of endoscopically obtained biopsies is that the depth of the biopsy generally is limited to the mucosa, and deeper layers may be predominantly involved in eosinophilic gastritis.

Laparotomy

- Exploratory laparotomy may show diffuse or focal thickening in affected regions of the stomach and GI tract.

- Diffuse involvement of the stomach wall or large focal granulomas may grossly resemble neoplasia.
- Regional lymphadenopathy is common.

Treatment

The treatment of choice for eosinophilic gastritis in dogs is glucocorticoid therapy combined with dietary management.

- If a broad-spectrum anthelmintic has not been administered recently, before initiating glucocorticoids, treat with fenbendazole (Panacur, Hoechst-Roussel Agri-Vet), 50 mg/kg daily for 3 days, to eliminate undetected GI parasites as a potential cause of the clinical signs.
- Treatment of eosinophilic gastritis in cats that is a manifestation of hypereosinophilic syndrome is discussed in Chapter 89. Eosinophilic gastritis or gastroenteritis in cats that is associated with focal GI involvement and resembles canine eosinophilic gastroenterocolitis can be managed as outlined next for dogs.

Anti-Inflammatory/Immunosuppressant Drug Therapy

- Administer prednisolone, 0.5–1 mg/kg q12h PO. Response is prompt and dramatic, usually occurring within 24–48 hours.
- Gradually taper the dosage over the following 6–8 weeks, decreasing to once daily (given in the morning) and then to alternate days. If the initial treatment period is too short, relapse may occur. If relapse does not occur while tapering the dosage, discontinue therapy at the end of the 6–8 week period. Continue to monitor for relapse.
- If side effects are a problem or if higher dosage or continued daily therapy is required, give azathioprine concurrently, as described previously for chronic gastritis.

Dietary Recommendations

- Because food hypersensitivity is a potential cause of eosinophilic gastritis, consider a trial with a hypoallergenic diet. Some dogs with eosinophilic gastritis may respond to a hypoallergenic diet alone. Institute a dietary trial even if corticosteroids are being given, because it may decrease the dose of corticosteroids required to control clinical signs.
- Suggested hypoallergenic diets (single protein or novel protein source) include home-cooked (boiled) lamb and rice in a 1:1 mixture, turkey and rice, or one part low-fat cottage cheese or tofu to three parts rice. Commercial hypoallergenic diets consisting of lamb and rice, egg and rice, fish and potato, or venison and rice are available.
  - Choose a protein and carbohydrate source that have not been a part of the animal's diet in the past 6 months.
  - Feed the diet exclusively for at least 3–4 weeks before determining effectiveness.
- If a hypoallergenic diet is ineffective, try a controlled diet that is easily digested, carbohydrate-based, and moderately fat-restricted.

Surgery

Perform surgical resection of obstructing granulomas at the antral and pyloric region and follow up with glucocorticoid therapy.

Prognosis

The prognosis for eosinophilic gastritis in dogs is good. Most dogs respond to therapy and many have complete resolution of clinical signs on a long-term basis. In others, relapses occur, and a hypoallergenic diet or corticosteroid therapy is required on a long-term basis.

GASTRIC OUTFLOW OBSTRUCTION

Etiology

Gastric outflow obstruction most commonly is caused by mural, mucosal, and luminal abnormalities involving the antral and pyloric regions of the stomach (see Table 87–1). External compression of the gastric outflow tract is identified less frequently. Common causes of outflow obstruction include the following:

- Foreign bodies often lodge in the pylorus and cause partial or complete outflow obstruction.
- Chronic hypertrophic pyloric gastropathy (CHPG) is a benign disorder of middle- to older-aged small-breed dogs that frequently results in outflow obstruction. (See discussion later in this chapter under Hypertrophic Gastropathy.)
- Pyloric stenosis is hypertrophy of the circular muscle fibers of the pylorus. Congenital pyloric stenosis occurs in young dogs and cats. Acquired muscular pyloric stenosis is sometimes a component of CHPG in older animals.
- Chronic gastritis, especially eosinophilic gastritis and granuloma, that involves the antral and pyloric region can result in outflow obstruction.
- Obstructing granulomas may be a manifestation of fungal gastritis caused by pythiosis or histoplasmosis.
- Gastric ulcers at the pylorus may cause outflow obstruction.
- Gastric neoplasia, especially adenocarcinoma, can obstruct outflow (see under Gastric Neoplasia).
- Gastric dilatation-volvulus is a well-recognized cause of acute outflow obstruction and is discussed later in this chapter.
- Extrinsic outflow compression may be caused by hepatic or pancreatic inflammation, abscesses, and neoplasia; marked regional lymphadenopathy; and diaphragmatic hernia with gastric displacement.

Clinical Signs

- Vomiting is a consistent sign of gastric outflow obstruction. Typically, undigested food is present in the vomitus greater than 12 hours after eating (the stomach normally empties by 8–10 hours after eating).
  - Bile-staining of vomitus is usually absent.
  - Projectile vomiting suggests outflow obstruction.
  - Complete obstruction results in severe, profuse vomiting.
- Abdominal distention caused by an enlarged fluid- or food-filled stomach may occur, especially after eating.
- Anorexia may occur because of a sense of fullness from gastric overdistention.
- Belching may indicate an attempt to release gas from the stomach.
- Weight loss and dehydration may result from chronic vomiting.

Diagnosis

History and Signalment

The history and signalment often indicate a possible underlying cause.

- In young animals, persistent vomiting since weaning suggests congenital pyloric stenosis.
- Acute onset of vomiting in young animals may indicate a foreign body.
- Chronic vomiting with hematemesis is seen with gastric neoplasia, chronic gastritis, and gastric ulcer.
- Chronic intermittent vomiting over weeks to months in middle-aged and older small-breed dogs is consistent with CHPG.
- Acute onset of nonproductive retching and gagging accompanied by abdominal distention in large-breed dogs suggests gastric dilatation-volvulus.

Physical Examination

- The examination may be unremarkable.
- Potential findings include abdominal distention and signs associated with metabolic abnormalities secondary to profuse vomiting such as weakness and dehydration.

Laboratory Evaluation

- Laboratory findings usually are unremarkable unless profuse vomiting results in fluid, electrolyte, or acid-base imbalances such as dehydration, hypokalemia, hyponatremia, hypochloremia, or metabolic alkalosis.
  - Always consider gastric outflow obstruction in animals with hypochloremic metabolic alkalosis.
- Other laboratory findings are variable and depend on the underlying cause of obstruction.

Radiography and Ultrasonography

Survey Abdominal Radiography
- The finding of a distended fluid-filled stomach or food present in the stomach greater than 12 hours after eating suggests delayed gastric emptying. The stomach normally empties by 8–10 hours after eating; however, emptying times up to 16 hours are normal in some dogs, especially when fed dry food.
- Identification of the underlying cause of delayed gastric emptying requires further evaluation with contrast radiography, ultrasonography, endoscopy, or exploratory laparotomy.

Contrast Gastrography
- A contrast gastrogram is useful to further evaluate gastric emptying. Liquid barium normally begins to

leave the stomach in 5–15 minutes and the stomach is usually empty in 30–60 minutes in cats and 1–2 hours in dogs.
- The presence of barium in the stomach after 12–24 hours confirms delayed gastric emptying.
- If the lesion affects the emptying of food more than that of liquids, emptying studies using contrast material mixed with canned food may be helpful (see Chap. 4).
- Contrast studies can provide important information about the cause of delayed gastric emptying. Potential findings include foreign bodies, thickening or mass lesions of the antral and pyloric region, and narrowing of the pyloric canal (the "beak" sign).

Fluoroscopy/Ultrasonography
- Fluoroscopy and ultrasonography may provide information about the outflow tract including intrinsic thickening of the wall of the pyloric antrum or extrinsic compression of the antrum and pylorus by hepatic and pancreatic lesions.

Endoscopy

Endoscopy is useful to identify and remove foreign bodies and to evaluate the antral and pyloric region for outflow obstruction.

- Fast the patient with suspected delayed gastric emptying for at least 24 hours before endoscopy to ensure that the stomach is empty. If large volumes of fluid are still present, aspirate the fluid through the endoscope to improve visualization.
- Foreign bodies, masses, mucosal proliferations (e.g., CHPG) or thickenings, and ulcers can readily be identified at endoscopy.
- Endoscopic biopsies of affected tissues can be obtained; however, if mechanical outflow obstruction is detected, immediate surgical relief of obstruction and full-thickness biopsies are preferred.
- If the outflow area looks normal and the endoscope is readily passed through the pylorus into the duodenum, mechanical outflow obstruction is much less likely. However, extrinisic compression of the outflow region cannot be fully appreciated with endoscopy and may require an exploratory laparotomy.
- An alternative consideration when the pylorus appears normal is that delayed gastric emptying is caused by a motility disturbance (see under Gastric Motility Disorders) of the stomach rather than by mechanical outflow obstruction.

Treatment

- Give appropriate fluid therapy to correct fluid, electrolyte, and acid-base disturbances before general anesthesia for surgery or endoscopy. Because metabolic imbalances are variable, base the choice of fluid composition on results of electrolyte and blood gas analysis (see previous discussion of fluid therapy under Vomiting).
- Metabolic alkalosis may occur secondary to outflow obstruction; manage with nonalkalinizing solutions such as 0.9% saline and Ringer's solution, supplemented with potassium chloride, as described in Chapter 5.
- Surgery is indicated for definitive treatment of gastric outflow obstruction (see Chap. 88).
- If gastric stasis persists after surgical relief of outflow obstruction, give metoclopramide or cisapride to improve gastric emptying (see Fig. 87–1). Promotility drugs such as these are contraindicated in the presence of mechanical outflow obstruction.

GASTRIC MOTILITY DISORDERS

Gastric motility disorders that result in weak or ineffective gastric contractions can cause delayed gastric emptying in dogs and cats. These disorders are not well documented in veterinary medicine. Currently, the diagnosis of a gastric motility disorder is presumptive and is based on clinical findings consistent with delayed gastric emptying in the absence of an obstructive lesion.

Etiology

The causes and pathophysiologic mechanisms of gastric motility disorders are poorly understood. Gastric motility is dependent on normal electrical and mechanical activity of the stomach. Control of gastric motility and emptying is influenced by hormones, autonomic nervous input, and the composition of the food. Emptying is prolonged as the the fat and protein content, acidity, osmolality, and viscosity of the gastric contents increase.

The following factors may be associated with functional delays in gastric emptying.

- Drug therapy with anticholinergic drugs or narcotic analgesics can delay gastric emptying.
- Inflammatory lesions such as gastritis, gastric ulcers, Physaloptera infection, and parvoviral gastroenteritis are associated with gastric motility disorders.
- Nervous inhibition associated with stress, trauma, pain, or psychogenic input may cause a transient delay in gastric emptying due to increased sympathetic stimulation.
- Metabolic disturbances such as hypokalemia, uremia, hepatic encephalopathy, and hypothyroidism may delay gastric emptying.
- Prolonged gastric obstruction may be complicated by secondary motility dysfunction.
- In many cases, functional gastric emptying disorders are idiopathic. These disorders may be associated with abnormal gastric electrical conduction disturbances such as tachyarrhythmias.
- Chronic trichobezoar formation in cats may be related to abnormal migrating motor complexes that impair gastric emptying of indigestible material during fasting.

Clinical Signs

The clinical signs of a gastric motility disorder causing delayed gastric emptying are similar to those of gastric outflow obstruction. These include:

- Vomiting with undigested food present in the vomitus greater than 12 hours after eating
- Abdominal distention and discomfort after eating
- Anorexia and belching

Diagnosis

History

Perform a complete history to determine if anticholinergics or narcotics are currently being administered or if other predisposing influences on gastric motility are present.

Laboratory Evaluation

Perform routine screening tests including a CBC, biochemical profile, and urinalysis to detect predisposing metabolic abnormalities.

- The finding of neutropenia in a young dog with acute onset of vomiting and bloody diarrhea suggests parvoviral gastroenteritis as a cause of gastric retention.

Radiography

- Perform abdominal radiographs. Delayed gastric emptying is suggested by the finding of a distended fluid-filled stomach or food present in the stomach greater than 12 hours after eating.
- Perform a contrast gastrogram to assess gastric emptying, as described previously under Gastric Outflow Obstruction. Normal gastric emptying of barium does not exclude a gastric motility disorder because it evaluates only the ability of the stomach to empty liquids and not solids. In functional gastric motility disorders, the gastric outflow region appears normal, but barium may not leave the stomach in a timely fashion.
- Commercially available barium-impregnated plastic spheres (BIPS) have also been used to evaluate gastric emptying time.

Endoscopy

- Endoscopy is a useful noninvasive method to exclude mechanical outflow obstruction as a cause of delayed gastric emptying.
- Fast the patient for at least 24 hours before endoscopy to ensure that the stomach is empty. Large volumes of fluid are often present and should be aspirated through the endoscope to improve visualization.
- In idiopathic gastric motility disorders, the gastric mucosa and pyloric outflow area appear normal. If gastritis is a predisposing cause, gross and microscopic changes will be detected.

Electrogastrograms

Electrogastrograms have been used on a research basis to document abnormal gastric electrical rhythms and may have clinical applications in the future.

Treatment

Whenever possible, identify and correct the underlying cause of a gastric motility disorder. For example, discontinue any anticholinergic drug therapy.

Fluid Therapy

Institute fluid therapy as needed. (See previous discussion of fluid therapy under Vomiting.)

Dietary Management

This is an important aspect of treatment for gastric motility disorders.

- The diet should be low in fat, high in digestible carbohydrate, and fed in small amounts at frequent intervals.
- The consistency of the diet can be altered. In many instances, the more liquid the diet, the better it empties from the stomach.

Promotility Drug Therapy

The treatment of choice for idiopathic gastric motility disorders is a motility modifier such as cisapride or metoclopramide (see Table 87–3). The effects of promotility drugs on the stomach are shown in Figure 87–1. Cisapride (Propulsid, Janssen), a newly available prokinetic drug, stimulates gastric emptying in dogs and cats and may be more effective than metoclopramide; however, cisapride lacks the broad-spectrum central antiemetic effects of metoclopramide.

- Administer cisapride one-half hour before meals at 0.25–0.5 mg/kg PO q8h in dogs; and in cats at 1.0 mg/kg q8h or 1.5 mg/kg q12h PO.
- Administer metoclopramide one-half hour before meals, 0.2–0.4 mg/kg PO q8h.
- The H_2 blockers, ranitidine and nizatidine, have mild gastric prokinetic effects.
- The antibiotic erythromycin has a prokinetic effect on the stomach of dogs, mimicking the effects of the hormone motilin. The promotility effect occurs at lower doses (0.5–1.0 mg/kg PO or IV q8h) than the antimicrobial effect.

HYPERTROPHIC GASTROPATHY

The term *hypertrophic gastropathy* is used to describe a heterogeneous group of poorly understood disorders associated with focal, multifocal, or diffuse hypertrophic changes of the gastric mucosa of dogs. Hypertrophic gastropathy appears to be quite rare in cats. Various other names have been used, including chronic hypertrophic pyloric gastropathy, hypertrophic gastritis, gastric polyps, and acquired pyloric stenosis or hypertrophy. These disorders may be variations of the same disease process. Microscopic changes are variable and include hyperplasia of mucosal epithelial cells, glandular hypertrophy, variable inflammatory infiltrates, and mucosal ulceration.

The most commonly recognized form of hypertrophic gastropathy in dogs is a benign disorder associated with mucosal hypertrophy of the antral and pyloric region, resulting in gastric outflow obstruction. Some affected dogs have a component of pyloric muscular hypertrophy. This disorder has been termed *chronic hypertrophic pyloric gastropathy* (CHPG).

Etiology

Little is known about the underlying etiology and pathophysiologic mechanisms of hypertrophic gastropathy. Environmental, hormonal, genetic, and immune-mediated mechanisms may play a role.

- Chronic irritation associated with aspirin therapy can result in focal gastric hypertrophy.
- Hormones such as gastrin, cholecystokinin, acetylcholine, and histamine can be trophic to the gastric mucosa. Causes of hypergastrinemia such as chronic renal failure, chronic gastric distention, gastrin-secreting tumors, and idiopathic hypertrophy of the antral G-cells (gastrin-secreting cells) may be important considerations in some cases.
- Basenji dogs have hypertrophic gastritis in association with immunoproliferative enteropathy; genetic, immune-mediated, and hormonal (gastrin) factors may play a role.
- Hypertrophic gastritis involving the body of the stomach has been described in the Drentse patrijshond breed of dog. Affected dogs also have red blood cell stomatocytosis and hemolytic anemia.
- Hyperplastic polyps involving the pylorus have been described in young, related French bulldogs with chronic vomiting and gastric outflow obstruction.
- CHPG is most common in highly excitable, nervous small-breed dogs; underlying neuroendocrine or stress-related mechanisms have been proposed.

Clinical Signs

- Chronic vomiting is the most consistent clinical sign. Vomiting occurs at variable intervals after eating.
  - If hypertrophic changes cause outflow obstruction, undigested food may be present in the vomitus greater than 12 hours after eating.
  - Hematemesis and melena may be detected in association with mucosal ulceration.
  - Dogs with CHPG often are otherwise healthy and are presented because of chronic intermittent vomiting for a duration of weeks to months (sometimes years).
- Anorexia, weight loss, abdominal distention, and belching are less frequent signs.
- Basenji dogs with immunoproliferative enteropathy and hypertrophic gastritis usually have concurrent chronic diarrhea, anorexia, and weight loss.

Diagnosis

History and Signalment

- CHPG is most common in middle-aged or older small-breed dogs such as Lhasa apsos, Shih Tzus, and miniature poodles.

- Males are affected more commonly than females.
- A history of chronic intermittent vomiting is typical.

Physical Examination

- Potential findings include weight loss and abdominal distension due to a fluid- or food-filled stomach.
- If significant gastrointestinal blood loss occurs, pale mucous membranes due to anemia may be detected.

Laboratory Evaluation

- Laboratory evaluation often is unremarkable.
- If profuse vomiting has occurred, laboratory findings may reflect dehydration or electrolyte imbalances. Metabolic alkalosis may occur secondary to gastric outflow obstruction.
- If hypertrophic gastropathy is associated with gastric ulceration, evaluate serum gastrin concentration to detect underlying hypergastrinemia (e.g., gastrinoma).
- Iron deficiency anemia may result from chronic GI blood loss.

Radiography and Ultrasonography

- Perform survey abdominal radiographs to detect a fluid-filled distended stomach or food remaining in the stomach greater than 12 hours after eating. These findings are consistent with a gastric retention disorder.
- Perform a contrast gastrogram (see under Gastric Outflow Obstruction).
  - Findings consistent with CHPG include delayed gastric emptying, filling defects in the antral and pyloric region due to hypertrophied mucosa, and narrowing of the pyloric canal.
  - With other types of hypertrophic gastropathy, potential findings include focal, multifocal, or diffusely thickened gastric rugae.
  - Radiographic features of hypertrophic gastropathy are not specific and mimic other inflammatory and infiltrative disorders.
- Ultrasonography can demonstrate thickening of the gastric wall at the antral and pyloric region.

Endoscopy

- Endoscopy can confirm focal, multifocal, or diffusely thickened mucosal folds. Moderate gastric distention with air is required so that normal-sized gastric rugal folds do not appear falsely thickened.
- With CHPG, the lesion predominantly involves the antrum and pyloric region, causing partial or complete pyloric obstruction. Mucosal ulceration or hemorrhage is not typical.
- Endoscopically obtained biopsies are inadequate to diagnose hypertrophic gastropathy because they are too superficial to demonstrate the lesion.

Surgery

- Definitive diagnosis of hypertrophic gastritis requires full-thickness biopsies obtained surgically.

- Excisional biopsies are indicated when possible to help relieve the obstruction.

Treatment

- Surgical excision of abnormal tissue and relief of outflow obstruction is the treatment of choice for CHPG (see Chap. 88). Response to surgery is usually good to excellent and most dogs are clinically normal after relief of obstruction. If gastric atony persists after surgery, a trial of cisapride or metoclopramide may be warranted.
- If hypertrophic gastropathy is associated with gastric erosions or ulcerations, institute antiulcer therapy with H_2 blockers and sucralfate as described under Gastroduodenal Ulceration.
- When hypertrophic gastropathy is accompanied by a significant inflammatory infiltrate, consider treatment with prednisolone as described under Chronic Gastritis.
- For treatment of Basenji dogs with hypertrophic gastritis and immunoproliferative enteropathy (see Chapter 89.)

GASTRIC NEOPLASIA

The clinical presentation of gastric neoplasia in dogs and cats is influenced by the size and location of the tumor, whether it is benign or malignant, and whether it is associated with outflow obstruction, altered gastric motility, or mucosal ulceration and bleeding.

Etiology

Malignant Neoplasia

▼ *Key Point* Gastric adenocarcinoma is the most common gastric neoplasm in dogs.

- In dogs, gastric adenocarcinoma occurs most commonly in the antral and pyloric region and may appear as a raised plaque or mass with a central ulcerated area or as diffuse infiltration of the gastric wall. Metastases to the regional lymph nodes, liver, adrenals, and lungs are common. Gastric adenocarcinoma is rare in cats.

▼ *Key Point* Lymphoma is the most common malignant gastric neoplasm in cats.

- Cats with gastric lymphoma usually are FeLV-negative. Lymphoma may appear as multiple, raised white masses or as diffuse infiltration of the gastric wall. Mucosal ulceration is common.
- Other, less common primary malignant neoplasms include leiomyosarcoma and fibrosarcoma.

Benign Neoplasia

- Benign adenomatous polyps occur infrequently in dogs and cats. Polyps probably develop in response to chronic gastric mucosal damage or irritation. They appear as single or multiple, pedunculated or polypoid nodules that vary in size from millimeters to centimeters. A predilection for the proximal duodenum within 1 cm of the pylorus has been noted in cats. Clinical signs usually are absent unless pyloric obstruction occurs. Polyps usually are an incidental finding at endoscopy or necropsy.
- Leiomyomas are the second most common gastric tumor in dogs. These tumors arise from the muscle layers of the gastric wall; clinical signs may be absent unless the mechanical effects of the mass alter motility or cause outflow obstruction. A predilection for the gastroesophageal junction has been noted. Mucosal ulceration occasionally occurs.

Clinical Signs

Malignant Neoplasia

- Dogs and cats with malignant gastric neoplasia are usually presented because of chronic progressive vomiting.
- If pyloric outflow obstruction occurs, clinical signs reflect delayed gastric emptying.
- Hematemesis and melena are common with adenocarcinoma because of mucosal ulceration. Other signs include anorexia, weight loss, and chronic debilitation.

Benign Neoplasia

- Clinical signs may be absent with benign neoplasms or polyps unless pyloric obstruction occurs.

Diagnosis

Gastric neoplasia is an important consideration in older dogs and cats with a history of chronic progressive vomiting and hematemesis.

Physical Examination

- Findings often include weight loss and cachexia.
- Palpable abnormalities of the stomach usually are absent, although, rarely, a gastric mass may be palpable.
- Pale mucous membranes and melena are consistent with mucosal ulceration and blood loss anemia.
- Gastric perforation and peritonitis are associated with abdominal distention, pain, collapse, and shock.
- Additional findings such as ascites, jaundice, and dyspnea reflect metastatic disease.

Laboratory Evaluation

Laboratory evaluation is variable and depends on secondary complications such as blood loss, perforation, metastatic disease, and metabolic complications of vomiting.

Radiography

- Survey films may be unremarkable or suggest outflow obstruction, a thickened gastric wall, or mass lesions.
- Contrast radiography is helpful to confirm mass lesions, filling defects, ulcers, and diffuse thickening of the gastric wall.

- Rigidity of the gastric wall when compared on multiple films suggests an infiltrative lesion.
- Delayed gastric emptying can result from pyloric outflow obstruction.
- Perform thoracic films to screen for pulmonary metastases.

Endoscopy

Endoscopy is useful to confirm lesions suggested on radiography and to obtain biopsies of affected tissues. Gastric neoplasia that does not involve the mucosa or result in a mass effect can be difficult to detect endoscopically, and a full-thickness biopsy obtained surgically is often necessary.

- Adenocarcinoma may appear as raised plaques, polypoid lesions, or a diffuse infiltrating lesion. Mucosal ulceration is common.
- Gastric lymphoma appears as multiple white nodules or diffuse infiltration of the mucosa with irregularity and thickening of the mucosal folds. With diffuse infiltration of the gastric wall, the stomach may lack distensibility.
- Leiomyomas are smooth mass lesions with a normal overlying mucosa unless complicated by ulceration.
- Polyps appear as small, smooth, or raspberry-like masses on a stalk.

Surgery

Surgical exploration is an important diagnostic method for gastric neoplasia.

- Palpate all areas of the stomach to identify affected areas.
- Obtain full-thickness biopsies.
- Evaluate regional lymph nodes and the liver for metastases.

Treatment

- The treatment of choice for gastric neoplasia is surgical resection of the tumor by partial gastrectomy (see Chap. 88). Because the antral and pyloric region are often involved, a gastroduodenostomy or gastrojejunostomy may be necessary (see Chap. 88).
- For treatment of lymphoma, surgical removal of large solitary masses can be followed by chemotherapy with cyclophosphamide, vincristine, and prednisone, as described in Chapter 24.

Prognosis

- The prognosis for benign neoplasms after surgical removal is good.
- The prognosis for adenocarcinoma is poor.
- Diffuse infiltration of the GI tract with lymphoma is not responsive to treatment and has a poor prognosis. However, some cats with lymphoma localized to the stomach may have a good to excellent response to chemotherapy.

GASTRIC DILATATION-VOLVULUS

Gastric dilatation-volvulus (GDV) is an acute, life-threatening disorder that is a medical and surgical emergency. Early recognition and treatment are essential for a successful outcome. Gastric dilatation refers to distention of the stomach, usually with swallowed air. Gastric dilatation may or may not be complicated by volvulus. GDV occurs when the stomach rotates on its long axis, resulting in complete gastric outflow obstruction. Concurrent obstruction of the gastroesophageal junction precludes relief of fluid and gas accumulation by vomiting or belching. Massive gastric distention impairs venous return through the portal vein and caudal vena cava, causing hypovolemic and endotoxic shock. Passive congestion of the abdominal viscera predisposes to local acidosis and disseminated intravascular coagulation (DIC). The spleen often is displaced concurrently, causing splenic vascular occlusion, congestion, and splenomegaly. Strangulation necrosis of the gastric wall occurs secondary to twisting of the stomach.

Etiology

The cause of GDV is unknown.

- An anatomic predisposition may play a role; large-breed, deep-chested dogs are most commonly affected, and the disorder is rare in small dogs and cats.
- Gastric dilatation due to excessive swallowed air is generally believed to precede volvulus; thus, causes of aerophagia such as gulping of food may be important.
- Delayed gastric emptying has also been suspected in some dogs with GDV.
- Overeating, postprandial exercise, and dry, cereal-based diets have been suggested to predispose to GDV but have not been substantiated clinically or experimentally.

Clinical Signs

- Acute onset of abdominal distention with tympany.
- Nonproductive retching.
- Salivating, restlessness, and respiratory distress.

Diagnosis

History and Signalment

- Consider GDV in the differential diagnosis of any large-breed, deep-chested dog with acute onset of abdominal distention.

Physical Examination

- Examination usually reveals abdominal distention and findings indicative of hypovolemia and/or shock, including increased heart rate, weak femoral pulses, decreased capillary refill time, and pale oral mucous membranes.

Laboratory Evaluation

- After initial stabilization (see later) submit blood for a CBC and biochemical evaluation to characterize secondary metabolic imbalances and to identify any other coexistent abnormalities.
- Hypokalemia is the most common electrolyte abnormality in dogs with GDV. Although serum potassium concentration may be normal initially, hypokalemia frequently develops after aggressive fluid therapy and, if surgery is necessary, postoperatively. Prevention of hypokalemia may decrease the frequency of postoperative cardiac arrhythmias and muscle weakness.
- Because a variety of acid-base imbalances may occur secondary to GDV, repeated laboratory assessment and frequent monitoring of blood gases and electrolyte concentrations are recommended.
  - Metabolic acidosis is most common and occurs because of decreased effective circulating blood volume, arterial hypoxemia, and lactic acid accumulation.
  - Metabolic alkalosis, respiratory alkalosis, respiratory acidosis, and mixed acid-base disorders may also develop.

Radiography

- Perform abdominal radiography only after the patient is stabilized medically (see below). Minimize stress to the patient during the procedure.
- Right lateral and ventral-dorsal abdominal radiographs are most useful to evaluate for GDV.
- Radiographic findings suggestive of GDV include:
  - Overdistention of the stomach with gas, pyloric displacement dorsally and to the left, and gastric fundic displacement caudally and to the right
  - Compartmentalization of the stomach on the lateral view
  - Splenomegaly
- Pneumoperitoneum suggests gastric perforation and requires immediate surgery.
- Thoracic radiography is not essential but may demonstrate microcardia due to hypovolemia, megaesophagus, or aspiration pneumonia.
- In cases of intermittent bloating or failure of surgical correction following tube decompression, perform a contrast gastrogram (see Chap. 4) to identify malposition of the stomach.

Initial Medical Management

Decompress the Stomach by Orogastric Intubation

- Sedation may be necessary to pass an orogastric tube. Give diazepam (0.1 mg/kg IV slowly) alone or in combination with butorphanol (0.5 mg/kg IV). An alternative is the combination of diazepam-ketamine (50:50), 1 ml/10 kg IV.
- Perform gastric decompression by passing a well-lubricated large-bore orogastric tube. Remove all air and fluid from the stomach and lavage the stomach with 4–5 L of warm saline or water. Repeat orogastric

decompression as needed during the stabilization period.
- If orogastric decompression is not possible with a tube, use several 18-gauge needles to trocarize the distended stomach. Following decompression with needle trocarization, a subsequent attempt to pass the orogastric tube often is successful.

Place an Intravenous Catheter and Administer Fluids

- While decompression is being performed, place a large-bore catheter in each cephalic vein.
- Give isotonic crystalloid fluids such as lactated Ringer's solution at an initial rapid rate of 90 ml/kg for the first hour. After shock is controlled and dehydration corrected, lower to a maintenance rate of administration. Add potassium chloride to the fluid (30–40 mEq KCl per liter of fluid) after the initial shock dose of fluids has been given. When blood gas analysis is not available, routine addition of NaHCO$_3$ to fluids is not recommended, because many dogs with GDV have relatively normal blood pH at presentation. Correction of volume depletion and mild metabolic acidosis by lactated Ringer's solution is sufficient unless severe metabolic acidosis is present.
- Alternatively, administer small-volume fluid therapy using 7% NaCl (5 ml/kg) in 6% dextran 70 (HS/D70). Give over 5–10 minutes and follow with 20 ml/kg/hour 0.9% NaCl.
- Place a Foley catheter in the bladder to monitor urine output.

Control Infection and Endotoxemia

- To treat endotoxemia, give prednisolone sodium succinate (10 ml/kg IV). Give a single dose of flunixin meglumine (Banamine, Schering), 1 mg/kg IV, during the initial phase of therapy.
- Give a broad-spectrum antibiotic (cefmetazole, 15 mg/kg IV) or combination drug therapy (cefazolin, 20 mg/kg IV, and gentamicin, 2 mg/kg IV).

Monitor and Treat Cardiac Arrhythmias

- Ventricular arrhythmias are the most common.
- To treat ventricular arrhythmias, give a bolus of lidocaine (1–2 mg/kg) IV while monitoring the electrocardiogram. If no conversion is noted within 3–5 minutes, repeat this dose. For a comprehensive discussion of diagnosis and treatment of arrhythmias, see Chapter 62.
- If only temporary conversion occurs, start a lidocaine drip. A maintenance effect is achieved with a constant rate infusion of lidocaine at 40–60 μg/kg/minute added to the IV fluids. Lidocaine's effectiveness may be impaired in the presence of hypokalemia.
- If lidocaine boluses are ineffective for controlling ventricular arrhythmias, consider giving procainamide (10–15 mg/kg IM q6h) or quinidine sulfate (6–15 mg/kg IM q6h). If arrhythmias are controlled with parenteral administration of procainamide or quinidine, an oral antiarrhythmic can later be substituted, as described in Chapter 62.

Surgical Management

The goals of surgical intervention for acute GDV include:

- Repositioning of the stomach and spleen
- Resecting devitalized gastric and splenic tissue
- Permanently fixing the stomach (pyloric antrum) to the right abdominal wall to prevent future occurrences of volvulus (see Chap. 88)

Prevention

If medical therapy alone is successful and no evidence of gastric volvulus is detected subsequently on a contrast gastrogram, there is still a 70–75% likelihood that the dog will have another episode of GDV. Owner education can help to lessen the probability of recurrence.

Instruct the owner to:

- Feed the dog frequent, small portions of food 3–5 times per day.
- Limit water intake and do not allow access to water for 1 hour after eating.
- Restrict exercise after eating, because this may predispose to GDV.
- Be aware of the early warning signs of GDV (e.g., depression, restlessness, belching, excessive flatulence, abdominal enlargement), especially when there is a change in the dog's environment—for example, when the dog is boarded or hospitalized, or when a new adult, child, or pet is introduced into the household.

SUPPLEMENTAL READINGS

Guilford WG, Center SA, Strombeck DR, et al., eds.: Strombeck's Small Animal Gastroenterology. Philadelphia: WB Saunders, 1996.

Orton EC: Gastric dilatation-volvulus. *In* Kirk RW, ed.: Current Veterinary Therapy IX. Philadelphia: WB Saunders, 1985, p 856.

Tams TR: Gastroscopy. *In* Tams TR, ed.: Small Animal Endoscopy, 2nd Ed. St Louis: Mosby, 1999, p 97.

Twedt DC: Diseases of the stomach. *In* Sherding RG, ed.: The Cat: Diseases and Clinical Management, Vol 2, 2nd Ed. New York: Churchill Livingstone, 1994, p 1181.

Whitney WO: Complications associated with the medical and surgical management of gastric dilatation-volvulus in the dog. Problems in Veterinary Medicine, Vol 1, No. 2. Philadelphia: WB Saunders, 1989, p 268.

Willard MD: Diseases of the stomach. *In* Ettinger SJ, Feldman EC, eds.: Textbook of Veterinary Internal Medicine, Vol 2, 4th Ed. Philadelphia: WB Saunders, 1995, p 103.

88 Surgery of the Stomach

Ronald M. Bright

Retrieval of foreign bodies is the most common reason for surgery on the stomach. Surgery of the pylorus is most often indicated for some forms of gastric outflow obstruction. The most common sign related to surgical disease of the stomach is emesis. The stomach has an excellent blood supply and heals rapidly (10–14 days).

ANATOMY

Stomach

- The stomach is a musculoglandular organ capable of undergoing a great amount of distention.
- The stomach is C-shaped and a partially coiled, bulging tube.
- The stomach lies in a transverse plane. The larger part of the stomach (fundus) lies to the left of the midline.
- The esophageal entrance and duodenal exit are dorsal—the former lying to the left of the midline, the latter to the right.
- In the fasting dog, the stomach does not extend caudally beyond the costal arch and is rarely palpable.
- The stomach is divided into four regions: cardia, fundus, body (corpus), and pylorus.
- The stomach has four tunics: mucosa, submucosa, muscularis, and serosa. The submucosa and mucosa layers are easily separated from the overlying seromuscular layers.
- The blood supply to the distal stomach is from a branch of the hepatic artery, giving rise to the right gastric and gastroepiploic arteries.
  - The splenic artery gives rise to the left gastroepiploic artery, which supplies the greater curvature.
  - The left gastric artery supplies blood to the lesser curvature of the stomach and the distal esophagus.
- Veins are satellites to the arterial branches. Most blood drains from the left side of the stomach via the gastrosplenic vein and from the right side via the gastroduodenal vein. These veins ultimately drain into the portal vein.
- The major innervation is parasympathetic from the vagi and sympathetic from the celiac plexus.

Omentum

- The greater omentum extends caudally from the greater curvature of the stomach to the urinary bladder, forming a double-layered cover of the small intestine.
- A splenic portion of the omentum attaches to the greater curvature to the spleen and a smaller portion attaches to the pancreas.
- The lesser omentum extends from the lesser curvature of the stomach and attaches to the diaphragm, liver, and duodenum.
- The hepatoduodenal and hepatogastric ligaments are loose attachments between the respective components.

Pylorus

- The pylorus is composed of two segments, the antrum and the canal. The antrum is a narrow funnel-shaped chamber leading to the narrowed pyloric canal.
- The inner circular muscle layer is thickened in the pyloric region and functions as a powerful sphincter. An outer longitudinal muscle layer is also present.
- The pylorus has two major functions—to control the emptying of solid food once it becomes reduced to an appropriate size and to prevent excessive duodenogastric reflux.

GASTROTOMY

Preoperative Considerations

▼ *Key Point* Serious water and electrolyte abnormalities often accompany conditions that affect the stomach and require gastrotomy. Initiate fluid and electrolyte resuscitation before gastrotomy.

- The most common indication for gastrotomy is to retrieve foreign bodies.
- Endoscopic retrieval of gastric foreign bodies is preferred. When this approach fails, a gastrotomy is indicated.

Surgical Procedure

Objectives

- Access to and exposure of intraluminal contents
- Collection of biopsy specimens
- Avoidance of contamination of the peritoneal cavity

Equipment

- General surgical pack
- Babcock forceps (optional)
- Abdominal self-retaining Balfour retractors
- Laparotomy pads

Technique

1. Make a cranial ventral midline abdominal approach, with the skin incision extending from the xiphoid to the umbilicus.
2. Exteriorize the stomach and isolate it from the other abdominal organs using moistened laparotomy pads.
3. Place two Babcock forceps or two stay sutures 10–15 cm apart on a hypovascular area of the stomach, halfway between the lesser and greater curvature.
4. Make a stab incision into the lumen with a #11 blade.
5. Use suction to remove liquids from the stomach.
6. Extend the stab incision with scissors.
7. Do a visual and tactile exploration of the entire stomach.

Closure

1. The first layer is a continuous inverting horizontal mattress (Connell) suture pattern involving only the submucosal and mucosal layers. A simple continuous suture pattern can be substituted. Synthetic 3-0 absorbable suture material is preferred. Use of chromic gut suture material is discouraged, because it breaks down too rapidly when coming in contact with the lumen of the stomach.
2. Close the second layer with a vertical (Lembert) or horizontal (Cushing) continuous inverting pattern.
3. If the gastrotomy closure is likely to incorporate diseased or devitalized tissue, suture a section of vascularized omentum or a serosal patch, employing a loop of jejunum over the wound for additional reinforcement.

Postoperative Care and Complications

Short-Term

- Give no food for 24 hours; water is allowed ad libitum.
- Monitor the patient for leakage, especially if the gastrotomy closure involves diseased tissue (neoplasia).
- Emesis may be noted once or twice following gastric surgery and treatment is usually not required.
- Systemic antacids are indicated if ulcers or severe gastritis is observed during surgery (see Chap. 87).

Prognosis

- Good to excellent if the reason for surgery is related to a foreign body.

PARTIAL GASTRECTOMY RELATED TO GASTRIC DILATATION-VOLVULUS

Preoperative Considerations

- Gastrectomy in patients with dilatation-volvulus is a high-risk procedure.

- Initially, attempt to stabilize metabolic abnormalities but rapidly proceed with surgery because gastric rupture may occur.

Surgical Procedure

Objectives

- Resect nonviable gastric tissue and restore gastric continuity.
- Use a stapling technique, if possible, to expedite this high-risk procedure.

Equipment

- General pack
- LDS stapler (U.S. Surgical, Norwalk, CT) (optional)
- TA stapler (U.S. Surgical, Norwalk, CT) (optional)
- Abdominal self-retaining retractor
- Laparotomy pads
- Noncrushing straight Doyen intestinal clamps

Technique

1. The approach to the stomach is similar to that for a gastrotomy.
2. Nonviable tissue is recognized by its lack of bleeding on cut surfaces, bluish-black or greenish discoloration, and severe thinning of the stomach wall on palpation.

▼ **Key Point** Do not rely on the appearance of the mucosa alone to determine if full-thickness stomach wall necrosis has occurred.

3. Ligate and divide the appropriate short gastric vessels. LDS stapler apparatus is optimal. This procedure may not be necessary because these vessels are frequently torn.
4. After placement of stay sutures, apply intestinal forceps 2 cm lateral to the junction of viable and nonviable tissue. The tips of the forceps meet at an approximate 45° angle.
5. Use a #10 scalpel blade to cut along the intestinal clamps, leaving a 1-cm margin of healthy tissue outside the intestinal clamps.

Alternate Method of Resection

1. Place a TA stapler parallel to the junction of viable and nonviable tissue, leaving a 1-cm width of normal tissue.
2. After the stapler is engaged and the staples are placed in the tissue, cut the stomach wall next to the blade of the stapler and remove the necrotic tissue.

Closure

1. Without a stapler, the closure is similar to that for a gastrotomy incision.
2. With a stapler, perform the closure before cutting the nonviable tissue away from the TA stapler's blade.
3. Close the abdomen routinely. If gastric rupture has occurred, the abdomen may be left partially open as in treating peritonitis (see Chap. 96).

Postoperative Care and Complications

Short-Term

- Refer to the discussion of gastric dilatation-volvulus surgery for postoperative management of metabolic problems.
- Delay feeding for 24 hours.
- Monitor very closely for signs of gastric leakage (fever, vomiting, pneumoperitoneum, peritonitis), especially during the first 96 hours postoperatively.

▼ *Key Point* When a partial gastrectomy is performed during surgical therapy for gastric dilatation-volvulus complex, the mortality rate ranges from 30–60%.

PARTIAL GASTRECTOMY (DISTAL STOMACH)

Preoperative Considerations

▼ *Key Point* Attempts to define the extent and nature of the disease (benign polyp, malignancy, fungal disease, chronic gastric ulcer) by radiography and endoscopic biopsy are extremely important when planning surgical therapy.

Many animals with gastric neoplasia are old and debilitated and are at greater risk during surgery than others.

Surgical Procedure—Partial Gastrectomy and Gastroduodenostomy (Billroth 1)

Objectives

- To remove diseased tissue that is benign or, if malignant, is limited to the antrum and/or body of the stomach
- To correct failed pyloroplasty procedures
- To maintain an adequate outflow lumen

Equipment

- Same as that for partial gastrectomy associated with the gastric dilatation-volvulus complex
- If a stapler technique is used, a GIA stapler (US Surgical, Norwalk, CT) is recommended.
- Large straight intestinal clamps

Technique

1. Place the dog in dorsal recumbency with surgical preparation similar to that for gastrotomy.
2. Stapling devices (e.g., the GIA stapler) can be substituted for more traditional suturing techniques.
3. If the diseased tissue is limited to the pylorus, a modification of a Billroth I (von Haberer) technique can be done (Fig. 88–1).
4. If a partial gastrectomy is performed to control ulcer disease, resect the entire antrum.
5. More extensive resection of the pylorus or distal stomach can be done and reconstructed with the original Billroth I (Shoemaker) procedure (see Fig. 88–1).

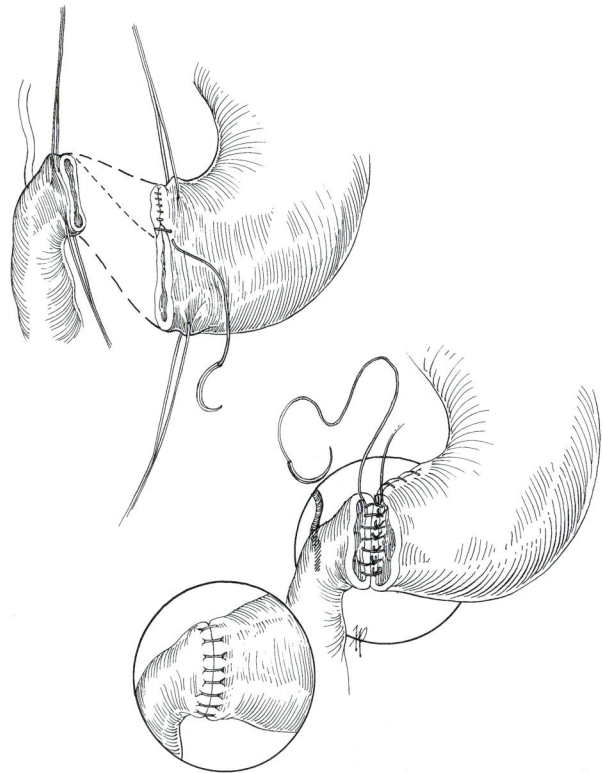

Figure 88–1. Partial gastrectomy with a Billroth I (gastroduodenostomy) repair. *Above,* Lesser curvature of the stomach is closed until lumen disparity is corrected. *Below,* Closure with single interrupted sutures.

6. After the line of resection is determined, ligate and divide the blood vessels supplying the lesser and greater curvature and attached omentum.
7. Mobilize the pylorus after incising the gastrohepatic ligament. Avoid cutting the common bile duct and hepatic arteries.
8. Isolate the area to be resected from the abdominal cavity with moistened laparotomy sponges.
9. Place large, straight noncrushing intestinal forceps above and below the proposed lines of incision.

Closure

1. Use a single-layer interrupted appositional suture pattern to appose the stomach and duodenum. With unequal lumen sizes, first close the lesser curvature side of the stomach until the lumen disparity is corrected (see Fig. 88–1, *top*).
2. Appose the back (far) wall first, placing the knots into the lumen. Synthetic 3-0 absorbable suture (e.g., polydioxanone [PDS]) is recommended.
3. Then appose the near wall.

Surgical Procedure—Partial Gastrectomy and Gastrojejunostomy (Billroth II)

Objectives

- Resect a significant portion of the diseased stomach and all or part of the duodenum.
- Remove the duodenum distal to the common bile duct opening.

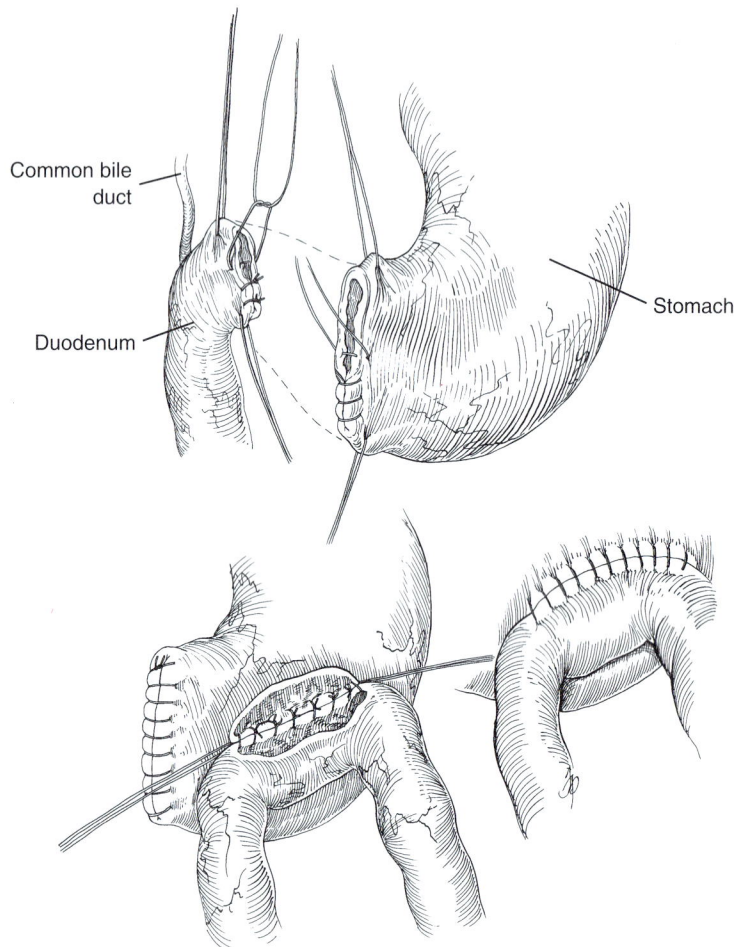

Figure 88–2. Billroth II procedure with side-to-side gastrojejunostomy.

- Reestablish continuity of the stomach with the small intestine with a gastrojejunostomy.
- Restore a biliary connection to the duodenal or jejunal stump via a cholecystenterostomy.

Equipment

Same as that for the Billroth I.

Technique

1. Ligate and divide the appropriate vessels and the common bile duct.
2. Close the duodenal or jejunal stump with a simple interrupted appositional suture pattern using 3-0 synthetic absorbable suture material or a TA stapler.
3. The original Billroth II reconstruction is done by closing the gastric stoma followed by a side-to-side anastomosis of the jejunum to an incision made in the ventral aspect of the stomach (Fig. 88–2).
4. Use a simple interrupted appositional suture pattern to appose the gastric and jejunal segments.
5. For more extensive resections, appose the entire width of the gastric stump to a longitudinal incision made in the jejunum (Fig. 88–3).
6. Use a suture pattern as described in Step 4 for closure.
7. Perform a cholecystenterostomy to complete the procedure (see Chap. 92).

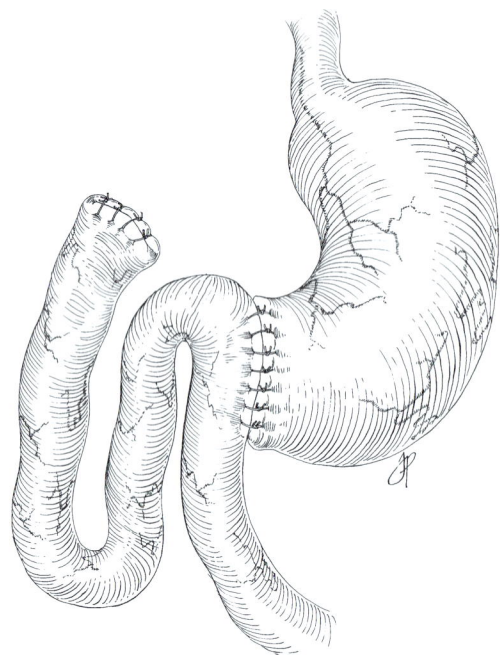

Figure 88–3. Billroth II with anastomosis of the entire gastric stump to a longitudinal incision of the jejunum.

8. Place a jejunostomy tube to provide nutrition in the debilitated patient.

Postoperative Care and Complications

Short-Term

- Monitor for fever and abdominal pain as early signs of leakage peritonitis.
- Withhold food and water by mouth for 24 hours.
- Offer small amounts of food by mouth (per os) 24 hours after surgery.
- Dumping syndrome (passage of undigested food directly into the jejunum) may initially be a problem.

Long-Term

- Dumping syndrome, due to disruption of the normal storage function of the stomach and rapid movement of ingested food into the small intestine, may cause chronic postprandial discomfort, vomiting, and diarrhea.
- Alkaline reflux gastritis may result from disruption of the pyloric sphincter.
- After extensive gastrectomy, multiple small feedings are necessary.

Prognosis

- Good—if the underlying disease is benign or inflammatory.
- Poor—if malignancy is the indication for surgery.

PYLOROMYOTOMY

Preoperative Considerations

- Delay pyloromyotomy until hypochloremic, hypokalemic metabolic alkalosis, which often accompanies the conditions requiring pyloromyotomy, is corrected.
- Direct fluid therapy toward restoring electrolyte *and* water abnormalities.
- In the younger dog or cat, add dextrose to the fluid therapy regimen in an attempt to maintain euglycemia.
- Food and water may be retained in the patient's stomach with outflow obstruction. Therefore, following sedation, place an orogastric tube into the stomach and evacuate the stomach contents.

▼ *Key Point* Pyloromyotomy will *not* effectively relieve outflow obstruction caused by mucosal hypertrophy. Pyloromyotomy is primarily indicated for dogs with muscular hypertrophy only (see Chap. 87).

Surgical Procedure

Objectives

- Increase the lumen diameter of the pylorus to enhance gastric emptying.

Equipment

- General surgery pack
- Abdominal self-retaining retractor
- Laparotomy sponges
- Babcock forceps

Technique

1. Place the dog in dorsal recumbency and aseptically prepare for a cranial midline abdominal incision.
2. Incise the skin and underlying tissues to allow an opening to the abdominal cavity extending from the xiphoid to 4–5 cm below the umbilicus.
3. Partially incise the gastrohepatic ligament to allow the pylorus to be mobilized.
4. Isolate the stomach with laparotomy sponges.
5. Place a stay suture or a Babcock forceps 3–5 cm proximal and distal to the pyloric ring.
6. Make an incision 4–5 cm long into a hypovascular area of the serosa overlying the pyloric antrum and canal and extend it distally into the proximal duodenum. The pylorus is at the midpoint of the incision (Fig. 88–4, *top*).
7. Gently incise or dissect away all muscle fibers, using a curved hemostat, to allow the submucosa and mucosa to bulge (see Fig. 88–4, *middle* and *bottom*).
8. Gently replace the stomach into the abdomen.
9. Perform routine ventral abdominal closure.

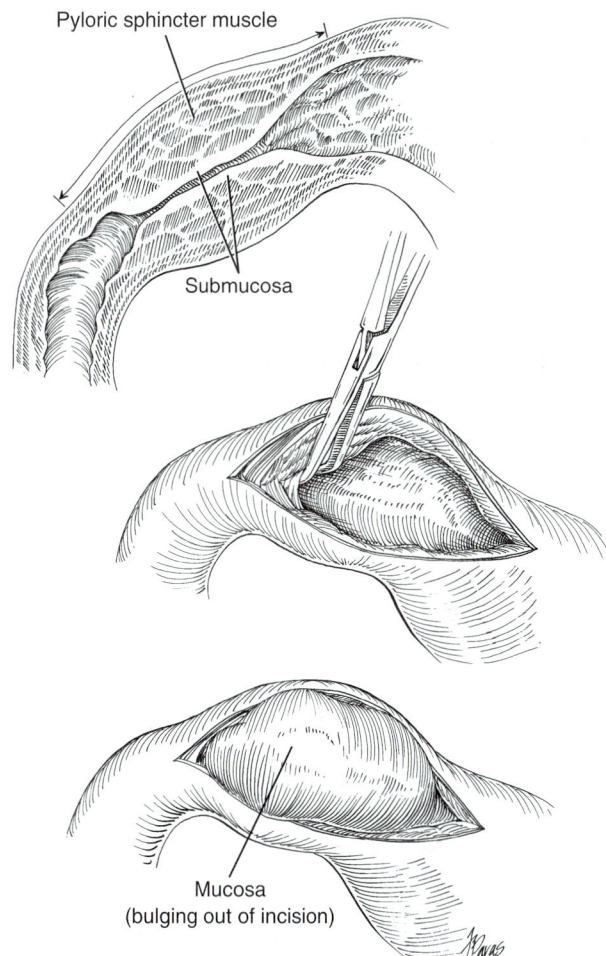

Figure 88–4. Technique for pyloromyotomy.

Postoperative Care and Complications

Short-Term

- Treat emesis lasting more than 6–8 hours postoperatively with metoclopramide, 0.2–0.4 mg/kg SC q6h as needed, or constant-rate IV infusion of metoclopramide at 1–2 mg/kg/day, which is most effective.
- Maintain fluid therapy for 36–48 hours postoperatively.
- Perform frequent monitoring of the packed cell volume, albumin, and blood glucose values, especially in the very young animal.
- Monitor electrolyte values closely in all animals for the first 24 hours.
- Begin feeding soft food 24 hours after surgery unless vomiting continues.

Long-Term

- Emesis may continue with little to no improvement noted. This sign may suggest a need to reoperate and perform a more extensive procedure (e.g., pyloroplasty).
- Signs of vomiting may recur several days or weeks following surgery. If other causes of vomiting are not identified, reoperation may be necessary.

Prognosis

Because the underlying disease in most cases is benign, the prognosis is good to excellent.

PYLOROPLASTY

Preoperative Considerations

- See under Pyloromyotomy.
- Pyloroplasty is indicated for pyloric hypertrophy involving muscle and mucosa or mucosa alone (see Chap. 87). Dogs with severe pyloric hypertrophy may require the Billroth I procedure (see previous discussion).
- Manual and visual inspection of the lumen of the distal stomach, pylorus, and proximal duodenum is possible with a pyloroplasty.

Surgical Procedure

Objectives

- Inspect the distal stomach and pylorus for abnormalities.
- Increase the diameter of the gastric outflow tract.

Equipment

See under Pyloromyotomy.

Heineke-Mikulicz Pyloroplasty

Technique

1. Place temporary stay sutures or Babcock forceps on the antrum and proximal duodenum proximal and distal to the pyloric ring.

2. Make a full-thickness stab incision into the pylorus using a #11 Bard-Parker scalpel blade. Place a suction tip into the stomach to evacuate contents and bile.
3. Extend the incision with scissors to 1–2 cm above and below the pylorus (Fig. 88–5).
4. Remove the stay sutures or Babcock forceps.
5. Close the longitudinal incision transversely with 3-0 synthetic absorbable sutures in a simple interrupted appositional pattern. Stay sutures can be placed on both sides of the incision to help orient the tissues for closure.
6. Routine abdominal closure follows warm saline lavage of the surgical site.

Y-U Pyloroplasty (Antral Flap Advancement)

Technique

1. Mobilize the pylorus as described under Pyloromyotomy.
2. Place temporary stay sutures 4–5 cm above and below the pylorus.
3. Make a Y-shaped incision through the seromuscular tissue overlying the pylorus and distal stomach (Fig. 88–6).
4. Each limb of the Y is approximately 3–4 cm in length depending on the size of the animal.
5. The base of the Y extends a small distance (3–4 mm) into the antrum proximal to the pylorus.

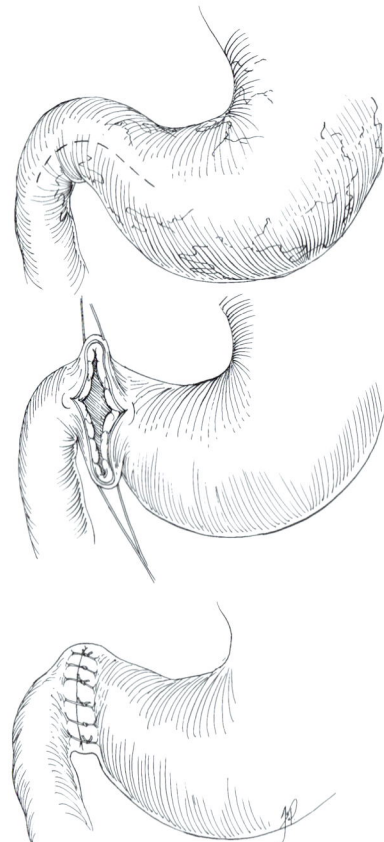

Figure 88–5. Technique for Heineke-Mikulicz pyloroplasty.

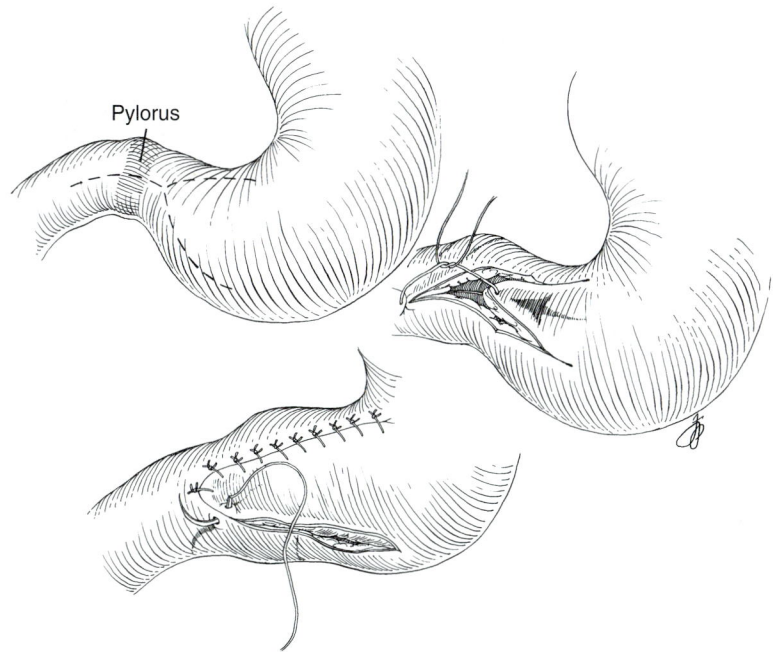

Pylorus

Figure 88–6.   Technique for Y-U pyloroplasty.

6. Trim the V-shaped antral flap to a U-shape. Save the resected tissue and submit for histopathology.
7. Thoroughly palpate and visually examine the stomach and proximal duodenum.
8. Excise hypertrophied tissue via a submucosal resection. Close adjacent mucosa/submucosa in a continuous pattern with 3-0 or 4-0 synthetic absorbable suture.
9. Begin pyloroplasty closure by suturing the base of the U-shaped flap distally to the proximal duodenum with 3-0 or 4-0 synthetic absorbable suture (see Fig. 88–6).
10. A simple interrupted appositional pattern is recommended. If necessary, preplace the sutures to ensure accuracy.
11. Appose the lesser curvature limb of the Y, followed by the greater curvature limb (see Fig. 88–6).

Postoperative Care and Complications

Short-Term

- Same as that for pyloromyotomy.

Long-Term

- Emesis containing a significant amount of bile several weeks after surgery may suggest duodenogastric reflux. Consider treatment with metoclopramide.
- Alkaline reflux gastritis resulting from duodenogastric reflux may require long-term therapy with metoclopramide or cisapride to promote normal gastric emptying and an H_2 blocker for acid control.

Prognosis

- Good—if the disease being treated is benign.

ACUTE GASTRIC DILATATION-VOLVULUS

Preoperative Considerations

- Aggressive fluid therapy, cardiac arrhythmia therapy, and orogastric decompression are necessary before any surgical intervention (see Chap. 87).
- Stabilization of most patients can be accomplished in 2–3 hours.
- Complicating gastric perforation is considered a surgical emergency.

Surgical Procedure

Objectives

- Reposition stomach and spleen to their normal anatomic relationship.
- Fix ("pexy") the stomach (pyloric antrum) to the right abdominal wall to prevent future episodes of volvulus.
- Resect devitalized tissue (spleen, stomach).

Equipment

- General surgical pack
- Self-retaining abdominal retractor (Balfour)
- Foley catheter (22–26 Fr.)
- Orogastric tube

Technique

1. Place the dog in dorsal recumbency and surgically prepare from the mid-sternum to 6–8 cm below the umbilicus. If a tube gastropexy is used, prepare the right side of the abdominal wall aseptically, halfway up the side of the thoracic and abdominal wall that corresponds with the length of the midline incision.

2. Gently place an orogastric tube into the esophagus and advance it until there is resistance.
3. Derotate the stomach by grasping the pylorus and duodenum, usually located near the gastro-esophageal junction, and elevating them to the right side of the body.
4. The fundus, usually on the right side, is depressed and rotated to the left side while the pylorus is being repositioned.
5. Place the orogastric tube within the stomach and perform stomach decompression.
6. Assess the viability of the stomach, and resect necrotic tissue if necessary (see discussion of Partial Gastrectomy Related to Gastric Dilatation-Volvulus).
7. Splenectomy is usually not done unless there is evidence of splenic torsion or necrosis.
8. Perform a gastropexy procedure on the right side of the dog (regardless of the technique employed). Each of the gastropexy techniques described subsequently is effective. The technique chosen depends on the surgeon's preference.

Tube Gastropexy (22–26 Fr. Foley Catheter)

Technique

1. Place a full-thickness pursestring suture in the mid-antrum area using 2-0 or 3-0 nonabsorbable suture. This suture is left untied (Fig. 88–7).
2. Pull the tip of a Foley catheter through a small right paracostal incision using Carmalt forceps, approximately 4 cm caudal to the costal arch and 4 cm lateral to the incision.
3. Make a stab incision into the middle of the pursestring suture area and advance the tip of the Foley catheter through this and into the stomach (see Fig. 88–7).
4. Inflate the balloon portion of the catheter.

5. Draw the pursestring suture tightly and tie it.
6. Move the stomach to the abdominal wall with traction on the Foley catheter.
7. Preplace six to eight interrupted sutures between the stomach, being sure to penetrate to the submucosa and the abdominal wall. Use nonabsorbable #1 or 1-0 suture material (see Fig. 88–7).
8. Tie the sutures starting dorsally and ending ventrally.
9. Affix the catheter to the skin with a traction suture.

Circumcostal Gastropexy

Technique

1. Place two retention sutures using 1-0 or 2-0 nonabsorbable suture material in the antrum approximately 6 cm apart and midway between the lesser and greater curvature.
2. Make a 3 × 3 cm incision through the seromuscular layer forming an I-shaped configuration (Fig. 88–8, *inset*).
3. The seromuscular flaps are formed by careful dissection between the muscular and submucosa tunics. Place two stay sutures on each flap.
4. Isolate the 11th or 12th rib ventral to the costochondral junction and rotate it laterally with two towel clamps placed 6 cm apart.
5. Expose a 4–5 cm length of the rib by incising through the peritoneum and muscle.

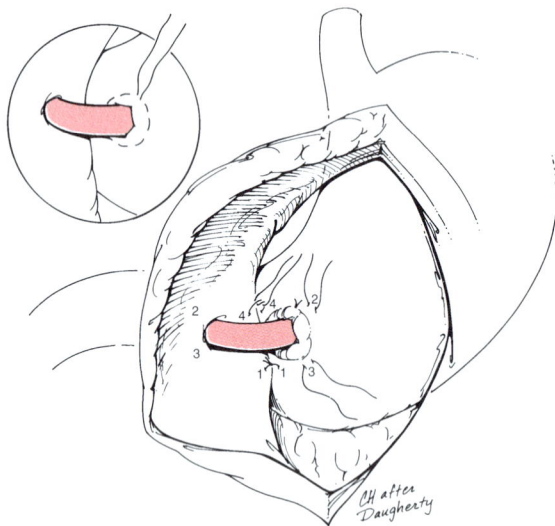

Figure 88–7. Technique for tube gastropexy in the treatment of gastric dilatation-volvulus. *Inset*, Place an untied pursestring suture in the midantrum area. Place a Foley catheter through the body wall, into the pyloric antrum. Connect the stomach and abdominal wall with interrupted sutures. In the figure, points 1 are connected, as are points 2 to each other, and so forth. (Drawing by Carol Haynes, after Daugherty.)

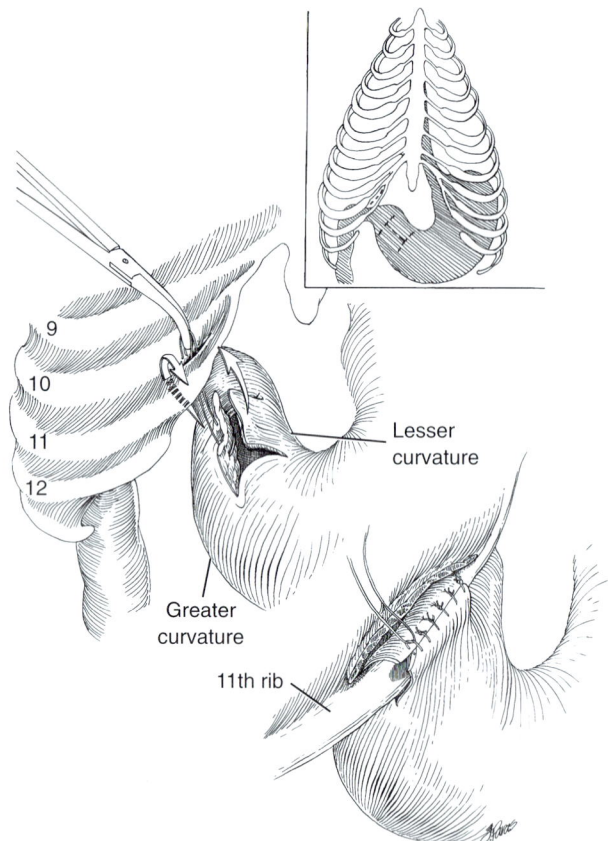

Figure 88–8. Technique for circumcostal gastropexy (for gastric dilatation-volvulus).

6. By blunt dissection remove all tissue attached to the rib.
7. Pass one arm of each stay suture under the rib.
8. Place another stay suture midway down the seromuscular flap found on the greater curvature side. This placement helps pull this flap around the exposed rib.
9. Once the flap is pulled around the rib, tie the two retention sutures.
10. Suture the seromuscular flap to the opposite flap using 2-0 synthetic absorbable or nonabsorbable suture (see Fig. 88–8). Use a simple interrupted full-thickness suture pattern.
11. Suture the peritoneum and musculature on the lateral aspect of the completed flap repair to the seromuscular layer of the stomach with six to eight sutures. This bridges and supports the seromuscular flap suture line.

Belt Loop Gastropexy

Technique

1. A belt loop of muscle is produced by making two parallel transverse incisions 2–3 cm apart and 2–3 cm in length through the peritoneum and fascia of the transversus abdominis muscle.
2. Bluntly separate the muscle fibers with scissors (Fig. 88–9A).
3. Make a 2 × 4 cm tongue-shaped seromuscular flap with the base of the flap along the greater curvature of the antrum (Fig. 88–9B).
4. A branch of the gastroepiploic artery is centered at the base of the flap.
5. When creating the flap, make the base is a little wider than the tip of the tongue-shaped flap.

6. Pass the stomach flap through the belt loop in a cranial-to-caudal direction (Fig. 88–9C).
7. The flap is now repositioned over its original anatomic location and reattached to adjacent seromuscular tissue with 1-0 monofilament synthetic absorbable or nonabsorbable suture (Fig. 88–9D).

Muscle Flap Gastropexy

Technique

1. Make a U-shaped incision through the peritoneum and transversus abdominis muscle caudal to the 13th rib on the right lateral side.
2. Undermine and reflect the muscle flap ventrally.
3. Preplace two horizontal mattress sutures using 1-0 nonabsorbable material from the base of the U through the seromuscular layer of the antrum and draw the antrum laterally to the right abdominal wall (Fig. 88–10A).
4. Tie the sutures and secure them against the body wall (Fig. 88–10B).
5. Secure the remaining base of the U to the stomach wall employing a simple continuous suture pattern (Fig. 88–10C).
6. Bring the muscle flap to the gastric surface, advancing it a few millimeters beyond the previous suture line.
7. Suture the flap with the same material to the stomach wall to close the myotomy (Fig. 88–10C).

Incisional Gastropexy

Technique

1. Refer to the incisional gastropexy procedure as described for hiatal hernia in Chapter 86.

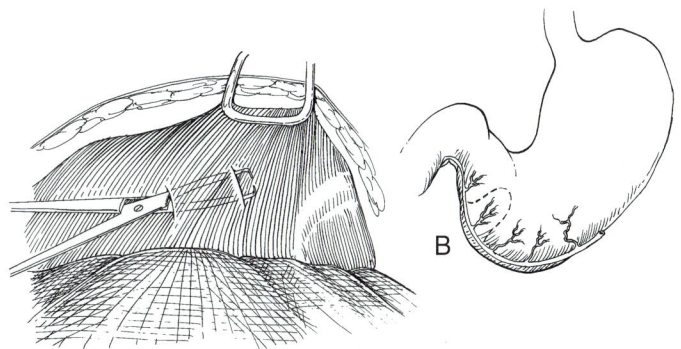

Figure 88–9. Technique for belt loop gastropexy (for gastric dilatation-volvulus). See text for details.

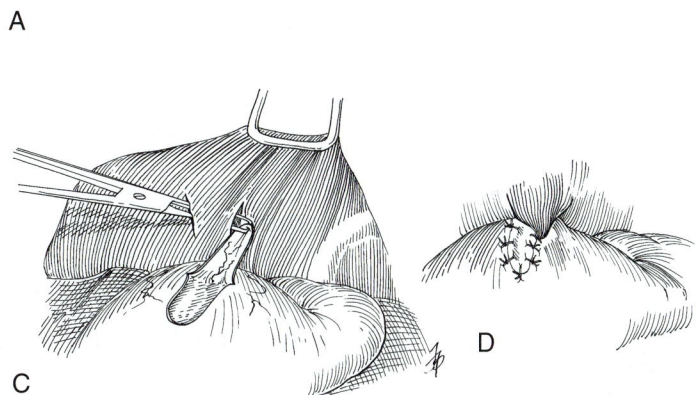

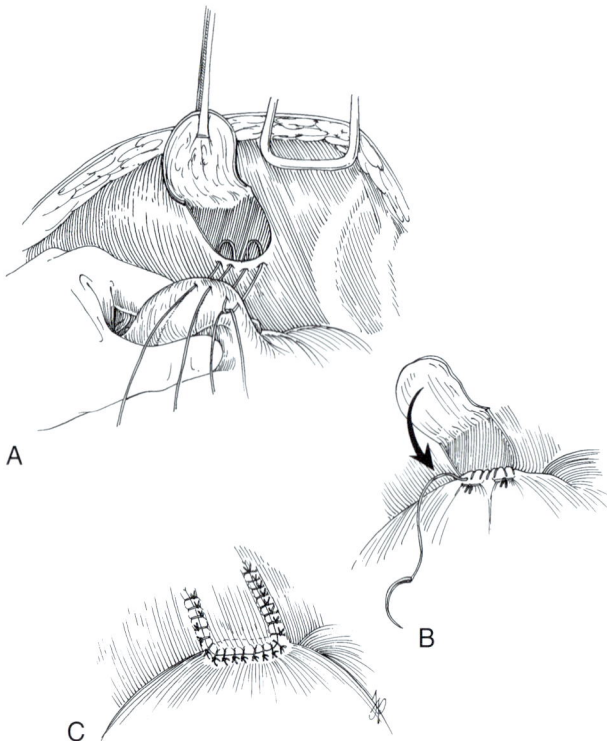

Figure 88–10. Technique for muscle flap gastropexy (for gastric dilatation-volvulus). See text for details.

2. An incisional gastropexy for gastric dilatation-volvulus differs by always being done on the right side (i.e., antrum to right side of body wall), as for the other gastropexy techniques described here.

Postoperative Care and Complications

Short-Term

- Monitor closely for a minimum of 4 days for cardiac arrhythmias, especially ventricular arrhythmias, (see Chap. 62 for details of treatment); hemodynamic abnormalities or circulatory collapse; recurrent gastric retention; and gastric perforation with subsequent peritonitis.
- Maintain fluid therapy and supplement with potassium for a minimum of 48 hours.
- Monitor serum electrolyte, blood gas, hematocrit, total protein, urinary output, and central venous pressure values as necessary.
- Promote gastrointestinal motility with metoclopramide, 0.2–0.4 mg/kg SC or PO q6–8h. Treat with systemic antacids and sucralfate (see Chap. 87) if ulceration or necrosis was present at surgery, or if vomiting of bloody fluid is present postoperatively.
- Maintain tube gastropexy under a soft padded bandage so that chewing or dislodgement of the tube is prevented.
- The tube can be used for decompression and administration of fluids, gruel, and medication.
- Feeding can resume 24–48 hours after surgery.

Long-Term

- Remove the tube (tube gastropexy) 5–7 days after placement. Allow the fistula to heal by second intention (contraction and epithelialization).
- Wean the animal slowly off antiarrhythmic drugs if cardiac arrhythmia was a problem and so treated.
- Encourage three to four feedings per day at home.

Prognosis

- Fair to good if partial gastrectomy is not indicated.
- Grave to poor when partial gastrectomy is done.

SUPPLEMENTAL READINGS

Gastrotomy

Arnockzy SP, Ryan WW: Gastrotomy and pyloroplasty. Vet Clin North Am 5:343, 1975.
Dulisch ML: Gastrotomy. Current Techniques in Small Animal Surgery II. Philadelphia: Lea & Febiger, 1983, p 157.

Partial Gastrectomy Related to Gastric Dilatation-Volvulus

Clark GN, Pavletic MM: Partial gastrectomy with an automatic stapling instrument for treatment of gastric necrosis secondary to gastric dilatation-volvulus. Vet Surg 20:61, 1991.
Matthiesen DT: Partial gastrectomy as a treatment of gastric volvulus: Results of 30 dogs. Vet Surg 14:185, 1985.

Partial Gastrectomy (Distal Stomach)

Ahmadu-Suka F, Withrow SJ, Nelson AW, et al.: Billroth II gastrojejunostomy in dogs: Stapling techniques and postoperative complications. Vet Surg 17:211, 1988.
Bright RM: Esophagus and stomach. *In* Harvey CE, Newton CD, Schwartz A, eds.: Small Animal Surgery. Philadelphia: JB Lippincott, 1990, p 323.

Pyloromyotomy

Fox SM, Burns J: The effect of pyloric surgery on gastric emptying in the dog: Comparison of three techniques. J Am Anim Hosp Assoc 22:783, 1986.
Matthiesen DT: Chronic gastric outflow obstruction. *In* Bojrab MJ, ed.: Current Techniques in Small Animal Surgery, 4th Ed. Baltimore: Williams & Wilkins, 1998, p 561.

Pyloroplasty

Bright RM, Richardson DC, Stanton ME: Y-U antral flap advancement pyloroplasty in dogs. Comp Cont Educ Pract Vet 10:139, 1988.
Stanton ME, Bright RM, Toal R, et al.: Chronic hypertrophic pyloric gastropathy as a cause of pyloric obstruction in the dog. J Am Vet Med Assoc 186:157, 1985.
Walters MC, Goldschmidt MH, Stone EA, et al.: Chronic hypertrophic pyloric gastropathy as a cause of pyloric obstruction in the dog. J Am Vet Med Assoc 186:157, 1985.

Gastric Dilatation-Volvulus (Surgery)

Fallah AM, Lumb WV, Nelson AW, et al.: Circumcostal gastropexy in the dog, a preliminary study. Vet Surg 11:9, 1982.
MacCoy DM, Sykes GP, Hoffer RE, et al.: A gastropexy technique for permanent fixation of the pyloric antrum. J Am Anim Hosp 18:763, 1982.
Schulman AJ, Lusk R, Lippincott CL, et al.: Muscular flap gastropexy: A new surgical technique to prevent recurrences of gastric dilatation-volvulus syndrome. J Am Anim Hosp Assoc 22:339, 1986.
Whitney WO, Scavelli TD, Matthiesen DT: Belt-loop gastropexy: Technique and surgical results in 20 dogs. J Am Anim Hosp 25:75, 1989.

Robert G. Sherding / Susan E. Johnson

DIARRHEA AS A CLINICAL SIGN OF INTESTINAL DISEASE

Diarrhea results from excessive fecal water content and is the most important clinical sign of intestinal disease in the dog and cat. It is characterized by an abnormal increase in the frequency, fluidity, and volume of feces. The pathogenesis involves derangement of transmucosal water and solute fluxes caused by abnormal digestion, absorption, secretion, permeability, or motility or a combination of these.

Acute versus Chronic Diarrhea

For initial management of diarrhea, determine if diarrhea is acute or chronic (based on history).

Acute Diarrhea

Acute diarrhea is a common clinical sign. It is characterized by sudden onset and short duration (3 weeks or less) of watery or watery-mucoid diarrhea that may be overtly bloody in severe cases. Inappetence, lethargy, and vomiting are frequent associated signs; fever, abdominal pain, and significant dehydration suggest more serious intestinal disease.

- Acute diarrhea in dogs and cats may be caused by dietary indiscretion or intolerance, drugs and toxins, intestinal parasites, infectious agents (viral, bacterial, rickettsial), and systemic or metabolic disturbances.
- Although there are exceptions, acute diarrhea associated with diet, parasites, and medications generally tends to be mild and self-limiting, whereas acute diarrhea that is severe and life-threatening occurs most frequently in young animals with infectious enteritis (e.g., parvoviral enteritis).
- Diagnostic evaluations in acute diarrhea need not be extensive. Because treatment is mainly supportive and nonspecific, many animals can be managed without determination of a definitive diagnosis. Nevertheless, it is important to identify parasites and enteropathogens that require specific treatments and to identify surgical diseases (e.g., foreign bodies, intussusception).
- Treatment of acute diarrhea is based on rehydration therapy and dietary restriction. Symptomatic therapy with antidiarrheal agents may be considered. Nonspecific or mild acute diarrhea often is self-limiting in

a day or two without treatment or with restriction of food intake.

Chronic Diarrhea

- Diarrhea is categorized as chronic if it has been persistent (3–4 weeks or longer) or has a pattern of episodic recurrence. Chronicity generally excludes simple dietary indiscretion, intoxication, and viral enteritis as causes.

▼ *Key Point* Base management of chronic diarrhea on diagnosis rather than symptomatic treatment. Specific intervention or treatment usually is necessary, requiring a specific diagnosis or histopathologic characterization.

- The first step in management is to classify the diarrhea as large or small bowel in origin, based on the history and physical examination. Diagnostic tests and procedures include routine hematologic and serum chemistry evaluations, tests of enteropancreatic function, fecal examinations, radiographic procedures, and endoscopic procedures. Biopsy of the small or large intestine often is necessary.

Small Bowel versus Large Bowel Diarrhea

The anatomic localization of the disease process to the small or large bowel is based on the fecal characteristics (frequency, volume, consistency, color, odor, composition) and defecation patterns (Table 89–1). This distinction is important because it determines the direction of subsequent diagnostic evaluations. Diffuse diseases of the gastrointestinal tract may produce concurrent small and large bowel signs and, sometimes, gastric signs such as vomiting.

Small Bowel Diarrhea

- Chronic small bowel diarrhea can be associated with maldigestion and malabsorption and is characterized by a high volume without urgency, tenesmus, or increased frequency. Weight loss and decline in body condition (malnutrition) may occur.
- Because of unabsorbed nutrients that are degraded and fermented by intestinal bacteria, the feces are rancid and foul-smelling. Increased production of luminal gas by bacteria results in excessive flatulence and borborygmus.

Table 89–1. DIFFERENTIATION OF SMALL BOWEL DIARRHEA FROM LARGE BOWEL DIARRHEA

Observation	Small Intestine	Large Intestine
Frequency of defecation	Normal to slightly increased	Very frequent
Fecal output	Large volumes	Small volumes frequently
Urgency or tenesmus	Absent	Present
Dyschezia	Absent	Present with rectal disease
Mucus in feces	Absent	Present
Hematochezia (red blood)	Absent (except in acute hemorrhagic diarrhea)	Present sometimes
Melena (digested blood)	Present sometimes	Absent
Steatorrhea	Present in maldigestive or malabsorptive disease	Absent
Flatulence & borborygmus	Present in maldigestive or malabsorptive disease	Absent
Weight loss	Present in maldigestive or malabsorptive disease	Rare
Vomiting	Present sometimes in inflammatory bowel disease	Rare

- Steatorrhea (feces containing an excess of unabsorbed fat) can be a prominent manifestation of small bowel diarrhea. In extreme cases, the feces may appear oily, greasy, and light in color. Hair around the perineum may also have an oily texture from contact with fatty feces.
- Small bowel diarrhea is generally free of grossly visible mucus or blood. When there is bleeding from a lesion in the proximal gastrointestinal (GI) tract, the luminal blood pigment produces dark black discoloration of the feces (melena) during transit. In the absence of gastric bleeding, melena generally indicates intestinal parasitism (hookworms), infection (viral, bacterial, fungal), ulceration (e.g., drug-induced), severe inflammation, or neoplasia.

Large Bowel Diarrhea

- Large bowel diarrhea is characterized by frequent urges to defecate (usually greater than three times normal frequency), each defecation producing small quantities of feces that contain excessive mucus and sometimes fresh red blood.
- Urgency resulting from irritability or inflammation of the distal colon causes frequent premature expulsions of small quantities of feces that would otherwise be insufficient to trigger the defecation reflex. Lapses in house-training ("accidents") may be caused by urgency and inability to control urges to defecate.
- Straining (tenesmus) may be noted as the animal remains in a squatting posture for an extended period of time after defecation or makes repeated attempts to defecate within a few minutes. These attempts may produce little or no feces, or sometimes a small amount of feces composed almost entirely of mucus, exudate, and blood.
- Because colonic diseases often are associated with mucosal injury, inflammation, or ulceration, abnormal fecal constituents frequently are present, including fresh red blood (hematochezia) that originates from sites of erosion or ulceration, mucus that originates from the abundant goblet cells in the colon that respond to mucosal injury by an outpouring of mucus, and exudate (leukocytes) that originates from the site of inflammation.

- Blood may coat the feces, streaks of blood may be mixed within the feces, or drops of blood may be passed at the end of defecation.
- Excessive mucus may give the feces a glistening or jelly-like appearance.
- Exudates are detected by the positive identification of fecal leukocytes, using cytology stains.

▼ *Key Point* Abnormal fecal constituents such as fresh red blood, mucus, and leukocytes are localizing signs indicative of colonic disease.

- Because the principal function of the colon is absorption of water and electrolytes rather than digestion and absorption of nutrients, nutrient malabsorption and steatorrhea are absent in large bowel diarrhea. Thus, dramatic weight loss and wasting are unlikely if the animal is eating, and the daily fecal output (volume or weight of feces) usually is only minimally increased.

Protein-Losing Enteropathy

Gastrointestinal loss accounts for approximately 40% of the normal daily turnover of plasma proteins. The term *protein-losing enteropathy* refers to a variety of intestinal diseases that are associated with hypoproteinemia caused by an accelerated loss of plasma proteins into the gut.

- Mechanisms of excessive enteric loss of protein include:
  - Impaired intestinal lymphatic drainage (e.g., lymphangiectasia) that results in extravasation of protein-rich lymph into the lumen
  - Disruption of the mucosal barrier (e.g., inflammation) that results in protein leakage from sites of exudation, bleeding, or increased permeability
- Protein-losing enteropathy occurs most frequently in association with chronic enteropathies such as:
  - Idiopathic canine intestinal lymphangiectasia
  - Chronic inflammatory small bowel diseases (lymphocytic-plasmacytic enteritis, granulomatous enteritis, eosinophilic enteritis, immunoproliferative enteropathy of basenjis

- Intestinal histoplasmosis
- Intestinal lymphoma

DIAGNOSTIC APPROACH TO DIARRHEA

History

The history is especially helpful for localizing the disease process to the small or large bowel. It also may indicate underlying extraintestinal causes of diarrhea (e.g., renal failure, hypoadrenocorticism, or hyperthyroidism) and identify important predisposing factors such as breed, diet, environmental factors, current medications, and exposure to parasites, infectious agents, and toxins. The following historical aspects of the diarrhea may be diagnostically useful:

- Mode of onset (abrupt versus gradual)
- Duration (acute versus chronic)
- Clinical course (intermittent, continuous, or progressive)
- Fecal characteristics (small bowel versus large bowel; see previous discussion)
- Correlation with diet (food intolerances, dietary indiscretions)
- Correlation with medication usage (drug side effects)
- Correlation with stressful events (psychogenic, anxiety or "irritability" factors)
- Response to previous treatments (prescribed diets, antibiotics, corticosteroids, anthelmintics)
- Association with other signs (weight loss, vomiting, dyschezia)

Physical Examination

A complete physical examination may reveal important clues about the severity, nature, and cause of diarrhea (Table 89–2), although in many patients the findings are nonspecific.

- Identify physical findings that may indicate underlying systemic disease that could be a cause or consequence of diarrhea.
- Identify abnormalities on abdominal palpation of the intestinal loops and digital palpation of the rectum.
- Inspect the fecal material obtained on the palpation glove for abrasive particles (such as bone chips), blood, and mucus. If indicated, examine the material microscopically for parasites, microorganisms, and inflammatory cells or submit for culture.

Routine Laboratory Tests

- Evaluate the complete blood count (CBC) for leukocyte responses and anemia that may be associated with intestinal disease (Table 89–3).
- Perform a serum biochemical profile and urinalysis to identify metabolic or systemic disorders that could cause or result from diarrhea (see Table 89–3).
- Measure serum thyroxin levels in older cats with diarrhea and weight loss to exclude hyperthyroidism as a cause (see Chap. 29).

Table 89–2. CLINICAL SIGNIFICANCE OF ABNORMAL PHYSICAL FINDINGS ASSOCIATED WITH INTESTINAL DISEASE

Physical Finding	Potential Clinical Associations
General Physical Examination	
Dehydration	Diarrheal fluid loss
Depression/weakness	Electrolyte imbalance, severe debilitation
Emaciation/malnutrition	Chronic malabsorption, protein-losing enteropathy
Dull unthrifty haircoat	Malabsorption of fatty acids, protein, and vitamins
Fever	Infection, transmural inflammation, neoplasia
Edema, ascites, pleural effusion	Protein-losing enteropathy
Pallor (anemia)	Gastrointestinal blood loss, anemia of chronic illness, or inflammation
Intestinal Palpation	
Masses	Foreign body, neoplasia, granuloma
Thickened loops	Infiltration (inflammatory, neoplastic)
"Sausage loop"	Intussusception
Aggregated loops	Linear intestinal foreign body, peritoneal adhesions
Pain	Inflammation, obstruction, ischemia
Gas or fluid distention	Obstruction, ileus, diarrhea
Mesenteric lymphadenopathy	Inflammation, infection, neoplasia
Rectal Palpation	
Masses	Polyp, granuloma, neoplasia
Circumferential narrowing	Stricture, spasm, neoplasia
Coarse mucosal texture	Colitis, neoplasia

Fecal Examinations

Fecal examinations are an important aspect of the diagnostic approach to diarrhea and may involve gross inspection (as previously described), parasite and microscopic examinations, quantitative fecal collection and analysis, chemical determinations, and cultures.

- Examination of feces for parasites should be part of the minimum database for all animals with diarrhea.
- In cases of chronic unresponsive diarrhea, expand the database to include microscopic examination of stained fecal smears for fat, starch, and leukocytes.
- If circumstances suggest infection, perform fecal culture for specific enteropathogenic bacteria (*Salmonella, Campylobacter*).
- Diagnostic methods for intestinal parasites and infectious agents are listed in Table 89–4.

Fecal Examinations for Parasites

- Perform conventional fecal flotations to identify metazoan ova.
- In warm, humid regions (e.g., southern United States) endemic for *Strongyloides* spp., perform a direct smear, sedimentation, or Baermann technique to identify larvae in feces.

Table 89–3. IMPLICATIONS OF VARIOUS LABORATORY FINDINGS IN INTESTINAL DISEASE

Abnormal Laboratory Findings	Clinical Associations
Hematologic Findings	
Eosinophilia	Parasitism, eosinophilic enteritis, hypoadrenocorticism
Neutrophilia	Bowel inflammation, necrosis, or neoplasia
Neutropenia	Parvovirus, endotoxemia, or overwhelming sepsis (e.g., leakage peritonitis from bowel perforation)
Monocytosis	Chronic or granulomatous inflammation (e.g., mycosis)
Lymphopenia	Loss of lymphocytes from intestinal lymphangiectasia
Anemia	Enteric blood loss, depressed erythropoiesis from chronic inflammation or malnutrition
Elevated hematocrit	Hemoconcentration from GI fluid loss
RBC microcytosis	Iron deficiency from chronic GI blood loss, portosystemic shunt
RBC macrocytosis	RBC regeneration, feline hyperthyroidism, feline leukemia virus, nutritional deficiencies (rare)
Serum Biochemical Findings	
Panhypoproteinemia	Protein-losing enteropathy
Hyperglobulinemia	Chronic immune stimulation, basenji enteropathy
Azotemia	Dehydration, primary renal failure
Hypokalemia	GI loss of fluid and electrolytes, anorexia
Hyperkalemia/hyponatremia	Hypoadrenocorticism, trichuriasis (rare)
Hypocalcemia	Hypoalbuminemia, lymphangiectasia, pancreatitis
Hypocholesterolemia	Lymphangiectasia, liver disease
Elevated liver enzymes/ bile acids	Liver disease
Elevated amylase/lipase	Pancreatitis, mild elevations in enteritis or azotemia
Elevated thyroxine (T4)	Feline hyperthyroidism

GI = gastrointestinal; RBC = red blood cell.

- *Giardia*, the most important protozoan parasite, is best diagnosed by identification of cysts using a zinc sulfate centrifugation-flotation method. Motile trophozoites of protozoan parasites, including *Giardia* spp., *Trichomonas* spp., *Entamoeba histolytica*, and *Balantidium coli*, can be identified microscopically in a drop of fresh feces suspended in a few drops of isotonic saline. The distinguishing characteristics of each of these protozoa are discussed in the section Protozoan Infections of the Intestines in this chapter.
- Use Sheather sugar flotation method to identify small coccidia such as *Cryptosporidium* spp.
- Diagnosis of occult parasite infections (e.g., *Giardia*, whipworms) can be based on response to a therapeutic trial.

▼ *Key Point* Intestinal parasitism can mimic virtually any of the more complex small and large bowel dis-

orders, and in many areas parasites are the most frequent cause of diarrhea. The most important enteropathogens are hookworms, whipworms, and *Giardia*.

Fecal Examinations for Infectious Agents

The diagnosis of infectious diarrhea often depends on the detection of the offending viral, bacterial, or fungal organisms in the feces. Details of diagnosis of these various enteric infections are found in the respective sections of this chapter.

Viruses. Viral diarrhea generally is acute and is confirmed by identification of virus in the feces serologically or by electron microscopy (see Chap. 12).

Bacteria. Specific enteropathogenic bacteria such as *Salmonella*, *Campylobacter*, *Clostridium*, and *Yersinia* can be isolated from fresh feces using specialized culture media. Such cultures are indicated when:

- Examination of fecal cytology preparations reveals the presence of numerous fecal leukocytes, *Campylobacter*-like bacteria, or a predominance of *Clostridium* spp. (large, gram-positive endospore-forming rods)
- There is an outbreak of diarrhea in groups of animals
- Feces may be assayed for the diarrheogenic enterotoxins of *Clostridium perfringens* and *C. difficile*.

Fungi. The diagnosis of fungal (*Histoplasma*, *Aspergillus*, *Pythium*, *Candida*) and protothecal infection usually is based on identification of the organisms in fecal cytologies or intestinal biopsies.

- Sabouraud's agar can be used to culture feces for *Histoplasma*, other fungi, and *Prototheca* (a rare cause of colitis), but culture growth is slow (up to 2 weeks) and the isolation rate is low.
- Serodiagnostic tests for histoplasmosis also are available (see Chap. 18).

Fecal Examination Using Special Stains

Feces can be examined microscopically for abnormal constituents using stains such as direct and indirect Sudan, Lugol iodine, Gram, and various other cytologic stains. In each test, 1–2 drops of feces and 1–2 drops of stain are mixed well on a microscope slide, coverslipped, and examined. In general, these procedures are only appropriate as initial screening tests because they are relatively insensitive and nonspecific and are dependent on the diet.

Sudan Stain

- *Direct Sudan Staining* (Sudan III stain) identifies excessive undigested (unsplit) fat in the feces as numerous, large, refractile orange droplets, indicating steatorrhea due to pancreatic maldigestion.
- *Indirect Sudan Staining* (Sudan stain with 36% acetic acid and heating) identifies unabsorbed fatty acids (split fat) as well as undigested fat. Thus, numerous large orange lipid droplets on an indirect Sudan stain in an animal with a negative direct Sudan stain

Table 89–4. DIAGNOSIS OF INTESTINAL PATHOGENS OF DOGS AND CATS

Pathogen	Method of Diagnosis
Helminths	
Ascarids *(Toxocara, Toxascaris leonina)*	Routine fecal flotation for ova
Hookworms *(Ancylostoma)*	Routine fecal flotation for ova
Whipworms *(Trichuris vulpis)*	Routine fecal flotation for ova; Rx trial
Tapeworms *(Taenia, Dipylidium caninum)*	Fecal proglottids or flotation for ova
Strongyloides	Fecal sediment or Baermann test for larvae
Others (flukes)	Zinc sulfate fecal flotation for ova
Protozoa	
Coccidia *(Isospora, Cryptosporidium)*	Sheather fecal flotation for oocysts
Giardia	Zinc sulfate fecal flotation for cysts; fecal smear for trophozoites; fecal ELISA; Rx trial
Pentatrichomonas hominas	Saline fecal smear for trophozoites
Entamoeba histolytica	Saline fecal smear for trophozoites
Balantidium coli	Saline fecal smear for trophozoites
Viruses	
Parvovirus:	
Canine parvovirus	Fecal ELISA for viral antigen; EM
Feline panleukopenia virus	Signs, leukopenia
Coronavirus:	
Canine coronavirus	Fecal EM
Feline enteric coronavirus, FIP	Signs, serology, fecal EM, PCR, biopsies
Rotaviruses	Fecal EM
Astrovirus	Fecal EM
Others:	
Canine distemper virus	Signs
Retroviruses (FeLV, FIV)	Signs, serology
Rickettsia	
Salmon poisoning disease *(Neorickettsiae helminthoeca)*	Operculated trematode eggs in feces; rickettsia in lymph node cytology (Giemsa stain)
Bacteria	
Salmonella	Fecal culture
Campylobacter jejuni	Fecal microscopy and culture
Yersinia enterocolitica, Y. pseudotuberculosis	Fecal culture
Bacillus piliformis (Tyzzer)	Biopsy (gut, liver) for filamentous bacteria; mouse inoculation
Mycobacteria	Biopsy for acid-fast bacteria
Clostridium perfringens, C. difficile (?)	Fecal microscopy, culture and toxin assays
Enteropathogenic *E. coli* (?)	Fecal culture and toxin assays
Fungi	
Histoplasma capsulatum	Fungi in biopsies/cytologies; serology
Pythium, Zygomycetes	Poorly septate hyphae in biopsies
Others *(Candida albicans, Aspergillus)*	Yeast or hyphae in biopsies
Algae (Prototheca)	Unicellular algae in cytologies or biopsies; fecal culture (Sabouraud's)

Rx = therapeutic response; ELISA = enzyme-linked immunosorbent assay; EM = electron microscopy; FIP = feline infectious peritonitis; FeLV = feline leukemia virus; FIV = feline immunodeficiency virus; PCR, polymerase chain reaction test.

suggest steatorrhea due to intestinal malabsorption of fatty acids.

Lugol Iodine Stain (2%). This method identifies excessive undigested starch in the feces (amylorrhea) as dark blue-black granules or identifies light brown, undigested striated muscle fibers in meat-fed animals; either of these findings suggest maldigestion due to pancreatic maldigestion. *Giardia* trophozoites and cysts also stain light brown with iodine.

Cytology Stain. Cytology staining (e.g., new methylene blue, Wrights, Diff-Quik) identifies fecal leukocytes that appear in exudative inflammatory bowel diseases when there is disruption of distal intestinal or colonic mucosa. Cytology may occasionally identify neoplastic cells or *Histoplasma* or *Prototheca* organisms. It is advisable to follow up patients that are positive for fecal leukocytes with colonoscopy and fecal cultures for invasive bacteria such as *Campylobacter* and *Salmonella*.

Gram Stain. Gram staining identifies an overabundance of large, gram-positive endosporulating rods (*Clostridia*) or *Campylobacter*-like organisms.

Tests for Fecal Occult Blood

These include a simple, in-office qualitative screening test (Hemoccult Test) and a more accurate, semiquantitative send-out test (HemoQuant; SmithKline). These tests are sensitive for detecting even very small amounts of gastrointestinal hemorrhage. Because of this sensitivity, it is recommended to exclude meat from the animal's diet for at least 3 days prior to testing to avoid false positive results.

- The presence of fecal occult blood signifies a bleeding lesion of the GI tract, which suggests an ulcerative, inflammatory, or neoplastic condition.
- The fecal occult blood test is also indicated to document GI bleeding as a cause of blood loss anemia.

Quantitative Fecal Fat Analysis

This can be used as an intestinal function test to confirm steatorrhea, but it is extremely cumbersome and impractical to perform and does not differentiate pancreatic maldigestion from intestinal malabsorption. Feces must be collected for a 24- to 72-hour period while the animal is confined and fed a standard diet. The feces are weighed and sent to a commercial laboratory for analysis. Normally, less than 10% of ingested fat is excreted in the feces, or less than 0.3 g/kg/d in dogs and less than 0.4 g/kg/d in cats.

Tests for Fecal Proteolytic Activity

Fecal proteolytic activity can be assayed as an indicator of pancreatic secretion of proteases (trypsin) for the diagnosis of exocrine pancreatic insufficiency (EPI). The serum trypsin-like immunoreactivity (TLI) assay is more accurate and is preferred for diagnosis of EPI (see Chap. 93).

Tests to Document GI Protein Loss

For the documentation of protein-losing enteropathy, GI loss of plasma proteins can be measured using the fecal excretion of intravenously administered radiolabeled proteins and macromolecules, such as ^{51}chromium-labeled albumin. However, these radiolabeled substrates are difficult to obtain and the procedures are impractical for use in the clinical setting.

Tests of Digestive and Absorptive Function

Exocrine Pancreatic Function Tests

Tests for exocrine pancreatic insufficiency (pancreatic maldigestion), such as serum TLI, oral bentiromide (BT-PABA) digestion, and fecal assays for proteolytic activity are described in Chapter 93.

Quantitative Fecal Fat Analysis

See preceding discussion.

Xylose Absorption Test

The xylose absorption test is the standard test for evaluating canine intestinal absorptive function; however, it is relatively insensitive and does not help to differentiate the numerous small intestinal diseases capable of causing malabsorption.

- In normal dogs, following a 12-hour fast and oral administration of xylose (0.5 g/kg as a 5–10% solution), plasma xylose concentration peaks at 60 mg/dL in 60–120 minutes. Intestinal malabsorption is indicated by an abnormally low plasma xylose level.
- In cats, the xylose absorption test provides inconsistent results; thus, the test is difficult to interpret and not recommended.

Serum Folate and Cobalamin Assays

Serum levels of folate and cobalamin (vitamin B$_{12}$) reflect intestinal absorptive function and the status of the intestinal flora. Serum folate levels (normal, 6.5–11.5 µg/L) depend on the absorptive function of the jejunum, whereas serum levels of cobalamin (normal, 300–700 ng/L) depend on secretion of pancreatic intrinsic factor and absorption in the ileum.

- Serum folate may be decreased in enteropathies that impair absorption in the proximal small intestine.
- Serum cobalamin may be decreased in exocrine pancreatic insufficiency and enteropathies that impair absorption in the distal small intestine.
- The levels of both vitamins may be decreased in diseases that cause diffuse intestinal malabsorption.
- In small intestinal bacterial overgrowth, serum folate levels may actually be increased due to synthesis of folate by the overgrown bacteria, whereas cobalamin may be decreased because bacteria can utilize or bind the vitamin, making it unavailable for absorption.

Radiography and Ultrasonography

Plain Abdominal Radiography

Plain radiography is indicated for detection of intestinal masses or abnormal gas-fluid patterns when mechanical or obstructive disorders are suspected (intestinal mass, foreign body, intussusception).

Upper GI Barium Contrast Radiography

This is indicated when other tests fail to determine the cause of small bowel diarrhea or when intestinal obstruction is suspected (see Chap. 4). The study may help to detect obstructive lesions, stagnant loops, and neoplastic or inflammatory lesions that cause an irregular mucosal pattern or distortion of the bowel wall. In most cases, however, diarrhea involves microscopic or functional changes in the bowel that are not detected by barium radiography.

Barium Enema Contrast Radiography

This may be useful in selected cases of large bowel diarrhea for evaluating the colon and cecum for intussusceptions, neoplasms, polyps, strictures, inflammatory lesions, and colonic displacement or shortening. Colonoscopy is generally preferred over barium enema for evaluating the colon because it yields more definitive diagnostic information.

Abdominal Ultrasonography

Ultrasonography can define intestinal and other abdominal masses and evaluate the mesenteric lymph nodes, pancreas, liver, biliary tract, and prostate (see Chap. 4).

Endoscopy

▼ *Key Point* Endoscopic examination with mucosal biopsy is required for definitive diagnosis or accurate characterization of the disease in most cases of chronic intractable diarrhea in which extraintestinal, dietary, parasitic, and infectious causes have been excluded.

Upper GI Endoscopy

- Duodenoscopy with a flexible fiberoptic endoscope can be performed in the anesthetized animal for visual examination of the duodenum, for duodenal aspiration (for quantitative bacterial culture or detection of *Giardia*), and for directed forceps biopsy of the intestinal mucosa (see Chap. 87 for a description of endoscopic equipment and discussion of gastroscopy).
- The normal duodenal mucosa appears pale pink with a uniformly granular villus pattern. Biliary and pancreatic duct papillae and Peyer lymphoid patches are normally seen. The mucosa is nonfriable and free of excessive granularity, ulcers, thickened folds, masses, or strictures.

Colonoscopy

- Colonoscopy allows direct visualization of the lumen of the colon, sampling of luminal content for culture and exfoliative cytology, and directed forceps biopsy of the ileocolonic mucosa.
- Suitable rigid colonoscopes are relatively inexpensive and easy to use. Because colonic diseases are often diffuse, examination of the descending colon with a rigid instrument is sufficient for diagnosis in many patients.
- When lesions are located predominantly in the ascending or transverse colon, areas inaccessible with a rigid colonoscope, use a flexible fiberoptic colonoscope. A flexible colonoscope often can be navigated through the ileocolic sphincter for examination and biopsy of the ileum in some animals.
- The normal colonic mucosa appears pale pink through the colonoscope and reflects light uniformly. It is nonfriable, thin enough that the submucosal vessels are visible, and free of ulcers, thickened folds, masses, or strictures.

Intestinal Biopsy

The least invasive and, in many cases, preferred method for procurement of intestinal biopsies is endoscopy; if this is unavailable or if endoscopic biopsies are inconclusive, consider full-thickness intestinal biopsy by laparotomy (see Chap. 90).

- Obtain multiple biopsies along the length of the gut even if no lesions are visible by gross inspection, which is often the case.
- Biopsy mesenteric lymph nodes and evaluate other abdominal organs, especially the pancreas, liver, and colon.
- Duodenal aspirates or duodenal mucosal impression smears may be examined for *Giardia* or cultured quantitatively for aerobic and anaerobic bacterial overgrowth.

NONSPECIFIC SYMPTOMATIC TREATMENT OF DIARRHEA

Dietary, supportive, and symptomatic therapy often is beneficial in diarrhea, especially acute diarrhea. In severe acute diarrhea, rehydration therapy can be lifesaving.

Diet

Acute Diarrhea

The initial goal is to allow the GI tract to rest by restricting food intake for at least 24 hours.

- When resuming feeding give bland low-fat foods in small amounts at frequent intervals. Examples of appropriate foods include boiled rice, potatoes, and pasta as carbohydrate sources combined with boiled skinless chicken, yogurt, or low-fat cottage cheese as protein sources. Ready-made commercial gastrointestinal diets can also be used.
- When the diarrhea has been resolved for 48 hours, gradually reintroduce the animal's regular diet.

Chronic Diarrhea

Divide daily food intake into 3 to 4 feedings; use low-fat diets with high digestibility for small bowel diarrhea, hypoallergenic diets for idiopathic inflammatory bowel diseases, and high-fiber diets for large bowel diarrhea (refer to respective disease sections of this chapter).

Fluid Therapy

- In severe acute diarrhea, such as occurs with parvoviral enteritis, fluid and electrolyte replacement is essential for management of intestinal fluid loss that may lead to serious dehydration, shock, and death (see Chap. 5).
- Parenteral methods of fluid therapy are preferred in most cases; however, over-the-counter oral glucose-electrolyte solutions are available for counterbalancing intestinal fluid losses in cases of mild diarrhea.

Antidiarrheal Drugs

Symptomatic treatment is based on drugs that modify motility and fluid secretion/absorption or that act locally within the lumen as protectants/adsorbents. In most cases, these drugs are reserved for short-term use, usually for periods of 5 days or less. Some commonly used antidiarrheal drugs and their dosages are listed in Table 89–5.

Opiate and Opioid Narcotic Analgesics

These are probably the most effective all-purpose antidiarrheal agents.

- Mechanism:
  - They inhibit intestinal fluid loss through modification of mucosal fluid and electrolyte transport.
  - They impede bowel transit by stimulating nonpropulsive contractions (segmentation) and decreasing propulsive motility (peristalsis), thereby allowing more contact time for absorption.
- Examples include paregoric, diphenoxylate (Lomotil), and loperamide (Imodium).

Table 89–5. DRUGS USED FOR SYMPTOMATIC TREATMENT OF DIARRHEA

Drug	Product (Manufacturer)	Preparation	Dosage	Frequency
Narcotic Analgesics*				
Diphenoxylate	Lomotil (Searle)	Tab—2.5 mg; Liq—0.5 mg/ml	0.1–0.2 mg/kg	q6–8h
Loperamide	Imodium A-D (McNeil)	Cap—2 mg; Liq—0.2 mg/ml	0.1–0.2 mg/kg	q6–8h
Codeine	Many	Tab; Cap; Liq	0.25–0.5 mg/kg	q6–8h
Anticholinergics/Antispasmodics				
Aminopentamide	Centrine (Fort Dodge)	Tab—0.2 mg, Inj—0.5 mg/ml	0.01–0.03 mg/kg	q8–12h
Dicyclomine	Generic	Tab—20 mg, Cap—10 mg,	0.2 mg/kg	q8–12h
Propantheline	Generic	Tab—15 mg	0.25 mg/kg	q8–12h
Hyoscyamine	Levsin (Schwarz)	Tab—0.125 mg; Liq—0.025 mg/ml, 0.125 mg/ml	0.003–0.006 mg/kg	q8–12h
Antisecretory/Protectant				
Bismuth subsalicylate†	Pepto-Bismol (Procter & Gamble)	Liq—9 and 16 mg salicylate/ml	0.5–1.0 ml/kg	q6–8h

*Narcotic analgesics are not recommended for cases of bacterial enteritis or liver disease.
†Avoid long-term (>3 days) use in cats because of low tolerance for salicylates.
Tab = tablets; Cap = capsules; Liq = elixir, suspension, or drops; Inj = injectable; CNS = central nervous system.

Anticholinergic/Antispasmodic Drugs

- Mechanism:
  - They inhibit intestinal fluid loss, presumably through an antisecretory effect.
  - They cause a generalized suppression of gut motility that may potentiate ileus; however, their "atropine-like" antispasmodic action may be beneficial for controlling the urgency and discomfort of colitis.
- Examples include dicyclomine (Bentyl), iso-propamide (Darbazine), aminopentamide (Centrine), and propantheline (Pro-Banthine).

Prostaglandin Inhibitors

- These drugs have an anti-inflammatory/antisecretory action.
- They can be used for intraluminal delivery of antiprostaglandin to the proximal GI tract (bismuth subsalicylate [Pepto-Bismol]) and to the lower GI tract or colon (sulfasalazine [Azulfidine], olsalazine, [Dipentum], mesalamine [Asacol]) for treatment of chronic colitis (see Chronic Inflammatory Bowel Disease later in this chapter).
- Avoid use of systemic prostaglandin inhibitors (non-steroidal anti-inflammatory drugs) because they tend to cause gastric ulceration.

Protectant/Adsorbent Drugs

- These oral agents are postulated to work in the lumen to adsorb injurious bacteria and toxins and to provide a protective coating on inflamed mucosal surfaces.
- The efficacy of these drugs remains unproven; large doses are often required, and they may be difficult to administer.
- Examples include kaolin-pectin, bismuth, activated charcoal, and barium.

Antibiotic Therapy

- Do not use antibiotics routinely as empirical therapy in cases of uncomplicated diarrhea of undetermined cause because of their adverse effects on the normal intestinal flora and their tendency to promote resistant strains of bacteria.
- Antibiotics are indicated when specific bacterial or rickettsial enteropathogens, such as *Salmonella, Clostridium,* or *Campylobacter,* are suspected causes.
- Antibiotics are appropriate in conditions associated with severe mucosal damage and a high risk of secondary sepsis or endotoxemia (e.g., parvoviral enteritis and hemorrhagic gastroenteritis). Thus, indications for antibacterial therapy in the animal with acute GI disease include bloody diarrhea, fever, leukocytosis, leukopenia, fecal leukocytes, and shock.

DIETARY DIARRHEA

Etiology

- Diarrhea as a result of indiscriminant eating and chewing behavior is particularly common in dogs. Dietary indiscretions include overeating, ingestion of spoiled garbage or decomposing carrion, and ingestion of abrasive or indigestible foreign material (e.g., bones, stones, hair, plants, wood, cloth, carpeting, foil, plastic) that can traumatize the GI mucosa.
- Diarrhea may result from an abrupt change in diet. Any change in the composition of the diet should be made in gradual increments over a period of several days to allow for adaptation.
- Animals may be intolerant of certain foods, such as lactose ingested as milk, fatty foods, spicy foods, and food additives found in certain commercial diets. Food hypersensitivity to specific protein sources is implicated as a cause of inflammatory bowel disease in dogs and cats.

Diagnosis

Dietary causes of diarrhea usually are identified by careful history-taking and the response to a restricted diet.

- Carefully question the owner about all aspects of diet and environment, including recent changes in type and brand of food, all supplemental feeding practices using "people foods," patterns of chewing behavior involving nonfood items (including toys, plants, haircoat), likelihood of garbage ingestion, and potential for unobserved indiscretions in free-roaming animals.
- Examine the feces for abrasive particles.

Treatment

Dietary diarrhea is self-limiting with feeding of a restricted diet, elimination of identifiable offending substances from the diet, and prevention of indiscriminant eating or chewing behavior. Management of dietary hypersensitivity is discussed under Chronic Inflammatory Bowel Disease later in this chapter.

DRUG AND TOXIN-INDUCED DIARRHEA

Etiology

- Diarrhea is a frequent adverse side effect of many medications, including nonsteroidal anti-inflammatory agents (NSAIDs) (e.g., aspirin, ibuprofen, indomethacin, phenylbutazone, flunixin meglumine), digitalis and other cardiac drugs, dithiazanine (Dizan), magnesium-containing compounds, lactulose (for hepatic encephalopathy), some anthelmintics, most anticancer drugs, and many antibacterial drugs (partly from adverse effects on the flora).
- Dexamethasone has been associated with hemorrhagic gastroenterocolitis characterized by erosion, ulceration, necrosis, and sometimes fatal colonic perforation, especially in dogs treated for intervertebral disc disease.
- Many exogenous toxins cause diarrhea, including biologic toxins such as the enterotoxin that causes staphylococcal food poisoning and various diarrheogenic chemical poisons such as heavy metals (lead, arsenic, thallium), insecticides (organophosphate dips, flea treatments), lawn and garden products (insecticides, herbicides, fungicides), and some houseplants.
- Free-roaming animals may drink from stagnant or run-off water polluted or potentially contaminated with toxic industrial, petroleum, or agricultural chemicals.

Clinical Signs

- Many medications and most toxins that cause diarrhea also cause vomiting.
- Some toxicities are associated with various extraintestinal signs (e.g., neurologic manifestations of lead and organophosphate toxicity).

Diagnosis

Suspect drug and toxin-induced diarrhea on the basis of history of exposure (or opportunity for exposure), clinical signs, and exclusion of other causes of diarrhea.

Treatment

- Drug-induced diarrhea usually resolves after discontinuation of the offending medication or a reduction in its dosage.
- Toxin-induced diarrhea resolves with symptomatic antidiarrheal therapy, prevention of further exposure to the toxin, and gradual elimination of the substance from the body. However, if the exact toxin is known, consult other sources of information for additional specific treatments and antidotes.

METAZOAN PARASITES OF THE INTESTINES

The majority of intestinal parasite infections are asymptomatic: when clinical signs do occur, diarrhea and weight loss are most common. Young growing animals generally are more frequently and severely parasitized, but never overlook endoparasitism as a possible cause of acute or chronic diarrhea of either the small or large bowel type in dogs and cats of all ages. Other intestinal diseases, such as viral or bacterial enteritis, often are complicated by intestinal parasite infection.

The diagnosis of parasitism depends on the identification of eggs, cysts, larvae, trophozoites, or proglottids in the feces (see Table 89–4). Parasites that are notorious for evading detection include *Giardia* in dogs and cats with small bowel diarrhea, and whipworms in dogs with large bowel diarrhea. In such cases, response to a therapeutic trial is an indirect method of diagnosis. Anthelmintics used to treat the common parasites are listed in Table 89–6.

Ascarids
Etiology

Ascarid nematodes are the most prevalent parasites of dogs and cats worldwide. The ascarids of the dog are *Toxocara canis* and the less common *Toxascaris leonina;* those in the cat are *Toxocara cati* and *T. leonina.*

Life Cycle

- Ascarid infection occurs by four routes:
  - Prenatal infection as a result of transplacental migration, which occurs only with *T. canis*
  - Milk-borne infection as a result of transmammary migration, which occurs with both *T. canis* and *T. cati*
  - Infection by ingestion of infective eggs, which occurs with all three ascarids (*T. canis, T. cati,* and *T. leonina*)
  - Infection by ingestion of a paratenic (transport) host (*T. canis, T. cati*) or intermediate host (*T. leonina*)

Table 89–6. ANTHELMINTICS FOR DOGS AND CATS

Drug	Product (Manufacturer)	Dosage	Efficacy			
			Ascarids	Hook-worms	Whip-worms	Tape-worms
Dichlorophene/toluene	Many products	Dog—capsule size as directed	++	++	−	+
Dichlorvos*	Performer (Performer)	Dog—27–33 mg/kg; cat & pups—11 mg/kg PO	++	++	++	−
Diethylcarbamazine (DEC)† plus	Many products	Dog—6.6 mg/kg daily or 110 mg/kg once PO	++	−	−	−
oxibendazole (OXI)†	Filarabits Plus (Pfizer)	Dog—6.6 mg/kg DEC & 5 mg/kg OXI daily PO	++	++	+	−
Epsiprantel	Cestex (Pfizer)	Dog—5.5 mg/kg PO; Cat—2.75 mg/kg PO	−	−	−	+++
Febantel (FEB) plus praziquantel (PRA)	RM-Parasitacide (Merial)	Dog/Cat—15 mg/kg FEB & 1.5 mg/kg PRA PO for 3 days	+++	+++	+++	+++
Febantel (FEB) plus praziquantel and pyrantel	Drontal-Plus (Bayer)	Dog/Cat—15 mg/kg (FEB)	+++	+++	+++	+++
Fenbendazole	Panacur (Hoescht-Roussel)	Dog/Cat—50 mg/kg PO for 3–5 days	+++	+++	+++	++‡
Ivermectin*†§	Heartgard Plus (Merial)	Dog—6 mcg/kg PO monthly	++	++	−	−
Milbemycin oxime†	Interceptor (Ciba-Geigy)	Dog—0.5 mg/kg PO monthly	++	++	++	−
Piperazine	Many products	Dog/Cat—110 mg/kg PO	++	−	−	−
Praziquantel	Droncit (Bayer)	Dog/Cat—See label; PO, SC, IM	−	−	−	+++
Pyrantel pamoate	Nemex (Pfizer)	Dog/Cat—10 mg/kg PO if <2.5 kg; 5 mg/kg PO if >2.5 kg	+++	+++	−	−

*Consult package insert because of special safety precautions or potential for serious side effects.
†Drugs used concomitantly as heartworm preventatives (see Chap. 68).
‡Efficacious for *Taenia* spp. of tapeworms only; not effective against *Dipylidium caninum*.

- Nearly all puppies are born infected with ascarids because of transplacental migration of the bitch's somatic *T. canis* larvae into the fetus (prenatal infection).
- Milk-borne infection during nursing is the major source of ascariasis in kittens.
- Three types of migration patterns occur when an animal is infected:
  - Liver-lung migration *(T. canis, T. cati)*
  - Migration within the wall of the GI tract (all three ascarids)
  - Somatic tissue migration *(T. canis, T. cati)*

Clinical Signs

- Signs of ascariasis occur most often in young puppies and kittens, in which the adult worms in the small intestine may cause abdominal discomfort, whimpering and groaning, potbellied appearance, dull haircoat, unthriftiness, stunted growth, and diarrhea. Worms frequently are passed in vomitus or diarrhea.
- Rarely, large tangled masses of worms occlude the lumen in young pups and cause death from intestinal obstruction, intussusception, or intestinal perforation.
- In the neonatal pup, the migration of large numbers of *T. canis* larvae through the lungs can cause severe damage and fatal pneumonia.
- In young animals with light infections and in adults, infection is most commonly asymptomatic, or evidenced merely by a loss of body condition.

Diagnosis

- The diagnosis of ascariasis is readily established by the identification of ascarid eggs in routine fecal flotation.
- Most pups begin passing large numbers of eggs in their feces at about 3 weeks of age and continue to shed eggs for most of early puppyhood (4–6 months) until treated.

Treatment

- Numerous effective anthelmintics for ascarids are available (see Table 89–6). Pyrantel pamoate is well tolerated in puppies and kittens and also is effective in controlling hookworms.
- Because most pups are born infected with *T. canis*, treatment is recommended at 2 weeks of age, before eggs are first passed in the feces, and repeated at 4, 6, and 8 weeks to kill all worms derived from prenatal, milk-borne, and ingestion routes of infection.
- Toxocaral visceral larva migrans (VLM) is a serious disease of humans (especially children) produced by the invasion of visceral tissues by migrating *T. canis;* thus, infected pups are considered public health hazards.

Hookworms

Etiology

- *Ancylostoma caninum*, the most common hookworm in the dog, is a voracious bloodsucker.

- *A. tubaeforme,* the common hookworm in the cat, is more of a tissue feeder than a bloodsucker and is far less pathogenic than *A. caninum* in dogs.
- *A. braziliense* (southern United States) and *Uncinaria stenocephala* (Canada) affect both dogs and cats but are less common than *A. caninum* and *A. tubaeforme* and are only mildly pathogenic.

Life Cycle

Hookworm infection can occur by five routes: prenatal, milk-borne, ingestion of infective larvae (L3), skin penetration by infective larvae, and ingestion of paratenic hosts. Ingestion and cutaneous migration probably are the most common routes of infection. With all routes of infection, eggs are passed in feces after 2–3 weeks.

Clinical Signs

Pathogenicity is directly related to the hookworm's bloodsucking activity and capacity for causing intestinal blood loss. Hookworms embed their mouthparts in the mucosa to suck blood and tissue fluid, leaving bleeding, punctiform ulcers as they "graze." Hence, an important consequence of severe hookworm infection is blood loss anemia.

- The clinical signs of ancylostomiasis include tarry (melena) or bloody diarrhea accompanied by pallor, weakness, emaciation, and dehydration.
- Rapidly progressive blood loss anemia may result in acute death of neonates. In other animals, chronic blood loss may cause iron deficiency anemia characterized by erythrocytes that show hypochromasia and microcytosis.
- Acute, pruritic dermatitis occasionally is associated with the active penetration of skin by hookworm larvae.
- Hookworm infections in mature animals often are asymptomatic.

Diagnosis

Young dogs are most often affected, and the diagnosis usually is readily established by identification of the characteristic strongyloid hookworm ova by routine fecal flotation. Ancylostomiasis often is associated with eosinophilia on the CBC.

Treatment

Anthelmintics effective for eradicating hookworms include pyrantel pamoate (safest for young animals), fenbendazole, febantel, butamisole HCl, mebendazole, and dichlorvos (see Table 89–6 for product names and dosages).

- In areas in which *A. caninum* is a frequent problem, routinely treat bitches and pups. Because of prenatal and milk-borne infection, initiate treatment of pups at 2 weeks of age, along with treatment for *T. canis.*

▼ *Key Point* Pyrantel pamoate suspension is an excellent anthelmintic for nursing pups because it is safe and active against both hookworms and ascarids.

- Severely anemic animals should receive whole blood transfusions, iron supplementation, and supportive therapy.

Prevention

- Parasite control is aided by good sanitation and impervious flooring in kennels and dog runs.
- Various commercial products have a combined effect as preventive agents against both heartworms and hookworms (e.g., oxibendazole and milbemycin; see Table 89–6).

Whipworms

Etiology

The canine whipworm, *Trichuris vulpis,* is a common cause of large bowel diarrhea in dogs in many areas. The adult nematode has a predilection for the proximal colon and cecum, where its distinctive threadlike head end, or "whip," firmly embeds deep within the mucosa to feed on blood and tissue fluids, thereby causing colitis and typhlitis.

The feline whipworms, *T. campanula* and *T. serrata,* are rare and usually are not associated with clinical signs.

Life Cycle

- Whipworm infections occur by ingestion of infective ova, and the life cycle is direct.
- The prepatent period is approximately 3 months. Ova may survive and remain infectious in the environment for 4–5 years; hence, contaminated ground is probably the major reservoir of infection.

Clinical Signs

- Whipworms infect dogs of all ages. Although there may be minimal clinical signs in light infestations, trichuriasis frequently causes acute, chronic, or intermittent signs of mucoid large bowel–type diarrhea with urgency and sometimes hematochezia.
- Pseudohypoadrenocorticism, characterized by hyperkalemia and hyponatremia in the presence of normal adrenal function, has been associated with severe whipworm diarrhea in several dogs.

Diagnosis

- Definitive diagnosis of whipworm infection requires identification of the characteristic brown, bipolar-operculated football-shaped ova by routine fecal flotation.
- Repeated fecal examinations may be necessary to identify ova because of the unusually long prepatent period and because it is not uncommon for active infection to be characterized by prolonged periods when ova are not shed in the feces.

- Alternative means of diagnosis of ova-negative, or so-called occult, infections, include:
  - Colonoscopic observation of adult whipworms in the bowel lumen
  - Resolution of signs in response to a therapeutic trial of an effective anthelmintic

Treatment

- Give fenbendazole (Panacur) or febantel (Rintal or Vercom) for 3 days (see Table 89–6). In refractory cases, a 5-day course is recommended. Routinely repeat treatment at 3 weeks and 3 months, because whipworms are difficult to eradicate.
- Other whipcidal anthelmintics include mebendazole (Telmintic), butamisole (Styquin), and dichlorvos (Task), but these drugs have less efficacy and greater toxicity (see Table 89–6) or are discontinued.
- Rarely, trichuriasis has been associated with severe transmural granulomatous typhlitis that may be palpable as a tender right-midabdominal mass. This lesion may be refractory to anthelmintics and require typhlectomy.

Prevention

- Because it is virtually impossible to eradicate the parasite from infected ground, frequent reinfection is a common problem. For this reason, collect and properly dispose of feces whenever possible.
- In dogs with frequent access to ground that has been heavily contaminated with whipworm ova (a common situation in many public parks and backyards), reinfection is so frequent that retreatment every 2–3 months may be necessary.
- Disinfect concrete runs with dilute sodium hypochlorite bleach.

Strongyloides spp.
Etiology

Strongyloides spp. are tiny (2 mm) rhabdoid nematodes found in warm, humid tropical regions such as the southern Gulf states of the United States.

- In dogs, strongyloidiasis is caused by *S. stercoralis,* a parasite that burrows in the mucosa of the proximal small bowel.
- In cats, strongyloidiasis is caused by *S. tumefaciens,* a parasite that burrows within the mucosa of the large intestine.

Life Cycle

- Infection with third-stage larvae is by the oral or cutaneous route, and adult worms develop in the small intestine following migration in the circulation and lung.
- Parthenogenetic female adults produce eggs that hatch within the gut lumen, so that first-stage (rhabdoid) larvae are passed in the feces. These larvae may develop into infectious third-stage (filariform) larvae or free-living adults.

Clinical Signs

- *S. stercoralis* is mainly a problem in pups, in which it causes acute hemorrhagic enteritis that is often fatal.
- *S. tumefaciens* infection in cats is usually asymptomatic, but in some cats the parasite causes peculiar tumor-like white nodular (2–3 mm) proliferations in the colonic mucosa and submucosa that are associated with chronic diarrhea and debilitation.

Diagnosis

- Ova containing first-stage *Strongyloides* larvae can be identified in feces by flotation techniques. Free larvae (0.8–1.6 mm long × 30–80 μm) may be identified by direct microscopic examination of fresh feces or by the Baermann technique.
- In cats, the diagnosis of *S. tumefaciens* also can be established by colonoscopic observation and biopsy of mucosal nodules filled with adult worms.

Treatment

Treat with fenbendazole (50 mg/kg/day PO for 5 days), diethylcarbamazine (100 mg/kg PO once), or pyrantel pamoate (20 mg/kg/day PO for 5 days).

Tapeworms
Etiology

- The most common tapeworm (cestode) of dogs and cats is *Dipylidium caninum.* Fleas and lice are intermediate hosts.
- Several species of *Taenia* can be acquired by dogs and cats (most commonly *T. pisiformis* in the dog, *T. taeniaeformis* in the cat) from ingestion of cysticercus-infected tissues from intermediate hosts (e.g., rabbits, rodents, sheep, and ungulates).
- Other cestodes that rarely cause infection include *Echinococcus, Multiceps, Mesocestoides,* and *Spirometra.*

Clinical Signs

- Tapeworms that parasitize the small bowel of dogs and cats are relatively harmless, rarely causing more than a subtle decline in body condition.
- The proglottids of *D. caninum* are highly motile and may cause anal pruritus as they crawl on the perineum; crawling proglottids are often detected by observant owners in the animal's stool or on the perineum.

Diagnosis

- Tapeworms are diagnosed by the identification of proglottids or ova in feces.
- *D. caninum* proglottids are distinguished from *Taenia* spp. by their barrel shape and double genital pore. Also, a proglottid can be squashed in a drop of water between a slide and coverslip to identify the characteristic *D. caninum* egg capsules that contain up to 20 eggs.

Treatment

- Praziquantel and epsiquantel are the most effective all-around drugs for treatment of cestodiasis (see Table 89–6).
- Mebendazole and fenbendazole are effective against *Taenia* spp. but not *Dipylidium caninum*.
- Flea and lice control is important for preventing *D. caninum* reinfection; control of predation and scavenging helps prevent infection with other cestodes.

PROTOZOAN PARASITES OF THE INTESTINES

Coccidia

Etiology

Canine and feline intestinal coccidia are protozoan parasites that belong to the genera *Isospora*, *Besnoitia*, *Hammondia*, *Sarcocystis*, *Neosporum*, *Toxoplasma*, and *Cryptosporidium*. Most enteric coccidial infections of dogs and cats are commensal and nonpathogenic.

- Primary enteric disease in small animals has been described only with *Isospora* and *Cryptosporidium*.
- *T. gondii* and *N. canis* cause multisystemic infection and are discussed in Chapter 19.
- *Isospora* spp. that infect dogs include *I. canis*, *I. ohioensis*, *I. burrowsi*, and *I. neorivolta*; *I. felis* and *I. rivolta* infect cats.

Life Cycle

- Infection occurs most commonly by ingestion of infective (sporulated) oocysts from a feces-contaminated environment.
- Infection occurs occasionally from ingestion of infective cyst-containing tissues of paratenic (transport) hosts such as rodents and other prey and ingestion of uncooked meat of herbivores.

Clinical Signs

- Coccidiosis in most animals is an asymptomatic, incidental infection.
- *Coccidia* are opportunists and clinical disease is usually related to massive oocyst ingestion in newborn animals and is associated with overcrowded, unsanitary, high-stress conditions in settings such as pet shops, kennels, pounds, catteries, and laboratory colonies. Concurrent disease, malnutrition, or immunosuppression are predisposing factors.
- Clinical disease usually is characterized by diarrhea that varies from soft to fluid and is occasionally mucoid or bloody. Other signs can include vomiting, lethargy, weight loss, and dehydration. *Isospora* spp. occasionally have been associated with chronic malabsorption.

Diagnosis

- Coccidiosis is diagnosed by the identification of oocysts in fresh feces.

- Because many normal dogs and cats harbor intestinal coccidia and these protozoa are generally regarded as minimally pathogenic, the clinical significance of finding coccidial oocysts often is questionable.
- *Cryptosporidium* oocysts can be isolated for identification from feces using concentration techniques such as Sheather's sugar flotation or formol-ether sedimentation, or by staining of feces with Kinyouin's carbol fuchsin stain or modified acid fast stain. Cryptosporidia oocysts are so small (as little as one-tenth the size of common *Isospora* oocysts) that careful examination of slides under oil immersion is necessary to visualize these tiny structures. Histologic or electron microscopic identification of *Cryptosporidium* in intestinal biopsies is another means of diagnosis.

Treatment

Identification of oocysts in a healthy animal with normal feces indicates a self-limiting commensal infection and does not necessarily warrant treatment, although treatment may help to reduce environmental contamination with oocysts.

If clinical signs are attributed to coccidiosis, as in young puppies and kittens with diarrhea, treat with one of the following coccidiostats:

- Sulfadimethoxine—50–60 mg/kg/day PO for 1–3 weeks
- Trimethoprim-sulfa—15–30 mg/kg q12–24h PO for 1 week
- Furazolidone—8–20 mg/kg/day PO for 1 week
- Amprolium (unapproved for use in dogs but often recommended for treating animals in kennels or other groups of dogs)—20% powder in gelatin capsules, 100 mg q24h for small-breed pups or 200 mg q24h for larger-breed pups, PO for 7–12 days; alternatively, ¼ tsp 20% powder per 4 pups mixed with puppy ration, or 1 ounce (30 ml) of 9.6%, solution per gallon of free-choice water

Treatment of Cryptosporidiosis

Cryptosporidiosis is generally self-limiting in immunocompetent hosts. The infection may be persistent in severely immunocompromised animals or humans. Spiramycin or a combination of quinine and clindamycin have been used to treat humans, but there is limited information on their use in cats. One infected cat with chronic diarrhea was unresponsive to clindamycin but responded to tylosin. Other suggested treatments include paromomycin (125–165 mg/kg PO q12h for 5 days), and azithromycin (7–15 mg/kg PO q12h for 5–7 days). Because *Cryptosporidium* are not species specific, zoonotic transmission between animals and humans can occur, sometimes with fatal consequences in the presence of severe immunosuppression. Case studies have implicated pets as a source of human infection.

Giardia spp.

Giardia spp. are pear-shaped, binucleated, flagellated protozoa that infect the small intestine, interfere with mucosal absorption, and sometimes produce diarrhea. There are two forms: motile trophozoites and non-motile infective cysts.

Life Cycle

The life cycle of *Giardia* is direct, and the usual source of infection is the ingestion of food or water contaminated with cysts. Wild animals are potential reservoirs.

Clinical Signs

- The majority of *Giardia* infections are subclinical, especially in mature animals.
- Clinically apparent giardiasis occurs most frequently in young dogs and cats and is characterized by intestinal malabsorption with large volumes of foul-smelling, light-colored, watery or "cow patty-like" diarrhea, steatorrhea, and weight loss. Diarrhea may be acute or chronic, intermittent or continuous, and self-limiting or persistent.
- The severity of giardiasis is enhanced by concomitant viral, bacterial, or helminth infections.

Diagnosis

- Definitive diagnosis of giardiasis depends on identification of cysts (oval; 8–12 μm × 7–10 μm) by zinc sulfate centrifugation-flotation of feces or of motile flagellated trophozoites (pear-shaped; 9–21 μm × 5–15 μm × 2–4 μm) in fresh diarrheic feces suspended in saline or in duodenal specimens (aspirates, brushings, or impression smears of mucosal biopsies).
- Negative fecal examinations do not exclude a diagnosis of giardiasis. When fecal examinations are negative, "occult" giardiasis may be diagnosed indirectly by the response to a therapeutic trial of an antigiardial drug such as fenbendazole or metronidazole.
- New methods of detecting *Giardia* by enzyme-linked immunosorbent assay (ELISA) and immunofluorescent antibody (IFA) techniques are becoming more available.

Treatment

Drugs currently available in the United States that are effective in the treatment of giardiasis include metronidazole, fenbendazole, albendazole, quinicrine, and furazolidone.

- Metronidazole (Flagyl; Searle) (25–30 mg/kg q12h PO for 5–10 days) usually is effective with minimal side effects, although up to one-third of infections may be metronidazole-resistant.
- Fenbendazole (Panacur) (50 mg/kg q24hr PO for 3 days) is very safe and effective for treating Giardia in dogs and probably cats.
- Albendazole (Valbazen) (25 mg/kg q12h PO for 5 days in cats and 2 days in dogs) is effective but has been associated with severe bone marrow toxicity. For this reason, fenbendazole is preferred.
- Furazolidone (Furoxone; SmithKline) (4 mg/kg q12h PO for 5 days) is effective and convenient for cats, as it is available in a suspension form.

Trichomonads

Pentatrichomonas hominas organisms are motile, pear-shaped, flagellated protozoa that inhabit the colon of dogs and cats. Trichomonads have been found in both normal and diarrheic feces, but pathogenicity is unproven.

Diagnosis

The diagnosis of trichomoniasis is based on identification in saline fecal smears of motile, pear-shaped, flagellated trophozoites with the characteristic wavelike motion of an undulating membrane and a constant erratic turning and rolling motion.

Treatment

Metronidazole (25–30 mg/kg q12h PO for 5 days) is an effective treatment.

Entamoeba spp.

E. histolytica, primarily a human pathogen, rarely may cause amebic colitis (bloody-mucoid diarrhea) in dogs and cats that drink polluted water.

Diagnosis

Diagnosis is based on identification of ameboid trophozoites with pseudopodial movement in saline smears of fresh diarrheic feces; amebic cysts in zinc sulfate flotation of formed feces; or trophozoites in colon biopsies.

Treatment

Amebic colitis responds to metronidazole (25–30 mg/kg q12h PO for 5–10 days) or furazolidone (2.2 mg/kg q8h PO for 7 days).

Balantidium spp.

B. coli, a ciliated protozoan that primarily infects swine, is a rare cause of chronic ulcerative colitis in dogs.

Diagnosis

Diagnosis is based on identification of large (40–80 μm × 25–45 μm), oval, brown, rapidly swimming ciliated trophozoites with prominent macronuclei in saline suspensions of fresh feces or identification of protozoal cysts in zinc sulfate or sedimentation preparations of feces.

Treatment

Metronidazole (25–30 mg/kg q12h PO for 5–10 days) is effective.

VIRAL INFECTIONS OF THE INTESTINES

Canine Intestinal Viruses

- Canine parvovirus, canine coronavirus, and rotavirus cause viral enteritis and diarrhea in dogs. Canine parvovirus is an acute, severe, highly contagious enteritis that is prevalent worldwide. Coronavirus and rotavirus are less prevalent and cause relatively mild clinical signs except in neonates. For details concerning intestinal viruses, see Chapter 12.

- Because of its epitheliotropism, canine distemper virus also causes diarrhea (Chap. 11).

Feline Intestinal Viruses

- The most clinically important primary enteric virus is feline panleukopenia virus (FPV), a parvovirus. Other feline intestinal viruses include enteric coronavirus, rotavirus, and astrovirus (see Chap. 12).
- The intestine may be involved as part of generalized viral infections such as feline leukemia virus (FeLV; see Chap. 6), feline immunodeficiency virus (FIV; see Chap. 7) and feline infectious peritonitis (FIP), a coronavirus (see Chap. 8).

BACTERIAL INFECTIONS OF THE INTESTINES

Most enteropathogenic bacteria produce intestinal disease by invading the epithelium (invasive bacteria) or by remaining attached to the mucosal surface without penetrating it and liberating a diarrheogenic enterotoxin (noninvasive or enterotoxigenic bacteria).

Enteropathogenic bacteria of clinical importance include *Salmonella* spp., *Campylobacter jejuni*, and *Clostridium* spp. (*Yersinia* spp. and *Bacillus piliformis* are rare and are not discussed here.) These bacteria primarily invade the colon and distal small bowel, causing mucosal damage that leads to inflammation, exudation, mucus secretion, and bleeding. Thus, typical signs of large bowel diarrhea and hematochezia are characteristic of these infections. Bacterial enterotoxins may also play a role in the pathogenesis of diarrhea.

▼ *Key Point* Because *Salmonella, Campylobacter,* and *Yersinia* also are human pathogens, pets occasionally are reservoirs for human infection.

Salmonella
Etiology

- Salmonellosis is caused by gram-negative bacilli belonging to the genus *Salmonella* of the family Enterobacteriaceae. *Salmonella* spp. frequently are isolated from the feces of normal dogs and cats, but clinical signs of salmonellosis are uncommon, indicating a prevalent asymptomatic carrier state.
- *Salmonella* infection is transmitted by the feco-oral route, mainly through ingestion of contaminated food or water. The organisms can survive in the environment for long periods outside the host; thus, fomite transmission also can occur.
- Infection risk depends on infectivity of the strain, size of the inoculum, competition from the established flora, age of the host, and host defense factors. Infection rates are greatest in young animals and in group confinement situations with overcrowding and poor sanitation.

Clinical Signs

Manifestations of *Salmonella* infection may be categorized into three syndromes: the subclinical carrier state, enterocolitis, and enterocolitis with bacteremia.

- Clinical salmonellosis is relatively uncommon compared with the prevalence of the subclinical carrier state.
- *Salmonella* enterocolitis is characterized by acute watery or mucoid diarrhea (containing blood in severe cases), vomiting, tenesmus, fever, anorexia, lethargy, abdominal pain, and dehydration. Most animals recover in 3–4 weeks, although shedding of organisms often persists for up to 6 weeks, and sometimes longer.
- *Salmonella* can cause chronic or intermittent diarrhea in some animals.
- Rarely, *Salmonella* enterocolitis progresses to a potentially fatal bacteremia or endotoxemia with signs of endotoxic shock and disseminated intravascular coagulation (DIC).

Diagnosis

- Suspect the salmonellosis in animals that develop acute diarrhea and have identifiable risk factors, such as known or probable exposure, young age, immune deficiency, debilitating illness, or housing in overcrowded or unsanitary conditions.
- Nosocomial outbreaks with high morbidity and mortality have been recorded in hospitalized animals, the greatest risk occurring in animals:
  - With severe illness
  - Undergoing major surgery
  - Hospitalized for 5 or more days
  - Receiving glucocorticosteroids, anticancer chemotherapy, or oral antibiotics (especially ampicillin) that upset the normal flora
- Routine diagnostic tests usually are noncontributory, except that a degenerative neutropenia may be found in severe cases with bacteremia and endotoxemia.
- Confirmation of the diagnosis depends on isolation of *Salmonella* spp. from properly cultured fecal specimens or from blood cultures in bacteremic animals.

Treatment

The use of antibiotics in the treatment of salmonellosis is controversial. *Salmonella* invasion that is confined locally to the mucosa produces enterocolitis that is self-limiting and is not likely to be affected by antibiotics.

▼ *Key Point* Antibacterial therapy, especially oral nonabsorbable antibiotics that alter the flora, may actually prolong shedding of *Salmonella* organisms and encourage development of a prolonged convalescent carrier state.

Antibiotics are indicated when *Salmonella* invasion becomes severe or complicated by bacteremia and endotoxemia, as indicated by signs such as shock, dehydration, high fever or hypothermia, and extreme depression; or by laboratory findings such as azotemia, electrolyte imbalances, neutropenia, hypoglycemia, hypoproteinemia, or coagulopathy. Peracute onset and severe hematochezia may also be an indication of impending systemic invasion and should prompt antibiotic therapy.

- Base antibiotic selection on culture and sensitivity testing. Most isolates are susceptible to enrofloxacin (Baytril; Bayer) (5 mg/kg q12h PO) or trimethoprim-sulfa (15 mg/kg q12h PO). Administer antibiotics for 7–10 days and reculture feces 1 and 4 weeks after treatment.
- In addition to antibiotics, fluid and electrolyte replacement and identification and correction of underlying predisposing conditions are important aspects of therapy.
- Proper hygiene in handling of infected animals is necessary to prevent feco-oral or fomite transmission of infection to other animals or to humans.

Prognosis

The prognosis for most animals with salmonellosis is good, although the mortality rate can be high in outbreaks in extremely susceptible populations (e.g., hospital patients, neonates).

Campylobacter spp.

C. jejuni organisms are fastidious, microaerophilic, gram-negative, motile, slender curved bacteria that are important pathogens of animals and humans worldwide.

Etiology

Many clinically normal dogs and cats shed *Campylobacter* in their feces. Isolation rates vary widely, from less than 1% in confined pet populations to 50% or more in some animal pounds and shelters. Thus, conditions of close confinement and poor sanitation apparently provide the greatest opportunity for exposure.

Clinical Signs

Because it is difficult to produce enteritis with *Campylobacter* experimentally in dogs and cats and because many of the animals that harbor these organisms are asymptomatic, it has been debated whether *Campylobacter* by itself causes diarrhea in dogs and cats unless superimposed on other enteropathogenic infections with viruses, other bacteria, *Giardia,* or helminths.

- Clinical signs associated with *Campylobacter* infection in dogs and cats have been attributed to superficial erosive enterocolitis or enterotoxin-mediated secretory diarrhea and are characterized by watery-mucoid diarrhea lasting 5–15 days that occasionally contains blood and may be accompanied by vomiting or tenesmus.
- Fever is usually mild or absent.
- In some animals the diarrhea appears to be chronic or intermittent.

Diagnosis

- *Presumptive* diagnosis of campylobacteriosis can be made by fecal microscopy; however, this requires an experienced examiner, because spirochetes and

other motile bacteria that are part of the normal flora may be mistaken for *Campylobacter.* The presence of fecal leukocytes may also be noted.

▼ *Key Point* *Campylobacter* are identified as slender curved gram-negative rods that are characteristically W-shaped in stained fecal smears and as highly motile, darting, spiral, or S-shaped bacteria in fresh saline fecal smears examined by dark-field or phase-contrast microscopy.

- *Definitive* diagnosis requires isolation of *Campylobacter* from fresh feces using special selective media. Since *Campylobacter* organisms are microaerophilic and difficult to isolate, obtain fecal specimens directly from the rectum and culture or place in transport media immediately after collection.

Treatment

- The antibiotic of choice is erythromycin (10–15 mg/kg q8h PO for 7 days). Anorexia and vomiting are frequent side effects.
- Other effective oral antibiotics include neomycin (10 mg/kg q8h PO), enrofloxacin (Baytril, Bayer) (5 mg/kg q12h PO), chloramphenicol, furazolidone, and doxycycline.
- Antibiotics are rapidly effective for eliminating fecal shedding of the organisms. Repeat fecal cultures 1 and 4 weeks after treatment.
- Because contact with feces from infected animals is a potential source of infection for humans as well as other animals, advise owners of infected pets to take standard precautions such as proper disposal of potentially infectious feces, hand washing after handling infected animals, and separating infected animals from infants and small children until post-treatment cultures confirm that infection has been eliminated.

Prognosis

The prognosis is considered good, although rare fatalities in dogs and cats have been reported.

Clostridia
Etiology

- *Clostridium perfringens* is part of the normal anaerobic intestinal microflora in dogs and cats. These toxin-producing bacteria may be involved in acute and chronic diarrhea.
- *C. difficile* causes severe pseudomembranous colitis in humans, usually subsequent to antimicrobial suppression of the normal flora. Toxigenic *C. difficile* and its toxin have been isolated from normal dogs and cats and from a few dogs with chronic diarrhea, but the significance of this organism as a pathogen in dogs and cats remains to be established.

Clinical Signs

Clostridia have been associated with canine hemorrhagic gastroenteritis (see subsequent section), acute necrotizing hemorrhagic enterocolitis, acute nosocomial diarrhea, and chronic diarrhea, but the evidence implicating these bacteria as primary pathogens is only circumstantial.

- Clostridial diarrhea is watery or soft, with or without mucus, blood, and tenesmus.
- Onset is usually acute, although chronic and recurrent diarrhea have been attributed to *C. perfringens* in some animals.

Diagnosis

- Presumptive diagnosis of *C. perfringens* infection is based on identification of fecal leukocytes and predominance of large gram-positive rods with endospores by fecal cytology. Greater than 2–3 spores (identified on Diff-Quik or Wright staining by their "safety-pin" appearance) per high-power oil immersion field is considered abnormal.
- Definitive diagnosis is based on detection of enterotoxin by fecal assay.
- Diagnosis of *C. difficile* infection is based on a positive fecal assay for *C. difficile* toxin.

Treatment

Standard dosages of amoxicillin, ampicillin, metronidazole, tylosin, tetracycline, or chloramphenicol for 5–7 days are effective for treating *C. perfringens* infection. Most cases are self-limiting or responsive to antibiotics in 2–3 days; however, fatalities have been reported. Chronic *C. perfringens* diarrhea may require long-term treatment with antibiotics to prevent recurrences. *C. difficile* is susceptible to metronidazole, tetracycline, or vancomycin.

FUNGAL INFECTIONS OF THE INTESTINES

Mycotic infections of the bowel are uncommon; however, fungi are opportunists that capitalize on predisposing factors such as lowered host resistance, malnutrition, antecedent debilitating illness, and prolonged therapy with antimicrobials or corticosteroids. Fungi may cause acute, dysentery-like diarrhea or chronic diarrhea accompanied by emaciation.

Causes of mycotic intestinal disease include *Histoplasma capsulatum*, *Pythium* spp., *Aspergillus* spp., *Candida albicans*, and other saprophytes. Histoplasmosis is a multisystemic mycotic infection and is discussed in Chapter 18. Intestinal aspergillosis and candidiasis are rare and will not be discussed further.

Intestinal Pythiosis and Zygomycosis

Various poorly septate saprophytic molds and fungi that include *Pythium* spp. (pythiosis) and several genera of Zygomycetes (zygomycosis) can deeply invade the tissues of the gastrointestinal tract. These infections were formerly misnamed phycomycosis.

Pythiosis is most common in young, large-breed dogs that live in the southern Gulf states of the United States. Rare feline cases are characterized by ulcerative gastroenteritis.

Clinical Signs

Pythium and Zygomycetes can infect any part of the digestive tract, but lesions most commonly involve the stomach, small intestine, mesentery, and mesenteric lymph nodes, resulting in an extensive granulomatous tissue reaction.

- Signs include chronic intractable diarrhea and vomiting, anorexia, depression, and progressive weight loss.
- Bowel necrosis and ulceration may cause bloody diarrhea in some cases.
- Regions of extensive granulomatous inflammation may produce palpable enteromesenteric masses.
- The infection may disseminate beyond the GI tract to other abdominal viscera.

Diagnosis

- Physical examination may reveal an abdominal mass or marked regional thickening of the bowel.
- The CBC may reveal mild to moderate nonregenerative anemia and mild neutrophilia, with or without a left shift.
- Routine abdominal radiography frequently demonstrates an abdominal mass; barium contrast GI radiography often delineates a thickened, stenosed segment of bowel.
- Confirmation depends on histologic identification of broad, nonseptate or sparsely septate hyphae in biopsies of the stomach, intestine, or abdominal lymph nodes. The organisms stain with Gridley or methenamine silver stains and are found mostly within the necrotic regions of granulomas in the submucosa and muscularis mucosa.
- Differentiate intestinal pythiosis from other granulomatous and neoplastic proliferations of the GI tract, including histoplasmosis, lymphosarcoma, and regional (granulomatous) enteritis.
- The extensive tissue reaction can easily be mistaken for neoplasia at laparotomy (or necropsy); thus, careful histologic evaluation including use of fungal stains is essential for accurate diagnosis.

Treatment

Because these fungi are resistant to standard antifungal drugs, the most effective treatment is radical surgical excision of the severely involved segments of bowel (for surgical technique, see Chap. 90). Some animals have been treated successfully with lipid-complexed amphotericin B and itraconazole or ketoconazole as described in Chapter 18.

Prognosis

The prognosis is guarded.

INTESTINAL PROTOTHECOSIS

Etiology

Prototheca spp. are ubiquitous unicellular algae that may rarely colonize the lamina propria and submucosa of the intestinal tract of dogs and cause severe necrotizing or ulcerating enterocolitis.

Clinical Signs

- The algae appear to have a predilection for initially invading the colon, resulting in signs of chronic large bowel diarrhea with hematochezia.
- The organisms typically disseminate widely throughout the body and most frequently involve other visceral organs, the eyes, and the central nervous system (CNS).
- Only a cutaneous form has been described in cats.

Diagnosis

- Colonoscopy reveals thickened, corrugated mucosal folds that may be friable or ulcerated.
- Organisms can be identified in feces, cytology preparations (Wright or Gram stain), and biopsies (Gomori or periodic acid–Schiff stain) as clusters of endosporulated ovoid structures (5–16 μm in length).
- *Prototheca* can also be cultured on Sabouraud's cyclohexamide-free dextrose media.

Treatment

Successful treatment of systemic prototothecosis in animals is rare.

CANINE HEMORRHAGIC GASTROENTERITIS

Etiology

Hemorrhagic gastroenteritis (HGE) is a syndrome of unknown etiology characterized by sudden onset of vomiting, profuse bloody diarrhea, and marked hemoconcentration. Despite its name, HGE does not appear to be primarily an inflammatory disease but rather is a condition of altered intestinal mucosal permeability and perhaps mucosal hypersecretion.

Cultures of intestinal contents from dogs with HGE have yielded large numbers of *C. perfringens*, leading to speculation that this organism or its toxins are the cause.

Signalment

HGE has a predilection for toy and miniature breeds, particularly schnauzers and toy poodles, but any breed can be affected. Dogs of any age can be affected, but especially young adults 2–4 years of age.

Clinical Signs

The first signs are usually sudden onset of vomiting and severe depression, followed within hours by a profuse, bloody, fluid diarrhea with a fetid odor. Progressive prolongation of capillary refill time and other indicators of circulatory failure are noted as shock develops.

Diagnosis

- The diagnosis of HGE is suggested by evidence of extreme hemoconcentration (packed cell volume [PCV] > 60%, reaching 70–80% in some dogs) along with fetid, bloody diarrhea.
- Radiography and other laboratory findings are generally unremarkable, but they are useful for excluding other causes of bloody diarrhea.
- The high PCV and lack of fever or leukopenia help distinguish HGE from parvoviral enteritis; however, for greater certainty, a fecal test for parvovirus may be necessary.
- Evaluate dogs with HGE for *C. perfringens* (see previous discussion).

Treatment

The mortality from HGE is low if treated promptly by vigorous fluid volume replacement.

- Rapidly infuse a balanced multiple electrolyte solution, preferably by indwelling IV catheter, at a rate of 90 ml/kg/h until capillary refill time and PCV are normal; then continue IV fluids at a maintenance rate for the next 24 hours.

▼ *Key Point* Without volume expansion using IV fluid therapy, HGE can cause circulatory failure and death in <24 hours.

- Occasionally, if shock appears to be refractory to IV fluid therapy, a dose of corticosteroids may be needed during the initial hours.
- Use antibiotics effective against *C. perfringens*, such as ampicillin or amoxicillin, empirically.
- Restrict food and water initially until vomiting and bloody or fluid diarrhea have ceased; then feed small amounts of bland food. Nonspecific antidiarrheal and antiemetic therapy may be helpful.
- Most animals show marked improvement within hours, although the diarrhea may not subside for 24–48 hours. Failure of the animal to improve dramatically in 24–48 hours should prompt a search for other diseases that may mimic HGE (e.g., parvovirus, GI foreign body, intussusception, volvulus).

CHRONIC INFLAMMATORY BOWEL DISEASE

The term inflammatory bowel disease (IBD) refers to a diverse group of chronic enteropathies characterized by idiopathic infiltration of the GI tract mucosa and (sometimes) submucosa with inflammatory cells. The infiltration may involve the stomach, small intestine, colon, or a combination of these and is classified on the basis of the predominant cell type as lymphocytic-plasmacytic, eosinophilic, neutrophilic, granulomatous, or histiocytic. A mixture of inflammatory cells in some lesions makes classification difficult.

Lymphocytic-Plasmacytic IBD
Etiology

- Lymphocytic-plasmacytic IBD is by far the most common form of IBD in both dogs and cats. The etiology is not determined in most cases; however, genetic, dietary, bacterial, immunologic, and mucosal permeability factors have been suggested to play a role.

- The pathogenesis of lymphocytic-plasmacytic IBD may involve a hypersensitivity reaction to antigens (bacterial, food, or self-antigens) in the bowel lumen or mucosa. This may result from a primary disorder of the intestinal immune system or its regulation or from immune events that occur secondary to mucosal injury and permeability. Chronic inflammation of the bowel may become self-perpetuating when loss of mucosal integrity allows bacterial or dietary proteins to enter the lamina propria, where they incite further immune reaction and inflammation.
- Genetic factors appear to be involved in predisposing certain breeds to lymphocytic-plasmacytic IBD (e.g., basenji, soft-coated Wheaton terrier, and Shar pei). Basenjis develop a severe form of IBD (also called immunoproliferative enteropathy) that is thought to be related to a genetic disorder of immune regulation and that is progressive in nature and exacerbated by stress.

Clinical Signs

- *Lymphocytic-plasmacytic gastroduodenitis* causes intermittent vomiting and occurs most frequently in cats with IBD.
- *Diffuse lymphocytic-plasmacytic enteritis* causes chronic unresponsive small bowel diarrhea and progressive weight loss. Signs may be intermittent or persistent. In severely affected dogs, protein-losing enteropathy (ascites, hydrothorax, edema) can occur.
  - Some animals with a biopsy diagnosis of lymphocytic-plasmacytic enteritis that fail to respond to treatment or that later relapse and deteriorate rapidly are found to have diffuse intestinal lymphosarcoma.
- *Lymphocytic-plasmacytic colitis* causes chronic large bowel diarrhea characterized by increased frequency of defecation, urgency, tenesmus, increased fecal mucus, and hematochezia. Intermittent hematochezia may be the only sign of IBD in some cats.

Diagnosis

- In the diagnostic evaluation, exclude parasitic (*Giardia,* canine whipworms) and infectious (*Campylobacter, Salmonella, Histoplasma*) causes of IBD.
- The differential diagnosis of lymphocytic-plasmacytic IBD includes dietary hypersensitivity, bacterial overgrowth syndrome, intestinal lymphosarcoma, intestinal lymphangiectasia, and the other types of chronic inflammatory bowel disease.
  - To exclude dietary hypersensitivity as a cause of IBD, use a feeding trial with a controlled "hypoallergenic" diet as described under Treatment.
- Routine hematologic and biochemical parameters typically are unremarkable except for occasional nonspecific findings such as a stress leukogram, hypoproteinemia, hypokalemia, and mildly elevated serum liver enzymes. Basenji enteropathy is associated with hypoalbuminemia and hyperglobulinemia,

whereas affected soft-coated Wheaton terriers may have hypoalbuminemia with concurrent glomerulonephropathy.

- Radiography (including barium contrast) usually is unremarkable.
- Serum vitamin levels (cobalamin, folate, vitamin K) can be decreased from malabsorption. Bleeding and abnormal hemostasis have been associated with vitamin K deficiency in some cats with IBD. Markedly decreased serum cobalamin is common in affected Shar peis.
- Intestinal biopsy (usually via endoscopy) is required for definitive diagnosis.
  - Endoscopically, the mucosa in IBD often appears thickened, friable, and abnormally granular. In the colon there is decreased visibility of the submucosal vessels and replacement of the glistening appearance of the mucosa with a dry granular surface covered with strands of mucus. Ulceration is uncommon. Mild cases of IBD may appear endoscopically normal, such that lesions can only be detected histopathologically.
  - Histopathologically, the lesion of lymphocytic-plasmacytic IBD is characterized by diffuse infiltration of the mucosa with mature lymphocytes and plasma cells.
  - Additional findings can include atrophic or fused villi, fibrosis, epithelial abnormalities (hyperplasia, degeneration, erosion, ulceration, glandular dilation, loss of goblet cells), and mixed infiltration of other types of inflammatory cells (neutrophils, eosinophils, macrophages).

Treatment

The initial treatment strategy is directed toward dietary manipulation; if this is unsuccessful, medical therapy is usually required using anti-inflammatory-immunosuppressive drugs as single agents or in combination, such as 5-aminosalicylates (e.g., sulfasalazine, olsalazine, mesalamine), corticosteroids (prednisone), metronidazole (Flagyl), and azathioprine (Imuran). Motility-modifying antidiarrheal drugs may help to alleviate some of the clinical signs. Various drugs used to treat IBD and their suggested dosages are indicated in Table 89–7.

Dietary Therapy

In some dogs and cats with lymphocytic-plasmacytic IBD, dietary modification produces complete or partial resolution of the signs and sometimes even regression of the lesions. This suggests that dietary hypersensitivity may be involved in the pathogenesis of the disease in some animals. Other potential explanations for a beneficial response to dietary modification include the effects of the diet on bowel motility, composition of the flora, mucosal morphology and function, and exclusion of food-borne antigens or irritating additives.

The dietary approach to treatment of IBD is based on the controlled feeding of a well-defined, additive-free diet that contains a single highly digestible or novel source of protein combined with an easily assimilated carbohydrate such as white rice. Both homemade and

Table 89–7. DRUGS USED FOR TREATMENT OF IDIOPATHIC CHRONIC INFLAMMATORY BOWEL DISEASE

Drug	Product (Manufacturer)	Preparations	Dosage
Anti-Inflammatory/Immunosuppressives			
Prednisone†	Many	Tab—5, 10, 20, 50 mg	Dog—1–2 mg/kg PO q24h
			Cat—2–3 mg/kg PO q24h
Methylprednisolone acetate	Depo-Medrol (Upjohn)	Inj—40 mg/ml	Cat—20 mg IM q2–4wk
Azathioprine‡	Imuran (Burroughs Wellcome)	Tab—50 mg	Dog—1–2 mg/kg PO q24–48h
			Cat—0.3–0.5 mg/kg PO q24–48h
Colonic Anti-inflammatory Drugs			
Sulfasalazine*	Azulfidine (Kabi Pharmacia)	Tab—500 mg	Dog—10–30 mg/kg PO q8–12h
			Cat—10–20 mg/kg PO q12–24h
Olsalazine	Dipentum (Kabi Pharmacia)	Cap—250 mg	Dog—10–20 mg/kg PO q12
Mesalamine	Asacol (Procter & Gamble)	Tab—400 mg	Dog—10–20 mg/kg PO q8–12h
Anti-inflammatory Retention Enemas§			
5-Aminosalicylate	Rowasa (Reid-Rowell)	Enema—4 g/60 ml	Needs to be determined
Hydrocortisone	Cortenema (Reid-Rowell)	Enema—100 mg/60 ml	20–60 ml rectally q24h
Antibiotics			
Metronidazole	Flagyl (Searle)	Tab—250 mg, 500 mg	10–15 mg/kg PO q8–12h
Tylosin¶	Tylan-Plus (Elanco)	Powder—470 mg/tsp	Dog—20–40 mg/kg PO q12h
			Cat—10–20 mg/kg PO q12h

Tab = tablets; Liq = elixir, suspension or drops; Cap = capsules; Inj = injectable.

*Dosage may need to be increased to 25–50 mg/kg q8h to achieve effect in some dogs; may cause keratoconjunctivitis sicca in dogs and salicylate toxicosis in cats.

†In some cats with severe colitis, prednisone dosage may need to be increased to 5 mg/kg/day, divided bid. In dogs, if steroidal side effects become a problem, decrease dosage and combine with azathioprine or metronidazole or both.

‡May cause myelotoxicity, so monitor CBC; tablet can be crushed and added to VAL Syrup (Fort Dodge) for accurate dosing of cats.

§Retention enemas for topical therapy of the distal colon may relieve signs of tenesmus and urgency in some animals with proctitis.

¶Tylosin powder is bitter-tasting and thus best tolerated when mixed with food.

commercial lamb and rice diets are reported to maintain remission of lymphocytic-plasmacytic IBD in many dogs and cats, especially in those with colitis.

- Several specialized commercial diets are marketed for dietary hypersensitivity, but many of these are relatively new products that have not yet received enough clinical evaluation in the treatment of IBD to determine efficacy. Products include:
  - Egg-based diets (e.g., dry Canine Prescription Diet d/d, Hill's Pet).
  - Lamb-based diets (e.g., canned Canine Prescription Diet d/d and Feline Prescription Diet d/d, Hill's Pet; Natural Pack, Eagle; Lamaderm, Natural Life; Natural Choice, Nutro; Wayne Sensible Choice, Royal Canin; Anergen I, Wysong; and Nature's Recipe Lamb & Rice).
  - Rabbit-based diets (e.g., Nature's Recipe Rabbit & Rice; Protocol).
  - Venison-based diets (e.g., Nature's Recipe Venison & Rice).
- Homemade diets for a feeding trial can be made from one part low-fat cottage cheese, tofu, or lamb (cooked or baby food) combined with 3 parts rice.
- A cooperative and patient owner is needed for success; allow a minimum of 3–4 weeks for the trial feeding period; in some cases 6 weeks or more may be required before improvement is complete.
- Eliminate intake of all other foods or sources of antigen throughout the feeding trial, including table scraps, treats, dog biscuits, rawhide chew toys, and flavored medications such as vitamins and heartworm preventatives.

- If there is a substantial response to the dietary trial, the animal can be rechallenged with its original diet.
  - Recurrence of signs confirms dietary intolerance or hypersensitivity.
  - Once remission is restored with the controlled diet, the animal can then be challenged sequentially with individual dietary components to identify the specific offenders. To do this, individual components of the original diet are added one at a time to the controlled diet while the animal is in remission. With each challenge the animal is monitored for recurrence of signs for 7–10 days. If signs recur, that substance is implicated as an offender.
- After several weeks of remission on the controlled diet, some animals can be returned to their original diet and remain asymptomatic; however, most animals will need specially formulated or hypoallergenic diets indefinitely to prevent relapse.
- If there is no response to dietary management within 4–6 weeks, institute medical therapy.

Other Dietary Adjustments. In cases in which hypoallergenic diets are not effective, other dietary adjustments may be beneficial.

- Various special-formulation diets can be helpful in IBD, such as Eukanuba (Iams) for dogs and Prescription Diet c/d (Hill's Pet) for cats.
- In animals with colitis, fiber supplementation of the diet using soluble fiber such as psyllium (Metamucil; 1–2 tbsp per day added to a highly digestible diet), or feeding of a commercial high-fiber diet (e.g., Canine or Feline Prescription Diet w/d, Hill's Pet) may improve colonic function and control diarrhea.

- Animals with small intestinal disease may improve on a highly digestible low-fiber diet (e.g., Prescription Diet i/d, Hill's Pet).

5-Aminosalicylic Acid (5-ASA, Mesalamine Drugs)

These drugs exert an anti-inflammatory effect in colitis through local inhibition of mucosal leukotrienes and prostaglandins. In dogs with IBD, 5-ASA drugs are the initial drugs of choice when the colon alone is involved. Cats generally tolerate corticosteroids better than salicylates; thus, prednisone is the first choice for feline IBD, and 5-ASA drugs generally are reserved for steroid-resistant feline colitis. For 5-ASA drugs to be effective in treating colitis they must reach the lumen of the colon; thus, each orally administered 5-ASA drug has a delivery vehicle mechanism that prevents significant absorption during passage through the small intestine.

Sulfasalazine (Azulfidine; Kabi Pharmacia). In this drug, 5-ASA is combined with sulfapyridine by an azo bond that prevents significant absorption of the drug so that 75% of it reaches the colon, where the bacteria split the bond and release the 5-ASA for its local effect in the colon (see Table 89–7 for dosages).

- The most common adverse side effect of sulfasalazine is keratoconjunctivitis sicca. When it occurs, the decline in tear production is often irreversible. For this reason, it is recommended that a baseline Schirmer tear test be performed at the start of therapy and monitored subsequently at monthly intervals if treatment is long-term.
- Less common side effects include allergic dermatitis, nausea and vomiting, and cholestatic jaundice. Rarely, cats may develop anemia.
- Because up to 30% of the salicylate is absorbed and cats metabolize salicylates very slowly, use caution when treating cats with this drug in order to avoid salicylate toxicity.

Olsalazine (Dipentum; Kabi Pharmacia). This newer derivative, consisting of two molecules of azo-bonded 5-ASA, is poorly absorbed, so that 98% reaches the colon, where the two 5-ASA molecules are then released by the action of colonic bacteria on the azo bond (see Table 89–7 for dosages).

- The advantages of olsalazine over sulfasalazine are that olsalazine contains only 5-ASA (without sulfa) and that a greater percentage of the drug reaches the colon.
- Unfortunately, olsalazine is currently available only in 250-mg capsules, an inconvenient size for dosing most animals.

Polymer-Coated Mesalamine (Asacol; Procter & Gamble). A pH-sensitive coating prevents release of 5-ASA until the drug reaches the site of inflammation in the colon.

Mesalamine Suspension Enema (RowASA; Reid-Rowell). This form of 5-ASA is available for direct instillation into the rectum. In animals, enema administration of 5-ASA is probably not as effective as the oral route except when proctitis is the principal manifestation.

Corticosteroids

Oral prednisone is the preferred initial therapy for dogs with concurrent IBD of the small intestine and for all cats with IBD. In addition, dogs with severe colitis or colitis that is refractory to 5-ASA drugs alone may respond best to prednisone used as a single agent or in combination with a 5-ASA drug (e.g., sulfasalazine, olasalazine) or metronidazole.

- Clinical response, using the dosage in Table 89–7, should be noted within 1–2 weeks. After 2 weeks of remission, taper the dosage over an additional 4-week period to the lowest effective alternate-day dosage (usually about 0.25–0.5 mg/kg in dogs and 0.5–1.0 mg/kg in cats).
- In cats that are too difficult to medicate orally, periodic injections of methylprednisolone acetate may be used instead (see Table 89–7).
- Corticosteroid therapy may be discontinued on a trial basis after 8–12 weeks of remission; however, continuous therapy is required in many cases to prevent relapse.
- Hydrocortisone retention enemas (Cortenema) may be useful for controlling severe urgency or tenesmus associated with proctitis. One dose in the evening is usually adequate, but in cases of severe proctitis, treatment can be given q8h (see Table 89–7).

Antibiotics

- Antibiotics such as metronidazole (Flagyl) and tylosin (Tylan-Plus) are sometimes beneficial in animals with colitis (see Table 89–7). These can be used alone as single agents, but they are most effective in combination with the previously mentioned treatment measures.
- The beneficial effects of metronidazole, as shown in human patients and experimental animals with colitis, may be attributed to the drug's intraluminal antibacterial action (reduction of bacterial-derived antigens) or to its suppressive effect on cell-mediated immune responses in the colon.

Azathioprine

- In IBD patients refractory to 5-ASA drugs, prednisone, and metronidazole, the combination of azathioprine (Imuran) with prednisone may be a more effective immunosuppressive regimen for producing remission of the disease (see Table 89–7). In addition to treating refractory IBD, the addition of azathioprine enables use of a lower dose of corticosteroid to control the disease and thereby minimizes steroidal side effects.
- Azathioprine usually is given as a daily treatment until remission occurs and then decreased to an alternate-day treatment (alternating with every-other-day prednisone) for maintenance. Because of its myelosuppressive toxicity (leukopenia), periodically monitor the CBC of azathioprine-treated animals.

Motility-Modifying Antidiarrheal Drugs

Adjunctive use of colonic motility-modifying drugs may provide some symptomatic relief for animals with colitis (see Table 89–5 for dosages).

- Opioid drugs such as loperamide (Imodium) and diphenoxylate (Lomotil) may aid control of diarrhea by acting on colonic smooth muscle to inhibit propulsive movements and by inhibiting mucosal efflux of water and electrolytes.
- Anticholinergic antispasmodics such as dicyclomine (Bentyl) may be beneficial in colitis patients with severe tenesmus and urgency associated with rectocolonic spasm.

Prognosis

- Inform the owner that persistence or recurrence of IBD is likely despite therapy; thus, a realistic expectation is maintenance of remission or control of relapses rather than a permanent cure.
- The clinical course in basenjis, soft-coated Wheaton terriers, and Shar peis is often progressive despite treatment.

Eosinophilic Gastroenteritis

Eosinophilic gastroenteritis (EGE) is a relatively uncommon form of IBD that is characterized by diffuse or segmental infiltration of some portion of the GI tract with mature eosinophils, often accompanied by a peripheral eosinophilia.

Etiology

Allergy and parasitism have been proposed as causes, but in most patients evidence for these is lacking, and the disease must be considered idiopathic.

Clinical Signs

- One or more layers of the stomach, small intestine, or colon may be affected, resulting in clinical syndromes of chronic vomiting (eosinophilic gastritis, see Chap. 87), chronic small bowel–type diarrhea (eosinophilic enteritis), chronic large bowel–type diarrhea (eosinophilic colitis), or any combination of these.
- Diffuse infiltration of the intestinal tract with eosinophils may result in malabsorption (watery diarrhea and weight loss) or protein-losing enteropathy.
- Diarrhea or vomitus may contain blood from mucosal erosions or ulcers.
- Eosinophilic granuloma of the deeper layers of the bowel wall occasionally produces segmental tumor-like thickening that can cause partial intestinal obstruction.

Diagnosis

- The history may indicate dramatic responsiveness to prior glucocorticoid therapy.
- Palpation may reveal diffusely thickened intestinal loops or a tumor-like intestinal mass (eosinophilic granuloma).
- Laboratory evaluation may reveal peripheral eosinophilia (although not present in all cases), hypoproteinemia, or impaired absorptive function tests.
- Routine fecal flotation is indicated because parasitism can also cause eosinophilic inflammation; it is important to exclude occult whipworm or hookworm infection in dogs by response to a therapeutic trial of an anthelmintic such as fenbendazole (see Table 89–6).
- Barium radiography may be normal or may indicate thickening and irregularity (mucosal filling defects) of bowel loops, or may delineate sites of partial luminal obstruction caused by eosinophilic granulomas.
- The diagnosis is based on demonstration of eosinophilic inflammation in intestinal biopsies. The endoscopic appearance is similar to that described for lymphocytic-plasmacytic IBD except that mucosal ulceration is more common in EGE. Occasionally lesions are deep in the submucosa and found only by full-thickness biopsy.

Treatment

- Because food allergy is a potential cause of EGE in some animals, a feeding trial using an elimination or hypoallergenic diet (as described for lymphocytic-plasmacytic IBD) can be considered initially; however, dietary therapy alone is seldom effective.
- Oral prednisone usually is the most effective treatment for EGE, at an initial dosage of 1–2 mg/kg/day for dogs and 2–3 mg/kg/day for cats. Clinical signs typically improve rapidly, especially when infiltration is limited to the mucosa. When remission has been maintained for 2 weeks, gradually taper the dosage over an additional 2–4 weeks to the lowest effective maintenance dose.
  - In some animals the treatment can eventually be discontinued, but in others alternate-day maintenance therapy is required.
- In some patients it may be necessary to add azathioprine to the corticosteroid regimen (as described for lymphocytic-plasmacytic IBD) to facilitate reduction of corticosteroid dosage and side effects or to provide more effective control of the disease.
- Obstructing transmural eosinophilic granulomas involving a localized segment of bowel wall occasionally require surgical excision followed by corticosteroid therapy.

Feline Hypereosinophilic Syndrome

Feline hypereosinophilic syndrome (FHS), a rare disease of cats, is characterized by severe eosinophilic gastrointestinal infiltration accompanied by widespread infiltration of various other organs (liver, spleen, lymph nodes, bone marrow, lung, pancreas, adrenals, skin).

Etiology

The etiopathogenesis is not known. The aggressive course and high mortality associated with this syndrome indicate that it should be considered distinct from the more benign eosinophilic gastroenteritis that is confined to the GI tract; in fact, FHS in many ways resembles neoplasia more than an inflammatory bowel disease.

Clinical Signs

- Vomiting, diarrhea (sometimes bloody), anorexia, and weight loss are the most consistent clinical signs.
- Clinical deterioration is rapidly progressive and fatalities are common.

Diagnosis

- Abdominal palpation may reveal intestinal thickening, hepatosplenomegaly, or mesenteric lymphadenopathy because of the disseminated visceral infiltration of eosinophils.
- Persistent, severe eosinophilia is a consistent finding in affected cats.
- The diagnosis depends on histopathologic confirmation of tissue infiltration and effacement by eosinophils in biopsies of affected organs.

Treatment

- Use high-dose prednisolone (4–6 mg/kg/day for 2–4 weeks) to induce remission, followed by half this dose for 2–4 weeks, and then by 1–2 mg/kg daily or on alternate days for maintenance. Add azathioprine or alkylating cancer chemotherapeutics in refractory patients.

Prognosis

Unlike EGE confined to the GI tract, FHS has a poor prognosis despite treatment.

Regional Granulomatous Enterocolitis

Regional granulomatous enterocolitis (RGE) is an uncommon form of IBD characterized by transmural granulomatous inflammation that results in a stenosing, masslike thickening of a region of the bowel wall. The ileocolic junction is most often involved, and the mass may incorporate adjacent lymph nodes and mesentery. In some dogs the granulomatous lesion also contains numerous eosinophils (eosinophilic granuloma).

Clinical Signs

The principal clinical sign of RGE is chronic large bowel diarrhea containing mucus and fresh blood, sometimes accompanied by tenesmus and abdominal pain. Additional signs may include weight loss, anorexia, and depression.

Diagnosis

- The diseased segment of bowel may be palpable as a firm mass in the midabdomen. The adjacent intestinal loops and mesentery may also be thickened and regional lymph nodes may be enlarged.
- A routine CBC may reveal eosinophilia, neutrophilia, or monocytosis. Panhypoproteinemia due to excessive enteric loss of protein may be found in some animals.

- Barium contrast radiography of the ileum and colon may delineate a thickened or stenosed segment of bowel.
- Definitive diagnosis of RGE requires biopsy by colonoscopy or laparotomy. The key feature is transmural granulomatous inflammation. Fibrosis and aggregates of epithelioid cells, giant cells, and eosinophils often are found deep in the lesion. Deep ulceration is common.
- Differentiate RGE from intestinal neoplasia and infectious causes of granulomatous bowel lesions, such as histoplasmosis, pythiosis, and mycobacteriosis. Examine granulomatous lesions by special stains to detect fungi and acid-fast organisms. In cats, feline immunodeficiency virus (Chap. 7) and FIP (Chap. 8) occasionally are associated with pyogranulomatous IBD.

Treatment

- Medical treatment of regional granulomatous colitis is based on the use of anti-inflammatory and immunosuppressive agents such as olsalazine or sulfasalazine, prednisone, azathioprine, and metronidazole, as described for treatment of lymphocytic-plasmacytic IBD.
- If the degree of thickening and cicatrization of the affected segment of bowel produces severe stenosis and obliteration of the lumen, surgical excision of the lesion may be necessary, followed by medical therapy for 6–8 weeks or longer to prevent recurrence of the lesion at the surgical site.

Histiocytic Ulcerative Colitis

- Histiocytic ulcerative colitis is a chronic idiopathic IBD of young boxer dogs characterized by infiltration of the lamina propria and submucosa of the colon by distinctive histiocytes engorged with deposits that stain positive with periodic acid–Schiff (PAS) stain.
- In addition to boxers, there have been isolated case reports of histiocytic colitis in a cat and a French bulldog, but it is not known if this is the same disease that occurs in boxers.

Clinical Signs

- Affected boxers generally develop severe, unresponsive, bloody-mucoid large bowel diarrhea before 2 years of age.
- Severe weight loss and debilitation occur in dogs with long-standing disease.

Diagnosis

The diagnosis is based on the known breed predisposition and the presence of numerous PAS-positive histiocytes in a colonoscopic biopsy. A mixture of other types of inflammatory cells is also found in the lesion, and usually there is severe mucosal ulceration.

Treatment

- Give olsalazine or sulfasalazine, prednisone, azathioprine, and metronidazole in single-agent or combination regimens as described for lymphocytic-plasmacytic colitis (see Table 89–7); however, lifetime therapy is needed, and the probability of effective control of the disease is poor.

- In general, these dogs seem to have less diarrhea on a highly digestible diet than on a high-fiber diet.

Neutrophilic (Suppurative) Enterocolitis

Etiology

- Bacterial enterocolitis (see under Bacterial Infections of the Intestines)
- Idiopathic (i.e., neutrophilic IBD in the absence of an identifiable infectious cause)

Clinical Signs

- Large bowel diarrhea that can be either acute or chronic.

Diagnosis

- Colonoscopic biopsy shows infiltration of predominantly neutrophils, with variable mucosal ulceration, necrosis, or crypt abscesses.
- Diagnosis is based on tests to exclude bacterial enteropathogens (see under Bacterial Infections of the Intestines).

Treatment

Give antibiotics (e.g., trimethoprim-sulfa, enrofloxacin, chloramphenicol) or regimens consisting of sulfasalazine, metronidazole, or anti-inflammatory/immunosuppressive drugs, as described for lymphocytic-plasmacytic IBD (see Table 89–7).

IRRITABLE BOWEL SYNDROME

Etiology

Irritable bowel syndrome (IBS) is characterized by non-inflammatory mucoid large bowel diarrhea associated with episodic disturbances of colonic myoelectrical function (spastic colon). Psychological and emotional factors are implicated in humans afflicted with IBS.

Clinical Signs

- Signs associated with myoelectrical dysfunction in humans with IBS are alternating patterns of diarrhea, constipation, and abdominal cramping.
- Evidence for the existence of IBS in animals is circumstantial, but psychomotor diarrhea due to colonic motility dysfunction or IBS may be a consideration in animals that have intermittent mucoid diarrhea but lack evidence of organic disease.
- Large breeds, especially those used as working dogs (e.g., police dogs, Seeing Eye dogs), and temperamental or excitable dogs seem to be predisposed to IBS.

Diagnosis

- By definition, irritable bowel syndrome is a functional disorder lacking in any identifiable lesions; therefore, the diagnosis can be established only by normal colonoscopic biopsy and diligent exclusion of the other known causes of colonic disease such as dietary, parasitic, infectious, and idiopathic colitis (IBD).
- At colonoscopy, the colon may appear to be hypermotile or spastic. The mucosa appears normal except for increased intraluminal mucus.

Treatment

Dietary Modification. Supplementing dietary fiber in the form of psyllium (Metamucil) (1–5 tbsp per meal) or a commercial high-fiber diet (Prescription Diet w/d; Hill's Pet) can normalize colonic myoelectrical activity and decrease functional diarrhea in some dogs.

Motility Modification. If dietary fiber supplementation is unsuccessful, consider medication to alter motility. Anticholinergics (antispasmodics) such as propantheline, aminopentamide, or dicyclomine or opioid drugs such as loperamide can be used (see Table 89–5 for dosages).

Mood Modification. Light sedation during stressful times with acetylpromazine, chlorpromazine, or phenobarbital may be helpful in excessively nervous or excitable animals. Anticholinergic CNS depressant drug combinations such as clidinium-chlordiazepoxide (Librax) also can be effective.

INTESTINAL LYMPHANGIECTASIA

Etiology

Lymphangiectasia is a chronic protein-losing enteropathy in dogs, characterized by marked dilation and dysfunction of the intestinal lymphatic network. Impaired intestinal lymph drainage is presumably caused by obstruction to the normal lymphaticovenous flow. It leads to stasis of chyle within dilated lacteals and lymphatics of the bowel wall and mesentery. Overdistended lacteals release intestinal lymph into the gut lumen by rupture or extravasation, causing loss of the constituents of chyle—plasma proteins, lymphocytes, and lipid (chylomicrons).

Clinical Signs

- The presenting signs of lymphangiectasia usually are attributable to protein-losing enteropathy and include dependent pitting edema of subcutis and limbs, fluid distention of the abdomen (ascites), and respiratory distress (hydrothorax). These manifestations of fluid transudation are the result of hypoalbuminemia and reduced plasma colloidal osmotic pressure.
- Chronic intermittent or persistent diarrhea with a watery or semisolid consistency often is observed, but not all patients have diarrhea.
- Progressive weight loss is common. Clinical signs often develop insidiously.

Diagnosis

▼ *Key Point* Typical laboratory findings in intestinal lymphangiectasia include hypoalbuminemia, hypoglobulinemia, lymphocytopenia, hypocholesterolemia, and hypocalcemia.

- Differentiate protein-losing enteropathy from nonenteric causes of hypoproteinemia, such as liver failure (impaired hepatic synthesis of albumin) and renal disease (protein-losing glomerulonephropathies), through liver function testing (Chap. 91) and urine protein determinations (Chap. 97).
- Ancillary diagnostic procedures may be helpful:
  - Radiography can detect or confirm ascites and pleural effusion
  - Fluid analysis of body cavity effusions may be helpful. The effusion associated with lymphangiectasia is usually a transudate. Chylous ascites and chylothorax are found occasionally.
  - Cardiac evaluations can exclude right-sided congestive heart failure, which is a rare cause of lymphangiectasia.
- Definitive diagnosis of lymphangiectasia is based on identification of the characteristic lymphatic lesions in biopsies obtained via laparotomy, or less invasively by endoscopy or suction biopsy capsule. Laparotomy may reveal the mesentery and serosa to have a prominent, weblike network of distended, milky-white lymphatics along with small yellow-white nodules and foamy granular deposits (lipogranulomas) adjacent to lymphatics.

Treatment

The major goal in treating intestinal lymphangiectasia is to decrease the enteric loss of plasma proteins so that normal plasma protein levels can be restored and edema and effusions controlled. This is accomplished with dietary manipulation and anti-inflammatory therapy.

Dietary Therapy

Because absorption of dietary long-chain triglycerides (LCTs) is a major stimulus of intestinal lymph flow, restriction of dietary intake of LCTs may reduce lymph flow, lymphatic distention, and protein loss in lymphangiectasia.

- The ideal diet contains minimal fat (LCT) and provides an ample quantity of high-biologic quality protein; for example, Prescription Diet r/d (Hill's Pet) or a homemade diet consisting of one part low-fat cottage cheese or yogurt as the protein source and three parts rice or potatoes as the carbohydrate source. Supplement diets with fat-soluble vitamins.
- Low-fat diets are inherently low in calories, but another goal of therapy is to promote regain of lost weight. Medium-chain triglycerides (MCT Oil; Mead Johnson) 1–2 ml/kg, can be added to the diet to replace the calories lost by restriction of conventional fat (LCT). MCTs are hydrolyzed more rapidly and efficiently than LCTs and are absorbed directly into the portal venous system. MCTs do not entirely bypass the dysfunctional lymphatics as was once thought, based on cannulation studies of the thoracic duct that find substantial levels of MCT in thoracic duct chyle of normal dogs and cats.
- The plasma protein loss and diarrhea of lymphangiectasia often benefit from anti-inflammatory doses of corticosteroids (prednisone, 2–3 mg/kg/day PO). When remission has been achieved, adjust the dosage to the lowest effective maintenance level.

Prognosis

The prognosis and response to therapy is unpredictable. Many patients achieve a remission of months to years in duration with combined dietary and anti-inflammatory therapy. However, some animals fail to respond and many eventually relapse to finally succumb to severe protein-calorie depletion, incapacitating effusions, or intractable diarrhea.

VILLOUS ATROPHY

Etiology

Villous atrophy is a lesion of the small intestine characterized by short, blunted mucosal villi and is associated with intestinal malabsorption and chronic diarrhea. The forms of villous atrophy may be categorized as primary or secondary.

Primary Forms

- Wheat-sensitive enteropathy of Irish setters resembles gluten enteropathy of humans (celiac disease, nontropical sprue). This is apparently hereditary in Irish setters in Great Britain and is characterized by partial villous atrophy, deficiency or delayed development of specific microvillus enzymes, and dietary sensitivity to wheat.
- Idiopathic canine villous atrophy is recognized most often in German shepherds.

Secondary Forms

- Sequelae of diffuse infiltrative diseases of the intestines, such as chronic inflammatory bowel disease and lymphoma
- Sequelae of enteric infections, such as viruses (coronavirus, rotavirus), bacteria (small intestinal bacterial overgrowth syndrome), and parasites (*Giardia*)

Clinical Signs

Villous atrophy generally causes chronic small bowel–type diarrhea and weight loss. The severity of signs depends on the degree of disruption of the villous absorptive surface area.

Diagnosis

Histologic examination usually is adequate for documentation of villous atrophy. However, because this can be a nonspecific secondary lesion found in various enteropathies, the diagnosis is mainly based on:

- Breed predilection (German shepherd dogs, Irish setters in Great Britain)
- Response to withdrawal of wheat from the diet
- Tests or procedures to identify enteric infections (e.g., *Giardia*) or bacterial overgrowth
- Characterization of morphologic and biochemical abnormalities in jejunal biopsies

In some cases, infiltration of lymphocytes and plasma cells and fibrosis make it difficult to determine if the lesion should be categorized as a primary idiopathic villous atrophy or as a chronic inflammatory disease (lymphocytic-plasmacytic enteritis) with secondary villous atrophy (see under Lymphocytic-Plasmacytic Enteritis).

Treatment

Wheat-Sensitive Enteropathy

In wheat-sensitive Irish setters, the signs and lesions of villous atrophy promptly resolve with complete elimination of wheat and possibly other gluten-containing cereal grains from the diet. Most commercial dog foods contain gluten; however, diets that are based on rice or corn rather than wheat or gluten-containing grains are available (e.g., Hill's Pet Food products such as Prescription Diets d/d and i/d and Science Canine Growth Diet; and Iams Pet Food products such as Chunks, Plus, and Eukanuba). Wheat restriction must continue for life, and breeding of affected animals is discouraged.

Idiopathic Villous Atrophy

- Dietary management with a gluten-restricted hypoallergenic diet (e.g., Prescription Diet d/d; Hill's Pet) is sometimes beneficial.
- Vitamin therapy with folate (5 mg daily PO) and cobalamin (500 μg monthly IM for 6 months) is indicated if serum levels of these are low.
- Antibiotic therapy is sometimes beneficial, using antibiotics such as oxytetracycline, tylosin, or metronidazole to empirically treat bacterial overgrowth (see under Small Intestinal Bacterial Overgrowth).
- Prednisone as used for treatment of inflammatory bowel disease (1–3 mg/kg/day PO for 4 weeks, followed by tapering to lowest effective alternate-day dosage) may produce clinical improvement in dogs with idiopathic villous atrophy that fail to respond to dietary modification, vitamins, or antibiotics.

Prognosis

The prognosis is guarded, as diarrhea and weight loss often persist despite treatment.

SMALL INTESTINAL BACTERIAL OVERGROWTH

Bacterial overgrowth syndrome is an overproliferation of microflora within the proximal small intestine that results in malabsorption and diarrhea. Human criteria that define bacterial overgrowth as a fasting bacterial count in duodenal juice of greater than 10^5 organisms/ml of intestinal contents do not appear to be valid in dogs and cats; thus, definitive evidence of this syndrome in animals is lacking.

Etiology

The normal small intestinal microflora is a sparse but stable population of aerobic and facultative anaerobic bacteria whose growth is regulated and influenced by a combination of host factors, bacterial interactions, and dietary composition. Mechanical self-cleansing action of normal intestinal motility and continuous downstream flow of ingesta are especially important for preventing bacterial overgrowth.

Because documentation of bacterial overgrowth is difficult, the syndrome may occur more frequently in dogs and cats than is generally recognized. Development of an abnormal small bowel flora should be considered a potential secondary complication in the following situations:

- Intestinal surgery
- Stasis-producing mechanical obstructions such as chronic intestinal foreign bodies and stenosing neoplastic or inflammatory lesions of the gut
- Destructive lesions of the ileocecocolonic junction that allow colonoenteric reflux
- Motility disorders such as idiopathic intestinal pseudo-obstruction
- Immune deficiency states (proposed as the explanation for an apparent breed predilection for overgrowth in German shepherds, basenjis, and Shar peis)
- Conditions associated with hyposecretion of gastric acid
- Exocrine pancreatic insufficiency

Clinical Signs

- Bacterial overgrowth typically causes chronic, foul-smelling watery diarrhea, steatorrhea, and weight loss; however, additional presenting clinical signs can depend somewhat on the underlying cause of the abnormal proliferation of flora.
- Diarrhea caused by overgrowth usually does not contain blood or mucus.
- Bacterial overgrowth may be responsible for failure of some dogs with exocrine pancreatic insufficiency to respond adequately to enzyme supplementation.

Diagnosis

Definitive diagnosis of small intestinal bacterial overgrowth requires quantitative aerobic and anaerobic cultures that yield greater than 10^5 organisms/ml of duodenal juice. Duodenal culture specimens are taken by endoscopy, intestinal intubation, or laparotomy after an 18-hour fast. This is impractical for routine clinical application.

Indirect evidence of bacterial overgrowth in animals with unexplained small bowel diarrhea and malabsorption include the following observations:

- Responsiveness to antibiotics (e.g., tetracyclines, tylosin, or metronidazole)
- Delayed intestinal transit of barium on radiographs (obstruction or poor motility)
- Idiopathic pseudo-obstruction manifested by a dilated, hypomotile segment of gut
- Elevated serum folate and decreased serum cobalamin (because bacteria may synthesize folate and bind or compete for cobalamin)

- Minimal morphologic abnormalities in intestinal biopsies
  - Unlike many other enteropathies, mucosal morphology in bacterial overgrowth may be normal or characterized by mild atrophy of villi and minimal increase in mononuclear cells in the lamina propria.
- Failure to obtain the expected treatment response in other intestinal disorders known to be conducive to bacterial overgrowth (such as exocrine pancreatic insufficiency)

Treatment

- Identify and treat underlying disorders or predisposing factors. In animals with stasis caused by anatomic abnormalities, this may include surgery.
- Antibiotic therapy:
  - Oral broad-spectrum antimicrobials and those with activity against anaerobes are recommended, such as tetracycline, oxytetracycline, doxycycline, metronidazole, ampicillin, chloramphenicol, tylosin, and erythromycin.
  - Continue treatment for at least 10–14 days and repeat as necessary. Some animals need treatment at frequent intervals or even continuously, others may remain in remission for months after one course of antibiotics.
  - Clinical signs and abnormal function tests usually resolve within the first week of therapy, which in itself is good indirect evidence in support of the diagnosis.
- Treatment with *Lactobacillus* or live yogurt culture usually is not effective for altering the enteric microflora.

INTESTINAL NEOPLASIA

Benign tumors of the intestinal tract include adenomatous polyps, adenomas, and leiomyomas. In dogs these occur most commonly in the rectum and terminal colon. The most common malignant neoplasms of the intestinal tract are adenocarcinoma and lymphosarcoma. Less common malignancies include carcinoid tumors, leiomyosarcoma, fibrosarcoma, mastocytoma, hemangiosarcoma, and anaplastic sarcoma.

Adenocarcinoma

- Adenocarcinomas are locally invasive and slow growing and are usually seen in older animals. The most common sites in dogs are the duodenum and colon; in cats, the ileum and distal jejunum.
- Morphologically there are three forms of adenocarcinoma:
  - Infiltrative—thickened stenotic region of bowel that obstructs the lumen
  - Ulcerative—deep indurated mucosal ulcer with raised edges
  - Proliferative—lobulated expanding intestinal mass
- Mucosal ulceration is frequent, sometimes resulting in melena and blood loss anemia.

- Local invasion of the mesentery, omentum, and regional lymph nodes is common. More widespread metastasis also may occur.

Lymphoma

- GI lymphoma arises from B lymphocytes of the gut-associated lymphoid tissue (GALT) and is the most common extranodal lymphoma in dogs and cats (see Chap. 25).
- In cats, intestinal lymphoma occurs mostly over 8 years of age and is caused by feline leukemia virus (see Chap. 6), although as few as 30% are viremic.
- Morphologically there are two types of intestinal lymphoma:
  - Diffuse lymphoma—diffuse infiltration of the lamina propria and submucosa with neoplastic lymphocytes causes malabsorption and occasionally deep ulceration
  - Nodular lymphoma—expanding intestinal mass, most often in the ileocecocolic region, causing progressive luminal obstruction
- Metastasis to regional lymph nodes and other organs is common.

Clinical Signs

- Small intestinal neoplasia typically develops insidiously with initial vague signs of anorexia and lethargy, progressing to diarrhea and intermittent vomiting. Weight loss develops and progresses in severity in parallel with tumor growth. Melena, hematemesis, anemia, fever, icterus, and abdominal effusion may also occur.
- Colonic polyps and tumors cause hematochezia, dyschezia, and tenesmus, sometimes with mucoid diarrhea; thus, they are easily confused with inflammatory diseases of the colon.
- Multifocal GI lymphoma may invade the stomach, small intestine, or colon, in any combination, thereby varying the clinical presentation. Furthermore, signs of extraintestinal involvement of organs such as the liver, spleen, or kidney may add to the clinical signs and physical findings.

Diagnosis

- Abdominal palpation often detects intestinal neoplasia as a firm mid-abdominal mass, thickened intestinal loops, or mesenteric lymphadenopathy.
- Rectal palpation detects stenosing or polypoid rectal masses. Most adenomatous rectal polyps can be exposed at the anus by everting the rectal mucosa with gentle traction. Polyps usually appear dark red and lobulated, are extremely friable, and bleed easily.
- Laboratory evaluation may reveal blood loss anemia, neutrophilic leukocytosis with left shift, hypoproteinemia, or elevated serum hepatic enzyme concentrations.
- Radiography, particularly barium-contrast, can be helpful for delineating regions of mucosal irregularity, luminal narrowing, and intramural infiltration,

thickening, or nodularity. Thoracic radiography is indicated for detection of metastasis.

- Abdominal ultrasonography may be used to better define abdominal mass lesions.
- Surgical excision or biopsy of the affected segment of bowel provides a definitive diagnosis:
  - Gastric, duodenal, or colonic lesions are accessible to endoscopic biopsy.
  - Percutaneous fine-needle aspiration can be used to make a cytologic diagnosis in selected cases in which the neoplastic intestinal mass or loop can be well delineated and stabilized by palpation.

Treatment

- Surgical resection is the treatment of choice for benign tumors such as polyps and, when feasible, for adenocarcinomas and other nonlymphomatous tumors. Unfortunately, many malignant tumors of the intestinal tract are too advanced for successful resection by the time they are recognized clinically. Always submit excised tissue for thorough histopathologic examination, including evaluation of surgical margins.
- Intestinal lymphoma can be treated with anticancer chemotherapy (see Chaps. 24 and 25).
- Treatment strategy and prognosis may be affected by complications such as malabsorption, protein-losing enteropathy, intestinal blood loss anemia, intestinal obstruction, intussusception, intestinal perforation and peritonitis, and metastasis to the liver or kidneys.

INTESTINAL OBSTRUCTION

Etiology

Intestinal obstruction in dogs and cats may be caused by intraluminal objects, intramural thickening or stenosis, and extramural compression. Specific causes include:

- Foreign bodies (e.g., bones, toys, cloth, metallic objects, stones, peach pits, acorns, rubber nipples, rubber balls, and linear objects such as string and thread)
- Intussusception
- Volvulus
- Intestinal torsion
- Incarceration of bowel in a hernia (includes abdominal hernias of all types, diaphragmatic hernia, and internal herniation of gut loops through a tear in the mesentery)
- Adhesions or stricture (post-trauma or postsurgery)
- Intramural abscess, granuloma, or hematoma
- Congenital malformation (stenosis or atresia)
- Intestinal neoplasia

Pathophysiology

Proximal Versus Distal Obstruction

The more proximal and complete the obstruction, the more acute and severe the signs and the greater the likelihood of dehydration, electrolye imbalance, and shock.

- *Proximal obstructions* cause gastric outlet occlusion, leading to persistent vomiting, loss of gastric secretions (hydrochloric acid), and metabolic alkalosis.
- *Distal obstructions* cause varying degrees of metabolic acidosis. Distal and incomplete obstructions can be insidious, with vague, intermittent signs of chronic anorexia and occasional vomiting that span several days or even weeks, leading to progressive starvation.

Simple versus Strangulated Obstruction

Vascular compromise of obstructed bowel worsens the severity of the condition.

- *Simple obstructions* occlude the lumen without compromising vascular integrity.
- *Strangulated obstructions* cause vascular compromise of the obstructed bowel segment. This occurs most often with intussusception, volvulus, and incarcerated hernia. The sequence of events following strangulation are edema and engorgement of the affected loop, tissue hypoxia and infarction of the bowel wall, accumulation of gut bacteria and toxins in the peritoneal fluid, and rapidly progressive toxemia and shock, culminating in death.

Clinical Signs

The clinical manifestations and consequences of obstruction depend on its location, completeness, and duration, as well as the vascular integrity of the affected bowel segment.

- Acute onset of vomiting, anorexia, and depression are the most consistent clinical signs.
- Other signs may include abdominal distention, diarrhea (watery, hemorrhagic, or melenic), abdominal pain (restlessness, panting, or abnormal body posture), and shock (acute collapse).

Diagnosis

- Abdominal palpation may identify intestinal foreign bodies, intussusceptions ("sausage loop"), or gas- and fluid-distended loops of bowel proximal to the obstruction.
- Radiography often confirms the presence of obstruction and delineates the cause, especially when contrast studies are used.
  - Radiographic findings suggesting obstruction include gas or fluid distention (mechanical ileus) of the bowel, delayed transit of contrast material, fixation or displacement of gut loops, luminal filling defects, and foreign objects within the lumen.
- Cats commonly ingest radiolucent linear intestinal foreign bodies (e.g., thread, string, cloth, fishing line, dental floss, and decorative tinsel) that cause aggregation and plication of the bowel and have a distinctive radiographic pattern.
- Laboratory findings often reflect fluid, electrolyte, and acid-base derangements; these vary with location, completeness, and duration of obstruction.

- Leukocytosis with a left shift or degenerative leukopenia accompanied by septic abdominal effusion indicates intestinal ischemia or perforation with peritonitis (see Chap. 96).

Treatment

- Intestinal obstructions are treated surgically. Give close attention to supportive care, especially maintenance of fluid, electrolyte, and acid-base homeostasis before, during, and after surgery (for further information on intestinal surgery, see Chap. 90).
- Treatment includes management of complications such as necrosis or perforation of the bowel, peritonitis (see Chap. 96), and endotoxic shock (see Chap. 72).

SUPPLEMENTAL READINGS

Burrows CF: Medical diseases of the colon. *In* Jones BD, ed.: Canine and Feline Gastroenterology. Philadelphia: WB Saunders, 1986, p 221.

Leib MS, Hay WH, Roth L: Plasmacytic-lymphocytic colitis in dogs. *In* Kirk RW, ed.: Current Veterinary Therapy X. Philadelphia: WB Saunders, 1989, p 939.

Nelson RW, Stookey LJ, Kazacos E: Nutritional management of idiopathic chronic colitis in the dog. J Vet Intern Med 2:133, 1988.

Richter KP: Diseases of the large bowel. *In* Ettinger SJ, ed.: Textbook of Veterinary Internal Medicine, 3rd Ed. Philadelphia: WB Saunders, 1989, p 1397.

Sherding RG: Chronic diarrhea. *In* Ford RB, ed.: Clinical Signs and Diagnosis in Small Animal Practice. New York: Churchill Livingstone, 1988, p 473.

Sherding RG: Diseases of the intestines. *In* Sherding RG, ed.: The Cat—Diseases and Clinical Management. 2nd Ed. Philadelphia: WB Saunders, 1994, p 1211.

Sherding RG: Diseases of the small bowel. *In* Ettinger SJ, ed.: Textbook of Veterinary Internal Medicine, 3rd Ed. Philadelphia: WB Saunders, 1989, p 1323.

Strombeck DR, Guilford WG: Idiopathic inflammatory bowel diseases. *In* Small Animal Gastroenterology, 2nd Ed. Davis, CA: Stonegate Publishing, 1990, p 357.

90 Surgery of the Intestines

Ronald M. Bright

Surgical therapy is indicated for structural disease of the bowel. Most animals that require surgery of the small bowel are physiologically compromised. When obstruction of the small bowel is proximal in location (high obstruction), serious electrolyte and water abnormalities can place these patients at high risk.

Prophylactic antibiotics administered perioperatively are indicated in small bowel surgery.

- Before surgery of the upper and middle small bowel, give a first-generation cephalosporin such as cefazolin (20 mg/kg) IV initially; repeat IV 3 hours later.
- Before surgery of the distal small bowel and large intestine, give a second-generation cephalosporin such as cefmetazole (15 mg/kg) IV or cefoxitin (30 mg/kg) IV; repeat IV 3 hours later.

ANATOMY

- The small intestine extends from the pylorus to the cecum.
- The duodenocolic ligament restricts the movement of the distal duodenum.
- The jejunum is the major portion of the small bowel and is a very mobile structure.
- The major blood supply is from the cranial mesenteric artery.
- A portion of the proximal duodenum is supplied by the celiac artery and shares a source of blood with the right lobe of the pancreas via the pancreaticoduodenal artery.
- The tunica of the small intestine includes the mucosa, submucosa, muscularis, and serosa.
- The submucosal layer provides blood vessels, lymphatics, and nerves. It is also the support or "holding" layer for sutures.

ENTEROTOMY

Preoperative Considerations

- Give perioperative antibiotics, as previously described.
- Attempt to correct electrolyte and water abnormalities before surgery.
- Low albumin levels affect the choice of suture materials (nonabsorbable) and the need for suture-line reinforcement technique such as serosal patch techniques.

Surgical Procedure

Objectives

- Gain access to the lumen of the small bowel to remove a foreign body.
- Help define a disease by acquiring a full-thickness biopsy.
- Avoid contamination of the peritoneal cavity.

Equipment

- General surgical pack
- Babcock forceps
- Laparotomy sponges
- Doyen noncrushing intestinal clamps
- #11 Bard-Parker blade

Technique

1. Make a midline abdominal incision to allow access to the small bowel.
2. Isolate the segment of bowel to be entered with moistened laparotomy sponges.
3. Place a 3-0 silk stay suture at both ends of the proposed enterotomy incision (Babcock forceps may be substituted).
4. Milk bowel contents away from the proposed enterotomy site; place noncrushing intestinal forceps (or an assistant's fingers) across the bowel to minimize spillage.
5. Make a full-thickness stab incision into the lumen, using a #11 Bard-Parker scalpel blade. Place a suction tip in the bowel lumen and remove its contents. Enlarge the incision as needed with Metzenbaum scissors.
6. If removing a foreign body, perform the enterotomy over healthy bowel distal to the foreign body.
7. If a biopsy is needed, excise a 2–3 mm strip of bowel parallel to the enterotomy incision.
8. Trim any everted mucosa with scissors.
9. Close the enterotomy incision with 3-0 or 4-0 synthetic absorbable or monofilament nonabsorbable suture material on a swaged-on taper-point needle. A full-thickness, simple interrupted or continuous appositional suture pattern is preferred.

▼ *Key Point* To minimize tissue trauma, avoid repeatedly grabbing the intestinal wall with thumb forceps.

10. Rinse the enterotomy site thoroughly with warm saline.
11. Use omentum or a jejunal onlay patch to reinforce the suture line. The author prefers to use omentum, even in relatively healthy tissue.
12. Some severely debilitated animals may benefit from placement of a jejunostomy tube for postoperative enteral nutritional support (See Chapter 3 for nutritional support of critical patients.)
13. Perform routine closure of the abdomen.

Postoperative Care and Complications
Short-Term

- Monitor for signs of leakage peritonitis by abdominal palpation, body temperature measurements, and a complete blood count (CBC).
- Give food and water the day after surgery.
- Gradually taper off fluid and electrolyte therapy as the animal returns to normal eating and drinking.

Long-Term

- Strictures are rare unless an excessive amount of tissue was removed for biopsy and the lumen diameter was compromised.
- Slow leakage from an enterotomy site may become walled off and later be manifested as an abscess.

Prognosis

- The prognosis is good if the enterotomy was done for a foreign body.
- If biopsy indicates neoplasia, the prognosis is poor.
- If biopsy reveals a protein-losing enteropathy due to benign infiltrative disease, the prognosis is poor to guarded (see Chap. 89).

INTESTINAL RESECTION AND ANASTOMOSIS

Indications for intestinal resection and anastomosis include:

- Diseases causing bowel necrosis (e.g., foreign body, volvulus, trauma)
- Neoplasia
- Intussusception
- Severe, focal infiltrative bowel disease (e.g., phycomycosis pythiosis, zygomycosis)

Preoperative Considerations

- Administer perioperative antibiotics starting 20–40 minutes before surgery, as described previously.
- Although controversy surrounds the choice of suture pattern for intestinal anastomosis, any of several techniques probably is acceptable in the hands of a competent surgeon who follows sound intestinal surgery principles.

- The author prefers the simple interrupted appositional (SIA) suture pattern for intestinal (large or small) anastomoses. This noncrushing technique causes little compromise of the blood supply of the intestinal segments. (Disruption of vascularity is the most common biologic cause of failure of an anastomosis.)

▼ *Key Point* Accurate and atraumatic placement of sutures and gentle handling of the bowel gives the best results. Failure of an anastomosis usually is due to poor surgical technique.

- Assess bowel viability before determining the amount of bowel to be resected. Standard clinical criteria include color, peristalsis, and arterial pulsations.
- In the rare case in which standard criteria are not adequate to determine bowel viability, an intravenous fluorescein dye technique can be used.
  - Inject 2 ml of 5% fluorescein dye IV; in a darkened surgery room, evaluate the pattern of fluorescence using #3600 ultraviolet illumination (Wood's lamp).
  - A smooth, uniform green-gold color or a finely mottled pattern with no areas of nonfluorescence greater than 3 mm denotes acceptable bowel viability.

Surgical Procedure
Objectives

- Remove the diseased or nonviable segment of bowel and restore bowel continuity with an end-to-end anastomosis.
- Preserve lumen diameter and tissue blood supply.
- Avoid spillage of bowel contents.

Equipment

- General surgical pack
- Doyen noncrushing clamps
- Laparotomy pads
- Abdominal retractors

Technique

1. Make a midline abdominal incision long enough to accommodate a thorough abdominal exploratory procedure.
2. Isolate the affected bowel segment with saline-moistened laparotomy sponges.
3. Isolate and ligate the mesenteric vessels to the affected area. Ligate the arcadial vessels within the mesenteric fat similarly.
4. Place crushing clamps across the bowel at a 60° angle to the long axis of the bowel and just inside the arcadial vessels.
5. Milk the ingesta away from the crushing clamps. Place a noncrushing clamp across the viable segments of bowel to be anastomosed, or have an assistant gently hold the bowel segments during the anastomosis.
6. Excise the diseased bowel by incising between the crushing clamp and the arcadial vessel ligation.

7. The mucosal collar may evert around the ends of the transected bowel. This can be trimmed with scissors.

8. Correct lumen disparity by cutting the small lumen at a more acute angle, longitudinally incising the antimesenteric edge of the small end, or oversewing the larger end.

9. Use a 3-0 or 4-0 suture on a small taper-point needle to place the sutures. All knots are extraluminal.

10. Carefully place the first suture at the mesenteric border. The second suture apposes the antimesenteric border. Place sutures approximately 2–3 mm apart along the "near" side of the anastomosis. Include the entire thickness of the bowel. Pull down the sutures slowly so as to gently appose the edges of the bowel (SIA pattern).

11. Appose the "far" side or back wall similarly.

12. Gently flush warm sterile saline over the anastomotic site and adjacent lengths of bowel.

▼ *Key Point* Do not flush the entire abdominal cavity unless there is gross contamination from the surgery or preexisting peritonitis.

13. Wrap a piece of omentum around the line of anastomosis and gently tack it to the bowel above and below the anastomosis.

14. Close the defect in the mesentery with a continuous suture.

15. Use new gloves and a sterile set of instruments for abdominal wall closure.

16. If nutritional support is necessary, place a jejunostomy tube before closure of the abdomen.

Postoperative Care and Complications

- Maintain intravenous fluid and electrolyte supplementation until the animal is drinking water.
- Withhold food and fluids for 12–24 hours, after which the regular diet can be fed.
- Discontinue antibiotics 2–4 hours postoperatively, unless peritonitis was present. In this case, continue therapy, basing choice of antibiotic on bacterial culture taken at time of surgery.
- Monitor for signs of depression, high fever, excessive abdominal tenderness, vomiting, and ileus, which may indicate leakage peritonitis. If warranted, initiate appropriate diagnostic (e.g., abdominocentesis) and therapeutic measures (see Chap. 96).

ENTEROENTEROPEXY/ENTEROPEXY (COLOPEXY)

- Enteroenteropexy, or plication of loops of bowel, is done to prevent recurrence of intussusception and is usually performed at the time of definitive surgical repair of the intussusception.
- Enteropexy, or fixation of bowel to the abdominal wall, is done as part of a tube jejunostomy placement procedure, as a colopexy for treatment of rectal prolapse, or as an adjunctive procedure for correcting

rectal sacculation related to a perineal hernia (see Chap. 95).

- These procedures have limited use in dogs and cats.

Surgical Procedures

Objectives

- Prevent recurrent telescoping of bowel following surgical repair of intussusception.
- Diminish likelihood of leakage around a jejunostomy tube as it exits the bowel and enters the abdominal wall.
- Prevent caudal movement of the colon and rectum (colopexy).

Equipment

General surgical pack
Balfour abdominal retractor

Technique

Enteroenteropexy

1. Place loops of small bowel side by side to form a series of gentle loops. Suture loops to each other by engaging the seromuscular layers with monofilament nonabsorbable suture (Fig. 90–1). Place sutures approximately 6–10 cm apart.

2. The amount of bowel to include in the "pexy" procedure is controversial. Some surgeons include the entire small bowel, starting at the descending duodenum and finishing at the ileocecocolic junction. Others include only two or three loops of bowel above and below the point of intussusception. Another option is to include only the distal jejunum and ileum, because most intussusceptions involve the distal small bowel.

Colopexy

1. Reduce the rectal prolapse by placing gentle traction on the descending colon, pulling it cranially.

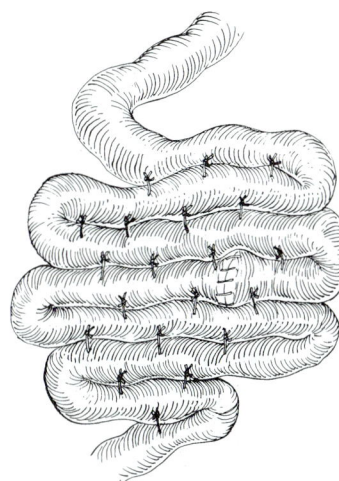

Figure 90–1. Jejunal enteroenteropexy to prevent intussusception via a ventral midline abdominal approach.

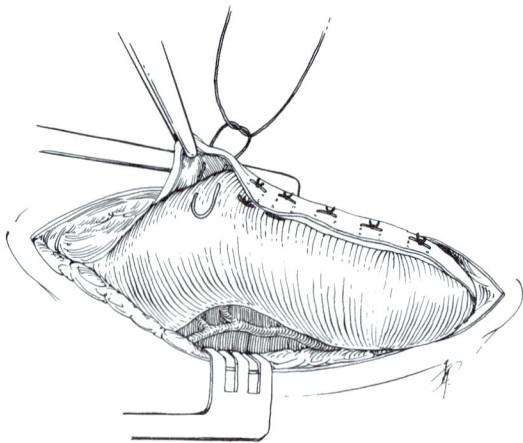

Figure 90–2. Technique for colopexy to prevent recurrence of rectal prolapse.

2. Scarify an 8–10 cm portion of the descending colon with a surgical blade along the antimesenteric border.
3. Alternately, make a longitudinal seromuscular incision along the antimesenteric border. This may result in a more consistent colopexy. Avoid entering the lumen.
4. Make an incision into the peritoneum and underlying musculature in the abdominal wall opposite the segment of prepared colon.
5. Preplace four to six horizontal mattress sutures between the colon and the exposed surface of the abdominal wall (Fig. 90–2). Monofilament nonabsorbable suture is preferred.
6. Tie the sutures to securely appose the fresh bleeding surfaces of the colon and abdominal wall (see Fig. 90–2).

Postoperative Care and Complications

- No special feeding limitations are necessary.
- Recurrence of intussusception (following enteroenteropexy) or rectal prolapse (following colopexy) suggests that the pexy site has broken down.

COLOTOMY

The most common indication for a colotomy is a full-thickness biopsy when diagnosis has eluded other diagnostic procedures. Whenever possible, colonoscopic methods of biopsy are preferred (see Chap. 89). Rarely, a colotomy is done to remove a foreign body.

Preoperative Considerations

- Surgical procedures involving the colon are more likely to be associated with dehiscence than those involving other portions of the gastrointestinal tract.

▼ **Key Point** Gentle handling of the colon and the prevention of excessive tension across the suture line will help preserve a good blood supply and promote ideal wound healing.

- The risk of a serious abdominal infection is considerable with colonic surgery.
- To reduce the risk of postoperative sepsis, administer perioperative antibiotics for gram-negative aerobes and anaerobes. Give cefmetazole (15 mg/kg) IV q1½h for 2 or 3 doses, starting 20–30 minutes before surgery. Cefoxitin (30 mg/kg) may be substituted.
- Preoperative mechanical cleansing of the colon via multiple enemas may be indicated. This can be especially helpful to improve exposure of colonic polyps or neoplasms during resection.

Surgical Procedure

Objectives

- Collect tissue for biopsy.
- Remove foreign body in cases of low bowel obstruction.
- Prevent spillage of colonic contents.

Equipment

- General surgery pack
- Babcock forceps
- Laparotomy sponges
- Doyen noncrushing intestinal clamps
- #11 Bard-Parker blade

Technique

1. Make a caudal midline abdominal incision for access to the colon.
2. Pack off the colon with laparotomy sponges at the proposed incision site.
3. Place stay sutures at both ends of the proposed colotomy incision (Babcock forceps can be substituted).
4. Milk the colonic contents away from the incision site and cross-clamp the bowel segment with Doyen clamps.
5. Using a #11 Bard-Parker surgical blade, stab into the lumen of the colon. Remove a full-thickness elliptical piece of tissue with Metzenbaum scissors.
6. Close the colotomy incision side-to-side with 3-0 or 4-0 synthetic absorbable suture (e.g., polydioxanone, PDS) in a simple interrupted appositional pattern. A nonabsorbable suture (e.g., polypropylene) may be substituted.
7. Gently irrigate the bowel immediately adjacent to the colotomy incision with warm saline before removing the laparotomy pad. Do not allow irrigation fluid to enter the peritoneal cavity.
8. Cover the colotomy incision line with omentum.
9. Perform routine closure of the abdomen.

Postoperative Care and Complications

Short-Term

- Monitor closely for signs of leakage peritonitis for 48 hours.
- Abdominal pain, an unusually high fever, and a neutrophilia with a left shift suggest a need for further diagnostic tests such as radiography and diagnostic peritoneal lavage.

Long-Term

- Strictures occur rarely.
- Slow-leakage peritonitis may be masked by antibiotics, or the infected area may be walled off, only to be manifested later as an abscess.

Prognosis

- The prognosis is good if the colotomy is done to remove a foreign body.
- If the biopsy suggests a non-neoplastic process, the prognosis depends on the underlying disease (see Chap. 89).

SUBTOTAL COLECTOMY

The primary indication for subtotal (90–95%) removal of the colon is for palliation of severe or recurrent constipation (obstipation related to megacolon). Idiopathic megacolon in the cat (see Chap. 89) is the most common disease for which surgery is indicated.

▼ *Key Point* Meticulous handling and careful apposition of tissue and a tension-free anastomosis are critical for the success of subtotal colectomy.

Preoperative Considerations

- In cats, the ileocolic valve can be resected with few postoperative problems. Reestablishing bowel continuity with an ileocolostomy versus a colocolostomy (when the ileocolic valve is preserved) is technically easier. However, it is preferable to preserve the ileocolic valve. The postoperative convalescent period is shorter and the likelihood of intractable diarrhea secondary to small bowel bacterial overgrowth is diminished.
- Administer prophylactic antibiotics, as described previously.
- Preoperative enemas are not necessary and, in fact, can complicate the surgery because of potential leakage of fluid from the colon.

Surgical Procedure

Objectives

- Palliate signs of constipation or obstipation that are associated with megacolon.
- Remove most of the colon with restoration of continuity by ileocolostomy or colocolostomy.
- Promote movement of bowel contents from the small bowel to the rectum.
- Prevent spillage of colonic contents.

Equipment

- General surgery pack
- Balfour abdominal retractors
- Laparotomy sponges
- Doyen noncrushing straight intestinal clamps
- Carmalt crushing forceps

Technique

1. Make a ventral midline abdominal incision, starting from midway between the xiphoid and umbilicus and coursing caudally to the brim of the pelvis.
2. Exteriorize and carefully isolate the colon and distal small bowel from the rest of the abdominal viscera outside the abdominal cavity.
3. Isolate the appropriate colic vessels approximately 1–2 cm from the mesenteric side of the colon. Ligate and divide these (Fig. 90–3).
4. If the ileocolic valve is being removed, ligate an additional set of vessels (ileocecocolic artery and vein) (see Fig. 90–3).
5. Caudally, ligate the caudal mesenteric artery and vein.
6. Milk the fecal contents toward the center of the segment of colon to be removed.
7. Place a noncrushing intestinal clamp across the distal colon approximately 1 cm cranial to the brim of the pelvis; if the ileocolic valve is being preserved, place another clamp across the short 1-cm segment of proximal colon remaining below the ileocolic valve.
8. If the ileocolic valve is being resected, place a noncrushing clamp across the ileum just proximal to the ileocolic valve.
9. Use crushing forceps to clamp the colon approximately 1 cm to the inside of the previously placed noncrushing clamps. Transect the colon next to the crushing forceps and the segment of bowel being removed (i.e., the crushing forceps come out with the resected bowel segment).
10. Perform an end-to-end anastomosis using 4-0 polypropylene or a monofilament synthetic absorbable suture in a simple interrupted, full-thickness, appositional suture pattern.

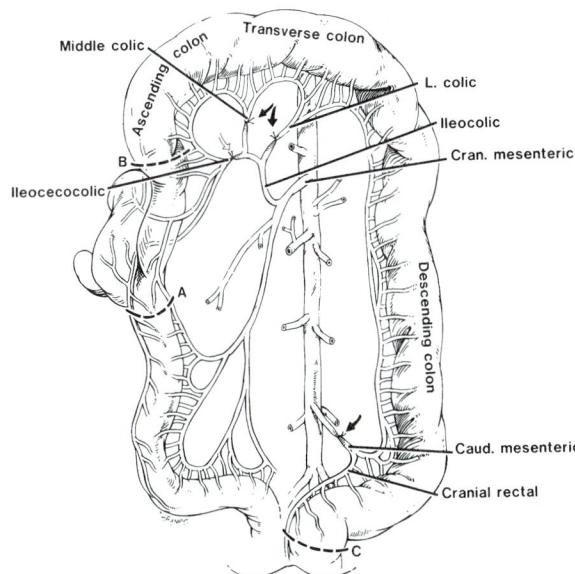

Figure 90–3. Subtotal colectomy. Sites of ligation of colic blood vessels before anastomosis and resection. Colonic resection can either include resection of the ileocecocolic valve (incision at *A*) or preserve the ileocecocolic area (incision at *B*). Distal incision (*C*) made in the colon.

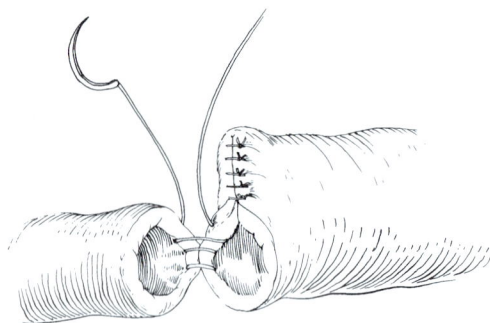

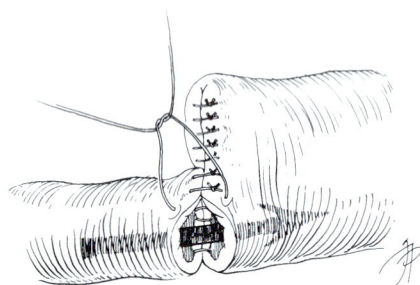

Figure 90–4. Subtotal colectomy. Correction of luminal disparity of the bowel by partial closure of larger segment before anastomosis.

11. Correct any lumen disparity by longitudinally incising the antimesenteric side of the bowel with the smaller lumen. Lumen disparity can also be corrected by partial closure of the larger colonic segment, using the same suture and pattern (Fig. 90–4).
12. Be careful to incorporate the serosa and to ensure accurate and gentle placement of all sutures. Place the sutures at 2–3 mm intervals.
13. Gently irrigate the anastomotic site and adjacent 4–5 cm of bowel with warm saline. Do not allow fluid to enter the peritoneal cavity.
14. Place an omental patch over the site of anastomosis and gently tack it with one or two sutures below the line of anastomosis.
15. Remove the laparotomy sponges and replace the bowel in the abdominal cavity.
16. Use new gloves and a sterile set of instruments for closure of the midline incision.

Postoperative Care and Complications

Short-Term

- Withhold food and liquids for 24 hours.
- Monitor closely for signs of leakage from the anastomosis for 48–72 hours.
- Some animals continue to have some tenesmus for 7–10 days after surgery.
- Loose stools and increased frequency of defecation occur but usually improve somewhat over a period of weeks to months.
- Continue intravenous fluids for 36–48 hours.

Long-Term

- The frequency of defecation generally increases by 30–50%.
- The stools remain soft indefinitely but often become less fluid and more semiformed within a few weeks.
- Cats do not need a special diet.
- It may be necessary to keep animals on a diet low in volume and high in caloric density for 10–14 days. Thereafter, feed a diet that minimizes diarrhea and results in solidly formed stools.

▼ *Key Point* Cats seem to adapt well to subtotal colectomy, whereas dogs may have persistent diarrhea postoperatively.

TYPHLECTOMY

Indications for typhlectomy, or surgical removal of the cecum, include:
- Typhlitis (cecal inflammation) caused by chronic whipworm infection
- Cecal inversion
- Cecal neoplasia

Preoperative Considerations

- If possible, evert the inverted cecum before its amputation.
- If manual reduction of cecal inversion is not possible because of adhesions, reduction may need to be done through a colotomy incision.
- The cecum is attached to the terminal ileum by the ileocecal fold, which consists of fascia and peritoneum.

Surgical Procedure

Objective

- Remove the cecum without interfering with ileocolic anatomy and function.

Equipment

- General surgery pack
- Doyen noncrushing straight intestinal forceps
- Abdominal retractor

Technique

1. Bluntly dissect the ileocecal fold to free the cecum from its attachments to the ileum.
2. Preserve the ileocecal vessels while ligating and dividing the cecal branches.
3. Carefully incise the remaining attachments of the cecum to the proximal colon.
4. When the cecum is isolated from its attachments and blood supply, double-clamp the base of the cecum with straight intestinal forceps.
5. Amputate the cecum between the two forceps.
6. Oversew the forceps remaining on the base of the cecum with 2-0 or 3-0 synthetic absorbable suture using a Parker-Kerr suture pattern.

7. Place a second layer of a continuous Lembert inverting suture.

Postoperative Care and Complications

Short-Term

Give food and liquids the day after surgery.

Long-Term

Complications are rare.

Prognosis

- The prognosis is good.

SUPPLEMENTAL READINGS

Enterotomy

Oates JA, Wood AJJ: Antimicrobial prophylaxis in surgery. N Engl J Med 315:1129, 1986.
Richardson DC: Intestinal surgery—a review. Comp Contin Educ Pract Vet 3:259, 1981.
Orsher RJ, Rosen E: Small intestine. *In* Slatter DH, ed.: Textbook of Small Animal Surgery, 2nd Ed. Philadelphia: WB Saunders, 1993, p 593.

Resection and Anastomosis

Bauer MS, Matthiesen DT: Complications and decision making associated with small intestinal surgery. Problems in Veterinary Medicine—Gastrointestinal Surgical Complications 1:316, 1989.
Ellison GW, Jokinen MP, Park RD: End-to-end approximating intestinal anastomosis in the dog: A comparison of fluorescein dye, angiographic and histopathologic evaluation. J Am Anim Hosp Assoc 18:729, 1982.
Richardson DC: Intestinal surgery—a review. Comp Cont Educ Pract Vet 3:259, 1981.
Sullins KE, Stashak TS, Mero KN: Evaluation of fluorescein dye as an indication of small intestinal viability in the horse. J Am Vet Med Assoc 186:257, 1985.

Wheaton LG, Strandberg JD, Hamilton SR, et al.: A comparison of three techniques for intraoperative prediction of small intestinal injury. J Am Anim Hosp 19:897, 1983.

Enteropexy, Enteroenteropexy, and Colopexy

Bauer MS, Matthiesen DT: Complications and decision making associated with small intestinal surgery. Problems in Veterinary Medicine—Gastrointestinal Surgical Complications 1:316, 1989.
Engen MH: Management of rectal prolapse. *In* Bojrab MJ, ed.: Current Techniques in Small Animal Surgery, 4th Ed. Baltimore: Williams & Wilkins, 1998, p 254.
Lewis DD: Intussusception in dogs and cats. Comp Cont Educ Pract Vet 9:523, 1987.
Orton EC: Enteral hyperalimentation administered via needle catheter—jejunostomy as an adjunct to cranial abdominal surgery in dogs and cats. J Am Vet Med Assoc 188:1406, 1986.

Colotomy

Orsher RJ: Problems and complications associated with colorectal surgery. Problems in Veterinary Medicine—Gastrointestinal Surgical Complications 1:243, 1989.
Richardson DC, Krahwinkel DJ: Surgery of the colon. *In* Bojrab MJ, ed.: Current Techniques in Small Animal Surgery II. Philadelphia: Lea & Febiger, 1983, p 162.

Subtotal Colectomy

Bright RM, Burrows CF, Goring R, et al.: Subtotal colectomy for the treatment of acquired megacolon in the dog and cat. J Am Vet Med Assoc 188:1412, 1986.
Richardson DC, Duckett KE, Krahwinkel DJ, et al.: Colonic anastomosis: Evaluation of an end to end crushing and inverting technique. Am J Vet Res 43:436, 1982.
Rosin E, Walshaw R, Mehlhaff C, et al.: Subtotal colectomy for treatment of chronic constipation associated with idiopathic megacolon in cats: 38 cases (1979–1985). J Am Vet Med Assoc 193:850, 1988.

Typhlectomy

Greiner T, Christie T: The cecum, colon, rectum, and anus. *In* Bojrab MJ, ed.: Current Techniques in Small Animal Surgery I. Philadelphia: Lea & Febiger, 1975, p 126.

91 Diseases of the Liver and Biliary Tract

Susan E. Johnson / Robert G. Sherding

DIAGNOSTIC STRATEGY FOR LIVER DISEASE

General Comments

The liver has many diverse functions related to hepatic blood flow; protein, carbohydrate, and fat metabolism; detoxification and excretion of drugs and toxins; and formation and elimination of bile. Consequently, the clinical and laboratory abnormalities associated with liver failure are diverse.

Overview of the Diagnostic Strategy

- Clinical, laboratory, and imaging studies to identify the presence of liver disease
- Characterization of the functional aspects of the hepatic disease
- Determination of an etiologic or histologic diagnosis, which usually requires a liver biopsy

Acute versus Chronic Disease

The clinical approach and management of patients with hepatic disease is dictated largely by the acute versus chronic nature of the hepatic disorder. Historical, physical, laboratory, and radiographic findings may suggest whether the hepatic disease is acute or chronic, but hepatic biopsy often is required for definitive evaluation. Classifying a disorder as acute or chronic has diagnostic, therapeutic, and prognostic implications.

- In acute hepatic failure, toxic or infectious causes are common, and intensive supportive care is warranted to allow time for hepatic regeneration. The long-term prognosis for recovery is favorable if the animal survives the initial stages.
- Chronic hepatic disorders are more likely to be accompanied by irreversible changes (cirrhosis); thus, the long-term prognosis may not be favorable.

Clinical Signs

Clinical signs of liver disease include those typically associated with hepatic dysfunction, such as jaundice, hepatic encephalopathy, ascites, and excessive bleeding, and nonspecific signs such as vomiting, diarrhea, anorexia, lethargy, and weight loss, which overlap with signs of other body system disorders.

Nonspecific Signs

- *Vomiting* is a common sign of liver disease. Hematemesis suggests gastroduodenal ulceration, a recognized complication of hepatobiliary disease.
- *Diarrhea* occurs less frequently than vomiting and is characteristically small-bowel diarrhea (see Chap. 89).
- *Anorexia* is a common but nonspecific sign of hepatobiliary disease.
- *Weight loss and stunted growth* are nonspecific signs that suggest chronic rather than acute hepatic disease.

Polyuria and Polydipsia

- Polyuria and polydipsia (PU/PD) may be important presenting clinical signs in dogs with liver disease. The mechanism is multifactorial and includes psychogenic polydipsia and renal concentrating defects.

Signs of Abnormal Bilirubin Excretion

- Pigmented urine *(bilirubinuria)* and *jaundice* (icterus) of the sclera, oral mucous membranes, and skin are classic signs of cholestatic liver disease. However, these findings are not specific for hepatobiliary disease and can also be caused by hemolytic disorders.
- *Acholic (gray) feces* occur secondary to severe cholestasis (usually from common bile duct obstruction), which prevents bilirubin in the bile from entering the intestinal tract and imparting the normal brown color to the feces.

Coagulopathy

- Excessive bleeding (i.e., hemorrhages of the skin and mucous membranes, melena, hematuria) occasionally is associated with liver disease, especially if hepatic damage is severe or is associated with common bile duct obstruction.
- Subclinical clotting abnormalities may become clinically apparent after liver biopsy, surgery, and development of gastroduodenal ulcers.
- Potential mechanisms for bleeding include disseminated intravascular coagulation (DIC), primary failure of the hepatocytes to synthesize clotting factors, and vitamin K deficiency (see Chap. 21 for additional details).

Hepatic Encephalopathy

- Hepatic encephalopathy is a metabolic encephalopathy that occurs secondary to severe liver disease or portosystemic shunting of blood.
- Clinical signs include depression, hypersalivation, behavioral changes, altered consciousness, motor disturbances, seizures, and coma. As with other metabolic encephalopathies, signs typically wax and wane and are interspersed with normal periods.
- Ammonia, mercaptans, short-chain fatty acids, gamma-aminobutyric acid (GABA), and endogenous benzodiazepines are potential encephalopathic toxins that are produced in the colon by bacterial action on various substrates. Because the liver normally detoxifies these substances, systemic concentrations are low. With severe liver disease or portosystemic shunting, these potential toxins reach high concentrations in the systemic circulation and the central nervous system (CNS), resulting in clinical signs.
- Exacerbation of encephalopathy occurs after eating a meal high in protein because protein is a substrate for toxins such as ammonia and mercaptans.
- It is important to differentiate hepatic encephalopathy from other metabolic encephalopathies and from primary CNS disorders.

Ascites

- Ascites is a common feature of severe chronic liver disease. Mechanisms of ascites and edema formation in liver disease include hypoalbuminemia, portal hypertension, and renal retention of sodium and water.
- Rupture of the biliary tract causing bile peritonitis also is associated with abdominal fluid accumulation.

Signalment and History

- The signalment often provides important clinical information, because breed predilections for specific liver diseases have been recognized, and young animals are more likely to be presented for congenital hepatic disorders such as portosystemic shunt.
- The history is helpful to characterize the clinical course of liver disease as acute or chronic. Recent onset of signs in an animal that was previously healthy suggests acute hepatic failure. However, because of the large functional reserve capacity of the liver, in occult chronic liver disease the clinical signs may be vague and may not be recognized by the owner until the final phase of hepatic decompensation.

▼ *Key Point* Chronic hepatic disease can be associated with recent onset of clinical signs and can initially seem to be an acute disease. However, persisting signs of weight loss and ascites and findings of hypoalbuminemia and microhepatica on subsequent diagnostic evaluation are indicative of chronic hepatic disease.

- The history may provide important information regarding the potential for exposure to known causes of hepatic injury such as drug therapy, surgical and anesthetic procedures, and toxins or infectious agents.
- Determine if the animal has a history of intolerance to drugs normally metabolized by the liver, such as sedatives, tranquilizers, anticonvulsants, and anesthetics.
- Determine the current vaccination status and exposure potential for infectious agents known to affect the liver, such as leptospirosis, infectious canine hepatitis, and feline infectious peritonitis (FIP).

Physical Examination

Skin and Mucous Membranes

- Evaluate the sclera, oral mucous membranes, and skin for jaundice. Jaundice is not clinically detectable until serum bilirubin concentrations are >2.5–3.0 g/dl. In cats, subtle jaundice often is best detected on the palatine mucosa.
- Evaluate the skin and mucous membranes for evidence of bleeding. Pallor may be detected with blood loss anemia.

Abdominal Palpation

- Palpate the abdomen carefully. The normal liver can be difficult to palpate in dogs and cats, and the edges are normally sharp, not rounded.
- Hepatomegaly is caused by passive venous congestion, diffuse inflammation, nodular hyperplasia, bile engorgement, and infiltration by fat, glycogen, and neoplastic cells.
- Pain on palpation of the liver (hepatodynia) usually indicates acute liver disease. The pain is caused by stretching of the liver capsule and must be differentiated from pain arising in the pancreas, stomach, or spleen.
- Moderate to severe abdominal effusion may be detected.

Neurologic Exam

- Perform a neurologic examination in animals with a history of neurologic signs. With hepatic encephalopathy, the neurologic examination may be normal or suggestive of diffuse cerebral disease (e.g., depression and dementia, disorientation, pacing, circling, head-pressing, hypersalivation, seizures, or coma).

Rectal Exam

- Perform a rectal examination and obtain a fecal sample to evaluate for melena (indicative of gastrointestinal bleeding) and acholic feces.

Laboratory Evaluation

Because clinical findings in hepatobiliary disease often are vague and nonspecific, hepatic disease may not be suspected until biochemical tests identify elevated liver enzyme activity or other evidence of hepatic dysfunction (e.g., hyperbilirubinemia, hypoalbuminemia).

Liver function studies such as serum bile acid (SBA) concentrations are used to:

- Identify occult liver disease
- Assess liver function when there is increased liver enzyme activity but normal serum bilirubin concentrations.
- Determine whether significant hepatic dysfunction is present to warrant performing a liver biopsy
- Monitor response to therapy

Findings consistent with liver disease on routine laboratory tests are described below.

Complete Blood Count (CBC)

- *Mild to moderate anemia* may occur secondary to liver disease because of blood loss (e.g., gastroduodenal ulceration, coagulopathy) or may be associated with normocytic-normochromic anemia of chronic disease.
- *Erythrocytic microcytosis* is a common finding in dogs and cats with portosystemic shunts. Decreased serum iron concentration, normal to increased serum ferritin concentration, and accumulation of stainable iron in the liver suggests that microcytosis is associated with abnormal iron metabolism (impaired iron transport or sequestration of iron), rather than absolute iron deficiency. Decreased availability of iron for hemoglobin synthesis appears to occur despite adequate tissue iron stores.
- *Target cells and poikilocytosis* (acanthocytes and elliptocytes) may occur in dogs and cats with various types of hepatic disease, due to altered red blood cell (RBC) membranes.

Urinalysis

- *Urine specific gravity* may be isosthenuric or hyposthenuric if liver disease is associated with PU/PD.
- *Bilirubinuria* is a sensitive indicator of abnormal bilirubin metabolism, and this finding precedes hyperbilirubinemia and jaundice. Bilirubinuria imparts a yellow-orange color to the urine. Bilirubin crystals may form in the presence of bilirubinuria.
  - Trace amounts of bilirubin may be found in concentrated urine of normal dogs (especially males).
  - Bilirubinuria is always abnormal in cats and suggests underlying hemolytic or hepatobiliary disease.
- *Urine urobilinogen* is a colorless product of enteric bacterial degradation of bilirubin that is absorbed from the gut. A small portion of urobilinogen escapes the enterohepatic circulation and is excreted in the urine. The finding of urobilinogenuria indicates an intact enterohepatic circulation of bilirubin pigments. The absence of urobilinogenuria in a jaundiced animal suggests common bile duct obstruction.
  - However, this test is not reliable in a clinical setting because many nonhepatic factors affect urine urobilinogen concentration, including altered intestinal flora, gastrointestinal bleeding, intestinal absorption, renal excretion, urine pH, urine volume, and urine storage.
- *Ammonium biurate crystals* are commonly detected in animals with portosystemic shunts.

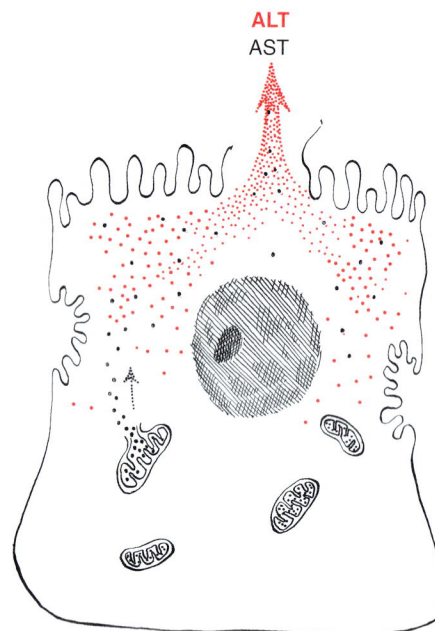

Figure 91–1. With hepatocyte injury, leakage of alanine aminotransferase (ALT) from the cytoplasm results in increased serum activity. Aspartate aminotransferase (AST) is primarily associated with mitochondria but is also present in the cytoplasm. Release of AST from the mitochondria requires a severe insult. Thus, with hepatocyte injury, ALT is more readily released and its activity level will usually be higher than that of serum AST.

▼ *Key Point* Suspect liver disease in any cat or non-Dalmatian dog with ammonium biurate crystalluria.

Liver Enzymes

Evaluation of liver enzyme activity in the serum is used as a screening test to detect liver disease. Increases in liver enzyme activity are not specific for the underlying hepatic disorder. However, liver enzymes can be used to categorize the underlying pathophysiologic mechanism. Increases in liver enzyme activity may occur secondary to hepatocellular injury and leakage (Fig. 91–1) or due to accelerated production stimulated by bile retention (cholestasis) or drug induction (Fig. 91–2).

Many systemic diseases can secondarily affect the liver, causing increased liver enzyme activity, but these are not necessarily associated with clinical liver disease. An important example is feline hyperthyroidism, which is commonly associated with increased liver enzyme activity without significant hepatic dysfunction.

▼ *Key Point* Liver enzymes do not evaluate liver function. Thus, severe hepatic dysfunction may coexist with normal liver enzyme activity; conversely, increased liver enzyme activity may be detected in animals without significant hepatic dysfunction.

Alanine Aminotransferase (ALT)*

- Increased ALT activity indicates hepatocyte injury with leakage of enzyme from the cytoplasm of the he-

---

*Formerly called serum glutamic pyruvic transaminase (SGPT).

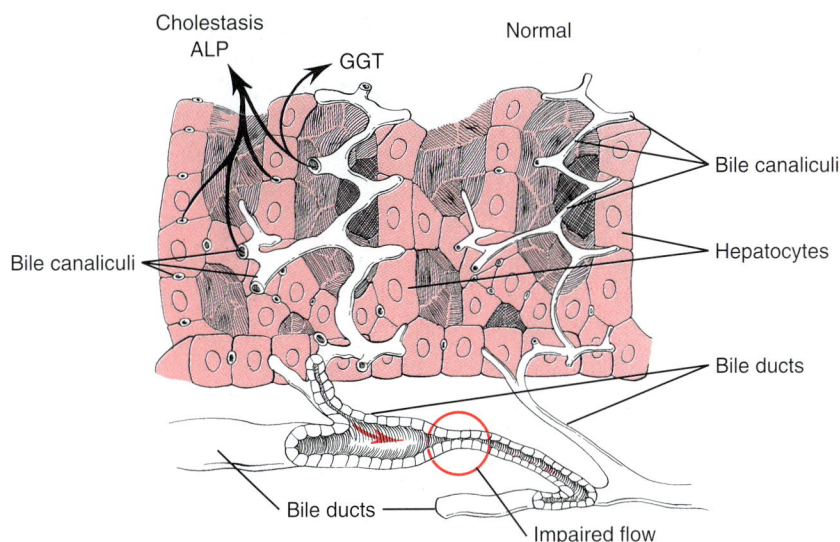

Figure 91–2. Impaired bile flow (cholestasis) causes increased synthesis of alkaline phosphatase (ALP) and gamma-glutamyltransferase (GGT). Alkaline phosphatase is a sensitive indicator of cholestasis in dogs but is less sensitive in cats (see text). With cholestatic disorders, increased ALP activity precedes hyperbilirubinemia. ALP and GGT lack specificity in differentiating between intrahepatic and extrahepatic cholestasis.

patocyte (see Fig. 91–1). The magnitude of ALT increase generally correlates with the number of injured hepatocytes.

- The largest increases in ALT activity occur with hepatocellular necrosis and inflammation (up to 100 times normal). Increases also occur with increased hepatocyte membrane permeability, such as that caused by hypoxia. Severe cholestasis can also cause secondary hepatocyte injury, with increases in ALT up to 20–40 times normal. Increased production of ALT by regenerating hepatocytes may account for persisting increases in enzyme activity after resolution of the initial injury.
- Anticonvulsant drug therapy (primidone, phenytoin, and phenobarbital) in dogs can be associated with mild increases in ALT activity (2 times normal) in the absence of obvious hepatocellular injury. Corticosteroid therapy or hyperadrenocorticism also is associated with mild to moderate (2–10 times normal) increases in ALT activity.
- Small amounts of ALT are present in canine skeletal muscle; it has been shown that severe skeletal muscle degeneration or necrosis (canine muscular dystrophy, necrotizing myopathy, polymyositis) may be associated with increases in ALT activity of 5–25 times normal (see Chap. 149). When increased ALT activity is caused by muscle injury, CK (creatine kinase) and AST activity are also markedly increased. Whether ALT is liver-specific in cats remains to be determined.

Aspartate Aminotransferase (AST)*

- Hepatocyte injury is associated with increased AST activity secondary to leakage from mitochondria and cytoplasm of hepatocytes (see Fig. 91–1).
- AST is not liver-specific in dogs and cats; it is present in significant quantities in hepatocytes and skeletal muscle tissue.

---

*Formerly called serum glutamic oxaloacetic transaminase (SGOT).

- Comparison of activities of ALT, AST, and CK, a muscle enzyme, can indicate whether AST activity is increased due to hepatic or muscle injury.

▼ **Key Point** Increased AST activity associated with hepatic injury generally parallels but is less than the increase in ALT activity, and CK is normal. Increased AST activity due to skeletal muscle injury is associated with increased CK activity and normal or mildly increased ALT activity.

- In some cats with liver disease, AST may be more sensitive than ALT in detecting hepatic disease.

Alkaline Phosphatase (ALP)

Increases in serum ALP activity are due to accelerated production of this enzyme, stimulated by cholestasis or drug induction (see Fig. 91–2). ALP is a membrane-associated enzyme present in many tissues; however, only liver, bone, and corticosteroid-induced isoenzymes contribute to serum ALP activity. Serum ALP activity in normal dogs and cats is usually due to the liver isoenzyme. An increase in this type of ALP activity indicates intrahepatic or extrahepatic cholestasis.

- Young growing animals or animals with severe bone disease may have mild increases in ALP activity due to the bone isoenzyme. Benign familial hyperphosphatemia was described in related Siberian husky puppies. The increase in ALP activity was >5 times the values for ALP in unaffected siblings and was attributed to the bone isoenzyme.
- Cats generally have smaller increases in serum ALP activity with hepatobiliary disease than do dogs, owing to a limited capacity for ALP production and a short serum half-life. Therefore, even small increases in serum ALP activity (2–3 times normal) in cats suggest significant cholestasis.
- Exogenous or endogenous glucocorticoids are associated with hepatic production of a novel isoenzyme of ALP, corticosteroid-induced ALP (CIALP), in

dogs, but not in cats. The isoenzyme of CIALP can be distinguished electrophoretically from bone and liver isoenzymes. In dogs with excess glucocorticoid levels, CIALP activity usually accounts for at least 50% of total serum ALP activity.

▼ **Key Point** Hypercortisolism caused by glucocorticoid therapy or hyperadrenocorticism (Cushing) is the most common cause of increased serum ALP activity in dogs; it is usually attributed to an increase in CIALP.

- Increase in ALP activity associated with corticosteroid therapy varies considerably with the individual animal and the drug, dose, and duration of therapy. Oral, systemic, and topical preparations (including ear and eye medications) are capable of inducing ALP activity. This increase does not necessarily imply the presence of iatrogenic hyperadrenocorticism, a suppressed pituitary-adrenal axis, or corticosteroid-induced hepatopathy, nor does it indicate that corticosteroid therapy must be discontinued.
- Increased CIALP activity is a sensitive but not specific test for exposure to excess glucocorticoids (iatrogenic or endogenous). Increases in CIALP activity may be detected with diabetes mellitus, anticonvulsant drug therapy, primary hepatic disorders including neoplasia, hypothyroidism, and chronic illnesses. In this setting, CIALP usually accounts for less than 50% of total ALP activity.
- Increased CIALP activity associated with exogenous or endogenous glucocorticoids may be accompanied by mild to moderate (2–10 times normal) increases in ALT activity that typically are of lesser magnitude than increases in ALP activity.
- Anticonvulsant drug therapy is associated with enzyme induction of the liver isoenzyme of ALP in dogs (but not in cats) in the absence of obvious hepatocellular injury. CIALP activity also may be increased in some dogs. Reported maximal increases for induced serum ALP activity include those caused by phenobarbital (30 times normal), primidone (5 times normal), and diphenylhydantoin (3 times normal).

Gamma Glutamyltransferase (GGT)

This membrane-associated enzyme is present in many tissues. Increased serum GGT activity usually reflects cholestasis and increased production by hepatocytes (see Fig. 91–2).

- Increased GGT activity parallels increased ALP activity in dogs, including increases associated with excess corticosteroids.
- Anticonvulsant therapy causes mild (2–3 times normal) increases in serum GGT activity in dogs.
- In cats, serum GGT activity exceeds serum ALP activity in most hepatobiliary diseases; an exception is hepatic lipidosis, in which GGT activity may be normal or mildly increased despite a moderate to severe elevation of serum ALP.

Other Biochemical Tests

Numerous biochemical tests can be altered by liver disease, including serum bilirubin, albumin, globulin, urea nitrogen, glucose, and cholesterol. Many of these parameters reflect some aspect of liver function; however, they lack sensitivity or specificity for liver disease.

Bilirubin

- Increased serum bilirubin concentration occurs secondary to hemolysis or cholestasis. Evaluate for underlying hemolytic disorders by performing a CBC to detect anemia.
- Fractionation of the total serum bilirubin into conjugated and unconjugated components (van den Bergh test) to distinguish the mechanism of hyperbilirubinemia is of little diagnostic value because there is considerable overlap in hemolytic, hepatocellular, and extrahepatic biliary disorders.
- Lipemia falsely elevates serum bilirubin concentration; the absence of concurrent bilirubinuria suggests pseudohyperbilirubinemia.

Albumin

- Albumin is synthesized exclusively by the liver. Because of a large reserve capacity for albumin production, hypoalbuminemia does not occur until the functional hepatic mass is reduced 70–80%. Hypoalbuminemia associated with hepatic disease implies chronicity because of the long half-life of albumin.
- With chronic liver disease, fluid retention and dilution of existing serum albumin may also contribute to hypoalbuminemia.
- When the serum albumin is <1.5 g/dl, hypoalbuminemia contributes to the development of ascites and edema.
- Hypoalbuminemia is not specific for liver disease, and other causes of hypoalbuminemia such as urinary and gastrointestinal (GI) loss must be excluded.

Globulin

- Hyperglobulinemia due to increased gamma globulins occurs in some dogs and cats with chronic liver disease. The most likely mechanism is a systemic response to antigens that escape from the GI tract because of impaired hepatic mononuclear phagocyte system function or portosystemic shunting.
- Significant hypoglobulinemia does not usually occur with liver disease despite the liver's role in the synthesis of alpha and beta globulins.

Blood Urea Nitrogen

- Blood urea nitrogen (BUN) concentration may be decreased secondary to liver disease because the liver is responsible for converting ammonia to urea. However, many nonhepatic factors (e.g., PU/PD, fluid diuresis, low-protein diet) can also decrease BUN levels.

Glucose

- Hypoglycemia may occur secondary to hepatic dysfunction because of impaired hepatic gluconeogenesis, decreased hepatic glycogen stores, and decreased hepatic insulin degradation. However, because <30% of liver function is sufficient to maintain euglycemia, hypoglycemia is an insensitive indicator of hepatic function.
  - Because it indicates severe liver dysfunction, liver-associated hypoglycemia is a poor prognostic factor, except in dogs and cats with congenital portosystemic shunts.
  - Some hepatic neoplasms such as hepatocellular carcinoma and adenoma, leiomyosarcoma, and hemangiosarcoma have been associated with profound hypoglycemia.
  - Also consider nonhepatic causes of hypoglycemia such as sepsis, hypoadrenocorticism, and insulinoma (see Chap. 33).

Cholesterol

- Hypercholesterolemia occurs with acute cholestatic disorders because of increased synthesis of cholesterol and decreased incorporation of cholesterol into bile acids; however, there are many nonhepatic causes of hypercholesterolemia.
- Although cholesterol is synthesized in the liver, hypocholesterolemia secondary to liver disease is rare; it has been noted with congenital portosystemic shunts and anticonvulsant-induced hepatic disease.

Electrolytes

- Serum electrolyte changes secondary to liver disease are variable. In acute liver failure, serum electrolyte concentrations are usually normal. With chronic liver disease, total body potassium depletion and sodium and water retention are common, and the serum sodium concentration is usually normal or decreased.

Liver Function Tests

Liver function tests can document clinically significant hepatic dysfunction when liver disease is suspected, based on historical, clinical, laboratory, and radiographic findings. SBA determinations have largely replaced the use of organic anion dyes such as sulfobromophthalein (Bromsulphalein; BSP) and indocyanine green (ICG). Blood ammonia concentration and ammonia tolerance tests can specifically evaluate the portal circulation (for portosystemic shunts) and detect hepatic encephalopathy.

▼ *Key Point* The test of choice for clinical evaluation of liver function is a combined fasting and 2-hour postprandial SBA concentration.

Serum Bile Acid (SBA) Concentrations

The normal physiology of bile acid metabolism is shown in Figure 91–3A. In health, bile acids are confined to the enterohepatic circulation, and systemic concentrations are low. SBA concentrations increase in the systemic circulation with all types of liver disease (Fig. 91–3B). Because the liver has a large reserve capacity for synthesis of bile acids, even severe hepatic dysfunction does not cause decreased SBA concentrations.

Fasting Serum Bile Acid (FSBA) Concentration

An FSBA concentration obtained after a 12-hour fast is a sensitive, specific measure of hepatobiliary function in dogs and cats.

- Increased concentrations occur with hepatocellular and cholestatic disorders that interfere with hepatic uptake or secretion of bile acids and with portosystemic shunting, in which bile acids are diverted directly into the systemic circulation (see Fig. 91–3B).
- Normal FSBA values in dogs and cats are <15 μmol/L. When concentrations exceed 30 μmol/L, a

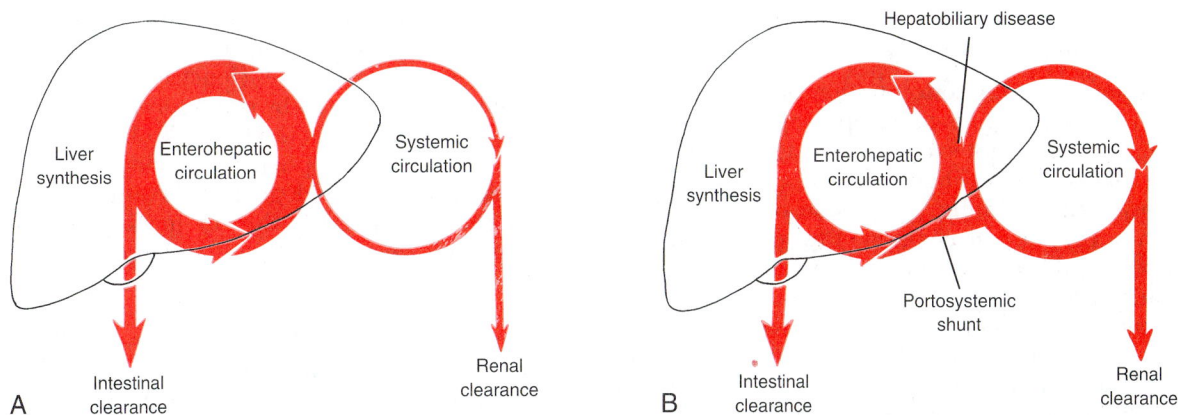

Figure 91–3. *A,* Bile acids are synthesized in the liver, secreted into the biliary system, and stored in the gallbladder during fasting. With ingestion of a meal, cholecystokinin release stimulates gallbladder contraction and entry of bile acids into the intestinal tract. Bile acids are efficiently reabsorbed in the distal ileum and carried in the portal blood back to the liver, thus completing the enterohepatic circulation. In the healthy animal, the liver removes 90 to 95% of bile acids from the portal circulation during the first pass of the enterohepatic circulation. This allows only small amounts of bile acids to escape to the systemic circulation. Normal serum concentrations are therefore low. (Fasting < 15 μmole/L; postprandial < 25 μmole/L). *B,* Hepatocellular dysfunction or cholestasis interferes with hepatic uptake, storage, and secretion of bile acids. Thus, impaired extraction of bile acids from the portal blood results in increased serum bile acid concentrations. With portosystemic shunting, bile acids in the portal blood are diverted directly into the systemic circulation.

liver biopsy may be warranted to evaluate the underlying liver disease.

Postprandial Serum Bile Acid (PPSBA) Concentration

PPSBA concentration is an endogenous challenge test of liver function. Whether PPSBA concentration is a more useful diagnostic test than FSBA concentration remains controversial. In dogs, similar information is provided by either test in most hepatobiliary disorders. Notable exceptions include dogs with portosystemic shunts or cirrhosis, because with these disorders, FSBA can be in the normal range. In cats, the diagnostic efficacy of PPSBA exceeds that of FSBA for all hepatic disorders including portosystemic shunts.

- To perform the PPSBA concentration test:
  - Obtain a serum sample for FSBA concentration, and then feed at least 2 teaspoons of food to small dogs and cats (<5 kg) and at least 2 tablespoons to larger patients.
  - To ensure gallbladder contraction, feed a diet high in fat (e.g., Prescription Diet p/d [Hill's Pet]; Prescription Diet c/d [Hill's Pet] for cats). For encephalopathic animals in which a high-protein diet is contraindicated, substitute a protein-restricted diet and add a few milliliters of corn oil per feeding.
  - Obtain a second serum sample 2 hours after feeding.
- *Results:* In normal dogs and cats, PPSBA concentrations are <25 µmol/L and peak 2 hours after a meal. A liver biopsy may be indicated when concentrations are >30 µmol/L.
- Healthy Maltese dogs have significantly higher PPSBA (mean 70 µmol/L ± 50; range 1–362 µmol/L) as measured by the enzymatic spectrophotometric method than when measured by HPLC, suggesting the presence of an additional reacting substance in their serum. However, a methodologic problem related to lipemia or hemolysis cannot be excluded.

Blood Ammonia (BA) Concentration

Ammonia is metabolized by the liver, and normal plasma concentrations are low.

- Measurement of BA concentration primarily is indicated to document hepatic encephalopathy. However, normal values do not exclude this diagnosis, because other toxins can contribute to the encephalopathy.
- Portosystemic shunting (congenital or acquired) is the most common mechanism of hyperammonemia, but severe, diffuse hepatic disease (especially acute hepatic necrosis) also increases BA concentrations.
- BA concentration is not a suitable screening test for congenital portosystemic shunt in young Irish wolfhounds since a transient metabolic hyperammonemia unassociated with liver disease occurs in this breed.
- Congenital urea cycle enzyme deficiency is a rare cause of hyperammonemia.

Ammonia Tolerance Test (ATT)

This is a more sensitive test than BA concentration for documenting portosystemic shunting. However, the ATT is contraindicated if resting ammonia levels are already increased, because no further diagnostic information will be obtained and performing an ATT can cause signs of hepatic encephalopathy. *Note:* The ATT is not recommended for use in cats.

- To perform the ATT:
  - Fast the dog for 12 hours, and then give 100 mg/kg of ammonium chloride (do not exceed a total dose of 3 g), either as a dilute solution by stomach tube or as a powder in a gelatin capsule.
  - Take a heparinized blood sample before and 30 minutes (stomach tube) or 45 minutes (capsule method) after administering the ammonium chloride. Vomiting may occur but does not invalidate the test.
- *Results:* In normal dogs, there is no increase in BA concentration or a mild increase (<2 times greater than baseline). In dogs with portosystemic shunting, results are consistently abnormal (up to 10 times baseline values); however, results may be normal in the presence of other hepatic disorders, especially those unaccompanied by portosystemic shunting.
- *Contraindications:* Measurement of ammonia is technically difficult, and appropriate sample handling requires heparinized blood samples to be stored immediately on ice, cold-centrifuged, and assayed as soon as possible. Because of these technical difficulties, the potential for exacerbation of hepatic encephalopathy, and the lack of sensitivity for detecting many hepatic disorders, SBA testing is preferable for assessing liver function in most clinical situations.

Parameters of Hemostasis

The liver plays a central role in the coagulation and fibrinolytic systems. The liver is responsible for synthesis of all coagulation factors except factor VIII, von Willebrand factor. Activated coagulation factors and fibrinolytic enzymes are also cleared by the liver.

- Mechanisms of excessive bleeding associated with hepatobiliary disease include primary failure of hepatocytes to synthesize clotting factors, DIC, and vitamin K deficiency. Vitamin K deficiency in hepatobiliary disease is usually caused by malabsorption of vitamin K secondary to complete bile duct obstruction. However, a vitamin K–responsive coagulopathy may sometimes be detected in dogs and cats with severe hepatic insufficiency, possibly due to marked intrahepatic cholestasis causing vitamin K malabsorption or from the inability of the liver to reactivate vitamin K from its inactive (epoxide) form.
- Clinical evidence of bleeding secondary to hepatobiliary disease is uncommon; however, the frequency of abnormal coagulation tests is much higher.
- Measure prothrombin time (PT) to evaluate the extrinsic coagulation system and activated partial thromboplastin time (APTT) to evaluate the intrinsic coagulation system. These tests can be abnormal in the presence of liver disease. Activated coagulation time (ACT) also can be used as a rapid screening test for abnormalities of the intrinsic coagulation

system. For further discussion of these tests, see Chapter 21.

- The PIVKA (proteins induced by vitamin K absence) clotting time is a more sensitive test than PT or APTT to detect bleeding tendencies in dogs and cats with liver disease. Normalization of PIVKA clotting time may occur after treatment with vitamin K_1
- Thrombocytopenia may occur secondary to splenic sequestration of platelets associated with portal hypertension or consumption of platelets from DIC. Platelet function defects also have been documented in dogs with liver disease, which may account for clinical bleeding tendencies in the presence of normal coagulation tests and platelet numbers. A mucosal bleeding time is useful for detecting platelet function abnormalities.
- The combination of prolonged PT and APTT, low plasma fibrinogen, increased fibrin degradation products, fragmented RBCs, and thrombocytopenia suggests DIC (see Chap. 21).

Blood Gas Analysis

Various acid-base imbalances may occur secondary to liver disease, including respiratory alkalosis, metabolic alkalosis, metabolic acidosis, and mixed acid-base disturbances.

Abdominal Fluid Analysis

- Ascitic fluid that accumulates secondary to liver disease and hypoalbuminemia is usually a transudate. With hepatic venous congestion from vena caval obstruction or cardiac causes, the fluid typically is a modified transudate with protein concentration >2.5 g/dl.
- Rupture of the biliary tract is associated with bile peritonitis. Grossly, the abdominal fluid appears yellow or green. Chemical tests for bilirubin are positive, and concentrations of bilirubin are higher in abdominal fluid than in serum. Cytologic examination reveals a mixed inflammatory infiltrate and bile-laden macrophages. Bacteria may be seen if bile peritonitis is complicated by sepsis.

Radiographic Evaluation

Survey Radiography

- Abdominal radiographs are useful to evaluate for:
  - Changes in liver size (hepatomegaly, microhepatica)
  - Altered tissue characteristics such as mineralized hepatic densities (choleliths) and radiolucencies (abscesses)
  - Presence of abdominal effusion
- If hepatic neoplasia is suspected, take thoracic films to evaluate for pulmonary metastases.

Ultrasonography

Ultrasonography can be used to image the liver noninvasively, especially when abdominal effusion precludes survey radiographic evaluation. A normal ultrasonographic appearance of the liver does not eliminate the possibility of significant hepatic pathology; however, ultrasonography is diagnostically useful to:

- Detect focal parenchymal abnormalities such as masses, abscesses, cysts, and regenerative nodules. The ultrasonographic appearance of these focal lesions often is similar, and biopsy is required for differentiation.
- Document that a palpable mass is associated with the liver.
- Investigate disorders of the biliary tract and gallbladder, such as biliary obstruction, cholelithiasis, and cholecystitis.
- Detect vascular lesions such as portosystemic shunts, hepatic arteriovenous fistulae, and hepatic venous congestion.
- Obtain percutaneous liver biopsies (see below).
- Identify abnormalities in other abdominal organs that may be a cause or effect of liver disease (e.g., pancreas, spleen, kidneys, bladder, GI tract, adrenal glands, and lymph nodes). For example, urate or uric acid urolithiasis may be detected in animals with portosystemic shunts; the primary tumor may be identified in animals with hepatic metastases; and identification of adrenal gland enlargement may help to diagnose steroid hepatopathy.

Angiography

Angiography is useful to diagnose vascular disorders involving the liver such as congenital and acquired portosystemic shunts, hepatic arteriovenous fistulae, and vena caval obstruction causing hepatic venous obstruction (see under Congenital Portosystemic Shunts).

Liver Biopsy

Liver biopsy often is required to definitively characterize the nature and severity of hepatic disease, to differentiate acute from chronic disorders, and to assess response to therapy. Selection of the best procedure for obtaining a liver biopsy depends on numerous factors including liver size, presence of coagulopathy, diffuse versus focal hepatic lesions, presence of biliary tract obstruction, presence of other intra-abdominal abnormalities, likelihood of surgical resection of a mass, tolerance of general anesthesia, available equipment, and expertise of the clinician.

▼ **Key Point** Perform a hemostasis screen prior to liver biopsy to detect coagulopathy. After the biopsy is performed, monitor for bleeding from the biopsy site.

Biopsy Methods

Fine-Needle Aspiration. Fine-needle aspiration for cytologic evaluation of the liver is most useful if the pathologic process is diffuse and architectural relationships (which can be obtained only by histopathology) are not essential to the diagnosis. Examples include feline hepatic lipidosis, hepatic neoplasia, and liver disease associated with infectious agents such as histoplasmosis.

Blind Percutaneous Needle Biopsy. Transabdominal and transthoracic needle biopsies are most likely to be successful when the liver is enlarged and pathologic changes are diffuse. The transabdominal approach is preferred, using a Tru-Cut (Travenol Labs) or Menghini (V. Mueller Co.) biopsy needle.

- The advantage of a percutaneous technique is that it requires minimal sedation and takes little time.
- Potential disadvantages are that trauma to adjacent organs may occur undetected, and an adequate tissue sample may not be obtained. Recognition of complications such as excessive bleeding or rupture of the biliary tract often is delayed.
- Feed a small quantity of corn oil (1 ml/kg body weight) 60 minutes prior to blind percutaneous needle biopsy to cause gallbladder contraction and minimize the likelihood of inadvertently puncturing the gallbladder.
- Blind biopsy procedures are contraindicated with suspected hepatic abscess or cyst, vascular tumors, bile duct obstruction, peritonitis, abdominal adhesions, and extreme obesity.

Ultrasound-Guided Needle Biopsy. This technique is the percutaneous procedure of choice, depending on the availability of equipment and clinician expertise.

- In addition to the advantages of the blind percutaneous technique, it is possible to obtain tissue from focal lesions, avoid structures adjacent to the liver, and monitor post-biopsy bleeding.
- Ultrasound-guided biopsy may be difficult if the liver is small or the ultrasonographer lacks experience.

Keyhole Needle Biopsy. Keyhole needle biopsy is performed under general anesthesia similarly to the percutaneous techniques. However, with this technique, a small abdominal incision is made, and a sterile, gloved finger localizes the liver lobe to be biopsied and helps guide the needle into the appropriate area.

Laparoscopy. Laparoscopy provides direct visualization of the liver and adjacent structures such as the pancreas and extrahepatic biliary tract. Biopsies also are obtained under direct visualization.

- When the liver is small, laparoscopy is a useful alternative method to ultrasound-guided needle biopsy.
- It is preferable to percutaneous techniques when excess bleeding is anticipated and to laparotomy when delayed wound healing (hypoalbuminemia) is anticipated.
- Laparoscopy requires heavy sedation or anesthesia and is subject to equipment availability and clinician expertise.

Laparotomy. Laparotomy is indicated for liver biopsy when a surgically correctable disease is suspected, such as extrahepatic biliary tract obstruction or a single, large hepatic mass (see Chap. 92 for description of the procedure for surgical biopsy).

- This technique makes it possible to:
  - Obtain large samples of liver tissue
  - Monitor for postbiopsy bleeding

- Disadvantages include:
  - The requirement for general anesthesia
  - A relatively high risk of complications
  - Delayed wound healing in hypoalbuminemic patients

Biopsy Analysis

- To prepare biopsy tissue for histopathology, place samples in 10% buffered formalin and allow to fix for 24 hours. The volume of fixative should be 20 times the volume of biopsy tissue.
- To prepare needle biopsy samples, gently remove liver tissue from the biopsy needle and place it on tissue paper; fold the paper and place it in a formalin jar.
- Perform routine light microscopy on liver tissue stained with hematoxylin and eosin (H&E).
- Additional stains may be requested, including trichrome for fibrous connective tissue; periodic acid–Schiff (PAS) for glycogen; rhodanine or rubeanic acid for copper; Prussian blue for iron; Congo red for amyloid; oil red O for fat; and silver or acid-fast stains for infectious organisms.
- Submit fresh liver tissue for bacterial and fungal culture as indicated.
- Perform quantitative copper analysis on fresh hepatic tissue.
- Place samples for electron microscopy in chilled, buffered 2.5% glutaraldehyde.

PRINCIPLES OF TREATMENT FOR LIVER DISEASE

Objectives

- Whenever possible, identify and eliminate the inciting or predisposing causes of liver disease. Identification of the underlying cause of hepatobiliary disease can provide insight into specific therapy, the likelihood and nature of potential complications, and the prognosis for recovery. (Therapy for individual hepatobiliary disorders is discussed later under specific diseases.)
- Prevent or manage complications of liver failure, including hepatic encephalopathy, ascites, GI ulceration, coagulopathy, infection, and endotoxemia.
- In patients in which hepatic regeneration and recovery are possible, supportive care allows time for this to occur. In other cases, clinical manifestations of hepatic failure may be minimized for variable periods.

Consider Drug Metabolism

The liver is a major site of drug metabolism, and liver disease may alter drug metabolism. In many cases, hepatic disease is associated with decreased hepatic clearance of a drug, with subsequent potential toxicity.

▼ *Key Point* Prior to administering any drug to a patient with hepatic disease, consider whether the drug is metabolized or excreted by the liver, is potentially hepatotoxic, or may exacerbate signs of liver failure.

Avoid drugs that:

- Are known to depend primarily on the liver for inactivation or excretion
- Are potential hepatotoxins such as thiacetarsamide
- May worsen signs of hepatic failure, such as methionine-containing products, tranquilizers, sedatives, analgesics, and diuretics (may exacerbate hepatic encephalopathy); and aspirin and corticosteroids (may cause GI bleeding and exacerbate hepatic encephalopathy).

Supportive Therapy for Liver Disease (Table 91–1)

Restore Fluid, Electrolyte, and Acid-Base Balance

- Maintain normal fluid balance to support hepatic blood flow and microcirculation and prevent complications such as hepatic encephalopathy, DIC, shock, and renal failure. The composition of the fluid to be given is influenced by the patient's electrolyte and acid-base status and the presence or potential for hypoglycemia (see Table 91–1 for guidelines).
- Avoid alkalinizing agents (e.g., lactate in lactated Ringer's solution; sodium bicarbonate) when hepatic encephalopathy is present or impending, because alkalosis augments the entry of ammonia into the CNS and can exacerbate signs of hepatic encephalopathy.

Give Nutritional Support

Nutritional support is important for promoting hepatic regeneration and maintenance of body weight.

- Modify the diet as needed to control complications of hepatic disease, such as hepatic encephalopathy, hypoproteinemia, and ascites (see Table 91–1).
- Supply the bulk of the calories by carbohydrates, which provide an easily assimilated source of nonprotein calories.
- Avoid high-protein diets that may exacerbate signs of hepatic encephalopathy. Indiscriminate protein restriction is discouraged, however, because adequate protein intake is important for normal hepatic regeneration and to counteract hypoproteinemia.
- When voluntary food intake is lacking, provide other methods of nutritional support, such as feeding through a gastrostomy tube (see Chap. 3).

Control Complications

Hepatic Encephalopathy

Goals for treatment of hepatic encephalopathy are summarized in Table 91–1.

- Restrict dietary protein intake. Increase dietary soluble fiber (see Table 91–1).
- Prevent formation and absorption of enteric toxins.
  - Give antibiotics (e.g., neomycin, metronidazole) to alter the urease-producing bacterial population in the colon, thus decreasing conversion of urea to ammonia (see Table 91–1).
  - Lactulose, a synthetic disaccharide, often is effective in controlling signs of hepatic encephalopathy and decreasing arterial blood ammonia concentrations through its actions as a cathartic and colonic

acidifier (see Table 91–1). It usually is given in combination with antibiotics.

▼ *Key Point* Detect and control GI hemorrhage, which could provide enteric bacteria with a source of protein for toxin production. Give fresh rather than stored blood if a transfusion is required, because stored blood contains substantial amounts of ammonia.

Ascites and Edema

Ascites in liver disease usually is associated with hypoalbuminemia, portal hypertension, and renal retention of sodium and water.

- For treatment of ascites, restrict dietary sodium and use diuretics to promote urinary sodium and water excretion (see Table 91–1).
- For temporarily supporting plasma colloid osmotic pressure in hypoproteinemic animals, consider plasma transfusion to supply albumin or volume expanders such as hetastarch or dextran (see Table 91–1; see Chap. 5).
- Avoid using abdominocentesis to treat ascites except when required for relieving respiratory distress.

Coagulopathy and Anemia

Hemostatic defects associated with hepatobiliary disease can be attributed to DIC, primary failure of hepatocytes to synthesize clotting factors, or vitamin K deficiency.

- Parenteral administration of vitamin K_1 corrects coagulopathy caused by vitamin K deficiency within 24–72 hours, but no response is seen when bleeding is caused by hepatocyte failure or DIC (see Table 91–1).
- For treatment of DIC and other coagulopathies, see Chapter 21.

Gastrointestinal Ulceration

Dogs with hepatobiliary disease are at increased risk to develop GI ulceration. Possible mechanisms include gastric acid hypersecretion, impaired gastric mucosal blood flow secondary to portal hypertension, and decreased gastric epithelial cell turnover.

- GI bleeding is deleterious in patients with hepatic encephalopathy because blood is a substrate for ammonia production.
- Manage GI ulceration with an H_2 blocker for control of acid secretion and with sucralfate for mucosal cytoprotection, as described in Chapter 87. Famotidine and nizatidine are preferable to cimetidine and ranitidine as H_2 blockers in animals with liver disease, because they do not inhibit hepatic microsomal enzymes.

Infection and Endotoxemia

An increased incidence of infection may be seen in animals with hepatic disease as enteric bacteria and endotoxins gain access to the systemic circulation as a result of impaired hepatic mononuclear phagocyte system

Table 91–1. GENERAL THERAPY OF HEPATIC FAILURE

Therapeutic Goals	Therapeutic Regimen
Fluid Therapy	
Maintain hydration	Use 0.9% NaCl or lactated Ringer's solution IV.* Use 0.45% NaCl in chronic disease.
Prevent hypokalemia	Add 20–30 mEq KCl to each liter of maintenance fluid. Monitor serum potassium daily and adjust as necessary.
Maintain acid-base balance	Avoid alkalosis in HE. Give $NaHCO_3$ rather than lactated fluids for treatment of severe metabolic acidosis.
Prevent or control hypoglycemia	To treat hypoglycemia, give 50% dextrose (0.5–1 ml/kg) IV to effect. To maintain normoglycemia, add dextrose to fluids to achieve 2.5–5.0% solution.
Nutritional Support	
Maintain caloric intake	Provide 60–100 kcal/kg/d of good-quality diet.
Provide adequate vitamins and minerals	Add B-vitamins to fluids of anorexic cats. For long-term therapy, give oral vitamin-mineral (especially B-vitamin) supplement. Give parenteral vitamin K_1 (3 mg/kg q12h IM or SC [dogs]; 1 mg/kg q12h IM or SC [cats]) in biliary obstruction or severe cholestastic liver disease.
Modify diet to control complications	See specific complications (e.g., HE, ascites).
Control Hepatic Encephalopathy	
Modify diet	Give NPO in initial stages of HE. For long-term management, provide a reduced-protein (dairy or vegetable source protein preferred; avoid meat or egg protein), easily digested, high-CHO diet. Recommend moderate protein restriction of 18–22% dry matter (dogs) or 30–35% dry matter (cats). Increase dietary soluble fiber (psyllium 1–3 tsp/d).
Prevent formation and absorption of enteric toxins	*In hepatic coma,* give warm water cleansing enema initially (10–25 ml/kg) until fluid is clear, followed by retention enema, 5–10 ml/kg, q8–12h containing: lactulose† (30% lactulose with 70% water) and neomycin (22 mg/kg) and held for 20–30 minutes or povidone iodine solution (diluted 1:10 with water; 50–200 ml total; flush out within 10 minutes). *For maintenance therapy,* give neomycin (22 mg/kg q8–12h PO) or metronidazole (7.5 mg/kg q12h, PO), or amoxicillin (22 mg/kg PO q12h) and lactulose† (0.25 to 0.5 ml/kg q8–12h PO to achieve 2–3 soft stools/d). When lactulose is used in combination with antibiotics, check the fecal pH after 7–14 d. If pH is <6, lactulose is being adequately degraded by enteric bacteria. If pH >7, increase lactulose dose or discontinue antibiotic.
Control gastrointestinal hemorrhage	Correct coagulopathy; treat GI parasites; treat gastric ulcer (famotidine and sucralfate‡); avoid drugs that exacerbate GI hemorrhage (e.g., aspirin and other NSAIDs, glucocorticoids).
Correct metabolic imbalances (e.g., dehydration, azotemia, hypokalemia, alkalosis, hypoglycemia)	See Fluid Therapy above.
Avoid drugs or therapies that exacerbate HE.	When possible, avoid sedatives, tranquilizers, anticonvulsants, analgesics, anesthetics, methionine-containing products, diuretics, stored blood, or commercial protein hydrolysates.
Control seizures	Use intravenous phenobarbital (monitor serum concentrations to adjust the dose) or oral loading doses of bromide (60–100 mg/kg q6h for 24 h, then 20–40 mg/kg q24h) for refractory seizures and status epilepticus. Avoid benzodiazepines. General anesthesia with pentobarbital or propofol may be required to control seizures. Intubate and use mechanical respirator to maintain Po_2 and Pco_2. Give mannitol (0.5–1 gm/kg by rapid IV bolus) for suspected cerebral edema. For chronic, stable seizure management or long-term therapy, give bromide (20–40 mg/kg q24h, PO in food). Monitor serum concentrations to adjust the dose.
Control infection	Give systemic antibiotics (see below).
Control Ascites and Edema	Give low-sodium diet; spironolactone (1–2 mg/kg q12h, PO),§ spironolactone/hydrochlorothiazide (Aldactazide¶ 2 mg/kg q12h, PO) or furosemide (1–2 mg/kg q12h, PO),§ paracentesis for relief of dyspnea or extreme abdominal distention; plasma transfusion or colloids such as hetastarch (10–20 ml/kg IV given over 6–8h; 2 doses, 12–24h apart) or dextrans (10–20 ml/kg/d to effect).
Control Coagulopathy and Anemia	Give vitamin K_1 (3 mg/kg q12h IM or SC [dogs]; 1 mg/kg q12h IM or SC [cats]); give fresh plasma or blood transfusion. For DIC, give heparin (50–75 IU/kg q8–12h SC).
Control Gastrointestinal Ulceration	Give famotidine (0.5–1.0 mg/kg q12–24h PO or IV) or nizatidine (2.5–5.0 mg/kg q24h PO); and give sucralfate‡ (1-g tablet/25 kg q8h PO)
Control Infection and Endotoxemia	Give systemic antibiotics (e.g., amoxicillin, ampicillin, penicillin, cephalosporins, aminoglycosides, metronidazole**).

*May be given subcutaneously if animal is mildly dehydrated and is not vomiting.

†Crystalline lactulose (powder) (Kristalose) is now available as 10- or 20-g packets (syrup concentration is 10 g/15 ml), distributed by Bertek Pharmaceuticals.

‡Beware of drug-associated constipation, which may worsen HE.

§Dose may be doubled if there is no effect in 4–7 d.

¶GD Searle & Co.

**Partially metabolized by liver. Use reduced dose (7.5 mg/kg q12hr PO) in animals with liver failure.

HE = hepatic encephalopathy; NPO = nothing by mouth; GI = gastrointestinal; DIC = disseminated intravascular coagulation.

Adapted from Johnson SE: Liver and biliary tract. *In* Anderson NV (ed.): Veterinary Gastroenterology, 2nd Ed, Lea & Febiger, Philadelphia, 1992, p 504.

function or portosystemic shunting. Septicemia and endotoxemia may, in turn, perpetuate liver injury.

- Give systemic antibiotics to control extrahepatic infections or sepsis. Penicillins, cephalosporins, or aminoglycosides are good choices because they are eliminated primarily by renal mechanisms.

Renal Failure

Renal dysfunction and azotemia may complicate liver disease, especially chronic liver dysfunction, and can be prerenal, primary renal, or both.

- Prerenal mechanisms that decrease effective circulating volume and renal perfusion include dehydration (including that induced by diuretics), hypoalbuminemia, ascites, and overzealous abdominal paracentesis. Appropriate fluid therapy is essential to avoid prerenal azotemia.
- Primary renal failure may occur with pre-existing renal disease or may result from infectious or toxic agents (e.g., leptospirosis) that affect the liver and kidneys concurrently or secondary to advanced liver disease.

ACUTE HEPATIC FAILURE

Acute hepatic failure occurs when a sudden severe insult to the liver compromises at least 70–80% of functional hepatic tissue. The clinical manifestations and laboratory findings associated with acute hepatic failure reflect general liver failure and are not specific for the underlying cause of injury.

Etiology

Causes of acute hepatic failure in dogs and cats include hepatotoxins, infectious and parasitic agents, and miscellaneous disorders (Table 91–2). In many cases, a specific cause cannot be identified.

Toxin-Induced Injury

- Hepatic injury may occur after exposure to a wide variety of industrial chemicals, organic solvents, pesticides, heavy metals, and biologic toxins (see Table 91–2). Exposure can be unobserved in a free-roaming animal that drinks from a contaminated water source.
- When hepatic necrosis is severe and widespread, rapid deterioration and death in 3–4 days often occur. With less extensive damage, complete recovery is possible.

Drug-Induced Injury

Drug-induced injury is a recognized cause of acute hepatic failure in dogs and cats. The incidence of drug-induced hepatic disease is unknown but is probably underestimated, based on the fact that 25% of human cases of fulminant hepatic failure and 5% of all human cases of jaundice are attributed to adverse drug reactions. Hepatic drug reactions are categorized as *intrinsic* or *idiosyncratic.*

Intrinsic Hepatotoxins. These hepatotoxins predictably damage the liver in an exposed population.

The effect is dose-related and reproducible experimentally. An example is thiacetarsamide, the arsenic compound used to treat adult heartworms.

Idiosyncratic Hepatotoxins. These hepatotoxins cause hepatic injury in only a small number of individuals that are unusually susceptible. The mechanism may be an allergy-like response or a unique metabolic pathway whereby the drug is metabolized to a toxic intermediate. The hepatotoxic effect is not time- or dose-dependent. Because of the unpredictability of an idiosyncratic reaction, a cause-and-effect relationship is difficult to establish. Examples include halothane and methoxyflurane, anticonvulsants, carprofen, mebendazole, oxibendazole, trimethoprim-sulfadiazine, and methimazole.

Drugs that have been incriminated as potential hepatotoxins include analgesics, anthelmintics, anticonvulsants, and antimicrobials (see Table 91–2). Specific clinical details regarding known drug reactions in dogs and cats are summarized in Table 91–3.

Infectious Agents

Infectious causes of acute hepatic failure (see Table 91–2) include leptospirosis (see Chap. 17), toxoplasmosis (see Chap. 19), histoplasmosis (see Chap. 18), FIP virus (see Chap. 8), and infectious canine hepatitis virus (see Chap. 14).

Miscellaneous Systemic Diseases

Hepatic injury can occur secondary to various systemic conditions, including those discussed below.

Hemolytic Anemia. Hemolysis, especially immune-mediated hemolytic anemia in dogs, can be complicated by centrilobular necrosis attributed to acute hepatocellular hypoxia or DIC-induced sinusoidal thrombosis. The hepatic injury generally resolves with resolution of the anemic crisis.

Anesthesia, Surgical Hypotension, Hypoxia, and Shock. Conditions that decrease liver blood flow can lead to hypoxia and hepatic damage. In the postoperative period it is difficult to differentiate hepatic damage or jaundice caused by the hypoxic effects of anesthesia and surgery from other potential causes, such as toxic injury induced by anesthetic agents (e.g., halothane, methoxyflurane) and other drugs, postoperative infections, and endotoxemia, or a combination of these factors.

Acute Pancreatitis. Pancreatitis in dogs and cats often is characterized by increased serum concentrations of liver enzymes resulting from secondary hepatic injury from released toxins, enzymes, and vasoactive substances (see Chap. 93). Hepatic lesions usually resolve with resolution of the pancreatitis and require no special treatment. Less commonly, jaundice results from partial to complete obstruction of the common bile duct associated with peripancreatic inflammation, pancreatic abscess, or pancreatic healing by fibrosis. Surgical intervention to relieve biliary obstruction is indicated in animals with pancreatic abscess or if jaundice persists after resolution of acute pancreatitis, which usually indicates pancreatic fibrosis as a cause of biliary obstruction (see Chap. 93).

Table 91–2. CAUSES OF ACUTE HEPATIC DISEASE IN DOGS AND CATS

Hepatotoxins		Infectious or Parasitic Agents (Refer to Section 2)
Drugs and Anesthetics		**_Viral_**
Acetaminophen	(D&C)	Infectious canine hepatitis (adenovirus I)
Aspirin	(D&C)	Canine herpesvirus
Amiodarone		Feline infectious peritonitis (coronavirus)
Anticonvulsants*		**_Bacterial_**
phenobarbital	(D)	Cholangiohepatitis
phenytoin	(D)	Leptospirosis
primidone	(D)	Liver abscess
valproic acid	(D)	_Bacillus piliformis_ (Tyzzer disease)
diazepam	(C)	_Salmonella_ spp.
Aprindine	(D)	_Francisella tularensis_ (tularemia)
Azathiaprine	(D)	**_Fungal_**
Carprofen	(D)	_Histoplasma_
Glipizide	(C)	_Coccidioides_
Griseofulvin	(C)	_Blastomyces_
Halothane	(D)	Others
Itraconazole	(D)	**_Protozoal and Parasitic_**
Ketoconazole	(D&C)	_Toxoplasma_
Mebendazole	(D)	_Babesia_
Megestrol acetate	(C)	_Cytauxzoon felis_
Methimazole	(C)	_Dirofilaria_ (postcaval syndrome)
Methotrexate	(D)	**_Rickettsial_**
Methoxyflurane	(D)	_Ehrlichia canis_
Mibolerone	(D)	_Rickettsia rickettsii_
Mithramycin	(D)	**Systemic or Metabolic Disorders**
Oxibendazole-diethylcarbamazine	(D)	Acute pancreatitis
Phenazopyridine	(C)	Acute hemolytic anemia
Tetracycline	(D&C)	Extrahepatic infection, septicemia and endotoxemia
Thiacetarsamide	(D)	Idiopathic feline hepatic lipidosis
Tolbutamide	(D)	Inflammatory bowel disease
Trimethoprim-sulfadiazine	(D)	Subcutaneous injection of intranasal vaccine (_Bordetella bronchiseptica_—canine
Biologic Substances		parainfluenza vaccine)
Aflatoxin		**Traumatic, Thermal, or Hypoxic Injury**
Amanita mushrooms		Abdominal trauma
Blue-green algae		Diaphragmatic hernia with liver entrapment
Cycadaceae (_Zamia floridana_, sago palms)		Heat stroke
Hymenoptera toxins (hornet sting)		Liver lobe torsion
Indigofera sp. (toxic plant)		Shock
Pennyroyal oil		Surgical hypotension and hypoxia
Chemicals		
Carbon tetrachloride		
Dimethylnitrosamine		
Galactosamine		
Metals (copper, iron, phosphorus)		
Organochloride pesticides		
Salt poisoning		
Zinc phosphide		
Many others		

*Usually causes chronic rather than acute hepatic disease except for diazepam in cats.
D = dog, C = cat.

Extrahepatic Bacterial Infections. Septicemia and endotoxemia associated with infections such as pneumonia, pyometra, peritonitis, and abscesses can cause jaundice, mild to moderate increases in liver enzyme activity (especially ALP), and increased SBA concentration. Liver biopsy reveals intrahepatic cholestasis without significant necrosis or inflammation. The hepatic injury resolves when the infection is controlled.

Clinical Signs

Clinical signs of acute hepatic failure often are nonspecific and overlap signs of disorders of other body systems. Clinical signs reflect general hepatic dysfunction rather than the specific underlying cause. Signs of extrahepatic or multisystemic disease often provide important diagnostic clues when hepatic injury occurs secondary to acute pancreatitis, hemolytic disease, septicemia/endotoxemia, and many infectious diseases.

- Acute onset of anorexia, lethargy, vomiting, and diarrhea are the most common presenting signs of acute hepatic failure.
- Other potential findings include PU/PD, jaundice, excessive bleeding, and hepatic encephalopathy.

Table 91-3. SELECTED HEPATOTOXIC DRUG REACTIONS IN DOGS AND CATS

Drug(s)	Species	Onset of Signs and Key Features	Hepatic Lesions	Suggested Mechanism	Comments
Analgesics					
Acetaminophen (Tylenol)	Canine and feline	Initial toxicity is cyanosis and methemoglobinemia, especially in cats.	Centrilobular necrosis and congestion; vacuolar hepatopathy and bile stasis	Intrinsic	Dose-related injury (dosages exceeding 200 mg/kg in dogs and 120 mg/kg in cats). Phenazopyridine causes toxicity by similar mechanism in cats. Treatment: N-acetylcysteine (140 mg/kg PO initially, then 70 mg/kg q6hr for 36 hr total) and ascorbic acid (30 mg/kg q6h for 36 h). Cimetidine (5–10 mg/kg IV q8–12h for at least 3 days); inhibits hepatic P-450 enzymes and prevents further conversion of acetaminophen to toxic product.
Carprofen (Rimadyl)	Canine	Acute hepatic failure[a] within 5–30d after starting drug. Labrador retrievers at increased risk.	Hepatocellular necrosis, ballooning degeneration, cholestasis	Idiosyncratic	Preexisting liver disease may be exacerbated by carprofen therapy; concurrent renal tubular necrosis and glucosuria may occur. Evaluate liver and kidney function prior to starting treatment. Rapid recovery in Labradors after stopping drug and giving supportive care; 50% mortality in non-Labrador breeds.
Anesthetics					
Halothane (Fluothane) and methoxyflurane (Metofane)	Canine	Acute hepatic failure* within 1 wk of most recent exposure.	Centrilobular necrosis	Idiosyncratic	Rare reaction in clinical veterinary medicine; difficult to separate from other potential causes of injury (e.g., other drugs, surgical trauma, hypoxia, concurrent infection). Multiple exposures may predispose. Potential for concurrent renal damage.
Anthelmintics					
Mebendazole (Telminic)	Canine	Acute hepatic failure* 1–14 d following administration.	Centrilobular necrosis	Idiosyncratic	High mortality.
Oxibendazole plus diethylcarbamazine (Filaribits Plus)	Canine	Acute hepatic failure* 2–4 wk after starting drug	Periportal hepatitis and vacuolar hepatopathy	Idiosyncratic	Clinical signs improve within days of stopping drug. Biochemical abnormalities may persist >6 mo.
		Chronic hepatic disease after 2–10 mo of drug therapy (especially Doberman pinscher); anorexia, lethargy, weight loss, ascites, increased liver enzymes, possible jaundice and seizures.	Periportal hepatitis, fibrosis, biliary hyperplasia	Idiosyncratic	Clinical improvement likely after discontinuing drug. Persistent hepatic damage is common despite clinical and biochemical improvement.
Thiacetarsamide (Caparsolate)	Canine	Acute hepatic failure* after 1–2 injections	Centrilobular or massive necrosis; intrahepatic cholestasis	Intrinsic	Dogs more susceptible to hepatic injury than cats. Can readminister uneventfully in 2–4 wks.
Anticonvulsants					
Primidone, phenytoin, phenobarbital, or combinations	Canine	Chronic liver disease and cirrhosis; anorexia, lethargy, weight loss, PU/PD, icterus, ascites, encephalopathy. ↑ ALP, ↑ ALT, ↑ GGT, ↑ total bilirubin, ↑ SBA and BSP. Coagulopathy.	Hepatocellular hypertrophy; intrahepatic cholestasis, lobular hepatitis, bridging necrosis, cirrhosis	Idiosyncratic or intrinsic†	Liver disease most likely with chronic administration of primidone or combination of primidone and phenytoin at higher doses. Phenobarbital alone may cause chronic liver disease and cirrhosis especially at higher doses (serum concentrations > 40 µg/ml). Dogs with phenobarbital hepatotoxicity may improve when dosage is decreased to therapeutic range as determined by serum phenobarbital levels or when potassium bromide therapy is substituted for phenobarbital. Incidence of chronic hepatic disease from long-term anticonvulsant therapy is approximately 6–14%.

Table continued on following page

Table 91-3. SELECTED HEPATOTOXIC DRUG REACTIONS IN DOGS AND CATS *Continued*

Drug(s)	Species	Onset of Signs and Key Features	Hepatic Lesions	Suggested Mechanism	Comments
Diazepam	Feline	Acute hepatic failure* within 4–11d of starting oral drug administration.	Diffuse hepatic necrosis	Idiosyncratic	Most cats with hepatotoxicity die within 15 days of initial administration of drug. In cats treated with oral diazepam, monitor baseline liver enzymes before and within 5 days after starting therapy; if enzymes are increased, discontinue drug and give supportive therapy.
Antimicrobials					
Ketoconazole (Nizoral)	Canine and feline	Asymptomatic with ↑ ALT, ↑ ALP or acute hepatic failure.*	Not characterized	Idiosyncratic‡	May be dose-related phenomenon: >40 mg/kg/d in dogs. In humans, asymptomatic serum enzyme elevations are considered harmless and enzymes usually return to normal despite continued therapy. Therapy should be discontinued if clinical signs or jaundice occurs. Recovery is usually uneventful.
Tetracycline	Canine	Not characterized	Vacuolar hepatopathy	Intrinsic	Experimental hepatic injury induced by high doses given IV. Avoid in animals with PSS. Unlikely to be clinically important as a hepatotoxin.
Trimethoprim-sulfadiazine	Canine	Acute hepatic failure* 3–28 d after starting therapy.	Massive necrosis or periportal hepatitis and intrahepatic cholestasis	Idiosyncratic	Multiple exposures may predispose to reaction; in dogs with intrahepatic cholestasis, rapid recovery after drug withdrawal. High mortality with massive hepatic necrosis.
Steroids					
Glucocorticoids (various types)	Canine	Chronic hepatopathy but hepatic failure rare. Signs indicative of hypercortisolism (e.g., PU/PD, polyphagia, hepatomegaly, lethargy). ↑↑ ALP usually with induction of steroid isoenzyme of ALP. Mildly ↑ ALT; normal total bilirubin. SBA WNL or mildly ↑ (<60 μmol/L)	Centrilobular vacuolization due to glycogen accumulation	Intrinsic but considerable individual variation	Lesions reversible after treatment discontinued. Rare in cats.
Megesterol acetate (Ovaban)	Feline	Chronic liver disease, jaundice	Not characterized	Idiosyncratic	Rare
Mibolerone (Cheque)	Canine	Chronic liver disease, jaundice	Not characterized	Idiosyncratic	Rare
Miscellaneous					
Methimazole (Tapazole)	Feline	Acute hepatic failure* within 2 months of starting therapy.	Necrosis and cholestasis	Idiosyncratic	Clinical signs resolve within 7 days of stopping therapy. Biochemical resolution by 45 days

*Typical manifestations of acute hepatic failure include anorexia, depression, vomiting, and jaundice accompanied by ↑ ALT, ↑ ALP, and ↑ serum bilirubin.
†See text for further information.
‡For drug reaction accompanied by clinical signs and hyperbilirubinemia.
PU/PD = polyuria/polydipsia; ALT = alanine aminotransferase; GGT = gamma glutamyltransferase; SBA = serum bile acids; BSP = Bromsulphalein sulfobromophthalein; PSS = portosystemic shunt.

Diagnosis

- When acute hepatic failure is diagnosed, attempt to identify the underlying cause with a complete history, ancillary diagnostic testing, and, if indicated, a liver biopsy. In many cases, a specific cause cannot be identified.
- When acute hepatic failure is accompanied by jaundice, consider diseases of the extrahepatic biliary tract such as biliary obstruction and rupture. Surgical intervention may provide both diagnostic and therapeutic benefit.

History

Attempt to document recent or potential exposure to any drug, toxin, or infectious disease, especially those listed in Table 91–2.

- Suspect a drug- or toxin-induced cause of acute hepatic failure when clinical and biochemical evidence of acute hepatic dysfunction is associated with recent exposure to a potential hepatotoxin.
- Consider toxin-induced injury in the absence of known exposure to toxins, because potential hepatotoxins can be present in contaminated dog food (aflatoxins), pond water (cyanobacteria ["blue-green algae"]), and many other unobserved sources.
- Although numerous drugs have been incriminated (see Tables 91–2 and 91–3), remember that an idiosyncratic reaction can occur with *any* drug. With most drug- and toxin-induced disorders, the diagnosis is presumptive and cannot be proved.
- To confirm the diagnosis:
  - Discontinue the drug and observe for clinical improvement, which usually occurs within several weeks, even after chronic drug administration.
  - Recurrence of hepatic damage after a challenge dose of the same drug (or inadvertent reexposure) supports the diagnosis of drug-induced hepatotoxicity. *Note:* This is not recommended as a diagnostic procedure because it is potentially dangerous, especially with a drug that causes hepatic necrosis.
- Determine if there is a history of recent surgical or anesthetic procedures that may be associated with drug- or hypoxia-related hepatic damage.
- Evaluate the animal's vaccination status for infectious diseases that can involve the liver, such as leptospirosis and infectious canine hepatitis.
- Determine if there are any subtle chronic signs of illness that suggest that the underlying liver disease may be chronic rather than acute and that the current illness may be exacerbation or decompensation of chronic liver disease.

Physical Examination

Physical findings often reflect general hepatic dysfunction rather than the specific etiology (see previous discussion of physical examination findings under Diagnostic Strategy for Liver Disease).

- Hepatodynia may occur with any cause of acute hepatic injury that results in swelling and stretching of the liver capsule.

- Findings of weight loss and ascites are indicative of a chronic rather than an acute process.
- Signs of extrahepatic or multisystemic disease may be important clues when liver injury occurs secondary to systemic disorders.
  - For example, fever may be present with infectious causes of hepatic injury such as leptospirosis, infectious canine hepatitis, bacterial cholangiohepatitis, liver abscess, systemic mycoses, and extrahepatic infections that secondarily involve the liver.
  - Fever and acute abdominal pain are presenting signs of acute pancreatitis but can also occur with cholangiohepatitis and hepatic abscess.
  - When jaundice is accompanied by pallor, consider immune hemolytic anemia.

Laboratory Evaluation

Acute hepatotoxicity frequently is associated with abnormal serum biochemical analyses, liver function tests, and urinalysis.

- Because diffuse hepatic necrosis is the most common lesion associated with acute hepatic failure, increased ALT activity is the most consistent finding, and values are often markedly increased. Increased ALP activity may also occur.
- Other potential findings include hyperbilirubinemia, increased serum bile acid concentrations, hypoglycemia, hyperammonemia, and coagulopathy. Hypoalbuminemia usually suggests chronic rather than acute liver disease.
- Some hepatotoxins (e.g., thiacetarsamide, carprofen, inhalation anesthetics) and infectious agents (e.g., leptospirosis) may concurrently damage the kidneys; thus, biochemical evidence of concomitant renal failure may be present.
- An inflammatory CBC suggests possible acute pancreatitis or underlying infectious disease. Evaluate serum amylase and lipase to diagnose acute pancreatitis.

Radiography

- Liver size usually is normal to increased unless massive hepatic necrosis causes parenchymal collapse and microhepatica.
- A small liver suggests chronic rather than acute hepatic disease.
- Additional radiographic findings may be noted, depending on the underlying disorder (Table 91–4).

Liver Biopsy

Perform a liver biopsy when the cause of acute hepatic failure is not suggested by preliminary laboratory evaluation.

- Histopathologic examination of hepatic tissue can help to establish the cause and to distinguish between acute and chronic liver disease. Diffuse hepatic necrosis is the histologic lesion most consistently associated with acute hepatic failure.
- If overt bleeding is present, liver biopsy may be contraindicated.

Table 91–4. ANCILLARY DIAGNOSTIC EVALUATIONS FOR HEPATOBILIARY DISEASE

Diagnostic Evaluation	Intended Diagnosis (Rule Out)
Bacterial cultures:	
Liver, gallbladder, bile	Bacterial cholangiohepatitis, cholecystitis, hepatic abscess
Blood, urine, infected tissues	Extrahepatic infections and sepsis
Serologic tests (antibody titers)	Leptospirosis
	Mycoses (histoplasmosis, coccidioidomycosis, blastomycosis)
	Toxoplasmosis
	Feline infectious peritonitis
Microfilaria exam	Heartworm disease
Fecal sedimentation (formalin-ether technique)	Liver fluke infection
Serum amylase and lipase	Acute pancreatitis in dogs
Serum trypsin-like immunoreactivity (TLI)	Pancreatitis in cats
Serum thyroxin (T4)	Feline hyperthyroidism
Coombs test	Immune hemolytic anemia
Lymph node aspiration cytology	Mycoses
	Lymphoma
Hepatic fine-needle aspiration cytology	Infectious agents (e.g., mycoses)
	Neoplasia (e.g., lymphoma)
	Idiopathic feline hepatic lipidosis
	Hepatic abscess (ultrasound-guided)
Abdominocentesis and fluid analysis	Ruptured biliary tract
	Feline infectious peritonitis
	Neoplasia
Thoracic radiography	Mycoses
	Toxoplasmosis
	Heartworm disease
	Metastatic neoplasia
	Diaphragmatic hernia
Abdominal radiography	Hepatic abscess
	Emphysematous cholecystitis
	Cholelithiasis
	Pancreatitis
Abdominal ultrasonography	Focal and diffuse hepatic parenchymal abnormalities
	Biliary or gallbladder disease
	Portosystemic shunt(s)
	Hepatic arteriovenous fistula
	Pancreatic disease
	Diaphragmatic hernia
Angiography	
Portography	Portosystemic shunt(s)
	Portal vein obstruction
Hepatic venography	Obstruction of caudal vena cava and hepatic veins
Celiac arteriography	Hepatic arteriovenous fistula
Nuclear imaging (transcolonic portal scintigraphy)	Portosystemic shunt(s)

Modified from Johnson, SE: Diseases of the liver. *In* Ettinger SJ, Feldman EC (eds.). Textbook of Veterinary Internal Medicine, 4th Ed., Vol II, WB Saunders, Philadelphia, 1995, p 1316.

Ancillary Diagnostic Procedures

Perform ancillary diagnostic procedures (see Table 91–4) to diagnose underlying causes of acute hepatic failure.

Treatment

- Management of the patient with acute hepatic failure is first directed toward supportive therapy (see Table 91–1). In many cases, even though the cause remains unidentified or specific therapy is unavailable, supportive care alone may allow adequate time for hepatic regeneration to occur.

- Maintenance of fluid, electrolyte, and acid-base balance is the cornerstone of supportive therapy (see Chap. 5).
- Prevent or control complications such as hypoglycemia, hepatic encephalopathy, coagulopathy, and endotoxemia (see section, Principles of Treatment for Liver Disease).
- Whenever possible, institute specific treatment for the underlying cause; for example, administer injectable penicillin or amoxicillin for treatment of leptospirosis. Although specific antidotal therapy usually is not available for drug-induced liver damage, discontinuing use of the suspect drug will prevent fur-

ther hepatic injury and may be associated with clinical improvement.

INFECTIOUS AND PARASITIC HEPATIC DISEASE

The liver can be involved in many systemic infections (Table 91–5). In some disorders, such as leptospirosis and infectious canine hepatitis, the liver is a target organ, and evidence of liver failure dominates the clinical presentation. In other infections, such as many of the systemic protozoal infections, the liver is involved as a result of widespread invasion of organs with a large mononuclear phagocyte population, such as the spleen, lymph nodes, and bone marrow (see Table 91–5). Signs of hepatic dysfunction may or may not be present and may be overshadowed by more obvious extrahepatic involvement. Liver cytology and biopsy can be diagnostically useful for identification of these organisms.

Systemic infections are covered in detail elsewhere in this book. Infections localized to the hepatobiliary tract are covered in greater detail here.

Hepatic Abscess

Hepatic abscesses from bacterial infection of the liver occur rarely in dogs and cats. Multifocal microabscesses or discrete unifocal abscesses may develop.

Table 91–5. INFECTIOUS DISEASES WITH POTENTIAL HEPATOBILIARY INVOLVEMENT*

Disease	Agent	Refer to
Viral		
Infectious canine hepatitis (ICH)	Canine adenovirus I	Chap. 14
Systemic neonatal herpesvirus	Canine herpesvirus, feline herpesvirus	Chap. 14
Canine acidophil cell hepatitis	Unknown	Chap. 14
Feline infectious peritonitis	Feline coronavirus	Chap. 8
Bacterial		
Leptospirosis:	*Leptospira interrogans:*	Chap. 17
Acute hepatic failure	Serovars *L. icterohemorrhagiae* and *L. canicola*	
Chronic hepatitis	Serovar *L. grippotyphosa* and others	
Tyzzer disease	*Bacillus piliformis*	Chap. 89
Nocardiosis	*Nocardia* spp.	Chap. 17
Actinomycosis	*Actinomyces* spp.	Chap. 17
Tuberculosis	*Mycobacterium tuberculosis, M. bovis, M. avium*	Chap. 17
Salmonellosis	*Salmonella typhimurium*	Chap. 89
Brucellosis	*Brucella canis*	Chap. 17
Hepatic abscess	*Staphylococcus* spp. (dogs)	
	Streptococcus spp. (cats)	
	Escherichia coli, anaerobes	
Cholangitis/cholangiohepatitis	Gram-negative bacteria (esp. *E.coli*), anaerobes	
Cholecystitis	Gram-negative bacteria (esp. *E.coli*), *Clostridium* spp., *Campylobacter jejuni*	
Yersiniosis	*Yersinia pestis*	Chap. 17
Tularemia	*Francisella tularensis*	Chap. 17
Mycobacterial infections	*Mycobacterium* spp.	Chap. 17
Fungal		
Histoplasmosis	*Histoplasma capsulatum*	Chap. 18
Blastomycosis	*Blastomyces dermatitidis*	Chap. 18
Coccidioidomycosis	*Coccidioides immitis*	Chap. 18
Aspergillosis	*Aspergillus terreus*	Chap. 18
Protozoal		
Toxoplasmosis	*Toxoplasma gondii*	Chap. 19
Neosporosis	*Neospora caninum*	Chap. 19
Babesiosis	*Babesia canis, B. gibsoni*	Chap. 20
Cytauxzoonosis	*Cytauxzoon felis*	Chap. 19
Hepatozoonosis	*Hepatozoon canis*	Chap. 19
Leishmaniasis	*Leishmania* spp.	Chap. 19
Encephalitozoonosis	*Encephalitozoon cuniculi*	Chap. 19
Rickettsial		
Ehrlichiosis	*Ehrlichia* spp.	Chap. 15
Rocky Mountain spotted fever	*Rickettsia rickettsii*	Chap. 15
Algal		
Protothecosis	*Prototheca* spp.	Chap. 89
Parasitic		
Canine schistosomiasis	*Heterobilharzia americana*	
Visceral larval migrans	*Toxocara canis*	
Liver flukes	*Platynosomum concinnum* (feline)	
	Amphimerus pseudofelineus (feline)	

*Not necessarily associated with clinical hepatobiliary disease.

Etiology

- Potential sources of bacteria include hematogenous spread, ascension via bile ducts, penetrating abdominal and caudal thoracic wounds, and direct extension from local suppurative diseases. Umbilical infections are the most common cause of hepatic abscesses in puppies *(Staphylococcus)* and kittens *(Streptococcus)*.
- Hypoxia of hepatic tissue caused by hepatic neoplasia or trauma may predispose to abscess formation, because small numbers of anaerobes (e.g., *Clostridium* spp.) normally are present in the liver and can proliferate under these conditions.
- Systemic diseases that are associated with immunosuppression (e.g., feline leukemia virus [FeLV], feline immunodeficiency virus [FIV]) or that predispose to infection (e.g., diabetes mellitus) may predispose to hepatic abscesses.
- Systemic infections (urinary tract infection, pneumonia, pancreatitis), liver lobe torsion, gallbladder rupture, and previous surgical liver biopsy have also been associated with hepatic abscesses.

Clinical Signs

- Signs are attributed to sepsis, inflammation, and hepatic dysfunction and include anorexia, lethargy, fever, vomiting, and diarrhea.
- Rupture of a hepatic abscess leads rapidly to peritonitis, septic shock, and death.

Diagnosis

- Physical examination findings are often vague but may include depression, fever, hepatomegaly, abdominal tenderness, and abdominal effusion.
- Potential laboratory findings include neutrophilia with a left shift (or neutropenia and degenerative left shift if rupture occurs), thrombocytopenia, markedly increased ALT and ALP activity (although they may be in the normal range), hyperglobulinemia, hyperbilirubinemia, hypoglycemia, and septic suppurative abdominal effusion.
- Radiolucent areas may be seen on abdominal radiographs when gas-producing organisms are involved. Ultrasonography may reveal one or more parenchymal abscess cavities. Ultrasound-guided fine-needle aspiration for cytology and culture may be diagnostic.
- Diagnosis often is established at exploratory laparotomy to determine the cause of septic peritonitis.
- Perform aerobic and anaerobic cultures of abdominal effusion, blood, and hepatic tissue.

Treatment

- Treatment of large, unifocal hepatic abscesses requires surgical excision of affected liver lobe (see Chap. 92).
- Ultrasound-guided percutaneous abscess drainage has been advocated for medical management of single lesions. No complications were observed in one series of cases.
- Initiate broad-spectrum antibiotics such as intravenous penicillin combined with an aminoglycoside (e.g., gentamicin, amikacin) while awaiting culture results. Monitor renal function during aminoglycoside therapy, and base further therapy on results of sensitivity testing. Give long-term antibiotic therapy (but not aminoglycosides) for at least 6–8 weeks.

Feline Inflammatory Liver Disease: Cholangiohepatitis and Lymphocytic Portal Hepatitis

Cholangiohepatitis is an inflammatory disorder of the bile ducts and adjacent hepatocytes. The term *cholangitis* is used when inflammation is confined to the bile ducts; the term *cholangiohepatitis* implies secondary hepatocyte involvement. Cholangiohepatitis is one of the most common hepatobiliary disorders of cats but is recognized much less frequently in dogs. Cholangiohepatitis can be separated into acute (suppurative) and chronic (nonsuppurative) forms.

- *Acute cholangiohepatitis* is characterized by large numbers of neutrophils within and around the bile ducts, disruption of the periportal limiting plate, and periportal necrosis.
- *Chronic cholangiohepatitis* is characterized by a mixed inflammatory response (neutrophils, lymphocytes, and plasma cells) into portal areas and bile ducts, periportal necrosis, biliary hyperplasia, and portal fibrosis. Chronic cholangiohepatitis may progress to biliary cirrhosis.
- *Lymphocytic portal hepatitis* has been proposed as a distinct entity from either acute or chronic cholangiohepatitis because some cats have lymphocytes and plasma cells in portal areas with a distinct lack of neutrophilic inflammation or bile duct inflammation, and the periportal limiting plate is intact. Fibrosis and bile duct proliferation may also occur. Lymphocytic portal hepatitis is more common in old cats (>10 years) and does not progress to pseudolobule formation or biliary cirrhosis.
- A severe form of chronic cholangiohepatitis, called *sclerosing cholangitis,* is characterized by the disappearance of small bile ducts and replacement with an "onion-skin" layering of connective tissue.

The following discussion focuses on cholangiohepatitis in cats; however, similar principles of diagnosis and therapy apply to cholangiohepatitis in dogs.

Etiology and Clinical Associations

- Bacterial infection is a possible cause when there is histologic evidence of suppurative inflammation. Gram-negative bacteria (especially *Escherichia coli*) are most commonly cultured from the bile of affected cats. Their role has yet to be defined; it is unknown whether they initiate cholangiohepatitis or are a secondary complication. Factors that predispose to bacterial infection include biliary obstruction and bile stasis, cholelithiasis, inflammatory bowel disease, pancreatitis, splenic abscesses, and anatomic malformations of the biliary tract.

- Infectious agents infrequently associated with lesions of cholangiohepatitis in cats include liver flukes (see the following discussion), *Toxoplasma*-like organisms, and *Hepatozoon canis*.
- The cause of nonsuppurative cholangitis/cholangiohepatitis is unknown. It may be a later stage of acute cholangiohepatitis (especially when a mixed pattern of inflammation including neutrophils is present), or it may represent immune-mediated disease.
- In cats, lesions of acute and chronic cholangiohepatitis commonly are associated with pancreatitis, cholecystitis, and inflammatory bowel disease. The triple combination of idiopathic inflammatory disease in adjacent areas of the biliary tract, duodenum, and pancreas has been called "triaditis" (i.e., cholangiohepatitis, duodenitis, and pancreatitis). Associated cholelithiasis and sludging of bile may cause partial or complete biliary obstruction.
- Cats with cholangiohepatitis occasionally develop secondary hepatic lipidosis, possibly related to anorexia and weight loss.

Clinical Signs

- Common signs include anorexia, depression, weight loss, intermittent vomiting, and jaundice. Hepatic encephalopathy, ascites, and excessive bleeding are uncommon unless cholangiohepatitis has progressed to biliary cirrhosis.
- Signs may be acute or chronic, intermittent or persistent.

Diagnosis

Suspect cholangiohepatitis in any cat with fever and jaundice (although not all cases are febrile). Definitive diagnosis requires liver biopsy to distinguish this disease from other hepatic disorders such as hepatic lipidosis, hepatic FIP, and neoplasia.

History and Physical Examination

- Persian cats may have a genetic predisposition for lymphocytic cholangitis.
- Cats with acute cholangiohepatitis may have a history of previous episodes responsive to antibiotic therapy. They are generally younger and have a more acute presentation (days or weeks).
- Physical examination findings include fever, jaundice, hepatomegaly, and dehydration. If chronic cholangiohepatitis has progressed to cirrhosis, ascites may occur.

Laboratory Evaluation

- Findings include a neutrophilia and left shift with acute cholangiohepatitis; hyperbilirubinemia and bilirubinuria; increased ALP, ALT, AST, and GGT activity; and increased FSBA and PPSBA concentrations. Hyperglobulinemia is found in more than 50% of cats with chronic cholangiohepatitis.
- A coagulopathy may occur secondary to vitamin K malabsorption or hepatocyte failure.

- Hypoalbuminemia, decreased BUN, and hyperammonemia suggest advanced disease.
- The feline trypsinogen assay (TLI test) should be considered to identify cats with concurrent or underlying pancreatitis.
- In tropical locations, fecal exams or a therapeutic trial of praziquantel should be considered to rule out liver flukes.

Radiography and Ultrasonography

- Radiographic features of cholangiohepatitis include hepatomegaly and, in some cases, cholelithiasis.
- Ultrasonography is useful to evaluate concurrent abnormalities of the extrahepatic biliary system, such as cholecystitis, cholelithiasis, sludging of bile, common bile duct obstruction, and pancreatic abnormalities. The hepatic parenchyma may have diffuse hypoechogenicity and prominent portal vasculature.
  - *Note:* a small amount of sludged bile may be detected ultrasonographically in anorectic, sick animals that do not have biliary tract disease.

Liver Biopsy

- If concurrent biliary obstruction occurs, obtain a liver biopsy specimen and aerobic and anaerobic bile cultures at laparotomy during surgical relief of the obstruction (see Chap. 92). Duodenal and pancreatic biopsies are also indicated.
- At laparotomy, the gallbladder and common bile duct frequently are thickened, firm, and distended. Inspissated bile and choleliths may be present.
- In the absence of obstruction, percutaneous liver biopsy is adequate for diagnosis.

Treatment

General Supportive Care

- Supportive treatment of cholangiohepatitis should include fluid therapy, nutritional support, and supplementation of potassium and B vitamins. Give vitamin K_1 (1 mg/kg SC or IM, q12 hours for three doses) if hemostasis evaluation suggests vitamin K deficiency.

Antibiotics

Antibiotics are the primary therapy for acute (suppurative) cholangiohepatitis. They are also used in the initial therapy of chronic cholangiohepatitis prior to initiating glucocorticoid therapy, in order to eliminate any bacterial component. Antibiotics are given for a minimum of 6–8 weeks, especially in acute cholangiohepatitis. In some cats with persistent elevation of serum bilirubin and liver enzymes, antibiotic therapy should continue 3–6 months. If possible, base the choice of drug on culture and sensitivity testing results; otherwise, consider the following recommendations:

- Consider ampicillin (20–40 mg/kg PO, IV, IM, SC q8 hours), amoxicillin (10–20 mg/kg PO, IV, SC q8–12 hours), amoxicillin-clavulanate (62.5 mg/cat PO q12 hours), or a cephalosporin as an initial choice. Combine one of these with metronidazole (7 mg/kg PO q12 hours) for broader spectrum against anaerobes as well as modulation of cell-mediated immunity and treatment of concurrent IBD.

- For refractory cases, enrofloxacin (2.5 mg/kg, PO or IM q12 hours) or a 1-week course of an aminoglycoside should be considered.

Immunosuppressive Therapy

Prednisone is used empirically in the treatment of (1) chronic cholangiohepatitis that does not respond to antibiotic therapy, (2) sclerosing cholangiohepatitis, and (3) lymphocytic portal hepatitis, because of its anti-inflammatory and immunosuppressive properties.

- Give 2 to 4 mg/kg/day prednisone (once daily or divided) until clinical remission, then taper over 6–8 weeks to 0.5 to 1.0 mg/kg/day or every other day.
- For cats that are resistant to prednisone (especially those with sclerosing cholangitis), low-dose pulse oral methotrexate in combination with prednisone, metronidazole, and ursodeoxycholic acid has been recommended. A suggested total dose is 0.4 mg methotrexate/cat divided into three doses over a 24-hour period (i.e., 0.13 mg at 0, 12, and 24 hours). This dose is repeated every 7–10 days, or if there is no response after several months, consider increasing the dose to 0.26 mg at 0 hour, while continuing 0.13 mg at 12 and 24 hours. Potential side effects include leukopenia, vomiting, diarrhea, and hepatotoxicity.

Ursodiol

Ursodiol, also known as ursodeoxycholic acid (Actigall, 10–15 mg/kg PO q24 hours), is recommended in all cats with cholangiohepatitis, once extrahepatic biliary obstruction is eliminated. Ursodiol, a hydrophilic bile acid, is believed to be beneficial by expanding the bile acid pool and displacing potentially hepatotoxic hydrophobic bile acids that may accumulate in cholestasis. It also has membrane-stabilizing, cytoprotective, and immunomodulatory effects on liver cells. It is a choleretic, which promotes increased fluidity of biliary secretions to treat or prevent bile sludging. It is well tolerated and safe in cats for long-term use.

Surgery

Indications for surgical intervention in the treatment of cholangiohepatitis include:

- Biliary decompression for extrahepatic biliary obstruction
- Sludge removal and bile duct and gallbladder irrigation
- Cholelith removal
- Cholecystectomy for necrotizing cholecystitis
- Splenectomy for complicating splenic abscesses that are sometimes seen.

Prognosis

The prognosis is variable. Many cats continue to have chronic smoldering disease requiring continuing treatment for many months. Persistence of lymphocytic in-

flammatory disease for several years has been documented in some cats. Other cats return to normal clinically and biochemically, especially cats with acute suppurative inflammation. Future recurrences sometimes occur in recovered cats.

Cholecystitis

Cholecystitis, or inflammation of the gallbladder, is a clinical problem that occurs uncommonly in both dogs and cats. Cholecystitis may be associated with cholangitis, cholangiohepatitis, cholelithiasis, and choledocholithiasis. Acute necrotic cholecystitis in dogs frequently is complicated by rupture of the gallbladder and septic bile peritonitis.

Etiology

- Bacteria appear to play an important role in cholecystitis. An enteric origin of bacteria seems most likely, because isolates are usually aerobic gram-negative bacteria (especially *E. coli*, but also *Klebsiella*, *Pseudomonas*, and *Salmonella* spp.) or anaerobes (*Clostridium* spp.). Intestinal bacteria may be refluxed into the gallbladder or they may be blood-borne from the hepatic circulation.
- *Campylobacter jejuni* bacteremia and acute cholecystitis have been documented in dogs. Although the gastrointestinal tract was suspected to be the source of the bacteria, diarrhea was not a presenting clinical sign.
- Gas-producing organisms, such as *E. coli* and *Clostridium*, can cause emphysema of the gallbladder wall. Emphysematous cholecystitis is recognized most frequently in diabetic dogs.
- Cholelithiasis can predispose to cholecystitis by obstructing the cystic duct, causing gallbladder overdistension and stasis, which enables proliferation of anaerobic organisms.
- Anatomic malformations of the gallbladder, biliary obstruction from any cause, and biliary surgery also predispose to biliary infections.

Clinical Signs

- Signs include anorexia, lethargy, fever, abdominal pain, hepatomegaly, vomiting, diarrhea, and jaundice.
- Acute rupture of the gallbladder with septic bile peritonitis causes abdominal distension, collapse, and septic shock.
- Signs may be acute or chronic, persistent or episodic.

Diagnosis

Differentiate cholecystitis from other cholestatic hepatobiliary disorders that are characterized by fever, inflammation, and similar clinical findings, such as acute pancreatitis or pancreatic abscess, cholangiohepatitis, cholelithiasis, hepatic abscess, and septicemia/endotoxemia.

Physical Examination

Physical examination findings include fever, cranial abdominal pain, jaundice, and shock (bile or septic peritonitis).

Laboratory Evaluation

- Laboratory findings are characteristic of severe cholestatic hepatobiliary disease, including hyperbilirubinemia, markedly increased ALP and GGT activity, increased ALT activity, increased serum bile acid concentrations, and hypercholesterolemia. Other findings suggestive of inflammation or sepsis are neutrophilia with a left shift and hypoglycemia.
  - Increased amylase and lipase levels have been reported in dogs with cholecystitis in the absence of clinical pancreatitis.
  - Prolonged PT and APTT occur if chronic biliary obstruction causes vitamin K malabsorption.
  - Other laboratory findings reflect dehydration and electrolyte and acid-base imbalances secondary to vomiting, dehydration, and sepsis.
- If cholecystitis is complicated by rupture of the gallbladder or biliary tract, abdominal fluid analysis is consistent with septic bile peritonitis. For a general discussion of peritonitis, see Chapter 96.

Radiography and Ultrasonography

- Potential radiographic findings include cholecystolithiasis, emphysema of the gallbladder wall, and, if perforation occurs, abdominal effusion.
- Ultrasonographic findings include distension of the gallbladder and cystic duct, increased echogenicity or hypoechoic thickening of the gallbladder wall, cholecystoliths, and increased echogenicity of gallbladder bile, with or without bile sludge. Small amounts of abdominal effusion not evident on survey radiographs may also be identified.
- Ultrasonographic-guided percutaneous cholecystocentesis by a transhepatic puncture has been recommended to obtain bile for cytology and culture (aerobic and anaerobic). Perform blood cultures to isolate bacteria associated with bacteremia and acute cholecystitis. Culture for *Campylobacter jejuni* requires selective culture techniques.

Surgery

- Findings at exploratory surgery include thickening, necrosis, and rupture of the gallbladder, localized or generalized peritonitis, and calculi or inspissated bile in the gallbladder, cystic duct, or bile duct. Previous gallbladder rupture may be associated with omental or hepatic adhesions.
  - Obtain aerobic and anaerobic cultures of the gallbladder mucosa and bile.
- Histologic examination of the gallbladder reveals varying degrees of necrosis, inflammation, and fibrosis.

Treatment

- Give parenteral vitamin K_1 prior to surgery to correct coagulopathy (see Table 91–1).
- Administer antibiotic therapy effective against aerobic gram-negative and anaerobic bacteria, as described previously for bacterial cholangitis and cholangiohepatitis. For acute cholecystitis with bacteremia or necrotic cholecystitis with septic peritonitis, combine amoxicillin or cephalosporin with an aminoglycoside or enrofloxacin. Long-term treatment (6–8 weeks) is indicated.
- Cholecystectomy is required in most cases (see Chap. 92). Surgically manage complications such as biliary obstruction, cholelithiasis, inspissated bile, and abdominal drainage for septic bile peritonitis (see Chap. 96).

Postoperative Care and Complications

- Correct all fluid, electrolyte, and acid-base imbalances.
- Common postoperative complications include vomiting, diarrhea, anorexia, hypoproteinemia, and hypokalemia.

Prognosis

- Death usually is attributed to sepsis and peritonitis.
- If the animal survives the immediate postoperative period, the long-term prognosis is good, and recurrence of biliary or hepatic disease is unlikely.

Liver Fluke Infection

Liver fluke infection is uncommon in cats and rare in dogs. Infection usually is asymptomatic but may cause clinical biliary tract disease when associated with marked biliary fibrosis, cholangitis, cholangiohepatitis, or extrahepatic bile duct obstruction. Cholangiocarcinoma has been reported in cats chronically infected with *Platynosomum concinnum*.

Etiology

- *P. concinnum (P. fastosum)* is the most important liver fluke in cats and is found in tropical and subtropical geographic areas, including Hawaii, Florida, and the Caribbean. In endemic areas, the prevalence of infection is high.
- Other liver flukes that have been identified in cats include *Amphimerus pseudofelineus (Opistorchis pseudofelineus)*, *O. tenuicollis*, *O. sinensis*, and *Metorchis conjunctus (M. complexus)*.
- Liver flukes require two intermediate hosts for their life cycle. Adult flukes reside in the gallbladder and bile ducts. Embryonated eggs are shed in the feces and ingested by a snail, the first intermediate host for all liver flukes. The house gecko, skink, lizard, and Bufo toad are second intermediate hosts for *P. concinnum;* fish are second intermediate hosts for the other species of flukes.

Clinical Signs

- Most infected cats are asymptomatic for liver fluke infection.
- Liver fluke infection occasionally is associated with anorexia, weight loss, diarrhea, vomiting, jaundice, hepatomegaly, abdominal distention, and death.

Diagnosis

- Operculated fluke eggs can be identified in feces by a formalin-ether technique (a sedimentation procedure). Routine methods for flotation do not consistently identify eggs. With complete bile duct obstruction, no eggs will be passed in the feces. Eggs may be identified on cytological examination of the bile.

- Other laboratory findings are inconsistent and often unremarkable. Eosinophilia, hyperbilirubinemia, and increased serum ALP and ALT activity is sometimes detected.
- A possible relationship between positive feline immunodeficiency virus status and infection with *Amphimerus pseudofelineus* has been suggested.
- At laparotomy or necropsy, the bile ducts and gallbladder may be distended and thick-walled and contain inspissated bile and small (<12 mm long) adult flukes. The liver frequently is enlarged. In many cases, no visible abnormalities are present.

Treatment

Little information is available about treatment of liver flukes.

- Praziquantel (Droncit), 20 mg/kg, given orally or parenterally once a day for three consecutive days, has been suggested. Drugs used unsuccessfully include mebendazole, levamisole, thiabendazole, diamphenethide, and rafoxanide. At least one follow-up fecal examination by formalin-ether sedimentation should be performed 30 days following treatment.
- Manage complications such as biliary obstruction and secondary bacterial cholangitis/cholangiohepatitis as described elsewhere in this chapter.

ANTICONVULSANT-ASSOCIATED HEPATIC DISEASE

Long-term anticonvulsant therapy for control of seizures has been associated with hepatic injury in dogs (see Table 91–3). Severe hepatic dysfunction is estimated to develop in 6–14% of dogs treated with anticonvulsants for more than 6 months. Two types of hepatotoxic injury have been identified: hepatic cirrhosis and cholestatic hepatopathy.

Etiology

- Long-term therapy with primidone, alone or in combination with other anticonvulsants, and with phenobarbital have been associated with cirrhosis and liver failure. Phenobarbital hepatotoxicity appears more likely when high oral dosages are used and serum concentrations are maintained at ≥40 μg/ml. Idiosyncratic hepatotoxicity is suspected.
- High-dose phenytoin therapy, in combination with primidone or phenobarbital, has been associated with a cholestatic hepatopathy and hepatic failure. Hepatic damage is reproducible experimentally in dogs, suggesting intrinsic hepatotoxicity.

Clinical Signs

- Clinical signs are those of chronic hepatic disease and include anorexia, lethargy, weight loss, weakness,

polydipsia, polyuria, and jaundice. Signs of overdosage (sedation and ataxia) are consistent findings in dogs with phenobarbital hepatotoxicity. Ascites and hepatic encephalopathy are most likely with advanced hepatic disease.
- When impaired hepatic inactivation of phenobarbital causes increased blood levels, seizure frequency may decrease.
- Increased frequency of seizures may be related to the development of hepatic encephalopathy or to failure of the liver to convert primidone to its active anticonvulsant metabolites (phenobarbital and phenylethylmalonic acid).

Diagnosis

Suspect anticonvulsant-associated hepatopathy in any dog with a history of chronic anticonvulsant therapy and clinical and biochemical evidence of hepatic injury.

Laboratory Evaluation

▼ *Key Point* To detect early evidence of hepatic damage, routinely monitor liver enzymes (serum ALP and ALT), total serum bilirubin, cholesterol, albumin, and phenobarbital levels at least every 6 months in all dogs on chronic anticonvulsant therapy.

- Phenobarbital, phenytoin, and primidone are potent inducers of serum ALP activity (see Diagnostic Strategy section). Increased ALP activity occurs in the absence of morphologic evidence of hepatic injury. Increases usually are due to induction of the liver isoenzyme of ALP but sometimes are the result of increased corticosteroid-induced isoenzyme. Increases in ALT activity (up to 2 times normal) with anticonvulsant therapy are less consistent. A proportionately greater increase in ALT activity than ALP activity may suggest hepatocellular injury.
- Findings of hyperbilirubinemia, hypoalbuminemia, and hypocholesterolemia suggest hepatic failure and should be further pursued with a liver function test such as FSBA and PPSBA. Increased SBA concentrations are a consistent finding in anticonvulsant-induced hepatic disease.

Radiography and Ultrasonography

- Radiographic findings may suggest microhepatica with cirrhosis, or hepatomegaly with phenytoin-induced cholestatic hepatopathy.
- Ultrasonography is useful to further characterize liver changes and to evaluate for other hepatic disorders.

Liver Biopsy and Histopathologic Evaluation

Perform liver biopsy when SBA concentrations are increased, liver enzyme activities are greatly increased, or clinical signs of hepatic dysfunction are present.

- The most consistent histologic finding in dogs on anticonvulsant therapy is hepatocellular hypertrophy with a ground-glass appearance of the cytoplasm. Hypertrophy is due to hyperplasia of smooth endoplasmic reticulum. This finding is commonly identified in dogs without clinical or biochemical evidence of hepatic dysfunction and does not warrant a change in drug therapy.

- Cirrhosis is characterized by biliary hyperplasia, nodular hyperplasia, and fibrosis. A mild inflammatory infiltrate (neutrophils, lymphocytes, plasma cells) is often present.
- Features of cholestatic hepatopathy include intrahepatic cholestasis, biliary hyperplasia, cytoplasmic vacuolization, disorganization of hepatocellular plates, and small, multifocal areas of necrosis.

Treatment

- If possible, discontinue or modify anticonvulsant therapy in dogs with biochemical and histologic evidence of hepatic disease (see Chap. 146). In dogs with phenobarbital-associated toxicosis, clinical, biochemical, and histologic improvement can occur if phenobarbital is discontinued or used at a reduced dosage before severe, end-stage liver disease occurs. Improvement in clinical signs can be noted within days to weeks of decreasing serum phenobarbital levels.
- Consider using potassium bromide (22–40 mg/kg PO q24 hours with food) as an anticonvulsant in dogs with anticonvulsant-associated hepatotoxicity because of its lack of hepatic metabolism or hepatotoxicity. With the addition of bromide, the phenobarbital dosage can be decreased or discontinued. If potassium bromide is used alone, a higher dosage may be necessary (50–80 mg/kg/day). Monitor serum levels of bromide to adjust the dose. Bromide is not an approved drug.
- Despite evidence for hepatotoxicity, phenobarbital is still the drug of choice for long-term control of seizures in dogs. Adjust the dosage by determining the serum phenobarbital concentration. To decrease the likelihood of hepatotoxicity, serum concentrations should not exceed 35 µg/ml.
- Additional supportive measures are important in managing dogs with anticonvulsant-induced hepatic disease. Control complications such as ascites and hepatic encephalopathy, as discussed previously (see Table 91–1).

CORTICOSTEROID-INDUCED HEPATOPATHY (STEROID HEPATOPATHY)

Corticosteroid-induced hepatopathy, or steroid hepatopathy, is a commonly recognized sequela of glucocorticoid administration in dogs. Glucocorticoids cause hepatic glycogen accumulation and hepatomegaly (see Table 91–3). Steroid hepatopathy is a benign, reversible hepatic lesion that, with rare exceptions, is not associated with clinical liver dysfunction. The most important clinical significance of this disorder is that it can easily be mistaken for a more serious hepatic disease.

▼ *Key Point* To avoid unnecessary diagnostic and therapeutic measures, be aware that increased serum ALP activity and hepatomegaly are commonly caused by glucocorticoid therapy in dogs.

Recognition of steroid hepatopathy often alerts the clinician to the presence of previously unsuspected spontaneous hyperadrenocorticism in dogs without a history of glucocorticoid therapy (see Chap. 31).

Cats are resistant to the hepatic effects of glucocorticoids, and development of steroid hepatopathy is very rare.

Etiology

- Steroid hepatopathy has been associated with numerous glucocorticoids including cortisone, prednisone, prednisolone, dexamethasone, and triamcinolone. Lesions of steroid hepatopathy can develop within 2 days of corticosteroid administration.
- Endogenous production of excess glucocorticoids caused by spontaneous hyperadrenocorticism also results in steroid hepatopathy. Hepatic lesions are identical to those seen with exogenous administration of glucocorticoids.
- Individual variation in susceptibility to steroid hepatopathy also appears to play a role.
- Dogs that are chronically stressed due to other illnesses (e.g., severe dental disease, chronic inflammation or infection, or neoplasia) may also develop this hepatic lesion, presumably due to stress-induced endogenous glucocorticoid release.

Clinical Signs

- Clinical signs reflect the systemic effects of hypercortisolism rather than hepatic disease and include PU/PD and polyphagia in an otherwise healthy dog.
- Dogs with other illnesses causing chronic stress are not typically PU/PD but may show signs pertaining to their underlying disorder.

Diagnosis

Suspect steroid hepatopathy in any dog with hepatomegaly and increased serum ALP activity that has a history of recent glucocorticoid therapy and/or clinical signs of hyperadrenocorticism.

History and Physical Examination

- Evaluate for previous glucocorticoid therapy within the past 3 months.
  - *Note:* Significant amounts of glucocorticoid can be absorbed from topical and ocular medications as well as from oral and injectable preparations.
- Hepatomegaly, which may be quite massive, frequently is detected.
- Other findings in dogs with hyperadrenocorticism or exogenous glucocorticoid administration include abdominal distention and thinning of the skin and hair coat.

Laboratory Evaluation

- Increased serum ALP activity is the most consistent biochemical abnormality detected in dogs with this hepatic lesion. After glucocorticoid administration, the initial increase in ALP activity is attributed to the liver isoenzyme rather than the corticosteroid-induced isoenzyme (CIALP; see previous discussion). This increase can occur after 5 days of glucocorticoid therapy and often is as high as 150 times normal. After 7–10 days the ALP elevation becomes progressively more attributable to increased CIALP. The increase in CIALP can persist for several months after exposure to corticosteroids.

- In contrast, ALT activity is normal or only mildly increased.
- Other biochemical tests that may be abnormal include serum GGT activity, BSP dye excretion, and SBA concentrations, which, however, generally are lower ($<60 \mu$mol/L) than those obtained in dogs with other hepatic disorders.
- Total serum bilirubin, serum albumin, blood ammonia concentration, and hemostatic tests typically are normal.
- Other findings characteristic of hypercortisolism include mature neutrophilia, lymphopenia, eosinopenia, monocytosis, and hypercholesterolemia.

Radiography and Ultrasonography

- Hepatomegaly usually is detected on abdominal radiographs.
- Ultrasonography reveals hepatomegaly and diffuse or multifocal increase in liver echogenicity.

Liver Biopsy

- Grossly, the liver is enlarged, smooth, pale, and friable. Microscopically, hepatic lesions are characterized by severe, vacuolated ballooned hepatocytes in a patchy distribution.
- Periodic acid–Schiff (PAS) staining of alcohol- but not formalin-fixed tissue reveals that hepatic vacuoles contain glycogen granules. In most cases, special stains are not required for the experienced pathologist to diagnose this lesion.
- When hepatic biopsy suggests steroid hepatopathy and a history of glucocorticoid administration is lacking, perform diagnostic tests for endogenous hyperadrenocorticism (see Chap. 31). If tests for hyperadrenocorticism are negative, evaluate for other chronic illnesses that may be associated with chronic stress.

Treatment

- Steroid hepatopathy is reversible after withdrawal of exogenous glucocorticoids or treatment of spontaneous hyperadrenocorticism.
- The length of time required for complete resolution is unpredictable, varying from weeks to months.

CHRONIC HEPATITIS

Chronic hepatitis is a heterogeneous group of necrotizing inflammatory diseases of the liver. The clinical signs of chronic hepatitis initially are vague and nonspecific,

such as anorexia, weight loss, and depression; however, as hepatitis becomes advanced, signs of liver failure develop, including jaundice, ascites, coagulopathy, or hepatic encephalopathy.

With few exceptions, the cause, pathogenesis, natural history, and optimal treatment of these disorders in dogs is unknown. Because the laboratory and histopathologic features often fail to determine the definitive etiology, combined clinical and histologic criteria rather than etiologic classifications generally are used to categorize patients with chronic hepatitis.

Idiopathic Chronic Hepatitis

Idiopathic chronic hepatitis is characterized by clinical signs and persistent laboratory indicators of hepatic disease in association with chronic portal inflammation, piecemeal hepatic necrosis, and fibrosis that frequently progresses to cirrhosis and liver failure.

Etiology

The disease must be considered idiopathic in most dogs; however, it is probable that after an initial inciting hepatocyte injury, immune mechanisms are involved in perpetuating the inflammation.

Signalment and Clinical Signs

- The incidence of idiopathic chronic hepatitis appears to be highest in female dogs.
- The mean age of onset is 5–6 years, but adult dogs of any age or breed can be affected.
- Common signs include anorexia, depression, weakness, PU/PD, ascites, jaundice, weight loss, and vomiting.

Diagnosis

The diagnosis is suggested by the clinical signs in conjunction with elevation of serum liver enzyme concentrations. The diagnosis can be confirmed only by liver biopsy. Historical and physical findings are consistent with chronic liver disease.

Laboratory Evaluation

- Serum ALT activity usually is >10 times normal, reflecting ongoing hepatic injury (inflammation). Serum ALP activity is usually >5 times normal, reflecting intrahepatic cholestasis. Hyperbilirubinemia and bilirubinuria also are common.
- Liver function tests such as SBA concentration, BSP dye excretion, and ammonia tolerance frequently are abnormal, reflecting the degree of liver dysfunction.
- Less consistent findings include hypoalbuminemia, hyperglobulinemia, mild nonregenerative anemia, and abnormal hemostasis. Ascitic fluid, when present, typically is a transudate or modified transudate.

Radiography and Ultrasonography

- Radiographically the liver may appear small, and on ultrasonography nonspecific changes in echogenicity may be detected.

Liver Biopsy

Liver biopsy and histopathology confirm the diagnosis.

- The liver often is small and nodular because of the fibrosis and nodular regeneration of cirrhosis.
- The primary lesion is portal inflammation consisting primarily of lymphocytes and plasma cells and occasional neutrophils and macrophages. The inflammation extends into the hepatic lobule, causing piecemeal necrosis of hepatocytes. These lesions are essential criteria for categorization as idiopathic chronic hepatitis.
- Fibrosis usually is present.

Differential Diagnosis

When chronic hepatitis has been confirmed histologically, look for potential inciting or perpetuating factors. If none are found, then idiopathic chronic hepatitis is the diagnosis. Recognized types of chronic hepatitis are listed in Table 91–6.

Treatment

Treatment includes drug therapy, discussed below, and supportive measures, previously described under Principles of Treatment for Liver Disease.

Prednisolone

- Give 2 mg/kg/day PO for immunosuppression until clinical remission occurs; then taper down to 0.5 mg/kg or the lowest effective alternate-day maintenance dose.
- Monitor serum biochemistries every 1–2 weeks in the initial stages of treatment.
- A follow-up liver biopsy, performed 2–3 months after starting therapy, is required to ensure that the disease is in remission.

Azathioprine

When prednisolone alone is ineffective or side effects become objectionable, consider combination therapy using azathioprine and prednisolone (at a lower dose if side effects are a problem).

- Give azathioprine (Imuran) at 1–2 mg/kg/day PO for induction therapy; for maintenance, give the same dose once every other day while giving prednisolone on the alternate days.
- Because azathioprine may cause bone marrow suppression, monitor periodically with a CBC.

Ursodiol

Ursodiol (Actigall) is a synthetic bile acid that has been useful in the treatment of humans with chronic hepatitis. Its use in conjunction with immunosuppressive therapy in dogs with chronic hepatitis appears promising.

- Ursodiol, a hydrophilic bile acid, is believed to be beneficial by expanding the bile acid pool and displacing potentially hepatotoxic hydrophobic bile acids that may accumulate in cholestasis. It also has membrane-

Table 91–6. CANINE CHRONIC HEPATITIS

Familial Predisposition
Bedlington terrier
Cocker spaniel (American and English)
Doberman pinscher
Skye terrier
West Highland white terrier

Infectious
Infectious canine hepatitis
Acidophil cell hepatitis
Leptospirosis
   Serogroup *Grippotyphosa* (serovar *grippotyphosa*)
   Serogroup *Australis* (serovars *australis, bratislava, muenchen*)

Drug-induced
Anticonvulsants
Oxibendazole/diethylcarbamazine
Carprofen(?)

Lobular Dissecting Hepatitis

Idiopathic Chronic Hepatitis

stabilizing, cytoprotective, and immunomodulatory effects on liver cells and promotes choleresis.
- No signs of toxicity have been noted when ursodiol is given to dogs at a dose of 15 mg/kg/day PO q24 hours.

Antioxidants

- Free radicals may be generated in chronic hepatitis and they may cause hepatic injury. Antioxidants, such as vitamin E, are important to scavenge free radicals and prevent oxidative injury.
- Vitamin E at 400–600 IU/day is recommended. Absorption of fat-soluble vitamins may be decreased in chronic cholestatic hepatobiliary disorders. In this setting a water-soluble form of vitamin E (Nutr-E-Sol, Advanced Nutritional Technology) may be preferable.

Prognosis

The response to treatment of idiopathic chronic hepatitis is variable, which is expected because it probably represents a heterogeneous group of diseases.

- Some dogs eventually can be taken off medication and remain in remission, but more often therapy must be continued indefinitely.
- Other dogs fail to respond, especially those that have advanced disease and cirrhosis (the treatment of cirrhosis and its complications is discussed elsewhere in this chapter).

Hepatic Copper Accumulation and Chronic Hepatitis

Copper accumulation in the liver can be associated with significant hepatic injury resulting in acute hepatitis, chronic hepatitis, and cirrhosis. It is one of the few well-documented causes of chronic hepatitis in the dog. The severity of hepatic injury is related to the amount of accumulated copper. Hepatic copper concentration in normal dogs is less than 400 μg/g dry weight. Hepatic damage does not consistently occur until the copper concentration exceeds 2000 μg/g dry weight.

Copper accumulation in the liver may be a cause or an effect of chronic hepatitis.

- Inherited metabolic defects in biliary copper excretion cause chronic hepatitis in Bedlington terriers and West Highland white terriers. Copper concentrations range from 850–12,000 μg/g in affected Bedlingtons and up to 3,500 μg/g in West Highland white terriers.
- Because copper normally is excreted in the bile, hepatic copper accumulation can also occur secondary to any cholestatic hepatobiliary disorder (such as idiopathic chronic hepatitis) that impairs bile flow.
  - Although not proven, Doberman pinschers with chronic hepatitis (copper concentration 300–4000 μg/g) probably have copper accumulation as an effect rather than a cause of chronic hepatitis. An alternative explanation is that Doberman pinschers may develop hepatic injury at lower hepatic copper concentrations than Bedlington terriers.
  - Whether secondary copper accumulation can further contribute to hepatic injury is unclear, but this is an important question since the role of copper chelator therapy in this situation is controversial.
- Other breeds of dogs occasionally are diagnosed with chronic hepatitis and cirrhosis accompanied by increased hepatic copper concentrations. At this advanced stage of disease, it is difficult to know whether copper accumulation is a cause or an effect of the chronic hepatitis. As a general rule, the higher the copper content, the more likely it is to be a primary problem.

Copper-Associated Hepatitis in Bedlington Terriers

Etiology

- Bedlington terriers have a hereditary (autosomal recessive) inability to excrete copper in the bile that is associated with progressive hepatic copper accumulation and chronic liver disease. Hepatic copper content increases with age. Because of extensive inbreeding, the prevalence within the breed is quite high.
- Excess copper is stored in hepatic lysosomes. When hepatic copper accumulation is >2000 μg/g, progressive hepatic injury occurs, including focal hepatic necrosis, chronic hepatitis, and eventually, cirrhosis. This disease is similar but not identical to Wilson's disease in humans.

Clinical Signs

Clinical signs and presentation vary widely, depending on the stage of disease.

- Most affected dogs are presented as young or middle-aged adults of either sex with signs of hepatic failure of varying severity, including lethargy, depression, weight loss, vomiting, and jaundice. Acute fulminant hepatic failure with rapid deterioration and death occurs in rare instances.

- Some middle-aged and older dogs are presented initially with end-stage liver disease and cirrhosis. In these animals there is a more chronic insidious clinical course, with similar but less severe signs. In the advanced stages of disease, cachexia, jaundice, ascites, and hepatic encephalopathy can occur.
- Affected dogs may be asymptomatic, especially young dogs in which copper is accumulating but has not yet reached toxic hepatic concentrations.

Diagnosis

Suspect copper-associated hepatitis in any Bedlington terrier with historical, physical, or biochemical evidence of hepatic disease or with vague, unexplained illness. Asymptomatic dogs can be identified only by routine biochemical screening or liver biopsy. Definitive diagnosis requires liver biopsy.

History

- Acute, recurrent episodes are common in many affected dogs. Stressful events such as whelping, showing, shipping, or a change in environment can precipitate these episodes.
- Dogs initially presenting with end-stage cirrhosis often have no history of previous episodes of hepatitis.

Physical Examination

- Findings in dogs with acute hepatitis include depression, lethargy, and dehydration. Hepatomegaly may occur. Jaundice may be detected within 48 hours of onset. Acute copper-induced hemolytic anemia may be a contributing factor.
- With advanced disease, dehydration, emaciation, ascites, hepatic encephalopathy, and jaundice may be detected. The liver is small and not palpable.
- Asymptomatic dogs are normal on physical examination.

Laboratory Evaluation

- Biochemical findings vary with the stage of disease. Increased serum ALT activity is probably the most sensitive laboratory indicator of this disease, although up to a third of affected dogs will have normal ALT values. These are mostly younger dogs that are in the early stages of the disease.
- Other serum biochemical abnormalities typical of hepatic dysfunction eventually develop, such as hyperbilirubinemia, bilirubinuria, hypoalbuminemia, increased SBA levels, and prolonged PT and APTT.
- Acute release of copper from necrotic hepatocytes occasionally causes hemolytic anemia. Laboratory findings include low packed cell volume (PCV), hemoglobinemia, and hemoglobinuria. Plasma copper levels are increased during episodes of hemolysis.

Radiography and Ultrasonography

- Abdominal radiographs are unremarkable except when advanced stages of disease are accompanied by microhepatica or ascites.

- Ultrasonography of the liver may be normal in the early stages. As the disease progresses, findings are indicative of diffuse liver disease or microhepatica and cirrhosis.

Liver Biopsy

Liver biopsy is indicated for definitive diagnosis and staging of the disease. Perform liver biopsies in all dogs being considered for breeding. Dogs should be older than 1 year of age to ensure adequate time for copper accumulation. The spectrum of gross and microscopic features in the liver parallels the variable expression of the disease.

- The liver can be grossly normal or swollen and smooth with accentuation of the lobules. As cirrhosis develops, the liver decreases in size and there is a mixture of fine and coarse nodules.
- Histologically, H&E-stained hepatic tissue reveals dark granules in hepatocyte cytoplasm. In the early stages, centrilobular hepatocytes are most affected, but later the distribution is diffuse.
- Histochemical stains for copper such as rhodanine and rubeanic acid are positive. These stains consistently detect copper in liver biopsies when amounts are >400 µg/g dry weight. Hepatic biopsies stored in formalin for more than 6 months lose their ability to pick up these stains.
- Associated histologic hepatic damage is variable. In the most mildly affected animals, only centrilobular copper granules are detected. This progresses to focal hepatitis, lesions of chronic hepatitis, and eventually cirrhosis.

Hepatic Copper Analysis

Perform quantitative copper analysis on fresh hepatic tissue. Copper analyses are available to veterinarians through the Veterinary Diagnostic Laboratories of Michigan State University and Colorado State University. Affected dogs have hepatic copper concentrations of 850–12,000 µg/g dry weight.

Treatment

Specific measures to control hepatic copper accumulation are summarized in Table 91–7. Base the choice of therapy for an individual patient on the severity of existing hepatic damage.

Management of the acute hepatic crisis also involves symptomatic and supportive care to control electrolyte, acid-base, and fluid imbalances and hepatic encephalopathy (see Table 91–1). Treatment of hemolytic anemia may require a blood transfusion.

Chelator Therapy

- Treat affected dogs with copper accumulation and chronic hepatitis with a copper chelator such as penicillamine or trientine hydrochloride, which promotes urinary copper excretion (see Table 91–7).
- For treating an acute hemolytic crisis, trientine hydrochloride (but not penicillamine) may be effective in chelating copper in the circulation.

- Lifelong therapy is necessary because copper reaccumulates if treatment is stopped.
- Preliminary clinical evaluation suggests that hepatic copper concentrations decrease about 750–1000 µg/g dry weight per year with chelator therapy.
- There may be other protective effects of penicillamine besides depletion of hepatic copper, because many Bedlington terriers on long-term therapy do not develop hepatic failure despite continued elevated copper levels and ongoing hepatic damage. Penicillamine may induce hepatic metallothionein, which binds and sequesters copper in a nontoxic form. Additional effects that may be beneficial include inhibition of collagen deposition, stimulation of collagenase activity, immunosuppression, and immunomodulation.

Zinc Therapy

- Zinc may be added to the chelator therapy but should not be used alone in dogs with active hepatitis. Whether zinc alone will be useful for long-term therapy is not known. Zinc appears to be most useful to prevent copper accumulation in the liver but preliminary information in Bedlington terriers and West Highland white terriers suggests it may also deplete hepatic copper concentrations (see Table 91–7). A major advantage of zinc over penicillamine and trientine hydrochloride is that it is less expensive.

Dietary Therapy

Low copper diets are of little value once hepatic copper accumulation has occurred (see Table 91–7).

Vitamin E Therapy

Administer vitamin E in all dogs with hepatic copper accumulation, (see Table 91–7). Hepatic injury associated with hepatic copper overload in Bedlington terriers appears to involve free radical damage to hepatic mitochondria. Vitamin E therapy protects against copper-induced hepatic damage experimentally.

Prognosis

- Dogs with mild to moderate acute hepatic failure usually respond to supportive care.
- If this disease is detected before severe hepatic failure occurs, many dogs can live out their lives with penicillamine therapy.
- The prognosis is poor if there is fulminant hepatic failure or chronic end-stage cirrhosis and failure.

Prevention

- Treatment of affected dogs with minimal hepatic injury is recommended in the hope of preventing acute hepatitis or progression to cirrhosis.
- Zinc therapy is a promising and less expensive alternative to penicillamine in this setting.
- Young dogs (less than 1 year) may be less responsive to chelator therapy than older dogs.

Table 91-7. TREATMENT OF HEPATIC COPPER (Cu) ACCUMULATION

Product	Formulation	Dose	Side Effects	Comments
Chelate Systemic Cu				
Penicillamine (Cuprimine, MSD; Depen, Wallace)	Cuprimine: 125- and 250-mg caps Depen: 250-mg tabs	10–15 mg/kg q12hr PO given on an empty stomach to improve absorption; do not give concurrently with any medication, including zinc* or vitamin/mineral supplement.	Anorexia and vomiting† are common; dermatologic drug eruption or autoimmune-like vesicular lesions of mucocutaneous junctions‡; reversible renal disease.‡	Causes systemic Cu chelation and urinary excretion. Indicated when hepatic Cu >2000 μg/g. Takes months to years to produce significant decrease in hepatic Cu concentration (900 μg/g/yr).§ but may produce subjective clinical improvement after a few weeks. May have protective effect in liver beyond chelation: induces hepatic metallothionein, which binds and sequesters Cu in nontoxic form. Not effective for treatment of Cu-associated hemolysis.
Trientine dihydrochloride¶ (Syprine, MSD)	250-mg caps	10–15 mg/kg q12hr PO; give 1 hr before meals; do not give concurrently with any medication, including zinc* or vitamin/mineral supplement.	None noted as yet	Use as an alternative to penicillamine if vomiting occurs; may be useful for treatment of hemolysis by chelating Cu in blood; more expensive than penicillamine.
2,3,2-Tetramine	Not commercially available	15 mg/kg PO	None noted as yet	Derivative of trientine that is 4–9 times as potent; thus, lowers hepatic Cu concentrations more rapidly than penicillamine or trientine.
Decrease Intestinal Cu Absorption				
Zinc acetate, sulfate, gluconate, or methionine	Many available	5–10 mg elemental zinc/kg q12hr. Use high end of dose for 3 mo, then 50 mg PO q12hr for maintenance. Separate administration from meals by 1–2 hr.	Vomiting,** zinc-induced hemolysis at plasma levels >1000 μg/dl	Induces intestinal metallothionein, which binds Cu and zinc and prevents absorption; takes 3–6 mo to obtain therapeutic zinc plasma levels. Do not use zinc alone in dogs with active hepatitis (add Cu chelator). Monitor plasma zinc every 2–3 mo to maintain level of >200 but <400 μg/dl by adjusting dose.
Decrease Cu Intake				
Low-copper diet	None commercially available	<0.5 ppm Cu in diet		Low-copper diet may slow further Cu accumulation but won't "decopper" the liver. Most commercial diets exceed the NRC requirement for Cu. Even Cu-restricted diets such as Hill's Prescription Diet u/d (4 ppm) are too high. Homemade low-Cu diet is most beneficial for managing young dogs with inherited hepatic Cu metabolism defect to slow hepatic Cu accumulation. Avoid high-Cu foods such as liver, shellfish, organ meats, chocolate, nuts, mushrooms, cereals, mineral supplements.
Antioxidant Therapy ***				
Vitamin E	Many available	400–600 IU/d, PO	None noted as yet	Oxidative damage occurs in Cu-associated liver disease. Vitamin E protects the liver against oxidant damage.

*Penicillamine and trientine will theoretically chelate zinc (and decrease its absorption) when given concurrently. Staggered oral administration is recommended.
†Often resolves after several weeks; start at reduced dose and increase to maintenance after a few days. Giving with food will decrease absorption, but a small amount of milk, cheese, or bread given concurrently may decrease vomiting.
‡Rare complications; renal compromise more likely with Depen.
§In Bedlington terrier; more rapid response in Doberman pinscher and other breeds.
¶Availability limited; may require a special order direct from manufacturer.
**Zinc methionine may be less irritating to the stomach than other formulations. To minimize vomiting, open capsule and mix contents with small amount of tuna or hamburger.
***Although vitamin C has antioxidant effects, it should be avoided in dogs with Cu accumulation because it increases Cu's oxidative damage to the liver.

- Bedlington terriers used in breeding programs can be certified free of disease through either the Canine Liver Registry at Purdue University or the Liver Registry of the Orthopedic Foundation for Animals in Columbia, Missouri.

Chronic Hepatitis in Doberman Pinschers

Chronic hepatitis in Doberman pinschers is associated with histologic features of chronic hepatitis and cirrhosis. Hepatic copper concentrations are increased in most but not all affected dogs.

Etiology

- The underlying etiopathogenic mechanisms are unknown, but a genetic basis is suggested by the high incidence in this breed. The wide age range (1.5–11 years) suggests that environmental influences modify a genetic predisposition.
- The significance of the increased hepatic copper concentration has not been determined. Copper accumulation secondary to chronic hepatitis and cholestasis appears most likely because of the low magnitude (300–4000 μg/g) of copper detected. Alternatively, excess hepatic copper concentrations may make these dogs more susceptible to hepatic injury, hepatic injury may occur at lower hepatic copper concentrations than in Bedlington terriers, or copper accumulation may be incidental.

Clinical Signs

- Females are predominantly affected.
- Clinical signs may be mild or absent when the disease is fortuitously diagnosed in the early stages. However, most dogs are diagnosed in the advanced stages of hepatic failure.
- Signs include anorexia, weight loss, lethargy, PU/PD, vomiting, diarrhea, ascites, and jaundice.
- Evidence of excessive bleeding (gingival bleeding, epistaxis, and melena) may be found.
- Signs of hepatic encephalopathy often predominate in the terminal stages.

Diagnosis

Suspect chronic hepatitis in any Doberman pinscher (especially females) with clinical and biochemical evidence of hepatic disease. Definitive diagnosis requires liver biopsy. Consider concurrent von Willebrand disease, because of its prevalence in this breed (see Chap. 21), in affected dogs with a bleeding disorder.

- Common physical examination findings include ascites, jaundice, weight loss, and encephalopathy. Splenomegaly (associated with portal hypertension) is common. The liver is small and not palpable.
- Laboratory findings frequently include increased ALP and ALT activity, hyperbilirubinemia, bilirubinuria, hypoalbuminemia, increased SBA levels, hyperammonemia, and prolonged BSP retention. Coagulopathy and thrombocytopenia are common in the advanced stages.

- Radiographic and ultrasonographic findings of microhepatica and ascites are consistent with chronic liver disease and cirrhosis.
- Liver biopsy and histopathologic evaluation
  - Grossly the liver is small with micro- or macronodular cirrhosis.
  - Histologically, the earliest lesion is inflammation and fibrosis around the small hepatic vein branches. As the disease progresses, fibrous tissue septa radiate from hepatic vein branches to the portal areas. In the late stage of the disease, lymphoplasmacytic inflammation occurs around larger hepatic veins and portal tracts. Fibrosis and architectural distortion consistent with cirrhosis are present.
  - Rhodanine and rubeanic acid stains usually are positive for copper, especially in centrolobular regions. Stains for hepatic iron usually are positive.
- Quantitative copper analysis reveals normal to moderate copper accumulation (400–4000 μg/g).

Treatment

Effective treatment has not been established.

- Institute, as needed, symptomatic and supportive therapy for complications of hepatic failure, including correction of fluid, electrolyte, and acid-base balance, and treatment of ascites, hepatic encephalopathy, and coagulopathies (see Table 91–1 and the Principles of Treatment section).
- Therapy with immunosuppressant drugs such as prednisolone with or without azathioprine may be given, as described previously for idiopathic chronic hepatitis. The efficacy of this treatment remains to be determined, but generally the response is poor, possibly because most dogs are presented in advanced stages of liver failure.
- The use of copper chelating agents is controversial, but consider copper chelator therapy in Doberman pinschers with chronic hepatitis and hepatic copper concentrations >1000 μg/g dry weight. Sporadic reports suggest that treatment of affected Dobermans with penicillamine decreases hepatic copper concentrations to <400 μg/g after 3–12 months of therapy (see Table 91–7). This is a notable difference from Bedlington terriers with copper accumulation, which may never achieve normal copper levels even with lifelong penicillamine therapy. Despite a decrease in hepatic copper content, it appears that hepatitis in Dobermans is progressive, suggesting that copper accumulation is secondary and not the cause of hepatic injury.
- Ursodeoxycholic acid and vitamin E are also recommended as described earlier for idiopathic chronic hepatitis.

Prognosis

- Treatment usually is unsuccessful. Most dogs die within weeks to months.
- The prognosis may be more favorable if the disease is detected in the early stages.

Copper-Associated Hepatitis in West Highland White Terriers

Etiology

West Highland white terriers are at increased risk to develop chronic hepatitis and cirrhosis. Increased hepatic copper concentration (2000–6800 μg/g dry wt) appears to be a factor in some but not all dogs with chronic hepatitis. Many West Highland white terriers have hepatic copper concentrations ranging from 200–1500 μg/g, but rarely does the value exceed 2000 μg/g, and clinical illness associated with excess hepatic copper accumulation is uncommon. Increased hepatic copper accumulation is a familial trait but the mode of inheritance has not been established.

As with Bedlington terriers, evidence of hepatic damage is not noted until values are >2000 μg/g. However, there are notable differences from the disease in Bedlingtons, such as:

- West Highland white terriers do not accumulate copper continuously throughout life. Peak hepatic copper concentrations occur by 6 months of age and may even decrease after 1 year of age.
- The magnitude of copper increase generally is lower than in Bedlingtons.
- West Highland white terriers with chronic hepatitis but without toxic hepatic copper levels (<2000 μg/g) may have idiopathic chronic hepatitis.

Clinical Signs

- Affected animals in the early stages of copper accumulation or those with focal hepatitis are usually asymptomatic.
- When widespread necrosis occurs, nonspecific signs of liver disease include anorexia, vomiting, diarrhea, lethargy, and jaundice.
- With advanced disease, jaundice and ascites are common.

Diagnosis

Episodes of hepatic necrosis may be precipitated by stressful events such as whelping or showing.

- The earliest biochemical abnormality associated with hepatic necrosis is increased ALT activity.
- With advanced disease, laboratory findings include increased liver enzyme activity, hyperbilirubinemia, increased SBA levels, impaired BSP excretion, hyperammonemia, and hypoalbuminemia. Copper-associated hemolytic anemia has not been documented.
- Liver biopsy for histopathology and quantitative copper analysis are required for definitive diagnosis. Histologic features include copper granules (which are initially centrilobular but become diffusely distributed with time), multifocal hepatitis, and postnecrotic cirrhosis.

Treatment

- The principles of therapy are similar to those described for Bedlington terriers (see Table 91–7).

- Because hepatic copper accumulation is not continuous throughout life, mature dogs with <2000 μg/g may not require chelator therapy. Treatment for copper accumulation is indicated when copper concentrations are >2000 μg/g or when active hepatic necrosis is evident.
- Preliminary evidence suggests that both penicillamine and zinc acetate can decrease hepatic copper concentrations in West Highland white terriers, when given on a long-term basis (see Table 91–7).

Copper-Associated Hepatitis in Skye Terriers

Chronic hepatitis and cirrhosis associated with hepatic copper accumulation (358–2257 μg/g) has been described in genetically related Skye terriers.

- In the early stages, copper accumulation is absent, and biopsy findings indicate hepatocellular degeneration with cholestasis and mild inflammation.
- Chronic lesions are associated with intracanalicular cholestasis, chronic hepatitis, and cirrhosis.
- Skye terrier hepatitis is speculated to be a result of disturbed bile secretion with secondary accumulation of copper.

Chronic Hepatitis in Cocker Spaniels

American and English cocker spaniels have an increased incidence of chronic hepatitis. The cause is unknown. Hepatic accumulation of alpha-1 antitrypsin appears more likely in Cocker spaniels with chronic hepatitis than other breeds and may play a role in this disorder.

Clinical Signs

- Young male cocker spaniels are most commonly affected (1.5 to 4 years old). Despite the chronicity of the underlying hepatic lesions, most affected dogs have a short duration of clinical illness, usually 2 weeks or less. Ascites is the most consistent presenting complaint. Other nonspecific signs of liver disease include depression, mild jaundice, melena, dehydration, subcutaneous edema, and coma.

Diagnosis

- Laboratory findings include mild anemia, mild to moderate increases in serum liver enzyme activity (although some dogs have normal values), and hypoalbuminemia, which is often profound (mean of 1.7 g/dl). The total serum bilirubin concentration is normal or mildly increased, supporting that cholestasis is not a key feature of the disorder. Fasting and postprandial SBA concentrations are increased.
- Ascitic fluid analysis is consistent with a transudate or modified transudate.
- Radiographic findings include microhepatica and ascites. On ultrasonography, a diffuse increase in echogenicity is usually noted, although some dogs have a normal-appearing liver.
- Liver biopsy reveals chronic periportal hepatitis (lymphocytes, plasma cells, and lesser numbers of neu-

trophils), with variable portal fibrosis. Other features include bridging fibrosis, piecemeal necrosis, hepatocyte vacuolar change, bile duct duplication, and micro- or macronodular cirrhosis.

- Hepatic copper accumulation does not appear to be a consistent feature (200 to 550 µg/g).

Treatment

- Treatment for cocker spaniels with chronic hepatitis consists of general supportive therapy for the complications of liver failure (see Principles of Treatment section; Table 91–1). The prognosis is poor and most dogs die within a month of diagnosis. Corticosteroid therapy may be beneficial in this disorder. Early diagnosis appears to be the key to long-term survival.

Lobular Dissecting Hepatitis

- Lobular dissecting hepatitis is a specific histologic form of chronic hepatitis that occurs in young dogs. The median age of 21 affected dogs was 11 months, with 54% of dogs being 7 months or younger.
- The lesion is characterized histologically by lobular hepatitis; inflammation (lymphocytes, plasma cells, macrophages, and neutrophils) is scattered throughout the hepatic lobule rather than concentrated in periportal regions. Bands of collagen and reticulin fibers dissect around single or small groups of hepatocytes and disrupt hepatic lobular architecture. Copper stains are negative or moderately positive, consistent with secondary copper accumulation. The liver is shrunken, pale to tan, with an almost smooth surface and occasional hyperplastic nodules. Multiple acquired portosystemic shunts are present.
- It has been suggested that this is a specific reaction pattern of the liver in neonatal and juvenile dogs to a wide variety of hepatic insults. Standard poodles may be at increased risk for this form of chronic hepatitis.
- Clinical features are those of advanced hepatic failure and portal hypertension. The most consistent clinical finding is ascites. Liver enzymes are typically increased. Hypoalbuminemia and increased serum bile acid concentrations are common. Diagnosis requires liver biopsy. An attempt should be made to identify other causes of chronic hepatic disease (see Table 91–6).
- Specific treatment has not been reported, but general measures for management of chronic liver failure are appropriate (see Table 91–1).

Acidophil Cell Hepatitis

Acidophil cell hepatitis has been described in Great Britain and is caused by an unidentified transmissable agent that is probably viral but distinct from canine adenovirus I (see Chap. 14).

- It is characterized by acute or chronic hepatitis with slow progression to cirrhosis. Acidophils, which are a consistent histologic feature of the disease, represent dying hepatocytes.
- Signs usually are typical of chronic liver failure.

- Specific treatment has not been described, but general measures for management of chronic liver failure are appropriate.

HEPATIC CIRRHOSIS AND FIBROSIS

Cirrhosis is characterized by diffuse fibrosis and replacement of liver tissue with structurally abnormal regenerative nodules.

Etiology

- Cirrhosis is the irreversible end stage of chronic hepatic injury caused by infection, hepatotoxins (e.g., copper, anticonvulsants), immunologic injury (chronic hepatitis), chronic cholestasis (chronic cholangiohepatitis in cats), and hypoxia. The common denominator is hepatocyte death, which leads to repair by fibrosis and nodular regeneration.
- These processes further compromise adjacent normal hepatocytes, intrahepatic blood flow, and intrahepatic bile flow; thus, cirrhosis eventually reaches a point at which it is self-perpetuating.
- When cirrhosis is fully developed, the histologic features of the original inciting injury often are obscured by the cirrhotic changes.

Clinical Signs

Cirrhosis causes generalized hepatic dysfunction; thus, the clinical signs are those of chronic hepatic failure. A combination of jaundice, ascites, and hepatic encephalopathy is highly suggestive of cirrhosis.

Diagnosis

Laboratory Evaluation

Laboratory evidence of liver disease usually precedes the development of cirrhosis but may go undetected because signs at that stage may be insidious and vague.

- Serum liver enzymes usually are increased, although more modestly than during the active injury stage of liver disease.
- Circulating bilirubin, ammonia, and bile acids usually are increased, whereas serum albumin usually is decreased. Hyperglobulinemia is sometimes seen.
- Hemostatic abnormalities may reflect DIC, impaired hepatic synthesis of coagulation factors, or vitamin K deficiency due to cholestasis (least likely).

Radiography and Ultrasonography

- Microhepatica is common in dogs with cirrhosis, whereas most cats with biliary cirrhosis have hepatomegaly.
- Ultrasonography findings include microhepatica, irregular hepatic margins, focal lesions representing regenerative nodules, and increased parenchymal echogenicity associated with increased fibrous tissue. Splenomegaly and secondary portosystemic shunts also may be detected.

Liver Biopsy

Definitive diagnosis of cirrhosis requires liver biopsy.

- Laparotomy or laparoscopy provides a better appreciation for the gross nodularity of the liver than can be ascertained from blind percutaneous needle biopsy.
- Microscopic features include fibrosis, regenerative nodules, and disruption of normal hepatic architecture.
- Concurrent inflammation may be detected, especially when the inciting cause of cirrhosis is chronic inflammation.

Treatment

- Because cirrhosis is essentially irreversible, treatment is mainly supportive, emphasizing measures that control complications of severe generalized liver failure, such as ascites, encephalopathy, gastric ulcers, coagulopathies, and infection (see Table 91–1 and General Principles of Treatment section).
- If a probable cause or category of injury can be determined, specific treatment directed at preventing further injury may slow progression of cirrhosis. If an underlying cause can be determined (or is suspected), refer to the appropriate section of this chapter for specific details regarding treatment. For example:
  - Adjust the drug regimen of dogs receiving anticonvulsants.
  - Treat dogs with copper-positive biopsies with a chelating agent such as penicillamine.
  - Treat dogs with histologic features of chronic hepatitis with immunosuppressive drugs.
- Penicillamine and prednisolone also have antifibrotic properties; however, the benefits of corticosteroids may be outweighed by the risk. These include a tendency for GI ulceration and bleeding, increased body catabolism that may exacerbate hepatic encephalopathy, and sodium retention that may exacerbate ascites and edema.
- Colchicine, an antifibrotic drug, has been used to treat humans with cirrhosis. Colchicine is a microtubule inhibitor, stimulant of collagenase activity, and inhibitor of collagen deposition. Its benefit in dogs with cirrhosis is unproven.
  - The recommended dose is 0.025–0.03 mg/kg/day PO.
  - The major side effects in dogs are nausea, vomiting, and diarrhea. In humans, other side effects include bone marrow toxicity and myoneuropathy.

FELINE HEPATIC LIPIDOSIS

Hepatic lipidosis is an excessive accumulation of triglyceride in the liver that occurs when there is an imbalance between the rates of deposition and mobilization of fat from the liver. It is the most common liver disease in cats and is associated with severe intrahepatic cholestasis and hepatic failure. Mortality is high if the disorder is untreated.

Etiology

General mechanisms of hepatic lipidosis include nutritional, metabolic, hormonal, toxic, and hypoxic liver injury. Diabetes mellitus is a well-recognized and easily diagnosed cause of hepatic lipidosis. Drug- (tetracycline) or toxin-induced injury can also cause histologic lesions of lipidosis. Hepatic lipidosis may occur secondary to other disorders, especially cholangiohepatitis, inflammatory bowel disease, and pancreatitis. The term *idiopathic hepatic lipidosis* is used when no other associated illness is identified.

The following mechanisms may be important in the development of idiopathic hepatic lipidosis:

- Persistent anorexia and rapid weight loss are hallmark features. Severe hepatic lipidosis most commonly develops in overweight cats that experience prolonged inappetence (sometimes triggered by a stressful event), usually lasting 2 weeks or longer. Obese cats do not seem to be able to adapt to metabolism of fat for energy during periods of starvation.
- Accumulation of lipids in hepatocytes can result from disruption of normal fat metabolism at any of the following steps:
  - Excess mobilization of fat from peripheral stores, which may overwhelm hepatic fat dispersal and metabolism (may explain predilection in obese cats)
  - Increased hepatic synthesis of triglycerides (currently appears unlikely)
  - Inability of the liver to adequately oxidize fatty acids (possibly due to relative deficiency of carnitine)
  - Inability to synthesize or secrete lipoproteins (due to protein deficiency)
- Arginine deficiency may be important, because cats with lipidosis have decreased serum arginine concentrations and arginine is an essential amino acid in the cat that is required for normal urea cycle function and ammonia detoxification.
- Taurine deficiency may contribute to intrahepatic cholestasis, because serum taurine concentrations are low and taurine is required for hepatic bile acid conjugation and normal bile acid metabolism in cats.

Clinical Signs

- Idiopathic hepatic lipidosis has no age, breed, or gender predilection. Many but not all affected cats are obese prior to the onset of disease.
- Prolonged anorexia, often of several weeks' duration, is the most consistent clinical sign.
- Other findings include lethargy, vomiting, constipation or diarrhea, and weight loss. Weight loss can be dramatic and may exceed 25% of the previous weight.
- Overt signs of hepatic encephalopathy such as hypersalivation, head pressing, dementia, and seizures are uncommon. However, nonspecific signs such as anorexia, lethargy and vomiting may be subtle signs of encephalopathy.
- Overt bleeding occurs in 20% of cases.

- Ventroflexion of the neck occurs in some cats and may represent muscle weakness associated with hypokalemia, hypophosphatemia, thiamine deficiency, or hepatic encephalopathy.

Diagnosis

Clinical findings and laboratory evaluation in cats with idiopathic hepatic lipidosis suggest hepatic disease, but liver biopsy is required to distinguish hepatic lipidosis from other causes of hepatic disease such as cholangiohepatitis, FIP, and neoplasia. When hepatic lipidosis occurs secondary to another disorder, additional testing is required to identify the primary disease (e.g., trypsin assay for pancreatitis; GI endoscopy and biopsy for inflammatory bowel disease).

History

- The history may reveal precipitating causes of anorexia such as stressful events (e.g., boarding, surgery, change in living arrangements), a diet change for weight reduction, and nonhepatic diseases associated with anorexia.

Physical Examination

- Findings include hepatomegaly, jaundice, muscle wasting, pallor, and seborrhea.

Laboratory Evaluation

- Hematologic findings are nonspecific and include a nonregenerative, normocytic, normochromic anemia with poikilocytosis and a normal WBC count. Hemolysis may occur secondary to severe hypophosphatemia or excessive treatment with vitamin K.
- Serum ALP, ALT, and AST activities, fasting and postprandial SBA concentrations, and total serum bilirubin concentration usually are increased. Increases in liver enzymes precede increases in total bilirubin and bile acids. Serum ALP activity generally is higher in cats with lipidosis than with other hepatic diseases. Serum GGT activity, which usually parallels or exceeds serum ALP activity in most feline hepatic diseases, is normal or only mildly increased in hepatic lipidosis.
- Other potential findings include hypokalemia, prolonged BSP retention, hyperammonemia, hypoalbuminemia, and decreased BUN. Many affected cats have abnormal coagulation tests, especially PIVKA (proteins induced by vitamin K absence) values and hypofibrinogenemia. In one study, PIVKA values improved in 50% of the cats treated with vitamin K, suggesting acquired vitamin K deficiency.

Radiography and Ultrasonography

- Radiographically, the liver is normal to increased in size.
- Ultrasonographic findings include hepatomegaly and diffuse increased echogenicity of the liver compared with falciform fat.

Fine-Needle Aspiration Cytology

- Fine-needle aspiration cytology is a less invasive alternative to liver biopsy that can provide similar information. Results of fine-needle aspiration cytology occasionally can be misleading because the small sample size may not be representative of the pathologic process in the liver.
- On cytologic evaluation, hepatocytes are foamy and vacuolated, and inflammatory cells are absent.

Liver Biopsy

Liver biopsy is required for definitive diagnosis.

- Grossly, the liver is enlarged, yellow, greasy, and friable with rounded edges. Biopsy specimens usually float in formalin.
- On routine H&E staining, severe vacuolization of hepatocytes in a micro- or macrovacuolar pattern is noted.
- Oil red O stain performed on nonparaffin embedded formalin-fixed tissue can confirm excess fat in the vacuoles.
- Inflammation or necrosis usually is absent.

Treatment

Because of lack of information regarding the underlying cause, treatment is primarily supportive. The greatest success has been with aggressive nutritional support.

Nutritional Therapy

- Provide the daily caloric requirement (60 kcal/kg body weight/day) by force-feeding or via nasogastric, esophagostomy, or gastrostomy tube. An endoscopically placed gastrostomy tube is preferable because long-term nutritional therapy (at least 3–6 weeks) usually is necessary. Nasogastric tubes are adequate for short-term management and are preferable to force-feeding. Techniques for placement of indwelling feeding tubes are described in Chapter 3.
  - Oral appetite stimulants are usually inadequate to achieve the consistent caloric intake required for treatment of lipidosis. Avoid benzodiazepines, in particular, because they can exacerbate hepatic encephalopathy and require the liver for metabolism.
- Administer balanced, canned commercial cat food with water to make a gruel that can be delivered through a tube in small feedings.
  - Initially, give one-fourth to one-half of the daily dietary caloric requirement through the tube, divided into 4–6 feedings per day. Gradually increase the total amount fed over 3–4 days until maintenance requirements are achieved. Commercial liquid diets such as CliniCare Feline Liquid Diet (Pet-Ag) can be used initially.
  - Use a restricted-protein diet only if hyperammonemia or overt signs of hepatic encephalopathy occur.
  - If vomiting or delayed gastric emptying is a problem, give metoclopramide (0.4 mg/kg SC q8 hours, 30 minutes before feeding). A liquid enteral diet can also be given by constant rate infusion into

the feeding tube to control vomiting in the initial stages of treatment. Dilution of the diet with water may also improve tolerance.

- A multiple-vitamin supplement can be given at double the daily maintenance dose. Consider thiamine supplementation, in particular, because prolonged anorexia can result in thiamine deficiency. Give 50–100 mg of thiamine q12 hours IM, SC, or PO for 3 treatments.
- Various dietary supplements have been recommended, based on the speculation that deficiencies may play a role in this disorder. However, feeding a balanced commercial cat food is usually adequate.
  - Taurine, 500 mg/day, is recommended by some clinicians for the first month.
  - Give arginine, 1 g/day, if a nonfeline liquid diet is used. Commercial feline diets are adequate in arginine.
  - L-Carnitine, 250–500 mg/day, is recommended by some clinicians in the belief that a relative deficiency of carnitine is present.

Fluid Therapy

- Intravenous fluid therapy with a balanced electrolyte solution supplemented with potassium chloride often is required in the initial stages of treatment (see Table 91–1). Hepatic lactate metabolism may be impaired in cats with hepatic lipidosis, suggesting that lactated Ringer's should be avoided.
- Avoid dextrose supplementation unless hypoglycemia is documented, because glucose may promote hepatic lipid accumulation if caloric needs are not being adequately met.
- Monitor serum phosphorus concentration and treat with IV potassium phosphate if levels decline to <2 mg/dl (see Chap. 5). Hemolysis may occur secondary to severe hypophosphatemia.

Control of Complications

- Abnormal blood coagulation test results and excess bleeding occasionally respond to vitamin K_1 therapy, suggesting severe cholestasis and vitamin K malabsorption (see Table 91–1). Fresh blood transfusion may be required for management of anemia.
- Hepatic encephalopathy is managed, as described in Table 91–1, with a low-protein diet, lactulose, and neomycin or metronidazole.
- Consider antibiotic therapy with amoxicillin to prevent infection secondary to compromised hepatic clearance of enteric organisms. Avoid tetracycline because it can predispose to hepatic lipid accumulation.

Response to Treatment and Prognosis

- With aggressive nutritional and supportive care, approximately 60–80% of cats with lipidosis respond within 3–6 weeks. Biochemical parameters are often normal by 4 weeks. Recurrence is rare and there is no evidence of residual hepatic damage.
- The earlier treatment is initiated, the better the prognosis. Thus, monitor serum liver enzyme levels and

institute nutritional support in any obese cat that becomes anorexic secondary to other disease processes.
- Consider the potential for lipidosis in any obese cat placed on a reducing diet. Monitor liver enzymes to evaluate for onset of lipidosis.

SUPERFICIAL NECROLYTIC DERMATITIS (HEPATOCUTANEOUS SYNDROME)

Superficial necrolytic dermatitis (SND), also called hepatocutaneous syndrome, necrolytic migratory erythema, or metabolic epidermal necrosis, is a crusting, ulcerative dermatopathy that appears to be a complication of hepatic or endocrine pancreatic disease in dogs and cats. In dogs it is most commonly associated with hepatic insufficiency but has also been described with a glucagon-producing pancreatic endocrine tumor, in the absence of liver disease. The hepatopathy is usually of unknown origin, although liver disease associated with anticonvulsant therapy and potential exposure to mycotoxins has been reported. Many dogs develop diabetes mellitus in the late stages of the disease. The syndrome has been reported in one cat with a pancreatic carcinoma.

Etiology

The etiology and pathogenesis of this syndrome are poorly understood. The dermatologic lesions are similar to necrolytic migratory erythema in humans, which is usually associated with hyperglucagonemia and hypoaminoacidemia secondary to a glucagon-secreting pancreatic tumor. Hyperglucagonemia is believed to cause severe hypoaminoacidemia by stimulating hepatic utilization of amino acids during gluconeogenesis, resulting in a metabolic or nutritional imbalance affecting the skin. Intravenous amino acid infusions can reverse the skin lesions in humans.

- Plasma glucagon levels are increased and most plasma amino acids are decreased in dogs with SND and an underlying pancreatic endocrine tumor. Dermatologic signs resolve if the tumor can be completely resected.
- Plasma glucagon levels are reported to be normal or only mildly increased in dogs with SND and hepatic insufficiency. However, many of these dogs have severe hypoaminoacidemia and some have responded to dietary supplementation with egg yolks, which are a rich source of amino acids. Hyperglucagonemia may still play a central role in this disorder because peripheral plasma glucagon levels are not a reliable indicator of increased pancreatic glucagon secretion, which controls hepatic gluconeogenesis.
- Other nutritional deficiencies such as biotin, essential fatty acids, or zinc have also been proposed.

Signalment and Clinical Signs

- SND is a disease of older dogs (mean age of 10 years), especially males. No breed predilection has been noted.

- Dogs are usually presented for dermatologic signs. They may or may not show signs of liver disease such as anorexia, polyuria, polydipsia, jaundice, lethargy, and weight loss.

Diagnosis

Physical Examination

SND is characterized by bilaterally symmetrical crusting or erosive lesions of the pads, mucocutaneous junctions, and pressure points (hocks and elbows). Jaundice may be detected in dogs with severe hepatic dysfunction.

Laboratory Evaluation

- Abnormalities may include nonregenerative anemia, abnormal red cell morphology (poikilocytes and target cells), increased serum liver enzymes (ALP, ALT, and AST), hyperglycemia, hypoalbuminemia, hyperbilirubinemia, and increased serum bile acid concentrations.
- Other potential findings include hypoaminoacidemia, hyperglucagonemia, and elevated insulin levels.

Ultrasonography

- Ultrasound examination of the liver may identify a unique "honeycomb" or "Swiss cheese-like" lesion consisting of 0.5–1.5 cm diameter hypoechoic regions surrounded by highly echogenic borders.
- The pancreas should be evaluated for nodules consistent with neoplasia.

Pathology

- Dermatohistopathology is pathognomonic for SND. Lesions consist of parakeratotic hyperkeratosis, interor intracellular edema, and epidermal hyperplasia. Bacteria, dermatophytes, and yeast can be secondary contaminants.
- The liver is usually normal to increased in size and has a striking nodular appearance that grossly mimics cirrhosis. However, the hepatic lesion is not true cirrhosis because microscopically, the fibrous tissue is actually condensed stroma secondary to parenchymal collapse and not due to increased collagen production. The hepatic lesion is characteristically a severe vacuolar hepatopathy with marked nodular regeneration. Hepatic necrosis and inflammation are absent. The hepatic lesion is most likely a reflection of underlying nutritional, hormonal, or toxic abnormalities.

Treatment

If a glucagon-producing pancreatic tumor is diagnosed, it should be surgically resected. When a toxic or metabolic cause of hepatic injury is identified (e.g., anticonvulsant therapy), there is the potential for resolution of the disorder if the cause can be removed.

Nutritional Considerations

- Despite underlying hepatic insufficiency, do not restrict protein intake unless overt hepatic encephalopathy occurs. A diet high in good-quality protein is preferred.
- Egg yolk supplementation may improve skin lesions (1 yolk per 4.5 kg/day) or consider oral amino acid supplementation (Pro-Mod, Ross Labs) 10 g/7kg (maximum of 40g) q24 hours. For severely debilitated animals, start IV hyperalimentation with a balanced amino acid solution.
- Administer an oral multivitamin supplement.
- Give zinc gluconate, 0.75 mg/kg PO q12 hours for possible zinc deficiency.
- Consider essential fatty acid supplementation.

Dermatologic Therapy

- Parenteral corticosteroids are contraindicated because of the diabetic or prediabetic state. Topical triamcinolone ointment q12 hours can be used on a short-term basis to decrease pain and inflammation associated with deep fissures.
- Manage secondary cutaneous bacterial and fungal infections appropriately.

Other Therapy

- Manage diabetes mellitus with insulin therapy and a high-fiber diet.
- Consider a long-acting somatostatin analogue (Octreotide; Sandostatin) to inhibit glucagon release.

Prognosis

The prognosis is poor unless a glucagon-producing pancreatic tumor is detected and removed. Most dogs die or are euthanized within 5 months of onset of the skin lesions.

CONGENITAL PORTOSYSTEMIC SHUNT (PSS)

Portosystemic shunts (PSS) are vascular communications between the portal and systemic venous systems that allow access of portal blood to the systemic circulation without first passing through the liver. Clinical signs of hepatic encephalopathy result from inadequate hepatic clearance of enterically derived toxins such as ammonia, mercaptans, short-chain fatty acids, gamma aminobutyric acid, and endogenous benzodiazepines. Decreased hepatic blood flow and lack of hepatotrophic factors result in hepatic atrophy. Urate urolithiasis is an important complication of PSS because of increased urinary excretion of ammonia and uric acid. Renal, cystic, and urethral calculi usually are green and contain an ammonia or uric acid component.

Etiology

PSS in dogs and cats can be congenital or acquired.

Congenital PSS

Congenital PSS is the most common and is categorized as single intrahepatic or single extrahepatic.

Intrahepatic

- Single intrahepatic shunts provide a communication between the portal vein and the caudal vena cava, often via the left hepatic vein. Failure of the fetal ductus venosus to close results in an intrahepatic shunt.
- This type of shunt is most common in large-breed dogs.

Extrahepatic

- Single extrahepatic shunts usually connect the portal vein or one of its tributaries (left gastric or splenic vein) with the caudal vena cava cranial to the phrenicoabdominal veins. Less frequently, the anomalous vessel will enter the azygous vein.
- This type of shunt is most common in small-breed dogs and cats.

Acquired PSS

Acquired PSS are collateral vessels that develop as a compensatory response to sustained portal hypertension. Disorders associated with portal hypertension and acquired (multiple) PSS are discussed elsewhere in this chapter.

- These shunts usually appear as a tortuous plexus of vessels that communicate with the caudal vena cava in the area of the kidneys.
- Diagnosis and therapy are directed toward the underlying liver disease.

The following discussion focuses on congenital PSS.

Clinical Signs

Clinical signs of congenital PSS are usually referable to the CNS, GI system, or urinary tract.

CNS Signs

- Signs of hepatic encephalopathy (HE) often predominate, including episodic weakness, ataxia, head-pressing, disorientation, circling, pacing, behavioral changes, amaurotic blindness, seizures, and coma.
- Hypersalivation, seizures, and blindness are more common in cats with PSS than in dogs.
- Clinical signs of encephalopathy tend to wax and wane and are often interspersed with normal periods, reflecting the variable production and absorption of neurotoxic enteric products.

GI Signs

- GI signs of intermittent anorexia, vomiting, and diarrhea are common and are not necessarily accompanied by overt signs of HE.

Urinary Signs

- Psychogenic polydipsia and subsequent polyuria are frequent findings in dogs.
- If urolithiasis is a complicating feature, pollakiuria, dysuria, and hematuria may occur.

Diagnosis

- Suspect congenital PSS in:
  - Young dogs and cats with intermittent CNS, GI, or urinary tract signs.
  - Dogs (except Dalmatians) or cats with urate urolithiasis.
  - Dogs and cats of any age with clinical and biochemical evidence of hepatic insufficiency (especially hepatic encephalopathy) and absence of histologic evidence of severe intrahepatic disease.
- Although congenital PSS may be suspected because of historical, physical, laboratory, and radiographic findings, a definitive diagnosis requires identification of a shunt by ultrasonography, contrast radiography, transcolonic portal scintigraphy, or exploratory laparotomy.
- In young animals with clinical features of a congenital PSS but without a demonstrable shunt on portography or transcolonic portal scintigraphy, consider hepatic microvascular dysplasia (see later in this chapter).

Signalment

- Congenital PSS is more common in purebred than mixed-breed dogs. The genetic basis is unknown, although an increased incidence has been recognized in miniature schnauzers, Yorkshire terriers, Irish wolfhounds, Cairn terriers, Maltese, Australian cattle dogs, Old English sheepdogs, Labrador retrievers, and golden retrievers.
- Domestic short-haired cats are affected more commonly than are purebred cats. Of affected purebreds, Persian and Himalayan cats are at increased risk.
- No sex predilection has been noted. Affected male dogs and cats commonly are cryptorchid.
- Age is an important diagnostic clue, because most animals develop signs by 6 months of age. A congenital PSS is also a diagnostic consideration in middle-aged and older dogs, because signs may be subtle and occasionally animals go undiagnosed until as old as 10 or 12 years of age.

History

- Many affected animals have a history of stunted growth or failure to gain weight compared with unaffected littermates.
- Prolonged recovery after general anesthesia or excessive sedation after treatment with tranquilizers, anticonvulsants, or organophosphates can be attributed to impaired hepatic metabolism of these substances.
- Signs of encephalopathy may be exacerbated by a protein-rich meal; GI bleeding associated with parasite infection, ulcers, or drug therapy; and administration of methionine-containing urinary acidifiers or lipotrophic agents.
- Clinical improvement after fluid therapy is common and most likely attributed to correction of dehydration and promotion of urinary excretion of ammonia and other toxins. Improvement with broad-spectrum antibiotic therapy reflects the effect of antibiotics on the toxin-producing intestinal flora.

Physical Examination

- Findings may be unremarkable except for small body stature or weight loss.
- The neurologic examination is normal or, if overt signs of HE are present, neurologic findings are consistent with diffuse cerebral disease.
- Ascites and edema are rare unless the shunt is complicated by hypoalbuminemia (less than 1 g/dl) or severe intrahepatic or extrahepatic portal atresia.
- Many affected cats have golden or copper-colored irises.

Laboratory Evaluation

Routine hematologic and biochemical findings often are unremarkable. Although individual parameters might be only mildly abnormal, test results often reflect a pattern suggesting hepatocellular dysfunction in the absence of significant cholestasis or hepatocellular necrosis.

- Hematologic findings include microcytosis, target cells, poikilocytosis (especially in cats), and mild nonregenerative anemia. Microcytosis is associated with abnormal iron metabolism (impaired iron transport or iron sequestration) rather than absolute iron deficiency. These RBC changes can be subtle but important diagnostic clues in an otherwise normal CBC.
- Urinalysis findings include dilute urine, ammonium biurate crystalluria, and mild bilirubinuria.
- Coagulation tests are normal. Mild thrombocytopenia occasionally is noted but does not appear to be clinically significant.
- Hepatocellular dysfunction is suggested by hypoproteinemia, hypoalbuminemia, hypoglobulinemia, hypoglycemia, decreased BUN, and mild hypocholesterolemia. Hypoalbuminemia is a consistent finding in dogs, but not in cats. Total serum bilirubin concentration is normal.
- Serum liver enzyme (ALP and ALT) levels are normal to mildly (2–3 times) increased, consistent with a lesion of hepatic atrophy and minimal hepatocellular injury or intrahepatic cholestasis. Increases in ALP activity in these young animals may actually be due to the bone isoenzyme.
- Measure SBA concentrations to document hepatic dysfunction in dogs and cats suspected of having congenital PSS. Fasting SBA concentrations may be normal or increased, but PPSBA concentrations are consistently abnormal and usually exceed 100 μmol/L.

▼ *Key Point* The pattern of normal FSBA concentration with markedly increased PPSBA level is characteristic of PSS. A consistently normal PPSBA concentration excludes a diagnosis of congenital PSS.

- Hyperammonemia is a common finding in animals with PSS, but fasting blood ammonia concentration may be normal. The ammonia tolerance test is consistently abnormal and is equal in sensitivity to PPSBA concentrations for detecting hepatic dysfunc-

tion associated with PSS (see Diagnostic Strategy for Liver Disease).

Radiography and Ultrasonography

- *Abdominal radiography* commonly reveals microhepatica in dogs, but not cats. Mild renomegaly of unknown clinical significance also is common. Intraabdominal detail may be poor because of lack of abdominal fat. Ammonium urate urinary calculi may be visible on survey radiographs if they contain substantial amounts of magnesium and phosphate.
- *Routine abdominal ultrasonography* may demonstrate intrahepatic and extrahepatic shunts. Intrahepatic shunts are more reliably detected with this procedure than are extrahepatic PSS. Urinary calculi also can be identified.
- *Transcolonic portal scintigraphy* using technetium 99m pertechnetate is a noninvasive test (available at some referral institutions) that can confirm whether a shunt is present; however, it does not provide reliable anatomic information such as the type and location of the shunt.
- *Positive-contrast portography* is the procedure of choice to accurately characterize the type and location of a PSS. Techniques include splenoportography, mesenteric (or jejunal) portography, and cranial mesenteric or celiac arterial portography. An operative mesenteric portogram is preferred because it allows evaluation of the entire portal vein, does not require special equipment, and results in few complications.
- Institute therapy for hepatic encephalopathy prior to giving anesthesia for portography or for surgical correction (see below).

Technique for Mesenteric Portography

1. Place the animal under general anesthesia (see Chap. 2 for anesthesia of the patient with liver disease).
2. Isolate a loop of jejunum through a ventral midline incision.
3. Place two ligatures around a jejunal vein, and place an over-the-needle catheter (Abbocath; Abbott) within the vessel. Tie the ligatures and secure the catheter to the vessel.
4. Temporarily close the abdominal incision.
5. Inject a water-soluble contrast agent (Conray, Mallinckrodt; or Iohexol, Winthrop) as a bolus (2 ml/kg) into the catheter.
6. If a rapid film changer is not available, take a lateral and ventrodorsal radiograph as the final milliliter is injected.

Interpretation

- If a single PSS is identified, it should be further characterized as intrahepatic or extrahepatic, because this has important surgical ramifications (see Chap. 92).
- If multiple extrahepatic PSSs are identified, portal pressure determination and gross and microscopic findings of the liver are used to distinguish between congenital and acquired causes (see next section).

- Failure to visualize the intrahepatic portal system is not a reliable indicator of vascular atresia but may correlate with a greater occurrence of postoperative complications after complete or partial shunt ligation.

Liver Biopsy

- The liver is grossly small but otherwise fairly normal in appearance.
- In some animals, biopsy findings are unremarkable.
- Liver biopsy most consistently reveals hepatocyte atrophy with small or absent portal veins. Varying degrees of sinusoidal congestion, biliary hyperplasia, arteriolar proliferation, lipogranulomas, and increased periportal connective tissue may be seen. Hepatocellular vacuolization is sometimes noted and may be severe.
- Microscopic CNS abnormalities include polymicrocavitation of the brain stem and cerebellum and an increased number of astrocytes in the cerebral cortex.

Treatment

Surgery

- The treatment of choice for dogs and cats with a single PSS is surgical attenuation or complete ligation of the shunt (see Chap. 92).
- Use of an ameroid constrictor for gradual occlusion of single extrahepatic shunts has recently become popular. Advantages of this procedure include gradual occlusion of the shunt over a 30–60 day period, decreased surgical and anesthetic time, and lack of need to monitor portal pressure during surgery.

Medical Therapy

Medical management of dogs and cats with PSS is palliative and is directed primarily at control of hepatic encephalopathy with a moderately protein-restricted diet supplemented with soluble fiber, lactulose, and neomycin (see Table 91–1).

- The short-term response to therapy for hepatic encephalopathy is often dramatic, and the animal usually is clinically normal even prior to surgical shunt ligation.
- If surgical shunt correction is not feasible or is declined by the owner, long-term medical management may control clinical signs for as long as 2–3 years. However, medical management of PSS does not reverse the progressive hepatic atrophy and alterations in carbohydrate, lipid, and protein metabolism.
- Acute decompensation of encephalopathy requires fluid therapy for correction of dehydration, correction of electrolyte and acid-base imbalances, and maintenance of blood glucose levels (see Table 91–1).
- When severe CNS depression or coma prevents the oral administration of lactulose and neomycin, administer these drugs via an enema (see Table 91–1).
- Identify and correct precipitating causes of encephalopathy whenever possible, such as hypoglycemia, GI bleeding from hookworm infection, and hypokalemia (see Table 91–1).

- Management of urate urolithiasis is discussed in Chap. 99.

Perioperative Complications

Seizures

- Occasionally, seizures or status epilepticus are a complication of surgical shunt ligation. Dogs older than 18 months of age may be at increased risk. The pathogenesis is obscure but seizures do not appear to be caused by simple hypoglycemia or hepatic encephalopathy. It is possible that the brain may have adapted to an altered metabolism.
- Evaluate for hyperammonemia, hypoglycemia, hypoxia, electrolyte imbalances, acid-base imbalances, and systemic hypertension. In addition to routine management of hepatic encephalopathy and correction of underlying metabolic imbalances (including thiamine administration in cats), manage seizures with IV phenobarbital or oral loading doses of potassium bromide (see Chap. 146).
- If seizures cannot be controlled, administer IV propofol to induce general anesthesia for 12–24 hours. An endotracheal tube is placed and a respirator is used to maintain pO_2 and pCO_2. Anesthesia can be maintained by propofol drip or isoflurane gas anesthesia. Mannitol (1 g/kg IV) may be indicated for control of cerebral edema.
- The prognosis for recovery from this complication is poor. Long-term anticonvulsant therapy is often required if the patient survives the acute postoperative period.

Other Complications

Other perioperative complications of shunt ligation include portal hypertension, intraoperative hypothermia and hypoglycemia, anesthetic complications, fever and positive blood cultures, portal vein thrombosis, acute pancreatitis, cardiac arrythmias, and hemorrhage.

Prognosis

- The prognosis in dogs for resolution of signs after total surgical ligation of the shunt is excellent if the dog survives the immediate postoperative period. In dogs with partial shunt ligation, the prognosis is not as good. Although clinical signs may resolve after surgery, and response appears favorable in the first few years, long-term follow-up (>3 years) suggests recurrence of signs will occur in 40–50% of dogs with partial shunt ligations. Based on this information, dogs who have previously undergone a partial ligation should be reevaluated by transcolonic portal scintigraphy. If shunting persists, surgical exploration to perform complete suture ligation or ameroid constrictor placement is indicated.
- The response to surgical correction of a congenital PSS in cats appears to be less encouraging than in dogs. With partial shunt ligation, clinical improvement is usually noted after surgery but relapse of clinical signs is common. Persistent seizures and

blindness are also more likely to occur when partial rather than total ligation is performed.

HEPATIC MICROVASCULAR DYSPLASIA

Hepatic microvascular dysplasia (HMD) refers to congenital histologic vascular abnormalities of the liver in dogs and cats that result in abnormally increased serum bile acid concentrations and may be associated with clinical signs of portosystemic shunting of blood. HMD may occur alone or with congenital PSS. The relationship between HMD and congenital PSS is unclear, but the increased incidence of HMD in breeds such as Cairn and Yorkshire terriers that are also at increased risk for PSS suggests that HMD and PSS are varying expressions of a more general portal vascular malformation. It is likely that most animals with PSS have some degree of HMD, which may explain the failure to normalize SBA concentrations and the persistence of histologic vascular lesions that sometimes occur despite complete surgical ligation of a PSS.

Etiology

Hepatic microvascular dysplasia has been studied extensively in Cairn terriers, where it is believed to be an inherited disorder. A polygenic mechanism of inheritance is suspected.

Clinical Signs

Clinical signs are not consistently seen in affected dogs and cats. This is especially true for Cairn terriers. In more severely affected animals, signs are similar to those seen with congenital PSS and include anorexia, lethargy, vomiting, diarrhea, hepatic encephalopathy, and dysuria and hematuria due to urate urolithiasis.

Diagnosis

Hepatic microvascular dysplasia should be considered in dogs and cats with clinical features of congenital PSS, increased SBA concentrations, and typical liver biopsy findings, and that do not have a demonstrable shunt. It is essential to rigorously pursue the diagnosis of congenital PSS in this setting because the clinical and histologic features of HMD alone are similar to those of congenital PSS, and specific surgical correction is available if a shunt is identified. Transcolonic portal scintigraphy is the most sensitive and least invasive method to detect a congenital PSS. A normal examination would make congenital PSS unlikely; however, false-negative results are possible.

Also consider the possibility that a dog or cat with increased SBA concentrations may have HMD and be asymptomatic for the disorder (especially Cairn terriers). An animal with HMD may have clinical signs due to an unrelated nonhepatic disease. Detection of increased SBA concentrations may focus diagnostic efforts on the liver, causing the clinician to overlook the true cause of the clinical signs.

Signalment

- Yorkshire terriers and Cairn terriers are most commonly affected. However, HMD has been diagnosed in many other small breeds of dogs such as Maltese, dachshund, poodle, Shih Tzu, Lhasa Apso, cocker spaniel, and West Highland white terrier.
- Domestic shorthair cats are at increased risk for HMD.
- Dogs with HMD tend to be older at presentation than dogs with congenital PSS.

Physical Examination

Physical examination is often within normal limits unless signs of hepatic encephalopathy are present.

Laboratory Evaluation

- Dogs with HMD consistently have increased SBA concentrations, but not as increased as in dogs with PSS. A shunting pattern is typically seen: normal or low FSBA concentrations with moderate to markedly increased PPSBA concentrations. Indocyanine green clearance values are also consistently abnormal.
- Dogs with HMD have higher values for MCV, total protein, albumin, creatinine, blood urea nitrogen, glucose, and cholesterol when compared with dogs with congenital PSS. Dogs with PSS have higher white blood cell count and higher ALP and AST activity.
- Hyperammonemia and ammonium biurate crystalluria rarely develop in dogs with HMD.

Radiography and Ultrasonography

- Radiographically the liver is usually normal in size but may be equivocally small in some cases.
- On ultrasonography the liver may be subjectively decreased in size and the portal vasculature may be decreased. Bladder or kidney stones are uncommon.
- Transcolonic portal scintigraphy is usually normal or only mildly abnormal, as opposed to the increased shunt fractions seen with congenital PSS.
- No large shunting vessel can be identified on a portogram. Cairn terriers with HMD have abnormal truncation of the terminal branches of the portal veins and delayed clearing of contrast, which gives the parenchyma a "blush" appearance.

Liver Biopsy

A wedge biopsy of the liver is preferred over a needle biopsy because it provides more hepatic lobules for evaluation.

- Grossly, the liver is normal in size and color compared with the small liver seen with congenital PSS.
- The histologic features of HMD are identical to those seen in dogs and cats with a congenital PSS or after experimental surgical creation of a PSS. Findings include hepatic arteriolar hyperplasia, small portal triads, increased smooth muscle thickness of hepatic venules, and an increase in small vascular structures in the periportal area.

- Histologic lesions vary between liver lobes with some lobes appearing very abnormal and others appearing normal. Thus, more than one lobe should be sampled.

Treatment and Prognosis

- No treatment is indicated for animals whose symptoms are subclinical.
- If clinical signs of hepatic encephalopathy are present, they can often be successfully managed with a moderately protein-restricted diet. Additional therapy with lactulose and neomycin (or metronidazole) is sometimes warranted (see Table 91–1).
- Follow-up in 11 dogs for a mean period of 15 months (range of 1 week–4.5 years) indicated a good clinical response to dietary therapy alone. Repeated SBA concentrations remained unchanged. Whether dogs who are asymptomatic for HMD will ever progress to have clinical signs remains to be determined.

MULTIPLE ACQUIRED PORTOSYSTEMIC SHUNTS

PSSs are extrahepatic collateral vessels that develop as a compensatory response to portal hypertension (PH). These acquired shunts are rudimentary nonfunctional microvascular communications between the portal and systemic veins that are present in normal dogs and cats. With sustained PH, these vessels enlarge and function to shunt blood into the lower-pressure systemic circulation, thus decreasing portal pressure. Multiple PSS usually connect the portal system and the caudal vena cava.

Etiology (Table 91–8)

Chronic End-Stage Liver Disease

- Chronic end-stage hepatic disorders such as chronic hepatitis, lobular dissecting hepatitis, cirrhosis, and hepatic fibrosis are the most common causes of portal hypertension and multiple PSS.
- Diagnosis of the underlying chronic liver disease requires liver biopsy.

Hepatic Arteriovenous (AV) Fistulas

These vascular communications between the hepatic artery and portal vein are a rare but important cause of severe PH and multiple PSS in young dogs and cats (see later section in this chapter).

Veno-occlusive Disease

- Veno-occlusive disease causing PH and multiple PSS has been described in four young related American cocker spaniels. Clinical signs were indicative of chronic liver disease.
- Liver biopsies revealed prominent smooth muscular sphincters, dilated central and portal veins, hepatocyte atrophy, and variable fibrosis. Similar histologic features are noted with portal vein hypoplasia and id-

iopathic noncirrhotic portal hypertension (see below), and these disorders may all be related.

Portal Vein Hypoplasia

- Portal vein hypoplasia (atresia) was diagnosed in 42 young dogs with portal hypertension, multiple PSS, and signs of chronic liver disease, especially ascites and hepatic encephalopathy. The extrahepatic portal vein was patent but underdeveloped in 13 of 42 dogs.
- Microscopically, all dogs had small portal veins. Other features included normal lobular architecture with hepatocyte atrophy, absence of inflammation, and variable arteriolar hyperplasia, bile duct proliferation, and portal fibrosis (which was sometimes severe). Whether hypoplasia of the portal system is the primary event or a response of the portal system secondary to decreased perfusion remains to be determined.
- The prognosis was poor—most dogs died or were euthanized within a few weeks of diagnosis.

Idiopathic Noncirrhotic Portal Hypertension

This is a syndrome of portal hypertension and multiple PSS in young dogs without an AV fistula, portal vein hypoplasia, or significant intrahepatic fibrosis or inflammation.

- The mean age is around 2 years. Medium- or large-breed dogs appear to be at increased risk. In one study, three related and one unrelated Doberman pinschers were reported.
- Common clinical findings include ascites, polydipsia, vomiting, and diarrhea. Signs of HE are uncommon.
- Laboratory findings are consistent with hepatic dysfunction and include microcytosis, hypoalbuminemia, decreased BUN, increased SBA, and mild increases in ALP and ALT (2–3 times normal).
- Findings on portography include multiple extrahepatic PSS, patency of the extrahepatic portal vein, and presence of intrahepatic portal vasculature.
- Findings on liver biopsy are similar to those changes seen in dogs with single congenital PSS and portal vein hypoplasia and include hepatocellular atrophy, arteriolar hyperplasia, mild portal fibrosis, muscular hypertrophy of central veins, and inconspicuous portal venules in some cases.
- The mechanism for PH in these dogs is unknown. Portal hypertension could be caused by severe intrahepatic portal vascular hypoplasia. However, dogs with single congenital PSS also have varying degrees of intrahepatic portal vascular atresia, yet PH and ascites are not typical features.
- The long-term prognosis is variable, but some dogs can live for years on a protein-restricted diet.

Other Causes of Portal Hypertension

Other causes of PH and multiple PSS include chronic partial occlusion of the portal vein, caudal vena cava, or main hepatic veins. PH also occurs as a postoperative complication of congenital PSS surgery (see Table 91–8).

Table 91-8. DISORDERS ASSOCIATED WITH MULTIPLE ACQUIRED PORTOSYSTEMIC SHUNTS

Chronic hepatitis and cirrhosis
Lobular dissecting hepatitis*
Hepatoportal fibrosis*
Congenital hepatic arteriovenous fistula*
Veno-occlusive disease of cocker spaniels*
Portal vein hypoplasia/atresia*
Idiopathic noncirrhotic portal hypertension*
Postoperative complication of congenital PSS ligation*
Portal vein obstruction (thrombosis, neoplasia, extraluminal compression)
Caudal vena cava or main hepatic vein obstruction (kinking, thrombosis, neoplasia)

*More common in young animals.

Clinical Signs

The clinical signs in dogs with multiple PSS are nonspecific and reflect PH, portosystemic shunting, or the underlying hepatic disorder.

- Because PH is the mechanism for secondary shunt formation, ascites is a common clinical sign.
- Hepatic encephalopathy can also complicate any disorder associated with multiple PSS because there is inadequate hepatic removal of toxins originating from the gastrointestinal tract when portal blood bypasses the liver and is shunted directly into the systemic circulation.

Diagnosis

History and Physical Examination

The most common findings include ascites, weight loss, and neurologic findings consistent with hepatic encephalopathy. Additional clinical findings reflect the underlying disorder. For example, with chronic end-stage liver disease, physical examination may reveal icterus.

Laboratory Evaluation

- Microcytosis, a common finding in dogs with congenital PSS, is also seen with primary hepatic disorders that are accompanied by PH and multiple PSS.
- A pattern of normal to mildly increased FSBA concentrations accompanied by markedly increased postprandial SBA values is consistent with portosystemic shunting, regardless of the underlying mechanism for shunt formation.
- Hyperammonemia and an abnormal ammonia tolerance test are also consistent features. Ascitic fluid is typically a transudate.
- Additional clinical and laboratory findings reflect the underlying disorder. For example, with chronic end-stage liver disease, laboratory findings may include increased serum liver enzyme activity, hyperbilirubinemia, hypoalbuminemia, and coagulopathy.

Ultrasonography

- Multiple PSS can be seen ultrasonographically, where they appear as enlarged tortuous vessels caudal to the liver. Other features of PH such as dilated portal veins, ascites, or splenomegaly may also be detected.
- Additional ultrasonographic findings are dependent on the underlying cause of PH. With chronic end-stage liver disease, the liver may be small and hyperechoic, with multiple regenerative nodules. Hepatic AV fistulas appear as tortuous, anechoic tubular structures in the liver.

Laparotomy and Contrast Portography

- Multiple PSS can be confirmed by contrast portography, or at exploratory laparotomy (or necropsy). Multiple PSS usually appear as multiple tortuous vessels that communicate with the caudal vena cava in the area of the left kidney. The portal pressure can be measured to document PH (normal portal pressure is 6-13 cm H_2O).
- When multiple extrahepatic PSS are identified, further diagnostic efforts should be directed toward identifying the underlying cause of PH, because the shunts are only a secondary phenomenon.
  - Liver biopsy is essential to evaluate for primary intrahepatic disorders.
  - Congenital hepatic AV fistulas can be diagnosed by celiac arteriography or exploratory laparotomy.
  - Portal vein obstruction or compression can be demonstrated by mesenteric portography or at surgery or necropsy.

Treatment

- Appropriate management of diseases complicated by PH and multiple PSS depends on identifying the underlying cause or mechanism. Symptomatic therapy is instituted to control the consequences of PH and multiple PSS such as ascites and hepatic encephalopathy (see Table 91-1 and Principles of Treatment section).
- Surgical ligation of multiple acquired PSS is contraindicated. Ligation may result in fatal PH because shunts form as a protective compensatory response to PH. Caudal vena caval banding is not recommended.

HEPATIC ARTERIOVENOUS FISTULA

Intrahepatic arteriovenous (AV) fistulas are vascular communications between the hepatic artery and portal vein that result in portal hypertension, ascites, and secondary portosystemic shunts. They occur rarely in dogs and cats.

Etiology

Intrahepatic AV fistulas may be congenital, which is most common, or acquired as a result of abdominal trauma, hepatic surgery, hepatic neoplasia, cirrhosis, or rupture of a hepatic artery aneurysm.

Clinical Signs

Signs are similar to those of congenital PSS and include anorexia, lethargy, vomiting, diarrhea, PU/PD, and encephalopathy in a young animal (usually less than 1.5 years).

Diagnosis

History and Physical Examination

- Historical and physical findings are similar to those in congenital PSS, with the notable exception that marked ascites is a consistent finding with hepatic AV fistulas but is uncommon with congenital PSS.
- Other causes of ascites to be differentiated include hypoproteinemia and right-sided congestive heart failure and other causes of portal hypertension and multiple PSS (see preceding section and Table 91–8).
- Auscultate the abdominal wall over the area of the liver for a continuous murmur (bruit) caused by runoff of arterial blood into the portal system.

Laboratory Evaluation

- Laboratory abnormalities are similar to those seen in congenital PSS and include hypoproteinemia, normal or mildly increased serum liver enzyme activity, and abnormal liver function tests including FSBA and PPSBA, blood ammonia and ATT, and BSP retention.
- Ascitic fluid typically is a transudate.

Radiography and Ultrasonography

- Survey radiographs show marked ascites.
- On abdominal ultrasonography, hepatic AV fistulas appear as tortuous, anechoic tubular structures in the liver. Multiple extrahepatic PSSs may also be identified.

Laparotomy

- The diagnosis is confirmed by celiac arteriography or exploratory laparotomy. Grossly, AV fistulas appear as thin-walled, tortuous, pulsating vascular channels that distort the hepatic parenchyma and elevate the overlying hepatic capsule.

Treatment

- Partial hepatectomy is indicated for treatment of hepatic AV fistulas involving one liver lobe (see Chap. 92). Dearterialization is required if multiple lobes are involved.
- Despite resection of involved liver lobes, hepatic function may not return to normal because of persistent shunting of portal blood through acquired PSS.
- Medical management of hepatic encephalopathy with a moderately protein-restricted diet, lactulose, and neomycin is indicated (see Table 91–1).

HEPATOBILIARY NEOPLASIA

Neoplasms involving the liver can be categorized as primary hepatic tumors (of either epithelial or mesodermal origin), hemolymphatic tumors, or metastatic tumors (Table 91–9). Hemolymphatic tumors (especially lymphoma and myeloproliferative disorders) are the most common type of neoplasia involving the liver of cats. Metastatic tumors to the liver are most common in dogs, especially hemangiosarcoma, islet cell carcinoma, pancreatic carcinoma, and fibrosarcoma. Hepatic lymphoma also occurs frequently in dogs.

Primary hepatic tumors occur infrequently in dogs and cats. They are usually of epithelial origin and are derived from either hepatocytes or biliary epithelium. They can be either benign or malignant.

- A benign tumor of the hepatocytes is called a *hepatocellular adenoma* (or hepatoma), and its malignant counterpart is called a *hepatocellular carcinoma*. Hepatocellular carcinoma is the most common primary hepatic tumor in dogs.
- A benign tumor arising from the biliary epithelium is called a *biliary adenoma*. The malignant form is called

Table 91–9. HEPATIC NEOPLASIA IN DOGS AND CATS

Primary Hepatic Neoplasia

Epithelial Origin

Hepatocellular carcinoma
Hepatocellular adenoma
Biliary carcinoma (cholangiocarcinoma, biliary cystadenocarcinoma)
Biliary adenoma (including biliary cystadenoma)
Hepatic carcinoid

Mesodermal Origin

Hemangiosarcoma
Hemangioma
Leiomyosarcoma
Fibrosarcoma
Fibroma
Osteosarcoma

Hemolymphatic Tumors

Lymphoma
Mast cell tumor
Myeloproliferative disorders
Myeloma
Thymoma

Metastatic Hepatic Neoplasia

Hemangiosarcoma
Islet cell carcinoma
Pancreatic carcinoma
Fibrosarcoma
Osteosarcoma
Transitional cell carcinoma
Intestinal carcinoma
Renal cell carcinoma
Pheochromocytoma
Thyroid carcinoma
Mammary carcinoma

a *biliary carcinoma*. Biliary carcinomas may be intrahepatic, extrahepatic, or within the gallbladder. The intrahepatic form is most common in dogs and cats. Biliary carcinomas and adenomas are the most common primary hepatic tumors in cats. Cystic forms of these tumors (cystadenocarcinoma, cystadenoma) have also been described.

- Hepatocellular carcinoma and bile duct carcinoma occur in three pathologic forms: (1) solitary—a single large mass in one liver lobe with or without smaller masses in other lobes; (2) multifocal nodular—discrete nodules of varying sizes in several liver lobes; and (3) diffuse—infiltration of large portions of the liver with nonencapsulated, highly invasive neoplastic tissue. Solitary masses are most likely to be successfully resected surgically. In dogs with hepatocellular carcinoma, approximately half of the tumors are solitary and half are multifocal or diffuse. Biliary carcinomas are more likely to be the multifocal or diffuse form.
- *Nodular hyperplasia* of the liver is a common postmortem finding in dogs more than 8 years of age. Nodular hyperplasia is not usually associated with clinical signs, but it can cause mild to moderate increases in serum ALP and ALT activity. Multiple hyperplastic nodules are often found in a random distribution throughout the liver lobes. These benign lesions should be considered in the differential diagnosis when hepatic nodules are identified during ultrasonography, laparoscopy, or surgery. Occasionally single hyperplastic nodules can become quite large and mimic a hepatocellular adenoma both clinically and microscopically.

Etiology

The cause of spontaneous primary hepatic neoplasms in dogs and cats is not usually determined. Some potential causes based on reports of experimental and spontaneous hepatic tumors include aflatoxins, nitrosamines, aramite, liver flukes (*Clonorchis* spp. *Platynosomum concinnum*), and radioactive compounds such as strontium-90 and cesium-144. In contrast to humans, no association between viral infections has been identified in spontaneous tumors of dogs and cats.

Clinical Signs

Dogs and cats with hepatic neoplasia usually show vague nonspecific signs of hepatic dysfunction that often do not appear until the more advanced stages of hepatic disease.

- The most consistent signs in dogs are anorexia, lethargy, weight loss, polydipsia, polyuria, vomiting, and abdominal distention. Other signs include jaundice, diarrhea, and excessive bleeding.
- Signs of CNS dysfunction such as depression, dementia, or seizures can be attributed to hepatic encephalopathy, hypoglycemia, or CNS metastases.

- Anorexia and lethargy are the most common presenting signs in cats; ascites and vomiting are uncommon in cats as compared with dogs.
- When the liver is secondarily involved with metastases, the clinical signs may reflect the primary tumor location or other metastatic sites rather than the hepatic involvement.

Diagnosis

Suspect hepatobiliary neoplasia in any older animal with clinical and biochemical evidence of hepatic disease accompanied by hepatomegaly.

Signalment

- Primary hepatic neoplasms are most common in dogs and cats that are older than 10 years of age.
- Labrador retrievers were found to be disproportionately represented in one study of dogs with biliary carcinoma.
- Male dogs and cats may be at increased risk for hepatocellular carcinoma.
- Male cats and female dogs have an increased risk for biliary carcinoma.

Physical Examination

- Findings often include a cranial abdominal mass or marked hepatomegaly. Hepatomegaly is less likely with metastatic tumors.
- Ascites or hemoperitoneum may contribute to abdominal distention. Tumor rupture and hemorrhage is most likely with hepatocellular adenoma, hepatocellular carcinoma, and hepatic hemangiosarcoma.
- Anemia and pale mucous membranes may be attributed to excessive hemorrhage from a ruptured neoplasm or anemia of chronic disease.
- Jaundice is a less frequent finding with hepatic tumors unless the tumor mass causes obstruction of the common bile duct.
- Severe weight loss and cachexia are common but nonspecific findings.
- Myasthenia gravis was suspected to be a paraneoplastic syndrome in a dog with biliary carcinoma.

Laboratory Evaluation

Hematologic and biochemical findings in animals with hepatic neoplasia are not specific and are indicative of hepatic disease and its complications.

- Potential hematologic findings include anemia and leukocytosis. Anemia is usually nonregenerative but may be regenerative if associated with excess bleeding or tumor rupture. When hematopoietic or lymphoid malignancies secondarily involve the liver, abnormal cells or pancytopenia may be detected on peripheral blood smears because of concurrent bone marrow involvement.
- Mild to marked increases in serum liver enzyme (ALT and ALP) activity are common in dogs with primary hepatic tumors (60–100%), but less so with

metastatic neoplasia. In contrast, most cats with non-hematopoietic hepatic neoplasms have increased serum ALT or AST activity, but serum ALP activity is usually normal. Increased serum AST activity may be the most sensitive indicator of metastatic hepatic disease in dogs (80% of cases) but lacks specificity.

- Hyperbilirubinemia appears to be a more frequent finding in dogs with metastatic neoplasia than in those with primary hepatic tumors (59% versus 25%).
- Hypoglycemia, sometimes severe, occasionally is noted in dogs with hepatocellular carcinoma and less frequently with hepatocellular adenoma, leiomyosarcoma, and hemangiosarcoma. Serum insulin concentrations are normal to decreased. Potential mechanisms of hypoglycemia include excess utilization of glucose by the tumor, release of insulin-like factors from the tumor, release of other substances from the tumor such as somatostatin, and secondary hepatic parenchymal destruction with impaired glycogenolysis or gluconeogenesis.
- Other biochemical findings are quite variable and include hypoalbuminemia, hyperglobulinemia, prolonged BSP dye retention, and increased SBA concentrations. The magnitude of increase in SBA concentrations in dogs with hepatic neoplasia can be quite small; SBA concentrations are often within normal limits.
- Although clinical evidence of impaired hemostasis is infrequent, prolongation of the PT and APTT may be identified in dogs with hepatic neoplasia.
- Analysis of abdominal fluid usually indicates a transudate or modified transudate; however, neoplastic cells or a bloody effusion are occasionally noted.
- Increased serum alpha-fetoprotein concentration (>250 ng/ml by enzymetry) may be an indicator of hepatocellular carcinoma and biliary carcinoma in dogs. Increased alpha-fetoprotein secretion also occurs with marked hepatic regeneration. Alpha-fetoprotein concentrations in cats with hepatic neoplasia have not been reported.

Radiography

- Abdominal radiographic findings in animals with hepatic neoplasia include symmetric or asymmetric hepatomegaly and ascites.
- Perform thoracic radiographs to detect pulmonary metastases.

Ultrasonography

The diagnosis of hepatic neoplasia cannot be made based on ultrasonographic findings alone; however, ultrasonography often reveals focal, multifocal, or diffuse changes in hepatic echotexture.

- Hepatocellular carcinoma usually appears as a focal hyperechoic mass.
- Primary or secondary neoplasia and nodular hyperplasia often appear as focal or multifocal hypoechoic or mixed echogenic lesions.
- "Target lesions," consisting of an echogenic center surrounded by a more sonolucent rim, are often neoplastic.

- Hepatic lymphoma is quite variable and may appear as a mild diffuse hyper- or hypoechogenicity, multifocal hypoechoic lesions, or a mixed echogenic pattern, or the appearance may be normal.

Liver Biopsy

Definitive diagnosis of hepatic neoplasia requires liver biopsy and histopathologic evaluation.

- *Laparotomy* is the procedure of choice for a single large hepatic mass because excision of the mass can also be performed concurrently.
- *Ultrasound-guided biopsy* is useful to diagnose focal or diffuse hepatic involvement, but the small size of the biopsy can make differentiation of nodular hyperplasia versus primary hepatic neoplasia difficult. A wedge biopsy obtained at surgery is often necessary.
- *Blind percutaneous needle biopsy* and *fine-needle aspiration* cytology are most useful for diagnosis of diffuse hepatic neoplasias such as lymphoma, myeloproliferative disorders, and mast cell tumor.

Treatment
Surgery

Surgical removal of the affected liver lobe is the treatment of choice for primary hepatic neoplasms such as hepatocellular adenoma or carcinoma that involve a single lobe (see Chap. 92). Early detection prior to metastasis to other liver lobes affords the best chance for surgical control.

Make a complete evaluation of the abdominal cavity for evidence of metastases, and biopsy hepatic lymph nodes.

When all lobes are affected, the prognosis is poor.

Chemotherapy

- Chemotherapy is not an effective means of control for primary liver tumors in dogs and cats.
- Secondary hepatic neoplasms such as lymphoma, mast cell tumor, or myeloproliferative disease might temporarily respond to chemotherapeutic intervention (see Chaps. 24 and 25).

HEPATIC CYSTS

Single or multiple diffuse hepatic cysts occasionally are identified in the liver of dogs and cats, usually as incidental findings at necropsy, but occasionally in the live animal.

Etiology

Hepatic cysts can be congenital or acquired, although the distinction is often difficult to make. In general, acquired cysts are usually solitary and congenital cysts are often multiple.

- Congenital polycystic disease of the liver and kidneys has been reported in Cairn terriers and West Highland white terriers.

- Polycystic renal disease in cats has been associated with cystic dilation of the intrahepatic bile ducts (see Chap. 97).
- Acquired cysts may represent benign bile duct adenomas or biliary cystadenomas or may occur secondary to trauma.

Clinical Signs

- Most solitary hepatic cysts do not cause any clinical signs unless they compress or displace adjacent structures. Signs are more likely to occur when congenital polycystic disease is accompanied by dilation of the extrahepatic biliary tract.
- Abdominal enlargement secondary to an enlarged cyst or abdominal fluid accumulation can be a presenting sign.

Diagnosis and Treatment

- Hepatic cysts should be considered in the differential diagnosis of any cavitated hepatic mass lesion detected on palpation, radiography, or ultrasonography.
- Surgery can confirm the diagnosis and allow excision of large solitary cysts.

CHOLELITHIASIS

Cholelithiasis occurs infrequently in dogs and cats. Choleliths may be present in the gallbladder (cholecystolithiasis), common bile duct (choledocholithiasis), or rarely, in the hepatic and lobar ducts. Most choleliths in dogs and cats consist of insoluble bile pigments. Minor components such as calcium, bile salts, protein, magnesium, phosphorus, iron, carbonate, and cholesterol also have been identified. Cholesterol choleliths, the most common type of stone in humans, are less likely to form in dogs because the cholesterol content of dog bile is lower than that in humans, and dogs have a better capacity for maintaining biliary cholesterol in solution. Little is known about the cholesterol content of cat bile, but cholesterol choleliths have been reported.

Etiology

The cause of spontaneous cholelithiasis in dogs and cats often cannot be determined. It is generally believed that gallstone formation requires initial nidus formation, retention of particles in the gallbladder, and then sustained growth of the cholelith. The following factors may be important in the development of pigment stones.

- Bile stasis and sludged bile is primarily composed of mucin, which subsequently binds calcium bilirubin pigments and cholesterol crystals.
- Increased gallbladder mucin acts as a nidus for cholelith formation.
- Cholecystitis and cholangiohepatitis can be associated with cholelithiasis, especially in cats (see Cholangiohepatitis section). It is difficult to determine whether choleliths were formed as a consequence of bile stasis, inflammation, and bacterial infection, or whether cholelithiasis initiated the inflammation, which led to secondary biliary stasis and infection.
- Bacteria such as *E. coli* contain beta-glucuronidase, which can deconjugate bilirubin to a less soluble form that precipitates with calcium.
- Dietary factors are unlikely with balanced diets; however, dogs fed an experimental diet that is low in protein and fat, high in carbohydrates, and supplemented with cholesterol will form pigment stones. This diet is deficient in taurine, which may contribute to cholelithiasis by precipitating bile acids.

Clinical Signs

- Dogs and cats with cholelithiasis often are asymptomatic. Clinical signs are most likely when cholelithiasis is complicated by bacterial infection, extrahepatic bile duct obstruction, perforation of the gallbladder or bile ducts, or secondary hepatic involvement (cholangiohepatitis or biliary cirrhosis).
- Common signs include vomiting, anorexia, weakness, polyuria/polydipsia, jaundice, weight loss, and dehydration.
- Signs may be acute or chronic, intermittent or persistent. An acute onset is most likely with sudden obstruction of the cystic or common bile duct by the cholelith or rupture of the gallbladder.

Diagnosis

Although it is uncommon, consider cholelithiasis in the differential diagnosis of any dog or cat with cholestatic hepatobiliary disease.

History and Physical Examination

- Aged, small-breed female dogs appear to be at increased risk.
- A long-standing history (months to years) of intermittent jaundice and vomiting is present in some affected animals.
- Physical examination may be unremarkable or findings may include jaundice, abdominal discomfort, hepatomegaly, fever, and abdominal distention. Fever is usually indicative of concurrent biliary bacterial infection or septic or bile peritonitis. Abdominal distension due to fluid accumulation is seen with secondary rupture of the biliary tract.
- Excessive bleeding may be noted with chronic common bile duct obstruction.
- Acholic feces are indicative of complete bile duct obstruction.

Laboratory Evaluation

- Laboratory findings may be unremarkable.
- Biochemical evaluation of symptomatic patients is not specific for cholelithiasis but is indicative of cholestatic hepatobiliary disease. Findings include moderate to marked increases in serum ALP and GGT activity and in cholesterol, SBA, and total serum bilirubin concentrations. Serum ALT activity usually

is increased, indicating secondary hepatocyte damage associated with severe cholestasis.

- Potential hematologic findings include neutrophilia with a left shift, usually indicating bacterial cholangiohepatitis or cholecystitis or complications such as a ruptured gallbladder. A mild, nonregenerative anemia is common. With chronic extrahepatic bile duct obstruction, coagulation tests may be affected by vitamin K malabsorption.
- With biliary rupture, abdominocentesis reveals bile peritonitis.

Radiography

- On routine abdominal radiographs, choleliths may appear as radiopaque densities in the area of the gallbladder or bile ducts. However, pigment stones are usually radiolucent unless they contain calcium. Hepatomegaly is common.
- Other findings are determined by the presence of complications such as obstruction (a distended gallbladder), emphysematous cholecystitis (gas density in the area of the gallbladder), and peritonitis (loss of abdominal detail).

Ultrasonography

- Ultrasonography detects both radiolucent and radiopaque choleliths as hyperechoic densities in the gallbladder and bile ducts. Choleliths are differentiated from mural masses by the presence of acoustic shadowing and movement of the density with changes in position of the animal.
- Inspissated or sludged bile also appears in the gallbladder as an echogenic substance, but sludge does not cause acoustic shadowing. Sludged bile may indicate biliary stasis but can also be seen in sick, anorexic animals without clinical biliary tract disease.
- Complications of cholelithiasis can be identified ultrasonographically, such as distention of the gallbladder and bile ducts with cystic or common bile duct obstruction, thickening of the biliary tract associated with inflammation, abdominal fluid accumulation with rupture of the gallbladder, and absence of the gallbladder.

▼ *Key Point* Because the majority of choleliths do not cause clinical signs, surgical removal may not always be warranted.

Laparotomy

Exploratory laparotomy generally is required for definitive diagnosis and treatment of cholelithiasis.

- Pigment choleliths usually are greenish-brown to black and may be single or multiple. Bile sludge appears grossly as viscous, greenish black bile containing sand-like gritty material.
- Perform the following diagnostic and therapeutic procedures during exploratory laparotomy:
  - Evaluate the patency of the gallbladder and bile ducts

- Remove choleliths for chemical analysis and bacterial culture
- Identify and repair secondary biliary rupture
- Collect samples of affected tissue (liver, gallbladder) and bile for aerobic and anaerobic bacterial culture and biopsy.

Histopathologic Evaluation

- Histopathologic changes in the gallbladder, bile ducts, and liver may be absent with uncomplicated cholelithiasis. However, mild cholangitis (cholangiohepatitis) and cholecystitis are common.

Treatment

- Institute supportive therapy to correct fluid, electrolyte, and acid-base imbalances prior to surgery.
- If a coagulopathy is detected, give vitamin K_1 for 24–48 hours prior to surgery (see Table 91–1).
- Administer systemic antibiotics in animals with inflammatory biliary tract disease and cholelithiasis. Ideally, base the choice of antibiotic on culture and sensitivity testing of bile and hepatic tissue obtained at surgery. See the discussion of antibiotic therapy of biliary infections under Cholangiohepatitis.
- Management of complications of cholelithiasis, such as ruptured gallbladder, biliary obstruction, and rupture of the biliary tract, is discussed later in this chapter.
- Surgery of the biliary tract is discussed in Chapter 92.

Prognosis

Little is known about the likelihood of recurrence of cholelithiasis in dogs and cats.

- If the underlying mechanism of cholelith formation is not reversed, recurrence is possible.
- A well-balanced commercial diet is recommended.
- Manage persistent cholangitis or cholangiohepatitis as described previously in this chapter.

EXTRAHEPATIC BILIARY OBSTRUCTION

Extrahepatic biliary obstruction of the common bile duct or large hepatic ducts interrupts bile flow into the intestine.

Etiology

Biliary obstruction can be a complication of primary biliary tract disorders such as cholelithiasis or biliary tumors or can be caused by extrahepatic disorders such as pancreatic fibrosis and pancreatic or duodenal masses (Table 91–10).

Clinical Signs

- Signs of biliary obstruction include anorexia, vomiting, jaundice, weight loss, abdominal pain, diarrhea, acholic feces, and excessive bleeding.
- Diarrhea and steatorrhea are characterized by tan-colored feces and are attributed to failure to secrete

Table 91–10. CAUSES OF EXTRAHEPATIC BILIARY OBSTRUCTION

Cholelithiasis
Inspissated (sludged) bile
Cholangitis and cholecystitis
Gallbladder mucocele
Acute pancreatitis, pancreatic abscess, chronic pancreatitis, pancreatic fibrosis
Biliary, hepatic, pancreatic, and duodenal neoplasia
Biliary stricture
Biliary hematoma
Liver flukes
Diaphragmatic hernia with entrapment of the gallbladder

bile acids, which results in malabsorption of fat and fat-soluble vitamins such as vitamin K.

- With prolonged extrahepatic biliary obstruction, vitamin K malabsorption and the subsequent decreased synthesis of vitamin K–dependent factors results in a coagulopathy.
- With complete biliary obstruction, the feces may become clay colored (acholic) because of a lack of bile pigments.

Diagnosis

The diagnostic strategy is to identify that biliary obstruction is present and then to identify the underlying cause of obstruction.

Physical Examination

- Findings include jaundice and hepatomegaly due to bile engorgement of the liver.
- A firm, distended gallbladder occasionally is palpated.
- Other findings are dependent on the underlying cause of obstruction, such as palpation of an abdominal mass (pancreatic or biliary neoplasia) and abdominal pain (acute pancreatitis, peritonitis).
- Fever may suggest bacterial cholecystitis or cholangiohepatitis, biliary rupture with peritonitis, pancreatitis, or pancreatic abscess.

Laboratory Evaluation

- Biochemical findings reflect marked cholestasis, including increased serum concentrations of ALP, GGT, cholesterol, bile acids, and bilirubin. Unfortunately, biochemical findings cannot distinguish whether cholestasis is caused by intrahepatic or extrahepatic mechanisms. In general, values for total bilirubin and ALP activity tend to be higher with extrahepatic biliary obstruction. Serum ALT and AST activity are concurrently increased due to secondary hepatic damage.
- On the CBC, a mild neutrophilia and mild, nonregenerative anemia are common. Neutrophilia with a left shift suggests the possibility of acute pancreatitis or abscess, bacterial cholangitis/cholecystitis, or biliary rupture.
- Findings on urinalysis include bilirubinuria and absence of urobilinogen.

- With vitamin K malabsorption, findings include prolonged PT, APTT, and activated clotting time (ACT). Platelet function defects have also been documented in dogs with biliary obstruction.

Radiography

Abdominal radiography is frequently nondiagnostic.

- Occasionally, a large, fluid-filled gallbladder can be seen superimposed over the liver. The liver may be normal to increased in size. Chronic biliary obstruction in dogs may lead to biliary cirrhosis and microhepatica.
- Other radiographic findings depend on the underlying cause of obstruction and may include cholelithiasis, emphysematous cholecystitis, pancreatitis, and mass lesions.

Ultrasonography

Ultrasonography is helpful to confirm extrahepatic biliary obstruction and to evaluate the underlying cause.

- In normal dogs, the cystic duct, common bile duct, and intrahepatic ducts are not visible. The common bile duct may be visible in some normal cats but is usually ≤4 mm. A common bile duct >5 mm is suggestive of extrahepatic biliary obstruction.
- With biliary obstruction, the biliary system, including the gallbladder, cystic duct, common bile duct, and intrahepatic ducts, becomes progressively dilated. The earliest detectable change is distension of the gallbladder and cystic duct, which occurs within 24 hours. By 48 hours, the common bile duct also is distended. Distention of intrahepatic ducts is not detected until 4–7 days after obstruction. Dilated hepatic biliary ducts are differentiated from hepatic and portal veins by their tortuosity and irregular branching patterns.
- Ultrasonographic evaluation of gallbladder emptying after cholecystokinin injection may be helpful to confirm biliary obstruction.
- Ultrasonography may identify underlying causes of biliary obstruction such as cholelithiasis, pancreatitis, or mass lesions.

Hepatobiliary Scintigraphy

Hepatobiliary scintigraphy may be used to confirm biliary obstruction but is available only at tertiary referral centers.

Laparotomy

Exploratory laparotomy usually is required to confirm extrahepatic biliary obstruction and to identify the underlying cause. Perform the following diagnostic procedures:

- Evaluate bile duct and gallbladder patency.
- Identify location and cause of obstruction.
- Evaluate for evidence of secondary rupture of the biliary tract.

- Collect a sample of bile for aerobic and anaerobic bacterial cultures.
- Perform a liver biopsy.

Treatment

Surgery

Specific therapy requires surgery to correct the underlying cause of obstruction (see Chap. 92).

- Prior to surgery, stabilize the patient with fluid therapy. Give vitamin K_1 parenterally for 24–48 hours prior to surgery to correct a coagulopathy.
- With complete biliary obstruction, antibiotics do not enter the bile.

Medical Therapy

If biliary obstruction occurs secondary to acute pancreatitis, manage the pancreatitis medically (see Chap. 93) and reserve surgery for those patients in which biliary obstruction does not resolve with resolution of pancreatic inflammation.

BILIARY RUPTURE

Leakage of bile into the abdominal cavity results in chemical peritonitis that can be complicated by sepsis.

Etiology

- Biliary tract rupture is commonly caused by blunt or sharp abdominal trauma from automobile-induced injuries, gunshot injuries, and bite wounds. Rupture of the common bile duct is most likely with blunt abdominal trauma.
- Necrotizing cholecystitis causes gallbladder rupture.
- Other causes of gallbladder rupture include cholelithiasis, biliary neoplasms, and iatrogenic puncture during percutaneous liver biopsy.

Clinical Signs

- When gallbladder rupture occurs secondary to cholecystitis or cholelithiasis, acute onset of anorexia, vomiting, diarrhea, jaundice, abdominal pain, fever, and shock may occur.
- Signs of biliary duct rupture secondary to trauma tend to be chronic and develop more slowly than with rupture of the gallbladder. With traumatic biliary rupture, early signs such as abdominal pain and vomiting are frequently overshadowed by more immediate signs of shock, fractures, and other injuries.
- Other signs, such as anorexia, listlessness, weight loss, jaundice, ascites, and acholic feces, do not occur until days or weeks following the traumatic event.

Diagnosis

History and Physical Examination

- A history of recent abdominal trauma and progressive jaundice and abdominal distention suggests the possibility of biliary rupture.

- Physical examination findings consistent with biliary rupture include jaundice, abdominal distension, and acholic feces.
- Abdominal pain is most likely with acute rupture or septic peritonitis.
- Fever may occur with septic peritonitis or cholecystitis.

Laboratory Evaluation

- Laboratory findings include hyperbilirubinemia and increased ALP, ALT, and SBA concentrations.
- Abdominal fluid appears yellow or green. Chemical tests for bilirubin are positive and concentrations of bilirubin are at least two times higher in the abdominal fluid than in the serum.
- Cytologic examination reveals a mixed inflammatory infiltrate and bile-laden macrophages.
- Bacteria may be seen if bile peritonitis is complicated by sepsis.

Radiography and Ultrasonography

- Abdominal radiographs reveal poor abdominal contrast due to fluid accumulation.
- On ultrasonography, the gallbladder may not be visible, and even a small amount of abdominal fluid may be detected.
- Other radiographic and ultrasonographic findings depend on the underlying cause of rupture, such as cholelithiasis, cholecystitis, and biliary neoplasia.
- When trauma is suspected as the cause of biliary rupture, take thoracic films to detect other complications such as pneumothorax, diaphragmatic hernia, and bile pleuritis.

Laparotomy

Confirm rupture of the biliary tract by laparotomy.

- Rupture of the gallbladder secondary to cholecystitis may be acute or chronic. With chronic gallbladder rupture, omental and hepatic adhesions are common. Biliary fistulas may develop from the gallbladder to other abdominal structures such as the diaphragm.
- Submit abdominal fluid and affected biliary tissue for aerobic and anaerobic bacterial culture.

Treatment

Surgery is required to repair the biliary rupture and is discussed in Chapter 92.

- Prior to surgery, stabilize the patient with fluid therapy and give vitamin K_1 parenterally for 24–48 hours and antibiotics.
- Open abdominal drainage is not necessary for dogs with sterile biliary effusions but may be helpful in managing dogs with septic peritonitis (see Chap. 96).

Prognosis

Prognosis is guarded. Dogs with septic peritonitis (positive bacterial cultures of the biliary effusion) are less likely to survive than are dogs with negative culture results.

SUPPLEMENTAL READINGS

Center SA, Johnson SE, Bunch SE: Pathophysiology, laboratory diagnosis, and diseases of the liver. *In* Ettinger SJ, Feldman EC, eds.: Textbook of Veterinary Internal Medicine, Vol 2, 4th Ed. Philadelphia: WB Saunders, 1995, p 1261.

Fossum TW, Willard MD: Diseases of the gallbladder and extrahepatic biliary system. *In* Ettinger SJ, Feldman EC, eds.: Textbook of Veterinary Internal Medicine, Vol 2, 4th Ed. Philadelphia: WB Saunders, 1995, p 1393.

Guilford WG, Center SA, Strombeck DR, et al. eds.: Strombeck's Small Animal Gastroenterology, 3rd Ed. Philadelphia: WB Saunders, 1996.

Day DG: Diseases of the liver. *In* Sherding RG, ed.: The Cat: Diseases and Clinical Management, Vol. 2. New York: WB Saunders, 1994, p 1297.

92 Surgery of the Liver and Biliary Tract

Stephen J. Birchard

Surgery of the liver and biliary tract is commonly performed in small animals and can be very challenging. Animals frequently are presented with surgical diseases of these organs, such as liver tumors and obstruction or infection of the biliary system. Some of the procedures described in this chapter require specialized training and facilities. Others, such as liver biopsy, partial hepatectomy, and simple exploration of the biliary tract, can be performed in a standard veterinary practice. Regardless of the procedure, preparation for the surgery by reviewing anatomy, pathophysiology, and specific techniques is very important for a successful outcome. Preparation of the patient prior to surgery also is extremely important because most of these diseases have serious metabolic effects.

SURGERY OF THE LIVER

Anatomy

Liver Lobes

- The liver is divided into six lobes: the right lateral, right medial, caudate, quadrate, left medial, and left lateral.
- The caudate lobe is divided into the caudate process and the papillary process.

Liver Attachments

- The major liver attachments to other organs and the body wall are the triangular, hepatogastric, and hepatoduodenal ligaments.
- The falciform ligament extends from the liver to the diaphragm and ventral abdominal wall. This mesenteric remnant can be quite large and fat-filled in obese animals. Consider removing this structure during liver surgery to gain better exposure of important structures.
- The hepatorenal ligament is a thin fold of peritoneum that extends from the renal fossa of the caudate lobe to the ventral surface of the right kidney.

Blood Supply

Portal Vein

- The portal vein receives blood from the spleen, pancreas, and intestines.

- The major hepatic branches of the portal vein are the right lateral trunk, right medial branch, and left lateral trunk.
- The portal vein is the combination of the cranial and caudal mesenteric veins and the splenic vein.
- The portal vein can be seen at the base of the mesoduodenum. It forms the ventral boundary of the epiploic foramen.
- The portal vein eventually empties into the liver and supplies approximately 80% of the blood flow of the liver. The remaining 20% comes from the hepatic arteries.
- In the fetus, the ductus venosus connects the portal vein to the caudal vena cava, allowing blood to bypass the liver. This vessel closes soon after birth in normal dogs. If it remains patent, it is called a patent ductus venosus and is one of the several types of portosystemic shunts.

Hepatic Arteries and Veins

- The hepatic artery is a branch of the celiac artery. Variable numbers of hepatic artery branches supply the liver lobes. The hepatic arteries are located in the vicinity of the hepatoduodenal ligament and are adjacent to the common bile duct. The cystic artery, which supplies the gallbladder, is a branch of the left branch of the hepatic artery.
- Six to eight large hepatic veins drain the liver lobes to the caudal vena cava.
- The hepatic veins enter the vena cava at the hilus of the liver and are obscured by the liver parenchyma.

Preoperative Considerations

Liver diseases cause a variety of significant hematologic and metabolic disorders in animals. Prior to surgery, perform appropriate diagnostics to confirm the disease and check for involvement of other organs. (See Chap. 91 for diagnosis of liver problems.)

Of particular concern to the surgeon are the following potential problems:

- *Hypoproteinemia*—Evaluate serum proteins and consider administration of plasma or hyperalimentation if significantly low.
- *Anemia*—Evaluate the animal's hemogram and establish a baseline packed cell volume so that changes can be kept in perspective. Blood loss before, during, and after liver surgery is common and should be monitored closely.

- *Coagulopathy*—Analyze the animal's coagulation profile and correct abnormalities if possible (see Chap. 21). Fresh whole blood transfusion before or during surgery may be necessary.
- *Diffuse disease*—Hepatic neoplasia may result in metastatic lesions. Thoracic and abdominal radiography and abdominal ultrasonography are helpful in determining the extent of disease.
- *Impaired liver function*—Manage hepatic encephalopathy, if present, medically (see Chap. 91) to stabilize the animal prior to surgery.
- *Hypoglycemia*—Consider giving the animal intravenous (IV) fluids supplemented with glucose before and during surgery (e.g., 5% dextrose in lactated Ringer's solution).

▼*Key Point* Diffuse hepatic disease may cause serious metabolic problems that can be compounded by anesthesia and surgery. Analyze liver function tests, such as serum bile acid and blood ammonia concentrations (see Chap. 91) to determine the animal's ability to undergo anesthesia and surgery.

- *Liver trauma*
  - Thoroughly evaluate all animals with a history of trauma to rule out thoracic trauma such as pneumothorax, pulmonary contusions, and other cardiopulmonary problems. Evaluate for damage to other organs such as the urinary tract, gastrointestinal tract, and neurologic and skeletal systems.
  - Animals with liver trauma usually have hemoperitoneum. Severe blood loss will cause clinical signs of shock and should be treated (see Chap. 72 for treatment of hypovolemic shock).

▼*Key Point* Most animals with liver trauma can be treated conservatively (e.g., IV fluids, whole blood transfusion, or autotransfusion of abdominal blood if not contaminated with bacteria or neoplastic cells).

Liver Biopsy and Partial Hepatectomy—Surgical Procedure

Objectives

- Examine the entire liver for grossly evident abnormalities.
- Obtain tissues for biopsy or completely remove the lesion by partial hepatectomy.
- Minimize intraoperative blood loss.

Equipment

- Standard general surgery pack and suture
- Balfour and malleable retractors
- Tru-Cut biopsy needle, Anchor Soft Tissue Biopsy Device (Anchor Products Co., Addison, IL) or skin punch biopsy instrument
- Tissue stapling device (e.g., Autosuture TA, U.S. Surgical, Norwalk, CT) (optional)
- Gelfoam

Technique

1. Place the animal in dorsal recumbency and prepare the entire ventral abdomen and caudal one-third of the sternum for aseptic surgery.
2. Perform a standard ventral midline abdominal approach. If additional exposure is necessary, also perform a left or right paracostal abdominal incision or a median sternotomy.
3. Use laparotomy sponges to protect the abdominal wall and place Balfour retractors to expose the liver and associated viscera.
4. Identify areas of liver to be removed or biopsied. If necessary, mobilize involved liver lobes by incising the triangular ligaments. Greater exposure of the liver can be achieved by placing a laparotomy sponge between it and the diaphragm.
5. Liver biopsy can be achieved by a variety of techniques:
   a. Obtain tissue samples from the periphery of the lobe, using the "guillotine" technique.
   b. Use absorbable suture to surround a small segment of liver and tie the suture tight to cut through the parenchyma and strangulate the blood vessels and bile ducts (Fig. 92–1). Alternatively, place the suture in a horizontal mattress pattern.
   c. Excise the tissue distal to the ligature, using a scalpel or Metzenbaum scissors. Check for bleeding and, if necessary, place a small piece of Gelfoam over the cut surface for hemostasis.
   d. Alternatively, use the Tru-Cut needle or skin biopsy punch to obtain small pieces of liver tissue. These are especially helpful if the lesion is centrally located in the liver lobe rather than pe-

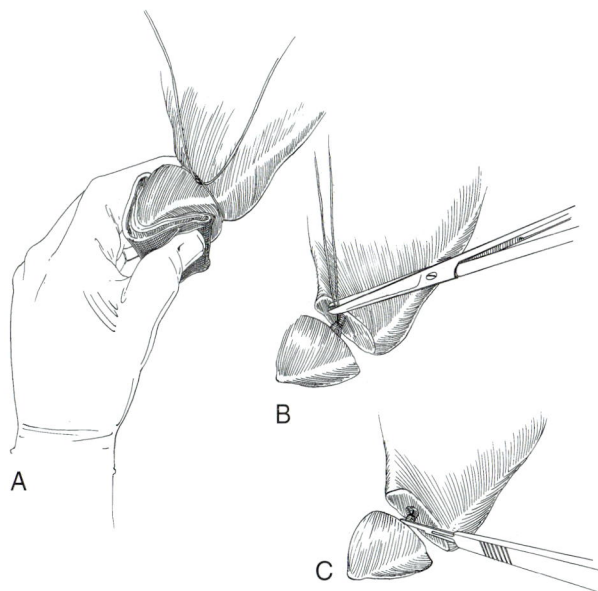

Figure 92–1. Guillotine method for intraoperative liver biopsy. Place a loop of absorbable suture around the tip of a liver lobe and tie tightly to cut through the liver parenchyma, ligating the vessels. Cut the suture ends and then cut the vessels to allow removal of the biopsy specimen.

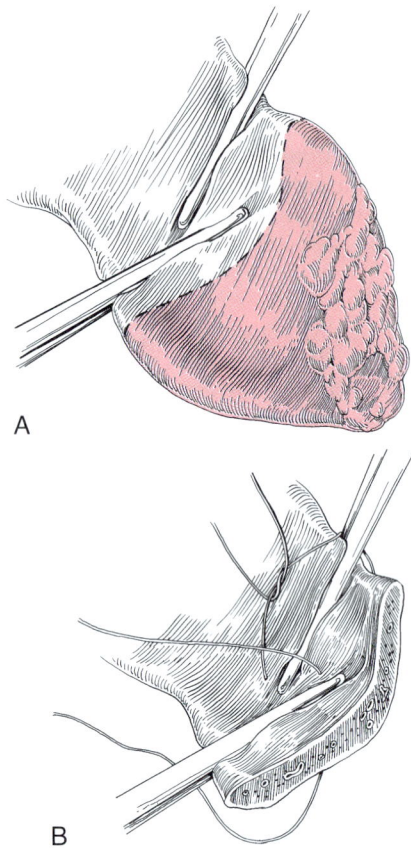

Figure 92–2. Partial hepatectomy. Lesions at the periphery of the liver lobe can be removed by placing crushing clamps across the lobe, proximal to the lesion, and then cutting distal to the clamps. Use absorbable sutures to ligate vessels proximal to the clamps. Tie these ligatures tightly as in the guillotine method for liver biopsy (see Fig. 92–1).

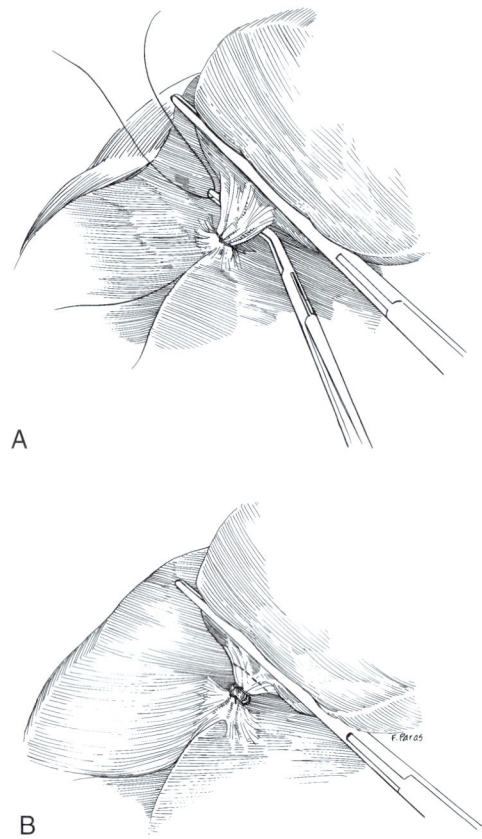

Figure 92–3. Double ligation *(A)* and transection *(B)* in total liver lobectomy.

ripherally. Be sure to include some normal tissue in the biopsy specimen.

6. Remove large lesions by partial hepatectomy (Fig. 92–2):
   a. Divide the liver parenchyma proximal to the lesion, using large crushing clamps or finger fractionation. Ligate the ducts and vessels with absorbable sutures (e.g., 3-0 or 4-0 chromic catgut).
   b. Alternatively, use surgical staples (e.g., U.S. Surgical Autosuture TA) to crush the tissue and ligate the vessels in one step.
   c. Complete removal of an entire liver lobe requires carefully placed ligatures to attenuate the large arteries and veins at the liver hilus. Oversew or transfix the vessels to prevent ligature slippage. Place large clamps on the vessels prior to resection of the lobe to prevent cranial retraction of the vessel (Fig. 92–3).

Postoperative Care and Complications

- Monitor for postoperative hemorrhage (oozing of blood from the incision, distention of the peritoneal cavity, pale mucous membranes). Administer blood transfusion if the hematocrit drops below 20%.
- Give supportive therapy with IV fluids and glucose until oral intake of food and water resumes.

- Monitor for evidence of pancreatitis (vomiting, abdominal pain, increased serum amylase and lipase). Delay resuming oral intake and keep on intravenous fluid therapy until this resolves.
- After massive liver resection, monitor liver function by evaluating bilirubin and serum bile acid concentrations or use the ammonia tolerance test. Liver function reportedly becomes abnormal after resection of 60% or more of the liver.

SURGERY FOR PORTOSYSTEMIC SHUNTS

Portosystemic shunts are abnormal vascular communications between the portal vein and a systemic vein. Diagnosis and medical treatment of this condition are discussed in Chap. 91. Animals with portosystemic shunts can initially improve with medical management. However, the definitive and most effective therapy for long-term resolution of clinical signs is surgical attenuation of the shunt vessel. With recent advances in the intraoperative and postoperative management of these animals, morbidity and mortality rates associated with surgery have decreased to very acceptable levels.

Anatomy

Portosystemic shunts are divided anatomically into *extrahepatic* and *intrahepatic* (Fig. 92–4). Definition of shunt anatomy preoperatively is important because intrahepatic shunts are much more difficult to correct

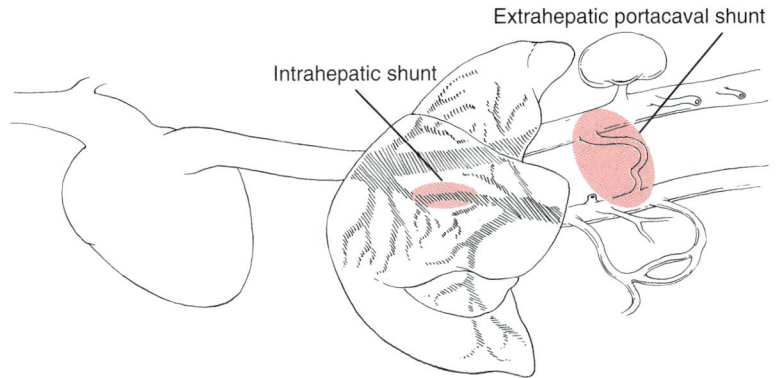

Figure 92–4. Schematic representation of an extrahepatic portacaval shunt and an intrahepatic portacaval shunt.

surgically than are extrahepatic shunts. Also, familiarity with the anatomy helps decrease surgical time and patient morbidity.

Extrahepatic Shunts

Extrahepatic shunts are caudal to the liver. These are vascular communications that usually occur between the portal vein and the caudal vena cava (portacaval shunt) or the azygos vein (portoazygos shunt). Extrahepatic portacaval shunts frequently join the caudal vena cava just adjacent to the epiploic foramen. Shunts involving the left gastric vein can be found near or on the lesser curvature of the stomach.

Intrahepatic Shunts

Intrahepatic shunts communicate with the caudal vena cava within or cranial to the liver parenchyma and can involve either the right or left branches of the hepatic portal vein.

Preoperative positive contrast portography helps differentiate between intrahepatic and extrahepatic shunts. Using these studies, the portal vein can be correlated to the thoracolumbar spine. The first branch of the hepatic portal vein (the right lateral trunk) is located at the 12th thoracic vertebra. If any part of the shunt is caudal to the 13th thoracic vertebra (T13), it is probably extrahepatic. If the entire shunt is cranial to T13, it is probably intrahepatic.

Preoperative Considerations

- Stabilize the animal by medically treating the hepatic encephalopathy for 1–2 weeks (see Chap. 91).
- Treat hypoglycemia, if present, with a 5% dextrose drip administered IV.
- If the animal is anorexic, consider giving nutritional support via nasogastric tube or some other feeding device and use a low-protein diet.
- Avoid lactated Ringer's solution for maintenance fluid administration. Lactated Ringer's can make the animal alkalotic and worsen the hepatic encephalopathy.

Anesthesia

▼ *Key Point* Animals with portosystemic shunts have markedly reduced capacity to metabolize anesthetic drugs in the liver.

- Avoid using drugs such as the barbiturates and phenothiazine derivatives.
- Use diazepam (at a reduced dosage; see Chap. 2) as a premedicant, if needed.
- Induce anesthesia via mask induction with isoflurane and oxygen or ketamine/diazepam combination (see Chap. 2).
- Maintain anesthesia with isoflurane and oxygen via endotracheal tube.
- In addition to routine monitoring, monitor blood pressure because changes may occur during manipulation of the shunt.
- Administer a 5% dextrose in 0.9% saline drip IV during anesthesia and surgery to prevent severe hypoglycemia.

Surgical Procedure

Objectives

- Place a jejunal vein catheter to monitor portal pressures.
- Identify and attenuate the portosystemic shunt to redirect portal blood flow to the liver.
- Avoid causing portal hypertension.

Equipment*

- Standard general surgery pack and retractors (Balfour, malleable)
- Over-the-needle intravenous catheter (e.g., Sureflo, Terumo Medical, Elkton, MD), water manometer, IV extension set, three-way stopcock, heparinized saline
- Small and large right-angled forceps
- DeBakey tissue-holding forceps

Technique

1. Place the animal in dorsal recumbency and prepare the entire ventral abdomen and caudal one-third of the sternum for aseptic surgery.
2. Perform a routine ventral midline abdominal approach. If the shunt is intrahepatic, it also may be necessary to perform a caudal sternotomy.
3. Isolate a loop of jejunum and place two stay sutures (4-0 silk) around the jejunal vessels. Place an over-

---

*Also see equipment listed under Median Sternotomy, which may be needed if the shunt is intrahepatic (Chap. 83).

the-needle catheter in the jejunal vein and ligate in place with the silk suture. Place an additional suture around the catheter and either the intestinal serosa or the mesentery to prevent slippage.

4. After flushing the catheter with heparinized saline, connect an extension set and water manometer to the jejunal vein catheter. Measure preligation portal pressure (normal is 8–10 cm H_2O).
5. Explore the abdomen and identify the shunt.
   a. *Extrahepatic shunts* usually are found by retracting the duodenum ventrally and to the left, and then following the mesoduodenum cranially and dorsally to the level of the epiploic foramen. Ventral retraction of the lesser omentum usually exposes the shunt entering the caudal vena cava. Be careful not to injure the hepatic arteries, which lie adjacent to the shunts located in this position. Some shunts can be found by creating a small window in the greater omentum and looking in the vicinity of the splenic vein or by making a window in the lesser omentum and looking craniodorsal to the lesser curvature of the stomach. Shunts in other locations require careful exploration of the cranial abdomen for location. It may be necessary to locate other branches of the portal vein, such as the splenic vein or the left gastric vein, in order to find the shunt.
   b. The location of *intrahepatic shunts* varies. Exposure may be facilitated by median sternotomy and ventral-to-dorsal division of the diaphragm. The intrahepatic shunt may be seen entering the caudal vena cava cranial to the liver. These shunts are usually closely adherent to the peritoneal surface of the diaphragm. Alternatively, the shunt or the branch of the portal vein entering the shunt may be seen and dissected caudal to the liver.
6. Carefully skeletonize a small portion of the shunt vessel and pass a silk ligature around it.

▼*Key Point* During shunt ligation, do not allow portal pressure to rise >10 cm above the preligation value or to reach an absolute value >20 cm H_2O.

7. Slowly ligate the shunt while monitoring portal pressure. Carefully observe the abdominal viscera, especially the pancreas and intestine, for evidence of portal hypertension (e.g., bluish color and congestion of venous vessels). Use both the portal pressure values and tissue appearance to be sure that portal hypertension is not developing during ligation.
   a. Reduce the degree of attenuation if there is any evidence of portal hypertension.
   b. Complete ligation is possible in rare cases; however, many animals respond well to only partial ligation of the shunt.
8. Alternatively, use an ameroid constrictor (Research Instruments and Manufacturing, Corvallis, OR) to attenuate the shunt. This device gradually occludes the shunt vessel over weeks, thereby reducing the

risk of acute portal hypertension. (See Supplemental Reading for more information.)
9. Remove the jejunal catheter and ligate the jejunal vein if necessary.
10. Close the abdominal incision in a routine fashion.

Postoperative Care and Complications

- Monitor for portal hypertension.
  - *Acute* portal hypertension is a life-threatening complication that may develop any time from immediately to several hours postoperatively. Watch for the following clinical signs of postoperative portal hypertension: acute collapse, severe abdominal pain, abdominal distention (ileus), pale mucous membranes, slow capillary refill, and diarrhea with frank blood.

▼*Key Point* If acute portal hypertension is suspected, reoperate immediately to remove the shunt ligature.

- - *Chronic* portal hypertension usually is manifested by ascites. Treatment generally is not necessary, and the ascites usually resolves in 1–3 weeks.
- Prevent hypoglycemia by giving 5% dextrose in saline until the animal resumes oral feeding.
- Add potassium to the fluid to prevent hypokalemia (see Chap. 5 on fluid therapy).
- Continue medical management of hepatic encephalopathy (see Chap. 91).
  - If the animal is doing well clinically, discontinue the lactulose and neomycin after 2–4 weeks.
  - Continue feeding a low-protein diet (e.g., Prescription Diet k/d [Hill's]) until liver function improves significantly. Measure pre- and postprandial serum bile acid concentrations 3 and 6 months postoperatively to evaluate improvement in liver function. If no clinical improvement is seen, consider follow-up portography and religation of the shunt vessel if continued shunting of blood is seen.

SURGERY OF THE BILIARY TRACT

Anatomy

Gallbladder

- The gallbladder is a pear-shaped sac located between the quadrate and right medial lobes of the liver.
- In a medium-sized dog, it has a capacity of 15 ml.
- Bile drains from the gallbladder to the cystic duct, and then to the common bile duct.
- The gallbladder is divided anatomically into three parts: the fundus (blind end), body (middle portion), and neck.
- Histologically, the gallbladder wall consists of a mucosal lining, layer of smooth muscle fibers, submucosal layer, and serosal covering.
- Blood supply is via the cystic artery, a branch of the hepatic artery.

Bile Ducts

- Hepatic cells discharge bile into minute canaliculi, which coalesce to form interlobar ducts and then hepatic ducts.
- Hepatic ducts and the cystic duct drain into the bile duct (or common bile duct).
- The common bile duct is present in the lesser omentum, and the free portion is about 5 cm in length. It then travels through the duodenal wall as an intramural portion that is 1.5–2.0 cm in length, and empties into the major duodenal papilla. The minor pancreatic duct in dogs empties immediately adjacent to the opening of the bile duct at the major duodenal papilla. In cats, the common bile duct and major pancreatic duct join and subsequently enter the duodenum at the major papilla as a common duct.

Preoperative Considerations

- Correct dehydration and serum electrolyte imbalances before surgery.
- If the animal is not already being treated for infection, administer prophylactic antibiotics (directed toward gram-negative and anaerobic bacteria) (see Chapter 91).

▼ *Key Point* If the bile duct is totally obstructed, coagulopathy may be present because of decreased absorption of vitamin K–dependent clotting factors (II, VII, IX, X).

- Give vitamin K_1 (Veda-K_1, Vedco) at 1–3 mg/kg divided q12h SC, 36 hours before surgery if necessary. If immediate surgery is required, give a fresh whole blood transfusion.

Cholecystectomy—Surgical Procedure

Cholecystectomy is indicated for severe diseases of the gallbladder, such as damage secondary to trauma, severe cholecystitis, neoplasia, and irreparable damage to the cystic duct.

Objectives

- Remove the gallbladder while minimizing trauma to surrounding tissues.
- Prevent leakage of bile to the peritoneal cavity.
- Avoid damage to the remainder of the biliary duct system.

Equipment

- Standard general surgery pack and suture
- Small and large gallbladder and other right-angled forceps
- Hemostatic stainless steel clips
- Sterile cotton-tipped applicators

Technique

1. Prepare the animal as previously described for liver biopsy and hepatic surgery.
2. Isolate the gallbladder from the remainder of the peritoneal cavity with moistened laparotomy sponges.
3. Dissect the gallbladder from the fossa by blunt dissection. Sterile cotton-tipped applicators are helpful to separate the gallbladder from the surrounding hepatic tissue. Babcock forceps or stay sutures can be used to manipulate the gallbladder during this dissection.
4. Isolate and double-ligate the cystic duct and cystic artery with absorbable sutures or hemostatic clips.
5. Place gallbladder forceps and incise the cystic duct and artery just distal to the forceps. Remove forceps and gallbladder.
6. Submit the gallbladder for aerobic and anaerobic bacterial culture and histopathology.
7. Close the abdominal incision in a routine fashion.

Cholecystotomy—Surgical Procedure

Cholecystotomy is indicated to remove biliary calculi or to flush the gallbladder of inspissated or infected bile. The gallbladder should be reasonably healthy and have a good blood supply to ensure satisfactory healing.

Objectives

- Open and inspect the gallbladder and its contents.
- Avoid spillage of bile into the peritoneal cavity.
- Provide a watertight seal of the cholecystotomy incision using absorbable suture material.
- Submit samples of tissue, calculi, and/or bile for analysis and culture.
- Thoroughly flush the gallbladder and biliary ducts to remove stones and infected material.

Equipment

Equipment is the same as for cholecystectomy plus:
- Fine absorbable suture with taper or taper-cut needle (4-0, 5-0 polydioxanone or polyglactin 910).
- Infant feeding tube or small (#5 Fr.) Brunswick rubber catheter.

Technique

1. Prepare and position the animal as previously described for liver biopsy and hepatic surgery. The surgical approach is the same as for a cholecystectomy.
2. Isolate the gallbladder from the remainder of the peritoneal cavity with laparotomy sponges.
3. Use stay sutures (5-0 silk) on the gallbladder on either side of the proposed incision.
4. Incise the gallbladder fundus, using a #11 scalpel blade and Metzenbaum or tenotomy scissors. Evacuate the contents and save samples of bile or calculi for analysis and culture.
5. Flush the gallbladder with warm, sterile saline.
6. To ensure patency, cannulate and flush the cystic and common bile ducts with an infant feeding tube or #5 Fr. Brunswick catheter.
7. If necessary, perform a duodenotomy approximately 2–4 cm distal to the pylorus to pass a catheter retrograde into the common bile duct through the major duodenal papilla. Place a stent catheter if recurrent

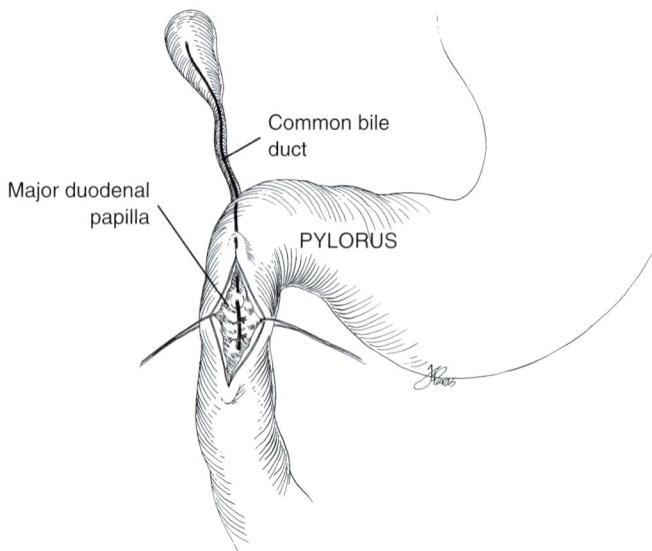

Figure 92–5. Placement of an indwelling stent catheter in the common bile duct. The catheter is placed via a duodenotomy. Insert the catheter retrograde through the major duodenal papilla and into the gallbladder. Leave the end of the catheter in the duodenal lumen and ligate in place with 4-0 or 5-0 catgut; close the duodenotomy incision.

bile duct obstruction is expected or to stent a ruptured biliary duct (Fig. 92–5).

8. Close the gallbladder incision in a one- or two-layer inverting pattern (e.g., Cushing and/or Lembert), using 5-0 or 4-0 absorbable suture and a taper needle.
9. Close the abdominal incision in a routine manner.

Cholecystoenterostomy—Surgical Procedure

Cholecystoenterostomy is surgical anastomosis of the gallbladder to the intestinal tract. The major objective is to bypass the cystic and common bile ducts when these ducts are irreversibly obstructed. Examples of indications are severe scar tissue in the bile ducts (sequela of cholangitis), nonresectable neoplasia, severe cholangiohepatitis with sludged bile (in cats), and large bile duct calculi that cannot be dislodged. The gallbladder can be anastomosed to the duodenum (cholecystoduodenostomy) or to the jejunum (cholecystojejunostomy).

Objectives

- Diversion of bile from the gallbladder directly to the duodenum or jejunum to bypass the cystic and common bile duct.
- Maintain sufficient lumen size to allow free flow of bile from the gallbladder to the intestine.
- Prevent bile or intestinal leakage.
- Provide a tension-free anastomosis.

Equipment

Equipment is the same as for cholecystotomy.

Technique

1. Prepare and position the animal as previously described for liver biopsy and hepatic surgery. The surgical approach is identical to that for cholecystectomy.
2. Using blunt dissection, gently free the gallbladder from the surrounding liver tissue.
3. Bring a loop of duodenum or jejunum close to the gallbladder and place stay sutures in both structures.

4. Incise the gallbladder along the fundus and the intestine on its antimesenteric surface.
5. Perform a two-layered anastomosis, using absorbable suture for the inner layer and a nonabsorbable monofilament suture for the outer layer. Make sure the anastomosis is at least 2.5 cm in diameter. This large opening helps prevent sequestration of intestinal contents in the gallbladder that could result in severe cholecystitis and cholangitis.
6. Close the abdominal incision in a routine manner.

Surgical Repair of Traumatic Biliary Rupture

Rupture of the biliary tract causes severe chemical and possibly septic peritonitis. Diagnosis and initial management of animals with bile peritonitis is discussed in Chapter 96. Perform surgical correction of bile leakage promptly because metabolic consequences are serious and life-threatening.

Objectives

- Evaluate the entire liver and biliary tract for evidence of damage.
- Identify the source of bile leakage and control it.
- Treat the peritonitis with copious lavage and abdominal drainage.
- Maintain competency of major biliary pathways.
- Provide nutritional access for hyperalimentation in patients in critical condition.

Equipment

Equipment is the same as for cholecystotomy, plus:

- Stent tubing (e.g., #5 Fr. Brunswick catheter, infant feeding tube, or Silastic tubing)

Technique

1. The preparation of the animal and surgical approach are the same as for cholecystectomy.
2. Evacuate fluid from the peritoneal cavity.

3. Examine the entire liver and biliary system for evidence of trauma and injury. Examine the remainder of the abdominal organs for abnormalities.
4. Find the source of bile leakage:
   a. If the gallbladder is intact, express it and look for leakage.
   b. If the above is unsuccessful, perform a duodenotomy over the major duodenal papilla and catheterize the common bile duct, using a #5 Fr. Brunswick catheter or infant feeding tube. Flush the bile duct with sterile saline and look for leakage.
5. Correct the leakage.
   a. Suture the rent if it is in the gallbladder or a large bile duct. Use fine absorbable suture material (4-0 or 5-0 polydioxanone).
   b. If primary closure is not possible, stent the torn duct by passing a soft catheter up the common bile duct through the major duodenal papilla. Make sure that the end of the catheter is at least 2–3 cm proximal to the rent. Secure the catheter to the duodenal mucosa by placing one or two ligatures of 5-0 catgut. Cut the catheter, leaving 2–3 cm in the lumen of the duodenum, and close the duodenal incision in a routine manner. In 1–2 weeks, the catheter will dislodge and be passed through the intestinal tract.
6. Lavage the abdomen with copious amounts of warm, sterile saline.
7. Close the abdomen routinely.

Postoperative Care and Complications

- Maintain IV fluid therapy until oral intake resumes.
- Monitor for evidence of bile peritonitis: painful abdomen, fever, leukocytosis, icterus, and bile-stained fluid on abdominal tap.

- If cultures from the biliary tract are positive, administer long-term (6 weeks) antibiotic therapy.

▼ *Key Point* Mortality associated with bile peritonitis is significantly higher if bacterial contamination is also present.

- Monitor for evidence of pancreatitis; withhold food and water if it occurs (maintain the animal on IV fluids).
- Reevaluate every 3–6 months for recurrence of biliary obstruction or ascending infection of the biliary tract after cholecystoenterostomy.

SUPPLEMENTAL READINGS

Breznock EM, Whiting PG: Portacaval shunts and anomalies. *In* Slatter DH, ed.: Textbook of Small Animal Surgery. Philadelphia: WB Saunders, 1985, p 1156.

Evans HE: The digestive apparatus and abdomen. *In* Evans HE, Christensen GC: Miller's Anatomy of the Dog, 3rd Ed. Philadelphia: WB Saunders, 1993, p 385.

Ludwig LL., McLoughlin MA, Graves TK, Crisp MS: Surgical treatment of bile peritonitis in 24 dogs and 2 cats: a retrospective study (1987–1994). Vet Surg 26:90, 1997.

Martin RA: Liver and biliary system. *In* Slatter DH, ed.: Textbook of Small Animal Surgery, 2nd Ed. Philadelphia: WB Saunders, 1993, p 645.

Vogt JC, Krahwinkel DJ, Bright RM, et al.: Gradual occlusion of extrahepatic portosystemic shunts in dogs and cats using the ameroid constrictor. Vet Surg 25:495, 1996.

93 Diseases and Surgery of the Exocrine Pancreas

Robert G. Sherding / Stephen J. Birchard / Susan E. Johnson

The pancreas is a V-shaped gland in the cranial abdomen composed of an exocrine portion (the acinar cells) and an endocrine portion (the islets of Langerhans). The normal functions of the exocrine pancreas are summarized in Table 93–1. The principal disorders of the exocrine pancreas include pancreatitis, exocrine pancreatic insufficiency, and neoplasia. (Diseases of the endocrine pancreas are discussed in Chaps. 32 and 33.)

PANCREATITIS

Pancreatitis is an acute or chronic inflammatory condition of the pancreas that develops when intrapancreatic activation of enzymes results in progressive autodigestion of the gland. The clinical forms of pancreatitis are categorized in Table 93–2.

Etiology

In most animals with spontaneous pancreatitis, an etiology is not identified and the pathogenesis is poorly understood. Based on clinical associations found in naturally occurring cases and on various experimental models for producing pancreatitis in dogs, the following have been proposed as etiologic or predisposing factors:

- Obesity and long-term intake of high-fat diets
- Ingestion of a fatty meal—e.g., meat trimmings
- Hyperlipidemia—e.g., as a result of intake of a fatty meal, hyperadrenocorticism, diabetes mellitus, hypothyroidism, or idiopathic hyperlipidemia of miniature schnauzers
- Corticosteroid therapy and hyperadrenocorticism
- Reflux of duodenal contents (bile, activated enzymes, bacteria) into the pancreatic duct
- Pancreatic duct obstruction—e.g., as a result of duodenitis, edema, spasm, calculi, neoplasia, metaplasia, or aberrant parasite migration

Table 93–1. FUNCTIONS OF THE EXOCRINE PANCREAS

Secretory Products	Functions
Digestive enzymes*	
Trypsins	Protein digestion
Chymotrypsins	Protein digestion
Elastases	Protein digestion
Carboxypeptidases	Protein digestion
Amylase	Polysaccharide digestion
Phospholipase	Lipid digestion
Lipase	Lipid digestion
Colipase	Coenzyme facilitator of lipase
Bicarbonate†	Neutralization of gastric acid entering duodenum
Pancreatic trypsin inhibitor	Protection against autodigestion
Pancreatic intrinsic factor	Facilitation of cobalamin (vitamin B_{12}) absorption
Miscellaneous	Facilitation of zinc absorption
	Antibacterial (inhibits intestinal bacterial overgrowth)
	Trophic effect on intestinal mucosa

*Acinar cells secrete enzymes in response to cholecystokinin (CCK), which is released into the blood from the proximal intestine when partially digested food enters the duodenum from the stomach. Proteolytic enzymes are secreted as inactive precursors (zymogens) that are not activated until they enter the intestinal tract. Enteropeptidase from the duodenal mucosa activates trypsinogen to active trypsin; trypsin then activates the other proteases and phospholipase.

†Centroacinar and duct cells produce bicarbonate-rich secretion in response to secretin released into the blood from the proximal intestine when acid enters the duodenum from the stomach.

Table 93–2. CATEGORIES OF PANCREATITIS

Acute Pancreatitis

(Abrupt onset; acute episodes may recur)

Mild (Edematous)
Self-limiting
No vascular compromise
No multisystem failure or complications
Uncomplicated recovery

Severe (Hemorrhagic)
Self-perpetuating (progressive)
Vascular compromise
Severe complications
Multisystem failure
Guarded prognosis

Chronic Pancreatitis

(May be continuous and "smoldering" or recurrent and episodic)

Mild
Minimal morphologic damage
Absence of complications

Severe
Progressive irreversible destruction of acinar and islet cells
Severe pancreatic fibrosis
Complications:
  Exocrine pancreatic insufficiency
  Diabetes mellitus
  Extrahepatic bile duct obstruction

- Biliary tract disease—e.g., pancreatitis associated with cholangiohepatitis in cats
- Infection—e.g., ascending enteric bacteria, parvovirus, and aberrant intestinal parasite migration; rarely feline infectious peritonitis virus, toxoplasmosis, and the pancreatic fluke *Eurytrema procyonis*
- Hypercalcemia—when total serum calcium exceeds 15 mg/dl, as can occur in hypercalcemia of malignancy, hyperparathyroidism, and vitamin D intoxication
- Abdominal trauma or surgery
- Hyperstimulation—by agents such as scorpion venom, cholinesterase inhibitors, cholinergic agonists, and cerulein (an analogue of cholecystokinin)
- Pancreatic ischemia—e.g., hypovolemia, thrombosis, local stasis of pancreas microvasculature
- Pancreatic neoplasia

Pathogenesis

The initiating events of pancreatitis are not fully understood, but acinar cell membrane damage (permeability) and intrapancreatic activation of trypsinogen are involved. Activated trypsin then activates other digestive enzymes, resulting in a progressive cascade of intrapancreatic enzyme activation and pancreatic autodigestion. Once initiated, amplification and progression of pancreatitis involves factors such as oxygen-derived free radicals, activated complement, the kallikrein-kinin system, disseminated intravascular coagulopathy (DIC), bacterial endotoxins, and pancreatic ischemia (Table 93–3).

▼ *Key Point* Activation of trypsin and other pancreatic enzymes is critical to the development of pancreatitis. Impaired pancreatic microcirculation is a key factor in the progression of mild edematous pancreatitis to severe necrotizing pancreatitis.

Clinical Signs and Manifestations

Clinical signs of acute pancreatitis are extremely variable, ranging from vague and nonspecific signs to obvious signs of an "acute abdomen" crisis. In chronic pancreatitis, episodic signs may correspond to periodic flare-ups of inflammation. In some cases, clinical signs are dominated by secondary complications (e.g., DIC) or sequelae (e.g., diabetes mellitus).

Canine Pancreatitis

- Vomiting (most consistent sign, but can be absent in some cases), anorexia, depression, and dehydration
- Cranial abdominal pain, varying from mild to intense (manifested as restlessness, panting, trembling, hunched-up abdomen, praying position of relief, seeking of cool surfaces, and pain on palpation)
- Diarrhea (sometimes hemorrhagic)
- Fever (can be solely due to inflammation and does not necessarily imply infection)
- Weakness or, in severe cases, acute collapse from shock

Feline Pancreatitis

- Cats are more likely to have smoldering, low-grade chronic interstitial pancreatitis, manifested by vague, nonspecific signs of lethargy, anorexia and weight loss, with or without vomiting. The disorder often goes unrecognized until discovered at necropsy.
- Concurrent cholangitis/cholangiohepatitis frequently is found; this may be related to the anatomic arrangement of the bile and pancreatic ducts that join and have a common opening into the duodenum in cats.

Table 93–3. FACTORS INVOLVED IN THE PATHOGENESIS OF PANCREATITIS

Factor	Proposed Role in Pathogenesis
Pancreatic Enzymes	
Trypsin	Perpetuates proteolytic damage of pancreatic tissue (autodigestion)
	Perpetuates activation of more trypsin and other proteases
	Consumption of plasma protease inhibitors
	Coagulation/fibrinolysis (DIC)
	Activates kinin system and releases histamine from mast cells, contributing to edema and hemorrhage
Phospholipase A	Cell membrane damage (necrosis, noncardiogenic pulmonary edema)
	Liberation of toxins (e.g., myocardial depressant factor)
Elastase	Vascular damage (progression of edematous to hemorrhagic pancreatitis)
Chymotrypsin	Activation of xanthine oxidase (generation of oxygen-derived free radicals; see below)
Lipase	Local fat necrosis (peritonitis; "calcium soaps"; hypocalcemia)
Inflammatory Mediators	
Oxygen-derived free radicals	Damage of tissues by disrupting cell membranes through peroxidation of lipids in the membrane
	Endothelial cell injury (pancreatic edema and hemorrhage; DIC)
Kallikrein-kinin system	Vasodilation, hypotension, and shock
Complement	Local inflammation and aggregation of leukocytes; peritonitis
Coagulation/Fibrinolysis	DIC
	Thrombosis of pancreatic blood vessels
	Ischemic pancreatic necrosis

DIC, disseminated intravascular coagulopathy.

Acute Complications

- Shock, collapse, and hypothermia (due to hypovolemia and endotoxemia)
- Peritonitis (sterile exudate) and intra-abdominal fat necrosis
- Sepsis
- DIC—bleeding, thrombosis, infarction
- Jaundice (intrahepatic cholestasis, hepatocellular necrosis, biliary obstruction)
- Acute oliguric renal failure
- Intestinal hypomotility (ileus)
- Hypocalcemia (tetany is rare)
- Hyperglycemia (due to hyperglucagonemia and hypoinsulinemia)
- Cardiac arrhythmias (myocardial depressant factor; myocardial ischemia or necrosis)
- Respiratory distress (rarely, noncardiogenic pulmonary edema or pleural effusion)

Chronic Complications and Sequelae

- Pancreatic pseudocysts and abscesses, characterized by persistence or recurrence of signs associated with development of a cavitated pancreatic mass containing liquefied necrotic debris, which can be sterile (pseudocyst) or infected (abscess)
- Chronic relapsing pancreatitis, characterized by chronic smoldering disease with periodic flare-ups
- End-stage pancreatic fibrosis and atrophy, manifested as diabetes mellitus or exocrine pancreatic insufficiency or both
- Liver disease, resulting from common bile duct obstruction due to chronic fibrosing pancreatitis

Diagnosis

Clinical Signs and Physical Findings

- Suspect pancreatitis in animals presented for vomiting, depression, anorexia, and abdominal pain.
- Identifiable risk factors increase the index of suspicion (e.g., obesity, schnauzer breed, recent fatty meal, evidence of corticosteroid excess).
- A palpable right cranial abdominal mass or fluid suggests a pancreatic lesion.

Serum Amylase and Lipase

Dogs. The clinical diagnosis of acute pancreatitis usually is based on elevated serum concentrations of amylase and lipase. Serum enzyme concentrations often are normal in chronic pancreatitis except during acute flare-ups of inflammation. Although serum amylase and lipase concentrations are sensitive indicators of pancreatitis, they lack specificity because elevated enzyme levels are frequent in nonpancreatic diseases. However, nonpancreatic elevations do not usually exceed two to three times the upper limit of normal. There is an inconsistent correlation between the degree of enzyme elevation and the severity of the pancreatitis or the prognosis.

- Delayed renal clearance of enzymes combined with increased secretion due to hypergastrinemia can cause elevations in azotemic patients. This can be a diagnostic dilemma because acute pancreatitis often causes prerenal azotemia and sometimes overt oliguric renal failure. Urinalysis is helpful in these situations.
- Amylase and lipase may sometimes be increased in gastrointestinal, liver, and neoplastic disease. Normal circulating amylase originates from nonpancreatic sources, especially the intestinal mucosa; thus, enteritis can increase serum amylase.
- Corticosteroids in high doses can cause a significant increase (up to five-fold) in lipase concentrations in the absence of pancreatitis while amylase decreases or remains normal.
- Amylase and lipase usually increase in parallel, but not always; therefore, evaluation of both amylase and lipase together is more diagnostic than evaluating either one alone. One or both enzymes can be normal in the presence of severe pancreatitis, presumably due to depletion of stored enzymes in the pancreas.

Cats. Cats with pancreatitis often have minimal or no increase in amylase and lipase; thus, these enzymes are of no value in the diagnosis of feline pancreatitis. In experimental pancreatitis in cats, serum lipase concentration increases while that of amylase decreases or remains within normal limits.

Amylase Assay Methods

- Catalytic methods—the amyloclastic method is valid for dogs, but the saccharogenic method is not.

▼ **Key Point** Amylase cannot be measured by saccharogenic methods used for humans because dog serum contains high levels of maltase and glucoamylase that yield falsely elevated amylase values.

- Immunoassay methods are reliable but are also species-specific.

Serum Trypsin-Like Immunoassay (TLI)

- Detects increased circulating trypsinogen and trypsin associated with leakage from the inflamed pancreas.
- Feline-specific TLI (fTLI) is useful for diagnosing pancreatitis in cats. Normal fTLI is 17–49 $\mu g/L$, and in cats with pancreatitis fTLI ranges from normal to > 500 $\mu g/L$ (mean, 100 $\mu g/L$).
- TLI is available at the Gastrointestinal Laboratory, Department of Small Animal Medicine and Surgery, College of Veterinary Medicine, Texas A&M University, College Station, TX.

Other Pancreatic Tests

These require further clinical evaluation before they can be recommended.

- Amylase isoenzyme analysis (for pancreas-specific isoenzyme)
- Assay for serum phospholipase A_2
- Plasma protease inhibitor consumption (alpha$_1$-antitrypsin, alpha-macroglobulin)
- Assay for trypsin-antiprotease complexes in plasma

Ancillary Laboratory Findings

- Fasting hyperlipemia and icteric serum are common in patients with pancreatitis.
- The complete blood count (CBC) usually reveals neutrophilia, with or without a left shift. Severe necrosis, peritonitis, sepsis, or endotoxemia can sometimes cause neutropenia with a degenerative left shift. Hemoconcentration (elevated packed cell volume [PCV]) from dehydration is typical; occasionally anemia occurs. Red blood cell (RBC) fragments and macroplatelets are consistent with subclinical DIC.
- Elevated serum liver enzymes (alkaline phosphatase [ALP], alanine aminotransferase [ALT]), and bilirubin can result from hepatocellular injury (due to ischemia, sepsis, or toxins from the pancreas) and biliary obstruction.
- Azotemia (increased blood urea nitrogen [BUN] and creatinine) is common and can result from dehydration and hypovolemia (prerenal) or from renal damage and acute oliguric renal failure.

▼ *Key Point* Because elevated levels of amylase, lipase, BUN, and creatinine are common in both renal failure and pancreatitis, assess the urine specific gravity (SG) as a reflection of renal concentrating ability; SG > 1.025 indicates adequate tubular function.

- Hyperglycemia (usually transient, but some animals are diabetic after recovery)
- Hypocalcemia (usually subclinical; tetany is rare)
- Fasting hyperlipemia (hypertriglyceridemia and hypercholesterolemia)
- Hemostatic abnormalities consistent with DIC: prolonged activated partial thromboplastin time (APTT) and one-stage prothrombin time (OSPT), decreased platelets, decreased fibrinogen, and increased fibrinolytic products
- Abdominal fluid analysis (brownish-red exudate; increased enzyme activity relative to blood; possible sepsis)
- Methemalbumin formation (human test is not very applicable to dogs because of hemin complexes with serum proteins other than albumin in dogs)

Radiography

- Increased density and loss of abdominal contrast and detail in the right cranial abdomen (localized peritonitis; ground-glass appearance)
- Displacement of the descending duodenum to the right and the pyloric antrum to the left, producing a widened angle or mass effect between the antrum and duodenum on ventrodorsal radiographs (on lateral views, the duodenum may be displaced ventrally)
- Gastric distention and static gas pattern (ileus) in the duodenum or transverse colon
- Delayed passage of barium from the stomach and through the duodenum; also, thickening, corrugation, or spasticity of the duodenum
- Possible complicating pulmonary edema or pleural effusion seen on thoracic radiography

Ultrasonography

- Irregular pancreatic enlargement, decreased or mottled echogenicity of the pancreas, hyperechoic peripancreatic mesentery, and peripancreatic effusion suggest pancreatitis.
- Pancreatic pseudocysts and abscesses can be identified as pancreatic cavitations.

Medical Treatment

Mild acute pancreatitis often is self-limiting and may resolve spontaneously in a few days. Severe acute pancreatitis is a life-threatening multisystem crisis that requires intensive therapy. The goal of treatment is to rest the pancreas, provide supportive care, and control complications as they arise in order to allow time for the pancreatic inflammation to subside. Surgical intervention may be required when abscessation occurs.

▼ *Key Point* Correction of hypovolemia by IV fluid therapy and prevention of pancreatic stimulation by temporary restriction of all oral intake are the most important therapeutic measures for acute pancreatitis.

Control Hypovolemia and Maintain Pancreatic Microcirculation

- Fluid Volume Replacement:
  - Administer a balanced electrolyte solution (e.g., lactated Ringer's). To treat *shock*, give up to 85 ml/kg IV in the first hour (see Chap. 72). To provide *rehydration* and *maintenance*, give 60 ml/kg/24h plus deficit plus extra losses (for a detailed discussion of fluid therapy, see Chap. 5).
  - Monitor urine output (for oliguria) and respiratory function (for pulmonary edema).
  - Consider transfusion of plasma or whole blood (10–20 ml/kg) for maintenance of normoalbuminemia and plasma oncotic pressure in hypoproteinemic patients (when serum albumin is <2.0 g/dl). This enhances pancreatic microcirculation and reduces pancreatic edema and helps to prevent renal failure, pulmonary edema, and pleural effusion. Plasma or whole blood can replace antiproteases (alpha-macroglobulins) that are consumed in pancreatitis. Use fresh whole blood plus heparin to treat overt DIC.
- Potassium supplementation: Add 20–30 mEq KCl/L of maintenance fluids and frequently monitor serum K^+.
- Acid-base status is unpredictable in pancreatitis; avoid excessive bicarbonate administration if unwarranted, because this can precipitate hypocalcemia.
- Use glucocorticoids only in patients presented in shock and only short-term (1–2 doses, as described for treatment of shock in Chap. 72). Glucocorticoids may impair clearance of circulating protease complexes.
- Control DIC to prevent pancreatic microthrombi (see Chap. 21).
- Other unproven agents to promote pancreatic microcirculation include vasopressin (5 units in oil) and glucagon.

Prevent Stimulation of Pancreatic Secretion

- In dogs, restrict oral intake to place the pancreas at "rest"; however, feed cats with pancreatitis if they are not vomiting, to prevent hepatic lipidosis.
  - Nothing per os usually is required for 3–4 days or longer. Food (especially fats and proteins) stimulates pancreatic secretion through cholecystokinin (CCK) release. Even fluids can stimulate pancreatic secretion through gastric distention and release of gastrin.
  - When vomiting has ceased for ≥24–48h, offer small amounts of water PO. If water is tolerated, then gradually reintroduce food, initially using a carbohydrate diet (e.g., rice, pasta) restricted in fat and protein to minimize pancreatic stimulation. Then gradually resume normal maintenance feeding of a balanced, moderately fat-restricted diet.
  - Prolonged restriction of oral intake (1–2 weeks) is required for some patients, which may necessitate feeding of elemental nutrients by jejunostomy catheter or total parenteral nutrition, provided that an ICU facility is available.
- Avoid anticholinergics; they are of questionable benefit and potentiate ileus of the intestinal tract.
- Inhibition of gastric acid secretion with drugs like cimetidine is of unproven benefit.
- Experimental treatment modalities include CCK inhibitors, glucagon, somatostatin, and enzyme inhibitors.

Promote Removal of Activated Enzymes

- Promote plasma antiprotease activity.
  - Alpha$_2$-macroglobulin binds circulating activated enzymes for removal by the mononuclear phagocyte system. Plasma or whole blood transfusion may benefit patients with fulminant pancreatitis by supplying macroglobulin (also supplies colloid in the form of albumin).
  - Avoid glucocorticoids because they may have a detrimental effect on removal of macroglobulin-enzyme complexes.
- Peritoneal lavage using a dialysis catheter can help to remove intraperitoneal enzymes, inflammatory mediators, and toxins. Although it is not practical to recommend as a routine method of treatment, it can be beneficial in cases of pancreatitis with abdominal effusion.

Control Abdominal Pain

- Rest and confinement help to minimize pain.
- If analgesia is needed, use butorphanol (Torbugesic, Fort Dodge) (0.1–0.4 mg/kg q4–6h SC, IM, IV) or oxymorphone (0.05–0.2 mg/kg q2–6h; SC, IM, IV), beginning at the lower dosage range in cats or with IV use, and titrating higher as needed.
- Oral pancreatic enzyme supplements (Viokase) and insulin have been beneficial for pain relief in humans with chronic pancreatitis, but this effect has not been evaluated in animal patients.

Control Acute Complications

- Control sepsis (and prevent pancreatic abscessation):
  - For prevention, administer ampicillin (20 mg/kg q8h IM) or a cephalosporin (e.g., cephalothin, cephazolin) (20 mg/kg q6–8h IV).
  - If sepsis or peritonitis occurs or is suspected, add gentamicin (Gentocin; 2 mg/kg q8h SC or IM) or amikacin (Amikin; 5 mg/kg q8h IM or IV). However, if renal failure is present, adjust the aminoglycoside dosage or choose an alternative antibiotic.
- Control DIC:
  - Prevent by IV fluid therapy to promote perfusion of the microcirculation.
  - To prevent microthrombi, give minidose heparin (10 units/kg q8h SC)
  - To treat overt DIC, see Chap. 21.
- Control oliguria:
  - Prevent by vigorous IV fluid therapy to control hypovolemia.
  - If oliguria occurs (<1 ml urine/kg/h), give furosemide (Lasix; 2 mg/kg IV; repeat once or twice at up to 4–6 mg/kg, if necessary). For refractory oliguria, give a constant-rate infusion of dopamine as described in Chapter 97.
- Control hyperglycemia (if glucose exceeds 300 mg/dl) with short-acting regular crystalline zinc insulin (see Chap. 32).
- Control cardiac arrhythmias if they occur (see Chaps. 62 and 63).
- Control noncardiogenic pulmonary edema if it occurs (see Chap. 78).

Treat Chronic Complications and Sequelae

- Surgical intervention is indicated for management of septic peritonitis (see Chap. 96), for drainage or excision of pancreatic abscesses, and for cholecystoduodenostomy (after active pancreatitis is resolved) to relieve persistent biliary obstruction.
- Insulin is indicated if persistent hyperglycemia consistent with diabetes mellitus occurs (see Chap. 32).
- Pancreatic enzyme supplementation is indicated for exocrine pancreatic insufficiency (see discussion later in this chapter).

Prevent Recurrences

- Identify and control underlying risk factors (see previous discussion under Etiology).
- Feed a fat-restricted diet and avoid "treats."

Surgical Treatment of Pancreatitis

Medical treatment, as outlined in this chapter, is preferred for most animals with pancreatitis. However, surgery may be appropriate in certain situations. The decision to operate on an animal with pancreatitis is very difficult because such patients frequently are poor anesthetic and surgical risks. The surgical procedure may cause the animal's overall condition to worsen. Consider all options and thoroughly discuss the prognosis and potential complications with the owner prior to surgery.

Indications for Surgery

- *Failure to respond to appropriate medical therapy*—Assuming an accurate diagnosis, consider an exploratory laparotomy if the patient's condition deteriorates or does not improve with medical treatment.
- *Presence of a pancreatic abscess or other mass*—Consider surgery if repeated ultrasonographic examinations reveal persistence or enlargement of a pancreatic abscess or other mass and if the patient's condition dictates aggressive action.
- *Severe icterus due to extrahepatic biliary obstruction*—As previously discussed, inflammation and tissue swelling associated with pancreatitis can cause biliary obstruction. Ultrasonography is helpful in making this diagnosis. If the obstruction and associated icterus does not improve with medical therapy, surgical exploration and biliary decompression may be necessary.
- *Severe pancreatitis and septic peritonitis*—Severe peritonitis may occur with pancreatitis (see Chap. 96). Surgical lavage and drainage may be necessary.

Preoperative Considerations

- Thoroughly assess the animal and review the history and clinical course of events.
- Consider patient factors that may increase the complication rate, such as age, debilitation, sepsis, hypoproteinemia, DIC, diabetes mellitus, and disorders of other organ systems.
- Determine the coagulation status in animals with severe pancreatitis and possible DIC.

Surgical Procedure

Objectives

- Surgically expose the pancreas and determine type and extent of disease; remove devitalized tissue.
- Thoroughly explore the abdominal cavity for evidence of associated lesions or other problems.
- Lavage the peritoneal cavity to remove necrotic tissue debris, toxins, enzymes, and exudate.
- Provide drainage in cases of severe peritonitis.

Equipment

- Standard general surgery pack and suture
- 5 Fr. infant feeding tube or red rubber tube

Technique

1. Aseptically prepare the ventral abdomen.
2. Perform a standard ventral midline abdominal approach from the xyphoid to the pubis.
3. Expose the pancreas by exteriorizing the small intestine and retracting the duodenum ventrally. Expose the left limb of the pancreas by retracting the transverse colon caudally.
4. Carefully and gently examine the pancreas for masses, abscesses, inflammation, and necrosis.
5. Gently break down adhesions and open areas of abscessation digitally to establish ventral drainage. Obtain samples of fluid or tissue for bacterial culture. Carefully and judiciously debride necrotic pancreatic tissue and fat. Do not disrupt the pancreatic blood supply during dissection (see Chap. 33 under description of partial pancreatectomy). Minimize trauma to normal or non-necrotic pancreatic tissues. Submit all tissues for histopathology.
6. Consider omentalization of large pancreatic abscesses or cysts. Grasp the caudal edge of the greater omentum and place it into the abscess cavity. Place several tacking sutures (synthetic nonabsorbable) from the omentum to the edges of the abscess cavity. As in omentalization of prostatic abscesses (see Chap. 105), the omentum will provide increased blood flow and lymphatic drainage, and fill dead space.
7. Carefully examine the gallbladder and biliary ducts for evidence of obstruction.
   a. Gently squeeze the gallbladder to determine if bile is expressible through the common bile duct.
   b. Consider retrograde catheterization of the common bile duct, using an infant feeding tube, if complete obstruction is suspected. A stent catheter can be left in the common bile duct if necessary (see Chap. 92). This procedure is somewhat risky because a duodenotomy is necessary and duodenal healing may be impaired by the severe local inflammation created by the pancreatitis.
8. Thoroughly lavage the peritoneal cavity with warm sterile saline.
9. Establish abdominal drainage by leaving the abdomen open (see Chap. 96) if severe peritonitis is present or if abscesses were opened during the pancreatic exploration. Otherwise, close the abdomen routinely.

Postoperative Care and Complications

- Maintain all aspects of medical therapy for pancreatitis (see previous discussion in this chapter). Consider plasma transfusions for hypoproteinemia and whole blood transfusions for postoperative anemia (PCV <20%).
- See Chap. 33 for postoperative care of the partial pancreatectomy patient.
- See Chap. 96 for postoperative care of peritonitis.
- Consider total parenteral nutrition for animals with severe pancreatitis and open abdominal drainage.
- See under Medical Treatment in this chapter for dietary recommendations.
- Complications include septic shock, hypoproteinemia, worsening of pancreatitis and peritonitis, abdominal pain, and dehiscence of intestinal incisions.

Prognosis

Although most patients recover, pancreatitis is a life-threatening disease that frequently has a prolonged and unpredictable clinical course; thus, a guarded prognosis is warranted. The prognosis is poor when pancreatitis is complicated by septic shock, DIC, acute renal failure, or bowel infarction.

EXOCRINE PANCREATIC INSUFFICIENCY

Exocrine pancreatic insufficiency (EPI) occurs when severe progressive loss of acinar tissue from atrophy or inflammatory destruction results in insufficient secretion of digestive enzymes and clinical signs of malabsorption.

Etiology

Juvenile Pancreatic Acinar Atrophy

The most common cause of EPI is noninflammatory pancreatic acinar atrophy (PAA) of young dogs. The etiology of PAA is not known. Many breeds can be affected, especially large breeds. The highest incidence is in the German shepherd, in which the predisposition to PAA may be inherited as an autosomal recessive trait.

Chronic Relapsing Pancreatitis

The end stage of slowly progressive inflammatory destruction of the pancreas is fibrosis and atrophy, which can result in EPI. Substantial islet destruction can result in concurrent diabetes mellitus. Any breed of dog can be affected, but most are smaller breeds and are middle-aged or older. Chronic pancreatitis or pancreatic duct occlusion can cause EPI in cats but is very rare.

Clinical Signs

The pathogenesis of malabsorption in EPI may involve not only impaired intraluminal digestion but also altered intestinal mucosal function and morphology, as well as overgrowth of bacteria within the lumen of the small intestine in many cases.

- Onset of signs in dogs with PAA is typically before 2 years of age, although occasionally it can occur later than this. Pancreatitis-induced EPI can occur at any age but most often is recognized in middle-aged and older dogs.
- Weight loss or failure to gain weight can occur despite a ravenous appetite and increased food intake. Intense hunger may cause pica and coprophagia in some dogs.
- Diarrhea from maldigestion and malabsorption of fat, carbohydrates, and protein is characterized by large volumes of soft, semi-formed or unformed, fatty feces with a rancid odor. The diarrhea may improve substantially with fasting or with feeding of a highly digestible or fat-restricted diet.
- Borborygmus and flatulence may occur.
- The hair coat is dull and poor in quality, with excessive shedding and greasy, oily hair around the perineum.

Diagnosis

- Diarrhea and weight loss are nonspecific signs that must be differentiated from other causes of intestinal malabsorption.
- Routine CBC, serum chemistries, urinalysis, and radiographs are generally unremarkable in EPI.
- For a discussion of the differential diagnosis of chronic diarrhea, see Chap. 89.

Fecal Microscopy

The examination of Sudan and iodine-stained fecal smears for steatorrhea (excessive fat in the feces) and amylorrhea (excessive undigested starch in the feces) can be used as preliminary in-office screening procedures; however, sensitivity and specificity are fairly low.

- Direct Sudan stain—Detects excessive undigested fat (neutral, unsplit) as numerous large refractile orange droplets, indicating steatorrhea of pancreatic maldigestion.
- Indirect Sudan stain—The addition of acetic acid and heating renders fatty acids (split fat) stainable as well; thus, numerous droplets in a fecal specimen that is negative by direct Sudan staining suggest steatorrhea caused by malabsorption of fatty acids.
- Lugol iodine stain—Detects undigested starch as blue-black granules, suggesting amylorrhea of pancreatic maldigestion.

Serum Trypsin-like Immunoreactivity (TLI) Assay

The serum TLI assay is highly sensitive and specific for detection of EPI. This test measures total circulating trypsinogen and trypsin in a single fasted serum sample and is available on a mail-out basis at selected veterinary laboratories (Table 93–4).

▼ *Key Point* The serum TLI assay is the test of choice for confirmation of EPI. In normal dogs and in dogs with intestinal disease, serum TLI is 5 to 35 μg/L. In dogs with EPI, serum TLI is consistently <2.5 μg/L. In cats with EPI, serum fTLI is <8.0 μg/L (normal, 7–49 μg/L).

Oral Bentiromide Digestion Test

The oral bentiromide (N-benzoyl-L-tyrosyl-P-aminobenzoic acid, or BT-PABA) test is not as accurate or easy to perform as the TLI assay. After administration of the bentiromide test substrate, a chymotrypsin-labile peptide (Chymex; Adria Labs.) (16.7 mg/kg PO), serum

Table 93–4. NORMAL VALUES FOR PANCREATIC FUNCTION TESTS

Test	Canine	Feline
Serum TLI assay*	5–35 μg/L	17–49 μg/L
Bentiromide test (peak PABA)	≥5.0 μg/ml	≥2.0 μg/ml
Radial enzyme diffusion (3-day mean)*	6–24 mm	6–17 mm
Azocasein hydrolysis (3-day mean)	19–200 ACU/g	29–207 ACU/g
Serum cobalamin*	225–660 ng/L	200–1680 ng/L
Serum folate*	6.7–17.4 μg/L	13.4–38.0 μg/L

*Available as mail-in test through Gastrointestinal Laboratory, Department of Small Animal Medicine and Surgery, College of Veterinary Medicine, Texas A&M University, College Station, TX.

TLI = trypsin-like immunoreactivity; PABA = para-aminobenzoic acid; ACU = azocasein units.

samples are taken at 60 and 90 minutes and assayed for free PABA (see Table 93–4).

- Dogs with EPI, because they secrete very little chymotrypsin, develop a negligible rise in plasma PABA; however, false-positive and false-negative results sometimes occur.
- In cats, PABA levels are lower and less consistent than in dogs, but nevertheless a minimal rise in plasma PABA suggests EPI (see Table 93–4).

Assays of Fecal Proteolytic Activity

Assays of fecal proteolytic activity by azocasein hydrolysis or radial enzyme diffusion are indirect methods of evaluating pancreatic function.

- Because the serum TLI assay is more reliable and practical, it is preferred over fecal proteolytic assays for diagnosis of EPI.
- Fecal specimens are collected on each of 3 consecutive days and immediately frozen for shipment to the laboratory (see Table 93–4).

Measurement of Serum Folate and Cobalamin

Serum folate and cobalamin (vitamin B_{12}) levels reflect intestinal absorptive function and the status of the intestinal flora. In addition, normal pancreatic secretions may have an influence. For normal values, see Table 93–4.

- Serum folate and cobalamin levels may be decreased in cats with EPI. This occurs in enteropathies that cause intestinal malabsorption.
- In small intestinal bacterial overgrowth, which commonly occurs in dogs with EPI, serum folate levels may be increased due to synthesis of folate by the overgrown bacteria, and cobalamin may be decreased because bacteria can utilize or bind the vitamin, making it unavailable for absorption.
- Deficiency of pancreatic intrinsic factor in EPI may contribute to the frequent finding of low cobalamin levels; enhanced folate absorption due to intestinal acidification may contribute to an increased serum folate.

Treatment

Pancreatic Enzyme Replacement

- Dried bovine or porcine pancreatic extracts are available commercially as tablets, capsules, powders, granules, and enteric-coated preparations; enzyme content and bioavailability varies widely.
- Pancreatin powder preparations are recommended (Viokase-V, Fort Dodge; Pancrezyme, Daniels). Add 1–2 tsp per meal to the food just prior to feeding and divide the daily food intake into 2–3 meals per day.
- When the diarrhea is in remission and the animal is gaining weight, titrate to the minimum effective maintenance dose (1 tsp added to each of two meals daily is adequate for most dogs).

- In cats that refuse food with commercial pancreatic extracts, give 1–3 oz. of chopped raw bovine pancreas with each meal.

▼ *Key Point* The effectiveness of enzyme supplementation is not increased by concurrent use of antacids, sodium bicarbonate, bile acids, or preincubation of enzymes with the food prior to feeding. Enteric-coated preparations and uncrushed tablets are less effective than powdered pancreatic extracts.

Diet

- Most dogs with EPI can be fed a maintenance diet; however, if the response to enzyme supplementation is incomplete, substitute a diet that is highly digestible, low in fiber, and mildly restricted in fat (e.g., Prescription Diet i/d; Hill's Pet).
- In treated dogs that fail to gain desired weight, provide supplemental calories in the form of medium chain triglycerides (MCT Oil, Mead Johnson; 1–2 ml/kg per day added to meals). Unlike conventional dietary fat, MCTs do not require lipolysis by pancreatic lipase for absorption. Discontinue MCT if it impairs appetite.
- Consider multivitamin supplementation, especially the fat-soluble vitamins (A, D, E, and K). Cobalamin and tocopherol are often severely depleted in dogs with EPI; thus, give high dosages initially for repletion: cobalamin (vitamin B_{12}), 500 μg, SC once or twice per month for 2–3 months; and tocopherol (vitamin E), 500 units PO daily for the first month. Cats are given cobalamin, 100–250 μg SC weekly for 6–8 weeks. Vitamin K–responsive coagulopathies have been reported in cats with EPI.

What to Do if There Is Failure to Respond

- *Step 1:* Adjust diet and enzyme brand, form, and dosage according to the above recommendations; if there is no response, go to Step 2.
- *Step 2:* Administer antibiotics (e.g., doxycycline, metronidazole, tylosin) for small intestinal bacterial overgrowth (see Chap. 89). If there is no response, go to Step 3.
- *Step 3:* Administer an oral H_2-receptor blocker with meals, such as, cimetidine (Tagamet, 10 mg/kg) or ranitidine (Zantac, 2 mg/kg), to reduce acidic inactivation of enzymes. These reduce activity of gastric lipase and may not be effective for improving overall digestion. If there is no response, go to Step 4.
- *Step 4:* Reassess diagnosis and evaluate for intestinal mucosal disease via endoscopic biopsy.

PANCREATIC NEOPLASIA

Pancreatic neoplasms can be hormone-secreting tumors that arise from islet cells (insulinoma and gastrinoma are discussed in Chap. 33), or they can arise from the exocrine pancreas as adenomas or adenocarcinomas of acinar or duct cell origin. Exocrine pancreatic adenomas are rare and usually unassociated with clinical signs. Exocrine pancreatic adenocarcinomas are more common and are discussed here. These are highly malignant and metastasize early to the liver, regional lymph nodes, mesentery, duodenum, stomach, and occasionally the lungs, often prior to the onset of clinical signs.

Clinical Signs

- Clinical signs are usually insidious and nonspecific, often mimicking chronic pancreatitis. Vomiting, anorexia, depression, and abdominal pain are usually noted first.
- Bile duct obstruction or extensive liver metastases may lead to jaundice.
- Duodenal invasion and obstruction may lead to persistent intractable vomiting.
- Peritoneal carcinomatosis may lead to peritoneal effusion.

Diagnosis

- Suspect pancreatic adenocarcinoma when a right cranial abdominal mass is identified by palpation, abdominal radiography, or abdominal ultrasonography in an animal with signs of chronic pancreatitis or obstructive hepatopathy. Serum bilirubin and liver enzymes usually are elevated.
- Exploratory laparotomy and surgical biopsy are usually required for definitive diagnosis. Because chronic pancreatitis and pancreatic adenocarcinoma can have a similar gross appearance, histopathologic evaluation is necessary.

Treatment

Attempted surgical resection (pancreatectomy; see Chap. 33) is sometimes palliative (e.g., for relief of bile duct or duodenal obstruction); however, in most cases surgery is not beneficial and virtually is never curative. Adjunctive chemotherapy can be used, but it also is of minimal benefit and efficacy.

SUPPLEMENTAL READINGS

The pancreas. *In* Guilford WG, Center SA, Strombeck DR, et al (eds): Strombeck's Small Animal Gastroenterology, 3rd Ed. Philadelphia, WB Saunders, 1996, p 381.

94 Anorectal Diseases

Robert G. Sherding

The presenting signs of anorectal disease can include any of the following: dyschezia, hematochezia, constipation, anal discomfort (licking, scooting), ribbon-like feces, fecal incontinence, anal discharge, foul perianal odor, matting of perianal hair, and perianal dermatitis. Physical examination establishes the diagnosis of anorectal disease in most cases. In many anorectal diseases, surgery is required for effective treatment.

CONSTIPATION

Constipation is a clinical sign characterized by absent, infrequent, or difficult defecation associated with retention of feces within the colon and rectum. When feces are retained for a prolonged period of time they become progressively harder and drier and, eventually, impacted as the mucosa continues to absorb water from the fecal mass. Terms associated with constipation are defined below.

Obstipation. A condition of intractable constipation in which the colon and rectum become so impacted with excessively hard feces that defecation cannot occur.

Dyschezia. A clinical sign often associated with constipation, characterized by difficult or painful evacuation of feces from the rectum and usually associated with lesions in or near the anal region.

Tenesmus. A clinical sign characterized by straining to defecate, usually ineffectively or painfully; thus, it usually accompanies dyschezia.

Megacolon. A disorder (not a sign) in which the colon becomes severely and irreversibly dilated and hypomotile. Megacolon usually is idiopathic and is an important cause of chronic constipation and obstipation in cats. It can also occur secondary to chronic pelvic canal stenoses.

Etiology

Underlying causes of or predisposing factors for constipation are listed in Table 94–1 and include dietary factors, environmental factors, painful defecation, anorectal or colonic obstruction, neuromuscular diseases, fluid and electrolyte disturbances, and drug-related effects.

- *Ingested foreign material,* such as indigestible fibrous material (especially hair in cats from their grooming behavior) and abrasives (especially bones in dogs), may become incorporated in the fecal mass and result in the formation of hard fecal impactions that are difficult and painful to evacuate from the colon.

- *Environmental factors* that are not conducive to defecation or that vary from the daily routine to which the animal is accustomed may cause the animal to inhibit the urge to defecate, leading to constipation. For example, this may occur when an animal is kept in strange surroundings, such as in a kennel or veterinary hospital, or when its daily outdoor exercise routine is changed. Cats often suppress the urge to defecate when their litter box is dirty.

- *Painful defecation* caused by anorectal diseases (anal sacculitis, perianal fistulas) or orthopedic disorders that limit positioning for defecation (diseases of the pelvis, spine, or hips) often result in voluntary inhibition of defecation and lead to constipation.

- *Anorectal or colonic obstruction* that mechanically impedes the passage of feces may result from intraluminal causes, such as foreign bodies, perineal hernia, and stenosing neoplastic or inflammatory lesions, or from extraluminal causes, such as prostatic enlargement, compressive pelvic fractures, and pseudocoprostasis (feces matted in perianal hair).

- *Neuromuscular disorders* may lead to constipation by interfering with colonic innervation or smooth muscle function or the ability of the animal to assume the normal defecation stance. For example, this may occur in association with disease or injury of the lumbosacral spinal cord (canine intervertebral disc disease), spinal deformity (e.g., in Manx cats), endocrine disease (hypothyroidism), and dysautonomia, a progressively fatal autonomic polyneuropathy of young cats. When innervation of the anus is also impaired, fecal incontinence may be an associated clinical sign. The pathogenesis of idiopathic megacolon is poorly characterized but probably involves a primary or secondary dysfunction of colonic smooth muscle.

- *Fluid and electrolyte disorders* may predispose to constipation. Dehydration can cause the feces to become excessively dry and hard. Hypokalemia and hypercalcemia can affect colonic smooth muscle function. A combination of these may explain the frequent constipation seen in chronic renal failure patients.

- *Drug-induced constipation* may be a side effect of motility-modifying drugs (anticholinergics, opiates, opioids), antihistamines, barium sulfate, aluminum hydroxide, and diuretics.

Table 94–1. CLASSIFICATION AND CAUSES OF CONSTIPATION

Category	Cause
Dietary	Ingested foreign material mixed with feces (hair, bones, cloth, garbage, cat litter, rocks, plant material)
	Inadequate water intake
Environmental/ psychological	Dirty litter box
	Prolonged inactivity
	Confinement (hospitalization, boarding)
	Change in habitat or daily routine
Painful defecation	Anorectal disorders:
	Anal sac impaction, infection, or abscess
	Anorectal stricture, tumor or foreign body
	Myiasis
	Perianal fistulae
	Perianal bite wound cellulitis or abscess
	Pseudocoprostasis
	Orthopedic disorders
	Spinal disease or injury
	Injuries of the pelvis, hip joints, or pelvic limbs
Rectocolonic obstruction	Extramural
	Prostatic hypertrophy, tumor, abscess, or prostatitis
	Paraprostatic cyst
	Pelvic fracture (malunion)
	Pelvic collapse due to nutritional bone disease
	Perianal tumor
	Pseudocoprostasis
	Intramural or intraluminal
	Rectocolonic stricture, tumor, or foreign body
	Rectal diverticulum or perineal hernia
	Rectal prolapse
	Fecolith
Neuromuscular dysfunction	Lumbosacral spinal cord disease (injury, deformity, degeneration, neoplasia)
	Bilateral pelvic nerve injury
	Dysautonomia (Key-Gaskell syndrome)
	Hypothyroidism
	Idiopathic megacolon
Fluid and electrolyte abnormalities	Dehydration (e.g., chronic renal disease)
	Hypokalemia
	Hypercalcemia (hyperparathyroidism)
Drug-induced	Anticholinergics
	Adrenergic blockers
	Calcium channel blockers
	Phenothiazines and benzodiazepines
	Opiates and opioids
	Diuretics
	Antihistamines
	Aluminum hydroxide antacids
	Sucralfate
	Kaolin-pectin
	Barium sulfate
	Iron
	Laxatives (chronic overuse)

Clinical Signs

- Constipated animals are usually presented because of failure to defecate over a period of days. The owner may notice tenesmus or frequent attempts to defecate with little or no passage of feces.
- Dyschezia usually indicates anorectal disease. The animal first may cry out as it attempts to defecate, usu-

ally with straining (tenesmus) during the attempt; then it may cease the effort, walk around anxiously, and repeatedly try again.
- Mucosal irritation caused by impacted feces may provoke a secretion of fluid and mucus, which bypasses the retained fecal mass and is expelled paradoxically as diarrhea during attempts to defecate.
- Other signs may include anorexia, lethargy, vomiting, dehydration, and a hunched-up appearance caused by abdominal discomfort.
- Constipation tends to be a recurrent problem.

Diagnosis

▼ **Key Point** The presence of constipation usually is determined from the history and confirmed by rectal and abdominal palpation of colonic distention with hard feces. The goal of diagnosis is to identify predisposing factors (see Table 94–1).

History

Identify dietary, environmental, behavioral, psychological, and medication-related factors or predispositions.

Physical Examination

- Perform a digital anorectal examination to detect painful or obstructive lesions of the anorectum.
- Perform a neurologic examination (see Chap. 144) to identify any underlying neurologic causes of constipation.
- Evaluate the pelvic limbs, coxofemoral joints, pelvis, and lumbosacral spine for orthopedic problems that could cause difficulty maneuvering into the defecation stance or painful defecation.
- In cats with constipation caused by dysautonomia (Key-Gaskell syndrome), additional manifestations of progressive autonomic failure that may be seen include urinary and fecal incontinence, megaesophagus, bradycardia, mydriasis, decreased lacrimation, and prolapse of the nictitating membranes.

Routine Laboratory Evaluations

Perform a serum biochemical profile, urinalysis, and complete blood count (CBC) to:

- Evaluate animals with recurrent constipation to identify underlying systemic disease (e.g., chronic renal failure) that could cause constipation due to dehydration or electrolyte disturbances.
- Evaluate severely constipated or obstipated animals, especially those that are vomiting or markedly depressed, in order to detect the metabolic consequences of prolonged fecal retention, such as fluid and electrolyte imbalances, endotoxemia, and azotemia, and to guide supportive treatment.

Thyroid Function Testing

Evaluate thyroid function in dogs with recurrent constipation and other signs compatible with hypothyroidism (see Chap. 29).

Abdominal Radiography

Perform abdominal radiography to:

- Confirm the extent of colonic impaction with densely packed feces.
- Identify the extreme dilation of the colon that indicates megacolon.
- Identify radiopaque foreign material (e.g., bone chips) in the retained feces that indicates a dietary cause of constipation.
- Identify pelvic, coxofemoral, or spinal lesions that can cause constipation.
- Identify underlying prostatic enlargement that might cause constipation.

Barium Enema Contrast Radiography or Colonoscopy

Perform after removal of retained feces to evaluate the lumen of the colon when intraluminal obstructive lesions are suspected.

Myelographic and Electrodiagnostic Evaluation

Perform to evaluate the lumbosacral spinal cord and spinal nerves (see Chaps. 144 and 147) in selected patients in which impaired anorectal innervation is suspected.

Treatment

- Mild constipation resolves spontaneously or is treated on an outpatient basis by dietary adjustments and oral or suppository laxatives.
- Severe constipation initially may require evacuation of impacted feces from the colon (using enemas or manual extraction or both) along with correction of complicating dehydration and electrolyte imbalances.
- Additional therapeutic goals are to eliminate or control any underlying causes of constipation (see Table 94–1) that are identified and to prevent recurrences using dietary adjustments and laxative therapy as needed.
- Obstructing neoplasms, strictures, and many anorectal disorders require surgical correction.
- Long-term management of megacolon or recurrent obstipation that is unresponsive to medical therapy in the cat may require subtotal colectomy (see Chap. 90).

Oral Laxative Therapy

Oral laxative medications and dietary supplements can be prescribed as needed for control of constipation (Table 94–2). Laxatives act on intestinal mucosal fluid transport and colonic motility and are classified by their properties and mechanisms of action as bulk-forming, lubricant, emollient, osmotic, or stimulant. The use of an oral laxative often must be individualized by adjusting the dose until the desired frequency of defecation and fecal consistency is obtained.

High-Fiber Bulk-Forming Laxatives.   These laxatives are added to food to promote soft feces and normal colonic motility as the initial approach for long-term control of constipation. These bulk-forming agents are nonabsorbable polysaccharide and cellulose derivatives that exhibit hydrophilic properties within the bowel.

This method of treatment is available as commercially prepared high-fiber diets (e.g., Prescription Diet w/d, Hill's Pet Products) or as fiber additives for the regular diet, such as unprocessed wheat bran, pumpkin pie filling, or commercial sources of psyllium (see Table 94–2).

Lubricant Laxatives.   Laxatives such as mineral oil and petrolatum products are used to soften and lubricate the feces to facilitate evacuation (see Table 94–2).

- Administer lubricants between meals so that they do not interfere with the absorption of fat-soluble vitamins.
- Avoid using mineral oil because its tastelessness can lead to inhalation lipid pneumonia; if necessary to use, always add flavoring and administer cautiously.

Emollient Laxatives.   Docusate sodium (available in enema and oral forms), docusate calcium, and docusate potassium are mild laxatives that promote water penetration into the feces, thereby softening the feces (see Table 94–2).

- Do not mix docusate and mineral oil.

Osmotic Laxatives.   These laxatives consist of poorly absorbed disaccharides (e.g., lactose or lactulose), ions (e.g., magnesium hydroxide, magnesium citrate), or inert osmotic agents (e.g., polyethylene glycol) that osmotically retain water in the bowel lumen to produce soft or fluid feces.

- A mild osmotic laxative effect can be produced in some animals by the addition of milk (lactose) to the diet in a quantity that exceeds the digestive capacity of small intestinal lactase, or by the administration of the nonabsorbable disaccharide lactulose (see Table 94–2). Excessive amounts of fermentable carbohydrates can cause abdominal discomfort and flatulence.

▼ *Key Point* Lactulose is an excellent choice as a safe and effective all-purpose laxative for both dogs and cats. Lactulose can be expensive for long-term use in large-breed dogs.

- Magnesium hydroxide is available as an over-the-counter drug (see Table 94–2). Magnesium is contraindicated in patients with renal failure.
- Magnesium citrate and polyethylene glycol-electrolyte solutions (see Table 94–2) are used as cathartics for preparation of the bowel for colonoscopy. The large doses required depend on administration by orogastric intubation, which limits their use for routine treatment of constipation.

Stimulant Laxatives.   Stimulant laxatives increase propulsive motility of the bowel. They are contraindicated in the presence of an obstructive lesion.

- Cisapride (see Table 94–2) is the most effective prokinetic drug for stimulating colonic motility.
- Ranitidine and nizatidine (see Table 94–2) are H_2-blockers that also stimulate GI and colonic motility through inhibition of synaptic acetylcholinesterase which increases acetylcholine.

Table 94–2. LAXATIVE THERAPY FOR CONSTIPATION

Treatment	Product (Manufacturer)	Dose Regimen
Oral Cathartics		
Bulk-forming laxatives		
Coarse bran	All-Bran (Kellogg) and others	1–5 tbsp daily with food
Canned pumpkin	Pie filling (Libby)	1–5 tbsp daily with food
Psyllium	Metamucil (Searle)	1–5 tsp daily with food
High-fiber diet	Prescription Diet w/d (Hill's)	Use as daily food source
Lubricant-laxatives		
White petrolatum	Laxatone (EVSCO)	1–5 ml daily PO
Mineral oil*	Many	5–25 ml daily (flavored)
Emollient laxatives		
Docusate sodium	Colace (Mead Johnson)	*Cat:* 50 mg daily PO
		Dog: 50–200 mg daily PO
Docusate calcium	Surfak (Hoechst-Roussel)	*Cat:* 50–100 mg daily PO
		Dog: 100–240 mg daily PO
Saline laxative		
Magnesium hydroxide	Phillips Milk of Magnesia (Glenbrook)	2–8 tablets daily PO
Osmotic laxatives		
Lactose	Milk	Add to diet to effect
Lactulose	Duphalac Syrup (Reid-Powell); Cephulac (Marion Merrell Dow)	0.5–1.0 ml/kg; q8–12hr PO
Polyethylene glycol and electrolytes†	Colyte (Reed & Carnick); GoLYTELY (Braintree)	25–40 ml/kg PO; repeat in 2–4hr (for bowel prep)
Motility stimulant laxatives		
Bisacodyl	Dulcolax (Boehringer Ingelheim)	*Cat:* 5 mg daily, PO
		Dog: 5–20 mg daily, PO
Cisapride	Propulsid (Janssen)	*Cat:* 1.0 mg/kg q8h or 1.5 mg/kg q12h, PO
		Dog: 0.25–0.5 mg/kg q8-12h PO
Ranitidine	Zantac (Glaxo)	*Cat:* 3.5 mg/kg q12h PO
		Dog: 2.0 mg/kg q12h PO
Nizatidine	Axid (Eli Lilly)	2.5 mg/kg q24h PO
Castor oil†	Many	5–30 ml, PO (bowel prep)
Enemas and Suppositories		
Enemas		
Warm tap water		5–10 ml/kg
Isotonic saline solution		5–10 ml/kg
Docusate sodium	Colace (Mead Johnson)	5–30 ml
Mineral oil	Many	5–30 ml or 1–2 ml/kg
Sodium phosphate‡	Fleet Children's Enema (Fleet)	1–2 ml/kg or 1 enema unit
Bisacodyl	Fleet Bisacodyl Enema (Fleet)	1–2 ml/kg or 1 enema unit
Rectal suppositories		
Glycerin	Many	1–3 pediatric
Docusate sodium	Colace (Mead Johnson)	1–3 pediatric
Bisacodyl	Dulcolax (Boehringer Ingelheim)	1–3 pediatric

Caution: may cause lipid aspiration pneumonia and may interfere with absorption of fat-soluble vitamins; combination with docusate may cause undesirable absorption of mineral oil.

†Used mainly to prepare the colon for radiography or endoscopy.

‡Do *not* use in cats or small dogs.

- Bisacodyl (see Table 94–2) works by stimulating colonic smooth muscle and the myenteric plexus. Although beneficial on a short-term basis in conjunction with measures to soften the feces, long-term use may damage the myenteric plexus.
- Castor oil is hydrolyzed in the intestines to ricinoleic acid, which stimulates colonic motility and secretion. Castor oil is not very useful for outpatient treatment because of poor patient acceptance, but it is effective for preparing the bowel for radiographic or endoscopic procedures.

Enema Therapy

Enema solutions are used to soften hard impacted feces and promote evacuation. Warm the enema solution prior to instillation and administer the calculated dose slowly so as not to induce vomiting. Commonly used enema solutions (see Table 94–2) include:

- Warm isotonic saline or tap water (5–10 ml/kg body weight), with or without the addition of a mild soap to stimulate defecation by an irritant effect (soap must not contain hexachlorophene because of its neurotoxicity)
- Docusate as an emollient
- Mineral oil as a lubricant
- Sodium phosphate solution, which has softening, bulk-producing, and irritant effects (safe to use only in medium-sized and large dogs with normal renal function)

▼ *Key Point* Caution! Never use phosphate enemas in cats or small dogs because they may cause dangerous hypernatremia, hyperosmolality, hyper-phosphatemia, and hypocalcemia. Do not mix mineral oil and docusate; docusate promotes mucosal absorption of mineral oil, whereas mineral oil coats the feces, reducing the emollient effect of docusate.

Manual Evacuation of Impacted Feces

- In severe constipation or obstipation, restore fluid and electrolyte balance parenterally and evacuate the colon manually under general anesthesia using a combination of:
  - Colonic irrigation with warm isotonic saline as an enema solution to soften the impacted feces
  - Extraction of retained fecal masses by gentle transabdominal manipulation to milk the feces into the distal rectum for digital or forceps removal (can use a sponge or whelping forceps)
- To avoid excessive bowel trauma in animals with extensive fecal impaction, it may be advisable to evacuate the colon manually in stages over a period of 2–3 days.

Prevention and Ancillary Treatment

Following evacuation of retained feces from the colon, institute measures to prevent and control recurrences of constipation. Identify and eliminate or correct underlying causes or predisposing factors (see Table 94–1).

- Prevent ingestion of constipating or abrasive materials such as bones.
- Prevent hair ingestion by adopting a routine of regular grooming to remove loose hair from the animal's hair coat before it can be ingested.
- Provide dogs a daily exercise routine and frequent opportunities to defecate.
- Provide cats with clean litter at all times to encourage regular defecation.
- Provide access to fresh water at all times to encourage water intake.
- Adjust or discontinue the use of any medications that promote constipation.
- Treat predisposing prostatic, endocrine (hypothyroidism), spinal, and orthopedic disorders.
- Correct, whenever possible, painful or obstructing anorectal lesions, by surgery if necessary (see Chap. 95).

▼ *Key Point* For severe recurrent constipation, obstipation, or megacolon that is unresponsive to medical management in the cat, subtotal colectomy is an effective method of treatment (see Chap. 90).

PSEUDOCOPROSTASIS

Etiology

Pseudocoprostasis is a condition of obstruction of the anal opening when the surrounding hair becomes densely matted with feces. It occurs most often in long-haired breeds of dogs and cats, especially during bouts of diarrhea.

Clinical Signs

The anal obstruction leads to anal irritation, inability to pass feces, and constipation.

- The animal usually is restless and attempts to bite or lick the anal region.
- The owner may complain of an unexplained foul odor from the animal.

The matted hair often results in an underlying dermatitis and in warm weather attracts flies that may produce a maggot infestation (myiasis) of the anal area.

Diagnosis

Examination of the anal region is sufficient for diagnosis.

Treatment

- Clip hair mats, cleanse the underlying irritated skin, and apply a topical antibiotic ointment. When the obstructing hair mats are removed, defecation should occur normally.
- If the animal has severe colonic impaction of feces, measures to evacuate the colon may be required (see under Constipation).

PROCTITIS

Proctitis, or inflammation of the rectum, can cause tenesmus, diarrhea, and hematochezia. Therefore, it must be differentiated from other anorectal diseases. Because proctitis usually is a component of colitis, it is discussed under Colitis in Chap. 89.

ANORECTAL PROLAPSE

Etiology

Anorectal prolapse usually is a consequence of an underlying disorder that produces persistent straining; thus it is associated with:

- Intestinal diseases that cause diarrhea and tenesmus
- Anorectal diseases that cause dyschezia
- Lower urinary tract and prostatic diseases that cause stranguria
- Dystocia

Clinical Signs

- Partial prolapse involves only the rectal mucosa and appears as a red, swollen, doughnut-shaped ring of prolapsed mucosa.
- Complete prolapse involves all layers of the rectal wall and appears as an edematous cylindrical-shaped mass. The prolapsed tissue may be viable (pink or red and moist) or necrotic (blackened and dry).

Diagnosis

Insert a thermometer or finger in the space between the prolapsed tissue and anal sphincter to probe for a cul-de-sac. If there is none and resistance is not met, the prolapsed tissue is an intussusception of ileum or colon (see Chap. 89), rather than an anorectal prolapse.

Treatment

Successful management of anorectal prolapse includes repair of the prolapse and identification and treatment of the underlying cause. Evaluate the anus, rectum, intestines, and urogenital tract by palpation, urinalysis, fecal examinations, proctoscopy, and radiographic studies, as appropriate.

- Treat minor prolapse in which the tissue is viable by reduction and medical therapy to reduce tenesmus and prevent recurrence. Treatment may include:
  - Anticholinergic-antispasmodic drugs such as dicyclomine (Bentyl; Marion Merrell Dow), 0.15–0.20 mg/kg q8–12h PO or SC
  - Hydrocortisone retention enema (Cortenema; Reid-Rowell), 10–60 ml q12–24h
  - Mesalamine retention enema (RowASA; Reid-Rowell) for dogs only, at an empirical dosage of 10–60 ml q12–24h
  - Mild sedation
- A temporary (2–3 days) anal pursestring suture may be required in animals with persistent straining that produces recurrence of the prolapse. Leave the pursestring suture loose enough to allow passage of feces.
- Perform amputation when the prolapsed tissue is nonviable.

Colopexy

Consider prophylactic colopexy for recurrent prolapse.

Technique

1. Perform colopexy via a ventral midline abdominal approach.
2. Place gentle traction on the descending colon to reduce the prolapse.
3. Perform the "pexy" by scarifying the serosa of the descending colon in 3 or 4 small areas (0.5–1.0 cm diameter) and scarifying corresponding areas of the peritoneal surface of the left body wall.
4. Appose the scarified areas of colonic serosa to the peritoneum using 2-0 or 3-0 monofilament nonabsorbable sutures.

PERINEAL HERNIA

Etiology

Perineal hernia occurs when weakness of the pelvic diaphragm muscles fails to support the rectal wall, resulting in persistent rectal distention and impaired defecation. The pathogenesis of the weakened pelvic diaphragm is poorly understood; male hormones have been implicated because the disease is extremely rare in castrated dogs. Aged, intact male dogs are almost ex-

clusively affected, although perineal hernia has been reported in a few cats.

The hernia usually contains outpouched rectum and can be unilateral or bilateral; unilateral hernias are predominantly right-sided. The hernia sac may also contain retroperitoneal fat, prostate gland, and, rarely, abdominal organs such as the urinary bladder or intestine. The rectal defects associated with perineal hernia have been classified as follows:

Sacculation. Unilateral loss of support allows expansion of the rectal wall to one side.

Dilation. Bilateral loss of support allows generalized distention of the rectum.

Deviation or Flexure. The rectum curves or bends to one side within the hernia sac.

Diverticulum. An outpouching of mucosa through a defect in the rectal wall.

Clinical Signs

- Clinical signs include constipation, obstipation, dyschezia, and tenesmus.
- Stranguria may occur with herniation of the urinary bladder and associated urethral obstruction.

Diagnosis

Diagnosis is based on palpation of a reducible swelling ventrolateral to the anus and rectal palpation of the weakened pelvic diaphragm and rectal dilation.

Treatment

The goal of initial treatment is evacuation of retained feces from the rectum (see under Constipation). Urethral catheterization or cystocentesis also may be necessary initially to relieve urinary obstruction.

- In some dogs with perineal hernia, normal defecations can be maintained by laxative therapy and stool-softening diets (see under Constipation).
- Castration of dogs with mild perineal hernia may prevent progression of the disorder.
- Perineal herniorrhaphy surgery combined with castration provides the best long-lasting results in most cases (see Chap. 95).

▼ *Key Point* Always perform castration as an adjunct to perineal hernia repair.

ANORECTAL FOREIGN BODIES AND FECOLITHS

Etiology

- Ingested foreign bodies such as bones, toys, sticks, and sewing needles can sometimes pass unobtrusively through the gastrointestinal tract and become lodged transversely within the rectum or at the anal sphincter.
- Foreign objects occasionally are inserted into the anus of an animal by a malicious or deranged person.
- Aged cats sometimes present because of inability to pass a firm lump of feces (fecolith) that is lodged in

the anal canal between the internal and external sphincter.

Clinical Signs and Diagnosis

When a foreign body or fecolith is lodged in the anal canal or rectum, defecation becomes painful or impossible, and dyschezia, tenesmus, and secondary fecal impaction occur. Diagnosis is by rectal examination.

Treatment

- Most anorectal foreign bodies and fecoliths can be detected and removed by rectal palpation; sedation or anesthesia may be necessary. In some cases a proctoscope may facilitate foreign body extraction.
- There are two potentially serious complications of anorectal foreign bodies:
  - Rectal laceration resulting in retroperitoneal cellulitis
  - Anorectal stricture (see below).

ANORECTAL STRICTURE (STENOSIS)

Etiology

Strictures of the anus or rectum can result from the following causes:

- Trauma caused by passage of sharp foreign bodies (especially bones).
- Postsurgical scarring after anorectal surgery
- Chronic inflammation associated with anal sac disease, perianal fistulas, or proctitis.

Clinical Signs and Diagnosis

Anorectal strictures cause dyschezia, tenesmus, hematochezia, and secondary constipation. The stricture can usually be identified by digital rectal palpation, proctoscopy, or barium enema contrast radiography.

Treatment

Anorectal strictures usually require surgical correction (see Chap. 95).

ANAL SPASM

Etiology

This rare idiopathic form of severe dyschezia occurs when the anal sphincter contracts in spasm when the animal attempts to defecate.

Clinical Signs

When attempting to defecate, the animal may cry out in pain, move about frantically before stopping to make another attempt to defecate, turn and stare at its hindquarters, and appear extremely anxious. There appears to be a cycle of painful defecation, leading to defensive contraction of the anal sphincter, leading to more pain.

Diagnosis

- Most affected dogs are German shepherds of temperamental disposition.
- Digital palpation of the rectum is vigorously resented, and the anal sphincter muscle feels hypertrophied and tightly contracted in spasm. Visually, the external sphincter muscle appears hypertrophied.
- To attribute dyschezia to anal spasm it is important to rule out structural causes of dyschezia (e.g., anal sac disease, perianal fistulas) and to exclude anal stricture (stenosis) by thorough rectal examination under anesthesia.

Treatment

- Conservative treatment using anal sac evacuation, topical analgesics, antispasmodics, sedatives and stool softeners has not been very successful.
- Resection of one or both anal branches of the pudendal nerve is required for palliation in most dogs. Fecal incontinence often is a postoperative problem.

IMPERFORATE ANUS AND RECTAL AGENESIS

Etiology

Imperforate anus and rectal agenesis are rare congenital malformations of cloacal development that result in an absence of a patent anal opening for defecation.

Clinical Signs

Within days or weeks of birth, the affected puppy or kitten develops signs of abdominal distention and discomfort, tenesmus, restlessness, vomiting, and loss of appetite.

Diagnosis

- The diagnosis is established by absence of an anal opening. Variations in the malformation range from an imperforate anal membrane covering the anal opening (atresia ani) to varying degrees of rectal agenesis (rectal atresia) in which the rectum ends in a blind pouch at some distance cranial to the anus.
- The terminal end of the rectum can be delineated radiographically by the intraluminal air when a lateral radiograph is exposed with the animal's hind end slightly elevated.
- In some animals, imperforate anus is associated with genitourinary defects such as rectovaginal fistula.

Treatment

The treatment for atresia ani is surgical opening and removal of the retained anal membrane, usually producing favorable results (see Chap. 95). For rectal atresia, surgical correction is more difficult and requires combined abdominal surgery and rectal pull-through; thus, the prognosis is guarded.

RECTOVAGINAL FISTULA

Rectovaginal fistula is a rare congenital malformation of females characterized by passage of fecal material through the vaginal opening. In many cases there also is an imperforate anus. Persistent fecal incontinence through the vagina leads to perivulvar dermatitis. Colonic distension usually occurs when the puppy or kitten begins eating solid food. The defect can be surgically corrected but the prognosis is guarded (see Chap. 113). Other related, rare anorectal anomalies include rectovestibular fistula, anovaginal cleft, and recto-urethral fistula.

ANAL SAC DISEASE

Anal sac disorders are the most common problem of the anal area in small animals, especially dogs. Anal sac disease has been classified as impaction, inflammation (sacculitis), infection, abscess, and rupture:

- *Impaction* usually is bilateral and indicated by a sac that is distended, mildly painful on palpation, and not readily expressed. The impacted contents are thick and pasty and dark brown or grayish brown.
- *Anal sacculitis* is associated with moderate or severe pain on palpation; the sacs contain a thinner than normal, yellowish or blood-tinged purulent fluid.
- *Anal sac abscess* usually is unilateral and characterized by marked distention of the sac with pus, cellulitis of surrounding tissues, erythema of the overlying skin, and fever.
- *Rupture*—Abscessed anal sacs may rupture through the adjacent skin, producing a draining fistulous tract.

These probably represent a continuum, in that impacted anal sacs tend to become inflamed and infected, and the infection may lead to abscessation and, finally, to rupture or fistulation.

All breeds of dogs can be affected. Anal sac disease is uncommon in cats and usually involves only impaction.

Etiology

The specific cause of anal sac disease is poorly understood. It is believed to be associated with conditions that promote inadequate emptying of the sacs, which should normally occur during defecation when feces of normal consistency are forced through a normally functioning anal sphincter. Abnormal retention of anal sac secretions leads to the impaction-inflammation-infection cycle.

Clinical Signs

- The most frequent clinical signs of anal sac disease are related to anal discomfort and include scooting, tenesmus, and licking and biting the anal area, perineum, or base of the tail.

- Chewing and licking may result in areas of self-inflicted (pyotraumatic) dermatitis.
- Tail chasing, malodorous perianal drainage, and change in temperament may be noted.

Diagnosis

The diagnosis of anal sac disease is based on the clinical signs and examination of the anal sacs. Examine the anal sacs by palpation with a gloved index finger inserted in the rectum and a thumb compressed against the skin ventrolateral to the anus.

Treatment

- *Anal sac impaction and sacculitis*—Manual evacuation of the sac contents to reestablish drainage is all that is required in many animals.
  - Follow-up examination and expression of the anal sacs again in 1–2 weeks is advisable.
  - A high-fiber diet (see Table 94–2) may help to prevent recurrence.
- *Recurrence of impaction or sacculitis*—Irrigation with povidone-iodine solution using a lacrimal needle and instillation of an antibiotic (e.g., otic or ophthalmic antibiotic ointment) into the sac may be helpful, along with expression of the sacs every 3–4 days.
  - Consider culture and sensitivity testing of the sac contents for animals with troublesome recurrences.
- *Abscesses*—Drain, irrigate with povidone-iodine solution, and treat with systemic antibiotics.
  - Treat recurrent anal sacculitis or abscess by surgical excision of the sacs (see Chap. 95). Delay anal sacculectomy until the severe inflammation associated with abscessation has resolved.

PERIANAL FISTULAS

This chronic progressive disease is characterized by deep ulcerating fistulous tracts and suppuration in the perianal tissues. Fistulas occur primarily in German shepherds, although they have been reported sporadically in Irish setters, Labrador retrievers, and various other breeds.

Etiology

The proposed pathogenesis includes infection and abscessation of the various glandular elements in and around the anus, promoted by the moist, contaminated environment of the area and a broad-based, low-slung tail conformation.

Clinical Signs

- Dogs with perianal fistulas usually present with signs of anal discomfort (licking the anal area, scooting, dyschezia, tenesmus).
- Hematochezia, constipation, fecal incontinence, and foul-smelling purulent perianal discharge may be present.

Diagnosis

Examination of the perianal area establishes the diagnosis.

- The fistulae first appear as small, draining puncture holes in the perianal skin; there is inflammation and hyperpigmentation of the surrounding skin.
- These small tracts enlarge and coalesce to form large, interconnecting fistulas and areas of ulceration and granulation tissue. The fistulous tracts may extend deep into the perirectal tissues, and the anal sacs may be infected or ruptured.
- Histopathological findings include hidradenitis, chronic necrotizing pyogranulomatous inflammation of skin and hair follicles, cellulitis, necrosis, and fibrosis.

Treatment

Surgery is the most traditional treatment for perianal fistulas (see Chap. 95). Surgical techniques have been advocated, including varying degrees of excision and debridement of diseased tissue, chemical and electrocautery, cryosurgery, and tail amputation. It is advisable to tailor the aggressiveness of the technique to the extensiveness of the lesions and to preserve as much normal tissue and anal function as possible.

Medical Therapy

- Cyclosporin (Sandimmune; Novartis), 1.75–3 mg/kg PO q12h produces a high rate of healing within 16 weeks, although the recurrence rate is 40%, necessitating additional treatment or surgery.

Prognosis

- Postoperative complications such as fecal incontinence, anal stenosis, and recurrence of the lesions can lead to an unacceptable outcome.
- Early diagnosis and cyctosporin treatment or surgical intervention allows a less radical excision than required in advanced disease, which in turn means less risk of postoperative complications and a better prognosis.

PERIANAL DERMATITIS

Anal irritation often causes licking and biting the anal area that leads to perianal dermatitis.

- Any pruritic skin condition (most notably from fleas) may cause local dermatitis in this area.
- The mucocutaneous junction of the perianal skin and anal mucosa may be severely inflamed and ulcerated like other mucocutaneous junctions of the body in any of the systemic mucocutaneous dermatologic disorders (e.g., pemphigus vulgaris, bullous pemphigoid, systemic lupus erythematosus, candidiasis, cutaneous drug eruption.
- Eosinophilic granuloma complex of cats may involve the perianal region.

Perianal dermatitis often can be treated topically; however, the key is to recognize that it is usually secondary to another anorectal or dermatologic disorder that must be identified and treated. For information regarding specific dermatologic disorders, see the respective chapters.

ANAL AND PERIANAL TUMORS

The most common tumor of the anal region is benign perianal (circumanal) gland adenoma of dogs. Other benign tumors of the anal area are rare and include lipoma and leiomyoma. The two most common anal malignancies are perianal (circumanal) gland adenocarcinoma and apocrine gland (anal sac, anal gland) adenocarcinoma. Other malignant tumors of the anal region include squamous cell carcinoma, melanoma, lymphoma, and mast cell neoplasia.

Perianal (Circumanal) Gland Adenoma

Etiology and Clinical Signs

- These androgen-dependent tumors occur most often in older, intact male dogs and they usually appear as small, firm well-circumscribed nodules in the skin surrounding the anus.
- Perianal gland adenomas may be incidental findings unassociated with clinical signs or they may cause anal irritation with scooting and licking at the anal area. In addition, they sometimes ulcerate and periodically bleed.

Treatment

- The treatment of choice is excision (see Chap. 95) and adjunctive castration because of their hormone-dependency. Castration alone can produce regression of these tumors; however, excisional biopsy at the time of castration is necessary to rule out malignancy.
- Estrogens are inhibitory for perianal gland adenomas; however, they cannot be recommended for prolonged use because of their myelotoxic effects.

Perianal Gland Adenocarcinoma

Etiology and Clinical Signs

- These tumors occur most often in aged male dogs and may resemble an ulcerated perianal gland adenoma, except that they are locally invasive and may cause diffuse thickening of surrounding tissues.
- The tumors eventually metastasize to regional lymph nodes (sublumbar) and beyond.
- Their appearance can be confused with a perianal fistula lesion or a ruptured anal sac.

Diagnosis and Treatment

- For potentially malignant lesions of the perianal area, excisional biopsy is the diagnostic procedure of choice (see Chap. 95). First perform thoracic and abdominal radiography and abdominal ultrasonography to evaluate for lung or lymph node metastasis.

- Early excision of malignant tumors of the anal region can be effective; however, when extensive local invasion or regional lymph node metastasis has occurred, the prognosis for a cure is poor.
- Repeated partial excisions, radiation therapy, cryosurgery, and chemotherapy have been used for palliative therapy in patients with inoperable malignancies of the anal region.

Apocrine Gland Adenocarcinoma

Etiology and Clinical Signs

- Apocrine gland adenocarcinoma arises in the anal sac and most often affects spayed older female dogs. These tumors are unique in that they can be an ectopic source of parathyroid hormone–like activity; thus, even very small apocrine gland adenocarcinoma nodules often produce a hypercalcemia of malignancy syndrome with polyuria and polydipsia.

- Metastasis to lungs and/or regional lymph nodes (sublumbar) may occur.

Treatment

- Surgical excision is the treatment of choice.
- For medical treatment of associated hypercalcemia, see Chap. 30.
- Adjunctive chemotherapy may be necessary for incompletely excised or metastatic tumors (see Chap. 24).

SUPPLEMENTAL READINGS

Sherding RG: Management of constipation and dyschezia. Comp Contin Educ Pract Vet 12:677, 1990.

Sherding RG: Diseases of the colon, rectum, and anus. *In* Tams TR, ed.: Manual of Small Animal Gastroenterology. Philadelphia: WB Saunders, 1996, p 321.

95 Anorectal Surgery

Ronald M. Bright

Surgery of the rectum and anus is associated with a high rate of complications. The high bacterial population of the rectum increases the risk of wound infection and dehiscence. Bowel preparation with multiple enemas can mechanically remove large numbers of bacteria; however, enemas should not be done within 8 hours of anorectal surgery. Synthetic absorbable sutures or monofilament nonabsorbable sutures are recommended for surgery of the rectum and anus.

ANATOMY

The rectum begins at the brim of the pelvis and joins the anal canal just inside the anal opening. The anal canal is approximately 1–2 cm in length. The circumanal glands, anal glands, and anal sacs are associated with the anus.

The rectum receives its blood supply from the caudal mesenteric artery and its branch coursing caudally, the cranial rectal artery. This artery forms anastomoses with the middle and caudal rectal arteries, which arise, in the male, from the prostatic artery, and in the female, from the internal pudendal arteries. At the caudal demarcation of the rectum are two anal sphincters (internal and external). Fecal continence is maintained by these sphincters, and surgery in this area always threatens their integrity.

RECTAL PROLAPSE

Rectal prolapse is almost exclusively limited to young dogs and cats. The most common cause is straining to defecate, associated with severe colitis or proctitis due to endoparasites. Other causes include foreign bodies, rectal neoplasia, dystocia, and, in the cat, persistent straining related to urethral obstruction or cystic calculi.

Differentiate this condition from prolapsed intussusception. In the latter condition, a probe can be inserted and advanced cranially into a space between the cylindrical mass and the edge of the anus. This cannot be done with rectal prolapse.

Preoperative Considerations

- Treat underlying diseases (e.g., parasitism) while attempting conservative management of rectal prolapse.

- Initial management consists of cleaning and lubricating the prolapse, determining viability of the tissue, then manually reducing the prolapsed tissue followed by a loose pursestring suture. The pursestring suture should be loose enough to allow passage of loose feces, but tight enough to keep the prolapsed tissue reduced.
- Feed a digestible low-fiber diet for 7–8 days while the pursestring suture is in place.
- Failure of conservative management may necessitate a surgical procedure.
- The preferred surgical procedure is colopexy (see Chap. 90), unless there is nonviable tissue within the prolapsed segment of rectum that requires resection and anastomosis.

Resection and Anastomosis
Objectives

- Remove devitalized tissue involved in the rectal prolapse.
- Remove excessive rectal tissue that continues to prolapse in spite of manual reduction or use of the pursestring suture technique alone or in conjunction with a colopexy.

Equipment

- General surgery pack
- A 3-cc syringe case

Technique

1. Place the animal in sternal recumbency in a perineal stand.
2. Insert a well lubricated 3-cc syringe case into the rectum.
3. Place three or four stay sutures around the circumference of the prolapsed tissue through all the layers of tissue. The needle should be against the syringe case at its deepest penetration (Fig. 95–1A).
4. Resect the prolapse around 180° of the circumference, caudal to the stay sutures (Fig. 95–1B).
5. Place synthetic absorbable sutures (3-0 or 4-0) through the full thickness of the incised bowel, being sure to incorporate the serosal layers. A simple interrupted appositional pattern is preferred (Fig. 95–1C).
6. Incise the remaining 180° and suture as described in Step 5. Push the rectum cranially into the pelvic canal.

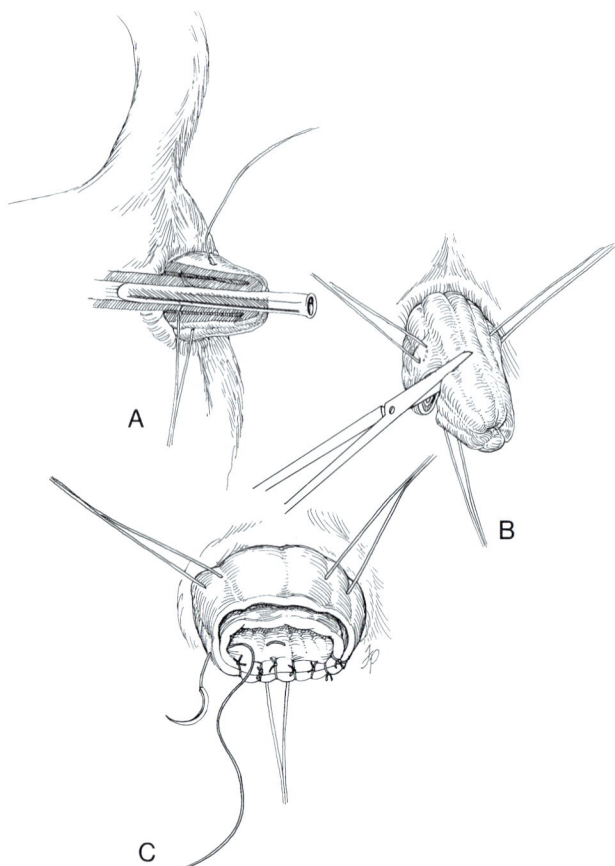

Figure 95-1. Resection and anastomosis of rectal prolapse.

Postoperative Care and Complications
Short-Term

- Give a stool softener (see Chap. 94) with food, which is offered the day after surgery. Continue giving the stool softener for 2 weeks.
- Closely monitor for leakage from the anastomotic site for at least 48 hours by observing the animal's temperature, level of activity, eating habits, and signs of excessive pain around the anorectal region. Be careful when placing a rectal thermometer.
- Recurrence of rectal prolapse may occur. A purse-string suture may have to be used again or a colopexy performed if it has not been done previously.

Long-Term

Long-term complications can include:

- Recurrence of rectal prolapse
- Fecal incontinence
- Anorectal stricture

ANORECTAL STRICTURE

Causes of anorectal stricture can be benign (e.g., inflammation) or malignant (e.g., adenocarcinoma):

- Inflammatory causes include perianal fistulas, prior anorectal surgery (including cryosurgery), and accidental trauma.

- Adenocarcinoma of the rectum and anus is the most common cause of stricture, resulting in a scirrhous, annular ring-type lesion.

Preoperative Considerations

- Simple, annular non-neoplastic lesions that are not too cranial in location may respond to a series of bougienage or balloon dilations. During this therapy, give prednisolone for 10–14 days (1 mg/kg q12h).
- For other lesions (e.g., adenocarcinoma), resection/anastomosis (described below) is the treatment of choice.

Surgical Procedure (Resection/Anastomosis with Rectal Pull-Through)
Objective

- Restore bowel lumen size that will accommodate the passage of feces with minimal resistance while preserving competence of the anorectal sphincter.

Equipment

- General surgery pack
- Senn retractors

Technique

1. Clip and aseptically prepare the perineal region.
2. Place a pursestring suture in the anus.
3. When the lesion is cranial to the anorectal junction, make an incision circumferentially around the anal ring.
4. Continue the perirectal dissection to normal tissue just cranial to the stricture ring. Avoid trauma to the sphincter muscles.
5. Place four stay sutures circumferentially through the normal rectal wall just ahead of the stricture.
6. Resect the diseased rectal tissue.
7. Pull the healthy tissue being held by the stay sutures caudally and appose to the anus. Avoid suturing under tension; mobilize more rectal tissue if necessary.

Postoperative Care and Complications
Short-Term

- Feed the animal the following day.
- Give stool softeners (see Chap. 94) for 2 weeks following surgery.
- Monitor for leakage from the anastomotic site, especially during the first 48 hours.
- Fecal incontinence may occur.

Long-Term

- A pelvic abscess due to earlier leakage from the anastomosis can occur.
- Postoperative stricture can occur, especially if tension was present at the suture line.

Prognosis

The prognosis is poor if the stricture is due to an adenocarcinoma. It is poor to guarded if the stricture is related to an inflammatory process.

ANAL STRICTURE LIMITED TO THE ANAL RING

Causes, preoperative considerations, and objectives are similar to those for anorectal strictures, as described in the previous section.

Surgical Procedure

Technique

1. Cut the stricture in four places around the anal ring at 3, 6, 9, and 12 o'clock.
2. Make the incisions perpendicular to the ring. Extend one-half of each incision outward into the skin and the other half inward through the fibrotic mucosa.
3. Suture the incisions in the opposite direction to the edge of the anal ring.

ATRESIA ANI

This condition exists in several forms, the most common being type I (imperforate anus) and type II, in which the rectal pouch is located cranial to the membrane overlying the anus. Regardless of the type, the main problem is loss of continuity between the rectum and anus during embryonal development of the cloacal membrane.

Preoperative Considerations

- Plain film radiography of the abdomen and pelvis with the animal standing helps to differentiate between type I and type II.
- Because the patient usually is only days or weeks old, there is a relatively high anesthetic risk.

Surgical Procedure

Objective

- Relieve the obstruction of feces in the rectum by opening the anus and reconstructing the anorectal junction.

Equipment

- General surgery pack
- Iris scissors
- Fine mouse-tooth thumb forceps

Technique

Type I

1. Incise the skin overlying the anus in a cruciate pattern.
2. Protect the anal sphincter.
3. Incise the rectal pouch just under the incision in a cruciate pattern.
4. Suture the rectal circumference to the subcutaneous tissues and skin with 4-0 or 5-0 nylon in a one-layer simple interrupted appositional pattern using monofilament nonabsorbable suture.

Type II

1. Incise the membrane overlying the anus in a cruciate pattern.
2. Continue the perirectal dissection cranially until the rectal pouch is identified.
3. Incise the blind pouch as described in Step 3 for type I.
4. Rectocutaneous apposition is achieved as described in Step 4 for type I.

Postoperative Care and Complications

Short-Term

- Monitor closely for suture line breakdown and infection of the surgical site.
- Because of the young age of these patients, give aggressive fluid therapy (including dextrose to prevent hypoglycemia) during surgery and well into the postoperative period.
- Initially, fecal incontinence often is a problem but resolves spontaneously in some animals.

Long-Term

- Fecal incontinence may continue indefinitely.
- Stricture is a possible sequela to anorectal surgery.
- Megacolon that sometimes accompanies atresia ani may be permanent and constipation may be an ongoing problem.

PERIANAL FISTULAE

Perianal fistulae are multiple draining tracts that surround the anus and are chronic in nature. German shepherds and Irish setters are affected most commonly (see Chap. 94 for a complete description of this disease).

Preoperative Considerations

- Consider conservative therapy, consisting of perianal cleansing with an antiseptic solution and application of hot packs.
- Antibiotic therapy for 2–3 weeks may ameliorate the pain associated with this condition. Medical therapy using cyclosporine is reported to cure perianal fistulas in many dogs (see Chap. 94).
- In some cases, surgical intervention will be necessary. Regardless of the procedure, surgical excision of diseased tissue is a compromise between complete excision and minimization of trauma to spare the external anal sphincter.
- An anal sacculectomy should accompany any excisional procedure.

Surgical Procedure

Objective

- Remove diseased tissue around a portion of the anus and, if necessary, around its entire circumference.

Equipment

General surgery pack

Technique

1. Make a skin incision to incorporate all the diseased tissue surrounding the anus.
2. Dissect and continue into the deeper tissues until the cranial extent of the fistulous tracts is determined.
3. Take care to prevent damage to the external anal sphincter muscle or its innervation.
4. In some instances, a portion of the sphincter muscle may be removed coincidentally when attempting to excise the diseased tissue.
5. In severe cases, remove a doughnut-shaped piece of tissue, leaving healthy rectal tissue underneath.
6. Transversely incise the rectum to allow removal of the anus and diseased tissue.
7. Suture the rim of rectal mucosa directly to the skin, using 3-0 monofilament nonabsorbable suture.

Postoperative Care and Complications

- Keep the incision and underside of the tail clean, using hydrotherapy twice a day. A thin layer of petroleum jelly placed around, but not in, the incision is helpful for preventing fecal soiling and irritation.
- Give stool softeners for 1–2 weeks.
- Incisional dehiscence may occur but is usually treated conservatively (let heal by second intention).
- Fecal incontinence may occur after extensive resections.
- Recurrence of fistulas can occur. Treat by excision of affected tissues.

PERINEAL HERNIA

Perineal hernia results from weakening of the perineal muscles (i.e., the levator ani and lateral coccygeus) and external anal sphincter. Hernias may result in rectal sacculation and herniation of prostate, fat, urinary bladder, or bowel (see Chap. 94). The exact cause is uncertain but is thought to be related to any condition that causes chronic tenesmus (constipation, prostatomegaly). Other possible causes include hormonal imbalance and degenerative changes to the levator ani musculature.

Preoperative Considerations

- Castration usually accompanies a herniorrhaphy. It is thought to help prevent recurrence by decreasing tenesmus related to prostatomegaly.
- Urethral obstruction secondary to bladder entrapment requires emergency treatment (cystocentesis and placement of a urethral catheter).

Surgical Procedure

Objectives

- Replace contents of hernial sac into the peritoneal cavity.
- Reconstruct the pelvic diaphragm.
- Prevent deviation of the rectum and retroflexion of the bladder and prostate gland.

Equipment

- General surgery pack.
- Self-retaining retractors.
- ¼″ Penrose drain.

Technique

1. Place the animal in sternal recumbency and secure the tail forward over the back.
2. Place a pursestring suture around the anus.
3. Make a half-curved or a curvilinear incision, beginning just lateral to the base of the tail and extending ventrally below the perineal bulge.
4. Using blunt dissection, remove the tissue overlying the hernia sac; open the sac with scissors.
5. Gently replace the herniated viscera into the abdominal cavity.
6. Dissect the tissue overlying the external anal sphincter, exposing the muscle striations.
7. Identify dorsolaterally the levator ani and lateral coccygeal muscles.
8. Palpate the sacrotuberous ligament and use it as the lateral landmark.
9. Carefully isolate the neurovascular bundle containing the pudendal nerve and the internal pudendal vessels and place a ¼-inch Penrose drain around it to identify its presence as sutures are placed.
10. Repair the dorsal aspect of the hernia first by preplacing three or four sutures between the coccygeal musculature and the external anal sphincter. Monofilament nonabsorbable sutures or synthetic absorbable sutures such as PDS or Maxon are preferred (Fig. 95–2A).
11. The sacrotuberous ligament may be incorporated with the coccygeal muscle when insufficient musculature is present. The sutures are then tied.
12. Identify the obturator muscle and isolate by bluntly dissecting the overlying tissue.
13. Incise the caudal border of the internal obturator muscle and elevate the muscle with a periosteal elevator until the caudal border of the obturator foramen can be seen (Fig. 95–2B).
14. Partially or completely incise the tendon of the obturator muscle to allow the muscle to be drawn dorsomedially (Fig. 95–2C).
15. Preplace similar sutures between the obturator muscle and the external anal sphincter. Avoid penetrating the rectum. Knot the sutures after gently apposing the tissues.

Postoperative Care and Complications

Short-Term

- Straining to urinate or hematuria suggests iatrogenic trauma to the urethra by a misplaced suture.
- Rectal prolapse may occur, especially if a bilateral repair was done. Staging the repair of right and left sides several weeks apart usually eliminates this complication.
- Fecal incontinence may result from damage to the pudendal or caudal rectal nerves or to the sphincter

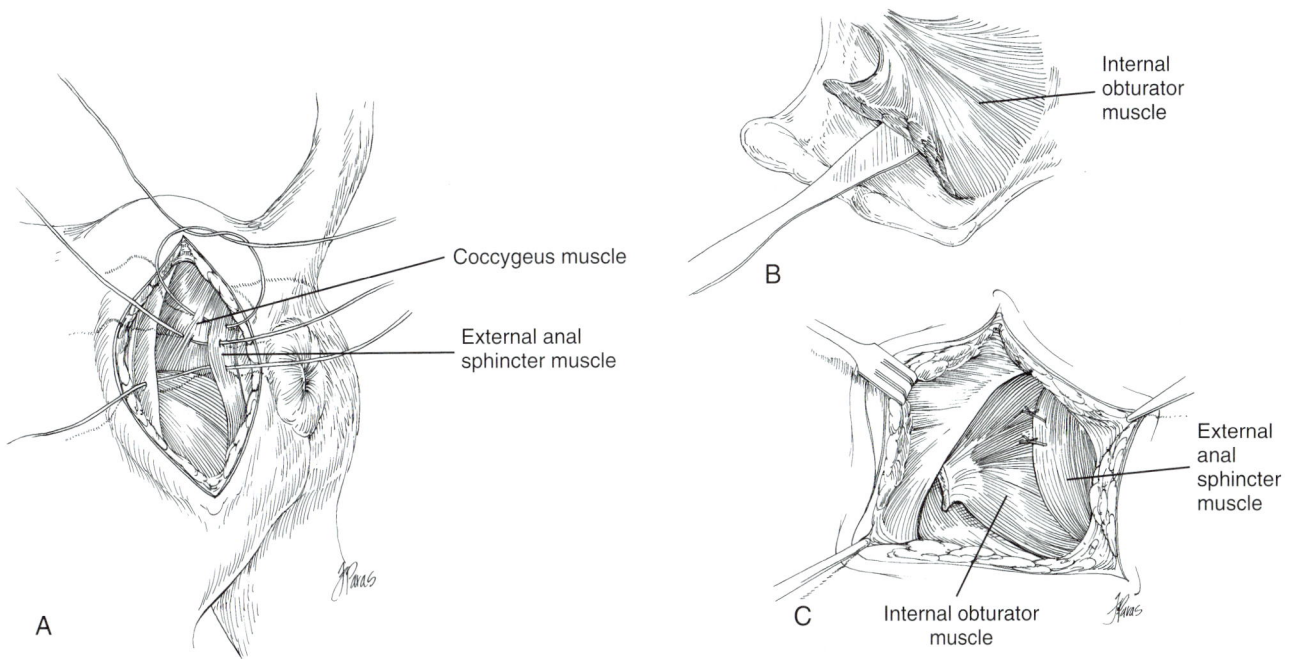

Figure 95–2. Repair of perineal hernia. Close the dorsal portion using the coccygeus and external anal sphincter muscles *(A)*. Close the remainder of the defect by elevating the internal obturator muscle *(B)* and suturing it to the external anal sphincter muscle *(C)*.

muscle itself. If damage to innervation is bilateral, the animal usually will not regain continence.

- Urinary incontinence sometimes occurs postoperatively but is infrequent. It appears to be associated with bladder retroflexion before surgery.
- Wound infection may result because of improper suture placement through the rectal wall, penetration of the anal sac, or contamination. This usually is seen in the first 48–72 hours postoperatively.

Long-Term

- Fecal or urinary incontinence may persist for weeks or months and sometimes indefinitely.
- Recurrence is directly correlated with the skill of the surgeon and the severity of the hernia. Castration may help to decrease recurrence regardless of the skill level of the surgeon.
- Colopexy and vas deferens pexy can be performed on recurrent hernias or if the initial hernia is severe. The colopexy procedure is described in Chapter 90. See Supplemental Readings for more information on the vas deferens pexy.

Prognosis

- If the surgery is performed by an experienced surgeon, the prognosis is good.
- Use of the obturator flap technique is believed to be associated with fewer problems postoperatively and with a lower recurrence rate.

ANAL SACCULECTOMY

The primary goal of anal sac surgery is correction of long-standing anal sac infection (see Chap. 94) that is refractory to conservative therapy.

Preoperative Considerations

- Do not perform anal sacculectomy during the acute inflammatory stage of infection.
- Administer antibacterial therapy, flush the anal sacs with antiseptic solutions, and use hot packs to control the sacculitis.
- Tumors of the apocrine glands of the anal sac are an indication for surgery. If neoplasia is suspected, obtain thoracic and abdominal radiographs (or abdominal ultrasound) to check for evidence of metastasis.

Surgical Procedure

Objectives

- Remove the entire anal sac.
- Preserve anorectal function by carefully avoiding excessive trauma to the external anal sphincter muscle and its corresponding innervation.

Equipment

- General surgery pack
- Electrocautery
- Iris scissors (optional)

Technique

1. Place a scissors blade into the duct of each anal sac (Fig. 95–3A).
2. Use thumb forceps to place countertraction on the duct before cutting so that all structures can be exposed.
3. After incising the sac, identify the lining by its gray color.
4. Place mosquito forceps at opposite ends of the anal sac lining.
5. Use small Metzenbaum or iris scissors to bluntly dis-

sect the sac free of its attachments, including the fibers of the external anal sphincter (Fig. 95–3B).

6. When dissecting medial to the anal sac duct, preserve the caudal rectal artery.

7. Use fine, nonabsorbable sutures to close the incision after flushing thoroughly with saline.

Postoperative Care and Complications

Short-Term

* Hemorrhage due to inadequate hemostasis may continue after closure of the skin.
* Rarely, temporary or permanent fecal incontinence may result.
* Wound infection is more likely because of the location of the surgical site.
* Tenesmus or dyschezia may occur for a few days but usually resolves spontaneously.

Long-Term

* Fistulous tracts may form after sacculectomy and are the result of incomplete excision of the anal sac lining.
* Wounds that do not heal after surgery may indicate a concurrent anal sac tumor.

Prognosis

The prognosis is good with complete excision of the sac lining and preservation of the external anal sphincter.

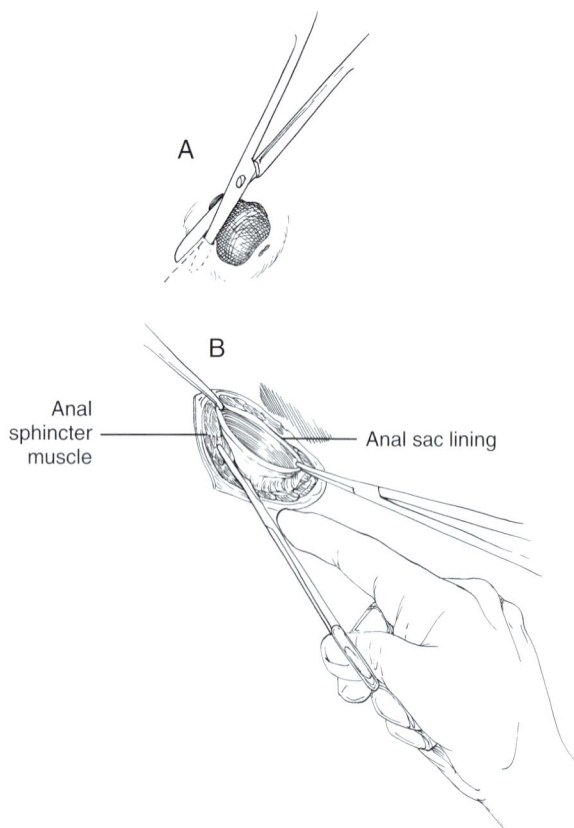

Figure 95–3. Surgical technique for resection of the anal sac.

SUPPLEMENTAL READINGS

Rectal Prolapse

Bright RM: Diseases of the anus and perianal area. *In* Morgan R, ed.: Handbook of Small Animal Practice. New York: Churchill Livingstone, 1988, p 479.

Engen MH: Management of rectal prolapse. *In* Bojrab MJ, ed.: Current Techniques in Small Animal Surgery, 4th Ed. Baltimore: Williams & Wilkins, 1983, p 254.

Anorectal Stricture

Bright RM: Diseases of the anus and perianal area. *In* Morgan R, ed.: Handbook of Small Animal Practice. New York: Churchill Livingstone, 1988, p 479.

Walshaw R: Rectoanal strictures in the dog. *In* Bojrab MJ, ed.: Current Techniques in Small Animal Surgery II. Philadelphia: Lea & Febiger, 1983, p 201.

Atresia Ani

Bright RM: Diseases of the anus and perianal area. *In* Morgan R, ed.: Handbook of Small Animal Practice. New York: Churchill Livingstone, 1988, p 479.

Matthiesen DT, Manfra-Marretta S: Diseases of the anus and rectum. *In* Slatter DH, ed.: Textbook of Small Animal Surgery, 2nd Ed. Philadelphia: WB Saunders, 1993, p 627.

Perianal Fistulae

Bloomberg MS: The clinical management of perianal fistulas in the dog. Comp Contin Educ Pract Vet 2:615, 1980.

vanEe RT: Tail amputation for treatment of perianal fistulas in dogs. J Am Anim Hosp Assoc 23:95, 1987.

Perineal Hernia

Anderson MA, Constantinescu GM, Mann FA: Perineal hernia repair in the dog. *In* Bojrab MJ, ed.: Current Techniques in Small Animal Surgery, 4th Ed. Baltimore: Williams & Wilkins, 1998, p 555.

Bilbrey SA, Smeak DD, DeHoff W: Fixation of the deferent ducts for retrodisplacement of the urinary bladder and prostate in canine perineal hernia. Vet Surg 19:24, 1990.

Hardie EM, Kolata RJ, Early TD, et al.: Evaluation of internal obturator muscle transposition in treatment of perianal hernia in dogs. Vet Surg 12:69, 1983.

Anal Sacculectomy

Manfra-Marretta S: Anal sac disease. *In* Bojrab MJ, ed.: Current Techniques in Small Animal Surgery, 4th Ed. Baltimore: Williams & Wilkins, 1998, p 283.

96 Peritonitis

Stephen J. Birchard

Peritonitis is a common problem in small animals. Primary peritonitis can occur in cats (feline infectious peritonitis; see Chap. 8), but other forms of peritonitis in dogs and cats are usually secondary to other diseases or injuries. Advances in the diagnosis and treatment of peritonitis have lowered mortality rates.

▼ *Key Point* The single most important recent advance in the surgical treatment of peritonitis is open abdominal drainage.

Open abdominal drainage allows more effective and complete drainage of the peritoneal cavity and has increased survival, even in cases of severe peritonitis. However, peritonitis continues to be a serious and life-threatening condition that requires aggressive management.

In this chapter the general topic of peritonitis is discussed. For more detailed information on the treatment of the specific causes of peritonitis, refer to appropriate chapters.

ANATOMY

The peritoneum is a serous membrane composed of mesothelial cells. It consists of the parietal peritoneum that lines the abdominal cavity and the visceral peritoneum that covers the abdominal viscera. The peritoneum has tremendous surface area (i.e., 50–100% of body surface area). The peritoneal cavity is closed in the male but open in the female through the reproductive tract. A small amount of fluid that lubricates the abdominal viscera is produced by the peritoneum.

ETIOLOGY

Viral

Feline infectious peritonitis is an example of primary peritonitis (see Chap. 8).

Bacterial

Gastrointestinal Perforation or Leakage

▼ *Key Point* Loss of bowel wall integrity accounts for the majority of cases of bacterial peritonitis in dogs and cats.

Leakage of bowel contents allows release of bacteria, predominantly anaerobes and gram-negative aerobes. Fluid and ingesta may also leak if gross bowel wall disruption occurs, resulting in a complex interaction of bacterial, chemical, and foreign body factors in the pathogenesis of peritonitis.

Bowel leakage can occur by a variety of mechanisms:

- *Perforation*—The bowel can be penetrated by external objects such as gunshot or a sharp object.
- *Neoplasia*—Leakage from a necrotizing gastrointestinal neoplasm (carcinoma, lymphoma) can occur.
- *Corticosteroids*—Colonic perforation can occur secondary to the administration of high doses of corticosteroids in animals with spinal compression.
- *Foreign bodies*—Sharp intestinal or linear foreign bodies frequently cause perforation (see Chap. 89). Also, intraluminal pressure on the intestinal wall by a foreign body can eventually lead to ischemic necrosis and leakage.
- *Blunt trauma*—Devitalization of the bowel can occur secondary to tearing of the mesenteric blood supply.
- *Strangulation*—Any process causing obstruction of the intestinal blood supply causes loss of mucosal integrity and eventually full-thickness necrosis (see Chap. 89). Loss of the so-called mucosal barrier can result in translocation of bacteria and/or endotoxins into the peritoneal cavity.
- *Dehiscence*—Unsatisfactory healing of a gastrointestinal incision may result in leakage through the wound and subsequent peritonitis.

Pyometra

Bacterial infection of the uterus can lead to peritonitis by leakage through the fallopian tubes or overt rupture of a pus-filled uterus (see Chap. 110).

Prostatic or Liver Abscess

Abscesses of the prostate gland (see Chap. 104) or liver (see Chap. 91) may leak bacteria to the peritoneal cavity spontaneously or iatrogenically during surgical exploration.

Surgical Contamination

A breakdown in aseptic technique can result in contamination of the peritoneal cavity and peritonitis.

Chemical

Urinary Tract

Leakage of urine from any part of the urinary tract can cause chemical peritonitis. Disruption of the urinary system may occur as the result of spontaneous or iatrogenic trauma.

- Causes of urinary tract disruption include trauma (blunt or penetrating), bladder or urethral rupture due to obstruction, and traumatic catheterization (see Chaps. 97, 99, and 101). Urinary tract disruption frequently is associated with pelvic and sacral fractures or luxations.
- Bacterial peritonitis can complicate the chemical peritonitis from urine leakage if urinary tract infection was present before the leakage occurred.

Biliary Tract

- Trauma to the biliary tract can cause leakage of bile due to rupture of the gallbladder or one of the bile ducts.
- Spontaneous leakage of bile can occur with necrotizing cholecystitis. Bacterial peritonitis may also complicate this situation.
- Bile is irritating to the peritoneum. However, several days may elapse before an affected animal is presented for clinical signs of peritonitis and biliary disease.

▼ *Key Point* A recent clinical study in dogs and cats found a grave prognosis for animals with combined bacterial and bile peritonitis.

Gastrointestinal Tract

- Gastric fluid contains hydrochloric acid and therefore is very irritating to the peritoneum. Proximal intestinal fluid contains bile and pancreatic enzymes that may cause a combination of chemical and bacterial peritonitis.
- Leakage of gastric fluid may occur due to trauma or any of the other causes of tissue breakdown listed under Gastrointestinal Perforation or Leakage.
- Gastric fluid may leak secondary to perforating ulcers or necrotizing gastric neoplasms (see Chap. 87).
- Tissue necrosis secondary to gastric dilatation-volvulus can cause leakage of gastric contents.
- Gastric contents are not always sterile. Bacterial contamination associated with leakage of ingesta can complicate the peritonitis and result in a combination of chemical and septic peritonitis.

Chyle

- Disruption of the mesenteric lymphatics, lymph nodes, or cysterna chyli can cause leakage of chyle into the peritoneal cavity.
- Neoplasia or other diseases causing erosion or obstruction of the lymphatics are more likely causes than disruption due to trauma.
- Chyle is irritating to the peritoneum, although in some animals it is reabsorbed by the abdominal lymphatics.

Pancreatitis

- Leakage of pancreatic enzymes and various chemical mediators of inflammation from the inflamed pancreas causes peritonitis (see Chap. 93).
- Local peritonitis is very common with pancreatitis. Severe, necrotizing pancreatitis or pancreatic abscess may cause generalized peritonitis.

Traumatic

Penetrating trauma that involves the peritoneal cavity, such as a gunshot or knife wound, will cause peritonitis even if the viscera are not injured.

Iatrogenic (Surgical)

- Varying degrees of peritonitis result from surgical manipulation of the peritoneum or abdominal structures.
- Analysis of peritoneal fluid after routine abdominal surgery shows increased neutrophils. Also, serum lipase concentrations significantly increase after abdominal exploration, suggesting pancreatic inflammation.
- Typically, peritonitis from routine visceral manipulation is clinically insignificant. Poor surgical technique, such as rough handling of tissues, allowing tissues to become desiccated, and lack of aseptic technique, can result in more serious peritonitis.

Foreign Body

Sutures

- Implantation of excessive sutures or large sutures can result in focal peritonitis.
- Nonabsorbable braided sutures (e.g., Braunamid, B. Braun Melsungen AG) that are contaminated can cause chronic focal peritonitis and resultant sinus tracts and abscesses.

Surgical Sponges

- Failure to remove surgical sponges can result in focal or diffuse peritonitis. Even sponges considered to be sterile can cause a significant foreign body reaction. Contaminated sponges cause abscesses and possibly severe, septic peritonitis.
- Prevention of this complication is essential.
  - Count surgical sponges before and after surgery to be sure that none have been left in the abdomen.
  - Use sponges that contain a radiopaque marker to allow diagnosis of a sponge foreign body with abdominal radiography.

Other

- Failure to remove surgical instruments can cause a foreign body reaction, irritation of viscera, and strangulation of blood supply to structures.
- Talc used on surgical gloves can cause a foreign body, granulomatous peritoneal reaction. After donning surgical gloves, rinse with sterile saline before opening the peritoneal cavity.

- Bacterial peritonitis is a frequent complication of peritoneal dialysis caused by contamination during the procedure or ascending infection via the indwelling dialysis catheter.

DISTRIBUTION AND LETHAL FACTORS

Local Peritonitis

- Local peritonitis is common and usually does not require aggressive surgical management.
- The abdominal structures, such as the omentum and mesentery, are able to "wall off" inflammatory processes and prevent spread to the entire cavity.
- The production of fibrin by the peritoneum is also an important process in confining bacteria and debris to an isolated area of the peritoneal cavity.
- Permanent adhesions can be a sequela of local peritonitis, but they rarely cause a significant clinical problem in small animals.

Diffuse Peritonitis

- Diffuse or generalized peritonitis occurs when the processes of confinement are overwhelmed and the entire cavity is affected.
- Diffuse peritonitis is a serious condition that requires aggressive medical and usually surgical therapy.
- Movement of the diaphragm, intestinal peristalsis, and gravity encourage dissemination of bacteria throughout the peritoneal cavity.
- Surgical manipulation of contaminated tissues can convert local to diffuse peritonitis.

Lethal Factors

Certain substances or combinations of substances have been shown to be especially devastating to the animal with peritonitis.

▼ *Key Point* The addition of blood, fluid, or barium (or other foreign material) to bacterial contamination of the peritoneum can cause severe, frequently fatal peritonitis.

- Hemoglobin, in addition to bacteria, creates a lethal combination in peritonitis. Hemoglobin tends to reduce the ability of the neutrophils to phagocytize bacteria.
- Barium sulfate, in addition to bacteria, has the same effect as hemoglobin.
- Excessive peritoneal fluid acts as an adjuvant in peritonitis. Fluid causes dissemination of bacteria and interferes with neutrophil migration along visceral and peritoneal surfaces.
- Contamination of the peritoneal cavity with multiple species of bacteria, such as occurs with bowel leakage, causes a more severe peritonitis than that due to one species.
- The combination of chemical and bacterial peritonitis is especially devastating. Proteolytic and lipolytic enzymes cause tissue necrosis, an ideal medium for bacterial growth.

CLINICAL SIGNS

Pain

The peritoneum is a very sensitive membrane. Irritation of the peritoneum can cause abdominal discomfort.

- The mildly affected animal is resistant to abdominal palpation.
- Signs of severe pain include reluctance to move and tachycardia and tachypnea.
- The animal may assume the "praying mantis" posture in an attempt to alleviate peritoneal pain.
- Peritoneal pain may cause the animal to contract the abdominal muscles, giving the abdomen a "tucked up" appearance.

Fever

- Pyrexia may or may not be present.
- Fever does not always imply sepsis but is more likely when bacterial contamination complicates peritoneal inflammation.
- An animal with overwhelming peritonitis, dehydration, and shock may have a subnormal temperature.

Vomiting

Vomiting may result from irritation of serosal surfaces, ileus, or the primary disease causing peritonitis.

Dehydration

- The peritoneum responds to inflammation by producing large amounts of protein-rich fluid.
- Loss of fluid from the peritoneum, inadequate intake of water and food, vomiting, and fever rapidly causes significant dehydration and hypovolemia.

Shock

- Hypovolemic shock can develop rapidly with peritonitis as a result of the processes described under Dehydration, as well as the sequence of events described in Chapter 72 on shock.
- Septic shock also is possible with diffuse peritonitis owing to release of bacteria to the peritoneal cavity, followed by absorption to the systemic circulation. Lysis of gram-negative bacteria that have leaked from the bowel causes endotoxemia. These endotoxins have a direct cytotoxic effect, as well as causing many systemic changes such as vasodilation and blood pooling, hypoglycemia, and acidosis.

DIAGNOSIS

History

- Thoroughly review the animal's history to gain clues to the presence of peritonitis and possible etiologies.
- Give special attention to any history of trauma or prior abdominal surgery.

- Determine if the animal recently ate any foreign bodies that could have caused bowel perforation.
- Determine if the animal has had any signs of gastric or colonic ulceration. A history of hematemesis, melena, or hematochezia is indicative of a more serious lesion of the gastrointestinal (GI) tract and increases the suspicion of perforation.
- Determine if the signalment and history are typical of pancreatitis.

Physical Examination

- Look for the clinical signs listed previously.
- Carefully palpate the abdomen for evidence of pain, fluid, ileus, or masses.
- Evaluate for fever.

Diagnostic Tests

Fluid Analysis

Abdominocentesis. See Chapter 3 for a description of the technique for abdominocentesis.

- Animals with peritonitis will have many neutrophils (> 500/μl) and may have bacteria on cytologic examination. Absence of bacteria suggests a sterile peritonitis, such as can occur with chemical peritonitis.
- The presence of bacteria within phagocytes confirms septic peritonitis. Bacteria within and outside phagocytes suggest that the infection is overwhelming the defense mechanisms. The presence of cocci and rods indicates mixed infection, such as can occur with GI perforation. Gram stain of the fluid can differentiate gram-negative rods (usually aerobes such as *Escherichia coli*) from gram-positive rods (usually anaerobes such as *Clostridium* spp.).
- Large numbers of red blood cells (RBCs) indicate hemorrhage associated with the peritonitis. This can occur with trauma, bleeding tumors, or disseminated intravascular coagulation.

Diagnostic Peritoneal Lavage (DPL). See Chapter 3 for a description of the technique for DPL.

- Observe the gross appearance of the fluid. Opaque fluid is likely from animals with peritonitis.
- Analyze the fluid for neutrophils (> 500/μl is considered a positive finding), toxic neutrophils, bacteria, bilirubin, creatinine higher than serum concentration, amylase > 200 IU, and vegetable fibers.
- Animals that have had recent surgery normally have a high number of nucleated cells in the peritoneal cavity (> 6000/μl).

Hematology

- Neutrophilia may be present with or without toxic neutrophils. A left shift (increase in number of band neutrophils) indicates more significant inflammation. A degenerative left shift (more bands than segmented neutrophils) indicates an overwhelming, life-threatening inflammatory process.
- Chronic blood loss or chronic infection may result in anemia.

- Hypoproteinemia due to loss or sequestration of albumin is very common in peritonitis.

Serum Chemistry Profile

- Many parameters may be altered, depending on the type of peritonitis and the associated clinical signs.
- Electrolytes (sodium, potassium, and chloride) may be depleted in animals that are vomiting. Acidotic animals may be hyperkalemic. Dehydration can artificially elevate electrolyte concentrations.
- Hypoglycemia may be present in animals with septic peritonitis.
- Serum urea nitrogen is elevated in animals with uroperitoneum and in animals suffering from prerenal azotemia due to dehydration or shock.
- Serum pancreatic enzymes (amylase, lipase, trypsin) frequently are mildly elevated in all types of peritonitis, and they are moderately to markedly elevated when underlying pancreatitis is the cause of peritonitis.
- Serum liver enzymes and bilirubin are variably increased in all types of peritonitis and may be markedly increased in sepsis, biliary tract rupture, liver abscess, and pancreatitis.

Radiography

Plain Radiography

- Plain abdominal radiography usually reveals a loss of contrast and lack of soft tissue detail either focally or throughout the abdomen. Fluid may be present in the peritoneal cavity.
- Pneumoperitoneum may be seen if any portion of the GI tract has perforated or there has been penetrating abdominal trauma. Radiographs obtained using horizontal projection can confirm air in the peritoneal space, because it rises to the dorsum of the cavity.
- Ileus may be present.

Contrast Studies

- Perform positive-contrast urethrography, cystography, and/or intravenous pyelography if uroperitoneum is suspected (see Chap. 4).
- Perform positive-contrast gastrointestinal studies to diagnose perforation (see Chap. 4). Avoid using barium as the contrast agent when perforation is suspected, because barium leakage into the peritoneal cavity can be devastating (treat with immediate laparotomy, peritoneal lavage, and drainage). Instead, use a water-soluble nonionic iodinated contrast agent, such as iohexol (Omnipaque).

Ultrasonography

- Ultrasonography can confirm the presence of peritoneal fluid. It is especially valuable for evaluating the pancreas as a potential cause of peritonitis.
- Soft tissue masses or abscesses may be detected (see Chap. 4).

TREATMENT

Management of peritonitis consists of supportive care and definitive measures to eliminate or correct the cause. The decision to treat the animal medically or surgically depends on the cause and the animal's response to treatment. If a surgical disease is not suspected and the peritonitis is mild, medical treatment alone may suffice. However, promptly initiate surgical treatment if the peritonitis is moderate or severe, is not improving with medical treatment, or is due to a surgical lesion such as a perforated intestine or biliary or urinary rupture.

Medical Management

Fluids

Intravenous (IV) fluids are probably the most important supportive treatment. The type of fluids used depends on the type of peritonitis and the metabolic alterations present in the patient.

- In most cases, use lactated Ringer's solution supplemented with potassium to prevent or correct hypokalemia.
- After correcting the dehydration, give fluids at a maintenance rate, plus continuing losses, until the animal is able to maintain hydration with oral intake. (See Chap. 5 for fluid therapy details.)

Antibiotics

Systemic antibiotics are indicated in bacterial peritonitis. Choose antibiotics based on culture and sensitivity testing of peritoneal fluid.

- In the absence of culture results, use broad-spectrum bactericidal drugs. Results of Gram stain of abdominal fluid (see under Diagnosis) can be used to guide antibiotic choice.
- Combinations of antibiotics may be necessary if a mixed population of bacteria are present. For example, combine ampicillin or one of the cephalosporins (e.g., cefazolin) with an aminoglycoside (e.g., amikacin or gentamicin) for peritonitis due to a mixed bacterial population. Other options include penicillins, clindamycin, or metronidazole for anaerobes, and fluoroquinolones for gram-negative rods.

Lavage and Drainage

▼ **Key Point** One of the most important treatments for peritonitis is drainage of fluid and debris from the peritoneal cavity.

Abdominal drains such as Penrose drains or sump drains (e.g., a fenestrated Brunswick catheter inside a fenestrated Penrose drain) are ineffective for draining the entire peritoneal cavity for any longer than a few hours. However, these types of drains can be effective for the initial drainage of the abdomen or for animals that are producing large amounts of abdominal fluid.

- Open abdominal drainage has been used successfully in experimental and clinical peritonitis and is described under Surgical Management.
- Lavage of the peritoneal cavity has been recommended but is controversial. Addition of fluid to the peritoneal cavity may potentiate generalized peritonitis and should only be used when all of the lavage fluid can be drained. Therefore, lavage should be reserved for those patients that undergo surgical treatment of the problem. Lavage consists of copious amounts of warm, sterile saline. Continue lavage until the fluid removed from the peritoneal cavity appears clear.
- Addition of antibiotics or antiseptics to the lavage fluid has *not* been shown to have any benefit over the use of saline alone in conjunction with systemic antibiotics.
  - Do not use aminoglycosides in peritoneal lavage during anesthesia, especially if neuromuscular blocking agents are being used. Aminoglycosides can potentiate the effect of these agents. Also, aminoglycosides will be absorbed and can reach toxic blood levels if they also are being given parenterally.
  - Avoid using povidone-iodine (Betadine) in lavage fluid in animals with peritonitis, because it can also be absorbed and cause severe toxicity, possibly due to absorption of large amounts of iodine.

Surgical Management

Correction of lesions resulting in peritonitis is covered in the appropriate chapters. Open peritoneal drainage as a general treatment for peritonitis is discussed here.

Preoperative Considerations

- As discussed under Medical Treatment, correct fluid and electrolyte disorders, when possible, before surgery.
- Begin antibiotic treatment before surgery if contamination is present or is likely to occur during the surgery.

Technique for Open Peritoneal Drainage

1. After the laparotomy has been performed and the cause of the peritonitis has been corrected, lavage the abdominal cavity with warm, sterile saline. Use copious amounts of saline to flush bacteria and debris from the cavity. Discontinue flushing when the lavage solution appears clear on removal from the abdomen.
2. Partially close the abdominal incision. Place large horizontal mattress or simple continuous sutures of monofilament polypropylene or nylon (1-0 or 2-0) in the linea alba to reduce the incisional gap to approximately 3–4 cm in width. Leave the remaining tissue layers open (Fig 96–1A).
3. Cover the incision with a sterile dressing consisting of (from inside out) sterile petrolatum-impregnated gauze, sterile laparotomy sponges or towels, cotton, conforming gauze, and tape. Make the bandage large

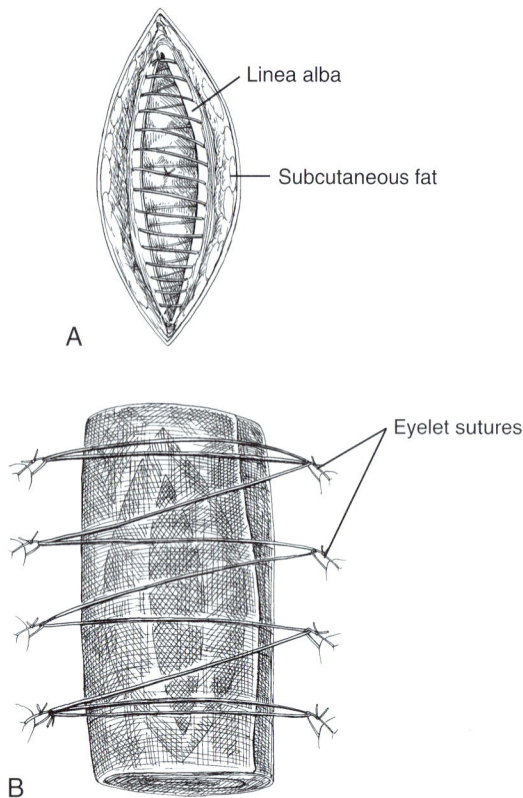

Figure 96–1. Partial closure technique for open abdominal drainage. *A,* Partially close the linea alba with a loosely placed simple continuous suture using a non-absorbable material. *B,* To hold the primary layer of the abdominal bandage in place, put several eyelet sutures in the skin, then use umbilical tape to "lace" through the eyelets, over the abdominal sponge.

enough to extend several centimeters beyond the cranial and caudal aspect of the incision and construct it so that slippage will not occur.
   a. Large polypropylene sutures can be used as "laces" to hold the laparotomy pads or towels in place (Fig. 96–1).
4. Change the bandage aseptically two or more times daily, depending on the quantity of fluid drainage. Omental or falciform ligament adhesions to the sutures can be gently broken down with a sterile-gloved hand between bandage changes. If necessary, obtain samples of peritoneal fluid periodically for cytology and culture.
   a. Weigh the bandage before and after placement on the animal to estimate fluid loss (500 ml = 1 lb). Use this information to help calculate fluid requirements and to monitor the trend of abdominal fluid production.

5. In most patients, the abdomen is closed within 5–7 days of the original surgery (see below). Perform abdominal closure by removing the original horizontal mattress sutures in the fascia and proceeding with a routine closure. Additional culture samples from the peritoneum may be obtained just before closure.

The decision on when to close the abdominal incision is subjective. I base this decision on several factors:

- Overall progress of the patient
- Quantity and character of fluid drainage from the abdomen
- Resolution of fever and neutrophilia with a left shift

Postoperative Care and Complications

- Keep the bandage as clean as possible. Urinary catheterization may be necessary in male dogs, or the animal can be kept on an elevated grate to prevent urine soaking of the bandage.
- Open drainage of the abdomen can cause several complications:
  - Loss of fluid and protein from the peritoneal cavity—Supportive care with IV fluids is very important. Hyperalimentation (or total parenteral nutrition) also is necessary if the animal is not eating adequately (see Chap. 3 for nutritional management of the critical care patient).
  - Electrolyte depletion, especially potassium—Supplement IV fluids with potassium if necessary (see Chap. 5).
  - Discomfort from the peritonitis and from open abdomen—Administer analgesics as necessary (e.g., morphine, butorphanol, buprenorphine, or oxymorphone).
- Herniation of abdominal viscera or omentum—This may occur if the bandage slips or is damaged by the animal. Gently lavage any tissue that becomes contaminated with sterile saline or remove surgically. Restrict exercise.

SUPPLEMENTAL READINGS

Bjorling DE, Crowe DT, Kolata RJ, Rawlings CA: Penetrating abdominal wounds in dogs and cats. J Am Anim Hosp Assoc 18:742, 1982.
Bjorling DE, Latimer KS, Rawlings CA, et al.: Diagnostic peritoneal lavage before and after abdominal surgery in dogs. Am J Vet Res 44:816, 1983.
Crowe DT, Bjorling DE: Peritoneum and peritoneal cavity. *In* Slatter DH, ed.: Textbook of Small Animal Surgery, 2nd Ed. Philadelphia: WB Saunders, 1993, p 407.
MacCoy, D: Peritonitis. *In* Bojrab MJ, ed.: Pathophysiology in Small Animal Surgery. Philadelphia: Lea & Febiger, 1981, p 142.

8 Disorders of the Urogenital System

Daniel Smeak

97 Diseases of the Kidney and Ureter

S. Dru Forrester

ACUTE RENAL FAILURE

Acute renal failure (ARF) is a syndrome caused by an abrupt decline in renal function that occurs over a period of hours to days. Clinical signs result from inability of the kidneys to excrete metabolic wastes and adequately regulate fluid, acid, base, and electrolyte balance. Consistent laboratory findings include azotemia with decreased urine concentrating ability (urine specific gravity usually <1.025).

▼ *Key Point* When azotemia is identified, it is important to distinguish between prerenal, renal, and postrenal causes.

Prerenal azotemia can result from any disorder that decreases renal perfusion (e.g., dehydration, heart failure, hypovolemia) or that results in increased production of urea (e.g., gastrointestinal hemorrhage). With few exceptions (Table 97–1), dogs and cats with purely prerenal causes of azotemia produce concentrated urine (i.e., specific gravity >1.035 in dogs and >1.040 in cats). In addition, prerenal azotemia quickly resolves when the cause of decreased renal perfusion is corrected (e.g., fluid therapy).

Renal azotemia is caused by renal failure and occurs when 75% of nephrons are nonfunctional. Dogs and cats with renal failure have concomitant azotemia and inability to adequately concentrate urine. Isosthenuria

(specific gravity of 1.008–1.012) often exists and urine specific gravity is almost always <1.025, although some cats with renal failure maintain ability to concentrate urine up to 1.035. In contrast with prerenal causes, renal azotemia usually does not resolve quickly with treatment.

Postrenal azotemia results from decreased elimination of urine from the body, most often due to urethral obstruction or a ruptured urinary bladder. There usually is something in the history (e.g., trauma, stranguria) or physical examination (e.g., abdominal fluid, swelling or discoloration of the perineal area, or masses within the prostate, urethra, or urinary bladder) that suggests a postrenal cause of azotemia. Additional tests such as radiography (plain and contrast), ultrasonography, and abdominal fluid analysis are helpful for confirming postrenal azotemia. Postrenal azotemia also rapidly resolves after correction of the underlying cause.

Etiology

Acute renal failure in dogs or cats results from acute tubular necrosis (i.e., nephrosis) and less frequently from renal inflammation (i.e., nephritis). Acute tubular necrosis is caused by nephrotoxins or renal ischemia (Table 97–2). Nephritis usually is due to infectious diseases in small animals.

Toxins. Renal tubular toxins are responsible for about 20–25% of cases of ARF. Ethylene glycol is responsible for the overwhelming majority of ARF cases

913

Table 97–1. DISORDERS THAT MAY BE ASSOCIATED WITH AZOTEMIA AND INADEQUATE URINE CONCENTRATION DESPITE NORMAL RENAL FUNCTION IN DOGS AND CATS

Drugs
Corticosteroids
Diuretics
Fluid therapy

Endocrine Diseases
Diabetes mellitus (ketoacidosis)
Hyperadrenocorticism
Hyperthyroidism
Hypoadrenocorticism

Other Disorders
Hepatic disease
Hypercalcemia
Pyometra
Urinary obstruction (postrenal azotemia)

due to toxins. Less commonly, drugs (e.g., aminoglycosides) are a cause of ARF.

Ischemia. Renal ischemia probably causes ARF more often than was once considered. Approximately one-third of dogs with ARF have a condition that predisposes to renal ischemia. In general, renal ischemia is most likely to cause ARF in patients that have preexisting renal disease or that have multiple, concomitant disorders that cause renal injury.

Nephritis. Nephritis causes ARF in a small number of cases, probably less than 10%. Leptospirosis is the most common infectious cause of ARF (see Chap. 17), but pyelonephritis also may cause ARF, especially if concomitant urinary obstruction exists. Rarely, ARF occurs in dogs with rickettsial infections such as Rocky Mountain spotted fever (see Chap. 15).

Table 97–2. CAUSES OF ACUTE RENAL FAILURE IN DOGS AND CATS

Nephrotoxicosis	Renal Ischemia
Therapeutic Agents	*Hypovolemia*
Aminoglycosides	Dehydration
Amphotericin-B	Hemorrhage
Tetracycline (IV)	Hypoadrenocorticism
Cisplatin	
Thiacetarsamide	*Decreased Cardiac Output*
	Congestive heart failure
Endogenous Substances	Arrhythmias
Hypercalcemia	Inhalational anesthesia
Hemoglobinuria (intravascular	
hemolysis)	*Renal Vasoconstriction*
	ACE inhibitors
Other Substances	NSAIDs
Ethylene glycol	
Iodinated contrast agents (IV)	*Renal Thrombosis*
New methylene blue (IV)	Bacterial endocarditis
	Systemic thromboembolism
	Disseminated intravascular
	coagulation

Idiopathic. Even after thorough evaluation, a cause for ARF cannot be identified in approximately 20–25% of patients.

Clinical Signs

Clinical findings in patients with ARF are nonspecific and include lethargy, depression, inappetence, vomiting, and diarrhea. Urine volume varies, and in most cases the patient is presented for other signs before the owner has a chance to observe a change in urinary habits. Most patients with ARF have normal to decreased urine output, although some have polyuria (e.g., aminoglycoside toxicosis).

Diagnosis

▼ *Key Point* It is very important to distinguish between acute and chronic renal failure because ARF is a potentially reversible condition that requires aggressive treatment initially.

It usually is possible to distinguish between acute and chronic renal failure on the basis of findings from history, physical examination, and routine laboratory evaluation (Table 97–3). Evaluation of renal size by abdominal radiography or ultrasonography also is helpful. In some cases, a renal biopsy is necessary to make a definitive diagnosis of acute or chronic renal failure.

History

- Carefully question owners about potential for exposure to nephrotoxins. Ethylene glycol toxicosis cannot be excluded in any patient that is allowed outdoors, especially in free-roaming pets. Ask the owner if the animal has been given any over-the-counter medications such as nonsteroidal anti-inflammatory drugs (ibuprofen, aspirin).
- Ask about the patient's urine volume. Many dogs and cats with chronic renal failure have a history of polyuria/polydipsia (PU/PD), whereas oliguria or anuria usually indicates ARF.

Physical Examination

- Nonspecific findings on physical examination of patients with ARF include depression, dehydration, hypothermia, and oral ulcerations.
- Abdominal palpation may reveal enlarged, painful kidneys in patients with ARF, whereas finding small, irregularly shaped kidneys suggests CRF.
- Fever may be present in patients with ARF due to infectious diseases such as leptospirosis or pyelonephritis.
- Icterus in a patient with ARF suggests multisystemic disease such as leptospirosis, Rocky Mountain spotted fever, or disseminated intravascular coagulation.

Laboratory Evaluation

Hemogram

- Hemogram changes in patients with ARF usually are nonspecific and may include leukocytosis, with or without a left shift, and monocytosis. Increased hematocrit and plasma protein are consistent with

Table 97–3. DIFFERENTIATION BETWEEN ACUTE AND CHRONIC RENAL FAILURE

	Acute Renal Failure	Chronic Renal Failure
Clinical Findings	Acute onset of inappetence, depression, and vomiting	Chronic history of inappetence, vomiting, depression, and weight loss
	Urine volume often decreased	Polyuria or polydipsia common
	Good body condition	Poor body condition
	Kidneys often enlarged and painful	Kidneys often small, irregular, and "lumpy-bumpy"
	Bone density normal	Bone density decreased (rubber jaw)
Laboratory Findings	Normal or increased hematocrit	Nonregenerative anemia common
	BUN and serum creatinine previously normal but increase progressively	BUN and serum creatinine previously increased and typically stable
	Normal to increased serum potassium	Normal to decreased serum potassium, especially in cats
	Moderate to severe metabolic acidosis	Mild to moderate metabolic acidosis
	Active urine sediment sometimes observed with proteinuria and casts	Inactive urine sediment unless there is concomitant infection

dehydration. Mild anemia may occur secondary to gastrointestinal hemorrhage or hemodilution after fluid therapy. Finding a normocytic, normochromic, nonregenerative anemia (PCV <30%) is common in patients with CRF.

Biochemistries

- Serum chemistry abnormalities include azotemia and hyperphosphatemia. Hyperkalemia is very suggestive of ARF because patients with CRF usually have a normal or low serum potassium. Some patients with ARF, especially due to ethylene glycol intoxication, may have hypocalcemia.
- Blood gas evaluation most often shows metabolic acidosis. Calculate the anion gap $[(Na + K) - (Cl + HCO_3)]$ to help characterize metabolic acidosis; normal values for anion gap are 12–18 mEq/L. An increased anion gap may occur with CRF, ARF, diabetic ketoacidosis, or lactic acidosis, but values >40 are almost always due to ethylene glycol intoxication or salicylate poisoning, which can be ruled out from the history.

Urinalysis

Analysis of urine, collected by cystocentesis where possible, should include evaluation of urine specific gravity, routine dipstick tests, and sediment examination.

- Urine specific gravity (USG) in patients with ARF is either isosthenuric (1.007–1.012) or minimally concentrated (usually <1.025).
- Dipstick analysis may reveal proteinuria or glucosuria due to renal tubular damage.
- Examine urine sediment for pyuria, bacteriuria, crystalluria, or cylindruria (renal casts).
  - Pyuria or bacteriuria suggests urinary tract inflammation or infection, respectively, and indicates the need for bacterial urine culture.
  - Hippurate or calcium oxalate crystals in patients with ARF suggest ethylene glycol intoxication.
  - White or red blood cell casts indicate renal inflammation or hemorrhage, respectively. However, most patients with pyelonephritis do not have white blood cell casts.
  - Renal epithelial cellular casts occur in patients with ARF due to acute tubular necrosis (i.e., nephrotoxicosis or ischemia).

Urine Culture

- Culture of urine collected by cystocentesis is indicated in patients with ARF to rule out urinary tract infection, a potentially reversible cause of renal injury.

Abdominal Radiography

- Plain radiographs of the abdomen help to objectively evaluate renal size and identify radiopaque uroliths that may be associated with urinary obstruction or infection.
- Contrast radiography may be indicated to help identify urinary tract rupture or obstruction as a cause of postrenal azotemia (see Chap. 4).
  - Excretory urography is indicated for evaluation of the kidneys and ureters. To avoid additional renal injury, establish adequate hydration prior to administration of IV contrast agents. Except for identifying rupture or obstruction of the upper urinary tract, excretory urography is of limited value in patients with renal failure because the kidneys cannot excrete contrast material well enough to produce useful images.
- Perform contrast urethrocystography when obstruction or rupture of the urinary bladder or urethra is suspected.

Ultrasonography

- Abdominal ultrasonography is helpful for evaluating renal size and architecture and for identifying uroliths and signs of urinary tract obstruction (hydroureter, hydronephrosis). Ultrasonography is preferred over excretory urography for evaluation of the kidneys in patients with ARF.

Renal Biopsy

- Collection of renal tissue for histologic evaluation is unnecessary in most cases of well-defined ARF.
- Renal biopsy may, however, be helpful:
  - When it is not possible to distinguish between ARF and CRF on the basis of clinical and laboratory findings.
  - When the cause of ARF is not apparent and the mechanism of renal injury seems to be ongoing.
  - When response to treatment is inadequate and expensive forms of treatment such as dialysis are being considered.
- Renal biopsy is contraindicated in patients with coagulopathies (thrombocytopenia), renal cysts or abscesses, or hydronephrosis. Use caution in patients that have only one kidney.

Ancillary Tests

- If leptospirosis is suspected, submit serum samples for determination of *Leptospira* titers (see Chap. 17 for guidelines on interpreting results of titers).

Treatment

▼ *Key Point* Objectives of treating ARF are to minimize additional renal injury, promote diuresis if oliguria exists, and combat metabolic consequences of uremia.

With time, renal injury in patients with ARF may be repaired so that there is adequate renal function to maintain homeostasis. This requires 2–4 weeks of aggressive medical treatment in many patients.

Discontinue all potentially nephrotoxic drugs to avoid additional renal injury; if a potentially nephrotoxic drug must be administered, adjust the dosage appropriately.

Rapidly correct all prerenal factors (dehydration, decreased cardiac output) so that renal perfusion is maintained.

Administer treatment as necessary to control consequences of uremia such as vomiting, metabolic acidosis, hyperkalemia, and hyperphosphatemia.

If an underlying cause of ARF or renal injury can be identified (pyelonephritis, leptospirosis), administer specific treatment to eliminate the disorder.

Initial Patient Management

- Determine baseline values for packed cell volume (PCV), plasma or total protein, blood urea nitrogen (BUN), serum creatinine, phosphorus, potassium, calcium, sodium, and total carbon dioxide (CO_2).

- Record values for body weight and hydration status. Use body weight after rehydration as a reference for future comparisons.
- Aseptically place an indwelling IV catheter, preferably in a jugular vein. In addition to convenience for the patient, jugular catheters allow for collection of blood, measurement of central venous pressure, and IV administration of hypertonic solutions (see Chap. 5).
- If oliguria (i.e., urine volume <1 ml/kg/hr) persists after apparent rehydration, place an indwelling urinary catheter so that urine volume can be objectively measured. Connect the urinary catheter to a closed collecting system. Unless absolutely necessary, avoid administering antimicrobials to patients with indwelling urinary catheters because it may predispose to developing resistant urinary tract infection.

Fluid Therapy

A comprehensive discussion of fluid therapy is provided in Chapter 5.

Initial Treatment

- Calculate the dehydration deficit using the following formula to determine volume of fluids (ml) to correct dehydration initially:

$$\% \text{ dehydration} \times \text{body weight (kg)} \times 1000$$

- If cardiac function is normal, correct dehydration within 6 hours by administering fluids IV.
- Ideally, select the type of fluid on the basis of serum electrolyte concentrations and acid-base status. It usually is safe to use lactated Ringer's solution in most patients unless hyperkalemia exists. If serum potassium concentration is unknown, initial administration of 0.9% sodium chloride is more appropriate.
- Clinical dehydration may not be apparent in all patients with ARF; however, most of these patients have a history of inappetence, vomiting, and/or diarrhea. Therefore, it generally is safe to assume subclinical dehydration (3–5% of body weight) and treat accordingly. In most cases, it is better to cause slight overhydration than to risk persistent mild dehydration, which may contribute to prerenal azotemia and potentiate renal injury.

Maintenance Treatment

- After rehydration, the volume of fluids to administer IV for maintenance needs equals the sum of ongoing losses (e.g., vomiting or diarrhea), insensible losses, and urine volume.
- Select a fluid such as Plasma-Lyte M or Normosol-M to facilitate maintenance of normal serum electrolytes. Avoid lactated Ringer's solution and 0.9% sodium chloride because they contain too much sodium and too little potassium to be maintenance solutions. If a maintenance fluid is not available, alternate lactated Ringer's solution with 5% dextrose to avoid hypernatremia; add potassium to fluids as

needed to maintain serum potassium concentration, especially during the recovery phase of ARF.

- Depending on the severity of renal injury, IV fluid therapy may be necessary for 1–3 weeks.

Discontinuing Fluids

- Gradually taper the volume of fluids administered to patients with ARF, once BUN and serum creatinine return to normal or oral intake of fluid is tolerated without vomiting.
- Provide unlimited access to water and decrease the patient's daily fluid volume administered IV by one-half every 24 hours.
- Monitor hydration (body weight, skin turgor, moistness of mucous membranes) closely while IV fluids are gradually discontinued.
- Monitor BUN, serum creatinine, and electrolytes every 1–2 days to detect need for additional treatment.

Reversing Oliguria

▼ *Key Point* Do not attempt to stimulate diuresis in patients that are dehydrated or that have nonoliguric renal failure. This may worsen or cause dehydration and electrolyte disturbances, which adversely affect renal function.

If oliguria (<1 ml urine/kg/hr) persists after correction of dehydration, additional treatment is indicated to increase urine production. Urine formation does not necessarily indicate improved renal function; however, it generally is easier to maintain serum electrolytes and acid-base balance in patients that are not oliguric. If there is any doubt whether oliguria exists, place an indwelling urinary catheter so that urine output can be measured.

IV Fluid Therapy

- Intravenous administration of balanced electrolyte solutions promotes diuresis in normal patients and those with nonoliguric renal failure but usually is not effective in patients with ARF.
- Fluids should be administered to correct dehydration or cause slight volume expansion (3–5% of body weight) only and not at 1.5–3 times maintenance volumes. Patients with ARF cannot adequately handle excessive IV fluids because of acute renal tubular dysfunction and are predisposed to overhydration, which may cause peripheral and pulmonary edema.

Osmotic Diuretics

Osmotic diuretics often are used initially to stimulate urine production in patients that remain oliguric after rehydration. Selection of which agent to use is personal preference. To avoid thrombophlebitis in peripheral veins, administer hypertonic solutions (>10%) through a jugular vein.

- *Mannitol (20 or 25%)*
  - Initially, administer 0.25–0.5 g/kg IV over 5–10 minutes. If treatment is effective, increased urine production begins within 15 minutes. The goal is to produce 1–2 ml of urine/kg/hour.
  - Continue mannitol every 6–8 hours as needed or administer 5–10% mannitol diluted in IV fluids at a constant rate of 2–5 ml/minute.
  - If urine flow does not increase after initial treatment, repeat the dose every 15 minutes up to a total dose of 1.5 g/kg. Do not administer additional mannitol because vascular overload may occur.
- *Dextrose (20%)* may be used instead of mannitol.
  - Administer 0.5–1.5 g/kg IV over 15–20 minutes (20% dextrose = 0.2 g of dextrose per ml).
  - If adequate diuresis occurs, repeat the dose every 8–12 hours as needed and administer maintenance fluids between doses. Alternately, administer a maintenance infusion containing 10% dextrose for 12–24 hours.
  - If adequate urine flow (1–2 ml/kg/hour) is not observed within 60 minutes of initial infusion, discontinue dextrose to avoid vascular overload.

Furosemide

- Loop diuretics, such as furosemide, may be administered to promote diuresis when an osmotic diuretic has been unsuccessful. Do not use furosemide in patients with aminoglycoside-induced ARF, because it can worsen renal injury.
- Administer furosemide at a dose of 2.2 mg/kg IV initially. If urine production increases, continue every 8 hours.
- If urine production does not increase within 30–60 minutes, administer a dose of 4.4 mg/kg IV. If there still is no response, administer furosemide 6.6 mg/kg IV. If the third attempt is unsuccessful, additional furosemide treatment is unlikely to be effective.

Dopamine

- Dopamine often is used to stimulate urine production when patients do not respond to other treatment. Infusion of low doses of dopamine causes dilation of renal vasculature and increased urine production.
- Dilute dopamine in 0.9% saline or 5% dextrose and infuse at a rate of 1–3 µg/kg/minute using an infusion pump or pediatric infusion set.
- Ideally, a separate IV line should be used so that changes in rate of dopamine infusion can be made without interfering with administration of other IV fluids. However, patients with severe oliguria may need to receive dopamine mixed in a small volume of fluids to avoid overhydration.
- Monitor patients during infusion of dopamine, preferably by continuous electrocardiography, to detect tachycardia or cardiac arrhythmias, which indicate the need to slow the rate of infusion.
- If urine production increases, continue dopamine for 12–24 hours or until urine flow can be maintained with IV fluids.
- Continued infusion of dopamine after 6 hours is likely to be ineffective if urine production does not increase.

Furosemide/Dopamine Combination

- There is some evidence to suggest that concomitant treatment with furosemide and dopamine may be more effective than either drug used alone.
- The author prefers to use both drugs simultaneously by administering dopamine as directed and also giving furosemide at a dose of 1 mg/kg IV every hour.
- Treatment beyond 6 hours is unlikely to be beneficial.

Dialysis

If oliguria persists despite measures to stimulate urine production, other treatment such as dialysis is indicated to maintain homeostasis. This requires an intensive care facility. For financial reasons and because of the guarded to grave prognosis for recovery, most owners elect euthanasia at this point.

Managing Electrolyte Disturbances

Hyperkalemia

Hyperkalemia is a potentially life-threatening electrolyte abnormality that occurs in patients with oliguria.

- Serum potassium concentrations between 6 and 8 mEq/L usually do not cause clinically important problems and are best treated by IV administration of 0.9% sodium chloride.
- If serum potassium concentration exceeds 8 mEq/L or if signs of cardiotoxicosis occur (bradycardia, prolonged P-R intervals, absent P waves, tall and peaked T waves, widened QRS complexes, ventricular arrhythmias) other treatment is indicated in addition to IV fluids. Administer sodium bicarbonate (0.5–1.0 mEq/kg) IV over 15–20 minutes. Sodium bicarbonate may be preferred in patients with ARF because they often have concomitant acidemia. Sodium bicarbonate causes potassium to move into the cells, which lowers serum potassium concentration for several hours.
- Alternatively, administer 20 or 25% dextrose (2–4 ml/kg) IV or a continuous infusion of 5–10% dextrose. This stimulates release of insulin, which also causes potassium to shift inside the cells.
- If life-threatening cardiac arrhythmias exist, administer 10% calcium gluconate (0.5–1.0 ml/kg IV over 10–15 minutes) to effect. During treatment, monitor the ECG for shortening of the QT interval and progressive bradycardia and slow or discontinue calcium infusion if these occur. Calcium gluconate directly antagonizes effects of hyperkalemia on the myocardium for 10–15 minutes. It does not affect serum potassium; therefore, concurrent treatment with either bicarbonate or dextrose is indicated to lower serum potassium.

Hypokalemia

- Hypokalemia may occur during the recovery phase of ARF due to excessive urinary losses and decreased oral intake. Therefore, monitor serum potassium every 1–2 days to detect hypokalemia.
- Add potassium chloride to IV fluids to correct hypokalemia (see Chap. 5 for specific guidelines).

Hyperphosphatemia

Hyperphosphatemia occurs secondary to decreased renal elimination of phosphorus in patients with ARF.

- Intravenous administration of fluids helps lower serum phosphorus.
- Additional treatment to control hyperphosphatemia (i.e., feeding a phosphate-restricted diet and administering phosphate binders) can be instituted when the patient tolerates oral feeding.

Correction of Acid-Base Abnormalities

Metabolic acidosis is the most common and clinically important acid-base disturbance that occurs in patients with ARF. Acidosis occurs because of the kidneys' inability to reabsorb bicarbonate and excrete hydrogen ions.

- Patients with blood pH values above 7.2 or a total CO_2 >12 mEq/L usually respond to IV administration of fluids alone.
- If blood pH is less than 7.2 or the total CO_2 is <12 mEq/L, administer sodium bicarbonate to help normalize acid-base status.
  - Calculate the initial bicarbonate dose (mEq) using the formula:
    (base deficit) $\times$ (body weight in kg) $\times$ (0.3)
    If base deficit is unknown, substitute the value for [20 − total CO_2].
  - Administer one-quarter to one-half of the deficit over the first 1–2 hours and add the remaining volume of bicarbonate to calcium-free IV fluids and administer over the next 12 hours.
  - Reassess blood gas data or total CO_2 to determine the need for additional bicarbonate therapy. If these values are not available, add bicarbonate at a dosage of 1–5 mEq/kg, depending on severity of initial acidemia, to IV calcium-free fluids to be administered over the next 12–24 hours.
- Refer to Chapter 5 for a detailed discussion of managing acid-base abnormalities.

Control Vomiting

Vomiting is a common complication of ARF due to effects of uremic toxins on the chemoreceptor trigger zone and emetic center, and due to gastrointestinal ulceration, which results from decreased renal elimination of gastrin and subsequent gastric hyperacidity.

- Administer an H_2-receptor antagonist to help control uremic gastritis.
  - Administer cimetidine (Tagamet, SmithKline Beecham) IV initially at a dose of 10 mg/kg q12h. As uremia resolves, decrease the dose to 5 mg/kg IV q12h.
  - Alternatively, administer ranitidine (Zantac, Roche) at a dose of 2 mg/kg IV q8h in dogs and 2.5 mg/kg IV q12h in cats.
- If vomiting persists, administer a centrally acting antiemetic.

- Metoclopramide (Reglan, Robins) may be administered at a dose of 0.2–0.4 mg/kg IV q6–8h. Because it is a dopamine antagonist, do not use it concomitantly with dopamine.
- Alternatively, administer chlorpromazine (Thorazine) at a dose of 0.25–0.5 mg/kg IV or IM q6–8h. Because chlorpromazine may cause hypotension and decrease renal perfusion, avoid using it in patients that are dehydrated. Do not combine chlorpromazine and metoclopramide as this can potentiate neurologic side effects.
- Refer to Chapter 87 for other recommendations for treating gastritis and the control of vomiting.

Monitoring Patients

The objectives of monitoring patients are to evaluate response to treatment, avoid potential complications, and help establish a prognosis. Patients generally are monitored more frequently during initial treatment or when life-threatening complications such as severe metabolic acidosis or hyperkalemia exist and less often when there is improvement or stabilization of the patient's condition. Parameters that are evaluated include hydration status, body weight, urine volume, and laboratory values.

- Record body weight and hydration status 2–4 times daily. Because clinical estimation of hydration status and fluid losses can be inaccurate, use changes in body weight to help guide fluid therapy. Once a patient is rehydrated, rapid changes in body weight generally reflect net fluid losses or gains and signal the need for a change in the rate of fluid administration.
- Measure hematocrit and total protein values daily to help evaluate hydration status.
- Measure serum chemistries and electrolytes daily for the first 4–7 days or until values begin to decline.
- Monitor blood gas values or total CO_2 and serum potassium several times daily if severe metabolic acidosis or hyperkalemia exists.
- To prevent overhydration, monitor changes in central venous pressure in patients with cardiac disease or persistent oliguria. In addition, a system of measuring "ins" and "outs" helps guide fluid therapy in these patients (see Chap. 5).
- Place an indwelling urinary catheter in patients that appear to have anuria or oliguria after rehydration. This helps determine the need for measures to stimulate urine production and guides fluid therapy to prevent overhydration.

Treatment of Underlying Diseases

Leptospirosis

- Administer penicillin (20,000–40,000 U/kg IV q12h) or ampicillin (22 mg/kg IV q8h) initially. When vomiting resolves, administer amoxicillin (22 mg/kg PO q12h) for 2 weeks.
- After treatment with a penicillin derivative, additional treatment may be needed to eliminate the carrier state of leptospirosis. Dihydrostreptomycin (15 mg/kg IM or SC q12h for 2 weeks) has been recom-

mended but has several disadvantages including the need for parenteral administration, unavailability, and potential for causing nephrotoxicosis. The author prefers to administer doxycycline (5 mg/kg PO q12h) for 2 weeks.

Ethylene Glycol (Antifreeze) Toxicosis

If a patient is presented within 6 hours of ingesting ethylene glycol, induce vomiting, lavage the stomach, and administer activated charcoal. If it has been less than 24 hours since ingestion, administer agents to prevent conversion of ethylene glycol to its toxic metabolites. Unfortunately, most patients with ethylene glycol intoxication are presented after ARF develops and the following treatments are not effective.

- *Ethanol*
  - Ethanol (20%) acts as a substrate for alcohol dehydrogenase and prevents metabolism of ethylene glycol.
  - In dogs, administer 5.5 ml/kg IV q4h for five treatments, then q6h for four additional treatments.
  - In cats, administer 5 ml/kg IV q6h for five treatments, then every 8 hours for four additional treatments.
- *4-Methylpyrazole*
  - 4-Methylpyrazole (5%) inhibits alcohol dehydrogenase and does not cause central nervous system depression like ethanol. It is the preferred treatment for ethylene glycol intoxication in dogs.
  - Administer 0.4 ml/kg IV initially, then 0.3 ml/kg IV at 12 and 24 hours after ingestion, and then a final dose of 0.1 ml/kg IV at 36 hours after ingestion.
  - 4-Methylpyrazole is not effective for treatment of ethylene glycol intoxication in cats.

Prevention

Because of expensive treatment and a guarded prognosis, make every effort to prevent ARF whenever possible.

- Warn owners about the danger of ethylene glycol if their pet lives outdoors.
- Do not use nephrotoxic drugs unless absolutely necessary (use enrofloxacin instead of aminoglycosides for severe gram-negative infections). If a nephrotoxic drug must be used, make sure the patient is well hydrated prior to treatment.
- Older patients often have chronic renal disease and are very susceptible to acute renal injury associated with dehydration or hypotension. Avoid stress and make sure the pet has access to fresh water at all times. Tell owners to avoid administering over-the-counter pain medications such as aspirin or ibuprofen. If general anesthesia is planned, administer IV fluids before and during anesthesia to maintain renal perfusion.

CHRONIC RENAL FAILURE

Chronic renal failure (CRF) is a syndrome characterized by inability of the kidneys to perform excretory, regulatory, and synthetic functions due to a loss of nephrons over a period of months to years. Loss of excretory function causes retention of urea nitrogen, creatinine, phosphorus, and other substances that are eliminated by glomerular filtration. Decreased ability of the kidneys to regulate fluid, electrolyte, and acid-base balance causes polyuria and/or polydipsia, hypokalemia, and metabolic acidosis, as well as other abnormalities. Failure of the kidneys to synthesize erythropoietin and calcitriol causes nonregenerative anemia and renal secondary hyperparathyroidism, respectively.

Etiology

Some breeds are predisposed to development of CRF due to congenital or familial renal disease; however, most dogs and cats with CRF are older and have acquired disease. Although many disorders may predispose to development of CRF in middle-aged to older patients, an underlying cause often is not identified. Regardless of the inciting cause, CRF tends to be a progressive and irreversible disorder.

- *Congenital and familial diseases* that cause CRF in dogs and cats are listed in Table 97–4.
- *Infectious and inflammatory disorders* may cause glomerular or tubulointersitial damage that progresses to CRF. Immune-mediated glomerular injury (e.g., glomerulonephritis) secondary to infectious or inflammatory diseases often progresses to cause CRF, especially in dogs. Tubulointerstitial inflammation associated with pyelonephritis, leptospirosis, or feline infectious peritonitis may progress to cause CRF.
- *Amyloidosis* may cause CRF in dogs secondary to deposition of amyloid in glomeruli, and in cats due to deposition of amyloid in the renal medulla.
- *Neoplasia* of the kidneys infrequently causes CRF. Renal lymphoma in cats is probably the most common neoplastic cause of CRF.
- *Nephrotoxic substances* (drugs, toxins, hypercalcemia) usually cause ARF; however, CRF may persist after recovery from the acute insult.
- *Hyperthyroidism* in cats is often associated with CRF. Although the relationship is not yet fully understood,

renal arteriolar hypertension is thought to play a role (see Chap. 29).

- *Idiopathic* glomerular or tubulointerstitial disease is the most common cause of CRF in dogs and cats. Despite thorough diagnostic evaluation, most patients do not have evidence of an inciting cause of renal injury.

Clinical Signs

Clinical signs in patients with CRF depend on the degree of renal insufficiency and the underlying cause.

- Lethargy, depression, and weight loss are nonspecific signs that often occur.
- Gastrointestinal signs such as inappetence, vomiting, and diarrhea often occur in uremic patients; oral ulcerations also may be observed. Constipation is common in cats with CRF.
- Weakness and exercise intolerance may result from anemia.
- Polyuria and polydipsia often are reported by owners and may be the first abnormality noted.

Diagnosis

▼ *Key Point* Try to identify any concomitant disorders that may contribute to progression of CRF; these include pyelonephritis, hypertension, hyperthyroidism, hypercalcemia, renal neoplasia, and urinary obstruction.

History

- Ask owners about potential for exposure to nephrotoxic substances, including any over-the-counter medications.
- To help distinguish between CRF and ARF, ask how long clinical signs have been present. Most patients with CRF have changes in appetite, body weight, urine volume, and/or water consumption that have been present for several weeks to months, whereas clinical signs in patients with ARF have been present for <1 week.

Physical Examination

- Assess hydration status by evaluating skin turgor and moistness of mucous membranes.
- Examine the oral cavity for ulcerations that occur with uremia and pale mucous membranes that may be associated with anemia.
- Perform ophthalmic evaluation to detect changes consistent with hypertension including retinal hemorrhages or detachments, or tortuous vessels.
- During abdominal palpation, try to evaluate renal size and consistency. Both kidneys usually can be palpated in cats, whereas in dogs only the left kidney can reliably be identified on physical examination. Small, firm, and/or "lumpy-bumpy" kidneys are typical of CRF, although kidneys in patients with CRF also may be of normal size and consistency. Enlarged kidneys most often occur with ARF, especially in dogs. In cats, however, renomegaly may result from disorders that

Table 97–4. BREEDS WITH CONGENITAL OR FAMILIAL RENAL DISEASE

Breed	*Renal Disease*
Abyssinian cat	Renal amyloidosis
Basenji	Renal tubular dysfunction
Beagle	Unilateral renal agenesis
Cairn terrier	Polycystic renal disease
Cocker spaniel	Tubulointerstitial fibrosis
	Renal cortical hypoplasia
Doberman pinscher	Glomerulosclerosis
Domestic longhaired and Persian cats	Idiopathic polycystic kidney disease
Lhasa apso	Renal dysplasia
Norwegian elkhound	Tubulointerstitial fibrosis
Pembroke Welsh corgi	Telangiectasia
Samoyed	Glomerular atrophy
Shih tzu	Renal dysplasia
Soft-coated Wheaten terrier	Renal dysplasia

cause CRF such as hydronephrosis, feline infectious peritonitis, renal lymphoma, and polycystic kidney disease.
- Ascites, and less frequently peripheral edema, may be observed in patients with hypoalbuminemia due to severe glomerular disease.
- In cats, palpate the neck region for thyroid nodules.
- In dogs, perform a rectal examination to identify any potential causes of post-renal azotemia such as urinary bladder, urethral, or prostatic masses.

Laboratory Evaluation

- Hemogram often reveals nonregenerative anemia in patients with CRF. Infectious, inflammatory, or neoplastic diseases may cause hyperproteinemia.
- Serum chemistry abnormalities include azotemia and hyperphosphatemia.

▼ **Key Point** Approximately 75% of nephrons must be nonfunctional before azotemia occurs. This means that BUN and serum creatinine are insensitive indicators of renal function, and patients may have severe renal disease in the absence of azotemia.

- Hypokalemia often occurs in cats with CRF.
- Urinalysis shows decreased renal concentrating ability and isosthenuria (urine specific gravity of 1.008–1.013) in most patients. Some cats with CRF may retain concentrating ability with values for urine specific gravity up to 1.035.

Urine Culture

- Culture urine obtained by cystocentesis to rule out urinary tract infection in all patients with CRF.

Radiography

- Survey abdominal radiographs are helpful for evaluating renal size and identifying other abnormalities of the urinary tract such as radiopaque uroliths.
- Excretory urography may be indicated for evaluation of suspected pyelonephritis, hydronephrosis, and obstructive uropathy; however, reduced renal excretory function often limits usefulness of this technique.

Ultrasonography

- Ultrasonography is the preferred technique for identifying abnormalities in renal size and architecture.
- This can also be useful for diagnosing obstructive nephropathies and nephrolithiasis.

Renal Biopsy

- Consider collection of renal tissue for histologic evaluation when results could alter treatment or help give the owner a more accurate prognosis (biopsy techniques are described in Chap. 98).
- Disorders in which a renal biopsy may provide useful information include glomerular diseases (glomerulonephritis, amyloidosis) and renal neoplasia.

Systemic Blood Pressure

- Measurement of systemic blood pressure is indicated because 50–90% of dogs and cats with CRF are hypertensive.
- Indirect measurement of blood pressure using Doppler ultrasonic or oscillometric (e.g., Dinamap) techniques are the most practical and convenient for the clinical setting.
- Generally, it is recommended to collect three consecutive measurements of systolic, mean, and diastolic pressures and use the mean of these values.
- Hypertension is defined as systolic pressure greater than 180 mm Hg, mean pressure >150 mm Hg, or diastolic pressure >100–120 mm Hg. Hypertension is also discussed in Chapter 69.

Treatment

Because CRF is an irreversible disorder that usually has no identifiable underlying cause, the goals of treatment are to make the patient more comfortable and slow the progression of disease, if possible. This is accomplished by the following measures.

- Control the clinical signs of uremia.
- Maintain fluid, electrolyte, and acid-base balance.
- Provide adequate nutrition.
- Minimize the progression of renal failure by treating concomitant disorders such as urinary tract infection and hypertension.

Dietary Management

Dietary management of patients with CRF consists of feeding a diet that is moderately restricted in the amount of protein, phosphorus, and sodium while providing adequate amounts of nonprotein calories, vitamins, and minerals.

Protein Restriction

- The primary beneficial effect of feeding a restricted amount of high-quality protein (contains only essential amino acids) is to control clinical signs of uremia by reducing the amount of nitrogenous wastes that result from protein catabolism.
- Currently recommended protein levels for dogs (2.0–2.2 g/kg/d) and cats (3.3–3.5 g/kg/d) may be achieved by feeding commercial or homemade diets.
- Adjust protein intake to prevent malnutrition as evidenced by hypoalbuminemia, worsening anemia, or weight loss.
- Severely restricted protein diets (1.25 g/kg/d) that are used to treat patients with urolithiasis should be reserved for patients that continue to have signs of uremia after moderate protein restriction and even then should be used carefully because of potential for protein malnutrition.

Phosphorus Restriction

- Feeding a phosphate-restricted diet also may lessen signs of uremia and could prevent progression of CRF by blunting renal secondary hyperparathyroidism and decreasing renal mineralization. Most protein-restricted diets are also phosphate-restricted.

Sodium Restriction

- Restriction of dietary sodium may help control hypertension in patients with CRF.
- Gradually restrict sodium intake by changing to the new diet over a 2- to 4-week period to allow the kidneys time to adapt to changes in sodium intake. A sudden decrease in dietary sodium could precipitate hypovolemia, which could worsen renal function.
- Avoid severely restricted sodium diets such as those used to treat patients with congestive heart failure because they may cause volume depletion and renal hypoperfusion.

Managing Fluid/Electrolyte/Acid-Base Disorders

Fluid Balance

Because of tubular dysfunction, patients with CRF cannot adequately produce concentrated urine and have primary polyuria. Fluid balance is maintained by increased water consumption.

- Therefore, it is very important that patients with CRF always have unlimited access to fresh water at all times.
- If water intake is not adequate to maintain hydration, as is often the case in cats, owners can administer supplemental fluids subcutaneously at home.

Potassium Balance

Hypokalemia is the most common abnormality of serum potassium in patients with CRF; it is more common in cats than dogs. Hypokalemia most likely results from decreased oral intake as well as excessive urinary loss of potassium.

- If the patient is not vomiting, oral administration of potassium is preferred.
  - Administer potassium gluconate (Tumil-K) at a dose of 2–6 mEq/cat once or twice daily, depending on severity of hypokalemia and the cat's size.
  - Initially, monitor serum potassium weekly to determine the appropriate maintenance dose; 2–4 mEq/cat once daily often is adequate.
- If parenteral potassium is necessary due to vomiting or severe hypokalemia, administer potassium chloride with IV fluids (see Chap. 5 for details).

Metabolic Acidosis

Metabolic acidosis is the most common acid-base abnormality in patients with CRF. Treatment generally is indicated if blood pH is <7.2 or total CO_2 is <12 mEq/L.

- Administer sodium bicarbonate at a dose of 8–12 mg/kg PO q8–12h (1 teaspoon of baking soda = 2000 mg sodium bicarbonate); start at the lower dose and give several times daily to avoid fluctuations in blood pH.
- Alternatively, administer potassium citrate at a dose of 0.3–0.5 mEq of potassium/kg PO q12h. One advantage of potassium citrate is that it can be used to treat both hypokalemia and metabolic acidosis, which may be present together.
- Monitor total CO_2 in 10–14 days and try to maintain values within the normal range (e.g., 18–24 mEq/L).
- Avoid administering urinary acidifiers or feeding diets that are intended to acidify urine because they may worsen metabolic acidosis.

Controlling Hyperphosphatemia

Dietary phosphate restriction usually is successful for controlling hyperphosphatemia initially; however, as renal failure progresses, additional measures are necessary. Administer phosphate binders with a phosphate-restricted diet to provide additional control.

- Aluminum hydroxide (Amphojel), calcium carbonate (Tums E-X, Rolaids, Cal Carb-HD), and calcium acetate (PhosLo, Phos-Ex) are effective phosphate binders.
- Administer aluminum hydroxide at an initial dose of 100 mg/kg/day.
- Alternatively, administer calcium carbonate (100 mg/kg/d) or calcium acetate (60 mg/kg/d) if hypercalcemia does not exist.
- Phosphate binders are most effective when the daily dose is divided and administered three to four times daily with meals.
- Monitor serum phosphorus and calcium concentrations every 2–4 weeks initially and adjust the dose of phosphate binder as needed to maintain normophosphatemia.
- Side effects of phosphate binders include constipation with aluminum hydroxide and diarrhea or hypercalcemia with calcium-containing products.

Treatment of Anemia

Treatment of anemia may be indicated when hematocrit is <25% in cats and <30% in dogs or when clinical signs such as fatigue, depression, weakness, or respiratory distress occur. It is likely that anemia is responsible for many of the signs of CRF that have been attributed to uremia. This is supported by the observation that correction of anemia is associated with substantial clinical improvement and quality of life despite continued or worsening azotemia.

Transfusion

- Administration of whole blood or packed red cells generally is reserved for patients with severe clinical signs (dyspnea, extreme lethargy) due to anemia. Because of cost, limited availability of blood products, and inconvenience of repeated transfusions, this is not an option for long-term maintenance of hematocrit in dogs and cats with CRF.

Anabolic Steroids

- Anabolic steroids have been used to treat anemia associated with CRF but are typically ineffective. If other treatments are contraindicated or cost-prohibitive for the owner, administration of androgens can be attempted.

- Orally administered androgens such as stanozolol (Winstrol-V) at a dose of 1–4 mg/dog or 1 mg/cat q12h or oxymetholone (Anadrol) at 1–5 mg/kg q24h have produced inconsistent results.
- Parenteral androgens such as nandrolone (Deca-Durabolin) at 1.0–1.5 mg/kg IM every 7–10 days may be more effective.
- Side effects of androgens include development of prostatomegaly, hepatotoxicosis, and perianal adenoma.

Erythropoietin

- At this time, administration of recombinant human erythropoietin (Epogen) is the most reliable method for correcting anemia due to CRF in dogs and cats. It may be cost-prohibitive for some owners and has potentially significant side effects; however, its beneficial effects exceed its disadvantages for patients with severe anemia due to CRF. Because erythropoietin is a human drug and is not approved for use in veterinary patients, obtain informed consent from owners before treatment.
- Prior to using erythropoietin, measure blood pressure and control hypertension.
- Evaluate iron status by measuring serum iron and total iron-binding capacity (TIBC) and calculating percent saturation (serum iron divided by TIBC). If iron deficiency is detected (see Chap. 20), it should be corrected before administration of erythropoietin.
- Administer erythropoietin (75–100 U/kg SC three times weekly) until hematocrit reaches 37–45% in dogs and 30–40% in cats; this usually requires 8–12 weeks of treatment, depending on severity of anemia and individual patient response.
- Because of the time required to reach a normal hematocrit, it may be more cost-effective to administer a transfusion, especially in larger patients, and then begin treatment with erythropoietin.
- Once hematocrit reaches the low normal range, decrease frequency of treatment with erythropoietin to twice weekly. If anemia recurs during twice weekly treatment, administer erythropoietin three times weekly again. Most patients can be maintained with a dose of 75–100 U/kg, two or three times per week.
- Because of tremendous demand for iron during treatment with erythropoietin, there is great potential for developing iron deficiency. Therefore, it may be best to administer iron to all patients receiving erythropoietin. Oral ferrous sulfate has been recommended for cats (50–100 mg/cat/d) and dogs (100–300 mg/dog/d); however, iron products often are unpalatable and cause gastric irritation. One over-the-counter ferrous sulfate product (Slow Fe) appears to be less likely to cause gastric irritation and may be suitable for veterinary patients.
- Monitor patients carefully during treatment with erythropoietin to determine efficacy and detect side effects.
  - Measure hematocrit weekly until it reaches the normal range and remains stable for 4 weeks on a maintenance dosage and then every 1–2 months.
  - Determine iron status 1 month after beginning treatment and every 2–3 months thereafter. Increase iron supplementation if serum iron is <84 µl/dl or percent saturation is <20%.
  - Measure blood pressure once monthly during initial treatment, then every 1–2 months thereafter. If hypertension exists, monitor blood pressure more frequently.
- In addition to seizures and exacerbation of hypertension, the most clinically important side effect of treatment is development of antibodies against erythropoietin. This is reported to occur in 25–30% of veterinary patients. Development of antibodies is characterized by a precipitous drop of hematocrit that is preceded by erythroid hypoplasia of bone marrow. If this occurs, discontinue erythropoietin. These patients become transfusion-dependent because the antibodies also form against endogenous erythropoietin, and hematocrit often is lower than before treatment with erythropoietin.

Controlling Hypertension

Because of the potential for serious consequences (blindness, worsening of renal failure), treat hypertension whenever it is identified in a CRF patient. The goal is to maintain normal systemic blood pressures (systolic <160 mm Hg, diastolic <90 mm Hg).

- Feed a diet that is moderately restricted in sodium; most diets formulated for patients with CRF fit this criterion.
- Hypertension in patients with CRF usually does not respond to dietary sodium restriction alone and also requires administration of antihypertensive drugs. Avoid administering drugs to control hypertension if blood pressure cannot be adequately monitored. It is best to start with a single drug at the lowest dose and gradually increase the dose; however, it is not uncommon for hypertensive dogs and cats to require multiple drugs administered simultaneously to control hypertension (see Chap. 69 for additional treatment recommendations).
- *Beta blockers* appear to decrease blood pressure by decreasing cardiac output, inhibiting renin release, or decreasing sympathetic activity. They often are used for initial treatment of hypertensive patients. Atenolol (0.25–1.0 mg/kg q8–12h PO) is preferred in patients with respiratory disease because it is a cardioselective beta blocker and does not cause bronchoconstriction like propranolol (0.25–1.0 mg/kg q12–24h PO).
- *Angiotensin-converting enzyme (ACE)* inhibitors such as enalapril (0.25–0.5 mg/kg q12–24h) also may be used initially to control hypertension. They prevent formation of angiotensin II resulting in arteriolar dilation and venodilation and decreased blood pressure. Because ACE inhibitors can worsen renal function, it is important to start with a low dose and gradually increase while monitoring renal function. If azotemia develops or worsens, discontinue ACE inhibitors.
- *Calcium channel blockers* such as diltiazem (Cardizem) cause vasodilation and decreased blood pressure and

are effective antihypertensive agents. The dose of diltiazem for dogs is 0.5–1.5 mg/kg PO q8–12h and for cats is 1.0–2.25 mg/kg PO q8–12h. Amlodipine (Norvasc) is a long-acting calcium channel blocker that has been used effectively to treat hypertension in cats at a dose of 0.625 mg/cat PO q24h.

- To determine efficacy of treatment, monitor blood pressure every 1–2 weeks until pressures stabilize within the normal range and then every 1–3 months indefinitely.

Monitoring Patients

Monitor patients with CRF to determine efficacy of treatment and need for adjustments in therapy. Frequency of evaluation depends on severity of metabolic complications and the patient's overall condition. Those with severe abnormalities obviously need more frequent monitoring than stable patients.

- Evaluate stable patients (those that are eating, drinking, and maintaining body weight) every 2–4 months.
- Perform physical examination to detect changes in body weight, hydration status, and general condition.
- Perform laboratory evaluation including CBC, serum chemistries, electrolytes, and urinalysis to determine need for adjusting treatment.

PYELONEPHRITIS

Pyelonephritis implies inflammation of the renal pelvis and kidney; however, it usually is used to describe bacterial infection of the kidneys. Altered host defense mechanisms (diabetes mellitus, hyperadrenocorticism, hydroureter, ectopic ureters, nephrolithiasis) predispose to development of pyelonephritis, although not all patients have an identifiable cause. In general, urinary tract infections, including pyelonephritis, occur more often in dogs than cats. For additional information on urinary tract infections see Chap. 99.

Etiology

▼ *Key Point* Ascending infection from the urinary bladder is the most common route of renal infection.

Organisms that most often cause urinary tract infection in dogs and cats include *Escherichia coli, Staphylococcus, Streptococcus, Klebsiella pneumoniae, Pseudomonas aeruginosa, Proteus,* and *Enterobacter.*

Clinical Signs

- Acute pyelonephritis often is associated with lethargy, depression, dehydration, fever, and abdominal pain.
- Chronic pyelonephritis usually is subclinical or is characterized by vague signs such as weight loss, inappetence, and polyuria or polydipsia.
- Patients with pyelonephritis may have concomitant signs of lower urinary tract infection such as pollakiuria, stranguria, and dysuria.

- Discolored urine (hematuria) or malodorous urine also may be noted.

Diagnosis

Because there is no specific test that is diagnostic of pyelonephritis, a presumptive diagnosis usually is made on the basis of clinical findings and results of laboratory evaluation and diagnostic imaging.

History

- Clinical signs may be apparent from the history; however, many patients with pyelonephritis have no clinical signs.

Physical Examination

- Palpate the kidneys to detect enlargement or pain, which may occur with acute pyelonephritis.
- Physical examination usually is unremarkable in patients with chronic pyelonephritis.

Laboratory Evaluation

- *Serum chemistries* often are normal unless concomitant renal failure exists, causing azotemia and hyperphosphatemia.
- *Hemogram* changes may include leukocytosis characterized by mature neutrophilia with or without a left shift.
- *Urinalysis* may show decreased urine specific gravity, proteinuria, hematuria, pyuria, and/or bacteriuria. Although white blood cell casts are diagnostic of renal inflammation, they often are not observed in patients with pyelonephritis.

Urine Culture

- Quantitative culture of urine collected by cystocentesis is indicated in patients with suspected pyelonephritis.
- A positive urine culture indicates urinary tract infection, but it must be interpreted with clinical findings and results of other diagnostic tests to make a presumptive diagnosis of pyelonephritis. For additional information on urine culture see Chap. 99.
- Some patients with chronic pyelonephritis may have a negative urine culture because infection has been treated previously or resolved.

Radiography

- Results of excretory urography help support a diagnosis of pyelonephritis but changes are neither sensitive nor specific (see Chap. 4).
- Dilation of ureters and renal pelves and decreased opacity of contrast media in the collecting system may be observed in patients with pyelonephritis. Predisposing factors may also be identified (nephroliths, malformations).

Ultrasonography

- Ultrasonography is an excellent noninvasive method for evaluating patients with suspected pyelonephritis (see Chap. 4).

- Ultrasonographic findings of pyelonephritis include dilation of the renal pelvis and proximal ureter and generalized hyperechogenicity of renal cortices. Predisposing factors may also be identified (nephroliths, malformations).

Treatment

Treatment of patients with pyelonephritis includes correction of abnormal host defenses if possible and administration of appropriate antimicrobials.

- Ideally, selection of an antimicrobial is based on results of urine culture and susceptibility.
  - Because treatment of patients with acute pyelonephritis must begin before culture results are available, select an antimicrobial such as ampicillin that is effective against many of the organisms that cause urinary tract infection and can be administered parenterally.
  - If life-threatening septicemia is suspected, administer a broad-spectrum combination such as ampicillin and enrofloxacin.
- Administer parenteral antimicrobials to patients with acute pyelonephritis until systemic signs such as fever, pain, and inappetence resolve (usually 2–3 days).
- Administer oral antimicrobials to patients with chronic pyelonephritis for a minimum of 6–8 weeks (Table 97–5).
- Monitor effectiveness of treatment by performing urine cultures 7–10 days after beginning treatment and 5–7 days after completing treatment.
- To detect relapsing or recurrent infections, repeat urine cultures every 4–8 weeks until negative findings are obtained from three consecutive cultures.

GLOMERULAR DISORDERS

Glomerular disorders are characterized by significant proteinuria that causes hypoalbuminemia. Glomerulonephritis and amyloidosis are the two most common disorders that cause glomerular disease in dogs and cats. In general, glomerular disorders are more commonly diagnosed in dogs than cats.

Etiology

- Any systemic infectious or inflammatory process may cause production of immune complexes that adhere to glomeruli (i.e., glomerulonephritis) or that stimu-

Table 97–5. ANTIMICROBIAL DOSAGES USED TO TREAT PYELONEPHRITIS

Drug	Dosage (mg/kg)	Frequency
Ampicillin/amoxicillin	25	q8hr
Cephalexin	18	q8hr
Tetracycline	18	q8hr
Trimethoprim sulfa	15	q12hr
Amoxicillin/clavulanic acid	16.5	q8hr
Enrofloxacin	5	q12hr

Table 97–6. CONDITIONS ASSOCIATED WITH GLOMERULONEPHRITIS IN DOGS AND CATS

Familial
Doberman pinscher
Samoyed
Bull terrier

Infectious
Bacterial endocarditis
Infectious canine hepatitis
Brucellosis
Dirofilariasis
Ehrlichiosis
Borreliosis (Lyme disease)
Systemic mycoses
Pyometra
Feline infectious peritonitis
Feline leukemia virus infection

Miscellaneous
Hyperadrenocorticism
Chronic glucocorticoid treatment

Neoplastic
Lymphoma
Mast cell tumor
Many others

Inflammatory
Systemic lupus erythematosus
Chronic pancreatitis
Chronic pyoderma
Polyarthritis

late production of amyloid, which deposits in glomeruli (Table 97–6).
- Some breeds of dogs have a familial predisposition to development of glomerular disease.

Clinical Signs

- Signs that may result from hypoalbuminemia include weight loss, peripheral edema, and ascites. The combination of ascites or edema and hypoalbuminemia, proteinuria, and hypercholesterolemia is referred to as *nephrotic syndrome*.
- Inappetence, vomiting, and diarrhea may occur in patients that have developed CRF and azotemia secondary to glomerular disease.
- Some patients may have severe proteinuria and no clinical signs.

Diagnosis

▼ *Key Point* Look for historical, physical, and laboratory findings that might suggest the underlying cause of glomerular disease such as infectious, immune-mediated, parasitic, or neoplastic conditions.

History

- Try to determine potential for exposure to infectious diseases by asking owners about travel history, environment, and tick control. Certain infectious diseases are more common in some geographic areas and in pets that live outdoors or are housed in kennels or catteries.
- Ask owners about vaccination, heartworm preventive, and feline leukemia virus status.
- If the patient is an intact female, consider pyometra as a potential cause of glomerulonephritis and determine when the last heat cycle occurred.

Physical Examination

- Some patients with glomerular disease develop peripheral edema or ascites.

- Thin body condition, decreased muscle mass, and poor haircoat are common but nonspecific findings.
- Carefully examine patients for any signs of systemic infectious, inflammatory, or neoplastic disorders that may predispose to development of glomerular disease. These signs include:
  - Fever
  - Anterior uveitis or chorioretinitis
  - Dermatologic lesions such as chronic pyoderma or mucocutaneous ulcerations
  - Lymphadenopathy
  - Hepatomegaly or splenomegaly
  - Icterus
  - Abdominal pain
  - Enlarged uterus or other abdominal masses
  - Joint swelling, pain, or reluctance to walk
  - Signs consistent with hyperadrenocorticism such as thin skin, abdominal distention, and hyperpigmentation

Laboratory Evaluation

- *Hematologic abnormalities* are nonspecific and may include nonregenerative anemia, hypoproteinemia, and leukocytosis. Some infectious, inflammatory, or neoplastic disorders may be associated with thrombocytopenia. Occasionally, hyperproteinemia is observed because of increased globulins.
- *Serum chemistry abnormalities* may include hypoalbuminemia, hypercholesterolemia, and/or hyperglobulinemia. Azotemia and hyperphosphatemia are present in patients with CRF.
- *Urinalysis*

▼ *Key Point* The hallmark of glomerular disease is the presence of significant proteinuria in the absence of hematuria, pyuria, and bacteriuria.

Urine specific gravity values are variable; most patients with glomerular disease retain the ability to concentrate urine unless CRF has developed.

Assessment of Proteinuria

- Dipstick analysis of urine protein is a semiquantitative test that is affected by urine concentration. Finding a 1+ protein in urine with a specific gravity >1.035 probably is not significant, but a 2–4+ proteinuria probably is significant at any urine specific gravity.
- Measurement of urine protein and creatinine for calculation of the protein:creatinine ratio is the most practical test for confirming significance of proteinuria.
  - In the absence of pyuria, hematuria, and bacteriuria, a urine protein:creatinine ratio >1 indicates significant proteinuria.
  - In general, values for protein:creatinine ratios are highest in patients with amyloidosis, although patients with severe glomerulonephritis may have similar values.

Ancillary Tests

▼ *Key Point* Because glomerular diseases may be associated with potentially treatable underlying disorders, perform diagnostic tests to help identify these conditions.

- *Ophthalmic examination* to detect lesions such as anterior uveitis or chorioretinitis, which suggest active infectious, inflammatory, or neoplastic disease
- *Serologic tests* (as indicated by other clinical findings) to exclude occult heartworm disease, rickettsial diseases, feline leukemia and immunodeficiency virus infection, systemic mycotic infections, and systemic lupus erythematosus
- *Serum protein electrophoresis* to characterize hyperglobulinemia as polyclonal or monoclonal
- *Thoracic and abdominal radiographs* to detect signs of occult heartworm disease, systemic fungal infection, primary or metastatic neoplasia, and pancreatitis
- *Abdominal ultrasonography* to help identify pyometra and hepatic, splenic, or lymph node enlargement
- *Fine-needle aspiration cytology* to evaluate lymphadenopathy, splenomegaly, or hepatomegaly
- *Arthrocentesis* if there is lameness, joint swelling or pain, stiffness or reluctance to move, or there is no obvious cause for persistent fever

Renal Biopsy

- A renal biopsy is indicated if the results will change treatment or provide additional prognostic information.

▼ *Key Point* The only method for distinguishing between glomerulonephritis and amyloidosis is to obtain renal tissue for microscopic examination.

- The distinction between amyloidosis and glomerulonephritis is important because amyloidosis has no reliable treatment and rapidly progresses to terminal renal failure. In contrast, glomerulonephritis tends to progress more slowly and may even resolve if the underlying infectious, inflammatory, or neoplastic disease can be eliminated.
- The most reliable methods for obtaining samples of renal tissue are percutaneously by ultrasound guidance or keyhole technique or at exploratory laparotomy (see Chap. 98 for discussion of renal biopsy techniques).
- Contact the laboratory to determine the appropriate medium in which to submit samples. In most cases, it is appropriate to place samples for routine histologic evaluation in formalin and samples for immunofluorescence in Michel's solution.
- Findings on routine histologic evaluation usually are sufficient to diagnose either glomerulonephritis or amyloidosis. Special stains such as Congo red may be used to help identify amyloid.
- Immunofluorescent studies are done to identify glomerular immune complexes; however, their presence is not specific for glomerulonephritis. Findings

must be interpreted with results of clinical signs, laboratory tests, and routine histologic studies of the kidney.

Treatment

Management of Glomerulonephritis

Predisposing Causes

Eliminate any disorders that may predispose to additional glomerular injury.

- Treatment of some diseases (e.g., pyometra, heartworm disease, hyperadrenocorticism) often is associated with resolution of proteinuria.
- In many cases, however, a cause for glomerular disease cannot be identified or is not amenable to treatment (e.g., feline leukemia virus infection, neoplasia, feline infectious peritonitis).

Immunosuppressive Therapy

- In general, avoid immunosuppressive treatment (e.g., prednisone, azathioprine, cyclophosphamide) of patients with glomerular diseases. At present, no studies have documented the efficacy of immunosuppressive agents for treatment of dogs or cats with glomerular disease, and these agents may actually worsen proteinuria and signs of renal failure.
- However, immunosuppressive drugs are indicated if an underlying disorder (e.g., systemic lupus erythematosus, leukemia, lymphoma) is amenable to such treatment.

Antiplatelet Therapy

- Because of the role of platelet aggregation in the pathogenesis of glomerulonephritis, antiplatelet drugs may be helpful.
- Consider administering a low dose of aspirin (for dogs: 0.5–5 mg/kg PO q12–24h) to inhibit cyclooxygenase and prevent platelet aggregation.
  - Although studies to document beneficial effects of aspirin in dogs or cats with glomerulonephritis are lacking, a low dose probably is unlikely to produce serious side effects.
  - Use caution when administering any nonsteroidal anti-inflammatory drugs (NSAIDs) such as aspirin to patients with CRF because they can cause acute worsening of renal function.
- Thromboxane synthetase inhibitors have been shown to lessen severity of proteinuria in dogs with experimentally induced and naturally occurring glomerulonephritis. These agents inhibit production of thromboxane, a potent inducer of platelet aggregation. At this time, however, thromboxane synthetase inhibitors are not routinely available.

Management of Amyloidosis

▼ *Key Point* No reliable treatment exists for patients with amyloidosis and most progress rapidly to develop terminal renal failure.

- Treatment with dimethyl sulfoxide (DMSO) has been associated with improvement in some dogs with amyloidosis.
  - Because the drug has few serious side effects and for lack of any other effective treatment, a therapeutic trial with DMSO may be warranted.
  - Dosage regimens have included 125 mg/kg twice daily and 80 mg/kg three times weekly; DMSO can be administered either orally or subcutaneously.
- Avoid administering immunosuppressive agents to patients with amyloidosis because they may potentiate renal amyloid deposition.

Dietary Management

- The ideal diet for dogs and cats with glomerular disease is unknown at this time.
- Currently, a diet that is moderately restricted in protein and sodium, similar to that for treatment of CRF, is recommended for patients with glomerular disease.
  - Moderate protein restriction may lessen severity of proteinuria.
  - Restriction of sodium intake probably is beneficial because most patients with glomerular disease are also hypertensive.
- Avoid dietary protein supplementation because this may actually increase glomerular injury and worsen proteinuria.
- Carefully monitor patients for signs of protein malnutrition (continued weight loss, worsening hypoalbuminemia and proteinuria, anemia), worsening renal function, and increased proteinuria.
  - Measure BUN, serum creatinine, serum albumin, and protein : creatinine ratio 2 weeks after changing diets.
  - Continue dietary protein restriction if renal function has not deteriorated, magnitude of proteinuria is reduced or unchanged, and serum albumin has remained stable or has increased.

Managing Complications

Renal Failure

- Renal failure is a common complication of glomerular disease (see previous section in this chapter for recommendations on treatment of patients with CRF).

Ascites and Edema

- Ascites and peripheral edema may occur in patients with glomerular disease secondary to hypoalbuminemia and renal retention of excessive sodium and water.
- Avoid removing fluid from body cavities unless it significantly interferes with respiration. Removing fluid potentiates hypovolemia, protein loss, and formation of additional edema or ascites.
- Enforce cage rest for 2–3 days until ascites or edema decreases or resolves.
- Administer loop diuretics such as furosemide (2–4 mg/kg PO q8–12h for dogs; 1–2 mg/kg PO q12–24h

for cats) cautiously and only if edema or ascites inter-feres with vital functions. Gradually taper the dose and discontinue when edema resolves.

Hypertension

- Measure blood pressure and treat patients with hypertension to avoid additional worsening of renal function (see previous section in this chapter and Chap. 69 for guidelines on treatment of hypertension).

Thromboembolism

- Thromboembolism, especially of pulmonary vessels, is a potential complication of glomerular disease. Factors that contribute to a hypercoagulable state in glomerular disease include platelet hyperaggregability and glomerular loss of antithrombin.
- Because of the guarded to grave prognosis associated with thromboembolism, consider preventive measures to minimize its occurrence.
  - Reduce magnitude of proteinuria.
  - Treat any underlying inflammatory condition.
  - Avoid indwelling intravenous catheters.
  - Maintain adequate hydration.
  - Avoid excessive use of diuretics.
  - Avoid treatment with corticosteroids.
- For additional information on management of patients with thromboembolic disease, see Chap. 69.

RENAL TUBULAR DISORDERS

Renal tubular disorders are caused by functional tubular defects that produce altered urine, and in some instances abnormal plasma concentrations, of some substances.

Etiology

Renal Tubular Acidosis

- Renal tubular acidosis (RTA) may be acquired or congenital and rarely is observed in small animals.
- Proximal RTA (type II) is characterized by wasting of bicarbonate. It occurs as part of the Fanconi-like syndrome in certain breeds of dogs. Type II RTA has been associated with gentamicin-induced nephrotoxicosis in dogs.
- Distal RTA (type I) is characterized by inability of the distal tubule to secrete hydrogen ions and produce acidic urine. Type I RTA has been reported in a cat with pyelonephritis and in another cat with hepatic lipidosis.

Fanconi-like Syndrome

- Fanconi-like syndrome is characterized by multiple proximal tubular dysfunctions, which cause glucosuria, proteinuria, and phosphaturia.
- It is suspected to be an inherited disorder and has been observed in basenjis, Norwegian elkhounds, Shetland sheepdogs, and schnauzers.

- Acquired Fanconi-like syndrome has been reported in dogs treated with aminoglycoside antibiotics.

Renal Glucosuria

- Primary renal glucosuria is characterized by defective proximal tubular transport of glucose. It is an inherited defect in Norwegian elkhounds but has been observed in other breeds.

Cystinuria

- Cystinuria is characterized by defective tubular transport of the amino acid cystine and other amino acids.
- It occurs most often in dachshunds but has been observed in other breeds such as English bulldogs.
- Cystine is sparingly soluble in urine, and animals with cystinuria are predisposed to development of cystine urolithiasis (see Chap. 99 for discussion of urolithiasis).

Nephrogenic Diabetes Insipidus

- Nephrogenic diabetes insipidus is characterized by failure of the kidneys to concentrate urine because of renal tubular inability to respond to normal amounts of antidiuretic hormone.
- It usually is an acquired disorder that occurs secondary to disorders (pyometra, hyperadrenocorticism, pyelonephritis, hypercalcemia) that interfere with renal tubular response to antidiuretic hormone; however, it also is a rare congenital defect in dogs.

Clinical Signs

Clinical findings vary depending on the renal tubular defect that exists.

- Signs of lower urinary tract disease such as stranguria, dysuria, and pollakiuria may occur with urolithiasis (e.g., cystinuria).
- Polyuria or polydipsia may occur with glucosuria, Fanconi-like syndrome, or nephrogenic diabetes insipidus.
- Stunted growth and weight loss may be observed in patients with glucosuria, congenital nephrogenic diabetes insipidus, and RTA.
- Vomiting often occurs due to gastric distention with water associated with severe polydipsia in animals with congenital nephrogenic diabetes insipidus.
- Some metabolic disorders (glucosuria, cystinuria) may not be associated with clinical signs.

Diagnosis

History

- History identifies breeds at risk as well as clinical findings that occur with metabolic disorders.

Physical Examination

- Physical examination findings often are nonspecific but may include decreased muscle mass, muscle weakness, distended urinary bladder, and palpable urocystoliths.

Laboratory Evaluation

- *Hemogram* results usually are normal.
- *Serum chemistries* may be abnormal.
  - Hypokalemia may occur in RTA and Fanconi-like syndrome.
  - Hyperchloremia may be observed in RTA.
  - Hypophosphatemia may develop in patients with Fanconi-like syndrome.
- *Urinalysis*
  - Normoglycemic glucosuria occurs in patients with renal glucosuria and Fanconi-like syndrome.
  - Proteinuria occurs in Fanconi-like syndrome.
  - Urine specific gravity shows hyposthenuria (<1.008) in patients with congenital nephrogenic diabetes insipidus and ranges from 1.001–1.018 in dogs with Fanconi-like syndrome.
  - Cystine crystals may be observed in urine of dogs with cystinuria; these crystals are colorless and hexagonal and are most likely to form in concentrated, acidic urine.
  - Urine pH values >6 often occur in patients with RTA. In the presence of metabolic acidosis, patients with proximal RTA can produce acidic urine (pH <6), whereas patients with distal RTA cannot.
- *Blood gas evaluation* reveals hyperchloremic metabolic acidosis with a normal anion gap in patients with RTA.

Ancillary Tests

- Infuse sodium bicarbonate to help distinguish between proximal and distal RTA. Animals with proximal RTA respond with increased urine pH and fractional excretion of bicarbonate, whereas those with distal RTA do not.
- Confirm presence of Fanconi-like syndrome by performing renal clearance studies that show excessive urinary losses of protein, amino acids, glucose, bicarbonate, phosphate, and potassium.
- Perform a modified water deprivation test to confirm nephrogenic diabetes insipidus (see Chap. 34 for details on performing water deprivation tests).

Treatment

Renal Tubular Acidosis

- Identify and eliminate any underlying causes.
- Administer sodium bicarbonate (1–2 mEq/kg PO) to control acidemia; higher doses may be needed for patients with proximal RTA. Adjust dosage on the basis of response to treatment.
- Administer supplemental potassium if hypokalemia exists (see previous discussion in this chapter).

Fanconi-like Syndrome

- Discontinue drugs that might cause acquired disease.
- Try to maintain a plasma bicarbonate of 12–18 mEq/L by administering sodium bicarbonate as needed.
- Administer supplemental potassium as needed to correct hypokalemia.

- Monitor patients for development of severe acidosis, hypokalemia, or decreased renal function.
- Allow unlimited access to fresh water at all times.

Primary Renal Glucosuria

- This condition does not require any treatment.

Cystinuria

- Monitor patients for development of cystine uroliths and remove them surgically or employ medical treatment to promote dissolution (see Chaps. 99 and 100).

Nephrogenic Diabetes Insipidus

- Treat the underlying cause if acquired diabetes insipidus exists.
- For congenital diabetes insipidus feed a low-sodium diet and administer chlorothiazide (Diuril) at 20–40 mg/kg q12h PO. This diuretic enhances proximal tubular reabsorption of sodium, chloride, and water, which decreases urine volume.

CYSTIC RENAL DISEASE

Cysts are epithelium-lined cavities that contain fluid. Renal cysts are dilated nephron segments that may be single or multiple (i.e., polycystic). Pseudocysts are accumulations of fluid that collect outside the renal parenchyma. They are not lined by epithelium, and, therefore, are not true cysts.

Etiology

- *Familial* polycystic disease has been reported in Cairn terriers and longhaired cats. This disease is inherited as an autosomal dominant trait in Persian cats.
- *Acquired* cystic disease may develop in animals with any type of chronic renal disease.
- *Perinephric pseudocyst* is an uncommon condition reported mainly in cats. Pathogenesis is unknown.

Clinical Signs

- Progressive abdominal enlargement is the most common clinical sign. This generally is the only sign in cats with perinephric pseudocysts.
- Vomiting, anorexia, weight loss, and polyuria or polydipsia occur secondary to renal failure in animals with familial polycystic renal disease.
- Solitary or multiple cysts that do not enlarge are usually of little clinical significance.

Diagnosis

History

- *History* identifies the clinical signs of cystic renal disease, especially in breeds with familial predispositions. Question the owner about an affected dam, sire, or sibling.

Physical Examination

- *Physical examination* findings include abdominal enlargement and nonpainful renomegaly.

Laboratory Evaluations

- *Hemogram* may show increased erythropoiesis in long-haired cats with idiopathic polycystic renal disease, possibly due to hypoxia-induced release of erythropoietin.
- *Serum chemistry profile* abnormalities include increased BUN and serum creatinine concentrations and hyperphosphatemia in renal failure.
- *Urinalysis*
  - Isosthenuria occurs in renal failure.
  - Bacteriuria and pyuria occur if secondary urinary tract infection is present.

Urine Culture

- *Culture the urine* if urinary tract infection is suspected.

Excretory Urography

- *Excretory urography* (see Chap. 4) confirms renomegaly in animals with polycystic renal disease and may show the cysts as multiple radiolucent areas in the renal parenchyma. In animals with perinephric pseudocyst, the kidney is demonstrated within the fluid-filled structure.

Ultrasonography

- *Ultrasonography* (see Chap. 4) is quite useful for detection and characterization of fluid-filled renal lesions. Their number, size, and anatomic relationships can be assessed.

▼ *Key Point* Ultrasonography is the procedure of choice for reliable diagnosis of polycystic kidneys and perinephric pseudocyst.

Aspiration

- *Aspirate the cyst* if necessary to confirm that it is a fluid-filled structure.

Treatment

- No specific treatment of cystic renal disease now exists. Bilateral polycystic kidneys result in CRF. A unilateral polycystic kidney can be treated by unilateral nephrectomy (see Chap. 98), providing normal renal function is documented in the unaffected kidney.
- If renal failure exists, treat it medically (see CRF).
- Treatment for perinephric pseudocyst is surgical drainage and resection of the cyst walls. (See Chap. 98 for a general discussion of renal surgery.)

Prognosis

- The prognosis for animals with perinephric pseudocysts is good after surgical treatment
- The prognosis for progressive bilateral polycystic kidney disease is poor. Advise the owner of the potential

genetic aspects (autosomal dominant in Persian cats) of the disease.

NEPHROLITHIASIS AND URETEROLITHIASIS

Uroliths are polycrystalline concretions that are composed mainly of organic or inorganic crystalloids (90–95%) and a smaller but essential amount of organic matrix (5–10%). Uroliths form in the urinary space within the excretory pathway, and they usually are classified according to mineral composition.

▼ *Key Point* In dogs and cats, the majority of uroliths are found in the urinary bladder or urethra (see Chap. 99). Fewer than 10% are found in the renal pelvis.

Occasionally, nephroliths pass from the kidney and become ureteroliths.

Etiology

- *Urinary tract infection* (UTI) by bacteria that hydrolyze urea (e.g., *Staphylococcus, Proteus*) is the most common cause of magnesium ammonium phosphate (struvite) urolithiasis in dogs. UTI also may occur secondary to urolithiasis that initially developed in the absence of infection.
- *Metabolic disorders* that cause excessive urinary excretion of sparingly soluble compounds may predispose an animal to urolithiasis.
  - Inborn errors of metabolism predispose Dalmatians to urate urolithiasis, dogs with cystinuria to cystine urolithiasis, and animals with RTA to calcium phosphate urolithiasis.
  - Portal vascular anomalies predispose affected dogs and cats to the development of urate urolithiasis because of hepatic dysfunction (see Chap. 91).
  - Acquired metabolic disorders that predispose animals to urolithiasis include hyperparathyroidism (see Chap. 30), which may lead to the formation of calcium phosphate uroliths.
- *Dietary factors*
  - High-magnesium alkalinizing diets promote struvite urolithiasis in cats.
  - Diets containing large amounts of corn gluten or soybean hulls have been associated with formation of silica uroliths.
  - Excessive dietary calcium or phosphorus intake may promote formation of calcium phosphate uroliths.
- *Idiopathic conditions* often cause urolithiasis. The pathogenic mechanisms of urolith formation in animals with calcium oxalate, sterile struvite, and silica urolithiasis are poorly understood.

Clinical Signs

- Clinical signs associated with renal and ureteral uroliths are diverse and primarily depend upon the following:

- Size, number, and location of the stones.
  - Presence (degree and duration) or absence of obstruction to urine flow.
  - Presence or absence of UTI.
- Hematuria and signs of sublumbar or abdominal discomfort may be observed.
- Bilateral obstruction or unilateral obstruction with inadequate renal function in the contralateral kidney causes vomiting, anorexia, and depression, owing to postrenal azotemia/uremia.
- Urine may have a foul odor if UTI exists.
- An affected animal may have subclinical disease.

Diagnosis

History

- *History* identifies the breed predispositions (see Chap. 99) and clinical signs associated with nephrolithiasis and ureterolithiasis.

Physical Examination

- *Physical examination* abnormalities may include sublumbar or abdominal pain and/or renomegaly. Fever may be found in a patient with UTI causing nephritis, especially with concurrent obstruction.

Laboratory Evaluations

- *Hemogram* usually is normal. Leukocytosis may be found when UTI causes pyelonephritis, especially with concurrent obstruction.
- *Serum chemistry panel*
  - Increased BUN, serum creatinine, and serum phosphorus concentrations accompany renal failure, bilateral ureteral obstruction, or unilateral obstruction of a single functioning kidney.
  - Hypokalemia, hyperchloremia, and metabolic acidosis may occur in cases of urolithiasis associated with renal tubular acidosis (see previous discussion).
  - Hypercalcemia occasionally is found in animals with calcium-containing uroliths; however, most of these animals are normocalcemic.
- *Urinalysis*
  - Hematuria is a common finding.
  - Suspect UTI when pyuria or bacteriuria is found.
  - Urine pH tends to be alkaline with struvite uroliths and acidic with cystine uroliths. Urate and calcium oxalate uroliths may be associated with either alkaline or acidic urine.
  - Examine sediment for struvite, ammonium urate, cystine, or calcium oxalate crystals. Crystalluria represents a risk factor for urolithiasis; however, do not presumptively identify the mineral content of uroliths solely on the type of crystalluria.

Urine Culture

- *Urine culture* is indicated in all patients with uroliths.

Radiography

- Confirm the presence, location, density, size, and number of uroliths with abdominal radiography.

- Urolith density is quite variable; however, oxalate, struvite, calcium phosphate, and silica uroliths usually are more radiodense than urate and cystine uroliths.
- Confirm the presence of nephrolithiasis and ureterolithiasis and the degree of urinary obstruction by excretory urography (see Chap. 4). Consider cystourethrography to identify concomitant lower urinary tract uroliths (see Chap. 4).

Ultrasonography

- *Ultrasonography* helps to confirm the presence and location of uroliths, identify radiolucent uroliths, and assess the degree of obstruction.

Urolith Analysis

- *Quantitative (crystallographic) urolith analysis* is required to accurately determine mineral composition of uroliths.

▼ **Key Point** A tentative diagnosis of urolith composition often can be made using information from the clinical, laboratory, and radiographic findings.

Treatment

The goals of treatment are to correct any predisposing factors if possible, eliminate existing calculi by surgical or medical treatment, and prevent recurrence. Refer to Chapter 99 for discussion of treatment for urolithiasis.

Nonobstructing, sterile nephroliths that do not increase in size, do not cause significant hematuria, and do not produce deterioration in renal function can be monitored without treatment. However, even for seemingly innocuous nephroliths, consider medical dissolution therapy if the mineral composition (struvite, urate, cystine) can be estimated with confidence.

Correct Underlying Causes

- When concomitant UTI exists, administer an appropriate antimicrobial drug and continue for 2–3 weeks after dissolution or removal of uroliths.
- Correct portosystemic shunts surgically, when possible (see Chap. 92).
- Remove parathyroid adenomas in patients with primary hyperparathyroidism (see Chap. 30).

Medical Treatment

- This is not effective for calcium oxalate, calcium phosphate, or silica uroliths. Struvite, urate, and cystine uroliths may respond partially or completely to medical calculolytic therapy (see Chap. 99, for description of protocols).
- *Monitor* the patient to determine efficacy of medical dissolution therapy efforts.
  - Reassess the size and location of uroliths using radiography and/or ultrasonography every 4–6 weeks.
  - Perform urinalysis periodically (every 4–6 weeks).
  - Crystalluria must be absent for medical dissolution therapy to be effective.

- Perform urine culture periodically (every 4–6 weeks) to verify continuing control of UTI.
- If uroliths enlarge or fail to steadily decrease in size, verify compliance with intended treatment instructions and based on that consider other treatment options. The original assessment of urolith mineral type might be incorrect, or the urolith might be composed of more than one mineral.
- As nephroliths decrease in size, they may move into the ureter causing partial or complete obstruction.

Surgical Treatment

- *Surgical treatment* is required in some situations (see Chap. 98).

▼ *Key Point* Nephroliths or ureteroliths that obstruct urine flow to any substantial degree are surgically removed with little delay.

- If treatment of uroliths composed of calcium oxalate, calcium phosphate, or silica is required, surgical removal is indicated.
- Uroliths that fail to dissolve when treated with appropriate medical strategies may also require surgical removal.

Prevention

Prevention of recurrent urolithiasis depends upon the mineral type involved (see Chap. 99).

RENAL PARASITISM

Etiology

Dioctophyma renale is the canine kidney worm. *D. renale* infection is a rare condition. Dogs become infected by ingesting the larvae or by ingesting a paratenic host, usually a fish, that contains encysted larvae.

Clinical Signs

- Dogs often are asymptomatic. Signs of renal failure do not occur with unilateral involvement.
- Abdominal enlargement may occur if the worm migrates into the peritoneal cavity and causes peritonitis.
- Hematuria may be observed.

Diagnosis

History

- *History* identifies clinical findings and potential for exposure to a paratenic host.

Physical Examination

- *Physical examination* findings may be normal, or abdominal enlargement may be found.

Laboratory Evaluations

- *Hemogram:* eosinophilia, basophilia, and hyperproteinemia may be observed.

- *Serum chemistries:* azotemia does not occur unless both kidneys are affected or unless one kidney is affected and the other kidney is impaired owing to some other cause.

Urinalysis

- The diagnosis is confirmed by observing characteristic double operculated ova in urine sediment. Renal infestation is required for a patent infection.
- Hematuria, pyuria, and proteinuria may occur secondary to urinary tract inflammation.

Abdominal Fluid Analysis

- With peritoneal involvement, findings are consistent with peritonitis (see Chap. 96).
- Look for parasitic ova in abdominal fluid.

Treatment

- No medical therapy is effective.
- Surgical Treatment
  - Perform a nephrectomy if severe unilateral renal infection exists and a nephrotomy if bilateral renal infection exists. (Surgical techniques for nephrectomy and nephrotomy are described in Chapter 98).
  - If peritonitis is present, perform an exploratory procedure to identify and remove all parasites.

Prevention

Do not allow dogs to ingest paratenic hosts or infected water.

RENAL NEOPLASIA

Etiology

Primary Tumors

- Renal cell carcinoma, transitional cell carcinoma, and embryonal nephroblastoma are the most common primary renal tumors in dogs. A syndrome of dermatofibrosis and renal cystadenocarcinoma occurs primarily in female German shepherd dogs and may be a heritable trait.
- Renal cell carcinoma is the most common primary renal tumor in cats.
- Renal tumors in dogs and cats are usually malignant.

Metastatic Tumors

- Metastatic neoplasia is more common than primary renal neoplasia.
- The kidneys are often involved in patients with lymphoma, especially cats.
- Hemangiosarcomas, melanomas, mast cell tumors, and carcinomas also may metastasize to the kidneys.

Clinical Signs

- Clinical signs usually are vague and nonspecific. Lethargy, anorexia, and progressive weight loss may occur.

- Anorexia, vomiting, and polyuria or polydipsia may occur in patients that develop renal failure.
- Hematuria of renal origin may be observed.

Diagnosis

History

History identifies the clinical signs of renal neoplasia.

Physical Examination

- Palpate the kidneys for renomegaly.
- Examine for tumors or masses in other organ locations.

Laboratory Evaluations

- *Hematology:* polycythemia may occur with some renal tumors (e.g., carcinoma, fibrosarcoma) presumably owing to inappropriate production of erythropoietin.
- *Serum chemistries:* azotemia and hyperphosphatemia due to renal failure may occur with bilateral renal neoplasia, especially in cats with lymphoma.
- Hematuria and proteinuria may be observed.

▼ *Key Point* Feline leukemia virus status is determined in cats with renal lymphoma. About 50% of affected cats are positive for FeLV by ELISA test.

Radiography

- Survey abdominal radiographs may reveal unilateral or bilateral renomegaly. An abdominal mass that cannot be identified as kidney sometimes is seen.
- When a renal mass is suspected, perform excretory urography to confirm renal involvement (see Chap. 4).
- Radiography of the thorax is needed to look for possible metastasis. This finding is most likely with renal cell carcinoma.

Ultrasonography

Ultrasonography of the abdomen helps confirm renal mass lesions.

Renal Biopsy

- In cats with bilateral renomegaly, cytologic examination of a fine-needle aspirate sample from a kidney often is diagnostic of lymphoma and eliminates the need for renal biopsy.
- For other neoplasms, perform a renal biopsy. Tissue for histologic evaluation is submitted to determine definitive diagnosis. Surgical biopsy may be necessary to allow direct exposure of the neoplasm.

Treatment

Chemotherapy

- Treat lymphoma with combination chemotherapy (see Chap. 25).

Surgery

- Evaluate the function of the contralateral kidney prior to nephrectomy.

- With the exception of lymphoma, surgical excision of the neoplastic kidney and its ureter is the treatment of choice (see Chap. 98). Consider adjunctive treatment (see Chaps. 24 and 25).

Prognosis

The prognosis is guarded to poor for patients with malignant renal neoplasms.

RENAL AND URETERAL TRAUMA

Because of their location in the abdominal cavity, traumatic injury to the kidneys and ureters is uncommon in small animal patients. See Chapters 99 and 101 for discussion of bladder and urethral trauma.

Etiology

- *Blunt trauma* may be caused by vehicular injuries and falls from heights.
- *Penetrating trauma* may result from fight wounds, gunshot injuries, and other objects.

Clinical Signs

- In most cases, renal and ureteral trauma is mild and self-limiting.
- Rupture of the renal capsule, pelvis, or mid to upper ureter causes extravasation of urine into the retroperitoneal space, which is associated with vague nonspecific signs including abdominal pain and fever.
- Rupture of the distal ureter causes leakage of urine into the abdominal cavity. Clinical findings result from peritonitis and uremia and may include abdominal enlargement and pain.
- Macroscopic hematuria occurs frequently.
- Severe bruising to the ventral abdominal wall is often, but not always, seen with traumatically induced uroabdomen.
- Normal urination may be seen with unilateral ureteral rupture.

Diagnosis

▼ *Key Point* Suspect renal or ureteral trauma when there are vague signs of abdominal discomfort; macroscopic hematuria; or fractures of the caudal ribs, vertebrae, or pelvis, particularly.

History

- Question the owner about the possibility of trauma.

Physical Examination

- Observe for any external signs of trauma.
- Palpate the abdomen to detect evidence of pain and fluid accumulation.

Laboratory Evaluations

- *Hemogram* is usually normal.
- *Serum chemistry panel* may reveal azotemia if the injury is not acute and significant urine leakage has occurred.
- *Urinalysis* may show hematuria.

Abdominal Fluid Analysis

Note: Urine leakage may remain confined to the retroperitoneal space and not result in uroabdomen.

- Perform cytologic evaluation. Nonseptic inflammation occurs most often with uroabdomen.
- Determine creatinine concentration in abdominal fluid.
  - When urine leaks into the abdominal cavity, the creatinine concentration of the peritoneal fluid is greater than that of the serum initially.
  - Urea is a small molecule; therefore, its concentration rapidly equilibrates with that of serum, making its measurement less useful for diagnosis of uroabdomen.

Radiography

Radiography provides the most useful information regarding the location of ureteral rupture.

- *Survey abdominal radiographic* findings are rarely diagnostic of renal or ureteral trauma.
  - Signs suggestive of trauma include displacement, asymmetry, and inability to visualize one or both kidneys.
  - Urine leakage into the retroperitoneal space causes increased opacity and streaky, hazy areas in the retroperitoneum.
  - Loss of abdominal contrast occurs when urine leaks into the peritoneal space.
- *Contrast radiography*

▼ *Key Point* Excretory urography is the diagnostic test of choice for patients with renal and ureteral trauma.

- Look for an accumulation of contrast material in the area of suspected leakage.
- If a kidney is not visualized, perform renal arteriography to evaluate the kidney's vascular supply.
- Perform thoracic radiography in all trauma patients to evaluate for consequences of thoracic trauma.
- Ultrasonography may be helpful to delineate the kidneys and retroperitoneal space.

Treatment
Supportive

- Stabilize the patient by administering fluids and employing other shock treatment measures as needed (see Chap. 72).
- Observe the animal for evidence of a ruptured urinary tract. Other injuries may be self-limiting (e.g., renal contusions, hematoma).
- Provide abdominal drainage in animals with uroabdomen to stabilize them prior to surgery (see Chap. 96).

Surgery

- After stabilization and diagnostic evaluation, consider surgical treatment (see Chap. 98).
- Indications for surgery include leakage of urine into the abdomen or retroperitoneal space and crushing injury to the kidney or its vascular supply.

ECTOPIC URETER

Etiology

- Ureteral ectopia is a congenital abnormality whereby one or both ureters do not terminate in the trigone of the urinary bladder.
- In females, ectopic ureters may terminate in the vagina, urethra, or uterus. In males, ectopic ureters end in the pelvic urethra.

Clinical Signs

- Urinary incontinence is usually observed by the owner around the time of weaning. Incontinence can be continual or intermittent.
- Animals with ureteral ectopia usually retain the ability to urinate normally. (see Chap. 103, for discussion of micturition disorders.)
- Urine may have a foul odor if a urinary tract infection exists.
- Soiling of the perineal hair and skin with urine may cause dermatitis.

Diagnosis
History

- Identify urinary incontinence in a young animal. (For a discussion of diagnostic approach and differential diagnosis for incontinence, see Chap. 103.)
- Female dogs are affected most frequently; however, male dogs and cats may also have ectopic ureters.

Physical Examination

- Verify urinary incontinence by urine-soaked perineal area or after observation during hospitalization.
- Look for other congenital defects.

Laboratory Evaluations

- These are usually normal with the exception of urinalysis. Pyuria and bacteriuria often occur secondary to urinary tract infection.

Urine Culture

- *Perform urine culture* to rule out urinary tract infection.

Contrast Radiography

- *Excretory urography* (see Chap. 4).
  - Usually confirms the diagnosis of ureteral ectopia.
  - Dilated ureters and hydronephrosis may occur secondary to urinary tract infection.

- Inflating the bladder with room air or CO_2 helps improve visualization of terminal ureters, and oblique films may be indicated to outline individual ureters.
- *Retrograde contrast urethrography* or *vaginography* may help to localize the site of ureteral termination.

Vaginoscopy and Cytoscopy

- Vaginoscopy or cytoscopy may be helpful to locate the terminal ureteral orifice and to evaluate for ureteral abnormalities.
- Surgical exploration occasionally is required to achieve a definitive diagnosis if cytoscopy is not available. Cytoscopy allows for evaluation of ureteral orifice location. Intramural ectopic ureter may enter the bladder in a normal trigonal position.

Treatment
Surgical Treatment

- *Surgical correction* is the treatment of choice (see Chap. 98 for description of techniques).

▼ *Key Point* Surgical correction cures about 50% of patients with ectopic ureter; incontinence continues in approximately 50%. One-third of these animals respond to medical treatment.

Medical Treatment

- Treatment of urinary tract infection is indicated.
  - Culture urine to determine the species of infecting organism.
  - If pyelonephritis is suspected, administer an antimicrobial agent for 6–8 weeks.
  - Reculture urine 3–5 days after beginning treatment and again 5–7 days after discontinuing treatment.
- Adrenergic stimulants (agonistic) may reduce incontinence following surgery (see Chap. 103).

Prevention

- Counsel the owners regarding possible inheritance of ectopic ureter.
- Consider neutering the animal.

URETERAL OBSTRUCTION

Etiology

- *Neoplasia*
  - Primary ureteral tumors include leiomyosarcoma and leiomyoma.
  - Any abdominal tumor may compress a ureter, causing extramural obstruction.
  - Extension of tumors from the bladder (e.g., transitional cell carcinoma, rhabdomyosarcoma) and prostate (e.g., adenocarcinoma) may obstruct the ureters.
- *Uroliths* formed in the kidney may enter a ureter, causing obstruction (see discussion of calculi of kidney and ureter).

- *Blood clots* may lodge in the ureter secondary to renal hematuria.
- *Strictures* may be congenital or occur secondary to inflammation or surgery.

Clinical Signs

- Partial and unilateral obstruction may be subclinical. Bilateral obstruction causes signs of renal failure (see previous discussion).
- Signs may result from the underlying disease.
  - Hematuria and stranguria may occur with urinary bladder neoplasia and prostatic disease.
  - Straining to defecate may be observed with prostatic disease.
  - Ureterolithiasis may cause pain and abdominal discomfort.

Diagnosis
History

- Look for clinical signs of ureteral obstruction.
- Determine the possible history of abdominal surgery or trauma, urolithiasis, and neoplasia.

Physical Examination

- Palpate the abdomen for evidence of pain and abdominal masses.
- Perform a rectal examination to evaluate the prostate gland, pelvic urethra, and sublumbar lymph nodes.
- Palpate the urinary bladder to detect a mass.

Laboratory Evaluations

- *Hemogram* may be normal or show an inflammatory response (e.g., pyelonephritis).
- *Serum chemistry panel* is usually normal. Azotemia may occur if both kidneys are affected.
- *Urinalysis* may show hematuria or pyuria associated with inflammation, neoplasia, or urolithiasis.

Radiography

- *Survey abdominal radiographs* may demonstrate radiopaque ureteroliths or compressing masses.
- *Excretory urography* confirms the presence and location of ureteral obstruction. Dilation of the ureter proximal to the obstruction and hydronephrosis often occur.

Ultrasonography

- Noninvasively detects changes (e.g., hydronephrosis) consistent with ureteral obstruction.
- Preferred over excretory urography in patients with compromised renal function.
- Normal findings do not rule out a diagnosis of obstruction.

Treatment

The goals of treatment are to provide supportive care and to remove the underlying cause, if possible.

Medical Treatment

- If the obstruction is partial, urine is sterile, and the cause of obstruction may resolve spontaneously (e.g., blood clot), monitor the animal for a period of weeks to months.
- If partial obstruction occurs because of urolithiasis (e.g., struvite, urate), attempt dissolution of the urolith.

Surgical Treatment

- Surgery is indicated with evidence of progressive renal damage, persistent urinary tract infection, and no response to medical therapy.
- If ureteral neoplasia or stricture exists, surgical excision is the treatment of choice.
- If possible, remove extramural masses that compress the ureter. Severe renal damage from chronic obstruction and/or pyelonephritis with concurrent ureteral obstruction is treated by nephrectomy-ureterectomy, provided that the contralateral kidney is functioning adequately.

SUPPLEMENTAL READINGS

Acute Renal Failure

Forrester SD: Diseases of the kidney and ureter. In Leib MS, Monroe WE, eds.: Practical Small Animal Internal Medicine. WB Saunders, 1997, p 283.
Grauer GF, Lane IF: Acute renal failure. In Ettinger SJ, Feldman EC, eds.: Textbook of Veterinary Internal Medicine. WB Saunders, 1995, p 1720.
Rentko VT, Clark N, Ross LA, et al.: Canine leptospirosis: A retrospective study of 17 cases. J Vet Intern Med, 1992;6:235.

Chronic Renal Failure

Cowgill LD: CVT update: Use of recombinant human erythropoietin. In Kirk RW, Bonagura JD, eds.: Current Veterinary Therapy XII. Small Animal Practice. Philadelphia: WB Saunders, 1995, p 961.
Lulich JD, Osborne CA, O'Brien RD, et al.: Feline renal failure: Questions, answers, questions. Compend Contin Educ Pract Vet 1992:14:127.
Polzin DJ, Osborne CA, Bartges JW, et al: Chronic renal failure. In Ettinger SJ, Feldman EC, eds.: Textbook of Veterinary Internal Medicine. Philadelphia: WB Saunders, 1995, p 1734.
Polzin DJ: Chronic renal failure: Improving therapeutic response with patient monitoring. In Kirk RW, Bonagura JD, eds.: Current Veterinary Therapy XII. Small Animal Practice. Philadelphia: WB Saunders, 1995, p 948.
Polzin DJ, James KM, Osborne CA: Metabolic acidosis in renal failure: Consequences, diagnosis, and treatment. In Kirk RW, Bonagura JD, eds.: Current Veterinary Therapy XII. Small Animal Practice. Philadelphia: WB Saunders, 1995, p 956.

Pyelonephritis

Lees GE, Rogers KS: Diagnosis and localization of urinary tract infections. In Kirk RW, ed.: Current Veterinary Therapy IX. Small Animal Practice. Philadelphia: WB Saunders, 1986, p 1118.
Lees GE, Forrester SD: Update: Bacterial urinary tract infections. In Kirk RW, Bonagura JD, eds.: Current Veterinary Therapy XI. Small Animal Practice. Philadelphia: WB Saunders, 1992, p 909.
Lulich JP, Osborne CA: Bacterial infections of the urinary tract. In Ettinger SJ, Feldman EC, eds.: Textbook of Veterinary Internal Medicine. Philadelphia: WB Saunders, 1995, p 1775.

Glomerular Diseases

Grauer GF, DiBartola SP: Glomerular disease. In Ettinger SJ, Feldman EC, eds.: Textbook of Veterinary Internal Medicine. WB Saunders, 1995, p 1760.
Hurley KJ, Vaden SL: Proteinuria in dogs and cats: A diagnostic approach. In Kirk RW, Bonagura JD, eds.: Current Veterinary Therapy XII. Small Animal Practice. Philadelphia: WB Saunders, 1995, p 937.
Lulich JP, Osborne CA: Interpretation of urine protein-creatinine ratio in dogs with glomerular and nonglomerular disorders. Compend Contin Educ Pract Vet 1990;12:59.

Renal Tubular Disorders

Bovee KC: Canine cystine urolithiasis. Vet Clin North Am (Sm Anim Pract) 16:211, 1986.
Breitschwerdt EB: Nephrogenic diabetes insipidus. In Kirk RW, ed.: Current Veterinary Therapy X. Small Animal Practice. Philadelphia: WB Saunders, 1986, p 1140.
Brown SA: Fanconi's syndrome. In Kirk RW, ed.: Current Veterinary Therapy X. Small Animal Practice. Philadelphia: WB Saunders, 1989, p1163.
Brown SA, Rakich PM, Barsanti JA, et al.: Fanconi syndrome and acute renal failure associated with gentamicin therapy in a dog. J Am Anim Hosp Assoc 22:635, 1986.
Polzin D, Osborne C, O'Brien T: Diseases of the kidneys and ureters. In Ettinger SJ, ed.: Textbook of Veterinary Internal Medicine, 2nd ed. Philadelphia: WB Saunders, 1989, p 1962.

Cystic Renal Disease

Crowell WA: Polycystic renal disease. In Kirk RW, ed.: Current Veterinary Therapy IX. Small Animal Practice. Philadelphia: WB Saunders, 1986, p 1138.
Lulich JP, Osborne CA, Walter PA, O'Brien TD: Feline idiopathic polycystic kidney disease. Compend Contin Educ Pract Vet 10:1030, 1988.
Polzin D, Osborne C, O'Brien T: Diseases of the kidneys and ureters. In Ettinger SJ, ed.: Textbook of Veterinary Internal Medicine, 2nd ed. Philadelphia: WB Saunders, 1989, p 1962.

Nephrolithiasis and Ureterolithiasis

Ling GV: Nephrolithiasis: Prevalence of mineral type. In Kirk RW, Bonagura JD, eds.: Current Veterinary Therapy XII. Small Animal Practice. Philadelphia: WB Saunders, 1995, p 980.
Ling GV, Sorenson JL: CVT update: Management and prevention of urate urolithiasis. In Kirk RW, Bonagura JD, eds.: Current Veterinary Therapy XII. Small Animal Practice. Philadelphia: WB Saunders, 1995, p 985.
Osborne CA, Unger LK, Lulich JP: Canine and feline nephroliths. In Kirk RW, Bonagura JD, eds.: Current Veterinary Therapy XII. Small Animal Practice. Philadelphia: WB Saunders, 1995, p 981.
Osborne CA, Lulich JP, Thumchai R: Feline calcium oxalate uroliths. In Kirk RW, Bonagura JD, eds.: Current Veterinary Therapy XII. Small Animal Practice. Philadelphia: WB Saunders, 1995, p 989.
Lulich JP, Osborne CA: Canine calcium oxalate uroliths. In Kirk RW, Bonagura JD, eds.: Current Veterinary Therapy XII. Small Animal Practice. Philadelphia: WB Saunders, 1995, p 992.

Renal Parasitism

Brown SA, Prestwood AK: Parasites of the urinary tract. In Kirk RW, ed.: Current Veterinary Therapy IX. Small Animal Practice. Philadelphia: WB Saunders, 1986, p 1153.

Renal Neoplasia

Hammer AS, LaRue S: Tumors of the urinary tract. In Ettinger SJ, Feldman EC, eds.: Textbook of Veterinary Internal Medicine. WB Saunders, 1995, p 1788.
Klein MK, Cockerell GL, Harris CK, et al.: Canine primary renal neoplasms: a retrospective review of 54 cases. J Am Anim Hosp Assoc 24:443, 1988.

Mooney SC, Hayes AA, Matus RE, MacEwen EG: Renal lymphoma in cats: 28 cases (1977–1984). J Am Vet Med Assoc 191:1473, 1987.

Renal and Ureteral Trauma

Forrester SD: Diseases of the kidney and ureter. *In* Leib MS, Monroe WE, eds.: Practical Small Animal Internal Medicine. WB Saunders, 1997, p 283.

Pechman RD: Urinary tract trauma in dogs and cats. J Am Anim Hosp Assoc 18:33, 1982.

Zenoble RD, Pechman RD: Urinary tract trauma. *In* Kirk RW, ed.: Current Veterinary Therapy IX. Small Animal Practice. Philadelphia: WB Saunders, 1986, p 1155.

Ectopic Ureters

Faulkner RT, Osborne CA, Feeney DA: Canine and feline ureteral ectopia. *In* Kirk RW, ed.: Current Veterinary Therapy VIII. Small Animal Practice. Philadelphia: WB Saunders, 1983, p 1043.

Forrester SD: Diseases of the kidney and ureter. *In* Leib MS, Monroe WE, eds.: Practical Small Animal Internal Medicine. WB Saunders, 1997, p 283.

Ureteral Obstruction

Polzin D, Osborne C, O'Brien T: Diseases of the kidneys and ureters. *In* Ettinger SJ, ed.: Textbook of Veterinary Internal Medicine, 2nd ed. Philadelphia: WB Saunders, 1989, p 1962.

98 Surgery of the Kidney and Ureter

Dale E. Bjorling

Biopsy of the kidney often gives the most reliable information regarding the presence of disease and the prognosis for improvement. When renal calculi are removed surgically, a nephrotomy is usually performed. When the renal pelvis and proximal ureter are dilated, a pyelolithotomy may be performed to remove calculi. Removal of the kidney (nephrectomy) is often considered because of severe damage due to trauma, neoplasia, infection, or obstruction of the ureter. Reattachment of the ureter to the renal pelvis is extremely difficult without magnification and is infrequently attempted in veterinary practice. This disorder is more commonly treated by unilateral nephrectomy and ureterectomy. A ureterotomy may be performed to remove calculi or other objects from the lumen of the ureter. Ureteral anastomosis is a challenge for the veterinarian in small dogs and in cats. Magnification is strongly encouraged during this procedure to improve outcome. Ureteroneocystostomy is a feasible treatment option for lesions of the distal ureter and is considered for ectopic ureter.

ANATOMY

Kidney

- The kidneys are normally found in the retroperitoneal space in a sublumbar location. The cranial pole of the right kidney may be in contact with the liver, and the left kidney may usually be found several centimeters caudal to the liver.
- The renal arteries divide into dorsal and ventral branches after arising from the aorta. Each branch divides into five to seven interlobar arteries. The interlobar arteries branch into arcuate arteries at the corticomedullary junction and ultimately give rise to the interlobular arteries. Multiple renal arteries may occur on the left side in up to 13% of all dogs but are rare on the right side. Multiple renal arteries are extremely uncommon in cats. The renal artery may give rise to the ovarian artery, and the ovarian vein occasionally drains into the renal vein.

Ureter

- The ureter is a muscular tube that lies within the retroperitoneal space. The ureter carries urine to the bladder by coordinated peristaltic contractions.

- The arterial blood supply of the ureter is longitudinal. Do not disturb the arterial blood supply during dissection of the ureter.
- The ureter approaches the bladder at an oblique angle and passes submucosally within the bladder wall toward the neck of the bladder. A valve-like function is provided by the submucosal location of the ureters, which decreases vesicoureteral reflux of urine.

RENAL BIOPSY

Preoperative Considerations

- Platelet count and coagulation function must be normal prior to undertaking renal biopsy.

▼ **Key Point** Hemorrhage is a common occurrence after renal biopsy. Evaluate coagulation function before surgery. Apply pressure to the biopsy site until bleeding has stopped.

- If unilateral disease is present and if a percutaneous biopsy is to be performed, identify the site of disease before performing the biopsy.

Surgical Procedure

Objectives

- Obtain a representative sample of renal tissue.
- Avoid damage to major vasculature or the renal pelvis.
- Control hemorrhage.

Equipment

- Standard surgical instruments and suture
- Vim-Silverman or Tru-Cut biopsy needle (or other biopsy needle of the surgeon's preference)
- Balfour self-retaining retractor for the celiotomy approach.

Technique

Perform kidney biopsy through a percutaneous, "keyhole," approach, or through celiotomy. The celiotomy approach is described.

1. Place the animal in dorsal recumbency.
2. Aseptically prepare the ventral abdomen for a standard celiotomy incision.

3. Make a ventral midline approach to the abdominal cavity and extend the incision cranially to the xiphoid process to facilitate exposure of the kidneys.
4. Place a self-retaining Balfour retractor to maintain exposure of the abdominal cavity.
5. Examine and palpate the kidneys. If an isolated lesion is present, select an appropriate biopsy site.
6. Obtain single or multiple biopsy samples using a biopsy needle, or perform a nephrotomy to collect a wedge or slice of renal tissue. The technique for biopsy during nephrotomy is discussed in this chapter under Nephrotomy.
7. When a biopsy needle is used, direct the needle away from the pelvis to avoid damaging this structure and large vessels, and obtain at least two samples to be sure that a representative one has been taken. Apply pressure to the biopsy site for 5 minutes to promote hemostasis. If bleeding persists, tack the omentum onto the biopsy site with one or two sutures to act as a patch.

Postoperative Care and Complications

- Establish diuresis by intravenous (IV) administration of a balanced electrolyte solution at a rate of 90 ml/kg/24 hr for 8–12 hours. This helps prevent the formation of blood clots within the renal pelvis.
- Hematuria is occasionally observed after renal biopsy and is usually self-limiting.
- Hemorrhage after renal biopsy can become life-threatening. If this occurs, surgically expose the kidneys via celiotomy, and place sutures in a mattress pattern through the capsule and superficial parenchyma to control hemorrhage. Tighten sutures just enough to stop bleeding but avoid capsular tearing. On rare occasions, uncontrollable hemorrhage necessitates nephrectomy.

NEPHROTOMY

Preoperative Considerations

- Nephrotomy is most often performed for removal of renal calculi. Investigate for other calculi within the urinary tract with excretory urography or ultrasonography before surgery.
- Remove large solitary calculi that result in extensive dilation of the renal pelvis by pyelolithotomy (described in other texts).
- If possible, evaluate coagulation function before surgery. Abnormal coagulation may result in prolonged hemorrhage after surgery. Correct fluid deficits and serum electrolyte abnormalities, if possible, before surgery.
- If bilateral renal calculi are present, perform nephrotomy as a staged procedure. Perform the second surgery approximately 1 month after the first. Because of a transient decrease in renal function after nephrotomy, absent or decreased function of the contralateral kidney may preclude nephrotomy. In these instances, pyelolithotomy is greatly preferred.

Surgical Procedure

Objectives

- Remove renal calculi.
- Obtain a renal biopsy or microbial culture specimen.
- Confirm patency of the ureter.

Equipment

- Standard surgical instruments and suture
- Balfour self-retaining retractor
- Catheters of appropriate diameter to pass into the ureter (3.5 Fr. or 5 Fr.)
- Vascular forceps or Rommel tourniquet

Technique

1–4. Refer to Renal Biopsy; Technique, Steps 1–4.
5. Examine and palpate the kidneys. Free the affected kidney of its peritoneal attachments, and identify and isolate the renal vasculature.
6. Apply a Rommel tourniquet or vascular forceps to the renal artery and vein. The time at which the vasculature is occluded is noted, and ischemia of the kidney is limited to 30 minutes or less.
7. Make an incision through the renal capsule on the greater curvature of the kidney (Fig. 98–1A). The incision is of adequate length to allow exposure of the renal pelvis after the renal parenchyma has been divided or incised. Sharply incise the renal parenchyma with a scalpel.

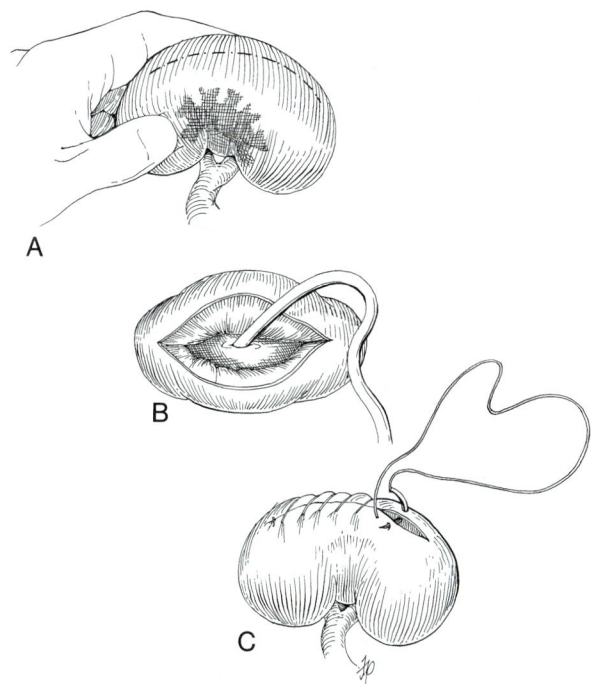

Figure 98–1. Nephrotomy. *A,* Make an incision through the renal capsule. Limit the length of the nephrotomy incision to the dimensions of the renal pelvis. *B,* Remove calculi from the renal pelvis, and pass a catheter through the ureter. *C,* Close the nephrotomy incision by placing sutures through the renal capsule and superficial parenchyma. (From Stone EA: Canine nephrotomy. Compend Contin Ed Pract Vet 9:883, 1987.)

8. Remove calculi from the pelvis and diverticula of the kidney. Submit the calculi for analysis.

▼ *Key Point* After removal of renal calculi, irrigate the renal pelvis and ensure that no calculi fragments are present in the ureter.

   Obtain samples for microbial culture. Pass a catheter through the ureter into the bladder to assess patency (Fig. 98–1*B*).

9. If a biopsy is to be done, remove a wedge or slice of tissue 2 to 4 mm in thickness with a scalpel from the surface of the nephrotomy incision through the renal parenchyma. Take care to avoid damaging the pelvis or diverticula.

10. Appose the exposed surfaces of the renal parenchyma, and hold them in this position with digital pressure as the tourniquet or vascular forceps is removed. Maintain pressure for 5 minutes to allow clotting to occur.

11. Close the nephrotomy incision by placing a single layer of absorbable suture in a simple continuous pattern through the renal capsule and superficial parenchyma (Fig. 98–1*C*).

12. If calculi are present in the bladder, perform a cystotomy to remove them.

13. Return the kidney to its normal position within the abdominal cavity, and close the body wall, subcutaneous tissues, and skin in a routine manner.

Postoperative Care and Complications

• Initiate and maintain diuresis by IV administration of a balanced electrolyte solution at a rate of 90 ml/kg/24 hr. Continue this for at least 12–24 hours. Monitor urine output to be sure that the kidneys are functioning satisfactorily.

• Hematuria is usually observed macroscopically for 1–3 days and microscopically for up to 1 week.

• Institute appropriate therapy to treat infection and prevent reformation of the calculi.

NEPHRECTOMY

Preoperative Considerations

▼ *Key Point* Function of the remaining kidney must be sufficient to support life.

• Preoperative evaluation of the function of a single kidney is often difficult. Common laboratory tests (determination of blood urea nitrogen, serum creatinine, serum potassium concentrations) are only relative indicators of renal function. Distinguish among prerenal, renal, and postrenal causes of azotemia. Concentration and excretion of a radiopaque dye on excretory urography demonstrates that the vascular supply to the kidneys is intact and that the kidneys are capable of extracting the dye from the blood and excreting it. This finding is only a relative indicator of renal function. Renal function is best evaluated by measuring the clearance of an indicator (e.g., creatinine,

inulin, radioisotopes). Nuclear scan of the kidney allows determination of unilateral renal function, whereas determination of single kidney clearance of other indicators requires ureteral catheterization and collection of the urine from that kidney. See Chapter 97 for additional information on renal function testing. In general practice, excretory urography and standard clinical pathology testing are routinely done and usually provide adequate information.

• If possible, correct metabolic and hydration imbalances before performing surgery.

Surgical Procedure

Indications for nephrectomy are listed in the introduction to this chapter.

Objectives

• Remove the diseased kidney and associated ureter.
• Control hemorrhage.

Equipment

• Standard surgical instruments and suture
• Balfour retractor
• Vascular forceps (optional)

Technique

1–4. Refer to Renal Biopsy; Technique, Steps 1–4.
5. Examine and palpate the kidneys. Obtain biopsy samples of the kidney to be preserved to be sure that it is free of disease.
6. Release the diseased kidney of its attachments. Apply a vascular forceps or tourniquet to the renal vessels or ligate these vessels before dissection to minimize hemorrhage.
7. Ligate the renal vasculature with nonabsorbable suture or surgical staples or clips. Doubly ligate the renal vessels.
8. Ligate the ureter near the bladder with absorbable suture material, and remove the entire ureter. Leaving a segment of ureter may promote subsequent urinary tract infection by urine's being retained within the ureteral remnant.
9. Examine the renal bed for hemorrhage before closure of the abdominal wall.
10. Close the abdominal wall, subcutaneous tissues, and skin in a routine manner.

Postoperative Care and Complications

• If the function of the remaining kidney is in doubt, initiate and maintain diuresis by IV administration of a balanced electrolyte solution at a rate of 90 ml/kg/24 hr until renal function and urine output appear satisfactory. (See Chap. 97 for more information on diuresis.)

• Observe the patient for 24 hours for hemorrhage due to displacement of ligatures, vascular staples, or clips.

• Warn the owner that continued renal disease in the patient may result in irreversible injury to the remaining kidney.

URETEROTOMY AND URETERAL ANASTOMOSIS

Preoperative Considerations

- Ureterotomy is most often performed for removal of calculi that have lodged within the ureter and cannot be dislodged by flushing and/or catheterization. Prolonged obstruction of the ureter by calculi results in necrosis of the ureteral wall and leakage of urine. Lesions of the distal ureter are best treated by ureteroneocystostomy.
- Ureteral obstruction or disruption most often is diagnosed by excretory urography.
- When ureteral calculi are diagnosed, carefully examine the kidneys and bladder for additional calculi.
- Warn the owner of the potential for stricture formation after ureteral surgery.

Surgical Procedure

Objectives

- Relieve ureteral obstruction.
- Ensure patency and integrity of the ureter.

Equipment

- Standard surgical instruments and suture
- Balfour retractor
- Magnification loupes are highly desirable, and an operating microscope is optional.
- Small (6-0 to 8-0) monofilament absorbable suture (polydioxanone [PDS] or polyglyconate [Maxon])
- Catheters of appropriate size (3.5 or 5 Fr.)

Technique

1–4. Refer to Renal Biopsy; Technique, Steps 1–4. The incision is extended caudally to a few centimeters cranial to the pubis.
5. Examine and palpate the kidneys, ureters, and bladder.
6. To perform ureterotomy, identify the site of the ureterotomy and make a longitudinal incision over the area of obstruction. Remove the calculi, and pass a catheter through the ureterotomy site to the kidney and to the bladder to ensure patency of the ureter. In extremely small patients, use a large suture (1 or 0 polypropylene or nylon) instead of a catheter. Close the ureterotomy incision transversely with small (6-0 to 8-0) absorbable suture in an interrupted or continuous pattern. The transverse configuration of the closure increases the ureteral diameter at the site of the ureterotomy. This maneuver is achieved by initially opposing the midpoint of the proximal and distal ends of the ureterotomy incision with a single suture.
7. If necessary, resect the devitalized portion of the ureter and identify the lumen of the proximal and distal remnants of the ureter. Make a linear incision 3 to 5 mm in length in the ends of the ureter to increase the circumference of the anastomosis. Per-form the anastomosis with small, absorbable suture placed in an interrupted or a continuous pattern.
8. A catheter can be passed through the urethra, bladder, and ureter to divert the flow of urine past the ureterotomy or anastomotic site for 10–14 days if leakage is considered a possibility. The placement of a catheter (stent) following surgery is controversial, and some believe this practice may predispose the patient to stricture formation in the ureter.
9. Close the abdominal wall, subcutaneous tissue, and skin in a routine manner.

Postoperative Care and Complications

- Stricture formation is common after ureteral surgery, particularly in cats and small dogs. Reevaluate the patient 3–4 weeks after surgery by excretory urography. If ureteral obstruction is observed, consider resecting the affected area of the ureter and performing an anastomosis or implanting the proximal portion of the ureter into the bladder (ureteroneocystostomy).

URETERONEOCYSTOSTOMY (URETERAL REIMPLANTATION)

Preoperative Considerations

- This procedure is performed most often for treatment of ectopic ureter. Inform the owner that incontinence associated with an ectopic ureter may or may not resolve after ureteroneocystostomy. Incontinence that persists after this procedure may be the result of developmental abnormalities of the urethral sphincter or the presence of the remnant of the distal ureter within the sphincter mechanism.
- Ureteroneocystostomy may also be performed to treat disorders resulting in destruction or loss of function of the distal ureter and is preferable to resection and anastomosis of the distal ureter because a lower complication rate is observed after ureteroneocystostomy.

Surgical Procedure

Objectives

- Restore flow of urine from ureter into the bladder.
- Treat incontinence associated with ectopic ureter.

Equipment

- Standard surgical instruments and suture
- Balfour retractor
- Magnification is extremely helpful with small patients but optional with large patients.
- Fine-gauge (5-0 to 7-0) absorbable suture.

Technique

1–4. Refer to Renal Biopsy; Technique, Steps 1–4. Continue the incision caudally to the pubis.
5. Examine and palpate the kidneys, ureters, and bladder.

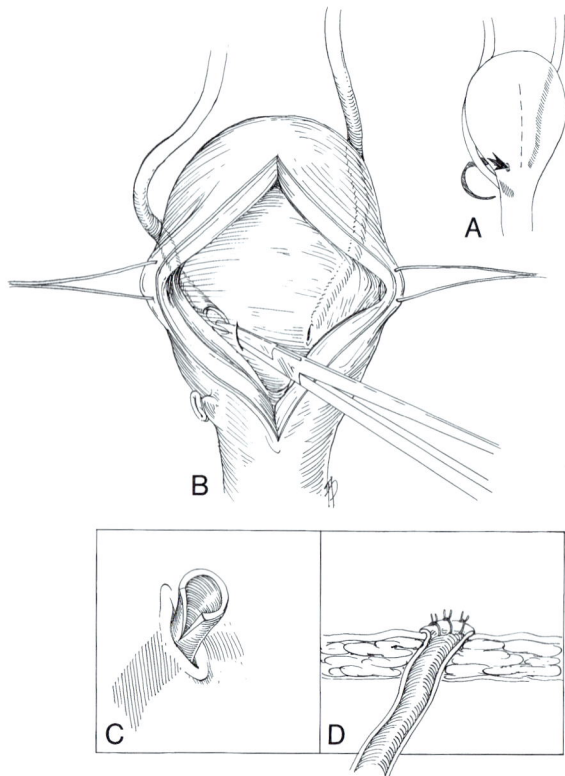

Figure 98–2. Ureteroneocystostomy. *A,* Isolate, ligate, and divide the distal ureter and perform a ventral cystotomy. *B,* Create a circular defect in the bladder mucosa, and pass forceps through the bladder wall to grasp the end of the ureter. *C,* Debride and spatulate the end of the ureter. *D,* Suture the ureter to the bladder mucosa. (From Rawlings CA: Repaired ectopic ureter. *In* Bojrab MJ, ed.: Current Techniques in Small Animal Surgery, 3rd ed. Philadelphia: Lea & Febiger, 1990, p 374.)

6. Identify the distal ureter and isolate it by dissection. Take care to preserve the longitudinal blood supply of the ureter. If the ureter is in an ectopic location, ligate the distal continuation (Fig. 98–2*A*). Preserve a sufficient length of ureter to allow implantation into the bladder under minimal tension.

7. Perform a ventral cystotomy and create a circular defect 5–10 mm in diameter in the cranial aspect of the mucosa of the dorsal wall of the bladder (Fig. 98–2*B*). Pass a forceps from the lumen of the bladder at an oblique angle in a caudal-to-cranial direction. Grasp the distal end of the proximal remnant of the ureter, or preferably a suture attached to this end of the ureter with the forceps, and draw the ureter through the bladder wall (Fig. 98–2*B*). As the ureter is drawn through the bladder wall,

take care to avoid twisting the ureter, because this may obstruct the ureter or its blood supply.

8. Make a longitudinal incision 5–10 mm in length in the ventral aspect of the end of the ureter (Fig. 98–2*C*). Secure the ureter to the edge of the defect created in the bladder mucosa with small (5-0 to 7-0) synthetic absorbable sutures in an interrupted pattern (Fig. 98–2*D*). A ureteral catheter is not maintained after surgery.

9. Alternatively, create a new opening into the bladder by making an incision through the bladder mucosa overlying an intramural ectopic ureter into the lumen of the ureter. Suture the ureteral mucosa to the bladder mucosa with fine-gauge absorbable suture, and excise the distal ureter.

10. Close the cystotomy incision in a standard manner (see Chap. 100).

11. Close the abdominal wall, subcutaneous tissue, and skin in a routine manner.

Postoperative Care and Complications

- Obstruction of the ureteroneocystostomy or leakage of urine from the site of ureteral reimplantation is extremely uncommon.
- Treat urinary incontinence that persists after surgery with alpha-agonists in an attempt to increase urethral sphincter tone (see Chap. 103). Warn the owner that incontinence due to ectopic ureter may or may not improve in the patient after surgery and medical therapy.
- Perform excretory urography 4 weeks after surgery to assess the shape and function of the ureter.

SUPPLEMENTAL READINGS

Christie BA, Bjorling DE: Kidneys. *In* Slatter DH, ed.: Textbook of Small Animal Surgery, 2nd Ed. Philadelphia: WB Saunders, 1993, p 1428.

Christie BA, Bjorling DE: Ureters. *In* Slatter DH, ed.: Textbook of Small Animal Surgery. Philadelphia: WB Saunders, 1993, p 1443.

Gahring DR, Crowe DT, Powers TE, et al.: Comparative renal function studies of nephrotomy closure with and without sutures in dogs. J Am Vet Med Assoc 171:537, 1977.

Mason LK, Stone EA, Biery DN, et al.: Surgery of ectopic ureters: Pre- and postoperative radiographic morphology. J Am Anim Hosp Assoc 26:73, 1990.

Stone EA, Mason AK: Surgery of ectopic ureters: Types, method of correction, and postoperative results. J Am Anim Hosp Assoc 26:81, 1990.

Stone EA, Barsanti JA: Urologic Surgery of the Dog and Cat. Philadelphia: Lea & Febiger, 1992, pp 161–210.

99 Diseases of the Urinary Bladder

Joseph W. Bartges

Urolithiasis and bacterial urinary tract infection (UTI) are the most common urinary bladder diseases in any age dog, but neoplasia is more common in older animals. The most common urinary bladder diseases of cats include idiopathic feline lower urinary tract disease (IFLUTD), urolithiasis, and bacterial UTI. In younger cats urolithiasis and IFLUTD are most common, whereas bacterial cystitis is seen more often in older cats.

DIAGNOSTIC TESTING FOR BLADDER DISEASE

The primary function of the urinary bladder is to store and expel urine in coordination with urethral relaxation. Thus, clinical signs of urinary bladder disease are often manifested as disruption in the micturition process.

Urinalysis

Collection and analysis of urine are essential for the confirmation and diagnosis of urinary bladder disease. Perform a complete urinalysis including microscopic examination of a sample following centrifugation. Examine urine sediment for red blood cells, white blood cells, casts, crystals, and bacteria. Occasionally other infectious agents (such as fungi) or neoplastic cells may be observed. Abnormalities in a urinalysis may result from upper urinary tract, lower urinary tract, or reproductive tract disease.

Urine Culture and Sensitivity

If bacterial UTI is suspected, submit urine collected by cystocentesis for culture. Urine collected by cystocentesis should not contain bacteria, whereas urine collected by catheterization or catching of a midstream voided sample may contain bacteria normally present in the distal urogenital tract.

▼ *Key Point* Confirmation of bacterial UTI is best made by culturing urine samples collected by cystocentesis.

Complete Blood Cell Count (CBC) and Serum Biochemical Analysis

In the absence of kidney disease, obstruction, or internal urine leakage, CBC and serum biochemical analysis are usually normal.

- Azotemia may be observed with urethral obstruction or rupture of the urinary bladder.
- Evidence of sepsis (neutrophilic leukocytosis with left shift, hypoalbuminemia, increased alkaline phosphatase activity, low blood urea nitrogen [BUN] concentration) may be observed with severe urinary tract infections.
- Hypercalcemia may be observed in some cases of calcium oxalate urolithiasis or with certain neoplasms of the urogenital tract.
- Hyperuric acidemia, hyperammonemia, a low BUN concentration, and microcytosis may be observed with ammonium urate uroliths that form in association with portosystemic shunts (PSS). Hyperuric acidemia may be observed with urate uroliths that form in animals that do not have portosystemic shunting of blood.

Radiography

- *Survey abdominal radiography* may be beneficial in the diagnosis of diseases of the bladder that are associated with densities different from soft tissue (such as uroliths). It may also be used to evaluate the location of the bladder (e.g., with perineal or inguinal herniation, or pelvic bladder) or for evaluation of bladder integrity (e.g., small urinary bladder with fluid density in the abdominal cavity may be observed with rupture of the urinary bladder).
- *Contrast radiography* may help to delineate diseases associated with mural thickening (either diffuse or localized), abnormal storage volumes, bladder rupture, uroliths, or anatomic abnormalities (e.g., urachal diverticulum or pelvic location of the bladder).

Ultrasonography

Ultrasonography may provide the same information that contrast radiography provides without the necessity to sedate or anesthetize the animal or breach the host's bladder defense mechanisms with a urinary catheter. Although ultrasonography may be helpful in diagnosing urolithiasis, it is not helpful in estimating the mineral content of the urolith(s) or in determining the number of uroliths present. It is not possible to assess the entire urethra with abdominal ultrasonography.

Cystoscopy

Cystoscopy may be of benefit in the diagnosis of urolithiasis, polyps, mucosal lesions, neoplasia, and foreign bodies. It confirms disease processes and may allow further diagnostics, such as biopsy, to be performed.

Detrusor Function Testing

Cystometrometry is a specialized test that is useful in determining abnormalities of storage of urine, and in the response of the bladder to distention (see Chap. 103).

Determination of Residual Volume

Some diseases of the bladder may be associated with abnormal residual volume following voiding. Measure residual volume by first allowing the animal to finish voiding voluntarily. Pass a catheter into the bladder, and measure the volume of remaining urine. Normal residual volumes in cats are less than 2–3 ml. In female and male dogs, normal residual volume is 5–10 ml and 10–20 ml, respectively.

DEGENERATIVE DETRUSOR DISEASE

Detrusor areflexia or atony and detrusor hyperreflexia and decreased bladder capacity are degenerative diseases of the detrusor muscle that cause abnormal micturition. These are discussed in Chapter 103.

CONGENITAL DISEASES

Bladder Anomalies
Etiology

Complete agenesis of the urinary bladder is extremely rare. Bladder hypoplasia has been reported more frequently, but is also rare. Bladder hypoplasia may be seen in animals with ectopic ureters. Urinary bladder duplication and colourocystic fistula have also been rarely observed. These conditions occur in younger animals. Rule out ureteral or urethral abnormalities that do not allow the bladder to store urine.

Clinical Signs

Incontinence and recurrent or persistent UTI are the most common clinical signs.

Diagnosis

Physical Examination. Abdominal palpation may reveal a small bladder or absent bladder.
Urinalysis. Normal unless UTI is present.
Urine Culture. Negative unless UTI is present.
CBC and Serum Biochemical Analysis. Normal unless azotemia is present.
Radiography and Ultrasonography. Radiography and ultrasonography may confirm a small bladder or the absence of a bladder.

Treatment

Treatment of the primary disease is not possible (unless ectopic ureters are the primary disease). Control of UTI may be beneficial. Some animals with bladder hypoplasia and ectopic ureters may show improvement in continence when ectopic ureters are repaired surgically.

Patent Urachus

The urachus is a fetal conduit that allows urine to pass from the developing urinary bladder to the placenta. It usually atrophies completely and is nonfunctional at birth. The atrophied urachus is typically seen as a fibrous connective tissue remnant at the bladder apex.

Etiology

Incomplete atrophy of urachus after birth

Clinical Signs

Urine leakage from the umbilical area, and occasionally incontinence.

Diagnosis

History. Usually is diagnosed in young animals.
Physical Examination. Urine may be observed to collect or leak on ventral abdominal wall around the umbilicus.
Urinalysis. Normal unless a UTI is present.
Urine Culture. Negative unless a UTI is present.
CBC and Serum Biochemical Analysis. Usually normal.
Radiography and Ultrasonography. Plain radiography is usually normal; however, contrast cystography or ultrasonography may reveal the patent urachus.

Treatment

Resect the patent urachus (see Chap. 100).

Urachal Diverticulum
Etiology

A urachal diverticulum is a small outpouching of tissue at the bladder apex. It may represent a microscopic lesion that becomes macroscopic in association with bladder disease, such as urolithiasis or infection.

Clinical Signs

Usually no clinical signs are observed with a small urachal diverticulum. It may be observed as an incidental finding radiographically or ultrasonographically in association with other bladder disease. If there is a large urachal diverticulum, it may become a nidus of infection and cause recurrent UTI or urolith formation.

Diagnosis

History. Often there is a history of lower urinary tract disease associated with the primary disease.
Physical Examination. Findings consistent with the primary disease.
Urinalysis. Normal, or inflammation, crystalluria or UTI may be observed.

Urine Culture. Positive with a UTI; otherwise negative

CBC and Serum Biochemical Analysis. Usually normal.

Radiography and Ultrasonography. A diverticulum may be observed on survey radiographs; however, usually it is diagnosed with contrast cystography or ultrasonography. Look for a small pouch or outpocketing of the bladder apex.

Treatment

For a documented urachal diverticulum and secondary UTI, surgical resection may be necessary if associated with recurrent disease.

UROCYSTOLITHIASIS (BLADDER CALCULI)

Uroliths or calculi are concretions of minerals that form in the urinary tract. The urinary bladder is the most common site of urolith formation.

Etiology

Uroliths form when urine is oversaturated with minerals. Supersaturation occurs when the amount and concentration of calculogenic minerals are increased, factors such as urine pH favor a decrease in solubility of the calculogenic minerals, and promoters or lack of inhibitors of crystallization is present. Uroliths may be composed of different types of minerals (Table 99–1); struvite is the most common urolith in dogs. Although struvite once was the most common urolith in cats, currently calcium oxalate is most common. UTI with urease-producing microbes promotes formation of struvite because it results in alkaline urine and increased levels of ammonium ion in urine. Some types of uroliths form because of metabolic disease such as urate-containing calculi in Dalmatians, and calcium-containing uroliths in animals with hyperparathyroidism. Additional risk factors for urolith formation include breed, gender, age, and diet. Once initiation of urolith formation has occurred, the nidus must be retained within the urinary tract, and conditions must favor continued precipitation of minerals to promote growth of the urolith.

Clinical Signs

Animals affected with urocystoliths present for signs of lower urinary tract disease including dysuria, stranguria, pollakiuria, and hematuria. If uroliths are small enough to move out of the urinary bladder but too large to pass through the urethra, urethral obstruction will occur. Because bacterial UTI may be associated with urocystoliths, urine may be cloudy or have an abnormal odor. In some animals, urocystoliths may not be associated with any clinical signs.

Diagnosis

History. Signs consistent with lower urinary tract disease are often, but not always, present. Animals may have a history of passing uroliths or of previous urolith episodes.

Physical Examination. Often normal unless urethral obstruction is present. Urocystoliths may be palpated in approximately 20% of the cases; it is more difficult to palpate urocystoliths in dogs, particularly large breeds, than in cats. Animals that form ammonium urate urocystoliths in association with PSS may be stunted in

Table 99–1. MINERAL COMPOSITION OF 30,749 CANINE UROLITHS AND 6336 FELINE UROLITHS EVALUATED BY QUANTITATIVE METHODS* AT THE MINNESOTA UROLITH CENTER† FROM 1981 TO 1994

Predominant Mineral Type	Canine Uroliths		Feline Uroliths	
	Number	Prevalence (%)	Number	Prevalence (%)
Struvite	16,542	53.8	3413	53.9
Newberyite	2	<0.1	16	0.3
Calcium oxalate	8557	27.8	2037	37.2
Calcium phosphate	237	0.8	68	1.1
Urate	2130	6.9	432	6.8
Xanthine	30	<0.1	9	0.1
Cystine	485	1.6	22	0.3
Silica	356	1.2	0	0
Mixed‡	623	2.0	118	1.9
Compound§	1755	5.7	115	1.8
Matrix	32	0.1	106	2.0
Total	30,749	100	6336	100

*Uroliths analyzed by polarized light microscopy and x-ray diffraction methods.
†Minnesota Urolith Center, College of Veterinary Medicine, University of Minnesota, 1352 Boyd Avenue, St. Paul, MN 55108.
‡Uroliths did not contain at least 70% of mineral type listed; no nucleus or shell detected.
§Uroliths contained an identifiable nucleus and one or more surrounding layers of a different mineral type.

Table 99–2. CHARACTERISTICS OF URINE CRYSTALS

Type	Appearance	Acid	Neutral	Alkaline
		pH Where Commonly Found		
Ammonium urate	Yellow-brown spherulites, thorn apples	+	+	±
Bilirubin	Reddish brown needles or granules	+	−	−
Calcium oxalate dihydrate	Small colorless envelopes (octahedral form)	+	+	±
Calcium oxalate monohydrate	Small spindles, "hemp seeds" or dumbbells	+	+	±
Calcium phosphate	Amorphous, or long thin prisms	±	+	+
Cholesterol	Flat, colorless plates with corner notch	+	+	−
Cystine	Flat, colorless hexagonal plates	+	+	±
Hippuric acid	4- to 6-sided colorless elongated plates or prisms	+	+	±
Leucine	Yellow-brown spheroids with radial and concentric laminations	+	+	−
Struvite	3- to 6-sided colorless prisms	+	±	+
Tyrosine	Fine colorless or yellow needles arranged in sheaves or rosettes	+	−	−
Uric acid	Diamond or rhombic rosettes, or oval plates, structures with pointed ends; occasionally 6-sided plates.	+	−	−

± = Crystals may occur at this pH, but are more common at the other pH.

growth or exhibit signs of hepatoencephalopathy. Dogs and cats with infection-induced struvite urocystoliths may exhibit more severe signs due to the bacterial UTI.

Urinalysis. Examination of urine may reveal hematuria, pyuria, bacteriuria, and/or crystalluria (Table 99–2). Urine pH may aid in predicting the possible mineral composition of the uroliths; if a UTI with urease-producing bacteria is present, the urine pH will be alkaline.

▼ **Key Point** Although struvite urolith formation is induced by UTI in most dogs and in some cats, the presence of a UTI does not prove that uroliths are composed of struvite.

Infection with a urease-producing organism is required for infection-induced struvite uroliths to form.

Urine Culture. A urine culture should be positive with a urease-producing organism (usually *Staphylococcus* spp. or *Proteus* spp., occasionally *Streptococcus* spp., *Klebsiella* spp., or *Ureaplasma* spp.) with infection-induced struvite uroliths. Urine cultures may be positive with any urolith in which a secondary bacterial UTI has occurred.

CBC and Serum Biochemical Analysis. CBC and serum biochemical analysis are usually normal. Hypercalcemia may be observed in approximately 4% of dogs and 35% of cats with calcium oxalate uroliths. A low BUN concentration, hyperammonemia, and hyperuric acidemia may be observed in animals with ammonium urate uroliths that form in association with PSS. Hyperuric acidemia is also observed in dogs with urate uroliths that do not have PSS.

Radiography and Ultrasonography. Survey radiography may reveal uroliths if they are radiodense (Table 99–3). Urate uroliths and occasionally cystine uroliths are not always observed because of their poor mineral density. Double-contrast cystography will reveal urocystoliths. Additionally, small uroliths may be retrieved during the procedure and submitted for quantitative analysis. Ultrasonography may demonstrate the presence of urocystoliths. Only the proximal urethra may be evaluated by ultrasonography.

Additional Laboratory Testing. Submit urocystoliths that are retrieved for quantitative analysis. Assess liver function in animals with ammonium urate uroliths (other than in Dalmatian dogs) to determine if a PSS is

Table 99–3. TYPICAL RADIOGRAPHIC CHARACTERISTICS OF UROLITHS COMMONLY ENCOUNTERED IN DOGS AND CATS

Mineral Type	Degree of Radiopacity	Shape
Cystine	+ to ++	Smooth; usually small; round to oval
Calcium oxalate dihydrate	++++	Often rough; round to oval (occasionally jackstone)
Calcium oxalate monohydrate	+++	Often smooth, round (occasionally jackstone)
Struvite	+ to ++++	Smooth; round or faceted; sometimes assume shape of renal pelvis, ureter, bladder, or urethra; sometimes laminated
Calcium phosphate	++++	Smooth; round or faceted
Urate	0 to ++	Smooth but occasionally irregular; round or oval
Silica*	++ to ++++	Typically jackstone
Mixed and compound	+ to ++++	Varies with composition; may have detectable nucleus and shell
Matrix	0 to +	Usually round, but may be influenced by location

*Not observed as a primary mineral in cats.

Table 99–4. CHECKLIST OF FACTORS THAT SUGGEST THE PROBABLE MINERAL COMPOSITION OF UROLITHS

1. Urine pH
   a. Struvite and calcium apatite uroliths—usually alkaline; sterile struvite uroliths may be observed when urine pH is 6.5 or higher
   b. Ammonium urate uroliths—acid to neutral
   c. Cystine uroliths—acid*
   d. Calcium oxalate—often acid to neutral*
   e. Silica—acid to neutral (only in canine)*
2. Identification of crystals in uncontaminated fresh urine sediment, preferably at body temperature (see Table 99–2)
3. Type of bacteria, if any, isolated from urine
   a. Urease-producing bacteria, especially staphylococci and less frequently *Proteus* spp., are typically associated with canine struvite uroliths; ureaplasma may cause struvite uroliths in dogs
   b. Urinary tract infections often are absent in patients with calcium oxalate, cystine, ammonium urate, and silica uroliths
   c. Calcium oxalate, cystine, ammonium urate, and silica uroliths may predispose patients to urinary tract infections; if infections are caused by urease-producing bacteria, struvite may precipitate around these metabolic uroliths
4. Radiographic density and physical characteristics of uroliths (see Table 99–3)
5. Serum chemistry evaluation
   a. Hypercalcemia may be associated with calcium-containing uroliths
   b. Hyperuricemia may be associated with uric acid or urate uroliths
   c. Hyperchloremia, hypokalemia, and acidemia may be associated with distal renal tubular acidosis and calcium phosphate or struvite uroliths
6. Urine chemistry evaluation
   a. Patient should be consuming a standardized diagnostic diet, or the diet consumed when uroliths formed
   b. Excessive quantities of one or more minerals contained in the urolith are expected; the concentration of crystallization inhibitors may be decreased
7. Breed of dog and history of occurrence of uroliths in patient's ancestors or littermates
8. Quantitative analysis of uroliths fortuitously passed during micturition, or collected via catheterization

*Concomitant infection with urease-producing microbes may result in formation of alkaline urine.

---

present (see Chap. 91). Consider intravenous pyelography in animals with nephroliths or ureteroliths, or in animals with recurrent bacterial UTI.

Estimation of Urolith Composition. In order to determine if medical dissolution of urocystoliths may be beneficial, estimate the mineral composition using several parameters (Table 99–4).

Treatment

Consider risks and benefits of medical versus surgical (see Chap. 100) therapy of urocystoliths. Uroliths that cause repeated urethral obstruction, unacceptable clinical signs, or in which the owners do not wish to attempt medical dissolution should be removed surgically. Urocystoliths that are smaller than the smallest diameter of the urethra may be retrieved using voiding urohydropropulsion or catheter-assisted retrieval technique.

▼ *Key Point* Because many types of urocystoliths are recurrent, surgical removal or medical dissolution of urocystoliths is not the end point of therapy. Institute appropriate preventive measures and follow-up evaluations.

Infection-Induced Struvite Urocystoliths

Medical dissolution of infection-induced struvite uroliths is possible using appropriate antimicrobial therapy and a diet designed for struvite dissolution (Table 99–5). A diet for struvite dissolution should be protein and magnesium restricted, and should induce an acid urine pH. Average dissolution time is 8–10 weeks.

Sterile Struvite Urocystoliths

Dissolution of sterile struvite uroliths is accomplished in a manner similar to infection-induced struvite uroliths except that antimicrobial therapy is not necessary (see Table 99–5). Average dissolution time is 2–4 weeks.

Calcium Oxalate Urocystoliths

There is no medical therapy available for dissolution of calcium oxalate uroliths; therefore, removal remains the treatment for uroliths that are causing clinical problems (Table 99–6).

Ammonium Urate Urocystoliths

Associated with PSS

Medical dissolution of ammonium urate uroliths in animals with PSS has not been successful; therefore, surgical removal remains the treatment of choice if uroliths are causing clinical problems. Uroliths may be removed at time of surgical ligation of the shunt. Theoretically, uroliths may dissolve after the shunt is corrected.

Not Associated with PSS

Urate uroliths may be dissolved using allopurinol (15 mg/kg PO q12h) and a low protein, alkalinizing diet (Table 99–7). Average time for dissolution is 4 weeks. Medical dissolution is successful in approximately 50% of cases. No effective protocol has been formulated for dissolution of urate uroliths in cats; how-

---

Table 99–5. PROTOCOL FOR MEDICAL DISSOLUTION OF STRUVITE UROLITHS

Adult Dogs and Cats with Infection-Induced Struvite Uroliths

1. Perform appropriate diagnostic studies including complete urinalysis, quantitative urine culture, and diagnostic radiography; determine precise location, size, and number of uroliths. The size and number of uroliths are not a reliable index of probably efficacy of therapy.
2. Determine mineral composition of uroliths.
3. Consider surgical correction if uroliths are obstructing urine outflow, and/or if correctable abnormalities predisposing to recurrent urinary tract infection are identified by radiography or other means.
4. Eradicate or control UTI with appropriate antimicrobial agents. Maintain antimicrobial therapy during, and for 3–4 weeks following, urolith dissolution.
5. Initiate therapy with calculolytic diets. No other food or mineral supplements should be fed to the patient. Compliance with dietary recommendations is suggested by reduction in BUN concentration (usually <15 mg/dl).
6. Monitor efficacy of therapy:
   a. Avoid diagnostic follow-up studies that require urinary catheterization. If they are required, give appropriate pericatheterization antimicrobial agents to prevent iatrogenic UTI.
   b. Evaluate serial urinalyses. Urine pH, specific gravity, and microscopic examination of sediment for crystals are especially important. Remember that crystals formed in urine stored at room or refrigeration temperatures may represent in vitro artifacts.
   c. Perform serial radiography at monthly intervals to evaluate stone location(s), number, size, density, and shape.
   d. If necessary, perform quantitative urine cultures. They are especially important in patients that are infected prior to therapy, and in patients that are catheterized during therapy.
   e. Feed patients calculolytic diet for one month following disappearance of uroliths.
   f. If uroliths increase in size during dietary management or do not begin to decrease in size after approximately 4–8 weeks of appropriate medical management, alternative methods should be considered. Difficulty in inducing complete dissolution of uroliths by creating urine that is undersaturated with the suspected calculogenic crystalloid should prompt consideration that (1) the wrong mineral component was identified, (2) the nucleus of the uroliths is of different mineral composition than other portions of the urolith, and (3) the owner or the patient is not complying with medical recommendations.
7. Consider administration of acetohydroxamic acid (Lithostat; 25 mg/kg/d divided into 2 equal doses) to dogs with persistent uroliths and persistent urease-producing bacteriuria despite use of antimicrobial agents and calculolytic diets.

Adult Dogs and Cats with Sterile Struvite Uroliths

1. Follow the protocol described above, but do not administer antimicrobial agents or Lithostat.
2. Periodically culture urine specimens obtained by cystocentesis to detect secondary urinary tract infections. If UTI develops, initiate antimicrobial therapy.

Immature Dogs and Cats with Struvite Uroliths

1. Pending further studies, surgery remains the safest means of removing uroliths from immature animals.
2. Use caution in the use of protein-restricted diets in growing animals.
3. Short-term therapy with calculolytic diets may be considered. If initiated, monitor the patient for evidence of nutritional deficiencies (especially protein malnutrition).
4. Acetohydroxamic acid has not been evaluated in growing animals.

Table 99–6. PROTOCOL FOR MEDICAL TREATMENT OF CALCIUM OXALATE UROLITHS

1. Perform appropriate diagnostic studies including complete urinalysis, quantitative urine culture, serum biochemical profile, and diagnostic radiography or ultrasonography. Determine precise location, size, and number of uroliths, and patency of excretory pathway.
2. If available, determine mineral composition of uroliths. If unavailable, estimate their composition by evaluation of appropriate clinical data (see Table 99–4).
3. Determine urine concentrations of appropriate metabolites (if possible), especially calcium, oxalate, magnesium, uric acid, and citrate.
4. Consider immediate surgical correction if uroliths thought to be composed of calcium oxalate are causing intolerable clinical signs. Uroliths also may be removed by catheter-assisted retrieval or by voiding urohydropropulsion.
5. If necessary, eradicate or control secondary urinary tract infections with appropriate antimicrobial agents.
6. Hypercalcemic hypercalciuric patients:
   a. Approximately 35% of cats and 4% of dogs with calcium oxalate uroliths are hypercalcemic.
   b. Have a high index of suspicion of primary hyperparathyroidism. If confirmed, surgically correct abnormality of parathyroid glands. This is a rare cause of calcium oxalate uroliths.
   c. If uroliths are symptomatic, consider surgical removal.
   d. Avoid thiazide diuretics because they may aggravate hypercalcemia.
   e. Induce polyuria (but avoid excessive dietary sodium supplements).
   f. High-fiber diets appear to decrease the degree of hypercalcemia and should be used with potassium citrate (initial dose: 75 mg/kg PO q12hr; adjust dose to induce a urine pH of 7.0–7.5).
7. Normocalcemic patients with active calcium oxalate urolithiasis:
   a. Induce diuresis, but avoid excessive dietary supplementation with sodium.
   b. Consider oral administration of potassium citrate (see above).
   c. Consider change to a diet that does not contain excessive oxalate, sodium, or protein.
   d. Avoid dietary or therapeutic supplements of ascorbic acid and vitamin D.

Table 99–7. PROTOCOL FOR TREATMENT OF AMMONIUM URATE UROLITHIASIS NOT ASSOCIATED WITH PORTOSYSTEMIC SHUNTS IN DOGS

1. Perform appropriate diagnostic studies, including complete urinalysis, quantitative urine culture, and diagnostic radiography. Determine precise location, size, and number of uroliths. The size and number of uroliths are not a reliable index of probably efficacy of therapy.
2. If available, determine mineral composition of uroliths. If unavailable, estimate their composition (see Table 99–4).
3. Consider surgical correction if uroliths are obstructing urine outflow.
4. Determine baseline pretreatment serum uric acid concentrations and 24-hour excretion of urine uric acid.
5. Initiate therapy with a low-protein, alkalinizing diet. No other food supplements should be fed to the patient. Compliance with dietary recommendation is suggested by reduction in BUN (usually <10 mg/dl).
6. Initiate therapy with allopurinol at a dosage of 15 mg per kg q12hr (a lesser dose will be required in azotemic patients).
7. If necessary, administer potassium citrate orally in order to eliminate aciduria. Strive for a urine pH of approximately 7.
8. If necessary, eradicate or control urinary tract infections with appropriate antimicrobial agents. Maintain antimicrobial therapy during, and for an appropriate period following, urate urolith dissolution.
9. Devise a protocol to monitor efficacy of therapy:
   a. Try to avoid diagnostic follow-up studies that require urinary catheterization. If they are required, give appropriate pericatheterization antimicrobial agents to prevent iatrogenic urinary tract infection.
   b. Evaluate serial urinalyses. Urine pH, specific gravity, and microscopic examination of sediment for urate crystals are especially important. Remember that crystals formed in urine stored at room or refrigeration temperatures may represent in vitro artifacts.
   c. Serially evaluate the serum uric acid concentrations and (if possible) fractional excretion of urine uric acid.
   d. Evaluate urolith(s) location(s), number, size, density, and shape at approximately monthly intervals. Intravenous urography may be utilized for radiolucent uroliths located in the kidneys, ureters, or urinary bladder. Double-contrast cystography may be required for radiolucent uroliths.
   e. If necessary, perform quantitative urine cultures. They are especially important in patients that are infected prior to therapy, and in patients that are catheterized during therapy.
10. Continue calculolytic diet, allopurinol, and alkalinizing therapy for approximately 1 month following disappearance of uroliths as detected by radiography.

---

ever, we have successfully treated urate uroliths in cats using allopurinol (7.5 mg/kg PO q12h) and a low-protein, alkalinizing diet.

Cystine Urocystoliths

Dissolution may be accomplished in dogs using 2-mercaptopropionol glycine (15 mg/kg PO q12h) and feeding a low-protein, alkalinizing diet. Average time for dissolution is 4–6 weeks.

Others

Other mineral types such as calcium phosphate and silica cannot be dissolved.

Prevention

Most types of urocystoliths are recurrent; therefore, institute preventive measures. Production of dilute urine is beneficial in all urolith types except for infection-induced struvite; therefore, induce diuresis. Dilute urine is a predisposing risk factor for UTI; therefore, it may predispose to infection-induced struvite urolith formation. Because uroliths are recurrent, recommend frequent reexaminations.

Infection-Induced Struvite

Because this type of struvite urolith forms as a result of a UTI with urease-producing bacteria, prevention is dependent upon preventing recurrence of the infection. Treat any causes of recurrent UTI, such as hyperadrenocorticism. If necessary, use low-dose antibiotic therapy as prophylaxis. Modification of the diet is not necessary.

Sterile Struvite

Prevention of sterile struvite uroliths involves modification of the diet. Because struvite is more soluble in acidic urine (pH <6.8), prevention involves feeding a diet that produces urine pH between 6.1 and 6.5. Diets that produce a urine pH less than approximately 6.1 may induce metabolic acidosis. Dietary magnesium restriction may also be of benefit.

Calcium Oxalate

The cause of calcium oxalate urolith formation is not completely known. No treatment has been shown to be completely effective (see Table 99–6). In dogs, feeding a protein-and-sodium-restricted, alkalinizing diet has been shown to delay recurrence. If a neutral to slightly alkaline urine pH is not accomplished by diet, give potassium citrate (initial dose: 75 mg/kg PO q12h; adjust to induce a urine pH of 7.0–7.5). Although similar recommendations have been made for cats with calcium oxalate uroliths, prevention in cats appears to be more successful when feeding a higher-fiber diet, and administering potassium citrate (initial dose: 75 mg/kg PO q12h; adjust to induce a urine pH of 7.0–7.5). Other treatments that have been proposed include vitamin B$_6$ (2 mg/kg PO q24h) and hydrochlorothiazide (2–4 mg/kg PO q12h). Because calcium oxalate uroliths are highly recurrent, perform serial monitoring of urinalyses and survey abdominal radiographs.

Ammonium Urate

Associated with PSS

If the shunt can be repaired, the risk of ammonium urate urolith formation should decrease. No further treatment may be indicated. If the shunt is not repairable, then feeding a low-protein, alkalinizing diet may be of benefit. Allopurinol is not effective in animals with PSS.

Not Associated with PSS

In dogs, feeding a low-protein, alkalinizing diet has been successful in preventing recurrence in approximately 80% of cases. If urate crystalluria persists despite feeding an appropriate preventive diet, administer allopurinol (7–10 mg/kg PO q12–24h). In cats, feeding a low-protein, alkalinizing diet has been nearly 100% successful. Do not use allopurinol until safety and efficacy studies are done.

Cystine

Feeding a low-protein, alkalinizing diet is highly successful in preventing formation of cystine uroliths. Cystine solubility increases in alkaline urine; therefore, maintaining a urine pH of >7.5 is important. If the urine pH is not >7.5, administer potassium citrate (initial dose: 75 mg/kg PO q12h; adjust dose to induce a urine pH >7.5). Alternatively, administer 2-mercaptopropionol glycine (15 mg/kg PO q24h) with alkalinization therapy without modifying diet. Do not feed ultra-low-protein diets to English bulldogs because of an association with urate or cystine urolithiasis and dilated cardiomyopathy.

URETHRAL PLUGS IN MALE CATS

Etiology

Matrix-crystalline plugs may form in male cats and cause urethral obstruction. Matrix-crystalline urethral plugs represent part of the spectrum of lower urinary tract disease in cats. Formation of matrix by an infectious agent or by an inflammatory process in a cat with concomitant crystalluria may lead to formation of a plug. Approximately 87% of matrix-crystalline urethral plugs contain minerals, primarily struvite; however, 13% of plugs contain only matrix and inflammatory cells. Approximately 20% of cats under 10 years of age with lower urinary tract disease have matrix-crystalline plugs; however, only 5% of cats over 10 years of age with lower urinary tract disease have urethral plugs.

Clinical Signs

Male cats with urethral obstruction require emergency treatment. If untreated, death may occur within 2–3 days due to postrenal azotemia, electrolyte imbalances, and severe metabolic acidosis. A cat with urethral obstruction may attempt to urinate without voiding urine and may appear to be in pain. As the obstruction persists, signs of postrenal azotemia (anorexia, vomiting) may occur.

Diagnosis

History. Usually there is a history of the cat attempting to urinate without passing urine. Occasionally, owners may find a cat with urethral obstruction that is stuporous, comatose, or dead.

Physical Examination. Palpation of a large urinary bladder that is not easily expressed indicates urethral outflow obstruction. Abdominal fluid may be palpated if the urinary bladder has ruptured. Bradycardia occurs if the cat is hyperkalemic. Dehydration is usually present.

Urinalysis. Inflammation and hematuria, and occasionally crystalluria, are present.

Urine Culture. Negative in most cats.

CBC and Serum Biochemical Analysis. Can be normal. However, azotemia, hyperkalemia, hyperphosphatemia, and metabolic acidosis may be found if the urethra has been obstructed for >12 hours.

Radiography and Ultrasonography. A large urinary bladder is usually observed; however, if the bladder has ruptured, abdominal effusion may be observed. The mineral component of the plug may be observed in the distal urethra. Survey radiography is a useful procedure because 10–20% of cats with lower urinary tract disease have urolithiasis. Contrast radiography is not usually necessary unless difficulty is encountered while trying to unobstruct the cat or if a perineal urethrostomy (PU) is considered. Ultrasonography may reveal a distended bladder with a thickened wall. A urachal diverticulum may be observed. If the bladder has ruptured, abdominal fluid may be observed.

Additional Laboratory Testing. If hyperkalemia is present, electrocardiography may reveal prolonged P-R interval (potassium concentration 6–8 mEq/L), dropped P waves and bradycardia (potassium concentration 8–10 mEq/L), and premature ventricular contractions or ventricular tachycardia (potassium concentration >10 mEq/L).

Treatment

Establishment of urethral patency is imperative (see Chap. 101). A cystocentesis may be performed prior to establishing urethral patency for a diagnostic sample, and to relieve pressure. Administer IV fluids to correct dehydration (see Chap. 5). If urethral obstruction is recurrent, and the obstruction occurs in the distal penile urethra, consider doing a PU after appropriate radiographic studies (see Chap. 102). If the urinary bladder has ruptured, establish urethral patency and place an indwelling urinary catheter. Surgical closure is indicated in bladder tears unless very small.

Prevention

Feeding an appropriate diet that minimizes struvite formation often may modify the mineral component of matrix-crystalline plugs (see section on Urolithiasis and Table 99–5). Because >70% of urethral plugs contain struvite, feeding an acidifying, magnesium-restricted diet is recommended. Cats that have a PU are at greater risk for bacterial UTI—20–50% of cats with PU develop bacterial UTI compared with 1–2% of cats with lower urinary tract disease that do not have PU. Monitor PU cats for recurrent infection and stricture (see section on Bacterial Urinary Tract Infections).

NEOPLASTIC DISEASE

Etiology

Neoplasms of the urinary bladder are the most frequently identified urinary tract tumor in dogs and cats; however, they account for <1% of all neoplasms. Bladder neoplasms tend to occur in older animals and are more frequently observed in female dogs. Bladder neoplasia is very rare in cats. The most common neoplasm of the urinary bladder is transitional cell carcinoma, a malignant epithelial tumor. Neoplasms of other tissue types including lymphomas, fibromas, myosarcomas, and adenocarcinomas occur less frequently.

Clinical Signs

Regardless of the type of tumor, clinical signs relate to signs of cystitis including hematuria, pollakiuria, and stranguria. Animals may not show any clinical signs in the early stages of the disease. In older animals that present for UTI, particularly if recurrent, bladder cancer should be suspected. If the neoplasm involves the trigone region, urethral or ureteral obstruction may occur, resulting in azotemia.

Diagnosis

History. May have a history of persistent or recurrent UTI or hematuria. Signs of uremia may also be observed.

Physical Examination. A large bladder, if the urethra is obstructed, or a large kidney, if a ureter is obstructed, may be palpated. Occasionally, the bladder tumor may be palpated. Perform a rectal examination in older dogs because extension of the mass into the urethra may be palpable.

Urinalysis. Usually hematuria is observed. A UTI may also be present. Occasionally neoplastic cells may be observed in the urine sediment.

Urine Culture. Negative unless a UTI is present.

CBC and Serum Biochemical Analysis. Usually normal. A mild normocytic, normochromic anemia consistent with chronic disease may be present. Azotemia may be present if the urethra or both ureters are obstructed.

Radiography and Ultrasonography. Survey radiography may be normal, although a large urinary bladder or a large kidney may be observed. Sublumbar lymphadenomegaly may be observed if the cancer has metastasized. Perform contrast cystography or ultrasonography to confirm bladder masses or thickening and to delineate location and size of lesions.

Additional Diagnostics. A fine-needle aspirate of the bladder mass may reveal neoplastic cells. A biopsy of the mass(es) may be obtained via cystoscopy or laparotomy.

Treatment

The prognosis for most animals with bladder neoplasia is poor. Surgical excision is the treatment of choice for solitary benign tumors (see Chap. 100). Partial cystec-tomy or total cystectomy with urinary diversion may be considered for malignant tumors but results are mostly unrewarding. Neoplasms that are responsive to chemotherapy, such as lymphoma, should be treated appropriately (see Chap. 25). Transitional cell carcinomas are not usually resectable and do not respond to chemotherapy. Piroxicam (dogs: 0.3 mg/kg PO q48h; cats: dosage undetermined) may be used as palliative therapy. If urethral obstruction occurs, but the animal's quality of life is good, consider placing a cystostomy catheter (see Chap. 100).

Prevention

Because no etiologic agent has been determined for bladder cancers, no preventative recommendations can be made. In older animals, particularly female dogs, that have persistent or recurrent hematuria or UTI, perform a thorough diagnostic work-up.

BLADDER INFECTION

Bacterial UTI is the most common infectious disease of the urinary bladder. Fungal cystitis is occasionally observed, particularly in animals that are immunosuppressed; however, many cases are self-limiting. Parasitic cystitis occurs rarely, and is usually asymptomatic.

Etiology

Bacterial Cystitis

The body has many defense mechanisms to prevent bacterial invasion of the urinary bladder, which does not normally contain bacteria. Natural resistance factors, inherent to the urinary tract, include complete and frequent unidirectional voiding of urine, mucosal defense barriers, and antimicrobic properties of urine. Acquired resistance factors are activated only after infection with bacteria. Immune responses to bacterial infection are an example of acquired resistance. Therefore, any breach in these defense mechanisms may result in bacterial colonization of the urinary bladder.

- Bacterial cystitis is one of the more common causes of lower urinary tract disease in dogs. The most common organisms causing bacterial cystitis include *Escherichia coli, Staphylococcus* spp., *Proteus* spp., *Streptococcus* spp., and *Enterobacter* spp., with the incidence of *E. coli* being 40–50% of the cases.
- In cats less than 10 years of age, bacterial cystitis occurs in 1–2% of cases of lower urinary tract disease; however, in cats older than 10 years, bacterial cystitis may occur in approximately 50% of cases. Renal failure is the most common disease associated with bacterial cystitis in older cats. Causative bacteria are similar to those observed in dogs.

Fungal Cystitis

Yeast and fungi in urine usually represent contamination of the sample. Infections with *Candida albicans* and *Torulopsis* spp. may occur, especially in patients with resistant UTI that have been unsuccessfully treated with a variety of antimicrobial agents for prolonged periods, or in patients that are immunocompromised. On occasion, fungi (e.g. *Blastomyces, Cryptococcus*) may be observed in urine of patients with polysystemic fungal diseases.

Parasitic Cystitis

Rarely, parasitic ova are observed in urine samples. *Dioctophyma renale* is a parasite of the kidneys, but if a gravid female worm is present in the kidney, ova may be observed in urine.

Capillaria plica may be found in the urinary bladder of dogs and cats, and *Capillaria feliscati* may be found in cats. Ova are passed in urine. The first-stage larvae develop in approximately 1 month but do not hatch unless they are ingested by an earthworm. The definitive host becomes infected by eating earthworms that harbor the first-stage larvae.

Clinical Signs

Bacterial cystitis is usually associated with signs of hematuria, dysuria, and pollakiuria. Animals may also display inappropriate urination. Occasionally it does not cause clinical signs, particularly when an infection occurs in association with polyuric states or immunosuppressive disease. Fungal and parasitic cystitis are usually asymptomatic; however, clinical signs similar to bacterial cystitis may occur.

Diagnosis

History

The animal may not have a history of disease or there may be recurrent or protracted disease. Polyuria and polydipsia may be observed with underlying renal failure, hyperthyroidism, diabetes mellitus, hyperadrenocorticism, or glucocorticoid therapy. Skin, oral, or respiratory infections may be observed with immunosuppressive therapy or disease.

Physical Examination

Physical examination may be normal. Examination findings that relate to the predisposing cause may be observed (e.g., prostatic mass; hepatomegaly and alopecia with hyperadrenocorticism; weight loss, uveitis, harsh lung sounds, and draining skin lesions with systemic mycosis).

Urinalysis

The infectious agent (bacterium, fungus, yeast, or parasitic ova) is usually observed on urine sediment examination. Signs of inflammation are often present with bacterial cystitis, but usually not with fungal or parasitic cystitis. Signs of inflammation may be absent if the animal is immunocompromised (e.g., hyperadrenocorticism, glucocorticoid therapy, feline leukemia virus, or immunodeficiency virus infection). Nitrate and leukocyte pads on urinalysis strips are not accurate for use in dogs and cats. Examine urine sediment to identify inflammation and an infectious agent. Evaluate for glucosuria indicative of underlying diabetes mellitus.

Urine Culture

Perform aerobic bacterial culture of urine in suspected cases of bacterial cystitis. Submit urine collected by cystocentesis for culture. Quantitation of the number of bacterial colony forming units may be of benefit (Table 99–8). If there is difficulty in obtaining adequate urine culture results, submit a urine sample and inoculate on a blood agar plate or place in transport media.

Select antimicrobial agents on the basis of culture and sensitivity results. The agar-gel disk diffusion method is most commonly used. It is based on expected serum drug concentrations, not urine concentrations (which tend to be higher for many drugs), and thus underestimates the effectiveness of some drugs. If sensitivities are established by determining the minimum inhibitory concentration (MIC), select antibiotics that reach urine concentrations four times the MIC.

Urine may be submitted for a fungal culture as well, although a diagnosis of mycotic infection is often made on sediment examination.

CBC and Serum Biochemical Analysis

Rule out cystitis associated with a systemic disease (such as renal failure or hyperadrenocorticism).

Radiography and Ultrasonography

Perform to rule out primary bladder or other urogenital diseases.

Additional Laboratory Testing

Perform endocrine testing in dogs suspected of having hyperadrenocorticism or cats with hyperthyroidism.

Table 99–8. INTERPRETATION OF QUANTITATIVE URINE CULTURES (NUMBERS OF BACTERIA PER ML OF URINE)

Collection Method	Significant		Suspicious		Probable Contaminant	
	Dog	Cat	Dog	Cat	Dog	Cat
Cystocentesis	>1000	>1000	100–1000	100–1000	<100	<100
Catheterization	>10,000	>1000	1000–10,000	100–10,000	<1000	<100
Voluntary void or Manual compression	>100,000	>10,000	10,000–90,000	1000–90,000	<10,000	<1000

Table 99-9. GUIDELINES FOR TREATMENT OF URINARY BACTERIAL PATHOGENS*

Pathogen	Drug(s) of Choice	Alternatives
Enterobacter spp.	Trimethoprim-sulfa, fluoroquinolones	Cephalosporins (1st, 2nd generation), chloramphenicol, nitrofurantoin, gentamicin
Escherichia coli	Trimethoprim-sulfa, fluoroquinolones, nitrofurantoin	Cephalosporins (1st, 2nd, 3rd generations), chloramphenicol, gentamicin
Klebsiella spp.	Cephalosporins (1st generation), fluoroquinolones	Trimethoprim-sulfa, cephalosporins (2nd, 3rd generation), fluoroquinolones
Mycoplasma, Ureaplasma	Fluoroquinolones	Chloramphenicol, doxycycline, erythromycin, tetracycline
Proteus spp.	Ampicillin, amoxicillin, penicillin G, fluoroquinolones	Cephalosporins (1st, 2nd, 3rd generations), chloramphenicol, nitrofurantoin, trimethoprim-sulfa, gentamicin
Pseudomonas aeruginosa	Tetracycline, fluoroquinolines	Trimethoprim-sulfa, cephalosporins (3rd generation), gentamicin
Staphylococcus intermedius	Penicillin G, ampicillin, amoxicillin, fluoroquinolones	Cephalosporin (1st generation), chloramphenicol, nitrofurantoin, trimethoprim-sulfa
Streptococcus	Penicillin G, ampicillin, amoxicillin	Cephalosporin (1st generation), chloramphenicol, nitrofurantoin, trimethoprim-sulfa

*Prior treatment with antimicrobial drugs may alter the susceptibility of bacterial pathogens to these drugs.

Perform feline leukemia virus antigen test and a feline immunodeficiency virus antibody test in cats with UTI.

Treatment

Bacterial Cystitis

Select antimicrobic agents on the basis of culture and sensitivity results (Table 99–9).

- Treat uncomplicated cystitis with the appropriate antimicrobial for at least 14 days. Perform a second urinalysis and, optimally, a culture and sensitivity 4–7 days after cessation of treatment.
- Bacterial cystitis is complicated if it is recurrent or associated with an underlying risk factor. Give antimicrobial therapy for 3–4 weeks followed by a urinalysis and possibly a urine culture 3–5 days after beginning therapy to ensure bacterial eradication. Perform a second urine culture 4–7 days after cessation of therapy. Identify risk factors and treat accordingly.
- *Relapses* (i.e., recurrence with the same bacteria following eradication) require reassessment of antimicrobial choice based on culture and sensitivity results, and treatment of any complicating factors (Table 99–10). A deep-seated infection could require a second, longer course of therapy.

- *Reinfection* (i.e., recurrence with a different organism within a few weeks to months following eradication) requires reevaluation and treatment for complicating risk factors. Treat each episode based on results of urine culture and sensitivity testing.
- Consider long-term, low-dose antibiotic therapy to treat animals with frequent relapses or reinfections. This involves administering $\frac{1}{3}$ to $\frac{1}{2}$ of the recommended therapeutic dose of the antimicrobial once a day, preferably at night to allow excretion and collection of the antimicrobial in the urinary bladder.
- Bacterial cystitis may occur as a result of urinary catheterization. If a catheter is passed only once into the urinary bladder, pericatheterization treatment with amoxicillin or a cephalosporin should prevent infection. If an indwelling catheter is placed, do not administer antimicrobials while the catheter is in place. Instead, a urine sample should be evaluated once the catheter is removed. If a bacterial cystitis is present at that time, treat appropriately.

Fungal Cystitis

Treat fungal cystitis only if the animal is symptomatic. Alkalinization of urine to >7.5 using potassium citrate (initial dose: 75 mg/kg PO q12hr; or sodium bicarbo-

Table 99-10. SUMMARY OF OBJECTIVES FOR TREATMENT OF PERSISTENT OR RECURRENT URINARY TRACT INFECTIONS

1. Identify and eliminate or control predisposing or complicating causes of the urinary tract infection (e.g., hyperadrenocorticism, urolithiasis, anatomic defects).
2. Identify causative pathogens by qualitative and quantitative culture, and select antimicrobial drugs on the basis of antimicrobial susceptibility tests. Ideally, the agent chosen should have the narrowest possible spectrum of antimicrobial activity.
3. If sepsis is present, treat aggressively with appropriate dosages of antimicrobials.
4. Although usually unnecessary, urine pH can be altered to enhance antimicrobial activity.
5. Reculture urine 3–5 days following initiation of therapy to check efficacy of the antimicrobial agent in sterilizing urine.
6. Continue antimicrobial therapy beyond chemical and laboratory evidence of response.
7. Anticipate, prevent, and treat as necessary symptomatic or asymptomatic recurrences because they may be associated with irreversible and potentially progressive disease.

nate: 12 mg/kg PO q8h) may result in eradication of the fungal organism; however, this is not usually successful. In animals that have persistent or recurrent signs of cystitis due to a fungal infection, administer ketoconazole (30 mg/kg PO q24h), itraconazole (5 mg/kg PO q24h), or amphotericin B (see Chap. 18).

Parasitic Cystitis

Because many animals with parasitic cystitis are asymptomatic, treatment may not be warranted. For urinary capillariasis, give levamisole (2.5 mg/kg/d PO for 5 days). Use of fenbendazole (25 mg/kg PO q12h for 3–10 days) has been reported, but it does not appear to be as effective as levamisole. Dogs with urinary capillariasis may be treated with albendazole (50 mg/kg PO q12h for 10–14 days) or a single dose of ivermectin (0.2 mg/kg SC).

Prevention

Prevention of infectious cystitis is dependent upon identifying and eliminating or controlling the underlying disease.

Emphysematous Cystitis

Emphysematous cystitis is rarely seen as a complication of a bacterial urinary tract infection.

Etiology

Occurs when bacterial cystitis is caused by a gas-producing bacterium such as *Clostridium* spp.

Clinical Signs

Clinical signs are similar to other forms of cystitis.

Diagnosis

History. There may be a history of clinical signs consistent with diabetes mellitus, hyperadrenocorticism, or administration of immunosuppressive or chemotherapeutic agents.

Physical Examination. The urinary bladder is usually small and firm on palpation.

Urinalysis. Urinalysis shows inflammation; the agent may not be observed.

Urine Culture. Aerobic cultures may be negative if an anaerobic organism is responsible.

CBC and Serum Biochemical Analysis. Usually normal, unless associated with a metabolic disease such as diabetes mellitus or hyperadrenocorticism. Evidence for sepsis may be present. Evidence for bone marrow suppression may be present if associated with administration of chemotherapeutic agents.

Radiography and Ultrasonography. Radiography and ultrasonography reveal air trapped in the wall of the urinary bladder.

Treatment

Administer an appropriate antimicrobial (e.g., ampicillin, amoxicillin, or amoxicillin-clavulanate) for 3–6 weeks. Treat the underlying predisposing disease, if possible. If the animal is receiving immunosuppressive or chemotherapeutic agents, consider temporarily stopping the the drug or decreasing the dosage.

Prevention

Identifying animals at risk for infectious cystitis is important. Monitor animals known to have a disease that compromises their local or systemic defenses or animals receiving immunosuppressive or chemotherapeutic drugs for UTI periodically. Many of these animals may not demonstrate clinical signs but may have evidence of UTI on urinalysis.

IDIOPATHIC FELINE LOWER URINARY TRACT DISEASE

Idiopathic feline lower urinary tract disease (IFLUTD) has also been called feline urologic syndrome (FUS) and feline interstitial cystitis (FIC) because of many similarities with human IC.

Approximately 1–2% of cats in the United States are affected with lower urinary tract disease. In 50–70% of these cats that are less than 10 years of age, no definable cause can be found. In cats older than 10 years of age, IFLUTD is diagnosed in approximately 5% of the cases; therefore, a more extensive diagnostic work-up would be expected to identify a primary disease.

Etiology

The cause of IFLUTD is not known, but possibilities include viral cystitis, neurogenic inflammation, abnormal glycosaminoglycans lining the urinary bladder mucosa, unidentified bacterial infection, and mast cell–related disease. Since the cause of IFLUTD has not been identified, expect a variable clinical course.

Clinical Signs

Clinical signs associated with IFLUTD include hematuria, dysuria, and inappropriate urination which usually resolves in 5–7 days; however, in some cats, signs may last for weeks or wax and wane chronically. Urethral obstruction may occur in male cats (see section on Urethral Plugs in Male Cats).

Diagnosis

History. Clinical signs may be observed for a period of days before the cat is examined. There may or may not be a previous history of lower urinary tract disease.

Physical Examination. If urethral obstruction is not present, the urinary bladder will be small on palpation.

Urinalysis. Hematuria and possibly crystalluria is present.

Urine Culture. Urine culture is negative.

CBC and Serum Biochemical Analysis. Normal.

Radiography and Ultrasonography. A small urinary bladder is observed on survey radiography. Contrast radiography and ultrasonography may be normal or may reveal a thickened bladder wall.

Cystoscopy. The hallmarks of IFLUTD are mucosal

edema, glomerulations, and increased vascularity. Cystoscopy is valuable for ruling out other causes of lower urinary tract signs in cats with chronic or recurrent problems.

Treatment

Specific Treatment

No specific treatment recommendation can be made because the cause of IFLUTD is unknown. There are no proven effective treatments for IFLUTD. Antibiotics are not warranted without evidence of bacterial cystitis (see previous discussion). In two studies, antibiotics administered to cats with nonobstructive IFLUTD were no more effective than a placebo. Glucocorticoids administered to cats with IFLUTD have also not been more effective than placebo, and therefore are not indicated.

Symptomatic Treatment

- Recommend measures to encourage increased water intake.
  - Add water to the food.
  - Provide access to fresh water at all times.
  - Consider providing bottled or distilled water.
  - Offer "wet" foods (broth, tuna water, clam juice).
  - Make ice cubes out of meat or fish broth to add to the water bowl for flavoring.
  - Try running water, such as a pet fountain or a dripping faucet, into a sink or bowl.
- Antispasmodics (propantheline bromide: 5–7.5 mg PO q8h or 7.5 mg PO q72h; or oxybutynin: 0.5–1.25 mg PO q8–12h) and/or urethral relaxing agents (phenoxybenzamine: 2.5–10 mg PO q24h; diazepam: 2.5–5.0 mg PO q8h; dantrolene: 0.5–1.0 mg/kg PO q12h; or nicergoline: 1–5 mg PO q8h) may be of benefit.
- Torbugesic (0.3 mg/kg PO q8h) may be useful as an analgesic.
- Amitriptyline, a tricyclic antidepressant (2.5–12.5 mg PO q24h administered at night; adjust dose to produce a calming effect) has been used empirically with variable success in chronic or highly recurrent cases of IFLUTD.
- Because the glycosaminoglycan layer of the bladder is abnormal, reestablishment of a normal glycosaminoglycan layer may be of benefit, and is under investigation.
- No dietary change is necessary unless crystalluria is present. Recommend a commercial acidifying diet, and encourage water intake in cats with struvite crystalluria, especially males because of the risk of urethral matrix–crystalline plug formation.

Prevention

The biologic behavior of IFLUTD is variable. There are no proven effective preventive treatments. If crystalluria is present without urolith or urethral plug formation, consider special diets (see section on Urolithiasis). Stress may be an inciting cause of IFLUTD; therefore, avoidance of stress or use of anxiolytic drugs (such as diazepam) may be of benefit.

POLYPLOID CYSTITIS

Etiology

Polyps may be observed in animals with urinary bladder disease. They may represent benign or malignant neoplasia (see section on Neoplasia); however, they may also represent an inflammatory response to an underlying condition.

Clinical Signs

Polyps may be subclinical or they may cause hematuria, dysuria, pollakiuria, and possibly inappropriate urination.

Diagnosis

History. Usually, there is a history of lower urinary tract disease, particularly recurrent or persistent disease.

Physical Examination. Usually normal. Check for evidence of neoplasia by doing careful abdominal and rectal palpation.

Urinalysis. Hematuria, pyuria, and bacteriuria are often observed.

Urine Culture. Usually positive.

CBC and Serum Biochemical Analysis. Usually normal.

Radiography and Ultrasonography. Survey radiography is usually normal unless radiodense uroliths are present. Contrast radiography and ultrasonography reveal the polyps as being confluent with the bladder wall.

Treatment

Treatment of the underlying disease will usually result in resolution of the polyps if they are inflammatory in origin. Surgical excision may be indicated if the polyps persist and are associated with recurrent bladder disease.

Prevention

Prevention of inflammatory polyps is dependent upon preventing the primary disease.

CYCLOPHOSPHAMIDE-INDUCED CYSTITIS

Etiology

Cyclophosphamide, an alkylating agent, is used to treat various neoplasms and immune-mediated diseases. Approximately 30% of dogs receiving cyclophosphamide, usually for >2 months, develop a sterile hemorrhagic cystitis. Acrolein, a metabolite that is excreted in urine, is thought to cause mucosal ulceration, necrosis of smooth muscle and small arteries, hemorrhage, and edema.

Clinical Signs

Signs are similar to other causes of cystitis.

Diagnosis

History. Occurrence of clinical signs is variable in relation to receiving the drug, although it more commonly occurs after chronic administration.

Physical Examination. Pain is elicited on bladder palpation.

Urinalysis. Hematuria is present; pyuria and bacteriuria may be present.

Urine Culture. Usually negative unless a secondary bacterial infection is present.

CBC and Serum Biochemical Analysis. Usually normal unless bone marrow suppression has occurred due to chemotherapy

Radiography and Ultrasonography. Usually a small bladder with thickened walls. Contrast radiography and ultrasonography reveal irregular mucosa.

Treatment

Inducing diuresis appears to be the only effective means of treating cyclophosphamide-induced cystitis. Although instillation of medications such as DMSO and formaldehyde has been recommended, they are unproved. Systemic anti-inflammatory therapy is also unproved. If a secondary UTI is present, treat with an appropriate antibiotic.

Prevention

If possible, discontinue cyclophosphamide therapy. Substitute another alkylating agent if chemotherapy or immunosuppressive therapy is continued. If cyclophosphamide cannot be discontinued, then administer the drug and induce diuresis (see Chap. 97). Or administer at a time of day when the animal is likely to void shortly after receiving the drug (i.e., in the morning rather than in the evening). Owners should wear gloves because the active drug and metabolite are present in urine.

BLADDER TRAUMA

Etiology

The urinary bladder may be damaged by blunt trauma, such as being hit by a car; by penetrating objects, such as a bite wound or gunshot; or from other diseases, such as urolithiasis. The urinary bladder may also be damaged or ruptured due to improper urinary catheterization.

Clinical Signs

Clinical signs may be limited to hematuria and dysuria; uremia may be present if the bladder ruptures.

Diagnosis

History. There may be a history of the cause of the trauma, such as being hit by a car.

▼ *Key Point* Normal urination does not rule out a ruptured bladder.

Physical Examination. Inguinal bruising may be seen. Pain may be elicited on bladder palpation. Fractures and other organ injury may be present. If the urinary bladder is ruptured, abdominal distention due to urine and the absence of a palpable bladder may be found.

Urinalysis. If urine can be collected, it will often be hemorrhagic.

CBC and Serum Biochemical Analysis. May be normal or may reveal postrenal azotemia (increased BUN first, followed by increased creatinine), hyperphosphatemia, and metabolic acidosis. Hyperkalemia from uroperitoneum and elevated creatine phosphokinase activity due to muscle injury may occur. Other changes may be present depending on the severity of the trauma, and whether sepsis is present.

Radiography and Ultrasonography. The bladder may be small, present in the inguinal or perineal region if herniated, or not visible. If it has ruptured, abdominal fluid may be present. Consider contrast radiography to confirm bladder rupture.

Abdominocentesis. If abdominal fluid is present, perform abdominocentesis. Assess urea nitrogen and creatinine concentration of the abdominal fluid. The creatinine concentration will be higher in the fluid than in blood if the fluid is urine.

Treatment

If a small rupture has occurred evidenced by minimal leakage on positive contrast cystogram, place a urethral catheter and a closed collection system for 3–7 days. Repeat the cystogram to confirm healing of the rent. If a large rupture has occurred, then surgical repair is indicated (see Chap. 100).

Prevention

Prevent unnecessary iatrogenic trauma to the bladder. Use soft red rubber urinary catheters rather than rigid polypropylene catheters, and pass the catheter slowly to minimize catheter-induced trauma. When urine is observed to flow through the catheter, do not advance the catheter any farther. Carefully palpate the bladder in animals with urethral obstruction.

SUPPLEMENTAL READINGS

Kruger JM, Osborne CA, Lulich JP: Inherited and congenital disease of the lower urinary tract. *In* Osborne CA, Finco DR, eds.: Canine and Feline Nephrology and Urology. Media, PA: Williams & Wilkins, 1995, p 681.

Lane IF: Disorders of Micturition. *In* Osborne CA, Finco DR, eds.: Canine and Feline Nephrology and Urology, Media, PA: Williams & Wilkins, 1995, p 693.

Ling GV: Lower Urinary Tract Diseases of Dogs and Cats. St. Louis: Mosby–Year Book, 1995, p 1.

Osborne CA, Kruger JM, Lulich JP: Disorders of the feline lower urinary tract I. Vet Clin North Am Small Anim Pract 1996;26:169.

Osborne CA, Kruger JM, Lulich JP: Disorders of the feline lower urinary tract II. Vet Clin North Am Small Anim Pract 1996;26:423.

Osborne CA, Kruger JM, Lulich JP, Polzin DJ: Disorders of the feline lower urinary tract. *In* Osborne CA, Finco DR, eds.: Canine and Feline Nephrology and Urology. Media, PA: Williams & Wilkins, 1995, p 625.

Osborne CA, Lees GE: Bacterial infections of the canine and feline urinary tract. *In* Osborne CA, Finco DR, eds.: Canine and Feline Nephrology and Urology. Media, PA: Williams & Wilkins, 1995, p 759.

Osborne CA, Lulich JP, Bartges JW, et al.: Canine and feline urolithiasis: Relationship of etiopathogenesis to treatment and prevention. *In* Osborne CA, Finco DR, eds.: Canine and Feline Nephrology and Urology. Media, PA: Williams & Wilkins, 1995, p 798.

100 Surgery of the Urinary Bladder

Roger B. Fingland

Cystotomy is the most common surgical procedure on the urinary bladder in small animals. Subtotal or total cystectomy may be indicated for management of benign or malignant urinary bladder neoplasms. Incised bladder wall heals quickly and regains nearly 100% of original tissue strength after healing. The mucosal lining of the bladder is quite delicate and easily becomes edematous, necessitating meticulous tissue handling and proper suture placement. Intramural absorbable suture placement is ideal because material exposed to the bladder lumen may act as a nidus for calculi formation.

ANATOMY

- The urinary bladder is divided into three regions: (1) the cranial portion is the apex, (2) the caudal portion that joins the urethra is the neck, and (3) the segment between the apex and neck is the body.
- The ureteral openings and the urethral orifice form a triangular area on the dorsal aspect of the bladder called the trigone.
- The three ligaments of the bladder are composed of double layers of peritoneum. The ventral ligament extends from the ventral surface of the bladder along the ventral midline of the abdominal wall to the umbilicus. The ventral peritoneal ligament contains the urachus in the fetus. The urachus is an embryologic structure that connects the urinary bladder and the allantoic sac. The urachus closes and atrophies soon after birth, leaving a small scar at the apex of the urinary bladder. The lateral ligaments connect the lateral aspects of the bladder to the pelvic canal and enclose the ureters, deferent ducts, and umbilical arteries.
- The major blood supply to the bladder comes from the caudal vesical artery—a branch of the internal pudendal artery that lies in the pelvic fascia. The pelvic plexus of nerves is located dorsal to the bladder. The cranial vesical artery, present in only 50% of adult dogs, supplies the cranial aspect of the bladder. Venous blood drains into the internal pudendal veins. Bladder lymphatics drain into the hypogastric, sublumbar, and median iliac lymph nodes.
- Sympathetic innervation to the bladder is via the hypogastric nerve, and parasympathetic innervation is via the pelvic nerves. The hypogastric and pelvic nerves reach the bladder through the lateral ligaments near the caudal vesical arteries.

ANOMALIES OF THE URACHUS

Preoperative Considerations

- Persistent urachus results when the entire urachal canal remains patent after birth. Urine is voided through the urachal opening at the umbilicus. Vesicourachal diverticulum results when the origin of the urachus at the bladder apex fails to close. The diverticulum forms a pocket of stationary urine, predisposing the animal to recurrent bacterial urinary tract infections (UTI).
- A persistent urachus is removed surgically.
- Vesicourachal diverticula often are diagnosed by contrast radiography in young animals with persistent UTI. Diverticula may be diagnosed fortuitously during abdominal surgery. Diverticulectomy is indicated in animals with persistent UTI. Diverticula discovered during abdominal surgery may be removed to reduce the likelihood of recurrent UTI. Urachal scars commonly are observed at the dome of the bladder and seldom cause a problem. In contrast to urachal scars, diverticula are discrete pouch or sac openings from the bladder lumen.

Persistent Urachus—Surgical Procedure
Objectives

- Remove the patent urachus.
- Obtain specimens for bacterial culture and histopathologic analysis.

Equipment

- Standard general surgery instrument pack and suture
- Balfour retractor
- Laparotomy sponges

Technique

1. Place the animal in dorsal recumbency.
2. Prepare the ventral abdominal region for aseptic surgery.
3. Perform a routine ventral midline celiotomy from approximately 3 cm cranial to 3 cm caudal to the umbilicus.

4. Make an elliptical incision around the umbilical opening. Dissect the urachus from surrounding tissues, from umbilicus to the urinary bladder.
5. Place a Balfour retractor and isolate the urinary bladder with moistened laparotomy sponges.
6. Place stay sutures in the bladder to facilitate retraction.
7. Create a full-thickness elliptical incision in the bladder around the origin of the patent urachus.
8. Submit the patent urachus for histologic analysis.

▼ *Key Point* Resect the urachus, rather than just ligating it at the bladder apex, because this may result in a vesicourachal diverticulum and predispose the animal to persistent urinary tract infection.

9. Submit samples of the excised vesicourachal junction for bacterial culture and susceptibility testing.
10. Remove the stay sutures and laparotomy sponges, and close the bladder, as described later under Cystotomy, Technique.
11. Close the abdominal wall routinely.

Postoperative Care and Complications

- Postoperative complications are rare.
- Administer antibiotics based on the results of bacterial culture and susceptibility testing. Prolonged (>4 weeks) antibiotic therapy may be necessary to reduce the risk of recurrent UTI.
- See Cystotomy, Postoperative Care and Complications, for routine patient care.

Vesicourachal Diverticulum Excision— Surgical Procedure

Objectives

- Remove the vesicourachal diverticulum.
- Obtain samples for bacterial culture and susceptibility testing and histologic analysis.

Equipment

- Standard general surgery instrument pack and suture
- Balfour retractor
- Laparotomy sponges

Technique

1. Patient positioning and surgical approach are the same as those described under Persistent Urachus.
2. Do not make an elliptical incision around the umbilicus; instead, use the approach recommended for cystotomy.
3. Isolate the urinary bladder with moistened laparotomy sponges.
4. Place stay sutures to facilitate retraction.
5. Make a full-thickness elliptical incision in the bladder wall around and approximately 5 mm from the edge of the diverticulum.
6. Divide the excised diverticulum in half.
7. Submit samples for histologic analysis and bacterial culture and susceptibility testing.

8. Remove stay sutures and laparotomy sponges.
9. Close the bladder as described under Cystotomy, Technique.
10. Close the abdominal incision routinely.

Postoperative Care and Complications

- Postoperative complications are rare. Recurrent infections after removal of the diverticulum are uncommon.
- Administer antibiotics based on the results of bacterial culture and susceptibility testing. Prolonged antibiotic therapy (>4 weeks) may be necessary.
- See Cystotomy, Postoperative Care and Complications, for routine patient care.

CYSTOTOMY

Preoperative Considerations

- Cystotomy in small animals is indicated most commonly for removal of cystic calculi.
- Neoplasia of the urinary bladder and ureteral reimplantation also may require cystotomy.
- Antibiotics are not administered preoperatively unless prior urine culture indicates UTI. Otherwise, administer antibiotics intraoperatively after specimens for culture and susceptibility testing have been obtained.

Surgical Procedure

Objectives

- Open the urinary bladder to remove calculi, reimplant ureters, or explore the bladder lumen.
- Obtain samples for bacterial culture and susceptibility testing and histopathologic analysis.
- Prevent urine leakage into the peritoneal cavity.

Equipment

- Standard general surgery pack and suture
- Balfour retractor
- Laparotomy sponges
- Urinary catheter (male dogs)
- Human gallbladder scoop or sterile teaspoon to aid in stone removal
- 12-ml syringe
- 22-gauge needle
- Soft urethral catheter for patients with cystic calculi

Technique

1. Place the animal in dorsal recumbency.
2. Prepare the ventral abdominal region and vulvar area in the female for aseptic surgery. Irrigate the prepuce with antiseptic solution and include it in the aseptic field to enable intraoperative urethral catheterization, if necessary.
3. Incise the skin and subcutaneous tissue on the ventral abdominal midline.
4. In male dogs, incise the skin and subcutaneous tissue parallel and adjacent to the prepuce. Identify

and ligate the preputial branches of the caudal superficial epigastric vessels in the subcutis.

5. Incise the linea alba from the umbilicus to the pubis. (Incise from xyphoid to pubis if a full abdominal exploratory is necessary.) The paramedian approach can be used in male dogs.
6. Position the Balfour retractor. Explore the abdomen for associated abnormalities of the kidneys, ureters, prostate, urethra, and iliac lymph nodes.
7. Isolate the urinary bladder with moistened laparotomy sponges.
8. Place stay sutures at each end of the proposed cystotomy incision to facilitate retraction and atraumatic manipulation (Fig. 100–1A).
9. Remove urine from the bladder by cystocentesis.
10. Orient the cystotomy incision to avoid major vessels and provide optimal exposure for the procedure. Dorsal or ventral cystotomy incisions can be used for removal of calculi. A ventral incision is preferred for routine cystotomy and for exposure of the ureteral openings.

▼ *Key Point* A ventral cystotomy incision has no greater risk of leakage or adhesion formation than does a dorsal incision. In addition, the ureters are located well away from the ventral region, reducing inadvertent damage.

11. Plan the cystotomy incision to remove a vesicourachal diverticulum, if present.
12. Make a stab incision into the bladder with a scalpel (Fig. 100–1B).

13. Extend the incision proximally and distally with Metzenbaum scissors.
14. Avoid "corkscrewing" the incision around the bladder.
15. Avoid the trigone and ureters.
16. Remove uroliths with the gallbladder scoop or sterile teaspoon.

▼ *Key Point* Always submit uroliths to the laboratory for stone analysis.

17. Retrograde flushing may be required to remove small calculi from the proximal urethra in male dogs. Pass a sterile urinary catheter retrograde (from outside the penis) to the level of the os penis, occlude the end of the penis, and flush vigorously with sterile saline.
18. Pass the catheter throughout the entire length of the urethra and feel for grit or roughness.
19. Do not close the bladder until absolutely certain that all stones have been removed.
20. Incise a 4-mm × 1-cm full-thickness wedge of bladder wall from the edge of the cystotomy incision.
21. Submit half the wedge for histopathologic analysis and half for bacterial culture and susceptibility testing.

▼ *Key Point* If the animal has been on antibiotics, submit a full-thickness wedge of bladder wall for bacterial culture and susceptibility testing even if urine has been submitted for culture.

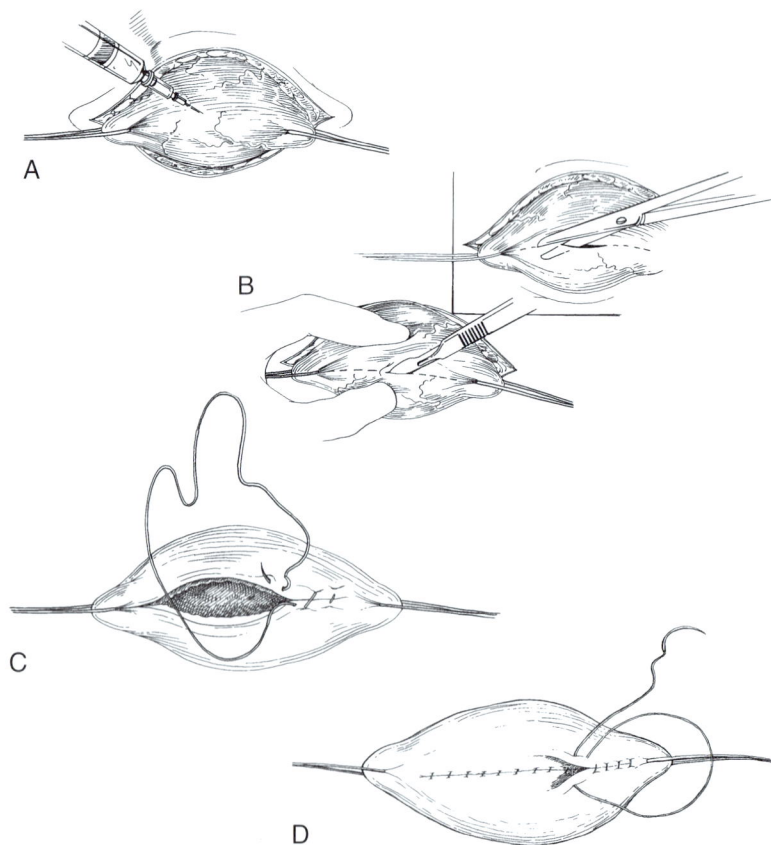

Figure 100–1. Cystotomy. *A,* With stay sutures in place, remove urine from bladder. *B,* Make stab incision with scalpel and extend with Metzenbaum scissors. *C,* After uroliths are removed and biopsy samples taken, place a Cushing pattern incorporating all tissue layers except the mucosa. *D,* Oversew the Cushing pattern with a Lembert pattern.

22. If a female dog requires an indwelling urinary catheter postoperatively (e.g., for maintaining bladder decompression or monitoring urine output), place the catheter before closing the bladder.
23. Pass a catheter normograde through the urethra and out the vulva.
24. Attach the end of a sterile Foley catheter to this catheter.
25. Pull the Foley catheter retrograde into the bladder lumen.

▼ *Key Point* Avoid incorporating the ureters in the bladder closure, especially with dorsal incisions.

26. Close the cystotomy (see subsequent description).
27. Remove stay sutures and laparotomy sponges.
28. Close the abdominal wall routinely.

Classically, cystotomy incisions are closed with a two-layer continuous inverting pattern. Synthetic absorbable suture material (3-0 to 4-0) with a swaged-on urogenital tapered needle is an ideal choice. A Cushing pattern, incorporating all tissue layers except the mucosa, is used for the first layer, followed by a Lembert pattern (Fig. 100–1*D*).

The bladder wall may be quite thick in animals with chronic cystitis, making inversion of the wall difficult.

In this situation, choose single-layer or double-layer continuous or interrupted appositional suture patterns. An appositional pattern is necessary when the cystotomy incision extends so far distally that inversion might result in occlusion of the ureters or narrowing of the urethra.

Postoperative Care and Complications

- Hematuria for 12–36 hours after surgery is common.
- If a transurethral catheter was placed, connect it to a closed collection system.
- Long-term (≥4 weeks) antibiotic and dietary therapy, based on results of bacterial culture and susceptibility testing and stone analysis findings, is necessary in animals with urolithiasis.
- Although rare, urine leakage from inadequate bladder closure may occur, particularly if obstruction develops distally. Monitor urine production.
- Observe for stranguria.
- Obtain abdominal radiographs after surgery, if multiple radiopaque stones were present, to confirm complete stone removal.

BLADDER TRAUMA

Preoperative Considerations

- See Chapter 99, Diseases of the Urinary Bladder, for a discussion of etiology, pathophysiology, clinical signs, laboratory abnormalities, and diagnosis of ruptured bladder.
- Contusions, partial-thickness lacerations, and iatrogenic ruptures during catheterization usually heal spontaneously and are managed medically. Consider urinary diversion (transurethral catheterization or

tube cystostomy) and antibiotic therapy until healing is complete.
- Intraperitoneal rupture of the urinary bladder may heal spontaneously. This outcome is inconsistent and unpredictable. Surgical repair is the treatment of choice.

▼ *Key Point* Fluid, electrolyte, and acid-base disorders (dehydration, hyperkalemia, acidosis, azotemia) must be managed prior to anesthetizing an animal for repair of a ruptured bladder.

- Animals with a ruptured bladder that cannot be anesthetized because of fluid, electrolyte, and acid-base abnormalities may be treated initially by temporary urinary diversion. Place large Penrose drains transabdominally to drain urine from the peritoneal cavity.
- Administer intravenous fluid therapy with isotonic saline, antibiotics, and sodium bicarbonate therapy if necessary.

Surgical Procedure

Objective

- Remove urine from the peritoneal cavity.
- Repair the ruptured bladder.
- Identify and treat other intra-abdominal injuries.

Equipment

- Standard general surgery instrument pack and suture
- Balfour retractor
- Laparotomy pads
- Suction device
- Foley catheter (if tube cystostomy is indicated).

Technique

1. Place the animal in dorsal recumbency.
2. Prepare the ventral abdominal region for aseptic surgery.
3. Perform a routine ventral midline celiotomy from the umbilicus to the pubis.
4. Perform an abdominal exploratory.
5. Isolate the urinary bladder with moistened laparotomy sponges.
6. Locate the rupture in the urinary bladder.
7. Place stay sutures to facilitate exposure of the rupture.
8. Liberally debride nonviable tissue from the edges of the rent.
9. Approximate the viable edges of the rent with 3-0 synthetic absorbable suture material using an inverting or approximating suture pattern.
10. Remove the stay sutures.
11. When the viability of the bladder wall is questionable, resect the nonviable region if possible. Alternatively, cover the area with omentum or, preferably, a serosal patch using jejunum.
12. Manage other intra-abdominal injuries.
13. Lavage the peritoneal cavity with copious amounts of warm, sterile, physiologic saline solution.

14. Remove residual abdominal fluid.
15. Submit samples of peritoneal fluid for bacteriologic culture and susceptibility testing.
16. Consider placing a sterile transurethral catheter to keep the bladder decompressed if the repair is tenuous or the viability of the bladder wall is questionable. Urinary diversion seldom is necessary following proper repair of ruptured bladder.
17. Close the abdominal wall routinely.

Postoperative Care and Complications

- Administer broad-spectrum antibiotics in animals with extensive tissue trauma until culture and susceptibility results can be used to direct antibiotic therapy.
- The animal may be hematuric and pollakiuric for 12–48 hours after surgery.
- Continue to monitor and manage fluid, electrolyte, and acid-base imbalances after surgery. Monitor urine output.
- If a transurethral catheter is in place to decompress the bladder when the repair is tenuous, remove it 2–3 days after surgery.
- See Cystotomy, Postoperative Care and Complications, for routine patient care.

SUBTOTAL CYSTECTOMY

Preoperative Considerations

- Subtotal cystectomy is performed most commonly in an attempt to cure or palliate an animal with bladder neoplasia. Subtotal cystectomy may be indicated to remove benign lesions, such as traumatic or congenital diverticula (see under Anomalies of the Urachus), polyps, intramural granulomas, and devascularized areas of bladder wall.
- Therapeutic results are related to the size and location of the bladder neoplasm and the presence or absence of metastasis. Animals with bladder neoplasia must undergo thorough diagnostic testing, including thoracic and abdominal radiography, contrast radiographic studies, and cytologic evaluation prior to surgical intervention.
- Neoplasms located in accessible areas of the bladder can be removed by partial cystectomy. Subtotal cystectomy is not considered when there is extensive involvement of the neck or trigone of the bladder or when a large portion of the bladder wall is affected.

▼ **Key Point** A substantial portion of the nontrigone bladder, perhaps greater than 75%, can be excised with few untoward effects.

Surgical Procedure
Objective

- Remove abnormal section of bladder wall.
- Biopsy a bladder mass.
- Maintain reservoir function of bladder.

Equipment

- Standard general surgery instrument pack and suture
- Balfour retractor
- Sterile urinary catheter

Technique

1. Patient positioning, surgical approach, and isolation of the bladder are as described previously under Cystotomy, Technique.
2. Locate the area to be removed by gentle palpation.
3. Excise the abnormal bladder wall, including at least 1 cm of normal-appearing tissue on all sides.
4. Wide surgical margins (>3 cm) are not necessary if the disease process is benign.
5. Ureteral transplantation may be necessary. Refer to Chapter 98.
6. Close the bladder with 3-0 or 4-0 synthetic absorbable suture material in an appositional or inverting pattern (see Cystotomy, Technique).
7. If neoplasia is suspected, explore the entire abdomen for metastasis. Biopsy regional lymph nodes.
8. Close the abdomen routinely.

Postoperative Care and Complications

- Adjunct radiotherapy or chemotherapy may be beneficial following subtotal cystectomy for bladder neoplasia.
- Hematuria and pollakiuria are commonly observed after subtotal cystectomy.
- Frequent voiding may persist due to loss of reservoir volume.
- The reservoir function of the bladder returns, at least partially, by 3 months.
- See Cystotomy, Postoperative Care and Complications, for routine patient care.

TUBE CYSTOSTOMY

Preoperative Considerations

- Tube cystostomy is indicated for temporary diversion of urine from the urethra.
- Dogs with metabolic alterations resulting from obstruction to urine outflow frequently are unable to tolerate general anesthesia.
- When transureteral catheterization is not possible or desired, diversion of urine via tube cystostomy permits delay of definitive repair of urethral trauma or removal of urethral calculi until metabolic alterations are corrected.
- Tube cystostomy is a practical means of temporary urine diversion when the bladder has lost contractile function.
- A permanent cystostomy catheter can be placed to relieve urine outflow obstruction in a dog with inoperable bladder neoplasia. Relatively long-term (months) palliation can be achieved with minimal complications.

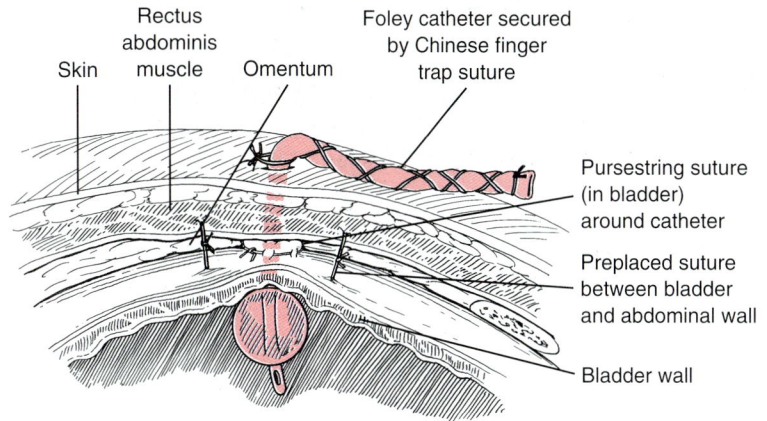

Figure 100–2. Suture and tube placement for tube cystotomy.

- General anesthesia usually is not needed for tube cystostomy. Narcotic analgesics, such as oxymorphone combined with local infiltration of lidocaine, are adequate.

Surgical Procedure

Objective

- Divert the flow of urine from the urethra via a Foley catheter placed into the bladder.

Equipment

- Standard general surgery instrument pack and suture
- 8 Fr. Foley catheter with intact balloon
- Small Gelpi or Weitlaner retractor

Technique

1. Administer oxymorphone, 0.1–0.3 mg/kg IV, or other appropriate analgesic, if necessary.
2. Position the animal in dorsal recumbency.
3. Prepare the ventral abdominal region for aseptic surgery.
4. Infiltrate the abdominal wall with lidocaine in the area of the planned paramedian incision—approximately 3 cm lateral to the midline at the level of the prepuce.
5. Make a 4-cm paramedian incision through the abdominal wall. Avoid incising the distended urinary bladder. Place the self-retaining retractor.
6. Pass the Foley catheter through the abdominal wall via a paramedian stab incision made adjacent to the celiotomy incision.
7. Place a pursestring suture in the wall of the bladder on the ventral side near the apex. Use 3-0 synthetic absorbable suture material with a swaged-on taper needle.
8. Pass the Foley catheter into the bladder through a stab incision in the center of the pursestring suture.
9. Tighten and tie the pursestring suture. Do not occlude the catheter.
10. Inflate the balloon of the Foley catheter with sterile saline.
11. Preplace four sutures of 2-0 or 3-0 synthetic absorbable material between the bladder and the abdominal wall, where the Foley catheter exits.
12. Secure the bladder to the body wall by tying the preplaced sutures.
13. The potential for intraperitoneal leakage of urine may be lessened by placing omentum around the catheter between the bladder and body wall prior to tying the preplaced sutures (Fig. 100–2).
14. Close the paramedian incision routinely.
15. Secure the Foley catheter to the skin using the Chinese finger trap knot (see Chap. 3).

Postoperative Care and Complications

- The Foley catheter can be attached to a closed sterile urine collection system (preferred) or capped and drained intermittently.
- Place an Elizabethan collar or side brace on the animal to prevent mutilation of the system.
- Administer a broad-spectrum antibiotic.
- Deflate the balloon and withdraw the catheter when it is no longer needed. If the catheter has been in place for approximately 7 days, the stoma will heal spontaneously. Earlier removal may require surgical closure of the bladder and abdominal wall.
- Rarely, adhesions between the bladder and peritoneum from tube cystostomy can inhibit complete bladder emptying. Placement of the Foley catheter in the body of the bladder rather than the apex helps prevent this problem.

SUPPLEMENTAL READINGS

Osuna DJ: Postoperative management of urinary tract surgical patients. Compend Cont Ed 9:873, 1987.

Smith JD, Stone EA, Gilson SD: Placement of a permanent cystostomy catheter to relieve urine outflow obstruction in dogs with transitional cell carcinoma. J Am Vet Med Assoc 206:496, 1995.

Stone EA: Surgical therapy for urolithiasis. Vet Clin North Am Sm Anim Pract 14:77, 1984.

101 Diseases of the Urethra

Donald R. Krawiec

CONGENITAL URETHRAL DISORDERS

Congenital urethral disorders appear to occur only sporadically in the dog and rarely in the cat. Although no comprehensive retrospective or prospective studies have been reported, congenital urethral disorders tend to occur more frequently in male dogs than in females.

Etiology

- Apenia, megalopenis (due to excess testosterone), and micropenis (due to testosterone deficiency) are anomalies of the penis that also affect the urethra (see Chap. 108).
- Urethral anomalies include urethral agenesis, urethral stricture and stenosis, urethral diverticulum, urethral duplication, accessory meatus, urethral ectopia, anterior or posterior urethral valves, urethrorectal and vesicorectal fistulas, hypospadias, and epispadias.
- Hypospadias is a consequence of incomplete fusion of urethral grooves and usually appears as urethral openings on the ventral side of the penis.
- Epispadias occurs in both males and females and results in a dorsally displaced urethra.

Clinical Signs

- Clinical signs depend on the anomaly.
- Some anomalies are simply an anatomical abnormality and cause no clinical signs.
- Other anomalies that result in urine scalding, incontinence, and recurrent bacterial cystitis are surgically treated.
- Animals with urethral-rectal fistula urinate through their rectum.
- Congenital urethral anomalies may cause urethral obstruction and may cause signs of uremic crisis.

Diagnosis

- Congenital urethral anomalies are usually identified on physical examination (including rectal examination).
- Contrast radiographic examination and/or endoscopic procedures are also helpful in locating and defining the urethral abnormality.

Treatment

▼ *Key Point* Treatment consists of surgical correction of anomalies only if they are causing *cosmetic or clinical problems.*

- Surgically correct strictures and fistulas (see Chap. 102).
- Treat secondary cystitis with an appropriate antibiotic based on urine culture and susceptibility results (see Chap. 99).
- Surgically correct urethral obstruction after the animal has been stabilized.
- Medical therapy for incontinence may be necessary (see Chap. 103).

Treatment for Hyospadias

- Castrate animals with urethral openings cranial to the scrotum and perform a scrotal urethrostomy (see Chap. 102).
- Perform perineal urethrostomy on animals with urethral openings in the perineal region if the urine stream is causing dermatitis.
- In either case remove the prepuce and penis if necessary.

Treatment for Urethrorectal Diverticulum

- Perform enemas the day before surgery to help evacuate the colon and rectum.
- Administer antibiotics that have anaerobic and aerobic activity the day before and 24 hours after surgery.
- Through a perineal surgical approach, identify the fistula and ligate and sever near the urethra.
- Approximate the urethral mucosa with fine absorbable sutures.

URETHRITIS

Bacterial Urethritis

Etiology

- Bacterial urethritis usually occurs with cystitis (see Chap. 99) or prostatitis (see Chap. 104).

Clinical Signs

- Clinical signs of bacterial urethritis may include dysuria, hematuria, stranguria, pollakiuria-type urinary incontinence, and urethral obstruction.

Diagnosis

- Identifying pathologic bacteria in the urethra is difficult because the urethra is contaminated with commensal bacteria.
- It is rarely necessary to identify specific bacteria within the urethra causing urethritis because it is almost always associated with cystitis.
- As a general rule, assume bacteria cultured from the bladder are also affecting the urethra.

Treatment

- Administration of a systemic antibiotic that is effective for the treatment of bacterial cystitis is usually successful for treatment of bacterial urethritis (see Chap. 99).
- If the inflammatory disease is causing significant urethral obstruction, place an indwelling urinary catheter until specific treatment is effective in reducing inflammation and urethral spasm.
- The urethral catheter is usually left in for 3–7 days.
- Consider giving prednisolone in the acute phase of urethritis to decrease inflammation.
- Continue antibiotics for 2–3 weeks after corticosteroids are discontinued. Ensure sterile urine following antibiotic treatment.
- Phenoxybenzamine may be used as a smooth muscle relaxant and diazepam may be used to decrease urethral skeletal muscle tone in animals that have urethral spasm due to inflammation (see Chap. 103).

Granulomatous Urethritis

Etiology

- Granulomatous urethritis occurs most commonly in older female dogs and is believed to be an immune-mediated infiltrative disease.
- Granulomatous urethritis is possibly due to an allergic reaction to commensal bacteria and it is currently not known if it is associated with chronic urinary tract infection.

Clinical Signs

- Clinical signs of granulomatous urethritis are dysuria, hematuria, stranguria, pollakiuria, urinary incontinence, and urethral obstruction.
- Animals with granulomatous urethritis often present with urethral obstruction. Urethral neoplasia is the primary rule-out.

Diagnosis

- Palpate the urethra via the rectum. Granulomatous urethritis and neoplasia feel like a ropy thickened tube on the ventral pelvic floor.
- Remove samples of urethra mucosal and submucosa via urethroscope or traumatic urethral lavage. Diagnose granulomatous urethritis by identifying a mononuclear cell infiltration of urethral mucosa or submucosa from cytologic and histologic biopsy samples.

Treatment

- Treat granulomatous urethritis with antibiotics if there is concurrent urinary tract infection.
- This disease responds to anti-inflammatory agents such as prednisolone and immunosuppressive agents such as cyclophosphamide.
- Antibiotic treatment is generally continued for 2 or 3 weeks after the anti-inflammatory treatment is stopped.

Chlamydial Urethritis

Etiology

- Chlamydial urethritis is caused by the same organism that produces keratoconjunctivitis and rhinitis in cats (see Chap. 9).

Clinical Signs

- Clinical signs may include dysuria, hematuria, stranguria, pollakiuria, urinary incontinence, and urethral obstruction.

Diagnosis

- Clinical signs of all urethral inflammatory disorders are similar. Base diagnosis on response to treatment, evaluation of cytology and biopsy samples, and urethral culture results.

Treatment

- Chlamydial urethral infections are usually successfully treated with standard dosages of doxycycline, tetracycline, or chloramphenicol.

URETHRAL OBSTRUCTION

Etiology

- Urethral obstruction may be due to a structural or functional impairment of urine flow.
- Structural obstructions are most often caused by either urolithiasis or strictures but can also be caused by urethral plugs (mucus and crystals), neoplasia, and blood clots.
- Functional obstructions are most often caused by neurologic disorders or inflammation.

Clinical Signs

- Incomplete outflow obstruction may result in dysuria, urinary incontinence, and hematuria.
- Complete outflow obstruction results in uremia in 3–4 days and death in 5–6 days.

- Urinary tract infection in the face of obstructive uropathy can result in pyelonephritis, acute renal failure, septicemia, and a rapidly fulminating course leading to death.

Diagnosis

- Suspect urethral obstruction in animals straining to urinate with an inability to empty their bladders.
- A large distended bladder in an animal that cannot void is highly suggestive of urethral obstruction.
- Clinical signs of uremia in an animal with a distended bladder are also suggestive of urethral obstruction.
- Perform a rectal exam to palpate the urethra and locate or identify a possible cause.
- Also palpate the urethra in the perineal and penile regions.
- Gently compress the bladder to assess urethral patency.
- Catheterize the urethra to localize the problem.
- Resistance in urethral catheterization usually means there is a physical urethral obstruction.
- Easy catheterization in an animal that has difficulty voiding usually indicates an inflammatory condition that is resulting in urethral spasm.
- Radiograph the caudal abdomen, including the perineal region, to identify obstructing radiopaque calculi.
- Consider performing contrast urethrography to identify radiolucent calculi or stricture if survey radiographs fail to reveal a physical obstruction.
- Perform a complete blood count, serum chemistry profile, and urinalysis and culture before fluids are administered, if possible.
- Animals with urethral obstruction may have hyperkalemia, metabolic acidosis, and azotemia (see Chap. 97).

Treatment

Initial Treatment

- Immediately decompress the bladder with an appropriate catheter if possible or, alternately, via cystocentesis.
- Collect urine for urinalysis and culture.
- Give polyionic isotonic fluids IV to correct dehydration and to balance the solute diuresis that will occur after relief of the obstruction. Use normal saline (fluids that do not contain potassium) until serum chemistry results are obtained.
- Calculate the fluid rate so the animal will be rehydrated in 4 to 6 hours (see Chap. 5).
- Both hyperkalemia and acidosis rapidly correct themselves after the obstruction is relieved if appropriate fluids are administered.

Treating Hyperkalemia Associated with Urethral Obstruction

- Rehydrate with potassium-free fluid (e.g., saline).
- Give sodium bicarbonate at a dose of 2 mEq/kg body weight slowly over 30 minutes.

- Give dextrose as a 20–30% solution to effect.
- Both sodium bicarbonate and dextrose therapy will drive potassium intracelluarly.
- Consider administration of a 10% calcium gluconate solution IV over 10–15 minutes if the patient is in danger of imminent death. Calcium protects the heart from the toxic effects of potassium.

Unobstructing the Urethra

- Attempt to establish urethral patency only after the bladder has been decompressed and fluids are being administered.
- If anesthesia is needed for relieving the obstruction, titrate drugs to effect. Uremic animals generally require smaller doses of anesthetic agents then normal animals.
- If a calculus can be palpated rectally, gently manipulate the stone and attempt to push it into the bladder. This technique is especially useful in female dogs.
- Male dogs and cats generally require some form of urethral hydropropulsion to dislodge an obstruction and push it into the bladder.

Technique for Urethral Hydropropulsion

- Place a sterile mixture of 50% saline and 50% sterile lubricant in a 12–20 ml syringe.
- Use this solution to both lubricate the obstruction and propel the obstruction into the bladder.
- The most common site of obstruction is the distal penis of male cats and just behind the os penis in male dogs.
- *In male cats* place a urethral catheter (tomcat catheter) in the urethral orifice and gently flush the lubricant mixture into the urethra. Flush the plug out of the urethral orifice and into the bladder. Gently advance the catheter until it is in the bladder.
- *In male dogs* urethral propulsion of calculi usually requires urethral dilation.
  - Advance an appropriate size polyurethane urethral catheter to the area of obstruction.
  - Compress the pelvic urethra with a gloved finger in the rectum. Hold off the urethral orifice and flush.
  - After the urethra is dilated, stop compression of the pelvic urethra, and the stone usually follows in the direction of the flush up the dilated urethra.
  - Perform urethra hydropropulsion as many times as needed to remove the obstruction.

Postobstruction Care

- Leave the indwelling catheter in place if urine output requires monitoring or reobstruction is a concern.
- Once the obstruction is relieved and the animal is stable, treat the underlying cause of the obstruction.
- If bacterial cystitis is present, treat with an appropriate antibiotic for 3–4 weeks (see Chap. 99).

Prevention of Recurrence

- Submit calculi removed from the urethra or bladder for quantitative analysis and begin measures to prevent recurrence (see Chap. 99).

- Perineal urethrostomies in cats will usually prevent recurrence of obstruction (see Chap. 102).
- Scrotal urethrostomies in male dogs help prevent recurrence of obstruction due to calculi (see Chap. 102).

URETHRAL TRAUMA

Etiology

- Urethral trauma may be caused by pelvic fractures, urethral catheterization, bite wounds, and other penetrating trauma.
- Trauma may induce bruising, mild hemorrhage, and partial to complete urethral rupture.
- Ruptures result in leakage of urine into muscle and subcutaneous tissue surrounding the tear. Periurethral inflammation may result in stricture formation.
- Urethral lacerations near the trigone of the bladder may result in uroabdomen.

Clinical Signs

- Mild urethral trauma without mucosal defects may result in no signs or in mild signs of dysuria and stranguria.
- Urethral tears with urine escaping into surrounding tissues will result in severe inflammation and necrosis. Inguinal and abdominal bruising is common. The inflammation can be severe and may induce profound swelling and extreme irritation of the affected tissues.
- Extravasation of urine into the abdominal cavity causes ascites, postrenal azotemia, and uremia (see Chaps. 97 and 99).

Diagnosis

- Suspect urethral trauma on physical examination in animals with evidence of trauma in the pelvis or perineum.
- Animals with hind limb and perineal swelling, pain, and superficial skin bruising and swelling may have a ruptured urethra, or only soft tissue trauma and hemorrhage.
- Abdominal distention following trauma could indicate hemoabdomen or uroabdomen.
- Diagnose urethral tears radiographically by demonstrating contrast media escaping into surrounding tissues during contrast urethrography. If the urine in the abdomen is due to urethral laceration, positive contrast cystography may be normal. However, contrast media will be identified flowing into the abdominal cavity when a positive contrast urethrogram is performed.
- Uroabdomen may be identified by performing abdominocentesis. Urea nitrogen and creatinine concentrations in the ascitic fluid will exceed blood concentrations, especially for creatinine (see Chap. 96).

Treatment

- Treat partial urethral tears by placing a soft (preferably Silastic) indwelling urethra catheter. Catheter size should be close to normal urethral lumen size.

Maintain the catheter in place for 7–21 days depending on the severity of the urethral trauma.
- Treat complete ruptures by careful surgical anastomosis or permanent urethrostomy proximal to the damage (see Chap. 102).

Prevention

- Prevent urethral trauma caused by urinary catheterization by careful technique as well as by using less irritating silicone, soft Teflon-coated latex, or polyvinylchloride catheters.

URETHRAL STRICTURE

Etiology

- Stricture may be a sequela to urethral trauma or chronic inflammation.
- Chronic inflammatory conditions that might result in stenosis include severe granulomatous or bacterial urethritis, lodged urethral calculi, or neoplasia.

Clinical Signs

- Urethral stricture may cause a poor urine stream, dysuria, stranguria, oliguria, and urinary incontinence.
- Severe stricture may produce a chronically distended bladder, hydroureter, hydronephrosis, postrenal azotemia, and uremia.

Diagnosis

- Distal urethral strictures may be detected on physical examination.
- Differentials for the clinical signs associated with urethral strictures include other obstructive disorders like urethral neoplasia, calculi, and severe inflammation.
- Diagnose by positive contrast urethrography or urethroscopy.

Treatment

- Urethral stenosis may be treated with balloon dilation techniques or permanent urethrostomy proximal to the lesion (see Chap. 102).
- Bladder atony may be a long-term complication if the stricture was chronic (see Chap. 99).

URETHRAL PROLAPSE

Etiology

- Urethral prolapse is idiopathic and often occurs in young male brachycephalic breeds.
- This condition may occur secondary to sexual excitement or urethritis, especially if it is diagnosed in other dog breeds.

Clinical Signs

- Clinical signs may include dysuria, urinary incontinence, and often blood dripping from the urethral meatus.

Diagnosis

- Urethral prolapse is diagnosed by extrusion of the penis. Diagnose urethral prolapse by identifying a characteristic doughnut-shaped protrusion of urethral mucosa from the penis (retract the prepuce to expose the penile tip)

Treatment

- Conservative treatment consists of sedating the animal and reducing the prolapse, but this is generally unsuccessful long-term.
- The resulting inflammation sometimes fixes the urethra to surrounding tissue during healing.
- If the prolapse recurs or if the tissue is necrotic, perform surgical resection (see Chap. 102).
- Place an Elizabethan collar to prevent the dog from traumatizing the penis.
- Ancillary medical therapy includes tranquilization, antispasmotics, and anti-inflammatory agents, which may help prevent irritation and inflammation-induced straining.
- Antibiotics may be used if bacterial urethritis is present.

URETHRAL NEOPLASIA

Etiology

- Primary tumors of the dog and cat urethra are rare but appear to be more common in the female than in the male.
- Mean age of occurrence has been reported to be 10.4 years and beagles reportedly are at increased risk.
- Prolonged urethral irritation may be a risk factor.
- Transitional cell carcinoma and squamous cell carcinoma are the most frequently identified urethral tumors. Prostatic adenocarcinoma can extend down the urethra.
- Urethral tumors are most common in the prostatic portion of the male urethra and tend to grow slowly, invade surrounding tissue, and metastasize to lymph nodes and/or the lung in about 30% of cases.

Clinical Signs

- Chronic dysuria is the most common sign associated with urethral neoplasia.
- Occasionally, the first sign observed may be urethral obstruction.
- Hematuria and urethral incompetence may also be seen.

Diagnosis

- Identify urethral masses by rectal palpation (a thickened, irregular urethra in females; may not be palpable in males).
- Caudal abdominal masses, or in cases of urethral obstruction, distended bladders may also be palpated. Severely enlarged sublumbar lymph nodes may be palpated through the abdominal wall or via rectal palpation.
- Vaginoscopy may reveal a mass protruding from the urethral orifice or into the urethral lumen.
- Abdominal ultrasound or radiography may reveal a caudal abdominal mass.
- Use positive contrast urethrography to localize the mass in the urethra.
- Definitive diagnosis of neoplasia requires cytologic or histologic verification.
- Evaluate biopsies of the urethra obtained via catheterization by cytology or by histology if the sample is large enough.
- Consider surgical exploration of the urethra to obtain a diagnostic sample, if biopsies cannot be obtained through uninvasive means.
- Radiograph the thorax to stage the disease process.

Treatment

- In most instances urethral neoplasia is diagnosed only after the neoplasia is in an advanced stage.
- Surgical excision and a permanent urethrostomy can be used in dogs that are obstructed with distal lesions.
- Surgery and radiation therapy have not been shown to increase survival time over surgery alone.
- Consider palliative tube cystostomy if an owner wants to prolong an animal's life (see Chap. 100).

SUPPLEMENTAL READINGS

Krawiec DR: Urethral diseases of dogs and cats. *In* Osborne CA, Finco DR, eds.: Canine and Feline Nephrology and Urology. Williams & Wilkins, 1995, p 718.

Kruger JM, Osborne CA, Lulich JP: Inherited and congenital disease of the lower urinary tract. *In* Osborne CA, Finco DR, eds.: Canine and Feline Nephrology and Urology. Williams & Wilkins, 1995, p 681.

Klausner JS, Caywood DD: Neoplasms of the urinary tract. *In* Osborne CA, Finco DR, eds.: Canine and Feline Nephrology and Urology. Williams & Wilkins, 1995, p 903.

Ling GV: Lower Urinary Tract Disease of Dogs and Cats. St. Louis, Mosby–Year Book, 1995.

Wingfield WE, Van Pelt DR, Barker S: Physical injuries to the urinary tract. *In* Osborne CA, Finco DR, eds.: Canine and Feline Nephrology and Urology. Williams & Wilkins, 1995, p 895.

102 Surgery of the Urethra

Dale E. Bjorling

Urethral disorders in dogs and cats frequently result in partial or complete obstruction. Emergency care may be required to restore the flow of urine and to treat metabolic imbalances. Calculi within the urethra are often accompanied by urinary tract infection (UTI) and cystic calculi. Aggressive medical and dietary management is required after surgery to prevent recurrence. Be careful during surgical manipulation of the urethra to minimize the potential for postoperative scar tissue formation and subsequent urethral obstruction.

▼ *Key Point* Correct metabolic imbalances in an animal with urethral obstruction prior to performing general anesthesia and prolonged operative procedures.

ANATOMY

Male Canine Urethra

- The urethra in the male canine is divided into three parts: the prostatic, membranous, and cavernous or penile portions.
- The urethral sphincter is not a discrete structure in the dog. Urethral pressure profiles demonstrate a zone of increased pressure that extends from the prostatic urethra into the membranous urethra. Of the components of the urethral sphincter closure mechanism (fibroelastic tissue, smooth muscle, striated muscle), smooth muscle is probably primarily responsible for maintaining tone in the resting state. Therefore, alpha-adrenergic agonists may be successful in the treatment of sphincter incompetence.
- The smooth muscle of the urethra is innervated by autonomic nerves arising from the pelvic plexus. The striated musculature receives innervation from branches of the pudendal nerve.
- The distal portion of the penile urethra lies within the os penis. Dilation of the urethra is limited within the os penis and in the perineal portion of the urethra, as it curves around the ischium. These are common locations for calculi to become lodged within the urethra.

Male Feline Urethra

- The male feline urethra consists of three parts: (1) the preprostatic, which lies between the bladder and the prostate gland and is relatively longer than the corresponding portion of the male canine urethra; (2) the prostatic part, which extends from the prostate to the bulbourethral glands; and (3) the penile urethra. Immediately caudal to the bulbourethral glands, the urethral lumen rapidly narrows from approximately 4 mm in diameter to 1 mm. This diameter is maintained through the remainder of the penile urethra. When the penis is retracted, the prostatic and proximal penile urethra may assume the appearance of a flattened or gentle "s," which complicates urethral catheterization unless the penis is manually extended.
- An area of increased pressure thought to correspond to the sphincter mechanism is found in the urethra caudal to the prostate. Despite a decrease in intraurethral electromyographic activity after perineal urethrostomy in male cats, urinary incontinence is an uncommon occurrence. This may be due to the smooth muscle fibers as well as the remaining striated fibers of the urethral sphincter, which results in resting urethral pressure greater than intravesicular pressure during bladder distension.
- The urethra is innervated by branches of the pudendal nerve and receives autonomic fibers from the pelvic plexus.

Female Canine and Feline Urethra

- The urethra in the female dog and cat is relatively short in comparison to the male and corresponds to the portion of the male urethra found cranial to the level of the mid prostate. The female urethra is also relatively larger in diameter and more distensible than the corresponding male urethra.
- It appears unlikely that a discrete urethral sphincter is present in either dogs or cats. The urethral pressure profile does not demonstrate a discrete increase in pressure, but the major increase in urethral pressure develops in the mid urethra of the female dog. A localized area of increase in urethral pressure has been observed in female cats associated with striated musculature near the external urethral orifice.
- The female urethra is innervated by autonomic fibers of the hypogastric and pelvic nerves and sensory and motor fibers from the pudendal nerve.
- Obstruction of the female urethra is extremely uncommon because of its short length, wide diameter, and relative distensibility.

URETHRAL ANASTOMOSIS

Preoperative Considerations

- Perform urethral anastomosis for treatment of urethral disruption, prostatectomy, stricture formation, or removal of granulomatous or neoplastic masses.
- Perform retrograde positive contrast urethrocystography to identify the location of obstruction or disruption.
- Treat animals that are uremic as a result of urethral obstruction or leakage of urine into the periurethral tissues prior to inducing anesthesia and performing surgery.

▼ *Key Point* Incomplete lacerations or defects (discussed later in this chapter) may be satisfactorily treated by placing an indwelling urethral catheter to divert the flow of urine for 2 to 3 weeks. This form of treatment will be successful only when intact urethral mucosa bridges a portion of the injured area.

Surgical Procedure

Objectives

- Remove diseased tissue.
- Restore urethral continuity.
- Minimize the potential for postoperative stricture formation.

Equipment

- Standard surgical instruments and suture
- Urinary catheters of appropriate diameter and length
- Gelpi or Weitlaner self-retaining retractors
- Monofilament nonabsorbable suture (4–0 or 5–0) or synthetic absorbable suture (4–0 or 5–0)
- Magnification (optional)
- Penrose drains, if cellulitis or tissue necrosis due to extravasation of urine has occurred.

Technique

1. The positioning of the animal (dorsal recumbancy or ventral recumbancy in a perineal stand) depends upon the portion of the urethra to be operated upon.
2. With the animal positioned appropriately, prepare the overlying skin for aseptic surgery.
3. Pass a sterile urethral catheter from the external urethral orifice in a retrograde direction to facilitate identification of the proximal end of the distal portion of the urethra.
4. If the distal end of the proximal portion of the urethra cannot be identified, perform a cystotomy and pass a urethral catheter in an antegrade direction.
5. Excise the damaged portions of the urethra. Although it is critical that a tension-free anastomosis be performed, do not be reluctant to debride

and resect an adequate amount of urethra to properly treat the disease process.

▼ *Key Point* If the urethra cannot be reconstructed without undue tension across the anastomotic site, consider alternatives, such as prepubic urethrostomy.

6. With the urethral catheter in place, perform the anastomosis by placing full-thickness sutures in a simple interrupted pattern.
7. Place the first suture through the dorsal aspect of the urethra.
8. Cut the ends of the suture at a sufficient length so that they may be grasped by a forceps.
9. Gently rotate the urethra to facilitate placement of subsequent sutures. Preplacement of sutures may help to ensure accurate placement of sutures.
10. Place sutures evenly; six to eight sutures are usually sufficient to perform a satisfactory anastomosis.
11. Maintain a soft, loose-fitting urethral catheter connected to a sterile urine collection bag for 7–10 days after surgery.
12. If necessary, use an Elizabethan collar or a body brace to prevent catheter displacement. Alternatively, place a cystostomy catheter to divert the flow of urine from the urethra (see Chap. 100).
13. Close the wound in a standard manner.

Postoperative Care and Complications

- If the urethral catheter is removed prematurely, a decision must be made regarding whether or not to replace the catheter. If resistance is encountered during attempts to pass the urethral catheter, replacement is abandoned.
- Monitor the animal carefully for evidence of urine leakage.
- Warn the owners of the potential for postoperative stricture, and advise them to carefully observe the animal during urination for evidence of urethral obstruction.
- Perform a retrograde positive contrast urethrocystogram 2–3 months after surgery to evaluate the urethral diameter at the anastomotic site.
- Treat infection or urinary calculi appropriately.

URETHROTOMY IN THE DOG

Preoperative Considerations

- Perform this procedure to remove urethral calculi lodged caudal to the os penis or in the perineal urethra and to temporarily divert the flow of urine.
- If the animal is azotemic and depressed, perform this procedure without sedation by infiltrating the tissue overlying the urethra with local anesthetic.
- If calculi remain in the kidneys, ureters, bladder, or urethra after urethrotomy, perform definitive surgery to remove the calculi after the animal is stabilized.

- Perform urethrotomy only after attempts to pass a urethral catheter or to flush calculi in a retrograde direction into the bladder have failed.

Surgical Procedure

Objectives

- Relieve urethral obstruction.
- Remove urethral calculi.
- Pass urethral catheter.
- Allow patient stabilization prior to definitive repair.

Equipment

- Scalpel, hemostats, thumb forceps, Metzenbaum scissors
- Urethral catheter
- Suture to secure the urethral catheter

Technique

1. Restrain the dog in dorsal (prescrotal urethrotomy) or lateral recumbency (perineal urethrotomy). Prescrotal urethrotomy is the preferred technique.
2. Infiltrate the skin and subcutaneous tissues overlying the urethra with local anesthetic.
3. Prepare the skin overlying the intended site of urethrotomy for aseptic surgery.
4. Make an incision 1–2 cm in length over the urethra at the level of obstruction.
5. Using a combination of blunt and sharp dissection, expose the appropriate area of the urethra.
6. In the prescrotal location, identify the retractor penis muscles and retract them laterally. The urethra appears as a purple structure on the midline flanked on either side by the white penile tunic.

▼ *Key Point* Take care to incise the urethra on the midline. The urethra is a highly vascular structure and will bleed briskly when incised.

7. Remove calculi from the urethra with forceps.
8. Pass a urethral catheter from the urethrotomy site into the bladder. Catheterize the distal urethra (retrograde and/or antegrade) to ensure patency.
9. Maintain the urethral catheter after surgery to monitor urine output and diminish the likelihood of subsequent urethral obstruction prior to surgical removal of cystic calculi.
10. Leave the urethrotomy open to heal by second intention or suture with 4–0 monofilament synthetic absorbable suture in a simple interrupted or simple continuous pattern.

Postoperative Care and Complications

- Hemorrhage may be observed intermittently, usually associated with urination, for 7–14 days after surgery. The flow of urine dislodges clots, and urokinase (a plasminogen activator found in urine) interferes with clot formation. This complication may be minimized by suturing the urethrotomy site.

- If the urethrotomy site is sutured, seroma or abscess formation may occur.
- On rare occasion, a stricture may form at the urethrotomy site. This is more likely when the urethral mucosa has sustained significant damage.
- Treat UTI and calculi with appropriate antibiotic and dietary therapy and other interventions to prevent reformation of calculi. Inform the owner that surgery will not cure this problem, and appropriate medical therapy is critical to a satisfactory outcome.
- If large calculi from the bladder pass into the urethra, urethral obstruction may recur despite the urethrotomy.
- If the skin incision is made too close to the scrotum, the testes may prolapse through the skin incision. Treat this prolapse by suturing the caudal aspect of the incision.
- Swelling and edema of the scrotum and testes may be observed because of inflammation associated with the urethrotomy or subcutaneous accumulation of urine. Subcutaneous accumulation of urine occurs infrequently if the urethrotomy incision is made near the caudal end of the os penis.
- Prolonged urethral obstruction and distension of the bladder may cause a loss of detrusor function of the bladder, resulting in loss of contractile function of the bladder.

URETHROSTOMY IN THE MALE DOG

Preoperative Considerations

- Urethrostomy results in a permanent opening for the urethra and is performed proximal to the site of narrowing, obstruction, or destruction of the urethra. Perform a urethrostomy in the male dog in the perineal, scrotal, prescrotal, or prepubic location.
- Urethrostomy is most often performed in the scrotal position, because the urethra is wide and superficial at this location. Minimal hemorrhage occurs, and a cosmetic result is achieved. Avoid urethrostomy in the perineal position because of the potential for urine scalding of the caudal surface of the thighs. Prepubic urethrostomy is discussed further in this chapter.

▼ *Key Point* Inform the owner that urethrostomy will not cure urinary tract infection or urinary calculi. In fact, urethrostomy may predispose the animal to urinary tract infection. However, the overall incidence of urinary tract infection after urethrostomy in male dogs is low.

- Urethrostomy decreases the potential for urethral obstruction due to passage of calculi but does not eliminate it. Calculi of sufficient diameter may still become lodged in the urethra proximal to the site of urethrostomy.

▼ *Key Point* Scrotal urethrostomy necessitates castration of the animal. Inform the owner prior to undertaking surgery.

- Stabilize animals that have azotemia because of urethral obstruction prior to undertaking a prolonged anesthetic and operative procedure.

Surgical Procedure—Scrotal Urethrostomy

Objectives

- Allow discharge of urine proximal to the site of urethral obstruction or destruction.
- Diminish the possibility of urethral obstruction due to urinary calculi.

Equipment

- Standard surgical instruments and suture
- Monofilament nonabsorbable suture (4–0 or 5–0) and synthetic absorbable suture (2–0 or 3–0) with swaged taper or taper-cut needle (preferred).
- Urethral catheter

- Delicate forceps for grasping and holding the urethra (optional)
- Magnification (optional)

Technique*

1. Place the dog in dorsal recumbency.
2. Prepare the caudal ventral abdomen, prepuce, scrotum, and ventral perineal region for aseptic surgery.
3. Make a circumferential incision around the scrotum at the point of reflection of the skin from the ventral body wall (Fig. 102–1A). Preserve enough skin to minimize tension on the suture line.
4. Isolate, ligate, and divide the spermatic cords and

---

*The procedure for scrotal urethrostomy is described. A similar technique is used to create a urethrostomy in the perineal or prescrotal position.

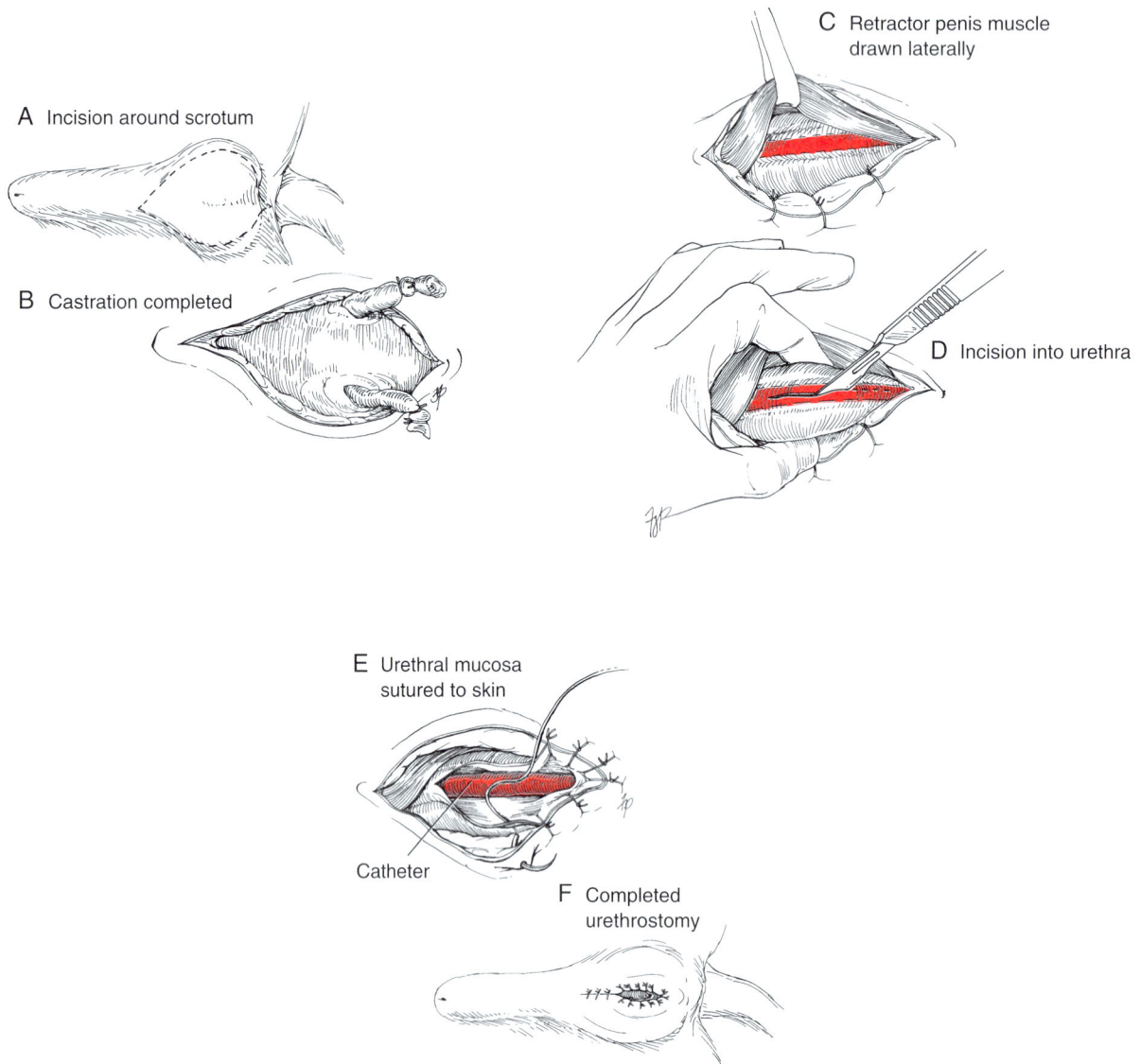

Figure 102–1.   Scrotal urethrostomy. *A,* Make an incision encircling the scrotum. *B,* Ligate and sever the spermatic cord and vessels and remove the scrotum and testes. *C,* The retractor penis muscles are drawn laterally, secure the subcutaneous tissues to the tunica albuginea. *D,* Make an incision on the ventral midline of the urethra. Placement of a catheter facilitates identification of the urethra. *E,* Suture the urethra to the skin. *F,* The cranial opening of the urethra at the urethrostomy site remains open. (From Smeak DD, Fingeroth JM: Scrotal urethrostomy. *In* Bojrab MJ, ed.: Current Techniques in Small Animal Surgery, 3rd Ed. Philadelphia: Lea & Febiger, 1990, p 381.)

vessels by a combination of sharp and blunt dissection.

5. Free the scrotum and testes of their attachments to the ventral abdomen and penis and remove them (Fig. 102–1*B*).

6. Retract the paired retractor penis muscles laterally.

7. Secure the tunic of the penis to the subcutaneous tissues with four to six interrupted sutures of absorbable material (2–0 or 3–0) (Fig. 102–1*C*).

8. Place these sutures in such a manner that an adequate amount of skin is available to be sutured with minimal tension to the site of incision in the ventral urethra.

9. Make an incision in the ventral surface of the urethra for the length of the urethrostomy site (approximately 5 cm) (Fig. 102–1*D*).

▼ *Key Point* Make the urethral incision on the ventral midline to facilitate urethrostomy closure.

10. If tension is encountered as the skin is drawn towards the edge of the urethra, adduct the stifles. This usually diminishes the amount of tension placed on the skin in this position.

11. Suture the skin to the edge of the urethra with 4–0 or 5–0 monofilament nonabsorbable suture in an interrupted or continuous pattern (Fig. 102–1*E* and *F*). The distal continuation of the urethra into the os penis remains open.

Postoperative Care and Complications

- Apply an Elizabethan collar or a body brace to prevent postoperative self-mutilation.

- Hemorrhage may be observed intermittently from the urethrostomy site. This is particularly noticeable when the animal urinates. In the immediate postoperative period, treat this by application of pressure or a cold compress. Sedation of the animal, particularly with acepromazine (which may decrease the systemic blood pressure), may also decrease the incidence of hemorrhage. Warn the owner that hemorrhage may occur for up to 2 weeks after the surgery. Recent clinical studies have found decreased postoperative hemorrhage with the continuous suture pattern.

- Remove sutures 2 weeks after surgery. Sedate animals that are difficult to handle for suture removal.

▼ *Key Point* Inform the owner that the removal of the sutures may result in intermittent hemorrhage from the urethrostomy site for 2 to 3 days.

- Treat UTI and urinary calculi by appropriate antibiotic, dietary, and medical therapy (see Ch. 99). Inform the owner that urethrostomy will not treat UTI or prevent calculi formation and that urethral obstruction may recur if calculi form.

- Leakage of urine into the subcutaneous tissues is uncommon.

- Stricture formation is extremely uncommon but may occur. If this happens, reconstruct the urethrostomy and carefully appose the mucosa to skin without tension.

- Scalding of the inner surface of the thighs by contact of the skin with urine is extremely uncommon. Apply petroleum jelly to the skin surrounding the stoma to reduce this problem until sutures are removed.

- Prolonged urethral obstruction and distention of the bladder may result in a loss of detrusor function of the bladder.

- Urinary incontinence due to surgery has not been reported.

PERINEAL URETHROSTOMY IN THE MALE CAT

Preoperative Considerations

- This procedure is performed most often in cats that suffer recurrent urethral obstruction because of idiopathic lower urinary tract disease, also referred to as feline interstitial cystitis (FIC) and feline urologic syndrome (FUS). Improved dietary management of this disorder has greatly decreased the need for urethrostomy in cats.

▼ *Key Point* Performance of perineal urethrostomy (PU) will not cure FIC or FUS, and signs of this disorder may persist after surgery. Inform the owner that the surgery is performed to diminish the probability of urethral obstruction and not to cure FIC or FUS.

- This procedure can be used to treat any form of urethral obstruction due to lesions of the urethra distal to the bulbourethral glands.

- Castration and amputation of the distal penis are necessary for PU in cats. Inform the owner of these procedures.

Surgical Procedure

Objectives

- Create a cutaneous opening of the urethra of satisfactory diameter near the bulbourethral glands.

- Minimize tension across the suture line to decrease the potential for stricture formation.

- Preserve urethral sphincter function.

Equipment

- Standard surgical instruments and suture
- Delicate instruments to handle the urethra
- 3.5 Fr. catheter
- Fine periosteal elevator (Freer)
- Monofilament suture (4–0 or 5–0), taper-cut needle

Technique

1. Place the cat in ventral recumbency with the hindquarters slightly elevated.
2. Secure the tail in a forward position.
3. Place a pursestring suture around the anus.
4. Completely evacuate urine from the bladder.
5. Prepare the perineal area surrounding the scrotum and prepuce for aseptic surgery.
6. If the cat is intact, make an incision at the reflection of the scrotum from the surrounding skin.

This incision encircles the scrotum and continues ventrally along the line of reflection of the prepuce from the perineal skin.

7. If the cat has previously been castrated, make an incision encircling the prepuce and scrotal remnant. Ventrally, the incision comes to a point.

8. Isolate, ligate, and divide the spermatic cords and vessels.

9. Sharply divide the ventral attachments of the penis to the pelvic floor near their attachment to the penis.

10. Continue sharp and blunt dissection circumferentially adjacent to the penis until the ischiocavernosus muscles are identified. Take care to restrict dissection to the area immediately adjacent and ventral to the penis.

11. Divide or free the ischiocavernosus muscles and penile ligament of their attachments to the ischium to allow the penis to be drawn caudally. The muscles will bleed profusely if incised.

12. Incise the fascia overlying the attachment of the ischiocavernosus muscles to the ischium.

13. Sever the attachment of the ischiocavernosus muscles to the ischium with a periosteal elevator. This usually results in minimal hemorrhage.

14. Continue blunt dissection in a cranial direction until the penis is freed of its ventral attachments and the caudal aspect of the bulbourethral glands lies at the level of the skin incision.

15. Limit dorsal dissection to minimize the potential for incontinence. If exposure of the proximal, dorsal urethra is inadequate, careful dissection of dorsal urethra tissues may be necessary.

16. Retract the penis in a caudal direction, and pass a catheter into the urethra.

17. Identify the retractor penis muscle on the dorsal aspect of the penis and excise it.

18. Excise the distal penis and prepuce and discard, along with the scrotum and testes.

19. With the urethral catheter in place, make an incision in the dorsal aspect of the urethra to the level of the bulbourethral glands.

▼ *Key Point* Continue the incision cranially until the portion of the urethra that enlarges in diameter is reached.

20. Secure the tunic of the penis distal to the bulbourethral glands to the subcutaneous tissues by a few (two to four total) interrupted sutures of synthetic absorbable material (3–0 or 4–0). Place these sutures so that the skin may be brought to the edge of the urethral incision without tension across the suture line.

▼ *Key Point* Ensure that the urethral mucosa is well apposed to the skin to prevent stricture formation.

21. Suture the skin to the edge of the urethra. Place the first suture through the apex of the incision through the urethra and the most dorsal aspect of the skin incision.

22. Place interrupted sutures on either side from dorsal to ventral to create a satisfactory urethrostomy opening. Use monofilament nonabsorbable suture (4–0 or 5–0).

23. After sutures have been placed along the urethra for a distance of approximately 1.5 cm, excise the remaining penis.

24. Place and tighten an encircling absorbable suture submucosally around the exposed end of the penis. This will diminish hemorrhage from the body of the penis.

25. Close the remainder of the skin incision with nonabsorbable suture in an interrupted or continuous pattern.

26. Remove the urethral catheter upon completion of the surgery.

27. Remove the pursestring suture around the anus.

Postoperative Care and Complications

- An Elizabethan collar is often used to prevent self-inflicted damage of the urethrostomy site. Some surgeons, however, prefer to allow the cat access to the operative site to keep it clean.
- Hemorrhage is frequently observed after surgery. In the early postoperative period, control this by application of pressure or cold compresses (ice packs). Tranquilization of the animal may be helpful in controlling prolonged hemorrhage.
- Stricture of the urethrostomy site is one of the most commonly observed complications.
  - This complication most often results from failure to satisfactorily free the penis from its attachments within the pelvic canal, causing tension on the suture line; poor mucosa-to-skin apposition; or failure to continue the urethral incision far enough cranially.
- Subcutaneous leakage of urine may result in cellulitis and abscessation. This leakage usually results from poor mucosa-to-skin apposition, especially at the proximal aspect of the urethrostomy.
- Urinary or fecal incontinence is infrequently observed after perineal urethrostomy in cats.
- The overall incidence of UTI in cats after perineal urethrostomy is low; however, it is more commonly observed in these cats than in male cats that have not undergone the procedure.
- Perineal hernia has been reported after perineal urethrostomy in male cats but is rare.
- Obstruction of the urethra may occur after perineal urethrostomy because of the persistence of FIC/FUS or the development of urinary calculi.
- Prolonged urethral obstruction and bladder distension may result in a loss of detrusor function of the bladder.

PREPUBIC URETHROSTOMY

Preoperative Considerations

- Perform this procedure for treatment of diseases that cause a loss of urethral function distal to the prostatic and pelvic portions of the urethra.

- This procedure can be performed in male or female animals.
- If a sufficient length of urethra and the associated innervation remain intact, the animal retains urinary continence.
- If this procedure is to be performed in a male dog with an enlarged prostate, a partial prostatectomy may also be necessary. This prevents the enlarged prostate within the subcutaneous tissues from interfering with the appropriate placement of the stoma.

Surgical Procedure

Objectives

- Create a new urethral opening on the ventral abdominal surface using the remaining length of urethra.
- Retain urinary continence.

Equipment

- Standard surgical instruments and suture
- Balfour retractors
- Monofilament nonabsorbable suture (4–0 or 5–0)
- Urethral catheter
- Magnification (optional)

Technique

1. Place the animal in dorsal recumbency.
2. Prepare the caudal surface of the ventral abdomen for aseptic surgery.
3. Make an incision on the ventral midline of the abdomen from the umbilicus to the pubis in female dogs and cats and male cats, and in a parapreputial location in male dogs.
4. Examine the bladder, prostate (in male dogs), and urethra.
5. Identify the diseased portion of the urethra.
6. Transect the urethra, retaining the maximal amount of normal proximal urethra.
7. Resect the affected urethra if neoplasia is present.
8. Ligate vessels leading to the distal portion of the urethra and associated tissues.

▼ *Key Point* Take care during dissection to preserve the innervation and vascular supply of the bladder neck and proximal urethra.

---

9. If difficulty is encountered in identifying the lumen of the proximal urethra, pass a catheter in a retrograde direction or perform a cystotomy to allow passage in an antegrade direction.
10. Bring the proximal urethra and adjacent structures to the level of the skin incision, and select an appropriate site to create the stoma.
11. Create the stoma on the ventral midline in female dogs and cats and male cats and in a parapreputial position in male dogs. The stoma can be placed in the incision through which the abdominal cavity was entered. Position the stoma to allow the urethra to curve in a gentle arc through

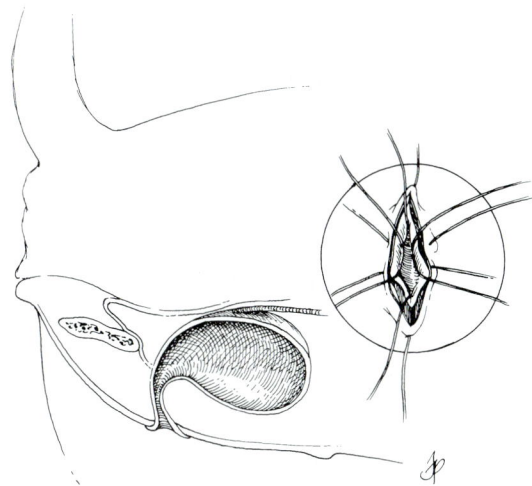

Figure 102–2. Prepubic urethrostomy. The urethra is brought across the body wall at a "gentle angle" to prevent urethral obstruction. Make an incision on the ventral surface of the urethra, and suture the urethra to the skin. (From Bjorling DE: Traumatic injuries of the urogenital system. Vet Clin North Am Small Anim Pract 14:61, 1984.)

the ventral abdominal wall to avoid kinking or obstructing the urethra (Fig. 102–2).
12. Avoid twisting the urethra when passing it through the abdominal wall.
13. Close the abdominal wall in a standard manner, leaving 1.5–2.0 cm of the distal end of the proximal urethra exposed. The abdominal wall is not tightly closed in the area through which the urethra passes.
14. Secure the adventitia surrounding the urethra to the subcutaneous tissues with two absorbable sutures.
15. Make an incision 1.5–2.0 cm in length on the ventral surface of the distal end of the proximal urethra. This is done to increase the diameter of the stoma.
16. Close the subcutaneous tissues in a standard manner.
17. Suture the cut edge of the urethra, including the mucosa, to the skin with monofilament nonabsorbable suture (4–0 or 5–0) in an interrupted pattern to create the urethrostomy opening.
18. Close the remainder of the skin incision in a standard manner.
19. Catheterization of the urethra may facilitate accurate placement of sutures through the wall of the urethra.
20. Do not leave the catheter in place after surgery unless monitoring of urine output is necessary.

Postoperative Care and Complications

- Use an Elizabethan collar or a body brace to prevent trauma after surgery.
- Leakage of urine into the subcutaneous space or abdominal cavity will result in cellulitis or peritonitis. Prevent this by accurate suture placement during the operative procedure.

- Stricture formation is an unusual complication of this procedure. When stricture occurs, revise the opening.
- If the procedure is performed appropriately and a satisfactory length of proximal urethra is available, urinary continence is retained. If urinary continence is lost, treatment with alpha-agonists (see Ch. 103) can be instituted to increase urethral tone. This therapy may or may not be successful if nerve or muscle function is lost.
- Prepubic urethrostomy predisposes an animal to ascending UTI. Frequent reevaluation and urine culture is recommended after the surgery.
- Loss of urinary continence predisposes to scalding of the ventral abdominal surface with urine.
- In obese animals or animals with redundant skin in the area of the urethral stomas, resection of skin and fat may be required to prevent obstruction of the stoma by adjacent skin folds.
- Urethral obstruction may occur if the position of the stoma results in an acute angle in the urethra relative to the bladder neck.

URETHRAL PROLAPSE IN THE MALE DOG

Preoperative Considerations

- Urethral prolapse occurs most often in young brachycephalic dogs.
- The most common complaint of the owner is that the dog develops hematuria when it urinates or becomes excited. Hemorrhage is usually self-limiting.
- After the exposed urethral tissue has been traumatized, hemorrhage may recur during or following urination because of dislodgement of blood clots by the flow of urine.
- Diagnosis of urethral prolapse is made by direct observation of exposed urethral tissue that appears as a fleshy ring surrounding the external urethral orifice. Extrude the penis from the prepuce to observe urethral prolapse.
- If the animal is not to be used for breeding, castration may help control urethral prolapse.

Surgical Procedure

Objectives

- Prevent hemorrhage from the tip of the penis.
- Excise exposed urethral tissue and prevent recurrence.
- Maintain an adequate urethral lumen.

Equipment

- Standard surgical instruments and suture
- Tourniquet or Penrose drain
- Urethral catheter
- Monofilament nonabsorbable suture (4–0 or 5–0)

Technique

1. Place the dog in dorsal recumbency.
2. Prepare the interior of the prepuce and the penis for aseptic surgery.
3. Extrude the penis from the prepuce.
4. Pass a urethral catheter into the urethra until the tip lies approximately at the level of the scrotum.
5. Apply a tourniquet to the penis caudal to the os penis. The tourniquet will maintain the penis in an exteriorized position and minimize hemorrhage. Use a commercial tourniquet or a tourniquet created with a forceps and Penrose drain.
6. Partially excise the exposed urethral mucosa. Incise through the distal extent of the penile tunic and urethra, extending around half the circumference of the distal penis. This incision is proximal to damaged urethral mucosa and provides an exposed edge of the penile tunic, which is subsequently sutured to the urethra.
7. Suture the cut edge of the urethra to the tunic of the penis with monofilament nonabsorbable suture (4–0 to 5–0) in an interrupted or continuous pattern. If a continuous pattern is used, avoid creating a "purse-string" effect.

▼ *Key Point* The purpose of initiating closure prior to complete excision of the urethral tissue is to prevent retraction of the urethral tissue within the penis and to facilitate accurate suture placement.

8. After the incision that has been made is partially closed, excise the remainder of the exposed urethral tissue by continuing the incision circumferentially.
9. Close the remainder of the defect with monofilament nonabsorbable suture with a similar pattern.
10. Remove the tourniquet and urethral catheter.

Postoperative Care and Complications

- Intermittent hemorrhage may persist for 2–3 days (or longer) after surgery. This is usually associated with urination or excitement. If hemorrhage is excessive, re-examine the tip of the penis. Active bleeding from gaps in the closure may require placement of additional sutures. Tranquilization (e.g., with acepromazine) of the dog may decrease hemorrhage.
- Recurrence of urethral prolapse is uncommon. If this occurs, repeat the surgery and strongly recommend castration.
- Mutilation may occur and is discouraged by placing an Elizabethan collar or a body brace or by using sedation.
- Sedate the dog for suture removal.
- Urethral prolapse rarely occurs in older animals. If observed in older animals, rule out a tumor at the tip of the penis. If the surgeon has any concern that the tissue excised may be neoplastic, submit this tissue for histopathologic evaluation. Tumors of the distal urethra and penis are extremely uncommon.

SUPPLEMENTAL READINGS

Anson Al W: Urethral trauma and principles of urethral surgery. Compend Cont Ed Pract Vet 9:981, 1987.

Bradley RL: Prepubic urethrostomy: An acceptable urinary diversion technique. Probl Vet Med 1:120, 1989.

Newton JD, Smeak DD: Simple continuous closure of canine scrotal urethrostomy: results in 20 cases. J Am An Hosp Assoc 32:531, 1996.

Smith CW: Surgical diseases of the urethra. *In* Slatter D, ed.: *Textbook of Small Animal Surgery,* 2nd ed. Philadelphia: W. B. Saunders, 1993, p 1462.

Stone EA, Barsanti JA: Urologic Surgery of the Dog and Cat. Philadelphia: Lea & Febiger, 1992.

Weber WJ, Boothe HW, Brassard JA, Hobson HP: Comparison of the healing of prescrotal urethrotomy incision in the dog: Sutured vs. nonsutured. Am J Vet Res 46:1309, 1985.

Yoshioka MM, Carb A: Antepubic urethrostomy in the dog. J Am Anim Hosp Assoc 18:290, 1982.

103 Disorders of Micturition

Mary Anna Labato

Micturition is a two-stage process involving the passive storage and the active voiding of urine. Processes that interfere with the storage and voiding of urine are termed micturition disorders. The loss of voluntary control of micturition is defined as urinary incontinence.

Most cases of micturition disorders have been reported in middle-aged and geriatric dogs. The clinical importance of these disorders is twofold:

- Incontinence is unacceptable to most owners; if not adequately treated, this disorder may result in euthanasia of the pet.
- Micturition disorders may lead to unresponsive urinary tract infection, resulting in an ascending pyelonephritis.

It is critical that the etiology of micturition disorders be diagnosed correctly in order to properly implement treatment.

NORMAL ANATOMY AND PHYSIOLOGY OF THE URINARY BLADDER

In order to recognize the many possible manifestations of micturition disorders it is imperative to understand the anatomy of the bladder, its functional composition, and the neurophysiology of micturition.

Bladder Function

Bladder function is primarily under the influence of smooth muscle. The body of the bladder contains smooth muscle, referred to as the detrusor muscle. The outlet conduit is composed of the trigone and proximal urethra. The smooth muscle fibers of the detrusor continue into the proximal urethra, forming a functional internal urethral sphincter. The distal urethra is composed of striated skeletal muscle, and functions as an external sphincter.

During the storage phase of micturition the bladder functions as a low-resistance, high-capacity vessel. The urethra functions as a high-resistance barrier. The reverse is true during the voiding phase. The bladder acts as a muscular pump and the urethra is a low-resistance vessel.

Nervous Control

Nervous control of the bladder and urethra is a combination of autonomic and somatic interactions. The micturition reflex is integrated by numerous interneurons and synapses between the sympathetic and parasympathetic systems.

Parasympathetic Innervation

Parasympathetic innervation is supplied to the detrusor by the pelvic nerve, which arises from sacral spinal cord segments (S1–S3). Stimulation of the pelvic nerve results in detrusor contraction.

Sympathetic Innervation

Sympathetic innervation is supplied via the hypogastric nerve, which is composed of preganglionic fibers exiting the lumbar spinal cord (L1–L4) and synapses in the caudal mesenteric ganglion. Sympathetic innervation is supplied to both the detrusor and urethral smooth muscles and facilitates the storage phase of micturition. Alpha-adrenergic fibers synapse in smooth muscle in both the trigone and urethra. Stimulation results in contraction of these muscles and forms a functional internal urethral sphincter. There are also alpha-adrenergic fibers that have a modulating effect on the external urethral sphincter. Beta-adrenergic fibers synapse in the detrusor muscle; stimulation results in relaxation.

Somatic Innervation

The pudendal nerve, which arises from sacral spinal cord segments (S1–S3), provides somatic stimulation to the striated urethral musculature.

Higher Centers of Innervation

For voluntary control of micturition to occur there must be integration between the cerebral cortex, pons, and the spinoreticular tract. A second pathway from the cerebral cortex to the sacral nuclei coordinates voluntary sphincter control. Additionally, cerebellar neurons inhibit nervous transmission to the reticulospinal pathways in the pons.

ETIOLOGY OF MICTURITION DISORDERS AND INCONTINENCE

Disorders of micturition and continence can be divided broadly into two types: neurogenic and non-neurogenic (Table 103–1).

Table 103–1. DISORDERS OF MICTURITION

Type of Disorder	Diagnostic Features	Treatment
Neurogenic		
Lower motor neuron bladder	Distended, easily expressed bladder Continuous incontinence—dribbling of urine No perineal or bulbospongiosus reflex No detrusor reflex	No effective therapy Manual expression q8h Trial with bethanechol chloride Concurrent antibiotics
Upper motor neuron bladder	Large, turgid bladder Difficult manual expression Increased sphincter tone ± detrusor reflex	Aseptic intermittent catheterization initially Concurrent antibiotics Long-term management usually frustrating
Detrusor-urethral dyssynergia	Large, nonexpressible bladder Initiation of urine stream with abrupt disruption of urination Intact spinal reflexes Bladder easily catheterized	Phenoxybenzamine Baclofen Diazepam Dantrolene
Non-neurogenic		
Hormone-responsive incontinence	Older, neutered animal Voluntary control of urination with intermittent incontinence Incontinence usually when relaxed or asleep	Diethylstilbestrol (females) Testosterone (males) Phenylpropanolamine
Urethral incompetence	Loss of voluntary control when placed in a stressful situation or at rest Ability to urinate voluntarily	Phenylpropanolamine Ephedrine Imipramine
Urge incontinence (detrusor hyperreflexia)	Frequent small urinations Urine spraying Stranguria Hyperreflexive detrusor	Treat cystitis Propantheline bromide Flavoxate Oxybutynin Dicyclomine
Atony from overdistention	Large, flaccid bladder Large residual urine volume Continuous incontinence Intact perineal and bulbospongiosus reflex No detrusor reflex	Remove mechanical obstruction Indwelling catheterization Bethanechol chloride
Paradoxical incontinence	Stranguria Persistent urine dribbling Large, turgid bladder that is difficult to express	Remove obstruction Indwelling catheterization Surgical exploration
Ectopic ureter(s)	Continuous dribbling of urine Ability to urinate voluntarily	Surgical transposition of ureters Phenylpropanolamine

From Handbook of Small Animal Practice. New York: Churchill Livingstone, 1992. Reprinted with permission from Churchill Livingstone.

Neurogenic Disorders

There are three types of neurogenic disorders: lower motor neuron, upper motor neuron, and detrusor-urethral dyssynergia.

Lower Motor Neuron Disorders

Lower motor neuron, or atonic, bladder results from lesions involving the sacral spinal cord segments or pelvic nerve, including intervertebral disc disease, cauda equina syndrome, sacroiliac luxations, sacrococcygeal fracture/separation, and tumors (e.g., spinal lymphoma). This type of disorder causes both detrusor and sphincter areflexia. Dribbling of urine with the bladder remaining full is often referred to as overflow incontinence.

Upper Motor Neuron Disorders

Upper motor neuron, or automatic, bladder results from a lesion involving the spinal cord above the sacral spinal cord segments, such as intervertebral disc disease, tumor, or trauma. This disorder causes incomplete reflex detrusor contraction and spasticity of the urethral sphincter, with resulting incomplete emptying of the bladder.

Voluntary control is lost and manual expression is difficult if not impossible. After a period of days to weeks the spinal reflexes resume. Nonvoluntary micturition is initiated when the threshold capacity of the bladder is reached (automatic bladder).

Detrusor-Urethral Dyssynergia

In this condition, the initiation of the detrusor reflex resulting in voiding is followed by an involuntary contraction of the urethral sphincter. Detrusor-urethral dyssynergia refers to involuntary contraction of the external urethral sphincter in the postprostatic urethra (detrusor-striated muscle sphincter dyssynergia) or contraction of smooth muscle in the bladder neck and prostatic urethra (detrusor-smooth muscle sphincter dyssynergia) during detrusor contraction. It results from lesions or partial lesions (masses, degeneration) of the reticulospinal tract. Increased sympathetic activity of both the smooth and striated urethral musculatures may result from a lesion cranial to or involving the caudal mesenteric ganglion.

Non-Neurogenic Disorders

A number of disorders resulting in urinary incontinence are non-neurogenic in origin. A brief description of each disorder follows.

Hormone-Responsive Incontinence

Hormone-responsive incontinence is one of the most frequently diagnosed disorders. It is a disorder of older animals (mean age of occurrence is 8 years); however, it has been documented in animals as young as 8–9 months.

Hormone-responsive incontinence is seen primarily in spayed female dogs, who may be predisposed because of decreased sex hormone believed to contribute to normal urethral muscle tone and mucosal integrity.

Occasionally hormone-responsive incontinence occurs in castrated male dogs, and it has been reported infrequently in neutered male and female cats.

Urethral Incompetence (Stress Incontinence)

This is the most common nonhormonal cause of urinary incontinence in small animals. Stress incontinence is a syndrome reported in women that consists of involuntary release of urine secondary to an increase in intra-abdominal pressure without detrusor atony or detrusor hyperreflexia. Urethral incompetence is the veterinary counterpart of stress incontinence. The cause is thought to be urethral smooth muscle incompetence or urethral malposition.

Urge Incontinence (Detrusor Hyperreflexia)

Urge incontinence is due to involuntary detrusor contractions resulting in frequent voiding of small volumes of urine. The condition may result from an inflamed or irritated bladder or occasionally from partial spinal long tract or cerebellar involvement. The syndrome is commonly seen in cats that suffer from cystitis or "feline urologic syndrome." An idiopathic form has been documented in cats and dogs without any evidence of cystitis.

Detrusor Atony from Overdistention

This results from a mechanical or functional outflow obstruction, causing separation of the tight junctions of the detrusor muscle. Subsequent contractions of the detrusor muscle are weak and ineffectual. A functional outflow obstruction may have a neurogenic component. It usually is the result of excessive sympathetic stimulation to the urethra, resulting in increased urethral tone. Common examples of mechanical obstruction are:

- Urethral obstruction (especially in cats)
- Cystic and urethral calculi

- Neoplasia of the trigone or urethra
- Severe urethritis
- Stricture of the urethra
- Prostate disease

Obstruction causes an increase in urine volume until the intravesicular pressure can overcome the urethral resistance. Once the urethral pressure has been overcome, dribbling of urine occurs because of ineffectual detrusor contractions.

Paradoxical Incontinence

This is similar to overflow incontinence from detrusor atony. It is involuntary dribbling of urine associated with an outflow obstruction. It often results from a partial urethral obstruction caused by urethral calculi, neoplasia, or urethritis. The difference between the two conditions is a matter of duration and whether the atony is temporary or permanent. Paradoxical incontinence is of a shorter duration. When the partial obstruction is relieved, normal function returns, and the detrusor contracts effectively.

Ectopic Ureter(s)

Ectopic ureter and other congenital urethral malformations are a common cause of urinary incontinence. The abnormal entry of the ureter(s) into the distal urethra or vagina from a congenital malformation results in continuous or intermittent dribbling of urine (see Chap. 97).

CLINICAL SIGNS

- *Incontinence*—dribbling of urine, loss of voluntary control, and urine-scald dermatitis
- *Abnormal micturition*—inability to urinate, disruption of the urine stream, stranguria, dysuria, and abdominal pain or discomfort
- *Lower motor neuron bladder*—dribbling of urine and a large distended bladder that is easily expressed by manual compression
- *Upper motor neuron bladder*:
  - A full bladder that is difficult to express initially
  - Voluntary control is lost
  - After a period of days to weeks, the spinal reflexes resume and nonvoluntary micturition is initiated when the threshold capacity of the bladder is reached
  - Incomplete and inappropriate urination is the result
- *Detrusor-urethral dyssynergia* (differentiate from mechanical obstruction): Initiation of voiding, often after a period of hesitation, which then is abruptly disrupted
  - Stranguria
- *Hormone-responsive incontinence*—normal voluntary urination with involuntary dribbling when the animal is relaxed or asleep
- *Urethral incompetence (stress incontinence)*—signs similar to hormone-responsive incontinence; also involun-

tary loss of urine when placed in a stressful or new situation
- *Detrusor hyperreflexia*—frequent small urinations, stranguria, and urine spraying in cats; small bladder (compare with detrusor atony from overdistention)
- *Detrusor atony from overdistention*—stranguria, dysuria, persistent urine dribbling; large distended bladder
- *Paradoxical incontinence*—same clinical signs as detrusor atony
- *Ectopic ureter(s)*:
  - Continuous or intermittent dribbling of urine usually with the ability to urinate appropriately and voluntarily
  - Most commonly diagnosed in young dogs and cats

DIAGNOSIS

History

The history is of the utmost importance; include the following items:

- Reproductive status
- If animal was neutered, age at neutering
- Age at onset of problem
- Previous medical problems, especially those involving the urogenital system
- Previous history of trauma
- Description of the abnormality
- If the problem is incontinence, ask:
  - Is it continuous or intermittent?
  - What is the amount of urine passed?
  - Is the animal aware that urine is being passed?
- If the animal has difficulty urinating, ask:
  - How frequent is urination?
  - Is there nocturia, dysuria, or hematuria?

Physical Examination

Perform a general examination, with particular attention to the urogenital system, and perform a neurologic examination (see Chap. 144).

- Palpate the bladder carefully prior to and immediately following voiding to evaluate the extent of distention, tone, and ease with which the bladder may be manually expressed.
  - Lower motor neuron lesions generally are associated with easy manual expression and reduced sphincter tone.
  - Upper motor neuron lesions generally are associated with difficult manual expression and increased sphincter tone.
- In the neurologic examination, evaluate the innervation of the urogenital system.
  - The perineal reflex evaluates the pudendal nerve. Pricking or pinching the skin of the perineum should result in anal sphincter contraction.
  - The bulbospongiosus reflex evaluates the integrity of both the pudendal nerve and sacral spinal segments. Squeezing the distal portion of the penis or vulva will cause anal sphincter contraction.
- Perform a rectal examination to evaluate the prostate gland, the pelvic diaphragm, and anal tone.

▼ *Key Point* Observe the animal when urinating to verify the micturition abnormality.

- Measure the residual urine volume. Allow the animal to void until urine is no longer passed; catheterize the bladder and collect and measure any residual urine. In a normal animal, the residual urine volume should not exceed 0.4 ml/kg.
- Perform cystoscopy or vaginoscopy if ectopic ureters are suspected. Cystoscopy is often diagnostic for ectopic ureter but requires specialized equipment.

Laboratory Evaluation

- Evaluate renal function by determining blood urea nitrogen (BUN) and serum creatinine concentration.
- To evaluate for associated urinary tract infection, perform cystocentesis and submit urine for urinalysis, culture, and sensitivity. If possible, do this before any bladder catheterization.

Radiographic Examination

Both survey and specialized studies may be useful.

- Use survey radiographs to evaluate any obvious abnormalities in the bladder, urethra, pelvis, or spine.
- Use contrast radiographic studies (intravenous urography, retrograde urethrocystography, and vaginourethrography; (see Chap. 4) to evaluate for:
  - Ectopic ureters
  - Bladder wall thickening
  - Calculi
  - Urachal diverticulum
  - Prostatic enlargement
  - Urethral strictures
  - Skeletal abnormalities in the pelvis

Urodynamic Studies

Urodynamic studies to evaluate micturition disorders routinely consist of the cystometrogram and urethral pressure profile; electromyography also may be a part of the study. These specialized modalities are readily available at most veterinary institutions and are becoming increasingly common in private referral practices.

- The cystometrogram is a pressure-volume recording that measures bladder tone and volume, threshold volume and pressure, maximum contraction pressure, and the detrusor reflex.
- The urethral pressure profile measures intra-urethral resistance and identifies and localizes areas of increased or decreased resistance.
- Electromyography can evaluate coordination of muscular activity between the detrusor and urethral sphincter. Electromyography is usually performed on the anal sphincter; however, using specialized catheters that incorporate electrodes it can also be performed directly on the urethral sphincter.

Diagnosis of Individual Disorders

Lower Motor Neuron Bladder

- The bladder typically is large, distended, and easily expressed.
- The incontinence is continuous.
- There is a loss of perineal, bulbospongiosus, and detrusor reflexes.

Upper Motor Neuron Bladder

- The bladder is large, turgid, and initially extremely difficult to express.
- There is a history of an inability to urinate.
- Frequently there is concomitant hindquarter paresis or paralysis.

Detrusor-Urethral Dyssynergia

- Diagnosis is made by observation; commonly there is stranguria, initiation of voiding, and then abrupt disruption of the urine stream.
- Palpation often reveals a large, nonexpressible bladder.
- The bladder is easily catheterized.
- There is no evidence of stricture or obstruction when a retrograde contrast cystourethrogram is performed. A cystometrogram reveals an intact pelvic nerve; however, the urethral pressure profile reveals increased resistance.

Hormone-Responsive Incontinence

- There is a history of neutering and subsequent intermittent incontinence.
- Palpation commonly reveals a small bladder.
- Urinalysis may or may not show evidence of cystitis.
- Typically there is response to sex hormone supplementation.

▼ *Key Point* Urinary tract infection results in an exaggeration of the incontinence; if infection is present, resolve it before making a diagnosis of hormone-responsive incontinence.

Urethral Incompetence (Stress Incontinence)

- There is a history of intermittent incontinence when the animal is at rest or placed in a stressful situation.
- Palpation reveals a small bladder.
- The animal is able to urinate voluntarily.
- There is no evidence of infection on urinalysis.
- There are no radiographic abnormalities.

Urge Incontinence or Detrusor Hyperreflexia

- The bladder is small on physical examination.
- Cystometrography reveals involuntary smooth muscle contractions during the filling phase of micturition. Contractions can be spontaneous or provoked but cannot be suppressed.
- Urodynamically, detrusor instability usually appears as a rapid, involuntary increase of >15 cm of water pressure during the filling phase of the cystometrogram. However, there is voluntary control of urination.
- In cases associated with cystitis, there may be a history of urine spraying or infection, and there is evidence of inflammation on urinalysis. A urine culture may be positive or negative.
- With cystitis, the bladder may be thickened on palpation, and a contrast cystourethrogram may reveal bladder wall thickening.
- In idiopathic detrusor hyperreflexia there is no evidence of cystitis and no abnormalities on contrast cystourethrograms.

Detrusor Atony from Overdistention

- There is a history of continuous incontinence and urine outflow obstruction.
- Abdominal palpation reveals a large, flaccid bladder.
- Neurologic examination reveals intact perineal and bulbospongiosus reflexes; yet there is an absent or weak detrusor reflex.
- There is a large residual urine volume.
- Urodynamic studies may help rule out a neurogenic component.

Paradoxical Incontinence

- Base the diagnosis on the results of a urinalysis, plain, and often contrast, radiographs.

Ectopic Ureters

- Make a definitive diagnosis by intravenous urography and retrograde cystourethrography.
- Consider cystoscopy to identify abnormal ureteral openings.
- There usually is a history of continuous incontinence with ability to urinate voluntarily. Usually a small bladder is revealed on abdominal palpation.
- On the physical examination, urine-soaked fur often is seen along the rear legs.
- The animal typically is young when the diagnosis is made.

TREATMENT

Individual Disorders

Individual disorders are discussed in terms of their treatment modalities. See Table 103–2 for details of treatment, including drug dosages.

▼ *Key Point* Remember that urocystitis commonly is associated with micturition disorders. Treat the underlying infection as well as the individual disorders.

Lower Motor Neuron Bladder

- Manually express the bladder three or four times daily.
- Long-term therapy for this disorder has not been successful.

Table 103–2. PHARMACOLOGIC MANAGEMENT OF MICTURITION DISORDERS

Agent	Class	Indications	Dosages	Side Effects	Contraindications
Baclofen (Lioresal; Geigy)	Skeletal muscle relaxant	Detrusor-urethral dyssynergia	Dogs: 1–2 mg/kg q8h PO	General muscle weakness Gastrointestinal upset	
Bethanechol chloride (Urecholine; Merck Sharp & Dohme)	Parasympathomimetic	Detrusor atony	Dogs: 2.5–25 mg q8h PO Cats: 2.5–5.0 mg q8h PO	Vomiting Diarrhea Salivation Anorexia	Urethral obstruction
Dantrolene (Dantrium; Norwich Eaton)	Skeletal muscle relaxant	Functional urethral obstruction due to increased external urethral tone	Dogs: 3–15 mg divided q8–12h PO	Generalized muscle weakness Hepatotoxicity	
Diazepam (Valium; Roche Products)	Skeletal muscle relaxant	Functional urethral obstruction due to increased external urethral tone	Dogs: 2–10 mg q8h PO	Sedation	
Dicyclomine (Bentyl; Marion Merrell Dow)	Anticholinergic, direct-acting smooth muscle relaxant	Detrusor hyperreflexia Urge incontinence	Dogs/Cats: 10 mg q6–8h PO	Diarrhea Sedation	Obstructive uropathy Hyperthyroidism Cardiac disease Prostatic hypertrophy
Ephedrine (various brand names and manufacturers)	Alpha-adrenergic agonist	Urethral sphincter incompetence	Dogs: 5–15 mg q8h PO Cats: 2–4 mg q8h PO	Restlessness Excitability Hypertension	Hypertension
Estrogen (Diethylstilbestrol; various veterinary compounding pharmacies)	Female sex hormone	Hormone-responsive incontinence	Dogs: 0.1–1.0 mg/day for 3 days, then 1.0 mg once weekly PO	Induces signs of estrus Bone marrow toxicity	
Flavoxate (Urispas; Smith Kline & French)	Anticholinergic, smooth muscle relaxant	Detrusor hyperreflexia Urge incontinence	Dogs/Cats: 100–200 mg q6–8h PO	Vomiting Increased intraocular pressure Tachycardia	Glaucoma
Imipramine (Tofranil; Geigy)	Tricyclic antidepressant	Urethral incompetence	Dogs: 1 mg/kg q8h PO Cats: 2.5–5.0 mg q12h PO	Tachycardia Tremors Hyperexcitability Seizures	

Table continued on following page

Table 103–2. PHARMACOLOGIC MANAGEMENT OF MICTURITION DISORDERS *Continued*

Agent	Class	Indications	Dosages	Side Effects	Contraindications
Oxybutynin (Ditropan; Marion Merrell Dow)	Anticholinergic, smooth muscle relaxant	Detrusor hyperreflexia	Dogs/Cats: 5 mg q8–12h PO	Diarrhea Sedation	Hyperthyroidism Cardiac disease Prostatic disease
Phenoxybenzamine (Dibenzyline; Smith Kline & French)	Alpha-adrenergic blocker	Functional outflow obstruction	Dogs/Cats: 0.25–0.5 mg/kg q8hr PO Dogs (alternate): 2.5–20.0 mg/day PO	Nausea Hypotension Increased intraocular pressure	Glaucoma Diabetes mellitus
Phenylpropanolamine (various brand names and manufacturers)	Alpha-adrenergic agonist	Urethral sphincter incompetence Hormone responsive incontinence	Dogs: 1–2 mg/kg q12h PO Cats: 1 mg/kg q12h PO	Restlessness Excitability Hypertension	Hypertension
Prazosin (Minipress; Pfizer)	Alpha-adrenergic blocker	Functional outflow obstruction	Dogs: 0.5–2.0 mg q12–24h PO Cats: 0.5–1.0 mg q12–24h PO	Hypotension Syncope Nausea/Vomiting Diarrhea	Glaucoma Diabetes mellitus Caution with concurrent phenobarbital or sulfonamides
Propantheline bromide (Pro-Banthine; Schiapparelli Searle)	Anticholinergic	Detrusor hyperreflexia Urge incontinence	Dogs: 7.5–30.0 mg q8–24h PO start low Cats: 7.5 mg q24–72h PO	Vomiting Xerostomia Sedation Constipation Increased intraocular pressure	Glaucoma
Testosterone Testosterone cypionate (DEPO-testosterone: Upjohn)	Male sex hormone	Hormone-responsive incontinence	Dogs: 1–2 mg/kg q2–4wk IM	Prostatic enlargement Male sexual characteristics	
Testosterone propionate			Dogs: 0.5–1.0 mg/kg, 2–3 × per week SC or IM		

From *Handbook of Small Animal Practice.* New York: Churchill Livingstone, 1992. Reprinted with permission from Churchill Livingstone.

- Bethanechol may be administered to increase detrusor contractions. Side effects such as vomiting, diarrhea, salivation, and anorexia may limit the drug's usefulness.
- Complications include urine scalding, decubital ulcers, and recurrent urinary tract infections.
- Agents that have been used experimentally to treat an atonic or hypocontractile bladder include metoclopramide, which has been reported to directly stimulate detrusor contractions in humans and dogs, and prostaglandins E_2 and F_2, which have been shown to stimulate both detrusor and urethral smooth muscle.

Upper Motor Neuron Bladder

- Initially it is difficult to express the bladder manually. Because of the risk of bladder rupture, do not attempt this until manual evacuation of the bladder is tolerable.
- Instead, aseptically catheterize the patient at least three times daily to completely empty the bladder. Avoid using an indwelling catheter because of the risk of urinary tract infections.
- Perform frequent urinalyses with culture and sensitivity testing.
- Antibacterial agents may be indicated, especially with long-term intermittent catheterization.

Detrusor-Urethral Dyssynergia

Treat by decreasing sympathetic tone or with muscle relaxants (see Table 103–2):

- Consider using alpha-adrenergic blocking agents, such as phenoxybenzamine, prazosin, and terazosin, to decrease internal sphincter resistance.
- In addition to its alpha-1 antagonism in urethral smooth muscle, prazosin can cause a centrally mediated decrease in somatic input to the external urethral sphincter.
- Consider diazepam and dantrolene as skeletal muscle relaxants to decrease external sphincter resistance.
- Baclofen is a skeletal muscle relaxant that decreases muscle tone by a depressive effect on the central nervous system (CNS). The drug inhibits medullary interneurons and spinal reflexes. Baclofen decreases muscle spasticity by reducing the activity of gamma efferent neurons, which decrease the sensitivity of muscle spindles that initiate striated muscle stretch reflexes.

Hormone-Responsive Incontinence

Replacement of the sex hormone is necessary for successful treatment (see Table 103–2).

- Treat female dogs with diethylstilbestrol or alpha-adrenergic agonist.

▼ *Key Point* Estradiol cypionate is not recommended because of the potential for bone marrow suppression.

- Testosterone cypionate may be used in male dogs. Minimal side effects have been noted except for prostatic enlargement.
- In some instances, animals develop a tolerance for hormonal replacement. Additional therapy with a sympathetic alpha-agonist that increases urethral tone is then indicated (see Table 103–2).

Urethral Incompetence (Stress Incontinence)

Treat with drugs that increase urethral tone (see Table 103–2).

- The most successful drugs are the sympathomimetic alpha-adrenergic agonists, which directly increase urethral smooth muscle tone. The drug of choice is phenylpropanolamine; an alternate drug is ephedrine.
- Imipramine is a tricyclic antidepressant agent that causes inhibition of norepinephrine re-uptake at the synaptic level and results in increased urethral tone.

Urge Incontinence (Detrusor Hyperreflexia)

Treat with drugs that reduce detrusor hyperspasticity and relax smooth muscle (see Table 103–2).

- Propantheline bromide is an anticholinergic drug that decreases detrusor hyperspasticity. Start with the lowest possible dosage and slowly increase until signs are alleviated or side effects are encountered.
- Direct-acting smooth muscle relaxants are promising in the treatment of this syndrome. These drugs also have a mild anticholinergic effect. Recommended drugs include flavoxate, oxybutynin, and dicyclomine.

Detrusor Atony from Overdistention

This is the single disorder in which indwelling urinary catheterization for up to 7–14 days is indicated to keep the bladder as small as possible in order to reestablish tight junction connections in the detrusor muscle. When indwelling catheterization cannot be accomplished, tube cystostomy is an alternative (see Chap. 100).

- Remove the obstruction or primary cause. Occasionally anti-inflammatory therapy is indicated.
- Perform frequent urinalyses and administer appropriate antibiotics, based upon susceptibility results.
- The cholinergic drug bethanechol has been used successfully to stimulate detrusor contractions in both neurogenic and non-neurogenic atonic bladders (see Table 103–2). It is effective for postobstructive atony; however, be careful to ensure urethral patency.
- When the overdistension is caused by increased urethral resistance, administer an alpha-adrenergic blocker prior to giving the bethanechol.

Paradoxical Incontinence

Treat by relieving the obstruction. Retropulsion of calculi or urethrostomy (e.g., urethritis) or surgical exploration (e.g., neoplasia) (see Chap. 102) may be required.

- In some instances indwelling catheterization may be indicated (e.g., severe urethritis) until the inflammation resolves.

Ectopic Ureter(s)

Treat by surgical transposition of the ureter(s) to the trigonal area (see Chap. 98).

- Ectopic ureters are often associated with other urinary tract abnormalities (urethral incompetence) that may be treated with alpha-adrenergic agonists.

Endoscopic Injections

Teflon

Teflon injections have been used experimentally for the treatment of urethral sphincter incompetence in dogs (Arnold et al., 1989). A Teflon paste is injected cystoscopically into urethral and periurethral tissues. This procedure inflates the tissues and compresses the urethral lumen at the site of injection.

Collagen

Teflon products have been supplanted by collagen-based agents. A study looking at the submucosal injection of glutaraldehyde cross-linked collagen was undertaken (Arnold et al., 1996). The results are promising, with 75% of the dogs becoming continent after one or two injections. No complications were observed in the present study. Consider this treatment for dogs that are not responsive to pharmacologic treatment.

Surgical Techniques

Surgery for disorders of the urinary system and micturition are discussed elsewhere in this text (see Chaps. 98, 100, and 102).

Several surgical treatments for incontinence have been described in the veterinary literature and include sling urethroplasty, colposuspension, and urethral compression (cystourethropexy or urethral banding). Initial studies with a prosthetic sphincter made of Silastic

(a polymeric silicone product) have been promising. Surgical techniques may be used as a last resort therapy when medical management has failed, or when owners are unable or unwilling to administer medications indefinitely.

SUPPLEMENTAL READINGS

Anderson K: Current concepts in the treatment of disorders of micturition. Drugs 35:47, 1988.

Arnold S, Jager P, DiBartola SP, et al.: Treatment of urinary incontinence in dogs by endoscopic injection of Teflon. J Am Vet Med Assoc 195:1369, 1989.

Arnold S, Hubler M, Lott-Stolz G, et al.: Treatment of urinary incontinence in bitches by endoscopic injection of collagen. J Small Anim Pract 37:163, 1996.

Dean PW, Novotny MJ, O'Brien DP: Prosthetic sphincter for urinary incontinence: Results in three cases. J Am Anim Hosp Assoc 25:447, 1989.

Gookin JL, Bunch SE: Detrusor-striated sphincter dyssynergia in a dog. JVIM 10(5):339, 1996.

Gookin JL, Stone EA, Sharp NJ: Urinary incontinence in dogs and cats. Part II. Diagnosis and Management. Comp of Cont Educ 18(5):525, 1996.

Labato MA: Disorders of micturition. In Morgan RV, ed.: Handbook of Small Animal Practice. New York: Churchill Livingstone, 1992, p 611.

Lappin MR, Barsanti JA: Urinary incontinence secondary to idiopathic detrusor instability: Cystometrographic diagnosis and pharmacologic management in two dogs and a cat. J Am Vet Med Assoc 191:1439, 1987.

Lovering JS, Tallett SE, McKendry JBJ: Oxybutynin efficacy in the treatment of primary enuresis. Pediatrics 82:104, 1988.

Marks SL, Straeter-Knowlen IM, Moore M, et al.: Effects of acepromazine maleate and phenoxybenzamine on urethral pressure profiles of anesthetized, healthy, sexually intact male cats. Am J Vet Res 57(10):1497, 1996.

Moreau PM, Lappin MR: Pharmacologic management of urinary incontinence. In Kirk, RW, ed.: Current Veterinary Therapy X. Philadelphia: WB Saunders, 1989, p 1214.

Ruffman R: A review of flavoxate hydrochloride in the treatment of urge incontinence. J Int Med Res 16:317, 1988.

Sackman JE, Sims MH: Electromyographic evaluation of the external urethral sphincter during cystometry in male cats. Am J Vet Res 51:1237, 1990.

Straeter-Knowlen IM, Marks SL, Rishniw M, et al: Urethral pressure response to smooth and skeletal muscle relaxants in anesthetized, adult male cats with naturally acquired urethral obstruction. Am J Vet Research 56:919, 1995.

104 Diseases of the Prostate Gland

Nancy D. Kay

Diseases of the prostate gland are common in middle-aged and older dogs. Medium and large breed dogs (especially Doberman pinschers) are more commonly affected. Although cats have prostate glands, for unknown reasons feline prostatic disease is extremely rare. This chapter discusses canine prostatic disease only.

ETIOLOGY

Several types of prostatic disease exist and some may occur simultaneously (e.g., prostatic cyst with abscessation, prostatic neoplasia with bacterial prostatitis).

Benign Prostatic Hyperplasia

To some degree, both hypertrophy (increased size) and hyperplasia (increased numbers) of prostatic cells account for enlargement of the gland in all middle-aged and older noncastrated dogs.

▼ *Key Point* Benign prostatic hyperplasia is the most common disorder of the prostate gland.

- Causes of benign prostatic hyperplasia include an imbalance in the ratio of androgens to estrogens, increased numbers of androgen receptors, and increased tissue sensitivity to androgens.
- Dihydrotestosterone is the main androgen that promotes prostatic hyperplasia.

Squamous Metaplasia

This morphologic alteration of prostatic epithelial cells is caused by estrogen stimulation arising from an exogenous or endogenous (e.g., Sertoli cell tumor) source.

Cystic Hyperplasia

This condition refers to multiple fluid-filled cavities within the prostatic parenchyma that result from the obstruction of glandular excretory ducts.

- Cystic hyperplasia commonly is associated with benign prostatic hyperplasia and squamous metaplasia.

Paraprostatic Cysts

These fluid-filled structures develop adjacent to the prostate gland and result from fluid accumulation within embryologic vestiges (uterus masculinis). The cystic lining may become calcified.

Prostatic Infection

- Bacterial prostatitis occurs when normal host resistance is altered.
  - Predisposing causes include disruption of normal glandular architecture (benign hyperplasia, squamous metaplasia, neoplasia), urethral diseases, urinary tract infections, alterations in urine flow, altered prostatic secretions, and host immune dysfunction.
  - Infection usually occurs by an ascending route, although hematogenous spread of bacteria also may occur.
  - The most common pathogens are *Escherichia coli*, *Staphylococcus*, *Proteus mirabilis*, *Streptococcus*, and *Mycoplasma*. Less common isolates include *Klebsiella*, *Brucella canis*, *Pseudomonas*, and *Ureaplasma*. Anaerobic infections are rare.
- In rare cases, disseminated (systemic) mycotic infections, such as *Blastomyces*, *Cryptococcus*, or *Coccidioides*, can cause prostatitis (see Chap. 18).

Idiopathic Prostatitis

Idiopathic (nonbacterial) prostatitis has been documented in dogs.

- Clinical signs are similar to those associated with chronic bacterial prostatitis.
- The etiology of the inflammation is uncertain.

Prostatic Abscesses

Prostatic abscesses are either extensions of bacterial prostatitis in which obstruction of an excretory duct has occurred, or secondary infection of a preexisting cyst.

Prostatic Neoplasia

Neoplasia is relatively rare compared with other forms of canine prostatic disease.

- Prostatic adenocarcinoma and transitional cell carcinoma are most common.
- Previously, castration was thought to prevent the development of prostatic cancer. In one study (Obradovich et al., 1987), 19 of 43 dogs had been castrated at least 3 years before the development of prostatic disease. More recent studies have also con-

cluded that castration at any age has no sparing effect on the development of prostate cancer. Tumors from neutered dogs tend to be more highly undifferentiated and often metastasize to the lung. This may reflect a more aggressive neoplastic process or delayed detection of the disease.

- Development of prostatic cancer in dogs may not be hormonally mediated or may be influenced by hormones of nontesticular origin. Hormones produced by the adrenal and pituitary glands may play a significant role.
- Metastasis is common. Frequent sites of metastasis include lymph nodes (regional and distant), bones (near and distant), and visceral organs.

CLINICAL SIGNS

Clinical signs associated with canine prostatic disease are variable. Depression, anorexia, and vomiting are systemic manifestations of bacterial prostatitis or prostatic abscessation. Other clinical signs do not correlate well with etiology (Table 104–1). Hematuria and blood dripping from the prepuce are the most frequent signs seen with most types of prostatic disease. In animals with uncomplicated benign prostatic hyperplasia, however, clinical signs frequently are absent until prostatomegaly becomes severe.

- *Hematuria* is caused by reflux of blood from the prostatic urethra into the bladder. It also may be associated with a concurrent bacterial cystitis.
- *Urethral discharge* results from the exudation of blood, pus, and/or prostatic fluid into the prostatic urethra. This fluid drips passively from the penile urethra and is often blood-tinged.
- *Stranguria* is present if partial or complete urethral obstruction results from prostatic enlargement.
- *Fecal tenesmus* or a *change in stool diameter* occurs when prostatic gland enlargement encroaches on the rectum. *Constipation* may be secondary to avoidance of pain associated with defecation.
- *Fever, depression, anorexia, vomiting,* and *diarrhea* are signs of systemic involvement and are most com-

monly associated with bacterial prostatitis or prostatic abscessation.
- *Recurrent urinary tract infection* in a male dog may be associated with nonresolving or recurrent bacterial prostatitis.
- *Abdominal distention* may be caused by a paraprostatic cyst or prostatic abscess.
- *Caudal abdominal pain, lumbar pain,* and/or *hindlimb stiffness* may be associated with metastasis of prostatic neoplasia to bone or muscle or with peritonitis associated with prostatic abscess.
- *Hypertrophic osteopathy* may occur secondary to prostatic disease such as tumors.
- *Hindlimb pitting edema* may occur secondary to lymphatic invasion by metastatic tumors.
- *Urinary incontinence* can be caused by impingement on the pelvic nerves by an adjacent prostatic mass (tumor or abscess) or from inflammation of the urethra from urinary tract infection.
- Other clinical conditions that may be associated with prostatic disease include *impaired libido, infertility, sepsis, ketoacidotic diabetes mellitus, perineal hernia,* and *testicular tumor.*

DIAGNOSIS

Localizing and defining the etiology of diseases of the prostate gland can be a challenging task. Until recently, few diagnostic techniques have combined reliability and specificity of results with safety and ease of application. The ideal method for the diagnosis of prostatic disease should localize the disease to the prostate gland and eliminate other parts of the urinary and reproductive tracts as sources of the disease.

Physical Examination

Abdominal palpation in dogs with prostatic disease may reveal abdominal pain, abdominal distention, or the presence of an abdominal mass.

▼ *Key Point* A rectal examination is essential in the diagnosis of prostatic disease.

Table 104–1. INCIDENCE OF CLINICAL SIGNS ASSOCIATED WITH PROSTATIC DISEASE

Prostatic Disease (No. of Cases)*	Hematuria	Blood Dripping from Prepuce	Stranguria	Tenesmus	Depression/ Anorexia	Vomiting	Diarrhea	Abdominal Pain	Hindlimb Deficit	Chronic UTI
Bacterial prostatitis (12)	4	3	2	2	3	2	2	1	0	2
Nonbacterial prostatitis (7)	1	2	0	0	0	0	0	1	0	3
Hyperplasia (16)	7	6	1	1	0	0	1	0	0	4
Neoplasia (4)	3	3	2	3	0	0	0	0	1	0
Squamous metaplasia (2)	2	0	1	0	0	0	0	0	0	1

UTI, urinary tract infection.
*Some prostate glands were affected by more than one disease process.
Kay ND, Ling GV, Johnson DL: Clinical diagnosis of canine prostatic disease using a urethral brush technique. J Am Anim Hosp Assoc 25:517–526, 1989.

- In rectal examination, palpate ventrally for the prostate gland and dorsally for iliac lymph node enlargement or lumbar pain.
- Evaluate the prostate gland for location, size, symmetry, surface contour, consistency, movability, and pain. The normal prostate gland is bilobed, intrapelvic, symmetric, smooth, movable, and nonpainful.
- As the prostate gland enlarges with disease, it may move cranially over the pelvic brim. Therefore, simultaneous rectal and caudal abdominal palpation may be helpful.

▼ *Key Point* The prostate gland of a normal Scottish terrier may be up to four times larger than those of other breeds.

Imaging Studies
Abdominal Radiography

Abdominal radiography rarely determines the specific etiology of prostatic disease, but it can reveal various associated abnormalities, including:

- Prostatomegaly
- Prostate gland asymmetry
- Abnormal fluid-filled mass in the caudal abdomen
- Prostate gland mineralization
- Iliac lymph node enlargement
- Vertebral or pelvic bone periosteal reactions
- Decreased soft tissue detail in the caudal abdomen due to tissue inflammation
- Urine or fecal retention

▼ *Key Point* Prostate gland mineralization and iliac lymph node enlargement are often but not always associated with prostatic neoplasia.

Urethrography

Positive-contrast retrograde urethrography may help to localize the disease process. However, there is no correlation between urethroprostatic reflux and the type of prostatic disease. Reflux may be observed in some dogs without prostatic disease.

Ultrasonography

Ultrasonography can be used to evaluate the prostate and to guide percutaneous needle aspiration or needle core biopsy. Ultrasound observations may include:

- Prostatomegaly
- Intraprostatic cyst or abscess (appears as focally hypoechoic or anechoic)
- Paraprostatic cyst
- Focal or multifocal areas of increased echogenicity (may represent bacterial prostatitis or neoplasia)
- Shadowing (may represent bacterial prostatitis or neoplasia)
- Prostatic calculi
- Iliac lymphadenopathy

Laboratory Studies
Complete Blood Count and Serum Biochemistry

- Hemogram abnormalities do not consistently correlate with the occurrence of infectious or noninfectious prostatic diseases. An exception is neutrophilic leukocytosis, which is consistently associated with acute, fulminant bacterial prostatitis.
- A mild to moderate nonregenerative anemia may occur in chronic inflammatory or neoplastic prostatic disease.
- An increase in serum alkaline phosphatase commonly accompanies bacterial prostatitis and prostatic neoplasia. It is not known which alkaline phosphatase isoenzyme is responsible.

Urinalysis and Urine Culture

- Bacterial cystitis and bacterial prostatitis may occur independently.
- Urinalysis and urine culture are always indicated for animals with signs of urinary tract disease. However, they may not be useful in the diagnosis of prostatic disease.
  - For example, urine sediment examination is not reliable for the diagnosis of prostatic neoplasia, and urine cultures can be negative in dogs with bacterial prostatitis or prostatic abscess.
  - For this reason, in addition to urine, evaluate prostatic fluid or tissue or both in dogs suspected of prostatic disease.

Prostatic Fluid or Tissue Culture

This procedure is necessary for documentation of bacterial prostatitis. *Mycoplasma* organisms require specialized culture media (pleuropneumonia-like organism [PPLO] agar); therefore, specifically request this culture (see Specimen Collection section for techniques for collection of microbiology specimens).

Prostatic Fluid Cytology

Cytologic studies may identify benign prostatic hyperplasia, squamous metaplasia, bacterial prostatitis, nonbacterial prostatitis, and prostatic neoplasia (see Specimen Collection section for techniques for collection of cytology specimens).

Serum and Seminal Plasma Markers

- Prostate-specific antigen is not detected in canine serum or seminal plasma.
- Serum and seminal acid phosphatase activities do not differ between normal and diseased dogs.
- Serum canine prostate-specific esterase activity is higher in dogs with benign prostatic hyperplasia than in normal dogs.

Specimen Collection
Ejaculate Specimen

For ejaculate collection, handle the dog in a quiet environment. Many dogs are more responsive if exposed to

---

Table 104–2. TECHNIQUE FOR COLLECTION OF EJACULATE SPECIMEN

1. Retract the prepuce and gently cleanse the tip of the glans penis with a sterile gauze sponge.
2. Apply digital pressure with one hand at the base of the penis proximal to the bulbus glandis.
3. With the other hand, manipulate the penis within the sheath.
4. Collect the specimen in a sterile container.
5. The first two components of the ejaculate (presperm and sperm) are milky in appearance. Separate these from the third component, which is clear prostatic fluid, by collecting into two different sterile containers.
6. Perform a bacterial culture on the prostatic fluid.

---

a female in estrus or to vaginal swabs obtained from a female in estrus (Table 104–2).

Advantages

- It is relatively easy to perform.
- It is safe.
- It can be done without chemical restraint.
- It is inexpensive.
- It provides specimens for bacterial culture.

Disadvantages

- Success depends on the animal's compliance, which may be diminished if the animal is old, ill, weak, nervous, overexcited, or in pain.
- It is difficult to effectively separate the prostatic fluid component from the presperm and sperm components.
- A positive bacterial culture fails to localize the disease process. Potential sources of infection include the testes, epididymides, deferent ducts, prostate gland, and urethra. A distal urethral culture with quantitation of organisms collected before ejaculation is useful in interpreting ejaculate specimen culture results.
- The ejaculate specimen is not useful for cytology.

Prostatic Wash Specimen

A prostatic wash specimen has potential microbiologic and cytologic applications (Table 104–3).

Table 104–3. TECHNIQUE FOR PERFORMING PROSTATIC MASSAGE

1. Pass urethral catheter into the bladder and remove all urine.
2. Flush bladder with 5 ml sterile physiologic saline solution and save fluid. Label this specimen Sample 1.
3. Retract catheter tip and align it with the caudal pole of prostate gland (positioning is determined via rectal palpation).
4. Massage prostate gland for 1 minute.
5. Flush 5 ml sterile physiologic saline solution slowly through catheter while the urethral orifice is occluded around catheter to prevent retrograde loss of sample.
6. Advance catheter into bladder as fluid is aspirated. Save fluid and label Sample 2.
7. Quantitate bacterial numbers in both specimens to ascertain significance of bacterial growth in prostatic fluid specimen (Sample 2).

Advantages

Advantages of this technique are similar to those of ejaculate specimen collection.

Disadvantages

- Results may be inaccurate due to urine and urethral contamination as well as volume dilution by urine. Microbiology results are noninterpretable in cases with concurrent bacterial cystitis.
- The prostate gland may not be within reach for effective rectal massage (abdominal prostatic massage may be effective).
- Overzealous massage can rupture a prostatic abscess or cause sepsis in dogs with acute bacterial prostatitis.

Urethral Brush Specimen (Figs. 104–1 and 104–2)

This technique uses a 90-cm microbiology specimen brush designed for bronchoscopic use (Microbiology Specimen Brush, Microvasive, Watertown, MA) (Table 104–4).

Advantages

Advantages of this technique are similar to those of ejaculate specimen collection and prostate wash, *plus:*

- The disease process is localized to the prostate gland; urethral contamination is minimized because of the plug in the tip of the catheter.
- Useful cytologic and microbiologic information is obtained.

Disadvantages

- The specimen brush cannot be reused, which makes the procedure relatively expensive.
- The prostate gland may not be within reach for effective rectal massage (prostate massage through the abdominal wall may be effective).
- Overzealous massage can rupture a prostatic abscess or cause sepsis in dogs with acute bacterial prostatitis.

Ultrasound-Guided Prostatic Aspirate

This technique uses ultrasonography to guide the insertion of a needle into the prostate gland. Its docu-

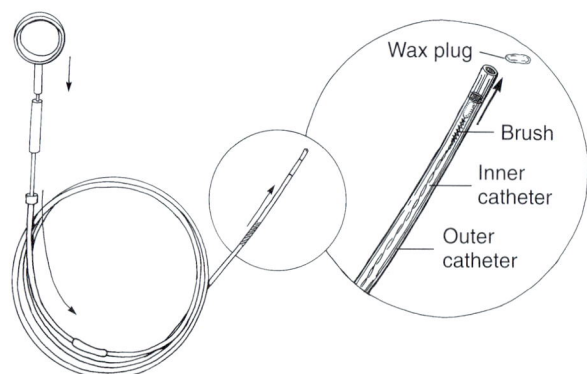

Figure 104–1. The microbiologic specimen brush used for obtaining prostatic urethral specimens.

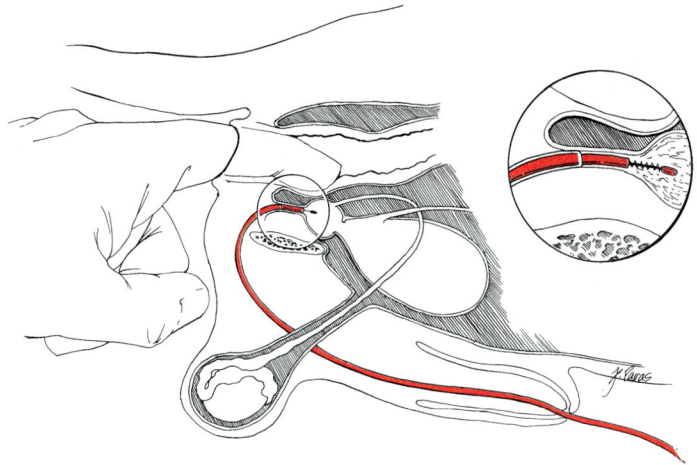

Figure 104–2. With the catheter positioned in the prostatic urethra, advance and retract the brush five or six times *(inset)*.

Table 104–4. TECHNIQUE FOR OBTAINING URETHRAL BRUSH SPECIMEN

1. Place animal in lateral recumbency.
2. Retract prepuce and cleanse end of glans penis with sterile swab.
3. Advance a sterile, 90-cm microbiologic specimen brush (Microbiology Specimen Brush, Microvasive, Watertown, MA) into urethra (see Fig. 104–1).
4. Direct an assistant to use rectal palpation to align tip of catheter with the caudal pole of prostate gland (see Fig. 104–2). The catheter is then held in this position.
5. Have the assistant massage prostate gland per rectum for 1 minute.
6. Advance the inner catheter approximately 1 cm within the urethra, thereby dislodging the absorbable catheter plug (see Fig. 104–1).
7. Advance and retract microbiologic brush 5 or 6 times within prostatic urethra for sample collection (see Fig. 104–2).
8. Following sample collection, retract brush and inner catheter and remove apparatus from urethra.
9. Expel any fluid within catheter into a test tube containing 3 ml sterile lactated Ringer's solution.
10. Extend brush, remove with sterile scissors, and drop into the same test tube.

---

mented use is for the diagnosis of bacterial infection and possibly neoplasia.

Advantages

- It is a safe procedure in noninfectious conditions.
- It accurately localizes the source of bacterial infection to the prostate gland.

Disadvantages

- Specialized equipment and skills are required.
- Chemical restraint usually is necessary.
- Aspiration of a prostatic abscess has the potential to result in peritonitis; seeding of the abdomen with neoplastic cells may occur with prostatic neoplasia.

Prostate Gland Biopsy

- Before performing biopsy, evaluate the animal for normal coagulation status.
- Several techniques have been described for prostate biopsy, including transperineal, transrectal, transab-

dominal, ultrasound-guided, and biopsy via laparotomy (see Chap. 105).
- Ultrasound-guided prostate gland biopsy uses ultrasonography to assist in directing the biopsy instrument into the gland.
  - The frequency of complications is less than with some other biopsy techniques, and the success of obtaining a definitive diagnosis is enhanced because focal lesions can be identified ultrasonographically.
  - Chemical restraint as well as specialized skill and equipment are necessary.
- If ultrasonography is not available, biopsy via laparotomy is the most accurate, although the most invasive, technique.
- Several complications from prostate gland biopsy are possible (Table 104–5).

TREATMENT

Treatment of canine prostatic disease is based on the specific diagnosis. Conservative management (castration and drug therapy) of canine prostatic disease is discussed in this chapter. Surgical management of prostatic disease is discussed in Chapter 105.

Benign Prostatic Hyperplasia and Sterile Cystic Hyperplasia

Therapy may not be indicated if clinical signs are absent. However, it is advisable to caution owners that problems associated with prostatomegaly may develop.

A description of various treatment modalities follows.

Table 104–5. COMPLICATIONS ASSOCIATED WITH PROSTATE GLAND BIOPSY

Periprostatic hemorrhage	Hematuria
Perineal hematoma	Septicemia
Urethral perforation	Fever
Perineal abscessation	Peritonitis
Dissemination of neoplastic cells	Urethral fistula formation

Castration

- Castration (see Chap. 107) is the treatment of choice in dogs not intended for breeding.
- A significant decrease in prostate gland size occurs within 1–4 weeks following castration.

Estrogen Therapy

- Theoretically, estrogen acts to decrease prostatic tissue mass by decreasing the concentration of gonadotropin-releasing hormone, which, in turn, decreases the concentration of testosterone. In fact, however, estrogen may act directly on the prostate gland to cause stromal hypertrophy and squamous metaplasia.
- It also may alter prostatic secretions and increase the gland's susceptibility to infection.
- Bone marrow suppression is a potential serious side effect.

▼ **Key Point** Because of potentially serious side effects, estrogen is contraindicated for the treatment of benign prostatic hyperplasia.

Megestrol Acetate

- Megestrol acetate interferes with the conversion of testosterone to dihydrotestosterone, the main androgen that promotes prostatic hyperplasia. This drug is also thought to increase metabolic clearance of androgens as well as cause direct pituitary suppression.

▼ **Key Point** Megestrol acetate effectively decreases the size of the prostate gland without impairing fertility in cases of benign prostatic hyperplasia.

- Administer 0.55 mg/kg q24h PO for 4 weeks; then give the same dosage once a week. Do not use for longer than 32 consecutive days.
- This drug reportedly produces a decrease in the size of the prostate gland without decreasing the number of spermatozoa. Thus, a treated animal subsequently may be used for breeding purposes.

Delmadinone Acetate

- Delmadinone acetate (Tardak, Syntex Laboratories) is an androgen inhibitor licensed for use in dogs in some countries other than the United States and Canada.
- It is recommended for the treatment of benign prostatic hyperplasia, perianal tumors, and hypersexuality.
- Delmadinone acetate is administered SC or IM at 1.5–2.0 mg/kg for dogs less than 10 kg, 1.0–1.5 mg/kg for dogs 10–20 kg, and 1.0 mg/kg for dogs greater than 20 kg; subsequent doses at 3–4 week intervals usually are necessary.
- Effects are observed within 2–4 days. A second treatment is recommended at 8 days if no improvement is noted.
- Concurrent use of other steroid drugs should be avoided, and this drug is contraindicated in dogs

with a history of decreased fertility or lack of libido if they are to be used for breeding.

Other Hormone-Manipulating Drugs

New drugs, which work either by lowering serum testosterone (flutamide), blocking conversion of testosterone to dihydrotestosterone (finasteride), or decreasing gonadotropin-releasing hormone (leuprolide) may show promise in the future for treating benign prostatic hypertrophy. However, minimal information is currently available regarding use of these drugs in dogs.

Squamous Metaplasia

- Discontinue any source of exogenous estrogen.
- Castration is the treatment of choice. Examine the testicles histopathologically for the presence of an estrogen-secreting Sertoli cell tumor.

Bacterial Prostatitis

Principles of Antibiotic Therapy (see Table 104–6 for specific drugs and dosages)

- Select an antibiotic based on urine or prostatic fluid culture and susceptibility results.

▼ **Key Point** The ideal antibiotic for bacterial prostatitis is lipid-soluble and therefore capable of penetrating the blood-prostate barrier. Antibiotics of choice include erythromycin, chloramphenicol, trimethoprim-sulfa, clindamycin, oleandomycin, and enrofloxacin.

- The ideal antibiotic has a relatively low degree of protein binding, which allows greater drug availability for diffusion into the prostate gland. Chloramphenicol is highly protein bound; therefore, it should be used at the higher end of the recommended dosage range (see Table 104–6).
- In cases of bacterial prostatitis, the pH of the prostatic fluid is usually acidic. Antibiotics that work best in an acidic environment are erythromycin, enrofloxacin, clindamycin, trimethoprim-sulfa, and chloramphenicol. Ciprofloxacin and norfloxacin do not

Table 104–6. ANTIBIOTICS RECOMMENDED FOR THE TREATMENT OF BACTERIAL PROSTATITIS

Drug	Dosage
Trimethoprim-sulfa (multiple manufacturers)	15 mg/kg q12h PO or SC
Chloramphenicol (multiple manufacturers)	50 mg/kg q8h PO, IV, SC, or IM
Erythromycin (multiple manufacturers)	10 mg/kg q8h PO
Clindamycin (Antirobe, Upjohn)	5–10 mg/kg q8h PO, IV, or IM
Enrofloxacin (Baytril, Bayer)	5 mg/kg q12h PO*

*This is twice the manufacturer's current recommended dosage.

appear to penetrate into the prostate gland as readily as enrofloxacin.

- Continue antibiotic therapy for a minimum of 4 weeks. Reculture the prostatic fluid 5–7 days after the onset of therapy to document the in vivo effectiveness of the antibiotic, and again in 2–3 weeks following discontinuation of therapy.
- If initial culture and susceptibility results cannot be obtained, a good initial treatment choice is trimethoprim-sulfa, chloramphenicol, or enrofloxacin.

Treatment of Concurrent Septicemia or Peritonitis

- Obtain abdominal fluid and/or blood for bacterial culture and susceptibility testing and select an appropriate antibiotic.
- Obtain a blood specimen for bacterial culture and susceptibility.
- Monitor the patient for hypoglycemia.
- Administer IV fluids and parenteral antibiotics.
- If a prostatic abscess is thought to be the source of septicemia, surgical drainage is indicated (see Chap. 105).
- Treat peritonitis as described in Chapter 96.

Castration

Castration diminishes the potential for recurrence of bacterial prostatitis, but do not perform castration until the patient is clinically stable and has been on antibiotic therapy for at least 1–2 weeks. Rule out the presence of a prostatic abscess or paraprostatic cyst, because castration alone typically is not curative for these conditions.

Idiopathic Prostatitis

- Because idiopathic prostatitis in dogs has only recently been described and the etiology is unknown, effective therapy has not been reported. Castration is likely to be beneficial.
- Treatment of idiopathic prostatitis in humans has included tetracycline, corticosteroids, anticholinergic drugs, and muscle relaxants. No consistently positive results have been reported.

Paraprostatic Cysts and Prostatic Abscesses

- Medical therapy consists of antibiotics if infection is present and treatment of concurrent septicemia, peritonitis, or hypoglycemia.
- Paraprostatic cysts and prostatic abscesses are indications for surgical therapy (see Chap. 105).

Prostatic Neoplasia

Multiple therapeutic modalities exist; however, the prognosis in cases of prostatic neoplasia is poor.

Radiation Therapy

- Intraoperative radiation therapy is currently the treatment of choice. It is well tolerated by the patient and has few side effects.
- Radiation therapy is not indicated if metastasis is detected. The most common site for metastasis is the iliac lymph nodes. Other sites include lungs, omentum, mesentery, pelvis, and lumbar vertebrae.

Prostatectomy

Prostatectomy (see Chap. 105) is associated with complications, especially urinary incontinence, but can be offered if the tumor is small and has not metastasized.

Noninvasive Ultrasonic Subtotal Ablation

This experimental technique uses high-intensity focused ultrasound to ablate the prostate gland without damaging surrounding tissues.

Chemotherapy

No known protocols have any documented efficacy.

Castration

Castration is of questionable benefit. The cancer growth may not be hormonally mediated or it may be affected by nontesticular hormones (adrenal androgens or estrogens, luteinizing hormone [LH], follicle-stimulating hormone [FSH], prolactin, or growth hormone).

Estrogen Therapy

Estrogen therapy suppresses gonadotropin secretion by the pituitary gland, which, in turn, decreases the level of testicular testosterone secretion. As with castration, nontesticular hormones are unaffected.

Total Androgen Blockade

The advantage of a total androgen blockade over castration is that all sources of androgen production are affected rather than just testicular androgens.

- Luteinizing hormone–releasing hormone (LH-RH) agonists cause a transient rise followed by a paradoxical decrease in FSH, LH, and testosterone release. This decrease may be due to downregulation of, or a decrease in, the number of pituitary LH-RH receptors. There is minimal information about use of these drugs in veterinary medicine.
- Ketoconazole (see Chap. 31 for details of ketoconazole therapy) inhibits testicular and adrenal testosterone synthesis and decreases the testosterone level to that of a castrated dog in 24–48 hours. The dosage range in humans is 400–1200 mg/day. Currently, a dosage for the treatment of canine prostatic neoplasia has not been determined, but dosages reported in limited studies vary from 20–30 mg/kg/day.
  - Ketoconazole has been shown to have a significant effect on hormonal production by the adrenal gland in the treatment of canine hyperadrenocorticism at an oral dose of 30 mg/kg PO once daily or divided b.i.d. A similar dosage may be effective in the treatment of canine prostatic neoplasia.
  - Dosages of 10–30 mg/kg/day are tolerated by most dogs when used for antifungal therapy.

SUPPLEMENTAL READINGS

Bell FW, Klausner JS, Hayden DW, et al.: Clinical and pathologic features of prostatic adenocarcinoma in sexually intact and castrated dogs: 31 cases (1970–1987). J Am Vet Med Assoc 199:1623, 1991.

Bell FW, Klausner JS, Hayden DW, et al.: Evaluation of serum and seminal plasma markers in the diagnosis of canine prostatic disorders. J Vet Intern Med 9:149, 1995.

Feeney DA, Johnston GR, Klausner JS, et al.: Canine prostatic disease—comparison of ultrasonographic appearance with morphologic and microbiologic findings: 30 cases (1981–1985). J Am Vet Med Assoc 190:1027, 1987.

Hargis AM, Miller LM: Prostatic carcinoma in dogs. Compend Contin Educ 5:647, 1983.

Kay ND, Ling GV, Nyland TG, et al.: Cytological diagnosis of canine prostatic disease using a urethral brush technique. J Am Anim Hosp Assoc 25:517, 1989.

Kay ND, Ling GV, Johnson DL: A urethral brush technique for the diagnosis of canine bacterial prostatitis. J Am Anim Hosp Assoc 25:527, 1989.

Kincaide LF, Sanghui NT, Cummings O, et al.: Noninvasive ultrasonic subtotal ablation of the prostate in dogs. Am J Vet Res 57:1225, 1996.

Krawiec DR, Heflin D: Study of prostatic disease in dogs: 177 cases (1981–1986). J Am Vet Med Assoc 200:1119, 1992.

Obradovich J, Walshaw R, Goullaud E: The influence of castration on the development of prostatic carcinoma in the dog. J Vet Intern Med 1:183, 1987.

Olsen PN, Wrigley RH, Thrall MA, et al.: Disorders of the canine prostate gland: Pathogenesis, diagnosis, and medical therapy. Compend Contin Educ 9:613, 1987.

Turrel JM: Intraoperative radiotherapy of carcinoma of the prostate gland in ten dogs. J Am Vet Med Assoc 190:48, 1987.

105 Surgery of the Prostate Gland

Harry W. Boothe

Surgical procedures of the prostate gland include biopsy, drainage procedures (including drain tube placement, omentalization, and marsupialization), and prostatectomy (partial or complete). Perform orchidectomy of the patient with prostatic disease either before or at the time of prostatic surgery (see Chap. 107 for castration technique). Prostatic disorders that may require surgery include hyperplasia, trauma, infection (abscess), cyst formation, and neoplasia. A thorough understanding of prostatic anatomy is necessary before performing surgery. Information in this chapter refers only to the dog because prostatic disease is extremely rare in cats. See Chapter 104 for additional information on prostatic diseases.

ANATOMY

- The prostate gland completely encompasses the proximal portion of the male urethra at the neck of the bladder.
- The position of the prostate is age-dependent; the prostate is confined to the pelvic cavity until about 4 years of age and is essentially totally within the abdomen by 10 years of age.
- The dorsal prostatic surface is flattened and has a mid-dorsal sulcus. The gland has a relatively thick capsule and is divided into right and left lobes by a prominent median septum.
- The two deferent ducts enter the craniodorsal surface of the prostate.
- The blood supply is closely allied to the nerve supply, with both being located in the lateral pedicles and entering the prostate dorsolaterally. The prostatic artery gives off branches to the ductus deferens, urethra, urinary bladder, ureters, and rectum. Damage to branches of the prostatic artery may result in devascularization of surrounding structures.
- The hypogastric (sympathetic) and pelvic (parasympathetic) nerves follow the vasculature.

▼ *Key Point* The hypogastric and pelvic nerves are required for micturition and continence. Avoid iatrogenic trauma to these structures.

- The prostatic lymph vessels empty into the median iliac lymph nodes.

BIOPSY

Preoperative Considerations

- Accurate preoperative assessment of prostatic size, consistency, and location is important. Palpation (both rectal and abdominal), radiography (including contrast radiography), and ultrasonography are helpful in gaining this information.
- Adequate immobilization of the prostate gland during biopsy is indicated, particularly when using needle biopsy techniques.

▼ *Key Point* Perform aspiration of the prostate before needle biopsy to exclude abscessation.

Procedure for Percutaneous Needle (Punch) Biopsy

Objectives

- Obtain a representative sample of the prostate gland for histologic and microbiologic evaluation.
- Avoid entering the prostatic urethra.
- Minimize blood loss and potential dissemination of infection.

Equipment

- Tru-Cut biopsy needle (one-handed model) or Franklin-Silverman needle
- Scalpel blade and handle

Technique

1. Place the dog in sternal recumbency with the tail positioned over the back.
2. Prepare the perineal region from the base of the tail to ventral to the level of the ischial tuberosities.
3. Direct an assistant to exert gentle pressure on the caudal abdomen to move the prostate gland into the pelvic inlet.
4. Perform rectal examination to define the position of the prostate gland.
5. Incise the perineal skin (5 mm long) just off the midline midway between the anus and ischial tuberosity.
6. Insert the biopsy needle in the closed position through the prostatic capsule under digital control within the rectum by the other hand.

7. Fully insert the inner cannula into the prostate gland and, while holding the inner cannula stationary in its extended position, sharply advance the outer cannula over the inner rod.
8. Remove the biopsy needle in a closed position.
9. Verify that an adequate biopsy has been obtained by seeing prostatic tissue in the specimen notch.
10. Place the biopsy sample in the appropriate containers for histologic and microbiologic testing.

Procedure for Wedge Biopsy

Equipment

- Standard general surgical pack and suture
- Laparotomy sponges
- Balfour retractors

Technique

1. Place the dog in dorsal recumbency on a level surgery table.
2. Aseptically prepare the ventral abdominal region from the xiphoid process to caudal to the pubic brim.
3. Incise the skin and ventral abdominal wall from the umbilicus to the pubis while avoiding the prepuce. Use a midline abdominal approach. Alternately, a paramedian approach to the caudal abdomen can be used.
4. Gently retract the urinary bladder cranially using a stay suture. Isolate the prostate gland with moistened laparotomy sponges.
5. Excise a representative wedge of prostatic tissue, while avoiding the urethra on the midline, using a scalpel blade.
6. Close the prostatic defect (simple interrupted or continuous pattern, absorbable suture).
7. Routinely close the ventral abdominal incision in three layers.

Postoperative Care and Complications

Short-Term

- Closely monitor for hemorrhage, including hematuria, infection, and urine leakage.
- Monitor for postoperative orchitis and scrotal edema.

Prognosis

- The prognosis depends on the disease process(es) present.
- Prostatic biopsy is usually associated with minimal patient morbidity.

DRAINAGE PROCEDURES

Preoperative Considerations

- Distinguish between infectious and noninfectious causes of fluid retention within or near the prostate gland.

- Perform microbiologic testing of prostatic fluid to assist in selection of an antimicrobial agent.
- Perform ultrasonography to determine the degree and location of cavitation within the prostatic parenchyma.
- When prostatic abscessation is present, drainage, omentalization, or resection of diseased parenchyma is indicated.
- Perform orchidectomy before or at the time of a prostatic drainage procedure.

▼ *Key Point* Always biopsy and obtain culture samples from the prostate as part of the drainage procedure.

- Choice of drainage procedure (i.e., placement of drain tubes, omentalization, or marsupialization) depends on the size and location of prostatic cavitation. Large cystic lesions may be more amenable to partial resection and omentalization.

Objectives

- Create a common cavity to provide ventral drainage.
- Thoroughly lavage the cavity at the time of drainage.
- Avoid entering the prostatic urethra if possible.
- Minimize blood loss and dissemination of infection.

Procedure for Placement of Drain Tube(s)

Equipment

- Standard general surgical pack and suture
- Red rubber urethral catheter(s) or Penrose drain(s)
- Suction apparatus, tubing, and tip
- Laparotomy sponges
- Balfour retractors

Technique

1. Place the dog in dorsal recumbency. Catheterize the urethra.
2. Aseptically prepare the ventral abdominal region from the xiphoid process to caudal to the pubic brim.
3. Incise the skin and ventral abdominal wall from the umbilicus to the pubis while avoiding the prepuce.
4. Isolate the prostate from the rest of the peritoneal cavity, using laparotomy sponges.
5. Incise the ventrolateral aspect of the prostatic lobe(s) containing the fluid. Avoid vessels and nerves contained in the lateral pedicles.
6. Remove fluid, using suction and lavage after digitally creating a common cavity. Obtain biopsy and culture samples.

▼ *Key Point* Creation of a common prostatic cavity during any drainage procedure improves drainage and decreases the probability of recurrence.

7. Place one or more drains into the prostatic cavity while avoiding the urethra as follows:
   a. Pass Penrose drain(s) (¼ inch) through the cavity to exit on the ventrolateral aspect of each lobe (Fig. 105–1), or

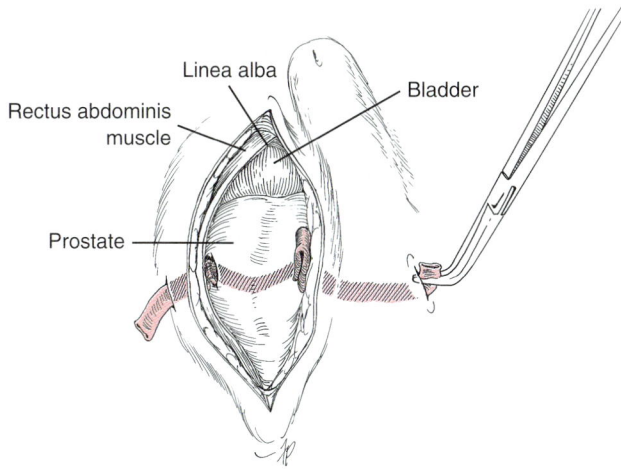

Figure 105–1. Prostatic drainage procedure. A single Penrose drain has been placed within the abscess cavity of the prostate and exits on the ventrolateral aspects of the gland. The ends of the drain are placed through the body wall and skin on each side of the prepuce.

b. Position a single red rubber catheter to permit continuous drainage of the prostatic cavity.

8. Exteriorize the end(s) of the drain tube(s) through the body wall approximately 2 cm lateral to the prepuce, and suture the drain to the skin.

9. Routinely close the ventral abdominal incision.

Procedure for Omentalization

Equipment

- Standard general surgical pack and suture
- Suction apparatus, tubing, and tip
- Laparotomy sponges
- Balfour retractors

Technique

1. Refer to steps 1–4 under Procedure for Placement of Drain Tube(s).
2. Incise the lateral aspects of each prostatic lobe.
3. Remove fluid, using suction and lavage after digitally creating a common cavity. Obtain biopsy and culture samples.
4. Introduce the greater omentum through one capsulotomy wound by using a forceps, which is placed through the contralateral prostatic wound (Fig. 105–2).
5. Pass the omentum around the prostatic urethra and

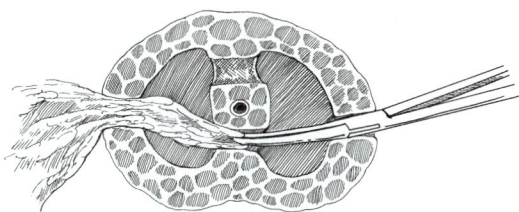

Figure 105–2. Intracapsular omentalization procedure. The greater omentum is introduced into the dorsal abscess cavities by using a forceps. (From White RAS, Williams JM: Intracapsular prostatic omentalization: A new technique for management of prostatic abscesses in dogs. Vet Surg 24:392, 1995.)

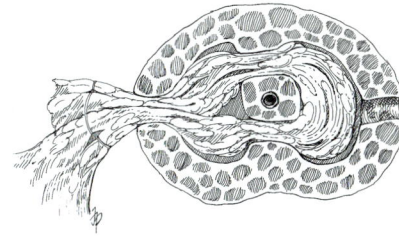

Figure 105–3. The omentum has been packed in the prostate gland encircling the urethra and has been sutured to itself. (From White RAS, Williams JM: Intracapsular prostatic omentalization: A new technique for management of prostatic abscesses in dogs. Vet Surg 24:393, 1995.)

exit it through the same capsulotomy wound through which it was introduced.

6. Suture the omentum to itself (horizontal mattress pattern, absorbable suture; see Fig. 105–3).
7. Routinely close the ventral abdominal incision.

Procedure for Marsupialization

Equipment

- Standard general surgical pack and suture
- Suction apparatus, tubing, and tip
- Laparotomy sponges
- Balfour retractors

Technique

1. Refer to steps 1–4 under Procedure for Placement of Drain Tube(s).
2. Incise the ventrolateral aspect of the fluid-filled prostate and evacuate fluid, using suction and lavage after digitally creating a common cavity. Obtain biopsy and culture samples.
3. Incise the skin (5 cm long), subcutaneous tissue, and abdominal musculature just lateral to the prepuce on the side opposite the original skin incision.
4. Place the walls of the prostatic cavity near the skin incision and appose the wall adjacent to the prostatic incision to the external rectus fascia (simple continuous pattern, absorbable suture) and the incised prostatic edges to the skin (simple interrupted pattern, nonabsorbable suture).

▼ **Key Point** If a paraprostatic cyst is present and can be dissected free from surrounding tissues, resection of all or most of the cyst is indicated. Pack the cyst remnant with omentum. This eliminates the complications associated with marsupialization.

5. Routinely close the ventral abdominal incision.

Postoperative Care and Complications

Short-Term

- Prevent self-inflicted trauma to the drain(s) or the stoma site by using a side brace or Elizabethan collar until the drain tubes are removed.
- Continuous suction drainage using a single red rubber catheter and a suction reservoir may be more effective in evacuating prostatic cavities than simple

gravity drainage; however, such drainage requires more conscientious postoperative patient observation and care.

- Passage of urine through the drainage tubes may occur but usually resolves in a few days.
- Prostatic abscessation requires aggressive medical therapy to eliminate infection and usually responds better to omentalization or drain tube placement than to marsupialization.
- Remove drains about 3 weeks after surgery.
- Administer an appropriate antibiotic (see Chap. 104) to patients with prostatic abscessation for 2–4 weeks after the hospitalized period.

Long-Term

- Long-term complications of prostatic tube drainage procedures include urinary incontinence (46% incidence), recurrent urinary tract infection (30% incidence), recurrence of prostatic abscessation (18% incidence), and urethrocutaneous fistula formation (2% incidence).
- Carefully monitor response to therapy through urine or prostatic fluid culture and susceptibility testing, as well as ultrasonography, if available, after discontinuing antibiotics.

Prognosis

- Paraprostatic cysts respond best to complete or partial surgical removal, because recurrence following drainage is relatively common.
- Prostatic abscessation has the potential for significant morbidity and mortality, and immediate postoperative mortality may approach 25%.
- The incidence of postoperative sepsis and shock approximates 33%. Rupture of a prostatic abscess results in a mortality rate of approximately 50%.
- Patients with prostatic abscessation that survive the initial 2 weeks after surgery will likely make a satisfactory recovery.

PARTIAL (SUBTOTAL) PROSTATECTOMY

Preoperative Considerations

- Be familiar with the vascular and regional anatomy of the prostate and surrounding structures.
- Perform partial prostatectomy for stable patients with recurrent abscessation and for dogs with cystic disease that have not responded to more conservative methods (i.e., orchidectomy).

▼ *Key Point* Complete rather than partial prostatectomy is indicated for prostatic neoplasia.

- Pass a urethral catheter to the urinary bladder to aid in identification of the urethra.

Surgical Procedure

Objectives

- Remove as much diseased prostatic tissue as possible while maintaining urinary continence.

- Avoid traumatizing the prostatic urethra.
- Maintain the blood supply to the prostatic urethra and adjacent organs.

Equipment

- Standard general surgical pack and suture
- Electrocoagulation unit with both coagulation and cutting capabilities
- Laparotomy sponges
- Balfour retractors

Technique

1. Refer to steps 1–4 under Procedure for Placement of Drain Tube(s).
2. Isolate and ligate all major vessels leading to the prostate, while staying immediately adjacent to the prostate gland.
3. Incise and remove the prostate to within approximately 5 mm of the lateral aspect of the prostatic urethra, using either scissors and electrocoagulation, cutting electrocoagulation, or an ultrasonic surgical aspirator (Fig. 105–4).
4. Routinely close the ventral abdominal incision.

Postoperative Care and Complications
Short-Term

- Submit excised tissue for histologic and microbiologic evaluation.
- Maintain urinary diversion (i.e., indwelling urethral catheter) for approximately 5 days.
- Prevent self-inflicted trauma to the urinary catheter by using a side brace until the catheter is removed.
- Shock, urine leakage, and urinary incontinence are potential short-term complications of partial prostatectomy.

Long-Term

- Nocturnal urinary incontinence has been identified as a long-term complication of partial prostatectomy in approximately 50% of patients.

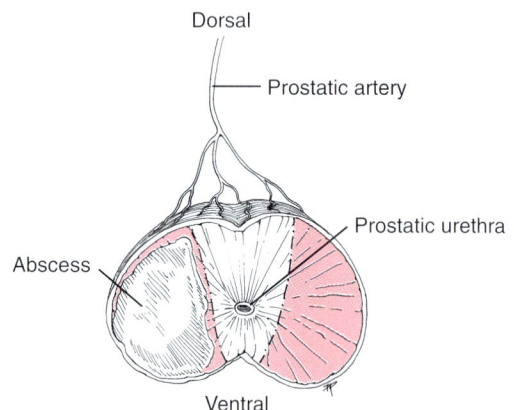

Figure 105–4. Partial (subtotal) prostatectomy technique. The shaded area denotes the prostatic parenchyma to be removed to within approximately 5 mm of the prostatic urethra using sharp dissection and/or an ultrasonic surgical aspirator.

Prognosis

- The prognosis depends on the disease process(es) present.
- Resolution of prostatic and urinary tract infection is likely following partial prostatectomy and appropriate antimicrobial therapy.

TOTAL PROSTATECTOMY

Preoperative Considerations

- Indications for total prostatectomy include severe trauma, neoplasia with no apparent metastasis, and recurrent prostatic abscessation unresponsive to other less invasive surgical procedures.

▼ *Key Point* Urinary incontinence is a common complication of total prostatectomy.

Surgical Procedure

Objectives

- Remove the entire prostate gland.
- Preserve the blood supply to the urinary bladder and urethra.
- Preserve as much urethra as possible.
- Perform an accurate urethral anastomosis.

Equipment

- Standard general surgical pack and suture
- Electrocoagulation unit
- Laparotomy sponges
- Urethral catheter
- Balfour retractors

Technique

1. See steps 1–4 under Procedure for Placement of Drain Tube(s).
2. Expose the prostate by careful dissection through the periprostatic fat as close to the prostate as possible.
3. Ligate and divide the prostatic vessels and ductus deferens close to the gland.
4. Carefully dissect the prostatic tissue from the urinary bladder and urethra, using sharp and blunt dissection.
5. Transect the urethra as close to the prostate and as far from the bladder neck as possible.
6. Transect the urethra as close to the caudal extent of the prostate as possible.
7. Remove the prostate by slipping it off the urinary catheter, and reposition the catheter into the urinary bladder. Submit the gland for histologic and microbiologic evaluation.
8. Approximate the urethral ends in an end-to-end fashion (simple interrupted pattern, synthetic absorbable suture), starting at the dorsal aspect of the urethra. Temporarily leave suture tags long and use them to help rotate the urethra to facilitate the anastomosis.
9. Thoroughly lavage the abdomen before closure.
10. Provide urinary diversion by performing a prepubic tube cystostomy (see Chap. 100) or by maintaining placement of the urethral catheter for approximately 2 weeks (longer if delayed healing is expected).
11. Routinely close the ventral abdominal incision.

Postoperative Care and Complications

Short-Term

- Prevent self-inflicted trauma to the catheter by using a side brace or Elizabethan collar.
- Complications include urinary incontinence, urine leakage at the urethral anastomosis, and urethral stricture.

Long-Term

- Urinary incontinence may be a long-term complication. Attempt control using drugs to increase proximal urethral tone (see Chap. 103).

Prognosis

- Prostatic neoplasia in the dog is most commonly malignant (adenocarcinoma or transitional cell carcinoma), metastasis is most common to the median iliac lymph nodes, periprostatic tissue, urinary bladder, pelvic structures, and lung.
- Successful treatment of prostatic neoplasia is difficult because of its aggressive biologic behavior; micrometastasis to adjacent tissues is probable, even when no gross evidence of metastasis exists.

SUPPLEMENTAL READINGS

Basinger RR: Surgical management of prostatic diseases. Compend Contin Educ Pract Vet 9:993, 1987.

Basinger RR, Robinette CL, Hardie EM, et al.: The prostate. *In* Slatter D, ed.: Textbook of Small Animal Surgery, 2nd Ed. Philadelphia: WB Saunders, 1993, p 1349.

Bray JP, White RAS, Williams JM: Partial resection and omentalization: A new technique for management of prostatic retention cysts in dogs. Vet Surg 26:202, 1997.

Evans HE, Christensen GC: Miller's Anatomy of the Dog. Philadelphia: WB Saunders, 1979, p 565.

Hardie EM, Barsanti JA, Rawlings CA: Complications of prostatic surgery. J Am Anim Hosp Assoc 20:50, 1984.

Hardie EM, Stone EA, Spaulding KA, et al.: Subtotal canine prostatectomy with the neodymium:yttrium-aluminum-garnet laser. Vet Surg 19:348, 1990.

Mullen HS, Matthiesen DT, Scavelli TD: Results of surgery and postoperative complications in 92 dogs treated for prostatic abscessation by a multiple Penrose drain technique. J Am Anim Hosp Assoc 26:369, 1990.

Rawlings CA, Crowell WA, Barsanti JA, et al.: Intracapsular subtotal prostatectomy in normal dogs: Use of an ultrasonic surgical aspirator. Vet Surg 23:182, 1994.

Weaver AD: Transperineal punch biopsy of the canine prostate gland. J Small Anim Pract 18:573, 1977.

White RAS, Williams JM: Intracapsular prostatic omentalization: A new technique for management of prostatic abscesses in dogs. Vet Surg 24:390, 1995.

106 Diseases of the Testes and Scrotum

Susan F. Soderberg

Diseases of the testes and scrotum may cause discomfort with an acute injury or infection or may cause systemic effects with an endocrinopathy. Most dogs with testicular diseases have no clinical signs. Expect infertility, with or without testicular atrophy, if the disease is chronic.

▼ *Key Point* Early diagnosis and therapy of testicular disease are critical to preserving reproductive function.

ETIOLOGY

Congenital Diseases

Congenital diseases of the testicles are detectable prior to puberty.

- *Cryptorchidism* is the failure of one or both testes to descend into the scrotum. Normal descent of the testes into the scrotum is complete by 6–8 weeks of age but occasionally is delayed to as late as 6 months of age.
  - The undescended testis may be found within the abdominal cavity, the inguinal canal, or lateral to the penis.
  - This defect is considered hereditary in most breeds and is a sex-linked, autosomal recessive trait.
- *Testicular hypoplasia* results from abnormal development of the seminiferous tubular germinal epithelium. This development leads to significant reduction in sperm number and infertility. A significant decrease in the size of one or both testicles is present at the time of puberty.
- *Aplasia of the testicular duct system* results in impaired transport of sperm to the urethra, accumulation of sperm proximal to the obstruction, potential development of sperm granuloma, and subsequent testicular degeneration. This defect is commonly unilateral.
- *Female pseudohermaphrodites* have the external genitalia of a male but generally have more than a single X chromosome. These individuals frequently have an XXY karyotype.
- *Male pseudohermaphrodites* have testicular hypoplasia, cryptorchidism, or abnormal development of the penis or prepuce.
- *Scrotal hernia* (herniation of abdominal organs or omentum through the inguinal canal into the scrotum) may be congenital or traumatic in origin.

Infectious and Inflammatory Diseases

Infections of the testes and scrotum are often detected by swelling, pain, and enlargement of the affected area.

Scrotal Dermatitis

- Local irritation can be an acute reaction from contact with chemical irritants, such as soaps, dips, or disinfectants, or from insect bites, such as fly strike.
- Acute orchitis causes dermatitis by stimulating excessive licking of the scrotum.
- Abrasions and other traumatic insults, such as surgical preparation, can also initiate scrotal dermatitis.
- The scrotum can be involved in any generalized dermatitis.

Orchiepididymitis

- *Acute orchiepididymitis* may develop from several routes.
  - Direct trauma, especially a puncture wound, can initiate bacterial infection in the testis.
  - Bacterial septicemias, originating in other organ systems, may spread to the testicles via the lymphatics.
  - Bacterial prostatitis or cystitis can initiate infection by descent down the vas deferens.
  - *Brucella canis* or distemper virus can cause orchiepididymitis.
  - Bacterial infections can cause suppurative inflammation that results in abscess formation, which may rupture and drain through the scrotal skin.
- *Chronic orchiepididymitis* may develop secondary to acute infection.
  - Orchiepididymitis may appear in an animal with no previous history of or owner's awareness of an inflammatory testicular problem.
  - Slow, progressive, low-grade, nonsuppurative inflammation with fibrosis may be caused by *B. canis, Escherichia coli,* or canine distemper virus.

Trauma

Traumatic injury to the testes and scrotum can result in abrasion, contusion, hematoma, laceration, or edema. All such lesions require prompt treatment to avoid acute or chronic orchiepididymitis.

Adverse Drug Reactions

Many drugs, toxins (e.g., lead), and irradiation are capable of causing damage to the seminiferous epithelium and subsequent deterioration in semen quality. Some of the agents that can adversely affect semen quality include amphotericin B, anticancer drugs, and cimetidine. Deleterious drugs are withdrawn as soon as possible to allow recovery of the seminiferous epithelium before severe or permanent damage occurs.

Endocrine Diseases

Spermatogenesis is altered by endocrinopathies, such as hypothyroidism and diabetes mellitus, or abnormally high or low concentrations of glucocorticoid, estrogen, androgen, or gonadotropin. Such conditions alter the metabolism of the gonadal hormones and gradually cause deterioration of the seminiferous epithelium.

Immune-Mediated Diseases

Immune-mediated orchitis develops subsequent to exposure of spermatozoal antigens to the immune system. Normally, a blood-testis barrier prevents such exposure. Traumatic and infectious diseases of the epididymis or testis can damage this barrier and result in exposure of spermatozoal antigens to the general circulation and immune system. Invasion of the interstitial tissues of the testes and epididymis with lymphocytes and plasma cells follows. This infiltrate results in deterioration of the seminiferous epithelium.

Neoplasia

- Scrotal tumors most commonly include mast cell tumors (see Chap. 26) and melanomas (see Chap. 28). These tumors have a high potential for malignant behavior and require radical therapy.
- Primary testicular neoplasias include Sertoli cell tumors, interstitial cell tumors, and seminomas.
  - When these tumors occur in scrotal testes, they are most often benign.
  - If Sertoli cell tumors and seminomas are located within the abdominal cavity they may be malignant.
  - These tumors compromise testicular integrity and function by invading or compressing seminiferous tubules or by producing abnormally elevated levels of estrogen or testosterone.
  - Elevations in testosterone levels (interstitial cell tumors) can contribute to benign prostatic hyperplasia, perineal hernia, or perianal adenoma.
  - Elevations in estrogen levels by Sertoli cell tumors can contribute to squamous metaplasia of the prostate gland, feminization, and myelotoxicity.

Idiopathic Diseases

- *Testicular torsion* occurs most often in an enlarged, neoplastic abdominal testis. Rarely, testicular torsion occurs in a scrotal testis and, usually, after a traumatic incident. The testis rotates on its horizontal axis, resulting in torsion of the spermatic cord. Occlusion of venous and lymphatic drainage from the testis causes testicular engorgement and eventual necrosis.
- *Spermatocele* is a cystic distention in the testicular duct system that contains sperm.
- *Sperm granuloma* is an accumulation of sperm in the duct system that generates a chronic, inflammatory process. These granulomas develop slowly; fertility is maintained until total obstruction occurs. The degree of compromise in semen quality depends on whether the obstruction is in a major duct or is unilateral or bilateral and whether an immune-mediated disease develops.
- *Varicocele* is a dilation and subsequent thrombosis of a spermatic vein. This condition results in disruption of normal blood flow and thermoregulation of the testis.

CLINICAL SIGNS

Acute, inflammatory diseases of the testes and scrotum are most commonly characterized by pain, swelling, and licking of the scrotum. Anorexia, listlessness, fever, reluctance to walk, or a stiff and stilted gait is intermittently reported. Acute abdominal pain may occur with testicular torsion. Changes in testicular size, testicular consistency, or semen quality is more commonly detected with chronic disease.

DIAGNOSIS

History

Historical information, including duration of clinical disease, is important in determining an accurate diagnosis.

- Determine the disorders of other organ systems and previous systemic illnesses.
- Determine whether exogenous administration of drugs has occurred that could adversely affect testicular function.
- Determine whether traumatic episodes or periods of serious stress are involved.
- Determine the breeding management practices and housing facilities.

Perform a complete physical examination in order to recognize underlying problems in other organ systems and to evaluate the scrotum and testes.

Physical Examination

Scrotum

The scrotum should be uniform in thickness.

- Chronic or severe scrotal inflammation may alter normal thermoregulatory processes, which can alter spermatogenesis and/or spermatozoal storage in the epididymis.
- Scrotal swelling may be the result of diffuse thickening of the scrotum; edema from local inflammation;

testicular or epididymal enlargement; inguinoscrotal hernia; or systemic edematous conditions, such as hypoalbuminemia or vasculitis.

Testicles

Note the location of the two testicles. Both testicles should be located within the scrotum by 4–6 months of age. Palpate the testicles for size, shape, and consistency.

- The normal testicle is oval with a smooth, regular outline.
- The two testicles should be approximately the same size, comfortably filling the scrotal cavity.
- An irregular surface, nodule, or adhesion to the scrotum may be the result of chronic inflammation, infection, or neoplasia.
- Soft, spongy, or doughy testicles are indicative of a degenerative process.
- Firm, hard testicles result from neoplasia or acute orchitis.
- Testicular pain on palpation suggests acute orchitis or testicular torsion, especially if the testis is enlarged.

Ultrasound

Testicular and scrotal ultrasound may help diagnose testicular neoplasia, abscess, testicular torsion, and scrotal hernia.

Semen Evaluation

Perform a semen evaluation as part of the reproductive examination to determine the male's fertility status and to provide samples for cytology and culture. The technique for collection of ejaculate is described in Chapters 104 and 114. Perform the microscopic examination of sperm immediately after collection. Semen evaluation determines the following:

Color

- Semen is normally white to opalescent and opaque.
- Semen that has a green tint, with or without clumps, clots, or flakes, is found with infection in the reproductive tract.
- Red semen is generally the result of hemorrhage from the prostate gland or from a traumatized engorged penis.
- Any agent (urine, purulent debris, blood) that contaminates the semen can affect the concentration, motility, and life of the sperm.

Motility

- A normal semen sample contains greater than 70% of sperm progressing in a forward direction.
- Spermatozoa moving in circles or in a side-to-side motion, without forward progress, are not normal.
- The percentage of actively motile sperm is reduced when the semen is exposed to temperature extremes, water, urine, purulent debris, blood, or lubricants.

Sperm Number

- The number of sperm in an ejaculate varies, depending in part on the age, testicular weight, sexual activity, and possibly season of the year. Sperm are counted using a hemocytometer.
- Normal fertility is thought to be possible when the sperm count is over 200 million in an ejaculate.
- When damage occurs to the seminiferous tubules from scrotal or testicular disease, the sperm count drops for a period of weeks to months.

Interpretation

- No single characteristic is an accurate measure of fertility.
- For a male to be considered acceptable for breeding, the semen evaluation exceeds the minimum criteria suggested for percentage of progressive motile sperm, sperm concentration per ejaculate, and sperm morphology.
- Reevaluate several semen samples over 6 months before permanent infertility is diagnosed.

Bacterial Culture and Brucella Testing

- Bacterial cultures from deep draining wounds identify the causative organism(s). Superficial wounds are often contaminated with organisms from the environment.
- Culture of the sperm-rich fraction of the ejaculate identifies the organisms that originate in the testes and prostate.
- Culture of the prostatic fraction is more specific for prostatic organisms (see Chap. 104).
- If each fraction is cultured separately, the sperm-rich fraction and prostatic fraction yield less than 100 bacteria/ml in normal dogs.

▼ *Key Point* Test all males presented for reproductive failure, chronic scrotal dermatitis, or orchitis for *B. canis.*

- *B. canis* infections may cause orchitis, epididymitis, testicular atrophy, discospondylitis, generalized lymphadenopathy, or fever of unknown origin. Use serum agglutination tests to screen for *B. canis*. False-positive findings are possible with this test. Confirm the diagnosis with the cytoplasmic antigen agar-gel immunodiffusion test or blood culture (see Chap. 17).

Cytology

Fine-needle aspiration along with cytology of the testes and scrotum is a rapid and inexpensive method for diagnosis.

- Impression smears of scrotal lesions can uncover fungal elements, neoplastic cells, or other infiltrates.
- Fine-needle aspiration of the epididymis is indicated when palpation of the epididymis is abnormal or when azoospermia is present. The aspirate is evaluated for live motile sperm, inflammatory cells, and bacteria.

- Fine-needle aspiration of the testicle should demonstrate mature spermatozoa and all phases of maturing seminiferous epithelium. Inflammatory cells, bacteria, or neoplastic cells might also be detected.

Biopsy

A testicular biopsy is indicated to assess histology when reduction or lack of sperm in the ejaculate persists. The purpose of the biopsy is to identify the etiology of the problem, to formulate a rational therapeutic plan, and to provide a prognosis. The technique for testicular biopsy is described in Chapter 107. Complications as the result of a testicular biopsy are uncommon but include immune-mediated orchitis or testicular atrophy.

Other Tests

When testicular atrophy is discovered, endocrinopathy due to testicular neoplasia or hormone-producing organs may be responsible.

- Hypothyroidism adversely affects reproductive function. Evaluate thyroid hormone levels in any male showing poor libido and lethargy (see Chap. 29).
- Abnormal cortisol levels (excessive or deficient) also adversely affect reproductive function (see Chap. 31).
- Testosterone levels can become elevated with interstitial cell tumors. Testosterone deficiency may be detected in a female pseudohermaphrodite.
- Estradiol elevations may be detected with Sertoli cell tumors or with seminomas.
- Variation in luteinizing hormone (LH) levels have not been correlated with specific changes in testicular function or disease.
- Follicle-stimulating hormone (FSH) concentrations have been found to become elevated in direct proportion to the amount of histologic damage to the seminiferous epithelium. The highest levels are found when the seminiferous tubules contain only the Sertoli cells.
- Karyotyping is used to determine the chromosomal composition of a suspected intersex abnormality (XXY) (Chap. 114).

TREATMENT

Remove the causative agent of disease whenever possible.

- Discontinue exposure to all drugs whenever they are not required for the long-term well-being of the individual.
- Scrotal irritants such as soaps, detergents, and disinfectants that are used in the cages and kennels must be diluted and rinsed well after use.
- Do not apply topical insecticide sprays, dips, or grooming products to the scrotum.

If an endocrinopathy has been identified in the diagnostic workup, institute appropriate therapy. The semen quality does not show improvement for several months after control of these endocrinopathies has been achieved.

Cryptorchidism

Treatment of choice for cryptorchidism is bilateral castration (see Chap. 107).

- Surgical therapy to place a retained testis into the scrotum is an unethical practice and is not offered as an option.

Superficial Scrotal Lesions

Topical therapy can prove beneficial for superficial scrotal lesions.

- Careful daily rinsing and cleansing along with judicious use of topical ointments (e.g., Panolog, Solvay) prove most helpful.
- An Elizabethan collar is often necessary to prevent further irritation caused by licking.
- Scrotal swelling and inflammation are reduced as rapidly as possible with cold water or ice to minimize heat damage to the testes.

Septic Orchiepididymitis

Systemic therapy is required for septic orchiepididymitis.

- In dogs with acute orchiepididymitis—when maintaining fertility is not a concern—treatment is aimed at stabilization with IV fluids and broad-spectrum antibiotics. The antibiotic of choice, before culture results are available, is trimethoprim-sulfadiazine most commonly, or an aminoglycoside. Resistant *Staphylococcus* infections may require treatment with a cephalosporin or oxacillin. Orchiectomy is performed once stabilization has been achieved.
- If the owner desires reproductive function maintained in the animal with acute orchiepididymitis, therapy is expanded beyond supportive care with intravenous fluids and systemic antibiotics. Cold compresses are placed on the scrotum to minimize thermal damage to the germinal epithelium. An anti-inflammatory agent, such as corticosteroid or aspirin, may be used to control inflammation, local hyperthermia, and exposure of the immune system to spermatozoal antigens following disruption of the blood-testis barrier. Unilateral orchiectomy may be necessary to prevent damage to an unaffected testis. The prognosis for maintaining normal fertility is guarded.
- If chronic orchiepididymitis is diagnosed, the prognosis for fertility is guarded to poor. When a positive culture occurs, administer appropriate antibiotic therapy for a minimum of 3 weeks. If plasmacytic lymphocytic infiltration is identified histologically, immunosuppressive drugs (e.g., prednisone, cyclophosphamide, or azathioprine) may be beneficial.
- Do not use a dog positively diagnosed with *B. canis* as a breeding animal, because it is a potential source of infection for other dogs and for humans. Neuter or euthanize affected animals. Treatment attempts can be expensive and offer little hope for cure. Persistent bacteremia may be eliminated during antibiotic therapy but often recurs in 1–3 months after therapy. An-

tibiotics that have been recommended are minocycline, which is very expensive, and doxycycline or tetracycline, in combination with an aminoglycoside (see Chap. 17).

Other Diseases

Perform orchiectomy for conditions that have no treatment protocol or for which treatment has failed (see Chap. 107). Orchiectomy is indicated with testicular torsion, testicular hypoplasia, and testicular ductular aplasia or for cryptorchid dogs over 6 months of age. Orchiectomy may also be necessary to correct scrotal hernias. After removal of the testicle and spermatic cord, ligate the hernial sac with a transfixing ligature. Consider unilateral orchiectomy when there is unilateral trauma, infection, or tumor in a male that is intended to continue breeding. Remove the testicles of infertile males to reduce the risk of androgen-induced conditions (prostatitis, neoplasia, perineal hernia).

Submit abnormal testicles for histopathologic evaluation following surgery.

SUPPLEMENTAL READINGS

Barsanti JA: Abnormalities of the external genitalia. *In* Lorenz MD, Cornelius LM, eds.: Small Animal Medical Diagnosis. Philadelphia: JB Lippincott, 1987, p 366.

Cox VS: Cryptorchidism in the dog. *In* Morrow DA, ed.: Current Therapy in Theriogenology 2, Philadelphia: WB Saunders, 1986, p 541.

Feldman EC, Nelson RW: Disorders of the testes and epididymides. *In* Feldman EC, Nelson RW, eds.: Canine and Feline Endocrinology and Reproduction, 2nd Ed. Philadelphia: WB Saunders, 1996, p 697.

Johnson CA: Disorders of the canine testicles and epididymides. *In* Morrow DA, ed.: Current Therapy in Theriogenology 2. Philadelphia: WB Saunders, 1986, p 551.

Seager SWJ: Semen collection and evaluation in the dog. *In* Morrow DA, ed.: Current Therapy in Theriogenology 2. Philadelphia: WB Saunders, 1986, p 539.

107 Surgery of the Testes and Scrotum

Harry W. Boothe

Orchidectomy is the most commonly performed surgical procedure of the testis. The technique depends, in part, on species and location of the testes (i.e., ectopic or scrotal). Indications for performing orchidectomy are listed in Table 107–1. Testicular biopsy may be part of a fertility examination. Scrotal ablation may be part of a routine orchidectomy or for neoplasia resection, especially in older dogs. It is also performed at the time of scrotal urethrostomy and feline perineal urethrostomy.

▼ *Key Point* Obtain owner consent before performing orchidectomy as a primary procedure or concurrently with another surgical procedure.

ANATOMY

- The testes are positioned obliquely within the scrotum, with their long axis directed dorsocaudally.
- The scrotal testis is covered by peritoneum (parietal and visceral vaginal tunics) and a dense, white, fibrous capsule (tunica albuginea).
- The testis and epididymis are connected to the parietal vaginal tunic by the caudal ligament of the epididymis.
- The arterial and venous patterns are similar, with the right testicular artery originating from the abdominal aorta cranial to the left and the veins forming an extensive pampiniform plexus in the spermatic cord.
- The right testicular vein empties into the caudal vena cava, whereas the left terminates in the left renal vein; testicular lymphatics drain to the median iliac lymph nodes.
- The canine scrotum is located more ventrally than the feline.

Table 107–1. INDICATIONS FOR PERFORMING ORCHIDECTOMY IN THE DOG AND CAT

Sterilization	Prostatic cyst
Modification of behavior patterns	Perineal adenoma
Testicular neoplasia	Perineal hernia
Severe testicular or scrotal trauma	Scrotal urethrostomy (canine)
Refractory orchitis/epididymitis	
Benign prostatic hyperplasia	Perineal urethrostomy (feline)
Suppurative prostatitis	

- The scrotal wall consists of the skin and dartos, a layer of smooth muscle and elastic fibers.
- The external spermatic fascia attaches to the caudal aspect of the scrotum as the scrotal ligament.
- Blood supply to the scrotum is principally via branches of the external pudendal artery; lymphatic drainage is to the inguinal lymph nodes.

TESTICULAR BIOPSY

See Chapter 114 for indications.

Preoperative Considerations

- Usually only one testis is sampled.
- Incisional techniques usually provide the best tissue samples for analysis.
- Fixation of specimens in Bouin's, Zenker's, or Stieve's fixative is preferable to formalin fixation because of better preservation of architectural detail.

Surgical Procedure

Objectives

- Obtain a representative sample of the testis for histologic evaluation.
- Minimally disrupt the testicular architecture.

Equipment

- Standard general surgical pack and suture
- Sterile, thin razor blade
- Bouin's, Zenker's, or Stieve's fixative

Technique

1. Place the animal in dorsal recumbency and aseptically prepare the prescrotal area.
2. Incise the skin just cranial to the scrotum and place the testis with the epididymis away from the incision.
3. Incise the tunics with a scalpel blade and the tunica albuginea with a sterile, thin razor blade, while avoiding blood vessels.
4. Excise the bulging testicular tissue using the razor blade, or, if testicular tissue does not bulge, excise a wedge of testicular parenchyma. The razor blade's sharp, flat blade makes it ideal for this procedure.
5. Close the tunica albuginea and the tunics separately (simple interrupted pattern, 4-0 absorbable suture).

6. Routinely close the skin (simple interrupted pattern, nonabsorbable suture).

Postoperative Care and Complications

- Uncommon complications include hemorrhage, infection, scarring, adhesions, and atrophy.
- A temporary slight decrease in sperm count may occur.

Prognosis

- The prognosis depends on the disease process(es) present.
- Minimal patient morbidity is expected.

ORCHIDECTOMY IN THE DOG

Preoperative Considerations

- Determine the location of the testes before surgery.
- Remove scrotal testes using either the closed or open method (choice of technique is surgeon's preference).
- Approach an abdominal testis through a parapreputial skin incision, and an extra-abdominal ectopic testis by incising directly over the testis.
- Histologically examine all ectopic and grossly abnormal testes.

Surgical Procedures

Objectives

- Remove both testes.
- Minimize postoperative complications and patient morbidity.

Equipment

- Standard general surgical pack and suture

Technique for Scrotal Testis (Closed Technique)

1. Place the dog in dorsal recumbency and aseptically prepare the prescrotal area. Avoid clipping and scrubbing the scrotal skin to minimize dermal irritation.
2. Incise the prescrotal skin on the midline while gently pushing one testis toward the skin incision.
3. Incise the subcutaneous tissue and spermatic fascia over the testis to expose the parietal vaginal tunic.
4. Exteriorize the tunic-covered testis and, using scissors, incise the spermatic fascia and scrotal ligament close to the testis.
5. Reflect the fat and fascia surrounding the parietal vaginal tunic using a gauze sponge to enable maximal exteriorization of the spermatic cord.
6. Double-ligate the intact spermatic cord and vaginal tunics using transfixation ligatures of absorbable suture material (Fig. 107–1).
7. Transect the spermatic cord and cremaster muscle distal to the ligatures and return them to the inguinal region.

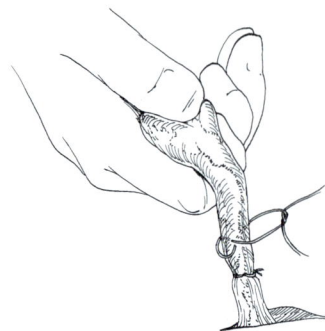

Figure 107–1. Transfixation (double) ligation of the intact spermatic cord. The suture needle is carefully passed through the spermatic cord between the cremaster muscle and the ductus deferens. The entire spermatic cord is enclosed in the ligature.

8. Routinely close the subcutaneous tissue (simple interrupted pattern, absorbable suture) and skin (simple continuous intradermal pattern, absorbable suture or routine skin closure with monofilament nonabsorbable suture).

Technique for Scrotal Testis (Open Technique)

1. Exteriorize the testis as described for the closed technique.
2. Incise the parietal vaginal tunic where ligatures are to be placed on the spermatic cord.
3. Double-ligate the spermatic cord using transfixation ligatures of absorbable material.
4. Alternatively, incise the parietal vaginal tunic over the testis, and then double-ligate the spermatic cord using transfixation ligatures of absorbable material.
5. Ligate the parietal vaginal tunic and cremaster muscle using a transfixation ligature; transect the spermatic cord and cremaster muscle, and return them to the inguinal region.
6. Routinely close the subcutaneous tissue (simple interrupted pattern, absorbable suture) and skin (simple continuous intradermal pattern, absorbable suture or routine skin closure with monofilament suture).

Technique for Abdominal Ectopic Testis

1. Place the dog in dorsal recumbency and aseptically prepare the ventral abdominal region from the xiphoid process to caudal to the pubic brim.
2. Incise the skin and ventral abdominal wall from the umbilicus to the pubis while avoiding the prepuce. A midline abdominal approach is used.
3. Locate the ectopic testis by tracing one of the following:
   - Ductus deferens from its prostatic termination
   - Testicular artery from its aortic origin
   - Testicular vein from its termination in the caudal vena cava (or left renal vein)
   - Gubernaculum testis to the testis
4. Double-ligate the testicular vessels and ductus deferens.
5. Transect the vessels and ductus deferens; remove the testis and submit it for biopsy.
6. Routinely close the abdominal wall.

Technique for Extra-Abdominal Ectopic Testis

1. Place the dog in dorsal recumbency and prepare the pubic region.
2. Incise the skin and subcutaneous tissue directly over the testis. Remove any loose connective tissue to expose the spermatic cord.
3. Double-ligate and transect the spermatic cord.
4. If the testis is not found subcutaneously, extend the incision into a paramedian approach to the abdomen and find the testis, as previously described.
5. Routinely close the subcutaneous tissue (simple interrupted pattern, absorbable suture) and skin (simple interrupted pattern, nonabsorbable suture).

Postoperative Care and Complications

Short-Term

- Scrotal bruising and inflammation, particularly following the open technique.
- Hemorrhage, which may be serious. Severe scrotal swelling from hemorrhage may necessitate scrotal ablation.
- Scrotal infection, which may require drainage or scrotal ablation.
- Use an Elizabethan collar to help prevent self-inflicted trauma. Intradermal skin closure also helps to prevent self-trauma to the incision.
- Inadvertent prostatectomy has been reported as a complication of removal of abdominal ectopic testes.

Prognosis

- Prognosis following orchidectomy of the cryptorchid dog is generally favorable even with testicular neoplasia, which usually is benign.

ORCHIDECTOMY IN THE CAT

Preoperative Considerations

See Orchidectomy in the Dog.

Surgical Procedure

Objectives

See Orchidectomy in the Dog.

Equipment

- Standard minor surgical pack

Technique

1. Position the cat in dorsal recumbency with the rear limbs pulled cranially, and aseptically prepare the perineal region.
2. Incise the scrotum over each testis and expose the testis.
3. Grasp the parietal vaginal tunic with hemostats, separate it from the testis, and excise it.
4. Separate the ductus deferens from the rest of the spermatic cord and separate it from the testis.

5. Tie two square knots in the spermatic cord, using the ductus deferens and spermatic vessels as separate strands, and transect the spermatic cord distal to the knots.
6. Alternatively, ligate the spermatic cord using an instrument-tied overhand knot with absorbable suture material.
7. Do not suture the scrotal incision.

▼ *Key Point* The traction avulsion technique of feline orchidectomy is *not* advisable because of the potential for significant postoperative complications, including hemorrhage and urethral avulsion.

Postoperative Care and Complications

See Orchidectomy in the Dog.

Prognosis

See Orchidectomy in the Dog.

SCROTAL ABLATION

Preoperative Considerations

- Indications include severe trauma, neoplasia, ischemia, scrotal abscess, orchidectomy in old dogs with pendulous scrotums, scrotal urethrostomy, and feline perineal urethrostomy.

▼ *Key Point* Plan the skin incisions to leave sufficient skin for tension-free closure.

Surgical Procedure

Objectives

- Reduce postoperative problems following orchidectomy in the dog.
- Allow incision into the urethra and subsequent urethrostomy.
- Remove redundant scrotal tissue.

Equipment

- Standard general surgical pack and suture

Technique

1. Place the animal in dorsal recumbency and prepare the periscrotal region.
2. Incise the skin in an elliptical, curvilinear fashion near the base of the scrotum, with the incisions curved toward the scrotum (Fig. 107–2).
3. Transect the scrotal septum after orchidectomy and routinely close the subcutaneous tissue (simple interrupted pattern, absorbable suture) and skin (simple interrupted pattern, nonabsorbable suture).

Postoperative Care and Complications

Short-Term

- Prevent self-inflicted trauma to the incision. This may require an Elizabethan collar.

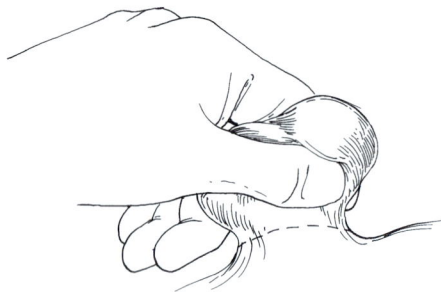

Figure 107–2. Ablation of the scrotum in the dog. The curved scrotal skin incision curves toward the scrotum to ensure tension-free closure of the incision. (From Harvey CE: Scrotal ablation and castration in the dog. J Am Anim Hosp Assoc 9:170, 1973.)

- Common complications include hemorrhage, particularly associated with urethrostomy procedures (see Chap. 102), infection, and dehiscence.

Prognosis

- Minimal patient morbidity is expected.

SUPPLEMENTAL READINGS

Boothe HW: Penis, prepuce, and scrotum. *In* Slatter D, ed.: Textbook of Small Animal Surgery, 2nd Ed. Philadelphia: WB Saunders, 1993, p 1336.

Boothe HW: Testes and epididymides. *In* Slatter D, ed.: Textbook of Small Animal Surgery, 2nd Ed. Philadelphia: WB Saunders, 1993, p 1325.

Crane SW: Orchiectomy of descended and retained testes in the dog and cat. *In* Bojrab MJ, ed.: Current Techniques in Small Animal Surgery, 4th Ed. Philadelphia: Lea & Febiger, 1998, p 517.

Evans HE, Christensen GC: Miller's Anatomy of the Dog, 3rd Ed. Philadelphia: WB Saunders, 1993, p 504.

Harvey CE: Scrotal ablation and castration in the dog. J Am Anim Hosp Assoc 9:170, 1973.

Larsen RE: Testicular biopsy in the dog. Vet Clin North Am Small Anim Pract 7:747, 1977.

Millis DL, Hauptman JG, Johnson CA: Cryptorchidism and monorchism in cats: 25 cases (1980–1989). J Am Vet Med Assoc 200:1128, 1992.

Pettit GD: There's more than one way to castrate a cat. Modern Vet Pract 62:713, 1981.

Phillips JT, Leeds EB: A closed technique for canine orchiectomy. Canine Pract 3:23, 1976.

Romagnoli SE: Canine cryptorchidism. Vet Clin North Am Small Anim Pract 21:533, 1991.

108 Diseases of the Penis and Prepuce

Susan F. Soderberg

Diseases of the penis and prepuce are most commonly characterized by abnormal discharges at the preputial orifice. Alternatively, defects may be present which do not allow for the normal movement of the prepuce over the penis. These defects may not allow the penis to be extended from the prepuce, causing pain and inability to breed, or the penis may become trapped outside the prepuce, resulting in compromised venous return and traumatic injury from exposure.

ETIOLOGY

Underlying causes of disease found in the penis and prepuce include:

- Congenital defects
- Balanoposthitis
- Traumatic injuries
- Foreign material
- Neoplasia

Congenital Defects

Congenital diseases of the penis and prepuce include hypospadias, penile hypoplasia, persistent penile frenulum, preputial stenosis, and phimosis. These defects are responsible for compromising the normal movement of the penis in or out of the prepuce.

Hypospadias. Hypospadias and/or failure of preputial closure is the result of failure of the genital folds and/or genital swellings to fuse during fetal development. This failure results in abnormal development of the penile urethra, penis, prepuce, or scrotum.

- Most commonly, the urethral opening is found to be abnormally positioned ventral and caudal to its normal opening at the tip of the penis.
- Occasionally, the urethral opening will be found in the perineal region.
- The penis commonly is underdeveloped, and the prepuce is incomplete ventrally.

Penile Hypoplasia. Penile hypoplasia is an underdevelopment of the penis such that it is much shorter than the prepuce. Urine may pool within the prepuce, often causing irritation of the preputial lining and infection.

- This defect is most frequently found in the Great Dane, collie, Doberman pinscher, and cocker spaniel.

- Penile hypoplasia may be an indication of female pseudohermaphroditism.

Persistent Penile Frenulum. This is a band of connective tissue extending from the ventral tip of the penis to the prepuce. The band unites the penis and prepuce during fetal development.

- Normally the penile frenulum ruptures before puberty as a result of normal mechanical stress.
- When the connective tissue persists, it hinders extrusion of the penis from the prepuce and causes deviation of the penile tip in a ventral or lateral direction.

Preputial Stenosis. In this condition, the preputial opening is extremely small, compromising the extrusion of the penis (phimosis) and/or the flow of urine. If urine cannot escape, infection is a common sequela.

- In neonates, septicemia may result and cause death by 10 days of age.
- This severe neonatal defect is most frequently found in the German shepherd dog and golden retriever.

Os Penis Deformity. Deformity of the os penis results in deviation of the penis, occasionally causing inability to retract the penis fully into the prepuce.

- A congenitally shortened os penis may result in excessive flaccidity of the penile tip, causing impaired copulation.

Balanoposthitis

Balanoposthitis is inflammation of the penile and preputial mucosa.

- The most common cause is bacterial infection. Other sporadic infectious causes include canine herpesvirus and fungi such as *Candida* and *Blastomyces*.
- Mild infection causing a small amount of yellow-green discharge from the preputial opening is so common in dogs that it generally is considered normal.
- Copious amounts of purulent discharge require further investigation and treatment.

Trauma

Causes of trauma to the penis and prepuce include a fall, a blow to the inguinal region, or injuries inflicted by fighting.

- Traumatic injury may result in contusion, hematoma formation, laceration, or fracture of the os penis.

Foreign Body

Foreign bodies may be accidentally or maliciously lodged within the prepuce or around the penis.

- Grass awns, other plant material, or small objects may be entrapped in the preputial cavity, often causing balanoposthitis.
- Preputial hair or rubber bands may be wrapped around the penis, causing venous engorgement that prevents the penis from retracting back into the prepuce (paraphimosis).

▼ *Key Point* If the penis becomes trapped outside the prepuce, severe injury, desiccation, and necrosis of the penis may rapidly occur.

- Urethral obstruction can occur secondary to paraphimosis.

Neoplasms

Neoplasms involving the mucosa of the prepuce and penile surface include transmissible venereal tumors, papillomas, and carcinomas.

- Urethral neoplasms such as transitional cell carcinoma, squamous cell carcinoma, and rhabdomyosarcoma occasionally extend to the penis.
- Transmissible venereal tumor (TVT) is a contagious tumor found on the external genitalia of male and female dogs.
  - It is spread primarily by sexual contact but can also spread by licking and other forms of contact.
  - In the male, it is most often found as a fleshy, friable mass at the base of the penis.

CLINICAL SIGNS

- *Purulent preputial discharge* in copious amounts occurs with balanoposthitis, urine pooling in the prepuce, foreign bodies, and occasionally neoplasms. Discomfort and excessive licking often are exhibited when purulent discharges are present.
- *Hemorrhagic discharge* can occur with traumatic injuries, neoplasms, and bleeding in the urinary tract. Lesions of the urinary tract that may cause hemorrhage from the prepuce include prostatitis, urethral prolapse, calculi, trauma, and neoplasia. Clinical signs when hemorrhagic discharge is present include excessive licking and discomfort.
- *Urine scalding of the abdomen and perineum* may occur with hypospadias and penile hypoplasia.
- Urinating in unexpected directions (e.g., on the rear feet) may be noticed with a persistent penile frenulum, causing deviation of the penile tip.
- *Unwillingness or inability to copulate* due to pain when attempting an erection or the inability to extend the penis can be signs of persistent penile frenulum, deformity of the os penis, or preputial stenosis.
- *Absence of clinical signs* despite the presence of disease is common.

DIAGNOSIS

History

Obtain a complete history and determine the duration of events associated with the onset of signs.

▼ *Key Point* Determine if there is a history of systemic illness, traumatic episodes, or breeding problems in animals with penile or preputial diseases.

Physical Examination

Perform a complete physical examination before investigating the source of the complaint.

- Visually inspect the prepuce, penis, and urethral orifice.
- Normal findings include the following:
  - The prepuce is complete ventrally and completely covers the penis in its normal position.
  - A small amount of yellow-green discharge is found at the preputial orifice in dogs.
  - The prepuce moves freely over the penis and the penis is easily exposed by pulling the prepuce caudally over the bulbus glandis.
  - The penile mucosa is pinkish white, smooth, and nonpainful to the touch.
  - The urethral orifice is located at the tip of the penis.
- Hyperplasia of the lymphoid follicles in the area of the bulbus glandis and preputial mucosa is common in many male dogs.
- Palpate the penis and os penis to the brim of the pelvis. Swellings may be caused by a urolith, foreign body, hematoma, fracture of the os penis, or neoplasm.
- Perform a rectal examination to rule out prostatic disease and diseases of the pelvic urethra.
- Catheterize the urethra if trauma or obstruction is suspected.

Imaging Studies

- Radiography may be used to detect congenital defects of the os penis, fractures of the os penis, and defects of the pelvis and pelvic canal.
- Contrast urethrography may be performed to identify obstructive lesions, diverticula, and traumatic damage of the urethra.

Laboratory Studies

Cytology

Cytology of preputial discharges and masses can help to determine their etiology.

- Cytology of the normal preputial discharge contains variable numbers of epithelial cells, inflammatory cells (primarily neutrophils), and extracellular bacteria.
- Balanoposthitis is characterized by large numbers of toxic neutrophils, often containing bacteria.
- Causative agents (foreign material or fungi) may also be detected by cytologic inspection of the discharge.

- Cytology of TVT reveals large round cells with numerous mitotic figures. The cells resemble lymphoblasts.
- Perform histopathologic diagnosis of all neoplasms in order to formulate the best therapeutic plan.

Culture and Sensitivity Testing

- To determine the most effective therapy for bacterial infections, perform culture and susceptibility testing of all preputial discharges.
- Culture for herpesvirus usually is unsuccessful; however, a fourfold rise in serum neutralization titers may indicate a diagnosis of herpesvirus. Herpesvirus infection usually has no clinical signs in adult dogs (see Chap. 14).

Cytogenetic Evaluation

- To detect female pseudohermaphrodites, perform cytogenetic karyotype evaluation in dogs with hypospadias or penile hypoplasia.

TREATMENT

The objectives of medical therapy are:

- Elimination or prevention of infection
- Prevention of adhesion formation
- Reduction of inflammation

Medical Therapy

Trauma

- In animals with traumatic injury to the penis and prepuce, apply local pressure to control hemorrhage, and then cleanse and debride the wounds. Be certain the urethra has not been compromised.
- Sutures may be necessary, depending on the nature of the wound.
- After the wounds are repaired, extrude the penis from the prepuce twice daily in order to apply an antibiotic ointment and prevent adhesions.

Balanthoposthitis

- Apply specific topical antibacterial ointments and administer broad-spectrum systemic antimicrobial drugs, such as trimethoprim-sulfadiazine, after foreign bodies or other predisposing factors are eliminated.
- Remove copious preputial discharges and foreign debris with a douche of 10% povidone-iodine (Betadine).

Paraphimosis

- Treat paraphimosis promptly to prevent further trauma and vascular compromise to the exposed penis.

- Heavy sedation or anesthesia may be necessary to provide adequate therapy.
- Thoroughly cleanse, lubricate, and replace the penis into the prepuce. Cool water soaks or hypertonic dextrose solutions may be applied to reduce edema.
- Remove any foreign material such as preputial hair constricting the penis.
- If the penis cannot be replaced into the prepuce, the preputial orifice may need to be enlarged (see Chap. 109).
- If severe necrosis of the penis has developed from prolonged exposure and vascular compromise, amputation of the penis may be necessary (see Chap. 109).

Transmissible Venereal Tumor

- Transmissible venereal tumors are treated most successfully with chemotherapeutic regimens. Vincristine (Oncovin, Lilly) is effective administered at a dosage of 0.5 mg/m^2, IV, once a week for 3–6 weeks.

Surgical Therapy

- Surgical correction of congenital or acquired conformational defects is indicated if the dog has clinical signs.
- Conditions that require surgical intervention include hypospadias, penile hypoplasia, preputial stenosis, deviation or fractures of the os penis, or a persistent penile frenulum. (Specific reconstructive techniques are discussed in Chap. 109).
- Surgical resection of carcinomas should be radical whenever possible. Amputation of the penis and sheath may be necessary for complete tumor removal (see Chap. 109).

SUPPLEMENTAL READINGS

Barsanti JA: Vaginal and preputial discharges. *In* Lorenz MD, Cornelius LM, eds.: Small Animal Medical Diagnosis. Philadelphia: JB Lippincott, 1987, p 359.

Feldman EC, Nelson RW: Disorders of the penis and prepuce. *In* Feldman EC, Nelson RW, eds.: Canine and Feline Endocrinology and Reproduction, 2nd Ed. Philadelphia: WB Saunders, 1996, p 691.

Hornbuckle WE, White ME: Preputial discharge in the dog. *In* Kirk RW, ed.: Current Veterinary Therapy X. Philadelphia: WB Saunders, 1989, p 1259.

Johnston SD: Disorders of the canine penis and prepuce. *In* Morrow DA, ed.: Current Therapy in Theriogenology 2. Philadelphia: WB Saunders, 1986, p 549.

Surgical procedures of the penis and prepuce include:

- Penile amputation to treat traumatic or neoplastic lesions
- Enlargement of the preputial orifice to treat phimosis or paraphimosis
- Cranial advancement of the prepuce to treat minor deficiency in preputial length
- Severance of persistent penile frenulum

Diagnosis and medical treatment of penile problems are discussed in Chapter 108.

ANATOMY

Penis

- The feline penis is shorter, directed caudally, and covered with small papillae compared with its canine counterpart, but both species have three principal penile divisions: root, body, and distal portion (glans).
- The penile corpora contain enlarged venous spaces and have two principal divisions: the corpora cavernosa and the corpus spongiosum.
- Each corpus cavernosum (right and left) arises from the ischial tuberosity, continues distally in the dorsolateral part of the penile body as far as the os penis, and is covered by the tunica albuginea.
- The corpus spongiosum originates within the pelvic cavity, surrounds the penile urethra throughout its course, and supplies both the bulbus glandis and pars longa glandis in the distal penis.
- The os penis is located in the penile body and is attached to the bulbus glandis, pars longa glandis, and tunica albuginea.
- The four paired extrinsic penile muscles in the dog are retractor penis, ischiocavernosus, bulbospongiosus, and ischiourethralis.
- The principal blood supply to the penis is from three branches of the artery of the penis, which are continuations of the internal pudendal artery: artery of the bulb, deep artery of the penis, and dorsal artery of the penis.
- Venous drainage occurs via the internal and external pudendal veins. Lymphatic drainage is to the inguinal lymph nodes.
- See Chapter 102 for penile anatomy associated with perineal urethrostomy in cats.

Prepuce

- The canine and feline prepuce covers the nonerect penis.
- Paired preputial muscles extend from the xiphoid cartilage to the dorsal preputial wall.
- Blood supply is via the caudal superficial epigastric artery and dorsal artery of the penis; lymphatic drainage is to the inguinal lymph nodes.

PENILE AMPUTATION

Preoperative Considerations

- The location and extensiveness of traumatic or neoplastic penile lesions determine the site of penile amputation. Animals with urethral prolapse that recurs after attempts to resect urethral mucosa may require partial penile amputation. Nonsurgical management of certain neoplasms of the penis (e.g., transmissible venereal tumor) may be preferable (see Chap. 108).
- Preputial shortening may be indicated after partial penile amputation.
- Bilateral orchidectomy, scrotal ablation, and either scrotal (preferred) or perineal urethrostomy are indicated following extensive penile amputation.

Surgical Procedure

Objectives

- Provide hemostasis by ligation of blood vessels and closure of the tunica albuginea.
- Create a permanent urethrostomy by suturing urethral mucosa to either penile mucosa or skin.
- Avoid an osteotomy by positioning the amputation site either cranial or caudal to the os penis.

Equipment

- Standard general surgical pack and suture
- Penrose drain tubing for temporary tourniquet application

Technique—Partial Amputation

1. Place the dog in dorsal recumbency, prepare the preputial cavity by multiple flushes with chlorhexidine solution (Nolvasan; Fort Dodge), and catheterize the urethra.

2. Maintain penile exteriorization from the prepuce by placing Penrose drain tubing in tourniquet fashion around the penis as far caudally as possible.
3. Create bilateral flaps of the tunic and cavernous tissue, using sharp dissection, proximal to the os penis while leaving the urethra intact.
4. Dissect the urethra and transect it just distal to the proposed amputation site.
5. Transect the os penis, if necessary, with bone-cutting forceps at the base of the flap.
6. Identify and ligate blood vessels after loosening the tourniquet and appose the tunica albuginea and flaps of erectile tissue (simple interrupted pattern, absorbable suture).
7. Suture urethral mucosa to penile mucosa over the ventral portion of the end of the penile stump (simple interrupted, absorbable suture) after incising the urethra along its ventral midline (Fig. 109–1).

Technique—Subtotal Penile Amputation

1. Place the dog in dorsal recumbency and prepare the ventral abdominal and perineal regions.
2. Incise the skin in a curvilinear fashion from just cranial to the prepuce, along each side of the prepuce to an appropriate level on the perineal midline.
3. Isolate and temporarily encircle the penis cranial to the scrotum, using a heavy ligature proximal to the initial transection site.
4. Transect and remove the penis, prepuce, testes, and scrotum.
5. Exteriorize the proximal portion of the penis through a separate midline perineal skin incision or through the caudal aspect of the original skin incision. Remove the temporary ligature, provide definitive hemostasis, and close the tunica albuginea over

the end of the penis (simple interrupted pattern, absorbable suture).
6. Perform a scrotal or perineal urethrostomy proximal to the penile amputation site (simple interrupted or continuous pattern, nonabsorbable sutures) (see Chap. 102).
7. Routinely close the ventral abdominal incision.

Postoperative Care and Complications

- Hemorrhage and/or hematoma formation may occur at the penile amputation or urethrostomy site.
- Prevent self-inflicted trauma with an Elizabethan collar or a side brace.

Prognosis

- The prognosis depends on the disease process(es) present.
- Urethral stricture may occur if healing is complicated (e.g., urethral mucosal dehiscence occurs).
- Minimal long-term patient morbidity is expected.

ENLARGEMENT OF THE PREPUTIAL ORIFICE

Preoperative Considerations

- Use this procedure to correct phimosis (multiple attempts may be necessary in the young dog) or paraphimosis. Position the incision on the dorsal aspect of the prepuce to avoid persistent exposure of the glans penis.
- Castration of the patient as well as preputial orifice reconstruction is recommended to reduce the possibility of paraphimosis recurrence following erection.

Surgical Procedure
Objectives

- Enlarge the preputial orifice to allow unrestricted movement of the penis in and out of the prepuce.
- Minimize fibrous tissue formation by accurately apposing tissues.
- Completely excise neoplasms, if present.

Equipment

- Standard general surgical pack and suture

Technique

1. Position the dog in dorsal recumbency and aseptically prepare the parapreputial area.
2. Depending on the degree of phimosis, either excise a wedge-shaped segment of skin, or make an incision through the subcutaneous tissue and preputial mucosa on the dorsal surface of the prepuce to enable exteriorization of the end of the penis.
3. Appose the preputial mucosa to the skin (simple interrupted pattern, nonabsorbable sutures).

Postoperative Care and Complications

- Prevent self-inflicted trauma to the surgical site (an Elizabethan collar may be necessary).

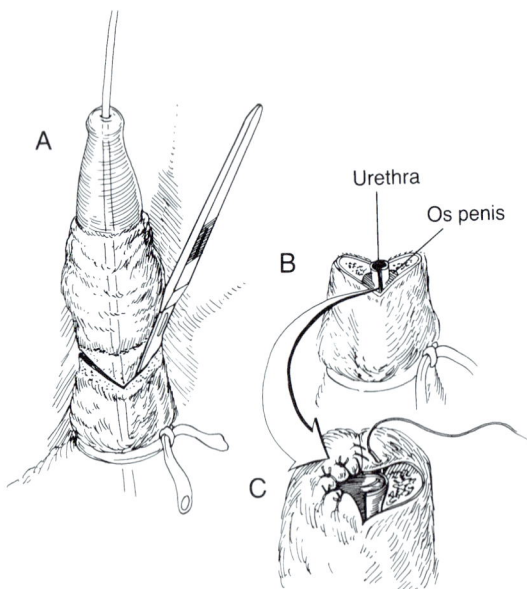

Figure 109–1. Closure of the end of the penis following partial penile amputation. The urethral mucosa is sutured to penile mucosa near the ventrum of the incision, while the remainder of the end of the penis is closed.

- Postoperative fibrosis may create an insufficient preputial orifice.
- Patient growth may necessitate another surgical procedure.

Prognosis

- If a tumor was present, the prognosis generally is good, provided there was a complete excision.

CRANIAL ADVANCEMENT OF THE PREPUCE

Preoperative Consideration

- This procedure is indicated in dogs with incomplete preputial coverage of the penis in order to prevent penile desiccation and irritation. Only minor deficiencies (<1–2 cm) in preputial length can be corrected by advancing the prepuce cranially along the abdominal wall.

Surgical Procedure

Objective

- Achieve complete coverage of the distal penis.

Equipment

- Standard general surgical pack and suture

Technique

1. Place the dog in dorsal recumbency and aseptically prepare the ventral abdomen.
2. Make a U-shaped incision in the skin immediately cranial to the prepuce.
3. Dissect this part of the prepuce from the abdominal skin, advance the prepuce cranially until the penis is covered, and mark this point on the skin.
4. Make a U-shaped incision in the skin at the mark and excise the skin between the two incisions.
5. Suture the prepuce to its cranial position (two-layer closure: subcutaneous tissue with simple interrupted, absorbable suture; skin with simple interrupted, non-absorbable suture).

Postoperative Care and Complications

- Although adequate penile coverage may be achieved at surgery, exposure of the distal penis may recur postoperatively.
- Prevent self-inflicted trauma.

Prognosis

- Repair of congenital preputial defects has a guarded prognosis.
- An extensive preputial deficiency may require partial or subtotal penile amputation (preferred) or preputial reconstruction.

SEVERANCE OF PERSISTENT PENILE FRENULUM

Preoperative Considerations

- The penile frenulum normally ruptures by puberty.
- The persistent penile frenulum usually is composed of minimally vascular connective tissue.

▼ *Key Point* Diagnose persistent frenulum by extruding the penis manually or by observing penile deviation during erection.

Surgical Procedure

Objective

- Sever the persistent penile frenulum to enable painless extrusion of the penis from the prepuce.

Equipment

- Standard minor surgical pack

Technique

1. Place the dog in lateral recumbency and aseptically prepare the preputial cavity.
2. Exteriorize the penis and excise the penile frenulum with scissors. Control hemorrhage with local pressure.

Postoperative Care and Complications

- Prevent self-inflicted trauma.

Prognosis

- The prognosis is good.

SUPPLEMENTAL READINGS

Boothe HW: Penis, prepuce, and scrotum. *In* Slatter D, ed.: Textbook of Small Animal Surgery, 2nd Ed. Philadelphia: WB Saunders, 1993, p 1336.

Evans HE, Christensen GC: Miller's Anatomy of the Dog. Philadelphia: WB Saunders, 1979, p 554.

Hayes AG, Pavletic MM, Schwartz A, et al.: A preputial splitting technique for surgery of the canine penis. J Am Anim Hosp Assoc 30:291, 1994.

Hobson HP: Surgical pathophysiology of the penis. *In* Bojrab MJ, ed.: Disease Mechanisms in Small Animal Surgery, 2nd Ed. Philadelphia: Lea & Febiger, 1993, p 552.

Hobson HP: Surgical procedures of the penis. *In* Bojrab MJ, ed.: Current Techniques in Small Animal Surgery, 4th Ed. Philadelphia: Lea & Febiger, 1998, p 527.

Smith MM, Gourley IM: Preputial reconstruction in a dog. J Am Vet Med Assoc 196:1493, 1990.

110 Diseases of the Ovaries and Uterus

Amy M. Grooters

DISEASES OF THE OVARIES

Primary ovarian disease is uncommon in the dog and cat and includes ovarian cysts and ovarian neoplasia. For information concerning infertility in the bitch and queen, see Chapter 114.

Cystic Ovarian Disease

Ovarian cysts may be normal structures, including vesicular follicles and cavities within immature corpora lutea, or abnormal structures, including follicular cysts and luteinized cysts. Remnant ovarian tissue resulting from incomplete ovariohysterectomy may also become cystic.

Clinical Signs

Signs associated with abnormal ovarian cysts are due to excess sex hormone secretion by the cystic structure or decreased function of the remaining ovarian tissue.

Persistent Anestrus

Persistent anestrus or an increased interestrous interval is the most common clinical sign associated with follicular and luteinized cysts.

- When associated with nonfunctional follicular cysts, this is probably the result of a mass effect of the cystic structure, causing a decrease in the surrounding functional ovarian tissue.
- Luteinized cysts prolong anestrus through persistent progesterone secretion.

Persistent Estrus

The duration of estrus in the bitch usually is 5–9 days and is considered abnormal if it lasts >3 weeks.

- Persistent estrus can be caused by continued secretion of estrogen by follicular cysts, or it can be caused by functional ovarian tumors.
- Persistent estrus may be identified by the owner as behavior consistent with estrus or as persistent hemorrhagic vaginal discharge.
- Differentiate this condition from *split estrus,* which may be seen in young bitches. Split estrus occurs when follicular development is followed by follicular regression instead of progressing to ovulation, result-

ing in clinical signs of proestrus that are not followed by signs of estrus until the bitch enters estrus during a subsequent cycle (usually 2–12 weeks later).

Diagnosis

- Perform *vaginal cytology* to confirm estrogen influence in a bitch displaying signs consistent with persistent estrus. A majority of superficial cells is expected (see Chaps. 112 and 114 for vaginal cytology techniques).
- Measure *plasma estrogen concentrations* to confirm excess estrogen secretion; however, normal concentrations do not rule out functional ovarian cysts.
- *Abdominal ultrasonography* may be used to identify cystic ovarian structures; however, this modality cannot definitively differentiate normal follicles from abnormal cystic structures.
- *Surgical exploration* provides a definitive diagnosis.

Treatment

Surgery

- Ovariohysterectomy (see Chap. 111) is the treatment of choice for nonbreeding animals and is curative.
- Surgical removal of an ovarian cyst or the affected ovary often results in complete resolution of signs and a good prognosis for the future fertility of the bitch.
- Submit excised ovarian tissue for histologic evaluation to differentiate follicular cysts from functional ovarian neoplasia.

Medical Therapy

Pharmacologic agents to induce luteinization of the cysts may be attempted in breeding bitches. The following drugs have been used:

- Gonadotropin-releasing hormone (Cystorelin, Ceva), given IM once at a dosage of 50 µg per bitch.
- Human chorionic gonadotropin (HCG), given once at a dosage of 22 units/kg IM.
- Poor response to treatment and recurrence of cystic disease are possible following medical therapy. Insufficient information is available to evaluate response and recurrence rates or to predict fertility following treatment.
- When medical therapy is successful, response is expected in 2–3 weeks and indicated by a change in vaginal cytology from cornified to noncornified cells.

Spontaneous Regression

- Follicular cysts may undergo atresia or become luteinized without treatment.
- Monitor ovarian cysts using ultrasonography, vaginal cytology, and serum progesterone concentrations if treatment is delayed.

Ovarian Neoplasia

Tumors of the ovary are uncommon in the bitch and queen and are classified according to their embryologic origin as epithelial, germ cell, or sex-cord stromal tumors. The most common ovarian tumors in the bitch are epithelial and granulosa cell tumors.

Classification

Epithelial Tumors

- *Papillary adenoma* is a benign tumor that often occurs bilaterally and is one of the most common ovarian neoplasms seen in the bitch.
- *Papillary adenocarcinoma* is a malignant tumor that frequently is bilateral. Metastasis is common through the ovarian bursa to the abdominal cavity, as well as to regional lymphatics and distant sites. Abdominal cavity metastasis may result in peritoneal effusion. Adenocarcinoma is the most common malignant tumor of the ovary in the bitch.
- *Cystadenoma* is a less common benign epithelial tumor that consists of multiple thin-walled cysts.

Sex-Cord Stromal Tumors

▼ *Key Point* Granulosa cell tumors occur frequently in the bitch and are the most common ovarian tumor in the queen.

- *Granulosa cell tumors* are usually large unilateral tumors that are often palpable, can cause abdominal distention, and may produce signs of hyperestrogenism including persistent estrus. These tumors commonly are malignant in the cat but often are benign in the dog, with metastasis occurring in only 10–25% of cases.
- *Thecomas* and *luteomas* are rare, but these cell types may be found in combination with granulosa cell tumors.

Germ Cell Tumors

- *Dysgerminomas* are uncommon. These large unilateral tumors have a metastatic rate of 10–20%.
- *Teratomas*, which develop as multiple tissue types (e.g., epithelium, cartilage, and bone), are large benign unilateral tumors that may cause a palpable abdominal mass or abdominal enlargement.

Diagnosis

Many ovarian tumors cause no clinical signs and may be incidental findings at necropsy or surgery.

- Most signs associated with ovarian neoplasia are related to a large abdominal mass, peritoneal effusion, local or distant metastasis, or hyperestrogenism.

- Abdominal radiography or ultrasonography can be used to confirm the mass but rarely allows determination of its origin.
- Establish a definitive diagnosis through exploratory laparotomy.

Treatment

Ovariohysterectomy

The treatment of choice for ovarian neoplasia is ovariohysterectomy, which is often curative if metastasis has not occurred. Avoid rupture of the tumor during removal.

- Exploration of the abdomen allows staging of the tumor. Biopsy local lymph nodes if they are enlarged.
- Chemotherapy may be used in addition to surgery for metastatic tumors, but this is only palliative. Cyclophosphamide ($50 \, mg/m^2$, PO, given three times a week) has been used in dogs for granulosa cell tumors and carcinomas.

DISEASES OF THE UTERUS

Pyometra

Pyometra in dogs and cats is the result of hormonally induced changes in the uterus that allow secondary infection to occur. The patency of the cervix (closed or open pyometra) is an important influence on the severity of the disease, its prognosis, and the treatment options that can be offered.

Etiology

Cystic Endometrial Hyperplasia

The first step in the development of pyometra is cystic endometrial hyperplasia (CEH), which is an exaggerated response of the endometrium to progesterone. The mechanism is as follows:

- Following ovulation, the intact female enters a luteal phase (diestrus) that is characterized by elevated plasma progesterone concentrations for 8–10 weeks.
- In preparation for a possible pregnancy, the uterus responds to increases in progesterone with glandular hypertrophy and increased endometrial secretory activity. Prolonged progesterone influence causes this glandular tissue to become cystic, edematous, and grossly thickened.
- Excessive secretions may accumulate within the uterus, providing an ideal environment for bacterial growth. This is complicated by the inhibition of myometrial contractility by progesterone, which decreases uterine drainage.

Exogenously administered progestins, such as megestrol acetate (Ovaban, Shering), result in similar endometrial changes that are especially severe with higher doses or prolonged administration.

Bacterial Infection

Secondary bacterial infections usually originate from contamination through the cervix, and may be facilitated by a progesterone-mediated inhibition of leukocyte function.

- *Escherichia coli*, the most common organism isolated, has a specific affinity for progesterone-sensitized endometrium, and can bind to the endometrium and myometrium through a specific antigen.

Exogenous Estrogens

Exogenous estrogens alone do not cause cystic endometrial hyperplasia, but they do potentiate the effects of progesterone on the uterus, thereby predisposing to pyometra.

▼ *Key Point* The use of estrogen to prevent pregnancy greatly increases the risk of developing pyometra and is a common cause of pyometra in young bitches.

Clinical Signs

Signalment

Pyometra occurs in older intact bitches and queens except when exogenous estrogens or progestins are given, in which case younger animals may be affected.

History

- Signs of pyometra usually occur 1–2 months after estrus or exogenous progesterone administration.
- Lethargy, depression, and anorexia are common; these signs are more severe in cases of closed-cervix pyometra. Vomiting and diarrhea also occur more often with closed pyometra.
- Vaginal discharge is present in most animals with open-cervix pyometra and typically is purulent but may contain blood or mucus.
- Polyuria and compensatory polydipsia may occur because of impairment of renal tubular concentrating ability. This is probably due to unresponsiveness of the tubules to antidiuretic hormone (ADH) mediated by *E. coli* endotoxin, although the exact mechanism is unknown.
- Cats with pyometra are sometimes presented primarily for evaluation of abdominal distention.

▼ *Key Point* Because pyometra is such a common disease, a high index of suspicion is warranted when an intact female animal is presented with nonspecific signs of illness.

Physical Examination

- Common findings in open-cervix pyometra include lethargy, dehydration, a palpable uterus, and vaginal discharge.
- Closed-cervix pyometra is more likely to result in septicemia, which may cause shock, hypothermia, and collapse.
- Fever is a variable finding and often is absent.

Diagnosis

Clinical Pathology

- *Hematology* typically reveals an inflammatory leukogram characterized by extreme neutrophilia with a left shift. In more severe cases, sepsis results in toxic changes in the neutrophils and a degenerative left shift. However, a normal leukogram can also occur with pyometra, and is usually associated with an open cervix. A mild nonregenerative anemia and hyperproteinemia are common.
- *Serum chemistry abnormalities* include hyperglobulinemia due to chronic antigenic stimulation and azotemia that usually is prerenal.
- Electrolyte abnormalities may be present if vomiting has been severe.
- *Urinalysis* may reveal isosthenuria caused by decreased concentrating ability, and proteinuria caused by immune complex glomerular damage or preexisting renal disease.
- Do not attempt cystocentesis when pyometra is suspected because of the possibility of inadvertent needle damage to the friable uterus and subsequent abdominal contamination.

Radiography and Ultrasonography

- Perform *abdominal radiography* to confirm an enlarged uterus and to evaluate for the possibility of uterine rupture and peritonitis. A normal nongravid uterus cannot be detected on abdominal radiographs.
- Pyometra results in a fluid-dense tubular structure in the caudal abdomen that often displaces bowel loops cranially and dorsally. However, this is also the appearance of a gravid uterus before fetal skeletal calcification (<42 days' gestation). Therefore, pyometra must be differentiated from pregnancy, which may also be associated with a vaginal discharge.

▼ *Key Point* Open-cervix pyometra may allow enough drainage to prevent radiographically detectable uterine enlargement; therefore, the inability to identify the uterus on abdominal radiographs does not rule out pyometra.

- Perform *abdominal ultrasonography* to differentiate pyometra from pregnancy.

Cytology and Culture

- Vaginal cytology and culture may be helpful in the diagnosis of pyometra but do not provide a definitive diagnosis.
- Cranial vaginal cultures may be used to choose an appropriate antibiotic if medical therapy is employed.

Treatment

The decision to treat pyometra surgically or medically depends on the condition of the animal at the time of presentation, its age, and the importance to the owner of preserving the animal's reproductive capacity.

- *Ovariohysterectomy* is the treatment of choice for pyometra.

- *Medical management* may be attempted in stable animals whose breeding potential is of utmost importance.

Surgical Management

Preoperative Considerations

- Institute fluid and antibiotic therapy before surgery in all cases. Animals with signs of sepsis or shock require very aggressive fluid therapy.
- Immediately administer broad-spectrum antibiotics intravenously (IV), such as cephalothin (Keflin, Lilly) (22 mg/kg q8h) and amikacin (Amiglyde-V; Fort Dodge) (5–10 mg/kg q12h).

▼ *Key Point* Because of their nephrotoxicity, use aminoglycosides such as amikacin cautiously in dehydrated animals or in those with questionable renal function.

- Surgically remove the uterus as soon as the animal is stable enough for anesthesia.

Surgical Procedure

- For a discussion of ovariohysterectomy, see Chapter 111.

Postoperative Considerations

- Continue supportive care with fluids and injectable antibiotics postoperatively, if necessary. However, most animals show great improvement following removal of the uterus if abdominal contamination has not occurred.
- Continue oral antibiotic therapy (e.g., cephalosporin or trimethoprim-sulfa) for 10–14 days after surgery. Quinolone antibiotics (e.g., enrofloxacin) are preferred in animals with severe gram-negative sepsis.
- The prognosis is good if there is no uterine rupture or other cause of abdominal contamination, with mortality rates below 10%.
- In animals with gross peritoneal contamination and resultant peritonitis, treat with open abdominal drainage (see Chap. 96).

Medical Management

Medical treatment of pyometra in the bitch and queen uses pharmacologic agents to reduce the plasma progesterone concentration, relax the cervix, and promote myometrial contraction, resulting in evacuation of the uterus. Several different drugs, including ecbolic and hormonal compounds, have been used in an attempt to treat pyometra. However, only prostaglandins produce a consistent response. Concomitant systemic antibiotics are used to prevent bacteremia during uterine evacuation.

Indications

- Reserve medical management for young breeding animals without signs of sepsis or severe illness.
- Both open- and closed-cervix pyometra can be treated with prostaglandins. However, medical treatment of closed-cervix pyometra has a guarded prognosis because of a low response rate and the potential for uterine rupture or retrograde movement of uterine contents through the oviducts into the abdominal cavity, causing peritonitis. Therefore, avoid medical therapy of closed-cervix pyometra. Recommend ovariohysterectomy on these animals.

Prostaglandin Therapy. Prostaglandin $F_{2\alpha}$ ($PGF_{2\alpha}$) acts by causing cervical dilation, myometrial contraction, and, at higher dosages, luteolysis.

- Naturally occurring and synthetic analogs of $PGF_{2\alpha}$ are available. However, use only the natural product (Lutalyse, Upjohn) because the synthetic analogs are highly potent compounds whose efficacy for pyometra in small animals has not yet been investigated. None of the prostaglandins currently are approved for use in small animals.
- *Protocol* (for bitches and queens): Administer 0.1–0.25 mg/kg $PGF_{2\alpha}$ SC once daily for 3–5 days. Lower doses can be used for the first 1–2 days to minimize adverse side effects. The duration of therapy is dictated by resolution of uterine discharge and decreased uterine size. The character of the vaginal discharge usually changes to serous or serosanguineous before it disappears.
- Clinical improvement is not apparent until 48 hours following the first prostaglandin injection. For this reason, medical therapy is a poor option for animals presented with evidence of sepsis or toxemia. If these signs occur during the course of prostaglandin treatment, consider ovariohysterectomy.
- Monitor all animals treated with prostaglandins, especially those with closed-cervix pyometra, for signs of abdominal contamination and peritonitis, necessitating surgery.
- Recheck the animal 2 weeks after prostaglandin therapy. If purulent vaginal discharge or uterine enlargement is still present, a second series of injections can be administered.
- *Side effects* of prostaglandin therapy are encountered routinely, especially with initial administration. They include restlessness, panting, vomiting, defecation, tachycardia, fever, abdominal pain, and salivation in both the bitch and queen; and vocalization, kneading, and grooming in the queen. These effects occur within 15–120 minutes after subcutaneous injection of $PGF_{2\alpha}$.
  - The severity of the reaction is dose dependent and decreases with subsequent injections, so that side effects are usually minimal by the fourth and fifth administrations.
  - Empirically, side effects may be reduced by walking the animal for 30 minutes after each injection, or by administering atropine (0.5 mg/kg IM) at the time of $PGF_{2\alpha}$ injection. Because of the likelihood of vomiting, do not feed an animal for 2–3 hours prior to $PGF_{2\alpha}$ administration.

Antibiotic Therapy

- Administer systemic broad-spectrum bactericidal antibiotics concurrent with prostaglandin therapy to prevent bacteremia during uterine evacuation. Base the choice of antibiotics on sensitivity testing results of cranial vaginal cultures. Continue oral antibiotics for 1–3 weeks following evacuation of the uterus.

Complications. Complications of medical therapy include uterine rupture, contamination of the peritoneal cavity, sepsis, and the side effects of the prostaglandin itself, as previously described.

- Evaluate animals treated with $PGF_{2\alpha}$ daily for signs of peritonitis and sepsis.

Prognosis

- Success rates for clinical resolution of open-cervix pyometra following prostaglandin treatment range from 76–93%. Approximately one-third of bitches treated successfully for open-cervix pyometra require two series of prostaglandin injections.
- The response of closed-cervix pyometra to medical therapy is poor, with 25–40% of bitches treated obtaining clinical resolution. The percentage of bitches with closed-cervix pyometra requiring two series of injections is higher than for those with open-cervix pyometra.
- Recurrence of pyometra after medical therapy is fairly common and is reported to be as high as 77% in bitches followed long-term. This may indicate that prostaglandin therapy does not totally resolve the uterine pathology but simply reduces it to a subclinical level. For these reasons, animals treated successfully with prostaglandins should be bred during the first subsequent estrus to maximize the chances of obtaining a litter.
- The percentage of successfully treated animals that go on to produce at least one normal litter is reported to be 40–82% (bitch) and 81% (queen).

Acute Metritis

Metritis is a severe postpartum bacterial infection of the uterus that may rapidly progress to sepsis and toxemia.

Etiology

The onset of metritis is almost always in the immediate postpartum period, although it may also occur after artificial insemination, natural breeding, or abortion.

- Ascending bacterial infection occurs secondary to a predisposing factor such as a retained placenta, retained fetus, or trauma from dystocia or obstetric manipulations.
- *E. coli* is the most common invading organism, but gram-positive bacterial infections also occur.

Clinical Signs

Acute metritis can occur in any postpartum bitch but most often is associated with a predisposing complication of parturition.

- The onset of clinical signs is acute and occurs within 1 week of parturition.
- Abnormalities reported in the history are consistent with systemic illness and include lethargy, anorexia, loss of maternal instinct, poor milk production, and vomiting.
- A foul-smelling vaginal discharge is typical.
- Physical examination reveals depression, dehydration, tachycardia, fever, and an enlarged turgid uterus.
- Metritis may rapidly progress to sepsis and subsequent shock and hypothermia.

Diagnosis

The diagnosis of acute metritis is usually based on the history and physical examination alone. Further diagnostics are useful to confirm the diagnosis and assess the severity of the accompanying sepsis.

Clinical Pathology. The hemogram reflects a severe bacterial infection with a neutrophilia with a left shift, or leukopenia with a degenerative left shift in septic animals. Serum chemistries usually are normal with the exception of prerenal azotemia.

Radiology and Ultrasonography. Perform abdominal radiographs or ultrasonography to confirm uterine enlargement and to check for retained fetuses. Ultrasonography may be useful to identify a retained placenta.

Cytology and Culture. Evaluation of the vaginal discharge can help to differentiate acute metritis from other causes of postpartum vaginal discharge such as hemorrhage and normal lochia.

- The discharge of acute metritis is septic, containing neutrophils, bacteria, and sometimes endometrial cells.
- Cranial vaginal cultures are not diagnostic for metritis but are useful in guiding antibiotic therapy.

Treatment

Because of its acute progressive nature, metritis necessitates immediate therapy. Administer IV fluids and antibiotics in conjunction with removal of the uterine contents through pharmacologic evacuation or ovariohysterectomy, depending on whether or not the animal will be used for breeding. Because of the debilitating nature of this disease and its effect on milk production, most bitches with acute metritis are unable to nurse their pups, necessitating bottle-feeding of the litter.

Medical Management

Fluid Therapy. Initiate fluid therapy on presentation. Septic animals may require shock doses of IV fluids (see Chap. 72).

Antibiotic Therapy. Administer broad-spectrum bactericidal IV antibiotics immediately.

- A combination of amikacin (Amiglyde-V, Fort Dodge) (5–10 mg/kg q12h IV) with cephalothin (Keflin, Lilly) (22 mg/kg q8h IV) or amikacin with sodium penicillin G (25,000 units/kg q6h IV) is often used if sepsis is suspected.
- *Note:* Because of their nephrotoxicity, use aminoglycosides such as amikacin cautiously in dehydrated animals or those with questionable renal function.

- Base the choice of antibiotic on sensitivity results from cranial vaginal cultures, once these are available.
- Continue oral antibiotics for 1–2 weeks following removal of the uterine contents.

Uterine Evacuation. This is accomplished pharmacologically with ecbolic agents to stimulate myometrial contraction and promote uterine involution. Uterine rupture is a potential complication of initiating contractions in a friable or obstructed uterus.

- Administer oxytocin, 0.5–1.0 units/kg (maximum 20 units), IM; repeat in 1–2 hours if needed.
- Administer prostaglandin $F_{2\alpha}$ (Lutalyse, Upjohn) once daily for 3–5 days at a dose of 0.25 mg/kg SC (see under Pyometra for details of prostaglandin therapy).

Uterine Infusion. If the cervix can be cannulated, an intrauterine infusion of 2% povidone-iodine solution or sterile saline may be helpful.

- Because of the friable state of the diseased uterus, uterine rupture is a potential complication. Therefore, perform catheterization cautiously.

Surgical Management

Indications for ovariohysterectomy (see Chap. 111) in the treatment of acute metritis include uterine rupture, retained fetuses, poor response to medical management, and animals not intended for future breeding.

Prognosis

- The prognosis is guarded with acute metritis because progression to sepsis and toxemia can rapidly cause life-threatening illness.
- Chronic metritis may result in infertility.

Subinvolution of Placental Sites

Normal uterine involution occurs to a large degree in the 4–6 weeks following parturition and is fully complete by 12 weeks post partum. During this time, sloughing of collagenous masses from placental sites and reconstruction of the endometrium result in a hemorrhagic vaginal discharge called lochia. This discharge is normally present for up to 6 weeks after parturition. Subinvolution of placental sites (SIPS) is a delay in the normal involution process that results in a persistent hemorrhagic postpartum discharge.

Etiology

- The cause of the failure of normal involution in SIPS is unknown.
- Histopathologically, SIPS is characterized by the invasion of trophoblast-like cells into the endometrium and myometrium, which may prevent involution.
- Lack of thrombosis in endometrial blood vessels results in persistent hemorrhage from the uterus.
- SIPS may involve all placental sites in the uterus, or only a portion of them, with the remaining sites showing normal involution.

Clinical Signs

- SIPS occurs most often in young (<3 years) female dogs of any breed that may be either primiparous or multiparous.
- Persistent hemorrhagic vaginal discharge lasting >6 weeks post partum is usually the only sign associated with SIPS, and affected bitches appear otherwise healthy on physical examination.
- Abdominal palpation may reveal distinct, firm round masses within the uterus.
- Very rarely is the amount of hemorrhage from the uterus enough to produce signs of anemia.

Diagnosis

- The diagnosis of SIPS usually is based simply on the presence of a persistent hemorrhagic postpartum discharge in an otherwise healthy bitch. Rule out other causes of hemorrhagic discharge following parturition, including metritis, retained fetal or placental tissues, coagulopathy, trauma to the genital tract, and chronic vaginitis.
- Abdominal palpation, radiography, and ultrasonography can aid in the differential diagnosis of SIPS.
- Vaginal cytology consists of erythrocytes, neutrophils, and parabasal cells. Occasionally, trophoblastlike cells are present in the discharge, suggesting SIPS.
- A definitive diagnosis of SIPS of placental sites can be made only on histopathology.

Treatment

- Most bitches with SIPS do not require treatment because spontaneous resolution of the discharge usually occurs.
- Ovariohysterectomy is the treatment of choice in nonbreeding animals.
- Monitor breeding animals with SIPS for potential complications, including perforation of the uterine wall, ascending metritis, and anemia.

Prognosis

- Because SIPS is self-limiting and complications are infrequent, the prognosis is good.
- There does not seem to be any decrease in fertility in bitches following spontaneous resolution of SIPS, and there is no predisposition for recurrence of subinvolution with future litters.

Uterine Prolapse

Uterine prolapse is a rare problem in the bitch and queen that usually occurs during or immediately after parturition but also can be seen following abortion.

- Prolapse may be associated with dystocia, forced fetal or placental extraction, or excessive straining due to retained tissues, metritis, or other causes. However, it may also occur with normal parturition.
- The diagnosis is made by identification of the prolapsed uterine tissue, which must be differentiated from vaginal hyperplasia and neoplasia (see Chap. 112).

- Treatment of uterine prolapse includes supportive fluid therapy and either reduction or amputation of the prolapsed tissue. If prolapse occurs as a complication of excessive straining, eliminate the cause of the straining.
  - For a discussion of manual reduction and surgical amputation for uterine prolapse, see Chapter 111.
  - If the uterus is replaced, administer systemic antibiotic therapy to treat metritis.

Uterine Torsion

Torsion of the uterus is uncommon in small animals and usually occurs near the end of gestation (although it can occur without pregnancy), resulting in dystocia.

- Clinical signs include abdominal distention, abdominal pain, and hemorrhagic vaginal discharge.
- Abdominal radiographs are consistent with either a gravid or fluid-filled uterus.
- Treatment of uterine torsion is ovariohysterectomy because the ischemic uterine tissue usually is devitalized.

Uterine Neoplasia

Tumors of the uterus are very rare in dogs and cats.

- Leiomyomas, which are benign tumors arising from the myometrium, account for the majority of uterine tumors.
- Leiomyosarcoma is the most common malignant uterine neoplasia in the bitch, whereas endometrial adenocarcinoma is most common in the queen.
- Other tumor types include fibrosarcoma, fibroma, lipoma, and adenoma.

Clinical Signs

- Many uterine tumors are not associated with clinical signs and are discovered as incidental findings at necropsy or during elective ovariohysterectomy.
- Large tumors may cause abdominal distention or compression of the gastrointestinal or urinary tracts, resulting in tenesmus and dysuria.
- Vaginal discharge, if present, is typically hemorrhagic.

Diagnosis

- The diagnosis of uterine neoplasia is supported by identification of a mass lesion on abdominal radiographs or ultrasonography.
- Vaginal cytology is rarely helpful because leiomyomas and leiomyosarcomas do not readily exfoliate neoplastic cells.
- Exploratory laparotomy is often necessary for definitive diagnosis.

Treatment

- Ovariohysterectomy is the only recommended treatment for uterine neoplasia. It is usually curative unless metastasis has occurred.

Abortion

Etiology

Abortion may be the result of fetal, maternal, or placental disorders. These disorders represent a variety of etiologies, including systemic or reproductive tract disease in the bitch or queen, fetal maldevelopment, and infectious agents.

Maternal Disorders

Maternal disorders that result in abortion may be systemic or may be confined to the reproductive tract. Any serious systemic illness potentially can result in abortion through secondary effects on the uterus and/or fetus. Disorders of the reproductive tract that result in abortion may be uterine or ovarian in origin.

- Uterine diseases that can cause abortion include chronic endometritis, cystic endometrial hyperplasia, and uterine adhesions.
- Ovarian diseases may result in abortion if the corpus luteum fails to secrete progesterone in amounts sufficient to maintain pregnancy (hypoluteoidism). Cases of primary hypoluteoidism in the bitch and queen have not been well documented.

Fetal Maldevelopment

Maldevelopment resulting in fetal death causes resorption or abortion, depending on the stage of gestation.

Infectious Agents

Organisms that can cause abortion in the bitch include *Brucella canis*, *Campylobacter*, *Streptococcus*, *Leptospira*, *E. coli*, *Toxoplasma*, canine herpesvirus, canine distemper virus, and *Mycoplasma*. Of these, *B. canis* and canine herpesvirus are probably the most important because of their impact on breeding programs. In the queen, viral agents such as feline leukemia virus, feline infectious peritonitis, and feline rhinotracheitis are most important.

Brucellosis. *B. canis* infection usually causes abortion in the third trimester of gestation, but it may also cause embryonic death and subsequent resorption early in pregnancy.

- Most dogs with brucellosis are not seriously ill, and many are asymptomatic carriers.
- In addition to abortion and resorption, *B. canis* infection is associated with infertility and pups that may be stillborn or bacteremic.
- *B. canis* infection is important because of its impact on breeding populations; it can have devastating results because it is a highly contagious organism for which there is no vaccine or effective treatment (see Chap. 17 for more information).

Canine Herpesvirus. Infection with canine herpesvirus has been reported to cause late gestation abortion, stillbirth, mummified fetuses, a decrease in the number of pups per litter, and infertility in the bitch. In addition, it causes an acute hemorrhagic septicemia in neonatal puppies of affected bitches (see Chap. 14 for more information).

Drugs. Drugs that have been associated with abortion in the bitch include glucocorticoids and chloramphenicol.

Clinical Signs

- Observable signs of abortion vary according to the etiology and time of gestation.
  - Early fetal resorption may occur without any clinical signs or may be associated with a vaginal discharge.
  - Animals aborting late in gestation may show signs consistent with normal parturition, such as restlessness and abdominal contractions.
- Signs of systemic illness such as anorexia, lethargy, vomiting, or diarrhea at any time during pregnancy may be an indication of recent or impending abortion and are an indication for thorough evaluation of the animal.
- Bitches with canine herpesvirus may develop vesicular or follicular lesions of the vaginal mucosa soon after they are infected. These lesions are transient and often recur during proestrus.

Diagnosis

A definitive diagnosis of abortion is difficult to make unless expulsion of fetuses is actually observed. Documentation of early pregnancy is difficult, so that early embryonic resorption may be clinically indistinguishable from infertility. Ultrasonography can be used to consistently demonstrate pregnancy in the bitch after 16 days' gestation. Radiographic detection is dependent on fetal skeletal calcification, which can be seen after 42 days' gestation.

General Diagnostics

- Give all animals suspected of aborting a pregnancy a thorough physical examination to evaluate for systemic illness.
- If signs of illness are detected, a hemogram, biochemical profile, and urinalysis are indicated.
- Rule out pyometra in any diestral animal with systemic signs of illness.
- Abdominal palpation may allow assessment of pregnancy status if the animal is in mid- or late gestation.

▼ *Key Point* Ultrasonography is an invaluable tool for assessing the status of pregnancy in the bitch and queen and is especially helpful in early gestation.

- In addition to evaluating the presence and viability of any fetuses in the uterus, ultrasonography may indicate uterine pathology in some cases. It is also useful for the identification of retained fetuses (either alive or dead) in an animal that is known to have aborted.
- If an aborted fetus and/or placenta is available, perform necropsy, histopathology, and culture.
- Samples from a cranial vaginal swab or from postabortion vaginal discharge may also be useful for culture.

Serology

Serologic tests for *B. canis* are indicated in any bitch suspected of abortion or fetal resorption. Several serologic tests are available for evaluation of canine brucellosis (see also Chap. 17).

- The rapid slide agglutination test (RSAT) is an excellent screening test because it gives very few false-negative results, and thus an animal with a negative RSAT is almost certainly free from infection.
- However, because false-positive results are fairly common, retest bitches with positive RSAT results with the more specific tube agglutination test (TAT), which has a low incidence of false-positive results.
- An agar gel immunodiffusion test is available for retesting of samples that were positive on the RSAT or TAT.

Plasma Progesterone

Plasma progesterone concentrations can be measured to document hypoluteoidism as a cause of abortion.

- Progesterone concentrations <2 ng/ml are inadequate to maintain pregnancy and are consistent with luteal failure.
- In some cases luteal regression and low progesterone levels may occur secondary to another primary disorder; therefore, a low plasma progesterone level does not definitively indicate primary hypoluteoidism.

Treatment

The objective of therapy for abortion is identification and treatment of the underlying etiology. Supportive care such as fluid therapy may be necessary in animals with signs of systemic illness.

Uterine Infections

For a detailed discussion of the management of uterine infections, see previous sections in this chapter.

- Pyometra is best treated with ovariohysterectomy, but may be managed medically in some bitches without severe illness.
- Retained fetal or placental tissues are best treated surgically but may respond to medical evacuation of the uterus in some cases.

Brucellosis

Medical Therapy. Currently no effective treatment protocols are available for the cure of canine brucellosis. Although treatment with combinations of tetracycline, dihydrostreptomycin, trimethoprim-sulfadiazine, and demeclocycline have been somewhat effective in transiently eliminating bacteremia, none have been able to completely eliminate the infection, and bacteremia can recur after therapy is discontinued.

▼ *Key Point* Owners should be made aware that, although neutering and antibiotic treatment of a *Brucella*-positive dog reduces the risk of transmission, the dog may still harbor and shed organisms, making it a potential source of infection to dogs and people.

- The most effective therapeutic regimen has been the combination of minocycline (25 mg/kg q12h PO) given for 2 weeks and streptomycin (22 mg/kg q24h IM, SC) given for the first week. Unfortunately, minocycline administered at this extremely high dose is prohibitively expensive.

Prevention. Because no vaccine is available, prevention of canine brucellosis can be accomplished only through identification and elimination of infected animals.

- In kennels that are free of brucellosis, isolate all new animals until they are brucellosis-negative on two tube agglutination tests at least 1 month apart.
- Include an RSAT for brucellosis screening in prebreeding examinations. Do not use any brucellosis-positive animal for breeding because of the likelihood of spread of the disease to other breeding animals and because pups born to that bitch are likely to be stillborn or bacteremic.

Hypoluteoidism

- Decreased luteal function because of primary ovarian failure can be treated with exogenous progesterone in some cases. This must be done with caution, however, for the following reasons:
  - Hypoluteoidism is not well understood in the bitch.
  - Low plasma progesterone concentrations may be a complication of an underlying disorder and may not always be an indication for progesterone therapy.
  - Progesterone administration predisposes to the development of pyometra in the bitch and queen.
- Despite these problems, exogenous progesterone has been used successfully in a few bitches with recurrent fetal resorption associated with consistently low plasma progesterone levels.

PREGNANCY TERMINATION

Unwanted pregnancy is a common problem presented to the small animal practitioner. The first step in evaluating the bitch presented for mismating is confirmation that mating has actually occurred. This assessment is based on a careful history and a vaginal smear. Vaginal cytology is used to identify the stage of estrus and to check for sperm. When a bitch is presented for pregnancy termination >3 weeks following an unplanned breeding, pregnancy should always be confirmed (ideally with ultrasonographic evaluation) before treatment is initiated. In one study of bitches presented for pregnancy termination 30–35 days after a single unplanned breeding, 62% were not pregnant.

- If a bitch presented for recent mating is found to be in proestrus or diestrus, it is unlikely that conception has occurred.

- Sperm or sperm heads are present for 24 hours in the vaginal cytology of 65% of bitches that have been bred, and for 48 hours in 50% of bitches. The presence of sperm confirms breeding, although lack of sperm does not rule it out.

Surgical Management

Ovariohysterectomy is the treatment of choice in bitches not intended for future breeding. Because a uniformly benign and effective medical alternative for termination of pregnancy is not currently available, ovariohysterectomy is recommended for an older bitch or one whose reproductive importance is questionable.

Medical Management

None of the protocols discussed here is always effective, and most are associated with significant side effects. Therefore, advise owners wishing to pursue medical treatment of unwanted pregnancy of the possibility of failure and the risks of potentially serious side effects. In some cases, it may be safer for the bitch to allow her to carry the litter to term instead of attempting medical termination of the pregnancy.

Estrogens

Estrogenic compounds traditionally have been used for termination of pregnancy in the dog and cat. However, the serious side effects produced by these agents severely limit their usefulness. In addition, because estrogens must be administered soon after mating, pregnancy cannot be confirmed; thus, treatment with estrogens unnecessarily exposes some animals to potentially life-threatening side effects.

Mechanism of Action

Exogenous estrogens delay the transport of fertilized ova through the oviducts and may stimulate contraction of the uterotubular junction. This prevents migration of the embryo into the uterus, where implantation normally occurs in the bitch on the 12th day of diestrus.

Estradiol Cypionate

- Estradiol cypionate (ECP), an injectable estrogen, is not approved for pregnancy termination in dogs or cats.
- ECP is used in the bitch at a dosage of 0.02 to 0.04 mg/kg (not to exceed 1 mg total dose), IM, given once within 3 days of mating. This protocol has been shown to be 50% to 100% effective in terminating pregnancy.
- Cats are given a total dose of 0.25 mg, IM, once within 3 days of mating.

▼ *Key Point* Never give ECP more than once in the same estrus or in total doses exceeding 1 mg in the dog or 0.25 mg in the cat.

▼ *Key Point* There is no dose of ECP that is consistently both safe and effective; therefore, the author recommends against its use.

Diethylstilbestrol

Diethylstilbestrol (DES) has been used in both injectable and oral forms. However, the injectable product is no longer available, and the oral form has demonstrated poor efficacy, with success rates as low as 8%.

Estrogen Side Effects

Because of their potentially life-threatening side effects, including bone marrow suppression and pyometra, even at recommended doses, estrogens are not recommended for pregnancy termination in the bitch or queen.

Bone Marrow Suppression

- Bone marrow suppression results in aplastic anemia, thrombocytopenia, and sometimes leukopenia, usually within 2–8 weeks of estrogen administration.
- The susceptibility of individual dogs to bone marrow suppression is extremely variable.
- Although most occurrences are associated with doses above the recommended range or repeated multiple times, suppression has also been documented in dogs given a single appropriate dose.
- Cats may also be affected by bone marrow suppression but appear to be somewhat more resistant than dogs.

Pyometra

- Although estrogens do not cause pyometra directly, they potentiate the effects of progesterone on the uterus, which may result in cystic endometrial hyperplasia and pyometra.
- The administration of estrogen for pregnancy termination is the most common cause of pyometra in young bitches (see previous discussion under Pyometra).

Prognosis for Future Reproduction

Estrogen administration may be associated with future infertility problems in the bitch. The mechanism of this effect is not well understood.

Prostaglandins

Although not approved for use in companion animals, prostaglandins have been increasingly advocated in recent years for pregnancy termination in dogs. Despite problems with side effects and resistance to luteolysis in early diestrus, prostaglandins may offer the best option for medical pregnancy interruption. Prostaglandins should only be used in young healthy bitches, and are contraindicated in animals with preexisting cardiovascular or respiratory problems.

Mechanism of Action

- The secretion of progesterone by the corpus luteum is required throughout gestation for the maintenance of pregnancy in the bitch. Prostaglandins terminate pregnancy through luteolysis and subsequent lowering of the plasma progesterone concentration.

Abortion occurs in the bitch if plasma progesterone concentrations remain <2 ng/ml for 36–48 hours.

- The corpus luteum of the bitch is not sensitive to the luteolytic action of prostaglandins throughout pregnancy; the immature corpus luteum is resistant to luteolysis for the first 2–3 weeks of gestation. Prostaglandins administered during this time often cause a transient fall in plasma progesterone concentration, which then returns to a normal gestational level, allowing maintenance of pregnancy. However, when administered after 25–30 days of gestation, prostaglandins can cause complete luteolysis.
- In addition to luteolysis, prostaglandins also have an ecbolic effect and possibly a direct embryotoxic effect, which may add to their effectiveness as abortifacients.

Natural Prostaglandin $F_{2\alpha}$

This has been used for abortion when given for 4–7 days (to effect) after day 25–30 of gestation in the bitch. Higher doses are required for pregnancy termination in early diestrus, whereas lower doses are reliably effective during the last half of gestation, with fewer side effects. Administration of $PGF_{2\alpha}$ three times daily may be more effective than twice daily.

- In bitches in the first half of gestation (but at least 5 days past onset of cytologic diestrus), administer $PGF_{2\alpha}$ (Lutalyse, Upjohn) at 250 μg/kg q12h SC for 4 days. Draw blood for serum progesterone at the time of the last injection; progesterone concentration <2 ng/ml confirms luteolysis. Reexamine the bitch 3–4 weeks later to confirm pregnancy termination. Because pregnancy is difficult to confirm prior to day 21 of gestation, confirmation of pregnancy may not be possible before using this protocol, resulting in some bitches being treated unnecessarily. In addition, at this stage of gestation it is difficult to confirm that abortion has occurred, necessitating reexamination at a later time. For these reasons, some clinicians recommend waiting until pregnancy can be confirmed 30 days after breeding before initiating prostaglandin therapy.
- In bitches in the second half of gestation, administer $PGF_{2\alpha}$ (Lutalyse, Upjohn) at 100 μg/kg q8h SC for 2 days, and then 200 μg/kg q8h SC thereafter to effect. This protocol has been reported to be 100% effective in terminating pregnancy in bitches treated 30–35 days after an unplanned mating. Alternatively, administer 250 μg/kg q12h SC until abortion is complete. Aborted tissues are passed vaginally within 3–9 days of starting treatment.
- Prostaglandins for pregnancy termination in cats have not been extensively studied. However, a $PGF_{2\alpha}$ dosage of 100–250 μg/kg q12h SC to effect has been reported to cause luteolysis in the cat when administered after day 33 of gestation.
- Hospitalize animals during prostaglandin therapy.
- Nesting behavior may be observed 1–2 days before abortion occurs, and a temperature drop (similar to that seen with normal parturition) occurs within 24 hours of abortion as a result of decreasing plasma progesterone concentration.

- Prostaglandin therapy may result in abortion of only part of a litter if treatment is discontinued at the onset of abortion. Evaluate the bitch ultrasonographically after abortion to ensure that no fetuses remain in the uterus that might be carried to term. Abdominal palpation is not reliable for confirming complete pregnancy termination.

Prostaglandin Analogs

Cloprostenol (Estrumate, Haver/Diamond) and other analogs have been studied for abortion in the bitch because they cause luteolysis at much lower doses than natural prostaglandins and may be associated with fewer side effects. However, until these compounds have been more thoroughly evaluated in the bitch, protocols for pregnancy termination cannot be recommended.

Side Effects

See the previous section on Medical Management under Pyometra.

Prognosis for Future Reproduction

- Prostaglandin therapy does not seem to alter future reproductive capability in the bitch.
- Shortening of the interestrous interval following prostaglandin-induced luteolysis has been noted consistently in bitches treated with $PGF_{2\alpha}$ for pregnancy termination. The normal anestrous period in the dog is 4–10 months. However, following $PGF_{2\alpha}$ therapy, it may be as short as 40 days.

Glucocorticoids

Dexamethasone can cause termination of pregnancy in mid- to late gestation, but does not appear to be as consistently effective as $PGF_{2\alpha}$. However, it offers a viable alternative for clients who cannot afford prostaglandin therapy, or who refuse to have their pet hospitalized. The mechanism through which glucocorticoids act to terminate pregnancy has not been well documented, but appears to be related to luteolysis.

- In 15 bitches that were at 28–34 days of gestation, dexamethasone terminated pregnancy when given orally for 7.5 days at a dosage of 0.1–0.2 mg/kg q12h for the first 3 doses, then 0.2 mg/kg q12h for the next 7 doses, and then tapering to 0.02 mg/kg over the last 5 doses.
- Uterine contents were either resorbed or aborted, or both (depending on the stage of gestation) by 2–16 days after initiating dexamethasone therapy.
- Side effects of polyuria and polydipsia resolve after completion of therapy.

DYSTOCIA

Abnormalities of parturition are common in veterinary medicine. Base the decision to intervene with parturition on historical, physical, and diagnostic information and a familiarity with the numerous causes of dystocia. Understanding the pattern of gestation and changes occurring during the stages of labor can help to determine whether a problem in parturition is imminent.

Normal Parturition

The length of gestation in the bitch and queen is 63 days from the time of ovulation. However, the time to parturition from any single breeding date may vary from 58 days to as long as 70 days because the signs of estrus (i.e., receptivity) may occur both before and after ovulation actually takes place. A more accurate whelping date can be calculated as 57 days after the onset of diestrus, which is marked by a change in the vaginal cytology to mostly noncornified cells. Parturition often occurs earlier in animals with large litters and later in those with small or single pup litters. A transient temperature drop occurs within 24 hours of the onset of parturition and may be detected with twice-daily monitoring.

Although the following description of parturition refers specifically to the bitch, normal parturition in the queen is very similar. Parturition in the bitch and queen consists of three stages.

Stage I Labor. Stage I is characterized by prepartum behavior changes including anxiety or restlessness, panting, anorexia, shivering, and sometimes vomiting. Nesting behavior is also evident. Uterine contractions begin during this stage but are not detectable externally. Stage I labor usually lasts 6–12 hours in the bitch and ends with complete dilation of the cervix.

Stage II Labor. This is the segment of parturition during which the fetus is expelled. It is characterized by visible uterine contractions and straining. The first fetus should be delivered within 1–2 hours of the onset of stage II labor. Following delivery of the fetus, the bitch will often enter a resting phase, which may last up to 4 hours. Active straining returns for 5–30 minutes before the expulsion of the next fetus. Two or more pups may be delivered in rapid succession, especially in bitches with large litters. A problem should be suspected if the resting phase lasts longer than 4 hours or if the bitch is actively straining for more than 30–60 minutes without producing a pup.

Stage III Labor. Stage III includes the expulsion of the placenta. This usually occurs within 5–15 minutes of the delivery of the fetus. Multiple placentas may follow the delivery of several pups if they are whelped within a short period of time. A greenish vaginal discharge is associated with placental separation and is a normal finding during and after delivery.

Etiology

The causes of dystocia can be classified as maternal, including uterine inertia and anatomic abnormalities, or fetal, due to malformation, malposition, or fetal death. In some cases, dystocia is caused by a combination of maternal and fetal factors.

Maternal Causes

Anatomic Abnormalities

- A narrow pelvic canal may be a congenital lesion in brachycephalic breeds and terriers or an acquired

problem in animals with previous pelvic fractures or neoplasia involving the pelvic canal.
- Uterine malposition can occur with a uterine torsion or from prolapse of the uterus through an inguinal hernia.
- Developmental abnormalities of the genital canal that result in dystocia include vaginal stenosis, vulvar hypoplasia, and persistent hymen in the form of a vertical band or annular fibrotic stricture (see Chap. 112).
- Insufficient strength of the abdominal muscles may prevent fetal expulsion in English bulldogs.

Uterine Inertia

Primary uterine inertia may be complete, resulting in a total absence of the signs of stage II labor, or partial, which occurs after part of a litter has been delivered. The primary types must be differentiated from secondary uterine inertia, which is the result of exhaustion from persistent straining against an obstruction. Secondary uterine inertia frequently is seen in small breeds of dogs.

- *Primary uterine inertia* is characterized by a gestation length of greater than 68–70 days in a bitch that has shown a temperature drop or has entered stage I labor and then fails to exhibit signs of stage II labor within 24–36 hours.
  - Causes of primary uterine inertia include insufficient stimulation for uterine contraction due to a small litter (especially single fetus litters), overstretching of the uterus due to a large litter, stress and anxiety in first-litter bitches, and underlying systemic disorders (e.g., hypocalcemia, hypoglycemia, sepsis).
- *Secondary uterine inertia,* which is secondary to persistent straining against an obstruction, can complicate obstructive dystocia and result in failure of the bitch to resume stage II labor after the obstruction has been corrected.
  - Diagnosis is made by identifying a loss of uterine contractions in association with an obstruction.
  - Secondary uterine inertia is never the only cause of dystocia.

Fetal Causes

- *Fetal oversize* may be absolute or relative to the size of the birth canal. Causes of a large fetus include a large sire, a single fetus litter, and prolonged gestation.
- *Fetal malposition* can result in obstructive dystocia. The orientation of the fetus during delivery is described in terms of presentation, position, and posture.
  - *Presentation* is cranial, caudal, or transverse, depending on which part of the fetus is delivered first. Cranial and caudal presentations are both normal in the bitch.
  - *Position* describes the area of the uterus which is adjacent to the dorsal surface of the fetus. A dorsal position is normal.
  - *Posture* describes the relationship of the pup's head and limbs to its body. Extended and flexed postures are both normal.
- *Fetal developmental abnormalities,* such as severe hydrocephalus, can cause obstruction.

- *Fetal death* can result in malpositioning of the fetus and may cause dystocia through secondary effects on the uterus.

Diagnosis

The diagnosis of dystocia can be difficult and necessitates a thorough history. It is based on the recognition of one or more of the following:

- Obvious structural abnormalities that prevent parturition, such as vaginal stenosis or previous pelvic fractures that have narrowed the pelvic canal.
- Prolonged gestation >70 days from the first breeding or >60 days from the onset of diestrus. A gestation length 65–70 days from first breeding, especially with a large litter, is questionable.
- Active straining for more than 30–60 minutes without expulsion of a fetus.
- A resting phase without signs of straining for >4 hours between deliveries, with known retained pups.
- Intermittent weak contractions for >2 hours without delivery of a fetus.
- Systemic signs of illness such as fever, profound weakness, and vomiting.
- Signs of pain during parturition such as crying out or biting at the vulvar area.
- Purulent or hemorrhagic vaginal discharge.
- Evidence of fetal death characterized radiographically by intrafetal gas patterns, collapse of the spinal column, or overlapping of the skull bones.

Treatment

Rule out obstructive dystocia as the first step in managing abnormal parturition. Perform a physical examination including vaginal palpation. Clip and cleanse the perineum before vaginal examination, which is done with sterile gloves and lubrication. Abdominal radiographs are used to help determine fetal number, position, and viability. If available, abdominal ultrasonography is an excellent tool for determining fetal viability. Evidence of systemic illness such as sepsis or hypoglycemia warrants appropriate treatment for the underlying problem. If uterine contractions are not present, medical or surgical treatment for uterine inertia is indicated. However, attempt medical therapy only after obstruction has been ruled out. Base the decision to manage the dystocia medically through manipulation or surgically on the history, physical examination, and radiography.

Medical Management
Tranquilization

Relief of stress may allow progression of stage II labor in a nervous first-litter bitch. Acepromazine at low doses (0.05 mg/kg IM) can be used safely in an otherwise healthy bitch.

Ecbolic Agents

These drugs stimulate uterine contractions. They may decrease postpartum hemorrhage, prevent retained fetal membranes, and facilitate uterine involution.

▼ *Key Point* Rule out an obstruction before administering ecbolic agents.

- *Oxytocin* is the agent used most commonly to stimulate uterine contraction. Because it may also cause cervical contractions, it should only be used if the cervix is dilated.
  - Give oxytocin initially at 5–20 units (bitch) or 3–5 units (queen), IM.
  - If there is no response to the first dose, repeat at intervals of 30–40 minutes for a total of up to three doses.
- *Ergonovine maleate* is a more potent ecbolic agent with a longer half-life than oxytocin. Because of the possibility of inducing uterine rupture, this drug is not recommended for routine use in the treatment of uterine inertia, but it may be used to help control postpartum hemorrhage.

Adjunct Medical Therapy

- *Calcium gluconate* given intravenously is indicated when hypocalcemia can be documented in a bitch with uterine inertia. It may also be helpful in animals with a normal serum calcium level and is often given 5–15 minutes before the second or third dose of oxytocin.
  - Give 2–10 ml of 10% calcium gluconate slowly IV.
  - Monitor for cardiac arrhythmias and stop administration if they occur.
- *Dextrose* is indicated for any animal with uterine inertia and confirmed hypoglycemia. It is more commonly used in conjunction with oxytocin therapy or after oxytocin has failed to stimulate uterine contractions.
  - Give 5–10 ml of 50% dextrose slowly IV.

Manipulation

Manual manipulation is used to assist the delivery of a fetus through the vaginal canal. It is useful in some cases of obstructive dystocia due to fetal malposition, slight fetal oversize, or fetal death, but is not indicated in obstructive dystocia once secondary inertia has occurred. Manual delivery may also be necessary to retrieve the last pup of a litter in cases of partial primary uterine inertia.

- Digital manipulation, when possible, is preferable to instrumental manipulation.

- Place the bitch in a standing position and use adequate sterile lubrication and sterile gloves.
- Attempt to determine the position of the fetus and correct any malposition through repulsion and repositioning.
- Once proper positioning is established, use gentle traction on the fetus in a caudodorsal direction until the puppy is exposed, then place traction caudoventrally. Gentle rotation or side-to-side motion may aid in delivery. Do not place traction on the fetal extremities.
- Use instrumental manipulation only when necessary, or when the fetus is dead. Do not use instrumentation on a fetus that cannot be palpated digitally.
  - Guide the instrument into place with a finger and palpate the area after placement to ensure that the vaginal mucosa is not included in the grasp of the forceps.

Surgical Management

Perform cesarean section to manage dystocia in cases of uterine inertia (especially cases unresponsive to medical treatment), obstructive dystocia that cannot be corrected through manipulation, and fetal death associated with putrefaction. For a discussion of the surgical management of dystocia, see Chapter 111.

SUPPLEMENTAL READINGS

Concannon PW: Use of progesterone-suppressing drugs for termination of unwanted pregnancy in dogs. *In* Bonagura JD, Kirk RW, eds: Current Veterinary Therapy XII. Philadelphia: WB Saunders, 1995, p 1075.

Davidson AP: Medical treatment of pyometra with prostaglandin $F_{2\alpha}$ in the dog and cat. *In* Bonagura JD, Kirk RW, eds: Current Veterinary Therapy XII. Philadelphia: WB Saunders, 1995, p 1081.

Feldman EC, Davidson AP, Nelson RW, et al.: Prostaglandin induction of abortion in pregnant bitches after misalliance. J Am Vet Med Assoc 202:1855, 1993.

Feldman EC, Nelson RW: Canine and Feline Endocrinology and Reproduction, 2nd Ed. Philadelphia: WB Saunders, 1996, p 572.

Gaudet DA, Kitchell BE: Canine dystocia. Comp Cont Ed 7:406, 1985.

Johnston SD: Subinvolution of placental sites. *In* Kirk RW, ed: Current Veterinary Therapy IX. Philadelphia: WB Saunders, 1986, p 1231.

Root MV, Johnston SD: Pregnancy termination in the bitch using prostaglandin $F_{2\alpha}$. *In* Bonagura JD, Kirk RW, eds: Current Veterinary Therapy XII. Philadelphia: WB Saunders, 1995, p 1079.

Zone M, Wanke M, Rebuelto M, et al.: Termination of pregnancy in dogs by oral administration of dexamethasone. Theriogenology 43:487, 1995.

111 Surgery of the Ovaries and Uterus

Roger B. Fingland

Surgical procedures performed on the uterus and ovaries include ovariohysterectomy, cesarean section, and, rarely, ovariectomy. Uterine surgery usually is straightforward but requires sound basic surgery skills and a thorough understanding of the anatomy and physiology of the reproductive tract.

ANATOMY (Fig. 111–1)

Ovaries

- The ovaries are located 1–3 cm caudal to the kidneys.
- The ovaries are attached to the abdominal wall by the mesovarium, a part of the broad ligament.
- The suspensory ligament is the cranial continuation of the broad ligament and extends between the ventral third of the last two ribs and the ventral surface of the ovary.
- The proper ligament is a continuation of the suspensory ligament and extends from the caudal end of the ovary to the cranial end of the uterine horn.
- The ovarian arteriovenous complex (OAVC) lies on the medial side of the broad ligament and supplies the ovaries and the cranial portion of the uterine tube. The distal two-thirds of the OAVC is convoluted in the dog, similar to the pampiniform plexus in males.
- The left ovarian vein drains into the left renal vein; the right ovarian vein drains into the caudal vena cava.

Uterus

- The uterus consists of the cervix, body, and two uterine horns. Oviducts (uterine tubes) connect the uterine horns and ovaries.
- The uterus is attached to the dorsolateral wall of the abdominal cavity and the lateral wall of the pelvic cavity by paired double folds of peritoneum called broad ligaments.
- The round ligament is the caudal continuation of the proper ligament. The round ligament extends caudally and ventrally in the broad ligament and passes through the inguinal canal, terminating subcutaneously near the vulva.
- The uterine branch of the internal iliac artery is the main artery to the uterus. The uterine branch of the urogenital artery supplies the caudal portion of the uterus, the cervix, and part of the vagina. The uter-

ine branch of the ovarian artery supplies the cranial part of the uterine horns.

OVARIOHYSTERECTOMY

Objective

- To remove the uterus and ovaries.

Preoperative Considerations

- Elective sterilization is the most common indication for ovariohysterectomy. Ovariohysterectomy is the treatment of choice for most uterine diseases including pyometra, uterine torsion, cystic endometrial hyperplasia, uterine rupture, and uterine neoplasia (see Chap. 110 for a description of these diseases).

▼ **Key Point** Ovariohysterectomy before the first estrus provides a definitive protective factor against development of mammary neoplasia.

Whether the procedure is elective or not, perform an appropriate preoperative evaluation, including a complete history, physical examination, and complete blood count (CBC).

Surgical Procedure

Equipment

- Standard general surgery instrument pack and suture
- Ovariohysterectomy (Snook) hook (optional)
- Chromic catgut (2-0 or 3-0) or synthetic absorbable suture material for all ligatures

Technique

1. After anesthetizing the animal, manually express the urinary bladder.
2. Position the animal in dorsal recumbency.
3. Prepare the entire ventral abdominal region for aseptic surgery.
4. Skin incision:
   a. *Dog:* Make a ventral midline incision extending from the umbilicus to a point halfway between the umbilicus and the brim of the pubis.
   b. *Cat:* Begin the ventral midline incision approximately 1–2 cm caudal to the umbilicus and extend the incision caudally 3–5 cm.

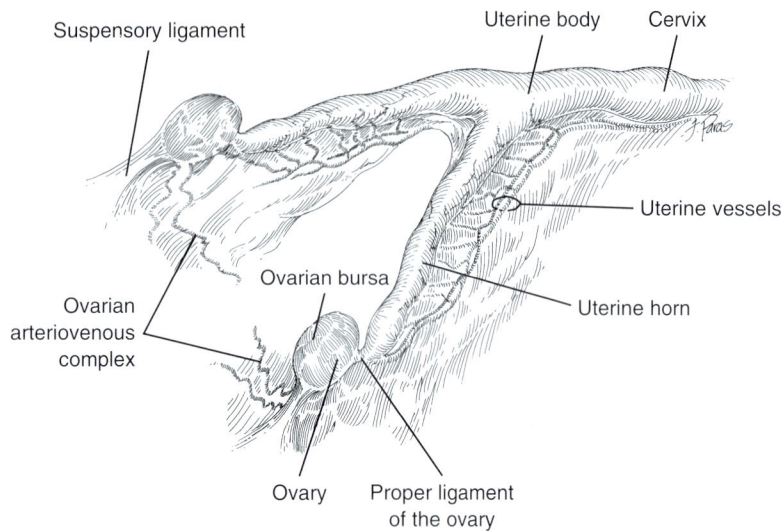

Figure 111-1. Anatomy of the uterus and ovaries.

c. A longer abdominal incision is required to remove an enlarged uterus (e.g., pyometra).

d. Attempt to incise exactly on midline in lactating bitches to avoid trauma to the mammary glands.

5. Enter the abdominal cavity through the linea alba.

6. Locate the left uterine horn using the ovariohysterectomy hook or index finger. Displace the omentum and bowel cranially if necessary to find the uterus.

7. Place a small hemostat across the proper ligament to aid in caudal retraction of the ovary.

8. Grasp the ovary between the thumb and middle finger. Place the index finger as far proximal as possible on the suspensory ligament (Fig. 111–2A).

9. Place tension on the suspensory ligament by rotating the index finger caudally. Gradually increase tension on the suspensory ligament until the ligament breaks.

▼ *Key Point* Avoid placing tension on the OAVC during manipulation of the suspensory ligament or when placing ligatures.

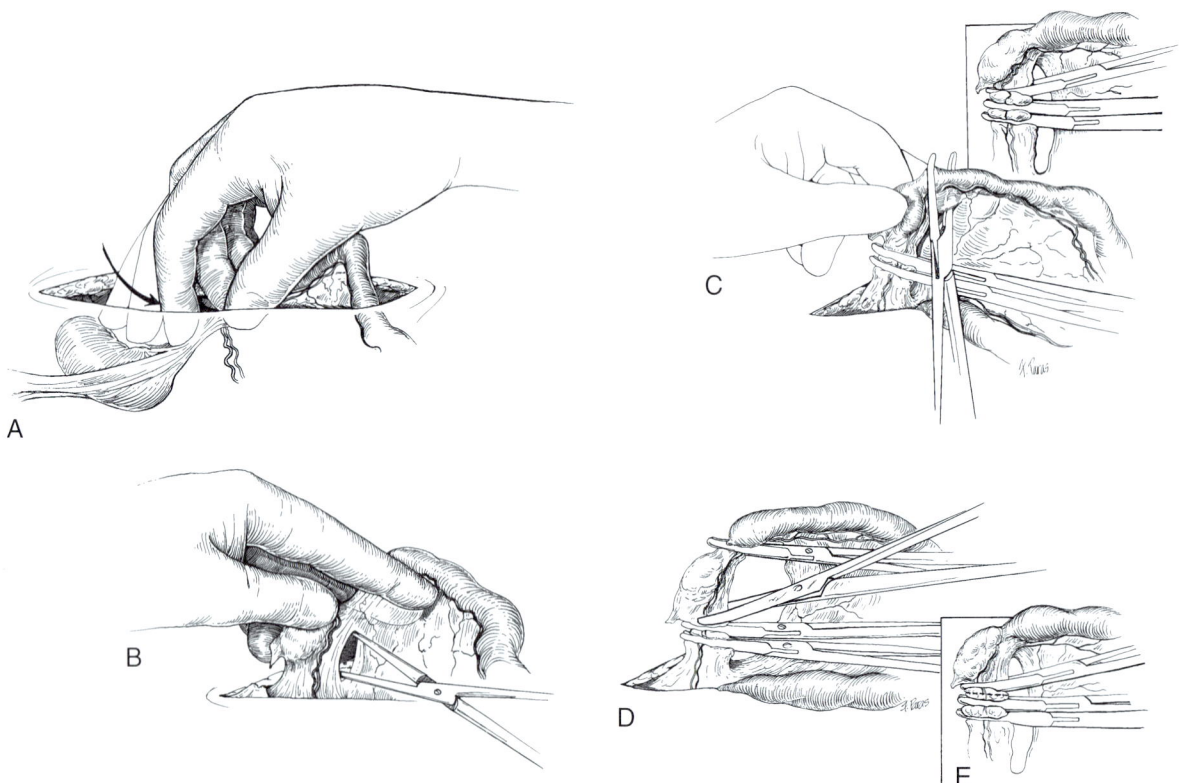

Figure 111-2. Ovariohysterectomy. *A,* Separate the suspensory ligament. *B,* Open the mesovarium immediately caudal to the ovarian arteriovenous complex (OAVC). *C,* Triple-clamp the OAVC. *D,* Transect the OAVC between the ovary and the clamp. *E,* Alternative clamp and transection method.

10. Identify the OAVC. Using a Rochester-Carmalt hemostatic forceps (clamp), make an opening in the mesovarium immediately caudal to the OAVC in an area clear of vessels and fat (Fig. 111–2*B*).
11. Triple-clamp and transect the OAVC (Fig. 111–2*C*).
    a. Double-clamp the OAVC with Rochester-Carmalt hemostatic forceps. Place the first clamp immediately proximal (toward the aorta) to the ovary and the second clamp approximately 5 mm proximal to the first. Place a third clamp across the proper ligament between the ovary and the uterine horn. Transect the OAVC between the middle clamp and the ovary (Fig. 111–2*D*).
    b. Alternatively, place all three clamps across the OAVC proximal to the ovary. Transect the OAVC between the middle clamp and the clamp adjacent to the ovary (Fig. 111–2*E*).

▼ *Key Point* Place the hemostatic forceps on the OAVC as close as possible to the ovary to prevent accidental inclusion of the ureter, but be sure to remove all of the ovarian tissue.

12. Loosely place a circumferential ligature around the proximal clamp. Tighten the ligature as the clamp is removed (Fig. 111–2*F*). In this manner, the circumferential ligature is tightened in the groove of crushed tissue created by the clamp (Fig. 111–2*G*).

▼ *Key Point* The clamp adjacent to the ligature may need to be loosened before knotting to ensure proper tightness of the knot.

13. Place a transfixing ligature between the circumferential ligature and the transected end of the OAVC (Fig. 111–2*H* and *I*). A full ligature (circumferen-

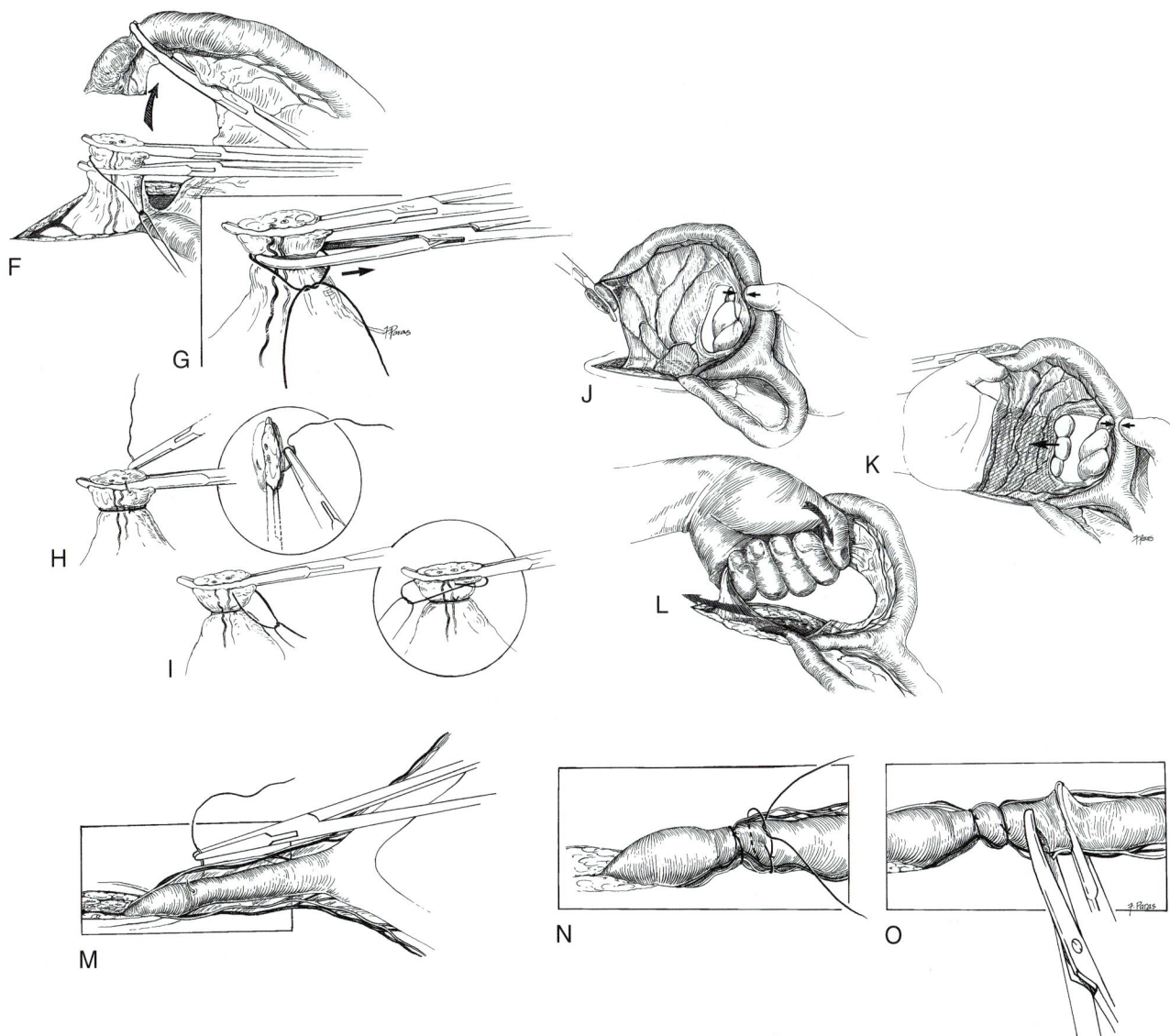

Figure 111–2. *Continued F,* Place circumferential suture around proximal clamp. *G,* Tighten suture in groove of crushed tissue. *H* and *I,* Ligature pattern for transfixing ligature. *J,* Open the broad ligament adjacent to the uterine artery and vein close to the cervix. *K,* Grasp the broad ligament. *L,* Pull the broad ligament cranially until it and the round ligament are free. *M,* Place first transfixing suture. *N,* Place second transfixing suture. *O,* Transect the uterine body.

tial) may be used instead of a transfixing ligature in young cats or small dogs.

▼ *Key Point* Never include ovarian tissue in the ligatures.

14. Grasp the OAVC (without grasping a ligature) with thumb forceps, remove the middle clamp, and inspect the OAVC for bleeding. If bleeding occurs, place a second circumferential ligature on the OAVC proximal to the first.
15. Follow the left uterine horn distally to the bifurcation, locate the right uterine horn, and follow the right uterine horn proximally to the right OAVC.
16. Ligate and transect the right OAVC, as described previously.
17. Transect the broad ligament.
    a. Mass ligation of the broad and round ligaments seldom is necessary. Individually ligate large vessels in the broad ligament.
    b. In most preparturient animals, the broad ligament can be manually separated. Make an opening in the broad ligament adjacent to the uterine artery and vein close to the cervix (Fig. 111–2*J*). Place four fingers through the opening in the broad ligament and grasp the entire broad ligament, including the round ligament (Fig. 111–2*K*). Pull the broad ligament cranially (not ventrally) until the broad ligament and the round ligament are free (Fig. 111–2*L*).
18. Exteriorize the uterine body and locate the cervix.
19. Divide the uterine body after two ligatures are placed (Fig. 111–2*M, N,* and *O*). The entire uterus proximal to the cervix should be removed during routine ovariohysterectomy.
20. Evaluate the OAVC pedicles and the uterine body for bleeding prior to abdominal closure. The left and right OAVC are located immediately caudal to the caudal pole of the respective kidney.
    a. Locate the left OAVC pedicle by retracting the descending colon medially, exposing the left paralumbar gutter.
    b. Locate the right OAVC pedicle by retracting the duodenum medially, exposing the right paralumbar gutter.
    c. Retroflex the bladder. The ligated uterine body lies ventral to the descending colon and dorsal to the bladder.
21. Close the abdominal incision routinely.

Postoperative Care

- Restrict exercise and monitor for wound complications or hemorrhage after ovariohysterectomy.
- Postoperative care following ovariohysterectomy for pyometra:
  - Dogs with pyometra frequently have renal dysfunction without associated morphologic abnormalities, and they may be azotemic, oliguric, or anuric. Monitor renal function and maintain hydration after surgery. Diuresis with crystalloid fluids administered intravenously for at least 24–36 hours after surgery is advisable.
  - Dogs with pyometra may be toxemic or septicemic (see Chap. 110). Administer broad-spectrum antibiotics during surgery, and continue antibiotics after surgery if the animal is toxemic or septicemic or if peritonitis was present at surgery.

Postoperative Complications

Complications following elective ovariohysterectomy are rare and may include the following.

Hemorrhage

- Hemorrhage is the most common complication following ovariohysterectomy in dogs weighing more than 25 kg.
- Common causes of hemorrhage include failure to adequately tighten circumferential or transfixion ligatures, tearing of the OAVC while breaking the suspensory ligament, failure to ligate large vessels in the broad ligament, tearing of the uterine artery due to excessive traction on the uterine body, premature removal of a clamp during ligation, or coagulation defects.
- The incidence of hemorrhage can be reduced by maintaining meticulous surgical technique. Avoid becoming complacent during routine ovariohysterectomy.

Uterine Stump Pyometra

Uterine stump pyometra can occur if a portion of the uterine body or uterine horn is not removed and the animal has an elevated serum progesterone level. The source of elevated serum progesterone can be endogenous from residual ovarian tissue or exogenous from progestational compounds administered for treatment of dermatitis.

▼ *Key Point* Complete excision of the uterine body and ovaries reduces the incidence of uterine stump pyometra.

Ovarian Remnant Syndrome (Recurrent Estrus)

- This condition results from retained functional residual ovarian tissue.
- Treatment is removal of residual ovarian tissue.

▼ *Key Point* To increase the likelihood of identifying residual ovarian tissue, perform exploratory celiotomy to find ovarian remnants when the dog is showing signs of recurrent estrus.

- If ovarian tissue is not located, identify both ureters and resect remnants of the OAVC pedicles bilaterally. Submit the tissue for histopathologic analysis.

Ligation of Ureter

- This condition is most likely to occur when the urinary bladder is distended and the trigone and ureterovesical junction are displaced cranially.
- Hydronephrosis and occasionally pyelonephritis can result.

- Ureteronephrectomy may be required.
- Avoid by careful placement of ligatures on the OAVC and uterine body.

Urinary Incontinence

- Causes include low systemic estrogen level, adhesions or granulomas of the uterine stump that interfere with urinary bladder sphincter function, and vaginoureteral fistula from common ligation of the vagina and ureter (very uncommon).
- Estrogen-responsive urinary incontinence in older female dogs spayed at an early age is uncommon and poorly understood. Prudent administration of exogenous estrogens or alpha-adrenergic drugs may be indicated (see Chap. 103).

Fistulous Tracts and Granulomas

- Sublumbar draining sinus tracts in spayed female dogs may develop when nonabsorbable multifilament suture material, such as polymerized caprolactam (Braunamid, B. Braun Melsungen AG) used for ligating the OAVC or uterine body becomes contaminated.
- Treatment is exploratory celiotomy and removal of suture material.

▼ **Key Point** Do not use nonabsorbable multifilament suture material for ligation of the OAVC or uterine body.

Body Weight Gain

Weight gain is common after ovariohysterectomy; the cause is poorly understood.

Eunuchoid Syndrome

This is a rare complication identified in working dogs after ovariohysterectomy. Clinical signs include decreased aggression, loss of interest in work, and decreased stamina.

Complications Related to Celiotomy

The most common complications associated with celiotomy are:

- Self-mutilation of the abdominal wound
- Seroma formation
- Dehiscence
- Failure to remove gauze sponges from the abdominal cavity
- Laceration of the spleen or urinary bladder

CESAREAN SECTION

Preoperative Considerations

Indications for Cesarean Section

- Dystocia from primary uterine inertia
- Protracted dystocia resulting in secondary uterine inertia

- Obstructive dystocia (oversized fetus or narrow pelvic canal)
- Prolonged gestation
- Dystocia from fetal malpositioning
- Fetal death with putrefaction

Certain breeds (chihuahuas, English bulldogs) frequently require cesarean section because of a high incidence of dystocia. (See Chap. 110 for further discussion of dystocia.)

Anesthesia

- Animals that require cesarean section often have fluid and metabolic disturbances that make them poor candidates for general anesthesia.
- Correction of fluid and metabolic abnormalities should be well underway prior to induction of anesthesia. Intravenous fluid therapy and prophylactic administration of a broad-spectrum antibiotic such as cefazolin, 25 mg/kg IV, are recommended.
- Various regimens for induction and maintenance of anesthesia (see Chap. 2 for general principles of anesthesia) have been recommended.
  - Intravenous narcotics combined with local anesthesia may be used in dogs.
  - Ketamine and local anesthesia may be used in cats.
  - Administer standard inhalation anesthesia after the puppies or kittens are removed.

▼ **Key Point** Minimize time from induction to delivery by fully preparing the surgical site prior to anesthesia.

- Induce anesthesia and intubate the animal on the surgery table, preferably after the initial skin preparation.

▼ **Key Point** Inform the owner prior to surgery that ovariohysterectomy may be necessary if the uterus is not viable.

Surgical Procedure

Objective

- To remove all fetuses from the gravid uterus as quickly and safely as possible.

Equipment

- Standard general surgery instrument pack and suture
- Laparotomy sponges
- Clean towels
- Doxapram (Dopram, Robins) and naloxone (Narcan, Elkins-Sinn) (if narcotics are used for induction)
- Incubator or heat lamp

Technique

1. Position the animal in standard dorsal recumbency. A 20° lateral tilt from dorsal recumbency is not necessary because supine hypotension syndrome does not occur in the parturient female dog.

2. Perform the final skin preparation and place surgical drapes.
3. Incise skin, subcutaneous tissue, and linea alba on the ventral midline beginning cranial to the umbilicus and extending as far caudally as necessary to exteriorize the uterus.

▼ *Key Point* Avoid incising mammary tissue when making the initial skin incision. Enter the abdominal cavity cautiously to avoid lacerating the gravid uterus.

---

4. Exteriorize the uterus.
5. Isolate the uterus from the abdominal viscera with moist laparotomy sponges.
6. Identify an avascular area on the dorsal or ventral midline of the uterine body. Make a small incision in the uterine body with a scalpel. Do not inadvertently lacerate a fetus with the scalpel.
   a. Extend the incision with Metzenbaum scissors to a sufficient length to accommodate the largest fetus. The uterus may tear during extraction of a fetus if the length of the incision is not adequate.
7. Move a fetus to the incision by gently squeezing the uterine horn (Fig. 111–3A).
8. Grasp the fetus and gently pull it from the uterus.
9. Break the amnionic sac as the fetus is removed (Fig. 111–3B). Direct fetal fluids away from the operative field to minimize contamination.
10. Clamp and transect the umbilical vessels approximately 2 cm from the fetal abdominal wall (Fig. 111–3C).
11. Place the neonate on a sterile towel and pass it to an assistant. Alternatively, the neonate can be passed to the assistant before the umbilical vessels are transected, leaving this responsibility to nonsterile operating room assistants.
12. Remove the placenta by gently pulling it from the endometrium. To decrease the potential for severe postoperative uterine hemorrhage, do not remove the placenta if placental separation is difficult.

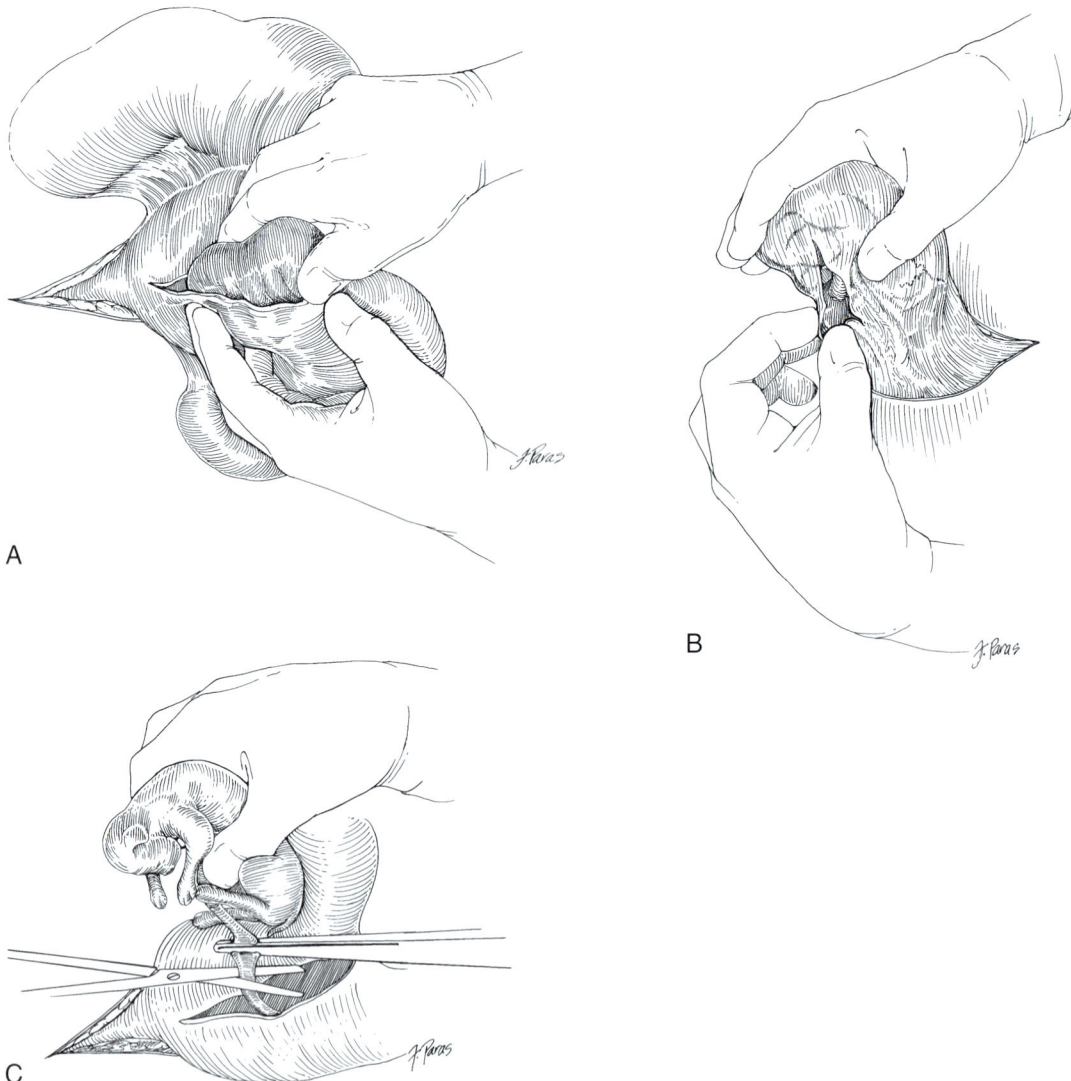

Figure 111–3. Cesarean section. *A,* Move fetus toward incision. *B,* Break amniotic sac as fetus is removed. *C,* Clamp and transect umbilical vessels.

13. Extract the remaining fetuses.
14. Palpate the uterus from the pelvic canal to the ovaries to make certain that no fetuses remain.
15. The uterus will contract rapidly after all fetuses have been removed, and occasionally during extraction of the last few fetuses. Administration of oxytocin rarely is necessary to initiate uterine involution.
16. Close the uterus with 2-0 or 3-0 chromic catgut or synthetic absorbable suture material in a one- or two-layer inverting suture pattern (e.g., Cushing and Lembert).
17. Locally lavage the uterus with warmed physiologic saline solution prior to returning it to the abdominal cavity.
18. Lavage the abdominal cavity with warm physiologic saline solution and aspirate all lavage fluid if contamination or spillage of uterine contents occurred.

▼ *Key Point* En bloc ovariohysterectomy (rapid removal of the uterus and ovaries before hysterotomy and removal of the neonates) is associated with a neonatal survival rate that is similar to other techniques for medical and surgical management of dystocia.

Postoperative Care and Complications

Care of Neonates

▼ *Key Point* Remove the fetal membranes from the neonate's mouth and nose immediately after delivery.

- Clamp the umbilical vessels and remove the fetal membranes if this was not done by the surgeon.
- Clear mucus from the mouth and nares with gentle suction or cotton swabs.
- Assess the viability of the neonate. Neonates often are bradycardic and apneic.
  - Dry the neonate briskly with a soft towel because skin stimulation reflexly stimulates respiration.
  - Mucus can be cleared from the upper airway by grasping the neonate firmly and slowly swinging it downward.
- Administer a respiratory stimulant such as doxapram (Dopram, Robins), 0.5–2.0 mg/kg PO or IM, if the neonate does not respond to mechanical stimulation.
- Poor neonatal viability can be due to anesthetic agents administered to the dam for induction of anesthesia. Administer a narcotic antagonist such as naloxone (Narcan, Elkins-Sinn), 0.01 mg/kg PO or IM, if the dam was given a narcotic for induction of anesthesia.
- Alternately, medications can be dropped on the neonate's tongue to be absorbed through the mucous membranes.
- Some neonates may not breathe spontaneously for 30–60 minutes after delivery. Be persistent with resuscitation efforts. Neonates that do not breathe spontaneously can be intubated with a sterile puppy feeding tube for assisted ventilation.
- Place neonates in an environmental temperature of approximately 32°C.
- Examine neonates for congenital abnormalities such as cleft palate, imperforate anus, hernias, and limb deformities.

Care of the Dam

- Clean residual antiseptic solution, blood, and fetal fluids from the dam's mammary glands prior to allowing the neonates to nurse.
- Place the dam with neonates after anesthetic recovery so that neonates receive colostrum as soon as possible after birth.
- Make certain that the dam has adequate milk and that each neonate nurses.
  - Oxytocin (0.5 units/kg IV or IM) can be administered to stimulate milk production.

▼ *Key Point* Ovariohysterectomy performed in conjunction with cesarean section should not interfere with the dam's mothering instincts or ability to produce milk. Ovarian hormones are not important for maintenance of lactation.

- Consider discharging the dam and neonates as soon as the dam has recovered from anesthesia and has demonstrated appropriate behavior toward the neonates.

Complications

Short-Term

- These include hemorrhage, hypovolemia, and hypothermia.
- Place the dam in a warm, quiet environment and administer crystalloid or colloid fluids, as needed.

Long-Term

- Potential long-term complications include peritonitis, wound dehiscence, agalactia, and uterine hemorrhage.
- Prolonged severe endometrial hemorrhage may require administration of oxytocin or, in nonresponsive cases, emergency ovariohysterectomy.
- Monitor serum calcium levels if hypocalcemia is suspected. See Chapter 30 for diagnosis and treatment of eclampsia.
- Although multiple cesarean sections can be performed on a dam, uterine scarring may prevent future placentation, and peritoneal adhesions may complicate subsequent celiotomies.

UTERINE PROLAPSE

Preoperative Considerations

- Uterine prolapse can occur any time during or up to several days after parturition.

- Animals presented with uterine prolapse may be clinically stable or may have mild to severe metabolic imbalances. Treat disturbances in fluid, electrolyte, or acid-base balance before managing the uterine prolapse.
- Assess the viability of the prolapsed uterus.
- Treatment options include manual reduction, manual reduction with immediate ovariohysterectomy, internal reduction via celiotomy, and amputation of the uterus externally.
  - Manual reduction of the prolapsed uterus is the treatment of choice, although an episiotomy may be required.
  - Ovariohysterectomy may be necessary after manual reduction if the uterus is devitalized.
  - Consider external amputation only if the uterus cannot be reduced. Then remove ovaries through a celiotomy incision.

Manual Reduction

Technique

1. Epidural anesthesia is preferred, but standard general anesthesia can be used.
2. Clean the uterus and wrap it with sterile gauze sponges soaked in physiologic saline. Soaking the sponges with a hypertonic dextrose solution may help to reduce swelling.
3. Apply sterile water-soluble lubricating jelly to the uterus and attempt gentle reduction with a gloved finger or with a sterile smooth syringe case.
4. If manual reduction is unsuccessful, prepare the perineum and the prolapsed uterus for aseptic surgery and perform an episiotomy (see Chap. 113 for technique). Reduction is facilitated by episiotomy. If manual reduction still is not possible, consider internal reduction via celiotomy, or external amputation.

Surgical Procedure for External Amputation of Prolapsed Uterus

Objectives

- Resect the prolapsed uterine horns and, if possible, the ovaries.
- Avoid contamination of the abdominal cavity.
- Minimize uterine hemorrhage.

Equipment

- Standard general surgical instrument pack

Technique

1. Administer epidural or general anesthesia.
2. Position the animal in dorsal recumbency with the rear limbs tied forward.
3. Prepare the ventral abdominal and perineal areas for aseptic surgery. Place a pursestring suture in the anus.
4. Incise the uterine body near the vulva. Place stay sutures in the incised proximal wall of the uterine body to prevent retraction into the vagina. Be careful not to damage the urethra if the vagina has prolapsed with the uterus.
5. Identify the uterine horns.
6. Apply gentle caudal traction on the uterine horns to expose the ovaries. Ligate the right and left OAVC.
7. If the ovaries cannot be exposed, place two circumferential ligatures around each uterine horn as far cranial as possible. Transect the uterine horns between the two ligatures.
8. Double-ligate and transect the uterine vessels.
9. Close the proximal stump of the uterine body with a synthetic absorbable suture material in a simple interrupted pattern and reduce the remaining tissue into the abdomen.
10. If the ovaries remain, perform a ventral midline celiotomy and bilateral ovariectomy.

Postoperative Care and Complications

- Recurrence after successful manual reduction of a uterine prolapse is rare.
- Complications seldom occur after manual reduction or external amputation of the uterus. Life-threatening hemorrhage can occur rarely after external amputation.

SUPPLEMENTAL READINGS

Berzon JL: Complication of elective ovariohysterectomies in the dog and cat at a teaching institution: Clinical review of 853 cases. Vet Surg 8:89, 1979.

Gaudet DA: Retrospective study of 128 cases of canine dystocia. J Am Anim Hosp Assoc 21:813, 1985.

Gaudet DA: Canine dystocia. Compend Contin Educ 7:406, 1985.

Robbins MA, Mullen HS: En bloc ovariohysterectomy as a treatment for dystocia in dogs and cats. Vet Surg 23:48, 1994.

Roberts DD, Straw RC: Uterine prolapse in a cat. Compend Contin Educ 10:1295, 1988.

112 Diseases of the Vagina and Vulva

Amy M. Grooters

DISEASES OF THE VULVA

The vulva or female external genitalia consists of the labia, clitoris, and vestibule (for a review of vulvar anatomy see Chap. 113). The vestibule, which connects the vagina to the external genital orifice, embryologically arises from the caudal portion of the urogenital sinus and fuses with the müllerian ducts to form the vestibulovaginal junction. The clitoris develops from the genital tubercle, whereas the labia are formed from the genital swellings.

Developmental Abnormalities

Vulvar anomalies usually are detected because of the secondary problems they cause. Diagnosis of these abnormalities often is made by physical examination and digital palpation.

Vulvar Hypoplasia

Etiology. A small vulva usually is the result of hypoplastic development in bitches spayed before reaching sexual maturity. The juvenile vulva often is recessed, resulting in urine pooling and moist dermatitis in the skin folds of the perivulvar region. This is a particular problem in obese, older animals.

Clinical Signs. Most signs of vulvar hypoplasia are related to secondary urine pooling and perivulvar dermatitis and include excessive licking of the vulva and malodor. Severe perivulvar dermatitis results in ulcerative lesions that can be very painful, making cleaning of the area difficult. Secondary vaginitis is common, and urine pooling also predisposes the animal to ascending urinary tract infection. Recurrent cystitis occurs in some cases (see Chap. 99).

Treatment. Medical therapy for the secondary dermatitis (see Chap. 35) and vaginitis (see later in this chapter) has limited success without concurrent surgical correction of the underlying anatomic abnormalities. Episioplasty is used to remove excessive perivulvar skin and to elevate the recessed vulva (see Chaps. 50 and 113). Weight reduction is important in obese animals.

Vulvar Stenosis

Etiology. Abnormal fusion of the genital folds and genital swellings results in stenosis of the vulva. This usually occurs at the vestibulolabial junction and is manifested as a narrowing of the canal in that region.

Clinical Signs. Affected animals may show signs of pain when mating is attempted.

If pregnancy does occur (either through natural breeding or artificial insemination), the stenosis may cause dystocia.

Treatment. Perform an episiotomy (see Chap. 113) to enlarge the canal temporarily to relieve dystocia.

Permanent vulvar canal enlargement (episiostomy) may be indicated in breeding animals. In episiostomy, an episiotomy incision is made and, instead of closing the midline incision in three layers, the mucosa is sutured to the skin along both sides of the incision, thereby permanently enlarging the canal.

Acquired Abnormalities

Clitoral Hypertrophy

Etiology
- Enlargement of the clitoris is associated with intersex abnormalities, in which case it is a developmental abnormality (see Chap. 114), with hyperadrenocorticism (see Chap. 31), and rarely with administration of anabolic (androgenic) steroids.

Clinical Signs
- The clitoris normally lies within the vestibule, but with hypertrophy it can protrude through the vulvar cleft.
- Vaginitis results from irritation and poor drainage caused by the enlarged clitoris. Abrasion and drying of the clitoris result from chronic protrusion.
- Affected animals may be asymptomatic or may show signs related to inflammation, including excessive licking and, infrequently, vaginal discharge.

Treatment
- Nonspecific therapy includes treatment of the secondary vaginitis and protection of the exposed clitoris with lubricants and topical antibiotic ointments. However, this rarely eliminates clinical signs without correction of the underlying cause.
- Withdrawal of anabolic steroids or treatment of hyperadrenocorticism often causes regression of the enlargement when either of these is the cause.
- Clitoral resection is indicated in hermaphrodites and pseudohermaphrodites with persistent clinical signs and may also be necessary in some animals with clitoral hypertrophy secondary to anabolic steroid ad-

ministration or hyperadrenocorticism (if conservative treatment fails), especially if an os clitoris is present.

- Remove the enlarged clitoris via an episiotomy (if necessary). Incise sharply around the base of the clitoris and control hemorrhage (usually profuse) with electrocoagulation. Appose the remaining vestibular mucosa with absorbable suture.
- Dogs with intersex abnormalities may have large "phalluses" containing a urethra. In correcting this abnormality spare the urethra during clitoral resection and spatulate and suture to the remaining vestibular mucosa.

Vulvar Enlargement

- Edema and swelling of the vulva occur in response to estrogenic stimulation. This is a normal finding in bitches in estrus, but if it is present for more than 14 days it may indicate persistent estrus due to estrogen-secreting ovarian neoplasia or cystic ovarian disease.
- Vulvar enlargement associated with estrus resolves when the bitch enters diestrus, although older intact females with numerous recurrent episodes may have chronic hypertrophy and thickening. Ovariohysterectomy (see Chap. 111) is the treatment of choice for vulvar enlargement caused by ovarian hormone imbalance.

Vulvar Neoplasia

For a discussion of tumors of the vulva, see Vaginal Neoplasia later in the chapter.

DISEASES OF THE VAGINA

The vagina develops from the complete fusion of the caudal portions of the paired müllerian ducts. These ducts unite with the caudal segment of the urogenital sinus to form the hymen at the vestibulovaginal junction. This membrane is gone by birth in the normal canine (for a review of vaginal anatomy see Chap. 113).

Developmental Abnormalities

Vaginal Stenosis and Persistent Hymen

Vaginal stenosis and persistent hymen are discussed together because clinical signs, diagnosis, and treatment of both disorders are similar.

Etiology
- *Vaginal stenosis* secondary to segmental hypoplasia or aplasia of the genital canal can occur at any point in the vagina or vestibule, but it is most common at the vestibulovaginal junction.
- *Persistent hymen* occurs as an incomplete perforation of the hymen (imperforate hymen) or as an incomplete fusion of the müllerian ducts resulting in a residual vertical membrane that divides the vagina sagittally.
  - *Incomplete perforation of the hymen* is caused by inadequate union of the müllerian ducts with the uro-

genital sinus. This results in hymenal remnant tissue at the vestibulovaginal junction in the form of either a vertical band or an annular fibrotic stricture.
- An *elongated vertical vaginal septum* results in partial or complete partitioning of the vagina along its long axis. If the partition is complete, a double vagina is formed.

Clinical Signs
Many animals with congenital vaginal defects do not show any clinical signs. When present, clinical signs associated with vaginal stenosis and the various forms of persistent hymen are similar and include breeding difficulty, chronic vaginitis, and intermittent positional dribbling of urine.

Dyspareunia
- Dyspareunia, or pain and difficulty during mating, may be the first indication of vaginal stenosis or persistent hymen. The bitch usually allows mounting, but the vaginal anomaly prevents intromission, causing signs of pain in the bitch and often in the sire as well. (See Chapter 114 for more discussion of breeding disorders.)
- Hymenal remnants or stenosis may result in dystocia if an affected bitch is able to mate normally or is artificially inseminated.

Chronic Vaginitis
- Chronic inflammation causes excessive licking of the vulva and occasionally a persistent vaginal discharge.

▼ *Key Point* Chronic vaginitis is a common complication of persistent hymen and responds poorly to medical therapy without surgical correction of the underlying anomaly.

Urine Pooling
- Urine pooling cranial to the vestibulovaginal junction occurs with annular fibrotic strictures, vertical bands, and vaginal stenosis. Chronic vaginitis as well as positional dribbling of urine that resembles incontinence may result (for differential diagnosis of urinary incontinence, see Chap. 103).
- The owner typically reports that the animal leaks urine when lying down.
- The static urine in the vagina predisposes to ascending urinary tract infection, a potential source of recurrent cystitis.
- Retention of fluids in the uterus and cranial vagina occurs with complete obstruction caused by vaginal aplasia and may be confused with pyometra.

Diagnosis
Digital Palpation

▼ *Key Point* Digital palpation is the most useful tool for diagnosis of congenital vaginal defects.

- The most common location for vaginal anomalies is the vestibulovaginal junction, which is just cranial to the external urethral orifice and is easily reached digitally.

- A single small central opening cranial to the vestibule is suggestive of an annular fibrotic stricture or vestibulovaginal stenosis. Often this opening is too small to allow digital penetration into the vagina.
- Two small openings, each lateral to a central membrane, are suggestive of a vertical band, elongated sagittal septum, or double vagina. Occasionally the band is so tense that it can be "strummed" with a finger.

- Do not confuse muscular contraction or spasm during palpation with stenosis.
- Because of the relaxation of the vestibulovaginal tissues that occurs during estrus, digital palpation at this time may reveal an increased diameter compared to that during diestrus.

Other Diagnostic Procedures

- Vaginoscopy with a speculum or endoscopic equipment is helpful for evaluating the cranial vaginal mucosa but often bypasses abnormalities at the vestibulovaginal junction.
- A vaginogram performed by infusing radiographic contrast through a Foley catheter may help to identify an elongated vaginal septum or to delineate the extent of segmental stenosis.

Treatment

- *Manual dilation* of the stenotic area under general anesthesia can be attempted in animals with segmental hypoplasia or imperforate hymen. Results with digital dilation or bougienage are inconsistent, and recurrence of a stricture or inadequate dilation is common.
- *Surgical excision* of remnant membranes is the treatment of choice for clinically affected breeding animals with persistent hymen (see Chap. 113).

Acquired Abnormalities

Acquired disorders of the vagina include vaginal hyperplasia, vaginal prolapse, vaginal neoplasia, and vaginitis.

Vaginal Hyperplasia

Etiology

- Estrogenic stimulation normally causes some degree of swelling and edema in the vulvar and vaginal tissues of the bitch.
- Vaginal hyperplasia is an exaggerated response to estrogen that results in excessive edema and enlargement of the mucosal folds of the vaginal floor.

Clinical Signs

- Vaginal hyperplasia occurs most often in young, intact, large-breed female dogs during proestrus or estrus.
- Rarely, it may be associated with parturition.
- Affected bitches often are presented because of the owner's observation of a mass at the vulva.
- Other signs include dysuria, excessive licking of the vulva, painful mating, and a bulging perineum. The protruding tissue has a mass-like appearance and may be traumatized.

- The clinical appearance of vaginal hyperplasia varies in severity.
  - In mild disease, the swelling is confined to the folds of the ventral vaginal floor cranial to the urethral orifice.
  - More severe hyperplasia may cause protrusion of these tissues as a tongue-shaped mass through the labia (depicted in Chap. 113, Fig. 113–2). It may also progress to a vaginal prolapse involving the full circumference of the vaginal wall.
- Vaginal hyperplasia begins during proestrus, enlarges throughout estrus, and subsides during diestrus. It tends to recur with each estrus.

Diagnosis

- The primary differential diagnosis for vaginal hyperplasia is vaginal neoplasia.
- Diagnosis of hyperplasia usually can be made based on the signalment, the appearance and origin of the protruding tissue, and stage of the estrous cycle.
- Vaginal cytology is useful to confirm the stage of estrus.
- Vaginal biopsy can be performed to definitively differentiate hyperplasia from neoplasia in questionable cases.

Treatment

Spontaneous Regression. Regression of the hyperplasia typically occurs when the bitch enters diestrus. Recurrence is common in subsequent estrus periods and can be prevented by ovariohysterectomy.

▼ *Key Point* Ovariohysterectomy is the treatment of choice for vaginal hyperplasia in nonbreeding animals.

Medical Therapy. Medical therapy for breeding bitches involves either conservative management of the exposed tissue until spontaneous resolution occurs, or hormonal manipulation to eliminate the estrogenic stimulation. Because it interferes with natural breeding, vaginal hyperplasia is a standard indication for artificial insemination in breeding bitches.

- Conservative management includes topical antibiotic ointment to minimize drying of mucous membranes and prevention of further trauma. Lubricate and reduce the everted tissue, if possible, and then keep it in place with retention sutures to narrow the vulvar cleft until it regresses during diestrus.
- Hormonal treatment is aimed at shortening the time to diestrus by inducing ovulation.
  - Gonadotropin-releasing hormone (Gn-RH) (Cystoreline, Abbott) (2.2 µg/kg IM) may induce ovulation during the follicular phase. However, many bitches have already ovulated by the time vaginal hyperplasia is diagnosed, in which case Gn-RH will not shorten the clinical course. Gn-RH may cause ovarian cysts or luteinization of immature follicles.
  - Megestrol acetate (Ovaban, Schering) has been used to prevent vaginal hyperplasia through estrogen antagonism; however, because ovulation is prevented through the same mechanism, it cannot

be used in bitches intended to be bred during that cycle.

Surgical Excision

- Surgical excision of exposed vaginal tissue (see Chap. 113 for description of the procedure) is indicated to:
  - Remove devitalized or severely traumatized tissue
  - Attempt to prevent recurrence of vaginal hyperplasia in subsequent cycles
- Surgical resection is often the best option for managing hyperplasia in breeding animals, but recurrence may continue to be a problem despite previous resection. Only ovariohysterectomy offers a permanent cure.

Vaginal Prolapse

- Prolapse of the vagina may occur as a consequence of severe vaginal hyperplasia, or may be associated with mechanical factors without any underlying vaginal pathology.
- Severe vaginal hyperplasia is the most common cause of vaginal prolapse and results in a "doughnut-shaped" mass protruding from the vulva (depicted in Chap. 113).
- Vaginal prolapse without vaginal hyperplasia is rare and may be associated with dystocia, tenesmus, or forced separation during mating.
- Management of vaginal prolapse associated with vaginal hyperplasia consists of supportive care and treatment of the underlying disorder (see Vaginal Hyperplasia).
- Vaginal prolapse that is not associated with vaginal hyperplasia may be treated successfully with manual reduction of the vaginal tissue and placement of temporary retention sutures in the vulva (see Chap. 113).
- Surgical excision of prolapsed tissue is sometimes required (see Chap. 113 for description of the surgical procedure).

Vaginal Neoplasia

The most common neoplasms of the canine vagina and vulva are leiomyomas and fibromas, which are benign tumors originating from smooth muscle or connective tissue. Other tumors include transmissible venereal tumors, leiomyosarcomas, and lipomas. Most vaginal and vulvar tumors in dogs and cats are benign.

Benign Tumors
Etiology

- *Leiomyomas* arise from the smooth muscle of the vaginal or vestibular wall. They are often pedunculated and do not readily exfoliate neoplastic cells. These tumors are noninvasive and do not metastasize, but may recur following surgical resection. Leiomyomas may be either intraluminal or extraluminal.
- *Lipomas* may occur in the vagina but are much less common.
  Signalment. Older intact female dogs are most often affected.

Clinical Signs

- Clinical signs include vaginal discharge or bleeding, protrusion of a mass through the vulvar cleft, excessive licking of the vulva, dysuria, dyschezia, and constipation due to rectal compromise if masses are extensive.
- Extraluminal leiomyomas and lipomas often cause perineal swelling.

Diagnosis

- Most vaginal tumors are identified by visual or digital examination (rectal and vaginal).
- Vaginoscopy may be useful for diagnosis of cranial vaginal tumors and can also facilitate biopsy.
- Vaginal cytology generally is not useful in the diagnosis of vaginal neoplasia because of the failure of these tumors to shed cells. However, fine-needle aspiration may be attempted with masses that are externally accessible.
- Perform exisional biopsy for definitive diagnosis of vaginal and vulvar tumors.

Treatment

- *Surgical resection* is the treatment of choice for benign vaginal and vulvar tumors. Adequate surgical exposure often requires an episiotomy (see Chap. 113). Recurrence of the tumor may follow resection.
- Consider *ovariohysterectomy* as an adjunct to surgical resection to lower the incidence of recurrence of benign vaginal tumors. This recommendation is based on the possibility that leiomyomas are estrogen-dependent tumors.

Malignant Tumors

- *Leiomyosarcoma* is the most common malignant tumor of the canine vagina. Others include squamous cell carcinoma, hemangiosarcoma, adenocarcinoma, and mast cell tumor.
- These tumors are less often pedunculated than benign tumors and have a greater tendency to recur following resection. There is no evidence for hormonal dependency of malignant vaginal tumors.

Transmissible Venereal Tumors

Canine transmissible venereal tumor (TVT) is a proliferative tumor of the vagina and vulva that is transmitted during sexual or social contact by the direct transplantation of neoplastic cells (see Chap. 108).

Signalment

TVT occurs in younger (mean age 4 years) sexually active male and female dogs. Incidence is higher in crowded urban populations.

Clinical Signs

- TVTs may be solitary or multiple and are friable, hemorrhagic, cauliflower-like masses that may be necrotic or traumatized.
- The most common site in the bitch is the caudal vagina or vestibulovaginal junction.
- Extragenital sites include the skin, oral cavity, nasal cavity, and perineum.
- Metastasis is rare but usually occurs in regional lymph nodes. Distant metastasis is possible.

Treatment

- *Surgical excision* is effective in some animals in which total resection is possible. However, the frequency of recurrence after surgery and the difficulty in obtaining complete excision in some locations make surgery a poor option in many cases. Surgery is not useful for metastatic TVT.

- *Radiation* is highly effective, and may be used either as the sole means of treatment or as an adjunct to surgery. Most dogs show a total response following a single dose.
- *Chemotherapy* is the treatment of choice for multiple or metastatic TVT and can also be used as a first-line treatment for solitary local tumors. Both single and multiagent protocols are effective.

▼ *Key Point* Vincristine is highly effective for treatment of transmissable venereal tumors.

- Single-agent therapy with vincristine at 0.025 mg/kg (maximum 1 mg) IV, once weekly for 3–7 weeks, appears to be as effective as combination therapy, with the advantage of having fewer side effects.
- Combination chemotherapy agents include vincristine, cyclophosphamide, and methotrexate.

Vaginitis

Etiology

Juvenile Vaginitis. This occurs commonly in female dogs less than 1 year of age. The cause of the vaginal inflammation is nonspecific, and it usually resolves spontaneously after the first estrous cycle.

Bacterial Vaginitis. Bacterial vaginitis is rarely a primary disorder but is commonly seen secondary to abnormalities of the genital or urinary tracts.

- Predisposing genital abnormalities may be congenital or acquired.
  - Developmental abnormalities include vaginal stenosis, persistent hymen, and vulvar hypoplasia.
  - Acquired abnormalities include clitoral hypertrophy, vaginal or vestibular foreign body, vaginal neoplasia, and vaginal trauma.
- Urinary tract disorders that may cause a secondary vaginitis are urinary tract infection and urinary incontinence.

Viral Vaginitis. Vaginitis caused by canine herpesvirus infection (see Chap. 14) may cause vesicular or follicular mucosal lesions in the vagina and vestibule of the bitch.

- Lesions are usually transient and may recur, often during proestrus.
- Bitches infected with herpesvirus may manifest infertility, abortion, and stillbirth.

Clinical Signs

- Animals with vaginitis are usually presented for vaginal discharge and/or excessive licking of the vulva. Other signs may include pollakiuria and increased attention from male dogs.
- Vaginitis must be distinguished from other causes of vaginal discharge.
  - Nonpathologic reasons for vaginal discharge include proestral discharge (serosanguineous), early diestral discharge (mucoid), and postpartum dis-

charge (dark brown or green), which may normally persist for 4–6 weeks following parturition.
  - Abnormal discharge may be the result of vaginal neoplasia or uterine disease (see Chap. 110), such as open pyometra, subinvolution of placental sites, acute metritis, and brucellosis (see Chap. 17).

Diagnosis

Digital Examination. Digital examination of the vulva and vagina is indicated in all cases of vaginitis to identify underlying anatomic anomalies.

Vaginal Cytology. Cytology is important in the differentiation of vaginitis from other causes of vaginal discharge.

- Perform vaginal cytology by placing a cotton-tipped applicator in the vagina and then rolling it on a slide. Stain the smear with Quik–Dip (Mercedes Medical; Sarasota, FL) or Wright's stain.
- Cytology consistent with vaginal inflammation shows large numbers of neutrophils that range from healthy to toxic in appearance and may contain phagocytized bacteria.
- Do not confuse vaginitis with the normal discharge of diestrus, which is characterized by moderate numbers of healthy neutrophils. Proestral discharge contains red blood cells and increasing numbers of keratinized squamous epithelial cells.

Bacterial Culture and Susceptibility Testing. Culture and susceptibility testing of the cranial vagina is indicated in cases of chronic vaginitis.

- Bacteria are found in the cranial vagina of 60% of normal bitches. The most common isolates include staphylococci, streptococci, *Escherichia coli*, and *Pasteurella*.
- Because these organisms cultured from bitches with chronic vaginitis are qualitatively the same as those found in normal bitches, culture results cannot be the sole basis for a diagnosis of bacterial vaginitis. However, they may be helpful in choosing a course of treatment.

Urinalysis. Urinalysis obtained by cystocentesis followed by urine culture and susceptibility testing, if indicated, is useful for identifying a predisposing or secondary urinary tract infection.

Abdominal Radiography and Ultrasonography. These modalities may help to distinguish vaginitis from uterine causes of vaginal discharge (see Chap. 4).

Treatment

Juvenile Vaginitis

- Usually no specific treatment is required; the condition resolves after the first estrus. Medical therapy does not appear to shorten the clinical course and therefore is not routinely indicated.

▼ *Key Point* Juvenile vaginitis usually resolves after the first estrous period and does not require treatment.

- Nonspecific vaginitis in young bitches that becomes chronic warrants further diagnostics including careful digital palpation for congenital anomalies. If no underlying problems are detected, institute medical management of the vaginitis with systemic and topical antimicrobials, as described for bacterial vaginitis.

Bacterial Vaginitis

- Ideally, treat through detection and resolution of the underlying primary genital or urinary abnormality.
- Most cases of secondary vaginitis resolve quickly with conservative medical therapy once the primary problem is corrected.
- Chronic vaginitis with no apparent predisposing cause is a frustrating problem and often is poorly responsive to medical management.
- Medical treatment consists of systemic antibiotic therapy and local (topical) therapy.
  - Base systemic antibiotic therapy on culture and susceptibility results, and continue treatment for 2–4 weeks. A good empirical choice is amoxicillin/clavulanate (Clavamox, Pfizer), 15 mg/kg q12h PO.
  - Local therapy includes topical antibiotics, antiseptic douches, and sometimes glucocorticoids (when antibiotic therapy is unsuccessful). Place 10–30 ml of a douche solution of 1:10 diluted chlorhexidine (Nolvasan, Fort Dodge), or povidone-iodine solution (Betadine Douche, Purdue Frederick) in the vagina with a bulb syringe, disposable enema bottle, or soft large-diameter catheter. Administer 1–3 times daily for 2–4 weeks.

Viral Vaginitis

- Treat viral vaginitis due to canine herpesvirus infection with nonspecific therapy, as no vaccine is available.
- Isolate bitches with evidence of infection. Instruct owners not to use these animals for breeding.

SUPPLEMENTAL READINGS

Calvert C, Leifer CE, MacEwen EG: Vincristine for treatment of transmissible venereal tumor in the dog. J Am Vet Med Assoc 181:163, 1982.

Johnson CA: Diagnosis and treatment of chronic vaginitis in the bitch. Vet Clin North Am Small Anim Pract 21:523, 1991.

Root MV, Johnston SD, Johnston GR: Vaginal septa in dogs: 15 cases (1983–1992). J Am Vet Med Assoc 206:56, 1995.

Thacher C, Bradley RL: Vulvar and vaginal tumors in the dog: A retrospective study. J Am Vet Med Assoc 183:690, 1983.

Wykes PM: Diseases of the vagina and vulva in the bitch. In Morrow DA, ed.: Current Therapy in Theriogenology 2. Philadelphia: WB Saunders, 1986, p 476.

113 Surgery of the Vagina and Vulva

Roger B. Fingland

The surgical procedures performed most commonly on the vagina and vulva are episiotomy, episioplasty, and excision of hyperplastic vaginal tissue. Episiotomy is performed to increase exposure for excision of vaginal or vestibular masses. Vaginal neoplasia is uncommon, and the majority of vaginal tumors are benign. Vaginal hyperplasia and vaginal prolapse are more common in intact females during estrus. Diseases of the external genitalia that require surgical intervention are rare in neutered females. See Chapter 112 for discussion of diseases of the vagina and vulva.

ANATOMY

Vagina

- The vagina is a musculomembranous distensible canal that extends from the uterus to the vulva.
- The caudal boundary of the vagina is located cranial to the urethral opening, a point demarcated from the vestibule by a transverse mucosal ridge. A hymen normally is not present at the vestibulovaginal junction in the adult, although a vestige is retained in some females.
- The vagina is quite long in dogs, necessitating episiotomy for adequate surgical exposure of the cranial aspect.
- The longitudinal folds (rugae) of the vaginal mucosa allow significant expansion in diameter during pregnancy and whelping.
- The dorsal median postcervical fold extends from the cervix and terminates caudally by blending with longitudinal folds of vaginal mucosa. This fold can be mistaken for the cervical os during vaginoscopy.
- Blood supply to the vagina is via the vaginal artery, a branch of the urogenital artery.

Vulva

The vulva (external genitalia) consists of three parts:

- The *vestibule* is the space between the vagina and the labia.
  - The urethral tubercle (papilla), a ridge-like projection on the ventral floor of the vestibule caudal to the vestibulovaginal junction, contains the external urethral orifice.

- The vestibulovaginal junction is readily identified because the vestibular mucosa is smooth, unlike the vaginal mucosa, which is thrown into distinct ridges.
- The *labia* form the external boundary of the vulva.
  - The right and left labia join dorsally and ventrally at the commissures.
  - The labia open to form the vulvar cleft.
- The *clitoris* is the homologue of the penis.
  - The clitoris normally does not contain structures comparable to the os penis or the urethra of the male.
  - An os clitoris may develop in response to altered hormone balance.

The vulva is surrounded by two striated circular muscles.

- The constrictor vestibule muscle fuses along its caudal surface to the external anal sphincter.
- The thinner constrictor vulvae muscle lies immediately caudal to the constrictor vestibule muscle.

Blood supply to the vestibule, labia, and clitoris is via branches of the urogenital arteries and the internal and external pudendal arteries.

EPISIOTOMY

Indications

- To resect benign or malignant vaginal masses
- To reduce a vaginal prolapse
- To resect vaginal strictures
- To manage dystocia resulting from vulvar stenosis
- To suture vaginal lacerations
- To expose the urethral papilla for catheterization

Surgical Procedure

Objective

- Temporarily enlarge the vulvar cleft to enhance exposure of the vestibule and vagina.

Equipment

- Standard general surgery instrument pack and suture
- Gelpi or Weitlaner retractor
- Sterile Foley catheter

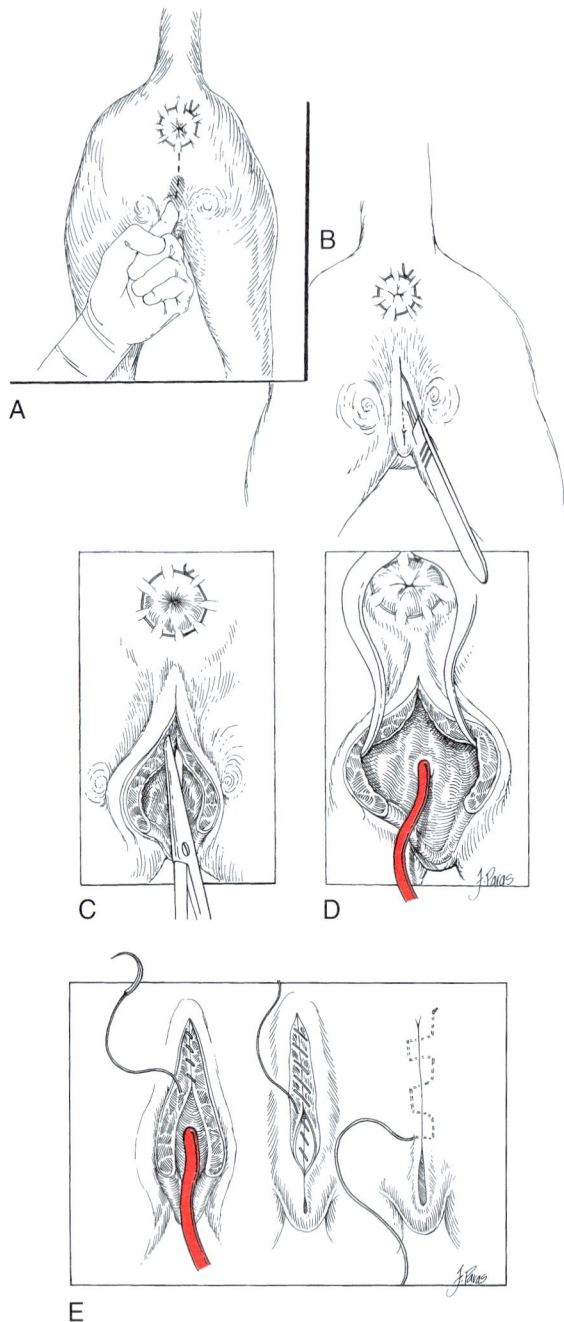

Figure 113–1. Episiotomy. *A*, After pursestring suture is placed around the anus, insert finger in the vestibule to identify the caudodorsal aspect of the vaginal canal. *B*, Incise from the caudodorsal aspect of the vaginal canal to the dorsal commissure of the vulvar cleft. *C*, Extend the depth of the incision with Metzenbaum scissors. *D*, Complete the procedure for which episiotomy is needed (in this case, bladder catheterization). *E*, Close in three layers.

Technique

1. Episiotomy can be performed under general, epidural, or local anesthesia.
2. Position the dog in ventral recumbency, preferably in a perineal stand.

▼ *Key Point* To avoid femoral nerve palsy, make certain the edge of the table or perineal stand is well padded when placing animals in the perineal position.

3. Place a pursestring suture in the anus and fix the tail in an upright and forward position.
4. Prepare the perineal region for aseptic surgery.
5. Flush the vestibule and vagina with dilute antiseptic solution (e.g., chlorhexidene).
6. Place a Foley catheter in the urinary bladder, using sterile technique.
7. Place surgical drapes so that the vulvar cleft and dorsal commissure are exposed. Exclude the anus from the surgical field.
8. Insert a finger in the vestibule and identify the caudodorsal aspect of the vaginal canal. This point represents the dorsal extent of the episiotomy incision (Fig. 113–1*A*).
9. Make a median skin incision, beginning at the point described above and extending ventrally to include the dorsal commissure of the vulvar cleft (Fig. 113–1*B*).
10. Using Metzenbaum scissors, complete the episiotomy by incising the muscular layer and the mucosa in the same plane as the skin incision (Fig. 113–1*C*).
11. Complete the procedure for which the episiotomy was performed (Fig. 113–1*D*).
12. Closure is in three layers (Fig. 113–1*E*).
    a. Appose the mucosal edges with 3-0 absorbable suture material in a simple continuous pattern with knots exposed to the lumen.
    b. Appose the muscular layer and subcutaneous tissue together with 3-0 absorbable suture material in a simple continuous pattern.
    c. Appose the skin edges with 4-0 absorbable suture material, using a continuous intradermal suture pattern.
13. Remove the pursestring suture from the anus.

Postoperative Care and Complications

* A side brace or Elizabethan collar may be necessary to prevent self-trauma.
* Clean the incision if it becomes soiled.
* Postoperative complications are uncommon and usually are related to poor surgical technique (e.g., carrying the incision too far dorsally or improper suture placement).

EPISIOPLASTY

Preoperative Considerations

* Episioplasty is indicated for aged, obese dogs with chronic perivulvar pyoderma resulting from redundant perivulvar skin and a recessed juvenile vulva. Juvenile vulva is common in dogs spayed before reaching sexual maturity.
* Manage severe perivulvar pyoderma medically before performing episioplasty (see Chap. 35). Administer systemic antibiotics based on culture and susceptibility testing.

Surgical Procedure

Objective

- Remove redundant perivulvar skin to reduce the incidence of skin fold pyoderma.

Equipment

- Standard general surgery instrument pack and suture

Technique

1. Episioplasty can be performed under general or epidural anesthesia. General anesthesia is preferred.
2. Position the dog in ventral recumbency in a perineal stand. (Pad the edge of the perineal stand.)
3. Place a pursestring suture in the anus.
4. Prepare the perineal region for aseptic surgery.
5. Determine the amount of perivulvar skin to be removed by plicating the redundant skin between the thumb and finger.
6. Make a crescent-shaped incision around the vulva, beginning lateral to the ventral commissure of the vulva, curving laterally and then dorsally to a point 1 cm dorsal to the dorsal commissure of the vulva (depicted in Chap. 50). Complete the crescent-shaped incision by making a mirror-image incision on the contralateral side.
7. Make a second crescent-shaped incision around the vulva. This incision begins and ends at the same points as the first incision. The second incision extends more dorsally than the first, creating a wider arc and including the redundant perivulvar skin.
8. Remove the perivulvar skin isolated by the two crescent-shaped incisions.
9. Remove excessive subcutaneous tissue.
10. Temporarily approximate the skin edges dorsal to the vulva. Remove additional skin dorsally if the skin folds are not eliminated or the vulva remains recessed. Do not alter the shape of the skin defect.
11. Control hemorrhage with ligation and electrocoagulation.
12. Closure may not be uniform because the incision nearest the vulva is shorter than the more dorsally placed incision. Follow these steps to avoid formation of "dog ears."
    a. Place an absorbable suture (simple interrupted pattern) in the subcutaneous tissue at the dorsal midpoint of the defect.
    b. Place additional subcutaneous sutures (simple interrupted pattern) at the midpoints of the remaining defects until the skin edges are apposed. (Bury all knots.)
    c. Place monofilament nonabsorbable skin sutures (simple interrupted pattern) at the 9, 12, and 3 o'clock positions. If there are discrepancies in the skin edges, place simple interrupted skin sutures closer together on the shorter (ventral) side of the defect than the longer (dorsal) side.
13. Remove the pursestring suture from the anus.

Postoperative Care and Complications

- See under Episiotomy.
- Continue systemic antibiotic therapy after surgery, as needed (usually 7–10 days), to manage residual pyoderma. Topical antibacterial therapy may be required to control pyoderma.
- Place obese dogs on a weight-reducing diet.
- Complications are rare with proper technique.
  - Perivulvar pyoderma may persist if the skin excision was insufficient.
  - Overzealous excision may result in excessive tension on the suture line and dehiscence. Ideally, dehiscence should be managed by wound debridement and primary closure. Keep the wound open if primary closure is not a viable option.

PERSISTENT HYMEN EXCISION

Preoperative Considerations

- A number of congenital abnormalities that obstruct or constrict the vestibulovaginal opening occur in animals, but not all represent persistent hymen. Incomplete perforation of the hymen in dogs usually is observed as a vertical septum or an annular fibrous constriction at the vestibulovaginal junction.
- Most animals with persistent hymen are asymptomatic. Symptomatic animals usually present for breeding or whelping problems or chronic vaginitis. Vaginitis results from inadequate drainage of vaginal or uterine secretions or urine pooling. Positional incontinence occasionally is observed in animals that pool urine.
- A digital vaginal examination usually is adequate to obtain a diagnosis of persistent hymen. Vaginal septa are palpated as firm central bands with small stoma on either side. A small central stoma that does not allow penetration of the finger represents an annular constriction. Vaginal examinations with specula or endoscopic equipment are helpful but can be difficult to interpret, leading to misdiagnosis. Contrast radiography of the vagina is seldom necessary.
- Per vagina resection or digital breakdown is possible when the persistent membrane is thin and located distally in the vaginal vault. More frequently the membrane is located at the vestibulovaginal junction, necessitating an episiotomy for adequate surgical exposure.

Surgical Procedure

Objective

Excise the persistent hymen or constriction.

Equipment

- Standard general surgery instrument pack and suture
- Gelpi or Weitlaner retractor
- Sterile Foley catheter

Technique

1. Perform an episiotomy, as described previously.
2. Expose the vestibulovaginal junction and place a self-retaining retractor.
3. Place a Foley catheter in the urethra to avoid inadvertent damage to the urethral papilla.
4. Identify and excise the vertical band or annular constriction.
   a. *Vertical band:* Place a curved instrument cranial to the band and retract the band caudally. Superficially transect the band at the dorsal and ventral attachments. Close the mucosal defects with 4-0 absorbable suture material in a simple continuous pattern.
   b. *Annular constriction:* Thin membranes can be circumferentially excised at the mucosal attachment. When submucosal fibrous tissue exists, make a circumferential incision in the mucosa adjacent to the membrane and submucosally dissect and excise the fibrous tissue band. Close the mucosal defect with 4-0 absorbable suture material in a simple interrupted pattern. Alternatively, suture the mucosal defect with short runs of a simple continuous pattern.

▼ *Key Point* Rarely, dogs have both a vertical band and annular constriction. Evaluate the diameter of the vaginal opening after resecting a vertical band and before closure.

5. Close the episiotomy incision, as described previously.
6. Remove the pursestring suture from the anus.

Postoperative Care and Complications

- A side brace or Elizabethan collar may be necessary to prevent self-trauma.
- Excision of persistent hymen often is curative.
- Rarely, dogs may require intermittent digital dilation to prevent fibrous narrowing after excision of annular constrictions. Permanent stenosis is possible in animals with this complication.

VAGINAL HYPERPLASIA EXCISION

Preoperative Considerations

- Refer to Chapter 112 for additional information on this condition.
- Application of a petroleum-based ointment or temporary labial closure with horizontal mattress sutures provides temporary relief of the hyperplasia. Resection of the redundant mucosa may be necessary in severe cases or in bitches used for breeding. Recurrence after resection may occur.
- Ovariohysterectomy prevents recurrence and can be used as the sole means of treatment if the vaginal hyperplasia and prolapse is small and not devitalized.

Surgical Procedure

Objective

- Excise redundant vaginal mucosa.
- Excise benign vaginal tumors (e.g., fibroma).

Equipment

- See under Episiotomy.

Technique

1. Perform an episiotomy, as described previously (Fig 113–2*A* and *B*).
2. Identify the margins of the redundant mucosa on the floor of the vagina.
3. Elevate the *mucosal* mass and identify the urethral papilla on the floor of the vagina caudal to the mass.

▼ *Key Point* Catheterize the urethra with a Foley catheter before excising the mucosal mass.

4. Make an elliptical superficial incision around the base of the mucosal mass.
5. Excise the mucosal mass. Electrocoagulate bleeding submucosal vessels. Do not extend the excision deeper than the mucosa (Fig. 113–2*C*).
6. Suture the mucosal defect with 3-0 absorbable suture material in a simple continuous pattern (Fig. 113–2*D*).
7. Close the episiotomy incision, as described previously.
8. Remove the pursestring suture from the anus.

Postoperative Care and Considerations

- A side brace or Elizabethan collar may be necessary to prevent self-trauma.
- Owners of breeding animals should be informed that vaginal hyperplasia may recur with subsequent estrus periods despite excision of redundant mucosa. Excision should be considered palliative rather than curative.

VAGINAL PROLAPSE EXCISION

Preoperative Considerations

- Refer to Chapter 112 for additional information on this condition.
- Vaginal prolapse may be partial or complete. Prolapse of the complete vaginal circumference through the labia results in the appearance of a doughnut-shaped mass ventral to the anus. This is in contrast to vaginal hyperplasia, in which redundant mucosa arises from the ventral aspect of the vagina. The urethral papilla may be observed on the prolapsed vaginal mucosa.
- Venous congestion can result in engorgement and discoloration of the prolapsed vaginal mucosa. Desiccation and self-trauma lead to ulceration and infection of the mass.

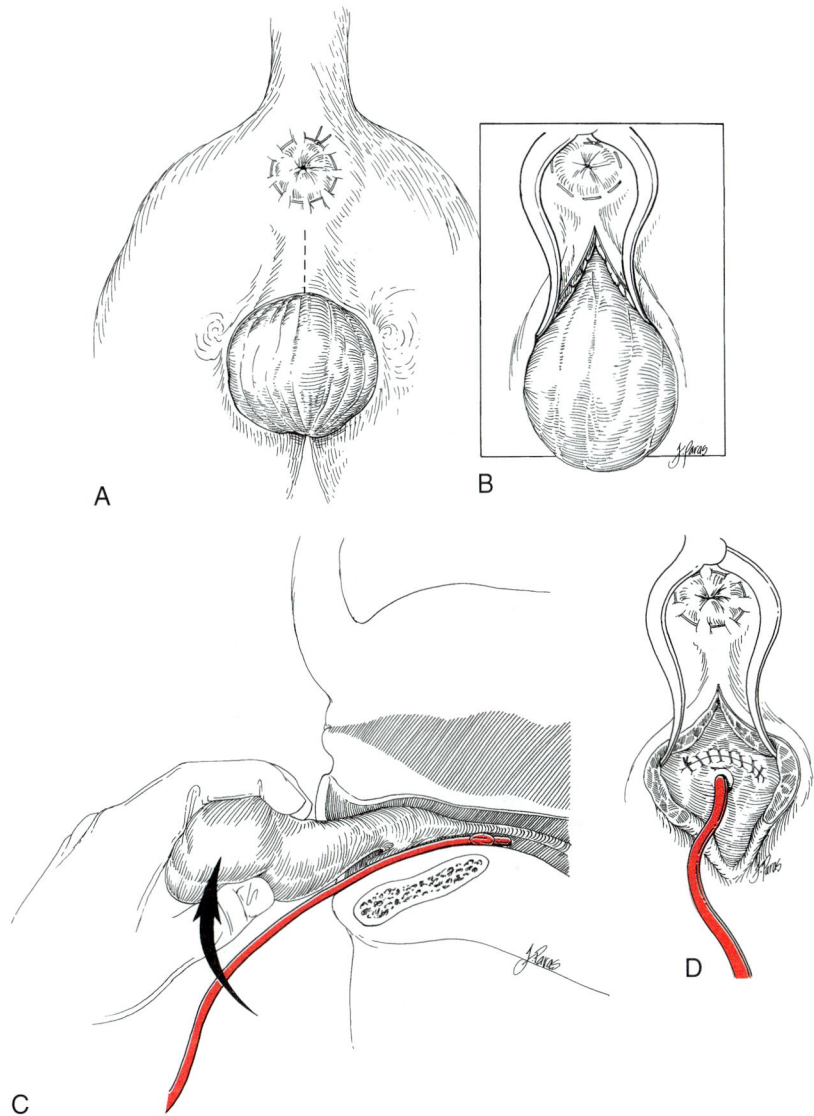

Figure 113–2. Excision of vaginal hyperplasia. *A,* Perform episiotomy as described previously. *B,* Retract skin to expose hyperplastic tissue. *C,* Elevate mass and identify urethral papilla. *D,* Suture mucosal defect in a simple continuous pattern (avoid penetrating the urethra).

- After a thorough cleaning, coat the mass with sterile lubricating jelly and gently replace the mass with a finger or appropriately sized syringe case. Place temporary nonabsorbable sutures (mattress pattern) across the vulva if the vagina tends to reprolapse.
- Consider general anesthesia followed by episiotomy if the prolapse cannot be replaced digitally in the awake dog. Manual replacement still may not be possible if a large part of the vagina is prolapsed or if there is extensive mucosal edema.
- Consider repositioning by cranial traction on the uterine body through a ventral midline celiotomy when repositioning via the vulvar approach is unsuccessful and the mucosa is healthy. Perform permanent hysteropexy by suturing the uterine body or horns to the abdominal wall.
- Excise the prolapsed portion of the vagina when repositioning is not possible because of extensive venous engorgement or ulceration and necrosis of the vaginal mucosa.

- As in vaginal hyperplasia, ovariohysterectomy is helpful in reducing recurrence.

Surgical Procedure

Objective

- Excise the prolapsed portion of the vagina.

Equipment

- Standard general surgery instrument pack and suture
- Sterile Foley catheter

Technique

1. Position the dog in dorsal recumbency with the rear legs tied forward (Fig. 113–3*A*).
2. Place a pursestring suture in the anus.
3. Gently clean the prolapsed vagina. Prepare the perineal region for aseptic surgery.

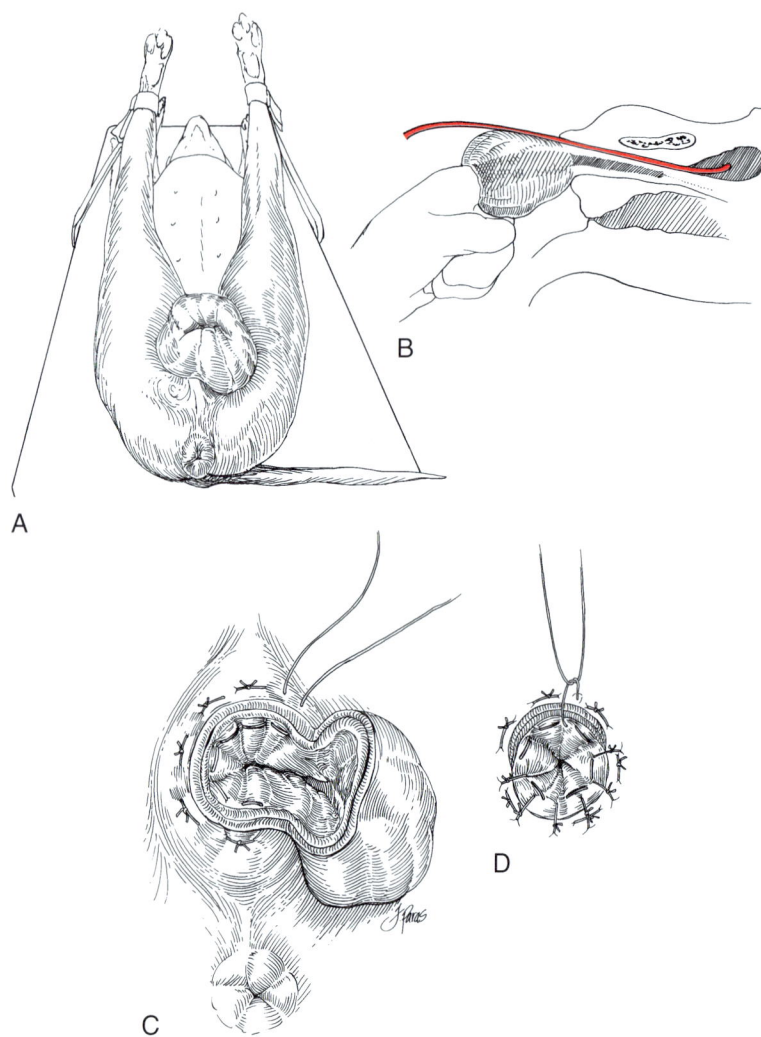

Figure 113–3. Correction of vaginal prolapse. *A,* Position dog in dorsal recumbency. *B,* Insert index finger or sterile syringe case into prolapsed opening to identify inner mucosal layer. *C,* Incise and suture the edges remaining after the prolapsed tissue is excised. *D,* Suture together the cut edges.

▼ *Key Point* Perform an episiotomy only if necessary to expose the base of the prolapsed vaginal tissue.

4. Identify the urethral papilla and place a Foley catheter in the urethra.
5. Identify the proposed line of excision at the base of the prolapsed portion of the vagina. Identify the urethra by palpating the Foley catheter through the vaginal wall.
6. Incise the outer mucosal layer for approximately 4 cm along the proposed line of excision. Dissect through all layers of the vaginal wall to the inner mucosal layer. Insert an index finger or sterile syringe case into the prolapsed vaginal opening to identify the inner mucosal layer (Fig. 113–3*B*). Carefully incise the inner mucosal layer, exposing the finger or syringe case.
7. Control hemorrhage with electrocoagulation or ligation.
8. Using 2-0 absorbable suture material, place horizontal mattress sutures in the vaginal wall between the mucosal surfaces, approximately 5 mm from the cut edge.

9. Continue this incision-suture technique in approximately 4-cm increments until the prolapsed tissue is excised (Fig. 113–3*C*).
10. Appose the cut edges of the inner and outer mucosal layers with 4-0 absorbable suture material in either a simple interrupted pattern or short runs of a simple continuous pattern (Fig. 113–3*D*).
11. Remove the pursestring suture from the anus.

Postoperative Care and Complications

- A side brace or Elizabethan collar may be necessary to prevent self-trauma.
- Mild vaginal bleeding may occur for 24–48 hours after surgery.
- Future breeding and whelping will not be impaired by this procedure. However, breeding of females prone to vaginal prolapse is ill-advised because the condition may be heritable.
- If labial sutures are placed, make certain that the animal is able to urinate spontaneously after surgery. Swelling around the urethral papilla may necessitate catheterization for several days after surgery.

SUPPLEMENTAL READINGS

Bilbrey SA, Withrow SJ, Klein MK, et al.: Vulvovaginectomy and perineal urethrostomy for neoplasms of the vulva and vagina. Vet Surg 18:450, 1989.

Kyles AE, Vaden S, Hardie EM, Stone EA: Vestibulovaginal stenosis in dogs: 18 cases (1987–1995). J Am Vet Med Assoc 209:1889, 1996.

Root MV, Johnston SD, Johnston GR: Vaginal septa in dogs: 15 cases (1983–1992). J Am Vet Med Assoc 206:56, 1995.

Wykes PM, Soderberg SF: Congenital abnormalities of the canine vagina and vulva. J Am Anim Hosp Assoc 19:995, 1983.

FEMALE

Appropriate breeding management techniques are crucial to allow animals with normal reproductive function to conceive and deliver viable young. Breeding management includes the provision of sanitary housing, optimal nutrition, proper preventive medical care, disease control, and proper timing of mating. The majority of females presented for evaluation of their fertility status have had deficient management practices. Breeding disorders result in failure to conceive or allow a pregnancy to continue to normal parturition. Such disorders commonly require the breeder and veterinarian to work together through one or more estrous cycles to determine an etiology and an appropriate treatment plan when possible.

Etiology

▼ *Key Point* The etiology of most breeding disorders is inappropriate breeding management.

When the animal is compromised by poor nutrition or disease, reproductive ability is impaired. Individuals with normal health and metabolism that have failed to conceive most commonly are bred at an inappropriate time. Less frequently, abnormalities of the female reproductive organs are the cause of infertility. Interestrous periods that are too long or too short are most indicative of diseases of the reproductive organs.

The underlying causes of canine infertility include:

Congenital Defects

These include abnormalities of sexual differentiation or developmental defects of the vagina, vestibule, or vulva. Animals with defects of sexual differentiation most often demonstrate persistent anestrus. Developmental defects of the vagina, vestibule, or vulva cause pain or difficulty with efforts to perform natural breeding.

Abnormalities of sexual differentiation may occur at the time of translation of chromosomal sex to gonadal sex, or at the time of development of the internal tubular tract of the bitch and the external genitalia into phenotypic sex. Individuals with such defects appear female externally, have primary or secondary anestrus,

and have sex chromosome monosomy (XO), trisomy (XXX or XXY), or chimerism (XX in some cells and XY in other cells). Animals that have errors in chromosomal sex may have gonads that are small, lack oocytes, or are composed of both ovarian and testicular tissue (true hermaphrodites).

Animals with errors in phenotypic sex have gonadal sex that matches chromosomal sex but fail to develop the appropriate internal tubular tract or external genitalia for the genotype. These include male pseudohermaphrodites, which may appear female externally but contain the XY sex chromosome complement and abdominal testes; such animals do not show signs of estrus.

Vaginal/vestibular barriers to breeding include persistent hymenal remnants, annular structures, vaginal hypoplasia, and vertical septa bifurcating part or all of the vagina. The stud or bitch may have difficulty breeding naturally due to pain caused by these barriers. If breeding efforts are successful, dystocia may occur during parturition.

Breeding Mismanagement

Breeding mismanagement is probably the most common cause of unsuccessful conception. Breeding management includes not only proper timing of breeding but also adequate and sanitary housing, nutrition, parasite control, and prevention or management of systemic disease.

Infectious Agents

Infectious agents that can cause infertility or abortion at some stage of pregnancy include: *Brucella canis, Mycoplasma, Ureaplasma, Escherichia coli, Staphylococcus* sp., and herpesvirus, as well as many other microorganisms.

Hormone Imbalances

Hormone imbalances may be caused by disease of the pituitary gland, follicular cysts, persistent corpora lutea, or abnormal function of the thyroid or adrenal glands.

Pituitary Insufficiency

Pituitary insufficiency is very rare in the dog. German shepherd dogs with hereditary dwarfism are most commonly identified. Affected animals retain the physical stature, haircoat, and dentition of puppies and have variable thyroid and adrenal gland function. Some of these animals have, however, shown reproductive cycling.

Thyroid Insufficiency

Thyroid insufficiency is a common endocrinopathy in many breeds of dog. It can be associated with primary or secondary anestrus, vague signs of heat (minimal bleeding, minimal vulvar swelling), prolonged proestrus, or ovulation failure. Most hypothyroid bitches demonstrate normal reproductive activity within 3–6 months of adequate replacement therapy.

Ovarian Dysfunction

Persistent corpora lutea or luteal ovarian cysts commonly cause primary or secondary anestrus with serum progesterone concentrations in excess of 2 ng/ml for more than the normal 2-month luteal phase.

Insufficient luteal phase is due to premature luteolysis or decline in serum progesterone concentrations to less than 1 ng/ml 2–4 weeks following breeding. This does not allow maintenance of pregnancy for a sufficient period of time or allow for adequate fetal development. Abortion is the most common result.

Follicular cysts generally cause persistent signs of estrus for longer than the normal 4–6 week period.

Neoplasia in the Reproductive Tract

Neoplasia in the ovaries may cause alteration of the reproductive hormone levels (see Chap. 110). Physical obstruction to breeding or implantation may occur with neoplasia in the uterus, cervix, or vaginal tract.

Clinical Signs in the Dog
Normal Estrous Cycle

The normal canine estrous cycle occurs approximately every 6 months but may vary between 4 and 18 months depending on the individual and family history. Clinical estrus is detectable for approximately 3 weeks, which includes proestrus, estrus, and early diestrus.

Proestrus

Proestrus lasts between 3 and 14 days. During proestrus, a bloody vaginal discharge is commonly observed with swelling of the vulva. Males are attracted but are not allowed to mate.

Estrus

Estrus averages 3–9 days. This is the period of female receptivity. At this time, the female stands for the male to mount and "flags" her tail. The vulva will soften and slightly decrease in size. The discharge may change from bloody to clear or straw color. It is not uncommon, however, for the discharge to remain bloody.

Diestrus

Diestrus signifies the end of the receptive period and the end of the fertile period. Progesterone levels rise and remain elevated for approximately 57 days whether pregnancy occurs or not. The vulva returns to normal size and turgor. Vaginal discharges are mucoid to mucopurulent in appearance.

Anestrus

Anestrus is the transition period between one cycle and the next. The quiescent period ranges from 4–12 months. Dogs require a minimum "repair" period of 4 months to allow for normal implantation on subsequent breedings. Normal dogs may have a family history of exceptionally long or short interestrous intervals.

Refusal to Breed

Females refusing to breed are usually presented to the male when not in estrus. Bitches in estrus may refuse to breed if they experience pain upon intromission due to restrictive vulvar or vestibulo-vaginal anomalies. Additionally, exceptionally heavy males or poor hip conformation may cause discomfort when mounting efforts are made. A female may also refuse to breed because she finds the male undesirable (color or personality) or is too uncomfortable in the male's environment.

Abnormally Long Anestrus

An abnormally long anestrus may be the only symptom in an otherwise normal female. Hypothyroidism may cause additional clinical signs, including a tendency toward obesity and possibly, alopecia (see Chap. 29). Unobserved estrus, luteal cysts, prior ovariohysterectomy, use of contraceptive agents, abnormalities of sexual differentiation, or ovarian hypoplasia are other causes of prolonged anestrus in an otherwise normal female.

Abnormally Long Estrus

An abnormally long estrus may be the only symptom in an otherwise normal female. This is most commonly associated with cystic follicles or tumors causing persistent estradiol production. Cystic follicles or ovarian tumors generating elevated estradiol concentrations cause a female to appear persistently in estrus.

A "split heat" might also be misinterpreted as an abnormally long estrus. In a split heat, during proestrus, vulvar swelling and vaginal bleeding occurs, followed by an apparent diestrus for 2–10 weeks. Proestrus is then again followed by estrus and ovulation. This is most common in the young female and is generally not associated with any underlying problem.

▼ *Key Point* Abnormal vaginal discharges associated with infertility are most commonly observed 3–8 weeks into diestrus.

Abnormal Vaginal Discharges

Mucopurulent vaginal discharges occur with endometritis and pyometra. Vaginitis rarely is associated with infertility unless the infection extends into the uterus or there is sufficient discomfort to discourage breeding attempts. Bleeding during anestrus may be an indication of abortion, prolonged estrogen influence, or an ulcerated neoplasm. Also consider coagulation disorders including von Willebrand disease (see Chap. 21).

Clinical Signs in the Cat

Normal Estrous Cycle

The feline estrous cycle is delineated by changes in behavior rather than clinically detectable changes in the genitalia or discharges from the reproductive tract. Cats are seasonally polyestrous with estrous cycles becoming apparent in January through March in response to the lengthening day after the winter solstice. They continue to cycle until October through December. Reproductive quiescence occurs in the interim. Artificial light can alter this pattern.

Proestrus

Proestrus is rarely apparent clinically with similar behavior to estrus, which includes rubbing, rolling, and vocalization. During proestrus, the male is attracted to a nonreceptive female. This stage lasts only ½–2 days.

Estrus

Estrus is the period when the female will allow the male to breed. In addition to rubbing, rolling, and vocalization, the female demonstrates lordosis and deviation of the tail to one side while allowing the male to mate. Estrus behavior lasts 1–21 days (average 7 days).

Diestrus

Diestrus is the phase of progesterone dominance. The queen must have coital contact or vaginal stimulation to induce ovulation before corpora lutea develop to secrete progesterone. Most queens ovulate after four or more copulations. A queen bred only once daily has a much lower incidence of ovulation induction than a queen bred 4–8 times every other day. Pseudopregnancy will last 35–50 days (average 45 days), during which breeding activity ceases. During pregnancy, breeding activity also ceases for approximately 60 days. Progesterone levels are higher in pregnant queens than in pseudopregnant queens.

Interestrous Period

Interestrous period in a female without corpora lutea producing progesterone lasts 3–15 days (average 8 days). The female returns to her normal personality and does not attract males during this time.

Abnormally Long Anestrus

Failure to cycle and prolonged interestrous intervals appear similar in that estrous behavior is not detected in an otherwise normal female. Systemic illness or disease will cause any variety of clinical signs, and as in the dog, the queen will fail to cycle. One should always consider the possibility of prior ovariohysterectomy or inability to detect estrus due to "subdued" behavior.

Abnormally Long Estrus

Prolonged sexual receptivity may be normal with overlapping cycles or may be secondary to follicular cysts.

Abnormal Vaginal Discharges

Abnormal vaginal discharges may be bloody or mucopurulent in nature. Bloody vaginal discharge may be secondary to metritis or abortion. Rule out bleeding disorders. Mucopurulent discharges are most commonly associated with endometritis.

Diagnosis

History

Dogs and cats presented for breeding disorders have generally been bred one or more times with unsatisfactory results. A thorough history of the timing of these breedings, method of breeding, detection techniques for ovulation and pregnancy, medical history (including medications and prior surgery), and results of the breedings direct the clinician to the most likely diagnostic path to pursue.

Physical Examination

Perform a thorough physical examination on all females presented for assistance with breeding management or suspected breeding disorders. Look for evidence of systemic disease and reproductive anomalies.

- The vulva should be normally positioned and of a size and character appropriate for the stage of the cycle. Similarly, any discharges when present should be appropriate for the phase of the cycle.
- The clitoris should be small and contained in the clitoral fossa. Enlargement of the clitoris should raise suspicion for a testosterone stimulus and further investigation.
- Perform a digital vaginal examination on all bitches larger than 10 pounds in order to assess vaginal size for normal copulation. Inspect the junction of the vestibule and vagina both visually and digitally to detect anomalies that could compromise breeding. Anomalies include strictures, hypoplasia, vertical vaginal bands, and double vaginas.
- The reproductive tract can rarely be examined digitally much beyond the caudal vagina in the normal individual. Use vaginoscopy, if necessary, to identify vaginal hyperplasia, polyps, or neoplasms.

Laboratory Evaluation

Submit samples for CBC, biochemical profile, urinalysis, heartworm check, and fecal study to detect occult disease, which could adversely affect conception. In cats, test for feline leukemia virus (FeLV), feline immunodeficiency virus (FIV), feline infectious peritonitis (FIP), and toxoplasmosis. Test females for *Brucella canis* prior to each breeding and males at least annually. Some clinicians recommend routine screening for hypothyroidism, *Mycoplasma*, canine herpesvirus, and bacterial cultures from the anterior vagina. These tests may not be necessary for normal individuals presented for routine prebreeding examination but are considered appropriate when infertility is suspected.

Vaginal Cytology

Vaginal cytology may be used to approximate the stage of the cycle in the dog and help determine when natural, multiple breedings are appropriate. A single examination of vaginal cytology is of no value in predicting when ovulation will occur. Breeding can only be recommended when maximal cornification is present.

A brief description of the characteristics of vaginal cytology during the various stages of the estrous cycle are as follows:

Canine

Proestrus: increasing cornification of the epithelial cells, many red blood cells, healthy neutrophils, and variable numbers of bacteria.

Estrus: maximal cornification of epithelial cells (superficial cells predominate), large numbers of bacteria without reactive neutrophils, and variable numbers of red blood cells.

Diestrus: decreased superficial cells, return of neutrophils in varying number with reduced numbers of bacteria.

Anestrus: parabasal cells predominating with few neutrophils, bacteria, or red blood cells.

Feline

Feline vaginal cytology is much more difficult to collect and one runs the risk of inducing ovulation due to stimulation of the cervix during collection. Changes in the vaginal epithelium may appear similar to those seen in the dog but develop at a much faster rate.

During proestrus, cornification is not yet obvious. The only hint of approaching estrus may be the liquefaction of vaginal mucus, seen as absence of precipitated, basophilic strands on the microscope slide, known as "clearing."

During estrus, the vaginal epithelium begins to demonstrate cornification, as in the dog. Typically, differential cell counts show a 60% rise in large superficial cells within 24 hours. Moderate to scant amounts of cloudy, pink fluid exudate from the vagina are present, but usually erythrocytes are not seen.

Detection of Ovulation

Determination of ovulation is critical in those instances where there are factors present that could adversely affect conception rates. These include use of chilled/extended semen, use of frozen semen, bitches with a history of apparent infertility, breedings with stud dogs with low semen quality, or limited access to the stud dog.

Timing of ovulation has become more sophisticated using hormone test kits. These test kits allow for hormone levels to be determined with the results available the same day. This helps identify the optimal fertile breeding time for the female. Prior to the development

of these kits, testing was possible but the results were available only for retrospective use. Currently, test kits are only available for dogs.

Progesterone and Luteinizing Hormone Assay

Canine Progesterone ELISA Assay (Status-Pro or Target Canine Ovulation Timing Test, ICG) detects the rise in progesterone, which begins on the day of the luteinizing hormone (LH) surge. Before the LH surge, progesterone levels are baseline. After the LH surge, progesterone begins to rise and continues to increase as the cycle progresses. Ovulation occurs 2 days after the LH peak. The LH peak can be determined directly using a semi-quantitative LH assay (Status LH, ICG). The eggs then take an additional 2–3 days to mature to support fertilization. These mature eggs remain viable for 48–72 hours. Thus, the fertile period of the bitch falls between days 4 and 7 after the LH peak with the most fertile days being on days 5 and 6 post–LH peak. For most natural mating or artificial insemination with fresh semen, breeding should begin 2–3 days after the LH peak and continue every 2–3 days until the end of the fertile period. When using chilled or frozen semen, or a stud dog with compromised semen quality, breeding should occur on the most fertile days (4, 5, and 6 post–LH peak).

Using both LH and progesterone assays improves ovulation timing accuracy.

Perform an initial progesterone test to establish a baseline level during the first 5 days of estrous activity. If testing is started after the onset of estrus, it is likely that the LH surge has already occurred and cannot be identified in retrospect. When vaginal cytology indicates 50% cornification, begin daily LH testing.

▼ *Key Point* Because the LH surge may occur within a 24-hour period, it is crucial that daily serum samples be tested.

When LH testing indicates a positive result, make preparations to breed. Perform an additional progesterone test 72 hours post–LH surge to confirm a rise in progesterone because small pulsate fluctuations in LH may occur during proestrus, while progesterone remains at low baseline levels. Progesterone rises, however, after the preovulatory surge in LH. By the third day post–LH peak, the majority of bitches will demonstrate a rise in progesterone levels above the 2 ng/ml level.

Urine Assay

A *home test on dog urine* for purposes of confirming ovulation is also available. This test detects a metabolite of progesterone that is present in the bitch's urine as the level of progesterone rises in the bloodstream, indicating that ovulation has taken place. Use of this test is designed for normal routine breedings where fresh semen is used. This necessitates that the stud and bitch be together at the same location. Breeding is recommended on the day of the first positive test. Repeat breeding every other day for a total of two to three breedings. This type of testing is not recommended for chilled, extended, or frozen semen breedings or any breedings where there is decreased longevity of the sperm.

Radiography

Radiographs are of little value in the nonpregnant normal female because ovaries and uterus of normal size are not visible. Fetal skeletons are sufficiently ossified to be visible radiographically after 42–45 days of gestation. Thus, an enlarged uterus appears similar in the bitch with either early pregnancy or endometritis. Radiography is more accurate than ultrasonography to determine whether the fetus is full term and to compare fetal size to the size of the maternal pelvis.

Ultrasound

Ultrasound, like radiography, does not readily detect the normal uterus or ovaries.

- The ultrasonic appearance of fetuses at the various stages of pregnancy has been well delineated. Photographic and written descriptions are readily available in ultrasound textbooks and atlases.
- When there is fetal resorption, the implantation site may be detected as a focal thickening of the uterine horn that persists to the end of gestation. When fetal death occurs in the third trimester, it may trigger early whelping or spontaneous abortion of the entire litter. Within 24–48 hours, the organs of a dead fetus appear hypoechoic and less defined due to autolysis. There is rapid resorption of fetal fluid, and the body of the dead fetus decreases in size. After several days, only skeletal structures may be recognized.
- Endometritis appears as a uterus with thickened walls. The lumen of the uterus contains variable amounts of fluid, which is either anechoic or echogenic. Ultrasound diagnosis of metritis and endometrial hyperplasia is not very accurate because the changes caused by these conditions are often subtle and inconsistent. Either of these conditions may enlarge uterine diameter, and the uterus may have "blotch" echogenicity, multiple 1–5 cm cysts, or a central echogenic layer. This layer could represent thickened endometrium or a small accumulation of bloody discharge, exudate, mucus, or necrotic debris.
- Mass lesions of the uterus are readily detected by ultrasound. Scar tissue and necrotic fat are usually hyperechoic and poorly marginated in appearance. Uterine polyps can appear as multicystic uterine masses. See Chapter 110 for more information on uterine disorders.
- Causes of ovarian enlargement can be differentiated with the aid of ultrasound. Fluid-filled follicular cysts are anechoic. Neoplasms are more apt to have a solid echogenic appearance.

Serology

Brucellosis (see also Chap. 17)

Perform testing for serum *Brucella canis* antibodies prior to each breeding, including in virgin animals since ingestion of the bacteria from an infected bitch is the most common mode of transmission. *B. canis* can cause infertility, abortion, or neonatal mortality. More important, *B. canis* is of zoonotic concern.

Canine Herpesvirus

Because the neonatal form of canine herpesvirus is fatal, prior to breeding isolate bitches with negative titers from other dogs during the final 3 weeks of pregnancy through the 3 weeks after parturition. Systemic canine herpesvirus causes placental infection and may cause abortion during the second trimester, stillborn pups, or neonatal death if disease is contracted during pregnancy. Most adult dogs have prior exposure to canine herpesvirus infection through aerosol spread. It is thought that positive titers are protective for developing fetuses and neonates.

Feline Viral Disease

Feline viral diseases including herpesvirus, feline leukemia virus (FeLV), feline immunodeficiency virus (FIV), feline infectious peritonitis (FIP), and toxoplasmosis are known to cause infertility, abortion, stillborn kittens, or neonatal death (see appropriate chapters in Section 2). Regular testing and quarantine of new individuals into the cattery are important to maintain a viable breeding program.

Culture

Aerobic Bacteria

Bacterial infections with beta-hemolytic streptococci, *Haemophilus canis*, *Escherichia coli*, species of *Pseudomonas*, *Proteus* spp., and other bacteria have been found to cause infertility. Although culture results can be an important part of an infertility evaluation, it is important to also understand their limitations. Over half of normal bitches harbor aerobic bacteria in the cranial vagina and most bitches harbor similar organisms in the caudal vagina. Recognize that male dogs harbor microorganisms in the prepuce and semen similar to those found in normal vaginal cultures. Thus, prebreeding cultures without signs of clinical disease are of little value.

Mycoplasma and Ureaplasma

Mycoplasma and ureaplasma can cause a syndrome of infertility characterized by poor conception, early embryonic death, embryonal or fetal resorption, abortion, stillborn pups, weak newborns, or neonatal death. Diagnosis is made by passing a guarded culture swab into the cranial vagina during anestrus, early proestrus, or whenever a mucopurulent discharge is present. Amies transport media without charcoal is recommended, but the author has had no problem recovering these microorganisms in pure culture if the sample arrives at the laboratory in a timely fashion and remains cool during transport. Request mycoplasma or ureaplasma isolation because they are rarely detected with routine culture techniques. Because of human health concerns, not all laboratories will attempt to isolate mycoplasma or ureaplasma. Because small numbers of mycoplasma and ureaplasma may be part of the normal flora, request a quantitative culture.

Endocrine Evaluation

Thyroid Hormone

Identify hypothyroid animals and treat with thyroid supplementation (see Chap. 29). Although normal estrous cycling and fertility will return within several months, the question as to whether to breed individuals with a potential hereditary predilection remains.

Pituitary Hormones

Both FSH and LH are persistently elevated when there is ovarian aplasia or hypoplasia, after ovariohysterectomy, and in some cases of premature ovarian failure.

Karyotyping

Diagnosis of all categories of abnormalities of sexual differentiation can be achieved with a 10-ml heparinized blood sample or a small skin biopsy for karyotyping. Commercial karyotyping is available at several colleges of veterinary medicine.

Histopathology

Biopsy of reproductive organs requires a laparotomy because the structure of the cervix does not allow easy access to the uterus of the dog or cat. Laparotomy allows for physical and visual inspection of the entire reproductive tract, which may reveal abnormalities not detected by other diagnostic tools (see Chap. 111).

Histopathology of the ovaries is required for definitive diagnosis of ovarian hypoplasia, luteal ovarian cysts, lymphocytic oophoritis, and ovarian neoplasms. Lymphocytic oophoritis is characterized by degenerating follicles with infiltration of lymphocytes, oocyte degeneration, and thickening and collapse of the zona pellucidae. Treatment with immunosuppressive agents is not commonly successful after diagnosis.

Histopathology of the uterus most often defines some degree of endometritis. Atrophy of the endometrial glands is diagnosed less often. Uterine neoplasia requires histopathology to determine if maintaining the remaining reproductive tract is appropriate.

Treatment

Improve Management Strategies

Provide breeding animals with optimal nutrition, comprehensive preventive medicine for disease and parasite control, and a sanitary, well-lit environment. When conventional methods to determine an appropriate time to breed have failed, perform progesterone measurement to determine ovulation followed by natural breeding or artificial insemination 2 days later.

Correction of Vaginal Anomalies

Correct vaginal anomalies whenever possible before breeding attempts are made. This eliminates both the frustration of not being able to accomplish a natural breeding at the appropriate time and the pain that the female and/or male might experience during breeding attempts.

Retained hymenal remnants and strictures can often be corrected with digital manipulation of the area with the aid of general anesthesia. Muscular vertical bands in the vagina often require removal through an episiotomy incision. Hyperplasia of the vagina also requires surgical removal of the excess tissue through an episiotomy incision (see Chap. 113).

Artificial Insemination

▼ *Key Point* The key to success with vaginal insemination is proper semen handling technique and placing the insemination pipette into the cranial vaginal canal.

Elevate the bitch's hind legs for 5–10 minutes to aid the pooling of semen around the cervix. Use a rigid insemination pipette.

It has been theorized that an increase in conception rate can occur if semen of poor quality is deposited directly into the uterus, thus bypassing the cervical barrier. Intrauterine insemination has also been recommended when using frozen semen, especially that of marginal quality after thawing. Cannulating the canine cervix is difficult, tedious, and potentially traumatic to the cervix. Performing intrauterine insemination by laparotomy can be performed safely, rapidly, and with maintenance of sterile technique.

Artificial insemination may be necessary when physical or psychological obstacles are encountered at the appropriate time to breed. Fresh semen should be inseminated soon after collection and microscopic evaluation to ensure motile sperm. Fresh semen of a normal, healthy stud may remain viable 5 or more days in the bitch. Therefore, semen inseminated a day or two before the fertile period should be viable at the time of peak fertility. Perform artificial insemination 2–3 days after ovulation.

Chilled, extended semen will usually live 2–4 days after collection. One day of this time is typically used for transport from the male to the location of the female. This reduced survival time requires that breeding be conducted closer to the short fertile period of the bitch. Perform two inseminations on days 3 and 5 or 4 and 6 post—LH surge.

Artificial insemination with frozen, thawed semen requires deposition of the semen into the uterine body for normal reproductive performance, because motile sperm that have experienced freezing and thawing appear unable to adequately traverse the cervix. Frozen, thawed dog sperm have short half-lives (less than 24 hours after thawing); therefore, insemination must be timed so that ova, ready for fertilization, are present in the oviducts. Best results occur with frozen semen inseminated 3–5 days following ovulation in the bitch.

Treatment of Infections

Some bitches with bacterial uterine infection have conceived and maintained a normal pregnancy when treated with antibiotics (3-week duration), starting in early estrus. Choose antibiotics, whenever possible, based on the results of culture and susceptibility with caution given to potential teratogenic effects of the selected medication. *Mycoplasma* infection of the uterus probably is best treated with enrofloxacin (2.5 mg/kg q12h PO for 2 weeks) or doxycycline (5 mg/kg q12h PO for 2 weeks). However, do not treat during pregnancy. Affected bitches should be treated at the time of diagnosis and should not be bred until the next cycle. If breeding has already taken place, treatment with erythromycin or ampicillin can be provided in early pregnancy. In the last half of pregnancy chloramphenicol has been used successfully.

Hormone Treatments

Ovulation Induction

In some bitches, persistent estrus ceases without treatment, implying that some estrogen-secreting follicles or follicular cysts undergo spontaneous atresia or luteinization. In breeding bitches, various regimens using gonadotropin-releasing hormone (GnRH) or human chorionic gonadotropin (hCG) have been recommended. Although ovulation may follow either therapy, it is unlikely, and mating is not recommended at this time. If estrus persists or recurs soon after GnRH or hCG therapy, increased suspicion of neoplasia is warranted. Ultrasound examination and surgical exploration are indicated.

Thyroid Hormone Supplementation

The only cause of primary or secondary anestrus in the bitch that is known to be reversible is thyroid insufficiency. This usually responds to administration of 0.02 mg/kg thyroxine q12h PO. Affected bitches usually will show improvement in coat and skin quality in 4–6 weeks and onset of a fertile estrous in 3–6 months (see Chap. 29).

Prolonged Anestrus

A potentially reversible cause of primary/secondary anestrus in the bitch is a luteal ovarian cyst, which may respond to the luteolytic action of prostaglandin F2-alpha or to surgical excision.

Before attempting to induce estrus, anestrus should be demonstrated for at least 18 months and confirmed with monthly serum progesterone measurement for 6 consecutive months. Progesterone rises to over 2 ng/ml for approximately 2 months after each estrus. If progesterone is found to be elevated, unobserved estrus is occurring. Several methods for rapid induction of fertile estrus in dogs have been described. These protocols can be laborious and provide variable response. Also, there are problems of availability, quality, and dependability of the necessary hormone preparations.

Short Anestrus

The canine endometrium is known to slough and regenerate during a 4-month period of anestrus. Bitches with normal follicular and luteal phases demonstrating estrus more frequently than every 4 months may benefit from mibolerone 2.6 µg/kg daily at least 30 days prior to the next anticipated proestrus to permit time for complete endometrial regeneration. Treatment with mibolerone for 2–6 months commonly results in conception on the subsequent estrus.

Infection

Treat infection in the reproductive tract with 2–6 weeks of appropriate antibiotics. Females with open pyometra also require treatment with prostaglandin F2-alpha to cause luteolysis and expulsion of uterine contents (see Chap. 110).

▼ *Key Point* Many bitches treated medically for pyometra conceive on the next estrus but are prone to develop pyometra on subsequent cycles.

Surgery for Neoplasia

Neoplasia and polyps that arise in the reproductive organs can be surgically removed to potentially allow fertility to resume. An ovariohysterectomy may be most appropriate if malignancy is demonstrated clinically or histologically (see Chap. 111).

MALE

The male reproductive tract is almost completely available for physical examination. Additionally, semen evaluation can usually indicate if fertility is likely. When infertility is demonstrated but physical examination is normal, review breeding management techniques so that adverse exogenous influences can be removed. Additionally, identify and treat systemic disease. When normal semen quality is demonstrated repeatedly, evaluate the timing of the breeding and the fertility of the female.

Etiology

For additional information, refer to Chapter 106 regarding diseases of the testes and Chapter 108 regarding diseases of the penis and prepuce.

Congenital Defects

Cryptorchidism is the failure of one or both testes to descend into the scrotum. The undescended testis may be found within the abdominal cavity, in the inguinal canal, or lateral to the penis. This defect is a sex-linked, autosomal recessive trait in most breeds; therefore, discourage breeding of affected animals.

Testicular hypoplasia results from abnormal development of the seminiferous tubular germinal epithelium. This leads to significant reduction in sperm number and infertility. A significant decrease in the size of one or both testicles is present at the time of puberty.

A *female pseudohermaphrodite* has the external genitalia of a male but generally has more than a single X chromosome. These individuals frequently have an XXY karyotype. Male pseudohermaphrodites have testicular hypoplasia, cryptorchidism, or abnormal development of the penis or prepuce.

Persistent penile frenulum is a band of connective tissue extending from the ventral tip of the penis to the prepuce. When the connective tissue persists, it hinders extrusion of the penis from the prepuce and causes deviation of the penile tip in a ventral or lateral direction.

Penile hypoplasia is an underdevelopment of the penis making it much shorter than the prepuce. Penile hypoplasia may be an indication of female pseudohermaphrodism.

Os penis deformity results in deviation of the penis, occasionally causing inability to retract the penis fully into the prepuce. A congenitally shortened os penis may result in excessive flaccidity of the penile tip, causing impaired copulation.

Breeding Mismanagement

The frequency of ejaculation has a direct effect on semen volume and concentration of spermatozoa. Collection of semen every second or third day allows for optimal semen quality. Collection of semen once or twice daily can cause significant reduction in spermatozoal concentration.

Avoid dramatic changes in environmental temperature. Preparation and handling of samples to be extended and cooled or frozen require special equipment and careful attention to recommended protocols. Sterilize equipment used for semen collection and artificial insemination if at all possible and remove all agents that could be spermicidal (water, powder, disinfectant residues, or lubricants).

Infectious Agents

Infectious agents can disrupt normal spermatogenesis subsequent to inflammation of the seminiferous tubules. Poor semen quality has been demonstrated with scrotal dermatitis, acute orchiepididymitis, chronic orchiepididymitis, and prostatitis (see Chaps. 104 and 106). The resulting subfertility or infertility associated with the poor semen quality may be temporary or permanent.

Hormone Imbalances

Endocrinopathies, such as hypothyroidism, diabetes mellitus, or abnormally high or low concentrations of glucocorticoid, estrogen, androgen, or gonadotropin alter spermatogenesis. Such conditions alter the metabolism of the gonadal hormones and gradually cause deterioration of the seminiferous epithelium.

Neoplasia in the Reproductive Tract

Neoplasia in the testes can cause infertility by hormone production (estradiol by Sertoli cell tumors and seminomas or testosterone by Leydig cell tumors). Tumors can also cause physical replacement of testicular tissue by the tumor's causing pressure necrosis or obstruction of the tubular network (see Chap. 106).

Neoplasia (or hyperplasia) of the prostate gland can obstruct the vas deferens and sperm flow (see Chap. 104).

Clinical Signs

Failure of Erection

Dogs who are fearful in unfamiliar surroundings (i.e., a veterinary hospital) will frequently fail to have an erec-

tion or produce an ejaculate. Some males are afraid of a selected mate, if she is dominant. Some males are afraid that breeding attempts will result in disciplinary action. When these individuals are moved away from the dominant owner, collection of an ejaculate occurs without difficulty. Inexperienced males who have never been bred or had semen collected with manual stimulation may be confused or afraid of what is happening.

Pain can cause an erection to cease. This pain may be caused by vigorous massage, a persistent frenulum causing pain with efforts to extrude the penis from the sheath, or engorgement of the bulbus glandis within the sheath. Pain from inflammation of the penile mucosa, preputial mucosa, or prostate gland may also cause cessation of an erection.

Reduced libido due to reduced androgen concentrations, elevated estrogen concentrations, or hypothyroidism can result in failure to generate an erection.

Erection Without Ejaculation

Obstructive lesions in the tubular outflow through the vas deferens or prostate gland can allow an erection to develop and often muscular pulsation to occur without producing an ejaculate. This obstruction may be due to edema secondary to inflammation, physical compression due to hyperplasia, or neoplasia or sperm granulomas in the epididymis.

Fear and pain can also allow an erection to develop without expulsion of a complete ejaculate.

Retrograde ejaculation into the urinary bladder can occur in some males with prostatitis, urethritis, or neuropathies. Most of the time the cause is not apparent. These individuals have a normal erection and pulsation but do not expel an ejaculate. If a urine sample is collected shortly after attempts to collect semen, a large number of sperm are found in the urine sample without sperm in the collected ejaculate.

Ejaculation with Normal Semen Quality

Nonconception using males that demonstrate normal ejaculation and semen quality suggest a problem with either the female or the timing of the breeding.

Many factors can adversely affect semen quality. Collect at least three samples over a period of several days, looking for a consistent abnormality.

Ejaculation with Abnormal Semen Quality

▼ *Key Point* Persistent conception failure with several females despite appropriate breeding management techniques suggests reduced spermatozoal longevity and survival. Perform careful review of the spermatozoal motility and morphology to ensure that it is indeed normal.

Sperm Function

Agglutination of the sperm may not allow for effective sperm motility. Diagnostic tests to assess sperm functional activity are routinely employed as part of fertility examinations in several other species. Such tests have yet to be developed for routine use in dogs and cats.

Sperm Numbers

Severe reduction in the numbers of spermatozoa in an ejaculate will certainly result in reduced conception rates. Although 200 million sperm is considered a normal number of spermatozoa in an ejaculate, it is uncertain at what point reduced conception is demonstrated. Reduced spermatozoal numbers in an ejaculate may be the result of an incomplete collection, reduced production by the seminiferous epithelium, or compromise of the outflow from at least one testis. When there is complete lack of sperm in an ejaculate from a male with normal-sized testes, measure the alkaline phosphatase in the collected sample. A true, complete ejaculate will have levels greater than 5,000 U/L, which is excreted into the semen in the epididymis. Samples with lower concentrations of alkaline phosphatase either produce an incomplete ejaculate or have an obstructive lesion past the level of the epididymis.

Sperm Motility

Abnormal motility of spermatozoa is thought to hinder the sperm's ability to reach the fallopian tube, where fertilization takes place. When a high percentage of sperm demonstrate a complete lack of motility, there may be environmental influences that affect the collected sperm. A male that has not had sperm collected for many months may have a large number of non-motile sperm due to prolonged storage in the epididymis. An elevated temperature in the epididymis due to environmental influence or inflammation in the surrounding tissues can result in "dead" sperm. If proper collection techniques are being utilized to prevent "cold shock," a second or third sample collected later that day or on subsequent days may demonstrate spermatozoa with normal motility. Extremes in the pH of the semen can also "kill" sperm. Infections in the reproductive tract or urine or blood in the semen could cause such extremes in pH. Foreign agents such as water, disinfectants, or lubricants can cause sperm death on contact.

Sperm Morphology

Primary defects of the spermatozoa in more than 20% of those sampled may result in infertility. Such defects include abnormal heads, necks, or tails. These are defects that occur in the seminiferous tubules during development. Suspect inflammatory disease in the testes and perform a testicular biopsy (see Chap. 107).

Secondary defects of the spermatozoa in more than 20% of those sampled may result in infertility. Review collection techniques when a large percentage of sperm demonstrate bent tails or coiled tails because these defects can develop after collection with cold shock. Large numbers of spermatozoa with distal cytoplasmic droplets may indicate abnormal epididymal function and warrant further investigation.

Other Abnormalities

Blood in the semen is most commonly from the prostate gland if surface trauma to the penis cannot be detected. The prostate gland may be inflamed with overstimulation, benign prostatic hyperplasia, infection, or neoplasia (see Chap. 104). Perform careful microscopic evaluation of the semen sample before insemination to ensure that infection is not present.

Diagnosis

History

Systemic disease or a history of infection in the reproductive or urinary tract may warrant further investigation or treatment. Identify medications that can reduce spermatogenesis. Ask about disinfectants used on the kennels if scrotal dermatitis is causing inflammation. Review breeding attempts and their subsequent results along with how the timing of the breedings was determined.

Physical Examination

Perform a thorough physical examination. Inspect the scrotum and its contents for position, consistency, size, and shape. Scrotal tenderness and thickening is most commonly seen with scrotal dermatitis of variable duration. Detection of scrotal neoplasia may require ultrasound and biopsy in chronic cases (see Chap. 107). Testicular atrophy is generally detected after a chronic influence has caused destruction of seminiferous epithelium. Pain and enlargement of the testes is most indicative of acute inflammatory disease. Palpate the prostate gland rectally and abdominally for size, shape, and tenderness. Persistent discharge from the penis and prepuce may reflect balanoposthitis or prostatitis and warrants further investigation.

Laboratory Analysis

Perform CBC, serum chemical profile, urinalysis, fecal study, serum thyroid concentrations, and heartworm check to ensure that systemic influences are not causing altered metabolism and infertility.

If abnormal libido is observed, measure serum testosterone levels. Testosterone is secreted in a pulsatile manner; therefore, do repetitive sampling or challenge testing. For a challenge test, obtain serum for baseline testosterone. Inject GnRH at 2 mg/kg IM and obtain postchallenge serum 1 hour later.

Radiography

Radiography is of little use in evaluation of the male reproductive tract. Only the size and shape of the prostate gland and the integrity of the os penis are visible.

Ultrasound

Ultrasound has been used to define the character of the prostate gland routinely. Hyperechoic tissue may represent hyperplasia or neoplasia. Cystic pockets may be identified with abscessation or cyst formation. Perform ultrasonic evaluation on the testes. An "offset pad" may be required. Small, nonpalpable tumors or granulomas may be identified.

Serology

Brucellosis

All males should be tested for *Brucella canis* once or twice a year if bred frequently, or before each breeding. Females presented for breeding should also have a negative test prior to breeding (see Chap. 17).

Canine Herpesvirus

Canine herpesvirus can cause infertility in both the male and female. Additionally, the male may show no clinical signs but transmit the virus to the female, resulting in neonatal death. Most commonly, the male has a herpesvirus titer performed only when a female has suspected infection or when persistent infertility is present.

Culture

1. Aerobic bacteria can cause infection of the scrotum, testes, epididymis, or prostate gland. Perform culture of the prostatic fraction of the ejaculate.
2. *Mycoplasma* and *Ureaplasma* can, as in the female, cause infertility. Perform quantitative culture of the prostatic fraction of the ejaculate.

Thyroid Hormone Measurement

As previously mentioned, hypothyroidism can cause infertility. If testicular atrophy has not yet developed, fertility can return in 3–12 months after instituting supplementation.

Karyotyping

Diagnosis of all categories of abnormalities of sexual differentiation can be achieved with a 10-ml heparinized blood sample or a small skin biopsy for karyotyping. Commercial karyotyping is available at several colleges of veterinary medicine.

Histopathology

Biopsy testes that have changed in size, shape, or consistency (see Chap. 107). Treat the specific cause. Removal of one testis with disease can occasionally save the integrity of the unaffected testis.

Biopsy abnormal prostate glands (see Chap. 105). As most of the fluid of the ejaculate comes from the prostate gland, removal of the gland will probably reduce fertility.

Treatment

Treat males with systemic disease appropriately. Discontinue medications that could adversely affect spermatogenesis whenever possible. Treat inflammation or infection in the reproductive tract as soon as possible to avoid chronic disease and permanent infertility. Progestin (Ovaban, Shering) therapy may be most appropriate for prostatic hyperplasia or prostatitis while allowing fertility to be maintained.

Spermatogenesis and epididymal maturation takes approximately 75 days in the dog, and it may take several cycles before sufficient numbers of functional sperm appear in the ejaculate. Therefore, allow sufficient time for this to occur.

Testosterone deficiency is difficult to correct because the testicular levels tend to be 50–100 times that of serum levels, and exogenous testosterone will inhibit any gonadal testosterone release due to negative feedback inhibition.

If hypothyroidism is identified, treat with appropriate supplements (see Chap. 29).

SUPPLEMENTAL READING

Davidson, AP, Feldman, EC: Ovarian and estrous cycle abnormalities in the bitch. *In* Ettinger SJ, Feldman EC, eds.: Textbook of Veterinary Internal Medicine. Philadelphia, WB Saunders, 1995, p 1607.

Hegstad, RL, Johnston, SD: Use of serum progesterone ELISA tests in canine breeding management. *In* Kirk RW, Bonagura JD, eds.: Current Veterinary Therapy XI. Philadelphia, WB Saunders, 1992, p 943.

Johnston, SD: Breeding management of the bitch. *In* Ettinger SJ, Feldman EC, eds.: Textbook of Veterinary Internal Medicine. Philadelphia, WB Saunders, 1995, p 1604.

Johnston, SD: Infertility in the bitch. *In* Kirk RW, Bonagura JD, eds.: Current Veterinary Therapy XI. Philadelphia, WB Saunders, 1992, p 954.

Meyers-Wallen, VN: Semen analysis, artificial insemination, and infertility in the male dog. *In* Ettinger SJ, Feldman EC, eds.: Textbook of Veterinary Internal Medicine. Philadelphia, WB Saunders, 1995, p 1649.

Oettle, EE: Sperm abnormalities and fertility in the dog. *In* Bonagura JD, Kirk RW, eds.: Kirk's Current Veterinary Therapy XII. Philadelphia, WB Saunders, 1995, p 1060.

Shille, VM, Sojka, NJ: Feline reproduction. *In* Ettinger SJ, Feldman EC, eds.: Textbook of Veterinary Internal Medicine. Philadelphia, WB Saunders, 1995, p 1690.

Yeager, AE, Concannon, PW: Ultrasonography of the reproductive tract of the female dog and cat. *In* Bonagura JD, Kirk RW, eds.: Kirk's Current Veterinary Therapy XII. Philadelphia, WB Saunders, 1995, p 1040.

Chapter 115 Fractures of the Skull

Mark M. Smith

Fractures of the zygomatic arch require surgery if they interfere with mastication or compress ocular structures. The most common extracranial fracture requiring surgery is a depression fracture of the frontal sinus. Intracranial fractures that require surgery are those that depress into brain parenchyma, causing significant compromise of cerebral function. Most skull fractures are amenable to conservative management.

Weigh the complications of general anesthesia in a neurologically compromised patient against the positive effects of surgical intervention. Fine motor movement is not necessarily required of small animal pets; therefore, intracranial surgery rarely is performed.

ANATOMY

Zygomatic Arch

- The cranial portion of the zygomatic arch is formed by the zygomatic bone and the caudal portion by the zygomatic process of the temporal bone.
- The zygomatic arch forms the ventral and lateral rim of the orbit.

Calvarium

- The dorsal sagittal crest courses craniocaudal over the calvarium.
- The nuchal crest courses mediolateral over the caudal edge of the skull.
- The frontal sinus of the frontal bone comprises the frontal encasement of the brain.
- The diploic calvarium has two distinct cortical bone layers between which is an interstitial layer of honeycombed bone and vessels.

- The brain is encased by the frontal, parietal, temporal, and occipital bones.
- The temporalis muscles cover almost the entire calvarium.

ZYGOMATIC ARCH FRACTURE

Preoperative Considerations

- Before anesthesia and surgery, perform a complete neurologic examination on all head trauma patients.
- General anesthesia may alter intracranial pressure (ICP), leading to exacerbation of intracranial edema and/or hemorrhage.
- To reduce ICP, consider hyperventilation (to reduce $PaCO_2$), osmotic agents, corticosteroids, and an anesthetic protocol including barbiturates.
- Obtain skull radiographs to document fracture displacement and to screen for other, less apparent fractures. If possible, perform radiography immediately before surgery, thus avoiding the necessity for, and risk of, two separate anesthetic procedures.
- Confirm the presence of an intact optic nerve and vision before surgery. Surgery for a zygomatic arch fracture may be contraindicated if ocular function is irreversibly impaired.

▼ *Key Point* Acepromazine may lower the central nervous system (CNS) seizure threshold, and ketamine increases cerebral blood flow. Do not use these drugs in patients with a history of brain trauma.

Surgical Procedure

Objectives

- Reduce fractures that can cause compression of the eye or cosmetic deformity.
- Avoid trauma to the zygomaticotemporal and zygomaticofacial nerves.

▼ **Key Point** Nondisplaced fractures of the zygomatic arch have a good prognosis for uncomplicated healing with conservative management.

Equipment

- Standard general surgical pack and sutures
- Gelpi or Weitlaner self-retaining retractors
- Sharp periosteal elevator
- Small Steinmann pins and orthopedic wire (multiple sizes, 18–24 gauge)
- Small malleable retractor

Technique

1. Place the patient in ventral recumbency with the head supported. Attach tape to the mandibular canines and the table to secure head position.
2. Prepare the periocular area for aseptic surgery. Ocular lubricating ointment avoids corneal damage from antiseptic agents.
3. Incise the skin directly over the zygomatic arch.
4. Incise and elevate the periosteum using a sharp periosteal elevator. Be careful to avoid the zygomaticotemporal and zygomaticofacial nerves (medial to the zygomatic bone).
5. Use a small malleable retractor to protect the orbit.
6. Reduce and secure fracture fragments using orthopedic wire (18–24 gauge, depending on the size of the animal). Small pins may be used to make holes in the bone for wire placement. Small orthopedic plates may be required to maintain reduction in extremely comminuted fractures or when cosmesis is of paramount importance.

▼ **Key Point** Do not use small pins as a component of the definitive repair, because pin migration following surgery may cause ocular and intracranial trauma.

7. Closure
   a. Appose subcutaneous tissues in a simple interrupted pattern (absorbable suture).
   b. Subcuticular sutures (absorbable suture) provide skin apposition and avoid suture irritation of ocular structures.

Postoperative Care and Complications

Short-Term

- Perform serial neurologic examinations to monitor changes in neurologic status.
- Monitor for clinical signs of seroma and infection.

Long-Term

- Excessive bony callus may compress ocular structures and interfere with mastication.
- Periarticular fractures may lead to degenerative joint disease of the temporomandibular joint (TMJ) and bony ankylosis.
- If normal function is inhibited or pain persists, resection of the affected segment of the zygomatic arch is indicated. Reconstruction of the muscle tissue provides acceptable appearance and function.

Prognosis

- The prognosis is good with conservative management.
- With operative management, the prognosis is good to excellent.

EXTRACRANIAL FRACTURES

Extracranial fractures include fractures of the nuchal crest, sagittal crest, and frontal sinus.

Preoperative Considerations

- See Zygomatic Arch Fracture.

Surgical Procedure

Objective

- Maintain reduction of severely displaced fractures of the nuchal crest, sagittal crest, and frontal sinus.

▼ **Key Point** The cranial muscle mass usually prevents severe fracture displacement and provides enough fracture stability to allow conservative management of most extracranial fractures.

Equipment

- Standard general surgical pack and sutures
- Gelpi or Weitlaner self-retaining retractors
- Sharp periosteal elevator
- Small Steinmann pins and orthopedic wire (multiple sizes, 20–24 gauge)

Technique

1. Place the patient in ventral recumbency with the head supported. Attach tape to the mandibular canines and table to secure the head position.
2. Prepare the fracture area for aseptic surgery.
3. Make a skin incision directly over the fractured bony prominence.
4. Elevate the periosteum to allow anatomic reduction.
5. Frontal sinus fractures usually are depressed, requiring elevation and fixation with orthopedic wire.
6. Reduce and fix nuchal and sagittal crest fractures with orthopedic wire.

▼ **Key Point** Do not use small pins as a component of the definitive repair because pin migration following surgery may cause ocular or intracranial trauma.

7. Appose muscle fascia and subcutaneous tissues in individual layers, using absorbable suture in a simple interrupted pattern.
8. Close the skin similarly, using nonabsorbable suture.

Postoperative Care and Complications

Short-Term

- Perform serial neurologic examination to monitor for change in neurologic status.
- Monitor for clinical signs of seroma and infection.
- Subcutaneous emphysema may occur secondary to frontal sinus fracture. Whether management of the fracture is surgical or conservative, a compressive bandage minimizes continued formation of subcutaneous emphysema until organized hematoma and fibrin deposition provide a functional barrier to air migration from the frontal sinus. Thus, bandaging is recommended for 2–4 days.

Long-Term

- Fractures usually heal without complications, providing acceptable cosmesis.
- Most complications are related to CNS trauma, such as seizures (see Chap. 146).

INTRACRANIAL FRACTURES

Preoperative Considerations

- Preoperative anesthetic and neurologic concerns are similar to those for zygomatic arch fractures.
- Fractures may be linear cracks, depressed bony fragments, or comminuted separate bony fragments.
- Intracranial fractures are usually closed fractures.
- Comminuted calvarial fractures may lacerate meninges, venous sinuses, or the cerebral cortex.
- Calvarial fractures usually are associated with CNS compromise. Medical management of CNS trauma is

indicated before diagnostic procedures requiring anesthesia.
- Progressive deterioration in CNS status despite intensive medical management is an indication for skull radiography to determine fracture severity.

Surgical Procedure

Objectives

- Elevate depressed calvarial fractures that may cause extensive functional loss of cerebral mass.
- Remove large comminuted fragments of the calvarium that may cause cerebral laceration.

▼ *Key Point* Linear and minor depressed intracranial fractures are best managed conservatively.

Equipment

- Standard general surgical pack and sutures
- Gelpi or Weitlaner self-retaining retractors
- Sharp periosteal elevator
- Pneumatic or electric bur drill

Technique

1. Place the patient in ventral recumbency with the head supported. Attach tape to the mandibular canines and table to secure the head position.
2. Prepare the dorsal skull area for aseptic surgery.
3. Make a dorsal incision (Fig. 115–1A).
4. Incise the superficial temporal fascia and elevate the temporalis muscle ventrally to expose the fracture area (Fig. 115–1B).
5. Drill multiple small bur holes through the calvarium around the periphery of the fracture area to allow elevation of the fracture fragments (Fig. 115–1C).
6. Elevate fragments with a small, blunt elevator (Fig. 115–1D).
7. Remove any large comminuted fragments that may cause laceration. Despite the potential for large cal-

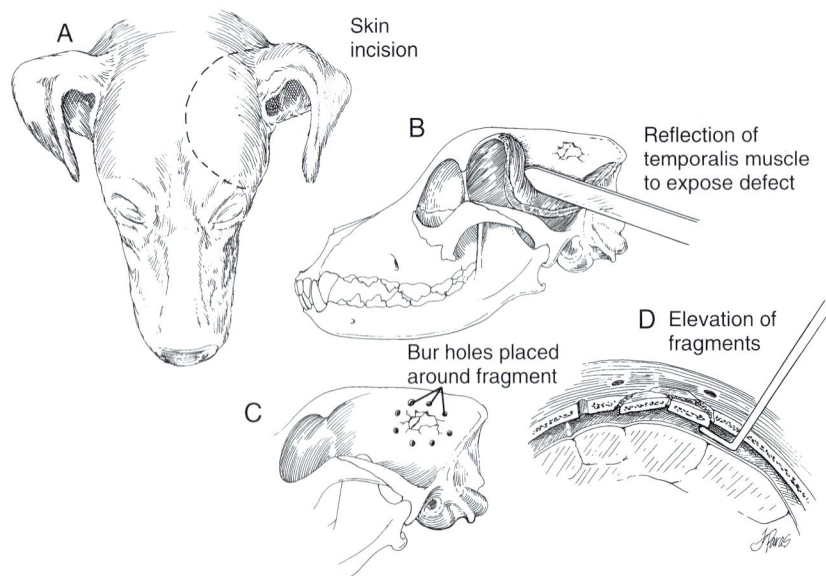

Figure 115–1. Procedure for repairing intracranial fracture. See text for explanation.

varial defects, replacement of the temporalis muscle provides adequate coverage.
8. Closure
   a. Replace the temporalis muscle and appose the superficial fascia using absorbable suture in a simple interrupted pattern.
   b. Close the subcutaneous layers similarly, followed by skin closure using nonabsorbable suture in a simple interrupted pattern.

▼ *Key Point* Meticulous, atraumatic surgical technique, prevention of cerebral edema, and removal of hematoma if calvarial fragments are removed are of the highest priority when operating on intracranial fractures.

Postoperative Care and Complications
Short-Term

- Perform serial neurologic examinations to monitor for change in neurologic status.
- Monitor for clinical signs of seroma and infection.

Long-Term

- Bony healing occurs without complication; however, neurologic recovery depends on the location and severity of the original traumatic incident.

Prognosis

- Cranial fracture repair—good prognosis.
- Neurologic recovery—guarded prognosis.

SUPPLEMENTAL READINGS

Dulisch ML: Skull and mandibular fractures. *In* Slatter DH, ed.: Textbook of Small Animal Surgery. Philadelphia: WB Saunders, 1985, p 2286.
Newton CD: Fractures of the skull. *In* Newton CD, Nunamaker DM, eds.: Textbook of Small Animal Orthopaedics. Philadelphia: JB Lippincott, 1985, p 287.
Oliver JE: Craniotomy, craniectomy, and skull fractures. *In* Bojrab MJ, ed.: Current Techniques in Small Animal Surgery. Philadelphia: Lea & Febiger, 1975, p 359.

116 Fractures and Dislocations of the Mandible

Paul E. Howard

Mandibular fractures are encountered commonly in small animal practice and can present a unique set of challenges to the veterinarian. Dislocations of the mandible are uncommon but can occur alone or in conjunction with a fracture. Many surgical and nonsurgical techniques have been described for mandibular fracture repair. Certain principles must be followed if clinical success is to be achieved on a consistent basis.

ANATOMY

The mandible is composed of two halves, divided into a horizontal component (body) and a vertical component (ramus). The two halves of the mandible, joined rostrally at the mandibular symphysis, compose the lower jaw.

- The alveolar border is that part of the body into which the tooth roots insert.
- The dorsal half of the ramus is the coronoid process.
- The mandibular foramen, located on the medial side of the ramus, is the caudal opening of the mandibular canal through which traverses the mandibular alveolar artery and vein and the mandibular alveolar nerve.
  - The mandibular canal opens cranially at the three mental foramina.
  - The mandibular alveolar nerve is a branch of the trigeminal nerve supplying motor and sensory innervation to the mandible.

The condyloid processes of the hemimandibles articulate with the mandibular fossae of the temporal bones to form the temporomandibular joints (TMJ), which permit considerable dorsal-ventral motion.

Mandibular fractures can be divided into three broad groups, based on anatomic location of the fracture:

- Mandibular symphysis—most common area fractured in cats, often an open fracture
- Mandibular body—most common area fractured in dogs, usually an open fracture
- Ramus—least common area fractured, owing to its protection by an adjacent muscle mass (masseter muscle).

OVERVIEW OF MANDIBULAR FRACTURES

Etiology

- The primary cause of mandibular fractures is trauma, including:
  - Being struck by a motor vehicle
  - Fighting
  - Gunshot injury
  - Falling from excessive heights (cat falling from high-rise building window)
- Iatrogenic fracture of the mandible may occur during overzealous attempts at tooth extraction in animals with severe periodontal disease and/or metabolic disease causing osteoporosis.

Clinical Signs

Clinical signs are variable and include:

- Crepitus on manipulation of the mandible
- Pain when jaw is opened
- Asymmetry of the jaw
- Nasal or oral hemorrhage
- Nasal obstruction

Diagnosis

- Diagnosis usually is not difficult and is based on a recent history of trauma, malocclusion, and, frequently, a palpable fracture.
- Oblique radiographs of the skull are helpful in identifying the fracture site and demonstrating the degree of fracture displacement.
  - Examine radiographs carefully for associated maxillary and other skull fractures.
  - When an animal presents with a mandibular symphyseal separation, evaluate the condyloid process radiographically for a fracture.

Complications

- The most common complication when considering all types of mandibular fractures is dental malocclusion.
- Other complications are osteomyelitis, nonunion, malunion, implant failure, and infection of soft tissues.

- Complications are more likely to occur in open fractures and in fractures requiring the removal of teeth at the time of fixation.

Surgical Procedures

Principles applicable to all fractures and dislocations of the mandible are discussed here. Techniques for the repair of specific problems are discussed with each condition further in the chapter.

Preoperative Considerations

- Because mandibular fractures are primarily an orthopedic problem, consider the following principles of orthopedic repair:
  - Anatomic reduction of the fracture ensures proper dental occlusion.
  - Rigid fixation of the fracture permits the earliest return to function.
  - Placement of fixation devices can be impeded by tooth roots.

▼ *Key Point* Avoid perforation of tooth roots and invasion of the mandibular canal.

- Perforation of tooth roots ultimately requires endodontic therapy or extraction of the involved tooth.
- If bone loss is present, the alignment of the teeth can be used as a template for fracture reduction. This is feasible only if teeth being used for alignment are not displaced.
- Treat fractures of the mandibular body as open fractures; thus, use antibiotic therapy. Fractures of the caudal aspect of the body are sometimes closed.
- Osteomyelitis is encountered infrequently, but, when present, it can be very difficult to eliminate.
- A tooth in a fracture line will not prevent fracture healing. In an experimental study, teeth adjacent to mandibular osteotomy sites retained their viability, were encased in new woven bone, and did not loosen.

▼ *Key Point* Do not remove a tooth in a fracture line if it aids in the reduction and stabilization of the fracture.

- Loss of teeth often makes anatomic reduction of the fracture more difficult. If indicated, extract the tooth when it is no longer needed for fracture repair.
- Provide means of delivering proper nutrition to the animal during the healing phase.
  - If the animal cannot receive food and water per os, consider placement of an esophagostomy or gastrostomy tube (see Chap. 3).
- Intubate animals during anesthesia and fracture repair to prevent aspiration of blood and irrigating solution.
  - In repair of severe mandibular fractures, place the endotracheal tube out from the side of the pharynx to permit unobstructed evaluation of occlusion during surgery.

- An alternative method, although less desirable, is to periodically remove the normally positioned endotracheal tube and assess occlusion.

▼ *Key Point* In some severe fractures of the mandible, adequate surgical repair may not be possible. In such cases, partial mandibulectomy may be the preferred method of treatment (see Chap. 118).

Objectives

- Reduce the bone fragments and maintain this position until adequate bone healing occurs. Determine if the mandible requires surgical reduction or if the fracture is sufficiently aligned to permit nonsurgical treatment.
  - Proper reduction ensures proper occlusion.
- Allow early return to normal function, primarily mastication, with rigid fixation.
- Maintain the animal's nutritional status at an optimal level.

Equipment

- Standard general surgical pack
- Wire twisters and wire cutters
- Orthopedic wire (18–24 gauge)
- Bone plates and screws
- External fixation devices
- Kirschner wires (K-wires)
- Acrylic or dental composite

Postoperative Care and Complications

- Feed the patient a gruel for 2 weeks. Feed canned food or dry food softened with water for an additional 4 weeks before returning to the usual diet.
- Prevent dogs from chewing bones, sticks, balls, and other hard objects that may disrupt the fracture repair during the healing phase.
- Daily oral flushing with chlorhexidine preparations may be beneficial in the immediate postoperative period in reducing oral bacteria in animals with open fractures.
- Evaluate animals no later than 2 weeks postoperatively to ensure that proper occlusion has been maintained.

MANDIBULAR SYMPHYSEAL FRACTURES

A mandibular symphyseal fracture is a commonly encountered unstable fracture that prevents normal mastication. This type of fracture is repaired easily with minimal equipment, most frequently with wire, although pins and screws can be used with equal success.

Wire Stabilization

Technique

1. Place the patient in dorsal recumbency and prepare the chin for aseptic surgery.
2. Make a midline stab incision in the skin slightly ros-

tral to the caudal extent of the mandibular symphysis.

3. Insert a hypodermic needle (larger than the anticipated wire size) through the skin incision, lateral to one hemimandible, and exit in the oral cavity immediately caudal to the canine tooth (Fig. 116–1*A*).
4. Insert a strand of orthopedic wire of appropriate size (24 gauge for cats and small dogs; 20 or 18 gauge for large dogs) through the distal end of the needle and remove the needle, leaving the strand in place (Fig. 116–1*B*).
5. Through the same stab incision in the skin, insert the needle lateral to the contralateral hemimandible and exit the needle caudal to the canine tooth (Fig. 116–1*C*).
6. Pass the end of the wire *that is in the mouth* into the end of the needle until it exits the needle hub. Remove the needle, leaving both wire ends exiting the stab incision in the chin.
7. Maintain proper alignment of the rostral ends of the hemimandibles, with digital pressure, and twist-tighten the wire to maintain anatomic reduction of the symphysis. Cut off the twisted wire, leaving at least three twists (Fig. 116–1*D*).

Postoperative Care and Complications

* Leave the wire ends exposed, and clean the area with warm water as necessary.
* Feed a soft diet until the wire is removed.
* Instruct owners to avoid the exposed end of the wire.
* Leave wire in place for 6–8 weeks. Remove by cutting the exposed wire in the patient's mouth; extract the cut ends through the skin incision by pulling on the twisted end. A short-acting general anesthetic facilitates the procedure and eliminates discomfort.

Alternative Techniques

* A noninvasive technique involves placing a piece of orthopedic wire around the base of the canine or incisor teeth and tightening the wire so that the wire twists are rostral to the incisor teeth.
* Wire may need to be secured with dental composite to avoid having the wire slip off the teeth.
* Interdental wiring techniques can be used instead of the wire loop technique.

ROSTRAL MANDIBULAR BODY FRACTURES

Repair of fractures behind the canine teeth or between the rostral premolar teeth is complicated because only a small amount of bone is available for implant insertion. The majority of the rostral mandible is composed of tooth root structure. Frequently this type of fracture occurs bilaterally, complicating the repair.

Tape Muzzle

Unilateral fractures of the rostral mandible often can be repaired satisfactorily with a tape muzzle. Tape muzzles are tolerated well by most dogs. Brachycephalic breeds and cats are less tolerant of the muzzle (see Chap. 117).

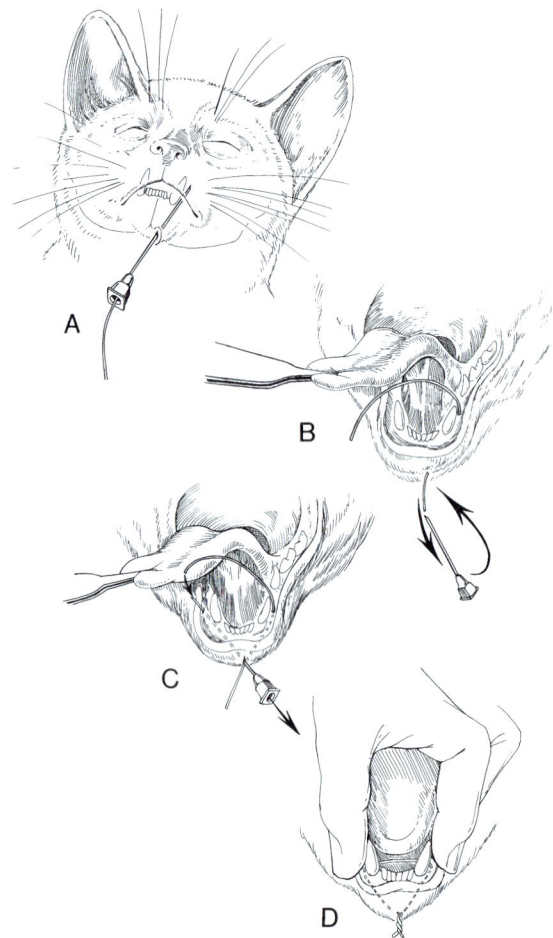

Figure 116–1.   Wire stabilization for mandibular symphyseal fracture. See text for details.

Figure-Eight Wire

This procedure is indicated in bilateral fractures.

Technique

1. Pass orthopedic wire around the canine teeth and between the roots of the first premolar teeth in the caudal fracture segments. Wire passage under the furcation of the tooth is facilitated if a pathway is first established with a K-wire. When stabilizing bilateral fractures, tighten the wires in unison to maintain equal compressive forces.
2. A secondary wire may be required through holes drilled in the ventral aspect of the mandible to prevent distraction of the fracture line due to the pull of the figure-eight wires.
3. To keep the wire passed around the canine teeth from slipping, cover the wire with composite material (see Chap. 117).
4. Alternatively, drill a hole in the mandible rostral to the canine tooth and pass the wire through this hole. Similarly, a hole can be drilled in the mandible rather than passing the wire through the premolar tooth furcation.

▼ *Key Point*   When drilling holes in the mandible, avoid tooth roots.

Cross-Pinning

- Use large K-wires or small intramedullary pins to stabilize bilateral fractures in selected cases. Avoiding tooth roots is often difficult using this technique.

CENTRAL MANDIBULAR BODY FRACTURES

These fractures offer the greatest number of repair options, including internal and external fixation, splinting devices, and muzzles. The choice of repair depends on a number of factors including available equipment, expertise of the veterinarian, and cost.

Plate Fixation

The method of choice is plate fixation because it provides rigid, anatomic reduction and maintains normal occlusion. This permits an early return to function without the need for external fixation devices or intraoral splints. The major drawbacks are the skill required for using plating equipment and the expense of the implants.

Technique

1. Place the patient in dorsolateral recumbency (dorsal recumbency if the fractures are bilateral).
2. Make a skin incision along the ventrolateral margin of the mandibular body.
3. Elevate the subcutaneous tissues with a periosteal elevator to expose the fracture site.
4. Conform the plate to fit as ventral as possible on the lateral aspect of the mandibular body to avoid placing screws through adjacent tooth roots and the mandibular canal. The plate should be long enough to permit two screws on each side of the fracture site.
   a. In complicated mandibular fractures, mandibular reduction forceps (Synthes, Paoli, PA) can aid in maintaining fracture reduction while the plate is being applied.
   b. Placement of plates on the dorsolateral surface of the mandible is not recommended, as it can result in gingival erosion, damage to tooth roots, and osteomyelitis.
5. Following plate application, close the subcutaneous tissues and skin. Intraoral approaches are recommended by some surgeons to avoid possible contamination and infection that may result from an approach through the skin. The author, however, prefers exposure through a skin incision because infection with this approach is uncommon, and exposure is better.

External Skeletal Fixation

In cases of severely comminuted body fractures, external skeletal fixation is an excellent method for maintaining spatial relationships and occlusion during fracture healing.

- Fix with conventional pins, clamps, and connecting bars, with screws and acrylic (biphase external fixa-

tion), or with intramedullary pins and acrylic (modified biphase external fixation).
- Advantage:
  - Dissection of soft tissue for the placement of the pins is minimal.
  - Fracture reduction can be fine-tuned without the need for removing pins previously placed into the bone.
  - Occlusion is maintained in fractures with bone loss.
  - Biphase or modified biphase splints can be contoured around the rostral end of the mandible.
- Disadvantages:
  - The protruding device can be dislodged.
  - Pin loosening can result in loss of fracture reduction.
  - Pin tract infection and drainage from tracts may be less desirable to owners.

Technique

▼ **Key Point** Do not insert pins rostral to the third mandibular premolar tooth, or the root of the canine tooth may be penetrated.

1. Make small stab incisions in the skin over the intended site of pin or screw placement. Bluntly dissect to the bone surface with a periosteal elevator.
2. After determining the number of pins to be used in the fracture repair (a minimum of three pins in each fracture segment is desirable), insert one pin in each fracture segment. Accurate pin placement can be facilitated by predrilling with a pin or drill bit that is smaller than the final pin.
3. After loosely joining the pins with clamps and a connecting bar, reduce the fracture, achieve normal occlusion, and tighten the clamps.
4. Insert additional pins into the mandible by first passing the pin through a clamp previously placed on the connecting bar. (Inserting pins in this manner ensures that all pins are placed in the same plane, negating the need for additional connecting bars that would add unnecessary weight to the fixation device.)
5. After the pins are placed and the clamps are tightened, evaluate the occlusion. If necessary, loosen the clamps to permit better reduction of the fracture to improve occlusion.

▼ **Key Point** Although this is sometimes recommended, do not cover the clamps and connecting bar with tape, but leave them exposed to facilitate cleaning.

6. An alternative to the use of clamps and a connecting bar is dental acrylic (see Chap. 84). Silastic tubing or other suitable material is impaled on the pins. The acrylic is injected into the tubing and, once hardened, fracture reduction is maintained. A disadvantage of acrylic is that, once the acrylic has hardened, adjustment of the fracture reduction and improvement of occlusion is not possible.

Postoperative Care and Complications

- Clean the sites where the pins or screws exit the skin daily with a disinfectant. This is easier if the external fixation device is not covered with tape or other material.
- Once a week, evaluate fixation devices that use clamps to be sure that the nuts are secure.
- The major complication is premature dislodging or loosening of the implant.

Intramedullary Pinning

- The use of IM pins for the repair of mandibular body fractures is not recommended, although there are reports of its successful use. The normal mandibular curvature makes it difficult to insert an IM pin into the mandibular body without invasion of the mandibular canal or damage to the tooth roots.
- Placement of IM pins into the mandibular canal has been done without apparent detrimental effects. Nevertheless, pin placement in this area is discouraged.
- Fractures repaired with IM pins have a high risk of nonunion or malunion with resultant malocclusion. This is because most IM pins have a tendency to resist bending to conform to the curved portion of the mandibular canal, resulting in distraction of the fracture.

Dental Composite or Acrylic

This technique requires no special equipment, is inexpensive, will not damage teeth, and can be used to treat fractures in all areas of the mandible.

- Advantages
  - Does not damage blood supply or teeth.
  - Can achieve proper occlusion in the presence of bony defects.
  - Can be used in cats and brachycephalic breeds.
- Disadvantages
  - Ideally requires four intact canine teeth; can be applied with only two intact.
  - Animal may overheat in warm environment.
  - May be difficult for animal to eat, necessitating feeding tube of some type.
  - Makes animal susceptible to aspiration pneumonia if animal vomits.

Technique

1. Intubate the anesthetized patient either per os or via a pharyngotomy incision. Pharyngeal intubation allows better evaluation of occlusion and is preferred.
2. Clean the teeth with scaler if calculus is present.
3. Acid-etch the teeth.
4. Align the fracture with the apices of the apposing canine teeth in close proximity to each other.
5. Apply composite to maintain fracture reduction and normal occlusion.
   a. Immobilize one side at a time.
   b. Apply additional layers of composite until sufficient strength and stability are present.

6. Remove dental composite with a bur after the fracture has healed.
7. Clean and polish the teeth after the composite is removed.
8. If using an esophagostomy tube, place it before the procedure.

Tape Muzzle

- A tape muzzle can be used as the sole means of stabilizing minimally displaced or nondisplaced fractures (see Chap. 117).
- Stresses on internal fixation devices can be reduced when used in combination with a tape muzzle.

CAUDAL MANDIBULAR BODY FRACTURES

- Treat minimally displaced fractures in this region with a tape muzzle (see Chap. 117).
- Stabilize displaced and unstable fractures with internal fixation methods such as bone plates and interfragmentary wiring.
- Some methods of fracture fixation are not suitable for caudal body fractures.
  - External fixation pins are difficult to position properly in the caudal fracture segment.
  - Insufficient-size teeth or lack of a suitable number of teeth in the caudal fracture segment prevents use of interdental wiring techniques.

MANDIBULAR RAMUS FRACTURES

The ramus is a thin bone in which improperly placed implants loosen prematurely. Complete surgical exposure of the ramus is difficult because of muscle attachment. The higher the location of the fracture on the ramus, the less critical the need for surgical intervention.

- Fractures of the ramus often are minimally displaced owing to the adjacent musculature, which aids in maintaining reduction and stability during fracture healing. Many of these fractures respond favorably if jaw motion is restricted with a tape muzzle.
- Animals with fractures of the lower ramus, especially when bilateral, benefit from fracture stabilization. Various methods can be used, including small plates, interfragmentary wiring, and K-wire fixation in combination with orthopedic wire.

Technique

Two approaches can be combined to provide greater exposure of the angular portion of the ramus and the TMJ.

1. Expose the angular portion of the ramus by making a skin incision along the ventrolateral border of the caudal mandible.
   a. Incise the platysma muscle to expose the digastricus muscle.
   b. Continue deeper dissection to expose the mandible and the masseter muscle, which is sub-

periosteally reflected dorsally to expose the masseteric fossa and the condyloid and angular processes.

2. Alternatively, expose the dorsal aspect of the ramus by making a skin incision along the caudoventral margin of the zygomatic arch.
   a. Incise the platysma muscle and reflect it ventrally, exposing the lateral surface of the TMJ and the condyloid process.
3. Apply the selected implant after fracture reduction.
4. Pin and wire combinations or interfragmentary wiring techniques work well in the lower part of the ramus, in which the bone is thicker than the dorsal aspect of the ramus.
5. Bone plates are the preferred method of stabilization of the ramus because of the thinness of the bone.
   a. Reconstruction plates (Synthes) can be contored in multiple planes and are well suited for use in this area.
   b. Use of a T-plate reduces the amount of surgical exposure required for plate application.

CONDYLOID PROCESS FRACTURES

Fractures of the condyloid process of the mandible occur infrequently and usually are minimally or nondisplaced. They usually occur in association with other mandibular fractures.

- Evaluate the TMJ radiographically when other mandibular fractures are identified.
- In younger animals, fractures of the condyloid process are more likely to heal and remodel without surgical intervention. For displaced fractures or condylar fractures in older animals, internal fixation may be of benefit.

Condylectomy

Condylectomy is recommended in animals with a nonreducible condyloid process fracture. This technique has several advantages:

- Normal dental occlusion and range of jaw motion is maintained and problems with mastication or degeneration of the contralateral TMJ are not encountered.
- Degenerative joint disease of the TMJ can develop subsequent to condyloid process fractures. In severe cases, a condylectomy can alleviate the discomfort or pain caused by degeneration of the joint.

Bilateral condylectomies should be avoided.

Technique

1. The approach to the TMJ is as previously described for mandibular ramus fractures.
2. Insert a K-wire or small intramedullary pin from the ventral surface of the mandible to a sufficient depth to maintain reduction. Avoid penetration of the articular surface of the condyloid process.

MANDIBULAR (TMJ) LUXATIONS

Luxation of the mandible occurs infrequently and can be an isolated injury or found in association with mandibular or maxillary fractures. Evaluate cats presented for mandibular symphyseal separations for possible luxation of the TMJ.

Etiology

Temporomandibular dysplasia is a nontraumatic cause of TMJ luxation and has been reported in American cocker spaniels, Basset hounds, Irish setters, and St. Bernards. This can result in open-mouth jaw locking, requiring manual reduction.

Diagnosis

Suspect TMJ luxation when malocclusion of the mandible exists without an identifiable fracture.

- TMJ luxation can be rostral or caudal as well as unilateral or bilateral. The direction often can be determined on physical examination. The mandible can deviate toward the normal side (rostral luxation) or the luxated side (caudal luxation).
- Confirm the diagnosis and direction of luxation radiographically.

Preoperative Considerations

- If the luxation is of traumatic origin, ensure a patent airway and identify potentially life-threatening injuries.
- Mandibular or maxillary fractures may hinder efforts to reduce the mandibular luxation.
- Evaluate the TMJ radiographically for fractures that may prevent reduction of the luxation.

Surgical Procedure

Objectives

- Reduce the mandibular luxation atraumatically to reestablish normal jaw motion and occlusion.
- In cases of open-mouth jaw locking, provide unrestricted movement of the ramus.

Equipment

- No special equipment is needed.

Technique—TMJ Luxation

1. Place the patient, under general anesthesia, in dorsal recumbency.
2. Place a small dowel or pencil across the last molars to act as a fulcrum.
3. Close the animal's mouth over the pencil and move the mandible in the appropriate direction to reduce the luxation.
   a. When reducing the luxation, open reduction may rarely be required. Exposure for open reduction is as previously described for the approach to the dorsal aspect of the ramus.

4. After reduction, apply a tape muzzle (see Chap. 117) to minimize reluxation and limit mouth opening during the healing phase.
5. Interarch wiring has been used as an alternative to the tape muzzle for preventing reluxation but has the following disadvantages:
   a. A long-term feeding tube is required.
   b. Wire stretching and breaking can occur.
   c. Aspiration pneumonia is possible.

Technique—Jaw Locking

Jaw locking occurs when the condyloid process of the ramus is trapped lateral to the zygomatic arch. This can occur when the mouth is opened widely, often when dogs yawn. Although some dogs are able to effect reduction unassisted by exaggerated jaw movements, many dogs require assistance in unlocking the jaw.

1. When the jaw is locked, there is a prominent bulge below the zygomatic arch on the locked side. Unlock the jaw by opening the jaw as far as possible and applying pressure over the prominent bulge.
2. While continuing to apply pressure, close the jaw.
3. In chronic cases, partially resect the zygomatic arch or condyloid process to prevent lateral fixation of the ramus.

Postoperative Care and Complications

TMJ Luxation

- Maintain the tape muzzle for 2–3 weeks.
- Feed a soft diet for 4–6 weeks with gradual reintroduction of a dry diet.
- Reluxation is possible. If reduction cannot be maintained, a mandibular condylectomy is indicated.

Jaw Locking

- No special care is necessary regarding feeding or activity.
- Complications are not reported.

SUPPLEMENTAL READING

Taylor RA: Mandibular fractures. *In* Bojrak MJ, ed.: Current Techniques in Small Animal Surgery. Philadelphia: Lea & Febiger, 1990, p 890.

117 Fractures of the Maxilla

Paul E. Howard

Maxillary fractures generally refer to any fracture of the upper jaw and adjacent bone.

ANATOMY

- The upper jaw is composed of paired maxilla and incisive bone (also called premaxilla) joined along the midline by their contralateral counterparts.
  - The maxilla contains the canine, premolar, and molar teeth. It varies greatly in form among different breeds of dogs (i.e., brachycephalic, mesocephalic, dolichocephalic).
  - The incisive bone joins caudally with the maxilla and contains the incisor teeth. The portion between the teeth and nasal cavity is very thin and can be damaged easily from trauma or during dental procedures involving the incisor teeth.
- The palatine bone is located caudomedial to the maxilla and forms the caudal part of the hard palate. Along its lateral suture, it joins with the maxilla to form the major palatine foramen.
  - The major palatine foramen is at the level of the distal margin of the maxillary fourth premolars.
  - The minor palatine foramen (occasionally two or more) is found caudal to the major palatine foramen.
- The bones of the upper jaw are covered with gingiva (the gums), which is composed of dense fibrous tissue covered by smooth vascularized mucosa. The gingiva extends around the necks of the teeth and into the alveolar sockets. It is continuous externally with the mucosa, and internally with the hard palate.
- The major blood supply to the upper jaw is provided by the pterygopalatine portion of the maxillary artery.
  - The minor palatine artery arises from the ventral surface of the maxillary or one of its terminal branches dorsal to the last maxillary molar tooth and supplies the adjacent soft and hard palate.
  - The major palatine artery arises rostral to the minor palatine artery from a common trunk with the sphenopalatine artery, exits through the major palatine foramen, and supplies the mucosa overlying the hard palate. This artery frequently anastomoses with its contralateral counterpart.

GENERAL PRINCIPLES OF FRACTURE FIXATION

Preoperative Considerations

- Diagnosis of maxillary and incisive bone fractures is usually not difficult. Direct observation and palpation often are sufficient for definitive diagnosis.
  - Consider any fracture of the maxilla in which the integrity of the gingiva is disrupted an open fracture. Antibiotic therapy is appropriate.
  - Evaluate maxillary fractures radiographically to assess the extent and severity of the injury.
- Maintenance of a patent and functioning airway is of primary importance. Respiratory distress can result from hemorrhage, edema, and soft tissue obstruction secondary to associated trauma.
- When the animal's condition is stabilized, evaluate the dental occlusion. The site of malocclusion and its severity can help the clinician identify the location and severity of the fracture.

▼ *Key Point* Restoration of normal anatomic alignment of the fracture ensures restoration of dental occlusion unless the teeth are traumatized or bone fragments are missing.

- Stable fixation of the teeth often provides suitable stabilization of the fractured bone.
- Stabilization of bone fragments can be difficult, owing to thinness of bone or the presence of tooth roots.
- Noninvasive methods of fracture fixation often result in satisfactory healing of the fracture and are preferred to invasive surgical procedures.
- Indications for open reduction of fractures:
  - Airway obstruction due to depression fractures (unreduced fractures of the nasal or maxillary bones can result in callus formation and later obstruction of the nasal passages)
  - Lack of alternative measures for acceptable dental occlusion or fracture stabilization
  - Presence of an oronasal defect, from either trauma or tooth loss
  - Severe facial deformity

Objectives

- Ensure a patent airway.
- Establish and maintain acceptable dental occlusion.
- Correct severe facial deformities.

Equipment

Specialized equipment is not required. Equipment needed varies, depending on the method of repair selected, and may include:

- Wire twisters and cutters
- Orthopedic wire of various sizes (18–24 gauge)
- Bone plates and screws
- External skeletal fixation devices
- Kirschner wires (K-wires) and small intramedullary pins
- Adhesive tape

GENERAL PRINCIPLES OF POSTOPERATIVE CARE AND COMPLICATIONS

- Feed a soft diet (gruel or liquid) until fractures are healed.
- Deny access to bones, balls, chew toys, and other hard objects to prevent dislodging the fixation device.
- Instruct the owner to examine the oral cavity once daily to ensure that proper dental occlusion is being maintained and that any external implants used are still in place. Instruct the owner to avoid excessive manipulation of the jaw.
- Radiographically evaluate fracture healing in 4–6 weeks. Remove exposed fixation devices when there is radiographic evidence of bony union.
- Continue postoperative restrictions for 3–4 weeks following radiographic evidence of bony union to ensure sufficient osseous healing before allowing resumption of normal activities and return to a normal diet.

Complications

Complications are infrequently encountered but may include the following:

- Infection—Severe periodontal disease can compromise fracture healing due to the large numbers of bacteria in the area of the fracture.
- Oronasal fistula
  - Chronic fistulas may lead to respiratory infection due to aspiration of food particles and saliva.
  - Although usually located at the site of a missing tooth, traumatically induced fistulas can exist anywhere between the oral and nasal cavities.
  - Conservative treatment usually is not successful and surgical intervention is required (see Chap. 84).
- Bone sequestration—rare due to the good vascular supply to the area.
- Chronic respiratory obstruction
  - Causes include malalignment of fracture fragments and callus produced as fracture healing progresses, occluding normal air flow.
  - Depending on the severity of the obstruction, surgical intervention to reestablish a patent air passage may be necessary (see Chap. 3).
- Malocclusion or tooth loss
  - Trauma to the maxilla can damage tooth structures, resulting in loss of tooth vitality.
  - Treat nonviable teeth endodontically to eliminate the potential for abscess formation (see Chap. 84).
  - Extract excessively loose or irreparably damaged teeth after they are no longer needed for fracture stabilization.
- Altered normal growth in young animals (<6 months of age).

PROCEDURES

Tape Muzzle

Indications

- Repair of nondisplaced or minimally displaced fractures involving the hard palate or teeth, in which normal dental occlusion can be established and maintained without other means of fixation
- An adjunct to fixation, used in combination with internal fixation, in which the purpose is to limit postoperative jaw motion
- Temporary means of reducing motion at the fracture site until definitive methods of repair are employed

Preapplication Considerations

- To properly evaluate alignment and stability, general anesthesia or heavy sedation may be required.
- If proper occlusion is present, maintain a 1-cm gap between the incisors as the tape muzzle is applied.
- If occlusion can be maintained only by holding the mouth completely closed with interdigitation of the teeth, apply the muzzle with the mouth closed.
  - Provide alimentation by esophagostomy tube or gastrostomy tube (see Chap. 3).
  - Be sure that the animal can breathe through its nose.

▼ *Key Point* If possible, avoid muzzling with the animal's mouth completely closed, because openmouth breathing and evaporation of saliva from the tongue play an important role in thermoregulation.

Technique

1. Place the first piece of tape around the posterior muzzle with the sticky side of the tape facing out. When the circle is complete, double back the tape on itself to cover the adhesive and prevent it from sticking to the animal.
2. Place a second ring of tape in the same manner and secure it snugly around the neck, immediately behind the ears (Fig. 117–1).

▼ *Key Point* An unanesthetized animal may resist attempts to apply the tape around the nose. Premeasure the animal's muzzle with your hands and make

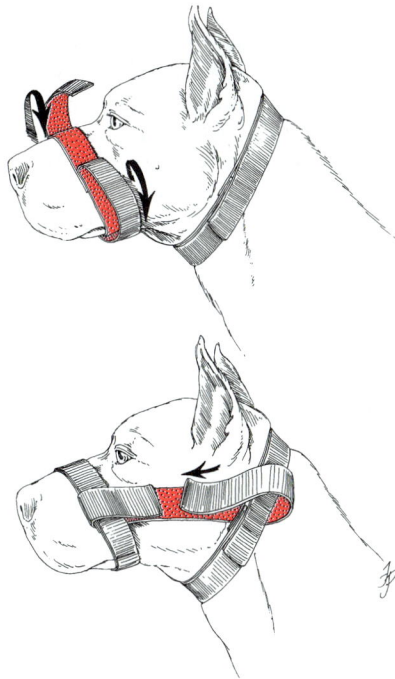

Figure 117–1. Procedure for creating a tape muzzle. See text for explanation.

a tape ring based on this measurement. Slip the ring over the animal's muzzle while an assistant holds the animal's mouth closed.

3. Join the two rings of tape with lateral straps, made by folding a piece of tape on itself with the adhesive side inward. Secure these to the rings by an additional layer of tape wrapped around the nose and neck rings. Excess tape is trimmed away. In cats and brachycephalic breeds, a strip of tape can be run between the tape rings along the dorsal midline of the skull to aid in keeping the muzzle in place.
4. Remove the muzzle by cutting the neck ring and slipping off the nose ring.

Postoperative Care and Complications

- If necessary use an Elizabethan collar to prevent attempts by the dog to remove the muzzle.
- Restrict diet to soft food; do not allow chewing of hard objects.
- Instruct the owner to examine the skin around the tape daily for signs of redness or discharge. Moist dermatitis may be encountered under the tape around the muzzle. The condition should resolve rapidly once the muzzle is removed.
- Muzzles used long-term may need to be replaced periodically.
  - Muzzles soiled from feed and water can cause irritation to the skin.
  - The tape rings will stretch slightly, permitting excessive jaw motion and requiring replacement of the tape.
- Leave the muzzle on until the fracture is stable (usually 4–8 weeks).

- Jaw motion following removal of the tape muzzle often is restricted. Normal range of motion returns in 1–3 weeks without the need for physical therapy.

Interdental Wiring

Interdental wiring is used as a primary method of fracture stabilization of fractures of the hard palate and alveolar bone or in conjunction with other fixation procedures. It is an excellent method for maintaining dental occlusion.

Technique

1. Use the largest-size orthopedic wire (usually 22- or 24-gauge) that can be passed between the involved teeth without distorting occlusion and that can be conformed intimately to the surface of the teeth.

▼ *Key Point* Wire not closely conformed to the teeth will not provide adequate stability.

2. Place the wire as close to the gingival margin as possible. Wire that tends to slip off owing to the conical shape of the tooth (e.g., canine tooth) can be kept in position by securing the wire in place with a small amount of composite material (see discussion of oral cavities in Chap. 84). In multirooted teeth, the wire can be placed through the furcation in preference to around the tooth.
3. Place wire twists on the buccal side of the teeth and bend the twisted end parallel to the long axis of the tooth to minimize soft tissue irritation.
   a. Covering twists with composite resin or brace wax reduces soft tissue irritation.
4. Incorporate teeth on each side of the fracture site in the wire pattern until the first tooth solidly embedded in alveolar bone can be included. Including additional teeth in the repair does not provide added stability.

Ivy Loop

This is a simple wiring pattern for stabilizing a fracture between two teeth that have remained firmly embedded in their respective alveolar sockets (Fig. 117–2).

Technique

1. Make a loop in the middle of the wire and place the wire between the two involved teeth, with the loop on the buccal surface of the teeth and the wire tails on the lingual aspect.
2. Pull one wire tail tightly around the distal aspect of the caudal tooth to the buccal surface where it is threaded through the wire loop.
3. Draw the other tail around the mesial aspect of the rostral tooth to the buccal surface of the tooth.
4. Cross and twist the two ends of wire on each other while applying firm traction to the wires, ensuring an even twist.
5. Cut the twisted wire, leaving three twists to prevent separation of the wire ends.

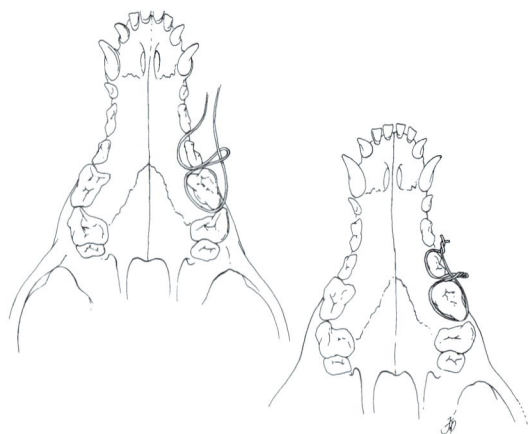

Figure 117–2.   Initial *(left)* and final *(right)* appearance of Ivy loop wiring pattern.

Stout Continuous Loop

This wiring pattern is indicated for stabilization of alveolar and palate fractures in which teeth adjacent to the fracture are loose. The pattern is continued until solidly embedded teeth are encountered on both sides of the fracture (Fig. 117–3).

Technique

1. Identify the teeth to be wired and place a piece of wire along the buccal aspect of the teeth. Measure and cut a small length of wire beyond the last tooth at one end, and leave a working length of wire at least 1½ times the distance between the teeth being wired.
2. Bring the working end of wire around the tooth to the lingual side and pass it through the interproximal space and under the wire lying on the buccal surface of the tooth. Bring the working wire over the stationary wire and pass it back through the interproximal space. Before pulling the wire tight, twist a single loop in the working wire where it passes over the stationary wire.
3. Continue this pattern the entire length of the teeth until the last solidly embedded tooth is encountered. Pull the wire around the last tooth to the buccal surface of the tooth.
4. Before twisting the wire ends together, apply traction to the stationary wire and twist each loop in the working wire tightly, beginning at the far end and working toward the free ends of wire.
5. After tightening all the working loops, twist the two ends of wire evenly on each other until tight and cut off the excess wire, leaving three twists.
6. In a modification of this technique, place the loops through the interproximal spaces and thread the stationary wire through the loops. Tighten the wire as previously described.

Interfragmentary Wiring

This is a potentially useful method for repairing comminuted fractures of the maxilla or incisive bone. Multiple wires can be used to stabilize hard palate fractures or transverse fractures of the maxilla. Small-diameter wire (22 or 24 gauge) is preferred because it conforms better to the thin bone than does heavier-gauge wire.

Technique

1. Drill small holes in the fragments and preplace the wire through drill holes in adjacent fragments. Each fragment requires a minimum of two wires to provide sufficient stability. In some cases, three or more wires may be placed through a single fragment.
2. Preplace all wires before tightening them to ensure proper positioning of all wires.
3. Discard very small pieces of bone rather than attempting to replace them. The resultant osseous defect will be covered with soft tissue and new bone formation can be expected if the periosteum is preserved.

Pin and Wire Fixation

The primary indication for pin and wire fixation is the stabilization of palate fractures in which interdental or interfragmentary wiring techniques alone do not provide adequate fracture stabilization.

Technique

1. Insert K-wires or small intramedullary pins, determined by the size of the animal involved, from the alveolar margin across the fracture, and exit on the opposite side. The pin actually traverses the floor of the nasal cavity.
2. Exercise care during pin placement to avoid penetrating tooth roots.

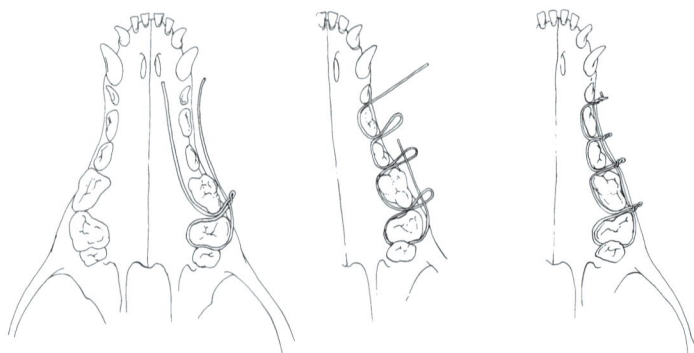

Figure 117–3.   Initial *(left)* and final *(center* and *right)* appearance of Stout continuous loop wiring pattern. Note that the working wire is *not* twisted lingual to the stationary wire.

3. Orthopedic wire is placed in figure-eight fashion around the ends of the pin and tightened. As the wire is tightened, compression is applied at the fracture site. The wire twists are positioned so as to minimize subsequent trauma to adjacent soft tissues.

EXTERNAL SKELETAL FIXATION

This often-described but infrequently used method of fixation uses external pins and acrylic to stabilize comminuted fractures of the nasal and maxillary bones. External skeletal fixation has the following disadvantages:

- The thinness of the bone makes it difficult to achieve secure retention of the pins long enough for fracture healing to occur.
- The external apparatus can be dislodged, resulting in loss of fracture reduction.

Technique

The principles of standard external skeletal fixation for stabilization of long bone fractures apply to this method.

1. Insert pins through stab incisions in the skin, minimizing the need for extensive soft tissue dissection.
2. When possible, place a minimum of two pins in each fracture fragment, to avoid rotation of the fragments.
3. Keep pin entry sites clean to minimize pin tract infections.
4. Connect the external pins with acrylic rather than external metal bars because the reduced weight is advantageous, and the acrylic permits the incorporation of pins of various sizes in multiple planes.

▼ *Key Point* Use an Elizabethan collar to protect the apparatus.

Plate and Screw Fixation

Plating maxillary fractures is seldom necessary, but this method of fracture fixation is used in selected cases.

- Comminuted fractures with a bony defect can be effectively stabilized with a plate.
- Transverse fractures of the premaxilla, which are difficult to stabilize with interfragmentary wires, are amenable to plate and screw fixation.

Technique

1. Because of the minimal soft tissue overlying the maxilla, use small, thin bone plates.
2. The thinness of the bone necessitates the use of short screws.
3. Because the maxilla has only a single cortex, maximize plate length and the number of screws.
4. Avoid tooth roots and the infraorbital foramen.
5. Reconstruction plates (Synthes, Paoli, PA) and plastic plates (Lubra, Fort Collins, CO) can be more easily contoured to the maxilla than conventional plates.

SUPPLEMENTAL READINGS

Bone DL: Maxillary fractures. *In* Bojrab MJ, ed.: Current Techniques in Small Animal Surgery. Philadelphia: Lea & Febiger, 1990, p 883.
Dulisch ML: Skull and mandibular fractures. *In* Slatter DH, ed.: Textbook of Small Animal Surgery. Philadelphia: WB Saunders, 1985, p 2286.

118 Neoplasia of the Maxilla and Mandible

Paul E. Howard

Neoplasms of the oral cavity and associated structures are encountered commonly in dogs and cats. The oral cavity is the fourth most common site of neoplasms, accounting for approximately 5% and 7% of malignant tumors in dogs and cats, respectively. Oral neoplasms in dogs often are malignant; in cats they are nearly always malignant.

▼ *Key Point* Squamous cell carcinoma is the most frequently identified neoplasm in cats; malignant melanoma, squamous cell carcinoma, and fibrosarcoma are the neoplasms diagnosed most often in dogs.

- Certain breeds of dogs appear to be predisposed to oral tumors, including boxers, German shepherds, German shorthaired pointers, golden retrievers, cocker spaniels, and Weimaraners.
- When oral tumors are considered collectively, male dogs are affected more frequently than female dogs.
- Small-breed dogs have a greater tendency to develop malignant melanoma; large-breed dogs are more prone to develop squamous cell carcinoma and fibrosarcoma.
- Dogs with heavily pigmented oral mucosa are predisposed to malignant melanomas.

TUMOR TYPES

Benign Nonodontogenic Neoplasms

Epulis

Epulides are fibromatous tumors of the periodontal ligament, differentiating them from odontogenic tumors. They are rarely seen in the cat but are among the most frequently observed oral tumors in the dog.

- There is an equal distribution between sexes.
- A familial predisposition has been noted in boxers.

Epulides are categorized into three different types based on histologic appearance.

Fibromatous Epulis

- This is a benign, noninvasive growth in which the periodontal ligament stroma is the dominant cell type.
- Fibromatous epulides appear as pedunculated masses that are usually multiple and grow by expansion.

- The enveloping nature of the lesion can cause interference with mastication. Treatment is necessary only if the lesion is causing clinical signs.

Treatment
- Surgical excision of only the visible portion of an epulis usually results in recurrence.

▼ *Key Point* Warn the pet owner that recurrence is likely if the lesion is only debulked.

- Because the origin of the lesion is the periodontal ligament, prevention of recurrence requires extraction of the involved tooth and curettage of the associated periodontal ligament.
- An alternative procedure is en bloc resection of the bone and involved tooth. In most instances, this option is not necessary.

Ossifying Epulis

- Biologic behavior is similar to that of fibromatous epulis, except that the tumor has an osteoid component.
- Malignant transformation to osteosarcoma has been reported.

Treatment
- Treatment, as described for fibromatous epulides, is necessary only if the tumor is causing clinical signs.
- The possibility of malignant transformation makes surgical excision of an ossifying epulis a prudent choice.

Acanthomatous Epulis

This locally invasive neoplasm causes destruction of adjacent alveolar bone and is found most often on the rostral mandible. It does not metastasize.

Treatment
A variety of treatments can be used.

- Simple local excision results in a high rate of recurrence.
- Wide surgical excision of affected bone (partial mandibulectomy or partial maxillectomy) is effective.
- Radiation therapy is effective and can be curative.
- Radiation often is combined with surgical excision of large tumors.
- Chemotherapy is not effective.

- Epulides rarely undergo malignant transformation and recur as squamous cell carcinoma, fibrosarcoma, or osteosarcoma.

Other Benign Nonodontogenic Neoplasms

These include fibroma, lipoma, hemangioma, chondroma, osteoma, and histiocytoma. They are seen less frequently than epulides. However, because of their similar clinical appearance to other tumors, biopsy and histopathologic evaluation are necessary.

Malignant Nonodontogenic Neoplasms

Malignant Melanoma

- Malignant melanoma (MM) is the most commonly diagnosed oral tumor in dogs but is rare in cats.
  - The incidence in male and female dogs is 4:1.
  - Animals with darkly pigmented oral mucosa may be at greater risk for the disease.
- MM is noted for its rapid local infiltration, frequent recurrence rate, and high likelihood of metastasis to regional lymph nodes and the lungs.
  - Amelanotic melanoma can be mistaken on gross observation for other oral neoplasms, indicating the necessity for histologic diagnosis.

Treatment
- Wide surgical excision (partial maxillectomies and mandibulectomies) currently appears to be the most effective method of treatment.
- Some success has been reported with high dose per fraction radiotherapy. Dogs in one study were alive 9–19 months after initiation of therapy.
- Chemotherapy and immunotherapy have been used to a minimal degree, and their efficacy is unknown at this time. Several different chemotherapy agents have been tried with varying degrees of success.

Prognosis. The prognosis for malignant melanoma is poor, with a 1-year survival rate of <10%.

Squamous Cell Carcinoma

- Squamous cell carcinoma (SCC) is the most common malignant tumor of the oral cavity in cats and the second most common malignant oral tumor in dogs.
  - In cats, differentiate SCC from inflammatory lesions such as eosinophilic granuloma and nasopharyngeal polyp.
- SCC can be classified as tonsillar and nontonsillar.
  - Both types occur with equal frequency in dogs.
  - In dogs, nontonsillar SCC occurs with equal frequency in males and females; tonsillar SCC occurs more frequently in males.
- Nontonsillar SCC is locally invasive but slow to metastasize to regional lymph nodes and lungs. It often invades bone, causing lysis of bone and loosening of teeth; the radiographic appearance can be confused with osteosarcoma and osteomyelitis.
- Tonsillar SCC is very aggressive and has a poor prognosis (see Chap. 84).

Treatment
- Wide surgical excision is the treatment of choice.
- Nontonsillar SCC is potentially sensitive to radiation therapy if treated aggressively.
- The current trend is to offer multimodality treatment, combining surgical excision with radiation therapy and some form of chemotherapy.

Prognosis
- The prognosis in cats is poor, because local recurrence is common.
- The prognosis in dogs is better; about 50% of treated dogs live for 1 year.

Fibrosarcoma

- In dogs, fibrosarcoma (FS) is diagnosed third most frequently after MM and SCC. It is the second most frequent malignant tumor in cats, but much less common than SCC.
- FS is seen twice as often in canine males as in females.
- It is more common in large-breed dogs than in small breeds.
- The FS tends to invade local tissues rapidly, causing bony destruction.
- Metastasis occurs late in the course of the disease, but local recurrence is very common.

Treatment
- Effective treatment of FS can be difficult, especially of tumors involving the hard palate.
- Wide surgical excision is the treatment of choice.
- Radiation therapy, chemotherapy, and immunotherapy are offered as adjunctive treatment modalities to surgery.
- Cryosurgery is not recommended because it is believed to stimulate recurrence.

Prognosis
- The prognosis is poor, owing to local recurrence and eventual metastasis.
- The 1-year survival rate is less than 20%.

Osteosarcoma

- Osteosarcoma is uncommon in dogs and cats.
- The initial presenting complaint is jaw pain, and radiographs obtained early in the course of the disease may be nondiagnostic.

Treatment
- Wide surgical excision of the involved bone in combination with chemotherapy is currently recommended, but the prognosis is poor.

Other Malignant Nonodontogenic Neoplasms

Less commonly seen tumors include adenocarcinoma, undifferentiated carcinoma, transmissible venereal tumor, mast cell tumor, hemangiosarcoma, and tonsillar lymphosarcoma.

Odontogenic Neoplasms

- Odontoma, a rare tumor of dental origin, can invade all of the dental tissues (enamel, cementum, dentin, and pulp).

- Ameloblastoma is a benign, slow-growing, invasive neoplasm of epithelial origin. It occurs most commonly in the mandible, grows by expansion, and metastasizes infrequently.

Treatment
- Because these tumors arise from deep alveolar bone, local, nonaggressive therapy often results in recurrence.
- Wide surgical excision usually is curative.
- Radiation can be used, but recurrence is likely.

CLINICAL SIGNS

- Clinical signs of benign and malignant oral neoplasms are similar and include excessive salivation, oral hemorrhage, reluctance to eat or difficulty eating, jaw pain, loose teeth, and facial asymmetry.
- Weight loss can occur secondary to the above clinical signs.

▼ *Key Point* Consider neoplasia in an animal that requires dental extraction because of excessive tooth mobility.

DIAGNOSIS

- Base a tentative diagnosis on the age, sex, and breed of the animal and the gross appearance and location of the lesion.
- Make a definitive diagnosis by histopathologic evaluation of a representative lesion specimen.
  - Obtain a specimen by incisional or excisional biopsy, depending on the nature and extent of the lesion.
  - Perform fine-needle aspiration of regional lymph nodes to evaluate for metastasis.
- Radiology
  - Radiographs of the skull assess the extent of bony involvement.
  - Multiple projections may be necessary to adequately assess bony changes.
  - Obtain thoracic radiographs in all cases of malignant oral neoplasia to determine distant metastatic lesions. Ideally, perform thoracic radiography before the animal is anesthetized for biopsy.
  - Inform owners that false-negative thoracic radiographs can occur.

PRINCIPLES OF THERAPY

- The goal of therapy is the elimination of neoplastic tissue while preserving function and, if possible, cosmetic appearance.
  - The severity of the lesion at the time of treatment may permit only palliative measures.
  - Slowly progressing, noninvasive neoplasms are more responsive to therapy than are rapidly growing, invasive tumors.

- No single treatment protocol is effective for all oral tumors (see Treatment in preceding discussion of specific neoplasms). Adapt protocols to the animal being treated, based on the following factors:
  - Tumor type and primary site
  - Age and overall health of the animal
  - Extent of tissue involvement
  - Presence of lung metastasis
  - Expertise of the veterinarian
  - Cost of treatment and owner preference

▼ *Key Point* Early, aggressive therapy of malignant oral tumors offers the best chance of success.

- In selected tumors, a combination of treatment modalities may be more effective than individual modalities.
- Aggressive surgical management improves success rates. Table 118–1 compares the responsiveness of various tumor types to surgery and radiation therapy.
- Cryotherapy (freezing of tissue to destroy tumor cells) is not recommended because of associated complications and poor results compared with surgery.

SURGICAL PROCEDURES

Surgical Excision

- Surgical procedures range from simple local excision to mandibulectomy and maxillectomy.
  - Hemimandibulectomy is partial or total removal of bone and associated teeth from one side of the mandible.
  - Hemimaxillectomy is the en bloc removal of the portion of the maxilla between the second and third premolars that is confined to one side of the maxilla (see Fig. 118–3).
  - Caudal hemimaxillectomy is the en bloc resection of the maxilla from the fourth premolar caudally.
- Local excision often is unsuccessful, owing to tumor recurrence at the primary surgical site.
- En bloc resection (mandibulectomy, maxillectomy) of the affected bone is recommended to prevent local tumor recurrence.

Table 118–1. RESPONSIVENESS OF COMMON ORAL TUMORS TO AGGRESSIVE SURGICAL EXCISION AND RADIATION THERAPY

Tumor Type	Surgery	Radiation
Epulis		
Fibromatous	+++	NI
Ossifying	+++	NI
Acanthomatous	++	+++
Malignant melanoma	+	+
Squamous cell	+++ (dogs)	+++ (rostral tumors)
carcinoma	+ (cats)	++ (caudal tumors)
Fibrosarcoma	++	++
Osteosarcoma	++	+

NI, not indicated; +, poor; ++, fair; +++, good.

- Stabilization of the hemimandibles using pins, screws, or bone grafts is unnecessary and is not recommended.

Anatomy

- The masseter muscle lies on the lateral surface of the ramus with some fibers of the superficial layer projecting around the ventral and caudal borders of the mandible to insert on the ventromedial surface.
- The temporalis muscle inserts on the coronoid process of the mandible, with some fibers inserting further down on the ventral margin of the masseteric fossa.
- The lateral pterygoid muscle inserts on the medial surface of the mandibular condyle.
- The medial pterygoid muscle inserts on the medial and caudal surfaces of the angular process of the mandible.
- The inferior alveolar artery and vein enter the mandibular foramen located on the medial side of the ramus at approximately the level of the last molar, midway between the cranial and caudal edges of the ramus. The artery exits at the mental foramen of the mandible.
- The blood supply to the maxilla is via the major and minor palatine arteries (which lie just deep to the mucosa of the hard palate) and the infraorbital artery (exits through the infraorbital foramen dorsal to the upper third premolar tooth). The infraorbital vein and nerve parallel this artery.

Preoperative Considerations

- Indications:
  - Evidence of malignancy or local invasiveness (bone involvement) in the absence of distant metastasis
  - Tumor recurrence
  - Radiation is ineffective (fibrosarcoma, malignant melanoma)
  - Small, mobile, and easily resectable mass
  - Palliation in tumors that are not resectable

▼ *Key Point* The first attempt at surgery offers the best chance at success. Local recurrence of the neoplasm often is due to an insufficiently aggressive excision of the initial lesion.

- When performing excision of mass lesions, include a margin of at least 1 cm of normal-appearing tissue.
- Show owners pictures of animals that have undergone mandibulectomy and maxillectomy to prepare them for the animal's postoperative appearance and to reassure them that gross deformities do not result.
- Reserve electrocautery for coagulation, and use it sparingly. Incisions made with electrocautery heal slowly and have a tendency toward dehiscence.
- The suture material of choice is a synthetic absorbable suture used with a cutting needle (e.g., polydioxanone [PDS], poliglecaprone [Monocryl, Ethicon, Inc., Somerville, NJ]).
- Drape the surgical site as well as possible; recognize that the procedure is not being performed in a sterile field.

- Administer intravenous (IV) broad-spectrum antibiotics at the time of anesthetic induction. It is rarely necessary to continue them postoperatively.

Positioning of the Animal

Good exposure is important, especially when considering surgery of the caudal aspect of the oral cavity.

Maxillectomy
- Place the animal in dorsal recumbency.
- Use sterile tongue depressors to keep the mouth open; this will cause minimal obstruction for the surgeon.
- Alternatively, use a sterile mouth speculum, or tape the dog's mouth open to an anesthetic screen or to IV stands placed on each side of the operating table.
- Tie the endotracheal tube to the mandible.

Mandibulectomy
- Surgery of the mandible is best accomplished with the dog in lateral recumbency or, when operating on the caudal mandible per os, in sternal recumbency.
- When the animal is placed in sternal recumbency, hold the jaw open by taping the maxilla to IV stands on both sides of the operating table.
- Rostral mandibulectomy is best performed in dorsal recumbency with the animal's mouth held open by an oral speculum.

Objectives

- Excise all neoplastic tissue.
- Reconstruct oral soft tissues to preserve function.

Equipment

- Standard surgical pack and sutures
- Oral speculum
- Electrocautery
- Bone saw and/or osteotome and mallet
- Bone wax

Unilateral Rostral Hemimandibulectomy
Technique

1. Incise the gingiva around the lesion while attempting to include a minimum of 1 cm of normal tissue (Fig. 118–1A). Reflect the lip ventrally.
2. Continue the dissection around the entire bone, incising the soft tissue attachments on the lingual side of the mandible.
3. Separate the mandibular symphysis with an osteotome and mallet. Use an oscillating saw to facilitate separation and osteotomy of the mandible.
4. The inferior alveolar artery and vein will be severed. Control resultant hemorrhage with electrocautery and bone wax.
5. Do not attempt to stabilize the hemimandibles.
6. Cover the bone and close the defect by suturing the labial gingival mucosa to the lingual mucosa in a single layer, using absorbable suture material (Fig. 118–1B).
7. To prevent the tongue from hanging out of the mouth, advance the commissure of the mouth by de-

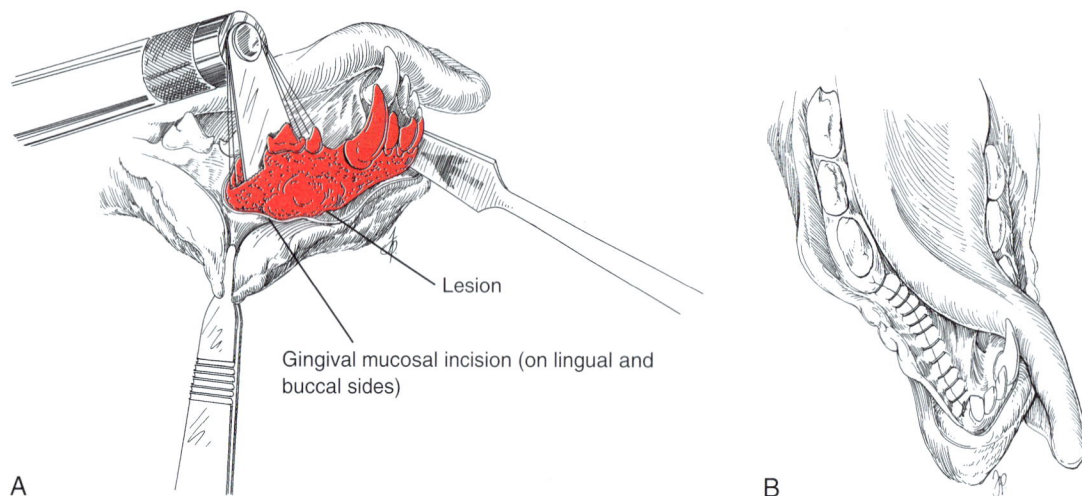

Figure 118–1. Unilateral hemimandibulectomy. *A,* Incise the gingiva around the lesion, keeping at least 1 cm of normal tissue around it. Separate the mandibular symphysis and continue the original incision through the bone. *B,* Cover the bone and close the incision.

briding the lips dorsally and ventrally and closing them up to the second premolar area.

Bilateral Rostral Hemimandibulectomy

Technique

1. Perform the same procedure as that described for unilateral hemimandibulectomy.
2. Resection of the mandibles caudal to the second premolar teeth necessitates resection of some skin to effect a cosmetic closure.
3. Stent sutures may be necessary to secure the remaining lower lip to the cut ends of the mandibles. Place these sutures through the skin, then through a hole made in the mandibular stump, then back out through the skin. Buttons or rubber tubing can be used to prevent skin necrosis.

Central Hemimandibulectomy

Technique

1. The procedure is similar to that for unilateral rostral hemimandibulectomy, except that a central portion of the mandible is removed, preserving the symphysis and temporomandibular joint (TMJ).
2. Osteotomize the bone slightly beyond the incisions in the mucosa. This allows normal gingival and oral mucosa to be pulled over the bone ends and sutured without tension.

Caudal Hemimandibulectomy

Technique

1. Make a skin incision paralleling the zygomatic arch.
2. Incise the periosteum and elevate the temporalis muscle subperiosteally from the zygomatic bone dorsally and medially.
3. Elevate the masseter muscles subperiosteally from their origin on the ventral zygomatic arch. Continue subperiosteal dissection until the zygomatic bone is freed completely of all muscle attachments.

4. Using an oscillating saw, transect the zygomatic arch at its rostral and caudal margins. Alternatively, resect the zygomatic bone with Gigli wire or a hobby saw.
   a. Do not use an osteotome and mallet because of the potential for splintering the bone.
   b. Wrap the zygomatic bone in a blood-soaked sponge in anticipation of replacing it during closure of the surgical wound.
5. Elevate the masseter muscle ventrally from the ramus and incise and elevate the temporalis muscle to expose the ramus.
6. Osteotomize the ramus with an oscillating saw.
   a. The location of the tumor determines if the TMJ can be preserved.
   b. If disarticulation of the TMJ is necessary, use sharp dissection to incise the joint capsule and soft tissue attachments. Avoid trauma to the maxillary artery located just medial to the TMJ. Ligate this vessel if necessary to remove the section of mandible.
7. Close the incision by securing the osteotomized zygomatic bone with orthopedic wire at each end.
8. Suture the masseter muscle to the zygomatic bone with nonabsorbable sutures passed through the muscle fascia and encircling the bone.
9. Appose and suture the subcutaneous tissues and skin routinely.

Premaxillectomy (for Lesions Rostral to the Second Premolar)

Technique

1. Make an incision at least 1 cm around the lesion (Fig. 118–2A).
2. Control hemorrhage, which often is profuse when the palate is incised, with temporary direct pressure or electrocoagulation.
3. Elevate the mucoperiosteum outward from the lesion in preparation for excising the diseased bone.
4. Using the incision line as a guide, cut the bone with an oscillating saw or side-cutting bur and free it from remaining soft tissue attachments.

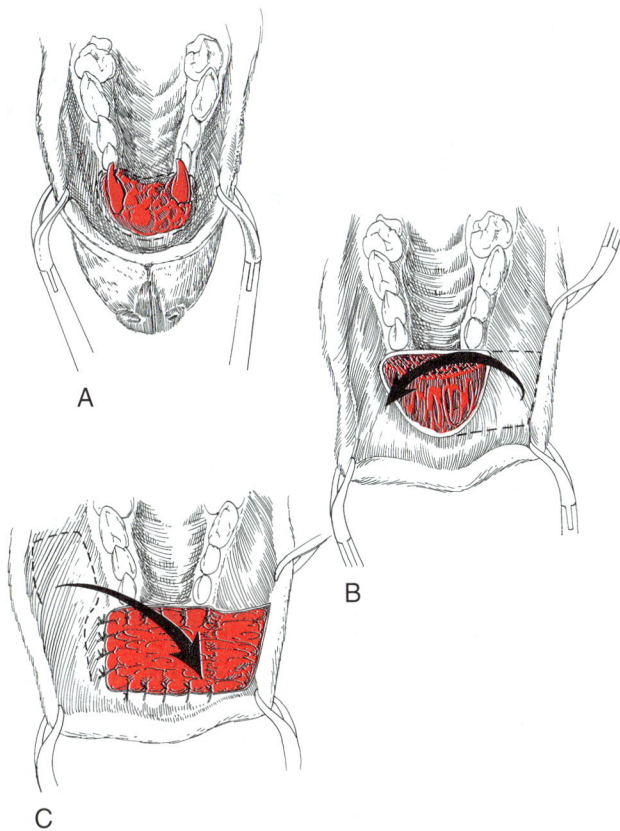

Figure 118–2. Bilateral premaxillectomy, double flap technique. *A,* Site of incision. *B,* First flap parallel to excised dental arch. This flap is flipped over (reversed) so that the labial mucosa is on the nasal cavity side of the defect. *C,* Second flap from opposite side of premaxilla.

5. Remove the mobilized section of bone en bloc, creating an oronasal defect.
   a. Exercise care when removing the bone to minimize damage to normal turbinate tissue. Remove diseased or damaged turbinates.
6. Create a labial flap adjacent to the defect of sufficient size to allow suturing the flap to the palatal mucosa without tension.
   a. The labial flap can be a sliding flap or a reversed flap (Fig. 118–2*B*) in which the mucosal surface is flipped over to form the floor of the nasal cavity.
   b. The sliding flap is less likely to fail because of vascular compromise. The length of the flap should not exceed three times the width of the flap base.
   c. Create a labial flap by undermining the tissue adjacent to the defect to include the mucosa, submucosa, and subcutaneous tissue.
   d. Allow the exposed surface of the reversed flap to heal by epithelialization, whisch usually is complete in 3–4 weeks.
7. Suture the labial flap to the palatal mucosa in two layers, using absorbable synthetic suture material on a cutting needle.
   a. Suturing the deep layer is facilitated by passing the suture through small drill holes (made with a Kirschner wire) in the hard palate.
   b. Suture the outer layer in a simple interrupted pattern. Alternatively, intersperse a "far-far-near"

near" suture pattern to disperse any tension on the suture line.
8. Large defects may require labial flaps on both sides that are sutured on the midline (problems with healing may be encountered).
9. To improve the postoperative cosmetic appearance of the nose, use a double flap technique in which the flaps overlap each other to provide additional soft tissue to support the nose.
   a. Create the first flap with the base of the flap paralleling the just-removed dental arch (Fig. 118–2*B*). Reverse the flap to place the mucosa on the floor of the nasal cavity, and suture this flap to the nasal mucosa and through holes previously drilled in the hard palate.
   b. Create a second, rostrally based, labial flap of similar size on the opposite side of the premaxilla (Fig. 118–2*C*). Rotate this flap over the first flap (without reversing) and suture in place as previously described.

Hemimaxillectomy

Technique

1. Make a mucosal incision around the lesion, attempting to leave at least 1 cm of normal tissue between the lesion and the incision (Fig. 118–3*A*).
2. Elevate the mucosa with a periosteal elevator to expose the underlying bone.

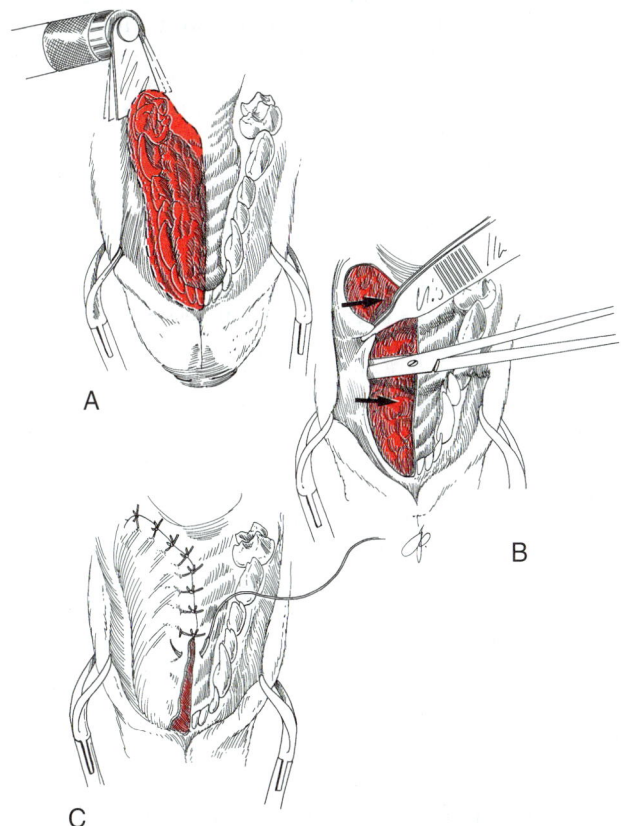

Figure 118–3. Hemimaxillectomy. *A,* Incise around lesion, then remove mass by ostectomy. Create (*B*) and close (*C*) labial flap.

3. Excise the mass by ostectomy of the involved bone. The ostectomy can be performed with an oscillating saw, side-cutting bur, or osteotome and mallet.
    a. If this equipment is not available, remove the diseased bone with bone rongeurs.
4. Control hemorrhage, which often is profuse when the palate is incised, with ligation or cautery after removal of the section of bone.
    a. Occlusion of the carotid arteries before performing surgery reduces the amount of hemorrhage during ostectomy of the diseased portion of the maxilla. This usually is not necessary, but it may be beneficial in dogs with a low preoperative packed cell volume (PCV) (see Chap. 76 for details of temporary carotid artery occlusion).
5. After mobilizing the bone, sever soft tissue attachments and remove the bone en bloc, exposing the nasal cavity.
    a. Remove nasal turbinates involved in the disease process or damaged severely during ostectomy via sharp dissection.
    b. Control hemorrhage with direct pressure, ligation, cautery, or placement of Gelfoam (Upjohn Co., Kalamazoo, MI). If necessary, pack the nasal cavity with sterile gauze strips (NuGauze, Johnson & Johnson Medical, Inc., Arlington, TX), which then exits the nose and is sutured to the nostril (see Chap. 76). Remove packing 24–48 hours postoperatively.
6. Base the labial flap created to close the defect (Fig. 118–3B and C) rostrally or caudally, with the flap rotated into position, along what was the mucogingival border, with the flap flipped over so the mucosa becomes the floor of the nasal cavity. Alternatively, dissect under the labial mucosa, along the lip margin, with the mucosa undermined sufficiently to be pulled over the defect.
    a. Flaps based along the lip margins tend to have a poor cosmetic appearance during the initial postoperative period. However, after healing is complete there is little noticeable cosmetic difference among the various techniques.
7. An alternative technique for small lesions is to mobilize the palatal mucosa and slide the mucosa to the incised buccal margin where the tissues are sutured. The exposed hard palate heals by epithelialization. The advantage of this technique is that the operated area is still covered with the normally thicker palatal mucosa.
    a. The major palatine artery may have to be ligated. Alternatively, the major palatine foramen can be enlarged with bone rongeurs or a bur, and the major palatine artery can be mobilized and preserved.

Caudal Hemimaxillectomy

Technique

1. The proximity of the palatine, lacrimal, and zygomatic bones may require their resection, depending on the extent of the disease process.

2. Ligate major vessels encountered during the resection.
3. Create labial flaps as described to close the defect.
4. When extensive disease in the caudal maxilla necessitates removal of the bone supporting the globe, postoperative sinking of the globe can be encountered.
    a. Procedures to support the globe, using synthetic materials or adjacent musculature, can be attempted.

POSTOPERATIVE CARE AND COMPLICATIONS

- Administer analgesics during the initial postoperative period.
- Elizabethan collars are occasionally necessary to prevent self-mutilation or disruption of skin incisions.
- Feed a liquid diet (water and gruel) on the day following surgery.
    - IV maintenance fluids may be necessary until the animal adapts to the loss of the rostral portion of the mandible or maxilla (1–3 days).
    - Consider esophagostomy or gastrostomy tubes (see Chap. 3) in those rare cases where oral intake is likely to be delayed for a considerable period (e.g., severe debilitation, lingual dysfunction).
- Evaluate animals as necessary for the first month following surgery. If there are no complications, the initial postoperative evaluation can be delayed until the end of the first month.
    - Subsequently, examine the animal every 3–4 months for evidence of tumor recurrence. If a mass is seen at the site of the previous surgery or elsewhere, obtain a biopsy immediately.
- Perform thoracic radiography every 6 months for evidence of tumor metastasis.
- Transient edema and ranula can occur following mandibulectomies but usually do not require treatment. Dehiscence of suture lines can be due to excessive tension on the excisional line, excessive use of electrocautery, constant licking by the animal, necrosis of the labial mucosa flap, animal debilitation, and tumor necrosis.
    - Examine the oral cavity to monitor incision line healing.
    - Postoperative nasal discharge may be a sign of maxillary suture line dehiscence.
- Allow minor wound dehiscence to heal by second intention. Resuture more severe breakdowns (e.g., where bone is exposed). Eliminate tension on the suture line.
    - In some instances, extraction of the tooth adjacent to the margin of the ostectomy site and elevation of the palatal and buccal mucosa provide adequate mobility of sufficient tissue to achieve healing at the ends of the ostectomy site.
- The cosmetic appearance of dogs and cats usually is good, even after major resection of bone and soft tissue.
- Tissue swelling, inversion of the upper lips, and drooling may occur for several days. These problems improve markedly in a few weeks.

- Protrusion of the tongue often is temporary following unilateral rostral partial hemimandibulectomy but may be permanent following bilateral rostral partial mandibulectomy.
- Removal of the TMJ in conjunction with the ramus causes some medial displacement of the mandible. Infrequently, it is necessary to lower the crown height of the lower canine tooth on the unoperated side to prevent chronic impaction into the oral mucosa of the hard palate, which could result in an oronasal fistula.
  - If the pulp canal is entered during this procedure, seal the pulp canal using a vital pulp canal procedure (see Chap. 84). Nasal discharge, noisy respirations, inappetence, and facial swelling may occur after premaxillectomy. With general medical support, these conditions improve in 5–7 days.

RADIATION THERAPY

Radiation therapy is efficacious in treatment of certain oral tumors. Major limitations are the limited number of radiation centers available and the cost.

Indications

- Radiosensitive neoplasms such as SCC and acanthomatous epulis.
- Cases in which surgical excision is:
  - Very difficult or impossible
  - Unsuccessful in removing all the neoplastic tissue
- Combined with surgical excision:
  - To kill residual tumor cells postoperatively
  - When radiation alone is not effective in treating the neoplasm

Complications

In most cases there is a narrow range between the radiation dose that is curative and one that can cause serious side effects.

- Common side effects include moist desquamation and mucositis. These problems resolve with supportive care.
- Hair loss is expected and often is permanent. Hair regrowth of a different color and texture sometimes occurs.
- Ocular pathology, including corneal ulcers, keratoconjunctivitis sicca, and cataracts, can occur when the irradiated area includes the eye.
- Improper dosing can cause radiation burns, resulting in severe tissue sloughing and bone necrosis.
  - This complication in the maxilla can result in an oronasal fistula that may respond poorly to aggressive surgical therapy.
- A long-term complication is recurrence of the tumor in the irradiated field.

SUPPLEMENTAL READINGS

Bradley RL, MacEwen EG: Mandibular resection for removal of oral tumors in 30 dogs and 6 cats. J Am Vet Med Assoc 184:460, 1984.

Salisbury SK, Lantz GC: Long-term results of partial mandibulectomy for treatment of oral tumors in 30 dogs. J Am Anim Hosp Assoc 24:285, 1988.

Salisbury SK, Thacker HL, Pantzer EE, et al.: Partial maxillectomy in the dog: Comparison of suture material and closure techniques. Vet Surg 14:265, 1985.

Salisbury SK, Richardson DC, Lantz GC: Partial maxillectomy and premaxillectomy in the treatment of oral neoplasia in the dog and cat. Vet Surg 15:16, 1986.

Withrow SJ, Holmber DL: Mandibulectomy in the treatment of oral cancer. J Am Anim Hosp Assoc 19:273, 1983.

119 Fractures and Dislocation of the Spine

Stanley D. Wagner

ATLANTOAXIAL INSTABILITY

Atlantoaxial instability can result in varying degrees of compression to the cervical spinal cord. Miniature and small-breed dogs are most often affected by absence, malformation, failure to ossify, and insufficient ligamentous support of the odontoid process. Fractures of the odontoid process or between the process and body of C2 can occur in dogs of all breeds.

Surgical Anatomy

- The atlantoaxial joint is a pivot joint that permits the head and atlas to rotate around a longitudinal axis.
- The dens or odontoid process is a peglike eminence along the ventral surface of C2 (axis) that projects rostrally to lie on the floor of C1 (atlas) in the spinal canal.
- The dens is secured to the ventral arch of the atlas by the transverse atlantal ligament, to the occipital condyles by the paired alar ligaments, and to the ventral aspect of the foramen magnum by the apical dental ligament. The dorsal arches of the atlas and axis are stabilized by the dorsal atlantoaxial ligament.

▼ *Key Point* Luxation with an intact dens, luxation resulting from congenital dens malformation, and fractures through the dens or body of the axis result in dorsal displacement of the axis and compression of the spinal cord (Fig. 119–1).

Clinical Signs and Diagnosis

- Clinical signs range from cervical pain to motor dysfunction in all four limbs.
- Lateral cervical radiography under general anesthesia may show widening of the atlantoaxial space (i.e., the space between the dorsal spine of the axis and the dorsal arch of the atlas). Ventrodorsal and open mouth radiography may outline the dens.

Surgical Procedures

Preoperative Considerations

- Be cautious when manipulating the neck, especially in flexion, to minimize further damage to the spinal cord.

- Ventilator assistance may be indicated if acute cord edema affects respiratory centers.
- The surgical procedures described here require advanced skills; therefore, these cases should be referred to a surgical specialist.

Objectives

- Stabilize the dorsal arch of the atlas to the dorsal spine of the axis with a prosthetic ligament.
- Stabilize fractures and/or remove malformed dens.
- Avoid further damage to the spinal cord.

Equipment

- Standard orthopedic and neurologic packs
- Gelpi or Weitlaner self-retaining retractors
- Cicherelli rongeurs or high-speed pneumatic drill and small round bur
- Bipolar cautery and suction setup
- Large-gauge (Number 2) monofilament synthetic suture material
- Kirschner wires (K-wires), small Steinmann pins or bone screws
- Rigid vacuum-type apparatus* for patient stabilization on operating room table
- Methylmethacrylate

Technique

Dorsal Approach

1. Place the animal in sternal recumbency with the front legs tied cranially and the head supported in a slightly flexed position.
2. Prepare the skin from the middle of the cranium to C7 for aseptic surgery.
3. Incise the skin on the dorsal midline from the external occipital protuberance to C3 or C4.
4. Palpate the transverse processes of C1 and the spinous process of C2.
5. Reflect the paravertebral muscles from the arches of C1 and the spinous process of C2 from the midline, and retract with self-retaining retractors. These muscles are the cervicoscutularis, cervicoauricularis superficialis, and platysma. Separate the paired cervicoscutularis and cervicoauricularis muscles, which join at a fibrous raphe.

---

*Vac-pac, Olympic Medical, Seattle, WA 98108.

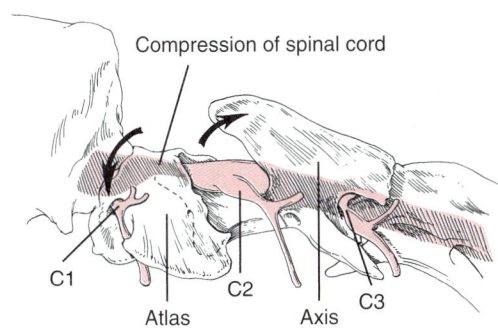

Figure 119–1. Dorsal displacement of the axis.

6. With deeper dissection, separate the paired bellies of the biventer cervicis, and elevate the rectus capitis dorsalis major muscle to expose the dorsal spinous process of the axis. Reflect the caudal capitis muscle from one side of the spinous process of the axis.

7. If dissection is to extend laterally, identify and preserve the paravertebral and cerebrospinal arteries and the first and second cervical nerves.

8. The spinal cord can be decompressed by hemilaminectomy, but this usually is not indicated. Perform decompression by removing the caudal arch of the atlas and cranial dorsolateral lamina of axis with Cicherelli rongeurs or a high-speed drill.

▼ *Key Point* Removal of too much dorsal arch will compromise dorsal fixation.

   a. Continuous downward pressure on the spine of the axis will reduce the luxation.

9. Drill two transverse holes (cranial and caudal) into the dorsal spine of the axis.

10. Insert a reversed swedged-on needle of adequate length, extradurally, starting at the caudal edge and under the dorsal arch of the atlas.

11. When the needle is identified at the atlanto-occipital space, form a retrieval loop from the accompanying suture material.

12. Pass the prosthetic suture material through the retrieval loop and pull the loop under the dorsal atlas arch.

13. Fashion the prosthetic ligament from nonmetallic, heavy-gauge monofilament suture material. Divide the prosthetic ligament suture, pass the ends through the holes in the axis, and tie securely.

14. Routinely close the incision with absorbable suture material in an interrupted pattern.

Ventral Approach

This approach is indicated when damaged dorsal structures cannot support a fixation device, when dorsal repair has failed, or when added support is needed.

▼ *Key Point* With the ventral approach, reduction of C2 can be more difficult than with the dorsal approach.

1. Place the animal in dorsal recumbency with the front legs tied caudally.

2. Prepare the ventral cervical region, from the caudal mandibles to the manubrium, for aseptic surgery; include an area on the proximal humerus for bone graft.

3. Incise the skin on the ventral cervical midline from the larynx to vertebra C4.

4. Separate the paired sternohyoideus muscles and retract with self-retaining retractors.

5. Identify, protect, and retract the trachea, esophagus, carotid sheath, and vagus nerve (away from the surgeon). Elevate the longus colli muscle from vertebral bodies.

6. Identify the C1–C2 joint caudal to the pointed ventral tubercle of C1.

7. If indicated, excise a malformed or fractured odontoid process through a burred slot made in the ventral arch of the atlas.

8. Remove the cartilage from the articular surfaces of the C1–C2 joint; drive transarticular pins from the ventral surface of the axis across the atlantoaxial joint into the atlas, medial to the alar notch.

9. Apply a small bleb of methylmethacrylate to the pins' cut ends to prevent migration.

10. An alternative to transarticular pins can be bone screws.

11. Collect cancellous bone from the proximal humerus and implant at the arthrodesis site.

12. Using absorbable suture material, close muscles and subcutaneous tissue routinely in a simple interrupted pattern.

Postoperative Care and Complications

- The respiratory center may be damaged at the time of injury or intraoperatively. Provide ventilatory assistance, gradually weaning from the ventilator by serial monitoring of arterial blood gases when the animal is exposed to short periods of room air.
- Support the surgical site with neck and body braces until bony fusion is radiographically evident.
- Restrict exercise for 4–6 weeks.
- Complications of the dorsal approach:
  - Suture breakage and reluxation
  - Insufficient bone to support the fixation device
  - Insufficient reduction
  - Suture material pulls out of bone
- Complications of the ventral approach:
  - Iatrogenic damage to the spinal cord with orthopedic appliance
  - Inadequate pin placement
  - Pin migration before bony fusion occurs

SPINAL FRACTURES AND DISLOCATIONS

Repair of spinal fractures and dislocations depends on the area of spinal cord involvement, neurologic signs, size of patient, the surgeon's expertise, amount of vertebral displacement, ventral stability, concurrent injuries, and continued neurologic deterioration despite medical management.

- Consider surgical stabilization for animals with spinal fractures or luxations that are unstable and are not responding to medical therapy.

▼ *Key Point* The thoracolumbar and lumbosacral junctions are prone to fracture and luxation because they are the sites of marked transition between the stiff and the mobile sections of the spine.

Surgical Anatomy

- Vertebrae vary in size and shape and consist of:
  - Body
  - Dorsal arch that forms the spinal canal
  - Paired lateral intravertebral foramina through which the spinal nerves, arteries, and veins pass
  - Single dorsal spines (other than C1) that vary in size
  - Cranial and caudal articular facets
  - Transverse, accessory, and mammillary processes for muscle attachment
  - Fibrocartilaginous disc interposed between vertebral endplates
- The ratio of vertebral canal diameter to spinal cord diameter is greater in the cervical area than other areas.
- The cervical dorsal spinous processes are poorly formed (short and thin), whereas the thoracic and midlumbar vertebrae have large uniform dorsal spinous processes that can support orthopedic devices. The dorsal spinous processes of L7 and S1 are small.
- The cervical vertebral bodies are flat ventrally and are suitable for the application of orthopedic appliances. Surgical exposure of the ventral cervical region generally is easier than with the dorsal approach.
- The lumbar vertebral bodies are long, allowing orthopedic appliance fixation on the dorsolateral surface if major nerve roots from L4–5 through L7–S1 can be avoided. The ventral approach to lumbar vertebrae for internal stabilization generally is not recommended.
- Lateral surgical exposure to the thoracic vertebrae is hindered by the rib head and the potential for entrance into the thoracic cavity. Hemilaminectomy or laminectomy of the thoracic vertebrae can be performed.

Surgical Procedures

Preoperative Considerations

- Recognition of clinical neurologic signs exhibited by the awake animal on physical examination is important for lesion location. Intact cerebral recognition of deep pain is important for the prognosis (see Chap. 147 for more information on spinal cord diseases).

▼ *Key Point* If cerebral recognition of pain is absent for 24 hours, the prognosis is poor.

- Take care that physical manipulation does not worsen compression of the spinal cord, especially in a sedated or anesthetized animal.

- Immobilize the animal to prevent additional spinal cord damage prior to surgery; use a small cage or body cast or strap the animal to a rigid board.
- Preoperative radiographs may not show the extent of spinal cord injury due to the fracture luxation.
- Myelography may be indicated to evaluate spinal cord compression at the fracture luxation site and to evaluate areas cranial and caudal to the traumatized area (see Chap. 4).

▼ *Key Point* Myelography is beneficial in determining if stabilization alone, decompression alone, or a combination of the two is warranted.

▼ *Key Point* Localize the lesion by neurologic examination prior to administering analgesics, sedation, or general anesthesia. Make a complete assessment of body systems (cardiovascular, urogenital, etc.), especially in cases of automobile accidents.

- Spinal fractures or luxations should be repaired by a surgical specialist.

Objectives

- Decompress the spinal cord, if indicated.
- Evaluate spinal cord integrity by durotomy, if indicated.
- Minimize additional trauma to spinal cord by fracture reduction and stabilization.

▼ *Key Point* No single internal fixation technique or surgical approach is adequate for all vertebral fracture luxations in small animals. Anatomy and lesion location dictate the choice of orthopedic implant.

Equipment

- Orthopedic and neurologic packs
- 2.7-mm and 3.5-mm bone plating sets and Lubra plates
- Assorted size intramedullary (IM) pins
- Methylmethacrylate
- Gelpi or Weitlaner self-retaining retractors
- Curved, sharp-point Lempert or Cicherelli rongeurs (6 1/2")
- Power drill
- Bipolar electrocautery and suction setup
- Scalpel blades (#10, 11, 15)
- High-speed pneumatic drill and associated bur sizes
- Gelfoam
- External fixator clamps (medium size)

Technique

Dorsal Approach to Midcervical Vertebrae

1. Place the animal in sternal recumbency, with the cervical neck supported in flexion.
2. Prepare the area from the external occipital protuberance to the first thoracic vertebrae for sterile surgery.
3. Make a midline skin incision.

4. Make a dorsal midline incision in the fibrous median raphe, from the aponeurosis of the platysma, cleidocervicalis, and trapezius muscles.
5. Expose the longitudinal yellow elastic fibers of the nuchal ligament, running from the axis to the first thoracic vertebra along the dorsal spinous processes.
6. Make an incision in the rectus capitis, spinalis and semispinalis cervicis, and multifidus cervicis muscles along one side of the nuchal ligament.
7. Control hemorrhage by direct pressure or bipolar cautery, or cover the area with a free piece of skeletal muscle or Gelfoam.
8. Spinal cord decompression by laminectomy or hemilaminectomy can be achieved through the dorsal approach.

▼ *Key Point* Dorsal stabilization of cervical fractures or luxations is difficult because the thin and inconsistent spinous processes in this area may not support dorsal spinous plates; vascular and neurologic structures also make dorsolateral plating difficult. Alignment and fixation of articular facets can be performed through this approach.

Dorsal Approach to the Caudal Cervical Vertebrae

1. Place the animal in sternal recumbency, with the cervical neck supported in flexion.
2. Prepare the dorsal cervical region from the external occipital protuberance to the fifth thoracic vertebrae for aseptic surgery.
3. Incise the skin on the midline from C2 to T1.
4. Incise and retract the midline raphe, which is composed of the aponeurosis of the trapezius muscle cranially and rhomboideus muscle caudally.
5. Expose the subscapularis laterally, the splenius cranially, and serratus dorsalis caudally.
6. Incise the splenius and serratus dorsalis muscles to expose the semispinalis capitis and longissimus cervicis muscles, along with the nuchal ligament.
7. Dissect the semispinalis capitis, longissimus cervicis, and multifidus muscles to expose the dorsal spinous processes.
8. Spinal cord decompression of the affected area is achieved by dorsal laminectomy or hemilaminectomy.

Ventral Approach to the Cervical Vertebrae

1. Place the animal in dorsal recumbency, with the front legs tied caudally and the neck extended.
2. Prepare the ventral cervical region from the caudal mandibles to the manubrium for aseptic surgery.
3. Incise the skin on the ventral cervical midline from the larynx to the manubrium.
4. Separate and retract the paired sternohyoideus and sternothyroideus muscles with self-retaining retractors.
5. Identify and retract the following structures: esophagus, carotid artery, jugular vein, vagosympathetic trunk, and recurrent laryngeal nerve.
6. Elevate the longus colli muscle from the ventral surface of the vertebral body.

7. If indicated, place a bone plate ventrally so that at least two screw holes engage on either side of the fracture luxation after the ventral spinous processes have been burred to provide a flat surface.
   a. Angle the screws in the plate away from the spinal cord.
   b. Plastic plates placed in this area are flexible so that the cancellous screws do not pull out of the bone, although the plate may break.
   c. If necessary, add cancellous bone graft from the proximal humerus to the fracture site to increase the chances of fusion.
8. If the plate cannot be applied ventrally, place two or more Steinmann IM pins or bone screws in each vertebra on both sides of the fracture luxation at angles of 25–30° to the midline and directed into the dorsolateral vertebral cortex.
   a. Align the fracture and apply methylmethacrylate in a circular mass to incorporate the Steinmann pins or screws.
   b. Be sure that the amount of bone cement applied to the orthopedic implants does not interfere with normal tracheal position or compromise soft tissue closure.
9. Close the ventral muscles and subcutaneous tissue routinely with absorbable suture material in a simple interrupted pattern.

Thoracolumbar Fracture Luxation

1. Place the animal in sternal recumbency and use a vacuum positioner (Vac-pac) to stabilize it in this position.
2. Prepare the area T8 through L7 for sterile surgery.
3. Make a midline to slightly lateral dorsal midline skin incision.
4. Expose the dense lumbodorsal fascia after incision of the fat.
5. Incise the supraspinous ligament around and between the tip of each dorsal spinous process.
6. Elevate the multifidus lumborum muscle from the spinous processes and vertebral arches laterally to the mammillary processes.
7. Incise the muscular aponeurosis on each mammillary and accessory process. Blood vessels will be encountered at each process.
8. Be careful to identify the dorsal branches of the spinal nerves at the intervertebral foramina.
9. Palpate rib 13 to use as a landmark to locate the area of trauma.
10. Perform laminectomy or hemilaminectomy if decompression is indicated.

Internal Fixation for Thoracolumbar Fracture Luxation Dorsolateral Vertebral Body Plate (Fig. 119–2)

1. Position the metal bone plate dorsal to the transverse process so that hemilaminectomy of the spinal cord can be performed without loss of fixation if indicated. Hemilaminectomy can also be done before applying the plate and will allow better exposure when drilling screw holes.
2. Limit plate application to the caudal thoracic and

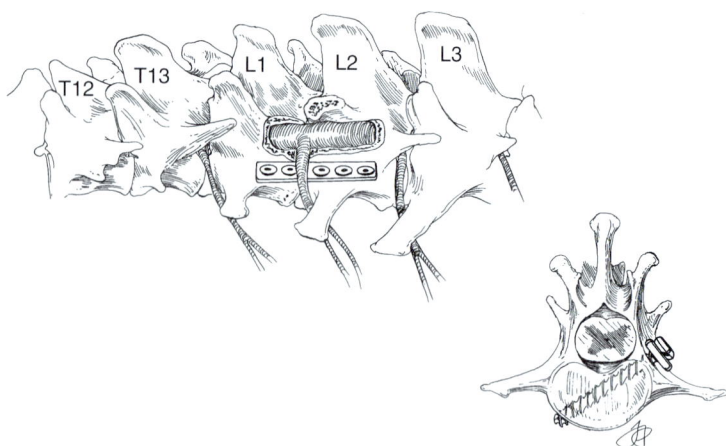

Figure 119-2. Dorsolateral vertebral body plate. Inset shows correct angle of body screws.

cranial lumbar region to avoid severing the femoral, sciatic, and pudendal nerves as they exit the caudal lumbar region.

3. Place bone screws into the vertebral bodies angled away from the spinal cord, but not in a ventral direction, to avoid vascular structures.
4. Plate application to caudal thoracic vertebrae requires dislocation of rib heads.

Dorsal Spinous Process Stabilization

Use this method to stabilize comminuted vertebral body fractures or fractures of the caudal lumbar spine when the major nerve roots do not allow vertebral body plating. The dorsal spinous processes must be present and intact.

1. "Sandwich" the dorsal spinous processes between two polyvinylidine fluoride plates (Lubra Plate) by a bolt, with washer and nut, that passes between the processes.
2. Distal to L4, the dorsal spinous processes may not be prominent enough to support this manner of fixation.
   a. Attach the caudal end of the plate to transilial pins.
   b. Use a combined dorsal spinal plate fixation and a type II external fixator (Kirschner-Ehmer).
   c. Repair fracture luxation of L7–S1 with transilial pins and prevent pin migration by application of external fixator clamp.

▼ *Key Point* In biomechanical studies applied to isolated canine lumbar spines, the combination of a dorsal spinous process plate and a dorsolateral vertebral body plate provided the most rigid stabilization.

Other Fixation Methods

Other methods of fixation, in decreasing order of stability and strength, are dorsolateral vertebral body plate, dorsal spinous process plate, polymethylmethacrylate-pin technique, and vertebral body cross-pins. Spinal stapling may be valuable but has not been biomechanically evaluated.

Postoperative Care and Complications

- Turn recumbent animals to avoid pressure sores. Use water bed or air mattress.
- Use manual urinary bladder expression or intermittent catheterization q8h for dogs unable to urinate. If using an indwelling catheter with closed drainage system, culture urine q48–72h.
- Administer broad-spectrum antibiotics, based on urine bacterial culture and sensitivity tests.
- To maintain hygiene and lessen muscle atrophy, give a whirlpool bath for 20 minutes q12h following incisional healing.
- Avoid gastrointestinal hemorrhage by avoidance or judicious use of glucocorticoids and minimize hospital stress. An oral H_2 antagonist (e.g., cimetidine) or a synthetic prostaglandin E1 analog (misoprostol) may be indicated to prevent gastrointestinal problems (see Chap. 87).
- Monitor for breakage or loosening of orthopedic implants before fracture luxation heals. Plastic plates may fail owing to fracture of plates or dorsal spinous process. A methylmethacrylate collar can fracture or loosen at the cement-orthopedic appliance interface.
  - Wound drainage and seroma formation will be evident if the plate loosens.
  - Reluxation or fracture failure can occur if orthopedic implants fail; at least 6 weeks is necessary for healing to occur.
  - If reduction is unstable, proliferative callus formation will encroach on the spinal cord, with subsequent worsening of clinical signs.

CAUDAL CERVICAL SPONDYLOMYELOPATHY

Caudal cervical spondylomyelopathy (wobbler syndrome) is a condition characterized by extradural spinal cord compression due to malformation of bony or ligamentous structures that react to instability or chronic disc disease. Affected animals may have neck pain, an abnormal gait most noticeable in the rear legs, or even tetraplegia. Great Danes and Doberman pinschers are most commonly affected, but the disorder may occur in other breeds. Great Danes are usually affected at a young age, Dobermans may not exhibit clinical signs until middle age. The compressive lesions can be static (constant pressure) or dynamic (intermittent pressure).

▼ *Key Point* The compressive lesion of caudal cervical spondylomyelopathy is usually hypertrophy of the dorsal annulus fibrosus secondary to chronic disc disease, vertebral malformation, or instability.

Anatomy

Cervical Spinal Canal

- Articular facets and joint capsule
- Vertebral canal
- The ligamentum flavum is located dorsal to the canal
- The dorsal longitudinal ligament and dorsal annulus fibrosus is located ventral to the canal
- Cervical vertebral bodies are rectangular in shape

Clinical Signs

- Signs include varying degrees of neurologic deficit, including pain, paraparesis, ambulatory tetraparesis, and nonambulatory tetraparesis.

Diagnosis

- Lateral radiography may show bony vertebral body changes, but myelogram is necessary to demonstrate sites and type of cord compression.
- Stress radiography (mild flexion, mild extension, or linear traction) during myelogram may differentiate static compression from dynamic compression on the cord.

▼ *Key Point* *Caution:* Flexion and extension stress radiography can worsen clinical signs.

- Myelography findings:
  - Ventral spinal cord compression from hypertrophied dorsal annulus fibrosus secondary to chronic type II disc disease (i.e., gradual protrusion of a disc into the spinal canal)
  - Dorsal spinal cord compression from hypertrophied ligamentum flavum
  - Dorsolateral compression from malformed articular processes
  - Compression from tipping of the craniodorsal edge of the caudal vertebral body and the caudodorsal lamina of the cranial vertebra

Preoperative Considerations

- Prior to surgery, wean animals from steriodal and nonsteroidal anti-inflammatory drugs (NSAIDs).
  - Aspirin can cause platelet dysfunction for the life of the circulating platelet (10 days).
  - Prolonged bleeding time due to platelet dysfunction makes surgery more difficult.
  - Consider performing von Willebrand assay in predisposed breeds (e.g., Dobermans).

Surgical Procedures

No single operative procedure can be recommended for all dogs. Because hypertrophy of the dorsal annulus fibrosus at C5–C6 and C6–C7 is relatively common, two methods of treatment for this condition are described in detail: ventral decompression alone and ventral distraction/stabilization technique. The procedures described should be performed by a surgical specialist.

Objectives and Indications

- Base the decision for surgery and choice of technique on stress myelography (flexion-extension) and on linear traction radiographic findings.
- Dorsal laminectomy with fat graft is indicated for static lesions such as ligamentum flavum hypertrophy, malformed articular processes, and vertebral canal stenosis.
  - Disadvantages include extensive muscle dissection, especially in large breeds, and the potential for fracture through the articular facets.
  - An advantage is that decompression can be done at multiple sites through a single surgical approach.
- Ventral decompression alone is indicated when a single disc space is involved, to remove disc material and the dorsal annulus fibrosus for decompression of the spinal cord.
- Ventral vertebral distraction is indicated for a compressive lesion that can be resolved by linear traction. Advantages include:
  - The dorsal annulus fibrosus is preserved.
  - The spinal canal is not entered.
  - Distraction can be maintained with a tibial cortical allograft or ulnar autograft held in position with a bone plate and screws, with Steinmann pins and a methylmethacrylate collar, or by interbody methylmethacrylate.

Equipment

- Orthopedic and neurologic packs
- Scalpel blades (#10, 11, 15)
- Gelpi retractors
- Suction and electrocautery setup
- Gelfoam or bone wax
- High-speed air drill and burs
- Lubra Plates, drill bits, screw taps, and bone screws
- Power drill
- Methylmethacrylate

Technique

Ventral Decompression

1. Place the animal in dorsal recumbency, with the front legs tied caudally and the neck slightly hyperextended.
2. Prepare the ventral cervical region from caudal mandible to manubrium for aseptic surgery.
3. Incise the skin from the wing of C1 to the manubrium.
4. Separate the paired sternohyoideus muscles.
5. Retract the trachea and esophagus to the left of the midline. To prevent tracheal collapse, be sure that the endotracheal tube extends to the thoracic inlet.
6. Elevate the longus colli muscles from the ventral aspects of the involved intervertebral space.
7. Use the transverse processes of C6 as landmarks to locate the involved disc space.

8. Bur out the disc space initially to visualize its cranial slope.
9. Outline the proposed slot with the bur: the slot should be one-half the length and width of the adjacent vertebral body; an oval or rectangular slot works well.
10. Remove the bone in three uniform layers, observing color changes to recognize when approaching the spinal canal.
11. Control bleeding from cancelleous bone by packing with gauze sponges, Gelfoam, muscle, or bone wax.
12. Remove the dorsal part of the annulus fibrosus, using blunt tartar scrapers, a #11 surgical blade, fine hemostats, or a small curet.
13. Avoid laceration of the vertebral sinus, which has been displaced. When suction is used, especially in small dogs, be careful that exsanguination does not occur from a lacerated sinus.
14. Flush the area with saline solution.
15. Close the muscle, including the longus colli, with absorbable suture material in an interrupted pattern.

Ventral Distraction with Vertebral Fusion

1. Make a ventral slot, using an approach similar to that described previously for ventral decompression, with the following exceptions:
   a. The spinal cord is not invaded.
   b. The depth of the slot is approximately three-fourths of the vertebral body width, measured radiographically.
2. Place a cortical allograft or autograft in the slot while applying linear traction on the animal's head and limbs.
   a. Alternatively, autogenous cancellous bone can be used to fill the slot.
   b. Gelpi retractors can be used as a vertebral spreader.
3. Hold the graft in place with a bone plate and four screws that engage the vertebral bone on either side of the slot (Fig. 119–3).
   a. Steinmann pins and a methylmethacrylate collar can be used instead of a bone plate.
4. Close the soft tissue as previously described for ventral decompression.

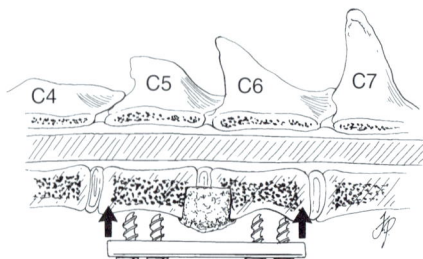

Figure 119–4. Insertion of polymethylmethacrylate plug (PMP) to maintain distraction. CG, cancellous bone graft; DAF, dorsal annulus fibrosus. (From Dixon BC, Tomlinson JL, Kraus KH: Modified distraction-stabilization technique using an interbody polymethylmethacrylate plug in dogs with caudal cervical spondylomyelopathy. J Am Vet Med Assoc 208:61, 1996.)

Ventral Distraction-Stabilization

1. Make a ventral slot as previously described.
2. Instead of using an autograft or allograft insert methylmethacrylate to maintain distraction (Fig. 119–4).
   a. When the methylmethacrylate powder and methylacrylate copolymer liquid are mixed, heat results. The soft tissues, especially the spinal cord, must be protected from the thermal reaction by sterile flush irrigation.
   b. Be sure to maintain sterility. Infected cement will require removal, which in this case would be catastrophic for the patient.
   c. Once cement has hardened, pack the area with cancellous bone.

▼ **Key Point** Ventral vertebral distraction is used for dynamic lesions in which traction will reduce ligamentous redundancy.

Postoperative Care and Complications

- Nursing problems in large dogs that are not ambulatory are common. Avoid pressure sores.
- Neck braces or body casts that extend to the thorax can be used for support.
- The condition may worsen as a result of surgical trauma, hemorrhage, inadequate tissue removal, inadequate reduction, and improper placement of orthopedic equipment.
- Long-term problems include:
  - Movement of the orthopedic implant
  - Failure of distraction devices with collapse of the disc space
- Accelerated degenerative changes in the disc spaces adjacent to the surgically fused area may cause recurrence of clinical signs (domino effect).

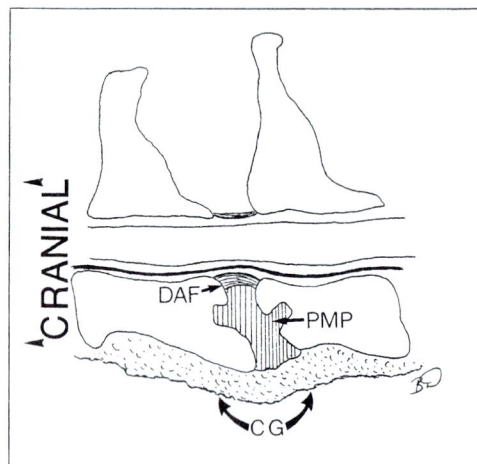

Figure 119–3. Ventral distraction and fusion of cervical vertebrae.

Prognosis

- The prognosis is better in animals presenting with pain alone, paraparesis, or ambulatory tetraparesis.
- Nonambulatory tetraparetic patients have a poor prognosis.

SUPPLEMENTAL READINGS

Dixon BC, Tomlinson JL, Kraus KH: Modified distraction-stabilization technique using an interbody polymethyl methacrylate plug in dogs with caudal cervical spondylomyelopathy. J Am Vet Med Assoc 208:61, 1996.

Hawthorne JC, Blevins WE, Wallace LJ, et al: Cervical vertebral fractures in 56 dogs: A retrospective study. J Am Anim Hosp Assoc 35:135, 1999.

Kraus, KH: Management of neurosurgical conditions. Sem Vet Med Surg (Small Animal) 11:1996.

Selcer RR, Bubb WJ, Walker TL: Management of vertebral column fractures in dogs and cats: 211 cases (1977–1985). J Am Vet Med Assoc 198: 1965, 1991.

Turner TM, Shires PK: Fractures of the skull, mandible, spine and ribs. *In* Olmstead ML, ed.: Small Animal Orthopedics, St. Louis, Mosby, 1995, p 171.

120 Neoplasia of the Axial Skeleton

Mark M. Smith

Osteosarcoma and chondrosarcoma are the two most common primary neoplasms affecting the axial skeleton. These neoplasms have a similar radiographic appearance, with osteolytic, osteoblastic, or mixed osteoblastic/osteolytic characteristics. Hemangiosarcoma and fibrosarcoma are other primary bone tumors that must be considered. Overall, these tumors more commonly affect the ribs and pelvis than the vertebrae. Multilobular osteoma (chondroma rodens) is the most common tumor of the skull.

Early recognition and accurate diagnosis are of paramount importance for client education and rationale for surgical intervention. Surgery may be diagnostic (vertebrae), palliative (pelvis), or curative (rib), depending on tumor invasiveness and location of axial skeletal involvement. Tumors of the mandible, maxilla, and nasal cavity are discussed in other chapters in this section. The types of neoplasms and principles of treatment discussed in this chapter are similar to those for tumors of the cranium. Removal of cranial tumors requires specialized equipment and skills and therefore is best handled by a surgical specialist. Tumors of the appendicular skeleton are discussed in Chapter 135.

HISTORY AND CLINICAL SIGNS

- Patients usually are presented for swelling over a bony prominence.
- Intrathoracic extension of neoplasia of the rib may cause respiratory compromise.
- Pain or an unusual gait secondary to neurologic dysfunction (transverse myelopathy) may be related to neoplasms of the vertebrae.
- Animals with skull tumors usually present because of a palpable mass. Neurologic signs may develop if brain impingement occurs.
- Constipation may result from pelvic tumors.

DIAGNOSIS

Pelvis and Ribs

- Include two radiographic projections of the lesion.
- Radiographic signs of primary bone neoplasms (e.g., osteosarcoma, chondrosarcoma) may range from primarily lytic to proliferative lesions.

- Polyostotic lytic lesions are seen with malignant lymphoma and multiple myeloma (see Chap. 25).

▼ *Key Point* Do not use radiography as the sole basis for determining tumor type.

- Determine if metastatic disease is present.
  - Perform palpation, and fine-needle aspiration of regional lymph nodes, if nodes are enlarged.
  - Perform abdominal palpation for mass lesions, vertebral palpation for metastasis-related pain, and a rectal examination for intrapelvic masses.
  - Evaluate three-projection thoracic radiographs (ventrodorsal, left, and right lateral) to detect pulmonary metastasis.

Skull and Vertebrae

- Survey radiographs of the spine often show osteolysis secondary to primary bone neoplasia or to invasion of soft tissue neoplasia.
- Osteosarcoma or multilobular osteoma of the cranium appears radiographically as a proliferative bony lesion of the flat bones.
- Perform cerebrospinal fluid (CSF) analysis to rule out infection and inflammation (see Chap. 144). CSF of patients with vertebral neoplasia may have increased levels of protein and elevated pressure.

▼ *Key Point* Because most tumors affecting the spinal cord are extradural, cytologic examination of the CSF may be normal.

- Myelography is important to detect the exact site of the vertebral tumor and the extent of spinal cord compression (see Chap. 4).

▼ *Key Point* Metastatic lesions from remote malignant tumors may mimic primary neoplasms of the axial skeleton. Histopathologic examination of biopsy tissue is required for differentiation.

- Computed tomography (CT) is useful to evaluate intracranial effects of skull tumors.

Bone Biopsy

Objectives

- Obtain multiple tissue samples of the tumor for histopathologic diagnosis.

- Avoid causing iatrogenic trauma to the vertebrae or skull, if they are involved.

Equipment

- Small suture pack and suture material
- Jamshidi-type biopsy needle or bone trephine
- Sterile ruler

Technique

1. Prepare the cutaneous area over the tumor site for aseptic surgery.
2. Make a skin incision large enough to introduce the biopsy instrument over the center of the lesion.
3. Measure the center of the tumor from the nearest prominent anatomic landmark.
4. Take a minimum of two biopsies: one from the center of the tumor and one from the center directed to the periphery. Use extreme caution when performing biopsy of tumors of the cranium.
5. Using a horizontal mattress pattern, place sutures of absorbable material in the subcutaneous or fascial layers to minimize hemorrhage from the biopsy site.
6. Close the skin with nonabsorbable suture material in a simple interrupted pattern.

▼ **Key Point** Biopsy of vertebral lesions is best performed during decompressive laminectomy or with the aid of fluoroscopy to guide biopsy needle placement.

▎ TREATMENT

Surgical Procedures for Rib Neoplasia: Resection and Thoracic Wall Reconstruction

Objectives

- Completely remove the thoracic wall mass.
- Attempt to obtain wide tumor-free margins.
- Minimize hemorrhage.
- Provide rigid reconstruction to prevent abnormal chest wall movement.
- Perform airtight closure to prevent pneumothorax.

Equipment

- Standard general surgical pack and suture material
- Two large Gelpi or Beckman self-retaining retractors
- Gigli wire or Liston bone cutters
- Chest tube, three-way stopcock, and large syringe
- Polypropylene mesh

Technique

1. Place the animal in lateral recumbency with the hindlimbs extended caudally and the forelimbs extended cranially.
2. Prepare the lateral chest wall for aseptic surgery.
3. Incise the skin over the mass. If the tumor is adhered to the dermis, make a large, elliptical skin incision around the tumor.

4. Incise or, preferably, reflect the latissimus dorsi muscle if it is not adhered to the tumor.
5. Incise all remaining muscle layers one intercostal space cranial and caudal to the mass.
6. Cut all involved ribs and intercostal muscles 2 cm dorsal and ventral to the tumor, using Liston bone cutters and Metzenbaum scissors.
7. Clamp and ligate the intercostal arteries and veins.
8. Place a chest tube a minimum of two intercostal spaces cranial or caudal to the resection site.

▼ **Key Point** Consider giving an intraoperative lidocaine intercostal nerve block to decrease pain during the acute postoperative period (see Chap. 83, Principles of Thoracic Surgery).

9. Use polypropylene mesh (e.g., Marlex) to reconstruct large thoracic wall defects.
10. Place polydioxanone or polypropylene sutures, using an interrupted horizontal mattress pattern, in a paracostal location to secure the mesh.
    a. A slight fold may be created along all borders of the mesh to provide a double-thickness layer for holding sutures.
11. Secure the mesh to the cut ribs with sutures of similar material, using a circumferential simple interrupted pattern. Create slight tension on the mesh to provide rigidity.
12. Suture the latissimus dorsi and external abdominal oblique muscles over the defect with absorbable suture material in an interrupted pattern to provide a tissue seal.
13. Close subcutaneous tissues with absorbable suture material in an interrupted pattern to minimize dead space.
14. Appose the skin routinely, using nonabsorbable suture material.
15. Use the chest tube system to reestablish negative intrathoracic pressure.

▼ **Key Point** Small thoracic wall defects may be closed using adjacent latissimus dorsi and external abdominal oblique muscles without the need for a mesh implant.

Postoperative Care and Complications

Short-Term

- Closely monitor for hemorrhage, seroma formation, and pneumothorax.
- Apply a light chest bandage to minimize seroma formation and air migration along the chest tube.

▼ **Key Point** Place the bandage loose enough to allow normal chest excursion and optimal pulmonary function.

- Analgesics that minimally affect pulmonary function (butorphanol, 0.4 mg/kg q6h IM) may be required in the acute postoperative period.

Long-Term

- Repeat physical and radiographic examinations every 4–6 months to monitor for recurrence or metastasis.

- Consider adjuvant chemotherapy if the tumor is malignant or if tumor cells are present in resected tissue margins (see discussion of chemotherapy in Chap. 24).

Prognosis

- Chest wall neoplasms usually are malignant and carry a poor prognosis if incompletely excised. This is especially true for osteosarcoma.
- The prognosis is guarded even if the tumor is completely resected because subclinical distant metastasis may have occurred before surgery.

Surgical Procedure for Pelvic Neoplasia: Resection of the Ilial Wing

Preoperative Considerations

Perform ilial wing resection for localized tumors. Invasive, malignant tumors may require hemipelvectomy, which involves resection of part of the lateral pelvis and hindlimb. Refer the patient to a surgical specialist for hemipelvectomy.

Objectives

- Completely remove the pelvic mass.
- Obtain wide, tumor-free margins.
- Minimize hemorrhage.
- Avoid damage to major pelvic limb nerve tracts in order to maintain limb function.

Equipment

- Standard general surgical pack and suture
- Two large Gelpi or Beckman self-retaining retractors
- Gigli wire or osteotome and mallet

Technique

1. Place the animal in lateral recumbency.
2. Prepare the lateral pelvic area and proximal hindlimb for aseptic surgery.
3. Incise the skin over the mass. If the tumor is adhered to the dermis, make a large elliptical incision around the tumor.
4. Incise through the superficial, middle, and deep gluteal muscles cranial to the acetabulum.
5. Incise the sartorius and tensor fascia lata muscles before their insertion on the ilium.
6. Incise the iliocostalis and longissimus muscles cranial to the pelvic mass.
7. Incise the quadratus lumborum and iliacus muscles before their insertion on the medial aspect of the ilium.
8. Cut the sacroiliac joint and ilial body using a Gigli wire or osteotome and mallet.
9. Elevate the other fascial attachments to free the proximal ilial segment.
10. Control hemorrhage with electrocoagulation or individual vessel ligation.

▼ *Key Point* Maintain wide margins of excision with no gross evidence of tumor.

11. Closure
    a. Appose the resected muscle ends by simple interrupted sutures of absorbable material placed in the fascia.
    b. Extensive resection may require Penrose drain placement to minimize potential dead space.

▼ *Key Point* Make separate small incisions in the surgical area for entrance and exit of drains, avoiding the primary wound incision.

    c. Close subcutaneous tissues with absorbable sutures in a simple interrupted pattern.
    d. Appose the skin similarly, using nonabsorbable sutures.

Postoperative Care and Complications

Short-Term
- Use a modified Robert Jones bandage to decrease the incidence of seroma. Bandage application and maintenance is more cumbersome in male dogs.
- Monitor the wound for signs of seroma and infection.
- Administer analgesic therapy (butorphanol, 0.4 mg/kg q6h IM) during the acute postoperative period.

Long-Term
- Repeat physical and radiographic examinations every 4–6 months to monitor for recurrence and metastasis.
- Consider adjuvant chemotherapy if the tumor was malignant or if tumor cells are present in resected tissue margins (see discussion of chemotherapy, Chap. 24).

Prognosis

Prognosis is the same as for rib neoplasia.

Surgical Procedure for Vertebral Neoplasia: Dorsal Laminectomy

Because laminectomy is a difficult surgical procedure that should be performed only by surgical specialists, only an overview of the procedure is given here. (See Chap. 147 for more information on principles of surgery of the spinal cord.)

Objectives

- Debulk the tumor.
- Decompress the spinal cord.
- Obtain tissue for histopathologic diagnosis.

Equipment

- Standard general surgical pack and suture material
- Two large Gelpi or Beckman self-retaining retractors
- Pneumatic or electric power equipment for laminectomy
- Kerrison or Lempert bone rongeurs
- Iris scissors

General Procedure

- Preoperatively administer dexamethasone (0.5 mg/kg IV) to decrease edema of the spinal cord related to surgical manipulation.
- Save adequate amounts of tumor tissue in 10% buffered formalin for histopathologic evaluation.
- The laminectomy procedure ends when the spinal cord is relieved of the compression effect of the tumor.
- Dorsal laminectomy can be combined with hemilaminectomy if additional lateral exposure is required.

▼ *Key Point* Iatrogenic vertebral fracture/luxation is unlikely, because reactive bone and scar tissue secondary to the neoplasm compensates for the destabilizing sequelae of laminectomy and tumor debulking.

Postoperative Care and Complications

Short-Term

- Monitor for seroma formation and infection at the wound site.
- Perform serial neurologic examinations to monitor neurologic status.
- Administer prednisolone (0.5 mg/kg q12h PO) for anti-inflammatory therapy (if necessary) until neurologic status is improved.
- Urine retention requires frequent manual decompression of the bladder or maintenance of a closed indwelling catheter system. Monitor for development of urinary tract infection.

- Turn the patient every 4 hours to prevent decubital ulcers secondary to prolonged recumbency.

Long-Term

- Supportive therapy and good nursing care are mandatory during the neurologic recovery period.
- Consider adjuvant chemotherapy and/or radiation therapy (see Chap. 24, based on the histopathologic diagnosis, because complete resection of the tumor is not possible.

PROGNOSIS

- The prognosis for malignant tumors of the vertebral axial skeleton is poor.
- Neoplasms secondarily affecting vertebrae (e.g., lymphoma) may warrant a guarded prognosis, based on responsiveness to chemotherapy.

SUPPLEMENTAL READINGS

Holiday TA, Higgins RJ, Turrel JM: Tumors of the nervous system. *In* Theilen GH, Madewell BR, eds.: Veterinary Cancer Medicine. Philadelphia: Lea & Febiger, 1987, p 601.

LaRue SM, Withrow SJ: Tumors of the skeletal system. *In* Withrow SJ, MacEwen EG, eds.: Clinical Veterinary Oncology. Philadelphia: JB Lippincott, 1989, p 234.

Orton C: Thoracic wall. *In* Slatter DH, ed.: Textbook of Small Animal Surgery. Philadelphia: WB Saunders, 1985, p 536.

Fractures of the shoulder, and particularly of the scapula, may be associated with concurrent thoracic trauma. This may range from nondisplaced rib fractures to more severe internal thoracic trauma such as lung contusions, pneumothorax, and hemothorax (see Chap. 82). Damage to neurologic structures such as the brachial plexus and peripheral nerve components, particularly the suprascapular nerve, may also occur with shoulder fractures. Therefore, a thorough preoperative evaluation of the thorax and neurologic function is mandatory before proceeding with definitive fixation.

ANATOMY

- The shoulder is a diarthrodial joint that is dependent on the surrounding supportive soft-tissue structures.
  - The primary stabilizing structures are the medial and lateral glenohumeral ligaments and the joint capsule.
  - The more "active" ligaments are the biceps tendon, supraspinatus tendon, infraspinatus tendon, subscapularis tendon, and teres minor tendon.
- The scapula is a broad, thin, expansive bone with a prominent spine along the central aspect of the scapular body.
- The greatest density of bone stock occurs along the line of reflection of the scapular spine from the body and in the region of the scapular neck and glenoid.
- The weakest area of the scapula is at the scapular neck.
- The suprascapular nerve lies along the cranial and lateral aspect of the scapular neck. Identify and protect this structure during the surgical approach and repair of fractures in this area.

FRACTURES OF THE SCAPULA

Preoperative Considerations

- Manage minimally displaced or nondisplaced fractures of the scapula by strict cage confinement or alternatively by placing the animal's limb in a modified Velpeau sling.
- Frequently, fractures involving the scapula tend to override, resulting in relative limb shortening and the potential for impingement on the brachial plexus and other neurovascular structures. Internal fixation of scapula fractures provides rigid stability, thus allowing a very rapid return to function.
- Because of the thinness of the scapula, stabilization of fractures generally is achieved with bone plates. In some fracture types, hemicerclage wires also may be advantageous.
- Assess the integrity of the ligamentous supporting structures and if damaged, repair them to maintain normal shoulder function.

Surgical Procedures

Objectives

- To stabilize the fracture fragments in an anatomic position in order to prevent limb shortening and malalignment, and to allow support of the glenoid, effecting return of joint function.
- To restore the articular surface of the glenoid to allow return of normal joint range of motion and function.

Equipment

- Standard orthopedic pack, periosteal elevators, bone fragment clamps and plate benders
- Orthopedic wire (0.8 mm and 1.0 mm in diameter) and wire twister (useful in some fractures)
- A wide variety of bone plates, including the 2.0-mm dynamic compression plate (DCP) or cuttable plate, 2.7-mm DCP standard plate and finger plate series (rarely, the 3.5-mm standard plate series may be used)

Preliminary Procedures

Technique

1. Place the patient in lateral recumbency with the limb prepared for aseptic surgery.
2. Use a standard lateral or craniolateral approach to the scapula for exposure of the specific area of the fracture.
3. Select an appropriate bone plate and contour with a plate bender to the specific area to be stabilized.

Scapular Spine Fractures (Fig. 121–1)

Technique

1. Contour a small finger plate (2.0 mm or 2.7 mm) to 90°, attach to the scapular spine, and then attach to the scapular body with appropriate screws.

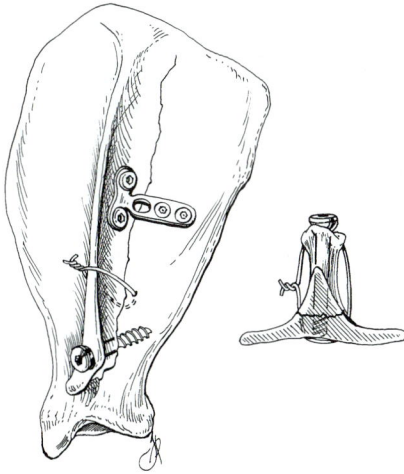

Figure 121–1. A fracture of the scapular spine can be stabilized using a T-plate and a lag screw through the acromion process into the body. Alternative fixation may be achieved using hemicerclage wires.

2. Alternatively, apply a series of two or more hemicerclage wires to stabilize the spine to the body.

Fractures or Osteotomy of the Acromion

Technique

1. If the fragment is of sufficient size, reattach to the scapular body using a lag screw (2.0 mm, 2.7 mm, or 4.0 mm) (see Fig. 121–1).
2. Alternatively, apply two or more hemicerclage wires to reattach the fragment.
3. As another alternative, stabilize the fracture with a figure-eight cerclage wire, with or without Kirschner pins, using a tension band technique (Fig. 121–2).

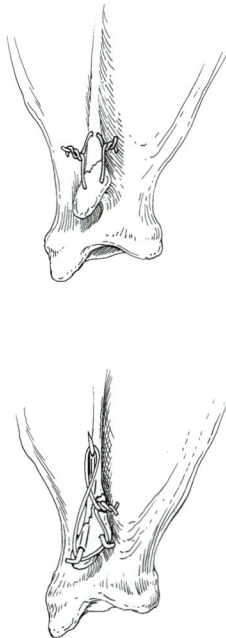

Figure 121–2. A fracture of the acromion process may be stabilized with two interfragmentary wires *(top)* or with a Kirschner wire and a figure-eight wire *(bottom)*.

Fractures of the Scapular Body

- Anatomic reduction of the fracture fragments involving the body is important to restore proper anatomic length.

Technique

1. To achieve fixation of the fracture fragments, apply a bone plate either cranial or caudal to the scapular spine.
2. Preferably, use three or more screws on either side of the fracture line.

▼ *Key Point* To obtain maximum thread purchase, direct screws obliquely into the region of the reflection of the scapular spine from the body.

3. Stabilize multiple fractures individually with a combination of small plates and hemicerclage wires.
4. Alternatively, place the fracture fragments in anatomic position and bridge the entire area with the plate serving as a buttress.

Scapular Neck Fractures (Fig. 121–3)

- Scapular neck fractures tend to override, owing to the distal pull of the deltoid muscles and the medial and proximal pull of the pectoralis muscles.
- Displacement of these fractures may result in impingement on the adjacent brachial plexus as well as

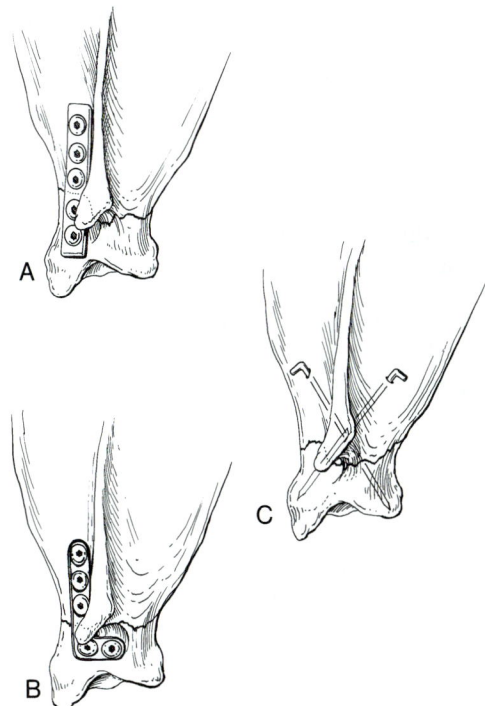

Figure 121–3. *A,* A scapular neck fracture may be stabilized with a 2.7 mm or 2.0 mm standard plate if at least two screws of purchase can be obtained in the glenoid fragment. Alternatively, the fracture may be stabilized using a finger plate *(B),* which allows two screws of purchase parallel to the articular surface, or two crossed Kirschner wires *(C).*

limb shortening and compromise of the range of motion of the shoulder.

Technique

1. Identify and protect the suprascapular nerve.
2. Use finger plate or mini-finger plate series and standard plates (2.0 mm and 2.7 mm) for stabilizing fractures in this area.
3. Alternatively, stabilize these fractures with two Kirschner pins inserted in a cross-pin technique.
   a. It may be difficult to insert the pins at a proper angle to achieve maximum purchase on either side of the fracture line.

Glenoid Fractures (Fig. 121–4)

Technique

1. Approach via an osteotomy of the acromion.

▼ *Key Point* Because they are intra-articular fractures, glenoid fractures always require open reduction and internal fixation. Accurate alignment of the articular surface is imperative to restore normal joint function.

2. Identify and protect the suprascapular nerve.
3. When the fracture fragments are anatomically repositioned and the articular surface is congruous, achieve fixation with a Kirschner pin inserted parallel to the articular surface.
4. Insert a lag screw parallel to the articular surface to obtain compression of the fracture site. The Kirschner pin may be retained to serve as supplemental fixation or, if sufficient bone stock allows, may be replaced with an additional lag screw.

Scapular Tuberosity Avulsions

- This fracture is an avulsion of the cranial aspect of the glenoid rim. The tuberosity is the site of attachment of the tendon of origin of the biceps muscle.
- This fracture occurs most frequently in immature animals.
- The fracture fragment usually is small, composed primarily of metaphyseal bone, and is distracted distally, owing to contracture of the biceps muscle.

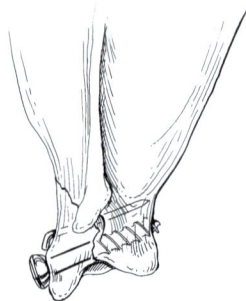

Figure 121–4. Stabilized glenoid fractures with a lag screw to compress the fracture site, obtaining supplementary fixation with a Kirschner wire.

Technique

1. Osteotomy of the greater tubercle of the humerus provides the best exposure for repair of this fracture (see description of osteotomy repair).
2. When anatomic reduction is achieved, stabilize the fracture using a single lag screw (2.7 mm or 4.0 mm).
3. Alternatively, stabilize the fracture with a tension band wire technique, using one to two Kirschner pins and a figure-eight wire.

▼ *Key Point* The avulsed fragment of bone usually is small and soft. Therefore, avoid overtightening the screw, which can result in iatrogenic fragmentation of the scapular tuberosity.

4. If the fracture cannot be anatomically reduced and stabilized, the tuberosity or biceps tendon may be transposed to the proximal diaphysis of the humerus and secured there with a lag screw (with or without a spiked washer).

T Fractures

- These fractures are a combination of a scapular neck fracture and a glenoid fracture. They are difficult to repair and generally require an acromion osteotomy.

Technique

1. Direct attention initially to reestablishing the articular surface of the glenoid fragments (see previous discussion of glenoid fractures).
2. Reattach the reconstructed glenoid fragment to the scapular body, using a standard plate or finger plate series (2.0 mm, 2.7 mm) (see previous discussion of scapular neck fractures).

Postoperative Care

- Restrict activity for 6 weeks or longer, depending on the healing of the fracture as well as the degree of comminution of the fracture fragments.
- Evaluate the fracture radiographically at 4–6 week intervals until it has healed.
- If pending failure is evident radiographically (e.g., loosened screws), institute one or more of the following measures:
  - Restrict the animal's activity further.
  - Apply coaptation splint support.
  - Place the limb in a non–weight bearing sling.
  - Perform an additional internal stabilization procedure.

Complications

- Malalignment at the articular surface is an important potential complication.
- Malalignment of the scapular body may lead to a valgus or varus position of the limb. Nonunion of fractures in these locations is rare.
- A more commonly encountered complication is injury to the suprascapular nerve, which can result in atrophy of the infraspinatus muscles.

Prognosis

- The prognosis is good provided technical principles of bone plate application are followed.
- The potential for restoration of shoulder joint range of motion is good.

PROXIMAL HUMERAL FRACTURES

See also Chapter 123, Fractures of the Humerus.

Preoperative Considerations

- Fractures of the proximal humerus occur with much less frequency than scapular fractures.
- Generally, these fractures occur in skeletally immature animals in the form of a Salter-Harris type I or II fracture (see Chap. 138) with involvement of the growth plate.

Surgical Procedures

- Physeal fractures generally require only a craniolateral approach to the shoulder.
- Complex fractures involving the humeral head require osteotomy of the acromion and a shoulder joint capsulotomy.
- Fractures involving the humeral head necessitate reestablishment of the articular surface in order to be congruent with the opposite glenoid cavity.

Objectives

- Restore anatomic alignment of the articular surface.
- Restore function by reestablishing joint congruency and stability.

Equipment

- Standard orthopedic pack and bone reduction forceps
- A selection of Kirschner and Steinmann pins
- Bone plate sets including 2.7-mm and 3.5-mm series (occasionally a 4.5-mm series)

Preliminary Procedures

Technique

1. Place the animal in lateral recumbency with the limb prepared for aseptic surgery.
2. Use a standard lateral or craniolateral approach for exposure of the specific area of the humeral fracture.

Fractures of the Proximal Epiphysis (Fig. 121–5)

Technique

1. In immature animals, stabilize the fracture using two or more smooth Kirschner or Steinmann pins inserted from the proximal aspect of the greater tubercle into the caudal cortex of the metaphyseal region.
2. Alternatively, stabilize the fracture fragment with Rush pins or pins inserted in a Rush pin technique.

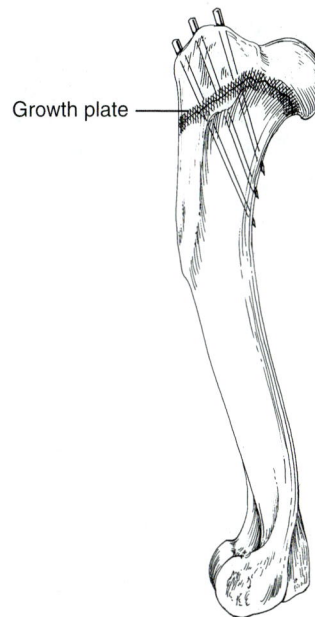

Figure 121–5. A Salter-Harris physeal fracture of the proximal humerus may be stabilized using two or three small-diameter pins or Kirschner wires.

Fractures or Osteotomy of the Greater Tubercle

Technique

1. In immature animals, stabilize the tubercle with two or more smooth Kirschner or Steinmann pins. Insert the pins through the tubercle into the caudal cortex.
2. In mature animals, stabilize the tubercle with two or more lag screws or pins.

Fractures of the Humeral Head

Technique

1. If only one fracture line is present, anatomically align and stabilize the fracture fragment with three smooth Kirschner pins; in mature animals, use lag screws.
   a. Avoid penetrating the articular surface of the humeral head.
2. If multiple fragments of the humeral head are present, reconstruct and stabilize them with appropriate Kirschner pins or lag screws, and then reattach to the proximal humeral metaphyseal region. If necessary, use a bone plate to support the reconstructed fragments.

Lesser Tubercle Fractures

- These fractures occur most frequently in immature animals.
- Use lag screw fixation for stabilization.

Fractures of the Humeral Neck (Fig. 121–6)

Technique

1. Anatomically align the fracture fragment and then stabilize it using a T-plate, with the horizontal aspect of the plate directed proximally, or a standard DCP

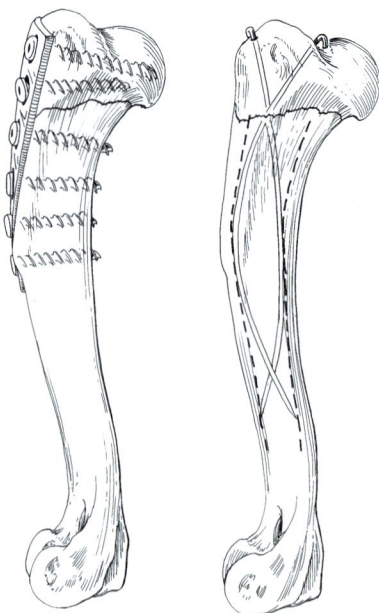

Figure 121–6. A fracture of the humeral neck may be stabilized with a standard dynamic compression plate (DCP) or T-plate, placing a minimum of two screws in the proximal fragment *(left)*, or with Rush pins or smooth pins inserted using a Rush pin technique *(right)*.

plate, with at least two screws of purchase in the proximal fragment.
2. Alternatively, stabilize the fracture using smooth Kirschner pins or small-diameter Steinmann pins inserted in a Rush pin technique.

Postoperative Care

- Obtain appropriate radiographs immediately postoperatively and at intervals of 4–6 weeks until the fracture is healed.

- Assess the shoulder joint by placing the shoulder through a range-of-motion exercise to be certain that metal does not protrude into the articular surface and that the shoulder is stable.

Complications

- Nonunion or malunion in this region occurs rarely.
- Premature closure of the proximal humeral growth occurs infrequently.

Prognosis

- Owing to the high density of cancellous bone and the large cross-sectional area present, these fractures usually heal consistently and rapidly.
- The prognosis is good for maintaining a normal range of motion of the shoulder, provided accurate alignment of the articular surface is achieved at the time of fracture stabilization.

SUPPLEMENTAL READINGS

Brinker WO, Hohn RB, Prieur WD: Manual of Internal Fixation in Small Animals. New York: Springer-Verlag, 1984, p 129.
Newton CD, Nunamaker DM: Textbook of Small Animal Orthopedics. Philadelphia: JB Lippincott, 1985, pp 333–343, 357.
Piermattei DL, Greely RG: An Atlas of Surgical Approaches to the Bones of the Dog and Cat, 2nd Ed. Philadelphia: WB Saunders, 1980, p 59.

Scapulohumeral Luxation

Robert A. Taylor

Scapulohumeral luxation is an uncommon clinical condition. Congenital and traumatic luxations occur; the latter is more common.

Medial luxation of the humeral head is most common, especially in smaller breed dogs. Lateral luxation of the humeral head, while less common, usually occurs in larger dogs (Fig. 122–1). Cranial and caudal luxations are rare.

ANATOMY

- The shoulder joint is a ball-and-socket joint. The articular surface of the scapula forms the concave glenoid and the convex humeral head articulates within. Although the joint is capable of movement in any direction, its major actions are flexion and extension.
- The joint capsule is continuous and blends with the medial and lateral glenohumeral ligaments (Fig. 122–2). These ligaments help to support the joint and may be 2.0 mm or greater in thickness.
- The subscapularis, supraspinatus, infraspinatus, and teres minor muscles provide periarticular support.
- The tendon of origin of the biceps brachii and its sheath join with the joint capsule on its cranial medial aspect and provide additional stability. The bicipital tendon is held in the bicipital groove by the small but sturdy transverse humeral ligament.
- Luxation is not possible unless the glenohumeral ligaments and joint capsule have been ruptured.

CLINICAL SIGNS

- The principal signs are varying degrees of lameness, depending on the severity of the luxation.

DIAGNOSIS

- Diagnosis is made by physical examination and confirmed by radiography.
- Careful palpation of the area between the acromion of the scapula and greater tubercle can be helpful.
  - In medial luxations, hold the elbow in a flexed position and abduct the lower limb.
  - In lateral luxations, hold the elbow in a flexed position and adduct the lower limb.

- Examine both shoulders simultaneously and use the normal limb for comparison.

PREOPERATIVE CONSIDERATIONS

- Radiograph the shoulder to rule out intra-articular fractures.
- Use general anesthesia for all shoulder reduction procedures, whether open or closed.
- Closed reduction is a nonsurgical treatment.

PROCEDURES FOR CLOSED REDUCTION

Procedure for Medial Luxation

1. Flex the elbow and pull the limb laterally while exerting digital pressure on the scapular spine.
2. Gently rotate the limb downward to reduce the luxation.
3. Place the limb in a Velpeau sling for 10–14 days.
4. If the joint is stable on removal of the sling, begin passive range-of-motion exercises. When possible, encourage swimming as an adjunct to physical therapy, but restrict exercise for 1 month.

Procedure for Lateral Luxation

1. Flex the elbow and extend the shoulder to reduce the luxation.
2. Gently rotate the humeral head upward to facilitate reduction.
3. Use a spica splint to support the joint for 10–14 days.

▼ *Key Point* Open reduction and stabilization are indicated for recurrent luxations or when closed reduction fails owing to interposed soft tissue or hematoma.

SURGICAL PROCEDURE FOR OPEN REDUCTION

Objectives

- Surgically repair the ruptured glenohumeral ligament and joint capsule.
- Stabilize the shoulder joint and prevent recurrent luxations.

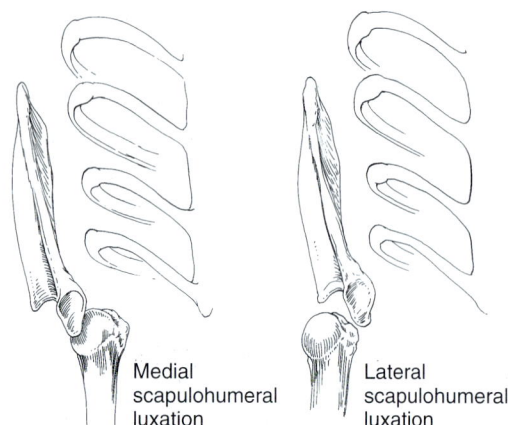

Figure 122–1. Medial *(left)* and lateral *(right)* luxations of the scapulohumeral joint.

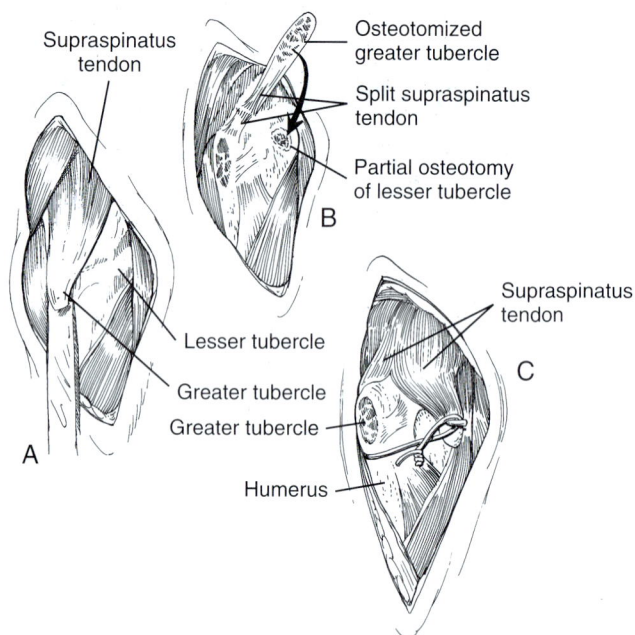

Figure 122–3. *A,* Use an oscillating bone saw or osteotome to partially osteotomize the greater tubercle. *B,* Split the supraspinatus tendon with a scalpel blade. *C,* Attach the split portion of the supraspinatus tendon to the region of the lesser tubercle.

Equipment

- Standard general surgical pack and suture material
- Standard orthopedic set
- Oscillating bone saw
- Osteotomes and mallet
- Kirschner wires and pin chuck
- Appropriate retractors

Surgical Repair of Medial Luxation

Technique

1. Place the dog in lateral recumbency with the affected leg up. After preparing the limb for aseptic surgery, place the distal extremity in a sterile stockinette so that it is accessible to intraoperative manipulation. Make an incision on the craniomedial aspect of the joint.
2. Reflect the skin and subcutaneous tissue and incise the brachiocephalicus muscle along its medial edge and retract it.
3. Incise the superficial and deep pectoral muscles near their point of insertion on the humerus. Be sure to separate the supraspinatus muscle from the deep pectoral muscle.
4. Using an osteotome or oscillating saw (Fig. 122–3A), partially osteotomize the greater tubercle of the humerus. Hold the osteotome on the crest of the greater tubercle and make the medial line of the cut

parallel to the humeral border of the transverse humeral ligament. Avoid cutting the infraspinatus tendon.
5. Using sharp dissection, carefully split the supraspinatus tendon (Fig. 122–3B).
6. Partially osteotomize the lesser tubercle and prepare it to accept the bony fragment of the greater tubercle. Secure the greater tubercle fragment (with the attached portion of the supraspinatous tendon) in place with two Kirschner wires (Fig. 122–3C). A tension band wire may be used.
7. Suture the deep pectoral muscle over the lesser tubercle. Advance the superficial pectoral muscle over the proximal cranial border of the humerus and suture it to the deltoideus muscle. Suture the brachiocephalicus muscle to the brachial fascia.
8. Close the subcutaneous tissue and skin routinely.

Monitor for signs of seroma formation, hemorrhage, and infection.

Repair of Lateral Luxation

Technique

1. Positioning and draping is similar to that for surgical repair of medial luxation.
2. Skin incision and tissue retraction are the same as for medial luxation repair.
3. Incise the superficial and deep pectoral muscles. Incise the deltoideus muscle near the point of insertion on the cranial lateral aspect of the proximal humerus.
4. Transect the transverse humeral ligament and free the bicipital tendon from the surrounding tissue (Fig. 122–4A).

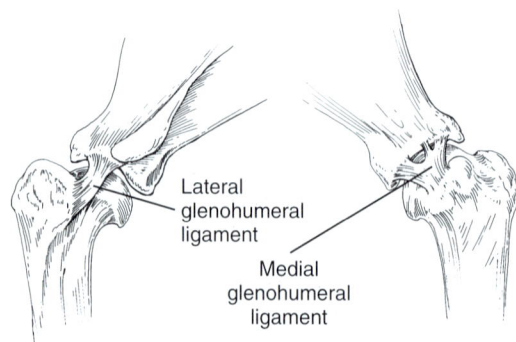

Figure 122–2. The glenohumeral ligaments.

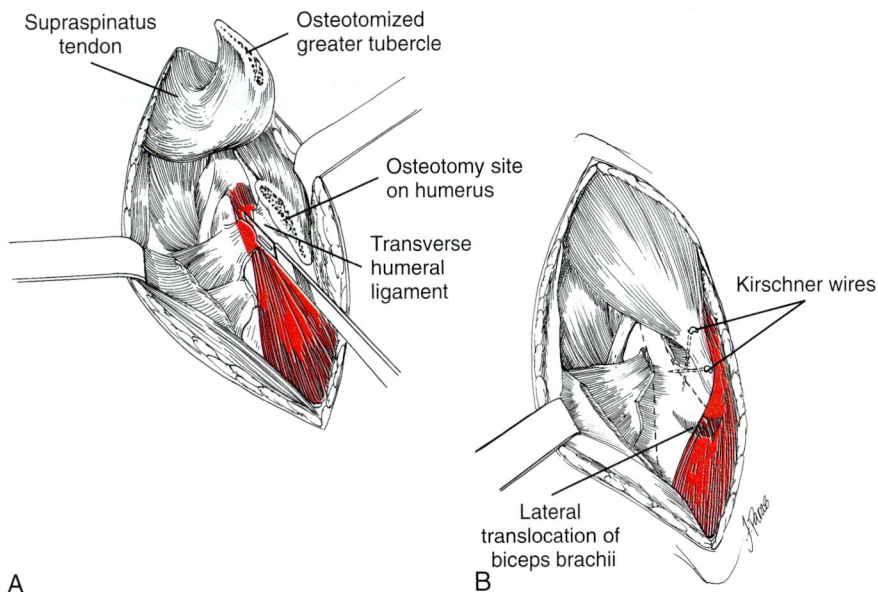

Figure 122–4. *A,* Transection of the transverse humeral ligament. *B,* Lateral translocation of the bicipital tendon. Use Kirschner wires to stabilize the greater trochanter back to its origin.

A

B

5. Completely osteotomize the greater tubercle to allow reflection of the intact tendon.
6. Translocate the bicipital tendon laterally on the opposite side of the osteotomized greater tubercle (Fig. 122–4*B*). Secure the greater tubercle with several Kirschner wires.
7. Reattach the muscles and close the skin and subcutaneous tissue routinely.

POSTOPERATIVE CARE

- Following medial luxation repair:
  - Support the limb in a Velpeau sling for 7–10 days; if the repair is stable, this may be unnecessary.
- Following lateral luxation repair:
  - If necessary, place the limb in a spica splint for additional support.
  - Strict cage rest for 7–10 days is advised, especially if the limb is not bandaged.
- Monitor for seroma formation, hemorrhage, and signs of infection.
- Begin physical therapy the first postoperative week with passive range-of-motion exercises. After suture removal, recommend swimming and partial weight bearing.

PROGNOSIS

The prognosis is good with adequate stabilization.

SUPPLEMENTAL READINGS

Craig E, Hohn RB, Anderson WD: Surgical stabilization of traumatic medial shoulder dislocation. J Am Anim Hosp Assoc 16:93, 1980.

Hohn RB, Rosen H, Bohning RH, et al.: Surgical stabilization of recurrent shoulder luxation. Vet Clin North Am Small Anim Pract 1:537, 1971.

Vasseur PB: Clinical results of surgical correction of shoulder luxation in dogs. J Am Vet Med Assoc 182:5, 1983.

Vasseur PB, Moore D, Brown SA: Stability of the canine shoulder joint: An in vitro analysis. Am J Vet Res 43:2, 1982.

Vasseur PB, Pool RR, Klein K: Effects of tendon transfer on the canine scapulohumeral joint. Am J Vet Res 44:5, 1983.

123 Fractures of the Humerus

Robert B. Parker

ANATOMY

- The proximal portion of the humerus is fairly strong and thick cranially and extends to the large deltoid tuberosity. The musculospiral groove starts caudally and twists cranially over the lateral aspect of the bone. The brachialis muscle and neurovascular structures, including the clinically significant radial nerve, lie within the musculospiral groove.
- When viewed cranially, the bone is essentially straight; however, the medullary canal runs slightly lateral to medial from proximal to distal. Distally, the medial condyle is larger than the lateral condyle, and is in a more direct line with the medullary canal. The lateral condyle has a thinner epicondylar attachment to the bone and is the main weight-bearing surface for the radial head.
- Important muscles to identify laterally are the lateral head of the triceps, the brachialis, the brachiocephalicus, and the acromial head of the deltoid. The radial nerve is important to identify laterally.
- Important medial soft tissue structures include the medial head of the triceps, the biceps brachii, and the median and ulnar nerves.

ETIOLOGY

- Most humeral fractures occur secondary to motor vehicle trauma or are caused by a fall from excessive height.

DIAGNOSIS

- Rule out injuries associated with thoracic trauma. Perform a complete clinical and radiographic examination to rule out pneumothorax, hemothorax, diaphragmatic hernia, rib fractures, chylothorax, and traumatic myocarditis.

▼ *Key Point* Consider thoracic radiography for all animals with humeral fractures.

- The neurovascular integrity of the limb is of paramount importance. Fully assess the injured forelimb.

- Obtain radiographs of the involved humerus to characterize the fracture(s). If necessary (e.g., for prebending bone plates), obtain radiographs of the normal humerus.

PRINCIPLES OF TREATMENT

- Because it is difficult to immobilize the shoulder joint with closed reduction and external fixation, most humeral fractures are treated by open reduction and internal fixation.

Equipment

- General surgical instrument pack
- Jacob's pin chuck and a complete assortment of Steinmann pins and Kirschner wires
- Bone-holding forceps
- Small and large reduction forceps with points
- Cerclage wire equipment
- Periosteal elevator
- Kirschner apparatus (external pin fixators)
- Additional (AO) equipment (Synthes, Wayne, PA) for plate and screw fixation (for selected fractures)

PROXIMAL HUMERAL PHYSEAL FRACTURES

Preoperative Considerations

- This type of fracture is seen infrequently in young dogs prior to physeal closure. Closure of the proximal physis occurs between 9 and 15 months of age.
- The fracture typically is complete, but incomplete and impaction fractures can also occur.
- Except for incomplete fractures, closed reduction is very difficult. Open reduction of complete fractures is recommended.
- In selected cases, use a Velpeau sling or spica cast to immobilize the shoulder joint.

Surgical Procedure
Objectives

- Provide stable fixation while allowing continued physeal growth.
- Provide early range of motion.

Technique

Open Reduction

1. After preparing the limb for aseptic surgery, use a cranial approach with cranial retraction of the brachiocephalicus muscle to elevate and expose the fragments.
2. Use small pointed forceps to carefully grasp the epiphysis and use the elevator to lever the fragments into reduction.
3. Achieve fixation with double Kirschner wires or Steinmann pins, beginning at the greater tubercle. To prevent compression of the physis, do not use a figure-eight tension band.
4. Cancellous lag screws have been used by some surgeons, but they can cause interfragmentary compression and premature physeal closure (see Chap. 121 for additional information on shoulder fractures).

Postoperative Care

- Encourage early range of motion exercise by allowing restricted activity.
- Remove fixation devices when healing is complete.

▼ *Key Point* Premature closure of the physis may occur as a result of the initial or surgical trauma; however, this rarely causes a clinical problem.

PROXIMAL DIAPHYSEAL FRACTURES

Preoperative Considerations

- Proximal fractures are the least common diaphyseal fractures owing to the comparative strength of the humerus in this area.
- Most proximal diaphyseal fractures occur just proximal to the deltoid tuberosity. The distal fragment is displaced cranially due to the pull of the deltoid muscle, and medially due to the pull of the pectoral muscle.
- Evaluate the brachial plexus and the radial nerve. Accurate reduction is important because excessive callus production can produce postoperative pressure on these neural structures.
- Many of these fractures occur secondary to metabolic bone disease. Carefully evaluate radiographs of the fracture for evidence of bone disease. Perform appropriate tests if metabolic disease is suspected.

Surgical Procedure

Objective

- Because closed reduction with external coaptation probably is not an option, perform open reduction with internal fixation.

Technique

Open Reduction

1. For open reduction, use a cranial approach. Incise the skin along the craniolateral aspect of the humerus, beginning at the scapular tuberosity. In-

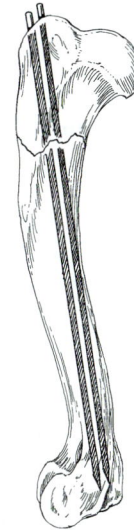

Figure 123–1. Steinmann pin placement for repair of a proximal diaphyseal fracture.

cise the fascial attachment of the brachiocephalicus muscle on the cranial aspect of the humerus to allow cranial retraction of the muscle. Elevate the deltoid muscle from the deltoid tuberosity and retract it caudally to gain access to the fracture site.
2. Place single or double Steinmann pins retrograde from the fracture site into the proximal fragment (Fig. 123–1).
3. Because the fractures often are transverse, a single intramedullary pin may not provide rotational stability. Use a type I external fixator (see Chap. 130) or hemicerclage wires to provide rotational stability in a transverse or short oblique fracture.
4. Alternatively, two Rush pins provide excellent rotational stability in fractures of this type.
5. In very large dogs, a bone plate applied to the cranial surface of the humerus is an excellent method of fixation. The basic principle of three screws (six cortices) above and three screws below the fracture site applies.

Postoperative Care

- External fixation is not desirable following internal fixation; however, if necessary, use a Velpeau sling or shoulder spica cast.
- Encourage early range of motion by allowing restricted exercise.

DIAPHYSEAL FRACTURES

Preoperative Considerations

- Muscle contracture causes overriding of the fragments.
- The fractures often are spiral or oblique and may entrap the radial nerve.
- Consider early closed reduction and closed normograde pinning. Attempt this only within the first few days following the injury.

Surgical Procedure

Objective

- Provide stable fixation without jeopardizing important neurovascular structures.

Technique

1. For open reduction, make a lateral approach to expose midshaft to distal fractures. Incise the fascia cranial to the lateral head of the triceps muscle to allow cranial retraction of the brachiocephalicus and superficial pectoral muscles, and caudal retraction of the triceps. At the distal one-third of the incision, use extreme care to identify the radial nerve as it crosses from caudal to cranial between the brachialis and lateral head of the triceps. Use the brachialis muscle as a cushion to protect the radial nerve. Retract the brachialis either proximally or distally to expose the fracture site. Reduction may be facilitated by careful myotomy of the brachialis.

2. Many humeral fractures in small to medium-sized dogs can be successfully repaired with a combination of pins, stacked pins, full or hemicerclage wires, or external skeletal fixation. This is especially true with oblique or spiral fractures.
   a. When using pin fixation, retrograde the pins into the proximal fragment from the fracture site. When the fracture is reduced, the pin should enter the medial condyle when driven into the distal fragment. Correct pin placement is slightly lateral to medial to engage the medial condyle (Fig. 123–2, *left*).

▼ *Key Point* Try to direct the pin slightly laterally when retrograding it into the proximal humeral fragment.

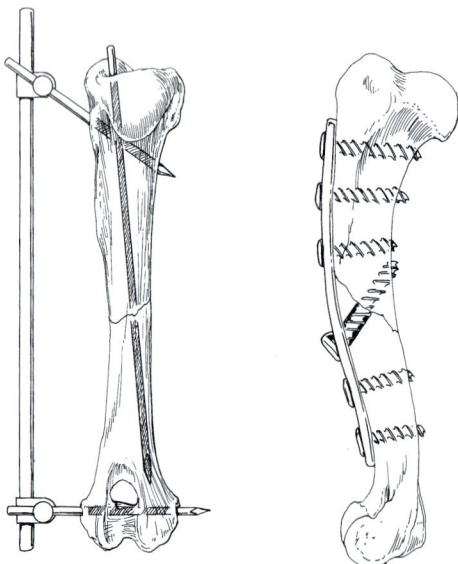

Figure 123–2. Fixation of diaphyseal fracture. *Left,* External skeletal fixation. *Right,* Internal cranial plate placement.

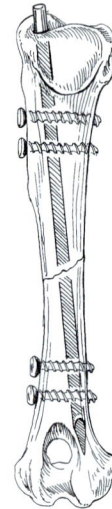

Figure 123–3. Cranio-caudal view of humerus with an interlocking nail and four locking screws.

   b. Rotational stability may not be achieved without additional pins, orthopedic wire, or external skeletal fixation.

3. Interlocking nails (Innovative Animal Products, Rochester, MN) have been successful in stabilizing diaphyseal fractures in larger breeds. By statically locking the nail both proximally and distally, rotational forces can be effectively neutralized (Fig. 123–3).

4. Because the humerus is difficult to expose and is anatomically a complex bone, the exposure for plate fixation can be difficult; however, cranial, lateral, or medial plate fixation can produce excellent results.
   a. Cranial plate placement is preferred for midshaft fractures. After exposure and reduction, contour an appropriately sized plate to fit the cranial aspect of the bone (Fig. 123–2, *right*). Protect the radial nerve distally. Freeing the origin of the extensor carpi radialis muscle may enhance distal exposure; however, the supratrochlear foramen may limit the distal extent of the plate.
   b. Lateral plate placement is difficult because of the contours of the musculospiral groove and lateral epicondylar ridge.
   c. Medial plate placement affords a fairly flat bony surface, and the plate can be contoured onto the medial condyle. Medial placement is especially useful for distal diaphyseal fractures. The medial approach involves a medial skin incision and careful division between neurovascular structures. Retract the biceps brachii muscle, the median and musculocutaneous nerves, and brachial artery and vein cranially, and retract the medial head of the triceps and ulnar nerve caudally. The pectoral muscles limit exposure proximally.

Postoperative Care

- Restrict activity, but encourage early range of motion.
- If external skeletal fixation is used to supplement rotational or axial stability, remove it in 4–6 weeks.

- Remove intramedullary pins following fracture healing; supplemental cerclage or Kirschner wires are usually left in place.
- Do not remove bone plates unless they are causing a problem.

SUPRACONDYLAR FRACTURES

Preoperative Considerations

- The supratrochlear foramen creates a weak point in the distal humeral metaphysis.
- The medial condyle is in a straight line with the diaphysis of the humerus. Additionally, the majority of the forces are transmitted through the lateral condyle, which articulates with the radial head. The lateral condyle junction with the shaft in the area of the supratrochlear foramen is smaller and weaker than the medial side.
- Rigid internal fixation generally is indicated. Excessive callus formation from inadequate immobilization can result in impairment of normal elbow function.

Surgical Procedure

Objective

- Provide stable internal fixation to allow early weight bearing and range of motion.

Technique

1. The surgical approach is similar to the previously described lateral and medial approaches.
    a. The caudal approach to the elbow joint by olecranon osteotomy also provides excellent exposure to the supracondylar area. This approach is particularly useful for comminuted fractures in this area in large breed dogs, when plating is anticipated.
2. Steinmann pin(s) placed well into the medial condyle, with an additional cross-pin from the lateral condyle to produce rotational stability, may provide adequate stability. A type I external fixator, using a transcondylar distal fixation pin, can provide additional fixation and rotational stability.
    a. To seat the Steinmann pin adequately in the medial condyle, initially retrograde the pin distally into the medial condyle from the fracture site. The pin exits the condyle medial to the ulna and can be withdrawn until the tip is flush with the fracture site. After reduction, advance the pin proximally to exit the humerus at the greater tubercle. Withdraw the pin proximally until the distal tip is flush with the medial condyle.
3. Alternatively, double Rush pins can provide excellent stability.
4. Because of the propensity for nonunion in medium- and large-sized dogs and in dogs with severely comminuted fractures, small bone plates can be applied to the caudal medial or lateral ridges of the epicondyles. This is usually done through a caudal approach (osteotomy of the olecranon).

Postoperative Care

▼ *Key Point* Physical therapy (e.g., active or passive elbow flexion and extension) is critical to prevent postoperative limitation of elbow function.

- See the previous discussion of Postoperative Care under Diaphyseal Fractures.

CONDYLAR FRACTURES

Preoperative Considerations

- About 90% of condylar fractures involve the lateral portion of the condyle.

▼ *Key Point* The lateral portion of the condyle (capitulum humeri) carries most of the force through the elbow joint by way of its articulation with the radial head. The capitulum humeri sits lateral to the humeral diaphysis when compared with the medial portion (trochlea humeri).

- Anatomic reduction is necessary to prevent secondary degenerative joint disease.
- The capitulum humeri generally is displaced distally owing to the pull of the extensor carpi radialis muscle.
- Spaniel-type dogs have been shown to have a heritable defect producing incomplete ossification of the humeral condyle, predisposing them to this injury.

Surgical Procedure

Objectives

- Achieve anatomic reduction and interfragmentary compression because the joint surface is involved.
- Restore range of motion of the elbow joint.

Technique

1. Open reduction and internal fixation usually are necessary. However, closed reduction maintained with a condyle clamp and fixation with a percutaneously applied transarticular lag screw has been described.
2. For open reduction, use a lateral or craniolateral approach.
3. Align intercondylar and supracondylar fracture lines perfectly and hold with a Vulsellum or AO pointed reduction forceps.
4. Use a transcondylar lag screw with an antirotation Kirschner wire to achieve interfragmentary compression (Fig. 123–4, *left*).
    a. The starting point for the drill bit is slightly distal and cranial to the most prominent point of the lateral epicondyle. Aim the drill at the corresponding point on the medial side. After measuring and tapping, place an appropriate screw.
    b. When using a fully threaded screw, overdrill the lateral fragment to achieve interfragmentary compression ("lag" effect).

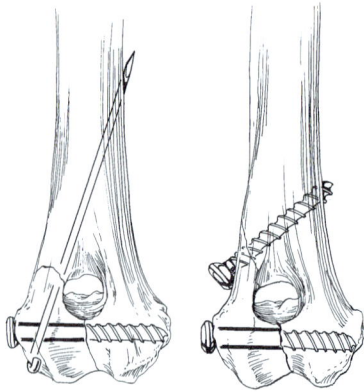

Figure 123–4. Fixation of condylar fractures. *Left,* Transcondylar lag screw and antirotation K-wire. *Right,* With oblique fractures, use two lag screws for increased stability.

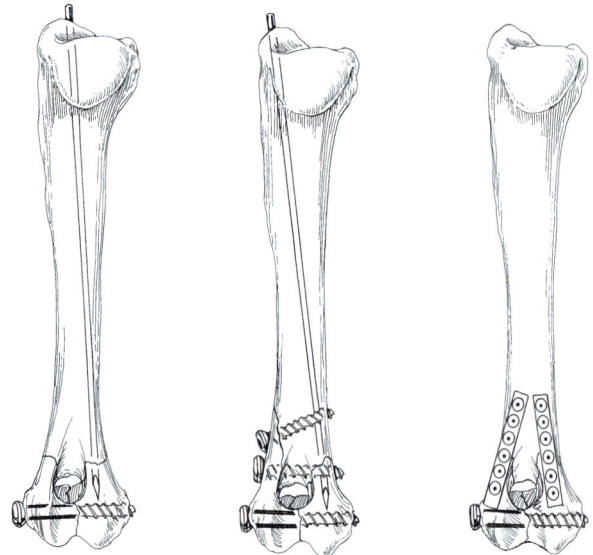

Figure 123–5. Fixation methods for intercondylar fractures. *Left,* Repair condyle with lag screw, then secure to humeral diaphysis with Steinmann pins. *Center,* Attach medial portion of the condyle to humerus with lag screw, then attach lateral portion of the condyle with lag screws and pin. *Right,* Caudal bone plates provide further stability.

c. As an alternative method of achieving precise screw location with a fully threaded screw, use the overdrill bit to make the gliding hole in the lateral condyle. Rotate the condyle laterally to expose the intercondylar fracture surface of the lateral condyle. Center the drill at the fracture surface and direct it laterally to exit the bone just distal and cranial to the lateral prominence. Then reduce the fracture and use a drill sleeve insert (in the drill hole in the lateral condyle) to direct the smaller drill (thread hole) into the medial condyle. Place the screw routinely.

d. Place an antirotational Kirschner wire across the condyles or across the distal diaphysis of the humerus (Fig. 123–4, *left*).

e. If the supracondylar portion of the fracture is oblique enough, place additional screws along this aspect for additional stability (Fig. 123–4, *right*).

f. Using crossed Kirschner wires to achieve intercondylar stability has not been successful in my experience.

Postoperative Care and Complications

- Encourage early range of motion.
- The lag screws usually are not removed.
- Reduced range of motion and arthritis of the elbow joint are the most common complications. Accurate alignment and apposition of fracture fragments reduces the incidence of these problems.

T OR Y (INTERCONDYLAR) FRACTURES OF THE HUMERAL CONDYLES

Preoperative Considerations

- In this type of fracture, both the lateral and medial portions of the condyle are fractured from the humeral metaphysis; in addition, an intra-articular fracture occurs, splitting the condyle.
- The basic principles of repair are the same as for supracondylar and single condylar fractures.

- These usually are very difficult to repair adequately. Consider referring these cases to an orthopedic specialist.

Surgical Procedure

Objective

- Achieve accurate anatomic reduction and stability in an unstable area.

Technique

1. Expose the fracture through a caudal approach via olecranon osteotomy.
2. Lag the condyles together initially to create a "two-piece fracture" (now similar to a supracondylar fracture) which is attached to the humeral diaphysis; or attach the medial condyle to the humerus; follow with lag-screw fixation of the lateral condyle to the medial condyle (Fig. 123–5, *left and center*).
   a. For more rigid stability, stabilize the supracondylar portion of the fracture with two small caudally placed bone plates (Fig. 123–5, *right*).

Postoperative Care and Complications

- Encourage early function or passive range of motion exercises.
- In one series, 46% of dogs regained moderate to normal limb function; 18% had severe lameness as a result of deformity and osteoarthritis.

SUPPLEMENTAL READINGS

Berzon JL: Humeral fractures. *In* Slatter DH, ed.: Textbook of Small Animal Surgery. Philadelphia: WB Saunders, 1985, p 2061.

Brinker WO, Piermattei DL, Flo GL: Handbook of Small Animal Orthopedics and Fracture Treatment. Philadelphia: WB Saunders, 1990, p 175.

Denny HR: Pectoral limb fractures. *In* Whittick WG, ed.: Canine Orthopedics. Philadelphia: Lea & Febiger, 1990, p 357.

Marcellin-Little DJ, DeYoung DJ, Ferris KK, et al: Incomplete ossification of the humeral condyle in spaniels. Vet Surg 23:475, 1994.

Nunamaker DM: Fractures of the humerus. *In* Newton CD, Nunamaker DM, eds.: Textbook of Small Animal Orthopedics. Philadelphia: JB Lippincott, 1985, p 357.

124 Fractures and Growth Deformities of the Radius and Ulna, Luxation of the Elbow

James Tomlinson

FRACTURES OF THE RADIUS AND ULNA

Fractures of the radius and ulna are commonly seen in small animal practice. Although most of these fractures occur as a result of automobile accidents, they also result from falling or jumping. Fractures of one or both bones and a wide variety of fracture types are seen. Open fractures of the distal one-half of the radius and ulna are common, owing to minimal soft tissue coverage. Complications include delayed union, nonunion, joint stiffness, and arthritis.

Anatomy

Radius

- The radius and ulna make up the antebrachium.
- The radius is the main weight-bearing bone of the antebrachium and is shorter than the ulna. The radius is composed of the head, neck, body, and distal extremity. The medullary canal is elliptical in shape owing to flattening of the radius.
- The radius is attached to the ulna by an interosseous ligament that helps to maintain their spatial relationship following fracture. The short radial collateral ligament runs from the styloid process of the radius to the radial carpal bone and provides medial support to the antebrachiocarpal joint.
- The cranial surface of the distal radius contains three grooves that contain (from medial to lateral) the tendons of abductor pollicis longus, extensor carpi radialis, and common digital extensor muscles.

Ulna

- The ulna is the longest bone in the body and is composed of the olecranon, trochlear notch, anconeus, body and the distal extremity called the styloid process.
- The olecranon has a strong muscular attachment, the triceps muscle.
- The ulnar body tapers as it crosses caudal to the radius to articulate with the palmarolateral aspect of the carpus. The medullary canal of the ulna functionally ends about one-third from the distal end.

- The strong, short ulnar collateral ligament runs from the tip of the styloid process of the ulna to the ulnar carpal bone, giving lateral support to the antebrachiocarpal joint.

Vascular Supply

- The radial and interosseous arteries provide the main arterial supply to the antebrachium and are subject to injury from trauma or surgery.
- The radial artery travels along the palmaromedial aspect of the radius just under the flexor carpi radialis muscle.
- The interosseous artery branches into other interosseous arteries that run in the space between the radius and ulna.

Nerve Supply

- The radial, median, and ulnar nerves supply the antebrachium and manus.

General Preoperative Considerations

- Evaluate the thorax for pulmonary contusions, pneumothorax, and diaphragmatic hernia with thoracic radiography. Evaluate for traumatic myocarditis with electrocardiography.
- Examine the animal for concurrent injuries; inspect other limbs for fractures or other significant injury.
- Inspect the antebrachium for evidence of wounds indicating an open fracture.
- Evaluate nerve function of the affected limb by testing reaction to a painful stimulus to the skin of the various dermatomes and by withdrawal of the limb.
- Initially place the limb in a Robert Jones bandage or splint to prevent further soft tissue damage and to prevent the fracture from becoming an open fracture.
- Obtain two radiographic views of the fractured limb to include the elbow and carpus.

General Objectives of Surgical Procedures

- Align and stabilize the fracture(s) to permit uncomplicated healing with normal joint and limb function.

1111

▼ *Key Point* Exact anatomic alignment and rigid fixation (compression) of articular fractures is imperative.

- Allow early return to weight bearing.
- Preserve neurovascular structures during repair.

General Postoperative Care and Complications for Radial and Ulnar Fractures

- Place the limb in a soft padded bandage for 3–10 days to reduce postoperative swelling. Provide more rigid external support if needed.
- Reevaluate the fracture radiographically every 3–4 weeks until the fracture has healed.
- Restrict activity until the fracture has healed.

Complications
- Delayed and nonunion healing (see Chap. 141), osteomyelitis (see Chap. 140), and implant failure may occur.
- Joint fractures are prone to subsequent degenerative joint disease and callus that interferes with joint mobility if anatomic alignment and rigid stability have not been achieved.
- Joint stiffness can develop with articular fractures. Rigid stability of the fracture allows early, controlled use of the joint.

▼ *Key Point* Radius and ulna fractures in immature animals may cause premature closure of the growth plates and synostosis of the radius and ulna. Both conditions cause growth deformities of the limb. Early recognition and intervention is necessary to minimize growth deformities.

Olecranon Fractures
Objective

- Counteract the distractive force of the triceps and convert it into a compressive force using the tension band principle.

Equipment

- General surgery pack and standard suture material
- Monofilament stainless steel surgical wire (20 and 18 gauge)
- Intramedullary pins and Kirschner wires (K-wires)
- Jacobs chuck or power drill
- Wire-tightening device (vise grips or wire twister)
- Pin and wire cutter
- Bone reduction forceps

Technique

1. Place the patient in lateral recumbency, with the affected leg up, and prepare the limb for aseptic surgery.
2. Make a caudolateral skin incision centered over the olecranon.
3. Reflect the skin and subcutaneous tissue to expose the olecranon and proximal shaft of the ulna. Sub-

periosteally elevate the extensor and flexor carpi ulnaris muscles from the proximal shaft of the ulna.
4. Reduce the fracture and hold it in reduction with bone reduction forceps.
5. Drive two K-wires or small intramedullary pins parallel from the tip of the olecranon across the fracture line and into the distal segment of the ulna (in very small animals, drive only one K-wire).
6. Drill a hole (perpendicular to the ulnar long axis) in the distal ulnar segment 1½–2 times the distance from the olecranon to the fracture line.
7. Insert surgical wire in the hole and place the wire around the pins in a figure-eight fashion.
8. Twist the wire to achieve equal tension on the wire.
9. Bend the pins over and cut them off short. Cut the wires leaving two to four twists and bend the wire tips over (Fig. 124–1).
10. Close the subcutaneous tissue and skin routinely.

Trochlear Notch Fractures
Objectives

- Maintain precise anatomic alignment of the fracture (because it is an articular fracture).
- Perform rigid fixation of the fracture to minimize periosteal callus.
- Counteract the distractive forces of the triceps muscle using the tension band principle.

Equipment

- Same as for olecranon fractures with the addition of bone plating equipment.

Technique

Small and Medium-Sized Dogs; Cats; No Fracture Comminution Present
1. Repair the fracture with a tension band wiring technique, as described previously under Olecranon Fractures.

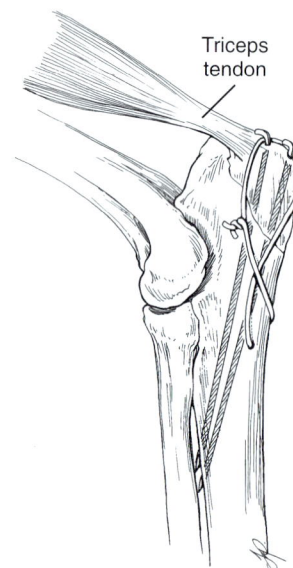

Figure 124–1. Pin and wire placement for olecranon fracture repair.

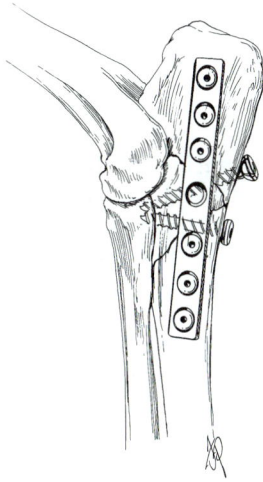

Figure 124–2. Bone plate and screw replacement for trochlear notch fracture repair.

2. Maintain anatomic alignment of the fracture while driving the pins and tightening the wire in a figure-eight configuration.

Large Dogs; Fractures with Comminution

1. Expose the trochlear notch, as described for olecranon fractures.
2. Reattach butterfly segments of bone with lag screws and Kirschner wires.
3. Contour a bone plate to the caudal or caudolateral side of the ulna and secure it to the ulna with bone screws (Fig. 124–2).
4. If comminution is not present, apply the plate with a compression technique. If comminution is present, apply the plate in a neutralization manner (e.g., no compression).

Radial Head Fractures

Objectives

• Perform precise anatomic reduction of the fracture with rigid fixation of the fragments.

Equipment

• General surgery pack and standard suture material
• Hohmann retractor
• Bone screws and bone screw insertion equipment
• Power drill and Jacobs pin chuck
• K-wires

Technique

1. Place the patient in lateral recumbency, with the affected limb up, and prepare the limb for aseptic surgery.
2. Incise the skin, beginning at the proximal end of the lateral epicondyle of the humerus and continuing distally over the radial head to the proximal one-fourth of the radius.
3. Incise the subcutaneous tissue and the antebrachial fascia along the same line to expose the extensor muscles of the antebrachium.

4. Dissect between the ulnaris lateralis muscle and the lateral digital extensor. Cut the ulnaris lateralis tendon, leaving sufficient tendon for suturing. If necessary, incise the anconeus muscle from the lateral epicondyle of the humerus.
5. Reflect the lateral digital extensor muscle cranially with a Hohmann retractor to expose the fracture.
6. Drive a K-wire across the fracture line to hold the fracture in reduction.
7. Insert a screw in "lag screw" fashion to compress the fracture line.
8. For small fragments, place two or three K-wires in a divergent pattern.
9. Reattach the ulnaris lateralis tendon with nonabsorbable monofilament suture material in a horizontal mattress pattern. Suture the muscle fascia and subcutaneous tissue in a simple continuous pattern, using absorbable suture material. Close the skin routinely.

Radial Neck and Proximal Physeal Fractures

Objectives

• Stabilize the fracture in immature animals without fracture compression to help prevent premature closure of the growth plate.
• Stabilize and align the radial head so that it articulates properly with the humeral condyle.

Equipment

• General surgery pack and standard suture material
• Jacobs pin chuck
• K-wires

Technique

1. Approach the fracture as described for radial head fractures, and reduce the fracture.
2. Stabilize the fracture with two K-wires placed in cross-pin fashion from the lateral side. Start one pin just below the articular surface of the radius and drive it distomedially. Start the second pin distal to the fracture and drive it proximomedially.
3. Bend the pins over and cut them off short.
4. Take care not to penetrate the articular surface of the radius.
5. Close the incision as described under Radial Head Fractures.

Postoperative Care

• Remove the K-wires in 3–4 weeks and monitor for premature closure of the growth plate.

Monteggia Fractures

This is a fracture of the ulna that can occur at various levels, with a radial head luxation.

Objectives

• Reduce and stabilize the radial head luxation.
• Align and stabilize the ulnar fracture.

Equipment

- General surgery pack and standard suture material
- Bone plating equipment
- Power drill
- Bone reduction forceps

Technique

1. Expose the ulnar fracture, as described under Olecranon Fractures and Trochlear Notch Fractures. Expose the ulna as far distally as needed.
2. Expose the radial head, as described under Radial Head Fractures, if the luxation cannot be reduced closed.
3. Reduce the ulnar fracture and hold it in reduction with bone reduction forceps.
4. If the annular ligament is ruptured, contour and apply a bone plate to the caudal aspect of the ulna. Insert a screw in "lag screw" fashion into the radius from the ulna through the plate to secure the radial head in position (Fig. 124–3).
5. If the annular ligament is intact, contour and apply a bone plate to the caudolateral aspect of the ulna.

Mid-Shaft Radial and Ulnar Fractures

Objectives

- Achieve healing of the fracture with proper angulation, rotation, and length of the limb.
- Prevent synostosis of the radius and ulna in immature animals.

Equipment

- Fiberglass casting tape, stockinette, 1 inch-wide medical tape
- General surgery pack and standard suture material
- Bone reduction forceps
- Jacobs pin chuck and power drill
- Kirschner-Ehmer apparatus
- Bone plating equipment

Closed Reduction and Cast Fixation for Minimally Displaced Transverse Fractures

Technique

1. Place 1 inch-wide medical tape stirrups on the dorsal and plantar surface of the foot.
2. Apply a snug-fitting double layer of stockinette over the limb. Make the stockinette long enough to extend 1 inch past the tip of the toes and as far proximal above the elbow as possible.
3. Reduce the fracture and position the limb for correct angular and rotational alignment.
4. Place the carpus in a slight varus position, flexed 5–10°.
5. Flex the elbow to a functional angle (approximately 140°).
6. After wetting, apply the fiberglass casting tape, starting at the tip of the second and fifth nails.
7. Overlap the casting tape 50% with each wrap, working from distal to as far proximal as possible above the elbow.
8. Apply four or five layers of fiberglass casting tape.
9. Reflect the stockinette and stirrups over the end of the cast and incorporate them into the final layer of cast material.
10. Hold the limb in the proper position until the cast has set.

External Skeletal Fixation for Comminuted Fractures and Simple Fractures

Technique

1. Reduce comminuted fractures closed.
2. Use a limited open approach if the fracture cannot be reduced closed.
3. Make small stab incisions in the skin before driving the transfixation pins.
4. Drive the most distal transfixation pin across the radius perpendicular to the long axis of the radius from medial to lateral and parallel to the radial

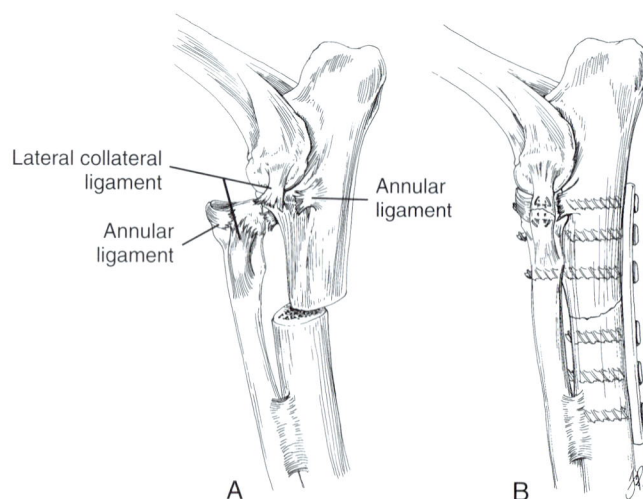

Lateral collateral ligament

Annular ligament

Annular ligament

A

B

Figure 124–3. Monteggia fracture repair. *A,* Anatomy of fracture and ligament damage; *B,* plate placement and ligament repair. See text for details.

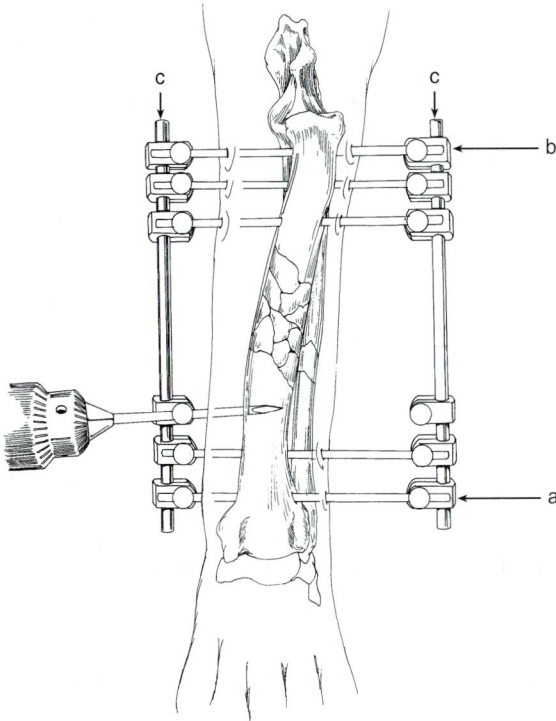

Figure 124-4. External skeletal fixation for radius and ulna fractures. See text for explanation.

carpal joint (Fig. 124–4, pin a). Drive the transfixation pins through the skin on both sides of the limb.

5. Drive the most proximal transfixation pin (Fig. 124–4, pin b) in a similar manner, parallel to the articular surface of the radial head.

6. Apply connecting bars (Fig. 124–4, pin c) to the transfixation pins on both the lateral and medial sides.

7. Place the appropriate number of single connecting clamps on the connecting bar.

8. Align the fracture and tighten the end connecting clamps to maintain reduction of the fracture.

9. Drive the remaining transfixation pins through the connecting clamps and tighten them (see Chap. 130).

10. If possible, place three or four transfixation pins on each side of the fracture line.

11. Cover the external skeletal fixation device with gauze and tape to protect the fixator and furniture surfaces. Clean pin tracts daily (see Chap. 130).

Plate Fixation for Distal Metaphyseal Fractures

These fractures occur primarily in small dogs. There is a high incidence of nonunion if these fractures are not treated correctly.

Objectives

- Achieve anatomic alignment with compression of the fracture.
- Insert a cancellous bone graft.

Equipment

- General surgery pack and standard suture material
- Mini-bone plating equipment (1.5 mm and 2.0 mm screws and plates)
- Power drill
- Curette (Brun 3-0)
- Small bone reduction forceps

Technique

1. Place the patient in lateral recumbency, with the affected leg up, and prepare the limb for aseptic surgery.

2. Make a skin incision on the dorsal aspect of the leg, starting at the cephalic vein and extending distally to the mid-metacarpus. Make the incision lateral to the cephalic vein.

3. Incise the subcutaneous tissue and fascia along the same line.

4. Identify the extensor carpi radialis and the common digital extensor tendons and subperiosteally elevate them from their grooves in the radius.

5. Incise the abductor pollicis muscle for additional proximal exposure.

6. Reduce the fracture and hold it in reduction with bone reduction forceps.

7. Contour a bone plate to the cranial surface of the radius and apply the plate. In small dogs, use a 1.5 mm or 2.0 mm bone plate.

8. Make a 2-cm long incision over the craniolateral aspect of the greater tubercle of the humerus.

9. Incise the subcutaneous tissue along the same line. Drill a small hole in the greater tubercle.

10. Use a #3-0 Brun curette to collect a cancellous bone graft from the greater tubercle. During the collection process, place the graft on a blood-soaked sponge.

11. Pack the bone graft around the fracture site.

12. Close the subcutaneous tissue and the skin incisions routinely.

13. After surgery, apply a soft padded bandage to the leg.

Fractured Styloid Process of Ulna

Objective

- Reduce and stabilize the fracture to reestablish lateral support to the carpus.

Equipment

- General surgery pack and standard suture material
- Surgical stainless steel wire (20 and 18 gauge)
- K-wires
- Jacobs pin chuck
- Wire tightening device (vise grips, wire twister)
- Pin and wire cutter
- Bone reduction forceps

Technique

1. Place the patient in lateral recumbency with the affected leg up and aseptically prepare the limb.

2. Make a skin incision over the lateral aspect of the sty-

loid process. Incise the subcutaneous tissue along the same line.

3. Dissect between and elevate the tendons of the lateral digital extensor and the extensor carpi ulnaris.
4. Reduce the fracture and drive a K-wire from the distal tip of the ulna just above the ulnar collateral ligament into the proximal segment.
5. Drill a hole in the proximal segment of the ulna and pass a wire through the hole.
6. Place the wire around the tip of the pin in a figure-eight configuration, and tighten the wire on both arms of the figure-eight.
7. Close the deep fascia and subcutaneous tissue with absorbable suture in a simple continuous pattern. Close the skin routinely.
8. Splint the fracture for 3–4 weeks postoperatively.

GROWTH DEFORMITIES OF THE RADIUS AND ULNA

Growth deformities of the radius and ulna result from trauma and disruption of the blood supply to the physis; retained cartilaginous cores (see Chaps. 136 and 138); and synostosis (bony bridging) of the radius and ulna. Specific treatment depends on the physis injured, the extent of deformity, and the age of the animal.

Anatomy

- The radius and ulna form the largest paired bones of the body. Abnormal growth of one bone may affect the other bone, elbow, or carpus.
- In dogs, the growth plates (physes) of the radius and ulna close about 7–9 months of age (see Chap. 138) for more information about physeal structure).
- The distal ulnar physis is conical in shape, making it vulnerable to crushing during trauma. The two radial physes are relatively flat.
- The distal ulnar physis contributes 85% to the longitudinal growth of the ulna; the proximal physis (olecranon) contributes 15%.
- The proximal and distal radial physes contribute 40% and 60%, respectively, to the longitudinal growth of the radius.
- The radius and ulna must grow in a synchronous manner to retain a normal shape and joint congruity. As the radius and ulna grow, they normally slide past each other.

Preoperative Considerations

- Early recognition and treatment of physeal injury of the radius and ulna is the key to prevention or minimization of deformities.
- Base treatment of a growth deformity on whether the dog is mature or immature (whether physes are still growing) and on the specific deformity.

▼ *Key Point* The general principles of treatment of growth deformities are prevention or correction of angular deformities and joint abnormalities and maintenance of acceptable leg length.

- Obtain lateral and craniocaudal radiographs of the affected and normal forelimbs. Include both the elbow and carpus.
- Preplan corrective procedures on paper or cleared radiographic film by making tracings and cutouts copied from the radiographs.

General Postoperative Care and Complications for Growth Deformities

- In immature dogs, splint the limb when ostectomy has been performed. The other intact bone will hypertrophy to withstand the added stress.
- Reevaluate the leg radiographically at least every 3 weeks until the dog has stopped growing.
- If bone bridges the ostectomized gap before growth has ceased, repeat the original surgery.
- If the procedure for immature dogs does not correct the deformity, perform the procedure recommended for mature dogs after bone growth stops.

General Prognosis

- The prognosis is guarded, especially for mature dogs with severe deformities.

Surgical Procedure to Correct Premature Closure of the Distal Ulnar Physis

Immature Dogs

Objectives

- Remove a section of the ulna to allow unrestrained growth of the radius.
- Prevent regrowth of the ulna by placement of a free fat graft.

Equipment

- General surgery pack and standard suture material
- Gigli wire saw or oscillating bone saw
- Gelpi retractor

Technique

1. Place the patient in lateral recumbency, with the affected leg up, and prepare the limb for aseptic surgery.
2. Make a 6-cm incision over the lateral aspect of the distal third of the ulna. Incise the subcutaneous tissue and antebrachial fascia along the same line.
3. Dissect between the extensor carpi ulnaris and the lateral digital extensor muscles to expose the ulna. Elevate the muscles and tendons from the ulna on top of the periosteum all the way around the bone.
4. Using the Gigli wire saw or the oscillating saw, ostectomize at least 2 cm of the ulna at the junction of the distal one-third and middle one-third of the bone.
5. Remove all the periosteum to prevent rapid bone regrowth.
6. Make a 3-cm incision over the flank just in front of the wing of the ilium.

7. Dissect down to the subcutaneous fat and collect a piece of fat large enough to completely fill the defect in the ulna.
8. Place the fat graft in the ulnar defect and close the antebrachial fascia in a simple continuous fashion with absorbable suture material.
9. Close the subcutaneous tissue and skin routinely.
10. Place the limb in a splint for the first month following surgery.

Mature Dogs

Deformities

- Cranial and/or medial bowing with lateral torsion of the radius
- Carpal valgus with external rotation
- Limb shortening
- Malalignment of radius and/or ulna in the elbow joint

Objectives

- Correct angular and rotational deformity
- Correct joint incongruity
- Maintain as much leg length as possible

Equipment

- General surgery pack and standard suture material
- Gigli wire saw or oscillating bone saw
- Kirschner-Ehmer fixation device
- Jacobs pin chuck or power drill

Technique

1. Place the patient in lateral recumbency, with the affected leg up, and prepare the limb for aseptic surgery.
2. Drive a transfixation pin across the most distal aspect of the radius, aligned parallel with the craniocaudal plane and mediolateral plane of the articular surface of the radius (Fig. 124–5).
3. Drive a second transfixation pin in the same manner as the first pin, except as far proximal as possible and parallel to the articular surface of the proximal radius.
4. Approach the radius as described previously in Plate Fixation for Distal Metaphyseal Fractures.
5. Perform an osteotomy of the radius at the point of maximal curvature of the radius.
6. Fracture the ulna at the same level, either manually or with a saw.
7. Connect the transfixation pins on the lateral and medial sides with single connecting clamps and connecting bars. Place the appropriate number of single connecting clamps on the connecting bars.
8. Manually align the proximal and distal transfixation pins so that they are parallel to each other in both planes. Tighten the connecting clamps to hold the proper alignment (Fig. 124–6).
9. If there is any concern over the alignment, obtain radiographs of the leg at this point.
10. Drive the remaining transfixation pins through the open single connecting clamps.

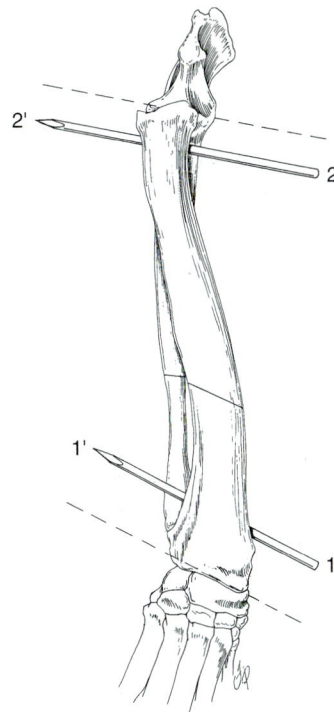

Figure 124–5. Pin placement for repair of premature closure of the distal ulnar physis. Place the first pin (1–1′) parallel to the cranial-caudal and medial-lateral plane of the articular surface of the radius. The second pin (2–2′) is parallel to the articular surface of the proximal radius.

11. Close the incisions routinely.
12. Cover the K-device with gauze and tape.
13. If elbow incongruity is not severe, it will resolve with weight bearing after the ulna is cut.

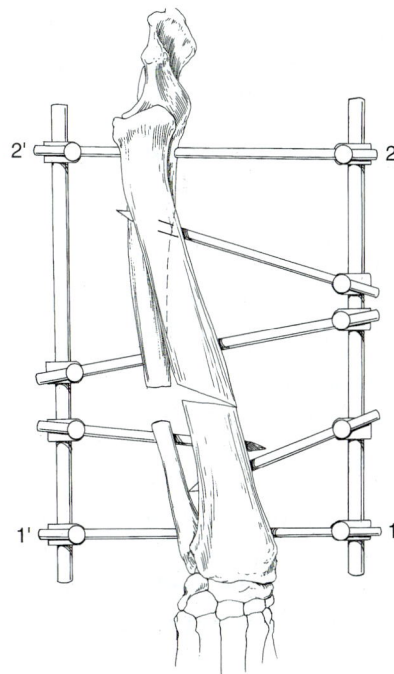

Figure 124–6. Final pin placement (see Fig. 124–5), osteotomy, and ulnar fracture for repair of premature closure of the distal ulnar physis.

Surgical Procedure to Correct Premature Closure of the Proximal Radial Physis

Generally this deformity is recognized after the bone growth of the radius is finished. If it occurs in an immature dog, use the technique described for complete premature closure of the distal radial physis in immature dogs.

Deformities

- There is distal luxation of the radial head from the humerus.
- Leg is straight.

Objective (Mature Dogs)

- Reposition the radial head into the elbow joint so that it articulates properly with the humerus and ulna.

Equipment

- General surgery pack and standard suture material
- Bone plating equipment
- Power drill
- Oscillating saw

Technique

1. Place the animal in lateral recumbency, with the affected leg up and prepare the limb for aseptic surgery.
2. Approach the radial head as described previously under Radial Head Fractures.
3. Approach the mid-shaft of the radius as described previously for mid-shaft radial fractures.
4. Perform a stepped radial osteotomy. Make the longitudinal arm of the osteotomy long enough to accept two bone screws (Fig. 124–7).
5. Slide the radial head proximally so that it articulates correctly with the humeral condyle and the ulna.
6. Place two screws, from medial to lateral, in "lag screw" fashion across the osteotomy site.
7. Apply a bone plate on the cranial aspect of the radius to further stabilize the osteotomy.
8. Collect a cancellous bone graft from the proximal humerus.
9. Place the bone graft in the defect in the radius.
10. Close the incisions routinely.
11. Place the leg in a soft padded bandage for 10–14 days postoperatively.

Surgical Procedure to Correct Premature Closure of the Distal Radial Physis

Premature closure of the distal radial physis can be complete or partial. If partial closure occurs, the lateral aspect of the physis usually is affected.

Complete Closure (Immature Dog)

Deformities

- Distal luxation of the radial head and elbow joint incongruity occur.

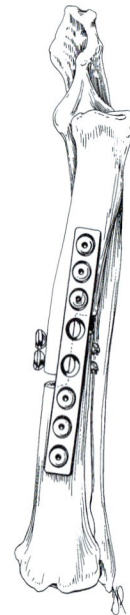

Figure 124–7.   Plate and screw placement for stepped radial osteotomy performed for repair of premature closure of the proximal radial physis.

- The limb is shortened.
- Usually the leg remains straight.
- Bowing of the radius and ulna occurs rarely.

Objectives

- Remove a section of the radius to allow unrestricted growth of the ulna.
- Prevent regrowth of the radius until the other growth plates have stopped growing.

Equipment

- General surgery pack and standard suture material
- Gigli wire saw or oscillating saw

Technique

1. Place the animal in lateral recumbency, with the affected leg down, and prepare the limb for aseptic surgery.
2. Approach the mid-shaft radius as described previously for mid-shaft radial fractures.
3. Ostectomize a 2-cm section of radius, including the periosteum. Protect the interosseous artery.
4. Collect a free fat graft from the flank, as described previously for premature closure of the distal ulnar physis in immature dogs.
5. Place the fat graft in the radial defect and close the antebrachial fascia with absorbable suture material in a continuous pattern.
6. Close the incision routinely from the toes to the distal humerus.
7. Place the leg in a splint postoperatively.
8. When the dog has stopped growing, reconstruct the defect in the radius with a cancellous bone graft.

Partial Lateral Closure (Immature Dog)

Deformities

- Carpal valgus with external rotation
- Cranial and medial bowing of the forelimb
- Shortening of the limb
- Elbow joint incongruity

Objectives

- Remove the closed portion of the distal radial physis
- Prevent bony bridging of the removed physis with a fat graft.

Equipment

- General surgery pack and standard suture material
- Curets

Technique

1. Place the patient in lateral recumbency, with the affected leg up, and prepare the limb for aseptic surgery.
2. Approach the distal radius as described previously for distal radial fractures.
3. Carefully expose the physis to minimize damage.
4. Probe the physis with a 25-gauge needle to determine the extent of the closure.
5. Use a curet to remove the closed section of the physis.
6. Place a free fat graft collected from the flank in the defect.
7. Close the incision routinely.
8. Splint the leg until bone growth is complete.
9. When bone growth is complete, remove the fat graft, if necessary, and graft the defect with cancellous bone.

Mature Dogs

Deformities

The deformities are the same as described for complete and incomplete closure in immature dogs.

Objectives

- Reestablish congruity to the elbow joint.
- Correct angular deformity of the limb.

Equipment

- Equipment is same as listed for premature closure of the proximal radius and distal ulna in maturedogs.

Technique

- If the radial head is luxated distally and the limb is straight, use the technique described previously for correction of premature closure of the proximal radius in mature dogs.
- If angular and rotation deformity is present, use the techniques described previously for correction of premature closure of the distal ulna in mature dogs.

TRAUMATIC LUXATION OF THE ELBOW

- Lateral luxation of the elbow is common because the medial condyle of the humerus is larger and is slightly beveled downward, preventing medial luxation of the radius and ulna.

Clinical Signs

- The animals present with acute non–weight bearing lameness.
- The foot and antebrachium are usually abducted, and flexion and extension of the elbow are not possible.

Diagnosis

- Radiographs of the elbow (lateral and anteroposterior) demonstrate the luxation.

Preoperative Considerations

- Most elbow luxations can be treated by closed reduction if the procedure is performed within the first 3 days after injury.
- If closed reduction is not possible, or if elbow fractures are present, open reduction is indicated. Open reduction of an elbow luxation can be a difficult procedure and is best handled by a surgical specialist.

Procedure for Closed Reduction

Objectives

- Reduce the luxation to reestablish normal function.
- Prevent recurrence of luxation with external coaptation.

Equipment

- Bandage material for constructing a spica, or lateral splint.

Technique

1. Place the animal in lateral recumbency with the luxated leg up.
2. Place the elbow joint in full flexion.
3. With one hand on the radius and ulna, and the other hand on the distal humerus, pull the radius and ulna distally along the lateral aspect of the humerus.
4. While continuing distal traction on the radius and ulna, rotate the radius and ulna inward to place the anconeal process over the lateral humeral epicondyloid crest.
5. Use the thumb of one hand to maintain lateral to medial pressure on the olecranon while slowly extending the elbow with the other hand.
6. Keep the elbow extended to maintain reduction.
7. Evaluate the joint for instability of the collateral ligaments.

Postoperative Care

- Obtain lateral and craniocaudal radiographs of the elbow to confirm reduction and evaluate for other injuries.

- Place the affected leg in a spica or lateral splint to keep the elbow in extension.
- Maintain the splint for 2 weeks, then allow leash walking only for another 2 weeks.
- Reevaluate at 2, 4, and 6 weeks postoperatively.
- If open reduction or ligament repair of the elbow is necessary, refer the patient to a surgical specialist.

SUPPLEMENTAL READINGS

Brinker WO, Hohn RB, Prieur WD: Manual of Internal Fixation of Fractures. New York: Springer-erlag, 1984, p 144.

Brinker WO, Piermattei DL, Flo GL: Fractures and corrective surgery in young growing animals. *In* Brinker WO, Piermattei DL, Flo GL, eds.: Handbook of Small Animal Orthopedics and Fracture Treatment. Philadelphia: WB Saunders, 1990, p 244.

Brinker WO, Piermattei DL, Flo GL: Fractures of the radius and ulna. *In* Brinker WO, Piermattei DL, Flo GL, eds.: Handbook of Small Animal Orthopedics and Fracture Treatment. Philadelphia: WB Saunders, 1990, p 195.

Johnson AL: Correction of radial and ulnar growth deformities resulting from premature physeal closure. *In* Bojrab MJ, ed.: Current Techniques in Small Animal Surgery. Philadelphia: Lea & Febiger, 1990, p 793.

Piermattei DL, Greeley RG: An Atlas of Surgical Approaches to the Bones of the Dog and Cat. Philadelphia: WB Saunders, 1979, p 108.

Probst CW: Stabilization of fractures of the radius and ulna. *In* Bojrab MJ, ed.: Current Techniques in Small Animal Surgery. Philadelphia: Lea & Febiger, 1990, p 783.

125 Fractures and Dislocations of the Carpus

Kurt J. Matushek

Injuries to the carpus consist of fractures, ligamentous damage due to luxations or subluxations, and combinations of the two.

Fractures of the carpus are rare and are seen most often in racing Greyhounds and working dogs.

▼ *Key Point* When managing fractures of the carpus, remember that most involve articular surfaces.

ANATOMY

Osseous Structures (Fig. 125–1)

- The carpus consists of seven bones arranged in two rows and a small sesamoid bone located in the tendon of insertion of the abductor pollicis longus muscle.
- The bones of the proximal row are the radial, ulnar, and accessory carpal bones.
  - The radial carpal bone, the largest of the carpal bones, is located on the medial aspect of the proximal row. It articulates proximally with the radius and distally with the four distal carpal bones.
  - The ulnar carpal bone is the lateral bone of the proximal row. It articulates proximally with the radius and ulna, distally with the fourth carpal bone and fifth metacarpal bone, and with the accessory carpal bone on the palmar aspect.
  - The accessory carpal bone is located on the palmar surface of the carpus. It articulates with the ulnar carpal bone and the styloid process of the ulna.
- The first, second, third, and fourth carpal bones make up the distal row.
  - The fourth carpal bone is the largest bone in the distal row. It articulates distally with the fourth and fifth metacarpal bones.

Articulations

- The carpal joints include the antebrachiocarpal, the middle carpal, and the carpometacarpal joints. The joints between the carpal bones of each row are called intercarpal joints.
- As a group, the carpal joints act to permit flexion and extension, with a small amount of medial and lateral movement.

- The greatest amount of motion occurs in the antebrachiocarpal joint. The middle carpal joint accounts for approximately 10–15% of carpal motion. Very little motion occurs in the carpometacarpal and intercarpal joints.

Ligamentous Structures

- No long collateral ligaments span all three joints of the carpus.
- Support to the carpus is provided by two sleeves of collagenous tissue with the tendons in between.
  - The superficial sleeve is a thickening of the deep carpal fascia.
  - The deep sleeve is a thickened fibrous layer of the joint capsule.
  - The two sleeves fuse laterally and medially to form short collateral ligaments.
- The flexor retinaculum, formerly called the transverse palmar carpal ligament, provides support to the palmaroproximal aspect of the carpus.
  - The flexor retinaculum attaches laterally to the accessory carpal bone and medially to the styloid process of the radius, the radial carpal bone, and the first carpal bone.
- The palmar carpal fibrocartilage crosses the palmar surface of the carpus and attaches to all the carpal bones except the accessory carpal bone.
  - The palmar carpal fibrocartilage is particularly heavy distally and attaches to the proximal ends of the third, fourth, and fifth metacarpal bones.
- The short radial collateral ligament consists of two parts, both originating from the styloid process of the radius: the straight portion, which inserts on the medial surface, and the oblique portion, which inserts on the palmaromedial surface of the radial carpal bone.
- The short ulnar collateral ligament originates on the ulnar styloid process and inserts on the ulnar carpal bone.
- The accessory carpal bone is stabilized distally by two ligaments, both of which originate from the free end of the accessory carpal bone. One ligament attaches to the fifth metacarpal bone, and the other to the fourth metacarpal bone.
- Other multiple small ligaments attach the carpal bones to each other and to the metacarpal bones.

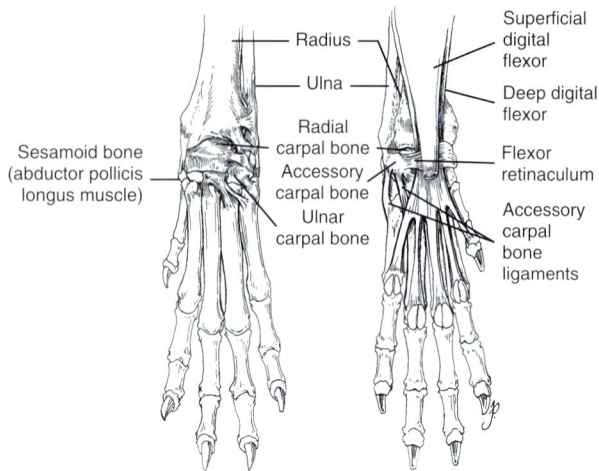

Figure 125–1.   Anatomy of the carpus. *Left,* Dorsal view; *right,* palmar view.

FRACTURES OF THE RADIAL CARPAL BONE

Preoperative Considerations

- Fractures occur because of
  - Hyperextension injuries, resulting in chip fractures of the proximal dorsal border.
  - A fall, resulting in slab fractures.
- Lameness usually is acutely severe; however, with chronic injuries, the injured limb may become partially weight bearing.
- Diagnosis may be difficult because the fragments usually are only minimally displaced.
  - High-detail radiographs are essential for diagnosis.
  - Oblique radiographic views often are necessary.
- Bone fragments tend not to reattach, resulting in synovitis and degenerative joint disease.

Surgical Procedure
Objectives

- Remove small chips that cannot be reduced and stabilized adequately.
- Stabilize larger fragments with lag screws or multiple Kirschner wires.

Equipment

- General surgery pack and standard suture material
- Bone-holding forceps
- Lag screws or Kirschner wires (K-wires)
- Esmarch bandage and tourniquet

Technique

1. Surgery is most often performed with a tourniquet in place; most fractures can be exposed through a dorsal approach (see description under Pancarpal Arthrodesis).
2. Alignment and reduction is achieved with small, pointed bone-holding forceps.
3. If lag screws are used, countersink the screw head to avoid interference with the movement of other structures.

Postoperative Care and Complications

- Place the limb in a splint for 1–3 weeks after surgery.
- Restrict exercise for 6–8 weeks or until there is radiographic evidence of union.
- Secondary degenerative joint disease is common, and intermittent lameness can occur.

FRACTURES OF THE ACCESSORY CARPAL BONE

Preoperative Considerations

- This type of fracture is common in racing greyhounds; it is rare in other breeds.
- When possible, internal fixation of fragments is preferable.

Surgical Procedure
Objectives and Equipment

- Same as for fractures of the radial carpal bone.

Technique

1. Use a palmarolateral approach to the accessory carpal bone.
2. Reduce and stabilize fracture, using screws placed in a "lag screw" fashion.

Postoperative Care and Complications

- Maintain the limb in a splint for 4–6 weeks after surgery.
- Resume training (in athletic dogs) in 12–16 weeks.

FRACTURES OF THE ULNAR CARPAL BONE AND CARPAL BONES 1–4

- Fractures of these bones are very rare.
- Most often these are small chip fractures of the dorsal surface, resulting from hyperextension injuries.
- Treatment consists of removal of the fragments followed by splintage for 2 weeks. Restrict exercise for 8 weeks.

LUXATIONS AND SUBLUXATIONS OF THE CARPUS—HYPEREXTENSION INJURIES

Luxations and subluxations are most commonly seen as a result of hyperextension injuries resulting from falling or jumping from a height. The hyperextension force causes tearing and rupture of the palmar joint capsule and ligaments and results in loss of support of any or all of the three carpal joints.

Clinical Signs and Diagnosis

- The injured limb usually is non–weight bearing if the animal is examined immediately after the injury. However, most animals begin walking on the leg in a relatively short period, although a limp is present.

- Mild tenderness and swelling of the carpus usually is present.
- A plantigrade stance is characteristic of a hyperextension injury. Most dogs walk on their carpal pads.
- Occasionally, the injury is bilateral. When this occurs, perform bilateral surgery.
- Standard radiographic views may not always demonstrate the lesion. A lateromedial projection taken with stress applied to the toes to create carpal hyperextension is necessary to determine which carpal joint is involved.
- In general, the antebrachiocarpal joint is injured 5–10% of the time; the middle carpal joint, 50–70%; and the carpometacarpal joint, 25–40%.

▼ *Key Point* External coaptation (splints or casts) is rarely if ever successful in treating hyperextension injuries. Many injuries appear improved immediately after the cast is removed but are worse in 1–2 weeks.

Preoperative Considerations

- Panarthrodesis has been advocated for hyperextension injuries regardless of the specific carpal joint involved.
  - Results have generally been good, with 74% of owners in one series of cases reporting normal use of the limb.
- Selective arthrodesis of the involved joints may be a better approach. Because 90% of the motion in the carpus occurs in the antebrachiocarpal joint, if this joint can be saved, very little alteration in gait would be expected.

Surgical Procedure

Objectives

- Follow the basic principles of joint fusion:
  - Remove all articular cartilage from the joint surfaces.
  - Use a cancellous bone graft.
  - Provide rigid internal or external fixation for a sufficient time to allow complete fusion.

Equipment

- General surgery pack and standard suture material
- Esmarch bandage and tourniquet
- Air-powered drill
- Bone curettes
- Steinmann pins
- Compression plates and screws
- Type II Kirschner-Ehmer device

Pancarpal Arthrodesis—Dorsal Approach

Technique

1. Place the patient in lateral recumbency, with the affected limb up, and prepare the limb for aseptic surgery.
2. Apply an Esmarch bandage and tourniquet to the limb to provide hemostasis.
3. Make a skin incision on the dorsal midline, extend-

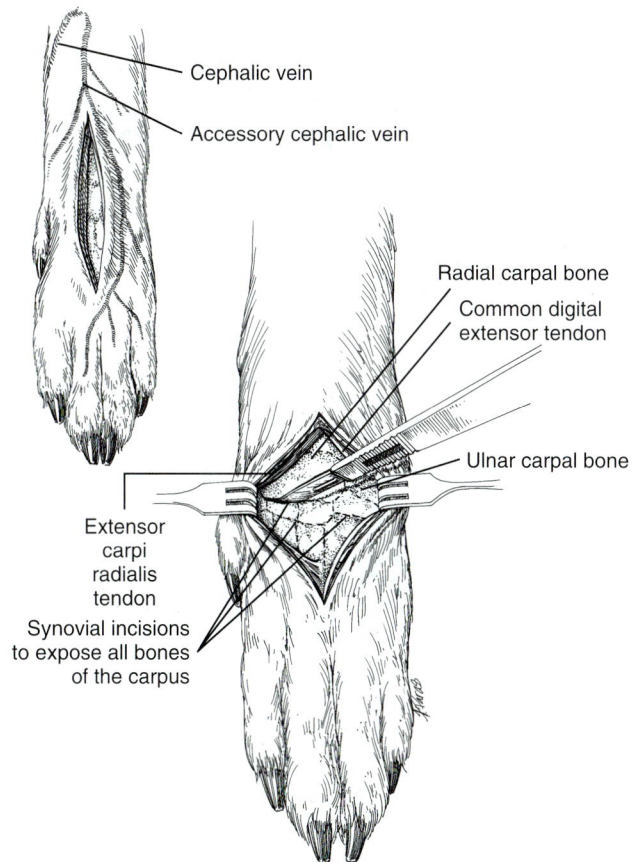

Figure 125–2. Dorsal surgical approach to the carpus. Avoid incising venous drainage *(top left)*.

ing from the junction of the cephalic and accessory cephalic veins to the mid-metacarpus (Fig. 125–2).
4. Incise the fascia between the tendons of the extensor carpi radialis and common digital extensor muscles and retract to expose the joint capsule.
5. Make incisions in the synovial membranes of the carpal joints to expose the articular surfaces.
6. Remove all articular cartilage, using an air-powered drill or bone curettes.
7. Use autogenous cancellous bone graft from the proximal end of the humerus or the wing of the ilium to pack all joint spaces.
8. Achieve rigid internal fixation with a seven-hole compression plate.
   a. Bend the plate to provide 5–10° of hyperextension.
   b. Place three screws in the distal part of the radius, one screw in the radial carpal bone, and three screws in the third metacarpal bone (Fig. 125–3, *top*).
9. Alternatively, stabilize the joint with a type II Kirschner-Ehmer device, placing two pins in the distal part of the radius and two pins in the third and fourth metacarpal bones (Fig. 125–3, *bottom*).

Postoperative Care

- Place the limb in a palmar splint for 6–8 weeks after surgery, or until radiographic union is evident.

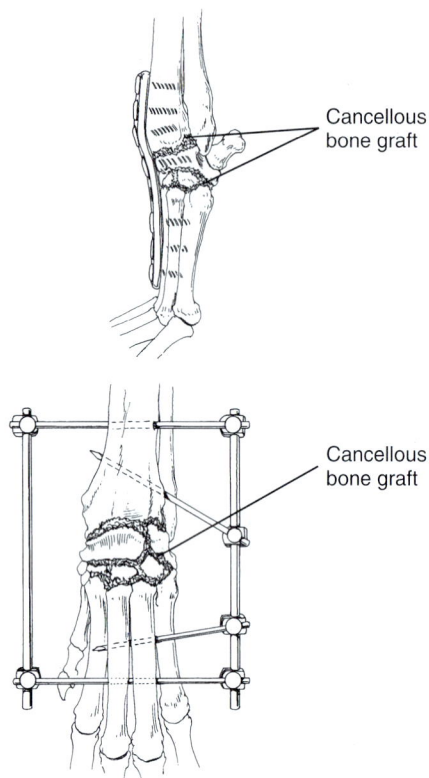

Figure 125–3.   Pancarpal arthrodesis, dorsal approach. *Top*, Plate stabilization; *bottom*, stabilization with Kirchner-Ehmer apparatus.

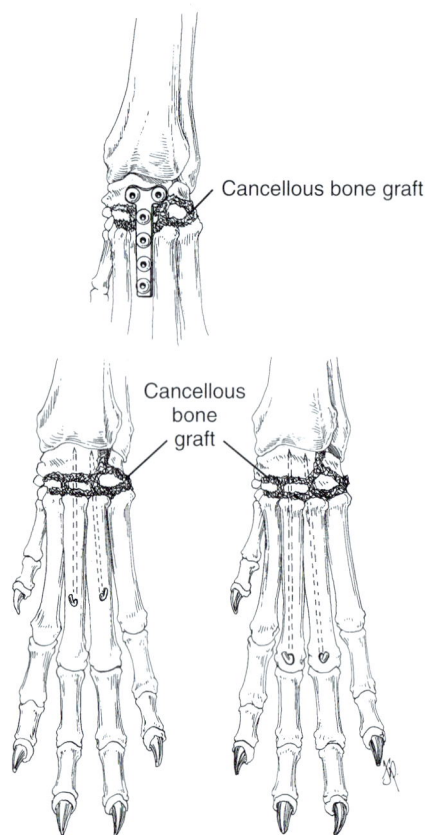

Figure 125–4.   Partial carpal arthrodesis. *Top*, Plate stabilization; *bottom*, stabilization with intramedullary pins.

Partial Carpal Arthrodesis

Technique

▼ *Key Point* Partial carpal arthrodesis is indicated when the antebrachiocarpal joint and its ligaments and the ligaments of the accessory carpal bone are intact.

1. Use a dorsal approach to the carpus, as described under Pancarpal Arthrodesis. However, remove the articular cartilage from the middle carpal and carpometacarpal joints only.
2. Pack a cancellous bone graft into the joint spaces.
3. Several techniques can be used to achieve stabilization.
   a. Apply a T- or L-plate to the dorsal aspect of the third or fourth metacarpal bone with the T or L portion attached to the radial carpal bone (Fig. 125–4, *top*). During extension, do not allow the plate to overlap the antebrachiocarpal joint. Place the limb in a palmar splint for 6 weeks after surgery, or until there is radiographic evidence of union.
   b. Alternatively, place Steinmann pins normograde from the third and fourth metacarpal bones and embed the pins in the radial carpal and ulnar carpal bones (Fig. 125–4, *bottom*). The pins originate from slots drilled into the dorsal surfaces of the metacarpal bones. Bend the pins upward to prevent pin migration and soft tissue trauma.

Place the limb in a palmar splint for 6–12 weeks after surgery, or until there is radiographic evidence of union. Remove the pins after healing is complete.
   c. For partial carpal fusion without the use of metallic implants, prepare the articular surfaces as described previously and pack a cancellous bone graft into the joint spaces. Place the limb in a splint immediately after surgery. When swelling from the surgery has decreased (approximately 3 days) apply a full cast to the limb from the elbow distally with the carpus in 5–10° of hyperextension. Change the cast every 4 weeks until union is evident radiographically (usually about 12 weeks).

Postoperative Complications

- Postoperative swelling caused by impairment of lymphatic or venous drainage is common and usually subsides within a few days.
- If fusion occurs, complications are rare.
- The most common reasons for arthrodesis failure are any one or a combination of the following:
  - Incomplete removal of articular cartilage
  - Inadequate bone grafting
  - Inadequate internal or external support for a sufficient period of time

SUPPLEMENTAL READINGS

Brinker WO, Piermattei DL, Flo GL: Handbook of Small Animal Orthopedics and Fracture Treatment. Philadelphia: WB Saunders, 1983, p 386.

Evans HE, Christensen GC: Miller's Anatomy of the Dog, 2nd Ed. Philadelphia: WB Saunders, 1979, pp 190, 248.

Gambardella PC, Griffiths RC: Treatment of hyperextension injuries of the canine carpus. Compend Contin Educ Pract Vet 4:127, 1982.

Johnson KA: Accessory carpal bone fractures in the racing greyhound: Classifications and pathology. Vet Surg 16:60, 1987.

Johnson KA, Dee JF, Piermattei DL: Screw fixation of accessory carpal bone fractures in racing greyhounds: 12 cases (1981–1986). J Am Vet Med Assoc 194:1618, 1989.

Slocum B, Devine T: Partial carpal fusion in the dog. J Am Vet Med Assoc 180:1204, 1982.

126 Fractures of the Pelvis

Peter Muir / Kenneth A. Johnson / Paul A. Manley

Pelvic fractures in dogs and cats occur most often as a consequence of severe trauma, and are frequently associated with other orthopedic injuries and injuries to other body systems. Decisions regarding management of pelvic fractures can be assisted by recognizing the types of pelvic fractures that have a higher priority for surgical treatment and by diagnosing concurrent injuries of other body systems.

SURGICAL ANATOMY

- Each half of the pelvis is composed of the ilium, ischium, pubis, and acetabulum, which are fused as the os coxae, or hip bone.
- The sacroiliac joint has a limited range of motion and is composed of a synchondrosis craniodorsally and a synovial articulation ventrally.
- The sacrotuberous ligament extends from the caudolateral part of the apex of the sacrum and the transverse processes of the first caudal vertebra to the lateral part of the ischiatic tuberosity. The sacrotuberous ligament is absent in the cat.
- The sacrum and pelvic bones form a complete bony canal. Therefore, pelvic fractures usually are multiple, or pelvic fracture may be accompanied by sacroiliac fracture or luxation. If a pelvic fracture appears to be single, examine radiographs carefully for evidence of additional undisplaced fractures.
- The major weight bearing regions of the pelvis are the sacroiliac joint, body of the ilium, and acetabulum.

DIAGNOSIS AND EVALUATION OF PELVIC FRACTURES

- Thorough physical examination may be difficult in injured animals that are in pain or shock. After emergency treatment, complete the general physical examination as soon as possible.
- Management of cardiopulmonary, neural, and certain soft tissue injuries may have a higher priority than that of orthopedic injury. Obtain thoracic and abdominal radiographs routinely in animals with suspected pelvic fractures. Obtain both left and right lateral radiographic views.
- Injury to intra-abdominal and intrapelvic organs such as the liver, spleen, urinary bladder, and urethra

commonly accompanies pelvic fractures. Surgical treatment of soft tissue injuries may take priority over pelvic fracture repair.
- When the patient is in stable condition, perform an orthopedic examination.
  - Carefully palpate the pelvic bones, manipulate the hip joints, and perform a rectal examination to detect pelvic fractures and to check for a palpable defect in the rectal wall.
  - Obtain radiographs of the pelvis in at least two projections to fully evaluate bone injury. Further radiographs, including contrast studies, may be necessary to evaluate soft tissue injury. If necessary, sedate or anesthetize the patient to obtain high-quality diagnostic radiographs.

▼ *Key Point* Although rectal tears are not commonly associated with pelvic fracture, failure to make an early diagnosis usually results in severe pelvic infection, sepsis, and patient death.

- Perform a neurologic examination to detect damage to the spinal cord, cauda equina nerve roots, and peripheral nerves.

CONSERVATIVE TREATMENT

In many animals with pelvic fractures, conservative treatment is all that is needed for successful fracture healing and normal pelvic limb function. However, careful nursing is required for several weeks, because multiple injuries are commonly present. Patient size is an important consideration in making the decision to manage pelvic fractures without surgery. Small dogs and cats are much easier to manage for extended periods of time.

The following measures are helpful in conservative therapy:

- Dogs and cats with pelvic fractures often are reluctant to stand and may be unable to turn over. Turn these animals regularly and use a padded bed to help prevent decubital ulcers.
  - Give analgesics as needed (see Chap. 2).
- Pain, bone instability, and neurologic injury may make it difficult for animals with pelvic fractures to urinate and defecate normally.
  - Empty the urinary bladder regularly by manual expression or catheter drainage, to prevent exces-

sive distention, overflow incontinence, and urine soiling.
- If necessary, give a mild laxative or stool softener to prevent constipation.
- Some patients are able to stand and walk within a few days; however, restrict activity to a cage for 4–6 weeks.
- If limb adduction is weak as a consequence of ventral pelvic fractures or muscle trauma, use a body sling or towel support around the abdomen as necessary to assist recovery.
- Obtain radiographs every 4–6 weeks during recovery to monitor fracture healing.

INDICATIONS FOR SURGERY

The main advantages of surgical treatment of pelvic fractures are reduced pain, early return to normal function, avoidance of fracture-associated disease, and minimal hospitalization time. Pelvic fractures may result in marked narrowing of the pelvic canal if left untreated, with the risk of consequent obstipation, dystocia, dysuria, or sciatic nerve entrapment. If operative treatment of pelvic fractures is delayed beyond 5 days, muscle spasm and fibrosis may make reduction of the fracture fragments difficult, because of the large muscle mass surrounding the pelvis.

Surgical treatment may be indicated for the following injuries:

- Fracture of the ilium with associated fracture of the pubis and ischium creating an unstable acetabulum
- Intra-articular fractures (acetabulum)
- Markedly displaced, unstable, or painful sacroiliac fracture or luxation
- Severe bilateral fractures of the pelvis or displaced pelvic fractures associated with an additional major orthopedic injury of a pelvic limb, such as hip luxation or fracture of the femur
- Fractures of the ischium that have an intra-articular component in the acetabulum, or that are suspected of entrapping the sciatic nerve
- Fracture of the pubis or separation of the pubic symphysis associated with abdominal wall rupture and herniation of abdominal or pelvic organs

FRACTURES OF THE ILIUM

Preoperative Considerations

- Fractures of the ilium are usually oblique and are often accompanied by fractures of other regions of the pelvis.

▼ *Key Point* If fracture displacement is present, the caudal fragment usually is displaced medially, and thus the pelvic canal is narrowed.

- Perform a thorough neurologic examination (see Chap. 144), particularly with markedly displaced fractures. Damage to the sciatic nerve may be present.
- Surgical repair of fractures of the ilium is generally

recommended because most fractures of the ilium are displaced or unstable. Surgical treatment may consist of more than one operation.
- Precontouring the bone plate to the ilium of an intact pelvis from a cadaver of similar size reduces operating time.
- Administer prophylactic antibiotics at the time of anesthetic induction.

Surgical Procedure

Objectives

- Anatomically reduce and stabilize the ilium.
- Relieve pain.
- Provide early restoration of pelvic limb function.
- Avoid iatrogenic sciatic nerve damage.

Equipment

- Standard general surgical pack and suture material
- Gelpi or Weitlaner self-retaining retractors
- Orthopedic surgical pack with AO-ASIF and Kern bone-holding forceps and Hohmann retractors
- Bone-plating equipment
- Periosteal elevator
- Suction and electrocautery setups

Technique

1. Place the animal in lateral recumbency and stabilize the pelvis by placing sandbags under the animal and securing the animal to the table.
2. Place a lubricated gauze sponge in the rectum, and place a pursestring suture in the anus.
3. Prepare the skin for aseptic surgery on the lateral and medial sides of the pelvic limb from the tarsocrural joint to the dorsal and ventral midline and from the mid-lumbar area to the base of the tail.
4. Use a ventrolateral (gluteal roll-up) approach to the ilium.
5. Make a skin incision from the iliac crest to the greater trochanter.
6. Incise and retract the cutaneous trunci muscle and subcutaneous fat to expose the pelvic musculature.
7. Obtain hemostasis by careful electrocoagulation.
8. Dissection and fracture stabilization
   a. Identify and separate the sartorius, the tensor fasciae latae, and middle gluteal muscles. Retract the sartorius muscle cranially. Retract the tensor fasciae latae muscle ventrally, and retract the middle gluteal muscle dorsally to expose the ilium. Subperiosteal reflection of the middle and deep gluteal muscles dorsally exposes the lateral surface of the body of the ilium.
   b. During exposure of the body of the ilium, it may be necessary to retract or transect branches of the cranial gluteal vein, artery, and nerve that supply the tensor fasciae latae muscle.
   c. Preserve the lateral circumflex femoral vessels immediately cranial to the acetabulum.

▼ *Key Point* Avoid damage to the sciatic nerve, which lies dorsomedial to the ilium during reduction and stabilization of the fracture.

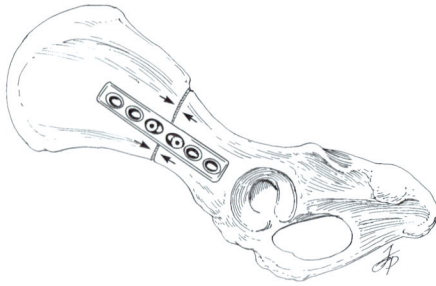

Figure 126–1. Slightly oblique fracture of the body of the ilium that has been reduced and stabilized with a six-hole dynamic compression plate. The screws have been loaded to produce compression of the fracture.

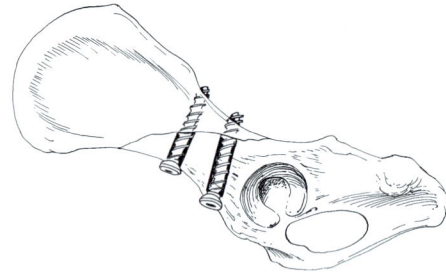

Figure 126–2. A long oblique fracture of the body of the ilium that has been stabilized with two fully threaded screws. The near cortex has been overdrilled to produce interfragmentary compression of the fracture as the screws are tightened.

d. After exposing the fracture, use AO-ASIF bone-holding forceps to manipulate and reduce the caudal fragment. Attaching bone-holding forceps to the greater trochanter or ischium is helpful in reduction of the caudal ilial fragment.

e. After reducing the fracture, contour a bone plate to the body of the ilium. Position the plate so that one screw in the cranial fragment can be placed in the body of the sacrum to engage more bone. The cranial part of the wing of the ilium is thin and screws may strip easily if the body of the sacrum is not engaged.

f. Initially, attach the plate to the caudal fragment. Lateral traction on the caudal fragment, greater trochanter, or ischium assists final reduction of the fracture and aids reduction of accompanying fractures in other regions of the pelvis.

g. If a dynamic compression plate (DCP) is used to stabilize a transverse fracture, compress the fracture by using the drill guide in the load position before screw placement (Fig. 126–1). If a bone plate is used, place at least three screws on each side of the fracture. Select implant sizes according to the guidelines in Table 126–1.

h. If fracture comminution is present, smaller fracture fragments may be stabilized with Kirschner wires (K-wires) or lag screws to further assist fracture reduction.

i. It may be possible to stabilize oblique fractures of the body of the ilium with bone screws alone, particularly in large dogs. Use the screws for lag effect by overdrilling the cortex closest to the head of the screw, or use partially threaded screws. The

fracture will be compressed as the screws are tightened (Fig. 126–2).

9. Closure
   a. Close the muscle and fascia (simple continuous pattern, absorbable suture), subcutaneous tissue (simple continuous pattern, absorbable suture), and skin (interrupted pattern, nonabsorbable suture) or skin staples.
   b. Remove the pursestring suture from the anus.

Postoperative Care and Complications

Short-Term

- Evaluate immediate postoperative radiographs for plate contouring and screw placement, particularly any screws inserted into the body of the sacrum.
- Closely monitor for hemorrhage and seroma formation.
- Good patient care is essential to encourage early mobility and return to normal function (see Conservative Treatment).
- Reassess the neurologic status of the patient.

Long-Term

- Restrict activity for 6–8 weeks to minimize the risk of fixation failure.
- If neurologic deficits are present, reevaluate these regularly.
- Obtain radiographs every 4–6 weeks to monitor fracture healing.
- Do not remove plate and bone screws unless there are clinical signs of implant-associated problems. Stress protection by the plate is not a recognized complication.

Prognosis

- The prognosis is good with anatomic reduction, stable fixation, and no neurologic damage. Pelvic fractures usually heal in 6–10 weeks. Delayed union or nonunion is uncommon because the pelvic bones have a large proportion of cancellous bone, and their extensive soft tissue coverage maintains a good blood supply to the fractured bone and also provides some degree of fracture stabilization.
- If neurologic deficits are present after surgery, the prognosis is fair to poor, and recovery of normal

Table 126–1. GUIDELINES FOR IMPLANT SIZES FOR FRACTURES OF THE ILIUM IN DOGS AND CATS

Body Weight (kg)	Plate Size (mm)
<10	2.0 DCP or 2.0/2.7 VCP
10–20	2.7 DCP or 2.7 RP
>20	3.5 DCP or 3.5 RP

DCP, dynamic compression plate; RP, reconstruction plate; VCP, veterinary cuttable plate.

function may be delayed by weeks to months, or may not occur at all.

- If the implant is too small or if insufficient screws are placed on each side of the fracture, plate breakage or screw loosening may occur.

FRACTURES OF THE ACETABULUM

Preoperative Considerations

- Fractures of the acetabulum are usually accompanied by fractures of other regions of the pelvis. If other major weight bearing regions of the pelvis are fractured, multiple surgical procedures may be necessary.
- Fractures of the acetabulum are classified by the anatomic region (cranial, central, or caudal acetabulum), the degree of comminution, and the degree of displacement.
- Conservative management has been advocated for undisplaced and caudal fractures of the acetabulum. However, the treatment of choice for all intraarticular fractures of the acetabulum is surgical stabilization, because this minimizes the severity of subsequent osteoarthritis.

▼ *Key Point* When it is not possible to reconstruct comminuted acetabular fractures anatomically, conservative management or stabilization of the major fragments, is indicated. After the fractures of the acetabulum have healed, femoral head and neck ostectomy or total hip arthroplasty may be performed to relieve residual hip pain.

- Damage to the joint capsule may be associated with fractures of the acetabulum, especially if the hip is luxated.
- Perform a thorough neurologic examination, particularly with displaced fractures of the caudal acetabulum. Damage to the sciatic nerve may be present.
- Administer prophylactic antibiotics at the time of anesthetic induction.

Surgical Procedure

Objectives

- Anatomically reduce and stabilize the acetabulum to restore joint congruity and limb function.
- Relieve pain.
- Provide early restoration of pelvic limb function.
- Avoid iatrogenic sciatic nerve damage.

Equipment

- Standard general surgical pack and suture material
- Gelpi or Weitlaner self-retaining retractors
- Orthopedic surgical pack with AO-ASIF and Kern bone-holding forceps and Hohmann retractors
- Bone-plating equipment including acetabular and reconstruction plates
- Periosteal elevator
- Suction and electrocautery setups

Technique

1. Place the patient in lateral recumbency and stabilize the pelvis by placing sandbags under the patient. Secure the patient to the table.
2. Place a lubricated gauze sponge in the rectum, and place a pursestring suture in the anus.
3. Prepare the skin for aseptic surgery on the lateral and medial sides of the pelvic limb from the tarsocrural joint to the dorsal and ventral midline and from the mid-lumbar area to the base of the tail.
4. For fractures of the central and caudal regions of the acetabulum, use a combined dorsal and caudolateral approach to the hip joint.

▼ *Key Point* Make a separate surgical approach to the ischium and elevate the internal obturator and gemelli muscles to expose the ramus of the ischium. Placement of a Kern bone-holding forcep on the ramus of the ischium allows manipulation of the caudal bone fragment, while minimizing risk of iatrogenic damage to the sciatic nerve. Precontour a bone plate to an intact pelvis of equivalent size cadaver to minimize operating time and risk of wound infection.

5. Make a curved skin incision, centered over the caudal surface of the greater trochanter, beginning close to the dorsal midline, and ending at the junction of the proximal and middle thirds of the femur. Obtain hemostasis by careful electrocoagulation.
6. Incise and retract the subcutaneous tissues to expose the underlying musculature.
7. Dissection and fracture stabilization
   a. Incise the fascia of the biceps femoris muscle along its cranial border.
   b. Free the cranial part of the origin of the biceps femoris muscle from the sacrotuberous ligament. Transect the insertion of the superficial gluteal muscle on the third trochanter, and retract this muscle dorsally. Retract the biceps femoris muscle caudally.
   c. Identify and avoid the sciatic nerve.
   d. Perform a dorsal approach to the hip by tenotomy of the middle and deep gluteal muscles. If preferred, osteotomy of the greater trochanter of the femur may be performed as an alternative. Transect the combined tendons of the internal obturator and gemelli muscles close to their insertion in the trochanteric fossa. Retract these muscles by the use of a stay suture in the tendons. Retraction of these muscles indirectly retracts the sciatic nerve caudally.
   e. Retract the gluteal muscles dorsally. Part of the origin of the deep gluteal muscle may need to be elevated to expose the more cranial region of the acetabulum.
   f. Preserve as much of the joint capsule as possible. Do not elevate it from the acetabular bone. To observe the joint surface, perform a small radial arthrotomy.
   g. After exposing the fracture, use AO-ASIF small

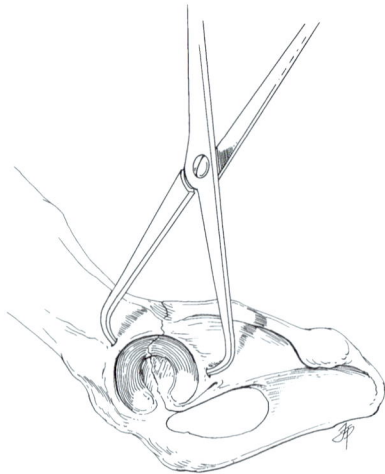

Figure 126–3. Two-piece fracture of the acetabulum that has been reduced with the aid of point-to-point bone-holding forceps, placed in a cranial-to-caudal direction in predrilled (1.5 mm) drill holes.

reduction forceps in combination with the Kern bone-holding forcep placed on the ischium to manipulate and reduce the fracture fragments. Bone-holding forceps placed on the greater trochanter also provide lateral traction and aid in manipulation of the femoral head for better identification of the fracture.

h. Fractures of the acetabulum are rarely stable immediately after reduction. Maintain reduction of the fracture by placing point-to-point bone-holding forceps craniocaudally across the acetabulum (Fig. 126–3). If necessary, place shallow drill holes (1.1 or 1.5 mm) in each fragment to prevent the point-to-point forceps from slipping. In addition, a 1.0-mm K-wire may be placed across the fracture.

i. After the fracture has been reduced, apply a precontoured bone plate. If interfragmentary compression is desirable, slightly overbend the plate.

j. Stabilize fractures of the acetabulum with an acetabular plate, a small DCP, or a reconstruction plate. Engage at least six cortices on each side of the fracture. Because of the thin cortical bone that is present in the pelvis, carefully drill and tap the screw holes. Select implants according to the guidelines in Table 126–2.

Table 126–2. GUIDELINES FOR IMPLANT SIZES FOR FRACTURES OF THE ACETABULUM IN DOGS AND CATS

Body Weight (kg)	Plate Size (mm)
<10	2.0 AP, 2.0 DCP, or 2.0 RP
10–20	2.0 or 2.7 AP, 2.7 DCP, or 2.7 RP
20–30	2.7 AP, 2.7 DCP, or 2.7 RP
>30	2.7 AP, 3.5 DCP, or 3.5 RP

AP, acetabular plate; DCP, dynamic compression plate; RP, reconstruction plate.

8. Closure
   a. If the joint capsule has been torn or incised, appose it with sutures in a simple interrupted pattern. Reattach the tendon of the internal obturator and gemelli muscles. Reattach the tendons of the gluteal muscles or stabilize the osteotomy of the greater trochanter of the femur with a tension band wire technique.
   b. Close the fascia (simple continuous pattern, absorbable suture), subcutaneous tissue (simple continuous pattern, absorbable suture), and skin (interrupted pattern, absorbable suture), or skin staples.
   c. Remove the pursestring suture from the anus.

Postoperative Care and Complications

See Fractures of the Ilium.

Prognosis

- The prognosis is good if anatomic reduction of the acetabulum is achieved, hip stability is maintained, and neurologic function is normal.
- If anatomic reduction is not achieved, the prognosis is fair to poor. Osteoarthritis is likely to develop, and further surgical or medical treatment may be necessary.
- The prognosis is guarded if femoral head excision is performed to repair a comminuted acetabular fracture.

SACROILIAC FRACTURE OR LUXATION

Preoperative Considerations

- If subluxation or luxation of the sacroiliac joint has occurred, craniodorsal displacement of the ilium is usually present, together with fractures in other regions of the pelvis. Bilateral sacroiliac joint separation may also occur.
- Perform a thorough neurologic examination, particularly when displacement of the fracture is marked or sacroiliac joint luxation is severe, because damage to the cauda equina nerve roots may be present.
- Because surgical treatment of sacroiliac fracture or luxation is technically difficult, undertake surgical treatment only after careful consideration of other options, including conservative management or referral.

▼ *Key Point* In many animals with sacroiliac luxation the displacement is not severe and the injury responds well to conservative management. However, successful reduction and stabilization of the sacroiliac joint relieves pain more quickly, allowing more rapid return to normal function. Anatomic reduction and rigid stabilization has a higher priority as a treatment option if neurological deficits are present.

- Administer prophylactic antibiotics at the time of anesthetic induction.

Surgical Procedure

Objectives

- Anatomically reduce and stabilize the sacrum and sacroiliac joints.
- Relieve pain.
- Provide early restoration of pelvic limb function.
- Avoid iatrogenic damage to the cauda equina nerve roots and sciatic nerve.

Equipment

- Standard general surgical pack and suture material
- Gelpi or Weitlaner self-retaining retractors
- Orthopedic surgical pack with AO-ASIF and Kern bone-holding forceps and Hohmann retractors
- Bone-plating equipment
- Periosteal elevator
- Suction and electrocautery setups

Technique

1. Place the patient in lateral or ventral recumbency, and stabilize the pelvis by placing sandbags under the patient. Secure the patient to the table.
2. Place a lubricated gauze sponge in the rectum, and place a pursestring suture in the anus.
3. Prepare the skin for aseptic surgery on the lateral and medial sides of the pelvic limb from the tarso-crural joint to the dorsal and ventral midline and from the midlumbar area to the base of the tail. With bilateral fracture or luxation, bilateral incisions may be necessary.
4. Use a dorsolateral or ventrolateral approach to the sacroiliac joint. (For the ventrolateral approach, see Fractures of the Ilium.) A dorsal approach may be used for bilateral sacroiliac fractures or luxations.
5. Make a skin incision for the dorsolateral approach over the crest of the ilium.
6. Incise and retract the cutaneous trunci muscle and the subcutaneous fat to expose the pelvic musculature.
7. Obtain hemostasis by careful electrocoagulation.
8. Dissection and fracture stabilization
   a. Incise the middle gluteal muscle along its origin at the cranial and dorsal borders of the wing of the ilium, and subperiosteally elevate it, beginning cranially.
   b. During dissection, protect and preserve the cranial gluteal artery, vein, and nerve, which cross medially to laterally over the caudal iliac spine, and enter the middle and deep gluteal muscles. The sacrospinalis muscle and dorsal sacroiliac ligament are usually disrupted and therefore require little additional dissection.
   c. Maneuver the ilium using Kern bone-holding forceps. Initially, displace the ilium ventrally and laterally to expose the articular surface of the sacrum.
   d. Place a drill hole in the body of the sacrum (Fig. 126–4). Align the drill hole perpendicular to the midsagittal plane, rather than perpendicular to the articular surface of the sacrum, in order to

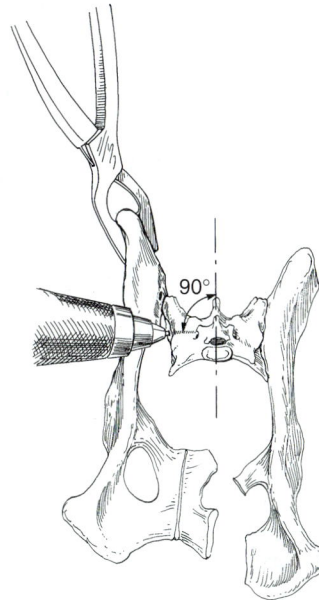

Figure 126–4. Surgical approach to sacroiliac luxation. Bone-holding forceps have been placed on the wing of the ilium to assist reduction. A hole has been drilled into the body of the sacrum in preparation for reduction of the luxation.

avoid misdirection of the screw dorsally or ventrally. Make the depth of the drill hole two-thirds of the width of the sacral body, and measure the hole with a depth gauge and tap the hole.
   e. The site on the medial surface of the ilium that corresponds to the drill hole in the sacrum determines the exact location of the drill hole on the lateral surface of the ilium. Overdrill the hole to allow compression of the sacroiliac joint with a fully threaded lag screw.
   f. Determine the length of the screw by adding the thickness of the ilium to the depth of the sacral drill hole. Select the size of the bone screw using the guidelines in Table 126–3.
   g. Place the screw into the ilium until the tip of the screw just protrudes from the medial surface. Reduce the sacroiliac joint and insert and tighten the screw to stabilize and compress the joint.
   h. If indicated, place a second screw just cranial and dorsal to the first to give two-point fixation. Determine the screw length by measurement from

---

Table 126–3. GUIDELINES FOR SCREW SIZES IN REPAIR OF SACROILIAC FRACTURE OR LUXATION IN DOGS AND CATS

Body Weight (kg)	Single Screw (mm)	Two Screws (mm)*
<10	2.7	2.7 and 2.0
10–20	3.5	3.5 and 2.7
20–30	4.5	4.5 and 3.5
>30	5.5	5.5 and 3.5

*Place the smaller screw craniodorsal to the larger screw, which is inserted into the body of the sacrum.

ventrodorsal radiographs, so that it does not penetrate the neural canal. A second screw may be necessary if the patient is a large dog, the sacrum is fractured, or the first screw is not ideally placed in the body of the sacrum.

i. With bilateral fractures or luxations, screw(s) may be placed bilaterally, or a single screw may be placed through both ilial wings and the sacral body. In the latter instance, use an aiming device to ensure that the drill hole is placed in the correct plane.

9. For closure, see Fractures of the Ilium.

Postoperative Care and Complications

Short-Term

- Because errors in screw placement are common, carefully evaluate immediate postoperative radiographs for screw placement.
- Closely monitor for hemorrhage and seroma formation.
- Good patient care is essential to encourage early mobility and return to normal function (see Conservative Treatment).

Long-Term

- If neurologic deficits are present, reevaluate the animal regularly for improvement in function. Intensive patient care may be necessary for a number of weeks after surgery.
- Obtain postoperative radiographs to monitor joint and fracture healing.
- Do not remove the bone screws from animals that have no clinical signs of implant-associated complications.

Prognosis

- The prognosis is good with correct positioning of the bone screws and no neurologic damage.
- If the bone screws do not correctly engage the sacral body, fixation failure is more likely.
- If neurologic deficits are present after surgery, the prognosis is guarded.

FRACTURES OF THE ISCHIUM

- Fractures of the ischium are usually associated with fractures of other major weight bearing regions of the pelvis. If appropriate surgery is performed to anatomically reduce and stabilize other, functionally more important fractures, additional fixation of ischial fractures is unnecessary.
- Fractures of the ischium are usually displaced ventrally as a consequence of tension created by the caudal thigh muscles (the biceps femoris, semitendinosus, and semimembranosus muscles).
- Occasionally, isolated fractures of the ischium may be encountered. If severe pain is associated with the fracture(s) or if displacement of the fracture fragments is such that the function of the hip joint is im-

paired, internal fixation may be indicated (see Fractures of the Acetabulum).

▼ **Key Point** Surgical repair of fractures of the ischium is usually unnecessary.

FRACTURES OF THE PUBIS

- Fractures of the pelvic symphysis, which is composed of the pubic and ischial symphyses, may be associated with fractures of other regions of the pelvis. This problem is more common in young animals in which bony union of the pelvic symphysis has not yet occurred.
- Anatomic reduction and stabilization of the other, functionally more important pelvic fractures usually makes surgical treatment of the pubic fracture unnecessary. However, internal fixation of pubic fractures may occasionally be indicated.
- If pubic fractures are associated with a caudal abdominal wall rupture and herniation of abdominal or pelvic organs, surgical repair of the hernia may be assisted by internal fixation of the fractures. Cerclage wire is usually the preferred method for fixation.

NARROWED PELVIC CANAL ASSOCIATED WITH HEALED PELVIC FRACTURES

- Obstipation and dystocia are occasionally associated with healed pelvic fractures and a narrowed pelvic canal. This problem is most commonly encountered in cats and small dogs whose pelvic fractures are more likely to be managed conservatively.
- Manage dystocia by cesarean section or ovariohysterectomy.
- Operations designed to widen the pelvic canal have been described. Osteotomy of the ilium, the ischium, and the pubis, and lateralization of the caudal fragment with a plate is the preferred method.
- In dogs and cats with obstipation as a consequence of a narrowed pelvic canal, subtotal colectomy may be necessary (see Chap. 90), because colonic dysfunction is not always relieved by corrective osteotomy and use of a motility modifier such as cisapride.

▼ **Key Point** If obstipation has been present for several months, normal colonic motility does not always return after the bony pelvic canal has been widened, and obstipation can continue to be a problem.

SUPPLEMENTAL READINGS

Brinker WO, Piermattei DL, Flo GL: Handbook of Small Animal Orthopedics and Fracture Treatment, 3rd Ed. Philadelphia: WB Saunders, 1997.

DeCamp CE, Braden TD: The surgical anatomy of the canine sacrum for lag screw fixation of the sacroiliac joint. Vet Surg 14:131, 1985.

Olmstead ML: Small Animal Orthopaedics. St. Louis: CV Mosby, 1995.

127 Disorders of the Coxofemoral Joint

Marvin L. Olmstead

The coxofemoral joint is the most proximal of the free-moving joints of the pelvic limb. Surgery is frequently performed on or near this joint to treat conditions such as coxofemoral luxations and hip dysplasia. Avascular necrosis of the femoral head, which occurs infrequently, also can be treated surgically.

Anatomic considerations, pathophysiology, and treatment of these conditions of the coxofemoral joint are discussed in this chapter.

ANATOMY

- The coxofemoral joint is a ball-and-socket joint made up of the femoral head and the acetabulum.
- In a normal animal, the joint capsule attaches to the rim of the acetabulum and around the circumference of the femoral neck just distal to the junction of the head and neck. When the limb is taken through range-of-motion exercises, the joint capsule maintains joint congruency.
- The ligament of the head of the femur runs between the acetabular fossa and the fovea capitis of the femoral head.
  - The fovea and the fossa are sometimes mistakenly identified as radiographic abnormalities.

▼ *Key Point* The fovea causes a natural flattened area on the femoral head that can be mistaken for the flattening associated with hip dysplasia. The fossa creates a shadow that can be mistaken for a fracture line.

- The blood supply to the femoral head is extensive.
  - Small arterial loops arise from the iliolumbar artery cranially; the lateral circumflex femoral artery dorsally, cranially, and ventrally; and the medial circumflex femoral artery dorsally, caudally, and ventrally. They all penetrate the femoral head at the joint capsule attachment.
  - No significant blood vessels penetrate the femoral head from the ligament of the head of the femur.
- Several surgically important muscles have their insertions or origins close to the coxofemoral joint, either on the proximal femur or the pelvis.
  - The middle and deep gluteal muscles originate on the wing of the ilium and insert on the dorsal and cranial border of the greater trochanter.

- The superficial gluteal muscle originates on the sacrum and the first coccygeal vertebra and inserts on the third trochanter.
- The internal and external obturator and gemelli muscles insert in the caudal trochanteric fossa.
- The vastus lateralis and intermedius muscles originate on the cranial aspect of the femur, whereas the rectus femoris originates on the pelvis cranial to the acetabulum.
- The tensor fascia lata muscle originates along the caudolateral edge of the femur, covering the vastus lateralis muscle, and along the cranial edge of the biceps femoris muscle via three or more tissue slips.
- The origin of the pectineus muscle is just ventral to the acetabulum.
- Two angles of surgical significance have been described in the proximal femur:
  - When the femur is viewed from a cranial position, the *angle of inclination* is the angle formed between a line that bisects the long axis of the femur and a line that bisects the femoral neck. In the normal dog, this angle is 135–145°.
  - When the femur is viewed from a straight lateral position, the axis of the femoral neck is displaced cranially in reference to the femoral shaft. This is the torsion angle and in dogs this angle is positive and called anteversion. One method of measuring this angle involves taking radiographs of the femur with the dog on its back with the long axis of the femur positioned 90° to the radiographic plate and the stifle flexed 90°. The radiographic beam must pass directly down the center of the femur, parallel to its long axis. One line is drawn parallel to the caudal edge of the femoral condyles, and a second bisects the femoral head and neck. The angle created by the intersection of these two lines is the *anteversion angle*, which, in normal dogs is 20–27°.
  - Abnormal alterations can occur in these angles during hip development, resulting in pathology in the hip or further distally in the limb.

COXOFEMORAL LUXATIONS

Most coxofemoral luxations are craniodorsal displacements of the femoral head; almost all others are caudoventrally displaced. Usually these are associated with motor vehicle accidents; thus, full evaluation of other organ systems for trauma (see Chaps. 3 and 82), as well as coxofemoral joint evaluation, is indicated in these patients.

Diagnosis

▼ *Key Point* The evaluation of the coxofemoral joint for luxation includes gait analysis, manipulation of the hip, comparison of hindlimb lengths, and two radiographic views of the pelvis.

- Animals with a luxated hip usually will not bear weight on the affected limb. If a craniodorsal luxation is present, the limb may be externally rotated and adducted.
- Range-of-motion evaluation of the hip may reveal grating and/or pain in the area of the coxofemoral joint.
- Evaluate the relationship between the caudal edge of the greater trochanter and the cranial edge of the ischiatic tuberosity to determine the position of the proximal femur.
  - If a caudoventral luxation is present, there will be no space between these two structures.
  - If a craniodorsal luxation is present, there will be a wide space that does not close (as in the normal animal) when the limb is externally rotated.
- When both hindlimbs are pulled directly caudally, they will be equal length in a normal animal. If they are uneven in length, this is a strong indication that the coxofemoral joint is dislocated.
- The primary method of diagnosis is radiography of the coxofemoral joint to
  - Rule out fractures of the proximal femur which can mimic a luxation on physical examination.
  - Evaluate the acetabulum for an avulsion fracture from the femoral head (an absolute indication for surgery) or acetabular fracture.

Closed Reduction

If there is no avulsion fracture, perform closed reduction of the joint under general anesthesia.
- To perform reduction for a craniodorsal luxation
  - Grasp the foot just distal to the talocrural joint and externally rotate the limb.
  - Then externally rotate the femoral head.
  - Apply distal traction to the limb until the femoral head is even with the acetabulum; and then rotate the femoral head internally, causing it to drop into the acetabulum (Fig. 127–1).
- Reduction of a caudoventral luxation is accomplished by abducting and externally rotating the limb.
- The longer the femoral head is luxated craniodorsally, the more damage that is done to the dorsal joint capsule. An intact joint capsule is helpful in maintaining reduction.
- If the reduced hip easily luxates again, perform open reduction.
- If the reduced hip snaps solidly into position, place the hip in a flexion sling for a craniodorsal luxation;

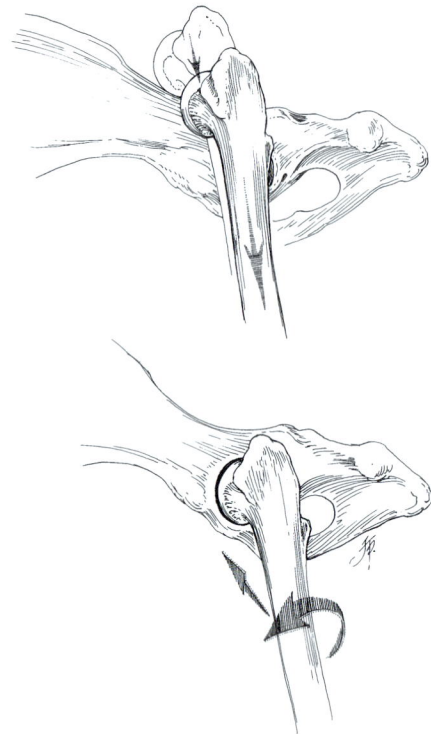

Figure 127–1. Closed reduction of the coxofemoral joint. External rotation and distal traction of the limb *(top)* is followed by internal rotation of the femoral head *(bottom).*

place the legs in hobbles for a caudoventral luxation (Fig. 127–2). Apply these restriction bandages for 10–14 days in the adult and 7–10 days in the immature animal. Limit exercise during this period, and for an additional 2–4 weeks.
- Examine the reduced hip physically on a daily basis or instruct the owner to do this, until the restriction bandage is removed.
  - If there is any question about the hip's position, reevaluate with lateral pelvic radiographs. If the hip is reluxated, perform an open reduction.

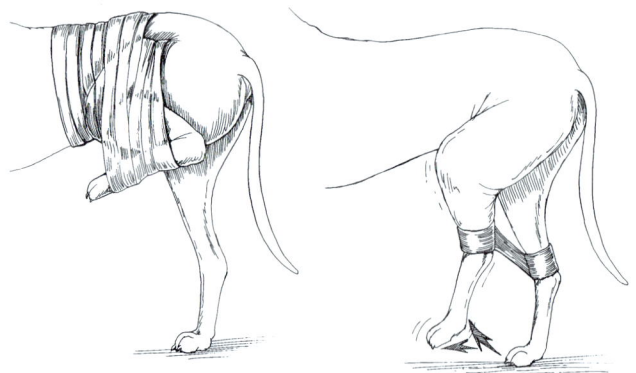

Figure 127–2. After reduction, use a flexion (Ehmer) sling for a craniodorsal luxation *(left)* and hobbles for a caudoventral luxation *(right).*

Open Reduction—Surgical Procedures

Objectives

- Reduce the luxated coxofemoral joint.
- Reconstruct as much soft tissue as possible.
- Remove fibrous tissue from the acetabulum, remnants of the ligament of the head of the femur, and avulsed bone fragments that cannot be stabilized.

Equipment

- Standard surgery pack and suture material
- Special equipment as needed for specific procedures (noted in following text)

Techniques

1. The standard approaches used for surgical repair of luxations are the cranial lateral approach to the hip and the trochanteric osteotomy approach. Occasionally a caudal approach (caudal to the greater trochanter of the femur) to the coxofemoral joint may be used.
2. Initially, assess the overall damage and the status of supporting tissues, clean out the acetabular cup, and reduce the femoral head into the acetabulum.
3. Once reduced, use one or more stabilization techniques to secure the femoral head into the acetabulum.
4. If the joint capsule is minimally damaged and adequate capsular tissue is present on either side of the tear, suture the capsule (this may be the only support necessary).
   a. Use an absorbable monofilament suture of significant size (2-0, 0, or 1, depending on the animal's size), placed in a cruciate pattern.
   b. If adequate capsule is attached to the acetabular rim but not enough solid capsule is attached to the femoral neck, drill an anchor hole with lateral to cranial orientation in the proximal femur. Pass one-half of the suture strands through the hole and tie them tightly to the other half of the strands (Fig. 127–3).

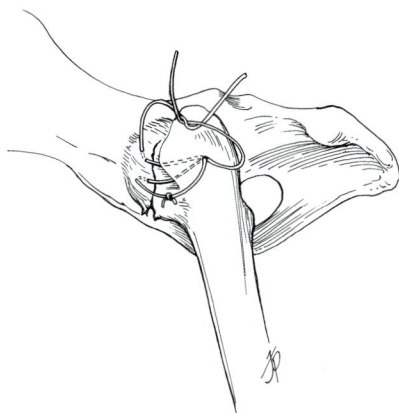

Figure 127–4. Suture support for coxofemoral luxation with a damaged joint capsule.

5. The capsule may be so severely damaged that it cannot hold a conventionally placed suture. (This may occur if there is a long delay between the time of injury and repair.)
   a. In these cases suture support can be provided by making anchor points for the sutures. Drill a hole (as described in Step 4b above) for an anchor site in the femur. Place one to three bone screws (usually a 3.5-mm cortical screw) in the dorsal rim over the acetabulum as anchor points on the pelvis. Place the suture support between these to form a dorsal reinforcement (Fig. 127–4).
   b. Alternatively, place a temporary intramedullary pin in the proximal femur, parallel with the neck axis, and through the acetabular fossa. Be sure that the pin does not extend too far into the pelvic canal (Fig. 127–5). Keep the limb immobile with a flexion sling until the pin is removed, 7–10 days after surgery.
   c. Another alternative is to place a toggle pin through a hole in the acetabular fossa with suture attached to it. This creates an artificial ligament between the head of the femur and the acetabulum. Pass the suture through a hole drilled, from lateral to medial, in the proximal femur. The

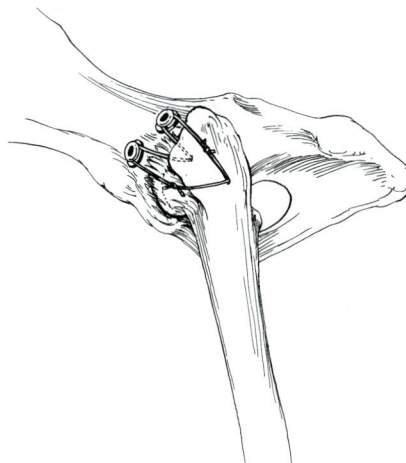

Figure 127–3. Surgical repair of luxation if adequate capsule remains attached to the acetabular rim. An anchor hole has been drilled in the proximal femur.

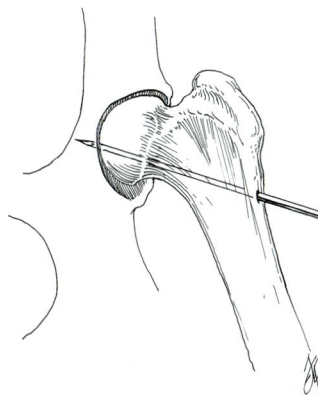

Figure 127–5. Temporary intramedullary pin for open reduction of coxofemoral joint.

hole enters the femur just dorsal to the third trochanter and exits at the insertion point of the ligament of the head of the femur on the femoral head. Pull all the suture strands through this hole, and then pass half the suture strands through a second hole in the femur drilled in a cranial to caudal direction. Tie the two sets of suture strands together.

6. Rotate the femoral head inwardly, and tighten the gluteal muscle pull on the femur by moving the greater trochanter to a position caudal and distal to its original location. This technique can be used with a trochanteric osteotomy approach.

    a. Do not depend on this technique as the sole means of stabilization.

    b. Any positional changes in gait caused by this relocation are temporary, because the gluteal muscles eventually will stretch.

7. If the femoral head does not remain in the acetabulum even with the application of support techniques, consider a primary salvage procedure such as excision arthroplasty or total hip replacement.

Postoperative Care and Complications

- If there is any doubt about the strength or security of the stabilization, place the limb in an immobilization sling or bandage for 7–14 days.
- Examine the sling or bandage and the visible parts of the limb daily for odor, chewing, swelling, pressure sore development, and slippage.
- Check the spatial relationship between the greater trochanter and the ischiatic tuberosity daily. If this changes, evaluate the position of the femur with lateral radiography of the pelvis. This can be accomplished without removing the sling.
- Restrict the animal's activity (leash walking only) for 1 month after the surgery.
- The most common complication following surgery or closed reduction is reluxation. If reluxation occurs after open reduction, consider excision arthroplasty or total hip replacement.

AVASCULAR NECROSIS OF THE FEMORAL HEAD

- This condition (also known as Legg-Perthes or Legg-Calvé-Perthes disease, osteochondritis juvenilis, and coxa plana) is most commonly found in adolescent, small-breed dogs of either sex; occasionally it occurs in large breeds.
- Trauma is not usually associated with the onset of lameness, and the lameness can progress to non–weight bearing.
- The condition occurs bilaterally in about 15% of the animals.
- Changes in the proximal femur seen radiographically and grossly are the result of collapse and remodeling of the trabecular bone of the femoral head following the avascular episode.

- It is not clear what causes the femoral head to become avascular; following this, the bone revascularizes and remodels as the dead bone undergoes resorption.
- Weight bearing causes the weakened subchondral bone to collapse, which, in turn, leads to fracture of the cartilage.

Diagnosis

- Base the diagnosis on physical examination and radiographic findings. Abduction of the limb often elicits a pain response, even before radiographic signs are evident. Crepitus is sometimes observed with flexion and extension of the joint.
- The limb may be shortened and the muscles atrophied.
- Radiographs are needed for a definitive diagnosis. The ventrodorsal straight-leg view of the pelvis is the most helpful in assessing the femoral heads.
    - The joint space may be widened, and numerous foci of decreased bone density may be seen in the femoral head and neck.
    - In advanced stages, there may be irregular indentations, flattening, and possibly fragmentation of the femoral head. Osteophytes on the acetabular rim and secondary osteoarthritis in the joint may also be seen.

Supportive Treatment

Some dogs respond to nonsurgical treatment including limited activity and analgesics. However, in most cases surgery is ultimately necessary.

▼ *Key Point* Surgical treatment of avascular necrosis of the femoral head has a much higher success rate than nonsurgical treatment.

Surgical Procedures

Objectives

- Eliminate painful bone-to-bone contact.
- Preserve hip motion as close to normal as possible.

Equipment

- Standard surgical pack and suture material
- Specialized equipment, depending on the specific procedure

Preoperative Considerations

- Because most of the dogs with this condition are small breeds, excision arthroplasty (discussed below) is the most common procedure performed for this disease.
- In large dogs, consider total hip replacement (see next section) as an option.

HIP DYSPLASIA

Hip dysplasia is a faulty development of the hip joint characterized by varying degrees of joint laxity that permit subluxation early in life. As the condition progresses, deformation of the architecture of the acetabulum and femoral head is accompanied by the development of degenerative joint disease.

▼ *Key Point* Hip dysplasia is the most prevalent disorder of the canine hip and the most important cause of osteoarthritis in that joint.

- Although almost all breeds are at risk, hip dysplasia most commonly affects large- and giant-breed dogs, and its mode of inheritance is polygenetic.
- Joint instability occurs as muscle development and maturation lag behind the rate of skeletal growth.
  - The first 60 days of life are the most critical period for the developing soft tissue structures.
  - When the stress and weight exerted at the hip joint exceed the strength limits of the supporting soft tissues, joint instability results.

Diagnosis

Base the diagnosis of hip dysplasia on the history, physical examination, and radiographic evaluation of the coxofemoral joints.

Physical Examination

- Lameness of the hindlimb and gait abnormalities frequently are seen, especially after exercise periods; motion of the coxofemoral joint often is limited because of joint pain.
- Joint laxity and pain may be elicited by examination of the range of motion of the coxofemoral joint. Joint laxity is present in mild to moderately dysplastic animals.
- Ortolani sign: With a hand placed on the knee of the affected limb, apply dorsal pressure to the femur while moving the bone from an adducted to an abducted position.
  - The click or pop that is heard or felt as the femoral head reenters the acetabulum is a positive Ortolani sign and an indication of joint laxity.
  - If the hip is normal or if arthritic changes in the acetabulum preclude movement of the femoral head in and out of the acetabulum, the Ortolani sign is negative.

Radiography

Radiographs are needed for a positive diagnosis of hip dysplasia.

- In early cases, proper positioning of the ventrodorsal view is extremely critical; in advanced stages, the changes are pronounced and positioning is less important.
- Radiographic changes associated with hip dysplasia range from subluxation of the femoral head to severe secondary degenerative joint disease, with marked alterations in the architecture of the femoral head and the acetabulum.

Nonsurgical Therapy

Nonsurgical therapy is recommended for animals mildly affected by hip dysplasia and those with an initial episode of lameness.

- Restrict activity to allow the inflammatory response within the joint capsule to subside.
- Give medication to relieve pain and reduce the inflammation associated with the degenerative joint disease. Aspirin (20 mg/kg q12h) or carprofen (2.2 mg/kg q12h PO) is sometimes adequate.

▼ *Key Point* When nonsurgical therapy is no longer effective or if the patient is constantly disabled over an extended period, consider one of the following surgical therapies.

Surgical Procedures—Overview

Various surgical procedures that have been effective in the treatment of hip dysplasia are discussed. An improved quality of life for the patient is the ultimate goal. The procedures are not listed in any order of preference.

Triple Pelvic Osteotomy

Preoperative Considerations

- In the ideal candidate for the procedure, there is some coverage of the femoral head by the acetabulum, the Ortolani sign is positive, and there are no signs of degenerative joint disease in the hip.
- Most dogs that meet the above criteria are 5–11 months of age.
- The animal should show clinical signs associated with hip dysplasia.

Objectives

- Increase the amount of acetabular coverage over the femoral head by rotating the acetabular portion of the pelvis.
- Maintain the normal architecture and congruency of the femoral head and acetabulum.
- Prevent or minimize the development of degenerative joint disease.

Equipment

- Standard surgical pack and suture material
- Equipment necessary to insert bone screws
- Bone plates designed for pelvic osteotomy (e.g., pelvic osteotomy plate; Synthes USA, Paoli, PA; Slocum Enterprises, Inc., Eugene, OR)
- Orthopedic wire
- Oscillating bone saw
- Osteotomes

Technique

1. Expose the ilium, pubis, and ischium
   a. Make a lateral approach to the wing of the ilium with dorsal elevation of the middle and deep gluteal muscles (see Chap. 126).
   b. Approach the pubis through a second incision over the pectineus muscle or through the lateral approach to the ilium by retracting the vastus muscles caudally and the rectus femoris muscle cranially.

c. The approach to the ischium depends on the site of the osteotomy. If the osteotomy is performed from the ischial tuberosity cranial to the obturator foramen, make an approach directly over the tuberosity. If the osteotomy is performed just caudal to the acetabulum, extend the lateral incision and reflect the biceps femoris muscle caudally.

2. Perform osteotomies at the ilium, pubis, and ischium so that the acetabulum can be rotated in a manner that provides more dorsal coverage of the femoral head.

3. Hold the tilt on the acetabulum in place with bone plates if a transverse osteotomy has been performed, or with screws and orthopedic wire if a stair-step osteotomy is done.

4. The osteotomy of the ischium may be stabilized with orthopedic wire.

5. Close the incisions routinely.

Postoperative Care and Complications

- Restrict activity for 8 weeks.
- Immediate postoperative radiographs may indicate no apparent change in the acetabular coverage of the femoral head. In some cases, subsequent radiographic evaluations reveal improved acetabular coverage and a femoral head well seated in the acetabulum.
- Occasionally, the desired amount of femoral head coverage is never achieved. This most often occurs when a patient has a totally luxated hip or when many degenerative changes are present at the time of surgery.
- If the acetabulum is rotated too far at the time of surgery, extension of the coxofemoral joint will be limited and result in a gait alteration.

Femoral Head and Neck Excision Arthroplasty

Preoperative Considerations

This salvage procedure can be performed in dogs of all ages; it is most successful in dogs weighing less than 18 kg.

Objectives

- Remove the femoral head and neck.
- Eliminate painful contact points in the joint.
- Allow a fibrous tissue joint ("false joint") to replace the ball and socket joint.

Equipment

- Standard surgical pack and suture material
- Mallet and osteotome, oscillating bone saw, or bone cutter
- Rongeur or rasp

Technique

1. Use a cranial lateral approach or a ventral approach (pectineal myotomy near its origin on the prepubic tendon).

2. Perform osteotomy of the femoral neck by cutting the bone from the lateralmost edge of the tro-

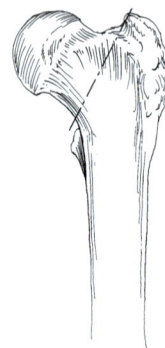

Figure 127-6. Site of osteotomy for femoral head and neck excision arthroplasty.

chanteric fossa to a point just dorsal to the lesser trochanter (Fig. 127-6).

3. Remove the femoral head and neck. It may be necessary to incise the ligament of the head of the femur. If using a ventral approach, this is done following osteotomy of the femoral neck. If using a cranial lateral approach, this is done before osteotomy so that the head and neck can be better exposed by rotating the femur externally 90° and luxating the femoral head from the acetabulum.

4. Examine the remaining portion of the proximal femur for rough areas or bone spurs and remove any, if present.

5. Close the incision routinely.

Postoperative Care and Complications

- Encourage use of the operated limb 3–7 days postoperatively. Use passive range-of-motion exercise on patients that do not willingly use the limb.
- Obtain radiographs to document the amount and configuration of the remaining bone.
- On the average it will take 2–3 months for the limb to reach its satisfactory functional level. In some animals the gait is indistinguishable from normal; in others an obvious gait abnormality is present.
- Because a false joint is formed after surgery, all animals have a limited range of motion. The clinical significance of this limitation depends on the activity of the animal, the animal's size, and the amount of restrictive scar tissue that is present.
- Because normal muscle mass is not regained there may be marked atrophy of the limb.
- The femur may displace dorsally relative to the pelvis. If the displacement is large, a post-legged gait with the stifle at nearly full extension can result.

Pectineal Myectomy

Preoperative Considerations

- This procedure can be done on dogs of all ages.
- Performance of this procedure does not exclude attempting other procedures, should this be unsuccessful.
- This procedure does not alter the progression or intensity of changes in the joint caused by hip dysplasia, but may palliate joint pain.

Objectives

- Remove all of the belly of the pectineus muscle bilaterally.
- Decrease tension on the medial aspect of the coxofemoral joint capsule.

Equipment

Standard surgical pack and suture material

Technique

1. Place the patient in a dorsal recumbent frog-leg position.
2. Make an incision 10–16 cm long over the pectineus muscle on the medial aspect of the thigh.
3. Isolate and incise the muscle at its origin proximally and its muscle-tendon junction distally. Take care to avoid the femoral artery and vein that pass lateral to the middle of the muscle belly.
4. Close the dead space tightly by meticulous suture of the fascia and subcutaneous layers.

Postoperative Care and Complications

- Restrict activity for 2 weeks.
- The most common postoperative complication is seroma formation. This requires aspiration or drainage only if the seromas become very large. Usually the fluid is absorbed and no treatment is needed.
- In some dogs, the gait is noticeably improved and there seems to be marked pain relief. The length of time for which this relief persists varies.

Intertrochanteric Osteotomy

Preoperative Considerations

- Patient selection is important. Qualifications include:
  - A marked increase in the angle of anteversion and/or inclination (see previous discussion under Anatomy)
  - No degenerative changes in the joint
  - Age close to skeletal maturity (6–8 months) or older
  - Clinical signs associated with hip dysplasia

Objectives

- Decrease the angles of inclination and anteversion.
- Position the femoral head more deeply in the acetabular cup.

Equipment

- Standard surgical pack and suture material
- Intertrochanteric osteotomy bone plates and 3.5-mm cortex screws (Synthes)
- Intertrochanteric osteotomy instrument set (Synthes)
- Oscillating bone saw

Technique

1. Approach the femur craniolaterally, exposing the cranial surface of the femoral neck.
2. Perform a transverse intertrochanteric osteotomy.

3. Perform a second osteotomy along a preplanned line that allows removal of a wedge of bone and a decrease in the angle of inclination to less than normal, thus creating a coxa vara position.
4. Decrease the angle of anteversion to normal by rotating the proximal femur caudally.
5. Rigidly fix the bone segments in position with a 3.5-mm hook plate (Synthes) or with standard bone plates.
6. Close the incision routinely.

Postoperative Care and Complications

- Restrict activity for 8 weeks.
- A significant number of patients are pain-free and function with normal mobility.
- Degenerative joint disease continues to develop in most patients.

Total Hip Replacement

This procedure, which provides an artificial femoral head and artificial acetabular cup, demands a high degree of technical proficiency and strict adherence to good aseptic and surgical techniques. Referral to an experienced specialist is recommended.

Preoperative Considerations

- The growth plates must be closed before this procedure can be performed; thus, the animal must be at least 9 months of age. There is no upper age limit, but older animals should be fully evaluated for systemic disease.
- Depending on the size of the femur and the depth of the acetabular cup, the minimum weight of the animal is 13–18 kg.
- Consider total hip replacement when a disabling condition of the hip exists with no other systemic or hindlimb pathology. The dog must be totally free of infection anywhere in the body.

Objectives

- Replace the degenerative coxofemoral joint with a high-density polyethylene cup and a cobalt chrome femoral prosthesis.
- Provide a mechanically sound, pain-free joint that will last the dog's life.

Equipment

- Standard surgical pack and suture material
- Reaming and implantation instruments designed specifically for canine total hip replacements (BioMedtrix, Allendale, NJ)
- Ultra-high-density polyethylene cup, a cobalt chrome femoral head, and a cobalt chrome femoral stem (BioMedtrix)
- Oscillating bone saw
- Power drill

Technique

1. Approach the coxofemoral joint through a craniolateral approach.

2. Remove the femoral head and a portion of the neck along an osteotomy line that parallels the collar of the prosthesis, and ream the acetabular cup to the medial pelvic wall. Ream and broach the medullary cavity of the femur to accept a trial femoral stem.

3. Cement the prosthetic acetabular cup and the femoral stem into position with polymethylmethacrylate (Howemedica).

4. After the femoral head is secured onto the stem, reduce it into the cup.

5. Close the joint capsule tightly; close the remaining tissues in layers.

Postoperative Care and Complications

- Restrict activity to leash walking for 3 months, after which the dog can return to full activity, even if it includes vigorous work.

- Over 95% of dogs treated with this procedure have satisfactory function if established techniques are followed. Increased muscle mass, extended exercise tolerance, and improved hip motion commonly are observed.

- Although degenerative joint disease usually is present in both hips, 80% of dogs receive sufficient relief that the other hip does not need to be replaced. The limb with the hip replacement becomes dominant, thus reducing the unoperated limb's weight bearing load.

- Complications include infection, implant loosening, luxations, fractures, and neurapraxia. The majority of these can be successfully treated.

SUPPLEMENTAL READINGS

Brinker WO, Piermattei DL, Flo GL: Diagnosis and treatment of orthopedic conditions of the hindlimb. *In* Brinker WO, Piermattei D, Gretchen F: Handbook of Small Animal Orthopedics and Fracture Treatment, 2nd Ed. Philadelphia: WB Saunders, 1990, p 341.

Hauptman J: The hip joint. *In* Slatter D, ed.: Textbook of Small Animal Surgery. Philadelphia: WB Saunders, 1985, p 2135.

Olmstead ML: The canine cemented modular total hip prosthesis: Surgical technique and preliminary clinical results. J Am Anim Hosp Assoc 31:109, 1995.

Schrader SC: Triple pelvic osteotomy of the pelvis as a treatment for canine hip dysplasia. J Am Vet Med Assoc 178:39, 1981.

128 Fractures of the Femur

Peter Shires

Surgery of the femur usually is performed to repair fractures. Biopsy of tumors or cysts or obtaining samples for bone cultures are less common reasons for femoral surgery. The femur is the bone most commonly associated with traumatic fractures in the dog. Surgical repair of femoral injuries may be divided into surgery of the proximal, diaphyseal, and distal femur.

PROXIMAL FEMUR

Anatomy

- The proximal femur includes the femoral head, the femoral neck, the trochanters, and their attachments to the femoral shaft.
- The ligament of the head of the femur runs from the fovea capitis of the femoral head to the acetabular fossa.
- The articular surface and epiphysis of the femoral head are separated from the femoral neck by the capital physis.
- The joint capsule of the hip joint inserts at about the midpoint of the femoral neck.
- The primary blood supply to the epiphysis of the femoral head is through vessels running longitudinally in folds of the joint capsule (Fig. 128–1).
- The greater trochanter is the point of attachment for the deep and middle gluteal muscles and the piriformis muscle (Fig. 128–1).
- The trochanteric fossa is the site of insertion of the internal obturator, external obturator, and the gemelli muscles.
- The articularis coxae inserts on the cranial aspect of the femoral neck.
- The lesser trochanter on the medial aspect of the proximal femur is the site of insertion of the iliopsoas muscle.
- The third trochanter (lateral and distal to the greater trochanter) is the site of insertion of the superficial gluteal muscle and the origin of the quadratus femoris muscle and part of the vastus lateralis muscle.
- The proximal femur is the site of origin of the vastus lateralis, vastus medialis, vastus intermedius, quadratus femoris, and adductor longis muscles and of the proximal part of the adductor magnus and adductor brevis muscles.

- The deep muscles of the femur are covered by the tensor fasciae latae and biceps femoris muscle confluence.
- The sciatic nerve runs caudal to the hip on top of the gemelli, internal obturator, and quadratus femoris muscles. It is covered by the biceps femoris and the superficial gluteal muscles.
- The femoral artery, nerve, and vein are very superficial in the femoral triangle on the medial aspect of the proximal to midfemur.
- The nutrient artery for the femur enters caudally just distal to the greater trochanter as a branch of the medial circumflex femoral artery.

TREATMENT OF PROXIMAL FEMORAL FRACTURES

Preoperative Considerations

▼ *Key Point* Evaluate the entire patient for trauma-related problems; neurologic, urologic, and intrathoracic injuries are common with blunt trauma.

- Stabilize the patient before considering surgery.
- Obtain a minimum of two radiographic views to evaluate the proximal femur.
- Give intraoperative broad-spectrum antibiotics IV (at induction of anesthesia; repeat if necessary) if the surgery will take longer than 2 hours.
- Continue treatment with systemic antibiotics if the fracture is open (see Chap. 140).

Surgical Procedure

Objectives (for all proximal femoral injuries)

- Expose the femoral neck.
- Osteotomize the femoral neck.
- Repair fractures of the capital physis and femoral neck.
- Expose the greater trochanter for osteotomy and fixation.
- Expose the proximal femur for fracture repair.

Equipment

- Standard general instrument pack and suture material

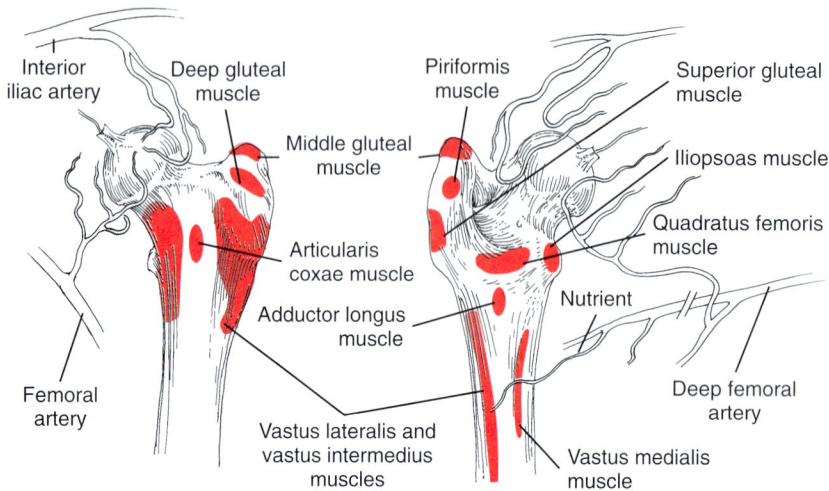

Figure 128–1. *Left,* Cranial view; *right,* caudal view. Proximal femur showing the muscle attachments and main blood supply.

- Orthopedic instruments, as required (e.g., for fracture fixation, ostectomy, subtrochanteric derotational osteotomy), including:
  - Intramedullary pins
  - Orthopedic and Kirschner wires (K-wires)
  - Osteotomes and mallet or oscillating bone saw
  - Plates and screws
  - Bone reduction forceps
- Self-retaining retractors (e.g., Gelpi, Weitlaner)
- Hohmann retractors (for femoral head ostectomy)

Operative Techniques

Techniques are similar for all objectives listed. Increased exposure is necessary to accomplish more complicated procedures. Techniques are described in order of procedure completion.

Common (Craniolateral) Approach

Technique

1. Prepare the affected leg for aseptic surgery.
2. Make a linear or slightly curved skin incision centered over the cranial aspect of the greater trochanter, starting near the dorsal midline and ending on the cranial aspect of the proximal one-third of the femur.
3. Incise the subcutaneous tissue to expose the tensor fasciae latae muscle. Incise two layers of the fasciae latae along the cranial border of the biceps femoris muscle to expose the underlying vastus lateralis muscle.
4. Extend the fascial incision proximally through the gluteal fascia along the cranial border of the superficial gluteal muscle.
5. Bluntly dissect the loose connective tissue between the vastus lateralis muscle and the gluteal muscles to allow insertion of self-retaining retractors to expose the joint capsule.

▼ *Key Point* Several vessels, including the cranial femoral artery and vein and the branches of the femoral nerve, crisscross the connective tissue and will be significantly damaged if dissection is rough.

6. Using a scalpel, incise through the joint capsule from the acetabulum, longitudinally along the femoral neck, to the proximal femur at the insertion of the vastus lateralis muscle.
7. If necessary, partially incise the tendon of insertion of the deep gluteal muscle and the origin of the vastus lateralis muscle to increase exposure of the femoral neck.

Femoral Head and Neck Ostectomy

See Chapter 127.

Femoral Neck/Capital Physeal Fracture Repair

Technique

1. Rotate the femur outward to expose the fractured surface.
2. Retrograde a K-wire of appropriate size through the femoral neck fracture surface to exit the lateral surface of the proximal femur.
3. If a compression (lag) screw is used, drill a gliding hole through the center of the femoral neck to exit the lateral surface of the proximal femur.
4. If multiple K-wires are used, preplace them all through the femoral neck, using the same technique as described in Step 2 above.
5. Withdraw the wires from the lateral surface until the pinpoints are flush with the fracture surface.
6. Rotate the femur inward to reduce the fracture.
7. Rotate the femoral head until the fracture is anatomically aligned.
8. Advance one K-wire into the femoral head without penetrating the articular surface (Fig. 128–2, *left*).
9. If a compression screw is used, insert a drill sleeve into the gliding hole and drill into the femoral head. The articular cartilage should not be penetrated. Measure and tap the hole and place a screw of suitable length. Compress the fracture without penetrating the articular surface with the screw (Fig. 128–2, *right*).
10. If K-wires are used, drive these individually into the head without penetrating the articular cartilage.

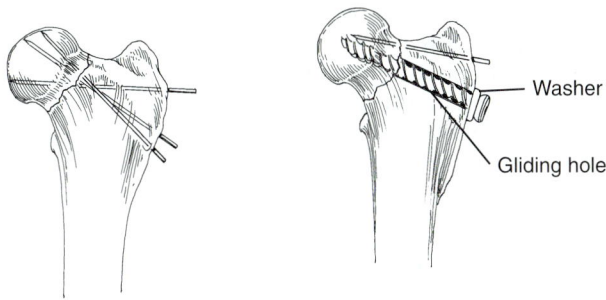

Figure 128–2. Fixation of femoral neck fractures. *Left,* Multiple Kirschner wires; *right,* compression screw and Kirschner wire.

▼ *Key Point* Lifting and rotating the proximal femur allows limited examination of the femoral head surface to check for penetration by the implants. Movement of the femur should be unrestricted and smooth and should not produce crepitation.

11. Bend the K-wires over close to the lateral aspect of the trochanter and cut them off as short as possible.

Trochanteric Osteotomy

This technique is used for exposure of the hip joint as part of open reduction of coxofemoral luxation or as an approach to acetabular fractures (see Chap. 127).

Technique

1. Incise the tendon of the superficial gluteal muscle near the third trochanter.
2. Retract the belly of the superficial gluteal muscle proximally.
3. Incise the proximal origin of the vastus lateralis muscle and elevate the muscle to expose the trochanteric osteotomy (or fracture) site, or the femoral neck fracture site.
4. If necessary for exposure, incise and elevate the adductor muscle origin caudally.
5. If a trochanteric osteotomy is planned, pass a curved Kelly forceps under the deep gluteal insertion.
6. Using the curved Kelly forceps as a guide, direct the osteotome (or pull the Gigli wire through), and osteotomize the trochanter off the proximal femur, leaving the medial and deep gluteal muscles attached to the osteotomized bone.

▼ *Key Point* Identify and protect the sciatic nerve, which is caudal to the femur and can be traumatized by excessive manipulations.

Trochanter Fracture Osteotomy Repair

Technique

1. Drill a hole transversely through the femur at least 1 cm distal to the osteotomy (fracture) site.
2. Thread a strand of 18-gauge orthopedic wire through the hole.
3. Clamp the proximal fragment in its anatomic position with a small-fragment bone reduction forceps.

4. Drive two appropriate-size K-wires from the proximal end of the trochanter, across the osteotomy (fracture) line, and into the femur until they are seated in compact bone.
5. Pass one free end of the orthopedic wire proximal to the pins and under the gluteal tendons (Fig. 128–3).

▼ *Key Point* Form a figure-eight configuration (tension band wire) around the pin ends and through the hole.

6. Twist the free ends of wire together and twist a loop of wire on the other crossover strand.
7. Tighten both twists evenly until the osteotomy (fracture) is securely closed.
8. Bend the pin ends over laterally and cut off the excess.
9. Cut the twisted wire, leaving two twists in place.

Proximal Femoral Shaft Fracture Repair

Technique

1. Extend the subperiosteal/subvastus lateralis dissection distally and elevate the adductor caudally until the fracture is adequately exposed.

▼ *Key Point* Both muscles (vastus lateralis and adductor) can be entirely released if necessary, but they must be reattached.

2. Repair the fracture(s) with appropriate orthopedic techniques and implants.
3. Use cerclage wires, hemicerclage wires, pins, K-wires, skewers, and lag screws to rebuild the fragments into a two-piece fracture.
4. Stabilize the fracture with a plate and screws.

▼ *Key Point* The femoral neck and trochanters provide excellent anchors for screw fixation.

5. Place an autogenous cancellous bone graft harvested from another site (e.g., proximal tibia or wing of ilium) around the fracture to aid in healing.
6. Reattach the vastus lateralis and adductor muscles to their origins with absorbable sutures.
   a. If necessary, elevate the periosteum to obtain enough tissue for suturing.

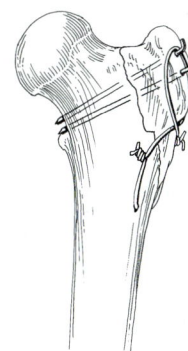

Figure 128–3. Tension band fixation of trochanter fracture or osteotomy.

b. Alternatively, use surrounding musculature or drill holes in the femur to anchor the proximal ends of these muscles.

Closure

1. Close the incised tendon of the superficial gluteal muscle with several mattress sutures using absorbable suture material.
2. Close the fascia of the gluteal muscles to the cranial edge of the superficial gluteal muscle with a simple continuous absorbable suture.
3. Close the fascia of the tensor fasciae latae muscle to the cranial edge of the biceps femoris muscle with a simple continuous absorbable suture.
4. Close the subcutaneous tissue with a simple continuous absorbable suture.
5. Close the skin with simple interrupted, monofilament, nonabsorbable sutures.

Postoperative Care

Femoral Neck/Capital Physeal Fracture Repair

- Take two radiographic views of the repair.
- Restrict activity (cage rest) for 3 days, and then allow leash walking only for 2–3 weeks.
- Perform non–weight bearing physical therapy (swimming, passive flexion-extension exercises).
- Repeat radiographs of the fracture at 4 weeks to evaluate healing.
- If healed, start a gradual return to full function.
- Remove pins (K-wires) if palpable, any time after 6 weeks if the bone has healed radiographically.
- Remove screws and plate only if causing a problem and only after 6 months.

Trochanteric Osteotomy/Fracture

- Recommendations are the same as for femoral neck/physeal fracture repair, except
  - Restrict activity (cage rest) for at least 24 hours.
  - Repeat radiographs at 6 weeks to evaluate healing.

Proximal Femur Fracture

- General recommendations are the same as for femoral neck/physeal fracture repair, except
  - Remove implants, if indicated, after 3–6 months.
- The proximal femur is subject to considerable and variable stresses that jeopardize all fixations. If any doubt exists as to the stability of a fracture fixation, a conservative postoperative approach is recommended.
  - Apply an Ehmer sling (see Chap. 127) to prevent weight bearing during the initial 1–2 weeks of healing.
  - Start physical therapy (non–weight bearing) and gradually increase controlled activity from week 2 to week 4.
  - After week 4 obtain repeat radiographs before starting significant activity levels.

Postoperative Complications

- Femoral neck/physeal fracture healing includes a period during which increased vascularity causes

bone demineralization of the femoral neck. This "apple coring" effect is transient and of no significance unless the fracture is unstable or infected. Monitor with serial radiographs if necessary.
- Implant failure and improper selection or application of orthopedic techniques can lead to failure of healing.

FEMUR DIAPHYSIS

Anatomy

- The shaft of the femur has muscle attachments on its caudal and medial aspects. Proximally and laterally, the adductor muscles are attached to most of the length of the femur. The origin of the vastus medialis muscle is found medial and proximal, whereas the insertion of the pectineus muscle is medial and distal. The insertion of the semimembranosus muscle is distal and medial.
- The femoral shaft is encased in a sheath of muscles including the vastus medialis, lateralis, and intermedius; rectus femoris; semimembranosus; semitendinosus; and pectineus muscles.
  - On the lateral aspect, this muscle mass is surrounded by a fascial compartment made up of the tensor fasciae latae and biceps femoris muscle sheaths. Medially the sartorius muscle continues this fascial sheath.
  - The femoral artery and nerve pass medially down the length of the shaft within this compartment.
- The sciatic nerve is lateral to the semimembranosus muscle and caudal to the vastus lateralis muscle.

TREATMENT OF FEMORAL SHAFT FRACTURES

Preoperative Considerations

- See under Proximal Femur.

Surgical Procedure

Objectives

- Expose the femoral shaft.
- Repair fractures of the femoral shaft.

Equipment

- Standard general instrument pack and suture material
- Orthopedic instruments as required for pinning, wiring, and plating.
- Self-retaining retractors (e.g., Gelpi, Weitlaner) or an assistant with hand-held retractors (e.g., Army-Navy).
- Several bone-holding forceps (e.g., Self-Retaining Speed Lock, Synthes; Lane, Kirschner).

Technique

1. Prepare the patient's leg for aseptic surgery.
2. Incise the skin from the trochanter to the patella on the cranial lateral aspect of the femoral shaft.

3. Expose the tensor fasciae latae muscle where it joins the biceps femoris muscle aponeurosis.
4. Incise both fascial layers, from the trochanter to the patella.
5. Retract the biceps femoris muscle caudally and the vastus lateralis muscle cranially.
6. Incise the intermuscular septum between the vastus lateralis and the biceps femoris muscles to expose the femoral shaft.
7. Bluntly separate the vastus intermedius muscle from the cranial aspect of the femur (Fig. 128–4).
8. Elevate (only as much as necessary) the adductor muscles subperiosteally on the caudal aspect of the femur; minimal elevation helps to preserve the blood supply to the bone.
9. Isolate the bone fragments and clean the fracture surfaces carefully.

▼ *Key Point* Remove fragments that are without muscle attachments and wrap them in blood-soaked sponges; maintain all soft tissue attachments to the remaining fragments.

10. Rebuild the proximal and distal fragments with the appropriate orthopedic devices until a two-piece fracture remains. A combination of cerclage, hemicerclage, and K-wires and interfragmentary screws, skewer pins, and figure-eight wire can be used to achieve a stable, two-piece fracture.
11. Use avascular bone fragments only if they are necessary to obtain stability in the fracture. These fragments must be securely fixed in order to be incorporated into the healing callus.
12. Reduce and align the two major fragments and apply the appropriate orthopedic fixation device to maintain these in alignment under stable conditions.

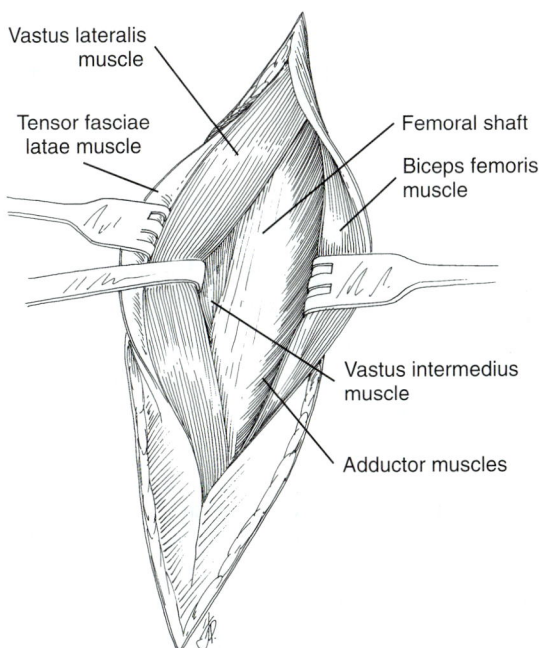

Figure 128–4. Lateral approach to the midshaft of the femur.

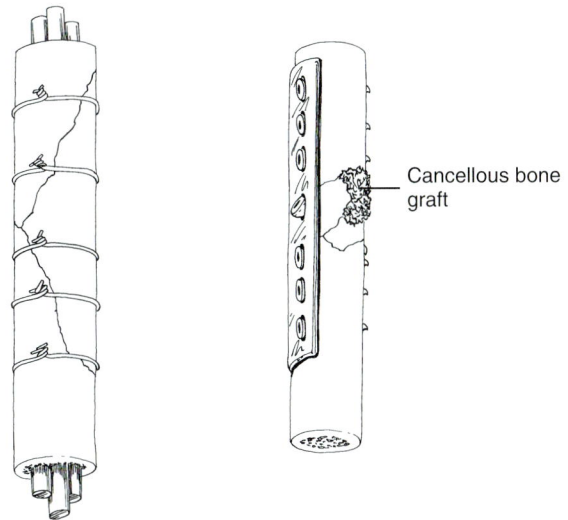

Figure 128–5. Diaphyseal femoral fracture fixation. *Left,* Simple long oblique fracture repaired with cerclage wires and intramedullary pins; *right,* comminuted transverse fracture repaired with a plate, screws, and cancellous bone graft.

13. In general, a two- or three-piece fracture with long oblique fracture lines can be rebuilt with cerclage wire and supported with one or more normograde (driven proximal to distal) intramedullary pins Fig. 128–5, *left*. Intramedullary pins also can be driven retrograde from the fracture site to the proximal femur.

▼ *Key Point* Extend and adduct the hip joint while driving the intramedullary pin through the proximal femur to avoid trauma to the sciatic nerve.

   a. Reduce the fracture and drive the pin into the distal fragment.
   b. Highly comminuted fractures are relatively unstable after being rebuilt and require added fixation devices to maintain alignment and stability. In these less stable situations, plating techniques or a combination of intramedullary and external skeletal fixation may be necessary to achieve stability (Fig. 128–5, *right*).

▼ *Key Point* All implants should lie directly against the bone; hence limited local muscle elevation is necessary to attach wires and plates.

14. Harvest autogenous cancellous bone graft from another site and pack around the fracture before closure. This is especially prudent if defects are present after reconstruction.
15. Flush the area copiously with warm normal saline solution *before* placing the cancellous bone graft in defects.

Closure
1. Close the fascia of the tensor fasciae latae to the biceps femoris with absorbable sutures in a simple interrupted pattern.
2. Close the subcutaneous tissue and skin routinely.

Postoperative Care

- General measures are the same as for femoral neck/physeal fracture except
  - Use a non–weight bearing sling if the fixation is unstable in any respect.
  - Start leash walking at 3–5 days if the fixation is stable. Increase exercise slowly over a 4-week period.
  - Repeat radiographs at 6 weeks to evaluate fracture healing.
  - Remove implants, if indicated (e.g., intramedullary pins usually are removed), when there is radiographic evidence of healing; with intramedullary pins this is generally 6–8 weeks postoperatively.

Postoperative Complications

- Orthopedic implant failure, improper implant selection, and improper use of implants are the most common causes of fracture collapse, malunion, and nonunion (see Chap. 141). Osteomyelitis may result from contamination.
- Large devitalized bone fragments that are not stabilized can lead to chronic draining tracts and osteomyelitis.
- Extensive subperiosteal dissection and rough handling of bone can produce an excessive periosteal reaction and large callus formation.

DISTAL FEMUR

Anatomy

- The distal femur includes the metaphysis, condyles, trochlea, and patella.
- The quadriceps muscle group inserts on the proximal tibia through the patellar tendon, which includes the patella within it.
- The two heads of the gastrocnemius muscle originate on the distal, caudal aspects of the medial and lateral metaphyses, and include the fabellae in their tendons of origin.
- The superficial digital flexor muscle originates just medial to the lateral head of the gastrocnemius muscle next to the fabella.
- The long digital extensor muscle originates in a fossa on the distal lateral condyle.
- The popliteus muscle originates on the caudal lateral condyle.
- The joint capsule on the stifle extends from above the trochlea, around both condyles, and underneath the fabellae bilaterally.
- The aponeuroses of the biceps femoris muscle laterally and the sartorius muscle medially blend with the fibrous joint capsule over the distal femur.
- The femoral artery divides into the popliteus and saphenous arteries, which run laterally and medially, respectively, on the caudal aspect of the distal femur.
- Several small branches of these two arteries supply the femur, the patella, and the vastus lateralis muscle.
- The muscular branch of the caudal femoral artery bridges the fascial separation between the biceps femoris muscle and the vastus lateralis muscle just above the lateral fabella.
- The peroneal and saphenous nerves supply the lateral and medial aspects of the distal femur, respectively, and run caudal to the femur.

TREATMENT OF FRACTURES OF THE DISTAL FEMUR AND PATELLA

Preoperative Considerations

- Obtain a minimum of two radiographic views for evaluation of the distal femur.
- Palpate joint stability with the animal under sedation or anesthesia to investigate the possibility of simultaneous ligamentous injuries in the stifle.
- The age of the patient influences choice of implant for repair of distal femoral fractures. In young animals, bone is softer, and healing is more rapid than in older animals (see Chap. 138).
- The majority of distal femoral fractures are physeal fractures; warn owners of the consequences of physeal closure in younger animals.

Surgical Procedure

Objectives

- Expose the distal femur and repair fractures of the metaphysis and epiphyses of the distal femur.
- Expose the articular surface of both distal femoral condyles for accurate intra-articular fracture reconstruction.
- Expose the patella and repair fractures of the patella.

Equipment

- Standard general instrument pack and suture material
- Orthopedic instruments as required for specific procedures, including pinning, wiring, and screw fixation.

Technique

1. Prepare the patient's leg for sterile surgery.
2. Expose the distal femur and patella using a lateral, medial, or cranial approach. For patient positioning convenience, the lateral approach is most frequently used.
3. Extensive reconstruction of the articular surface may require an osteotomy of the tibial crest for added exposure of the distal femur.

Lateral Approach

1. Make a slightly curved skin incision from the distal one-third of the femur to the tibial crest just lateral to the patella.
2. Incise the subcutaneous tissue to expose the fascial layer.
3. Incise the fibrous joint capsule and fascia starting at the tibial plateau just lateral to the patella tendon

and extending proximally, parallel to the patellar tendon and the patella.

4. Follow the border of the vastus lateralis muscle caudally to the septum between the biceps femoris and the vastus lateralis muscles. Separate these two muscles, double-ligating the muscular branch of the caudal femoral artery that bridges them distally.
5. Bluntly elevate the quadriceps muscles from the distal femur and luxate the patella medially to expose the distal femur (Fig. 128–6).
6. Expose and gently clean the fracture ends.

▼ *Key Point* Handle the metaphyseal bone gently, especially in young animals.

7. Apply the appropriate orthopedic implants as indicated by the fracture type. For simple physeal fractures, cross-pinning, multiple pinning, and modified Rush pinning techniques are appropriate.
   a. Start the pins from the fracture line and retrograde distally out through the epiphysis, avoiding the articular surface; or start from the caudolateral and caudomedial aspect of the epiphysis and drive (normograde) pins to the fracture line.
   b. With retrograde pinning, adjust the pins until the pinpoint is flush with the fracture line, realign the fracture anatomically, and drive the pins proximally up the shaft of the femur in one of the previously mentioned configurations (Fig. 128–7).
   c. Cut off the pins flush with the condyles and lavage the joint copiously with saline solution before closure.

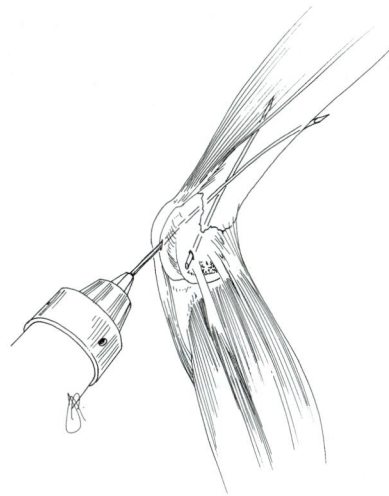
Figure 128–7. Cross-pinning of a distal femoral physeal fracture using a lateral approach.

Medial Approach

1. The technique is basically identical to that for the lateral approach except that it is made on the medial aspect of the distal femur.
2. In addition, one may substitute medial for lateral (vastus medialis muscle for vastus lateralis muscle, and cranial sartorius muscle for biceps femoris muscle) to achieve medial exposure of the distal femur.

Cranial Approach

1. Incise the skin from the lateral distal one-third of the femur to the medial aspect of the proximal tibia.
2. Separate the fascia as described for the medial and the lateral approaches, which are combined to give wider bilateral exposure of both condyles.

Tibial Crest Osteotomy

1. A tibial osteotomy can be combined with any of the previously described approaches to achieve additional exposure for complicated fractures.
2. Isolate the patellar tendon through the original skin incision.
3. Place an osteotome under the patellar tendon, aimed distally, and osteotomize the tibial crest free from the proximal tibia.

▼ *Key Point* Be sure to remove enough bone to facilitate fixation when reattaching the tibial crest.

4. Retract the quadriceps muscle proximally to fully expose the joint.
5. Repair intra-articular fractures with good visibility of the critical articular surface.
6. Compression (lag) screw fixation of intra-articular fracture fragments is recommended to allow accurate reconstruction and avoid movement, thus reducing the potential for arthritis.
7. Repair the osteotomy by pinning the tibial crest into position with two large K-wires transversely placed

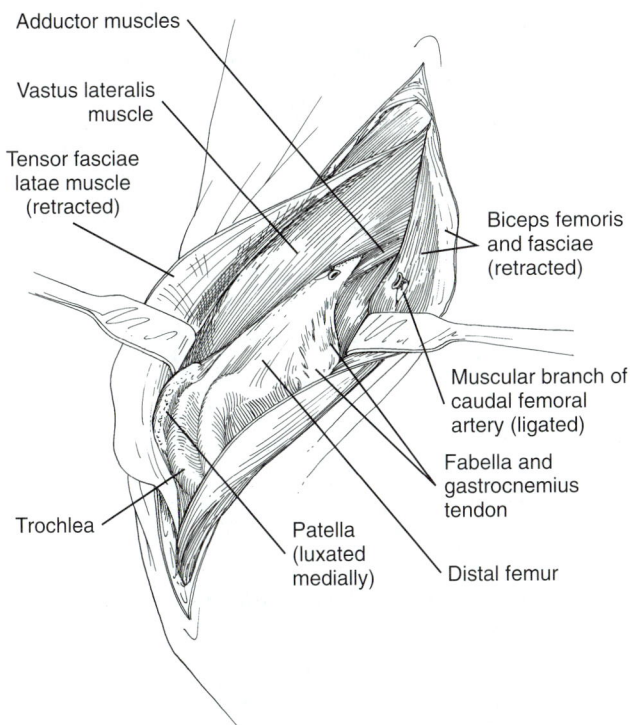
Figure 128–6. Lateral approach to the distal femur.

through the osteotomized bone fragment and into the proximal tibia. Place a figure-eight tension band wire around the base of the pins and through a hole in the cranial tibia, distal to the osteotomy site.

Patella Fracture Repair

1. Expose the patella via the lateral approach, as previously described. Identify the patella by rotating the distal quadriceps muscle.
2. Pass two K-wires lengthwise through the patella across the fracture line.
3. Rotate the quadriceps muscle back to its normal position and loop a figure-eight orthopedic wire around the pin ends on the cranial surface of the patella.
4. Twist both long strands of the figure-eight wire to tighten the tension band apparatus and close the fracture line of the patella.
5. Cut the pin ends as short as possible. Cut the twisted wire, leaving two twists.

Closure

1. Close the joint capsule with monofilament absorbable suture in a simple continuous pattern.
2. Close the fascial layer with absorbable sutures in a simple interrupted pattern.
3. Close the subcutaneous tissue and skin routinely.

Postoperative Care

- General recommendations are the same as for femoral neck/physeal fracture except:
  - Restrict activity (cage rest) for at least 24 hours.
  - If fixation is judged to be stable, start leash walking 1–2 days postoperatively.
  - If fixation is unstable, support the leg in a flexion sling.

Postoperative Complications

- Quadriceps tie-down (contracture) occurs when adhesions form between the healing fracture callus and the overlying quadriceps muscle and the patella tendon. This is most likely to happen if the leg is fixed in an extended position (e.g., with a Thomas splint). Tie-down can be prevented by early mobilization and/or a flexion sling for support.

▼ *Key Point* To help avoid quadriceps tie-down, do not apply splints that place the stifle in extension.

- If intra-articular fractures are not reduced anatomically, degenerative joint disease and postoperative joint pain can result. Accurate reduction and stable fixation is essential.
- If the animal is very young at the time of the physeal fracture, femoral shortening is to be expected if premature physeal closure occurs. If shortening is less than 20% compared with the normal leg, clinical signs are unlikely.

SUPPLEMENTAL READINGS

Aron JN, Kaddatz LA, Dueland R: A review of reduction and internal fixation of proximal femoral fractures in the dog and man. J Am Anim Hosp Assoc 15:455, 1979.

Berg JR, Egger EL, Konde LJ, et al.: Evaluation of prognostic factors for growth following distal femoral physeal injuries in 14 dogs. Vet Surg 13:142, 1984.

Brinker WO, Piermattei DO, Flo GL: Handbook of Small Animal Orthopedics and Fracture Treatment. Philadelphia: WB Saunders, 1983.

Evans HE, Christensen JC: Miller's Anatomy of the Dog, 2nd Ed. Philadelphia: WB Saunders, 1979.

Newton CD, Nunamaker DM: Textbook of Small Animal Orthopedics. Philadelphia: JB Lippincott, 1985.

Piermattei DO: An Atlas of Surgical Approaches to the Bones of the Dog and Cat, 3rd Ed. Philadelphia: WB Saunders, 1993.

Shires PK, Hulse DA: Internal fixation of physeal fractures using the distal femur as an example. Compend Contin Educ Small Anim Pract 2:854, 1980.

Slatter DH: Textbook of Small Animal Surgery, Vols 1 and 2, 2nd Ed. Philadelphia: WB Saunders, 1993.

Sumner-Smith G: Decision Making in Small Animal Orthopedic Surgery. Toronto: BC Decker, 1988.

129 Orthopedic Disorders of the Stifle

R. Tass Dueland

Common traumatic and congenital/developmental conditions of the stifle include patella luxation, cruciate disruptions, meniscal problems, collateral ligament injuries, and stifle luxation. The first three listed (excluding fractures) comprise 95% of stifle disorders in dogs and cats.

ANATOMY

Cranial Stifle

- The quadricep muscles, patella, trochlear groove and notch, patellar tendon, and tibial tuberosity are linearly aligned with the coxofemoral joint, talocrural joint, and paw. Normally there is no medial or lateral deviation of these structures.
- Craniomedial and caudolateral ligamentous bundles constitute the cranial cruciate ligament, which originates on the caudomedial aspect of the lateral femoral condyle and inserts centrally on the tibial plateau caudal to the cranial intermeniscal ligament (Fig. 129–1).
- The caudal cruciate ligament originates on the craniolateral aspect of the medial femoral condyle and inserts on the caudocentral tibial plateau and medial popliteal notch.
- The fat pad lies caudal to the patella tendon.
- The long digital extensor tendon originates on the lateral femoral condyle cranial to the lateral collateral ligament and popliteus muscle.
- Retinacular fibrous tissue overlies the craniolateral and craniomedial aspects of the stifle joint.
- The trochlear notch is the more distal non–weight-bearing portion of the trochlear groove.

Caudal Stifle

- Medial and lateral fabellae articulate intracapsularly with the femoral condyles and have strong fabellofemoral ligaments (Fig. 129–2).
- The medial meniscus is attached to the tibia and to the medial collateral ligament whereas there are tibial and femoral attachments of the lateral meniscus.
- The popliteus muscle courses under the lateral collateral ligament.
- Neurovascular structures run longitudinally and centrally close to the caudal joint capsule.

GENERAL PREOPERATIVE CONSIDERATIONS

- Client communication and cooperation and a successful return to function by the patient are enhanced by meticulous evaluation of the stifle joint preoperatively and intraoperatively. This facilitates an accurate diagnosis and selection of the appropriate procedure(s).
- Radiography is useful:
  - To confirm the diagnosis
  - For comparison with the opposite joint
  - For medical and legal documentation
- Perform a thorough orthopedic examination, including the joints, bones, and muscles of the affected extremity.

Orthopedic Evaluation

Include the following maneuvers in palpation of the stifle:

- Palpation of the patellar tendon and parapatellar tissue should reveal a distinct "sharp" feel to the tendon edges. If they feel indistinct or "doughy," this indicates stifle effusion, which is often associated with cranial cruciate rupture or DJD secondary to rupture.
- Perform gentle full range of stifle motion in normal flexion and extension; then repeat with internal and external rotation.
  - Often, clicks caused by meniscal pathology and crepitation from osteoarthritis can be detected.
- With the femur held motionless with one hand and the proximal tibia held securely by the other hand, attempt cranial movement of the tibia after placing the stifle in slight to moderate flexion (drawer sign or Lachman test).
- With a finger held over the tibial tuberosity and the femur held securely, flex the hock to detect cranial movement of the tibia (tibial compression test).
  - This test (and the Lachman test) indicates laxity of the cranial cruciate ligament.
- With the femur held motionless, determine internal and external movement of the tibia on the femur by grasping the hock and rotating the tibia. Normal range of motion is 20–30° of internal rotation and 5–10° of external rotation with the stifle in flexion.

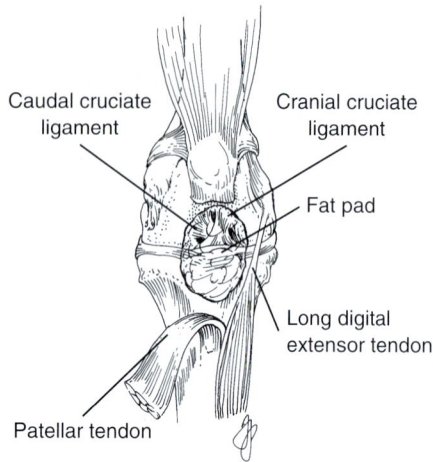

Figure 129-1. Anatomy of the cranial stifle.

- Exert medial and lateral digital pressure on the patella while putting the stifle through range of motion to detect any patellar luxation.
- Exert pressure with the thumbs on the lateral side of the femoral condyle and proximal tibia, and then repeat on the medial side. Laxity of the collateral ligaments is detected by increased laxity of the joint space.
- Exert deep pressure of the stifle area with a fingertip to ascertain focal points of pain from soft tissue tears and bone bruises.

▼ *Key Point* Perform the tests sequentially while the animal is conscious, and repeat when the animal is sedated or anesthetized. Plan appropriate surgical procedures based on this diagnostic information.

GENERAL PRINCIPLES OF STIFLE SURGERY

1. For the majority of the surgical procedures, place the dog in dorsal recumbency with the forelegs and unaffected rear limb secured. This gives good access

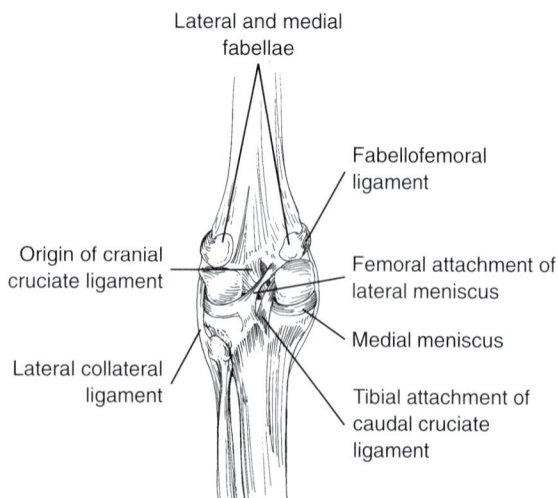

Figure 129-2. Anatomy of the caudal stifle.

to both sides of the stifle in a comfortable operating position. Place the instrument table over the dog's trunk.
2. Perform an arthrotomy of sufficient length to facilitate luxation of the patella and, using flexion and retraction, identify, inspect, and assess the articular surfaces of the patella, trochlear groove, tibial plateau, pericondylar, and supracondylar areas of the femur, patellar tendon, fat pad, and long digital extensor tendon.
   a. When operating alone, place the sterile, covered paw on your (gowned) abdomen.
   b. By moving your body forward and backward you can adjust the amount of flexion of the stifle.
3. Place a small, sharp rake retractor (Senn) deeply behind the fat pad; retract cranially and inspect both cruciates.
4. Place a second retractor on either side of the first to examine the menisci.
   a. To see the caudal horns well, place the tip of a narrow Hohmann retractor (Synthes 399.18) or curved hemostat just behind the tibial plateau. Positioning the instrument against the trochlear notch acts as a lever to move the tibia forward and increase exposure.

PATELLAR LUXATION

Medial and lateral patellar luxations affect miniature breeds commonly and large and giant breeds less often. Patellar luxations generally are congenital or developmental. Contributing factors include structural abnormalities such as coxa vara and coxa valgus (decrease and increase, respectively, in the angle formed by the head and neck of the femur and the axis of its shaft), bowing or torsion of the distal portion of the femur, shallow trochlear groove, increased internal or external tibial rotation, and a malpositioned tibial tuberosity.

Patellar luxations are classified as:

- Grade I: The patella lies in the trochlear groove but can be manually subluxated or luxated.
- Grade II: Spontaneous luxation occurs clinically. The patella can be luxated manually but reduces spontaneously or with gentle manipulation.
- Grade III: The patella is luxated most of the time but can be reduced manually.
- Grade IV: The patellar luxation cannot be reduced manually. Often, flexure contracture has occurred and limb use is minimal.

Diagnosis

- History usually reveals intermittent rear leg lameness. The lameness classically is characterized by rapidly alternating use and disuse of the limb, particularly during exercise.
- Definitive diagnosis is based on physical examination. Palpate the patella while placing the stifle through full range of motion. In a Grade I or II patellar luxation, the patella can often be luxated when the stifle is in extension.

Preoperative Considerations

- Evaluate the maximum internal and external rotation of the tibia on the femur. An increase in internal rotation >30° (often occurring in miniature breeds) indicates lateral retinacular laxity and the need for lateral imbrication.
- Patellar luxation procedures vary; some animals require only one step whereas others need combined procedures.
  - In some cases, combined parapatellar arthrotomy/release is necessary (to release means to diminish the pull or tension on tissue, often accomplished by incising perpendicularly to the line of tension).
  - In other cases, combined arthrotomy/imbrication is needed (to imbricate means to tighten, either by suturing alone or by excision and subsequent closure of tissue).

Surgical Procedures

Objective

- Stabilize the patella anatomically in the trochlea while maintaining full range of pain-free motion.

Equipment

- Standard orthopedic surgical pack and suture material
- Preferably, power-bur, oscillating saw, and drill *or*
- Double-action rongeurs, bone curets, and fine hand saw (hacksaw or Exacto saw #236), file, or rasp
- Sharp osteotomes and mallet

Surgical Principles

- Reduce the patellar luxation and determine whether the tissues are tight on the side toward which the patella luxates and whether the tissues opposite the luxated side are very lax.
  - If the former is present, perform combined parapatella arthrotomy/release to diminish the pull of the tissues.
  - If the latter is present, a combined arthrotomy/imbrication is indicated to tighten the lax side.
- With an adequately deep trochlear groove and no excessive tibial rotation, a release may be the only step needed to maintain the patella in its anatomic position.
- With a shallow trochlea, deepening can be accomplished by trochleoplasty, chondroplasty, or wedge resection. Techniques in which the articular cartilage is preserved (e.g., wedge resection) are preferred over those in which articular cartilage is not preserved.
- Correct excessive medial rotation of the tibia with a lateral antirotational nylon suture (fabella to tibial tuberosity drill hole, Fig. 129–7) or by translocation of the tibial tuberosity laterally.

Techniques

Trochleoplasty

1. Following arthrotomy and inspection of the stifle, mark the medial and lateral boundaries of the planned trochlear groove by longitudinal cuts in the trochlear cartilage, using a scalpel blade. To prevent fracture, try to obtain as much width and height as possible without weakening the remaining condylar bone.
2. Remove the articular cartilage within the marked lines by power burring or with a rongeur.
3. Reduce the luxated patella for a trial fit and, if necessary, smooth the new surface with a fine half-round file or rasp. The depth of the new trochlea should accommodate the patella so that one-half to two-thirds of the patella's height is in the groove.
4. Verify depth, smoothness, and stability by palpating the patella while putting the joint through its range of motion (flexion and extension with internal and external rotation of the tibia).
5. Close the synovia and joint capsule with appropriately sized monofilament nylon sutures in an interrupted cruciate pattern. If possible, perform partial-thickness closure whereby the suture is not within the joint. Close skin and subcutis routinely.

Postoperative Care

- Begin physical therapy, consisting of ice packs and gentle, passive flexion and extension to half the normal range of motion on the day of surgery. Twenty repetitions, four to six times daily is recommended. Swimming after suture removal is permitted.
- Restricted activity (leash walking only, no stairs, no ball playing, etc.) for 1 month.
- Give analgesics (e.g., butorphanol, 0.2 mg/kg IM; Bufferin, 10 mg/kg PO, bid with food or carprofen [Rimadyl] 2.2 mg/kg PO bid) as needed.

Chondroplasty

1. Make a trochlear outline, as described for trochleoplasty, down to subchondral bone (Fig. 129–3).
2. Using a thin, sharp, curved osteotome (Zimmer #2881–00–01, #2881–00–02) perform an osteotomy and create a rectangular cartilage flap with the hinge either proximally or distally. Include 1–2 mm of bone in the thickness of the flap.

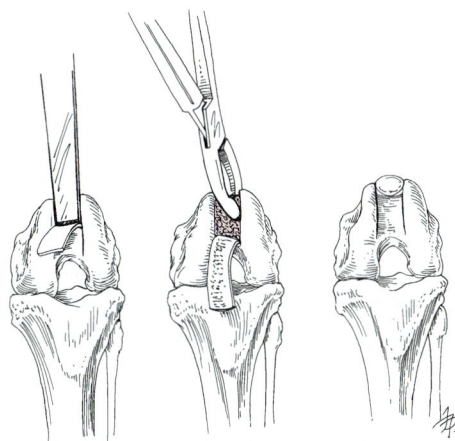

Figure 129–3. Chondroplasty procedure. See text for details.

3. Remove underlying bone with power burring, a bone curet, or rongeurs.
4. After adequate depth is obtained, press the flap manually into the new groove. Pressure from the patella helps keep the flap in position.
5. Close the skin and subcutis routinely.

▼ *Key Point* This technique is best used in dogs less than 6 months of age in which the mineralized tissue is relatively soft and pliable for creating a flap.

Postoperative Care

• Perform physical therapy and administer analgesics, as described previously for trochleoplasty.

Wedge Resection

1. Make a trochlear outline as described for trochleoplasty.
2. With a power saw or fine hand saw, make two pie-shaped cuts at the peripheral borders previously outlined. Medial and lateral condylar osteotomies should meet centrally. Remove this central piece of bone and articular cartilage and place it in a blood-soaked sponge.
3. The shallowness of the trochlea determines the width of the next two saw cuts, which are parallel and peripheral to the first cuts. Remove these two pieces of bone. Place the trochlear segment with its intact cartilage into the recess; this results in a deeper trochlea with preservation of most of the articular surface.
4. Pressure of the articulating patella ensures good contact of the osteotomized segment. If stability of the segment is questionable, drive small Kirschner wires horizontally through the condyles into the reinserted segment, although this is not usually necessary.
5. Close the skin and subcutis routinely.

Postoperative Care

• Perform physical therapy and administer analgesics, as described for trochleoplasty.

▼ *Key Point* Use caution with this technique in immature animals with open physes. Premature closure may occur; therefore it is better suited for animals more than 8 months of age.

Patelloplasty

1. Occasionally, after deepening and widening of the trochlea, the patella is still too large for the groove. Pivot the patella on edge.
2. With a power bur or rongeurs, remove bone from the medial and lateral surfaces of the patella until it fits well into the trochlear groove.

Postoperative Care

• Perform physical therapy and administer analgesics, as described previously for trochleoplasty.

Imbrication

After the depth of the trochlear groove is reestablished, reevaluate the status of tibial rotation. If there is medial or lateral rotary instability, perform imbrication of the lax side, using one of several techniques.

Techniques

1. DeAngelis technique (fabella to patellar tendon Fig. 129–7, *left*): Using nonabsorbable monofilament suture, place mattress pattern sutures around the medial and lateral fabellae and running extracapsularly, engaging the distal patellar tendon.
2. Flo technique (Fig. 129–7, *right*): Place the proximal aspect of the sutures similarly, but distally engage the proximal tibia through a transverse drill hole in the tibial tuberosity.
3. Place additional sutures, if needed, in a fan-like pattern, originating at the fabella and engaging the parapatellar tissue.
4. Alternatively, scarify the retinacular tissue with the scalpel blade and use a Lembert suture pattern to place several bilateral parapatellar sutures.
5. If there is redundant tissue on one side of the patella after reduction, make two elliptical incisions through retinaculum, capsule, and synovia. Remove the redundant tissue and imbricate using routine closure or a vest-over-pants suture pattern.

▼ *Key Point* As a rule, when suturing is the main component of imbrication, physical therapy should be gentle to diminish stress upon the suture material, and allow adequate time for tissue healing.

Tibial Tuberosity Translocation
Equipment

• Osteotome and mallet or a dental molar cutter
• Orthopedic Kirschner wires

Technique

1. Perform medial and lateral parapatellar arthrotomies. For lateral translocation, reflect cranial tibial muscle.
2. With an osteotome/mallet or molar cutter, make an osteotomy of the tibial tuberosity, leaving the soft tissue still attached distally if possible (Fig. 129–4, *center*).
3. Hold the osteotomized tibial tuberosity in position with a bone clamp (Synthes 399.07), after creating a bed in the tibia by roughening the site with a rongeur or curette.
4. Using a power or hand drill, make two small holes through the newly positioned osteotomized segment and through the base of the tibial tuberosity (Fig. 129–4).
5. Place an appropriately sized (20–22 gauge) orthopedic wire through the holes in a mattress pattern and twist tightly medially to secure the bone in the new site. Cut the wire, leaving two to three twists. The new location of the insertion of the patellar

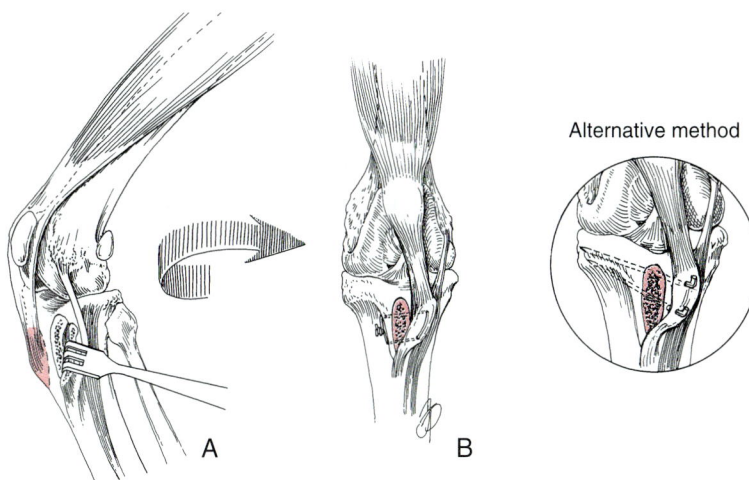

Figure 129-4. Alternate fixation method A, B: Kirschner wires holding osteotomized tibial tuberosity in transposed position. Tibial tuberosity transposition. *Left,* Area of partial osteotomy of tibial tuberosity is shown in color; the cranial tibial muscle is reflected. *Right,* The newly positioned segment is wired in place.

Alternative method

tendon should realign the forces to maintain the patella in position, assuming other disruptive forces have been corrected.

6. If the new position is not closely adjacent to the osteotomy site, insert Kirschner wires (Fig. 129-4*A* & *B*), a tension band, or a lag screw obliquely for stable fixation.

▼ *Key Point* Exercise great care in young animals not to cause physeal growth arrest by inappropriate placement of Kirschner wires through the proximal tibial growth plate.

- If the wire ends cause skin irritation, they may be removed after bony union has occurred.

▼ *Key Point* Because medial and lateral rotary instability/laxity contributes significantly to malalignment of the tibial tuberosity, correction of the laxity by imbrication (Flo) technique may eliminate the need for transposition of the tuberosity.

CRANIAL CRUCIATE LIGAMENT (CL) RUPTURE

Diagnosis

- The history usually reveals an acute onset of rear limb lameness, particularly during exercise. Lameness may partially or completely resolve, then recur with exercise.
- Chronic and persistent lameness may also be seen, especially in older, overweight dogs.
- Firm swelling of the medial aspect of the joint can be palpated when a chronic CL rupture is present.

Diagnostic Manipulations

Two diagnostic manipulations can confirm abnormal cranial movement of the tibia at the stifle.

Cranial Drawer

- Position the thumbs on the caudolateral aspect of the stifle so that the lower thumb engages the head of the fibula while the upper thumb is placed in the region of the lateral fabella or the edge of the lateral femoral condyle.
- Wrap the other fingers of the upper hand around the cranial aspect of the lower thigh, keeping the femur motionless and the patella in the trochlea groove.
- Test the cranial laxity of the stifle joint with the tibia in full extension, in modest flexion (15–30°) (Lachman test), and in 45–90° (or more) of flexion (cranial drawer sign).
  - With complete rupture of both bands of the cranial CL, cranial laxity is detectable at each position.
  - With partial rupture, laxity may be detectable at only one of these positions.
- Severity of laxity is subjectively ranked in 2-mm increments (e.g., 1+ = 2 mm; 2+ = 4 mm; 3+ = 6 mm; 4+ = 8 mm) of cranial displacement (translation) of the tibia on the femur.

Tibial Compression

- Use one hand to hold the femur motionless, with the index finger resting on the tibial tuberosity; gently dorsiflex the hock with the other hand.
- The gastrocnemius muscle will tighten and, when cranial CL laxity is present, the tibia can be felt to move cranially under the index finger.

In the author's experience the cranial drawer/Lachman test is more consistent than the tibial compression test. However, both tests should be done. A diagnostic impression is obtainable in 90% of unanesthetized dogs if proper positioning and a calm approach are used.

Preoperative Considerations

- Preoperative stifle radiographs are useful to document joint effusion, extent of the degenerative joint disease, normal fabellae, and avulsions of ligamentous attachments.
- To rule out predisposing or concurrent diseases, consider obtaining a routine laboratory database of complete blood count (CBC), serum chemistry profile, and urinalysis.

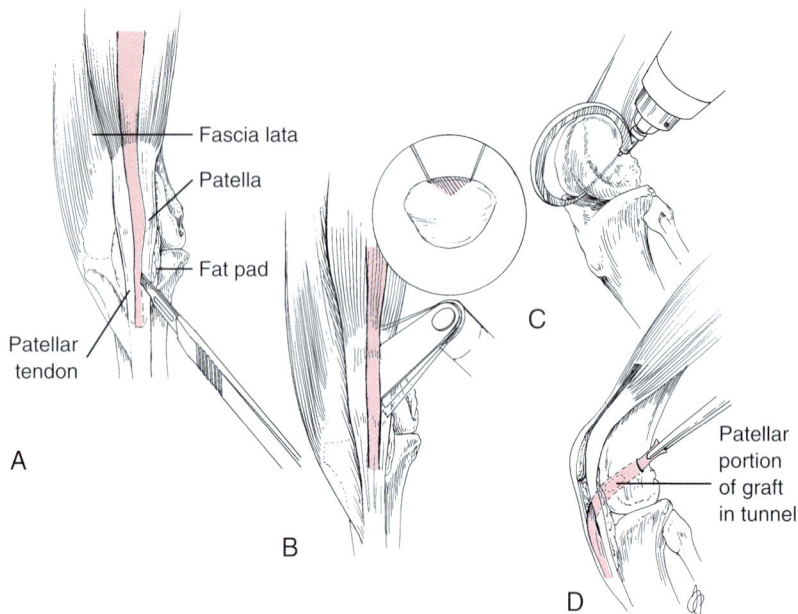

Figure 129–5. Patellar tendon technique for repair of cranial cruciate rupture. See text for details.

Surgical Procedures

Objectives

- Visually assess the extent of joint damage.
- Slow the progression of degenerative joint disease by stabilizing the joint.
- Reduce or eliminate the drawer sign.
- Debride the joint and replace the damaged cranial CL with an autogenous graft.
- Inspect the meniscus for tears (usually caudal horn of medial meniscus).

Patellar Tendon Procedure (For Dogs Weighing 25–175 lb)

Equipment

- Standard orthopedic pack including 2 Senn retractors (1 each, sharp and dull)
- C-clamp drill guide (Synthes #312.47), with 3.2-mm and 4.5-mm drills and drill sleeve inserts (312.45, 312.32)
- Alligator forceps or suture passer
- Power saw/drill (e.g., 3M minidriver) or Steinmann pin/hand chuck, Exacto saw #236 (1.25″) or hack saw*
- Osteotomes 1.0″ and 0.75″ and mallet

Technique

1. Place the dog in dorsal recumbency and prepare the stifle for aseptic surgery.
2. Make a cranial skin incision extending from 2 inches above the patella to the tibial crest. Suture a sterile stockinette to the incision.
3. Incise the superficial fascia and fatty layers longitudinally on the midline, exposing the deeper fascia,

the cranial head of the sartorius muscle (medially), the patella, and the patellar tendon (Fig. 129–5).

▼ **Key Point** If the cranial CL rupture diagnosis is uncertain preoperatively, perform arthrotomy or arthroscopy and joint inspection before creating a new ligament.

---

4. Make two parallel incisions through the first layer of the fascia lata/quadriceps fascia starting 2–3 mm lateral to the cranial head of the sartorius muscle and continuing distally over the patella, through the patellar tendon, to the tibial tuberosity. Make the width of these incisions uniform and equal to the middle third of the patellar tendon (generally 4–6 mm in a 40–70 lb dog) (Fig. 129–5A).
5. Free the fascial and patellar tendon portions of the graft from the underlying tissue. Cut the most proximal (fascial) end of the graft transversely, leaving the distal (patellar tendon portion) graft still attached to the tibial tuberosity. Be careful to cut through the full thickness of the patellar tendon, but do not cut into the underlying fat pad, to avoid unnecessary bleeding.
6. Make converging saw cuts into the patella from the previous guiding incisions made over the patella. The bone cuts join in the outer third of the patella and do not reach the articular surface of the patella (Fig. 129–5B). If these pie-shaped cuts are made properly, one or two taps with an osteotome and mallet will dislodge the bony segment of the graft. To ensure preservation of insertions of the fascia proximally and patellar tendon distally to the patellar wedge, make the saw cut 3–4 mm deep.
7. Using a scalpel, make a final dissection to free up the graft. Use Metzenbaum scissors to trim the soft tissue of the graft to uniform dimensions. If the patellar wedge is oversized, reduce it with rongeurs or a power bur.

---

*Government surplus rotary dental saws are reasonably priced and serve well for this procedure.

8. Perform a lateral parapatellar arthrotomy and luxate the patella medially to expose the stifle joint. Perform a thorough inspection of the stifle, as previously described. Remove the remnants of the ruptured cranial CL with sharp dissection, using a #15 scalpel blade. If necessary, perform corrective surgery for meniscal problems (see later in this chapter), cartilaginous defects, and exostosis removal to complete the joint debridement.

9. Place the C-clamp drill guide at the anatomic origin of the cranial CL, drilling a tunnel through the lateral femoral condyle from exterior to interior. For dogs 25–60 lb, use a 3.2-mm drill; for larger dogs, use a 4.5-mm drill. Make the tunnel longitudinally oblique to prevent bony edges from eroding the graft (Fig. 129–5C).

10. Reduce the patella, and with a curved hemostat placed through the void made in the patellar tendon, create a tunnel through the fat pad. Grasp the proximal end of the graft with a hemostat and bring it through the patellar tendon defect and into the stifle via the fat pad tunnel. Place an alligator forceps into the stifle joint via the lateral condylar tunnel. With the jaws grasping the proximal (fascial) end of the graft, pull the graft through the condylar tunnel without twisting it. A small thumb forceps may be needed to guide the patellar portion of the graft into the bony tunnel. Occasionally, enlargement of the tunnel with bone curettes or redrilling is necessary. Postoperatively, the patellar portion of the graft lies entirely in the condylar tunnel and is firmly incorporated in the tunnel, providing permanent stability of the cruciate graft (Fig. 129–5D).

11. After thorough lavage of the joint, suture the fascial defect, patellar tendon defect, and arthrotomy incisions using 00–1 monofilament nylon in a cruciate pattern. Secure the graft last, after adjusting tension as necessary by incorporating the proximal fascial portion of the graft into the arthrotomy closure with three to four nylon sutures. A very minimal drawer sign (trace to 1+) is acceptable at closure because the joint usually tightens in the postoperative period. Routinely close the subcutaneous tissue and skin. Supplemental imbrication (Flo or DeAngelis technique) sutures are unnecessary.

12. If a power saw/drill and a C-clamp drill guide are not available, the procedure can be performed with minor modification of the above technique:
   a. Make a medial (not lateral) arthrotomy in order to drill the tunnel with a Steinmann pin and hand chuck. If a C-clamp drill is not available, it is easier and more accurate to make the tunnel from the interior of the stifle to the exterior.
   b. Luxate the patella laterally; this makes it possible to line up the drill hole without interference from the reflected soft tissue. Make a small separate lateral incision to accept the passage of the graft and facilitate suturing of the graft.
   c. Patellar osteotomies can be made with an Exacto saw or a hacksaw. Other aspects of the surgery are the same.

Postoperative Care

Apply a sterile Robert Jones bandage (RJB), supplemented with a 3–4″ wide, full-length cranial fiberglass slab and secure the bandage to the body with a belly band.

▼ **Key Point** Do not remove the RJB prematurely; it can be replaced but not removed!

- Replace the bandage as necessary but use for 1 month to prevent stifle motion in order to allow bony incorporation of the patellar segment in the condylar tunnel with resultant strong graft fixation.

▼ **Key Point** Inform owners that autogenous tissue graft used to replace the cranial cruciate ligament is biomechanically weaker than the original ligament, and that during the first 3 months after surgery the graft is undergoing revascularization and needs protection from stress. Recommend restricted, leash-only exercise and no use of stairs.

- Gradually increase exercise after 3 months, with return to full function in 6–9 months.
- Excess graft tension diminishes revascularization and normal healing of the graft.

Prognosis

- The author has been very satisfied with the results of this technique, having used and refined it for more than 35 years. On the few occasions when the stifle was later operated, the graft appeared strong and stable.

Fascial Strip Over-The-Top Procedure (For Dogs Weighing 15–25 lb)

Equipment

- Standard orthopedic pack and suture material

Technique

1. Place the dog in dorsal or lateral recumbency and prepare the stifle for aseptic surgery.
2. Make a craniolateral skin incision similar to that in the patellar tendon technique but slightly more lateral.
3. Perform a craniolateral arthrotomy with formation of a distally based fascial strip. For adequate biomechanical strength, make the width of the strip two to three times the width of the patellar tendon. The length needed is twice the distance from the proximal patella to the tibial tuberosity. The base of the strip is at the level of the joint line.
4. Cut the fascial strip proximally and insert it, lateral to medial, through a fat pad tunnel made with a hemostat (Fig. 129–6). Then, enter the caudolateral joint capsule caudal to the lateral fabella and gently advance the hemostat through the intercondylar notch, keeping the hemostat tip lateral to the caudal cruciate ligament. Grasp the proximal end of the graft in the joint and pull it through the intercondylar notch lateral to the

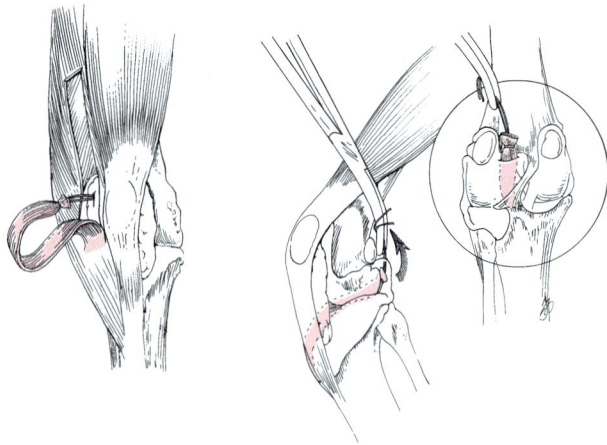

Figure 129-6. Fascial strip over-the-top technique for repair of cranial cruciate rupture. See text for details.

caudal CL and over the top of the lateral condyle. Make a small incision through the joint capsule, pull the fascial strip through it, and secure it to the capsular reflection onto the lateral femoral condyle with six to eight monofilament nylon sutures (2-0) with the appropriate tension to achieve a minimal drawer sign.

5. Close the arthrotomy incision with nonabsorbable nylon suture. Complete closure may not be possible distally, depending on the width of graft harvested. Use a lateral imbrication suture of monofilament nylon (see imbrication technique) from fabella to distal patellar tendon for temporary stabilization of the joint until healing occurs.

6. Routinely close the remaining tissues.

Imbrication Procedure (For Dogs Weighing Less Than 25 lb)

Equipment

- Standard orthopedic pack and suture material

Technique

1. Place the dog in lateral recumbency and prepare the stifle for aseptic surgery.
2. Make a lateral parapatellar skin incision.
3. Perform a lateral arthrotomy.
4. Debride the joint and close the arthrotomy incision as previously described for the fascial strip over-the-top procedure.
5. Prepare the tibial tuberosity by incising the cranial origin of the cranial tibial muscle at the lateral aspect of the tibial tuberosity. Reflect the muscle caudally from the tibia with a periosteal elevator.
6. Drill a hole transversely (mediolaterally) through the proximal tibia approximately 1 cm distal to the joint and 1 cm caudal to the cranial edge of the tibial tuberosity. Drill a second hole approximately 1 cm distal to the first one. The holes should be large enough to accommodate passage of the needle and suture.
7. Anchor extracapsular lateral imbrication nylon su-

tures from around the lateral fabella or through the fabellofemoral ligament (See Fig. 129-7). (Sterilized 50-, 80-, and 100-lb test monofilament nylon has provided good results.)

8. The author finds it easiest to place the suture needle around the fabella using a caudal to cranial motion, "walking" the tip of the needle up the caudal aspect of the femur until the proper angle is attained and the needle can be brought through the tissue. A sturdy needle assists the maneuver.
   a. Pull firmly on the suture to confirm that suture placement is correct and that the fabella has been properly engaged.
   b. If the fixation feels inadequate, incise the fascia to better identify the fabella.
9. The previously placed lateral fabellar suture is now passed below the fascia, but remains extracapsular and is passed under the cranial tibial muscle so that the needle exits from the muscle along the tibial tuberosity at the level of the first drill hole.
10. Pass the needle and suture lateral to medial through the proximal drill hole and then medial to lateral through the distal drill hole.
11. Cut the suture from the needle, leaving two distinct sutures. Use the needle to similarly bring the two proximal suture ends distally under the cranial tibial muscle. Tie the first suture with the tibia externally rotated and the stifle in extension. Tie the second suture with external tibial rotation and moderate stifle flexion. Five to six throws are used for the knots, which are buried under the cranial tibial muscle. Routinely close the incision.

▼ **Key Point** Size of monofilament nylon suture is important. Use #1 for small dogs <10 kg, 50-lb test line for dogs up to 20 kg, 80-lb test for dogs up to 30 kg, and 100-lb test for dogs >30 kg.

Postoperative Care

- No bandage or splint is required.
- Restrict exercise as for previously described techniques for several months until adequate fibrosis and healing occurs.

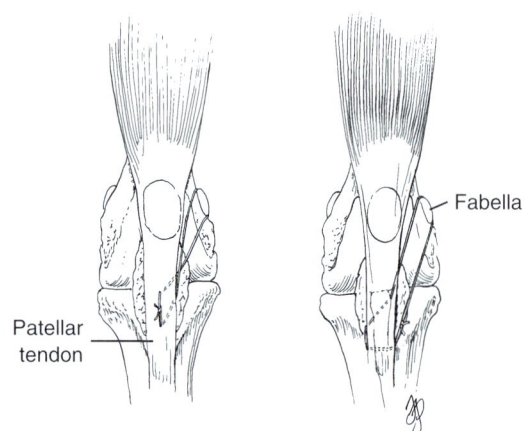

Figure 129-7. Imbrication techniques of DeAngelis (*left*) and Flo (*right*). These techniques are used for cruciate stabilization and also for antirotation purposes with patella luxations.

CAUDAL (POSTERIOR) CRUCIATE LIGAMENT (CL) RUPTURE

The importance of the caudal CL is controversial in both dogs and humans. A study in humans (Clancy et al., 1983) indicated severe pathology results with time. In dogs, isolated rupture of the caudal CL without bony avulsion is, in the author's experience, extremely rare.

Diagnosis

Diagnosis is based on:

- A history of acute lameness and caudal drawer sign tested at 90° of stifle flexion
- A caudal sag of the proximal tibia, compared with the normal, opposite side, viewed on a lateral radiographic projection
- Avulsion of the bony attachment

Surgical Procedure

Objectives

- Similar to those for cranial CL except rupture repair

Equipment

- Similar to that for the patellar tendon procedure for cranial CL rupture

Technique

1. Make a cranial skin incision extending from 4 cm above the patella to 4 cm below the tibial tuberosity.
2. Perform a medial arthrotomy and debridement of the caudal CL.
3. Drill two tunnels. Extend one tunnel from the origin of the caudal CL at the nonarticulating portion of the trochlear groove, exiting on the medial side of the medial femoral condyle. Extend the second tunnel from a point approximately 2 cm below the tibial plateau just medial of the midline, directed caudally to exit just below the centromedial portion of the tibial plateau.
4. Harvest a patellar tendon graft as in the cranial CL patellar tendon procedure; in addition, obtain a piece of tibial tuberosity bone (4 mm wide × 6 mm long × 2 mm thick), including its patellar tendon insertion (i.e., making a free graft). Drill holes in each of the patellar and tuberosity pieces of bone and pass long nylon suture strands through the holes.
5. Using a suture passer, introduce the sutures that are attached to the patellar segment into the tibial tunnel in a cranial to caudal direction, and pull the patellar portion of the graft through, leaving the tibial graft segment in the tibial tunnel. Similarly, draw the patellar piece into the femoral tunnel.
6. Insert partially threaded 4-mm Synthes screws, with the far cortex engaged, near the cranial tibial tunnel and at the exit of the femoral tunnel. Use these to anchor the tuberosity and patellar sutures after adjusting the graft to its proper tension.
7. Close the incision and tissues routinely. Place the

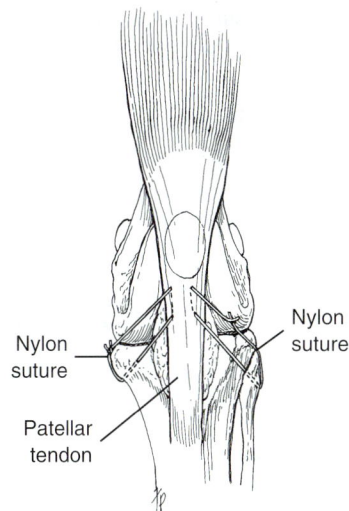

Figure 129–8. Imbrication technique for rupture of caudal cruciate ligament.

limb in a RJB for 1 month, as described in the patellar tendon procedure for cranial CL rupture repair.

8. An alternate technique for caudal cruciate rupture is to place two imbricating nylon sutures (Fig. 129–8). Place the first suture from the proximal patellar tendon to a drill hole through the proximal head of the fibula. Place the second suture from the proximal patellar tendon through a drill hole in the caudomedial aspect of the proximal tibia. Tighten these sutures with the stifle held in slight extension.
9. For bony avulsion injuries, if the bony portion is large enough, drill holes in the *bony* segment (lag screws or a Bunnell suture pattern can be used). Pass the suture through the ligament using a Bunnell pattern, and pass the suture ends through the bony drill holes. This gives firm fixation of the sutures to the ligament.
   a. Make two drill holes through the avulsion site, exiting on the medial side of the femur or on the cranial surface of the tibia.
   b. Using a suture passer, pass the sutures through the drill holes and tie them securely; this anatomically reduces the avulsion fracture and restabilizes the caudal CL.

MENISCAL PROBLEMS

Preoperative Considerations

- An isolated meniscal tear or laxity is rare in dogs, compared with humans. More commonly, meniscal pathology is associated with a partial, or a complete cranial cruciate tear.
  - Secondary meniscal damage can occur in the weeks and months following an unrecognized or untreated cruciate injury.
- The resultant craniocaudal and rotational laxity allows the femoral condyles to traumatize the caudal horn of the medial meniscus (Fig. 129–9A). A com-

Normal position of
medial meniscus

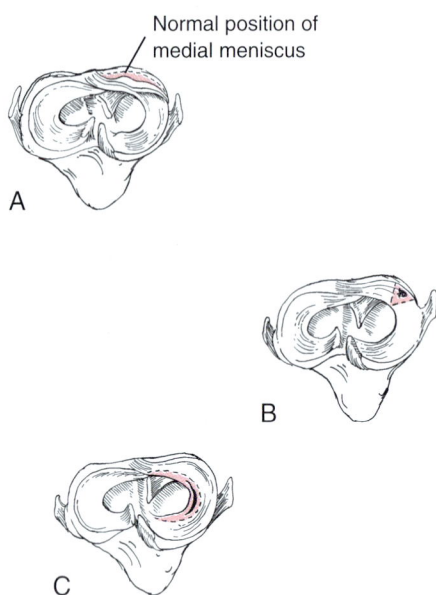

Figure 129–9.   Repair of medial meniscal injuries. See text for details.

mon lesion is a folding cranially of the caudal horn of the medial meniscus.

- Diagnose by palpating a click or clunk during range of motion as the femoral condyle slips over the double thickness of the folded meniscus.
- Total (complete) meniscectomy is not advised unless there is severe damage of both caudal and cranial horns.

Surgical Procedure

Objectives

- Remove or repair damaged portions of the menisci

Equipment

- Standard orthopedic pack and suture material
- Narrow Hohmann retractor (Synthes #399.18)
- Scalpel blade (#15)

Technique

1. Place the dog in dorsal recumbency with the forelegs and unaffected rear limb secured. Perform sterile preparation, stockinette, draping, and suturing in of stockinette to the skin incision.
2. Because meniscectomy usually is performed in conjunction with CL reconstruction, use the arthrotomy approach (medial or lateral) appropriate for the cruciate technique. Make the arthrotomy of sufficient length to permit adequate retraction and exposure of both menisci.
3. After dislocating the patella from the trochlea, insert a small, sharp Senn retractor behind the fat pad and exert traction cranially. Keep the retractor in position until all internal joint manipulation is completed.

   a. Avoid unnecessary trauma to the fat pad with retractors to prevent damage to the vascular supply.
4. Debride cruciate and meniscal remnants, as necessary, and evaluate all joint structures for damage.
5. Place a second, dull Senn retractor on the medial side of the central Senn retractor to identify the medial meniscus, and then place it laterally to observe the lateral meniscus.
6. To facilitate exposure of the caudal horns, insert a narrow Hohmann retractor or hemostat to gently pry the tibial plateau forward (see General Principles of Stifle Surgery in this chapter).
7. Use a probe to determine laxity of the menisci and the extent of any tears.
8. Grasp the partially detached, forward-displaced caudal horn with a hemostat at the midportion. Often, the medial caudal horn is still attached peripherally to the medial collateral ligament and to the caudal tibial insertion.
9. With traction on the caudal horn use a #15 scalpel blade to make a perpendicular cut to sever the caudal horn from the normally attached cranial horn. The meniscal-medial collateral attachment is usually cranial to the folded caudal horn.
10. Cut the remaining attachment (to the tibia) by placing the blade horizontally under the remaining caudal horn, and remove the caudal horn.

    a. Be careful to avoid cutting into the cartilage of the condyle or tibial plateau or lacerating the caudal CL or popliteal vessels caudal to the meniscus.
11. Flush the joint well with sterile Ringer's lactate solution, reposition the patella and run the joint through a range of motion. No crepitation or clicks should be felt.
12. Remove any areas of localized injury or tears with a scalpel and create a vascular access channel running from the peripheral synovium (see Fig. 129–9*B*). In "bucket handle" tears (see Fig. 129–9*C*), the vascularity of central area (shaded area, see Fig. 129–9*C*) is compromised and therefore is removed by sharp dissection.

COLLATERAL LIGAMENT DISRUPTIONS

Preoperative Considerations

- Collateral ligament injuries usually occur as a result of severe medial (varus) or lateral (valgus) stress to the stifle by blunt force to the joint with the paw fixed during weight bearing.
- Collateral ligament strains are graded as to severity:
  - First degree—stretching and minor disruption of collagen fibers
  - Second degree—partial tearing
  - Third degree—complete discontinuity of the substance of the ligament or avulsion of a bony attachment.
- Animals usually are presented with acute lameness.

- Verify joint instability with stress radiographs.
- First- and second-degree injuries respond well to rest, restricted exercise, or a modified RJB.
- Third-degree injuries require surgical repair and partial immobilization for a few weeks, using a modified Robert Jones bandage.

Surgical Procedure

Objectives

- Restore the integrity of the injured ligament and the stability of the stifle.

Equipment

- Standard orthopedic pack and suture material
- Power drill
- Spiked washers/screw

Technique

1. Surgical approach is directly over the damaged ligament.
2. For complete ligament tears, use a Bunnell, locking loop, or triple pulley suture pattern (see Chap. 134) for primary repair.
3. For bony avulsion, use a screw and spiked washer (Synthes #219.9, 219.93–95) if the bony portion is large enough to accept a screw. When the bony portion is small, use a ligament fixation plate (Synthes #65.00.1, 65.00.10, 65.00.11).
4. Reinforce a severely traumatized ligament by forming a supplemental fascial strip with two parallel incisions cranial and caudal to the involved collateral ligament: then suture the fascial strip to the repaired collateral ligament; or a fascial strip can be folded down and sutured to the ligament to reinforce the primary repair (see Fascial Strip Over-the-Top Procedure).
5. Alternatively, place screws at the origin and insertion of the collateral ligament and make a prosthetic ligament by looping monofilament nylon (or #1- to 50-lb test, depending on the size of the dog) in a figure-eight pattern around the screws. The wire or nylon usually breaks with time, but enough scar tissue forms to stabilize the joint.

STIFLE LUXATION

Preoperative Considerations

- Severe trauma is necessary for complete stifle luxation to occur. The condition is more common in cats.
- Physical examination reveals total laxity in all directions: cranial, caudal, and rotational; the medial and lateral aspects of the stifle joint open up excessively.
- Usually, the patellar tendon is not disrupted; however, the popliteus and long digital extensor tendons may be torn, as well as both cruciates, both collaterals, and, in varying degrees, the meniscal attachments.

Surgical Procedure

Objectives

- Repair ligaments and tendons to reestablish joint stability.

Equipment

- Standard orthopedic pack and suture material
- Power drill/drill bits
- Kirschner-Ehmer pins and clamps

Technique

1. Make a long lateral parapatellar skin and arthrotomy incision and assess the damage to ligaments, tendons, menisci, and cartilage.
2. If possible, stabilize the menisci by suturing peripheral attachments; otherwise, perform meniscectomy.
3. Repair the long digital extensor tendon, popliteus, and collateral ligaments with locking tendon loop, pulley, or Bunnell suture patterns; spiked washer and screw; or fascial reinforcement as described previously under collateral ligament repair.
4. Cruciate stabilization may be done by intracapsular replacement or extracapsular imbrication techniques as previously described in this chapter.

Postoperative Care

- To allow adequate healing, place a transarticular external skeletal fixation device, placing pins in the distal femoral and proximal tibia. This device is maintained for 3–4 weeks, followed by gradual motion using an RJB for 2 weeks and then a light wrap for 2 weeks. An alternative to the transarticular ESF would be a full cast.
  - With any form of immobilization of the stifle, place the joint in a functional (partially flexed) position.
- Some limitation of joint range of motion is acceptable and preferable to instability.

▼ **Key Point** For complete, multiple, midsubstance ligament disruptions, apposition of ligament ends is important for healing to occur; however, early mobilization also is important for complete biomechanical recovery.

SUPPLEMENTAL READINGS

Arnoczky SP, Marshall JL: The cruciate ligaments of the canine stifle: An anatomical and functional analysis. Am J Vet Res 38:1807, 1977.

Brinker WO, Piermattei DL, Flo GL: Handbook of Small Animal Orthopedics and Fracture Treatment, 2nd Ed. Philadelphia: WB Saunders, 1990, p 403.

Chiroff RT: Experimental replacement of the anterior cruciate ligament: A histological and microradiographic study. J Bone Joint Surg 57-A:1124, 1975.

Clancy WG, Narechania RG, Rosenberg TD, et al.: Anterior and posterior cruciate ligament reconstruction in Rhesus monkeys. J Bone Joint Surg 63-A:1270, 1981.

Clancy WG, Shelbourne KD, Zoellner GB, et al.: Treatment of knee joint instability secondary to rupture of the posterior cruciate ligament. J Bone Joint Surg 65-A:310, 1983.

Clancy WG, Thomsen E, Dueland RT, et al.: Anterior cruciate and posterior cruciate ligament reconstruction with patella tendon utilizing a medial vascular graft, lateral vascular graft, and free patella tendon graft. Trans Orthop Res Soc 12:70, 1987.

Dueland RT: A recent technique for reconstruction of the anterior cruciate ligament. J Am Anim Hosp Assoc 2:1, 1966.

Woo SL-Y, Inoue M, McGurk-Burleson E, Gomez MA: Treatment of the medial collateral ligament injury. II: Structure and function of canine knees in response to differing treatment regimens. Am J Sports Med 15:22, 1987.

130 Fractures of the Tibia and Fibula

Erick L. Egger

Fractures of the tibia and fibula compose a significant proportion (15–20%) of all long bone fractures in small animals. In addition, the minimal soft tissue coverage of these bones increases the incidence of contamination of open fractures, which may result in infection and healing complications. Proper treatment of tibial and fibular fractures requires:

- An understanding of the disruptive biomechanical forces that must be controlled to promote the healing process
- Selection of a fixation technique that will control these forces
- Application of fixation without damaging the fracture healing process or compromising the function of the limb.

ANATOMY, FUNCTION, AND BIOMECHANICS OF THE TIBIA AND FIBULA

The anatomy of the tibia and fibula can be divided into regions based on their location, function, architecture, and the forces acting on them.

Epiphysis

Location and Function

Proximally the epiphysis consists of:

- The tibial plateau, which provides support for the articular cartilage of the distal stifle joint (for information concerning the stifle joint, see Chap. 129)
- The fibular head, which serves as the distal attachment for the lateral collateral ligament
- The tibial tubercle, which is the insertion point of the patellar tendon of the quadriceps muscle

Distally, the epiphyseal region consists of:

- The cochlea tibia, which supports the distal articular cartilage and articulates with the tibial tarsal bone
- The medial malleolus, which is the proximal attachment of the medial collateral tarsal ligaments
- The fibular epiphysis (lateral malleolus), which acts as the proximal attachment of the lateral collateral tarsal ligaments

Biomechanics

- The epiphyseal regions of the tibia and fibula are primarily composed of loosely woven, trabecular bone

surrounded by a thin shell of dense cortex. This architecture limits the holding power of fixation implants, requiring extra care in their application.
- The epiphyseal regions that serve as ligament and tendon attachments are subjected to distractive forces. Consequently, repair of avulsion fractures of these areas must control these tensile forces.
- The epiphyseal regions that support articular cartilage are subjected to compressive loads that tend to separate the fragments, resulting in articular incongruity, instability, and eventually degenerative arthritis. Fixation of these fractures must provide anatomic reduction and rigid immobilization so that the fracture will heal with minimal callus formation, and so that early joint motion can be initiated to avoid joint stiffness.

Physis

- The physeal regions of the tibia and fibula are located adjacent to the epiphysis and exist only in growing immature animals.
- The hypertrophied layer and calcifying layers of the physis are relatively fragile, and are commonly fractured with trauma.
- Because the cartilage layers are irregular and transverse, fractures tend to interdigitate well when reduced and require only control of bending forces.

Metaphysis

- The metaphysis is an indistinct region of bone located between the physis and the diaphysis (central shaft).
- The function of the metaphysis in the mature animal is the gradual alteration of the general construction of the bone from the wide-diameter thin cortex of the epiphysis to the narrow-diameter thick cortex of the diaphysis. The biomechanics and architecture of these regions change along their length.

Diaphysis

- The diaphysis is the central portion of the tibia and makes up the majority of its length.
- The tibial diaphysis is subjected to severe bending and torsional forces, in addition to axial compressive loads. Its hollow tubular construction of relatively thick cortical bone maximizes its effectiveness in resisting these forces.

PREOPERATIVE CONSIDERATIONS

General Considerations

- Examine the animal carefully for nonorthopedic injuries.
  - Evaluate cardiovascular status. If cardiopulmonary problems are suspected, radiograph the thorax.
  - Evaluate neurologic status. Determine deep pain perception in the fractured limb for local nerve damage, and proprioceptive and sensory perception in the other limbs for evidence of nerve or spinal cord trauma.
- Examine the animal carefully for concurrent musculoskeletal injuries.

▼ *Key Point* Nearly all small animals with tibial and/or fibular fractures are able to support themselves on the remaining three limbs. If not, suspect additional injuries.

- Determine the extent of soft tissue injury and fracture contamination.
  - Cover all open fractures with sterile bandages to prevent further contamination, and debride as soon as possible.
  - Broad-spectrum antibiotics are indicated if the fracture is open. Obtain samples for culture and sensitivity testing from the fracture site before beginning antibiotic therapy.
  - Until definitive treatment is possible, support all tibial fractures with a compressive wrap (Robert Jones bandage) or splint to prevent additional soft tissue injury.

Specific Considerations in Selecting a Fracture Fixation Technique

- Determine the potential axial stability of the reduced fracture based on preoperative fracture radiographs.
  - Stable fractures generally are simple transverse or short oblique. They tend to impact and become more stable upon weight bearing.
  - Unstable fractures have patterns, such as long oblique or comminuted, which tend to override or collapse upon axial loading.
- Perform rigid fixation of extensively contaminated open fractures. However, avoid placing large implants in the fracture site.
- Fractures in immature animals heal quickly, but:
  - Premature physeal closure can occur with or without internal fixation.
  - Immature animals rapidly develop joint stiffness with limb immobilization.
  - Implants quickly loosen in the soft bone of immature animals.
- Fractures in very old animals heal slowly.
  - Brittle bone in older animals often splinters when implants are applied.

SURGICAL PROCEDURES

Objectives

- Provide adequate stability for fracture healing to occur while causing minimal damage to the biologic healing process.
- Restore normal limb function by minimizing joint stiffness and muscle atrophy and avoiding subsequent degenerative joint disease.

Pin and Tension Band Wire Fixation

Indications

- Avulsion fractures of the fibular head
- Avulsion fractures of the lateral (fibular) malleolus and medial (tibial) malleolus (Fig. 130–1)
- Avulsion fractures of the tibial tubercle

Equipment

- General orthopedic pack:
  - Standard surgical pack
  - Bone and fracture reduction forceps
  - Periosteal elevator
  - Jacob hand chuck
  - Wire pliers and cutters
- Stainless steel monofilament orthopedic wire (18–22 gauge)
- Kirschner wires (0.035–0.062 inch)

Technique

1. Incise the skin directly over the affected bone.
2. Reduce and stabilize fracture with small fragment reduction forceps.
3. Create a transverse hole through the intact tibia approximately equidistant from the fracture line with the hand chuck and a Kirschner wire.

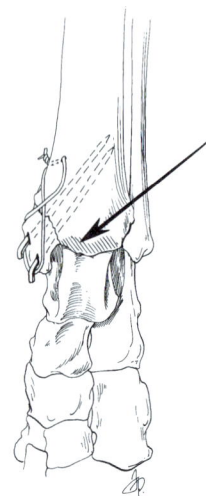

Figure 130–1. Pin and tension wire fixation of a medial malleolar avulsion fracture. Do not violate the cochlear articular surface with the Kirschner wire *(arrow)*.

4. Insert two parallel Kirschner wires through the fragment, across the fracture, and into the parent bone.

▼ *Key Point* In the treatment of malleolar fractures, avoid penetrating the articular surface of the distal cochlea.

5. Pass orthopedic wire (18 gauge for most dogs, 20–22 gauge for small dogs and cats) through the transverse hole, cross the wire over the fracture site, and pass one end under the ligament or tendon attachment.
6. Twist both ends of wire together to form a figure eight. Tighten the wire just enough to compress the fracture (see Fig. 130–1).
7. Cut off excess orthopedic and Kirschner wires. Bend the Kirschner wires over and embed them in the soft tissues to trap the orthopedic wire loop and minimize soft tissue irritation.
   a. In the treatment of tibial tubercle fractures, if the animal still has significant growth potential, do not use tension band wires because this procedure can induce premature physeal closure. If necessary, use additional Kirschner wires oriented perpendicular to the physis for fixation stability.
8. Close soft tissues routinely.

Interfragmentary Lag Screw Fixation

Indications

- Intra-articular fractures of the proximal epiphysis (tibial plateau) and distal epiphysis (tibial cochlea)
- Reconstruction of comminuted shaft fractures prior to neutralization plating (see Fig. 130–7)

Equipment

- General orthopedic pack
- Bone screws and application instrumentation
- Power drill
- Kirschner wires

Technique

1. Manipulate fragments to obtain anatomic reduction of the intra-articular portion of the fracture and temporarily stabilize with fracture forceps.
2. Insert an interfragmentary screw and compress the intra-articular fracture line, using either a partially threaded screw or over-drilling the near fragment to create a gliding hole for fully threaded screws. Orient the screw perpendicular to the fracture line.
3. Insert additional screws or cross pins, depending on the fragment size, to prevent rotation around the first screw and to provide additional support.

Cross-Pin and Rush Pin Fixation

Indications

- Transverse fractures of the epiphysis (may be combined with interfragmentary lag screw technique if the fracture extends into a joint)
- Axially stable fractures of the metaphysis (Fig. 130–2)
- Salter I and II fractures of the proximal and distal physis

Equipment

- General orthopedic pack
- Kirschner wires or small Steinmann pins (1/16–1/8″ in diameter)
- Pin cutter

Technique

1. Manipulate the fracture and reduce through an open approach. Medial approach to the tibial shaft is preferred owing to relative lack of soft tissues.
2. Select the proper pin diameter (approximately 15% of bone diameter for cross pins, 10% for pins placed in the Rush technique).
3. With a hand chuck (a power drill can be used for cross pins), insert pins from the medial and lateral aspect of the fragment across the fracture into the medullary canal of the parent bone.
4. Orient cross pins obliquely to the long axis (35–45°) so that they penetrate the far cortex (parent bone) when inserted (see Fig. 130–2).

▼ *Key Point* Cross-pins provide excellent fracture fixation, but because they can interfere with normal function of the growth plate, use them with caution in immature animals.

5. Orient pins placed in the Rush technique more parallel (25–35°) to the long axis. During insertion they bounce off the inner cortex of the medullary canal and are driven in to impact into the trabecular bone of the distant metaphysis.
   a. Pins placed in the Rush technique may be preferable for physeal fractures because of their smaller

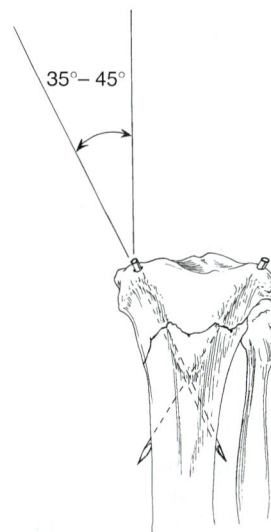

35°– 45°

Figure 130–2. Fracture of the proximal tibial metaphysis fixed with cross pins. Note the angle of pin insertion and penetration of the parent diaphyseal cortex.

diameter (resulting in less damage to the proliferative zone of the physis) and because of their more perpendicular orientation to the physis (allowing sliding of the physis along the pins as it grows).

    b. Prebend the pins to facilitate reflection of the pins off the inner cortical wall as they are inserted.

6. Cut off excess pin length and countersink the ends below bone level (if the pins will not be removed) or bend the ends over to avoid soft tissue interference.

Intramedullary (IM) Pin and Wire Fixation

Indications

- Simple, axially stable fractures of the tibial diaphysis
- Other selected reducible tibial diaphyseal fractures

Contraindications

- Infected or significantly contaminated open (grade 3) fractures (see Chap. 139)
- Fractures that cannot be reconstructed

Equipment

- General orthopedic pack
- Steinmann pins
- Pin cutter

Technique

IM Pinning Technique for Simple, Axially Stable Tibial Fractures

1. Select a pin diameter 50–60% of the smallest medullary canal diameter.
2. Reduce the fracture, usually by manipulation through a medial open approach.
3. Insert the pin at a point midway between the tibial tubercle and medial collateral ligament along the edge of the tibial plateau (slightly distal to the articular surface).
4. Drive the pin distally (normograde) down the proximal fragment and across the fracture to impact into the distal metaphyseal bone.
5. Determine the pin insertion length by comparison with a second pin, identical in length, held along the side of the bone.

▼ *Key Point* Avoid driving IM pins through the articular cartilage of the cochlea, because this can result in development of significant arthritis.

---

6. Remove excess pin length with a pin cutter.
7. Determine rotational stability. If significant rotational motion persists, apply interfragmentary wire or a two-pin external fixator.
    a. Two-pin fixation is similar to type I external skeletal fixation (described later) but uses only two pins, one above and one below the fracture.

Technique

Wiring Techniques for Fracture Reconstruction Prior to IM Pinning

With Cerclage Wires

Cerclage wires can be used only on long oblique fracture lines (fracture line length ≥2 × bone diameter) (Fig. 130–3).

1. Use large (18 gauge for medium and larger dogs; 22 gauge for toy breeds and cats) monofilament wire.
2. To control motion, at least two wires must cross the complete fracture line.
3. Orient wires perpendicular to the long bone axis, space apart at least one-half bone diameter, and twist to tighten.
4. Use cerclage wires for fissure fractures as necessary.
5. Always use an IM pin in addition to the cerclage wires to control bending forces.

With Interfragmentary Wires

Use interfragmentary wires to stabilize short oblique patterns (fracture length <2 × bone diameter) when only one wire can be applied.

1. Create holes in each bone fragment with a hand chuck and Kirschner wire. Position the holes so the wire crosses the fracture perpendicular to the fracture line, thus providing maximum interfragmentary compression when the wire is tightly twisted.
2. Thread the wire through the holes and incorporate the IM pin that has been inserted to the level of the fracture as described previously.

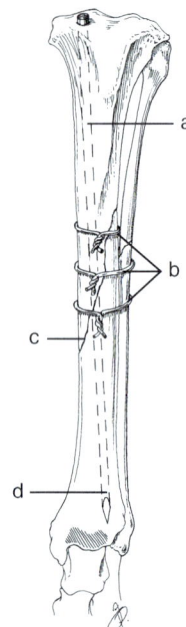

Figure 130–3. Use of cerclage wire to prevent axial collapse of a long oblique fracture stabilized with an intramedullary (IM) pin. (a) Pin diameter equals 50–60% of the medullary canal; (b) wires must be perpendicular to bone axis and ½ bone diameter apart; (c) fracture length must be ≥2 × bone diameter; (d) stop pin insertion short of cochlea.

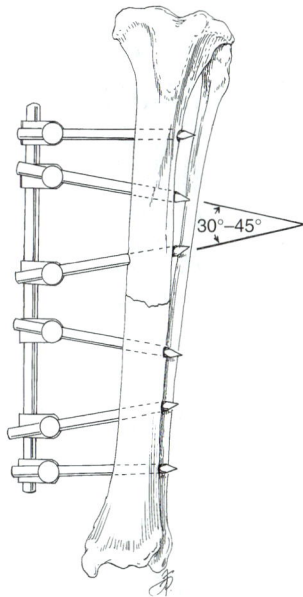

Figure 130–4. A six-pin type I (unilateral) external skeletal fixator applied to the medial side of a relatively stable tibial fracture. Addition of a lateral connecting bar would convert this to a type II (bilateral) fixator.

3. Reduce the fracture, complete the IM pin insertion, and tighten the interfragmentary wire.

External Skeletal Fixation (ESF)

Indications

- Stable, reducible, and nonreducible fracture patterns depending on ESF frame configuration:
  - Type I (unilateral) frames are relatively flexible in axial bending. Therefore, they are appropriate for relatively stable fractures (Fig. 130–4).

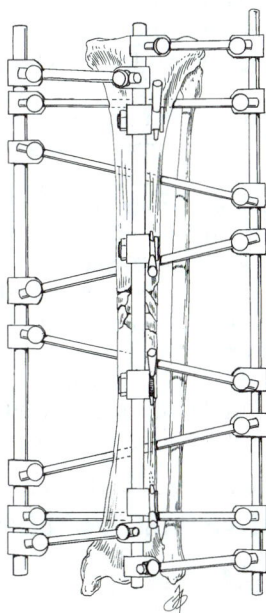

Figure 130–5. A very rigid type III (trilateral) external skeletal fixation (ESF) configuration applied to a nonreconstructible diaphyseal fracture.

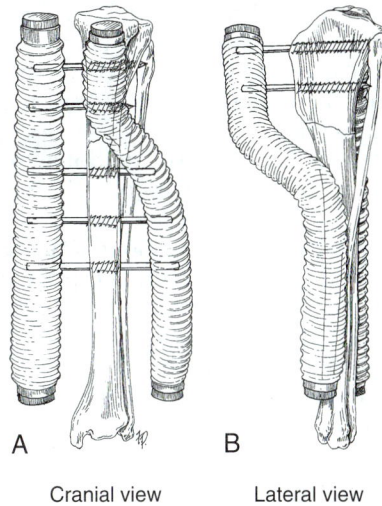

Cranial view   Lateral view

Figure 130–6. Biplanar configurations allow placement of an adequate number of pins in short metaphyseal fragments.

- Type II (bilateral) and type III (trilateral) configurations (Fig. 130–5) have axial rigidity comparable to that of plates.
  - Biplanar configurations (Fig. 130–6) allow placement of an adequate number of pins in short metaphyseal fragments.
- Open fractures with significant soft tissue damage or infected fractures, because rigid fixation can be obtained without large implants (e.g., IM pins, plates) in the fracture site.
- Contraindications
  - Intra-articular fractures
  - Avulsion fractures of ligament and tendon epiphyseal attachments

Equipment

- General orthopedic pack
- Low-speed power drill
- Kirschner apparatus is available in three sizes for small animal application
- Acrylic pin external fixator (APEF) system available in three sizes.

Technique for Kirschner External Fixator

1. Fixation usually is placed on the medial side of the tibia. However, it can be oriented laterally or cranially to avoid soft tissue injuries.
2. Hold the fracture in approximate reduction, and insert the most proximal and distal fixation pins through small skin incisions into each fragment, using a low-speed power drill. Predrill holes with a drill bit 90% pin diameter before inserting threaded pins. Threaded pins reduce the incidence of loosening of pins.
3. Slide a connecting bar with the appropriate number of clamps onto the end fixation pins (at least three pins in each fragment).
4. Reduce the fracture, using closed manipulation on more comminuted fractures or a limited open approach on simpler fractures, and tighten the end clamps.

5. Insert fixation pins through the remaining open clamps into the bone and tighten each connecting clamp when placing the pin. If threaded pins are not used, obtain a 30° angle between at least two of the pins in each fragment.

6. For unstable fractures, insert additional pins and bars in other planes to create more rigid frame configurations.

7. Collect autogenous cancellous bone graft from the proximal medial tibial tuberosity, and place it in any bony defects remaining after open fracture reduction.

8. Do not completely close incisions or wounds of open or infected fractures (see Postoperative Care and Complications).

Technique for APEF System Application

1. Insert fixation pins (usually a combination of threaded pins for optimal bone-pin integrity, and nonthreaded pins for economy) in the bone fragments oriented to best meet the mechanical needs of the fracture and minimize soft tissue tethering.

2. Attach the APEF alignment frame to pins on both sides of the fracture close to the skin level. Reduce the fracture (using closed manipulation or open reduction), and bone clamps may be used to temporarily maintain reduction.

3. Close open reduction incisions or pack open wounds aseptically. Adequacy of closed reduction can be checked with radiographs.

4. Cut pins approximately 4–5 cm from the skin level.

5. Impale the acrylic column molding tubes on the pin ends and position the tubes adjacent to the alignment frame, parallel to the limb about 2–3 cm from the skin.

6. Plug the most dependent end of each molding tube.

7. Premeasured acrylic is mixed for 2–3 minutes to a smooth consistency.

8. Cut a corner of the bag with scissors, then pour the acrylic into the open end of each tube.

9. Allow the acrylic to cure (10–12 minutes).

10. Remove the alignment frame, plugs, and excess molding tube.

Plate and Screw Fixation

Indications

- The stabilized limb is needed for immediate weight bearing because of orthopedic or neurologic injuries to the other limbs.
- Restricted activity or adequate postoperative care is not possible.
- Rigid fixation is necessary (e.g., in large, very active dogs).

Equipment

- General orthopedic pack
- Plates, screws, and specialized instrumentation for their implantation
- Power drill

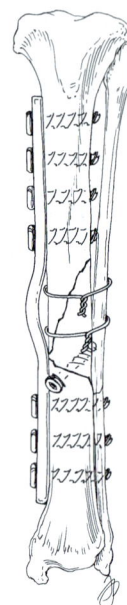

Figure 130–7. Use of a plate to protect a reconstructed comminuted tibial fracture from excessive bending forces. The screw and wires maintain reduction, and the plate "neutralizes" the weight-bearing forces.

Technique

1. Contour an appropriate-size plate to the shape of the intact bone and apply the plate to the medial (tensile) side of the tibia.

2. If the fracture pattern is axially stable, compress the fracture by applying the plate in the compression mode. When using dynamic compression plates, compression is achieved by drilling screw holes such that the screw slides toward the fracture line.

3. Initially, rebuild long, oblique, and reducible comminuted fractures with interfragmentary lag screws and/or wires. Apply a plate to the tibia without compression to protect the interfragmentary fixation from bending forces (i.e., neutralization mode) (Fig. 130–7).

4. To prevent collapse under loading, apply a heavy plate in the buttress mode for nonreducible fractures.

    a. Add cancellous autograft to the fracture to stimulate rapid formation of load-sharing callus.

    b. Alternatively, remove detached bone fragments (break into small pieces and add to bone graft), transversely osteotomize fragment ends, and collapse the fracture to reestablish good cortical contact and a stable repair. As much as 20% of the tibial length may be removed without causing permanent dysfunction.

POSTOPERATIVE CARE AND COMPLICATIONS

Immediate Postoperative Care

- Apply a compressive wrap (Robert Jones bandage) for 3–5 days to prevent soft tissue swelling and to protect the incision.

- Use gauze and tape to cover the connecting bars and clamps of external fixators. This decreases the incidence of the fixator "hanging up" on objects in the environment and protects the opposite limb.

▼ *Key Point* Do not primarily close infected and severely open fractures. Lavage and debride the wound q 24–48 hr until healthy granulation tissue covers the wound (7–10 days). Complete wound closure at that time or allow healing by second intention if there is tension at the wound margins.

- Where using ESF, clean around pin-skin junction daily with hydrogen peroxide.

Implant Removal

- Do not routinely remove small implants such as cross pins, cerclage wires, lag screws, and tension band wires unless they cause problems such as joint interference and chronic drainage.
- Remove large IM pins unless the proximal pin end has been buried by tibial growth.
- Partially disassemble (destabilize or dynamize) rigid external fixation frames to a flexible configuration after early osseous bridging has occurred (about 6 weeks postoperatively). This increases fracture loading, stimulating callus hypertrophy and remodeling while protecting the fracture from excessive forces that might cause refracture. Remove the balance of the fixator when fracture healing is complete.
- Remove bone plates in the following situations:
  - Animal with short hair coat develops pain in limb when exposed to cold ambient temperatures.
  - Stiff plate design induces bone atrophy due to stress protection.
  - Chronic infection and drainage does not resolve.

Complications

Nonunion

- Hypertrophic nonunion:
  - There is exuberant callus proliferation without fracture bridging because of inadequate fracture immobilization. These fractures are biologically active and require only adequate immobilization.
  - Augment existing fixation or replace with a more rigid fixation technique to allow the fracture to heal.
- Atrophic nonunion:
  - There is lack of callus production, bone sclerosis, and bone resorption, reflecting a loss of biologic healing potential. These nonunions usually result from significant vascular damage from the trauma, surgical manipulation, or unstable fixation.
  - Treatment includes resection of nonviable bone, reestablishment of vascularity, control of infection, rigid fixation, and induction of new bone proliferation with an autogenous cancellous bone graft.

Malunion

- Malunion occurs when the fracture heals but poor alignment results in abnormal limb function. This may reflect inadequate initial reduction or loss of reduction owing to inadequate fixation.
- Treatment includes osteotomy, realignment, and adequate fixation.

Infection

- Acute infection of a tibial fracture occurs when bacterial proliferation overwhelms the body's defense mechanisms.
- Clinical signs include pain, swelling, and erythema that reflect the underlying accumulation of exudate and necrotic tissue.
- Immediate aggressive treatment is indicated to avoid progression to chronic osteomyelitis and nonunion:
  - Open the incision and extend the margins, if necessary, to ensure adequate drainage.
  - Culture the wound for aerobic and anaerobic organisms to determine specific antibiotic sensitivity.
  - Repeatedly lavage and debride the fracture site to remove exudate and necrotic soft tissue.
  - Initiate systemic broad-spectrum antibiotic therapy (e.g., cephalothins) until culture and sensitivity testing indicate specific therapy.
- See Chap. 140 for management of chronic osteomyelitis.

Growth Deformities

Growth deformities can result from trauma to the proliferative layer of one of the physes, or from application of fracture fixation that limits physeal elongation. Angular deformities become apparent about 3 weeks after physeal injury; arthritic changes follow if the condition is not corrected. Treatment depends on the cause of physeal dysfunction and the animal's maturity.

- In actively growing animals:
  - Resect the osseous bridge crossing the physis and replace with autogenous fat graft.
  - Remove fixation implants that might be inhibiting physeal growth.
- In mature animals:
  - Perform corrective osteotomy and articular realignment.

SUPPLEMENTAL READINGS

Aron DN, Palmer RH, Johnson AL: Biologic strategies and a balanced concept for repair of highly comminuted long bone fractures. Compend Contin Educ Pract Vet 17:35, 1995.

Chan KL, Leung YK, Cheng JC, Leung PC: The management of Type III open tibial fractures. Injury 16:157, 1984.

Coombs R, Green SA, Sarmiento A: External Fixation and Functional Bracing. London: Orthotext, 1989, p 13.

Egger EI, Histand MB, Norrdin RW, et al: Canine osteotomy healing when stabilized with decreasingly rigid fixation compared to constantly rigid fixation. U.C.O.T. 6:182, 1993.

Johnson AL, Seitz SE, Smith CW, et al.: Closed reduction and type-II external fixation of comminuted fractures of the radius and tibia in dogs: 23 cases (1990–1994). JAVMA 209:1445, 1996.

Piermattei DL: An Atlas of Surgical Approaches to the Bones of the Dog and Cat, 3rd Ed. Philadelphia: WB Saunders, 1993, p 298.

Robertson WW: Newest knowledge of the growth plate. Clin Orthoped Rel Res 253:270, 1990.

131 Luxation, Subluxation, and Shearing Injuries of the Tarsal Joint

Dennis N. Aron

Luxation, subluxation, and shearing injuries of the tarsus involve damage to the supporting ligaments of the joint. Treatment and prognosis of these injuries depend on the location of the ligament damage and subsequent joint instability. Subluxations can be caused by spontaneous overstress or external trauma. Vehicular trauma usually causes luxations and shear injuries. Conservative treatment of most of these injuries with external coaptation is not advised, because continued instability and the development of degenerative joint disease are the likely outcome.

▼ *Key Point* Surgical stabilization gives the most consistent results in repair of luxation, subluxation, and shearing injuries of the tarsus.

SURGICAL ANATOMY AND SPECIAL CONSIDERATIONS

General

- The tarsus consists of the tibia, fibula, metatarsal bones, and seven specific tarsal bones orderly stacked in levels (Fig. 131–1).
- A multiple complex arrangement of ligaments connects the bones of the joint and helps to prevent luxation (Fig. 131–2).
- The *tarsocrural* joint is formed by the tibia and fibula at the proximal level and by the talus and calcaneus at the distal level.
- The *intertarsal* joints are all the articulations between the tarsal bones. Several of these joints are named and include the
  - Talocalcaneal joint—between the talus and calcaneus
  - Talocalcaneocentral joint—between the talus and central tarsal bone (includes a small communication with the calcaneus)
  - Calcaneoquartal joint (proximal intertarsal joint)—between the calcaneus and fourth tarsal bone
  - Centrodistal joint (distal intertarsal joint)—between the central tarsal bone and distal numbered tarsal bones
  - Tarsometatarsal joints—between the distal tarsal and metatarsal bones

Tarsocrural Joint

- Synonyms for this joint are the tibiotarsal, talocrural, and hock joint.
- Most luxations, subluxations, and shear injuries directly involve this joint.
- The major ligaments providing stability on the medial side of the joint are the long medial ligaments and tibiotalar short component ligament (Fig. 131–3A).
- The major ligaments providing stability on the lateral side of the joint are the long lateral ligament and the calcaneofibular short component ligament (Fig. 131–4A).
- The components of the medial and lateral ligaments complement each other in maintaining the talus in the mortise provided by the tibia and fibula.
- Certain parts of the ligament complexes are tighter in extension (long lateral and medial ligaments) or flexion (calcaneofibular and tibiotalar short component ligaments).
- The tibiotalar and calcaneofibular short component ligaments of the medial and lateral sides, respectively, are especially important for maintaining stability of the joint. The joint capsule and malleoli also contribute to joint stability.
- The gross anatomy of the medial and lateral collateral ligament complexes is similar (see Figs. 131–3 and 131–4). The components cross at the tarsocrural joint space, providing the greatest amount of ligament and an advantageous spatial arrangement directly over the joint.

▼ *Key Point* In the reconstruction of the collateral ligamentous supporting structures of the tarsocrural joint, consider the complementary nature of ligamentous structure and function.

Intertarsal and Tarsometatarsal Joints

- The most common injury is damage to the plantar ligaments and tarsal fibrocartilage (see Fig. 131–2).
- The plantar ligaments and tarsal fibrocartilage limit extension of the intertarsal joints.
- Most of the intertarsal joint stability is provided by three distinct plantar ligaments. These ligaments fuse, with a thickening of the joint capsule (the tarsal fibrocartilage) at the tarsometatarsal joint.

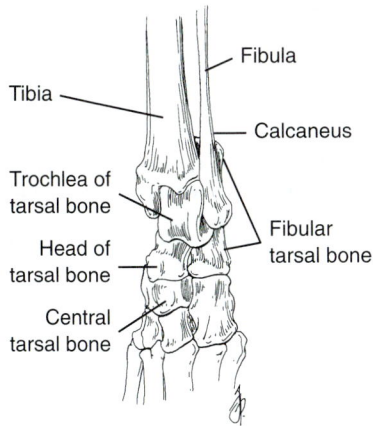

Figure 131–1.   Anatomy of the bones of the tarsus.

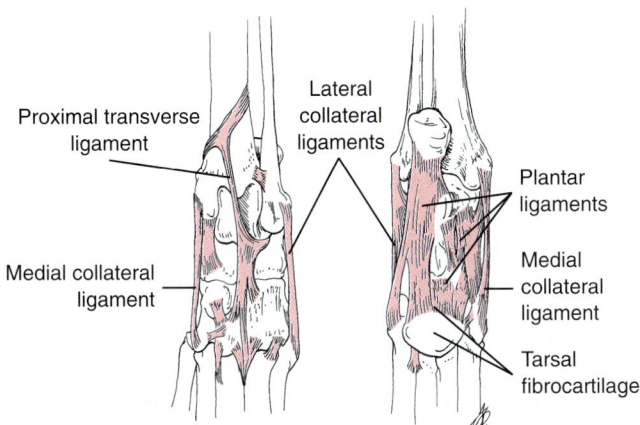

Figure 131–2.   Cranial (*left*) and caudal (*right*) views of the ligamentous anatomy of the tarsus.

- The first ligament originates from the plantar surface of the sustentaculum tali and attaches to the central tarsal bone and tarsometatarsal joint capsule.
- The second ligament originates from the plantar-lateral surface of the calcaneus. It joins with the long component of the lateral collateral ligament complex and attaches to the base of the fifth metatarsal bone.

- The third ligament originates from the body of the calcaneus and attaches to the fourth tarsal bone and the base of the fourth and fifth metatarsal bones.

TARSOCRURAL LUXATION AND SUBLUXATION

Surgical methods are recommended for treatment of luxation or subluxation injuries of the tarsocrural joint. Luxation and subluxation usually are the result of rupture of the medial or lateral collateral ligament complex.

Double-Prosthesis Replacement

- Double-prosthesis replacement (described later) closely reproduces the components of the intact medial and lateral collateral ligament complexes, thus allowing nearly normal joint stability to be maintained throughout a functional range of motion.
- Similar to the components of the normal collateral ligaments, double-suture prostheses become taut and lax with flexion and extension. Because of this, wire is not useful. Certain sutures (see later) give more successful results, most likely owing to the retention of elasticity upon cyclic loading.
- Clinically, double-ligament replacement gives results superior to conservative management with splints or nonanatomic single ligament replacement methods. The prognosis is good for long-term function with most closed luxation and subluxation injuries, depending on timely repair (within 5 days of injury) and absence of articular damage.

Preoperative Considerations

- Tarsocrural luxation results from different combinations of injuries including:
  - Fractures of both malleoli
  - Fracture of one malleolus and damage to the contralateral ligament complex
  - Fracture of the fibula and damage to the medial ligament complex
  - Uncommonly, damage to both the lateral and medial collateral ligament complexes and no fractures

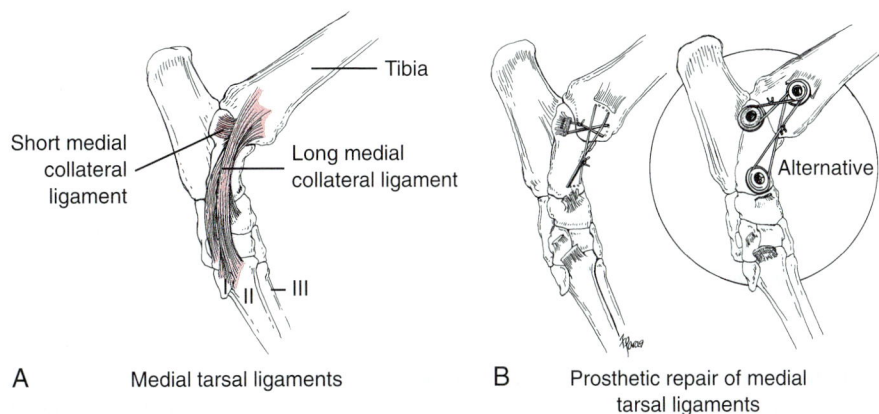

Figure 131–3. *A,* Medial ligamentous anatomy of the tarsus. *B,* Suture prosthesis repair of medial ligament injury. Tunnel sutures through the bones at points where the ligaments attach. Alternatively, place bone screws at these points and pass sutures around them.

A   Medial tarsal ligaments

B   Prosthetic repair of medial tarsal ligaments

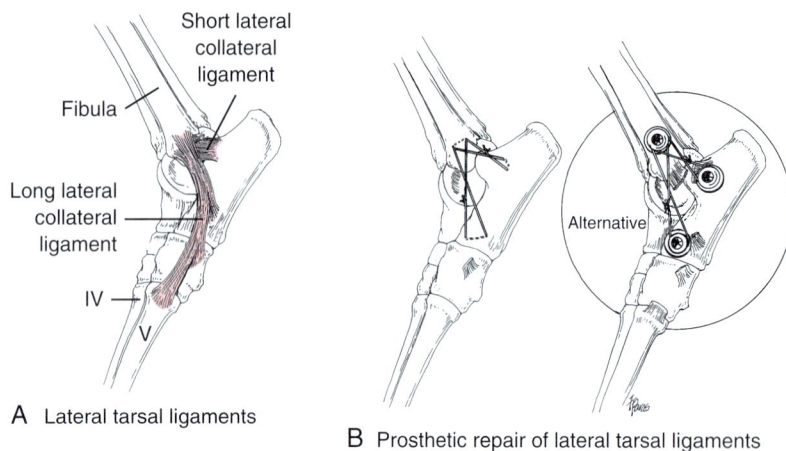

A Lateral tarsal ligaments

B Prosthetic repair of lateral tarsal ligaments

Figure 131–4. *A,* Lateral ligamentous anatomy of the tarsus. *B,* Suture prosthesis repair of lateral ligament injury. Tunnel sutures through the bones at points where the ligaments attach. Alternatively, place bone screws at these points and pass sutures around them.

- Tarsocrural subluxation usually results from complete rupture or avulsion of either the lateral or medial collateral ligament complex.
  - In medial ruptures, the paw tilts abnormally toward the lateral direction with a laterally (valgus) applied force.
  - In lateral ruptures, the tilt is in a medial direction with a medially (varus) applied force.
- Occasionally, there is rupture of only the long or short components of the medial or lateral ligament complexes. Less joint laxity makes these subluxation injuries more difficult to diagnose. Determine joint laxity using the following methods:
  - Place lateral and medial tilt forces on the hock at different joint angles: Laxity in extension but not flexion suggests major damage to the long medial ligament, or long lateral ligament; laxity in only flexion suggests that most damage is isolated to the tibiotalar or calcaneofibular short components.
  - Make a dorsoplantar (stress) radiograph while applying lateral and medial tilt forces on the hock: Take the stress radiograph at the tarsocrural joint angle that produces the subluxation; for subtle subluxations, compare this radiograph with a similar radiograph of the contralateral (normal) hock.

▼ *Key Point* Routine dorsoplantar and lateral radiographic views are always needed to check for concomitant tarsal injuries. Stress radiographs are useful to confirm the diagnosis but are not always necessary.

Surgical Procedure

Objectives

- Stabilize the joint.
- Maintain an adequate range of motion.
- Avoid trauma to the articular surfaces.
- Achieve pain-free weight bearing.
- Minimize patient morbidity and owner expense.

Equipment

- Standard orthopedic instrument pack and suture material

- Gelpi self-retaining retractors
- Small periosteal elevator
- Orthopedic drill (power drill preferred)
- Orthopedic screws, washers, and insertion equipment
- Kirschner wires (K-wires)
- Assortment of straight and curved needles
- Coaptation splint
- Braided polyester*

Technique

1. Clip the injured limb from the level of the proximal femur, extending distally to include the paw. Include the paw in the sterile field to allow direct manipulation.
2. Place the patient in lateral recumbency, with the injured limb up for lateral replacement or down for medial replacement, and prepare the limb for aseptic surgery.
3. Expose the subluxation through a curved skin incision centered over the medial or lateral malleolus.
   a. Begin from the distal one-fourth of the tibia and continue to the proximal metatarsal bones.
   b. Locate the medial or lateral collateral ligament complex along the same line by incising the subcutaneous tissue and deep fascia.
4. Inspect the components of the ligament complexes for damage.
   a. To help assess the damage, stress the ligament components with a varus or valgus tilt in both flexion and extension.
   b. It is unlikely that there will be a totally isolated injury to only one component of the ligament complex. The ligaments can appear intact but may have lost considerable function owing to internal derangement of the collagen fibers.

▼ *Key Point* Usually, the ligament components are too badly damaged to allow primary suturing of the torn ends or reattachment to bone. Replace irreparable ligaments and protect repaired ligaments with prosthetic sutures.

---

*Polydek or Tevdek, Deknatel, Inc., Queens Village, NY 11429

5. Replace or protect the medial or lateral ligament complexes with two figure-eight heavy sutures anchored to the bone directly or with bone screws.
   a. Drill bone tunnels in the malleolus in locations similar to the origins of the components of the ligament complex (see Figs. 131–3 and 131–4). Bone tunnels serve as anchors for the suture prostheses.
   b. Secure the suture prosthesis that mimics the lateral or medial short components to tags of the torn ligament at the insertion site. Use a locking loop suture pattern to grip the torn ligament (see Chap. 134). A bone screw (see Shear Injury) may be needed to fix the prosthesis to the insertion site (see Figs. 131–3B, 131–4B).
   c. Secure the suture prosthesis that mimics the lateral or medial long components to a drill hole in the tubercle of the distal talus or distal calcaneus (see Figs. 131–3B and 131–4B). A bone screw (see Shear Injury) may be used to fix the prosthesis (see Figs. 131–3B and 131–4B).

6. Use one or two (for large patients) strands of #1–5 braided polyester sutures for prosthetic replacement or protection.
   a. Set the sutures in a figure-eight pattern.
   b. Do not use absorbable sutures.
   c. Do *not* use monofilament nylon and monofilament polypropylene for sutures. They tend to stretch permanently and are better suited for primary repair of torn ligaments.

7. Tie the long and short suture prostheses.
   a. Tie the short prosthesis with the tarsocrural joint held in approximately 90° flexion for dogs and 70° for cats.
   b. Tie the long suture prosthesis with the joint in a functional standing angle of 135° for dogs (varies with breed) and 120° for cats.
   c. After the sutures are tied, tighten the screws against the bone.

8. Expose the luxation injury through separate surgical incisions on the medial and lateral sides of the joint.
   a. Fix the malleolar fracture with a tension band technique.
   b. Replace or protect the contralateral ligaments.

9. To manage luxations due to fracture of the fibula and damage to the contralateral ligament complex
   a. Replace or protect the medial ligaments.
   b. Stabilize the fibula by fixing the limb in a long, rigid coaptation splint. Extend the splint from above the stifle to the paw and position the stifle and hock joints in a functional angle. Maintain for 4–6 weeks.

Postoperative Care

- Immobilize the tarsocrural joints with a short, semi-rigid coaptation splint.
  - Extend the splint from just below the stifle distally to include the digits.
  - Place the hock in a functional standing angle.
  - Provide semirigid softcast coaptation with a full circular cast.*

---

*Softcast (3M Center, St. Paul, MN).

- Maintain the semirigid softcast coaptation splint for 4–12 weeks; the length of time depends on the amount of initial trauma and joint instability. A longer time is required for luxation and major subluxation injuries, a shorter time for incomplete tears and partial injuries.
  - The semirigid softcast allows for controlled mobilization by progressive unwrapping of layers to increase tissue microstrain as healing advances.
  - Once all coaptation is removed, continue progressive controlled mobilization by slowly increasing the animal's activity over another 4–8 week period. During this period, if the animal shows signs of increased lameness or pain, progress more slowly with controlled mobilization in a manner that does not create lameness or discomfort.

▼ *Key Point* Do not allow immediate uncontrolled activity of an animal after removal of coaptation.

SHEAR INJURY

Preoperative Considerations

- Shear injury usually occurs when an animal is trapped by a moving vehicle, resulting in shearing by the road surface of supporting ligaments, joint capsule, and malleolus.
- The medial side of the joint is injured more commonly than the lateral side of the joint.
- Perform wound management and ligament replacement when the bone and cartilage damage is mostly isolated to the malleolus. Severe soft tissue damage makes stabilization difficult and prolongs healing.
- Although a successful ligament replacement gives better results than a tarsocrural joint arthrodesis, consider joint arthrodesis if there is extensive bone and cartilage damage.

Surgical Procedure

Objectives

- Prevent infection.
- Anatomically stabilize the tarsocrural joint, eliminate pain, and maintain a functional range of motion.
- Avoid trauma to the articular surfaces.
- Attain wound coverage with a full-thickness skin graft.
- Minimize patient morbidity and owner expense.

Equipment

- Equipment is the same as for tarsocrural luxation and subluxation plus
  - External skeletal fixator
  - Wound dressing materials

Wound Management and Debridement

Technique

1. Before debridement and ligament replacement, cover the shear wound with a temporary sterile

dressing and apply a temporary splint to prevent further damage to the unstable joint. Exteriorized material will contaminate deeper recesses if replacement into the wound is attempted.

  a. Do not push or "stuff" extruded soft tissue, bone, or cartilage back into the wound.
  b. Do not soak the wound.

2. Perform debridement as soon as the animal is a stable candidate for surgery, ideally within 6 hours from the time of injury, and preferably sooner.

▼ *Key Point* Ligament reconstruction and wound closure can be delayed but do not delay wound debridement.

  a. Anesthetize the animal and remove the temporary splint.
  b. Keeping the wound covered, clip the limb, and cleanse with an appropriate antiseptic.
  c. Remove the dressing and thoroughly irrigate the wound with copious amounts of a prewarmed balanced electrolyte solution (see Chap. 52).
  d. Obtain cultures of the joint surface for identification of contaminating organisms and their sensitivity to antibiotics. A Gram stain may be helpful in identifying bacteria type.

3. After moving the animal to the operating area, perform a final surgical scrub and drape the limb.

4. Debride the wound of all visible necrotic tissue and debris. Be careful to avoid damage to articular surfaces.

  a. During the debridement process, lavage continuously with copious amounts (1 L or more) of a balanced electrolyte solution such as lactated Ringer's, using a moderate amount of pressure, through a 30- to 60-ml syringe and 18- or 19-gauge needle or catheter. Pulsatile suction and lavage is ideal.

5. Perform ligament replacement at this time or delay for repeat wound debridement or orthopedic referral. If delaying replacement:

  a. Cover the wound with an absorbent dressing to keep the wound moist (e.g., wet-to-dry dressing; see Chap. 52).
  b. Stabilize the joint with a rigid coaptation splint.
  c. Change the dressing once a day or more frequently if necessary.

6. Repeat wound debridement if necrotic tissue is left in the wound after the first procedure. Continue this process until only viable tissue is present in the wound.

Ligament Replacement

The ligament replacement technique usually requires three bone screws and two figure-eight heavy sutures.

Technique

1. Use 4.0-mm partially threaded cancellous screws or 2.7-mm cortical screws with 2.7-mm spiked washers,*

---

*Synthes Ltd., Wayne, PA 19087.

depending on the size of the animal. Place the screws as close as possible to the origin and insertion of the components of the ligament complex (see Figs. 131–3*B* and 131–4*B*).

2. Position the origin screw in the distal tibia for the medial ligament or the distal fibula and tibia for the lateral ligament. Direct this screw slightly proximal to avoid penetrating joint cartilage and to obtain maximum bony purchase.

3. Position the insertion screw for the medial tibiotalar short ligament in the proximoplantar quadrant of the medial trochlear facies of the talus.

4. Position the screw corresponding to the insertion of the medial long ligament through the tubercle at the plantar base of the talus. Direct this screw slightly proximodorsally.

5. Position the screw corresponding to the insertion of the calcaneofibular short ligament proximoplantar to the base of the lateral articular facies of the tuber calcis.

6. Position the insertion screw for the long ligament through the tubercle at the dorsal extent of the base of the calcaneus. Direct this screw slightly proximoplantar.

7. Using one or two (for large patients) strands of #1-5 polyester sutures as prosthetic replacements, place suture(s) around the origin screw and the short insertion screw, and separate suture(s) around the origin screw and long insertion screw.

  a. Set the sutures in a figure-eight pattern.
  b. Tie taut the tibiotalar or calcaneofibular short suture prosthesis with the tarsocrural joint held in approximately 90° flexion for dogs and 70° for cats. Tie taut the medial long or lateral long suture prosthesis with the tarsocrural joint in a functional standing angle of 135° for dogs (varies for some breeds) and 120° for cats.
  c. Tighten the screws against the bone.

▼ *Key Point* Never perform primary soft tissue closure over a shear injury.

8. If possible, allow second intention healing; alternatively, perform delayed closure or apply a skin graft (see Chaps. 52 and 53) after all surfaces of the wound and prosthetic sutures are covered with healthy granulation tissue.

Postoperative Care

- Immobilize the tarsocrural joint for 2–4 weeks, using transarticular external skeletal fixation (see Chap. 130).
  - Use the fixator to provide consistent stability during serial debridement and general wound management and following prosthetic replacement.
  - Remove the fixator when the wound appears healthy and the prosthetic sutures are sufficiently covered by granulation tissue and wound contraction.
- After the fixator is removed, immobilize the hock for an additional 4–12 weeks with a short semirigid soft-cast coaptation splint. This gives less stability than the

fixator but does not risk failure of the prosthetic sutures.
- During use of the semirigid softcast coaptation splint, perform controlled mobilization by progressively unwrapping layers to increase tissue microstrain as healing advances.
  - Once all coaptation is removed, continue progressive controlled mobilization by slowly increasing the animal's activity over another 4–8 week period. During this period, if the animal shows signs of increased lameness or pain, progress more slowly with controlled mobilization in a manner that does not create lameness or discomfort.

Prognosis

The prognosis is good to guarded for long-term pain-free function if there is no damage to the articular surfaces other than the malleolus.

TARSOCRURAL JOINT ARTHRODESIS

Tarsocrural joint arthrodesis can be done by tarsocrural joint fusion or pantarsal fusion.

- Pantarsal arthrodesis includes fusion not only of the tarsocrural joint but also of the intertarsal and tarsometatarsal joints.
- Pantarsal arthrodesis gives more consistent functional results and there is less patient morbidity.

Preoperative Considerations

Indications for performing tarsocrural joint arthrodesis instead of ligament replacement include:

- Moderate to severe osteochondral damage to the joint mortise
- Prolonged tarsocrural joint subluxation or luxation causing moderate to severe degenerative joint disease
- Failure of reconstructive surgery or postoperative development of painful degenerative joint disease

Surgical Procedure (Pantarsal Arthrodesis)
Objectives

- Fuse the tarsocrural, intertarsal, and tarsometatarsal joints.
- Fuse the hock at a functional angle.
- Allow pain-free use of the limb.
- Minimize patient morbidity and owner expense.

Equipment

- Standard orthopedic instrument pack and suture material
- Gelpi self-retaining retractors
- Power drill
- Power saw or osteotome and mallet
- Pneumatic surgical bur (optional)
- Bone curettes
- K-wires

- Bone plates, screws, and application equipment
- Coaptation splint

Technique

1. Approach the joint dorsally from the distal one-third of the tibia, extending over the tarsal bones and ending at the proximal one-third of the third metatarsal bone.
2. Using a power saw or osteotome, cut the articular cartilage from the distal tibia and trochlea of the talus.
   a. Cut the distal tibia perpendicular to the longitudinal axis.
   b. Cut the trochlea of the talus at an appropriate angle, allowing the distal tibia to rest flush on the talus and form the proper weight bearing angle at the hock. Before surgery, use the animal's contralateral limb to determine the correct weight bearing angle (approximately 140° for dogs (varies with certain breeds) and 120° for cats).
3. Match the tibia to the talus at the appropriate angle and temporarily fix the two bones with K-wires.
4. With a bone curette or pneumatic bur, remove as much cartilage as possible from the intertarsal and tarsometatarsal joints.
5. Obtain autogenous cancellous bone from the ipsilateral greater tubercle of the humerus and proximal tibia. Pack cancellous bone into the intertarsal and tarsometatarsal joints and around the tarsocrural joint.
6. Apply a bone plate to the dorsal surface of the distal tibia, tarsus, and third metatarsal bone (Fig. 131–5).
   a. Bend an appropriately sized eight- to ten-hole plate to the proper fit.
   b. Fix three cortical screws and the plate to the tibia, two or three screws to the tarsal bones, and three screws to the third metatarsal bone.
   c. Alternatively, do not place screws in the tarsal bones, and pack this area with cancellous bone.
7. Remove the temporary K-wires, pack more cancellous bone around the tarsocrural joint, and perform routine closure.

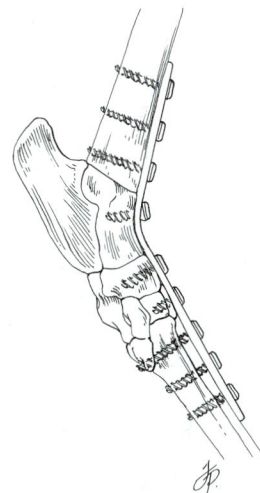

Figure 131–5. Pantarsal arthrodesis by dorsal application of a bone plate.

Postoperative Care

- Apply a short, rigid coaptation splint or full cylinder cast from the foot to just below the stifle until there is radiographic evidence of bone fusion.
- Remove the bone plate after there is complete bone union, usually in 6–9 months.
- Protect the arthrodesis for 6 weeks following plate removal with a semirigid softcast coaptation splint; restrict exercise.

OVERVIEW OF INTERTARSAL LUXATION AND SUBLUXATION INJURIES

- Many intertarsal ligament injuries are a result of daily activity and occur without known trauma.
- Acute loading (e.g., with jumping) can damage plantar ligaments and cause a hyperextension injury.
- Affected animals usually are non–weight bearing or walk plantigrade, have variable swelling in the tarsal region, and have instability of the tarsus.
- Palpation and stress radiographs (see Chap. 4) usually can localize the area of injury.
- Hyperextension injuries are repaired by arthrodesis or tension band wire stabilization.
- Because surgery is performed only on the low-motion intertarsal or tarsometatarsal joints, the prognosis usually is excellent for pain-free normal function.

PROXIMAL INTERTARSAL SUBLUXATION WITH PLANTAR INSTABILITY

Preoperative Considerations

- Injury to the plantar ligaments of the calcaneoquartal and talocalcaneocentral joints results from excessive dorsiflexion; the hock collapses and the animal walks plantigrade.
- A traumatic episode usually is not identified.
- Diagnose by palpation and stress radiographs (see Chap. 4).
- This condition does not respond to conservative management with coaptation splints. Treat surgically by arthrodesis of the calcaneoquartal joint.

Surgical Procedure

Objectives

- Fuse the calcaneoquartal joint.
- Avoid trauma to the tarsocrural joint.
- Achieve pain-free, normal weight bearing.
- Minimize patient morbidity and owner expense.

Equipment

- Standard orthopedic instrument pack and suture material
- Gelpi self-retaining retractors
- Intramedullary pins
- Bone curettes or pneumatic bur
- Bone drill and assorted drill bits
- K-wires
- Orthopedic wire (18 or 20 gauge)
- External coaptation devices

Technique

1. Expose the joint plantar-laterally with medial retraction of the tendon of the superficial digital flexor (SDF). This may entail incising the lateral retinaculum, which normally secures the SDF tendon to the lateral process of the calcaneal tuber.
2. Using a bone curette or pneumatic bur, remove articular cartilage from the surfaces of the calcaneus and fourth tarsal bone.
3. Insert an appropriate-size single intramedullary pin ($\frac{5}{64}$–$\frac{1}{8}$ inch) from the proximal calcaneus down the shaft.
   a. Drill a pilot hole in the (very hard) calcaneus before inserting the intramedullary pin.
   b. Position the pin in the calcaneus.
4. Obtain autogenous cancellous bone from the ipsilateral greater tubercle of the humerus and pack it into the joint space.
5. Reduce the joint, drive the intramedullary pin across the joint, and fix the pin in the distal end of the fourth tarsal bone (Fig. 131–6).
6. Retract the intramedullary pin slightly, cut it short, and countersink it beneath the cartilage of the tuber calcis.
7. Drill a transverse hole across the distal portion of the fourth tarsal bone and the middle section of the calcaneus.
8. Place an orthopedic tension band wire (18 or 20 gauge) in a figure-eight pattern through the drilled holes (see Fig. 131–6).
   a. Set the wire directly against the bone under all soft tissue.
   b. Tighten the wire evenly with a double-twist method and bend the twists over to rest against bone.
9. Reduce the superficial digital flexor tendon and suture the lateral retinaculum to stabilize the tendon.
10. Close the subcutaneous tissue and skin routinely.

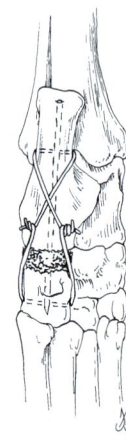

Figure 131–6. Fusion of the calcaneoquartal joint via pin and tension band wire fixation and cancellous bone graft.

Postoperative Care

- Place a short (from the proximal tibia to the paw) semirigid softcast coaptation splint for 4–8 weeks. Perform progressive controlled mobilization with the softcast.
- Restrict activity until bony fusion of the joint is evident on radiographs (usually 6–8 weeks).

PROXIMAL INTERTARSAL LUXATION WITH PLANTAR INSTABILITY

Preoperative Considerations

- This condition occurs infrequently, compared with subluxation injury.
- Trauma results in a high-energy hyperextension injury. There is more joint displacement and instability than with subluxation injury.
- Because of the severe instability in this condition, perform arthrodesis of the intertarsal joint with a bone plate rather than with a less rigid pin and wire tension band technique.

Surgical Procedure

Objectives

- Fuse the proximal intertarsal joint. Otherwise, objectives are the same as for proximal intertarsal subluxation.

Equipment

- Standard orthopedic instrument pack and suture material
- Gelpi self-retaining retractors
- Bone curettes or pneumatic bur
- Power drill
- Bone plates, screws, and application equipment
- External coaptation devices

Technique

1. Make a lateral approach from the tuber calcis, extending over the calcaneus and fourth tarsal bone and ending over the proximal one-third of the fifth metatarsal bone.
2. Using a bone curette or pneumatic bur, remove articular cartilage from the bones of the proximal intertarsal joint.
3. Place autogenous cancellous bone in the joint space. Reduce the joint.
4. Place a bone plate on the lateral aspect of the calcaneus, fourth tarsal bone, and proximal fifth metatarsal bone (Fig. 131–7).
   a. Shape the bones slightly to accommodate the plate.
   b. Secure an appropriate-size seven-hole plate with two screws in the calcaneus, one in the calcaneus and talus, one in the fourth and central tarsal bones, and three in the fourth and fifth metatarsal bones.

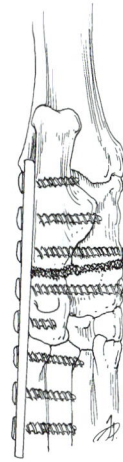

Figure 131–7. Proximal intertarsal joint fusion via lateral application of a bone plate and cancellous bone graft.

   c. Alternatively, do not place the screw in the fourth and central tarsal bones, and pack this area with cancellous bone.
5. Close the tissue and skin routinely.

Postoperative Care

- Protect the arthrodesis with a short semirigid softcast coaptation splint. Remove the splint when there is radiographic evidence of bony fusion.
- Remove the bone plate after the arthrodesis is complete. If retained, the plate usually loosens, causing pain and lameness.

DISTAL INTERTARSAL (TARSOMETATARSAL) SUBLUXATION WITH PLANTAR INSTABILITY

Preoperative Considerations

- This condition is less common than proximal subluxation injury.
- The cause is tearing of the plantar tarsal fibrocartilage and usually is associated with trauma.
- A few days after the injury the animal attempts weight bearing and walks plantigrade.
- Consistent with hyperextension injuries, surgical arthrodesis is the treatment of choice.

Surgical Procedure

Objectives

- Fuse the distal intertarsal joint. Otherwise, objectives are the same as for proximal intertarsal subluxation.

Equipment

- See Proximal Intertarsal Subluxation with Plantar Instability.

Technique

1. Expose the injury by an incision over the plantar-lateral calcaneus, fourth tarsal bone, and metatarsal bones.

2. Retract the superficial and deep digital flexor tendons medially and laterally to expose the joints.
3. Remove articular cartilage from the distal intertarsal joint surfaces.
4. Pack autogenous cancellous bone into the joint space.
5. Use a pin and tension band wire technique similar to that described for proximal intertarsal subluxation with plantar instability, but slightly modified.
   a. Insert an appropriate size intramedullary pin ($\frac{5}{64}$–$\frac{1}{8}$ inch) down through the calcaneus; extend through the fourth tarsal bone and continue into the distal one-half of the fourth metatarsal bone.
   b. Drill transverse holes for the tension band wire (18 or 20 gauge) in the distal one-third of the calcaneus and the bases of two or three of the metatarsal bones.
   c. Place the wire in a figure-eight pattern under the superficial digital flexor tendon.
6. Alternatively, perform the tarsometatarsal arthrodesis with a bone plate. Use bone screws to secure two holes of a five-hole plate to the fourth and central tarsal bones and distal tarsal bones proximal to the subluxation, and three holes to the metatarsal bones distal to the subluxation.

Postoperative Care

Maintain a short semirigid softcast coaptation splint until there is radiographic evidence of bony fusion.

OTHER INTERTARSAL-TARSOMETATARSAL SUBLUXATION INJURIES

Proximal Intertarsal Subluxations with Dorsal Instability

- Physical examination findings include:
  - Primary damage of the dorsal ligaments and dorsal joint capsule
  - Frequently, concurrent lateral or medial instability
  - Usually, no evidence of external trauma
- The animal places full weight on the limb with only periodic lameness, which is made worse by coincident lateral or medial instability.
- Diagnose by palpation and stress radiographs.
  - Slight dorsal swelling and increased flexion and opening of the dorsal joints are seen.
  - Lateral or medial instability may be concurrent with dorsal laxity.

Treatment

- If possible, manage the instability with rigid coaptation splints.
- Surgical repair may be necessary if
  - Injuries are severe.
  - The instability does not respond to splinting.
  - Dorsal ligament damage is associated with lateral or medial damage.
  - The affected animal is a large, athletic dog.

Surgical Technique and Postoperative Management

1. Fix the dorsal instability with a neutralization bone screw placed from the medial side of the head of the talus, diagonally into the distal tarsal bones.
2. Remove articular cartilage before screw placement.
3. Supplement with an appropriately positioned figure-eight tension band wire for concurrent lateral or medial instability; a neutralization screw may not be needed.
4. Postoperatively, maintain a semirigid softcast coaptation splint for 6 weeks.
   a. Perform progressive controlled mobilization with the softcast.
   b. Remove the screw or tension band wire if it loosens.

Distal Intertarsal Subluxation with Dorsomedial Instability

- This type of subluxation can occur alone or combined with other areas of instability involving the tarsus.
- Diagnose by palpation and stress radiographs.
  - Valgus deformity and dorsomedial instability are seen.
- Stabilize with a medially positioned tension band wire.

Stabilization Technique and Postoperative Management

1. Place a bone screw in the central and fourth tarsal bones proximally, and a second screw in the second, third, and fourth tarsal bones distally.
2. Secure a figure-eight wire (20 or 22 gauge) around the screws.
3. Postoperatively maintain a semirigid softcast coaptation splint below the stifle for 6 weeks. Perform progressive controlled mobilization with the softcast.

Tarsometatarsal Subluxation with Dorsomedial Instability

- Stabilize with a medially positioned tension band.

Stabilization Technique and Postoperative Management

1. Place a bone screw in the central and fourth tarsal bones proximally, and a second screw in the second and fourth metatarsal bones distally.
2. Secure a figure-eight wire around the screws.
3. Postoperatively, maintain a semirigid softcast coaptation splint below the stifle for 6 weeks. Perform progressive controlled mobilization with the softcast.

Tarsometatarsal Subluxation with Dorsal Instability

- This is a subtle injury that requires stress radiographs to confirm the diagnosis.
- If possible, stabilize with rigid coaptation splints.
- Injury in a large dog or chronic injury may require surgical arthrodesis, using a pin and tension band wire or bone plate technique.

- Alternatively, the arthrodesis can be done by inserting cross-pins from the proximal metatarsal bones into the distal tarsal bones.
- Postoperatively, maintain a semirigid softcast coaptation splint below the stifle for 6 weeks. Perform progressive controlled mobilization with the softcast.

Luxation of the Head of the Talus, the Central Tarsal Bone, and the Talocalcaneus

- These types of luxation occur as an isolated injury or with concomitant tarsal joint instability. Usually, luxation of the head of the talus and the talocalcaneal luxation are the result of relatively high-energy trauma.

Technique and Postoperative Management

1. Reduce the luxated tarsal bone(s) and stabilize with a cortical bone screw.
   a. For luxation of the head of the talus or talocalcaneal luxation, insert a neutralization screw from the talus to the calcaneus.
   b. For the central tarsal bone luxation, insert a neutralization screw from the central tarsal bone to the fourth tarsal bone.
   c. Place the screw so that the luxated bones are held in position (neutralized). Do not compress the bones.

2. Postoperatively, maintain a semirigid softcast coaptation splint below the stifle for 6 weeks. Perform progressive controlled mobilization with the softcast.

SUPPLEMENTAL READINGS

Aron DN: Prosthetic ligament replacement for severe tarsocrural joint instability. J Am Anim Hosp Assoc 23:41, 1987.

Aron DN: Management of open musculoskeletal injuries. Semin Vet Med Surg 3:290, 1988.

Aron DN: Tendons. *In* Bojrab MJ, ed.: Current Techniques in Small Animal Surgery, 3rd Ed. Philadelphia: Lea & Febiger, 1990, p 549.

Aron DN, Purinton PT: Collateral ligaments of the tarsocrural joint: An anatomic and functional study. Vet Surg 14:173, 1985.

Aron DN, Purinton PT: Replacement of the collateral ligaments of the canine tarsocrural joint: A proposed technique. Vet Surg 14:178, 1985.

Brinker WO, Piermattei DL, Flo, GL: Handbook of Small Animal Orthopedics and Fracture Treatment, 2nd Ed. Philadelphia: WB Saunders, 1990, p 435.

Matthiesen DT: Tarsal injuries in the dog and cat. Compend Contin Educ Small Anim Pract 5:548, 1983.

Rytz U, Aron DN, Foutz L, Thompsons A: Mechanical evaluation of softcast and conventional rigid and semirigid coaptation methods. Vet Comp Orthop Traumatol 9:14–21, 1996.

Swaim SF, Henderson RA: Small Animal Wound Management. Philadelphia: Lea & Febiger, 1990.

132 Orthopedic Disorders of the Distal Extremities

Steven C. Budsberg

Disorders of the extremities distal to the carpus and tarsus usually result from direct trauma. Most abnormalities involve bone fracture and/or ligament damage associated with joint instability. The majority of fractures involve the metacarpal and metatarsal bones. Animals are usually presented with acute, non–weight bearing lameness. Regardless of the bone being managed, internal fixation, external coaptation, or a combination of both can be used. If fractures are open, proper open wound management is required before fracture fixation. It is essential to follow the generally accepted principles of fracture repair, including adequate reduction, alignment, and stable fixation, for the successful management of these injuries.

METACARPAL AND METATARSAL FRACTURES

Anatomy

The metacarpal and metatarsal bones are numbered 2 to 5, from medial to lateral. There are usually five metacarpal and four metatarsal bones. The third and fourth bones bear most of the forces transmitted through the foot.

Each bone is divided into the proximal base, middle body, and distal head.

Body Fractures

Body fractures may involve one or more bones. Racing animals may develop stress fractures of these bones. Closed reduction and coaptation usually are effective, but internal fixation may be required in cases involving multiple limb trauma, multiple bone fractures, and comminuted, severely displaced, or unstable fractures.

Preoperative Considerations

- Rule out associated injuries with a thorough physical examination and appropriate diagnostic tests.
- Identify the bone and region involved.
- Determine the type of injury (e.g., soft tissue, open or closed fracture, degloving injury).
- The number of bones involved affects treatment.
- Indications for external coaptation include:
  - Single bone fractures

- Multiple, nondisplaced fractures without other limb trauma
- In combination with appropriate internal fixation (e.g., intramedullary pins, screws, plates)
- Indications for internal fixation include:
- Multiple bone fractures with severe displacement
- Combined fractures of the third and fourth bones
- Additional limb injury
- Fracture in working or show dogs
- Open fractures
- Articular fractures

Surgical Procedure
Objectives

- Reduce and stabilize the fractures.
- Maintain viable soft tissues.
- Preserve joint function.

Equipment

- Standard surgical pack and suture material
- Kirschner wire (K-wire) (various sizes)
- Mini-fragment plates and screws (1.5, 2.0, and 2.7 mm)
- Small self-retaining retractors
- Small bone-holding forceps

Technique

1. Place the patient in dorsal recumbency, clip the hair, and prepare the extremity for aseptic surgery.

▼ *Key Point* Because of the central (metacarpal, metatarsal) and digital pads, surgical approach via the palmar or plantar surfaces of the metacarpal and metatarsal bones is contraindicated.

---

2. Make a dorsal incision directly over the affected bone or joint.
   a. To approach a single bone, make a longitudinal incision directly over the bone. To expose adjacent bones, make the incision between them, if necessary.
   b. To approach multiple bones, make two parallel longitudinal incisions or a curved incision incorporating the entire dorsal region (Fig. 132–1).

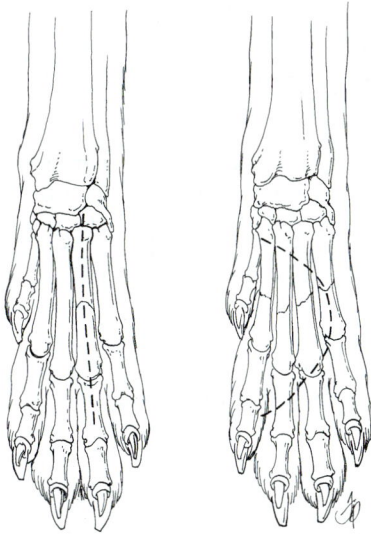

Figure 132–1. Dorsal incision lines for metacarpal fractures of a single bone *(left)* or multiple bones *(right)*.

3. Incise the deep fascia directly over the bone.
   a. In the metacarpus, identify and retract the major tendons (i.e., the tendons of the common digital extensor and lateral digital extensor muscles).
   b. In the metatarsal region, take care to protect the tendon of the long digital extensor muscle (Fig. 132–2).
4. Intramedullary pinning for fracture repair:
   a. Antegrade the pins from distal to proximal through a predrilled hole in the dorsal surface (Fig. 132–3). (Make the predrilled guide hole with a pin one size larger than the intended intramedullary pin.) Bend the pin ends slightly to facilitate removal and to avoid entering the metacarpo(tarso)phalangeal (MP) joint.

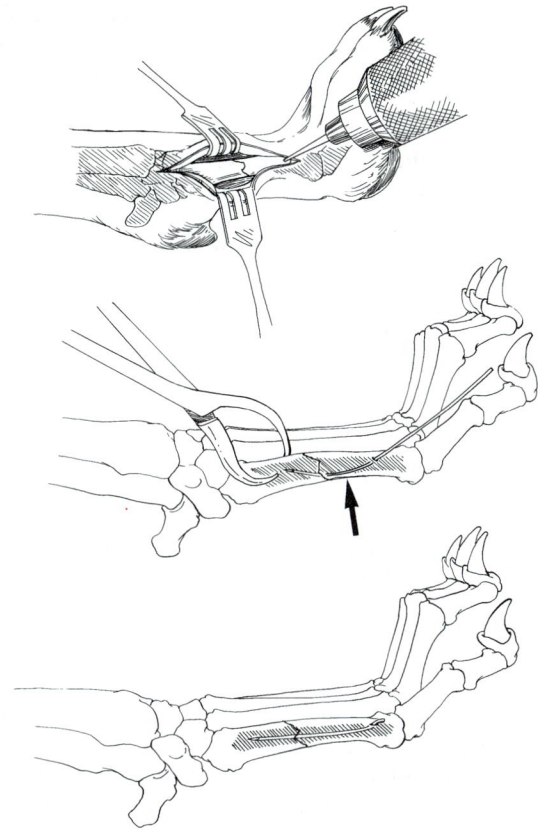

Figure 132–3. Placement of an intramedullary pin for repair of a metacarpal fracture. The center view shows how the pin is "bounced off" the palmar cortex *(arrow)*.

▼ *Key Point* When passing pins in an antegrade fashion, use a hand drill rather than a power drill to allow the pins to "bounce off" (instead of penetrating) the palmar/plantar cortex.

   b. Alternatively, retrograde the pins from the fracture site to the predrilled hole in the dorsal cortex, reduce the fracture, and seat the pins in the proximal segment (Fig. 132–4).

▼ *Key Point* Fixation with single intramedullary pins can accomplish reduction and alignment; however, this procedure does not provide rotational stability to the fracture.

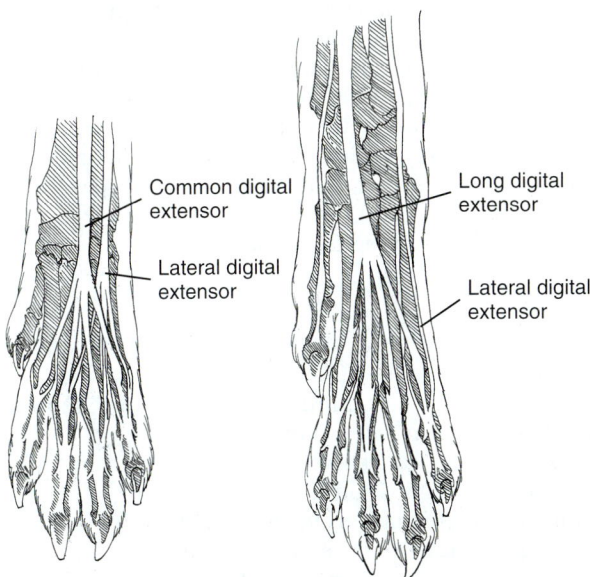

Common digital extensor

Lateral digital extensor

Long digital extensor

Lateral digital extensor

Figure 132–2. Important tendons of the metacarpus *(left)* and metatarsus *(right)*.

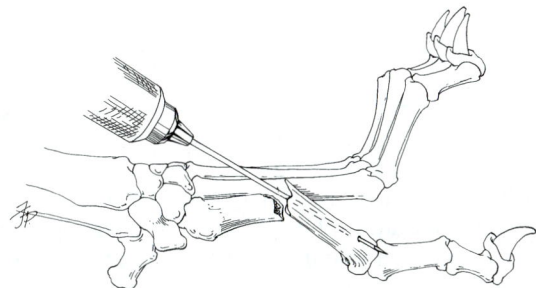

Figure 132–4. Retrograde placement of an intramedullary pin from the fracture site to a predrilled hole in the dorsal cortex.

c. Use supplementary external coaptation of fiberglass (molded half-circumference cast) or metal (palmar/plantar splint) to augment internal fixation.

5. Plate fixation:
   a. For fixation of the third and fourth bones, place the plates on the dorsal surface. For fixation of the second and fifth bones, place the plates on the medial and lateral surfaces, respectively, or dorsally.
   b. A minimum of four cortices of screw purchase above and below the fracture is required.
   c. Perform supplementary external coaptation, as described previously.

6. Lag screw fixation:
   a. Use in oblique fractures, primarily the first, second, and fifth metacarpals and the second and fifth metatarsals.
   b. Perform supplementary external coaptation.

7. Close the incision routinely.

Base and Head Fractures

Preoperative Considerations

- Base fractures usually involve the second and fifth metacarpals, owing to ligamentous attachment; avulsion fractures commonly are seen. Valgus and varus displacement often is noted.
  - Internal fixation is strongly recommended.
  - Nondisplaced fractures may be treated with a palmar splint; however, some displacement usually occurs. Delayed union may be a problem because of the motion from ligamentous attachment.
- Head (articular) fractures usually have concurrent subluxation or complete luxation of the MP joint owing to the collateral ligament attachment.
  - Reconstruction of the articular surface is required.

Surgical Procedure

Objectives

- Reduce and stabilize the fracture.
- Repair or reconstruct ligament instability of the joint.
- Reconstruct the articular surface, if necessary.

Equipment

- Same as for body fractures, described previously

Technique

1. The approach is the same as for body fractures, described previously.
2. In base fractures, fix with lag screws or a tension band technique. Supplementary external coaptation is required.
3. In head fractures, use Kirschner and cerclage wires or a combination K-wire and hemicerclage technique. Supplementary external coaptation is required.
4. Close the incision routinely.

Postoperative Care and Complications

▼ *Key Point* Management of soft tissue injuries in open fractures is as important as internal fixation.

- Maintain external coaptation in combination with intramedullary pins and lag screw fixation until there is clinical union of the fracture. Animals with plate fixation require coaptation for approximately 4 weeks.
- Remove intramedullary pins following clinical bone union. In working dogs, also remove plates. Lag screws and plates in nonworking animals may be left in permanently.
- If postoperative bleeding is anticipated, apply a pressure bandage for 48–72 hours to minimize hemorrhage.
- In all cases, control and limit exercise until clinical bone union (usually 6–10 weeks).
- Rarely, delayed union and nonunion may result from inadequate stabilization. Excessive proliferative callus formation may cause tendon entrapment and/or pain.
- Valgus or varus deviation may result from undetected or untreated concurrent collateral ligament damage.
- If joint surfaces are involved, degenerative joint disease may develop.
- Treat tissue swelling with warm compresses or hydrotherapy.

PHALANGEAL FRACTURES

Phalangeal fractures are similar to metacarpal and metatarsal fractures. They usually are single injuries; however, they may occur in association with other, more severe multiple injuries to the paw.

Anatomy

- Each digit consists of a proximal phalanx and a distal phalanx. The phalanges are numbered similar to the metacarpals and metatarsals.
- The proximal and middle phalanges are divided into a proximal base, middle body, and distal head.
- The distal phalanges are approximately the same size in all digits and are partially covered by the nails.
- *Dewclaw* is the term applied to the variably developed first digit of the hind paw.
- Polydactyly (extra digits) is common in cats.

Preoperative Considerations

- Same considerations as metacarpal and metatarsal fractures
- Open, severely comminuted fractures may require digit amputation (see Chap. 133).
- Most fractures can be reduced closed and immobilized in a fiberglass splint.
- Some of the indications for internal fixation include:
  - Large working dogs or racing animals
  - Articular fractures involving the base or head
  - Failed external coaptation

Surgical Procedure

Objectives

- See under Metacarpal and Metatarsal Fractures.

Equipment

- The same as for metacarpal and metatarsal fractures, discussed previously.

Technique

1. Make an incision directly over the affected bone.
2. Articular fractures require anatomic reduction and fixation with lag screws, orthopedic wire sutures, K-wire, or a combination of these.
3. Treat body fractures with miniplates or (for oblique fractures) cross-pins and lag screws.

Postoperative Care and Complications

- See Metacarpal and Metatarsal Fractures.
- External coaptation is required until clinical bone union.

PALMAR AND PLANTAR SESAMOID INJURIES

Fractures of the sesamoid bones of the MP joints usually are seen in racing greyhounds. However, they can cause lameness in any dog, particularly large-breed animals. Signs include sudden lameness with swelling and pain on palpation. Injuries of the second and seventh sesamoids are reported to be the most common.

Anatomy

- The sesamoid bones are numbered 1 to 8 medial to lateral (two for each MP joint).
- The sesamoid bone articulates primarily with the head of the metacarpal/metatarsal bone and secondarily with the palmar tubercles of each proximal phalanx.
- Occasionally, bipartite sesamoid bones are present and may be mistaken for fractures.

▼ *Key Point* Old sesamoid fractures or bipartite sesamoid bones may be mistaken as the cause of lameness.

Preoperative Considerations

- An acute injury requires external coaptation. The foot is splinted in slight flexion.
- Recurrent lameness requires surgical intervention.

Surgical Procedure

Objective

- Remove the damaged sesamoid.

Equipment

- Standard surgical pack and suture

Technique

1. Make an incision adjacent to the metacarpal/metatarsal pad, with the middle of the incision directly over the MP joint.
2. Slightly undermine the pad to allow retraction and further deep dissection of the affected sesamoid bone.
3. Identify the distal venous arch on the proximal aspect of the incision.
4. Dissect directly over the sesamoid bone and move the flexor tendon to the side if necessary.
5. Transect the sesamoid ligaments and remove the offending fragments.
6. If less than one-third of the total bone is fragmented, leave the larger fragment and remove the smaller one.
7. Close each incised fascial plane with simple interrupted sutures of an absorbable suture material.
8. Close the remainder of the incision routinely.

Postoperative Care and Complications

- Place a snug padded bandage on the paw for 7–10 days.
- Limit exercise for 2 weeks and gradually increase to normal by 6 weeks.
- Complications are rare.

SUPPLEMENTAL READINGS

Benedetti LT, Berry K, Bloomberg M: A technique for intramedullary pinning of metatarsals and metacarpals in cats and dogs. J Am Anim Hosp Assoc 22:149, 1986.

Bennett D, Kelly DF: Sesamoid disease as a cause of lameness in young dogs. J Small Anim Pract 26:567, 1985.

Dee JF, Dee LG, Early TD: Manual for Internal Fixation in Small Animals. Berlin: Springer-Verlag, 1984, p 206.

Evans HE, Christensen GC: Miller's Anatomy of the Dog. Philadelphia: WB Saunders, 1979, p 192.

133 Amputation of the Digit

Paul A. Manley

ANATOMY

Distal Phalanx (Cats)

- The distal phalanx (P3) of the cat is made up of a bony component and the claw (Fig. 133–1).
- The distal end of P3 is composed of an ungual crest and an ungual process.
- The ungual crest encircles the base of the third phalanx and projects into the claw.
- The stratum basale contains the germinal cells of the claw and extends into the ungual crest.

Dewclaw (Dogs)

- The dewclaw is the medial or first digit of the rear limb in the dog. Often, P1 and P2 are missing, and P3 and the claw are attached only by skin and fibrous tissue.
- In some breeds, there are multiple dewclaws.
- The dewclaw articulates with metatarsal bone I, which is often small and may be fused to tarsal bone I.
- If two dewclaws are present, there may be complete duplication of the phalanges and metatarsal bone I.
- Blood supply to the first digit is via the dorsal metatarsal artery and the lateral dorsal proper digital artery (a branch of the dorsal pedal artery).

Digits (Dogs and Cats)

- The digits consist of three phalanges (P1, P2, and P3) and a nail or claw. The first digit in the front foot does not have a middle phalanx (P2); the first digit in the rear foot is the dewclaw.
- The superficial digital flexor tendon attaches to the proximal end of P2; the deep digital flexor attaches to P3; the common digital extensor tendon attaches to the extensor process of P3.
- A digital pad is located on the palmar and plantar aspect of the distal interphalangeal joint of each digit, except for the first one. Metacarpal and metatarsal pads are located on the palmar and plantar aspects, respectively, of the metacarpophalangeal and metatarsophalangeal joints.
- Blood supply is via dorsal and palmar (or plantar) digital arteries; venous drainage is via dorsal and palmar (or plantar) digital veins.

ONYCHECTOMY (CATS)

Onychectomy often is performed on house cats as an elective procedure; however, it may be necessary to perform this procedure when a claw is severely traumatized or infected.

Preoperative Considerations

- Avoid damage to the digital pad when removing the claw.
- Inform owners that most cats should be kept indoors as house pets after declawing.
- It is seldom necessary to remove the claws of the rear limbs.

▼ *Key Point* The germinal cells of the claw extend into the ungual crest. To prevent claw regrowth, completely remove the ungual crest.

Surgical Procedure

Objectives

- Completely remove the claw(s).
- Prevent regrowth of a deformed claw.
- Protect the digital pad.
- Prevent excessive blood loss.

Equipment

- Penrose drain or appropriate tourniquet
- Scalpel blade (#12)
- Curved Kelly forceps
- Nail trimmers (Resco or White)

Technique

1. Place a tourniquet above the elbow.
2. Prepare the entire foot with a germicidal soap and solution.
3. Extend the claw by grasping the claw with forceps or by pushing up on the digital pad.
4. Position the nail trimmer so that one blade rests dorsally at the distal interphalangeal joint and the other blade rests at the distal margin of the digital pad (see Fig. 133–2). Close the blades and, with a slight twisting motion of the wrist, remove the claw and P3.
   a. Alternatively, a #12 scalpel blade may be used to disarticulate the distal interphalangeal joint.

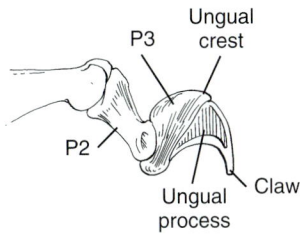

Figure 133–1. Distal phalanx of the cat. Note the position of the ungual crest relative to the claw.

5. When using nail trimmers, it is common to leave a small portion of the palmar aspect of P3. Grasp this with forceps and remove with a scalpel. If the piece is very small, removal is unnecessary (Fig. 133–2).
6. Following declawing, apply a snug-fitting bandage to the level of the distal antebrachium. Avoid excessive tightness of the proximal portion of the bandage to ensure adequate blood supply to the paw.
7. Remove the tourniquet.

Postoperative Care and Complications

Short Term

- Bleeding after bandage removal occasionally is a problem. If necessary, replace the bandage, and then remove in 2–3 days.
- Keep the cat indoors, and use shredded paper as cat litter for 2 weeks after surgery.
- Commercial cat litter may work its way into the wound and irritate the declawed area.

Long Term

- Treat infection by establishing drainage at the distal extremity and administering systemic antibiotics.
- Regrowth of a deformed nail can result from incomplete removal of the ungual crest. Perform disarticulation of the distal interphalangeal joint with a scalpel.
- Chronic lameness may result from incomplete removal of the ungual crest or trauma to the digital pad.

DEWCLAW REMOVAL (DOGS)

Dewclaw removal is usually an elective procedure, although the claw may become traumatized, especially if it is only loosely attached to the skin.

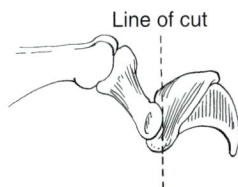

Figure 133–2. Distal phalanx of the cat (see Fig. 133–1). This line of excision ensures complete removal of the ungual crest, although a small piece of P3 is left behind.

Preoperative Considerations

- Removal of the dewclaw for cosmetic reasons is best performed in the neonate.

Surgical Procedure

Objectives

- Remove dewclaw and minimize scarring on the medial aspect of the foot.

Equipment

- Standard surgical pack and suture material
- Bone cutters

Technique

Neonates

1. Surgically scrub the dewclaw and surrounding area.
2. Grasp the nail with small forceps and abduct it from the metatarsal bone.
3. With scissors, cut the dewclaw from its attachment to the metatarsal bone.
4. Use a single absorbable suture to close the skin.

Older Animals

1. Anesthetize the animal and prepare the foot for aseptic surgery.
2. Make an elliptical incision around the base of the dewclaw.
3. Ligate the metatarsal and the dorsal proper digital arteries.
4. If only soft tissue attachment exists from the dewclaw to the metatarsal bone, remove the dewclaw and close the skin. If a bony attachment exists, disarticulate P1 from metatarsal bone I.
5. Alternatively, use bone cutters to transect P1 close to its base.
6. Close the skin routinely.

Postoperative Care and Complications

- In neonates, a bandage is not necessary. In older dogs, place a bandage over the foot for 5–7 days.
- Scar formation at the site may be caused by the animal removing sutures prematurely, leading to wound dehiscence. Stainless steel sutures, an Elizabethan collar, or a bandage may prevent this complication.

DIGIT REMOVAL (DOGS AND CATS)

Digit amputation in dogs and cats usually is performed because of severe trauma, osteomyelitis, or neoplasia. The level of amputation depends on the condition and the site of involvement. The digit may be removed at the metacarpophalangeal joint, metatarsophalangeal joint, proximal interphalangeal joint, or distal interphalangeal joint or by osteotomy of the bones of the affected digit.

Preoperative Considerations

- Digit amputation proximal to the distal interphalangeal joint may necessitate digital pad removal. In performance animals, it may be preferable to maintain the digital pad.
- The primary weight bearing digits are the third and fourth.

Surgical Procedure

Objectives

- Remove the digit.
- Minimize blood loss.

Equipment

- Same as for dewclaw removal

Technique

1. Prepare the limb for aseptic surgery.
2. For digit removal distal to mid-P2, make a transverse incision on the dorsal aspect of the digit around to the digital pad.
   a. Ligate the digital arteries and veins.
   b. Disarticulate the digit at the distal interphalangeal joint, after transecting the flexor and extensor tendons. Alternatively, use bone cutters and transect P2.
   c. Suture the subcutaneous tissue of the pad to the extensor tendon with absorbable suture material and close the skin routinely.
3. For digit removal proximal to mid-P2, make an elliptical incision at the base of the digit.
   a. Ligate the vessels and disarticulate the digit with a scalpel or bone cutters (see Step 2b previously).
   b. A proximal extension of the elliptical skin incision usually facilitates cosmetic closure of the skin (Fig. 133-3).
   c. Close the subcutaneous and skin layers routinely.

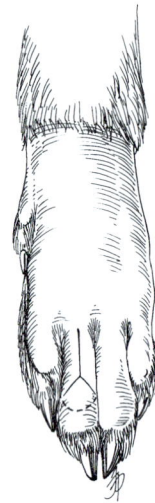

Figure 133-3.   Skin incision *(arrow)* for digit removal proximal to mid-P2.

Postoperative Care

- Apply a bandage to the foot for 7–10 days. Keep the bandage clean and dry.
- Remove skin sutures 10–14 days postoperatively.

SUPPLEMENTAL READINGS

Dee JF, Dee LG, Earon-Wells RD: Injuries of high performance dogs. *In* Whittick WG, ed.: Canine Orthopedics. Philadelphia: Lea & Febiger, 1990, p 519.

Krahwinkel DJ, Bone DL: Surgical management of specific skin disorders. *In* Slatter DH, ed.: Textbook of Small Animal Surgery. Philadelphia: WB Saunders, 1985, p 509.

134 Surgery of Skeletal Muscle and Tendons

Steven W. Petersen

Surgery of skeletal muscle usually is indicated for repair of injuries such as muscle belly rupture and laceration. Accordingly, the decision for surgery depends on the chronicity of the injury and the potential for lost function with scar tissue healing. Occasionally, an orthopedic surgical approach necessitates the transection of a muscle belly to gain improved exposure to a long bone fracture or joint.

Tenorrhaphy is primary suture apposition of severed tendons. Indications for tenorrhaphy are similar to those described for skeletal muscle repair. Tendon lacerations are common; tendon ruptures are seen less frequently. Several orthopedic surgical approaches use tendon transection to achieve exposure to various joints.

ANATOMY

Skeletal Muscle

- Skeletal muscle is composed of bundles or fascicles of muscle fibers, each enveloped in their own connective tissue sheath. Each muscle fiber consists of multiple individual myofibrils, the fundamental subunit of skeletal muscle.
- Muscle fibers gradually terminate at the proximal and distal ends of most muscle bellies, and connective tissue continues on as the tendon of origin or insertion, respectively. Some muscles attach directly to bone periosteum without this connective tissue interface.
- The vascular supply of muscle is well developed in order to provide for its high metabolic needs. Arteries branch from neighboring vessels and enter the muscle belly at distinct locations. Veins and nerves accompany arteries. Locations for entrance of these neurovascular bundles remain relatively constant in different animals.

Tendons

- Tendon superstructure resembles that of muscle. Collagen fibers are arranged in bundles and surrounded by a loose connective tissue sheath, the endotenon. Intrinsic blood vessels, nerves, and lymphatics are carried within the endotenon.

- The epitenon is a connective tissue sheath that surrounds the entire tendon and is, in turn, enveloped by the paratenon, which is the outer connective tissue layer that covers the tendon.
- Tendon vascularity is sparse compared with that of muscle. Vessels entering at the musculotendinous junction are the predominant blood supply. Distally, the tendon is supplied by vessels that enter at the osseous tendon insertion. Extrinsic vessels that travel along the paratenon supply the middle portion of the tendon.

SURGERY OF SKELETAL MUSCLE

Preoperative Considerations

- Muscle injuries in which wound edges are not apposed heal by deposition of fibrous scar tissue.
  - Myofibrils cannot penetrate the thick band of scar tissue that forms between unapposed muscle wound edges.
  - As interposed scar tissue remodels and elongates, muscle function is lost because the muscle belly is no longer able to fully contract.
- Myofibril regeneration can occur to a limited extent with direct wound edge apposition.
  - Small numbers of myofibrils are able to penetrate the smaller connective tissue scar that forms at the junction of apposed muscle edges.

▼ *Key Point* Complete muscle tissue regeneration does not occur across the scar.

- Experimentally, complete muscle belly lacerations that have been surgically repaired regain only 50% of their ability to produce tension and only about 80% of their ability to shorten.

Surgical Procedure
Objectives

- To provide muscle-to-muscle appositional anastomosis
- To thoroughly excise all preexisting scar tissue
- To preserve blood supply by delicately handling tissues.

Equipment

- Standard instrument pack
- Self-retaining and hand-held retractors
- Synthetic nonabsorbable monofilament suture
- Penrose drains, rubber tubing, Silastic buttons

Technique

▼ **Key Point** When incising muscles, make incisions parallel to the muscle fibers.

1. Thoroughly debride wound edges to remove scar tissue and hematomas.
2. Place sutures within the dense outer fascial sheath and/or deeper, inner belly fascial layers, using simple interrupted cruciate or horizontal mattress patterns (Fig. 134–1, *left*).
3. Use sections of Penrose drains, rubber tubing, or Silastic buttons as stents to prevent deeper tension sutures from pulling out (Fig. 134–1, *right*).

Postoperative Care and Complications

- Completely immobilize affected limb and muscle for 2–3 weeks.
- Gradually return the animal to normal activity over the ensuing 4–6 weeks.
- Use physiotherapy (passive range of motion with progressively increased flexion/extension) as the animal is allowed to return to activity.
- The primary complication is loss of function resulting from muscle atrophy and/or excessive scar tissue deposition.

SURGERY OF TENDONS

Preoperative Considerations

- Selection of correct suture pattern and material is fundamental to the success of the repair.
- Manage deep tendon lacerations with a contaminated wound by delayed primary tenorrhaphy.
  - Tag severed tendon ends with small-diameter nonabsorbable sutures.
  - Immobilize the limb to prevent further tendon segment distraction (e.g., transarticular external skeletal fixator).

- Treat contaminated wounds in an "open" manner with sterile dressings, daily wound debridement, and lavage (see Chap. 52).
- Proceed with tenorrhaphy, as described subsequently, and delay wound closure until healthy granulation tissue is present.

Surgical Procedure

Objectives

- Anatomically align the tendon ends.
- Delicately manipulate tissues to avoid iatrogenic injury to the tendon ends.
- When planning the surgical approach, allow ample space for identification and debridement of the tendon ends.

▼ **Key Point** Minimize gap formation at the tenorrhaphy site.

- In contrast to muscle, make incisions in tendons perpendicular to tendon fibers.

Equipment

- Same as for muscle, described previously

Technique

1. Meticulously debride traumatized edges, scar tissue, and hematoma at severed tendon ends.

▼ **Key Point** Use synthetic, nonabsorbable, monofilament, nonreactive suture material such as nylon or polypropylene for anastomosis.

2. Select the largest-diameter suture that will pass atraumatically through the tendon.
3. The suture pattern of choice is the three-loop pulley tenorrhaphy (Fig. 134–2):
   a. Place each loop of the pattern in a different plane of tissue, rotating approximately 120°.
   b. Place sutures alternately in a near-far (loop #1), middle-middle (loop #2), and far-near (loop #3) manner.

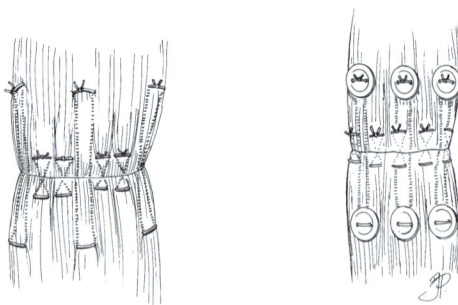

Figure 134–1. Suture patterns for muscle apposition. *Left,* Interrupted cruciate sutures with interposed deeper horizontal mattress sutures. *Right,* Silastic buttons prevent deep tension sutures from pulling out.

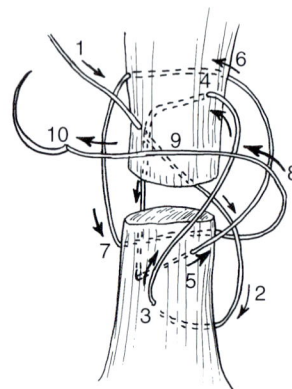

Figure 134–2. Three-loop pulley tenorrhaphy suture pattern. Needle passes follow numbered sequence and alternate in a near-far, middle-middle, and far-near pattern. Loops are oriented in separate planes of tissue and rotate approximately 120° from each other.

c. Minor alteration in the degree of rotation between loops allows use of this pattern for tenorrhaphy in tendons of all shapes and diameters.

4. In the common calcaneal and triceps tendons, which are composed of several smaller tendons, suture each tendon individually, using the three-loop pulley pattern.

5. Anastomose the paratenon of larger composite tendons with fine sutures in an interrupted pattern.

6. If necessary, use adjoining fascia to reinforce the tenorrhaphy in large-diameter tendons.

Postoperative Care and Complications

▼ *Key Point* Staged return to activity is critical for a successful repair.

- Restrict activity, allowing gradual return to normal function:
  - Completely immobilize the limb with a full cast or transarticular external skeletal fixator (no stress across the tenorrhaphy) for the first 3–4 weeks.
  - During the second 3–4 weeks, use a partial cast or splint to allow minimal weight bearing (limited longitudinal stress across the tenorrhaphy will allow collagen fibers to realign along lines of tension). A bivalved cast allows the suture line to be inspected during the extended healing/immobilization period without having to apply a new cast.
  - During the final 3–4 weeks place a padded bandage (modified Robert Jones) to allow increased weight bearing (permitting increased stress across the tenorrhaphy and tendon axis).
- Premature weight bearing with excessive stress across the tenorrhaphy may result in suture pullout or failure with secondary disruption of the repair.
- Manage failed tenorrhaphy as described for the initial procedure.

SUPPLEMENTAL READINGS

Aron DN: Tendons. *In* Bojrab JM, ed.: Current Techniques in Small Animal Surgery, 3rd Ed. Philadelphia: Lea & Febiger, 1990, p 549.

Berg JR, Egger EL: In vitro comparison of the three loop pulley and locking loop suture patterns for repair of canine weight bearing tendons and collateral ligaments. Vet Surg 15:107, 1986.

Bloomberg M: Muscles and tendons. *In* Slatter DH, ed.: Textbook of Small Animal Surgery. Philadelphia: WB Saunders, 1985, p 2331.

Chaplan A, Carlson B, Faulkner J, et al.: Skeletal muscle. *In* Woo SLY, Buckwalter JA, eds.: Injury and Repair of the Musculoskeletal Soft Tissues. Park Ridge, IL: American Academy of Orthopaedic Surgeons, 1988, p 213.

Easley KJ, Stashak TS, Smith FW, Vanslyke G: Mechanical properties of four suture patterns for transected equine tendon repair. Vet Surg 19:102, 1990.

Jann HW, Stein LE, Good JK: Strength characteristics and failure modes of locking loop and three loop pulley suture patterns in equine tendons. Vet Surg 19:28, 1990.

Morshead D, Leeds EB: Kirschner-Ehmer apparatus immobilization following Achilles tendon repair in six dogs. Vet Surg 13:11, 1984.

135 Neoplasia of Thoracic and Pelvic Limbs

Bernard M. Bouvy

ETIOLOGY

Neoplasia of the appendicular skeleton can affect bones primarily or secondarily. Tumors that arise from bone include osteosarcoma (intraosseous or parosteal), osteoma, chondrosarcoma, chondroma, osteochondroma (including multiple cartilaginous exostoses), enchondroma, fibrosarcoma, hemangiosarcoma, malignant mesenchymoma, liposarcoma, plasma cell myeloma (multiple myeloma), lymphosarcoma, and giant cell tumor (osteoclastoma).

In the dog, osteosarcoma accounts for up to 85% of malignancies originating in the skeleton, with the highest incidence in the distal radius and proximal humerus. It is classically a cancer of large and giant breeds. Body size seems to be a more important predisposing factor than breed. Only 5% of osteosarcomas occur in dogs weighing less than 15 kg. Canine osteosarcomas are aggressive tumors that rapidly metastasize to the lungs. In cats osteosarcomas account for 70–80% of all primary malignant cancers. Primary lesions occur more often in hindlimbs, and the disease is far less metastatic than in dogs.

Soft tissue tumors may infiltrate underlying bone; these include squamous cell carcinoma, malignant melanoma, and connective tissue tumors such as synovial cell sarcoma (malignant synovioma), rhabdomyosarcoma, and fibrosarcoma. On rare occasions, metastases to bone from primary neoplasia elsewhere in the body occur. Carcinomas are most likely to metastasize to limb bones. Tumors that metastasize to bone usually are diaphyseal, whereas primary bone tumors usually are metaphyseal.

CLINICAL SIGNS

- Clinical signs can vary from a nonpainful swelling to non–weight-bearing lameness.
- Conditions that are most often mistaken on radiography for bone neoplasia are hypertrophic osteodystrophy, osteomyelitis (bacterial or mycotic), and traumatic injury.
- Dogs rarely have respiratory signs as the first clinical evidence of pulmonary metastasis.

DIAGNOSIS

Radiography of the affected bone is indicated. Primary bone tumors may cause bony proliferation, lysis, or a combination of both.

- The definitive diagnosis cannot be substantiated by radiography alone. A representative biopsy for histopathologic and microbiologic evaluation often is necessary for distinction.
- Obtain biopsies by wedge resection (soft tissue tumor) or by using a bone marrow biopsy needle (Jamshidi).

TREATMENT

- In rare instances, benign tumors and soft tissue tumors not involving bone can be treated successfully by local resection.

▼ *Key Point* In most cases, local control of the tumor requires partial or complete amputation of the affected limb.

- Despite the poor long-term survival associated with most limb malignancies, amputation has important immediate advantages, including relief of pain, improvement of attitude and mobility, and improved quality of life.
- Limb-sparing procedures are complicated and are briefly described at the end of this chapter.
- Consider adjuvant treatment to prolong survival time (3–6 months with amputation alone).

SURGICAL ANATOMY

Anatomy relevant to limb amputation includes the major blood vessels to be ligated. Accurate identification of these vessels can limit significant blood loss.

Thoracic Limb

- The axillary artery extends from the cranial border of the first rib to the joint tendinous insertion of the

teres major and latissimus dorsi muscles. It lies deep to the brachial plexus.
- Major veins include the cephalic vein (deep to the cleidobrachialis muscle), the brachial vein, and the axillary vein (caudal and cranial to the axillary artery, respectively).

Pelvic Limb

- The femoral artery lies superficially in the femoral triangle between the caudal belly of the sartorius muscle and the pectineus muscle.
- The femoral vein lies caudal to its satellite artery.

LIMB AMPUTATION

Preoperative Considerations

- Radiograph the thorax to rule out gross metastasis to the lungs (VD or DV view and *both* right and left lateral views).

▼ *Key Point* Although less than 5% of dogs affected with osteosarcoma have radiographically detectable pulmonary metastasis at presentation, approximately 90% will die with lung metastatic disease within 1 year when amputation is the only treatment.

- Coexisting cardiomyopathy or any degree of heart failure may lead to serious complications, particularly with fluid diuresis during administration of cisplatin chemotherapy.
- Perform a thorough evaluation of the lymph nodes (including cytology, if they are enlarged), all extremities (including bone radiologic survey, if indicated), spine, and abdominal cavity for metastasis.
- Perform a complete blood count (CBC), serum biochemical panel, and urinalysis to assess the animal's overall condition.
- Obtain a representative biopsy to confirm neoplasia. Osteosarcoma can sometimes be an exception to this rule when radiologic features (severe cortical lysis and new bone formation such as "sunburst" or "Codman" triangle) of involved bone do not support other pathologies.

▼ *Key Point* Using closed technique and a Jamshidi bone marrow biopsy needle, obtain bone core biopsies *from the center and margin* of the suspected area to ensure diagnostic sampling (Fig. 135–1).

- Jamshidi needle biopsy has an accuracy rate of 91.9% for detection of tumor versus other disorders and an 82.3% accuracy rate for diagnosis of specific tumor subtype.
- Base indications for partial or total amputation on location and biological behavior of the tumor or on poor prognosis for a functional limb because of uncontrollable pain or irreversible damage.
- Assess gross margins of bone involvement on orthogonal fine-detail radiographs to determine the extent of surgery necessary to excise the neoplasm.

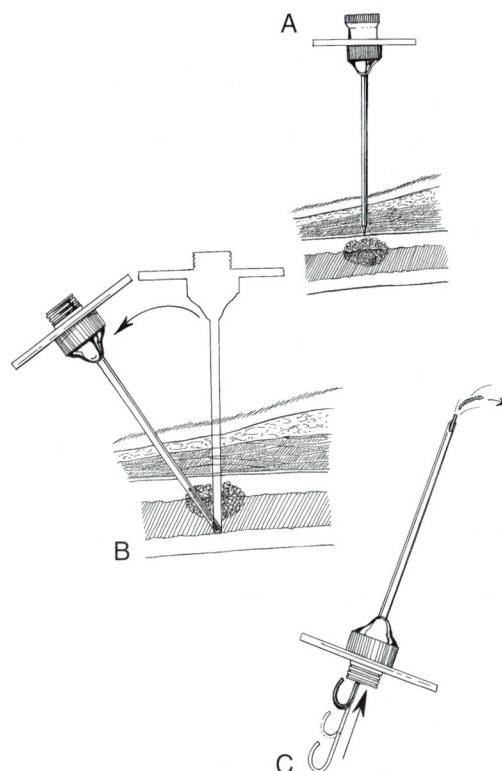

Figure 135–1. *A,* Biopsy of bone by closed technique with a Jamshidi needle. *B,* With the stylet locked in place, advance the cannula through soft tissue until bone is reached. *C,* Remove the stylet and penetrate the one cortex with the cannula. Withdraw the cannula and repeat the procedure with redirection of the needle.

▼ *Key Point* Perform the amputation at least one joint above involved bone.

- Amputation of a limb is difficult for an owner to accept. Prior to surgery, explain the functional and cosmetic changes resulting from amputation.
- Assess the other legs to be sure they can support the animal's weight after amputation. Radiograph the pelvis before rear leg amputation in dogs predisposed to hip dysplasia.
  - In the case of aggressive neoplasia, amputate the affected limb regardless of these findings.
- In animals with malignant tumors, especially osteosarcoma, be sure that owners have a realistic view of the treatment objectives and realize that cure is unlikely.

Surgical Procedures for Amputation
Objectives

- Achieve local tumor control by complete resection of tumor with wide margins of normal tissue.
- Minimize blood loss.

▼ *Key Point* To avoid pooling of a large amount of blood in the limb, double-ligate arteries before veins (use reverse procedure if dissemination of disease is a major concern). Achieve systematic hemostasis throughout the procedure.

- Preplan skin and soft tissue incisions to allow cosmetic closure of the wound after amputation.
- Preserve the vascular supply to the remaining skin and muscles.
- Eliminate dead spaces during closure and do not close tissues under tension.

▼ *Key Point* Close in multiple layers using "walking" suture patterns. Place Penrose drains in the wound if significant dead space remains.

- Achieve a short amputation stump to avoid trauma resulting from attempted use.

Equipment

- Standard general surgical pack
- Electrocautery unit
- Bone-cutting device (oscillating saw, Gigli wire, or osteotome)
- Elastic compression bandage

Technique

Thoracic Limb Amputation with Removal of the Scapula

Use this technique when the tumor involves the humerus or scapula. Disarticulation of the shoulder is sometimes performed when the scapula is not involved but is not recommended because it is technically more difficult than removal of the scapula. Partial scapulectomy can be performed for small noninvasive tumors of the most proximal aspect of the scapula.

1. Place the dog in lateral recumbency and aseptically prepare the entire leg and chest wall for surgery.
2. Incise the skin along the spine of the scapula to the greater tubercle of the humerus. Carry the incision circumferentially to the medial side of the shoulder joint.
3. Ligate and divide the cephalic vein as it runs deep to the cleidobrachialis muscle.
4. Sharply separate the omotransversarius and the cervical and thoracic trapezius muscles from the scapular spine.
5. Subperiosteally elevate the rhomboideus and serratus ventralis muscles from the medial aspect of the scapula, and abduct the latter from the chest wall.
6. Sever the common insertion of the latissimus dorsi, teres major, and cutaneous trunci muscles from the teres tubercle of the humerus.
7. Ligate and divide the thoracodorsal artery and vein and cut their satellite nerve. Further abduct the scapula and rotate it medially.
8. Ligate and divide the axillary and lateral thoracic arteries and the brachial and axillary veins.
9. Transect the brachial plexus of nerves with scissors or scalpel.
10. Complete the amputation by cutting the pectoral and cleidobrachialis muscles away from the humerus.
11. Routinely close the muscles, subcutaneous tissues, and skin.

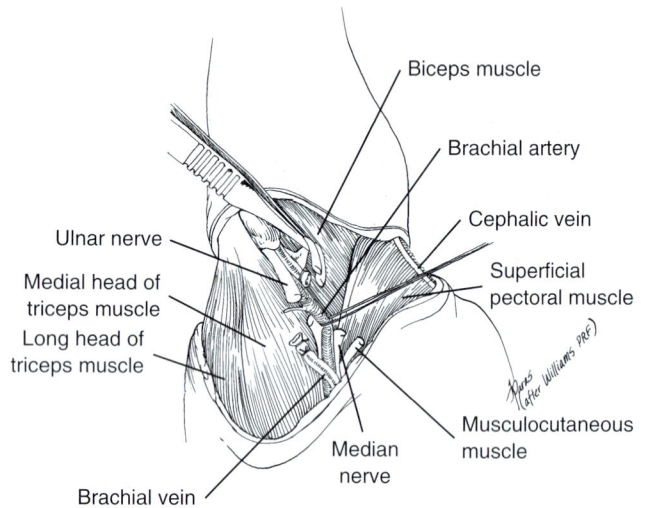

Figure 135–2. Medial dissection of vessels and nerves for thoracic limb amputation at midhumerus.

▼ *Key Point* In all amputation procedures, eliminate dead space during closure and do not close tissues under tension.

12. Apply a soft padded compressive bandage around the chest.

Technique

Thoracic Limb Amputation at the Midhumerus

Use this method when there is no tumor involvement of the humerus or scapula. This technique is faster and causes less blood loss than removal of the scapula because it requires transection of insertions of only three muscles and requires no major muscle belly transection.

1. Place the dog in lateral recumbency and aseptically prepare the entire leg for surgery.
2. Incise the skin circumferentially at the junction of the middle and distal thirds of the humerus, curving laterally as low as the epicondylar ridge.
3. Expose, ligate, and divide the brachial artery and vein (Fig. 135–2).
4. Sever the median, ulnar, and musculocutaneous nerves.
5. Isolate and transect the triceps tendon at the level of the olecranon (Fig. 135–3).
6. Tenotomize the biceps and brachialis muscles at their distal insertion on the medial aspect of the radius and ulna.
7. Ligate and transect the cephalic vein at the distal one-third of the humerus. Sever the radial nerve at the same level.
8. Reflect the three severed tendons proximally to subperiosteally elevate the brachiocephalic muscle from the humerus.
9. Complete the amputation with osteotomy of the humerus, leaving the proximal one-third of this bone.

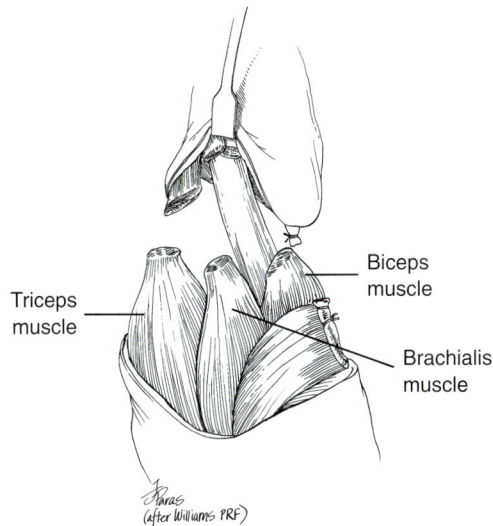

Figure 135–3. Transection of muscles for thoracic limb amputation at midhumerus.

10. Cover the humeral stump by suturing the three cut muscles together.
11. Routinely close subcutaneous tissues and skin.

Technique

Pelvic Limb Amputation at the Midfemur

Use this technique when the tumor does not involve the femur. This method has the advantage of lateral protection of the genitalia in males.

1. Place the dog in lateral recumbency and aseptically prepare the entire leg and hemipelvis for surgery.
2. Incise the skin in two connected semicircles; ventrolaterally from the tuber ischii down to the patella and up to the flank and ventromedially from the ends of the lateral incision down to midthigh.
3. Transect the caudal belly of the sartorius and gracilis muscles at midthigh.
4. Isolate, ligate, and divide the saphenous nerve and the femoral artery and vein.
5. Transect the pectineus muscle at its insertion on the femur, and the cranial sartorius and quadriceps muscles proximal to the patella.
6. Incise the tensor fasciae latae and biceps femoris muscles along the skin incision.
7. Isolate the sciatic nerve trunk and sever it at the greater trochanter.
8. Transect the abductor cruris caudalis, semitendinosus, semimembranosus, and adductor magnus et brevis muscles at midthigh.
9. Complete the amputation by osteotomy of the femur, leaving the proximal one-third of this bone.
10. Routinely close the muscles, subcutaneous tissues, and skin.

Technique

Pelvic Limb Amputation by Hip Disarticulation

Use this technique when there is tumor involvement of the femur. Tumors of the proximal femur may require en bloc resection of the acetabulum (subtotal hemipelvectomy) with the femur to ensure complete removal.

1. Place the dog in lateral recumbency and aseptically prepare the entire leg and pelvis for surgery.
2. Incise the skin in two connected semicircles, ventrolaterally from the tuber ischii down to the midthigh and up to the flank, and ventromedially from the ends of the lateral incision down to the inguinal fold.
3. Isolate, ligate, and divide the femoral and superficial circumflex femoral arteries and femoral vein.
4. Transect the sartorius, pectineus, gracilis, and adductor magnus et brevis muscles 2 cm from their origin (Fig. 135–4A and B).
5. Ligate and divide the medial circumflex femoral artery and vein.
6. Elevate the iliopsoas muscle from the lesser trochanter of the femur.
7. Sever the saphenous and femoral nerves.
8. Cut the medial coxofemoral joint capsule and round ligament.
9. Transect the tensor fasciae latae, biceps femoris, abductor cruris caudalis, semitendinosus, and semimembranosus muscles in their proximal one-third.
10. Sever the sciatic nerve distal to its branches to the upper thigh muscles (Fig. 135–4C).
11. With the leg in flexion and abduction, sever the hip rotator muscles, including the internal and external obturator and the gemellus muscles.
12. Complete the amputation by severing the three gluteal muscles (superficial, middle, and deep), and the lateral joint capsule and by elevating the rectus femoris muscle from the iliopubic eminence (Fig. 135–4D).
13. Routinely close the muscles, subcutaneous tissue, and skin.

Postoperative Care and Complications

Short Term

- Submit the amputated limb or the entire diseased area for histopathologic confirmation of the preoperative diagnosis. On the basis of preoperative biopsy alone, osteosarcoma can be confused with other primary bone tumors.
- Closely monitor for hemorrhage and hypovolemic shock.
- Treat seroma formation by pressure bandages, and treat infection with antibiotic therapy. Drain large seromas or abscesses by opening part of the incision or placing a Penrose drain.
- Beginning 24 hours after surgery, apply hot packs to the surgical site three to four times daily until suture removal.
- Assist walking with towel support until dog has adapted to amputation.

Long Term

- Frequently (every 8–12 weeks) reevaluate the dog clinically and radiographically for detection of tumor at the amputation stump and in the chest.

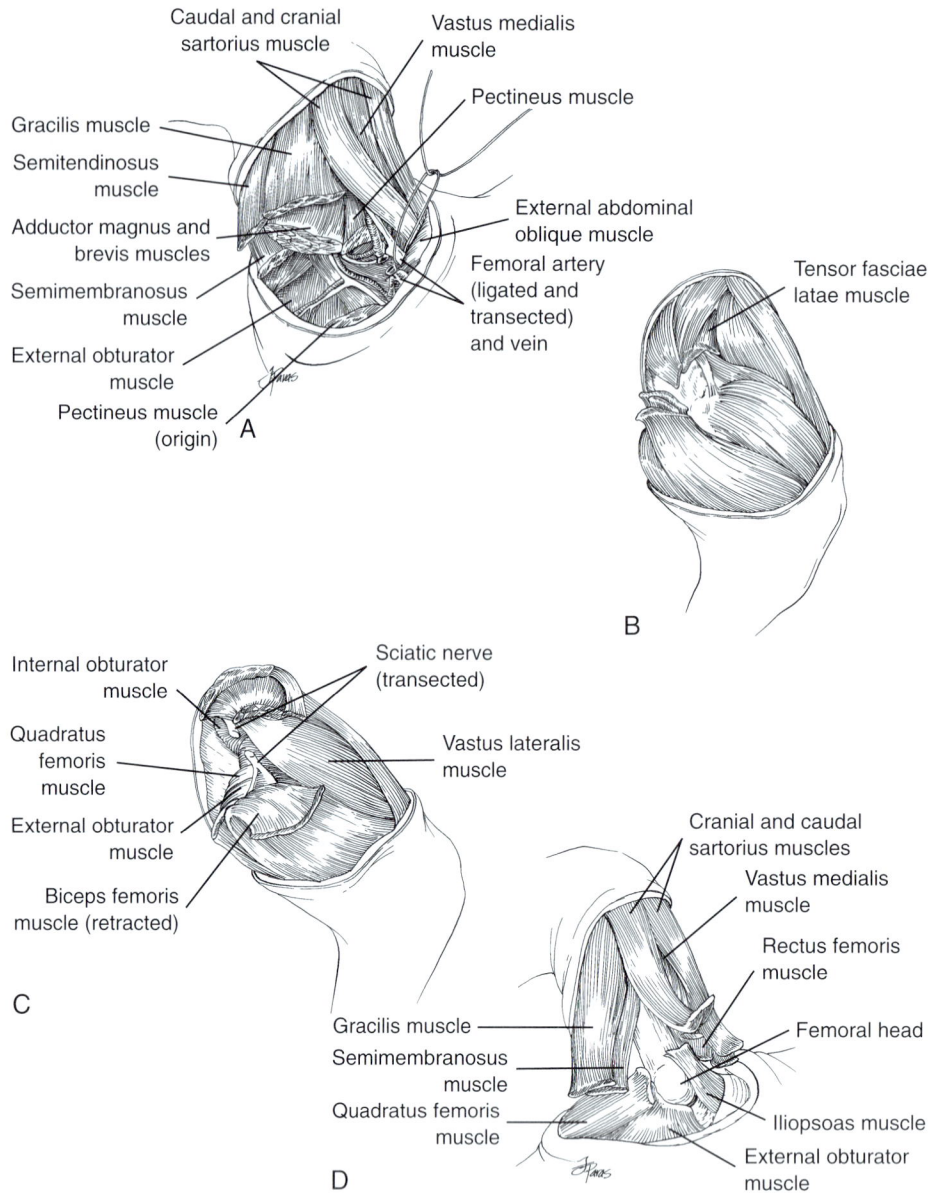

Figure 135–4. Dissection of muscles, vessels, and nerves for pelvic limb amputation by hip disarticulation. *A* and *D*, medial views; *B* and *C*, lateral views.

- Advise strict weight control for large dogs, especially after forelimb amputation.

Adjuvant Treatment

Adjuvant Treatment (see Chap. 24 for general principles of Chemotherapy)

- Use the following adjunctive chemotherapy for canine osteosarcoma.

Cisplatin

- Administer cisplatin at a dose of 70 mg/m² IV as soon as possible following surgery (ideally at the time of amputation); repeat at 21-day intervals for three to six treatments.

- There is a trend for dogs receiving higher cumulative doses to have longer survival times (50 mg/m² IV of cisplatin up to nine occasions).
- Myelosuppression and renal toxicity are potential serious and life-threatening complications.
- Saline diuresis helps prevent nephrotoxicity. The protocol recommended is that described by Straw and Withrow (1996).
- For safe administration of cisplatin, dogs should have >3000 PMN leukocytes per μl, >150,000 platelets per μl, a normal BUN and creatinine, and urine specific gravity of 1030 with no proteinuria or casts in the urine sediment.
- Clinical oncologic research at major veterinary schools has shown benefit from the administration of macrophage activators (muramyl dipeptide derivatives) in addition to IV cisplatin (Wisconsin) and

from drug delivery systems (polylactic acid polymers) for slow topical release of cisplatin (Colorado).

Carboplatin

- Carboplatin is less nephrotoxic than cisplatin with apparently similar antimetastatic effects.
- It can be given IV without the saline diuresis necessary for cisplatin administration.
- Administer 300 mg/m^2 IV at amputation; repeat at 21-day intervals for three treatments provided there are no signs of severe bone marrow suppression.

Radiation

- Consider radiation therapy for radiosensitive neoplasms (e.g., mast cell tumors; see Chap. 26)

Prognosis

- The prognosis is good if the tumor was benign.
- The prognosis is fair if the tumor was malignant and completely excised and there is no preoperative evidence of distant metastasis. With adjunctive chemotherapy, the median survival time for dogs with osteosarcoma is approximately 10–13 months.
- If the tumor is biologically aggressive, incompletely excised, or has spread to distant organs, the prognosis is poor. Survival time usually is less than 6 months.
- In cats the median survival after amputation alone is 24 months.

Metastatic Disease

- Pulmonary metastatectomy for canine osteosarcoma can significantly prolong survival time
- Absolute selection criteria includes:
  - Primary tumor in complete remission preferably for >300 days
  - No more than two nodules visible on plain thoracic radiographs
  - Cancer found only in the lung (negative bone scan or survey)
- The median survival time in 36 dogs after pulmonary metastatectomy was approximately 6 months.

▼ *Key Point* Chemotherapy appears to be ineffective for the treatment of *measurable* metastatic osteosarcoma in the dog.

LIMB-SPARING PROCEDURES

Limb sparing is a complicated process that requires a supply of allograft (bone bank) and, more important, a coordinated team effort among surgical and medical oncologists, radiologists, pathologists, and technical staff.

Objectives

- Obtain local tumor control.
- Provide a pain-free and functional limb.
- Enhance long-term survival.

Chemotherapy and Radiation

Chemotherapy and radiation usually are administered before surgical debulking to promote tumor necrosis.

Bone Allograft

Bone allograft techniques should be performed by a trained surgical specialist. Some referral centers possess banks of frozen or gas-sterilized bones.

- Consider bone allograft in cases of limb neoplasm if one or more of the following conditions apply:
  - The tumor is confined to less than 50% of the length of a long bone, with minimal or no soft tissue involvement.
  - No evidence of metastasis, infection, or concurrent disease is present.
  - Sufficient healthy bone stock remains for internal fixation with screws and plate.
  - Preoperative biopsy reveals a benign or nonaggressive neoplasm.
  - The owner refuses limb amputation.
  - A sterile allograft from a healthy animal is available.
- The most suitable cases for limb sparing are dogs with tumors in the distal radius and ulna.
- Postoperative complications may include infection, sequestration, fracture, fixation failure, and tumor recurrence either locally or from metastases.
- For the more than 200 limb-sparing procedures performed at Colorado State University through 1994, limb function has been good to excellent in 80% of the animals, and survival has not been adversely affected by removing the primary tumor with marginal resection as compared with amputation (radical margins).

SUPPLEMENTAL READINGS

Bergman PJ, MacEwen EG, Kurzman ID, et al.: Amputation and carboplatin for treatment of dogs with osteosarcoma: 48 cases (1991–1993). J Vet Int Med 10:76–81, 1996.

Bone DL, Aberman HM: Forelimb amputation in the dog using humeral osteotomy. J Am Anim Hosp Assoc 24:525, 1988.

Evans HE, Christensen GC: Miller's Anatomy of the Dog. Philadelphia: WB Saunders, 1979.

Kirpensteijn J, Straw RC, Pardo AD, et al.: Partial and total scapulectomy in the dog. J Am Anim Hosp Assoc 30:313, 1994.

O'Brien MG, Straw RC, Withrow SJ, et al.: Resection of pulmonary metastases in canine osteosarcoma: 36 cases (1983–1992). Vet Surg 22:105, 1993.

Slatter DH: *Textbook of Small Animal Surgery*. Philadelphia, WB Saunders, 2nd Ed. 1993.

Straw RC, Withrow SJ, Powers BE: Partial or total hemipelvectomy in the management of sarcomas in seven dogs and two cats. Vet Surg 21:183, 1992.

Straw RE, Withrow SS: Treatment of canine osteosarcoma. *In* Bonagura JD, ed: Kirk's Current Veterinary Therapy XII. Philadelphia, WB Saunders, 1996, pp 506–511.

Withrow SJ, MacEwen EG: Small Animal Clinical Oncology. 2nd Ed. Philadelphia: WB Saunders, 1996, pp 234–252.

136 Miscellaneous Diseases of Bone

James K. Roush

Some of the diseases affecting bone are discussed in this chapter. See respective chapters for other bone and cartilage diseases, such as hip dysplasia, avascular necrosis of the femoral head, and osteochondrosis.

PANOSTEITIS

Panosteitis is a disease of young large-breed dogs manifested by intermittent lameness of one or more limbs. Onset usually occurs in the first year of life. The disease is self-limiting but clinical signs may persist in one or more limbs for months. Differentiate panosteitis from other causes of lameness in young dogs, such as hip dysplasia and osteochondritis dissecans.

Etiology

- The etiology of panosteitis is unknown.
- Panosteitis may have a polygenetic origin, because German shepherd dogs are commonly affected.
- Contributing causes include stress, transient vascular abnormalities, metabolic disorders, allergies, hyperestrogenism, and autoimmune reaction following viral infection.
- The characteristic histopathologic lesion is degeneration of medullary adipocytes, followed by stromal cell proliferation, intramembranous ossification, and regeneration of the adipose bone marrow.

Clinical Signs

Signalment

- Panosteitis usually is seen in large and giant-breed dogs, most often 5–12 months of age; however, it has been reported in dogs up to 5 years of age.
- Male dogs are affected more frequently than females (4:1 ratio). In females, the first episode of the disease often occurs in association with the first estrus.
- Panosteitis has been reported in the German shepherd, Great Dane, Irish setter, St. Bernard, Doberman pinscher, Airedale, basset hound, and miniature schnauzer.

Lameness

- There is acute onset of weight bearing lameness without a history of recent trauma.

▼ *Key Point* Lesions often resolve in one bone and develop in another, resulting in the classic history of "shifting leg" lameness.

- Pain due to the disease is of intermittent duration and severity, but the dog rarely, if ever, is completely non–weight bearing on the affected limb or limbs.
- Lameness or radiographic lesions may occur simultaneously in multiple limbs or bones, or lameness may resolve for a period of time, only to recur in another limb. After a bone passes through the lesion cycle, it is unlikely that it will be affected again, but lameness may occur in that limb if the disease affects another bone in the limb.
- Clinical signs often continue for several months and usually resolve by 18–20 months of age.

Diagnosis

▼ *Key Point* Diagnosis of panosteitis is established by eliciting pain on firm palpation of a long bone and by characteristic radiographic lesions.

Physical Examination

- Applying firm pressure to the diaphyses of the affected bone results in clinical signs of discomfort.

Laboratory Evaluation

- Hematology and serum chemistry profiles usually are normal.
- Eosinophilia occurs inconsistently (this disease was previously referred to as eosinophilic panosteitis).

Radiography

Confirm suspected cases by survey radiography of the affected bone(s).

- Early radiographic lesions are characterized by areas of increased density and accentuated trabecular pattern within the medullary cavity (Table 136–1).
  - These areas may be focal or multifocal and commonly occur near the nutrient foramen.
  - Bone cortices may be thickened, and progressive mottling and opacification of the medullary cavity occur.
  - A smooth, linear periosteal proliferation may develop.

Table 136–1. CHARACTERISTIC RADIOGRAPHIC LESIONS SEEN IN DISEASES AFFECTING BONE

Disease	Lesion
Panosteitis	Increased opacity in medullary cavity of diaphysis
Hypertrophic osteodystrophy	Radiolucent metaphyseal line adjacent to physis
Hypertrophic osteopathy	Periosteal reaction beginning on metacarpals or metatarsals, bilaterally symmetric
Craniomandibular osteopathy	Bony proliferation on ventral mandible and skull
Cartilaginous exostosis	Large, smooth bony protuberance in metaphyseal area
Bone cyst	Well-circumscribed, radiolucent metaphyseal defect
Retained enchondral cartilaginous core	Longitudinal, linear radiolucent defect in distal ulna

- During resolution, sclerotic areas gradually decrease in size and density. Radiographic signs may persist for several months after lameness resolves.
- There is no correlation between the radiographic lesions and severity of clinical signs.

Differential Diagnoses

- Differentiate panosteitis as a cause of lameness from other diseases that are characterized by onset during or shortly after the rapid-growth phase in large-breed dogs.
  - In particular, eliminate hypertrophic osteodystrophy, osteochondritis dissecans of the shoulder or elbow (see Chap. 137), ununited anconeal process (see Chap. 137), and hip dysplasia (see Chap. 127) as a cause of lameness before ascribing clinical signs to panosteitis.

Treatment

▼ *Key Point* Panosteitis is a self-limiting disease.

- No specific therapy for panosteitis exists.
- Administer buffered aspirin (10–25 mg/kg q8h PO) or carprofen (2.2 mg/kg q12h PO), as needed, to alleviate pain.
- Restrict exercise in severely affected animals.
- Inform clients that the lameness may shift to other limbs and that the animal may be intermittently lame for 6–18 months.

HYPERTROPHIC OSTEODYSTROPHY

Hypertrophic osteodystrophy (HOD) is a developmental disease of young, rapidly growing large and giant-breed dogs. Dogs with HOD exhibit lameness in one or more limbs in association with swelling and inflammation of the metaphyseal regions of long bones. The incidence of the disease has declined in recent years. Complications related to prolonged recumbency,

anorexia, and hyperthermia have been reported in severely affected animals. The overall prognosis for HOD is guarded. Although many dogs recover spontaneously, permanent bone changes and physical deformities may develop.

Etiology

- The etiology of HOD is unknown.
- Historically, the disease has been attributed to vitamin C deficiency, but decreased levels of ascorbic acid in the serum or urine do not appear to be related to the disease.
- Skeletal lesions similar to those of HOD have been produced experimentally by feeding a free-choice diet abnormally high in protein, calories, and calcium.
- Canine distemper virus may be involved as a causative agent.

Clinical Signs
Signalment

▼ *Key Point* HOD occurs only in growing animals with open physes.

- Onset of clinical signs usually occurs at 3–4 months of age (range, 2–8 months).
- HOD has been reported in the Great Dane, Irish wolfhound, St. Bernard, Irish setter, Labrador retriever, basset hound, greyhound, German shepherd, German short-haired pointer, borzoi, boxer, Dalmatian, Weimaraner, Doberman pinscher, and collie.

Systemic Signs

- The severity of HOD varies, ranging from an absence of systemic signs to severe anorexia, weight loss, fever, and depression.
- Clinical signs are episodic in nature, and lameness often is bilaterally symmetric.

Lameness

- Lameness varies from a mild limp in minimally affected dogs to non–weight bearing lameness in severely affected animals.
- Affected long bone metaphyses are extremely swollen, warm, and painful in animals with severe disease.
- Multiple long bones and limbs are affected, and, in extreme cases, dogs are reluctant to stand or move.

Diagnosis
History/Physical Examination

- The history may include recent weight loss, reluctance to move, and anorexia.
- Affected metaphyses are warm and swollen on palpation.
- Signs of pain may be elicited on palpation of the metaphyseal areas.
- Pyrexia of up to 106°F may be present.

Laboratory Evaluation

- Laboratory data are normal or mild abnormalities related to anorexia and stress may be present.

Radiography

- Radiographic changes usually occur in the metaphyses of the long bones and are bilaterally symmetric. Other bones, including the mandible, ribs, and scapula, may be affected.
- The characteristic radiographic lesion is generalized sclerosis and enlargement of the metaphysis.

▼ *Key Point* Radiolucent areas form in the metaphysis and coalesce to form an area of radiolucency parallel to the growth plate, called a double physeal line (Fig. 136–1).

- Irregular widening of the physis may be seen in later stages of the disease.
- Subperiosteal or extraperiosteal bone formation is seen in metaphyseal regions and may involve the diaphysis.

Differential Diagnoses

- Differentiate HOD from other causes of lameness in immature large or giant-breed dogs.
  - Other diseases that result in metaphyseal swelling or in signs of pain during palpation of long bones include panosteitis, bone-associated neoplasms, and hypertrophic osteopathy. Radiographic lesions in these diseases are distinct and allow easy differentiation; the last two diseases are unlikely to be the cause of lameness in young dogs.

Treatment

▼ *Key Point* There is no specific treatment for HOD.

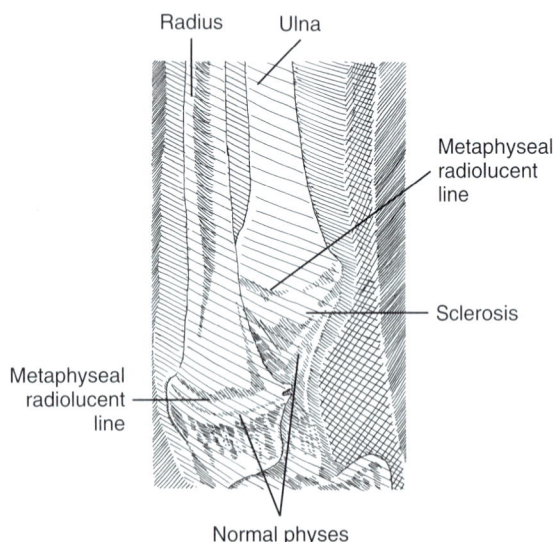

Figure 136–1. Metaphyseal radiolucent lines and metaphyseal sclerosis proximal to distal radial and ulnar physis in a dog with hypertrophic osteodystrophy.

- In mild or moderately affected dogs, there is often spontaneous remission.
- Correction of dietary imbalances and decreased caloric intake may be beneficial.
- Good supportive care of severely affected dogs is essential to prevent decubital ulcers, provide nutrition (see Chap. 3) and maintain hydration (see Chap. 5).
- Give nonsteroidal analgesics, as needed, to relieve discomfort (buffered aspirin, 10–25 mg/kg q8h PO or carprofen (2.2 mg/kg q12h PO).
- Severely affected animals may require nutritional intake via force-feeding or gastrostomy tube (see Chap. 3). Parenteral fluids may be needed to prevent dehydration in these animals (see Chap. 5).
- There is no evidence that mineral, vitamin C, or vitamin D supplements are beneficial; these substances actually may accelerate the rate of dystrophic calcification.

HYPERTROPHIC OSTEOPATHY

Hypertrophic osteopathy (HO) is a pathologic disease process affecting long bones secondary to a space-occupying mass in the abdominal or thoracic cavities. The disease has been reported in many species, including dogs, cats, and humans. HO is characterized by bilateral symmetric swelling of the distal limbs accompanied by periosteal bone formation. HO has been referred to as hypertrophic pulmonary osteoarthropathy, pulmonary osteoarthropathy, and hypertrophic pulmonary osteopathy. Hypertrophic osteopathy is the term that most accurately reflects the rare joint involvement and the variable site of the primary space-occupying lesion.

Etiology

- Hypertrophic osteopathy occurs secondary to a variety of diseases and occurs in dogs and cats of all breeds and ages.
- HO is most often secondary to metastatic pulmonary neoplasia, although it has been reported with primary pulmonary neoplasia, pulmonary abscesses, pulmonary tuberculosis, chronic bronchopneumonia, spirocercosis, dirofilariasis, rib tumors, bacterial endocarditis, hepatic adenocarcinoma, and various primary bladder neoplasms (neurofibrosarcoma, botryoid rhabdomyosarcoma, and transitional cell sarcoma).
- The pathogenic mechanisms underlying the bone pathology are unknown. Evidence points to an increased peripheral vascular supply secondary to the pulmonary lesion. This increased peripheral blood flow has been observed both in dogs and humans and may be related to irritation of afferent nerve pathways and stimulation of a nervous reflex.

Clinical Signs

▼ *Key Point* Signs of HO may be present months before onset of clinical signs relating to the underlying disease; early recognition is important for diagnosis and treatment of the primary disease.

Signalment

- Dogs and cats with HO may be of any breed and usually are affected late in life.
- A reported increased incidence of the disease in female and large-breed dogs may be due to the increased incidence of mammary tumor metastasis in female dogs, and of primary bone tumors in large-breed dogs.

Lameness

- Most animals present with acute or gradual lameness of all four limbs and with reluctance to move.

Diagnosis

Physical Examination

- The distal limbs are swollen, firm, and warm.
- Signs of pain may be elicited on deep palpation of the long bones.

Laboratory Evaluation

- Laboratory findings reflect the underlying disease process and are not characteristic of HO.

Radiography

- Survey radiographs demonstrate a bilateral, symmetric, generalized periosteal proliferative reaction affecting the long bones of the appendicular skeleton (Fig. 136–2). Endosteal bone proliferation does not occur.
- Distal portions of the limbs, especially the metatarsals and metacarpals, are involved first, but periosteal proliferation eventually may involve the more proximal long bones and occasionally the mandible, pelvis, ribs, and vertebrae.
- In very early cases, periosteal new-bone formation is not evident, but symmetric soft tissue swelling is present.

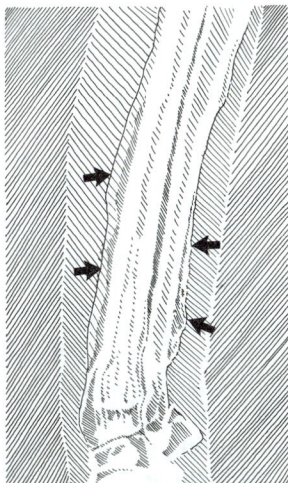

Figure 136–2. Smooth periosteal proliferation *(arrows)* on radius and ulna characteristic of hypertrophic osteopathy.

- If the primary disease resolves, the bony and soft tissue radiographic abnormalities regress.

▼ *Key Point* Thoracic and abdominal radiographs are essential to evaluate the underlying disease process and to confirm the diagnosis of HO. Abdominal ultrasound may also be helpful in identifying a mass lesion.

Differential Diagnoses

The bony periosteal reactions of hypertrophic osteopathy are similar to those of panosteitis and hypertrophic osteodystrophy, but HO will not exhibit the increased medullary opacities of panosteitis, nor the radiolucent metaphyseal line characteristic of HOD. It is rare to see HO in a young (adolescent) animal.

Treatment

▼ *Key Point* Removal of the underlying primary lesion usually results in regression of the lameness and distal limb lesions.

- Resection of primary or metastatic pulmonary neoplasms provides temporary relief of signs related to HO, but long-term survival is dependent on the type of neoplasm.
  - Appropriate treatment of dirofilariasis, spirocercosis, and primary lung disease may increase the chances for long-term survival.
- Inflammation and clinical signs of pain resolve 1–2 weeks after removal of the thoracic or abdominal mass. Periosteal reactions regress in 3–4 months, but residual radiographic changes may persist in severe cases. Lameness may persist in some animals even after removal of the mass.
- When resection of the primary mass is not feasible, unilateral vagotomy (on the side of the lesion) may provide temporary regression of clinical signs.

CRANIOMANDIBULAR OSTEOPATHY

Craniomandibular osteopathy (CMO) is a nonneoplastic, noninflammatory proliferative bony disease in growing dogs that affects bones of endochondral origin, most commonly the mandibles, occipital bones, or temporal bones. Bony lesions are bilateral and symmetric. CMO occurs predominantly in terriers, especially Scottish, West Highland white, and Cairn terriers, but the disease also has been reported in the boxer, Labrador retriever, Great Dane, and Doberman pinscher.

Etiology

- The etiology of CMO is unknown.
- Osteoclastic resorption of mandibular bone occurs, followed by production of woven bone on both the periosteal and endosteal surfaces of the bone. Cyclic episodes of bone resorption and proliferation result in the formation of mature fibrous bone that may remain permanently.

Clinical Signs

- Disease onset occurs at 4–10 months of age. Both sexes are affected equally.
- Presenting clinical signs include pain on manipulation or opening of the mouth, mandibular swelling, ptyalism, inability to open the mouth, intermittent fever, and lethargy.

Diagnosis

Physical Examination

Signs of pain are elicited during direct palpation of the swelling or attempts to open the mouth. In advanced cases, the clinician may be unable to open the mouth more than 1 or 2 cm. Dogs may be febrile during the period of bone proliferation. Lymphadenopathy or temporal muscle atrophy may be present.

Radiography

Diagnosis of CMO is confirmed by radiographic evidence of the bony proliferative lesions.

- Obtain survey radiographs of the skull and mandible, including oblique, dorsoventral, and lateral views, to assess the extent of the disease.
- A non-neoplastic, bilaterally symmetric bony proliferation is seen projecting from the periosteal surfaces of the mandible or other bones of the cranium (Fig. 136–3).
- Angular processes of the mandible and bullae may fuse and obstruct jaw motion. Lesions may also involve the occipital bone, parietal bone, frontal bone, maxilla, and appendicular bones.
- The proliferation of new bone decreases as growth slows, and becomes radiographically static when the animal is approximately 1 year old. Partial or complete regression of bony lesions occurs, but moderate or severe cases result in permanent bone proliferation to varying degrees.
- The prognosis is poor for dogs with radiographic evidence of partial or complete bony ankylosis of the temporomandibular joints (TMJs).

Differential Diagnoses

- Lesions of CMO in the appendicular skeleton may appear radiographically similar to HOD, but CMO lacks the metaphyseal radiolucent line of HOD.

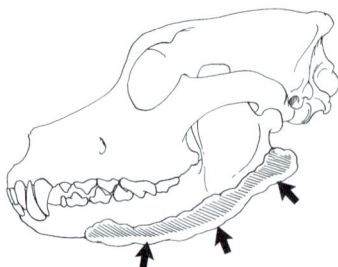

Figure 136–3. Bony proliferation (*arrows*) on the ventral mandible of a dog with craniomandibular osteopathy.

- Radiographic appearance differentiates CMO from bony neoplasia and osteomyelitis.

Treatment

- There is no specific therapy for CMO.
- Administer analgesic therapy (buffered aspirin, 10–25 mg/kg q8h PO or carprofen, 2.2 mg/kg q12h PO), as needed.
- Nutritional support by gastrostomy or enterostomy tube or parenteral supplementation may be necessary (see Chap. 3). As the condition stabilizes, most animals have impaired mouth function but are capable of maintaining normal nutritional status.
- Surgical intervention to reduce new bone mass and increase TMJ range of motion has met with limited success.

MULTIPLE CARTILAGINOUS EXOSTOSIS

Multiple cartilaginous exostosis (MCE) is a disease of dogs and cats in which multiple ossified protuberances arise from the bone in metaphyseal regions. Vertebrae, ribs, and long bones commonly are affected. The exostosis ceases to grow when the physis nearest the exostosis ossifies.

Etiology

MCE probably is heritable in dogs, horses, and humans.

The accepted pathogenesis is that the exostosis is derived from displaced chondrocytes that separate from the physis during development.

Clinical Signs

- The animal often is presented with a firm, distinct swelling on the involved bone.
- Lameness or limb dysfunction develops only when adjacent structures such as the tendons or nerves are compressed or mechanically distorted by the exostoses.
- Other clinical signs, including pain, lameness, mechanical dysfunction, and neurologic deficits, depend on the structure affected.

Diagnosis

Physical Examination

- A smooth, immovable bony swelling is visible and palpable near a metaphysis.
- Pain may be elicited on palpation of the mass or surrounding soft tissues.

Radiography

- Obtain skeletal survey radiographs of animals with suspected cartilaginous exostosis.
  - Radiographic lesions are juxtacortical masses at or adjacent to the metaphysis.
  - Large, scattered radiolucent areas of hyaline cartilage may be present within the exostosis. The exos-

totic growths may involve any bone except the skull.

- Surgical biopsy of the lesion confirms the diagnosis.

Treatment

▼ *Key Point* Removal of the exostosis relieves associated pain, mechanical dysfunction, and neurologic deficits.

- Removal of MCE sometimes is requested to improve cosmetic appearance.
- Malignant transformation of exostoses to chondrosarcomas or osteosarcomas has been reported. Continued growth of the exostosis after the animal is mature suggests malignant transformation.
- In general, the prognosis is good after removal of uncomplicated MCE.

BONE CYSTS

Bone cysts are smooth radiolucent cavities found rarely in the long bones of dogs. Flat bones (e.g., mandible, ribs) also may be affected. Four types of bone cysts have been described in dogs:

- Monostotic (affecting one bone)
- Polyostotic (affecting more than one bone)
- Aneurysmal
- Subchondral

Aneurysmal bone cysts are extremely rare in dogs and are locally aggressive. Bone cysts, found in young, large-breed dogs usually do not produce clinical signs until they attain a large size.

Etiology

- The etiology of monostotic, polyostotic, and aneurysmal bone cysts is unknown.
- Subchondral bone cysts often are not primary lesions and may be the result of chronic degenerative joint disease or diseases leading to degenerative joint disease (e.g., rheumatoid arthritis, systemic lupus erythematosus).

Clinical Signs

Signalment

- The age of affected animals ranges from 4–30 months, but most animals are less than 1 year of age.
- Breeds reported to develop bone cysts include the German shepherd, Weimaraner, Irish wolfhound, Afghan, saluki, Great Dane, and Doberman pinscher.

Presentation

- Pain, swelling, and stiffness of the nearest joint may be present.
- Acute lameness or swelling may occur at the site of the cyst owing to a pathologic fracture.

Diagnosis

Radiography

- Survey radiographs establish a diagnosis of bone cysts. A benign, expansive, radiolucent area in the metaphysis is characteristic.
- The metaphyseal cortex may be thinned by expanding cysts.
- Pathologic fractures may be evident radiographically.

Histopathology

- The cyst is lined by fibrous connective tissue.
- Aneurysmal bone cysts are filled with blood, and the blood spaces are lined by connective tissue trabeculae. Multinucleate giant cells and mature bone may be present in these cysts.
- Monostotic and polyostotic cysts may fill with blood after pathologic fracture.

Differential Diagnoses

- Differentiate bone cysts from more aggressive lesions such as chondrosarcoma, osteosarcoma, and giant cell tumors.

Treatment

- Curettage of the walls and filling of the defect with cancellous bone is the definitive treatment in most animals.
- Treat pathologic fractures through cysts by debridement of the cyst wall, cancellous graft, and fracture fixation.
- Consider cyst resection if the lesion is located in flat bones (e.g., rib resection or mandibulectomy).

RETAINED ENCHONDRAL CARTILAGINOUS CORES

Retained enchondral cartilaginous cores occur in the distal ulnar metaphysis of young, large-breed dogs. Radiographically, the retained enchondral cartilage is seen as a central, longitudinal radiolucent cone in the distal ulnar metaphysis and usually is an incidental finding of no clinical significance. These lesions, however, may interfere with normal growth of the ulna, resulting in forelimb deformities.

Etiology

- The etiology is unknown.

Clinical Signs

- Signs may include valgus deviation, external rotation of the carpus, and cranial bowing of the radius.

Diagnosis

- Survey radiographs establish the diagnosis in animals with appropriate forelimb deformities.
- The lesion also may be an incidental finding unrelated to clinical lameness if normal growth of the ulna is apparent.

Treatment

- No treatment is necessary for animals without forelimb deformity.
- Immature animals with forelimb deformities may benefit from distal ulnectomy, which may allow spontaneous correction of radial and ulnar deformities during continued growth (see Chap. 124).
- Mature animals require ulnar and radial osteotomies to correct forelimb deformity (see Chap. 124).

SUPPLEMENTAL READINGS

Alexander JW: Selected skeletal dysplasias: Craniomandibular osteopathy, multiple cartilaginous exostoses, and hypertrophic osteodystrophy. Vet Clin North Am Sm Anim Pract 13:55, 1983.

Alexander JW: Orthopedic diseases. *In* Slatter DH, ed.: Textbook of Small Animal Surgery. Philadelphia: WB Saunders, 1985, p 2312.

Goldschmidt MH, Biery DN: Bone cysts in the dog. *In* Newton CD, Nunamaker DM, eds.: Textbook of Small Animal Orthopaedics. Philadelphia: JB Lippincott, 1985, p 611.

Lenehan TM, Fetter AW: Hypertrophic osteodystrophy. *In* Newton CD, Nunamaker DM, eds.: Textbook of Small Animal Orthopaedics. Philadelphia: JB Lippincott, 1985, p 597.

Lenehan TM, Fetter AW: Hypertrophic osteopathy. *In* Newton CD, Nunamaker DM, eds.: Textbook of Small Animal Orthopaedics, 1st Ed. Philadelphia: JB Lippincott, 1985, p 603.

Lenehan TM, Van Sickle DC, Biery DN: Canine panosteitis. *In* Newton CD, Nunamaker DM, eds.: Textbook of Small Animal Orthopaedics. Philadelphia: JB Lippincott, 1985, p 591.

Muir P, Dubielzig RR, Johnson KA, Shelton GD: Hypertrophic osteodystrophy and calvarial hyperostosis. Compend Cont Ed Pract Vet 18:143, 1996.

Riser WH, Newton CD: Craniomandibular osteopathy. *In* Newton CD, Nunamaker DM, eds.: Textbook of Small Animal Orthopaedics. Philadelphia: JB Lippincott, 1985, p 603.

137 Osteochondrosis

Timothy M. Lenehan / Josh Jackson

Osteochondrosis is a pathological condition of rapidly growing cartilage that develops due to a disturbance in endochondral ossification. Multiple theories have been developed concerning the etiology of osteochondrosis, including nutrition (increased calcium or quantity of diet), trauma, ischemia, and hereditary abnormalities of ossification. Likely, the etiology is a combination of these factors. Typically, large or giant breeds are affected, with males affected more frequently than females.

- Disruption of endochondral ossification in the articuloepiphyseal complex results in osteochondritis dissecans (OCD), which is most commonly reported in the caudal aspect of the humeral head, the medial humeral condyle, the medial and lateral femoral condyles and trochlear ridges of the talus.
- Disturbances of endochondral ossification in the metaphyseal growth plate can result in focal growth plate thickening (retained endochondral cartilage cores of the distal ulna), cartilage retention nests (femoral epiphyses), physeal slowing (radius curvus), and "slippage" of metaphyseal growth plates (ununited anconeal process [UAP], proximal calcaneus).

In the elbow joint, three disorders are believed to be related to osteochondrosis: UAP, fragmented coronoid process (FCP), and OCD.

- Dogs with FCP or OCD of the distal medial humeral condyle present with similar clinical symptoms; their diagnosis and treatment can be approached identically. However, these two entities can occur alone, together, individually with UAP, or both together with UAP.
- UAP describes a radiologic diagnosis pertaining to the failure of a specific growth plate in the elbow to close completely.

UNUNITED ANCONEAL PROCESS

Anatomy and Pathophysiology

- In the dog, the anconeal process develops from a separate center of ossification and unites with the proximal ulna at 20–24 weeks of age (physeal closure). Therefore, diagnosis of UAP before 24 weeks of age may be premature.
  - If in doubt, radiograph the contralateral elbow for comparison (the incidence of bilateral UAP is approximately 30% in dogs).

- Union of the anconeal process to the ulna initially occurs at the distal aspect of the physis and then progresses proximally along the growth plate.
- Incomplete endochondral ossification can result in foci of retained cartilage within an otherwise closed physis; such retention nests can mimic UAP.
- An intact anconeal process provides stability to the elbow joint, particularly in extension (weight bearing phase). Failure of union of this process results in foreign body irritation, mild to moderate elbow instability (depending on the size of the UAP), and subsequent osteoarthritis.
- Blood supply to the anconeal process is via the dorsal periosteal capsular attachments; the bone can remain viable and capable of endosteal callus formation unless completely separated from these attachments.
- In chondrodystrophic breeds, UAP may accompany (or result from) premature closure of the distal ulna and asynchronous growth of the radius and ulna.

Ununited Anconeal Process in Immature Dogs (<1 Year)

Clinical Signs

- Dogs with UAP present with varying degrees of lameness that usually worsens with exercise.
- Pain may be elicited with extension or flexion of the elbow.

Diagnosis

- Detailed preoperative radiographs of the elbow are mandatory. The following views are helpful:
  - *Straight lateral*—to evaluate all compartments of the joint, assess relative bone lengths (radius/ulna), and observe for panosteitis lesions.
  - *Flexed lateral*—facilitates detailed evaluation of the region between the anconeal process and the ulna.
  - *Craniocaudal*—to examine the medial joint compartment for concurrent arthritis, FCP, and OCD of the medial aspect of the humeral condyle.
  - *Craniocaudal medial oblique*—to evaluate for FCP not visible on a standard craniocaudal view.
- Assess the elbow for
  - Panosteitis in adjacent bones
  - Coexistent FCP or OCD lesions in the elbow joint
  - The degree of osteoarthritis present in the elbow
  - The type of UAP

- Incongruities indicating a radioulnar growth inequity

▼ *Key Point* If panosteitis is present, a "radiographic" UAP may be clinically silent; alternatively, there may be two (or more) clinically significant problems.

Preoperative Considerations

- Concomitant FCP, OCD of the medial aspect of the humeral condyle, or both may dramatically change the prognosis, both with and without surgical intervention.
- Factors determining the surgical approach include the number of lesions present and the type of UAP. Four categories can be defined:
  - *Cartilage retention nest*—In this lesion (usually an incidental finding), the anconeal process is united. It is unlikely to be the cause of the lameness.
  - *Delayed union*—A normal union proceeds distoproximally. Confine/rest animals with a delayed union and radiograph the elbow monthly until there is evidence of union.
  - *Nondisplaced nonunion*—The anconeal process is apposed to the proximal ulna by collagenous tissue or fibrocartilaginous interface. Such fragments may be successfully reconstructed, depending on the bone density (screw-holding power), viability of the tissue interface, degree of compression achieved with the lag screw, and degree of radioulnar asymmetry.
  - *Displaced nonunion*—The anconeal process is physiologically (lack of blood supply or viable interface tissue) or anatomically separated from the proximal ulna and acts as a foreign body that interferes with normal joint function. Optimally, these "joint mice" should be removed. In some cases, the anconeal process becomes lodged in the olecranon fossa, thus minimizing the irritant effect.

▼ *Key Point* Theoretically, surgical reconstruction is preferable to removal because reconstruction maintains elbow stability, thereby diminishing the potential for subsequent arthritis.

- An elbow with a displaced, free-floating nonunion benefits from surgery, as the "joint mouse" is removed. However, joint incongruity, and subsequent arthritic progression, will remain.

Surgical Procedures

Objectives

- Remove or reconstruct the UAP.
- Address concurrent disease in the medial elbow compartment (OCD/FCP).

Equipment

- Standard surgical pack and suture material
- Gelpi self-retaining retractors
- Suction and cautery
- Bone elevator (Sayre) and rongeurs (medium)
- Drill, bits, taps, and screws
- Small bone curette

Technique

1. Place the patient in lateral recumbency, with the affected limb up, suspended, and prepared from carpus to shoulder for aseptic surgery.
2. Make a lateral approach to the elbow, placing the incision in the anconeus muscle closer to the ulna than to the humeral condyle.
3. Using the Gelpi retractor, retract the lateral head of the triceps and anconeus muscles.
4. Slightly flex the elbow and externally rotate the antebrachium for the best identification of the anconeal process and its tissue interface with the ulna.
5. If a displaced nonunion is present, remove the process.
6. If the nonunion is not displaced, determine the chances for successful reconstruction
   a. Assess the vascular supply to the process.
   b. Assess mobility at the nonunion site.
   c. Assess the shape of the anconeal process for elbow congruency.
7. If in doubt, attempt lag screw fixation of the UAP.
   a. Drill the thread hole either freehand, entering at the apex of the anconeal process and exiting at the caudal ulna; or by entering at the caudal ulna and exiting at the apex of the anconeal process (the latter may require a C-clamp drill guide).
   b. Overdrill the ulnar hole.
   c. Tap the anconeal drill hole.
   d. Place the lag screw from caudal to cranial and observe the degree of compression (Fig. 137–1).
   e. Do not let the screw tip protrude beyond the tip of the process.
8. Do not hesitate to remove the process if:
   a. Technical difficulties prevent successful reconstruction.
   b. Bone quality (screw purchase) is poor and the nonunion site will not compress.

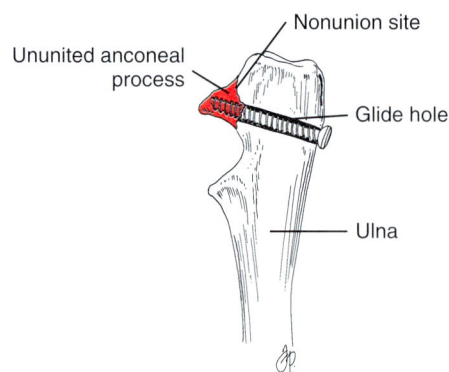

Figure 137–1. Place the lag screw in a caudo-cranial direction across the nonunion site and compress the nonunion. Placement in this direction facilitates removal at a later date and keeps metal out of the joint.

c. Joint congruency is disrupted by the repaired process.

9. Lavage the joint thoroughly and routinely close the muscle, fascia, and subcutaneous tissues (absorbable sutures, simple interrupted pattern), and skin.

10. If radioulnar growth disparity is suggested radiographically, a proximal diaphyseal ulnar osteotomy releases pressure on the anconeal process and may facilitate union.

Postoperative Care and Complications

Short-Term

- Apply a light, modified Robert Jones bandage from the digits to above the incision site and leave in place for 10–14 days to minimize swelling and seroma formation and to discourage excessive use of the limb.
- Remove sutures in 10–14 days.
- If the anconeal process has been removed, no further restriction is necessary.

Long-Term

- Confine the dog to house and leash walking only for 6–8 weeks.
- Obtain follow-up radiographs at 4 and 8 weeks to assess union of the process.
- Surgical nonunions require subsequent screw and anconeal process removal.
- Animals with union may experience low-grade lameness until the screw is removed.

Prognosis

- The prognosis is excellent if surgical reconstruction is successful.
- In animals with process removal, the prognosis is good to fair; most animals begin to show lameness related to osteoarthritis at 6–7 years of age.

Ununited Anconeal Process in Mature Dogs (>1 Year)

Diagnosis

- Obtain detailed preoperative radiographs of the elbow. Use the radiographic views and guidelines to assess the elbow listed previously under Ununited Anconeal Process in Immature Dogs. Determine whether the anconeal process is lodged in the olecranon fossa (and hence immobile) or whether the UAP is free-floating.
- In animals greater than 1 year of age, cartilage retention nests, delayed union, and nondisplaced nonunion are rare. Displaced nonunion is commonly seen. The UAP may be free-floating or lodged in the olecranon fossa. It is unlikely that a UAP lodged or ankylosed in the olecranon fossa is the cause of lameness.
- Differential diagnoses include:
  - Hyperextension/flexion injury resulting in fractured osteophytes and inflamed capsular tissue; signs include pain in the elbow with mild to moderate joint effusion.
  - Displaced nonunion; signs include pain in the elbow and mild joint effusion.
  - Septic arthritis; signs include pain in the elbow with varying degrees of effusion.
  - Immune-mediated joint disease (see Chap. 143).

OSTEOCHONDROSIS (OSTEOCHONDRITIS DISSECANS/FRAGMENTED CORONOID PROCESS) OF THE ELBOW

Anatomy and Pathophysiology

- OCD and FCP affect the medial joint compartment of the elbow; UAP affects the caudal joint compartment (Fig. 137–2). All three problems eventually lead to arthritic changes in all joint compartments.
- Joint congruency hinges on uniform growth of the humeral, radial, and ulnar bony components.
- A defect in endochondral ossification, uneven joint loading due to asymmetric growth of the radius and ulna, or both, can cause two problems:
  - Joint mice (FCP, OCD)
  - Incongruent joint surfaces
- In young dogs, the age at closure for growth plates around the elbow varies:
  - Anconeal process: 5–6 months
  - Proximal radius: 8–9 months
  - Olecranon: 8–9 months
  - Distal humeral condyles: 7–8 months
- The lateral aspect of the joint is relatively free of major neurovascular structures. The medial aspect of the elbow, however, is rich in major nerves (median and ulnar) and vascular structures (brachial artery and vein).

▼ **Key Point** Clinical diagnosis of OCD/FCP often is made before growth plate closure; therefore, avoid surgical approaches requiring osteotomies.

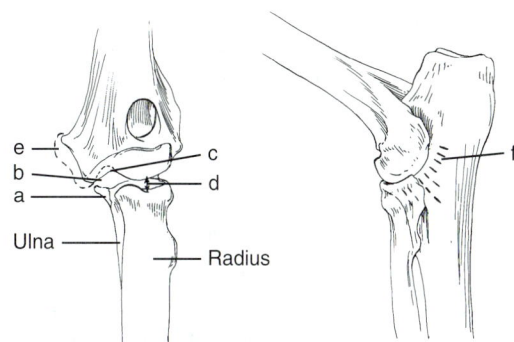

Figure 137–2. Anteroposterior *(left)* and lateral *(right)* views of the elbow demonstrate a fragmented coronoid process (FCP) fragment (a), osteochondritis dissecans (OCD) flap (b), OCD flap bed (or FCP kissing lesion) (c), increased humeroradial joint space (d), elongated medial humeral condyle (e), and increased radioulnar sclerosis (f) seen in dogs with OCD/FCP.

Osteochondritis Dissecans/Fragmented Coronoid Process in Immature Dogs (<1 Year)

Diagnosis

For accurate preoperative diagnosis, detailed preoperative radiographs are mandatory. Table 137–1 lists typical radiographic changes seen in OCD/FCP.

- Using the radiographic views and guidelines described previously (see Ununited Anconeal Process in Immature Dogs), perform the following evaluations:
  - Rule out panosteitis, UAP, and radioulnar growth disparities.
  - Assess the degree of arthritis present.
  - Attempt to differentiate FCP and OCD (Fig. 137–2).
- FCP and OCD can be difficult to differentiate radiographically in young dogs. Radiographic changes usually are not evident before the animal is 7–8 months old.
- Although it cannot differentiate OCD from FCP, nuclear scintigraphy has been useful to localize the source of obscure lameness to the medial compartment of the elbow joint.
- MRI or computed tomography, if available, may be the imaging modality of choice to diagnose FCP and detect cartilaginous defects preoperatively.
- Diagnosis also can be difficult because both conditions may occur concurrently. For example,
  - Osteophytes on the medial coronoid process may mimic FCP fragments.
  - A radiographically indistinct FCP may appear as a humeral condylar "kissing lesion" that mimics an OCD lesion.

Preoperative Considerations

▼ **Key Point** Often an accurate diagnosis of OCD or FCP is made only during surgery.

Table 137–1. RADIOGRAPHIC FINDINGS SEEN IN ANIMALS WITH OSTEOCHONDRITIS DISSECANS/FRAGMENTED CORONOID PROCESS

Findings Typical of FCP

Fragment in medial joint compartment (AP view)
Widened humeroradial joint space (AP view)

Findings Typical of OCD

Flap in medial humeral joint compartment (AP view)
"Divot" or flap bed in medial humeral condyle (AP view)
Flattened, elongated medial humeral condylar joint surface (AP view)

Findings Common to OCD and FCP

Fuzziness and periosteal proliferation on the dorsal anconeal process (flexed lateral view) and in the medial joint compartment (craniocaudal view)
Increased radioulnar interface sclerosis (lateral view)

OCD, osteochondritis dissecans; AP, anteroposterior; FCP, fragmented coronoid process.

- A similar surgical approach can be used for OCD and FCP.

Surgical Procedure

Objectives

- Remove the fragment and/or flap of the OCD/FCP lesion, while minimizing trauma to the young, growing joint.
- Curette the flap bed (or kissing lesion) to stimulate neochondrogenesis.

Equipment

- Same as for Ununited Anconeal Process in the Immature Dog

Technique

▼ **Key Point** There is no easy method for observation of all joint compartments using a single surgical approach.

1. Place the patient in lateral recumbency, with the affected limb down, suspended and prepared from the carpus to the axilla for aseptic surgery.
2. Make a medial approach to the elbow through the skin and deep antebrachial fascia. Separate the pronator teres from the flexor carpi radialis at their origins on the medial epicondyle, holding them apart with Gelpi retractors (Fig. 137–3).
3. Make a transverse cut in the joint capsule caudal and cranial to the collateral ligament. Carry this incision as far cranial as practical, taking care not to damage the median nerve or brachial vessels.

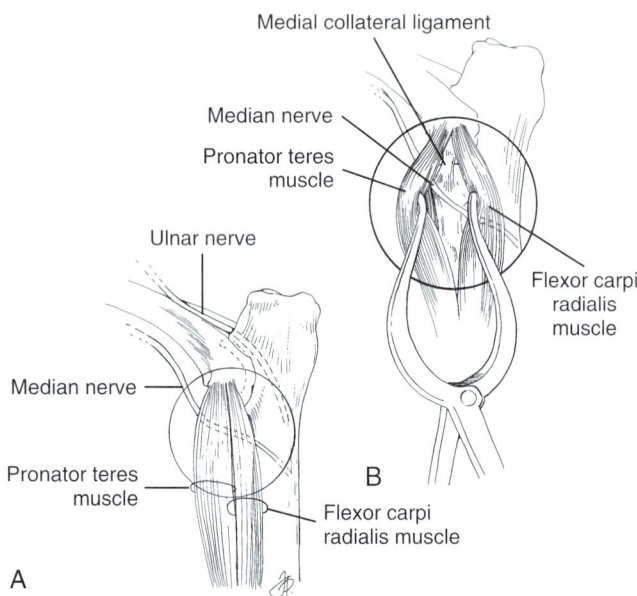

Figure 137–3. Medial approach to the elbow. *A*, Identify the pronator teres and flexor carpi radialis muscles and the median nerve. *B*, In separation of the flexor carpi radialis and pronator teres muscles with a Gelpi retractor, make a transverse cut in the joint capsule to expose the medial aspect of the elbow joint.

4. Using the edge of the table as a fulcrum and the antebrachium as a lever, open the medial joint compartment.
5. Locate the coronoid process and, if it is fragmented, remove it.
   a. FCP removal can usually be accomplished through a capsulotomy, with or without a partial desmotomy (division of the ligaments).
6. If present, remove the OCD flap.
   a. If further exposure is needed, a medial collateral desmotomy may be followed by a pronator teres tenotomy.
   b. OCD flap removal and curettage generally necessitate a complete desmotomy. Curette the OCD flap to healthy, bleeding bone so that a clot forms a base for neochondrogenesis.
7. Thoroughly lavage the joint with sterile saline solution.
8. Close the desmotomy and tenotomy with a locking loop or horizontal mattress suture pattern (2-0 polypropylene/nylon), followed by 2-0 polyglactin 910/polydioxanone closure of the capsule, and all other tissue planes.
9. Arthroscopic removal of of both OCD and FCP has been described. This may become the technique of choice as the equipment becomes more available.

Postoperative Care and Complications

- Apply a light, modified Robert Jones bandage from the digits to above the incision site and leave in place for 7 days (capsulotomy) to 14–21 days (desmotomy).
- Remove sutures in 10–14 days.
- Confine the dog to the house and restrict activity to leash walking for 4 weeks; allow access to the yard for the next 4 weeks before resumption of full activity.

Prognosis

- The degree of elbow incongruity, arthritis at the time of surgery, the size of the flap/fragment, and the surgical technique determine outcome.

▼ *Key Point* It is unrealistic to expect dogs with advanced arthritis and large lesions to benefit significantly from surgery.

Osteochondritis Dissecans/Fragmented Coronoid Process in Mature Dogs (>1 Year)

Anatomy

- See Osteochondritis Dissecans/Fragmented Coronoid Process in Immature Dogs.

Treatment

- Surgical procedures are generally not warranted in older animals for uncomplicated FCP/OCD lesions. In most animals with FCP/OCD that are greater than 1 year of age arthritic changes are too extensive to warrant surgical intervention.
- Differential diagnosis for acute lameness is similar to that for older animals with UAP, and includes hyperextension/flexion injury and septic arthritis.

- Diagnosis and treatment are similar to that described for Ununited Anconeal Process in Mature Dogs.
- Salvage procedures for dogs that have extensive arthritic changes and fail to respond to medical management include elbow arthrodesis or elbow arthroplasty.
- Medical management is discussed in Chapter 142.

OSTEOCHONDRITIS DISSECANS/FRAGMENTED CORONOID PROCESS/UNUNITED ANCONEAL PROCESS IN THE SAME ELBOW

Anatomy

See Ununited Anconeal Process and Osteochondrosis (OCD/FCP) of the Elbow.

Preoperative Considerations

- The diagnosis is based on detailed preoperative radiographs (as described previously).

▼ *Key Point* Multiple lesions in the elbow reduce the likelihood of surgical success.

Surgical Procedure

Objectives

- Remove or reconstruct the UAP.
- Address any concurrent disease in the medial elbow compartment (FCP/OCD).

Equipment

- Same as for Ununited Anconeal Process in The Immature Dog *plus*
- Osteotome/mallet or oscillating saw

Technique

1. In young dogs with open physes, make two separate approaches to the elbow:
   a. A lateral approach for the UAP.
   b. A medial approach to treat the FCP/OCD.

▼ *Key Point* Advantages of a dual surgical approach include minimal invasiveness; disadvantages include having to turn the animal and repeat preparation and draping of the limb for surgery.

2. If the physes around the elbow are closed, make an approach to the elbow using a proximal ulnar diaphyseal osteotomy (Fig. 137–4).
   a. Make a lateral approach to the elbow extending distally to the caudolateral surface of the ulna through the skin and superficial fascia.
   b. Following incision of the anconeus and lateral triceps muscles, reflect the extensor carpi ulnaris and abductor pollicis longus muscles laterally, while elevating the flexor carpi ulnaris and deep digital flexors from the medial aspect of the ulna, exposing the annular and interosseous ligaments.

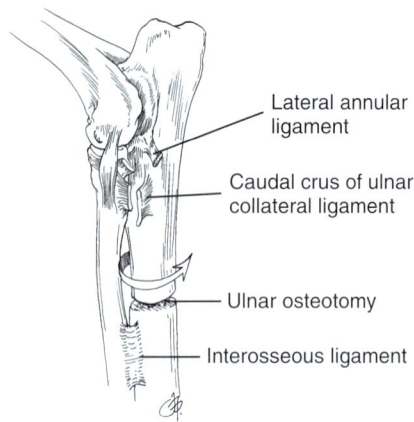

Figure 137-4. A proximal ulnar diaphyseal osteotomy allows observation of all compartments of the elbow in the mature dog.

   c. Perform a transverse osteotomy of the ulna below the level of the radial head, followed by transection of the lateral annular ligament, and caudal crus of the ulnar collateral ligament.

   d. Externally rotate the proximal ulna to allow exposure of the entire elbow joint.

3. Following correction of the UAP/FCP/OCD, thoroughly lavage the joint with sterile saline solution and realign the ulna.

4. Stabilize the ulnar osteotomy using two pins and a figure-eight tension band wire. Suture the annular ligament, and close all muscle and fascial planes in layers.

Postoperative Care and Complications

- Apply a light, modified Robert Jones bandage from the digits to above the incision site and leave in place for 10–14 days.
- Remove sutures in 10–14 days.
- Restrict activity to the house and leash walking only for 6–8 weeks.
- Obtain follow-up radiographs at 4 and 8 weeks to assess osteotomy healing.
- Ulnar nonunions most commonly result from the use of small pins or wires of inadequate strength.

Prognosis

- The greater the number of problems and the more radical the surgical technique, the more guarded is the prognosis.

OSTEOCHONDRITIS DISSECANS OF THE SHOULDER, STIFLE, AND HOCK

In dogs, OCD can occur not only in the elbow but also in the shoulder, stifle, and hock.

Anatomy

- See respective chapters on shoulder, stifle, and hock injuries (Chaps. 121, 129, and 131).

Pathophysiology

- A basic defect in endochondral ossification results in abnormal subchondral bone development and often results in formation of a cartilage flap in the overlying area.
- The size of the flap can be quite variable, and in some joints the flap has, as a component, some underlying bone (OCD tarsus). Thus, OCD results in two distinct joint abnormalities: a joint mouse and resultant joint incongruity. Neither problem can be "cured."
- Removal of the flap/fragment removes the source of irritation.
- Curettage of the flap bed results in neochondrogenesis, but the material properties of the resulting fibrocartilage are not equal to those of hyaline cartilage, and the new cartilage rarely grows to a height or density that reestablishes full joint congruency (particularly in the hock).
- In a complex joint such as the elbow, the existence of a flap/concave bed may inhibit or modify normal development of impinging structures (opposing joint surfaces). Hence, while surgery can remove the joint mouse and stimulate some neochondrogenesis, it cannot fully resolve the residual joint incongruity.
- Removal of the joint mouse may significantly slow down *but not completely arrest* arthritic progression. This has been demonstrated clinically and experimentally in the shoulder of the dog.

Preoperative Considerations

- As the size of the flap/fragment increases in relation to joint surface area, the residual joint incongruity following fragment removal similarly increases. Hence, a small OCD lesion has less impact on a simple, large surface area joint (shoulder) than on a smaller (tarsus) or more complex joint (stifle, elbow).
- Clinically, dogs with OCD of the hock seem to fare equally well with or without surgery; this may be related to the small joint/large fragment ratio.
- Surgical intervention typically helps but does not entirely alleviate clinical symptoms in dogs with OCD of the stifle and elbow (complex joints, variably sized fragments). Optimal results can be expected in a large joint with a small lesion; suboptimal results in a complex, small joint with a large lesion.
- The degree of osteoarthritis present at the time of diagnosis is important. As the degree of arthritis progresses, the benefits of surgical intervention diminish.
- Ideal surgical candidates are young dogs with small flaps/fragments and no arthritis.
- Old (and young) dogs with severe arthritis and large fragments/flaps are unlikely to benefit from surgical intervention.

Surgical Procedures

- Surgical objectives are similar to those described for OCD of the elbow.
- See respective chapters on shoulder, stifle, and hock injuries for description of surgical approaches (Chaps. 121, 129, and 131).

Postoperative Care and Complications

- See respective chapters on shoulder, stifle, and hock injuries.
- Also see postoperative care for OCD of the elbow.

Prevention

Prevention should be aimed at not breeding affected individuals or their parents. Owners of large, rapidly growing breeds should be warned to avoid overfeeding, calcium supplementation, and excessive rough play.

SUPPLEMENTAL READINGS

Lenehan TM, Nunamaker DM: Lateral approach to the canine elbow by proximal ulnar diaphyseal osteotomy. J Am Vet Med Assoc 180:523, 1982.

Lenehan TM, van Sickle DC: Ununited anconeal process, ununited medial coronoid process, ununited medial epicondyle, patella cubiti, and sesamoidal fragments of the elbow. *In* Newton CD, Nunamaker DM, eds.: Textbook of Small Animal Orthopaedics. Philadelphia: JB Lippincott, 1985, p 999.

Probst CW, Flo G, McLaughlin M, DeCamp C: A simple medial approach to the canine elbow for treatment of fragmented coronoid process and osteochondritis dissecans. J Am Anim Hosp Assoc 25:331, 1989.

138 Pediatric Fractures

Paul A. Manley

The majority of fractures in immature animals involve the metaphyseal area of the long bones. The metaphyseal area is the site of the growth plate, which is weaker than the surrounding bones and supporting ligaments. Occasionally, the diaphysis of the long bones is fractured in immature animals. Principles for management of these diaphyseal fractures are the same as for adult animals.

ANATOMY

Metaphyseal Growth Plate (Physis)

- The metaphyseal growth plate (MGP) (also called the physis) separates the epiphysis from the metaphysis and is the major site of longitudinal bone growth.
- The MGP has a cartilage component composed of developmental zones, a bony component composed of trabecular bone, and a fibrous component composed of fibroblasts, fiber bundles and connective tissue.
- Blood supply to the metaphysis and epiphysis is separated by the MGP until closure of the growth plate occurs. The epiphyseal vessels supply the germinal cells; the metaphyseal vessels supply the metaphyseal side of the MGP.
- The zones of the MGP, from superficial to deep, are reserve, proliferative, hypertrophic, ossification, and metaphyseal.
  - The *reserve zone* contains several layers of randomly arranged chondrocytes. These chondrocytes function to store nutrients.
  - The *proliferative zone* is the growth zone of the MGP. The chondrocytes divide and form palisades of cells at right angles to the long axis of the bone. Longitudinal growth occurs as a result of active cell division and matrix production by these chondrocytes.
  - The chondrocytes enlarge in the *hypertrophic zone* by storing calcium and increasing their fluid intake. It is more appropriate to refer to this area as the zone of cellular swelling, because the cells swell rather than hypertrophy. As the cells enlarge, the matrix is squeezed into longitudinal septae. Near the bottom or deep portion of this zone, the cells begin to degrade and deposit calcium in the matrix.
  - Vessels from the metaphyseal capillaries invade the deep portion of the hypertrophic zone and result

in mineralization of the matrix. This results in the formation of primary and secondary spongiosa in the *ossification zone.*
  - The *metaphyseal zone* is characterized by remodeling of the primary and secondary spongiosa.
- Although most of the longitudinal growth of long bones comes from the MGP, the epiphysis of immature animals has an epiphyseal growth plate that gives rise to some increase in bone length.

Classification of Injuries

▼ *Key Point* Physeal fractures usually occur through the hypertrophic zone of the physis, because the cells are large and there is very little supporting matrix.

- Many fractures in the immature animal involve the metaphyseal growth plate. These fractures have been classified into five types by Salter and Harris (Fig. 138–1):
  - Type I is a separation of the epiphysis from the metaphysis through the hypertrophic zone of the physis.
  - Type II is a fracture through the hypertrophic zone with fracture of a portion of the metaphysis.
  - Type III is a fracture that extends from the joint surface to the metaphyseal growth plate and along the metaphyseal growth plate to the periphery.
  - Type IV is a fracture that extends from the joint surface through the metaphyseal growth plate and through a portion of the metaphysis.
  - Type V is a crushing injury to some or all of the MGP. In this injury there is a high incidence of premature physeal closure because the germinal cells of the physis are injured by direct trauma.

PREOPERATIVE CONSIDERATIONS

Tissue Handling

- The bone of immature animals is very soft and can be fractured easily during reduction attempts.
- In fractures of the MGP, the germinal cells are usually with the epiphyseal fragment; be especially careful when manipulating this segment of bone.
- Early treatment of the fracture usually facilitates easy reduction.

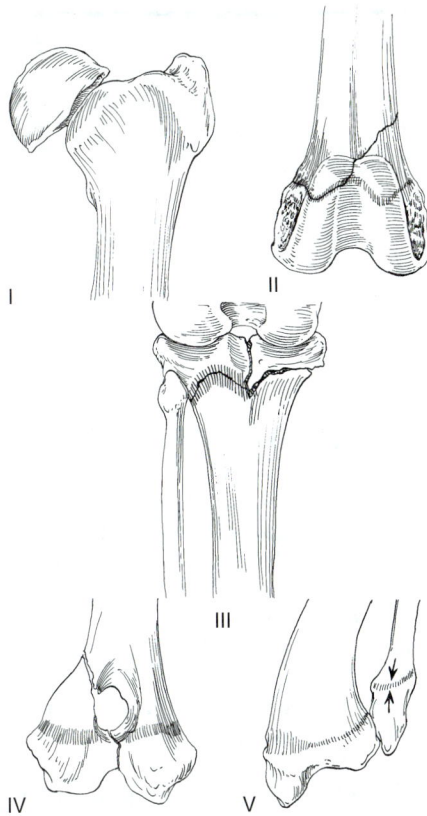

Figure 138–1. Five different types of growth plate fractures. See text for explanation.

Growth Potential

- The prognosis depends on the type of injury, location of the fracture, type of repair, and growth potential remaining in the MGP at the time of injury.
- Premature physeal closure of a single bone may result in limb shortening or an angular limb deformity if only a portion of the physis is affected.
- Premature physeal closure of one of a pair of bones (e.g., radius and ulna; see Chap. 124) may result in angular limb deformity and joint subluxation.

SURGICAL PROCEDURES

General Considerations

- If the fracture is <48 hours old, and is a type I or II growth plate fracture, it may be possible to reduce closed and stabilize with external coaptation.

- If internal fixation is necessary in a growth plate fracture, the method chosen should provide adequate stabilization and minimize further damage to the physis.
- Regardless of the type of growth plate fracture, the method of internal fixation should not span the MGP if there is growth potential left.
- Single or paired pins or Kirschner wires are the implants of choice for fractures involving the MGP.
- Pins, cerclage wires, external fixators, plates, and screws are appropriate methods of internal fixation for diaphyseal fractures in immature animals. (See appropriate chapters for details on surgical management of specific diaphyseal fractures).

POSTOPERATIVE CARE AND COMPLICATIONS

- Obtain follow-up radiographs at 2–3 week intervals for signs of premature growth arrest.
- Remove implants that cross the growth plate in 2–3 weeks to decrease their effects on potential growth.
- Loss of bone length may result in altered gait; however, most animals have the ability to compensate fairly well unless >25% of the bone length is lost.
- Premature closure of the physis of one of a pair of bones (e.g., radius and ulna) usually results in significant angular deformity and joint incongruity. Single or multiple osteotomies may be necessary to correct the deformities.
- It may be necessary to perform multiple osteotomies in young animals to allow for continuous growth.

SUPPLEMENTAL READINGS

Brinker WO, Piermattei DL, Flo GL: Handbook of Small Animal Orthopedics and Fracture Treatment, 2nd Ed. Philadelphia: WB Saunders, 1990.

Manley PA, Henry WB, Wilson JW: Diseases of the epiphysis. *In* Whittick WG, ed.: Canine Orthopedics, 2nd Ed. Philadelphia: Lea & Febiger, 1990.

Rang ME: The Growth Plate and Its Disorders. Edinburgh: Livingstone, 1969.

Salter RB, Harris WR: Injuries involving the epiphyseal plate. J Bone Joint Surg 45A:487, 1963.

139 Open Fractures

Charles E. DeCamp

An open fracture is one that has been exposed to the environment and contaminated by or infected with bacteria. The soft tissue injury that accompanies an open fracture may be a simple puncture wound or a complex injury with vascular compromise and tissue necrosis. Successful management of open fractures depends on proper treatment of soft tissue wounds and fracture fixation. If soft tissue wounds are properly managed, the morbidity of wound infection is reduced and fracture healing can proceed at a normal rate.

CLASSIFICATION OF OPEN FRACTURES

Open fractures are classified as type I, II, or III, based on the mechanism and severity of soft tissue injury (Fig. 139–1). The purpose of classification is to determine the likelihood of serious infection. The type of wound management and the choice of fracture fixation partly depend on the classification.

- Type I develops when a fracture fragment penetrates the skin, exposing the fracture to bacterial contamination. Soft tissue injury is minor, and wound infection is unlikely with proper care.
- Type II develops when an external object forcefully penetrates the skin and soft tissues, creating a fracture and contaminating the wound. Fracture severity is highly variable, but soft tissue injury is relatively minimal and usually is not complicated by vascular compromise and tissue necrosis. Bacterial contamination generally is more extensive than for type I injuries.
- Type III develops when an external object forcefully penetrates the skin and soft tissues, creating a fracture, contaminating the wound, and severely damaging the soft tissues. The ability of the body to combat soft tissue infection commonly is complicated by vascular compromise and necrosis. The risk of bacterial infection is very high.

▼ *Key Point* Type I open fractures are least likely to develop wound infections; type III open fractures almost always have some level of infection.

- In all fracture types, if the wound has been neglected and infection develops, manage the injury as though it were a type III injury.

PREOPERATIVE CONSIDERATIONS

- The diagnosis of an open fracture may be made by direct inspection, palpation, and radiography.
- If skin penetration, laceration, or avulsion is present, assume that the fracture is open and contaminated until proven otherwise.
- Cover all open wounds with a sterile dressing.
- Obtain radiographs after dressing placement.
  - Radiographic signs of air within the soft tissues adjacent to a fracture is diagnostic of an open fracture.
- Use aseptic technique when manipulating the wound.

▼ *Key Point* Violating the rules of strict asepsis during early wound management increases the probability of nosocomial infection.

- If preparation of the wound cannot proceed immediately, use external coaptation for temporary stabilization of the fracture. Apply a reinforced Robert Jones bandage for injuries below the stifle or elbow. Use a spica splint for open fractures of the femur or humerus.
- To prepare the wound, remove the sterile bandage and carefully clip surrounding hair to avoid contamination. If necessary, cover the wound with sterile gauze sponges moistened with sterile saline to prevent introduction of the clipped hair into the wound.
- Lavage the wound with copious amounts of sterile saline or lactated Ringer's solution to wash small particulate matter from the wound interstices (see Chap. 52).
- Betadine and alcohol may be used on the skin surrounding the wound; however, avoid contact of detergents or alcohol with the open wound.
- Remove a sample of fluid from the fracture site for laboratory tests, using a swab if the size and type of wound permit its introduction. Base definitive antibiotic treatment on culture and sensitivity tests. A Gram stain may reveal the organism type and aid in the initial choice of antibiotics.
- Consider giving broad-spectrum systemic antibiotics.

▼ *Key Point* Systemic antibiotics are less important than proper wound care for prevention and treatment of wound infection.

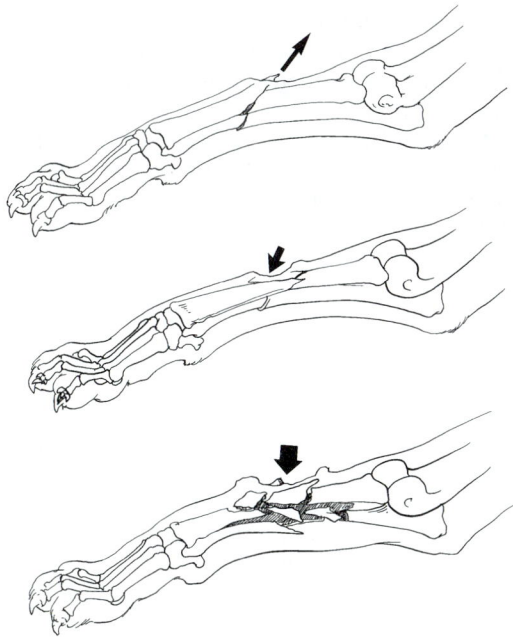

Figure 139–1. Types of open fractures. Type I *(top):* fracture fragment penetrates skin. Type II *(center):* penetrating object causes minor injury to soft tissue. Type III *(bottom):* penetrating object causes extensive damage to soft tissue.

SURGICAL DEBRIDEMENT, FRACTURE FIXATION, AND SOFT TISSUE RECONSTRUCTION

Objectives

- Improve wound environment to reduce the risk of infection.
- Reconstruct soft tissue to cover bone and provide limb function. It may be necessary to defer this aspect if a large tissue defect or necrosis is present.
- Provide temporary or definitive fracture fixation.

Equipment

- Two standard general orthopedic packs and suture material
- Bone curette and brush
- Scalpel blades
- Sterile saline or lactated Ringer's solution
- Fracture fixation equipment:
  - Materials for external coaptation
  - External skeletal fixation pins and clamps
  - Power drills
  - Bone plating equipment

Surgical Debridement

Technique

Type I Open Fracture

1. Little or no surgical debridement is required.
2. If the bone is not visibly exposed and the wound is small, copiously lavage the wound with sterile lactated Ringer's solution.

3. Sharply excise necrotic tissue, if present, from the wound before fracture fixation.

Type II Open Fracture

1. Surgical debridement generally is not extensive; however, be careful to remove all nonviable tissue.
2. Copiously lavage the wound with sterile lactated Ringer's solution before fracture fixation.

Technique

Type III Open Fracture (Extensive Debridement and Lavage)

1. Prepare the limb and wound for aseptic surgery. If a surgical approach to a bone is anticipated, extend the skin preparation to the appropriate anatomic field.
2. Drape the limb using standard aseptic technique, using water-impermeable drapes.
3. Sharply excise necrotic skin, fat, fascia, and muscle from the wound.
4. Remove any loose, dirty, small fragments of bone.
5. To preserve the blood supply and prevent development of bone sequestra, maintain tissue attachments to bone fragments.

▼ *Key Point* Clean *large,* attached bone fragments with a bone curette or brush if necessary. *Do not remove them.*

6. Clean, but do not debride, tendons, ligaments, intact blood vessels, and nerves unless they are necrotic.
7. If necessary, extend access to the bone by a surgical approach for fracture fixation. If severe contamination or infection is present, apply external skeletal fixation with minimal or no surgical approach (see Chap. 130).

Fracture Fixation

- Do not carry out fracture fixation until initial wound management is complete (as described previously).
- If the fracture is stable and nonarticular and involves a bone distal to the stifle or elbow joint, external coaptation may be effective. Most other fractures require surgically applied orthopedic fixation.

Technique

1. If a surgical approach is made, obtain samples of fluid from the fracture site and submit for culture and sensitivity.

▼ *Key Point* To avoid bacterial contamination from debrided tissues, use a new, sterile pack for the surgical approach and fracture fixation.

2. *Type I open fractures*—Repair with the appropriate method of external or internal fixation.
   a. If a surgical approach is made to the bone, avoid contact with the traumatic wound to prevent bacterial contamination. Skin drapes may be used.

b. After fracture fixation, close the wound routinely. Penrose drains or delayed wound closure techniques usually are not necessary.

3. *Type II open fractures*—Repair with the appropriate method of external or internal fixation.

a. If a surgical approach is made to the bone, avoid contact with the traumatic wound. Skin drapes may be used.

b. Because bacterial contamination of the wound can be more severe than for type I fractures, provide proper drainage of exudates.

c. If the surgical wound is closed, place Penrose drains to exit the wound at a site ventral to the surgical incision.

d. If bacterial contamination is severe, perform delayed or partial wound closure to ensure proper drainage (see Chaps. 51 and 52).

▼ *Key Point* Treatment of most type III open fractures proceed in the following order: wound care, fracture fixation, and skin reconstruction.

4. *Type III open fractures*—Carefully choose a method that reduces the risk and severity of wound infection.

a. In general, do not use metallic implants at the fracture site unless adequate wound drainage is assured. Intramedullary pins are not recommended because of the difficulty in providing surgical drainage from the medullary canal.

b. Bone plates may be used in conjunction with delayed or secondary wound closure techniques, unless severe infection is present.

c. External skeletal fixation (see Chap. 130) is recommended because a fixator may be constructed that avoids placement of metallic implants directly in the fracture site. However, anatomic considerations may contraindicate their use.

▼ *Key Point* Regardless of the type of orthopedic implant, rigid fixation is mandatory for definitive treatment of the fracture.

d. If an external fixator cannot be used, type I external fixator, transarticular external fixator, or external coaptation may be used as temporary fixation so that local wound care and resolution of infection may proceed. When the wound environment has improved, other methods of internal fixation such as bone plates and lag screws may be applied with less risk of infection.

RECONSTRUCTIVE SOFT TISSUE SURGERY

- Primary, delayed primary, or secondary closure techniques (see Chaps. 51 and 52) may be used to treat traumatic wounds in open fractures.
- Wounds may be allowed to heal by second intention.
- Some wounds may not heal because of their large size, or because they are located at a site of active motion or pressure point (e.g., elbow). In these cases, reconstruct the skin wound with a skin flap or graft (see Chap. 53).

- Skin flaps or grafts may be constructed at the time of fracture fixation but often are delayed until a healthy bed of granulation tissue indicates that wound infection is resolved.
- If arthrodesis is the primary method of orthopedic fixation for the carpus or tarsus, perform skin reconstruction 1 month before arthrodesis. This allows full resolution of soft tissue infection and good soft tissue cover over the proposed arthrodesis site.

Postoperative Care

- Proper postoperative wound care is mandatory to prevent and control infection.
- Keep open wounds bandaged, and replace the bandage daily to prevent accumulation of exudates at the wound site.
- Lavage open wounds daily with sterile saline or lactated Ringer's solution, until healthy granulation tissue indicates resolution of infection.
- Restrict activity, depending on the fracture type and method of fixation.
- Use an Elizabethan collar, if necessary, to prevent the animal from licking its wounds or removing the bandages.
- Stage implant removal to provide optimal bone healing and minimize risk of long-term wound or bone infection.
- Perform a physical examination and obtain radiographs at appropriate intervals to evaluate proper bone healing and resolution of infection.

Complications

- Continued infection suggests the presence of necrotic soft tissue or bone, an unstable fracture site, or unstable orthopedic implants.
- Delayed healing of a fracture may develop from prolonged infection at the fracture site, poor reduction, unstable fixation, or bone loss due to trauma or infection.

▼ *Key Point* Most complications can be avoided with proper wound management, orthopedic fixation, and postoperative care. Serial examinations to assess progress are essential to avoid development of major problems.

SUPPLEMENTAL READINGS

Brinker WO, Piermattei DL, Flo GL: Handbook of Small Animal Orthopedics and Fracture Treatment. Philadelphia: WB Saunders, 1990, p 50.

Dueland RT: Open (compound) fractures. *In* Brinker WO, Hohn RB, Prieur WD, eds.: Manual of Internal Fixation in Small Animals. Berlin: Springer-Verlag, 1984, p 108.

Nunamaker DM: Open fractures and gunshot injuries. *In* Newton CD, Nunamaker DM, eds.: Textbook of Small Animal Orthopaedics. Philadelphia: JB Lippincott, 1985, p 481.

Richardson DC: Fracture first aid: The open (compound) fracture. *In* Slatter DH, ed.: Textbook of Small Animal Surgery. Philadelphia: WB Saunders, 1985, p 1945.

140 Osteomyelitis

Kenneth A. Johnson

Osteomyelitis implies inflammation of bone and the soft tissue elements of marrow, endosteum, periosteum, and vascular channels. It is caused most often by infectious organisms. Bacterial osteomyelitis is classified as:

- Acute, with systemic illness and no radiographic alteration in the bone in the first 5–10 days *or*
- Chronic, with radiographic signs of progressive destruction and proliferative osseous change that become evident after 10–20 days.

Traditionally, osteomyelitis has been considered to have a poor prognosis; however, with improved understanding of pathophysiology and proper surgical treatment, it is sometimes curable. Osteomyelitis can mimic panosteitis (see Chap. 136), hypertrophic osteodystrophy (see Chap. 136), and neoplasia (see Chap. 135), complicate a fracture; or cause nonunion (see Chap. 141). It must be differentiated from these diseases.

ETIOLOGY

Bacteria

- Bacterial infections are acquired by direct inoculation, by extension of existing infection, or hematogenously (Table 140–1).

▼ *Key Point* Although the type, virulence, and quantity of bacteria are important, bacteria alone will not necessarily cause osteomyelitis. Initiating factors include altered blood flow, soft tissue injury, impaired host tissue defenses, bone necrosis, fracture instability, foreign material, and radiation necrosis of bone (Fig. 140–1).

- Infections with β-lactamase-producing *Staphylococcus* organisms predominate. Other organisms include *Streptococcus* spp., *Brucella canis*, gram-negative bacteria (*Escherichia coli*, *Proteus* spp., *Klebsiella*), and anaerobic bacteria (*Bacteroides* spp., *Actinomyces viscosus*, *Clostridium* spp.).
- Bacteria colonize the surface of implants and sequestra, producing a coating of mucopolysaccharide called glycocalyx. Glycocalyx prevents resolution of chronic osteomyelitis by protecting bacteria from the actions of phagocytes, antibiotics, and antibodies.

Fungi

- Fungal infections often are multicentric and disseminate hematogenously after pulmonary inoculation (see Chap. 18). Most infections involve the metaphyses, flat bones, vertebral bodies, and discs.
- *Coccidioides immitis*, *Blastomyces dermatitidis*, *Histoplasma capsulatum*, *Cryptococcus neoformans*, and *Aspergillus* spp. can cause fungal osteomyelitis.

Corrosion of Implants

- Corrosion occurs in implants composed of dissimilar metals, such as spring-loaded intramedullary Jonas pins and vitallium plates with stainless steel screws. A sterile inflammatory response occurs, with localized bone lysis and a draining tract. Secondary bacterial infection subsequently develops.

CLINICAL SIGNS

- Osteomyelitic lesions invariably are painful and cause lameness, disuse atrophy, and occasional neurologic deficits. Bone fractures may contribute to these signs.
- Excessive pain, inflammation, or exudation may be the first sign of acute osteomyelitis in the first week following orthopedic surgery or trauma.
- In chronic osteomyelitis, single or multiple sinus tracts intermittently open and drain mucopurulent exudate.
- Other nonspecific signs include anorexia, lethargy, and depression.

DIAGNOSIS

▼ *Key Point* The diagnosis of osteomyelitis usually is based on history, radiology, or microbiology findings or a combination of these.

History

- Osteomyelitis may be preceded by trauma, open fracture, orthopedic surgery, or travel in an endemic fungal region.

Physical Examination

- Palpate the musculoskeletal system to localize the involved bone(s).

Table 140–1. ROUTES OF INFECTION IN OSTEOMYELITIS

Open reduction and internal fixation of fractures; other orthopedic intervention
Open fractures
Extension from soft tissue infection (periodontal disease, rhinitis, otitis media)
Traumatic injuries and bite wounds
Penetrating foreign bodies including sticks and grass awns
Gunshot injury
Hematogenous
Prosthetic joint replacement surgery

- Heat, swelling, redness, and tenderness are present in the acute phase.
- Muscle atrophy, fibrosis, and contracture are features of chronic disease. Enlarged regional lymph nodes may be palpable.
- Limb angulation, shortening, instability, and crepitus can be present when fracture or nonunion (see Chap. 141) coexists with osteomyelitis.
- Perform a neurologic examination (see Chap. 144) to identify concomitant involvement of spinal cord or peripheral nerves.
- Sinus tracts follow fascial planes and emerge distal or dependent to chronically infected bone (see Fig. 140–1). Yellow-brown mucopurulent exudate drains intermittently. Inactive tracts are closed by scar tissue.

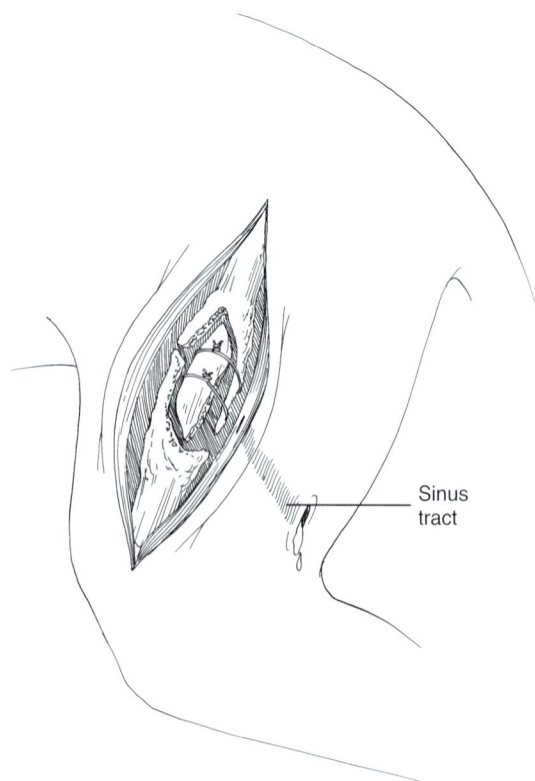

Sinus tract

Figure 140–1. Chronic osteomyelitis with sequestrum, loose unstable implants, and involucrum walling off the focus of infection. These conditions favor chronic bacterial infection, and purulent exudate drains through a dependent sinus.

- Scarring of the skin and underlying tissues is evidence of previous incisions, drainage, open fracture, trauma, foreign body penetration, fracture surgery, or bone fixation by intramedullary pins or external fixators.
- Thoracic auscultation and radiography are essential if pulmonary involvement is a possibility.

Hematology

- Results may be consistent with systemic infection (neutrophilic leukocytosis) in acute osteomyelitis but usually are unremarkable in patients with chronic osteomyelitis.

Radiography and Radionuclide Imaging

Radiography is an important means of evaluating the extent of osteomyelitis, sequestra (dead, avascular bone that has become separated from the viable bone), involucrum (bony proliferation around a sequestrum), and concomitant fracture.

Survey Radiography

- In acute osteomyelitis, only soft tissue swelling is seen initially.
- Depending on age of the animal, bone resorption, sclerosis, and periosteal new bone are seen after 5–10 days.
- Bone sequestra are diagnostic of chronic osteomyelitis.
- Fracture nonunion due to instability (see Chap. 141) can be difficult to distinguish from nonunion due to infection.
- Fungal osteomyelitis lesions tend to affect the metaphyses and may be multiple, with a lytic, proliferative, or mixed appearance.
- Deep postoperative wound infections are indistinguishable from acute osteomyelitis because there are minimal radiographic changes.

Contrast Radiography

- This modality is useful in some animals for delineation of the course and extent of sinuses and radiolucent foreign bodies.
- Perform a sinogram (or fistulogram) with water-soluble contrast media (e.g., Urografin 76%) injected slowly through a Foley catheter inserted in the sinus. Inflate the balloon to prevent leakage.

Radionuclide Imaging

- Imaging of the bone after indium-111 labeling of leukocytes is the most sensitive and specific noninvasive means of detecting osteomyelitis; however, it rarely is needed in routine cases. Specialized equipment is necessary.

Laboratory Evaluation

Cytology

- Use sterile aspiration to detect and drain fluid accumulations.

- Stain smears of fluid with Diff-Quik (Dade AG, Düdingen, Germany) to look for toxic neutrophils, phagocytized bacteria, and fungal organisms.

Bacteriology

▼ *Key Point* Results of tests of cultures from externally draining tracts are an inaccurate representation of causative organisms, as these tracts are often colonized by skin organisms.

- Obtain aerobic and anaerobic cultures of fluid collected by sterile aspiration from deep within the wound or, preferably, from samples of fluid, necrotic tissue, and sequestra collected at the time of surgical debridement.

Histopathology

- Histopathologic examination of tissue and bone biopsies is essential if neoplasia (see Chap. 135) is suspected.
- Analysis of methenamine silver and periodic acid–Schiff stained tissue sections can demonstrate fungal hyphae.

TREATMENT

Plan the treatment regimen according to the etiology, chronicity, location, and severity of the osteomyelitis lesion. The majority of osteomyelitis cases are bacterial in origin and chronic. Acute osteomyelitis is diagnosed much less frequently. However, treat soft tissue infections associated with open fractures, trauma, bites, and surgery as if acute osteomyelitis exists, because delays in appropriate treatment invariably lead to chronic osteomyelitis. Manage fungal osteomyelitis as a part of the overall systemic mycotic disease (see Chap. 18).

Surgical Procedures

Objectives

- Identify pathogenic organisms.
- Determine antibiotic sensitivity.
- Drain infected tissue.
- Remove avascular bone (sequestrectomy).
- Stabilize the fracture.
- Implant a bone graft to aid osseous union of fractures.

Equipment

- Standard surgical pack and suture material
- Volkmann curette
- Gelpi or Volkmann retractors
- Silver probe
- Fracture instruments (external fixator or plate and screws)
- Bone graft collection instruments

Acute Osteomyelitis

The major objectives of surgery are to debride infected tissue, provide drainage, and stabilize fractures.

Preoperative Considerations

- Begin antibiotic therapy after collection of samples for microbiology. The initial choice of antibiotic is empiric.
  - Administer cloxacillin (30 mg/kg q6h PO) or amoxicillin-clavulanate (20 mg/kg q8h PO) for suspected β-lactamase-producing *Staphylococcus* infections.
  - Give metronidazole (15 mg/kg q12h PO) for suspected anaerobic infections.
  - Give ciprofloxacin (5–11 mg/kg q12h PO) for suspected gram-negative infection.

▼ *Key Point* The ultimate choice of an antibiotic depends on results of microbiologic tests.

Technique

1. Aseptically prepare the region for surgery and cover with water-impervious drapes.
2. Expose focal osteomyelitic lesions by removal of overlying normal cortical bone with a drill or Volkmann curette, to allow drainage.
3. Open infected surgical wounds extensively by removal of sutures. Debride necrotic muscle, fascia, hematoma, foreign material, and nonfunctional sutures. Collect samples for microbiologic tests.
4. Open and drain traumatic wounds (e.g., bites) with a surgical incision that allows dependent drainage.
5. Keep wounds open to permit adequate drainage and irrigation.
6. Cover exposed bone with viable muscle.
7. Metallic implants can be left exposed, but cover the wound with a sterile dressing.

▼ *Key Point* Closed suction drainage systems and Penrose drains are contraindicated because they provide ineffective drainage and potentiate ascending infections and abscesses.

8. If the fracture fixation is stable, treat osteomyelitis without removal of the implants, until healing or loosening of implants occurs.

▼ *Key Point* Bone can heal in the presence of infection, provided there is stable fixation.

9. Loose implants lead to the triad of fracture instability, persistence of infection, and bone resorption (Fig. 140–2). Remove loose implants immediately, and stabilize the fracture with another device.
10. External skeletal fixation is the preferred method for providing both temporary and definitive fracture stability in the tibia, mandible, and radius-ulna, where active osteomyelitis exists.
    a. The large muscle groups surrounding the femur and humerus allow application of only type I or biplanar (pins placed laterally and cranially) external fixation. These configurations may not provide sufficient stability for healing, owing to excessive pin-bone stress, soft tissue necrosis around pins, pin tract osteomyelitis, and premature pin loosening.

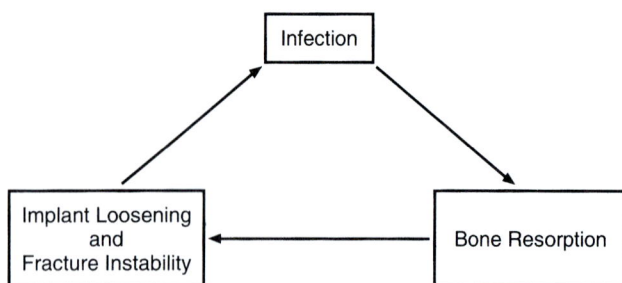

Figure 140–2. The unhappy triad of osteomyelitis.

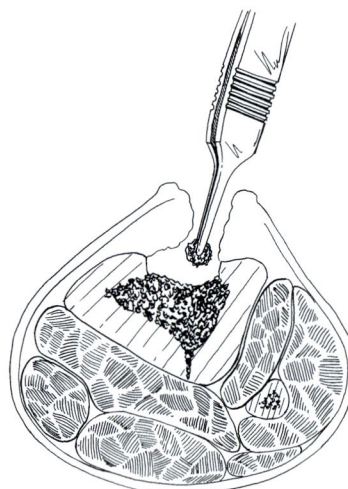

Figure 140–3. Autologous cancellous bone grafting of fractures and bone deficits in chronic osteomyelitis after the infection is controlled and healthy granulation tissue fills the wound. Insert the graft by elevation of granulation tissue or via a separate approach through normal tissues.

   b. Use plates if external skeletal fixation is inappropriate or secondarily after the infection becomes quiescent, and when an external fixator is no longer effective.

11. Irrigate wounds intraoperatively with 1–2 L of sterile physiologic saline, under pressure with a 60-ml syringe or suction-lavage unit.

Postoperative Care and Complications

- Pack dressings of sterile, dry gauze or paraffin-impregnated gauze into the wound. Cover this with a layer of cast-padding and conforming cotton bandage and adhesive elastic bandage.
- Protect incisions on the trunk or upper limbs with a tie-over bandage (extend over the dorsum of the animal).
- Elizabethan collars provide further wound protection until healing is complete.
- Repeat daily irrigation, using sterile technique, until infection is controlled.
- After 3–5 days, wound closure with granulation tissue begins to occur. Reopen the wound if drainage and irrigation are not possible.
- Select antibiotics on the basis of bacteriologic findings, and administer for 4–6 weeks.
- Obtain radiographs at intervals of 7–14 days to evaluate fracture fixation and healing, and progress of osteomyelitis.

Chronic Osteomyelitis

Preoperative Considerations

Assess soft tissue in regard to vascularity, peripheral nerve injury, muscle contracture, joint stiffness, and pain to determine if a cure is feasible or if amputation is indicated. In animals with phalangeal osteomyelitis, immediate digit amputation (see Chap. 133) is an acceptable treatment.

Technique

1. Expose the infected bone, using an appropriate approach, to remove sequestra and debride necrotic tissue and bone.

▼ *Key Point* Careful search for and removal of sequestra is crucial for success of surgical treatment of chronic osteomyelitis.

   a. Sequestra may migrate and become trapped in a draining sinus some distance from the original infection.

   b. Elevate extensive involucrum with a chisel or rongeurs to reach sequestra and establish drainage.

2. To prevent a pathologic fracture, support bone weakened by extensive debridement with external skeletal fixation (see Chap. 130) or a splint.

3. Chronic osteomyelitis may be a sequela of unstable internal fixation of fractures. Stabilize these fractures to allow healing (see Acute Osteomyelitis).

4. Remove implants composed of dissimilar metals that are responsible for corrosion and osteomyelitis. Provide alternative stable fixation if the fracture is ununited.

5. Keep wounds open and irrigate with sterile saline solution (see Acute Osteomyelitis).

6. After 7–10 days, graft bone defects caused by debridement, osteomyelitis, or fracture with autologous cancellous bone, when granulation tissue permits rapid vascularization and incorporation of the graft (Fig. 140–3). Cancellous bone grafts are not at risk for sequestration.

Postoperative Care and Complications

- Select antibiotics on the basis of the bacteriology and administer for 4–6 weeks.

▼ *Key Point* It is useless to proceed with treatment of chronic osteomyelitis with antibiotics, unless microbiologic culturing, surgical drainage, sequestrectomy, and fracture stabilization are meticulously performed.

- Obtain radiographs at intervals of 7–21 days to assess progression of healing and resolution of infection.

- If there is lack of response to treatment or recurrence of osteomyelitis, one or more of the following may be necessary:
  - Reexamine for sequestra.
  - Repeat debridement.
  - Reestablish drainage.
  - Reevaluate fracture stability.
  - Perform a bone graft.
  - Repeat microbiology tests.
  - Change the type of antibiotic.
- Use skin grafts (see Chap. 53) or myocutaneous flaps to cover extensive open wounds on the distal limbs that fail to close by second intention healing.
- Implant removal is necessary after healing of fractures.

SUPPLEMENTAL READINGS

Brinker WO, Olmstead ML, Sumner-Smith G, Prieur WD: Manual of Internal Fixation in Small Animals, 2nd ed. Berlin: Springer-Verlag, 1998, p 115.

Johnson KA: Osteomyelitis. *In* Olmstead ML, ed.: Small Animal Orthopedics. St. Louis: CV Mosby, 1995, p 261.

Weber BG, Cech O: Pseudarthrosis, Pathophysiology, Biomechanics, Therapy, Results. Bern: Hans Huber, 1976.

141 Delayed Unions, Nonunions, and Malunions

Randy J. Boudrieau

DELAYED UNION AND NONUNION

Healing times for similar fractures in any single group of patients are fairly uniform; however, a small number of fractures have longer than "normal" healing times, or may fail to heal at all. The particular type of fracture (comminuted or simple), the bone involved, the location (distal radius/ulna or midshaft humerus), the age of the animal, and the type of fixation use all influence normal healing times.

- Classification:
  - When the fracture requires longer than normal time to heal but shows definitive signs of progression in healing, it is classified as a *delayed union*.
  - A fracture that does not heal over a similar period and that has no tendency toward further healing is classified as a *nonunion* (Table 141–1).

Other classifications are based on fracture site, fragment displacement, and presence or absence of infection.

Delayed Union

Delayed union usually needs no other therapy than continuation of ongoing treatment of the fracture.

Table 141–1. EXPECTED APPROXIMATE HEALING TIMES OF UNCOMPLICATED DIAPHYSEAL FRACTURES WITH MINIMAL LOSS OF CORTICAL BONE

Age of Animal	External Skeletal and Intramedullary Pin Fixation	Bone Plate Fixation*
<3 mo	2–3 wk	4 wk
3–6 mo	4–6 wk	2–3 mo
6–12 mo	5–8 wk	3–4 mo
>1 yr	7–12 wk	5–8 mo

*Fractures stabilized by this method may not be considered clinically healed (have sufficient strength) as early as fractures stabilized by other means of fixation, because direct cortical union (primary bone healing by haversian remodeling) is not supported by periosteal callus. This is of primary importance when considering timing of implant removal. Clinical function is not adversely affected by this method of fixation because plates provide rigid fixation.

Continued immobilization *(assuming stable fixation)* allows healing to occur in the majority of cases. A delayed union may, however, be preliminary to a nonunion.

Nonunion

Most fractures unite within a reasonable time despite systemic factors such as malnutrition, generalized metabolic or endocrine abnormalities, and acute or chronic generalized disease states. Nonunion, therefore, results from local factors at the fracture site. In most cases, these local factors can be identified (Table 141–2). Nonunion requires some form of surgical intervention in order for healing to progress.

▼ *Key Point* The most common cause of delayed union or nonunion is inadequate fixation and instability at the fracture site.

Problems Related to Nonhealing Fractures

Patients with nonhealing fractures may have additional problems related to function, such as disuse muscle atrophy, decreased range of joint motion and stiffness related to scar tissue contraction, neurovascular dysfunction, and limb angulation and/or shortening.

Bone Healing

- Bone heals by either primary (haversian remodeling) or secondary (periosteal callus) union.
- Secondary bone healing, with formation of visible periosteal callus, begins with connective tissue formation that progresses to form fibrocartilage and finally bone.
- Primary bone healing occurs without formation of connective tissue; bone deposition occurs directly (fracture gaps <0.8 mm) without any visible callus. Familiarity with these concepts allows accurate sequential evaluation of the healing process.

Histology

- The most notable histologic feature of a delayed union or nonunion is increased periosteal cartilage in the callus in lieu of bone formation.
- Persistent fracture gaps at the bone ends (sometimes greater than that present at the time of the original fracture) are filled with fibrous tissue/fibrocartilage callus.

Table 141–2. FACTORS ASSOCIATED WITH DELAYED UNION AND NONUNION

Local Factors*

Fracture location
Fracture gap
    Soft tissue interposition
    Bone loss secondary to trauma
Soft tissue trauma
    Loss of blood supply as a result of initial trauma
Contamination, infection
Neoplasia

Treatment Factors†

Malposition (inadequate reduction)
Fracture gap
    Soft tissue interposition
    Distraction (by implants or external fixation devices)
    Bone loss due to intraoperative removal
Soft tissue trauma
    Loss of blood supply due to surgical trauma
Inadequate fixation (internal or external)‡
    Instability
Postoperative infection

*Related to the fracture.
†Related to reduction and fixation.
‡Most common factor.

- Sclerosis of the bone ends at the fracture site also may occur, effectively sealing the medullary cavity (and access to the medullary circulation).

Clinical Signs

- Pain usually is present at the level of the fracture, and movement of this area may be detected clinically (occasionally these areas are relatively stable and are not overly painful).
- Palpable enlargement of the fracture area is present.
- Muscle atrophy and joint stiffness are likely sequelae to limb disuse.
- The patient is usually lame on the affected limb, and may be non–weight bearing.

Diagnosis

Radiographic Evaluation

- Radiographic signs vary, depending on the extent of healing (delayed union versus nonunion) and the type of delayed or lack of healing observed; classification of these events is the basis for treatment.
- Radiography allows sequential evaluation of healing:
  - *Delayed union:* There is continued healing, albeit slow, as indicated by progressive callus formation and resorption of dead bone. A persistent fracture line with evidence of some nonbridging callus is characteristic. The marrow cavity remains open without evidence of significant sclerosis of the bone ends.
  - *Nonunion:* There is no evidence of progression of fracture healing (i.e., little or no change on sequential radiographic evaluation). Smooth fracture surfaces (no periosteal "irritation") are typi-

cal, with evidence of sclerosis at the bone ends and sealed marrow cavities.
- Evaluate the "treatment factors" (Table 141–2) that may be contributing to the delayed union or nonunion. The fracture fixation is the most common source of the problem. For example, a small, radiolucent halo around any of the implants (screws, wires, etc.) indicates a loose device. A change in the position of the implants on serial radiographs also indicates implant instability.

▼ *Key Point* Differentiation of a delayed union vs. a nonunion is not only based on time but, more specifically, on serial radiographic evaluation.

Surgical Plan

- Always prepare for at least one autogenous cancellous graft donor site.
- Obtain tissue (preferably bone) from the fracture site for aerobic and anaerobic bacterial culture and sensitivity testing.
- Administer perioperative antibiotics (cephazolin, 22 mg/kg IV *after* cultures have been obtained; continue IV administration q2h during the surgical procedure). Continue the antibiotics (cephazolin, 22 mg/kg q8h SC) until culture results and sensitivity testing are available. Further antibiotic therapy depends on the culture results.
- If grossly apparent infection is present (see Chap. 52), consider open wound management (and secondary wound closure with an autogenous cancellous bone graft at a later date).
- If primary closure is performed, consider closed suction drainage of the fracture site.
- Decide whether to increase the stability of the fixation without disturbing the fracture site (delayed union) or to debride the fracture site and add an autogenous cancellous bone graft in addition to increasing the stability of the fixation (nonunion).

▼ *Key Point* If necessary, change the fixation to obtain rigid stability.

- Rigid stability is best achieved with screw and plate fixation. Place the plate under tension in order to compress the fracture fragments and thus use the frictional forces generated at the point of bone fragment contact to increase stability.
- Consider options for treatment of soft tissue complications (e.g., joint stiffness, contracture).

Surgical Procedure

Objectives

- Increase the stability of the fracture site by increasing or changing the fixation (compression plate fixation).
- Debride the fracture site as necessary to provide restimulation for fracture healing.
- Perform autogenous cancellous bone grafting, if gaps are present, to provide further stimulation for bone formation and promote osseous union.

- Restore satisfactory function of the affected limb (*aggressive* physical therapy).

Equipment

- Standard orthopedic pack and suture material
- Implants, usually screws and plates (occasionally may necessitate a separate tension device in order to obtain greater compression at the fracture site)
- Oscillating saw (for making osteotomy cuts)
- Bur set or rongeurs (for debriding fragment ends)
- Curettes for procurement of cancellous grafts
- Closed suction drainage system

Technique

1. Prepare the affected limb for aseptic surgery. Aseptically prepare a separate suitable donor site for harvest of autogenous cancellous bone. Usually the wing of the ilium and the proximal humerus yield a large amount of bone graft.
2. Make a standard anatomic approach to the affected bone, preserving all soft tissue structures. A large amount of fibrous connective tissue probably is adhered to the overlying muscle bellies; identification of the various tissue planes generally is difficult and requires *sharp* dissection. Exercise caution when approaching sites of major neurovascular structures.
3. Obtain samples of bone for aerobic and anaerobic bacterial culture and sensitivity testing of the fracture site.
4. *Delayed union:* Increase the stability of the fixation with implants such as additional intramedullary pins or an external skeletal fixator (see Chap. 130), or change the implant device (e.g., type III external skeletal fixator or bone plate placed under tension).
5. *Nonunion:*
   a. Debride the fracture site. Remove any loose metal, dead bone (sequestra) and infected tissue.
   b. Remove the fibrous connective tissue in the fragment gap by local debridement (bur or rongeurs) or transverse ostectomy (1–2 cm) of the entire nonunion site (Fig. 141–1). *Note:* The latter tech-

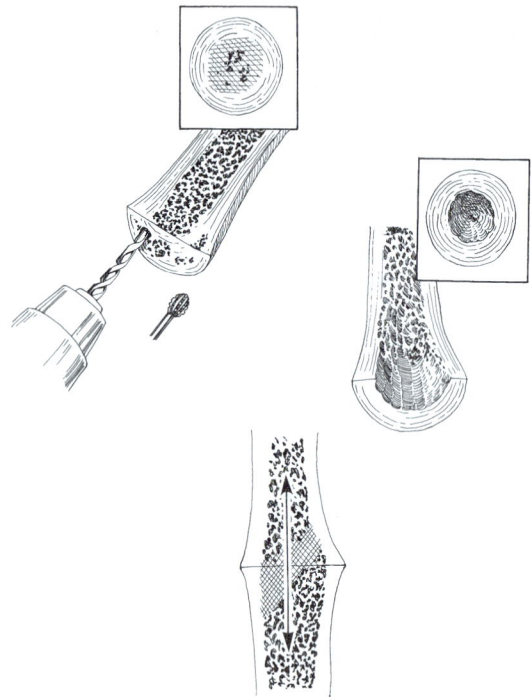

Figure 141–2. After an osteotomy or debridement of the fracture site, the medullary canal may remain sealed by the remaining sclerotic bone at this level. *Top left,* Medullary continuity is reestablished by drilling from the fracture site into the medullary canal or by using a bur. *Center right,* the end of this process is shown. *Bottom,* Both fracture fragments are reapposed and medullary continuity is reestablished *(arrow).* Insets show cross sections of bone. Hatched areas depict removed sclerotic bone.

nique creates a small amount of limb shortening, but this generally is not a functional problem in animals, owing to their flexed joint stance.
   c. Reestablish medullary continuity (and therefore the medullary circulation) by drilling the sclerotic bone ends (Fig. 141–2).
   d. Further "stimulation" of the fracture site may be obtained by the Judet technique (Fig. 141–3) of creating "shingles" of bone (this usually is not necessary with the osteotomy technique).
   e. Place an autogenous cancellous bone graft around the debrided fracture site. To prevent possible contamination of the donor site, use separate sterile instruments to procure the entire graft. Bone grafts may not be necessary in cases in which the nonunion site has been ostectomized back to healthy bone, and circumferential fragment contact is ensured under stable, compression plate fixation. Add a cancellous graft if any doubt concerning healing exists.
   f. When using plate fixation, a separate tension device may be required in order to achieve adequate fragment compression if greater than 4.0 mm of compression is desired (not necessary with the osteotomy technique).
6. If the tissues grossly appear healthy, routinely close the incision. Place closed suction drains if any question of contamination/infection exists or if dead space with continued diffuse bleeding is present.

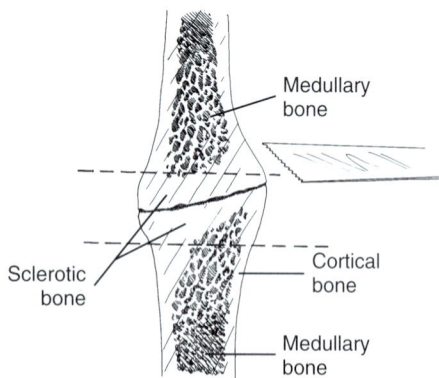

Figure 141–1. Nonunion with sealed medullary cavity (sclerotic bone at fracture margin). Dotted lines indicate level of osteotomy cuts made to remove 1–2 cm of bone, essentially removing the entire nonunion site.

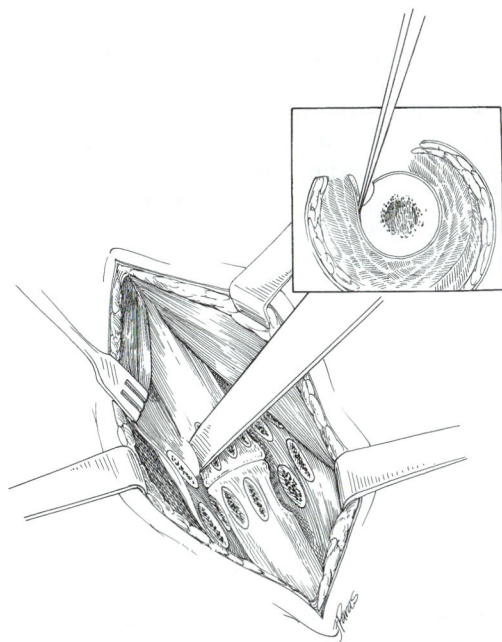

Figure 141–3. Elevate small cortical chips of bone from the shaft but maintain attachments to the surrounding soft tissues (Judet technique). Use a chisel *(inset)* to elevate these fragments of bone after the periosteum is split longitudinally with a scalpel.

7. Open wound management is indicated if tissues appear grossly infected; perform delayed primary closure and autogenous cancellous bone grafting at a later date after a healthy granulation tissue bed has developed.
8. Healing *will proceed* in the presence of infection *provided* the fixation is stable.

Postoperative Care and Complications

Physical Therapy

- Perform passive range of motion of joints adjacent to the surgical site *immediately* after surgery (30–50 flexions-extensions 3–4 times daily). Analgesics may be required in the first 2–4 days postoperatively. (The degree of stability obtained with plate fixation allows this level of activity without major patient discomfort.)
- Perform or encourage active range of motion exercises (controlled) such as short walks and swimming (the benefits of the latter cannot be overemphasized).
- Encourage controlled weight bearing. Limb use favors improved circulation and exercise of the musculature, which in turn improves the local fracture environment.

Open Wound Management

- Change bandage(s) at least once daily (pack entire wound with wet-to-dry gauze; see Chap. 52). Keep the soft tissues and (more important) bone moist. The goal is establishment of a healthy granulation tissue bed to cover both bone and implant.

- Perform delayed primary closure, usually with the addition of an autogenous cancellous bone graft. Consider using closed suction drains if dead space is present.
- Following apparently successful open wound management of infected wounds, persistent drainage and local or diffuse incisional dehiscence (usually over the implant) may occur. Continued wound management is required during fracture healing, and the implants are left in position to maintain stability. Subsequent implant removal is necessary to finally eliminate the infection.

Prognosis

- Satisfactory bone healing usually occurs within a relatively short time frame (8–12 weeks).
- Prognosis ultimately is limited only by the magnitude of the soft tissue problems associated with limb dis use. The prognosis generally is good, provided a severe functional deficit (joint contraction, etc.) or overwhelming infection is not present at the onset of treatment.
- Limb shortening with the osteotomy technique usually does not result in a major functional abnormality if not more than 20–30% of length is lost; however, the gait will be altered due to a slight mechanical lameness.

MALUNION

Many fractures heal with some degree of deformity without significant effect on function or appearance. These are not considered "true" malunions. Malunion implies a union with deformity sufficient to cause a functional and/or cosmetic defect. Malunion can occur as a result of untreated or improperly treated fractures.

Malunion may result in angular and rotational deformities, limb shortening, and soft tissue adhesions. These problems may directly affect adjacent joint function by alteration of the articular surfaces and/or supporting ligamentous structures. They also may affect the adjacent joints indirectly through changes in the functional angles placed on the joint and the abnormal stresses thus placed on the ligaments and joint capsule. Joint involvement, either direct or indirect, may result in decreased range of joint motion and degenerative joint disease (see Chap. 142). Correction of the malunion is accomplished by osteotomy through the area of greatest deformity, followed by realignment with stable skeletal fixation.

Precise fracture management can prevent malunion. Serial radiographic evaluation of the fracture throughout the healing period is essential to ensure continued appropriate fragment apposition and alignment. If a deformity is identified early, immediate corrective measures may prevent further complications.

Diagnosis

- Carefully evaluate the entire limb for bone and joint problems. Define the area of the long bone with the greatest amount of deformity: bowing of the bone in the cranial-caudal aspect, varus/valgus angulation, or rotational abnormalities along the axis of the bone. For example, a distal radial malunion resulting from premature distal ulnar physeal growth arrest (see Chap. 124) results in cranial bowing, carpal valgus, and external rotation of the distal radius.

- Define the orientation of the adjacent joints. All axes of joint rotation should be parallel to the weight bearing surface (in the example cited above of a distal radial malunion the radiocarpal joint surface angles cranially and medially; depending on the duration of the deformity, severe derangements of the intercarpal joints may be present).

- Assess adjacent structures to the malunion for abnormalities of orientation and function (e.g., degenerative joint disease, joint contraction, altered range of motion).

▼ *Key Point* Undertake surgical therapy for malunion only when the procedure is justified by the impairment of function or cosmetic defect.

Surgical Plan

- Determine the amount of angulation present in the awake, weight bearing animal and compare with that of the opposite normal limb.
- Determine the amount of angulation observed on radiographic evaluation of the involved limb and compare with radiographs of the opposite normal limb. Carefully determine joint axis orientation.
- Compare and collate information derived from the physical examination and the radiographic evaluation to determine the amount of correction (angle) of osteotomy required.
- Using a duplicate radiograph of the involved limb, draw the limb and joint axes and plot the angle of correction at the area of greatest deformity.
  - Cut the radiograph along the predrawn lines and place in the corrected position to evaluate the planned osteotomy cut and the expected result, making adjustments as necessary.
  - This two-dimensional radiograph allows correction to be planned in only *two* planes: cranial-caudal and medial-lateral. Determine the remaining rotational deformity by observation at the time of surgery. (See Chapter 124 for more information about growth deformities of the radius and ulna.)

Surgical Procedure

Objectives

- Straighten the limb by corrective osteotomy.
  - The closing wedge osteotomy is the most versatile and easy to use technique. The loss of bone length is approximately equal to the width of wedge removed.
  - Other osteotomy techniques (reverse wedge, oblique, and dome) are more difficult to perform and/or less precise in the correction of the malunion.

- A newer technique using distraction osteogenesis may be used to gradually correct the deformity after a single osteotomy cut.
- Provide stable fixation.
  - Apply a plate with bone fragments placed under tension for maximal stability.
  - Alternatively, apply an external skeletal fixator (see Chap. 130) when a very short fragment must be stabilized adjacent to a joint.

Equipment

- Standard orthopedic pack and suture material
- Implants (preferably screws and plates, external skeletal fixator, K-wires)
- Oscillating saw
- Goniometer (for measuring and confirming angles of correction intraoperatively)

Technique (Closing Wedge Osteotomy)

1. Determine the angle of correction, based on the previously evaluated radiographs and physical examination.
2. Prepare the affected limb for aseptic surgery. Consider aseptic preparation and full draping of the opposite normal limb within the operative field for use as a comparison (especially important with chondrodystrophic-breed dogs).
3. Perform a standard surgical exposure to the bone at the level of greatest deformity.
4. Perform wedge osteotomy of the affected bone to correct the deformity.
5. Reduce both bone fragments (full contact with both osteotomy surfaces) and temporarily secure with two small cross-pins (K-wires). Make any necessary further adjustments at this time (by removing the cross-pins and shaving additional bone as necessary).
6. Apply plate fixation to both bone fragments under tension (standard ASIF [Association for the Study of Internal Fixation] technique, including prestressing of the implant), and then remove cross-pins.
7. Close the surgical wound routinely.

Postoperative Care and Complications

- Provide standard postoperative care as for any fracture fixation, including exercise restriction and physical therapy. Evaluate the postoperative conformation and gait.
- Persistent, mild cosmetic disfiguration requires no further therapy.
- Continued functional problems require further, more precise surgical correction.
- Complications include:
  - Inadequate or overcorrection of the deformity
  - Continued functional problems due to other, previously unrecognized abnormalities (e.g., degenerative joint disease, abnormal range of joint motion)
  - Slightly decreased range of joint motion when the fixation device is placed immediately adjacent to the joint (generally not a functional limitation)

- Slight limb shortening (generally not a functional limitation)
- Infection (as can occur after any surgical procedure)
- Delayed union or nonunion

Prognosis

- The prognosis generally is good with proper case selection.

SUPPLEMENTAL READINGS

Binnington AG: Delayed union and nonunion. *In* Slatter DH, ed.: Textbook of Small Animal Surgery. Philadelphia: WB Saunders, 1985.

Brinker WO, Hohn RB, Prieur WD, eds.: Manual of Internal Fixation in Small Animals. Berlin: Springer-Verlag, 1984.

Newton CD: Principles and techniques of osteotomy. *In* Newton CD, Nunamaker DM, eds.: Textbook of Small Animal Orthopaedics. Philadelphia: JB Lippincott, 1985.

Piermattei DL: An Atlas of Surgical Approaches to the Bones of the Dog and Cat, 3rd Ed. Philadelphia: WB Saunders, 1993.

Rudy RL: Corrective osteotomy for angular deformities. Vet Clin North Am 1:549, 1971.

Weber BG, Cech O: Pseudoarthrosis: Pathology, Biomechanics, Therapy, Results. Bern: Hans Huber, 1976.

142 Osteoarthritis

Callum W. Hay / Paul A. Manley

Osteoarthritis (OA) is the term commonly used in describing the pathologic process of cartilage degeneration in mammalian diarthrodial joints. The term osteoarthrosis is preferred by those who wish to stress the noninflammatory nature of this disease. Degenerative joint disease (DJD) is a term used to encompass all changes seen in OA. For practical purposes, the terms can be used interchangeably. Even though aging results in articular cartilage changes of reduced tensile strength, OA is not recognized frequently as a result. The purpose of this chapter is to discuss the etiology, diagnosis, and treatment of small animal OA.

▼ *Key Point* Osteoarthritis is diagnosed in dogs far more frequently than cats.

ANATOMY AND PHYSIOLOGY

- Diarthrodial joints consist of articular cartilage lubricated by synovial fluid that is secreted by the synovial membrane lining. The synovial membrane secretes synovial fluid, provides a boundary to the joints, and contains pain receptors. Articular cartilage is aneural and receives nourishment by diffusion from the joint fluid.
- Eighty percent of articular cartilage is composed of water, with most of the remainder composed of type II collagen and proteoglycan matrix, which is synthesized by chondrocytes (Fig. 142–1).

▼ *Key Point* In normal articular cartilage, chondrocytes continually synthesize and degrade proteoglycan. Type II collagen is degraded only during disease processes, and then type I collagen is synthesized.

- Proteoglycan consists of many repeating chains of glycosaminoglycans (mainly chondroitin sulfate and keratin sulfate). Glycosaminoglycans are bound to a protein core, which in turn is bound to hyaluronate by a link protein, to form a macromolecular structure called aggrecan (Fig. 142–1).
- Glycosaminoglycans are negatively charged, causing them to repel one another and maintain the aggrecan in an expanded state. The negative charges bind water and cations, while the expanded state imparts stiffness to the cartilage matrix.

▼ *Key Point* As compressive loads move the glycosaminoglycan chains together, displacing water, the negative charge resists further compression. In this way, cartilage is viscoelastic and is able to deform and re-form with normal repetitive loading.

ETIOLOGY

- OA can be caused by primary or secondary disorders. Primary causes are rarely recognized in clinical practice. Secondary causes due to altered joint biomechanics account for most cases of OA in veterinary patients.
- Secondary causes of OA include developmental disorders, such as osteochondritis dissecans or hip dysplasia, and acquired causes, such as cranial cruciate ligament injury, patellar luxation, joint instability due to ligament sprain, and malunion of intra-articular fractures.

PATHOPHYSIOLOGY

▼ *Key Point* In dogs and cats OA usually results from a disruption of normal joint homeostasis by an overriding biomechanical force.

- Cartilage derangements observed in OA include increased synthesis and degradation of proteoglycan, increased cartilage hydration, loss of collagen integrity, loss of tensile strength, fibrillation, and eburnation.
- Synovial membrane derangements observed in OA include synovitis, mainly from mononuclear cell infiltration, which releases inflammatory mediators into synovial fluid.

▼ *Key Point* The release of degradative cartilage enzymes (metalloproteinases) is pivotal in the pathology of OA and results in irreversible cartilage damage. Metalloproteinases can arise from both chondrocytes and synovial membrane.

- Cytokines such as interleukin-1 (IL-1) and tumor necrosis factor-α (TNF-α) cause catabolic cartilage changes by promoting degradative cartilage enzyme production. Other mediators such as insulin-like growth factor (IGF), transforming growth factor-β

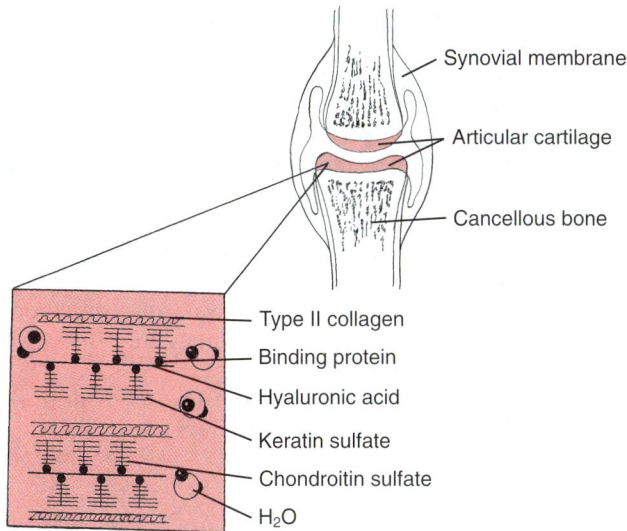

Figure 142–1. Schematic representation of cartilage structure.

(TGF-β), and interleukin-6 (IL-6) are associated with increased proteoglycan synthesis.
- The sources of inflammatory mediators include chondrocytes, synovium, and mononuclear inflammatory cells.

▼ *Key Point* Although there is increased proteoglycan synthesis in OA, there is increased destruction and a net loss of proteoglycan from matrix, leading to loss of structure and function.

CLINICAL SIGNS

- Morning stiffness, which improves with gentle exercise (animal "warms" out of it).
- Lameness worsens after heavy exercise.
- Lameness in one or more legs, with occasional or persistent non–weight bearing.

DIAGNOSIS

A suspicion of OA will be present after history and physical examination. Radiographs and rarely joint fluid analysis confirm the diagnosis. It is rare to confuse OA with polyarthropathy due to noninfectious or infectious causes.

History and Physical Examination

- Any age, breed, or sex of dog or cat can be affected with OA. Younger animals tend to have developmental disease. Adolescents and older dogs tend to have acquired conditions.
- A history of previous trauma that might lead to joint instability or disturbance of the articular surface is important.
- While the animal is standing, palpate for joint effusion especially in the knees, hocks, elbows, and carpi. Muscle atrophy around the thighs and over the spine

of the scapula can also be better appreciated in standing animals.
- Complete the rest of the examination with the animal on its side.

▼ *Key Point* Gentle restraint in lateral recumbency works best with sedation, depending on the animal's temperament.

▼ *Key Point* Reduced range of motion and/or joint effusion are good indicators of a joint problem.

- Palpate for pain and crepitus (a grinding feeling when joints are flexed and extended).
- Palpate for joint laxity, which may be especially prevalent in the hip and knee.

Radiographic Examination

▼ *Key Point* Good-quality radiographs with correct exposure for bone and joint evaluation and proper developing technique are essential in detecting subtle evidence of OA. Radiographic abnormalities include joint effusion, osteophytes at the site of capsular attachment, subchondral bone sclerosis, and bone remodeling.

Joint Fluid Analysis

- Rarely needed in diagnosing OA.
- In most cases of OA, joint fluid yields a noninflammatory, mononuclear cell population.
- See Chapter 143 for a discussion on joint fluid analysis.

TREATMENT

OA is a progressive disease, cannot be reversed, and is generally not arrested by medical therapy. Decide if a particular patient needs to be treated surgically or medically. Many cases of OA can be managed surgically with a good prognosis for improvement in function.

Medical Treatment

There are two general groups of small animal patients that may be treated medically.

Group 1. Older dogs with OA in which surgery will not help because OA is advanced or surgery is risky due to concurrent medical problems or those dogs in which surgery is declined by the owners for financial or emotional reasons. (These patients usually have advanced OA in the hips, knees, or elbows.)

Group 2. Dogs in which surgery may be part of the treatment.

▼ *Key Point* Often weight loss (in overweight animals) and lifestyle modifications are the only treatments necessary for an animal with OA.

- Gentle exercise is beneficial at maintaining joint mobility. Swimming and controlled leash walks work best. Generally, avoid heavy activity. Counsel owners to identify activities that exacerbate their pet's problem. Such activities are Frisbee catching, rigorous hunting, or excessive agility exercises.

- Supporting joints with external coaptation (i.e., for OA in the carpus or tarsus) may have a short-term benefit for dogs with acute exacerbations. Soft padded bandages or a support splint could be used.

Nonsteroidal Anti-Inflammatory Drugs

- NSAIDs are the mainstay of managing OA.
- Some of the pain in OA comes from prostaglandin release. By inhibiting cyclooxygenase, NSAIDs reduce prostaglandin production, alleviating pain and inflammation. Some NSAIDs (e.g., acetaminophen) have anti-inflammatory and analgesic action not attributable to cyclooxygenase inhibition; little is known about these mechanisms. It is likely that some of the NSAIDs used in small animal practice also have analgesic actions not attributable to cyclooxygenase activity.

▼ *Key Point* Most NSAIDs used in small animal practice inhibit proteoglycan synthesis and worsen the pathology of OA. Many NSAIDs have undesirable gastric and renal side effects. Management of OA with NSAIDs is a tradeoff between pain relief and deleterious cartilage effects and/or gastric or renal toxicity. Pain relief does not necessarily equate with chondroprotection.

- It is increasingly apparent that at least two categories of cyclooxygenase enzymes exist. Cyclooxygenase 1 (cox 1) is present in vascular tissue and is responsible for normal vascular homeostasis. Cyclooxygenase 2 (cox 2) is induced by cytokines and may have a role in OA.

▼ *Key Point* Inhibition of cox 1 leads to gastric ulceration and nephrotoxicity. Different classes of NSAIDs have varying abilities to inhibit cox enzymes, which dictates their efficacy and side effects. The ideal NSAID is one that inhibits cox 2 preferentially and has no deleterious effect on proteoglycan synthesis. Newer NSAIDs have been developed with these principles in mind.

- Use the lowest possible dose of NSAIDs to minimize gastric and renal side effects and minimize cartilage damage.

NSAIDs for Use in All Dogs (Groups 1 and 2)

▼ *Key Point* Managing OA in dogs is a balance among effective pain relief, minimal side effects, and owner satisfaction with treatment. Proper owner education about NSAIDs is essential to the harmony of this process.

Buffered Aspirin

- Often chosen first, due to economy and effectiveness.
- Analgesic dose is 10–25 mg/kg q8–12h PO; anti-inflammatory dose is 20–40 mg/kg q8–12h PO in dogs.

- Buffered aspirin works better than nonbuffered products. Absorption of enteric-coated aspirin can be erratic and may give variable results.
- Inhibits cox 1 more than cox 2, so gastrointestinal (GI) side effects (ulceration) may occur.
- If aspirin is not tolerated due to vomiting, the gastric side effects can be alleviated with misoprostol (a prostaglandin E_2 analog) at 2–5 µg/kg q8h PO. Alternatively, change to a less ulcerogenic NSAID.
- Although human buffered aspirin products are not licensed products for animals, we prescribe them commonly. Several preparations marketed for small animals are available.
- Use aspirin with extreme caution in cats. A dose of 10 mg/kg q52h PO is suggested.

Carprofen

- Carprofen may be used as a first choice over aspirin because of its proven effectiveness in pain relief, and less chance of gastric side effects.
- Dose is 2.2 mg/kg q12h PO.
- Carprofen is a carboxylic acid related to ibuprofen, but it inhibits cox 1 less relative to cox 2, so GI side effects are less than aspirin and its relative, ibuprofen.
- Carprofen is licensed for use in dogs but not in cats.
- Rare and reversible hepatic toxicity has been associated with carprofen administration in dogs.

Etodolac

- Etodolac is a pyranocarboxylic acid which has selective cox 2 inhibition and possibly direct cellular anti-inflammatory activity.
- Etodolac undergoes extensive enterohepatic recirculation, so administer once daily at 10–15 mg/kg PO.

Phenylbutazone

- A commonly used alternative to aspirin due to better pain relief and tolerance.
- Dose is 10–15 mg/kg q8h PO (maximum dose is 800 mg/day regardless of body size).
- Side effects such as GI irritation and bone marrow suppression can occur. Try to taper to lowest possible dose.
- It is licensed for small animal use.
- Do not use in cats, due to adverse side effects.

NSAIDs for Use in Group 1 Dogs

- These drugs carry higher risks of gastrointestinal side effects, but they provide good pain relief and may be necessary for long-term use in patients in which surgery is not an option.

Piroxicam

- Is generally very effective for pain relief.
- Dose is 0.3 mg/kg q24–48h PO. It comes in capsule form, so in smaller patients breakage and division of the capsule contents is necessary to prevent overdosing.
- May not depress proteoglycan synthesis as much as other NSAIDs, based on in vitro studies.

- Gastric ulceration may occur.
- Not licensed for small animal use.

Meclofenamic Acid

- Is generally effective for pain relief.
- Dose is 1.1 mg/kg q24h PO for 4–7 days then 0.5 mg/kg q24h PO.
- Watch for gastrointestinal side effects.
- Is licensed for dogs.

Ibuprofen

- Do not use ibuprofen due to potential side effects (such as gastric or colonic perforation) and the availability of suitable licensed alternatives.

Other NSAIDs

- Flunixin, ketoprofen, and meloxicam are licensed for small animal use in other countries but were not currently licensed in the United States at the time of publication. The recommended dose of flunixin is 0.5–2.2 mg/kg q24h IM or IV or 1–2 mg/kg q24h PO for a maximum of 3 days. Do not use in cats or for long-term therapy in dogs due to potential gastrointestinal or renal side effects.

Other Drugs for Group 1 Dogs

Corticosteroids

- Unlike NSAIDs, corticosteroids severely depress synthesis of proteoglycan, even in normal articular cartilage.
- Use corticosteroids judiciously at the lowest possible dose. Corticosteroids should be used for very short-term (weeks) therapy *only*.
- Combination preparations with aspirin are available, although it is best to administer each drug separately so the dose of steroid can be reduced individually.
- Steroids tend to cause significant pain relief due to their potency; however, this does not equate with long-term benefit to the patient. It also makes it difficult to wean a patient with OA off steroids because of the apparent improvement in their condition.
- Steroid therapy in surgical patients (group 2) is not advisable, since steroids may hamper any beneficial outcome of surgery.

Chondroprotective Agents

- The precise mechanism(s) of action of these drugs is still under investigation. They reportedly promote cartilage preservation through stimulation of proteoglycan synthesis and inhibition of degradation.

Polysulfated Glycosaminoglycans

- These have been shown to provide improvement in pain and function in dogs with OA, especially hip dysplasia.
- If needed in group 2 patients, surgery is the best option.

- Dose is 5–7 mg/kg IM once every 4 days for 7 injections. Then repeat 1–2 times monthly as needed.
- Initially, intra-articular use was recommended but is rarely done now because of the effectiveness of intramuscular administration and the increased risk of joint infection associated with intra-articular injection.

Glucosamines (Nutraceuticals)

- The hypothesis for their use is that incorporation of glucosamine into glycosaminoglycan is a rate-limited step in OA, and thus by supplementation with glucosamine, more proteoglycan will be produced.
- Most compounds are oral supplements.
- Their use is currently being evaluated and may be beneficial in some cases.
- Be aware that they are licensed as nutritional supplements and not pharmacologic agents.

Shark Cartilage and Fish Cartilage Supplements

- These are marketed similarly to nutraceuticals.
- Many over-the-counter preparations are available.
- Anecdotally, they help some animals and have minimal side effects.

Vitamin C

- This is often used as a treatment for many orthopedic disorders.
- The benefit in OA is questionable but it appears to do no harm.

Surgical Treatment

- Surgical management of certain cases of secondary OA should be considered. These include osteochondritis dissecans (shoulder, elbow, tarsus, stifle), cranial cruciate ligament disease, patellar luxation, and hip dysplasia. (See respective chapters for more information on these disorders.)
- Surgery can be expected to slow down the progression of OA and improve lameness.
- Salvage surgical procedures, such as total hip replacement and carpal arthrodesis, can provide excellent results.
- Salvage arthrodesis procedures for other joints give variable results.

SUPPLEMENTAL READINGS

Beale BS, Goring RL: Degenerative joint disease. *In* Bojrab MI, ed: Pathophysiology in Small Animal Surgery, 2nd Ed. Philadelphia: Lea & Febiger, 1993, pp 727–736.

Manley PA: Treatment of degenerative joint disease. *In* Bonagura JD, ed: Kirk's Current Veterinary Therapy, 12th Ed. Philadelphia: WB Saunders, 1995, pp 1196–1199.

May SA: Degenerative joint disease (osteoarthritis, osteoarthrosis, secondary joint disease). *In* Houlton J, Collinson R, eds: Manual of Small Animal Arthrology. Ames, Iowa State University Press, 1994, pp 62–74.

143 Immune-Mediated Arthritis

Callum W. Hay / Paul A. Manley

Immune-mediated arthropathies are inflammatory, noninfectious, and considered either nonerosive or erosive, depending on the effect on articular cartilage. The arthropathies are characterized by synovitis and articular cartilage damage. Erosive arthritis is characterized by articular cartilage loss, and nonerosive arthritis is not. Nonerosive forms are more common in small animal practice. These conditions are not curable but can be treated to improve quality of life.

ETIOLOGY

▼ *Key Point* The initial site for the pathology of immune-mediated arthritis is in the synovium, rather than in the articular cartilage as in osteoarthritis (OA).

- The etiology of immune-mediated arthritis is often unknown.
- Little investigation of cytokines has been done in immune arthropathies in dogs and cats. It is well established that interleukin-1 (IL-1) and tumor necrosis factor-α (TNF-α) activate metalloproteinases and cause cartilage degeneration. These cytokines diffuse from synovial membrane to articular cartilage (and vice versa). Studies in humans have shown higher levels of IL-1 and TNF-α in inflammatory arthropathies compared to osteoarthritis. Future investigation in small animals will probably show that these cytokines are involved in the pathology of both nonerosive and erosive inflammatory arthritis.

Nonerosive Forms

- The nonerosive arthropathies are characterized by antigen-antibody deposition in the synovium.
- Antigen-antibody complexes (type III hypersensitivity reaction) are potent stimuli for inflammatory mediator release, through complement fixation and subsequent infiltration of synovium by inflammatory cells. This inflammatory process releases cartilage-degrading enzymes (metalloproteinases) and leads to a self-perpetuating process of synovial inflammation and cartilage degradation. When such complexes involve antinuclear antibodies, this disease is termed systemic lupus erythematosus (SLE).

Erosive Forms

In rheumatoid arthritis, host IgG becomes antigenic, with rheumatoid factor (IgM antibody) being formed in response. The binding of IgM with IgG triggers inflammatory mediator release, similar to the pathology of the nonerosive forms. It is ill-defined, however, which factor is responsible for the development of articular cartilage erosion.

▼ *Key Point* A polyarthropathy is swelling of six or more joints. Swelling of more than one and less than six joints is termed pauciarthropathy.

CLINICAL SIGNS

Canine Nonerosive Arthritis

- This form usually affects larger-breed dogs with an average age of 5–6 years.
- The signs may be acute onset of lameness, fever, lethargy, and swelling, especially of the distal joints.
- Initially, the range of motion in the joints may be decreased due to swelling, and later the joints may become unstable due to ligamentous damage.

▼ *Key Point* The nonerosive arthropathies are more commonly seen in veterinary patients and have been classified into four groups.

- Type I—These have idiopathic causes and account for 50% of small animal cases.
- Type II—These are associated with remote infection from sites other than joints, e.g., bacterial endocarditis or any other focus of infection that could act as a source of antigens. The joints are usually not infected; rather, immune complexes between host antibody and bacterial components cause the problem. Type II accounts for 25% of small animal cases.
- Type III—These are associated with chronic gastrointestinal disease and are also called enteropathic arthritis. They account for 15% of small animal cases.
- Type IV—These are associated with neoplasia remote to joints and account for the remaining 10% of small animal cases.

Nonerosive Arthritis Syndromes

- Several disease syndromes that do not fit in the above classification include:

Systemic Lupus Erythematosus

- Characterized by autoimmunity to body tissues and immune complex disease. Clinical problems include thrombocytopenia, hemolytic anemia, neutropenia, dermatitis, glomerulonephritis, and polyarthritis.

Juvenile-Onset Polyarthritis Syndrome in Akitas

- Affects Akitas less than 1 year of age. Clinical signs include cyclic pain, fever, lymphadenopathy, and occasionally nonseptic meningitis. A heritable component is suspected.

Inflammatory Arthritis of Chinese Shar-Peis

- Affects Shar-Peis of any age. The arthropathy is characterized by episodic fever and swelling, mainly of the hocks. It is usually associated with renal amyloidosis and is also known as Shar-Pei fever.

Polyarthritis/Polymyositis

- Affects spaniel breeds. Clinical signs include muscle pain, atrophy, and contracture along with pyrexia and polyarthropathy. High levels of creatine phosphokinase may be seen, due to muscle involvement.

Polyarthritis/Meningitis

- Affects Bernese mountain dogs, beagles, boxers, German shorthaired pointers and Weimaraners. Clinical signs include cyclic fever and neck pain lasting 3–7 days. Joint swelling may be seen but is not the primary feature of the disease.

Idiopathic Drug-Induced Polyarthritis

- Most commonly seen secondary to administration of antibiotics such as sulfonamide drugs and less commonly erythromycin, lincomycin, cephalosporins, and penicillins. Doberman pinschers have been identified as being particularly susceptible to the effects of sulfonamide drugs. The mechanisms of drug-induced polyarthritis could include a hapten reaction or direct immune complexes of host-produced antibody with the drug.

Canine Erosive Arthritis

Rheumatoid Arthritis

- Most commonly recognized canine erosive arthropathy, but is rarer than nonerosive arthropathies.
- This form affects smaller-breed dogs of any age.
- The signs may be more insidious than in the nonerosive forms and may be associated with fever, lethargy, swollen joints, and shifting leg lameness.
- Angular deformities may occur especially in the carpi as a result of ligamentous destruction around the joints.

Greyhound Polyarthritis

- Affects young greyhounds and has been described in Australia and the United States. The cause is unknown, but *Mycoplasma spumans* has been suspected.

- The disease may have an insidious or acute onset characterized by joint swelling, pyrexia, weight loss, pneumonia, and diarrhea. The articular cartilage pathology observed includes erosion and pannus.

Inflammatory Arthropathies of Cats

▼ *Key Point* Inflammatory arthropathies in cats are recognized less frequently than in dogs.

Nonerosive Forms

- The Type I to IV classification described in dogs also holds true for cats.
- With polyarthropathy in cats, bone marrow neoplasia (type IV) should be suspected, with lymphoma or multiple myeloma being the cause.

Feline Progressive Polyarthritis

- This is described in both nonerosive and erosive forms. The nonerosive form, also known as the periosteal proliferative form, is most common.
- The nonerosive form occurs almost exclusively in male cats. Clinical signs include stiffness, pyrexia, and lymphadenopathy. Commonly, the tarsi and/or carpi are affected.
- Feline syncytia-forming virus and feline leukemia virus have been implicated as the causal agent.

Erosive Forms

- This is the less common form of feline progressive polyarthritis.
- Chronic onset of stiffness involving the carpi and/or tarsi may be seen.
- The disease often progresses to subluxation and luxation of the carpi, tarsi, and phalanges.

DIAGNOSIS

Unfortunately, no one diagnostic test is specific for a certain type of immune-mediated polyarthropathy. Extensive diagnostic testing may yield confusing results. Infectious agents such as rickettsiae, *Borrelia burgdorferi*, mycoplasma, bacteria, and fungi can cause polyarthropathy. They may be ruled in or out with a variety of serologic tests and/or cultures.

History/Physical Examination

- Signalment and history help determine if breed-specific causes may be present.
- A thorough physical examination is necessary because of the wide range of causes of polyarthritis.
- Joint swelling and reduced range of motion or laxity, especially of the carpi and tarsi, may be appreciated on physical examination.
- Peripheral lymphadenopathy and splenomegaly may be present.
- About 30% of dogs with the nonerosive form have dermatitis, or focal alopecia.
- Elevated rectal temperature can be present.

Radiography

Nonerosive Forms

- Early-stage nonerosive arthropathies may show joint swelling and minimal radiographic signs of osteophytes. Osteophytes may be present later in the disease.

Erosive Forms

- Erosive arthropathies show small or large lytic areas of subchondral bone and osteophytosis.

▼ *Key Point* It may be difficult to radiographically distinguish long-standing nonerosive disease (with secondary joint destruction) from erosive disease.

Laboratory Evaluation

- Obtain a complete blood count, serum chemistry profile, and urinalysis. In conjunction with history and physical examination, prioritize the rule-out list and identify concurrent diseases.
- The presence of an inflammatory leukogram and hyperglobulinemia suggests inflammation.
- Over 50% of patients with nonerosive polyarthropathies are proteinuric, so hypoalbuminemia may be seen as a result of renal damage.
- Consider a rheumatoid factor (RF) test. Dogs with rheumatoid arthritis may periodically have positive or negative RF tests and dogs without rheumatoid arthritis may have a positive RF test.
- Antinuclear antibody (ANA) is helpful in supporting a diagnosis of SLE. A lupus erythematosus (LE) preparation is an in vitro test used to identify polymorphonuclear cells that have phagocytosed nuclear material. This test may be considered when the ANA test is positive and the diagnosis of SLE is elusive.

▼ *Key Point* In diagnosing rheumatoid arthritis, the most reliable criteria include the following combination of clinical findings: erosive changes on radiographs, a positive RF test (present in up to 75% of cases), and inflammatory synovial fluid (see Table 143–1). A biopsy to identify histologic synovial membrane changes consistent with canine rheumatoid arthritis may be helpful in elusive cases.

Joint Fluid Analysis

- Aseptic percutaneous needle arthrocentesis under heavy sedation or, preferably, anesthesia is necessary to evaluate joint fluid.
- Clip the hair around the joint and prepare with a disinfectant scrub.
- Use a 20- or 18-gauge needle and 5-cc or 12-cc syringe and aspirate gently.
- Remove the syringe before withdrawing the needle. This prevents iatrogenic blood contamination of the sample from the subcutaneous tissue due to negative pressure in the syringe as the needle is removed.
- Submit synovial fluid (in order of priority) for cytology, total cell count, protein levels, and mucin clot. Save some synovial fluid for aerobic culture. Before submitting to a laboratory by mail, make two slides (one for cytology, one for a Gram stain) and place some synovial fluid in a blood culture bottle to enrich small numbers of bacteria that may be present if sepsis is suspected. Then place the rest of the synovial fluid in a blood tube with ethylenediaminetetraacetic acid (EDTA) shaken out (frequently the synovial fluid volume is small, so there is a relative excess of EDTA). EDTA interferes with the mucin clot test, making interpretation difficult.
- The predominant cell type seen on cytology in immune arthropathy is usually nondegenerate neutrophils, but mononuclear cells can sometimes be predominant.
- See Table 143–1 for comparison of joint fluid analysis in various arthropathies.

Synovial Biopsy

- May be indicated in diagnostically challenging cases of immune-mediated joint disease.
- Requires open biopsy using strict aseptic technique.
- Harvest synovium at the cartilage-bone margin.
- Histology shows plasma cell and lymphocyte infiltration.

TREATMENT

A dilemma in the treatment of polyarthropathy is whether the process is infectious or noninfectious. The treatment for a noninfectious problem (i.e., immunosuppression) exacerbates an infectious cause of poly-

Table 143–1. JOINT FLUID ANALYSIS IN DIFFERENT CLASSES OF JOINT DISEASE*

Disease	Mucin Clot	Appearance	WBC Count (mm³)
Normal	+	Clear	0–2900
Osteoarthritis	+	Clear	<3000
Immune-mediated	±	Turbid	>5000; neutrophils are well preserved
Septic arthritis	−	Very turbid	Usually >60,000; degenerate neutrophils

*Isolation or observation of significant numbers of any microorganism from joint fluid is highly supportive of an infectious or septic etiology, regardless of cell count. Cell counts in immune-mediated and septic joints may be similar in many cases.

WBC, white blood cell; +, positive; ±, can be positive or negative; −, negative.

arthropathy. If intracellular bacteria are seen on synovial fluid analysis or if bacterial culture is positive, then the process is likely septic. However, in endemic areas for Lyme disease and ehrlichiosis it can be difficult to distinguish these from immune-mediated joint disease. Some prefer to initially treat with tetracyclines (e.g., for 1 week) and change to corticosteroids if no response is seen, or after results of diagnostic testing are available. The cyclic nature of many of the immune-mediated diseases, however, makes interpreting a response to treatment difficult.

Nonerosive Forms

▼ *Key Point* The initial treatment for all nonerosive immune-mediated arthropathies is similar. Use either nonsteroidal anti-inflammatory drugs (NSAIDs) or corticosteroids.

- The lowest dose of drugs to control signs should be used.
- Recurrences are possible after cessation of therapy.

Initial Therapy (2–4 weeks of therapy)

- Buffered aspirin at the higher (anti-inflammatory) dose range (25–40 mg/kg q8h PO) could be tried. Carprofen (2 mg/kg q12h PO) could be administered as an alternative because of its lower risk of gastrointestinal side effects.
- If sepsis has been ruled out, prednisone at 1–3 mg/kg q12h PO may be given.
- It is best to use NSAIDs or steroids, not both. The higher doses of these drugs together may potentiate each other's side effects. It is feasible to use prednisone on alternate days with NSAIDs, at low doses.
- Besides clinical signs, repeat aspiration of joint fluid may allow monitoring of the effectiveness of therapy. A cell count of less than $4000/mm^3$ is ideal. In cases in which the cell count does not decrease and the clinical signs are present, other immunosuppressive drugs may be needed (see Table 143–2).

Long-Term Therapy (months to years)

- Preferably, the patient should be weaned off therapy after 2–4 months of treatment.
- If signs reappear after several attempts to discontinue therapy, the patient will likely require long-term corticosteroid therapy at the lowest possible dose. Base the decision to proceed with long-term therapy on the severity of the problem. Cases nonresponsive to glucocorticoids may require more aggressive immunosuppression as outlined in the next section.

Erosive Forms

▼ *Key Point* Canine rheumatoid arthritis usually requires immunosuppression in addition to prednisone for a response.

- Cyclophosphamide is often used along with prednisone in treating rheumatoid arthritis.
- The side effect of hemorrhagic cystitis associated with cyclophosphamide can be devastating to the patient. Discontinuing cyclophosphamide after 4 months of therapy minimizes the chances of hemorrhagic cystitis.
- Note that cyclophosphamide is used for 4 days during each week of therapy.
- Gold sodium thiomalate can be used to maintain remission after cessation of cyclophosphamide. Gold salt is a slow-acting antirheumatic drug and is unsuitable for inducing remission.
- Azathioprine can be used instead of cyclophosphamide to induce remission in dogs only, since it is toxic to cats.
- Additional treatment information is in Table 143–2.

Surgery

- Surgery has a limited role in managing immune-mediated arthropathies.
- Pancarpal arthrodesis could be considered in some patients with localized disease to the carpi.

Table 143–2. DRUG REGIMENS USED FOR CONTROL OF IMMUNE-MEDIATED ARTHRITIS

Drug	Dose	Action	Comments
Acetylsalicylic acid (aspirin)	25–40 mg/kg q8h PO	Analgesic; anti-inflammatory	Generally more effective for degenerative joint disease
Glucocorticoids (prednisone, prednisolone)	1–3 mg/kg q12h PO until remission achieved; then decrease to lowest effective maintenance dose	Anti-inflammatory; immunosuppressive	First choice for nonerosive forms; can be used alone or in combination with other drugs
Cyclophosphamide* (Cytoxan, Mead Johnson)	1.5–2.5 mg/kg PO q24h 4 days/week	Immunosuppressive	Monitor WBC count; watch for hemorrhagic cystitis
Azathioprine† (Imuran, Burroughs Wellcome)	*Dogs:* 2 mg/kg q48h PO	Immunosuppressive	Monitor WBC count; relatively toxic in cats
Gold sodium thiomalate (Solganal, Schering)	0.5–1 mg/kg IM once weekly	Unknown	Used in erosive forms; limited clinical experience

*Glucocorticoids are commonly administered concurrently with this drug.
†Glucocorticoids are commonly administered on alternating days with this drug.
WBC, white blood cell.

- Surgery for cranial cruciate ligament rupture in immune-mediated polyarthropathies should be considered with a very guarded prognosis due to ongoing joint destruction.

Supportive Care

- As in osteoarthritis, lifestyle modification, weight reduction, and exercise restriction aid in managing immune-mediated arthropathies.

PROGNOSIS

Nonerosive Forms

The prognosis for type I to III forms is favorable; it is guarded for type IV due to the presence of neoplasia. The breed-specific diseases differ in prognosis. The arthritis of Akitas and Shar-Peis has a poor prognosis. SLE patients may frequently relapse. The polyarthritis-myositis syndrome of spaniels has a guarded to good prognosis and the polyarthritis-meningitis syndrome in other dogs has a good prognosis. Drug-induced polyarthropathies usually respond to cessation of drug therapy. The nonerosive form of feline progressive polyarthritis has a guarded prognosis.

Erosive Forms

Canine rheumatoid arthritis can be difficult to treat successfully and may be expensive, especially if gold salt therapy is needed. Greyhound polyarthritis and the erosive forms of feline progressive polyarthritis have poor prognoses.

SUPPLEMENTAL READINGS

Bennet D: Treatment of the immune-based inflammatory arthropathies of the dog and cat. *In* Kirk RW, ed.: Current Veterinary Therapy: Small Animal Practice, 12th Ed. Philadelphia: WB Saunders, 1995, pp 1188–1195.

Bennet D: Immune-based non-erosive inflammatory joint disease of the dog. Part 3: Canine idiopathic polyarthritis. J Small Anim Pract 28:909, 1987.

Goring RL, Beale BS: Immune-mediated arthropathies. *In* Bojrab MJ, ed.: Pathophysiology in Small Animal Surgery, 2nd Ed. Philadelphia: Lea & Febiger, 1993, pp 742–757.

10 Nervous System

Michael Podell

144 Diagnostic Approach to Neurologic Disease

William R. Fenner

PRINCIPLES OF NEUROLOGIC EXAMINATION

Objectives

- Confirm that neurologic disease is present.
- Localize the site of any lesion(s).
- Determine the extent to which the nervous system is involved.
- Guide the choice of diagnostic aids.
- Determine the prognosis.

Approach

- Perform the examination in a logical, methodical, and consistent manner.
- Develop a consistent sequence and follow it with all patients.
- Begin with the general and advance to the specific.
- Perform painful portions of the examination last.

PROCEDURES FOR THE NEUROLOGIC EXAMINATION

General Observations

Mental Status

Mental status is regulated by the brain stem and cerebrum and consists of level and content of consciousness.

- Begin by evaluating the level of consciousness. A normal animal is alert; an abnormal animal is depressed, stuporous, or comatose, depending on the severity of the mental depression. Abnormal levels of consciousness may result from lesions of the brain stem or diffuse cerebral disease.
- In addition to the level of consciousness, evaluate the patient for mentational disorders. Behavior of a normal animal is described as appropriate; an animal with abnormal behavior is considered demented.
  - A demented animal is unaware and unconcerned with its surroundings. It may head-press, walk off tables, and in other ways show a complete disregard for its own safety and well-being.
  - Dementia is a sign of a cerebral disorder.

Head Posture

Head posture is regulated by the vestibular system and strength of neck muscles.

- A normal animal holds its head in a plane parallel to the ground.
- If an animal holds one ear closer to the ground than the other ear, it is described as having a head tilt, which suggests a vestibular injury.
- In some animals, the chin is tucked under or pulled tightly toward the sternum; this postural abnormality (ventroflexion) may be seen in cats with polymyopathies (e.g., hypokalemia) or thiamine deficiency and in dogs with atlanto-axial-occipital malformations.

Coordination of Head Movement

This is regulated primarily by the cerebellum. Disturbances of head coordination appear as head tremors.

Circling

Circling is a nonspecific finding in animals with brain disease.

- A lesion in any part of the brain may cause circling; the animal usually circles toward the diseased side.
- Circling in brain stem and cerebellar injury usually is a result of a vestibular dysfunction; therefore, circling is accompanied by a head tilt.
- Animals with cerebral injury circle, but they rarely have head tilts.

Gait and Stance

Gait

A normal gait requires integration of almost the entire nervous system; therefore, abnormal gaits may result from injury to almost any part of the nervous system.

- Sensory disturbances, such as loss of proprioception, usually result in ataxia or loss of coordination of limb movements. Signs of loss of coordination of the limbs include swaying, veering, crossing over of the limbs, and scuffing of the toes.

▼ **Key Point** Ataxia may be seen with disease or injury of the cerebellum, brain stem, spinal cord, and injuries to peripheral nerves such as the spinal nerves or cranial nerve 8 (vestibular nerve). Cerebral lesions rarely cause ataxia.

- Cerebellar lesions cause ataxia in most patients.
- Cerebral lesions produce weakness characterized by stumbling, falling, tripping, and inability to initiate or sustain activity. Weakness may be caused by an injury to the cerebrum, brain stem, spinal cord, or peripheral spinal nerves. When classifying the weakness, also consider the resting muscle tone in the limbs.
- Spasticity is an increase in muscle tone resulting in decreased flexion of the limbs during movement. The resultant gait is rigid and choppy.
  - Spasticity implies a lesion of the upper motor neuron (UMN), and may be seen with injuries to the cerebrum, the brain stem, and some levels of the spinal cord.

Stance

Normal animals stand with their limbs at about shoulder or hip width, with the weight equally distributed on all four limbs.

- Abnormal posture may be caused by diminished position sense (proprioception), weakness, or pain.
- Many animals present with abnormal posture as the result of pain from orthopedic disorders rather than neurologic disturbances.

Tests of Postural Reactions

Attitudinal and postural (A-P) reactions test the integrity of the interconnecting pathways that regulate posture and movement as an extension of the evaluation of gait and stance. These tests evaluate the proprioceptive fibers of peripheral nerve, spinal cord, brain stem, cerebrum, and cerebellum. Some tests also evaluate special proprioception. The upper motor neurons and their connections to lower motor neurons are also evaluated.

Because so many portions of the nervous system are evaluated, A-P reactions are good screening tools for detecting nervous system disorders but are not very helpful with specific localization.

- With lesions of the cerebrum, the clinical deficit normally is seen in the limbs on the opposite side of the body (contralateral) from the diseased hemisphere.
- With brain stem lesions, the clinical signs usually are bilateral but are worse on the same side (ipsilateral) as the brain stem injury.
- With lesions of the cerebellum, spinal cord, and peripheral nerves, the clinical signs are almost always on the same side of the body as the nervous system injury.
- With cerebellar injuries, A-P reactions usually are present but are ataxic.
- With peripheral vestibular injuries, A-P reactions are preserved, but the animal tends to lean, fall, and roll to the diseased side when the maneuvers are performed.
- With lesions in other regions in the nervous system, A-P reactions generally are lost or absent.

Proprioceptive Positioning

Abnormally abduct or adduct a limb, or turn the paw so that the animal bears weight on the dorsal surface of its paw (stands knuckled over). If A-P reactions are intact, the animal briskly brings the limb back to a normal resting position.

Hemihopping

Hold the limbs on one side off the ground while the patient is hopped sideways on its other two limbs. A normal animal has no trouble maintaining itself during this test.

Wheelbarrowing

Hold the thoracic or pelvic limbs off the ground while the patient is walked forward and then backward on its other two limbs. A normal animal has no trouble maintaining itself and walking normally during this test.

Other A-P Reactions

Additional A-P reactions include the extensor postural thrust reaction, righting reaction, visual placing reactions, tactile placing reactions, and tonic neck reactions. All these tests evaluate the same basic pathways, although each may test one portion of the nervous system more completely than another. These tests are well described in standard neurology texts.

Cranial Nerve (CN) Examination

The CN examination tests the function of each CN. Often a CN deficit confirms the presence of a lesion above the foramen magnum. The CN examination allows precise localization of intracranial diseases in many cases. Because many CNs supply only the motor or the sensory component of a CN reflex, but not both, the testing of a CN reflex generally involves testing more than one nerve. This is unlike spinal reflexes in which generally the sensory and motor components of a reflex are both carried by the same nerve.

Many of the CN reflexes also are under higher control. Therefore, a CN reflex evaluates:

- two peripheral CNs (one motor and one sensory)
- a central connection (usually the brain stem)
- a higher regulatory center (usually the cerebrum)

A lesion in any one of these sites may cause loss of the reflex being tested. For a more complete review of the neuroanatomy of CNs, consult a neuroanatomy textbook.

Menace Response (Also see Chap. 160)

The menace response tests CN2 (sensory) and CN7 (motor) and their central connections in the brain stem and cerebrum. The test is performed by making a menacing gesture toward an animal. The normal response is an avoidance response (for example, an eye blink or turning of the head).

- Loss of the menace response normally indicates a lesion in one of the following sites: retina (ipsilateral), optic nerve (ipsilateral), optic tract (contralateral), cerebrum (contralateral), brain stem (ipsilateral), or facial nerve (CN7) (ipsilateral).
- Some animals with cerebellar disorders may have an ipsilateral loss of the menace response as well.
- False-positive menace responses also occur, most commonly when the movement of the hand produces air currents that stimulate the corneal reflex.
- Sounds and other distractions may make the menace response difficult to evaluate.

Pupillary Light Reflex (PLR) (Also see Chap. 160)

This tests the reflex portion of the optic nerve (CN2) and the visceral function of the oculomotor nerves (CN3). The test is performed by illuminating the eye with a bright light source. The normal response is rapid constriction of both pupils.

The pupillary constriction in the eye being illuminated is called the *direct pupillary response*. The constriction in the opposite pupil (the one being illuminated indirectly) is called the *consensual response*. Failure of one or both pupils to constrict is an abnormal PLR.

- A lesion of CN2 produces loss of constriction in both pupils when the affected eye is illuminated; however, when the normal eye is illuminated, both pupils constrict.

- If the lesion is in CN3 or the brain stem, the affected pupil fails to constrict regardless of which eye is being illuminated, but the unaffected eye constricts normally when each eye is illuminated.
- Because ophthalmic diseases such as posterior synechia or severe iris atrophy may also produce loss of pupillary responsiveness, a thorough eye examination is essential in any patient with abnormal pupils.
- Other causes of a misleading PLR are increased sympathetic tone and a weak light source, both of which will slow the PLR.

Pupillary Symmetry

In this test the eyes are observed for equal pupils.

- If CN3 and the sympathetic nerve to the eye are normal, the two pupils will be equal in size.
- If the pupils are unequal (anisocoria), this indicates possible damage to one of these two nerves.
  - If CN3 is abnormal, the large pupil is denervated and the PLR will be absent in that eye.
  - If the sympathetic nerve is abnormal, the small pupil is abnormal and the PLR will be normal in both eyes.
- Cats may have mild physiologic anisocoria if one eye is receiving more light than the other. For this reason, ensure that both eyes receive equal illumination when evaluating for anisocoria.
- A number of ophthalmic disorders may produce anisocoria, including glaucoma, iritis, uveitis, and synechia. Because of this, perform a complete ophthalmic examination on all patients with anisocoria.

Pupillary Size

The size of the pupil is determined by the amount of ambient light (CN2) and the integrity of the innervation of the pupillary muscles (CN3 and sympathetic nerve).

- Abnormally large pupils may be caused by excitement (sympathetic stimulation), bilateral optic nerve injury, CN3 paralysis, or ophthalmic disease.
- Abnormally small pupils may be associated with loss of sympathetic tone, excess parasympathetic tone, or ophthalmic disease.

Ocular Position

In normal dogs and cats, both eyes look in the same direction at any given time (normally straight ahead). This normal resting position is determined by the influence of the cerebrum and CN8 on the extraocular muscles (CN3, 4, and 6). If one of these portions of the nervous system is not functioning, deviation of one or both of the eyeballs may occur.

Strabismus is deviation of only one globe.

- Medial strabismus may result from an injury to CN6 (abducens nerve).
- Ventrolateral strabismus may result from injury to CN3 or CN8 (vestibulocochlear nerve).
- A lesion to CN4 (trochlear nerve) results in intorsion (a form of rotation) of the eye, which can be recog-

nized only in animals with oval pupils or on ophthalmic examination.

- Passive deviation of both eyes in the same direction (gaze paresis) is sometimes seen in cerebral injuries.

Ocular Motility

Voluntary Eye Movement

Voluntary eye movement is initiated by cerebral stimulation of CNs 3, 4, and 6. As the animal looks around the examination room, observe to see if it appears unable to move the eyes in one or more directions.

- With a cerebral lesion, both eyes are involved, and there is a tendency for the eyes to look toward the diseased cerebral hemisphere.
- With a lesion of the cranial nerves, only one eye is involved. The involved eye will tend to have strabismus at rest and totally lack the ability to move.

Involuntary Eye Movements—Nystagmus

Involuntary rhythmic oscillations of the eyes, termed nystagmus, can be induced by turning the head. This maneuver stimulates CN8, which in turn stimulates CN3, 4, and 6, which innervate the extraocular muscles. This involuntary eye movement is called physiologic nystagmus.

Physiologic Nystagmus. Physiologic nystagmus is characterized by rhythmic oscillation of both eyes, first moving slowly away from the direction in which the head is turning, and then moving rapidly in the same direction. This recurring slow-fast, slow-fast oscillation continues as long as the head is moving.

- A lesion of CN8 or its central connections may result in loss of the ability to initiate physiologic nystagmus, so that neither eye will move.
- A lesion of one or more of the cranial nerves that innervate the eyeball itself (CN3, 4, or 6) paralyzes only that eye, resulting in loss of physiologic nystagmus in the paralyzed eye.

Pathologic Nystagmus. When a normal animal's head is not moving, it does not display any involuntary eye movements. If nystagmus is present when the head is at rest, this is a sign of nervous system disease and is called pathologic nystagmus. This usually is the result of an imbalance in the special proprioceptive system, which includes the inner ear, brain stem, cerebellum, and CN8. A lesion of any of these structures can cause pathologic nystagmus. Features of pathologic nystagmus that may help localize its origin include the *direction*, *method of induction*, and *persistence* of the nystagmus.

- Direction of nystagmus:
  - In *horizontal nystagmus*, the eyes move in a plane parallel to the head (i.e., the eyes move from side to side).

▼ *Key Point* Horizontal nystagmus is most commonly seen in peripheral vestibular disease (see Chap. 57). The "fast" component of the nystagmus usually is away from the diseased side.

- In *vertical nystagmus*, the eyes move in a plane perpendicular to the head (e.g., the eyes move up and down).

▼ *Key Point* Vertical nystagmus is most commonly seen in central vestibular disease. The fast component of the nystagmus is usually away from the diseased side; therefore, brain stem disease causes upgoing nystagmus, and cerebellar disease causes downgoing nystagmus.

- In *rotatory nystagmus*, the eyes rotate in a clockwise or counterclockwise direction in the orbit, with components of both horizontal and vertical movement. This type of nystagmus is not localizing; it may occur with a lesion anywhere in the special proprioceptive system.
- Method of induction of nystagmus:
  - *Resting nystagmus* occurs when the head is at rest and in a normal position. This type of nystagmus is most characteristic of peripheral vestibular disease.
  - *Positional or induced nystagmus* occurs when the head is still but is in an abnormal position (e.g., on its side or upside down). Positional nystagmus is most characteristic of central vestibular dysfunction (e.g., brain stem and cerebellar lesions). It is also seen during the recovery phase of peripheral vestibular diseases.
- Persistence of nystagmus:
  - *Permanent nystagmus* persists over time. It may have any direction and method of induction, but it is consistently present. Permanent nystagmus is characteristic of all brain stem diseases and of progressive peripheral vestibular and cerebellar diseases.
  - *Resolving nystagmus* disappears over a period of 10–14 days. It does not recur unless there is new damage to the vestibular system. Resolving nystagmus is characteristic of nonprogressive peripheral vestibular and cerebellar diseases. In this period, nystagmus may become positional (recovery phase).

Facial Symmetry

Facial weakness (CN7) may result from injury to the contralateral cerebrum, ipsilateral brain stem, and ipsilateral peripheral nerve.

- Clinical signs include drooping of the lip, deviation of the nasal philtrum, increases in palpebral fissure (pseudoptosis), and in some animals true ptosis (drooping of the eyelid).
- Confirm the diminished muscle function by testing the palpebral and/or corneal reflexes.

Palpebral Reflex

This reflex tests CN5 and its brain stem connection to CN7.

- Initiate the reflex by touching the palpebral margins, which produces an eye blink. Loss of the eye blink is usually complete.

- In some animals with incomplete paresis of CN5 or CN7, lagophthalmos or incomplete closure of the palpebral margins is observed.

Corneal Reflex

Like the palpebral reflex, this reflex tests CN5 and its brain stem connection to CN7.

- Initiate the reflex by lightly touching the cornea, which produces an eye blink.

Retractor Oculi Reflex

This reflex tests CN5 and its brain stem connection to CN6 (abducens nerve).

- Initiate the reflex by lightly touching the cornea, which produces retraction of the eye into the orbit.
- Lack of the reflex usually is a sign of neurologic dysfunction.
- In some animals with loss of the retrobulbar fat pad, the eye may be enophthalmic and incapable of retraction, whereas in others, a retrobulbar mass may prevent retraction.

Facial Sensory Examination

This tests CN5 and its cerebral connections.

- Lightly stimulate the nasal mucosa, which should produce an avoidance response such as head turning.
- The nasal mucosa is a more reliable site for stimulation than the lips, which are relatively insensitive in some animals.

Gag Reflex

The gag reflex, which is easier to test in dogs than in cats, tests CN9 (glossopharyngeal nerve) and CN10 (vagus nerve) and their brain stem connections.

- To initiate the test, lightly stimulate the oropharynx, which should produce a swallowing reflex. Loss of the reflex usually indicates brain stem or peripheral nerve dysfunction.
- Examine the pharynx for evidence of paralysis of the soft palate, and look at the larynx for evidence of laryngeal paralysis (may be difficult in an awake animal). Either condition may result from brain stem injuries or peripheral nerve injuries to CN9 or CN10.

Tongue Examination

- Look for atrophy of the tongue, which can be produced by brain stem or peripheral nerve injury to CN12.
- Also look for deviation of the tongue, which can be caused by cerebral injuries as well as brain stem and peripheral nerve injuries.

Spinal Reflex Examination

The spinal segmental reflexes directly test the reflex arcs of the spinal cord. They also indirectly test the higher centers in the brain that regulate the spinal reflexes.

▼ *Key Point* If an injury occurs within the reflex arc, it will cause loss of the reflex. Such a reflex loss allows precise localization of a nervous system injury. Because a lesion in the lower motor neuron (LMN) is involved, loss of reflexes is called an LMN sign or an LMN reflex change.

▼ *Key Point* If a lesion occurs cranial to a reflex arc, it disconnects the reflex from its higher (brain) regulation. This regulation tends to be inhibitory, and thus loss of regulation results in exaggeration of reflexes. Because this exaggeration reflects a lesion in the CNS, involving upper motor neuron (UMN) pathways, these reflex changes are called UMN signs or UMN reflexes.

UMN changes are not as precisely localizing as LMN reflexes. Spinal reflexes are classified into three groups:

- Proprioceptive reflexes
- Nociceptive reflexes
- Special (released) reflexes

This division is based on the type of sensory stimulation required to elicit the first two reflexes and on the special conditions required to elicit the third reflex.

Proprioceptive Reflexes

These myotatic reflexes are initiated by stretch of tendons or muscle spindles. They have a strong influence from the UMN and therefore are likely to be exaggerated with UMN lesions. Increases and decreases in the force of reflex activity are both components of proprioceptive reflexes; thus, be sure to grade the strength of these reflexes. A standard grading scale is:

0 = absent reflex
1 = diminished reflex
2 = normal reflex
3 = increased reflex
4 = increased reflexes with clonus

Thoracic Limb Proprioceptive Reflexes

Triceps Reflex. This tests the radial nerve and arises from spinal cord segments C7–T2.

- Elicit by striking the tendon of insertion of the triceps muscle. A normal response is a slight extension of the elbow.
- Often it is difficult to obtain and, when present, to interpret this reflex in normal animals.

Extensor Carpi Radialis Reflex. Like the triceps reflex, this tests the radial nerve and spinal cord segments C7–T2.

- Elicit by striking the muscle belly of the extensor carpi radialis muscle, which results in extension of the carpus.
- This reflex is easier to elicit than the triceps reflex.

Biceps Reflex. This reflex evaluates the musculocutaneous nerve, which arises from spinal cord segments C6–C7.

- Initiate by striking the tendon of insertion of the biceps tendon, causing a slight flexion of the elbow.
- This reflex is more difficult to obtain than the triceps reflex and is difficult to interpret.

Pelvic Limb Proprioceptive Reflexes

Patellar Reflex. This reflex tests the femoral nerve and its cord segments (L4–L6).

- Elicit by striking the patellar tendon, producing extension of the stifle.
- When testing this reflex, a phenomenon known as a *false localizing sign* sometimes occurs, because paralysis of the sciatic nerve results in a hyperactive patellar reflex. It may be due to functional loss of the antagonist muscles that oppose the extensors of the stifle.

Cranial Tibialis Reflex. This reflex tests the peroneal branch of the sciatic nerve, which originates from spinal cord segments L2–S2.

- Initiate by striking the belly of the cranial tibial muscle. The normal response is flexion of the tarsus.

Gastrocnemius Reflex. This reflex tests the tibial branch of the sciatic nerve, which originates from spinal cord segments L6–S2.

- Elicit by striking the belly of the gastrocnemius muscle or its tendon of insertion. The expected normal response is extension of the tarsus; however, many patients have flexion of the tarsus.

Nociceptive Spinal Reflexes

The nociceptive reflexes are initiated by nociceptive (painful) stimuli, such as pinching, compression, and pin pricks, that induce withdrawal of the limb or some other reflex action. These reflexes only test the integrity of a spinal reflex arc.

▼ *Key Point* The fact that reflex withdrawal is present tells nothing about the health of the nociceptive pathways traveling cranially to the brain. The most significant change seen is loss of a nociceptive reflex, which indicates an LMN lesion.

These reflexes do not have a large UMN influence; therefore, they do not normally become exaggerated with UMN lesions.

Thoracic Flexor Reflex. This reflex utilizes all the peripheral nerves of the thoracic limb and tests spinal cord segments C6–T2.

- Elicit by digital compression. The normal response is withdrawal of the limb from the source of the stimulus.
- Loss of the reflex indicates a lesion in the reflex arc.

Pelvic Limb Flexor Reflexes. These reflexes test the sciatic nerve and its branches and L6–S2 nerve roots, the fibers go to form the sciatic nerve.

- Initiate by digital compression. The normal response is withdrawal of the limb from the source of the stimulus.

- Loss of this reflex indicates a lesion in the reflex arc.

Perineal Reflexes. The most commonly used is the *anal reflex,* which tests the perineal and pudendal nerves, spinal cord segments S1–S3, and the cauda equina.

- Initiate by lightly pricking or stroking the perianal skin. The expected response is constriction of the anal sphincter and flexion of the tail.
- If a mild weakness is suspected, it is best to test the reflex during a digital rectal examination, in order to estimate the strength of contracture of the sphincter.

Special (Released) Reflexes

These are reflexes that are suppressed by the UMN in normal animals. When disconnection between the reflex arc and the UMN occurs, these reflexes become released or uninhibited. Thus, the presence of these reflexes indicates loss of UMN inhibition to a reflex arc.

Babinski Reflex. This occurs only in the pelvic limbs.

- Elicit by lightly stroking the plantar aspect of the metatarsus. In a normal animal, the toes either are unaffected or flex slightly.
- In the presence of UMN disease, the toes spread apart and elevate (dorsiflex), which is known as a positive Babinski reflex.

Crossed Extensor Reflex. This abnormal reflex may be seen in any limb.

- Initiate by eliciting a flexor response in an animal in lateral recumbency. In a normal animal, the limb being stimulated flexes and the contralateral, paired limb is unaffected.
- In UMN disease, when the stimulated limb flexes, the contralateral paired limb will involuntarily extend.

▼ *Key Point* The crossed extension reflex is a consistent sign of UMN dysfunction.

Nociceptive Evaluation

Nociceptive evaluation (testing pain responses) is a logical continuation of the flexor reflexes that tests for more than simple reflex withdrawal of the limbs. Cerebral recognition of pain perception is essential for a positive response to these tests.

Decreased Pain Perception

A mild loss in pain perception is called *hypalgesia* or *hypesthesia.* If the loss is total it is referred to as *analgesia* or *anesthesia.*

- Loss of pain perception is tested by producing enough pain so that cerebral recognition occurs and a reaction is produced.
- To elicit reaction, compress the digits vigorously. The expected response is turning of the head and/or vocalization.

This evaluation tests peripheral nerves, spinal cord, brain stem, and cerebrum. The cerebellum is not involved in the nociceptive pathways.

▼ *Key Point* Peripheral nerve lesions usually cause focal sensory loss, confined to the distribution of the involved nerve(s), Spinal cord lesions cause a bilateral, symmetric sensory loss proceeding caudally from the approximate level of the injury.

- Brain stem lesions rarely produce detectable analgesia, because a lesion of that severity would result in the death of the animal.
- Cerebral lesions produce only hypalgesia.
- The sensory deficit with a cerebral lesion is unilateral and is contralateral to the diseased hemisphere.

Increased Sensitivity or Exaggerated Response to Pain

Hyperesthesia refers to increased sensitivity; *hyperpathia* is an exaggerated response to pain. In veterinary medicine these two terms are used interchangeably.

Exaggerated responsiveness to pain is tested by digital manipulation of the paraspinal muscles, stimulation of the paraspinal region with a hemostat or safety pin, or a similar maneuver.

- The objective is to produce a recognizable stimulus that is not normally bothersome to the patient.
- This stimulus is applied up and down the spine, looking for an area where the patient shows an unusually acute response to the stimulus.

- An exaggerated response usually is an indication of a nerve root or meningeal lesion (e.g., herniated disc or meningitis).

▼ *Key Point* Paraspinal stimulation is valuable for localizing spinal cord lesions, because a hyperpathic response indicates that the problem is extramedullary and establishes the location of the lesion.

INTERPRETATION OF THE NEUROLOGIC EXAMINATION

Make a list of abnormal findings, along with a list of the anatomic regions of the nervous system. Mark each anatomic region where a lesion could produce the listed findings (Fig. 144–1), and then ask yourself the following questions:

- Does the patient have a neurologic disease?
  - If there are pluses after any of the listed findings, answer this question in the affirmative.
- Is the disease in the CNS or PNS?
  - If the animal has CN deficits, use your evaluation of the limbs and mental status to answer this question.
  - If there are only isolated cranial nerve deficits with no other signs, the lesion probably is in the PNS.
  - If there are CN deficits, plus limb signs, the lesion probably is in the CNS.

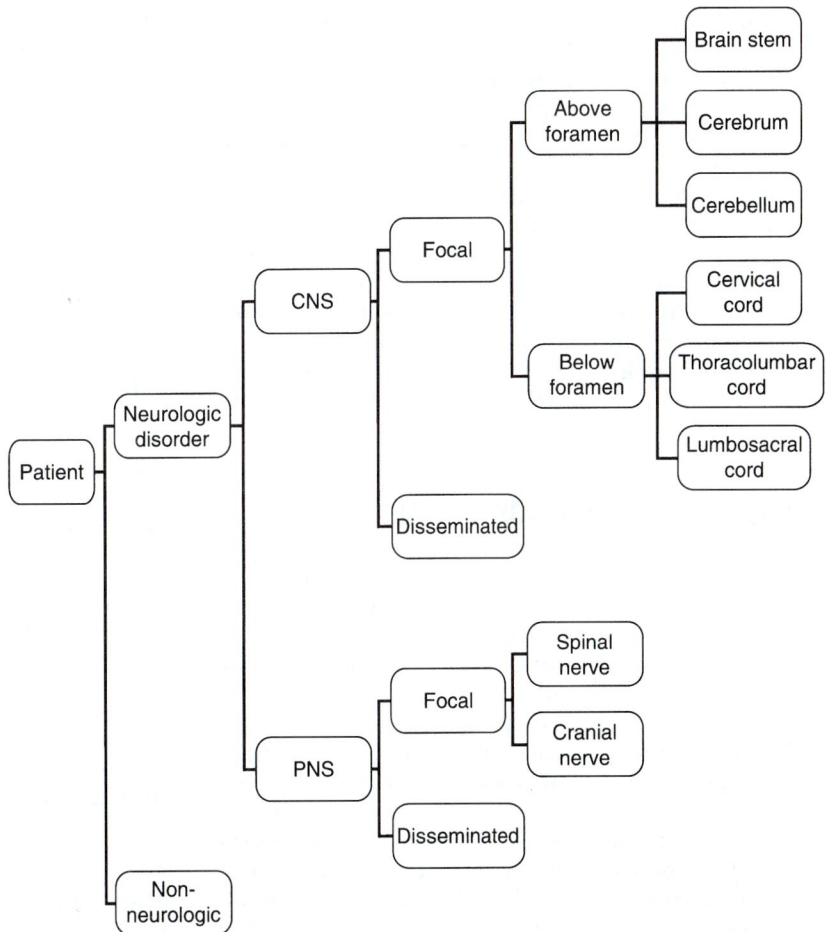

Figure 144–1. Localization flow chart. (CNS, central nervous system; PNS, peripheral nervous system.)

- If the disease is below the foramen magnum and UMN reflex changes are present, the lesion probably is in the CNS.
- If all spinal reflexes are LMN reflexes, the lesion probably is in the PNS.
- Is the disease above or below the foramen magnum?
  - If the animal has a CN abnormality, history of seizures, abnormal head posture, abnormal head coordination, or abnormal level of consciousness, the lesion is likely to be above the foramen magnum.
  - If the lesion involves the limbs alone, the lesion is most likely below the foramen.
- At this point in the interpretation of the neurologic examination, negative findings become as important as positive findings.
  - For example, a UMN tetraparetic patient may have a cerebral, brain stem, or cervical cord injury.
  - If the patient has no head signs, look for a cord lesion based on the negative head findings combined with the positive limb findings.
- After you have localized the lesion (above or below the foramen; CNS or PNS), try to localize the lesion more precisely.
- What do you gain by localizing the disease?
  - You will know whether the problem is focal or disseminated; the etiologies are different for each class.
  - Disseminated diseases usually are caused by inflammation, metabolic diseases, and degenerations.
  - Focal diseases usually are caused by masses, trauma, and vascular lesions.
  - Localization automatically eliminates some differentials from the diagnosis.
  - For example, a cat with signs suggesting a focal cerebral mass would not have an intervertebral disc extrusion as the cause of the problem.
  - Localization also helps in choosing diagnostic aids because certain diagnostic tools are only of value with lesions in certain anatomic regions.
  - An example is the electroencephalogram, which is helpful only in patients with cerebral injuries. Using this tool in a patient with peripheral nerve disease is a misdirected effort and a waste of the client's money.

SELECTION OF DIAGNOSTIC AIDS

Diagnostic aids are laboratory tests and procedures that help to determine which differential diagnosis is the most likely cause of the patient's signs. The primary purpose of a diagnostic aid is to provide etiologic information. As a consequence of establishing a diagnosis, these tests may also provide prognostic information. In addition, some tests provide anatomic information, allowing "fine-tuning" of the results of the neurologic examination.

Diagnostic aids used in evaluation of the nervous system include general screening tests such as routine serum biochemistries and blood counts, that identify metabolic and toxic injuries to the nervous system. Also included are specific tests of nervous system anatomy

(e.g., neuroradiology), function (e.g., cerebrospinal fluid analysis, electrodiagnostic tests), or both (e.g., electromyography).

To select the most appropriate diagnostic aids, combine historical information with neurologic examination findings. After interpreting results of the diagnostic aids, the diagnosis should be evident.

GENERAL SCREENING TESTS

Hematology

Limitations

In the majority of patients with nervous system disease, there are minimal hematologic changes. There are exceptions, such as encephalitis and systemic disease that secondarily affect the nervous system (e.g., lead poisoning).

Positive Results

White Blood Cell (WBC) Changes. Elevation of WBC numbers often indicates an inflammatory disease process; however, a low WBC count may be seen in viral infections.

Red Blood Cell (RBC) Changes. Anemia, if profound, may result in hypoxia and cerebral signs. An abnormally high RBC count (polycythemia) with increased serum viscosity can cause diminished blood flow to muscles and produce a myasthenia-like syndrome. It also may result in sludging of cerebral blood flow with subsequent CNS infarction.

Biochemical Tests

These tests help evaluate animals with metabolic illness. Because the cerebrum has very high metabolic demands, it is affected by many generalized metabolic disorders. The motor unit also appears susceptible to a wide variety of generalized metabolic insults. Examples of biochemical abnormalities that have an impact on the nervous system include hypo- and hyperglycemia, hypo- and hypercalcemia, hypo- and hyperkalemia, hypo- and hypernatremia, acidosis and alkalosis, uremia, hyperammonemia, hyperlipidemia, and hyperviscosity from dysproteinemia.

Urinalysis

Many metabolic diseases that affect the nervous system produce changes in the urine. In addition, many CNS infections affect the urinary system; therefore, evaluation of urinalysis may be helpful in CNS infections.

Fecal Analysis

Severe parasitism has been reported as a cause of CNS disease in young animals.

Serology

Many viral, fungal, and protozoal infections of the nervous system result in the development of antibodies. These antibodies may be assayed in the patient's serum or in CSF (refer to the chapters in the Infectious Disease section for specific information).

Immunofluorescence

Some viral infections that affect the nervous system may be diagnosed by using immunofluorescent techniques to detect antigen in CSF or nervous tissue (the latter is reserved for postmortem examination).

Toxicology

Blood can be assayed for many toxins known to affect the nervous system (e.g., lead poisoning).

NEURORADIOGRAPHY AND SPECIAL IMAGING

Radiography, with or without enhancing techniques, can be used to visualize the supporting structures of the nervous system and in some cases the nervous system itself. These studies provide information about CNS anatomy and can reveal structural abnormalities, but generally do not provide information about neurologic function (see Chap. 4 for additional information about neuroradiography).

Positioning of the animal, proper exposure techniques, and choice of contrast (when appropriate) are important when performing neuroradiography.

Positioning

At least two views at 90° angles are required for proper identification of abnormalities. Because of the irregular shape of most structures evaluated in neuroradiology, proper positioning is critical. Most neuroradiographs are taken with the patient under anesthesia.

Radiographic Density

The spinal cord and discs appear less dense because they are surrounded by bone; thus, in many cases disc and cord evaluation depend on identification of changes in supporting structures. A short scale of contrast is preferred for spinal radiographs (see Chap. 4).

Plain Radiography of the Spine

- *Indications:* to localize surgical lesions and to diagnose nonsurgical lesions of bone tissue.
- *Advantage:* noninvasive and allows diagnosis of bony lesions
- *Disadvantages:* requires anesthesia; false-negative results are common.

Myelography

- For myelography of the spine, inject positive (radiopaque) contrast material into the subarachnoid space to outline the spinal cord before taking radiographs (see Chap. 4).
- *Indications:* to localize surgical lesions and to diagnose nonsurgical lesions of soft tissue, such as intramedullary tumors or vascular lesions.
- *Advantage:* allows diagnosis of soft tissue lesions.

- *Disadvantages:* requires anesthesia; causes mild meningitis, and may worsen underlying cord injury; false-negative (degenerations and small mass lesions) and false-positive (air bubbles in dye column, extradural dye) results can occur.

Interpretation (Location of Lesions)

- *Extradural*—most common; usually a lesion involving the discs or vertebrae
- *Intramedullary*—cord swelling from any cause (e.g., edema, tumor, or hemorrhage)
- *Intradural and extramedullary*—quite rare; usually a tumor of the meninges or peripheral nerve sheath

Skull Radiography

The skull is a complex structure composed of about 50 different bones. There are three basic head shapes in dogs: brachiocephalic (short head), mesaticephalic (intermediate head), and dolicocephalic (long head).

Positioning

The normal bilateral symmetry of the skull is helpful in radiographic evaluation. Because good positioning is extremely important, obtain radiographs with the animal under anesthesia.

- On lateral views, elevate the nose to keep the skull parallel to the x-ray plate.
- Routine views of the skull include lateral and either ventrodorsal (VD) or dorsoventral (DV).
- Special views are taken for the tympanic bullae, foramen magnum, nasal passages, and teeth.
- See Chapter 4 for more details of skull radiography.

Normal Findings

The dorsal calvaria are of uniform thickness, with the thickness appropriate for the breed.

- Convolutional markings can be seen on the inside of the skull, which represent the normal indentations of the sulci and gyri of the brain.
- The nasal passages and frontal sinuses contain air outlining delicate bone turbinates.

Abnormal Findings

See Table 144–1.

Computerized Tomography (CT)

See Chapter 4.

Magnetic Resonance Imaging (MRI)

See Chapter 4.

CEREBROSPINAL FLUID (CSF) COLLECTION AND ANALYSIS

Factors Affecting CSF Production

- *Drugs:* Furosemide decreases the rate of production by 50%. Furosemide dosages of 0.9–2.0 mg/kg have

---

Table 144–1. RADIOGRAPHIC LESIONS OF THE SKULL AND SPINE SEEN ON RADIOGRAPHY

Congenital Lesions of the Skull
Hydrocephalus
Occipital dysplasia

Congenital Lesions of the Spine
Cervical vertebral instability (canine wobbler syndrome, spondylolisthesis)
Cervical vertebral stenosis
Atlantoaxial malformation

Traumatic Lesions
Skull: fractures
Spine: fractures, fracture-luxation

Infectious Lesions
Skull: middle ear infections, rhinosinusitis
Spine: discospondylitis

Neoplasia of the Skull or Spine

Degenerative Lesions of the Spine
Spondylosis
Spinal arthritis (spondylitis)
Degenerative intervertebral disc disease

Lesions Seen on Myelography
Intervertebral disc disease
Spinal vertebral body lesions (tumors or abscesses)
Spinal cord tumors
Spinal cord hemorrhage or edema

---

been reported to be effective in lowering CSF pressure.

- *Hydrostatic pressure:* Increases in CSF pressure have little effect on the rate or volume of CSF production.
- *Osmolality:* Acute serum hyperosmolality lowers production, whereas acute serum hypo-osmolality raises production. A 1% change in osmolality results in a 6.7% change in CSF production, either up or down.

Effects of Elevated Intracranial Pressure

Elevations of intracranial pressure, which produce elevations of CSF pressure, can have devastating effects both on the nervous system and systemically.

- *Nervous system effect*

▼ *Key Point* The most serious sequela to increased CSF pressure is the tendency for herniation of brain contents; this is generally fatal.

- *Systemic effects:* Cardiac arrhythmias, subendocardial hemorrhage, pulmonary edema, gastrointestinal hemorrhage, and gastrointestinal ulceration may occur with elevations of intracranial pressure.

CSF Collection

- *Purpose*
  - To obtain fluid for diagnostic evaluation
  - To introduce contrast agents into the spinal fluid
  - To introduce therapeutic agents into the spinal fluid
- *Indications:*
  - An abnormal neurologic examination
  - Epilepsy

- Recurring fevers
- Chronic pain
- *Contraindications:*
  - Recent CNS trauma
  - Rapidly declining level of consciousness
- *Advantages:* CSF taps are generally safe, inexpensive, and, when positive, very helpful.
- *Disadvantages:*
  - Anesthesia usually is required in small animals.
  - In spinal cord diseases, a lumbosacral tap is preferred, which is technically more difficult than a cerebellomedullary cistern tap.
  - CSF taps often are nondiagnostic except in inflammatory diseases.

Technique

1. Collect CSF for analysis at the cerebellomedullary cistern or by lumbar puncture.
   a. In small animals, the lumbar space is more difficult to enter, yields smaller volumes of fluid, and has a higher rate of blood contamination.
   b. The cerebellomedullary cistern is easier to enter in small animals, yields larger volumes of generally less contaminated fluid, but the resultant sample may not allow evaluation of the spinal cord.
2. The average distance between the skin and subarachnoid space in the cervical spine varies with the size of the patient. Reported distances for dogs and cats are ½ inch for cats and dogs <4.5 kg; ¾ inch for dogs 4.5 to 9.1 kg; 1 inch for dogs 9.1 to 22.7 kg; 1½ inches for dogs 22.7 to 50.9 kg; and 2 inches for dogs >50.9 kg.
3. Collect the CSF by allowing it to drip into a container.

Complications

- The most common complication is blood contamination. This can affect interpretation of results.
- The most serious complication is brain herniation. In the face of elevated intracranial pressure, the pressure shift created by the removal of CSF may precipitate a shift in intracranial contents. This sudden movement of intracranial contents (brain herniation) may result in death.

CSF Analysis

Analysis includes measuring CSF pressure, gross visual examination, cytologic analysis, biochemical analysis, and culture. In addition, serologic procedures may be indicated. There are slightly different normal values for fluid collected from cerebellomedullary and lumbar spaces; thus, note the collection site. Fluid from the cerebellomedullary cistern tends to have slightly more cells and lower protein than fluid from the lumbar space.

Pressure

Opening pressure (OP) is measured at the beginning of collection, using a manometer. Normal values for the dog are dependent on body weight (BW). The published formula for calculation of normal values based on body size for dogs under pentobarbital anesthesia is:

$$OP = 46.5 + 3.83(BW) - 0.048(BW)^2$$

with BW measured in kilograms. Normal pressures using this formula are 50–140 mm H_2O. When measuring CSF pressure, only elevations of pressure above normal are considered significant.

- Severe elevations are considered diagnostic of a space-occupying mass effect such as a tumor.
- Mild to moderate elevations may be seen with encephalitis, meningitis, and hydrocephalus.
- Normal CSF pressure doesn't exclude any of the aforementioned diseases, because pressure is only one piece of the diagnostic puzzle.

Gross Visual Examination

Normal CSF is clear and colorless.

- With inflammation, CSF generally becomes turbid and assumes an off-white to grayish color.
- Pink discoloration is usually caused by blood contamination. Spin the CSF sample down to separate RBCs and examine the supernatant.
- Yellow-orange colored CSF (xanthochromic) generally indicates either breakdown of hemoglobin from previous hemorrhage or severe elevations of CSF protein (>100 mg/dl).

Cytologic Evaluation

Cytologic evaluation consists of a total cell count on unconcentrated CSF, and preparation of a slide from a concentrated CSF sample for evaluation of cell types and differential numbers.

- Perform the total cell count quickly (within 1 hour or less) because cells from CSF begin to degenerate rapidly following collection.
- If the slides cannot be prepared immediately, refrigerate the sample.
- The type and number of cells reflect the cause of the inflammation and thus provide etiologic information.
- Normally there are <5 WBCs/µl.
- 5–10 WBCs/µl suggests disease; >10 WBCs/µl are definitively abnormal if no RBCs are present.
- 5–50 WBCs/µl suggests a mild inflammatory process as seen with viral diseases and some forms of trauma, vascular disease, and neoplasia.
- 50–200 WBCs/µl suggests a moderate inflammation, as seen with fungal, protozoal, and immune diseases, but may also be seen with meningiomas.
- >200 WBCs/µl indicates a marked inflammatory process, as seen with bacterial meningitis and some immune diseases.

Diagnostic Interpretation

Suppurative Meningitis. Suppurative meningitis is diagnosed if the number of cells in the CSF are increased and are predominantly neutrophils. Suppurative meningitis is the most common pathologic response to bacterial encephalitis, although it is also characteristic of acute, severe viral infections of the nervous system, idiopathic vasculitis/meningitis in young dogs, and some tumors (e.g., meningiomas).

Mixed (Granulomatous) Inflammation. Mixed inflammation is diagnosed when the increased number of cells in the CSF are composed of multiple cell types, including macrophages, lymphocytes, neutrophils, and sometimes plasma cells. Although a mixed cytology is generally the result of a granulomatous encephalitis, such as fungal, protozoal, and idiopathic diseases, this cytologic change may also be seen in chronic bacterial infections that are being inadequately treated.

Nonsuppurative Inflammation. Nonsuppurative inflammation is diagnosed when the numbers of cells in the spinal fluid are increased and are composed primarily of mononuclear cells, especially lymphocytes. It is most characteristic of viral and rickettsial infections. Although this type of CSF abnormality is least likely to be due to an acute bacterial infection of the nervous system, it may occur.

Prognostic Value of CSF Cytology. In humans and in experimental studies in animals with bacterial meningitis, there appears to be a correlation between the numbers of WBCs in pretreatment CSF cytology and prognosis. High initial WBC counts were associated with a favorable prognosis. Animals with continued high WBC counts after therapy had a poor prognosis.

Biochemical Evaluation

When evaluating the chemical composition of the CSF, remember that CSF is produced both by active transport and by ultrafiltration. As a result, CSF contains essentially the same constituents as plasma, but they are present in different concentrations. Generally the levels of CSF constituents are lower than the serum levels. The two constituents measured most commonly for diagnostic purposes are *protein* and *glucose.*

Protein Levels. The concentration of protein is quite low in CSF compared to plasma. In dogs and cats, protein from a cerebellomedullary cisternal tap is usually less than 25 mg/dl, whereas that from a lumbar puncture may be as high as 45 mg/dl. This elevation may be the result of an increase in the permeability of the blood-brain barrier, production of immunoglobulins in the intrathecal space, or a combination of both. Conditions known to elevate CSF protein include encephalitis, meningitis, neoplasms, CNS infarctions, and trauma. Analyze CSF protein qualitatively and quantitatively by electrophoresis or immunoelectrophoresis. In normal CSF, albumin composes about 75% of the protein, and most of the remainder is globulin. An increase in CSF globulin without a parallel increase in albumin suggests local immunoglobulin production and encephalitis; even if CSF WBC levels are normal.

Glucose. Normal CSF glucose levels are about 60–80% of those in blood. In humans, the ratio between blood glucose and CSF glucose is routinely lower in bacterial infections. There does not appear to be a similar relationship between bacterial encephalitis and decreased CSF glucose in dogs. Plasma glucose can decrease dramatically in the presence of septicemia and bacteremia. A meningitic patient that is also bacteremic will likely have a drop in CSF glucose.

CSF Serologic Examination

The CSF may be examined serologically for antibodies against infectious agents (as well as for bacterial antigens as mentioned above). Detection of antibodies may be helpful in the diagnosis of viral, fungal, and rickettsial diseases, but are less helpful in bacterial encephalitis. Little or no antibody is present in normal animals. In most circumstances, the presence of antibodies is an indication of local immunoglobulin production, indicating that the organism against which the antibodies are found is the cause of the encephalitis.

A limitation of serology is that paired titers are required for greatest accuracy.

False-Positive CSF Antibody Levels

- False-positive antibody levels can be caused by leakage of plasma proteins into the CSF. For example, in encephalitis, fever may transiently open the blood-brain barrier, resulting in some leakage of serum antibodies into the CSF. Those circulating antibodies may be the result of immunity from previous infections or vaccination.
- Increased albumin on CSF electrophoresis supports a false-positive diagnosis, as does comparison of CSF with simultaneous serum antibody titer measurement.

ELECTROENCEPHALOGRAPHY

Electroencephalography (EEG) is the graphic recording of shifts in resting membrane potential of the dendritic network in the superficial layers of cerebral cortex. This network is influenced and modulated by the activity of subcortical nuclear centers such as the reticular formation.

Evaluation of abnormal EEG patterns allows identification of the area of the brain where these patterns originate. This information can be used to differentiate between possible etiologies.

- *Indications:* EEG evaluation is indicated for patients suspected of having:
  - Any type of cerebral dysfunction
  - A multifocal disease, in order to discern if the cerebrum is involved.
- *Advantages:* EEG is noninvasive, is relatively inexpensive, and frequently can be performed without chemical restraint in the dog.
- *Disadvantages:*
  - EEG tracings can be artifact-laden and difficult to interpret.
  - Tracings may be affected by the patient's age, drugs, and normal variations in wakefulness.

Evaluation

The EEG can be a valuable tool if carefully performed (see Table 144–2). However, there is little hard data and

much artifact in animal EEGs. These two facts suggest caution when interpreting EEGs. Consider them to be a piece of data with no more significance than other laboratory tests.

BRAIN STEM AUDITORY EVOKED RESPONSE (BAER)

- *Indication:* This procedure is used to test the nervous system pathways for hearing. It may indirectly evaluate the vestibular system.

Technique

1. Place recording electrodes over the ear and the cerebrum and connect to an amplifier.
2. A sound made in the ear is a stimulus that triggers EEG recording of all brain activity that occurs during the 100 msec following the stimulus.
3. About 1000 stimuli are recorded, and the waveform patterns are compared by a data processor.
4. All random occurrences of waveforms are deleted, leaving only responses that appear consistently in every tracing. This "averaged response" is the BAER.

Diagnostic Interpretation
Conduction Deafness

There is loss of all waveforms on the BAER. This is the most common type of congenital deafness, and the BAER is widely used as a screening test in puppies.

Peripheral Vestibular Disease

- With otitis media/interna, there can be loss of all waveforms.
- With idiopathic vestibular disease, the BAER may not be affected, because it tests hearing but not balance.
- With brain stem vestibular diseases, often there are increased latencies, and sometimes actual loss, of later waveforms.

ELECTRODIAGNOSTIC EXAMINATION OF THE MOTOR UNIT

The electrodiagnostic examination of the motor unit consists of three parts:

- Needle electromyography (EMG)
- Nerve conduction studies (NCS)
- Repetitive nerve stimulation (RNS)

Each test evaluates different aspects of the motor unit. Interpretation of abnormal electrodiagnostic findings is summarized in Table 144–3 (also see Table 144–2).

Needle EMG

- *Indications:* EMG provides information about the functional status of motor unit innervation.

Table 144–2. DIAGNOSTIC STUDY FINDINGS IN VARIOUS CATEGORIES OF NEUROLOGIC DISEASE

Disease Category	Diagnostic Modality	Findings
Degeneration		
	Radiography	
	Plain	Usually normal; degeneration of supportive structures (i.e., discs) may be seen.
	Contrast	Usually not affected; may be decreased in size of NS with NS degeneration; may be compression with supportive structure (disc) degeneration.
	CSF analysis	Usually not affected; in future, may detect enzyme abnormalities.
	Electrodiagnostics	
	EEG	In cerebral degeneration: diffuse slowing of waves.
	EMG	In spinal gray matter degeneration: diffuse denervation.
	NCS	In PNS degeneration: slowed conduction and abnormal waveforms.
	RNS	In NMJ degeneration: delayed transmission and small-amplitude waveforms.
Anomalies		
	Radiography	
	Plain	Bony anomalies can be seen (e.g., hemivertebrae, occipital dysplasia); NS anomalies cannot be seen (e.g., hydrocephalus, spinal dysraphism).
	Contrast	Can reveal anomalies that change size of NS or its components (e.g., hydrocephalus causes increased size of ventricle).
	CSF analysis	Usually normal.
	Electrodiagnostics	
	EEG	In cerebral anomalies: slowing of waves over site of anomaly (e.g., diffuse with hydrocephalus).
	EMG	In spinal gray matter anomalies: denervation at site of gray matter destruction.
	NCS and RNS	Usually normal; PNS anomalies occur rarely.
Metabolic		
	Radiography	
	Plain	Not affected.
	Contrast	Usually normal.
	CSF analysis	Usually normal; in future, may detect chemical abnormalities (e.g., changes in neurotransmitter levels).
	Electrodiagnostics	
	EEG	In cerebral dysfunction: diffuse slowing of waves; abnormalities wax and wane.
	EMG	Usually normal; diffuse denervation can be seen if PNS is involved.
	NCS	In PNS dysfunction: slowed conduction and abnormal waveforms.
	RNS	In NMJ dysfunction: delayed transmission and small-amplitude waveforms.
	Blood testing	Most helpful diagnostic tool.
Neoplasia		
	Radiography	
	Plain	Usually normal, unless tumor involves bone.
	Contrast	May show NS swelling and/or compression at tumor site: injury to vascular supply; leakage from vessel due to blood-brain barrier injury.
	CSF analysis	Increased cells are seen only if tumor invades ventricles/subarachnoid space (e.g., lymphoma, choroid plexus tumor); protein increases due to blood-brain barrier injury.
	Electrodiagnostics	
	EEG	In cerebral neoplasia: focal slowing of waves over tumor; epileptic spikes due to irritation may be seen.
	EMG	In spinal cord neoplasia: focal denervation in muscle innervated by affected spinal segment.
	NCS and RNS	Usually normal.
Nutritional		
	Radiography	
	Plain	Usually normal; secondary bone changes may be seen.
	Contrast	Usually normal.
	CSF analysis	Usually normal; may be abnormal metabolite levels in some cases.
	Electrodiagnostics	
	EEG	In cerebral dysfunction: diffuse slowing of waves; abnormalities wax and wane.
	EMG	Usually normal; if PNS is involved, diffuse denervation may be seen.
	NCS	In PNS dysfunction: slowed conduction and abnormal waveforms.
	RNS	In NMJ dysfunction: delayed transmission and small-amplitude waveforms.
	Blood testing	May be helpful in some cases.
Inflammation		
	Radiography	
	Plain	Rarely helpful, unless there is bone infection.
	Contrast	Usually not helpful; may show spinal cord swelling at site of granuloma/abscess.
	CSF analysis	Usually increased WBCs; type (neutrophils, lymphocytes, eosinophils, etc.) reflects nature of etiology; protein is elevated as result of blood-brain barrier injury and also due to production of immunoglobulins.

Table continued on following page

Table 144–2. DIAGNOSTIC STUDY FINDINGS IN VARIOUS CATEGORIES OF NEUROLOGIC DISEASE *Continued*

Disease Category	Diagnostic Modality	Findings
	Electrodiagnostics	
	EEG	If cerebrum is involved: diffuse multifocal changes; seizure discharges also may be seen.
	EMG	If spinal cord is involved: multifocal areas of denervation.
	NCS	If PNS is involved: slowed conduction and abnormal waveforms.
	RNS	NMJ rarely is involved.
Infarct		
	Radiography	
	Plain	Usually normal.
	Contrast	Can show NS swelling and/or compression at infarct site; may show injury to vascular supply and leakage from vessels due to blood-brain barrier injury.
	CFS analysis	Cells are sometimes seen with hemorrhage; protein is increased due to blood-brain barrier injury.
	Electrodiagnostics	
	EEG	In cerebral infarcts: focal slowing of waves over infarct; epileptic spikes due to irritation may be seen.
	EMG	In spinal cord infarcts: focal denervation in muscle innervated by affected spinal segment.
	NCS and RNS	Usually normal.
Toxic		
	Radiography	
	Plain	Usually normal.
	Contrast	Usually normal.
	CSF analysis	Usually normal; may be abnormal metabolite levels in some cases.
	Electrodiagnostics	
	EEG	In cerebral dysfunction: diffuse slowing of waves; abnormalities wax and wane.
	EMG	Usually normal; if PNS is involved, diffuse denervation can be seen.
	NCS	In PNS dysfunction: slowed conduction and abnormal waveforms.
	RNS	In NMJ dysfunction: delayed transmission and small-amplitude waveforms.
	Blood testing	May be helpful in some cases.
Trauma		
	Radiography	
	Plain	Can show fractures and dislocations and evidence of joint instability (see Chap. 119).
	Contrast	Can show compression and areas of edema; may show vascular injury.
	CSF analysis	Cells usually are increased (especially RBCs); protein usually is increased due to blood-brain barrier injury.
	Electrodiagnostics	
	EEG	In cerebral injury: focal slowing of waves; epileptic spikes due to irritation may be seen.
	EMG	In spinal cord injury: focal denervation in muscle innervated by affected spinal segment.
	NCS	In PNS injury: slowed or blocked conduction resulting from focal/multifocal nerve damage.
	RNS	Rarely affected.

NS, nervous system; CSF, cerebrospinal fluid; EEG, electroencephalography; EMG, electromyography; NCS, nerve conduction studies; PNS, peripheral nervous system; NMJ, neuromuscular junction; RNS, repetitive nerve stimulation; WBCs, white blood cells; RBCs, red blood cells.

Table 144–3. INTERPRETATION OF THE ABNORMAL ELECTRODIAGNOSTIC EXAMINATION

Procedure	Abnormal Finding	Interpretation
Electromyography	Increased insertional activity	Neuropathies Myopathies Myotonia Cramps Electrolyte disorders
	Spontaneous activity	Myopathies Neuropathies (axon or cell body) Electrolyte disorders
Motor unit action potentials	Diminished size	Myopathies Acute denervation
	Increased size	Reinnervation Myopathies
Nerve conduction studies	Decreased velocity	Myelinopathies
Repetitive nerve stimulation	Incremental or decremental response	Junctionopathies

- *Advantage:* EMG is used primarily as a localizing tool, but it may indirectly provide etiologic information (e.g., in a suspected case of botulism, a positive EMG would exclude this disorder from further consideration).
- *Disadvantage:* False-negative results are common, and positive test results may be contradictory, confusing, or difficult to interpret.
- *Procedure:* A needle is inserted into a muscle and the muscle potentials are recorded and evaluated.

Diagnostic Interpretation

Motor Unit Action Potentials (MUAPs)

Acute Neurogenic Lesions. With acute lesions, there is a reduction in the number of available motor units; this reduction leads to reduced recruitment. Those MUAPs seen are normal in amplitude and duration.

Chronic Neurogenic Lesions. When the lesions become chronic, there is axon sprouting of the terminal branches of surviving neurons. These axon sprouts reinnervate some of the denervated muscle fibers. The MUAPs of the recruited muscles will then have a prolonged duration (temporal dispersion) and may become polyphasic.

Myopathic Lesions. With myopathic lesions (e.g., polymyositis), the recruitment pattern is normal but all MUAPs are reduced in size. In most neuromuscular junction (NMJ) disorders, MUAPs are normal or reduced in amplitude if they can be elicited. However, some myopathies (e.g., myotonia congenita) are characterized by bizarre discharges called myotonic discharges. These are high-frequency repetitive discharges that wax and wane in frequency and amplitude, causing a characteristic "dive-bomber" sound.

Spontaneous Activity

Spontaneous resting activity requires denervation. Denervation may be seen with motor neuron destruction, axonal transection, and inflammatory myopathies that produce segmental necrosis of muscle. Spontaneous depolarizations are known as fibrillation potentials or positive sharp waves (PSWs), depending on their size and shape.

Fibrillation Potentials. Fibrillation potentials reflect denervation hypersensitivity. They are 1–5 msec in duration, have an initial positive deflection, and may be biphasic or triphasic, with fibrillation amplitudes of 25–200 μV. Fibrillation potentials may be abolished by the use of curare.

PSW. PSWs are biphasic, with an initial positive deflection, 10–100 msec in duration, and amplitudes of 50–1000 μV. Because PSWs may be induced by needle movement in normal muscle, they are considered pathologic only if they persist after the needle has come to rest.

Nerve Conduction Studies

Nerve conduction studies measure latency or two-point nerve conduction velocities. Latency is the amount of time that elapses between stimulus and response.

- *Indications:* The speed of conduction primarily evaluates the health of the myelin sheath. The size and duration of MUAPs are indicative of the number of healthy fibers. This also evaluates the NMJ, because some junctionopathies may result in complete conduction blockade.

Procedures

Motor Nerve Conduction Testing. The M wave, also called the direct evoked compound muscle action potential, is the potential measured from a distal muscle after proximal stimulation of a nerve. This is best elicited with a supramaximal stimulus. It tests demyelination and the number of healthy axons.

Sensory Nerve Conduction. This procedure tests the sensory nerve and the dorsal root ganglion. The procedure is similar to motor nerve conduction testing, except that the stimuli are applied distally and the recordings are made directly from the nerve proximal to the site of stimulation.

Diagnostic Interpretation

Myelin Injuries. With injury to myelin, there is an increase in intranodal conduction time, leading to slowing of conduction velocities. Because not all fibers conduct at the same rate, there is temporal dispersion (prolonged duration) of the evoked potential as well.

Axonal Injuries. With axonal injury that spares the myelin sheath, the nerve conduction may be normal or mildly decreased. There is a reduction in the number of available motor units; this reduction leads to reduced size of the evoked potential. As the neurogenic lesion becomes chronic, there is axon sprouting of the terminal branches of surviving neurons. These axon sprouts reinnervate some of the denervated muscle fibers. The evoked potential will then have a prolonged duration (temporal dispersion) and may become polyphasic. This occurs because the axon sprouts conduct more slowly than the normal fibers, so that the muscle fibers receive their impulses at different times. In addition, because the motor unit now has more fibers, the evoked potential will be increased in amplitude.

Combined Injuries. There will be abnormalities in conduction velocity and in the amplitude of the evoked response. This occurs as a result of wallerian degeneration.

Repetitive Nerve Stimulation

Repetitive nerve stimulation (RNS) measures the amplitude of the motor unit potential during a supramaximal stimulus. RNS tests the health of the NMJ. If there is a progressive change in the amplitude during the first five stimuli, it is abnormal. An increase in amplitude is called an *incremental response;* a decrease in amplitude is called a *decremental response.* For a complete evaluation, RNS should be performed at both fast and slow rates.

Incremental Response. An incremental response is best seen on fast stimulation. It suggests a presynaptic disease such as botulism, myasthenic syndrome, aminoglycoside intoxication, hypocalcemia, and hypermagnesemia.

Most of the disorders that result in incremental responses appear to involve the role of calcium in the release of acetylcholine.

Decremental Response. A decremental response, especially to slow repetitions, suggests a postsynaptic disease, especially myasthenia gravis. Other conditions that may cause this response include myasthenic syndrome and botulism.

OTHER MOTOR UNIT TESTS

Tensilon Test

In myasthenia gravis, where the disorder is in the postsynaptic NMJ, anticholinesterase drugs can reverse the clinical symptoms. The most widely used of these drugs is Tensilon (edrophonium HCl), which has the advantage of a short (10 minutes) duration of action (see Chap. 149 for more information).

Muscle Enzymes

Any disease process that results in necrosis of the muscle cell membrane releases muscle enzymes into the systemic circulation. The most significant of these conditions is polymyositis. Because many incidental conditions (e.g., muscle trauma from an intramuscular injection), also release these enzymes, this must be taken into account when interpreting elevated serum levels of muscle enzymes.

Acetylcholine Receptor Antibodies

Serologic testing for antibodies against acetylcholine receptors is the diagnostic test of choice for acquired myasthenia gravis (see Chap. 149).

Muscle and Nerve Biopsy

Inflammatory and degenerative diseases of nerve and muscle are best diagnosed by biopsy (also see Chaps. 148 and 149). These procedures can now be done safely with minimal complications. The tissues require special handling and processing; therefore, arrangements should be made with the laboratory prior to collection of the samples. Analysis by a laboratory that is experienced in handling these biopsies will avoid erroneous results.

RESULTS OF DIAGNOSTIC STUDIES IN VARIOUS DISEASE CATEGORIES

Diagnostic study findings are listed by disease category in Table 144–2.

SUPPLEMENTAL READINGS

Chrisman CL: Problems in Small Animal Neurology, 2nd Ed. Philadelphia: Lea & Febiger, 1991.

Oliver JE, Lorenz MD, Kornegay JN: Handbook of Veterinary Neurology. Philadelphia: WB Saunders, 1997.

Wheeler SJ (Ed.): Manual of Small Animal Neurology, 2nd Ed. Cheltenham, British Small Animal Veterinary Association, 1995.

145 Diseases of the Brain

Philip A. March

The brain may be anatomically and functionally divided into three major compartments, the brain stem, cerebellum, and cerebrum. Cranial nerves have their cell bodies within the brain, but most of their nerve fibers course outside the brain. Diseases of the brain and cranial nerves may be neoplastic, infectious, idiopathic, vascular, traumatic, metabolic, toxic, congenital, or degenerative in origin. These disorders may result in dysfunction of a focal, regionally specific brain area or may produce more diffuse or multifocal deficits. Because many different diseases can affect similar areas causing very similar clinical signs, the first portion of this chapter discusses clinical signs of lesions in each brain region. The remainder of the chapter discusses important brain diseases within each etiologic category. Diagnosis of neurologic disease is discussed in Chapter 144, and management of seizures is discussed in Chapter 146.

CLINICAL SIGNS AND NEUROLOCALIZATION
(Refer also to Chap. 144)

Brain Stem Lesions

- Cranial nerve dysfunction is a common sign of brain stem disease. The brain stem contains cranial nerves (CN) 3 through 12. Multiple or single cranial nerves may be involved in a disease process; signs are typically asymmetrical. CN5 through 12 in the pons and medulla are more commonly affected than CN3 and CN4 in the midbrain.
- Central vestibular signs are usually present in diseases of the brain stem. Head tilt, circling, falling, disequilibrium, and nystagmus indicate damage to vestibular nuclei of CN8. Head tilts usually occur toward the side of the lesion. Paradoxical vestibular syndrome is characterized by a head tilt opposite the side of the lesion.
- Facial sensory (CN5) and motor (CN7) deficits are common. Disorders of swallowing (CN9 and 10), laryngeal function (CN9 and 10), and tongue mobility (CN12) can occur but are less common.
- Oculomotor weakness, strabismus, and resting pupillary changes occur with CN3, 4, and 6 involvement.
- Injury to ascending white matter tracts in the brain stem results in ipsilateral conscious proprioceptive deficits and other abnormalities in postural reactions. Occasionally, ataxia, dysmetria, and exaggerated postural reactions may be seen.
- Injury to descending upper motor neuron (UMN) nuclei and their tracts in the brain stem causes tetraparesis or paralysis characterized by increased extensor muscle tone and exaggerated reflexes. The weakness or paresis is usually more severe in limbs on the same side as the lesion.
- Severe brain stem lesions can result in disruption of the ascending reticular activating system. Clinical signs of progressively decreasing levels of consciousness (depression, obtundation, stupor, coma) correlate with the severity of the injury.
- Severe brain stem lesions can also affect the cardiovascular and respiratory regulation. Altered heart rate (bradycardia, supraventricular arrhythmias) and respiratory patterns (hyperventilation, ataxic respirations, apnea) are evident.

Cerebellar Lesions

- *Ataxia of gait:* Cerebellar lesions produce pronounced limb incoordination during voluntary movements. Exaggerated range and force of limb movement is common. Hypermetria and limb circumduction can be seen. Strength and conscious proprioception are preserved. Postural reactions often are preserved but exaggerated.
- *Truncal ataxia:* Truncal swaying and a wide-based stance are typical of cerebellar disease. Affected patients may fall to one side. Dysmetric head bobbing with overshooting and undershooting occurs. Forward and backward movements of the trunk (titubation) may be seen.
- *Intention tremor:* A fine oscillating tremor of the head and sometimes the body is seen during highly controlled movements, such as eating or visually fixating on an object.
- *Menace deficit:* The menace response is lost ipsilateral to the cerebellar lesion. Vision and facial nerve function are intact.
- *Anisocoria:* Mild mydriasis may be seen ipsilateral to the cerebellar lesion.
- *Vestibular signs:* The cerebellum contains the flocculonodular lobe, which is considered part of the vestibular system. Lesions in this area of the cerebellum may produce pathologic (and often positional) nystagmus, head tilt, and circling. Occasionally, a pendular nystagmus (rhythmic but rapid horizontal oscillation of the eyes) is seen with cerebellar disease.

- *Mental status* is normal in patients with isolated cerebellar injury.

Cerebral Lesions

- Cerebral diseases can affect the hemispheres either bilaterally (diffusely) or unilaterally (focally). Both diffuse and focal cerebral disorders can cause:
  - Seizures (generalized or partial)
  - Behavior/personality change
  - Dullness, agitation, or otherwise inappropriate responses to environmental stimuli (abnormal mentation or "dementia")
  - Contralateral visual deficits (loss of menace) with intact pupillary light reflexes
- Diffuse diseases of the cerebrum can also cause:
  - Generalized conscious proprioceptive deficits (all four limbs)
  - Stupor or coma with decreased to absent responses to painful stimuli
  - Generalized ataxia if an acute injury
  - Bilateral miosis with an intact pupillary light reflex
- Focal diseases of the cerebrum can cause:
  - Circling toward the side of the lesion
  - Contralateral conscious proprioceptive deficits and slow postural reactions
  - Contralateral facial sensory deficits (especially nares sensation)
  - Contralateral mild facial weakness
  - Hemi-inattention to stimuli on the side of the body opposite the lesion
- Cerebral diseases do not cause significant gait or strength abnormalities.

Manifestations of Systemic Metabolic Alterations

The above description of generalized and focal cerebral diseases applies to intracranial or structural disorders. Extracranial diseases (toxic, metabolic, and some nutritional disorders) may not produce actual structural lesions but may alter cerebral function enough to produce cerebral signs. Usually signs are diffuse in nature and mental status is altered. Seizures may be seen and may be either generalized or focal. Between seizures, lateralizing neurological deficits are not found. Other body systems are often affected concurrently by systemic extracranial disorders.

Herniation from Space-Occupying Brain Lesions

- Space-occupying lesions in the cerebrum and cerebellum may grow rapidly, may be accompanied by extensive edema, or may result in acute hemorrhage or infarction due to invasion of local blood vessels. Intracranial tissue and fluid compartments (parenchyma, blood, cerebrospinal fluid [CSF]) can compensate for space-occupying lesions up to a point. Beyond this critical threshold, brain shift or herniation occurs. Sudden changes in clinical signs not referable to the original neurolocalization suggests brain herniation and warrants emergency treatment.

The two most common types of herniation are caudal transtentorial herniation due to an expanding cerebral mass and foramen magnum herniation due to an expanding cerebellar lesion.

- Clinical signs of *transtentorial herniation* include extensor rigidity in all four limbs and cervical musculature (decerebrate rigidity), pupillary constriction followed by dilatation or fixed, mid-range pupils, loss of the vestibulo-ocular reflex (doll's eye reflex), and a stuporous or comatose state
- Clinical signs of *foramen magnum herniation* include opisthotonus (extended head and neck), thoracic limb rigidity usually with rigidity of the pelvic limbs, pupillary changes (usually miosis), and either severely irregular respirations or apnea.
- Appearance of these clinical signs indicates a severe brain injury and a need for immediate medical attention.

NEOPLASIA

Primary and secondary brain tumors most commonly affect middle-aged and older dogs and cats and can be located anywhere in the brain. Direct mechanical compression and necrosis of surrounding brain parenchyma, peritumoral edema, and blood vessel invasion with hemorrhage may all contribute to signs of a space-occupying mass. Clinical signs reflect location of the tumor in a specific brain area. As discussed above, when brain compensatory mechanisms are exhausted, brain herniation occurs and rapid clinical deterioration ensues.

Brain tumors can be *extra-axial*, arising from more superficial areas of the brain and compressing or invading the underlying parenchyma, or *intra-axial*, arising deep within the brain parenchyma and invading neural tissue surrounding them. Extra-axial masses tend to have a gradual onset and slow progression of signs. Intra-axial tumors tend to have a more rapid onset and progression.

Etiology

Primary Brain Tumors in the Canine

Primary tumors of the canine brain arise spontaneously and may grow slowly or rapidly: the two most common primary brain tumors in the dog are meningiomas and gliomas. Etiologic factors are not well understood. The glioma group includes astrocytomas, glioblastomas, oligodendrogliomas, ependymomas, and choroid plexus papillomas/carcinomas. Meningiomas arise from arachnoid cells of the meninges whereas gliomas arise from neuroectodermal supporting cells.

Meningiomas tend to occur in dolichocephalic breeds whereas gliomas tend to occur in brachycephalic breeds. Any dog, however, may develop either tumor. Meningiomas in the dog are often located in the olfactory/frontal lobe or over the convexities of the cerebrum but can occur on the floor of the intracranial vault (rostral, middle, or caudal fossae), in brain stem structures, or intraventricularly. Typically, they are well-circumscribed masses. Astrocytomas and oligodendrogliomas arise mostly from deep intra-axial locations in the cerebrum. Ependymomas are relatively uncommon and arise from cells lining any of the ventricular compartments. The lateral ventricles of the cerebrum are the most common sites for ependymoma formation. Choroid plexus papillomas and carcinomas develop in areas of the brain where choroid plexus is present. The most common site for a choroid plexus papilloma is the fourth ventricle/lateral aperture area. Choroid plexus carcinomas may metastasize to other central nervous system (CNS) areas by way of CSF pathways.

Primary Brain Tumors in the Feline

▼ *Key Point* The most common brain tumor of aged cats is the meningioma.

Most feline meningiomas are cerebrally located, extra-axial, and well encapsulated. They are frequently multiple and may occur anywhere along the falx, the tentorium cerebelli, and in the tela choroidea of the third ventricle. Gliomas in the cat are very uncommon but do occur. Primary CNS lymphoma may arise from brain structures, but most commonly arises in thoracolumbar spinal cord locations.

Secondary Brain Tumors in the Canine and Feline

Secondary tumors are either solitary or multiple. The two most common mechanisms of brain invasion are by hematogenous routes and by extension from surrounding tissues. Hemangiosarcoma, malignant melanoma, mammary adenocarcinoma, pulmonary adenocarcinoma, and multicentric lymphoma use the hematogenous route to metastasize to the brain. The most frequent metastatic location is the cerebrum. Tumors that invade the brain by local extension include nasal adenocarcinoma, pituitary macroadenoma and carcinoma, and bony tumors of the skull. Peripheral nerve sheath tumors of CN3 and 5 also tend to grow up their respective nerve trunks and invade the brain stem. Ganglioneuromas in young dogs behave similarly.

Many of the same tumors that secondarily invade the canine brain also occur in the feline. These include metastatic carcinomas, nasal carcinomas, and pituitary carcinomas. Squamous cell carcinomas can extend into the brain from middle ear locations.

Clinical Signs

- The onset and progression of clinical signs depend on the type of tumor and its location. Extra-axial meningiomas grow slowly and clinical signs are gradual in onset and progression. Intra-axial gliomas grow rapidly and cause a more rapid clinical deterioration. Secondary tumors also tend to progress rapidly. An exception to this is the trigeminal neurofibroma, which exhibits very slow growth (months to years).
- Early clinical signs may be vague and include increased irritability, behavior change, pacing, and increased lethargy.

- Some brain tumors may be clinically "silent" or may only cause seizures. These tumors can be located in the olfactory, temporal, or occipital cerebral lobes.
- Unilateral cerebral signs are characteristic. These include circling and contralateral conscious proprioceptive, visual field, and facial sensorimotor deficits.
- Diffuse cerebral signs may occur secondary to a tumor obstructing CSF flow. This results in fluid accumulation in the lateral ventricles of the cerebrum and secondary hydrocephalus.
- Herniation syndromes are common with tumors of the cerebral hemispheres or cerebellum (see under Herniation from Space-Occupying Brain Lesions).
- *Cerebellopontomedullary angle tumors* (choroid plexus papillomas, ependymomas, neurofibromas, meningiomas, and other tumor types) may invade the flocculonodular lobe of the cerebellum or the cerebellar peduncles. If this occurs, a "paradoxical vestibular syndrome" is seen. Signs are head tilt with possible circling and ataxia *away* from the side of the lesion. The fast phase of nystagmus is often toward the side of the lesion. Long tract signs (e.g., proprioception), however, are ipsilateral to the lesion. If other cranial nerves are involved (for example, CN5 and 7), those deficits will be on the same side as the lesion.
- *Cavernous sinus syndrome.* This is a sporadic syndrome due to a lesion in the cavernous sinus or orbital fissure along the floor of the rostral fossa (beneath the cerebrum). Neoplastic masses occupying this area will compress CN3, 4, and 6, the ophthalmic branch of CN5, and the sympathetic nerve going to the eye. The result is an ipsilateral miosis, absent corneal and eyelid sensation, and ocular immobility.

Diagnosis

Laboratory Testing

- Perform a complete blood count (CBC), chemistry profile, and urinalysis to rule out extracranial causes of brain dysfunction prior to pursuing tests for intracranial disease.
- Because most patients with brain tumors are older, run a geriatric screen of liver and kidney function.
- Perform an adrenocorticotropic hormone (ACTH) stimulation test and a low-dose dexamethasone suppression test if a pituitary mass is suspected.

Ophthalmic Exam

Perform a complete ophthalmologic examination to check for papilledema (a sign of increased intracranial pressure), uveitis, retinal hemorrhage, and other abnormalities.

Electrodiagnostic Testing

- An electroencephalogram (EEG) may detect asymmetries in brain activity or actual epileptiform complexes if a seizure focus is present. See Chapter 144 for a more thorough description of the EEG and its uses.
- A brain stem auditory evoked response (BAER) may aid in localizing a brain stem lesion. See Chapter 144 for additional information.

Radiography

- Usually not helpful in the diagnosis of a brain tumor.
- Skull radiographs may reveal a nasal or bony tumor with secondary brain invasion.
- An area of bone sclerosis or lysis may be visible in the skull immediately adjacent to a feline meningioma.
- Some feline meningiomas may have an area of dystrophic mineralization that is visible on skull radiographs.
- Perform thoracic radiographs to screen for metastasis.

Computed Tomography (CT) and Magnetic Resonance Imaging (MRI)

- CT and MRI have replaced older techniques such as ventriculography, cavernous sinus venography, cisternography, and scintigraphy.
- Tumor margins and neuroanatomic location can be more precisely defined. Peritumoral edema is also visible on both CT and MRI. Parenchyma definition, especially in brain stem areas, is best identified with MRI.
- Intravenous contrast agents (meglumine iothalamate for CT and gadolinium DTPA for MRI) highlight areas of blood-brain barrier disruption. Patterns of enhancement are not pathognomonic for tumor type but aid in making a tentative diagnosis.
- Inflammatory or other non-neoplastic lesions may mimic a neoplastic lesion on both CT and MRI. A CSF tap and biopsy of the mass are sometimes needed to confirm the underlying process.
- CT and MRI provide the precise neuroanatomic information needed for accurate biopsy, surgical, and/or radiation procedures.

CSF Analysis

(For CSF tap technique and normal values, see Chap. 144)

- CSF analysis may be useful in distinguishing inflammatory from neoplastic processes. Antibody and antigen titers for a variety of infectious agents can be checked (see Inflammatory Disease section). Rarely, an organism is visible cytologically.
- CSF pleocytosis may be seen if the tumor is necrotic and has a secondary inflammatory component. Many gliomas are characterized by no cytologic abnormalities. Neoplastic lymphocytes in CSF are typically seen with CNS lymphoma.
- Protein levels are usually elevated for all tumor types. Protein electrophoresis can be done on CSF and serum to determine the extent of blood-brain barrier disruption.
- CSF opening pressure measurements are of limited value. CT and MRI availability have made this procedure unnecessary.
- The CSF tap procedure is contraindicated in patients with elevated intracranial pressure. If clinical signs and/or CT or MRI suggest elevated intracranial pressure, mannitol, furosemide, and hyperventilation may lessen the risks of brain herniation.

Therapy

Corticosteroids

- Corticosteroids primarily help in resolving vasogenic edema and often benefit patients with peritumoral edema. If there is a rapid progression of signs due to a significant edema component, administer methylprednisolone sodium succinate (Solu-Medrol) at 30 mg/kg IV once followed by 15 mg/kg IV every 6 hours for 24–48 hours or dexamethasone at 1 mg/kg IV every 12 hours for 24 hours.
- Dog and cats with meningiomas may clinically respond to corticosteroids for a period of time.

Hyperosmotic Solutions and Diuretics

- Mannitol therapy is reserved for those patients with signs of increased intracranial pressure and/or herniation.
- In the euvolemic patient, mannitol at 1 g/kg IV over 20 minutes will draw fluid out of more normal areas of brain and temporarily lower intracranial pressure.
- Furosemide given 20 minutes after mannitol at 1–2 mg/kg IV will help to prolong the effects of mannitol. Furosemide may also decrease CSF production.

Anticonvulsant Therapy

Phenobarbital at 2 mg/kg PO every 12 hours is indicated if seizures are part of the clinical picture (see Chap. 146).

Specific Chemotherapy

- Controlled clinical trials in dogs and cats have not been done to assess the true efficacy of different chemotherapeutic agents in the treatment of brain tumors.
- Nitrosoureas (lomustine, carmustine) appear to be beneficial in the treatment of some canine gliomas and meningiomas. Longer survival and even temporary tumor regression have been reported. Nitrosoureas are unique in that they cross the blood-brain barrier, the limiting factor for most chemotherapeutic agents. Give 50–80 mg/m^2 of body surface area every 6–8 weeks.
- Cytosine arabinoside reaches therapeutic CSF concentrations after large intravenous doses in normal dogs. Intrathecal and IV infusions of cytosine arabinoside have been used in dogs with CNS lymphoma. Efficacy and dosage have not been clearly established.
- Tumor cell heterogeneity with respect to relative phase in the cell cycle diminishes the likelihood of a uniform tumor response to chemotherapeutic agents.

Surgery

- Craniotomy or craniectomy with tumor excision is a treatment option for extra-axial tumors involving the cerebrum or cerebellum.
- Survival rates are generally good to excellent when feline meningiomas over the cerebral convexities are

removed surgically. Up to 1-year survival periods are reported following meningioma excision in dogs. Postoperative irradiation may further extend the survival period in the canine.

- Tumors in more intra-axial and brain stem locations cannot be resected completely. Biopsy and irradiation (see below) can be performed.

Radiation Therapy

- External beam megavoltage irradiation for brain tumors appears to prolong survival more consistently than other modes of therapy. It is most effective if started within several days of surgical debulking. 45–48 Gy irradiation in 12 fractions over 4 weeks appears to be a well-tolerated treatment protocol.
- Longest survival times for dogs with meningiomas were obtained when radiation therapy was combined with surgery.
- Canine pituitary tumors are radiation sensitive. Long remission times have been achieved.
- Brain metastases may respond to irradiation.
- Complications of radiation therapy include ocular and dermatologic changes and rapid tumor necrosis with secondary hemorrhage. A potential late, delayed reaction may occur several months postirradiation and is characterized by white matter necrosis. Whole brain irradiation may also lead to decreased CSF absorption and a secondary hydrocephalus.

INFLAMMATORY BRAIN DISEASES

Inflammation of brain parenchyma and its meninges (meningoencephalitis) occurs secondary to infectious or idiopathic insults. Idiopathic disorders may have an immune-mediated component. Some diseases also cause an inflammation of blood vessels (vasculitis), which further compounds the injury. Most infectious agents reach the brain hematogenously. Local extension from extraneural sites, usually due to erosion through bone, is a mechanism used by some fungal and bacterial organisms. An unusual but important mode of entry into CNS is that used by rabies and pseudorabies viruses and by *Listeria* bacteria via retrograde axonal transport into the CNS.

The cascade of inflammatory changes that occurs after brain injury leads to a self-perpetuating process of brain tissue ischemia, necrosis, and edema. Inflammatory brain disorders are usually multifocal or diffuse in nature, with lesions often disseminated throughout the CNS. Clinical signs, however, may indicate a focal neurolocalization for the most prominent lesion. Some inflammatory disorders have a predilection for the cerebral cortex, whereas many others have a predilection for brain stem sites and frequently cause central vestibular signs. As in the case of neoplastic conditions, inflammatory diseases can lead to the formation of large, space-occupying lesions, increased intracranial pressure, and herniation of brain structures.

The onset and progression of clinical signs can vary, making the diagnosis of inflammatory brain disease a challenge. Infectious diseases may be accompanied by systemic signs, but idiopathic brain conditions are usually characterized by signs referable to the CNS only. CSF analysis remains an important means of distinguishing neoplastic from inflammatory lesions. Infectious agents can occasionally be seen in the CSF, antibody or antigen titers can be very useful, and features of white blood cell pleocytosis may more strongly suggest an inflammatory disorder (see Tables 145–1 and 145–2). Evidence of multifocal or diffuse heterogeneous contrast enhancement on CT or MRI suggests an inflammatory lesion, but focal inflammatory lesions (granulomas, abscesses) can appear identical to neoplastic foci using these two imaging modalities. Occasionally, a brain biopsy may be needed to make a definitive diagnosis.

Infectious Meningoencephalitis

Some of the more important causes of infectious meningoencephalitis and their clinical and clinicopathological features in the dog and cat are listed in Tables 145–1 and 145–2. Also refer to the Infectious Causes of Vasculitis section, later in this chapter. Additional information can be found in the following sections of this text:

- Feline Infectious Peritonitis (FIP): Chap. 8
- Cryptococcosis (and other fungal disorders): Chap. 18
- Toxoplasmosis: Chap. 19
- Feline Immunodeficiency Virus (FIV): Chap. 7
- Rabies and Pseudorabies: Chap. 13
- Canine Distemper Virus (CDV): Chap. 11
- Rocky Mountain Spotted Fever (RMSF) and Ehrlichiosis: Chap. 15

IDIOPATHIC INFLAMMATORY BRAIN DISORDERS

Granulomatous Meningoencephalomyelitis (GME)

Etiology

GME is an idiopathic condition in dogs characterized by pronounced inflammatory changes in the CNS. These changes tend to predominate in white matter areas of the brain and spinal cord. Perivascular accumulations of lymphocytes, plasma cells, and histiocytic-like cells are the hallmark of GME. Some of the perivascular cell aggregates may coalesce to form a space-occupying mass in the brain. GME should be distinguished from neoplastic reticulosis and from B-cell lymphoma in which homogeneous populations of neoplastic cells predominate. Whether inflammatory cells in GME eventually undergo neoplastic transformation to these cancerous phenotypes is still unknown. At present, the mixed granulomatous cell response is believed to represent a chronic immune response to a suspected but unconfirmed antigen.

Three forms of GME have been described. The *disseminated form* is characterized pathologically by multifocal perivascular cuffs throughout the brain and spinal cord and clinically by multifocal neurologic signs. The

Table 145–1. INFLAMMATORY BRAIN DISEASE CAUSED BY INFECTIOUS AGENTS IN THE CAT

Disease/Agent	Typical Age of Onset	Onset/ Progression	Typical Neurologic Signs	Typical CSF Characteristics	Treatment*
FIP (coronavirus)	Young (<2 yr)	Rapid or intermediate	Brain stem and cerebral (may be multifocal)	Suppurative or mixed; very high protein	Palliative only (corticosteroids, chlorambucil, cyclophosphamide, melphalan)
Cryptococcosis (*Cryptococcus neoformans*)	Any age	Intermediate to slow	Brain stem (may be multifocal)	Mononuclear or mixed; moderate protein; CSF antigen titer is diagnostic	Fluconazole (itraconazole, amphotericin B, ketoconazole, flucytosine)
Toxoplasmosis (*Toxoplasma gondii*)	Adult	Rapid to intermediate	Multifocal	Mild to moderate mononuclear; rare eosinophils; moderate protein; IgM or rising IgG titer	Trimethoprim-sulfadiazine, and pyrimethamine; clindamycin
FIV (lentivirus)	Adult	Slow	Cerebral (behavior change, dementia, roaming)	Mild lymphocytic; normal protein; FIV serum antibody titer positive	Experimental only (alpha-interferon, PMEA, AZT)
Rabies (rhabdovirus)	Any age	Rapid	Cerebral (behavior change, irritable, seizures); may be multifocal	Normal or mild lymphocytic; normal or mild protein	None

*Preferred treatment(s) listed first; other available drugs are listed in parentheses.

focal form is characterized by a focal neurolocalization due to the presence of a granulomatous mass. The focal form, however, is probably a variant of the disseminated form since histologic lesions can usually be identified postmortem all throughout the neuraxis. A more rare *optic form* with dense optic nerve infiltration by inflammatory cells is also recognized.

Clinical Signs

- GME is primarily a disease of toy and small breeds between 1 and 8 years of age. Large-breed dogs may occasionally be affected (e.g., Airedale terriers).
- Onset and progression of clinical signs may be more rapid in the disseminated form compared with the focal form, which tends to be more intermediate in progression.
- Initially, a mild fever, lethargy, and intermittent anorexia may be the only clinical signs seen.
- Neurologic signs often indicate a focal pontomedullary or cerebral lesion.
- Central vestibular signs are common and may be paradoxical (see Neoplasia section). Long tract signs and other cranial nerve deficits (CN5 and 7) may be present.
- Neck pain may be present and indicates meningeal involvement.
- Focal or multifocal areas of intramedullary spinal cord inflammation (myelitis) may cause tetraparesis or paraparesis.
- The optic form is characterized by a sudden onset of bilateral or unilateral blindness.

Diagnosis

- A marked mononuclear pleocytosis consisting of lymphocytes, plasma cells, monocytes, macrophages, and multinucleated giant cells is usually evident on CSF analysis. Neutrophils may be present. Rarely, CSF cytology is normal. Protein is usually elevated.
- CSF titers, cultures, and virus isolation studies are negative for any infectious etiology.
- CT or MRI may reveal a contrast-enhancing lesion (homogeneous or heterogeneous).
- GME is a diagnosis of exclusion. A predominant mononuclear CSF pleocytosis and negative tests for infectious agents (rickettsial, fungal, bacterial, protozoal, viral) suggest a diagnosis of GME. If the CSF is normal and a focal lesion is present, a brain biopsy is necessary to rule out neoplasia.

Treatment

- Prednisone 2 mg/kg every 12 hours for 2 weeks, then 1 mg/kg every 12 hours for 1 to 2 months followed by a gradual taper over several months will usually result in temporary remission of clinical signs in the focal form. The disseminated form has a less favorable response to therapy. The optic form, if treated in the early stages, can result in recovery of vision.
- Other therapies for GME include cyclophosphamide, azathioprine, lomustine, and cyclosporine. Azathioprine, 2 mg/kg PO every 24 hours for 7 days followed by the same dose every other day may be beneficial in some dogs when used in combination with prednisone therapy.

Table 145–2. INFLAMMATORY BRAIN DISEASE CAUSED BY INFECTIOUS AGENTS IN THE DOG

Disease/Agent	Typical Age of Onset	Onset/ Progression	Typical Neurologic Signs	Typical CSF Characteristics	Treatment*
CDV (paramyxovirus)	Young (<1yr)	Rapid or intermediate	Cerebral, brain stem, cerebellum or spinal cord) (may be multifocal)	Normal or mild mononuclear; mild protein; positive titer usually	None
Cryptococcosis	Any age; often young (<1yr)	Intermediate to slow	Brain stem (often multifocal brain stem signs)	Mixed or mononuclear or suppurative (rare eosinophils); high protein	Fluconazole (itraconazole, amphotericin B, ketoconazole, flucytosine)
RMSF (*Rickettsia rickettsii*)	Adult	Rapid	Diffuse or multifocal; often central vestibular component; neck pain	Mixed or suppurative; moderate protein; (paired serum titers to diagnose)	Doxycycline, (chloramphenicol, enrofloxacin)
Ehrlichiosis (*Ehrlichia canis*)	Adult	Rapid or intermediate	As for RMSF above	Mixed or non-suppurative or suppurative; moderate protein	As for RMSF above
Neosporosis (*Neospora caninum*)	Young (<1yr)	Rapid	Pelvic limb paresis, ataxia or ascending tetra-paresis; pelvic limb hyper-extension	Nonsuppurative; moderate protein (serum antibody titer or muscle biopsy to diagnose)	Trimethoprim-sulfadiazine and pyrimethamine; (clindamycin)
Rabies (rhabdovirus)	Adult	Rapid	Spinal cord, brain stem, and/ or cerebral signs (may be multifocal)	Normal or mild mononuclear; normal or mild protein	None
Pseudorabies (herpesvirus)	Any age	Rapid	Hyperesthesia; spinal cord and brain stem signs; often multifocal	Mild mononuclear; mild protein	None

*Preferred treatment(s) listed first; other available drugs are listed in parentheses.

- Radiation therapy for the focal form of GME may be of benefit as adjunctive therapy.

Prognosis

Relapses are common and may occur weeks to months (up to 48 months) following onset of therapy. Upon relapse, patients are often refractory to a second course of chemotherapy.

Pug Encephalitis

Etiology

Pug dog encephalitis is probably a variant of GME and bears many similarities to GME. Lymphocytes and histiocytes form large perivascular cuffs in cerebrum. Neuronal necrosis and malacia in both gray and white matter are more severe than in GME. A familial predisposition is probable, but this disorder is considered idiopathic.

Clinical Signs

- Age of onset of clinical signs is 9 months to 4 years.
- Seizures, neck pain, ataxia, and cortical blindness are seen in the acute form.

- Mild partial or generalized seizures that progress over weeks to more severe and frequent seizures are seen in the chronic form.
- Brain stem and cerebellar signs are also reported.

Diagnosis

A diagnosis of pug dog encephalitis is supported by clinical signs and a CSF mononuclear pleocytosis. Small lymphocytes predominate in some dogs. Protein levels are increased. The primary differential diagnoses are GME, infectious disease, and neoplasia.

Treatment

Immunosuppressive therapy as for GME.

Prognosis

The prognosis is poor even for short-term survival.

Necrotizing Meningoencephalitis of Maltese Dogs and Yorkshire Terriers

Etiology

This is a recently described clinical syndrome in the Maltese dog that is being seen with increased frequency. The pathological features are indistinguishable from those of pug dog encephalitis. Histologically, necrosis and nonsuppurative inflammation of cerebral gray and white matter predominate. Nonsuppurative meningitis is also a component of the lesion. Subcortical white matter atrophy can result in assymetrical dilatation of the lateral ventricles. A similar condition is seen in the Yorkshire terrier.

Clinical Signs

- Onset of signs between 9 months and 4 years of age.
- Seizures are the primary neurologic abnormality and can rapidly or slowly increase in frequency and severity.

Diagnosis

There is a mononuclear pleocytosis and increased protein levels on CSF analysis.

Prognosis

The prognosis is grave.

Generalized Idiopathic Tremors (Little White Shaker Syndrome) of Adult Dogs

Etiology

An acute onset of tremor in toy to small-breed dogs with white coat color (Maltese terrier, West Highland white terrier, poodle, bichon frise, samoyed) is recognized. Other breeds with other coat colors (beagle, miniature schnauzer, spitz, Yorkshire terrier, etc.) can also be affected. This syndrome was originally described by some authors as a "nonsuppurative encephalitis" or "cerebellitis" due to the occasional finding of a nonsuppurative meningoencephalitis involving the cerebellum and other brain areas. A demyelinating disorder, a neurotransmitter defect, and various other mechanisms have been hypothesized but not proven.

Clinical Signs

- Young adult dogs (less than 6 years of age) are affected.
- The onset is acute to peracute.
- Clinical signs are a severe coarse head and body tremor that worsens with stress, exercise, or handling. At rest or during sleep, the tremor diminishes. Animals maintain the ability to walk but continuous shaking makes ambulation difficult. The excessive muscle activity may cause hyperthermia.
- Disconjugate, jerky eye movements may be seen (opsoclonus).
- Dogs are alert and responsive and rarely have other neurologic deficits.

Diagnosis

- Differential diagnoses include neurotoxin exposure ("moldy cheese" toxicity), other inflammatory CNS diseases, and generalized seizures. Generalized tremors in the absence of other signs of epilepsy or systemic illness suggest a diagnosis of shaker syndrome.
- CSF may be normal or a mild lymphocytic pleocytosis may be seen.

Treatment

- Cool if hyperthermic.
- Diazepam, 0.5–1.0 mg/kg PO every 8 hours will help alleviate signs in the short term.
- Prednisone, 1 mg/kg every 12 hours for 4 weeks followed by a gradual taper over the next 8 weeks appears to be the most effective treatment. Some dogs may recover without therapy.

Prognosis

The prognosis is good for recovery. Relapses may occur.

VASCULAR DISEASES

Damage to brain vasculature can result in edema, hemorrhage, or infarction. An infarction is an area of brain necrosis due to loss of regional blood supply (ischemia). Loss of blood supply to a brain region can be secondary to blood vessel trauma, inflammation, or blockage by tumor emboli, infectious (septic) emboli, blood clots, or atherosclerotic lesions. Atherosclerosis has been associated with hypothyroidism in the dog. Edema or hemorrhage is usually due to blood vessel damage secondary to trauma, inflammation (vasculitis), or local tumor infiltration. Spontaneous hemorrhage also occurs secondary to systemic hypertension, arteriovenous malformations, or primary coagulopathies (rodenticide poisoning, disseminated intravascular coagulation, etc.). Acute vascular problems in dogs and cats are occasionally associated with cardiac arrhythmias, myocardial ischemia, or overt heart failure.

Traumatic injuries to the brain and its vessels are discussed in the Head Trauma section of this chapter. Other common causes of vascular disease in small animals are discussed below.

Feline Ischemic Encephalopathy

Etiology

This is an idiopathic syndrome of adult cats characterized by a peracute onset of unilateral cerebral infarction due to occlusion of the middle cerebral artery. The pathogenesis of this disease is not well understood. It is usually *not* associated with thromboembolic disease secondary to feline hypertrophic cardiomyopathy. An association between aberrant *Cuterebra* sp. migration in brain and possible middle cerebral artery vasospasm has been suggested because of the occasional finding of this parasite in the cranial vault. There is a higher incidence of this syndrome in late summer.

Clinical Signs

- Affected cats exhibit acute signs of unilateral cerebral dysfunction. Altered mentation, behavior change, circling visual field deficits, contralateral postural deficits, and seizures may occur.
- Signs may worsen slightly over 24–48 hours but then stabilize.
- If the injury is not fatal, signs may steadily improve over days to months.

- Seizures and altered personality may be long-term sequelae.

Diagnosis

- Rule out other causes of unilateral cerebral dysfunction and peracute vascular disease (cardiomyopathy-associated thromboemboli, hypertension, hypercoagulable states, vasculitis, neoplasia, trauma).
- CSF analysis may reveal a pleocytosis and elevated protein due to inflammatory changes induced by necrotic tissue.
- The peracute onset of signs in an otherwise healthy cat aids in making a tentative diagnosis.

Treatment

- There is no specific treatment.
- Corticosteroids do not alter the clinical course.
- Start anticonvulsant therapy (diazepam or phenobarbital) if seizures occur (see Chap. 146).

Prognosis

The prognosis for survival is fair to good. The prognosis for complete recovery is guarded.

Vasculitis of the Beagle, Bernese Mountain Dog, and German Shorthair Pointer

Etiology

A necrotizing vasculitis of young adult beagles, Bernese mountain dogs, and German shorthair pointers is frequently associated with neurologic signs. This is an idiopathic condition, but a genetic predisposition is suspected. The typical lesion is a fibrinoid necrosis and thrombosis of small- and medium-sized meningeal vessels with subsequent meningeal fibrosis. A marked inflammatory component to the lesion suggests an immune-mediated basis for the disease. Meningeal artery damage may lead to hemorrhage or thrombosis/infarction of adjacent neural parenchyma.

Clinical Signs

- Age of onset is 3–18 months of age.
- Signs of meningitis (neck pain and stiffness, stiff, stilted gait, fever) are common. "Painful" episodes may wax and wane. Clinical signs of meningitis are very similar to sterile suppurative meningitis of young, large-breed dogs.
- Secondary parenchymal involvement may result in conscious proprioceptive deficits and paresis. Rarely, cranial deficits occur.
- Blindness and seizures are seen secondary to an associated encephalitis in Bernese mountain dogs.
- Beagles may have neutrophilic polyarthritis and coronary arteritis associated with the neurologic disease.

Diagnosis

- CSF analysis is characterized by a marked neutrophilic pleocytosis and elevated protein levels. No infectious agents can be isolated and titers for infectious causes of meningitis (rickettsial, viral, bacterial, fungal, protozoal) are negative.
- GME can be ruled out based on the CSF findings.
- Intervertebral disc disease is ruled out by the demonstration of no compressive lesions on cervical myelography.
- Antinuclear antibody titers are negative and there is no evidence of neoplasia or a drug reaction.

Treatment

- Immunosuppressive doses of corticosteroids (2 mg/kg PO every 12 hours for 2 weeks with a very slow taper over 3–6 months) often results in a clinical response.
- Occasional patients are nonresponsive and may require other immunosuppressive agents.

Prognosis

The prognosis is fair to guarded. Some patients do not respond to therapy. Relapses can occur.

Infectious Causes of Vasculitis

Etiology

Many of the infectious causes of vasculitis have previously been discussed in the Inflammatory Brain Disease section (see Tables 145–1 and 145–2). Various fungal and protozoal agents may create secondary blood vessel inflammation with edema, hemorrhage, or infarction. Rickettsial disorders may produce an immune-mediated vasculitis and direct damage to endothelial cells due to intracellular replication. Bacterial vasculitis occurs most commonly as a sequela to sepsis. Bacterial toxins and inflammatory mediators released by neutrophils increase vascular permeability and cause edema and hemorrhage. Septic thromboemboli lead to multiple areas of infarction. Focal abscesses may form space-occupying masses within brain parenchyma.

Clinical Signs

- Diffuse or multifocal vasogenic edema can result in brain swelling and diffuse cerebral signs of dullness, dementia, head pressing, and pacing. Signs of brain herniation may be evident.
- Head and neck pain are common due to accompanying meningitis.
- Multifocal cranial nerve deficits and long tract signs reflect multifocal involvement of the brain stem and spinal cord. Rickettsial diseases are often associated with central vestibular signs.
- Focal or generalized motor seizures and other focal cerebral signs may be seen.
- Systemic signs of fever, lymphadenopathy, polyarthritis, uveitis, and peripheral edema are sometimes present.

Diagnosis

- CSF characteristics will depend on the inciting cause (see Inflammatory Disease section; Tables 145–1 and 145–2). The degree of pleocytosis is often determined by the degree of meningitis. Bacterial vasculitis is characterized by normal or neutrophilic pleocytosis and high protein levels.

- Xanthochromia, free blood, and erythrophagocytosis by neutrophils or macrophages are typical CSF findings in patients with previous hemorrhage.
- Gram stains and other special stains may demonstrate organisms.
- Appropriate CSF titers and cultures will often reveal the underlying pathogen.
- A complete blood count, chemistry profile, and other blood tests will frequently uncover abnormalities in other organ systems.

Treatment

- Treatment is directed at the underlying etiologic agent.
- Antimicrobial therapy for bacterial infections is based on culture and sensitivity results, the bacteriocidal versus bacteriostatic properties of the drug, and how effective the drug crosses the blood-brain barrier. See Table 145–3 for properties of specific antimicrobial agents.
- For bacterial causes, diffuse breakdown of the blood-brain barrier often already exists, so drug selection according to blood-brain barrier penetration may not be as critical. Intravenous ampicillin is often an effective treatment pending culture and sensitivity results.
- Third-generation cephalosporins (e.g., cefotaxime) or enrofloxacin are usually good choices for gram-negative infections.
- Prolonged corticosteroid use is contraindicated in the patient with infectious vasculitis and meningoencephalitis due to its immunosuppressive effect and its effect on decreasing blood-brain barrier permeability.

Prognosis

The prognosis will vary depending on the underlying pathogen, its sensitivity to chemotherapies, and the state of disease progression. Aggressive medical therapy is necessary to prevent irreversible brain injury.

BRAIN TRAUMA

Pathophysiology

Severe head trauma can result in acute brain injury. Primary mechanical injury to cell membranes and fiber tracts results in irreversible necrosis. This can take the form of a blunt contusion or a laceration. Secondary events are due to biochemical changes at the cellular level and increased intracranial pressure (ICP). Excitotoxins, free radicals, prostaglandins, and inflammatory cytokines fuel a self-perpetuating cycle of ischemia and necrosis in the traumatized brain. Intracranial edema and hemorrhage combine to raise ICP, exhaust compensatory mechanisms, and create conditions favorable for brain herniation. Elevated ICP may also lead to cardiac arrhythmias or failure (see Neoplasia for discussion), systemic hypertension, and neurogenic pulmonary edema. A final immediate or delayed consequence of brain trauma is epilepsy. Seizures can be seen up to months following head trauma.

Clinical Signs

- The signs of brain trauma will depend upon whether the lesion remains localized or progresses to involve other brain structures. If progression occurs, it will occur within the first 24–48 hours postinjury. For this reason, it is critical to perform serial neurological examinations every few hours in traumatized patients.

Table 145–3. ANTIMICROBIAL DRUGS FOR CNS INFECTIONS

Drug	BBB Penetration	Bacteriocidal vs. Bacteriostatic	Dose (mg/kg)	Route	Frequency (hours)
Amphotericin B	poor	static	0.15–0.5	IV	48
Ampicillin	intermediate	cidal	10–20	IV	6
Cefotaxime	good	cidal	25–80	IV or IM	6–8
Cephalexin	poor	cidal	10–30	PO	8
Chloramphenicol	good	static	15–25	PO	8–12
Clavamox	poor	cidal	10–20	PO	8–12
Clindamycin	poor	static	12.5–25	PO or IM	12
Doxycycline	intermediate	static	2.5–5	PO	12
Enrofloxacin	intermediate	cidal	2.5–5	PO	12
Fluconazole	good	static	5–10	PO	12–24
Flucytosine	intermediate	static	25–50	PO	8
Gentamicin	poor	cidal	2–4	IV or IM	8
Itraconazole	poor	static	5	PO	12–24
Ketoconazole	poor	static	5–20	PO	12–24
Metronidazole	good	cidal	10–15	PO	8–12
Penicillin G	intermediate	cidal	20,000–40,000 U/kg	IV	6
Tetracycline	poor	static	15–22	PO	8
Trimethoprim/ sulfadiazine	good	cidal	15–30	PO	12

BBB, blood-brain barrier; PO, per os; IM, intramuscularly; IV, intravenously.

- Focal signs may originate from injury to the cerebrum, cerebellum, or brain stem and will reflect dysfunction of the region involved.
- Signs of increased ICP, transtentorial herniation, and foramen magnum herniation are discussed in the first section of this chapter, under Herniation from Space-Occupying Brain Lesions. An orderly progression of signs due to increased ICP can be graded from mild to severe.
  - Motor activity tends to progress from normal ambulatory status to recumbency with progressive extensor rigidity.
  - Pupils initially appear miotic but soon become mydriatic or midrange and nonresponsive to light.
  - The oculovestibular reflex (doll's eye) is lost in the late stages of transtentorial herniation and is a poor prognostic sign.
  - Level of consciousness deteriorates from the alert state to depression, stupor, and coma. These states are defined by the patient's responsiveness to stimuli, including deep pain.
  - Hyperventilation may be seen with midbrain compression, whereas either an ataxic (irregular) respiratory pattern or apnea may be seen with medullary compression.

Diagnosis

- Clinical signs usually reflect the severity of the injury.
- The EEG and BAER can be used to localize areas of brain damage (see Chap. 144). The EEG can also be used to detect seizure foci.
- CT and MRI are usually not indicated due to prolonged anesthetic times required for imaging and the likelihood that the information obtained will not change therapy.
- A CSF tap is rarely necessary for the same reasons. It is contraindicated in the patient with increased ICP.

Treatment

- Correct hypovolemic shock, pneumothorax, cardiac arrhythmias, and other life-threatening non-neural injuries. When correcting for shock, do not overhydrate the patient (see Fluid Choices later).
- Elevating the head will facilitate venous return to the heart, enhance CSF resorption, and help to maintain cerebral blood flow. Avoid jugular vein compression when elevating the head.
- Hypercarbia will act to cause cerebral vasodilation and increased ICP. Intubation and hyperventilation will lower blood and brain carbon dioxide concentrations and stimulate vasoconstriction. Vasoconstriction of cerebral vessels will decrease intracranial blood volume, lower ICP, and raise cerebral perfusion pressure.
- Methylprednisolone sodium succinate (Solu-Medrol) may be of some benefit if administered at the time of or immediately following the trauma (within 1–2 hours). Administer methylprednisolone sodium succinate 30 mg/kg as an intravenous bolus, then give repeat boluses of 15 mg/kg IV at 2 hours and then every 6 hours for 1–2 days. After this, discontinue the steroids.

- Mannitol and furosemide are administered if signs of impending herniation are present. Administer a single (1 g/kg) IV bolus of mannitol as a 20% solution at a rate of 2 ml/kg/minute. Administer 0.7 mg/kg furosemide IV 15 minutes after mannitol. Furosemide will prolong the effects of mannitol and decrease CSF production. Mannitol may exacerbate pre-existing intracranial hemorrhage.
- Use hypertonic saline (7.5% as a 4 ml/kg IV bolus) with hydroxyethyl starch (20 ml/kg IV) in a patient that presents with both hypovolemic shock and head trauma/cerebral edema. Hypertonic saline will lower ICP as long as there is no bleeding from a major vessel. Hydroxyethyl starch will prolong the effects of the hypertonic saline. Follow these boluses with LRS at 40–50 ml/kg/hour. If there is significant bleeding, administer whole blood or plasma at 25 ml/kg over 1 hour (do not use hypertonic saline or mannitol). Follow with LRS at 40–50 ml/kg/hour. Fluid therapy is discussed in Chapter 5 and management of shock in Chapter 72.
- Administer intravenous diazepam to control seizures. Intravenous phenobarbital and other anticonvulsants may be needed in some cases (see Chap. 146). Oral anticonvulsant (phenobarbital) therapy should be instituted and not tapered or discontinued unless the patient remains seizure free for a minimum of 6 months.
- Supportive therapy: Fluid therapy should be monitored to prevent overhydration or dehydration (see Chap. 5). Patients should be turned and kept on padded bedding. Intermittent bladder expressions or catheterizations may be necessary. Parenteral or enteral nutritional support should be instituted (see Chap. 3).

METABOLIC ENCEPHALOPATHIES

The brain relies on the body's various homeostatic mechanisms to control extracellular osmolality, electrolyte concentrations, acid-base balance, oxygenation, and glucose levels. Potentially neurotoxic metabolites are continuously removed from the body by fully functional hepatic and renal systems. If homeostatic mechanisms are disrupted, normal brain function may be impacted and physical brain injury may occur. The cerebrum is often the major brain region affected by metabolic encephalopathies. Altered behavior, depressed mentation, and seizures are common manifestations of diffuse cerebral dysfunction. Table 145–4 lists important metabolic causes of brain disease, specific regional vulnerabilities, and clinical signs and treatment. Etiologies, pathogenic mechanisms, diagnosis, and further descriptions of each disorder are discussed in detail in other sections of this text. For additional information, refer to sections, or chapters listed below.

- Osmotic and ionic imbalances: Chapters 5 and 30.
- Acid-base imbalances: Chapter 5.
- Hypoglycemia: Chapters 32 and 33.
- Hypoxia: Section 6.
- Renal failure, uremia: Chapter 97.
- Hepatic encephalopathy/Liver failure: Chapter 91.

Table 145–4. IMPORTANT METABOLIC ENCEPHALOPATHIES IN SMALL ANIMALS

Condition	Causes	Brain Region Affected	Clinical Signs	Treatment
Global hypoxia/ischemia	Pulmonary disease; anemia; carbon monoxide; cyanide; shock; cardiac disease or arrest	Cerebrum (occipital region); cerebellum; hippocampus	Blindness; seizures; ataxia; memory loss; coma	Correct underlying cause; fluids; oxygen; mannitol and furosemide if edema
Hypoglycemia	Juvenile hypoglycemia; insulinoma; sepsis; severe liver disease; Addison's disease	Cerebrum; cerebellum; hippocampus	Ataxia; weakness; collapse; pupillary changes; depressed mentation; seizures; focal facial twitches	Correct underlying cause; see Chap. 33
Hypocalcemia	Eclampsia; hypoparathyroidism; renal failure; others	Cerebrum (neuromuscular junction)	Muscle tremors; spastic tetraparesis/tetany; behavior change; seizures; myoclonus	0.5–1.5 ml/kg up to 10 ml total of 10% calcium gluconate slow IV
Hypernatremia	Diabetes insipidus; severe dehydration; adipsia; primary hyperaldosteronism	Cerebrum	Ataxia; weakness; tremors; depression; seizures; coma	Slow correction with normal saline then half-strength saline
Hyponatremia	Diuretics; Addison's disease; inappropriate ADH secretion; water intoxication	Cerebrum	Depression; stupor; coma	Slow correction with normal saline then hypertonic saline; will induce pontine or thalamic myelinolysis if corrected too fast
Uremia	Acute renal failure (ARF); chronic renal failure (CRF)	Cerebrum	For ARF: seizures, tremors, myoclonus, non-fixed muscle twitches; for CRF: dementia, depression, coma	Correct underlying cause; anticonvulsants if seizures; oral phosphate binders; cimetidine; see Chap. 97
Hepatic encephalopathy	Portocaval shunt; acquired liver disease	Cerebrum	Episodic dementia; head pressing; pacing; ataxia; visual deficits; seizures; ptyalism	IV fluids with potassium; colon evacuation; lactulose or dilute Betadine enemas; metronidazole PO; low-protein, high-carbohydrate diet; surgery for shunt ligation; see Chap. 91

THIAMINE OR VITAMIN B₁ DEFICIENCY

Etiology

Thiamine is a water-soluble B-vitamin that is an essential dietary nutrient. Depleted body stores of thiamine may be a result of deficient thiamine in the diet, a prolonged period of anorexia, or chronic ingestion of all-fish diets containing thiaminase. Thiamine deficiency results in altered energy metabolism, decreased adenosine triphosphate (ATP) formation, and eventual cell death. Neurons in brain stem nuclei are most vulnerable to this energy deficit. Cats are much more frequently affected than dogs presumably because of lower body stores of the vitamin.

Clinical Signs

- Signs may be intermittent initially but are rapidly progressive once present. Affected cats are often either thin or on a poor diet.

- Head and neck ventroflexion and ataxia may progress to recumbency, extensor rigidity, opisthotonus, and coma.
- Ocular changes include mydriasis, sluggish to no pupillary light reflexes, blindness, and absence of the oculovestibular reflex.
- Positional vertical nystagmus is common. Seizures may be present.
- Sudden death can occur in 24–48 hours after onset of signs.

Diagnosis

- Rule out other causes of acute brain stem or central vestibular signs in the cat, including feline infectious peritonitis, cryptococcosis, toxoplasmosis, and vascular disorders.
- CSF may show a slight pleocytosis and protein elevation and/or xanthochromia due to ongoing necrosis and hemorrhage.
- Erythrocyte transketolase activity may be decreased and blood pyruvate and lactate levels may be increased.

- Blood thiamine levels may be normal or decreased.
- Response to therapy is the usual method of diagnosis.

Treatment

- Give parenteral thiamine 25–50 mg per cat intramuscularly or subcutaneously every 12 hours until signs resolve.
- Institute a balanced diet and supplement with B-vitamins for at least 2 weeks.
- A dramatic response to thiamine is usually seen in 24–48 hours.

Prognosis

The prognosis is good with prompt therapy. If pretreatment signs are severe, the response may be incomplete. The condition is fatal if no treatment is instituted.

NEUROTOXINS

A variety of toxins can affect the CNS in dogs and cats. Multisystemic signs may or may not be present. Any region of the neuraxis can be affected. Those neurotoxins that result in signs of brain dysfunction are discussed below.

For most ingested toxins, general treatment guidelines include:

- Induction of vomiting with 2 ml/kg of 3% hydrogen peroxide (except in comatose or obtunded patients or in the case of petroleum distillate or alkali ingestion) if less than 2 hours since ingestion.
- Gastric lavage under anesthesia if less than 2 hours since ingestion. Use 5–10 ml/kg of water for each lavage and lavage several times. Leave activated charcoal in the stomach after the final lavage.
- Administration of activated charcoal 2 g/kg orally by stomach tube.
- Administration of a cathartic (usually magnesium sulfate) at the same time as or 30 minutes following activated charcoal administration.
- Colonic lavage and enemas (especially for heavy metals)

Lead Poisoning

Etiology

Lead poisoning is a sporadic problem caused by ingestion of lead-containing paint chips, plaster board and sheetrock, grease, crankcase oil, linoleum, battery parts, solder, putty and caulking material, roofing material, and, occasionally, lead-contaminated soil. Younger animals are more frequently affected than older animals due to chewing tendencies, increased gastrointestinal absorption, and increased blood-brain barrier permeability. Acute toxicity is generally seen, but chronic exposure to low levels of lead may lead to a cumulative toxicity. Within the CNS, lead causes endothelial cell damage, edema, hemorrhage, and cerebrocortical laminar necrosis.

Clinical Signs

- Acute systemic signs of vomiting, diarrhea, anorexia, and abdominal pain may be seen. A rare finding is megaesophagus.
- Neurologic signs include hysteria, behavior change, pica, vocalization, and blindness.
- Either generalized or focal motor seizures may be present. "Chewing gum" seizures and myoclonus may be observed.

Diagnosis

- A blood lead level of greater than 40 μg/dl is suggestive of lead poisoning. A level greater than 60 μg/dl is diagnostic of lead poisoning.
- Urinary lead levels will be elevated approximately 24 hours after the start of chelation therapy.
- Abdominal radiographs may reveal radiopaque material in the gastrointestinal tract.
- Nucleated red blood cells and basophilic stippling are often evident on stained blood smears.

Treatment

- If lead is visible in the gastrointestinal tract, administer cathartics and enemas.
- Chelating drugs (any one of the following may be used):
  - Calcium disodium EDTA 25 mg/kg SC every 6 hours for 5 days. Prepare a 1% solution in 5% dextrose in water. Side effects are anorexia, diarrhea, and nephrotoxicity.
  - D-Penicillamine 110 mg/kg/day PO divided into three or four doses every 6–8 hours for 2 weeks. Gastrointestinal side effects are common.
  - 2,3-Dimercaptosuccinic acid 10 mg/kg/day PO for 10 days. Side effects are rare.
- Administer anticonvulsants for seizures (diazepam, phenobarbital; see Chap. 146).
- Treat suspected cerebral edema with mannitol and corticosteroids.

Prognosis

The prognosis is fair to good if neurologic debilitation is not severe. Residual neurologic deficits and seizures may be long-term sequelae.

Metaldehyde Poisoning

Etiology

Metaldehyde is a molluscide that can produce signs of neurotoxicity after oral ingestion. Metaldehyde produces a severe metabolic acidosis. Levels of the CNS neurotransmitters gamma-aminobutyric acid, norepinephrine, and serotonin are decreased in affected animals. The exact mechanism of neurotoxicity is unknown.

Clinical Signs

- Seizures, tremors, depression, salivation, tachycardia, hyperesthesia, hyperthermia, vomiting, and diarrhea are seen peracutely. Cats may also have nystagmus and ataxia. Respiratory failure may develop within 24 hours.

- If animals survive the initial toxic insult, hepatic failure occurs 3–4 days postingestion.

Diagnosis

- Compatible signs, acidosis, and a history of exposure are suggestive of metaldehyde intoxication.
- A definitive diagnosis can be made by chemical analysis of stomach contents, urine, or liver tissue.

Treatment

- Perform gastric lavage and administer activated charcoal if within 2 hours of ingestion.
- Use sodium bicarbonate to treat the acidosis.
- Anticonvulsants are indicated for seizure control (see Chap. 146).

Prognosis

The prognosis for recovery is poor.

Methylxanthine Toxicosis

Etiology

Ingestion of stimulants containing caffeine, theophylline, aminophylline, or theobromine may produce signs of methylxanthine toxicosis. Chocolate contains both caffeine and theobromine. Ingestion of 1 ounce of baker's chocolate per kilogram of body weight can be lethal in the dog. Although it is known that methylxanthines inhibit phosphodiesterases, increase calcium influx into cells, and enhance catecholamine release, the mechanism of its neurotoxicity is unknown.

Clinical Signs

- Tachycardia, cardiac arrhythmias, vomiting, polyuria and polydipsia, hyperthermia, respiratory paralysis, and cyanosis.
- Acute signs occur within several hours of ingestion and include seizures, hyperactivity, muscle tremors, ataxia, and coma.

Diagnosis

- Drug or chocolate exposure and clinical signs allow for a tentative diagnosis of methylxanthine toxicosis.
- Serum, stomach contents, and urine can be analyzed for methylxanthine levels.

Treatment

- Administer activated charcoal and promote diuresis with aggressive fluid therapy.
- Treat cardiac arrhythmias with antiarrhythmic agents (see Chaps. 62 and 63).
- Use diazepam for muscle tremors and seizures.

Prognosis

The prognosis is fair to good if treatment is instituted early.

Organophosphate and Carbamate Poisoning

Etiology

Both organophosphates and carbamates inhibit acetylcholinesterase, the enzyme that breaks down acetylcholine at muscarinic and nicotinic sites of the autonomic and somatic nervous systems. Usually signs of parasympathetic stimulation predominate, but signs of somatic, sympathetic, and CNS overstimulation may also be present. Delayed organophosphate neurotoxicity can cause an irreversible central-peripheral axonal degeneration. Chlorpyrifos, dichlorvos, fenthion, carbaryl, methonyl, aldicarb, and carbofuran are just a few of the insecticides that can be toxic after dermal application or following oral ingestion. Many of these insecticides are found in dips and sprays, flea collars, and wormers.

Acute Clinical Signs

- Muscarinic signs include salivation, vomiting, diarrhea, bronchial secretion, miosis, and bradycardia.
- Nicotinic signs are muscle tremors, neuromuscular weakness, and respiratory paralysis.
- CNS stimulation results in hyperactivity and seizures.
- Organophosphate toxicity in cats is characterized by pronounced muscle weakness, mydriasis, twitching, and anorexia, which may last for weeks.

Delayed Clinical Signs

- Exercise intolerance
- Neuromuscular weakness
- Muscle atrophy
- Self-mutilation behavior

Diagnosis

Exposure history, clinical signs, and low whole blood cholinesterase activity (less than 25% of normal) suggest toxicosis.

Treatment

- Induce vomiting if ingestion has occurred within 2 hours of presentation and the patient is asymptomatic. Provide a meal prior to giving an emetic. Follow with activated charcoal and a cathartic (may need to repeat every 8 hours).
- Bathe the animal in dishwashing detergent and water if exposure was by skin contact.
- Start anticonvulsants (IV diazepam, phenobarbital) if seizures occur (see Chap. 146).
- Administer 0.2 mg/kg atropine (0.05 mg/kg IV, 0.15 mg/kg SC); repeat as necessary for bradycardia, bronchoconstriction, respiratory depression, and other muscarinic signs.
- Use pralidoxime chloride (10–15 mg/kg IM or SC) for muscle tremors and nicotinic signs.
- Intravenous fluids, nutritional support, frequent turns, and padded bedding are recommended.
- No treatment for delayed organophosphate toxicity.

Prognosis

The prognosis is good with early treatment.

Metronidazole Toxicity

Etiology

Metronidazole (Flagyl) toxicosis is seen in the dog and cat following oral doses of 66 mg/kg/day for more than 7 days. The mechanism of toxicity is unknown. Lesions of the vestibular nuclei and Purkinje cells of the cerebellum are recognized.

Clinical Signs

- Severe ataxia, positional vertical or rotary nystagmus, opisthotonus, seizures, asymetrical upper motor neuron tetraparesis, and spastic muscle tremors may be seen acutely.
- Affected animals may exhibit a crouched posture in the pelvic limbs that is accentuated during ambulation.
- Many animals are disoriented to the point that they are recumbent, nonambulatory, and anorexic.

Diagnosis

Drug exposure and compatible clinical signs are suggestive of the diagnosis. Tests for inflammatory, neoplastic, or other causes of multifocal CNS disease are negative.

Treatment

Discontinuing the drug will result in gradual resolution of clinical signs over 1–2 weeks. Provide supportive care as necessary.

Prognosis

The prognosis is good if the drug is withdrawn.

Bromethalin Poisoning

Etiology

Bromethalin is a pelleted anticoagulant rodenticide that uncouples oxidative phosphorylation in CNS mitochondria. This results in a cellular ATP deficit, a sodium-potassium pump failure, and mild cerebral and spinal cord edema. Cats are more susceptible than dogs to the neurotoxic effects. Histopathological lesions are mild, indicating a functional deficit at the cellular level.

Clinical Signs

- Acute hyperexcitability, muscle tremors, hyperthermia, running fits, and focal or generalized seizures may be seen in dogs. Thoracic limb rigidity, nystagmus, anisocoria, and depressed levels of consciousness are also part of the acute syndrome in dogs.
- Chronic signs (1–4 days postingestion) in dogs include pelvic limb ataxia, paresis, and hyper-reflexia. This progresses to paraplegia and loss of deep pain. Cats exhibit very similar clinical signs 3–7 days postingestion.

Diagnosis

- Exposure history and appropriate clinical signs suggest bromethalin toxicity.
- Tissue chemical analysis is definitive but not widely available.

Treatment

- Induce vomiting, perform gastric lavage, and administer activated charcoal if less than 2 hours postingestion. Activated charcoal and a cathartic are recommended every 4–8 hours for at least four doses.
- Mannitol and dexamethasone do not appear to alleviate clinical signs.
- Control seizures with IV diazepam or phenobarbital (see Chap. 146).
- Provide supportive care; avoid overhydrating the patient with IV fluids.
- Monitor for 48 hours to evaluate for continued absorption or delayed onset signs.

Prognosis

The prognosis is poor once neurologic signs are seen.

Ethylene Glycol Poisoning

Ethylene glycol is a potent neurotoxin that can cause marked CNS depression. See Chapter 97 for additional information.

CONGENITAL MALFORMATIONS AND ANOMALIES

Most developmental defects of the brain affect either the cerebrum or the cerebellum. Clinical signs are usually present at birth and are nonprogressive. Congenital hydrocephalus can worsen postnatally with a gradual or sudden exacerbation of clinical signs. Although a majority of congenital malformations have a suspected genetic basis, a small number of disorders are due to in utero viral or toxic insults.

Hydrocephalus

Etiology

Primary hydrocephalus is a congenital disorder characterized by a pathologic accumulation of CSF within the ventricular system of the brain. Congenital hydrocephalus is recognized in the Maltese terrier, Yorkshire terrier, Chihuahua, Manchester terrier, Pomeranian, toy poodle, Cairn terrier, Shi Tzu, English bulldog, Boston terrier, Pekinese, Lhasa apso, and other breeds. Decreased CSF absorption at arachnoid villi or occlusion of the mesencephalic aqueduct are incriminated as potential causes, but frequently an underlying structural abnormality cannot be identified.

Clinical Signs

- Signs are usually seen in dogs less than 1 year of age, but trauma may precipitate signs in older dogs.
- Altered consciousness, head pressing, dementia, behavior changes, seizures, visual deficits, and ataxia are observed.

- Acute intraventricular hemorrhage can cause a sudden deterioration in neurologic status.
- Affected animals are frequently stunted, unthrifty, and poor-doers.
- Associated signs are an open fontanelle, a thinned and domed calvarium, and bilateral ventrolateral strabismus ("setting sun sign").

Diagnosis

- Differential diagnoses include hepatic encephalopathy due to a portosystemic shunt, encephalitis due to infectious or idiopathic causes, or toxin exposure (lead).
- Skull radiographs may demonstrate a large, thinned calvarium with loss of gyral markings.
- Ultrasonography through an open fontanelle allows visualization of dilated ventricles.
- Optimum visualization of ventricular dilatation and subcortical white matter atrophy is obtained by CT or MRI.
- Affected animals have normal (normotensive) or elevated (hypertensive) CSF pressures.

Treatment

- Provide therapy only if the patient has clinical signs of cerebral dysfunction. Many animals with ventriculomegaly are clinically normal and do not require therapy.
- Corticosteroids with or without furosemide benefit many patients in the short term.
- Mannitol is helpful if patients are exhibiting signs of acute intracranial pressure elevation.
- Anticonvulsant therapy is used for seizures (see Chap. 146).
- Ventriculoperitoneal or ventriculovenous shunts can be placed to promote drainage of CSF. This procedure has alleviated clinical signs in some cases; however, referral to a neurosurgery specialist is required.

Prognosis

The prognosis is fair with early diagnosis and treatment.

Lissencephaly

Etiology

Lissencephaly is a migration defect of neural cell precursors in the telencephalon characterized by an absence of cerebrocortical convolutions, thickened cortical gray matter, and thinned subcortical white matter. It is presumed to be an inherited defect in the Lhasa apso, wire-haired fox terrier, and Irish setter. Affected wire-haired fox terriers and Irish setters often have concurrent cerebellar hypoplasia.

Clinical Signs

- Neurologic signs are usually present at birth or within the first year of life.
- Behavioral changes, visual deficits, dementia, and seizures are seen.

Diagnosis

- Differential diagnoses are the same as for hydrocephalus (see above).

- CT or MRI reveals absence of gyri and sulci, thickening of the gray matter, and thinning of the white matter. Ventricular size is usually normal.

Treatment

- There is no specific treatment for this condition.
- Treat seizures symptomatically with anticonvulsants (see Chap. 146).

Prognosis

The prognosis is fair to poor. Seizures may be refractory to therapy.

Cerebellar Hypoplasia in Cats
Etiology

Cerebellar hypoplasia refers to a defect in cerebellar development leading to decreased neuronal numbers with or without a gross reduction in size. This condition in kittens is usually due to an in utero or early postnatal panleukopenia viral infection (see Chap. 12). Vaccination of pregnant queens with modified live panleukopenia virus vaccine may also produce this syndrome. Rapidly dividing cells in the developing cerebellum are killed by the virus.

Clinical Signs

- Severe ataxia, falling, hypermetria, head intention tremor, head bobbing, and loss of menace response are usually seen at 3–4 weeks of age when kittens begin to ambulate.
- Signs are nonprogressive.
- There may be fewer clinical signs with lesser degrees of cerebellar damage.
- Littermates may or may not be affected.

Diagnosis

- Differential diagnoses are other infectious causes of cerebellar disease, cerebellar abiotrophy, or lysosomal storage disease.
- Clinical signs of a nonprogressive, purely cerebellar disorder in kittens is strongly suggestive of a diagnosis of cerebellar hypoplasia.
- CT or MRI will often reveal a small cerebellum

Treatment

No treatment is available.

Prognosis

The prognosis is poor for clinical improvement. Many cats with cerebellar hypoplasia make functional pets.

Cerebellar Hypoplasia in Dogs
Etiology

Most of the canine forms of cerebellar hypoplasia have a genetic basis. An exception to this is cerebellar hypoplasia secondary to postnatal herpesvirus infection. Breeds affected include the chow chow, Airedale, Irish setter, wire-haired fox terrier, Boston terrier, bull terrier,

Weimaraner, dachshund, and Labrador retriever. The Irish setter and wire-haired fox terrier have concomitant lissencephaly. Selective involvement of the cerebellar vermis (vermian hypoplasia) is observed in the Boston terrier and bull terrier.

Clinical Signs

- Nonprogressive cerebellar signs are obvious at the time of ambulation but subtle deficits can be detected from birth.
- Truncal ataxia, disequilibrium, dysmetria, falling, intention tremor, and an absent menace response are seen to varying degrees.

Treatment

No treatment is available.

Prognosis

Strength, conscious proprioception, and personality are maintained. If coordination is not incapacitating, affected dogs can make acceptable pets.

DEGENERATIVE BRAIN DISEASE

Inborn errors of metabolism can lead to neural cell degeneration after normal differentiation and maturation. Neuronal or glial cell degeneration is termed *abiotrophy*. Neurodegenerative changes may occur within either the cell body or its processes. Although most abiotrophies affect the cerebellum, others may affect neurons in multiple brain regions. Clinical signs will reflect the brain region that is affected. A metabolic defect has not been identified in the vast majority of abiotrophies in animals.

Lysosomal storage diseases are autosomal recessive neurodegenerative disorders in which the cellular defect has been identified in most cases. Homozygous recessive individuals often exhibit a specific lysosomal hydrolase defect that leads to a cascade of structural and biochemical changes at the cellular level. The most obvious change is the accumulation of undegraded material within lysosomes, giving neurons a foamy, vacuolated, and swollen appearance. Other abnormalities include neuroaxonal dystrophy (axonal swellings), changes in synaptic connections, neurotransmitter and calcium imbalances, and, occasionally, cell death. Neuronal ceroid lipofuscinosis is unique in that massive neuronal cell loss and atrophy occurs in both cerebrum and cerebellum. Other lysosomal storage diseases do not share this feature.

Lysosomal storage disorders result in a slowly progressive neurologic disease with multifocal cerebellar, brain stem, and spinal cord signs. For reasons not well understood, the cerebellum is especially vulnerable and will often show the most severe pathologic changes early in the disease course. Consequently, early clinical signs in the majority of lysosomal storage diseases are predominantly cerebellar in origin. Differential diagnoses for cerebellar signs in young cats and dogs include infectious diseases (FIP, cryptococcosis, toxoplasmosis, canine distemper virus, etc.), cerebellar hypoplasia, or cerebellar abiotrophy. With the exception of globoid cell leukodystrophy, lysosomal storage diseases are also characterized by visceral storage of undegraded material. Storage in liver, pancreas, spleen, kidney, bone marrow, adrenal glands, ocular structures, and lymph nodes is commonly found but rarely causes organ dysfunction. Globoid cell leukodystrophy results in storage within cells of the nervous system only and eventually produces central and peripheral demyelination.

Cerebellar Abiotrophies

Etiology

Purkinje cell abiotrophies have been identified in many canine breeds and in the cat. Breeds affected include the beagle, samoyed, Irish setter, Kerry blue terrier, Gordon setter, rough-coated collie, Airedale, Finnish harrier, Bern running dog, Bernese mountain dog, Labrador and golden retrievers, cocker spaniel, Cairn terrier, Great Dane, Australian kelpie, Brittany spaniel, English springer spaniel, bull terrier, and German shepherd. Normal Purkinje cell formation is followed by premature degeneration and cell death. Cerebellar granule cell loss may also occur. Pathogenic mechanisms are largely unknown. An autosomal recessive mode of inheritance is proven in some breeds.

Clinical Signs

- Age of onset is usually between 4 and 10 weeks of age but some breeds show an earlier or later onset. Most dogs are normal at birth.
- Progression may be slow or rapid.
- Cerebellar signs of intention tremor and progressive ataxia and dysmetria are characteristic.

Diagnosis

- Other causes of progressive cerebellar disease in young dogs (infectious diseases, lysosomal storage disease, myelin disorder, medulloblastoma) should be ruled out.
- CT or MRI may reveal a smaller than normal cerebellum, but usually the cerebellum is normal in size.

Treatment

No treatment is available.

Prognosis

The prognosis is guarded to poor due to the progressive, debilitating nature of these disorders.

Multisystem Neuronal Abiotrophies

Multisystem neuronal abiotrophies are characterized by overt cell loss or chromatolytic change in multiple brain compartments. Breeds affected include the Kerry blue terrier, rough-coated collie, miniature poodle, cocker spaniel, and Cairn terrier. The primary lesion in Kerry blue terriers, rough-coated collies, and miniature poodles is cerebellar abiotrophy, but multiple brain stem nuclei, spinal cord neurons, and cerebrocortical neurons also degenerate. Affected cocker spaniels have cell loss in multiple regions and neuroaxonal dystrophy in cerebellar and cerebral white matter. Multisystem chromatolytic degeneration in Cairn terriers is characterized by chromatolysis of neurons in spinal cord, brain stem, and cerebellum. An autosomal recessive mode of inheritance has been demonstrated in some breeds.

Clinical Signs

- Onset of signs is between 4 and 16 weeks of age and clinical progression may be rapid (over weeks) or slow (over months).
- Kerry blue terriers and rough-coated collies exhibit primarily cerebellar signs.
- Miniature poodles have early cerebellovestibular signs at 3–4 weeks of age, followed by upper motor neuron tetraplegia at 4 months of age.
- Cocker spaniels show both cerebellar and cerebral signs at 1 year of age.
- Signs in Cairn terriers include cerebellar ataxia, paresis, and cataplexy.

Diagnosis

- Differential diagnoses include lysosomal storage disease and inflammatory CNS disease.
- A tentative diagnosis is based on signalment, clinical signs, and progression.
- A definitive diagnosis can only be made postmortem.

Treatment

No treatments are available.

Prognosis

The prognosis is poor.

Multisystem Neuroaxonal Dystrophy

Etiology

Primary neuroaxonal dystrophy refers to an inherited error of metabolism resulting in swellings or spheroids along any region of the axon. The distal axon and axon terminal are the most common cellular sites affected by this neurodegenerative disease. Any region of the CNS may be affected including cerebellum, cerebrum, and brain stem. Neuroaxonal dystrophy has been reported in the rottweiler, Jack Russell terrier, Chihuahua, collie-sheepdog mixed-breed, bull mastiff, Labrador retriever, and domestic shorthair cat. An autosomal recessive mode of inheritance is known or suspected in these breeds.

Clinical Signs

- Clinical signs are primarily cerebellar in origin in the majority of affected breeds.
- Cerebral signs are seen in the Labrador retriever.

Diagnosis

- Differential diagnoses include inflammatory, metabolic, toxic, and other congenital causes of cerebellar or cerebral disease.
- No specific diagnostic tests are available.

Treatment

No treatment is available.

Lysosomal Storage Disorders

See Table 145–5 for a list of the more important lysosomal storage disorders.

CRANIAL NERVE DISORDERS

Disorders of the peripheral portions of cranial nerves may occur secondary to neoplastic, inflammatory, idiopathic, congenital, and endocrine diseases. The most common cranial neuropathies affecting CN5, 7, or 8 are discussed below. Horner's syndrome is discussed in Chapter 160. Laryngeal paralysis is covered in Chapter 77. Megaesophagus is discussed in Chapter 85.

Idiopathic Disorders

Trigeminal Neuritis (Idiopathic Trigeminal Neuropathy, Dropped Jaw Syndrome)

Etiology

The etiology is unknown. A bilateral, nonsuppurative neuritis of CN5 and its ganglia is seen histologically. There is no breed predilection. Most dogs are middle-aged.

Clinical Signs

- An acute to peracute onset of a dropped jaw and inability to close the mouth are seen. The signs are nonprogressive and muscle atrophy rarely occurs.
- Animals have difficulty prehending and chewing food. Food and water fall out the sides of the mouth. Swallowing abilities are usually maintained if food is placed in the back of the mouth.
- A unilateral or bilateral Horner's syndrome may be seen in association with trigeminal neuritis.
- Sensation to the face is usually normal, and there are no long-tract signs or changes in mentation.
- Pain may be elicited upon palpation around the jaw.

Diagnosis

- Clinical signs of acute, severe mandibular paralysis in the absence of other neurologic deficits is usually pathognomonic for this disease.
- Lymphoma with nerve root involvement and rabies may rarely produce similar signs.

Treatment

- Therapy is strictly supportive. Maintaining hydration and nutrition is critical.
- Corticosteroid therapy is of no benefit.

Prognosis

The disorder is self-limiting with recovery taking place within 2–4 weeks after the onset of signs. The prognosis is excellent with adequate nutritional support.

Table 145–5. LYSOSOMAL STORAGE DISEASES IN DOGS AND CATS

Disease	Enzyme Defect	Breeds	Age of Onset	Clinical Signs	Diagnosis	Treatment
GM1 gangliosidosis	β-Galactosidase deficiency	Portuguese water dog, English springer spaniel, Siamese cat, DSH	2–4 mo	Cerebellar signs early; UMN tetraparesis, dementia, seizures, cranial nerve deficits, visual deficits ± hepatomegaly, skeletal deformities, corneal opacities	Enzyme assays on WBC, plasma, other tissues; vacuolated WBCs	BMT with limited effect
GM2 gangliosidosis	β-Hexosaminidase deficiency	Japanese spaniel, mixed-breed dog, DSH, Korat cat	2–4 mo (18 mo in dogs)	Cerebellar signs, UMN tetraparesis, blindness, seizures, dementia ± skeletal deformities, corneal opacities	WBC, plasma, tissue assays; WBCs with heterochromatic granules	BMT with no clinical effect
Niemann-Pick disease type A	Sphingomyelinase deficiency	Balinese cat, Siamese cat, miniature poodle	4–5 mo	Cerebellar signs, LMN tetraparesis ± hepatomegaly	WBC, plasma, tissue assays	Not attempted
Niemann-Pick disease type C	Cholesterol transport defect	DSH, boxer	2–4 mo	Cerebellar signs, UMN tetraparesis, mentation changes ± hepatomegaly	Cholesterol esterification assays on cultured fibroblasts	BMT with limited effect
Mucopolysaccharidosis I	α-L-Iduronidase deficiency	DSH, Plott hound	3–6 mo	No neurologic signs, skeletal deformities, stunted growth, corneal changes,	WBC and other tissue assays, urine screening test	BMT with moderate to marked effect
Mucopolysaccharidosis VI	Arylsulfatase B deficiency	DSH, Siamese cat, miniature pinscher	2–6 mo	See MPS-I above; paraparesis due to cord compression	WBC and other tissue assays, urine screening test	BMT with moderate to marked effect
α-Mannosidosis	α-Mannosidase deficiency	DSH, DLH, Persian	2–7 mo	Cerebellar signs ± cataracts, hepatomegaly, limb deformities	WBC and other tissue assays	BMT with marked clinical effect
Fucosidosis	α-Fucosidase deficiency	English springer spaniel	6–12 mo	Behavior change, cerebellar signs, dementia, visual deficits, jaw chomping	WBC, plasma, CSF, or tissue assays	BMT with moderate effect
Neuronal ceroid lipofuscinosis	Defect unknown (mitochondrial subunit accumulates)	English setter, Dalmation, border collie, Australian cattle dog, others	1–2 y	Behavior change, dementia, visual deficits, seizures ± cerebellar signs	Brain biopsy	BMT not effective or not attempted in many breeds
Globoid cell leukodystrophy	Galactocerebrosidase deficiency	WHWT, Cairn terrier, miniature poodle, bluetick hound beagle, others	2 and 4 mo	Cerebellar signs, paraparesis to tetraparesis	WBC and tissue assays; peripheral nerve biopsy	BMT not attempted in dog (moderate success in mouse)

DSH, domestic shorthair cat; DLH, domestic longhair cat; UMN, upper motor neuron; LMN, lower motor neuron; BMT, bone marrow transplantation; WBC, white blood cell; MPS, mucopolysaccharidosis.

Idiopathic Facial Paralysis/Palsy

Etiology

An idiopathic paralysis of the facial nerve occurs in dogs. There may be unilateral or bilateral involvement. Histologically, there is axonal degeneration with secondary demyelination of the facial nerve. There appears to be a high incidence in cocker spaniels.

Clinical Signs

- Signs are acute in onset and nonprogressive.
- Complete paralysis of the facial nerve results in a unilateral facial droop (lips, ears, etc.) and an inability to blink the eye. The palpebral fissure may be wider than normal.
- Food, water, and saliva tend to fall out the side of the mouth that is paralyzed.
- The nasal philtrum is deviated slightly toward the unaffected side due to unopposed nasal muscles.
- Denervation of the lacrimal gland may lead to decreased tear production.
- Facial contracture (lip retraction, deviation of the lip and nose toward the affected side) can be seen chronically.
- No other neurologic signs are usually present but involvement of the opposite facial nerve is not uncommon.

Diagnosis

- Differential diagnoses include otitis media/interna (see Chap. 57), hypothyroid neuropathy (see Chap. 29), a neuropathy associated with pituitary lesions, lead poisoning, neoplasia, and trauma.

Treatment

- There is no treatment. Artificial tears may be needed to prevent corneal lesions (see Chap. 158).

Prognosis

The prognosis for recovery of function is guarded to fair. Many dogs may recover partial function only.

Canine Idiopathic Vestibular Disease (Old Dog [Geriatric] Vestibular Syndrome)

Etiology

This is a disease of older dogs (average age of 12–13 years old) that occurs commonly in many different breeds. The pathogenesis is unknown. This condition can also occur in the cat at any age but usually occurs in young adult cats.

Clinical Signs

- Signs of vestibular imbalance are peracute and include head tilt, ataxia, circling, falling, rolling, and nystagmus (usually rotary) with a fast phase away from the side of the head tilt.
- Postural reactions and strength are preserved.
- Anorexia with or without vomiting is common.

- Signs are most severe at the onset and gradually improve over days to weeks.

Diagnosis

- Otitis media/interna, hypothyroidism, trauma, and neoplasia should be ruled out.
- There are no specific diagnostic tests.

Treatment

- There is no specific treatment.
- Nutritional and fluid support may be necessary if persistent nausea and anorexia are present.
- A padded, confined area may be needed to prevent self-injury.

Prognosis

The prognosis is good to excellent for recovery. Recurrences are uncommon, especially in the cat.

Neoplasia

Trigeminal Neurofibroma (Schwannoma, Nerve Sheath Tumor)

Etiology

The most common tumor that may involve CN5 is the neurofibroma or schwannoma. Lymphoma and meningioma may involve the trigeminal nerve less commonly. Trigeminal neurofibromas are invariably unilateral and usually originate peripherally with eventual encroachment on brain stem structures in the region of the cerebellopontomedullary angle. Nuclei of CN7 and 8 may secondarily be affected. This neoplastic disease occurs in middle-aged to old dogs.

Clinical Signs

- The onset and progression of signs are slow (over months).
- Marked unilateral temporalis and masseter muscle atrophy is seen initially.
- Jaw weakness is not clinically apparent.
- Muscle atrophy is followed by facial sensory loss.
- Brain stem involvement is indicated by the onset of ipsilateral vestibular signs, facial muscle weakness, and, occasionally, long-tract signs with ipsilateral hemiparesis and conscious proprioceptive deficits.

Diagnosis

- The main differential diagnosis is trauma to CN5. The progressive course of this disorder helps to rule out trauma.
- Electromyography and temporal muscle biopsies reveal signs of denervation.
- Contrast-enhanced MRI scanning is most sensitive in detecting the tumor location and extent.

Treatment

- Surgical excision is the treatment of choice.
- Presurgical MRI aids in surgical planning and may improve outcome.

Prognosis

The prognosis is guarded to poor, especially if brain stem involvement has occurred. Aggressive surgical management early in the disease course may prolong survival times.

Primary and Secondary Neoplasia Involving CN8

Etiology

Primary neurofibromas of CN8 are rare. Meningiomas in the caudal fossa may affect the extradural, intracranial portion of CN8. Secondary tumors affecting CN8 usually originate in the temporal bone or bullae and invade the nerve or its peripheral receptors by local extension. Squamous cell carcinoma, ceruminous gland adenocarcinoma, osteosarcoma, and chondrosarcoma are tumors in this category and do occur in the dog and cat. Middle ear polyps in cats may also secondarily involve vestibular and cochlear structures in the inner ear (see Chaps. 57 and 58).

Clinical Signs

- Slowly or rapidly progressive vestibular signs are observed.
- Horner's syndrome and other cranial neuropathies (especially of the facial nerve) may be seen concurrently.

Diagnosis

- Rule out otitis media/interna (see Chap. 57), idiopathic conditions, endocrine-related neuropathy.
- Otic examination and biopsy may reveal a neoplastic process.
- Bullae radiographs detect soft tissue opacities or bony lysis.
- CT is useful in identifying both bony and neural parenchyma involvement.

Treatment

- Total surgical resection is usually not possible, except in the case of a benign inflammatory polyp.

Prognosis

The prognosis is usually poor.

Congenital Degenerative Disorders

Congenital Sensorineural Deafness

Etiology

Postnatal cochlear hair cell and spiral ganglion degeneration occurs in many breeds including Dalmations, English setters, bull terriers, Old English sheepdogs, English bulldogs, Australian heelers, border collies, collies, Australian shepherds, Australian cattle dogs, catahoulas, Norwegian dunkerhounds, pointers, rottweilers, and white cats with blue irises. Cochlear structures develop normally but degeneration of the stria vascularis is soon followed by loss of cochlear hair cells. The pathogenesis is unknown. The method of genetic transmission is also poorly understood in most breeds.

Clinical Signs

- Deafness may not be clinically apparent until after 2–4 weeks of age. Owners may not recognize a deaf puppy for several months.
- Poor response to verbal commands and loud noises often indicates bilateral deafness.
- Unilaterally deaf pups may not orient to sounds properly or may appear completely normal.

Diagnosis

- Clinical signs may or may not be definitive.
- The brain stem auditory evoked response (BAER) will accurately detect unilaterally and bilaterally deaf animals.

Treatment

- There is no treatment for this degenerative disorder.

Prognosis

The prognosis is poor for recovery of hearing. Special behavioral training is often necessary for dogs with bilateral deafness.

SUPPLEMENTAL READINGS

Bagley RS, Kornegay JN, Page RL, et al.: Central nervous system. *In* Slatter D, ed.: Textbook of Small Animal Surgery, Vol. 2, 2nd Ed. Philadelphia, WB Saunders, 1993, p 2137.

Braund KG: The Clinical Syndromes in Veterinary Neurology, 2nd Ed. St. Louis, Mosby, 1994.

deLahunta A: Veterinary Neuroanatomy and Clinical Neurology, 2nd Ed. Philadelphia, WB Saunders, 1983.

Dow SW, LeCouteur RA, Poss ML, et al.: Central nervous system toxicosis associated with metronidazole treatment in dogs: Five cases (1984–1987). J Am Vet Med Assoc 195:365, 1989.

Fenner WR: Diseases of the brain. *In* Ettinger SJ, Feldman EC, eds.: Textbook of Veterinary Internal Medicine, Vol. 1, 4th Ed. Philadelphia, WB Saunders, 1995, p 578.

Hansen SR: Management of organophosphate and carbamate insecticide toxicoses. *In* Bonagura JD, ed.: Kirk's Current Veterinary Therapy XII: Small Animal Practice. Philadelphia, WB Saunders, 1995, p 245.

LeCouteur RA: Tumors of the nervous system. *In* Withrow SJ, MacEwen EG, eds.: Small Animal Clinical Oncology, 2nd Ed. Philadelphia, WB Saunders, 1996, p 393.

March PA: Degenerative brain disease. *In* Bagley RS, ed.: Veterinary Clinics of North America: Small Animal Practice, Intracranial Disease 26:4, 1996, p 945.

O'Brien DP, Kroll RA: Metabolic encephalopathies. *In* Kirk RW, Bonagura JD, eds.: Kirk's Current Veterinary Therapy XI: Small Animal Practice. Philadelphia, WB Saunders, 1992, p 998.

Summers BA, Cummings JF, deLahunta A: Veterinary Neuropathology. St. Louis, Mosby, 1995.

146 Seizures

Michael Podell

Any animal may be prone to have a seizure, often with little indication of when, why, or how often the seizures will occur. Moreover, most clinical signs of the disease are never observed by the veterinarian. This unpredictability and lack of direct connection with the disease is challenging to veterinarians trying to determine the appropriate diagnostic and therapeutic plan. The purpose of this chapter is to provide a perspective on how to identify and treat dogs and cats with a seizure disorder.

TERMINOLOGY (Fig. 146–1)

A *seizure* is a nonspecific, "sudden, often catastrophic event."

An *epileptic seizure* is the clinical manifestation of excessive and/or hypersynchronous abnormal neuronal activity in the cerebral cortex. Thus an epileptic seizure has a specific neural origin, which is not true of all seizures. Absolute confirmation that a seizure is epileptic may be difficult, as it requires simultaneous observation of behavioral and electroencephalographic changes. As a result, historical information is often used in veterinary medicine to diagnose an epileptic seizure.

Clinical Stages of Epileptic Seizures

- *Aura* is the initial manifestation of a seizure. During this time period, which can last from minutes to hours, animals usually exhibit a change in behavior. Some owners even report that they know that their pet is going to have a seizure days in advance by changes in the pet's behavior.
- *Ictal period* is the actual seizure event manifested by involuntary muscle tone or movement, and/or abnormal sensations or behavior lasting usually from seconds to minutes.
- *Postictal period* is the time immediately following the epileptic seizure. An animal can exhibit unusual behavior, disorientation, inappropriate bowel or bladder activity, excessive or depressed thirst and appetite, and actual neurologic deficits of weakness, blindness, and sensory and motor disturbances. The postictal period can last from minutes to days and rarely longer. Often owners only observe the postictal period as evidence that their pet has had a seizure.

Epileptic Seizure Types

Partial Seizures

Partial seizures are the manifestation of a focal epileptogenic event in the cerebral cortex. The focal nature of this seizure type is associated with a higher prevalence of focal intracranial disease.

- *Simple partial seizures* are characterized by asymmetric motor or sensory signs without a change in consciousness. Examples include facial focal seizures or excessive pawing or biting of a body part.
- *Complex partial seizures* are characterized by impaired consciousness, often with bizarre behavioral activity. Also termed psychomotor seizures, animals with these seizures may show "fly-biting" behavior patterns, become aggressive without provocation, howl incessantly, become restless, or exhibit a variety of motor disturbances.

Generalized Seizures

Generalized seizures originate from both cerebral hemispheres from the start. Unlike partial seizures, generalized seizures are not necessarily associated with focal cerebrocortical disease.

- *Generalized convulsive seizures* are the most common seizure type seen in veterinary medicine. These seizures are characterized by impaired consciousness coupled with bilateral motor signs of either a tonic-clonic, tonic, myoclonic, or even atonic nature.
- *Generalized nonconvulsive seizures* are rare in veterinary medicine, if they occur at all. The classic form is the "absence" variety manifested as impaired consciousness only.

Status Epilepticus

Status epilepticus is present when recurrent complex partial or generalized seizures prevent a return to normal consciousness in 30 minutes, or if simple partial seizures last for more than 30 minutes without any impairment in consciousness.

Primary, Secondary, and Reactive Seizures

- *Primary epileptic seizures (PES)* are diagnosed if no underlying cause for the seizure can be identified. Although this term is often reserved for inherited epilepsy in people, the author prefers to include all

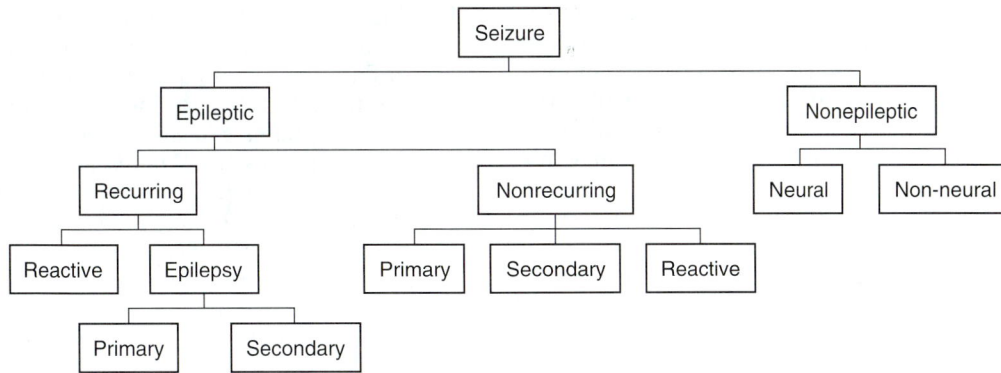

Figure 146–1.   Seizure classification chart for the terminology used in this chapter. Primary = idiopathic; Secondary = structural cerebral disease; and Reactive = normal brain reacting to abnormal stimulus (metabolic).

idiopathic epileptic seizures in this category, as the genetic component of epilepsy is difficult to ascertain in most animals. Primary genetic (breed-related inherited) epilepsy in the dog has been documented in the beagle, Belgian Tervuren, keeshound, dachshund, and British Alsatian. Other breeds with a high incidence of primary epilepsy suspected of having an inherited component are the German shepherd, border collie, Irish setter, and golden retriever.

- *Secondary epileptic seizures (SES)* are the result of structural cerebral disease.
- *Reactive epileptic seizures (RES)* are a reaction of the normal brain to a transient systemic insult or physiologic stress.

Epilepsy

Epilepsy is present if the animal has a chronic brain disorder characterized by recurrent epileptic seizures (PES or SES). A patient with recurring RES is not defined as having epilepsy, as there is not a primary chronic brain disorder underlying the seizure activity. Note that neither the terms seizure nor epilepsy connote the underlying etiology of the disorder.

Nonepileptic seizures are paroxysmal events with severe consequences to the body but without any epileptic electroencephalographic activity.

EPILEPTIC SEIZURES

Etiology

- Epilepsy represents a heterogeneous disease consisting of diverse etiologies, electrophysiologic and behavioral seizure patterns, and responses to therapy. Genetically determined "seizure susceptibility factors" play a crucial role in the brain's response to triggering or precipitating factors. Seizures in these individuals may be activated from unrecognized changes in neuronal activity, intrinsic neurochemical transmission, or by environmental stimuli that do not cause seizures in the normal brain.

▼ *Key Point* A basic mechanism of epilepsy is an imbalance in excitatory and inhibitory neurotransmission.

- A seizure develops when the balance shifts toward excessive excitation. Recruitment of a critical number of areas in the brain with synchronized depolarization will then lead to a seizure. Reasons for the progressive nature of epilepsy include:
  - Conditions leading to excessive excitation or loss of inhibition result in depolarization of neurons without normal regulatory feedback mechanisms.
  - The number of cells with an intrinsic pattern of high spontaneous firing activity ("pacemaker cells") increases in the epileptic focus.
  - A mirror focus of actively firing epileptogenic neurons may develop in a similar region on the opposite hemisphere. This enables the number of epileptic foci to multiply rapidly. As an animal continues to have seizures, an increased number of areas of the brain are randomly and spontaneously able to initiate a seizure.
- Refer to Chapter 145 for information regarding specific diseases of the brain.

Clinical Signs

A thorough and accurate history is essential for diagnosis of seizure patients.

- Obtain past historical information concerning pedigree information, vaccination status, travel, trauma and toxin exposure potential, previous medical and surgical problems, and drug history.
- Organize information about the actual seizure episode(s) by stage into the aura, ictal, postictal, and interictal periods.
- Record dates, times, duration, and description of each abnormality to assess progression and allow a comparison if medication is started.

▼ *Key Point* Evaluate the status of the pet's cerebrocortical function between seizures (after the postictal period) by asking questions concerning the animal's behavior, vision, gait, and sleep-wake patterns.

- Take a thorough neurologic history. For example, question if the dog is more withdrawn or attention seeking, shows any unusual episodes of aggression or irritability, or fails to follow simple commands. These would suggest a structural cerebral problem. Likewise, determine the presence of subtle gait abnormalities (stumbling up and/or down the stairs), visual disturbances (occasionally bumping into objects on one side), and restless sleep patterns that may indicate cerebral problems.

- Classify seizure type as partial or generalized (see Epileptic Seizure Types and Fig. 146–1).
  - Subcategorize partial seizures into simple partial (SP) and complex partial (CP) seizures.

▼ *Key Point* Whenever a partial seizure is suspected, the clinician should be suspicious of a focal cerebral disturbance and plan the diagnostic workup accordingly.

  - Subcategorize generalized seizures into convulsive ("grand mal") and nonconvulsive ("petit mal") seizures.
- Characterize postictal abnormalities.
  - Seizures can be isolated (one per 24 hours) or clustered (two or more in 24 hours). As a consequence of severe or prolonged seizure events, animals can develop detectable neurologic deficits during the immediate and extended postictal period. More severe immediate postictal abnormalities include vision loss, circling, paresis, profound disorientation, aggressive personality changes, and other dementing behaviors. Some of these changes may last for several days to weeks, a condition known as Todd paralysis when sensorimotor localizing deficits are found. Fortunately, practically all of these abnormalities are reversible.
- Characterize seizure-related interictal abnormalities.
  - With chronic seizure activity, changes in cellular physiology of the brain can lead to actual changes in neurologic function, especially persistent behavior disturbances. Dogs with recurrent epileptic seizures may also exhibit changes in personality. Lack of obedience, withdrawal activity, changes in socialization with other animals or people in the household, and unprovoked aggressive behavior can all occur as interictal manifestations of a chronic epileptic condition in the dog. Attributing these changes to the disease or the treatment can be difficult to discern.

Diagnosis

Differential Diagnosis

Dogs

▼ *Key Point* Carefully evaluate for an underlying identifiable etiology for seizures when dogs present <1 or >5 years of age, have an initial interictal interval <4 weeks, or have a partial seizure as the first observed seizure.

When approaching a differential diagnoses list, consider the signalment, history, physical and neurologic examination changes, and laboratory abnormalities.

- For dogs <1 year of age, seizures are most commonly secondary, in particular, caused by developmental and inflammatory diseases (Table 146–1). Specific diseases to include are canine distemper encephalitis and hydrocephalus. Specific breeds prone to congenital hydrocephalus are Maltese, Chihuahuas, Yorkshire terriers, and the brachycephalic breeds. Any breed of dog, however, may suffer from this disease.
- For dogs between 1 and 5 years of age, the most common cause of seizures is primary epilepsy. However, a proportion of dogs in this age category can suffer from a congenital brain anomaly that may be progressive in nature.
- For dogs >5 years of age that start to experience seizures, consider specific structural (e.g., SES) and metabolic diseases (e.g., RES). In particular, brain tumors appear to be more prevalent in dogs in this age category. Cerebrovascular disease is another consideration in the geriatric dog.

Cats

▼ *Key Point* Primary epilepsy is rare in the cat.

The diverse genetic background of cats has fortunately made primary epilepsy an uncommon diagnosis. Practically all cats have an underlying etiology for their seizure disorder. The differential diagnoses of seizure etiology for cats is listed in Table 146–2.

Diagnostic Approach

Refer to Chapter 144 for information on diagnostic evaluation of the patient with neurologic disease, and Chapter 145 for diagnostic parameters of specific diseases of the brain.

▼ *Key Point* The decision to pursue diagnostic testing should not be based on the number or severity of prior seizures. Rather, the decision should be based on the signalment, history, and initial neurologic examination.

Dogs

The goals of a diagnostic evaluation in a patient with seizures are to determine the underlying etiology, evaluate the prognosis for recurrence, and establish if antiepileptic medications are necessary for treatment. Most dogs have already suffered from more than one seizure by the time they are presented to a veterinarian. Furthermore, many dogs appear normal when examined during interictal periods. In a dog with a history of seizures, try to determine if the seizure will recur and whether a more serious underlying disease exists.

- A diagnosis of SES is more likely when:
  - A dog is <1 or >7 years old at the first seizure.
  - The first seizure is a partial seizure.
  - The interval between the first and second seizure event (an event being all seizures within a 24-hour period) was brief (<4 weeks).
  - The neurologic examination is abnormal.

Table 146–1. PRIORITIZED DIFFERENTIAL DIAGNOSES FOR SEIZURES ACCORDING TO AGE AT TIME OF FIRST SEIZURE IN THE DOG

<1 Year of Age	Between 1 and 5 Years of Age	5 Years of Age or Older
Anomaly Hydrocephalus	*Primary* Idiopathic	*Neoplasia* Primary Metastatic

Inflammatory
Infectious
   Viral: Canine distemper
   Parasitic
   Bacterial
   Fungal
Immune-mediated
	Inflammatory
	Infectious
	   Viral: Canine distemper
	   Parasitic
	   Bacterial
	   Fungal
	Immune-mediated
		Metabolic
		Hypoglycemia: Insulinoma
		Hepatic: Cirrhosis
		Electrolyte disturbances

Metabolic
Hepatic: Portosystemic shunt
Hypoglycemia
Electrolyte disorders
	Anomaly
	Hydrocephalus
		Vascular
		Focal ischemia
		   Thromboembolism
		   Vasospasm
		Hemorrhage
		   Hypertension
		   Vasculitis

Toxic
Lead
Drug-related
Other exposures
	Trauma
	Acute
	Delayed
		Inflammatory
		Infectious
		   Viral: Canine distemper
		   Parasitic
		   Bacterial
		   Fungal
		Immune-mediated

Trauma Acute Delayed	*Metabolic* Hepatic: Portosystemic shunt Hypoglycemia Electrolyte disorders	*Primary* Idiopathic
Degenerative Storage disorders	*Toxic* Lead Drug-related Other exposures	*Degenerative*
Primary Idiopathic	*Neoplasia* Primary Metastatic	*Toxic* Lead Drug-related Other exposures

- A diagnosis of RES is more likely when:
  - The interval between the first and second seizure event was brief (<4 weeks).
  - The animal is showing signs of systemic illness.
- A diagnosis of PES is more likely when:
  - The dog is between 1 and 5 years of age at the first seizure.
  - The dog is a large breed (>15 kg).
  - The interval between the first and second seizure event was long (>4 weeks).
- Diagnostic tests in dogs
  - Evaluate a minimum database consisting of a complete blood count (CBC), serum chemistry profile, and urinalysis to rule out possible metabolic causes. Unfortunately, these tests have a very low yield of positive findings in seizure patients.
  - If SES are suspected, consider computed tomography (CT) or magnetic resonance imaging (MRI). These offer the best opportunity to diagnose either an intracranial anomaly or primary neoplasia, which are the prevalent causes of seizures in dogs

<1 and >7 years of age, respectively. If negative scan results are found, then cerebellomedullary cerebrospinal fluid (CSF) should be collected for analysis.
- Collect CSF first if a multifocal disease or meningeal inflammatory process is suspected after the neurologic examination.
- Perform additional diagnostic testing in any dog with persistent interictal neurologic abnormalities. Select tests according to the history and clinical suspicions; for example, serum bile acids to evaluate liver function, serial fasting blood glucose paired with insulin levels to diagnose hyperinsulinemia, plasma lead concentration, and specific serum antibody titers for infectious diseases.

Cats

In cats, always consider an underlying cause for seizures, until proved otherwise. Consider the following diagnostic tests in cats.

Table 146–2. PRIORITIZED DIFFERENTIAL DIAGNOSES FOR SEIZURES ACCORDING TO AGE AT TIME OF FIRST SEIZURE IN THE CAT

<1 Year of Age	Between 1 and 7 Years of Age	>7 Years of Age
Inflammatory	*Inflammatory*	*Neoplasia*
Infectious	Infectious	Primary
Viral: FIP	Viral: FIP*	Metastatic
Parasitic	Parasitic	
Bacterial	Bacterial	
Fungal	Fungal	
Immune-mediated	Immune-mediated	
Anomaly	*Vascular*	*Vascular*
Hydrocephalus	Focal ischemic encephalopathy	Focal ischemic encephalopathy
	Thromboembolism	Thromboembolism
	Vasospasm	Vasospasm
	Hemorrhage	Hemorrhage
	Hypertension	Hypertension
	Vasculitis	Vasculitis
Metabolic	*Trauma*	*Metabolic*
Hepatic encephalopathy	Acute	Chronic renal failure
Hypoglycemia	Delayed	Endocrine: Hyperthyroidism
Electrolyte disorders		Hepatic encephalopathy
Thiamine deficiency		Electrolyte disturbances
		Hypoglycemia
Toxic	*Metabolic*	*Inflammatory*
Lead	Hepatic encephalopathy	Infectious
Drug-related	Hypoglycemia	Viral: FIP
Other exposures	Electrolyte disorders	Parasitic
	Thiamine deficiency	Bacterial
		Fungal
		Immune-mediated
Trauma	*Toxic*	*Toxic*
Acute	Lead	Lead
Delayed	Drug-related	Drug-related
	Other exposures	Other exposures
Degenerative	*Neoplasia*	*Degenerative*
Storage disorders	Primary	
	Metastatic	
Primary	*Primary*	*Primary*
Idiopathic	Idiopathic	Idiopathic

*FIP, feline infectious peritonitis.

- Evaluate a minimum database consisting of a CBC, serum chemistry profile, baseline thyroid level, and urinalysis to rule out possible metabolic causes.
- Collect CSF first if a multifocal disease or meningeal inflammatory process is suspected and/or in all cats <7 years of age.
- Perform CT or MRI scanning in all cats >7 years of age or in those cats with a normal CSF analysis. The combination of CT or MRI scanning and CSF analysis is often the most direct approach to a definitive diagnosis.
- Also consider specific serologic tests for infectious diseases (e.g., toxoplasmosis, feline immunodeficiency virus, feline leukemia virus), and serum bile acids to evaluate liver function.

Treatment

This section describes seizure control therapy. Refer to Chapter 145 for treatment of specific diseases of the brain.

Goals of Therapy

Prior to starting antiepileptic drug (AED) treatment, owners and veterinarians should have a realistic expectation of what to expect over the course of therapy.

- First and foremost is that seizure control does not equal elimination.
- Realistic goals are a decrease in the number and severity of seizures, fewer postictal complications, and an increase in the interictal period.
- Inform clients that this may be a lifetime, daily treatment regimen, there will be frequent reevaluations, there is a potential for emergency situations to arise, and there are inherent risks from the drugs.
- Single drug therapy for treating epilepsy is preferred because it reduces possible drug-drug interactions and adverse effects.

▼ *Key Point* The ultimate goal of antiepileptic therapy is to maintain a seizure-free status without unacceptable adverse effects.

Limitations of Antiepileptic Drugs

Unfortunately, several limitations exist in the selection of AEDs for use in veterinary medicine:

- *Toxicity*. Drugs with hepatic metabolism have the potential for hepatotoxic effects.
- *Tolerance*. This can be metabolic in origin in that progressively more drug is needed over time to maintain the same therapeutic serum concentration, or it can be functional in that cellular adaptations occur that prevent full efficacy of the drug.
- *Inappropriate pharmacokinetics*. Certain AEDs are metabolized too rapidly to allow a steady-state concentration to be achieved with normal-interval dosing (2–3 times per day).
- *Expense*. Lifetime drug administration and monitoring can be prohibitively expensive for some owners.

Deciding When to Start Treatment

▼ *Key Point* Instruct the owner to document seizures and other problems in a written log. This record provides the basis for initiating and adjusting AED therapy, and for determining the benefits of therapy.

Base the decision to initiate AED therapy on the underlying etiology, seizure type and frequency, and diagnostic evaluation. Initiate phenobarbital therapy in the following situations:

- An identifiable disease process is present.
- Status epilepticus has occurred.
- Two or more isolated seizures have occurred within a 6-month period.
- Two or more cluster seizure episodes have occurred within a 12-month period.
- The first seizure was within 1 week of trauma.

Phenobarbital Administration

Phenobarbital is the initial antiepileptic drug of choice because it is a relatively inexpensive, well-tolerated drug that effectively prevents seizures in animals when administered 2–3 times per day.

Phenobarbital in Dogs

▼ *Key Point* In the dog, give phenobarbital initially at least every 12 hours at a dosage of 2.5 mg/kg PO with subsequent increases in dosage most likely within 30 days to maintain a trough therapeutic serum concentration.

- In the dog, phenobarbital has a high bioavailability (between 86 and 96%). The drug is rapidly absorbed within 2 hours with a maximal plasma concentration obtained within 4–8 hours after oral administration. Almost one-half of the drug is protein-bound. The majority of phenobarbital is metabolized by the liver, with approximately one-third excreted unchanged in the urine. Phenobarbital is an autoinducer of hepatic microsomal enzymes (p-450 system), which can progressively reduce the elimination half-life with chronic

dosing. Elimination half-lives have been reported to range from 42–89 hours, with a significantly shorter half-life in beagles (32 hours). Thus, initial steady-state serum phenobarbital concentrations (Css) are achieved within a maximum of 18 days in dogs with the longest elimination half-life (five elimination half-lives). At 5.5 mg/kg/day dosing, Css and total body clearance are stable by 30 days.

Phenobarbital in Cats

▼ *Key Point* In the cat, give phenobarbital initially every 24 hours in the evening at a dose of 2.5 mg/kg with subsequent increases in dosing or frequency most likely within 30 days to maintain a trough therapeutic serum concentration.

- As in the dog, phenobarbital has a high bioavailability with rapid gastrointestinal absorption in the cat. Unlike the dog, the cat does not have significant autoinduction of the p-450 system with phenobarbital treatment. Thus, the elimination half-life of 40–60 hours does not appear to change significantly over time. This long half-life makes it possible to start once-a-day therapy. However, a wider fluctuation between the peak and trough daily serum concentration with once-a-day dosing may not provide adequate seizure control, necessitating dosing to be given in twice-daily intervals in some cats.

Intravenous Phenobarbital Loading

▼ *Key Point* Phenobarbital has the dual advantage of achieving high serum concentrations and reducing cerebral metabolic rate following intravenous (IV) dosing.

- The advantage of IV administration is the ability to achieve a therapeutic concentration in the brain very rapidly (see Hospital Emergency Treatment for Seizures). IV phenobarbital is rapidly distributed within 10 minutes in the dog and the cat; therefore, it provides a rapid, high drug concentration to stop seizures while serving as a cerebral protectant.
- To achieve a serum concentration of 25 μg/ml in the dog:

Total IV loading dose (mg) = (Body weight [kg])
$$\times \ (0.8 \ \text{L/kg}) \times (25 \ \mu\text{g/ml})$$

- To achieve a serum concentration of 20 μg/ml in the cat:

Total IV loading dose (mg) = (Body weight [kg])
$$\times \ (0.9 \ \text{L/kg}) \times (15 \ \mu\text{g/ml})$$

Give the total dose at a rate of <100 mg/minute.

Serum Monitoring of Phenobarbital

▼ *Key Point* Monitor trough serum concentrations of phenobarbital to determine if a therapeutic level is maintained at the time when the lowest serum concentration is present (i.e., immediately before the next dose). Animals will be most susceptible to seizure at this time.

Overall, phenobarbital is well tolerated at therapeutic serum concentrations in the dog and cat. The trough therapeutic concentration range of phenobarbital is between 20 and 40 µg/ml in the dog.

- The goal of any AED therapy is to achieve serum concentrations within the established therapeutic range for that drug. The major advantage of monitoring serial serum trough phenobarbital concentrations is to individualize treatment by documenting that an adequate amount of drug is being given while minimizing the potential for toxic effects.
- The lower limit of the therapeutic range is the minimal concentration at which 50% of animals will have any therapeutic benefit. Conversely, the upper limit is the maximal concentration at which 50% of animals will not have toxic adverse effects. Monitor the serum concentrations only after steady-state levels are reached. Furthermore, wide variations in serum concentration can occur in dogs and cats on similar oral doses of phenobarbital.

▼ *Key Point* Optimal seizure control with minimal toxicity can be obtained by maintaining the trough serum concentration of phenobarbital between 20 and 35 µg/ml in dogs, and between 15 and 30 µg/ml in cats.

- Measure trough serum concentrations of phenobarbital according to the following guidelines:
  - At 14, 45, 90, 180, and 360 days after the initiation of treatment.
  - At 6-month intervals thereafter.
  - At any time the pet has more than two seizure events between these times.
  - At any time cluster seizures or status epilepticus occur.
- Adjustments of the trough concentration can be calculated with the following formula:

$$\frac{\text{Desired concentration}}{\text{Actual concentration}} \times \text{no. mg PB per day}$$

$$= \text{Total no. mg PB per day}$$

This new value can then be divided either twice daily or three times daily. The only advantage of administration three times a day is less fluctuation between the peak and trough serum concentrations, which may be important in animals requiring tighter therapeutic windows. Note that no adjustment is made according to weight and no upper limit dosage is present. Each animal is treated as an individual with allowances for individual variations in metabolism.

- If concern arises about toxicity, obtain peak levels by measuring the concentration 4–6 hours after pill ingestion with once-daily or twice-daily administration and 4 hours after pill ingestion with three-times-a-day dosing.

- Evaluate serum chemistry profiles at 3 months and at 6-month intervals thereafter for evidence of toxicity. Evaluate complete blood counts at 3 months and at yearly intervals to check for drug-related blood dyscrasias.

Adverse Effects of Phenobarbital

▼ *Key Point* Do not lower the initial phenobarbital dose if signs of sedation or behavior changes are seen after starting treatment. These signs are transient adverse effects that typically disappear in 10–14 days.

Adverse effects of any AED can be broadly categorized into predictable and unpredictable (idiosyncratic) complications. Further subclassification can be based on transient versus chronic or progressive problems. Despite the long historical use of phenobarbital in veterinary medicine, few reports exist documenting the adverse effects of the drug in dogs and cats. Lack of reportable information may be due to overall safety of the drug, the difficulty in accurately documenting clinical adverse reactions, delay in detection of problems after onset of therapy, or a combination of these.

Idiosyncratic Drug Reactions

Idiosyncratic drug reactions to phenobarbital are usually associated with unusual behavioral changes after starting the drug. Hyperexcitability and restlessness are infrequent problems that do not appear to be dose-related. Acute toxic hepatopathy is infrequently associated with phenobarbital administration in the dog and cat.

Transient and Mild Effects

More predictable, dose-related transient adverse effects of a non–life-threatening nature can be categorized into:

- *Behavior changes.* Owners may complain that their pet is acting more sedate and lethargic after starting phenobarbital therapy. This change often dissipates after 1–2 weeks of treatment. Other potential transient complaints are polydipsia, polyuria, and polyphagia. On physical and neurologic examination, animals may demonstrate excessive somnolence, ataxia, and disorientation. Higher oral and IV doses can produce more profound behavioral changes. Polydipsia and polyphagia can also occur. Dogs may develop psychogenic polydipsia with associated polyuria. The polyphagia can lead to intense scavenging and begging behavior. This can lead to dietary indiscretion with subsequent serious problems of gastroenteritis, pancreatitis, or foreign body obstruction. Some owners also complain that their dog "just isn't the same pet" after phenobarbital therapy.
- *Physical examination changes.* The most common change with chronic phenobarbital therapy is weight gain. Most likely this is the result of increased appetite (with an increased food supply) coupled with a more sedentary lifestyle. Some dogs may develop

splenomegaly and/or hepatomegaly. Persistent neurologic deficits without underlying intracranial pathology are extremely uncommon.

- *Clinical laboratory changes.* Transient clinical laboratory changes are minimal. Urine specific gravity may decrease. The most common clinical laboratory change associated with chronic phenobarbital therapy is elevation of serum alkaline phosphatase (ALP) in the dog. This can occur as quickly as 2 weeks after therapy. Neither endogenous adrenocorticotrophic hormone (ACTH) nor exogenous response to ACTH is altered by phenobarbital. However, baseline serum thyroxine concentration is depressed in 60–70% of dogs on phenobarbital. These dogs have a normal response to thyroid-stimulating hormone (TSH). Thus, use TSH response to diagnose hypothyroidism in dogs on phenobarbital.

Life-Threatening Complications

Three serious and potentially life-threatening complications can occur with long-term phenobarbital therapy:

- *Physical dependence* on the drug develops over time. Withdrawal seizures can develop as serum phenobarbital concentration declines, especially during precipitous drops below 20 μg/ml (dog) or 15 μg/ml (cat).
- *Functional tolerance.* The loss of drug efficacy despite adequate serum concentration can develop as the result of altered transport of the drug through the blood-brain barrier, downregulation of receptors in the brain, and progression of epilepsy resulting in multiple seizure foci or changes in neurotransmission. The degree of functional tolerance to phenobarbital in the dog is not clear. In the author's experience, phenobarbital is less effective in the presence of underlying cerebral pathology, in dogs with primary (idiopathic) breed-related (hereditary) epilepsy, and in dogs with complex partial seizures, and/or cluster seizures as the first seizure event.
- *Drug-induced hepatotoxicity.* Hepatotoxicity to primidone (which is metabolized predominantly to phenobarbital), either alone or in combination with other AEDs, occurs in dogs. Phenytoin (Dilantin) treatment combined with primidone (or phenobarbital) causes a predictable hepatotoxic reaction leading to irreversible liver damage. Chronic phenobarbital therapy can also lead to hepatotoxicity, especially if serum trough levels are maintained above 35 μg/ml.

▼ *Key Point* Since both primidone and phenytoin have been proved not to provide effective seizure control and are potentially hepatotoxic in the dog, do not use these drugs to treat seizures in the dog.

Treatment of Refractory Epilepsy in Dogs

Approximately 20–50% of dogs treated for epilepsy at referral veterinary institutions are reported to not be well-controlled with medical management and thus become classified as refractory epileptics.

Criteria for Refractory Epilepsy

The author's criteria for classifying primary canine epileptics as refractory are:

- A primary etiology of seizures has not been identified.
- Phenobarbital has been administered for at least 3 months with all serum trough concentrations between 20–40 μg/ml, and a trough steady-state concentration ≥30 μg/ml without a subsequent change in dosage for at least 1 month.
- Seizure number and severity has not improved or has worsened for at least 3 months despite phenobarbital and/or other AED treatment.
- Status epilepticus has occurred.
- Hepatotoxicity is present.

▼ *Key Point* Consider adding a second anti-epilepsy drug in dogs whose seizures continue despite persistent trough serum phenobarbital concentrations >30 μg/ml for 1–2 months.

Bromide Therapy

Currently, the recommended second antiepileptic drug of choice in the dog is bromide (Table 146–3). Although bromide is proved effective in human and veterinary medicine, inorganic bromide is not approved for use as a medical therapy in any species in the United States. The Food and Drug Administration, Center for Veterinary Medicine, requires that written registration be acquired prior to dispensing bromide. The analytic chemical grade of potassium bromide can then be obtained from most major chemical companies.

- Although its exact mechanism of action is not completely understood, bromide appears to have a competitive interaction with chloride to hyperpolarize neuronal membranes in the brain. Thus, bromide is expected to have a synergistic effect with drugs that enhance chloride conductance, such as phenobarbital.
- Bromide is a unique AED in that it has a very long elimination half-life of about 25 days, and it takes about 120 days to achieve a steady-state serum concentration. Bromide, however, may still be an effective treatment during this time period when steady-state concentration is being reached.
- The protocol for potassium bromide administration and monitoring is as follows:
  - *Preparation.* Dissolve potassium bromide in double distilled water as a 200 mg/ml solution.
  - *Administration.* The initial dosage is 30 mg/kg/day orally in food (with concurrent phenobarbital administration). The solution can be placed directly on the dog's food. Give the drug once per day or divided every 12 hours. Dividing the dose allows for a better adaptation to the sedative effects of the drug.
  - *Monitoring.* Obtain trough serum concentrations of bromide at 30 days, 120 days, and every 6 months after initiation. The therapeutic range is 150–200 mg/dl (1.5–2.0 mg/ml) with concurrent phenobarbital administration (maintaining trough

Table 146–3. SUMMARY OF ANTIEPILEPTIC DRUG THERAPY IN THE DOG

Drug	Indications	Administration	Monitoring	Potential Adverse Effects
Phenobarbital	· Identification of a structural lesion · Status epilepticus · Two or more isolated seizures within a 6-month period · Two or more cluster seizure episodes within a 2-month period · The first observed seizure is within a week of head trauma · Prolonged, severe, or unusual postictal periods	Initial oral dose: 2.5 mg/kg q12h PO IV loading dose: Total mg IV = (Body weight [kg] × (0.8 L/kg) × (25 µg/ml)	· Measure trough serum phenobarbital · Therapeutic range is between 20–40 µg/ml · Evaluate serum chemistry panel at 45 days and every 6 mo	· Transient: lethargy, behavior change · Persistent: Polyuria, polydipsia, polyphagia, weight gain, excessive sedation · Severe: Hepatotoxicity
Potassium bromide	· Persistent seizure activity with steady-state trough serum phenobarbital concentration ≥ 30 µg/ml for at least 1 month · Hepatoxicity from phenobarbital or primary hepatic disease · Severe cluster seizures	Potassium bromide dissolved in double distilled water as 200 mg/ml solution Dose: 30 mg/kg/day orally in food as initial dose	Measure trough serum concentrations 30 days, 120 days, and every 6 months after initiation Therapeutic range is 150–200 mg/dl (1.0–2.0 mg/ml) with concurrent phenobarbital (25–30 µg/ml); 200–300 mg/dl as monotherapy	Lethargy Polydipsia Polyuria Pancreatitis Ataxia Stupor
Felbamate	· Complex partial seizures · Refractory to phenobarbital and bromide therapy	20 mg/kg q8h PO as initial dose; increase as needed up to a maximum of 3000 mg/day	No active drug metabolites are commercially measurable Monitor complete blood counts every 6–12 weeks to check for bone marrow suppression Monitor liver enzymes every 6–12 weeks to check for hepatotoxicity	Hepatotoxicity (people) Aplastic anemia (people)
Gabapentin	· Complex partial seizures · Refractory to phenobarbital and bromide therapy	Initial dose: 300 mg q12h PO Increase: Up to 1200 mg q8h PO over 4 wk	No active drug metabolites are commercially measurable	Sedation No organ toxicity reported
Diazepam per rectum	· Generalized cluster epileptic seizures · Status epilepticus	On phenobarbital: 2 mg/kg per rectum of diazepam parenteral solution (5 mg/ml) Without phenobarbital: use 1 mg/kg Administer at the onset of a seizure up to three times in 24 hr	Instruct owners to stay with pet for 1 hr after administration	Sedation

serum phenobarbital concentration at 25–30 µg/ml). Decrease the phenobarbital if hepatotoxicity occurs or if the dog is seizure-free for ≥6 months.

- *Dosage adjustments.* A linear relationship between bromide dose and serum concentration is not found in the dog. There is high variability in serum bromide concentrations in different dogs on equal dosages of the drug. The best method to adjust dosage is through gradual adaptation. Increasing by small increments (100–200 mg) on a weekly basis will often allow dogs to acclimate better to the adverse effects of sedation and weakness. Obtain follow-up serum concentrations 30 days after dosage adjustment.
- Bromide is indicated as a single-agent antiepileptic drug in the following situations:
  - Underlying liver disease (e.g., hepatotoxicity, portosystemic shunting), which prevents the use of phenobarbital.
  - Prolonged seizure-free status (>1 year) on combined phenobarbital and bromide therapy.
  - Unacceptable quality of life on combined phenobarbital and bromide therapy with a seizure-free status period of ≥3 months.
  - The optimal serum concentration when bromide is used as a single agent is > 200 mg/dl. Many dogs can adapt to serum concentrations of up to 300 mg/dl.
- *Adverse effects.* Bromide is generally well tolerated in the dog. The most common adverse effects seen with combination bromide and phenobarbital therapy are polydipsia, polyphagia, and increased lethargy. Pancreatitis has also been seen with combination therapy. Ataxia can also occur, particularly with trough serum concentrations approaching 200 mg/dl. Dogs with higher concentrations appear to be more severely affected, suggesting a dose-dependent effect. Bromide intoxication to the point of stupor is rare, especially with close monitoring of serum concentrations. Therapy of bromide intoxication consists of IV 0.9% saline administration to enhance bromide renal excretion. Carefully monitor dogs for increased susceptibility to seizure activity with lowering of the bromide serum concentration.

New Antiepileptic Drugs with Potential for Use in Dogs

Several new AEDs that have recently been approved for use in people offer exciting potential for use in dogs. Unfortunately, little to no information is available on the pharmacokinetic or therapeutic properties of these drugs in controlled studies in dogs. Furthermore, most of these medications are still quite expensive.

Felbamate (Felbatol)

This is a dicarbamate with proved ability to block seizures induced by a variety of methods in laboratory animal models. Felbamate is believed to increase seizure threshold and prevent seizure spreading by reducing excitatory neurotransmission in the brain. In clinical trials in people, felbamate has been shown to be most useful as monotherapy in the treatment of uncontrolled partial epilepsy.

- The author has successfully used felbamate to manage several dogs with complex partial and generalized seizures.
- The recommended dosage in dogs is 20 mg/kg q8h PO initially; increase as necessary up to a maximum of 3000 mg/day.
- Measure trough serum concentration of felbamate one week after initiation of treatment. The therapeutic range is 25–100 mg/L.
- A higher incidence of aplastic anemia and liver toxicity was found in people treated with felbamate compared with the general population. The author has not found similar problems in dogs. Monitor complete blood counts and serum liver enzymes every 6–12 weeks to check for bone marrow suppression and hepatotoxicity, respectively.
- Avoid concurrent use of felbamate and phenobarbital due to the possibility of increased hepatotoxicity and alteration of serum phenobarbital concentrations (felbamate increases serum phenobarbital concentration by 25%).

Gabapentin (Neurontin)

This is an interesting new AED whose mechanism of action is still not fully understood. Initially designed to mimic γ-aminobutyric acid (GABA) in the brain, gabapentin can readily pass through the blood-brain barrier. Once in the brain, however, gabapentin does not mimic the pharmacologic properties of GABA, nor does it bind to GABA receptors. A major benefit of the drug is that it is not metabolized by the liver; thus, it can be used in conjunction with drugs with hepatic elimination, such as phenobarbital.

- The recommended dosage is:
  - **Dogs < 10 kg:** 100 mg q8h PO; increase to 200 mg q8h PO after 1 week. Maximum dose is 600–900 mg q8h PO.
  - **Dogs > 10 kg:** 300 mg q8h PO; increase 600 mg q8h PO after 1 week. Maximum dose is 1200–1800 mg q8h PO.
- Serum drug monitoring is not needed. Monitor complete blood count and renal profile every 3–6 months.
- Toxic effects are mainly limited to excessive sedation.

Maintenance Antiepileptic Drugs to Avoid in Dogs

Phenytoin (Dilantin)

- High risk of hepatotoxicity with this drug.
- It is difficult to maintain adequate steady-state serum concentrations due to the very rapid elimination half-life (approximately 2 hours).

Diazepam (Valium)

- Functional tolerance develops very quickly to diazepam, which results in inability to use diazepam as an effective emergency drug to stop cluster seizures or status epilepticus.

- Potential for causing physical dependence and withdrawal seizures.
- It is difficult to maintain adequate steady-state serum concentrations.

Gamma-vinyl-GABA (Vigabatrin)

- Potential for causing hemolytic anemia.
- Potential for causing central nervous system vacuolation with chronic use.
- Ineffective for stopping seizures.

Treatment of Refractory Epilepsy in Cats

Since cats have an extremely high prevalence of secondary epileptic seizures, epileptic cats may not respond to phenobarbital alone. Moreover, the often focal nature of the underlying pathologic condition (e.g., meningioma, cerebrovascular accident) may predispose cats to partial seizure activity, which can be difficult to control with phenobarbital in the author's experience. Unfortunately, cats are quite sensitive to the sedative effects of many of the AEDs. Therefore, most combination therapies require a delicate balance of drug dosing. In the author's experience, cats are best controlled with a single AED. The following drugs may be tried in place of phenobarbital therapy in cats.

▼ *Key Point* Addition of a second antiepileptic drug or changing to a different therapy should be considered in cats whose seizures continue despite persistent trough serum phenobarbital concentrations above 25 µg/ml.

Potassium Bromide

- Use bromide as a combination therapy with phenobarbital initially, and possibly as monotherapy after seizures stop.
- Dosage: 30 mg/kg once per day in the evening. Use a capsule formulation. Obtain bromide capsules from a pharmacist specializing in compounding veterinary drugs.
- The elimination half-life of bromide is reported to be shorter in the cat than in the dog (about 16 days). Thus, steady-state serum concentrations can be obtained in 3 months.
- Monitor trough serum bromide concentrations 3 weeks and 2 months after initiation of treatment. A serum concentration between 100–150 mg/dl (1.0–1.5 mg/ml) often provides the best combination of seizure control and quality of life.
- Toxicity includes sedation, weakness, and inappetence.

Diazepam

- Cats appear to be resistant to developing functional tolerance to diazepam.
- *Dosage:* 0.5–2.0 mg/kg PO divided every 8 to 12 hours.
- Serum concentrations of nordiazepam can be monitored, but a therapeutic range has not been determined for the cat.

- Fatal, acute idiosyncratic hepatotoxicity after diazepam administration has been reported in the cat. Thus, obtain a liver chemistry panel in all cats 3, 7, 14 days, and then every 3–6 months after initiation of therapy.

Clorazepate

- Clorazepate is a long-acting benzodiazepine, similar in action to diazepam.
- *Dosage:* 2–3.75 mg q12–24h PO. Start at a low dose (1–2 mg) and gradually increase over time.
- Serum concentrations of nordiazepam can be monitored, but a therapeutic range has not been determined for the cat.
- As a benzodiazepine, monitor for acute idiosyncratic hepatotoxicity, as described for diazepam.

Hospital Emergency Treatment for Seizures

▼ *Key Point* A reliable protocol for rapid treatment is necessary for the emergency management of seizuring dogs.

The physiologic sequelae of frequent or continuous seizure activity (status epilepticus) leading to increased intracranial pressure and neuronal necrosis include systemic arterial hypertension, loss of cerebrovascular regulation, disruption of the blood-brain barrier, and cerebral edema. If not treated appropriately, the seizuring patient may develop serious neurologic complications due to these events.

Guidelines for When to Administer Emergency Therapy for Seizures

- A single seizure persists >1 minute from the time the seizure is identified.
- Status epilepticus.
- More than one seizure per hour occurs, regardless of seizure length.
- Three or more seizures per day occur, regardless of seizure length.

Protocol for Emergency Management of Seizures

A protocol for the emergency treatment of seizures in the dog is listed in Table 146–4. Two main components are listed in this protocol: restoring homeostatic conditions and providing specific seizure treatment. Many drugs used to control seizures have the potential to cause serious adverse effects, including death. Specific seizure treatment is divided into four successive phases.

- Phases 1 and 2 involve using a short-acting AED to stop immediate seizure activity and a long-acting AED to prevent further seizures. Diazepam is currently the drug of choice in treating prolonged seizures, including status epilepticus and cluster seizures.
- Phases 3 and 4 outline steps to follow if a dog continues to seizure despite prior treatment.
- To implement this protocol, be sure to have injectable diazepam, phenobarbital, pentobarbital, and a 24-hour monitoring facility.

Table 146–4. PROTOCOL FOR HOSPITAL EMERGENCY SEIZURE MANAGEMENT IN THE DOG AND CAT

Restore Homeostasis

1. Maintain a patent airway.
2. Administer IV thiamine (vitamin B₁) at 25–50 mg IM per animal. Administer before any dextrose-containing solution is given. Thiamine is an essential coenzyme in glucose utilization by the brain.
3. Evaluate STAT PCV, TP, blood glucose, BUN, and electrolytes (Na, K, Ca).
4. Administer dextrose at 500 mg/kg of 50% dextrose IV over 10 minutes if blood glucose is ≤ 60 mg/dl.
5. Administer IV isotonic saline solution with proper potassium chloride supplementation at a maintenance rate. Isotonic saline is chosen so that IV diazepam can be infused in the same line without the chance of microprecipitation.
6. Maintain normal body temperature. Animals may become hyperthermic with continuous or recurrent seizure activity. All cooling measures should be stopped when rectal temperature reaches 102°F to prevent rebound hypothermia.

Specific Seizure Therapy

Phase One

Use short-acting antiepileptic drugs with minimal side effects to immediately control the active seizures, while rapidly establishing serum levels of a maintenance drug to preserve control.

    A. Administer Diazepam. At 0.5 mg/kg IV bolus (maximum single dose = 25 mg IV). Diazepam is given at the time of a seizure episode if the episode lasts at least 1 minute, there have been two or more seizures, or an underlying intracranial etiology is suspected.

    B. Administer Phenobarbital (PB). The onset of action of this drug is about 15–30 minutes; therefore, PB is given simultaneously with the diazepam to provide sustained antiepileptic effect as the serum levels of diazepam decline.

        1. Naive Patients (no previous seizure treatment). A loading dose of PB is given to all naive patients to rapidly establish therapeutic drug levels using the formula:

$$\text{(Dog) Loading dose (total mg)} = \text{(Desired serum level } \mu g/ml) \times \text{(Body weight in kg)} \times (0.8 \text{ L/kg})$$

$$\text{(Cat) Loading dose (total mg)} = \text{(Desired serum level } \mu g/ml) \times \text{(Body weight in kg)} \times (0.9 \text{ L/kg})$$

            IV injection at a rate not greater than 100 mg/min:
                For dogs: Desired serum level = 25 μg/ml
                For cats: Desired serum level = 15 μg/ml

        2. Confirmed Epileptics. Review results of your STAT serum PB level prior to administering the PB. Administer PB at 1 mg/kg for each μg/ml that you wish to raise the patient's serum level.
            Dogs. Raise the serum concentration at increments of 5 μg/ml. If the PB level is ≥ 35 μg/ml, go to Phase Two.
            Cats. Raise the serum concentration at increments of 3 μg/ml. If the PB level is ≥30 μg/ml, go to Phase Two.

    C. Maintenance PB: All patients should be on maintenance antiepileptic drugs. Intramuscular PB can be given if the animal cannot take oral medication

        1. Naive Patients. After the IV loading dose, initiate oral therapy at 2.5 mg/kg every 12 hours started at the next time of administration.
        2. Established Epileptic Patients. Increase the dose to a level higher than that being administered on admission.
          Use the formula:

$$\text{(Desired Level/Established Level)} \times \text{Total mg PB} = \text{New Total mg PB/Day}$$

            Increase the desired level 5 μg/ml up to 40 μg/ml (dog) or 30 μg/ml (cat).

    D. Potassium Bromide (KBr) induction therapy: KBr loading

        1. Oral bromide loading can help achieve a more rapid rise in serum concentration. The time to reach a steady state serum concentration, however, may not be changed.
        2. Recommended dose is 100 mg/kg PO q6h as a 200 mg/ml solution dissolved in doubled distilled water administered either with food or via nasogastric tube.
        3. Gastric irritation may occur with loading dose, especially if given as a concentrated capsular formulation.
        4. Sodium bromide (NaBr) should be used in dogs with renal insufficiency or Addison's disease.
        5. Maintenance KBr therapy is administered as a 200 mg/ml solution dissolved in doubled distilled water at 30 mg/kg/day PO with food.
          • KBr is recommended therapy for dogs refractory to phenobarbital.
          • Monotherapy KBr is most effective in the epileptic dog after these dogs have been controlled with concomitant phenobarbital and KBr.

Phase Two

    A. Seizures Stop. If the seizures stop following the above therapy, continue to administer maintenance PB at the dose calculated PO or IM.
    B. Seizures Continue at Lower Frequency. If the seizures are continuing, but at a lower frequency than before, administer an additional IV dose of diazepam at that time, at a dose of 0.5 mg/kg. If the patient has more than three seizures after starting therapy, continue to Phase Three. Continue to administer maintenance PB at the calculated dose PO or IM.
    C. Continued High Frequency of Seizures. Proceed directly to Phase Three.

Phase Three

This phase of therapy is designed for the patients that failed to respond to the initial course of bolus doses of IV diazepam and phenobarbital.

    A. Step One. Continuous IV diazepam infusion: Administer diazepam at an initial rate of 0.1 mg/kg/hr in a 2.5% dextrose/0.9% NaCl drip at a maintenance rate. The dose can be increased up to 0.5 mg/kg/hr in both dog and cats. Seizures can occur with benzodiazepine withdrawal; therefore, the dosage rate should be decreased by 50% every 6 hours for at least two reductions before discontinuing the drug.

Table continued on following page

Table 146–4. PROTOCOL FOR HOSPITAL EMERGENCY SEIZURE MANAGEMENT IN THE DOG AND CAT *Continued*

    B. Step Two. Pentobarbital bolus
        1. If the patient has three or more seizures while on the diazepam infusion, administer pentobarbital IV. Give an initial bolus to induce general anesthesia. The recommended dosage is 2 mg/kg slowly IV, but if the patient has been on pentobarbital prior to admission, a higher dose of pentobarbital may be needed. Maintain the anesthesia for 4 hours, using additional boluses if required.
        2. Supportive patient care:
           Place an endotracheal tube in all patients under general anesthesia.
           Provide a padded area for the animal to lie on.
           Turn the patient to the opposite side every 4 hours.
           Start IV broad spectrum antibiotic treatment to control aspiration pneumonia.
           Monitor heart rate and temperature every hour.
    C. Step Three. Continuous pentobarbital infusion. Let the patient recover from the previous anesthesia. If any further seizures occur, start a continuous infusion of pentobarbital.
        1. Dosage: After an initial bolus sufficient to induce general anesthesia, start a continuous IV infusion of pentobarbital at a rate of 5 mg/kg/hr. If the patient has been on pentobarbital prior to admission, it may require much higher levels of pentobarbital to maintain a satisfactory plane of anesthesia. Once a dosage is found that maintains a satisfactory anesthesia, continue it for 6 hours. At the end of 12 hours, decrease the dose by 1 mg/kg/hr every 6 hours. Maintain the patient on pentobarbital for approximately 24 hours. Initiate supportive care as for Step Two. Administer maintenance pentobarbital therapy IM throughout the anesthesia.

Phase Four
Gas Anesthesia. Indications include seizures that are refractory to all of the above outlined steps, or contraindication to the use of benzodiazepine or barbiturate drugs (e.g., hepatotoxicity or hepatic encephalopathy)
    A. Anesthetic agent: Isoflurane. Provides a rapid induction and adjustable anesthetic depth with smooth emergence from anesthesia. Isoflurane offers the advantage of no hepatotoxicity, fewer perfusion problems, and less effect on elevation of intracranial pressure than halothane.
    B. Supportive patient care:
        1. Maintain endotracheal intubation.
        2. For optimal therapy, use a respirator throughout the anesthetic period to prevent atelectasis and maintain adequate perfusion-ventilation.
        3. Initiate broad-spectrum bactericidal IV antibiotic therapy.
        4. Monitor arterial blood gases every 4–8 hours to ensure adequate oxygenation.

At-Home Emergency Treatment for Seizures Using Diazepam per Rectum

Financial and emotional constraints of recurrent emergency therapy are often the limiting factor in an owner's decision to continue treating his or her animal. Per rectal administration of diazepam is a safe, affordable home treatment for cluster seizures that can reduce owner cost, decrease patient morbidity, and contribute positively to the overall AED therapy.

Per rectum administration of diazepam allows a rapid absorption of active drug into the bloodstream through the rectal mucosa in <15 minutes. Antiepileptic plasma concentrations are maintained for several hours after administration. In comparison, an intramuscular injection of diazepam results in an erratic absorption of the drug, and may take up to 30 minutes for peak concentrations to appear in the blood. Use rectal administration of diazepam for the emergency treatment of seizures in the dog according to the following recommendations. No information is available for the cat.

- *Indications:* History of generalized cluster epileptic seizures, status epilepticus, and underlying cerebral disease.
- *Administration:* Use a syringe through a plastic application tip (1⅓ inch J-12 teat infusion cannula) lubricated with a water-soluble jelly.
- *Dosage:*
  - If not on phenobarbital: 1 mg/kg per rectum of diazepam parenteral solution (5 mg/ml).
  - If on phenobarbital: 2 mg/kg per rectum of diazepam parenteral solution (5 mg/ml).
  - Do not exceed a maximum dose of 100 mg.
  - Administer at the onset of a seizure up to three times in 24 hours, but no closer than 15 minutes apart.
- *Toxicity:* Increased sedation.

NONEPILEPTIC SEIZURES DUE TO NARCOLEPSY AND CATAPLEXY

Nonepileptic seizures can be categorized into non-neurogenic and neurogenic causes. Many events may mimic epileptic seizures. Distinguishing nonepileptic seizures is important, because failure to do so could lead to failure to identify another serious medical condition, administration of unnecessary medication to the animal, and undue emotional and financial strain on the owner. This section discusses the nonepileptic seizures associated with sleep disorders—narcolepsy and cataplexy.

Etiology

Cataplexy is a brief, sudden episode of muscle weakness without loss of consciousness. The signs are due to motor inhibition only. *Narcolepsy* is a disorder of daytime somnolence characterized by excessive sleeping episodes. Narcolepsy and cataplexy can occur together.

The underlying cause is a neurochemical imbalance in the brain due to depression of serotonin metabolism and excitation of the cholinergic system. In general, the narcolepsy-cataplexy syndrome is thought to have an inherited basis.

- Breeds documented to have an autosomal inheritance are: Doberman pinscher, Labrador retriever, poodle, and dachshund.
- Several other breeds reported with narcolepsy-cataplexy include the Airedale, Afghan, Irish setter, malamute, Saint Bernard, rottweiler, English springer spaniel, Welsh corgi, and giant schnauzer.
- This disease is rare in cats.

Clinical Signs

In practically all instances, dogs with nonepileptic seizures do not exhibit postictal effects. Possible exceptions are dogs that exhibit autonomic release phenomena (e.g., urination) after a syncopal episode, and dogs with vestibular disease that continue to appear disoriented from their vertigo. The typical history and clinical signs of narcolepsy-cataplexy consist of:

- Onset usually by 6 months of age.
- Sudden, paroxysmal generalized muscle atonia lasting seconds to 10–20 minutes.
- Episodes often precipitated by excitement.
- Intact respirations, cough and swallow reflexes.
- Some animals aroused by external stimuli.
- Possible signs of rapid eye movement sleep (REM) with ocular motility, facial or eye muscle twitching, and whining.

Diagnosis
Differential Diagnosis

Non-Neurogenic Epileptic Seizures

- Syncope of cardiac origin
  - Arrhythmias
  - Right-to-left shunts (reverse patent ductus arteriosus; tetralogy of Fallot)
  - Cardiomyopathy
- Metabolic disturbances
  - Polycythemia
  - Hypoglycemia
  - Hypoadrenocorticism (Addison disease)
  - Pheochromocytoma

Neurogenic Epileptic Seizures

- Narcolepsy and cataplexy
- Vestibular disease (see Chap. 145)
- Myasthenia gravis (see Chap. 149)

Food-Elicited Test

The purpose of this test is to create an environment of excitement to induce an attack.

- *Protocol:* Place 10 pieces of palatable food approximately 1 cm³ in size in a row about 1 ft apart from each other. Record the time required to eat all of the

pieces and the number, type, and duration of the attacks.
- *Interpretation:* The normal dog will eat the food in < 1 minute and have no attacks.
- *Abnormal responses:*
  - The dog will take > 2 minutes to eat the food and have two or more attacks.
  - The animal drops to the ground with flaccid paralysis (complete attack).
  - Thoracic and/or pelvic limbs drop to the ground, but the head does not (partial attack).

Pharmacologic Testing

The purpose of these tests is to induce or reduce attacks with various central-acting drugs.

- *Yohimbine response test:* Give a 50 µg/kg IV bolus of yohimbine. A positive response is 75% reduction in the number or severity (time reduction) of attacks. Response occurs within 30 minutes and may last up to 4 hours.
- *Physostigmine challenge test:* Give 0.025 mg/kg physostigmine salicylate as an IV bolus. Follow each injection with a food elicited test in 10 minutes. Repeat the test with additional 0.025 mg/kg increments up to 0.10 mg/kg. In affected animals, signs increase in severity and frequency in a dose-dependent manner. The total effect of each dose will last 15–45 minutes.
- *Atropine response test:* Give atropine sulfate, 0.1 mg/kg, as an IV bolus, and follow each injection with a food elicited test in 10 minutes. In affected animals, signs decrease in severity and frequency.

Electrophysiologic Testing

The purpose of these tests is to confirm loss of muscle activity during an attack and absence of epileptic activity in the brain.

- Electroencephalographic recordings are consistent with acute onset of REM sleep during an attack without epileptiform activity.
- Concurrent electromyographic recordings from appendicular muscles show complete loss of activity during an attack.

Treatment
Yohimbine (Yobine)

- The drug of choice for narcolepsy and cataplexy.
- Dose: 50–100 µg/kg q8–12h SC.
- Minimal adverse effects.

Methylphenidate (Ritalin)

- Dose: 0.25 mg/kg, q24h or q12h PO.
- May cause inappetence, irritability, or altered sleep patterns.

Imipramine (Tofranil)

- Dose: 0.5–1.0 mg/kg q8h PO.
- Can be used in combination with methylphenidate.

Prognosis

Overall, the prognosis for a good life is fair to good. Dogs may improve as they get older. Alterations of lifestyle may be necessary to avoid precipitating events, such as reducing excitement or stressful events as much as possible.

SUPPLEMENTAL READINGS

Braund KG: Clinical Syndromes in Veterinary Neurology, 2nd Ed. Philadelphia: CV Mosby 1994.

Lane S, Bunch S: Medical management of recurrent seizures in dogs and cats. J Vet Intern Med 4:26, 1990.

Parent JML, Quesnel AD: Seizures in cats. Vet Clin North Am Small Anim Pract 26:811, 1996.

Podell M: The use of diazepam per rectum at home for the acute management of canine cluster seizures. J Vet Intern Med 8:68, 1995.

Podell M: Seizures in dogs. Vet Clin North Am Small Anim Pract 26:779, 1996.

Podell M: Seizure management in dogs. In Bonagura JD, ed.: Current Veterinary Therapy XIII. Philadelphia: WB Saunders, 1997.

Podell M, Fenner WR: Use of bromide as an antiepileptic drug in dogs. Compend Cont Educ 16:767, 1994.

Podell M, Fenner WR, Powers JD: Seizure classification in dogs from a nonreferral based population. J Am Vet Med Assoc 206:1721, 1995.

Quesnel AD, Parent JM, McDonell W, et al.: Diagnostic evaluation of cats with seizure disorders: 30 cases (1991–1993). J Am Vet Med Assoc 210:65, 1997.

Schwartz-Porsche D: Management of refractory seizures. In Bonagura J, ed.: Current Veterinary Therapy XI. Philadelphia: WB Saunders, 1992, p 986.

147 Disorders of the Spinal Cord

Patricia J. Luttgen

The term *spinal cord disorders* (see Table 147–1 for classification and examples) broadly refers to all diseases affecting the spinal cord. Clinically, spinal cord disorders cause dysfunction in one or more limbs and/or the tail.

▼ *Key Point* Disorders of the spinal cord do not cause signs referable to diseases above the foramen magnum, such as mentation change, cranial nerve deficits, and vestibular and cerebellar ataxia.

Differentiate spinal cord disorders from peripheral nerve disorders, which cause many of the same clinical signs (see Chap. 148). Disorders of the spinal cord can seriously impair the quality of life of afflicted animals.

ETIOLOGY

Spinal cord disorders can arise from numerous insults and may be associated with particular signalments (breed, age, sex) and neuroanatomic localizations. Many of these disorders cause relatively predictable patterns of onset (acute versus chronic) and clinical signs (progressive versus nonprogressive).

Degenerative Disorders

Degenerative conditions are usually insidious but progressive in nature.

- Many of these conditions are inherited and are seen in young animals (e.g., spinal muscular atrophy of Brittany spaniels and hereditary ataxia of Jack Russell and smooth-haired fox terriers).
- Other disorders seem to be related to aging and may be familial, such as the degenerative myelopathy seen in older, large-breed dogs, particularly the German shepherd.

Anomalies

Anomalies of the spinal cord usually are first recognized when ambulation begins. However, traumatically induced "decompensation" may be required for minor lesions to be recognized clinically.

- Spinal cord anomalies can be inherited, such as spinal dysraphism in Weimaraners, or congenital, such as myelomeningocele. The majority of these conditions are nonprogressive, but may become progressive if additional disease conditions are superimposed.
- Vertebral anomalies that compromise the stability of the vertebral column or the canal size may cause spinal cord dysfunction secondary to compression. For example, hemivertebra may lead to spinal luxation, and malarticulation/malformation of articular facets may lead to spinal canal stenosis.

Metabolic Conditions

Metabolic disorders that affect the nervous system generally are chronic and progressive, with signs referable to more than the spinal cord.

- However, dogs afflicted with globoid cell leukodystrophy may display signs of spinal cord disease prior to development of other neurologic signs.
- Hypervitaminosis A in cats may result in extensive cervical and thoracic vertebral new bone formation with secondary compression of the spinal cord.

Neoplasia

Neoplasia of the spinal cord can affect animals of all ages and breeds. Initial clinical signs vary, depending on the type and location of the tumor. Signs usually become progressive. Two major types of tumors affect the spinal cord: intramedullary and extramedullary.

- Intramedullary tumors such as astrocytoma and ependymoma arise from the spinal cord itself, causing damage by derangement of the normal anatomy.
- Extramedullary tumors arise from tissues surrounding the spinal cord and cause damage by compression. Extramedullary tumors can be located intradurally (e.g., meningiomas and nerve root tumors) or extradurally (e.g., vertebral osteosarcomas and multiple myeloma).
- See Chapter 120 for discussion of neoplasia of the axial skeleton.

Inflammation/Infection

Numerous infectious agents can affect the spinal cord and surrounding structures of animals of all breeds and ages. Clinical signs vary, depending on the inciting agent, the location of the lesion, and the degree of spinal cord involvement. Often inflammatory disease of the central nervous system (CNS) is not confined to the spinal cord, and clinical signs of brain involvement also will be present (see Chap. 145).

Table 147–1. CLASSIFICATION AND EXAMPLES OF SPINAL CORD DISORDERS

Category	Examples
Degenerative	Myelopathy of German shepherds
	Hereditary spinal muscular atrophy of Brittany spaniels
	Hereditary ataxia of smooth-haired and Jack Russell terriers
Anomalous	Spinal dysraphism
	Spina bifida
	Myelodysplasia
Metabolic	Globoid cell leukodystrophy
	Hypervitaminosis A in cats
Neoplastic	Intramedullary ependymoma
	Extramedullary intradural meningioma
	Extradural vertebral osteosarcoma
Inflammatory	Feline infectious peritonitis
	Canine distemper myelitis
	Toxoplasmosis
Granulomatous	Granulomatous meningoencephalitis
Immune-mediated	Steroid-responsive meningitis/vasculitis
Toxic	Tetanus
	Strychnine
Traumatic	Intervertebral disc herniation
	Fracture/luxation of spinal column
	Caudal cervical spondylomyelopathy
Vascular	Fibrocartilaginous embolization
	Progressive hemorrhagic myelomalacia
	Caudal aortic embolization

Bacterial

Primary bacterial meningitis or meningomyelitis is infrequently diagnosed in dogs and cats. Bacterial infection is most commonly introduced secondary to infection of surrounding tissues or to trauma.

- For example, bacterial discospondylitis causes discomfort from disc and vertebral body infection and, if extensive, secondary compression of the spinal cord.
- Infection of the lumbar epaxial muscles seen with grass awn migration can extend through the intervertebral foramen to cause secondary meningitis.

Viral

Viral myelitis is a relatively common problem in dogs and cats. Clinical presentation and neuroanatomic localization vary.

- Typically, encephalitic signs are associated with rabies infection, but this virus may also cause signs of myelitis (see Chap. 13).
- All ages of dogs are susceptible to canine distemper virus (CDV; see Chap. 11). Previous vaccination does not preclude "breaks" in immunocompetency due to other illnesses or disease states. Signs of spinal cord disorder without associated encephalitic signs may occur.
- In cats, coronavirus (feline infectious peritonitis) and retrovirus (feline leukemia virus and feline immunodeficiency virus) infections frequently cause signs of spinal cord disorder with or without signs of brain involvement (see Chaps. 6, 7, and 8).

- For a discussion of these viral diseases of dogs and cats, see appropriate chapters.

Fungal

Fungal myelitis has been reported in patients with cryptococcosis, blastomycosis, histoplasmosis, and coccidioidomycosis.

- Multiple levels of the nervous system usually are involved simultaneously (e.g., eyes, brain, spinal cord); however, signs are limited to the spinal cord in some patients.
- Systemic mycoses are discussed in Chapter 18.

Rickettsial

In addition to other clinical signs, the tickborne rickettsial diseases, ehrlichiosis and Rocky Mountain spotted fever (see Chap. 15), cause nervous system dysfunction.

- Signs referable to spinal cord dysfunction include ataxia, upper motor neuron limb dysfunction, and hyperesthesia resulting from meningitis and myelitis.

Protozoal

The main protozoal disease causing spinal cord disorders in dogs and cats is toxoplasmosis (see Chap. 19).

- Encephalitis, ocular involvement, and myositis may be present.
- Fortunately this rarely occurs in pet animals, owing to decreased predation of the intermediate hosts.

Granulomatous Meningoencephalitis

The cause of this disease is unknown, but an infectious agent that has not been definitively identified, immune-mediated disease, and a unique form of neoplasia have been proposed.

- Both acute and chronic onset of signs have been reported.
- The disease is invariably progressive in nature, and disseminated CNS involvement is the general rule (see Chap. 145); however, signs limited to the spinal cord have been reported. The cervical area seems to be the preferred site of involvement in the spinal cord.

Immune-Mediated Disorders

Immune-mediated steroid-responsive meningitis and/or meningeal-vasculitis has been reported in numerous dogs.

- Clinical signs are typical of spinal meningitis, including neck stiffness, hyperesthesia, and fever.
- Signs are usually acute in onset and are progressive if the dog is untreated.

Toxins

Strychnine and tetanus directly affect the spinal cord in dogs and cats.

- These toxins act in a similar manner: tetanus toxin decreases the release of the inhibitory neurotransmitters, γ-aminobutyric acid and glycine in the spinal cord, whereas strychnine competitively blocks the inhibitory effect of glycine.
- Clinical onset is usually acute, and the disease progresses to a state of severe tetany.

Trauma

Trauma is the most frequent cause of spinal cord disorders in dogs and cats.

- Trauma can arise from external sources (e.g., being hit by a car or a bullet) or from internal sources (e.g., disc herniation or a pathologically collapsed vertebra).
- Clinical signs are usually acute and nonprogressive. However, progressive signs may be seen if disc nucleus herniates slowly or instability of the spinal column allows further luxation to occur.

Vascular Disorders

Vascular conditions resulting in ischemia of the spinal cord most often cause acute nonprogressive spinal cord dysfunction.

- In dogs, fibrocartilaginous embolization seems to be the main etiologic agent.
- In cats, caudal aortic embolization secondary to cardiomyopathy is the most common cause.

CLINICAL SIGNS

▼ *Key Point* Ascending proprioceptive fibers in the spinal cord are the most sensitive to compressive lesions. Therefore, incoordination (sensory ataxia) of one or more limbs is commonly the initial sign of spinal cord disease.

- As compression increases, the descending upper motor neurons (UMNs) in the spinal cord are affected, resulting in a loss of muscle strength in one or more limbs.
- If the lesion is located in the cervical or thoracolumbar area, UMN signs of exaggerated myotatic reflexes (e.g., patellar reflex) will be apparent in the limbs caudal to the lesion.
- If the lesion is located in the cervicothoracic or lumbosacral area and it causes compression so severe that it damages the ventral horn cells in the ventrolateral gray matter of the spinal cord, lower motor neuron (LMN) signs of decreased or absent myotatic reflexes may be present in the corresponding limbs (cervothoracic lesion results in forelimb signs; lumbosacral lesion results in hindlimb signs).

▼ *Key Point* The ascending spinal cord pain fibers are the most resistant to compressive lesions. Therefore, lack of deep pain perception as demonstrated by no visible response to a noxious stimulus applied to a limb or tail caudal to a compressive lesion indicates severe damage to the spinal cord.

- **Deep Pain.** Test for deep pain by presenting a noxious stimulus to the affected limb or tail.
  - Deep pain perception is indicated by the animal's demonstration of conscious perception of the pain (e.g., crying, turning the head toward the leg.)
  - Withdrawing of the limb alone may be reflexive and is not evidence of deep pain perception.

DIAGNOSIS

History

In spinal cord disorders, key aspects of the history are signalment, nature of onset, and progression of clinical signs.

- Because many spinal cord disorders are relatively predictable in these areas, the history can identify general differential possibilities that should be considered before performing the physical examination.
- For example, chronic progressive disease in an old German shepherd suggests degenerative myelopathy, neoplasia, or chronic disc herniation. Acute nonprogressive disease in a young dog suggests trauma, such as disc herniation or vascular insult, such as fibrocartilaginous embolization.

Lesion Localization (Neurologic Examination)

The neurologic examination establishes the presence or absence of neurologic dysfunction (see Chap. 144). When dysfunction is established, localize the affected areas of the spinal cord. For this purpose, the spinal cord is divided into four major areas: cervical (C): C1–C5 cord segments; cervicothoracic (CT): C6–T2 cord segments; thoracolumbar (TL): T3–L3 cord segments; and lumbosacral (LS)-coccygeal: L4–S3 cord segments and caudal.

- C lesions classically cause UMN tetraplegia, or UMN hemiplegia if the lesion is asymmetric.
- CT lesions cause tetraplegia with LMN signs in the forelimbs and UMN signs in the hindlimbs. However, there are many exceptions because of the large amount of extradural space in the area. CT lesions may cause only UMN forelimb signs if not of sufficient severity to interrupt LMN cell body function. If the lesion affects the CT area of the spinal cord asymmetrically, one forelimb may show more dysfunction than the other or hemiplegia may be present.
- TL lesions typically cause UMN paraplegia (normal forelimb responses; UMN hindlimb responses).
- LS lesions cause LMN paraplegia (normal forelimb responses; LMN hindlimb and perineal responses). If coccygeal segments also are involved, the tail will show LMN motor dysfunction. LS lesions may affect only the sacral and/or coccygeal segments without affecting the lumbar cord segments that contribute to the femoral and sciatic nerves. In these cases, the animal will have LMN perineal and/or tail responses while maintaining motor function of the hindlimbs.

Minimum Database

Establishing a minimum database (MDB) is essential for assessment of the animal's overall health prior to general anesthesia for neurologic testing.

▼ *Key Point* The MDB for neurologic patients consists of a complete physical examination (including neurologic, otic, and ophthalmic evaluation), complete blood count (CBC), serum biochemical analysis, urinalysis, fecal analysis, and electrocardiogram. Routinely test for heartworms in endemic areas.

Specialized Laboratory Examinations

Specialized tests may be indicated, based on physical examination findings and/or MDB results. Examples include endocrine function tests, fine-needle aspiration cytology of enlarged lymph nodes, tests for infectious diseases (e.g., feline leukemia, feline immunodeficiency, feline infectious peritonitis, canine distemper, toxoplasmosis, erlichiosis, and fungal infections; see appropriate chapters in Section 2, Infectious Diseases).

Electrodiagnostic Tests

Electrodiagnostic tests useful in the diagnosis of spinal cord disease include electromyography (EMG), motor and sensory nerve conduction velocity (MNCV and SNCV, respectively) studies, spinal cord evoked potentials (SCEPs), and somatosensory evoked potentials (SSEPs). These evaluations generally require specialized equipment and referral to a veterinary neurologist.

- Epaxial and limb EMG is useful for verifying denervation potentials and more specifically for localizing lesions.
- MNCV and SNCV studies of peripheral nerves help to rule out peripheral nerve and muscle diseases that present with many of the same clinical signs as spinal cord disease (see Chaps. 148 and 149 for discussion of peripheral nerve and muscle disorders, respectively).
- SCEPs and SSEPs evaluate the integrity of the ascending spinal cord tracts to determine the extent of functional damage.

Imaging Techniques

▼ *Key Point* Neuroradiography is the single most important technique used for diagnosis of spinal cord disorders.

Spinal radiography is especially important if surgical treatment of the condition is being considered.

Plain Spinal Radiography

- Plain spinal films often are sufficient to diagnose problems such as vertebral fracture/luxation, disc herniation, vertebral neoplasia, vertebral anomalies, and discospondylitis.
- Refer to Chapter 4 for positioning and technique. Avoid causing further injury to the animal during

these procedures. When plain radiographs are inconclusive, use specialized procedures.

Myelography

- Myelography is the most commonly performed special neuroradiographic procedure and is particularly helpful in differentiating intramedullary and extramedullary spinal cord lesions.
- With the introduction of new contrast agents, postmyelographic complications, such as seizures and contrast-induced meningitis, have been markedly reduced. However, myelography is contraindicated in the presence of CNS inflammation (encephalitis, myelitis, meningitis) or if increased intracranial pressure is suspected.
- See Chapter 4 for myelography technique and interpretation.

Discography

- Discography, in which contrast media is injected into an intervertebral disc nuclear area, is useful in cases of LS stenosis if magnetic resonance imaging (MRI) is not available.
- Combined with EMG, this technique can add valuable information to confirm the presence of a chronic (type II) disc herniation at the LS junction.
- Fluoroscopic guidance is useful, but not absolutely necessary, to confirm needle placement prior to injection of contrast media.

Epidurography and Sinus Venography

These modalities are seldom performed and have limited diagnostic usefulness because of ready accessibility to more advanced imaging techniques at referral centers.

Specialized Imaging Techniques

Computerized fluoroscopy, computed tomography (CT), and/or MRI are now available through most neurologic referral centers. These modalities provide detailed information about the precise nature, location, and extent of conditions affecting the spinal cord.

- If the goal is to evaluate a suspected bony lesion, CT is the preferred imaging modality.
- If the spinal cord, discs, or other soft tissue structures need to be evaluated, MRI is by far the superior imaging modality. As availability grows, MRI is rapidly replacing myelography as the diagnostic procedure of choice, especially in large breed dogs.

Cerebrospinal Fluid Analysis

CSF analysis is the test of choice for establishing an inflammatory cause of spinal cord disease; furthermore, it provides nonspecific information that is helpful in the diagnosis of degenerative, metabolic, neoplastic, and vascular conditions, including the following:

- Degenerative, neoplastic, and occasionally vascular problems may cause albumino-cytologic dissociation of CSF (increased protein levels in the presence of normal cell counts).

- Neoplastic cells rarely are seen in the CSF of patients with CNS neoplasia. However, globoid cells may be identified in cases of globoid cell leukodystrophy.
- Inflammatory conditions of the spinal cord cause increases in CSF protein and variable increases in cell numbers and type, depending on the specific etiologic agent causing the insult.
- Etiologic agents (e.g., bacteria, rickettsiae, protozoa, fungi) are sometimes identified in CSF by culture (bacteria) or cytology. Comparative titers on simultaneously collected CSF and serum are also helpful for identifying active CNS infection with specific agents.

For further details concerning CSF collection technique and abnormalities in specific infectious and inflammatory conditions of the CNS, see Chapter 144.

TREATMENT

The management of spinal cord disorders depends on the causative agent and the degree of irreversible damage caused. Often only palliative treatment can be provided.

Medical Therapy

Spinal Cord Trauma

Medical therapy to combat the effects of acute spinal cord trauma (e.g., edema, ischemia) is based on the use of anti-inflammatory and hyperosmotic agents. However, the benefits of hyperoxygenation to reduce CNS edema should not be forgotten in the rush to the pharmacy shelf.

Anti-inflammatory Agents

Glucocorticosteroids are the most useful anti-inflammatory agents. Unfortunately, their vigorous use to "save" a spinal cord may result in significant hemorrhagic or ulcerative gastroenteritis and pancreatitis. Therefore, administer H_2-receptor antagonists (e.g., cimetidine or ranitidine) and cytoprotectants such as sucralfate (see Chap. 87 for dosages).

The two most commonly used glucocorticosteroids are dexamethasone and the newer and apparently superior agent, methylprednisolone sodium succinate (Solu-Medrol, Upjohn). The general principles of administration are similar for both drugs. Best results in spinal cord trauma are obtained when large doses are administered immediately after injury, followed by rapid dosage tapering. The maximum amount of time that glucocorticosteroids are beneficial following spinal cord injury appears to be 2–3 days; longer administration is of little benefit and enhances the likelihood of gastric ulcers, gastroenteritis, and pancreatitis.

Dexamethasone. The relative value of dexamethasone versus dexamethasone sodium phosphate is still being debated.

- For both types, administer 2–4 mg/kg IV immediately after severe trauma.

- Base the total dosage and tapering of dosage on the patient's response to therapy.

Methylprednisolone Sodium Succinate (Solu-Medrol). This highly soluble, fast-acting glucocorticosteroid is especially effective when administered immediately following spinal cord trauma.

- In experimental models, a dosage of 30 mg/kg administered during the first 12–24 hours following injury has shown remarkable sparing action on the spinal cord compared with dexamethasone, mannitol, dimethyl sulfoxide (DMSO), naloxone, and thyrotropin-releasing hormone.
- A clinically proved protocol in human medicine uses an initial dose of 30 mg/kg IV followed by a continuous infusion of 5 mg/kg/hr IV for 23 hours. This protocol is used if spinal injury occurred <1 hour previously. The benefit in veterinary patients is unproved.
- The dosage is usually tapered rapidly over the course of 2 days.
- If additional glucocorticosteroid therapy is necessary, methylprednisolone sodium succinate may be continued in reduced dosages, or less expensive dexamethasone or prednisone may be substituted.
- Use concurrent H_2-blocker therapy to reduce the potential for gastric ulceration with this potent glucocorticosteroid therapy.

Hyperosmotic Solutions

Hyperosmotic solutions have been widely used to combat post-traumatic brain edema, but their use in cases of spinal cord trauma does not appear to be as successful.

- *Mannitol* is the most commonly used hyperosmotic agent for CNS trauma. Give one or two doses of 1–2 g/kg IV. Be cautious when considering further administration, because of possible rebound paradoxical CNS edema.

Dimethyl Sulfoxide

This is used more commonly in large animal species for spinal cord trauma.

- DMSO appears to have many beneficial effects on damaged CNS tissues, including antiedema properties, stabilization of cell membranes, and reduction of metabolic demands of affected tissues.
- Recommended dosage is 0.5–2.5 g/kg q8h IV.

Other Drugs

Other investigated drugs for adjunctive therapy of spinal cord trauma, such as antioxidants, calcium channel blockers, and vasodilators, are not routinely recommended at this time.

Infection

Antimicrobial Agents

Antimicrobial drugs may be indicated if specific infectious agents are identified or suspected. Treatment of systemic mycoses, toxoplasmosis, and rickettsial infections are discussed in detail in Chapters 18, 19, and 15, respectively.

Myelitis and Spinal Meningitis. In cases of meningitis or myelitis, select antimicrobials that are known to cross the blood-brain barrier readily (i.e., highly lipid soluble in the nonionized state).

- Examples of antimicrobials with good penetrating abilities include trimethoprim-sulfonamide combinations, rifampin, metronidazole, chloramphenicol, and certain imidazoles such as fluconazole.
- Drugs with intermediate penetrating abilities in the normal CNS may have improved penetrating abilities when the CNS is inflamed. These include the penicillin family (e.g., amoxicillin, carbenicillin), quinolones (e.g., enrofloxacin), the newer-generation tetracyclines (e.g., doxycycline, minocycline), certain cephalosporins, and itraconazole.
- Avoid drugs that penetrate poorly, such as the aminoglycosides, amphotericin B, and ketoconazole.

Discospondylitis. Treatment of discospondylitis presents a unique challenge because of the difficulty of presenting sufficient antimicrobial concentrations to the affected disc space and vertebral bodies. *Staphylococcus* is the organism most frequently reported. *Brucella canis, Nocardia, Streptococcus canis, Corynebacterium diphtheroides,* and various fungi also have been isolated. Most infections arise via hematogenous spread from infected tissues.

- If possible, base selection of antimicrobial drugs on positive culture results (blood, urine, or the affected disc space) or a positive *Brucella* agglutination test. Otherwise, assume that the causative organism is coagulase-positive *Staphylococcus* and administer beta-lactamase–resistant antibiotics (e.g., cephradine, cloxacillin), which reach sufficient therapeutic levels in bone and pus.
- Clinical symptoms usually improve after only a few days of therapy, but several weeks of drug administration are required to effect a "cure."
- In some cases, antimicrobials alone are not effective, and surgical intervention is required. When surgery is required, remove the infected vertebral end plates and associated disc structures. Use a vertebral body bone plate to stabilize the area and fill in the defect with cancellous bone.

Degenerative Disorders/Neoplasia

- Glucocorticosteroids have been recommended in degenerative conditions for slowing the degenerative process and as chemotherapeutic agents in certain types of neoplasia such as lymphoma.
- Other chemotherapeutic agents usually are not effective in CNS neoplasia.
- Radiation therapy has been beneficial in the treatment of some types of neoplasia. The benefits must be weighed against the significant risk of radiation-induced spinal cord injury.

Intoxication

Tetanus. Penicillin, tetracycline, and metronidazole have been shown to be effective against *Clostridium* organisms and are used to treat tetanus.

- Administer penicillin G (20,000–100,000 IU/kg q6–12h IV or IM) as the first line of attack.
- Tetracycline (22 mg/kg q8h PO or IV) is recommended as an alternative because of the variable effect of penicillins on vegetative forms of the organism.
- Metronidazole (dog, 10 mg/kg q8h PO; cat, 250 mg total, q12–24h, PO) has shown excellent efficacy. It is bactericidal against most anaerobes and reaches effective levels in necrotic tissues.
- Equine tetanus antitoxin (100–1000 IU/kg IV, usually administered only once) may combat the neurotoxin if given early enough; however, anaphylactic reactions are common, necessitating an initial test dose (0.1–0.2 ml) given SC or ID (intradermally) 15–30 minutes prior to IV dosing.
- Chlorpromazine (0.5–2.0 mg/kg q8–12h, given IM, IV, or PO) is effective against the hyperexcitability sometimes observed.
- Diazepam (dog, 5–10 mg total, q2–4h, given PO, IV, or IM; cat, 2.5–5 mg total, q2–4h, PO) blocks the effect of the toxin on the spinal cord but has a very short duration of action.
- Barbiturates also may be used to combat the tetany. Phenobarbital (11–13 mg/kg, IV) can be given to immediately control seizure activity and generalized body stiffness, followed by oral maintenance therapy (2–4 mg/kg q12h PO).

Strychnine Intoxication. When strychnine intoxication is suspected, block further gastrointestinal absorption by aspiration of stomach contents and by oral administration of binding agents, such as activated charcoal, that prevent absorption of the toxin.

- Diazepam therapy also can be used to block the action of the toxin at the spinal cord level (see dosage used for tetanus).
- Barbiturates may be necessary to combat seizures (see Chap. 146 for dosage).

Principles of Surgical Treatment

Surgical intervention is most frequently effective in cases of compressive extramedullary spinal cord disease rather than in cases of intramedullary disease such as spinal cord laceration and neoplasia. The primary goals of neurosurgical intervention are:

- Decompression of the spinal cord and nerve roots.
- Stabilization of the vertebral column.

Criteria for Surgery

The decision for neurosurgical intervention is based on:

- A thorough understanding of the historical presentation of dysfunction (i.e., acute versus chronic onset, progressive versus nonprogressive course).
- The localization and extent of neurologic deficits.
- Radiographic or special imaging (CT, MRI) studies done under anesthesia.

Timing of Surgery

- When indicated, surgical intervention is most valuable in the early stages of a problem, especially in acute compressive conditions such as disc herniation, in which the functional outcome often parallels the speed with which surgical decompression is performed.

- In chronic progressive conditions, such as caudal cervical myelopathy, surgery performed in the early stages of disease is far more rewarding than surgery performed after significant dysfunction has been allowed to develop. Chronic compression causes irreversible damage to the spinal cord that surgery cannot correct and may even worsen by decompensating a chronically compensated condition.

▼ *Key Point* When recommending spinal cord surgery for a paralyzed animal, warn the owner that extensive postoperative physiotherapy and nursing care may be necessary.

Effect of Spinal Segment on Prognosis

How a particular extramedullary problem affects the spinal cord depends a great deal on the level of the spinal column involved. The spinal cord fills only approximately half of the available canal space in the cervical area, in contrast to the thoracolumbar area, where it fills almost the entire available canal space. There is also a great deal of extradural space in the last two lumbar canal spaces because of the tapering of the spinal cord into the cauda equina. Consequently, a spinal subluxation of one-fourth the canal space in the cervical area may cause very little if any clinical dysfunction, but significant hindlimb paralysis if the same degree of luxation occurs in the thoracolumbar area. (See Chap. 119 for details on treatment of spinal fractures and luxation.)

Effect of Extramedullary Versus Intramedullary Location on Prognosis

- In general, extramedullary compressive lesions have a better prognosis than intramedullary destructive lesions. It is possible to debulk some intramedullary tumors, but surgery has no application in the majority of intramedullary diseases (i.e., degenerative, anomalous, and infectious disorders; traumatic lacerations; vascular accidents).
- In comparison, there are many surgical alternatives for the treatment of compressive extramedullary disease such as disc herniation.

Prognostic Guide Using Clinical Signs

The long axonal tracts in the spinal cord vary in their sensitivity to pressure depending on their size. Clinical signs parallel the degree of compression and can be used as a prognostic guide.

- Sensory ataxia only in animals with non-neoplastic extramedullary compression is a good prognostic sign because it indicates compression affecting only the proprioceptive fibers. Most of these animals will not require surgery unless there is a fracture or other injury that may potentially destabilize the spinal column in the future, or unless chronic pain from nerve

root entrapment or irritation of the meninges is a problem.

- Paresis or more severe paralysis indicates a greater degree of spinal cord compression and a guarded prognosis is justified initially. Most of these patients improve if deep pain perception is still present and surgery is performed immediately.
- The prognosis usually is grave when superficial and deep pain perception are lost. However, transient loss of deep pain, which cannot be differentiated clinically from irreversible loss, can frequently be seen in the hours immediately following an acute insult to the spinal cord. In an animal with spinal fractures, if radiographs indicate severe vertebral displacement, it is likely that the neurologic deficit is irreversible; therefore, advise the owner that surgical intervention probably will not be beneficial. However, in cases in which radiography indicates that the spinal cord may be intact, a significant percentage will improve if surgery, combined with aggressive medical therapy, is performed within a few hours of injury. If deep pain has been absent for several hours to days, surgical decompression is of little value.

▼ *Key Point* Accurately assess for deep pain sensation prior to recommending surgery on paralyzed animals. The animal must exhibit conscious perception of pain, not just a withdrawal reflex.

Surgical Techniques

- Surgical decompression of the spinal cord usually is performed via hemilaminectomy or dorsal laminectomy in the thoracolumbar spine, depending on the site of the lesion.
- Cervical cord decompression for disc herniation usually is performed via ventral slot decompression (through the vertebral body). Dorsal decompression of the cervical cord is used less frequently.
- Disc fenestration is routinely performed by neurosurgeons as a prophylactic procedure to prevent recurrence of disc herniation. The efficacy of fenestration is supported by clinical observations. Disc fenestration does not decompress the spinal cord.
- Spinal cord surgery requires advanced skills and equipment, and can cause significant harm to the animal if improperly performed.

Physiotherapy and Nursing Care

▼ *Key Point* Regardless of the nature of the spinal cord disorder, physiotherapy and good nursing care are extremely important to avoid secondary problems and to hasten return to a functional state.

Physiotherapy

- Thermal applications—cold and hot packs
- Soft tissue mobilization—muscle massage
- Joint mobilization—limb manipulations
- Functional exercise training—towel walking, sit-to-stand, and so on
- Electrical stimulation of muscles
- Hydrotherapy—swimming

Nursing Care

- Perform frequent evacuation of the bladder (q4–6h) to prevent urinary tract infections and secondary bladder dyssynergia.
- Use a padded clean bedding or pet waterbed to prevent decubital ulceration.
- Give daily baths to prevent secondary dermatitis.

PROGNOSIS

The prognosis depends to a great extent on the etiologic agent involved.

- Degenerative conditions vary in the rate of progression but invariably lead to severe disability.
- Anomalous conditions usually have a nonprogressive course and thus their prognosis depends on the extent of spinal cord injury.
- Some metabolic conditions, such as globoid cell leukodystrophy, cannot be treated and lead to a chronic degenerative state; others, such as nutritional disorders, can be reversible if proper therapy is initiated promptly.

Neoplasia

The prognosis for neoplastic conditions varies greatly.

Intramedullary Tumors

Intramedullary tumors usually have a poor prognosis.

- Surgical removal is not possible or feasible in most cases.
- Chemotherapeutic agents, including glucocorticosteroids, may slow progression but do not effect a cure.
- Radiation therapy can provide some relief but seldom a cure, and may cause additional damage.

Nerve Root Tumors

Nerve root tumors have a variable prognosis depending on their location (intramedullary, extramedullary, or both) and extent of involvement.

- The prognosis is poor when multiple nerve roots are involved, but can be good if only one nerve root is involved and surgical removal can be performed. Even in these cases, however, the tumor often develops in the ventral horn cell area of the spinal cord and becomes an intramedullary problem.

Extramedullary Tumors

Some extramedullary tumors, including lymphoma and meningioma, are very sensitive to chemotherapy and/or radiation therapy. In combination with surgical debulking, good results can be obtained.

Vertebral Tumors

Vertebral tumors such as osteosarcoma and multiple myeloma have a poor prognosis.

- These tumors compromise the structural integrity of the spinal column, leading to secondary spinal cord compression from proliferative bone and/or pathologic collapse.
- Surgical and chemotherapeutic protocols may be used, but pathologic collapse of the spinal column is usually the end result. (See Chap. 120 for more information about tumors of the axial skeleton.)

Infection

In general, infectious problems have a guarded prognosis unless a specific causative agent can be identified and/or response to antimicrobial therapy occurs. Under the best of circumstances, it is difficult to obtain significant levels of appropriate antimicrobials in the CNS, disc space, and vertebrae, and prolonged administration usually is required. If the spinal cord parenchyma is directly involved, the prognosis is poorer.

- *Infectious myelitis and spinal meningitis* are treated with the appropriate antimicrobial agents, depending on the infectious agent (refer to the Infectious Disease section).
- *Granulomatous meningoencephalitis* is initially very steroid-responsive. Unfortunately, relapses are common and the disease usually proves fatal (see Chap. 145).
- Glucocorticosteroids are the therapy of choice for immune-mediated *meningitis/vasculitis,* but the results are highly variable.

Toxicity

- *Strychnine* toxicity can be fatal if aggressive therapy is not begun immediately.

Disc Herniation, Trauma, and Vascular Accidents

The prognosis in cases of spinal cord trauma from disc herniation or other causes is highly variable, as discussed previously. The same is true for vascular accidents. The prognosis depends on the location and extent of spinal cord involvement.

- The prognosis is good if the cervical or thoracolumbar area is involved (i.e., UMN paralysis and deep pain perception has been preserved).
- In patients with fibrocartilaginous embolization, the cervicothoracic and lumbosacral areas are predisposed sites (i.e., LMN paralysis of one or more limbs). As in caudal aortic embolization, which mainly affects the lumbosacral spinal cord, the prognosis is guarded to poor until response to therapy and time prove otherwise.

PREVENTION

In general, degenerative, anomalous, metabolic, neoplastic, and vascular disorders of the spinal cord cannot be prevented.

- Certain infectious conditions (e.g., canine distemper, feline leukemia) can be reasonably prevented by a regular vaccination program.

- Most cases of external trauma (hit by car) and toxicity can be prevented if pets are restricted to fenced backyards and leash walks.
- Keeping susceptible dogs from jumping excessively or becoming obese helps prevent disc herniations.

SUPPLEMENTAL READINGS

Greene CE, ed.: Infectious Diseases of the Dog and Cat, 2nd Ed. Philadelphia: WB Saunders, 1998.

LeCouteur RA, Child G: Diseases of the spinal cord. *In* Ettinger SJ, ed.: Textbook of Veterinary Internal Medicine, 4th Ed. Philadelphia: WB Saunders, 1995, p 629.

Luttgen PJ: Paraplegia. *In* Ford RB, ed.: Clinical Signs and Diagnosis in Small Animal Practice. New York: Churchill Livingstone, 1988, p 295.

Oliver JE Jr, Hoerlein BF, Mayhew IG: Veterinary Neurology. Philadelphia: WB Saunders, 1987.

148 Peripheral Nerve Disorders

Linda G. Shell/Karen Dyer Inzana

ANATOMY AND PHYSIOLOGY

The peripheral nervous system (PNS) is composed of 12 pairs of cranial nerves (see Chaps. 144 and 145) and 36 pairs of spinal nerves that arise from the spinal cord. Spinal nerve fibers give rise to the peripheral nerves, which usually are composed of both sensory and motor fibers. Sensory nerve fibers are activated by peripheral receptors (Fig. 148–1). Impulses are transmitted up the peripheral nerve to the spinal cord. Some disorders affect only the sensory nerve fibers or ganglia, causing clinical signs such as hyperesthesia and analgesia, proprioceptive deficits, and self-mutilation (Table 148–1). In many cases sensory losses may be difficult to detect.

Motor or efferent nerve fibers arise from nerve cell bodies in the gray matter of the spinal cord. They carry information from the central nervous system (CNS) to the striated muscles (Fig. 148–1). Motor deficits, characterized by limb weakness, muscle atrophy, and reduced spinal reflexes, occur with injury to any of the following: lower motor neuron in the gray matter of the spinal cord, ventral nerve root, spinal nerve, peripheral motor nerves, neuromuscular junction, and muscle (Fig. 148–1). Disorders of the neuromuscular junction and muscle are discussed in Chapter 149.

Neuropathy is a general term denoting pathologic changes and/or functional disturbances in the PNS. *Polyneuropathy* refers to involvement of several nerves, usually resulting in bilaterally symmetric signs.

CLINICAL SIGNS

Motor nerve disorders generally cause weakness and muscle atrophy. Sensory nerve disorders cause hyperesthesia or anesthesia, self-mutilation, and other abnormalities (Table 148–1). The clinical signs of motor nerve disorders are similar to those of muscle disorders and can be distinguished using muscle enzyme determinations and muscle and nerve biopsies (see Chap. 149).

▼ *Key Point* Many common peripheral nerve disorders are manifested as one of the following clinical problems: acute flaccid quadriplegia, chronic progressive quadriparesis, monoparesis or monoplegia, and sensory disturbances (Table 148–2).

PRINCIPLES OF DIAGNOSIS

History and Physical Examination

- The *history* allows classification of the disease process as acute or chronic and progressive or nonprogressive.
- Perform a careful *physical examination* to detect signs of involvement of other systems (e.g., endocrine disorders) that may influence the peripheral nerves.
- Perform a *neurologic examination* (see Chap. 144) to localize the process to the PNS if reduced muscle mass and tone and reduced spinal reflexes are found on the physical examination.

Laboratory Evaluation

- Initial studies usually consist of a hemogram, blood chemistry profile, and urinalysis to evaluate for metabolic, endocrine, and neoplastic disorders.
- Elevated serum concentrations of muscle enzymes (creatine kinase, aldolase, lactate dehydrogenase [LDH], and aspartate aminotransferase [AST]) suggest a muscle disorder.
- Low cholinesterase levels in whole blood or serum may indicate exposure to organophosphates.
- Blood and tissue samples can be analyzed for heavy metal levels.

Electrodiagnostics

- Use *needle electromyography (EMG) studies* to record electrical activity in skeletal muscle (see Chap. 144).
  - They are used to confirm the presence and distribution of peripheral nerve and muscle disorders and can be performed on a cooperative awake or anesthetized patient.
  - Spontaneous abnormal activity, such as fibrillations and positive sharp waves (denervation potentials), are found in many neuropathies.
- Use *nerve stimulation studies* to determine the location and nature of peripheral nerve abnormalities (see Chap. 144).
  - Reduction of the conduction velocity or a change in amplitude, duration, or waveform of the evoked action potential suggests pathologic conditions.
  - Nerve conduction studies are recorded using specialized electrodiagnostic equipment (usually by a

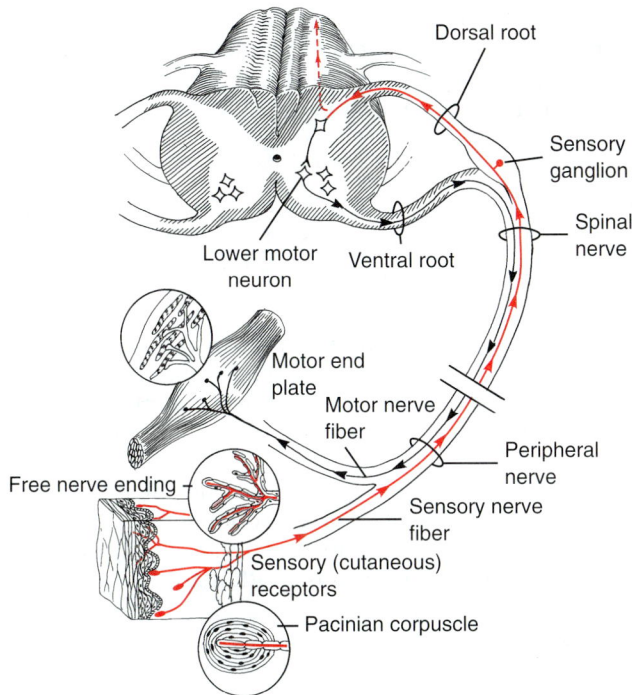

Figure 148–1. Impulse pathways in peripheral and spinal nerves.

specialist at a referral center) under general anesthesia. Both motor and sensory nerves can be evaluated.

Muscle and Nerve Biopsy

- *Muscle biopsy* specimens not only distinguish different muscle disorders but can also differentiate nerve from muscle disorders if histochemical staining is used (see Chap. 149).
- *Sensory and motor nerve biopsies* involve removing a fascicle of the nerve several centimeters in length, leaving the rest of the nerve intact. Because special handling and processing are required, these biopsies are probably best performed by a specialist at a referral center.
- *Spinal fluid analysis* occasionally is beneficial in diagnosis of disorders of the nerve roots such as acute polyradiculoneuritis and protozoal diseases.

Table 148–1. CLINICAL SIGNS OF MOTOR AND SENSORY NERVE DEFICITS

Motor Nerve Deficits
Weakness/paralysis
Muscle atrophy
Reduced reflexes
Reduced muscle tone

Sensory Nerve Deficits
Hyperesthesia/anesthesia
Self-mutilation
Loss of proprioception
Dysmetria
Reduced reflexes

Table 148–2. DIFFERENTIAL DIAGNOSIS BASED ON CLINICAL SIGNS OF NEUROPATHY

Problem	Differential Diagnosis
Monoparesis or Monoplegia	
Acute onset	Trauma to nerve root or peripheral nerve
	Fibrocartilaginous infarct
	Intervertebral disc herniation to lateral side
Chronic onset	Tumor of nerve root or peripheral nerve
	Intervertebral disc herniation to lateral side
	Joint disease
Acute Flaccid Quadriplegia	Acute polyradiculoneuritis (Coonhound paralysis)
	Tick paralysis
	Botulism
	Postvaccinal polyneuropathy
	Acute idiopathic polyneuropathy
	Protozoal neuritis/myositis
Chronic Progressive Quadriparesis	
Immature	Globoid cell leukodystrophy
	Giant axonal neuropathy (German shepherds)
	Progressive axonopathy (boxers)
	Hypertrophic neuropathy (Tibetan mastiffs)
	Motor neuron diseases (Brittany spaniels, pointers, rottweilers)
Mature	Chronic relapsing polyradiculoneuritis
	Distal denervating disease
	Distal polyneuropathy (Doberman pinschers)
	Distal symmetric polyneuropathy
	Metabolic neuropathy
	Neoplastic neuropathy
	Toxic neuropathy
	Nutritional neuropathy
	Various myopathies
Sensory Disturbances	
Immature	Acral mutilation in pointers
	Sensory neuropathy (longhaired dachshunds)
Mature	Sensory neuropathy (ganglioradiculoneuritis)

PRINCIPLES OF TREATMENT

▼ *Key Point* The key to treatment is to find the cause. Unfortunately, a specific cause of many of the acquired peripheral neuropathies may not be obvious even after extensive diagnostic evaluation.

Treatment often must rely on supportive care. In all peripheral nerve disorders that cause decreased mobility and muscle wasting, the following measures are important:

- Use waterbeds or heavily padded surfaces for bedding, to prevent decubital ulcer formation.

- Flex and extend the joints several times a day to prevent tendon and muscle contraction.
- Maintain proper nutritional intake.
- Ensure frequent and complete bladder evacuation.
- Use corticosteroids only for those neuropathies associated with immune-mediated diseases such as systemic lupus erythematosus.

SPECIFIC PERIPHERAL NERVE DISORDERS

A wide range of disease processes, varying from simple trauma to more complex inherited disorders, can affect the peripheral nerves. For the purpose of this discussion, peripheral nerve disorders are categorized according to their etiology, that is, anomalous/inherited/congenital, metabolic, nutritional, neoplastic, inflammatory/immunologic, idiopathic, traumatic, and toxic.

Anomalous, Inherited, and Congenital Disorders

Anomalous causes of peripheral nerve disease usually are noticed before 1 year of age. For each of the following anomalies, signalment and clinical signs are keys to a presumptive diagnosis, and thus only additional procedures are described under Diagnosis.

▼ *Key Point* Many anomalous causes of neuropathies are breed-specific and are not treatable.

Globoid Cell Leukodystrophy

This is caused by an inherited (autosomal recessive) deficiency of the enzyme beta-galactocerebrosidase that results in cell damage to oligodendrocytes and Schwann cells in the CNS and PNS, respectively.

- *Signalment:* West Highland white and Cairn terriers, beagles, poodles, Pomeranians, basset hounds, and cats <1 year of age.
- *Clinical Signs:* Pelvic limb ataxia progressing to tetraparesis, hyporeflexia, hypermetria, and head tremors. Nystagmus, blindness, and anorexia may develop prior to death.
- *Diagnosis:* Nerve biopsy demonstrating segmental demyelination, axonal degeneration, and endoneural globoid cell accumulation; biochemical evaluation of beta-galactocerebrosidase enzyme activity in leukocytes, brain, and spinal cord.

Giant Axonal Neuropathy in German Shepherds

This is an inherited (probably autosomal recessive) neuropathy characterized primarily by distal axonal swellings filled with neurofilaments in the PNS and CNS.

- *Signalment:* German shepherds 1–2 years of age.
- *Clinical Signs:* Progressive symmetric paraparesis followed by loss of patellar reflexes, distal muscle atrophy, hypalgesia in the pelvic limbs, weak bark, vomiting, regurgitation from megaesophagus, and aspiration pneumonia. Some dogs have a curly coat.

- *Diagnosis:* Spontaneous needle EMG activity in distal muscle groups; decreased amplitude of evoked action potential on nerve stimulation; giant axonal swellings on nerve histopathology.

Hypertrophic Neuropathy in Tibetan Mastiffs

This inherited (autosomal recessive trait) chronic demyelinating disease of the PNS is most likely due to an inability of the Schwann cells to form and maintain a myelin sheath.

- *Signalment:* Tibetan mastiffs 7–12 weeks old.
- *Clinical Signs:* Pelvic limb weakness that rapidly progresses to generalized weakness, hyporeflexia, hypotonia, and recumbency. Some dogs may regain some strength.
- *Diagnosis:* Occasional spontaneous needle EMG activity; slowed motor nerve conduction velocities; Schwann cell proliferation and relatively little axonal degeneration on nerve histopathology.

Progressive Axonopathy of Boxers

Progressive axonopathy is an inherited (probably autosomal recessive trait) neuropathy characterized by axonal degeneration and demyelination and remyelination in the PNS. The CNS also is affected, having large axonal spheroids.

- *Signalment:* Boxer dogs <1 year of age.
- *Clinical Signs:* Slowly progressive pelvic limb ataxia with a swaying hypermetric gait; hypotonia; loss of patellar reflex and conscious proprioception; and mild muscle atrophy. Thoracic limb involvement and mild cerebellar signs may occur late in the disease.
- *Diagnosis:* Normal or slightly reduced motor nerve conduction velocities; small or absent evoked muscle action potential; characteristic histopathologic changes on nerve biopsy (see earlier).

Acral Mutilation and Nociceptive Loss in Pointers

This is a suspected inherited (probably autosomal recessive) nociceptive defect.

- *Signalment:* Pointers 3–4 months to 1 year of age.
- *Clinical Signs:* Biting and licking at paws progressing to mutilation of paws; normal gait, posture, and spinal reflexes, with loss of pain sensation in digits of the pelvic limbs.
- *Diagnosis:* Normal EMG activity and sensory and motor nerve conduction velocities; pathologic changes of the primary sensory neurons include degeneration of nerve fibers in the dorsal roots and peripheral nerves and reduced number of cell bodies in spinal ganglia, with the remaining cell bodies appearing smaller than normal.

Sensory Neuropathy in Longhaired Dachshunds

This is a familial disorder (possibly autosomal recessive trait) characterized by degeneration of large and small, myelinated and unmyelinated, sensory and autonomic nerve fibers.

- *Signalment:* Young longhaired dachshunds. Signs begin at 2–3 months.
- *Clinical Signs:* Slowly progressive pelvic limb ataxia, urinary and fecal incontinence, loss of conscious proprioception, and decreased pain perception over the entire body; normal patellar reflexes but absent flexor reflexes.
- *Diagnosis:* Reduced sensory and normal motor nerve conduction velocities; loss of myelinated fibers in sensory nerves and widespread unmyelinated fiber pathology on nerve histopathology.

Motor Neuron Diseases in Brittany Spaniels, Pointers, and Rottweilers

These disorders are characterized by progressive degeneration and eventual loss of the motor neurons in the gray matter of the spinal cord and the motor nuclei of the brain stem.

- *Signalment:* Young Brittany spaniels, pointers, and rottweilers.
- *Clinical Signs:* Progressive weakness, muscle atrophy, and hyporeflexia.
  - Megaesophagus and head tremors have been observed in some affected rottweilers.
  - Three variants exist in Brittany spaniels; the accelerated form with signs at 6–8 weeks of age; the intermediate form with signs at 6–12 months of age; and the chronic form with milder signs at >1 year of age.
- *Diagnosis:* Histopathology of the spinal cord and brain.

Metabolic Disorders

Metabolic disorders do not always produce a clinically evident peripheral neuropathy; however, do not overlook the presence of hypothyroidism, hyperadrenocorticism, diabetes mellitus, hyperinsulinism, uremia, and hepatopathy. Additionally, there is increased incidence of neuropathies in patients with neoplasms.

▼ *Key Point* Evaluate all animals with signs of a chronic neuropathy for an underlying endocrine or metabolic abnormality.

Diabetes Mellitus

Diabetes mellitus can cause nerve fiber degeneration, although the exact pathophysiology is not fully understood. Clinical signs consist of weakness (especially of the pelvic limbs) and mild muscle atrophy. A plantigrade stance is common in cats. The diagnosis is based on clinical signs and laboratory evidence of diabetes mellitus (see Chap. 32), needle EMG, denervation potentials, decreased motor and sensory nerve conduction velocities, and demyelination and distal axonal loss on nerve histopathology. Neurologic signs usually improve over weeks to months with proper control of the diabetes mellitus (as described in Chap. 32).

Hypothyroidism

Hypothyroidism (see Chap. 29 for detailed description) occasionally is associated with polyneuropathies, but the pathophysiology is not understood. Most likely there is a relationship between thyroid hormone activities and neuronal metabolism.

- *Clinical Signs:* Slowly progressive weakness, muscle wasting, and normal or reduced spinal reflexes. Cranial nerve disturbances, such as facial paresis, laryngeal paralysis, or vestibular dysfunction, may also be found. Other clinical signs of hypothyroidism, such as obesity, mental depression, and dermatologic lesions, are not always present.
- *Diagnosis:* Needle EMG changes and decreased motor nerve conduction velocities; thyroid function testing (as described in Chap. 29).
- *Treatment:* Replacement hormone therapy (see Chap. 29) may improve the neurologic signs.

Hyperinsulinism

Hyperinsulinism results in hypoglycemia and most commonly is caused by pancreatic islet cell tumors. Profound hypoglycemia most frequently causes CNS disturbances such as seizures (see Chap. 33); however, a few cases of muscle atrophy and weakness due to a neuropathy have been documented. Because insulinomas generally are malignant, do not overlook the possibility that the neuropathy is the result of a paraneoplastic effect. (Diagnosis and treatment of hyperinsulinism are described in Chapter 33.)

Paraneoplastic Neuropathies

These neuropathies may occur more often than realized. The pathogenesis is poorly understood, but there is an unusually high incidence of peripheral neuropathy in humans with carcinomas.

- *Clinical Signs:* Weakness (especially in the pelvic limbs), decreased muscle tone, and reduced spinal reflexes. Decreased sensory and motor nerve conduction velocities also may be seen. Demyelination, ganglioneuritis, and axonal atrophy may be observed on nerve histopathology.
- *Diagnosis:* Identification of a primary neoplasm and the elimination of other causes.
- *Treatment:* Remove the underlying neoplasm if possible.

Nutritional Causes

Nutritionally induced neuropathies are uncommon in veterinary medicine; however, consider vitamin B deficiency, because of an inadequate diet or impaired intestinal absorption (e.g., malabsorption or small intestinal bacterial overgrowth), especially in idiopathic cases.

Neoplastic Causes

Progressive lameness or monoparesis resulting from neoplasia usually occurs in middle-aged and older patients. The nerves to the forelimb are most frequently affected.

Nerve Sheath Tumors

These are the most common primary tumors affecting the PNS. Schwannomas (malignant transformation of

Schwann cells) are the most common type; tumors arising from endoneural and epineural fibroblasts (neurofibromas, neurofibrosarcomas) also occur.

- *Signalment:* Mature dogs; rarely cats.
- *Clinical Signs:* Signs vary with tumor location. Spinal nerve roots of the brachial plexus are most susceptible. Nerve root tumors at C8–T2 often cause ipsilateral Horner syndrome and ipsilateral loss of the cutaneous trunci reflex. Neoplastic cells invade adjacent spinal nerve roots, causing dysfunction of multiple peripheral nerves. Proliferation of neoplastic cells within the spinal canal can result in a compressive myelopathy.

▼ *Key Point* Vague lameness progressing to weakness and muscle atrophy of the affected limb is the most common sign of a nerve sheath tumor.

- *Diagnosis:* Needle EMG denervation potentials; histopathology. If spinal nerve roots are involved, survey spinal radiographs may show an enlarged intervertebral foramen or myelography may show an intradural-extramedullary mass. Computed tomography (CT) or magnetic resonance imaging (MRI) scans may identify neoplastic nerve roots.
- *Treatment:* Surgical excision of the tumor and/or amputation of the affected limb. Recurrence is common.

Lymphoma

▼ *Key Point* Lymphoma is the most common tumor of non-neural origin affecting the PNS.

Lymphoma is more common in cats than in dogs. Clinical signs and diagnosis are similar to those of nerve sheath tumors except that other signs of multicentric lymphoma may be present. Treatment consists of chemotherapy (see Chap. 25) and/or surgical removal of the tumor. Peripheral nerve damage may be permanent.

Inflammatory and Immune-Mediated Disorders

These disorders can affect the neuromuscular junction, peripheral nerves, spinal nerves and roots, and ventral horn cells in the gray matter of the spinal cord.

Protozoal Neuritis/Myositis

Organisms such as *Toxoplasma gondii* and *Neospora caninum* can cause inflammatory and degenerative changes in peripheral nerves and dorsal and ventral nerve roots, as well as muscle. Dogs <4 months of age are frequently presented for hindlimb hyperextension, but others may be presented for acute or progressive flaccid weakness. (See Chap. 19 for diagnosis and treatment of protozoa infections.)

Acute Polyradiculoneuritis (Coonhound Paralysis)

This is one of the most common peripheral nerve disorders in dogs. It is characterized by a mild lymphocytic radiculitis with demyelination of the ventral (and occasionally the dorsal) spinal roots and mild axonal degeneration. Immune-mediated destruction of the myelin is suspected.

- *Signalment:* Adult dogs of any age, breed, or sex; frequently observed in hunting dogs 7–14 days after contact with a raccoon.
- *Clinical Signs:* Pelvic limb weakness progressing to hyporeflexic or areflexic quadriparesis or quadriplegia within 1–2 days; and rapid muscle atrophy. Voluntary tail movement is often unaffected. Thoracic limb weakness occasionally develops first. Responses to mild pain stimuli often are exaggerated. Some dogs develop facial paralysis, change in bark, and dysphagia. Respiratory muscle paralysis occurs occasionally, requiring the use of a respirator.
- *Diagnosis:* Needle EMG denervation potentials; normal or slowed motor nerve conduction velocities; increased spinal fluid protein.

▼ *Key Point* Differential diagnoses for coonhound paralysis include botulism, tick paralysis, and protozoal infection of nerve and muscle.

- *Treatment:* Supportive care (e.g., physical therapy, bladder evacuation). Recovery usually is complete but may take weeks or months. Complications include cystitis, aspiration pneumonia, tendon contracture, and decubital ulcers.

Brachial Plexus Neuritis

This is a rare weakness of the thoracic limbs that has been compared to serum neuritis in humans. In one case, a newly instituted horse meat diet was incriminated as the cause of the allergic neuritis. Flexor reflexes in the thoracic limbs are reduced or absent and muscle atrophy is present. Pelvic limb function is normal. Spontaneous recovery may take weeks to 4 months.

Postvaccinal Polyneuropathy

This disorder is rare and occurs 7–10 days after rabies vaccination. Clinical signs are similar in appearance to those of acute polyradiculoneuritis. Spontaneous recovery usually occurs over a period of weeks to months.

Idiopathic Disorders

The causes of many acquired peripheral nerve disorders often are unknown. There are many single case reports but very few series of cases for the majority of these disorders. To consolidate these disorders, they are grouped here according to the predominant site of pathology. Many of the cases described under a single heading actually may have multiple, but as yet unknown, causes.

Idiopathic Neuropathies Affecting the Neuronal Cell Body

Lower Motor Neuron Disease. This disorder, characterized by an acute loss of ventral horn cells within the spinal cord, has been reported in nine dogs in New Zealand.

- *Clinical Signs:* Acute onset of paraparesis or quadriparesis that progresses over 2–4 weeks until euthanasia is performed. Sensory and autonomic function are preserved.
- *Diagnosis:* Spinal cord histopathology

Sensory Neuropathy Ganglioradiculitis. This has been reported in several adult dogs with progressive ataxia and decreased patellar reflexes. Muscle tone and limb strength are preserved.

- Variable degrees of facial hypalgesia, dysphagia, and prehension difficulty may occur.
- Few to no needle EMG changes, normal to slightly reduced motor nerve evoked action potentials, and reduced sensory nerve evoked action potentials and conduction velocity are found in affected dogs.
- Histopathology shows degeneration of sensory neurons within dorsal root and cranial nerve ganglia.

Dysautonomia. Dysautonomia is characterized histopathologically by a loss of neurons in all autonomic ganglia, some cranial nerve ganglia, and occasionally ventral horn cells. It is more common in cats in the United Kingdom, but isolated cases have been observed in other countries. A disorder with similar features has been reported in dogs in the United Kingdom and United States.

- *Clinical Signs:* Mydriasis, megaesophagus, constipation, dry mucous membranes, bradycardia, and protrusion of the nictitating membrane. Pupillary pharmacologic testing showed increased sensitivity to direct-acting parasympathomimetics or sympathomimetics.
- *Treatment:* Recovery is possible after months to years of supportive care.

Idiopathic Neuropathies Affecting the Proximal Axon

Acute Idiopathic Polyneuropathy. This has been reported in 14 dogs.

- *Clinical Signs:* Acute onset of generalized flaccid paralysis, similar to that described for acute polyradiculoneuritis (coonhound paralysis) except that there is no known exposure to raccoons or other neurotoxins.
- *Treatment:* Most dogs recover spontaneously. Those that die have mononuclear inflammation of the nerve roots and extensive peripheral nerve demyelination.

Chronic Relapsing Polyradiculoneuritis. This chronic form of acute polyradiculoneuritis has been reported in both dogs and cats.

- *Clinical Signs:* Insidious onset of weakness in one or more limbs with periods of remissions and subsequent relapses; muscle atrophy and hyporeflexia is also seen.
- *Diagnosis:* Needle EMG changes; reduced motor and sensory nerve conduction velocities; demyelination and remyelination found on nerve histopathology.

Idiopathic Neuropathies Affecting the Distal Axon

Distal Denervating Disease. This disorder has been reported in 10 dogs with tetraparesis, diffuse muscle atrophy, and areflexia. Eight of the 10 dogs recovered spontaneously in 1–5 months. Needle EMG changes and abnormal motor nerve evoked action potentials were present. Histologically, distal degeneration of motor axons was found.

Distal Polyneuropathy in Doberman Pinschers (Dancing Doberman Disease). This chronic, progressive distal axonopathy begins with persistent rear limb flexion ("bicycling" motions) when the dog is standing. One or both rear limbs may be affected, and the gastrocnemius muscles are predominantly affected. Progression over months to years may produce generalized weakness, muscle atrophy, and proprioceptive deficits. Diagnosis is based on breed, clinical signs, EMG changes, and muscle histopathology.

Distal Symmetric Polyneuropathy. This disorder has been reported in adult large-breed dogs with progressive weakness and atrophy of limb muscles, especially those distal to the stifle and elbow. EMG changes are present. Evoked muscle action potentials are small. Muscle and nerve histopathology confirm denervation and distal axonopathy, respectively.

Traumatic Injury

Traumatic injuries to peripheral nerves are common causes of monoparesis or monoplegia.

Nerve Injuries

Nerve injury can occur from automobile trauma, intramuscular injections, fractures and repair of fractures, lacerations, and bite wounds. Tables 148–3 and 148–4 list the nerves that can be injured, their site of origin, and the clinical signs associated with each injury. Injuries are commonly classified as neurapraxia, axonotmesis, and neurotmesis.

Neurapraxia. Neurapraxia is a temporary loss of physiologic function without physical disruption of the nerve fibers. It results in weakness with intact pain perception. Motor function usually returns to normal within days to weeks.

Axonotmesis. Axonotmesis is severance of nerve fibers (axons) within a nerve, usually producing motor and sensory deficits. Following disruption of the axons, the distal axonal fragments degenerate. The proximal axonal segment must regrow along the intact connective tissue sheath at the rate of 1–3 mm/day or about 1 inch per month. Because the connective tissue sheath is intact, axonal regeneration may result in functional recovery, but this may take weeks to months, depending on the extent and the location of the injury. If the proximal axon segment is more than 12 inches from the muscle it innervates, it is unlikely that it will be able to make anatomic contact with the muscles because the connective tissue sheath shrinks and muscle fibers become fibrotic with time.

Neurotmesis. Neurotmesis is severance of axons and the connective tissue sheath. Axonal regeneration is

Table 148–3. SIGNS OF NERVE INJURY IN THE THORACIC LIMB

Nerve	Origin	Clinical Signs of Dysfunction	Reflexes Affected
Suprascapular	C6–7	No gait changes; pronounced atrophy of supraspinatus and infraspinatus muscles	None
Radial	C6–T1	*Injury proximal to branches that supply triceps muscle:* Unable to support weight; limb collapses; may carry the limb if musculocutaneous nerve is functional; atrophy of triceps muscle *Injury distal to branches that supply triceps muscle:* Can support some weight but knuckles on dorsum of paw	Reduced to absent triceps and extensor carpi radialis reflexes
Musculocutaneous	C6–C8	No gait changes; slight straightening of angle-to-elbow joint	Reduced withdrawal and biceps reflexes
Median and ulnar	C8–T2	Slight carpal extension ("dropped carpus")	Reduced carpal flexion on withdrawal reflex
Axillary	C6–C8	None	Reduced shoulder flexion on withdrawal reflex

hampered because there is no scaffold of connective tissue to guide the direction of growth of the axons. Without surgical intervention to appose the two severed ends of the nerve, it is unlikely that any function will return.

▼ *Key Point* The closer the injured nerve is to the muscle it innervates, the better the prognosis.

Nerve Root or Brachial Plexus Avulsions

These avulsions are common sequelae of road traffic accidents or jumping from moving vehicles. It is more common for the nerve roots to be torn or avulsed from the spinal cord than for the brachial plexus to be severed (injured). Occasionally motor nerve roots (ventral nerve roots) are affected and sensory nerve roots (dorsal nerve roots) are spared.

- *Clinical Signs:* Sudden onset of a combination of the nerve injuries to the forelimb as described in Table 148–3. Signs of radial nerve injury are almost always present.
  - Damage to the T1–T3 ventral nerve roots may cause an ipsilateral Horner's syndrome.
  - Damage to C8 and T1 nerve roots may result in loss of ipsilateral cutaneous trunci (panniculus) reflex.

- Damage to C5, C6, and C7 nerve roots may cause ipsilateral paralysis of the diaphragm.
- *Diagnosis:* History of trauma and clinical signs of monoparesis, needle EMG denervation potentials 5 days after injury; decreased motor nerve conduction velocity within 3 days of injury.
- *Treatment:*
  - Perform daily physical therapy to prevent tendon and muscle contraction.
  - Use a sock, boot, or bandage to prevent abrasions.
  - Regrowth of injured nerves (axonotmesis or neurotmesis) is slow and may take months. Perform monthly examinations.
  - Consider amputation if there is self-mutilation or unacceptable improvement in motor abilities after 6–8 months.

Toxic Neuropathies

Toxic neuropathies are diagnosed infrequently; however, the list of agents with the potential to cause neuropathies is quite extensive (Table 148–5). Suspect toxic causes when there is history of exposure.

Chemical Agents

Certain organophosphorus compounds can cause a delayed neuropathy in sensitive species.

Table 148–4. SIGNS OF NERVE INJURY IN THE PELVIC LIMB

Nerve	Origin	Clinical Signs of Dysfunction	Reflexes Affected
Femoral	L4–L6	Unable to support weight; limb collapses or may be carried; short stride; lack of pain perception on medial surface of thigh, stifle, leg, and paw; atrophy of quadriceps muscle	Reduced to absent patellar reflex
Sciatic	L6 to S1–S2	Supports weight on limb but knuckles on dorsum of paw; unable to flex or extend hock; atrophy of biceps femoris, semimembranosus, semitendinosus, cranial tibial, gastrocnemius and other muscles; lack of pain perception on caudal and lateral sides of leg	Reduced to absent withdrawal reflex
Peroneal	L6–S1	Straightening of hock; knuckles on dorsum of paw and fetlock	Reduced to absent hock flexion on withdrawal reflex
Tibial	L6–S2	Increased flexion to hock ("dropped" hock)	None
Obturator	L4–L6	Abduction of limb on slippery surface	None

Table 148–5. POSSIBLE CAUSES OF TOXIC NEUROPATHY IN HUMANS AND ANIMALS

Chemical Agents
  Organophosphorus compounds
    Parathion
    Malathion
    Tri-ortho-cresyl phosphate
    Di-isopropyl fluorophosphate
  Acrylamide
  Lindane
  Polychlorinated biphenyls
  Carbon tetrachloride
  Methylbutyl ketone
  Zinc pyridinethione
  Carbon disulfide
  N-hexane
  Chlorophenothane

Heavy Metals
  Arsenic
  Lead
  Gold
  Thallium
  Mercury

Drugs
  Vincristine
  Vinblastine
  Doxorubicin
  Chloramphenicol
  Ampicillin
  Erythromycin
  Tetracycline
  Nitrofurantoin
  Diphenylhydantoin

- *Clinical Signs:*
  - Signs of generalized motor unit disease develop within 2–3 weeks after exposure.

- Long, large-diameter axons in the peripheral nerves and the spinal cord undergo distal degeneration ("dying-back"), causing a mixture of lower motor neuron clinical signs (muscle atrophy, weakness, reduced spinal reflexes) and upper motor neuron signs (weakness, exaggerated spinal reflexes).
- *Treatment:* There is no treatment for the delayed neuropathy. Partial recovery may occur if the nerves regenerate.

Drugs

Nitrofurantoin, vincristine, vinblastine, and doxorubicin can have adverse effects on peripheral nerves; however, reports in veterinary literature are scant.

Heavy Metals

Arsenic, lead, and mercury appear to be uncommon causes of neuropathies in animals.

SUPPLEMENTAL READINGS

Braund KG: Peripheral nerve disorders. *In* Ettinger ST, Feldman EC, eds.: Textbook of Veterinary Internal Medicine, Vol 1, 4th Ed. Philadelphia: WB Saunders, 1995, p 701.
Duncan ID: Peripheral neuropathy in the dog and cat. Prog Vet Neuro 2:111, 1990.

149 Disorders of Muscle and Neuromuscular Junction

G. Diane Shelton

Neuromuscular disorders of dogs and cats are disorders of the motor unit. The motor unit is the morphologic and functional unit of skeletal muscle and includes:

- Motoneuron, consisting of the cell body and axon extending along a peripheral nerve
- Neuromuscular junction
- Myofibers innervated by the motoneuron

▼ *Key Point* Weakness is the clinical sign common to all neuromuscular disorders, with the clinical expression varying considerably in severity and distribution.

This chapter focuses on disorders of the neuromuscular junction and muscle. Disorders of peripheral nerves are discussed in Chapter 148.

ETIOLOGY

Underlying causes of disorders of muscle and neuromuscular transmission are listed in Table 149–1 and include hereditary or suspected hereditary disorders and acquired disorders with autoimmune, metabolic, endocrine, neoplastic/paraneoplastic, infectious, toxic or drug-induced, and ischemic etiologies.

Hereditary Disorders

Several neuromuscular diseases have a known or suspected genetic basis.

Canine X-Linked Muscular Dystrophy

Canine X-linked muscular dystrophy in golden retrievers has striking phenotypic and genotypic similarities to Duchenne muscular dystrophy (DMD) in humans. Onset of clinical signs in affected males is about 10 weeks of age. Affected animals show stunting, weakness, gait abnormalities, and muscle atrophy with hypertrophy of proximal limb muscles. Serum creatine kinase (CK) levels are dramatically elevated (>10,000 Units/L, compared with normal levels of <100 Units/L). As in humans with DMD, affected dogs lack the Duchenne gene transcript and its protein product, dystrophin. Similar X-linked myopathies have been reported in Irish terri-

ers, samoyeds, rottweilers, and in a miniature schnauzer.

Central Core Myopathy

Myopathy with pathological changes in the central region of muscle fibers has been reported in young Great Danes with progressive exercise intolerance. Excitement associated with feeding or exercise precipitates episodes of general body tremors and collapse. This condition is not pathologically analogous to the human disorder with this name. The precise biochemical defect requires further investigation.

Congenital Myasthenia Gravis

A congenital familial form of myasthenia gravis (MG), inherited as an autosomal recessive trait, is described in Jack Russell terriers, springer spaniels, and smooth fox terriers. Failure of neuromuscular transmission results from a deficiency in muscle acetylcholine receptor (AChR) content, but unlike the acquired form of MG, it is not related to autoantibodies to AChR.

Familial Canine Dermatomyositis

Familial canine dermatomyositis is well documented in young collies and less well characterized in Shetland sheepdogs. In collies the inheritance pattern appears to be autosomal dominant with variable expression. Initially there is a variably severe dermatitis on the skin of the face, ears, distal extremities over bony prominences, and tail tip that may be followed by an inflammatory myopathy of the masticatory muscles and muscles distal to the elbow and stifle. There is evidence of an immunologic pathogenesis in DM, but exact mechanisms are uncertain.

Feline Muscular Dystrophy

A lethal muscle hypertrophy has been described in young male cats associated with dystrophin deficiency. Clinically the cats have generalized skeletal muscle hypertrophy, glossal hypertrophy and dysfunction, and excessive salivation. Progressive hypertrophy of the diaphragmatic muscles may result in occlusion of the esophagus.

Table 149–1. CAUSES OF NEUROMUSCULAR DISEASES

Hereditary Disorders

Canine X-linked muscular dystrophy
  Golden retriever
  Irish terrier
  Rottweiler
Central core myopathy
  Great Dane
Congenital myasthenia gravis
  Jack Russell terrier
  Springer spaniel
  Smooth fox terrier
Familial canine dermatomyositis
  Collie
  Shetland sheepdog
Feline muscular dystrophy
Glycogen storage disorders (Glycogenoses)
  Acid maltase deficiency (Glycogenosis type II)
    Lapland dogs
  Branching enzyme deficiency (Glycogenosis type IV)
    Norwegian forest cat
  Debranching enzyme deficiency (Glycogenosis type III)
    German shepherd dog
  Phosphofructokinase (PFK) deficiency (Glycogenosis type VII)
    English springer spaniel
Hereditary myopathy of Labrador retrievers
Hereditary myotonia of Chows
Mitochondrial myopathy
  Clumber spaniel
  Sussex spaniel
  Old English sheepdog
Muscle hypertonicity in the Cavalier King Charles spaniel
Nemaline rod myopathy
  Cats
  Border collie

Acquired Disorders

Autoimmune
  Generalized myasthenia gravis
  Focal myasthenia gravis
  Masticatory muscle myositis
  Polymyositis
  Extraocular myositis
Metabolic
  Abnormalities of glycogen metabolism
  Abnormalities of lipid metabolism and oxidative phosphorylation
  Electrolyte alterations
  Hyperthermia; malignant and exercise-related
Endocrine
  Hypothyroidism
  Hypo- and hyperadrenocorticism
Neoplastic/paraneoplastic
Infectious
  Toxoplasma gondii
  Neospora caninum
  Hepatozoon canis
  Ehrlichia canis
  Feline immunodeficiency virus
Toxic or drug-induced
  Tick paralysis
  Botulism
  Organophosphate toxicity
  Drugs affecting neuromuscular transmission
Ischemia

Glycogen Storage Disorders (Glycogenoses)

Although rare in companion animals, disorders of lysosomal glycogenosis (acid maltase deficiency, an α-glucosidase that releases glucose from maltose, oligosaccharides, and glycogen) and nonlysosomal glycogenosis (branching enzyme deficiency, debranching enzyme deficiency, and phosphofructokinase (PFK) deficiency affecting glycogenolysis, glycolysis, or glycogen synthesis) have been described. In dogs, clinical presentations for the nonlysosomal glycogenoses are not usually specific to the neuromuscular system since glycolysis plays a relatively minor role in canine muscle energetics. In branching and debranching enzyme deficiencies, muscle involvement may be overshadowed by liver dysfunction, hypoglycemia, or cardiomyopathy. In PFK deficiency, chronic hemolytic anemia and episodic stress-related hemolytic crises without overt weakness may predominate.

Hereditary Myopathy of Labrador Retrievers

Although this disorder of Labrador retrievers is commonly referred to as type II myofiber deficiency or "muscular dystrophy," at present the underlying pathologic mechanism is unknown. The disorder typically presents as progressive muscle weakness with exercise intolerance and abnormalities of gait and posture. There is, however, a wide variation in clinical presentations and pathologic findings. This may be more than one disorder affecting young Labradors. The mode of inheritance is autosomal recessive. Within muscle biopsy specimens, variable morphologic features have been reported; some biopsies show changes typical of neuropathic disease, whereas others show myopathic changes. The fiber type proportions are also variable. To date, pathologic changes in the spinal cord and peripheral nerves have not been found, even in cases where histologic changes within the muscle biopsy suggest an underlying neuropathic disorder.

Hereditary Myotonia of Chows

Clinical signs, noted when pups first ambulate, are due mainly to a myotonia and include stiffness on rising and walking, especially after rest. The mode of inheritance is autosomal recessive.

Mitochondrial Myopathy

Although there has been an explosion of information related to mitochondrial-associated diseases in humans in the past 10 years, only a few case reports are in the veterinary literature regarding this potentially important group of disorders. In the mitochondrial myopathies, clinical presentation is for marked exercise intolerance with associated metabolic acidosis and excessive rise in lactate and pyruvate. In Clumber and Sussex spaniels, a deficiency of pyruvate dehydrogenase was reported. Although a similar exertional lactic acidosis has been reported in Old English sheepdog littermates, the exact biochemical defect has not been identified. Given the importance of oxidative metabolism in canine muscle energetics, additional reports of these disorders should be forthcoming.

Muscle Hypertonicity in the Cavalier King Charles Spaniel

Exercise-induced muscle hypertonicity has been reported in young related Cavalier King Charles spaniels. Exercise and excitement-induced collapse was preceded by a "deer-stalking" gait. Increased extensor tone of the muscles of all four limbs was evident during the period of collapse. Recovery of limb function required about 10 minutes. Treatment with diazepam (5 mg two or three times daily) did not result in improvement. While ultrastructural abnormalities of mitochondria and the sarcotubular system were described, the precise underlying abnormality has not been established.

Nemaline Rod Myopathy

Five related cats were described with an early onset of mild weakness with progression to tremors, reluctance to move, and a crouched, hypermetric gait. Muscle atrophy was progressive. Numerous nemaline rods were present within myofibers. A similar myopathy has been seen in a young Border collie.

Acquired Neuromuscular Disorders

Autoimmune

Some of the most commonly occurring neuromuscular disorders of dogs are in this group. Included are MG, masticatory muscle myositis, and polymyositis. Although considered in the hereditary group, dermatomyositis in collies and shelties is also postulated to have an autoimmune basis.

Acquired Myasthenia Gravis. Acquired MG is common in dogs but rare in cats. Acquired MG probably is the best defined of all the neuromuscular disorders with respect to mechanisms of injury and pathogenesis. It is now well documented that acquired MG is associated with autoantibodies directed against the nicotinic AChR on the postsynaptic membrane of the neuromuscular junction. As a consequence of autoantibody binding, there is loss of AChRs resulting in impaired neuromuscular transmission and marked muscle weakness. AChR loss is a result of

- Increased endocytosis due to cross-linking of AChRs by antibody
- Complement activation leading to focal lysis of the postsynaptic membrane
- Direct inhibition of AChR function by bound antibodies

Masticatory Muscle Myositis. Masticatory muscle myositis (MMM) is a focal inflammatory myopathy that selectively affects the muscles of mastication. This selective distribution may be attributed to histochemical and biochemical differences between canine masticatory and limb muscles that provide the basis for a selective immune-mediated response. Although the role of autoantibodies is not yet determined, autoantibodies against cytoplasmic and sarcolemmal proteins of masti-

catory muscle type 2M proteins have been demonstrated by immunocytochemical methods both within muscle biopsy sections and indirectly in the serum in cases of MMM.

Extraocular Muscle Myositis. Another focal inflammatory myopathy is described in which the cellular infiltration is localized to canine extraocular muscles with lack of involvement of the masticatory muscles. An immune-mediated condition is suggested by a marked lymphocytic cellular infiltrate, bilateral muscle necrosis, and a rapid response to corticosteroid therapy alone. Although the specific immune mechanism is not known for this disorder, myofiber-specific antigens may play a role in the selective involvement of the extraocular muscles.

Polymyositis. Not as common as masticatory muscle myositis, polymyositis (PM) is a generalized inflammatory myopathy in which muscle damage is probably the result of cell-mediated immunity. An association has been reported with systemic lupus erythematosus and with an immune-mediated arthritis/polymyositis complex (see Chap. 22). PM also may be associated with malignancies; it has been reported as a paraneoplastic disorder associated with thymoma.

Metabolic

Enzyme Deficiencies. Although neuromuscular disorders associated with defined enzyme deficiencies have an early onset and are associated with specific breeds, some abnormalities, in particular those associated with oxidative metabolism, may occur later in life. Some of these may need to be reclassified as heritable, while others may be the result of environmental influences, toxins or drugs that affect oxidative pathways. Reversible mitochondrial myopathies are well described in the human literature secondary to azidothymidine therapy. Several cases of lipid storage myopathy have been evaluated by this author in various breeds of dogs having an older age of onset. Canine lipid storage myopathy has been associated with intramyofiber lipid droplets in muscle biopsy samples, elevated lactate and pyruvate, and secondary carnitine deficiency.

Malignant Hyperthermia. This hypermetabolic disorder of skeletal muscles has been described in dogs and in one cat. Hyperpyrexia usually occurs following administration of certain anesthetic agents, particularly halothane and quaternary amide muscle relaxant drugs. An exercise-related hyperthermia is described in an English springer spaniel. An exercise-related hyperthermia may also occur in young Labrador retrievers; however, a recent study has demonstrated that following strenuous exercise, normal dogs may obtain body temperatures of greater than 42°C.

Electrolyte Imbalances. Alterations in the levels of serum K^+ and Ca^{2+} due to underlying metabolic disorders can affect the excitability of neurons and muscle fibers, resulting in an increase or decrease in membrane excitability and resultant episodes of muscle weakness. A condition analogous to hyperkalemic periodic paralysis in humans has been described in a young

American pit bull. Studies in cats have shown that certain diet types (e.g., acidifying diets containing insufficient potassium) and diseases (especially renal disease) are associated with an increased occurrence of hypokalemia and clinically evident weakness that resolves following potassium administration. Alterations in the levels of serum phosphate and magnesium may also result in neuromuscular dysfunction although they are poorly characterized. Electrolyte disorders and their therapy are discussed in Chapter 5.

Endocrine

Myopathies can be associated with endocrine disorders, especially hypothyroidism and glucocorticoid excess. In hypothyroidism (see Chap. 29), peripheral neuropathies and myopathies are reported to occur, whereas myopathy and myotonia are associated with hyperadrenocorticism (see Chap. 31). Muscle weakness, probably as a consequence of hyperkalemia, is frequently associated with hypoadrenocorticism (see Chap. 31).

Neoplastic/Paraneoplastic

An association between neoplasia and neuromuscular disorders is suspected but not proved. Thymoma is sometimes associated with MG and polymyositis. Thymoma may also be diagnosed after the diagnosis of MG is established and should be considered if AChR antibody titers remain elevated for long periods. Consider evaluating AChR antibody titers before surgery in all dogs with a suspected thymoma. Positive AChR antibody titers and clinical signs of MG have been reported in two cases of canine osteosarcoma and in single cases of cholangiocellular carcinoma and anal sac adenocarcinoma. Postulated mechanisms of paraneoplastic-associated muscle damage include:

- Autoantibodies produced against tumor antigens that cross-react with muscle components
- Release of myotoxic substances by the neoplasm
- The possibility that the neoplasm and the underlying muscle disorder have a common pathogenesis

Parasitic

Although not common clinically, parasitic myositis can be caused by protozoa such as *Toxoplasma gondii*, *Neospora caninum*, and *Hepatozoon canis*. Infection may be diagnosed on a muscle biopsy (further discussion of protozoa is found in Chap. 19). An association between polymyositis and *Ehrlichia canis* infection in dogs has been reported. Other parasites, such as *Trichinella spiralis*, *Sarcocystis*, and *Hammondia*, elicit minimal inflammation and may be found incidentally in muscle biopsies.

Viral

- Some strains of feline calicivirus are associated with transient myalgia.
- A generalized lymphocytic myositis has been reported in adult cats infected with feline immunodeficiency virus.

Toxic or Drug Induced

Neuromuscular blockade may be the result of various neurotoxins.

- Neurotoxins that inhibit the evoked release of acetylcholine (ACh) at the neuromuscular junction are secreted by ticks such as *Dermacentor* and *Ixodes* species, resulting in tick paralysis.
- Ingestion of the exotoxin of *Clostridium botulinum* results in clinical signs of botulism by a similar mechanism.
- Organophosphate insecticides containing long-acting anticholinesterases reversibly or irreversibly bind acetylcholinesterase (AChE), permitting continuous cholinergic stimulation with accumulation of ACh at central, muscarinic, and nicotinic cholinergic synapses. "Myasthenia-like" syndromes are reported with organophosphate intoxication.
- Several drugs have been shown to reduce the safety margin of neuromuscular transmission, including aminoglycoside antibiotics, antiarrhythmic agents, phenothiazines, methoxyflurane, and magnesium given parenterally or in cathartics. These agents can potentiate neuromuscular blocking agents used during surgical procedures and may worsen or unmask preexisting disorders of neuromuscular transmission.
- Polymyositis may occur rarely in association with certain drug therapies. In human medicine, the drug most often implicated has been D-penicillamine. Polymyositis can occur as part of a generalized allergic drug reaction in Doberman pinschers following trimethoprim-sulfadiazine administration; however, this has not been confirmed by muscle biopsies or electromyographic studies.
- MG has been documented to occur in hyperthyroid cats on methimazole therapy. The mechanism may be similar to D-penicillamine-induced MG described in humans.

Ischemic

Ischemia as a result of thromboembolic disease and vascular occlusion is the most common cause of ischemic myopathy and neuromyopathy in dogs and cats. Circulation may be partly or completely compromised; the severity of clinical signs varies with the degree of occlusion.

CLINICAL SIGNS

▼ *Key Point* Muscular weakness is the clinical sign common to all neuromuscular disorders. Expression of muscular weakness may be limited to certain muscle groups or may be generalized and is variable in severity.

Generalized signs of motor system involvement include:

- Gait abnormalities
- Paresis or paralysis
- Exercise-related weakness

Other clinical signs that may occur concurrently with generalized weakness or in the absence of detectable weakness include:

- Masticatory dysfunction
- Dysphagia (pharyngeal dysfunction)
- Regurgitation (esophageal dysfunction)
- Dysphonia and dyspnea (laryngeal dysfunction) indicating involvement of selected motor units serving visceral functions

DIAGNOSIS

A thorough history and careful general physical and neurologic examinations are critical to the evaluation of neuromuscular disorders. Perform routine and special diagnostic testing procedures based on the differential diagnosis. Following the examination, it should be possible to tentatively localize the disorder to the motor unit.

History

Evaluate for:

- Exposure to chemical agents
- Recent illnesses and recent medications
- Exposure to different geographic locations

Physical and Neurologic Examinations

Following a careful general physical examination including a thorough evaluation of the cardiovascular system, perform a complete neurologic evaluation, as described in Chapter 144.

- Weakness (motor sign) is common to all motor unit abnormalities.
- Evaluate muscle strength by observing the animal's gait as it walks and, if necessary, after more strenuous exercise.
- Examine for stiffness of movement, seen in inflammatory myopathies, myotonias, and MG.
- The presence of ataxia (sensory sign) suggests an underlying neuropathic disorder with involvement of large myelinated proprioceptive fibers or their cell bodies in sensory ganglia.
- Assess muscle tone and spinal reflexes.
- Note muscle atrophy or swelling.

Because the clinical expression of weakness varies considerably in severity and distribution, perform other tests such as wheelbarrowing, hopping, or hemiwalking.

Clinical signs such as dysphagia, regurgitation, dysphonia, and dyspnea may indicate selective involvement of motor units. These clinical signs may occur in the absence of generalized weakness and may indicate disorders of motor units originating in cranial nerves.

▼ *Key Point* Differentiate vomiting from regurgitation because a wrong assessment may lead to an inappropriate diagnosis.

Routine and Special Laboratory Examinations

Perform a complete blood count (CBC), serum chemistry profile (including electrolytes), and urinalysis in all cases to evaluate possible underlying metabolic abnormalities. Although not indicated in all instances, other laboratory assays may assist in obtaining a diagnosis.

Serum Creatine Kinase Assay

Serum CK levels are elevated in muscle disorders associated with damage to myofibers and membranes. Although CK is a sensitive indicator of the presence and severity of myonecrosis, it has not been reliable in the diagnosis of polymyositis. Modest elevations in CK can occur in neuropathies.

▼ *Key Point* An elevation of serum CK is not diagnostic of myositis. Perform a muscle biopsy to confirm the diagnosis.

Resting and Post-Exercise Plasma Lactate/Pyruvate Assays

Evaluate plasma lactate and pyruvate levels at rest and following 10 minutes of strenuous exercise to diagnose disorders of oxidative metabolism. Perform these evaluations in any animal with exercise intolerance. Collect blood for lactate analysis in sodium fluoride/potassium oxalate tubes (gray top), centrifuge immediately, then separate the plasma. Special handling is required for pyruvate analysis.*

Thyroid and Adrenal Function Tests

Myopathies can occur secondary to disorders of both the thyroid and adrenal gland. Hypothyroidism can occur concurrently with autoimmune neuromuscular disorders such as acquired MG and an optimal clinical response may rely on the treatment of both disorders.

Antinuclear Antibody Assay

A positive antinuclear antibody (ANA) titer in association with an inflammatory myopathy suggests an underlying systemic autoimmune disorder. A subset of canine patients with myasthenia gravis also have positive ANA titers.

Serologic Tests

- Serum *Toxoplasma gondii* and *Neospora caninum* titers, as described in Chapter 19, may be useful in the evaluation of inflammatory myopathies and peripheral neuropathies caused by protozoa. However, demonstration of the organism in a muscle biopsy specimen is diagnostic.
- Serum *Ehrlichia* titers may be indicated in dogs, as described in Chapter 15.

---

*Assays are available from the Comparative Neuromuscular Laboratory, Basic Science Building, Room 1057, University of California–San Diego, La Jolla, CA 92093-0612 (phone: 619-534-1537).

- Evaluate cats suspected of feline immunodeficiency virus–associated myopathy with FIV serology, as described in Chapter 7.

Plasma Cholinesterase Levels

Myasthenia-like syndromes and delayed neuropathies are associated with organophosphate toxicity.

Serum Antibodies Against Masticatory Muscle Type 2M Fibers

The demonstration of autoantibodies against masticatory muscle type 2M fibers in fresh-frozen muscle sections by immunocytochemical methods using the immunoreagent staphylococcal protein A–horseradish peroxidase is useful in the diagnosis of masticatory muscle myositis. Direct methods for demonstrating the antibodies bound to myofibers within a muscle biopsy and indirect methods for demonstrating antibodies circulating within the patient's serum are available.*

Serum Antibodies Against Nicotinic AChRs

Demonstration of autoantibodies against muscle AChRs by immunoprecipitation radioimmunoassay is the diagnostic test of choice* for acquired MG. This assay is sensitive and specific and demonstrates an immune response specifically against muscle AChRs. It is particularly valuable in cases of focal myasthenia in which muscle weakness is localized to pharyngeal or esophageal musculature in the absence of detectable generalized weakness. Serial serum antibody titers also are important in following clinical response to treatment because there is good correlation between serum titers and response to treatment.

▼ *Key Point* Previous corticosteroid administration can lower serum antibody levels in assays for masticatory muscle myositis and MG. Collect serum before corticosteroid therapy.

Edrophonium Chloride Challenge Test

A presumptive diagnosis of generalized MG in dogs and cats may be based on an increase in muscle strength following intravenous (IV) administration of edrophonium chloride (Tensilon, Roche) at a recommended dosage of 0.1–0.2 mg/kg. The most dramatic response to edrophonium chloride is in MG; however, responses are variable: some patients with MG fail to respond, whereas some patients with neuropathic disorders show an increase in muscle strength.

▼ *Key Point* Do not eliminate a diagnosis of MG based on a negative response to edrophonium. Serum AChR antibody titers can confirm the diagnosis.

- Perform an edrophonium challenge test in all cases of confirmed myasthenia gravis for determination of the correct treatment protocol. If there is a good response to edrophonium, there should be a good response to anticholinesterase therapy. If the response to edrophonium is negative, then corticosteroids may be the treatment of choice.
- In cases of focal MG, if the palpebral reflex is absent or decreased, administration of the edrophonium chloride may result in an improved blink.
- During treatment of generalized MG with anticholinesterase drugs, edrophonium chloride may be useful in differentiating a myasthenic crisis (underdosing) from a cholinergic crisis (overdosing).
  - In a myasthenic crisis, rapid improvement usually follows IV administration of edrophonium chloride.

Electrodiagnostic Evaluation

Electrodiagnostic testing is a valuable adjunct to the neurologic examination. It provides

- Information on the location of a lesion within the motor unit (e.g., axon, neuromuscular junction, or muscle)
- Information on the distribution and severity of the disease process
- Guidance to appropriate muscle groups and peripheral nerves for subsequent biopsy

Electrodiagnostic testing includes:

- Evaluation of muscles by electromyography
- Evaluation of peripheral nerves by measurement of motor and sensory nerve conduction velocities and compound muscle and nerve action potentials (see Chap. 148).
- Measurement of evoked potentials following repetitive nerve stimulation, which is useful in the diagnosis of disorders of neuromuscular transmission if performed appropriately

In normal dogs stimulus rates greater than 5/second resulted in large decrements and variations between dogs. Use of stimulus rates greater than 5/second is not recommended because it can result in an inaccurate diagnosis of MG.

Muscle Biopsy

Muscle biopsy allows direct examination of portions of most motor unit components (e.g., intramuscular nerve branches, neuromuscular junction, and myofibers) and of supportive, connective, and vascular tissues. Using fresh-frozen sections, histologic and cytologic detail is preserved, and many biochemical and immunochemical reactions within cells and tissues can be localized. Frozen sections also may be used in specific biochemical assays for enzymes and substrates.

▼ *Key Point* For maximum information from a muscle biopsy, specimens should be fresh-frozen in isopentane precooled in liquid nitrogen. Biopsy samples must be received cold for subsequent freezing at a laboratory specialized in processing muscle biopsies. Consult with the laboratory *before*

---

*Assays are available from the Comparative Neuromuscular Laboratory, Basic Science Building, Room 1057, University of California–San Diego, La Jolla, CA 92093-0612 (phone: 619-534-1537).

taking a muscle biopsy. Place a second muscle biopsy in fixative for subsequent ultrastructural examination if required.

Appropriate sampling and transport methods are essential to the diagnostic value of the muscle specimen. Selection of the muscle(s) for biopsy is also important.

- Sample an involved muscle; however, avoid end-stage muscle because essential diagnostic features may no longer be present.
- The site of a localized disorder determines which muscle(s) should be sampled; however, in generalized disorders (e.g., polyneuropathy and polymyositis), obtain samples from standard muscles (e.g., vastus lateralis in dogs and cats).
- Following collection, dip the muscle in saline, place in a watertight container, and transport on cold packs to the laboratory.
- Delivery to the laboratory for processing within 24 hours is critical for optimal results.

Carnitine Quantification in Plasma, Urine, and Muscle

Lipid storage myopathies may result from primary or secondary abnormalities of carnitine. If excessive lipid droplets are present within a muscle biopsy section, carnitine should be quantified for formulation of a treatment plan.

Contrast Radiographic Studies

Because dysphagia as a result of oropharyngeal dysfunction and megaesophagus is a major problem in certain neuromuscular disorders, contrast studies that evaluate the dynamic swallowing process and motility throughout the esophagus are indicated. These studies should be attempted only if appropriate fluoroscopy and video recording equipment is available. (See Chapter 85 for discussion of diagnosis and management of esophageal disease.)

▼ *Key Point* If a large air-filled pharynx or a megaesophagus is seen on plain radiographs, do not perform a barium swallow. If a contrast agent is absolutely necessary, use a small amount of dilute barium solution to minimize chances of barium aspiration.

TREATMENT

Selective breeding and prevention is the treatment of choice for the *hereditary* neuromuscular disorders. New techniques in molecular genetics, available at selected research centers, allow the identification of underlying genetic defects and carrier animals. Gene replacement therapies are currently in experimental testing stages and may be available in the future for treatment of some of these disorders. *Acquired* neuromuscular disorders in many instances are secondary to diverse underlying medical problems such as hypothyroidism (see

Chap. 29), adrenal gland dysfunction (see Chap. 31), electrolyte disorders (see Chap. 5), and protozoal infection (see Chap. 19). Whenever possible, treat the primary problem. Specific treatment is available for some neuromuscular disorders. These are described below.

Generalized Myasthenia Gravis

Anticholinesterase Drugs

These drugs are the cornerstone of treatment for MG. They inhibit enzymatic hydrolysis of ACh at the neuromuscular junction, thereby increasing the effective concentration of ACh and the duration of its effect in the synaptic cleft and prolonging the interaction of released ACh with remaining AChRs.

- If there was a positive response to edrophonium chloride testing and the animal can tolerate oral medication, administer pyridostigmine bromide syrup (Mestinon, Roche) diluted 1:1 in water at a dose of 0.5–3.0 mg/kg q8–12h PO beginning at the low end of the dosage scale and gradually increasing.
- In cases of focal MG without generalized weakness or a fatigable palpebral response, begin pyridostigmine bromide syrup at a dosage of 0.5–1.0 mg/kg q8–12h PO.
- If oral delivery of drugs is a problem owing to megaesophagus or pharyngeal dysfunction, give injectable neostigmine (Prostigmin, Roche) at a dosage of 0.04 mg/kg q6h IM until the animal is able to handle oral medication.
- Initiate concurrent treatment for aspiration pneumonia (see Chap. 79) as needed.

▼ *Key Point* In the treatment of MG, titrate dosages to fit each animal's needs; requirements may vary from day to day in response to activity levels and stress.

Corticosteroids

Do not use corticosteroids as initial therapy in MG unless there was a negative response to edrophonium chloride testing. Although it is true that MG is an autoimmune disease, clinical signs of weakness can be controlled in most cases with anticholinesterase drugs.

Contraindications
- Some dogs become weaker *with immunosuppressive dosages* of corticosteroids, possibly precipitating a myasthenic crisis.
- In many dogs with MG, there is spontaneous remission within variable periods of time; therefore, generalized immunosuppression may not be warranted, particularly in light of the side effects of these drugs in dogs.

Indications
- If muscle strength is not greatly improved following anticholinesterase treatment and aspiration pneumonia is not present, administer prednisone at 0.5 mg/kg q12h, gradually tapering to alternate-day dosage.
- Other autoimmune disorders, for which a specific treatment for the underlying clinical signs is not

available, may occur concurrently with MG. In these cases, immunosuppression with corticosteroids is warranted.

Other Immunosuppressive Treatments

Reserve agents such as azathioprine and cyclophosphamide for the rare refractory cases that do not respond to conventional therapy.

▼ *Key Point* Rare cases may present in myasthenic crisis with peracute onset of collapse and respiratory insufficiency. Anticholinesterase drugs may be of no benefit in these cases; thus, respiratory support and plasmapheresis may be necessary.

Management of Pharyngeal Dysphagia and Megaesophagus

▼ *Key Point* Early recognition of regurgitation due to megaesophagus is important in the successful management of MG; management includes alteration in methods of delivery of food and water.

- Administer anticholinesterase drugs 1 hour before feeding.
- Deliver food and water with the animal in an upright position (see Chap. 85).
- Ensure that the animal remains upright for at least 10 minutes following feeding.
- If upright feeding fails to control regurgitation, place a gastrostomy feeding tube, as described in Chapter 3, to bypass the dysfunctional pharynx and esophagus.

▼ *Key Point* In the absence of severe aspiration pneumonia and with appropriate management, the prognosis for complete remission of MG is good. In many animals, the megaesophagus resolves and regurgitation is eliminated. Continue treatment until serum AChR antibody titers are normal.

Focal Myasthenia Gravis

Megaesophagus and pharyngeal dysfunction in the absence of detectable generalized weakness may occur in MG. The diagnosis in these cases is made by demonstration of positive serum AChR antibody titers.

- The single most important part of treatment is elevation of food and water (see Chap. 85).
- The value of anticholinesterase drugs in focal MG is not known; however, lower doses may be of some benefit in controlling regurgitation. In the absence of generalized weakness, monitoring drug response is difficult and overdosages may occur.
- In the absence of aspiration pneumonia and pharyngeal weakness, a large percentage of dogs with the focal form of MG go into spontaneous remission. Although it is not known whether the benefits of corticosteroids outweigh the risks, in focal MG as in generalized MG the presence of concurrent autoimmune disorders without a specific therapy warrants the use of corticosteroids.

Immune-Mediated Inflammatory Myopathies

Masticatory Muscle Myositis

- During the acute stages of MMM, masticatory muscle swelling and trismus (spasm) usually resolve rapidly subsequent to immunosuppressive dosages of glucocorticoids (prednisone, 2–3 mg/kg q12h PO).
- Determine response to therapy by ability to open the jaw and by serial determinations of serum CK levels.
- If the response is favorable, decrease the dosage after 1–2 weeks to 1.0 mg/kg q12h PO; then gradually decrease to the lowest effective alternate-day dosage.
- Relapses are common.

▼ *Key Point* In acute MMM, glucocorticoids usually produce rapid resolution. In chronic MMM, glucocorticoid therapy may improve jaw mobility even though a significant proportion of muscle is replaced by fibrous connective tissue.

Polymyositis

- Treat dogs with polymyositis with immunosuppressive doses of corticosteroids in the absence of aspiration pneumonia or an underlying infectious agent. Initiate a treatment regimen similar to that for MMM.
- In refractory cases, use corticosteroids and other immunosuppressive agents such as azathioprine or cyclophosphamide concurrently.

Lipid Storage Myopathy

- Large intramyofiber lipid droplets within a fresh-frozen muscle biopsy sample is an indication of an underlying metabolic abnormality. Evaluate lactate, pyruvate, and carnitine status.
- Treat orally with L-carnitine (50 mg/kg q12h), coenzyme Q_{10} (100 mg q24h) and riboflavin (100 mg q24h) for a minimum of 2 months for determination of response. The treatment may need to be continued indefinitely.

SUPPLEMENTAL READINGS

Carpenter JL, Schmidt GM, Moore FM, et al.: Canine bilateral extraocular polymyositis. Vet Pathol 26:510, 1989.

Cooper BJ, De Lahunta A, Gallagher EA, Valentine BA: Nemaline myopathy of cats. Muscle Nerve 9:618, 1986.

Gashen FP, Hoffman EP, Gorospe JRM, et al.: Dystrophin deficiency causes lethal muscle hypertrophy in cats. J Neurol Sci 110:149, 1992.

Le Couteur RA, Dow SW, Sisson AF: Metabolic and endocrine myopathies of dogs and cats. Semin Vet Med Surg (Small Anim) 4:146, 1989.

Sharp NJH, Kornegay JN, Lane SB: The muscular dystrophies. Semin Vet Med Surg (Small Anim) 4:133, 1989.

Shelton GD: Disorders of neuromuscular transmission. Semin Vet Med Surg (Small Anim) 4:126, 1989.

Shelton GD: Canine myasthenia gravis. *In* Kirk RW, Bonagura JD, eds.: Current Veterinary Therapy XI. Philadelphia: WB Saunders, 1992, p 1039.

Shelton GD: Megaesophagus secondary to acquired myasthenia gravis. *In* Kirk RW, Bonagura JD, eds.: Current Veterinary Therapy XI. Philadelphia: WB Saunders, 1992, p 580.

Shelton GD: Canine lipid storage myopathies. *In* Kirk RW, Bonagura JD, eds.: Current Veterinary Therapy XII. Philadelphia: WB Saunders, 1995, p 1161.

Shelton GD, Cardinet GH III: Pathophysiologic basis of canine muscle disorders. J Vet Intern Med 1:36, 1987.

Shelton GD, Cardinet GH III: Canine masticatory muscle disorders. *In* Kirk RW, ed.: Current Veterinary Therapy X. Philadelphia: WB Saunders, 1989, p 816.

Shelton GD, Willard MD, Cardinet GH III, Lindstrom J: Acquired myasthenia gravis: Selective involvement of esophageal, pharyngeal, and facial muscles. J Vet Intern Med 4:281, 1990.

Targett MP, Franklin RJM, Olby NJ, et al.: Central core myopathy in a great dane. J Small Anim Practice 35:100, 1994.

Wright JA, Smyth JBA, Brownlie SE, Robins M: A myopathy associated with muscle hypertonicity in the Cavalier King Charles spaniel. J Comp Pathol 97:559, 1987.

11 Ophthalmology

David A. Wilkie

150 Ophthalmic Equipment and Techniques

David A. Wilkie

OPHTHALMIC EQUIPMENT

The instruments and other equipment necessary for ophthalmic examination and surgery can be generally categorized as basic and advanced.

Diagnostic Equipment

Basic

- Penlight
- Direct ophthalmoscope with Finnoff transilluminator
- Indirect lens (20 diopter)
- Tonometer (Schiøtz) or Tonopen (Mentor O&O)
- Miscellaneous
  - Schirmer tear test strips
  - Fluorescein stain
  - Nasolacrimal cannula (23 gauge)
  - Dilating agent (e.g., tropicamide)
  - Topical anesthetic (e.g., proparacaine)
  - Graefe forceps for third eyelid manipulation
  - Kimura spatula for cytology

Advanced

- Biomicroscope (slit lamp)
- Indirect ophthalmoscope
- Indirect lenses (15, 20, and 30 diopter)
- Applanation tonometer
- Gonioscopy lens
- Streak Retinoscope
- Ultrasound (7.5, 10.0 MHz)

- Fundus Camera
- Electroretinography

Surgical Equipment

Basic

- Magnifying loupes (4–6 ×)
- Colibri corneal forceps (0.3 mm teeth with tying platform)
- Bishop Harmon forceps (0.3- or 0.8-mm teeth)
- Barraquer needle holder (curved, without lock device; 9 mm × 0.85 mm jaws)
- Westcott tenotomy scissors
- Stevens tenotomy curved scissors
- Barraquer eyelid speculum
- Beaver blade handle
- Bard-Parker blade handle
- Desmarres chalazion clamp
- Strabismus hooks (two)
- Jamieson calipers
- Jaeger eyelid plate
- Irrigating cannula (23 gauge)

Advanced

- Operating microscope
- Right and left corneal section scissors
- Lens loop
- Angled tying forceps
- Carter sphere introducer
- Castroviejo cyclodialysis spatula
- Various intraocular forceps

- Diode or Nd:YAG laser
- Corneal trephines
- Phacoemulsification/Irrigation-Aspiration device

Other

- Suture material
  - 7-0, 8-0 Vicryl or Dexon—ophthalmic spatula needle
  - 9-0 nylon
  - 6-0 monofilament—ophthalmic cutting needle (nylon, Surgilene, prolene)
- Blades
  - #64, 63, and 65 Beaver blades
  - #11 and 15 Bard-Parker blades
- Irrigating solutions
  - Ophthalmic balanced salt solution (BSS)
  - Lactated Ringer's
- Weck-cel surgical spears
- Prosthesis implants (18–19 mm)

OPHTHALMOLOGY TECHNIQUES

The general veterinarian in private practice should be able to perform the following routine ophthalmic procedures:

- Culture of the eye
- Schirmer tear test
- Examination of the nictitating membrane (third eyelid)
- Direct ophthalmoscopy
- Indirect ophthalmoscopy
- Fluorescein stain of the cornea
- Nasolacrimal irrigation
- Tonometry (Schiøtz, Tonopen)
- Conjunctival/corneal cytology

To properly evaluate and treat the patient with ocular disease, the clinician must have an accurate understanding of ophthalmic anatomy (Fig. 150–1).

In addition, based on the information obtained by these diagnostic tests, the clinician should be able to arrive at a diagnosis and formulate a plan for further diagnostic tests or treatment.

Culture

Indications

- Chronic, nonresponsive corneal ulcer
- Acute, severe melting corneal ulcer
- Purulent ocular discharge
- Infectious blepharitis

Equipment

- A sterile, moist, synthetic culture swab is preferable but a sterile cotton swab can be used.

Technique

The general principles and techniques for obtaining a culture from the eye are the same as for other organs.

1. Using a sterile swab moistened in transport media, obtain the sample in an aseptic manner from the area of concern; for example:
   a. If the lesion is a corneal ulcer, touch the swab to the ulcer (do not place in the conjunctival fornix).
2. Do not use a topical anesthetic for this procedure because it may interfere with the growth of organisms.
3. Label the sample and submit for aerobic and possibly fungal culture and sensitivity testing. It should be streaked onto nutrient agar as soon as possible.

Schirmer Tear Test

Indications

- Assessment of normal aqueous tear production
- Chronic pigmentary keratitis
- Epiphora, including chronic mucoid epiphora

Equipment

- Commercially available Schirmer tear test strips

Technique

1. Place the notched end of the test strip in the lower conjunctival fornix. Do not touch this end.
2. Hold the eye closed and allow the strip to remain in place for exactly 1 minute. If convenient, both eyes may be tested at the same time.
3. Remove the strip and, using the standard measurement on the package, measure and record tear production. Normal dogs secrete 15 mm or more in 1 minute.
4. Do not use topical anesthetic for this test because the objective is to measure the response of the eye to an irritant. This requires the response of the ophthalmic branch of cranial nerve (CN) V as the afferent arm and the parasympathetic fibers in CN VII as the efferent arm.
5. In addition to the Schirmer tear test, evaluation of the tear breakup time (BUT) to assess the mucin portion of the precorneal tear film and corneal

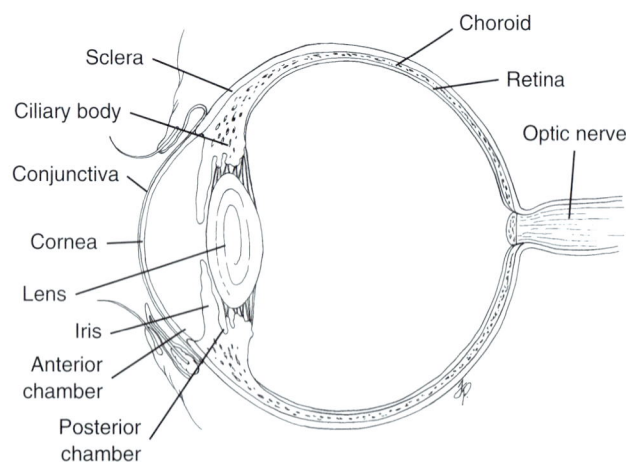

Figure 150–1. Normal ophthalmic anatomy.

staining with rose Bengal are also tools used in the assessment of the precorneal tear film and corneal surface health.

Examination of the Nictitating Membrane

Indications

- Chronic conjunctivitis
- Suspicion of a foreign body
- Mass lesion of the nictitating membrane (third eyelid)

Equipment

- Topical anesthetic
- Atraumatic forceps

Technique

1. Examine the palpebral surface of the third eyelid by gently retropulsing the globe and allowing the nictitating membrane to prolapse passively while the lower eyelid is retracted. This is useful for assessing the mobility of the third eyelid and for protecting the eye when obtaining a conjunctival scraping.
2. Examine the bulbar surface of the third eyelid. This requires topical anesthesia.
   a. The topical anesthetic of choice is proparacaine (Alcaine), which provides 10–15 minutes of anesthesia. Apply 2 drops of anesthetic and wait 2–3 minutes for the full effect.
   b. After anesthetizing the surface, gently grasp the leading edge of the third eyelid with small non-toothed forceps. Take care to avoid damaging the cornea.
   c. Gently pull the third eyelid up and out to allow examination of the posterior surface.
3. Examine all surfaces and the inner and outer fornices of the third eyelid for a foreign body and for lymphoid follicles, which indicate a chronic inflammatory process.

Direct Ophthalmoscopy

This technique provides an upright image of the fundus and associated structures and magnifies the image 15–18 times. In small animals, the field of view is narrow and therefore difficult to use for general screening of the eye.

Indications

- Examination of the ocular fundus
- Detailed examination with higher magnification of specific areas such as the optic nerve and blood vessels.

Equipment

- Dilating agent, (e.g., tropicamide)
- Charged, direct ophthalmoscope

Technique

1. Turn on the ophthalmoscope and use the rheostat to adjust the light intensity.
2. Turn the diopter wheel to the zero (0) setting. This usually is the proper setting to view the fundus.
3. Darken the examination room.
4. Place the ophthalmoscope to your eye, and from a distance of 12–24 inches obtain the tapetal reflection. While looking through the ophthalmoscope move toward the animal's eye, observing for any interference with the tapetal reflection, which may indicate opacity of the transmitting media, cornea, aqueous humor, lens, or vitreous. When you are 1–2 inches from the patient's cornea, the retina, optic nerve, retinal vessels, and tapetum will be clearly in focus.
5. Locate a blood vessel and follow it to the optic nerve. Evaluate the optic nerve and blood vessels and scan the fundus for abnormalities of color, clarity, size, and shape. Use the diopter wheel to adjust the focus, and to evaluate raised and depressed lesions (numbers in red indicate negative or deeper; those in black are positive or more superficial).

Indirect Ophthalmoscopy

Although practice is required to become proficient in this technique, once it is mastered it is more useful than direct ophthalmoscopy for screening the fundus in small animals. Also, the equipment needed is less expensive. Indirect ophthalmoscopy provides an inverted, reversed image magnified 3–5 times. This image, although of a lower magnification than with direct ophthalmoscopy, has a much larger field of view and is better for routine screening of the eye.

Indications

- Examination of the ocular fundus

Equipment

- Dilating agent (e.g., tropicamide)
- Light source (e.g., penlight)
- Indirect, handheld 20-diopter lens

Technique

1. Dilate the patient's pupil with 1–2 drops of tropicamide (Mydriacyl). Allow 10–15 minutes for complete dilation (the effect will last 8–12 hours in dogs).
2. Begin the examination at arm's length from the patient, having an assistant restrain the patient and hold the eyelids open.
3. Darken the examination room.
4. With a focal light source (e.g., a penlight or direct ophthalmoscope) held at arm's length from the patient, obtain the tapetal reflection.
5. Holding the lens in the other hand, place the lens 1–2 inches in front of the patient's eye, in the path of the light. The fundus should appear as a virtual image in front of the lens.
   a. Be sure to look at the image that is in front of the lens and not at the lens or the eye.

6. To view other areas of the fundus, you must move yourself, the light source, and the lens while keeping all of these in alignment. Remember that because the image is inverted you must move in the opposite direction to the image.

7. If the image is lost, move the lens out of the light beam and start again.

Fluorescein Stain of the Cornea

Fluorescein is a hydrophilic drug that binds to the corneal stroma, but not to the epithelium or to Descemet's membrane.

Indications

- Red or painful eye
- An obvious corneal irregularity
- Ocular trauma or a foreign body
- Assessment of nasolacrimal duct function

Equipment

- Prepackaged fluorescein strips (commercially available)
- Sterile ocular collyria (eyewash solution)
- Cotton balls

Technique

1. Remove the fluorescein strip from the package, holding it by the green end. Fold the strip lengthwise to create a trough.

2. Place 2–3 drops of sterile eyewash solution on the strip and tilt it to allow the stain to drip onto the eye. Do not touch the eye with the strip because this may result in an iatrogenic area of stain retention.

3. With the eyewash solution, gently irrigate excess stain from the eye onto a cotton ball; examine the eye for stain uptake, using a penlight. Identification of the fluorescein uptake is improved by using a blue or Woods light, which excites the fluorescein molecules, making them fluoresce green.

Assessment of Nasolacrimal Duct Function

1. To evaluate the patency of the nasolacrimal duct, perform the previously described steps, but do not rinse the fluorescein from the eye. The stain should appear at the nares within 5 minutes.

2. A positive test is definitive for a patent nasolacrimal duct but does not prove that both puncta are patent. A negative test suggests a problem, and irrigation of the duct is indicated.

Nasolacrimal Duct Irrigation

- This procedure can be performed on a minimally restrained dog, using only topical anesthesia.
- Sedation or general anesthesia usually is required for cats.

Indications

- Epiphora without an obvious etiology
- Failure of passage of fluorescein stain
- Mucopurulent ocular discharge

Equipment

- Topical anesthetic
- Syringe (3–6 ml)
- Nasolacrimal duct cannula (23 or 25 gauge)

Technique

1. Apply a topical anesthetic and connect a nasolacrimal duct cannula to a syringe filled with eyewash solution.

2. While an assistant restrains the animal's head, elevate and roll the upper eyelid in the medial canthus to expose the superior punctum.

3. Place the thumb or index finger on the plunger of the syringe, in preparation for injection. Hold the syringe loosely so that no injury will result if the patient should jerk its head.

4. Gently insert the cannula in the punctum and, without forcing, allow it to seat itself in the duct. Apply gentle pressure to the plunger and observe fluid emerging from the inferior punctum.

5. Occlude the lower punctum, tip the nose down, and continue flushing. Fluid should now appear at the nostril.

▼ **Key Point** Do not use excessive force when placing the catheter or when irrigating.

6. If a patent duct cannot be established and the epiphora is severe, consider medical therapy such as topical antibiotics or anti-inflammatories and repeated irrigation, or examine under general anesthesia to further pursue the problem.

Tonometry

Be sure to have a functioning tonometer and be familiar with its use. There are two specific ways to determine intraocular pressure (IOP): indentation tonometry and applanation tonometry.

Indications

- Diffuse corneal edema
- Anisocoria
- Fixed and dilated pupils
- Episcleral congestion
- Blindness
- Buphthalmos
- Anterior uveitis
- Breeds predisposed to primary glaucoma—annual IOP determination
- Monitoring of medically or surgically controlled glaucoma
- Evaluation of the contralateral eye in animals with unilateral primary glaucoma

Schiøtz Indentation Tonometry

The Schiøtz tonometer is an indentation tonometer and measures the amount of corneal indentation that occurs when a given weight is placed on the cornea. The result is inversely proportional to the intraocular pressure. Obtain the actual pressure from a table of values. The Schiøtz tonometer requires assembly, disassembly, and cleaning in order to ensure its accuracy. The foot plate is large and the patient must be cooperative in order to place the foot plate on the cornea in a vertical position. If the animal is fractious or the eye painful, it is unlikely that accurate placement will be obtained and erroneous values will result. The result is that glaucoma is not diagnosed or monitored accurately and IOP determination is not performed at the frequency indicated by the breed or clinical signs.

Equipment

- Topical anesthetic
- Calibrated Schiøtz tonometer
- Conversion chart

Technique

1. Anesthetize the cornea with topical proparacaine.
2. To assemble the tonometer, place the shaft in the housing and attach the 5.5-g weight. Hold the instrument vertically and check that the plunger slides freely within the hollow sleeve.
3. Use the metal calibration standard to test the accuracy of the tonometer. When the instrument is placed on the standard it should read zero (0) on the scale (i.e., the 5.5-g weight does not indent the metal standard).
4. While an assistant gently elevates the patient's nose, elevate the upper eyelid and place the tonometer foot plate on the cornea. Keep the tonometer vertical and on the center of the cornea. The tonometer should rest on the eye and does not need to be pushed down.
5. Take three readings and average them. Using the conversion chart, convert the averaged value to an approximation of the intraocular pressure, matching the weight used with the reading obtained.
6. Normal values for dogs are 15–27 mm Hg; the variation in both eyes should be no greater than 5 mm Hg.

Applanation Tonometry—Tonopen

Applanation tonometry determines IOP by evaluating the force required to applanate or flatten a given surface area of cornea. In recent years the Tonopen (Mentor O&O) has been evaluated and shown to be similar to other applanation tonometers in accuracy. It is lightweight, portable, accurate, self-calibrating, and averages several readings and gives a percentage error to ensure accuracy. In addition, the small footplate allows this tonometer to be used on painful eyes in less cooperative patients because only a small area of cornea is required to obtain a reading, and the position of the patient's head is not related to obtaining the reading.

Equipment

- Topical anesthetic
- Calibrated Tonopen

Technique

1. Anesthetize the cornea with topical proparacaine.
2. Activate the Tonopen and gently tap the transducer tip, which is protected by a sleeve, against the cornea. A gentle bouncing motion of the transducer tip against the cornea works best. The device will give an audible tone as each reading is accepted and a longer tone when enough readings have been averaged.
3. Obtain the patient's IOP from the digital reading at the Tonopen display window. The standard error bar should be over the <5% error. If there is a greater percent error, repeat the procedure until a reliable measurement is obtained.

Cytology

Cytology is a simple, fast, and inexpensive method for characterizing the type of inflammatory process and in many cases to obtain a diagnosis.

Indications

- Obtain a sample for Gram stain
- Characterize the type of inflammation, i.e., neutrophilic, lymphocytic, eosinophilic
- Aid in the diagnosis of feline conjunctivitis (e.g., for *Chlamydia, Mycoplasma*)
- Obtain samples for fluorescent antibody testing

Equipment

- Topical anesthetic
- Platinum spatula or other instrument suitable for sample collection
- Microscope
- Microscope slides
- Stain

Technique

1. Place a topical anesthetic in the animal's conjunctival sac.
2. Gently retropulse the globe and retract the lower eyelid, thus exposing the third eyelid.
3. Using a spatula or other suitable instrument, scrape the palpebral surface of the third eyelid and the adjacent palpebral conjunctiva. Avoid damaging the surface, but use sufficient force to exfoliate cells.
4. Place the cells on a glass slide and streak them to form a monolayer.
5. Submit the slide for Gram staining (to characterize the type of bacteria); for Giemsa, Wright, or Diff-Quik staining (to examine for cell type, inclusion bodies, etc.); for fluorescent antibody testing (*Chlamydia,* herpesvirus).

Table 150–1. OPHTHALMIC CLINICAL SIGNS ASSOCIATED WITH SYSTEMIC DISEASES

Ophthalmic Clinical Sign	Associated Systemic Disease
Keratitis sicca	Hypothyroidism Autoimmune disease Drug induced (sulfonamides) Facial nerve paralysis Otitis media/interna Canine distemper virus
Anterior uveitis/ chorioretinitis	Infectious (bacteria, rickettsia, mycoses, viruses) Trauma Neoplasia Autoimmune disease
Glaucoma	Anterior uveitis Neoplasia Trauma Hyphema
Cataract	Trauma Diabetes mellitus Nutritional disorder Radiation Inflammatory diseases (see anterior uveitis/ chorioretinitis)
Retinal detachment	Trauma Infectious (bacteria, rickettsia, mycoses, viruses) Neoplasia Autoimmune diseases Systemic hypertension (renal disease, pheochromocytoma, hyperthyroidism, idiopathic) Hyperviscosity
Blindness	Trauma Neoplasia Reticulosis Infectious (bacteria, rickettsia, mycoses, viruses) Autoimmune diseases Other central nervous system diseases
Horner's syndrome	Thoracic mass Spinal cord trauma (C1–T2) Neck trauma Otitis media/interna Orbital mass lesion
Hyphema	Coagulopathy Trauma Hypertension (renal disease, pheochromocytoma, hyperthyroidism, idiopathic) Infectious diseases Neoplasia

OCULAR MANIFESTATIONS OF SYSTEMIC DISEASE

Ophthalmic clinical signs frequently are manifestations of systemic disease (Table 150–1). For many of these ophthalmic signs, specific ocular causes must be differentiated from the systemic ones provided in Table 150–1. For a more complete discussion of these diseases and their treatment, refer to appropriate chapters in this book.

151 Diseases of the Eyelid

Susan E. Kirschner

Diseases of the eyelid result in a variety of clinical signs. Initially, the eyelids alone may be affected, but because of their close proximity to the cornea and conjunctiva, disease of these structures frequently results. Because corneal and conjunctival involvement is often more severe and more obvious, eyelid disease may be overlooked. Manage concurrent conjunctival and corneal disease as described in Chapters 152 and 153, respectively, in this section.

Diseases of the eyelid can be broadly categorized by their appropriate treatment (i.e., surgery or medical therapy), as listed in Table 151–1.

ANATOMY

- The eyelid functions to protect and moisten the cornea and to remove debris. The eyelid is covered by skin and lined internally by palpebral conjunctiva.
- The eyelid is closed by the orbicularis oculi muscle, which is innervated by the palpebral branch of the facial nerve. Paralysis of this nerve results in inability to close the eyelids. Spasm of the orbicularis oculi muscle results in spastic entropion.
- The eyelids are opened by the levator palpebrae and Mueller's muscle, which are innervated by the oculomotor nerve and by postganglionic sympathetic fibers, respectively. Paralysis of either of these nerves results in ptosis, or drooping of the eyelid.
- The meibomian glands line the conjunctival surface of the eyelid margin. They open onto the eyelid margin, where they secrete an oily fluid that helps prevent evaporation of the precorneal tear film. Distichia and ectopic cilia originate from the meibomian glands.

PRINCIPLES OF EYELID SURGERY

- The skin covering the eyelids is thin and easily traumatized. Perform clipping and aseptic preparation gently. A povidone-iodine solution diluted with saline solution to a 1:10 concentration is appropriate for preparing the eyelids for surgery.
- The eyelids have an extensive blood supply, and injured tissue heals well; therefore, remove only clearly necrotic tissue. Removal of excess tissue can result in abnormal lid function.

- Close eyelid skin incisions with 4-0 to 6-0 monofilament nonabsorbable suture in a simple interrupted pattern. Close conjunctival wounds with 6-0 to 8-0 absorbable suture material. Remove nonabsorbable sutures 2 weeks following surgery.
- An Elizabethan-type collar may be necessary to prevent self-trauma.

▼ **Key Point** Accurate closure of the eyelid margin is the most important component of eyelid defect repair.

ANKYLOBLEPHARON

Ankyloblepharon is a condition seen in neonatal puppies in which the eyelids do not open properly.

- This condition may result in a subpalpebral infection called ophthalmia neonatorum.
  - If infection occurs, gently massage the eyelids to open a portion of the palpebral fissure. Occasionally, scissors or a scalpel blade is required to partially open the eyelids.
  - Lavage the subpalpebral area with a 1% povidone-iodine solution and apply a topical antibiotic solution or ointment (e.g., triple antibiotic, erythromycin, gentamicin) three to four times daily.
- If the infection is left unattended, the cornea may ulcerate or perforate.
- If the entire palpebral fissure is opened prematurely, corneal damage may result from exposure and desiccation.
  - To protect against corneal desiccation, use an artificial tear ointment four to six times daily.

COLOBOMA

In this disorder, which affects kittens and occasionally puppies, a portion of the lid margin does not form.

- The major clinical signs are epiphora and blepharospasm.
- Coloboma may be confused with entropion because eyelid hairs often contact the cornea.
- Many cases can be corrected by slightly everting the lid with entropion correction surgery, thus preventing corneal trauma by facial hairs.

Table 151–1. CLASSIFICATION OF EYELID DISEASES ACCORDING TO TYPE OF THERAPY

Surgery
Ankyloblepharon
Coloboma
Entropion
Ectropion
Distichiasis/ectopic cilia
Lagophthalmos
Neoplasia

Medical Treatment
Bacterial blepharitis
Chalazion/hordeolum
Allergic blepharitis
Parasitic and fungal blepharitis

- Extensive colobomas require a pedicle flap or other reconstructive surgical procedure performed by a veterinary ophthalmologist.

ENTROPION

Entropion often is observed in young dogs and is common in the chow, Shar pei, and hunting breeds. It can also occur in cats.

- Clinical signs vary from conjunctivitis with mild serous discharge to severe blepharospasm with corneal ulceration and purulent discharge.
- Diagnosis is made by examination of the eyelids. When the eyelid is rolled inward, facial hairs often directly contact the cornea.
- Correct neonatal entropion in the Shar pei with temporary everting sutures at 3–5 weeks of age. Failure of this technique indicates the need for permanent surgical correction.

Classification

▼ *Key Point* Entropion may be anatomic, anatomic with secondary eyelid spasm, or primarily spastic.

Classification of entropion is made when the eyelids are relaxed. This may require topical anesthesia, palpebral nerve blocks, or general anesthesia.

- *Anatomic entropion*—The eyelid rolls inward even when the eyelids are relaxed. This may be from a defect in the eyelids themselves, or in the case of certain breeds such as the Shar pei and the bloodhound, from forehead or brow folds, which force the eyelids inward.
  - Surgical correction is indicated.
- *Anatomic entropion with secondary spasm*—Blepharospasm exaggerates entropion such that a portion of the rolling is from an anatomic abnormality, with the remainder due to squinting.
  - Surgically correct the anatomic portion of the entropion; additional temporary everting sutures may be required until the spasm cycle is broken.

- *Spastic entropion*—Blepharospasm results in rolling inward of the eyelid margin. Under anesthesia or when the eyelids are relaxed, the entropion resolves.
  - Correct with temporary everting sutures and treatment of the underlying cause of the spasm.

Surgical Techniques

Ventral or Dorsal Eyelid Entropion

1. Remove an ellipse of skin parallel to and 2–3 mm from the lid margin (Fig. 151–1). The amount of skin removed depends on the severity of the entropion.
2. Remove the tissue with a scalpel or by crushing the selected tissue with a hemostat and then removing the crimped tissue with scissors.
3. Close the skin routinely with monofilament nylon sutures (e.g., 4-0) in a simple interrupted pattern.

Lateral Entropion

1. Remove a V-shaped area of skin (Fig. 151–2A) at the lateral canthus.
2. If the lateral canthus is extremely lax, dissect the underlying orbicularis oculi muscle free (Fig. 151–2B) and suture it to the lateral orbital rim with 4-0 or 5-0 nonabsorbable monofilament suture material (Fig. 151–2C).
3. Close the skin with 4-0 or 5-0 nonabsorbable sutures in a simple interrupted pattern.

Medial Entropion

1. Evert the skin with an elliptical incision, as for ventral entropion.
2. Alternatively perform a medial canthoplasty. Make a V-shaped incision along the eyelid margin that encompasses the caruncle (Fig. 151–3A). Take care not to injure the underlying lacrimal canaliculi.
3. Close the incision by suturing the upper lid to the lower lid to create a horizontal closure (Fig. 151–3B and C). This has the effect of correcting the entropion and slightly shortening the palpebral fissure.

Temporary Everting Sutures for Spastic Entropion and for Neonatal Entropion in Shar Peis

1. Use minimal anesthesia for very young puppies (occasionally, light inhalation anesthesia via a mask is required).

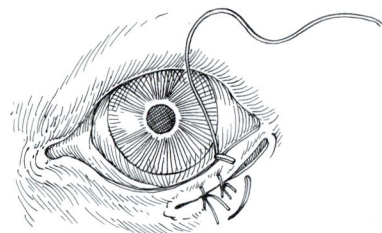

Figure 151–1.   Correction of ventral entropion.

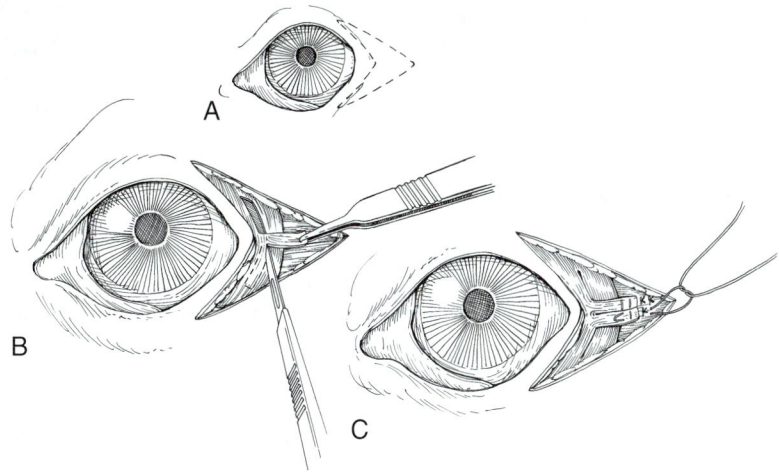

Figure 151–2. Correction of lateral entropion. *A,* Area of skin to be removed; *B,* orbicularis oculi dissected free; and *C,* orbicularis oculi sutured to the lateral orbital rim.

2. In older dogs, inject a short-acting anesthetic (see Chap. 2).
3. Place one to two 4-0 to 5-0 nylon sutures in a mattress pattern in each eyelid. Sutures should be partial thickness only. Make the first bite 1–2 mm from the eyelid margin. Place the second bite at a sufficient distance to cause eversion of the eyelid margin when the suture is tied (Fig. 151–4).
4. Leave the sutures in place for 3–4 weeks. Premature suture removal may result in recurrence of the entropion.

Entropion Caused by Heavy Brow Folds

1. The skin of the forehead may be removed en bloc, or the folds may be elevated.
2. To elevate the folds, use surgical mesh, such as mersilene, cut into strips 3–4 mm wide and 10–15 cm long, and a straight surgical needle with an eye capable of receiving the end of the mesh strip.
3. Make a horizontal skin incision 1–2 cm above the

lid margin, and a second one 8–12 cm higher on the brow.
4. Pass the mesh suture from the upper incision, beneath the skin to the lower incision, then horizontally through subcutaneous muscle, then beneath the skin back to the upper incision. Tighten to achieve the desired effect. Tie as with a typical suture.
5. Place two to six of these lifting sutures, as needed. Close the skin incisions with 3-0 to 4-0 nylon suture.

ECTROPION

- Ectropion may be caused by excessive eyelid length or by decreased tone of the eyelid muscles. This results in sagging of the lower eyelid, with exposure of conjunctiva. In addition, ectropion can result iatrogenically from overcorrection of entropion.
- Increased conjunctival exposure often results in chronic conjunctivitis or exposure keratitis. Poor lid-to-cornea fit may exacerbate keratoconjunctivitis sicca (KCS) because of abnormal tear distribution.
- Most cases of ectropion can be corrected by a full-thickness wedge resection of the affected portion of the eyelid (see under Neoplasia for procedure).

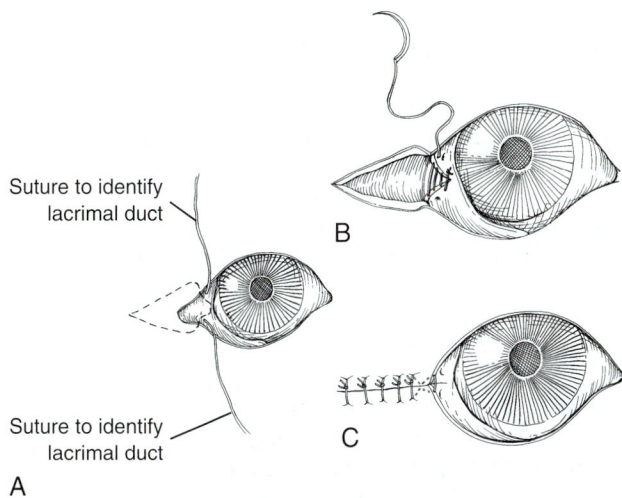

Figure 151–3. Correction of medial entropion by medial canthoplasty. *A,* Mark the lacrimal canaliculus with a suture—then make a V-shaped incision along the eyelid margin, encompassing the caruncle. *B* and *C,* Close the incision in two layers, creating horizontal closure.

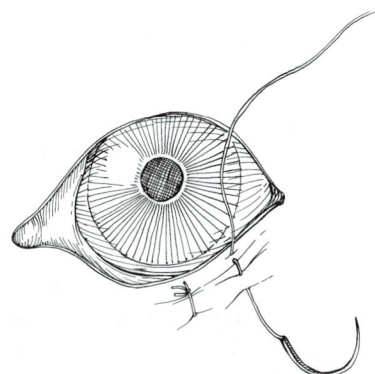

Figure 151–4. Temporary lid-everting sutures.

- Shortening of the palpebral fissure via a permanent lateral tarsorrhaphy is beneficial in many dogs.

DISTICHIASIS

Distichiasis is a condition in which hairs that originate from the meibomian glands and emerge from their ducts contact the cornea and cause irritation. It is common in cocker spaniel, golden retriever, and Shih Tzu breeds and occasionally is seen in Saint Bernards and other breeds.

▼ *Key Point* Reserve surgical removal for animals in which epiphora, blepharospasm, or corneal disease is a significant clinical sign and when other ocular disease has been ruled out.

- The most common complication of distichiasis surgery is recurrence 3–5 months postoperatively.

Surgical Technique

Cryoepilation

1. Evert and stabilize the lid with a chalazion clamp and freeze a 3-mm band along the base of the meibomian glands, on the conjunctival surface of the eyelid, below each abnormal cilium. Freeze time varies, depending on whether nitrous oxide or liquid nitrogen is used. In general, the ice ball should extend to the lid margin, taking care not to freeze the full thickness of the lid.
2. A double freeze-thaw cycle is most effective.

Electroepilation

Reserve this time-consuming technique for cases in which only a few hairs are to be removed.

1. Insert an electrolysis stylet along the hair shaft into the base of the follicle.
2. Apply low amperage (2–4 mA) coagulating current until a small amount of meibomian gland material bubbles out of the duct opening.

ECTOPIC CILIA

- Ectopic cilia are hairs originating from the meibomian gland that emerge through the conjunctival surface of the eyelid.
- The most common clinical signs are blepharospasm and corneal ulceration.
- The most common location is the central upper eyelid, 2–4 mm from the eyelid margin.

Technique for Removal

1. Excise the hair and its root en bloc with a #11 scalpel blade, leaving the eyelid margin intact.
2. Stabilize the eyelid during the procedure with a chalazion clamp.
3. The conjunctival wound may be left open.

LAGOPHTHALMOS

- Lagophthalmos is a condition in which the eyelids cannot completely close. The most common cause is anatomic exophthalmos, seen in brachycephalic breeds. In these breeds, blink frequency often is decreased, exacerbating the problem.
- It also is associated with buphthalmos (progressive enlargement of the eye), palpebral nerve palsy, and ectropion.
- Corneal disease, including ulceration, pigmentation, neovascularization, and keratinization, may result.
- Treat surgically by permanent closure of a portion of the palpebral fissure.

Technique

1. Excise the eyelid margin of the ventral and dorsal lids at the lateral or medial canthus.
2. Close the eyelids in two layers, as described for wedge resection under Neoplasia.

NEOPLASIA

Diagnosis

- The most common eyelid tumor in the dog is meibomian gland adenoma. Other tumors seen in the eyelids include papilloma, meibomian gland adenocarcinoma, melanoma, histiocytoma, squamous cell carcinoma, and basal cell tumors.
  - Meibomian gland tumors originate in the base of the gland but often emerge from the meibomian gland duct on the eyelid margin.
- Tumors occurring in the eyelids of cats include melanoma, fibrosarcoma, neurofibroma, and squamous and basal cell carcinoma.
  - Squamous cell carcinomas usually are seen in white cats and appear as nonhealing ulcerative lesions. They are locally aggressive and have a high recurrence rate.
  - Melanomas of the eyelids have been known to metastasize in cats.
- In dogs, most eyelid tumors are benign and are removed to prevent irritation or injury to the cornea or conjunctiva.
- In cats, most eyelid tumors are malignant and carry a guarded prognosis.
- For additional information on skin tumors in dogs and cats, see Chapter 28.

Preoperative Considerations

▼ *Key Point* One-fourth of the upper eyelid and one-third of the lower lid can be removed without severe distortion of the palpebral fissure.

- The most common cause of recurrence of meibomian gland adenoma is incomplete removal of the tumor. Keep in mind that even though the bulk of the tumor is at the eyelid margin, the tumor originates from the base of the meibomian gland.

Surgical Techniques

- A full-thickness wedge resection of the eyelid is sufficient to remove most tumors.
- Cryosurgery also can be used to treat many eyelid tumors.
  - Although there is a higher recurrence rate with this technique than with excision, it is a relatively safe, simple procedure that may be performed with local anesthesia combined with tranquilization.
- Submit all excised tissues for histopathology.

Wedge Resection

1. Using a scalpel blade, incise the skin in a pie-shaped wedge with the base at the eyelid margin. Alternatively, crush along the incision line with hemostats and cut along the crimped line with scissors. Use a tenotomy or Metzenbaum scissors to complete the incision.
2. Close the incision in two layers:
   a. Close the subconjunctival tissue with 6-0 or 7-0 absorbable sutures, with the knots buried within the eyelid.
   b. Close the skin with 4-0 to 6-0 sutures beginning at the lid margin (Fig. 151–5).
3. Close the eyelid margin with a figure-of-eight 4-0 to 6-0 suture, and the remainder of the skin with sutures in a simple interrupted pattern. Alternatively, a horizontal mattress or simple continuous pattern can be used to close eyelid margins.

Cryosurgery

1. Perform a double freeze-thaw cycle. Treat an area extending 3–5 mm beyond the tumor.
2. For meibomian gland tumors, place the probe on the conjunctival surface of the eyelid.

INFLAMMATORY EYELID DISEASES

Bacterial Blepharitis

- In blepharitis, the eyelids and lashes are crusted with mucopurulent discharge and are erythematous and swollen. The conjunctiva usually is inflamed, and there may be an associated nonulcerative keratitis.
- Blepharitis can also be a manifestation of various generalized inflammatory skin diseases (see the section on Skin and Ear Diseases), including pyoderma, atopy, dermatomycosis, demodicosis, and autoimmune diseases.

Treatment

- Apply a topical bactericidal ophthalmic solution or ointment (e.g., neomycin, bacitracin, polymyxin B) three to four times daily.
- Instruct the owner to give eyelid scrubs, using dilute baby shampoo once a day.

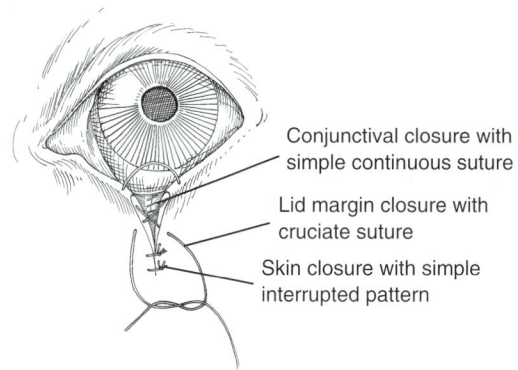

Figure 151–5. Closure for wedge resection of the eyelid. Close the subconjunctiva with 6-0 or 7-0 absorbable suture in a simple continuous pattern; the lid margin with a cruciate suture; and the remainder of the skin with 6-0 suture, in a simple interrupted pattern.

- In severe or chronic cases, give systemic antibiotics as described for pyoderma (see Chap. 35).
- If there is associated nonulcerative keratitis, consider giving topical corticosteroids or cyclosporine ointment once or twice a day.
- If associated with pruritus or other signs of atopy, give systemic antihistamines twice a day.
- If a good response is not seen within 2 weeks, swab the meibomian gland secretions or upper conjunctival cul-de-sac for culture and sensitivity testing, and perform thyroid function testing.

▼ **Key Point** Bacterial blepharitis can be difficult to cure. Inform the owner that some dogs require periodic eyelid scrubs and antibiotic therapy on a long-term basis.

Chalazion and Hordeolum

- *Chalazion* is a granuloma of the meibomian gland.
  - Treat with surgical curettage of the granuloma via the conjunctival surface of the eyelid.
- *Hordeolum* is an infection or abscess of a meibomium gland or of an eyelash that results in a focal swelling of the lid.
  - Treat with hot packs and systemic antibiotics.
  - To hasten resolution, apply a topical antibiotic/corticosteroid solution or ointment, such as dexamethasone 0.1%, neomycin, or polymyxin B, q6–8h.

Allergic Blepharitis

- The animal usually presents with swelling of the eyelids that may be pruritic but is rarely painful. There may be a serous to mucopurulent discharge.
- Chronic or recurrent allergic blepharitis may be a manifestation of atopy.
- Treat with systemic antihistamines such as diphenhydramine (Benadryl, 2–4 mg/kg q6–12h PO) or corticosteroids (Prednisone, 0.5–1.0 mg/kg q12–24h PO) and with topical corticosteroids.
  - Cold compresses help to decrease pruritus.
- For further information on allergy testing and treatment for atopy, see Chapter 41.

Parasitic or Fungal Blepharitis

- The eyelids may be infected by cutaneous parasites such as *Demodex* and *Sarcoptes* or by dermatophytes (ringworm).
- In dogs in which periocular alopecia and skin lesions are present but in which the conjunctiva is relatively spared, perform skin scrapings, dermatophyte cultures, and skin biopsies (see Chaps. 37, 38, and 39).

Granulomatous Blepharitis

- Dogs with this condition present with prominent multifocal firm swellings of the lid margins of both eyes, often associated with the meibomium glands. It is not usually painful. The skin in advanced cases may be ulcerated. Etiology is unknown.
- Mild cases may be treated with topical antibiotic-dexamethasone solution 4–8 times a day and oral corticosteroids (e.g., prednisone 0.5–1.0 mg/kg q12–24h). Oral antibiotic therapy is occasionally helpful.

- More severe cases may require oral azathioprine (2 mg/kg initially, then 0.5–2.0 mg/kg every 48 hours; CBCs should be run 2 to 4 times per month).
- Some cases are recurrent and require ongoing topical corticosteroids for control.

SUPPLEMENTAL READINGS

Bistner S, Aguirre G, Batik G: Atlas of Veterinary Ophthalmic Surgery. Philadelphia: WB Saunders, 1977, chs. 3–5.

Lavach JD, Gelatt KN: Diseases of the eyelids. Part II. Compend Contin Educ Pract Vet 1:485, 1979.

Roberts SM, Severin GA, Lavach JD: Prevalence and treatment of palpebral neoplasms in the dog: 200 cases (1975–1983). J Am Vet Med Assoc 189:1355, 1986.

Wheeler CA, Severin GA: Cryosurgical epilation for the treatment of distichiasis in the dog and cat. J Am Anim Hosp Assoc 20:877, 1984.

152 Diseases of the Conjunctiva

Cecil P. Moore

ANATOMY AND PHYSIOLOGY

- Conjunctival mucosa covers the inner aspect of the eyelids, the third eyelid, and the anterior sclera. Conjunctiva extends from the lacrimal caruncle medially to the lateral canthus temporally.
- Normal conjunctiva is semitransparent and appears moist and glistening. Numerous small, branching blood vessels are visible within the conjunctiva.
- Sensory innervation to the conjunctiva is via ophthalmic and maxillary branches of the trigeminal nerve.
- The conjunctiva serves as a protective external physical and immunologic barrier for the eye.
- Epithelial goblet cells within the conjunctiva produce mucus, which contributes to the preocular tear film, harbors immunoglobulin, and traps foreign material and debris.

The term *conjunctivitis* describes nonspecific inflammation of the ocular mucous membrane. Conjunctivitis is the most common cause of "red eye" in animals. To accurately assess the small animal patient presented with conjunctivitis, recognize inherent species differences in susceptibility and establish whether the disorder is primary or secondary. For example, feline conjunctivitis is generally caused by a primary ocular infection. Canine conjunctivitis, however, usually is secondary to ocular surface irritants, tear film deficiencies, or foreign bodies.

Additional pertinent information is found in other chapters in this text. Conjunctival disease is often associated with viral infections, diseases of the cornea (see Chap. 153), diseases of the lacrimal apparatus (see Chap. 158), and diseases of the eyelids (see Chap. 151).

ETIOLOGY OF CONJUNCTIVITIS

Causes of conjunctivitis are numerous. Frequently, more than one etiologic factor plays a role in the clinical course of the disease.

▼ *Key Point* Regardless of the primary cause, bacterial infection is a common complicating factor in conjunctivitis.

Infectious Agents

Infectious agents cause severe conjunctivitis in cats by infecting epithelial cells. Feline herpesvirus and *Chlamydia psittaci* cause the most serious and common ocular infections in cats (see Chap. 9). *Mycoplasma felis*, *Staphylococci* spp., *Streptococci* spp., and coliform organisms are bacterial causes of usually less severe forms of feline conjunctivitis.

Gram-positive aerobic bacteria are most commonly isolated from cases of canine conjunctivitis. Opportunistic bacterial infections are common in dogs following conjunctival irritation from other causes. Canine distemper virus (see Chap. 11) causes conjunctivitis and dacryoadenitis.

Tear Film Deficiency

Tear film deficiency results in dehydration with accompanying inflammation of the conjunctiva and cornea. Aqueous tear deficiency, or keratoconjunctivitis sicca, occurs more frequently in dogs than in cats (see Chap. 158). Although less common than aqueous deficiency, inadequacy of the lipid or mucous components may, when present, complicate the surface disease. Poor eyelid conformation, as with exophthalmos and lagophthalmos, potentiates exposure and drying and is a further complicating factor.

Foreign Bodies

Foreign bodies of the conjunctiva can include plant material, synthetic material, and metallic substances. Plant awns and weed seeds may become embedded in the fornices of the conjunctiva or migrate behind the third eyelid. Embedded plant material is quite reactive and stimulates an intense pyogranulomatous inflammation. By contrast, synthetic material, such as glass and plastic, or certain metals, such as lead and stainless steel, are minimally reactive. Depending upon the location and rigidity of the material, conjunctival foreign bodies may cause direct frictional irritation and result in surface ulceration.

Trauma

Trauma to the conjunctiva may be blunt, resulting in bruising of an intact membrane, or penetrating with puncture or laceration. In cases of conjunctival trauma, examine the eye thoroughly for the presence of foreign bodies and intraocular lesions.

Chemical Irritants

Chemical irritants that damage the conjunctiva include noxious gases, alkalis, and acids. Alkaline substances, e.g., lye, fresh lime, or ammonia, cause the most serious injuries. When chemical injury has occurred, flush the eye copiously and evaluate for associated corneal and/or anterior uveal involvement.

Environmental Irritants

Environmental irritants, such as dust, particles of sand or plant material, wind, and solar irradiation, are additional causes of conjunctivitis in small animals. These are particularly common causes in hunting dogs and outdoor working dogs.

Immune-mediated Conjunctivitis

Immune-mediated conjunctivitis results from acute allergic chemosis, atopy (see Chap. 41), follicular conjunctivitis, and conjunctivitis resulting from eosinophilic or plasmacytic infiltrates. An immune-mediated ulcerative conjunctivitis occurs in Doberman pinscher dogs.

Proliferative Diseases

Proliferative diseases are categorized as non-neoplastic or neoplastic.

Non-Neoplastic Disease

Episcleritis and idiopathic granulomatous disease are the main non-neoplastic proliferative disorders (see Chap. 153). Conjunctival epithelial hyperplasia, granulation tissue, and pigmentary infiltrates are additional examples of non-neoplastic proliferative conditions.

Neoplasia

Conjunctival neoplasms may be primary or secondary. Papillomas, squamous cell carcinomas, and hemangiomas are the most common primary tumors. Less common primary neoplasms are hemangiosarcomas, mastocytomas, and melanomas. Adenomas, adenocarcinomas, fibromas, fibrosarcomas, lymphosarcomas, and melanomas are tumors that may secondarily involve the conjunctiva.

Other Eye Diseases

Other eye diseases, either ocular surface disorders or intraocular diseases, are frequently associated with conjunctival inflammation. Surface diseases where conjunctivitis is prominent include episcleritis, keratitis, and eyelid disease (e.g., chalazia, entropion, ectropion, cilia disorders). Conjunctival inflammation occurs with uveitis and glaucoma, although deeper episcleral injection is a hallmark of these intraocular diseases.

Iatrogenically Induced Conjunctivitis

Iatrogenically induced conjunctivitis is caused when topically administered therapeutic agents or surgical manipulations cause conjunctival inflammation. A number of drugs may cause conjunctivitis because of irritation from their active ingredients, vehicles, or preservatives. Surgical procedures result in conjunctivitis from direct insult (e.g., manipulation, dissection, thermal injury, exposure during or following surgery).

CLINICAL SIGNS OF CONJUNCTIVITIS

- *Hyperemia* resulting from vasodilation of conjunctival vessels causes the appearance of a red eye. The redness is intensified when conjunctival hemorrhage or episcleral vascular injection is also present.
- *Ocular discharge* is characteristic of conjunctivitis and is serous, mucoid (catarrhal), or mucopurulent. The type of discharge may change as conjunctivitis progresses—from serous (mild) to mucopurulent (severe).
- *Chemosis* is swelling or "puffiness" of the conjunctiva caused by edema of the mucous membrane.
- *Pain* with conjunctivitis varies with the severity of the ocular disease. Squinting and tearing are characteristic of most cases of conjunctivitis. Photophobia and blepharospasm generally occur only when other eye disease is present, such as ulcerative keratitis or uveitis.
- *Tissue proliferation* is a variable finding of subacute or chronic conjunctival disease. Conjunctival lymphoid follicular hyperplasia may develop in dogs as a nonspecific immune response to persistent antigenic stimulation. In cats, conjunctival follicles are associated with chlamydial conjunctivitis (see Chap. 9). Diffuse thickening of the conjunctiva may occur from epithelial hyperplasia or from chronic inflammatory cell infiltrates. Focal, acquired, proliferative lesions may be either granulomas or neoplastic.

DIAGNOSIS OF CONJUNCTIVITIS

History

History pertinent to cases of conjunctivitis includes possible systemic illnesses; environment and habits; possible exposure to infectious or chemical agents; possible trauma; and previous ocular diseases, including the medications administered.

Physical Examination

Perform *physical examination* to rule out multisystemic diseases (see Chap. 150).

Cultures

Cultures are indicated for the definitive diagnosis of ocular infection. Subsequent susceptibility testing of aerobic bacterial isolates is important in selecting the optimal antimicrobial agent. When culturing for fungi, *Mycoplasma, Chlamydia,* or viral agents, consult with the laboratory in advance regarding any special requirements for submitting culture samples.

▼ *Key Point* When the need for cultures is anticipated, collect samples prior to applying topical agents or manipulating ocular surface tissues.

Ophthalmic Examination

Ophthalmic examination should be thorough and, in addition to confirming conjunctivitis, is aimed at identifying other forms of eye disease. Components of the complete ophthalmic examination are to:

- Inspect the external ocular surfaces and the anterior portion of the globe directly using a focal light source with magnification. The focused light is also used to check for pupil symmetry and light response.
- Perform the intraocular examination with a focused light and an ophthalmoscope. Opacities of the normally clear ocular media (cornea, intraocular chambers, lens) are noted. Perform funduscopy to determine if abnormalities of the retina, choroid, or optic nerve are present.
- Measure aqueous tear production with Schirmer tear test strips as described in Chaps. 150 and 158. Aqueous tear deficiency must be ruled out because this is a common occurrence in small animals, particularly in dogs, and results in chronic conjunctivitis with a tenacious mucopurulent ocular discharge.

▼ *Key Point* The Schirmer tear test strips measure reflex tear production. Evaluate prior to application of any local solutions including topical anesthetic agents.

- Apply fluorescein stain to determine if surface ulceration is present. Establish nasolacrimal duct patency by allowing fluorescein stain to gravitate into the external nares.
- Following application of a topical anesthetic, examine for foreign bodies. Use blunt-tipped forceps to probe the conjunctiva fornices and to lift the third eyelid allowing inspection of the posterior surface.
- Use tonometry to rule out other intraocular causes of red eye, e.g., glaucoma (elevated pressure) and uveitis (low pressure). Indentation (Schiøtz) or applanation tonometry produces accurate intraocular pressure readings in small animal patients (see Chaps. 150 and 156).

Cytology

Cytology of conjunctival scrapings may provide a definitive diagnosis of inflammatory or neoplastic disease. Immunofluorescence testing of cytologic specimens can confirm viral or chlamydial infection. Fine-needle aspirates of masses can also provide the cytologic material for a definitive diagnosis.

Polymerase Chain Reaction

Polymerase chain reaction (PCR) utilizes technology that allows detection of the DNA of ocular pathogens when present in very small amounts. In cases of feline conjunctivitis, the PCR procedure has been used successfully to diagnose feline herpesvirus-1 (FHV-1) infections. The sensitivity of PCR for FHV-1 diagnosis appears to be superior to other available methods. For the PCR test, place conjunctival swabs or scrapings in 1 ml phosphate buffered saline (PBS), frozen at −20°C, and submit for analysis.

Biopsy

Biopsy the conjunctiva when cytology has not allowed the differentiation of inflammatory from neoplastic processes. Conjunctival biopsy is also needed to determine goblet cell density in suspected cases of preocular mucin deficiency.

TREATMENT

The goals for therapy of conjunctival disease are as follows:

- Correct or remove the underlying cause
- Control secondary infection
- Remove exudates and clean the eye and periocular area
- Ensure a moist and well-hydrated ocular surface
- Reduce inflammation and discomfort

Treat Primary Cause

Because the primary causes of conjunctivitis in small animals are numerous, specific treatments vary considerably. Depending upon the circumstances, the following treatments may apply:

- Treat infection with a specific antimicrobial agent
- Remove foreign materials
- Surgically remove or correct for irritants (hairs or masses) that rub the eye
- Remove offending allergens when possible
- Treat for allergies (see Chap. 41)
- Treat tear deficiencies medically (see Chap. 158).

See Table 152–1 for more specific treatment recommendations.

▼ *Key Point* The following procedures are beneficial as symptomatic treatment and may be used as adjuncts when treating the primary disease, when awaiting results of diagnostic tests, or when treating empirically in nonspecific or undiagnosed cases of conjunctivitis.

Antimicrobial Therapy

To control or prevent secondary pathogenic or opportunistic bacterial infections, broad-spectrum antibiotic ophthalmic drops or ointments are applied topically. Avoid prolonged, indiscriminate application of topical antibacterial agents because this may encourage development of antibiotic-resistant bacterial strains or secondary fungal infections. This practice can predispose the animal to medication hypersensitivity.

Cleanse Discharges

Use an eyewash solution (e.g., Dacriose, Cooper-Vision) to irrigate the ocular surface, remove exudates, and

Table 152–1. TREATMENT OF SPECIFIC CAUSES OF CONJUNCTIVITIS

Causes	Treatments
Infectious Agents	
Bacterial	
Chlamydia felis	Tetracycline ointment (q6–8h × 14–28 d) (Terramycin, Pfizer; Achromycin, Lederle; Aureomycin, Lederle)
Mycoplasma felis	Tetracycline ointment (q6–8h × 10–14 d)
	or
	Erythromycin ointment (q6–8h × 10–14 d) (Erythromycin, Pharmafair)
	or
	Chloramphenicol ointment (q6–8h × 7 d) (Chlorbiotic, Schering-Plough)
Streptococcus spp.	Triple antibiotic (TA) ointment (q6–8h × 10–14 d) (Neobacimyx, Schering-Plough; TriOptic-P, SmithKline; or equivalent)
Staphylococcus spp.	TA or gentamicin (Gentocin, Schering-Plough) (as per TA above)
Gram-negative aerobes	TA, gentamicin, or ciprofloxacin (Ciloxan, Alcon) (as per TA above)
Viral	
Feline herpesvirus	Trifluridine (see Chap. 9 and Chap. 153)
	Symptomatic therapy (see text)
Canine distemper virus	Symptomatic therapy (see text)
Keratoconjunctivitis Sicca	Treat cause if determined (see Chap. 158)
Many causes	Topical cyclosporine (see Chap. 158)
	Topical antibiotics as needed
	Artificial tears (see Chap. 158)
	Lubricant ointments (see Chap. 158)
Foreign Bodies	Remove using magnification
	Irrigate eye
	Symptomatic therapy (see text)
	Complete eye examination
Trauma	
Bruise/focal puncture	Symptomatic therapy (see text)
Laceration	Symptomatic therapy (see text)
	±Surgical repair
Chemical Irritants	Copious irrigation
	Symptomatic therapy (see text)
Environmental Irritants	Flush eyes
	Topical corticosteroid (CS) (q6–8h reduced to q12h as response noted, then discontinue) only if fluorescein stain results are negative
	Lubricant ointment (q8h reduced to q24h as response noted, then discontinue)
	± Topical antibiotics
	Avoid reexposure
Immune-Mediated Disorders	
Acute chemosis	Topical and systemic CS
Atopy	Topical ± systemic CS, antihistamines, desensitization (see Chap. 41)
Follicular conjunctivitis	Topical ± intralesional CS, ± abrade follicles
Eosinophilic infiltrate	Topical ± intralesional CS (see Chap. 153)
Plasmacytic infiltrate	Topical ± intralesional CS (see Chap. 153)
Ulcerative conjunctivitis	Topical ± systemic CS, topical cyclosporine A (Optimmune, Schering-Plough)
Proliferative Diseases	
Inflammatory	Topical ± intralesional or systemic CS
Neoplastic	Surgery ± radiation or cryosurgery
Other Ocular Diseases	
Surface diseases	
Eyelid disorders	Medical ± corrective surgery (see Chap. 151)
Keratitis	Medical ± surgery (see Chap. 153)
Episcleritis	Topical ± intralesional or systemic CS (see Chap. 153)
Intraocular diseases	
Uveitis	Treat cause if determined (see Chap. 155)
	Topical CS and atropine
	Systemic anti-inflammatory agents
Glaucoma	Determine if primary or secondary (see Chap. 156)
	Topical hypotensive agents (see Chap. 156)
	Systemic hypotensive agents (see Chap. 156)
	Cycloablative or filtration surgery
Iatrogenic	
Topical agents	Discontinue use of irritating medications
Surgical procedures	Symptomatic treatment until surgical site heals

clean the eye and periocular area. Clip the periocular hairs. Use cotton swabs moistened with saline to soak and remove exudates.

Moisten/Hydrate Eye

Ensure that the conjunctival and corneal surfaces are kept moist. If applied three to four times daily, antibacterial ointments have sufficient lubricating property to ensure continuous moistening of swollen or injured conjunctival tissues. When severe chemosis results in exposure of swollen conjunctiva, temporary tarsorrhaphy sutures are placed until the acute swelling subsides (see Chap. 151). In cases in which the Schirmer tear test values are subnormal, apply artificial tear solutions topically four to six times daily. Lacrimostimulants may be indicated (see Chap. 158).

Anti-Inflammatory Therapy

Systemic anti-inflammatory drugs may be used in selected cases to minimize acute swelling, discomfort, and self-trauma. In cases of ocular trauma in dogs, systemic nonsteroidal anti-inflammatory drugs may be beneficial to reduce chemosis, hyperemia, and associated ocular pain. In dogs with normal renal function, flunixin meglumine (Banamine, Schering) may be given as a single dose IV of 0.5–1.0 mg/kg. This may be followed by oral aspirin at a dosage of 10 mg/kg q12h until signs of inflammation subside. Oral carprofen (2.2 mg/kg q12h) is also effective for controlling ocular inflammation. Monitor the animal closely for the side effects of gastritis and protect the stomach with an H_2-blocker, such as cimetidine (see Chap. 87). Flunixin and aspirin are not given to cases in which hemorrhage is the primary manifestation of the conjunctival disease.

Topical corticosteroids may reduce the swelling and hyperemia of an inflamed conjunctiva.

▼ *Key Point* Topical corticosteroids are contraindicated in cases of primary infectious conjunctivitis or corneal ulceration.

Topical 5% sodium chloride may be applied to reduce chemosis; however, it is not applied in eyes producing marginal amounts of aqueous tears because it will further dehydrate the ocular surface.

CONJUNCTIVAL SURGERY

Surgery of the conjunctiva may be performed for one of the following reasons:

- Trauma repair
- Diagnostic procedure
- Focal lesion resection
- Repair of fibrosis/adhesions
- Grafting procedure.

Because the last category applies primarily to the treatment of ulcerative keratitis, refer to Chapter 153 for a discussion of conjunctival flaps and grafts.

Laceration Repair

Preoperative Considerations

- Examine the eye carefully for other damage (e.g., corneal, scleral, intraocular lesions) and evaluate for retained ocular foreign bodies. Radiograph the head and orbit to check for radiopaque foreign bodies and to assess the extent of the trauma.

▼ *Key Point* If the traumatized eye is opaque, consider ultrasound imaging to determine the integrity of the globe and the extent of any intraocular damage.

- Because of the conjunctiva's rapid reparative characteristic, many punctures and small lacerations heal spontaneously without the need for suturing. Suture conjunctival lacerations 7–8 mm or greater or those associated with eyelid lacerations.

Surgical Procedure

Objectives

- Cleanse and disinfect the wound.
- Remove surface foreign material and tissue debris.
- Explore the wound to determine if a foreign body was retained and to determine if deeper structures were damaged.
- Suture the conjunctival wound, if necessary, to restore mucous membrane integrity and function.
- Prevent secondary infection.

Equipment

- Eyelid retractors (e.g., Barraquer wire speculum)
- Small rat-tooth forceps (e.g., Bishop-Harmon forceps)
- Ophthalmic needle holders (Castroviejo)
- Conjunctival or Stevens tenotomy scissors
- Braided 6-0 or 7-0 absorbable suture material (e.g., Dexon, Vicryl) with microcutting needle

Technique

1. Following general anesthesia, insert eyelid retractors and flush the conjunctiva with 1:50 betadine:saline solution; explore the wound for foreign bodies and for damage to deeper structures.
2. After assessing the extent of the conjunctival defect and confirming that surgical repair is needed, minimally debride the margins of the wound and gently undermine adjacent conjunctiva.
3. Close the conjunctival wound in a continuous pattern; space suture bites 2 mm apart.

Postoperative Care and Complications

- Apply topical antibiotics (e.g., neomycin, bacitracin, polymyxin B) three to four times daily for 10 days.
- Administer systemic antibiotics for 1 week.
- If the eye is painful, apply fluorescein stain to identify corneal erosion or ulceration.

Biopsy

Preoperative Considerations

- Conjunctival biopsy and histopathology results should distinguish inflammatory from neoplastic diseases and determine goblet cell densities in suspected cases of preocular mucin deficiency.
- In tractable animals, conjunctival biopsy procedures can usually be performed following serial applications of topical anesthetic (e.g., 0.5% proparacaine).
- Subconjunctival or intralesional local anesthetic may be injected for deeper biopsies or for lesions of the palpebral, perilimbal, or third eyelid conjunctiva. Sedation and systemic analgesia may be needed in some cases.

Surgical Procedure

Objectives

- Remove a representative sample of conjunctiva for histopathology.
- Minimize the resulting defect and avoid distorting the conjunctiva.

Equipment

- Small rat-tooth forceps
- Curved conjunctival or tenotomy scissors (e.g., Stevens, Westcott)
- Vial of 10% buffered formalin

Technique

1. Following local anesthesia, grasp the desired area of conjunctiva with a rat-tooth forceps and tent slightly.
2. Using small curved scissors excise a 3 mm × 4 mm specimen.
3. Gently spread the specimen onto a flat surface, such as a small Styrofoam pad or a section of wooden tongue depressor.
4. Immediately fix the specimen in 10% buffered formalin.

Postoperative Care and Complications

- A small amount of hemorrhage is anticipated but is usually minimal, as fibrin quickly seals the wound.
- Defects resulting from biopsy that are less than 4 mm × 4 mm usually heal uneventfully with topical antibiotic treatment. Larger defects should be sutured as described in the Laceration Repair section.
- Remove discharges and cleanse the eye as needed. This may be necessary three to four times the first day but is reduced over the following 5 days to once daily.
- Apply topical antibiotic ointment (e.g., neomycin, bacitracin, polymyxin B) to the affected eye three times daily for 7 days.

Mass Removal

Preoperative Considerations

- Surgical excision alone may be curative for cysts, dermoids, ectopic hairs, focal granulomas, and certain neoplasms of the conjunctiva (e.g., papillomas and adenomas).
- Surgical excision is an important adjunct in the treatment of inflammatory pseudotumors and more aggressive neoplasms, such as squamous cell carcinomas or adenocarcinomas.
  - Chemotherapy, immunotherapy, cryosurgery, hyperthermia, or beta-irradiation may be needed in addition to local excision.
  - Definitive therapy depends upon the specific diagnosis.
- General anesthesia is usually required for effective removal of conjunctival masses.

Surgical Procedure

Objectives

- Surgically remove conjunctival masses that interfere with ocular function, threaten preservation of the globe, or pose a threat to survival of the animal.
- Debulk a mass to increase efficacy of adjunctive treatments (e.g., cryosurgery, radiation, immunotherapy, hyperthermia, chemotherapy).

Equipment

- Same as that listed for Laceration Repair
- Vial of 10% buffered formalin

Technique

1. Grasp the mass with forceps and elevate; undermine and excise with small curved tissue scissors.
2. Small conjunctival wounds, i.e., less than 5 mm in diameter, generally do not require suturing and heal in 2–4 days.
3. Suture conjunctival wounds 5 mm in diameter or larger with 7-0 braided absorbable material (Vicryl) in a continuous pattern.
4. To allow primary closure for wounds greater than 5 mm in diameter, it may be necessary to undermine and slide adjacent conjunctiva.
5. Repair large defects by a pedicle graft of adjacent healthy conjunctiva similar to that of a swinging cutaneous pedicle graft.
6. For conjunctival mass lesions involving the cornea, see Figure 153–1, in Chapter 153.

Postoperative Care and Complications

- Remove discharges and cleanse the eye as needed.
- Apply topical antibiotic ointment (e.g., neomycin, bacitracin, polymyxin B) to the affected eye three times daily for 7 days.
- Prevent self-trauma with a restraint collar.
- Large defects of the conjunctiva that heal by second intention may result in extensive granulation and scarring, with possible symblepharon formation.

Symblepharon Repair

Preoperative Considerations

- Symblepharon results from the fibrosis of two apposing ulcerated epithelial surfaces.

- Neonatal conjunctivitis of kittens, caused by feline herpesvirus, is a common cause in cats (see Chap. 9).
- Postinflammatory adhesions may reduce or obliterate the conjunctival fornices resulting in immobility of the globe.
- Abnormal tear dynamics account for chronic epiphora.
- Corneal involvement results in scarring and opacification, which reduces vision.

Surgical Procedure

Objectives

- Remove scar tissue and free adhesions, thereby restoring normal anatomic relationships and functions of the ocular surface structures.
- Prevent readhesion and minimize postoperative scarring.

Equipment

- Colibri forceps
- Beaver blade (#64) with handle
- Instruments as listed for Laceration Repair

Technique

1. When extensive corneal opacification is present, perform a lamellar keratectomy (see Fig. 153–1, Chap. 153).
2. Incise the perilimbal bulbar conjunctiva with a #64 Beaver blade, undermine and free adhesions with small curved scissors, and elevate the conjunctiva as a mobile circumlimbal flap.
3. Perform sufficient dissection and removal of subconjunctival scar tissue to reestablish the conjunctival fornices.
4. Free the third eyelid by dissecting between the third eyelid, the globe, and the eyelids, if necessary.
5. Place a bandage soft contact lens over the corneal surface behind the third eyelid.
6. Apply a broad-spectrum antibiotic ophthalmic ointment into the conjunctival cul de sac.
7. Place a corneal-scleral conformer over the globe and the front side of the third eyelid.
   a. A conformer may be constructed using a commercially available corneal-scleral protector (Crouch corneal protector, Storz Instrument, St. Louis).
   b. The corneal protector may be reduced to an appropriate size by trimming the perimeter with utility scissors, smoothing the cut margins with a file or fine sandpaper, rinsing the plastic of sanded particles, and sterilizing with gas.
8. Secure the corneal protector with three temporary tarsorrhaphy mattress sutures.

Postoperative Care and Complications

- Place a restraint collar on the animal to prevent self-trauma.
- Immediately postoperatively, administer a mild sedative/analgesic.
- Remove discharges and cleanse the eye as needed.
- Tarsorrhaphy sutures prevent topical treatment of the eye; therefore, administer broad-spectrum systemic antibiotics (e.g., oral amoxicillin).
- Remove tarsorrhaphy sutures, conformer, and contact lens in 14 days.
- Following removal, irrigate the eye and initiate topical treatment with an antibiotic ointment three times daily for 1 week or until the ocular surface has a negative reaction to fluorescein stain.
- Initiate topical antibiotic/corticosteroid (e.g., neomycin, bacitracin, dexamethasone) treatment three times daily *after* the surface has completely healed (i.e., negative results with fluorescein stain).
- Gradually reduce the frequency of topical treatments, and discontinue after 3 weeks.
- Additional corneal scarring and readhesion of conjunctival surfaces are the main complications with symblepharon surgery; however, the contact lens and corneal conformer minimize these problems and result in marked improvement in ocular function.

Conjunctival Grafts

See Chapter 153.

SUPPLEMENTAL READINGS

Brooks DE: Veterinary Ophthalmology. Philadelphia: Lea & Febiger, 1991, p 290.

Gerding PA, McLaughlin SA, Troop M: Pathogenic bacteria and fungi associated with external ocular diseases in dogs: 131 cases (1981–1986). J Am Vet Med Assoc 193:242, 1988.

Hendrix DVH: Diseases of the canine conjunctiva. *In* Gelatt KN, ed.: Veterinary Ophthalmology, 3rd Ed. Hagerstown, MD: Lippincott Williams & Wilkins, 1999, p 619.

Nasisse MP: Veterinary Ophthalmology. Philadelphia: Lea & Febiger, 1991, p 529.

Nasisse MP, Weigler BJ: The diagnosis of ocular feline herpesvirus infection. Vet Compar Ophthalmol 7:44, 1997.

Ramsey DT, Ketring KL, Glaze MB, et al.: Ligneous conjunctivitis in four Doberman pinschers. J Am Anim Hosp Assoc 32:439, 1996.

153 Diseases of the Cornea and Sclera

Thomas J. Kern

Disorders of the cornea are common in veterinary practice. Acquired corneal disorders such as ulcerative keratitis, melanosis, and pannus are leading causes of preventable blindness in dogs and cats. The high frequency of corneal disorders should not lull practitioners into forgetting the importance of rigorous diagnosis and attentive management.

Disorders of the sclera are less common. Their diagnosis may be more difficult than corneal disorders and they may be presented at a more advanced stage.

CONGENITAL DISORDERS

Dermoids

Dermoids are islands of skin embryologically misplaced on the cornea (especially the temporal cornea) and conjunctiva and occasionally malpositioned on the eyelids. They contain epidermis, dermis, fat, sebaceous glands, and hair follicles.

Etiology

- In Burmese cats, dermoids are an inherited condition that frequently involves the eyelids.
- Dermoids are considered a spontaneous nonheritable condition in dogs, although some breeds (e.g., German shepherd) appear to be afflicted at a higher frequency than others; thus a genetic basis cannot be completely ruled out.

Clinical Signs

- Dermoids' surface irregularity promotes chronic blepharospasm and epiphora; the hairs cause corneal and conjunctival irritation.

Diagnosis

- On ocular examination, the typical appearance of skin on the cornea or conjunctiva is diagnostic.

Treatment

- Remove by keratectomy. If removal is complete, corneal scarring is present but minimal.
- If the conjunctiva also must be resected, suture the edges of the conjunctiva to the limbus, using 7-0 Vicryl, to discourage postoperative adhesion of the conjunctiva to the cornea.

Microcornea

Etiology

Microcornea usually is associated with complicated *microphthalmos,* a condition with both genetic and environmental causes.

- Inherited microphthalmos syndromes have been characterized in the Australian shepherd, collie, Shetland sheepdog, Old English sheepdog, Akita, American cocker spaniel, miniature schnauzer, Doberman pinscher, Samoyed, Cavalier King Charles spaniel, and Lancashire heeler.
- Multiple heritable ocular defects associated with partial albinism and deafness occur in the Great Dane and collie. Teratogenic influences on the dam during early pregnancy (e.g., viral or other illnesses, live virus vaccines, drugs) may be responsible.
- Microphthalmos occurs less frequently in cats than in dogs; its causes are poorly characterized.

Clinical Signs

- The cornea appears abnormally small and often is misshapen.

Diagnosis

- Measure the horizontal and vertical diameters of the cornea and compare with those of the normal contralateral eye, if present, or with the eye of a normal animal of similar breed.

Treatment

- Treatment is neither available nor warranted. If the condition is associated with microphthalmos, vision may be impaired.

Corneal Opacities

Persistent Pupillary Membrane-Associated Opacities
Etiology

- An embryologic cleavage defect results in strands of iris attached to the endothelial surface of the cornea. Where attachment occurs, endothelium is absent and Descemet membrane is abnormal, resulting in permanent nonprogressive opacity.
- The condition is inherited in basenjis and probably in other breeds; the mode of inheritance is uncertain (see Chap. 155).

Axial Geographic Subepithelial Opacities in Puppies

Etiology

- The cause(s) of these variably prominent, well-circumscribed corneal opacities is unknown.
- They are commonly noted during examination of certain breeds (collie, Shetland sheepdog, English springer spaniel) for inherited ocular disorders and thus have an uncertain genetic basis.

Clinical Signs

- Most obvious in the "exposure strip" of axial cornea, these superficial opacities are usually bilateral, relatively symmetric, painless, and irregular.
- Typical appearance is that of a nonulcerated geographic axial corneal opacity of variable density.

Diagnosis

- A typical corneal opacity in a dog less than 1 year of age suggests the diagnosis.
- The absence of fluorescein dye retention rules out ulcerative keratitis and lack of corneal vascularization rules out an old corneal scar.

Treatment

- Do not treat. Most opacities substantially disappear by maturity.
- A residual faint opacity may remain near the nasal and temporal limbus.

Colobomatous Defects of the Sclera

Etiology

- Scleral defects occur as part of the spectrum of inherited ocular anomalies in collies, Shetland sheepdogs, and Australian shepherds.
  - The collie/Shetland sheepdog anomaly is said to be due to a simple recessive gene with variable expression; a different mode of inheritance has been postulated for the colobomas.
  - The Australian shepherd defect is inherited as an incompletely penetrant recessive trait.
- Optic disk and peripapillary colobomas occur in basenjis; inheritance may be autosomal dominant.
- Great Danes that are the progeny of two harlequin parents are afflicted with colobomatous microphthalmos similar to that in Australian shepherds.
- Posterior pole colobomas of the optic disk and surrounding sclera of unknown cause are seen occasionally in domestic short- and longhaired cats.

Clinical Signs

- In collies and Shetland sheepdogs, the only commonly visible external sign of the defect is relative or absolute microphthalmos. Choroidal hypoplasia, scleral ectasia, optic nerve coloboma, and retinal detachment may be present in the fundus. Blindness is present with retinal detachment and/or optic nerve coloboma.
- Affected Australian shepherds (and Great Danes) usually have mostly white coat color and unilateral or bilateral microphthalmos. In many microphthalmic eyes there are large equatorial staphylomas (i.e., areas of pitted and thinned sclera posterior to the ciliary body). Iris anomalies (heterochromia, corectopia, persistent pupillary membranes, pseudopolycoria) often are present, as are cataracts, retinal dysplasia, and retinal detachment.
- Basenjis with optic disk colobomas have abnormal vision and may have persistent pupillary membranes, although the two defects may not be related.
- Cats afflicted with posterior segment optic nerve coloboma and scleral ectasia are blind in the affected eye, the external appearance of which is normal except for tonic mydriasis.

Diagnosis

- Indirect ophthalmoscopy provides panoramic views of the ocular fundus and is the most sensitive and practical means of diagnosis.

Treatment

- Therapy for these defects is neither indicated nor available.
- Discourage breeding of affected animals.

CORNEAL DEGENERATIONS AND DYSTROPHIES

▼ *Key Point* Corneal dystrophy is a congenital or acquired, usually bilateral, corneal opacity typically unassociated with neovascularization. Degenerations are often but not invariably unilateral abnormalities, frequently (but not necessarily) associated with neovascularization, which are secondary to other ocular or systemic disorders.

Corneal degenerations and dystrophies may affect epithelium, stroma, or endothelium (epithelial dystrophies are discussed under Corneal Ulceration). In some animals, differentiation between the two disorders is difficult.

Stromal Dystrophy

Etiology

- Stromal corneal dystrophy is a genetic disorder afflicting many breeds of dogs, including the collie, Siberian husky, Cavalier King Charles spaniel, beagle, Airedale terrier, cocker spaniel, Alaskan malamute, bearded collie, bichon frise, German shepherd, Lhasa apso, mastiff, miniature pinscher, Weimaraner, pointer, and Samoyed.
- One line of Manx cats was reported with an inherited bilateral stromal dystrophy.

Clinical Signs

- At least two forms of stromal dystrophy occur in dogs:
  - One form is a bilaterally symmetric oval axial or paraxial subepithelial/anterior stromal crystalline opacity.

- The second form, in which a deeper stromal opacity involves more peripheral portions of the cornea, occurs in Siberian huskies and occasionally in other breeds.
  - Corneal neovascularization is absent in both forms. Age of onset varies according to breed and individual animals, from 6 months to old age.
- Affected Manx cats developed progressive stromal edema leading to bullous keratopathy and recurrent epithelial erosion.

Diagnosis

- *Dogs:* The typical crystalline, usually bilateral, corneal opacity (fluorescein dye–negative) unassociated with corneal neovascularization or other corneal pathologic changes suggests stromal dystrophy.
  - Rule out causes of corneal degeneration, which may appear similar, including keratoconjunctivitis sicca (KCS), lagophthalmos, eyelid defects, and endocrinopathy (e.g., hypothyroidism).
- *Cats:* Progressive corneal edema in Manx cats suggests the diagnosis.

Treatment

- Treatment in dogs is rarely indicated or necessary. Keratectomy may remove superficial opacities, but recurrence is likely.
- Do not breed affected animals.

Stromal Degenerations
Etiology

Ocular causes of stromal degenerations include:

- Ulcerative and nonulcerative keratitis
- Corneal exposure
- Dryness secondary to keratoconjunctivitis sicca or lagophthalmos

▼ *Key Point* Systemic diseases suspected to cause degenerations include primary hyperlipidemia, secondary hyperlipidemia (especially associated with hypothyroidism), and hyperadrenocorticism (implicated in calcific degeneration or "band keratopathy").

Clinical Signs

- The central (axial) to paracentral opacities are often bilaterally symmetric and range from crystalline to dense yellow-white; they may be indistinguishable from primary corneal dystrophy.
- In calcific degeneration, the cornea feels "gritty" when touched with a cotton-tipped applicator.
- Neovascularization is often although not invariably present.

Diagnosis

- A typical lesion (with or without neovascularization) and/or with a history of a previous condition (e.g., ulcer, other keratitis, lagophthalmos) suggest degeneration rather than dystrophy.

▼ *Key Point* Do not assume that concurrent primary or secondary hyperlipidemia or hyperadrenocorticism is the cause unless ocular causes of degeneration have been ruled out. Even then, a causal relationship may be uncertain.

- Clinical differentiation of these two conditions frequently is difficult.

Treatment

- Treatment is rarely indicated or necessary.
- Consider keratectomy for large, dense axial lesions that interfere with vision.
  - Prognosis is guarded, as recurrence is possible; in addition, postoperative corneal opacity may be significant.
- For calcific degeneration, consider keratectomy for superficial lesions. Topical application of 1–4% EDTA q4–6h may be helpful.

Endothelial Dystrophy
Etiology

- Endothelial dystrophy is a breed-related, acquired disease resulting in premature loss of corneal endothelial cells to a level below that required to maintain normal corneal stromal deturgescence.

Clinical Signs

- *Dogs:* Progressive bilateral corneal edema may affect Boston terriers, Chihuahuas, and occasionally other breeds. It can begin focally or in a diffuse pattern and progress from the peripheral to the central cornea or vice versa.
  - Initially painless, the condition frequently results in recurrent corneal erosion when stromal and epithelial edema become extensive. Corneal neovascularization usually is absent.
- *Cats:* Endothelial dystrophy causing progressive bilateral corneal edema has been reported rarely in domestic shorthaired cats.

Diagnosis

- Endothelial dystrophy is presumptively diagnosed when bilateral corneal stromal edema is present unassociated with signs of uveitis or glaucoma.

▼ *Key Point* Determine intraocular pressure (IOP) to rule out uveitis (decreased IOP) or glaucoma (elevated IOP) (see Chaps. 155 and 156).

- Corneal ulceration, if present, usually is superficial and insufficient to cause the degree of stromal edema observed.

Treatment

- For severe stromal and epithelial edema, consider treatment with topical 5% sodium chloride (Muro-128) q4–6h to discourage corneal erosion.

- When erosions occur, debride nonadherent epithelium and administer topical broad-spectrum antibiotics and 1% atropine.

Endothelial Degeneration

Etiology

- Intraocular inflammation or hemorrhage, primary and secondary glaucoma, anterior lens luxation, and corneal injury may cause endothelial degeneration.
- Natural infection with canine adenovirus-1 (infectious canine hepatitis) or vaccination with modified live vaccines containing adenovirus-1 or adenovirus-2 may result in immune-mediated anterior uveitis and endothelial destruction 7–10 days following exposure (see Chap. 14).
  - The proportion of dogs affected can be high (in natural infection, about 20%), low (adenovirus-1 vaccination), or very low (adenovirus-2 vaccination).

Clinical Signs

- Chronic focal or diffuse corneal edema (giving the cornea a ground-glass appearance) with or without superficial or deep corneal neovascularization characterizes endothelial degeneration. If the edema resolves, only transient endothelial dysfunction occurs.

▼ **Key Point** Corneal endothelial cells in many adult domestic animals have little to no regenerative capacity. Repair occurs by hypertrophy and migration of remaining endothelial cells.

- Most dogs with adenovirus-mediated uveitis present with generalized corneal edema after resolution of transient uveitis.
  - A small proportion of affected dogs, especially sight hounds and Arctic breeds, quickly develop intractable secondary glaucoma.

Diagnosis

- Diffuse, moderate to severe generalized corneal edema strongly suggests endothelial dysfunction.
- Perform a careful ocular examination to rule out antecedent causes (e.g., inflammation, glaucoma, hyphema, lens luxation).

Treatment

- Direct treatment toward prevention by effectively controlling the causative or attendant conditions (e.g., glaucoma, uveitis, hyphema) before irreversible endothelial degeneration occurs.

Prognosis

- Most dogs with adenovirus-related endotheliopathy recover endothelial function, and the corneal edema resolves within a few weeks.
- Corneal edema secondary to other causes has a variable prognosis for resolution.

CORNEAL ULCERATION

Loss of one or more corneal epithelial layers commonly is termed *corneal erosion or abrasion*. Full-thickness loss of epithelium with at least some stromal loss is termed *ulceration*.

- *Simple corneal ulceration* is that which heals uneventfully in a normal amount of time (3–5 days).
- *Complicated corneal ulceration* involves delayed healing associated with infection or other pathologic processes.
- *Progressive corneal ulceration* involves a deepening or enlarging area.

Etiology

Traumatic Injury

This is probably the most common cause of ulcerative keratitis in dogs and cats.

- Blunt trauma may cause focal or diffuse damage to any or all corneal layers. Corneal laceration may be partial or full-thickness. Aqueous loss, anterior chamber collapse, and iris prolapse may ensue.
- Most traumatic corneal erosions and ulcers heal rapidly; however, some become persistent if epithelial basement membrane damage is severe or if a foreign body persists in the conjunctival fornix.
- Traumatic injury may begin a cascade of pathologic complications resulting in complicated ulceration.

Bacterial Infection

At least minor epithelial injury is required for colonization to occur; bacteria do not adhere to normal epithelial cell membranes.

- Pathogenic and normally nonpathogenic commensal organisms may infect the cornea. *Staphylococci* and *Streptococci* are the ocular bacterial organisms most frequently isolated from normal eyes of dogs and cats.
- Topical antibiotic or corticosteroid therapy may result in overgrowth of pathogenic fungi, yeasts, and bacteria. However, infection of corneal ulcers by fungi is rare in dogs and cats.

Pseudomonas

- *Pseudomonas* infection commonly results in corneal melting, perforation, and loss of the eye.
- Proteolytic enzymes produced by the bacteria, inflammatory cells, and response to infection by the cornea itself cause stromal proteoglycan and collagen destruction, giving the affected cornea a mucoid appearance as melting occurs.

Feline Herpesvirus (FHV)

- FHV infection is an important cause of corneal ulceration in cats (see Chap. 9). Superficial ulcers may be small, punctate, or linear branching fernlike figures classically described as dendrites. Larger, geographic superficial to deep ulcers form from coalescence of smaller focal ulcers. Stromal ulcers, descemetoceles (i.e., a circular loss of stroma down to Descemet membrane), and perforations may develop.

Epithelial Dystrophy (Erosion, Indolent Ulcer, Boxer Ulcer)

- An apparently inherited corneal epithelial basement membrane dystrophy has been recognized in boxers and probably occurs in other breeds. A different inherited epithelial dystrophy afflicts Shetland sheepdogs. Affected dogs are usually middle-aged or older.
- Trauma and chronic corneal inflammation may result in acquired epithelial basement membrane abnormalities.
- Endocrinopathies such as diabetes mellitus, hyperadrenocorticism, and hypothyroidism may be associated with fragile corneal epithelium that may be susceptible to injury and prone to delayed healing.

Neurotrophic Keratitis

This condition develops following denervation of the cornea's sensory nerve supply from the ophthalmic branch of the trigeminal nerve. Sensory nerves and the neurotransmitters and other substances involved have a beneficial influence on the maintenance of epithelial integrity.

Corneal Dryness

This condition occurs secondary to:

- Aqueous tear deficiency (KCS)
- Qualitative tear film abnormalities (mucin deficiency)
- Exposure from lagophthalmos due to conformational abnormalities of eyelid closure or facial nerve palsy (see Chap. 158)

Endocrinopathies

Endocrinopathies such as diabetes mellitus, hypoadrenocorticism, and hypothyroidism have been associated with corneal ulceration in dogs; a causative role in the development of ulcers has not been established.

Idiopathic Corneal Ulceration

An idiopathic form is unique to the cat and is associated with corneal sequestrum formation ("mummification").

- Following chronic, usually superficial, unilateral or bilateral corneal ulceration a brown or black discoloration of the stroma develops. The discolored plaques of degenerate cornea remain in place or slough away after weeks or months.
- A corneal sequestrum is associated with pain and corneal neovascularization.
- Concurrent herpesvirus infection has been demonstrated in some cats.

Clinical Signs

- *Blepharospasm, photophobia,* and *epiphora* are stimulated by painful sensations from damaged epithelium as well as from secondary ciliary muscle spasm.

- *Corneal opacity* results from stromal and epithelial edema and infiltration by inflammatory cells into the affected area.
- *Corneal surface depression* is present if stromal loss, including descemetoceles, has occurred.
- *Neovascularization* denotes complicated ulceration in which healing has been delayed by ocular (e.g., KCS, eyelid defects, infection) or nonocular factors (e.g., self-trauma, inappropriate medical therapy).
  - Superficial neovascularization usually suggests a corneal or external complicating factor and appears as tree-like individual vessels infiltrating focal sectors of cornea.
  - Deep (ciliary) neovascularization denotes intraocular inflammation and appears as an advancing ring of fine vessels evenly infiltrating the peripheral cornea for its entire circumference.
- In *epithelial dystrophy*, the fluorescein dye–positive stained area is surrounded by a halo of poorly adherent or nonadherent epithelium that stains less brilliantly than the center, where epithelium is absent.
  - Corneal neovascularization is absent unless previous traumatic manipulation (e.g., chemical cauterization) has been performed. This is in contrast to chronic corneal ulceration due to traumatic, infectious, and other causes, which routinely incite neovascularization.
  - Blepharospasm and photophobia, if present, frequently are minimal.
- *Miosis* occurs as an axon reflex from stimulation of corneal, conjunctival, and periocular branches of the ophthalmic nerve (see Chap. 155).
- *Aqueous flare* (i.e., the presence of large amounts of serum proteins in the anterior chamber) indicates iridocyclitis (anterior uveitis) with breakdown of the blood-aqueous barrier (see Chap. 155).
- *Hypotony* (reduced intraocular pressure) usually accompanies moderate to severe anterior uveitis and results from reduced aqueous production and, possibly, increased aqueous outflow.

Diagnosis

History

Important aspects include:

- Time and circumstances of onset
- Presence and duration of discharge and blepharospasm
- Change in the eye's appearance between onset and presentation
- Current and previously treated ocular disorders

Ocular Examination and Accessory Diagnostic Tests

- Collect samples for corneal culture before instilling any diagnostic solutions.
- The hallmark of corneal ulceration is retention of fluorescein dye, which stains corneal stroma, tear, and aqueous humor.
  - To rule out KCS, perform Schirmer tear test (Iolab Pharmaceuticals) before fluorescein dye application.

▼ *Key Point* Descemetoceles demonstrate an annular pattern of dye retention along their walls, but exposed Descemet membrane in the center does not stain.

- Before applying topical anesthesia, test corneal sensitivity with a cotton-tipped swab.
- Following topical anesthesia, obtain scrapings for cytology and Gram staining from ulcers showing rapid progression, soft edematous margins, or a yellow inflammatory cell infiltrate.
- Because sequestra have been noted in cats experimentally infected with FHV, submit diagnostic tests (viral isolation, polymerase chain reaction, or immunofluorescence testing of conjunctival scrapings; see Chap. 9) to rule out herpesvirus infection.
- The diagnosis of epithelial dystrophy is suggested by a chronic nonadherent epithelial margin with only mild discomfort.

Medical Treatment

▼ *Key Point* Ocular corticosteroid administration is contraindicated with corneal ulceration.

▼ *Key Point* Topical anesthetics for *diagnostic* purposes are safe; however, because they are toxic to corneal epithelium, their use in *treatment* is contraindicated.

Simple Erosions and Superficial Ulcers

- Instill topical broad-spectrum antibiotics (e.g., bacitracin, neomycin, polymyxin). Treat with ointments q6hr or with aqueous solutions at least q4h.
- Instill topical 1% atropine ointment or solution, to effect, to maintain mydriasis and, presumably, ciliary muscle paralysis (e.g., q6–8h initially, followed by q12–24h, and then every other day).
- Schedule follow-up examinations every few days until epithelialization is complete.

Deep and/or Progressive Ulceration

Base the choice of topical and subconjunctival antibiotics on corneal cytologic findings (Table 153–1).

- Supplement topical 1% atropine therapy with:
  - Topical fortified gentamicin or tobramycin drops (Tables 153–2 and Table 153–3) applied q1–2h
  - Subconjunctival antibiotic injection (see Table 153–1).
- Consider treatment of acetylcysteine or sodium EDTA (0.15 M) q1–2h if corneal melting is apparent or suspected. Efficacy of these drugs is uncertain.

Surgical Management

- Consider surgical options for treatment of corneal ulcers that are deep and progressive.
- Objectives
  - Prevent ulcer progression
  - Repair perforation
  - Protect the corneal surface
  - Retard melting

Protective Procedures

▼ *Key Point* Protective procedures do not provide blood supply or cells to aid in the healing of corneal ulceration. They do interfere with treatment and further evaluation of corneal ulceration.

- *Nictitans flap*—Indications include postproptosis corneal coverage and, possibly, conservative treatment of recurrent superficial erosion following debridement; contraindications include deep or infected ulcers, descemetoceles, and uncorrected perforations.
- *Temporary tarsorrhaphy*—Indications and contraindications are the same as for nictitans flap.

Supportive Procedures

Supportive procedures include conjunctival flap surgery and cyanoacrylate tissue adhesive application.

Table 153–1. ANTIBIOTIC SELECTION BASED ON GRAM STAIN OF CORNEAL SCRAPINGS

Gram Stain Finding	Antibiotics*		
	Topical	Subconjunctival	Systemic
Gram-positive cocci	Bacitracin (Neosporin; Burroughs Wellcome) or cefazolin (Kefzol; Eli Lilly)	Methicillin (Staphcillin; Squibb), 100 mg, or gentamicin (Gentocin; Schering), 10–40 mg, or tobramycin (Tobrex; Alcon Labs.), 10–30 mg	Ampicillin or gentamicin or cefazolin or tobramycin
Gram-negative rods	Gentamicin or tobramycin	Gentamicin, 10–40 mg, and/or carbenicillin, 250 mg, or tobramycin, 10–30 mg	Chloramphenicol or gentamicin or tobramycin
Mixed infections	Bacitracin and gentamicin	Methicillin, 100 mg, and gentamicin, 20 mg	Gentamicin or tobramycin

*Product name and manufacturer are given in parentheses following the first mention of the generic drug.
Modified from Kern TJ: Ulcerative keratitis. Vet Clin North Am [Small Anim Pract] 20(3):653, 1990.

Table 153-2. FORMULAS FOR FORTIFIED ANTIBIOTICS IN ARTIFICIAL TEARS

Drug	Form	Quantity of Antibiotic	Quantity of Artificial Tears (ml)	Final Volume (ml)	Final Concentration (mg/ml)
Gentamicin (Gentocin injectable; Schering)	100 mg/ml	2.5 ml (250 mg)	15	17.5	14
Gentamicin (Gentocin injectable; Schering)	50 mg/ml	5 ml (250 mg)	12.5	17.5	14
Tobramycin (Nebcin; Eli Lilly)	40 mg/ml	5.5 ml (220 mg)	15	20.5	11
Bacitracin (Bacitracin sterile USP; Quad Pharmaceuticals)	50,000 IU/vial	150,000 U (3 vials)	15	15.6	9600 IU/ml
Cefazolin (Kefzol; Eli Lilly)	1 g/vial	3 ml (1 vial)	15	18	50

Reprinted with permission from Kern TJ: Ulcerative keratitis. Vet Clin North Am [Small Anim Pract] 20(3):655, 1990.

Conjunctival Flap

Indications

Deep ulcers, infected ulcers following short-term intensive antibiotic therapy, descemetoceles, sutured corneal wounds that leak, and, rarely, recurrent epithelial erosions.

Type

Depending on the extent and location of the lesion, the flap may be a pedicle graft (Fig. 153–1), fornix-based hood (180°) flap (Fig. 153–2), or circumferential (360°) flap.

Technique

1. Carefully debride any necrotic or melting corneal stroma from the ulcer and its margin, using a #64 Beaver blade.
2. Form flaps by making a conjunctival incision at the limbus. Bluntly dissect the conjunctiva from the underlying connective tissue (episclera) using tenotomy scissors.
3. Free the conjunctival graft by cutting it from its limbal attachment.
4. Suture pedicle and hood grafts to the cornea, using 7-0 Vicryl or smaller suture material. Attempt to achieve epithelial to epithelial apposition of the conjunctiva and cornea. To relieve tension, the graft can be sutured to the limbus with two sutures.
5. Suture complete 360° flaps in a horizontal mattress pattern, top half to the bottom half, along the center of the cornea but not directly to the cornea.
6. Remove sutures in 10–14 days.
7. Separate the graft from its blood supply and trim points of adhesion of the flap to the previous corneal defect with tenotomy or iris scissors under topical anesthesia 1 week after suture removal.

Cyanoacrylate Tissue Adhesive Application

Indications

Small partial- or full-thickness perforations, small descemetoceles, and deep stromal ulcers.

Technique

1. Sedate or anesthetize the animal as necessary.
2. Debride the lesion as necessary to remove necrotic tissue, nonadherent epithelium, and adherent mucus.
3. Instill a topical anesthetic (Alcaine; Alcon, Inc.; Ophthaine; Solvay Animal Health, Inc.; Ophthetic; Allergan Pharmaceuticals).
4. Insert an eyelid speculum.
5. Dry the corneal site of application with a cotton-tipped swab or cellulose sponge.
6. Apply a very thin layer of adhesive (Ophthalmic Nexaband) through a 30-gauge needle. Application of excessive amounts of adhesive can result in failure of the plug to adhere to the cornea.

Table 153-3. FORMULAS FOR FORTIFIED FORMS OF PROPRIETARY TOPICAL OPHTHALMIC ANTIBIOTICS

Drug	Bottle Concentration (mg/ml)	Bottle Volume (ml)	Parenteral Antibiotic Added	Final Concentration (mg/ml)
Gentamicin (Gentocin ophthalmic solution; Schering)	3	5	50 mg (1 ml of 50 mg/ml solution)	11
Tobramycin (Tobrex; Alcon)	3	5	10 mg or 40 mg/ml	4 or 9

Reprinted with permission from Kern TJ: Ulcerative keratitis. Vet Clin North Am 3(20):565, 1990.

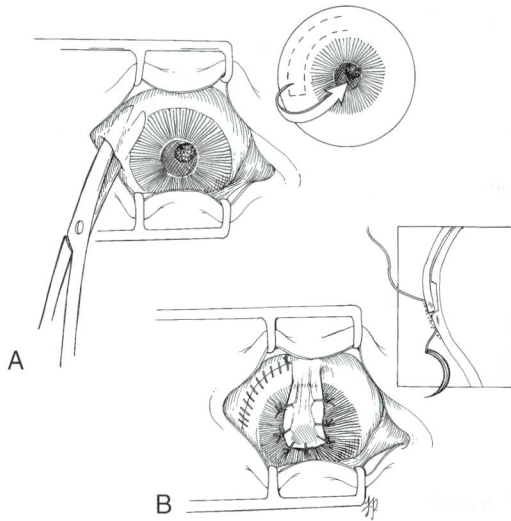

Figure 153–1. Pedicle graft. *A,* Using Stevens tenotomy scissors, elevate the bulbar conjunctiva, incise, and dissect free of the globe. Create and rotate a pedicle of conjunctiva, epithelial surface up, to cover the corneal defect.

B, Suture the conjunctival pedicle to the cornea, covering the defect, using simple-interrupted sutures. Appose the epithelial margins of the conjunctival graft to the cornea (see inset Fig. 153–2*B*).

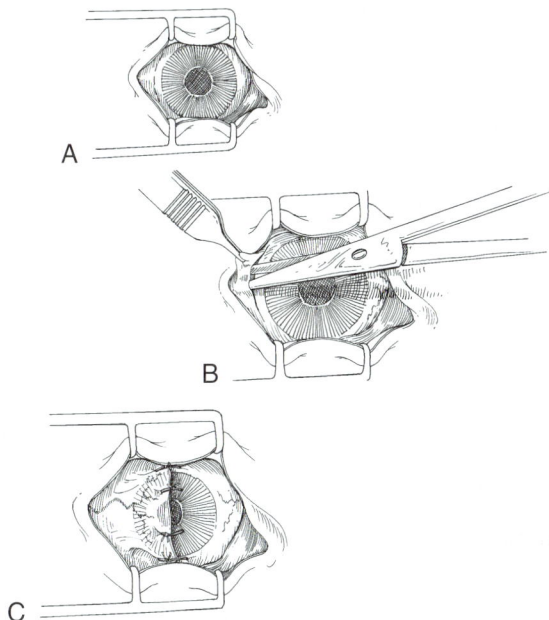

Figure 153–2. Fornix-based hood (180°) flap. *A,* A corneal ulcer is present and is to be repaired with a hood-graft from the adjacent bulbar conjunctiva.

B, Elevate the bulbar conjunctiva adjacent to the corneal defect and use Stevens tenotomy scissors to incise and dissect free this portion of conjunctiva. *C,* Advance the conjunctiva over the defect and suture in place using simple interrupted sutures. Place sutures in the cornea to stabilize the graft over the corneal defect and in the limbus to relieve tension.

7. Wait several minutes for the adhesive to polymerize before removing the speculum. Instill lubricant ointment until blinking returns.
8. Epithelialization occurs underneath the adhesive, which is extruded spontaneously by most animals within a few weeks. Excessive neovascularization may overgrow the plaque, necessitating manual removal under topical anesthesia.

Reconstructive Procedures

- Reconstructive procedures are indicated for descemetoceles and perforating corneal wounds. Commonly used types include sutures, pedicle flaps, and free conjunctival grafts.

Sutures

Technique

1. Suture perforating wounds and small descemetoceles directly with 7-0 to 9-0 absorbable (e.g., polyglactin 910—Vicryl, Ethicon) or nonabsorbable (monofilament nylon) sutures, using a horizontal mattress or simple interrupted pattern (Fig. 153–3).
2. Remove nonabsorbable sutures in 10–14 days.

Pedicle Flap

Technique

1. Raise a pedicle of bulbar conjunctiva, rotate, and then suture it to the edges of the deep corneal wound with absorbable suture material (e.g., polyglactin or polyglycolic acid-Dexon) (see Fig. 153–1).
2. After 2–4 weeks, trim adhered flap connection to the limbus, leaving an island of conjunctiva to be incorporated into the scar.

Free Conjunctival Graft

Technique

1. Dissect an island of conjunctiva slightly larger than the corneal defect from the bulbar or palpe-

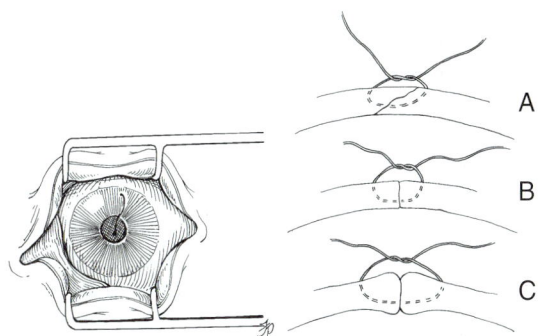

Figure 153–3. Repair of corneal laceration. Note that all sutures are placed to a depth of approximately ⅔ of the corneal thickness. *A,* Closure of oblique edges of the laceration. *B,* Closure of vertical wound edges. *C,* Closure of edematous wound margins. Be sure the sutures extend beyond the edematous edge and into healthy cornea.

bral conjunctiva, and suture it to the cornea directly over the defect.

2. The grafted conjunctiva will become incorporated as a translucent portion of the cornea.

Referral Reconstructive Procedures:

- *Corneoconjunctival transposition* and *autogenous corneal grafting* are forms of lamellar corneal graft requiring special instrumentation and expertise.
- *Penetrating keratoplasty (corneal transplant)* has few indications in veterinary medicine.

Treatment of Chronic Superficial Erosion

- After instilling a topical anesthetic, debride the nonadherent epithelium with a wet or dry cotton-tipped applicator back to the junction with normally adherent epithelium. Frequently, most of the corneal epithelium is removed in the process.

▼ *Key Point* Cauterants such as phenol, aqueous and tincture of iodine, trichloroacetic acid, and others are unnecessary and harmful. These agents incite excessive neovascularization that retards rather than accelerates epithelial healing.

- Instill topical broad-spectrum antibiotic drops (q3–4h) or ointments q6h, until healing is complete.
- To maintain mydriasis, administer topical 1% atropine drops or ointment to effect; apply q8h until dilatation occurs, followed by once daily to every other day.
- If the erosion has not healed, or nearly so, within 10 days, consider the following options:
  - Contact lenses and collagen shields
  - Keratotomy
  - Drugs

Contact Lenses and Collagen Shields

Insertion of a soft contact lens (Duragel; Veterinary Hydrophilics) or collagen shield (Opti-Cor; Pitman Moore) following simple debridement frequently is effective.

Indication:
Chronic corneal ("indolent") erosion

Contraindications:
KCS; bacterial keratitis

Technique
1. Following topical anesthesia, debride nonadherent epithelium with a cotton-tipped swab.
2. Insert soft contact lens or collagen shield (diameter, 15 mm; base curve, 8.4–8.8 mm). A partial temporary tarsorrhaphy is optional.
3. Administer a topical broad-spectrum antibiotic and 1% atropine solutions as described for simple erosions. Apply an Elizabethan collar.
4. Remove the contact lens weekly and stain with flu-

orescein to monitor ulcer healing. Reinsert the contact lens or insert a new one after cleaning and disinfection; repeat the process until the cornea is healed. Collagen shields degrade and disappear within a few days of insertion. Insert a new shield if erosion has not healed.

Superficial Punctate or Linear Keratotomy (Anterior Stromal Puncture)

The resultant small, visually insignificant scars are believed to secure the epithelium to the stroma.

Technique
1. Sedate the animal.
2. Instill a topical anesthetic to effect.
3. Debride nonadherent epithelium with a cotton-tipped swab.
4. Under magnification (Optivisor or similar device), make a series of shallow punctures or linear cuts with a sterile 25-gauge needle, spaced approximately 0.5 mm apart throughout the debrided area and extending 1 mm onto the surrounding epithelium.
5. Instill a topical broad-spectrum antibiotic and 1% atropine as described for simple erosions.

Superficial Keratectomy to Remove the Affected Area of Stroma, Epithelium, and Basement Membrane

Disadvantages include:

- The need for general anesthesia
- Proficiency in the surgical technique
- Possible permanent corneal thinning

Drugs

Drugs not yet commercially available but showing promise for medical management of chronic corneal erosions include epidermal growth factors, fibronectin, and aprotinin.

Surgical Management of Corneal Sequestra

- Perform keratectomy to remove sequestra that lie in the *superficial* half of the cornea; deeper keratectomy encourages iatrogenic corneal perforation.
- Sequestra may recur at the operated site or at other sites.
- For large or deep sequestra, consider performing a conjunctival pedicle graft to support and reconstruct the wound.

NONULCERATIVE CORNEAL DISORDERS

Chronic Superficial Keratitis (CSK)
Etiology

- The specific cause of CSK is unknown.
- Its predominance in a small spectrum of dog breeds (German shepherd, greyhound, occasionally others) and in mixed-breed dogs originating from these

strongly implicates a genetic predisposition for immune-mediated disease.

Clinical Signs

- Superficial, bilaterally symmetric neovascularization, usually beginning inferotemporally, with or without melanosis is a hallmark. Pain is not a common sign.
- Rarely, corneal ulceration develops.
- Corneal degeneration, manifested by oval crystalline opacities, may develop with chronicity.

Diagnosis

- Base diagnosis on typical corneal signs in a German shepherd, greyhound, or mixed-breed dog of their extraction, in the absence of other causes of chronic superficial keratitis (e.g., tear deficiency, eyelid abnormalities).

Treatment

- Administer corticosteroids topically (and, intermittently, subconjunctivally) to control this incurable condition.
  - For initial management administer a subconjunctival injection of 5 mg of betamethasone acetate and sodium phosphate (Betavet Soluspan; Schering Veterinary), triamcinolone acetonide (Kenalog-40; Squibb), or methylprednisolone acetate (Depo-Medrol; Upjohn).
  - Supplement with a topical corticosteroid ointment or solution on a regimen of reducing frequency (e.g., q3–4h tapering to q8h over 4 weeks).
  - Long-term topical therapy is essential to maintain control; even short periods of owner noncompliance will result in relapse.
  - Only neovascularization responds to this therapy; melanosis and corneal degeneration do not.
- Consider instillation of 1 drop of 2% cyclosporine in oil (see Chap. 158) q12h. Over many months, this may reduce corneal melanosis in many conditions, including CSK, by a poorly understood mechanism. CSK is believed to be a T-lymphocyte–mediated disease and has been reported to respond in some instances to cyclosporine therapy.
- Plesiotherapy with strontium-90–generated beta-radiation is an effective adjunctive treatment for neovascularization. However, this is only available through specialty practices and teaching institutions.

▼ *Key Point* Do not perform keratectomy for removal of corneal pigmentation. Complications include delayed epithelialization, recurrence of CSK, and corneal perforation.

Feline Eosinophilic Keratitis
Etiology

- The etiology is unknown.

Clinical Signs

- Corneal neovascularization, which is frequently bilateral and symmetric, leads to formation of a pink-white plaque covered by a granular, crumbled cheese–like material. The superior temporal, inferior temporal, and inferior nasal quadrants are most frequently involved.
- This lesion is unique to the cat.
- Corneal ulceration is present rarely.

Diagnosis

- Corneal scrapings contain combinations of eosinophils, mast cells, and mixed inflammatory cells.

▼ *Key Point* Identification of numerous eosinophils or mast cells in corneal scrapings is pathognomonic for feline eosinophilic keratitis.

Treatment

Corticosteroids

Intensive topical corticosteroid therapy frequently is successful.

- Give dexamethasone 0.1% (Decadron; Merck, Sharp and Dohme) or prednisolone 1% (Econopred Plus; Alcon) as an ointment or solution, q3–4h. Monitor progress closely if epithelial erosion was present.
- If needed, combine topical corticosteroids with subconjunctival betamethasone, triamicinolone, or methylprednisolone (3–6 mg per eye). This combination controls the condition in most cats.
- Once the disease is in remission, reduce frequency of topical therapy to minimal levels; discontinue if remission is maintained.
- Some affected cats will have relapses, requiring chronic topical corticosteroid administration at a minimal effective frequency.

Megestrol Acetate

- Administer megestrol acetate (Ovaban; Schering) (0.5 mg/kg q24h until effect, and then 1.25 mg 1–3 times weekly) *only* to cats that have not responded to topical and subconjunctival corticosteroids.
- Side effects of oral megestrol acetate include weight gain, behavior changes, diabetes mellitus, and mammary gland hypertrophy and neoplasia.

Corneal Melanosis
Etiology

- Among domestic animals, only dogs commonly develop corneal pigmentation, which apparently develops through migration of limbal melanocytes into the basal epithelial layers and anterior stroma.

▼ *Key Point* Melanosis develops in dogs in response to chronic irritation from many causes, including KCS, eyelid deformities, lagophthalmos, and chronic superficial keratitis.

Clinical Signs

- Superficial corneal pigmentation develops focally or over large areas. Corneal neovascularization usually precedes or accompanies melanosis.

Diagnosis

- The typical appearance of a variably melanotic cornea is diagnostic.
- Rarely, melanosis must be distinguished from iris prolapse (anterior synechiae are also apparent) or, at the limbus, epibulbar melanoma.

Treatment

- Identify and treat the underlying causes of melanosis if possible (e.g., KCS) or definitively correct them (e.g., entropion, nasal fold trichiasis).
- Rarely, perform superficial keratectomy to improve corneal clarity when vision is reduced, but only after correcting the inciting cause.
- Consider long-term topical therapy for KCS with 2% cyclosporine drops or 0.2% cyclosporine ointment (Optimmune, Schering-Plough) (see Chap. 158), which may retard or reduce corneal melanosis (evidence of benefit is anecdotal).

SCLERAL INFLAMMATION AND TRAUMA

Fibrous Histiocytoma; Proliferative Keratoconjunctivitis of Collies; Nodular Granulomatous Episclerokeratitis

Etiology

- This condition probably is a genetic disorder of collies, but has been noted in other breeds. Clinical and pathologic features of both inflammation and neoplasia are present.

Clinical Signs

- Bilaterally symmetric scleral/episcleral nodules, especially at the temporal limbus, are hallmarks.
- The eyelids, planum nasale, and other mucocutaneous junctions (lips, anogenital areas) may be involved.
- If the cornea is invaded, corneal opacity develops, often with a leading edge of crystalline corneal degeneration.

Diagnosis

- Typical lesions in a collie are presumptive evidence.
- Obtain a biopsy of atypical lesions.
- The histologic appearance is that of fibroplasia with extensive histiocytic proliferation.
- Differential diagnosis includes lymphoma and other neoplasms.

Treatment

- Corticosteroids are the initial treatment of choice. For dogs with ocular lesions only, combine intensive topical corticosteroid therapy (dexamethasone 0.1% or prednisolone 1%) with subconjunctival injection of 3–6 mg per eye of triamcinolone, betamethasone, or methylprednisolone acetate.
  - Long-term topical steroid treatment at the minimally effective frequency reduces recurrence.

- For dogs with ocular and oral, nasal, and/or genital lesions, administer oral prednisone (1.1 mg/kg q12h); taper to the effective minimal dose and frequency. Indefinite treatment may be required.
- For dogs with corticosteroid-unresponsive lesions, administer azathioprine (Imuran; Burroughs Wellcome) 2.2 mg/kg q24h PO for 14 days followed by 1 mg/kg every other day for 14 days; then give 1 mg/kg once weekly for 4 weeks and discontinue.
  - Indefinite treatment at a low frequency may be required.
  - Monitor leukocyte and platelet counts in animals on azathioprine therapy. Discontinue treatment if a significant reduction in either is observed.
- Discourage breeding of affected dogs.

Scleritis; Episcleritis; Ocular Nodular Fascitis

Etiology

- The cause is unknown; an immune-mediated etiology is suspected.

Clinical Signs

- Nodular, diffuse infiltrative, and necrotizing forms have been recognized.
  - Nodular lesions resemble fibrous histiocytomas, but often are unilateral and affect dogs other than collies.
  - Diffuse thickening and inflammation of the sclera may be associated with scleral necrosis and moderate to severe uveitis.

Diagnosis

- The diagnosis is based on clinical signs, histopathology, and response to therapy.
- Differential diagnosis includes lymphoma and other neoplasia.

Treatment

- Treatment plan is similar to that for fibrous histiocytoma.

Scleral Wounds

Etiology

Blunt or perforating trauma may cause rupture of the globe through the sclera while the cornea is spared.

Clinical Signs

- Chemosis, conjunctival or external ocular hemorrhage, hyphema, and eyelid swelling in a traumatized animal suggest scleral perforation.

Treatment

- Surgical repair of small wounds may result in preservation of the globe as well as vision if the repair is performed promptly.
- Enucleation or evisceration with intraocular prosthesis implantation is indicated if the scleral laceration is large or if other ocular injuries prevent comfortable retention of the globe.

CORNEOSCLERAL NEOPLASIA

Primary–Epibulbar Melanoma

Etiology

- These benign neoplasms probably arise from conjunctival or episcleral melanocytes.
- The German shepherd is a predisposed breed, but the disorder has been reported in numerous other breeds.

Clinical Signs

- A nonpainful, pigmented mass near the limbus, involving the sclera (and, later, adjacent cornea), slowly enlarges, expanding horizontally and vertically into the surrounding sclera.

Diagnosis

- The typical appearance suggests the diagnosis.
- Epibulbar melanomas should be distinguished (not always easily) from uveal melanomas, which are intraocular tumors that may expand through the sclera.

Treatment

- Small, superficial lesions may be resectable. Because scleral grafting may be necessary, consider referral to a specialist.
- Observe for a long period to assess the growth rate and characteristics of individual tumors.
  - In dogs, these normally benign neoplasms may be safely observed until/unless deeper extension causes uveitis or glaucoma, prompting enucleation.
  - Recommendations in cats are similar, although based on fewer reported cases.

Secondary Neoplastic Invasion of the Sclera

Etiology

- Primary or secondary intraocular neoplasms may extend through the sclera and into the orbit.

- Rarely, episcleral metastasis of a distant primary or multicentric neoplasm may occur.

Clinical Signs

- Masses may be obvious extensions of intraocular tumors. Episcleral masses may mimic episcleritis or fibrous histiocytoma.

Diagnosis

- Relationship to an intraocular tumor is presumptive evidence. Association of a scleral mass with a visible intraocular tumor suggests that the scleral mass is an extension of it.
- For histopathological evaluation, completely excise solitary masses.

Treatment

- Consider palliative and diagnostic enucleation of a painful globe.

SUPPLEMENTAL READINGS

Cooley PL, Dice PF: Corneal dystrophy in the dog and cat. Vet Clin North Am [Small Anim Pract] 20(3):681, 1990.

Dice PF, Cooley PL: Use of contact lenses to treat corneal diseases in small animals. Semin Vet Med Surg (Small Anim) 3:46, 1988.

Kern TJ: Ulcerative keratitis. Vet Clin North Am [Small Anim Pract] 20(3):643, 1990.

Kirschner SE: Persistent corneal ulcers: What to do when they won't heal. Vet Clin North Am [Small Anim Pract] 20(3):627, 1990.

Moore CP: Surgery of the conjunctiva. In Bojrab MJ, ed.: Current Techniques in Small Animal Surgery, 3rd Ed. Philadelphia: Lea & Febiger, 1990, p 76.

Munger RJ: The conjunctiva. In Slatter DH, ed.: Textbook of Small Animal Surgery. Philadelphia: WB Saunders, 1985, p 1469.

Slatter DH: Cornea and sclera. In Fundamentals of Veterinary Ophthalmology, 2nd Ed. Philadelphia: WB Saunders, 1990, p 257.

Slatter DH: Cornea and sclera. In Slatter DH, ed.: Textbook of Small Animal Surgery. Philadelphia: WB Saunders, 1985, p 1509.

Vestre WA: Surgery of the cornea. In Bojrab MJ, ed.: Current Techniques in Small Animal Surgery, 3rd Ed. Philadelphia: Lea & Febiger, 1990, p 947.

154 Diseases of the Lens

David A. Wilkie / Margi Gilmour

ANATOMY

The normal canine and feline lens is composed of an outer capsule, epithelial cells beneath the anterior capsule, and fibers formed by the migration of epithelial cells to the lens equator, where the cells elongate and create a regular arrangement of fibers. The regular arrangement of these fibers accounts for the transparency of the lens. The lens is posterior to the iris; anterior to the vitreous to which it is attached; and suspended by zonules, which arise from the ciliary body and attach to the lens capsule at the equator (see Fig. 150–1).

CONGENITAL ANOMALIES

Etiology

Lens development takes place early in embryogenesis and is complete in the dog by day 30 of gestation. Any genetic abnormality affecting lens development or any insult to the bitch or queen early in gestation, including infectious, nutritional, chemical, or drug-related, can result in congenital lens anomalies. These abnormalities are often associated with other congenital ocular anomalies, including microphthalmia (small globe), persistent pupillary membranes, persistent hyaloid artery, retinal dysplasia, retinal detachment, posterior coloboma/staphyloma, and optic nerve hypoplasia.

Clinical Signs

Examples and features of congenital lens anomalies include the following.

- *Microphakia* (small lens). With the pupil dilated, the equator of the lens and fine zonules, attaching at the equator and originating from elongated ciliary processes, are visible.
- *Coloboma* (notch defect). With the pupil dilated, a notch defect may be visible in any quadrant of the equatorial zone, with or without zonular attachments.
- *Cataract.* See the cataract discussion in this chapter.
- *Lens luxation.* Often associated with microphakia (see discussion in this chapter).

Diagnosis

- Clinical signs (see previous section)
- Present at birth. Microphakia and coloboma are always congenital. Cataract and lens luxation, unless associated with microphakia, may not be congenital. An accurate history and early examination are helpful in differentiating congenital from acquired abnormalities.

Treatment

- Determine concomitant ocular anomalies and their significance to vision.
- Microphakia and coloboma alone require no treatment.
- Cataract, if impairing vision, may be amenable to surgical removal once the integrity of the retina and optic nerve has been ascertained by fundic examination, electroretinogram, ocular ultrasound, and visual-evoked potential.
- Remove a luxated lens if it is inciting uveitis and/or glaucoma, impairing vision, or interfering with corneal endothelial cell function.

Prevention

Congenital anomalies are not necessarily inherited anomalies. Careful inquiry into affected littermates and prevalence of problems in previous matings may raise the suspicion for an inherited defect. If the cause of the abnormality cannot be determined, discourage the use of this and related animals for breeding.

CATARACT

Etiology

Cataract is an opacity of the lens resulting from pathologic changes in lens protein composition or disruption of lens fiber arrangement.

▼ *Key Point* Cataract must be distinguished from nuclear sclerosis. Nuclear sclerosis is a normal aging change seen in all dogs and cats 6 years of age or older, produced by compression of central lens fibers.

Etiologies of cataract development include the following:

- *Hereditary.* This is the most common cause of cataract in the dog (Table 154–1). Location, progression, and

Table 154–1. BREEDS OF DOGS WITH INHERITED OR FAMILIAL CATARACTS*

Afghan hound	French bulldog	Papillon
Alaskan malamute	German shepherd	Pembroke Welsh corgi
Beagle	German shorthaired pointer	Pointer
Bedlington terrier	Giant schnauzer	Pomeranian
Belgian Tervuren	Golden retriever	Poodle (toy, miniature, standard)
Bernese mountain dog	Great Dane	Puli
Bichon frise	Ibizan hound	Rhodesian ridgeback
Border collie	Irish setter	Rottweiler
Border terrier	Irish water spaniel	Saint Bernard
Borzoi	Irish wolfhound	Samoyed
Boston terrier	Italian greyhound	Schipperke
Bouvier des Flandres	Keeshond	Scottish terrier
Cairn terrier	Kerry blue terrier	Siberian husky
Cavalier King Charles spaniel	Labrador retriever	Silky terrier
Chesapeake Bay retriever	Lakeland terrier	Staffordshire bull terrier
Cocker spaniel	Lhasa apso	Standard schnauzer
Collie	Manchester terrier	Tibetan terrier
Curly-coated retriever	Miniature pinscher	Welsh springer spaniel
Dachshund	Miniature schnauzer	Welsh terrier
English cocker spaniel	Norfolk terrier	West Highland white terrier
English springer spaniel	Norwegian elkhound	Whippet
English toy spaniel	Norwich terrier	Wire fox terrier
Field spaniel	Old English sheepdog	Yorkshire terrier

*From Rubin LF: Inherited Eye Diseases in Purebred Dogs. Baltimore: Williams & Wilkins, 1989.

mode of inheritance of cataracts vary among breeds. The majority of inherited cataracts are bilateral but often asymmetric in onset and progression.

- *Inflammatory.* This is a common cause of cataract in the cat. Because the lens needs the aqueous and vitreous humors for nutrition and removal of metabolic wastes, intraocular inflammation can result in capsular and cortical opacities. Posterior synechia from anterior uveitis can result in anterior capsular cataracts.
- *Metabolic.* Diabetes mellitus in dogs frequently results in rapid (days to weeks) onset of bilateral cataracts, because of a shift in metabolic pathways, an accumulation of sorbitol causing an osmotic gradient, and a subsequent disruption of lens fibers. The cataracts are irreversible.
- *Traumatic.* Severe blunt trauma to the eye can result in cataract formation from concussive effects or can be secondary to inflammation and/or lens luxation. Penetrating injuries that puncture the anterior lens capsule (e.g., cat claw injuries) result in a focal or diffuse cataract, depending upon the severity of the capsular tear. Uveitis may occur secondary to rupture of the lens capsule.
- *Nutritional.* Puppies and kittens hand fed exclusively milk-replacement formula that is deficient in required amino acids, the most frequently cited being arginine, can develop bilateral cataracts.
- *Toxic.* Electric shock, radiation therapy involving the ocular region, and certain drugs have been reported to cause cataracts.

Clinical Signs and Diagnosis

▼ *Key Point* For a thorough examination of the lens, mydriasis is mandatory because some of the most significant changes occur in the extreme periphery (equatorial zone) of the lens. Topical tropicamide 1% (Mydriacyl, Alcon) results in mydriasis in 15–20 minutes and lasts 6–8 hours.

- Any *opacity,* anywhere in the lens or its capsule observed after dilation of the pupil, is a cataract.
- The degree of *visual impairment* is dependent upon the extent of cataract development in one or both eyes. In addition, the use of the animal must be considered. Incipient and immature cataracts are more significant in hunting and working dogs with respect to vision impairment.
- Differentiate cataracts from nuclear sclerosis. Nuclear sclerosis is a bilaterally symmetric, well-defined, homogeneous haze in the center of the lens observed in animals older than 6 years. Sclerosis is not a true opacity, and it does not obstruct a dilated examination of the fundus or cause clinically significant visual impairment.
- A focal cataract can be localized with respect to anterior or posterior by comparing the nasal/temporal direction of movement of the cataract with that of the eye. Anterior cataracts will move in the same direction as the globe; posterior cataracts will appear to move in the opposite direction of the globe. Thus—if the animal looks temporally—an anterior opacity will move temporally and a posterior opacity will move nasally. By localizing cataracts, one can help determine if they are inherited and predict progression. For example, nuclear cataracts are generally static, whereas equatorial cataracts, where new lens fibers are forming, are generally progressive.

Stage of Development

Incipient

Focal or multifocal opacities of the lens causing no clinical loss of vision and not impairing tapetal reflection or view of the fundus.

Immature

Significant lenticular opacity. Tapetal reflection remains, but an incomplete view of the fundus is present. Vision is affected depending upon the extent of lens involvement.

Mature

Dense lenticular opacity with no tapetal reflection or fundus visible, resulting in total vision loss in the affected eye.

Hypermature

As lens protein degenerates and liquefies the lens can become smaller in the anterior-posterior axis, resulting in a wrinkled anterior capsule and deep anterior chamber.

Resorbing

As lens protein degenerates and liquefies it can leak through the capsule. This is usually associated with hypermature cataracts but can occur in immature and mature cataracts as well. The process is faster in young dogs. A resorbing lens has varying amounts of clear, liquefied cortex with the remaining lens material often taking on a sparkling appearance. Although in some animals vision is regained by significant lens resorption, the process generally results in mild-to-severe lens-induced uveitis because of the antigenicity of the leaking lens protein.

Lens-Induced Uveitis

Exposure of excessive amounts of lens protein can overwhelm the normal low-dose T-cell tolerance resulting in both a humoral and cell-mediated immune response characterized by lymphocytes and plasma cells. This process is termed phacolytic or lens-induced uveitis (LIU). This may result in hypotony, miosis, flare, keratitic precipitates, synechia, retinal detachment, and glaucoma if allowed to persist (see Chap. 155). In addition, LIU may be associated with intraoperative complications during cataract surgery, a reduction in surgical success, and an increase in postoperative medication.

Phacoclastic uveitis is the result of rupture, spontaneous or traumatic, of the lens capsule. The resulting uveitis is much more severe than seen with phacolytic uveitis and results in secondary glaucoma, pupillary occlusion, and fibroplasia. The treatment of choice is immediate lens extraction once a lens capsule rupture is observed.

Treatment

▼ *Key Point* There is no medical treatment to eliminate cataracts. Surgical removal of cataracts is a referral procedure.

Previously, because of the risks associated with cataract surgery, the cost to the owner, and the ability of a blind dog to acclimatize to their environment, cataract surgery was an elective procedure reserved for those animals with bilateral, mature cataracts. Recently, the improved success rate of phacoemulsification, the availability of intraocular lens implants, and the increased success associated with early surgical intervention have resulted in cataract surgery being offered in cases of unilateral and immature cataracts. Regardless, cataract surgery remains an expensive and elective procedure, the exception being a traumatic cataract with secondary lens capsule rupture and impending phacoclastic uveitis. Owners should be aware that not removing a cataract may result in its progression and secondary LIU and associated complications.

Success rates for cataract surgery vary depending on preexisting uveitis, stage of the cataract, predisposition for glaucoma, surgical procedure used, and surgeon expertise. Success rates with phacoemulsification are reported to be 90–95% with little decline over time while success of the open-sky extracapsular technique is approximately 80% with a steady decline in success over time following surgery to less than 50%.

Preoperative Considerations

- For owners expressing an interest in cataract surgery, refer them to a veterinary ophthalmologist early, while the fundus is still visible and before lens-induced uveitis develops.
- The animal should be healthy. If diabetic, the condition should be well-regulated.
- The eyes are examined for concurrent uveitis, glaucoma, abnormal iridocorneal angle, keratitis, and retinal disease.
- If the fundus is not visible through the cataract, an electroretinogram is performed to evaluate for progressive retinal atrophy. An ocular ultrasound is carried out to evaluate for retinal detachment.

Surgical Procedures

- The most common technique for cataract removal in veterinary ophthalmology is phacoemulsification. This uses ultrasonic energy to drive a needle that emulsifies the lens and through irrigation-aspiration, removes the lens material from the lens capsule. This procedure requires a smaller incision, involves shortened surgical time, and maintains the anterior chamber, all of which result in improved success as compared with the technique of open-sky extracapsular extraction. The procedure requires a phacoemulsification device, an operating microscope, appropriate surgical equipment, and expertise. Therefore, it is a referral procedure.
- A 3.0-mm incision is made in the cornea at the limbus, the anterior chamber inflated using a viscoelastic material, a continuous tear anterior capsulorrhexis performed, and the lens removed by phacoemulsification. Care is taken to avoid traumatizing the iris, cornea, and remaining lens capsule. Once the lens is removed and the remaining lens cortex aspirated, some surgeons will also remove a circular portion of the posterior lens capsule to ensure a clear visual axis and minimize postoperative lens capsule fibrosis.

The corneal incision is then enlarged to allow insertion of an intraocular lens (IOL). The most common lens for replacement in the canine eye is a single-piece lens constructed of polymethylmethacrylate with a 7.0-mm optical portion, 15–17 mm haptic to haptic dimension, and a power of 41.5 diopters. This IOL is placed through the anterior capsule opening and into the remaining lens capsule, allowing the lens capsule to provide support and ensure position. The corneal incision is then closed. If the opposite eye also has a cataract, many surgeons will remove this lens and place an IOL at this time. The animal is then recovered. Failure to replace the cataractous lens with an IOL will leave the animal 14 diopters hyperopic (farsighted) and result in significant visual impairment.

Postoperative Considerations

Complications of cataract surgery can occur immediately to several years postoperatively. Evaluate patients frequently for several months following surgery. Maintain a long-term, 6-month reevaluation schedule for life.

- *Immediate postoperative complications* include anterior uveitis, glaucoma, luxation of the IOL, and retinal detachment.
- *Long-term complications* include chronic low-grade uveitis, glaucoma, corneal endothelial damage with associated corneal edema, fibrous metaplasia across the posterior capsule with opacification of the capsule, posterior synechia, production of new cortical material from remaining epithelial cells, IOL decentration, and retinal detachment.
- Reevaluation includes tonometry to determine intraocular pressure (IOP) and a dilated examination of the posterior capsule and fundus.

Prevention

- Incidence of inherited cataracts can be reduced by discouraging breeding of affected animals and carriers and by encouraging breeders to have yearly Canine Eye Registration Foundation (CERF) examinations.
- Inflammatory cataracts can often be prevented by prompt, appropriate treatment of uveitis (see Chap. 155).

LENS LUXATION

Etiology

- *Primary zonular degeneration.* This is an inherited trait in many terrier breeds and has familial tendencies in other breeds (Table 154–2). Lens luxation usually occurs at middle age with no predisposing ocular disease.
- *Glaucoma.* Chronic glaucoma results in a buphthalmic (enlarged) globe that can stretch and break the lenticular zonules, causing the lens to luxate.

▼ *Key Point* A primary lens luxation can also cause glaucoma, making it difficult to distinguish which occurred first in some cases.

- *Uveitis.* Chronic uveitis may weaken zonules owing to inflammatory cell infiltration.
- *Cataracts.* Advanced cataracts may cause degenerative changes in the zonules or zonular attachments.
- *Trauma.* Severe ocular trauma may cause lens luxation; however, it is not a common cause unless there is underlying zonule pathology.

Clinical Signs

- The clinical signs of lens luxation vary depending upon whether the lens luxates anteriorly or posteriorly. Many times it is the secondary ocular changes that result in the clinical presentation, rather than the lens luxation itself.
- In many eyes with luxated lenses, the vitreous will liquefy and can be found in the anterior chamber. Vitreous appears as filmy white material suspended in the aqueous humor. Its presence, in the absence of lens luxation, may indicate early zonular breakdown and subluxation or an animal's predisposition to lens luxation.

Anterior Lens Luxation

- A penlight beam directed parallel to the iris will reveal the lens positioned in the anterior chamber, anterior to the iris and often blocking the pupil.
- Blue light (Wood's lamp) will cause a clear lens to fluoresce, simplifying the examination.

Table 154–2. BREEDS OF DOGS WITH INHERITED OR FAMILIAL LENS LUXATION*

Australian cattle dog	Lakeland terrier	Sealyham terrier
Border collie	Manchester terrier	Siberian husky
Cairn terrier	Miniature schnauzer	Skye terrier
Cardigan Welsh corgi	Norfolk terrier	Smooth fox terrier
Chihuahua	Norwegian elkhound	Tibetan terrier
German shepherd	Norwich terrier	Welsh terrier
Greyhound	Pembroke Welsh corgi	West Highland white terrier
Irish setter	Poodle (toy)	Whippet
Jack Russell terrier	Scottish terrier	Wire fox terrier

*From Rubin LF: Inherited Eye Diseases in Purebred Dogs. Baltimore: Williams & Wilkins, 1989.

- A focal area of corneal edema may result from the lens' touching the posterior cornea and damaging the corneal endothelium. This may be a permanent change.
- Secondary glaucoma can occur from pupillary occlusion by the lens or attached vitreous or from occlusion of the aqueous outflow through the iridocorneal angle.

Posterior Lens Luxation

- The edge of the lens may be seen through the pupil, resulting in an "aphakic crescent" between the pupil margin and the edge of the lens.
- The lens may fall into the vitreous where it can be seen on the floor of the chamber, trapped in the vitreous, or adhered to the retina.
- Without support of the lens, the iris may tremble with eye movement (iridodonesis). The anterior chamber will be deep.

Diagnosis

- Based on ophthalmic examination
- Tonometry to identify primary or secondary glaucoma
- Ocular ultrasound (if intraocular structures cannot be observed because of corneal or aqueous opacity)

Treatment

- Treatment for lens luxation is surgical. Anterior lens luxation is a potential emergency and posterior lens luxation a more elective surgical procedure. If immediate referral for an anterior lens luxation is available, do not dilate the pupil. If referral is delayed, then some ophthalmologists may prefer the pupil be dilated to minimize corneal endothelial trauma and the risk of pupillary block glaucoma.
- Determine the intraocular pressure in all eyes with lens luxation.
- Remove a luxated lens through a large limbal corneal incision removing the lens and lens capsule intact, termed an intracapsular lens extraction. Minimize trauma to the vitreous and remove as little of it as possible. Removal of an anterior lens luxation is technically easier than a posterior luxation. The latter requires vitrectomy to gain access to the lens with an increased risk of intraoperative retinal detachment. Following intracapsular lens extraction, an intraocular lens can be placed to restore emmetropia. Unlike traditional cataract surgery where the IOL can be placed in the lens capsule, the IOL in this instance must be sutured in position. Using two to three 10-0 nylon sutures attached to the IOL haptics, a needle is passed ab interno behind the iris, through the ciliary sulcus, and out the sclera. This is repeated for each suture attached to the haptic. Position the lens posterior to the iris, anterior to the vitreous, and in the ciliary sulcus. Close the corneal incision and reinflate the anterior chamber. Using the sutures attached to the haptics the lens is manipulated into position in the pupillary opening and the 10-0 nylon sutures fixed to the sclera.
- Postoperative complications include retinal detachment, glaucoma, IOL decentration, dyscoria, uveitis, synechia, and vitreous entrapment in the corneal incision.
- If surgical removal is not possible, the lens is best kept in the vitreous chamber. Once there, topical miotics, such as 2% pilocarpine, can be used in an effort to trap the lens behind the iris. Follow-up care should include periodic determination of intraocular pressure. Lenses that are luxated and not removed will become cataractous.
- Examine the contralateral eye in instances of primary lens luxation and if unstable instruct the owner what to watch for as a sign of lens luxation. Alternately, some ophthalmic surgeons will offer to remove a lens due to instability, preferring to replace it with a sulcus-fixated IOL.
- If the lens luxation is secondary to buphthalmia and chronic glaucoma, therapy is directed toward the glaucoma (see Chap. 156).

Prevention

- Examine the contralateral eye carefully for evidence of lens subluxation, such as a deep or shallow anterior chamber, iris tremor, aphakic crescent, or vitreous in the anterior chamber.
- Advise owners to watch the animal's eye at risk for signs of lens luxation and to call immediately if noted.

SUPPLEMENTAL READINGS

Curtis R: Lens luxation in the dog and cat. Vet Clin North Am [Sm Anim Pract—Sm Anim Ophthalmol] 20:755, 1990.

Dziezyc J: Cataract surgery—current approaches. Vet Clin North Am [Sm Anim Pract—Sm Anim Ophthalmol] 20:737, 1990.

Glover TD, Constaninescu GM: Surgery for cataracts. Vet Clin North Am (Sm Anim Pract—Surgical management of ocular disease) 27:1143, 1997.

Gwin RM, Gelatt KN: The canine lens. In Gelatt KN, ed.: Veterinary Ophthalmology. Philadelphia: Lea & Febiger, 1981, p 435.

Nasisse MP: Surgery for lens instability. Vet Clin North Am (Sm Anim Pract—Surgical management of ocular disease) 27:1175, 1997.

Rubin LF: Inherited Eye Diseases in Purebred Dogs. Baltimore: Williams & Wilkins, 1989.

Wilkie DA, Peiffer RL: Must you do phacoemulsification to be a successful cataract surgeon? Vet Comp Ophthalmol 5:124, 1995.

155 Uvea

David A. Wilkie

ANATOMY AND PHYSIOLOGY

The uvea is the middle or vascular tunic of the eye. It is covered externally by the fibrous tunic and provides much of the blood supply to the inner nervous tunic (retina) (see Chap. 150).

The uvea is composed of *three regions:* the iris, ciliary body, and choroid (see Chap. 157).

Iris

- The iris is the anterior most portion of the uvea. It forms an incomplete diaphragm between the anterior and posterior chambers and regulates the amount of light entering the posterior portions of the eye.
- The color of the iris varies between species, within species, and even within the same animal. Heterochromia is a different color within or between irides.
- The iris contains a sphincter muscle controlled by parasympathetic fibers that travel from the Edinger-Westphal nucleus with the oculomotor nerve (CN3) to the ciliary ganglion where they synapse. The action of the sphincter muscle causes miosis. Intraocular inflammation will also result in contraction of the sphincter muscle. This results in the miosis and pain seen in anterior uveitis. The sphincter muscle can be paralyzed with parasympatholytic agents, causing dilation of the pupil. This is used clinically to better see the posterior portions of the eye and to treat anterior uveitis.

▼ *Key Point* The diagnostic parasympatholytic agent of choice is tropicamide (Mydriacyl), whereas the therapeutic parasympatholytic agent of choice is atropine 1%.

- The iris dilator muscle fibers are radially oriented and lie along the base of the posterior epithelium. The dilator muscle is under sympathetic control in mammals. The sympathetic fibers course along the spinal cord to T1–T3, leave in the ventral roots, course through the anterior mediastinum, and run anteriorly with the internal carotid to the cranial cervical ganglion where they synapse. They then travel to the eye in association with the ocular vascular supply (see Chap. 160). The action of the dilator muscle is to produce mydriasis.

Ciliary Body

The ciliary body is divided into the pars plicata and pars plana and is located posterior to the iris. The ciliary processes are folds of the ciliary epithelium with a vascular core and are the source of aqueous humor. The ciliary body is also the origin of the lenticular zonules, which serve to anchor the lens. Through these zonules and the ciliary musculature, accommodation occurs.

Choroid

The choroid is continuous anteriorly with the ciliary body and extends posteriorly to the optic nerve. The choroid lies external to the retina and serves to supply nutrition to the outer portions (rods and cones) of the retina in the dog and cat. The tapetum is located in the dorsal portion of the fundus and lies within the choroid (see Chap. 157).

CONGENITAL ABNORMALITIES

Persistent Pupillary Membranes

Etiology

These are persistent remnants of fetal blood vessels in the anterior chamber that originate from the collarette region of the anterior iris face. They may be seen alone or in association with other congenital abnormalities. Although persistent pupillary membranes (PPMs) are felt to have an inherited component (especially in basenjis), the mode of inheritance is not established in most affected breeds.

Clinical Signs

The clinical signs vary depending on where the PPM strands attach. In general, the color of the PPM will be similar to that of the iris. PPMs that bridge iris to iris generally result in no clinical signs, whereas those attaching to the anterior lens capsule or corneal endothelium are associated with focal opacities of these structures. Differentiate PPMs from anterior and posterior synechiae when attaching to the cornea or lens, respectively.

Diagnosis

Base the diagnosis on the clinical signs and breed. Perform a complete ophthalmic examination to detect other congenital ocular abnormalities.

Treatment

There is no treatment required and the lesion is nonprogressive. Council breeders about possible inheritance and discourage breeding of affected basenjis and corgis.

Coloboma

Etiology

A coloboma is a developmental anomaly in which a portion of the tissue, in this case the uvea, is absent. Colobomas can affect all three portions of the uvea and are often associated with other congenital anomalies such as PPMs, lens coloboma, or retinal detachment. Colobomas can be inherited or the result of a toxic insult to the developing eye during gestation.

Clinical Signs

Depending on which portion of the uvea is affected, clinical signs will vary. Colobomas of the iris result in dyscoria and may be associated with PPMs or lenticular abnormalities. Colobomas of the ciliary body or choroid are generally not noted by the owner and are seen on a routine ophthalmic examination or present as a result of other congenital abnormalities or from secondary changes such as retinal detachment. Posterior segment colobomas are seen as part of the collie eye anomaly (CEA) (see Chap. 157).

Diagnosis

Base the diagnosis on the clinical signs and breed. Perform a complete ophthalmic examination to detect other congenital ocular abnormalities.

Treatment

There is no treatment required and the lesion is nonprogressive. Council breeders about possible inheritance and discourage breeding of affected dogs.

Uveal Hypoplasia/Aniridia

A lack of complete development or absence of the affected portion of the uvea, iris hypoplasia, or aniridia is rare and usually associated with other congenital ocular abnormalities. Choroidal coloboma occurs in several breeds of dogs and is seen as part of CEA.

UVEAL CYST

Etiology

Uveal cysts arise from the posterior iris or ciliary body and can remain attached or break free and float in the anterior chamber. They arise as a primary disorder in certain breeds (golden retriever, Boston terrier) or can be secondary to anterior uveitis.

Clinical Signs

Uveal cysts are pigmented, attached to the posterior iris, or free-floating in the anterior chamber. They can rupture, depositing on the ventral corneal endothelium or anterior lens capsule. In dogs, iris cysts will transilluminate, facilitating diagnosis. In cats, however, cysts are more densely pigmented, often remain attached, and may not transilluminate, making diagnosis more difficult.

Diagnosis

Base the diagnosis on the clinical signs and breed. A free-floating, pigmented mass that transilluminates is a cyst. If the mass remains attached or fails to transilluminate, it must be distinguished from a uveal melanoma. Use ocular ultrasound to demonstrate the hollow appearance of a cyst and distinguish between a cyst and a melanoma.

Treatment

If the cyst is not interfering with vision, no treatment is required. Large or multiple cysts may require treatment if vision becomes impaired. In addition, in cats, large cysts can be associated with an increase in intraocular pressure, requiring intervention. Treatment includes mechanical aspiration of the cyst from the anterior chamber or diode or Nd:YAG laser photoablation of the cyst, resulting in the rupture and/or resorption of the cyst.

IRIS ATROPHY

Etiology

Iris atrophy is seen most often in aged animals, especially toy breed dogs and cats. Iris atrophy has been classified as primary, senile, and secondary. *Primary iris atrophy* is seen in Siamese cats, miniature schnauzers, poodles, and Chihuahuas. This is a slow progressive atrophy of the iris. *Senile iris atrophy* occurs in aged animals of all species and breeds. The distinction between these two forms of atrophy may not be significant. *Secondary iris atrophy* occurs as a sequela to chronic glaucoma, uveitis, or ocular trauma.

Clinical Signs

If the iris musculature is affected, the pupillary light response may be incomplete or absent and anisocoria may be noted. Atrophy of the pupil margin results in dyscoria. Thinning of the iris stroma appears as a focal color change or, if complete, as a hole in the iris.

Diagnosis

The diagnosis is made based on the clinical appearance and signalment. The differential diagnosis includes other internal or external causes of dyscoria, anisocoria, incomplete pupillary light response, or iris color changes. Measurement of intraocular pressure, a complete ophthalmic examination, and determination of afferent vs. efferent pupil response abnormalities are all indicated with iris atrophy (see Chap. 160).

Treatment

No treatment is required. However, differentiate iris atrophy from other pupillary response abnormalities.

ANTERIOR UVEITIS

Uveitis is inflammation of the uvea and is divided into anterior (iris and ciliary body), posterior (choroid), and panuveitis (all three portions of the uvea). Posterior uveitis is often called chorioretinitis because of the intimate association between the choroid and retina (see Chap. 157). Anterior uveitis is associated with pain and can be the result of both ocular and systemic factors. Because many etiologies of uveitis are systemic it is essential to ascertain the reason for the inflammation when presented with an animal with anterior or posterior uveitis (Table 155–1).

▼ *Key Point* If no primary ocular etiology of anterior uveitis can be ascertained, consider systemic disease. This approach applies whether the uveitis is unilateral or bilateral.

Etiology

Corneal Ulceration

Corneal ulceration often results in reflex anterior uveitis. Uveitis occurs due to stimulation of the ophthalmic branch of cranial nerve 5 (CN5) and does not indicate infectious keratitis.

Trauma

Trauma can result in anterior uveitis due to a direct penetration of the globe or a concussive effect. Uveitis may be associated with other ophthalmic abnormalities, such as corneal ulceration, hyphema, lens luxation, retinal detachment, proptosis, and globe rupture. See appropriate chapters for further discussion of these abnormalities.

Infection

Infectious causes of anterior uveitis are numerous and include bacteria, fungi, rickettsia, and protozoal organisms (see Table 155–1). These organisms result in anterior uveitis by direct infections of the eye, immune-mediated responses, or circulating endotoxins. Many of these infectious agents also cause posterior segment (retina, choroid) involvement (see Chap. 157). Direct infection of the eye can occur from penetrating trauma or blood-borne infection. Although anterior uveitis is commonly associated with infectious causes, the organism itself is generally not present within the anterior segment of the eye.

Lens-Induced Anterior Uveitis

Lens-induced anterior uveitis results from traumatic rupture of the lens capsule or from leakage of the lens material through an intact capsule as noted with a hypermature cataract. Lens protein is antigenic and, if released, will result in mild-to-severe anterior uveitis. Cataracts are discussed in Chapter 154.

Autoimmune Anterior Uveitis

Autoimmune anterior uveitis, unassociated with lens protein leakage, is observed in the uveodermatologic syndrome (formerly Vogt-Koyanagi-Harada syndrome or VKH). This syndrome is observed in dogs and results in anterior and posterior uveitis, poliosis (depigmentation of the hair), and vitiligo (depigmentation of the skin). See Chapter 43 for discussion of the dermatologic manifestations.

Clinical Signs (Table 155–2)

- *Miosis* is a smaller than normal pupil due to contraction of the iris sphincter muscle. Spasm of the iris sphincter muscle, along with the ciliary body musculature, results in pain, noted clinically as photophobia (intolerance of light).
- *Flare* results from a breakdown in the blood-aqueous humor barrier and a subsequent leakage of plasma protein (with or without cells) into the eye. It is observed clinically as a haze in the anterior chamber (Fig. 155–1).
- *Hypotony* is a decrease in the intraocular pressure below the normal range of 15–25 mm Hg—due to decrease in the production of aqueous humor.
- *Cells* are released into the anterior chamber in severe uveitis. The inflammatory cellular response can be polymorphonuclear or granulomatous. In addition, red blood cells (hyphema) or neoplastic cells can enter the anterior chamber. Cells can appear suspended in the aqueous humor, settled in the ventral anterior chamber (hypopyon), or as keratitic precipitates.

Table 155–1. SYSTEMIC INFECTIOUS ETIOLOGIES OF ANTERIOR UVEITIS*

Mycotic
  Blastomycosis, cryptococcosis, histoplasmosis, coccidioidomycosis, aspergillosis, others
Rickettsial
  Ehrlichiosis, Rocky Mountain spotted fever
Toxoplasmosis
Feline infectious peritonitis (FIP), feline immunodeficiency virus (FIV), feline leukemia virus (FeLV)
Lyme disease
Bacteremia/septicemia
Bartonella spp.
Brucellosis
Aberrant parasitic migration
  Heartworm, roundworm, hookworm, others
Canine distemper
Infectious canine hepatitis
Prototheosis
Mycobacteriosis
Leptospirosis
Leishmaniasis

*For a description of each disease see the appropriate chapters.

Table 155–2. CLINICAL SIGNS OF ANTERIOR UVEITIS

Discharge (serous, mucoid)	Redness
Blepharospasm	Photophobia
Miosis	Hypotony
Corneal edema	Aqueous flare
Keratitic precipitates	Hyphema
Hypopyon	Blindness

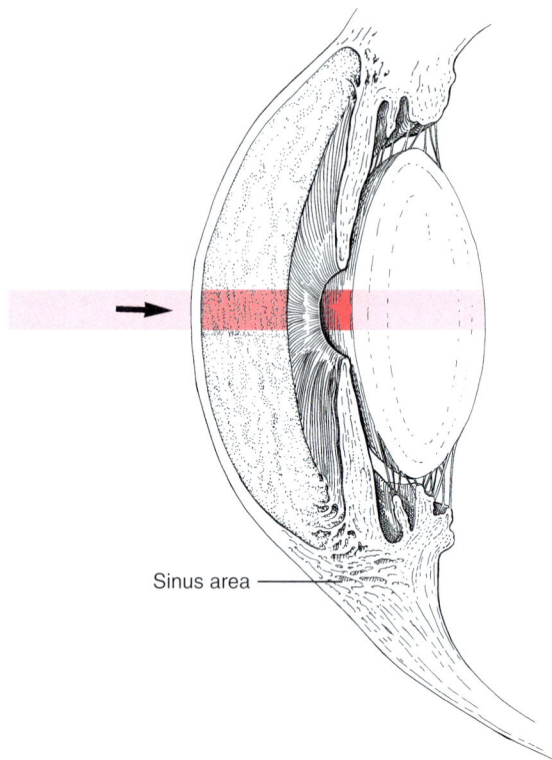

Figure 155–1. Using a bright, focused light source, aqueous flare is seen as a continuation of the light beam through the normally dark-appearing anterior chamber.

Keratitic precipitates appear as focal deposits on the ventral corneal endothelium. They are associated with a granulomatous uveitis and are accumulations of protein, macrophages, and lymphocytes and plasma cells. In the dog they are most often seen in association with lens-induced uveitis or disseminated mycosis and in cats in association with feline infectious peritonitis or toxoplasmosis.

- *Hyperemia* or redness may be seen on examination of the conjunctival, episcleral, and iris blood vessels in eyes with anterior uveitis.
- *Corneal edema,* associated with anterior uveitis, occurs from endothelial cell dysfunction/loss and is diffuse in nature. Diffuse corneal edema indicates intraocular disease and the need for measurement of intraocular pressure. If the edema is of a focal nature the cornea should be stained with fluorescein to rule out a corneal ulcer with secondary anterior uveitis.

Diagnosis

History

A complete *history* is essential to detect previous or concurrent problems that may be associated with anterior uveitis. The history includes both ophthalmic and systemic problems.

Physical Examination

Complete physical examination is an essential part of the diagnostic evaluation of a patient with anterior uveitis. Palpate all external lymph nodes, auscultate the car-diopulmonary system, palpate the abdomen, and determine the body temperature.

Penlight Examination

A *penlight examination* is performed to evaluate pupil size, symmetry, and response to light. Assess the severity and character of the uveitis by the degree of aqueous flare and the cellular response. Assess the clarity of the clear media of the eye, cornea, aqueous humor, lens, and vitreous. Evaluation of flare requires a bright focal light source, and a Finoff transilluminator works well for this purpose. All abnormalities are described and diagramed in the medical record.

Tonometry

Tonometry is the determination of the intraocular pressure (IOP). Eyes with anterior uveitis have a decreased IOP (hypotony). A normal or elevated IOP indicates the potential for, or the presence of, glaucoma. While previous recommendations suggested the Schiøtz tonometer was the most cost-effective tonometer for private practice, the Tonopen (Dan Scott and Associates) is a more portable, accurate, and user-friendly tonometer and will result in more frequent and more accurate intraocular pressure readings. It is also easier to use on painful eyes (see Chap. 156).

▼ *Key Point* The clinical signs of anterior uveitis and glaucoma can be similar. Both diseases can be present together in the same eye. Determination of IOP is therefore essential.

Fundic Examination

Perform *fundic examination,* either by direct or indirect ophthalmoscopy, to determine the presence or absence of posterior segment involvement. Anterior uveitis in combination with posterior uveitis is termed panuveitis and is strongly suggestive of systemic disease, especially those infectious in nature (see Table 155–1). Posterior segment changes indicating active inflammation include retinal hemorrhage, retinal detachment, vasculitis, and infiltration by granulomatous or neoplastic cells. If the posterior lesions are chronic, they will appear as tapetal hyper-reflectivity, pigment clumping and depigmentation of the nontapetal region, and atrophy of the retinal vasculature (see Chap. 157).

Fluorescein Stain of Cornea

Perform *fluorescein stain* to examine for a corneal ulcer. Corneal ulcers can result in a secondary anterior uveitis. If detected, the ulcer must be characterized with regards to depth, severity, and infection (see Chap. 153). In addition, determine the etiology and treat appropriately. Anterior uveitis, resulting from a corneal ulcer, resolves once the ulcer is healed.

Routine Laboratory Tests and Radiography

- Perform *biochemical profile, urinalysis,* and *complete blood count* on all patients with anterior uveitis of unknown cause and patients with concomitant systemic abnormalities.

- Perform *serology,* for the specific infectious diseases listed in Table 155–1, as indicated by the findings of the history, physical examination, ophthalmic examination, biochemical profile, urinalysis, and complete blood count.
- *Radiograph* the thorax and abdomen to evaluate for systemic mycosis, disseminated neoplasia, or other organ system involvement.

Cytology

- *Cytology* of intraocular or extraocular samples may be indicated in selected instances. Intraocular samples include both the aqueous and vitreous humors. Of these, the vitreous humor sample is the most diagnostic but also the most traumatic to obtain. Anterior chamber samples are frequently not diagnostic. The indication for vitreocentesis is panuveitis in a blind eye for which the diagnosis cannot be obtained by alternate methods.
  - Using general anesthesia, insert a 20-gauge needle 4–5 mm posterior to the corneal-scleral junction superior-temporally.
  - Direct the needle toward the center of the eye and aspirate 0.5–1.0 ml of fluid for culture and cytology.

- Extraocular cytology includes aspirates of regional lymph nodes or mass lesions.

Treatment

The treatment of anterior uveitis includes nonspecific approaches directed toward decreasing the inflammation and sequelae and specific ones directed toward eliminating the underlying etiology when one has been identified (Table 155–3).

Mydriatic-Cycloplegics

Use *mydriatic-cycloplegics* to paralyze the iris sphincter and ciliary body musculature. This effect will decrease the pain associated with anterior uveitis and the tendency toward formation of posterior synechia. The mydriatic-cycloplegic of choice is topical 1% atropine (parasympatholytic). Administer atropine to effect (pupil dilation) but not to exceed a treatment frequency of four times per day. This results in maximum drug effects with minimal side effects.

▼ *Key Point* Atropine is contraindicated in anterior uveitis when accompanied by secondary glaucoma.

Table 155–3. DOSAGES OF COMMONLY USED OCULAR ANTI-INFLAMMATORY AGENTS

Drugs	Trade Names	Dosages
Topical		
Corticosteroids		
1.0% Prednisolone acetate suspension	Econopred Plus	1–6×/d
0.1% Dexamethasone solution	Decadron	1–6×/d
0.05% Dexamethasone ointment	Decadron	1–6×/d
NSAIDs		
0.03% Flurbiprofen	Ocufen	4×/d
1.0% Suprofen	Profenal	4×/d
Atropine		
1.0% Atropine		1–4×/d
Systemic		
Corticosteroids		
Prednisolone/prednisone		*Dog*
Immunosuppressive		1.0 mg/kg PO q12h × 7–14 d, then taper
Anti-inflammatory		0.5 mg/kg PO q12h × 3–5 d, then taper
NSAIDs		
Acetylsalicylic acid	Aspirin	*Dog*
		10–25 mg/kg PO q12h
		Cat
		80 mg PO q48–72h
Flunixin meglumine	Banamine	*Dog*
		0.25–0.5 mg/kg IV single dose
		Cat
		Do not use
Phenylbutazone	Butazolidin	*Dog*
		13 mg/kg PO q8h × 48 h, then taper
		Cat
		10–14 mg/kg PO q12h
Immunosuppressive		
Azathioprine	Imuran	*Dog*
		2.2 mg/kg PO q48h, then taper
Cyclophosphamide	Cytoxan	*Dog*
		50 mg/m^2 PO q24h × 4 d/wk

Topical Anti-Inflammatory Drugs

Topical anti-inflammatory drugs include both corticosteroids and nonsteroidal agents (see Table 155–3). Topical medication does not penetrate beyond the iris and ciliary body. Use only for problems of the anterior segment of the eye.

Corticosteroids

The topical corticosteroid of choice for the treatment of anterior uveitis is 1% prednisolone acetate ophthalmic suspension (Econopred). This agent achieves the highest intraocular level of the ophthalmic corticosteroids. If unavailable, 0.1% dexamethasone solution or 0.05% dexamethasone ointment can be applied. The frequency of treatment varies according to the severity of the uveitis, ranging from one to six times a day.

▼ *Key Point* Topical corticosteroids delay healing and potentiate infection and collagenase ulceration. Topical corticosteroids are contraindicated for anterior uveitis associated with corneal ulceration.

Topical corticosteroids are also absorbed systemically and alter adrenal and hepatic function.

Nonsteroidal

The indications for topical nonsteroidal anti-inflammatory ophthalmic drugs are similar to those for topical corticosteroids. They are used as supplements to topical corticosteroids or as substitutes when topical corticosteroids are contraindicated (e.g., in diabetes mellitus). As with topical corticosteroids, nonsteroidal agents may delay the healing of a corneal ulcer. Administer four times a day.

Systemic Anti-Inflammatory Drugs

Systemic anti-inflammatory drugs include corticosteroids, nonsteroidal agents, and immunosuppressive drugs (see Table 155–3).

Corticosteroids

Systemic corticosteroids are indicated in the management of noninfectious posterior uveitis and in severe anterior uveitis as a supplement to topical corticosteroids. The dosage is dependent upon the underlying disease. An immunosuppressive dose is indicated for animals with uveodermatologic syndrome and an anti-inflammatory dose is indicated for most other cases (see Table 155–3). The side effects of systemic corticosteroids include polyphagia/polyuria/polydyspia, infection potentiation, altered carbohydrate metabolism, and adrenal suppression. Therapy with systemic corticosteroids begins at a high dose to achieve a response followed by a tapered dose to maintain effect and to decrease adverse side effects.

Nonsteroidal

Systemic nonsteroidal anti-inflammatory drugs (NSAIDs) include aspirin, flunixin meglumine, phenylbutazone, carprofen, and others. They are indicated to decrease inflammation and facilitate pupil dilation. In small animal ophthalmology, flunixin meglumine is administered as a single dose (0.25–0.5 mg/kg IV) prior to ocular surgery to decrease postsurgical ocular inflammation. If prolonged therapy with NSAIDs is required, aspirin is the drug of choice. Side effects of NSAIDs include gastrointestinal ulceration and hemorrhage and acute renal papillary necrosis. Systemic NSAIDs are not used in combination with systemic corticosteroids and must be used with caution in patients with questionable renal function.

Immunosuppressive Drugs

Systemic immunosuppressive therapy may be required when animals fail to respond to corticosteroids or NSAIDs or when the required levels of these drugs result in systemic toxicity.

Specific

Specific therapy is dependent upon the etiology of the uveitis. See appropriate chapters for treatment of the systemic diseases that cause anterior uveitis.

Sequelae

- *Secondary glaucoma* results from the obstruction of the outflow pathway of the aqueous humor. This can occur at the pupil from posterior synechia, at the drainage angle from anterior synechia, or in the trabecular meshwork from deposits of inflammatory debris and fibrosis. Control of this type of secondary glaucoma through medical therapy is often extremely difficult to achieve (see Chap. 156).
- *Synechiae* are adhesions from the iris to adjacent structures, such as the cornea or lens. Synechiae can result in abnormal pupillary light response, misshapen pupil, glaucoma, pigmentation of the cornea or lens, and blindness.
- *Cataracts* can occur subsequent to anterior uveitis. The lens is dependent upon the aqueous humor for nutrients and waste product removal. Anterior uveitis results in altered lens metabolism and a buildup of inflammatory by-products that may cause opacification of the lens and capsule (cataract) (see Chap. 154).
- *Corneal edema* occurs from the failure of the corneal endothelial cell pump/barrier. Corneal endothelial cells are responsible for the maintenance of corneal deturgesence, which is essential to corneal transparency. Endothelial cells need the aqueous humor for nutrients and waste product removal. Anterior uveitis may alter the function of these cells, resulting in diffuse corneal edema. Corneal endothelial cells in the adult dog and cat have little regenerative capabilities, thus damage may be permanent.

- *Blindness* secondary to severe anterior uveitis is common and results from secondary glaucoma, cataract formation, synechia, pigment migration, or posterior segment (retina, choroid) changes.
- *Phthisis bulbi* occurs as a result of atrophy of the ciliary body and a sustained decrease in aqueous humor production. Chronic hypotony (i.e., low IOP) results, and the eye decreases in size.

Prevention

Although prevention of anterior uveitis is usually not possible, the sequelae of anterior uveitis can be prevented by accurate diagnosis and appropriate and rapid treatment. Therapy directed towards the etiology will not only aid the management of the ocular disease but may also prevent the serious and life-threatening complications of the systemic disease.

UVEAL NEOPLASIA

Uveal neoplasms can be primary or secondary. Primary neoplasms include iris, ciliary body and choroidal melanomas, and ciliary body adenoma/adenocarcinoma. Secondary neoplasms include lymphoma and metastatic carcinomas (most common), or any disseminated neoplasm. Intraocular neoplasms result in damage to the eye through displacement of normal ocular structures, causing lens luxation, dyscoria, and retinal detachment. In addition to an intraocular mass lesion, glaucoma, uveitis, and hyphema are the most common presenting signs of intraocular neoplasia. In general, secondary neoplasms are more inflammatory and destructive as compared to primary neoplasms.

Primary Neoplasia

Of the primary neoplasms, anterior uveal melanoma is most common. Tumor behavior varies depending on the species.

Canine Melanoma

Canine anterior uveal melanomas are generally benign in nature with less than 5% metastatic potential. In addition, it appears that Labrador and golden retrievers and German shepherds may be predisposed to iridal melanomas. In these breeds the neoplasm may arise in a juvenile dog, and a suggestion of inheritance has been proposed. The best criterion for predicting malignancy of intraocular melanoma in the dog appears to be the mitotic index.

Feline Melanoma

In contrast to the dog, feline uveal melanoma has been reported to metastasize in 60% of affected cats. Pigmented lesions of the feline iris or ciliary body, especially those that are raised, displacing adjacent structures or resulting in other intraocular damage, should be removed by enucleation. In addition, perform a complete systemic evaluation including thoracic and abdominal radiographs and palpation of regional lymph nodes. No information exists to suggest that enucleation of these affected eyes affects the rate of metastasis, favorably or unfavorably.

Feline Spindle Cell Sarcoma

Intraocular spindle cell sarcoma can occur in the feline eye as a sequela to ocular trauma or uveitis. The period following ocular trauma or uveitis to the time of diagnosis of intraocular spindle cell sarcoma varies from 5 months to 12 years. These tumors are locally invasive, extending transsclerally or traveling along the optic nerve, and have the potential for metastasis. Enucleation or possibly orbital exenteration is the treatment of choice. Consider enucleation of severely traumatized or chronically inflamed, blind feline eyes to avoid the possible development of an intraocular spindle cell sarcoma.

Other Tumors

In addition to primary intraocular melanoma, ciliary body adenoma and adenocarcinoma, hemangiosarcoma, and astrocytoma have been reported in the dog and cat. These are often slow to metastasize, but can cause intraocular damage as they enlarge.

Treatment

The treatment of primary ocular neoplasms varies according to the species, location, and severity of the neoplasm, rate of progression, presence or absence of vision, intraocular pressure, and availability of treatment modalities. Enucleation, excisional biopsy with preservation of the globe and/or vision, and laser ablation are all used for primary intraocular neoplasms. Small masses with no associated secondary complications can be documented, followed, and then treated if found to be progressive. In addition, an en bloc excision in the form of a sector iridectomy or iridocyclectomy can be used to excise a mass, preserve vision, and obtain a biopsy. This is a referral procedure. Laser surgery is used most often for pigmented melanomas and uses a diode or Nd:YAG laser to achieve a thermal effect resulting in coagulation necrosis of the tumor mass.

Secondary Neoplasia

Lymphoma is the most common intraocular neoplasm in the dog and cat. In addition, adenocarcinoma, hemangiosarcoma, and several other neoplasms metastasize to the eye. The most common ocular abnormalities seen in association with secondary neoplasms include glaucoma, uveitis, hyphema, retinal detachment, and lens luxation. Treatment should be directed at finding the primary source of the neoplasia followed by systemic therapy including chemotherapy, surgery, and radiation. Additional therapy might include topical ophthalmic anti-inflammatory drugs and atropine for uveitis or topical and systemic medications aimed at reducing the intraocular pressure if secondary glaucoma is present. Topical therapy is often unrewarding.

Systemic treatment of the primary problem usually results in a greater ocular response. If the eye is painful, blind, or nonresponsive to systemic treatment, perform enucleation.

SUPPLEMENTAL READINGS

Blouin P: Uveitis in the dog and cat: Causes, diagnosis, and treatment. Can Vet J 25:315, 1984.

Crispin SM: Uveitis in the dog and cat. J Small Anim Pract 29:429, 1988.

Martin CL: Ocular signs of systemic disease. Mod Vet Pract 689, 799, 1982.

Morgan RV: Vogt-Koyanagi-Harada syndrome in humans and dogs. Compend Cont Ed Pract Vet 11:1211, 1989.

Patnaik AK, Mooney S: Feline melanoma: A comparative study of ocular, oral, and dermal neoplasms. Vet Pathol 25:105, 1988.

Peiffer RL: Inherited ocular diseases of the dog and cat. Compend Cont Ed Pract Vet 4:152, 1982.

Swanson JF: Uveitis. In Kirk RW, ed.: Current Veterinary Therapy X. Philadelphia: WB Saunders, 1989, pp 652–655.

Wilcock BP, Peiffer RL: The pathology of lens-induced uveitis. Vet Pathol 24:549, 1987.

Wilcock BP, Peiffer RL: Morphology and behavior of primary ocular melanomas in 91 dogs. Vet Pathol 23:418, 1986.

156 Glaucoma

David A. Wilkie

Glaucoma is an increase in the intraocular pressure (IOP) beyond that compatible with maintenance of normal ocular physiology and function.

ANATOMY

See Chapter 150.

ETIOLOGY

Primary Glaucoma

Primary glaucoma is not associated with any other event or problem within the eye. It is usually breed related and often hereditary in nature. A list of predisposed breeds is given in Table 156–1.

▼ *Key Point* When glaucoma is primary, the opposite, unaffected eye may also develop glaucoma. Studies indicate an incidence of 50% involvement of the contralateral eye within 2 years following the diagnosis of glaucoma in the first eye.

Secondary Glaucoma

Secondary glaucoma is the result of an antecedent event within the eye. The etiologies of secondary glaucoma include anterior uveitis, anterior lens luxation, hyphema, intraocular neoplasia, chronic retinal detachment, preiridal fibrovascular membrane, and trauma.

- *Anterior uveitis* can cause glaucoma through obstruction of the flow of aqueous humor. This results from peripheral anterior or posterior synechiae or from inflammatory debris in the iridocorneal angle. Anterior uveitis is discussed in Chapter 155.
- *Anterior lens luxation* can obstruct the flow of aqueous humor from the posterior to the anterior chamber or to the iridocorneal angle. The etiologies of anterior lens luxation include hereditary (in terriers), intraocular neoplasia, anterior uveitis, and trauma (see Chap. 154). Anterior lens luxation can also result from chronic glaucoma with enlargement of the globe (buphthalmos) and tearing of the lens zonules.
- *Intraocular neoplasia,* whether primary or secondary, can block the flow of aqueous humor through shedding of neoplastic cells into the iridocorneal angle or displacing of normal intraocular structures (see Chap. 155).
- *Hyphema* can result from trauma, systemic hypertension, congenital ocular anomalies, vascular disorders, or bleeding disorders (see Chap. 155). Red blood cells can obstruct the trabecular meshwork of the iridocorneal angle resulting in ghost cell glaucoma.
- *Trauma* can result in anterior uveitis, anterior lens luxation, hyphema, or damage to the iridocorneal angle, all of which may lead to secondary glaucoma.
- *Retinal detachment,* when chronic, may be associated with proliferation of a preiridal fibrovascular membrane arising from the anterior iris stroma and resulting in anterior and posterior synechiae and iridocorneal angle obstruction. Chronic uveitis and intraocular neoplasia can result in a similar change.

CLINICAL SIGNS

- *Acute glaucoma* is a true medical and ultimately a surgical emergency. The diagnosis is made based on history and clinical signs (Table 156–2). If in doubt, err on the side of a diagnosis of acute rather than chronic glaucoma.
- *Chronic glaucoma* implies ophthalmic changes that cause the irreversible loss of vision (Table 156–3).

Table 156–1. BREEDS PREDISPOSED TO PRIMARY GLAUCOMA

American and English cocker spaniel
English springer spaniel
Welsh springer spaniel
Miniature poodle
Beagle
Basset hound
Siberian husky
Norwegian elkhound
Samoyed
Malamute
Chow chow
Afghan
Akita
Cairn terrier
Dalmation
Bouvier des Flandres
Shar-Pei
Other

Table 156–2. CLINICAL SIGNS OF ACUTE GLAUCOMA

Episcleral hyperemia
Diffuse corneal edema
Dilated pupil
Slow-to-absent pupillary light response
Weak-to-absent menace response
Epiphora
Blepharospasm

The clinical changes most indicative of chronic glaucoma are retinal and optic nerve degeneration and buphthalmos.

DIAGNOSIS

▼ *Key Point* Although the history, breed, and clinical signs are all important in the diagnosis of glaucoma, definitive diagnosis can be made only through measurement of the IOP.

IOP measurement requires a tonometer. Digital tonometry is an inaccurate and unreliable method of IOP determination. While previous recommendations suggested the Schiøtz tonometer was the most cost-effective tonometer for private practice, the Tonopen (Mentor O&O, Inc.) is a more portable, accurate, and user-friendly tonometer and will result in more frequent and more accurate intraocular pressure readings. This in turn will improve the veterinarian's ability to make an early diagnosis and more accurately assess response to treatment (see Chap. 150). The Tonopen is lightweight, portable, accurate, self-calibrating, and averages several readings and gives a percentage error to ensure accuracy. In addition, the small footplate allows this tonometer to be used on painful eyes in less cooperative patients because only a small area of cornea is required to obtain a reading, and the position of the patient's head is not related to obtaining the reading. Normal IOP in the dog and cat is 15–25 mm Hg.

Once the diagnosis of glaucoma is made based on IOP, establish the etiology (i.e., primary vs. secondary) and the degree of ocular damage. Depending on the history and associated ocular changes, the glaucoma can be classified as either acute or chronic.

Table 156–3. CLINICAL SIGNS OF CHRONIC GLAUCOMA

Episcleral hyperemia
Diffuse corneal edema
Corneal striae
Dilated pupil
Absent pupillary light response
Absent menace response
Epiphora
Blepharospasm
Retinal degeneration
Optic nerve cupping
Buphthalmia

TREATMENT

▼ *Key Point* In order to treat glaucoma appropriately, answer two specific questions (Fig. 156–1). Is the glaucoma primary or secondary? Is the glaucoma acute or chronic?

Treatment can be grouped into medical and surgical approaches. If the glaucoma is acute, a return of a portion of, or all of, the animal's vision is then possible. In acute glaucoma, immediate aggressive medical therapy is required to reduce the IOP to within normal range. Failure of medical therapy to lower and maintain IOP at a normal level indicates the need for surgical intervention and the possible referral to a veterinary ophthalmologist.

The most appropriate treatment for chronic glaucoma is surgery, the goal of which is to reduce the IOP in order to relieve discomfort. Medical therapy of chronic glaucoma is neither effective nor cost effective over time. The surgery of choice is either placement of an intraocular silicone prosthesis or an enucleation.

Intravitreal injection of gentamicin or lidofovir (Vistide) designed to destroy the intraocular tissues is used by some to reduce intraocular pressure. This results in uveitis, cataract, and often phthisis bulbi and is cosmetically unappealing and unpredictable.

Medical

Medical therapy of acute glaucoma includes some, or possibly all, of the following agents (Table 156–4). The decision as to which medications to choose varies according to the severity of the glaucoma, the etiology, and the response to the initial therapy.

Osmotic Drugs

- *Osmotic agents* act to dehydrate the vitreous and aqueous humors and thereby decrease the IOP. In order to be effective, they require an intact blood-eye barrier and therefore may not work well in eyes with uveitis or hyphema.

▼ *Key Point* The initial drug of choice for rapidly decreasing IOP in the treatment of acute glaucoma is an osmotic agent. The osmotic agent of choice is 20% mannitol, administered intravenously (see Table 156–4).

- Water is withheld from the animal for 3–4 hours following osmotic administration. The IOP begins decreasing within 20 minutes, with the maximum effect at 2 hours—the duration of effect is approximately 6 hours. An alternative osmotic agent is oral glycerin, but emesis is a frequent side effect.

Carbonic Anhydrase Inhibitors

- *Carbonic anhydrase inhibitors* (CAIs) work to decrease the IOP by blocking the enzyme responsible for the active production of aqueous humor. The systemic CAIs of choice, based on their efficacy and low

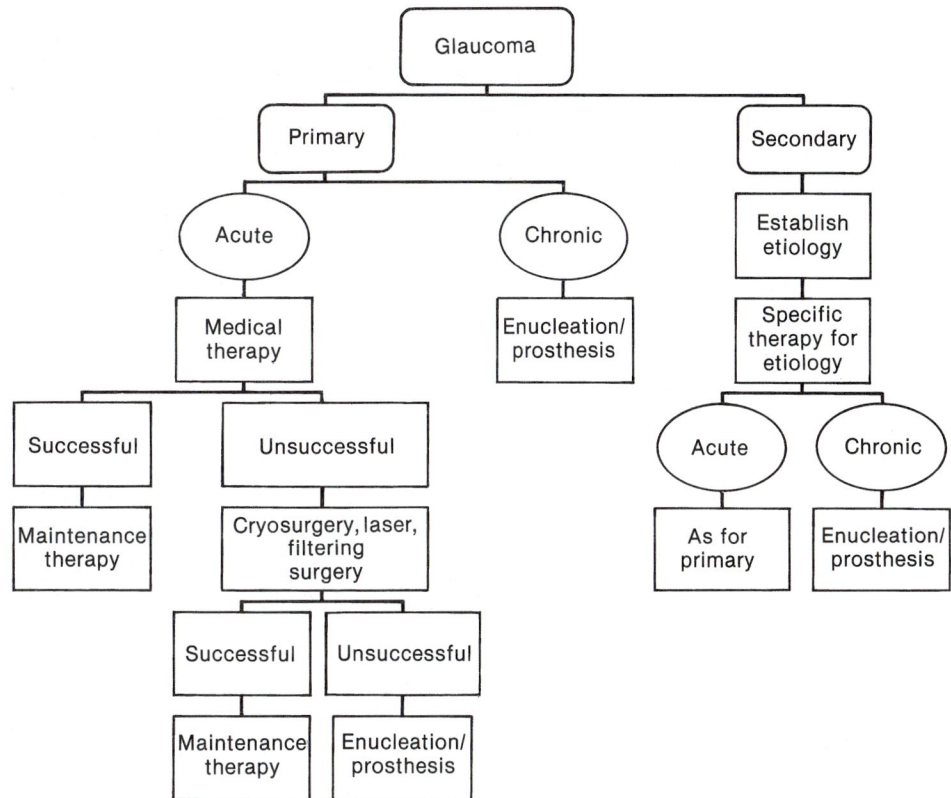

Figure 156–1. Treatment algorithm for glaucoma.

frequency of side effects, are dichlorphenamide and methazolamide. These are administered orally q8–12h (see Table 156–4).

- In addition to the eye, carbonic anhydrase can be found in the kidney, red blood cells, and lungs. Po-

tential side effects of oral carbonic anhydrase inhibitors include metabolic acidosis and hypokalemia, manifested as panting, depression, vomiting, diarrhea, and collapse. If any of these side effects are noted, CAI therapy is discontinued. Symptoms

Table 156–4. MEDICAL TREATMENT OF ACUTE GLAUCOMA

Drug/Concentration	Trade Name	Dose
Systemic		
Osmotic drugs		
Mannitol		0.5–1.0 g/kg IV
Carbonic anhydrase inhibitors		
Dichlorphenamide	Daranide	2–4 mg/kg, q8–12h PO
Methazolamide	Neptazane	2–4 mg/kg, q8–12h PO
Topical		
Carbonic anhydrase inhibitors		
Dorzolamide 2%	Trusopt	q8–12h
Parasympathomimetics		
Pilocarpine 2%	Isopto Carpine	q8–12h
Demecarium bromide		
0.125%/0.25%	Humorsol	q12–24h
Sympathomimetics		
Epinephrine 1–2%	Epifrin	q8–12h
Dipivefrin HCl 0.1%	Propine	q8–12h
Alpha-2 agonists		
Apraclonidine 0.5%	Iopidine	q12–24h
Brimonidine 0.2%	Alphagan	q12–24h
Combination		
Pilocarpine 2%: epinephrine 1%	E-Pilo-2	q8–12h
Dorzolamide: timolol maleate	Cosopt	q8–12h
Sympatholytics		
Timolol maleate 0.5%	Timoptic	q8–12h
Prostaglandins		
Latanoprost 0.005%	Xalatan	q12–24h

should resolve within 24 hours, and therapy can be reinstituted at a decreased dosage.

- A topical CAI, dorzolamide 2% (Trusopt, Merck & Co.), is also available. Administer q8–12 h; this drug does not cause the systemic side effects seen with oral CAI administration. Topical CAIs are indicated for treatment of glaucoma and have also become the drug of choice for prophylactic treatment of the contralateral eye.

Autonomic Drugs

- *Autonomic agents* include parasympathomimetics, sympathomimetics, and sympatholytics. All of these drugs are administered topically q8–12h (see Table 156–4). These drugs are synergistic and can, if needed, be applied to the same eye, provided their administration is 5–10 minutes apart.

Parasympathomimetics

- *Parasympathomimetics* result in contraction of the iris sphincter and ciliary body musculature. Contraction of the longitudinal ciliary musculature increases the outflow of aqueous humor. In addition, parasympathomimetics result in vasodilation of the conjunctiva and increased aqueous humor protein and may reactivate or exacerbate iritis.
- The parasympathomimetic of choice is 2% pilocarpine (see Table 156–4). Transient topical irritation is often exhibited following administration but resolves 24–48 hours following initiation of therapy. An alternative parasympathomimetic is demecarium bromide (Humorsol), a potent and long-acting cholinesterase inhibitor. This has the advantage of once daily administration.
- Parasympathomimetics are contraindicated in animals with active anterior uveitis that results in secondary glaucoma. Parasympathomimetics exacerbate the pain and symptoms of anterior uveitis.

Sympathomimetics

- *Sympathomimetics* increase the outflow of aqueous humor. Their mechanism of action differs from that of the parasympathomimetics and the two are synergistic.
- The sympathomimetic agent of choice is 0.1% dipivefrin HCl (Propine), a prodrug of epinephrine (see Table 156–4). Alternately, 1.0% epinephrine HCl can be administered either alone or in combination with 2% pilocarpine (E-Pilo-2).
- Side effects are minimal and include mild topical irritation, which is avoided with the use of 0.1% dipivefrin HCl.

Sympatholytics

- *Sympatholytics* decrease the active production of aqueous humor.
- The sympatholytic agent of choice is a nonselective beta-blocking agent, 0.5% timolol maleate (Timoptic). Although disagreement exists over the efficacy of topical timolol maleate in small animal patients, information indicates that it has some IOP-lowering ability. Side effects have not been observed in small animals, but potentially systemic absorption could cause bronchoconstriction and bradycardia, both of which are side effects in humans.
- New topical alpha-2 adrenoreceptor agonists, apraclonidine 0.5% and brimonidine tartrate 0.2%, serve to lower IOP by reducing the formation of aqueous humor and in addition, in the case of brimonidine, increasing uveoscleral outflow. Apraclonidine may also result in mydriasis in the dog and miosis in the cat. Both of these drugs have been associated with side effects such as bradycardia, vomiting, and even death, especially in cats.

Prostaglandins

Prostaglandins, administered topically in low concentration, have been found to lower IOP by increasing uveoscleral outflow. They are very species specific and while they appear to have efficacy in veterinary species, the work is still preliminary. Side effects in humans include iris hyperpigmentation and conjunctival and facial irritation.

Plan of Action for Medical Treatment

When presented with a patient with acute glaucoma, administer mannitol first, followed by maintenance therapy with an oral or topical CAI and topical pilocarpine, provided no contraindications for these medications are present. Monitor IOP every 2–4 hours for the next 24 hours. If, following the initial reduction in IOP with mannitol, the IOP increases and exceeds 30 mm Hg, repeat mannitol therapy. Medical therapy can be increased to include all of the aforementioned topical medications. When administering multiple topical medications, space each treatment 5 minutes apart. The failure of this aggressive, maximal therapy to lower and maintain IOP within the normal range indicates the need for surgical intervention (see following section).

In addition to therapy aimed at lowering IOP, attention is now focused on the resulting reperfusion injury that occurs to the retinal ganglion cells and axons of the optic nerve following rapid reduction of IOP. Newer therapies used in conjunction with pressure reduction are being examined and include calcium channel blocking agents, corticosteroids, and other potentially neuroprotective agents.

Surgical
Cyclocryosurgery

Cyclocryosurgery involves transscleral freezing of a portion of the ciliary body. This procedure selectively destroys an area of the ciliary processes, thereby decreasing the production of aqueous humor. It works best in conjunction with medical therapy and is indicated primarily in cases of acute glaucoma in which IOP is not effectively controlled with medical therapy alone.

Objectives

- Reduce the intraocular pressure to a level compatible with maintaining vision.
- Relieve the discomfort associated with glaucoma.

Equipment

- Liquid nitrogen *or* nitrous oxide cryogen unit with an ocular probe, 2.5 mm in diameter.

Technique

1. Place the anesthetized animal in lateral recumbency. Administer a single dose of systemic flunixin meglumine (Banamine) (0.25 mg/kg IV). Do not use systemic flunixin meglumine in combination with methoxyflurane anesthesia, because this may exacerbate its renal toxicity.
2. Use an eyelid speculum to obtain adequate exposure of the globe (Fig. 156–2).
3. Place the cryoprobe on the conjunctiva, 4–5 mm posterior to the limbus, in the superior or inferior temporal quadrant of the eye (see Fig. 156–2). Avoid the long posterior ciliary arteries found at the 3- and 9-o'clock positions.
4. Activate the cryoprobe and freeze the site. The actual freezing time varies according to the cryounit. Approximate freeze times and probe tip temperatures are for nitrous oxide, 2 minutes, −60 to −80°C, and for liquid nitrogen, until the ice ball extends 1 mm into the cornea (<30 seconds), −185°C.
5. Multiple sites are frozen. The number of freeze sites varies according to the severity of the glaucoma and the cryoprobe. In general, freeze four to eight sites with liquid nitrogen, fewer than are done with nitrous oxide.

Following surgery, monitor the IOP. Prescribe medical therapy for glaucoma, based on the response of the IOP to cryosurgery. Treat postoperative discomfort with oral nonsteroidal anti-inflammatory drugs, such as aspirin (10 mg/kg PO bid).

Transscleral Cyclophotocoagulation

This technique uses a contact or noncontact neodymium:yttrium-aluminum-garnet (Nd:YAG) or diode laser to deliver energy that destroys a portion of the ciliary body and reduces aqueous humor formation (Fig. 156–2). While the initial cost of these lasers is high, resulting in their being restricted to a referral-only procedure, the side effects are less than with cyclocryosurgery and the success is greater. The key to success appears to be early intervention, thus performing the cyclophotodestructive procedure prior to the development of acute congestive glaucoma. With the introduction of better prophylactic drugs and accurate IOP determination in practice using the Tonopen, early referral has become more common, with laser surgery performed at an IOP between 20 and 35 mm Hg. The procedure works best in these eyes and has minimal side effects. Postsurgical uveitis and a transient ocular hypertension are the most common side effects. Treatment of eyes with IOP greater than 50 mm Hg appears to be less effective for achieving long-term control. Cyclophotocoagulation should be used in conjunction with, not as a replacement for, medical therapy.

Filtering Procedures

These are designed to provide an alternate outflow pathway for the aqueous humor. The aqueous is usually redirected to the subconjunctival tissue space through either a filtering hole or an implantation of a filtering device. Although the initial success with this procedure may be high, most filtering procedures ultimately fail owing to fibrosis of the new outflow pathway. Filtering procedures work best in conjunction with medical and surgical therapies and for a short time only. Refer animals requiring a filtering procedure to an appropriate specialist.

Intraocular Prosthesis

Objectives

- Relieve pain associated with chronic glaucoma
- Maintain cosmetic appearance of the eye

▼ **Key Point** This procedure is indicated only for chronic glaucomatous eyes that are irreversibly blind. Intraocular prosthetic implants are contraindicated in cases of intraocular neoplasia, infectious

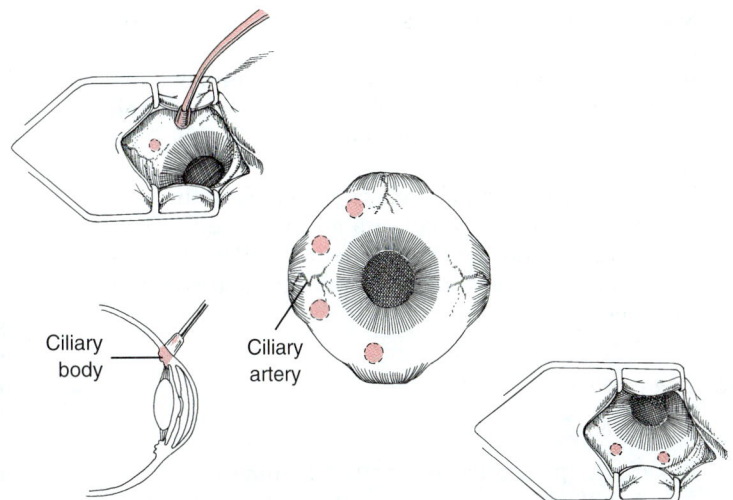

Figure 156–2. Cryosurgery or cyclophotocoagulation selectively destroys portions of the ciliary body (at areas indicated) and effects a decrease in the production of aqueous humor. Avoid damaging the long posterior ciliary arteries.

Ciliary body

Ciliary artery

panophthalmitis, and midstromal or deeper corneal ulceration.

Equipment

- Routine ocular surgical pack with a cyclodialysis spatula
- Sterile intraocular silicone implant (Jardon Corp.). The implant is 2 mm larger than the horizontal dimension of the cornea of the normal eye. In the dog, a 19-mm prosthesis generally is satisfactory.
- Sphere introducer

Technique

1. Place the anesthetized animal in lateral recumbency. Administer systemic flunixin meglumine as discussed in the cryosurgery section.
2. Use an eyelid speculum to obtain adequate exposure of the globe.
3. Make an incision in the superior conjunctiva, 4–5 mm posterior to the limbus (Fig. 156–3A). Continue the incision 120° around the globe.
4. Dissect the conjunctival and episcleral tissues to the level of the sclera.
5. Make an incision in the superior sclera, 4–5 mm posterior to the limbus.
6. Introduce a cyclodialysis spatula into the globe between the fibrous and vascular tunics and gently separate these tunics. Avoid injury to the cornea (Fig. 156–3B).
7. Enlarge the scleral incision (Fig. 156–3C).
8. Remove the intraocular contents (Fig. 156–3D), leaving only the fibrous tunic (cornea and sclera).
9. Place the silicone implant within the globe.
10. Close the sclera and conjunctival tissues with 6-0 absorbable suture (e.g., Vicryl, Ethicon) in simple interrupted and simple continuous patterns, respectively.

Postoperative Care

- Topical, broad-spectrum antibiotic ointment four times per day
- Warm, moist compresses twice daily for 5–7 days
- Systemic nonsteroidal anti-inflammatory agents as required
- As the surgical procedure removes the aqueous humor (the primary source of corneal nutrition) the cornea will vascularize over the 2–4 weeks following surgery.
- Evaluate the eye 2 weeks after surgery. Note the progression of corneal vascularization and the absence of corneal ulceration. Determine the IOP in the contralateral eye of patients with primary glaucoma at this time.

Enucleation

Objectives

- Relieve the pain associated with glaucoma

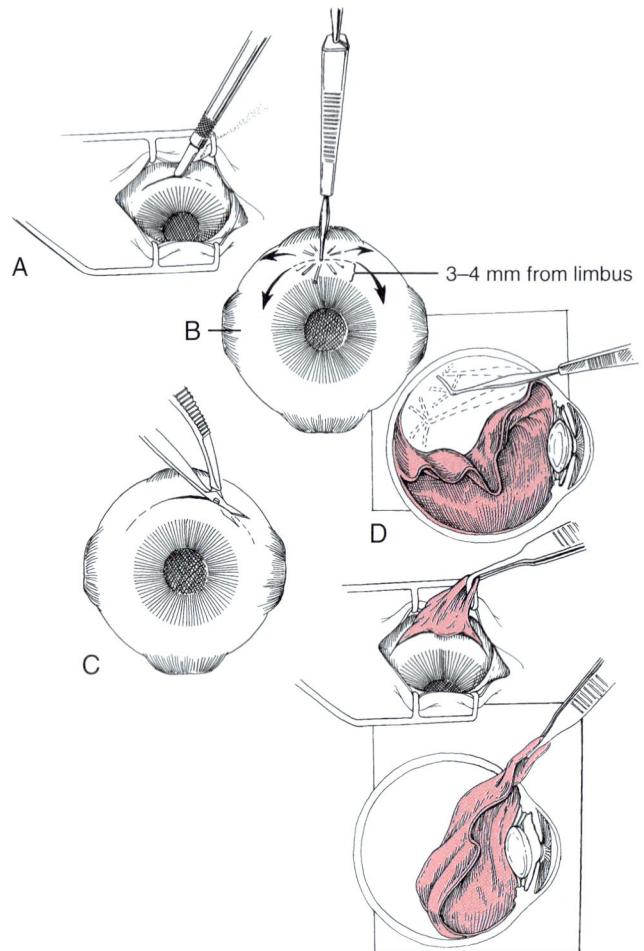

Figure 156–3. Preparation of globe for intraocular prosthesis. See text for details.

▼ *Key Point* An enucleation is indicated in animals with chronic glaucoma, causing irreversible blindness and in which an intraocular prosthetic implant is contraindicated.

Equipment

- Routine ocular surgical pack

Technique

1. Aseptically prepare and suture eyelids closed.
2. Incise the skin 5–6 mm away from the eyelid margin 360° around the eyelids. Using sharp dissection, continue the incision to the level of the extraocular muscles.
3. Sever the extraocular muscles at their attachment to the sclera.
4. Clamp and sever the optic nerve and blood vessels. Ligate the pedicle with 3-0 to 4-0 absorbable sutures.
5. If desired, insert an intraorbital silicone prosthesis to minimize the postsurgical "sunken" appearance of the orbit. A 24- to 34-mm prosthesis is used, nearly filling the orbital space.

6. Close the extraocular muscles, periorbita, subcutaneous tissues, and skin in a routine manner. Close the orbital space and subcutaneous tissues utilizing continuous 4-0 absorbable sutures and the skin utilizing 5-0 or 6-0 nonabsorbable sutures in an interrupted or continuous pattern.

Postoperative Care

- Administer postoperative systemic antibiotics for eyes enucleated for infectious panophthalmitis or penetrating keratitis.
- Submit all enucleated eyes to a qualified veterinary pathologist for examination.
- Remove sutures 10–14 days following surgery.

Pharmacologic Ablation

In my opinion, this is an unacceptable method for the management of glaucoma. It involves the intravitreal injection of a substance toxic to the eye in the hope that this approach will result in the destruction of the ciliary body, thereby lowering the intraocular pressure. This is an irreversible, inaccurate, and sometimes painful procedure. In addition, the end result is usually a noncosmetic phthisic globe, often requiring enucleation.

PREVENTION

- Evaluate IOP in all breeds predisposed to primary glaucoma, as part of the routine yearly physical examination. A sustained, gradual increase in IOP, even if still within normal limits, is sufficient cause to initiate preventive topical therapy.

- In an animal with primary glaucoma in one eye, examine the IOP in the opposite eye, every 2–4 months.
- In an animal with primary glaucoma in one eye, use preventive treatment in the opposite eye. This can consist of a systemic CAI administered to control the affected eye, which will also lower the IOP in the opposite eye. Alternatively, treat the unaffected eye topically, if systemic CAIs are not required for the affected eye.
- Measure IOP in all eyes with lens luxation or subluxation, anterior uveitis, or hyphema. If possible, the primary problem is eliminated in an effort to avoid secondary glaucoma.
- It is essential that owners understand that cure is not possible in most instances. Instead, control, management, and prevention are more appropriate terms to use when discussing glaucoma.

SUPPLEMENTAL READINGS

Brooks DE, Dziezyc J: The canine glaucomas: Pathogenesis, diagnosis, and treatment. Compend Cont Ed Pract Vet 5:292, 1983.

Nasisse MP, Davidson MG, MacLachlan NJ, et al.: Neodymium: yttrium, aluminum, and garnet laser energy delivered transsclerally to the ciliary body of dogs. Am J Vet Res 49:1972, 1988.

Ridgway MD, Brightman AH: Feline glaucoma: A retrospective study of 29 clinical cases. J Am Anim Hosp Assoc 25:485, 1989.

Roberts SM, Severin GA, Lavach JD: Cyclocryotherapy—Part I. Evaluation of a liquid nitrogen system. J Am Anim Hosp Assoc 20:823, 1984.

Roberts SM, Severin GA, Lavach JD: Cyclocryotherapy—Part II. Clinical comparison of liquid nitrogen and nitrous oxide cryotherapy on glaucomatous eyes. J Am Anim Hosp Assoc 20:828, 1984.

Whitley RD, Shaffer KW, Albert RA: Implantation of intraocular silicone prosthesis in dogs. Compend Cont Ed Pract Vet 7:802, 1985.

157 Diseases of the Retina, Choroid, and Optic Nerve

Nicholas J. Millichamp / Joan Dziezyc

EVALUATION OF THE POSTERIOR SEGMENT

The posterior segment of the eye includes the vitreous humor; the retina and its vasculature; and the choroid, sclera, and optic nerve. The fundus is the portion of the posterior segment that can be seen with an ophthalmoscope. Considerable variation exists in the appearance of the normal fundus in the dog and cat. To fully appreciate subtle differences in normal fundi, consult available atlases detailing their appearance.

Generally, the fundus is divided into the brightly colored and reflective tapetal region, occupying the upper and more temporal area, and the darkly pigmented nontapetal region, occupying the lower area and completely surrounding the tapetal area. Apart from these fundic regions, examine the retinal blood vessels and the optic nerve head (optic disk).

Ophthalmoscopy is the technique used to examine the fundus (see Chap. 150). The technique is ideally performed after dilating the pupil (except in an animal with ocular hypertension, glaucoma, or lens luxation) with a short-acting parasympatholytic drug such as tropicamide (Mydriacyl 0.5%, Alcon).

- *Direct ophthalmoscopy* with a hand-held ophthalmoscope is commonly used in practice. Unfortunately, this technique yields limited information about the fundic appearance even in the hands of experienced ophthalmologists. Small lesions and variations in contrast between normal and abnormal areas of the fundus are often overlooked when utilizing the direct technique.
- *Indirect ophthalmoscopy*, utilizing a 20D planoconvex lens held 2–3 inches from the animal's eye and illuminated with a penlight held at arm's length from the animal, is more useful as a diagnostic technique.

▼ *Key Point* Indirect ophthalmoscopy enables the examiner to quickly scan a large area of the fundus and to recognize obvious lesions.

- *Ocular ultrasonography* is utilized to evaluate the structures of the posterior segment when opacities of the ocular media prevent an ophthalmoscopic examination.

- *Electroretinography* employs a light stimulus of varying intensity and frequency to elicit a retinal response from rod and/or cone photoreceptors. This test evaluates the functional integrity of the retina and is a procedure that requires referral to a specialist.

DISEASES OF THE VITREOUS HUMOR

The vitreous is a gel composed mostly of water with lesser quantities of mucopolysaccharides and proteins. The normal adult vitreous is transparent and lacks blood vessels. The vitreous cannot itself become inflamed. However, products of inflammation or other abnormalities of adjacent tissues can result in exudate or hemorrhage that enters the vitreous and is seen by ophthalmoscopy.

Etiology

- *Retention of the fetal hyaloid artery* or its remnants may be seen in an adult dog as a fine gray strand arising from the optic disk or inserting onto the posterior pole of the lens.
- *Persistent hyperplastic primary vitreous/persistent tunica vasculosa lentis* is inherited in some breeds, notably the Doberman pinscher. The hyaloid artery is retained and is hyperplastic and associated with vessels that ramify over the posterior lens surface. Blood vessels and associated posterior lens capsular pigmentation and opacities (cataracts) or intralenticular hemorrhage is observed clinically. Surgical therapy yields poor results. Do not use these animals for breeding.
- *Asteroid hyalosis* is a unilateral or bilateral degenerative change associated with aging in dogs. Calcium-lipid complexes are deposited on the vitreous protein matrix. These appear as multiple white sparkles that oscillate slightly with eye movements. Asteroid hyalosis does not significantly impair vision, and no treatment is indicated.
- *Cholesterosis bulbi* or synchysis scintillans is a less common entity in which white cholesterol crystals are deposited in the vitreous secondary to intraocular inflammation. The vitreous often will become liquefied (*synersis*) as a result of posterior segment inflammation. The cholesterol deposits sink to the bottom of

the vitreous cavity. When the eye moves, the deposits swirl in the liquid vitreous before settling again under gravity. The initial cause of ocular inflammation and vitreous liquefaction may often have subsided by the time cholesterosis bulbi is detected. Vision is not affected by the cholesterosis bulbi per se, although it may be compromised by the underlying inflammatory disease.

- *Vitreous hemorrhage* most commonly occurs in the dog and cat as a sequel to ocular trauma, intraocular surgery, retinal detachment, or systemic coagulopathy. If the hemorrhage is severe, blindness may result.
- *Exudate and cellular infiltrate* appear as hazy, white, or gray material in the vitreous or on the posterior capsule of the lens. Pigment may also be deposited in the vitreous. Cellular infiltrate may become dense enough to obscure a view of the retina. Investigate for anterior uveitis or chorioretinitis.
- Other possible vitreous opacities include posterior lens luxation; retinal detachment; foreign bodies; parasites *(Dirofilaria);* and neoplasms arising from the ciliary body, retina, choroid, or optic nerve.

Clinical Signs

▼ *Key Point* Opacities of this otherwise clear medium are the most commonly observed clinical findings that indicate disease of the vitreous.

The effect on the animal's vision depends upon the severity and density of the opacities.

Diagnosis

- *Ophthalmoscopic examination* with a focal light source (penlight) or an ophthalmoscope will reveal the nature of the opacities (asteroid hyalosis, hemorrhage, pigment).
- *Submit blood for a clotting profile* when vitreous hemorrhage occurs unassociated with ocular trauma or intraocular surgery.
- *Perform physical examination, complete blood count,* and *serum biochemistry* and *serology evaluations* for infectious inflammatory disease (see Chorioretinitis) in cases in which vitreous exudate or cellular infiltrate is seen.
- *Perform ultrasonography* to rule out a diagnosis of coexisting retinal detachment, posterior segment neoplasia, or foreign bodies.

Treatment

- *Vitreous hemorrhage* resorbs slowly over the course of several weeks. Treat the coagulopathy systemically when possible.
- *Exudate and infiltrate* decrease by treating the underlying inflammatory disease with systemic antibacterial, antifungal, and nonsteroidal anti-inflammatory drugs (NSAIDs), as indicated. Corticosteroids can be used in dogs and cats once infectious etiologies are ruled out (prednisone or prednisolone, 1–2 mg/kg, q12–24h PO). NSAIDs (aspirin, 25 mg/kg q12h PO

in dogs only) often improve ocular inflammatory disease.

CONGENITAL DISEASES OF CHORIORETINA AND OPTIC NERVE

Etiology

Many of these diseases occur most frequently in dogs and are inherited. Other possible congenital causes include inflammation and necrosis in the developing retina in utero due to infectious diseases, radiation, and teratogens.

- *Collie eye anomaly (CEA)* is a disorder that occurs commonly in collies and less often in Shetland sheepdogs and some other breeds. CEA affects the retinal pigment epithelium; the choroid; and, in severe cases, the retina and optic nerve. The disease is usually asymmetric in the two eyes. The most characteristic lesion is choroidal hypoplasia, which appears as a pale area of fundus temporal to the optic nerve. The lesion is one of depigmentation of the retinal pigment epithelium and choroid, exposing hypoplastic choroidal blood vessels overlying the sclera. Occasionally, hazy white corneal opacities accompany the chorioretinal lesions. In severe cases, colobomas (gaps or holes due to incomplete development) may occur in the optic nerve or choroid. Retinal detachment or intraocular hemorrhage is found in the most severe cases.

▼ *Key Point* The developmental abnormalities do not worsen after birth. Retinal detachment associated with optic nerve colobomas, however, may occur at any age.

- *Retinal or vitreoretinal dysplasia* occurs in cats and dogs. The disease may be inherited (often recessively) in the dog or may be a sequel to intrauterine infection (canine herpesvirus, feline panleukopenia). In the dog, inherited retinal dysplasia may be manifested as bilaterally asymmetric, small focal folds in the outer layers of the retina that do not result in retinal elevation. These folds are observed in the cocker spaniel and the Labrador retriever. The folds may appear as small dark dots, streaks, or circles in the tapetal fundus and gray or dark spots or streaks in the nontapetal fundus. In some breeds (Sealyham and Bedlington terriers, Labrador retrievers, springer spaniel), the lesion is severe, and the dog is blinded by the retina lying unattached in abnormally formed vitreous.
- *Multiple ocular anomalies* are seen most commonly in Australian sheepdogs. Affected animals may have microphthalmia, iris colobomas, cataracts, retinal dysplasia or detachment, and uvea-lined defects (staphylomas) in the sclera.
- *Optic nerve hypoplasia,* if bilateral, may be noted by breeders or owners in animals a few weeks old. Affected eyes lack pupillary light reflexes and are blind. Ophthalmoscopy reveals a small optic nerve head with normal retinal vasculature.

Clinical Signs

Vision may be affected in dogs with severe congenital lesions. The pupillary light reflexes may also be variably affected, depending upon the severity of the lesions.

Diagnosis

Congenital abnormalities of the fundus are most readily diagnosed by the ophthalmoscopic appearance at 4–8 weeks of age.

Treatment and Prevention

The mode of transmission in the inherited diseases is often as an autosomal recessive trait (e.g., CEA and retinal dysplasia in most breeds). Prevent intrauterine infections by vaccination of breeding animals and by avoidance of infection and exposure of pregnant animals to ionizing radiation and teratogenic toxins.

▼ *Key Point* There is no treatment for congenital chorioretinal disease. Do not breed affected dogs.

ACQUIRED DISEASE OF THE CHORIORETINA AND OPTIC NERVE

Chorioretinal Degeneration

Etiology and Clinical Features

- *Progressive retinal atrophy (PRA)* includes several genetic retinal diseases in which the ultimate outcome is degeneration and loss of retinal structure with varying degrees of blindness. The different forms of PRA are all progressive and bilaterally symmetric. The disease occurs commonly in many purebred and mixed-breed dogs. The inheritance in most instances in the dog is autosomal recessive. PRA also occurs in various breeds of cat, although it has been best characterized in the Abyssinian.
- PRA may primarily affect the photoreceptors (rods/cones) or the adjacent layer of retinal pigment epithelium. Pigment epithelial dystrophy, or central PRA, is extremely rare in the United States and apparently on the decline in other parts of the world, including Europe. PRA affecting the rods or cones can be distinguished by the age of onset. In early-onset PRA (rod, rod-cone dysplasias), affected dogs show signs of night blindness during the first year of life. Affected breeds include the collie, Irish setter, miniature schnauzer, elkhound, and miniature dachshund. In late-onset PRA (progressive rod-cone degeneration), night blindness may be noticed at any age from 1 year on. Breeds affected include the miniature poodle, cocker spaniel, and Labrador retriever. The typical ophthalmoscopic appearance of diffuse retinal degeneration is an increased reflectance of light from the tapetal fundus (tapetal hyper-reflectivity). Retinal blood vessels are narrowed or lost, and depigmentation and patchy hyperpigmentation in the nontapetal fundus may be seen. In advanced cases, atrophy of the optic nerve occurs.

- *Sudden acquired retinal degeneration (SARD)* is a degeneration of the retina that occurs in dogs. The defect that causes the degeneration is unknown. Dogs of any age that are otherwise normal may be affected. Obese, middle-aged dogs are most prone to the disorder. The most characteristic feature of SARD is the rapid and complete loss of vision, often within a few days or at most weeks. The disease usually affects both eyes equally.

▼ *Key Point* In SARD, the photoreceptors are ultrastructurally abnormal at the time when blindness is first noted, although the fundus appears ophthalmoscopically normal.

Ophthalmoscopic signs of retinal degeneration (tapetal hyper-reflectivity, vascular attenuation) appear over several months. The electroretinogram is extinguished at the time of presentation, which distinguishes the disease from optic neuritis, pituitary neoplasia, and central nervous system blindness.

- *Nutritional deficiency* or taurine deficiency in the cat, especially in cats fed dog food that is deficient in taurine (an essential amino acid in the cat), results in feline central retinal degeneration (FCRD). The typical early lesion is a focal area of tapetal hyper-reflectivity in the temporal fundus. With progression of the lesion, a similar area appears nasally and the two patches join to form a horizontal band above the optic disk. Continued deficiency results in diffuse atrophy throughout the retina. Restoration of a taurine-rich diet halts the degeneration in the early stages, although the fundic lesion remains visible throughout the cat's life. Cats with taurine deficiency rarely show any evidence of blindness until the disease is advanced. For discussion of the cardiac effects of taurine deficiency in cats, see Chapter 66. FCRD also occurs in some cats on diets with adequate taurine. The cause in this situation is unknown.
- *Chronic glaucoma* results in diffuse retinal atrophy because of ischemia and pressure necrosis of initially the inner and later the outer retina (see Chap. 156).
- *Inflammation* that subsides or is successfully treated often results in focal lesions of chorioretinal degeneration in the affected areas. These lesions appear as focal hyper-reflective areas in the tapetal fundus or depigmented areas in the nontapetum. Vision is affected to an extent commensurate with the area and region of the fundus involved (central vs. peripheral retina).

Clinical Signs

- *Blindness* is a characteristic feature of retinal degeneration. Night blindness may be noted first in PRA that progresses to complete visual loss. Blindness may be sudden when caused by SARD and slowly progressive when caused by glaucoma.
- *Mydriasis* may be observed. Pupillary light reflexes may be incomplete and sluggish in advanced cases of PRA and can be absent in SARD.

Diagnosis

- *Ophthalmoscopy* identifies retinal degeneration when typical lesions are present.
- *Electroretinography (ERG)* may help one to make a diagnosis of PRA before typical ophthalmoscopic signs are seen and to confirm a diagnosis of SARD. ERG is a test of retinal function. Refer to a specialist.
- Genetic testing of blood samples is now available to diagnose PRA in selected breeds. Refer to a specialist.

Treatment

No treatment is available for PRA or SARD. Chorioretinal degeneration due to glaucoma (see Chap. 156) or inflammation (see Chorioretinitis) can be limited by controlling the primary disease process. A deficiency of taurine in the diet can be corrected to halt progression of the disease (see Chap. 66).

Prevention

Progressive retinal atrophy in either dogs or cats can be prevented by selective breeding of unaffected dogs and of those dogs believed not to be carriers of the PRA gene. Recommend yearly evaluations of all breeding purebred dogs by a board-certified veterinary ophthalmologist, and register these animals through the Canine Eye Registry Foundation (CERF) as phenotypically normal.

Chorioretinitis

Chorioretinitis is inflammation of the retina and choroid. Although inflammation may begin in either of the two layers, their proximity often results in spread and involvement of both. Clinically, the differentiation is of little importance.

Etiology

Numerous causes of, or diseases associated with, chorioretinitis are recognized in the dog and cat. Chorioretinitis may develop as an extension of anterior uveitis (see Chap. 155) or as an isolated entity. Systemic diseases that can cause unilateral or bilateral chorioretinitis are listed in Tables 157–1 and 157–2. Refer also to the appropriate chapters elsewhere in this book for specifics on these diseases.

Clinical Signs

- *Vision* may be affected in severe cases of chorioretinitis, especially with concurrent optic nerve inflammation. In mild cases of chorioretinitis, visual deficits may not be noticed.
- *The tapetal fundus* areas of chorioretinal exudate or edema appear as hazy gray areas that may have discrete borders and appear elevated. If cellular infiltrate is also present, the areas may appear darker and obscure the underlying tapetum.
- *The nontapetal fundus* areas of exudate or cellular infiltrate appear gray or white. Perivascular cuffing appears as a hazy white border to retinal vessels.
- *Hemorrhages* may be seen at various depths in the retina.

Table 157–1. DISEASES ASSOCIATED WITH CHORIORETINITIS IN DOGS

Viral	Distemper
Fungal	Blastomycosis
	Coccidioidomycosis
	Cryptococcosis
	Histoplasmosis
	Aspergillosis
	Geotrichosis
Bacterial	*Brucella canis*
	Borrelia burgdorferi
	Leptospirosis
Algal	Prototrichosis
Rickettsial	Ehrlichiosis
	Rocky Mountain spotted fever
Parasitic	Toxoplasmosis
	Neosporum caninum
	Leishmaniasis
	Migrating fly larvae
	Toxocara canis larva migrans
Immune-mediated	Autoimmune chorioretinitis
	Uveodermatologic syndrome
Neoplastic	Lymphosarcoma
	Multiple myeloma
	Metastatic neoplasia
Toxic	Miscellaneous toxins (often undiagnosed)

- *Exudative retinal detachments* may occur.
- *Associated ocular disease* may include anterior uveitis (see Chap. 155) and exudate or hemorrhage in the vitreous.

Diagnosis

▼ **Key Point** Unilateral or bilateral chorioretinitis indicates a systemic disease until proven otherwise.

- *Physical examination*—look for any evidence of inflammatory or neoplastic disease elsewhere in the body.
- *Evaluate complete blood count, serum biochemistry profile, and urinalysis* for evidence of underlying systemic disease.
- *Evaluate thoracic and abdominal radiography* for evidence of systemic mycosis or neoplasia.
- *Evaluate serology* to rule out the various infectious causes of chorioretinitis as described in the chapters

Table 157–2. DISEASES ASSOCIATED WITH CHORIORETINITIS IN CATS

Viral	Feline infectious peritonitis
	Feline leukemia virus
	Feline immunodeficiency virus
Bacterial	Tuberculosis
Fungal	Blastomycosis
	Cryptococcosis
	Histoplasmosis
Parasitic	Toxoplasmosis
	Migrating fly larvae
Immune-mediated	Autoimmune chorioretinitis
Neoplastic	Lymphosarcoma
	Metastatic neoplasia
Toxic	Miscellaneous toxins (often undiagnosed)

on viral diseases, systemic mycoses, and toxoplasmosis.

- *Evaluate lymph node aspirate and skin biopsy samples* in animals with lymphadenopathies or cutaneous lesions.
- *Evaluate vitreous by paracentesis* for cytology and culture, but *only as a last resort* in cases in which all other less invasive systemic diagnostic techniques have been performed and the eye is irreversibly blind.

Treatment

The retina and choroid are inaccessible to most topical medications.

▼ *Key Point* To effectively treat chorioretinitis, drugs must be given systemically.

Underlying systemic disease is treated appropriately (as described in the relevant chapters in this book). If all evidence of infectious disease is ruled out, systemic corticosteroids or NSAIDs are given to control the inflammation. Additional therapy with immunosuppressive drugs such as azathioprine (Imuran) may be indicated in immune-mediated chorioretinitis (see Chap. 155).

After achieving an initial improvement in chorioretinitis with a systemic corticosteroid (prednisone) and/or immunosuppressive drug (azathioprine), these drugs may be combined at half of their regular dose for long-term therapy. This may avoid development of side effects from each drug and result in better control of posterior segment inflammation.

Retinovascular Disease

The retinal or choroidal vasculature may be affected in the aforementioned congenital chorioretinal diseases, retinal degenerations, and chorioretinitis. Vascular disease also may occur unrelated to these other entities.

Etiology

- *Coagulopathies*, including canine ehrlichiosis, warfarin and aspirin toxicity, von Willebrand disease, autoimmune hemolytic anemia, and immune-mediated thrombocytopenia in dogs, may cause retinal hemorrhage (see Chap. 21).
- *Systemic hypertension* in dogs and cats may result in retinal hemorrhage and transudative retinal detachment (see Chap. 69).
- *Congenital cardiac anomalies* may cause engorgement of retinal venules (see Chap. 70).
- *Hyperviscosity syndrome* due to macroglobulinemia in dogs with myelomas and polycythemia causes engorgement of the retinal blood vessels.
- *Anemia* in cats has been associated with retinal hemorrhage.
- *Hyperlipidemia* in cats and dogs results in pink-colored retinal blood vessels.

Clinical Signs

Retinal and vitreous hemorrhage and retinal detachment may result in acute blindness and loss of the pupillary light reflex.

Diagnosis

- *Ophthalmoscopy* reveals retinal hemorrhage, vessel engorgement, increased tortuosity, and color change.
- *Clotting profile and complete blood count* assess clotting time, clotting factor deficiencies, thrombocytopenia, and anemia. Coagulopathies are described in Chapter 21.
- *Blood pressure measurement* (see Chap. 69) is indicated in any older dog or cat with retinal hemorrhage or detachment. Rule out renal disease, cardiac disease, and hyperthyroidism in animals with hypertension (see appropriate chapters for each).

Treatment

Direct therapy in all acquired forms of retinovascular disease at the underlying cause. In most cases, retinal hemorrhage resorbs spontaneously, during a few days to weeks, once the disease is under control.

Retinal Detachment

Retinal detachment is separation of the neural retina from the retinal pigment epithelium (RPE). Unilateral detachments may exist undetected.

▼ *Key Point* Retinal detachments are often caused by systemic disease in dogs and cats.

Detachments may be partial or complete (infundibular) and arise near the periphery of the retina or adjacent to the optic nerve.

Etiology

- *Congenital developmental disease* includes both CEA and retinal dysplasia.
- *Inflammation* results in accumulations of serous fluid or cellular infiltrate or granulomas between the retina and retinal pigment epithelium, causing detachment. The same causes of chorioretinitis apply to retinal detachment (see Tables 157–1 and 157–2).
- *Hypertension* (see Chap. 69) causes accumulation of transudate within and beneath the retina.
- *Tears* in the retina associated with cataract formation, intraocular surgery, or liquefaction of the vitreous may allow vitreous to penetrate between the retina and retinal pigment epithelium.
- *Traction* on the retina may result from fibrous tissue that forms in the retina or vitreous secondary to intraocular hemorrhage or chorioretinitis.
- *Neoplasia* or *granuloma* of the choroid or orbit may indent the sclera and detach the retina.
- *Ethylene glycol* toxicity in cats (see Chap. 97) may result in serous retinal folding and detachment.

Clinical Signs

- *Sudden blindness* occurs if bilateral; visual deficits occur if unilateral, depending upon the extent of the detachment.
- *The pupil is often dilated,* and the pupillary light reflexes are weak to absent.

- *A translucent, folded, gray or white sheet of tissue* with retinal blood vessels may be observed behind the lens.

Diagnosis

- *Ophthalmoscopy* reveals focal retinal detachment. Complete retinal detachment can usually be seen clearly with a focal light source.
- *Measure blood pressure* performed to diagnose hypertension (see Chap. 69).
- *Ultrasonography* may support the diagnosis of retinal detachment in cases of intraocular neoplasia or hemorrhage. It is also indicated to detect retinal detachment in eyes with opacities of otherwise clear ocular media (cornea, lens, vitreous).
- *Serology* is indicated if infectious disease is suspected.

Treatment

- *Appropriate therapy for a systemic disease* (hypertension) once diagnosed sometimes results in retinal reattachment, especially if the detachment is not chronic. This response may result in a return of vision and is more likely in dogs than in cats. Treat cats with hypertension with the calcium channel blocker amlodipine besylate (Norvasc), 0.14 mg/kg q12–24h, usually 0.625 mg/cat q24h. Often this will result in rapid resolution of retinal detachment and some restoration of vision.
- *Systemic corticosteroids* are used after infectious disease and hypertension have been diagnostically ruled out (see Chap. 155).
- *Systemic NSAIDs* are indicated in retinal detachment, although avoided in cases associated with intraocular hemorrhage (see Chap. 155).
- *Retinal reattachment surgery* is indicated in recent detachments associated with small retinal tears. Laser retinopexy may halt further detachment. Scleral buckling with or without vitrectomy or other retinal tamponade and retinopexy methods may be effective for some detachments and maintain vision. These procedures are performed at some referral centers. In retinal detachments with 360° tears, surgery is not indicated.

ACQUIRED DISEASE OF THE OPTIC NERVE

The optic nerve may be involved in several chorioretinal diseases, including chorioretinitis and retinal degeneration.

Optic Neuritis

Optic neuritis is inflammation of the optic nerve. The condition may be recurrent in nature and often results in atrophy of the optic nerve and permanent blindness, regardless of therapy.

Etiology

- *Inflammatory and infectious etiologies* are similar to those causing CNS disease (see Chap. 145) and chorioretinitis (see Tables 157–1 and 157–2).
- *Neoplasia* (canine GME, feline lymphosarcoma) affecting the CNS may cause optic neuritis (see Chap. 145).
- *Ocular trauma* (ocular proptosis) causes optic neuritis.
- *Orbital inflammatory disease* may, in severe cases, result in optic neuritis.
- *Immune-mediated optic neuritis* may be presumed in cases in which no underlying systemic cause can be identified.
- *Miscellaneous toxins* may potentially cause optic neuritis, although diagnosis is rarely possible.

Clinical Signs

- *Acute blindness* is present with bilateral optic nerve involvement, although no visual deficit may be noted if the neuritis is unilateral.
- *Mydriasis* and absence of the pupillary light reflex are evident.

Diagnosis

- *Ophthalmoscopy* allows the diagnosis of intraocular optic neuritis and helps differentiate optic neuritis from retinal detachment as a cause of sudden blindness.
- *The optic disk appears hazy, elevated, and edematous.* The edema often radiates into the peripapillary retina when the inflammation involves the intraocular portion of the nerve. Hemorrhages may be present at the disk or in the adjacent retina or vitreous. Vitreous exudate may obscure the optic disk.
- *Ophthalmoscopic signs may not be present* if the neuritis does not involve the optic disk.
- *Chorioretinitis* can be a concurrent finding.
- *Electroretinography* is indicated to rule out SARD in cases in which the optic nerve appears normal.
- *Ultrasonography* can detect nerve swelling when the retrobulbar nerve is involved.
- *Perform neurologic examination,* cerebrospinal fluid (CSF) analysis, and magnetic resonance imaging (MRI) to diagnose concomitant neurologic disease (see Chap. 144).
- *Evaluate the complete blood count and serology findings* for evidence of infectious etiologies.

Treatment

- Wherever possible, identify infectious etiologies and treat appropriately (see appropriate chapters).
- In cases in which infectious etiologies are ruled out, administer systemic corticosteroids (prednisone, 2 mg/kg q24h PO). Failure to limit the inflammation results in optic atrophy and vision loss.

Papilledema

Papilledema is the bilateral swelling of the optic nerve due to reduced blood and axoplasmic flow from the optic disk. The term is loosely applied in dogs and cats to any form of optic disk edema.

Etiology

- *Pressure applied to the optic nerve* by tumors or granulomas of the nerve or within the orbit can cause stasis of axoplasmic and optic nerve blood flow and can result in papilledema.
- *Neoplasia and inflammation of the CNS* can cause papilledema in dogs and cats by increasing CSF pressure and increasing pressure within and around the optic nerve.

Clinical Signs

- *Vision is usually unaffected*. However, blindness may occur in the absence of optic neuritis when inflammatory or neoplastic lesions significantly damage the central optic pathways, including the visual cortex (see Chap. 160).

Diagnosis

- Attempt to differentiate papilledema from optic neuritis.
- *Ophthalmoscopic appearance of a swollen optic disk, usually with normal vision*, is likely to indicate papilledema. This is unlike optic neuritis in which vision is affected.
- *The optic disk* protrudes into the vitreous. The retinal blood vessels leaving the optic disk appear to cascade over the edge of the disk. The margins of the optic disk appear hazy and indistinct. Hemorrhages may occasionally be observed in the adjacent retina.
- *Perform globe retropulsion* to determine whether a space-occupying lesion is present in the orbit.
- *Neurologic examination* can help localize CNS lesions.
- *Ultrasonography, radiology, and computed tomography (if available)* can be used to locate orbital space-occupying lesions.
- *Exploratory orbitotomy* is a difficult technique that can be employed to localize and diagnose any masses detected with the previous methods.

Treatment

- Because papilledema is often associated with CNS tumors, the prognosis is guarded to poor.
- Orbital tumors may occasionally be surgically removed during exploratory orbitotomy.
- *Perform exenteration of the eye and orbital contents* when a mass is localized near the globe.

Optic Nerve Atrophy

Atrophy of the optic nerve may occur as a sequel to other ocular diseases.

Etiology

- Advanced inherited retinal degenerations can occur.
- Glaucoma causes ischemia of the optic nerve at the scleral lamina cribrosa, resulting in atrophy and "cupping."
- Optic neuritis can be either severe or recurrent.
- Optic nerve trauma (traumatic ocular proptosis) can occur.
- Orbital inflammation or neoplasia may be noted.

Clinical Signs and Diagnosis

- Blindness is evident in the affected eye.
- The pupil is mydriatic, and the pupillary light reflexes are absent.
- Ophthalmoscopy confirms the diagnosis. The optic disk appears small and gray, with a loss of retinal blood vessels. The outline of the scleral lamina cribrosa may become visible, particularly in cats. In dogs, the margins of the disk may appear to spread from the disk owing to peripapillary gliosis (hypertrophy of neuronal supporting cells).

Treatment

No treatment is effective once the optic nerve undergoes atrophy.

NEOPLASIA OF THE POSTERIOR SEGMENT

Most tumors of the posterior segment in dogs and cats result from metastasis from other sites. The most common secondary tumor is malignant lymphoma. Primary tumors are rare but include malignant teratoid medulloepitheliomas, melanomas, and optic nerve meningiomas. Therapy entails enucleation or exenteration of the orbit, depending upon the localization of the tumor to the globe.

SUPPLEMENTAL READINGS

Barnett KC: Color Atlas of Veterinary Ophthalmology. Baltimore: Williams & Wilkins, 1990.

Curtis R, Barnett KC: Canine posterior segment. *In* Gelatt KN, ed.: Veterinary Ophthalmology, 2nd ed. Philadelphia: Lea & Febiger, 1991.

Millichamp NJ: Retinal degeneration in the dog and cat. Vet Clin North Am [Sm Anim Pract] 20:799, 1990.

Rubin LF: Atlas of Veterinary Ophthalmology. Philadelphia: Lea & Febiger, 1974.

Rubin LF: Inherited eye diseases. *In* Purebred Dogs. Baltimore: Williams & Wilkins, 1989.

Slatter D: Fundamentals of Veterinary Ophthalmology, 2nd ed. Philadelphia: WB Saunders, 1990.

Walde I, Schäffer EH, Köstlin RG: Atlas of Ophthalmology in Dogs and Cats. Philadelphia: BC Decker, Inc., 1990.

158 Diseases of the Lacrimal Apparatus

Renee L. Kaswan

Common disorders of the lacrimal apparatus include insufficient tearing (i.e., keratoconjunctivitis sicca), prolapse of the gland of the nictitating membrane (third eyelid), and overflow tearing (i.e., epiphora). Keratoconjunctivitis sicca (KCS) occurs when tear secretion is deficient and the cornea and conjunctiva become desiccated. Aqueous tear deficiency leads to excessive mucus buildup; secondary bacterial conjunctivitis; recurrent corneal ulcers; corneal pigmentation, vascularization, and keratinization; and dense corneal scars. Traditionally a difficult disorder to manage, KCS has been one of the most frequent causes of canine visual loss. Introduction of topical cyclosporine (Optimmune; Schering-Plough) has greatly reduced the morbidity of KCS and increased the convenience of treatment.

Cyclosporine restores secretion of physiologic tears and induces regrowth of the lacrimal glands when treatment is begun before the glands reach end-stage atrophy. Routine use of the Schirmer tear test allows for early diagnosis and treatment of KCS, preventing disease progression and sight loss.

Prolapse of the nictitating membrane gland is a cosmetic problem. The major significance of prolapse management is that the gland is replaced, not removed, to avoid KCS.

Epiphora, or overflow tearing, can be a cosmetic problem or an indication of ocular pain necessitating diagnosis. Irritation of the eye, distichiasis (eyelashes touching the eye), trichiasis (misdirected facial hairs touching the eye), entropion (inward rolling of the lid margin), and dacryocystitis (inflammatory blockage of the nasolacrimal drainage duct) cause epiphora.

ANATOMY AND PHYSIOLOGY

Lacrimal Glands

- There are two lacrimal glands in cats and dogs: the nictitans gland and the orbital lacrimal gland. They each produce approximately one-half of the tear volume.
- The *nictitans gland* is the lacrimal gland of the nictitating membrane. The nictitans gland is wrapped around the vertical cartilage of the third eyelid (Fig. 158–1).
- The *orbital lacrimal gland* lies internal to the lateral orbital ligament, directly below the zygomatic process of the frontal bone.

- Parasympathetic innervation of the lacrimal gland originates with the trigeminal nerve, courses through the inner ear with the facial nerve, and distributes superficially as divisions of the facial nerve.

Tear Film

- Tears provide the cornea with physical lubrication as well as essential proteins, vitamins, epithelial growth factors, and hormones. Because the cornea is avascular, the lacrimal glands have evolved to produce the nutrients and regulatory proteins necessary to sustain a healthy, transparent cornea.
- The tear film is composed of three transparent layers of fluid—inner mucus, middle aqueous, and outer lipid—which coat and protect the cornea.
- Tears flow from the excretory ducts of the lacrimal glands and coat all the exposed surfaces of the conjunctiva and cornea. The overflow exits through the nasolacrimal drainage system.

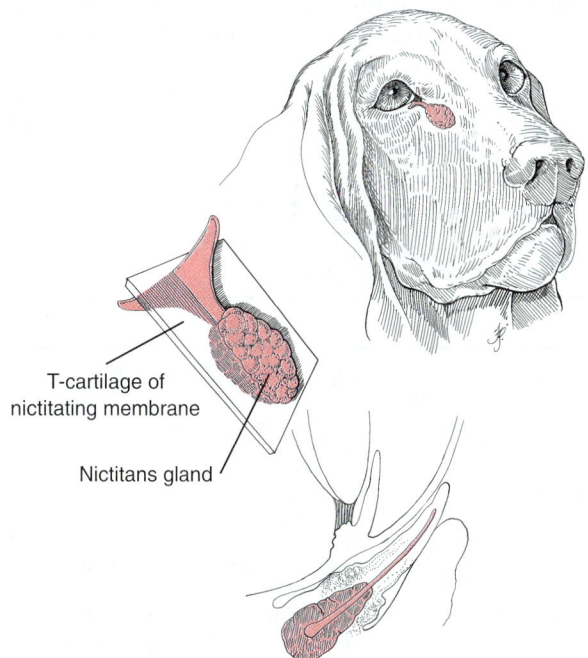

T-cartilage of
nictitating membrane

Nictitans gland

Figure 158–1. In situ representation of the nictitans gland. Note how it wraps around the vertical cartilage of the nictitating membrane or third eyelid (*below*).

KERATOCONJUNCTIVITIS SICCA

Etiology

▼ *Key Point* Despite a list of known etiologies of canine KCS (Table 158–1), in most animals KCS is considered to be either idiopathic or immune-mediated.

Serology has identified numerous KCS-affected dogs with positive rheumatoid factor, antinuclear antibodies, and hypergammaglobulinemia. Lacrimal gland biopsy specimens typically reveal multifocal to diffuse mononuclear cell infiltration, with varying degrees of fibrosis and atrophy. Paradoxically, many glands have few focal inflammatory lesions and large areas of apparently normal acinar tissue, except that the acinar cells have reduced numbers of secretory granules. These dysfunctional acini are one proposed target of cyclosporine intervention. Cyclosporine induces cellular changes leading to regrowth and normalization of the tear-secreting glands.

Clinical Signs

▼ *Key Point* KCS is the most common cause of canine conjunctivitis. Misdiagnosed cases treated with virtually any topical medication will show transient improvement, however. Suspect KCS in any dog with chronic or recurrent conjunctivitis, keratitis, or corneal ulceration.

- Chronic mucoid-to-mucopurulent discharge is the hallmark of KCS. Secondary bacterial overgrowth may be misleading and cause the primary diagnosis of KCS to be overlooked. If this problem occurs, the dog may be treated endlessly for conjunctivitis without resolution of the underlying cause.
- Clients often become frustrated when conjunctivitis treated with antibiotics relapses; they fail to return for necessary follow-up visits; KCS then progresses, often with sight loss. Educate the client to anticipate management for a lifelong ocular disorder.
- In KCS, blepharitis and conjunctivitis occur with hyperemia, chemosis, thickened conjunctiva, periocular crust, and pruritus.
- In chronic KCS the cornea appears dull and opaque. Corneal scarring varies in severity. Signs of scarring include vascularization, pigmentation, surface granulation, keratinization, and fibrosis. Exophthalmic breeds and highly pigmented dogs exhibit corneal scarring most severely.
- *Blindness commonly occurs because of corneal opacification.*
- Superficial or deep-melting ulcers may occur. Ulcers are more common in acute cases of KCS, in which the cornea has not become thick and keratinized.
- Pain is highly variable and warrants examination for corneal ulcers. Common signs of pain include blepharospasm, photophobia, and eye rubbing.
- KCS, less frequent in cats, occurs with similar but less dramatic signs. In cats, fright may cause transient sympathomimetic inhibition of tearing. This temporary condition must be distinguished from KCS by clinical signs.

Diagnosis

The Schirmer tear test (STT) is indicated in all animals suspected of keratoconjunctivitis, even when the cornea does not appear dry. Before administering any ocular drops, place the 5 × 30 mm commercial STT filter paper strip (Schering-Plough) in the medioventral cul-de-sac for 1 minute. Normal wetting for dogs and cats is 20 ± 5 mm/minute. Typically, KCS patients wet less than 10 mm/minute. Diagnosis of KCS can be made when decreased STT values occur together with mucopurulent conjunctivitis, corneal inflammation, ulceration, or pigment deposition.

Treatment

Traditionally, KCS management has focused on tear replacement, tear conservation, and neurologic tear stimulation. Surgical transposition of the parotid salivary duct to the eye is a last resort for medically unmanageable cases. A radically new management approach uses a topically applied immunosuppressive agent, cyclosporine, intended to reverse immune-mediated destruction of the lacrimal gland and restore normal tear production.

Topical Cyclosporine (Optimmune)

▼ *Key Point* The initial treatment of choice for KCS is topical cyclosporine, Optimmune.

Cyclosporine is a noncytotoxic (reversible) T-cell inhibitor used primarily for human organ transplantation. Unexpectedly, cyclosporine also increases tearing in animals with KCS associated with facial nerve paralysis, sulfonamide toxicity, nictitans gland removal ("cherry eye" surgery), and other causes.

Table 158–1. CHARACTERISTICS OF KERATOCONJUNCTIVITIS SICCA OF VARIOUS ETIOLOGIES

Cause	Common Characteristics
Idiopathic or immune-mediated	Frequently associated with atopy, otitis externa, hypothyroidism, rheumatic diseases, deficient salivation (xerostomia)
Congenital alacrima	Usually unilateral, extreme xerosis, small breeds
Neurologic	Associated with other neurologic signs (e.g., facial nerve loss, deficient blink, head tilt, lip droop); commonly associated with otitis media (see Chap. 57)
Drug-induced	Sulfadiazine, sulfasalazine, phenazopyridine, atropine (usually transient)
Distemper virus	In puppies with inadequate vaccinations; recent clinical infection (see Chap. 11)

Advantages

- *Production of natural tears.* Cyclosporine interrupts the pathologic process in the lacrimal glands, allowing them to resume tear production.

▼ *Key Point* Because tears contain antibodies, vitamins, amino acids, mucin, growth regulatory hormones, and many other constituents essential to corneal health, production of natural tears is a major advantage over artificial tears.

Comparison of tear composition in cyclosporine-treated dogs with that produced by normal dogs shows that major tear proteins are conserved by cyclosporine.

- *Anti-inflammatory effects.* Cyclosporine is an immunosuppressive drug that reduces corneal vascularization, granulation, pigmentation, and conjunctival inflammation—similar to the activity of corticosteroids. However, unlike corticosteroids, cyclosporine does not activate collagenase in the presence of corneal ulcers.

Administration

In wide-scale controlled clinical trials, 0.2% cyclosporine ointment was the most effective treatment for KCS, and compared favorably to other concentrations and vehicles. Administer cyclosporine ophthalmic ointment twice daily, usually for the lifetime of the patient. Although package instructions call for a ¼-inch strip, much of this dose will be wasted when the lids blink and expel it; therefore, application of a smaller amount is fiscally prudent and usually effective.

Teaching Ointment Administration

Many clients and dogs require training in the administration of ophthalmic ointments. An artificial tear ointment or triple antibiotic ointment is an inexpensive and useful medium for this practice. Demonstrate the administration of the ointment, advise giving dog treats for compliance, and encourage practice initially using an inexpensive ointment. For dogs that shy away from ocular medications, advise owners to position the dog in front of them and approach the eye from behind the dog's head, so that the dog doesn't readily see the treatment coming toward the eye.

Topical Antibiotic Administration

A short course of antibiotics is useful in dogs that have secondary bacterial infections associated with KCS, indicated by a purulent discharge. Most dogs will initially present with a secondary bacterial infection, which resolves more quickly when antibiotics are used concurrent with cyclosporine ophthalmic ointment, for the first 7–14 days. Triple antibiotic ophthalmic ointment, given q.i.d., is a practical choice.

Relapses

Over the lifetime of the dog, it is likely that the dog will have occasional relapses of conjunctivitis even while using cyclosporine. Pruritic dogs scratching infected ears or skin and then pawing their eyes often reinfect the eyes with pathogenic species of bacteria. Treatment of the concurrent surface infections may be required to keep the eyes infection free. A 7- to 14-day course of ocular antibiotics is appropriate whenever the dog has a relapse of purulent conjunctivitis. Continue topical cyclosporine concomitantly.

Monitoring

Reevaluate the animal using STT results and clinical signs, 2–4 weeks after beginning treatment, and then monthly, until clinical control is achieved. Following 6 weeks of treatment, if signs have not improved, increase dosing to q8hr. If the STT is greater than 20 mm/minute, on reevaluation, decrease to once daily or, occasionally, alternate-day dosing.

The rate of tear secretion often varies from day to day in any given patient. Occasional spuriously low or spuriously high STT test results can occur. Do not attach too much significance to this.

▼ *Key Point* Measure the STT approximately 3 hours after dosing cyclosporine because the effect on the STT is lost in most cases in 12–24 hours.

When treatment is interrupted for 24 hours, signs recur in 90% of dogs that have been treated for over a year. Recapture of cyclosporine efficacy occurs rapidly, with the STT increasing after approximately 3 hours and the keratitis decreasing, usually, within 1 week after resumption of treatment.

Response Rate

End-stage lacrimal gland pathology cannot be reversed with cyclosporine. The etiology of KCS does not accurately predict the response to therapy: positive responses have been seen in every known etiology. Treatment failure has, likewise, occurred in all types of KCS. Although investigated, no sex or breed predilection for response has been discerned.

About 70% of all dogs with KCS respond positively to cyclosporine treatment within 2–4 weeks. An additional 10–15% of dogs respond to long-term treatment, with the slowest reported onset of response being one dog who began tearing following 8 months of twice-daily treatment. About 10–15% of dogs will not tear; however, they may show resolution of corneal scarring and mucoid conjunctivitis. Approximately 10% of dogs do not benefit clinically, requiring return to traditional methods of treatment (as described in the sections that follow), such as artificial tears, corticosteroids, pilocarpine, acetylcysteine as needed, or parotid duct transposition surgery as a last resort.

▼ *Key Point* Increased lacrimation in response to cyclosporine therapy is related to the initial STT. Those dogs with STT of >2 mm/minute wetting had a much greater response (87–100%) than those with STT of <2 mm/minute (29–59%).

Artificial Tears

Artificial tears supplementation using primarily methylcellulose and polyvinyl alcohol increases artificial tear viscosity and surface tension, which increase ocular surface wetting time. Table 158–2 lists commonly used artificial tear preparations. In dogs, ointments are usually preferred to solutions because of their lower cost and decreased dosing frequency. Preservative-free products are also preferred. Artificial tears are applied as often as reasonably possible, from 4–12 times daily, depending upon the severity of disease and owner compliance.

Tear Stimulants

Pilocarpine 2% dosed at 1 drop/5 kg body weight twice daily on feed can be used to stimulate the parasympathetic supply to the lacrimal gland and maximize its output. If the initial dosage is ineffective, it may be increased by 1 drop per day to effect or until toxicity develops.

Table 158–2. ARTIFICIAL TEAR SOLUTIONS AND OINTMENTS

Product Names	Principal Ingredients	Preservatives
Solutions		
Adsorbotear	HEC, Adsorbobase	Thimerosal, EDTA
Akwa Tears	PVA	EDTA
Aquisite	PEG, Dex	No preservative
Bion Tears	Dex, HMC	No preservative
Comfort Tears	HEC	Benzalkonium Cl, EDTA
Isopto	HMC	Benzalkonium Cl
Celluvisc	CMC 1.0%	No preservative
Just Tears	PVA	Chlorbutanol
Murocel	HPMC 1.5%, DEX	Parabens
Teargard	HEC	EDTA
Tearisol	HPMC 1.0%	Benzalkonium Cl, EDTA
Tears Naturale	HMC, DEX	EDTA
Tears Naturale II	HMC, DEX	Polyquaternium-1
Tears Renewed	MC, DEX	Benzalkonium Cl, EDTA
Tears Naturale Free	HMC, DEX	No preservative
Vit-A-Drops	Vitamin A, PSB	EDTA
Hypotears	PVA 1%, HEC, DEX	Benzalkonium Cl, EDTA
Liquifilm Tears	PVA 1.4%	Chlorobutanol
Refresh	PVA 1.4%	No preservative
Tears Plus	PVA 1.4%	Chlorobutanol
Ointments		
Akwa Tears	Petrolatum, Lanolin	No preservative
Dry Eyes	Petrolatum	No preservative
Duratears	Petrolatum, Lanolin	No preservative
Hypotears	Petrolatum	No preservative
Lacri-Lube	Petrolatum, Lanolin	Chlorobutanol
Lacri-Lube S.O.P.	Petrolatum, Lanolin	No preservative
Refresh PM	Petrolatum, Lanolin	No preservative

CMC = carboxymethylcellulose, DEX = dextran, GEL = gelatine, HEC = hydroxyethyl cellulose, EDTA = ethylenediaminetetraacetic acid, HPMC = hydroxypropyl methyl cellulose, MC = methyl cellulose, PSB = polysorbate 80, PVA = polyvinyl alcohol, PG = propylene glycol.

▼ *Key Point* The first sign of pilocarpine toxicity is hypersalivation, followed by vomiting and diarrhea. Severe bradycardia and death can occur with overdosage.

Gastrointestinal discomfort is a side effect in humans that cannot be evaluated in dogs. Pilocarpine's effect diminishes over time. Treatment is long term. Approximately 20% of dogs respond positively.

Mucolytics

Acetylcysteine 5% (Mucomyst) (diluted 1;1 with artificial tears) solution may be applied topically once or twice daily to reduce the heavy mucus accumulation on the eye. Package directions indicate a shelf life of 5 days; however, it can be refrigerated and used longer, provided it is not discolored.

Topical Antibiotics

Use topical broad-spectrum *antibiotics* whenever corneal ulcers or secondary bacterial conjunctivitis, notably a purulent discharge, develops (see Chaps. 152 and 153). Because bacterial overgrowth rather than a specific pathogen is involved, ocular culture is rarely needed.

Topical Corticosteroids

Use topical *corticosteroids* judiciously to decrease inflammatory signs. Prior to application, evaluate a corneal fluorescein stain to ensure the absence of corneal ulceration. Because corneal ulcers can occur intermittently in KCS, and because corticosteroids activate collagenase that can melt an ulcer and cause ocular perforation, the high risk of steroids must be conveyed to the owner, balanced with the need for anti-inflammatory drugs. In general, topical cyclosporine is better as an anti-inflammatory agent, because it avoids the risk of a melting corneal ulcer that is associated with corticosteroids. Some ophthalmologists prefer concurrent cyclosporine and corticosteroids in patients with dense pigmentary keratitis.

Surgical Treatment

When medical management fails, the *parotid salivary duct can be surgically transposed* to the lateral conjunctival surface. Refer the animal to an ophthalmologist if this procedure is necessary.

PROLAPSE OF THE GLAND OF THE THIRD EYELID

Hypertrophy and prolapse of the nictitating membrane gland, i.e., gland of the third eyelid, also called "cherry eye," presents an unattractive appearance often accompanied by recurrent conjunctivitis.

▼ *Key Point* Removal of the third eyelid gland precipitates KCS in a predisposed animal. Because this gland provides half the lacrimation, do not remove it.

The gland can be repositioned surgically (Fig. 158–2). Alternatively, topical corticosteroids and antibiotics can be administered to combat the conjunctivitis, and the appearance can be ignored.

Surgical Procedure

Objectives

- Replace the gland of the nictitans to its normal position.
- Restore normal nictitans function.
- Preserve function of the gland of the nictitans.

Equipment

- Eyelid speculum
- Standard ophthalmic surgical pack (see Chap. 150)

Technique

1. Expose the globe for repositioning of the nictitating membrane and nictitans gland (see Fig. 158–2A).
2. Extend the nictitating membrane and incise the palpebral conjunctiva of the fornix (see Fig. 158–2B).
3. With 3-0 nonabsorbable monofilament suture, take a long bite of the periosteum along the orbital rim. The needle should traverse medially to laterally through the rim and not perpendicularly (toward the eyeball).
4. Pass the suture back through the incision, then dorsally through the prolapsed gland, exiting on the dorsal bulbar face (see Fig. 158–2C).
5. Reflect the nictitating membrane downward.
6. Pass the suture back through the exit hole in the apex of the gland, taking a horizontal bite through the dorsal prominence of the gland.

7. The final pass of suture begins again at the previous exit hole and passes ventrally through the gland, exiting through the conjunctival incision, within which both suture ends are securely tied (see Fig. 158–2D).
8. Alternatively, replace the gland using the "pocket" technique. See reference for details (Morgan, Duddy, McClurg).

Postoperative Care and Complications

- Administer topical broad-spectrum antibiotics four times daily for 7 days
- Complications are uncommon, but include reprolapse of the gland and infection of the surgical site. Reprolapse is treated surgically, repositioning the gland. Infection is managed with systemic antibiotics.

EPIPHORA

Epiphora is the overflow of tears down the face. It can be an important sign of ocular pain, or it can be a cosmetic problem (staining of facial hair) associated with nasolacrimal duct dysfunction.

When corneal ulceration or uveitis is present, investigate the underlying etiology as described in Chapter 153.

Aberrant Hair

Aberrant hair can also cause epiphora. When facial hairs lie in the tear film (trichiasis), they act like a wick and draw tears onto the face. Distichia (abnormal eyelashes) and entropion (rolling inward of the lid margin) also cause epiphora, and surgical correction is advised (see Chap. 151).

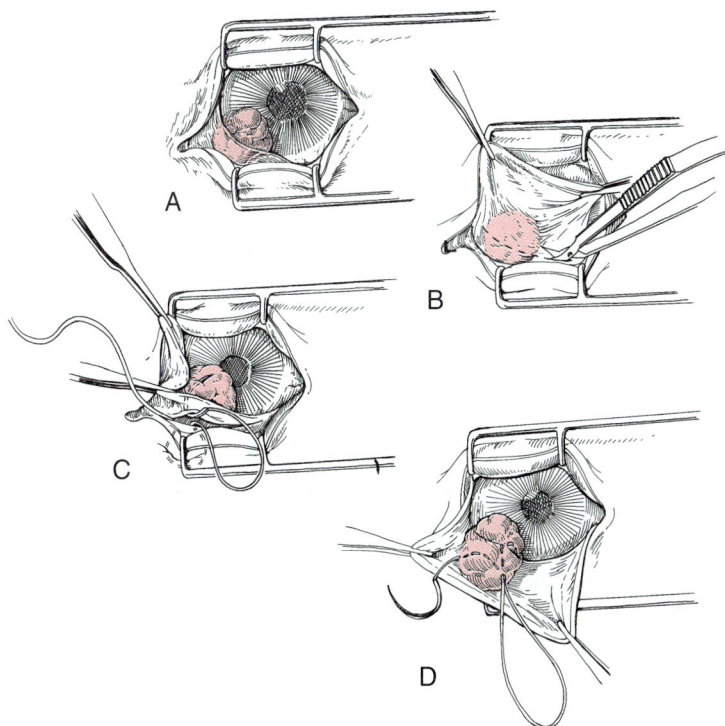

Figure 158–2. Procedure for repositioning of nictitating membrane and gland. See text for explanation. (From Kaswan RL, Martin CL: Surgical correction of the third eyelid prolapse in dogs. J Am Vet Med Assoc 186:83, 1985.)

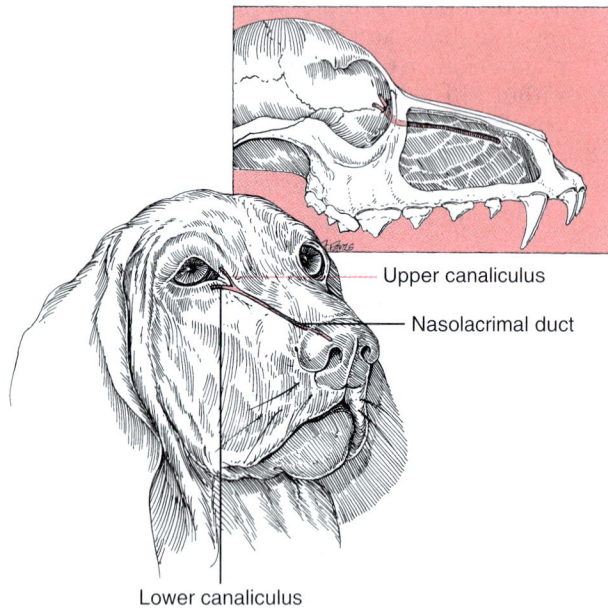

Figure 158–3. Anatomic representation of the canaliculi and nasolacrimal duct.

Dacrocystitis

Dacryocystitis, inflammation and obstruction of the nasolacrimal outflow duct (Fig. 158–3), may cause epiphora. Careful irrigation of the duct with a lacrimal cannula is advised (see Chap. 150). Topical antibiotic-corticosteroid preparations are indicated. In the case of recurrent nasolacrimal duct obstruction, anesthetize the animal and place an indwelling monofilament nylon suture (2-0 to 4-0, depending on size) for 2 weeks to maintain patency while using topical antibiotic-corticosteroid preparations.

Imperforate Inferior Punctum

Imperforate inferior punctum is seen in some dogs, especially cocker spaniels. The nasolacrimal system is normal except for a conjunctival membrane covering the inferior nasolacrimal canaliculus. Grasp the conjunctiva over this area and excise. Then irrigate the nasolacrimal system (see Chap. 150). This procedure can often be performed using topical anesthesia. Give topical antibiotic-corticosteroids for 5–7 days following the correction.

Nasolacrimal Punctal Malposition

Nasolacrimal punctal malposition may occur in exophthalmic dogs with prominent globes and tight lid conformation. With medial entropion, the ventral punctum may roll inward, such that the tears are not drained efficiently. Medial entropion correction can be used (see Chap. 151).

SUPPLEMENTAL READINGS

Lavach JD: The lacrimal system. *In* Slatter DH, ed.: Textbook of Small Animal Surgery, vol. II. Philadelphia: WB Saunders, 1985, p 1496.

Jensen HE: Keratitis sicca and parotic duct transposition. Compend Cont Ed Pract Vet 9:721, 1979.

Kaswan RL, Salisbury MA: A new perspective on canine keratoconjunctivitis sicca. Vet Clin North Am [Sm Anim Pract] 20:583, 1990.

Kern TJ: Disorders of the lacrimal system. *In* Kirk RW, ed.: Current Veterinary Therapy IX. Philadelphia: WB Saunders, 1986, p 634.

Morgan RV, Duddy JM, McClurg. Prolapse of the gland of the third eyelid in dogs: A retrospective study of 89 cases (1980–1990). J Am Anim Hosp Assoc 29:56, 1993.

159 Diseases of the Orbit

Mary B. Glaze

Disorders of the orbit are relatively uncommon in companion animals. Because the area cannot be directly examined without sophisticated imaging devices or complicated surgical procedures, even the simplest of lesions can pose a diagnostic and therapeutic challenge.

ORBITAL ANATOMY

Orbital Cavity

- The orbit is a cone-shaped cavity that surrounds the eye and its supporting structures.
- Only the medial wall and part of the orbital roof are bony in the dog and cat. The floor of the orbit is muscular, with the exception of a small shelf of maxillary bone in the cat. The lateral aspect is completed by a ligament that bridges the space between the frontal and zygomatic bones.
- Three prominent openings at the apex of the orbit permit the passage of its major vessels and nerves.
- When the mouth is opened, the dorsal aspect of the ramus of the mandible moves rostrally, compressing the orbital contents.
- Neighboring structures include the oral cavity, teeth, tongue, zygomatic salivary gland, mastication muscles, paranasal sinuses, and nasal turbinates. Diseases of these structures may extend into the orbit and must always be considered when evaluating orbital disease.

Orbital Contents

- The contents of the orbit are enclosed by a fibrous membrane, the periorbita, which attaches to the orbital wall at the optic foramen and extends to the orbital rim. The periorbita contains sympathetically innervated smooth muscle fibers.
- The anterior limit of the orbit is formed by a sheet of connective tissue, the orbital septum, which extends from the periorbita at the orbital margin to blend with the tarsus of the lid.
- Of the seven extraocular muscles, six originate at the orbital apex. The inferior oblique arises from the anteromedial orbital wall.
- The orbital fat pad cushions the orbital contents and is found between the periorbita and the surrounding structures. Fat is also located within the periorbita between the extraocular muscles.

- In addition to numerous arteries, veins, and autonomic nerves, the second, third, fourth, and sixth cranial nerves and the ophthalmic branch of the trigeminal nerve traverse the orbit.
- The nictitans occupies the ventronasal portion of the orbit and moves primarily in relation to globe movements.
- The lacrimal gland is contained within the periorbita near the superotemporal aspect of the globe.
- The zygomatic salivary gland occupies the lateral orbital floor, just behind the orbital margin and outside the periorbita.

ALTERATIONS IN THE GLOBE-ORBIT RELATIONSHIP

The position of the eye within the orbit depends upon the orbital dimensions, the relative globe size, and the volume of the other orbital contents. The normal brachycephalic dog or cat has a shallow orbit and prominent eye. Larger orbits and less prominent eyes are found in mesaticephalic and dolichocephalic breeds. As a general rule, the feline globe nearly fills the orbit and predisposes the animal to alterations in the globe-orbit relationship early in the course of orbital disease.

▼ *Key Point* The first clinical sign of orbital disease is often a change in the position or the direction of the globe relative to the orbital rim and to the other eye.

EXOPHTHALMOS

Exophthalmos refers to the abnormal protrusion of a normal-sized eye. The condition is distinguished from buphthalmos (enlarged eye) by comparing the corneal diameter of the animal's affected eye with the normal eye. Differentiate exophthalmos from contralateral enophthalmos, the exaggerated palpebral fissures of macroblepharon and facial paralysis, and the characteristically prominent globe of the brachycephalic dog and cat.

Causes of exophthalmos in dogs and cats encompass a spectrum of developmental disorders, inflammatory processes, neoplasias, traumatic lesions, cystic disorders, and skeletal diseases.

Developmental Disorders

Congenital Cysts

- Orbital cysts develop in association with other ocular anomalies, appearing as appendages of microphthalmic eyes or entirely supplanting a recognizable globe.
- These cysts are rare, nonheritable consequences of defective ocular organogenesis.
- If asymptomatic and cosmetically acceptable, no treatment is warranted. Excise large, exposed cysts to prevent secondary drying and irritation.

Craniofacial Deformities

- *Cyclopia* is a rare lethal anomaly in which the orbits and their contents are fused into a single structure. The anomaly is characterized by a single midline orbit and a dysplastic eye, which may appear as a single or bilobed sphere. The nose and maxilla are rudimentary. Obviously there is no treatment for this anomaly.
- *Orbital malformation* and a subsequent divergence of the ocular axes accompany hydrocephalus (see Chap. 145 for further discussion of hydrocephalus).

Arteriovenous Malformations

Etiology

Rarely, fistulas may develop between orbital or periorbital vessels. The cause is unknown.

Clinical Signs

Exophthalmos is associated with a pulsatile murmur auscultated over the orbit. The bruit diminishes when the carotid artery is compressed. The exophthalmos may exacerbate in response to postural changes, as when the animal lowers its head to eat.

Diagnosis

Confirm the malformation in the anesthetized patient using orbital ultrasonography, color Doppler imaging, or contrast venography. For venography, inject 5–10 ml of contrast medium into the angularis oculi vein, using a 21-gauge needle or catheter, immediately before and during radiography. Perform a contrast study on the normal side for comparison.

Treatment

Surgical attempts at ligation and resection are frequently unsatisfactory. One report described severe intraoperative hemorrhage and postoperative recurrence of the lesion in a dog.

Acquired Disorders

Acquired disorders are more common than congenital orbital diseases as causes of exophthalmos in dogs and cats. Acute lesions associated with discomfort and swelling of conjunctiva and eyelids are usually inflammatory, whereas slowly progressive, nonpainful disorders are secondary to space-occupying lesions.

▼ *Key Point* In instances of acquired exophthalmos, document the rapidity of onset and the presence or absence of pain, especially that noted upon opening the mouth.

Inflammatory/Infectious Disorders

Orbital Cellulitis/Orbital Abscess

Orbital inflammatory disease is a common cause of *acute, painful,* unilateral exophthalmos.

Etiology
Orbital inflammation is usually the result of trauma or infection or the extension of a disease process from neighboring structures.

- Trauma—Trauma produces both septic and nonseptic inflammation. Infections follow breaching of the oral mucosa or eyelids by bite wounds or foreign objects, such as bones. Blunt trauma may damage the osseous and soft tissues of the orbit. Iatrogenic injury may occur as a consequence of aggressive or improper dental extraction techniques. Occasionally, a foreign body will be retained within the orbit, causing recurrent inflammation.
- Infection—Bacteria, fungi, and parasites infect the orbit primarily or extend from the paranasal sinuses and nasal cavity. Orbital fungal pyogranulomas can occur with blastomycosis, cryptococcosis, and coccidioidomycosis. In cats, *Aspergillus* and *Penicillium* have been implicated in orbital cellulitis secondary to sinusitis. Larvae of *Dirofilaria immitis* and *Ancylostoma* species produce primary orbital cellulitis by invading canine orbital tissues. The nasal mite *Pneumonyssus caninum* is a documented cause of orbital cellulitis and sinusitis in a dog. Even *Cuterebra* larvae occasionally invade the orbit.
- Extension of Disease—Disorders of the teeth, frontal or paranasal sinuses, nasolacrimal system, temporal and pterygoid muscles, or zygomatic salivary and lacrimal glands may cause secondary orbital inflammation or infection. Inflammation of the posterior sclera may also affect adjacent orbital tissues.
- Rare proliferative inflammatory disorders referred to as pseudotumors may mimic orbital neoplasms and include fibrous histiocytoma, undifferentiated inflammatory pseudotumor, and eosinophilic granuloma.

Clinical Signs
Orbital inflammation is characterized by a relatively *acute* unilateral exophthalmos, with chemosis, third eyelid protrusion, and *pain on opening the mouth.* The animal may be febrile and exhibit an inflammatory leukogram. Abscesses may produce swelling or discoloration behind the last upper molar.

Diagnosis
Diagnosis is based upon history and physical examination, including a thorough evaluation of the oral cavity.

Consider sedation in animals in obvious pain. Hematology, radiography, cytology, and culture of orbital aspirates may be of benefit in some cases.

Radiographically localize orbital foreign bodies with four views: lateral, ventrodorsal, oblique, and frontal. Place a ring of wire around the limbus as a helpful point of reference.

Treatment

- Administer a broad-spectrum systemic antibiotic for at least 10 days. Response to antibiotic therapy is generally rapid, with resolution within 1 week.
- Protect the corneal surface with an antibiotic ophthalmic ointment in cases of extreme exophthalmos.
- Alleviate the acute swelling and discomfort with compresses and a systemic nonsteroidal anti-inflammatory agent (aspirin, 10–25 mg/kg q12h PO in dogs). Corticosteroid therapy is controversial owing to the potential for sepsis in some patients.
- If no response is seen within 24–48 hours, establish ventral drainage through the mouth.
- Incise the mucous membrane behind the last upper molar with a #15 Bard-Parker scalpel blade.
- Carefully insert a hemostat through the pterygoid muscle and open gently in the retrobulbar space. Insert a sterile, open-ended tomcat catheter through the mucosal opening to obtain aspirates for cytology and culture.

▼ *Key Point* This procedure can damage the optic nerve, globe, or major orbital vasculature and must be performed carefully.

Eosinophilic Myositis

Inflammation and swelling of the muscles of mastication may compromise the orbital space and push the globe forward.

Etiology

The finding of myofibril-specific antibodies in affected dogs suggests an autoimmune disorder.

Clinical Signs

Temporal and masseter muscle swelling causes fever, pain on opening the mouth, difficulty eating, and trismus (spasm of masticatory muscles). The German shepherd appears most susceptible. The condition is more often bilateral than unilateral. Acute episodes may last 10–20 days. Recurrences lead to muscle atrophy and decreased prominence of the globe. Blindness is a rare complication.

Diagnosis

Confirm the clinical diagnosis with temporal muscle biopsy samples, which demonstrate mononuclear and eosinophilic infiltrates (see Chap. 149). The finding of peripheral eosinophilia is inconsistent.

Treatment

Administer oral prednisone, beginning with a daily dose of 1 mg/kg for 1–2 weeks. Continue treatment for a total of 4–6 weeks, reducing the dose by half each week. Treatment must precede the onset of muscle atrophy to prevent recession of the globe into the orbit.

Bilateral Extraocular Polymyositis

This unusual myositis targets the extrinsic muscles of the eye in primarily young, large-breed dogs.

Etiology

A mononuclear infiltrate composed predominantly of T lymphocytes and localized to the extraocular muscle bellies suggests an immune mechanism directed at specific extraocular myofibers. The disorder is reminiscent of euthyroid Graves' ophthalmopathy in humans.

Clinical Signs

- Affected dogs range in age from 5–72 months, with a mean of 13.5 months. Females are affected twice as often as males. The golden retriever is the most commonly affected breed.
- Chemosis typically precedes the onset of bilateral, sometimes asymmetrical, nonpainful exophthalmos. The globes appear otherwise normal. Vision impairment occurs infrequently as a consequence of retinitis or compressive optic neuropathy.

Diagnosis

Document the extraocular muscle swelling with orbital echography, computed tomography, or magnetic resonance imaging. Confirm the clinical diagnosis with extraocular muscle biopsy to demonstrate the mononuclear cell infiltrate which stains positively with anti-CD3 antibody. Complete blood counts and serum chemistry values are normal.

Treatment

Administer oral prednisone, 1–2 mg/kg every 12 hours. Minimize recrudescences by continuing therapy for at least 21 days before tapering dosage. Topical corticosteroid therapy is not effective.

Prognosis

The mean duration of clinical signs from the onset of chemosis to resolution of exophthalmos is 5.8 weeks. Recurrences are likely. Strabismus and enophthalmos are uncommon sequelae.

Neoplasia

▼ *Key Point* Most orbital neoplasms are aggressive, malignant tumors that are diagnosed in the advanced stages of development.

Etiology

Both primary and secondary orbital tumors occur in dogs and cats. Primary neoplasms arise from an assortment of tissues within the orbit, including epithelium; bone; nerves; vessels; and connective, hemolymphatic, and glandular tissues. Secondary tumors extend from adjacent structures or metastasize from distant sites.

In dogs, 75% of orbital tumors are primary; 70% of feline tumors invade from adjacent tissues. In both species, 90% of orbital tumors are malignant.

Clinical Signs

Gradual, painless exophthalmos is accompanied by periocular swelling, third eyelid protrusion, and globe deviation. Secondary lagophthalmos may cause corneal drying. Compression of the globe can cause retinal detachment with subsequent abnormalities of the pupillary light response and blindness. Primary orbital neoplasia is typically unilateral. Metastatic disease may affect both orbits.

The mean age of dogs with orbital neoplasia is 8 years, ranging from 18 months to 15 years. Older cats experience a similar risk, yet orbital lymphosarcoma and multicentric fibrosarcoma occur in cats less than 2 years of age.

Diagnosis

- Perform a complete physical examination to evaluate for other neoplastic changes.
- Substantiate the clinical diagnosis with radiography and orbital ultrasonography.
- Evaluate adjacent structures, such as the nasal cavity and sinuses, radiographically.
- Perform thoracic radiography for metastatic disease.
- With the animal heavily sedated or anesthetized, obtain orbital aspirates for cytologic evaluation using a 1-inch, 22-gauge needle attached to a 12-ml syringe. The direction of deviation of the exophthalmic globe suggests the tumor's location and the site for needle entry. For example, lateral strabismus suggests a medial space-occupying mass. To reach the mass, insert the needle medial to the third eyelid, penetrate the conjunctiva, and aspirate gently along the medial orbital wall. Other orbital quadrants may be sampled in a similar manner. For masses directly behind the eye, surgically prepare the lateral aspect of the orbit and insert the needle just posterior to the angle formed by the lateral orbital ligament and the zygomatic arch. If available, ultrasound-guided orbital aspiration helps to minimize complications and ensure accurate needle placement.

Treatment

Surgical resection of the neoplasm is the treatment of choice. Orbitotomy and excision may be attempted in cases of circumscribed primary tumors. If the extent of involvement precludes total excision of the tumor, perform orbital exenteration (removal of the globe; adnexa, and orbital contents). Many tumors respond to adjunct chemotherapy or radiation therapy (see Chap. 24).

Surgical approaches to the orbit are described elsewhere. Refer patients requiring exploratory orbitotomy to a veterinary ophthalmologist or surgeon.

Prognosis

In a series of 23 patients, only 3 dogs with orbital neoplasia survived 3 years. The mean survival time after diagnosis in a series of 21 cats was only 1.9 months.

Orbital Trauma

Traumatic Proptosis

Complete displacement of the globe from the orbit is a true emergency. Treatment begins as soon as the animal's systemic condition allows.

Etiology

The depth of the orbit dictates the force necessary to displace the globe. Proptosis most commonly occurs in the brachycephalic dog because of its shallow orbit and exaggerated palpebral fissure. Excessive restraint may be sufficient to dislodge the globe. In contrast, the feline eye is rarely displaced from its well-proportioned orbit except in severe head trauma.

Clinical Signs

The globe rests in front of the eyelids, its proximity to the orbit determined by the extent of the extraocular muscle damage, the integrity of the optic nerve, and the degree of retrobulbar hemorrhage. Chemosis and subconjunctival hemorrhage are often present. Prolonged exposure of the cornea leads to ulceration.

Diagnosis

Perform a thorough physical examination to assess the other effects of head trauma. Examine the eye closely for intraocular damage. Palpate the orbital rim for fractures, and radiograph if indicated. Apply fluorescein dye to the cornea to document ulceration.

Treatment

Apply a bland ophthalmic ointment to the eye to protect the corneal surface from drying. Once the animal's general condition is stabilized from the effects of the trauma, reposition the eye as soon as possible. Reserve enucleation for ruptured globes or for those with severed optic nerves.

Surgical Procedure

Objectives

- Manipulate the eyelids to place them anterior to the globe.
- Protect the cornea from exposure.

Equipment

- Two strabismus hooks
- Ophthalmic forceps and needle holder
- Tubing or other material suitable for use as stents

Technique

1. Anesthetize the patient.
2. Irrigate the globe and surrounding tissues with sterile physiologic saline.
3. Elevate the eyelid margins with either a blunt probe, such as a strabismus hook, or simple interrupted 4-0 nonabsorbable suture material placed over stents. Sutures enter the eyelid 5 mm from the margin and exit through the meibomian gland openings to prevent corneal damage. As the eyelids elevate, apply gentle counterpressure against the cornea with a moistened cotton ball or the flat surface of a scalpel handle to replace the globe within the orbit.
4. Suture the eyelid margins together, leaving a slight separation at the medial canthus to facilitate topical therapy with broad-spectrum antibiotics and 1% atropine ointments two or three times daily.
5. Administer an oral broad-spectrum antibiotic, such as ampicillin, for 7 days. Avoid systemic sulfonamides, which may reduce tear production.
6. Administer an initial IV or IM injection of dexamethasone (0.2 mg/kg). Continue oral prednisone therapy (1.0 mg/kg) for 5 days to reduce orbital swelling.

▼ *Key Point* Do not inject medication into the retrobulbar area. Do not aspirate orbital contents or the globe itself.

---

7. Remove the eyelid sutures when the orbital swelling resolves, usually in 2–3 weeks. Orbital swelling is evaluated by retropulsing the globe. Use the unaffected eye for comparison.

Prognosis

An animal with an eye tightly positioned against the eyelids, a miotic pupil, a minimal amount of extraocular muscle damage, and an absence of hyphema has the best prognosis for salvaging the globe. Prognosis for vision is guarded at best.

Potential sequelae include lateral strabismus, chronic keratitis due to lagophthalmos or low tear production, phthisis bulbi, and blindness. A deviated globe may spontaneously realign as the extraocular muscles fibrose after several weeks to months.

Orbital Hemorrhage/Emphysema

Etiology

Less severe orbital trauma may result in lagophthalmos due to retrobulbar and subconjunctival hemorrhage. Fractures of the sinus wall may cause air to collect beneath the conjunctiva. Entry of air through the nasolacrimal duct may lead to orbital emphysema after routine enucleation.

Clinical Signs and Diagnosis

Mild-to-moderate exophthalmos is associated with lagophthalmos, chemosis, subconjunctival hemorrhage or emphysema, and lid swelling.

Treatment

Confine the patient to limit further hemorrhage. Use cold compresses to reduce acute swelling. Apply topical methylcellulose artificial tear ointments frequently (four to six times daily) to protect the corneal surface from drying. Administer oral or parenteral corticosteroids as described for the proptosed globe. Avoid nonsteroidal anti-inflammatory drugs, such as aspirin, which inhibit platelet function.

Arteriovenous Fistula

Orbital vascular fistulas may develop secondary to trauma. Clinical signs and diagnostic procedures are similar to those described for developmental vascular anomalies.

Cystic Diseases

Acquired orbital cysts are uncommon consequences of trauma to orbital glands and incomplete excision of secretory tissues during enucleation.

Zygomatic Mucocele

Leakage of saliva from the zygomatic salivary gland or its duct is an uncommon cause of exophthalmos in the dog.

Etiology

The condition may occur spontaneously or after orbital trauma.

Clinical Signs

A painless swelling beneath the inferior temporal or nasal conjunctival fornix is commonly associated with prominence of the third eyelid. The mucosa behind the last upper molar may protrude.

Diagnosis

Aspirate fluid from the lesion. The mucocele contains a clear, straw-colored, or blood-tinged tenacious material. Perform a zygomatic sialogram to confirm the clinical and cytologic diagnosis.

Treatment

The treatment is surgical and the location of the swelling dictates the approach for removal of the mucocele. Approach mucoceles beneath the inferior conjunctival cul-de-sac transconjunctivally, making an incision between the nictitans and the lower eyelid, or through the eyelid surface. Lateral mucoceles require a limited orbitotomy, the details of which are described in other texts.

Mucocele Following Enucleation

Cystic swelling of the orbit may follow enucleation if mucus or tear-producing tissues are not completely excised.

Etiology

Retained conjunctival goblet cells or glandular tissue from the third eyelid may cause cystic swelling of the orbit.

Clinical Signs

As fluid accumulates within the orbit, the overlying skin distends. A fistula may develop, draining seromucoid fluid.

Diagnosis

Clinical signs are suggestive. Perform aspiration cytology to rule out postsurgical infection.

Treatment

Explore the orbit to remove retained secretory tissue, approaching anteriorly through the eyelids.

Other Causes of Exophthalmos

Anecdotal reports attribute other causes of exophthalmos to the hormonal influences of estrus and to the edema caused by hypoproteinemia or systemic hypertension.

ENOPHTHALMOS

Enophthalmos refers to the recession of the eye within the orbit. Differentiate the condition from the relative enophthalmos that accompanies periorbital swelling or edema of the eyelids and conjunctiva.

Enophthalmos may be accompanied by mucoid-to-mucopurulent discharge, because of the exaggerated conjunctival cul-de-sac, and by ptosis and entropion, because of the eyelids losing the support of the underlying globe. With rare exception, restoration of the globe's normal position within the orbit is seldom successful.

Causes of enophthalmos include developmental abnormalities, retraction of the globe due to pain, atrophy of orbital tissues following debilitating disease or trauma, and loss of smooth muscle tone in the periorbita.

Developmental Disorders

Microphthalmos/Anophthalmos

The microphthalmic globe fails to develop to normal size in dogs and occasionally in cats. Anophthalmos refers to a rare condition in which all ocular tissues are absent.

Etiology

Microphthalmos is inherited in several breeds of dog, including the Australian shepherd, miniature schnauzer, Old English sheepdog, Akita, Cavalier King Charles spaniel, Samoyed, American cocker spaniel, Bedlington and Sealyham terriers, beagle, Labrador retriever, and Doberman pinscher. Multiple ocular defects, including microphthalmos, occur associated with partial albinism and deafness in the Great Dane and collie. Teratogenic influences during early pregnancy may affect ocular de-

velopment. Causes of microphthalmos in cats are poorly characterized.

Clinical Signs

The anomaly is characterized by varying degrees of enophthalmos. Because orbital development is influenced by globe size during skeletal maturation, the orbit may also appear small and the palpebral fissure narrowed. Accompanying ocular defects include persistent pupillary membranes, cataracts, colobomas, retinal dysplasias, and orbital cysts. Multiple ocular anomalies may render the globe sightless, but on occasion small globes may be structurally and functionally normal.

Diagnosis

Diagnosis is based upon clinical signs. Differentiate microphthalmos from phthisis bulbi, an acquired atrophy of the globe. Evidence of scarring, inflammation, and normal-sized orbit accompany atrophy. Anophthalmos is diagnosed only after serial histologic examination of orbital tissue has excluded the possibility of microphthalmos.

Treatment

There is no treatment for microphthalmos. Enucleate if chronic irritation and discharge accompany the condition. Eliminate affected animals from breeding programs.

Breed-Related Enophthalmos

Etiology

The large orbits and deeply set eyes inherited as conformational traits of dolichocephalic breeds, such as the Doberman pinscher, Irish setter, and golden retriever, may create a relative enophthalmos.

Clinical Signs and Diagnosis

The globe appears normal but deeply set within the orbit. The nictitans may be prominent. Mucoid-to-mucopurulent discharge, ptosis, and entropion are common sequelae.

Treatment

The condition is incurable. Manage secondary conjunctivitis with intermittent applications of topical antibiotic-corticosteroid ointment. Correct accompanying entropion.

Acquired Disorders

Acquired enophthalmos is common, particularly in response to ocular pain and as a consequence of severe or recurrent inflammation of the globe itself.

Ocular Pain

The retractor bulbi muscle pulls the eye into the orbit when pain is present. The phenomenon is more apparent in the dog than the cat.

Etiology

Any painful ocular disorder may cause enophthalmos, especially ulcerative keratitis, anterior uveitis, and acute glaucoma.

Clinical Signs

In addition to enophthalmos, the animal demonstrates other nonspecific signs of ocular pain: excessive tearing, eye rubbing, blepharospasm, photophobia, and nictitans protrusion.

Diagnosis

Examine closely for ectopic cilia, foreign body, corneal ulcer, or intraocular disease. Pain associated with ocular surface disorders, such as ulcers, may decrease following topical application of 0.5% proparacaine.

Treatment

Treat the underlying ocular disease.

Changes in Orbital Volume

Reduction in retrobulbar tissue mass or damage to the bony or soft-tissue structures forming the walls of the orbit causes the globe to recede. Orbital neoplasia occasionally produces enophthalmos, especially in cats.

Dehydration/Cachexia

Loss of retrobulbar fat causes a mechanical sinking of the globe into the orbit. Pronounced weight loss and dehydration secondary to vomiting, diarrhea, or other debilitating conditions decrease the retrobulbar fat pad. Reduced orbital tissue mass may also be a feature of aging. Correct dehydration is treated, but enophthalmos secondary to cachexia and loss of retrobulbar fat may not be reversible.

Atrophy Following Inflammation or Trauma

Reduction of the orbital tissue mass effectively enlarges the orbit, resulting in enophthalmos.

Etiology

Atrophy of the temporal, masseter, and pterygoid muscles is relatively common in dogs following myositis or as an idiopathic phenomenon (see Chap. 149). Brain stem infections or injuries may produce alterations in the trigeminal motor nucleus and result in atrophy of the muscles of mastication. Similar lesions may develop as a consequence of trauma to the trigeminal nerve at the base of the ear or fractures in the temporomandibular joint or skull at the oval foramen. Chronic or recurrent orbital inflammation may lead to atrophy of orbital contents; trauma or inflammation of the globe may lead to phthisis bulbi.

Clinical Signs and Diagnosis

Atrophy of the masticatory muscles alters the facial appearance, exaggerating the skull's bony protuberances. The animal is unable to open the mouth widely and often has difficulty prehending food. Enophthalmos and passive nictitans prolapse may cause visual impairment.

The phthisical globe is small and blind, with a thickened sclera, opaque cornea, and profound disorganization and scarring of the intraocular structures.

Treatment

Consult a veterinary ophthalmologist regarding autogenous fat transplants or implantable beads (strictly a cosmetic procedure) to modify the degree of postinflammatory or post-traumatic enophthalmos.

There is no effective treatment for phthisis bulbi. Control secondary conjunctivitis with regular irrigation and intermittent topical antibiotic-corticosteroid ophthalmic preparations. Enucleate phthisical globes in cats because of the potential for post-traumatic ocular sarcoma.

Orbital Fat Prolapse

Enophthalmos and nonpainful subconjunctival swelling are reported in dogs with prolapse of orbital fat. Subconjunctival fine-needle aspirates are diagnostic. Surgical resection of the displaced fat is curative.

Sympathetic Denervation

Horner syndrome and feline dysautonomia cause loss of sympathetic tone in the periorbita, with varying degrees of enophthalmos (see Chap. 160).

SUPPLEMENTAL READINGS

Gilger BC, Hamilton HL, Wilkie DA, et al.: Traumatic ocular proptoses in dogs and cats: 84 cases (1980–1993). J Am Vet Med Assoc 206:1186, 1995.

Gilger BC, McLaughlin SA, Whitley RD, et al.: Orbital neoplasms in cats: 21 cases (1974–1990). J Am Vet Med Assoc 201:1083, 1992.

Gilger BC, Whitley RD, McLaughlin SA: Modified lateral orbitotomy for removal of orbital neoplasms in two dogs. Vet Surg 23:53, 1994.

Kern TJ: Orbital neoplasia in 23 dogs. J Am Vet Med Assoc 186:489, 1985.

McCalla TL, Moore CP: Exophthalmos in dogs and cats. Compend Contin Educ Pract Vet 11:911, 1989.

O'Brien MG, Withrow SJ, Straw RC, et al.: Total and partial orbitectomy for the treatment of periorbital tumors in 24 dogs and 6 cats: A retrospective study. Vet Surg 25:471, 1996.

Ramsey DT, Gerding PA, Losonsky JM, et al.: Comparative value of diagnostic imaging techniques in a cat with exophthalmos. Vet Comp Ophthalmol 4:198, 1994.

Ramsey DT, Hamor RE, Gerding PA, et al.: Clinical and immunohistochemical characteristics of bilateral extraocular polymyositis of dogs. Proceedings, American College of Veterinary Ophthalmologists 26:130, 1995.

Ramsey DT, Marretta SM, Hamor RE, et al.: Ophthalmic manifestations and complications of dental disease in dogs and cats. J Am Anim Hosp Assoc 32:215, 1996.

160 Neuro-ophthalmology

Randall H. Scagliotti

Clinical signs of ocular dysfunction may appear as disorders in the neuroanatomic pathways that allow normal vision. Vision is optimal when sufficiently protected eyes receive the proper amount of light while holding images steady on the retina. Many complex neurologic systems are involved in vision, including the visual sensory system (retina to visual cortex), the autonomic nervous system (pupillary function and lacrimation), the ocular motor system (neural control of eyeball, eyelid, and third eyelid position and movement), and the trigeminal somatic sensory system (pain sensation) of the eye and adnexa.

The diagnosis of abnormal neuro-ophthalmic signs is dependent upon acquiring a solid base of knowledge about the various neural substrates that enable normal vision. How these neural substrates interact determines the normal physical reflexes and responses that are observed during examination of each of the above-mentioned neurologic systems. This chapter emphasizes the examination process for each system and the interpretation of normal and abnormal responses, and discusses diagnostic tests that can aid in lesion localization and diagnosis. Specific diseases of the eyes and nervous system that afflict each system are discussed in other chapters of this book.

NEURO-OPHTHALMIC ANATOMY

The cranial nerves that enable normal vision are summarized in Table 160–1. The nerves of the petrous temporal bone are of two types: those in transit through the bone and destined for distant locations that subserve the eye or some of its supporting functions like lacrimation, and those that mediate other functions like hearing or taste. Those in transit to and destined for the eyeball or to protective and supporting structures for vision (e.g., the adnexa or the vestibular apparatus for head-eye coordination) include cranial nerves (CNs) V, VII, VIII, postganglionic neurons of the sympathetic nervous system, and pre- and postganglionic fibers of the parasympathetic nervous system. The parasympathetic system (general visceral efferent or GVE fibers) of the glossopharyngeal nerve (CN IX) may be indirectly involved in ensuring ocular health and vision. The preganglionic parasympathetic fibers of CN IX synapse on a collection of cell bodies known as the *otic ganglion*, which lies within the ventrorostral petrous

temporal bone. This ganglion is the source of postganglionic parasympathetic neurons that innervate the parotid and zygomatic salivary glands. These glands may become denervated and dysfunctional (leading to xerostomia) by the same process and at the same time that lacrimation ceases or is diminished from the lacrimal gland (leading to keratoconjunctivitis sicca [KCS]). Be sure the parotid gland is normal before performing parotid duct transposition in cases of medically refactory KCS.

Two neuroanatomic pathways modulate the pupillary light responses, the pupillary light reflex (PLR) pathway and the efferent sympathetic pathway (Fig. 160–1). The afferent arm of the pupillary light reflex pathway from each eye is a three-neuron pathway. Each consists of a retinal chain neuron (photoreceptors and bipolar cells), optic nerve, and pretectal neuron that distribute information bilaterally (i.e., to both parasympathetic nuclei of the third nerve) as a result of the crossover that occurs at both the optic chiasm and the caudal commissure. *Note that the crossover of optic nerve fibers is unequal at the level of both the optic chiasm and caudal commissure.* The afferent arms of the PLR are part of the central nervous system (CNS). Each efferent arm of the PLR is a two-neuron pathway from the autonomic nervous system (ANS) and consists of preganglionic and postganglionic parasympathetic neurons that are distributed as part of the oculomotor nerve (CN III). The efferent arms of the PLR do not cross to the opposite side en route to the iris sphincter muscles (for pupil constriction) and therefore do not distribute information to both eyes. The other pathway that controls the iris is the efferent sympathetic pathway. This pathway, which originates centrally in the posterolateral hypothalamus, remains unilateral throughout its course. The central neuron pathway (which may actually consist of several linked pathways leaving the brain stem) proceeds down the lateral cervical spinal cord to synapse with preganglionic sympathetic fibers within the lateral-rostral thoracic spinal cord. After these fibers exit the vertebral column, they return to the head by ascending the neck in the vagosympathetic trunk, where they synapse on the cranial cervical ganglion medial to the tympanic bullae. The postganglionic sympathetic fibers course through the middle ear and base of the brain to reach the orbits from which they extend to the dilator muscle of the iris (for pupil dilation).

Table 160–1. SUMMARY OF NEUROANATOMY

Nerve	Nerve Type	Nerve Cell Body Location		Ganglion	Distribution	Function
		Gross	Micro			
Optic (CN II)	SSA	Retina	Ganglion cell Layer of retina	—	Lateral geniculate body	Vision
					Pretectal nucleus	Innervates parasympathetic nucleus of CN III (miosis)
Oculomotor (CN III)	SE	Ventral mesencephalon	Motor nucleus of oculomotor nerve	—	Medial, dorsal, ventral recti, ventral oblique Levator palpebrae muscle	Ocular motility
	GVE	Ventral mesencephalon	Parasympathetic nucleus of CN III	Ciliary ganglion	Iris sphincter muscle Ciliary muscle	Miosis Regulates lens curvature
Trochlear (CN IV)	SE	Dorsal mesencephalon	Motor nucleus of trochlear nerve	—	Dorsal oblique muscle	Ocular motility
Trigeminal (CN V)	SA	Cavum trigeminal of dura at apex of petrous temporal bone	Trigeminal ganglion (gasserian or semilunar)	—	Ophthalmic division— orbit Maxillary division— eyelids	Sensory to orbit, eyeball, and eyelid Sensory to eyelids
Abducens (CN VI)	SE	Ventral Metencephalon	Motor nucleus of abducens nerve	—	Lateral rectus muscle Retractor bulbi muscle	Ocular motility Globe retraction, third eyelid protrusion
Facial (CN VII)	SVE	Ventral Metencephalon	Motor nucleus of facial nerve	—	Orbicularis oculi Muscles of face	Eyelid closure Facial expression
	GVE	Ventral Metencephalon	Parasympathetic nucleus of CN VII	Pterygo-palatine ganglion	Lacrimal gland	Tear secretion
Vestibulo-cochlear (CN VIII)	SP	Myelencephalon	Vestibular ganglion	—	Semicircular canals, utricle, sacculus	Coordinates eye with head movement
Glosso-pharyngeal (CN IX)	GVE	Myelencephalon	Parasympathetic nucleus of CN IX	Otic ganglion	Parotid salivary gland	Salivary secretion, used for PDT

CN, cranial nerve; SE, somatic efferents; GVE, general visceral efferents; SVE, special visceral efferents; PDT, parotid duct transposition; SA, somatic afferents; SSA, special somatic afferents; SP (SSA proprio.), special proprioception.

CLINICAL SIGNS OF NEURO-OPHTHALMIC IMPORTANCE

- *Absence of reflex blinking.* Associated with eyelid closure abnormalities.
- *Ptosis or blepharoptosis.* Indicates insufficient opening of the eyelids. Differentiate from *pseudoptosis*, which occurs when the upper eyelid droops over an eye that is abnormal in size (microphthalmic), shape (keratoconus), or position (enophthalmic) (see Chap. 151).
- *Decreased tear production.* Schirmer tear test of less than 10 mm wetting/minute may indicate a disorder of either the afferent arm (trigeminal nerve) or the efferent arm (parasympathetic neurons of the facial nerve) of the trigeminolacrimal reflex. Differentiate injury along the trigeminolacrimal reflex pathway from injury to the lacrimal gland proper (see Chap. 158).
- *Decreased parotid salivary gland secretion.* Can result from denervation of the parasympathetic fibers of the glossopharyngeal (CN IX) nerve. Parotid secretion must be adequate in the event that the parotid salivary duct is to be transpositioned to an eye for treatment of KCS (see Chap. 158).
- *Loss of pain or tactile sensation to the eye and adnexa.* This sign occurs as a result of trigeminal sensory neuropathies. Differentiate ulcerative keratitis due to denervation of the trigeminal nerve (i.e., neuroparalytic keratitis) from other types of ulcerative keratitis.
- *Anisocoria.* Can result from developmental problems of the iris (e.g., aniridia) or acquired problems of the iris (e.g., posterior synechia). Differentiate from the anisocoria observed following neuropathology of the visual sensory system (CN II), pupillary light reflex pathway, or efferent sympathetic pathway.
- *Strabismus.* Indicates a problem with ocular alignment. This may occur due to a space occupying mass in the orbit, mechanical restriction of extraocular muscles, extraocular muscle myopathy or junctionopathy, or neurologic dysfunction to the extraocular muscles.
- *Nystagmus.* An involuntary, repetitive, to-and-fro movement of one or both eyes that includes smooth sinusoidal oscillations (pendular nystagmus) and alternation of slow drift and corrective quick phase

Binocular Overlap

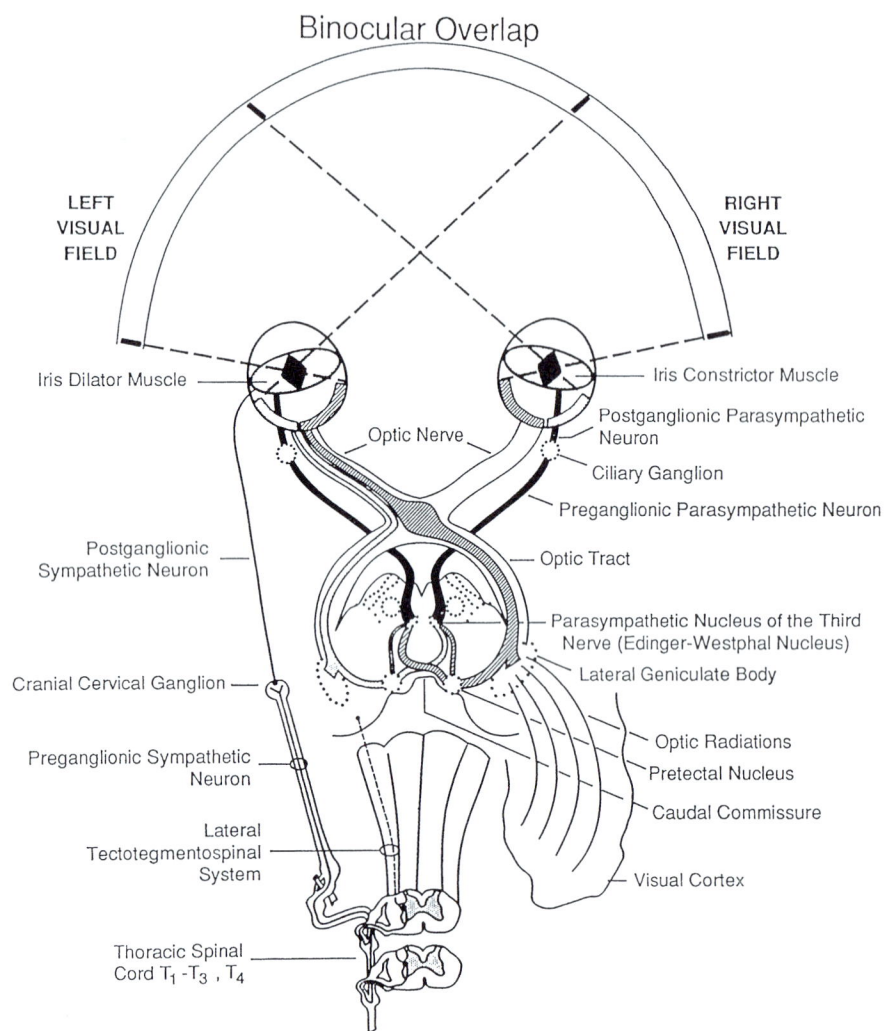

Figure 160–1. Pathways modulating the pupillary light response.

oscillations (jerk nystagmus). Nystagmus occurs in any plane, can be permanent or transient, and may be either acquired (vestibular disease) or congenital (animals born congenitally blind).

- *Blindness.* A congenital or acquired condition in which there is a complete loss of vision including all appreciation of or responses to light and dark. This may result from disorders of the eyes, visual pathways to the brain, or areas in the brain responsible for the sense of vision.

DIAGNOSIS

History

General History

Obtain information about prior neurologic disturbances, systemic illness, head or neck disease, and drug use. Rubbing at the face or eyes with the paws or floor or furniture surfaces may indicate ocular pain. Orbital and ocular pain often lead to altered patterns of behavior. Most often patients with pain become secretive and

reclusive; however, occasionally aggressive behavior is observed.

Ocular History

Establish the specific nature of any ocular secretion; inflammation about the eye, eyelids, and orbit; and abnormalities in globe position and motility. When vision loss is incomplete, owners may characterize specific types of vision abnormalities. These descriptions include having difficulty observing stationary versus moving objects, seeing near versus far, or having loss of night or day vision.

General Physical Examination

Perform a complete physical examination including a thorough neurologic examination as described in Chapter 144, with particular emphasis on CNS II through IX.

▼ *Key Point* Evaluate the ear, nose, mouth, pharynx, and paranasal sinuses, because they are intimately linked in disease to one another and to the eye.

Disease involving any one these regions may directly or indirectly cause abnormal neuro-ophthalmic signs.

Visual Sensory System Evaluation

Visual field testing, strictly speaking, cannot be performed in animals because their eyes will not hold a target (fixate) long enough to assess all visual fields. However, that should not preclude use of helpful clinical tests, albeit crude, to obtain information on vision quality or the integrity of the visual sensory system. Although no one test alone should be relied upon to determine either aspect, use results from all the tests to make a good estimate of the type or degree of vision loss or the location of the lesion.

Ocular Examination

Use focal illumination and magnification to assess the anterior segment, and direct or indirect ophthalmoscopy to examine the posterior segment.

Visual Placing Reaction

This is a visually dependent postural reaction. Lift and support the patient under the abdomen and thorax while holding the head in a forward stationary position and advance toward a table edge. Present the table edge frontally (perpendicular to the long axis of the head and body) and then laterally (parallel to the long axis of the head and body). The normal response of a sighted patient is the forward advancement and placement of both feet on the table when the table edge is presented head-on and a lateral reaching movement with the leg nearest the table edge when it is seen by the **nasal hemiretina** (extreme lateral visual field). In lateral placing, have the nose extend beyond the corner of the table to ensure that only the most extreme portion of the nasal hemiretina (i.e., the most rostral portion of the nasal hemiretina referred to as the monocular crescent) is stimulated. When testing the visual fields, present the table edge from the front and side (laterally) under monocular and binocular test conditions. Visual placing requires an intact rostral portion of the striate cortex and foreleg region of the motor cortex.

Visual Cliff

An indication of depth perception (stereopsis) ability can be obtained with a visual cliff. These are crudely created by using multiple variable height platforms or simply a table with variable height. A homogeneous texture and color has to cover all testing surfaces. Use a black-and-white checkered tablecloth. Normal dogs and cats will jump onto the lower platform (e.g., floor), whereas animals with poor depth perception will be unwilling to do so, will lower their bodies to the tabletop and slide off the table, or will crash their chins into the floor as they miscalculate the depth of the jump. Monocular testing provides a reasonable control for determining whether monocular depth perception cues

have been eliminated by the tablecloth. Most monocular patients are reluctant to jump, or they miscalculate the jump.

Visual Obstacle Course

Use an obstacle course with a standardized layout based on the examiner's preference for most effective geometric design. This will result in more reliable deductions about the performance differences between sighted and nonsighted animals. Use five or six gray polyurethane foam cylinders, 2 feet tall and 4 inches in diameter, rather than the unprofessional and possibly injurious furniture objects customarily used, to ensure a safe, effective course. Run the course under monocular and binocular conditions using photopic (ambient room light) and scotopic (with an incandescent red light bulb on a dimmer switch) illumination. Visually deficient animals will be reluctant to move in a strange environment under ambient light and/or scotopic light conditions, or will move slowly through the course with their noses to the floor (i.e., "pick" their way). A few of the visually impaired will perform in a bouyantly bold manner, yet run into many cylinders during each trial. Four or more trials through the obstacle course performed correctly under both photopic and scotopic illumination can be considered normal.

Dazzle Reflex

This is a *subcortical reflex*, manifested as a *bilateral partial eyelid blink* in response to a bright light shined in one eye at a time. It is present when the optic nerve is intact to the level of the midbrain. It also requires an intact facial nerve to elicit the blink. The closure is rapid and incomplete in the stimulated eye, and if present in the opposite eye, it is less extensive than in the stimulated eye Use a powerful light source (halogen power with a Finoff transilluminator or preferably a fiberoptic light).

Menace Response

The menace response is a *cortically mediated* eyelid closure (i.e., cortical blink) and occasional head withdrawal originating in the cerebral cortex in response to a sudden threatening gesture in the near visual field. This response is complex and not totally understood. It requires intact peripheral and central visual pathways, including the cerebellum and facial nerves. Evaluation of the visual sensory system (CN II and higher vision centers) requires isolating its function and integrity from the corneal blink reflex pathway (CN V–CN VII). If this is not achieved, a blink following a visual threat may elicit the corneal blink reflex afferently mediated by CN V, rather than the desired CN II–mediated menace response. Use a windshield (plastic shield or helmet visor) to block airwaves while still allowing the patient a view of the menacing threat. Menace the visual field of each eye (nasal and temporal hemiretina) after patching the other eye, which eliminates its participation in the response. Then evaluate the left and right binocular visual fields (i.e., the nasal hemiretina of one eye and temporal hemiretina of fellow eye) by eliciting the menace response without patching.

Specialized Diagnostics

- *Electroretinography (ERG).* This technique differentiates retinal pathology from disorders of postretinal anatomy (see Chap. 157).
- *Cerebrospinal fluid (CSF) pressure and analysis.* This invasive technique assesses the status of the CNS when lesions are thought to be central in origin (see Chap. 144).

Autonomic Nervous System Evaluation

Pupillary Responses

Pupillary Light Reflexes (see Fig. 160–1)

This exam is best conducted in darkened conditions using a powerful light source. A halogen-powered light is minimally required to adequately evaluate the pupillary light reflex, but a fiberoptic light source is best. The pupil under direct light stimulation (direct PLR) will constrict to a greater degree than the other eye. The constriction of the other eye is called the indirect or consensual light reflex. Thus, this pupil is said to react indirectly or consensually. Because the pupil receiving the direct light constricts to a greater degree than the other pupil (indirect pupil), an anisocoria exists during this active stimulation that is referred to as a dynamic contraction anisocoria. This is a normal physiologic response. Anisocoria is absent in ambient light unless there is heterochromia of the irides, iris disease, PLR pathway, or efferent sympathetic pupillary pathway pathology.

▼ *Key Point* Remember that iris muscle atrophy (as evidenced by light retroilluminating through holes in the iris) will weaken and, in some advanced cases, prevent the pupillary light reflex.

Measurement of Pupil Size and Symmetry

Pupillary symmetry is best obtained clinically using the direct ophthalmoscope as a crude pupillometer. Direct the light source at the interpupillary space on the bridge of the nose to observe the tapetal reflection of both eyes simultaneously. The overall size of the pupils and the existence of any inequality will be revealed quickly and accurately. Measure *pupil size* in ambient light using a hole sizing ruler or a caliper.

Swinging Flashlight Test

This test measures the integrity of the retina and prechiasmal optic nerve. Perform in a darkened room because the pupillary light reflex will be exaggerated. Immediately following direct light stimulation into one eye, swing the light source into the other eye, and then back again to the first eye directly stimulated. Repeat this procedure back and forth (thus the swinging flashlight) as often as necessary to be sure that both pupils constrict directly and indirectly. If a pupil dilates rather than constricts during direct stimulation immediately following its return from direct stimulation of the other eye, a unilateral retinal or prechiasmal optic nerve lesion exists. If dilatation of a pupil instead of pupil constriction occurs during the swinging flashlight test, this is referred to as positive for the dilating eye.

▼ *Key Point* A positive swinging flashlight test is pathognomonic for a unilateral retinal or prechiasmal optic nerve lesion.

Pharmacologic Testing

Use topical drugs in cases of anisocoria to differentiate anatomic problems in the iris (e.g., synechia or iris atrophy) from neurologic problems. Also use topical drugs to localize the lesion to pre- or postganglionic fibers within each of the two efferent pathways (the efferent sympathetic pathway and the efferent parasympathetic pathway of the PLR). In an injured nerve whose terminals are allowed to degenerate, the structure supplied by it becomes supersensitive to the transmitter substance released by the terminals. Use pilocarpine (2%) and physostigmine (0.5%) to test the parasympathetic system and phenylephrine (10%) and hydroxyamphetamine (1–5%) to test the sympathetic system.

Lacrimation

Schirmer Tear Tests (Schirmer 1 and 2) (see Chap. 158)

Use strips of Whatman paper to measure the autonomic innervation to the lacrimal gland (reflex tearing as measured by Schirmer 1 in the unanesthetized eye) and basal secretion from the lacrimal gland (by Schirmer 2 in the anesthetized eye). The contribution of the gland of the third eyelid is also figured into these measurements.

Trigeminolacrimal Reflex

This reflex is responsible for reflex tearing as measured by Schirmer 1 values. The reflex-induced amount of tears is the difference between Schirmer 1 and 2 values. This difference is not as significant in the cat. The sensory (CN V) nerve of the eye conducts noxious stimuli centrally; the efferent arm of the reflex arises in the parasympathetic nucleus of CN VII in the ventral metencephalon (see Table 160–1) to course with branches of the facial nerve within the petrous temporal bone in route to the orbit. The pterygopalatine ganglion within the extraperiorbital sheath area of the orbit gives rise to postganglionic parasympathetic fibers that course with the zygomaticotemporal nerve (a branch of the maxillary division of the trigeminal nerve) to innervate the lacrimal gland with postganglionic parasympathetic fibers. It is assumed that the same reflex pathway is involved in the tear contribution made by the gland of the third eyelid.

▼ *Key Point* Lacrimation may be affected when the preganglionic parasympathetic fibers within the petrous temporal bone or the postganglionic parasympathetic fibers within the orbit are damaged during infectious or inflammatory disease in these regions.

Ocular Motor System Evaluation

Eyelid Position and Movement

Voluntary Eyelid Movement and Position

Observing *voluntary movement* (blinks or eyelid elevation) in response to visual or auditory stimuli indicates much about normal eyelid closure and opening. Abnormal *eyelid position* is more easily observed because asymmetry of the palpebral fissures is more readily detected than eyelid movement. For instance, in facial paralysis, a lack of voluntary eyelid movement can be easily overlooked with certain head types (i.e., brachycephalic) that conceal the palpebral asymmetry associated with this disorder.

Eyelid Opening

Motoneurons of the oculomotor nerve (CN III) innervate the *levator palpebrae superioris muscle*, the main muscle of upper eyelid elevation. In the dog, the *levator anguli oculi medialis muscle* (innervated by CN VII) assists by elevating the medial portion of the upper eyelid and eyebrow. This muscle action is readily assessed by leading the eyeball into a dorsal and medial position (*intorsion*) within the orbit. In order for an eye looking up and medially to maximize its visual field, the medial upper eyelid must be moved out of the way, so the eyebrow elevates during this eyeball movement. Evaluate both sides in a like manner.

Eyelid Closure

The facial nerve and the *orbicularis oculi muscle*, mediate the final common neurologic pathway for all types of eyelid closure. The corneal blink reflex, dazzle reflex, and menace response all depend on a blink response and an intact facial nerve and afferent nerve supply. If any of the blinks are abnormal determine whether it is an afferent or efferent arm problem.

- *Corneal blink reflex.* The corneal blink reflex is a *subcortical reflex* closure of the eyelids in response to a tactile or painful stimulus on the unanesthetized cornea. This reflex is afferently mediated by the trigeminal nerve (corneal sensory nerve) and efferently by the facial nerve. Stimulation should come from outside the visual field to isolate this reflex from the menace response. A 3-ml syringe with a 27-gauge needle can provide a tight "air puff" stimulus across the corneal face outside the visual field.
- *Dazzle reflex.* See under Visual Sensory System Evaluation.
- *Menace response.* See under Visual Sensory System Evaluation.

▼ *Key Point* If all three types of blink responses are nonfunctional it is most likely due to facial nerve paralysis.

Third Eyelid Position and Movement

- *Trigeminoabducent reflex and the third eyelid protrusion sign (TEPS).* This reflex, in addition to protecting the eyeball by retraction (see trigeminoabducent reflex and the eyeball retraction response [ERR] below), is also responsible for the *active protrusion of the third eyelid* through abducent nerve innervation of the *lateral rectus muscle*, which sends a slip of skeletal muscle to the third eyelid.
- *Passive protrusion of the third eyelid.* The third eyelid will passively protrude secondary to a variety of disorders, such as dehydration, atrophia bulbi, space-occupying mass, or displacement fractures of the bony orbit.
- *Active third eyelid retraction.* Sympathetic tone on the third eyelid retains the third eyelid in a retracted state in the ventral medial canthus. This is the normal position for the third eyelid.

▼ *Key Point* Protrusion of the third eyelid is indicative of pathology within the orbit, third eyelid, conjunctival surfaces, eyeball, or its innervation.

Eyeball Position and Movement

Duction Test

The ability of one eye to rotate while it is viewing is referred to as a duction. Duction movements of an eye are evaluated by covering the other eye while the unpatched viewing eye is led through secondary and tertiary positions of gaze. Evaluate each eye in this manner for range of eye movement.

Version Test

The ability of both eyes to move conjugately is referred to as version movement. Observe the eyes for conjugate movement and range of movement as they are led through the secondary and tertiary positions of gaze.

Forced Duction Tests

These tests can be active or passive and are used in cases where there is restricted range of eyeball movement. These tests help differentiate mechanical limitation of motion from paralysis of the extraocular muscles. In a passive forced duction test, grasp the anesthetized eye at the limbus with forceps on the side opposite to the direction in which the eye is to be moved and forcibly move the eye in the direction of gaze limitation. If no mechanical limitation is present, the eye can be moved fully into the direction of limitation. This indicates that the restricted movement of the eye is secondary to neurologic paralysis. If mechanical limitation is present, the eye will resist attempts to rotate it into the field of limitation. In the active forced duction test, grasp the anesthetized eye on the side of the gaze limitation. Hold the eye while the patient is coaxed into looking into the direction of gaze limitation. A tug on the grasped eye is felt if the nerve supply to the muscle is intact.

Trigemino-abducent Reflex and the ERR

This reflex is responsible for the protective eyeball retraction into the orbit from noxious stimulation of the eye and adnexa. This retraction can be sustained as long as needed because the motorneurons of the abducent nerve are stimulating *retractor bulbi muscles,* which are skeletal muscles. This reflex also causes *active protrusion of the third eyelid.* The enophthalmos created by active retraction also causes partial *passive protrusion of the third eyelid* (see third eyelid position and movement discussion above).

Vestibulo-ocular Reflex (VOR)

This reflex maintains the eyes steady on a target during head rotation. This reflex is mediated through the vestibular apparatus, which compensates for the angular acceleration sensed by the semicircular canals. It is responsible for sustaining a clear visual image during head movement. It is often referred to as the doll's eye movement and is elicited by to-and-fro or up-and-down head rotation. One eyeball appears to move toward its medial canthus and the other eye simultaneously toward its lateral canthus during horizontal head rotation. During up-and-down movement of the head, both eyes will simultaneously move toward the center of the eyelids opposite the direction of the head movement.

Trigeminal Somatic Sensory System of the Eye and Orbit

- *Corneal blink reflex.* See eyelid position and movement above.
- *Corneal sensitivity.* The sensitivity of the cornea or the ability of the trigeminal nerve to feel and respond to discomfort is quantitatively measured with the Cochet and Bonnet aesthesiometer.

NEURO-OPHTHALMIC SYSTEM ABNORMALITIES

Abnormalities of the Visual Sensory System

Menace Response and Visual Fields

Loss of a hemivisual field (homonymous hemianopia) and menace response in that visual field occur as a result of lesions that affect the ipsilateral nasal hemiretina and contralateral temporal hemiretina or higher in the CNS, a unilateral lesion in the contralateral striate cortex. Lesions of the rostral portion of the nasal hemiretina of one eye produce loss of the menace response and blindness in the ipsilateral monocular segment of the visual field.

Blindness

Blindness broadly represents a loss of visual acuity and/or visual fields, and it may be complete or partial, unilateral or bilateral. Blindness can be categorized according to the location of the lesion. Lesions in the eye, brain stem, and cerebral cortex can result in blindness of neurologic origin.

Ocular Blindness

Ocular blindness is caused by any non-neurologic disorder that destroys the clarity of the ocular media (e.g., corneal scars or cataract) or any neurologic disorder (e.g., neuronal ceroid lipofuscinosis of the brain and retina) that interrupts the retinal processing of light. A lack of funduscopic abnormalities does not rule out the retina as the site of ocular blindness.

- Diseases of the retina can be divided into inherited and acquired. The inherited diseases are most frequently bilateral and may cause selective loss of vision (i.e., *nyctalopia* or *hemeralopia*) or progressive generalized loss of vision (i.e., generalized retinal atrophy and degeneration). Acquired retinal diseases (e.g., granulomatous meningoencephalitis [GME, reticulosis] of the ganglion cell layer and optic disk) may be unilateral or bilateral, and can result in only partial or temporary loss of vision. Use electroretinography to assist in the differentiation of retinal diseases (see Chap. 157).
- The essential features of *unilateral ocular blindness* of retinal or prechiasmal optic nerve origin include loss of the dazzle reflex, menace response, direct PLR, and indirect PLR in the other eye. *Static anisocoria* (i.e., anisocoria present in steady ambient room light) and *a positive swinging flashlight test* are present in unilateral retinal disease as well as in unilateral prechiasmal optic nerve disease. The above reactions (i.e., dazzle reflex, menace response, PLR, a positive swinging flashlight test) are lost in *advanced* bilateral retinal disease. In such advanced bilateral disease, the pupils are near maximum dilation and anisocoria may not be observed. In bilateral retinal disease at an *intermediate stage of progression,* the disease may be symmetric or asymmetric in its destruction of the retina, and therefore the reflexes will vary. The pupils will be larger than normal, with or without anisocoria (depending on the symmetry of retinal destruction), and the PLR can be *absent, sluggish and incomplete, or paradoxical* (see Anisocoria in Optic Nerve Dysfunction below). Ocular motility is normal in all positions of gaze.

Brain Stem Blindness

Blindness from acquired lesions in this region of the brain are the result of inflammation, infection, neoplasia, or vascular accidents. The areas of importance are those involved as vision relay centers (the dorsal lateral geniculate body) and visual pathways (the optic tracts, or optic radiations [cerebral cortex]), and those responsible for visually guided behavior (rostral colliculi).

- The essential neuro-ophthalmic abnormalities will be variable depending on the lesion location and extent. The clinical features may include loss of visually guided behavior, blindness, anisocoria, loss of the dazzle reflex and menace response, and abnormal pupillary light reflexes. Abnormal eye movement (gaze paresis) and eyeball position (strabismus) may be seen.

- Other neurologic signs referable to the brain stem may be present.

Cerebral Blindness

This is a generalized term describing the blindness that is caused by a disorder in any area of the cortex that plays a role in vision but that often results from a more rostral, cerebral cortical abnormality. In some cases cerebral blindness includes cortical blindness.

- The essential neuro-ophthalmic features may include complete loss of all visual sensation including that for light and dark, a loss of the menace response and visual placing reactions, and the ability to detect a visual cliff. The eyes retain normal pupillary light reflexes, dazzle reflexes, eye movements, and ocular alignment.

Cortical Blindness

This type of blindness indicates selective loss of the visual occipital cortex (striate cortex).

- The essential features include the loss of the menace response, problems with stereopsis, blindness in corresponding areas of the visual field, and abnormalities in the visual placing responses. The configuration of abnormalities is dependent upon the lesion site. The dazzle reflex (subcortical reflex) and pupillary light reflex (subcortical reflex) remain normal. Ocular motility appears clinically normal, although ocular alignment may be abnormal, especially if the vision abnormality is congenital. For example, some Siamese cats have a congenital striate cortex abnormality that results in congenital bilateral esotropia with or without a pendular nystagmus. Although they do not have motion or visual field blindness, they are stereoblind (i.e., lack depth perception) (see Table 160–3).

▼ *Key Point* Distinguish vision loss occurring from lesions in the striate cortex from lesions in the motor cortex. Lesions of the motor cortex result in behavioral responses (e.g., falling off a visual cliff, running into objects) that are clinically used to indicate whether vision is present.

- Unilateral lesions of the motor cortex in the regions for eyelid closure in response to a menace and in the region for visual placing in response to presentation of a table edge within the visual field result in the contralateral loss of the menace response and visual placing reaction. A loss of these responses usually is interpreted as a loss of vision. If the striate cortex is intact, both the menace and table are seen in the contralateral visual field, but the lesion in the appropriate areas of the motor cortex prevents the appropriate behavioral response, a blink, and placing reaction. For the same reason, a patient may fall off a visual cliff even if it is seen by the striate cortex. Thus, care must be taken in evaluating and defining the "blind" patient.

Abnormalities of the Autonomic Nervous System (Pupillary Light Reflexes and Lacrimation-Salivation)
Abnormalities of the Pupillary Light Reflexes

Lesions of the pupillary light reflex pathways result in all or some of the following clinically detectable disturbances, depending upon the lesion site and extent: abnormalities in pupillary diameters, and, in the cat, sometimes shape; abnormalities in response to dark adaptation; abnormalities in the pupillary light reflex; and abnormalities in vision (Table 160–2).

Anisocoria in Ambient Light

- Unilateral pupillary pathway (i.e., afferent or efferent pupillary light reflex pathway or efferent sympathetic pathway) lesions result in anisocoria of variable degrees. Some pupillary disorders that create anisocoria (e.g., feline spastic pupil syndrome and feline hemidilated pupil) also result in dyscoria.
- Unilateral lesions of the afferent arm of the pupillary light reflex, create subtle (i.e., the pupil size difference is very small) anisocorias and vision defects. The subtle anisocoria in Horner's syndrome is similar in appearance to those created by lesions in the afferent arm of the PLR. Differentiate on the basis of the associated clinical signs in Horner's syndrome (e.g., ptosis, reverse ptosis, enophthalmos, protruded third eyelid). Additionally, vision is not impaired in Horner's syndrome unless the extent of the third eyelid protrusion mechanically blocks vision. However, all lesions that occur in the afferent arm of the PLR result in a complete to partial vision loss. Horner's anisocoria partially or completely disappears in bright light, while afferent PLR defects do not.
- Anisocoria with *large differences* in pupil size occurs with unilateral lesions of the efferent arm of the PLR.

Anisocoria in Darkness

- All unilateral and bilateral lesions of the afferent arm of the pupillary light reflex dilate maximally and equally in darkness.
- In cats with lesions of the efferent arm (both pre- and postganglionic parasympathetic fibers) of the PLR, the pupils dilate maximally and equally in darkness. This occurs because the efferent arm, including the short ciliary nerves, consists of purely parasympathetic fibers up to the point of entering the sclera where they are joined by the long ciliary nerves (containing sensory trigeminal neurons and postganglionic sympathetics). Thus, injury to the short ciliary nerves rarely involves the sympathetic system in cats.

▼ *Key Point* Maximal and equal dilation in darkness distinguishes lesions of the afferent arm (dog and cat) of the PLR and efferent arm of the PLR (cats only) from all other pupillary abnormalities, including those caused by physical restriction of iris movement (synechia).

Table 160-2. NEUROPATHIC AND OTHER CAUSES OF ANISOCORIA: DIFFERENTIAL SIGNS AND TESTS

Diseases	Pupil Affected Side	PLR D	PLR I	SFT	Dazzle Reflex	Menace Response	DAD Test	Tonometry	PT	Diagnostic SLB	Funduscopy	Vision	Special Tests
Anterior uveitis	Miotic	±	±	−	+	±	Unequal	Hypo	No	+	−	Poor	−
Glaucoma (advanced)	Dilated (fixed)	−	−	−	−	−	Unequal	Hyper	No	±	+	Blind	−
Afferent arm lesions													
Retina/optic nerve	Dilated	−	±	+	−	−	Equal	Normo	No	−	±	Blind	−
Chiasm	±Dilated	±	±	−	±	±	Equal	Normo	No	−	−	Variable	−
Optic tract	Miotic	+	+	−	+	+	Equal	Normo	No	−	−	Homonymous hemianopia	−
Efferent arm lesions													
Atrophic iris disease	Dilated	−	+	−	+	+	Variable	Normo	Yes	+	−	Normal	PT
Traumatic iridoplegia	Dilated	−	+	−	+	+	Unequal	Hypo/normo	Yes	±	−	May be poor	PT
Pharmacologic blockade (atrophine-induced mydriasis)	Dilated	−	+	−	+	+	Equal	Normo	Yes	−	−	Normal	PT
Postganglionic denervation	Dilated	−	+	−	+	+	Dog, unequal Cat, equal	Normo	Yes	−	−	Normal	PT
Preganglionic/central denervation		−	+		+	+	Unequal	Normo	Yes	−	−	Normal	PT
Efferent sympathetic nerve lesions													
Preganglionic denervation	Miotic	+	+	−	+	+	Unequal	Normo	Yes	−	−	Normal	PT
Postganglionic denervation	Miotic	+	+	−	+	+	Unequal	Normo	Yes	−	−	Normal	PT
Polyneuropathy													
Spastic pupil syndrome	Variable	±	±		+	+	No	Normo	No	−	−	Normal	+FeLV

PLR, pupillary light reflexes; D, direct (in affected, stimulated eye) light reflex; I, indirect (in nonaffected, unstimulated opposite eye) light reflex; SFT, swinging flashlight test; DAD test, dark adaptation test; PT, pharmacologic test; SLB, slit lamp biomicroscopy; FeLV, feline leukemia virus; Hypo, <15 mm Hg; Hyper, 0.25 mm Hg; Normo, 15–25 mm Hg.

- In dogs with ciliary ganglion or short ciliary nerve injury, anisocoria persists in darkness because the short ciliary nerves in the dog are mixed nerves containing both sympathetic and parasympathetic postganglionic fibers in addition to sensory nerves. The smaller pupil is ipsilateral to lesions in the ciliary ganglion or short ciliary nerves.
- The anisocoria of Horner's syndrome becomes more pronounced in darkness because the intact innervation to the dilator muscle opens the normal eye in darkness, but not the Horner's pupil.
- Cats with the feline spastic pupil syndrome will retain their anisocoria and dilate minimally or not at all in darkness.

Anisocoria in Optic Nerve Dysfunction

- A complete unilateral prechiasmal lesion, which involves the retina or prechiasmal optic nerve, creates anisocoria with the smaller pupil contralateral to the side of the lesion (see previous discussion of anisocoria in darkness and Table 160–2).
- Lesions of the chiasm lead to anisocoria when the fiber destruction is asymmetric. The PLR may be paradoxical (i.e., the pupil of the eye opposite to that which is directly stimulated will constrict to a greater extent than the eye under stimulation). The reaction may still be paradoxical when the other eye is stimulated. The pupils are generally larger than normal in ambient light (see previous discussion of Anisocoria in Darkness and Table 160–2).
- A unilateral lesion of the optic (postchiasmal) tract always appears with a subtle anisocoria with the smaller pupil ipsilateral to the side with the lesion. (See Anisocoria in Darkness above and Table 160–2).

Anisocoria in Oculomotor Dysfunction

Injury to the oculomotor nerve's (CN III) pre- or postganglionic parasympathetic fibers (GVEs) that constitute the efferent arm of the PLR leads to anisocoria without any visual loss. The pupil on the affected side is widely dilated and fixed (will not move) to direct and indirect light (see Anisocoria in Darkness and Table 160–2).

Anisocoria in Oculosympathetic Dysfunction

Lesions in the efferent sympathetic pathway lead to the signs of Horner's syndrome, with anisocoria (miosis on the affected side) as its most diagnostic feature (see Table 160–2). Any or all of the other signs of Horner's syndrome, including the narrowed palpebral fissures from oculosympathetic ptosis (and reverse ptosis), the third eyelid protrusion, and enophthalmos, may be present.

Abnormalities of Lacrimation

Loss of reflex tearing, which results in decreased Schirmer 1 tear test values in the unanesthetized eye, occurs with disorders (e.g., inflammation, infection, neoplasia) of the trigeminal nerve (afferent arm of the trigeminolacrimal reflex) or of the preganglionic or postganglionic parasympathetic neurons of the facial nerve (efferent arm of the trigemino-lacrimal reflex) (see Chap. 158).

Topical Diagnosis of Lacrimation Disorders

- *Central facial nerve paralysis.* Paralysis of the proximal portion of the facial nerve containing the preganglionic parasympathetic fibers to the lacrimal gland may lead to a reduction of reflex tearing. The cerebellopontine angle and the petrous temporal bone are likely locations for nerve injury.
- *Otitis media.* Chronic middle ear disease can injure the *major petrosal nerve* containing the preganglionic parasympathetic fibers (GVEs) of the facial nerve, which innervate the lacrimal gland. This is a leading cause of KCS.
- *Pterygopalatine ganglion injury.* The cell bodies of the postganglionic parasympathetic fibers of the facial nerve are vulnerable to injury from penetrating foreign bodies to the floor of the orbit and from suppurative and nonsuppurative extraperiorbital sheath myositis (*temporalis and pterygoideus muscles*).
- *Lateral orbit injury.* Head trauma can injure the *zygomaticotemporal nerve,* an eyelid sensory nerve (a branch of the maxillary division of the trigeminal nerve) containing the postganglionic parasympathetic (GVEs of the facial nerve) innervation to the lacrimal gland.
- *Ophthalmic nerve.* Injury to this division of the trigeminal nerve results in corneal anesthesia, loss of the *trigeminolacrimal reflex,* and diminished Schirmer 1 tear test findings.
- *Xeromycteria.* A dry nasal mucosa occurs in some cases of KCS, leading to an accumulation of dried mucus at the nares on the affected side. This mucus accumulation is often erroneously thought to result from the exit of mucus from an eye with KCS via the nasolacrimal duct. In fact, it is the result of damage to the postganglionic parasympathetic fibers from the pterygopalatine ganglion that course with the *caudal nasal nerve* (maxillary branch of CN V) to innervate the *lateral nasal gland.* The lateral nasal gland located near the maxillary sinus functions as a thermoregulatory gland by keeping the nasal cavity moist. Denervation of the lateral nasal gland leads to compensatory hyperplasia and production of the mucus-producing glands within the nasal mucosa, just as the conjunctival goblet cells hypersecrete mucus with KCS. Only a small percentage of KCS cases have mucus collection about the nares as a result of xeromycteria.
- *Paradoxical gustolacrimal reflex.* Crocodile tears are unilateral profuse tearing in response to stimulation of the taste receptors.

Abnormalities of Salivation

The gustosalivary reflex is demonstrated by patients that have had a successful parotid duct transposition each time they eat. The profuse "tearing-salivation" is mediated afferently by taste receptors on the tongue and efferently by the parasympathetic nervous innervation of the parotid and zygomatic salivary glands. Medical treatment failure for KCS or for circumstances preventing its adequate medical therapy results in the need for parotid duct transposition to sustain a healthy cornea. The same conditions that cause a dysfunctional lacrimal gland may also affect the salivary glands, thereby rendering the parotid gland unsuitable for parotid duct transposition. Determine the health of the parotid gland by assessing parotid secretion prior to duct transposition. The bitter taste of atropine sulfate ophthalmic solution applied directly to the buccal mucosa immediately stimulates the gustosalivary reflex to elicit parotid gland secretion. A pulse-like squirting of parotid secretion from the parotid duct papilla is indicative of adequate secretion. If the parotid secretion slowly flows from the duct orifice without the pulse-like squirting, successful transposition is more problematic.

- *Otitis media.* Disease of the middle ear can injure the preganglionic parasympathetic fibers of the *minor petrosal nerve* and the *otic ganglion* and its postganglionic parasympathetic fibers located in the dorsolateral aspect of the auditory tube. These fibers lead to the parotid gland.
- *Otitis externa.* Diseases of the external ear, especially those that ossify the external auditory canal and lead to periauricular tissue damage, can injure the *auriculotemporal nerve*, a branch of the mandibular division of the trigeminal nerve. This sensory nerve conducts the glossopharyngeal postganglionic parasympathetic fibers arising from the otic ganglion to the parotid gland that is situated between the ear and the angle of the mandible.

▼ *Key Point* The otic ganglion and minor petrosal nerves lie close to the major petrosal nerve and may be injured in lesions that injure the major petrosal nerve. Lesions of the dorsorostral middle ear (e.g., from eustachian or auditory tube disease) will lead to KCS, xeromycteria, and xerostomia.

Abnormalities of the Ocular Motor System (Eyelid, Third Eyelid, and Eyeball)

Eyelid Position and Movement Abnormalities

Eyelid Closure Abnormalities

The eyelids will reflexly close to protect vision when the eyes are confronted with bright illumination (dazzle reflex), with a threatening image (menace response), and with noxious tactile stimulation (corneal blink reflex). The muscle responsible for all three closures is the *orbicularis oculi* innervated by the facial nerve. Observing voluntary eyelid closure prior to testing indicates the facial nerve and the *orbicularis oculi* are intact. Failure of one of the eyelid closure responses may result from a disrupting lesion of the afferent arms (optic nerve or trigeminal nerve) of these reactions. Denervation of the *orbicularis oculi* results in the absence of all three eyelid closure responses. Determine the cause for failure of reflex eyelid closure by separate testing of the various nerve components of the reflex in order to isolate each nerve.

- *Absent corneal blink reflex.* Test this reflex as described above for eyelid position and movement. Presenting the stimulus (noxious) outside the visual fields avoids stimulating the optic nerve (visual image) and therefore isolates the trigeminal nerve. If the corneal blink reflex is absent but a voluntary blink is present, the trigeminal nerve is dysfunctional (Table 160–3). Absence of voluntary blink suggests facial nerve dysfunction. When the corneal blink reflex is absent as a result of facial nerve paralysis, there frequently are associated deficits in some or all of the functions served by this nerve.
  - *Topical diagnosis of facial nerve disease.* Topical diagnosis along the facial nerve is beyond the scope of this chapter. Schirmer tear testing, facial nerve conduction studies, acoustic reflex testing (to evaluate the facial nerve at the level of the stapedius muscle in the middle ear), brain stem auditory evoked responses (BAER), and magnetic resonance (MR) imaging can be used to localize the lesion. The BAER is used because CN VIII is close to CN VII within the petrous temporal bone, and a lesion at CN VII may therefore be demonstrated by a BAER deficiency in CN VIII.
  - *Eyelid signs with facial nerve paralysis.* Denervation of eyelid closure leads to a widened palpebral fissure, an increased amount of visible sclera (i.e., scleral showing), and the illusion of proptosis.
- *Absent dazzle reflex.* The dazzle reflex is a *subcortical reflex* afferently mediated by the optic nerve and efferently by the facial nerve. It produces a *bilateral partial eyelid closure* (blink or squint) in response to a bright light shined in one eye at a time. To isolate the dazzle reflex (CN II–CN VII) from the corneal blink reflex (CN V–CN VII) avoid touching the cornea or eyelid hair when shining the stimulating light in each eye. The loss of the dazzle reflex when a voluntary blink or the corneal blink reflex is present indicates that the facial nerve is intact and that there is unilateral retinal disease or unilateral optic nerve disease along the afferent pathway to the midbrain (see Table 160–3).
- *Absent menace response.* The menace response is not a reflex, but rather a *cortically mediated* rapid eyelid closure response, with or without head withdrawal, in

---

Table 160–3. LESION DIFFERENTIATION BASED ON BLINK REFLEX

Lesion	Optic Dazzle Reflex*	Tactile Corneal Reflex†	Menace Response	Vision
CN II lesion	−	+	−	−
CN V lesion	+	−	+	+
CN VII lesion	−	−	−	+
Visual cortex lesion	+	+	−	−
Large cerebellum lesion	+	+	−	+

*The dazzle and corneal reflexes are subcortical responses.
†The menace response requires an intact visual cortex.

response to a threatening or unexpected image suddenly appearing within the near visual field. This response requires intact peripheral and central visual pathways, including the cerebellum and the facial nerves.

- In general, the menace response is abolished in the visual fields contralateral to unilateral lesions in specific areas of the cerebral cortex.
- Unilateral lesions in the caudal striate cortex, eyelid region of the motor cortex, and parietal lobe situated between the striate cortex and motor cortex will cause unilateral disappearance of the contralateral menace response (see Table 160–3).

▼ *Key Point* While all three cerebral cortex lesions cause loss of the menace response, only striate cortex lesions cause the ensuing hemianopia.

- Absence of the menace response resulting from destruction of the eyelid region of the motor cortex is due to a partial supranuclear facial palsy and loss of menace response. Parietal lobe lesions entail no visual disturbances or partial facial palsy (voluntary blink remains).
- In dogs, the ipsilateral menace response can be lost and vision retained with large unilateral cerebellar lesions. Diffuse cerebellar cortical degenerative lesions cause a failure of the menace response bilaterally, without any visual deficit. (see Table 160–3).

▼ *Key Point* The menace response (cortical) may be lost when the corneal blink and dazzle reflexes (subcortical) persist.

Eyelid Opening Abnormalities

Neuroanatomic diagnosis of ptosis is dependent upon clinical signs and evidence of neuropathic, neuromuscular, or myopathic disease. Consider the following types:

- *Oculomotor ptosis.* This ptosis results from injury to the oculomotor nerve at any level from the cerebral cortex to the *levator palpebrae superioris muscle.* Oculomotor ptosis is exaggerated in the lateral two-thirds of the eyelid during eyebrow elevation in the dog if the facial nerve, which innervates the *levator anguli oculi medialis muscle,* remains intact. This latter muscle assists in lifting the nasal portion of the eyelid and erects the long tactile hairs (pili supraorbitales) of the eyebrow. This muscle action is readily assessed by leading the eyeball into a dorsal and medial position *(intorsion)* within the orbit, which requires elevation of the eyebrow. Topical diagnosis of oculomotor lesions is enhanced when other functions (e.g., GVEs for PLR, motor fibers for ocular motility) of the oculomotor nerve are disturbed.
- *Oculosympathetic ptosis.* This is a component of Horner's syndrome and results from nerve damage along the efferent sympathetic pathway that innervates the smooth muscles of the eyelid. The lower lid often has an "upside down ptosis," which creates a narrowed palpebral fissure. Differentiate from oculo-

motor ptosis. It helps when all or some of the other signs of Horner's syndrome (ipsilateral miosis, enophthalmos, protrusion of the third eyelid) are present.
- *Myopathic ptosis.* This is usually an acquired condition caused by damage to the levator muscle by inflammation, infiltration, or orbital trauma.

Third Eyelid Position and Movement Abnormalities

- *Hyperactive trigeminoabducent reflex.* Painful stimulation of the eyeball and/or adnexal surface (e.g., ectopic cilia) or a trigeminal neuritis will lead to the ERR and third eyelid protrusion sign (TEPS), both mediated by the trigemino-abducent reflex. Third eyelid protrusion leading to TEPS is strictly *active protrusion.* Third eyelid protrusion may be assisted by active retraction of the eyeball(s) by the *retractor bulbi muscle* action causing an enophthalmos. The enophthalmos leads to *passive protrusion* of the third eyelid. Although the final common pathway for each reflex (i.e., third eyelid protrusion and eyeball retraction) is mediated by the CN VI, each acts independently of the other.
- *Denervation of third eyelid sympathetics (Horner's syndrome).* Denervation of sympathetic neurons to the third eyelid leads to *passive protrusion* of the third eyelid. This, like the complete Horner's syndrome, is usually unilateral.
- *Third eyelid dysautonomia (so-called Haw).* Any imbalance in the sympathetic-parasympathetic system that innervates the muscles of the third eyelid may lead to protrusion of the third eyelids. This condition is usually bilateral and the protrusion is usually partial, but it may be extensive enough to impair vision. It is more frequently seen in cats but can be seen in dogs, especially golden retrievers. The cause is unknown. Gastrointestinal dysfunction may antedate the protrusion of the third eyelids or be concomitant.
- *Third eyelid protrusion of tetanus.* Tetanus infections lead to contraction of the skeletal muscles, which is caused by the potent neurotoxin liberated by *Clostridium tetani.* The third eyelids protrude in tetanus as a result of contraction of the lateral rectus muscles, which *actively* protrude the third eyelids. Tetanus also causes contraction of the retractor bulbi muscles along with all the other extraocular muscles, which leads to enophthalmos and a *passive* protrusion of the third eyelids. The antagonistic contraction of the facial muscles, including the opposing muscles of the eyelid, the *orbicularis oculi muscle,* and *levator palpebrae superioris muscle,* creates a sardonic smile with almond-shaped eyelids.

Eyeball Position and Movement Abnormalities
Ocular Position and Alignment

Strabismus (abnormal eye position) may be congenital or acquired. It is the result of CNS dysfunction, as is commonly observed in Siamese cats, or from peripheral abnormalities to the motor nerves of the eye (CNs III, IV, and VI). Disorders of the neuromuscular junction and extraocular muscle myopathy may also result in strabismus.

- *Comitant strabismus.* This is an ocular deviation that does not vary with different positions of gaze or with either eye fixating.
- *Incomitant strabismus.* This ocular deviation varies when the direction of gaze changes and/or when either eye fixates.

Ocular Movement

- *Range of movement.* When the range of movement is restricted during version and/or duction movements, *restriction caused by muscle paresis must be distinguished from mechanical restriction.* Such differentiation is accomplished by performing passive and active forced duction tests (see Eyeball Position and Movement—forced duction tests).
- *Oculomotor nerve (CN III) dysfunction.* Damage to the oculomotor (CN III) motoneurons (somatic efferents) leads to ptosis and an inability to rotate the eye upward, downward, or inward. When the unaffected eye is fixating straight ahead (primary position of gaze), the eye is held in a position of divergent (outward and downward) strabismus. The eye can be returned to midline by having the gaze directed to the side opposite the paralysis. The strabismus therefore is incomitant.
- *Trochlear nerve (CN IV) dysfunction.* Trochlear nuclear lesions produce effects in the contralateral dorsal oblique muscle. Paralysis of the trochlear nerve results in extorsion (outward rotation) of the eye. This palsy can be readily seen in the cat because the dorsal apex of its elliptical pupil is tilted toward the lateral canthus (12 o'clock position of the eyeball is rotated temporally), whereas in species with round pupils like the dog, the dorsal retinal vessels can be used as one of the indicators of dorsal oblique dysfunction. Since the dorsal oblique muscle normally acts as a depressor on inward and downward gaze, in trochlear nerve dysfunction, leading the eye into this tertiary position of gaze reveals an inability to lower the eyeball in this direction of gaze. During normal outward movement the dorsal oblique muscle acts as an intorter (tilts the 12 o'clock eyeball position nasally). During outward gaze with trochlear palsy, the unopposed *ventral oblique muscle* exaggerates the extorsion of the eyeball.
- *Abducent nucleus and nerve (CN VI) dysfunction.* Abducent nerve (CN VI) lesions cause denervation of the *lateral rectus muscle* and ipsilateral palsy of horizontal gaze. This results in a convergent (incomitant type) strabismus when the normal eye is fixating in the primary position of gaze.
  - In abducent *nucleus* lesions, there is ipsilateral palsy of horizontal gaze during version movements toward the affected side. *Neither eye crosses the midline during such version movements.*
  - Lesions of the abducent *nerve* usually cause paralysis of both the lateral rectus and retractor oculi muscles. When the abducent *nerve* is damaged, the *contralateral eye now crosses the midline* during version movements toward the affected side.

- The *trigemino-abducent reflex* can be lost if the motoneurons to the retractor bulbi muscles are disturbed.
- The *vestibuloocular reflex* (see Chap. 144) is abnormal with a paralysis of any extraocular muscle.

Nystagmus

Nystagmus is a to-and-fro movement of the eyes and is a normal response to vestibular and optokinetic stimuli. Pathologic nystagmus occurs in disorders of the systems that stabilize images of objects on the retina during *head rotations* (vestibular system and optokinetic system) or stabilize images of moving objects on the retina (pursuit system).

Congenital Nystagmus

This type is caused by metabolic dysfunction or structural abnormalities of the brain or eye.

- *Sensory congenital nystagmus* is either of the jerk or pendular type and is associated with disease in the visual sensory system (cataracts, persistent hyperplastic primary vitreous, retinal detachment, aberrant sensory visual pathways). The nystagmus of some Siamese cats serves as an example of congenital sensory nystagmus.
- *Motor congenital nystagmus* is either of the jerk or pendular type and lacks any primary disease of the visual sensory system. Any decrease in vision is secondary to the nystagmus.

Acquired Nystagmus

This type of nystagmus is often associated with other neurologic signs. *Vestibular nystagmus* is an acquired jerk nystagmus caused by imbalance within the vestibular apparatus, with the corrective quick phases directed away from the side of the lesion.

- In *peripheral vestibular disease* the nystagmus is mixed because the axis around which the eye rotates relates to the geometric relationships of the semicircular canals. *Vertical-torsional nystagmus* indicates *posterior or anterior semicircular canal irritation* depending upon the direction of the corrective quick phase's vertical movement. *Horizontal-torsional nystagmus* occurs from *complete unilateral labyrinthitis.* Positional nystagmus can also be seen in peripheral vestibular disease.
- In central *vestibular disease,* the nystagmus is more purely torsional, horizontal, or vertical. Positional nystagmus can be present.

Abnormalities of the Trigeminal Somatic Sensory System of the Eye and Orbit

If the corneal blink reflex is absent but a voluntary blink is present, the trigeminal nerve is dysfunctional. Evaluate corneal sensitivity with a Cochet-Bonnet aesthesiometer to quantify the extent of sensory loss. Corneal denervation as a result of injury to the trigeminal nerve causes *neuroparalytic (neurotrophic) keratitis,* which results in ulcerative keratitis, corneal degenerative changes, and loss of corneal sensation. Head withdrawal during noxious stimulation of the cornea is also lost because the relay of ocular pain information to the cortex via the thalamus for conscious perception of pain is interrupted. The eyelid position in neuroparalytic keratitis is symmetric with the other eye. Absence of voluntary blink and the dazzle reflex, along with the loss of the corneal blink reflex, supports the diagnosis of facial paralysis.

TREATMENT

Treatment depends upon the type of pathology and the location, the extent, and the duration of the condition. Treatment often involves a combination of modalities, including both surgical and medical. Refer to other chapters in this text for specific treatment for the various afflictions of the eye and nervous system.

PROGNOSIS

In general, patients with diseases manifesting neuro-ophthalmic signs have a better prognosis if the pathology is only inflammatory. The prognosis in infectious diseases and cerebral vascular accidents is more guarded. Neoplastic conditions, although sometimes successfully treated, in general have a poor prognosis.

SUPPLEMENTAL READINGS

Scagliotti RH: Current concepts in veterinary neuro-ophthalmology. Vet Clin North Am (Sm Anim Pract) 10:417, 1980.
Scagliotti RH: Comparative Neuro-ophthalmology. *In* Gelatt KN, ed.: Textbook of Veterinary Ophthalmology, 3rd Ed. Philadelphia: Lippincott Williams & Wilkins 1999, p 1307.

12 Diseases of Avian and Exotic Pets

Barbara L. Oglesbee

161 Avian Techniques

Barbara L. Oglesbee

RESTRAINT

For General Physical Examination (Fig. 161–1)

- Hold the bird's head firmly with one hand, placing the thumb and second finger under the mandibles and the first finger on the crown.
- With the other hand, grasp the bird with a towel wrapped securely around the body.

For Radiography

- Anesthesia with isoflurane may be necessary and reduces stress from the procedure.
- Use an acrylic positioning board (Silverdust, El Granada, CA).

Dorsoventral View (Fig. 161–2A)

- Lock the head in an acrylic shield.
- Extend the wings fully and place masking tape proximal to the carpus and on the primary feathers.
- Tape the legs in full extension.
- Align the keel bone over the spinal column.

Lateral View (Fig. 161–2B)

- Position the bird with the right side down.
- Lock the head in an acrylic shield.
- Pull the wings dorsally and tape with masking tape proximal to the carpi.

- Tape the legs caudally, with the right leg slightly anterior to the left leg.
- Restrain the tail with masking tape.

OPENING THE MOUTH

- A mouth speculum (Lafeber Co., Odell, IL) can be used to keep the mouth open (Fig. 161–3A).

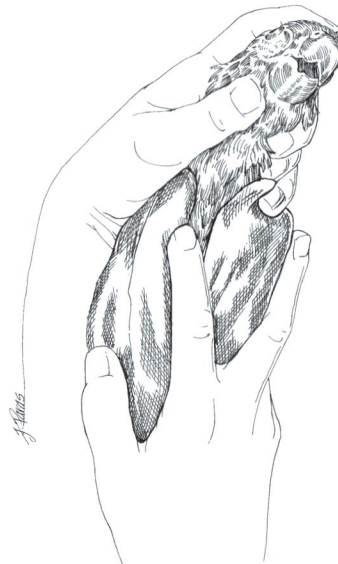

Figure 161–1. Restraint of parrot using towel.

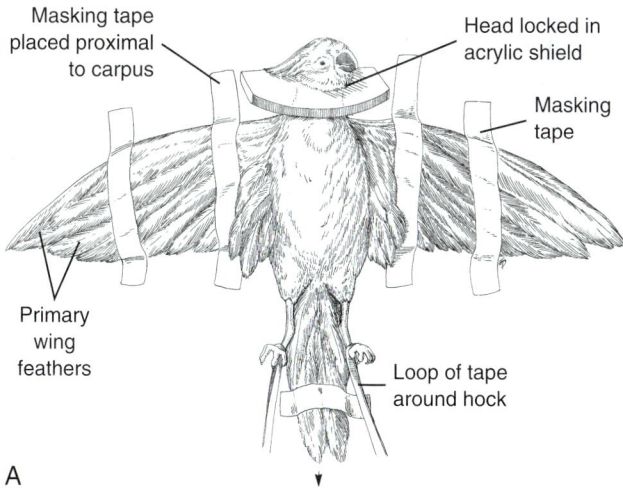

A

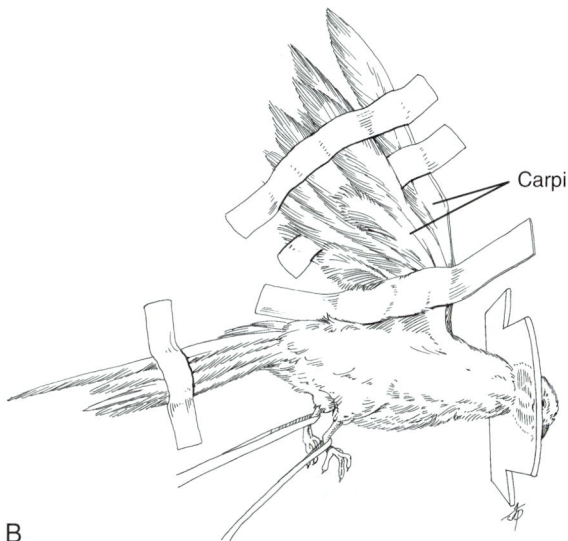

B

Figure 161-2. Restraint and positioning for radiography: *A,* dorsoventral view; *B,* lateral view.

- This procedure can cause cracking of the beak in some birds.
- Alternatively, loops of gauze can be used (Fig. 161-3*B*):
  - Restrain the bird in a towel with one hand (see Fig. 161-1); with the other hand, pull down on a gauze loop placed over the upper beak.
  - Instruct an assistant to pull a second gauze loop over the upper beak.

FORCED ALIMENTATION (GAVAGE FEEDING)

- Hold the bird in an upright position, using towel restraint if necessary (see Fig. 161-1).
- Hold the mouth open with a speculum or gauze loops (see Fig. 161-3).
- Gently pass a rigid feeding tube (Lafeber Co., Odell, IL) or soft rubber catheter with attached, gruel-filled syringe from the right side of the mouth into the crop (Fig. 161-4).

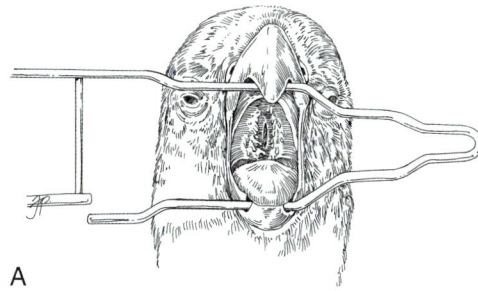

A

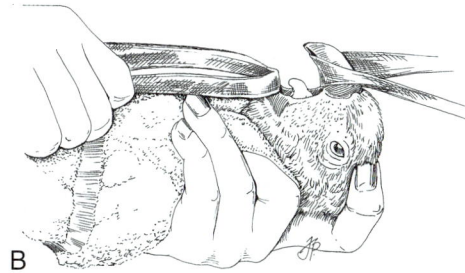

B

Figure 161-3. Opening the mouth using *(A)* a mouth speculum and *(B)* loops of gauze.

- Palpate the tube within the crop to check position.
- Expel the contents of the syringe while monitoring the pharynx for reflux of food.
- Withdraw the tube and immediately release the bird.
- The volume of gruel to be administered varies with the size and age of the birds. Suggested volumes: budgerigar, 1–3 ml; cockatiel, 3–6 ml; Amazon parrot, 15–35 ml; macaw 35–60 ml.

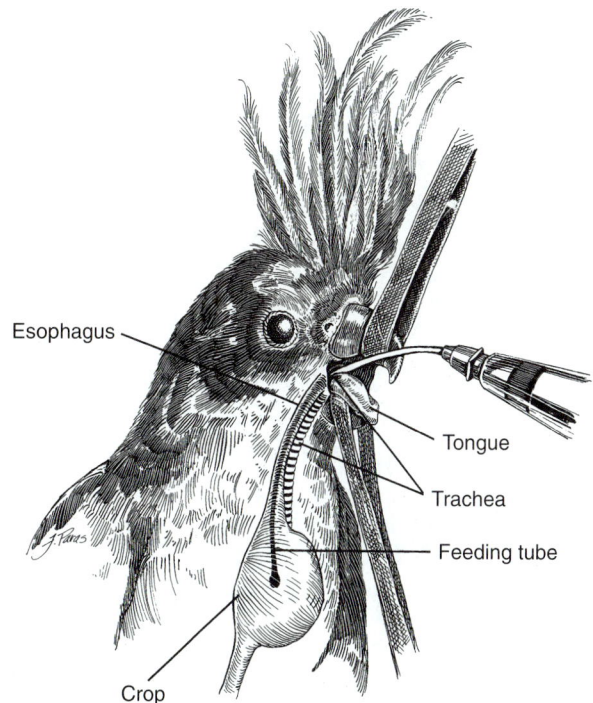

Figure 161-4. Forced alimentation.

- The same procedure may be used to perform a *crop wash* for diagnostic sample collection. In place of gruel, instill 0.5–1 ml of sterile saline into the crop, then aspirate immediately.

SUBCUTANEOUS FLUID INJECTION

- Use a 25-gauge needle.
- Always use warmed fluids, 0.9% NaCl or lactated Ringer's solution (98°F).
- Divide volume of fluid into two equal injections in the groin area (Fig. 161–5).
- Approximately 1–2 ml/100 g body weight (BW) of fluids may be administered; the larger volume is given to smaller birds.

COLLECTION OF SAMPLES FOR CULTURE

Via the Choana (Fig. 161–6*A*)

- Hold the bird upright and open its mouth with a speculum or gauze loops (see Fig. 161–3).
- Insert a cotton-tipped swab into the most rostral portion of the choana.

Via the Cloaca (Fig. 161–6*B*)

- Restrain the bird in a towel.
- To avoid trauma to the mucosa, moisten the cotton-tipped swab with transport media or sterile saline solution before insertion into the cloaca.

VENIPUNCTURE SITES

▼ *Key Point* To prevent hematoma formation, always apply firm pressure after venipuncture.

The following sites are recommended for blood collection and infusion of bolus fluids.

The volume of blood that may safely removed from a healthy bird for diagnostic sample collection is approximately 1% of body weight (e.g., 1 ml blood per 100 g BW).

Jugular Vein

This venipuncture site is preferred for psittacine birds because of the relatively large size of the vessel and decreased tendency toward hematoma formation.

Birds Under 200 g (Fig. 161–7*A*)

- Use a hypodermic needle (25 or 27 gauge) and syringe (1 ml) for blood collection.
- The jugular vein is highly movable; make sure that the neck is in full extension.

Larger Birds (Fig. 161–7*B*)

- If an assistant is not available, larger birds (e.g., parrots) may require anesthetization with isoflurane.

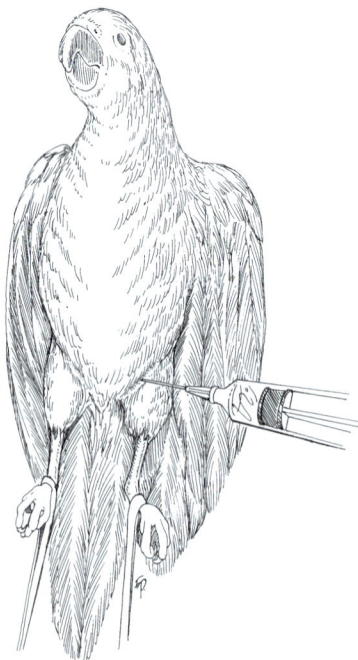

Figure 161–5. Subcutaneous fluid injection sites: interscapular region.

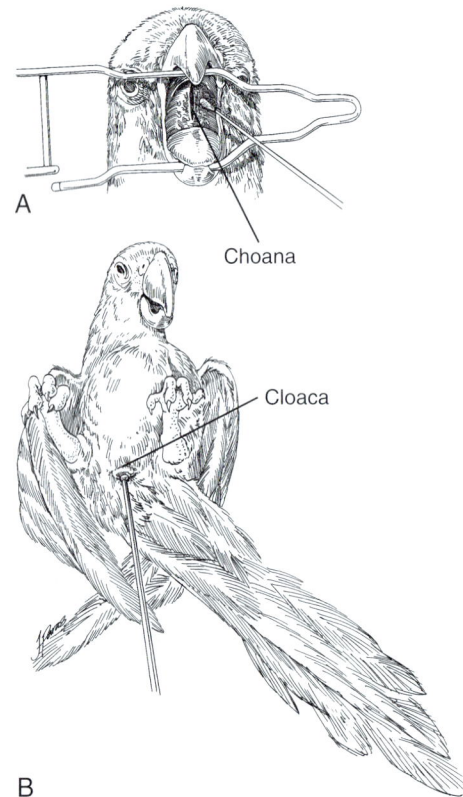

Figure 161–6. Collection of culture samples from (*A*) the choana and (*B*) the cloaca.

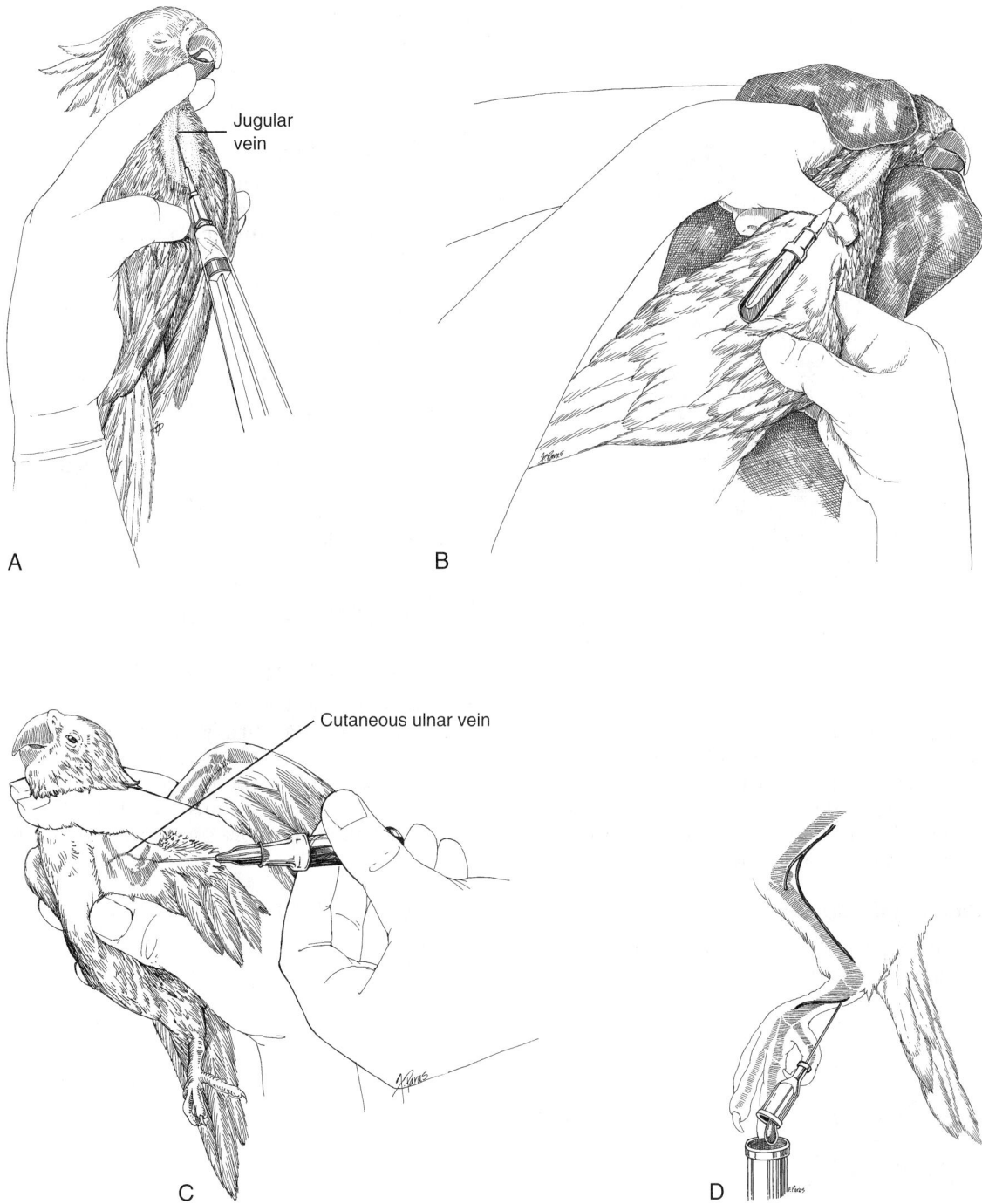

Figure 161–7. Venipuncture sites: *A*, jugular vein, birds weighing less than 100 g; *B*, jugular vein, larger birds; *C*, cutaneous ulnar vein; *D*, caudal tibial vein.

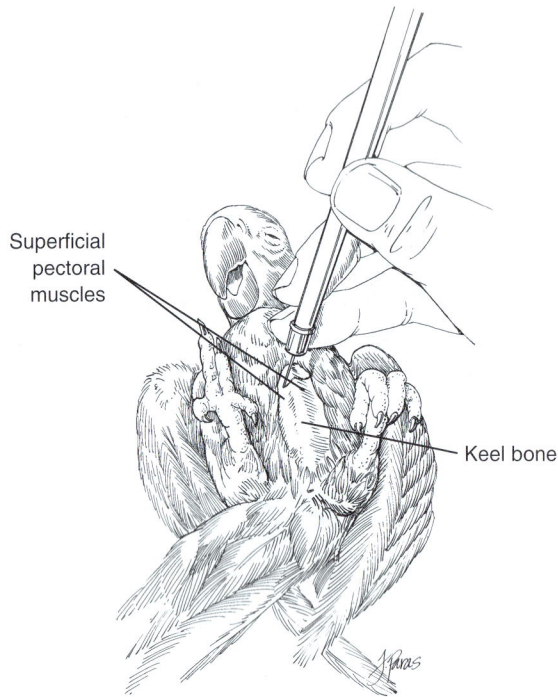

Figure 161–8. Intramuscular injection.

- With the right hand, the assistant holds the feet and the right wing pulled caudally; with the left hand, he or she restrains the bird's head.
- Using a larger needle (22–27 gauge) and syringe (3 ml) for blood collection, apply firm pressure to the right jugular vein at the thoracic inlet.

Cutaneous Ulnar Vein (Fig. 161–7C)

- The cutaneous ulnar vein crosses the ventral surface of the humeroradioulnar joint.

- To collect blood, cannulate the vessel with a 25-gauge needle and aspirate with a 1-ml syringe.
- This vein is prone toward significant hematoma formation.

Caudal Tibial Vein (Fig. 161–7D)

- The caudal tibial vein passes on the medial side of the tibiotarsus just above the tarsal joint.
- To collect blood, cannulate vessel with a 25-gauge needle and allow blood to flow into a microcollection tube (Microtainer; Becton-Dickinson, Rutherford, NJ).
- Apply firm pressure for several minutes until bleeding stops.

INTRAMUSCULAR INJECTION (Fig. 161–8)

- If necessary, use towel restraint (see Fig. 161–1).
- Inject into the superficial pectoral muscles on either side of the keel bone. Alternate sides with subsequent injections.

SINUS INJECTION/FLUSH

Sinus Injection/Aspirate (Fig. 161–9A)

- Restrain the bird in a towel.
- Restrain the head firmly in a normal upright position.
- Insert the needle percutaneously into the sinus slightly above the commissure of the beak, midway between the upper beak and the medial canthus of the eye.

Sinus/Nasal Flush (Fig. 161–9B)

- Restrain the bird in a towel over a sink or collection bowl.

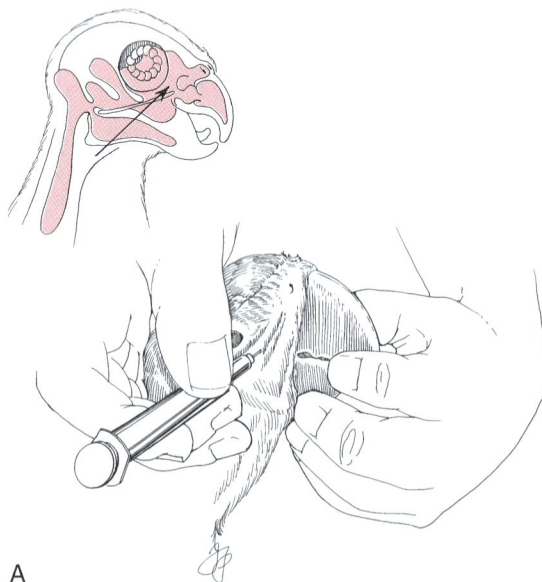

A

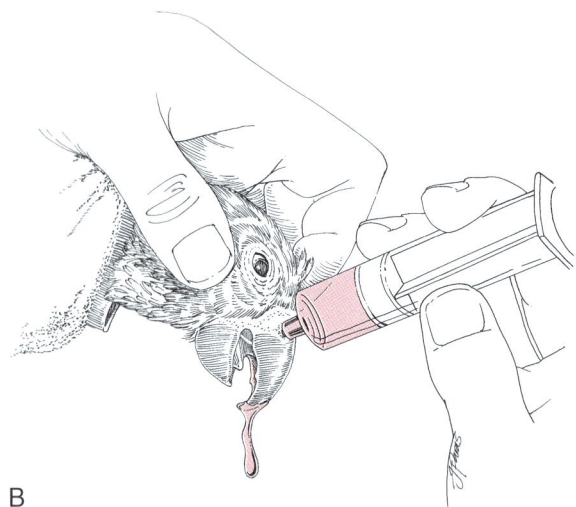

B

Figure 161–9. A, Sinus injection; *inset*, diagram of sinuses showing injection site *(arrow)*. B, Sinus flush.

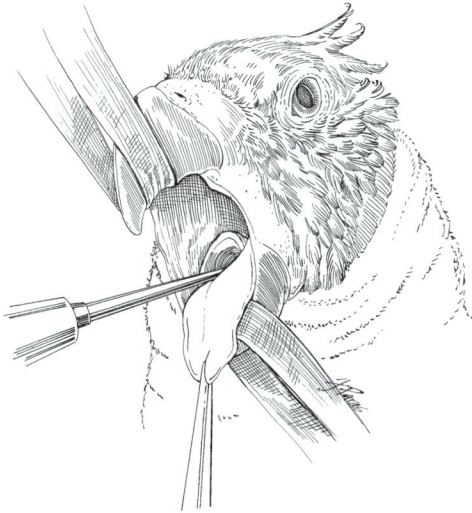

Figure 161–10. Tracheal injection/wash.

- Position the head so that it is slightly lower than the body, and restrain firmly.
- Press the syringe (without needle) against the nares opening.
- Inject 3–10 ml (depending on the size of the bird) of saline solution/antibiotic mixture into the nares with light pressure.
- If the flushing procedure is successful, the mixture will flow freely from the choana.
- Perform alternate flushes into each nares until all the mixture is used and/or no further exudate is produced.

TRACHEAL INJECTION/WASH (Fig. 161–10)

- Restrain the bird firmly.
  - For tracheal injection, the bird may be held with the face upward, if desired.
  - For tracheal wash, hold the bird in an upright position.
- Open the bird's mouth, using gauze loops or a speculum (see Fig. 161–1).
- Insert an open-ended tomcat catheter with attached syringe into the tracheal opening:
  - For tracheal injection—inject medication.
  - For tracheal wash—inject 1.0–2.0 ml of 0.9% NaCl/kg BW into the trachea, and then aspirate immediately.
- This method also may be used for tracheal endoscopy.

CROP SUPPORTER (Fig. 161–11)

- Cut Vetrap longitudinally on each end.
- Position the longitudinal cuts above and below each wing.
- Secure in back with tape.
- When applying the Vetrap, maintain slight pressure inward to aid in crop emptying.

PREPARATION FOR ENDOSCOPY OF THE ABDOMINAL AIR SAC (Fig. 161–12)

- Anesthetize the bird with isoflurane.
- Place the bird in lateral recumbency, right side down.
- Extend the wings out over the back; have an assistant hold them in this position.
- Pull the left leg as far caudally as possible.
- Push the right leg under the body to aid in maintaining true lateral recumbency.
- Pluck the area anterior to the proximal one-third of the femur free of feathers, and perform a sterile scrub.
- Apply clear drapes (3M, St. Paul, MN) over the area.
- Make a stab incision with a #15 scalpel blade through the skin anterior to the proximal one-third of the femur and caudal to the last rib.

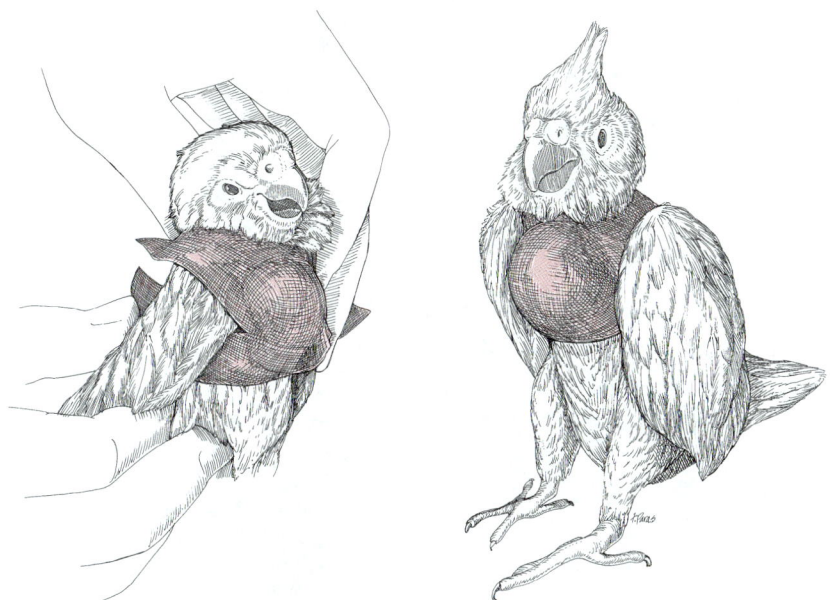

Figure 161–11. Crop supporter.

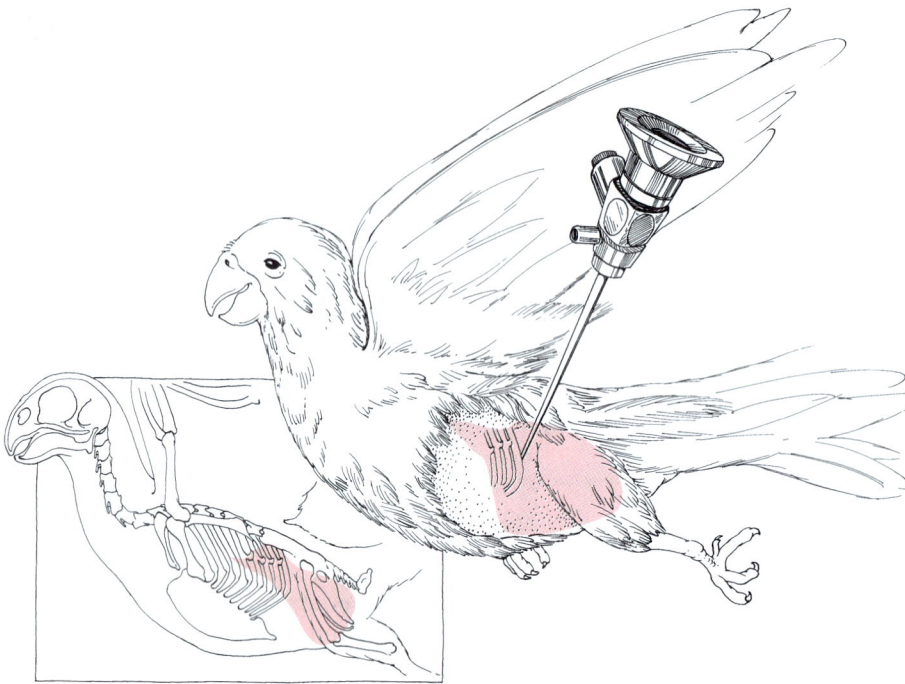

Figure 161–12. Preparation for endoscopy of the abdominal air sac; *inset*, trocar/cannula site.

- Bluntly separate the underlying musculature and peritoneum, using straight mosquito forceps.
- Introduce the trocar/cannula through the opened musculature to visualize the air sacs.

PLACEMENT OF ABDOMINAL BREATHING TUBE (Fig. 161–13)

- Enter the abdominal air sac using the technique described for endoscopy. Once the air sac is entered,

the bird will begin breathing normally through the opening.
- Hold open the abdominal musculature/peritoneum with the inserted mosquito forceps.
- Place a 1–2″ piece of a sterilized rubber catheter or shortened endotracheal tube in the opening and suture it in place with nonabsorbable suture material.
- The catheter can be left in place for up to 2 weeks. If obstruction with mucus or exudate occurs, flush with a 0.9% saline solution.

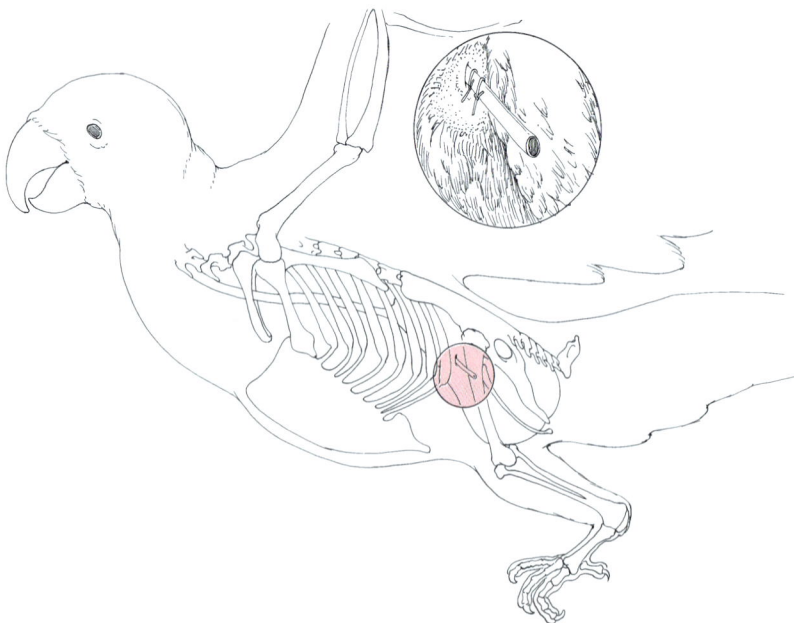

Figure 161–13. Abdominal breathing tube placement. Enlargement of placement site is shown in *inset*.

162 Avian Infectious Diseases

Barbara L. Oglesbee / Cynthia L. Bishop

ASPERGILLOSIS

Aspergillosis is an infectious but not contagious disease of pet and wild birds that is caused by the ubiquitous soil saprophyte *Aspergillus*. Infection generally occurs via inhalation of spores, resulting in primary lesions in the thoracic and abdominal air sacs and in the large airways (syrinx). Dissemination to other organ systems often occurs. Two forms of the disease, acute and chronic, commonly are seen.

- The *acute form*, which is seen most often in wild birds or psittacines under poor sanitary conditions, occurs after inhalation of an overwhelming number of spores. Severe dyspnea may result, with rapid progression to death.
- The *chronic form*, seen most often in psittacines, follows a stressful event or immunosuppressed state. Signs are often nonspecific and depend on the location of the infection and the immune status of the bird.
- The most common species isolated is *Aspergillus fumigatus. A. flavus, A. niger,* and other species play a lesser role.

▼ *Key Point* Aspergillosis is an opportunistic disease, requiring predisposing immunosuppressive factors such as stress, malnutrition, and environmental factors.

Etiology

Predisposing factors include the following:

- *Stress* may occur in shipping, quarantine, or movement to an unfamiliar environment. Stress also may result from a prolonged illness, such as chlamydiosis, or after a traumatic event such as an injury or smoke inhalation.
- *Malnutrition* or vitamin deficiencies, especially hypovitaminosis A, often occurs in birds on diets consisting of seed only.
- *Prolonged antibiotic or corticosteroid use* may cause underlying immunosuppression. For example, aspergillosis may occur after treatment for chlamydiosis owing to the immunosuppressive effects of tetracycline in conjunction with the debilitated state of a diseased bird.

▼ *Key Point* Suspect aspergillosis when respiratory signs do not respond to or worsen with antibiotic treatment.

- *Environmental factors:*
  - Poor ventilation in conjunction with damp litter (especially corn cob litter) soiled with feces promotes spore formation.
  - Poor sanitation, such as when nest boxes and incubators are cleaned inadequately, can predispose birds to aspergillosis.

Clinical Signs

Acute Form

- Signs include anorexia, dyspnea, and cyanosis.
- Sudden death may occur without signs.

Chronic Form

The onset is insidious, and signs vary, depending on the location of the infection.

- *Respiratory system*—Signs are common and depend on the area affected.
  - Signs include a change in voice, reluctance to talk, and a respiratory click that can be heard when lesions involve the main airways, especially the syrinx.
  - Severe dyspnea often occurs if the lesions are large enough to occlude the trachea or main stem bronchi. In some cases, these may be the only lesions present.
  - Mucoid to mucopurulent nasal discharge is occasionally seen with aspergillus infections.
  - Erosion of the nasal conchae and mis-shapened nares are seen in advanced cases of nasal aspergillosis.
  - The thoracic and abdominal air sacs may be involved, resulting in dyspnea or exercise intolerance.
  - In some cases, respiratory signs may be absent, even though lesions are seen on endoscopy or necropsy.
- *Liver and kidneys*—Diarrhea, anorexia, and polyuria may be seen. Green discoloration of the urates (biliverdinuria) and hepatomegaly occasionally are seen.
- *Nervous system*—Ataxia, torticollis, and paralysis may indicate central nervous system (CNS) involvement. Compression of the sciatic nerve by a granulomatous *Aspergillus* lesion has resulted in unilateral paralysis.

- *Nonspecific signs*—Weight loss, muscle wasting, depression, and lethargy often are the only clinical signs.

Diagnosis

History

- The history may identify an underlying environmental or immunosuppressive factor.

Physical Examination

- Examine the mouth and nares for mucus and exudates. Take samples from the trachea or choana for fungal culture.
- Palpate the breast muscles and weigh the bird for evidence of weight loss and muscle wasting.
- Palpate the abdomen for evidence of organomegaly.
- Auscultate the trachea and chest for abnormal chest sounds and a respiratory click.

Laboratory Tests

- A severe leukocytosis of 25,000–100,000 white blood cells (WBCs) per microliter is often present.
- The differential count usually reveals heterophilia, monocytosis, lymphopenia, and anemia of chronic disease. Occasionally, the CBC is normal.
- Increased serum total protein with an increased globulin portion is present in chronic disease.
- Aspartate aminotransferase (AST), lactate dehydrogenase (LDH), and creatine phosphokinase (CPK) levels usually are increased, especially with hepatic involvement.

Endoscopy

▼ *Key Point* Endoscopy is invaluable for the diagnosis of aspergillosis.

- When there are episodes of severe dyspnea, tracheal endoscopy may reveal a single lesion occluding the trachea or syrinx.
- If a thick, white discharge or plaque is seen in the trachea, obtain a sample for culture on Sabouraud's dextrose agar.
- Endoscopy of the abdominal air sacs may reveal diffuse cloudiness or white or yellow plaques. These plaques may become covered with a green/gray pigmented mold; obtain samples via air sac lavage for culture and cytology.
- Samples for culture and cytology may also be obtained by performing an air sac wash.

Radiography

- Radiographic changes often are not visible in early cases.
- In advanced disease, radiographic abnormalities can include loss of definition of the air sacs, asymmetry of the air sacs due to air sac collapse or hyperinflation, and focal densities in the lungs or air sacs.
- Hepatomegaly or renomegaly may be visible radiographically when there is involvement of these organs.

Treatment

Treatment is most successful when lesions are confined to the nares, trachea, syrinx, and main stem bronchi, and when aggressive treatment is instituted early.

Antifungal Agents

- Administer amphotericin B (Fungizone, Squibb), 1.5 mg/kg q8h, IV, for 3–7 days. Mask the bird with isoflurane anesthesia, and maintain an IV catheter for each injection.
  - If the main airways are involved, amphotericin B may be given by intratracheal injection, using a tomcat urinary catheter (Sherwood Medical) at a dosage of 1 mg/kg, q12h, for up to 1 month.
  - For nasal aspergillosis, a solution of 0.05 mg amphotericin B per milliter of sterile water may be used to flush the nares.
  - For mycotic air sacculitis, make a solution of 1 mg of amphotericin B per milliliter of sterile water and nebulize q12h for 15 minutes.
  - Amphotericin B is potentially nephrotoxic and may cause bone marrow suppression.
- Administer itraconazole (Sporanox, Janssen), 2.5–5 mg/kg for African gray parrots and 10 mg/kg q12h for other species, PO (with food) q12h, for 4–6 weeks in conjunction with or after amphotericin B treatment.
- Give fluconazole (Diflucan, Roerig), 5–15 mg/kg q24h, PO, for up to 6 weeks, with or after amphotericin B.
- Give 5-fluorocytosine (Ancobon, Roche Labs), 50–150 mg/kg q12h, PO, in conjunction with or after amphotericin B treatment. Give the higher dosage for active infections; use the lower dosage often prophylactically for 10–14 days in high-risk patients.

Antibiotic Therapy

- Antibiotic treatment based on culture and susceptibility testing may be necessary if a secondary bacterial infection is present.

Supportive Care

- Fluid therapy, forced alimentation (see Chap. 161), nebulization, and heat are imperative for successful treatment.

Prognosis

- The prognosis is poor to grave, depending on the severity of the disease.

Prevention

- Because *Aspergillus* is an opportunistic pathogen, attempt to reduce predisposing immunoppressive factors such as stress and malnutrition.
- Treat birds with prolonged antibiotic therapy or other birds at risk with 5-fluorocytosine prophylactically (as previously described).

▼ *Key Point* To avoid inhalation of an overwhelming number of *Aspergillus* spores, house birds in a well-ventilated area. Do not use organic materials as bedding in nest boxes.

CHLAMYDIOSIS

Avian chlamydiosis is known as psittacosis when occurring in psittacine species and ornithosis when occurring in passerine species. The incidence in pet birds is high and is reported at 15% to 30% of those tested.

Etiology

Avian chlamydiosis is caused by the obligate intracellular bacteria *Chlamydia psittaci*. The organism infects many species of wild, domestic, and exotic birds, domestic mammals, and humans. Manifestation of this disease varies from subclinical to fatal, depending on the strain of *C. psittaci* involved and the species of bird affected.

Life Cycle and Transmission

Chlamydiae have a biphasic life cycle.

- Infectious, extracellular *elementary bodies* are shed in oral/nasal secretions and feces and may survive outside the host for a month or longer. Dissemination may occur via shared food dishes or aerosolized fecal dust.
- Elementary bodies are inhaled or ingested and enter host cells where they undergo cellular rearrangement to form *reticulate bodies*, the replicating form of the organism.
- After replication, initial bodies reorganize to form *infectious* elementary bodies, which are released on rupture of the host cell. Elementary bodies then may be disseminated to cells of the liver, spleen, lungs, intestines, kidneys, gonads, and CNS.

Clinical Signs

▼ *Key Point* Clinical signs vary greatly, depending on the organ system affected, virulence of the organism, and immune status of the host.

- *Inapparent carriers* are common. These may be birds that have recovered from clinical illness or that may have never shown signs. High numbers of organisms may be shed intermittently from the feces or nasal/oral secretions, putting other pet birds and humans at risk.
  - Clinical signs may develop in these carriers when they are stressed or otherwise immunocompromised.

Acute Form

- The acute form of the disease is seen more often in young psittacines. Signs may include:
  - Liver/gastrointestinal (GI) signs, such as inappetence, green/gray diarrhea, biliverdinuria (lime-green urates), and occasionally vomiting or regurgitation
  - Respiratory signs, including serous to purulent nasal/ocular discharge, labored breathing, blepharitis, and conjunctivitis
  - Nonspecific signs, including ruffled feathers, weight loss, and depression
- Without treatment, signs may progress over a few weeks, leading to prostration and death.

Chronic Form

- Nonspecific signs such as muscle wasting and poor feathering may be the only signs.
- Recurent conjunctivitis and mild respiratory signs are often seen.
- Occasionally, CNS signs (e.g., torticollis, seizures, rear limb paresis/paralysis) may be seen alone.

Diagnosis

History

- Recently imported birds may be at higher risk because of the increased exposure and stress associated with quarantine.

▼ *Key Point* Recently acquired birds are not the only ones at risk; birds may harbor the disease for months and even years before manifestation of clinical signs.

Physical Examination

- Findings may be normal in inapparent carriers.
- Suspect chlamydiosis in birds with poor feathering, weight loss, or signs of GI or respiratory disease.

Laboratory Tests

- Leukocytosis, often > 40,000 WBC/μl demonstrating heterophilia with toxic heterophils, usually is seen in acute disease. Relative monocytosis and reactive lymphocytes and basophilia are often present.
- The WBC count may be normal in subclinical cases.
- A low packed cell volume (PCV) is common in both acute and chronic disease.
- Serum protein usually is elevated as a result of chronic inflammatory stimulation. Serum protein electrophoresis will demonstrate gammaglobulinemia.
- AST, LDH, bile acids, CK and/or uric acid levels may be elevated, depending on the organ system affected.

Radiography

- Hepatosplenomegaly is the most common radiographic feature.
- Diffuse clouding of the air sacs may be present with airsacculitis.
- Often, no radiographic abnormalities are seen with chronic disease.

Antigen Capture

Immunoassay

- An immunoassay (IDEIA antigen system, California Avian Laboratories, Citrus Heights, CA) may be used to detect chlamydial antigen in naso-ocular discharges, pharyngeal swabs, and feces. The chlamydial organisms do not have to be viable for antigen to be detected.
- Shedding of organisms is often intermittent, producing false-negative results.
- Shedding is inhibited temporarily in birds tested within 2–3 weeks of treatment with erythromycin

(e.g., Ornacyn, available in pet stores), doxycycline, tetracyclines, penicillins, chloramphenicol, tylosin, and quinolones.

- False-positive results also are common owing to cross-reactivity with some gram-negative bacteria. Confirm positive results using another method of testing.

Serology

Complement Fixation (CF)

- In the CF test (Texas Veterinary Medical Diagnostic Lab., College Station, TX), single serum samples are of value if the titer is sufficiently high.
- Titers up to 1:8 are considered negative, 1:16–1:32 is suspicious, and >1:64 is positive. A fourfold rise in titer over a 4-week period is considered most significant. Titers may remain high following successful treatment.
- Young birds, budgerigars, cockatiels, canaries, and finches with chlamydiosis may not produce antibody titers high enough to be detectable by CF, making negative results unreliable in these birds.
- False negatives may occur when birds are tested early in the course of the disease, before sufficient antibody formation.

Latex Agglutination

- This test detects serum IgM, which indicates a current infection.
- False-negative results are common in cockatiels, lovebirds, budgerigars, and some young birds, as well as in later stages of the disease.

Elementary Body Agglutination (Texas Veterinary Medical Diagnostic Lab)

- This test primarily detects IgM and is more sensitive than LA.
- An EBA titer of >80 suggests an active infection. Titers of 10–40 may be seen with low-grade infections, exposure, or recently treated infections.

Isolation on Culture

- Isolation requires live *Chlamydia* organisms.
- Success is highly dependent on proper transport medium, transport conditions, and previous antibiotic treatment.
- The chlamydial agent may be propagated in tissue culture, mice, or embryonated chicken eggs. Obtain postmortem samples from the spleen, liver, or air sacs.
- Isolation may be possible from antemortem exudate or fecal samples; however shedding often is intermittent. This is the most reliable postmortem confirmation.

▼ *Key Point* False-negative results are common when testing for *Chlamydia* organisms owing to intermittent shedding, administration of inhibitory antimicrobials, and production of low antibody titers in the face of active disease. Base the diagnosis of chlamydiosis on a combination of diagnostic tests, clinical signs, hematology, serum biochemical profile, and serum electrophoresis, and radiography.

Treatment

Tetracyclines are the most effective antibiotics against *Chlamydia.*

▼ *Key Point* Tetracyclines are effective only when the organism is actively dividing, necessitating a 45-day treatment regimen.

- Chlortetracycline (CTC)—medicated feed, achieving a therapeutic blood concentration of 1 µg/ml for 45 days, may be used for flock treatment.
  - CTC-impregnated pelleted food (Pretty Bird, Inc.) is commercially available, or a 1% CTC cooked mash may be prepared.
  - Reduce dietary calcium to 0.7% of the diet, because calcium interferes with CTC absorption.
  - This treatment regimen may not be effective, however, due to poor acceptance of these food mixtures.
  - Secondary enteric mycotic or bacterial infections owing to alterations of the normal enteric flora are a common problem.
- Doxycycline (Vibramycin syrup/suspension; Pfizer) appears to be more effective clinically than CTC. It is available only in an oral or intravenous (IV) form in the United States. The IV form should *not* be injected IM or subcutaneously.
  - Administer the oral form of doxycycline at a dose of 25 mg/kg q12h, or 50 mg/kg q24h for 45 days if this dosage is tolerated without vomiting.

Supportive Care

- Many birds with acute chlamydiosis are seriously ill and require supportive care such as fluid therapy, forced alimentation (see Chap. 161), and heat, as well as antibiotic therapy if secondary bacterial infection is present.

Prevention

- Because inapparent carriers are common and an accurate screening test is not available, it is difficult to prevent the introduction of *Chlamydia* organisms into a flock when purchasing new birds. A combination of serology and antigen capture to screen for chlamydiosis is recommended, with repeated yearly testing.

PSITTACINE VIRAL DISEASES

Psittacine Beak and Feather Disease (PBFD)

PBFD is an infectious, usually fatal disease characterized by feather loss, feather dystrophy, occasional beak deformity, and destruction of the thymus and bursa. Originally believed to affect only white and pink cockatoos and a few other South Pacific psittacine birds, the disease has been reported in more than 30 species of psittacines and is believed to be capable of causing disease in many others. Death is attributed to secondary bacterial, viral, or mycotic infections, or general debilitation, warranting euthanasia. Death typically occurs within several months after the onset of signs in the acute form; however, it may occur after several years with the chronic form of the disease.

Etiology

- PBFD is caused by a nonenveloped, single-stranded DNA virus (PBFDV) that is structurally similar to the porcine circovirus (PCV) and chicken anemia agent (CAA).
  - It has been proposed that these viruses be placed in a new family of animal viruses called *Circodnaviridae*.

Transmission

- Virus may be recovered in the feces, crop secretions, and feather dust of infected birds. Being nonenveloped, PBFDV is thought to be extremely stable in the environment and may be resistant to many disinfectants.
- Infection may occur by inhalation or ingestion of the virus.
- PBFDV is believed to spread throughout the body of an infected bird via circulating WBCs. There is evidence that inapparent carriers may exist.

▼ **Key Point** Feather dust is a major method of transmission and environmental persistence of PBFDV. Feather dust may be dispersed through natural air flow and may contaminate food dishes, cages, bird carriers, insects, and human clothing.

Clinical Signs

PBFDV may cause peracute, acute, or chronic disease.

Peracute Form

- This form is seen in neonates, most often cockatoos and African gray parrots, and may be associated with crop stasis, pneumonia, diarrhea, weight loss, and rapid death. There are few feather lesions.

Acute Form

This form is seen in birds as young as 30 days of age, when feathers begin to replace neonatal down.

- Feather lesions include fractures, necrosis, hemorrhage, curvature, and premature shedding of affected feathers.
- GI signs include diarrhea, crop stasis, and anorexia. There may be few feather lesions, especially in young cockatoos, lovebirds, and African gray parrots.
- Death may follow the onset of clinical signs within days to several weeks.

Chronic Form

- This form usually is recognized in psittacines younger than 3 years of age but has been reported in birds as old as 20 years of age. Birds may live for

months to years before succumbing to secondary infections or chronic debilitation.
- Progressive feather abnormalities may be accompanied by beak lesions.
  - Feather lesions include retained feather sheaths, bleeding within the pulp cavity, fractured feathers, clubbed feathers, circumferential constrictions within the feather shaft, curled or deformed feathers, and stress lines within feather vanes.
  - Feather loss typically begins with powder down feathers. Contour, crest, wing, and tail feather loss is roughly symmetric and progresses with each molt. Some birds become completely bald and remain so until death (months to years).
  - Beak lesions often occur in galahs and Mollucan and sulfur-crested cockatoos but are not routinely seen in other species. Lesions may include oral ulceration, and elongation and fractures of the beak, often accompanied by secondary mycotic or bacterial infections. Beak lesions usually occur after chronic feather loss but also can occur in birds with mild feather lesions. In cockatoos, the beak may appear shiny and black because of absence of powder that settles on the beak during preening.

Diagnosis

Histopathology

- In affected feathers, typically there are ballooning degeneration and necrosis of epithelial cells in the epidermal collar and in the epidermal basal and intermediate zones of the developing rachis.
- Nonsuppurative inflammation, characterized by perivascular accumulations of heterophils, plasma cells, lymphocytes, and macrophages, is the primary lesion seen in the feather pulp.
- Beak lesions histopathologically are similar to those seen in the feather shafts.
- The thymus and bursa typically are atrophied, with focal areas of necrosis and degeneration. These lesions are thought to cause immunosuppression.

Hematoxylin and Eosin (H&E) Stain

- Basophilic intranuclear and intracytoplasmic inclusion bodies may be seen with H&E staining in the feathers, pulp, and follicular epithelium. These were once considered diagnostic for PBFDV; however, other viruses (e.g., avian polyomavirus) may induce similar intranuclear inclusion bodies.

DNA Probe

- A highly sensitive and specific viral DNA probe for the detection of PBFDV infection is commercially available. Birds latently infected can be detected by submitting 0.2 to 0.5 ml of whole unclotted blood. This test allows veterinarians to screen for birds subclinically infected with PBFDV.*

---

*Positive results in birds with lesions suggest active infection. Birds without lesions are retested in 90 days. If positive, bird is considered a carrier; negative, virus is eliminated and bird is considered immune.

Treatment

- There is currently no effective treatment for PBFDV.
- Provide supportive care (e.g., good nutrition, debridement of lesions, beak trimming, heat) and antimicrobial therapy for secondary bacterial and fungal infections for chronically infected patients.

Prevention

▼ *Key Point* Using the DNA probe, test all birds for PBFDV prior to admission to the aviary.

- Isolate all birds testing positive for PBFDV to prevent contact with noninfected birds.
- Exercise care to prevent feather or fecal dust from infected birds contaminating noninfected birds, particularly psittacine neonates.

Polyomavirus

Polyomavirus is responsible for major economic losses in commercial budgerigar aviaries. Polyomavirus also has been reported to cause clinical disease in nearly all species of large psittacine birds and in passerine birds.

Budgerigars that survive BFD infection may develop feather abnormalities commonly referred to as "French molt." The lesions of French molt, however, also may be caused by PBFDV.

Transmission

- Polyomavirus may be present in feces, feather dust, and oronasal and oral secretions. These contaminated materials may be inhaled or ingested by susceptible birds.
- Infected hens may pass the virus to offspring through the egg.
- Latent infections are common in budgerigars and are believed to be responsible for spread of this virus. Clinically normal parents may transmit polyomavirus to their offspring, some of which also become inapparent carriers.
- There is currently no evidence to support the existence of persistent infections in larger psittacine birds. However, some psittacine birds may become infected without demonstrating clinical signs, and shed virus before eliminating the infection. Thus, birds with subclinical infections may be responsible for viral outbreaks, especially in pet stores and breeding facilities where susceptible neonates are exposed.

Clinical Signs

Hatchling Budgerigars < 15 Days Old

- Signs include abdominal enlargement, delayed crop emptying, subcutaneous hemorrhage, retarded growth, and abnormal feathers.
- Sudden death is common. Reported mortality rates vary from 30–100% of affected hatchlings.

Budgerigars > 15 Days Old

- Signs are similar to those described for hatchlings; however, the mortality rate is much lower.

Neonatal Parrots

Nonbudgerigar psittacine neonates are extremely susceptible to polyomavirus and are likely to develop clinical signs.

- Clinical signs usually develop at the time of weaning but may be seen anywhere from 14–150 days of age.
- Sudden death with and without clinical signs is common; birds that develop clinical signs usually die within 12–48 hours.
- Signs include diarrhea, delayed crop emptying, depression, anorexia, hemorrhage at the base of feathers and at injection sites, polyuria, and posterior paresis and paralysis.
- Unless immunosuppressed, adult nonbudgerigar psittacine birds demonstrate mild or no clinical signs, and eventually eliminate the virus. However, these birds are likely to shed virus before recovery and thus serve as a source of environmental contamination.

Diagnosis

- Gross pathologic changes include hydropericardium, cardiomegaly, pale kidneys, ascites, hepatomegaly, splenomegaly, and diffuse petechial and ecchymotic hemorrhages in the subcutis, intestines, myocardium, epicardium and serosal surfaces.
- Histopathologic demonstration of karyomegaly with basophilic intranuclear inclusion bodies in the kidneys, liver, spleen, heart or feather follicles suggests polyomavirus.
- Confirmatory diagnosis requires the identification of viral antigen using virus-specific antibodies or the detection of viral nucleic acid using virus-specific DNA probes.
  - Highly specific and sensitive viral DNA probes (Avian Research Associates, Inc. Laboratory, Milford, OH) can detect polyomavirus in infected tissue, cloacal swabs, and fresh feces of birds shedding virus. Identify birds that are shedding the polyomavirus by submitting a cloacal swab for testing. False-negative results may occur if the bird is not shedding virus at the time of testing.

Treatment

- Provide supportive care, as described for PBFD.

Prevention

▼ *Key Point* Quarantine all new birds for 30 days before entrance into an aviary. Perform DNA probe testing on all birds before entrance into an aviary. Isolate birds testing positive.

- Do not keep budgerigars in the vicinity of unvaccinated neonatal parrots.
- Do not mix neonates from different sources, or return a neonate to the nursery after exposure to other birds.
- Disinfection with chlorine solution (50 ml/liter of water) or prolonged contact with iodophors inactivates the virus.

Vaccination

A USDA-approved inactivated avian polyomavirus is considered safe and effective (Biomune, Inc., Lenexa, KS). Administer the vaccine subcutaneously. Mild injection site reactions have been reported but should resolve within 3–6 weeks after injection. Follow vaccination guidelines provided by the manufacturer.

Pacheco's Disease

Also known as *herpes hepatosplenitis,* Pacheco's disease (PD) causes an acute, necrotizing hepatosplenitis that usually is rapidly fatal. The hallmark of PD is sudden death in birds that appear clinically normal until just before death. All species of psittacines of all ages, both imported and domestically raised, are susceptible.

Etiology

- Several strains of antigenically unrelated herpesvirus (HV) may cause PD; HV persists by inducing latent disease, with periodic reactivation and shedding.

Transmission

- Although the exact route of PD virus transmission is unknown, this virus is present in high numbers in the feces and pharyngeal secretions of symptomatic and asymptomatic carrier birds. Thus, direct contact with contaminated aerosols and fecal-oral routes are the most likely routes of virus transmission.
- HV is an enveloped virus and is relatively unstable in the environment. Anecdotal reports suggest that humans can serve as vectors, even with relatively long time intervals between bird exposure. An incubation period of 3–7 days is common.

▼ *Key Point* Asymptomatic carriers of viruses that cause Pacheco's disease are common and often are incriminated in disease outbreaks. Any psittacine bird that has been exposed to or recovered from herpesvirus infection may potentially become a carrier.

Clinical Signs

- Sudden death without premonitory signs is encountered most commonly and has been reported most frequently in Amazon parrots, cockatoos, lovebirds, Pionus parrots and parakeets.
- Nonspecific signs, seen especially in macaws and conures, include lethargy, anorexia, vomiting, diarrhea (sometimes hemorrhagic), biliverdinuria, nasoocular discharge, and occasionally CNS signs.
- Signs often progress to death within several days; however, recovery has been reported in some birds with clinical signs consistent with PDV.

Diagnosis

Antemortem Diagnosis

- Virus isolation from feces may reveal infection; however, viral shedding may be intermittent, making it ineffective for the detection of carrier birds.
- Serologic testing is not commercially available.

▼ *Key Point* No reliable test is currently available for the identification of carrier birds with PD virus.

Postmortem Examination

- Gross lesions may include hepatomegaly, splenomegaly, hemorrhagic enteritis, sinusitis, pneumonia, airsacculitis, and congestion and hemorrhage in the spleen, liver, and kidneys. Gross lesions may not be apparent in birds with peracute death.
- Histopathologic lesions often include hepatic and splenic necrosis.
- Virus may be isolated from liver, spleen, small intestine, and pancreas.

▼ *Key Point* Basophilic and eosinophilic Cowdry type A inclusion bodies, often present in the liver, spleen, kidneys, and pancreas, suggest herpesvirus infection.

Treatment

- Oral administration of acylovir (Zovirax, Burroughs-Wellcome) (80 mg/kg q8h × 7d) or the IV form given IM (40 mg/kg q8h) has been reported to decrease morbidity and mortality during PD outbreaks.
- Supportive care, including fluids, heat, assisted alimentation, and antibiotic therapy for secondary infections, may be of some benefit.

Prevention

- Do not mix susceptible species with suspect carriers.
- Sanitation is critical in disease prevention because viral spread within an aviary occurs primarily by contact with contaminated feces and pharyngeal secretions.
  - Thoroughly clean water and feed dishes followed by treatment with a disinfectant. HV typically is inactivated by desiccation and through contact with most disinfectants.
  - Instruct all aviary personnel to practice sound hygiene by washing and disinfecting hands before entering the aviary and after handling individual birds or cages.
- Reduce stress to help prevent shedding and spread of the virus.

Vaccination

Provisionally licensed PD virus vaccine is currently available from Maine Biological Labs. (Waterville, ME) and Biomune, Inc. (Lenexa, KS). Two vaccinations subcutaneously in the inguinal area 4–8 weeks apart followed by yearly boosters are recommended. However, adverse reactions, such as granuloma formation, paralysis, and sudden death, have been reported.

Other Herpesviruses

Thirteen different herpesviruses are known to affect birds. The pathogenicity, host spectrum, and relation of these viruses largely are unknown.

- The only HV of known clinical significance in psittacine birds (besides those that cause PD) is Amazon tracheitis virus.
  - This virus causes a pseudomembranous tracheitis, pharyngitis, and sinusitis.
  - Signs include dyspnea, change or loss of voice, abnormal respiratory signs, and occasionally hemoptysis.
  - Base diagnosis on virus isolation or typical Cowdry type A inclusion bodies in the tracheal mucosa at necropsy.
  - Treatment is similar to that discussed for PDV.
- Based on histologic findings, another HV has been reported as the suspected etiology of wart-like lesions occurring on the feet of cockatoos.
  - Limited success has been reported in these cases with treatment with topical application of acyclovir cream.

Poxviruses

Poxvirus is commonly seen in canaries, pigeons and wild birds. It is less commonly seen in pet psittacine birds due to recent restrictions on importation of these birds.

Two forms of clinical disease caused by avian poxviruses commonly are encountered:

- Dry, or cutaneous, pox is characterized by discrete nodules on unfeathered skin.
- The more common wet, or diphtheritic, pox is characterized by fibronecrotic lesions in the respiratory system, conjunctiva, and pharynx.

The type of disease that develops may depend on the strain of infecting virus, route of infection and species, and age or condition of the host.

Recently imported Amazon parrots, especially blue-fronted Amazons and Pionus parrots, are among the most susceptible species, and typically, the diphtheritic form of the disease develops in these. Either form may develop in passeriformes (canaries, finches).

Etiology

- Avipoxviruses replicate in the cytoplasm of epithelial cells, inducing characteristic intracytoplasmic, lipophilic inclusion bodies called *Bollinger bodies*.
- Host susceptibility and virulence of the virus varies with the strain of avipoxvirus. Most poxvirus strains are relatively host-specific.

Transmission

- Poxvirus is incapable of penetrating intact epithelium. Entrance into the host is gained through pre-existing traumatic lesions or often is introduced into a flock via mosquito vectors.
- Virus is shed in epithelial crusts and exudates during active infection, and in feces, skin, and feather quills during recovery and in latent infections.
- Virus transmission may occur through direct contact with affected birds or through contact with contaminated soil, food, or cages.

- Aerosol transmission may be responsible for the diphtheritic (wet) form, whereas contamination of skin wounds or mosquito bites is most likely to result in the cutaneous (dry) form.
- Poxviruses are very resistant to desiccation, humidity, and light and may survive for up to 1.5 years in the environment.
- Recurrence of poxvirus lesions has been reported in some species.
- It is postulated that asymptomatic carriers of poxvirus may exist.

Clinical Signs

Diphtheritic (Wet) Pox

- Yellow to gray/brown fibronecrotic plaques may occur on the mucosa of the mouth, choana, beak, esophagus, and trachea.
  - Multiple plaques may coalesce, forming tightly adherent diphtheritic membranes, which, if forcibly removed, leave a raw, hemorrhagic surface.
- Respiratory epithelium may be affected, with resulting dyspnea, rales, serous to purulent naso-ocular discharge, lethargy, and anorexia.
- Death due to secondary bacterial bronchopneumonia is extremely common. Sudden death from septicemia occasionally is seen in recently imported Amazon parrots.

Cutaneous (Dry) Pox

- Signs include papules, pustules, and scabs on the unfeathered portions of the skin.
  - Secondary bacterial and fungal infections are common and may result in swelling or abscessation.
  - If no secondary bacterial infection occurs, the lesions may resolve without scarring in 10–14 days.
- In canaries and finches, wart-like lesions are common on unfeathered skin.

Diagnosis

- Clinical lesions suggest the diagnosis.
- Differential diagnoses for diphtheritic lesions include hypovitaminosis A, aspergillosis, and trichomoniasis (see Chap. 165).
- Epithelial hyperplasia with ballooning degeneration and intraepithelial vesicles seen on histopathologic examination suggest avian pox.
- Intracytoplasmic lipophilic Bollinger bodies are pathognomonic.

Treatment

Cutaneous Pox

- Treatment of secondary fungal or bacterial infections is based on culture and susceptibility testing.

Diphtheritic Pox

- Birds often have systemic illness, and mortality rates are high.

- Provide supportive care (see Chap. 161), such as supplemental heat, fluid therapy, and assisted alimentation, if mouth lesions are present.
- Prophylactic administration of systemic broad-spectrum antibiotics may prevent secondary bacterial infections.
- If bronchopneumonia is present, nebulization is recommended (see Chap. 164).

Prevention

Vaccination

Vaccines are available for psittacine birds, canaries, pigeons, and domestic fowl. Use of these vaccines is restricted to high-risk populations, such as recently imported birds or birds exposed to large numbers of mosquitos. Adverse reactions, including sudden death, have been associated with the vaccine.

Disinfection

Effective disinfectants include 1% potassium hydroxide (KOH), 2% sodium hydroxide (NaOH), and 5% phenol.

- To control an outbreak, replace all wood items in the aviary and clean and disinfect all equipment, nets, cages, and breeding containers.

Reoviruses

There are 11 avian serotypes of reoviruses that are antigenically distinct from each other and from reoviruses isolated from mammals. Of the common pet birds, African gray parrots are most commonly affected.

Etiology

- Avian reoviruses have been isolated or identified by electron microscopy from asymptomatic psittacine and passerine birds in quarantine stations.
- Infections in Old World species tend to be fatal, whereas New World species appear to be less susceptible to infections and often recover.

Transmission

- Both horizontal and egg transmissions of reovirus occur in chickens. However, little is known about transmission in psittacine birds; horizontal transmission through oral and respiratory routes is believed to occur.
- The incubation period in experimental studies is 2–15 days. After natural exposure, replication of the virus occurs in the GI mucosa, followed by viremia (24–48 hours) and spread to other organ systems.

Clinical Signs

- Severity of the disease, and thus clinical signs, varies, depending on the age of the host, the virulence of the virus, the route of infection, and the presence or absence of secondary infections.

- Signs include anorexia, depression, yellow-orange urates, diarrhea, dyspnea, and occasionally paresis, hindlimb paralysis, and bloody nasal discharge.

Diagnosis

- Gross pathologic changes include hepatosplenomegaly with pale yellow mottling and multifocal gray-white foci.
- The typical histologic lesion is disseminated or focal coagulative necrotizing hepatopathy.
- A tentative histologic diagnosis may be confirmed by isolating the virus in cell culture from feces, liver, or spleen.

Treatment

- Supportive care is the only treatment currently available.

▼ **Key Point** The prognosis for Old World avian species with clinical signs is poor. Death often occurs within 3–4 days after development of clinical signs. Infected New World species often survive with appropriate supportive care.

Prevention

- There currently is no serologic test or commercial vaccine available for reoviruses affecting pet birds.
- Strict quarantine of newly arrived birds, especially birds of African descent, may help to prevent flock exposure. However, epidemiologic evidence suggests the existence of an asymptomatic carrier state.
- Viral infectivity can be reduced by prolonged contact with phenols, aldehydes, ethanol, halides, 0.5% iodine solution, and a temperature of 158°F.

Adenoviridae

Adenovirus infections have been associated with depression, diarrhea, anorexia, and acute death in budgerigars, Amazon parrots, macaws, cockatoos, lovebirds, and parakeets. Adenovirus infections typically produce eosinophilic and basophilic intranuclear inclusion bodies.

Adenovirus infections in psittacines commonly are referred to as *inclusion body hepatitis* or *inclusion body pancreatitis*, depending on the predominant organ system involved.

Clinical Signs

- Signs generally are nonspecific and vary with the organ system affected. Signs include lethargy, depression, fluffed feathers, yellow urates, diarrhea, anorexia, and sudden death.

Diagnosis

- An enlarged, friable liver is the most consistent feature recognized on gross necropsy examination.
- Base definitive diagnosis on histologic examination of affected tissues from necropsy specimens. Histologically, there is diffuse necrosis of parenchymatous

organs with eosinophilic and basophilic intranuclear inclusion bodies.

Treatment

- There is no specific treatment.
- General supportive care may be beneficial (warmth, fluids, forced alimentation, and antibiotic therapy for secondary infection).

Prevention

- Disinfect cages and supplies with an aldehyde disinfectant (requires 1 hour of contact) to prevent spread of the disease.
- Quarantine all new birds and strictly isolate affected birds.

Newcastle Disease Virus (Paramyxovirus-1)

Newcastle disease virus (NDV) is of extreme economic importance to the poultry industry. Legally imported birds are placed in United States Department of Agriculture (USDA) quarantine stations for 30 days. These were created to prevent the introduction of virulent forms of this virus into the United States.

▼ **Key Point** Smuggling of birds into the United States is the main source of NDV-infected birds. Newcastle disease should not be a problem for the serious aviculturist who does not expose an aviary collection to birds of questionable origin.

Etiology

- There are nine serotypes of avian paramyxovirus (PMV). The most significant pathogens are virulent serotypes of PMV-1, which has been isolated from most species of domestic, aviary, and wild birds.

Transmission

- The respiratory and oral routes of transmission are equally important.
- Fecal contamination of eggshells may lead to viral spread. The virus infects the red blood cells and then is spread throughout the body.
- The incubation period typically is 4–7 days.

Clinical Signs

- Clinical signs depend on the virulence of the strain of virus involved.
- Predominant clinical signs in psittacine birds include fluffed feathers, conjunctivitis, and CNS signs (e.g., ataxia, wing and head tremors, paralysis of extremities).
- The mortality rate is 22% to 55% of affected birds.
- Chronic NDV infection may develop in survivors. Virus has been isolated from oral and cloacal swabs 84 days postexposure in conures, and 1 year postexposure in Amazon parrots.

Diagnosis

- Serologic testing using hemagglutination inhibition (HI), agar gel immunodiffusion (AGID), or ELISA can indirectly diagnose avian PMV infection. However, serology is less effective in diagnosing infections than viral isolation. Antibodies typically appear 8 days after infection.
  - HI is not specific for PMV-1 (cross-reaction may occur with other paramyxoviruses); however, suspect NDV in birds demonstrating high titers.
- Base definitive diagnosis on virus isolation from feces or oral secretions of live birds, or from infected organs at necropsy.

Treatment

- No treatment is available. Inform the USDA of any birds positively diagnosed with NDV.

Prevention

All birds legally presented for importation into the United States are placed in a USDA-approved quarantine station for 30 days, at which time samples are taken to detect hemagglutination (HA) viruses, including PMV and influenza. Birds with isolates of hemagglutination (HA) viruses that are pathogenic to chickens are refused entry.

▼ **Key Point** The best prevention against NDV in psittacine birds is avoidance of contact with birds that may have been smuggled into the country.

- No vaccine is available for psittacine birds.

SUSPECTED VIRAL DISEASES

Proventricular Dilatation Disease (PDD)

Other names for this disease include *myenteric ganglioneuritis, infiltrative splanchnic neuropathy,* and *macaw wasting disease.* The disease originally was seen only in macaws but has been reported in almost all psittacine species. Both ultrastructural findings and epidemiologic evidence suggest that PDD has a viral etiology. The disease appears to have a protracted course, with low virulence and extended incubation periods. The potential mode of transmission is unknown at this time.

Clinical Signs

- Signs include intermittent regurgitation, diarrhea, polydipsia/polyuria, depression, passage of undigested food, progressive weight loss, abdominal distension, and central and peripheral neurologic signs.
- In birds with a severely dilated proventriculus, secondary aspiration pneumonia may develop after repeated bouts of regurgitation.

▼ **Key Point** Once signs of PDD develop, the disease invariably is fatal.

Diagnosis

Antemortem Diagnosis

- A presumptive diagnosis may be based on clinical signs, radiographic identification of an enlarged proventriculus, and by ruling out other causes of proventricular dilatation.
  - Contrast radiography is usually necessary to positively identify a dilated proventriculus.
- Rule out other causes of regurgitation, proventricular dilatation, or passage of undigested food, such as GI foreign bodies, proventricular outflow obstruction (e.g., tumors, granuloma), heavy metal toxicity, proventriculitis, enteritis, crop disorders, impaction, pancreatitis, and liver and kidney disease.
- Definitive diagnosis requires the identification of typical histopathologic lesions on biopsy specimens. A biopsy of the crop is relatively noninvasive and may provide a diagnosis. When obtaining a biopsy, be certain to include mucosal blood vessels in the sample. This will increase the likelihood of obtaining a nerve, thus demonstrating histologic lesions. False-negative results are likely if nervous tissue is not obtained or if lesions are absent in the crop but present in other areas of the GI tract.
  - The CBC may demonstrate a leukocytosis and nonregenerative anemia.
- The serum biochemical profile may reveal increased CK and hypoproteinemia.

Postmortem Diagnosis

The diagnosis usually is made by identification of characteristic lesions on necropsy.

- Gross pathologic changes include proventricular dilatation, ventricular ulcers, and undigested food in the lower GI tract.
- Confirmation of the diagnosis requires identification of accumulated lymphocytes and plasma cells in the nerves of the GI tract, brain, or spinal cord.
  - GI lesions include endoventriculitis, muscle atrophy, lymphocytic leiomyositis, and smooth muscle degeneration.
  - Lesions may be found in the brain and peripheral nerves. Peripheral nervous tissue is affected most often, and lesions include lymphocyte and plasma cell infiltrates in the mesenteric plexus ganglia and in the intrinsic and extrinsic nerves of the proventriculus and ventriculus, and intranuclear and intracytoplasmic eosinophilic inclusion bodies in nerve cells of intestinal ganglia.
  - Other, less frequently encountered nervous tissue lesions include multifocal lymphocytic encephalitis with gliosis; neuronophagia and perivascular cuffing in the cerebellum, medulla oblongata, brain stem, cerebrum, spinal cord and meninges; visceral ganglioneuritis; and lymphocytic poliomyelitis.

Treatment

- There are some reports of prolonged survival with supportive care and a soft gruel diet. In most cases, however, PDD invariably is fatal.

Prevention

- Because an etiologic agent, its transmission mode, and incubation period have not been identified, prevention is difficult.
- Strictly isolate birds with confirmed PDD from direct or indirect contact with other birds.
- Quarantine birds exposed to confirmed cases for at least 6 months.

▼ *Key Point* Do not euthanize birds with radiographic evidence of proventricular dilatation unless a definitive, histologic diagnosis of PDD has been obtained. Rule out other causes of proventricular dilatation.

Papillomatosis

Papillomas are proliferative, wart-like lesions that may occur on mucosal surfaces of the intestinal tract, including the oral cavity, esophagus, crop, proventriculus, and cloaca. Lesions are most commonly identified on the cloacal mucosa. Macaws, Amazon parrots, and conures are the species most frequently affected. Cancer of the liver and pancreas are commonly associated with papillomatosis.

Etiology

- A viral etiology is suspected because papillomas often appear to spread through groups of birds, and it is known that papillomaviruses cause wart-like growths in other species.

Clinical Signs

Clinical signs vary with the location of the lesions.

- Signs of cloacal papillomas include straining to defecate, flatulence, malodorous and bloody stools, persistent enteric bacterial infections, and reduced fertility.
  - Cloacal papillomas may resemble granulation tissue and can be difficult to distinguish from cloacal prolapse.
- Oral papillomas may cause wheezing, dyspnea, excessive salivation, dysphagia, and persistent oral bacterial infections.
- Signs of esophageal, crop, and proventricular papillomas include vomiting, regurgitation, and weight loss.

Diagnosis

- Base the diagnosis on the appearance of the lesions, biopsy, and histopathology.

Treatment

In some cases, the size and appearance of lesions wax and wane without treatment. Treatment is indicated when clinical signs are evident, or, in the case of cloacal papillomas, if self-mutilation occurs.

- Cloacal papillomas may be gradually removed with chemical cauterization with silver nitrate sticks. Evert the papilloma from the cloaca, and roll a silver nitrate cautery stick onto the papilloma, taking extreme care not to cauterize normal mucosa. Rinse thoroughly with water. This procedure can be painful; therefore, anesthetize with isoflurane.

- Remove surgically by ligation and resection, electrocautery, or cryosurgery. The technique used depends on the extent of the lesion.
  - Circumferential lesions of the cloaca may require more than one procedure.
  - Take care to avoid the development of postoperative strictures.
- Treat secondary bacterial infections before surgical removal.

Prevention

- Because papillomas may be caused by an infectious agent, carefully examine the cloaca and mouth of all birds being added to a collection for the presence of papillomas. Those with lesions should be denied entry.
  - It may be difficult to detect birds that have had papillomas surgically removed. It is unknown whether a carrier state exists.

BACTERIAL DISEASES

Gram-Negative Infections

Bacterial infections requiring treatment commonly are encountered in avian medicine, especially in birds that have been stressed, are on a poor nutritional plane, or are housed in unsanitary conditions. Normal intestinal flora in most pet bird species consist primarily of gram-positive bacteria. Although small numbers of gram-negative bacteria may normally be found in healthy birds, most gram-negative bacteria are primary or potentially opportunistic pathogens. Normal psittacine flora include *Lactobacillus, Bacillus,* nonhemolytic *Streptococcus, Micrococcus, Staphylococcus, Corynebacterium,* and *Streptomyces* spp.

Etiology

Commonly encountered gram-negative pathogens include *Escherichia coli* and *Enterobacter, Klebsiella, Pseudomonas, Salmonella, Proteus, Pasteurella,* and *Campylobacter* spp.

Clinical Signs

Clinical signs depend on the organ system affected.

- Respiratory, GI, or nonspecific signs such as inappetence, lethargy, and ruffled feathers may be seen alone or concurrently.
- Septicemia, especially from invasion of enteric pathogens, is extremely common in pet birds.
  - Suspect septicemia in any severely depressed bird.

Diagnosis

- Perform a Gram stain and culture on samples collected from suspected sites of infection.
- CBC usually demonstrates leukocytosis, with a relative heterophilia. Toxic heterophils are often seen. With chronic disease, the serum protein elec-

trophoresis may demonstrate a hypergammaglobulinemia. The serum biochemical profile may be helpful in identifying hepatic or renal involvement.

Respiratory System

- The rostral-most portion of the choana is a readily accessible site for collecting specimens from the upper respiratory system.
- Other techniques for isolation of respiratory microbial agents include aspiration of the sinuses and tracheal washing (see Chap. 161).
- Direct culture of the air sacs or air sac flushing may be performed via laparoscopy.

Gastrointestinal System

- Readily accessible sites for isolation of microbial agents include the crop, cloaca, and fresh feces.
- In large birds, the proventriculus and ventriculus may be cultured directly using a rigid endoscope or pediatric bronchoscope.

Other Organ Systems

- Organ systems such as the urogenital tract and liver, both common sites of bacterial infection, are accessible only by more invasive techniques, such as laparoscopy or exploratory laparotomy.
- Septicemic birds often are severely depressed and are unable to withstand invasive procedures. Aggressive empirical treatment with antibiotics is indicated for these birds.

Treatment

Treatment is indicated when gram-negative bacteria are isolated from a bird with system-specific signs or signs of septicemia.

▼ **Key Point** Identification of gram-negative organisms on samples taken from clinically healthy birds does not necessarily warrant treatment. Monitor these birds for clinical signs and shifts in bacterial flora.

Selection of Antibiotics

Whenever possible, select antibiotics based on culture and susceptibility testing.

Kirby Bauer Susceptibility Test
- Bacterial isolates are classified as susceptible based on serum concentrations of antimicrobial agents that are achievable in humans.
  - Because it may not be possible to achieve these high levels in pet birds, this test may not accurately predict the efficacy of the antibiotic chosen in vivo.
- Determining the minimum inhibitory concentration (MIC) of antibiotics allows a more accurate assessment of antimicrobial efficacy in pet birds; however, this test is not readily available. For this reason, the Kirby Bauer test still is commonly used.
- When choosing an antibiotic based on standard Kirby Bauer testing:
  - The bacterial isolate should be susceptible to the antibiotic.

- The antibiotic preferably should be bactericidal, known to penetrate into the site of infection, and effective at very low serum concentrations.
- Antibiotics and dosages commonly used in pet birds are listed in Table 162–1.

Route of Administration

Oral Administration

- Direct oral administration of medications often is used in pet birds, especially for palatable solutions or suspension. However this method is difficult for some owners. Instruct owners on the proper restraint techniques. But even then, birds sometimes spit out the medication, and aspiration also is a possibility.
- Addition of medications to a favorite food is a stress-free method; however, the addition of food may decrease the drug's bioavailability.
- Administration of antibiotics via drinking water is the least preferred method because many antibiotics are unpalatable and are not water-soluble, and ingestion of the medication often is sporadic.
- Although there are several disadvantages to oral administration, in many flock situations, or when owners cannot hospitalize the bird or otherwise administer parenteral antibiotics, consider using one of the aforementioned methods.

- When a bird is hospitalized and the intestinal tract is functioning properly, oral medications may be administered via gavage tube.

Parenteral Administration

- Many antibiotics commonly used in avian medicine are poorly absorbed when given orally, necessitating parenteral administration.
- Use injectable antibiotics:
  - When a bird is unwilling to take oral medications
  - When gastrointestinal motility is altered
  - In critically ill or septicemic birds
- The advantages of this method include precise dosing, rapid development of therapeutic serum concentrations, and relatively stress-free administration.
- Many practitioners teach their clients to administer IM injections to their pets (the technique for IM injection is described in Chapter 161).

Monitoring

Assess antibiotic effectiveness by monitoring the resolution of clinical signs, serial hemograms, cytology, and culture. Serial fecal or cloacal Gram stains during and after antibiotic administration are important because development of secondary infections, especially yeasts, are common.

Table 162–1. ANTIBIOTICS FOR USE IN AVIAN PATIENTS

Generic Name	Product Name (Mfr)	Dose	Comments
Amikacin (250 mg/ml)	Amiglyde (Bristol)	20 mg/kg q12h IM	Potentially nephrotoxic Synergistic w/penicillins
Piperacillin (injectable)	Pipracil (Lederle)	100–200 mg/kg q6–8h IM, IV	Effective against most gram-negative bacteria Synergistic w/aminoglycosides Freeze after reconstitution until use Good activity against gram-negative bacteria
Cefotaxime	Claforan (Hoechst-Roussel)	75 mg/kg q6–8h IM	Broad-spectrum, low toxicity Good against getamicin-resistant gram-negative isolates
Ceftiofur	(Fortaz, Glaxo)	75–100 mg/kg q6–8h IM, IV	Synergistic w/aminoglycosides Reconstituted drug lasts 12 weeks in freezer, 10 days in refrigerator Broad-spectrum, penetrates into CNS
Cephalexin (suspension)	Keflex (Eli Lilly)	30–50 mg/kg q6h PO	Variable efficacy against gram-negative isolates Dosing schedule may be impractical
Ciprofloxacin (tablets)	Cipro (Miles)	20 mg/kg q12h PO	Broad-spectrum activity against gram-negative isolates, including *Pseudomonas* spp. Well absorbed orally Water-soluble—crush tablets and make into solution for direct oral dosing
Enrofloxacin	Baytril (Haver)	15 mg/kg q12h IM	Similar activity to Cipro Irritating when injected IM—do not use for > 3–5 days
Gentamicin	Gentocin (Schering)	10 mg/kg q12h IM 10 mg/kg q12h IT 1 ml/10 ml saline for neb	More nephrotoxic than amikacin when given IM Use IT or by neb as adjunctive therapy in respiratory infections (not absorbed)
Metronidazole	Flagyl (Searle)	50 mg/kg q12h	Effective against many anaerobic bacteria
Trimethoprim sulfamethoxazole (suspension)	Bactrim (Roche)	100 mg/kg q12h PO	Good against many gram-negative and gram-positive isolates Excellent for hand-feeding neonates May cause emesis in some birds, especially macaws

IM, intramuscularly; IT, intratracheally; neb, nebulization; PO, orally (per os).

Gram-Positive Infections

Gram-positive infections occur less frequently in pet birds. Pathogens include beta-hemolytic *Streptococcus*, *Staphylococcus aureus*, and *Clostridium* spp. Follow the same principles for diagnosis and treatment as outlined previously for gram-negative infections.

Avian Tuberculosis

Etiology

Tuberculosis in psittacines, unlike that in mammals, usually is a primarily alimentary disease.

- Although a few cases of *Mycobacterium tuberculosis* and *M. bovis* have been reported in pet birds, the causative agent usually is *M. avium*.
- These gram-positive, acid-fast granulated rods are capable of causing disease in birds, pigs, guinea pigs, rabbits, and humans.
- Brotorgeris parakeets (especially gray-checked parakeets) are particularly susceptible, followed by Amazon parrots, budgerigars, and Pionus parrots.

Transmission

- Transmission occurs primarily by ingestion of fecal-contaminated food, water, or soil; an aerosol route or wound contamination also is possible. The organism is capable of surviving in soil for up to 2 years.
- After ingestion, the organisms penetrate the GI mucosa and colonize under the serosa.
- A primary bacteremia occurs (usually without clinical signs), and the organisms are phagocytized (but not killed) by mononuclear phagocyte cells of the liver, spleen, and bone marrow. Multiplication within these cells causes a local reaction by the cell-mediated immune system, characterized by focal or diffuse infiltration of epithelioid cells and multinucleated giant cells. These nodules frequently contain necrotic centers, which may calcify with time.
- Release of the organisms from the liver results in a secondary bacteremia, with localization in lungs, kidneys, gonads, and intestines. Tubercles in the intestinal wall may open into the intestinal lumen, resulting in shedding of large numbers of organisms in the feces.

Clinical Signs

- Clinical signs include chronic weight loss (despite a good appetite), depression, chronic diarrhea, polyuria, and poor feathering.
- Abdominal distension due to hepatomegaly and dilated, fluid-filled, thickened intestines is common.
- Subcutaneous and periorbital masses may be seen.
- Lameness due to endosteal bone proliferation occasionally is reported.
- Signs often are nonspecific and slowly progressive.

Diagnosis

Hematology and Serum Biochemistry

- Severe leukocytosis (>20,000) with marked heterophilia and monocytosis is common.

- Anemia and polychromasia usually are present.
- Aspartate aminotransferase (AST) levels usually are elevated with hepatic involvement.

Histopathologic Lesions

- On postmortem examination, in addition to the grossly visible nodules previously described, diffuse infiltration of epithelioid or giant cells may result in a grossly thickened firm intestine, hepatomegaly, or splenomegaly.
- Histologically, the intestinal villi may be club-shaped and swollen and filled with epithelioid cells containing acid-fast rods.
- Definitive diagnosis is based on identification of acid-fast rods and epithelioid cells on biopsy or postmortem slide preparations. The liver is generally the most reliable source.
  - Acid-fast staining or culture of feces also may demonstrate the organism, although false-negative results are common owing to intermittent shedding of organisms.
  - Cultures require 3–6 weeks for results.
- Indirect diagnosis with intradermal tuberculin and slide agglutination tests also frequently produce false-negative results.

Treatment

- Euthanasia often is recommended because of the potential human health hazard, especially to immunocompromised owners.
- Successful treatment of pet birds with *M. avium*, mimicking human treatment protocols, has been reported.

SUPPLEMENTAL READING

Aguilar RF, Redig PT: Diagnosis and treatment of avian aspergillosis. *In* Bonagura JD, Kirk RW, eds: Current Veterinary Therapy XII, Small Animal Practice, Philadelphia, WB Saunders, 1995, pp 1294–1299.

Aranaz A, Liebana E, Mateos A, Dominguez L: Laboratory diagnosis of avian mycobacteriosis. Semin Avian Exot Pet Med, 6:9–17, 1997.

Cross GM: Viral diseases. Semin Avian Exot Pet Med, 4(2), 1995.

Dorrestein GM: Bacteriology. *In* Altman RB, Clubb SL, Dorrestein GM, Quesenberry K, eds: Avian Medicine and Surgery. Philadelphia, WB Saunders, 1997, pp 225–280.

Flammer K: Chlamydia. *In* Altman RB, Clubb SL, Dorrestein GM, Quesenberry K, eds: Avian Medicine and Surgery. Philadelphia, WB Saunders, 1997, pp 364–379.

Gerlach H: Viruses. *In* Ritchie BW, Harrison GJ, Harrison LR, eds: Avian Medicine: Principles and Application. Lake Worth, FL, Wingers Publishing, 1994, pp 862–948.

Gregory CR, Latimer KS, Niagro FD, et al: A review of proventricular dilatation syndrome. J Assoc Avian Vet, 8:69–75, 1994.

Ritchie BW: Papovaviridae. In Ritchie RW, ed: Avian Viruses: Function and Control. Lake Worth, FL, Wingers Publishing, 1995, pp. 127–170.

Ritchie BW: Herpesviridae. *In* Ritchie RW, ed: Avian Viruses Function and Control. Lake Worth, FL, Wingers Publishing, 1995, pp. 171–218.

VanDerHeyden N: New strategies in the treatment of avian mycobacteriosis. Semin Avian Exot Pet Med, 6:25–33, 1997.

163 Avian Dermatology

Elizabeth V. Hillyer

BASIC ANATOMY AND PHYSIOLOGY

An understanding of the structure and function of avian skin and feathers is necessary when working with avian dermatologic problems.

Skin

Avian skin, consisting of epidermis and dermis, is histologically similar to that of mammals but is relatively thin. It is devoid of true glandular structures.

Cutaneous Glands

There are four types of true cutaneous glands in birds:

- Meibomian glands of the eyelids
- Uropygial gland
- Glands of the external ear
- Mucus-producing glands around the vent

Uropygial Gland

The uropygial gland is a bilobed, holocrine gland located at the base of the tail.

- As birds preen, they spread uropygial gland secretions on the feathers; these secretions aid in waterproofing and in suppressing the growth of microorganisms.
- Amazon parrots and some other psittacines lack a uropygial gland.

Incubation Patch

- During the breeding season, most avian species develop an incubation or "brood" patch over the ventral abdomen. In this area, the feathers are sparse and the dermis becomes thickened and vascular to increase local body heat production for egg incubation.
- The brood patch may occur in one or both sexes, depending on the species of bird.

Feathers

Feather follicles are found in the dermis and may extend into the subcutis. The structure resembles that of hair follicles.

Adapted from Hillyer EV, Quesenberry KE, Baer K: Basic Avian Dermatology. Proceedings of the Association of Avian Veterinarians, Seattle, WA, 1989.

- Feathers of birds are specialized epithelial derivatives that provide flight, waterproofing, flotation, insulation, and display for breeding purposes. Feathers grow in tracts on the body called *pterylae;* the featherless tracts between pterylae are called *apteria.*
- There are seven types of feathers: contour, semiplume, down, powder down, hypopenna, filoplume, and bristle.
  - Contour feathers are the largest feathers and include the flight feathers and the external layer of feathering on the trunk.
  - Semiplume and down feathers provide thermal insulation.
  - Powder down feathers, which are found in many species of birds including psittacines, shed 1-mm granules of keratin, a white powdery substance that aids in waterproofing. Psittacines that produce a large amount of "powder" include many cockatoo species, cockatiels, and African gray parrots.

The Molt

- During the molt, the "old" feathers are pushed out by the growth of new feathers. After emergence of the new "pin" or "blood" feathers, the vascular pulp retracts back to the base of the follicle. Only the powder down feathers are continuously growing. Most species of birds molt once a year after the breeding season.
- Some species molt two or three times a year; other species molt continuously throughout the year.
- The molt is influenced by light exposure and controlled by hormones. Birds kept indoors may not show a regular molting pattern.
- The growth of new feathers results in an increase in protein mobilization and basal metabolic rate.

▼ *Key Point* The molting period is physically demanding for birds and may be a particularly stressful time for those receiving poor nutrition. Malnourished birds may not undergo normal molting.

- Dietary protein restriction during the molt in house sparrows has been shown to decrease intensity and duration of the molt.

Feather Color

- Feather color in birds is produced both by pigments and by what is termed *structural color.* Structural color

is produced by interference, resulting in iridescence, or by scattering of light which results in noniridescent color such as the blue of budgerigars.
- Pigmentary colors include melanins, carotenoids, and porphyrins.
  - Carotene pigments, which originate from plant material, are found in fat globules in the feathers. They are responsible for yellow, orange, and red colors; these bright colors are muted in the plumage of birds lacking a dietary source of carotenoids.
  - Dietary deficiencies that result in abnormal pigmentation of feathers include deficiencies in lysine, folic acid, iron, choline, and riboflavin.

Basic Recommendations for Healthy Skin and Feathers

1. Instruct clients on the proper diet for birds. The diet should contain good sources of carotenoids, such as mangoes, nectarines, and orange and dark green vegetables (e.g., carrots, sweet potatoes, squash, broccoli, watercress).
2. Do not keep birds in the kitchen because cooking fumes can coat the feathers.
3. Daily bathing or misting with warm water encourages normal preening and keeps the feathers healthy.

▼ *Key Point* Use only water on the feathers on a routine basis. Avoid using of commercial mite and lice sprays and other products that coat the feathers.

HISTORY

A complete history is important in the diagnosis of feather and skin disorders.

Diet

- Question the client about types, amounts, and frequency of food offered.
  - Is there a source of protein? of carotenoids?
  - Does the bird eat offered foods?

Environment

- Obtain a description of cage setup and surroundings.
- Determine the daily routine and the amount of interaction with people and with other birds.
- Is the bird getting adequate sleep (8–12 hours)?
- Has there been a change in routine?
- Does the bird have an adequately stimulating environment or outlet for normal chewing behavior?

Medical History

- Has the bird had previous medical problems or ongoing problems in addition to skin or feather abnormalities?
  - Does the bird show breeding behavior?
  - Important facts regarding the current dermatologic problem include duration of signs, initial ap-

pearance of lesions, progression of lesions, previous treatment, and response to same.
- Does the bird appear to be pruritic?
- Determine whether there is self-trauma. Ascertaining whether skin and feather lesions are self-induced helps to guide the differential diagnosis.
- Table 163–1 lists common dermatologic problems and their causes; Table 163–2 groups common problems by species.

FEATHER PROBLEMS

Pseudoproblems

The following normal avian behaviors and anatomic features often are perceived as abnormal by new bird owners.

- Normal molting mistaken for excessive feather picking:
  - During the molt, birds spend long periods preening to open up new feather shafts. Clues that a molt is under way are pin feathers on the head (where the solitary cage bird cannot reach to preen) and many feathers on the cage bottom. No

Table 163–1. CLASSIFICATION AND CAUSES OF DERMATOLOGIC PROBLEMS

Problem	Possible Etiologies
Feather loss without picking	*Knemidocoptes* mites, psittacine beak and feather disease, polyomavirus
	Genetic (e.g., baldness in Lutino cockatiels)
	Altered molt (e.g., with malnutrition)
	Endocrine abnormality
Feather picking	Behavioral/environmental problem
	Frustrated courtship/breeding behavior
	Primary skin disease
	Malnutrition causing pica
	Internal disease such as hepatopathy
Skin mass	Feather cyst/folliculoma
	Lipoma
	Xanthoma
	Other neoplasms
Uropygial mass	Gout tophi, abscess, or impaction
	Squamous cell papilloma
	Squamous cell carcinoma
	Adenoma/adenocarcinoma
Facial lesions	*Knemidocoptes* mite infection
	Poxvirus
	Trauma, insect bite
	Papillomavirus
Foot and leg lesions	*Knemidocoptes* mite infection
	Scaly leg syndrome of canaries
	Amazon foot skin necrosis syndrome
Granuloma (fungal/bacterial)	Pox-, polyoma-, and herpesvirus, Mycobacteria

Table 163–2. COMMON DERMATOLOGIC CONDITIONS IN DIFFERENT AVIAN SPECIES

Species	Dermatologic Condition
Canary *(Serinus canarius)*	*Knemidocoptes* mite infection
	Feather cysts
	Scaly leg syndrome
Budgerigar *(Melopsittacus unudulatus)*	*Knemidocoptes* mite infection
	Lipomas
	Fibrosarcoma
	Feather cysts
	Uropygial gland conditions
Cockatiel *(Nymphicus hollandicus)*	*Giardia* infection/featherpicking
	Genetic baldness in lutino cockatiels
	Feather cysts
Conures *(Aratinga* spp. and *Nandayus nenday)*	Feather picking
	Self-mutilation
Amazon parrot *(Amazona* spp)	Foot skin necrosis syndrome
	Lipomas
	Feather picking
Cockatoo *(Cacatua* spp.)	Feather picking
	Psittacine beak and feather disease virus
	Papillomas
Rose-breasted cockatoo *(Eolophus roseicapillus)*	Lipomas
Macaw *Ara* spp.	Feather picking
Lovebirds	Psittacine beak and feather disease virus
	Ulcerative dermatitis

featherless areas are grossly visable without evidence of pin feathers.
  • If the bird appears normal, with healthy skin and feathers, "excessive" feather picking probably is secondary to a normal molt.
• Dandruff:
  • Pieces of normal feather shaft, which fall to the cage bottom during preening of new feathers, may be misinterpreted as dandruff.
• Bare areas:
  • Sometimes the owner is concerned about the apteria (i.e., normal featherless areas) between the feather tracts.
• Dark or "bruised" skin:
  • Because avian skin is thin, the color of dark underlying muscle is visible through the skin; some owners become alarmed at this color.

Broken Blood Feather

▼ *Key Point* When a growing feather, or *blood feather,* breaks along the vascular shaft, it may continue to bleed until the feather is pulled from the base. Birds can die from blood loss due to a bleeding blood feather.

Instruct owners on how to pull a bleeding feather if there is not enough time to reach the clinic.

• Firmly stabilize the limb in one hand; then, using a hemostat or needle-nose pliers, firmly grasp the feather at the base and pull it out.

• The feather should separate at the epidermis; however, if the vascular dermis should tear, resulting in bleeding, apply pressure to the area until bleeding stops.

Feather Loss Without Plucking

This is less common than feather picking.

Etiology

Possible causes of spontaneous feather loss include:

• *Knemidocoptes* mite infection
• Previous damage to feather follicles
• Genetic causes (e.g., baldness in lutino cockatiels)
• Altered molt (e.g., with malnutrition)
• Abnormal growth of feathers, such as occurs with psittacine beak and feather disease virus (PBFDV) and polyomavirus infection (see Chap. 162)
• Endocrine disturbances such as hypothyroidism (uncommon in pet birds)

Clinical Signs

• Feather loss can occur anywhere on the body, including the head.
• The skin may be normal, or it may be thickened.
• The owner usually relates that the bird is not picking, scratching, or rubbing.

Diagnosis

• Obtain a thorough history including:
  • Rate and pattern of feather loss
  • Previous feather picking or self-trauma
  • Other medical problems
  • Specific details of diet and management
• Perform a thorough physical examination, paying particular attention to skin and feathers.
  • Examine pin feathers carefully for signs of abnormal growth, such as would occur with PBFDV.
• Consider a serum biochemical analysis, complete blood count (CBC), PBFDV testing, and whole body radiography to screen for systemic disease. Poor feathering may be a sign of chronic systemic disease.
• Perform skin biopsy (including several abnormal follicles) for diagnosis of PBFDV, hypothyroidism, malnutrition, and prior damage to follicles.

Feather Picking and Self-Mutilation

Feather picking refers to the plucking or mutilation of feathers by the bird. Psittacine birds are most commonly affected. Self-mutilation of skin and underlying muscle also can occur.

▼ *Key Point* Feather picking and self-mutilation are two of the most common, frustrating, and time-consuming conditions encountered by the avian practitioner.

Etiology

- Feather picking by psittacine birds, which are very social creatures, may be the result of jealousy, dominance behaviors, boredom, fear, frustration, and other emotions.
- Feather picking may begin as the result of a behavioral or medical problem and develop into a "vice."
- Feather picking that begins during the breeding season and involves the breast, abdominal, and leg regions may be a manifestation of exaggerated or frustrated courtship and brooding behavior. The role of sex hormones in eliciting true pruritus in birds has not been elucidated.
- True bacterial or mycotic folliculitis is rare in cage birds.
- Many bird owners worry about external parasites when they see their birds preening (normal) or feather picking (abnormal). Caution owners that commercial feather lice and mite spray is greatly overused and is ineffective.

▼ *Key Point* External parasites such as *Knemidocoptes* and feather lice are almost never a cause of feather picking.

- Malnutrition may result in pica, manifested as feather mutilation.
- Internal diseases such as intestinal parasitism, liver disease, and airsacculitis may result in feather picking.
  - Intestinal giardiasis is associated with feather picking in cockatiels. The mechanism is uncertain, but possible causes include a hypersensitivity reaction and malabsorption of essential nutrients.
  - Intestinal candidiasis as detected by fecal Gram's stain commonly is seen in association with feather picking. The cause and effect of this association is uncertain.
- Food allergy, especially to sunflower seeds, is suspected in some birds.
  - In one case, feather picking stopped when the owner eliminated the large quantity of oranges the bird was eating daily.

Diagnosis

▼ *Key Point* Investigate underlying medical problems before attributing feather picking to behavioral causes. The basic database ideally includes fecal parasite examination, fecal Gram's stain, CBC, serum biochemical analysis, whole-body radiography, and skin biopsy.

- Obtain a thorough history, including:
  - Diet and management practices
  - Any environmental changes
  - Behavior consistent with pruritis
  - Pattern and timing of feather picking
  - Other medical problems
- In the physical examination, look for the hallmark sign of feather picking: normal feathering on the head (inaccessible to the beak) with areas of feather loss or feather mutilation elsewhere on the body.
- Perform a fecal examination for intestinal parasites, including a direct fecal smear and fecal flotation. For cockatiels, a trichrome stain of the feces is useful to detect *Giardia* organisms.
- Obtain samples for fecal or cloacal Gram's stain. Submit a fecal culture if abnormal numbers of gram-negative bacteria are seen.
- Perform serum biochemical analysis and CBC to screen for systemic disease, especially if feather picking is chronic or if there is evidence of self-mutilation.
- Whole-body radiography is useful to evaluate internal organs.
- To perform a skin biopsy in birds:
  1. Make an elliptical incision with a #11 blade or obtain a sample with a biopsy punch (Acu-Punch, Acuderm, Inc., Ft. Lauderdale, FL).
  2. Close the incision with 5–0 absorbable suture in a simple continuous pattern.
- Elevated gamma globulins on serum protein electrophoresis (EPH) suggest an underlying infectious or inflammatory condition.
- If necessary, perform abdominal laparoscopy to investigate abnormalities seen on radiographs.
- A liver biopsy, via laparoscopy or keyhole skin incision, is useful if results of blood tests and radiography suggest liver disease.

Treatment

▼ *Key Point* There is no single effective treatment for feather picking. Tailor treatment to the individual bird and owner, and prepare the owner for the possibility of long-term therapy involving a series of therapeutic trials.

- If possible, identify and treat underlying medical problems.
- Consider treatment for giardiasis in all feather picking cockatiels, even if no *Giardia* organisms are found, because they are shed intermittently. Give metronidazole (50–60 mg/kg q12h, PO) for 7–10 days.
- Correct management practices when appropriate; for example:
  - Improve caging.
  - Move the cage to the center of family activity for a period of time each day.
  - Turn on the radio or television when leaving the bird alone.
  - Provide toys and "activity foods" such as chicken bones, corn on the cob, and pine cones.
  - Be sure that birds get 8–12 hours of sleep at night, and provide visual security in the form of hiding places during the day.
- Some birds, particularly cockatiels and conures, may benefit from a cagemate. However, warn the owner that the birds may not be socially compatible or the original bird may become less interactive with humans if it bonds with the new cagemate. Occasionally,

the feather-picking bird may "teach" the new bird to feather pick.

- Any new bird should be quarantined for a minimum of 30 days before introduction.
- Make any necessary diet corrections, including vitamin supplementation.
  - Supplementation with vitamin A is indicated if dietary modifications are difficult to institute.
- Antihistamines may relieve pruritus if present and have the additional benefit of causing mild drowsiness.
  - Give hydroxyzine hydrochloride (Atarax, Roerig) at a dose of 2 mg/kg q8h, PO, or 1.5–2.0 mg per 4 oz of drinking water daily; adjust the dosage as necessary to minimize drowsiness and maximize the antipruritic effect.
- Do not use tranquilizers such as diazepam and phenobarbital .
- Drugs used for neurodermatitis in humans and other mammals show some promise in birds. Varying degrees of success has been reported with administration of haloperidol (Haldol, DuPont) at 0.05–0.20 mg/kg PO q24h, doxepin (Sinequan, Roerig) at 0.5–1.0 mg/kg PO q12h, and clomipramine (Anafranil, Basel Pharmaceuticals) at 0.5–1.0 mg/kg PO q12h. Narcotic antagonists such as naltrexone (Trexan, DuPont) also has been used successfully at 1.5 mg/kg PO q24h. The safety and efficacy of any of these drugs have not yet been established in psittacine birds. Therefore, use these drugs with caution.
- Use anti-inflammatory and hormonal therapy with caution; avoid in birds with suspected liver disease.
  - Human chorionic gonadatropin (HCG) has been used successfully to treat feather picking in female birds. HCG is believed to cause an increase in endogenous progesterone.
  - Testosterone, megesterol acetate, or medroxyprogesterone may reduce feather picking in some birds. However, their use is discouraged because of the potential for serious side effects.
  - Side effects include hepatomegaly and anorexia. Corticosteroid administration can be fatal in some birds; the reason for this is not known.
- Use Elizabethan and tube collars with discretion because they can prevent normal preening and eating behaviors. These collars do not treat the underlying medical or behavioral problems that may lead to feather picking and often increase stress.
  - Hospitalize birds for 8–24 hours for observation; placement of a collar may elicit extreme listlessness and anorexia or, conversely, hyperexcitability.
  - Some birds will not tolerate a collar; others may benefit early in the course of treatment to prevent the development of feather picking into a "vice."
- Do not perform radical beak grinding or notching the upper beak. It interferes with a bird's ability to pull and mutilate feathers and is not recommended.

Prevention

- Owner education regarding nutrition, management, and the social needs of birds may help to reduce the incidence of feather picking. However, this disorder also is seen in apparently well-cared-for and socially well-adjusted birds.

INFECTIOUS DISEASES

Viral Diseases

Most viral diseases, such as PBFDV and avian polyomavirus, are in other chapters.

Herpesvirus

Herpesvirus (HV) is known to cause papilloma-like growths on the legs and feet of Moluccan and lesser sulfur-crested cockatoos. The lesions are self-limiting.

Bacterial Diseases

- Bacterial infection of the skin and feathers is uncommon in birds.
- Superficial infection may occur secondary to self-trauma.
- Base the diagnosis on skin biopsy and culture.

Bacterial Folliculitis

- Bacterial folliculitis is rare in birds.
- *Staphylococcus* spp. are believed to be the most common etiologic agent.
- One report describes *Aeromonas* folliculitis in a lovebird with acute pruritus on the ventral surface of the wings.

Septic Exudative Dermatitis

- This syndrome is characterized by epidermal erosion and ulceration with dermal hyperemia and edema focused primarily in the patagial area (the fold of skin that stretches from the carpus to the humeral region in birds).
- Staphylococci are the most common isolates on bacterial culture.
- Perform a skin biopsy and culture for diagnosis.
- Treat aggressively with systemic and local antibiotics; treatment may be unsuccessful because the self-mutilation that occurs as a result of scar formation and contraction.

Avian Tuberculosis

- A granulomatous dermatitis is seen in some cases of avian tuberculosis infection.
- On histopathology, large foamy macrophages containing *Mycobacterium avium* bacilli are seen in the dermis and subcutis.
- Systemic therapy for tuberculosis is necessary (see Chap. 162).

Parasitic Infection

Scaly Face and Leg Mite

▼ *Key Point* Scaly face and leg mite is the only external parasite seen commonly in cage birds.

Etiology

Knemidocoptes pilae is a mite that lives in the skin. It is seen most commonly in budgerigars and canaries but also has been reported in Lady Gouldian finches, cockatiels, Amazon parrots, and ringneck parakeets.

Canaries often are presented with thickened, erythematous scales on the legs and feet. This condition appears to be multifactorial; *Knemidocoptes* infection, low environmental humidity, and hypovitaminosis A and other nutritional deficiencies may all be contributory.

Clinical Signs

- Keratinaceous, proliferative, honeycomb-like lesions occur around the beak, cere, and vent and on the legs and feet. Lesions in canaries are predominantly on the legs and feet.
- In chronic infections, deformed growth of beak and nails may occur.

Diagnosis

- Infection can be latent for 2 years and longer.
- The history often does not include exposure to new birds.
- The gross appearance of the lesions usually is diagnostic.
- If necessary for confirmation, perform a gentle skin scraping of affected areas and examine them microscopically for the mite.

Treatment

- Ivermectin (Ivomec, Merck) is the treatment of choice.
  - For budgerigars and canaries, place 1 drop of the bovine preparation (Ivomec) on the skin over the jugular vein; the drug is absorbed percutaneously.
  - For larger birds, administer ivermectin, 200 μg/kg, SC or PO; repeat every 2 weeks for two to three applications.
- If lesions are proliferative, gently debride loose scales with mineral oil on a cotton swab.
- Clip nails and beak as necessary. Several corrective beak trims may be necessary.
- For scaly leg mite infection in canaries (see Etiology), consider vitamin A supplementation as well as ivermectin therapy.

Prevention

- Treat cagemates of affected birds.

Red Mite

Red mite infection is seen occasionally in cage birds. Canaries are affected most commonly. The mite may be found on budgerigars and other psittacines.

Etiology

Dermanyssus gallinae is a nocturnal feeder that leaves the host during the day.

Clinical Signs

- Signs include restlessness at night and manifestations of anemia, such as weakness, lethargy, and decreased appetite.

Diagnosis

- Cover the cage with a white cloth at night. In the morning, the mites, which appear red owing to the ingestion of blood, can be seen on the inner surface of the cover.

Treatment

- Remove the bird from the cage during the day and clean the cage and cage parts thoroughly.
- In cases of chronic infection, give general supportive care and, if indicated, treat for anemia with iron and vitamin supplementation.

Feather Lice

- Rarely, feather lice are found on cage birds. The lice are grossly visible on the feathers.
- Treat by dusting lightly with carbaryl powder (Sevin, Southern Agricultural Insecticides, Inc.).

ENDOCRINE DISEASES

Hypothyroidism

Several hypothyroid birds have been identified. All were older Amazon parrots with obesity, molting problems, and mild anemia. Dramatic feather loss or feather picking is not part of the presentation. Primary hypothyroidism also has been reported in a scarlet macaw demonstrating severe obesity, delayed molt, and lack of feather regrowth.

Etiology/Clinical Signs

- Because thyroid hormone plays an important role in the molt and in overall body metabolism, hypothyroidism in cage birds may contribute to an abnormal molt, dry skin, high serum cholesterol levels, enlarged fatty deposits, and lethargy.
- Budgerigars with iodine-deficiency goiter may become hypothyroid. However, clinical signs are usually the result of thyroid enlargement and include voice change, squeaking, and regurgitation.

Diagnosis

- Base the diagnosis of goiter in budgerigars on clinical signs and a positive response to iodine supplementation.
- Confirmation of hypothyroidism is difficult because thyoid-stimulating hormone (TSH) is no longer widely available. A presumptive diagnosis may be made based on history, clinical signs, skin biopsy, basal T_4 concentration, exclusion of other causes of feather loss, and response to therapy.

- Measurement of basal T_4 alone is not conclusive because low basal T_4 can result from a variety of illnesses, drugs, and stress.
- Perform a routine serum biochemical profile and CBC in birds suspected of being hypothyroid.
- Whole body radiography is helpful to rule out other, underlying disease.

Treatment

- Supplement iodine in budgerigars with goiter.
- No pharmacologic data are currently available to confirm the proper administration of thyroid hormone. Begin administration of L-thyroxine at a dosage of 0.01–0.02 mg/kg PO q12h. Monitor the bird and adjust the dosage based on postmedication T_4 concentrations, response to treatment or signs of toxicity.

▼ *Key Point* Hypothyroidism is an unusual cause of feather loss or feather picking. Carefully monitor all birds on thyroxine therapy. Serious side effects, such as hyperactivity, anorexia, cardiotoxicity and death commonly occur.

Prevention

- Routinely supplement iodine in all budgerigars.

Hyperadrenocorticism

Pituitary tumors have been reported in birds, but there are no clinical reports of spontaneous hyperadrenocorticism (Cushing's syndrome). However, iatrogenic Cushing's syndrome does occur.

▼ *Key Point* In psittacines and other avian species that have been studied, corticosterone (not cortisol) is the principal corticosteroid in adults.

Etiology

- In mammals, hyperadrenocorticism is the result of excessive production of cortisol by the adrenal cortex, either caused by a tumor or secondary to excessive production of adrenocorticotropic hormone (ACTH) by a pituitary gland tumor. Spontaneous hyperadrenocorticism in birds has not been reported.
- Iatrogenic Cushing's syndrome occurs secondary to the administration of systemic or topical corticosteroids. Clinical signs are the same as in spontaneous Cushing's syndrome; however, the adrenal glands are hypofunctional as the result of negative feedback from exogenous corticosteroids.
- The use of a cream or ointment containing triamcinolone acetate (Panolog, Solvay Animal Health, Inc.) for feather picking has been incriminated as a cause of iatrogenic Cushing's syndrome.

Clinical Signs

- Signs in birds with iatrogenic Cushing's syndrome include sparse feathering and increased subcutaneous

fat deposition. Polyuria-polydipsia (PU/PD) is common.

Diagnosis

- Determine whether the bird has PU/PD or shows other signs of Cushing's syndrome.
- Obtain a history of all treatments, including drug dosages and frequency of use.
- Perform a physical examination; give particular attention to the skin and feathers.
- In birds with PU/PD, perform a serum biochemical profile and CBC to check blood glucose levels, renal function, and hepatic values.

Treatment

- Discontinue exogenous corticosteroid therapy in birds with iatrogenic Cushing's syndrome.
  - Administer prednisone, starting at slightly less than the physiologic replacement dose (0.25 mg/kg q24h) and gradually taper the dose for 1–3 months.
  - Mineralocorticoid administration usually is not necessary.

Prevention

- Use systemic and topical corticosteroids with caution in avian patients.

Baldness in Canaries

A syndrome of testosterone-responsive baldness in male canaries has been reported. The incidence is as high as 60% in some flocks.

- Treatment consists of testosterone, 2.5 mg/kg, IM or PO, once weekly for 6 weeks.
  - Testosterone is contraindicated in birds with liver disease.

NUTRITIONAL DISEASES

A nutritionally complete diet is important in the normal molting process and for the health and coloration of the feathers and skin.

Etiology

Pet birds often are fed an all-seed diet without vitamin or mineral supplementation; as a result, adequate dietary protein, essential fatty acids, copper, zinc, and vitamins A, E, and B, may be lacking.

▼ *Key Point* Hypovitaminosis A is one of the most important nutritional deficiencies in pet birds.

Clinical Signs

- Dermatologic changes in malnourished birds include dull, ragged feathers and thickened, scaly skin, especially on the face, feet, and around the vent.

- Delay or interruption of the molt related to malnutrition results in feathers that are worn and frayed because they are not replaced.
- Malnourished birds are prone to reproductive disorders and upper respiratory and gastrointestinal infections.

Diagnosis

- Base the diagnosis on a complete dietary history.
- The physical examination demonstrates the aforementioned dermatologic changes.
- Evaluate a serum biochemical profile, CBC, and whole body radiographs to rule out underlying systemic diseases.

Treatment

- Educate the owner about proper management and feeding of pet birds.
  - Converting from an all-seed to a well-rounded diet often is a difficult and lengthy undertaking. Dispense high-quality avian vitamin and mineral supplements and instruct the owner on their proper use.
- Give oral vitamin A as beta-carotene (pro-vitamin A) via a proper diet.
  - For an average size Amazon parrot that refuses to eat vegetables, give 1 drop from a capsule of 5000 IU vitamin A once weekly for 4–8 weeks. Caution the owner against exceeding this dosage because of possible vitamin A toxicity.

NEOPLASTIC DISEASES

Cutaneous Papillomatosis

Cutaneous papillomas have been reported in African gray parrots, yellow-headed Amazons, cockatiels, budgerigars, and Quaker parakeets.

- Affected sites include head, neck, oral commissures, feet, and uropygial gland.
- Diagnosis and treatment is with excisional biopsy, if possible.

Squamous Cell Carcinoma

Squamous cell carcinoma (SCC) is a malignancy of squamous epithelial cells and can occur in the skin, oral cavity, crop, and esophagus.

- In birds, SCC is most common in the skin of the wing, beak, and uropygial gland.
- SCC is most common in older birds and has been reported in many species of psittacines.
- Cutaneous SCC usually appears as a poorly defined, raised, proliferative, and sometimes ulcerated cutaneous mass.
- Use exfoliative cytology or histopathology for diagnosis.
- Attempt complete excision of the tumor, if possible.

Uropygial Gland Adenoma and Adenocarcinoma

SCC is the most common neoplasm of the uropygial gland; however, adenomas and adenocarcinomas also occur.

- Adenomas are reported in budgerigars and canaries; adenocarcinomas have been seen in budgerigars, a yellow-fronted parrot, a peach-faced lovebird, and a plum-headed parakeet.
- Diagnosis of uropygial gland neoplasia is by exfoliative cytology or biopsy of the lesion.
- Surgically resect adenomas.
- The prognosis for birds with adenocarcinoma is poor, especially if there is radiographic evidence of metastasis or local bony invasion.
  - Consider surgical excision of uropygial gland adenocarcinoma if the lesion is amenable to total excision.

Lipoma

Lipomas occur most commonly in budgerigars and rose-breasted cockatoos and occasionally in Amazon parrots.

Etiology

- Lipomas are benign tumors arising from lipocytes; they may represent altered fat storage or lipocytic hyperplasia in the obese bird. High dietary fat levels or hypothyroidism may predispose obese birds to their development.

Clinical Signs

- Lipomas appear as smooth, raised masses growing in the subcutis; the yellow color is often visible through the skin. They occur primarily over the sternum and abdominal regions.
- Subcutaneous lipomas can become very large and may occur in multiple locations.

Diagnosis

- Establish the duration and rate of growth of the mass(es).
- Physical appearance of the tumor is usually diagnostic.
- If the diagnosis is questionable, perform fine-needle aspiration and cytology. However, there is no way to distinguish hyperplastic fat cells from lipoma cells on cytology (or histopathology).
- Rule out hypothyroidism as an underlying cause (see previous discussion under Hypothyroidism).

Treatment

- Dietary management may help to reduce the size of lipomas.
  - Gradually reduce the amount of oats offered to small seed eaters, such as budgerigars, and the amount of sunflower seeds offered to larger seed eaters, such as cockatoos.

- Provide supplemental iodine to budgerigars.
- Administer thyroxine to larger parrots only if a diagnosis of hypothyroidism has been determined (see Hypothyroidism section for dosage).
- Surgical removal of lipomas may be beneficial if the overlying skin is necrotic, if the bird picks at the area, or if a lipogranuloma is suspected. Weigh the risk of anesthesia and surgery against the benefits of surgical removal.

Prevention

- Recommend varied diets for pet birds; instruct owners to avoid offering a preponderance of oats or sunflower seeds.
- Provide supplemental iodine for budgerigars.

Liposarcoma

Liposarcoma, a malignant neoplasm of lipocytes, has been reported in budgerigars and cockatiels.

- Liposarcomas are less common than lipomas. They occur in similar areas but tend to be poorly encapsulated, firmer, and more highly vascularized than lipomas.
- Make a definitive diagnosis of liposarcoma by tissue biopsy; aspiration cytology may not be diagnostic.
- The treatment of choice is surgical excision; however, complete excision may be difficult because these tumors are locally invasive and there is a potential for metastasis.

Fibrosarcoma

- Fibrosarcoma is a malignant tumor of mesenchymal origin. This tumor is one of the most common malignancies of budgerigars; it also occurs in cockatiels, parrots, and macaws.
- Fibrosarcomas are locally invasive and may metastasize to the liver, lungs, and bones. They can occur anywhere on the body but often are found on extremities.
- Use aspiration cytology as an aid to diagnosis.
- The treatment of choice is total excision or amputation of the affected extremity.

Lymphohistiocytic Tumors

- Lymphoid neoplasms are relatively uncommon in cage birds. Cutaneous manifestations have been reported; the head and neck are the most common sites.
- Perform aspiration cytology for diagnosis. A full systemic medical evaluation is important.
- Possible treatments include excision and chemotherapy.

Xanthoma

Xanthoma ("yellow mass") is not a true neoplasm. Xanthomas have been seen in poultry, budgerigars, cockatiels, a rose-breasted cockatoo, a gray-cheeked parakeet, and a green-wing macaw.

Xanthomas are characterized microscopically by dermal infiltration with large numbers of macrophages containing lipid particles. There may be cholesterol clefts and multinucleated giant cells.

Etiology

- In dogs and cats, xanthomas usually are associated with abnormal concentrations or composition of plasma lipids, as with diabetes mellitus or hereditary hyperlipoproteinemia of cats.
- Toxic amounts or toxic substances in dietary fat may contribute to the development of xanthomatosis in birds.

Clinical Signs

- Xanthomas become a clinical problem if they are large or if the bird self-traumatizes the area.
- Xanthomas appear as yellow, thickened, featherless areas of skin that may be vascular and friable. The lesion may be discrete or diffuse (xanthomatosis).
- Xanthomas generally occur on the thigh, wingtip, or abdomen, but they can be found anywhere on the body and may overlie a tumor or lipoma.

Diagnosis

- Review the dietary history for evidence of overfeeding of foods high in fat. Determine whether there is self-trauma.
- The gross appearance of the tumor often is diagnostic.
- Perform tissue biopsy to make a definitive diagnosis.

Treatment

- No treatment is necessary for small xanthomas.
- If the xanthomas are large or bleeding, attempt surgical excision.
  - If surgical excision is not possible, consider low-energy radiation therapy (20–30 Gy) and hyperthermia.
- Although preexisting xanthomas probably will be unaffected, correction of the diet is important in long-term management.

Cutaneous Cysts

Cutaneous cysts are benign lesions defined as having an epithelial wall surrounding secretory or keratinaceous contents.

- *Follicular cysts,* also known as feather cysts, are much more common than epidermal cysts and occur in many passerine and psittacine species.
- *Epidermal cysts* are reported in budgerigars. These lesions are lined with stratified squamous epithelium filled with keratin and are found in the dermis or subcutis.

Etiology

- Follicular cysts are the result of congenital or acquired obstruction of follicular orifices, resulting in accumulation of keratinaceous debris in follicles. In some cases, the cyst actually may contain a feather shaft, representing an ingrown feather.

- Follicular cysts in canaries may have a hereditary basis because they occur most commonly in strains bred for dense and curled feathering, such as Norwich canaries.
- Microscopically, canary follicular cysts resemble benign neoplasms of follicular cells, and some authors have proposed calling them "folliculomas."

Clinical Signs

- Follicular cysts usually occur on the wings of psittacines and on the wings or dorsum of canaries.
- They appear as firm, raised, yellow skin masses that generally are movable over the underlying muscle.
- Self-trauma occurs in some instances.

Diagnosis

- Establish the duration and progression of the lesions and any history of self-trauma.
- The physical appearance of cutaneous cysts generally is diagnostic.
- Keratin debris is seen with aspiration cytology.
- Tissue biopsy is necessary for definitive diagnosis of follicular cysts and epidermal cysts.

Treatment

- If the cutaneous cysts are large or if the bird is picking at the area, surgical treatment is required.
  - Lancing or excision of the cyst can be performed under general anesthesia.
  - Careful hemostasis is important.
  - Recurrence is possible with either technique.

Lancing

- Lance the cyst and express its contents.
- Carefully curet and flush the cyst cavity.
- Leave open to heal.

Excision

- Excise the cyst and close the skin routinely.
  - In canaries, excision of an entire feather tract may be necessary.

GENETIC CONDITIONS

Two dermatologic conditions are thought to be hereditary: feather follicle cysts in canaries (see previous discussion) and a syndrome of baldness in Lutino cockatiels.

OTHER DISEASES

Allergies

Allergies in birds are difficult to prove. However, histopathologic lesions suggestive of hypersensitivity or allergic reaction have been seen. In many instances, feather picking has been attributed to food allergy to seeds, particularly sunflower seeds.

Amazon Foot Skin Necrosis Syndrome

Yellow-naped yellow-headed Amazon parrots are most commonly affected.

Etiology

- The cause of this disorder is unknown.
- Possible causes include bacterial or viral infection, allergy, sensitivity to cigarette smoke, and an immune-mediated disorder.

Clinical Signs

- This syndrome occurs in birds of all ages.
- Affected birds usually present for self-trauma to the feet.
- Irregular patches of erythema or brown or black discoloration occur on the unfeathered skin of the legs and feet.
- Bleeding and crusting of the feet occur secondary to self-trauma.

Diagnosis

- Obtain a history, giving particular attention to changes in diet, management, or environment that may have precipitated the problem. Often, no cause is identifiable.
- Physical examination is usually normal except for skin changes on the legs and feet.
- Base the diagnosis on the gross appearance of the lesions.
- Perform a serum biochemical profile and CBC to assess overall organ function.
- Consider whole-body radiography to evaluate for underlying disease.
- Biopsy of the affected skin usually is not possible because lesions are located on the extremities where there is minimal excess skin for closure of the surgical site.

Treatment

- Various treatment regimens have been used.
- Long-term management usually is necessary; recurrence is common after apparent recovery.
- There is no known prevention.

Systemic Drug Therapy

- Antipruritic drugs
  - Therapy with an antihistamine, hydroxyzine hydrochloride (Atarax, Roerig) has had some success; give 2 mg/kg q8h or 1.5–2.0 mg per 4 oz of drinking water, and adjust the dosage to minimize drowsiness but relieve pruritus.
  - Other antihistamines such as benadryl have minimal unwanted side effects and may be useful (extrapolate from canine and feline dosages).
  - Use corticosteroids with caution in birds.
- Administer broad-spectrum systemic antibiotics, such as trimethoprim/sulfadiazine, cefotaxime, enrofloxacin, or piperacillin.

Topical Therapy

- Topical disinfection with dilute chlorhexidine or dilute betadine can be used to clean the skin.
- Antibiotic and antifungal creams are preferred to ointments, which tend to coat the feathers.
- Use topical corticosteroids with caution.
- Leg and foot bandages may be necessary to minimize self-trauma.
- An Elizabethan collar helps to prevent self-trauma; however, this usually does not prevent self-trauma of the feet unless the collar is very wide.
- Instruct the owner on routine sanitation of the cage and environment.

Oiled Birds

Occasionally, the avian clinician is presented with a pet bird with oiled feathers. Generally this occurs because the bird accidentally landed in a household oil or because a well-meaning owner doused the bird with an oily substance because it was "picking at itself" (often normal preening behavior).

- A coating of oil disrupts the thermoregulatory and waterproofing functions of the feathers; ingestion of oil during preening may be harmful to the bird.
- Treatment consists of initial stabilization of the patient with heat, fluids, and nutritional support.
- Once the patient is stable, remove the oil using warm water and a dilute solution of a dishwashing detergent such as Dawn (Procter & Gamble) or Lux Liquid Amber (Lever).
  - After washing, blow-dry or towel-dry the bird carefully and place it in a warm environment until fully dry.

Glue Traps

Careless placement of pest control "glue traps" has resulted in unintended entrapment of pet birds.

- Instruct owners to bring trapped birds immediately into the veterinary hospital and to leave the bird attached to the trap unless it can be removed easily.
- On arrival, release the bird from the trap by gently pulling the feathers out of the glue, taking care not to rip the bird's skin.
- Remove the glue from the feathers; an automobile cleaner, Armor All Protectant (Armor All Products), is effective when sprayed onto the feathers and is relatively nontoxic.
  - Protect the eyes when spraying.
- Gently massage the feathers until the glue is removed; if necessary, rinse the feathers with warm water.

SUPPLEMENTAL READINGS

Bauck L: Avian dermatology. *In* Altman RB, Clubb SL, Dorrestein GM, Quesenberry K, eds: Avian Medicine and Surgery. Philadelphia, WB Saunders, 1997, pp 548–562.

Burgmann PM: Common psittacine dermatologic diseases. Semin Avian Exot Pet Med, 4:169–183, 1995.

Cooper JE, Harrison GJ: Dermatology. *In* Ritchie BW, Harrison GJ, Harrison LR, eds: Avian Medicine: Principles and Application. Lake Worth, FL, Wingers Publishing, 1994, pp 607–639.

Feldman EC, Nelson RW: Canine and Feline Endocrinology and Reproduction. Philadelphia: WB Saunders, 1987.

Galvin C: The feather picking bird. In: Kirk RW (ed): Current Veterinary Therapy VIII. Philadelphia: WB Saunders, 1983, p 646.

Johnson-Delaney C: Feather picking: Diagnosis and treatment. J Assoc. Avian Vet, 6:82–83, 1992.

Latimer KS, Rakich PM, Niagro FD, et al: Un updated review of psittacine beak and feather disease. J Assoc Avian Vet, 5:211–220, 1991.

Lightfoot TL: Clinical use and preliminary data of chorionic gonadotropin administration in psittacines. Proc Annu Conf Assoc Avian Vet, Tampa, FL 1996; pp 303–306.

Lothrop C: Personal communication, 1989.

Wilson L: Nonmedical approach to the behavioral feather plucker. Proc Assoc Avian Vet, 3–9, 1996.

Zenoble RD, Kemppainen RJ: Endocrinology of birds. In: Kirk RW, (ed): Current Veterinary Therapy IX. Philadelphia: WB Saunders, 1986, p 702.

GENERAL ANATOMIC CONSIDERATIONS

The avian respiratory system is a unique gas exchange system compared with that of other domestic animals.

- The lungs are tightly adhered to the body wall and have an essentially uniform volume throughout the respiratory cycle. This allows for more numerous, tightly packed air exchange surfaces, as compared with the mammalian lung.
- Air moves unidirectionally through a large portion of the lung, allowing a high efficiency of gas exchange.
  - The first passage of air through the trachea into the primary bronchus and lung enters the posterior air sacs.
  - The same air then re-enters the lungs, where most gas exchange takes place.
  - The "used" air moves to the anterior air sacs on the next inhalation and moves out the trachea on the subsequent exhalation.
- The high efficiency is derived from the action of the air sacs, unidirectional air flow through the lung, small air capillary diameter, a cross-current relationship between parabronchial gas and blood, countercurrent relationship between blood and air capillaries, and a high diffusion capacity of the lung for oxygen.
- Air sacs are hollow spaces divided by a thin layer of simple squamous epithelium supported by a small amount of connective tissue. They appear as clear, shiny membranes when healthy. Air exchange does not occur in the air sacs.
- Most birds have four paired and one unpaired pulmonary air sacs with diverticula. They also may have cervicocephalic, pharyngeal, and tracheal air sacs.
  - The cervicocephalic air sacs are located in the neck and head region and arise from the sinuses ventral to the tympanic area (Fig. 164–1).
  - The body air sacs are interconnected with the lungs and the pneumatic bones (ribs, vertebrae, humerus, coracoid, clavicle, sternum, ilium, ischium, and pubis).
- A diaphragm, which divides the thoracic and abdominal contents as in mammals, is not present in birds. Birds breathe by expanding and contracting the rib cage, which acts in conjunction with the air sacs, like a bellows.
- The complexity of the avian respiratory system must be considered when treating infections and administering inhalant anesthetics. Accessibility of drugs to all areas of the respiratory system can be limited, predisposing it to chronic disease and often necessitating concurrent systemic and topical (i.e., nebulization) treatment.

▼ **Key Point** Because of the high efficiency of the avian gas exchange system, inhalant anesthetic induction, changes in depth of anesthesia, and

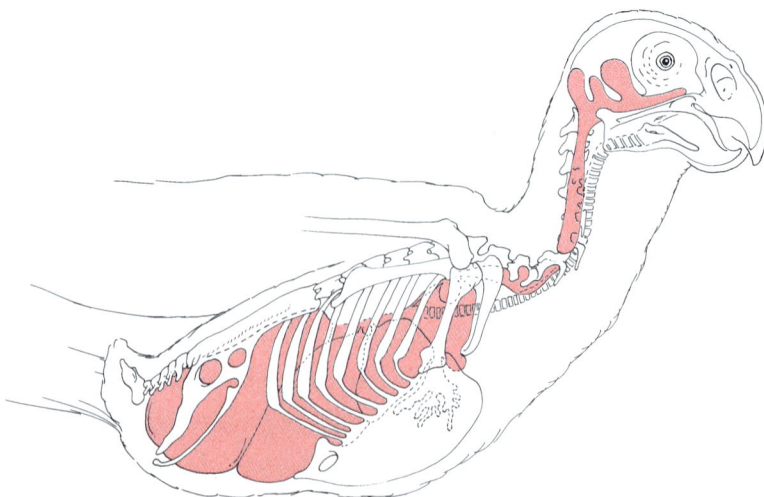

Figure 164–1. Air sac anatomy.

recovery all occur more rapidly in birds than in mammals.

DISEASES OF THE UPPER RESPIRATORY SYSTEM

The upper respiratory system includes the nares, nasal passages, paranasal sinuses (infra- and supraorbital), choana, pharynx, laryngeal prominence that contains the glottis, and the cervicocephalic air sacs.

Disorders of the Nares and Nasal Passages

Etiology

Underlying causes or predisposing factors leading to diseases of the nasal passages can be nutritional, mechanical, parasitic, environmental, infectious, traumatic, or neoplastic.

- *Hypovitaminosis A* is a common nutritional cause of nasal disease in birds. It is seen in birds fed inadequate diets, such as all-seed diets.
  - Hypovitaminosis A can cause squamous metaplasia of the respiratory epithelium, manifested clinically by secondary invaders such as gram-negative bacteria and fungi.
- *Mechanical obstruction* of the nares can be caused by dried exudates, foreign material, or thickening of the cere.
  - Introduction of foreign material (e.g., seeds, seed hulls, dust, feathers, air gun [BB] pellets) into the nares causes sneezing and nasal discharges.
  - Cere thickening (brown hypertrophy) can block the nares and obstruct nasal air movement. This benign thickening is believed to be the result of hormonal influences in older, laying budgerigar hens.
- *Parasites* such as *Cnemidocoptes pilae* mites can cause deposits of honeycomb crusts around the outside of the nares, sometimes obstructing air flow.
- *Environmental factors* such as airborne particles from smoking, cooking, heating and air-conditioning units, decreased humidity, perfumes, and aerosols can cause irritation of the nasal membranes.
- *Infectious agents* such as bacteria, fungi, *Chlamydia*, *Mycoplasma*, and viruses can attack the nasal membranes, causing sneezing, serous or mucous discharge, nasal obstruction (plugs), and distortion of the nares.
- *Trauma* to the nares or nasal passages can cause tissue damage and can lead to secondary infection or obstruction.
- *Neoplasia* of nasal membranes or nasal structures can cause signs of nasal disease. Tumor types reported include fibromas, fibrosarcomas, squamous cell carcinoma, adenosarcomas, and osteogenic sarcomas.
  - Nasal tumors in birds are frequently inoperable.

Clinical Signs

- Sneezing is usually the first sign of nasal irritation.
- Nasal discharge is the most common sign and can be present with or without sneezing and matting of the feathers around the nares.

- Chronic sinusitis can lead to changes in the size of the nares. Damage to the germinal layer of cells at the beak-cere border creates ridges or depressions in the surface of the beak.
- Anatomic distortion of one or both nares, common in African gray parrots, can cause mild to severe dyspnea.
  - Plugging of the nares with inspissated exudate, without any distortion, also may occur.
- Honeycomb crusting around the nares (which can extend to all nonfeathered areas around the head, feet, vent, and uropygial gland) usually is present with *C. pilae* infestation.

▼ *Key Point* Signs of nasal disease (rhinitis) usually are not indicative of systemic disease, but rather of inflammation of the upper respiratory system only. However, be sure to assess the health status of the entire bird.

Diagnosis

History

- Identify factors relating to dietary, environmental, traumatic, or mechanical causes.
- Determine potential exposure to infectious disease agents.

Physical Examination

- Examine the nares for the presence of nasal exudate.
  - An active discharge often stains or mats the feathers around the nares.
  - Pressure near the nasal opening may express exudate that was not previously visible.
  - Transillumination of the nasal passages with a bright focal light source may reveal the presence of fluid or solid tissue.
- Examine the choana for mucus and evidence of postnasal discharge. Also examine the connection between the nasal passages and the choana (i.e., the sphenopalatine cleft), which is visible at the most rostral portion of the choanal slit.
- Use a small, blunt thumb forceps or dental curette to remove caseous material or debris from the nasal opening. (Sometimes the material is solid tissue and cannot be removed in this way.)

Laboratory Studies

- After removal of nasal material, perform both fungal and bacterial culture and sensitivity tests, accompanied by a Gram stain; the sphenopalatine cleft appears to be a better location for culture specimens than the nasal passage. However, both locations may yield a potpourri of bacterial contaminants that are of no clinical significance.
- Cytology or microscopic evaluation of the nasal exudate can be helpful in ruling out fungi, *Chlamydia*, mycobacteria, yeasts, and foreign material. Scrapings of crusts from around the nares (or other featherless areas) reveal *C. pilae* mites.

- Histopathology of biopsied nasal tissue can help to identify neoplastic processes or deep infections, such as chronic fungal sinus infections.
- Perform a complete blood count (CBC) and serum chemistry profile to rule out systemic disease and infectious disease, and assess the chronicity of infection (if present).

Radiography

Radiography can identify metallic foreign bodies and space-occupying lesions in the nares or nasal passages.

Treatment

▼ *Key Point* In all birds with diseases of the nares or nasal passage, make necessary corrections in the diet when deficiencies are suspected, especially of vitamin A.

- Initially, an injection of a vitamin A supplement is helpful (Injacom, Morton & Pestle, Des Moines, IA) (0.1–0.2 ml/100 g body weight), followed by daily addition to the food of a powdered multivitamin product.
- When there are mild signs of nasal disease, flush the sinuses via the nares with 3–5 ml of a dilute solution of Nolvasan (30 ml per gal water) or sterile saline (with or without antibiotics) (see Chapter 161 for techniques). If foreign material is present, remove as much as possible before flushing.
- If bacterial rhinitisis is diagnosed, instill ophthalmic antibiotic ointments or drops (Gentocin Ophthalmic Ointment or Gentocin Durafilm, Schering) into the nares once or twice daily. Most cases of localized rhinitis respond to topical therapy alone.
  - For chronic or resistant infections, add systemic antibiotics to the treatment based on culture and sensitivity results.
- When the results of cultures are negative, nasal flushing as described previously, followed by a nasal decongestant, may be effective (1–2 drops of 0.25% Neo-Synephrine q12h).
- Remove any inciting environmental agents from the surroundings.
- Provide increased humidity with a humidifier or by placing the bird in a "steamed-up" bathroom. This is especially helpful in cases of acute sneezing or respiratory distress.
- If a fungal infection (e.g., aspergillosis) is diagnosed, use a topical antifungal amphotericin B ointment (Fungizone, Squibb) infused into the nares q12h. This can be accompanied by a systemic antifungal such as fluconazole (Diflucan, Roerig) at 20 mg/kg, PO, q48h, or Itraconazol (Sporanox) at 5–10 mg/kg PO q12h. See Chapter 162 for details on treatment of aspergillosis.
- For *C. pilae* mites, use 1% ivermectin (Ivomec, Merck) at a dosage of 200 µg/kg, PO, or topically over the jugular vein; repeat in 2–3 weeks.
- Flush traumatic wounds with antibiotics diluted in sterile saline and treat topically with ophthalmic antibiotic ointment. Leave the wounds open to allow healing by second intention.
- Because tumors of the nasal area are very vascular, surgical removal is difficult, if not impossible. Control of hemorrhage is the main problem.
- For chronic problems that do not respond to topical or systemic antimicrobial therapy, perform sinus trephination. (See appropriate text sources for surgical technique.)

Prevention

Education of the owner is the best prevention. Instruct the owner to:

- Provide food items high in vitamin A or add avian multiple vitamin supplements to the existing diet (see Chapter 165).
- Avoid exposure of the bird to airborne irritants.
  - Do not smoke in the same room as the bird.
  - Do not keep the cage in or near the kitchen. Use an air purifier or a fan with a filter. Sudden deaths have been attributed to overheating Teflon-coated pans, cooking gas, and electronic oven cleaning.
  - Do not house a susceptible bird with powder-producing birds such as cockatoos, cockatiels, and African gray parrots.
- Provide adequate humidity, preferably with a humidifying unit placed in the vicinity of the bird.
- Avoid traumatic injuries (e.g., choose the proper cage mate; do not allow the bird out of the cage unsupervised).

Disorders of the Paranasal Sinuses
Etiology

Underlying causes or predisposing factors leading to disease of the paranasal sinuses (infraorbital and supraorbital) include infections and neoplasia.

- *Infectious causes* include gram-negative bacteria, fungi, mycoplasma, and *Mycobacterium avium.*
- Neoplasms of the infra- or supraorbital sinus tissues are usually highly malignant and include undifferentiated sarcomas, fibrosarcomas, and osteogenic sarcomas.

Clinical Signs

- Swelling above or below the eye is the most common clinical feature.
- Occasionally, an ocular discharge accompanies the swelling.
- Exophthalmos may be present, with the eye displaced upward, downward, or outward. If the disorder is long-standing, the cornea may be dry and cloudy.

Diagnosis

▼ *Key Point* Paranasal sinus disease usually is determined from physical examination and confirmed by surgical exploration or aspiration of the affected sinus.

- Examine the periocular area for swelling; palpate to determine whether the swelling is solid, fluid, or air (most abscesses in birds are caseous and firm).
- Aspirate the swollen area for cytology and culture.
  - If air is obtained, this indicates a problem related to the cervicocephalic air sac system.
  - If a clear liquid is aspirated, as is the case with many canaries and budgies, a viral or mycoplasmal etiology is suggested, and cytology and culture usually are not rewarding.
- Surgical exploration (lancing and/or curettage) may provide a definitive diagnosis or differentiate an abscess from neoplasia.
- Perform culture and sensitivity testing of the sinus cavity for abscessation. Special stains may be required to rule out mycobacteria (acid-fast stain) and fungi (new methylene blue stain).
- Biopsy solid tissue masses for a definitive diagnosis and prognosis.
- Perform a CBC and serum biochemistry profile to rule out systemic disease and infectious disease and assess the chronicity of infection (if present). A serum protein electrophoresis may be helpful in diagnosing an underlying infectious disease.
- Diagnostic testing for *Chlamydia psittaci* also may be indicated.

Treatment

- Most paranasal sinus swellings require surgical intervention to remove caseated material, fluid, or isolated solid tissue masses.
  - To minimize swelling, use an electrosurgical wire to make an incision over the swelling.
  - After removal of the material, which may require curettage or dissection, flush the sinus once or twice daily with sterile saline (with or without antibiotics) or with a dilute solution of Nolvasan, then infuse the sinus with an appropriate ophthalmic antibiotic ointment. Aggressive flushing is necessary to keep the affected area open for treatment.
- If the causative agent is a fungus, administer an ointment containing an antifungal such as amphotericin B (Fungizone, Squibb).
  - Also treat with systemic antifungals, as described previously. See Chapter 162 for details on treatment of *Aspergillus*.
  - Prognosis for a cure is poor, and aggressive curettage or excision may be necessary.
- If mycobacteria are found to be the cause, excision of the affected tissue may not be possible because of the invasiveness of the disease (see Chap. 162 for treatment protocol).
  - The treatment of tuberculosis cases is controversial because of the possible health significance in humans. *M. avium* rarely been has reported to cause disease in humans, however, this is of increasing concern because of the rising prevalence of humans with immune-deficient diseases.
- Suspect mycoplasma infection when sterile fluid is present in the paranasal sinuses, especially in canaries and budgies.

- Remove the fluid, infuse with dilute Nolvasan, and administer tylosin (Tylan plus vitamins, Elanco) (½ g powder in 1 qt of water for 10 days). This has had good clinical results in many cases.

Disorders of the Oral Cavity
Etiology

Diseases of the oral cavity (choana, pharynx, laryngeal prominence with glottis) may obstruct the glottis or upper airway, causing respiratory distress or dyspnea. Underlying factors leading to diseases of the oral cavity and adjacent structures may be nutritional, infectious, parasitic, or neoplastic.

- A primary *nutritional factor* is hypovitaminosis A (as discussed previously for nasal disease).
- *Infectious agents*, including bacteria, fungi, yeasts, and viruses (e.g., avian pox), can cause conditions such as mechanical blockage in the oral cavity and adjacent structures that result in respiratory distress.
- *Parasites* (e.g., trichomonads) in the oral cavity can lead to inflammation and accumulation of caseated deposits around the glottis, causing dyspnea.
- *Neoplasms*, including oral papilloma (see Chap. 162), involving tissues in the oral cavity can cause signs of respiratory difficulty.

Clinical Signs

- Inspiratory or expiratory dyspnea manifested as open-mouth breathing, labored respiratory effort, horizontal posture, and tail bobbing
- Wasting or weight loss due to decreased appetite or inability to swallow food
- Crusty exudates at the commissures of the mouth
- Coughing and wheezing
- Abnormal respiratory sounds, such as squeaking, clicking, or moist sounds
- Distortion of the palate, tongue, or beak with abscesses, pustules, or keratin cysts

Diagnosis
History

- Identify predisposing or causative factors.
- Determine the duration of the problem and any previous treatment.
- Determine whether the bird is a new acquisition, caged alone, or previously owned.

Physical Examination

- Examine the oral cavity for exudates, abscesses, and keratin cysts.
- Palpate the breast musculature for evidence of muscle wasting (prominent keel bone), indicating chronic disease.
- Auscultate the chest for evidence of lower respiratory disease. Auscultation generally is unremarkable in birds with upper respiratory disease alone.

Laboratory Studies

- Culture and sensitivity testing along with a Gram stain is helpful in determining whether bacteria, fungi, or yeast are involved in the disease process.
  - Take samples from the choana, glottis, and any associated abscesses. Frequently, these apparent abscesses are sterile keratin cysts associated with hypovitaminosis A.
- Cytologic examination of oral deposits or plaques may reveal trichomonads in a wet mount preparation.
- Histopathologic examination is indicated for solid tissue masses.

Surgery

Surgical exploration of nodules in the oral cavity can differentiate abscesses from solid tumors.

Treatment

- Papillomas in the oral cavity usually involve the choana and glottis. Surgically excise these growths and submit for histopathology.
  - Apply silver nitrate to surface of tissue (3 to 4 treatments are adequate). Debulking with electrocautery also is recommended.
- Other neoplasms involving the oral cavity usually are not amenable to surgical excision. Tumors usually involve the palatine tissue and are highly malignant. Osteogenic sarcoma and fibrosarcomas frequently are seen.
- For palatine, lingual, or sublingual abscesses or keratin cysts, lance and curet the lesions (culture is optional).
  - After the removal of exudates, infuse the area with antibiotic ophthalmic ointment and inject an appropriate dose of vitamin A. Systemic antibiotics may be indicated by the overall condition of the bird.
- In trichomoniasis, the plaques of necrotic tissue containing the parasite usually extend deeply into the surrounding tissue and cannot be excised easily. Surgically debulk these lesions and then treat with metronidazole (Flagyl, Rhone-Poulenc), 10-30 mg/kg q12h, PO, for 10 days.
- Virus-induced lesions rarely cause respiratory difficulty unless they involve the glottis (as with avian pox). Symptomatic therapy (e.g., debridement) to provide an open airway and antibiotics to reduce secondary infection are necessary (see Chap. 162).

Disorders of the Cervicocephalic Air Sacs

Etiology

The principal manifestations of cervicocephalic air sac dysfunction are overinflation and rupture. Factors contributing to overinflation of the cervicocephalic air sacs can be infectious, traumatic, parasitic, or congenital.

- *Infectious agents* such as bacteria, viruses, fungi, mycoplasma, and yeasts can cause infections in the upper respiratory system that extend to the cervicocephalic air sacs.

- *Trauma* can lead to rupture of the air sacs and subcutaneous emphysema.
- *Parasites* (i.e., threadworms) have been reported in the cervical air sacs but were not incriminated as a cause of clinical problems.
- *Congenital anomalies* are suspected in neonates with rupture or overinflation of the cervicocephalic air sacs, although bacteria and yeasts occasionally have been cultured from affected birds.

Clinical Signs

- The skin over the head and/or neck is distended with air.
- Depending on the degree of distension, there may be dyspnea.

Diagnosis

- Diagnosis is made by visual observation of the distended skin.
- Confirm the presence of air by needle aspiration.
- Culture the affected air sac to rule out infectious causes.

Treatment

- Surgical correction:
  - Needle aspiration provides immediate relief and, when repeated as needed, may resolve the condition in some birds.
  - Excision of a circular piece of skin over the inflated area (2 cm or larger) and leaving it open gives longer-lasting results than aspiration.
  - Placement of a permanent valve (a small piece of Silastic tubing sutured to the skin) also has been successful.
  - Microsurgical repair of the infraorbital sinus/ cervicocephalic junction has been suggested; however, this is a difficult procedure, requiring the skill of an experienced microsurgeon.
  - The prognosis for these surgical procedures providing a permanent cure is guarded.
- If cultures are positive, institute appropriate antimicrobial therapy.

DISEASES OF THE TRACHEA AND SYRINX

The trachea is composed of complete cartilaginous rings (unlike the mammalian trachea) and resists compression or crushing.

Etiology

The underlying causes or factors leading to diseases of the trachea and syrinx may be mechanical, nutritional, infectious, parasitic, traumatic, or neoplastic.

- *Mechanical factors* include inhalation of foreign material, usually food-related (such as gavage, seeds, or seed hulls) but occasionally pieces of hyperkeratotic plaque that have been dislodged from the oral or tracheal mucosa. Dried mucus plugs, at the level of the syrinx, have been reported. The presenting sign is a sudden and severe dyspnea.

- Extrarespiratory causes such as thyroid hyperplasia or enlargement due to infection or neoplasia are common causes of progressive dyspnea.
- *Nutritional factors* center around hypovitaminosis A and subsequent squamous metaplasia. This can lead to hyperkeratotic plaques on the tracheal mucosa or thickened deposits at the level of the syrinx.
- *Infectious agents* include bacteria, viruses, fungi, and yeasts, which can cause inflammation and exudate formation, resulting in narrowing of the main airway and respiratory difficulty.
  - Specific agents include *Chlamydia* spp, diphtheritic avian pox, Amazon tracheitis virus, Newcastle disease virus and other avian paramyxoviruses, and *Aspergillus* and *Candida* spp. (see Chap. 2).
- *Parasitic organisms* of clinical significance that invade the trachea include tracheal and air sac mites *(Sternostoma tracheacolum)* and gapeworms *(Syngamus trachea)*.
- *Trauma* to the trachea can cause damage to the tracheal rings and narrowing of the airway, leading to dyspnea.
- *Neoplasia* of the trachea and syrinx is rare.

Clinical Signs

- Acute, sudden onset of severe inspiratory dyspnea; sometimes open-mouth breathing (gasping)
- Gradual onset of inspiratory or expiratory dyspnea; characteristic expiratory squeak in thyroid hyperplasia
- Coughing and wheezing
- High-pitched, or sucking, or clicking respiratory sounds
- Change in or loss of voice

Diagnosis

History

- If possible, identify predisposing or causative factors.
- Determine the duration of the problem and exposure to possible sources of infection.
- Always question the quality of the diet.

Physical Examination

▼ *Key Point* If the patient is dyspneic, administer oxygen therapy for 10–20 min before performing the physical examination. During the examination, keep restraint to a minimum, and return the bird to oxygen when necessary.

- Evaluate the severity of the dyspnea and assess the urgency of therapy.
- In small, light-skinned birds, the trachea can be transilluminated.
- In cases of tracheitis, auscultate for moist rales from excess mucus in the trachea and oral cavity.

- Examine the nares and choana for discharge. Observe the head for evidence of periorbital swelling.

Laboratory Studies

- Obtain specimens for culture and sensitivity testing of the trachea, using a small, sterile cotton-tipped swab (Calgi-Swab, Spectrum Labs). Introduce the swab through the glottis and into the trachea.
  - When the procedure is accompanied by a Gram stain, the presence of bacteria (gram-negative), yeasts, and fungal hyphae can be determined.
- Airway cytology of tracheal washings or exudate (see Chapter 161 for techniques) may reveal inflammatory cells, degenerate epithelial cells, and possibly the causative agent.
- Perform a CBC and serum biochemistry profile.

Radiography

- If indicated, obtain radiographs to determine the presence of material at the level of the syrinx, ascertain the architecture of the trachea, and assess involvement of lower respiratory structures.

Endoscopy

- In birds with acute respiratory distress, endoscopy of the trachea and syrinx may reveal obstruction of the airway by accumulation of exudates, which can occur with hypovitaminosis A, aspergillosis, certain viral infections, inhalation of foreign material, and damage to the tracheal rings.
- Endoscopy can be performed quickly under isoflurane anesthesia, or an abdominal breathing tube can be placed (see Chap. 161).

Treatment

▼ *Key Point* In cases of acute inspiratory dyspnea, which is a life-threatening condition in birds, institute immediate therapeutic measures.

- For acute dyspnea, immediate action is required.

Inhalation of Foreign Material

- Foreign material in the trachea of birds smaller than cockatiels frequently causes death.
- In cockatiels, in which surgical removal is not possible, attempt to push the foreign body into the thoracic cavity with a small cotton-tipped swab such as a Calgi-swab (Spectrum Labs); follow with long-term systemic antibiotic therapy.
- In larger birds, identify foreign bodies by endoscopy and remove with long alligator forceps or biopsy forceps. If this is not possible, surgical removal is indicated.
  - Use an abdominal breathing tube to maintain anesthesia.
- Suction can be attempted using an open-end urinary catheter or appropriately-sized red rubber feeding tube.

Surgical Technique

1. The surgical approach for removal of tracheal foreign bodies is cranial or caudal to the foreign body.
   - For foreign material in the syrinx, make the approach through the distal trachea.
2. Make a transectional incision, separating the tracheal rings. Avoid cutting the rings longitudinally, which can lead to tearing and, on closure, stricture.
3. Close the incision with fine 5–0 or 6–0 suture material such as Vicryl, Maxon, or PDS, using a simple interrupted pattern.
4. An abdominal breathing tube, used during surgery, can be left up to 7 days.

Infection

- Treat infections of the trachea (tracheitis) by placing the bird in a nebulizer (therapy unit plus nebulizing chamber; Corners Ltd.) with the appropriate solution for 30 minutes twice daily.
  - For suspected bacterial infections, begin nebulization with 10 ml sterile saline, 1 ml gentamicin (Gentocin) (50 mg/ml) or an appropriate antibiotic as determined from culture/sensitivity, and 0.5 ml acetylcysteine (Mucomyst).
  - For severe inflammation, add 0.25 ml dexamethasone (2 mg/ml).
  - For fungal infections, add amphotericin B instead of Gentocin (see Chap. 162 for treatment of aspergillosis).
  - For viral tracheitis, reduce inflammation and keep the trachea open. Death due to asphyxiation by excess mucus accumulation is common in birds with acute viral infections.
- Nebulization can be accompanied by intratracheal injections of appropriate antimicrobial agents diluted in saline. For noninfectious tracheal or syringeal deposits, injections of sterile saline alone may be effective (see Chap. 162 for intratracheal injection technique).
- Treat chronic infections with aggressive application of nebulization and systemic antibiotics.
  - If fibrinous exudates are present in the trachea or syrinx, attempt to remove them surgically, as previously described.
- For parasitic infections, give ivermectin (Ivomec, MSD Agvet), 200–400 µg/kg, PO or SC.

Neoplasms

- For neoplasia of the trachea or syrinx, euthanasia is recommended because surgical incision is not possible.

Nutritional Deficiency

- If an underlying nutritional deficiency is suspected, treat hypovitaminosis A with Injacom (Morton & Pestle, Des Moines, IA), 10,000–20,000 IU/kg IM.

DISEASES OF THE LOWER RESPIRATORY SYSTEM

The lower respiratory system includes the major bronchi, lungs, air sacs (excluding the cervicocephalic sacs), and pneumatic bones. Because the air sacs are poorly supplied with blood and lack cilia and glandular secretions to aid in removal of infectious agents and foreign material, they are relatively susceptible to disease. Note that air sacs do not communicate directly with one another.

Etiology

Underlying causes or predisposing factors leading to diseases of the bronchi, lungs, and air sacs may be mechanical, environmental, infectious, parasitic, or neoplastic.

- *Mechanical factors* include inhalation of foreign material (e.g., blood, gavage solution, hand-rearing formula), resulting in acute dyspnea.
  - With aspiration of large volumes of material, death usually is instantaneous. Smaller volumes can cause aspiration pneumonia or airsacculitis.
- *Environmental factors* include airborne irritants and toxins. The resultant inflammation can cause excess mucus production, chronic lung changes (e.g., thickening of bronchi and parabronchi), and airsacculitis.
  - Inhalation of toxins (e.g., carbon monoxide, polymer fumes from Teflon) can cause acute pulmonary hemorrhage and death.
  - Allergies can cause inflammation of lung tissue, with peribronchial thickening and edema.
- *Infectious agents* such as gram-negative bacteria, viruses, fungi, and mycobacteria can lead to pneumonia and pulmonary or air sac granulomas.
- *Parasites* in the bronchi, lungs, and air sacs may cause coughing, wheezing, and abnormally slow, deep respirations.
- *Neoplasia* of the bronchi and lungs is uncommon but should be considered. Rhabdomyoma/sarcoma, leiomyoma/sarcoma, fibrosarcoma, and mesotheliomas of lung tissue have been reported. Metastatic disease is also possible.

Clinical Signs

- Acute or severe dyspnea with horizontal posture, tail bobbing, and accentuated breathing movements
- Coughing and wheezing
- Audible moist rales or dull breathing sounds
- Concurrent upper respiratory problems

Diagnosis

History

- Identify factors related to possible mechanical, environmental, infectious, or parasitic causes.
- Determine whether the bird recently has been hand- or gavage-fed or recently has undergone laparoscopy.

- Determine if the bird recently has been exposed to other birds.

Physical Examination

- The bird usually is fluffed and in a slumped or horizontal posture.
- There may be audible respiratory sounds.
- Breathing movements may be obvious and can be very exaggerated, depending on the severity of the problem.
- Extrarespiratory factors may contribute to the dyspnea because of compression of the air sacs.
- Auscultation may help to identify fluid movement in the airways, although referred upper respiratory sounds frequently complicate the interpretation of auscultated sounds. Inflamed air sacs frequently make a crackling sound like crumpled cellophane.

▼ *Key Point* Many diseases that create respiratory symptoms are extrarespiratory; because birds lack a complete diaphragm. Organomegaly, ascites, tumors, or egg binding may cause mild to severe respiratory distress.

Laboratory Studies

- Clinical pathology aids assessment of severity: A high white blood cell (WBC) count, degenerative cell changes, and anemia can indicate the severity and duration of the illness.
- Perform serology (e.g., for *Aspergillus*, *Chlamydia*) or other tests to rule out psittacosis and aspergillosis.
- Cytology of air sac smears is useful for identification of bacteria (e.g., *Chlamydia*, *Mycobacterium* spp.) and fungi.
- Histopathology of birds necropsied from multiple-bird facilities with a history of respiratory disease can be useful. For example, moist or wet avian pox can be diagnosed (see Chap. 162).

Radiography

- Radiography is the most important diagnostic tool to assess the integrity of the lower respiratory system.
- Evaluate the lungs and bronchi for anatomic changes such as pulmonary densities and bronchial and peribronchial thickening.
- Radiographic changes indicating air sac disease may be subtle (e.g., diffuse densities, feathery-appearing densities, rounding of the caudal air sac borders); or the changes may be obvious, including discrete densities (granulomas), thickening of air sacs seen as definite lines, and hyperinflation of one side indicating disease on the other.
- Assess changes in extrarespiratory structures (heart, liver, spleen, kidneys, proventriculus and gizzard, reproductive organs, and intestines) to rule out other causes of respiratory signs; for example, heart disease can cause pulmonary edema.

Endoscopy

- Endoscopy can be used to examine the caudal borders of the lungs and the abdominal air sacs. During this procedure, obtain samples for culture, cytology, and biopsy.
  - The point of entry for the endoscope is the abdominal air sac (see Chap. 161 for technique).

Treatment

- Tailor treatment for lower respiratory diseases to the suspected cause as determined by diagnostic evaluation. While waiting for laboratory results, treat the symptoms.
  - Initially, administer a broad-spectrum antibiotic such as cefotaxime (Claforan, Hoechst-Roussel) (50–100 mg/kg q6–8h), enrofloxacin (Baytril, Haver/Diamond) (15–25 mg/kg, q12h, IM or SC), or piperacillin (Pipracil, Lederle, 100–200 mg/kg q12h).
  - If a fungal infection is suspected, give an antifungal agent such as fluconazole tablets at 20 mg/kg q48h or itraconazole at 5–10 mg/kg q12h with food. See Chapter 162 for details on treatment of aspergillosis.
  - If dyspnea is severe, administer nebulization with saline or antibiotic/antifungal combinations (as described earlier) for 20–30 min twice a day.
  - Confirm suspected mycoplasmal infections by response to treatment with tylosin powder ½ g. powder/qt. water (Tylan, Elanco) or doxycycline 100 mg/kg (100 mg/ml; Mortar & Pestle); culture and isolation frequently are unrewarding.
- If radiology and endoscopy identifies an isolated granulomatous mass, success of treatment depends on the specific location of the mass.
  - If the mass is in the lung tissue proper, surgical removal is difficult, if not impossible.
  - Granulomas in the air sacs offer a better prognosis if surgical removal is possible.
- The cause of the granulomas is an important factor in deciding treatment and predicting outcome (for suggested therapy for aspergillosis and chlamydiosis see Chap. 162).
- If acute dyspnea is caused by inhalation of gavage material, attempt to clear the airways with air via an endotracheal tube or by flushing saline into the trachea (5–10 ml have been used without any problems in Amazon parrots). Follow with oxygen therapy using a face mask.
  - Inhalation of large volumes of gavage material, usually is fatal; if only a small amount of material is aspirated, administer long-term antibiotic therapy in the hope that the body will wall off the inhaled material.
- Treat respiratory parasites with ivermectin (Ivomec, MSD Agvet) at a dosage of 200–400 μg/kg, PO or SC. This eliminates air sac mites and lung worms.
- Control exposure to environmental factors such as smoking; dust from heating or air conditioning ducts; dust from birds such as cockatoos, cockatiels,

and African gray parrots; cooking odors; and aerosols.

- Primary neoplasia of the lung is uncommon. Surgical removal of pulmonary tumors is risky because of inaccessibility and risk of blood loss.

Disorders of the Pneumatic Bones

- The pneumatic bones (ribs, vertebrae, humerus, coracoid, clavicle, sternum, ilium, ischium, and pubis) connect with the major air sacs; although extension of infection from these sacs may occur, it is uncommon and is not clinically significant.
- Infections within the pneumatic bones appear to have a hematogenous origin.

EXTRARESPIRATORY DISEASES

Various conditions in extrarespiratory organs may mimic respiratory disease; for example, thyroid and ultimobranchial body disorders, heart-base tumors, cardiomegaly, hepatomegaly, splenomegaly, gonadal conditions (disease and nondisease), and pancreatic and kidney diseases (see Chap. 165).

SUPPLEMENTAL READINGS

Altman RB et al: Avian Medicine and Surgery. Philadelphia: WB Saunders, 1996, pp 387–411.

Arnall L, Petrak ML: In Petrak ML (ed): Diseases of Cage and Aviary Birds. Philadelphia: Lea & Febiger, 1982, p 395.

Graham DL: The avian respiratory system: AAV Proceedings. Conference proceedings of the Association of Avian Veterinarians 1987, p 143.

Harrison GJ, Harrison LR: Clinical Avian Medicine and Surgery. Philadelphia: WB Saunders, 1986.

McDonald SE: Anatomical and physiological characteristics of birds and how they differ from mammals. AAV Proceedings, 1990, p 372.

Ritchie BW, Harrison GJ, Harrison LR: Avian Medicine: Principles and Application. Lake Worth, FL, Wingers Publishing, 1994, pp 556–581.

Rosskopf WJ, Woerpel RW: Diseases of Cage and Aviary Birds. Baltimore: Williams and Wilkins, 1996, p 415.

Rupley, Agnes: Manual of Avian Practice. W.B. Saunders Co. 1997, pp. 55–90.

Walsh M: Upper respiratory diseases in avian species: The rhinal cavities, sinuses, and cervicocephalic air sac system. AAV Proceedings, 1984, p 151.

Walsh MT, Martinez D: Lower respiratory system of psittacines. AAV Proceedings, 1985, p 155.

165 Avian Digestive System Disorders

Barbara L. Oglesbee / Scott McDonald / Ken Warthen

DISORDERS OF THE BEAK

General Principles

Normal Structure and Function

- The beak includes the bones of the upper and lower jaws and their keratinized sheaths or rhamphotheca. This horny covering functionally replaces the lips and teeth of mammals.
- The shape of the beak varies, depending on how the species feed and live.
  - In psittacines, the upper beak is massive and curved, and the lower beak is small and horseshoe-shaped (this is why psittacines are called hook-bills).
- The beak is adapted to cracking large nuts and seeds as well as tearing and shredding wood from trees to provide nest sites.
- Histologically, the horny beak resembles skin and consists of dermis and modified epidermis. The stratum corneum of the epidermis is very thick.
  - The horny tissue of the beak is continuously replaced during normal wear and tear.

Normal Beak Growth

- Many bird owners erroneously believe that the upper beak grows only from the cere and continues to the tip (or edges), where it is then worn off (and that the process is similar in the lower beak). On the contrary, beak tissue grows continuously outward (toward the surface) over much of the beak.
  - As the keratinized epithelium reaches the surface, it is worn off or may move distally a short distance before it is shed.
  - Beak tissue truly moves rostrally only toward the edges and tip.

Beak Overgrowth

Many pathologic conditions can change the normal outward appearance of the beak, adversely affecting its primary functions of food gathering, prehension, preening, and protection. Regardless of the etiology, overgrowth may take various forms, the most common of which are listed here.

- The tip of the upper beak, lower beak, or both, may be overgrown.

- The edge of one side of the beak is overgrown.
- Malocclusion of the beak causes the upper beak to angle off to one side, whereas the lower beak is in the opposite direction. The condition is referred to as *scissors beak*. The tips and outer edges usually are overgrown owing to a lack of occlusal wear.
- The upper beak is shortened and does not extend out over the tip of the lower beak (prognathism).
- An area of the beak may appear bulged or swollen because of buildup of covering horn. This commonly is seen in birds lacking access to rough surfaces.

Beak Trimming

- Severe malocclusions, such as scissors beak, require surgical correction. See Supplemental Readings at the end of this chapter.
- When the underlying condition has been identified and treated, corrective beak trimming may be necessary.
  - Mild overgrowth or a buildup of covering horn may be trimmed if it is interferring with the function of the beak. Depending on the size of the bird, use human fingernail trimmers, cuticle nippers, Roscoe nail trimmers, or an electric hobby tool (Dremel) with a coarse sanding bit.
  - Anesthesia usually is not required; however, be aware that some birds stress easily during this procedure, especially when a hobby tool is used, and deaths have been reported.

Nutritional Disorders

An *all-seed diet* is deficient in vitamin A, which is important in maintaining the health and integrity of epithelial tissues. Hypovitaminosis A may cause hyperkeratosis of epithelial surfaces.

Clinical Signs

- Signs include beak thickening and overgrowth. The surface of the beak is hard and thickened and appears flaky and chipped instead of smooth.

Diagnosis

- Base the diagnosis on clinical signs and a history of a seed-based diet.

Treatment

▼ *Key Point* Place all pet birds on a commercial pelleted diet whenever possible.

- Supplement this diet with fruits, vegetables, whole-grain baked goods or cereals, and small amounts of lean cooked meats or eggs.
- If the bird will not convert to a commercial diet, then use a commercial avian vitamin supplement.
- Perform beak trims as necessary.

Bacterial and Mycotic Infection

Superficial or deep bacterial and mycotic infections occasionally are seen. These usually are secondary to trauma, psittacine beak and feather disease virus (PBFDV), chronic rhinitis, or other systemic diseases. Gram-negative enteric organisms (e.g., *Pseudomonas, Escherichia coli, Klebsiella* spp) are the most common bacteria isolated. *Aspergillus fumigatus* is the mycotic agent most commonly identified. PBFDV and *Knemidokoptes* mites (in budgerigars) are among the most common causes of beak deformity.

Clinical Signs

- The surface of the beak appears brittle and crumbly instead of smooth and hard. This may involve the entire beak or may be localized.
- The bird is reluctant to eat, crack seeds, or play with toys. The beak may seem painful.
- Areas of localized necrosis may be found on the beak surface or on the underside of the upper beak.

Diagnosis

- Perform Gram and new methylene blue stains of lesions.
- Obtain bacterial and fungal cultures of lesions.

Treatment

▼ *Key Point* Bacterial and mycotic infections of the beak usually are secondary to systemic disease or nutritional deficiencies. Whenever possible, identify and treat the primary disease.

- Debride localized necrotic areas with the bird under anesthesia.
- Base antibiotic therapy on culture and sensitivity testing. Pending culture results, begin antibiotic therapy with a broad-spectrum antibiotic such as cefotaxime (Claforan, Hoechst-Roussel) or enrofloxacin (Baytril, Haver/Diamond) (see Chapter 162 for dosages). Long-term systemic therapy usually is required in addition to local debridement.
  - The poor success rate may be due in part to the sparse vascular supply to the horny layers of the beak.
- For localized *Aspergillus* infection, see Chapter 162 for diagnosis and treatment. Treatment for months may be required.
  - The prognosis is guarded if the fungal disease is systemic.

Trauma

Beak damage from trauma can occur in all species and often is the result of aggressive behavior between individual birds housed together, flying into walls or windows, or struggling after beak entrapment. A split lower beak may result from a fall, injury from another bird, biting with excessive force, or beak trimming.

Clinical Signs

- An inability to eat and manipulate food or toys may be the only presenting signs. Thoroughly inspect the beak to identify trauma because some injuries are not obvious.
- The beak may seem painful.
- Look for hemorrhage, cracks, punctures, avulsions, or complete amputation.

Treatment

Treatment varies with the type of injury. If the bird is reluctant to eat, forced alimentation may be necessary until the beak is healed sufficiently.

Cracked Upper Beak Tip

- Remove the tip with nail clippers or grind it with a hobby tool.
- Apply ammonium sulfate or ferric subsulfate powder to control hemorrhage.

Split Lower Beak

- If the crack extends throughout the entire length of the beak, dividing it into two movable segments, nothing can be done to permanently fuse the pieces back together.
  - Wire and dental acrylics can only temporarily repair the crack.
- Birds can eat a normal diet with this condition; cracking seed or pellets is not a problem.
- Occasional trimming of the lower beak segments may be necessary because of inadequate occlusion with the upper beak.

Puncture Injury Penetrating the Horny Layer

- Initially treat as an open wound and debride damaged and necrotic areas with the bird under general anesthesia.
- Administer topical and systemic antifungal or antibiotic agents, based on culture and sensitivity testing.
- Defects in the horny layer may be filled or patched later with acrylic compounds.

Beak Avulsions

- Avulsion of the distal one-third:
  - Treat initially as an open wound (as described previously).
  - Cover the open end with acrylics as a temporary patch if necessary.
  - Regeneration of the beak is possible, but the beak may never appear totally normal.
- Damage to the proximal one-third of the beak usually is not reversible.

- If the injured birds can be kept alive with forced alimentation, the damaged beak may scar over and the bird may adapt to a soft-food diet.
- Avulsion of the entire upper or lower beak is not reversible. Affected birds usually die of starvation or secondary infection, or require euthanasia.
  - Successful use of beak prosthetic devices has been reported but is rare.

Prevention

- Do not leave birds uncaged unless they are closely supervised.
- Keep apart birds that exhibit obvious aggressive tendencies toward each other. This is a common problem in breeding pairs of cockatoos. Sexually active males may attack females that are not sexually receptive, and beaks commonly are bitten. Preventive measures include:
  - Large flight cages
  - Clipping wings of male but not female bird
  - Nest boxes with two separate entrances

Neoplasia

Neoplasia of the beak is encountered infrequently, usually in older birds. Fibrosarcoma, fibroma, and squamous cell carcinoma are the most common types.

Clinical Signs

- *Fibrosarcoma* usually appears as a well-demarcated, fleshy protrusion from the horny layer.
- *Squamous cell carcinoma* appears as a focal area of hemorrhage or ulceration.
- Common signs include weight loss and inability to eat.

Diagnosis

Base the diagnosis on histopathologic examination of excised tissues.

Treatment

- Surgical excision or debulking of beak tumors is rarely successful.
- Cryosurgery or radiation therapy may be beneficial, but the prognosis is guarded.

Environmental Factors

- To maintain a normal appearance of the beak, chewing on hard objects and rasping of the outer horny layer of the beak is necessary.
- Lack of access to materials necessary for normal beak wear can result in beak overgrowth or a flaky, chipped surface.
- Provide ample amounts of wood for the bird to chew on. This may be in the form of perches, nest boxes, or wood toys.
- Other items suitable for chewing include rawhide, concrete perches, lava stones, mineral blocks, and leather.

Growth and Developmental Abnormalities

These conditions usually are seen in preweaned or recently weaned birds. The exact causes are unknown.

- The most common presentations are:
  - *Scissors beak,* a lateral deviation of the upper beak seen most often in macaws
  - *Prognathism,* which affects the architecture of the upper beak and is seen most often in cockatoos
- Treatment by construction and application of a simple, durable prosthesis allows the redirection of beak growth (see Supplemental Readings).

DISORDERS OF THE ORAL CAVITY

Normal Structure and Function

- Because birds lack a soft palate, which separates the nasal and oral parts of the pharynx in mammals, the oral cavity and pharynx of birds form a single cavity called the *oropharynx.*
- The roof of the mouth, or hard palate, is located immediately behind the upper beak.
  - Rostrally, the palate resembles a hard, fleshy cushion against which the tongue can manipulate objects.
  - Caudally, the palate is divided into two folds containing numerous caudally directed papillae, which are referred to as the *choana.* The choana communicate directly with the nasal passageway.
- The floor of the oropharynx is occupied by the tongue and the glottis.
  - The psittacine tongue is thick, blunt, and dextrous.
  - The glottis lies on the midline directly behind the tongue.
  - Papillae are distributed over the laryngeal prominence and posterior floor of the pharynx. Birds do not have an epiglottis.
- The surface of the oropharynx is lined by stratified squamous epithelium that is keratinized in regions subject to abrasion, such as the papillae.
  - *Salivary glands* are not visible grossly and are distributed over the palatine folds, base of the tongue, laryngeal prominence, and pharynx. These glands primarily produce mucus and thus often are referred to as mucous glands.
  - The large amount of watery saliva produced in mammals is not present in psittacines. Therefore, the oral mucosa is normally only slightly moist, and the tongue is dry.

▼ *Key Point* Because diseases of the oral cavity are common in psittacine birds, routinely inspect the mouth during examination.

Hypovitaminosis A

Hypovitaminosis A, which is generally the result of an unsupplemented all-seed diet, can cause squamous metaplasia of the oral epithelium and subsequent hyperkeratosis of the mucous glands. Keratin-filled cystic structures may be found on the palatine folds, base of the tongue, laryngeal prominence, and pharynx. These lesions often coalesce and become secondarily infected to form large abscesses.

Lesions are more likely to be seen in large psittacines (e.g., Amazon and African gray parrots, macaws, cockatoos) than in small species (e.g., budgerigars, cockatiels).

Clinical Signs

- Signs include white or yellow cysts and abscesses in the oral mucosa.
- If the lesions become secondarily infected, anorexia, general malaise, and weight loss may be present.
- Accompanying signs include blepharitis, conjunctivitis, uveitis, rhinitis, sinusitis, and dyspnea.

Diagnosis

- The diagnosis usually is based on the history and physical examination.
- Perform biopsy to confirm keratin-filled cysts and squamous metaplasia of the mucous glands.

Treatment

- Change the diet as previously described under Nutritional Disorders.
- Lance and drain oral abscesses and perform a Gram stain and bacterial and fungal culture on the abscess contents; perform curettage of lesions under isoflurane anesthesia.
- Administer systemic antibiotic or antifungal agents, as indicated by culture.
- Provide supportive therapy, such as forced alimentation and fluid therapy, as needed.

Prevention

- Provide a diet adequate in vitamin A or add vitamin supplementation, as described under Nutritional Disorders.
  - Dark green and yellow vegetables are good sources of vitamin A.

Psittacine Pox

- See Chapter 162 in this section for discussion of this disorder.

Oral Candidiasis

Candida albicans is a secondary invader that affects the mouth, esophagus, and crop. Factors predisposing to oral candidiasis include poor sanitation, malnutrition, coexisting disease, and prolonged antibiotic therapy. Cockatiels and macaws are affected most commonly.

Clinical Signs

Clinical signs vary with the severity of the disease and include:

- Anorexia, general malaise, and weight loss
- Vomiting, regurgitation, and mucus evident on the feathers of the head
- Wet feathers surrounding the mouth, halitosis, and oral hemorrhage
- Poor feeding response in hand-fed baby birds

Diagnosis

- Examine the oral mucosa for lesions that typically appear as a thickening of the oral mucosa associated with a mucoid exudate.
  - Lesions may progress to focal or widespread mucosal necrosis, forming diphtheritic membranes or white caseated plugs.
- Perform a Gram or new methylene blue stain on exudate from oral lesions; look for budding yeasts.
- Perform a fungal culture of oral lesions.

Treatment

▼ **Key Point** Candidiasis is usually a secondary invader. Correct predisposing factors in conjunction with specific antifungal treatment.

- In mild cases, birds may respond to nystatin (Mycostatin, Squibb), 1 ml/300 g q8h, PO.
- More often, systemic therapy with one of the azole antifungal agents is necessary. Administer ketoconazole (Nizoral, Janssen), 20–30 mg/kg q12h, PO, or fluconazole (Diflucan, Roerig), 2–5 mg/kg q24h.
- Continue treatment until all lesions are healed (usually 1 month or longer).

Prevention

- Provide a clean environment, including food and water. Do not leave moist foods in the cage for longer than 2 hours.
- Thoroughly disinfect utensils when feeding baby birds. Soak utensils in chlorhexidine solution (Nolvasan, Fort Dodge), 2 oz/gallon of water.
- Do not save powdered baby foods once they are reconstituted beyond one feeding because the number of yeast and bacterial colonies is greatly increased.
- If long-term antibiotic therapy is indicated (e.g., to treat chlamydiosis), give antifungal agents such as nystatin and ketoconazole prophylactically.

Bacterial Infections

Bacterial infections of the mouth are unusual and are secondary to predisposing conditions that encourage the growth of *C. albicans*. Common pathogens include *E. coli* and *Salmonella, Proteus, Pseudomonas, Enterobacter,* and *Citrobacter* spp.

Clinical Signs

- Lesions are variable but can appear similar to those of candidiasis (e.g., mucoid exudate, abscess formation).

Diagnosis and Treatment

Perform a Gram stain and bacterial culture on any exudate found in the mouth.

- Large numbers of enteric bacteria present in clinically ill psittacines with accompanying oral lesions are significant.
- Administer systemic antibiotic therapy, based on susceptibility testing.

Prevention

- Treat underlying systemic disease.
- Provide a clean environment and offer fresh food, as described previously under Oral Candidiasis.

Oral Papillomas

See discussion of oral papillomas in Chapter 162 in this section.

Trichomoniasis

Trichomonas gallinae is a flagellated protozoan parasite. Trichomoniasis usually occurs in aviaries with many birds and rarely is seen in individual pet birds. Infection may extend into the esophagus, crop, lungs, and oral cavity. The budgerigar is the most common psittacine affected. Outbreaks are reported in neonatal Amazon parrots, conures, and cockatiels.

Clinical Signs

- White, sticky plaques may coalesce to form yellow, caseous masses on the choana, tongue, or pharyngeal mucosa.
- Common signs include anorexia and weight loss.
- Moisture around the beak and halitosis may occur.

Diagnosis

- Perform a saline wet mount of oral exudate for microscopic examination.
  - Organisms are flagellated and pear-shaped and move in a spiral motion. Thousands may be seen on one slide.
  - In psittacine birds, organisms often are not present on wet mounts of oral exudates, especially in the early stages.
- High numbers of organisms are found on wet mount smears from lungs of recently deceased birds.

Treatment

Give metronidazole (Flagyl-Searle), 30 mg/kg, q12h PO, for 10 days. Crush the tablets and mix with a palatable liquid.

▼ *Key Point* Treat birds with oral lesions that suggest trichomoniasis with metronidazole, even when this organism is not positively identified.

Prevention

- In an aviary, quarantine and examine all new budgerigars for organisms in the pharynx and crop before introduction to the flock.

Trauma

Trauma to the mouth is rare, but when it occurs, lacerations or bite wounds to the tongue are most common. The next most common injury is laceration or crushing injury to the intermandibular space as a result of the bird's being hooked or caught on items such as chains or toys.

▼ *Key Point* Hemorrhage in tongue lacerations can be profuse and life-threatening. Immediate treatment is required.

Treatment

- Anesthesia may be required; use isoflurane via an endotracheal tube.
- Control hemorrhage via direct pressure or cauterization.
- Clean, debride, and suture injuries, as required.
- Administer systemic broad-spectrum antibiotics prophylactically.

DISORDERS OF THE ESOPHAGUS AND CROP

Normal Structure and Function

The Esophagus

- The avian esophagus is thin-walled and distensible. It courses down the right side of the neck, the opposite to that of mammals.
- The esophagus is lined by incompletely keratinized, stratified squamous epithelium, with numerous subepithelial mucous glands.

The Crop

- The crop is a dilatation of the esophagus found in many (but not all) species of birds. It is prominent in psittacines.
- The crop is located just cranial to the thoracic inlet. It is firmly attached to the underlying skin and thus can easily be seen and palpated externally.
  - The crop in parrots is oriented transversely across the neck. Food enters from the right side and exits caudally on the midline.
- When the proventriculus and ventriculus are full, food may be stored in the crop. Stored food undergoes softening and swelling, but no chemical digestion takes place.
  - Food eventually is moved caudally from the crop by powerful smooth muscle contractions of the crop and the esophageal wall.
- The crop (and proventriculus) is much larger in preweaned psittacines than in adults to accommodate the large volume of food required for rapid growth.
  - As a bird is weaned, it is not uncommon for it to lose 10–15% of its body weight because of shrinkage of these organs and the change in diet.

Crop Stasis

Many environmental, dietary, and systemic conditions can lead to crop stasis.

- Management factors include dehydration, low ambient temperature, change in formula or in the consistency or amounts being fed, and unsanitary feeding methods.
- Medical conditions that cause crop stasis include bacterial or fungal ingluvitis (inflammation of the crop), heavy metal toxicity, foreign bodies, tumors (including

papillomas), obstruction within the alimentary tract distal to the crop, and ileus due to generalized systemic disease (e.g., polyomavirus infection, proventricular dilatation disease).

- *Sour crop* refers to crop stasis in baby birds with bacterial or yeast overgrowth.

Clinical Signs

Hand-Fed Chicks

- The crop may be enlarged and pendulous and may fail to empty or may do so extremely slowly.
- Feeding response varies from normal to absent.
- Vomiting or regurgitation may occur.
- Initially, birds are alert and active, but depression and listlessness occur as the disease progresses.
- There is failure to gain weight or loss of body weight.
- The number of droppings decreases.
- There may be discoloration or necrosis of the skin overlying the crop.
- Complete crop fistulas result in leakage of formula.

Adult Birds

- The enlarged crop fails to empty or does so slowly.
- Varying degrees of weight loss, weakness, depression, and anorexia are seen.
- Vomiting may occur; expelled food may collect on feathers of the head and neck.

Diagnosis

History

- Question the owner regarding husbandry practices (housing, ambient temperature, humidity, and diet) and possible exposure to infectious diseases.

Physical Examination

- Palpate the crop to determine the amount and consistency of its contents, degree of thickness, muscle tone, fibrous or necrotic areas, and abscesses.
- Examine the skin over the crop for discoloration and necrosis.
  - Transillumination of the crop may reveal its contents.
  - The lower esophagus extends through the thoracic inlet and cannot be examined externally.
- Examine the mouth for oral lesions, which, if present, often extend into the esophagus and crop. This is often the case with bacterial and yeast infections, trichomoniasis, and occasionally papillomas.
- Endoscopy can be used to examine the interior of the crop and esophagus, but general anesthesia is required. This is not a routine procedure because the exposure is limited by mucus and fluids and rarely provides information not evident on external examination.
- In birds larger than 800 g, direct endoscopic examination of the proventriculus (i.e., with a pediatric bronchoscope) may identify proventriculitis, tumors, and foreign bodies that can cause crop stasis.
- Perform a Gram stain and culture of exudate or food material from the esophageal or crop wall.

- Large numbers of gram-negative bacteria and budding yeasts are abnormal.
- Perform a complete blood count (CBC) and serum chemistry profile to rule out systemic disease.
- Obtain blood samples for determination of blood lead and zinc concentrations to rule out heavy metal toxicity.
- Radiographs (plain films or contrast studies) may reveal obstruction caused by foreign bodies or tumors or the presence of heavy metals.
- Histopathologic examination of tissues from chicks at necropsy can be important in the management and treatment of outbreaks of disease in aviaries. Biopsy of individual birds is of limited value.

Treatment

The primary goal of therapy is to alleviate crop stasis which, if not corrected, leads to dehydration, starvation, secondary infections, and eventually, death. Treatment and management in neonates can be extremely labor-intensive and time-consuming. If at all possible, evaluate and stabilize these birds in the hospital, and then instruct the client in home treatment. Most clinics simply do not have the personnel, housing, or time to provide 24-hour nursing care.

▼ *Key Point* Regardless of the cause of crop stasis, do not feed solid food (adult birds) or formula (chicks) until crop motility returns.

Measures to Restore Crop Motility

- Add warm water or lactated Ringer's solution to the crop to break down impacted food. This may stimulate emptying of the crop.
- If crop motility does not return, manually empty the crop contents.
  - Insert a large catheter (metal or rubber) into the crop via the mouth and aspirate the contents. Be careful not to aspirate the mucosal lining of the crop during this procedure.
- Save samples of aspirated material for cytologic examination and bacterial or fungal culture.
- Rinse the crop with several flushes of normal saline or warm water after emptying contents.
- To treat dehydration, administer 25–50 ml/kg of subcutaneous fluids daily until crop motility returns.
- With severe dehydration or in critically ill birds, interosseous or intravenous fluids are indicated.
- Administer oral fluids such as lactated Ringer's solution and Pedialyte (Ross Labs.) in place of solid food or formula until motility begins to return. Frequent dosing of small amounts is recommended so as not to stretch the crop.
  - If the crop fails to empty adequately during this time, remove the solution contents once daily to prevent putrefaction.
  - If gastrointestinal obstruction has been ruled out, administer metoclopramide (Reglan, Robins) 0.5 mg/kg q12h, IM or IV or cisapride (Propulsid, Janssen) 0.5 mg/kg q8h, PO.

- As motility begins to return, add formula to the oral fluids. Begin with a very dilute solution and gradually increase the concentration until a normal consistency is achieved.
- Administer broad-spectrum antibiotic and antifungal agents as indicated by Gram staining or to prevent secondary infections.

Environmental Factors

- House well-hydrated birds in an incubator or brooder (95–98°F for hatchlings; 94–97°F for neonates up to 7 days old; 90–94°F, up to 14 days old; 85–90°F for chicks more than 14 days old).
- Maintain relative humidity above 50%.
- Feed birds a consistent formula type or brand. Formula temperature should be approximately 98–100°F.

▼ *Key Point* Identification and treatment of any underlying disorders are essential in the treatment of crop stasis.

Prolonged Crop Stasis

- Overfeeding or prolonged stasis in neonates can result in a pendulous, atonic crop.
- Use a crop supporter to provide support for the crop and facilitate emptying (see Chap. 161).

Prevention

- To prevent crop stasis in hand-fed neonates, provide a clean, warm brooder, feed a good hand-feeding formula, and practice sanitary handling techniques:
  - Clean the brooder daily; follow ambient temperature guides as previously described.
  - Use a commercial hand-feeding formula or a proven home recipe. Do not switch arbitrarily from one formula to another.
  - Feed birds on a regular schedule.
  - Feed amounts appropriate for the size of the bird; do not overfill the crop.
  - Maintain consistent formula viscosity and temperature.
  - Make fresh formula for each feeding.
  - Disinfect utensils and bowls used for food preparation and delivery after each feeding.
  - Use separate feeding syringes for each bird.
  - Instruct caretakers to wash hands before handling each bird.
- If there is a history of candidiasis in the aviary or for an individual bird, administer nystatin prophylactically until weaning.
- Correct other predisposing factors for bacterial and fungal infections, as previously described.

Foreign Bodies

The powerful beaks and persistent chewing habits of psittacines can lead to ingestion of foreign bodies, which may lodge in the crop.

Clinical Signs

- Crop stasis or delayed crop emptying may be seen.
- Regurgitation or repeated attempts at regurgitation may occur.

Diagnosis

- Palpate the crop. Many rigid objects large enough to lodge in the crop are palpable externally.
- Transillumination of the crop may reveal its contents.
- A small rigid endoscope may be used to examine the crop and remove foreign bodies.
- Radiograph the cervical area. In some cases, contrast (barium or air) radiography may be necessary to visualize the object.

Treatment

- Retrieve smaller foreign bodies by passing a forceps into the crop through the mouth or by percutaneously manipulating the object into the esophagus for removal through the mouth.
  - General anesthesia with isoflurane usually is required in all birds except neonates.
- Surgical removal via *ingluviotomy* (incision into the crop) may be required to remove the object.
  - Close the crop wall with 4–0 to 6–0 polydioxanone (PDS) sutures in an inverting, interrupted Lembert pattern.
  - Close the skin using a simple interrupted suture pattern.

Goiter

Etiology

- Iodine-deficient thyroid dysplasia may develop in budgerigars fed a seed diet without vitamin/mineral supplementation.

Clinical Signs

All clinical signs are attributed to the space-occupying effects of the enlarged glands; excessive thyroid hormone is not produced. Signs include:

- Regurgitation
- Crop stasis or delayed crop emptying
- Respiratory click

Diagnosis

Base the diagnosis on the clinical signs and history.

- The thyroid glands cannot be palpated externally because they are contained within the thoracic cavity.

Treatment

- Inject sodium iodide (Butler), 0.02 ml/30 g, IM, if birds are severely dyspneic.
- Maintain budgerigars on oral Lugol's iodine (Strong Iodine solution, Humco) in the drinking water. Mix 2 mL Lugols with 20 mL H_2O, then add 1 drop/oz of water daily for 1 week, and then once weekly thereafter.

Prevention

- For budgerigars, switch to a commercial pelleted diet, or supplement the existing diet with a commercial avian vitamin/mineral preparation.

Thermal Burns

Crop burns in neonates are caused by feeding hand-rearing formula at a temperature greater than 105°F. The formula usually was heated in a microwave oven and not sufficiently stirred or tested for temperature.

Clinical Signs

- Birds usually remain bright and alert and maintain a normal feeding response despite full-thickness necrosis of the crop and overlying skin. Therefore, these birds usually are not presented for evaluation until the caretaker notices formula leaking from the crop fistula onto the chest feathers.
- Necrosis and fistula formation may not be seen until several days after the burn occurs.

Diagnosis

- Base the diagnosis on the clinical signs and history.

Treatment

▼ *Key Point* Do not attempt surgical debridement or removal of scabs until wound contracture is complete and the crop begins to leak. Premature debridement may cause excessive loss of viable tissue.

- After anesthetizing the bird with isoflurane, debride all necrotic edges of the skin and crop.
- Close the crop wall and skin as described for ingluviotomy under Foreign Bodies.
- Administer prophylactic antibiotic therapy using enrofloxacin, trimethoprim-sulfa or cefotaxime.

DISORDERS OF THE PROVENTRICULUS AND VENTRICULUS

Normal Structure and Function

Proventriculus

- The proventriculus, or glandular stomach, is continuous with the esophagus at the level of the base of the heart and contains digestive (pepsinogen-secreting) and mucous glands.
- A strong muscular sphincter separates the proventriculus from the ventriculus.

Ventriculus

- The ventriculus, or muscular stomach (also known as the "gizzard"), contains two opposing sets of muscles used for grinding food.
- The epithelium secretes keratinous fluid that hardens to provide a surface against which food may be ground. Grit within the proventriculus aids in this grinding action; however, in most psittacines, grit is not essential for digestion of food.
- Contractions of the proventriculus and ventriculus are coordinated to provide adequate mixing and grinding of gastric contents and digestive enzymes.

Foreign Body Impaction

Ingested objects small enough to bypass the thoracic inlet may lodge in the proventriculus or ventriculus. The pyloric sphincter, a valve-like structure separating the ventriculus from the duodenum, helps to restrict larger solid objects from leaving the ventriculus. Small objects tend to collect in the ventriculus, owing to its blind pouch-like relationship to the remainder of the digestive tract.

Etiology

- Unweaned chicks typically are presented for ingestion of nesting substrates such as wood chips and shavings (especially young macaws), or for accidental swallowing of feeding instruments (e.g., tubes, spoons, gavage needles).
- In weaning-age chicks, there may be impaction of seed hulls and other food objects that have been swallowed whole.
- Adults commonly present with a history of ingesting toys, cage parts, perch materials, or carpet fibers.
- Overconsumption of grit can cause impaction. If grit is provided, a small amount (10–20 pieces) given every few months is adequate.

▼ *Key Point* Do not offer gravel or grit free-choice to pet birds. Ill or otherwise stressed birds may overconsume grit, causing impaction of the ventriculus. Do not offer whole seeds or other hard foods to weaning birds.

Clinical Signs

- Early signs include crop stasis, decreased fecal output, and regurgitation.
- If the impaction is partial, chronic regurgitation, weight loss in adults, and decreased weight gain in neonates may be seen.
- Endotoxemia and hypoglycemia may lead to anorexia, lethargy, depression, seizures, and death.

Diagnosis

- Rule out crop impaction and foreign bodies (described previously).
- Obtain radiographs of the abdominal area. Some objects may be visible on scout films, but contrast radiography often is necessary, using barium sulfate administered at 25 ml/kg into the crop via a gavage tube. The entire gastrointestinal (GI) tract should be delineated by the barium within 2½ hours.
- It may be possible to identify and retrieve the object via rigid endoscopy. Insert the endoscope through the crop via an ingluviotomy at the level of the thoracic inlet and direct it through the esophagus into the proventriculus.

- In larger birds, a flexible endoscope can be inserted through the oral cavity.

Treatment

- If the foreign body consists primarily of cellulose-containing materials (e.g., wood) the impaction may respond to cellulase-containing digestive enzymes.
- Small nontoxic objects lodged in but not obstructing the ventriculus may be ground down and enzymatically digested by natural processes. Limited amounts of fine gravel grit can expedite the process.
- If the object is visible via endoscopy, it usually can be removed using blunt-jawed grasping forceps.
- Gastric lavage may be used to flush out many objects lodged in the proventriculus.

Technique

1. Anesthetize the bird using isoflurane, intubate, pack the choana with gauze, and place the bird in lateral recumbency.
2. Fully extend the head and neck and insert a well-lubricated, soft rubber catheter through the mouth and down into the proventriculus.
3. Position the head so that it is lower than the body and attempt to flush the foreign material out through the mouth, using warm water or saline solution.

- Proventriculotomy may be necessary to remove larger foreign bodies.

Prevention

- In neonates, use only large, noningestible or, alternatively, easily digestible nesting substrates. Also, use only long, flexible feeding tubes to allow easy retrieval if syringe disconnection should occur.
- Monitor parent-reared chicks for signs of nestbox substrate ingestion.
- When chicks begin feeding on their own, do not feed seeds. Offer only small particles of fresh soft foods.
- Restrict adult birds from access to toys, cage parts, and other miscellaneous small objects. Remove coarse, shaggy bark from perches.
- Avoid feeding chitinous insects to pet birds.

Proventricular Dilatation Syndrome (PDS)

See Chapter 162 in this section for a discussion of PDS.

Papillomatosis

See Chapter 162 in this section for a description of this disorder.

Candidiasis

Etiology

Candida albicans is a secondary invader, primarily of the mouth, esophagus, and crop, and has been discussed previously as a cause of oral lesions and crop stasis. This mycotic overgrowth also may occur in the lower digestive tract, particularly in the proventriculus. Lesions usually are not found in the lower digestive tract alone but are an extension of esophageal or crop candidiasis.

Clinical Signs

Common signs include delayed crop emptying, vomiting, diarrhea, and weight loss.

Diagnosis

- Endoscopic examination of the proventriculus (described previously) may reveal rough, thickened, white mucosa characteristic of candidiasis. Similar gross lesions usually are visible in the crop.
- Perform a Gram stain and fungal culture on samples obtained from the crop and fresh feces or from the proventriculus during endoscopic examination.
  - Although *C. albicans* may be part of the normal intestinal flora, large numbers of budding yeasts on Gram stains of these samples are abnormal and warrant treatment.

Treatment

- See Treatment under Oral Candidiasis.

Bacterial Proventriculitis

Common pathogens of bacterial proventriculitis include *E. coli* and *Klebsiella, Enterobacter,* and *Salmonella* spp.

Clinical Signs

- Signs include vomiting, regurgitation, delayed crop emptying, and weight loss.

Diagnosis

- Perform the diagnostic procedures outlined under Oral Candidiasis.
- The CBC may demonstrate leukocytosis with heterophilia.

For further discussion of bacterial infections, see Chapter 162 in this section.

DISORDERS OF THE INTESTINES

Infectious Diseases

Bacterial enteritis, *Mycobacterium avium,* and viral enteritis are common causes of diarrhea, vomiting, and weight loss in pet birds (see Chapter 162).

Giardiasis

Etiology

The trophozoite and cyst forms of the flagellated protozoan parasite *Giardia* are found in the crop and duodenum.

- The incidence is estimated to be 20–50% in cockatiels, budgerigars, and lovebirds.
- Giardiasis occurs less frequently in conures, Amazon parrots, cockatoos, and macaws.

Clinical Signs

- Diarrhea (often voluminous), mucus-covered feces, or the passing of undigested food may be seen because of malabsorption caused by giardiasis.
- Weight loss may be gradual or sudden, with losses of 20–30% of body weight.
- Pruritus, especially along the wing webs, axillary region, and back, is a common finding in cockatiels with intestinal giardiasis. This often is manifested by feather picking and occasionally self-mutilation.
  - Although the exact relationship is unknown, a hypersensitivity reaction is believed to be responsible.
  - Relief from pruritus often is noted within hours of treatment for giardiasis.
- Paresis/lameness has been reported in birds with heavy *Giardia* infections. Malabsorption of vitamin E and selenium is the suspected cause.

Diagnosis

- Perform a direct saline smear assay on fresh feces immediately after collection to identify *Giardia* trophozoites and cysts. Staining with carbolfuchsin or iodine may aid in visualization of organisms.

▼ *Key Point* Because *Giardia* organisms are shed intermittently, false-negative test results are common.

- If a direct fecal examination cannot be performed immediately, collect feces in polyvinyl alcohol and then stain them with trichrome stain (California Avian Laboratories, Citrus Hill, CA).
- The CBC may demonstrate a peripheral eosinophilia.
- Hypoproteinemia may be noted on the serum biochemical profile as a result of intestinal malabsorption.

Treatment

- Give metronidazole (Flagyl, Searle), 30 mg/kg q12h, PO, for 7–10 days. Crush the tablets and mix with a palatable liquid.
- If lameness or paresis is present, give vitamin E/selenium (Seletoc, Schering), 0.1 mg/kg, IM, every 14 days.

Helminthiasis

Intestinal helminths are most frequently a problem in newly imported birds or birds in captive breeding colonies.

Etiology

- Ascarids commonly are found in cockatiels, cockatoos, budgerigars, and other Australian parakeets. Ascaridiasis can be a persistent problem in captive breeding colonies, particularly if the birds have access to a wood or concrete floor. The life cycle is direct, as in mammals.
- *Capillaria* spp. (intestinal threadworm) can be found in all species of pet birds but is most common in macaws, conures, and Australian birds. The worms

may be found in the mouth, esophagus, and small intestines. The life cycle is direct.
- Cestodes are found primarily in Old World psittacines (e.g., cockatoos, African gray parrots). They may be responsible for hemorrhagic enteritis and chronic wasting in African gray parrots. They have an indirect life cycle, with arthropod or annelid worms as intermediate hosts.

Clinical Signs

- Clinical signs are generally nonspecific, with weight loss, diarrhea, and general unthriftiness predominating.

Diagnosis

- Avian helminth eggs are detected by routine salt/sugar fecal flotation, as for dogs and cats.

Treatment

- Ivermectin (Ivomec 1% solution, Merck) is effective against intestinal nematodes when given at a dose of 200 µg/kg, IM, or diluted 1:9 with propylene glycol and given at 0.2 mg/kg, PO, every 2 weeks.
- Levamisole (Tramisol, American Cyanamid) is effective against most intestinal nematodes when given at 10–20 mg/kg, SQ, every 2 weeks, or as a solution of 10 ml/gallon drinking water if treating an entire flock (use as only source of drinking water for 1–3 days).
- For cestodes, give praziquantel (DroncitI, Haver/Diamond) at a dose of 10–20 mg/kg, PO, repeat in 10–14 days.
- Administer fenbendazole (Panacur Paste, Hoechst-Roussel) at a dose of 20–50 mg/kg, PO, once daily for 3–5 days.

DISORDERS OF THE LIVER

Infectious Diseases

Etiology

Infectious disorders such as chlamydiosis, viral disease, bacterial hepatitis, and occasionally *Mycobacterium avium* are the most common causes of liver diseases in pet birds. This is especially true in larger psittacines such as parrots, macaws, and cockatoos, although cockatiels and budgerigars also may be affected.

Diagnosis

- Indicators of liver disease include green-yellow urates (biliverdinuria), hepatomegaly (palpable or radiographically evident), and serum biochemical profile indicators such as increased levels of serum, bile acids, lactic dehydrogenase (LDH), and aspartate aminotransferase (AST). AST values may be elevated with either liver or muscle damage. Concurrent elevation in serum AST and creatine kinase (CK) values indicates muscle damage. Decreased serum albumin levels often are seen with liver disease.

- Liver biopsy often is necessary for definitive diagnosis with identification of a specific etiologic agent.
- See Chapter 162 for specific diagnostic tests, treatment, and prevention of infectious disease.

Fatty Liver Syndrome

Fatty liver syndrome (FLS), or hepatic lipidosis, commonly is seen in budgerigars, cockatiels, and some Amazon parrots. Gradual excessive triglyceride accumulation in the liver may cause the destruction of normal liver cells and lead to cirrhosis.

Etiology

- The etiology of FLS is unknown; however, malnutrition appears to play a major role.
  - Most birds with FLS are obese and on a high-fat diet consisting primarily of seeds.
- Unlike FLS in cats, anorexia does not appear to play a role in the development of this disorder.

Clinical Signs

- Signs often include diarrhea, biliverdinuria, obesity, poor feathering, and abdominal enlargement.
- Budgerigars frequently have overgrown, soft, friable beaks, with focal areas of hemorrhage.
- Sudden death has been reported in budgerigars, cockatiels, and Amazon parrots, with hepatic lipidosis as the only identifiable lesion on necropsy.

Diagnosis

- Palpate and, if indicated, obtain radiographs of the abdomen to detect hepatomegaly.
- Increased AST, bile acids, LDH, and cholesterol levels may be present on the serum biochemistry profile.
- Liver biopsy is necessary to confirm the diagnosis.

Treatment

- Administer intravenous or interosseous fluids to critically ill birds. If anorexic, forced alimentation with a low-fat gruel is indicated.
- Place the bird on a strict low-fat diet. Eliminate seeds from the diet.
  - For large birds, add more cereal grains.
  - Ideally, a commercial avian pellet formula should make up at least 40% of the diet, the remainder consisting of vegetables, fruits, and grains/legumes.
- Lactulose (Cephulac, Marion Merrell Dow), given at a dose of 0.3 ml/kg q8–12h, PO, may help to stimulate the appetite and decrease the colonic absorption of toxins that cause hepatic encephalopathy.

Hepatic Fibrosis

Etiology

- Hepatic fibrosis is a common sequela to chronic liver disease.
- The primary insult can be infectious (e.g., bacterial, viral, chlamydial) or noninfectious (e.g., FLS). Fibrosis can persist after elimination of the primary insult.

Diagnosis

- Liver biopsy is required for definitive diagnosis of hepatic fibrosis.

Treatment

- Colchicine has been reported to decrease clinical signs of chronic liver disease by interfering with collagen precursor synthesis.

Aflatoxicosis

Etiology

- Avian aflatoxicosis is caused by the ingestion of toxic metabolites from molds such as *Aspergillus flavus* and *A. parasiticus*. Foods in which these molds may be found include peanuts and peanut products, cereals, breads, cheeses, beans, and meat.
- Aflatoxins frequently are hepatoxic and may be carcinogenic.

Clinical Signs

- Signs generally are nonspecific and include anorexia, weight loss, and depression.

Diagnosis

- Base the diagnosis on history, clinical signs, and fungus isolation from feed or the GI tract.
- Gross and histopathologic lesions from postmortem or liver biopsy confirm the diagnosis.
  - Chronic lesions include biliary hyperplasia, cirrhosis, generalized fatty degeneration, and portal fibrosis.
  - Acute lesions include massive hepatocyte necrosis and hepatic hemorrhage.

Treatment

- No specific therapy is available.
- Activated charcoal may help to eliminate the toxin from the intestinal tract.
- Oral selenium may act as a competitive inhibitor of aflatoxins in the liver.
- Vitamin A is believed to provide some protection prophylactically against aflatoxins.

Hemochromatosis

Etiology

Hemochromatosis, defined as excessive deposition of iron in hepatic parenchymal cells with resultant cellular damage, is common in mynahs and toucans. Iron normally is absorbed from the intestines at a rate dependent on the body's needs and then recycled with minimal excretion from the body.

- In hemochromatosis, there is excessive uncontrolled absorption and storage of iron.
- The mechanism of this defect in iron metabolism is not understood, but affected birds absorb and store even small amounts of iron in the diet.

Clinical Signs

- Signs include weight loss, dyspnea, and abdominal swelling from severe hepatomegaly and ascites.

Diagnosis

- Diagnosis is based on clinical signs, elevated AST and LDH levels, serum iron levels in excess of 150 μg/100 ml are occasionally detected.

Treatment

- For symptomatic control of ascites, periodically remove abdominal fluid and administer diuretics.
- Successful long-term treatment has been reported with weekly phlebotomies.

Prevention

Many commercial mynah pellets contain excessively high levels of iron.

- Place mynahs and toucans on a diet consisting of a low-iron (< 100 PPM) kibbled dog food such as Science Diet Senior or Maintenance dog food (Hill's Pet) or with freshly diced fruits such as grapes, apples, and melons.

Neoplasia

Primary and metastatic neoplasms have been reported in all psittacines; they are particularly prevalent in budgerigars and Amazon parrots.

- An increased incidence of hepatic neoplasia has been noted in birds with papillomas.
- Primary tumors seen include bile duct carcinoma, hepatocellular carcinoma, hepatoma, fibrosarcoma, and hemangiosarcoma.
- Hepatomegaly usually is palpable or visible on radiographs.
- Diagnosis is confirmed by biopsy.
- Treatment is ineffective.

DISORDERS OF THE PANCREAS

Etiology

- As in liver disease, many infectious agents (e.g., bacteria, *Chlamydia*, viruses) may target the pancreas alone (e.g., many viral infections) or concurrently with other organ systems (see Chapter 161).

- Noninfectious causes of pancreatitis include nutritional factors; pancreatitis may be seen secondary to egg yolk peritonitis (see Chapter 166).
- In some cases, pancreatitis diagnosed at necropsy showed an intense inflammatory process without infectious etiology in birds on high-fat (seed) diets.
- There is a possible correlation between hypercalcemia occurring in hens in breeding condition (serum calcium levels usually are 20 times normal before ovulation) and the onset of pancreatitis (hypercalcemia is known to be a cause of pancreatitis in humans).

Clinical Signs

- Signs include anorexia, polyuria-polydipsia, diarrhea, and listlessness.

Diagnosis

- Serum amylase levels may be consistently elevated, and lipemia, hypercalcemia, and hyperglycemia may be present.
- Radiography may reveal decreased abdominal detail.
- In one confirmed case, an abdominal tap revealed blood and serum in the abdomen.

Treatment

- Treatment is similar to that for dogs and cats, and includes fluid therapy (nothing per os), antibiotic therapy, and maintenance on a low-fat diet.

SUPPLEMENTAL READINGS

Clipsham R: Surgical beak restoration and correction. Proc Ann Conf Assoc Av Vet, 1989, p 164.

Gould J: Liver disease in psittacines. Proc Ann Conf Assoc Av Vet, 1989, p 125.

Harrison GJ: Selected surgical procedures. *In* Harrison GH, Harrison LR, eds.: Clinical Avian Medicine and Surgery. Philadelphia: WB Saunders, 1986, p 577.

Hillyer EV: Bile duct carcinoma in two of ten Amazon parrots with cloacal papillomas. J Assoc Avian Vet 5(2):193, 1991.

Hoefer HL: Hepatic fibrosis and colchicine therapy. J Assoc Avian Vet 5:193, 1991.

Hoefer HL, Moroff S: The use of bile acids in the diagnosis of hepatobiliary disease in the parrot. Proc Ann Conf Assoc Av Vet, 1991, p 118.

Oglesbee BL: Mycotic diseases. *In* Altman RB, Clubb SL, Dorrestein GM, et al, eds.: Avian Medicine and Surgery. Philadelphia: WB Saunders, 1997, p 323.

Worell A: Phlebotomy for treatment of hemochromatosis in two sulfur-breasted toucans. Proc Ann Conf Av Vet, 1991, p 9.

166 Avian Obstetric Medicine

Walter J. Rosskopf / Richard W. Woerpel

This chapter describes the problems encountered in female pet avian species while forming, developing, and delivering eggs. Obstetric problems are common in birds (Table 166–1).

ANATOMY OF THE FEMALE REPRODUCTIVE TRACT

The gross anatomy of the female reproductive tract is relatively simple (Fig. 166–1).

Ovary

- In most pet bird species, only the left ovary is functional.
  - The inactive ovary is a miniature white botryoid organ; the cortex consists of a wall of small, white developing follicles, and a medulla of highly vascular connective tissue.
  - The active ovary contains numerous follicles containing varying amounts of yolk material.
- The ovary is associated intimately with the ventral surface of the cranial pole of the left kidney.
- The size and appearance of the ovary varies, depending on the physiologic state of the bird.

Oviduct

- Usually, the left oviduct is functional and the right side is vestigial.
- Anatomically, the oviduct is divided into five parts: the infundibulum, magnum (pars albuginea), isthmus, shell gland (pars calcigerous), and vagina (pars terminalis). The term *uterus* has been used synonymously for the term *oviduct* in birds; others consider the *shell gland* the uterus.
- The size of the oviduct varies, depending on the physiologic state and age of the bird.
  - The virgin oviduct may be microscopic in size; the mature oviduct is considerably larger.
  - A gravid oviduct may occupy much of the abdominal cavity.
- The oviduct is suspended by a cranial ligament and a caudal ligament, through which it receives its well-developed blood supply.

NORMAL EGG FORMATION

- The *development of ova* is influenced by several factors. When sexual maturity has been achieved, most avian species respond to increasing periods of daylight with follicular maturation.

Table 166–1. COMMON OBSTETRIC PROBLEMS BY SPECIES

Condition	Species*											
	1	2	3	4	5	6	7	8	9	10	11	12
Metritis				C		C		C				
Egg peritonitis			C	O	C		C	C	R	C	C	R
Egg binding			C	C	C	R	C	C	R	O		R
Cloacal prolapse		R	O			C						
Cloacal papilloma		C									C	O
Lipomatosis			C		C	C						
Abdominal hernia			C	R	C		O	O				
Other tumors	R	R	C									
Prolonged egg laying			C	O	C		C	C		C		
Ectopic eggs	R		R									
Oviduct prolapse			O	O	R	O		R				

R, rare; O, occasionally seen; C, commonly encountered.
*1 = African gray parrots; 2 = Amazon parrots; 3 = budgerigars; 4 = canaries; 5 = cockatiels; 6 = cockatoos; 7 = ducks; 8 = finches; 9 = gray-cheeked parakeets; 10 = lovebirds; 11 = macaws; 12 = conures.

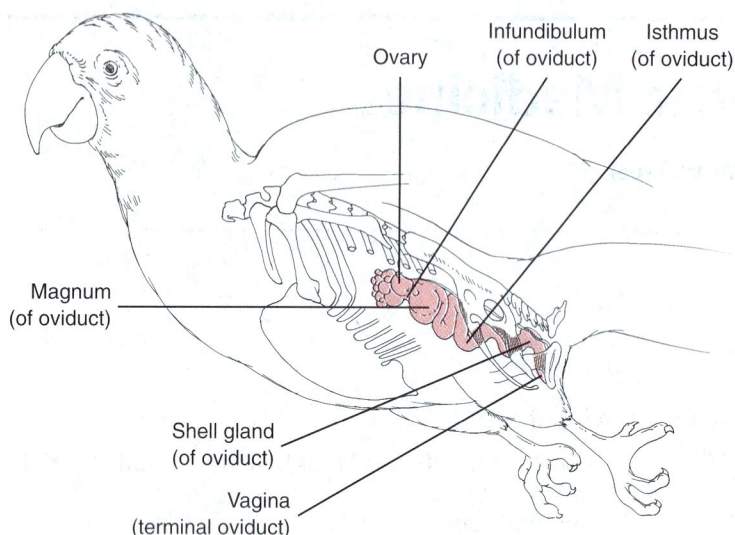

Figure 166-1. Reproductive anatomy of the female bird. The shell gland is equivalent to the uterus.

- *Follicular growth* is controlled by follicle-stimulating hormone (FSH). After an ovum begins growing within a follicle, maturation takes several days. Yolk is deposited as concentric rings, representing daily maturation.
- *Ovulation* is controlled by luteinizing hormone (LH). No structure analogous to a mammalian corpus luteum develops.
- The funnel-shaped *infundibulum* is closely associated with the ovary. It engulfs the extruded ova, and fertilization occurs here. The infundibulum propels the ovum down the oviduct.
  - If the engulfing procedure does not occur (injury, disease, drug therapy, obstruction, or other cause of nervous dysfunction), the ovum falls into the body cavity or is resorbed.
- The longest portion of the oviduct is the highly glandular *magnum*. Pressure on the secretory glands causes the magnum to secrete mucin and albumin around the ovum.
- The ovum next is propelled into the short, nonglandular *isthmus*, where the two shell membranes are secreted loosely around the ovum and albumin.
- The *shell gland* is a comparatively short, dilated portion of the oviduct, with glandular mucosa. Albumin also is secreted here, along with the shell and shell pigments (if present).
  - While the egg is in the shell gland and before calcification proceeds further, water, vitamins, and mineral salts pass through the semipermeable egg membranes into the egg and migrate toward the yolk, the site of lowest water concentration.
- The terminal portion of the oviduct, the *vagina*, is a muscular portion that communicates with the cloaca. This area is responsible for forcefully expelling the ova and is calcium- and oxytocin-responsive.
- Oviduct disease can be transferred to the egg contents (bacteria, fungi, viruses). Hypermotility of the oviduct and uterus, or calcium deficiencies, can result in a soft-shelled egg.
- *Egg transit time*—In most bird species, the ovum spends about 15 minutes in the infundibulum, 3 hours in the magnum, 1½ hours in the isthmus, and 20–21 hours in the shell gland and passes through the vagina almost instantly.

▼ *Key Point* Egg formation usually only takes 24–26 hours.

PHARMACOLOGIC INFLUENCES ON EGG PRODUCTION

There are no anatomic structures to prevent the egg from undergoing reverse peristalsis. Physical disturbance of a laying hen and certain drugs can result in egg peritonitis or eggs that are soft-shelled, shell-less, or misshapen.

- Adrenergic drugs cause relaxation of the oviduct, and cholinergic drugs cause constriction.
- Acetylcholine, oxytocin, and vasotocin produce expulsion of uterine eggs.
- For a shell to be produced, metabolic CO_2 must be converted to HCO_3^- within the shell gland catalyzed by carbonic anhydrase.
  - Drugs such as sulfonamides and acetazolamide inhibit carbonic anhydrase and result in eggshell thinning.

NUTRITIONAL INFLUENCES ON EGG PRODUCTION

Nutritional status has profound effects on egg producing and laying.

- *Protein deficiency* may result in reduced numbers of eggs and in high chick mortality.
- The formation of specialized medullary bone in the tibia and femur of females is stimulated by the action of estrogens and androgens; as a result, more calcium is made available for eggshell formation. However, breeding birds fed a *calcium-deficient* diet may

pass thin-shelled eggs and have an increased incidence of egg binding.

- Calcium also has profound effects on *uterine contractibility*. Calcium used for eggshell formation may result in borderline hypocalcemia with insufficient calcium available for uterine contraction.
- *Vitamin D₃ deficiency* may exacerbate signs of calcium deficiency and may be associated with poor bone development and splay legs.

DISEASES THAT AFFECT EGG PRODUCTION

Chronic Disease

- Overt disease may be precipitated by the production of ova or egg laying in female birds with borderline health status.
- A chronically ill bird is less likely to form ova, but surprisingly, many seriously ill birds, especially small birds such as budgerigars, cockatiels, and lovebirds, continue to lay eggs. In contrast to mammals, female birds tend to sacrifice themselves in egg laying. It is theorized that this phenomenon occurs because male birds can successfully raise young alone.

Bacterial Metritis

- Low-grade bacterial metritis, often secondary to systemic disease, may result in the death of neonates.
- Such infections can have adverse effects on shell formation and uterine contractility. Egg binding, uterine rupture, and septicemia may result.

Egg Peritonitis

- Egg peritonitis (see section in this Chapter) may result in ineffective contraction of the uterus (i.e., the inflammatory response interferes with the peristaltic and expulsive ability of the oviduct).
- Recovered birds may have adhesions and abdominal distension, influencing subsequent egg-laying efforts.

Cloacal Abnormalities

Cloacal abnormalities that may impair the ability to normally pass ova include weak cloacal musculature, papillomatosis, and cloacal strictures and scar formation.

- *Weak cloacal musculature* or *internal attachments*—A weakened cloaca may prolapse after the expulsive efforts of egg laying. The degree of cloacal prolapse varies.
  - Treatment of prolapse is described in detail later in this chapter.
- *Papillomatosis* (see Chap. 28) can be a problem in obstetrics. It is believed to be viral in origin and may have a venereal route of transmission.
- *Cloacal strictures* and *scar formation* can occur after egg laying, infection, injury, papilloma surgery, episiotomy, and cloacoliths.
  - Examine the vent and cloaca during prebreeding examination.

Abdominal Hernias

- In birds that have had previous heavy egg-laying episodes, large abdominal hernias may develop, interfering with subsequent egg laying; the abdominal musculature may completely separate. This is particularly common in cockatiels.
- Imbrication of abdominal musculature may be necessary. Remove an elliptical area of skin from sternum to vent, and suture the peritoneum and skin together, effectively tightening the area.
- Achieving muscle-to-muscle repair may be impossible if the condition is chronic and contraction of muscle tissue is severe.

Abdominal Tumors

- Lipomas and xanthomas that involve the abdomen are common in budgerigars and cockatiels.
- Massive lipomas are common in rose-breasted cockatoos. These growths may damage abdominal muscle tone and can influence egg laying, resulting in egg binding.
- Tumors of the kidneys and gonads may push the gizzard ventrally, mimicking the appearance of an egg.
  - In some birds, both abdominal masses and eggs may be present; radiographs of the abdomen can differentiate abdominal masses from retained eggs, unless the eggs have no shells.

Recurrent Reproductive Problems

- Carefully observe birds with a history of previous egg-laying problems.
- Recurrences of uterine or cloacal prolapses, egg peritonitis, or ectopic eggs are common.

Miscellaneous Problems

- Conditions that may influence obstetric procedures include congenital deformities, injuries (e.g., leg injury), previous egg-laying status (heavy egg layers tend to repeat), age (e.g., very old, very young), uterine structural status (e.g., strictures), nutritional status, and general health.

EXCESSIVE EGG LAYING

Excessive egg laying is a common problem in cockatiels, lovebirds, and budgerigars. This process can be detrimental. For instance, some cockatiels lay up to 30 eggs in 1½ months. Certain individual birds tend to be multiple egg layers; others of the same species rarely or never lay eggs.

Etiology

- Extremely close attachment of the bird to an owner, with a resultant display of masturbatory activity, may stimulate the process, especially if the owner encourages it.
- *Double clutching effect*—Usually, when the number of eggs laid constitute a clutch, hormonal levels change

and the female shifts into "broodiness" until the eggs are ready to be hatched, completing the cycle. Continuous removal of eggs as they are laid disrupts this cycle, causing repeated laying.

Treatment

Behavioral Modification

- Discourage mating behavior with the owner.
- Do not remove eggs until brooding is complete (usually 21 days).
- Change the bird's environment (e.g., move to another room); the mild stress may stop the egg-laying cycle. Consider moving the cage position daily. Try turning the lights out earlier to influence the photoperiod effect.

Medical Therapy

- If behavioral methods are ineffective, consider administration of human chorionic gonadotropin (HCG) (Pregnyl, Organon, Inc., West Orange, NJ) to break the egg-laying cycle. Treatment is most effective when the female is not paired with a male.
  - HCG has been effective in decreasing egg laying when administered at a dosage of 500–1000 IU/kg IM. If another egg is laid after injection, the dosage may be repeated 2 days after the first injection. Some birds may require a third injection 1 week later. HCG is safe but often requires repeat administration. Many clinicians routinely give injections on days 1, 3, and 7.

Medroxyprogesterone (Depo-Provera, UpJohn) also may inhibit egg laying, but is used less often because it has been associated with serious side effects such as depression, polyuria, weight gain, liver compromise with elevated serum glutamate oxaloacetic transaminase (SGOT) levels, lowered resistance to disease (with latent problems becoming overt) and, in rare cases, diabetes mellitus. Depo-Provera, if used properly, still has its uses. Some of the reported side effects may be due to overuse or from using doses that are too high.

Surgical Treatment: Hysterectomy

Hysterectomy is the method of choice for permanent alleviation of chronic egg laying. However, initially attempt conservative methods because clients may be concerned about surgical risk, loss of "intactness" of the bird, and loss of breeding potential.

In most birds, ovarian development is under uterine control, and removal of the uterus inhibits future follicle release; however, continued production of ova and subsequent yolk peritonitis occasionally occur after simple hysterectomy. In psittacines, partial hysterectomy (i.e., removal of ⅔ of uterus) is usually effective.

Indications

Consider hysterectomy if:

- The bird is refractory to administration of HCG.
- There are concurrent problems, such as severe uterine disease, repeated egg binding or a life-threatening egg-binding episode, and recurring or chronic peritonitis.

▼ *Key Point*   Most small birds normally experience "menopause" and stop laying eggs after a few years, but this varies.

Technique

1. Perform a left lateral laparotomy approach. To avoid hemorrhage, leave the ovary intact.
2. Bluntly dissect the infundibulum away from the ovary.
3. Ligate the artery leading to the ovary. Place a ligature around the uterus at the junction of the uterus with the cloaca.
4. Transect the uterus after tying off or cauterizing any other vessels contained in the suspensory ligaments.
   a. Electrocautery is a necessity in most small birds. In larger birds, blunt dissection and simple ligation may suffice.
5. Close the abdominal wall with absorbable sutures in a simple interrupted pattern.
6. Close the skin with absorbable or nonabsorbable sutures in a simple continuous pattern.
7. Administer HCG or Depo-Provera to stop egg formation until hormonal control ceases.

EGG PERITONITIS (YOLK PERITONITIS)

Peritonitis due to the escape of yolk material into the peritoneal cavity is a common condition in many avian species, including cockatiels, budgerigars, lovebirds, ducks, and macaws. Generalized peritonitis may result, with adhesions between the various organs, especially between loops of intestine. Subsequent inflammation may occur in vital areas such as the adrenal glands, liver, and pancreas.

Etiology

- It has been postulated that yolk excites only a mild histiocytic response and gradually is resorbed by the peritoneum and that yolk peritonitis occurs when the yolk (a good bacterial growth medium) becomes contaminated by bacteria.
- Alternatively, the yolk may cause a foreign body reaction or is itself caustic.
- Peritonitis can occur when ova extruded from the ovary fail to enter the infundibulum of the oviduct.
- Rupture of the oviduct may result from infection of surrounding tissues and weakening of the ovarian wall, stasis of normal or abnormal eggs, obstruction of the oviduct (egg binding, mechanical blockage as from cystic hyperplasia of the oviduct or neoplasia of the oviduct), or, in rare cases, injury.
- Reverse peristalsis of the oviduct may occur. In many apparently normal cockatiels, egg peritonitis develops immediately after egg laying. An ovum just starting to enter the infundibulum is driven into the body cavity when the expulsive egg-laying process is occurring simultaneously.

Clinical Signs

- Common signs include abdominal distension, depression, lethargy, and anorexia.

Diagnosis

Base the diagnosis of egg peritonitis on clinical signs, a complete blood count (CBC), radiography, abdominocentesis, and laparotomy.

- A history of egg laying may be helpful; however, egg peritonitis can occur just before the onset of laying.
- Abdominal radiographs often reveal a typical "ground glass" appearance. Calcified egg material is rarely present within the peritoneal cavity.
- A CBC is useful for diagnosing egg peritonitis. A severe inflammatory response (marked leukocytosis, heterophilia with a left shift, toxic heterophils) often mimicks chlamydiosis, septicemia, tuberculosis, or generalized aspergillosis. Table 166–2 lists typical hemograms seen in confirmed cases.
- Perform abdominocentesis if ascites is present. Aspirated fluid may contain yolk material, heterophils, macrophages, and bacteria.
- Laparotomy, which often is necessary for treatment (discussed later), can confirm the diagnosis.

Treatment

- If yolk peritonitis is mild, most birds recover with initial corticosteroid therapy and broad-spectrum antibiotics, and supportive care (e.g., vitamins, forced alimentation, heat, and fluids as indicated).
- Aspirin is an effective anticoagulant in birds. Dissolve one 5-grain tablet in 30 ml of water or juice.
  - A typical dose is 0.05 ml of the mixture given q8h to a 100-g bird.
- If massive amounts of yolk collect, laparotomy may be required after medically stabilizing the patient. Surgery may be postponed for long periods while the patient's condition stabilizes.
  - A scarlet macaw (see Table 166–2) was presented with a degenerative left shift and was near death from yolk peritonitis. After stabilization (e.g.,

WBC = 12,000 µl, PCV = 47%, no toxic heterophils), several inspissated yolks were removed and a large opening in the oviduct was closed.
- Birds with chronic peritonitis may require prolonged treatment; monitor with hematology and microbiology.
  - Warn owners that future problems may occur because of uterine and abdominal damage.
- Treat diabetes with long-term insulin therapy, if indicated.

Complications

- *Diabetes mellitus* may be an aftermath of yolk peritonitis, especially in cockatiels. Transient diabetes may occur, in which resolution appears to correlate with cessation of pancreatic inflammation.
- Yolk in serum, or *yolk emboli*, appears to have been responsible for stroke-like symptoms seen in several cockatiels with yolk peritonitis.
  - Lipemia and liver damage may be associated with this phenomenon.
  - Most cases resolve after a week or so with supportive care alone.

EGG BINDING

▼ *Key Point* Egg binding is one of the most common emergency conditions encountered in pet birds.

Birds may be presented in various stages of this condition, ranging from slight distress to moribund.

Etiology

- The obstruction may be caused by developing or fully formed eggs, concretions of egg material, calculi, or excessive secretions from the mucosa of the oviduct itself.
- Obstruction by a developing egg is the condition most frequently seen in clinical practice.
  - Inability to expel the egg may be due to low blood calcium levels, resulting from a calcium-deficient

Table 166–2. TYPICAL HEMOGRAMS OF BIRDS WITH CONFIRMED EGG PERITONITIS

	Budgerigar	Cockatiel	Scarlet Macaw	Scarlet Macaw
WBC (per µl)	29,000	24,000	120,000	2000
Bands (%)	3		6	6
Heterophils (%)	87	90*	75*	92*
Lymphocytes (%)	8	8	14	2
Monocytes (%)	2		5	
Eosinophils (%)		2		
Basophils (%)				
PCV (%)	55	60	48	31
SGOT (µ/L)	850	1750	1200	2300
Outcome	Resolved	Resolved	Died postoperatively	Degenerative picture; resolved after surgery

*Toxic heterophils.
WBC, white blood cells; PCV, packed cell volume; SGOT, serum glutamate oxaloacetic transaminase.

diet or from overproduction of eggs that drain calcium reserves.
- Other causes include uterine damage from peritonitis, infection, or injury.
- Occasionally, a larger-than-normal egg or an egg presented laterally is the cause.
- The most commonly affected species are budgerigars, canaries, finches, cockatiels, and lovebirds; however, any species is susceptible.

Clinical Signs

Signs depend on the species of bird and the position of the egg.

- Most egg binding occurs at the distal part of the oviduct (the uterus).
- Eggs trapped below the pelvis may crush the kidneys or cause intestinal blockage. The lack of "give" between the surface of the egg and the pelvic outlet makes this condition potentially life-threatening in a short period of time (Fig. 166–2).
- In small birds such as canaries or finches, sudden death without prior clinical signs is common.
- Larger birds may perch unsteadily with ruffled feathers and half-closed eyes. Birds may make frequent tail-wagging and abdominal straining movements and may move back and forth to the nest.
- Eventually, because of complications from intestinal blockage, kidney compromise, or ureter blockage, there are signs of pain, and the bird moves to the cage bottom.

Diagnosis

Diagnosis usually is made by clinical signs, palpation, and radiography.

- If an egg is palpable in a heavily producing cockatiel found on the bottom of the cage, it is usually easy to diagnose egg binding.

- In large birds such as parrots, macaws, and cockatiels, eggs can be distinguished easily by digital palpation against the pelvic girdle.
- In small birds such as canaries and finches, normal soft tissue structures such as the gizzard may be pushed downward, making palpation difficult.
- Differentiating an egg from an intra-abdominal mass, ascites, hernias, or lipomas may be difficult; in these cases perform abdominal radiography.
- If an egg is not easily palpable, consider yolk peritonitis, septicemia from stress of overproduction, leg injuries, and other causes in a "downer" egg-producing female.
- The presence of an egg is not conclusive evidence of egg binding.
  - Observe the bird for clinical signs of egg binding before undertaking corrective measures.

Treatment

Treatment and manipulative procedures in egg binding vary with the severity of the condition and the location of the egg (Fig. 166–3).

- Choose a treatment procedure that will induce the least amount of stress and shock potential.
- Because the condition may have been unattended for a long time, there may be difficult manipulative and surgical problems.
- For purposes of discussion of treatment, egg binding is divided into the following categories:
  - Cloacal binding
  - Oviduct (precloacal) binding
  - Egg binding with prolapsed oviduct.

▼ *Key Point* Avoid the use of anesthesia, which is unnecessary in the early stages of egg binding and can be dangerous in birds in late, critical stages. If an anesthetic is necessary, isoflurane is the agent of choice.

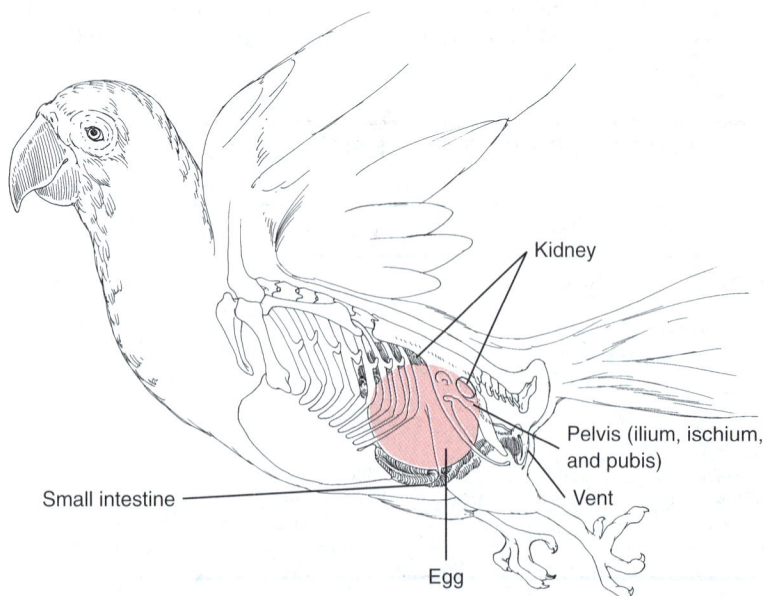

Figure 166–2. Anatomic landmarks associated with egg binding.

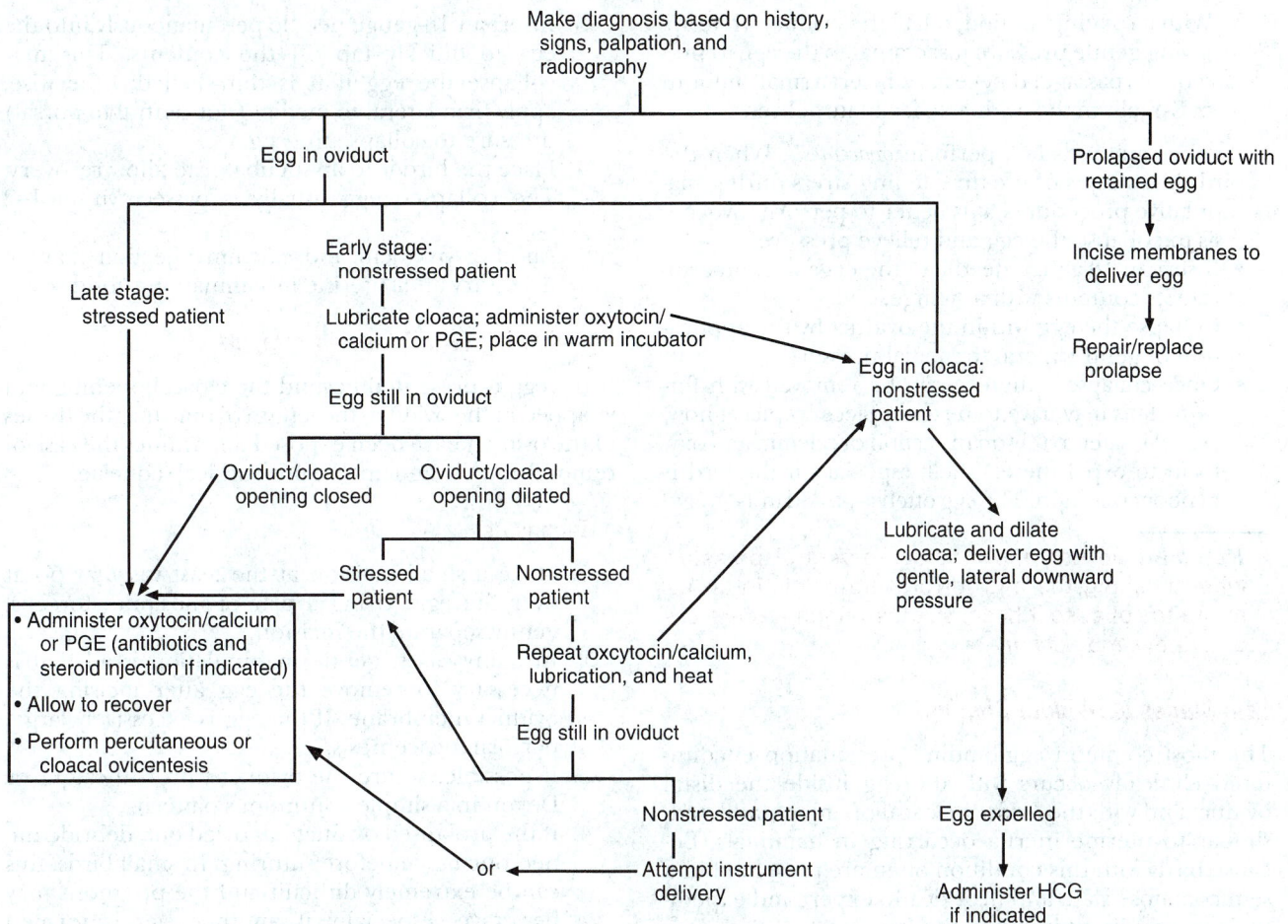

Figure 166–3. Flow chart for the treatment of egg binding.

Many birds that are not egg-bound show discomfort in the laying process, similar to labor in mammals.

Early Stages of Cloacal Binding

Birds in the early or incipient stages of cloacal binding are not immediately at risk.

- Briefly attempt to deliver the egg by working the thumb and forefinger between the egg and rib cage and then pushing outward and downward. Outward pressure prevents pain and shock from pressure on the kidneys.
- Relax the vent by gentle steam heat or use K-Y jelly to lubricate the cloaca.
- To stimulate uterine contraction and prevent hemorrhage, administer an intramuscular injection of calcium (Calphosan, Glenwood), 0.15–0.25 ml/100 g, and oxytocin, 0.025 ml/100 g 20 USP units/ml).
- If indicated, give antibiotics and corticosteroids prophylactically.

Early Stages of Oviduct Binding

In the early stages of oviduct binding, only mild signs of distress are present, and the bird is alert and active. However, because symptoms may be masked and rapid deterioration can occur, immediate medical therapy is recommended.

- Place the bird in a warm environment (e.g., incubator).
- Administer calcium and oxytocin at the dosages given previously for early stages of cloacal binding.
  - Alternatively, administer prostaglandin E (PGE) topically in the cloacal lumen.
  - In mild cases of uterine inertia, an egg is produced within 20–30 minutes.
- If an egg is not produced in 1 hour, the egg has not moved appreciably, and the bird does not demonstrate signs of further distress, repeat treatment.
- After careful observation, perform the manipulative procedures described previously for cloacal binding, if indicated.
- If gentle manual pressure does not produce results, attempt an instrumental delivery.

Technique

(Instrument Delivery)

1. Clean the cloaca and dilate it with a hemostatic forceps or small vaginal speculum.
2. When the oviduct is identified, insert a sterile probe between the oviduct and eggshell.

3. With a rotating motion, dilate the oviduct while applying gentle pressure just cranial to the egg to promote its passage. If necessary, insert a small amount of K-Y jelly in the oviduct to facilitate delivery.

- If other methods fail, perform *ovocentesis*. When the bird shows signs of life-threatening stress during manipulative procedures, it is better to perform ovocentesis to collapse the egg and relieve pressure.
  - Insert an 18-gauge needle in the eggshell and aspirate its contents with a syringe.
  - Collapse the egg within the oviduct by the application of gentle lateral to medial pressure.
  - Once collapsed, the egg can be removed with forceps. This may have to be done piece by piece; however, it is safer to rely on the action of calcium and oxytocin to expel the eggshell, especially if the bird is in poor condition. The egg often is passed in 1–2 days.

▼ *Key Point* Do not apply dorsal-to-ventral pressure when pushing the egg toward the pelvis in an attempt to collapse it because crushing of the ureters or kidneys may occur.

Late Stages of Oviduct Binding

The most common egg-binding presentation encountered clinically occurs with the egg inside the distal oviduct and with the oviduct-cloacal opening undilated, similar to uterine inertia occurring in mammals. Because birds with this condition often are presented in a semicomatose state and near death, expert and expeditious management is imperative.

Attempts to dislodge the egg can result in near-collapse and severe stress with panting. Surgical correction (e.g., laparotomy), requiring anesthesia and extensive manipulation, is dangerous. As an alternative to these methods, the following approach is recommended. This sequence relieves pressure on vital organs with a minimum of shock potential in an already compromised animal and is preferable to invasive techniques such as laparotomy and episiotomy.

- Handling the bird as little as possible, administer the following drugs intramuscularly:
  - An antibiotic such as piperacillin (Pipracil, Lederle), 100 mg/kg q12h
  - Dexamethasone (Azium, Schering), 2–4 mg/kg
  - Calcium (Calphosan, Glenwood), 0.15–0.25 ml/100 g
  - Oxytocin (20 USP units/L), 0.025 ml/100 g (to control hemorrhage) or PGE, as described previously.
- To treat dehydration, administer parenteral or intravenous fluids (see Chapter 161).
- Place the bird in an incubator for a few minutes to allow recovery from stress.
- Perform *percutaneous ovocentesis*.

Technique

(Percutaneous Ovocentesis)

1. Wipe the abdomen with alcohol.
2. Push the egg ventrally toward the abdominal wall, so that the skin is stretched taut over the egg.

3. Insert an 18-gauge needle percutaneously into the egg to quickly tap off the contents. This may collapse the egg if it is thin-shelled; otherwise, apply firm lateral-to-medial (not ventral-to-dorsal) pressure to collapse the egg.
4. Place the bird into an incubator to allow recovery. The collapsed egg usually is passed within 1–2 days.
5. Another oxytocin and calcium injection may be necessary after uterine inflammation subsides.

Egg Binding with Uterine Prolapse

If the egg is presented beyond the cloacal opening and wrapped in the oviduct, the length of time that the tissues of the oviduct have been exposed determines the ease of removal and the anticipated postsurgical sequelae.

Technique

1. Make a small incision at the least vascular point over the egg. Using a pair of mosquito forceps, gently separate the incision.
2. In many cases, gentle manipulation is all that is necessary to remove the egg after incising the oviduct membrane. If the egg is excessively large, perform ovocentesis.
3. If possible, suture the oviduct with 6–0 catgut or Dexon in a simple continuous pattern.
4. If the prolapsed oviduct has dried out, debride the necrotic tissue before suturing. In small birds, this can be extremely difficult and the prognosis may be grave, especially if another egg is formed quickly and travels through the injured oviduct.
   - Ectopic eggs (described later) and egg peritonitis with soft or nonshelled yolks released into the abdomen are common sequelae.
5. Using a saline-soaked cotton swab, manipulate the oviduct back into position through the oviduct-cloacal opening.
6. Administer oxytocin at the dosage previously given for early stages of cloacal binding to promote uterine shrinkage, control bleeding, and expel accumulated blood from the oviduct.

Episiotomy

Perform this procedure if the egg is valuable and egg aspiration and collapse or purposeful breaking of the egg must be avoided.

Technique

1. Incise the vent opening laterally on one side only.
2. Remove the egg and suture the incision with 4–0 Dexon on a tapered needle.
3. Use careful technique to prevent stricture formation postoperatively.

ECTOPIC EGGS

Ectopic eggs (eggs free within the peritoneal cavity) occur occasionally, especially in small birds such as budgerigars and cockatiels. Diagnosis usually is made by laparotomy after all the usual methods to cause expulsion of the egg have failed.

OVIDUCT PROLAPSE

Oviduct prolapse (uterine prolapse) after egg laying is a common problem in budgerigars, cockatoos, and, occasionally, other birds. The oviduct may prolapse alone, or concurrent with cloacal prolapse.

Oviduct Prolapse with Intact Cloaca

- If the mucosa appears healthy, thoroughly clean exposed tissues with normal saline solution. Push the oviduct back through the cloaca into the body cavity with a lubricated cotton swab.
  - Administer oxytocin (see Early Stages of Cloacal Binding for dosage) to hasten oviduct shrinkage.
- If the oviduct has become desiccated or necrotic, a full or partial hysterectomy (see Oviduct Prolapse with Cloacal Prolapse) may be necessary.

Oviduct Prolapse with Cloacal Prolapse

Usually, simple replacement of the cloaca and oviduct is insufficient because the oviduct has become desiccated or necrotic or because the cloacal-oviduct opening is damaged, resulting in continual prolapse of the oviduct back into the cloaca after cloacal replacement or repair.

- The prolapse may not be visible externally, and the oviduct will undergo necrosis if the condition is not recognized. For this reason, perform a *partial hysterectomy*. This technique has worked well as a salvage operation in inexpensive pet birds.

Technique

1. Apply overlapping mattress sutures through the viable part of the exposed uterus. (See Chapter 113 for surgical treatment of vaginal prolapse in dogs and cats.)
2. Using a lubricated cotton swab, debride necrotic tissue and reposition the partial uterus.

- In some cases, a laparotomy may be performed to replace the oviduct so that a complete hysterectomy can be performed.
- If the bird is too ill to be considered a surgical candidate, the uterus may be replaced inside the cloaca and held in place by transverse sutures in the cloaca until it is considered safe to perform laparotomy.
  - Carefully observe the bird to make sure that its droppings are passed regularly during this stabilization period.

▼ *Key Point* If it is safe to administer the drug, give HCG (see previous section on medical therapy of prolonged egg laying) after any serious obstetric problem to prevent ovulation.

CLOACAL PROLAPSE

Minor Prolapses

- Minor prolapses of the cloaca often are held in place with pursestring or two transverse stay sutures placed perpendicular to the vent (Fig. 166–4). Be careful to leave an opening large enough to allow feces to pass normally.
  - Sutures may be wire, silk, Vetafil, or other nonabsorbable material.
- Remove sutures after 3 days.
- Once tissue swelling has subsided, the oviduct and/or cloaca may heal.

Cloacopexy

If serious damage has occurred to the cloacal attachments, prolapse of the cloaca and oviduct may continue after suture removal. In these cases, perform cloacopexy. This technique effectively prevents recurrence of the prolapse. Birds can return to immediate reproductive activity. However, if the uterus is very thin-walled, permanent repair is much more difficult to achieve.

Technique

1. Make a midline abdominal incision.
2. Outline the cloaca by having an assistant, wearing a finger cot, push the cloaca into the incision site.
3. Dissect the fat pad (analogous to the falciform ligament in the dog) away from the cloacal wall.
4. Suture the anterolateral walls of the ventral cloaca with 3–0 Vicryl to the posterior ribs and, if necessary, to the cartilage of the ventral sternum. Apply sufficient tension to slightly invert the vent opening.
5. Suture the lateral and ventral cloaca to the abdominal musculature with 3–0 Vicryl in a simple interrupted pattern.

Complications

Failure may occur if:

- The adipose pad is not dissected away
- The lumen of the cloaca is not penetrated
- Rapidly absorbed suture material is used
- The ribs or ribs plus sternum are not used to anchor at least two sutures
- The sutures tear through a thin-walled cloaca

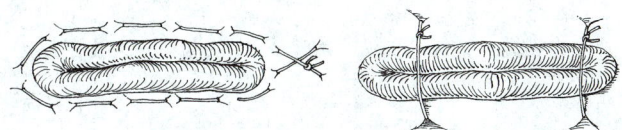

Figure 166–4. Cloacal suturing techniques. *Left,* Pursestring suture; *right,* transverse suture.

CLOACAL MUCOSAL RESECTION

Cloacal mucosal prolapse with necrotic or desiccated tissue is common in cockatoos and is seen in other avian species. Treatment consists of mucosal resection as performed in mammals.

SUPPLEMENTAL READINGS

Joyner KL, Theriogenology. *In* Ritchie BL, Harrison GJ, Harrison LR, eds.: Avian Medicine: Principles and Application. Lake Worth, Wingers Publishing, 1994, p 748.

Smith RE: Reproductive disorders in birds. *In* Rosskopf W, Woerpel R, eds.: Diseases of Cage and Aviary Birds, 3rd ed. Baltimore: Williams & Wilkins, 1996, p 499.

Speer B: Diseases of the urogenital system. *In* Altman RB, Clubb SL, Dorrestein GM, et al, eds.: Avian Medicine and Surgery. Philadelphia: WB Saunders, 1997, p 625.

167 Avian Neurologic Disorders

Katherine Quesenberry

Neurologic disease is common in cage and aviary birds. Methods of diagnosis and treatment in birds are limited by anatomic variations, patient size, and lack of reference values to interpret test results. Although many possible causes of neurologic disease exist, certain syndromes and diseases occur relatively frequently. Diagnosis of these more common syndromes is based on history, clinical signs, selected diagnostic tests, and response to therapy.

GENERAL HISTORY AND CLINICAL SIGNS

History

Several important points should be included in the general history of a bird with neurologic disease.

- Dietary history is important because nutritional deficiencies are factors in many diseases. Ask for specific details, such as:
  - What is the regular diet?
  - Which vitamin and mineral supplements are being given?
  - Is adequate calcium provided for heavy egg layers?
- What is the home environment of the bird, especially as related to exposure to trauma and toxins?
  - Is the bird always caged or is it allowed free flight in the house?
  - Does the bird chew on any painted surfaces, metal objects, or plants?
  - What type of toys are kept in the cage?
- Is the bird a recent purchase or a long-term pet? Is there exposure to other birds?
- When was the onset of the disorder and what has been the duration and progression of clinical signs?

Clinical Signs

Clinical signs associated with neurologic disease in birds are similar to those seen in mammals.

- The most common clinical signs are seizures, ataxia, paresis, paralysis, head tilt, circling, abnormal mentation, nystagmus, intention tremors, and visual deficits. Weakness and ataxia can be manifested as falling off the perch.
- It may be difficult to distinguish weakness secondary to severe systemic disease from that associated with neurologic disease.

- The presence or absence of other neurologic deficits may be helpful in determining which body system is involved.
- Unilateral or bilateral lameness or wing droop may indicate a peripheral nerve deficit. Rule out fractures and other musculoskeletal abnormalities as a cause.

Neurologic Evaluation

Assessment of cranial nerve function is basic to a thorough neurologic examination.

- Assess vision in each eye by slowly moving a hand or an object toward the bird from behind on each side. A bird with visual deficits does not react until the object is very close or its face is touched.
- The pupillary light reflex is difficult to evaluate because of the presence of striated muscle in the iris. A widely dilated pupil that reacts minimally to changes in light intensity may indicate a visual deficit.
- Check facial sensation by touching various parts of the face with hemostats. Assess the palpebral reflex as in mammals.

PRINCIPLES OF TREATMENT

▼ *Key Point* Special nursing care is necessary for birds with neurologic disease.

- Birds with neurologic disease usually require special *nursing care* in the hospital and at home.
  - Keep ataxic birds or birds having seizures in cages without perches. Provide soft bedding.
  - Use small, shallow, or covered water bowls to prevent accidental drowning.
  - Remove sharp objects, chains, and potentially dangerous toys from the cage.
  - Make food easily accessible by spreading it on the floor or by providing several large containers in the cage.
- *Supplemental fluids* and *gavage feeding* are necessary for anorexic birds (see Chap. 161) and birds that are unable to eat because of tremors or ataxia.
- Give *antibiotics* if bacterial disease is suspected or if a risk of secondary bacterial infection exists. If possible, use antimicrobials that cross the blood-brain barrier (e.g., trimethoprim-sulfa, chloramphenicol).

- Administer *antifungal* agents if fungal infection of the CNS is a differential diagnosis. Fluconazol (Pfizer, Roerig Division, NY, NY 10017) (2–5 mg/kg q24h) reaches therapeutic concentrations in the brain parenchyma and the cerebral spinal fluid.
- *Anti-inflammatory drugs* (corticosteroids) usually are beneficial in the treatment of acute head trauma. Be conservative in administration because of the potential for adrenal suppression and immune compromise.
- Give *supplemental calcium* if the diet is deficient in calcium or if blood calcium concentrations are below normal.
- Administer *chelating agents* such as calcium ethylenediaminetetraacetic acid (edetic acid [EDTA]) in birds with suspected heavy metal toxicosis, such as lead or zinc. With lead toxicosis, birds often clinically improve within 24–48 hours. Side effects are rare, and birds can be treated with calcium disodium edetate (CaEDTA) on an emergency basis until results of tests for blood lead or zinc concentrations are known.
- *Anticonvulsants* such as diazepam (Valium) (0.5–2.0 mg/kg, IM or IV) are sometimes helpful in controlling seizures. Continual IV drips of diazepam sometimes are needed.
- Give parenteral *vitamins* to birds with suspected vitamin deficiencies. Vitamin D$_3$ is especially important in African gray parrots and birds with hypocalcemia. Give multivitamin B-complex and thiamine if birds are anorexic or thiamine deficiency is suspected. Supplement with vitamin E/selenium if muscular weakness is present.

METABOLIC/NUTRITIONAL DISORDERS

Hypocalcemia

▼ *Key Point* African gray parrots are predisposed to a hypocalcemic syndrome.

Hypocalcemia is associated with neurologic abnormalities, especially in African gray parrots. However, this syndrome is less common than in previous years, probably because many bird owners are better educated about nutrition and the use of pelleted avian diets is more widespread.

Etiology

- The exact cause of this syndrome in African gray parrots is not known. A common history in many birds with hypocalcemia is an all-seed diet with little or no vitamin supplementation, suggesting that a lack of vitamin D$_3$ may be a factor. Intake of dietary calcium may or may not be adequate.
- Other possible etiologic factors include abnormal osteoclast function and abnormal or dysfunctional parathyroid glands in affected birds.

Clinical Signs

- Common neurologic signs include seizures, weakness, paresis, ataxia, head tilt, circling, visual deficits, abnormal mentation, and anorexia.
- Seizures are the most common clinical sign and may be triggered by sudden noise and excitement. The

seizure lasts several seconds and occurs as an acute onset of tetanic spasms with extensor rigidity, wing flapping, vocalizations, and, occasionally, nystagmus.
- Skeletal abnormalities, including pathologic fractures and nutritional bone disease, usually are associated with calcium deficiency. However, these abnormalities rarely are seen in African gray parrots.

Diagnosis

Base the diagnosis on the history, clinical signs, results of plasma biochemical analysis, and response to therapy.

- To determine proper treatment, a plasma biochemical analyses, including calcium concentration, is necessary.
  - The total serum calcium concentration is usually very low in affected birds (1.5–6.0 mg/dl).
- Obtain whole-body survey radiographs to identify soft tissue or bone abnormalities and to detect any metal objects in the gastrointestinal (GI) tract or soft tissues that may indicate lead toxicosis.
  - The proventriculus and intestinal loops may appear slightly dilated on radiographs. Calcium deficiency may cause decreased smooth muscle contraction and motility of the GI tract.
  - Radiographs usually are unremarkable in African gray parrots with hypocalcemia.
- Consider and investigate other potential causes (e.g., lead toxicosis, systemic fungal infection).

Treatment

- Give supplemental calcium orally or parenterally.
  - In severely debilitated birds, start treatment with calcium gluconate, 100 mg/kg, SC, q6–24h.
  - If seizures are infrequent and the danger of aspiration during seizures is minimal, give calcium supplements orally, such as Neo-calglucon (Sandoz), 1 ml/30 ml of drinking water or crush Tums® tablets over food one to two times weekly.
- During initial therapy, give supplemental vitamin D$_3$ (500–1000 IU D$_3$/100 g IM of compounded emulsion [10,000 IU D$_3$/ml]); repeat in 3–4 days.
- Provide general supportive care and control continuous or severe seizures with diazepam (Valium) as needed, at a dose of 0.5–2.0 mg/kg, IM or IV.
- Correct the diet to provide adequate calcium and vitamins.

Prognosis

- The prognosis is good in most birds; however, African gray parrots with blood calcium concentrations less than 2.0 mg/dl usually respond poorly to treatment. Improvement usually is slow and gradual.

Miscellaneous Disorders

Gout

Gout can cause peripheral gait abnormalities that may appear as neurologic deficits. Gout is most common in old parakeets but also occurs in other species.

- Ataxia, weakness, and a stiff gait are common signs. Clinical signs usually occur before uric acid deposits (tophi) are visible as subcutaneous deposits in the joints and legs.

- The plasma uric acid concentration may be moderately to significantly high.

Liver Disease

- Weakness, ataxia, and abnormal mentation are seen occasionally with severe *liver disease* (see Chapter 165).

Hypoglycemia

- Hypoglycemia can cause severe weakness, lethargy, and neurologic deficits.

▼ *Key Point* Measure whole-blood glucose concentration by rapid Chemstrip analysis in any bird that is collapsed, weak, having seizures, or comatose.

Lipemia

- Signs of central neurologic abnormalities can occur in birds with severe *lipemia*.
  - The cause of the hyperlipidemia is not known, but this syndrome is seen most frequently in reproductive hens and obese birds. In the hens, it may be related to the egg-laying cycle.

Yolk Emboli

- Yolk emboli to the central nervous system (CNS) may result in neurologic abnormalities (see Chapter 166)
  - Hens usually remain alert but are ataxic and have a head tilt.
  - Treatment with niacin (50 mg/kg q8h) and gemfibrozil (Lopid, Parke-Davis; 30 mg/kg q8h) is sometimes effective in controlling clinical signs. Hens gradually improve over weeks to several months.

Other Nutritional Factors

- Deficiencies in vitamins E, B-complex, C, and A and selenium are related to neurologic disorders.
- Because specific vitamin deficiencies are difficult to confirm, give supplemental multivitamins if a deficiency is suspected.

IDIOPATHIC EPILEPSY

Idiopathic epilepsy has been described as a clinical syndrome in lovebirds and red-lored Amazon parrots.

- Phenobarbital, available as an elixir (4 mg/ml), is variably effective in controlling clinical signs.
  - Give in the drinking water, 1.5–2.5 ml/4 oz of water, or 2–3 mg/kg q12h PO.

NEOPLASIA

Central Nervous System Neoplasia

Primary tumors of neural tissue origin develop infrequently in birds and are most common in budgerigars and cockatiels. Meningiomas, pituitary adenomas, and glioblastomas have been reported.

Clinical Signs

- Common signs include ataxia, weakness, wide-based stance, and postural abnormalities.
- Depression, nystagmus, abnormal mentation, and visual deficits often are present.

Diagnosis

- Clinical diagnosis of a CNS tumor is extremely difficult. Static or progressive clinical signs indicating CNS system involvement with failure to respond to therapy suggest neoplasia.
- In large birds, computed tomography (CT) of the brain can be diagnostic.
- Diagnosis usually is determined by results of necropsy.

Treatment and Prognosis

- No treatment is available.
- The prognosis is poor.

Paresis Secondary to Renal or Gonadal Neoplasia

▼ *Key Point* Tumors of renal tissue origin are common in budgerigars 4 years of age and older and are associated with progressive unilateral limb paresis.

Gonadal tumors are less common than renal tumors; clinical signs may resemble those of renal neoplasia.

Etiology

- The cause of renal tumors in budgerigars is not known.

Clinical Signs

- Progressive paresis or paralysis of the leg on the ipsilateral side develops from pressure of the tumor on the sciatic nerve.
- Muscle atrophy may be severe in the affected leg.
- Polyuria may be an early or late clinical sign.

Diagnosis

Base the diagnosis on history, clinical signs, and physical examination.

- Palpate the abdomen carefully on the affected side to detect the presence of a smooth soft tissue mass.
- Obtain radiographs of the abdomen to identify a soft tissue mass in the area of the kidney.
  - Barium contrast radiography may reveal ventral or lateral displacement of bowel loops in the area of the kidney or gonad.

Treatment and Prognosis

- No treatment is available.
- Parakeets usually die within several months of the onset of clinical signs.

INFECTIOUS DISEASES

Viruses

Several viruses affect the avian nervous system (see Chapter 162).

- *Paramyxovirus* causes neurologic disease in many species of wild and domestic birds.
- Proventricular dilatation syndrome or disease (PDS or PDD) is a common cause of neurologic signs in psittacine species. (See Chapter 162 for details.)
- Neurologic deficits are sometimes seen in birds with *polyomavirus*.
- Other suspected viral causes of neurologic disease have been reported but are uncommon.
  - Budgerigar *encephalitis* has been reported in Germany. An adenovirus is the suspected cause.
  - *Reovirus* affects several avian species. Ataxia, paresis, and paralysis can occur, along with the typical signs of depression, swollen abdomen, diarrhea, biliverdinuria, edema, and weight loss.

Bacteria/Fungi

Neurologic disease resulting from bacterial or fungal infection sometimes is seen.

- Bacterial encephalitis secondary to systemic infection can result in multifocal neurologic disease.
  - Neurologic signs secondary to salmonellosis are common in pigeons.
- Neurologic signs are seen with fungal infections affecting the central or peripheral nervous system. Clinical signs vary from paralysis or paresis to generalized weakness, ataxia, or seizures. *Aspergillus* spp. most commonly are implicated, but infections with other fungi do occur.
- *Chlamydia psittaci* (psittacosis) can cause CNS lesions and neurologic signs. Typical signs of psittacosis (see Chapter 162) may be present.
- Infection with *Mycobacterium* spp. can result in neurologic signs, either as a result of direct involvement of the nervous system or secondary to weakness associated with systemic disease.

Parasites

Parasitic causes of neurologic diseases are rare in birds.

- Possible causes include microfilaria, protozoa (e.g., *Plasmodium, Atoxoplasma* spp), sporozoa (*Sarcocystis, Toxoplasma* spp.) and nematode migration.
- Diagnosis usually is based on results of necropsy and histologic examination of tissue samples.

TOXICOSES

Lead Toxicosis

Lead toxicosis is a common cause of neurologic disease in caged birds. Other aspects of lead toxicosis, as pertaining to dogs and cats, are discussed elsewhere.

▼ *Key Point* Sources of lead that are potentially toxic include surfaces or objects painted with lead-based paint, stained glass, mirror backing, champagne bottle foil, lead-weighted objects (curtain weights, some bird toys), and some ceramic or glazed dishes.

Clinical Signs

- Signs of acute lead ingestion include depression, anorexia, gastroenteritis (usually hemorrhagic), crop stasis, regurgitation, dehydration, and hemoglobinuria.
- Neurologic signs may be acute or latent in onset. Latent signs include seizures, ataxia, weakness, paresis, paralysis, circling, head tilt, nystagmus, blindness, and severe depression.

Diagnosis

Establish the diagnosis based on the history, clinical signs, supportive diagnostic tests, and response to therapy.

- Measure blood lead concentration. Lead concentrations of 15 µg/dl or greater suggest lead toxicosis.
- Although this test is not widely available, measurement of δ-aminolevulinic acid dehydratase enzyme activity is a highly specific test for lead toxicosis. Because lead inhibits this enzyme, levels of less than 86 units indicate lead exposure.
- Obtain radiographs to screen for metal objects in the GI tract or soft tissues. The presence of metal in a bird with typical clinical signs suggests lead toxicosis.
  - The absence of metal in the GI tract does not exclude a diagnosis of plumbism because small amounts of lead may be absorbed before the onset of clinical signs.
- Birds with lead toxicosis have mild to severe anemia. Measure packed cell volume (PCV) in birds that appear anemic before collecting blood for routine tests. Basophilic stippling is seen uncommonly in avian red blood cells (RBCs).

Treatment

- Chelation therapy is indicated in any bird with suspected lead toxicosis. CaEDTA is effective and is the most commonly used chelating agent.
  - Give CaEDTA, IM or SC, after diluting with saline, at a dosage of 30–50 mg/kg q12h for 5 days.
  - Persistence of a high blood lead level or clinical signs indicate that a second course of therapy is needed.
- Other chelating agents are potentially useful in birds.
  - Dimercaptosuccinic acid (DMSA), which can be given orally, chelates lead in soft tissues more quickly than EDTA.
  - D-Penicillamine, another chelating drug administered orally can be used for chelation therapy. However, GI side effects (e.g., vomiting) sometimes occur and therapy must be discontinued.

- Magnesium sulfate (Epsom salts) given orally may help to bind lead particles in the GI tract and inhibit further absorption. Dosage is empirical (e.g., a pinch dissolved in dextrose or added to food given q12h).
- Supportive therapy includes supplemental fluids, antibiotics, iron supplementation, vitamins, and tube feeding.
- Anticonvulsants are rarely necessary to control seizures.

Prognosis

- Birds with lead toxicosis usually respond quickly to chelation therapy. Clinical signs may diminish significantly after 1–2 days of therapy.
- Monitor progress by repeating tests for blood lead concentration. If results remain high, repeat chelation treatment for another 5 days and recheck the blood lead concentration.

Other Toxicoses

- Other heavy metal toxicosis, such as zinc, occasionally are associated with neurologic disease in cage birds.
- Exposure to organophosphates and other pesticides may cause incoordination, severe depression, and diarrhea.
- Toxicoses from exposure to marijuana, alcohol, and other drugs have been reported.
- Neurologic signs may be seen immediately before death caused by exposure to fumes from polytetrafluoroethylene (Teflon) (see Chap. 164).

TRAUMATIC INJURY

Head Trauma

- Head trauma can cause mild to severe neurologic signs.

- Treatment depends on the severity of clinical signs.
  - Administer anti-inflammatory doses of corticosteroids to birds with acute trauma.
- Provide general supportive therapy as needed.
- The prognosis depends on the severity of the injury and the response to therapy.

Peripheral Nerve Trauma

- Musculoskeletal injury can result in peripheral nerve damage.
- Treatment and prognosis depend on the extent of tissue damage.

SUPPLEMENTAL READINGS

Clippinger TL, Bennett RA, Platt SR: The avian neurologic examination and ancillary neurodiagnostic techniques. J Avian Med Surg 10:221, 1996.

Gaskin JM: Psittacine viral diseases: A perspective. J Zoo Wildlife Med 20:249, 1989.

Gerlach H: Viral diseases. *In* Harrison GJ, Harrison LR, eds.: Clinical Avian Medicine and Surgery. Philadelphia: WB Saunders, 1986, p 408.

Labonde J: Pet avian toxicology. AAV Proceedings, 1988, p 159.

Lyman R: Neurologic disorders. *In* Harrison GJ, Harrison LR, eds.: Clinical Avian Medicine and Surgery. Philadelphia: WB Saunders, 1986, p 486.

Mautino M: Avian lead intoxication. AAV Proceedings, 1990, p 245.

McDonald S: Lead poisoning in psittacine birds. In: Kirk RW (ed): Current Veterinary Therapy IX. Philadelphia: WB Saunders, 1986, p 713.

Rosenthal K: Disorders of the avian nervous system. *In* Attman RB, Clubb SL, Dorrestein GM, et al, eds.: Avian Medicine and Surgery. Philadelphia: WB Saunders, 1997, p 461.

Rosskopf WJ, Woerpel R: Epilepsy in red-lored Amazons (*Amazona autumnalis*). AAV Proceedings, 1985, p 141.

Rosskopf W, Woerpel R: Epilepsy in peach-faced and pied peach-faced lovebirds. AAV Proceedings, 1988, p 225.

Quesenberry KE, Hillyer EV: Neurologic disorders in caged birds: A retrospective review of cases. AAV Proceedings, 1988, p 170.

Walsh MT: Seizuring in pet birds. AAV Proceedings, 1985, p 121.

Elizabeth V. Hillyer / Susan A. Brown

Clinical Techniques

Elizabeth V. Hillyer

RESTRAINT

- Because most pet ferrets are gentle and tractable, it is possible to use *minimal restraint* when performing a physical examination; this is preferable because ferrets (like cats) are calmer on the examination table when light restraint is used.
- Use *firm restraint* to administer vaccinations and perform procedures such as ear cleaning.
  - Control the head by a circumferential grip around the caudal aspect of the mandibles, by holding the scruff of the neck, or by placing the index and middle fingers on either side of the neck so the ferret cannot turn its head. Restrain the hindquarters tightly on the table with the ferret's hind legs underneath; do not pull the legs back.
  - Alternatively, suspend the ferret in the air by the scruff (Fig. 168–1). Stroke the abdomen with a downward motion to relax the ferret. This hold has

a calming effect on most ferrets, although very young ferrets and some females may resist.
- *Aggressive* ferrets, such as nursing females, kits, or ferrets raised with little human contact, are uncommon.
  - Restrain these ferrets by the scruff of the neck, using the techniques previously described.
  - Avoid using leather gloves, which are awkward; use sedation, if necessary.

DIAGNOSTICS

Blood Collection

There are several suitable sites for blood collection in ferrets:

- Cephalic vein
- Lateral saphenous vein
- Jugular vein
- Cranial vena cava
- Ventral tail artery

Do not perform cardiac puncture or retro-orbital bleeding.

Indications

- Perform cephalic or lateral saphenous venipuncture to obtain small amounts of blood for rapid determination of packed cell volume (PCV) or blood glucose or complete blood cell count (CBC).
- Use the jugular vein, cranial vena cava, cephalic vein, or ventral tail artery for blood collection for a complete blood count (CBC) and biochemical analysis.
- Use the jugular vein to collect blood for transfusion.

Other Considerations

- Sedation:
  - Sedation rarely is required for venipuncture of cephalic, lateral saphenous, or jugular veins.
  - Collection of blood from the cranial vena cava, and occasionally from the ventral tail artery, may require sedation or the assistance of two persons for restraint in addition to the person drawing blood.
- If necessary, clip the hair over the venipuncture site to see the vein.

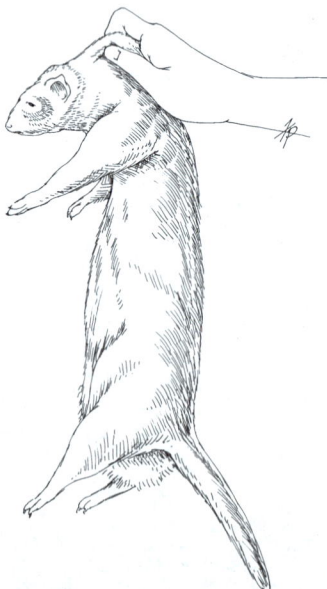

Figure 168–1. "Scruffing" a ferret for restraint.

- Because the normal hematocrit of ferrets is high, draw three times as much blood as the volume of plasma or serum required. See Tables 168–1 and 168–2 for blood values reported in normal ferrets.
- In ferrets, the PCV, red blood cell (RBC) count, hemoglobin, white blood cell (WBC) count, and plasma proteins fall rapidly after induction of isoflurane anesthesia.

Techniques

Cephalic Vein

- Collect blood from the cephalic vein in ferrets using the same restraint technique as for dogs and cats.
- Use Lo-Dose U-100 insulin syringe (Becton Dickinson, Rutherford, NJ) with a 28-gauge needle to obtain 0.3–0.4 ml of blood.
- Alternatively, place a 25-gauge needle in the vein and collect blood directly from the hub into small blood collection tubes.
- Collect a larger volume of blood, using a 25-gauge needle and 1- or 3-ml syringe.

Lateral Saphenous Vein

- The lateral saphenous vein in ferrets has the same orientation as in dogs and cats; however, it lies more distally, just proximal to the hock.
- Use a Lo-Dose insulin syringe as aforementioned to obtain a small blood sample.

Jugular Vein

- Position the ferret in sternal recumbency at the edge of the table. Extend the ferret's head dorsally with the front legs held down out of the path of the venipuncturist.
- Another technique is to wrap the ferret in a towel and position it in dorsal recumbency.
- Use a 3-ml or larger syringe with a 22- to 25-gauge needle.

Collection of Blood for Transfusion

The jugular vein is the preferred site for collection of large volumes of blood for transfusion.

Table 168–1. REFERENCE RANGES FOR HEMATOLOGIC VALUES IN FERRETS

Value	Sex	Fitch Ferrets* Range	Fitch Ferrets* Mean	Albino Ferrets† Range	Albino Ferrets† Mean
Hematocrit (%)	♂	46–57	49.1	44–61	55.4
	♀	47–51	48.4	42–55	49.2
Hemoglobin (g/dl)	♂	15.2–17.7	16.1	16.3–18.2	17.8
	♀	15.2–17.4	15.9	14.8–17.4	16.2
Red blood cells ($\times 10^6$/μl)	♂			7.30–12.18	10.23
	♀			6.77–9.76	8.11
Reticulocytes (%)	♂			1–12	4.0
	♀			2–14	5.3
White blood cells ($\times 10^3$/μl)	♂	5.6–10.8	7.3	4.4–19.1‡	9.7
	♀	2.5–8.6	5.9	4.0–18.2‡	10.5
Neutrophils	♂	616–7020/μl	2659/μl	11–82%	57.0%
	♀	725–2409/μl	1825/μl	43–84%	59.5%
Lymphocytes	♂	1728–4704/μl	3791/μl	12–54%	35.6%
	♀	1475–5590/μl	3426/μl	12–50%	33.4%
Monocytes	♂	0–432/μl	176/μl	0–9%	4.4%
	♀	100–372/μl	263/μl	2–8%	4.4%
Eosinophils	♂	112–768/μl	378/μl	0–7%	2.4%
	♀	50–516/μl	214/μl	0–5%	2.6%
Basophils	♂	0–112/μl	50/μl	0–2%	0.1%
	♀	0–172/μl	48/μl	0–1%	0.2%
Bands	♂	0–972/μl	233/μl		
	♀	0–248/μl	99/μl		
Platelets ($\times 10^3$/μl)	♂			297–730	453
	♀			310–910	545
Mean corpuscular volume (μm³)	♂				54
	♀				61
Mean corpuscular hemoglobin (pg)	♂				17.6
	♀				19.9
Mean corpuscular hemoglobin concentration (%)	♂				32.2
	♀				32.8

*Males all castrated.
†Males all intact.
‡These white blood cell counts are higher than those currently seen in clinical practice. At our laboratories, the normal white blood cell count is $3–8 \times 10^3$/μl, and most are $4–6 \times 10^3$/μl.

Adapted with permission from Lee EJ, Moore WE, Fryer HC, Minocha HC: Hematological and serum chemistry profiles of ferrets *(Mustela putorius furo)*. Lab Anim 16:133–137, 1982; and Thornton PC, Wright PA, Sacra PJ, Goodier TEW: The ferret, *Mustela putorius furo*, as a new species in toxicology. Lab Anim 13:119–124, 1979. Copyrights 1979 and 1982, Macmillan Magazines Limited.

Table 168–2. REFERENCE RANGES FOR SERUM BIOCHEMISTRY VALUES IN FERRETS

Value	Albino*	Fitch†
Total protein (g/dl)	5.1–7.4	5.3–7.2
Albumin (g/dl)	2.6–3.8	3.3–4.1
Glucose (mg/dl)	94–207	62.5–134
Fasting glucose (mg/dl)		90–125‡
Blood urea nitrogen (mg/dl)	10–45	12–43
Creatinine (mg/dl)	0.4–0.9	0.2–0.6
Sodium (mmol/L)	137–162	146–160
Potassium (mmol/L)	4.5–7.7	4.3–5.3
Chloride (mmol/L)	106–125	102–121
Calcium (mg/dl)	8.0–11.8	8.6–10.5
Phosphorus (mg/dl)	4.0–9.1	5.6–8.7
Alanine aminotransferase (U/L)		82–289 78–149§
Aspartate aminotransferase (U/L)	28–120	57–248§
Alkaline phosphatase (U/L)	9–84	30–120 31–66§
Bilirubin (mg/dl)	<1.0	0–0.1§
Cholesterol (mg/dl)	64–296	119–209§
Carbon dioxide (mmol/L)	16.5–28	16–28§

*Combined values of male (N = 40) and female (N = 24) ferrets from Thornton PC, Wright PA, Sacra PJ, Goodier TEW: The ferret, *Mustela puforius furo*, as a new species in toxicology. Lab Anim 13:119–124, 1979.

†Combined values of intact male, female, and castrated male ferrets (total N = 13, aged 4–8 mo) from Lee EJ, Moore WE, Fryer HC, Minocha HC: Haematological and serum chemistry profiles of ferrets (*Mustela putorius furo*). Lab Anim. 16:133–137, 1982, except where noted.

‡From Brown S: Personal communication, 1995.

§Combined values from cardiac and orbital venipuncture of male ferrets (N = 16) from Fox JG: Normal clinical and biologic parameters. In: Fox JG (ed): Biology and Diseases of the Ferret. Philadelphia: Lea & Febiger, 1988, pp 159–173.

- Although the normal blood volume of ferrets has not been reported, a conservative estimate is 60 ml/kg. Therefore, it is safe to draw 12 ml/kg from healthy ferrets.
- Sedate and place the donor ferret in dorsal recumbency.
- Using a butterfly catheter, collect the blood into a syringe with acid-citrate-dextrose (ACD) solution added as an anticoagulant (1.0 ml of ACD per 6 ml of blood).
- Transfer the blood immediately to the recipient.

Cranial Vena Cava

▼ *Key Point* Blood collection from the cranial vena cava requires complete immobilization of the ferret; otherwise, do not attempt the procedure.

- Use sedation or the help of two assistants for restraint.
- Do not use this site if intrathoracic disease (e.g., mediastinal mass, mega-esophagus) is suspected.

Technique
1. Place the ferret in dorsal recumbency with one assistant holding its head and neck extended and the forelegs caudally against the body and a sec-

ond assistant holding the hindquarters without pulling the rear legs back. Precise positioning facilitates the procedure.
2. Palpate the manubrium and locate the notch on both sides between the manubrium and the first rib.
3. Using a 3-ml syringe with a 25-gauge, ⅝-inch needle, enter the skin at either notch and direct the needle at a shallow angle toward the opposite hip.
4. Insert the needle, then locate the vein by gently aspirating while withdrawing the needle.

Ventral Tail Artery

Technique
1. Place the ferret in dorsal recumbency and prepare the site aseptically. Wrapping it in a towel may help with restraint. Venipuncture at this site may be painful.
2. Using a 22- to 25-gauge needle, collect 1–3 ml of blood from the artery that runs along the ventral midline of the tail.
3. Insert the needle approximately 2–3 cm from the anus and direct the needle toward the body at a 30° angle to the skin.
4. Gently insert the needle to the bone; withdraw it slowly while applying a slight vacuum to the syringe.

Radiography

- Use standard radiographic techniques. Sedation may be necessary for correct positioning. High detail radiography is recommended.
- When interpreting films, it helps to consider the ferret an "elongated cat."
- The kidneys are relatively short (about two lumbar vertebrae in length).
- Splenomegaly is a common radiographic finding.
- For barium-contrast radiography of the gastrointestinal (GI) tract, give 15 ml/kg of a 20% barium solution PO by syringe or by gavage tube. Normal GI transit time is about 3–4 hours.

Ultrasound

- Echocardiography is used to evaluate the heart in ferrets with suspected cardiac disease (see section on Cardiovascular Diseases).
- Other uses of ultrasound in ferrets, as in dogs and cats, include investigation of intra-abdominal or intrathoracic masses or organomegaly and paraurethral prostatic cysts.

Bone Marrow Aspiration

- The indications, guidelines, and techniques for bone marrow sampling are the same as for dogs and cats.
- Potential sites include the iliac crest, proximal femur, and humerus; the first two sites are preferable.
- After sedating the animal, use a 20- or 22-gauge spinal needle with stylet to aspirate the bone marrow.

Splenic Aspiration

Fine-needle aspiration of the spleen is a rapid means of evaluating splenic cytology. In ferrets, as in dogs, the only contraindication is suspected hemangiosarcoma of the spleen. The procedure has been performed successfully in ferrets. Sedation is rarely necessary.

Techniques

1. Place the ferret in dorsal recumbency.
2. Palpate the spleen and position it against the ventral or left lateral body wall.
3. Clip and prepare the site aseptically.
4. Using a 25-gauge needle attached to a 3-ml syringe, enter perpendicular to the skin and aspirate from the spleen.
5. When a small amount of bloody fluid is seen in the needle hub, withdraw the needle and prepare slides routinely for cytology.

Cystocentesis

- Use the same technique as for cats; a 25-gauge needle is preferable.

THERAPEUTIC TECHNIQUES

Intravenous Therapy

- For *small-volume* (0.3–0.4 ml) intravenous therapy, use a Lo-Dose insulin syringe and inject into the cephalic or lateral saphenous vein. Sedation rarely is needed for a single injection.
- A *butterfly catheter* can be used to administer larger, single volumes into the cephalic vein.
- An *indwelling catheter* can be placed in the cephalic, lateral saphenous, or jugular vein. Sedation may be necessary.
  - Because of the ferret's small size, flush with small volumes of heparinized saline solution to keep the catheter patent.
- *Peripheral catheters* can be placed more rapidly than jugular catheters and are useful in emergency situations and for surgery.

Technique for IV Catheter

1. Clip and prepare the site aseptically.
2. Tent the skin over the vein and make a small hole in the skin with a 22-gauge needle, taking care to avoid the vein.
3. Insert a short, indwelling catheter (20–24 gauge) through the hole and into the vein and tape it in place routinely.

- Placement of a *jugular catheter* generally requires sedation.
- Place the ferret in dorsal recumbency and clip and prepare the site aseptically. Make a small skin hole over the jugular vein as described previously.
- Either a short or long catheter can be used; 20-gauge or smaller is suitable.
- Ferrets often poorly tolerate jugular catheters.

Intraosseous Catheters

- An intraosseous catheter placed in the proximal femur is useful for fluid therapy. See Supplemental Readings.

Subcutaneous and Intramuscular Injections

- Administer subcutaneous and intramuscular injections in the same sites and using the same techniques as for dogs and cats. A scruff hold often facilitates administration.

Fluid Therapy

- The daily fluid requirement for ferrets has not been reported but can be estimated at roughly 70–100 ml/kg/day. Adjust for dehydration and fluid loss.
- Administer fluids SC over the dorsal cervical and thoracic region.
- Intravenous therapy in the ferret is used in a wide range of medical and surgical situations.

Blood Transfusions

- Indications for blood transfusions in ferrets are the same as for dogs and cats (see Chap. 20). Calculate the required blood transfusion volume using the same formula.
- Draw blood for transfusion purposes from the jugular vein of the donor (described earlier) and transfer immediately to the recipient.
  - As many as three transfusions from the same donor, as well as transfusions from multiple donors, are considered safe; blood groups have not been identified in ferrets.
- Administer fresh blood transfusions through an indwelling catheter or via a butterfly catheter into the cephalic or jugular vein. If a vein is inaccessible, administer into the peritoneal cavity or via the intraosseous route into the proximal femur.
  - Before transfusion, give a rapid-acting corticosteroid, such as dexamethasone sodium phosphate, 6–8 mg/kg once, IV, or prednisolone sodium succinate (Solu-Delta-Cortef; Upjohn), 22 mg/kg once, IV, as a slow bolus infusion.

Oral Therapy

- Oral medications are most easily given to ferrets in liquid form.
- Crush medications formulated only in tablet or capsule form and mix with a sweet-tasting substance, such as Nutri-Cal (Evsco Pharmaceuticals), feline hairball laxative, or fruit-flavored syrup, and administer by syringe. Ferrets suffering from insulinoma should not be given sugar-based treats or medications if at all possible.
- Alternatively, hide medications in fatty acid supplements, vegetable oil, whipping cream, or meat baby food.

Nutritional Support

- Most ferrets must be force-fed dietary supplements by syringe. Once they acquire a taste for a given supplement, it may be possible to offer it in a bowl.

- When indicated, give nutritional support as an adjunct to specific medical therapy.
- Foods useful for force-feeding include the following: high-energy paste supplements (e.g., Nutri-Cal; use only for ≤1 day); liquid soy-based formulas (e.g., Deliver 2.0, Mead Johnson Nutritionals); meat baby food; moistened, slurried cat or ferret food; whipping cream; and Science Diet A/D.

Drug-Dosing Guidelines

- Use feline dosages (scaled down for size) to calculate most drug dosages in ferrets, with the following exceptions:
  - Give chloramphenicol at a dose of 50 mg/kg q12h, IV, SC, IM, or PO.
  - Give aspirin at a dose of 10–25 mg/kg q8–24h (canine dosage).
  - Most ferrets can become lethargic on enalapril (Enacard, Merck Agvet). Start with a very low dose, such as 0.5 mg/kg q48h PO. Some ferrets cannot tolerate more than every-other-day therapy with enalapril.
  - Give ivermectin at a dose of 0.006 mg/kg q30d PO—heartworm prevention; 0.5 mg/kg—heartworm microfilaricide, 3–4 weeks after adulticide treatment; 0.50–1.0 mg/kg PO, SC, topically—for sarcoptic mites, repeat in 14 days; for otodectes, apply topically in ears and repeat in 14 days.

Urinary Catheterization

Sedation or isoflurane anesthesia facilitates urinary catheterization. The procedure may be difficult in ferrets with urethral disease.

- Position females in ventral recumbency with the hindquarters elevated and use a tomcat or #3.5-Fr. feeding catheter with or without stylet. Catheterize the urethra blindly or after identification using a vaginal speculum.
- To catheterize a male ferret, use an open-ended tomcat catheter, a small-gauge canine urinary catheter, a feeding catheter (#3.5 Fr), or a short, small-gauge IV catheter. A wire stylet may be useful. Prolapse the penis and find the urethral opening, which lies ventral to the tip of the penis.
  - In ferrets with urethral disease, usually the catheter passes only part way into the urethra (often to the pelvic flexure). This may be sufficient to allow retrograde flushing of urethral calculi into the bladder or to empty the bladder of a ferret with urethral obstruction secondary to prostatic enlargement.

Sedation

Doses for injectable agents used in ferrets are listed in Table 168–3.

- Acepromazine is useful for sedation. A combination of ketamine and acepromazine is effective and safe

Table 168–3. DRUGS RECOMMENDED FOR CHEMICAL RESTRAINT AND ANALGESIA OF FERRETS

Drug	Dosage (mg/kg)	Route
Chemical Restraint		
Acepromazine	0.1–0.3	IM, SC
Ketamine	25–35	IM, SC
plus acepromazine*	0.2–0.3	
Ketamine	25–35	IM
plus diazepam	2–3	
Ketamine	10–25	IM
plus xylazine	1–2	
Analgesics		
Buprenorphene	0.01–0.03 mg/kg q8–12h	SC, IM, IV
Butorphanol tartrate	0.05–5.0 mg/kg q8–12h	SC, IM
Carprofen	1 mg/kg q12–24h	PO
Flunixin meglumine	0.5–2.0 mg/kg q12–24h	IM, IV

*Use this combination for minor surgery.
IM, intramuscular; SC, subcutaneous.

for minor surgery. Ketamine alone does not produce effective muscle relaxation.
- A tiletamine-zolazepam preparation (Telazol, Fort Dodge) gives variable muscle relaxation but is useful for immobilization for procedures such as venipuncture, radiography, and electrocardiography.
- Isoflurane administered (Aerrane, Anaquest) by face mask is the most convenient method to immobilize a ferret for procedures such as venipuncture and radiography. Induction and recovery are rapid.

Anesthesia

- Isoflurane and halothane are useful gas anesthetics for surgery. Isoflurane is preferred because of more rapid induction and recovery and greater safety for human handlers.
- Use chamber or face-mask induction followed by endotracheal intubation.
- A 2.5–3.5 mm endotracheal tube usually is suitable.
  - Follow basic principles of anesthesia for small animals, and provide supplemental heat during surgery; administer an IV drip with isotonic electrolyte solution supplemented with 2.5% dextrose during long procedures and for insulinoma surgery.

Infectious Diseases of the Ferret

Susan A. Brown

VIRAL DISEASES

Canine distemper and influenza are the two most common viral diseases in the ferret. Influenza is transmissible between humans and ferrets. Canine distemper is nearly 100% fatal in the ferret; distemper vaccination of ferrets is imperative.

Canine Distemper

Etiology

Canine distemper virus (CDV), a large RNA paramyxovirus, can be transmitted to ferrets directly from affected animals of any species and through contact with fomites such as in shoes or clothing. The normal incubation period for CDV in the ferret is 7–10 days; however, incubation for some strains of CDV may take up to 21 days. For discussion of CDV in dogs, see Chapter 11.

Clinical Signs

- Early in the disease the only sign may be a mild conjunctivitis, either unilateral or bilateral.
- As the disease progresses, signs include a high fever (>40°C), anorexia, and profuse mucopurulent naso-ocular discharge.

▼ *Key Point* Ferrets develop a distinct pattern of thickening and crusting of the integument of the chin and lips and a pronounced hyperkeratosis of the footpads. Crusting also may include the rectal and inguinal area.

- Other signs include central nervous system (CNS) disturbances, diarrhea, and severe depression.

Diagnosis

▼ *Key Point* Diagnosis of CDV is based primarily on the signs, which are unlike those of any other disease in the ferret.

- Differential diagnoses early in the disease include influenza and bacterial conjunctivitis. Once the disease has progressed, concurrent integumentary lesions around the chin and lips are pathognomonic.
- The history usually reveals that the animal is unvaccinated, improperly vaccinated, or overdue for booster vaccination. There may be no evidence of direct exposure to another affected animal because fomite transmission can occur.
- Physical examination findings include the clinical signs previously described.
- A fluorescent antibody test can detect CDV antigen in blood smears and conjunctival scrapings, but it is a moderately insensitive test.

Treatment

▼ *Key Point* Treatment for canine distemper is rarely effective. Euthanize all but very mild cases.

- In a multiple animal household, remove all clinically affected animals. Vaccinate the remaining animals immediately.
- Disinfect the household thoroughly using 0.2% Roccal (Upjohn), 0.75% phenol, or 2–5% sodium hydroxide.

Prevention

▼ *Key Point* Vaccination is the most effective prevention for canine distemper in ferrets.

- Vaccinate all ferrets in the household or facility using an attenuated canine distemper vaccine of chick embryo tissue culture origin. FerVac-D (United Vaccine) is the only USDA-approved vaccine for ferrets at the time of this writing. Give 1 ml, SC, using the following schedule:
  - If the dam is vaccinated, vaccinate the kit initially at 8 weeks of age and repeat vaccination every 3–4 weeks until the kit is 16 weeks of age.
  - If the dam is unvaccinated, vaccinate the kit initially at 6 weeks of age and repeat as aforementioned.
- Revaccinate annually. Although some sources claim immunity for 3 years, outbreaks have been known to occur 18 months after vaccination.
- Alternately, check serum distemper virus titers to determine the need to revaccinate.
- Do not use CDV vaccines that contain parvovirus, adenovirus, or other viruses because the ferret is not susceptible to these diseases. Also, it is not necessary to vaccinate for leptospirosis unless there is exposure to wild rodents.
- Vaccinate any new animals brought into a facility or household containing ferrets immediately and quarantine for 4 weeks before exposure to the other animals.

Influenza

Etiology

The domestic ferret is susceptible to the same influenza viral strains that affect humans. Influenza virus from affected humans and other ferrets can infect ferrets by contact with naso-ocular discharges and inhalation of aerosolized droplets. Ferrets can transmit influenza to humans.

Clinical Signs

▼ *Key Point* Influenza generally causes only mild illness and discomfort in ferrets and is self-limiting in an otherwise healthy animal.

- Clinical signs are essentially the same as in humans with influenza and include any combination of the following:
  - Sneezing with a clear, serous nasal discharge
  - Mild conjunctivitis with serous ocular discharge and, rarely, crusting around the eyes
  - Nonproductive coughing that occurs more frequently at night and may be loud and paroxysmal.
  - Diarrhea and, rarely, vomiting
  - Listlessness, fever, and poor appetite (rarely, anorexia)
- The clinical course of the disease is 7–14 days.

- Severe illness or death may occur in neonates and in ferrets with concurrent immunosuppressive disease such as lymphosarcoma.
- Evaluate ferrets that have repeat influenza episodes for lymphosarcoma with a CBC and peripheral lymph node biopsy.

Diagnosis

Diagnosis is based primarily on the history and physical examination.

- Differential diagnoses include the very early stages of canine distemper, GI rotavirus infection, and lymphosarcoma.
- The history usually indicates recent exposure to a human or another ferret with influenza (the incubation period is 2–10 days).
- Physical examination reveals the clinical signs previously described.
- The overall physical condition remains good, although slight or moderate dehydration may be present if the animal is not eating or drinking normal amounts.
- If mucopurulent ocular or nasal discharge is noted, consider early CDV or a secondary bacterial infection.

Treatment

- *Supportive care* generally is sufficient.
  - Encourage the ferret to eat and drink. Offer strained meat baby food or Science Diet A/D if the animal refuses the regular diet.
  - If indicated, give an oral electrolyte solution that is palatable to ferrets.
- If sneezing or coughing is excessive and interferes with eating or sleeping, give an *antihistamine* such as chlorpheniramine, 1.0–2.0 mg/kg q8–12h PO, or diphenhydramine, 0.5–2.0 mg/kg q8–12h PO.
- Antibiotics are *not* necessary unless secondary bacterial infection is present.

Prevention

Good hygiene is the key to prevention.

- If influenza is present in ferrets or humans, advise clients to wash their hands frequently and to avoid holding the ferret near the face because transmission can occur in either direction.
- In the veterinary hospital, do not allow influenza-infected personnel to handle ferrets, especially if the animal is debilitated by serious disease.

Rabies

Etiology

Rabies is caused by a rhabdovirus that results in a fatal disease in ferrets. It is transmitted through contact with an infected animal's saliva (see Chap. 13).

Clinical Signs

▼ *Key Point* Very little is known about rabies in naturally infected ferrets.

It is known that ferrets may become naturally infected; however, there is some question about how easily they can contract the disease and the length of the incubation period. Information about clinical signs is derived primarily from experiments with laboratory-infected ferrets. Signs are variable and include:

- Behavioral abnormalities that range from hyperactivity and anxiety to lethargy
- Posterior paresis

Diagnosis

Diagnosis is based on a history of known or potential exposure to rabies and clinical signs.

- Euthanize the suspect animal to protect humans and other animals in its environment.
- Differential diagnoses include brain hypoxia from severe seizures, insulinoma, Aleutian disease, intervertebral disc disease, and botulism.
- History may include possible exposure to a rabid animal.
- The ferret usually is unvaccinated; however, vaccination breaks have been known to occur in other species.
- The physical examination reveals the clinical signs previously described.
- Postmortem laboratory testing confirms the diagnosis by examination of the brain tissue with fluorescent antibody staining (FAS) or virus isolation, as in dogs and cats (see Chap. 13).

Treatment

- There is no treatment for rabies.
- Euthanize a clinically ill animal suspected to have rabies and have the brain examined as previously described.

▼ *Key Point* Most public health facilities now recognize and accept the 10-day quarantine period. It has *not* been demonstrated by the most recent research that ferrets are *carriers* of rabies.

Prevention

- Vaccination is the only prevention. Immunity is excellent.
- Administer Imrab 3 (Rhone Merieux), an inactivated rabies vaccine approved for use in ferrets, at a dose of 1 ml SC.
- Vaccinate initially at 3 months of age and revaccinate annually.

Aleutian Disease

Etiology

Several strains of a parvovirus known as the Aleutian disease virus (ADV) affect both mink and ferrets. Transmission is by direct contact or through fomites contaminated with any infected body fluid, including blood.

ADV produces a progressive immune complex-mediated disease with antigen-antibody complex deposition in various organs of the body. The lesions caused by these deposits include inflammation and lymphocyte and plasma cell infiltration of tissues.

The disease is prevalent in the ferret population, but the percentage of ferrets in which clinically evident illness develops is low. In a survey of 700 ferrets, 10% were serologically positive, but only two animals developed clinically active disease. Some ferrets may have natural immunity to the disease.

Clinical Signs

▼ *Key Point* The clinical signs of Aleutian disease are extremely variable, and the incubation period can be as long as 200 days. Some ferrets become asymptomatic carriers.

- Posterior paresis may be the initial presenting sign. Initially, the ferret appears bright and alert. As the disease progresses, the paresis affects the forelimbs, and wasting occurs that may continue for weeks or even months.
- Dark, tarry stools; lethargy; and urinary incontinence are seen in later stages of the disease.
- Appetite is not lost unless the ferret is severely debilitated.
- A slow wasting disease exists without neurologic signs in ferrets.

Diagnosis

- Diagnosis is based primarily on clinical signs and a positive ADV test result.
- Differential diagnoses include lymphosarcoma, gastric foreign body, tuberculosis, intervertebral disc disease, systemic mycoses, and rabies (in cases with behavioral changes and sudden paralysis).
- The history is of little value because the presence of asymptomatic carriers makes it difficult to detect specific exposure to the disease.
- The physical examination reveals the signs previously described.
- FAS serum is the test of choice for antemortem diagnosis. The FAS technique developed for ADV in mink appears to be accurate for diagnosis in ferrets.
  - This test may be used in clinically normal animals for detection of inapparent carriers, but false-positive and false-negative results are possible occasionally. Retesting in 2 to 4 weeks is necessary in suspected cases.
- Serum protein electrophoresis may demonstrate hypergammaglobulinemia > 20% of the total serum protein.
- Histopathology, particularly of the kidney, liver, lymph nodes, and spleen, shows lymphocytic plasmacytic infiltration and perivascular cuffing.

Treatment

▼ *Key Point* There is no effective treatment for Aleutian disease. Euthanasia is recommended for most clinically affected animals. However, healthy animals that test FAS-positive do not need to be euthanized because they may never become clinically ill.

- Corticosteroid therapy and supportive care have prolonged the life of some ADV-infected ferrets, but clinically active disease is invariably fatal.

Prevention

- Breeding colonies
  - Test all ferrets and remove serologically positive animals from the population.
  - Quarantine and test any new additions.
  - Because of potentially long incubation period, retest ADV-negative animals in 6 months before adding them to the colony.
- Pets
  - It is not necessary to test a ferret kept as a pet unless it has been exposed to a clinically ill animal.
  - Retest ADV-positive animals in 6 months because occasionally a positive result may revert to a negative titer.
  - It is unnecessary to euthanize an ADV-positive nonbreeding ferret or remove it from contact with other ferrets if it is clinically normal. Advise the client, however, that there is a slight possibility that the pet may become clinically ill.
- Do not house ferrets in close proximity to mink.

Rotavirus

Rotavirus infects the GI tract and causes a bright green or yellowish-green diarrhea. Rotavirus is described under Gastrointestinal System in this chapter.

Lymphosarcoma

A viral agent is being sought for this disease, and it is discussed elsewhere in this chapter.

BACTERIAL DISEASES

Common Bacterial Infections

Etiology

Staphylococcus, Streptococcus, Escherichia coli, and other common bacteria from the environment can be introduced through penetrating wounds, punctures, abrasions, and contact with mucous membranes by inhalation or ingestion.

- Abscessation is an uncommon form of bacterial infection in ferrets. An abscess may occur in any part of the body, including the subcutis, mouth, vagina, anal glands, prostatic tissue, and mucous membranes.
- Deeper infections may occur in the uterus, mammary tissue, and lungs, primarily from *E. coli.*

Clinical Signs

- Body temperature may be greater than 40°C in bacterial sepsis.

- The total WBC count may be greatly elevated (>10,000).
- Bacterial vaginitis causes a thick mucopurulent yellow-to-green vaginal discharge with little odor. Fever is absent, and the animal does not appear systemically ill.
- Bacterial metritis may or may not cause a vaginal discharge; depression, fever, and partial or total anorexia are present.
- Bacterial mastitis causes depression, fever, and anorexia. One or more mammary glands are swollen, discolored, and warm to the touch. Mastitis occurs primarily in the lactating female.
- Bacterial pneumonia causes lethargy, fever, anorexia, and eventually dyspnea, sometimes accompanied by mucopurulent nasal discharge and coughing.
- Bacterial conjunctivitis causes a thick mucopurulent ocular discharge and swelling of the conjunctiva; corneal ulcerations may be present.
- Bacterial dermatitis causes thickened, irritated areas of skin. The ferret frequently licks and chews at these areas until they become denuded and ulcerated.

Diagnosis

- Diagnosis is based primarily on clinical signs and demonstration of bacteria on routine bacterial cultures.

Treatment

- Treatment consists of appropriate antibiotic therapy and, if necessary, surgical drainage or excision of the affected tissue.
- Initially, before culture and sensitivity testing results are available, or when obtaining a culture is not feasible, use a broad-spectrum antibiotic.
- Provide supportive treatment as needed, such as fluid therapy and nutritional support.

Specific Treatment

Abscesses

- Lance and thoroughly flush *cutaneous abscesses* with an antiseptic solution. Keep the area open and flush twice daily until healing by second intention occurs.
  - Administer oral antibiotics for 7–10 days.

Mastitis

- Infected mammary glands frequently require surgical removal.
  - If the jill continues to lactate, leave the kits with her, supplementing them with a milk replacer if necessary. Fostering the kits with another jill may result in mastitis in the foster jill.
  - Give oral antibiotics to the affected female and apply hot packs to the abdominal area two or three times daily for 2 days.
  - If there is no clinical response to medical therapy, consider surgical removal of the affected mammary tissue. Because of potential for severe toxicity and life-threatening disease, do not delay sur-

gery if there is no improvement with medical therapy.
  - Do not breed females with a history of mastitis.
- To prevent abrasions to mammary tissue and nipples that can cause *mastitis,* provide an opening with smooth edges into the nest box that is large enough for the ferret to pass through easily.

Uterine Infections

- For *metritis* and *pyometra,* perform ovariohysterectomy.

Pneumonia

- For *pneumonia,* start oral antibiotic therapy immediately.
  - If possible, first perform a tracheal culture.
  - If pleural effusion is evident on radiography, perform thoracic aspiration for culture and sensitivity testing and cytology.

Conjunctivitis

- For *conjunctivitis,* use a broad-spectrum ophthalmic ointment.
  - Perform fluorescent corneal stain tests to detect corneal ulcers.

Anal Gland Infection

- For *anal gland infection,* initially give oral antibiotics for 3–7 days until the swelling subsides, then excise both anal glands.

Campylobacteriosis Infection

- *Campylobacter* organisms primarily cause GI disease (see Gastrointestinal System in this chapter).

Salmonellosis

Salmonella organisms are gram-negative bacteria that rarely cause gastroenteritis in ferrets (see Salmonella under Gastrointestinal System in this chapter).

Botulism

- Botulism is a rarely encountered disease in the domestic ferret caused by the ingestion of food contaminated with the *Clostridium botulinum* toxin. *C. botulinum* is commonly found in the soil.
- Food contaminated with soil or uncooked food can be the source of the infection.

Tuberculosis

- Clinical cases of tuberculosis in the ferret are reported infrequently; however, ferrets are susceptible to bovine, avian, and human *Mycobacterium tuberculosis* infections.
- The disease can be transmitted by ingestion of contaminated meat (poultry or beef) or milk, or by con-

tamination of food from the droppings of infected wild or pet birds (see Chap. 17 for information about tuberculosis in dogs and cats).

FUNGAL INFECTIONS

Dermatomycoses

Etiology

Microsporum canis and *Trichophyton mentagrophytes* are the most common causes of superficial mycotic infections in ferrets. Dermatophytes are transmitted by direct contact with infected animals or contaminated bedding, caging, and other materials.

▼ *Key Point* Ferrets usually are not carriers of these organisms; the most common source of infection of the pet ferret is the household cat.

Clinical Signs

Like other species, young ferrets are infected more commonly than mature ferrets.

- The lesions are consistent with those seen in other species (see Chap. 37). Circular areas of alopecia are thickened, scaly, and inflamed and may be pruritic.

Diagnosis

- Diagnosis is based on the identification of the fungal agent on skin scrapings, fungal culture, or a positive Wood's light examination (see Chap. 37).

Treatment

- Dermatomycosis usually is self-limiting and resolves without therapy.
- In refractory cases, treat with lime-sulfur dips weekly and give griseofulvin (Fulvicin, Schering), 25 mg/kg q24h, PO (see Chap. 37 for details of management of dermatophyte infections).

Other Fungal Infections

Blastomycosis, histoplasmosis, cryptococcosis, coccidioidomycosis, and aspergillosis have been reported in domestic ferrets but are rare diseases in this species.

- Consider these infections in the differential diagnosis of any systemic disease that involves wasting, granulomatous lesions, persistent or recurring draining wound tracts, and chronic respiratory disease refractory to treatment.
- Diagnosis is based on the demonstration of the fungal organism by histopathology or cytology from biopsies or aspirates (see Chap. 18).
- Complement fixation and precipitation tests have been used with varying success.
- Treatment is the same as described for the dog and cat (see Chap. 18).

Hematopoietic System

Elizabeth V. Hillyer

SPLENOMEGALY

The spleen is readily palpable in most ferrets, and splenomegaly (enlarged spleen) is a frequent finding. Splenomegaly can be an incidental finding in an otherwise healthy animal, or it may occur in association with a wide variety of nonsplenic disease conditions.

▼ *Key Point* Splenomegaly is a common finding in ferrets and may be associated with other diseases. Primary disease of the spleen is uncommon. Perform a complete medical evaluation in all splenomegaly cases.

Etiology

- It is not known why splenomegaly develops so commonly in ferrets.
- Splenic histopathology in most cases reveals extramedullary hematopoiesis (also seen in normal spleens) and congestion. Neoplasia is less common but is usually lymphoma when it occurs.
- Splenomegaly can occur in conjunction with infectious, endocrine, and systemic conditions including (but not restricted to) influenza, enteritis, GI obstruction, cardiomyopathy, insulinoma, and adrenal tumors. The relation between splenomegaly and these diseases is uncertain.
- Idiopathic hypersplenism has been reported but is rare.

Clinical Signs

- Clinical signs usually result from the primary disease condition; for example, ferrets with insulinoma and splenomegaly have signs referable to the insulinoma.
- Abdominal discomfort due to splenomegaly, which occurs in dogs, is uncommon in ferrets.
- Abdominal distention may occur.

Diagnosis

- Diagnosis is based on evaluation of the spleen in addition to a search for other diseases.
- Monitor asymptomatic ferrets with splenomegaly with periodic CBC evaluation and splenic aspiration.

Differential Diagnosis

- Perform a CBC and platelet count to evaluate for cytopenia(s), which may accompany lymphoma or other neoplasia.
  - There is one reported case of idiopathic hypersplenism in ferrets.
- Perform a fine-needle aspiration of the spleen using a 25-gauge needle and submit it for cytologic evaluation (see Clinical Techniques in this chapter).

- Do not perform splenic aspiration if splenic *hemangiosarcoma* is suspected; however, this is rare in ferrets.
- The choice of other tests depends on the clinical signs and includes serum biochemical profile, fasting blood glucose assay, urinalysis, serum insulin assay, thoracic and abdominal radiography, echocardiography, abdominal ultrasonography, and bone marrow aspiration.
- Perform a splenic biopsy during abdominal exploratory surgery, particularly if the spleen is irregular or discolored.

Treatment

Treatment depends on the primary disease condition. Usually splenectomy is *not* necessary.

- Indications for splenectomy are the same as for other species and include hypersplenism, splenitis, splenic abscess, torsion, rupture, neoplasia, and discomfort caused by excessive splenic size.
- To perform splenectomy, follow the surgical guidelines for splenectomy in dogs and cats (see Chap. 23).
- Administer antibiotics and fluid therapy pre- and postoperatively.

ANEMIA

The clinical approach to anemia in ferrets is the same as for other species. Anemias are classified as regenerative or nonregenerative; treatment is aimed at the specific cause.

Etiology

There are many causes of anemia in ferrets, as in other companion animal species.

- *Regenerative anemias* usually are the result of blood loss or hemolysis.
  - The most common causes of blood loss in ferrets are trauma, external parasites such as fleas, and GI bleeding due to ulcers, foreign bodies, or enteritis/colitis.
  - Hemolysis is rare. Theoretically, lead or zinc toxicity can cause hemolysis in ferrets. Autoimmune diseases are not documented and would be difficult to diagnose because of lack of ferret-specific reagents.
- *Nonregenerative anemia* occurs when bone marrow hematopoiesis is disrupted.

▼ *Key Point* The most common cause of nonregenerative anemia in ferrets is estrogen toxicity due to persistent estrus. Ferrets are very sensitive to estrogen myelotoxicity, which can occur from 4 weeks after the onset of estrus. An estrogen-secreting ovarian remnant or adrenal tumor also may cause estrogen toxicity. All cell lines are affected, resulting in anemia, leukopenia, and thrombocytopenia.

Anemia is worsened because of bleeding from thrombocytopenia.

- Bone marrow infiltration by neoplastic cells (e.g., in lymphoma) can result in nonregenerative anemia.
- Anemia of chronic disease is seen in ferrets. Potential causes are similar to those in other species.

Clinical Signs

Clinical signs include weakness, lethargy, and inappetence.

- A swollen vulva is present in ferrets with persistent estrus and in some cases of adrenal neoplasia (see Neoplasia in this chapter).
- An observant owner may report melena if GI bleeding is present.

Diagnosis

▼ *Key Point* Anemia in an intact female ferret with a swollen vulva for more than 4 weeks most likely is due to estrogen toxicity.

History

- Obtain a careful history regarding possible blood loss, toxicity, and foreign body ingestion. Determine the duration of vulvar swelling (if present).

Physical Examination

- Mucous membranes are pale; jaundice may be seen with hemolysis.
- A soft systolic murmur is common in anemic ferrets.
- Examine females for a swollen vulva, an external indication of estrus, or elevated serum estrogens.
- Ferrets with estrogen toxicity also have signs of thrombocytopenia such as petechiae, ecchymoses, and melena. When anemia is severe, it usually is the result of blood loss from thrombocytopenia.
- Hair loss is common, especially on the shoulders and flanks in hyperestrogenism.
- Palpate the spleen. Splenomegaly may indicate hypersplenism and subsequent anemia.
- Check carefully for fleas.

Laboratory Studies

- Evaluate the packed cell volume (PCV) and RBCs on a peripheral blood smear as a minimum data base. If possible, obtain a CBC, platelet count, and reticulocyte count.
- If the anemia is not too severe, draw blood for serum biochemical analysis to check for chronic renal or metabolic disease. (Remember that less blood is needed to get a given amount of serum because of the lower PCV.)
- Perform bone marrow aspiration (see Clinical Techniques in this chapter), particularly if the anemia is nonregenerative, to identify infiltrative processes and assess the morphology of RBC precursors.

- Draw a blood lead level if lead poisoning is suspected.

Radiography

Consider:

- Thoracic radiography to identify intrathoracic neoplasia
- Abdominal radiography if intra-abdominal neoplasia or GI bleeding or obstruction is suspected
- Abdominal ultrasonography to diagnose an adrenal tumor

Treatment

The objectives of treatment are:

- Treat the anemia
- Treat the cause of the anemia

General Treatment of Anemia

- Give supportive care such as oxygen therapy, subcutaneous fluids, and nutritional supplementation.
- Provide oral iron supplementation.
- Treatment with erythropoietin may stimulate erythropoiesis in ferrets with poorly regenerative anemia. Administer 50–150 U/kg SC 3 times per week until desired PCV is reached, then administer once weekly as necessary.
- Use standard criteria to determine whether a blood transfusion is necessary (i.e., status of the patient, acuteness of blood loss, PCV). Consider a transfusion if the PCV is less than 15% (see Clinical Techniques in this chapter for blood transfusion techniques).

Treatment of the Cause of Anemia

- Arrest external bleeding.
- Treat fleas with any product that is safe for use in cats (see Chap. 40).
- Correct the underlying cause of GI bleeding, including medical therapy for GI ulceration (see Gastrointestinal System in this chapter), surgery to remove GI foreign body, and antibiotics and supportive care for enteritis/colitis.
- Treat lead poisoning after the same protocols recommended for cats (see Chap. 20).
- For diagnosis and treatment of adrenal tumors, see discussion of neoplasia in ferrets.
- Anemia secondary to neoplasia is associated with a poor prognosis. Some cases of lymphoma may respond to treatment (see Neoplasia in this chapter).
- For anemia of chronic disease, treat the underlying primary disease process.
- To correct estrogen toxicity, terminate estrus and provide supportive care until the bone marrow is functional. Broad-spectrum antibiotic therapy is important for control of sepsis in leukopenic patients.

▼ *Key Point* In ferrets with estrogen myelotoxicity, ovariohysterectomy can be performed to terminate

estrus if the PCV and platelet count are adequate; however, the safest method is hormonal stimulation of ovulation.

Termination of Estrus

- Administer human chorionic gonadotropin (hCG) in a single injection of 100 IU (or 1000 USP), IM. Repeat this dose in 1–2 weeks if vulvar swelling has not diminished.
- Alternatively, give gonadotropin-releasing hormone (GnRH) at a dose of 20 μg, IM or SC; repeat in 2 weeks if necessary.
- GnRH and hCG are effective only after the 10th day of estrus. Bone marrow toxicity is not immediately reversible with termination of estrus; the PCV continues to fall for a few days to weeks.
- Monitor the PCV as a useful guide to therapy and prognosis:
  - PCV > 25%—the prognosis is good and termination of estrus is the only therapy required.
  - PCV 15–25%—the prognosis is guarded because the PCV level can decrease further after termination of estrus.
  - PCV < 15%—the prognosis is poor, and aggressive supportive care is indicated, including multiple blood transfusions until bone marrow function is restored.

Prevention

- Some causes of anemia in ferrets can be prevented. Instruct owners about proper husbandry techniques to avoid trauma, foreign body ingestion, and flea infestation.

▼ *Key Point* To prevent estrogen myelotoxicity, spay all female ferrets not used for breeding.

Neoplasia

Elizabeth V. Hillyer / Susan A. Brown

INSULINOMA

Insulinoma, or pancreatic beta-cell tumor, is one of the most common tumors in ferrets, particularly in those that are 2–7 years of age. Adrenal neoplasia (discussed later) is found concurrently in most of these animals.

Etiology

The cause(s) of the high incidence of insulinomas in ferrets is unknown.

- Possible etiologies include genetics (ferrets in the United States come from a small gene pool) and diet.

Histology

- Histologic examination may reveal multiple tissue changes including hyperplasia, adenoma, and adenocarcinoma of beta cells, even within a single tissue specimen.

Clinical Signs

- Episodic lethargy, depression, "stargazing," and posterior paresis may be seen during periods of hypoglycemia. Because various counter-regulatory mechanisms compensate for hypoglycemia, early signs may be subtle and transient.
  - As the disease progresses, and in periods of inadequate feeding, signs become more pronounced and may progress to stupor or coma. Seizures also can occur.
- One of the most alarming clinical signs during episodes of hypoglycemia is profuse hypersalivation and pawing at the mouth, which are indicative of nausea.
- Splenomegaly is common; the mechanism for this is not known (see Splenomegaly under Hematopoietic System in this chapter).

Diagnosis

The differential diagnosis for hypoglycemia in ferrets includes hepatic insufficiency, starvation, and laboratory error.

Fasting Serum Glucose

- A carefully monitored fast of 4–6 hours is sufficient.
- Normal fasting serum glucose is 90–110 mg/dl. Ferrets with insulinoma may have a fasting serum glucose of 20–85 mg/dl.
- If necessary, obtain several samples over a period of several days.

▼ *Key Point* Do not fast the animal for more than 6 hours because prolonged fasting may cause collapse, coma, or even seizures in an affected animal. Feed the ferret a high-protein and high-fat meal as soon as possible after collection of blood.

Blood Insulin Values

- Values greater than 275 pmol/liter (or 38 μU/ml) are considered elevated in ferrets. However, because insulin and glucose are in a constant dynamic state, a random insulin value may be normal (relative rather than absolute hyperinsulinemia), especially if the ferret is severely hypoglycemic at the time.

▼ *Key Point* Base a presumptive diagnosis of insulinoma on clinical signs and hypoglycemia in the absence of other causes of hypoglycemia and with elevated or normal insulin levels. Make a definitive diagnosis with surgical removal and histopathology of a pancreatic tumor.

Serum Biochemical Profile and Complete Blood Count

- These values usually are normal except for low blood glucose levels.

- A slight elevation in alanine aminotransferase (ALT) levels (180–250 IU/L) may be seen; the cause is unknown.

Treatment

▼ *Key Point* Insulinoma is a progressive disease in ferrets, requiring constant monitoring and adjustment of medication. Instruct owners on how to recognize the signs of hypoglycemia and how to manage hypoglycemia at home (see Medical Therapy).

Surgical Removal

Surgical removal or debulking of pancreatic tumors is palliative and may provide at best only temporary remission of signs.

- Follow canine protocols (see Chap. 33), taking care to avoid hypoglycemia by fasting the ferret only 4–6 hours or by administering 2.5% dextrose during longer fasts.
- Administer IV dextrose (2.5–5.0%) during anesthesia and surgery.
- Gently palpate to locate tumor nodules, which are firmer than the surrounding tissue; nodules may be solitary or multiple.
  - Nodules may be removed individually or a partial pancreatectomy may also be performed
  - If no visible or palpable nodules are found, perform a pancreatic biopsy to look for random neoplastic cells.

▼ *Key Point* Perform a complete abdominal exploratory; insulinomas can metastasize to the regional lymph nodes, liver, and spleen (uncommon). Concurrent adrenal tumors (discussed later) are common.

- If the spleen is enlarged and appears irregular or mottled, consider performing splenectomy and submit for histopathology.

Complications

- *Iatrogenic pancreatitis* is rarely a problem in ferrets; however, as a precaution, withhold food and water for 12 hours postoperatively; give 2.5–5.0% dextrose as an intravenous drip during fasting.
  - Monitor blood glucose 1–4 times daily, depending on physical examination findings.
- *Transient diabetes mellitus* may occur postoperatively. Hyperglycemia and glucosuria may be present for several days to 3 weeks after surgery; generally no treatment is required.

Medical Therapy

Medical treatment is necessary as the disease progresses. Frequent feeding is the first step in treatment. Add prednisone and diazoxide as clinical signs necessitate. Corticosteroids promote hepatic gluconeogenesis and antagonize the effects of insulin at the cellular level. Ferrets appear to tolerate corticosteroids well; side effects are minimal at lower dosages.

- Feed frequent, high-quality protein and fat meals, especially after exercise or a long sleep. Avoid foods containing sugar or excessive carbohydrates (except to treat hypoglycemic episodes) because these foods cause short energy bursts followed by a period of hypoglycemia 1–2 hours later.
- Chromium has been reported to stabilize blood glucose and insulin levels in humans. Brewer's yeast, which is a rich source of chromium, has been beneficial in some ferrets with insulinoma.
  - Give ⅛–¼ tsp of brewer's yeast q12h in soft food such as strained meat baby food or canned.
- When frequent feedings no longer control clinical signs, give prednisone or prednisolone suspension or tablets at a starting dosage of 0.1–0.5 mg/kg q12h PO. As clinical signs worsen, increase the dosage gradually as needed to control signs.
- Add diazoxide (Proglycem, Baker Norton Pharmaceuticals) when frequent feedings and glucocorticoids no longer control clinical signs or when beginning glucocorticoid therapy. Administer diazoxide at 10 mg/kg/day, PO, divided q8–12h. Gradually increase diazoxide dosage to 60 mg/kg/day, divided q8–12h, as needed.
  - Diazoxide is not palatable for some ferrets and is expensive. Moreover, it can cause hypertension, lethargy, depression, anorexia, and nausea.

Treatment of Acute Hypoglycemic Episodes

Hypoglycemic episodes require specific therapy.

- Mild to moderately severe hypoglycemic episodes often can be treated successfully at home. Instruct the client to give the ferret honey or corn syrup.
  - If the ferret has collapsed, rub honey or corn syrup on the gingiva (taking care not to be bitten).
  - Once the animal is stabilized, feed a high-protein meal.
- Severe hypoglycemic episodes that do not respond to home therapy or that result in seizures require treatment in a hospital (see Chap. 33 for treatment of hypoglycemia in dogs and cats).
  - Administer a slow IV bolus of 50% dextrose (0.5–2 ml) until the ferret responds. Give no more than necessary to stop seizures. If the ferret is having seizures or remains comatose, place an IV catheter and administer fluids and a corticosteroid and begin an infusion of 5% dextrose.
  - Anticonvulsant therapy (diazepam 1–2 mg IV to effect) is rarely necessary. If the ferret is in status epilepticus, follow anticonvulsant protocols for dogs and cats (see Chap. 145) and correct hypoglycemia.
  - Control with a combination of medication, diet and possible surgery.

Prognosis

- The prognosis is guarded, but with surgery and medical treatment, ferrets have had a good quality of life for more than 1 year after diagnosis of insulinoma. The median survival time was 17 months (range, 0.5–40 mos) in one study of 53 ferrets treated with surgery, medical management, or both.

ADRENAL NEOPLASIA

Adrenal tumors are common in ferrets, occurring with approximately the same frequency as insulinomas and often concurrently. Adrenal tumors have been found in ferrets as young as 1 year of age, although typically they occur between 2 and 5 years of age.

Etiology

- Adrenal tumors in ferrets most commonly arise from adrenocortical tissue; hyperplasia, adenomas, and adenocarcinomas are seen.
- The etiology is unknown; however, possible causes of the high incidence of adrenal neoplasia in this species include early neutering, inbreeding, and lack of exposure to normal seasonal photoperiods.
- Hyperadrenocorticism in ferrets causes a variety of clinical signs (see following section) and probably is the result of excessive secretion of more than one adrenocortical hormone or hormones other than cortisol. Pituitary-dependent hyperadrenocorticism has not been documented in ferrets.

Clinical Signs

- Signs include bilaterally symmetric alopecia, usually starting at the tail base and progressing cranially. There may be a history of alopecia and spontaneous hair regrowth.
- Pruritus often is reported, along with excessive dryness of the skin and small excoriations. Thinning and softening of the skin are common.
- An enlarged vulva, mimicking estrus, may be the only sign in spayed females. Mucoid to mucopurulent vulvar discharge may be present. Castrated males may resume sexual activity and have the strong body odor and oily hair coats of intact males. Mammary hyperplasia can occur in either sex.
- Male ferrets may present with urinary obstruction secondary to urethral narrowing caused by hyperplasia or cystic changes, or both, of paraurethral prostate tissue.
- Atrophy of abdominal musculature and mobilization of fat to the ventral abdomen, leading to a pendulous appearance, may be seen.
- Atrophy of hindlimb musculature and rear limb paresis can occur.
- Polyuria/polydipsia is uncommon.
- Collapse, anemia, and petechiation, mimicking estrogen toxicity, are seen in some ferrets with advanced adrenal disease (see discussion of Anemia under Hematopoietic System in this chapter).

Diagnosis

▼ *Key Point* A history of symmetric truncal hair loss, with or without pruritus, suggests the diagnosis.

- Changes in plasma steroid hormones are indicative of the diagnosis, which then is confirmed at surgery.

- Levels of one or more plasma steroids may be elevated, including androstenedione, dehydroepiandrosterone sulfate, estradiol, and 17-hydroxyprogesterone (Table 168–4). Submit plasma for analysis at the Clinical Endocrinology Laboratory, College of Veterinary Medicine, University of Tennessee (423-974-5638).
- On physical examination, an enlarged left adrenal may be palpable cranial and medial to the left kidney; right adrenal tumors are more difficult to palpate.
- Ultrasonography can identify a mass in the region of the adrenal gland; in addition, the liver often is hyperechoic.
- The CBC usually is normal except for a mild thrombocytopenia in some ferrets. Rarely, the CBC shows leukopenia, anemia, and thrombocytopenia, probably resulting from estrogen myelotoxicity.
- The serum biochemical profile usually is normal except for low blood glucose levels in animals with concurrent insulinoma (discussed previously).
- Protocols for the adrenocorticotropic hormone (ACTH) stimulation test and the low-dose dexamethasone suppression test have been reported in ferrets; however, these are not useful in diagnosing adrenal tumors because cortisol is not the primary hormone secreted by most of these tumors.
- Adrenal mineralization has not been seen on abdominal radiography, as occurs in dogs.
- Perform exploratory surgery to confirm the diagnosis.

Treatment

Adrenal tumors can be managed medically or surgically. Surgical management is recommended.

Adrenalectomy

Follow the protocol described for dogs (see Chap. 31).

- Use a ventral midline abdominal approach.
- Palpate both adrenal glands carefully for firm, nodular changes.
  - The right adrenal gland lies cranial and medial to the right kidney and is adhered to the vena cava under the right liver lobe.
  - Visual changes, such as dark circular lesions and small raised cysts, may be present instead of gross enlargement.

Table 168–4. STEROID HORMONE CONCENTRATIONS IN FERRETS

Steroid	Range
Androstenedione (nmol/L)	0–15
Estradiol (pmol/L)	30–180
17-hydroxyprogesterone (nmol/L)	0–0.8

From Clinical Endocrinology Laboratory, University of Tennessee College of Veterinary Medicine

- Adrenal changes may be subtle, especially in younger ferrets and because the adrenal glands are surrounded by fat.
- One or both adrenal glands may be affected. If only the left adrenal gland is affected, removal is relatively straightforward. If the tumor is right-sided, removal can be difficult because of the proximity of the vena cava and the aorta. If both adrenal glands are affected, resect the left adrenal gland and debulk the right adrenal gland.

▼ *Key Point* Always perform a complete abdominal exploratory. Observe and palpate the pancreas at surgery for insulinomas, which often are found concurrently with adrenal neoplasia.

Medical Therapy

Medical treatment is an alternative when surgery is unsuccessful or is not possible, if the ferret is young (especially if adrenal hyperplasia is suspected), or if there is bilateral adrenal involvement. Response to mitotane is variable and difficult to prove because spontaneous remission of disease is possible. Response is poor in ferrets with large adrenal tumors or long-term hair loss.

- Perform a fasting blood glucose test before starting mitotane therapy. Do not use it if blood glucose is low (indicative of concomitant insulinoma).
- Give mitotane (also known as o,p′-DDD) (Lysodren, Bristol-Myers Oncology) at 50 mg/kg, q24h, PO, for 7 days, then q48h until clinical signs start to resolve, and then q72h until signs are resolved. Thereafter, maintain the ferret on 50 mg/kg once per week to once per month, as necessary.
  - Have the dosage prepared by a pharmacist by mixing the crushed tablets with cornstarch and dividing them into 50-mg aliquots in #1 capsules.
  - To administer, coat the capsules with vegetable oil, push into the back of the throat, and follow with a palatable liquid or blenderized cat food to promote swallowing.

▼ *Key Point* If an insulinoma is present, cortisol levels drop with treatment and serum glucose levels also may fall, causing a hypoglycemic crisis.

- The most common side effect of mitotane in ferrets is hypoglycemia. Teach owners to recognize the signs of hypoglycemia; and have prednisone available at home.
  - If side effects occur, discontinue mitotane and administer prednisone, 1.0–1.25 mg, PO. If continuation of mitotane therapy is desired after a hypoglycemic crisis, administer concomitantly with prednisone (see previous section on Insulinoma).

Postoperative Care and Complications

- Monitor fasting serum glucose levels every 1–3 months during Lysodren therapy and after adrenalectomy, even if no pancreatic nodules were evident during surgery.

Prognosis

Adrenal tumors appear to have a very low rate of metastasis in ferrets.

- With proper treatment, a full resolution of clinical signs can be expected.
- Even without treatment, ferrets may survive up to 2 years or longer after diagnosis, although the hair loss is generally progressive.
- Hair loss may resolve spontaneously, only to recur the following year.
- The second adrenal gland eventually also may become involved.

LYMPHOSARCOMA

Lymphosarcoma (lymphoma) is common in ferrets of all ages. Similar to the disease in cats and dogs (see Chap. 25), lymphoma in ferrets may be solid, disseminated, or leukemic. The most commonly involved organs are the spleen, liver, GI tract, cranial mediastinum, and lymph nodes.

Etiology

- A viral etiology is suspected, and research is currently under way to isolate the causative agent.

Clinical Signs

Clinical signs are variable, depending on the organ system involved.

- Lymphoma tends to be a more acute, fulminant disease in younger animals.
- Some ferrets are totally asymptomatic; lymphoma may be an incidental finding during evaluation for another medical problem.
- Common signs include:
  - Weight loss despite a normal appetite
  - Splenomegaly
  - Lethargy and inappetence
  - Dyspnea, tachypnea, and exercise intolerance with mediastinal and sternal lymph node involvement
  - Peripheral lymphadenopathy
  - Acute collapse, often with pyrexia
  - Cutaneous masses
  - Chronic diarrhea
  - Rectal prolapse

Diagnosis

The method of diagnosis depends on the organ system involved.

- Perform a thorough history and physical examination.
- Evaluate a serum biochemistry profile, CBC, and platelet count. If the ferret is anemic, perform a reticulocyte count.
  - The serum chemistry profile may disclose elevated liver enzymes if the liver is involved; paraneoplastic syndromes are uncommon in ferret lymphoma.

- The CBC may be normal or may reveal an absolute or relative lymphocytosis, occasionally with abnormal lymphocytes. Anemia, leukopenia, and thrombocytopenia also are seen. Persistent absolute lymphocyte counts greater than 3500 or a relative lymphocytosis ($\geq$60%) are considered suspicious; follow with lymph node biopsy if lymphadenopathy is present.
- Perform thoracic and abdominal radiography and ultrasonography to evaluate for intrathoracic and intra-abdominal masses.
- Perform a biopsy, if possible, or fine-needle aspiration, of affected tissues for histologic and cytologic examination.
  - Fine-needle aspiration of the spleen frequently is inconclusive.
  - The popliteal lymph node is the most accessible peripheral node for biopsy, which is the most helpful diagnostic tool for peripheral lymphadenopathy or when no masses are evident.
- Perform bone marrow aspiration to identify infiltration by neoplastic cells and stage II disease (see Clinical Techniques in this chapter).

Treatment

Splenectomy

- If the spleen is involved, perform a splenectomy (see Chap. 23) to reduce the overall tumor load.

Chemotherapy

Chemotherapy for lymphoma may be successful. In general, protocols have been adapted from feline medicine (see Chaps. 24 and 25).

- IV chemotherapeutic agents are given via butterfly catheter or small-gauge needle with the ferret under sedation; face-mask administration of isoflurane is the most convenient and rapid method.
- One protocol is outlined in Table 168–5.

Table 168–5. CHEMOTHERAPY PROTOCOL II FOR LYMPHOMA*

Week	Drug	Dose
1	Vincristine	0.07 mg/kg, IV
	Asparaginase	400 IU/kg, IP
	Prednisone	1 mg/kg, PO, q24h and continued throughout therapy
2	Cyclophosphamide	10 mg/kg, SC
3	Doxorubicin	1 mg/kg, IV
4–6	As weeks 1–3 above but discontinue asparaginase	
8	Vincristine	0.07 mg/kg, IV
10	Cyclophosphamide	10 mg/kg, SC
12	Vincristine	0.07 mg/kg, IV
14	Methotrexate	0.5 mg/kg, IV

IV, intravenously; IP, intraperitoneally; PO, per os (by mouth); SC, subcutaneously.
*Protocol is continued in sequence biweekly after week 14.
From Rosenthal KE: Ferrets. Vet Clin North Am 24:19–20, 1994.

▼ *Key Point* Monitor the CBC weekly. If the white blood cell (WBC) count falls below 2000 WBCs/μl, or the RBC count falls below 4 million/L, discontinue vincristine for 1 week or more until the WBC count increases to at least 3000 WBCs/μl.

OTHER TYPES OF NEOPLASIA

- Tumors of the *reproductive tract* in ferrets include granulosa cell tumors, luteomas, and leiomyomas in intact females and in remnant tissue in spayed females. Sertoli cell tumors have been seen in intact males.
- *Hepatic hemangiosarcomas* and *hemangiomas* occur in ferrets.
- Tumors of the *GI tract* are uncommon.
- Tumors of the *skin* and *subcutis* are discussed in Dermatologic Diseases in this chapter.
- Other tumors reported in ferrets include chordoma (a malignant tumor arising from the embryonic remains of the notochord), chondroma, osteoma, osteosarcoma, mesothelioma, thymoma, schwannoma, renal and pancreatic carcinoma, and fibroma fibrosarcoma.

Dermatologic Diseases

Susan A. Brown / Elizabeth V. Hillyer

SEASONAL CHANGES IN THE SKIN AND HAIR COAT

Ferrets may have dramatic seasonal changes in the hair coat length, thickness, and color triggered by photoperiod changes. This is particularly true in intact animals. If one is unfamiliar with these changes, normal coat alterations may be interpreted incorrectly as a medical problem.

▼ *Key Point* Although individual animals may exhibit different patterns of coat change each successive year, ferret coats generally get shorter and darker in the summer months and longer, thicker, and lighter in the winter months.

Hair Coat

- Hair thinning (along with up to 40% weight loss) occurs in the spring when the photoperiod is increasing. There may be a 1-day dramatic loss of the undercoat or, more commonly, gradual hair loss and regrowth.
  - The coat also may change color, and facial masks may appear or disappear.
- Normal thinning of the hair coat in spring and summer is diffuse and related to the loss of the undercoat, without any areas of focal alopecia. This condi-

tion is retained through the summer, with regrowth of the undercoat in the fall.
- Females in estrus and males "in season" may show an even more marked hair loss but should not have areas of alopecia.
  - Males typically lose hair in the inguinal area because of constant rubbing to mark territory; the mid- and caudal abdomen is often wet with urine.
- Neutered animals can experience the same coat cycles, although somewhat less dramatically. There may be no coat changes in neutered animals or in animals kept under unchanging lighting conditions.
- Neutering or spaying a ferret can cause dramatic, but temporary, hair thinning postoperatively, particularly if the animal was reproductively active at the time of surgery. The preoperative color pattern may not return.
- At any time of the year, regrowth of hair that has been shaved for medical procedures is slow in ferrets, but it is particularly so in the winter and summer, when no active hair growth is occurring.

Skin

- Ferrets in estrus may exhibit a bluish discoloration of the skin, most noticeable on the abdomen and the face. This discoloration is caused by new hairs growing through the dermis.
  - If ovariohysterectomy is performed while a ferret is in estrus, the discoloration may occur within 10 days after surgery.
- In ferrets with alopecia of any cause, hair regrowth often is preceded by a blue to purple discoloration of the skin that can alarm the owner.
- Hyperkeratosis of the foot pads severe enough to result in growth of pseudonails may occur in ferrets older than 2 years of age. It is seen most often in animals that are housed on carpeting or linoleum surfaces.
- A small amount of petroleum jelly or vitamin E oil rubbed into the pads daily is helpful.

INFECTIOUS DISEASES

Bacterial Infections

Cutaneous bacterial infections in ferrets usually are manifested as abscesses or a diffuse, ulcerative pyoderma.

Abscesses

- Abscesses usually occur as the result of a puncture wound or a serious bite but also may develop in the inguinal fat after a traumatic injury, (e.g., being stepped on).
- Diagnosis and treatment of abscesses are discussed in Infectious Diseases in this chapter.

Ulcerative Pyoderma

Ulcerative pyoderma is the second most commonly encountered form of bacterial dermatitis in the ferret.

Etiology

- Various bacteria can cause ulcerative pyoderma; however, the most common agents are *Staphylococcus* and *Streptococcus* spp.

Clinical Signs

- Focal alopecia with diffusely hyperemic, thickened ulcerated skin may occur over any area of the body.

Diagnosis

- Perform a cutaneous punch biopsy (see Chap. 49) to rule out diffuse cutaneous mast cell tumor, which may have a similar gross appearance.
- Perform a bacterial culture for susceptibility testing.

Treatment

- Administer systemic antibiotics based on culture and susceptibility testing. Antibiotics effective in the treatment of pyoderma in ferrets include amoxicillin-clavulanate (Clavamox, SmithKline), 13–25 mg/kg q12h PO and cephalosporins (use feline dosages).
- Topical treatment may include twice-weekly cleansing with an antibacterial shampoo containing chlorhexidine or benzoyl peroxide. Daily application of an antibacterial cream may be beneficial if the lesion is small and localized.

Canine Distemper Virus (CDV) Infection

Dermatologic lesions are quite prominent with CDV infection in ferrets.

- Dermatologic signs begin with hyperemia of skin around the lips, chin, eyes, and sometimes the inguinal area. With time, crusts and skin thickening may appear.
- Hyperkeratosis of the foot pads occurs as the disease progresses.
- See Infectious Diseases in this chapter for a detailed discussion of CDV in ferrets.

Dermatomycoses

- *Microsporum canis* and *Trichophyton mentagrophytes* are the most common causes of superficial mycotic infections in the ferret.
- See Infectious Diseases in this chapter for diagnosis and treatment.

EXTERNAL PARASITES

Fleas

- Flea infestation is the most common external parasite problem encountered in pet ferrets. Clinical signs are similar to those seen in cats (see Chap. 40).
- All flea products approved for use in cats are safe to use in ferrets, with the exception of flea collars, because they come off easily and small pieces can be ingested.

Ear Mites

Ear mite infection in ferrets is caused by *Otodectes cyanotis*, the same parasite that infects cats and dogs.

Clinical Signs

- Ferrets, unlike dogs and cats, rarely exhibit pruritus, even with heavy mite infestation.
- Ferrets typically have a large volume of dark reddish brown ear wax, mimicking the character of wax present with *O. cyanotis* infestation in cats. However, with heavy infestations wax production may be excessive and cause plugging of the external ear canal.
- Occasionally, *O. cyanotis* infestation may be exacerbated by a secondary bacterial infection. If the ear drum is ruptured, otitis media and interna may result, accompanied by head tilt, circling, and pain (see Chap. 57 for management of otitis media as in cats).
- With chronic ear mite infestation, a bluish pigment may appear on the inner surface of the pinnae. There may be thickening of the tissue in the areas of pigmentation. This pigmentation is not harmful, is a response to chronic irritation, and usually fades after the mites are "exterminated."

Diagnosis

- Examine all ferrets for mites because the incidence of infestation is high in some populations.
  - Mites in the ear canal frequently can be observed with the naked eye, using a bright light source.
  - Otoscopic examination is often difficult because of the uncooperative nature of the patient and small ear canal.
- Confirm the diagnosis by microscopic examination of ear wax.

Treatment

- Thoroughly clean the ears. Divide 1 mg/kg of ivermectin into two doses and instill into each ear. Repeat in 2 weeks.
  - Bathe the animal within 24–48 hours after treatment. Wash all bedding and treat any other affected mammals in the household (see Chap. 55).
- Other ear mite remedies approved for use in cats also may be used in ferrets (see Chap. 55). These treatments usually involve daily topical application, a task often difficult for clients to perform.

Sarcoptic Mange

Etiology

Sarcoptes scabiei mites are transmissible between dogs and ferrets. Transmission is by direct contact with infected hosts or their bedding. See Chap. 39 for discussion about sarcoptic mange in dogs and cats.

Clinical Signs

- Lesions commonly are confined to the feet, which become hyperemic, swollen, and intensely pruritic, with crusting around the nails and toes.

- Generalized alopecia, scaling, and pruritus occur rarely.

Diagnosis

- As in other mammals, diagnosis is based on a positive skin scraping. Several areas should be scraped.
- A common differential diagnosis is contact allergy. Similar lesions have been observed on the feet of ferrets housed in plastic-floor cages. These resolve when the cage bottom is changed to one of wire or wood.

Treatment

- Give ivermectin (Ivomec, Merck-Sharp & Dohme Agvet), 0.5 mg/kg, SC, once every 2 weeks for three treatments.
- Wash all bedding and treat all potential contact hosts in the household.

ENDOCRINE ALOPECIA

Tail Alopecia

Etiology

The etiology of tail alopecia in the ferret is unknown but is suspected to be caused by hormonal fluctuations because the disease responds to changes in the photoperiod. Hair loss occurs most commonly at the time of the fall molt, when the photoperiod is becoming shorter, but may be seen any time of year under artificial lighting conditions. Hair regrowth usually occurs in 2–8 weeks. The same pattern of alopecia is not always repeated annually.

Clinical Signs

- Hair loss, ranging from diffuse hair thinning to complete alopecia, occurs from the base to the tip of the tail.

▼ *Key Point* Alopecia occurs only on the tail. If alopecia extends to the body, suspect another form of endocrine disease.

- Comedones and a brown, waxy scale may accompany the alopecia.

Diagnosis

- Diagnosis is based on clinical signs.
- Differential diagnoses include the early stages of other endocrine alopecias; however, these conditions include hair loss on the body as well as the tail.

Treatment

- No treatment is necessary because hair regrowth occurs when the photoperiod changes. Artificially lengthening the photoperiod may speed hair regrowth in some cases, although not reliably.
- If the tail exhibits excessive amounts of waxy scaling or comedones, clean the tail weekly with a mild shampoo.

Estrus Alopecia

Alopecia may be seen in intact females that have been in estrus for 1 month or longer.

Clinical Signs

- Hair loss is bilaterally symmetric, beginning over the shoulders and flanks, and eventually may progress to involve the entire body. Hairs epilate easily, and the underlying skin appears normal.
- A grossly enlarged vulva indicates a state of estrus. Be aware that the ferret also may be anemic and thrombocytopenic (see Anemia in this chapter).

Diagnosis

- Diagnosis is based in clinical signs in an intact female.

Treatment

- Perform an ovariohysterectomy if the ferret can tolerate the procedure; otherwise induce ovulation with hCG (see section on Termination of Estrus under Anemia in this chapter).
- Hair regrowth is rapid after surgery or ovulation; however, changes in hair length, color, or thickness are common.

Adrenal Neoplasia

- Bilaterally symmetric alopecia is a common sign of adrenal neoplasia in ferrets (see Adrenal Neoplasia in this chapter).

Hypothyroidism

- Hypothyroidism has not been documented in ferrets.

NEOPLASIA

Neoplasia of the skin and subcutaneous tissues commonly occurs in ferrets 1 year of age and older. Because metastasis is a possibility, complete removal (preferred) or biopsy is recommended as soon as possible.

Mast Cell Tumors

Mast cell tumors are the most common skin tumors and are frequently benign in ferrets.

- Individual tumors appear most commonly as slightly raised, flat, button-like cutaneous masses typically ranging in size from 2–10 mm. The tumors are tan in color or may become hyperemic with a dark flaky crust because of scratching if pruritus is present. They also may appear as raised, ulcerated areas or as diffuse areas of erythema and crusting.
- Mast cell tumors occasionally have been associated with patchy or generalized alopecia that resolves with surgical removal of the tumor.
- See Chapter 26 for information about mast cell tumors in dogs and cats. Remove these tumors because of possible metastasis. Metastasis is rare but has been seen in the lung and gallbladder.

Sebaceous Epitheliomas

- These tumors have been variously called haral cell tumors and sebaceous adenomas and are also common in ferrets.
- Tumors can be wart-like, ulcerated, or cystic and range in size from 0.5–2 cm.
- Excision is usually curative. Recurrence is rare, and metastasis is not reported.

Other Neoplasms

- Other less common neoplasms of the skin and subcutaneous tissues include hemangioma, squamous cell carcinoma, basi-squamo-sebaceous carcinoma, sebaceous gland adenocarcinoma, basal cell carcinoma, myxosarcoma, perianal gland adenocarcinoma, neurofibrosarcoma, leiomyosarcoma, lymphoma, and histiocytoma.
- Adenocarcinomas often metastasize to regional lymph nodes, liver, and lungs. Remove promptly and completely.
- Diagnosis, treatment, and prognosis for these tumors in ferrets are the same as for dogs and cats (see Chap. 28).

Cardiovascular Diseases

Elizabeth V. Hillyer

CHARACTERISTICS OF THE NORMAL FERRET HEART

- The heart extends from the sixth rib to the caudal border of the seventh or eighth rib (compared with cats where it extends from the second to the sixth rib).
- Cardiac auscultation therefore is centered more caudally in the thorax than in cats.
- The heart rate averages 180–250 beats per minute.
- A pronounced sinus arrhythmia is common; temporary bradycardia is common during auscultation, almost to the point of transient sinus arrest.

Cardiomyopathy

Cardiomyopathy most frequently affects ferrets 2 years of age or older. Dilated (congestive) and hypertrophic forms can occur; the dilated form is more common.

Etiology

The causes of cardiomyopathy in ferrets are not known. Nutritional deficiencies may play a role.

Clinical Signs

- Ferrets appear to compensate well for early cardiac insufficiency, perhaps because a slight decrease in activity is not readily apparent to owners.

- A cardiac murmur or radiographic evidence of cardiomegaly may be detected as an incidental finding before the development of clinical signs.
- Ferrets in heart failure generally present with tachypnea and dyspnea.
- Weight loss is common, and anorexia and lethargy occur late in the disease.
- Coughing generally is not noted.
- Abdominal distention due to ascites may be present.

Diagnosis

- Obtain a dietary history as part of the clinical history.
- Perform a complete physical examination:
  - Evaluate for sluggish capillary refill time.
  - Auscult the heart for murmurs or arrhythmias.
  - Observe for tachypnea or dyspnea and auscult the lungs for crackles or wheezes.
  - Palpate the abdomen and examine for ascites.

▼ *Key Point* Proceed with further testing only if the ferret is stable. Otherwise, administer furosemide and oxygen therapy. If there is pleural effusion, thoracocentesis may be necessary.

- Obtain thoracic radiographs to evaluate the heart and lungs. The heart may be globoid in shape, with rounded right and left ventricles.
  - Pulmonary edema and pleural effusion may be present.
- Perform abdominal radiography and ultrasonography to evaluate the size of the liver and spleen and to detect abdominal effusion.
- Evaluate a serum biochemical profile, CBC, and urinalysis to detect other systemic diseases and electrolyte abnormalities.
- Perform standard six-lead electrocardiography (ECG) if possible (Table 168–6 lists normal ferret ECG parameters). Sedation may be necessary.
  - Sedation with ketamine or a ketamine-diazepam combination (see Table 168–3) raises the heart rate. The heart rate tends to decrease with ketamine-xylazine sedation; therefore, avoid using xylazine in ferrets with suspected cardiac disease.
- If thoracic or abdominal effusion is present, submit fluid for cytologic examination. Perform centesis as in cats; however, take into consideration the relatively caudal position of the heart in ferrets.
- The most useful diagnostic tool in ferrets with myocardial disease is echocardiography.
  - Contractility, wall thickness, and chamber size can be examined (Table 168–7).
  - Valve function and blood flow can be evaluated using various Doppler techniques.

Treatment

Treatment depends on diagnostic (especially echocardiographic) findings. Base the treatment protocol on the same parameters for cats (see Chap. 66).

- Consider oxygen therapy for ferrets that are dyspneic.
- If necessary, perform thoracocentesis and abdominocentesis to relieve dyspnea. Administer sup-

Table 168–6. ELECTROCARDIOGRAPHIC DATA FOR 52 CLINICALLY NORMAL FERRETS*

Parameter	Mean ± SD (Range)† (n = 25)	Value‡ (n = 27)
Age (mo)	10–20	Average, 5.2
Male:female ratio	All male	1.25
Body weight (kg)	1.4 ± 0.2	NA
Heart rate (beats/min)	196 ± 26.5 (140–240)	233 ± 22
Rhythm		
Normal sinus	NA	67%
Sinus arrhythmia	NA	33%
Frontal plane MEA (degrees)	+86.13 ± 2.5 (79.6–90)	+77.22 ± 12
Lead II		
P amplitude (mV)	NA	0.122 ± 0.007
P duration (s)	NA	0.024 ± 0.004
PR interval (s)	0.056 ± 0.0086 (0.04–0.08)	0.047 ± 0.003
QRS duration (s)	0.044 ± 0.0079 (0.035–0.06)	0.043 ± 0.003
R amplitude (mV)	2.21 ± 0.42 (1.4–3)	1.46 ± 0.84
QT interval (s)	0.109 ± 0.018 (0.08–0.14)	0.12 ± 0.04

NA, not available; MEA, mean electrical axis.

*All ferrets were sedated with ketamine-xylazine.

†Data from Bone L, Battles AH, Goldfarb RD, et al: Electrocardiographic values from clinically normal, anesthetized ferrets (*Mustela putorius furo*). Am J Vet Res 49:1884–1887, 1988.

‡Data adapted from Fox JG: Biology and Diseases of the Ferret. Philadelphia, Lea & Febiger, 1988, p 170; and Edwards J: Unpublished data, 1987.

portive care such as subcutaneous fluids (e.g., 0.45% saline and 2.5% dextrose) and nutritional support for ferrets that are inappetent.

Drug Therapy

- Ferrets tolerate diuretics well. Administer furosemide 1–4 mg/kg PO, IV, IM, or SC, q8–12h; increase or decrease the dosage as necessary. In severe cases, consider using hydrochlorothiazide diuretics at feline dosages.
- If cardiac contractility is poor, administer digoxin (Lanoxin, Burroughs Wellcome) (0.01 mg/kg q24h); start at 75% of lean body weight (as for dogs) and watch for potential side effects (see Chap. 63).
- Vasodilator therapy with enalapril (Enacard, Merck Agvet Division) may be useful, although ferrets are sensitive to the drug's hypotensive effects. Start at a low dosage: 0.5 mg/kg q48h. If possible, gradually increase the dosage—that is, give 0.5 mg/kg q24h.
- For hypertrophic cardiomyopathy and tachycardia, give a beta blocker such as atenolol, 6.25 mg PO q24h, or a calcium channel antagonist such as diltiazem, 3.75–7.5 mg PO q12h.

Table 168–7. MEAN ECHOCARDIOGRAPHIC VALUES FOR 34 NORMAL ADULT FERRETS

Parameter	Mean Value
Left ventricle, end-diastolic	11.0 mm
Left ventricle, end-systolic	6.4 mm
Left ventricular posterior or free wall	3.3 mm
Fractional shortening	42%
End-point septal separation	None

From Sitinas N, Beeber N, Skeels M: Unpublished data, 1992.

- If the diet is deficient in taurine, although supplementation is not harmful, its benefit is doubtful.
- Salt-free diets may be beneficial; however, they are unpalatable to ferrets. Instead, instruct the owner to avoid feeding snacks, treats, or food items with a high-salt content.

Prevention

There are no means of preventing cardiomyopathy other than ensuring that ferrets are fed a good diet.

Prognosis

- The prognosis depends on the severity of disease and the initial response to treatment.
- Many ferrets do well for months on the appropriate medications.
- Ferrets with dilated cardiomyopathy respond better to treatment than canine patients with similar echocardiographic findings.

Other Cardiac Diseases

As experience with pet ferrets increases, different types of cardiac disease are likely to be recognized. Third-degree heart block (of unknown etiology) and various forms of valvular disease, including mitral and tricuspid insufficiency and endocarditis, have been seen in ferrets.

- The approach to these conditions in ferrets is the same as for other companion animals; use the drug dosages given previously for cardiac myopathies.

Heartworm Disease

Natural and experimental heartworm infections have been reported in ferrets (see Chap. 68). The disease in ferrets resembles the canine form. However, because of the ferret's small size, the presence of even one adult worm in the heart can be lethal. Reported adult worm burdens range from 1 to 10.

Etiology

- Heartworm disease in ferrets is caused by *Dirofilaria immitis*, the canine heartworm. *D. immitis* is a filarial nematode that is transmitted via mosquitoes.
- Ferrets that are housed outdoors in endemic areas are at greatest risk of infection; however, ferrets kept indoors also can become infected.

Clinical Signs

- Presenting signs include lethargy, inappetence, coughing, dyspnea, abdominal distension secondary to ascites, and melena. Sudden death is common.

Diagnosis

- If the history is compatible with cardiac failure, inquire about possible mosquito exposure.
- Physical examination findings are referable to heart failure and include depression, dehydration, pale or cyanotic mucous membranes, systolic murmur, dyspnea, moist lung sounds, ascites, and hypothermia. Black, tarry feces may be seen.

▼ *Key Point* Minimize stress in ferrets suspected of heartworm disease. Delay further diagnostic tests until heart failure is stabilized (see previous discussion about cardiomyopathy).

- Thoracic radiographs may show right ventricular enlargement, enlarged main pulmonary artery, tortuous pulmonary arteries, pulmonary infiltrate (edema), and pleural effusion.
- Abdominal radiographs may show hepatomegaly, splenomegaly, and ascites.
- If possible, draw blood for the modified Knott's test for microfilaria and for an enzyme-linked immunosorbent assay (ELISA) for *Dirofilaria* antigen.
  - Reported incidence of microfilaremia in infected ferrets ranges from 2% in a group of naturally infected ferrets to 50% in a group of experimentally infected ferrets.
  - The ELISA test is more useful. A commercial assay (Snap Heartworm Antigen Test Kit; IDEXX Laboratories Inc., Portland, ME) has detected infections in ferrets.
- If possible, evaluate a serum biochemical profile, CBC, and urinalysis to detect other systemic disease.
- If pleural or abdominal effusion is present, submit fluid for cytology. A modified transudate is found with cardiac failure.
- Echocardiography may enable visualization of the worm(s); nonselective venous angiography is a more invasive means of visualizing *Dirofilaria* but may be helpful if the ferret is stable enough to tolerate the procedure.

Treatment

- Treatment of heartworm disease in ferrets is difficult and entails early diagnosis, supportive care, and long-term antithrombotic therapy in conjunction with adulticide therapy.
- Keep the ferret confined to a cage for the first 3 weeks of treatment.
- The initial goal of treatment is stabilization of the patient's heart failure (see previous discussion of cardiomyopathy).
  - Oxygen therapy, furosemide, aminophylline, and thoracocentesis may be helpful.
  - Also, consider subcutaneous fluid therapy and supportive care.
- Use thiacetarsamide (Caparsolate, Sanfi) or melarsomine (Immiticide, Rhone Merieux, Inc.) as an adulticide; give prednisone for antithrombotic effects.
  - Administer thiacetarsamide 2.2 mg/kg q12h, IV by cephalic catheter for 2 days (4 doses). Alternatively, administer Immiticide at the canine dosage and treat as a grade III based on package insert, namely, one IM injection followed by two IM injections 1 month later. Follow package insert instructions regarding injection technique. In ferrets, the semimembranosus-semitendinosus muscles are often a better injection site than the lumbar musculature (which may be small in ferrets).
  - Administer prednisone 1 mg/kg q24h PO, beginning at time of adulticide therapy and taper off gradually when the ELISA result becomes negative.
  - Begin heartworm prevention 1 month after adulticide treatment.
  - Evaluate the effectiveness of treatment by repeating the heartworm ELISA 3 months after beginning therapy and monthly thereafter until results are negative.

Prevention

▼ *Key Point* Because of the high mortality associated with heartworm disease in ferrets, prevention is imperative in endemic areas, even for indoor ferrets.

- House all ferrets in endemic areas in structures with mosquito-proof screening.
- Follow the same guidelines for heartworm prevention in ferrets as for dogs.
  - Ivermectin 0.02 mg/kg once monthly suppresses the maturation of *D. immitis* in ferrets. Administer liquid ivermectin 1% diluted in propylene glycol (0.3 ml ivermectin to 1 oz propylene glycol—dose at 0.2 ml/kg PO once per month). Keep solution in amber glass bottle out of sunlight. Alternatively, administer feline Heartgard (Merck Agvet), dosing as for a 1- to 5-lb cat. Administer once monthly for a period beginning 1 month before and continuing to 2 months after possible mosquito exposure.
  - A daily dose of diethylcarbamazine (DEC; Dec Tabs, Wendt) of 5–11 mg/kg also is effective. Do not give DEC to microfilaremic ferrets.

Gastrointestinal System

Elizabeth V. Hillyer

CHARACTERISTICS OF THE NORMAL FERRET DIGESTIVE TRACT

Teeth

- The permanent teeth erupt between 50 and 74 days of age. The dental formula for the permanent teeth is 2(I3/3, C1/1, Pm3/3, M1/2).
- All premolars and molars have two roots, except for the third upper premolar, or carnassial tooth, which has three roots, and the second lower molar, which has one root.

Gastrointestinal Tract

- The GI tract is that of a carnivorous animal with a simple stomach and a relatively short small intestine.
  - The duodenum ends at the jejunoileum; there is no gross anatomic distinction between the jejunum and the ileum.
  - Ferrets do not have a cecum.
  - The junction of the jejunoileum and the colon is gauged by the pattern of anastomosis of the jejunal artery with the ileocolic artery.
- GI transit time for food is approximately 3–4 hours.

Anal Sacs

- The anal sacs lie between the external and internal anal sphincter muscles; the ducts open at 4 and 8 o'clock near the mucocutaneous junction.

Nausea and Vomiting

- Ferrets, like other carnivores, are able to vomit. Ferrets are prone to experiencing nausea as the result of GI diseases such as gastric ulcers and GI foreign bodies. Hypoglycemia also can cause signs of nausea (see discussion of insulinoma).
- Signs of nausea include hypersalivation and pawing at the mouth.
- Tooth grinding may indicate abdominal discomfort.

DENTAL DISEASE

- Dental tartar and periodontal disease are common, especially in older ferrets on a soft diet.
- Dental abscesses are seen, even in young ferrets.
- Follow basic medical and surgical treatment principles for dental diseases in dogs and cats (see Chap. 84).

SALIVARY MUCOCELE

The five major salivary glands are parotid, submandibular, sublingual, molar, and zygomatic.
- Salivary mucoceles usually cause a soft to firm swelling in the region of the orbit, oral commissure,

or mandibular lymph node. Aspiration of the mass reveals a clear to serosanguineous, mucinous fluid is aspirated from the mass; microscopic examination shows amorphous debris and occasional RBCs.
- Treatment: lance the mucocele, leaving the incision open for drainage and flushing as needed until healed.

MEGAESOPHAGUS

Megaesophagus is rare in ferrets.

- The etiology of megaesophagus in ferrets is unknown (see list of possible causes in dogs in Chap. 85).
- Presenting signs are the same as for dogs with megaesophagus.
- The diagnosis is generally evident on thoracic radiography.
- Follow canine treatment protocols. The prognosis is poor.

GASTROINTESTINAL PARASITES

- Although GI parasites are uncommon in ferrets, perform routine fecal testing, especially in young animals and those with diarrhea or rectal prolapse.

Etiology

- Coccidiosis is seen most frequently in immature animals and may cause severe diarrhea and dehydration.
- *Giardia* spp. are seen occasionally in ferrets. Although their clinical significance is not known, treatment is recommended.
- Ascarids are rare.

Treatment

- Treat with anthelmintics, following protocols and dosages for cats (see Chap. 89).

GASTRIC AND DUODENAL ULCERS

Gastric and duodenal ulcers have been reported in laboratory ferrets and are seen occasionally in pet ferrets. Clinical signs are often vague, and the diagnosis is difficult.

Etiology

- The etiology is not known; however, environmental stress may be a predisposing factor.
- Bacteria (*Helicobacter mustelae*) have been associated with the disease. A similar organism (*H. pylori*) is associated with gastric ulcer disease in humans.

Clinical Signs

- Clinical signs include anorexia, lethargy, hypersalivation, tooth grinding, vomiting, and melena.

Diagnosis

- A barium series may demonstrate an ulcer. Gastrotomy or endoscopic examination of the stomach with biopsy may be necessary for a definitive diagnosis. A positive response to therapy provides a presumptive diagnosis.
- Other causes of nausea and upper GI bleeding should be considered, such as viral or bacterial gastroenteritis or a GI foreign body, the latter of which is much more common than gastric ulcers in ferrets.

Treatment

- Severely affected ferrets may require hospitalization for supportive care in addition to ulcer therapy.
- Administer the following three drugs concurrently for at least 2 weeks ("triple therapy"):
  - Amoxicillin 10 mg/kg q12h SC or PO
  - Metronidazole 20 mg/kg q12h PO
  - Bismuth subsalicylate (Pepto-Bismol, Procter & Gamble) interferes with *H. pylori* colonization in humans. In ferrets, give 0.25 ml/kg q4–6h, PO.
- Feed bland foods such as strained meat baby food and meat baby food mixed with Deliver 2.0 (Mead Johnson Nutritionals). Most ferrets accept these foods after an initial period of force-feeding by syringe. Alternative foods include Science Diet A/D and Eukanuba Total Recovery diet.

GASTROINTESTINAL FOREIGN BODIES

GI obstruction caused by foreign body ingestion or hairballs is one of the most common problems in pet ferrets.

Etiology

- Foreign bodies generally are found in ferrets younger than 1 year of age; hairballs are common in ferrets older than 2 years of age.

▼ **Key Point** Until proved otherwise, suspect the presence of a GI foreign body in any young ferret presented for anorexia—even if no vomiting is reported. Rubber objects are the most common foreign bodies.

- Obstruction with a hairball (older ferrets), cloth, or plant material also may occur.

Clinical Signs

- One or several episodes of vomiting may be reported; however, vomiting often is not observed. Other signs of nausea include hypersalivation and pawing at the mouth.
- Intermittent or total anorexia occurs in ferrets with GI foreign bodies. Sometimes chronic wasting is the only clinical sign.
- Signs include lethargy, hindlimb weakness, dehydration, infrequent defecation and small stools; and melena may occur.

Diagnosis
History

- Identify any possibility of foreign body ingestion. Question whether hairball prevention is used.

Physical Examination

- Palpate the abdomen thoroughly to detect intestinal gas, a firm mass, or a painful area.

Laboratory Studies

- The serum biochemical profile, urinalysis, and CBC usually are normal except for evidence of dehydration. Anemia is seen in some ferrets with melena.

Abdominal Radiography

- Look for radiodense foreign material in the GI tract. To improve identification of a suspected foreign body, be sure to fast the ferret (≤6 hours) before radiography.
- Excessive gas and intestinal distension may indicate GI obstruction.
- Diagnosis is generally evident from physical examination and plain radiographs; thus, barium contrast radiography is rarely necessary.

Treatment

Surgical removal is the treatment of choice. If the ferret is ill, do not delay surgery.

Surgery

- Follow routine preoperative, operative, and postoperative procedure principles to perform gastrotomy or enterotomy (see Chaps. 88 and 90). Ferret tissues are thinner than those of a puppy or kitten of equivalent weight. Use 4–0 or 5–0 suture material to close the GI tract.

Prevention and Prognosis

▼ **Key Point** Instruct owners to "ferret proof" the house if ferrets are allowed to roam. In particular, restrict access to rubber toys and rubber objects.

- To prevent trichobezoar formation, administer a feline hairball laxative product (2–4 cm) two or three times a week, PO.

Prognosis

- The prognosis is good with prompt therapy.

EPIZOOTIC CATARRHAL ENTERITIS

A highly infectious enteritis, epizootic catarrhal enteritis (ECE), dubbed "green slime disease," first appeared in 1993. Thought to be caused by a coronavirus or rotavirus, ECE currently occurs on the East coast and in the midwestern United States. ECE spreads rapidly through a ferret population, typically affecting 100% of ferrets within 48 hours. It causes voluminous green, watery diarrhea and occasional vomiting followed in some ferrets by chronic wasting. Histologic changes include lymphoplasmacytic enteritis with villous atrophy and blunting.

- Three clinical syndromes are seen:
  - In young ferrets with no underlying disease, ECE causes relatively mild diarrhea lasting several days.
  - In older ferrets or those with concomitant disease, ECE causes severe diarrhea for several days that may be followed by acute onset of severe bloody diarrhea, resulting in anemia.
  - In ferrets that recover from the diarrheal phase, a wasting disease with abnormal stools and gradual weight loss may develop despite a high-calorie diet.

Treatment

- Administer supportive care, including fluid therapy.
  - No one specific treatment is consistently effective.
  - Administer fluids PO, SC, or IV, depending on the ferret's status.
  - Intestinal adsorbents or protectants (e.g., Kaopectate, UpJohn) may help in some ferrets.
  - Administer broad-spectrum, parenteral antibiotics to ferrets with bloody diarrhea.
  - Feed a bland, high-calorie diet (e.g., Deliver 2.0, Mead Johnson Nutritionals). For ferrets with wasting, feed high-calorie supplements, such as heavy cream, blenderized beef liver, or Science Diet A/D.
  - Loperamide (Imodium A-D, McNeil Consumer) at 0.2 mg/kg (1 ml/kg) PO q12h for 1–3 days may slow gut motility and may be helpful early in the disease or in ferrets with severe, bloody diarrhea.
- The disease may recur in previously affected ferrets, and an asymptomatic carrier state appears to be possible.
  - Do not house ferrets that have had ECE with ferrets that have not had the disease.

ROTAVIRUS

- Rotavirus causes diarrheal illness in the young of several species, including humans, cattle, swine, sheep, and rats.
- Rotavirus has caused several outbreaks of diarrhea with high mortality among ferret kits 2–6 weeks of age, and has been named "ferret kit disease."
- In adult ferrets, rotavirus infection is rarely fatal but causes bright green diarrhea with mucus for several days.
- There is no readily available antemortem test for the disease, although rotavirus particles can be identified in feces by electron microscopy.

Treatment

- Treatment includes supportive care, especially fluid therapy, and antibiotics to prevent secondary bacterial infection.

SALMONELLA

Salmonella typhimurium infection generally is acquired through exposure to contaminated raw meat and meat by-products. It is uncommon in pet ferrets.

- Clinical signs include lethargy, anorexia, fever, and diarrhea that usually is bloody. Conjunctivitis and anemia also are seen.
- Diagnosis of salmonellosis is based on clinical signs and a positive fecal culture.
- Treatment includes supportive care and antibiotic therapy guided by results of culture and sensitivity testing.
  - Intravenous fluids and therapy with rapidly acting intravenous corticosteroids may be necessary for ferrets that are presented in shock.
- Other details of salmonellosis, including its public health significance, are discussed elsewhere in this text.

EOSINOPHILIC GASTROENTERITIS

This is a recently recognized syndrome of unknown etiology in ferrets. Extensive microscopic studies have failed to identify an etiologic agent.

- Clinical signs include intermittent vomiting, inappetence, diarrhea, weight loss, and skin lesions.
- On physical examination, mesenteric lymph nodes may be enlarged and the intestines may feel thickened.
- A marked peripheral eosinophilia is present. If eosinophilic gastroenteritis is suspected, perform abdominal exploratory surgery because definitive diagnosis depends on intestinal biopsy.
- Treat with two doses (400 μg/kg SC) of ivermectin (Ivomec, Merck-Sharp & Dohme Agvet) given 2 weeks apart.
- If ivermectin is ineffective, consider prednisone, which is the treatment of choice for dogs and cats with eosinophilic enteritis.
- One of the authors (SAB) has seen several ferrets with erythema and crusting of feet, ears, and face, in which histologic lesions were consistent with allergic dermatitis. These ferrets had eosinophilia (up to 40% eosinophils). They responded to corticosteroids. One responded to diet change.

PROLIFERATIVE BOWEL DISEASE (PBD)

Proliferative colitis in ferrets was first reported in 1982; a similar disease currently is recognized to affect the jejunoileum. A disseminated form of PBD with lesions in extraintestinal sites also has been reported. This is a disease primarily of young ferrets 4–14 months of age. PBD was relatively common in the late 1980s and early 1990s; currently, it is relatively uncommon.

Etiology

Intracellular bacteria called *Lawsania intracellularis* are seen with silver staining in the apical portion of colonic crypt epithelial cells.

Clinical Signs

- Acute and chronic forms of the disease can occur.
- Diarrhea, often with mucus and blood, is a constant finding. Defecations are frequent and small; ferrets often cry out when they defecate. The rectum may be partially prolapsed.
- Other signs include lethargy, depression, inappetence, weight loss, dehydration, and pyrexia.
- Neurologic signs such as ataxia and muscle tremors also may be present.

Diagnosis

- The colon or jejunoileum may be palpably thickened on physical examination.
- Perform direct fecal exam and fecal flotation tests to rule out GI parasitism.
- A tentative diagnosis of proliferative bowel disease is based on clinical signs and physical examination. Definitive diagnosis requires intestinal or colonic biopsy, but this rarely is warranted because response to therapy usually is good if initiated early.

Treatment

Treat mild cases on an outpatient basis. Hospitalization for supportive care may be necessary with severe disease.

- Chloramphenicol is the drug of choice (50 mg/kg q12h, PO, IV, IM, or SC). Treat for at least 2 weeks; longer therapy often is necessary to prevent relapse.
- Metronidazole (20 mg/kg q12h, PO) may be efficacious.
- Supportive care, including subcutaneous fluids and nutritional support, is necessary for dehydrated and debilitated ferrets.

Prevention and Prognosis

- There is no prevention.
- The prognosis is good with timely therapy.
- Some ferrets improve temporarily and then relapse at the end of the treatment period. Use a long-term course of antibiotic therapy in these animals.

RECTAL PROLAPSE

Rectal prolapse is common in younger ferrets.

- Diarrhea often is seen in conjunction with rectal prolapse.
- Causes include GI parasitism (e.g., coccidiosis), proliferative colitis, and other diseases that may cause straining or diarrhea. Other differentials include GI lymphoma, benign intestinal polyps, and postoperative complication of anal gland removal.
- Perform direct fecal and fecal flotation tests to screen for parasites.

- Medical treatment is similar to that for other species, namely anthelmintics and antibiotics; chloramphenicol is the drug of choice if proliferative bowel disease is suspected. Surgical correction is usually unnecessary.
- Perform a biopsy of the prolapsed tissue if lymphoma is a possibility.

Surgical Correction—Techniques

1. Flush the prolapsed tissues and replace them into the rectum.
2. Place a pursestring suture in the anus with a small opening to allow passage of feces. Keep the pursestring suture in place for 2–5 days.
   - Small prolapses of less than 5 mm often resolve on medical therapy without the need for a pursestring suture.
3. For ferrets with chronic prolapsed rectum, surgery may be necessary to reduce the size of the anal opening. Excise a small triangular wedge of anal mucosa and routinely close the defect by suturing.

ANAL SAC ABSCESS

- Clinical signs and physical findings in ferrets with an abscessed anal sac are the same as in dogs and cats.
- The recommended treatment is lancing and drainage of the abscess or surgical removal of both anal sacs (see Chap. 95).

Anal Sacculectomy

Perform anal sac removal to decrease the musky odor or as treatment for anal sac abscesses. For odor reduction, neutering is done simultaneously because the scent glands in the skin and the perianal sebaceous and apocrine glands are under hormonal control. Some clinicians believe that neutering is sufficient to decrease odor and that routine anal sacculectomy should be discouraged.

Technique

1. Grasp the anal sac opening and hold it closed with mosquito forceps. Make a circumferential skin incision around the duct opening.
2. Applying gentle caudal traction to the anal sac, use a scalpel blade or gauze to tease away the surrounding fascia.
3. Do not suture the incisions.

Alternative Techniques

1. Make small, arc-like incisions just lateral to the duct openings.
2. Dissect the subcutaneous tissues bluntly to reveal the neck of the anal sac; grasp the opening and hold it closed with mosquito forceps.
3. Dissect the sac free of surrounding tissues, using gentle traction.
4. Do not suture the incisions.

Urogenital System

Elizabeth V. Hillyer

REPRODUCTIVE SYSTEM

Characteristics of the Normal Ferret Reproductive System

Ferrets reach sexual maturity during the first breeding season after birth. The breeding season runs from March to August under natural lighting conditions.

Males

- Males (hobs) have a large, J-shaped os penis.
- Prostatic tissue is located at the base of the urinary bladder surrounding the urethra and may be difficult to identify in young males.
- During the breeding season, testicle size is twice that in the fall and winter months.

Females

- A swollen vulva is an external sign of estrus.
- Female ferrets (jills) are seasonally polyestrous and are induced ovulators.
- If mating is unsuccessful, pseudopregnancy results, lasting 41–43 days.
- Females may remain in heat if they are not bred. Because the resulting prolonged elevation of serum estrogens can cause bone marrow toxicity and pancytopenia (see discussion of Anemia under Hematopoietic System in this chapter), termination of estrus is recommended.

Estrus Termination

- Terminate estrus after day 10 by administration of a single intramuscular injection of 100 IU units (or 1000 USP) of hCG; repeat this dose, if necessary, 1–2 weeks later.
- Alternatively, give GnRH at a dose of 20 µg, IM or SC, following the same schedule.
- Submit blood for a CBC and platelet count if the ferret has been in estrus for more than 28 days.

Castration and Ovariohysterectomy

- Follow the same protocols and procedures as for cats (see Chaps. 107 and 111).
- Castration can be open or closed; use scrotal incisions.
- Note that the ovarian pedicles contain large amounts of fat.

Pyometra

- Pyometra is uncommon in pet ferrets in the United States because they are usually neutered before being sold as pets.
- Persistent estrus may predispose ferrets to pyometra; therefore, screen affected females for evidence of es-

trogen toxicity, especially to detect thrombocytopenia preoperatively, before treatment (see discussion of Anemia under Hematopoietic System in this chapter).
- Clinical signs, diagnosis, and treatment are the same as for dogs and cats (see Chap. 101).

Vulvar Swelling in "Spayed" Females

As previously mentioned, vulvar swelling is an external sign of estrus in female ferrets.

- In a female that purportedly is spayed, a swollen vulva indicates a remnant of ovarian tissue or another source of estrogens and estrogen precursors such as an abnormal adrenal gland (see Endocrine Diseases in this chapter).

Diagnosis

See diagnosis of Adrenal Neoplasia under Neoplasia section of this chapter.

- Run plasma steroid level test.

Pregnancy Toxemia (Eclampsia)

Pregnancy toxemia, or eclampsia, is a condition that occurs in late pregnancy and most commonly affects primiparous females.

- The cause of eclampsia in ferrets is not known.
- Affected ferrets usually are presented in an acute state of shock.
- Administer aggressive supportive care and perform an emergency cesarean section.
- The disease results in high mortality of jills and kits.

Mastitis

- See Dermatologic Diseases in this chapter.

URINARY SYSTEM

Characteristics of the Normal Ferret Urinary System

- The normal urine pH is 6.0 for ferrets on a meat-based diet.
- Normal values for urine specific gravity have not been reported.
- There is evidence that proteinuria may be normal in ferrets (7–33 mg/dl in males; 0–32 mg/dl in females) and that bilirubinuria can occur in the absence of liver disease.

Polycystic Kidneys

Unilateral or bilateral polycystic kidneys are relatively common in ferrets (see Chap. 97 for a description of this disease in dogs and cats). The condition usually is discovered as an incidental finding in middle-aged and older ferrets, although clinical signs can be present at any age, including early in life.

Etiology

- The cause of polycystic kidneys in ferrets is unknown. The disorder is usually congenital, as in other species.

Clinical Signs

- Usually no clinical signs are apparent.
- In ferrets with severe renal involvement, clinical signs are the result of renal insufficiency and include lethargy, inappetence, polyuria/polydipsia, vomiting, and melena.

Diagnosis

- Palpate the kidneys for irregular shape.
- Perform a serum biochemical profile, CBC, and urinalysis if renal disease is suspected.
- Abdominal radiography usually is not helpful unless the kidneys are very irregular.
- Intravenous pyelography may be helpful.
- Abdominal ultrasonography is the most useful tool for detection of polycystic kidneys and to rule out other conditions, such as renal neoplasia.
- Renal cysts may be an incidental finding during abdominal surgery.

Treatment

- No treatment is necessary in asymptomatic cases.
- If the affected kidney becomes very enlarged, consider unilateral nephrectomy (if the opposite kidney is functional).
- Supportive care such as subcutaneous fluid administration may temporarily improve the status of azotemic animals. Other therapy for chronic renal failure in dogs and cats may be helpful.
- The prognosis is grave if the ferret is in renal failure.

Hydronephrosis

- Hydronephrosis is uncommon in ferrets. Iatrogenic hydronephrosis may occur as the result of inadvertent ligation of a ureter during ovariohysterectomy (see Chap. 97 for information about hydronephrosis in dogs and cats).

Cystitis

- Bacterial cystitis without urinary calculi is rare in pet ferrets. Follow treatment protocols for cystitis in dogs (see Chap. 99).

Urolithiasis

Urinary tract calculi composed of struvite (magnesium ammonium phosphate hexahydrate) can occur in pet ferrets. Cysteine calculi also have been reported.

Etiology

- The cause of urinary calculi in ferrets, including the role of nutritional factors, is not known. However, most affected ferrets were being fed commercial dog food or low-quality cat food or ferret chow. Diets containing plant proteins as the main source of protein (rather than meats) are implicated most commonly in struvite urolithiasis because they promote an alkaline urine, which provides struvite crystallization. Calculi are rare in ferrets fed a high-quality meat-based feline or ferret diet.
- The cause of cysteine calculi is not known.
- Usually no growth occurs on bacterial culture.

Clinical Signs

Clinical signs depend on the location of the urolith(s):

- Cystic calculi result in dysuria and hematuria.
- Urethral calculi may cause obstruction in both male and female ferrets.
- Renal calculi may be asymptomatic or may result in renal failure.

Diagnosis

- On physical examination, cystic calculi are often palpable. The urinary bladder wall may be thickened; in cases of obstruction, the bladder is distended and firm.
- Abdominal radiography can confirm the presence of urinary tract calculi (struvite calculi are radiodense), although cysteine calculi are radiolucent.

Treatment

▼ *Key Point* The bladder is very fragile in ferrets. Handle ferrets with obstruction gently to avoid bladder rupture.

- Treatment of urinary obstruction may be difficult because urinary catheters are difficult to pass in ferrets.
  - If attempts at catheterization are unsuccessful, perform transabdominal cystocentesis to empty the bladder.
  - Consider a cystotomy for anterograde urethral catheterization and flushing. A perineal urethrotomy may be necessary.
- Remove cystic calculi surgically using the same technique as for dogs and cats (see Chap. 100).
  - Close the bladder with 4-0 or 5-0 absorbable suture material.
  - Submit the calculi for analysis and culture; results guide subsequent therapy.

Prevention

- Feed a high-quality, meat-based feline or ferret diet.
- Postoperative care and prevention of urolithiasis in ferrets may include antibiotic therapy. Begin treatment with either trimethoprim sulfate (15–30 mg/kg q12h SC or PO), chloramphenicol (50 mg/kg q12h IV, SC, IM, or PO), or amoxicillin-clavulinic acid (Clavamox, SmithKline).
  - Adjust antibiotic selection and dosage according to culture and sensitivity test results.

PARAURETHRAL CYSTS AND URINARY TRACT OBSTRUCTION

Urethral obstruction in male ferrets may occur secondary to extraluminal pressure from cystic enlargement of paraurethral tissue seen in association with adrenal disease. The cysts are thought to arise from prostatic tissue or urogenital glands or ducts.

Etiology

- Abnormal steroid hormone production by an adrenal tumor is thought to stimulate cystic changes of paraurethral tissue. Secondary bacterial infections and abscessation may occur.
- Prostate abscesses also have been reported in association with transitional cell tumor of the bladder.

History and Clinical Signs

- The history and clinical signs are compatible with urinary tract obstruction.
- A history of hair loss or other signs of adrenal disease may be evident.

Physical Examination

- On physical examination, a large, firm, caudal abdominal mass is palpable. With careful palpation, this mass is found to be bilobed, representing the urinary bladder and a cystic structure.
- Hair loss and other signs of adrenal neoplasia are usually present.

Diagnosis

- Evaluate abdominal radiographs to rule out obstruction from cystic calculi.

- If available, perform ultrasonography to evaluate adrenals and any masses. Cystocentesis may be necessary to empty the urinary bladder.
- Perform abdominal exploratory surgery for a definitive diagnosis.

Treatment

The cystic tissue typically regresses in size after adrenalectomy.

- Perform adrenalectomy of affected gland(s) (see Adrenal Disease section).
- The abnormal tissue is usually nonresectable because of size and position near the urethra and ureters.
  - Typically, the structures are cavitary with multiple small pockets of cystic or purulent material.
  - If an abscess is present, it may be necessary to marsupialize the abscess cavity.
  - On biopsy, these structures are composed of cystic or abscessed glandular tissue.

Prognosis

- The long-term prognosis is good if the paraurethral cysts regress after the adrenal gland disease is controlled.

SUPPLEMENTAL READINGS

Anderson NL: Intraosseous fluid therapy in small exotic animals. In: Bonagura JD, Kirk RW (eds): Current Veterinary Therapy XII. Philadelphia, WB Saunders, 1997, pp 1331–1335.

Fox JG: Biology and Diseases of the Ferret. Philadelphia: Lea & Febiger, 1988.

Hillyer EV, Quesenbery KE (eds): Ferrets, Rabbits, and Rodents: Clinical Medicine and Surgery. Philadelphia: WB Saunders, 1997.

Rosenthal K: Ferrets. Vet Clin North Am Sm Anim Pract 24:1, 1994.

Rabbits are popular pets for both children and adults. They are easily litter trained and require minimal maintenance. Management of diseases in pet rabbits differs from that of laboratory rabbits in the emphasis on individual animals and the approach to therapy. This chapter stresses diagnosis and management of problems commonly encountered in pet rabbits. Refer to the Supplemental Readings for more comprehensive information.

BIOLOGIC CHARACTERISTICS

Rabbits, hares, and pikas are members of the order Lagomorpha. Lagomorphs have six incisors in contrast to the closely related rodents, which have four incisors. The additional incisors (peg teeth) are small, rounded teeth located directly behind the upper incisors.

- All domestic rabbits are descendants of European wild rabbits, *Oryctolagus cuniculus*.
- The two main genera of rabbits are *Oryctolagus*, the European wild rabbits, and *Sylvilagus*, the cottontail rabbits. These genera differ in chromosome number and cannot interbreed.
- Currently, more than 50 breeds of rabbits are recognized.
  - Giant breeds, which average more than 5 kg in body weight, include the American Checkered Giant, the Flemish Giant, and the Giant Chinchilla rabbits.
  - Medium breeds, which average from 3.5 to 5 kg in body weight, include the Californian, the Silver Marten, and the Rex rabbits.
  - Small breeds, which average less than 3.5 kg in body weight, include the Netherland Dwarf, the Jersey Wooly, and the Polish rabbits.
  - Specific information concerning breeds can be obtained from the American Rabbit Breeders Association, 1925 S. Main, P.O. Box 426, Bloomington, IL 61702.

Anatomic and Physiologic Characteristics

- Females of several breeds of rabbits have a pendulous dewlap. This area is a frequent site of moist dermatitis, especially in obese rabbits kept in humid, warm environments.
- Teeth are open rooted and grow continuously. The dental formula is 2/1 incisors, 0/0 canines, 3/2 pre-

molars, and 2–3/3 molars. Malocclusion and overgrowth of the incisors, premolars, and molars are common.
- The gastrointestinal (GI) tract has a simple glandular stomach, a long intestinal tract, and a large cecum.
  - The cecum is the site of bacterial synthesis of B-vitamins.
  - About one-third of the normal stool output is composed of soft stools called cecotrophs. Cecotrophs are consumed primarily at night by domestic rabbits as an important source of B-vitamins, electrolytes, and nitrogen.
- The skeletal system is light and delicate compared with most mammals. The skeleton makes up 8% of the total body weight in rabbits, as opposed to 13% of the total body weight in cats.
- Inguinal canals remain open throughout life.
- Female rabbits (i.e., does) have four to five pairs of mammary glands and nipples.

▼ *Key Point* Red, pink, or orange discoloration of the urine occurs periodically in healthy rabbits. The color may be caused by porphyrin pigments or food-related metabolites excreted in the urine.

- Calcium and phosphorus are excreted primarily through urine in rabbits. Calcium is excreted in the bile in most other mammals.
- In rabbits, high total leukocyte counts may not be characteristic of acute inflammation from infectious causes. Instead, the distribution of the white blood cells (WBCs) shifts from a normally high lymphocyte/low neutrophil ratio to neutrophilia and lymphopenia.

Reproductive Characteristics

- Females mature sexually at 4 to 8 months of age, depending on breed. Males mature at 6 to 10 months of age.
- Females have a silent estrus and are induced ovulators.
- Gestation lasts for an average of 30 to 33 days.
- Pseudocyesis may last 17 days.
- Litters are usually born (i.e., kindled) at night. Litter size averages 4 to 10 young (i.e., kits).
- Does normally nurse their young once or twice daily. Weaning occurs at 4 to 6 weeks of age.
- Rabbit milk is approximately 13% protein, 9% fat, and 1% lactose.

Normal Parameters

Reference ranges for physiologic values are listed in Table 169–1. Reference ranges for hematology, serum biochemical analysis, and urinalysis are listed in Tables 169–2, 169–3, and 169–4.

PATIENT MANAGEMENT

Caging

- Cages or hutches can be purchased or constructed. Cages should be large enough to allow free movement. Small breeds, which weigh up to 2 kg, require a minimum of 1.5 ft^2 of floor space per animal. Large breeds, which weigh 5 kg or more, require at least 5 ft^2 of floor space per animal. Cages should be easy to clean.
- Both wire and hard flooring may predispose rabbits to sore hocks. If mesh flooring is used, either $1 \times \frac{1}{2}$ in^2 or $\frac{5}{8}$-in^2 mesh is recommended. Be sure there are no rough edges in the cage. Provide clean, soft bedding, such as straw, in one area of the cage.
- Rabbits can be housed indoors or outdoors at temperatures ranging from 40° to 80°F. Rabbits are very susceptible to heat stroke in ambient temperatures above 85° F. If outdoor housing is used, provide ventilation or protection from direct sunlight. In temperatures below 40°F, provide heat or protection from cold.

Restraint

▼ *Key Point* Restrain rabbits gently but firmly for most procedures. Inadequate restraint can result in a spinal fracture in the rabbit if it is allowed to kick with its hind legs.

- Carry the rabbit with its head tucked under one arm while supporting the body with the forearm; stabilize the rump with the other hand.
- Grasp the rabbit with the hindquarters supported in one arm and the rear legs held firmly between the fingers. Hold the rabbit firmly by the scruff at the base of the neck with the other hand.
- For examination or treatment, hold the rabbit to the table with firm, gentle downward pressure at the pelvic and thoracic girdles (Fig. 169–1).

Table 169–1. REFERENCE RANGES FOR PHYSIOLOGIC VALUES IN RABBITS

Temperature	38–40° C
Heart rate	130–325 beats/min
Respiratory rate	32–60/min
Life span	5–9 yrs
Blood volume	55–65 ml/kg
Food consumption	50 g/kg/day
Water consumption	
General population	50–100 ml/kg/day
Breeding does	<900 ml/kg/day

Table 169–2. REFERENCE RANGES FOR HEMATOLOGIC VALUES IN RABBITS

Erythrocytes	$5.1–7.9 \times 10^6$m^3
Hematocrit	33–50%
Hemoglobin	10.0–17.4 g/dl
Mean corpuscular volume	57.8–66.5 μm^3
Mean corpuscular hemoglobin	17.1–23.5 pg
Mean corpuscular hemoglobin concentration	29–37%
Platelets	$250–650 \times 10^3$/mm^3
Leukocytes	$5.2–12.5 \times 10^3$/mm^3
Neutrophils	20–75%
Lymphocytes	30–85%
Monocytes	1–4%
Eosinophils	1–4%
Basophils	1–7%

- The ventrum and anal area can be examined by cradling the rabbit on its back in one arm. Hold the rear legs firmly between the fingers of one hand and the forelegs between the fingers of the other hand (Fig. 169–2).
- For jugular venipuncture, restraint is similar to that for a cat. Extend the neck up and the forelegs down over a table edge. Press the pelvic girdle firmly to the table to control the rear legs.

Diagnostic Techniques

- Measure physical values, including heart rate, temperature, and respiratory rate. Auscultate the lungs and palpate the abdomen thoroughly.
- Check feet and hocks for evidence of erythema and ulceration.
- Check the incisors for overgrowth. Examine the molars with an otoscope for evidence of malocclusion.

Blood Collection

- Rabbit veins are thin and fragile. Use a small-gauge needle (i.e., 25-gauge or smaller) for venipuncture of

Table 169–3. REFERENCE RANGES FOR SERUM BIOCHEMICAL VALUES IN RABBITS

Albumin	2.4–4.6 g/dl
Alkaline phosphatase	4–16 U/L
Amylase	166.5–314.5 U/L
Bicarbonate	16–38 mEq/L
Blood urea nitrogen	13–29 mg/dl
Calcium	5.6–12.5 mg/dl
Chloride	92–112 mEq/L
Cholesterol	10–80 mg/dl
Creatinine	0.5–2.5 mg/dl
Globulin	1.5–2.8 g/dl
Glucose	75–155 g/dl
Glutamic-oxaloacetic transaminase	14–113 U/L
Glutamic pyruvate transaminase	48–80 U/L
Lactic dehydrogenase	34–129 U/L
Phosphorus	4.0–6.9 mg/dl
Potassium	3.6–6.9 mEq/L
Serum protein	5.4–8.3 g/dl
Sodium	131–155 mEq/L
Total bilirubin	0.0–0.7 mg/dl
Total lipids	243–390 mg/dl

Table 169–4. REFERENCE RANGES FOR URINALYSIS IN RABBITS

Urine volume	
Large breeds	20–350 ml/kg/day
Average breeds	130 ml/kg/day
Specific gravity	1.003–1.036
Average pH	8.2
Crystals present	Ammonium magnesium phosphate, calcium carbonate monohydrate, anhydrous calcium carbonate
Casts, epithelial cells, or bacteria present	Absent to rare
Leukocytes or erythrocytes present	Occasional
Albumin present	Occasional in young rabbits

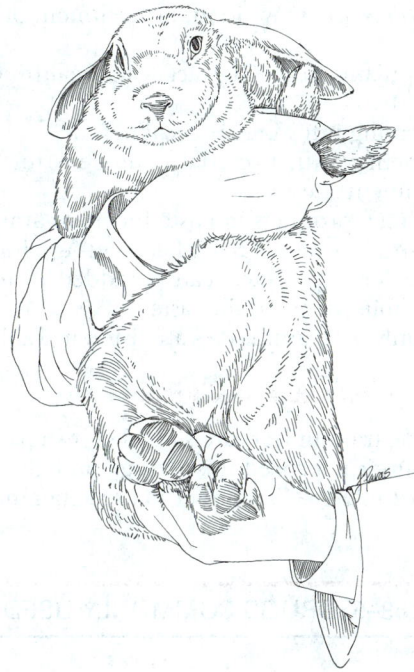

Figure 169–2. To examine the ventrum and anal area, cradle the rabbit as shown. Be sure to provide support to the hind limbs.

peripheral veins to prevent hematoma formation. Apply direct pressure for several minutes after venipuncture.

- Blood is collected easily from the lateral saphenous vein. This vein lies in the middle portion of the lateral aspect of the tibia.
- Plucking the hair over the vein is easier than shaving fine fur.
- The lateral ear vein can be used for blood collection in some large rabbits. Some clinicians use a vacutainer system for rapid withdrawal. In most medium- and small-breed rabbits, the ear vein is very small and is easily damaged by venipuncture. Thrombosis of the vein may lead to local sloughing of the pinna.
- The jugular vein can be used for venipuncture in many rabbits. Jugular venipuncture is sometimes difficult in females with heavy dewlaps. The vein usually is not visible; it lies superficially in the jugular furrow. Pluck or shave the hair from the midneck region and extend the head up for venipuncture as described under restraint. Alternatively, with the rabbit anesthetized, lay the rabbit on its back with its head and neck extended down over a table edge to expose the jugular veins.

Treatment Techniques

- Subcutaneous administration of fluids is acceptable in noncritical cases and may be the only practical route of fluid administration in small rabbits. Estimate daily maintenance fluids at 100-150 ml/kg/24 hours.
- An indwelling catheter is preferred in critical cases.
  - Small-gauge catheters (i.e., 24-gauge) can be placed in the cephalic or lateral saphenous vein in most rabbits.
  - Jugular catheters can be difficult to insert and may require a cutdown procedure.
- Medications can be administered orally into the lateral cheek pouch. Use liquid or paste preparations when possible because rabbits have a long, narrow oropharynx that makes pill administration difficult.
- Force-feed anorexic animals with a paste nutritional supplement (e.g., Nutri-Cal, Evsco Pharmaceuticals, Buena, NJ), a commercial nutritional formula, vegetable baby food, a gruel made of moistened rabbit pellets, or a mixture of any of these.
- Place nasogastric tubes in medium-to-large rabbits that require long-term nutritional support or that have had extensive oral surgery. The technique that follows is similar to that for placing a tube in a cat.
  - With manual restraint, place two to three drops of a topical anesthetic (Ophthaine, Solvay Veterinary, Inc., Princeton, NJ) in the mucosa of one nostril. Wait 5 minutes, then repeat application.
  - Lubricate the tip of a small infant feeding tube (e.g., 5 Fr., Bard-Parker, Becton-Dickenson and Company, Rutherford, NJ) with topical lidocaine (Xylocaine) jelly. Pass the tube medially along the nasal passage to the level of the last rib. The tip of the tube is located in the distal esophagus.
  - Secure the free end of the tube to the skin above the nose and eye with a butterfly tape and suture. An Elizabethan collar may be necessary to prevent the rabbit from dislodging the tube.

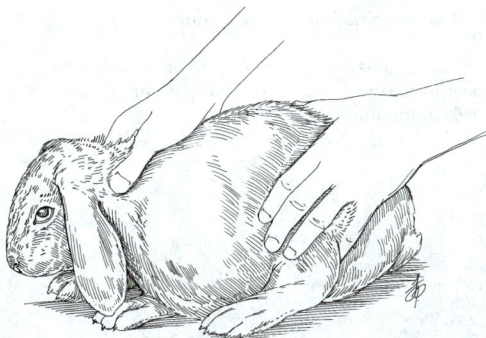

Figure 169–1. Proper method for restraining a rabbit.

- *Lactobacillus* spp. may aid in the treatment of enteritis by:
  - Repopulating the GI tract with healthy bacterial flora
  - Decreasing intestinal or cecal pH
  - Competing with bacterial pathogens for mucosal attachment sites
- Commercial products in paste form are available for administration (e.g., Bene-Bac, Pet-Ag, Inc, Elgin, IL). Powdered products can be added to food, but many rabbits object to the taste.
- Commonly used antibiotics are listed in Table 169–5.

Tranquilization and Anesthesia

- Injectable tranquilizers are suitable for short diagnostic or surgical procedures. Drugs and dosages are listed in Table 169–5. I prefer to use ketamine and diazepam or midazolam (Versed, Roche Pharmaceuticals, Inc., Manati, DR) in combination given IM or IV.
- Use inhalant anesthesia for long or painful surgical procedures. Clinically, isoflurane is very safe and is the preferred inhalant anesthetic. Halothane is potentially hepatotoxic and is associated with anesthetic-related deaths.
- Anesthesia in rabbits can be induced by face mask or in an induction chamber. Premedicate with ketamine, midazolam or diazepam, and glycopyrrolate. Gradually increase the concentration of isoflurane over several minutes until a surgical plane of anesthesia is reached. Anesthesia usually is maintained at 1.5–2% isoflurane in oxygen.

▼ *Key Point* Intubation is most successful in large rabbits; consider intubating medium-sized rabbits for

Table 169–5. DRUGS COMMONLY USED IN RABBITS

Drug	Dose	Comments
Antimicrobials		
Benzathine, penicillin G (Benza-Pen, SmithKline Beecham, Exton, PA)	84,000 IU/kg q7d × 3 treatments SC	For treatment of *Treponema cuniculi*
Chloramphenicol	25 mg/kg q12–8h PO 30 mg/kg q12–q8h IV, IM	
Ciprofloxacin (Cipro, Miles Pharmaceuticals, West Haven, CT)	5–15 mg/kg q12h PO	Have a suspension made by a compounding pharmacist for easy administration
Enrofloxacin (Baytril, Haver/Diamond Scientific, Shawnee, KS)	5–15 mg/kg q12h PO, IM	Manufacturers recommend one time only use of injectable formulation
Gentamicin	5–8 mg/kg total daily dosage; divided q8–24h IM, IV, SC	
Griseofulvin (Fulvicin, Schering-Plough, Kenilworth, NJ)	25 mg/kg divided q12h PO × 4–6 weeks	If using Gris-PEG, decrease dose by 50%
Procaine penicillin	40,000 IU/kg q24 hr SC	
Sulfadimethoxine	50 mg/kg PO first dose, then 25 mg/kg q24h PO × 5–20 days	For treatment of coccidiosis
Tetracycline	50–100 mg/kg q8h PO	
Trimethoprim/sulfa	15–30 mg/kg q12h PO, IM, SC	
Anthelmintics/Insecticides		
Lime sulfur solution	2% dip 1–2 times/week × 4 weeks	Used in young animals for treatment of mites, fleas, fungal dermatitis
Ivermectin	400 µg/kg q8–10d × 2–3 treatments	Effective against ear and fur mites
Piperazine	200 mg/kg; repeat in 2–3 weeks	
Pyrantel pamoate	5–10 mg/kg; repeat in 2–3 weeks	
Tranquilizers/Premedications		
Acepromazine	0.5–1 mg/kg IM/SC	
Diazepam	1–4 mg/kg IV, IM	Used in combination with ketamine
Glycopyrrolate	0.01–0.02 IM or SC	
Ketamine HCl	25–40 mg/kg IM 5–20 mg/kg IV	Use in combination with diazepam, midazolam, or acepromazine; ketamine/diazepam provides good relaxation and sedation
Midazolam (Versed)	1–2 mg/kg IM or slow IV	
Tiletamine-zolazepam (Telazol, Fort Dodge, IA)	5 mg/kg IM	
Analgesics		
Aspirin	100 mg/kg q4–6h PO	
Buprenorphine	0.01–0.05 mg/kg q8–12h SC, IM	
Butorphenol	0.1–0.5 mg/kg q2–4h SC	
Flunixin	0.3–2.0 mg/kg q12–24h PO, deep IM	
Ibuprofen	7.5 mg/kg; PO prn	

long surgical procedures. However, repeated attempts to intubate can damage the larynx, causing soft tissue trauma or laryngospasm that can be fatal after the rabbit is extubated. If laryngeal trauma occurs during intubation attempts, abandon the procedure and use a face mask, or postpone the procedure to another day. Corticosteroids may or may not be helpful in decreasing inflammation of the larynx and tracheal mucosa.

- The long, narrow oropharynx and the propensity for laryngospasm make intubation extremely difficult. The following technique can be used.
  - Induce anesthesia with isoflurane. Give a low IV dose of ketamine and diazepam in combination after the rabbit has begun to relax (2–10 mg/kg and 0.5–1.0 mg/kg, respectively).
  - Place the rabbit in sternal recumbancy. Extend the neck straight up and forward.
  - Place the tip of the short, flat-blade laryngoscope blade (i.e., Miller blade), at the base of the tongue. Hook the base of the blade against the top front incisors, and use the blade as a lever to see the glottis.
  - Pass a small endotracheal tube along the blade into the opening of the glottis. Depending on their size, most rabbits require a 2.5- to 5.0-mm endotracheal tube. The glottis cannot be seen while trying to pass the tube.
- Use a face mask to maintain anesthesia during short procedures or if intubation attempts are unsuccessful.
- Monitor all rabbits closely during any anesthetic episode.

NUTRITION

Nutritional Requirements

Most rabbits are fed a balanced commercial ration. Consequently, specific nutrient deficiencies are rare. The nutritional requirements of rabbits are published by the National Research Council (NRC) in the series Nutrient Requirements for Domestic Animals. Further research indicates that high levels of dietary fiber (20–25%) are needed for optimum health. Recommendations for the percentages of dietary protein, fiber, fat, and energy vary during growth, lactation, reproduction, and maintenance (Table 169–6).

Table 169–6. NUTRITIONAL RECOMMENDATIONS IN RABBITS

Stage	Crude Protein (%)	Fat (%)	Crude Fiber (%)
Maintenance	13	3	15–25
Lactation	18	5	12
Pregnancy	18	3	14
Growth	15	3	14

▼ *Key Point* Insufficient indigestible dietary fiber is a significant underlying factor in many disease problems.

- Inadequate fiber causes decreased colonic-cecal motility, slowing overall GI transit time. Decreased motility and prolonged retention of food material in the cecum may lead to enteritis and diarrhea.
- High-starch, low-fiber diets provide high levels of fermentation products for cecal bacteria. The number of bacterial pathogens may increase, resulting in increased toxin production.
- Hairballs (i.e., trichobezoars) are common in rabbits that are fed inadequate amounts of roughage. Fiber stimulates GI motility and mechanically helps to move fur through the upper GI tract. Fur-chewing or barbering is common in rabbits on low-fiber diets.

Some commercial rations have as little as 12% crude fiber. Add dietary fiber by feeding free-choice grass hay (e.g., timothy, orchard grass) or legume hay (e.g., alfalfa, clover). High-fiber, timothy-based pelleted feeds, which are 29% fiber, are available (Oxbow Hay Company, Murdock, Nebraska).

- If both alfalfa hay and alfalfa-based pellets are fed, dietary calcium intake may be too high in house rabbits, resulting in hypercalciuria or urinary calculi. Therefore, timothy hay may be the best choice for mature house rabbits.

DERMATOLOGIC PROBLEMS

Dermatitis/Alopecia

Etiology

- Mange, fur, and ear mites cause localized or diffuse dermatitis and/or alopecia. The area involved depends on the type of mite (see Ear Mites; Fur and Mange Mites).
- Dermatophytosis is associated with alopecia and a scaly dermatitis, particularly around the head and ears (see Superficial Mycosis).
- Fur-barbering is common in rabbits on diets deficient in roughage. A high incidence of barbering in does is seen during breeding season; this probably is related to hormonal influences.
- Ptyalism, alopecia, and dermatitis around the mouth are associated with malocclusion.
- Moist dermatitis of the dewlap is common in females during breeding season, especially when they are kept in warm or humid environments.
- Moist dermatitis with erythema and ulceration of the ventral abdomen and perineal area results from urine scald. Urine scald is associated with urinary incontinence, cystitis, excessive calcium in the urine, uterine adenocarcinoma, or poor management and unclean caging.
- Treponematosis (*Treponema cuniculi*) causes a scaly dermatitis in the genital area. The nose, lips, and periorbital area are less commonly involved.

Clinical Signs

- Mite infestations produce clinical signs characteristic of the mite involved (see Ear Mites; Fur and Mange Mites). Pruritis is common with sarcoptic mite infestations.
- Dermatophytes cause a partial alopecia with slight scaliness and erythema. Rabbits are usually pruritic.
- Fur-barbering is characterized by alopecia of the dewlap, back of the neck, and paws. The underlying skin is normal.
- Moist dermatitis of the dewlap or ventral abdomen is typically erythematous with scaling and ulceration. The fur around the alopecic areas is moist. Rabbits sometimes self-mutilate this area; use a collar to prevent further trauma.

Diagnosis

Determine the primary cause of the alopecia to make a diagnosis.

- Examine skin scrapings of scaly areas for evidence of adult mites or eggs.
- Obtain samples of fur and keratin debris for fungal culture.
- Submit a skin biopsy specimen for histologic examination if the etiogenic agent cannot be determined by other diagnostic tests.
- Examine the teeth in rabbits with excessive ptyalism and alopecia around the mouth (see Malocclusion).
- Obtain radiographs of rabbits with urine scald for evidence of cystic calculi.
- Submit a urine sample for urinalysis and bacterial culture and sensitivity testing.
- Submit a blood sample for serum biochemical analysis to check for high serum calcium, blood urea nitrogen, and creatinine concentrations.

Treatment

Treatment is directed toward the primary cause (see Ear Mites; Fur and Mange Mites; Hairballs; Malocclusion; Treponematosis; Cystitis; Superficial Mycosis).

- Correct the diet to include adequate roughage if fur-barbering is suspected. Perform ovariohysterectomy in females with a suspected hormonal basis for fur-barbering.
- Treat adult rabbits with suspected mite infestations with ivermectin (see Table 169–5).
- Steroids rarely are used for pruritic dermatitis in rabbits.
- Treat treponematosis with penicillin (see Treponematosis).
- Treat dermatophytosis with antifungal agents administered topically or orally depending on the extent of lesions.

Ear Mites *(Psoroptes cuniculi)*

Etiology

- Ear mites are common ectoparasites in both pet and laboratory rabbits.
- *Psoroptes cuniculi* is a large, nonburrowing mite that spends its 3-week life cycle on the host rabbit.

- Mites have biting mouthparts and cause inflammation by biting and chewing the epithelial surface of the skin.

Clinical Signs

- Infestation with psoroptic mites usually is confined to the inner epithelial surface of the ear. Lesions begin in the concha and eventually extend to the inner surface of the pinna. Other areas, such as the dewlap and feet, sometimes are involved.
- Lesions consist of thick, dry, flaky, gray-to-tan crusts on the inner surface of the ear pinna. The underlying epithelial surface is raw, inflamed, and hemorrhagic.
- Psoroptic mites cause intense pruritus. Affected rabbits shake their heads or scratch their ears with the rear feet.

Diagnosis

- Psoroptic mites are large and sometimes visible with the unaided eye.
  - Use an otoscope to detect movement of the mites within the ear canal.
  - Microscopic examination of crusts and exudate usually reveals mites and eggs.
- Check rabbits with mild cases of otitis for the presence of mites.

Treatment

- Clean the ears of all crusts and exudate. Use a mild otic cleansing agent to soften the crusts before removal.
  - Lesions are usually very painful.
  - Tranquilization is sometimes necessary for cleaning.
- If ivermectin is used, ears can be cleaned in 1 to 2 weeks after pain subsides and lesions heal.
- Psoroptic mites are susceptible to topical acaricides (e.g., Mitox Liquid, SmithKline Beecham, Exton, PA). Continue treatment for at least 3 weeks.
- Apply an antibiotic cream topically if a secondary bacterial infection is present. Topical application of anti-inflammatory agents may be beneficial once bacterial infection is under control.
- Ivermectin is effective against ear mites (see Table 169–5). Repeat treatment in 3 weeks. A combination therapy of ivermectin and topical acaricides can be used for severe infestations.

Prevention

- Psoroptic mites are transmitted easily between rabbits. Isolate affected rabbits from healthy rabbits.
- Keep cages and bedding clean to minimize spread through contaminated fomites.

Fur and Mange Mites

Etiology

- *Cheyletiella parasitivorax* is the common fur mite of rabbits. Infestations with other species of *Cheyletiella* occasionally occur. *Listrophorus gibbus* is a less common fur mite and is considered nonpathogenic.

- Cheyletid mites are nonburrowing, obligate parasites with an approximate 35-day life cycle.
- Infestation can be inapparent.
- Cheyletid mites may cause a self-limiting, transitory dermatitis in humans.
- The cheyletid mite is a known vector of rabbit myxomatosis in Australia.
- Mange mites (e.g., *Sarcoptes scabiei, Notedres cati*) occur infrequently in rabbits.

Clinical Signs

- Lesions produced by cheyletid mites consist of a scaly dermatitis with a flaky grayish-white exudate. Mites primarily inhabit the dorsal trunk and scapular region. The underlying skin may appear erythematous and inflamed. Pruritus is not a major clinical sign.
- Other areas of the body can be involved in severe infestations. Rabbits may act as if they are depressed and in pain.
- Mange mites produce a crusty dermatitis with alopecia.
- Intense pruritus results from mites burrowing in the epidermis.

Diagnosis

- Identify cheyletid mites through microscopic examination of skin scrapings. Alternatively, press a strip of cellophane tape to the skin and fur in scaly areas and examine it under a microscope.
- Deep skin scrapings are necessary to find mange mites. Results are sometimes falsely negative. Differential diagnosis then is based on the typical clinical signs of each type of mite.

Treatment

- Topical acaricides, including pyrethrins, carbamates, and lime sulfur solution dips (see Table 169–5), are effective against fur and mange mites. Products and treatment regimens that are safe for use in cats are usually safe for use in rabbits.
- Ivermectin is effective against mange and fur mites (see Table 169–5).
- The treatment period should extend through the life cycle of the mite.
- Cheyletid mites can exist off the host for short periods. Treat the home environment with parasiticides and eliminate potential fomites. Examine or treat any cats kept in contact with infested rabbits.

Myiasis (Cuterebriasis)

Etiology

Myiasis (fly larval infestation) is common in rabbits kept outdoors. Incidence is highest in the summer and fall.

- Several species of *Cuterebra* affect rabbits. Cuterebrid larvae burrow into subcutaneous tissue and migrate to preferred body sites. Areas commonly involved include the ventral cervical region (*Cuterebra horripilum*) and the inguinal, hindquarter, and axillary regions (*Cuterebra buccata*).
- Blowflies or screwworms invade preexisting wounds. These species include *Cochliomyia, Callitroga,* and *Wohlfahrtia.*

Clinical Signs

- Rabbits may appear to be in pain, reluctant to move, or lame.
- One or more firm, fistulated, subcutaneous swellings are found on physical examination. Frequently, the larvae are seen in the fistula surrounded by necrotic tissue.
- Secondary bacterial infections of the lesions are common.
- The eye also can be involved; this is known as ophthalmomyiasis.
- Severe infestation with multiple cuterebrid larvae can cause extreme debilitation and death.

Diagnosis

Diagnosis is based on a history of outdoor housing, clinical signs, and presence of larvae in wounds.

Treatment

- Remove larvae intact with hemostats if possible. Avoid rupture of the larvae. Ether can be applied topically to anesthetize the larvae before removal.
- Thoroughly debride wounds of necrotic tissue. Daily cleaning and debridement is usually necessary until healing occurs. With large wounds, perform complete excision of the necrotic area.
- Observe affected rabbits carefully for several weeks for additional lesions.
- Antibiotic therapy is recommended for secondary bacterial infections.

Prevention

- Keep outdoor rabbits in screened hutches, especially during summer and fall.

Superficial Mycosis

Etiology

- *Trichophyton mentagrophytes* is the most common dermatophyte affecting rabbits. Infections with *Microsporum* spp. and other dermatophytes are much less frequent.
- Infection occurs by direct contact with infected animals, contaminated fomites, or asymptomatic carriers.

Clinical Signs

- Lesions usually appear on the head and ears and can extend to the feet, neck, and other areas.
- Lesions consist of areas of alopecia with erythema and scaly dermatitis. Rabbits are usually pruritic. Alopecic areas may be circular with slightly raised edges.

Diagnosis

Dermatitis resulting from dermatophytosis must be differentiated from other possible causes, including mites, fur-barbering, and bacterial dermatitis.

- Submit samples of fur from the edge of the lesion for fungal culture.
  - *T. mentagrophytes* does not fluoresce with ultraviolet light.
- The organisms can be demonstrated with either PAS or silver stains in histologic sections of skin biopsy specimens of affected rabbits.

Treatment

Treatment of dermatophytosis is directed toward elimination of the organism while preventing spread of disease. Other animals and humans, especially children, are susceptible to infection.

- Apply topical antifungal agents, such as Conofite (Pitman-Moore, Mundelein, IL), daily for 3 to 4 weeks.
- Lime sulfur solution dips (2–3%) given every 5 to 7 days are often effective for treating fungal dermatosis. Continue treatment for 4 weeks.
- Griseofulvin is effective if given daily for 4 weeks or until the infection clears (see Table 169–5). Give griseofulvin with fats to enhance absorption. Gris-PEG (Allergen, Inc.), an ultramicronized formulation for improved absorption, is given at one-half the normal dose.
- Instruct owners to wear gloves when handling or treating affected animals because of the zoonotic disease potential.
- Check other animals in the household for evidence of dermatophytosis.

Prevention

- Prevent contact with infected animals.
- Have owners practice strict sanitation to eliminate spread through fomites.

Sore Hocks/Ulcerative Pododermatitis
Etiology

- Sore hocks usually develop as a result of management-related problems. Soiled or wet bedding, abrasions from flooring, sedentary behavior caused by excessive weight, small cages that restrict movement, and abrasions from thumping are predisposing factors.
- Lesions involve the plantar surface of the hocks and may be unilateral or bilateral. Forepaws are less commonly affected.
- Secondary bacterial infections are common with severely ulcerated lesions.

Clinical Signs

- Early lesions are areas of erythema and thinning fur on the plantar surface of the hock.
- Lesions progress to raw, ulcerative sores with scabs. Mucoid or purulent exudate is present with secondary bacterial infections.
- Severe lesions cause lameness and reluctance to move. Rabbits may be anorexic and depressed.

Diagnosis

Diagnosis is based on clinical signs. If wounds appear infected, submit samples for bacterial culture and sensitivity testing.

Treatment

- Correct the predisposing management and environmental factors.
- Thoroughly clean and debride wounds. A nonocclusive antibiotic cream can be applied topically.
- Topical astringents such as Domeboro solution (Miles, Inc., West Haven, CT) are beneficial in treating moist wounds. Apply the solution daily until the wound appears dry.
- Protect wounds with sterile, soft, padded bandages.
- Healing is often prolonged. Clean the wound with an antibacterial soak, topical antibiotics, and bandaging, daily or every other day.
- Systemic antibiotics may be necessary if cellulitis is present.

Prevention

- Wire flooring should be smooth, nonabrasive, and of sufficient width to prevent abrasions. Place soft, dry bedding, such as hay or several thicknesses of newspaper, in one area of the cage.
- Cages should be clean and of sufficient size to allow free movement.
- Check the feet and hocks periodically for signs of inflammation.

RESPIRATORY DISEASE

Respiratory disease is common in pet rabbits and usually is associated with pasteurellosis. However, respiratory disease can result from many interrelated factors and is precipitated by stress.

Rhinitis/Paranasal Sinusitis/Conjunctivitis
Etiology

- The primary infectious agent of paranasal sinusitis and rhinitis in rabbits is *Pasteurella multocida* (see Pasteurellosis). Other bacterial species less commonly involved include *Bordetella bronchiseptica* and *Staphylococcus aureus*.
- Infections can be transmitted from the doe to offspring or by direct contact with infected rabbits. Infection also may be spread through airborne transmission.
- Intermittent episodes of rhinitis with mucopurulent nasal discharge are common with pasteurellosis. Chronic disease may be subclinical and precipitated by stress.

Clinical Signs

- Nasal discharge may be serous or mucopurulent.
- Accompanying acute or chronic conjunctivitis with a serous-to-mucopurulent ocular discharge is common. One or both eyes may be affected.
- Many rabbits have no other clinical signs. Rabbits with severe disease may be anorexic and lethargic.

Diagnosis

Diagnosis of rhinitis is based on clinical signs and isolation of the causative agent through bacterial culture and sensitivity testing.

- Submit a swab of nasal or conjunctival exudate for bacterial culture and sensitivity testing. Small-tipped culturette swabs are convenient for sample collection (e.g., Mini-tip Culturettes, Becton Dickinson, Cockeysville, MD). Culture of nasal exudate in *Pasteurella*-infected rabbits is frequently negative.
- An antibody enzyme-linked immunosorbent assay (ELISA) for *Pasteurella* is available (see Pasteurellosis).

Treatment

▼ *Key Point* Treatment of upper respiratory disease secondary to pasteurellosis can be frustrating, especially with chronic infections (see Pasteurellosis).

- Give antibiotics at the first signs of respiratory disease (see Table 169–5). Choose an antibiotic effective against *Pasteurella* until culture results are known. The antibiotic choice may change based on results of bacterial culture and sensitivity testing.
- If conjunctivitis is present, flush the nasolacrimal duct of the affected eye or eyes. A topical ophthalmic anesthetic is necessary for this procedure. Repeated flushes of the nasolacrimal duct daily for 2–3 days or every 3 days for four or five treatments is most effective. Apply an ophthalmic antibiotic solution such as ciprofloxacin (Ciloxan, Alcon Laboratories, Fort Worth, TX) gentocin, or chloramphenicol four to six times daily for 14–21 days.
- Long-term therapy may be necessary with chronic disease.

Prevention

General preventive measures are described in the following section on Pasteurellosis.

Pasteurellosis
Etiology

- Pasteurellosis is an endemic bacterial disease of rabbits. It is caused by *Pasteurella multocida*, a small, gram-negative, bipolar-staining rod.
- Infection is spread by direct contact with infected rabbits or contaminated fomites, aerosolization, or from does to offspring during birth and nursing.
- Bacteria colonize the soft palate and nasal turbinates and may produce a lifelong infection. Infection may

be subclinical with intermittent episodes of mucopurulent nasal discharge, usually precipitated by stress.
- Spread from the nasal cavity can occur through several routes:
  - The eustachian tube to the middle or inner ear, meninges, and brain
  - The nasolacrimal duct to the conjunctival sac
  - The trachea to the lungs
  - The lymphatics vessels or blood stream to the peripheral lymph nodes, reproductive tract, or other organs

Clinical Signs

Clinical signs of disease depend on the site and chronicity of infection.

- Respiratory signs associated with pasteurellosis include rhinitis, conjunctivitis, and pneumonia.
- Abscesses of the joints and mandible and subsequent osteomyelitis are common.
- Neurologic signs, including head tilt, torticollis, nystagmus, and facial nerve deficits, can be seen with infections of the middle or inner ear, meninges, or brain.
- Abscesses can occur in various organs and in subcutaneous tissue. Exudate is typically white, thick, and caseous.
- Peracute death may occur from septicemia or pneumonia in young and weanling rabbits.

Diagnosis

- Submit samples from exudate, blood, or tissue for bacterial culture and sensitivity testing. Isolation of *P. multocida* is sometimes difficult. Many carrier animals have negative cultures of nasal swab samples.
- Several laboratory animal research centers have developed an ELISA to detect antibodies to *P. multocida*. The test requires whole blood or serum and is reported as positive, negative, or suspect. One laboratory offering the test is the AnMed.

Treatment

▼ *Key Point* Successful treatment of pasteurellosis can be difficult, especially in rabbits with advanced disease.

- Fluorinated quinolones are the most effective clinically in the treatment of rabbits with pasteurellosis. Give enrofloxacin (Baytril, Bayer Corporation, Shawnee Mission, KS) (5–15 mg/kg q12–24h) by injection or administer the injectable solution orally. The pills can be crushed and mixed with water or jam for oral administration. Ciprofloxacin (Cipro, Bayer Corporation, West Haven, CT) is easier to make into a suspension; have it compounded in cherry syrup by a compounding pharmacist and administer it at the same dosage as enrofloxacin.
  - Continue treatment for 14 to 30 days. Long-term therapy may effectively rid the animal of *Pasteurella* organisms.

- Other antibiotics have been used with varying success. Chloramphenicol, trimethoprim/sulfa, penicillin, and aminoglycosides may be effective. Base the choice of antibiotic on culture and sensitivity testing.
- Rabbit colonies have been treated with tetracycline added to drinking water at 300 mg/L. Feed additives also have been used (e.g., sulfaquinozaline at 225 g/ton, furazolidone at 50 g/ton). Success has been variable.
- Debride abscesses and drain them surgically. If possible, do a complete excision of subcutaneous abscesses.
- Mandibular or joint abcesses require extensive debridement and wound care (see Mandibular and Joint Abscesses).
- Daily management includes thorough cleaning and flushing until healing is well advanced.
- Debilitated rabbits require supplemental fluids, force-feeding, and general nursing care.

Prevention

- Pasteurellosis is an endemic disease in rabbits, and control is difficult. Colonies are kept *Pasteurella*-free through serologic testing and strict isolation and sanitation procedures.
- Prevention involves isolation of healthy animals from rabbits with clinical signs of disease. Eliminate rabbits with evidence of disease from breeding colonies.
- Closely examine pet rabbits for signs of respiratory disease before purchase.

Pneumonia

Pneumonia can be acute or chronic and may occur alone or accompany upper respiratory disease.

Etiology

- Pasteurellosis is the most common cause of pneumonia in rabbits. The infection spreads to the lungs from the upper respiratory tract through the trachea or, less frequently, through the bloodstream.
- Other less common causes of bacterial pneumonia include *B. bronchiseptica* and *S. aureus*.
- Stress is an important factor in disease. Sudden temperature changes, poor sanitation, or poor ventilation in high-ammonia areas contribute to the development of disease.

Clinical Signs

- Chronic pneumonia is characterized by labored breathing, weight loss, cachexia, and anorexia.
- Clinical signs are often inapparent until disease is advanced.
- Acute death is common in young rabbits.

Diagnosis

Diagnosis of pneumonia is based on clinical signs and supportive diagnostic tests.

- Auscultate the chest for crackles, expiratory wheezes, or decreased lung sounds over areas of consolidation or abscess.

- Thoracic radiographs may reveal lung lobe consolidation, air bronchograms, or well-delineated soft-tissue opacities if pulmonary abscesses are present.
- Results of a complete blood count may reveal a relative increase in heterophil numbers or a reversal of the lymphocyte/heterophil ratio, indicating an inflammatory response.
- Tracheal washes are very difficult in rabbits because of the anatomy of the oropharynx.
- Postmortem lesions may include acute fibrinopurulent pneumonia, pleuritis, and septicemia.

Treatment

- Parenteral antibiotic therapy is preferred in rabbits with severe pneumonia.
- Supportive therapy includes supplemental fluids, vitamins, and force-feeding of anorexic animals.
  - If an indwelling catheter can be placed, give fluids intravenously. Administer subcutaneous fluids if catheter placement is too stressful.
- Force-feed anorexic animals. Hold recumbent animals sternal while feeding.
- Additional supportive measures include providing oxygen therapy in severely dyspneic rabbits, periodic turning of recumbent animals to prevent hypostatic congestion, and application of ophthalmic ointments.

The prognosis of rabbits with pneumonia is extremely guarded to poor.

- Euthanasia often is elected for severely debilitated rabbits with advanced disease.

GASTROINTESTINAL DISEASES

Diarrhea/Enteritis

Etiology

- Dietary factors

▼ *Key Point* Lack of roughage in the diet is a major predisposing factor in diarrhea.

- Diets high in digestible carbohydrates contribute to overgrowth of pathogenic bacteria by supplying a ready source of fermentable products. Toxins produced by these bacteria are primary factors in enterotoxemia.
- Bacterial pathogens
  - *Clostridium spiroforme*, a gram-positive, anaerobic, spore-forming rod, is the primary pathogen implicated in bacterial enteritis in rabbits. It can be present as normal GI flora. However, with a ready supply of fermentation products, *C. spiroforme* produces iota toxin, which causes severe enterotoxemia.
  - *Escherichia coli* is the second important pathogen associated with enteritis in rabbits. *E. coli* is not part of the normal gut flora but often is found in large numbers in the cecum of rabbits with diarrhea. The bacteria attach to the mucosal epithelium,

causing necrosis and disruption of normal intestinal and cecal function.

- *Clostridium piliforme* (formerly *Bacillus piliformis*), which causes Tyzzer disease, is associated with acute diarrhea and death, primarily in young weanling rabbits. *C. piliforme* may be a subclinical inhabitant of the gut. With stress, the bacteria proliferate and cause severe epithelial necrosis of the cecum, colon, and distal ileum.
- A *Campylobacter*-like bacteria has been associated with proliferative enterocecocolitis in rabbits.
- Viruses
  - Rotavirus may be present as normal flora. Occasionally, the virus may act as a mild pathogen by destroying cells that produce disaccharidases and by contributing to carbohydrate overload.
- Parasites
  - Intestinal coccidiosis is primarily a disease of young rabbits. Several species of intestinal *Eimeria* infect rabbits. Diarrhea secondary to intestinal coccidiosis is usually mild; however, coccidia may predispose rabbits to bacterial enteritis (see Coccidiosis). The highly pathogenic *Eimeria stieda* infects the liver.
  - Helminthic parasites are rarely a problem in domestic rabbits. The only parasite that occurs commonly is the pinworm, *Passalurus ambigus*.
- Management-related factors
  - Antibiotic therapy can cause suppression of normal gut flora and overgrowth of pathogenic bacteria. Diarrhea is associated with antibiotics that are active against gram-positive aerobes and selective gram-negative anaerobes. Antibiotic-induced diarrhea has been associated with lincomycin, clindamycin, erythromycin, ampicillin, amoxicillin, cephalexin, and penicillin.
  - Stress is a major factor in diarrhea. Stress-related hormonal release may have a direct effect on intestinal motility and digestion, allowing overgrowth of pathogenic organisms.
  - Hairballs (trichobezoars) are associated with diarrhea. Hairballs slow GI motility, prolonging retention of fermentable food.

Clinical Signs

- The severity of diarrhea varies from chronic, soft stool to profuse, liquid, malodorous feces.
- Rabbits with mild diarrhea may be otherwise normal. Severe diarrhea may be accompanied by lethargy, weight loss, anorexia, and dehydration.
- Intestinal gas often is detected on abdomial palpation.
- Sudden death may be the only clinical sign in peracute disease.

Diagnosis

Diagnosis of the primary cause is based on clinical signs, history, and specific tests.

- Dietary history is very important. Determine the fiber content of the normal feed and the amount of supplemental roughage.

- Identify bacterial pathogens by submitting fecal samples for aerobic and anaerobic bacterial culture and sensitivity testing.
- Do a direct fecal smear or fecal flotation to check for coccidiosis, especially in young rabbits.
- Results of serum chemistry analysis often reveal electrolyte and metabolic abnormalities in animals with moderate-to-severe diarrhea.

Treatment

- Correct the diet in animals on marginal or deficient dietary fiber levels.
- Give dietary *Lactobacillus* supplements daily (see Treatment Techniques).
- Broad-spectrum antibiotics, such as the fluorinated quinolones, trimethoprim/sulfa, or chloramphenicol, are indicated if bacterial enteritis is suspected. Oral administration is effective in mild-to-moderate diarrhea. Give antibiotics parenterally in rabbits with severe clinical signs. Avoid antibiotics that may induce enteritis.
- Give supportive fluid therapy for rabbits with moderate-to-severe diarrhea. Oral electrolyte-replacement formulas are used by some clinicians.
- Force-feed anorexic animals.
- If young rabbits test positive for coccidiosis, administer appropriate therapy (see Coccidiosis).

Prevention

- Instruct owners to feed their rabbits proper diets with an adequate content of indigestible fiber.
- Minimize stress in young or weanling rabbits. Sudden temperature changes, changes in food, overcrowding, or poor sanitation contribute to disease.
- Isolate diseased animals from healthy rabbits.
- Screen young rabbits for coccidiosis or give prophylactic therapy.

Anorexia/Refusal to Eat
Etiology

▼ *Key Point* Malocclusion and gastric hairballs are the two most common causes of anorexia in rabbits.

- Anorexia may accompany any systemic infectious disease, especially enterotoxemia or pasteurellosis.
- Metabolic abnormalities such as kidney disease often are accompanied by anorexia.
- Anorexia and lethargy can be seen with lead poisoning and other toxicoses.

Clinical Signs

Clinical signs vary according to the specific cause (see Malocclusion; Hairballs).

- Rabbits with malocclusion, hairballs, and occasionally lead poisoning often have no other clinical signs. Most remain alert and active.
- Excessive salivation is common in rabbits with malocclusion.

- Some rabbits with hairballs become depressed, lethargic, dehydrated, and develop diarrhea.

Diagnosis

- Perform a thorough oral examination in all anorexic rabbits. Examine the back molars with an otoscope. Sedation is not usually necessary.
- A hairball is often palpable as either a soft and compressible or a firm mass in the cranial abdomen.

Treatment

- Incisors can be cut with a diagonal cutter, rongeur, or, preferably, a dental drill. Both pairs of upper incisors should be clipped.

▼ *Key Point* Do not use Resco-type nail clippers to cut incisors because excessive trauma and loosening of the roots can result.

- Molar malocclusion requires dentistry with sedation. The procedure is usually short and can be done with an injectable tranquilizer. Gas anesthesia requires a face mask or endotracheal tube, making it difficult to work in the very limited space in the oral cavity.
  - Place the rabbit in sternal recumbency with an assistant extending the neck and head forward.
  - Loop strips of gauze around both upper and lower incisors to hold the mouth open. The assistant holds the gauze around the lower molars in one hand. The second hand is placed on top of the rabbit's head, holding the gauze looped around the top incisors and forcing the head and neck into extension. Make sure the nostrils are not occluded and the neck is extended or the rabbit will have difficulty breathing.
- Use a short vaginal speculum to spread open the oral cavity. Check both lateral and medial edges of upper and lower molars. A nasal speculum with an attached light source is ideal for this procedure.
- A small bone rongeur can be used to clip the sharp edges of the cheek teeth. Use a tongue depressor to push the tongue to one side while clipping the medial edges of the lower cheek teeth. This method is quick and easy but leaves rough edges and may cause fractures of the teeth.
- A dental drill rounds and smoothes sharp edges but must be used with care. Use a tongue depressor or the vaginal speculum to isolate the arcade and prevent damage to the tongue or buccal mucosa.
- Root elongation of the premolars and molars can develop. Elongated roots of the mandibular teeth can be palpated as firm bony nodules on the ventral mandible. Roots of the maxillary teeth can invade the nasal passages, sometimes causing obstruction and resulting in inspiratory stridor. The roots often become infected, resulting in mandibular maxillary, or retrobulbar abscesses (see Mandibular and Joint Abscesses).

Prevention

- Most rabbits with incisor malocclusion need their incisors clipped every 4–8 weeks. Many owners prefer to do this procedure at home.
- Check rabbits with molar malocclusion every 2–3 months. Dentistry may be needed as often as every month or only once yearly.
- Rabbits with malocclusion should not be bred.

Hairballs (Trichobezoars)
Etiology

▼ *Key Point* Inadequate dietary roughage is associated with gastric hairballs in rabbits.

- Other factors may contribute to formation of hairballs. Long-haired breeds may consume large amounts of hair while grooming during shedding. Hormonal influences in breeding season may contribute to aggression and fur-barbering. Mineral deficiencies may cause pica of hair. Boredom also may be a factor in fur-barbering.
- Rabbits are unable to vomit, contributing to accumulation of hair in the stomach.

Clinical Signs

- Anorexia is the primary clinical sign associated with trichobezoars. Often rabbits remain alert and active, with no other signs.
- With chronic problems, weight loss, depression, and palpable intestinal gas are present. Fecal pellets may appear small, the amount of pellets passed may be less than normal, and hair may be visible in the pellets, causing them to "string" together.
- Diarrhea may be present in some animals (see Diarrhea/Enteritis).
- Acute pyloric obstruction causes severe depression, lethargy, bloating, dehydration, hypothermia, and shock.

Diagnosis

▼ *Key Point* Suspect a hairball in an anorexic but otherwise alert rabbit with a history of inadequate dietary fiber and excessive shedding.

- Palpation of a soft mass in the stomach area in an anorexic rabbit is evidence of a hairball. The stomach of a healthy rabbit is normally full. However, a rabbit that has been anorexic for several days should have an empty stomach.
- Radiographs are not necessary but may be used to confirm a diagnosis. An enlarged stomach may be visible on plain radiographs. Contrast radiography of the upper GI tract may outline the hairball. Give barium at a standard small-animal dose of 10–14 ml/kg orally into the cheek pouch.
- Ultrasound examination can be used to detect a mass in the stomach area.

- A complete blood count and serum biochemical analysis may be indicated in dehydrated, severely ill, or debilitated animals.

Treatment

▼ **Key Point** Providing adequate dietary roughage and making sure that the rabbit is hydrated are extremely important for successful treatment of hairballs.

- Medical management is successful in most rabbits. Although a few clinicians advocate routine surgical removal of hairballs, the risk of surgical or anesthetic complications is high considering the debilitated condition of most of these rabbits.
  - Direct treatment at hydrating the rabbit, providing dietary roughage, and stimulating GI motility. Give supplemental fluids subcutaneously or by intravenous catheter in debilitated animals. Continuous rate infusion of crystalloid fluids at maintainence requirements (approximately 100-150 ml/kg/day) through an indwelling catheter works well.
  - Stimulate GI mobility by encouraging the animal to move around. Provide a large hospital cage and allow the rabbit out of the cage once or twice daily to exercise. Administer cisapride (Propulsid, Janssen Pharmaceutica, Titusville, NJ) if no intestinal blockage is suspected and gut motility is poor.
  - Give the rabbit oral lubricants used to treat furballs in cats (e.g., Laxatone, Evsco Pharmaceuticals, Buena, NJ) at 1–2 ml/day for 3–5 days to aid in fur passage.
  - Offer free-choice hay and fresh vegetables at all times.
  - Force-feed nutritional supplements or slurried rabbit pellets until the rabbit's appetite returns.
  - The proteolytic enzymes bromelin and papain have been used anectdotely by owners to treat rabbits with furballs. These enzymes are present in fresh (not heat-processed) pineapple juice. Pineapple juice is given orally at 10 ml/day for 3–5 days in a medium-sized rabbit. Repeat the treatment in 3–5 days if anorexia has not resolved. As an alternative, bromelin or papain enzyme tablets can be purchased from a health-food store and administered orally. Dosage is empirical at 1–2 tablets daily for 3–5 days.
- Perform surgical removal in rabbits with clinical signs of acute pyloric obstruction. In my experience, the mortality rate in rabbits with pyloric obstruction is very high, even with surgery.

Prevention

▼ **Key Point** Correct the diet to include adequate dietary fiber (see Nutrition). Provide tree-choice timothy hay and fibrous vegetables. Feed rabbit pellets that have a high-fiber content (20–25%).

- Routinely brush long-haired rabbits or heavy shedders.

- Some owners administer a petrolatum-based cat laxative to their rabbits every 1–2 months.
- Encourage rabbits to exercise. Prevent obesity by restricting the amount of pellets fed and not feeding sweet "treats."

Coccidiosis

Etiology

- Coccidia are host-specific protozoan parasites.
- At least 10 different species of intestinal *Eimeria* infect rabbits. Pathogenicity varies according to species. *Eimeria magna* is the most pathogenic species affecting the small intestine.
- Hepatic coccidiosis results from infection with the highly pathogenic *Eimeria stieda*.
- Coccidiosis is primarily a disease of young and weanling rabbits. Natural immunity develops against each *Eimeria* species after exposure. No cross-protection in immunity exists between different *Eimeria* species. Adult animals can become ill if exposed to a species against which they have no immunity.
- The severity of disease is determined by the age at time of exposure, the species of *Eimeria* involved, the number of oocysts ingested, and the environmental stress factors.

Clinical Signs

- Intestinal coccidiosis is often subclinical or causes only mild-to-moderate diarrhea. However, coccidia may predispose the rabbit to bacterial enteritis (see Diarrhea/Enteritis).
- Severe diarrhea and death may occur with heavy infections.
- Hepatic coccidiosis is associated with anorexia, weight loss, abdominal enlargement, diarrhea, icterus, and acute death.

Diagnosis

Diagnosis is based on identification of *Eimeria* oocysts in a fecal sample.

Treatment and Prevention

The age of the host and the severity of clinical signs are factors to consider in treatment. Animals with light parasite burdens usually become immune and recover without therapy.

- Therapy with coccidiostats is more prophylactic than therapeutic. Coccidia are susceptible to treatment only during a specific period in the protozoan life cycle. Clinical signs are usually inapparent during this period.
- Coccidiostats may slow multiplication until host immunity develops.
- Sulfonamides are effective in prophylaxis. Sulfaquinoxaline is the only drug approved for use in commercially raised rabbits in the United States; however, other drugs are more effective.

- Give sulfadimethoxine orally at 50 mg/kg once, then at 25 mg/kg daily for 21 days.
- Add amprolium (9.6% solution) to the drinking water at 5 ml/gallon for 21 days.
- Add sulfamethazine to the feed at 0.05–1.0%.
- Administer sulfaquinoxaline in the feed at 0.025–0.03% continuously for 4–5 weeks during weaning or add it to the drinking water at 0.025–0.1% in alternating 2-week periods for 4–8 weeks during weaning.
- Sanitation is of utmost importance for effective therapy and prevention. Routinely disinfect cages, food bowls, and water bottles.
- Screen rabbits for shedding of coccidial oocysts. Separate or cull carriers from colonies.
- Check all young rabbits for coccidia.

UROGENITAL/REPRODUCTIVE DISEASES

Uterine Adenocarcinoma/Hyperplasia
Etiology

▼ *Key Point* Uterine adenocarcinoma is the most common tumor in domestic rabbits.

- Adenocarcinoma rarely occurs in does younger than 3 years of age. The incidence in rabbits older than 3 years of age ranges from 50–80% in certain breeds. Uterine adenocarcinoma is rare in Rex, Belgian, and Polish breeds, suggesting a genetic component to the disease.
- Endometrial changes resulting from senile atrophy of the glandular epithelial cells and stroma may precede neoplasia, although a direct association has not been proved. Estrogen may play a role in enhancing tumor growth.
- Endometrial changes that may precede neoplastic changes include endometriosis, endometritis, and papillary, cystic, or adenomatous hyperplasia.

Clinical Signs

- Uterine adenocarcinoma is a slow-growing tumor with a 5- to 24-month clinical course. Metastasis occurs late in the clinical course, after 10 to 12 months. Metastasis occurs locally to the peritoneum, lymph nodes, and liver before hematogenous spread.
- Clinical signs are usually inapparent during the early hyperplastic stages. Owners may notice increased aggressiveness in some does.
- Decreased reproductive performance is an early sign in breeding rabbits. Small litter size, stillbirths, dystocia, litter desertion, and infertility are seen.
- Pet owners may notice blood in the urine or a bloody discharge from the vaginal area.
- Cystic mastitis is associated with uterine changes in many does.

Diagnosis

- An enlarged, thickened uterus or multiple rounded caudal abdominal masses may be palpable on physical examination. It is sometimes difficult to differentiate a mass from abdominal fat in small does.
- An enlarged uterus usually is observed on abdominal radiographs.
- Abdominal ultrasonography also can be used to identify an enlarged uterus or uterine masses and to detect metastases.

Treatment

- Ovariohysterectomy is successful if done before metastasis has occurred.
- Prognosis is poor after metastasis has occurred. Euthanasia is recommended.

Prevention

- Consider ovariohysterectomy in does older than 3 years of age with evidence of cystic mastitis or increased aggressive behavior.
- Some clinicians recommend routine ovariohysterectomy of does before 3 years of age, excluding breeds with very low incidence (Belgian, Rex, and Polish breeds).

Mastitis
Etiology

Mastitis in rabbits can be either septic or nonseptic.

- Septic mastitis is most common in lactating does. Trauma to the mammary gland and poor sanitation predispose to infection.
- *Staphylococcus* and *Streptococcus* spp are the most commonly isolated bacteria. *E. coli* and *Pseudomonas, Pasteurella,* and *Klebsiella* spp also may cause mastitis.
- Nonseptic, cystic mastitis is seen in nonbreeding females. It may be associated with high estrogen levels, uterine hyperplasia, and uterine adenocarcinoma.

Clinical Signs

- With septic mastitis, the affected gland is swollen, erythematous, and warm to the touch. The tissues later become cyanotic. Infection spreads until all glands are affected.
- Systemic signs of septic mastitis include pyrexia, depression, anorexia, death of neonates, and death of the doe.
- In cystic mastitis, glands became swollen, firm, and bluish in color with a clear-to-dark serosanguineous discharge from the teats. Rabbits are not systemically ill.

Diagnosis

- Diagnosis of septic mastitis is based on clinical signs, history of lactation or pseudocyesis, and isolation of bacteria on culture of gland tissue or exudate.
- Diagnosis of cystic mastitis is based on history of a nonbreeding doe, usually older than 3 years of age, with no known trauma to the glandular tissue. Culture and sensitivity testing of the discharge is negative for bacterial growth.

Treatment

- Administer antibiotics. Base therapy on results of bacterial culture and sensitivity testing. Warm compresses 2 to 3 times daily also may be helpful. Consider surgical drainage or excision for mammary abscesses.
- Cystic mastitis resolves with ovariohysterectomy. Severely affected glands may be excised surgically.

Prevention

- Keep lactating does in a clean environment. Make sure no sharp surfaces or wire edges are present that can traumatize the teats.
- Routinely examine lactating does for evidence of inflammation or teat injuries.
- Cystic mastitis can be prevented by routine ovariohysterectomy.

Dysuria/Hematuria

Etiology

- Red, pink, or orange discoloration of the urine occurs periodically in healthy rabbits. The color may be the result of porphyrin pigments or food-related metabolites excreted in the urine.
- Thick, white urine indicates the presence of large quantities of mineral precipitates. Unlike other mammals, calcium absorption and blood calcium concentration are directly related to dietary calcium intake in rabbits. Excessive calcium intake results in excretion of large amounts of calcium in the urine. Calcium is excreted in the bile in other mammals.
- Hematuria occurs commonly with cystitis. Frank blood independent of or at the end of urination may indicate uterine adenocarcinoma.
- Cystic calculi occur in both male and female rabbits. Calculi usually are composed of calcium carbonate or calcium oxalate and may be associated with high dietary calcium intake.

Clinical Signs

- Rabbits with urinary pigment changes or excessive calcium in the urine usually have no other clinical signs.
- Dysuria and stranguria may accompany cystitis and cystic calculi.
- Lethargy, anorexia, and depression may be seen in rabbits with cystitis or cystic calculi.

Diagnosis

- Differentiate hematuria from pigment changes in the urine by simple dipstick analysis. If urine discoloration is intermittent, dispense dipsticks for owners to check the urine at home.
- Measure blood calcium concentrations in rabbits excreting large amounts of urinary calcium. Blood calcium concentrations often reach as high as 19 mg/dl.
- Perform urinalysis, serum biochemical analysis, complete blood count (CBC), and urine culture in rabbits with clinical signs of cystitis, cystic calculi, or hematuria.
- Distinguish between hematuria and hemorrhagic vaginal discharge occurring secondary to uterine adenocarcinoma by physical examination, history, and urinalysis. Uterine adenocarcinoma is likely in a doe older than 3 years of age with a thickened uterus or multiple abdominal masses.
- Obtain abdominal radiographs if cystic calculi are suspected. Calculi are usually radiopaque and therefore visible in the bladder or urethra. Calculi may also be visible in the ureters or kidneys. Large amounts of calcium sediment may be visible in the bladder in rabbits excreting large amounts of calcium.

Treatment

Treatment is not necessary in rabbits with pigment-based changes in urine color.

- Attempt to lower dietary calcium levels in rabbits with consistently high blood calcium concentrations. Grass hay (e.g., timothy) has a lower calcium content than legume hay (e.g., alfalfa). Decrease the amount of pelleted feed, which is alfalfa-based, and substitute greens and grass hay.
- Treat rabbits with simple bacterial cystitis with antibiotics. A 3-week course of chloramphenicol or trimethoprim/sulfa is usually effective. Submit a second urine sample for bacterial culture and sensitivity testing after 4 to 6 weeks.
- Cystic calculi must be removed surgically (see Chap. 100). Submit calculi for stone analysis. Decrease dietary calcium after surgery to help prevent recurrence.

Prevention

For prevention, decrease dietary calcium, especially in mature or aged rabbits. Most pelleted diets exceed dietary calcium requirements. Substitute grass or timothy hay for alfalfa hay in the diet. Discontinue any supplemental vitamins.

Treponematosis

Etiology

- *Treponema cuniculi* is the causative agent of rabbit syphilis.
- *T. cuniculi* is a spiral-shaped bacterium transmitted by direct contact between breeding rabbits or from doe to offspring.
- Cold environmental conditions may predispose to development of the disease.

Clinical Signs

- Most lesions develop on the external genitalia. The nose, eyelids, lips, and perineal area are less commonly involved. Lesions initially consist of erythematous vesicles that progress to papules, ulcerations, scaliness, and dry crusty lesions.

- Nasal lesions in pet rabbits are commonly mistaken for dermatophyte lesions.
- Rabbits remain alert, responsive, and active.
- The incidence of abortions, metritis, and infertility may increase in breeding females.

Diagnosis

Diagnosis is based on history, clinical signs, and response to therapy. Supportive diagnostic tests are done as needed.

- Submit fur samples for fungal culture and do skin scrapings to rule out dermatophytes and ectoparasites.
- *Treponema* organisms can be identified by darkfield microscopic examination of skin scrapings. The organisms also can be demonstrated histologically with silver stains of skin biopsy sections.
- Serologic tests are available to determine the presence of antibodies against *T. cuniculi*. These include the rapid plasma reagin (RPR) test, the Venereal Disease Research Laboratory (VDRL) slide test, and the Wasserman complement fixation test.
  - A fluorescent antibody test against treponemal antigen also is used. An ELISA is available from some laboratories to screen for antibodies against *Treponema*. These tests are used for screening in rabbit-breeding colonies.

Treatment

- *T. cuniculi* is susceptible to penicillin. Give injections of benzathine penicillin G (a long-acting penicillin) at 42,000 to 84,000 IU/kg IM three times at weekly intervals. Response is rapid; lesions dramatically regress, usually after one injection.

Prevention

- Screen rabbits in breeding colonies for treponematosis.
- The incidence of disease in pet rabbits is low. Preventive serologic screening is not necessary.

NEUROMUSCULAR/SKELETAL DISEASES

Mandibular and Joint Abscesses
Etiology

- Abscesses of the mandible and joints occur frequently in pet rabbits and usually are caused by *Pasteurella multocida*. Bacteria spread hematogenously from the initial infection site (see Pasteurellosis).
- Overgrowth of the cheek teeth sometimes may accompany mandibular abscesses. Infection may spread from the oral cavity along the tooth root.
- Soft-tissue abscesses occasionally occur in the oral cavity secondary to a penetrating wound from a foreign body.

Clinical Signs

- Joint abscesses are most frequent in the distal limb joints. The swellings are large, firm, and warm to the touch. Rabbits may be lame, depending on which joints are involved.
- Mandibular abscesses occur as firm swellings in the ventral facial area. Abscesses are sometimes quite large before they are apparent to the owner. Excessive ptyalism may be an early symptom.
- Affected rabbits may refuse to eat if mandibular abscesses are accompanied by dental disease.
- Many rabbits remain active and alert with no other clinical signs.

Diagnosis

- Thick, white purulent exudate is present on fine-needle aspirate of the swelling. Cytologic examination of the exudate shows neutrophils and proteinaceous debris; bacteria may or may not be visible.
- Obtain radiographs to check for bone involvement.
- Perform bacterial culture and sensitivity testing of tissue samples if treatment is elected. Submit samples at the time of surgical debridement.

Treatment

▼ *Key Point* Simple lancing of mandibular abscesses is ineffective because of the thick, viscous nature of the exudate.

- Surgically debride the area aggressively with the rabbit under general anesthesia. Remove any molars or premolars that are loose or that have radiographic evidence of extensive infection of the roots. Flush the soft tissue with copious amounts of sterile saline. Usually, the wound can be closed if the debridement is thorough.
  - Recently, the use of Consil (Nutrimax Laboratories, Baltimore, MD) has improved the success rate of surgical treatment of mandibular abscesses. This product is synthetic bone graft particulate and can be used in infected tissue to encourage new bone growth.
- Serial surgical debridements are usually necessary.
- Joint abscesses are difficult to debride surgically and drain because of the caseous nature of the exudate.
  - Amputation of the affected limb may be the most effective therapy for abscesses involving the joint and surrounding bone. Rabbits adapt well to amputation of either a fore or rear limb.
  - Disease may recur in other joints, even if amputation of the affected limb has been performed. Hematogenous spread of the bacterial infection to other joints may occur at any time during the clinical course.
- Long-term antibiotic therapy is necessary. Some rabbits respond to fluoroquinolone therapy in combination with surgical debridement or amputation.
- Owners must be able to do extensive nursing care at home. Have the owners flush the wounds with sterile saline once or twice daily. Provide sterile swabs for owners to debride the open wounds.

The prognosis for successful therapy is guarded. With bony involvement, the prognosis is poor.

Torticollis/Head Tilt/Ataxia

Etiology

- Bacterial infection of the inner ear, middle ear, or meninges is the most common cause of torticollis in pet rabbits. The primary causative agent is *Pasteurella multocida*.
- *Encephalitozoon cuniculi* is another common cause of torticollis and incoordination in rabbits.
- Vascular lesions, infection with herpesvirus, cerebral nematodiasis, hypovitaminosis A, and toxicoses (e.g., lead poisoning) are less common causes of head tilt and incoordination.

Clinical Signs

- Onset may be acute or slowly progressive. The head tilt may be mild or accompanied by torticollis, incoordination, and the inability to stand.
- Some rabbits have no other clinical signs. Other rabbits become depressed, anorexic, and lethargic.
- Rabbits with severe depression, positional nystagmus, and facial nerve deficits may have brain or meningeal lesions.

Diagnosis

Diagnosis is based on clinical signs. Establishing the exact cause may be difficult.

- Carefully examine both ear canals for evidence of infection.
- Results of a CBC may reveal an inflammatory response, which may indicate an infectious cause.
- Skull radiographs may aid in diagnosis. Anesthesia is usually necessary for proper positioning. Bony changes in the bulla may indicate osteomyelitis.
- Serologic tests can be used to detect antibodies against *E. cuniculi* or *P. multocida*. A positive result is not diagnostic of the specific agent but is helpful in ruling out some possible causes.
- Often, the etiology cannot be established, and a tentative diagnosis is based on response to therapy. Rabbits with pasteurellosis often improve with long-term antibiotic therapy and supportive care. Rabbits with parasitic migrations may remain unchanged or improve gradually. Rabbits with clinical signs secondary to encephalitozoonosis are usually unresponsive to treatment or they deteriorate clinically.
- The cause sometimes is determined only on postmortem examination.

Treatment

- Give antibiotics for 4 to 6 weeks. Choose an antibiotic that penetrates the blood-brain barrier and is effective against pasteurellosis (e.g., chloramphenicol and enrofloxacin).
- If exudate is visible in the ear canal, clean and flush the ear thoroughly. Tranquilization or anesthesia may be necessary. Administer a topical antibiotic in the ear canal 3 to 4 times daily. Administer systemic antibiotics.
- Adminster a *Lactobacillus* supplement given orally during long-term antibiotic therapy.
- Supportive care is necessary in rabbits that are laterally recumbent or that have severe torticollis. Recumbent rabbits should be turned every 6 to 8 hours or propped up sternally to prevent hypostatic congestion of the lungs. Apply eye lubricants several times daily if the blink reflex is diminished. Hand-feeding may be required. Keep rabbits on clean, dry bedding to prevent urine scalding and contact dermatitis.
- Inform owners about the amount of supportive care needed in recumbent rabbits. Many owners elect euthanasia when faced with the difficulties and the time required for long-term nursing care.
- Steroids sometimes are used if other treatments fail or if diagnostic test results are negative for pasteurellosis. Give prednisolone orally (0.25–0.5 mg/kg) q12h for 3 days, then q24h for 3 days, then on alternate days. Give antibiotics concurrently.
- Euthanasia often is selected in debilitated rabbits if no clinical improvement is seen after several days of therapy.

Encephalitozoonosis (Encephalitozoan cunuculi)

Etiology

- *E. cuniculi* is an obligate intracellular microsporidian parasite prevalent in domestic and wild rabbits. The organism infects mice, rats, hamsters, and guinea pigs less commonly.
- The major route of transmission is ingestion of spore-contaminated urine. Vertical transmission through the placenta is suspected.
- The organism becomes established in the kidney 30 to 40 days after ingestion. Signs of kidney disease are not evident. Infection progresses to the brain after several weeks, at which time neurologic signs may be evident.

Clinical Signs

- Infections are usually chronic and latent. Diagnosis usually is confirmed on necropsy.
- In some rabbits, clinical signs of torticollis, ataxia, seizures, paresis, and death may occur.

Diagnosis

Diagnosis is based on clinical signs and results of diagnostic testing of rabbits exhibiting neurologic signs or results of necropsy.

- Serologic tests are available through laboratory animal research centers to detect the presence of *E. cuniculi*. These include a complement fixation test, an indirect fluorescent antibody test, and an India ink immunoreaction test. An ELISA also has been developed for detection of antibodies against the organism.
- If serologic testing is not available, presumptive diagnosis is made based on clinical signs and response

to therapy. Clinical signs of encephalitozoonosis are similar to those of the neurologic form of pasteurellosis. However, rabbits with encephalitozoonosis usually decline rapidly despite aggressive antibiotic therapy and supportive care. Death often occurs within several days of onset of clinical signs. If more than one rabbit is exposed, multiple deaths may occur.

Treatment

- There is no effective therapy for encephalitozoonosis.

Prevention

- Identify carriers in rabbit colonies and breeding facilities through serologic testing and culling of animals that test positive.
- Eliminate urine contamination between cages through proper sanitation procedures.
- Prevent possible contact between pet rabbits housed outdoors and wild rabbits or rodents by elevating cages off the ground or housing pets in a rodent proof enclosure.

Vertebral Fractures

Etiology

- The rear leg muscles of rabbits are well developed for strong kicking and thumping.

▼ *Key Point* If rabbits are restrained poorly with inadequate control of the rear legs, animals may kick suddenly, resulting in fracture of their spinal vertebrae.

Clinical Signs

- Clinical signs of a fractured back include partial or complete paralysis of the rear legs and loss of normal bladder and bowel function.
- Signs are acute in onset and directly related to a traumatic incident.
- Other disease problems may cause clinical signs similar to a vertebral fracture. Multifocal infection of the spinal cord secondary to pasteurellosis, parasite migration, or vascular thrombosis within the cord can cause neurologic deficits; however, the clinical onset is usually more chronic and slowly progressive than that in a fracture.

Diagnosis

- Diagnosis is based on history and clinical signs.
- Obtain radiographs of the vertebral column confirm a fracture.

Treatment

- If a diagnosis is made within 6–12 hours of the time of the fracture, administer methylprednisolone sodium succinate (Solu-Medrol, UpJohn, Kalamazoo, MI) (suggested dosage: 30 mg/kg IV, then 15 mg/kg IV

q6h × 4 total doses). Alternatively, administer prednisolone sodium succinate (Solu-Delta-Cortef, UpJohn) or dexamethasone at shock dosages.
- If steroids are given, use anti-inflammatory dosages on a decreasing dosing schedule as outlined in the section on Torticollis.
- Attempts to stabilize the fracture surgically are usually not practical because of the poor prognosis and degree of nursing care necessary.
- Some owners try long-term supportive care to see whether neurologic function returns. They must be instructed on manual expression of the bladder and general nursing care.
- Prognosis for recovery is guarded to poor. Euthanasia usually is recommended in rabbits with complete rear limb paralysis and urinary and fecal incontinence.

Prevention

- See Figs. 169–1, 2 for proper restraint of rabbits.

Long Bone Fractures/Joint Luxations

Etiology

- The skeleton of the rabbit is light and fragile. The tibia, radius, and ulna fracture easily with trauma.
- Traumatic joint luxations of the elbow or stifle joint occasionally occur.

Clinical Signs

- Rabbits with long bone fractures or luxations are acutely lame.
- Fractures are usually palpable on physical examination. Joint luxations are palpable as firm swellings.

Diagnosis

- Diagnosis is based on history, clinical signs, and physical examination.
- Obtain radiographs to evaluate fractures for surgical repair or to confirm joint luxations.

Treatment

- Splints used in combination with padded bandages are usually adequate to stabilize metatarsal, metacarpal, and phalangeal fractures. Bandage the foot in a functional position. Contour a moldable splint or casting material (e.g., Hexcelite NS, Hexcel Medical, Dublin, CA) along the plantar surface.
- With joint luxations, anesthesia is needed to manipulate the joint into normal position. A lateral or caudal splint then is applied. Many luxations are unstable and do not remain in normal position. Surgery may be elected to stabilize the joint. However, many rabbits compensate well with a permanently luxated joint.
- Long bone fractures are more difficult to manage. Surgical reduction and stabilization are sometimes successful, but complications can occur because of the fragility of the bones. Bones may splinter or shatter

during attempted reduction. Surgical procedures may need to be modified and used in combination with restricted cage rest until healing occurs. Severely comminuted or open fractures sometimes are managed best with limb amputation.

SUPPLEMENTAL READINGS

Cheeke PR: Rabbit Feeding and Nutrition. Orlando: Academic Press, 1987.

Cheeke PR, Patton NM, Lukefahr SD, et al: Rabbit Production. Danville: The Interstate Printers and Publishers, 1987.

Harkness JE, Wagner JE: The Biology and Medicine of Rabbits and Rodents. Philadelphia: Lea & Febiger, 1989.

Hillyer EV, Quesenberry KE (eds): Ferrets, Rabbits, and Rodents: Clinical Medicine and Surgery. Philadelphia: WB Saunders, 1997.

Kraus AL, Weisbroth SH, Flatt RE, et al: Biology and diseases of rabbits. In: Fox JG, Cohen BJ, Loew FM (eds): Laboratory Animal Medicine. Orlando: Academic Press, 1984, p 207.

National Research Council (NRC): Nutrient Requirements of Rabbits. Washington, D.C.: National Academy of Sciences, 1977.

Schoeb TR, Fox JG: Enterocecocolitis associated with intraepithelial *Campylobacter*-like bacteria in rabbits *(Oryctolagus cuniculus)*. Vet Pathol 27:73, 1990.

Toth LA, Krueger JM: Hematologic effects of exposure to three infective agents in rabbits. J Am Vet Med Assoc 195:981, 1989.

Weisbroth SH, Flatt RE, Kraus AL (eds): The Biology of the Laboratory Rabbit. New York: Academic Press, 1974.

170 Pet Rodents

Nancy L. Anderson

Many small rodents commonly are kept in peoples' homes for companionship and enjoyment. This chapter provides the information needed to treat the most frequently encountered pet rodents and includes mice, rats, gerbils, hamsters, guinea pigs, and chinchillas.

HUSBANDRY

Caging and Sanitation

Cages should be made of stainless steel, hard plastic, or glass. These materials are cleaned and sanitized easily and are resistant to gnawing or corrosion from urine and fecal matter. Minimum floor space and height requirements are listed for each species in Table 170–1. With the exception of guinea pigs, all cages need secure lids.

Guinea pigs can be housed in open-topped enclosures with walls higher than 10 inches. Ensure that dogs, cats, wild animals, and small children do not have unsupervised access to these cages.

Clean cages as needed, usually 1–3 times per week for most rodents. A scrub brush, dish soap, and water work well. If cages are not kept clean, ammonia, other irritants, moisture, and bacteria rise to harmful levels, predisposing the animals to disease.

Disinfect the cage twice a month with one part sodium hypochlorite (household bleach) mixed in 30 parts water. Let the bleach solution stand for at least 15 minutes. Rinse the cage well afterward.

All solid floored cages need bedding. Shredded paper, nonresinous wood shavings, wood wool, and corn cobs are all acceptable. Provide at least 2 inches of bedding. Most rodents enjoy burrowing in deeper bedding when it is provided in one corner of a cage. Do not, however, fill the entire cage with deeper bedding. This usually leads to poor sanitation resulting from owners' failure to recognize buildup of hidden wastes such as moisture from leaking water bottles, cached foods, urine, and feces.

Successful use of wire mesh floors is dependent on the dimensions of the mesh. Size the openings to be just large enough for an adult to retract a tarsal joint back through the mesh. Larger holes make it difficult for the animals to walk and cause pressure sores. Smaller openings may cause injuries such as tibial fractures and self-mutilation during struggles to free trapped appendages. Bedding above the wire keeps waste from dropping through the wire and therefore is not recommended. Wire bottom cages do not work well for breeding animals because neonatal rodents must be surrounded by nesting material to maintain moisture in the nest and prevent dehydration. Young rodents often cannot walk correctly on mesh sized for adult feet.

All pet rodents require visual security. Tubes, jars, or cans made of nontoxic, nonabrasive substances work well for this purpose. Also provide objects for gnawing. Rodents possess open-rooted teeth, and constant wear is necessary to maintain normal dentition. Mice, rats, gerbils, and hamsters enjoy and benefit from exercise wheels.

A good room temperature range for most pocket pets is 70–75°F. Keep rodents with disease at 85–90°F unless hyperthermia is of concern (some chinchillas).

- Provide 10–12 hours of darkness to 12–14 hours of light. This light cycle is essential if breeding is desired.

Table 170–1. CAGING AND ENVIRONMENTAL REQUIREMENTS FOR POCKET PETS

Requirement	Rat	Mouse	Guinea Pig	Chinchilla	Hamster	Gerbil
Air changes/hour	10–15	10–15	10–15	> 6	> 6	> 6
Minimum cage floor space/animal (square inches)	35	15	101	288	20	36
Minimum cage height (inches)	> 6	> 5	> 10	> 12	> 6	> 6
Recommended room temperature (°C)	21.1–26.6	21.1–29.4	18.3–23.8	15.5–21.1	18.3–23.8	21.1
Maximum-minimum room temperature (°C)	18.3–29.4	18.3–31	12.7–32.2	10–23.8	12.7–23.8	18.3–29.4
Room humidity (%)	50–70	30–70	40–70	40–60	30–70	30–50
Cage-cleaning frequency (days)	2–7	2–7	3–4	7	3–7	14
Light cycle-hours light : hours dark	12–14:10–12	12:12	12:12	> 12.5:11.5	12:12	12:12

- Hamsters, guinea pigs, and chinchillas that are exposed to temperatures below 65°F may hibernate for a few days or until the ambient temperature rises. Heart rates may be less than 5 bpm during hibernation.

Nutrition

▼ *Key Point* Feed pet rodents laboratory animal chow appropriate for their species (Table 170–2). Seed diets are deficient in protein and contain excessive fat.

Seeds, as well as vegetables and other foods, may be fed as treats but not to provide more than 15% of calories. Intermittent exposure to vegetables and seeds causes mild, transient diarrhea.

Supplementation of vitamin C is recommended for all guinea pigs.

Adult chinchillas that are not obese should be fed high quality, fresh grass hay ad libitum. Obese animals may need to have the hay rationed. Chinchillas require ⅛- to ¼-cup of fresh pellets per animal each day. Feeding pellets free choice leads to obesity, and the high protein and calcium levels in these diets may predispose animals to urinary tract disease. Most pellets also do not provide sufficient fiber to maintain normal gastrointestinal (GI) motility.

- Store food in tightly sealed containers at less than 60°F; keep food refrigerated if possible.

Feed all diets within 90 days of milling to ensure the highest nutritional value. Encourage owners to check dates on packages and ask pet store managers about providing dates on bulk items.

If possible, feed pet rodents except guinea pigs from overhead racks. These devices reduce wastage and eliminate fecal contamination of food. Covered hoppers, heavy crocks, or stainless steel bowls that are attached to the side of the cage to eliminate spillage are acceptable and recommended for guinea pigs.

Feed breeding females and their litters from the floor of their cages until the young are large enough to reach overhead feeders or crawl in and out of crocks.

Cannibalism of neonates commonly occurs as the result of stress associated with cage cleaning. To minimize cannibalism, clean the cage and provide a 10- to 13-day food supply 1–2 days before parturition.

Water

▼ *Key Point* Provide fresh water in clean containers daily.

Do not provide water in open crocks. These are contaminated or spilled easily and are a common cause of dehydration and poor sanitation. Sipper tubes and water bottles work well. Clean with dish soap and water daily and disinfect them weekly. Guinea pigs blow food into their sipper tubes. This practice necessitates more frequent cleaning. Some water bottles have special valves to minimize backflow. Supplement guinea pigs' water daily with 200 mg vitamin C/L. If the water is not dechlorinated, it will inactivate the vitamin C.

Quarantine

Quarantine all newly acquired animals in a different room from current pets for a minimum of 30 days. Feed and handle quarantined animals last. Recommend that caretakers wash their hands and change clothes before handling current pets. Avoid the introduction of adult animals because this frequently results in fighting. Instead, place animals together while young and allow

---

Table 170–2. DIETARY INFORMATION FOR POCKET PETS

	Rat	Mouse	Guinea Pig	Chinchilla	Hamster	Gerbil
Recommended diet	Laboratory rodent chow	Laboratory rodent chow	Guinea pig chow	Chinchilla chow	Hamster chow	Laboratory rodent chow
Supplements and treats	< 15% of calories, avoid seeds	< 15% of calories, avoid seeds	Vitamin C 200 mg/L, drinking water, cabbage/kale	Ad lib grass, hay	< 15% of calories, avoid fats and seeds	< 15% of calories, avoid fats and seeds
Food consumption (g food/100 g body weight/day)	5–10	15	3–6	3–6	10–12	5–8
Water consumption (ml water/100 g body weight/day)	10–12	15	10–40		8–30	4–7
Recommended protein (%)	12–27	16–20	18–30		15–25	16–22
Recommended fat (%)	5–25	5–25			3–5	2–4
Recommended carbohydrate (%)		45–55	16		8	
Recommended minimum fiber (%)			16–18			

Table 170–3. NORMAL PHYSIOLOGIC DATA FOR POCKET PETS

	Rat	Mouse	Guinea Pig	Chinchilla	Hamster	Gerbil
Life span (yrs)	2–4	1–3.5	3–6	8–10	1.5–2.5	3–5
Heart rate (bpm)	250–600	325–780	150–400	40–100	250–600	360
Respiratory rate (breaths/min)	33–127	60–230	42–130	40–80	33–155	70–120
Body weight (g)						
Male	300–520	38–42	900–1200	450–600	85–110	60–110
Female	250–300	30–35	700–900	550–800	95–120	50–80
Birth weight (g)	5–6	0.5–1.5	60–115	30–50	2–3	2.5–3
Body temperature (°C)	35.9–38.2	35.5–38	37.2–40	36.1–37.8	36.2–37.5	38.1–38.4
Gender determination in neonates	At 7 days, the anogenital distance of males is 5 mm; of females, 2.5 mm Females show nipples at 8–15 days	Identify testicles through skin in neonates	Anogenital distance in males is 10 mm; in females, 5 mm			

them to mature together. Avoid keeping more than one male per cage because this also usually leads to fighting.

HISTORY AND PHYSICAL EXAMINATION

A systematic history and physical examination are mandatory. Many syndromes are the result of poor husbandry and ignorance by the owner. Pets that have been kept isolated from other rodents or acquired from a private breeder are less likely to harbor infectious disease than animals obtained from a pet store, laboratory, or wholesaler. See Table 170–3 for normal physiologic data.

Obtain the following information:

- Species, age, sex (species and sex may not be obvious or the owner may not know this information)
- Origin (e.g., private individual, breeder, pet shop, research laboratory, supply house)
- Length of ownership, owner's previous experience
- Environment, caging (ask owner not to clean cage before coming to hospital), cleaning, temperature, humidity, photoperiod, person responsible for care
- Diet: brand, dating on packages, storage, supple-

ments, type of feeder and waterer and method/frequency of cleaning, feeding schedule, person responsible for feeding
- Cagemates, other pets, quarantine history, presence of aggressive behavior
- Dates of unusual activity: breeding, parturition (Table 170–4), cannibalism, abnormal urination or defecation
- Medical history, previous weights
- Purpose for ownership: pet, breeder, display, education
- Purpose for visit: purchase examination, checkup, problem

Become familiar with normal behavior, locomotion, haircoat, and stools of each of the pet rodent species.

Observe the pet in its cage for mentation, activity, locomotion, dyspnea, head posture, haircoat, and any grossly observable abnormalities.

Note respiratory and heart rates before restraint when possible. Observe the condition of cagemates.

▼ *Key Point* If dyspnea or severe depression is detected, warn the owner that the animal is critically

Table 170–4. REPRODUCTIVE DATA FOR POCKET PETS

	Rat	Mouse	Guinea Pig	Chinchilla	Hamster	Gerbil
Age at puberty						
Males	42–110	35–50	60–120	240–540*	45–98	70–85
Females	42–110	50–60	60–90	240–540*	30–84	65–85
Length of estrous cycle (days)	4–5	4–5	15–17	41	4	4–6
Gestation (days)	21–23	19–21	63–68	105–115	15–18	24–26
Average litter size	6–14	10–12	3–4	2–3	6–8	4–6
Age at weaning (days)	21	18–28	14–28	36–48	20–25	20–30
Litter development	Eyes open 12–17 days	Eyes open 10–14 days	Precocious; eats solid food by 5 days	Precocious	Ears open 4–5 days; eyes open 14–16 days	Eyes open 16–20 days

*Fall babies breed 1 year later. Normal breeding season is November through May.

ill and could die of stress brought on by an examination.

Handle such animals as little as possible. Initially, treat severely ill animals symptomatically, then perform a complete physical examination after the pet's condition has stabilized.

Evaluate the cage:

- Note the type of diet and bedding as well as the level of sanitation and compare these with what was described in the history.
- Observe quantity and quality of feces and urine. Diarrhea, soft stools, absence of stools, copious urine, and discolored urine all can be signs of illness.
- Coprophagy is a normal behavior in rodents.
- Check the diet and water supply for freshness, quantity, source, and accessibility.
- Evaluate the presence and suitability of cage furniture. Adequate visual security and the ability to exercise and gnaw are extremely important.

Examine the animal itself.

- An accurate weight in grams is extremely important for evaluating an animal's body condition, calculating drug dosages, and monitoring treatment. The easiest method of weighing a pet rodent is to place it in a box and then subtract the weight of the container.

Restraint

Restraint of pet rodents is easy with experience. Pets that have been handled frequently and gently by the owners require only minimal restraint. Gentle pressure directs the animal as needed. Grasp less cooperative patients (except chinchillas and guinea pigs) by the scruff over the back of the neck with thumb and forefinger (Fig. 170–1). Take care to pinch enough skin to prevent the animal from turning around, yet leave enough slack for respiration. Hold the base of the tail, if present, between the fourth and fifth fingers to provide additional restraint on small specimens.

Hold docile guinea pigs with the palm of one hand supporting the chest while the other hand supports the hind quarters (Fig. 170–2). Place the thumb and fore-

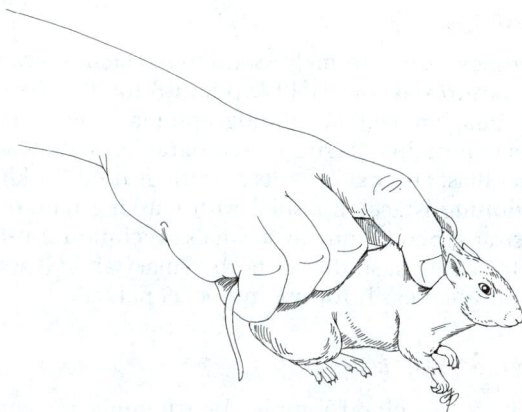

Figure 170–2.   Proper method for restraint of guinea pig.

finger of the first hand in the axillas for additional control.

Take care to minimize damage to the fur when handling chinchillas because they lose hair easily. Grasp the animal by the tail and scoop it up into the palm of the same hand (Fig. 170–3). If necessary, grasp the thorax just behind the axillas.

Appropriately sized towels placed over the head are especially effective in calming uncooperative rodents. Many physical examinations are completed by wrapping a patient in a towel and exposing only needed areas. Even oral, ophthalmic, and aural examinations can be accomplished with minimal effort if the animal is given the chance to relax in its new "burrow."

Remove particularly aggressive patients from their cages by scooping them up in a can or bucket; then slide them out onto a slick surface and pick them up or transfer them to a holding area or scale.

▼ *Key Point* Lift the hind quarters of mice and rats by the base of their tails to facilitate scruffing. Never use the tip of the tail for restraint, or the skin of the tail may slough.

Physical Examination

Once the animal is restrained properly, examine the head. Assess the cranial nerves. Check the nose for presence and character of discharge. Examine the

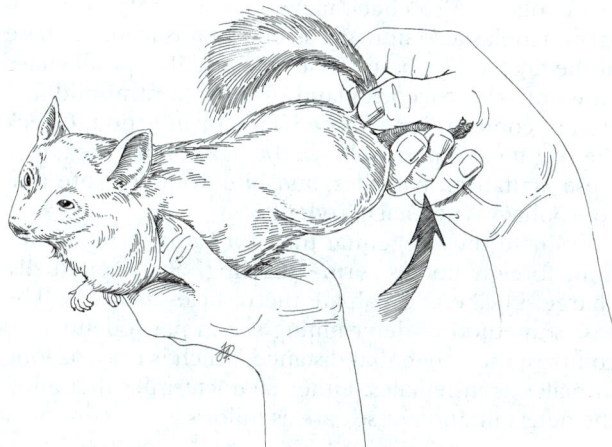

Figure 170–1.   "Scruffing" a mouse.

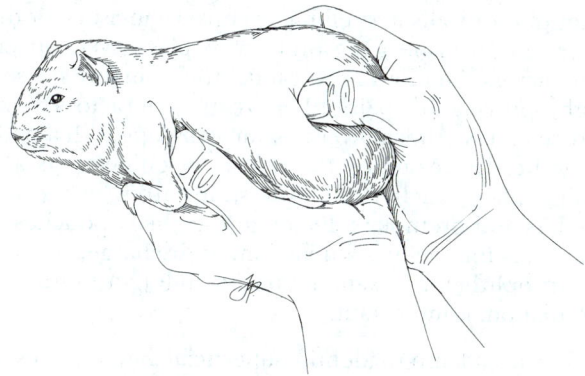

Figure 170–3.   Proper method for restraint of chinchilla.

mouth for ptyalism, swelling, overgrown incisors, or discharges. To inspect the oral cavity, place avian speculum across the mouth just caudal to the incisors. Use a light source and a pair of hemostats as retractors to improve access. Alternatively, use an otoscope with a pediatric head to examine the molars of guinea pigs and chinchillas, which commonly suffer from overgrown molars and premolars. Examine the cheek pouches of hamsters for swelling, impaction, or discharge.

An ophthalmic examination, including a fundic examination, is important.

- Use a slit lamp to identify superficial pathology, especially corneal ulcers or foreign bodies.
- If indicated, perform fluorescein stain and conjunctival scrapings or cultures.
- Note the presence of conditions such as discharge, asymmetry, and exophthalmos.

▼ **Key Point** Gerbils, rats, and mice produce red tears (chromodacryorrhea) with stress or disease. Do not confuse them with hemorrhage.

- Guinea pigs suffering from hypovitaminosis C often produce dry, white tears.

Check ears for discharge, foreign bodies, and mites. Bluish discoloration of the ears is a sign of cyanosis. Bright red injected coloration is associated with septicemia. Sores behind the ears and on the neck are often a sequela of aural disease.

Evaluate submandibular, axillary, inguinal, and popliteal lymph nodes for size and consistency. Enlargements usually indicate infectious or neoplastic disease.

Reevaluate respirations and heart rate after the stress of handling and compare them with the resting rate noted when the animal was in the cage. Note dyspnea or respiratory sounds. Auscultate animals weighing more than 200 g. Counting every third or fourth beat and multiplying by the appropriate factor allows recording of heart rates up to 500 bpm.

Palpate the abdomen. Pay special attention to differentiating pregnancy from the bladder, kidneys, abdominal masses, enlarged cecum, and fecal balls in the colon. While palpating the abdomen, examine the mammary chain of all female rodents for signs of mastitis, lactation, or neoplasia. Also check male mice and rats for mammary neoplasia. Mammary tissue extends from the base of the neck to the base of the tail. Gerbils typically have an elliptical sebaceous gland on their ventral midline. Do not confuse this with neoplasia or infection. Check the rectum and perineal area for signs of diarrhea, prolapse, irritation, parasites, and bite wounds. Note that coprophagy is normal in rodents.

Evaluate the urogenital tract for signs of inflammation, foreign bodies, urine scalding, and vaginal discharge. Locate and palpate the testicles in males. The easiest method of determining sex in pet rodents is to compare the anogenital distance, which is twice as long in males as in females. Other characteristics that allow the determination of sex are as follows:

- Visualization or palpation of testicles or extrusion of the penis from the prepuce indicates a male.

- The presence of two external openings (i.e., anus and urethra) indicates a male.
- The presence of three openings (i.e., anus, vagina, and urethra) indicates a female.

Examine the skin and fur for conditions such as crusts, alopecia, masses, herniations, and wounds.

Check tail and feet for swellings, coloration, sores, length of toenails, and condition of footpads.

Evaluate the extremities for trauma or other abnormalities.

DIAGNOSTICS

Skin and Ear

Apply cellophane tape to crusted areas of the skin and view under a microscope as an aid in diagnosing ectoparasites such as lice, mites, and fleas. Skin scrapings are beneficial in detecting mites and dermatophytes. Dermatophytes are diagnosed best through culture of broken hairs or crust on dermatophyte test medium.

Use tracheal swabs to obtain ear swabs from animals weighing more than 25 g. Mix debris with mineral oil and view under low magnification to test for ear mites, or roll onto a glass slide and Gram stain to look for bacterial or yeast infections.

Urine and Fecal Collection

Collect urine by placing the rodent in a clean mesh-bottomed cage with a plastic liner. After enough urine has been produced, collect it off the bottom of the cage with hematocrit tubes or a syringe and a 25-gauge needle. Perform cystocentesis on nonpregnant animals weighing more than 100 g with a 25- to 27-gauge needle.

Collect feces over several hours to provide a volume sufficient for fecal flotation. Flotation allows the detection of nematodes and some trematodes and cestodes. Cellophane tape applied to the perineal area and then viewed under a microscope often reveals oxyurid eggs. Use a fresh saline smear or fecal sedimentation to diagnose protozoal parasites. Fecal cultures are useful in diagnosing bacterial diarrhea.

Radiology

Radiology is an extremely useful tool. Machines capable of exposures as low as 40 kvp and 3 to 10 MAS effectively image mice. Most radiograph machines are capable of generating diagnostic radiographs of guinea pigs, chinchillas, and mature rats at settings used for kittens. Positioning is accomplished with masking tape or Velcro straps. Sedate unruly animals. Techniques used in cats for contrast studies of both urinary and GI systems are modified easily for use in pocket pets.

Blood Samples

Obtain small blood samples by trimming a clean toe nail close to the quick and collecting blood into hematocrit tubes.

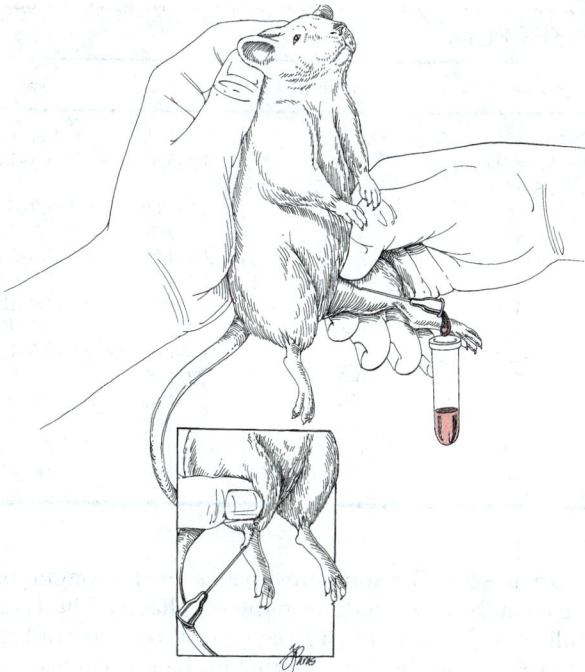

Figure 170-4. Medial saphenous venipuncture; *inset,* lateral tarsal venipuncture.

Use lateral or medial saphenous veins to obtain larger samples in animals heavier than 100 g. Liberally clip the area to allow exposure of the vessel before attempting venipuncture. Place a 25- to 27-gauge needle in the vein and collect blood into microtainers or hematocrit tubes as it drips from the hub of the needle (Fig. 170-4). Take extreme care not to collapse and lacerate the vein with overzealous aspiration if a syringe is attached to the needle.

- It is also possible to use the cephalic vein in guinea pigs.
- Jugular veins are good alternatives in thin individuals under sedation.
- An alternative technique that is useful in smaller animals is to coat the skin over the vein with a thin layer of petroleum jelly and then to puncture the vessel. Blood is collected with a hematocrit tube as it exits the wound. Samples up to 1% of the animal's weight are considered safe, even in stressed animals.

▼ *Key Point* Attempt tail or orbital sinus bleeding only as a last resort in mice, rats, gerbils, and hamsters. These techniques often are not acceptable to owners.

To bleed the tail, warm the tail with water or compresses to dilate the tail vessels. In large rats, perform venipuncture with a needle and obtain blood in the usual fashion. In smaller animals, lacerate or amputate the tip of the tail. Blood from the wound is collected as described previously. Orbital bleeding works best in mice. A microhematocrit tube is used to puncture the conjunctiva at the medial canthus. Aim the tip caudomedially and advance 1–3 mm. If blood does not begin to fill the tube immediately, abort the attempt. Reserve cardiac samples for extreme emergencies and perform this procedure only using sedation. See Tables 170–5 and 170–6 for hematology and chemistry values.

ROUTINE PROCEDURES

Oral Medications: Nutritional Support

Incorporate oral medications into a treat, or administer them in liquid form. If the medication is palatable, administer it by placing the tip of a dosing syringe into the diastema.

▼ *Key Point* Take care not to place the tip into the contralateral cheek pouch, or the patient may store the medication and expel it later.

Administer medication in small amounts. Ensure that the animal swallows the medication in its mouth before more is administered. This technique is useful for force-feeding pellet gruels to anorexic pets if the caregiver is patient. Medication or food that is administered too quickly will be spit out or aspirated.

For rodents that are intractable or for administration of unpalatable substances, pass a stomach tube per os.

- Metal feeding needles, red Brunswick urinary catheters, or infant feeding tubes work well. Selection is based on the size of the animal and individual

Table 170–5. NORMAL HEMATOLOGIC VALUES FOR POCKET PETS

Indices	Rat	Mouse	Guinea Pig	Chinchilla	Hamster	Gerbil
Erythrocytes ($\times 10^6$/mm^3)	7–10	7–12.5	4.5–7	5.2–10.7	4.0–10	7.0–10
Packed cell volume (%)	35–49.3	35–49	37–55	27–54	31–57	41–52
Hemoglobin (mg/dl)	11–18	10–20	11–16.5	8–15.4	10–19	12.1–16.9
Leukocytes ($\times 10^3$/mm^3)	5–17.2	4–12	7–19	4–11.5	3–11	4.3–12
Neutrophils (%)	9–50	5–40	15–60	9–45	10–42	3–41
Lymphocytes (%)	50–85	30–90	30–72	19–98	50–95	32–97
Monocytes (%)	0–5.0	0–10	3–12	0–6	0–3	0–9
Eosinophils (%)	0–6.0	0–8.0	1–5.0	0–9.0	0–4.5	0–4.0
Basophils (%)	0–1.5	0–1.5	0–3.0	0–1.0	0–1.1	0–2.0
Total protein (g/dl)	5.6–7.6	3.5–7.2	4.4–6.2	5.0–6.0	4.5–7.5	4.3–12.5
Platelets ($\times 10^3$/mm^3)	500–1300	100–1000	250–850	254–740	200–670	400–638

Table 170–6. NORMAL SERUM CHEMISTRIES FOR POCKET PETS

Indices	Rat	Mouse	Guinea Pig	Chinchilla	Hamster	Gerbil
Sodium (mEq/L)	135–155	112–193	132–156	130–155	128–144	144–158
Potassium (mEq/L)	4–8	5.1–10.4	4.5–8.9	5–6.5	3.9–5.5	3.8–5.2
Chloride (mEq/L)		82–114	98–115	105–115		
Calcium (mg/dl)	5.3–13	3.2–8.5	3–12	5.6–12.1	5–13.2	3.7–6.2
Phosphorus (mg/dl)	5.3–8.3	2.3–10.4	3–12	4–8	3–9.9	3.7–7.0
Albumin (g/dl)	3.4–4.8	2.5–4.8	2.1–3.9	2.5–4.2	2.6–4.9	1.8–5.5
Globulin (g/dl)	1.3–3.0	0.6	1.7–2.6		2.7–4.2	1.2–60
Glucose (mg/dl)	50–217	60–250	60–125	60–120	40–200	50–135
Blood urea nitrogen (mg/dl)	6–23.9	17–28	9–31.5	10–25	12–25	17–27
Creatine (mg/dl)	0.2–0.8	0.3–1.0	0.5–2.2		0.1–1.0	0.6–1.4
Alanine aminotransferase (IU/l)	16–89	26–77	10–25	10–35	22–128	
Aspartate aminotransferase (IU/l)		54–269		96	28–122	
Alkaline phosphatase (IU/l)	16–125	45–222	18–28	3–47	45–187	
Total bilirubin (mg/dl)	0.2–0.6	0.1–0.9	0.3–0.9	0.4	0.1–0.9	0.2–0.6
Cholesterol (mg/dl)	40–130	25–82	20–66	40–100	25–180	90–150

preference. Metal feeding needles with ball tips frequently are used in patients weighing less than 100 g (Fig. 170–5). The metal provides the necessary stiffness to pass a tube of small diameter. The ball at the end of the needle makes it difficult (but not impossible) to pass the tube into the trachea. These tubes have the potential to create esophageal tears with improper restraint or when excessive force is applied.

• Measure the length from the tip of the nose to the last rib. Ventroflex the head slightly, and place the tip of the tube through the diastema and over the tongue. If the tube does not pass easily down the esophagus to the premeasured distance, check the tube size and/or reposition the tube before attempting further advancement. The needle is easily palpable percutaneously if it is placed correctly. It is usually safe to administer up to 3 ml/100 g body weight.

A flexible catheter is ideal for use as a stomach tube in larger rodents (Fig. 170–6). Use a speculum to prevent chewing on the tube. An otoscope head, avian speculum, or piece of wood or plastic with a hole drilled in the center works well. Measure and mark the tube for the distance from the tip of the nose to the last rib. Place the speculum in the mouth and over the tongue. Pass the tube while holding the speculum in place and slightly ventroflexing the head. Resistance is encountered if the tube is malpositioned or is an inap-

propriate size. The tube must pass over the tongue before it can be advanced down the esophagus. This is difficult in some animals. Palpate the throat to confirm the presence of the feeding tube in the esophagus.

▼ *Key Point* Because the placement of a stomach tube is a blind procedure, administer a small volume of sterile saline into the tube before administering the medication to ensure that the tube is not in the trachea. Misplaced medications are fatal.

This method is also useful for administration of nutrition to anorexic patients. Place a pharyngostomy tube if repeated dosing is necessary, using the technique for cats. Flush pharyngostomy tubes with water at least every 4–6 hours. Nasogastric tubes are not recommended because they are difficult to place and maintain patency because of their small size. Securely suture all tubes to the skin. Place a tube collar made of radiographic film or use rear leg hobbles to prevent removal of tubes.

Nutritional support is critical in rodents because of their high metabolic rate. Provide supplements in animals that are anorexic for longer than 12 hours. If the GI tract is capable of digestion, use a slurry of pellets mixed with a high-calorie supplement. If the tube diameter is too small for this mixture, use avian hand-feeding formula or a mixture of vegetable and cereal

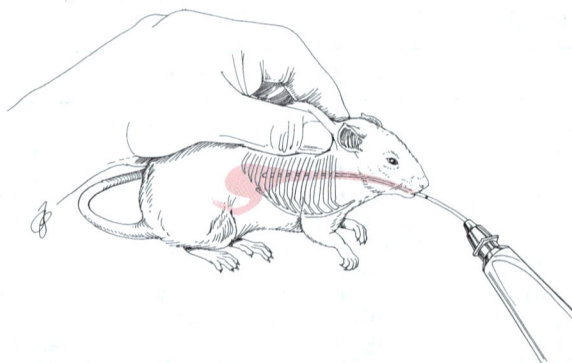

Figure 170–5. Proper placement of a metal feeding tube.

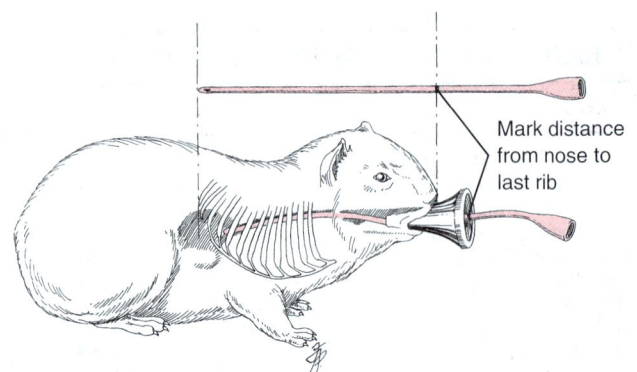

Mark distance from nose to last rib

Figure 170–6. Measurement and use of a flexible catheter as a feeding tube.

baby foods in place of the pellets. If the ability of the GI tract to tolerate enteral feeding is questionable, first try isotonic electrolyte or dextrose solutions. Parenteral nutrition is used successfully in research animals and may be feasible in select pet cases.

Subcutaneous (SC) Injections

Administer injectable medications or fluids over the shoulder blades or in folds of skin on the flank.

- Avoid irritating substances in rats and mice because their mammary tissue extends into these areas. The resulting inflammatory response is thought to increase the occurrence of mammary cancer.

▼ *Key Point* In general, avoid streptomycin and the carrier procaine in all pet rodents because of a high incidence of toxicity and hypersensitivity reaction.

Intramuscular (IM) Injections

Give intramuscular injections in the semimembranous and semitendinous muscles. Inject only small volumes of nonirritating substances, or tissue damage with resulting self-mutilation may occur. Use the epaxial or triceps muscles if repeated injections are necessary.

Intraperitoneal (IP) Injections

▼ *Key Point* Use intraperitoneal injections only as a last resort for large volumes of fluids or for irritating injections that cannot be administered via an intravenous or intraosseous route.

Express the bladder and aseptically prepare the abdomen.

Restrain the rodent with its head down to move the abdominal organs cranially. Give the injection 0.5–2 cm lateral to the midline in the caudal abdomen. Aspirate before injecting to ensure that the injection is not being given into the bladder or bowel. Never use this technique in pregnant animals.

Intravenous (IV) Injections

Give injections into any of the veins as previously described. In addition, the penile vein may be used in hamsters and guinea pigs. Placement of intravenous catheters is possible in animals heavier than 100 g.

For small rodents, give a bolus of fluids every 2–4 hours, followed by a diluted heparin flush. A pediatric intravenous pump is used for continuous infusion of fluids to larger animals. Maintenance of catheters in active animals is extremely difficult.

Intraosseous (IO) Injections

Place a spinal needle into the proximal tibia or femur following the technique used for placing an intramedullary pin. Once the needle is seated, remove the stylet. Aspirate and check the hub of the needle for bone marrow. The tip of the needle should be in the bone marrow cavity that directly drains into the central venous system in normal bones (i.e., the cortex must be intact). Administer drugs, blood, or fluids at a rate similar to that used for intravenous catheters.

ANESTHESIA

Premedication and Patient Preparation

In chinchillas and guinea pigs, withhold food for 6 hours before anesthesia. Withhold food from smaller, mature rodents for 2 hours. Fast immature animals for up to ½ hour depending on age and condition.

Use heat lamps and heating pads to prevent hypothermia. Have a prewarmed incubator available for recovery. Preoperative or intraoperative warmed subcutaneous or intravenous fluids are strongly recommended. Place intravenous or intraosseous catheters whenever possible.

Administer atropine preoperatively to reduce airway secretions. Acepromazine or diazepam work well as premedications for other anesthetics. Avoid acepromazine in gerbils because it potentiates seizures. See Table 170–7 for anesthetic drugs and dosages.

Monitoring

Surgical anesthesia is reached when toe, tail, and ear pinch fail to generate a withdrawal reaction.

Depth of anesthesia is best monitored by pulse and respiratory rate and character. Pulses drop to within normal ranges after induction. Further reduction, especially to less than 80% of the original stabilized value, is an indication to lighten the plane of anesthesia. Monitor the electrocardiogram (ECG) of small patients by clamping the alligator clips onto the hubs of all-metal 27-gauge needles or steel sutures placed through the skin at the usual sites. Tape cables to the table to maintain placement. Doppler units taped over the chest also provide accurate heart rates. Pulse oximeters are easier to use, more sensitive, and more expensive than the instruments mentioned previously. These instruments are easily taped to the patient's ear, foot, or tail and provide heart rates as well as information regarding oxygenation.

Respirations are often shallow and rapid during induction. They become deep and regular as a surgical plane of anesthesia is reached.

The corneal reflex varies markedly between individuals and anesthetic agents. If the animal has a corneal reflex after induction and then loses it, reduce the anesthetic.

Inhalation Anesthesia

Induction

Induce gas anesthesia using small face masks purchased from laboratory supply houses or make them from syringe cases and latex gloves (Fig. 170–7). Induction in an anesthetic chamber is also possible.

All rodents induced and maintained on gas anesthesia require some form of non-rebreathing system. Usual induction is achieved between 2–3% for isoflurane and

Table 170–7. INJECTABLE ANESTHETIC DRUG DOSAGES FOR POCKET PETS

Agent (Effect)	Rat	Mouse	Guinea Pig	Chinchilla	Hamster	Gerbil
Atropine sulfate (parasympatholytic)	0.04 mg/kg, SC	0.04–0.1 mg/kg, IM	0.1–0.2 mg/kg, IM, SC	0.2 mg/kg, IM, SC	0.04 mg/kg, IM, SC	0.04 mg/kg, IM, SC
Acepromazine (sedation)	1–2 mg/kg, IM				0.5–1.0 mg/kg IM	DO NOT USE
Diazepam (sedation)	3–5 mg/kg, IM	3–5 mg/kg, IM	0.5–3 mg/kg, IM		3–5 mg/kg, IM	3–5 mg/kg, IM
Ketamine hydrochloride (light sedation)	22 mg/kg, IM	22 mg/kg, IM	22–64 mg/kg, IM	40 mg/kg, IM	40 mg/kg, IM	40–60 mg/kg, IM
Ketamine hydrochloride (heavy sedation)	25–40 mg/kg, IM	44 mg/kg, IM	44–256 mg/kg, IM*		40–150 mg/kg, IM*	70–200 mg/kg, IM*
Ketamine hydrochloride/ xylazine (anesthesia)	60–80 mg/kg/7–12 mg/kg, IP, IM	80 mg/kg/16 mg/kg, IP, IM	35–40 mg/kg/4–8 mg/kg, IP, IM	35–40 mg/kg/ 4–8 mg/kg, IM	50–100 mg/kg/10 mg/kg, IP	50 mg/kg/2 mg/kg, IP
Ketamine hydrochloride/ acepromazine/xylazine (anesthesia)	22 mg/kg/0.75 mg/kg/2–5 mg/kg, IM	44 mg/kg/0.75 mg/kg/2–5 mg/kg, IM	22–64 mg/kg/ 0.75 mg/kg/2–5 mg/kg, IM	40 mg/kg/0.5 mg/kg/0 mg/ kg, IM		DO NOT USE
Ketamine hydrochloride/ diazepam (anesthesia)			35–40 mg/kg/5–10 mg/ kg, IM			
Nalorphine (reverses fentanyl)	2–5 mg/kg, IV					
Pentobarbital sodium (anesthesia)§	25–40 mg/kg, IP, IV	40–80 mg/kg, IP, IV	30–40 mg/kg, IP, IV	30 mg/kg, IV 35–40 mg/kg, IP	50–90 mg/kg, IP	30 mg/kg, IV 40–60 mg/kg, IP
Thiopental sodium (anesthesia)§	25–50 mg/kg, IP	25 mg/kg, IV 50 mg/kg, IP	20 mg/kg, IP		20–40 mg/kg, IV	

IM, intramuscular; IP, intraperitoneal; IV, intravenous; SC, subcutaneous.
*Wide dosage ranges are due to marked individual variation. Use lower dosages first.
§Dilute concentration to 10 mg/ml before injection.

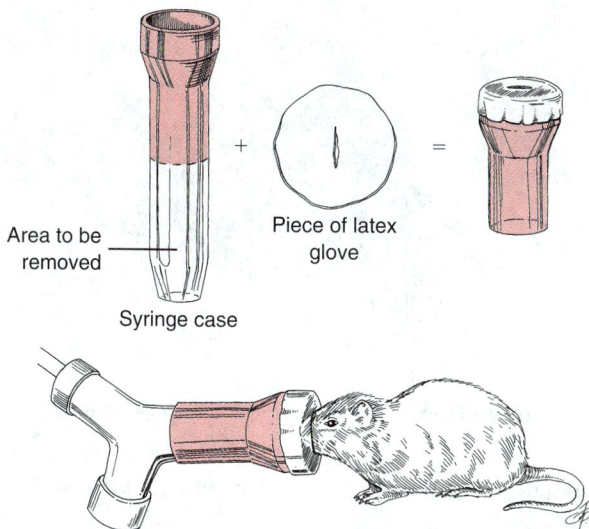

Figure 170–7. A nose cone for anesthesia delivery can be made from a cut-down plastic syringe case and material from a latex glove. Syringe cases from 12 to 60 cc can be used, depending on the size of the patient.

2–4% for halothane. Maintenance for isoflurane and halothane varies from 0.25–2%. There is marked individual variation in the amount of anesthetic required for induction and maintenance. Use of 50% nitrous oxide in oxygen reduces anesthetic concentration requirements for other gases.

▼ **Key Point** Some chinchillas and guinea pigs hold their breath while being induced with gas anesthetics and then take deep rapid breaths. If the concentration of anesthetic gases is high enough, this behavior results in death.

The risk of this behavior is reduced by premedication with tranquilizers, initial induction with nitrous oxide with later addition of primary anesthetic gas after relaxation, and low induction settings. Changes in respirations, especially erratic or apneustic patterns and decreased respiratory rates, indicate deepening anesthesia.

Endotracheal Intubation

Most pet rodents are not intubated for anesthesia because of their small size. When necessary, as in prolonged oral and other procedures, endotracheal intubation is accomplished with the animal in dorsal or ventral recumbency, depending on the clinician's preference. Small noncuffed or Cole endotracheal tubes work well. A stylet usually is required to provide enough stiffness for the tube to pass the larynx. Extend the animal's head and neck. Grasp the tongue with forceps and use gentle traction. The tip of the tube then is advanced above the tongue and just past its base. The hard palate is used to deflect the tip of the tube ventrally into the glottis. This is a blind procedure that is difficult to master. Use of a laryngoscope is helpful in larger rodents.

Another technique is to place an over-the-needle catheter in the trachea and move it up retrograde through the larynx to act as a guide. The catheter is removed after the endotracheal tube is in place.

▼ **Key Point** If endotracheal intubation is performed, it is extremely important that the tube be checked for patency. Rodents produce copious respiratory secretions, which frequently clog endotracheal tubes.

The small diameter allows these tubes to collapse or kink, resulting in asphyxiation of the patient. Check patency at least every 2 minutes by applying positive pressure ventilation at 10–15 cm water and watching for excursion of the chest wall. If extending the head and neck does not result in air flow, suction the tube. If this is either not successful or impossible, remove the tube and continue anesthesia with a mask or reintubate the animal with a new tube. Because of the small diameter of the trachea, endotracheal tube-induced tracheitis and subsequent swelling of the trachea may become a life-threatening situation.

Injectable Anesthesia

Doses and routes for injectable anesthetics are listed in Table 170–7. Needed doses for injectable anesthetics are tremendously variable among species and individuals. Most injectable anesthetics provide safe sedation for minor procedures, but very few induce a safe surgical plane of anesthesia on a consistent basis.

- Ketamine in combination with diazepam is easily obtainable, is given intramuscularly, and has a wide margin of safety, but it does not provide good analgesia.
- Intraperitoneal injections of barbiturates provide surgical anesthesia but have a low margin of safety and a significant mortality rate. Barbiturate anesthesia can result in fatal ileus.

EUTHANASIA

Euthanasia is performed easily by induction of inhalant anesthetic through a mask or chamber followed by an overdose of barbiturates given intraperitoneally, intravenously, or intracranially. Euthanasia by IP injection of barbiturates alone causes pain in some animals.

SURGERY

Hemostasis

- Surgical techniques for pet rodents are similar to those used in cats and birds.
- Hemostasis is critical because of small blood volumes.
- Electrosurgery for incisions and cautery is highly recommended.
- If necessary, give fresh blood transfusions drawn from a donor of the same species and mixed with sodium heparin (1000 IU/ml) at a rate of 0.005 ml/1 ml of blood directly into an intravenous or intraosseous line.
- The lack of a filter creates a potential for thrombosis.
- Transfusion reactions are possible.

Common Procedures

The most common surgeries are laceration repair and removal of dermal or subcutaneous masses.

- Most rodents will not gnaw on skin sutures.
- If this occurs, use steel sutures, subcuticular sutures, or tissue glue.
- If an animal still chews at its suture line, physical restraint, such as a tube or an Elizabethan collar, is required.

Castration

Castration is a common procedure in guinea pigs. This usually is performed when owners want to house more than one male together or do not wish to breed their female any longer.

Technique

1. Make a skin incision over each testicle or one incision on the midline just cranial to the prepuce.
2. Remove the testicles via a closed technique. All rodents possess open inguinal rings and can eviscerate if a closed technique is not used.
3. Close the skin incision with a subcuticular pattern using 4-0 synthetic absorbable suture.

Some surgeons partially suture the rings closed for extra security. This technique is also applicable to other rodent species.

Abdominal Surgery

Common abdominal surgeries include cystotomy for urolith removal in guinea pigs and rats, and cesarean section (C-section) in guinea pigs and chinchillas because of dystocia.

Use a technique similar to those described for dogs and cats. Preplaced stay sutures are recommended to define incision edges for closure. Use 4-0 polyglactin 910 or chromic gut swaged on a taper needle and suture in a simple continuous pattern to close the body wall. Close the skin with a subcuticular suture (absorbable) or interrupted skin monofilament, nonabsorbable suture.

Fracture fixation is accomplished best with intramedullary pinning or Kirschner apparatus. Rodents gnaw on bandages until they remove them. If they are unable to remove a splint, self-mutilation often results in self-amputation. If a cast or splint is necessary, physical restraint often is required. Healing usually takes 3–6 weeks.

Dental Procedures

Incisors can be trimmed with nail trimmers, but this technique often fractures the tooth, causing abscesses of the root. Instead, use a high-speed dental burr or a flat cutting disk on a Dremel hand tool. Trim molars with a high-speed drill or pediatric rongeurs. A mouth speculum that deflects the tongue and other soft tissues is essential to prevent lacerations and provide working space (Fig. 170–8). Intubate the trachea to prevent aspiration pneumonia when working on molars.

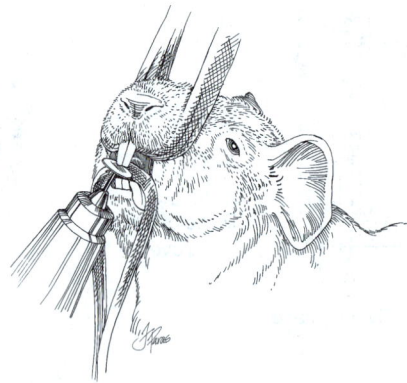

Figure 170–8. Proper technique for dental trimming.

If a tooth is abscessed, extract both it and the occlusal tooth.

- If necessary, approach cheek teeth via an incision through the cheek.
- Use a fine dental elevator to loosen the teeth.
- Patience and firm but gentle pressure are needed, or the root or surrounding bone may fracture.
- The roots of the maxillary incisors curve dramatically back into the head. Take care to follow the curve of the tooth.
- Packing an infected tooth socket with a calcium hydroxide paste may decrease the occurrence of persistent infection. Remove the paste in 3–4 days.

In chinchillas with dental malocclusion, the roots of the molars can become impacted, causing swelling of the mandible or exophthalmos and epiphora. These teeth are extremely difficult to extract without causing extensive bony and soft tissue damage. Discourage breeding of animals with malocclusion, unless it was acquired as a result of trauma or infection, because this trait is hereditary.

MOUSE

Most pet and laboratory mice are derived from *Mus musculus*, which is the common house mouse. Mice sold in the pet trade are randomly bred and less likely to suffer from the genetic problems associated with inbred laboratory rodents. Mice possess brown fat tissues between their scapulae that also are known as hibernating glands; these are thought to provide an energy store. The spleen in male mice is 50% larger than that of females.

Dermatology

Ectoparasites

Ectoparasites usually are found in new acquisitions.

Clinical Signs

- Alopecia and pruritus, especially on the back of the head and dorsal midline, usually are associated with lice (*Polyplax serrata*), mites, or fleas.

- Mite infestation (e.g., *Mycoptes musculinus*, *Myobia musculini*, *Radfordia affinis*) often causes a greasy haircoat and folliculitis.

Transmission of lice and mites occurs via direct contact. Fleas are transmitted by other household pets, such as cats and dogs.

- Diagnosis is based on clinical signs, history, visualization of parasite, skin scrape, and cellophane tape test.
- Pyrethrin powder is used to treat fleas and lice. Ivermectin is recommended for treatment of mites (Table 170–8).
- Change the bedding and thoroughly clean the cage between treatments to prevent reinfestation. Occasionally, the surrounding environment needs to be treated with a premises spray used for killing fleas.

Dermatophytosis

- Alopecia also may be the result of dermatophytes (see Chapter 37). Lesions are often hyperkeratotic.
- Diagnosis is made by skin scrape or isolation on culture. Most dermatophytes found in pet rodents do not fluoresce under a Wood's lamp.
- Treatment is with lime-sulfur dip or griseofulvin (Table 170–9).

Bacterial Disease

- Ulcerative dermatitis is a common syndrome caused by *Staphylococcus aureus* characterized by pododermatitis, mastitis, and abscesses in other areas.
- Administer antibiotics based on culture and sensitivity tests. Chloramphenicol is recommended pending culture results (see Table 170–9). The application of

Table 170–8. PARASITICIDE DOSAGES FOR PET RODENTS

Agent	Rat	Mouse	Guinea Pig	Chinchilla	Hamster	Gerbil
Fenbendazole	20 mg/kg q24h for 5 days	see rat	see rat	see rat	see rat	see rat
Flea powders	3–5% Malathion or 0.5% Pyrethrin powder 3 times per wk for 3 wks	see rat	5% carbaryl powder or 0.1% pyrethrin powder 1 time per wk for 3 wks	see guinea pig	see rat	see rat
Ivermectin	200–400 µg/kg, q7d for 3 wks SQ, PO	see rat	see rat	see rat	200–500 µg/kg q14d for 3 treatments, SC, PO	see rat
Lime-sulfur dip	Dilute 1:40. Dip q7d for 6 wks	see rat	see rat	see rat	see rat	see rat
Malathion	0.5% spray or 2% dip q7d for 3 wks	see rat	see rat	see rat	see rat	see rat
Mebendazole	40 mg/kg q7d PO for 3 wks	see rat				
Methyridine	100 mg/kg, SC					
Niclosamide	100 mg/kg repeat in 2 wks, PO	see rat	see rat	200 mg/kg, repeat in 2 wks, PO	see rat	see rat
Piperazine adipate	200 mg/kg, q24h for 7 days, wait 7 days and repeat, PO, or 0.5 g/L drinking water for 3 wks					200–600 mg/kg, q24h for 7 days, wait 7 days and repeat, PO
Piperazine citrate	2–5 mg/ml drinking water for 7 days, wait 7 days and repeat	see rat	see rat	see rat	see rat	see rat
Praziquantel	30 mg/kg q14d for 6 wks, PO	see rat	6–10 mg/kg q7d for 3 wks, PO	see guinea pig	see guinea pig	see rat
Quinacrine HCl	75 mg/kg, q8h					
Thiabendazole	200 mg/kg, q24h for 5 days, PO	100 mg/kg q7d for 4 treatments, PO	100 mg/kg q24 h for 5 days, PO	100 mg/kg q24 h for 5 days, PO	100 mg/kg q24 h for 5 days, PO	100 mg/kg q24 h for 5 days, PO

PO, by mouth (per os); SC, subcutaneous.

Table 170–9. ANTIBIOTIC, ANTIFUNGAL, AND ANTIPROTOZOAL DOSAGES FOR PET RODENTS

Agent	Rat	Mouse	Guinea Pig	Chinchilla	Hamster	Gerbil
Amikacin	2–5 mg/kg q 8–12h, SC, IM, IV, IO	2–5 mg/kg q 8–12h, SC, IM, IV, IO	2–5 mg/kg q8–12h, SC, IM, IV, IO	2–5 mg/kg q8–12h, SC, IM, IV, IO	2–5 mg/kg q8–12h, SC, IM, IV, IO	2–5 mg/kg q8–12h, SC, IM, IV, IO
Ampicillin	20–100 mg/kg, BID, IM, SC, PO	20–100 mg/kg, BID, IM, SC, PO	DO NOT USE	DO NOT USE	DO NOT USE	6–30 mg/kg, TID, PO
Carbenicillin	100 mg/kg, BID, PO	100 mg/kg, BID, PO				
Cephaloridine	10–25 mg/kg, SID, IM, SC	10–25 mg/kg, SID, IM, SC	10–25 mg/kg, SID-TID, IM		10–25 mg/kg, SID, IM	
Chloramphenicol palmitate	50 mg/kg, TID, PO	50 mg/kg,TID, PO	50 mg/kg, TID, PO	50 mg/kg, TID, PO	50 mg/kg, TID, PO	50 mg/kg, TID, PO
Chloramphenicol succinate	30 mg/kg, TID, IV, IM	30 mg/kg, TID, IV, IM	30 mg/kg, TID, IV, IM	30 mg/kg, TID, IV, IM	30 mg/kg, TID, IV, IM	30 mg/kg, TID, IV IM
Enrofloxacin	2.5–5.0 mg/kg q12h SC, IM, PO	2.5–5.0 mg/kg q12h SC, IM, PO	2.5–5.0 mg/kg q12h SC, IM, PO	2.5–5.0 mg/kg q12h SC, IM, PO	2.5–5.0 mg/kg q12h SC, IM, PO	2.5–5.0 mg/kg q12h SC, IM, PO
Gentamicin	5 mg/kg, SID, IM, SQ	5 mg/kg, SID, IM, SQ	5 mg/kg, SID, IM, SQ	5 mg/kg, SID, IM, SQ	5 mg/kg, SID, IM, SQ	5 mg/kg, SID, IM, SQ
Griseofulvin	25–50 mg/kg q12h, PO	25–50 mg/kg q12h, PO	25–50 mg/kg q 12h, PO	25–50 mg/kg q12h, PO	25–50 mg/kg q12h, PO	25–50 mg/kg q12h, PO
Metronidazole	40 mg/kg q24h, PO	40 mg/kg q24h, PO	10–40 mg/kg q24h, PO	50–60 mg/kg q24h, PO	70 mg/kg, q24h, PO	40 mg/kg q24h, PO
Neomycin	2.6 mg/ml drinking water = 10 g/gallon = 2650 mg/L	2.6 mg/ml drinking water = 10 g/gallon = 2650 mg/L	12–16 mg/kg, BID, PO	15 mg/kg q24h, PO	100 mg/kg, PO, SID or 0.5 mg/ml drinking water = 500 mg/L = 1.9 g/gallon	2.6 mg/ml drinking water = 10 g/gallon = 2650 mg/L
Oxytetracycline	3–5 mg/ml drinking water	3–5 mg/ml drinking water	Do not use oral 5 mg/kg, BID, IM		3–5 mg/ml of drinking water	10 mg/kg q8h, PO
Sulfamethazine or sulfamerazine	1 mg/ml drinking water	1 mg/ml drinking water	1 mg/ml drinking water	1 mg/ml drinking water	1 mg/ml drinking water	0.8 mg/ml drinking water
Sulfadiazine and trimethoprim	30 mg/kg, SID-BID, PO, SC	30 mg/kg, SID-BID, PO, SC	30 mg/kg, SID, SC	30 mg/kg, SID, SC	30 mg/kg, SID, SC	30 mg/kg, SID, SC
Sulfamethazole and trimethoprim PO			15 mg/kg, BID, PO	15 mg/kg, BID, PO	15 mg/kg, BID, PO	15 mg/kg, BID, PO
Tetracycline	20 mg/kg, BID, PO	20 mg/kg, BID, PO	20 mg/kg, PO, BID 0.2–0.35 mg/ml drinking water	20 mg/kg, PO, BID	55–65 mg/kg, TID, PO 0.4 mg/ml drinking water	15–20 mg/kg, TID, PO 20 mg/kg, SID, IM
Tylosin	10–20 mg/kg, SID, IM 10 mg/kg, PO, SID-BID	10–20 mg/kg, SID, IM 10 mg/kg, SID-BID, PO	DO NOT USE	10 mg/kg q24h, PO SC, IM	DO NOT USE	10 mg/kg q24h, PO, SC, IM

BID, twice a day; IM, intramuscular; IO, intraosseus; IV, intravenous; PO, by mouth (per os); SC, subcutaneous; SID, once a day; TID, three times a day.

hot packs, local drainage, and topical medications are also beneficial in selected cases.

- Mastitis also may be caused by *Escheria coli* or *Pasteurella, Klebsiella, Pseudomonas,* or *Streptococcus* species. Mastitis usually is caused by poor sanitation, abrasive bedding, or overly aggressive young.
- Preputial gland abscesses are fairly common in males and are usually caused by *E. coli* or *S. aureus*. Local flushing and topical treatment are usually adequate.
- Subcutaneous abscesses can be the result of the aforementioned bacteria or *Actinobacillus* spp. or *Corynebacterium kutscheri. Corynebacteria* is associated with widespread abscesses, septic arthritis, gangrene, and ulcerated draining tracts. Diagnosis is based on finding gram-positive pleomorphic rods on Gram stain and isolation on culture.
- The bacteria are usually sensitive to ampicillin, chloramphenicol, and tetracycline (see Table 170–9).

Neoplasia

- Lymphoma and mammary neoplasia are common causes of subcutaneous masses. Mammary neoplasia is usually malignant in mice, and metastasis to the lungs is common. (Mice have five pair of mammary glands—three thoracic and two abdominal.)
- Consider thoracic radiographs before surgery.
- Give a guarded prognosis for long-term survival.
- Other possibilities for subcutaneous masses are fungal granulomas, nodules from the *Psorergates simplex* mite, hematoma, hernia, non-neoplastic lymphadenopathy, or emphysema.

Otitis

- Otitis externa usually is caused by ear mites, although bacteria or fungi also may cause primary or secondary otitis.
- Clinical signs include erythema, pruritus, waxy debris, and excoriations behind the ears.
- Mites may be diagnosed by identification on otoscopic examination or microscopic examination of ear swabs (see Techniques).
- Treatment requires cleaning debris from ears with a commercial ear cleanser followed by administration of three doses of ivermectin at 2-week intervals or topical acaricides used daily for 3–4 weeks (see Table 170–9).
- Bacterial and fungal otitis is diagnosed by identification of organisms or Gram-stained specimens and isolation on culture.
- Treatment is similar to that used in cats.
- Otitis media/interna usually are caused by hematogenous spread or local invasion of bacteria from a primary abscess.
- Clinical signs include head tilt, circling, facial nerve paralysis, and otitis externa.
- Rule out mouse hepatitis virus as the cause of the head tilt (see Gastroenterology).
- If treatment of the primary disease is successful, the otitis media usually resolves, although a residual head tilt may persist.
- If a cluster of *Pseudomonas* infections occurs in a population, evaluate the water source and produce for contamination. Use sodium hypochlorite in the drinking water at 10 ppm to control an outbreak while water quality is being restored.
- Damage to the pinnae can be associated with trauma, dermatitis, pox virus, hypersensitivity reactions, and vasculitis. Dry gangrene is a common sequela and is usually self-limiting.

Miscellaneous

A steroid-responsive pruritus has been observed in pet mice by the author. The pruritus is severe enough to result in significant self-mutilation. This condition has been nonresponsive to treatment with ivermectin, lime-sulfur dips, griseofulvin, multiple antibiotics, oral prednisolone, and antihistamines. Attempts at bacterial and fungal culture have failed to identify a pathogen. An inflammatory response is observed on histologic examination. Mice with this condition respond to repository methylprednisolone injections every 2–4 weeks (1.0 mg/kg IM). Most owners have not elected to continue injections for longer than a few months. Once the injections are stopped, the pruritus returns, often requiring euthanasia of the affected mouse.

- Bilateral alopecia found around the muzzle associated with no other abnormalities usually is caused by friction from overhead feeders.
- Alopecia occurring in smaller, weaker individuals is often the result of barbering. Removal of the mice in best condition from the cage results in normal appearance of barbered mice in 2–3 weeks.
- Tailhead alopecia and scabbing are usually the result of aggression. Separate affected animals, or additional trauma may occur.
- Other rare causes of alopecia are endocrinopathies, leprosy, and hereditary alopecia in nude mice.

Ophthalmology
Epiphora

- Epiphora is a common condition of pet mice. The most common causes in pets owned for longer than 2 months are ammonia fumes and overgrown incisors.
- Ammonia causing contact irritation is diagnosed by examining an uncleaned cage and checking for odor.
- Treatment is improved sanitation.
- Overgrown incisors are diagnosed easily by oral examination. Treat by trimming the affected teeth and providing opportunities for gnawing.
- Foreign bodies and the resultant corneal ulcers can cause epiphora. An eye examination, including fluorescein stain, is indicated. Treat by removing the foreign body and administering an ophthalmic antibiotic (gentamicin, tetracycline, or chloramphenicol in affected eye, q8h–q6h).
- In newly acquired pets, epiphora is often the first clinical sign of an upper respiratory infection. *Pasteurella pneumotropica* is the most common pathogen, although *Salmonella* spp., mycoplasma, Sendai virus, lymphocytic choriomeningitis, and mouse pox also may cause epiphoria. The ocular discharge later appears mucopurulent (see the following Respiratory section).

Retinal Degeneration

Retinal degeneration can be either hereditary or (in albino mice) may be caused by exposure to high-intensity lighting. The resulting blindness often goes undetected because patients adapt well and behave normally in their cages.

Miscellaneous

- Cataracts are usually hereditary or postinflammatory.
- Other hereditary conditions are posterior lens capsule rupture, eyelid malformation, optic nerve hypoplasia, microphthalmos, and retinal dysplasia.

Respiratory

Pneumonia

- *Murine respiratory mycoplasmosis* (MRM) is one of the most common respiratory diseases in pet mice. It is caused by *Mycoplasma pulmonis*. The infection remains dormant for long periods of time and is activated by stress. There are many asymptomatic carriers, and transmission is by aerosol and direct contact. Spread of infection can be hematogenous, causing abscess of the middle ear, uterus, or joints.
- Clinical signs include dyspnea (often described as chattering), mucopurulent oculonasal discharge, hunched posture, and anorexia. Animals with a chronic history of this disease are often cachexic.
- Radiology aids in determination of the extent and severity of the pneumonia and the absence or presence of distant foci of infection.
- Treatment with tylosin is successful in controlling the disease if it is not too advanced. Tetracycline, enrofloxacin, and chloramphenicol also have been used (see Table 170–8).
- Many patients need nutritional support.
- Mice with pyometra or other abscesses require surgical debridement.
- Recovered animals are carriers and stress elicits clinical signs. Strictly quarantine these animals.

Sendai Virus

A common cause of pneumonia in newly acquired mice is Sendai virus. Acute fatalities are seen in suckling or weanling mice.

- Transmission is by aerosol or direct contact.
- Clinical signs in adults are caused by secondary bacterial infections and are similar to those in MRM.
- Diagnosis is based on clinical signs and serologic testing.
- Treat with antibiotics to control the secondary bacterial infection and provide supportive care as needed.
- Prohibit breeding for 4–6 weeks.
- A killed vaccine is available.
- Recovered animals are resistant to new infection.

Bacterial Pneumonia

Common primary or secondary pathogens causing respiratory signs in mice are *Streptococcus pneumoniae,* *Corynebacterium kutscheri, Pasteurella pneumontropica, Pseudomonas aeruginosa,* and *Klebsiella pneumoniae.* Treatment is empiric or based on culture and sensitivity of a tracheal swab sample.

Neoplasia

Dyspnea often is caused by metastasis to the lungs from mammary adenocarcinomas. Primary lung tumors, especially pulmonary adenomas, also occur frequently.

Other

Although not frequently diagnosed, cardiac disease can result in signs of respiratory disease. Diagnosis is based on radiographic evidence of cardiomegaly and pulmonary edema.

Gastroenterology

Parasites

- Tapeworms usually do not cause clinical signs. Occasionally, heavy burdens may cause diarrhea or weight loss. The chief concern is the zoonotic potential of one species, *Hymenolepis nana,* which is directly transmissible to humans.
- Diagnosis is made from visualization of eggs in the feces. Treat with praziquantel or niclosamide (see Table 170–8). Improve sanitation, and remove indirect hosts (e.g., fleas, beetles, roaches).
- Pinworms (*Syphacia obvelata, Aspiculuris tetraptera*) may cause anal pruritus and, in severe cases, rectal prolapse.
- Diagnosis is based on clinical signs and observation of eggs on cellophane tape after application to the perineal region. Treat with piperazine or mebendazole every 7–10 days for three treatments or with fenbendazole once daily for 5 days (see Table 170–8) and provide improved sanitation.
- The protozoal parasite *Spironucleus muris* causes diarrhea and slow growth associated with a pot-bellied appearance in young mice.
- Diagnosis is by fecal wet mount, although false-negative findings are common.
- Treat with oxytetracycline (see Table 170–9). Supportive care to combat dehydration and hypothermia is extremely important.
- Control is achieved with improved sanitation.
- *Giardia* spp. and, rarely, *Eimeria falciformis* show signs similar to *Spironucleus.* Giardiasis is zoonotic. Treat with metronidazole. Treat *Eimeria* with sulfadiazine/trimethoprim (see Table 170–9). Most other protozoa are considered nonpathogenic.
- *Cysticercus fasciolaris* causes nonpathologic cysts of the liver. These cysts are the infective form of *Taenia taeniaformis* in carnivores.

Diarrhea

Viral Diseases

- Diarrhea in mice 10–20 days old usually is caused by lethal intestinal virus of infant mice (LIVM).
- This virus may be a variant of mouse hepatitis virus. The mortality rate can reach 80%.

- Clinical signs are yellow diarrhea that mats on the perineal region, causing obstipation and perineal necrosis, anorexia, and stunted growth.
- Transmission is aerosol or feco-oral from the mother.
- Treat supportively, and quarantine survivors.
- Epizootic diarrhea of infant mice (EDIM) is clinically similar to LIVM. This disease usually affects mice younger than 2 weeks of age but can occur in mice up to 21 days of age.
- There is low mortality, and nursing continues through the infection.
Transmission is feco-oral.
- Diagnosis is based on clinical presentation.
- Treat supportively. Survivors usually are growth-stunted. Quarantine them from other mice.
- Mouse hepatitis virus is a corona virus. Most infections are latent. Outbreaks of yellow diarrhea and encephalitis secondary to viral hepatitis occur in mice 7–13 days of age. Older animals show clinical signs of infertility, jaundice, and hemoglobinuria as a result of a slowly progressive hepatitis.
- Diagnosis is based on clinical presentation, serology, and presence of syncytial giant cells in the epithelium of the small intestine.
- Treat supportively, and quarantine affected individuals. The prognosis is grave.
- Although less commonly seen in pet mice, reovirus occurs in older suckling mice. It is characterized by an oily diarrhea, which results in a greasy haircoat. Other signs are conjunctivitis, stunted growth, and tremors. Transmission is by ingestion.
- Diagnosis is based on clinical signs, histology, and serology.
- Treat supportively. The long-term prognosis is grave. Initial survivors are weak and jaundiced, suffer from alopecia, and eventually die.

Bacterial Diseases

- Transmissible murine colonic hyperplasia (MCH) caused by *Citrobacter freundii* is characterized by diarrhea followed by rectal prolapse and stunted growth. Transmission is feco-oral.
- Diagnosis is made by clinical signs and fecal culture.
- Treat with neomycin, tetracycline, or sulfamethazine until sensitivity results are available (see Table 170–9). Severe thickening of the distal half of the colon is observed at necropsy.
- Salmonellosis, also known as mouse typhoid, is transmitted by latent carriers or contaminated feed or bedding. Incubation lasts for 3–6 days.
- Clinical signs are lethargy, anorexia, purulent conjunctivitis, arthritis, and diarrhea.
- Diagnosis is based on clinical signs and fecal culture. Treat supportively. Use of antibiotics is controversial.
- Quarantine survivors.
- Sanitation is extremely important because *Salmonella* spp. are zoonotic. On gross postmortem examination, erythema of distal ileum and congestion of the spleen and liver are seen. With more chronic infections, necrotic foci are seen in the liver, spleen, and lymph nodes. Prevent infection by feeding a fresh laboratory chow from a reputable source. Thor-

oughly wash all produce and then dip it in a diluted bleach solution. Rinse completely before feeding.
- Tyzzer disease is caused by *Bacillus piliformis*. Transmission is feco-oral.
- Clinical signs are precipitated by stress and consist of anorexia, diarrhea, and high mortality in weanlings.
- Diagnosis is made by clinical signs or isolation on culture. Enteritis and multiple gray-yellow necrotic foci in the liver are seen on gross postmortem examination.
- Administer tetracycline for 4–5 days (see Table 170–9) and reduce stress to control the disease.

Theriogenology

Breeding systems vary; from one to six females may be placed with one male. All animals are housed together, and the young are removed after weaning. Females in proestrus have swollen vulvas. Vaginal plugs are present postcopulation.

Female mice that have been bred within 4 days abort if a new male is placed in the cage. Inappropriate light cycle, inappropriate age, crowding, and poor nutrition are the most common causes of infertility in pet mice. Pyometra due to *Pasteurella pneumontropica*, *Mycoplasma* spp., or other bacteria is also common.

Desertion of litters is usually a result of stress, lack of nesting materials, agalactia, or mastitis.

Urology

- Urethral obstruction from proteinaceous plugs of inspissated ejaculum may develop in aged male mice. *Pseudomonas*, *E. coli*, or *Proteus* are the most frequently cultured pathogens. Before complete obstruction, chronic hematuria may be noticed by the owner.
- Antibiotics, which are chosen based on the results of urine culture, are often curative with early presentation. Complete obstruction requires surgical removal.
- Glomerulonephritis is very common in geriatric mice. It frequently is secondary to chronic viral infection. Clinical signs are anorexia, lethargy, dehydration, and cachexia. Urinalysis demonstrates proteinuria. As the disease progresses, the urine becomes isosthenuric, the blood urea nitrogen (BUN) and creatinine levels rise, and other electrolyte abnormalities typical of chronic renal failure occur. Treat supportively. Prognosis for long-term survival is grave.
- Coccidia (e.g., *Klosseilla muris*) occasionally is found in the urine. The clinical significance of its presence is unknown.
- Mice can be asymptomatic carriers of leptospirosis; however, this is rarely seen in pet mice.
- Diagnosis is based on darkfield microscopy of urine, serology, or histopathology. Euthanasia of carriers is recommended.

Musculoskeletal

- Infectious polyarthritis or mouse rheumatism is caused by *Streptobacillus moniliformis*. In humans, it is known as rat bite or Havernill fever. Transmission is by direct contact. Clinical signs are cachexia, keratitis, edema and ulceration of the appendages, and ankylosing arthritis.

- Diagnosis is based on the bacterial culture findings or the presence of caseous pericarditis and arthritis on necropsy.
- Treat with antibiotics chosen through the results of culture and sensitivity tests. Use penicillin while awaiting results. Supportive care is important. Animals that recover remain arthritic. Control is achieved through quarantine and sanitation.

Neurology

- The most frequently diagnosed neurologic disease in pet mice is head tilt resulting from bacterial otitis media (see Otitis). The second most common cause of neurologic signs is trauma.
- Diagnosis is based on history and clinical signs. Consider neoplasia in aged mice with slowly progressive signs.
- Lymphocytic choriomeningitis is a zoonotic arenavirus. Transmission is airborne, transplacental, or by direct contact, fomites, or insect vectors. Acute signs usually occur in mice that are 3–6 weeks old. Approximately 20% of infected individuals show acute clinical signs, which include lethargy and photophobia followed by convulsions and paralysis. In animals that are latently infected, glomerulonephritis develops later. Mice infected after weaning and before 1 year in age lose weight, appear arthritic, and show signs of conjunctivitis and photophobia. The virus runs its course in several weeks. Animals that recover show no residual signs.
- Diagnosis is based on clinical signs and the presence of immunofluorescent antibody (IFA). Pleural effusion, splenomegaly, and hepatic lipidosis are found on necropsy. Treat supportively. House survivors separately.
- Prevent the disease by improving sanitation, providing pest control, and cleaning produce. Consider euthanasia because of the zoonotic potential of the virus.
- Mouse poliomyelitis/encephalomyelitis, also known as Theiler disease, causes clinical signs in 1:10,000 infected mice. Two-thirds of healthy mice are carriers. Transmission is by oral or respiratory routes. Mice younger than 4 weeks of age show signs of encephalitis. Animals that are 6–10 weeks old are weak in the rear legs and progress to paralysis. The tail may remain mobile. Affected mice continue to eat and be alert. Albino mice are predisposed to show clinical signs.
- Diagnosis is based on clinical signs, serology, or histopathology that shows necrosis of the ganglionic cells of the anterior horn of the spinal cord.
- Treat supportively. Consider euthanasia because of poor prognosis.
- Seizures in mice commonly result from otitis media, trauma, liver or kidney failure, toxin, bacterial meningitis, neoplasia, or viral encephalitis.

Hematology

- Leukemia in mice is usually viral in origin. Transmission is transmammary or transplacental.

- Clinical signs are anemia, dyspnea (with thymic involvement), and those signs that are compatible with chronic disease.
- Diagnosis is based on complete blood count (CBC), bone marrow aspirate, or histopathology. Prognosis is grave.
- *Eperythrozoon coccoides* is a rickettsial red blood cell (RBC) parasite of mice. Affected mice are usually asymptomatic. Occasionally, fever, anemia, and splenomegaly develop in infected animals. Transmission is through the louse *Polyplax serrata*. Control is by extermination of the louse.
- Treat with tetracyclines.

RAT

Pet rats are derived from the Norwegian or brown rat (*Rattus norvegicus*), which did not originate from Norway, but from Asia. Breeds of rats are called strains when they are inbred extensively and stocks when strains are hybridized. Rats have brown fat, as discussed in the section on mice. They do not possess a gallbladder. Their mandibular symphysis is articulated normally. Rats are neophobic; therefore, make gradual changes in food or environment when possible.

Dermatology

- Fleas, mites (e.g., *Radfordia ensifera*, *Ornithonyssus bacoti*), lice (i.e., *Polyplax spinulosa*), ear mites (i.e., *Notoedres muris*), and dermatophytes cause similar signs in both mice and rats. Treatment also is similar (see Mouse).
- Subcutaneous masses in rats are similar to mice. *Pasteurella pneumotropica* is a very common pathogen in mastitis and subcutaneous abscesses.
- Treat with chloramphenicol until culture results are available (see Table 170–9).
- Mammary cancer develops in 50–90% of adult female rats and in approximately 15% of male rats. Always submit biopsy specimens for histologic examination. Most, but not all, of these tumors are fibroadenomas, which are benign. Prognosis for long-term survival after surgical removal is good. Other common neoplasms include interstitial cell tumors of the testes, which cause subcutaneous swellings in the inguinal region, and squamous cell carcinomas of the Zymbals gland of the external ear canal.
- Ulcerative dermatitis occurs in rats as well as mice. *Staphylococcus aureus* is the causative agent. *C. kutscheri* follows a similar course in rats and mice (see Mouse).
- Ringtail is the formation of constrictive bands of fibrous tissue around the tail in nestling rats. These bands result in gangrene of the distal tail. This disease occurs when environmental humidity is less than 40%.
- Treat by making a longitudinal incision of the ring to release the stricture and apply topical dimethyl sulfoxide (DMSO), steroid, and antibiotic solution

(10 ml DMSO, 6 ml 50 mg/ml amikacin, 4 ml 2 mg/ml dexamethasone) four times daily.

- To prevent keep humidity above 50%, use solid-bottom cages and provide ample nesting material. Prognosis for life is excellent. Prognosis for retention of the distal tail is guarded.

Ophthalmology

- Epiphora and blepharospasm are caused mostly by ammonia fumes, overgrown incisors, or foreign bodies (see Mouse).
- Sialodacryoadenitis virus is a coronavirus that is endemic in many rat populations.
- Clinical signs vary from mild keratoconjunctivitis to blepharospasm, chromodacryorrhea, severe uveitis, hyphema, buphthalmos, periorbital swelling, and pneumonia. The clinical course of the disease lasts 10–14 days. Rats maintain normal activity levels and appetite.
- Treatment is not necessary for mild infections. Place rats showing marked ocular disease or discomfort on the appropriate ophthalmic ointments (e.g., atropine, antibiotic, steroid) based on presentation. Administer parenteral antibiotics to animals that show signs of respiratory problems. Recovery is usually complete unless the eye ruptures or self-mutilation occurs.
- Control is achieved by not introducing new animals for 4 weeks.
- In contrast to mice, Sendai virus rarely causes clinical signs in rats.
- Mucopurulent ocular discharge also may be caused by infection with mycoplasmosis, *Streptococcus pneumoniae*, *Pseudomonas* spp., and other less common bacterial or viral agents that cause pneumonia.
- Cataracts are primary hereditary defects or occur secondary to severe uveitis or diabetes mellitus. Retinal dystrophy and colobomas are also inheritable traits in rats. Retinal degeneration occurs in rats housed under intense lighting.

Respiratory

- MRM is extremely common in pet rats. Its presentation is similar to the disease in mice (see Mouse).
- *Streptococcus pneumoniae* is normal flora for rats. However, during stressful situations, bacteremia may occur, resulting in pneumonia. Clinical signs are similar to MRM. Differentiation is based on culture and the presence of extensive fibrinopurulent pleural effusion on necropsy.
- Ampicillin controls clinical signs if treated early in the course of disease (see Table 170–9). Prevent the condition by minimizing stress.
- *Corynebacterium kutscheri* and *Pasteurella pneumotropica* cause signs similar to MRM (see Mouse). There is a serologic test for *C. kutscheri*. See the Mouse section for a discussion of *Pseudomonas aeruginosa*.
- *Pneumocystosis carinii* is an uncommon protozoa that infects the lung. Cysts and trophozoites live in the alveoli. Clinical signs occur only in immune-compromised or geriatric individuals. Signs are cachexia, cyanosis, and dyspnea.
- Diagnosis is based on clinical signs, tracheal wash, response to therapy, or histologic examination.
- Treat with sulfadiazine/pyrinrethamine (see Table 170–9).

Cardiovascular System

- Myocardial degeneration and subsequent congestive heart failure are fairly common in geriatric rats. Diagnosis is based on radiographs of the thorax and clinical signs. Treat supportively, and use furosemide and digitalis at cat dosages to alleviate pulmonary edema.
- Polyarteritis nodosa is an idiopathic condition of geriatric rats that results in thickening and tortuosity of arteries, especially in the mesentery, pancreas, and testicles. Affected areas are predisposed to clot formation and aneurysms.

Gastroenterology

Parasites

- Nematode (*Syphacia muris*), cestode, and intestinal protozoal parasite infestations are similar to those in mice.
- *Capillaria hepatica* has no clinical significance. Yellow streaks on the liver are an incidental finding at necropsy.

Dental

The causes and treatment of malocclusion are similar to those for mice.

Diarrhea

- Epizootic diarrhea of suckling rats is a viral disorder found in rats 7–14 days old. The infection causes a mild diarrhea. Most animals recover. Occasionally, stunting occurs. Treat supportively.
- Salmonellosis in rats is similar to that in mice.

Theriogenology

- If breeding is desired, take females showing signs of estrus (e.g., lordosis, hyperactivity, quivering ears, and swollen vulva) to a male rat's cage for 24 hours, or keep one male in a cage with up to six females. Check females for a postcopulatory plug to confirm breeding. Remove females just before parturition, and house females individually while raising the young. A vaginal discharge is seen 1.5–4 hours before labor. Parturition is accompanied by stretching and extension of the rear legs. All neonates usually are delivered within 1–2 hours.
- Infertility is usually the result of age, malnutrition (e.g., protein, vitamin E), uterine infection, or improper light cycle, temperature, or humidity.
- Litter desertion is usually the result of stress. Inadequate nesting material or agalactia are other significant causes of abandonment and death.

▼ *Key Point* To prevent cannibalism, remove male rats from the cage before parturition and do not return them until after weaning is complete.

- Rat virus infection is a parvovirus that is usually inapparent unless individuals are infected in utero. Small litters or jaundiced, stunted neonates are often the only clinical signs. Transmission is both vertical and horizontal.
- Diagnosis is by serologic testing and characteristic histologic findings. Permanently quarantine all in-contact animals.

Urology

- Urolithiasis commonly occurs in older rats. Uroliths usually are composed of ammonium magnesium phosphate or calcium carbonate.
- Clinical signs include anorexia, stranguria, hematuria, and abdominal distention. Urinary obstruction can occur.
- Diagnosis is based on clinical signs, urinalysis, and radiographs. Treat by surgically removing uroliths and providing antibiotics based on culture and susceptibility testing.
- Two extremely common conditions in geriatric rats are nephrocalcinosis and chronic progressive nephropathy. Clinical signs are compatible with those of chronic renal failure. Enlarged or small irregular kidneys may be found on physical or radiographic examination. Isosthenuria and marked proteinuria are found in urinalysis.
- Definitive diagnosis is based on renal biopsy.
- Treat supportively. Prognosis for long-term survival is grave.
- *Trichasomoides crassicauda* is an uncommon parasite of the urogenital tract. The adult worms usually reside in the kidney, but they occasionally may wander into the genital tract. The ova are passed in the urine.
- Clinical signs are hematuria and stranguria. Proliferative mucosa of the bladder occasionally may be palpated as an abdominal mass.
- Treatment is somewhat successful with methyridene (see Table 170–8). Sanitation is critical in control of this disease.
- *Klossiella muris* is an incidental coccidia of the urinary tract.

Neurology

- Many geriatric pet rats have chronic progressive radiculoneuropathy.
- Clinical signs are compatible with cauda equina syndrome, including posterior paresis progressing to paralysis, urine retention, and incontinence. Prognosis is grave.
- Treat supportively or euthanize.
- *Streptobacillus moniliformis*, a normal bacteria found in the oral, nasal, and pharyngeal cavities of rodents, is isolated from 43% of middle ear infections and 35% of chronic pneumonias in rats. The bacteria is non-pathogenic for gerbils and guinea pigs.

- Clinical signs vary with the site of infection. Head tilt and circling, septic arthritis, and respiratory disease commonly are seen.
- Diagnosis is based on isolation on culture. The clinical signs mimic many other diseases, especially MRM and *Pseudomonas* infection (see Mouse).
- Head tilt in rats also may be the result of trauma or neoplasia, especially pituitary adenomas.

Hematology

- *Hemobartonella muris* is an RBC parasite of rats that is nonpathogenic unless the rat is immunocompromised or splenectomized. Transmission is through the louse *Polyplax spinulosa*.
- Clinical signs result from hemolytic anemia and hemoglobinuria.
- Treat with tetracyclines (see Table 170–9).

HAMSTER

Mesocricetus auratus, better known as the golden or Syrian hamster, is a primarily nocturnal rodent that originated in the Middle East. Almost all hamsters in the United States are the offspring of three siblings imported in the 1930s. Many color variations are available. Long-haired hamsters are called "teddy bear" hamsters. The stomach has two compartments, a nonglandular forestomach, which functions like a rumen, and a glandular stomach. Hamsters are very territorial. They possess flank glands, which are larger in males, that are rubbed against objects to mark their territory. Females are larger than males. Except during estrus, they use this size advantage to attack males. Do not allow groups to estivate together or recently awakened animals may cannibalize sleeping hamsters.

▼ *Key Point* Hamsters are extremely sensitive to antibiotics.

Penicillins, clindamycin, lincomycin, streptomycin, tylosin, erythromycin, and cephalosporins eliminate the normal intestinal flora, allowing overgrowth of pathogenic bacteria, particularly *Clostridium difficile*. Diarrhea, which is almost always fatal within 3–7 days, subsequently occurs. Even antibiotics considered to be safe can have this effect. Treat by discontinuing antibiotics, providing a *Lactobacillus* supplement, and giving supportive therapy.

Dermatology

- Hamsters are susceptible to *Demodex criceti* and *D. aurati* mites. *D. criceti* is limited to skin folds. *D. aurati* causes hyperpigmentation, alopecia, and seborrhea sicca affecting the dorsal midline. *Demodex* is carried by many normal-appearing hamsters.
- Clinical signs occur in immunosuppressed animals, as would occur with stress, chronic infection, pregnancy, or malnutrition.
- Diagnosis is based on clinical signs and deep-skin scrapings.

- Treat with amitraz every 2 weeks for two treatments past two consecutive negative skin scrapings. Use the manufacturer's recommended dilution for dogs.
- *Sarcoptes* mites infrequently cause facial alopecia. Diagnosis is based on skin scraping. Treat with ivermectin (see Table 170–8). Do not confuse this condition with alopecia caused by contact with feeders or barbering.
- *Notoedres* mites affect only the external ear canal in female hamsters but may affect the ears, feet, genitalia, and tail in males. Diagnosis is made by observation of mites on samples from ear swabs, skin scrapings, or both. Treat with ivermectin (see Table 170–8).
- Other less common causes of alopecia in hamsters are dermatophytosis, endocrinopathies, and genetic defects.
- Dermal subcutaneous masses are usually abscesses caused by *Pasteurella pneumotropica, S. aureus,* or *Streptococcus* spp. Treatment is based on results of culture and susceptibility testing. Use chloramphenicol until culture results are available. Other frequent causes of subcutaneous swellings are distended cheek pouches and testicles, mastitis, hernias, neoplasia, and lymphadenopathy.

Ophthalmology

- Epiphora and conjunctivitis are caused most frequently by increased environmental ammonia concentrations, incisor overgrowth, foreign body, or lymphocytic choriomeningitis (see Rat; Mouse).
- Mucopurulent discharge is caused by secondary infection by *Pasteurella* or *Streptococcus* spp.
- Hamsters are predisposed to rupture of the eye following trauma or infection. Surgical enucleation is advised. Electrosurgery is extremely helpful in controlling bleeding but do not apply heat to the stump of the optic nerve or vessels, or thermal injury to the brain may result. Place gelfoam in the socket to enhance clot formation.

Respiratory

- Hamsters are susceptible to viral respiratory infections of humans.
- Clinical signs include nasal discharge, sneezing, otitis media, fever, and pneumonia. Uncomplicated cases last 5–7 days. Complications are usually the result of secondary bacterial infections.
- Treat supportively. Use of antibiotics is indicated if copious nasal discharge, dyspnea, anorexia, or marked lethargy is observed. Overuse of antibiotics may cause diarrhea-related death in hamsters that might have recovered uneventfully if left untreated.
- Most dyspnea in hamsters is caused by blunt thoracic trauma. Hamsters often bite when startled. Reflex actions on the part of humans, especially children, cause hamsters to be flung against hard objects.
- Diagnosis is by history and presence of fresh epistaxis.
- Treat supportively. Emergency shock therapy, consisting of supplemental heat, oxygen administration,

parenteral fluids, and glucocorticoids, frequently is required.
- Sendai virus can cause death in suckling hamsters housed with mice. Adults show no clinical signs (see Mouse).
- Primary bacterial pneumonia most frequently is caused by *Yersinia pseudotuberculosis, Pasteurella pneumotropica,* or *Streptococcus.* Clinical signs are compatible with those of pneumonia seen in other species, as well as weight loss and conjunctivitis. All three agents have a tendency to form distant abscesses, especially in the uterus.
- Diagnosis is based on clinical signs and isolation on culture.
- Treat with chloramphenicol until antibiotic susceptibility results are available. Abscesses require surgical debridement; however, anesthesia in affected animals is very risky. Recovered hamsters are carriers and must be quarantined from other rodents. Prognosis is guarded.

Cardiology

- Cardiac thrombosis is seen in 73% of geriatric hamsters. Most thromboses occur in the left atrium and are secondary to degenerative cardiomyopathy, cardiac amyloidosis, sepsis, or calcification of the great vessels. Congenital myocardial necrosis also occurs.
- Clinical signs include cyanosis, dyspnea, and acute death. Enlargement of the cardiac silhouette and pulmonary edema sometimes can be seen on thoracic radiographs.
- Furosemide and digitalis (using standard cat doses) may temporarily alleviate clinical signs.

Gastroenterology

Parasites

- Hamsters can carry the zoonotic tapeworm *H. nana* (see Mouse).
- Treat with niclosamide or praziquantel (see Table 170–8) and provide improved sanitation.
- Pinworms *(Aspicularis tetraptera, Syphacia muris, S. obvelata)* occur in hamsters as well as in mice.
- Treat with fenbendazole (see Table 170–8).

Dental/Oral

- Hamsters are predisposed to dental caries. A large percentage of affected teeth become abscessed, causing facial swelling, ptyalism, and anorexia.
- Diagnosis is based on clinical signs, oral examination, skull radiographs, and isolation on culture.
- Extract the tooth and administer antibiotic therapy based on results of susceptibility testing. Prognosis is variable depending on the condition of the animal, tooth affected, and extent of the abscess (see Mouse).
- Overgrown incisors also occur, as in mice.
- The cheek pouches are very distensible. Impaction of the pouches occurs on occasion.
- Clinical signs vary from ptyalism to swelling from abscess. In simple cases, removal of the material from

the pouch with fine forceps is sufficient. Sedation usually is not required.

- If a fungal or bacterial infection of the pouch is present, remove the exudate, submit samples for Gram staining and bacterial or fungal culture, and flush the pouch with diluted iodine solution. If cellulitis is present, administer systemic antibiotics as well. Fistulas often heal spontaneously.

Diarrhea

- Proliferative ileitis (i.e., wet-tail disease) is thought to be caused by a *Campylobacter*-like organism with or without concurrent bacterial or viral infections. More than 90% of animals with clinical signs die. The highest morbidity and mortality rates occur in hamsters 3–8 weeks of age. Teddy bear hamsters may be more susceptible to infection than shorter-haired varieties. Transmission is feco-oral.
- Clinical signs include diarrhea, which mats on the ventrum and perineum, anorexia, dehydration, and a hunched posture. The abdomen frequently seems painful on palpation. Bowel loops often are distended on palpation because of ileal obstruction or intussusception. Rectal prolapse usually occurs.
- Administer neomycin, gentamicin, metronidazole, or tetracycline (see Table 170–9). Supportive care is critical. Prognosis is grave, even with treatment. Gross postmortem findings include gas and yellow diarrhea in the distal intestinal tract, mucosal thickening in the ileum and distal jejunum, peritonitis, and liver abscesses.
- Other common causes of bacterial diarrhea include *E. coli,* Tyzzer disease, or *Salmonella* spp. (see Mouse).

Liver

In hamsters older than 1 year of age, liver cysts that are derived from the biliary duct often develop. Less frequently, similar cysts arise from the pancreas, epididymis, and seminal vesicles. This syndrome is called *polycystic disease.* No clinical signs are associated with cysts in these structures, which are an incidental finding on abdominal palpation. No treatment is recommended.

Theriogenology

- Timing is critical to prevent injury to the male when breeding hamsters. Transfer the female to the male's cage in the early evening 3 days after a creamy, viscous vaginal discharge is noticed. Monitor the pair carefully. Remove the male immediately if the female is aggressive. Remove the male after mating or after 1–2 hours even if mating has not occurred. Two days after successful copulation, a gray malodorous vaginal discharge is observed. Pregnancy is highly likely if there is no translucent vaginal discharge 5–9 days postbreeding. Pseudopregnancies last 8–12 days. Normal gestation is 15–16 days. Before parturition, a hemorrhagic vaginal discharge appears, and the female may pant. Hamsters rarely suffer from pregnancy toxemia (see Guinea Pig).

- Infertility may be caused by pyometra (see *P. pneumotropica* and lymphocytic choriomeningitis).
- Cannibalism is most frequently a result of stress or mastitis.

Urology

- In almost 90% of geriatric hamsters, renal amyloidosis develops. The disease tends to develop more rapidly in females.
- Clinical signs include edema and ascites due to protein loss in the urine, as well as the typical signs of chronic renal failure.
- Treat supportively. Prognosis for long-term survival is grave.

Neurology

- Head tilt is usually secondary to otitis media. Also consider lymphocytic choriomeningitis or neoplasia as differential diagnosis (see Rat).
- In hamsters fed all-seed diets and deprived of exercise, cage paralysis syndrome often develops. Usually pets are presented for acute posterior paresis which, in reality, was slowly progressive. The distinction is important in ruling out trauma. In mild cases, the hamster is able to move its hind limbs but unable to support weight. Vitamin D and E supplementation, along with nutritional improvement and providing exercise, is curative in 1–2 weeks. In severe cases, recovery is negligible or incomplete.

Hematology/Oncology

Lymphoma and lymphosarcoma may be viral in origin. Diagnosis is made by biopsy or fine-needle aspiration of affected lymph nodes. Rule out lymphadenopathy caused by lymphadenitis from infection with *Streptobacillus moniliformis* (see Rat). Although many hamsters initially respond well to chemotherapy protocols established for cats and dogs, prognosis for long-term survival is grave.

GERBIL

The Mongolian gerbil *(Meriones unguiculatus)* originates from the deserts of Mongolia and northern China. Gerbils alternate between periods of activity and rest throughout the day. Peak periods of activity are in the late evening. Seed storage and burrowing are important natural behaviors. Most gerbils are brown with cream-colored abdomens (i.e., agouti). Several color variations are available (black, black and white). Gerbils drum their hind legs when alarmed. In general, gerbils are nonaggressive. However, introduction of unfamiliar adults results in fighting.

Dermatology

- Rarely, *Demodex* spp. mites cause alopecia in gerbils.
- Diagnosis is based on skin scraping.

- Treat with rotenone ointment or amitraz dips every 2 weeks for three to six treatments. Use manufacturer's recommended dilution for dogs.
- Acute moist dermatitis usually is caused by *S. aureus* infection. Infection on the face often begins with the harderian glands. The gland secretion is viscous and causes matting, with secondary *staphylococcal* infection occuring under the mats. Attempts at grooming spread the infection to the feet and abdomen.
- Diagnosis is based on clinical signs and isolation on culture.
- Administer enrofloxacin, tetracycline, or chloramphenicol and apply warm, moist compresses to remove dried debris. Remove possible irritants from cage (e.g., pine or cedar shavings, ammonia). Occasionally, surgical removal of a chronically infected or inflamed gland is needed.
- Alopecia of the facial area, especially when it is symmetric, is usually the result of self-trauma from feeders, cage bars, or overzealous burrowing.
- Treat by changing cage construction or providing better visual security.
- Gerbils that catch their tails in crevices or are restrained inappropriately by their tails often are presented for avulsion of the skin from their tails.
- Treat initially by controlling hemorrhage and hypovolemic shock.
- Amputate the tail after patient stabilization to prevent ascending infection. In some animals, the infection is localized to the distal tail, which is sloughed in approximately 3–4 weeks.
- Generalized alopecia is normal in some weanling gerbils. The hair grows in as the animals mature.
- Melanomas are found most frequently on the ears, feet, or base of the tail.
- Diagnosis is based on biopsy.
- Treat by surgical removal.
- Sebaceous gland disease is usually the result of bacterial infections or neoplasia.
- Diagnosis is based on cytologic examination, culture, histologic examination, and response to antibiotic therapy.
- Treat bacterial infections with parenteral or topical antibiotics based on the severity of signs.
- Sebaceous gland adenomas, basal cell tumors, and squamous cell carcinomas are the most frequently encountered neoplasms.
- Treat by surgical excision.
- Radiograph the thorax to diagnose metastases. Prognosis for long-term survival is based on tumor type, stage, and character.

Ophthalmology

Chromodacryorrhea and epiphora occur as in mice.

Gastroenterology

Parasites

Tapeworms (i.e., *H. nana* and *H. diminuta*) and pinworms (i.e., *Syphacia obvelata*, *Dentostomella translucida*, and *Aspicularis tetraptera*) occur as in mice.

Dental

Incisor overgrowth occurs as in mice.

Diarrhea

- *Salmonella* spp. cause transient diarrheas in gerbils. The source of infection is usually unwashed greens, contaminated feed, or carrier rodents of another species. Most recover. Animals that die have a fibrinosuppurative peritonitis.
- Treat supportively. Use antibiotics in severe cases based on results of culture and susceptibility testing.
- Tyzzer disease, caused by *Bacillus piliformis*, is seen most often in weanlings at 3–7 weeks of age and postpartum females.
- Clinical signs include anorexia, lethargy, rough haircoat, and sometimes diarrhea. Gross postmortem findings include yellow-gray nodules in the liver and hemorrhage at the ileocecal junction.
- Diagnosis is based on postmortem examination or response to therapy.
- Treat with oxytetracycline (see Table 170–9) and supportive care.

Liver

Hepatic lipidosis and gallstones are frequent sequela to lipemia in gerbils fed diets with excessive fat.

Theriogenology

- Breeding is most successful if animals are paired at weaning and kept in these pairs. Male gerbils aid in raising the young. Pairing older animals causes fighting. An average of 20% of neonates fail to survive to weaning. This is usually the result of agalactia and crushing.
- Chronic hemorrhagic discharge from the vulva is usually the result of cystic ovaries or ovarian tumors. Most tumors occur in animals older than 2 years of age and consist of granulosa cell tumors or theca cell tumors. Leiomyomas of the uterus also cause similar clinical signs.
- Rule out urinary tract disease by performing a urinalysis via cystocentesis. Large masses may be visualized on abdominal ultrasound. Definitive diagnosis is based on vaginal cytology followed by exploratory laparotomy.
- Ovariohysterectomy is curative for cystic ovaries and tumors if they have not metastasized.

Urology

- Chronic renal failure develops in most gerbils older than 2.5 years of age.
- Clinical signs are polyuria, polydypsia, weight loss, and anorexia. Urinalysis demonstrates proteinuria, hematuria, casts, and an increase in white and red blood cells.
- Treat supportively. Prognosis for long-term survival is grave.

Neurology

- Up to 50% of gerbils in certain family lines suffer spontaneous epileptiform seizures. The seizures are induced by stress and are self-limiting. Seizures usually start as the gerbil reaches 2 months of age.
- Treatment is unnecessary.

CHINCHILLA

Chinchilla laniger and *C. brevicaudata* are nocturnal rodents from the Andes mountains in South America. Most animals kept in the United States are the descendants of 11 animals. Aside from pets, chinchillas are raised commercially for their pelts. The most common pelt color is gray; the most valuable coat color is black.

▼ *Key Point* Chinchillas are sensitive to antibiotics (see Hamster); therefore, avoid use of penicillins, lincomycin, erythromycin, and cephalosporins.

House chinchillas in a cool environment because they are prone to overheating. If heat stroke occurs, treat with tepid water baths and supportive therapy.

Dermatology

- Chinchillas require dust baths to keep their skin in condition. Use commercially available chinchilla dust only. Sand substitutions do not condition the coat and occasionally cause conjunctivitis. Offer dust at least once a week.
- Dermatophytosis occurs as in guinea pigs.
- Fur chewing is a serious problem in chinchillas that are farmed for pelts and often is seen in pet chinchillas that are recent culls from a ranch. The etiology of fur chewing is unknown. Some cases seem to be related to chronic disease, malnutrition, poor caging, or stress. Theories for undiagnosed cases include genetic abnormality; undiagnosed dermatophytosis; or adrenal, pituitary, or thyroid gland abnormalities.
- Diagnostics such as skin scrape, fungal culture, fecal, CBC, profile, and biopsy are recommended. In general, if changes in diet and husbandry do not elicit a response or an underlying treatable disease condition is not discovered, prognosis for cure is grave.
- One source advocates plucking all remaining underfur in chewed areas in an attempt to stimulate new hair growth. Place collars after this procedure until the fur has grown in completely.
- Cystic subcutaneous masses may be caused by the intermediate stage of *Multiceps serialis*. Transmission is by ingestion of feed contaminated with canine feces.
- Diagnosis is made by histopathologic or cytologic examination of tissue samples. Treat by surgical removal of the masses.
- Otitis caused by *Pseudomonas* spp. occurs as in rats.

Mastitis

- Clinical signs include hot, swollen mammary glands. Suspect mastitis if previously healthy neonates become restless, then lethargic.

- Perform bacterial cultures on milk samples, and treat with antibiotics based on susceptibility testing. Administer sulfa drugs until susceptibility results are available. Local hot packing is also beneficial. Occasionally, surgical drainage is required. Foster neonates to another female if possible, or use puppy or kitten milk replacers to hand-raise babies.

Ophthalmology

- Conjunctivitis occurs as in mice.
- Cataracts are congenital or developmental.
- Asteroid hyalosis occurs as a degenerative change.

Respiratory

Pneumonia occurs as in guinea pigs.

Gastroenterology
Parasites

Tapeworms (i.e., *H. nana*) occur as in mice.

Dental

Malocclusion of incisors and cheek teeth occurs as in guinea pigs.

Diarrhea

- Diarrhea is caused most often by *Coccidia* or *Giardia* spp. or a bacterium.
- Clinical signs range from soft stools and weight loss to fluid diarrhea, dehydration, bloating, septicemia, and sudden death.
- The protozoal parasites are best diagnosed on fresh saline smear or necropsy.

Bacterial diarrhea is most often caused by contaminated feed and is diagnosed by isolation on culture. *Clostridium* spp., *Pseudomonas aeruginosa*, *E. coli*, *Salmonella enteritidis*, and *Pasteurella* spp. are the most common isolates.

- Treat supportively and use appropriate antiprotozoal or antibiotic drugs.
- *Pasteurella pseudotuberculosis* causes acute deaths from septicemia or a chronic weight loss with intermittent diarrhea. Enlarged mesenteric lymph nodes are a hallmark of this disease.
- Diagnosis is based on clinical signs, histopathologic examination of tissue samples, and isolation on culture. Treat with sulfa drugs until sensitivity results are available. Prognosis for recovery is poor. Gross postmortem examination reveals yellow to white necrotic foci in the liver.

Theriogenology

- Check male chinchillas four times per year for penile hair rings. Roll back the prepuce and expose the penis. Roll hair rings off the penis after application of a water soluble lubricant. Treat ulcerations topically or systemically as needed.

- Dystocia is fairly common in chinchillas (see Guinea Pig).
- Metritis is suspected when postpartum vaginal discharge, failure to return to a normal estrus cycle, anorexia, weight loss, polydypsia, polyuria, and chewing at flank and abdomen are present.
- Diagnosis is based on history, physical examination, abdominal radiographs, culture, ultrasound, and CBC. It usually is caused by bacteria introduced by the male or spread from an internal abscess. Retained placentas, macerated fetuses, and dystocia are predisposing factors toward metritis.
- Treat with ovariohysterectomy after stabilization. Females used only for breeding purposes may be treated with antibiotics alone, but the prognosis is poor.
- Female chinchillas are aggressive toward male chinchillas when not in estrus. Breeding operations usually have separate cages for females and an interconnecting run for the male. Females are kept out of the male's run by their larger size or collars. The young are precocious and do not need a nest. Chinchillas only produce two litters per year.

Neurology

- Chinchillas seem to be particularly sensitive to *Listeria monocytogenes*. Clinical signs can mimic *P. pseudotuberculosis* and include anorexia, lethargy, abortion, generalized central nervous system (CNS) signs, hepatitis, mild enteritis, and mild emphysematous pneumonia. Necropsy shows yellow foci in the liver.
- Diagnosis is based on isolation on culture.
- Treat with sulfa drugs (see Table 170–9) until sensitivity results are available. The prognosis is poor.
- Other less common causes of neurologic disease in chinchillas include lymphocytic choriomeningitis, *Streptococcus* spp., *Balisascaris procyonis* (i.e., aberrant migration of raccoon roundworm), lead poisoning, and thiamine deficiency.

GUINEA PIG

Guinea pigs *(Caviae porcellus)* are nocturnal rodents that originated in the Andes mountains. They are known for their dietary need for vitamin C. They are used as a food source in their native lands. There are three basic types: English, which have short hair; Abyssinian, which have short, cowlicked hair; and Peruvian, which have long hair. Male guinea pigs are known as boars and the females as sows.

Guinea pigs become neophobic as they mature. Offer a variety of foods early in life and make changes in diet or environment gradually. Guinea pigs stampede when excited. Square cages and strategically placed barriers on external walls prevent the trampling of small or weak animals.

The smooth muscle of the bronchial tree is quite developed in guinea pigs. This places them at high risk for asthmatic-type anaphylactic reactions.

Both male and female guinea pigs have one pair of inguinal mammary glands; however, only the female's are well developed.

▼ *Key Point* Antibiotic toxicity (see Hamster): guinea pigs also may be sensitive to tetracyclines.

Dermatology

- Fleas occur as in mice.
- Lice (i.e., *Gliricola porcelli, Gynopus ovalis*) usually cause no clinical signs except occasional alopecia, seborrhea, and trauma secondary to pruritus.
- Diagnosis is made by observation of lice on skin scraping.
- Treat with ivermectin, 5% malathion dust, or pyrethrin shampoo (see Table 170–8).
- The mite *Trixacarus caviae* causes severe pruritus and is zoonotic. It mainly affects the dorsal midline and is difficult to find on skin scraping. It occurs most frequently in recently postpartum females, in which alopecia is the predominant clinical sign. Treat with excellent sanitation and ivermectin (see Table 170–8).
- *Chirodiscoides caviae* lives on the hair shaft of the perineal regions. It does not cause clinical signs.
- Treat with 5% carbaryl or lime-sulfur dip (1:40) (see Table 170–8). Sanitation is critical in preventing reinfestation.
- About 6–13% of guinea pigs are carriers of *Trichophyton mentagrophytes*.
- Clinical signs are alopecia and seborrhea sicca, usually starting on the face and spreading along the dorsum.
- Treat with lime-sulfur dips or griseofulvin (see Table 170–9) combined with topical povidone iodine or chlorhexadine shampoos.
- Other causes for alopecia are barbering, alopecia of the flanks in late-gestation females, and generalized alopecia of young at weaning. Subclinical hypovitaminosis C causes a poor hair coat and seborrhea sicca, as well as anorexia and large, malodorous stools.
- "Lumps" is the lay terminology for cervical lymphadenitis, which is characterized by lymphadenopathy in the ventral neck region. *Streptococcus zooepidemicus* and *Streptobacillus moniliformis* are the two most frequently cultured pathogens. Transmission is through abrasions of the oral mucosa. The enlarged lymph nodes are filled with purulent exudate.
- Treat with chloramphenicol or sulfa drugs until culture results are available. If surgery is required, attempt to remove encapsulated abscesses intact. If this is not possible, excellent drainage is required. The infection may spread, causing otitis, arthritis, or upper respiratory tract infection. Recovered individuals are carriers. Quarantine both sick and recovered animals.
- Mammary tumors occur in the inguinal areas. About 30% are adenocarcinomas; the rest are usually benign fibroadenomas. Other possible causes of masses under the skin include hernias, neoplasias, granulomas, hematomas, or other abscesses.

- Diagnosis is based on cytologic or histopathologic examination of tissue samples. Use thoracic radiographs to determine the presence of metastases.
- Pododermatitis and sore hocks are very common in guinea pigs. Predisposing factors are untrimmed toe nails, poor sanitation, and wire flooring. *S. aureus* is the most commonly cultured pathogen.
- Clinical signs range from small ulcers on the soles of the feet to abscesses and gangrene. Radiography is essential in determining whether bony involvement is present. Untreated pododermatitis usually develops into osteomyelitis, which is very difficult to cure.
- Treat mild cases by improving sanitation and grooming. Place affected individuals in solid-floored cages with paper bedding. Use sulfa drugs (see Table 170–9) until results of susceptibility testing are available. Surgically remove or curette abscesses, and apply topical therapy and hot packing. Amputation may be necessary when severe osteomyelitis exists.

Ophthalmology

- Conjunctivitis and epiphora occur as in mice.
- Inclusion body conjunctivitis is caused by *Chlamydia psittaci* and is self-limiting in 3–4 weeks.
- White, dry ocular discharge is an early sign of hypovitaminosis C.
- "Pea-eyes" is the lay terminology for subscleral fatty deposits or protrusion of the lacrimal gland through the lower conjunctiva. The condition is thought to be hereditary. Treatment is not required.
- A conjunctival scraping should be used to differentiate inflammatory conjunctivitis secondary to infection from allergy. An idiopathic, topical steroid-responsive lymphoplasmacytic conjunctivitis has been observed by the author in guinea pigs.
- Cataracts occur and are either congenital or developmental.
- Corneal or scleral calcification is usually an incidental finding. A thorough workup, including serum chemistry profile and radiographs, is recommended to ensure that generalized metastatic calcification is not present.
- Diabetes mellitus in guinea pigs also may cause cataracts. Usually, no other clinical signs are present and urine glucose is greater than 100 mg/dl whereas blood glucose remains within normal limits.
- No treatment is necessary, but strictly quarantine all contact animals because this syndrome appears to be contagious.

Respiratory

- Pneumonia in guinea pigs usually is caused by infection with *S. pneumoniae*, *S. zooepidemicus*, or *Bordetella bronchiseptica*. *S. aureus*, *P. aeruginosa*, *Klebsiella pneumoniae*, and *Pasteurella multocida* also are cultured frequently. Transmission is by direct contact, fomites, or aerosol. Hypovitaminosis C and stress often predisposes guinea pigs to bacterial respiratory infections. Weanlings are particularly susceptible. Clinical signs and diagnosis are similar to other small mammals (see Mouse).

- Take radiographs to rule out abscesses, pleural effusion, or pericardial effusion in refractory cases.
- Treat with chloramphenicol, sulfa drugs, or enrofloxacin (see Table 170–9) and vitamin C (Table 170–10) until results of culture and susceptibility testing are available. Cats, dogs, rabbits, and rats are reservoirs for *Bordetella* spp. As in other rodents, respiratory infections may lead to otitis interna/media. *Bordetella* spp. also cause pyometra and abortions.
- Nasal discharge is most frequently a sign of upper respiratory tract infection but also may be associated with allergies or volatile irritants.
- The diagnosis of allergic rhinitis is made by exclusion and through response to antihistamines or environmental changes.
- Bronchogenic papillary adenoma develops in approximately 30% of guinea pigs older than 3 years of age.
- Diagnosis is often an incidental finding when thoracic radiography is performed for another problem.
- Occasionally, clinical signs are seen as a result of pressure on the heart or great vessels.
- Dyspnea most frequently is caused by heat stress or trauma. Other causes are pregnancy toxemia, gastric bloat, volatile irritants, pleural effusion, pneumonia, or pulmonary edema.

Cardiology

Rhabdomyomatosis is a common necropsy finding. Gross lesions appear as pale foci located on the endomyocardium and valves. Histologic examination reveals myocardial cells that have stored excessive glycogen. Do not confuse these areas with thrombi, abscesses, or neoplasia. Their clinical significance is unknown.

Gastroenterology

Parasites

- *Paraspidodera ucinata* is the cecal pinworm of guinea pigs. They are generally asymptomatic, but heavy infestations can cause diarrhea and weight loss.

Table 170–10. MISCELLANEOUS INJECTABLE MEDICATIONS FOR USE IN PET RODENTS

Butorphanol	1–2 mg/kg q4h IM, PO
Cimetidine	5–10 mg/kg q6–12h, PO, SC
Dexamethasone	0.6 mg/kg IM
Furosemide	4–10 mg/kg q12h, IM, PO
Flunixin meglumine	2.5 mg/kg q12–24h, SC
Prednisone	0.5–2.2 mg/kg IM, SC
Oxytocin	0.2–3.0 IU/kg, IV, IM, SC
Vitamin A	500–5000 IU/kg, IM, SC
Vitamin B complex	0.02–0.2 ml/kg, IM, SC
Vitamin C	20–200 mg/kg, IM, SC
Vitamin D	200–400 IU/kg, IM, SC
Vitamin E/Selenium*	0.1 ml/100–250 g of body weight, SC
Vitamin K	1–10 mg/kg, SC

IM, intramuscular; PO, by mouth (per os); SC, subcutaneous.
*Bo-Se: 2.19 mg sodium selenite and 50 mg vitamin E per ml (Schering-Plough Animal Health Corp., Kenilworth, NJ).

- Diagnosis is based on fecal examination or cellophane tape test.
- Treat with piperazine or fenbendazole (see Table 170–8).
- Coccidiosis caused by *Eimeria caviae* is a fairly common cause of diarrhea in guinea pigs recently purchased from pet stores.
- Clinical signs are tenesmus, diarrhea, dehydration, and death.
- Diagnosis is based on fecal examination. On gross postmortem examination, petechiation and thickening of the colon are seen.
- Treat supportively and administer sulfa drugs (see Table 170–9).
- *Cryptosporidium wrairi* and *Giardia* spp. are found rarely. They cause a chronic enteritis. *Balantidium* spp. are thought to be nonpathogenic.

Dental

- Malocclusion in guinea pigs is diagnosed on oral examination.
- Clinical signs are ptyalism and anorexia. The premolars are the most commonly affected teeth.
- Gingivitis secondary to hypovitaminosis C causes similar clinical signs, but the teeth appear normal.
- Long-standing hypovitaminosis C predisposes guinea pigs to malocclusion.
- Treat malocclusion as in other rodents (see Dental Procedures).

Diarrhea

- Hypovitaminosis C (i.e., scurvy) is associated with soft, malodorous feces. Degeneration of the epithelium of the intestinal tract adversely affects digestion and absorption and allows secondary bacterial infections.
- Diagnosis of scurvy is based on clinical signs, the exclusion of other causes of diarrhea, and response to vitamin C therapy (see Table 170–10).
- Salmonellosis usually is contracted through contaminated feed.
- Clinical signs range from sudden death to diarrhea and anorexia. The diarrhea is frequently light-colored. Sepsis is common and may cause conjunctivitis, shock, pneumonia, abortion, and neurologic symptoms.
- Diagnosis is based on isolation on culture of feces or other appropriate tissue samples.
- Treatment is controversial because recovered individuals remain carriers. Use sulfa antibiotics or enrofloxacin (see Table 170–9) until sensitivity testing results are available. Supportive care is essential.
- *E. coli*, *Arizona*, and *Clostridium* are other commonly cultured diarrhea-causing organisms. *Clostridium* are diagnosed most easily by finding large numbers of spores on a Gram stain fecal specimen. Treat with metronidazole (see Table 170–9).
- *Yersinia pseudotuberculosis* either causes an acutely fatal diarrhea or localizes into regional lymph nodes.
- Diagnosis is based on culture.
- Treat by surgical removal or drainage of abscessed lymph nodes. Mesenteric lymph node involvement necessitates abdominal surgery. Treat with sulfa drugs or enrofloxacin until susceptibility testing results are available (see Table 170–9).

Theriogenology

- One male usually is housed with four to six females for breeding purposes. Signs of estrus are vulvar swelling, lordosis, and opening of the vaginal closure membrane. Fetuses are palpable at 4–5 weeks of gestation. Parturition occurs within 48 hours after the pubic symphysis has reached 15 mm. Neonates weighing less than 60 g have a grave prognosis for survival even with intensive care. Neonates normally do not nurse for the first 12–24 hours. Litters with five or more fetuses usually result in abortion.
- Dystocia commonly occurs in females bred after the age of 6–9 months. After this age, the symphysis fuses and is unable to open the 2–3 cm required to allow passage of a fetus. Dystocia in younger guinea pigs may be caused by obesity, large fetal size, fetal malpresentation, subclinical ketosis, or uterine inertia. On presentation, check the pelvic symphysis. If active contractions are present and the symphyseal gap is less than 2 cm, perform a C-section. Normal parturition is very rapid, with a rest of only 3–7 minutes between fetuses.
- Perform a C-section if active straining does not produce a fetus within 15–20 minutes. Radiograph sows with a history of weak contractions to determine the stage of pregnancy and evaluate the size of the fetuses. If well-developed skeletons of appropriate size are seen and the pubis has not yet fused, give oxytocin and calcium (see Table 170–10). If no fetuses are produced within 15–20 minutes, perform a C-section.
- If poorly developed fetuses are seen radiographically, consider fetal death, ketosis, or a nonreproductive disorder as possible causes of dystocia.

▼ *Key Point* Pregnancy toxemia usually is seen in obese sows with large litters in late pregnancy. Other risk factors include systemic disease or diet change causing anorexia, genetics, stress, and first litter.

- Clinical signs are tachypnea, depression, malodorous breath, seizures, and icterus. A urine pH of less than 6 with marked proteinuria is compatible with pregnancy toxemia. A marked hyperkalemia and elevation of liver enzymes often occurs. Thrombocytopenia may be present.
- Treat with intravenous or intraosseous saline, dextrose, glucocorticoids, and calcium. Surgical abortion of the fetuses may be attempted, but the anesthesia risk is quite high. Prognosis for survival is grave. Do not rebreed affected females. Do not breed sows heavier than 500–900 g.
- Large litters can cause a hemorrhagic syndrome. Compression of the portal vein and liver causes hepatic dysfunction, which results in vitamin K and clotting factor deficiency.
- Treat with vitamin K supplementation (see Table 170–10). Response is poor in severely compromised

patients. Affected individuals are at risk of ketosis developing. Prognosis is guarded.

- Vaginitis in guinea pigs frequently is caused by foreign bodies, usually bedding.
- Diagnosis is made on vaginal examination.
- Treat by flushing the vagina to remove the foreign material.
- Vaginal discharge also can be caused by pyometra, uterine torsion, urinary tract infection, or urogenital neoplasia.
- Diagnosis is based on findings on abdominal palpation, vaginal cytology and culture, urinalysis, abdominal radiographs, ultrasound, and exploratory.
- Treatment varies with the condition and is similar to that used in cats.
- Ovarian teratomas and uterine tumors occasionally are diagnosed and usually resolve with ovariohysterectomy.
- A symmetric alopecia with concurrent abdominal enlargement may be seen in female guinea pigs with cystic ovaries.
- Diagnosis is based on abdominal palpation, cytology, and ultrasound.
- Treat by performing an ovariohysterectomy. If the guinea pig is not a good candidate for surgery, human chorionic gonadotropin (hCG, 1000 USP units IM, repeat in 1 week) may temporarily resolve clinical signs.
- Male guinea pigs are prone to preputial foreign bodies. A preputial discharge is the usual presenting complaint.
- Diagnosis is based on physical examination.
- Treat by removing foreign bodies and performing local flushing. Chronic problems require a change in bedding.
- Male guinea pigs produce sebaceous secretions in the folds around their perineal area. Clean these areas with soap and water semiannually to prevent localized pyoderma.
- If pyoderma occurs, treat with topical therapy and oral antibiotics.

Urology

Bacterial cystitis and urolithiasis are relatively common in guinea pigs. Diagnosis is based on a history of stranguria, hematuria, painful abdomen, and anorexia, in addition to abdominal palpation, urinalysis, urine culture, abdominal radiographs, and ultrasonography.

Treatment consists of antibiotics based on results of culture and susceptibility testing and surgical removal of calculi, if present. Prevention of recurrence is difficult if the calculi are not caused by a bacterial infection. Addition of vitamin C to the drinking water as well as changing the brand of diet are sometimes helpful in preventing recurrence of metabolic stones.

Klossiella cobayae is a coccidia that lives in the renal tubules. It has no clinical significance.

Musculoskeletal

The most common orthopedic problem seen in guinea pigs is overgrown toenails. This leads to pododermatitis and sore hocks as well as to degenerative joint disease and a predisposition to tibial fractures.

Tibial fractures are the most common fracture seen in guinea pigs. They most frequently occur after foot entanglement. Internal fixation with an IM pin or application of a Kirschner apparatus is the repair of choice.

▼ *Key Point* Signs of hypovitaminosis C or scurvy start to develop in guinea pigs as early as 10–15 days if they are placed on diets 100% deficient in vitamin C.

Early signs are soft malodorous stools, weight loss, poor hair coat, and anorexia. Later, petechia, gingivitis, cutaneous and oral sores, swollen costochondral junctions, joint pain and hemorrhage resulting in lameness, and conjunctivitis become apparent. Treat supportively and administer parenteral vitamin C (25 mg/day).

Neurology

- Lymphocytic choriomeningitis occurs as in mice.
- Guinea pig paralysis syndrome starts with mild pyrexia and urinary incontinence, followed by weight loss and posterior paresis that progresses to paralysis. Currently, the etiology is unknown, but it does not appear to be contagious.
- Treat with supportive care. Prognosis for long-term survival is grave.
- Head tilt is usually the result of otitis or trauma (see Mouse).

Hematology

Cavian leukemia has a viral etiology. The liver, spleen, and lymph nodes are the primary organs involved. There is no current treatment. Quarantine exposed individuals. Death usually occurs within 5 days after discovery of lymphoblasts in the peripheral blood.

Neutrophils normally have red granules. Kurloff bodies are normally occurring eosinophilic intracytoplasmic inclusion bodies that are found in mononuclear cells. They are seen most frequently in females and appear to correspond positively with estrogen levels.

Metastatic calcification occurs in most guinea pigs older than 1 year of age. It is more severe in females than in males. The stomach is one of the first organs affected. Dysfunction in motility causes obstruction. The tendency appears to be exacerbated by high calcium and low phosphorus diets.

SUPPLEMENTAL READINGS

Carpenter JW, Mashima TY, Rupiper DJ. Exotic Animal Formulary. Manhattan, KS: Greystone Publications, 1996.

Harkness JE, Wagner JE. The Biology and Medicine of Rabbits and Rodents, 4th ed. Philadelphia: Williams & Wilkins, 1995.

Quesenberry KE, Hillyer EV (eds): Veterinary Clinics of North America: Small Animal Practice Volume 24. Philadelphia: WB Saunders, 1994.

Seminars in Avian and Exotic Animal Medicine. Philadelphia: WB Saunders, 1992–1996.

171 Basic Husbandry and Medicine of Pet Reptiles

Nancy L. Anderson / Raymund F. Wack

Boas, pythons, king snakes, rat snakes, and milk snakes (all in the order "squamata") are the most common snakes kept as pets. Iguanas, geckoes, monitors, and anoles are frequently encountered pet lizards. Amphisbaenians are small, worm-like reptiles not commonly found in the pet trade. The order chelonia has approximately 235 species and consists of turtles, tortoises, and terrapins. Of the chelonians, box turtles, red-eared sliders, and a variety of tortoises are kept most commonly as pets. The order crocodilia has only 21 species, including alligators, crocodiles, caimans, and gharials.

PET INDUSTRY

Determine whether an animal is captive bred or wild caught. Captive-born animals have been somewhat genetically selected to tolerate manufactured environments and accept domestic sources of food. In general, they are less likely to be harboring overwhelming numbers of infectious agents (especially parasites) than their wild-caught counterparts. Most wild-caught animals have been collected overseas, then housed in inadequate, overcrowded facilities, and finally shipped to suppliers without having eaten. The ones that survive often are severely dehydrated and immunosuppressed. Some imported reptiles are injected prophylactically with antibiotics, which, in combination with dehydration, predisposes them to renal failure. Because of the slow metabolic rate of reptiles, many animals survive this abuse for many months before demonstrating obvious clinical signs.

▼ *Key Point* Encourage novice potential reptile owners to buy their pets only from reputable breeders.

COMPARATIVE ANATOMY AND PHYSIOLOGY

Body Temperature

Most reptiles need to maintain their core body temperature well above ambient temperatures for at least part of the day and generally achieve this by absorbing radiant heat. Reptiles can minimize body temperature fluctuations by modifying behavior. Reptiles that become too cool seek an elevated area to bask, lay perpendicular to the sun's rays, maximize their surface area by expanding their rib cage, and darken the pigment of their skin to increase heat absorption. If no sunlight is available, some reptiles burrow into warm soil or lay on an object that was warmed by the sun.

- Overheated reptiles place themselves parallel to the sun's rays, seek shade, pant, lighten skin color, and burrow into cool soil to decrease body temperature.
- Overall, reptiles have a limited ability to control their core body temperature. If they are unable to cool themselves, death due to thyroid dysfunction and/or hyperthermia may occur.
- When the body temperature falls below a critical point, enzymes are unable to function. Digestion then ceases or becomes incomplete, immunity is impaired, and reproductive function declines.
- Chilled animals are at high risk of disease, and if they become chilled for a long period, they fall into torpor. Under natural conditions, some reptiles hibernate, but in captivity, reptiles are unable to prepare for hibernation on their own.
- Hibernation is a period of dormancy marked by a decrease in metabolic rate. Before hibernation in the wild, most reptiles have completed metabolically taxing activities (such as reproduction) and have accumulated energy reserves. A period of reduced food sources then begins, resulting in a fast that empties the gastrointestinal (GI) tract just before hibernation.
- In captivity, this energy loading to provide fat stores and the subsequent fast must be duplicated, thus preventing putrefaction of undigested food. The most common mistake made by pet owners attempting to hibernate their reptile is to cool the animal into torpor (i.e., it cannot eat) but not enough to truly slow metabolism. In this state, the reptile often slowly starves. Systemic infections are also common while in torpor. Metabolic processes are too slow to allow proper immune function, and microorganisms still proliferate. Females cannot successfully hibernate if they are in the process of producing eggs or offspring.
- The ideal temperature range for a reptile is referred to as its *preferred optimum temperature*. This range in-

Table 171–1. PREFERRED OPTIMUM TEMPERATURE BASED ON HABITAT

Habitat	Temperature Range (°F)
Tropical	85–100
Desert	80–102
Lowland temperate	70–90
Mountain temperate	70–85

cludes all the temperatures that a reptile needs to maintain optimal body function. The cage should contain areas with both the high and low ends of the animal's preferred optimum temperature range so that it has an opportunity to self-regulate, much as it would in the wild. Suggested guidelines for temperature ranges based on natural habitats and common pet species are listed in Tables 171–1 and 171–2.

Circadian and Annual Rhythms

Tropical animals in the wild are exposed to very little variation in environmental temperature and therefore are not tolerant of large fluctuations. This is in contrast to desert animals that endure and require high daytime temperatures with an evening cooldown period. Reptiles from temperate climates can be very tolerant of temperature extremes (within reason) if they are free of disease. These species experience seasons in the wild and require seasonal changes in light cycle, temperature, and water or food availability to stimulate behaviors such as hibernation and breeding.

Skin and Sense Organs

Turtle Shells

The upper half of the shell is referred to as the carapace. The bottom half is the plastron. The shell is composed of bone and incorporates the sternum, vertebrae, ribs, and pelvis. Bone is covered by epidermal scales or skin.

Speculum

The speculum or spectacle is a clear epithelial covering that lies over the cornea of snakes and some lizards, such as Tokay geckoes. Speculums should be shed with the skin at ecdysis. Abnormal retention of these structures is a common problem in snakes. Topical ophthalmic preparations do not penetrate through the speculum.

Table 171–2. PREFERRED OPTIMUM TEMPERATURE FOR COMMON REPTILES

Common Species	Temperature Range (°F)
Boas and pythons	75–95
Rat/milk/king/garter snakes	68–95
Desert tortoises	65–100
Painted turtles	55–85
Box turtles	65–85
Anoles	70–90
Chameleons	55–75
Green iguanas	75–100

Oral/Nasal Salt Glands

Salt glands are located in the nares or on the tongue. The glands excrete excess salt and allow conservation of water. Salt is excreted by burrowing or sneezing. Pet green iguanas often are presented for sneezing small amounts of clear fluid that dries to crystals on the walls of the cage. Do not confuse this normal salt elimination with a respiratory infection.

In snakes, the vomeronasal organ is a highly innervated area used in the sense of smell. It is located on the roof of the mouth within the vomer groove and is an extremely sensitive organ.

Parietal Eye

The "third" or parietal eye appears as a grey dot on the forehead of green iguanas. The organ is an evagination of the thalamus and is connected to the pineal gland via the parietal nerve. It aids in regulation of circadian and annual rhythms.

Gastrointestinal Tract

The hyoid apparatus is very well developed in most reptiles. In snakes, it usually extends to the 10th cervical vertebra, allowing the tongue to be extremely mobile. This enables the snake to breathe directly through its glottis even while swallowing prey. In chameleons, the hyoid apparatus extends the full length of the abdomen to the cloaca. This structure allows their long, well-developed tongues the motility and strength necessary to catch flying insects.

▼ *Key Point* In snakes, restrain the head only by its dorsal surface to avoid damage to the hyoid apparatus and subsequent loss of tongue function. Avoid restraint that places pressure on the ventral cervical region.

Snakes possess an open mandibular symphysis and flexible rami that allow them to swallow large, intact prey. These features also make iatrogenic injury to the mandibles common, especially while performing an oral examination.

▼ *Key Point Never* force open a snake's mouth. To open the mouth, place a plastic credit card or hard rubber spatula at the corner or front of the mouth and use gentle, prolonged pressure combined with a slight wiggling motion. Once the mouth is opened, slide the card or spatula across the jaws (Fig. 171–1).

Snakes typically have four rows of teeth in their upper jaw. The teeth of snakes and lizards are fragile and curved caudally to aid in pulling food into the mouth. Be careful not to catch materials on teeth. If items such as swabs or gauze become caught, push caudally to disentangle the fibers before pulling out, or the teeth may break. Broken teeth cause oral pain and anorexia until a new tooth emerges.

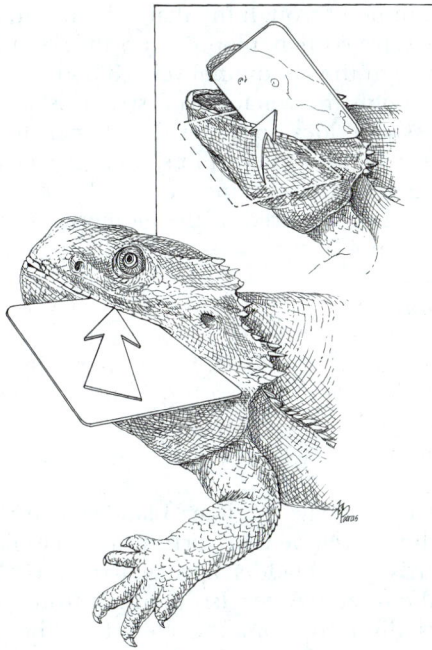

Figure 171–1. To open the mouth, place a plastic credit card or hard rubber spatula at the corner or front of the mouth and use gentle, prolonged pressure combined with a slight wiggling motion.

Chelonians do not have teeth but rather a horny beak made of keratin similar to birds. Treatment of beak problems is similar to beak repair in birds.

The esophagus is lined liberally with mucous glands. Although the musculature surrounding the esophagus is extremely strong in snakes to move whole prey caudally, the esophagus itself is thin and tears easily.

▼ *Key Point* When performing stomach intubation in snakes, the esophagus "grabs" the tube. Use liberal amounts of water-soluble lubricating jelly and gentle, constant pressure to pass the tube smoothly. If firm resistance is felt, redirect the tube. Never force a stomach tube because perforation may occur.

In many species of turtles, the esophagus makes a 90° turn before entering the stomach. Place medications administered by stomach tube in the distal esophagus. Use small volumes to prevent regurgitation. Also, in chelonians, the pancreatic and bile ducts enter the pylorus instead of the duodenum.

When present, the gallbladder usually is found near the liver in lizards and chelonians but is located caudal to the stomach in snakes. This is an important difference to recognize when performing surgery or diagnostics in this region.

The reptilian pancreas, although sometimes structurally different than in the mammal, is functionally similar. The pancreas usually is located between the ascending and descending portion of the duodenum in chelonians and lizards. In snakes, the pancreas is located caudal to the pylorus in the region of the gallbladder and spleen. In some snakes, the pancreas and spleen are fused.

The cecum is rudimentary in carnivorous reptiles such as snakes, crocodilians, and monitors. The cecum is present in chelonians and herbivorous lizards and functions in postgastric fermentation in these species.

The cloaca is a common collecting chamber for wastes from the colon and ureters and for the reproductive tract. The cloaca also receives urine from the bladder in species that possess a bladder. In males, the hemipenes or phallus everts from the caudal aspect of the cloaca. In some aquatic species, oxygen can be exchanged across the cloaca. Obstruction of the cloaca affects *all* the aforementioned systems and is therefore much more detrimental than mere constipation affecting the GI system in mammals.

Respiratory System

All reptiles possess a cleft palate (choana) that is necessary for nasal breathing. In contrast to birds, which have a single central cleft, reptiles have paired paramedian clefts. These clefts allow passage of air from the nares into the oral cavity and trachea.

Most reptiles lack a diaphragm, and breathing is accomplished by expansion of the chest wall by intercostal muscles except turtles, pectoral limb movement (except snakes), and smooth muscle contraction in the lung. Crocodilians also use movement of the liver to create negative pressure. Chelonians use movement of front limbs and visceral organs instead of excursion of the chest wall, which is impossible because of their rigid shell. A minimal amount of oxygen can be extracted from water through the skin in certain species of all reptilian orders. Some aquatic turtles can exchange dissolved oxygen across their pharynx and cloaca while submerged, although these sources only provide maintenance levels of oxygen.

- In crocodilians, the pharynx has a membrane that can be constricted to allow breathing while the mouth is full of water or food. This membrane must be pushed dorsally to place an endotracheal or stomach tube.
- The glottis in most species is located at the base of the tongue. This makes endotracheal intubation extremely easy. The glottis is very mobile in snakes to allow for respirations while swallowing whole prey.
- The tracheal rings are covered dorsally by smooth muscle in squamates. The rings are complete in chelonians and crocodilians. Therefore, use noncuffed endotracheal tubes in reptiles. The trachea is lined with many goblet cells that produce thick secretions, which may clog endotracheal tubes. Atropine administration appears to make secretions even more viscous. In some crocodiles, the trachea is bent on itself, making intubation difficult and bronchoscopy impossible. The trachea bifurcates more cranially in chelonians than in other orders, and a short endotracheal tube is needed to ensure aeration of both lung fields.
- The reptilian lung is composed of open-ended sacs lined with alveoli, structurally supported by smooth muscle. Each sac connects directly to a bronchus or to secondary bronchi in more developed species. In many species, the lungs end in thin-walled air sacs. Air sacs aid in respiration and can be inflated for use

as a defense mechanism or buoyancy control device. Vipers possess a tracheal lung, which is a collection of alveolar tissue on the dorsal portion of the trachea. This allows for gas exchange even when large swallowed prey compress the lungs. In most species of snakes, the right lung is larger than the left.

Cardiovascular

Reptiles (except for crocodilians) have a three-chambered heart with two atria and one common ventricle. Deoxygenated blood from the body empties into the right atrium via the sinus venosus. The left atrium receives oxygenated blood from the lungs. In non-crocodilians, both atria open on the left side of the ventricle. Blood from the right atrium tends to stay on the right side of the ventricle and enter the pulmonary artery. Reptiles have two aortic outflow tracts, the right and the left aortas, which combine caudal to the heart into a common aorta. The left aortic arch comes from the right side of the ventricle, carrying less-oxygenated blood. The right aortic arch comes from the left side of the ventricle, which has richly oxygenated blood. The right aortic arch supplies oxygenated blood to the head region before it combines with the left aortic arch.

- Diving causes increased pulmonary resistance, which causes more deoxygenated blood to be shunted into the left aortic arch. This results in increased mixing of oxygenated and deoxygenated blood.
- To shed the skin around the head region, squamates use a vascular phenomenon called the "swell mechanism." Blood pools in the vessels around the head, resulting in swelling of the head area to split the skin.
- The central ventral vein is a large vessel that runs down the ventral midline of squamates. Avoid this vein during laparotomy. Do not use this vein for venipuncture because life-threatening hematoma formation can occur.
- Paramedian vessels run as pairs parallel to the ventral midline under the shell in chelonians. During celiotomy, use a midline approach to avoid these vessels. These vessels may be ligated if needed.

Renal System

Most aquatic reptiles excrete ammonia, urea, and uric acid as nitrogenous waste products. Urea and ammonia require more water for their excretion compared with uric acid excretion. Terrestrial animals excrete mostly uric acid. However, sea turtles excrete almost exclusively ammonia or urea; semiaquatic turtles excrete 0% ammonia, 40–50% urea, and 50–60% uric acid; and desert tortoises excrete more than 90% uric acid.

Reptiles can only produce isosthenuric urine. The reptilian nephron contains no loop of Henle and therefore lacks the ability to concentrate urine. If renal blood flow is diminished below a critical level (as in dehydration), urates precipitate in the nephron, causing irreversible obstruction.

Reptiles possess a renal portal system that allows blood from tissues caudal to the kidneys to be shunted directly to kidneys. A valve exists at the junction of the abdominal and femoral veins. When the valve is closed, blood is shunted through the iliac vein into the kidney. When the valve is open, blood enters the systemic circulation through the abdominal vein. Blood entering the kidney through the renal portal system is supplied to the tubules and does not enter the glomerulus. Therefore, drugs, such as penicillins, that are cleared via tubular secretion are removed by the renal portal system, but drugs cleared by the glomerulus (e.g., gentamicin) are not.

▼ *Key Point* Do not administer drugs that are cleared by tubular secretion in the caudal half of the body. These drugs may be cleared before achieving therapeutic levels or, if the drug is nephrotoxic, may reach the kidneys in concentrations high enough to cause toxicity.

Not all reptiles have a urinary bladder. The bladder is most highly developed in terrestrial chelonians and some lizards. The bladder acts as a reservoir to store urine and conserve water. Isosthenuric urine from the kidneys is diverted from the cloaca to the bladder, where water is reabsorbed. The concentrated urine then is routed back to the cloaca for excretion. In reptiles without a bladder, diluted urine is moved from the cloaca into the large colon for water absorption. Salts also may be reabsorbed.

Reproductive System

Male Reproductive System

All reproductive organs, including the phallus in most species, are paired. Chelonians and crocodilians are the exception and have a single phallus. The phallus of adult crocodilians is fibrocartilagenous and is therefore palpable in the cloaca. This is a common sex determination technique used in this genera. The male copulatory organs of squamates are paired and are composed of highly vascular fibrocartilaginous and elastic connective tissue called *hemipenes*. Erection occurs secondary to engorgement with blood and contraction of the propulsor muscle, causing eversion of the organ. Hemipenes may be ossified in some monitors and geckoes; sex determination of these individuals can be performed radiographically. Hemipenes frequently have keratin spicules to aid in maintenance of copulation. Only one hemipene is used at a time and it may prolapse after prolonged use.

Seasonal variation in testicular size exists in most species. This is caused by an increase in the number of interstitial androgen-producing Leydig cells during breeding season. Spermatozoa move through the seminiferous tubules and are stored in the epididymis. During breeding, spermatozoa leave via the vas deferens, cloaca, and then hemipene or phallus. The male copulatory organs of reptiles do not carry nitrogenous wastes. Therefore, amputation does not affect urination but does affect breeding ability in animals with nonpaired organs.

Female Reproductive System

The right ovary is located cranial to the left in snakes. Fertilization occurs in the upper portion of the oviduct.

Crypt-like pits in the oviduct can store sperm for up to 6 years in some species. Reproduction may be oviparous (egg-layers), ovoviviparous (hold eggs in oviducts until they hatch), or viviparous (live-bearers), depending on the species. The oviduct produces albumin, shell membranes, and the shell. In viviparous species, a placenta-like structure is formed.

Environment for Egg Laying

Many reptiles indefinitely delay oviposition until the right conditions for egg laying occur. These conditions vary with the species. In aquatic turtles, this may be as simple as providing a moist sand pit of sufficient depth for the turtle to dig a nest. In other cases, a female in a multiple-specimen cage may not lay her eggs unless she is housed singly. Certain environmental clues may be required to trigger hormonal cycles necessary to stimulate egg laying. The absence of the proper environmental triggers may lead to dystocia.

Sex Determination in Common Pet Reptiles

Snakes

Females have short, abruptly tapering tails; males have longer, thicker tails necessary to accommodate the hemipenes. In very young snakes, a finger can be rolled from the mid-tail region toward the cloaca in an attempt to evert the hemipenes. This technique is only moderately reliable, and there is a significant risk of injuring a hemipene.

- Another technique for sexing snakes is commonly referred to as "probing." Commercially available metal probes or small red rubber feeding catheters are used to explore the caudal lateral aspect of the cloaca. In females, the probe falls into a scent gland and advances caudally two to four scales past the vent. In males, the probe enters the inverted hemipene and usually advances at least seven to eight scales caudal to the vent.
- There have been occasional reports of damage to the hemipene using this technique. In boas and pythons, male snakes have more developed paracloacal spurs than females.

Tortoises

In general, female tortoises and box turtles have a flat plastron with a notched caudal region to allow for the passage of eggs. Most females have short, poorly developed tails. The males have a concave plastron to allow for balancing on the female. Males also have long, well-developed tails to allow for copulation and storage of the phallus. Female box turtles have brown to orange irises, whereas male box turtles have bright red irises.

Water Turtles

It is more difficult to differentiate sex in water turtles than in their land counterparts. The females usually have shorter tails than the males. Because the water in the environment bears the male's weight, male water turtles usually do *not* have concave plastrons. In the *Emydoidea* genus, males have very long front claws that they wave in front of females during courtship.

Lizards

In general, males become more brightly colored during the courtship season. Males have more highly developed dorsal spines, dewlaps, and horns. Male iguanas produce keratinaceous plugs along the insides of their thighs from glands called femoral pores. Their function is unknown, but they are thought to be used for marking territories and to stimulate females by rubbing (scratching) the femoral pores over the female's hind quarters. Females have smaller versions of these pores. Only males of some gecko species have preanal pores that appear as little black pores located near the vent.

Immune System

- Reptiles do not have well-defined lymph nodes but do possess lymphoid aggregates. Lymphatic vessels exist and are well developed. Lymphocytes congregate in a bursa of the cloacal wall, thymus, and spleen. The thymus in chelonians is a distinct lobulated organ in the cervical area adjacent to the parathyroid glands. The spleen may be contiguous with the pancreas in chelonians and snakes.

Endocrine System

- Most reptiles have one to two pairs of parathyroid glands containing a cell type similar to mammalian chief cells. The glands are located at the base of the heart or along the carotid or jugular vessels. They are imbedded in the thymus in chelonians.
- The thyroid, when visible, is found at the base of the heart. The thyroid gland controls both metabolism and ecdysis.

The adrenal glands usually are located just cranial to the kidneys. In the green iguana, the left adrenal gland lies in the mesovarium and must be avoided during ovariectomy. The cortex contains chromaffin cells that produce neuroactive substances. The more centrally located population of cells produce adrenocorticosteroids. The structural architecture of these glands varies tremendously from species to species.

Special Sense Organs

Reptilian ears have no incus, malleus, or cochlea. In snakes and some lizards, the cavity of the middle ear and the tympanic membrane are vestigial. There is no external auditory opening in snakes. In these species, the stapes articulates directly with the quadrate bone. This mechanism picks up low-frequency sound and vibrations. Crocodilians have a movable ear flap that is located just behind the eye. They are able to open and close this flap to keep water out of their ears.

The eyes of most reptiles (except snakes) are similar to those of mammals with a few exceptions. Bony scleral ossicles support the globe. The iris and ciliary body are composed of striated muscle and do not respond to mydriatics. The retina contains a darkly pigmented projection called the conus papillarus, similar to the pecten in birds.

- Color vision is present in varying degrees in chelonians and lizards.
- In lidless lizards, a spectacle is present. Lidless lizards have long tongues, which are used to clean their eyes.

Snake eyes are unique among the animal kingdom and are thought to be the result of redevelopment of once rudimentary eyes. The lens accommodates by moving forward and backward. The eyes are covered by a spectacle that is impervious to topical ophthalmic preparations. The retina does not have a conus papillarus but is covered by a thin mat of vessels called the membrana vasculosa.

▼ *Key Point* The nasolacrimal ducts drain tears from the subspectacular space of the eye into the oral cavity. Infections in the oral cavity often ascend this duct. Always examine the mouth whenever a snake is presented for ocular disease.

Miscellaneous

Depot fat is stored in fat bodies within the abdominal cavity. These can be quite large and may be detected during abdominal palpation. A lack of fat bodies at surgery or necropsy is a strong indication of starvation.

HUSBANDRY

▼ *Key Point* The principal cause of disease and death in reptiles is poor husbandry.

Caging

Terrestrial Animals

Cages should be nonabrasive, escape proof, well insulated, easy to disinfect, and roomy. Aquariums, plastic sweater boxes, and polyurethane-sealed wood and glass cages work well.

Size

Cramped quarters induce stress. Snakes need room to stretch out to at least two-thirds of their length. For lizards, provide a minimum of 6 square inches of cage per inch of body size. Tortoises require a minimum of three times their body area. These are minimum areas for solitary animals. To reduce the chance of cagemate aggression, increase the cage size for more than one animal and for breeding.

Interior

Cage wall surfaces should be smooth to prevent abrasions, particularly to the nose. A rough branch or stone can be placed in the cage to aid in shedding. Provide cage "furniture," such as plastic containers, clay pots, and plastic plants, to provide visual security. Access to these hiding places allows reptiles to relax and prevents

cage pacing. Provide additional furniture that provides a varied terrain, without hazards, to stimulate activity.

Substrates

The ideal cage liner is paper, such as newspaper. It is nontoxic, inexpensive, and disposable. Change cage papers at least once daily. Artificial turf is a good alternative to newspaper. Change the turf as soon as it is soiled. It requires 48 hours to completely clean and dry turf, so make plenty of replacement pieces available. Remove loose strings to prevent foreign bodies. Rabbit or guinea pig pellets or recycled paper bedding may be used as cage substrates for herbivorous reptiles if they are replaced at least two times per week. Large stone gravel and bark chips also can be used but are less desirable because they can be ingested and harbor bacteria, parasites, and moisture. Change substrates at least once a month (can be expensive).

▼ *Key Point* Do *not* use kitty litter, small gravel, or corncobs as cage liners. These materials often are ingested and cause GI impactions or can be associated with skin infections.

Sand is recommended for desert species only. Other species soil sand quickly and are prone to GI sand impactions. Dry sand potentiates low environmental humidity, which is ideal for desert species but causes dehydration in nondesert species. If sand is used for burrowing desert species, it must be changed frequently to prevent buildup of wastes.

Humidity

The environmental humidity should be kept low for most species, because high humidity predisposes animals to disease. Excellent sanitation prevents buildup of wastes, and adequate ventilation allows evaporation of residual moisture, thus keeping the humidity low. Ventilation holes or screening on the top of cages is usually adequate. However, screen lids do not work well for animals that pace in their cage. These animals often rub their noses along the lid, resulting in severe nasal abrasions. Cages used to house animals that produce copious stools, require moisture-laden food, or have high water consumption may need shielded fans.

Temperature Regulation

Maintain the ambient cage temperature as a gradient incorporating as much of the preferred optimum temperature (POT) range as possible. One of the easiest methods of accomplishing this is to place a heat source at one end of the enclosure. The heat source should be able to heat the entire cage to a temperature within the POT range.

Thermal burns occur commonly. To decrease the possibility of thermal burns if heater malfunctions occur, be certain that the surface temperature at the hottest spot is slightly *less* than the high end of the POT range. Heating pads or heating tape are the safest to use. Place the cage on blocks to create an airspace between the cage floor and these heat sources.

Heat lamps also can be used successfully if care is taken to prevent thermal burns. Radiant heat actually is required by many large herbivorous lizards, such as adult green iguanas. To prevent burns, check the temperature by placing a hand directly under the heat lamp for 15 minutes after the lamp has been on for 2–3 hours. If it is uncomfortable to leave your hand in one spot, the lamp light is too intense. Also, place a thermometer on the surface to ensure that the POT has not been exceeded. Hot rocks are unreliable and only provide enough heat for small species.

▼ *Key Point Any* heating elements that have the potential to attain temperatures greater than 105°F must be shielded. *Routinely* test the thermostats on heating devices. Malfunctioning thermostats cause animal deaths and fires.

Annual and daily temperature fluctuations may be required by some species to maintain health and stimulate breeding.

Arboreal Animals

For arboreal animals, caging is similar to terrestrial animals but incorporates more vertical space and objects for climbing. Do not place climbing structures over water or food containers to prevent fecal contamination. Willow, bamboo, oak, birch, beech, and fruit trees provide safe branches.

Aquatic

▼ *Key Point* Strict attention to water quality is essential. A filter system or *frequent* water changing is absolutely necessary.

Never use an under-gravel filter because these may cause anaerobic toxins to accumulate in the gravel. Disturbance of the gravel or an overturn of tank water allows release of these toxins and may kill tank inhabitants. An out-of-tank biologic filter works best. Flush the sand, gravel, or fibers in these systems frequently to remove gross debris. Even these systems often cannot handle both fecal and discarded food loads. Therefore, offer food for limited periods in a separate tank, then return the reptile to its usual enclosure. The feeding tank does not need a filter because the water is changed completely before and after each feeding session and/or group of animals. Disinfect the tank and allow it to dry after feeding to prevent waste buildup and transmission of disease.

Overpopulation exacerbates water quality problems. A rule of thumb is 1 gallon of water per square inch of turtle carapace.

All aquatic reptiles except sea snakes and sea turtles need adequate basking space. Most "water" turtles drown because of exhaustion if not allowed to rest out of the water. In group tanks, this is often the cause of unexplained deaths of smaller animals. These losses often are eliminated by adding several basking areas, which allows the smaller reptiles to rest even when dominant individuals are defending their territories. Basking also is needed to allow drying of the skin and shell. An increased incidence of skin disease also is seen in reptiles not allowed to bask under ultraviolet (UV) light.

Maintaining appropriate water temperature is very important. A *reliable* waterproof heater is essential. Electric shock from nonwaterproof heaters kills not only animals in the tank but also human caretakers. In addition, malfunctions resulting in overheating or failure to heat a tank may kill aquatic animals. In small tanks, an aquarium heater with an *in-water* thermostat works well. Heaters with thermostats above the surface may under- or overheat the water because the thermostat measures the air temperature and not the water temperature.

Take care to ensure tank inhabitants will not burn themselves if they decide to wrap around the heater. This is accomplished most easily by screening the heater. Water temperature in larger enclosures can be maintained by keeping the room temperature at the lower end of the POT range and using infrared lights or heaters at one end to maintain a gradient. Temperature gradients over the basking areas are controlled as in terrestrial cages.

Ultraviolet Light

Many herbivorous and insectivorous reptiles require ultraviolet light (280–315 nm) to synthesize vitamin D_3. This spectrum of light is best provided by *unfiltered* sunlight (i.e. *not* passing through glass or plastic). Most plant lights do *not* provide adequate light in the appropriate spectrum. Vita-lite (Durotest, Fairfield, NJ), Chroma (General Electric, Fairfield, CT), TL-09 and TL-12 (Philips Electronics, Amsterdam, The Netherlands), and Ultra-Vitalux (Osram Sylvania, Danvers, MA) are products that produce the appropriate wavelengths. The intensity of all these lights is much less than that produced by natural sunlight. These lights produce UV radiation in the appropriate spectrum for only 2–4 months. Black lights also may be used, but the potential for damage to human as well as reptile vision has not been evaluated. Provide UV light at a rate of 20 watts/3–6 cubic feet. Place a basking area 18–24 inches from the source. Shield the light from direct animal contact. Provide UV light 8–10 hours a day. Constant UV light overstimulates the pineal gland and destroys normal circadian rhythms, which can lead to anorexia and disease.

Light Cycle

Provide 10–14 hours of light *and* dark daily. Base the proportion of light to dark on seasonal variations in the animal's natural habitat. Room light or light from an incandescent bulb used for heating left on at night does not provide adequate darkness. Only use infrared or ceramic bulbs if heating lamps must be used for 24 hours. If lights must be on in a room into the dark part of the cycle, cover the cage.

Sanitation

Reptiles rarely come in contact with their excrement in the wild. In captivity, the goal is to minimize this contact and the chance of spreading disease when contact occurs. The most important part of sanitation is mechanical removal of fecal material, urates, and leftover food. This can be as simple as removing a soiled sheet of paper, or as time consuming as scrubbing stones. Only after gross debris is removed can disinfectants destroy microbes that cannot be killed by cleaning alone. Disinfection is not a substitute for cleaning.

▼ *Key Point* Phenolic cleaners such as Lysol® and Pine-Sol® can be toxic to reptiles. Bleach (sodium hypochlorite) diluted 1:30 with water is an excellent, safe, and inexpensive disinfectant. It is inactivated by organic matter. Chlorhexidine and Roccal also can be used safely.

Nonsealed and porous surfaces cannot be disinfected thoroughly. Therefore, discard items such as wood, pottery, artificial turf, porous rocks, and bedding if they become soiled. Do not transfer these items from one group of animals to another.

Cage Density

Plenty of space and visual security is essential when housing more than one animal in an enclosure. Signs of inadequate space are cagemate aggression, disease, high parasite loads, starvation, and cannibalism. Some animals naturally prey on cagemates. These animals should be housed alone or at least with nonprey species.

Mixed-Species Enclosures

Do not mix species. Mixing genuses is often disastrous because organisms that are symbiotic or cause only mild diseases in one species may be fatal to another. An example is amebiasis, which causes a mild disease in turtles but may be fatal in snakes.

Quarantine

New animals should be quarantined in a separate building for at least 90 days. If the ideal situation is not possible, quarantine animals in separate rooms. Service new animals last and make sure that clothes are not contaminated. Dispose of wastes and wash hands thoroughly. Clean and disinfect food and water dishes at a separate location from the food preparation area. Animals should be tested for parasites and infectious disease before entering the main collection.

Nutrition

Clean Water

Change water at least every 24 hours. Clean water containers with soap and water daily and disinfect weekly. Large, shallow water dishes that allow reptiles to soak and defecate are preferred. Some lizards (e.g., chameleons, anoles) will not drink from bowls and require a mist sprayed on plants or the side of the cage.

Carnivore

Providing a complete and balanced diet is accomplished more readily in carnivorous reptiles compared with herbivorous or omnivorus ones. Most wild carnivorous reptiles eat whole animals (usually rodents or small birds), which are easily supplied in captivity. When they are fed whole prey, few nutritional deficiencies or excesses occur in this group of reptiles. Severe nutritional disease is seen in animal mistakenly fed only animal parts (e.g., all muscle, liver, etc.).

- Feed carnivores frozen and thawed (to 100°F) or freshly killed prey animals. Live prey may attack and seriously injure reptiles. Domestic animals fed as prey should simulate prey eaten in the wild as much as possible.
- Food animals should be raised on excellent diets because they are the only source of nutrients for the reptile. Do not offer obese prey animals because the excess fat may cause steatitis. Supplements for reptiles eating warm-blooded prey usually are not recommended.

▼ *Key Point* Some carnivores such as king snakes only eat other snakes. Be sure that these snakes used as prey are free from disease and parasites. If the snake eats thawed, frozen prey, it is recommended to freeze all feeder snakes for at least 30 days before feeding to prevent transmission of parasites. Good-quality feeder snakes can be difficult to obtain. Some snake eaters accept mice stuffed into a shed snake skin.

Some carnivores eat only amphibians or small reptiles of various genera. Freezing to prevent disease transmission is extremely important in these species as well. Some amphibian eaters can be trained to eat mice by placing a mouse inside a fresh frog skin or smearing a mouse with frog slime. Be careful not to attempt to feed amphibians, which produce toxic skin secretions.

Some snakes and monitors eat mostly eggs. Ideally, these eggs should be fertilized and contain embryos at different stages of development. Reptiles fed only unfertilized hen eggs suffer many nutritional deficiencies.

Some reptiles only eat crustaceans, gastropods, worms, or other specialized diets. Special attention needs to be paid to the natural history of reptiles needing specialized diets. If the suitable prey items cannot be obtained year-round, do not keep the animal in captivity.

Crocodilian

Nutritional diseases such as secondary hyperparathyroidism commonly occur when owners feed their crocodiles hamburger or table scraps. Feed only whole-animal diets (e.g., whole fish, rats, chickens, rabbits) to prevent nutritional diseases. Feed crocodilians individually whenever possible to prevent feeding frenzies and subsequent cagemate trauma.

Insectivore

Crickets, mealworms, and inch worms commonly fed to reptiles in captivity are deficient in nutrients. Provide an excellent diet for these insects to replace missing nutrients. To maximize their nutritional worth and provide extra nutrients from the intestinal contents of the insect, raise these insects on a high-calcium medium such as chicken layer mash. Before feeding the reptile, dust crickets and mealworms with a vitamin and calcium supplement. Large insectivores may accept young, hairless mice (commonly called "pinkies") or earthworms as an additional source of nutrients. Feed juvenile crickets, mealworms, or wingless fruit flies, which are small and lack chitin, to small or neonatal insectivores. Some insectivores require highly specialized diets.

Herbivore/Omnivore

Adult herbivores, such as green iguanas, should receive 90–98% of their calories from plants. Ninety percent of the plant diet should consist of a mixture of dark leafy greens, with 10% mixed vegetables and fruits. Many adult herbivorous tortoises require high-fiber diets, such as high-quality grass hay or fresh grass. Omnivores or young herbivores should receive 70–95% of their calories from plants. Most herbivores and all omnivores require the addition of some protein to their diets. Good sources of protein are crushed hard-boiled egg (with shell), trout chow, pinkie mice, alfalfa pellets, tofu, or cooked white meats. Dog food or monkey chow should not be fed. These foods contain excessive amounts of vitamin D and may cause metastatic calcification of soft tissues when fed extensively. Although some experts believe that feeding *any* animal protein to herbivores may cause renal disease, I believe that renal disease is related to the *quantity* rather than the source of protein.

- Vitamin and calcium supplements may be used in moderation, but avoid calcium supplements that contain phosphorus and extra vitamin D. These supplements also may cause metastatic calcification, and as a rule, most reptile diets are already too high in phosphorus from meat and fruit. Use Neo-calglucon syrup (Sandoz Pharmaceuticals) as a calcium supplement. This syrup is free of phosphorous, is highly palatable, and is readily lapped from a syringe or dropper, allowing individual dosing. Alternatively, crushed *boiled* egg shells or oyster shells are other excellent sources of phosphorus-free calcium. Healthy, adult herbivorous reptiles on excellent diets and provided adequate UV light usually only require vitamin and mineral supplements four to six times per month.

RESTRAINT

Lizards and Crocodilians

Restrain small lizards and crocodilians by using the thumb and forefinger to grasp the caudal mandibular area. Cradle the dorsal body in the palm of the same hand. Control the abdomen, chest, and pelvis with the

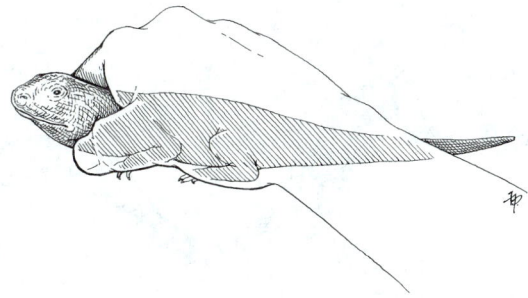

Figure 171–2. One-handed technique for proper restraint of a small lizard.

remaining fingers, thus allowing for respiration (Fig. 171–2.)

Grasp medium-sized lizards and crocodilians over the dorsal surface of the head and neck with one hand, and grab the base of the tail and pelvis with the other hand (Fig. 171–3). Wrap the reptile securely in a towel to prevent the back legs from scratching. Restrain the back legs by taping to the tail. To capture mildly aggressive animals, use a towel as a blind to hide the restrainer's hand from view. If an aggressive animal is brought in a sack, use the sack as a blind and grasp the head through the sack. Peel the sack away from the body without losing control of the head. A snare or snake hook can be used to pin the head if the animal is extremely aggressive. Care must be taken to use just enough pressure to prevent escape but not enough to cause trauma. Large lizards and crocodilians can inflict serious bites and often use their powerful tails as whips. Tape the snout of aggressive crocodilians shut with duct tape. The masseters are extremely strong; the digastricus, which opens the jaw, is very weak.

Stroking the ventral midline or pushing on the eyes of some lizards induces vagovagal response and a short trance-like state.

▼ **Key Point** Large reptiles can inflict serious damage, even death, to the handler. Attempt to handle these animals only if you are experienced and have adequate assistance.

Snakes

Most nonaggressive snakes may be picked up mid-body and allowed to glide from hand to hand. Some snakes

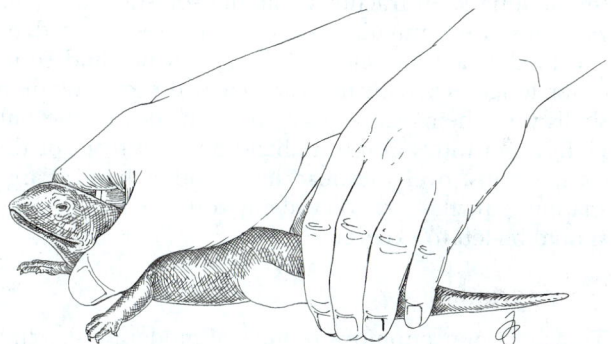

Figure 171–3. Proper restraint of a medium lizard.

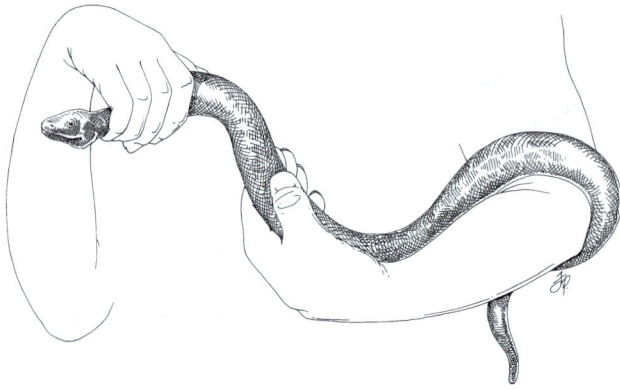

Figure 171–4.   Proper restraint of a nonaggressive, nonvenomous snake.

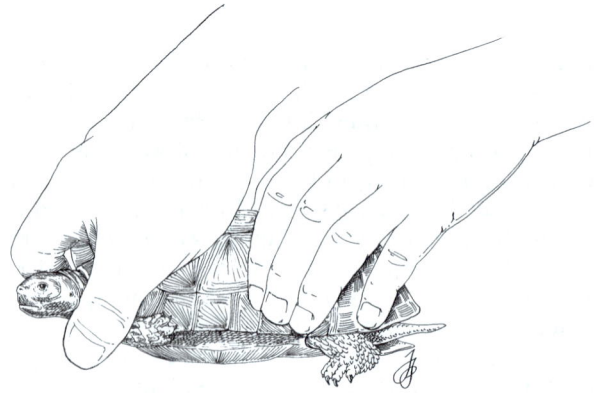

Figure 171–5.   Proper restraint of a turtle.

are more secure if allowed to coil around an arm (Fig. 171–4). Most snakes struggle less when handled with minimal restraint. Never let any snake near your face or around your neck!

▼ *Key Point* Never pick a snake up only by its head only because serious damage to the spine may occur. Reptiles only have one occipital condyle, making it relatively easy to luxate the spine from the head. Always support the body.

If an aggressive, nonvenomous snake arrives in a bag, grasp the head through the bag. Pin the head of free individuals with a snake hook or snare. Alternatively, grab the snake using a towel as a blind.

Large snakes can be very dangerous and may require up to four to six experienced people to restrain. Squeeze cages and sedation may be required to safely handle extremely large or aggressive individuals.

▼ *Key Point* Do not ever handle venomous reptiles without expert assistance and the appropriate antivenin. Any mistake made by the veterinarian, a technician, or the owner may result in human death.

Chelonians

Hold chelonians by the dorsal caudal portion of the shell (Fig. 171–5). This placement makes it difficult for the animal to reach around and bite, or to scratch with its rear feet. Be sure to have a firm grip, especially if the turtle is wet. Dropping a turtle may cause severe life-threatening shell fractures. Handle soft-shelled turtles with rinsed examination gloves, thus preventing damage to the delicate shell. Snapping turtles and some other long-necked turtles can reach the rear of their shells with their beaks. Grasp these turtles by the tail. Hold them with tail in one hand and the front of the carapace just over the head in the other hand. Large snapping turtles are very dangerous to handle and should be left to experts.

Transportation

Transport nonvenomous reptiles of moderate size in a tied cloth sack placed in a styrofoam cooler containing air holes. Chelonians do not need to be placed in a

sack. Coolers can be fitted with space for hot or cold water bottles or chemical packs if extreme temperatures are anticipated. These methods are to be used for transporting animals a short distance only.

History

▼ *Key Point* For most reptiles, improper husbandry is the primary predisposing factor for many diseases. Unless the diet and environment are improved, the best treatment plan will fail.

Ask the owner about the following:

- Species, age, sex
- Origin: initially, wild caught or captive bred; recently, pet shop or supply house
- Length of ownership, previous experience
- Environment, caging, cleaning, temperature, humidity, photoperiod, UV light source
- Diet: supplements, appetite, last meal, last stool
- Dates of unusual activity, breeding, egg laying, shedding
- Cagemates, quarantine history, aggressive behavior
- Medical history, previous weights
- Purpose of ownership: pet, breeder, display, education

Physical Examination

Observe the animal's behavior in the cage before handling. If necessary, observe healthy animals to become familiar with normal behavior, locomotion, weight, skin tone, and color. All terrestrial lizards (legged) and chelonians normally can lift their bodies off the ground when they walk. Fork-tongued reptiles frequently should flick their tongues to sample the air. Prolonged head tilts are abnormal. Legs and/or epaxial muscles should be full and have good tone. The skin should have a healthy color and texture, without moist, discolored, or ulcerated areas. Dyspnea is abnormal, but do not mistake hissing for dyspnea. Examine the stools for abnormal color, consistency, urates, grossly visible parasites, and polyuria.

Develop a routine, systematic technique when performing the physical examination, such as working from head to tail. Check the nose for abrasions or discharge.

Perform a thorough oral examination. Look for cyanosis, hyperemia, ulcers, discharge, abscesses, broken teeth, or parasites. Take samples of the choana or tracheal swabs for Gram staining or culture. Clear, viscous saliva is normal. Examine the mandibles for evidence of fibrous osteodystrophy or trauma. Examine the underside of the jaw and the periocular area for parasites. Look for retained spectacles when appropriate, and use a slit lamp and ophthalmoscope to examine the interior of the eyes. Examine the tympanic membrane, when present, which should be pliable with no exudate.

The heart of most herbivorous and insectivorous lizards is located under the pectoral girdle. To auscultate the chest, place a moistened gauze sponge between the bell of the stethoscope and the skin, thus minimizing sounds from scales rubbing. The technique can be applied to turtles and crocodiles, but the shell of chelonians and the thick skin of crocodilians make interpretation more difficult.

Palpate the abdomen to detect masses, eggs, bladder, and feces. In snakes, start cranially and move caudally, letting abdominal organs slip through your hands. A mass is less likely to be overlooked when this method is used.

Check the cloaca for tone. This is an excellent time to obtain cloacal samples for Gram staining or culture and to examine the cloaca for parasites. It is normal for stressed turtles to urinate, providing an opportunity to collect a urine sample. If a turtle does not urinate, this may be a sign of dehydration.

Palpate all extremities and check the skin for lesions. Especially examine the leg cavities in chelonians for external parasites and the ventral surface of all reptiles for signs of cutaneous lesions.

TECHNIQUES

Oral Examination

Snakes and Lizards

Use caution when opening the mouth. The teeth are sensitive and fragile, and broken teeth can cause prolonged anorexia. A snake's mandibles are very flexible and have an open symphysis. The jaws therefore are fractured easily if too much pressure is applied. Support the cranial cervical region to immobilize the head, and use the maxilla as a leverage point. Support the neck to minimize trauma to the cervical spinal cord. Use a thin plastic card or hard rubber spatula as a wedge in the corner of the mouth to gently pry open the mouth. Place pressure only on the gum line and never on the teeth. Once the mouth opens a little, slip the card across the mouth (see Fig. 171-1). A wedge or speculum may be necessary to hold the mouth open if the animal is large. Dewlaps, if present, may be used to provide downward traction.

Chelonians

To capture the head, wait until the turtle extends its head beyond the edge of its shell and quickly grasp the base of the head from over the top of the shell, using the shell as a blind. If a land turtle refuses to open its shell, it can be submerged in water to cover the opening to their shell. The head then can be grasped as it is extended to breathe. Once the turtle is caught, extend the neck and restrain the head from the sides just behind the mandibles. Do not grasp the dorsal or ventral surfaces of the neck because the trachea or hyoid apparatus may be crushed. Pry the beak open with a thin metal spatula. An avian mouth speculum then may be placed across the mouth. Always use a metal speculum if soft materials such as rubber catheters are going to be placed into the mouth. Use caution when opening the beak of an ill or malnourished turtle because beaks are often friable and easily damaged. Gauze strips may be useful in keeping the beak open and will not damage the beak. Some chelonians, especially tortoises, seal up in their shells, thus requiring sedation to extract their heads.

Venipuncture

Lizards and Snakes

Use the tail vein to draw blood from lizards, large snakes, and chelonians (Fig. 171-6). In snakes and lizards, the vein usually runs just ventral to the spine. In males, be sure to insert the needle caudal to the hemipenes. Insert the needle in a cranial direction at a 45-60° angle. After the needle contacts the vertebral body, withdraw it 1-2 mm while aspirating until blood is seen in the hub of the needle. Aspirate gently to prevent collapse or laceration of the vein. In all species, lymphatic vessels run parallel to the tail veins. Mixing of lymph and blood significantly alters hematology and some chemistry results.

Alternatively, open the mouths of boas and pythons with a soft spatula or tongue depressor to collect blood from the buccal veins on the inside of the mouth (Fig. 171-7).

Chelonians

Collect blood from the jugular vein whenever possible (Fig. 171-8). The vein is very mobile, so position the neck in a straight line. Hold off the vein at the base of the neck and locate the jugular vein visually or by palpation. Holding the turtle in a head-down position helps with filling of the vein. These vessels have a tendency to spasm; use atraumatic technique. Occlude the

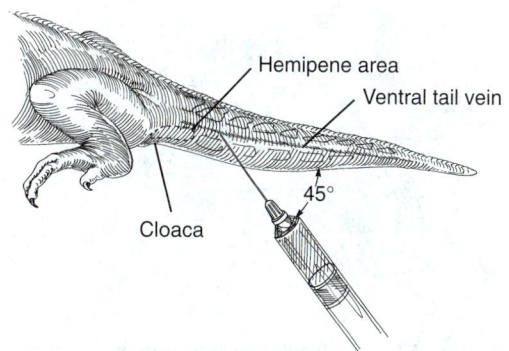

Figure 171-6. Venipuncture of ventral tail vein of a lizard.

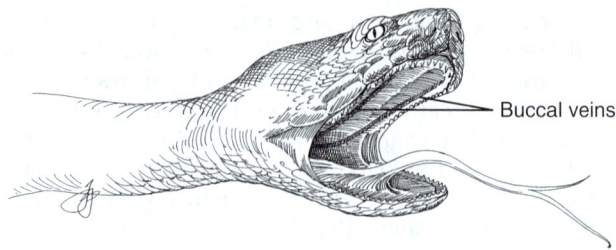

Figure 171–7. Venipuncture sites for the dorsal buccal veins of a snake.

vessel for at least 2 minutes after venipuncture to prevent hematoma formation. Alternatively, blood may be collected from the tail vein, which is located on the dorsal surface of the spine.

Stomach Intubation

Non-Chelonians

- Warm fluids or formulas to 80–90°F.
- To minimize regurgitation, administer no more than 1–6 ml/100g per feeding.
- Measure the distance from the tip of the nose to the last rib in lizards and crocodilians, or from the tip of the nose to the first 10% of the body length past the heart in snakes.
- Open the mouth as described previously.
- Visualize the glottis at the base of the tongue. Avoiding the glottis, pass a flexible tube to the premeasured distance. Be certain the tube is not in the trachea and identify the glottis before administering any medication. If the glottis is not visible, palpate the neck for both the trachea and feeding tube, and administer sterile saline first.
- In animals with jaws strong enough to sever a stomach tube, use an avian speculum, a block speculum with a hole drilled in the center, or a sized-down Frick tube to protect the feeding tube.

▼ *Key Point* Medications given inadvertently in the trachea are usually fatal.

Chelonians

- Turtles are more difficult to intubate because their glottis frequently is hidden by the tongue. Some

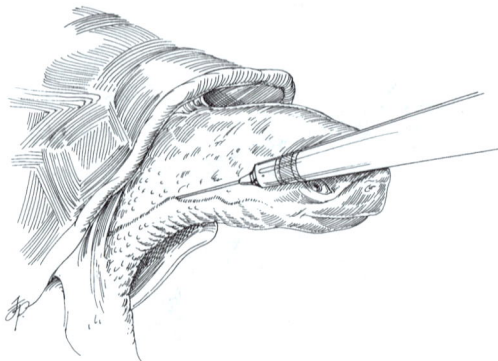

Figure 171–8. Jugular venipuncture site in a turtle.

species possess a 90° turn in the esophagus just cranial to the stomach.
- Measure the distance from the nose to halfway down the plastron.
- After placing a speculum, aim the tip of the tube toward the dorsocaudal pharynx. Let the tube follow the dorsal wall down into the esophagus. Try to identify the glottis by gently pushing up on the hyoid apparatus. This pushes the tongue forward. If the glottis still is not visible, palpate the neck for both the trachea and feeding tube. Check tube placement with sterile saline before administering medications.

▼ *Key Point* Never force a stomach tube because this may create an esophageal tear.

- If regurgitation occurs, cover the end of the tube to prevent dribbling and withdraw the tube. Turn the animal's head down and wipe out the mouth with paper. (Cotton or cloth will entangle on squamate teeth.) Wait until the animal is recovered and less stressed before making a second attempt, and halve the volume to administer. If no regurgitation occurs, slowly increase the volume over several tubings to the desired amount.

Perform a *stomach wash* on all vomiting reptiles. Intubate the stomach as aforementioned with a red rubber feeding tube, and give warmed 0.9% NaCL (3–6 ml/100 g body weight). Gently massage the stomach and aspirate the fluid. Use the fluid for bacterial or fungal cultures, cytologic examination, Gram staining, or direct saline smear for evidence of parasites.

Enema

Administer a mixture of 50% K-Y jelly and 50% 80°F water into the cloaca/colon at a rate of 1–3 ml/100 g body weight. Excellent restraint is essential. Select a red rubber urinary catheter that is approximately 0.25 times the size of the vent opening. In very small animals, tomcat catheters may be used to provide rigidity. The catheter is lubricated with a water-soluble lubricating jelly. Start the catheter at a 90° angle to the body. After the tip of the catheter passes the opening of the vent, aim it cranially, parallel to the colon, and advance. Never force the catheter or fluid into the cloaca, or cloacal perforations may occur. Never use high pressure to inject fluid into the cloaca. This may cause feces to be forced into the ureters or oviducts, resulting in life-threatening infection.

Injections

Always administer injections cranial to the kidneys to avoid the renal portal system (Fig. 171–9).

Subcutaneous

In nonchelonians, administer fluids or other therapeutic agents over the paralumbar region as in mammals. In turtles, use the skin folds located around the front and rear legs. If using the inguinal region, be sure not

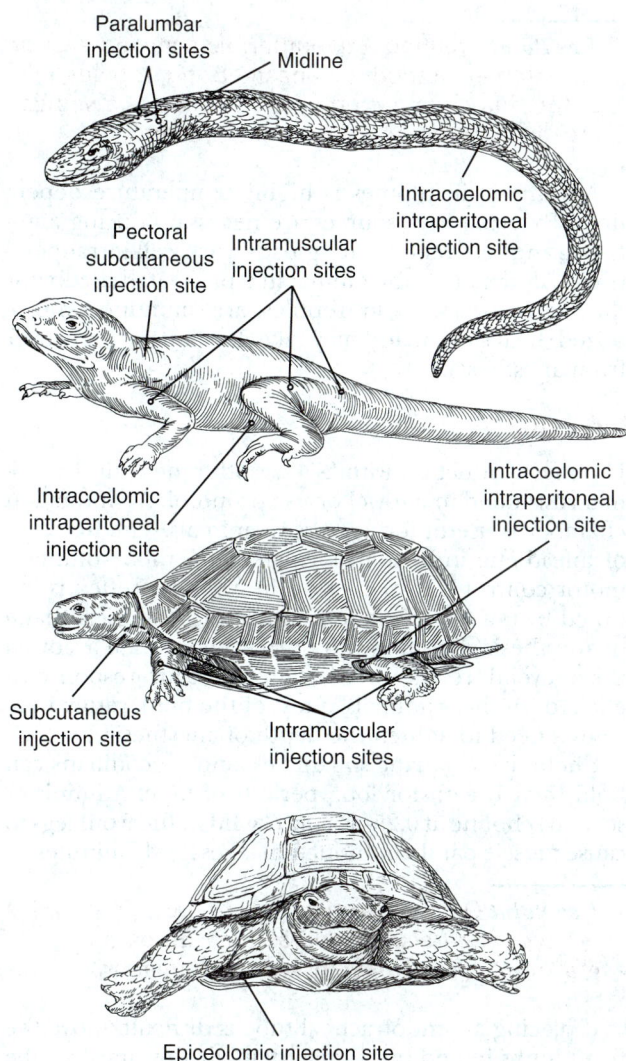

Figure 171–9.   Common injection sites in a snake *(top)*, lizard *(center)*, and turtle *(below)*.

to puncture through the body wall. Fluids should be warmed to 80–95°F.

Epicoelomic

This region is medioventral to the front legs and is used to administer fluids to chelonians. Absorption is excellent in animals with adequate perfusion (see Fig. 171–9).

Intramuscular

In snakes and legless lizards, administer intramuscular (IM) injections into the epaxial muscles. In all other reptiles, use the muscles of the front legs. The rear legs and the epaxial muscles of the tail may be used for injection of non-nephrotoxic drugs. Insert the needle between scales to minimize damage to the skin. With the bevel of the needle pointing up, aim proximally using a 45° angle. Always aspirate before injecting.

Intraosseous

Because most reptilian veins are not easily accessible, it may be necessary to use an intraosseous (IO) route to

administer medications and fluids. In lizards, try the distal femur, proximal tibia, proximal humerus, or distal radius.

- Surgically prepare the entry site.
- Choose a spinal needle that is 33–66% the diameter and length of the chosen bone.
- Identify the tibial crest or the dorsal midline of the distal femur just proximal to the condyles. Advance the tip of the needle through the skin at a 45–90° angle until the tip of the needle is through the cortex of the bone.

▼ *Key Point* It is extremely important to keep the needle straight while boring through the cortex to avoid extravasation of fluids.

- A sudden lack of resistance is felt once the tip of the needle enters the marrow cavity. At this point, angle the needle down the length of the bone and advance it until the hub is seated against the skin. The needle should advance easily.
- Once the needle is seated, remove the stylet. Attach a syringe and aspirate. In most cases bone marrow can be seen in the hub of the needle. If no marrow is identified on cytology, obtain radiographs to ensure appropriate placement of the catheter. Flush the intraosseous catheter with heparinized saline. Secure it to the skin with sutures.
- Although it is wise to avoid caustic substances, treat the catheter as if it were an intravenous catheter. Catheters can be maintained for 72 hours.
- In turtles, administer intraosseous fluids into a thickened area of bone that underlies the shell where the plastron and carapace meet (Fig. 171–10). Use a spinal needle.

Intracoelomic

▼ *Key Point* Intraperitoneal injections have the potential for causing peritonitis or respiratory compromise. Always prepare the area with a surgical scrub.

Use this technique for administration of fluids when other routes are not possible. Warm fluids to 80–85°F.

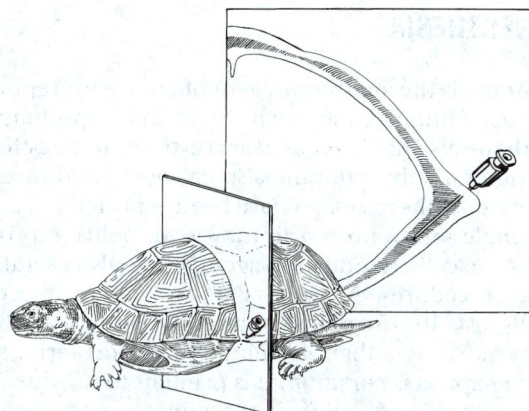

Figure 171–10.   Interosseus injection site of the turtle.

Avoid caustic substances because they can cause chemical peritonitis. In chelonians, give injections just cranial to the rear legs. Extend the rear legs and administer the injection with the animal in held in a head-down position. In snakes and lizards, inject fluids slightly off the ventral midline in the caudal third of the abdomen. Hold the head in a downward position while injecting (see Fig. 171–9). Always aspirate to ensure that the injection is not being given into the bladder, oviduct, or bowel.

- Do not use this technique in gravid females. Exceeding 2–3% of the body weight in fluids may result in respiratory compromise.

Radiography

Diagnostic radiographs require a machine capability of at least 200 ma and exposure times of less than $\frac{1}{60}$ of a second. Use rare earth screens when possible. Diagnostic radiographs require two views. Dorsal ventral views and standing lateral views are easier to obtain and interpret than ventral dorsal or lateral recumbent films.

To evaluate the lungs of turtles with suspected pneumonia, obtain an anterior/posterior horizontal beam view in addition to those aforementioned.

Contrast Radiography

Gastrointestinal transit times in reptiles are normally prolonged compared with those of mammals. Therefore, contrast studies have limited use. When 20–50 ml/kg of barium is administered to carnivorous lizards, it may take 3–6 days to reach the cloaca. When this dosage is administered to snakes, crocodilians, and herbivorous lizards, it may take up to 30 days. At a dosage of 20 ml/kg, barium requires 40 days to reach the cloaca in tortoises. Always ensure that the animal is well hydrated before the administration of barium, or it may become desiccated in the bowel, often requiring surgical removal. I have had excellent results using a 1:3 dilution of iohexol:saline as a contrast agent.

For evaluation of the coelomic cavity, ultrasound is an extremely useful diagnostic technique. A 5.0, 7.5, or 10 mHz transducer is necessary.

ANESTHESIA

Isoflurane is the anesthetic agent of choice for reptilian patients. Although the recovery period is prolonged, halothane also has been used successfully for anesthesia in reptiles. Methoxyflurane also has been used successfully, but deaths in snakes have been reported.

A single intravenous or intraosseous bolus of propofol is an excellent induction agent and is also useful for short procedures. Anesthesia from a single injection usually lasts 10–15 minutes and reptiles are usually fully recovered in less than 40 minutes. A short-term, self-limiting apnea is common. It is prudent to provide positive pressure ventilation if the apnea persists longer than 2 minutes.

▼ *Key Point* Creating a hypothermic state is never an acceptable method of anesthetizing reptiles. Hypothermia does not provide analgesia, slows healing, and depresses the immune system.

Anesthesia in reptiles is highly temperature dependent. External heat sources are necessary during anesthesia and recovery. Heating pads work well intraoperatively. Always place the animal in a preheated incubator during recovery. Cold reptiles are immunocompromized, heal slower, and may take days longer to recover from anesthesia.

Induction

Use mask induction with 2–4% isoflurane with the animal restrained in a towel or use propofol. An induction chamber is useful for aggressive animals. The first sign of anesthetic induction is excitement, then voluntary motor control is lost. Loss of the righting reflex is followed by muscle relaxation, indicating a surgical plane of anesthesia. Reptiles with third eyelids retain a slowed third eyelid reflex even when no pain response is elicited. In these animals, a loss of the blink reflex indicates a need to lighten the depth of anesthesia.

Chelonians, aquatic squamates, and crocodilians can hold their breath for long periods of time. Administer succinyl choline at 0.25–1.5 mg/kg IM in the front legs to cause muscle paralysis. Induction takes 20–45 minutes.

▼ *Key Point* Once relaxation occurs and the muscles of respiration also are paralyzed, intubate the animal and begin positive pressure ventilation.

If placing an endotracheal tube is difficult, move the front limbs in and out to maintain air flow until a tube is placed. Succinyl choline does not provide analgesia, so inhalant anesthesia must be used for painful procedures. If kept warm, most chelonians do not require assistance with respirations after 1 hour postinjection. Never repeat succinyl choline within a 24-hour period. Ketamine can be used to sedate large or aggressive individuals (see Injectable Anesthetics).

Intubation

Inflatable cuffs are not recommended for small animals. Inflating the cuff may cause tracheal inflammation severe enough to occlude the trachea. Endotracheal tubes for small individuals can be fashioned from catheters and infant feeding tubes. Because most reptiles become apneic during anesthesia, always have the animal intubated to provide positive pressure ventilation. Ventilate animals at a rate of 3–6 breaths per minute.

Maintenance

Maintain anesthesia at 1–2% isoflurane at 1 L of oxygen per 0.3–1 kg of body weight. Larger reptiles usually require 1 L per 5–10 kg of body weight. Be sure to monitor heart and respiratory rates. A marked reduction in either of these two values is an indication to lighten anesthesia.

Recovery

When isoflurane is used, animals may recover within 20 minutes. Many other anesthetics (and occasionally isoflurane) may cause prolonged recovery periods, lasting hours to days. Assisted ventilation is required until spontaneous respirations occur. Be prepared to offer ventilatory assistance as long as necessary, even if the reptile takes hours to breathe on its own. To speed recovery times, place the animal in a warm environment and continue fluid therapy during recovery. Ventilating with room air or providing small levels of carbon dioxide (such as exhaled air) instead of 100% oxygen will sometimes stimulate the respiratory centers.

Injectable Anesthetics

Isoflurane or propofol should be used for anesthesia whenever possible because recovery times are prolonged and dosage titration can be difficult when using injectable anesthetics.

Ketamine Hydrochloride

Most reptiles require 20–60 mg/kg IM or 5–15 mg/kg IV. Crocodilians often require the higher end of the dose range. Ketamine provides marginal relaxation and analgesia. It may be used for as sedation for nonpainful procedures or as a preanesthetic for reptiles that cannot be induced with a gas anesthetic.

Tiletamine Hydrochloride

The dose for tiletamine is 10–40 mg/kg IM in squamates, 15 mg/kg IM in crocodilians, and 5–15 mg/kg IM in chelonians. Induction usually requires less than 30 minutes. At safe levels of anesthesia, the righting reflex is slowed but not eliminated. Expect bouts of paddling and head pressing and expect the palpebral reflex to be unaffected. The recovery period lasts an average of 3 hours. This drug is not recommended for surgical procedures.

SURGERY

Suture Materials and Suture Placement

- Reptiles do not possess the enzymes needed to absorb gut sutures. Polydioxanone is the absorbable suture of choice. Polyglactin 910 also may be used.
- When closing the coelomic cavity, the skin is the holding layer.
- The skin must be closed in an everting pattern to allow dermis-to-dermis contact. Nonabsorbable sutures, such as nylon, should be removed after two sheds have occurred.

Approach to the Coelomic Cavity

A perimedian approach is necessary in non-chelonian species to avoid the central ventral vein. In snakes, the location for the approach is usually one to two scale rows dorsal to the belly scute. This site avoids the central ventral vein and the ribs and prevents placement on a surface in constant contact with the ground.

DRUG THERAPY

The use of various drugs in reptiles is similar to that in other genera with application of the following guidelines:

- Maintain reptiles at the high end of POT to enhance normal metabolism of drugs.
- Pay attention to species differences. A snake is less related to a turtle than a cat is to a cow. Drug clearances and toxicities are often species related.
- When available, use published dosages based on pharmacokinetic studies. Be aware that metabolic scaling is not always accurate.
- Weigh all animals before dosing drugs. Accurate dosages based on body mass are extremely important in avoiding side effects.
- When in doubt about renal clearance or hydration status, institute fluid therapy.
- Use bactericidal versus bacteriostatic antibiotics whenever possible.

▼ *Key Point* Never use ivermectin in chelonians. It is toxic and is associated with neurologic dysfunction and possible death.

- See Table 171–3 for dosages of common chemotherapeutic agents used in reptiles.

COMMON DISEASES OF REPTILES

Failure to adapt to captivity is the principal cause of death in captive reptiles. The captive environment is so alien to a wild-caught reptile that stress induces immunosuppression and anorexia. Secondary infections and starvation cause death of the animal.

▼ *Key Point* Most diseases of reptiles are secondary to poor husbandry and nutrition.

Bacterial Infections

Both enteric commensal bacteria and pathogenic bacteria are usually gram negative. Large numbers of monomorphic gram-negative bacteria or identification of intracellular bacteria on Gram-stained specimens are suggestive of bacterial disease. Perform bacterial cultures on samples collected from suspected infection sites. Anaerobic bacteria are common pathogens found in reptiles with lower respiratory infections.

▼ *Key Point* Reptiles are known carriers of leptospirosis and *Salmonella* spp. Inform clients of potential zoonoses. *Salmonella* spp. live in the intestines and are transmitted to people when fecal material is handled.

Many species of reptiles have adapted to some strains of *Salmonella* spp. These bacteria do not cause disease and may be necessary components of the normal intestinal flora. *Salmonella* spp. in this category may or

Table 171–3. REPTILE CHEMOTHERAPEUTICS

Species	Drug	Dosage	Comment
T	Acyclovir	80 mg/kg PO q24h × 10 days	Herpesvirus
S, L	Amikacin	2–4 mg/kg IM q72h	Use fluid therapy, excellent Gram (−)
T		2.25 mg/kg IM q96h	
U	Amoxicillin	10–22 mg/kg IM q12–24h	Anaerobes
S, L	Ampicillin	8 mg/kg IM q12–24h	Anaerobes
T, WT		20 mg/kg IM q12h	
S, L, T, WT	Carbenicillin	100–400 mg/kg IM q24–48h	Often combine with aminoglycoside
S	Ceftazadime	20 mg/kg IM q72h	
T, WT	Ceftiofur	2–4 mg/kg IM q24h	
S		2 mg/kg q48h	
S	Cephalothin	20–40 mg/kg IM q12h	
S, L, T, WT, C	Chloramphenicol	20–40 mg/kg IM q12–24h	Static
U	Clindamycin	2.5–5.0 mg/kg PO q12h	Anaerobes
S, L	Enrofloxacin	2.5 mg/kg IM q24h for 72 hrs, then q48h	May cause skin discoloration
U		5–10 mg/kg IM or PO q24h	
S, L, WT	Gentamicin	2–4 mg/kg IM q72h	Renal toxicity, recommend use amikacin instead
		6 mg/kg IM q96h	
S	Piperacillin	50–100 mg/kg IM q48h	Often use with aminoglycoside
S, L	Trimethoprim/ sulfadiazine	30 mg/kg IM q24h, then q48h 15 mg/kg PO q24h	Use fluid therapy
Antifungals and Antiprotozoa			
L	Fluconazole	5 mg/kg PO q24h	
T	Ketoconazole	15–25 mg/kg PO q24h	
C		50 mg/kg PO q24h	
S, L	Nystatin	100,000 IU/kg PO q24h	Not absorbed systemically
Anthelmintics			
All	Fenbendazole	50–100 mg/kg PO, repeat in 2 wks q24h for 3–5 days	Nematodes Extremely safe For resistant nematodes
All but turtles	Ivermectin	0.2 mg/kg IM repeat in 2 wks	Ectoparasites, nematodes *never* in chelonians
S, L	Levamisole	10 mg/kg IM or IP, repeat in 2 wks	Resistant nematodes Beware of toxicity
WT, T		5 mg/kg IM or IP	
S, L, WT	Mebendazole	20–25 mg/kg PO repeat in 2 wks	Resistant nematodes
All	Metronidazole	100 mg/kg PO, (40 mg/kg in milk and indigo snakes), repeat in 2 wks	Protozoa
		50 mg/kg PO q24–48h	Anaerobes
U	Paromomycin	30–60 mg/kg PO q24h	Protozoa, ± *Cryptosporidium*
U	Praziquantel	8 mg/kg IM or PO, repeat in 2 wks	Cestodes, ± trematodes
U	Pyrantel pamoate	5 mg/kg PO, repeat in 2 wks	Nematodes
S, L	Sulfadiazine, sulfamerazine, sulfamethazine	25 mg/kg PO q24h for 7 days–3 wks	*Coccidia*, avoid in dehydrated animals or animals with renal disease
U	Vapona strip	6 mm/10 ft³ cage for 3 days	Mites, caution toxicity
Miscellaneous			
L	Allopurinal	10 mg/kg PO q24h	Gout
S		20 mg/kg PO q24h	
L	Aminophylline	2–4 mg/kg IM	
L	Atropine sulfate	0.04 mg/kg IM or IV	
U	Butorphanol	0.2 mg/kg IM	Analgesia
L	Calcitonin	50 IU/kg IM q14d	Nutritional bone disease, ensure normocalcemia
U	Calcium glubionate	10 mg/kg PO q12h	Calcium supplement
L	(Neo-Calglucon, Sandoz)	0.25–1.0 ml/kg PO q24h: induction q7–14d: maintenance	
L	Calcium lactate/ glycerophosphate (Calphosan, Glenwood)	0.5–1.0 ml/kg SC q7d	Calcium supplement
U	Cimetidine	4 mg/kg PO or IM q8–12h	Gastric ulcers
U	Cisapride	0.5–2.0 mg/kg PO q24h	Improves intestinal motility
L	Dexamethasone	0.125–0.625 mg/kg IV or IM	Causes prolonged immune suppression
U	Doxapram	5 mg/kg IV	Stimulates respiration
U	Flunixin meglumine	0.1–1.0 mg/kg IM or IV q12–72h	Anti-inflammatory

C, crocodilian; IM, intramuscular; IP, intraperitoneal; IV, intravenous; L, lizard; PO, by mouth (per os); S, snake; SC, subcutaneous; T, land turtle; U, unspecified; WT, water turtle.

Table 171–3. REPTILE CHEMOTHERAPEUTICS *Continued*

Species	Drug	Dosage	Comment
L	Furosemide	5 mg/kg IM or IV q12–24h	Watch hydration No loop of Henle
T	Iodine	2–4 mg/kg PO q24h, for 3 wks, then q7d	Goiter
T	Levothyroxine	0.02 mg/kg PO q48h	Hypothyroidism/goiter
T	Metoclopramide	0.06 mg/kg PO q24h	Improves gastric motility
L	Oxytocin	1–10 IU/kg	After calcium for uterine inertia
U	Sodium bicarbonate	0.5–1.0 mEq/kg IV	Acidosis
L	Arginine vasotocin	0.01–1.0 µg/kg IV or IP	After calcium for uterine inertia
L	Vitamin A	1500–2000 IU/kg IM, SC q7d × 2–6 wks	Watch for signs for toxicity
U	Vitamins A, D$_3$, E (Vital E-A&D, Schering)	0.15 ml/kg IM	Malnutrition
L	Vitamin B complex	0.5 ml/kg IM	
L	Vitamin C	10–20 mg/kg IM	

may not cause disease in humans or other species of reptiles. However, certain serotype of *Salmonella* are highly pathogenic and may cause diarrhea, pneumonia, or septicemia. Fecal cultures do not distinguish pathogenic from nonpathogenic *Salmonella* serotype. Consider *Salmonella* spp. to be a significant pathogen when isolated directly from a grossly visible lesion, the respiratory tract, or intestinal tract of animals demonstrating clinical signs of enteric disease. Prophylactic treatment with antibiotics does not eliminate carrier stages.

It is almost impossible to eradicate *Salmonella* from pet reptiles. The following recommendations are aimed at controlling the spread of *Salmonella* and its ability to cause disease.

1. Minimize stress. Keep reptiles in the best husbandry situation possible. Avoid mixing species.
2. Proper hygiene is essential. Disinfect and clean cages regularly, but do not clean cages in food preparation areas (kitchens). Wash hands/equipment between animals, after handling, and before eating or smoking.
3. Perform a necropsy on all dead animals.
4. Reptiles are not recommended pets for immunocompromised people, such as infants, toddlers, elderly people, chemotherapy recipients, and people with acquired immuneodeficiency syndrome (AIDS).

COMMON DISORDERS IN BOAS, PYTHONS, AND LIZARDS

Anorexia in Boas and Pythons

Etiology

Anorexia may occur with or without obvious weight loss. Obtain a thorough history. Often there are no other signs of disease. Inadequate husbandry, particularly in the areas of temperature gradient, seclusion, selection of prey item (e.g., color, size, temperature if thawed, species, attack), light cycle, crowding, and adequate hydration or access to water, are the most common causes of anorexia.

Diagnosis

If husbandry problems are found and the animal appears otherwise healthy, perform a fecal float and fecal direct smear to rule out intestinal parasitic infections.

If the animal has not eaten for more than 2 months and has lost significant body condition, consider further diagnostics such as hematology, serum chemistry, cultures and radiographs.

Treatment

Treatment is based on improving husbandry and removing any parasites. Common helpful recommendations include:

- Use a thermometer to accurately measure the temperature gradient in the cage.
- Provide a hide box and feed stunned prey in the hide box.
- Monitor the light cycle. Ensure a 12-hour-to-12-hour light-dark cycle.
- Try another species, color, or different size prey.
- Feed when quiet or dark. Do not handle snakes for 1 week after feeding.
- Provide a water dish large enough for the snake to sit in.
- Feed stunned prey instead of dead if dead prey are not accepted.

If the reptile appears ill, assume that it also is dehydrated. Rehydrate with intraosseous (non-snakes), subcutaneous, or oral fluids depending on the state of hydration. Pass a stomach tube and administer warmed isotonic fluids to prepare the gut to receive solid food. Later, add glucose or electrolyte powders to increase the osmolality. Once this solution is tolerated, the formula may be changed to an avian hand-feeding formula. Start with a dilute mixture and slowly increase the concentration. Once full-strength hand-feeding formula is accepted, add meat baby food to the mixture to begin to introduce solid foods to carnivores. For herbivores or omnivores, use a mixture of alfalfa pellets and water to increase the fiber load. When ready to feed prey to carnivores, offer pinkies or small rodents first, and slowly increase the size of the prey. Begin feeding soft insects to insectivores. Place a pharyngotomy tube in animals requiring long-term tube feeding.

Respiratory Disorders

Pneumonia

Etiology

Pneumonia is most frequently secondary to poor husbandry, bacterial septicemia, or lung parasites.

Clinical Signs

The clinical signs of pneumonia include nasal discharge, gurgling, bubbling, open-mouthed breathing, and anorexia. Concurrent eye and mouth infections are common.

Diagnosis

Diagnosis usually is based on tracheal cytology and cultures. Other useful diagnostic tests include fecal flotation, hematology, bronchoscopy, and radiography.

Treatment

Administer antibiotics based on culture and sensitivity testing, or anthelmintic or antifungal drugs if indicated. Increase the environmental temperature to the high end of the POT. Parenteral vitamin C, fluid therapy, and nebulization therapy may be necessary.

Nebulize warmed saline to loosen debris in the bronchi. Antibacterial or antifungal medications may be added. A crude but apparently effective form of nebulization can be accomplished by the owner at home by using a hot shower to fill a bathroom with steam for 1 hour daily. Severely dyspneic individuals may require oxygen therapy. The long-term prognosis for these animals is grave.

Pentastomids

Etiology

Pentastomids are degenerate arthropod parasites of reptiles that resemble segmented worms. Infection occurs through an indirect life cycle involving insects and mammals. The parasites may live anywhere in the body but prefer the lungs and subcutaneous space.

Clinical Signs

Clinical signs in severely affected animals include dyspnea, hemoptysis, and cachexia.

Diagnosis

Diagnosis is based on fecal examination, tracheal cytology, or bronchoscopy.

Treatment

There is no effective treatment for pentastomids. High doses of ivermectin or levamisole have been anecdotally reported to suppress egg production. Because this parasite is zoonotic and is not readily treatable, euthanize infected animals. Infection can be avoided in captive reared animals by feeding only domestically reared prey items.

Infectious Stomatitis (Mouth Rot, Ulcerative Stomatitis)

Etiology

Mouth rot is usually secondary to poor husbandry, trauma from cage rubbing, or trauma from a rodent bite. The most common bacterial agents are *Aeromonas* and *Pseudomonas*, although other bacteria and fungi also are involved frequently. Neoplasia, mycotic infections, parasitic granuloma, or mandibular fractures also may cause stomatitis.

Clinical Signs

Early signs of mouth rot include oral petechia, ptyalism, and anorexia. As the infection progresses, caseous exudate, tooth loss, and osteomyelitis may be present. Mouth infections are frequently the nidus for concurrent eye infections and pneumonia.

Diagnosis

Perform a thorough oral examination and collect samples for cytologic examination. Obtain samples for bacterial culture and sensitivity testing, especially if caseous debris is found. The most accurate culture samples are obtained by making a small slit in the gum and swabbing the underlying tissues. In advanced cases, perform skull radiographs to determine the extent of osteomyelitis. If animals are anorexic, collect blood samples for hematology and blood chemistries.

Treatment

In mild cases in which petechia and ptyalism are present without anorexia, apply topical iodine, chlorhexadine solution, or hydrogen peroxide twice daily and instruct owners to improve husbandry. Reptiles with stomatitis should be housed at the high end of the POT. In more advanced cases, surgical debridement of the caseous debris, nutritional support, fluid therapy, and systemic antimicrobials may be required. Administer a combination of enrofloxacin and amoxicillin until culture results are available (see Table 171–1).

Prognosis

In mild cases, the prognosis is excellent if husbandry improves. The prognosis is guarded for cases with significant caseous debris and grave for reptiles with significant osteomyelitis.

Gastrointestinal Disorders

Regurgitation in Boas and Pythons

Vomitus often looks like a stool containing no urates. Use pH papers to identify vomitus if necessary. Fresh vomitus has an acid pH whereas feces are basic.

Old vomitus becomes alkaline with bacterial decomposition. The regurgitation of only mucus is a grave sign.

Poor Husbandry

Excessive handling of snakes within 48 hours of ingesting a meal may result in regurgitation. In these animals, regurgitation occurs shortly after handling. Base the diagnosis on history, lack of other clinical signs, and radiographic evidence of calcified remains of a meal in the stomach for more than 50 hours postprandially.

Diagnosis

A low body temperature inhibits the action of digestive enzymes, resulting in putrefaction of the ingested meal. In these snakes, regurgitation usually occurs 3–5 days postprandially. The diagnosis is based on history and a lack of other clinical signs.

Treatment

Treat by providing an adequate, safe heat source 24 hours a day.

Obstruction

Foreign bodies usually are ingested with prey items and include cage substrates, cage furniture, and foreign bodies inside of prey items. Clinical signs include regurgitation, absence of fecal material, abdominal swelling, and anorexia. Diagnosis is similar to that for mammals and includes plain radiography or endoscopy. Perform hematology and blood chemistries on systemically ill animals.

Treatment

Treatment is similar to mammals. In mild cases in which the obstruction consists of small pieces of granular material, administer saline or mineral oil via stomach intubation. Parenteral fluids are also helpful. If a large foreign body is located in the stomach, remove it via endoscope. Gastrotomy or enterotomy may be required to remove large objects or objects distal to the stomach.

Similar clinical signs may be seen in animals with intraluminal or extraluminal GI masses. Causes include neoplasia, abscess, or granuloma of the GI tract or other nearby organs, parasitic blockage, or organomegaly. Diagnosis is based on radiographs, ultrasound, fine-needle aspirate for cytologic examination and culture, or laparotomy and biopsy. Hematology or blood chemistries usually are indicated.

Diarrhea

Etiology

Gastroenteritis may be caused by enteric parasitic infections, gram-negative bacterial or clostridial infection, viral infections, or enteric fungi.

Diagnosis

- To rule out parasitic infections, perform fecal flotation, a fecal wet mount, and stomach wash, especially if diarrhea is accompanied by vomiting. Fecal sedimentation may be required if trematodes are suspected. Most cysts, eggs, and larvae can be identified to taxonomic family to direct anthelmintic treatment.
- Clinical bacterial or mycotic enteritis is often secondary to significant parasite infestations. Perform a fecal Gram stain to diagnose clostridial overgrowth or enteric yeasts. High numbers of monomorphic gram-negative rods are supportive of a diagnosis of bacterial enteritis (see Bacterial Infections). Routine culture techniques are not reliable in detecting *Salmonella*.
- Other diagnostic tests that may be useful include hematology, serum biochemistry, peritoneal lavage, and endoscopy.
- Other causes of diarrhea include foreign body, ruptured coelomic abscess, septicemia, and liver or pancreatic disease.

Treatment

- Administer fenbendazole for the prophylactic treatment of intestinal parasites.
- Administer praziquantel if cestodes or trematodes are suspected or found on fecal examination.
- Levamisole or ivermectin may be effective against acanthocephalans. Ivermectin is toxic to chelonians.
- Pending bacterial culture results, administer fluid therapy and parenteral antibiotics. In mild cases of dehydration, subcutaneous lactated Ringer's solution is an excellent choice. Fluid volumes should be calculated as for mammals, incorporating fluid losses from vomiting and diarrhea as well as maintenance needs. In severely dehydrated reptiles, use intraosseous fluids when possible. Administer half-strength lactated Ringer's solution or saline with 2.5% dextrose for the first 4 hours, followed by lactated Ringer's solution alone. Monitor serum or plasma potassium levels and add potassium to the fluids as needed.
- Parenteral administration of antibiotics is necessary in reptiles with GI disease. A combination of enrofloxacin and amoxicillin or ampicillin is usually effective in the treatment of most gram-negative, gram-positive, and anaerobic bacterial pathogens. This combination does not appear to have detrimental effects on GI flora when administered parenterally and has low potential for nephrotoxicity in dehydrated reptiles.

Cryptosporidium

Etiology

- *Cryptosporidium* is a protozoal parasite of snakes and some lizards. The parasite infects the stomach and large and small intestines, causing atrophy of intestinal villi and hypertrophy of the stomach wall.

Clinical Signs

- Clinical signs include diarrhea, regurgitation 2–3 days postprandially, and marked gastric distention causing a visible fusiform swelling in the stomach region. Chronic disease causes anorexia and weight loss. A subclinical carrier state exists.

Diagnosis

- Diagnosis is confirmed by identification of cysts on cytologic examination of fluid obtained from a stomach wash or stomach biopsies. Cysts occasionally are seen in feces. Cysts are 2.6–6.0 μm in diameter and stain blue on Giemsa stain. Yeasts can look very similar. If in doubt, stain the slide with iodine. Yeast turns brown and cysts remain colorless. Alternatively, *Cryptosporidium cysts* stain positive with acid fast stains, whereas yeasts do not. In the future, an enzyme-linked immunosorbent assay (ELISA) test may become available.

Treatment

- There is no effective treatment for cryptosporidiosis. Recommend euthanasia because animals remain carriers and there is a potential risk of zoonosis.

Amebiasis

Etiology

Amebiasis caused by *Entamoeba invadens* is diagnosed commonly in recently acquired carnivores. The likelihood of infection increases if the carnivores previously were exposed to chelonians. The parasite causes a hemorrhagic gastroenteritis and liver necrosis.

Clinical Signs

Clinical signs include anorexia in early infestations, followed by regurgitation and hematochezia.

Diagnosis

Diagnosis is based on identification of cysts or tropozoites on cytologic examination of fluid obtained from a stomach wash or fecal smear.

Treatment

Administer metronidazole and initiate supportive therapy as needed. Prognosis for early infections is excellent but for severe infestations is grave.

Constipation

Etiology

Many underlying causes for constipation exist, including exposure to cool temperatures, ingestion of foreign material (especially bedding), and an abrupt dietary change to more fibrous food. There is often a history of recent escape. Constipation also can occur secondary to compression of the colon by extraluminal masses such as eggs, organomegaly, granulomas, or uroliths. In chronic cases, renal failure may occur secondary to compression of the ureters by clocaliths (inspissated feces and urates in the cloaca).

Clinical Signs

Clinical signs of constipation vary from decreased stool production alone to signs of GI obstruction such as anorexia and vomiting. The animal may be cachexic if anorexic for long periods of time. Most affected animals are chilled and dehydrated.

Diagnosis

In early cases, abdominal palpation reveals a firm-to-doughy mass in the cloacal region. In chronic cases, the mass is hard and firm, and the animal may be bloated from retained ingesta. Radiographs and, if necessary, ultrasound may delineate the obstruction.

Treatment

If signs of systemic illness are not present, treat simple constipation at home with 1-hour warm water (85°F) body soaks administered 2 to 3 times over a 24-hour period. If defecation is not induced, administer an enema consisting of warm water/water soluble lubricating jelly enemas (see Techniques section). If treatment is effective, some stool should be passed after one to three enemas. If the impaction has been long-standing and large amounts of ingesta are present, consider giving an enema every 2–3 days until all the material is expelled. In chronic cases in which stool will not pass and in cases in which the obstruction is secondary to a foreign body or extramural compression of the colon, perform a laparotomy. Because these patients usually are debilitated, surgery is risky. Strict attention to aseptic technique is essential to avoid peritonitis or abdominal abscesses. The surgical approach to the colon is similar to that in mammals.

Cloacal Prolapse

Etiology

- Prolapsed cloacas usually are the result of straining due to enteritis, cloacitis, or dystocia.
- Pinworms are the most common cause of cloacal prolapse in green iguanas.

Diagnosis

Hyperemic, inflamed tissue is observed protruding from the vent on physical examination. Active straining may be present. The prolapse of other organs, such as the hemipene or oviduct, or cloacal neoplasia may appear similar. Use digital manipulation to determine the source of the prolapsed tissue. If in doubt, perform contrast radiography using iohexol (diluted 1:3 with warm water) administered as an enema to delineate the source of the tissue. Determine the primary cause of the straining. Fecal flotation, direct fecal wet mounts, and fecal Gram stains are the minimum diagnostic tests necessary to rule out parasites or clostridial or gram-negative bacterial enteritis.

▼ *Key Point* Diagnose and treat the underlying cause of cloacal prolapse to prevent recurrence.

Treatment

Clean the cloaca with warmed sterile saline. Avoid abrading the tissue. Use light sedation with isoflurane, propofol, or ketamine if the animal appears in pain or is difficult to restrain. Once the debris is cleaned from the tissue, determine whether the tissue is in fact the cloaca, and if it is intact. Ensure that the proximal colon is not involved in the prolapse. Until the primary cause for the prolapsed cloaca can be controlled, keep the cloaca in correct anatomic position.

If only the cloaca is involved, lubricate the tissue with water-soluble jelly and replace the cloaca with digital pressure. The application of topical hemorrhoidal medications or 50% dextrose may help reduce edema. If the cloaca is too small for digital pressure, use a well-lubricated cotton swab. Be sure to invert the cloaca entirely into its original position. Place a large horizontal mattress suture at the opening of the cloaca. Pass the needle perpendicular to the cloaca. Leave the ends of the suture long to adjust tension. In general, for reptiles less than 100 g, the opening should allow the passage of one lubricated cotton swab. Reptiles larger than 500 g usually require an opening large enough to accommodate four to six swabs. Adjust the tension so that the animal can defecate through the reduced opening, but the cloaca remains in normal position.

Instruct owners to watch for normal volumes of feces. Sutures are usually left in place 7–14 days. Feed a low residue diet for 2 weeks. If necessary, mix mineral oil with baby food and administer orally to soften the feces.

If the proximal colon is involved in the prolapse, perform surgical correction and cloacopexy. The technique is similar to that used in mammals. If the cloaca is damaged severely, amputation can be attempted as long as the ureters are left intact.

Prognosis

The prognosis is guarded. For severely traumatized prolapses in compromised animals, euthanasia may be the most humane alternative.

Reproductive Disorders
Dystocia

Dystocia is the inability to expel term eggs (oviposition) or fetuses. This is in contrast to retained ovarian follicles (see Green Iguanas).

Etiology

Dystocia usually results from inadequate husbandry, such as inadequate nutrition (especially calcium), temperature, lighting, seclusion, physical activity, or sub-strate on which to lay. Dystocia also can result from infections of the oviduct or other abdominal disease.

Clinical Signs

Clinical signs include anorexia, partial lay, or straining to lay with no result. The history may suggest that the snake is overdue for oviposition based on previous laying dates. Some species of reptiles normally harbor eggs internally; therefore determine that dystocia is actually present.

Diagnosis

Diagnosis is based on abdominal palpation and history. Radiographs and/or ultrasound may demonstrate mature eggs or fetuses in oviducts. Large or misshapen eggs are strong evidence of dystocia. In most gravid reptiles, serum calcium, phosphorus, cholesterol, and total protein levels are higher than concentrations seen in mammals or nongravid, healthy reptiles. Differential diagnosis for the abdominal masses and clinical signs include granuloma, neoplasia, intestinal obstruction, metastatic calcification, or gout.

Treatment

▼ *Key Point* Always determine whether dystocia is present. If the animal is not showing signs of being obstructed or critically ill, try modifying the environment. Provide a warmer temperature, a hide box, and an adequate moistened laying substrate, such as sand or soil.

If young are not produced within 2–3 days, administer parenteral calcium and either vasotocin or oxytocin. Drugs may be administered every 3–4 days as long as a few eggs are passed until all eggs are expelled. Do not give oxytocin or vasotocin daily or if no eggs are produced consistently, or oviductal rupture may occur. If the aforementioned steps are unsuccessful, attempt gentle manual expression. This may be effective if only a few eggs are left. Use copious lubrication. Oviductal rupture is a common sequela. If a large or misshapen egg is palpated, the contents of the egg may be aspirated percutaneously via an 18-gauge needle and syringe. The resulting reduction in size sometimes allows these eggs to pass. There is a risk of oviductal rupture and peritonitis with this procedure.

- Oviductectomy or oviductotomy frequently is required. If performed before severe systemic illness, the prognosis for life is excellent and for fertility (with oviductotomy) is good. If the animal is systemically ill, stabilize the patient with intraosseous or intravenous fluids and antibiotics before surgery. Correct electrolyte imbalances and perform surgery as quickly as possible.
- If the oviducts have ruptured and yolk is in the abdomen, the prognosis for long-term recovery is grave. Egg yolk peritonitis not only affects the GI tract but also often induces liver failure. Egg yolk

frequently embolizes and can cause infarcts in any tissue. If infection is present in the oviducts, submit the contents for bacteria culture and remove the oviducts and ovaries.

Prolapsed Hemipenes or Paraphimosis

Etiology

Prolapsed hemipenes usually occur after prolonged breeding. In chelonians, phallus prolapse occurs secondary to trauma by cagemates.

Clinical Signs

A prolapsed male copulatory organ is observed protruding from the cloaca. Most snake hemipenes have bristles. In all species, the appearance of the hemipenes is sufficient to be differentiated from a prolapsed cloaca or oviduct.

Treatment

Clean the tissue with saline and lubricate with water-soluble jelly. If the tissue is swollen, hemorrhoidal ointments can be used to reduce swelling. Replace the hemipene using gentle digital pressure, inserting the organ through the cloaca in a caudal direction. Place a horizontal mattress suture around the vent to keep the organ in place. In case of recurrent prolapse, a hemipene or phallus can be amputated without affecting urination, because they only transmit sperm. Amputation is accomplished by ligating the proximal portion of the organ with horizontal mattress sutures and using sharp dissection to remove the distal portion.

Dermatologic Disorders

Mites

- *Ophionyssus natricus,* or the snake mite, can be seen macroscopically as 0.5-mm black dots on the animal or on paper bedding. Look closely at the spectacle, in the gular fold, and around the vent. Mites can cause anemia and debilitation. They are also vectors for bacteria such as *Aeromonas* as well as viruses and blood parasites.
- Green iguanas have their own species of mite, which is red or gray in color. This mite causes spreading black patches of hyperkeratosis and can be diagnosed with skin scrapings.

Treatment

Treatment with ivermectin is usually effective. Never give ivermectin to turtles.

- Be sure to clean and disinfect the cage. In severe infestations, treat the entire room with a pyrethrin flea product. Treat all animals and the environment every 2 weeks for three treatments. Discard any porous substances such as wood, paper, plants, or nonglazed pottery.

Ticks

Ticks are large enough to be observed macroscopically, with their heads buried under scales. They can be well camouflaged and tend to congregate under the jaw and around the vent in snakes and in the axilla or groin in tortoises and lizards. As with mites, ticks can carry blood parasites, viruses, and bacteria.

Treatment

Spray a pyrethrin flea spray that is labeled safe for use in kittens on a cotton swab and apply it directly to the head region of the tick. Once the tick is stunned, remove it using forceps. Be careful to remove the tick's head to avoid abscessation.

▼ **Key Point** Many ticks are imported with the reptile from regions of the world that have serious zoonotic diseases that can be transmitted by ticks. Always use gloves or forceps when removing ticks. Dispose of the remains as biohazardous waste.

Blister Disease

Etiology

Blister disease is a lay term for vesicular dermatitis. It is most frequently caused by a bacterial infection resulting from unsanitary and high humidity conditions. Occasionally, vasculitis from a viral or bacterial septicemia causes similar clinical signs.

Clinical Signs

Fluid-filled vesicles or brown desiccated areas may be found on the ventral surface of the abdomen. These lesions may progress to ulcerations.

Diagnosis

Obtain a sample of the fluid within a vesicle for cytologic examination and bacterial fungal culture.

If the reptile is systemically ill, further diagnostics such as hematology and blood chemistries are recommended.

Treatment

Improve sanitation. Apply topical diluted iodine, and administer parenteral antibiotics. Administer parenteral amoxicillin and enrofloxacin until culture results are available. Nutritional and fluid support is essential in severe cases because these animals may lose large amounts of serum through the vesicles.

Thermal Burns

Etiology

Burns are usually the result of contact with a heat lamp or a "hot rock."

Treatment

Administer parenteral antibiotics to prevent secondary bacterial infections. Apply topical diluted iodine and topical silver sulfadiazine cream daily. Monitor for secondary fungal infections. If large, full-thickness burns are present, fluid and protein losses can be excessive. If the patient becomes dehydrated, administer appropriate fluid therapy. It may be necessary to supplement protein with injectable amino acids or plasma transfusion. If large areas of skin slough, apply a self-adhesive burn dressing such as Tega derm (3-M Corporation Minneapolis, MN). This dressing provides the equivalent of a second skin and encourages healing while decreasing pain and fluid losses.

▼ *Key Point* Treat thermal burns as soon as possible to decrease the risk of bacterial septicemia and excessive fluid or protein losses. Instruct owners to bring the animal in for treatment as soon as the burn is discovered.

Abscesses

Etiology

Abscesses may be secondary to either external trauma or bacterial septicemic emboli. If the abscess is secondary to septicemia, the primary infection also must be treated.

Diagnosis

Examine the skin for evidence of a firm swelling in the dermis. Palpate the abdomen to detect firm masses. Aspirate the swelling for cytologic examination and culture to confirm the diagnosis. Cultures taken from the edge of an abscess are the most useful. Most abscesses consist of gram-negative or anaerobic bacteria. Other differentials include neoplasia, fungal granuloma, foreign body, parasites, or cyst.

Treatment

Reptilian abscesses contain caseous exudate, which does not drain well. Surgically remove the abscess with the capsule remaining intact whenever possible. If the entire abscess is not resectable, curette the remaining lesion until only healthy tissue remains. Use local or general anesthetic for this procedure. After surgery, leave the abscesses open to heal by second intention. Flush the lesion with dilute iodine every 6–8 hours until completely healed. Enzymatic ointments may be helpful in breaking down caseous debris. In addition to topical treatment, use parenteral amoxicillin and enrofloxacin or amikacin pending culture results.

Nasal Trauma

Reptiles that are kept under inadequate husbandry conditions often pace their cages, resulting in injury to the rostral jaws. Excitable reptiles also may run into walls, which results in trauma to the same area.

Infectious stomatitis is a frequent secondary problem. Treatment is similar to that for abscesses and infectious stomatitis.

▼ *Key Point* Providing adequate husbandry is critical. Provide visual security, a smooth cage interior, screening, and as many corners as possible.

Gangrene or Abscesses of Extremities

Avascular Necrosis

Etiology

The most common cause of toe loss in lizards is avascular necrosis. Necrosis results from the formation of constricting bands when shedding of the skin on the toes or tail is incomplete. These bands usually form under conditions of low humidity and poor nutrition.

Diagnosis

Diagnosis is based on clinical signs.

Treatment

Amputation of the affected extremity usually is required. To prevent future lesions, educate the owner about proper husbandry. Recommend warm water soaks to soften and remove dry skin on the extremities.

Trauma Etiology

A second common cause of avascular necrosis is trauma due to tail thrashing or catching a toe in a screen. Open or closed contusions, lacerations, or fractures are apparent on physical examination. If the wounds are old, they may be infected or gangrenous.

Treatment

Treat with topical or parenteral antimicrobials. Cultures are indicated if the wound is old. Amputation usually is required. Modify the environment to minimize the chances of trauma's recurring.

Vasculitis

Etiology

Occasionally, gangrene of extremities is seen in reptiles with no known history of trauma. Often, these patients are systemically ill. The lesions are usually caused by vasculitis secondary to septicemia, mycobacteriosis, viral or fungal infection, gout, or ingestion of mycotoxin. Diagnosis is based on cytology, including special stains for mycobacteria and fungi, culture and sensitivity, hematology, blood chemistry, histopathology, or feed analysis for mycotoxins.

Treatment

Treat supportively and with appropriate antimicrobials. Surgical amputation of affected extremities almost always is required. Because the disease is usually systemic, prognosis is guarded to grave. Treatment for mycobacteria is difficult, and the zoonotic potential must be considered.

Ocular Disorders

Retained Spectacles

Etiology

Retained spectacles are associated with dysecdysis (abnormal shedding). Poor husbandry, especially low humidity and low temperature, usually is the cause. This condition commonly occurs in pet snakes.

Clinical Signs

Clinical signs include cloudy eyes after a recent shed or a silvery, wrinkled appearance to the eye. If more than a few spectacles are retained, the snake experiences blindness and stops eating. A subspectacular or eye infection may occur below the spectacle.

Treatment

Soak the animal in a warm water bath for 1–3 hours. Once softened, the eye cap can be removed by rubbing with a wet cotton ball or with fine forceps. If the spectacle cannot be removed after soaking for a few hours, soak the animal right before next full shed. If the spectacle persists, refer the animal to a hospital equipped to perform microsurgical removal.

▼ *Key Point* If the spectacle does not lift easily do *not* force removal, or the primary spectacle may be avulsed, leaving the cornea unprotected. Loss of the eye may ensue.

Subspectacular Infection

Etiology

This is the most common ophthalmic infection in snakes. These infections almost always are associated with stomatitis. The bacteria ascend the nasolacrimal duct, which empties into the space between the spectacle and the cornea.

Clinical Signs

The eye appears to be cloudy. Further inspection reveals that the fluid is under the speculum and there is distention of the subspectacular space. A 27- to 25-gauge needle may be used to aspirate fluid from the space for cytologic examination and culture.

Treatment

Treatment with parenteral antibiotics is usually curative. Do not use topical medications because these cannot penetrate the spectacle. In severe cases in which the cornea is in danger of perforation, remove a wedge from the ventral spectacle to allow drainage, flushing, and administration of topical medications. Flush the subspectacular space with saline until all debris is removed, then apply an appropriate topical ophthalmic

drop through the wedge. Once this surgery is performed, the cornea is exposed for approximately 2 weeks or until the snake next sheds. Therefore, apply ophthalmic lubricants until the new spectacle forms.

Neuromuscular Disorders

Viral Associated Encephalitis of Snakes

Etiology

This disease is believed to be caused by a retrovirus. Transmission may be vertical, by direct contact, from fomites, and from mites. Burmese pythons and boa constrictors seem to be particularly susceptible.

Clinical Signs

Snakes, especially pythoboids, demonstrate neurologic signs such as head tilt, ataxia, opisthotonos, anisocoria, and muscle tremors. Often, the front half of the snake coils in loops. Some snakes present for chronic regurgitation with no neurologic component. In general, the virus is slowly progressive.

Diagnosis

Diagnosis currently requires histopathologic observation of inclusion bodies. Submit esophageal lymphoid aggregates, kidney, pancreas, liver, and stomach samples. Snakes with neurologic signs may have lesions limited to the central nervous system, which makes premortem diagnosis difficult. The main differential diagnosis includes bacterial meningoencephalitis and paramyxovirus.

Treatment

I have provided supportive care to several boa constrictors that seemed to return to normal after 2–3 months of therapy. All affected snakes should be considered carriers. A *minimum* of a 90- to 180-day quarantine is recommended for all snakes entering a new collection.

Adenovirus of Bearded Dragons

Etiology

Adenovirus in bearded dragons causes acute hepatic coagulation necrosis.

Clinical Signs

Clinical signs occur in neonates and young adults and include seizures, muscle tremors, opisthotonos, lethargy, and icterus.

Diagnosis

Diagnosis is based on clinical signs and inclusion bodies in the liver and GI tract. The main differential diagnosis for seizures in bearded dragons is hypocalcemia, a common problem in animals fed an all-cricket diet.

Treatment

There is no effective treatment. The morbidity rate appears to be 50–60%. With supportive care, 30% of animals showing clinical signs survive. Many have residual neurologic deficits. Quarantine survivors and siblings permanently. Do not use these animals for breeding.

Spondylitis in Snakes

Etiology

Spondylitis is caused most commonly by infection with *Salmonella* spp., although other bacteria have been described. Snakes with spondylitis appear to be stiff or fall off a snake hook.

Diagnosis

Physical examination reveals segmental fused vertebrae and crepitus of the spinal column. In chronic cases, intestinal impaction due to loss of intestinal innervation is palpable. Radiograph the spine to look for lesions suggestive of discospondylitis. Neoplasia should be considered as a differential diagnosis.

Treatment

The prognosis for cure is grave. Progression can be arrested temporarily with parenteral antibiotics based on culture and sensitivity. Surgery can be used to decompress spinal nerves but is not strongly recommended as clinical signs.

Paramyxovirus Infections in Snakes

Etiology

Clinical signs vary from peracute death to death after a 24- to 48-hour progressive course of paresis. The snake tends to lie stretched out initially, then open-mouthed breathing occurs. Frequently, brown liquid is expelled from the mouth shortly before death. A more chronic form has been diagnosed that is characterized by a proliferative pneumonia, head tremors that can progress to seizures, mydriasis, loss of righting reflex, opisthotonos, and, many times, death.

Diagnosis

Diagnosis is based on clinical signs, necropsy, and a hemaglutination inhibition test offered by the University of Florida Veterinary Medical Teaching Hospital.

Treatment

Snakes with the chronic form may respond temporarily to supportive care and antimicrobial therapy only to relapse weeks to months later.

NUTRITIONAL DISORDERS

Secondary Nutritional Hyperparathyroidism of Green Iguanas

Etiology

The physiology of secondary nutritional hyperparathyroidism (SNHP) in reptiles is similar to that of mammals. Inadequate calcium, vitamin D_3, or UV light source in addition to excess phosphorus (usually from protein and fruits) are the main husbandry problems contributing to SNHP. Primary renal or parathyroid disease also can cause hyperparathyroidism.

Clinical Signs

- Clinical signs include pliable, thickened mandibles, folding fractures of extremities, posterior paresis due to hypocalcemia or fractured spine, kyphosis, ileus from denervation or hypocalcemia leading to impaction and/or incontinence, seizures, dystocia, anorexia, and general malaise.

Diagnosis

- The diagnosis is based on history and physical examination. Serum calcium concentration may be normal even if body stores are low. Radiographic evidence of decreased bone density occurs only in advanced cases. Other causes of seizures include trauma, neoplasia, or toxin.

Treatment

- Administer injectable calcium initially, followed by oral supplementation.
- An oral source of vitamin D_3 also is recommended.
- The owner *must* make appropriate environmental changes such as light cycle, UV light, and temperature gradient. Without these changes, medical therapy will fail. Many animals are chronically ill and on the verge of starvation. Tube-feed anorexic animals until their appetite returns, which may take several weeks. Most fractures heal on their own, without internal stabilization. Splinting rear legs against the tail may aid in stabilizing fractures.
- Avoid rough handling, and remove cage furniture to decrease the probability of future fractures. In mild cases, the prognosis is good if owners comply with recommended treatment. If posterior paresis is the result of a spinal fracture, the prognosis for normal ambulation is grave to guarded.
- Calcitonin has a bone-sparing effect, and some practitioners advocate its use *after* the serum calcium concentration has returned to normal. I hesitate to use this drug unless the mandibles are so soft that it is difficult for the iguana to eat on its own.

Hypocalcemia

- Reptiles with clinical hypocalcemia present with muscle tremors or seizures. A presumptive diagnosis is based on a history of inadequate diet and husbandry and physical examination findings that support SNHP.

Treatment

- If the animal is having seizures, administer calcium gluconate or calcium chloride IV or IO to effect. Diazepam may be necessary to control seizures.
- If muscle tremors without seizures are present, obtain a blood sample for serum or plasma calcium concentrations, then administer an IM calcium supplement while awaiting laboratory results.
- For long-term care, see the SNHP section.

Hypervitaminosis D3

- Metastatic calcification of soft tissues frequently is seen in herbivores, omnivores, and insectivores that are oversupplemented with calcium and vitamin D_3. The disease is seen most frequently in 4- to 6-year-old male green iguanas that were fed dog, cat, or monkey chow as a major proportion of the protein in their diet.
- Clinical signs are variable but usually include general malaise followed by anorexia. If the kidneys are mineralized, there are signs consistent with renal failure.
- Diagnosis is based on radiographic evidence of soft tissue mineralization. Diagnosis is difficult if radiographs do not reveal mineralization of soft tissues because serum concentrations of calcium and phosphorus may be within normal limits. Provide supportive care and eliminate the vitamin D_3 supplement from the diet.

Thiamine Deficiency

- Thiamine deficiency occurs in carnivores fed a diet high in fatty fishes such as goldfish and smelt. It also occurs in lizards fed muscle meat as a sole food source.
- Clinical signs include paralysis, paresis, pulmonary edema, dyspnea, tremor, cerebral edema, dehydration, enteritis, and blindness.
- Diagnosis is based on history and clinical signs.
- Administer thiamine at 25 mg/kg PO or SC q24h for 3–7 days.
- To prevent hypothiaminosis, feed a fresh, varied diet or add 1.1 mg thiamine per kg of fish fed.

Biotin Deficiency

- Biotin deficiency occurs in lizards fed a diet of raw infertile eggs.
- Clinical signs are similar to thiamine deficiency.
- Treat with injectable vitamin B complex.
- Prevent by feeding fertile eggs at different stages of development as well as whole-animal prey. A biotin supplement also can be offered.

URINARY SYSTEM

Gout

Etiology

Gout is the abnormal deposition of uric acid crystals into soft tissue. Gout usually occurs as one of two forms, visceral or articular. In visceral gout, the uric acid precipitates on internal organs, whereas articular gout occurs when uric acid tophi occur within and around joints and tendons. Gout occurs as a result of poor husbandry, dehydration, high-protein diets, and use of aminoglycoside antibiotics. In many cases, however, no recognizable risk factor is apparent.

Clinical Signs

- Clinical signs are variable and range from lethargy and anorexia to sudden death. If articular gout is present, affected joints are swollen and painful. In visceral gout, clinical signs are related to failure of the organ affected by the uric acid crystals.

Diagnosis

- Diagnosis is based on physical examination and identification of the uric acid crystals via cytologic or histopathologic examination of tissue samples (do not use formalin as a fixative). Gross lesions may be visible during laparoscopy or laparotomy. Uric acid deposits are sometimes visible on ultrasound or radiographs. Serum uric acid concentrations may be elevated; however, not all reptiles with gout have elevated serum uric acid concentrations.

Treatment

- Administer supportive care, especially fluid therapy. Improving temperature, humidity, and access to water is critical.
- Avoid high-protein diets (especially those high in purine) and nephrotoxic drugs.
- Avoid use of furosemide because it may inhibit renal excretion of uric acid.
- Antihyperuricemic drugs such as allopurinol, probenecid, sulfinpyrazone, and colchicine can be used to control, but not cure, gout.
- The prognosis for long-term survival is grave.

Urolithiasis

Urolithiasis is seen most frequently in land turtles and lizards fed high-protein diets without adequate access to water.

- Clinical signs include anorexia, straining, or abdominal distension.
- Uroliths are palpable as caudal abdominal masses.
- If necessary, confirm the diagnosis with ultrasound. Radiographs may not be diagnostic if the calculi consist of uric acid, which is of soft tissue density.

Treatment

After stabilizing the patient, perform a cystotomy to remove the calculi.

- Culture the calculi. They sometimes are associated with bacterial cystitis.
- Decrease the protein content of the diet and encourage water consumption.
- Avoid use of nephrotoxic drugs.

DISEASES OF CHELONIANS

Chelonians can acquire most of the disorders described for snakes and lizards. See the previous section for details.

Mycoplasma Pneumonia

Etiology

Mycoplasma and secondary *Pasteurella testudinis* infections are a common cause of upper and lower respiratory tract disease in tortoises.

Clinical Signs

- Clinical signs include nasal and ocular discharge, dyspnea, anorexia, and dehydration.
- Historically, the signs are often unresponsive or only partially responsive to typical antibiotic therapy.

Diagnosis

- Diagnosis is based on clinical signs, culture for *Mycoplasma*, routine bacterial culture and sensitivity, and tracheal cytology. Anemia; elevated sodium, blood urea nitrogen (BUN); aspartate transaminase (AST); and cholesterol; and decreased phosphorus levels often are seen.
- Differential diagnosis should include bacterial, viral, parasitic, aspiration, or fungal pneumonia, and neoplasia or foreign body.

Treatment

- Treat with enrofloxacin or tylosin and with fluid and nutritional support.
- Survivors may always be carriers; quarantine them for life.

Nutritional Disorders

Vitamin A Deficiency

Etiology

Vitamin A deficiency is seen most frequently in juvenile, semiaquatic turtles older than 6 months of age. Before this age, the remnants of the yolk sac provide adequate levels of vitamin A. Affected animals usually have been fed high-protein, unbalanced diets such as raw hamburger. Vitamin A deficiency results in squamous meta-

plasia of the glandular structures of the eye, oral cavity, respiratory passages, and genitourinary tract, as well as decreased local immunity. Changes in the kidney predispose animals to gout, particularly if they are on a high-protein diet.

Clinical Signs

- Clinical signs include conjunctivitis, pneumonia, stomatitis, and hyperkeratotic eyelids.

Diagnosis

- Diagnosis is based on history, clinical signs, and biopsy samples, which demonstrate lesions compatible with epithelial squamous metaplasia.

Treatment

- In most cases, oral supplementation of vitamin A is sufficient and safe. Treat with parenteral vitamin A only in severe cases. Long-term improvement of the diet is essential.

Vitamin A Toxicity

Vitamin A toxicity is seen within 2 weeks of administration of parenteral vitamin A. Toxic levels of vitamin A cause xeroderma initially and necrotizing dermatitis with long-term toxicity.

- Clinical signs include severe sloughing of epidermis, especially in the cervical region.
- Treatment consists of supportive care. Give fluid therapy to replace fluid losses from defects in the dermis and exposed muscle. Apply dressings to open wounds as needed.

▼ *Key Point* Never give injectable vitamin A unless there is a history of dietary deficiency and clinical signs of hypovitaminosis A are severe.

Hypothyroidism (Iodine Deficiency)

Hypothyroidism resulting from goiter is recognized in tortoises suffering from iodine deficiency. Iodine is bound by nitrates and compounds found in cabbage, kale, brussels sprouts, and uncooked soybeans.

- Clinical signs include myxedema and goiter.
- Treat with iodine and dietary modification.

Diseases of the Shell

Shell Trauma

The most common causes of shell trauma in turtles are accidental drops, car or lawn mower collisions, and attacks by dogs.

Treatment

- Stabilize the patient and stop all hemorrhage before attempting to repair the shell.

- If possible, draw blood for baseline complete blood count (CBC) and profile.
- Lavage the peritoneum and clean all cracks.
- Bandage full-thickness cracks or openings with nonstick dressings, then wrap the shell in plastic wrap to prevent contamination and loss of peritoneal fluids.
- Administer IV, IO, or SC fluids as needed. If the turtle is in shock, administer one dose of dexamethasone (0.5–1.0 mg/kg).
- Keep the patient warm and administer prophylactic antibiotics.
- Once the patient is stable, treat minor, relatively stable cracks by cleaning with iodine q12h, apply topical antibiotic cream, and stabilize the crack with bandages or steel wires as necessary.
- Most animals heal in 2–3 weeks.
- Unstable cracks or large shell defects must be repaired with fiberglass or acrylic resins or UV light-cured polymers.
- Allow ample time for underlying soft tissues to heal before attempting repair.
- Debris or microbes caught under the patch cause granulomas or abscesses.
- Once the wound is clean and has developed a healthy granulation bed, apply silver sulfadiazine cream to the wound.
- Apply Tegaderm (3M Corporation) over exposed soft tissues to provide protection from the polymers to be applied later.
- Clean the scutes adjacent to the defect with ether or acetone.
- Apply a thin layer of epoxy to the shell, then place nylon or fiberglass screening over the defect.

▼ *Key Point* Do not let the epoxy come in contact with bone or soft tissue. Also ensure that the epoxy or screening does not create a barrier to prevent granulation tissue from filling in the defect.

- Epoxy can be painted on top of the screen.
- Keep the animal out of water at least 24 hours to allow curing. Use only marine epoxies on aquatic turtles. Ensure adequate hydration for aquatic turtles by providing oral, SC, or IP fluids and a high relative humidity in their enclosure.
- Patches need to be removed in fast-growing animals.
- Complete healing takes 6–18 months.

Shell Rot

Healthy shell scutes are periodically shed in rapidly growing chelonians. Normal scute sheds should appear as clear keratin.

- Most shell infections are secondary to poor husbandry and are caused by bacteria or fungi.
- Occasionally, algae can cause erosions.
- Clinical signs of shell rot include petechia, sloughing of discolored, soft scutes, erosions, hyperemia, and fluffy or granulomatous growths. Dermatitis and septicemia are common.

Diagnosis

- Diagnosis is based on cytologic examination of shell scrapings or biopsy and bacterial or fungal culture and sensitivity. Differential diagnosis includes infections secondary to trauma, foreign body, or neoplasia.

Treatment

- Administer diluted topical iodine soaks for at least 1 hour daily. Dry the shell by keeping it out of water for at least 1 hour.
- Monitor for dehydration during this period.
- Use a sharp, clean knife to pare away dead sections of shell and expose the infected tissues.
- Many early cases of shell rot respond to treatment with iodine, desiccation, and improvement of husbandry.
- Turtles with deep erosions or septicemia need to be treated with systemic antimicrobials based on culture and sensitivity.
- If bone is exposed, the prognosis is guarded to grave.
- Severe erosions must be treated similar to thermal burns.

Pyramiding of Shell

Pyramiding of the scutes of the carapace or doming of the carapace are clinical signs of secondary nutritional hyperparathyroidism. The diet of affected turtles is often high in lettuce, melon, tomatoes, or protein. The shell also may appear to be small for the body in turtles fed too much protein. Concurrent beak deformities are often present.

- Similar lesions can occur in adult chelonians with systemic disease, particularly liver or renal disease.
- If caught early, the defects can be minimized with proper nutrition (see section on SNHP).
- More severely affected animals will be permanently disfigured.

Myiasis

Myiasis may occur in any reptile species but is most common in chelonians. Flies lay eggs into a wound.

- Maggots usually hatch in 12–24 hours.
- Remove the maggots and treat similar to mammals. Do not use ivermectin flushes in turtles. Provide supportive care as needed.

▼ *Key Point* Ivermectin is toxic to turtles and tortoises.

DISEASES OF CROCODILIANS

Hypoglycemia

Hypoglycemia is seen in stressed alligators, especially when malnutrition, cold temperatures, and high population density are present.

- Clinical signs include tremors, torpor, loss of righting reflex, generalized weakness, mydriasis, and catatonia.

- Diagnosis is based on low glucose levels on blood chemistry. To treat, administer 3 g/kg glucose PO and improve husbandry.

Vitamin K Deficiency

- Vitamin K deficiency can occur in alligators fed marginal diets and placed on long-term antibiotics. Clinical signs are similar to clotting deficiency in mammals.
- Gingival bleeding is an early sign.
- Treat with vitamin K and improve diet. Stop administration of antibiotic if possible.

Caiman Pox

Caiman pox is seen in caimans and Nile crocodiles. It is caused by a pox virus. Clinical signs include gray-white, circular, multifocal "pox-type" lesions that can be widespread on integument. Lesions may coalesce into diffuse necrotizing patches and cause digital necrosis. Proliferative oral lesions also can be seen.

- Diagnosis is made on histopathology in which large intracytoplasmic inclusions bodies are visualized in the epithelial cells.
- No treatment, other than supportive care, is available. Quarantine individuals with active lesions.

Coccidia: Eimeria spp.

- *Coccidia* causes necrotizing enteritis in young crocodiles.
- Diagnosis is made on routine fecal or cloacal swab. Treat with a sulfa antibiotic. Mortality can be high in dense populations.

SUPPLEMENTAL READINGS

Carpenter JW, Mashima TY, Rupiper DJ: Exotic Animal Formulary. Manhattan, KS: Graystone Publications, 1996.
Mader DR, Reptile Medicine and Surgery. Philadelphia: WB Saunders Co, 1996.

Appendix

Drug Dosage Guidelines
for Dogs and Cats

Acepromazine
0.05–0.2 mg/kg IV, 0.1–0.3 mg/kg, IM, SC (maximum 3 mg)
0.5–2.0 mg/kg q6–8h PO

Acetazolamide
Diamox
5–10 mg/kg q8–12h PO
Glaucoma: 4–8 mg/kg q8–12h PO

Acetylcysteine
Mucomyst
Antidote: 140 mg/kg (loading dose) PO, IV, then 70 mg/kg q4h for 5 doses
Eye: 2% solution topically q2h

Acetylsalicylic acid (aspirin)
Analgesic:
    Dog: 10–25 mg/kg q8–12h PO
Anti-inflammatory:
    Dog: 20–40 mg/kg q12h PO
    Cat: 10–20 mg/kg q48h PO
Antiplatelet:
    Dog: 5–10 mg/kg q24–48h PO
    Cat: 80 mg q48h PO

ACTH
See Corticotropin gel (ACTH)

Actinomycin D
Cosmegen
0.7 mg/m^2 IV (consult anticancer protocol for intervals)

Activated charcoal
See Charcoal, activated

Albendazole
Valbazen
    Dog: 25 mg/kg q12h PO for 2 days for giardia

Allopurinol
Zyloprim
10 mg/kg q8h then reduce to 10 mg/kg q24h

Aluminum carbonate gel
Basaljel
Phosphate binder: 10–30 mg/kg q8h PO (with meals)

Aluminum hydroxide gel
Amphojel
Phosphate binder: 10–30 mg/kg q8h PO (with meals)

Amikacin
Amiglyde-V
5–10 mg/kg q8h IV, IM, SC

Aminopentamide
Centrine
    Dog: 0.01–0.03 mg/kg q8–12h IM, SC, PO
    Cat: 0.02 mg/kg q8–12h IM, SC, PO

Aminophylline
    Dog: 10 mg/kg q8h PO, IM, IV
    Cat: 6.6 mg/kg q12h PO

5-aminosalicylic Acid
See Mesalamine; Osalazine sodium

Amitraz
Mitaban
Make a 0.025% solution (1 vial of Mitaban/2 gallons of water). Apply every 2 weeks until no viable mites are found (see Chapter 38).

Amitryptyline
Elavil
    Dog: 1–2 mg/kg q12h PO
    Cat: 5–10 mg/cat q12–24h PO

Amlodipine
Norvasc
    Cat: 0.625–1.25 mg/cat q24h PO
    Dog: 0.1–0.2 mg/kg q24h or divided q12h PO

Ammonium chloride
    Dog: 100 mg/kg q12h PO
    Cat: 800 mg/cat (approximately ¼ tsp) mixed with food daily

Amoxicillin
Amoxi-tabs
Amoxi-drops
11–22 mg/kg q8–12h PO

Amoxicillin plus clavulanate
Clavamox
    Dog: 12.5–25 mg/kg q12h PO
    Cat: 62.5 mg/cat q12h PO

Amphotericin B deoxycholate
Fungizone
0.25–0.5 mg/kg q48h IV (slow infusion), 3 times per week to a cumulative dose of 8–12 mg/kg in dogs and 4–8 mg/kg in cats

Amphotericin B lipid complex
AmBisome, Amphocil, Abelcet
1.0 mg/kg q48h IV, 3 times per week to a cumulative dose of 12 mg/kg

Ampicillin
Omnipen
10–20 mg/kg q6–8h IV, IM, SC (ampicillin sodium)
Principen
20–40 mg/kg q8h PO

Ampicillin trihydrate
Polyflex
6.5 mg/kg q12h, IM, SC

Amprolium
Amprol
Corid
1.25 g of 20% amprolium powder added to daily feed, or 30 ml of 9.6% amprolium solution to 3.8 L of drinking water for 7 days

Amrinone lactate
Inocor
1–3 mg/kg IV (loading dose) followed by 30–100 μg/kg/min IV infusion

Antacid drugs
See Aluminum hydroxide gel; Calcium carbonate; Magnesium hydroxide

Apomorphine hydrochloride
0.02–0.04 mg/kg IV, IM; 0.1 mg/kg SC; or instill 0.25 mg in conjunctiva of eye (dissolve 6-mg tablet in 1–2 ml of saline)

Ascorbic acid (vitamin C)
Diet supplement or for copper toxicity 100–500 mg/animal qd
Acetaminophen toxicity 30 mg/kg q6h for seven treatments, PO, SC

L-Asparaginase
Elspar
10,000–30,000 IU/m² IM, SC, or IP as needed (pretreat with antihistamines, steroids); see Chapter 24.

Aspirin
See Acetylsalicylic acid

Atenolol
Tenormin
    Dog: 6.25–25 mg/dog q12h PO
    Cat: 6.25–12.5 mg/cat q24h PO

Atracurium besylate
Tracrium
0.2 mg/kg IV initially, then 0.15 mg/kg q30min (or IV infusion at 3–8 μg/kg/min)

Atropine
0.02–0.04 mg/kg q6–8h IV, IM, SC
Organophosphate and carbamate toxicosis: 0.2–0.5 mg/kg (as needed)

Auranofin (triethylphosphine gold)
Ridaura
0.1–0.2 mg/kg q12h PO

Aurothioglucose
Solganal
    Dog <10 kg: 1 mg/dog IM first week, 2 mg/dog IM second week, 1 mg/kg/wk maintenance
    Dog >10 kg: 5 mg/dog IM first week, 10 mg/dog IM second week, 1 mg/kg/wk maintenance
    Cat: 0.5–1 mg/cat IM every 7 days

Azathioprine
Imuran
    Dog: 2 mg/kg q24h PO initially, then 0.5–1.0 mg/kg q48h
    Cat: 0.3–0.5 mg/kg PO, q24–48h (q48h is preferred)

AZT (azidothymidine)
See Zidovudine

BAL
See Dimercaprol

Benazepril
Lotensin
    Dog: 0.5 mg/kg q12–24h PO

Betamethasone
Celestone
Betasone
0.1–0.2 mg/kg q12–24h PO

Bethanechol chloride
Urecholine
    Dog: 2.5–25.0 mg/dog q8h PO
    Cat: 2.5–5.0 mg/cat q8h PO

Bicarbonate
See Sodium bicarbonate

Bisacodyl
Dulcolax
    Dog: 5–20 mg qd PO
    Cat: 5 mg qd PO

Bismuth subcarbonate
0.5–3.0 g q4h PO

Bismuth subsalicylate
Pepto-Bismol
1–3 ml/kg/d (in divided doses) PO

Bleomycin sulfate
Blenoxane
10 U/m² IV or SC for 3 days, then 10 U/m² weekly (maximum cumulative dose: 200 U/m²)

Bromide
See Potassium bromide

Bunamidine
Scolaban
20–50 mg/kg PO

Bupivacaine hydrochloride
Marcaine
0.5 mg/kg epidural

Buprenorphine
Temgesic
0.005 mg/kg q4–8h IV, IM

Buspirone
BuSpar
Cat: 2.5–5 mg/cat q12–24h PO

Butorphanol
Torbutrol
Torbugesic
>   Dog: Analgesic: 0.1–0.2 mg/kg IV, 0.1–0.4 mg/kg
>   IM or SC Antitussive: 0.55–1.1 mg/kg PO
>   q6–12h, 0.055–0.11 mg/kg SC q6–12h
>   Cat: Analgesic: 0.05–0.2 mg/kg IV, 0.1–0.3
>   mg/kg IM, SC

Calcitonin
Calcimar
4–6 IU/kg SC initially q12h, then q8h for
    hypercalcemia

Calcitriol
Rocaltrol
2–3 ng/kg/d divided q12h for 3–4 days, then 1–2
    ng/kg/d maintenance

Calcium carbonate
25–50 mg/kg/d PO
Camalox
60–100 mg/kg/d (in divided doses) as phosphate
    binder

Calcium chloride (10% solution)
Hypocalcemia: 5–15 mg/kg/h IV

Calcium citrate
>   Cat: 10–30 mg/kg q8h (with meals) PO

Calcium disodium EDTA
See Edetate calcium disodium (CaNa$_2$, EDTA)

Calcium gluconate (10% solution)
0.5–1.5 ml/kg IV (slowly)
Calcium gluconate tablets
25–50 mg/kg/day PO

Calcium lactate
25–50 mg/kg/d PO

Captan
0.25% solution topically, 2–3 times/wk

Captopril
Capoten
>   Dog: 0.5–2.0 mg/kg q8–12h PO
>   Cat: 3.12–6.25 mg/cat q8h PO

Carbenicillin disodium
Geopen
Pyopen
40–50 mg/kg q6–8h IV, IM, SC

Carbenicillin indanyl sodium
Geocillin
Urinary tract infections: 10 mg/kg q8h PO

Carbimazole
Neo-mercazole
>   Cat: 5 mg/cat q8h PO (induction), followed by 5
>   mg/cat q12h PO

Carboplatin
Paraplatin
>   Dog: 250–300 mg/m^2 q3wk IV
>   Cat: 150–250 mg/m^2 q4wk IV

Carnitine
See Levo-carnitine

Carprofen
Rimadyl
>   Dog: 2 mg/kg q12h PO

Castor oil
>   Dog: 8–30 ml/dog qd PO
>   Cat: 4–10 ml/cat qd PO

Cefadroxil
Cefa-Tabs
Cefa-Drops
>   Dog: 22 mg/kg q12h PO
>   Cat: 22 mg/kg q24h PO

Cefazolin sodium
Ancef
Kefzol
20–25 mg/kg q6–8h IV, IM

Cefmetazole sodium
Zefazone
15 mg/kg q8h IV, IM, SC

Cefotaxime sodium
Claforan
20–80 mg/kg q6h IV, IM

Cefoxitin sodium
Mefoxin
15–30 mg/kg q6–8h IV

Cephalexin
Keflex
10–30 mg/kg q6–12h PO

Cephalothin sodium
Keflin
10–30 mg/kg q4–8h IV, IM

Cephapirin sodium
Cefadyl
10–30 mg/kg q4–8h IV, IM

Cephradine
Velosef
10–25 mg/kg q6–8h PO

Charcoal, activated
Acta-Char
SuperChar Vet/Powder or Vet/Liquid
Toxiban
1–4 g/kg PO (granules)
6–12 ml/kg PO (suspension)

Chlorambucil
Leukeran
2–4 mg/m^2 q48h PO (see Chap. 24)
>   Cats (FIP):   20 mg/m^2 q2–3 wk PO
>   Chronic lymphocytic leukemia
>   20 mg/m^2 q1–2wks PO or 6 mg/m^2/day

Chloramphenicol
Chloromycetin
>   Dog: 30–50 mg/kg q6–8h IV, IM PO
>   Cat: 30–50 mg/cat q12h IV, IM PO

Chlorothiazide
Diuril
20–40 mg/kg q12h PO

Chlorpheniramine maleate
Phenetron
Chlor-Trimeton
    Dog: 0.4 mg/kg q8–12h PO
    Cat: 2 mg/cat q12h PO

Chlorpromazine
Thorazine
0.5 mg/kg q6–8h IM, SC, PO
Prior to cancer chemotherapy: 2 mg/kg q3h SC

Chlortetracycline
25 mg/kg q6–8h PO

Cholecalciferol (vitamin D$_3$)
500–2000 U/kg/d PO (1 mg = 40,000 U)

Chorionic gonadotropin
See Gonadotropin, chorionic (hCG)

Cimetidine
Tagamet
5–10 mg/kg q6–8h IV, IM, PO
Renal failure: 2.5–5.0 mg/kg q12h IV, PO

Ciprofloxacin
Cipro
5–15 mg/kg q12h PO

Cisapride
Propulsid
    Dog: 0.25–0.5 mg/kg q8–12h PO
    Cat: 1.0 mg/kg q8h, or 1.5 mg/kg q12h, PO

Cisplatin
Platinol
50–70 mg/m^2 q3wk IV drip (requires aggressive
    diuresis); do not use in cats

Clarithromycin
Biaxin
5 mg/kg q12h PO

Clavamox
See Amoxicillin plus clavulanate

Clavulanate
See Amoxicillin plus clavulanate

Clemastine
Tavist, Contac 12-Hr Allergy
    Dog: 0.05–0.1 mg/kg q12h PO

Clindamycin
Antirobe
Cleocin
    Dog: 5–10 mg/kg q8h PO, IV, IM
    Cat: 5.5 mg/kg q12h, or 11 mg/kg q24h
        (staphylococcal infections) PO; 11 mg/kg q12h,
        or 22 mg/kg q24h PO(anaerobic infections) PO
    Toxoplasmosis: 25–50 mg/kg/d PO (in divided
        treatments) for 2–3 weeks

Clomipramine
Anafranil, Clomicalm
1 mg/kg q12–24h PO up to a maximum dose of 3
    mg/kg q12–24h PO

Clonazepam
Klonopin
0.5 mg/kg q12h PO

Clorazepate dipotassium
Tranxene
2 mg/kg q12h PO

Clotrimazole (1%)
Lotrimin
Topical intranasal infusion; 50–60 ml per side over 1
    hour via indwelling catheter (for aspergillosis,
    penicilliosis)

Cloxacillin sodium
Cloxapen
Orbenin
Tegopen
20–40 mg/kg q8h PO

Cod liver oil
1 tsp/10 kg once daily PO

Codeine
Dog: Analgesic: 0.5–1.0 mg/kg q6–8h PO
Antitussive: 1–2 mg/kg q6–12h PO

Colchicine
0.025–0.03 mg/kg q24h PO

Corticotropin gel (ACTH)
Acthar
Response test: collect pre-ACTH sample and inject 2.2
    IU/kg IM; collect post-ACTH sample at 2 hours in
    dogs and at 1 and 2 hours in cats

Cosyntropin
Cortrosyn
Response test: collect pre-ACTH sample and inject
    0.25 mg IV in dogs and 0.125 mg IV in cats; collect
    post-ACTH sample at 1 hour

Cyanocobalamin (vitamin B$_{12}$)
    Dog: 100–200 µg/dog qd PO
    Cat: 50–100 µg/cat qd PO

Cyclophosphamide
Cytoxan
Anticancer therapy: 50 mg/m^2 q48h PO, or 50 mg/m^2
    once daily 4 days/week PO, or 100–300 mg/m^2 IV
    and repeat in 21 days (see Chap. 24)
Immunosuppressive therapy: 50 mg/m^2 q48h PO (see
    Chap. 22)
    Cat: 200 mg/m^2 q2–3wk PO (see Chap. 22)

Cyclosporine
Sandimmune, Neoral, Optimmune ointment
    Dog: 10 mg/kg q12h PO
    Cat: 5 mg/kg q12h PO to 15 mg/kg q24h (adjust
        dose via monitoring)
Perianal fistulae: 1.75–3.0 mg/kg q12h PO
Topical treatment for keratoconjunctivitis sicca: 1–2%
    solution in oil: instill 1 drop in eye q12hr

Cyclothiazide
Anhydron
0.5–1.0 mg/kg q24h PO

Cyproheptadine
Periactin
Antihistamine: 0.5–1.0 mg/kg q12h PO
Appetite stimulant in cat: 2 mg/cat q12h PO

Cytosine arabinoside
Cytosar
>Dog: 100 mg/m² once daily for 4 days IV, SC
>   (lymphoma) q3–4wk (see Chap. 24)
>Cat: 100 mg/m² IV or SC once daily for 2 days
>   (see Chap. 24)

Dacarbazine
DTIC
>Dog: 1000 mg/m² IV drip for 6–8 hours, repeat
>   q3wk (see Chap. 28)

Danazol
Danocrine
5–10 mg/kg q12h PO

Dantrolene sodium
Dantrium
>Dog: 1–5 mg/kg q8h PO
>Cat: 0.5–2.0 mg/kg q12h PO

Dapsone
1.1 mg/kg q8h PO

Deferoxamine mesylate
Desferal
10 mg/kg IV, IM q2h for 2 doses, then 10 mg/kg q8h
   for 24 hours

Delta-Albaplex (novobiocin plus prednisolone plus tetracycline hydrochloride)
>Dog 3–7 kg: 1–2 tablets/d PO
>Dog 7–14 kg: 2–4 tablets/d PO
>Dog 14–27 kg: 4–6 tablets/d PO
>Dog >27 kg: 6–8 tablets/d PO
>Cat: 1 tablet q12h PO

Deprenyl (L-deprenyl, selegiline)
Anipryl
>Dog: 1 mg/kg q24h PO

Derm Caps (omega fatty acid)
1 capsule/9.1 kg daily PO

Desmopressin acetate
DDAVP
Diabetes insipidus: 2–4 drops q12–24h intranasally
von Willebrand's disease: 1.0 µg/kg SC, IV, diluted in
   20 ml saline over 10 minutes

Desoxycorticosterone pivalate (DOCP)
Percorten-V
1.5–2.2 mg/kg q25d IM

Dexamethasone
Azium
Anti-inflammatory: 0.1–0.2 mg/kg q12–24h IV, IM, PO
Shock: 2.2–4.4 mg/kg IV

Dexamethasone sodium phosphate
Shock: 1–2 mg/kg IV

Dextran-70
Gentran-70
10–20 ml/kg IV q24h to effect

Dextromethorphan
Benylin DM and others
0.5–2.0 mg/kg q6–8h PO

Dextrose (5% solution)
40–50 ml/kg q24h IV

Diazepam
Valium
Preanesthetic: 0.1–0.25 mg/kg IV, IM, SC
Status epilepticus: 0.25–0.5 mg/kg IV; repeat if
   necessary; 1 mg/kg rectally
Appetite stimulant in cat: 0.1–0.2 mg/kg IV
   (q12–24h as needed)
Functional urethral obstruction in dogs:
   2–10 mg/dog q8h PO
Urinary disorder in cat: 1.25–2.5 mg/cat q8–12h PO

Diclorophene
See Toluene

Dichlorphenamide
Daranide
2–4 mg/kg q8–12h PO

Dichlorvos
Performer
>Dog: 26.4–33 mg/kg PO
>Cat: 11 mg/kg PO

Dicloxacillin
Dynapen
11–55 mg/kg q8h

Diethylcarbamazine
Caricide
Filaribits
Heartworm prophylaxis: 6.6 mg/kg q24h PO

Diethylstilbestrol (DES)
Urinary incontinence (dog): 0.1–1.0 mg/dog q24h PO
   for 3 days, then 1 mg/wk PO

Digitoxin
Crystodigin
0.02–0.03 mg/kg q8h PO

Digoxin
Lanoxin
Cardoxin
>Dog: 0.22 mg/m² q12h PO, 0.0055–0.01 mg/kg
>   q12h PO, (reduce dose by 10% for elixir)
>Cat: 0.01 mg/kg q48h, 0.007 mg/kg q48h (with
>   Lasix and aspirin)

Dihydrotachysterol (vitamin D)
Hytakerol
DHT
Initial: 0.02–0.03 mg/kg/day PO
   maintenance: 0.01–0.02 mg/kg q24–48h PO

Diltiazem hydrochloride
Cardizem
>Dog: 0.5–1.5 mg/kg q8h PO
>Cat: 1.75–2.4 mg/kg q8–12h PO
Dilacor XR
>Cat: 30 mg/cat q12–24h PO
Cardizem CD
>Cat: 10 mg/kg q24hr PO

Dimenhydrinate
Dramamine (U.S.)
Gravol (Canada)
>Dog: 4–8 mg/kg q8h IV, IM, PO
>Cat: 12.5 mg q8h IV, IM, PO

Dimercaprol
BAL in oil
4 mg/kg q4h IM

Dinoprost tromethamine
See Prostaglandin $F_{2\alpha}$

Dioctyl calcium sulfosuccinate
See Docusate calcium

Dioctyl sodium sulfosuccinate
See Docusate sodium

Diphenhydramine hydrochloride
Benadryl
2.2 mg/kg q8–12h IV, IM, PO

Diphenoxylate hydrochloride
Lomotil
> Dog: 0.1–0.2 mg/kg q8–12h PO
> Cat: 0.05–0.1 mg/kg q12h PO

Diphenylhydantoin
See Phenytoin

Diphosphonate disodium etidronate
See Etidronate disodium

Dipyridamole
Persantine
4–10 mg/kg q24h PO

Disopyramide phosphate
Norpace
> Dog: 6–15 mg/kg q8h PO

Dithiazanine iodide
Dizan
6.6–11.0 mg/kg q24h PO for 7–10 days

Divalproex sodium
Depakote
Equivalent to valproic acid (see Valproic acid)

Dobutamine
Dobutrex
Prepare 250 mg in 1 L 5% dextrose
> Dog: 2.5–20 μg/kg/min IV infusion
> Cat: 2.5–5.0 μg/kg/min IV infusion

Docusate calcium
Surfak
Doxidan
> Dog: 50–100 mg/dog q12–24h PO
> Cat: 50 mg/cat q12–24h PO

Docusate sodium
Colace
> Dog: 50–200 mg/dog q8–12h PO
> Cat: 50 mg/cat q12–24h PO

Dopamine hydrochloride
Intropin
2–10 μg/kg/min IV infusion (prepare 40 mg in 500 ml lactated Ringer's solution)

Doxapram hydrochloride
Dopram
5–10 mg/kg IV
Neonate: 1–5 mg SC, sublingually, or via umbilical vein

Doxorubicin
Adriamycin
> Dogs ≤ 10 kg and cats: 20–25 mg/m^2 IV q3wk
> Dogs > 10 kg: 30 mg/m^2 IV q3wk (maximum cumulative dose 180–240 mg/m^2) (see Chap. 24)

Doxycycline
Vibramycin
3–5 mg/kg q12h PO
Lyme borreliosis:
10 mg/kg q12h PO

Edetate calcium disodium (CaEDTA)
Havidote
25 mg/kg q6h SC for 2–5 days

Edrophonium chloride
Tensilon
> Dog: 0.11–0.22 mg/kg IV
> Cat: 2.5 mg/cat IV

Enalapril maleate
Vasotec
> Dog: 0.5 mg/kg q12–24h PO
> Cat: 0.25–0.5 mg/kg q12–24h PO

Enflurane
Ethrane
2–3% (induction); 1.5–3% (maintenance)

Enilconazole
Imaverol
Nasal aspergillosis: 10 mg/kg q12h instilled into nasal sinus for 10–14 days (10% solution diluted 50:50 with water)
Dermatophytes: solution diluted to 0.2% and lesion washed with solution 4 times at 3- to 4-day intervals

Enrofloxacin
Baytril
2.5–5.0 mg/kg q12h PO, IM, SC, or 5–10 mg/kg q24h PO, IM

Ephedrine
Urinary incontinence
> Dog: 5–15 mg/dog q8h PO
> Cat: 2–4 mg/cat q8h PO
Bronchodilator: 1–2 mg/kg q8h PO

Epinephrine
Adrenalin
20 μg/kg, or 0.1–0.5 ml of 1:1000 (1 mg/ml) solution; or 1–5 ml of a 1:10,000 (0.1 mg/ml) solution IV, IM, SC, IC, intratracheally

Epsiprantel
Cestex
> Dog: 5.5 mg/kg PO
> Cat: 2.75 mg/kg PO

Epsom salt
See Magnesium sulfate

Ergocalciferol (vitamin D$_2$)
Calciferol
Initial: 4000–6000 U/kg/d PO
Maintenance: 1000–2000 U/kg q24h–q7d PO (see Chap. 30)

Erythromycin
Antibiotic: 10–20 mg/kg q8–12h PO
Promotility: 0.5–1.0 mg/kg q8h PO

Erythropoietin (r-HuEPO)
Epogen
75–100 U/kg SC 3 times weekly (adjust dose to reach
and maintain hematocrit of 30–34%)

Essential fatty acids
(See also Omega fatty acids)
EFA-Z Plus
<6.7 kg: 3.7 ml/d PO
6.7–22.5 kg: 7 ml/d PO
>22.5 kg: 14 ml/d PO

Estradiol cypionate (ECP)
Depo-Estradiol
    Dog: 0.02–0.04 mg/kg IM (total dose not to
       exceed 1.0 mg) within 3 days of mating
    Cat: 0.25 mg/cat IM within 3 days of mating
Use of ECP for mismating is discouraged

Ethanol (20%)
For ethylene glycol toxicity:
    Dogs: 5.5 ml/kg IV q4h for 5 treatments, then
       q6h for 4 treatments
    Cats: 5.0 ml/kg IV q6h for 5 treatments, then
       q8h for 4 treatments

Ethoxzolamide
Cardrase
Glaucoma: 4 mg/kg q8–12h PO

Etidronate disodium
Didronel
5–10 mg/kg q12–24h PO

Etodolac
    Dog: 10–15 mg/kg q24h PO

Etomidate
1–4 mg/kg IV

Etretinate
Tegison
    Dog: 0.75–1 mg/kg q24h PO
    Cat: 2 mg/kg q24h PO

Famotidine
Pepcid
0.5–1.0 mg/kg q12–24h IM, SC, IV, PO

Febantel
Rintal
10 mg/kg q24h for 3 days PO

Febantel plus praziquantel
RM-Parasitacide; Drontal-Plus
15 mg/kg FEB + 1.5 mg/kg PRA, PO, for 3 days

Felbamate
Initially 20 mg/kg q8h PO (maximum dose: 3000
mg/d) (see Chap. 146)

Fenbendazole
Panacur
    50 mg/kg/d for 3 days PO

Fentanyl
Sublimaze
0.02–0.04 mg/kg IV, IM, SC, or 0.01 mg/kg IV, IM, SC
(with acetylpromazine or diazepam)
Analgesia: 0.002–0.005 mg/kg IV; 0.004–0.008 mg/kg
IM, SC

Fentanyl transdermal patch
Duragesic
    Dog: <10 kg, 25 µg/h, q72h
           10–20 kg, 50 µg/h, q72h
           20–30 kg, 75 µg/h, q72h
           >30 kg, 100 µg/h, q72h
    Cat: 25 µg/h, q118h

Ferrous sulfate
    Dog: 100–300 mg/dog q24h PO
    Cat: 50–100 mg/cat q24h PO

Fluconazole
Diflucan
2.5–5.0 mg/kg q12–24h PO or IV (double loading
dose on day 1)
(for CNS Cryptococcus: 10–15 mg/kg q12–24h)

Flucytosine
Ancobon
Cryptococcosis: 50 mg/kg q8h or 75 mg/kg q12h, PO
combined with Amphotericin B

Fludrocortisone acetate
Florinef Acetate
    Dog: 0.2–0.8 mg/dog (0.02 mg/kg) q24h PO
    Cat: 0.1 mg/cat q24h PO

Flumethasone
Flucort
    Dog: 0.0625–0.25 mg/dog q24h IV, IM, SC, PO
    Cat: 0.03–0.125 mg/cat q24h IV, IM, SC, PO
Anti-inflammatory: 0.15–0.3 mg/kg q12–24h IV, IM,
SC, PO

Flunixin meglumine
Banamine
1.1 mg/kg once IV, IM, SC, or 1.1 mg/kg/d for
3 days/wk PO
Ophthalmic: 0.5–1.0 mg/kg once IV

Fluorouracil
5-Fluorouracil
    Dog: 150–200 mg/m^2 q7d IV
    Cat: do not use

Fluoxetin
Prozac
    Dog: 0.5–1.0 mg/kg q24h PO
    Cat: 0.5–4 mg/cat q24h PO

Folic acid
Folvite
    Dog and cat: 0.004–0.01 mg/kg/d (4–10
      µg/kg/d)

Follicle-stimulating hormone (FSH)
See Urofollitropin

Furazolidone
Furoxone
4 mg/kg q12h for 7–10 days PO

Furosemide
Lasix
  Dog: 2–6 mg/kg q8–12h (or as needed) IV, IM, SC, PO
  Cat: 1–4 mg/kg q12h IV, IM, SC, PO

Gentamicin sulfate
Gentocin
  Dog: 2–4 mg/kg q6–8h IV, IM, SC, or 6 mg/kg q24h
  Cat: 3 mg/kg q8hr IV, IM, SC

Glipizide
Glucotrol
  Cat: 2.5–5 mg/cat q8–12h with food

Glucosamine chondroitin sulfate
Cosequin and others
  Dog: 1–2 RS (Regular Strength) capsules/d (2–4 capsules of DS (Double Strength) for large dogs)
  Cat: 1 RS capsule/d

Glyburide (Glibenclamide)
Diaβeta
Micronase
0.2 mg/kg daily PO

Glycerin
Glyrol
Osmoglyn
Glaucoma: 1–1.5 gm/kg PO initially, then 500 mg/kg q8h; or 1–2 ml of 50% solution q8h

Glycopyrrolate
Robinul-V
0.005–0.01 mg/kg IV, IM, SC q8–12h as needed

Gold sodium thiomalate
Myochrysine
Immune-mediated arthritis: 1 mg/kg once weekly IM

Gonadorelin (GnRH, LHRH)
Factrel
  Dog: 50–100 µg/dog q24–48h IM
  Cat: 25 µg/cat once IM

Gonadotropin, chorionic (hCG)
Follutein
  Dog: 22 U/kg q24–48h IM, or 44 U/kg once IM
  Cat: 250 U/cat once IM

Gonadotropin-releasing hormone
See Gonadorelin

Griseofulvin (microsize)
Fulvicin U/F powder or tablets
50 mg/kg q24h PO (maximum dose: 110–132 mg/kg/d in divided treatments)

Griseofulvin (ultramicrosize)
Fulvicin P/G
5–10 mg/kg/d PO (in divided treatments)

Growth hormone
0.1 U/kg 3 times/wk for 4–6 weeks

Halothane
Fluothane
3% (induction); 0.5–1.5% (maintenance) (see Chap. 2)

Heparin sodium
Liquaemin (U.S.)
Hepalean (Canada)
100–200 U/kg IV, loading dose; then 100–300 U/kg q6–8h SC (monitor clotting profiles)
Low-dose therapy (dog and cat): 70 U/kg q8–12h SC

Hetacillin potassium
Hetacin-K
20–40 mg/kg q8h PO

Hetastarch
See Hydroxyethyl starch

Hydralazine
Apresoline
  Dog: 0.5 mg/kg (initial dose), titrated to 0.5–2.0 mg/kg q12h PO
  Cat: 2.5–5 mg/cat q12–24h PO

Hydrochlorothiazide
Hydrodiuril
2–4 mg/kg q12h PO

Hydrocodone
Hycodan
  Dog: 0.22 mg/kg q6–12h PO

Hydrocortisone
Cortef
Replacement therapy: 1 mg/kg q12h PO
Anti-inflammatory: 2.5–5.0 mg/kg q12h PO

Hydrocortisone sodium succinate
Solu-Cortef
Shock: 50–150 mg/kg IV

Hydroxyethyl starch
Hetastarch
  Dog: 20 ml/kg/24h (5 ml/kg over 15 min for hypovolemia) (see Chap. 5)
  Cat: 10 ml/kg/24h (2.5 ml/kg over 15 min for hypovolemia) (see Chap. 5)

Hydroxyurea
Hydrea
For polycythemia vera: 30 mg/kg/d for 1 week, then 15 mg/kg/d until remission

Hydroxyzine
Atarax
  Dog: 2.2 mg/kg q8–12h PO
  Cat: 10 mg/cat q12h PO

Imidocarb
5 mg/kg IM SC once and repeated in 14 days

Imipramine
  Dog: 1 mg/kg q8h PO
  Cat: 2.5–5.0 mg/cat q12h PO

Insulin (NPH isophane)
  Dog: 0.5–1.0 U/kg q12–24h SC (to effect)
  Cat: 1–5 U/cat q12h SC (to effect)
    (see Chap. 32)

Insulin (PZI)
  Dog: 0.5–1.0 U/kg q12–24h SC (to effect)
  Cat: 1–5 units/cat (0.2–1.0 U/kg) q12–24h SC
    (adjust with monitoring)
    (see Chap. 32)

Insulin (regular crystalline)
Ketoacidosis:
 See Chapter 32 for complete treatment protocol

Insulin, ultralente
 Dog: 0.5–1.0 U/kg q12–24h SC (to effect)
 Cat: 1–5 U/cat q12–24h SC (to effect) (see
 Chap. 32)

Interferon-alpha
Roferon A; Intron A (dilute to 30 U/ml)
 Cat: 30 U/cat q24h for 7 days on alternating
 weeks

Iodide
See Potassium iodide

Ipecac syrup
 Dog: 1–2 ml/kg up to 15 ml PO
 Cat: 2–6 ml/cat PO

Iron
See Ferrous sulfate

Isoflurane
3.5% (induction); 1.5–2.5% (maintenance)
(see Chap. 2)

Isoproterenol
Isuprel
0.04–0.09 µg/kg/min IV; 0.1–0.2 mg/dog q4–6h
 IM, SC

Isosorbide dinitrate
Isordil
Sorbitrate
2.5–5 mg/animal q12h PO

Isotretinoin
Accutane
1–3 mg/kg/d (maximum dose: 3–4 mg/kg/d) PO

Itraconazole
Sporanox
 Dog: 5 mg/kg q12–24h PO
 Cat: 5–10 mg/kg q12h PO, or 20 mg/kg q24h

Ivermectin
Heartgard
Ivomec
Heartworm preventive in dog: 6 µg/kg q30d PO
 Cat: 24 µg/kg q30d PO
Microfilaricide in dog: 50 µg/kg PO 3–4 weeks after
 adulticide therapy
Ectoparasite therapy: 300–600 µg/kg q24h IM, SC, PO
 (do not use in collie and sheltie dogs)
Respiratory parasites: 200–400 µg/kg weekly SC, PO
 (do not use in collie and sheltie dogs)

Kanamycin sulfate
Kantrim
10 mg/kg q6–8h IV, IM, SC

Kaolin plus pectin
Kaopectate
1–2 ml/kg q2–6h PO

Ketamine
Ketalar
Ketaset
 Cat: 4–10 mg/kg IV, 10–20 mg/kg IM, SC (see
 Chap 2)
 Dog: 1 ml/10 kg IV of ketamine:diazepam
 mixture (50:50)

Ketoconazole
Nizoral
 Dog: 10–15 mg/kg q12h PO (*Malassezia canis*
 infection: 10 mg/kg q24h or 5 mg/kg q12h PO)
 Hyperadrenocorticism: 15 mg/kg q12h PO
 Cat: 5–10 mg/kg q8–12h PO

Ketoprofen
Ketofen
 Dog: 1.1 mg/kg q24h IV, PO for up to 5 days

Lactated Ringer's solution
40–50 ml/kg/d IV for maintenance requirements
Shock therapy:
 Dog: 90 ml/kg IV
 Cat: 60 ml/kg IV

Lactulose
Cephulac; Duphalac
Constipation: 1 ml/4.5 kg q8h PO (to effect)
Hepatic encephalopathy
 Dog: 0.5 ml/kg q8h PO
 Cat: 2.5–5.0 ml/cat q8h PO

Leucovorin (folinic acid)
Wellcovorin
With methotrexate administration: 3 mg/m² IV, IM,
 PO
Antidote for pyrimethamine toxicosis: 1 mg/kg q24h
 PO

Levamisole
Levasole
Tramisol
 Dog: 5–8 mg/kg PO once, up to 10 mg/kg PO
 for 2 days (hookworms); 10 mg/kg q24h PO for
 6–10 days (microfilaricide); 0.5–2.0 mg/kg
 3 times/wk PO (immunostimulant)
 Cat: 4.4 mg/kg PO once

Levo-carnitine
 Dog: 50 mg/kg q8h PO
 Cat: 250–500 mg/cat qd PO

Levodopa (L-dopa)
Larodopa
Hepatic encephalopathy: 6.8 mg/kg initially, then 1.4
 mg/kg q6h

Levothyroxine sodium
Soloxine
Thyro-Tabs
Synthroid
 Dog: 0.01–0.02 mg/kg q12h, PO
 Cat: 0.01–0.02 mg/kg q24h, PO

Lidocaine
Xylocaine
    Antiarrhythmia in dog: 2–4 mg/kg IV
        (maximum dose: 8 mg/kg over 10 min);
        25–75 µg/kg/min IV infusion;
        6 mg/kg q1.5h IM
    Cat: 0.25–0.75 mg/kg IV, slowly

Lime sulfur (2–3% solution)
Topically once/wk for 4–6 weeks

Lincomycin
Lincocin
15–25 mg/kg q12h IV, IM, PO

Liothyronine
Cytobin or Cytomel
4.4 µg/kg q8h PO
Suppression testing: See Chapter 29 for protocol

Lisinopril
Prinivil
    Dog: 0.25–0.5 mg/kg q12–24h

Lithium carbonate
Lithotabs
    Dog: 10 mg/kg q12h PO
    Cat: not recommended

Loperamide
Imodium
    Dog: 0.1–0.2 mg/kg q8–12h PO
    Cat: 0.1–0.3 mg/kg q12–24h PO

Lufenuron
Program
Flea control
    Dog: 10mg/kg q30d PO
    Cat: 30mg/kg q30d PO
Coccidioidomycosis
5 mg/kg PO q24h

Luteinizing hormone
See Gonadorelin

Magnesium citrate
Citroma, Citro-Nesia (U.S.)
Citro-Mag (Canada)
2–4 ml/kg PO

Magnesium hydroxide
Milk of Magnesia
Antacid: 5–10 ml per dog or cat PO
Cathartic:
    Dog: 15–50 ml/dog PO
    Cat: 2–6 ml/cat q24h PO

Magnesium sulfate
    Dog: 8–25 g/dog q24h PO
    Cat: 2–5 g/cat q24h PO

Mannitol
Osmitrol
Diuretic: 1 g/kg of 5–25% solution IV
Glaucoma or CNS edema: 0.5–1.0 g/kg of 15–25%
    solution over 15–60 minutes IV (repeat in 4–6 hours
    if necessary)

Marbofloxacin
Marbocyl, Zeniquin
    Dog: 2.75–5.55 mg/kg q24h PO

Mebendazole
Telmintic
22 mg/kg (with food) q24h for 3 days

Meclizine hydrochloride
Bonine
    Dog: 25 mg/dog q24h PO (motion sickness:
        administer 1 hour before traveling)
    Cat: 12.5 mg/cat q24h PO

Meclofenamic acid
Meclomen
Meclofen
Arquel
    Dog: 1 mg/kg/d for 5 days, then 0.5 mg/kg
        q24h PO

Medetomidine
Domitor
    Dog: 0.007–0.02 mg/kg IV; 0.01–0.04 mg/kg IM,
        SC
    Cat: 0.01–0.03 mg/kg IV; 0.03–0.08 mg/kg IM,
        SC

Medium-chain triglycerides (MCTs)
MCT oil
1–2 ml/kg daily in food

Medroxyprogesterone acetate
Depo-Provera
1.1–2.2 mg/kg q7d IM

Megestrol acetate
Ovaban
    Dog: Proestrus: 2.2 mg/kg q24h PO for 8 days
        Anestrus: 0.55 mg/kg q24h PO for 30 days
        Behavior problems: 2–4 mg/kg q24h for 8 days
        (reduce dose for maintenance)
    Cat: dermatologic therapy or urine spraying:
        2.5–5.0 mg/cat q24h PO for 1 week, then
        reduce to 2.5–5.0 mg once or twice/wk; suppress
        estrus: 5 mg/cat for 3 days, then 2.5–5 mg
        once/wk for 10 weeks

Melarsomine
Immiticide
    Dog: 2.5 mg/kg, IM, q24h for 2 doses,
        Alternate: 2.5 mg/kg, IM once; then after 1–2
        months give 2.5 mg/kg IM, q24h for 2
        additional doses

Melphalan
Alkeran
2–4 mg/m^2 q24–48h PO (see Chap. 24)

Meperidine
Demerol
    Dog: 0.4–2 mg/kg IV, 1.0–4.0 mg/kg IM, SC

6-Mercaptopurine
Purinethol
50 mg/m^2 q24h PO

Mesalamine
Asacol; Pentasa
    Dogs: 20 mg/kg q8–12h PO
(See also Osalazine sodium; Sulfasalazine)

Metaproterenol
Alupent
Metaprel
0.325–0.65 mg/kg q4–6h PO

Metaraminol bitartrate
Aramine
0.1 mg/kg IM, SC

Methazolamide
Neptazane
 2–4 mg/kg q8–12h PO

Methenamine hippurate
Hiprex
 Dog: 500 mg/dog q12h PO
 Cat: 250 mg/cat q12h PO

Methenamine mandelate
Mandelamine
10–20 mg/kg q8–12h PO

Methimazole
Tapazole
 Cat: 2.5 mg/cat q8–12h PO (initial), increase to
  5–10 mg/cat q8–12h PO by monitoring T4

Methionine (L-methionine, DL-methionine)
Uroeze
Methio-Form
 Dog: 150–300 mg/kg/d PO
 Cat: 1000–1500 mg/cat PO (added to food each
  day) (use in adult cats only)

Methocarbamol
Robaxin-V
44 mg/kg q8h PO on the first day, then 22–44 mg/kg
 q8h PO

Methotrexate (MTX)
2.5 mg/m^2 q24h PO; or 2–3 times per week;
15–20 mg/m^2 IV q3wk (see Chap. 24)

Methoxamine
Vasoxyl
200–250 µg/kg IM, or 40–80 µg/kg IV

Methoxyflurane
Metofane
3.5% (induction); 0.5–1.5% (maintenance)
(see Chap. 2)

Methscopolamine bromide
Pamine
0.3–1.0 mg/kg q8h PO (use cautiously in cats)

Methylene blue (1% solution)
 Dog: for pancreatic tumor identification:
  3 mg/kg IV slowly, diluted in isotonic saline
  (can cause hemolytic anemia)
 Cat: do not use

Methylprednisolone
Medrol
 Dog: 0.22–0.44 mg/kg q12–24h PO

Methylprednisolone acetate
Depo-Medrol
 Dog: 1 mg/kg IM q1–3 wk
 Cat: 10–20 mg/cat IM q1–3wk

Methylprednisolone sodium succinate
Solu-Medrol
For spinal cord trauma: 30 mg/kg IV, repeat at 15
 mg/kg IV in 2–6 hours

4-Methylpyrazole (fomepizole)
Antizol-Vet
20 mg/kg initially IV, then 15 mg/kg at 12- and
 24-hour intervals, then 5 mg/kg at 36h.

Methyltestosterone
Android
Fluoxymestrone
 Dog: 1.0 mg/kg q48h PO
(see also Testosterone cypionate; Testosterone
 propionate), for sex hormone dematoses in dogs: 1
 mg/kg (up to 30 mg total dose)
 Cat: 1.0–2.5 mg/cat q48h PO

Metoclopramide
Reglan
Maxolon
0.2–0.5 mg/kg q6–8h IV, IM, SC, PO, or 1–2 mg/kg
 q24h via continuous IV infusion

Metoprolol tartrate
Lopressor
 Dog: 5–50 mg/dog q8h PO
 Cat: 2–15 mg/cat q8h PO

Metronidazole
Flagyl
 Dog: for giardia: 50–65 mg/kg q24h PO for 5-7
  days; Antibacterial: 10–15 mg/kg q8–12h PO
 Cat: for giardia: 50 mg/kg q24h PO for 5 days;
  Antibacterial: 10 mg/kg q8h or 15 mg/kg
  q12h PO

Mexiletine
Mexitil
 Dog: 5–8 mg/kg q8–12h PO (use cautiously)

Mibolerone
Cheque
 Dog: (2.6–5.0 µg/kg/d PO)
  0.45–11.3 kg: 30 µg
  11.8–22.7 kg: 60 µg
  23–45.3 kg: 120 µg
  >45.8 kg: 180 µg
 Cat: safe dose not established

Midazolam
Versed
0.1–0.25 mg/kg IV, IM, or 0.1–0.3 mg/kg/h IV
 infusion

Milbemycin oxime
Interceptor
 Dog: 0.5 mg/kg q30d PO

Milk of magnesia
See Magnesium hydroxide

Minocycline
Minocin
5.0–12.5 mg/kg q12h PO

Misoprostol
Cytotec
 Dog: 3–5 µg/kg q6–8h PO

Mitotane (*o,p'*-**DDD**)
Lysodren
For pituitary-dependent hyperadrenocorticism: 50
  mg/kg/d PO (may be given in divided doses) for
  5–10 days, then 50–70 mg/kg/wk PO
Adrenal tumor: 50–75 mg/kg/d for 10 days PO, then
  75–100 mg/kg/wk PO (see Chap. 31)

Mitoxantrone
Novantrone
5–6 mg/m² IV q3wk

Morphine
  Dog: 0.2–0.6 mg/kg IM, SC (as needed); 0.1
    mg/kg epidural
  Cat: 0.1 mg/kg IM, SC (as needed)

Nadolol
Corgard
0.25–0.5 mg/kg q12h PO

Nafcillin sodium
Unipen
10 mg/kg q6h IM, PO

Nalbuphine
  Dog: 0.5–2.0 mg/kg IV, IM, SC
  Cat: 0.5–1.5 mg/kg IV, IM, SC

Nalorphine
Nalline
0.44 mg/kg IV, IM, SC (1 mg for every 10 mg of
  morphine)

Naloxone
Narcan
0.003–0.01 mg/kg IV, IM, for opiate reversal

Naltrexone hydrochloride
Trexan
Behavior problems: 2.2 mg/kg q12h PO

Nandrolone decanoate
Deca-Durabolin
  Dog: 1.0–1.5 mg/kg qwk IM
  Cat: 1 mg/cat qwk IM

Neomycin
Biosol
10–20 mg/kg q6–12h PO

Neostigmine bromide
Prostigmin bromide
2 mg/kg/d PO (in divided doses, to effect)

Neostigmine methylsulfate
Prostigmin
Antimyasthenic: 10 µg/kg IM, SC, as needed (atropine
  may be administered to counteract side effects)
Antidote for curiform block: 40 µg/kg IM, SC
  (administer with atropine)
Diagnostic aid for myasthenia gravis: 40 µg/kg IM, or
  20 µg/kg IV

Nitrofurantoin
Furadantin
Macrodantin
4 mg/kg q8h PO

Nitroglycerin ointment
Nitrol Ointment
Nitro-Bid Ointment
Nitrostat Ointment
(1 inch of ointment is approximately 15 mg)
  Dog: ½–1½ inch topically q12–24h
  Cat: ¼ inch topically q12–24h

Nitroprusside
Nipride
2.5–15 µg/kg/min constant IV infusion

Nizatidine
Axid
2.5–5 mg/kg q24h PO

Norfloxacin
Noroxin
22 mg/kg q12h PO

Novobiocin
See Delta-Albaplex

Olsalazine
Dipentum
  Dog: 20–30 mg/kg q8–12h PO

Omega fatty acids
See also Derm Caps
1 capsule q12h PO (see also Essential fatty acids)

Omeprazole
Prilosec
  Dog: 20 mg/dog or 0.7–1.0 mg/kg q24h PO
  Cat: Not recommended

Ondansetron
Zofran
0.1–0.5 mg/kg q6–12h IV, SC
0.5–1.0 mg/kg q6–12h PO

***o,p'*-DDD**
See Mitotane

Ormetroprim
See Primor

Oxacillin
Prostaphlin
Bactocill
22–40 mg/kg q8h PO

Oxazepam
Serax
Appetite stimulant: 2.5 mg/cat q12h PO

Oxtriphylline
Choledyl SA
  Dog: 47 mg/kg (equivalent to 30 mg/kg
    theophylline) q12h PO

Oxybutynin chloride
Ditropan
5.0 mg/dog q8–12h PO

Oxymetholone
Anadrol
1–5 mg/kg q24h PO

Oxymorphone hydrochloride
Numorphan
Analgesia:
    Dog: 0.05–0.1 mg/kg IV
        0.1–0.3 mg/kg IM, SC
    Cat: 0.01–0.04 mg/kg IV
        0.05–0.1 mg/kg IM, SC
For preanesthesia or sedation: see Chapter 2

Oxytetracycline
Terramycin
20 mg/kg q8h PO; 7.5–10.0 mg/kg q8h IV

Oxytocin
    Dog: 5–20 units/dog IM, repeat q30min for
        primary inertia
    Cat: 3–5 units/cat IM

2-PAM
See Pralidoxime chloride

Pancreatic enzyme (pancrelipase)
Viokase
Pancrezyme
2 tsp per 20 kg body weight, or 1–3 tsp/0.45 kg of
    food, mixed with food 20 minutes prior to feeding

Pancuronium bromide
Pavulon
0.1 mg/kg IV

Paregoric
Corrective Mixture
0.05–0.06 mg/kg q12h PO (5 ml of paregoric
    corresponds to approximately 2 mg of morphine)

D-Penicillamine
Cuprimine
10–15 mg/kg q12h PO

Penicillin G potassium
20,000–40,000 U/kg q6–8h, IV, IM

Penicillin G procaine
20,000–40,000 U/kg q12–24h IM

Penicillin G sodium
20,000–40,000 U/kg q6–8h IV, IM

Penicillin V
10 mg/kg q8h PO

Pentazocine
Talwin
    Dog: 1.65–3.3 mg/kg q4h IM
    Cat: 2.2–3.3 mg/kg IV, IM, SC

Pentobarbital
Anesthesia: 25–30 mg/kg IV (first ½ of the dose
    administered rapidly, then remaining administered
    to effect)

Petrolatum, white (flavored)
Laxatone
    Cat: 1–5 ml/cat q24h PO

Phenobarbital
Luminal
    Dog: 2–8 mg/kg q12h PO
    Cat: 1–2 mg/kg q12h PO
    For seizures: Initially: 2.5 mg/kg q12h PO (see
        Chapter 146) and adjust by plasma
        concentration
    Status epilepticus (dog or cat): 10–20 mg/kg IV
        (to effect) or IV loading protocol (preferred;
        see Chapter 146)

Phenoxybenzamine hydrochloride
Dibenzyline
    Dog: 0.25–0.5 mg/kg q8h PO
    Cat: 2.5 mg/cat q8–12h PO

Phentolamine mesylate
Regitine (U.S.)
Rogitine (Canada)
0.02–0.1 mg/kg IV (as needed to maintain normal
    blood pressure)

Phenylbutazone
Butazolidin
    Dog: 10–15 mg/kg q8h PO (maximum dose: 800
        mg)
    Cat: not recommended

Phenylephrine hydrochloride
Neo-Synephrine
0.01 mg/kg q15min IV
0.1 mg/kg q15min IM, SC

Phenylpropanolamine hydrochloride
Propagest
Dexatrim
    Dog: 1–2 mg/kg q12h PO
    Cat: 1 mg/kg q12h PO

Phenytoin
Dilantin
Antiepileptic in dog: 20–35 mg/kg q8h PO
Antiarrhythmic in dog: 30 mg/kg q8h PO or 10
    mg/kg IV over 5 minutes

Phytonadione
See Vitamin K$_1$

Phytomenadione
See Vitamin K$_1$

Piperazine
44–66 mg/kg PO once

Piroxicam
Feldene
    Dog: 0.3 mg/kg q48h PO (use cautiously)
    Cat: dosage not established

Polyethylene glycol electrolyte solution
GoLYTELY
25 ml/kg, then repeat in 2–4 hours PO

Polysulfated glycosaminoglycans
Adequan
1–2 mg/kg IM once every 4 days for 7 injections

Potassium bromide
    Dog and cat: 30 mg/kg q24h PO (in food) (see
        Chap. 146)

Potassium chloride
0.5 mEq/kg/d (do not administer at a rate faster than 0.5 mEq/kg/h)
10–40 mEq/500 ml of fluids, depending on serum potassium (see Chap. 5)

Potassium citrate
Urocit-K
    Dog: 50–75 mg/kg q12h PO

Potassium gluconate
Kaon elixir
Tumil-K
2.2 mEq/100 kcal of energy/day PO
    Cat: 2–6 mEq/cat daily PO

Potassium iodide
30–100 mg/cat daily (in single or divided doses) for 10–14 days

Potassium (or sodium) phosphate (potassium or sodium)
0.01–0.03 mmol phosphate/kg/hr for 3–6 hours (or, 2.5 mg/kg over 6 hours) (3 mmol/ml or 93 mg/ml phosphate)

Pralidoxime chloride (2-PAM)
Protopam Chloride
Organophosphate toxicosis: 20 mg/kg q8–12h (initial dose slow IV, or IM; subsequent doses IM, SC)

Praziquantel
Droncit
    Dog (PO):
        <6.8 kg: 7.5 mg/kg once
        >6.8 kg: 5 mg/kg once
    Dog (IM, SC):
        ≤2.3 kg: 7.5 mg/kg once
        2.7–4.5 kg: 6.3 mg/kg once
        ≥5 kg: 5 mg/kg once
    Cat (PO):
        <1.8 kg: 6.3 mg/kg once
        >1.8 kg: 5 mg/kg once
    Cat (IM, SC): 5 mg/kg IM, SC
        paragonimiasis: 25 mg/kg q8h for 2 days
        Liver flukes: 20 mg/kg qd for 3 days; PO, SC

Prazosin
Minipress
0.5–2.0 mg/animal q8–12h PO

Prednisolone
Anti-inflammatory:
    Dog: 0.5–1.0 mg/kg q12–24h IV, IM, PO initially then taper to q48h
    Cat: 2.2 mg/kg q12–24h IV, IM, PO initially, then taper to q48h
Immunosuppressive (dog and cat): initially 2.2–6.6 mg/kg/d IV, IM, PO, then taper to 2–4 mg/kg q48h

Prednisolone sodium succinate
Solu-Delta-Cortef
Shock: 15–30 mg/kg IV, then repeat in 4–6 h
CNS trauma: 15–30 mg/kg IV, then taper to 1–2 mg/kg q12h

Prednisone
See Prednisolone

Primidone
Mylepsin
Mysoline
Initial dosage: 5–10 mg/kg q8h PO

Primor (ormetroprim plus sulfadimethoxine)
25 mg/kg on first day, followed by 12.5 mg/kg q24h PO

Procainamide
Pronestyl
    Dog: 10–20 mg/kg q6h PO (maximum dose: 40 mg/kg); 8–20 mg/kg IV, IM; 25–50 µg/kg/min IV infusion
    Cat: 3–8 mg/kg IM, PO q6–8h

Procainamide (extended-release tablets)
Procan-SR
    Dog: 20–50 mg/kg q8h PO
    Cat: 62.5 mg/cat q8h PO

Prochlorperazine
Compazine
0.25–0.5 mg/kg q6–8h IM, SC

Progesterone, repositol
See Medroxyprogesterone acetate

Promazine
Tranquazine
1–2 mg/kg q6–8h IV, IM, PO

Promethazine hydrochloride
Phenergan
0.2–0.4 mg/kg q6–8h IV, IM, PO (maximum dose: 1 mg/kg)

Propantheline bromide
For detrusor hyperreflexia and urge incontinence:
    Dog: 7.5–30.0 mg/dog q8–24h PO (start low)
    Cat: 7.5 mg/cat q24–72h PO

Propofol
2–6 mg/kg IV for anesthesia (see Chap. 2)

Propranolol hydrochloride
Inderal
    Dog: 20–60 µg/kg over 5–10 min q8h IV, 0.2–1.0 mg/kg q8h PO
    Cat: 2.5–5.0 mg/cat (0.4–1.2 mg/kg) q8–12h PO

Prostaglandin E
See Misoprostol

Prostaglandin F$_{2\alpha}$
Lutalyse
Pyometra: Dog: 0.1–0.25 mg/kg, once daily for 3–5 days SC (see Chap. 110)
Abortion:
    (See Chapter 110 for protocol)

Psyllium
Metamucil
1–2 tbsp/d (added to food)

Pyrantel pamoate
Nemex, Strongid
    Dog: < 2.5 kg: 10 mg/kg PO
           > 2.5 kg: 5 mg/kg PO
    Cat: 20 mg/kg PO

Pyridostigmine bromide
Mestinon
Regonol
Antimyasthenic: 0.02–0.04 mg/kg q2h IV, or 0.5–3.0 mg/kg q8–12h PO
Antidote (curariform): 0.15–0.3 mg/kg IM, IV

Pyrimethamine
Daraprim
    Dog: 1 mg/kg q24h PO for 14–28 days (5 days for *Neosporum caninum*)
    Cat: 0.5–1.0 mg/kg q24h PO for 14–28 days

Quinacrine hydrochloride
Atabrine hydrochloride
    Dog: 6.6 mg/kg q12h PO for 5 days
    Cat: 11 mg/kg q24h PO for 5 days

Quinidine gluconate
Quinaglute
Duraquin
    Dog: 6–20 mg/kg q6h IM; 6–20 mg/kg q6–8h PO (of base)
(324 mg quinidine gluconate = 202 mg quinidine base)

Quinidine polygalacturonate
Cardioquin
    Dog: 6–20 mg/kg q6h PO (of base)
(275 mg quinidine polygalacturonate = 167 mg quinidine base)

Quinidine sulfate
Clin-Quin
Quinora
    Dog: 6–20 mg/kg q6–8h PO (of base)
(300 mg quinidine sulfate = 250 mg quinidine base)

Ranitidine
Zantac
    Dog: 2 mg/kg q8–12h IV, PO
    Cat: 2.5 mg/kg q12h IV; 3.5 mg/kg q12h PO

Retinoids
See Isotretinoin; Retinol; Etretinate

Retinol
Aquasol-A
625–800 IU/kg q24h PO

Riboflavin (vitamin B$_2$)
    Dog: 10–20 mg/d PO
    Cat: 5–10 mg/d PO

Rifampin
Rifadin
10–20 mg/kg q24h PO

Ringer's solution
40–50 ml/kg/d IV, SC, IP for maintenance requirements

Salicylate
See Acetylsalicylic acid (aspirin)

Selegiline
See Deprenyl (Anipryl)

Senna
Senokot
    Cat: 5 ml/cat q24h (syrup); ½ tsp/cat q24h with food (granules)

Sodium bicarbonate (NaHCO$_3$)
Acidosis: 0.5–1.0 mEq/kg IV, monitor blood gases (8.5% solution = 1 mEq/ml of NaHCO$_3$)
Renal failure: 10 mg/kg q8–12h PO (adjust as necessary)
Alkalinization of urine: 50 mg/kg q8–12h PO (1 tsp is approximately 2 g)

Sodium chloride (0.9%)
40–50 ml/kg/d IV, SC, IP

Sodium chloride 7% (hypertonic saline)
2–8 ml/kg/ IV for shock therapy

Sodium iodide (20%)
20–40 mg/kg q8–12h PO

Sodium nitroprusside
See Nitroprusside sodium

Sodium thiomalate
See Gold sodium thiomalate

Spironolactone
Aldactone
1–2 mg/kg q12h PO

Stanozolol
Winstrol-V
    Dog: 1–4 mg/dog q12h PO; 25–50 mg/dog/wk IM
    Cat: 1 mg/cat q12h PO; 25 mg/cat/wk IM

Sucralfate
Carafate
    Dog: 0.5–1.0 g/dog q8–12h PO
    Cat: 0.25 g/cat q8–12h PO

Sufentanil
Sufenta
2 μg/kg IV, up to a maximum dose of 5 μg/kg (premedicate with acepromazine)

Sulfadiazine
100 mg/kg IV, PO (loading dose), followed by 50 mg/kg q12h IV, PO (see also Trimethoprim)

Sulfadimethoxine
Albon, Bactrovet
55 mg/kg PO (loading dose), followed by 27.5 mg/kg q12h PO (see also Primor)

Sulfaguanidine
100–200 mg/kg q8h PO for 5 days

Sulfamethazine
100 mg/kg PO (loading dose), followed by 50 mg/kg q12h PO

Sulfamethoxazole
Gantanol
100 mg/kg PO (loading dose), followed by 50 mg/kg q12h PO

Sulfamethoxazole plus trimethoprim
Bactrim
Septra
See Trimethoprim plus sulfadiazine

Sulfasalazine (Sulfapyridine plus mesalamine)
Azulfidine (U.S.)
Salazopyrin (Canada)
>   Dog: 10–30 mg/kg q8–12h PO
>   Cat: 10–20 mg/kg q12–24h PO
(See also Mesalamine, Olsalazine)

Sulfisoxazole
Gantrisin
50 mg/kg q8h PO (urinary tract infections)

Taurine
>   Dog: 250–500 mg/dog q12h PO
>   Cat: 250 mg/cat q12h PO

Telezol
See Tiletamine plus zolazepam

Temaril-P (Trimeprazine plus prednisolone)
0.7–1.1 mg/kg (of trimeprazine) q12–24h PO

Terbutaline
Brethine, Bricanyl
>   Dog: 2.5–5.0 mg/dog q8h SC, PO
>   Cat: 0.625 mg/cat q12h SC, PO

Testosterone cypionate
Andro-Cyp
1–2 mg/kg q2–4wk IM (see also Methyltestosterone)

Testosterone propionate
Testex
Malogen
0.5–1.0 mg/kg 2–3 times/wk IM (see also
   Methyltestosterone)

Tetanus toxoid (equine antitoxin)
100–500 U/kg (maximum 20,000 U); IV slowly over
   5–10 minutes

Tetracycline
Panmycin
Achromycin
15–22 mg/kg q6–8h PO
4.4–11.0 mg/kg q8–12h IV, IM
(See also Oxytetracycline, Doxycycline, Minocycline)

Theophylline
>   Dog: 8 mg/kg q6–8h PO
>   Cat: 4 mg/kg q8–12h PO
(See also Aminophylline)

Theophylline (long-acting)
Theo-Dur
Slo-bid Gyrocaps
>   Dog: 20 mg/kg q12h PO (Theo-Dur)
>   30 mg/kg q12h PO (Slo-bid)
>   Cat: 25 mg/kg q24h PO at night

Thiabendazole
Omnizole
Equizole
>   Dog: 50 mg/kg q24h for 3 days, repeat 1 month
>   Cat *(Strongyloides):*   125 mg/kg q24h for 3 days

Thiacetarsamine sodium
Caparsolate
2.2 mg/kg IV twice daily for 2 days

Thiamine (vitamin B$_1$)
>   Dog: 10–100 mg/dog/d PO
>   Cat: 5–30 mg/cat/d PO (up to a maximum dose
>   of 50 mg/cat/d)

Thiomalate sodium
See Gold sodium thiomalate

Thiopental sodium
Pentothal
>   Dog: 6–10 mg/kg IV (to effect)

Thiotepa
0.2–0.5 mg/m^2 intracavitary or IV

Thyroid hormone
See Levothyroxine, Liothyronine

Thyrotropin (TSH)
Thytropar
>   Dog: collect baseline sample, followed by 0.1
>   IU/kg IV (maximum dose is 5 IU); collect post-
>   TSH sample at 6 hours
>   Cat: collect baseline sample, followed by 2.5
>   IU/cat IM and collect post-TSH sample at 8–12
>   hours

Ticarcillin
Ticar
33–50 mg/kg q4–6h IV, IM

Tiletamine plus zolazepam
Telezol
0.5–4.0 mg/kg IV, 4–10 mg/kg IM, SC

Tobramycin
Nebcin
2 mg/kg q8hr IV, IM, SC

Tocainide
Tonocard
>   Dog: 10–20 mg/kg q8h PO

Toluene
267 mg/kg PO (of Toluene), repeat in 2–4 weeks

Triamcinolone
Vetalog
Aristocort
Anti-inflammatory: 0.5–1.0 mg/kg q12–24h PO, taper
   dose to 0.5–1.0 mg/kg q48h PO

Triamcinolone acetonide
Vetalog
0.1–0.2 mg/kg IM, SC, repeat in 7–10 days
Intralesional: 1.2–1.8 mg, or 1 mg for every cm
   diameter of tumor q2wk

Tribrissen: see Trimethoprim sulfadiazine

Trientine hydrochloride
Syprine
10–15 mg/kg q12h, PO (1 hr before meals, do not give
   concurrently with other medications).

Triflupromazine
Vesprin
0.1–0.3 mg/kg IM, PO q8–12h

Tri-iodothyronine
See Liothyronine

Trimeprazine
Panectyl
0.5 mg/kg q12hr PO (also see Temaril-P)

Trimethobenzamide
Tigan, Trimazide
>   Dog: 3 mg/kg q8h IM, PO
>   Cat: not recommended

Trimethoprim plus sulfadiazine

Tribrissen

15 mg/kg q12hr IM, PO, or 30 mg/kg q12–24h SC, PO
(for Toxoplasma: 30 mg/kg q12h PO)

Tripelennamine

Pelamine

1 mg/kg q12h PO

TSH (thyroid-stimulating hormone)

See Thyrotropin

Tylosin

Tylocine, Tylan

20–40 mg/kg q12h PO

Urofollitropin

Metrodin

Cat: 2 mg/cat q24h IM

Ursodiol (ursodeoxycholate)

Actigall

10–15 mg/kg q24h PO

Valproic acid

Depakene

Dog: 60–200 mg/kg q8h PO; or 25–105 mg/kg
q24h PO when administered with phenobarbital

Vancomycin

Vancocin

Dog: 15 mg/kg q6–8h IV

Cat: 12–15 mg/kg q8h IV

Vasopressin (ADH)

Pitressin

Aqueous (20 U/ml): 10 U IV, IM (see also
Desmopressin acetate)

Verapamil

Calan

Isoptin

Dog: 0.05 mg/kg q10–30 min IV (maximum
cumulative dose is 0.15 mg/kg); oral dose is not
established

Cat: 1.1–2.9 mg/kg q8h PO

Vermiplex

See Toluene

Vinblastine

Velban

2 mg/m^2 q7–14d IV

Vincristine

Oncovin

Antitumor: 0.5–0.75 mg/m^2 q7d IV

Thrombocytopenia: 0.025 mg/kg once/wk IV

Viokase

(See Pancreatic enzyme)

Vitamin A (Retinoids)

See Isotretinoin (Accutane), Retinol (Aquasol A), or
Etretinate (Tegison)

Vitamin B complex

Dog: 0.5–2.0 ml q24hr IV, IM, SC

Cat: 0.5–1.0 ml q24hr IV, IM, SC

Vitamin B$_1$

See Thiamine

Vitamin B$_2$

See Riboflavin

Vitamin B$_{12}$

See Cyanocobalamin

Vitamin C

See Ascorbic acid

Vitamin D

See Dihydrotachysterol; Ergocalciferol

Vitamin E (Alpha tocopherol)

Aquasol E

100–400 IU q12h PO (or 400–600 IU q12h PO for
immune-mediated skin disease, hepatitis, and
copper-associated liver disease)

Vitamin K$_1$

AquaMEPHYTON

Mephyton

Short-acting rodenticide toxicity: 1 mg/kg/d SC, PO
for 10–14 days; long-acting rodenticide toxicity: 3–5
mg/kg/d SC, PO for 3–4 weeks; birds: 2.5–5.0
mg/kg q24h

Severe cholestatic liver disease: 1 mg/kg q12hr SC or
IM

Warfarin

Dog: 0.1–0.2 mg/kg q24h PO (adjust dose by
monitoring clotting time)

Cat: 0.06–0.1 mg/kg (monitor clotting time)

Xylazine

Rompun

Dog: 0.3–0.8 mg/kg IV, 0.5 –1.5 mg/kg IM, SC

Cat: 0.4–1.0 mg/kg IV, 0.8–1.8 mg/kg IM, SC

Yohimbine

Yobine

For xylazine reversal: 0.1–0.4 mg/kg IV

Zinc

Liver copper chelation: 5–10 mg/kg q12hr PO (1–2
hr separate from meals)

Zidovudine (AZT)

Retrovir

Cat: 15 mg q12h to 20 mg/kg q8h PO

Zolazepam

See Tiletamine plus zolazepam

Index

Note: Page numbers in *italics* indicate figures; those followed by t indicate tables.

ISBN 0-7216-7078-4